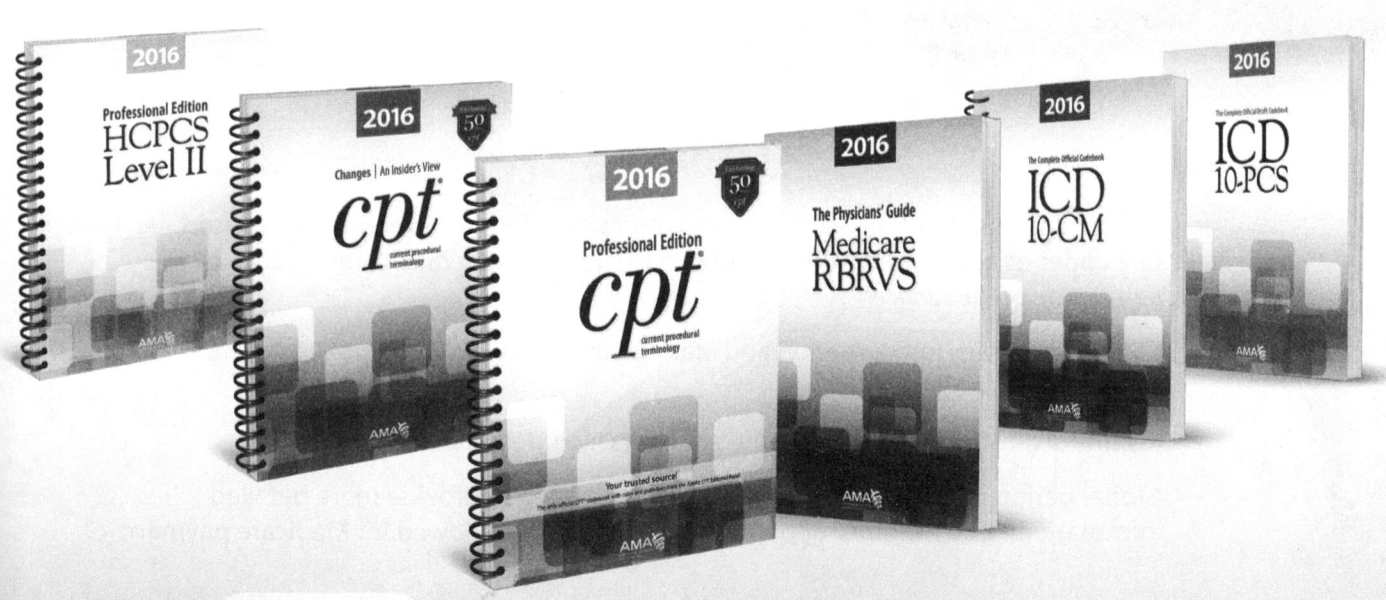
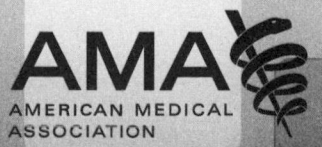

AMA|store

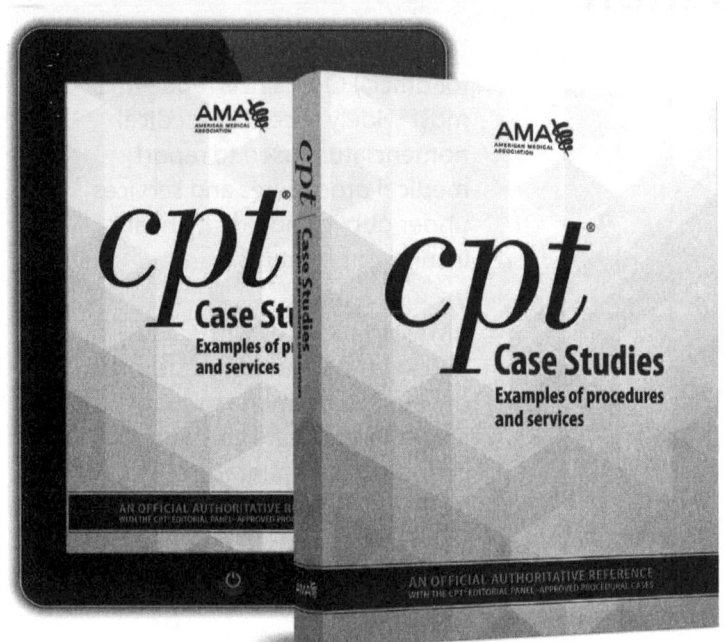
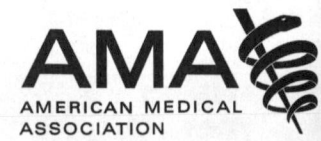

The Complete Official Codebook

ICD 10-CM

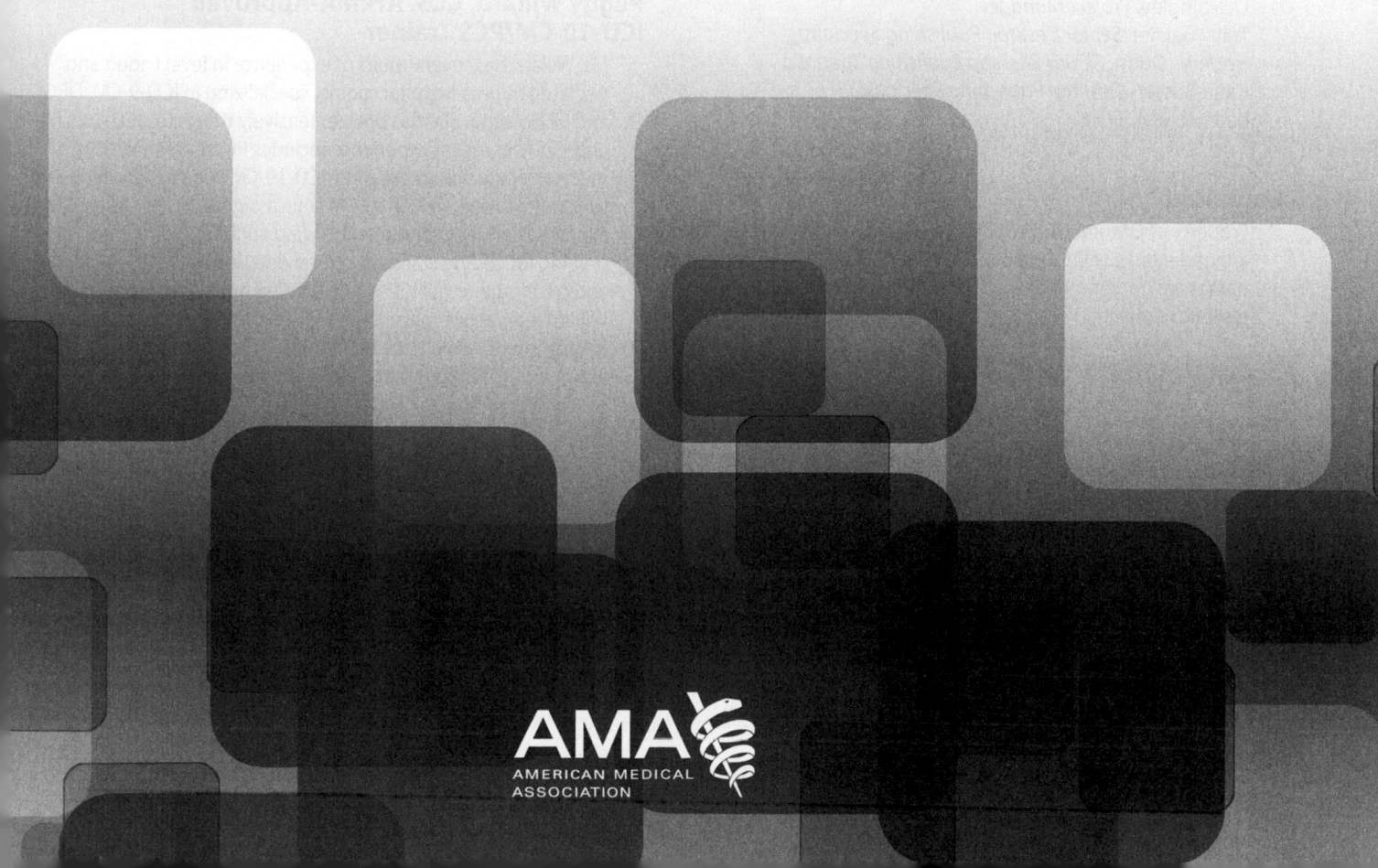

AMA
AMERICAN MEDICAL
ASSOCIATION

Publisher's Notice

The *ICD-10-CM: The Complete Official Codebook* is designed to be an accurate and authoritative source regarding coding and every reasonable effort has been made to ensure accuracy and completeness of the content. However, the AMA makes no guarantee, warranty, or representation that this publication is accurate, complete or without errors. It is understood that the AMA is not rendering any medical, legal or other professional services or advice in this publication and that the AMA bears no liability for any results or consequences that may arise from the use of this book. If medical, legal or other expert advice is required, the services of a competent professional should be sought.

Our Commitment to Accuracy

The AMA is committed to producing accurate and reliable materials.

To report corrections, please call the AMA Unified Service Center at (800) 621-8335.

Acknowledgments

Lauri Gray, RHIT, CPC, AHIMA-Approved ICD-10-CM/PCS Trainer, *Product Manager*
Karen Schmidt, BSN, *Technical Director*
Anita Schmidt, BS, RHIT, AHIMA-Approved ICD-10-CM/PCS Trainer, *Clinical Technical Editor*
Peggy Willard, CCS, AHIMA-Approved ICD-10-CM/PCS Trainer, *Clinical Technical Editor*
Karen Krawzik, RHIT, CCS, AHIMA-Approved ICD-10-CM/PCS Trainer, *Clinical Technical Editor*
Stacy Perry, *Manager, Desktop Publishing*
Lisa Singley, *Project Manager*
Tracy Betzler, *Senior Desktop Publishing Specialist*
Hope M. Dunn, *Senior Desktop Publishing Specialist*
Katie Russell, *Desktop Publishing Specialist*
Kate Holden, *Editor*

Copyright

Anita Schmidt, BS, RHIT, AHIMA-Approved ICD-10-CM/PCS Trainer

Ms. Schmidt has expertise in level I adult and pediatric trauma hospital coding, specializing in ICD-9-CM, DRG, and CPT coding. Her experience includes analysis of medical record documentation and assignment of ICD-9-CM codes and DRGs, and CPT code assignments for same-day surgery cases. She has conducted coding training and auditing, including DRG validation; conducted electronic health record training; and worked with clinical documentation specialists to identify documentation needs and potential areas for physician education. Ms. Schmidt is an active member of the American Health Information Management Association (AHIMA) and the Minnesota Health Information Management Association (MHIMA).

Karen Krawzik, RHIT, CCS, AHIMA-approved ICD-10-CM/PCS Trainer

Ms. Krawzik has expertise in ICD-10-CM, ICD-9-CM, and CPT/HCPCS coding. Her coding experience includes inpatient, ambulatory surgery, and ancillary and emergency room records. She has served as a DRG analyst and auditor of commercial and government payer claims, and as a contract administrator. Most recently she was responsible for the conversion of the ICD-9-CM code set to ICD-10 and for analyzing audit results, identifying issues and trends, and developing remediation plans. Ms. Krawzik is credentialed by the American Health Information Management Association (AHIMA) as a Certified Coding Specialist (CCS) and is an AHIMA-approved ICD-10-CM/PCS trainer. She is an active member of AHIMA and the Missouri Health Information Management Association.

Peggy Willard, CCS, AHIMA-Approved ICD-10-CM/PCS Trainer

Ms. Willard has several years of experience in level I adult and pediatric trauma hospital coding, specializing in ICD-9-CM, DRG, and CPT coding. She has been extensively trained in ICD-10-CM and PCS. Her recent experience includes in-depth analysis of medical record documentation, ICD-10-CM code assignment, and DRG shifts based on ICD-10-CM code assignment. Ms. Willard's expertise includes conducting coding audits, conducting coding training for coding staff and clinical documentation specialists, and creating internal ICD-10-CM coding guidelines/tips. Ms. Willard is an active member of the American Health Information Management Association (AHIMA) and the Minnesota Health Information Management Association (MHIMA).

Contents

Preface iii

Introduction v
   History of ICD-10-CM ....

How to Use ICD-10-CM: The Complete Official Codebook 2016 vi
   Steps to Correct Coding vi
   Organization vi

Overview of ICD-10-CM Official Conventions vii
   Format vii
   Punctuation vii
   Abbreviations vii
   General Notes vii

Additional Conventions ix
   Additional Characters Required ix
   Italics ix
   Color Coding ix
   Medicare Code Edits.. ix
   Other Notations in the Tabular ix
   Other Notations in the Alphabetic Indexes x

ICD-10-CM Official Guidelines for Coding and Reporting 2016 .... Coding Guidelines – 1

ICD-10-CM Index to Diseases and Injuries 1

ICD-10-CM Neoplasm Table 321

ICD-10-CM Table of Drugs and Chemicals 339

ICD-10-CM Index to External Causes............................... 387

ICD-10-CM Tabular List of Diseases and Injuries 423
   Chapter 1   Certain Infectious and Parasitic Diseases (A00-B99) 423
   Chapter 2   Neoplasms (C00-D49) 444
   Chapter 3   Diseases of the Blood and Blood-forming Organs and Certain Disorders Involving the Immune Mechanism (D50-D89) 478
   Chapter 4   Endocrine, Nutritional and Metabolic Diseases (E00-E89) 486
   Chapter 5   Mental, Behavioral, and Neurodevelopmental Disorders (F01-F99) 504
   Chapter 6   Diseases of the Nervous System (G00-G99) 522
   Chapter 7   Diseases of the Eye and Adnexa (H00-H59) 540
   Chapter 8   Diseases of the Ear and Mastoid Process (H60-H95) 572

   Chapter 9   Diseases of the Circulatory System (I00-I99) 583
   Chapter 10 Diseases of the Respiratory System (J00-J99) 617
   Chapter 11 Diseases of the Digestive System (K00-K95) 630
   Chapter 12 Diseases of the Skin and Subcutaneous Tissue (L00-L99) 648
   Chapter 13 Diseases of the Musculoskeletal System and Connective Tissue (M00-M99) 665
   Chapter 14 Diseases of the Genitourinary System (N00-N99) ...746
   Chapter 15 Pregnancy, Childbirth and the Puerperium (O00-O9A) 760
   Chapter 16 Certain Conditions Originating in the Perinatal Period (P00-P96) 795
   Chapter 17 Congenital Malformations, Deformations and Chromosomal Abnormalities (Q00-Q99) 806
   Chapter 18 Symptoms, Signs and Abnormal Clinical and Laboratory Findings, Not Elsewhere Classified (R00-R99) 821
   Chapter 19 Injury, Poisoning and Certain Other Consequences of External Causes (S00-T88) 839
   Chapter 20 External Causes of Morbidity (V00-Y99)................... 1035
   Chapter 21 Factors Influencing Health Status and Contact With Health Services (Z00-Z99) 1104

Appendixes Appendixes-1
   Appendix A: 10 Steps to Correct Coding Appendixes–1
   Appendix B: Valid 3-character ICD-10-CM Codes.........Appendixes–3
   Appendix C: Pharmacology List 2016............................Appendixes–5
   Appendix D: Z Codes for Long-Term Drug Use with Associated Drugs Appendixes–13
   Appendix E: Z Code Only as a Principal Diagnosis List Appendixes–15

Illustrations Illustrations-1
   Peripheral Nervous System...............................Illustrations–1
   Brain...Illustrations–2
   Cranial Nerves Illustrations–2
   Eye..Illustrations–3
   Lacrimal System Illustrations–3
   Ear and Mastoid Illustrations–3
   Middle Ear Illustrations–3
   Arteries...Illustrations–4
   Veins Illustrations–5
   Anatomy of Heart...Illustrations–6
   Arteries of Heart...Illustrations–6
   Cerebrovascular Arteries Illustrations–6
   Veins of Head and Neck....................................Illustrations–6
   Lymphatic System of Head and Neck................Illustrations–6
   Lymph Nodes Illustrations–6
   Respiratory System Illustrations–7

Paranasal Sinuses Illustrations–7

Oral Cavity Illustrations–7

Pancreas Illustrations–7

Gallbladder and Bile Ducts Illustrations–7

Liver Illustrations–7

Gastrointestinal System Illustrations–8

Endocrine System Illustrations–9

Dorsal View of Parathyroid Gland Illustrations–9

Kidney Illustrations–9

Urinary System Illustrations–9

Male Pelvic Organs Illustrations–9

Female Genitourinary System Illustrations–9

Shoulder (Anterior View) Illustrations–10

Shoulder (Posterior View) Illustrations–10

Elbow (Anterior View) Illustrations–11

Elbow (Posterior View) Illustrations–11

Hand Illustrations–11

Hip (Anterior View) Illustrations–12

Hip (Posterior View) Illustrations–12

Knee (Anterior View) Illustrations–13

Knee (Posterior View) Illustrations–13

Right Foot Illustrations–13

Bones/Joints Illustrations–14

Muscles Illustrations–15

Preface

ICD-10-CM Official Preface

This 2016 update of the International Classification of Diseases, 10th revision, Clinical Modification (ICD-10-CM) is being published by the United States government in recognition of its responsibility to promulgate this classification throughout the United States for morbidity coding. The International Statistical Classification of Diseases and Related Health Problems, 10th Revision (ICD-10), published by the World Health Organization (WHO), is the foundation of ICD-10-CM. ICD-10 continues to be the classification used in cause-of-death coding in the United States. The ICD-10-CM is comparable with the ICD-10. The WHO Collaborating Center for the Family of International Classifications in North America, housed at the National Center for Health Statistics (NCHS), has responsibility for the implementation of ICD and other WHO-FIC classifications and serves as a liaison with the WHO, fulfilling international obligations for comparable classifications and the national health data needs of the United States. The historical background of ICD and ICD-10 can be found in the Introduction to the International Classification of Diseases and Related Health Problems (ICD-10), 2008, World Health Organization, Geneva, Switzerland.

ICD-10-CM is the United States' clinical modification of the World Health Organization's ICD-10. The term clinical is used to emphasize the modification's intent: to serve as a useful tool in the area of classification of morbidity data for indexing of medical records, medical care review, and ambulatory and other medical care programs, as well as for basic health statistics. To describe the clinical picture of the patient the codes must be more precise than those needed only for statistical groupings and trend analysis.

Characteristics of ICD-10-CM

ICD-10-CM far exceeds its predecessors in the number of concepts and codes provided. The disease classification has been expanded to include health-related conditions and to provide greater specificity at the sixth and seventh character level. The sixth and seventh characters are not optional and are intended for use in recording the information documented in the clinical record.

Introduction

History of ICD-10-CM

The ICD-10-CM classification system was developed by the National Center for Health Statistics (NCHS) as a clinical modification to the ICD-10 system developed by the World Health Organization (WHO), primarily as a unique system for use in the United States for morbidity and mortality reporting. Although ICD-10 replaced ICD-9 for use in coding and classifying mortality data from death certificates beginning January 1, 1999, ICD-10-CM implementation was postponed many years until legislation to replace ICD-9-CM, volumes 1 and 2, with ICD-10-CM was approved.

ICD-10 is the copyrighted product of the World Health Organization (WHO), which has authorized the development of a clinical modification (CM) of ICD-10 for use in the United States. However, all modifications to the ICD-10 must conform to WHO conventions for ICD. The development of ICD-10-CM included comprehensive evaluation by a Technical Advisory Panel and extensive consultation with physician groups, clinical coders, and other industry experts.

The ICD-10-CM draft and crosswalk between ICD-9-CM and ICD-10-CM were made available on the Centers for Medicare and Medicaid Services (CMS) website for public comment. The initial public comment period extended from December 1997 through February 1998. A field test for ICD-10-CM was conducted in the summer of 2003 jointly by The American Hospital Association (AHA) and the American Health Information Management Association (AHIMA). Public comments and suggestions were reviewed and additional modifications to ICD-10-CM were made. Revisions were made to ICD-10-CM based on the established update process for ICD-10-CM (the ICD-10-CM Coordination and Maintenance Committee) and the World Health Organization's ICD-10 (the Update and Revision Committee).

These revisions to ICD-10-CM have included:

- information relevant to ambulatory and managed care encounters
- expanded injury codes
- creation of combination diagnosis/symptom codes to reduce the number of codes needed to fully describe a condition
- the addition of 6th and 7th character classifications
- incorporation of common 4th and 5th character classifications
- classifications specific to laterality
- classification refinement for increased data granularity

This new structure allows for further expansion than was possible with the ICD-9-CM classification system.

The Department of Health and Human Services (HHS) published the final rule regarding the adoption of both ICD-10-CM and ICD-10-PCS in the January 16, 2009, Federal Register (45 CFR part 162 [CMS—0013—F]). The initial compliance date for implementation of ICD-10-CM and ICD-10-PCS as a replacement for ICD-9-CM was set at October 1, 2013. On April 17, 2012, the Department of Health and Human Services (HHS) released a notice to postpone the date by which certain health care entities have to comply with International Classification of Diseases, 10th Revision diagnosis and procedure codes (ICD-10). The compliance date for implementation of ICD-10-CM and ICD-10-PCS as a replacement for ICD-9-CM was changed to October 1, 2014. On April 1, 2014, Congress enacted the Protecting Access to Medicare Act of 2014, which contained a provision to delay the implementation of ICD-10-CM/PCS by a least one year prohibiting the Department of Health and Human Services (HHS) from adopting the ICD-10-CM/PCS code sets as the mandatory standard until October 1, 2015.

ICD-10-CM: The Complete Official Code Set

ICD-10-CM: The Complete Official Code Set 2016 edition includes many of the enhancements described below in direct response to requests from our subscribers. Users will find many of the conventions, icons, color bars, and other enhancements familiar since many of these features are similar to the hallmark color coding and symbols of our ICD-9-CM code books.

As you review the content, you will find the following:

- Exclusive feature — Check Placeholder Alert symbol, indicating the need for one or more "filler" x character assignments in the 5th and/or 6th character position, in order to appropriately assign a required character in the 7th character position

- Exclusive feature — Key word differentiation by the use of a green font that highlights the differentiating terms in similar code descriptions in a given category

- Exclusive color coding, symbols, and footnotes that alert coders to coding and reimbursement issues, including the majority of the Medicare code edits

- Exclusive feature — Exclusive *following* references and Check Additional Character symbol in the indexes. The *following* references help coders locate those alphanumeric codes that are out of sequence in the tabular section.

- Exclusive feature — Exclusive shaded guides in the index help users easily follow the indent levels for the subterms under a main term.

- Illustrations at the back of the book feature anatomy and terminology included in the ICD-10-CM classification system

- Exclusive feature – Detailed muscle/tendon tables that correspond to codes in chapters 13 and 19

- The complete ICD-10-CM official guidelines for coding and reporting, published by the U.S. Department of Health and Human Services and approved by the cooperating parties (American Health Information Management Association, National Center for Health Statistics, Centers for Medicare and Medicaid Services, American Hospital Association)

- Exclusive feature – Official chapter-specific guidelines with coding examples at the beginning of each chapter

- All the official ICD-10-CM codes, indexes, notes, footnotes, and symbols

- Icons and definitions to differentiate between the two types of Excludes notes

- Check 4th, 5th, 6th, and 7th character symbols identify codes that require the addition of a 4th, 5th, 6th, or 7th character for code specificity and validity

- Color coding and symbol legend at the bottom of each page

Please review "How to Use *ICD-10-CM: The Complete Official Codebook*" in this section to learn about the features that will help you assign and report correct codes, ensuring appropriate reimbursement.

How to Use ICD-10-CM: The Complete Official Codebook 2016

This International Classification of Diseases, 10th Revision, Clinical Modification (ICD-10-CM) is being published by the United States Government in recognition of its responsibility to promulgate this classification throughout the United States for morbidity coding. This code book represents an adaptation of ICD-10 which was created specifically for use in the United States. Future revisions to ICD-10-CM will be made based on the established update process for ICD-10-CM (the ICD-10-CM Coordination and Maintenance Committee) and the World Health Organization's ICD-10 (the Update and Revision Committee). ICD-10-CM has been approved for implementation on October 1, 2015.

Steps to Correct Coding

1. Before beginning to use this code book, review section I.A., "Conventions for the ICD-10-CM" and section I.B., "General Coding Guidelines" of the ICD-10-CM Official Guidelines for Coding and Reporting 2016.

2. Look up the main term in the alphabetic index and scan the subterm entries as appropriate. Review continued lines and additional subterms that may appear in the next column or on the next page.

3. Note all parenthetical terms (nonessential modifiers) that help in code selection but do not affect code assignment. Shaded vertical guidelines in the Index are provided to help determine the indentation level for each subterm in relation to the main terms.

4. Pay close attention to the following instructions in the Index:

   - "see," "see also," and "see category" cross-references

   - "with"/"without" notes

   - "omit code" notes

   - "due to" subterms

   - other instructions found in note boxes, such as "code by site"

   - *Following* references and Check Additional Character symbol in the indexes. The *following* references help coders locate those alphanumeric codes that are out of sequence in the tabular section.

5. Do not code from the alphabetic index without verifying the accuracy of the code in the tabular list. Locate the code in the alphanumerically arranged tabular list.

6. To determine the appropriateness of the code selection and proper coding, read all instructional material:

   - "includes" and both types of "excludes" notes

   - "use additional code" and "code first underlying disease" instructions

   - "code also"

   - 4th, 5th, and 6th character requirements and 7th character extension requirements

   - age and sex symbols

7. Consult the official ICD-10-CM guidelines, which govern the use of specific codes. These guidelines provide both general and chapter-specific coding guidance.

8. Confirm and assign the correct code.

Organization

This book is organized in the following manner:

Introduction

The introductory material in this book includes the ICD-10-CM Official Preface, the history and future of ICD-10-CM as well as an overview of the classification system.

Official ICD-10-CM Conventions and Guidelines

This section provides an explanation of the conventions and guidelines regulating the appropriate assignment and reporting of ICD-10-CM codes. This coding guidance is presented by the National Center for Health Statistics (NCHS), a governmental agency of the Centers for Disease Control and Prevention (CDC), within the United States Department of Health and Human Services (DHHS).

Alphabetic Index to Diseases

The alphabetic index to diseases is arranged in alphabetic order by disease — by specific illness, injury, eponym, abbreviation, or other descriptive diagnostic term. The Index also lists diagnostic terms for other reasons for encounters with health care professionals.

Neoplasm Table

The Neoplasm Table provides the proper code based upon histology of the neoplasm and site.

Table of Drugs and Chemicals

The Table of Drugs and Chemicals is also included within the alphabetic index.

The Table of Drugs and Chemicals lists the drug and the specific codes that identify the drug and the intent. No additional external cause of injury and poisoning code is assigned in ICD-10-CM.

Index to External Causes

The alphabetic index to external causes of injuries is arranged in alphabetic order by main term indicating the event.

Tabular List of Diseases

ICD-10-CM codes and descriptors are arranged numerically within the tabular list of diseases within 21 separate chapters according to body system or nature of injury and disease. Classifications which were previously considered supplemental to ICD-9-CM (e.g., V codes and E codes) are incorporated into the tabular listing of ICD-10-CM as individual chapters. Chapters 20 External Causes of Morbidity and 21 Factors Influencing Health Status and Contact with Health Services include chapter-specific guidelines.

Appendixes

The additional resources described below have been included as appendixes for the *ICD-10-CM: The Complete Official Codebook.* These resources are designed to further instruct the professional coder on the appropriate application of the ICD-10-CM code set.

Appendix A: 10 Steps to Correct Coding

This step-by-step tutorial walks the coder through the process of locating the correct code in the Alphabetic Index and verifying it in the tabular section while following applicable conventions and guidelines. Detailed examples are provided and explained along with advice for proper sequencing.

Appendix B: Valid 3-character ICD-10-CM Codes

The user may consult this table to confirm that no further specificity, such as the use of 4th, 5th, 6th, or 7th characters or placeholders (x), is necessary. All ICD-10-CM codes that are valid at the three-character level are listed.

Appendix C: Pharmacology List 2016

This reference helps users select the most accurate code for drug classifications for adverse effects and poisonings, in addition to alerting the coder of potential chronic conditions in a patient record by identifying various medications used and their actions. This list is not all-inclusive but discusses many commonly used drugs.

Appendix D: Z Codes for Long-Term Drug Use with Associated Drugs

This resource correlates Z codes that are used to identify current long term drug use with a list of drugs that are typically categorized to that class of drug.

Note: These tables are not all-inclusive but list some of the more commonly used drugs.

Appendix E: Z Code Only as Principal Diagnosis List

Chapter 21, "Factors Influencing Health Status and Contact with Health Services," contains codes describing encounters for circumstances other than a disease or injury. Many of these codes may be reported *only* as the principal/first-listed diagnosis. This resource lists all of these codes in one table for quick and easy reference to ensure accurate reporting.

Illustrations

This section includes illustrations of normal anatomy with ICD-10-CM specific terminology.

Use of Official Sources

The *ICD-10-CM: The Complete Official Codebook* contains the official U.S. Department of Health and Human Services, Tenth Revision, Clinical Modification, ICD-10-CM codes, effective for the current year.

The color-coding, footnotes and symbols, which identify coding and reimbursement issues, are derived from official federal government sources, including the Integrated Outpatient Code Edits (IOCE), version 16.2.

Overview of ICD-10-CM Official Conventions

This is an overview of the ICD-10-CM official conventions, which are general rules for the use of the classification system, independent of the guidelines. The official conventions and instructions of the classification, which take precedence over the guidelines, are incorporated within the Alphabetic Index and Tabular List as instructional notes and are applicable regardless of the health care setting. For the full version of the official conventions, see the ICD-10-CM Official Guidelines for Coding and Reporting 2016, section I.A., which is included in this book.

Format

ICD-10-CM is divided into two main parts: the Index, an alphabetical list of terms and their corresponding code, and the tabular list, a sequential, alphanumeric list of codes divided into chapters based on body system or condition. The Index contains the Index to Diseases and Injuries (main index) and the Index to External Causes of Injury. Also included in the main Index is the Neoplasm Table and a Table of Drugs and Chemicals.

The tabular list contains categories, subcategories, and valid codes. ICD-10-CM is an alphanumeric classification system. The 1st character of a three-character category is a letter. The 2nd and 3rd characters may be numbers or alpha characters. A three-character category without further subclassification is equivalent to a valid three-character code. Subcategories are either four or five characters. Subcategory characters include either letters or numbers. Codes may be three, four, five, six, or seven characters in length, in which each level of subdivision after a category is a subcategory. The final level of subdivision is a valid code. The final character in a code may be either a letter or a number.

The ICD-10-CM uses the letter "X" as a place-holder. A placeholder "X" is used as a 5th character place-holder at certain six-character codes to allow for future expansion, without disturbing the 6th character structure. For instance, an initial encounter for accidental poisoning by penicillin is coded to T36.0X1A. The "X" in the 5th character position is a place-holder, or filler character.

Similarly, certain categories have applicable 7th character extensions. In these cases, the 7th character extension is required for all codes within the category, or as otherwise instructed in the tabular list notations. 7th character extensions must always be the last character in the data field. If a code is not a full six characters in length, a dummy place-holder "X" must be used to fill in the empty characters when a 7th character extension is required.

Punctuation

[ ]   In the tabular list, brackets are used to enclose synonyms, alternative wording, or explanatory phrases. In the Index, brackets are used to identify manifestation codes.

( )   Parentheses are used in both the Index and tabular list to enclose nonessential modifiers; supplementary words that may be present or absent in the statement of a disease or procedure without affecting the code number to which it is assigned.

:   Colons are used in the tabular list after an incomplete term that needs one or more of the modifiers following the colon to make it assignable to a given category.

Abbreviations

NEC

The abbreviation NEC, "Not elsewhere classifiable" represents "other specified" in the ICD-10-CM. An index entry that states NEC directs the coder to an "other specified" code in the tabular list. Codes titled "Other" or "Other specified" in the tabular list (usually a code with a 4th or 6th character 8 and 5th character 9) are for use when the information in the medical record provides detail for which a specific code does not exist.

NOS

The abbreviation NOS, "Not otherwise specified," in the tabular list may be interpreted as "unspecified." Codes in the tabular list with "Unspecified" in the title (usually a code with a 4th or 6th character 9 and 5th character Ø) are for use when the information in the medical record is insufficient to assign a more specific code.

Typeface

Boldface

Boldface type is used for main term entries in the alphabetic index, and all codes and descriptions in the tabular list.

General Notes

The following conventions and notes appear only in the tabular list of diseases:

Includes Notes

The word INCLUDES appears immediately under certain categories to further define, clarify, or give examples of the content of a code category.

Inclusion Terms

Lists of inclusion terms are included under certain codes. These terms indicate some of the conditions for which that code number may be used. Inclusion terms may be synonyms with the code title, or, in the case of "other specified" codes, the terms may also provide a list of various conditions included within a classification code. The inclusion terms are not exhaustive. The Index may provide additional terms that may also be assigned to a given code.

Excludes Notes

ICD-10-CM has two types of excludes notes. Each note has a different definition for use. However, they are similar in that they both indicate that codes excluded from each other are independent of each other.

Excludes 1

An EXCLUDES 1 note is a "pure" excludes. It means "NOT CODED HERE!" An Excludes 1 note indicates mutually exclusive codes; two conditions that cannot be reported together. For example, a congenital form of a disease may not be reported with the acquired form of the same condition. The code excluded should never be reported with the applicable codes listed above the excludes notation.

Excludes 2

An EXCLUDES 2 note means "NOT INCLUDED HERE." An Excludes 2 note indicates that although the excluded condition is not part of the condition it is excluded from, a patient may have both conditions at the same time. Therefore, when an Excludes 2 note appears under a code, it may be acceptable to use both the code and the excluded code together if supported by the medical documentation.

Default Codes

In the index, the default code is the code listed next to the main term. The default code represents the condition most commonly associated with the main term. This code may be assigned when documentation does not facilitate reporting a more specific code. Alternately, it may provide an unspecified code for the condition.

Syndromes

Follow the alphabetic index guidance when coding syndromes. In the absence of index guidance, assign codes for the documented manifestations of the syndrome.

And

When the term "and" is used in a narrative statement or code title, it may be interpreted as "and/or."

With

The word "with" should be interpreted to mean "associated with" or "due to" when it appears in a code title, the Alphabetic Index, or an instructional note in the Tabular List.

Instructional Notes Used in the Tabular List

In the tabular section, the following instructional notes appear in red type for emphasis:

Code First/Use additional code:

These instructional notes provide sequencing instruction. They may appear independently of each other or to designate certain etiology/manifestation paired codes. These instructions signal the coder that an additional code should be reported to provide a more complete picture of that diagnosis.

In etiology/manifestation coding, ICD-10-CM requires the underlying condition to be sequenced first, followed by the manifestation. In these situations, codes with "In diseases classified elsewhere" in the code description are never permitted as a first-listed or principal diagnosis code and must be sequenced following the underlying condition code.

Code Also:

A code also note alerts the coder that more than one code may be required to fully describe the condition. Code sequencing is discretionary. Factors that may determine sequencing include severity and reason for the encounter.

Additional Conventions

Color-coding and symbols are included to alert the coder to important reimbursement issues affected by the diagnosis code assignment. Some codes may carry more than one color and/or symbol. For a quick reference to the color codes and their meanings, refer to the color/symbol legend located at the bottom of each page in the tabular listing.

Additional Characters Required

√4ᵗʰ This symbol indicates that the code requires a 4th character.

√5ᵗʰ This symbol indicates that the code requires a 5th character.

√6ᵗʰ This symbol indicates that the code requires a 6th character.

√7ᵗʰ This symbol indicates that the code requires a 7th character.

√x7ᵗʰ This symbol indicates that the code requires a 7th character following the placeholder X. Codes with fewer than six characters that require a 7th character must contain placeholder "X" to fill in the empty character(s).

Italics

Italicized type is used for all exclusion notes and to identify manifestation codes, those codes that should not be reported as first-listed (principal) diagnoses.

Color Coding

Note

The term "Note" appears enclosed within a red icon and precedes the instructional information. These notes function as an alert, to highlight coding instruction within the text.

Key Word

Green font is used throughout the tabular list of diseases to differentiate the key words that appear in similar code descriptions in a given category or subcategory.

For example, refer to the list of codes below from category C7A:

C7A.020   Malignant carcinoid tumor of the **appendix**

C7A.021   Malignant carcinoid tumor of the **cecum**

C7A.022   Malignant carcinoid tumor of the **ascending colon**

C7A.023   Malignant carcinoid tumor of the **transverse colon**

C7A.024   Malignant carcinoid tumor of the **descending colon**

C7A.025   Malignant carcinoid tumor of the **sigmoid colon**

C7A.029   Malignant carcinoid tumor of the large intestine, **unspecified portion**

The portion of the code description that appears in bold font above appears in green font in the tabular list, to assist the coder in quickly identifying the key terms and in identifying the correct code. This convention is especially useful when the codes describe laterality, such as the following codes from category H40.22:

H40.221   Chronic angle-closure glaucoma, **right** eye

H40.222   Chronic angle-closure glaucoma, **left** eye

H40.223   Chronic angle-closure glaucoma, **bilateral**

H40.229   Chronic angle-closure glaucoma, **unspecified** eye

The key word convention is only used in those categories in which there are multiple codes with very similar descriptions with only a few words that differentiate them.

Medicare Code Edits

Medicare administrative contractors (MACs) and many payers use Medicare code edits to check the coding accuracy on claims. The coding edit information in this manual, effective from October 1, 2015, to September 30, 2016, reflect those edits used for physician office encounters. This ICD-10 version of the Integrated Outpatient Code Editor (IOCE) is version 16.2.

Manifestation Code

These codes appear in italic type, with a **_blue color bar_** over the title. A manifestation code cannot be reported as a first-listed or principal diagnosis. By definition, a manifestation code represents a demonstration of some aspect of an underlying disease, which is separately classifiable. In the alphabetic index, these codes are listed as the secondary code in brackets. The underlying disease code is listed first.

Age and Sex Edit Symbols

The age and sex edits below are used to detect inconsistencies between the patient's age and/or sex and the patient's diagnosis. The following edit symbols appear in the tabular list of diseases to the right of the code description.

Newborn Age: 0   **N**
These diagnoses are intended for newborns and neonates and the patient's age must be 0 years.

Pediatric Age: 0-17   **P**
These diagnoses are intended for children and the patient's age must between 0 and 17 years.

Maternity Age: 12-55   **M**
These diagnoses are intended for childbearing patients between the age of 12 and 55 years.

Adult Age: 15-124   **A**
These diagnoses are intended for the patients between the age of 15 and 124 years.

Male diagnosis only   ♂

Female diagnosis only   ♀

Other Notations in the Tabular

Other Specified Code

These codes will appear with a **gray color bar** over the code description. Use these codes when the documentation indicates a specified diagnosis, but the ICD-10-CM system does not have a specific code that describes the condition. These codes may be stated as "Other" or "Not elsewhere classified (NEC)."

Unspecified Code

These codes will have a **yellow color bar** over the code description. Use these codes when neither the diagnostic statement nor the documentation provides enough information to assign a more specific diagnosis code. These codes may be stated as "Unspecified" or "Not otherwise specified (NOS)." Note: Do not assign these codes when a more specific diagnosis has been determined.

PDx Symbol

`PDx`

This symbol identifies a Z code that generally is for use as a first-listed (or primary) diagnosis only but may be used as an additional diagnosis if the patient has more than one encounter on the same day or there is more than one reason for the encounter.

The instructions for Z code use contained in the ICD-10-CM official coding guidelines identify those Z codes that can only be used as a PDx. All other Z codes may either be SDx or PDx, depending upon circumstances of the encounter, by meeting the definition of first-listed or principal diagnosis, and by following any specific Z code guidelines in section I.C.21 a-c. The responsibility of those assigning the Z codes as PDx is to make sure the circumstances of the encounter meet the definition of first-listed or principal diagnosis, follow all coding instructions, and follow the Z code specific guidelines. This codebook does not include any SDx edit since there is no official source for it and the Z code use is determined by circumstances of the encounter.

Note: Please note that the symbols indicating the Z code "principal or first-listed only" designation and the Z codes that may be principal or first-listed diagnoses included in the official coding guidelines [Section I.C.21.c.16] are consistent with reporting guidelines for health care encounters *excluding acute care inpatient admissions*. These Z code edits are often in conflict with the inpatient prospective payment system (IPPS) edits. For example, code Z34.90 Encounter for supervision of normal pregnancy, unspecified, unspecified trimester, may be an appropriate primary reason for an outpatient encounter. However, supervision for a normal pregnancy is not an acceptable principal diagnosis or reason for an inpatient admission and will have an unacceptable principal diagnosis edit under inpatient prospective payment system (IPPS).

Muscle and Tendon Table

ICD-10-CM categorizes certain muscles and tendons in the upper and lower extremities by their action (e.g., extension or flexion) as well as their anatomical location. The Muscle/Tendon Table is provided at the beginning of chapter 13 and chapter 19 as a resource to help users when code selection depends on the action of the muscle and/or tendon. The categories and/or subcategories that relate to this table are identified by a purple diamond icon [✦], which refers the user to a footnote at the bottom of the page indicating the use of the table. Please note that this table is not all-inclusive and proper code assignment should be based on the provider's documentation.

Other Notations in the Alphabetic Indexes

▼   Subterms under main terms may continue to next column or page. This warning statement is a reminder to always check for additional subterms and information that may continue onto the next page or column before making a final selection.

Following References

The index includes *following* references to assist in locating "out-of-sequence" codes in the tabular list. "Out-of-sequence" codes contain an alphabetic character (letter) in the 3rd or 4th character position. These codes are placed according to the classification rules — the placement of the codes according to condition — not according to alphabetic or numeric sequencing rules.

Example:

Carcinoma (malignant) (*see also,* Neoplasm, by site, malignant)
    neuroendocrine (*see also* Tumor, neuroendocrine)
        high grade, any site C7A.1 (*following* C75)
        poorly differentiated, any site C7A.1 (*following* C75)

In the tabular rubric, C7A is included after rubric C75 and before C76.

Gout, chronic (*see also* Gout, gouty) M1A.9
    drug-induced M1A.20 (*following* M08)
        ankle M1A.27-(*following* M08)
        elbow M1A.22-(*following* M08)

In the tabular rubric, M1A is included after rubric M08 and before M10.

ICD-10-CM Official Guidelines for Coding and Reporting 2016

Narrative changes appear in **bold** text.

Items <u>underlined</u> have been moved within the guidelines since the 2014 version.

Italics are used to indicate revisions to heading changes.

The Centers for Medicare and Medicaid Services (CMS) and the National Center for Health Statistics (NCHS), two departments within the U.S. Federal Government's Department of Health and Human Services (DHHS) provide the following guidelines for coding and reporting using the International Classification of Diseases, 10th Revision, Clinical Modification (ICD-10-CM). These guidelines should be used as a companion document to the official version of the ICD-10-CM as published on the NCHS website. The ICD-10-CM is a morbidity classification published by the United States for classifying diagnoses and reason for visits in all health care settings. The ICD-10-CM is based on the ICD-10, the statistical classification of disease published by the World Health Organization (WHO).

These guidelines have been approved by the four organizations that make up the Cooperating Parties for the ICD-10-CM: the American Hospital Association (AHA), the American Health Information Management Association (AHIMA), CMS, and NCHS.

These guidelines are a set of rules that have been developed to accompany and complement the official conventions and instructions provided within the ICD-10-CM itself. The instructions and conventions of the classification take precedence over guidelines. These guidelines are based on the coding and sequencing instructions in the Tabular List and Alphabetic Index of ICD-10-CM, but provide additional instruction. Adherence to these guidelines when assigning ICD-10-CM diagnosis codes is required under the Health Insurance Portability and Accountability Act (HIPAA). The diagnosis codes (Tabular List and Alphabetic Index) have been adopted under HIPAA for all healthcare settings. A joint effort between the healthcare provider and the coder is essential to achieve complete and accurate documentation, code assignment, and reporting of diagnoses and procedures. These guidelines have been developed to assist both the healthcare provider and the coder in identifying those diagnoses and procedures that are to be reported. The importance of consistent, complete documentation in the medical record cannot be overemphasized. Without such documentation accurate coding cannot be achieved. The entire record should be reviewed to determine the specific reason for the encounter and the conditions treated.

The term encounter is used for all settings, including hospital admissions. In the context of these guidelines, the term provider is used throughout the guidelines to mean physician or any qualified health care practitioner who is legally accountable for establishing the patient's diagnosis. Only this set of guidelines, approved by the Cooperating Parties, is official.

The guidelines are organized into sections. Section I includes the structure and conventions of the classification and general guidelines that apply to the entire classification, and chapter-specific guidelines that correspond to the chapters as they are arranged in the classification. Section II includes guidelines for selection of principal diagnosis for non-outpatient settings. Section III includes guidelines for reporting additional diagnoses in non-outpatient settings. Section IV is for outpatient coding and reporting. It is necessary to review all sections of the guidelines to fully understand all of the rules and instructions needed to code properly.

Section I. Conventions, general coding guidelines and chapter specific guidelines 3

A. Conventions for the ICD-10-CM 3
1. The Alphabetic Index and Tabular List 3
2. Format and Structure 3
3. Use of codes for reporting purposes 3
4. Placeholder character 3
5. 7th Characters 3
6. Abbreviations 3
   a. Alphabetic Index abbreviations 3
   b. Tabular List abbreviations 3
7. Punctuation 3
8. Use of "and" 3
9. Other and Unspecified codes 3
   a. "Other" codes 3
   b. "Unspecified" codes 3
10. Includes Notes 3
11. Inclusion Terms 3
12. Excludes Notes 3
   a. Excludes1 3
   b. Excludes2 4
13. Etiology/manifestation convention ("code first", "use additional code" and "in diseases classified elsewhere" notes) 4
14. "And" 4
15. "With" 4
16. "See" and "See Also" 4
17. "Code also note" 4
18. Default codes 4
B. General Coding Guidelines 4
1. Locating a code in the ICD-10-CM 4
2. Level of Detail in Coding 4
3. Code or codes from A00.0 through T88.9, Z00-Z99.8 4
4. Signs and symptoms 4
5. Conditions that are an integral part of a disease process 4
6. Conditions that are not an integral part of a disease process 4
7. Multiple coding for a single condition 4
8. Acute and Chronic Conditions 5
9. Combination Code 5
10. Sequela (Late Effects) 5
11. Impending or Threatened Condition 5
12. Reporting Same Diagnosis Code More than Once 5
13. Laterality 5
14. Documentation for BMI, Non-pressure Ulcers, and Pressure Ulcer Stages 5
15. Syndromes 5
16. Documentation of Complications of Care 5
17. Borderline Diagnosis 5
18. Use of Sign/Symptom/Unspecified Codes 5
C. Chapter-Specific Coding Guidelines 6
1. Chapter 1: Certain Infectious and Parasitic Diseases (A00-B99) 6
   a. Human immunodeficiency virus (HIV) infections 6
   b. Infectious agents as the cause of diseases classified to other chapters 6
   c. Infections resistant to antibiotics 6
   d. Sepsis, severe sepsis, and septic shock 6
   e. Methicillin resistant *Staphylococcus aureus* (MRSA) conditions 7
2. Chapter 2: Neoplasms (C00-D49) 8
   a. Treatment directed at the malignancy 8
   b. Treatment of secondary site 8
   c. Coding and sequencing of complications 8
   d. Primary malignancy previously excised 8
   e. Admissions/Encounters involving chemotherapy, immunotherapy and radiation therapy 8
   f. Admission/encounter to determine extent of malignancy 9
   g. Symptoms, signs, and abnormal findings listed in Chapter 18 associated with neoplasms 9
   h. Admission/encounter for pain control/ management 9
   i. Malignancy in two or more noncontiguous sites 9
   j. Disseminated malignant neoplasm, unspecified 9
   k. Malignant neoplasm without specification of site 9
   l. Sequencing of neoplasm codes 9
   m. Current malignancy versus personal history of malignancy 9
   n. Leukemia, multiple myeloma, and malignant plasma cell neoplasms in remission versus personal history 9
   o. Aftercare following surgery for neoplasm 9
   p. Follow-up care for completed treatment of a malignancy 9
   q. Prophylactic organ removal for prevention of malignancy 9
   r. Malignant neoplasm associated with transplanted organ 10
3. Chapter 3: Disease of the blood and blood-forming organs and certain disorders involving the immune mechanism (D50-D89) 10
4. Chapter 4: Endocrine, Nutritional, and Metabolic Diseases (E00-E89) 10
   a. Diabetes mellitus 10

5. Chapter 5: Mental, Behavioral and Neurodevelopmental disorders (F01 – F99) 10
    a. Pain disorders related to psychological factors 10
    b. Mental and behavioral disorders due to psychoactive substance use 10
6. Chapter 6: Diseases of Nervous System (G00-G99) 11
    a. Dominant/nondominant side 11
    b. Pain - Category G89 11
7. Chapter 7: Diseases of Eye and Adnexa (H00-H59) 11
    a. Glaucoma 11
8. Chapter 8: Diseases of Ear and Mastoid Process (H60-H95) 12
9. Chapter 9: Diseases of Circulatory System (I00-I99) 12
    a. Hypertension 12
    b. Atherosclerotic coronary artery disease and angina 12
    c. Intraoperative and postprocedural cerebrovascular accident 12
    d. Sequelae of cerebrovascular disease 13
    e. Acute myocardial infarction (AMI) 13
10. Chapter 10: Diseases of the Respiratory System (J00-J99) 13
    a. Chronic Obstructive Pulmonary Disease [COPD] and Asthma 13
    b. Acute Respiratory Failure 13
    c. Influenza due to certain identified influenza viruses 13
    d. Ventilator associated pneumonia 14
11. Chapter 11: Diseases of the Digestive System (K00-K95) 14
12. Chapter 12: Diseases of the Skin and Subcutaneous Tissue (L00-L99) 14
    a. Pressure ulcer stage codes 14
13. Chapter 13: Diseases of the Musculoskeletal System and Connective Tissue (M00-M99) 14
    a. Site and laterality 14
    b. Acute traumatic versus chronic or recurrent musculoskeletal conditions 14
    c. Coding of Pathologic Fractures 14
    d. Osteoporosis 14
14. Chapter 14: Diseases of Genitourinary System (N00-N99) 15
    a. Chronic kidney disease 15
15. Chapter 15: Pregnancy, Childbirth, and the Puerperium (O00-O9A) 15
    a. General Rules for Obstetric Cases 15
    b. Selection of OB principal or first-listed diagnosis 15
    c. Pre-existing conditions versus conditions due to the pregnancy 16
    d. Pre-existing hypertension in pregnancy 16
    e. Fetal conditions affecting the management of the mother 16
    f. HIV Infection in pregnancy, childbirth and the puerperium ..16
    g. Diabetes mellitus in pregnancy 16
    h. Long term use of insulin 16
    i. Gestational (pregnancy induced) diabetes 16
    j. Sepsis and septic shock complicating abortion, pregnancy, childbirth and the puerperium 16
    k. Puerperal sepsis 16
    l. Alcohol and tobacco use during pregnancy, childbirth and the puerperium 16
    m. Poisoning, toxic effects, adverse effects and underdosing in a pregnant patient 16
    n. Normal delivery, code O80 16
    o. The peripartum and postpartum periods 17
    p. Code O94, Sequelae of complication of pregnancy, childbirth, and the puerperium 17
    q. *Termination of Pregnancy and Spontaneous abortions* 17
    r. Abuse in a pregnant patient 17
16. Chapter 16: Certain Conditions Originating in the Perinatal Period (P00- P96) 17
    a. General Perinatal Rules 17
    b. Observation and Evaluation of Newborns for Suspected Conditions not Found 18
    c. Coding Additional Perinatal Diagnoses 18
    d. Prematurity and Fetal Growth Retardation 18
    e. Low birth weight and immaturity status 18
    f. Bacterial Sepsis of Newborn 18
    g. Stillbirth 18

17. Chapter 17: Congenital malformations, deformations, and chromosomal abnormalities (Q00-Q99) 18
18. Chapter 18: Symptoms, signs, and abnormal clinical and laboratory findings, not elsewhere classified (R00-R99) ..18
    a. Use of symptom codes 18
    b. Use of a symptom code with a definitive diagnosis code 18
    c. Combination codes that include symptoms 18
    d. Repeated falls 18
    e. Coma scale 18
    f. Functional quadriplegia 18
    g. SIRS due to non-infectious process 18
    h. Death NOS 19
19. Chapter 19: Injury, poisoning, and certain other consequences of external causes (S00-T88) 19
    a. Application of 7th Characters in Chapter 19 19
    b. Coding of injuries 19
    c. Coding of Traumatic Fractures 19
    d. Coding of burns and corrosions 19
    e. Adverse effects, poisoning, underdosing and toxic effects 20
    f. Adult and child abuse, neglect and other maltreatment 21
    g. Complications of care 21
20. Chapter 20: External Causes of Morbidity (V00-Y99) 21
    a. General External Cause Coding Guidelines 21
    b. Place of Occurrence Guideline 22
    c. Activity code 22
    d. Place of occurrence, activity, and status codes used with other external cause code 22
    e. If the reporting format limits the number of external cause codes 22
    f. Multiple external cause coding guidelines 22
    g. Child and adult abuse guideline 22
    h. Unknown or undetermined intent guideline 22
    i. Sequelae (Late Effects) of External Cause Guidelines ...22
    j. Terrorism guidelines 22
    k. External cause status 23
21. Chapter 21: Factors influencing health status and contact with health services (Z00-Z99) 23
    a. Use of Z codes in any healthcare setting 23
    b. Z Codes indicate a reason for an encounter 23
    c. Categories of Z Codes 23

Section II. Selection of Principal Diagnosis **27**
    A. Codes for symptoms, signs, and ill-defined conditions ... 27
    B. Two or more interrelated conditions, each potentially meeting the definition for principal diagnosis 27
    C. Two or more diagnoses that equally meet the definition for principal diagnosis 28
    D. Two or more comparative or contrasting conditions 28
    E. A symptom(s) followed by contrasting/ comparative diagnoses 28
    F. Original treatment plan not carried out 28
    G. Complications of surgery and other medical care 28
    H. Uncertain diagnosis 28
    I. Admission from observation unit 28
        1. Admission Following Medical Observation 28
        2. Admission Following Post-Operative Observation 28
    J. Admission from outpatient surgery 28
    K. Admissions/Encounters for Rehabilitation 28

Section III. Reporting Additional Diagnoses **28**
    A. Previous conditions 28
    B. Abnormal findings 28
    C. Uncertain Diagnosis 28

Section IV. Diagnostic Coding and Reporting Guidelines for Outpatient Services **29**
    A. Selection of first-listed condition 29
        1. Outpatient surgery 29
        2. Observation stay 29
    B. Codes from A00.0 through T88.9, Z00-Z99 29
    C. Accurate reporting of ICD-10-CM diagnosis codes 29
    D. Codes that describe symptoms and signs 29
    E. Encounters for circumstances other than a disease or injury 29
    F. Level of Detail in Coding 29
        1. ICD-10-CM codes with 3, 4, 5, 6 or 7 characters 29
        2. Use of full number of characters required for a code 29

G. ICD-10-CM code for the diagnosis, condition, problem, or
    other reason for encounter/visit 29
H. Uncertain diagnosis 29
I. Chronic diseases 29
J. Code all documented conditions that coexist 29
K. Patients receiving diagnostic services only 29
L. Patients receiving therapeutic services only 30
M. Patients receiving preoperative evaluations only 30
N. Ambulatory surgery 30
O. Routine outpatient prenatal visits 30
P. Encounters for general medical examinations with
    abnormal findings 30
Q. Encounters for routine health screenings 30
Appendix I. Present on Admission Reporting Guidelines 30
**Categories and Codes Exempt from Diagnosis Present on
   Admission Requirement 31**

Section I. Conventions, general coding guidelines and chapter specific guidelines

The conventions, general guidelines and chapter-specific guidelines are applicable to all health care settings unless otherwise indicated. The conventions and instructions of the classification take precedence over guidelines.

A. Conventions for the ICD-10-CM

The conventions for the ICD-10-CM are the general rules for use of the classification independent of the guidelines. These conventions are incorporated within the Alphabetic Index and Tabular List of the ICD-10-CM as instructional notes.

1. **The Alphabetic Index and Tabular List**
   The ICD-10-CM is divided into the Alphabetic Index, an alphabetical list of terms and their corresponding code, and the Tabular List, a structured chronological list of codes divided into chapters based on body system or condition. The Alphabetic Index consists of the following parts: the Index of Diseases and Injury, the Index of External Causes of Injury, the Table of Neoplasms and the Table of Drugs and Chemicals.

   See Section I.C2. General guidelines

   See Section I.C.19. Adverse effects, poisoning, underdosing and toxic effects

2. **Format and Structure**
   The ICD-10-CM Tabular List contains categories, subcategories and codes. Characters for categories, subcategories and codes may be either a letter or a number. All categories are 3 characters. A three-character category that has no further subdivision is equivalent to a code. Subcategories are either 4 or 5 characters. Codes may be 3, 4, 5, 6 or 7 characters. That is, each level of subdivision after a category is a subcategory. The final level of subdivision is a code. Codes that have applicable 7th characters are still referred to as codes, not subcategories. A code that has an applicable 7th character is considered invalid without the 7th character.

   The ICD-10-CM uses an indented format for ease in reference.

3. **Use of codes for reporting purposes**
   For reporting purposes only codes are permissible, not categories or subcategories, and any applicable 7th character is required.

4. **Placeholder character**
   The ICD-10-CM utilizes a placeholder character "X". The "X" is used as a placeholder at certain codes to allow for future expansion. An example of this is at the poisoning, adverse effect and underdosing codes, categories T36-T50.

   Where a placeholder exists, the X must be used in order for the code to be considered a valid code.

5. **7th Characters**
   Certain ICD-10-CM categories have applicable 7th characters. The applicable 7th character is required for all codes within the category, or as the notes in the Tabular List instruct. The 7th character must always be the 7th character in the data field. If a code that requires a 7th character is not 6 characters, a placeholder X must be used to fill in the empty characters.

6. **Abbreviations**
   a. **Alphabetic Index abbreviations**
       NEC   "Not elsewhere classifiable"

This abbreviation in the Alphabetic Index represents "other specified". When a specific code is not available for a condition, the Alphabetic Index directs the coder to the "other specified" code in the Tabular List.

   NOS   "Not otherwise specified"
           This abbreviation is the equivalent of unspecified.

   b. **Tabular List abbreviations**
       NEC   "Not elsewhere classifiable"
               This abbreviation in the Tabular List represents "other specified". When a specific code is not available for a condition the Tabular List includes an NEC entry under a code to identify the code as the "other specified" code.
       NOS   "Not otherwise specified"
               This abbreviation is the equivalent of unspecified.

7. **Punctuation**
   [ ] Brackets are used in the Tabular List to enclose synonyms, alternative wording or explanatory phrases. Brackets are used in the Alphabetic Index to identify manifestation codes.

   ( ) Parentheses are used in both the Alphabetic Index and Tabular List to enclose supplementary words that may be present or absent in the statement of a disease or procedure without affecting the code number to which it is assigned. The terms within the parentheses are referred to as nonessential modifiers. The nonessential modifiers in the Alphabetic Index to Diseases apply to subterms following a main term except when a nonessential modifier and a subentry are mutually exclusive, the subentry takes precedence. For example, in the ICD-10-CM Alphabetic Index under the main term Enteritis, "acute" is a nonessential modifier and "chronic" is a subentry. In this case, the nonessential modifier "acute" does not apply to the subentry "chronic".

   :   Colons are used in the Tabular List after an incomplete term which needs one or more of the modifiers following the colon to make it assignable to a given category.

8. **Use of "and"**
   See Section I.A.14. Use of the term "And"

9. **Other and Unspecified codes**
   a. **"Other" codes**
       Codes titled "other" or "other specified" are for use when the information in the medical record provides detail for which a specific code does not exist. Alphabetic Index entries with NEC in the line designate "other" codes in the Tabular List. These Alphabetic Index entries represent specific disease entities for which no specific code exists so the term is included within an "other" code.

   b. **"Unspecified" codes**
       Codes titled "unspecified" are for use when the information in the medical record is insufficient to assign a more specific code. For those categories for which an unspecified code is not provided, the "other specified" code may represent both other and unspecified.

       See Section I.B.18 Use of Signs/Symptom/Unspecified Codes

10. **Includes Notes**
    This note appears immediately under a three character code title to further define, or give examples of, the content of the category.

11. **Inclusion Terms**
    List of terms is included under some codes. These terms are the conditions for which that code is to be used. The terms may be synonyms of the code title, or, in the case of "other specified" codes, the terms are a list of the various conditions assigned to that code. The inclusion terms are not necessarily exhaustive. Additional terms found only in the Alphabetic Index may also be assigned to a code.

12. **Excludes Notes**
    The ICD-10-CM has two types of excludes notes. Each type of note has a different definition for use but they are all similar in that they indicate that codes excluded from each other are independent of each other.

    a. **Excludes1**
        A type 1 Excludes note is a pure excludes note. It means "NOT CODED HERE!" An Excludes1 note indicates that the code excluded should never be used at the same time as the code above the Excludes1 note. An Excludes1 is used when two conditions cannot occur together, such as a congenital form versus an acquired form of the same condition.

b. **Excludes2**

A type 2 Excludes note represents "Not included here". An excludes2 note indicates that the condition excluded is not part of the condition represented by the code, but a patient may have both conditions at the same time. When an Excludes2 note appears under a code, it is acceptable to use both the code and the excluded code together, when appropriate.

13. **Etiology/manifestation convention ("code first", "use additional code" and "in diseases classified elsewhere" notes)**

Certain conditions have both an underlying etiology and multiple body system manifestations due to the underlying etiology. For such conditions, the ICD-10-CM has a coding convention that requires the underlying condition be sequenced first followed by the manifestation. Wherever such a combination exists, there is a "use additional code" note at the etiology code, and a "code first" note at the manifestation code. These instructional notes indicate the proper sequencing order of the codes, etiology followed by manifestation.

In most cases the manifestation codes will have in the code title, "in diseases classified elsewhere." Codes with this title are a component of the etiology/ manifestation convention. The code title indicates that it is a manifestation code. "In diseases classified elsewhere" codes are never permitted to be used as first-listed or principal diagnosis codes. They must be used in conjunction with an underlying condition code and they must be listed following the underlying condition. See category F02, Dementia in other diseases classified elsewhere, for an example of this convention.

There are manifestation codes that do not have "in diseases classified elsewhere" in the title. For such codes, there is a "use additional code" note at the etiology code and a "code first" note at the manifestation code and the rules for sequencing apply.

In addition to the notes in the Tabular List, these conditions also have a specific Alphabetic Index entry structure. In the Alphabetic Index both conditions are listed together with the etiology code first followed by the manifestation codes in brackets. The code in brackets is always to be sequenced second.

An example of the etiology/manifestation convention is dementia in Parkinson's disease. In the Alphabetic Index, code G20 is listed first, followed by code F02.80 or F02.81 in brackets. Code G20 represents the underlying etiology, Parkinson's disease, and must be sequenced first, whereas codes F02.80 and F02.81 represent the manifestation of dementia in diseases classified elsewhere, with or without behavioral disturbance.

"Code first" and "Use additional code" notes are also used as sequencing rules in the classification for certain codes that are not part of an etiology/ manifestation combination.

See Section I.B.7. Multiple coding for a single condition.

14. **"And"**

The word "and" should be interpreted to mean either "and" or "or" when it appears in a title.

For example, cases of "tuberculosis of bones", "tuberculosis of joints" and "tuberculosis of bones and joints" are classified to subcategory A18.0, Tuberculosis of bones and joints.

15. **"With"**

The word "with" should be interpreted to mean "associated with" or "due to" when it appears in a code title, the Alphabetic Index, or an instructional note in the Tabular List.

The word "with" in the Alphabetic Index is sequenced immediately following the main term, not in alphabetical order.

16. **"See" and "See Also"**

The "see" instruction following a main term in the Alphabetic Index indicates that another term should be referenced. It is necessary to go to the main term referenced with the "see" note to locate the correct code.

A "see also" instruction following a main term in the Alphabetic Index instructs that there is another main term that may also be referenced that may provide additional Alphabetic Index entries that may be useful. It is not necessary to follow the "see also" note when the original main term provides the necessary code.

17. **"Code also note"**

A "code also" note instructs that two codes may be required to fully describe a condition, but this note does not provide sequencing direction.

18. **Default codes**

A code listed next to a main term in the ICD-10-CM Alphabetic Index is referred to as a default code. The default code represents that condition that is most commonly associated with the main term, or is the unspecified code for the condition. If a condition is documented in a medical record (for example, appendicitis) without any additional information, such as acute or chronic, the default code should be assigned.

B. General Coding Guidelines

1. **Locating a code in the ICD-10-CM**

To select a code in the classification that corresponds to a diagnosis or reason for visit documented in a medical record, first locate the term in the Alphabetic Index, and then verify the code in the Tabular List. Read and be guided by instructional notations that appear in both the Alphabetic Index and the Tabular List.

It is essential to use both the Alphabetic Index and Tabular List when locating and assigning a code. The Alphabetic Index does not always provide the full code. Selection of the full code, including laterality and any applicable 7th character can only be done in the Tabular List. A dash (-) at the end of an Alphabetic Index entry indicates that additional characters are required. Even if a dash is not included at the Alphabetic Index entry, it is necessary to refer to the Tabular List to verify that no 7th character is required.

2. **Level of Detail in Coding**

Diagnosis codes are to be used and reported at their highest number of characters available.

ICD-10-CM diagnosis codes are composed of codes with 3, 4, 5, 6 or 7 characters. Codes with three characters are included in ICD-10-CM as the heading of a category of codes that may be further subdivided by the use of fourth and/or fifth characters and/or sixth characters, which provide greater detail.

A three-character code is to be used only if it is not further subdivided. A code is invalid if it has not been coded to the full number of characters required for that code, including the 7th character, if applicable.

3. **Code or codes from A00.0 through T88.9, Z00-Z99.8**

The appropriate code or codes from A00.0 through T88.9, Z00-Z99.8 must be used to identify diagnoses, symptoms, conditions, problems, complaints or other reason(s) for the encounter/visit.

4. **Signs and symptoms**

Codes that describe symptoms and signs, as opposed to diagnoses, are acceptable for reporting purposes when a related definitive diagnosis has not been established (confirmed) by the provider. Chapter 18 of ICD-10-CM, Symptoms, Signs, and Abnormal Clinical and Laboratory Findings, Not Elsewhere Classified (codes R00.0 - R99) contains many, but not all codes for symptoms.

See Section I.B.18 Use of Signs/Symptom/Unspecified Codes

5. **Conditions that are an integral part of a disease process**

Signs and symptoms that are associated routinely with a disease process should not be assigned as additional codes, unless otherwise instructed by the classification.

6. **Conditions that are not an integral part of a disease process**

Additional signs and symptoms that may not be associated routinely with a disease process should be coded when present.

7. **Multiple coding for a single condition**

In addition to the etiology/manifestation convention that requires two codes to fully describe a single condition that affects multiple body systems, there are other single conditions that also require more than one code. "Use additional code" notes are found in the Tabular List at codes that are not part of an etiology/manifestation pair where a secondary code is useful to fully describe a condition. The sequencing rule is the same as the etiology/manifestation pair, "use additional code" indicates that a secondary code should be added.

For example, for bacterial infections that are not included in chapter 1, a secondary code from category B95, Streptococcus, Staphylococcus, and Enterococcus, as the cause of diseases classified elsewhere, or B96, Other bacterial agents as the cause of diseases classified elsewhere, may be required to identify the bacterial organism causing the infection. A "use additional code" note will normally be found at the infectious disease code, indicating a need for the organism code to be added as a secondary code.

"Code first" notes are also under certain codes that are not specifically manifestation codes but may be due to an underlying cause. When there is a "code first" note and an underlying condition is present, the underlying condition should be sequenced first.

"Code, if applicable, any causal condition first", notes indicate that this code may be assigned as a principal diagnosis when the causal condition is unknown or not applicable. If a causal condition is known, then the code for that condition should be sequenced as the principal or first-listed diagnosis.

Multiple codes may be needed for sequela, complication codes and obstetric codes to more fully describe a condition. See the specific guidelines for these conditions for further instruction.

8. Acute and Chronic Conditions

If the same condition is described as both acute (subacute) and chronic, and separate subentries exist in the Alphabetic Index at the same indentation level, code both and sequence the acute (subacute) code first.

9. Combination Code

A combination code is a single code used to classify:

> Two diagnoses, or
>> A diagnosis with an associated secondary process (manifestation)
>> A diagnosis with an associated complication

Combination codes are identified by referring to subterm entries in the Alphabetic Index and by reading the inclusion and exclusion notes in the Tabular List.

Assign only the combination code when that code fully identifies the diagnostic conditions involved or when the Alphabetic Index so directs. Multiple coding should not be used when the classification provides a combination code that clearly identifies all of the elements documented in the diagnosis. When the combination code lacks necessary specificity in describing the manifestation or complication, an additional code should be used as a secondary code.

10. Sequela (Late Effects)

A sequela is the residual effect (condition produced) after the acute phase of an illness or injury has terminated. There is no time limit on when a sequela code can be used. The residual may be apparent early, such as in cerebral infarction, or it may occur months or years later, such as that due to a previous injury. Examples of sequela include: scar formation resulting from a burn, deviated septum due to a nasal fracture, and infertility due to tubal occlusion from old tuberculosis. Coding of sequela generally requires two codes sequenced in the following order: the condition or nature of the sequela is sequenced first. The sequela code is sequenced second.

An exception to the above guidelines are those instances where the code for the sequela is followed by a manifestation code identified in the Tabular List and title, or the sequela code has been expanded (at the fourth, fifth or sixth character levels) to include the manifestation(s). The code for the acute phase of an illness or injury that led to the sequela is never used with a code for the late effect.

See Section I.C.9. Sequelae of cerebrovascular disease

See Section I.C.15. Sequelae of complication of pregnancy, childbirth and the puerperium

See Section I.C.19. Application of 7th characters for Chapter 19

11. Impending or Threatened Condition

Code any condition described at the time of discharge as "impending" or "threatened" as follows:

> If it did occur, code as confirmed diagnosis.

> If it did not occur, reference the Alphabetic Index to determine if the condition has a subentry term for "impending" or "threatened" and also reference main term entries for "Impending" and for "Threatened."

> If the subterms are listed, assign the given code.

> If the subterms are not listed, code the existing underlying condition(s) and not the condition described as impending or threatened.

12. Reporting Same Diagnosis Code More than Once

Each unique ICD-10-CM diagnosis code may be reported only once for an encounter. This applies to bilateral conditions when there are no distinct codes identifying laterality or two different conditions classified to the same ICD-10-CM diagnosis code.

13. Laterality

Some ICD-10-CM codes indicate laterality, specifying whether the condition occurs on the left, right or is bilateral. If no bilateral code is provided and the condition is bilateral, assign separate codes for both the left and right side. If the side is not identified in the medical record, assign the code for the unspecified side.

14. Documentation for BMI, Non-pressure ulcers, and Pressure Ulcer Stages

For the Body Mass Index (BMI), depth of non-pressure chronic ulcers and pressure ulcer stage codes, code assignment may be based on medical record documentation from clinicians who are not the patient's provider (i.e., physician or other qualified healthcare practitioner legally accountable for establishing the patient's diagnosis), since this information is typically documented by other clinicians involved in the care of the patient (e.g., a dietitian often documents the BMI and nurses often documents the pressure ulcer stages). However, the associated diagnosis (such as overweight, obesity, or pressure ulcer) must be documented by the patient's provider. If there is conflicting medical record documentation, either from the same clinician or different clinicians, the patient's attending provider should be queried for clarification.

The BMI codes should only be reported as secondary diagnoses. As with all other secondary diagnosis codes, the BMI codes should only be assigned when they meet the definition of a reportable additional diagnosis (see Section III, Reporting Additional Diagnoses).

15. Syndromes

Follow the Alphabetic Index guidance when coding syndromes. In the absence of Alphabetic Index guidance, assign codes for the documented manifestations of the syndrome.

Additional codes for manifestations that are not an integral part of the disease process may also be assigned when the condition does not have a unique code.

16. Documentation of Complications of Care

Code assignment is based on the provider's documentation of the relationship between the condition and the care or procedure. The guideline extends to any complications of care, regardless of the chapter the code is located in. It is important to note that not all conditions that occur during or following medical care or surgery are classified as complications. There must be a cause-and-effect relationship between the care provided and the condition, and an indication in the documentation that it is a complication. Query the provider for clarification, if the complication is not clearly documented.

17. Borderline Diagnosis

If the provider documents a "borderline" diagnosis at the time of discharge, the diagnosis is coded as confirmed, unless the classification provides a specific entry (e.g., borderline diabetes). If a borderline condition has a specific index entry in ICD-10-CM, it should be coded as such. Since borderline conditions are not uncertain diagnoses, no distinction is made between the care setting (inpatient versus outpatient). Whenever the documentation is unclear regarding a borderline condition, coders are encouraged to query for clarification.

18. Use of Sign/Symptom/Unspecified Codes

Sign/symptom and "unspecified" codes have acceptable, even necessary, uses. While specific diagnosis codes should be reported when they are supported by the available medical record documentation and clinical knowledge of the patient's health condition, there are instances when signs/symptoms or unspecified codes are the best choices for accurately reflecting the healthcare encounter. Each healthcare encounter should be coded to the level of certainty known for that encounter.

If a definitive diagnosis has not been established by the end of the encounter, it is appropriate to report codes for sign(s) and/or symptom(s) in lieu of a definitive diagnosis. When sufficient clinical information isn't known or available about a particular health condition to assign a more specific code, it is acceptable to report the appropriate "unspecified" code (e.g., a diagnosis of pneumonia has been determined, but not the specific type). Unspecified codes should be reported when they are the codes that most accurately reflects what is known about the patient's condition at the time of that particular encounter. It would be inappropriate to select a specific code that is not supported by the medical record documentation or conduct medically unnecessary diagnostic testing in order to determine a more specific code.

C. Chapter-Specific Coding Guidelines

In addition to general coding guidelines, there are guidelines for specific diagnoses and/or conditions in the classification. Unless otherwise indicated, these guidelines apply to all health care settings. Please refer to Section II for guidelines on the selection of principal diagnosis.

1. **Chapter 1: Certain Infectious and Parasitic Diseases (A00-B99)**
   a. **Human immunodeficiency virus (HIV) infections**
   1) **Code only confirmed cases**
      Code only confirmed cases of HIV infection/illness. This is an exception to the hospital inpatient guideline Section II, H.

      In this context, "confirmation" does not require documentation of positive serology or culture for HIV; the provider's diagnostic statement that the patient is HIV positive, or has an HIV-related illness is sufficient.

   2) **Selection and sequencing of HIV codes**
      (a) **Patient admitted for HIV-related condition**
         If a patient is admitted for an HIV-related condition, the principal diagnosis should be B20, Human immunodeficiency virus [HIV] disease followed by additional diagnosis codes for all reported HIV-related conditions.

      (b) **Patient with HIV disease admitted for unrelated condition**
         If a patient with HIV disease is admitted for an unrelated condition (such as a traumatic injury), the code for the unrelated condition (e.g., the nature of injury code) should be the principal diagnosis. Other diagnoses would be B20 followed by additional diagnosis codes for all reported HIV-related conditions.

      (c) **Whether the patient is newly diagnosed**
         Whether the patient is newly diagnosed or has had previous admissions/encounters for HIV conditions is irrelevant to the sequencing decision.

      (d) **Asymptomatic human immunodeficiency virus**
         Z21, Asymptomatic human immunodeficiency virus [HIV] infection status, is to be applied when the patient without any documentation of symptoms is listed as being "HIV positive," "known HIV," "HIV test positive," or similar terminology. Do not use this code if the term "AIDS" is used or if the patient is treated for any HIV-related illness or is described as having any condition(s) resulting from his/her HIV positive status; use B20 in these cases.

      (e) **Patients with inconclusive HIV serology**
         Patients with inconclusive HIV serology, but no definitive diagnosis or manifestations of the illness, may be assigned code R75, Inconclusive laboratory evidence of human immunodeficiency virus [HIV].

      (f) **Previously diagnosed HIV-related illness**
         Patients with any known prior diagnosis of an HIV-related illness should be coded to B20. Once a patient has developed an HIV-related illness, the patient should always be assigned code B20 on every subsequent admission/encounter. Patients previously diagnosed with any HIV illness (B20) should never be assigned to R75 or Z21, Asymptomatic human immunodeficiency virus [HIV] infection status.

      (g) **HIV infection in pregnancy, childbirth and the puerperium**
         During pregnancy, childbirth or the puerperium, a patient admitted (or presenting for a health care encounter) because of an HIV-related illness should receive a principal diagnosis code of O98.7-, Human immunodeficiency [HIV] disease complicating pregnancy, childbirth and the puerperium, followed by B20 and the code(s) for the HIV-related illness(es). Codes from Chapter 15 always take sequencing priority.

         Patients with asymptomatic HIV infection status admitted (or presenting for a health care encounter) during pregnancy, childbirth, or the puerperium should receive codes of O98.7- and Z21.

      (h) **Encounters for testing for HIV**
         If a patient is being seen to determine his/her HIV status, use code Z11.4, Encounter for screening for human immunodeficiency virus [HIV]. Use additional codes for any associated high risk behavior.

         If a patient with signs or symptoms is being seen for HIV testing, code the signs and symptoms. An additional counseling code Z71.7, Human immunodeficiency virus [HIV] counseling, may be used if counseling is provided during the encounter for the test.

         When a patient returns to be informed of his/her HIV test results and the test result is negative, use code Z71.7, Human immunodeficiency virus [HIV] counseling.

         If the results are positive, see previous guidelines and assign codes as appropriate.

   b. **Infectious agents as the cause of diseases classified to other chapters**
      Certain infections are classified in chapters other than Chapter 1 and no organism is identified as part of the infection code. In these instances, it is necessary to use an additional code from Chapter 1 to identify the organism. A code from category B95, Streptococcus, Staphylococcus, and Enterococcus as the cause of diseases classified to other chapters, B96, Other bacterial agents as the cause of diseases classified to other chapters, or B97, Viral agents as the cause of diseases classified to other chapters, is to be used as an additional code to identify the organism. An instructional note will be found at the infection code advising that an additional organism code is required.

   c. **Infections resistant to antibiotics**
      Many bacterial infections are resistant to current antibiotics. It is necessary to identify all infections documented as antibiotic resistant. Assign a code from category Z16, Resistance to antimicrobial drugs, following the infection code only if the infection code does not identify drug resistance.

   d. **Sepsis, severe sepsis, and septic shock**
      1) **Coding of sepsis and severe sepsis**
         (a) **Sepsis**
            For a diagnosis of sepsis, assign the appropriate code for the underlying systemic infection. If the type of infection or causal organism is not further specified, assign code A41.9, Sepsis, unspecified organism.

            A code from subcategory R65.2, Severe sepsis, should not be assigned unless severe sepsis or an associated acute organ dysfunction is documented.

            (i) Negative or inconclusive blood cultures and sepsis
               Negative or inconclusive blood cultures do not preclude a diagnosis of sepsis in patients with clinical evidence of the condition, however, the provider should be queried.

            (ii) Urosepsis
               The term urosepsis is a nonspecific term. It is not to be considered synonymous with sepsis. It has no default code in the Alphabetic Index. Should a provider use this term, he/she must be queried for clarification.

            (iii) Sepsis with organ dysfunction
               If a patient has sepsis and associated acute organ dysfunction or multiple organ dysfunction (MOD), follow the instructions for coding severe sepsis.

            (iv) Acute organ dysfunction that is not clearly associated with the sepsis
               If a patient has sepsis and an acute organ dysfunction, but the medical record documentation indicates that

the acute organ dysfunction is related to a medical condition other than the sepsis, do not assign a code from subcategory R65.2, Severe sepsis. An acute organ dysfunction must be associated with the sepsis in order to assign the severe sepsis code. If the documentation is not clear as to whether an acute organ dysfunction is related to the sepsis or another medical condition, query the provider.

(b) Severe sepsis

The coding of severe sepsis requires a minimum of 2 codes: first a code for the underlying systemic infection, followed by a code from subcategory R65.2, Severe sepsis. If the causal organism is not documented, assign code A41.9, Sepsis, unspecified organism, for the infection. Additional code(s) for the associated acute organ dysfunction are also required.

Due to the complex nature of severe sepsis, some cases may require querying the provider prior to assignment of the codes.

2) Septic shock

(a) Septic shock generally refers to circulatory failure associated with severe sepsis, and therefore, it represents a type of acute organ dysfunction.

For cases of septic shock, the code for the systemic infection should be sequenced first, followed by code R65.21, Severe sepsis with septic shock or code T81.12, Postprocedural septic shock. Any additional codes for the other acute organ dysfunctions should also be assigned. As noted in the sequencing instructions in the Tabular List, the code for septic shock cannot be assigned as a principal diagnosis.

3) Sequencing of severe sepsis

If severe sepsis is present on admission, and meets the definition of principal diagnosis, the underlying systemic infection should be assigned as principal diagnosis followed by the appropriate code from subcategory R65.2 as required by the sequencing rules in the Tabular List. A code from subcategory R65.2 can never be assigned as a principal diagnosis.

When severe sepsis develops during an encounter (it was not present on admission) the underlying systemic infection and the appropriate code from subcategory R65.2 should be assigned as secondary diagnoses.

Severe sepsis may be present on admission but the diagnosis may not be confirmed until sometime after admission. If the documentation is not clear whether severe sepsis was present on admission, the provider should be queried.

4) Sepsis and severe sepsis with a localized infection

If the reason for admission is both sepsis or severe sepsis and a localized infection, such as pneumonia or cellulitis, a code(s) for the underlying systemic infection should be assigned first and the code for the localized infection should be assigned as a secondary diagnosis. If the patient has severe sepsis, a code from subcategory R65.2 should also be assigned as a secondary diagnosis. If the patient is admitted with a localized infection, such as pneumonia, and sepsis/severe sepsis doesn't develop until after admission, the localized infection should be assigned first, followed by the appropriate sepsis/severe sepsis codes.

5) Sepsis due to a postprocedural infection

(a) Documentation of causal relationship

As with all postprocedural complications, code assignment is based on the provider's documentation of the relationship between the infection and the procedure.

(b) Sepsis due to a postprocedural infection

For such cases, the postprocedural infection code, such as T80.2, Infections following infusion, transfusion, and therapeutic injection, T81.4, Infection following a procedure, T88.0, Infection following immunization, or O86.0, Infection of obstetric surgical wound, should be coded first, followed by the code for the specific infection. If the patient has severe sepsis, the appropriate code from subcategory R65.2 should also be

assigned with the additional code(s) for any acute organ dysfunction.

(c) Postprocedural infection and postprocedural septic shock

In cases where a postprocedural infection has occurred and has resulted in severe sepsis the code for the precipitating complication such as code T81.4, Infection following a procedure, or O86.0, Infection of obstetrical surgical wound should be coded first followed by code R65.20, Severe sepsis without septic shock. A code for the systemic infection should also be assigned.

If a postprocedural infection has resulted in postprocedural septic shock, the code for the precipitating complication such as code T81.4, Infection following a procedure, or O86.0, Infection of obstetrical surgical wound should be coded first followed by code T81.12-, Postprocedural septic shock. A code for the systemic infection should also be assigned.

6) Sepsis and severe sepsis associated with a noninfectious process (condition)

In some cases a noninfectious process (condition), such as trauma, may lead to an infection which can result in sepsis or severe sepsis. If sepsis or severe sepsis is documented as associated with a noninfectious condition, such as a burn or serious injury, and this condition meets the definition for principal diagnosis, the code for the noninfectious condition should be sequenced first, followed by the code for the resulting infection. If severe sepsis is present, a code from subcategory R65.2 should also be assigned with any associated organ dysfunction(s) codes. It is not necessary to assign a code from subcategory R65.1, Systemic inflammatory response syndrome (SIRS) of non-infectious origin, for these cases.

If the infection meets the definition of principal diagnosis, it should be sequenced before the non-infectious condition. When both the associated non-infectious condition and the infection meet the definition of principal diagnosis, either may be assigned as principal diagnosis.

Only one code from category R65, Symptoms and signs specifically associated with systemic inflammation and infection, should be assigned. Therefore, when a non-infectious condition leads to an infection resulting in severe sepsis, assign the appropriate code from subcategory R65.2, Severe sepsis.

Do not additionally assign a code from subcategory R65.1, Systemic inflammatory response syndrome (SIRS) of non-infectious origin.

See Section I.C.18. SIRS due to non-infectious process

7) Sepsis and septic shock complicating abortion, pregnancy, childbirth, and the puerperium

See Section I.C.15. Sepsis and septic shock complicating abortion, pregnancy, childbirth and the puerperium

8) Newborn sepsis

See Section I.C.16. f. Bacterial sepsis of Newborn

e. Methicillin resistant *Staphylococcus aureus* (MRSA) conditions

1) Selection and sequencing of MRSA codes

(a) Combination codes for MRSA infection

When a patient is diagnosed with an infection that is due to methicillin resistant *Staphylococcus aureus* (MRSA), and that infection has a combination code that includes the causal organism (e.g., sepsis, pneumonia) assign the appropriate combination code for the condition (e.g., code A41.02, Sepsis due to Methicillin resistant *Staphylococcus aureus* or code J15.212, Pneumonia due to Methicillin resistant *Staphylococcus aureus*). Do not assign code B95.62, Methicillin resistant *Staphylococcus aureus* infection as the cause of diseases classified elsewhere, as an additional code because the combination code includes the type of infection and the MRSA organism. Do not assign a code from subcategory Z16.11, Resistance to penicillins, as an additional diagnosis.

See Section C.1. for instructions on coding and sequencing of sepsis and severe sepsis.

(b) **Other codes for MRSA infection**

When there is documentation of a current infection (e.g., wound infection, stitch abscess, urinary tract infection) due to MRSA, and that infection does not have a combination code that includes the causal organism, assign the appropriate code to identify the condition along with code B95.62, Methicillin resistant *Staphylococcus aureus* infection as the cause of diseases classified elsewhere for the MRSA infection. Do not assign a code from subcategory Z16.11, Resistance to penicillins.

(c) **Methicillin susceptible *Staphylococcus aureus* (MSSA) and MRSA colonization**

The condition or state of being colonized or carrying MSSA or MRSA is called colonization or carriage, while an individual person is described as being colonized or being a carrier. Colonization means that MSSA or MSRA is present on or in the body without necessarily causing illness. A positive MRSA colonization test might be documented by the provider as "MRSA screen positive" or "MRSA nasal swab positive".

Assign code Z22.322, Carrier or suspected carrier of Methicillin resistant *Staphylococcus aureus*, for patients documented as having MRSA colonization. Assign code Z22.321, Carrier or suspected carrier of Methicillin susceptible *Staphylococcus aureus*, for patient documented as having MSSA colonization. Colonization is not necessarily indicative of a disease process or as the cause of a specific condition the patient may have unless documented as such by the provider.

(d) **MRSA colonization and infection**

If a patient is documented as having both MRSA colonization and infection during a hospital admission, code Z22.322, Carrier or suspected carrier of Methicillin resistant *Staphylococcus aureus*, and a code for the MRSA infection may both be assigned.

2. **Chapter 2: Neoplasms (C00-D49)**

General guidelines

Chapter 2 of the ICD-10-CM contains the codes for most benign and all malignant neoplasms. Certain benign neoplasms, such as prostatic adenomas, may be found in the specific body system chapters. To properly code a neoplasm it is necessary to determine from the record if the neoplasm is benign, in-situ, malignant, or of uncertain histologic behavior. If malignant, any secondary (metastatic) sites should also be determined.

Primary malignant neoplasms overlapping site boundaries

A primary malignant neoplasm that overlaps two or more contiguous (next to each other) sites should be classified to the subcategory/code .8 ('overlapping lesion'), unless the combination is specifically indexed elsewhere. For multiple neoplasms of the same site that are not contiguous such as tumors in different quadrants of the same breast, codes for each site should be assigned.

Malignant neoplasm of ectopic tissue

Malignant neoplasms of ectopic tissue are to be coded to the site of origin mentioned, e.g., ectopic pancreatic malignant neoplasms involving the stomach are coded to pancreas, unspecified (C25.9).

The neoplasm table in the Alphabetic Index should be referenced first. However, if the histological term is documented, that term should be referenced first, rather than going immediately to the Neoplasm Table, in order to determine which column in the Neoplasm Table is appropriate. For example, if the documentation indicates "adenoma," refer to the term in the Alphabetic Index to review the entries under this term and the instructional note to "see also neoplasm, by site, benign." The table provides the proper code based on the type of neoplasm and the site. It is important to select the proper column in the table that corresponds to the type of neoplasm. The Tabular List should then be referenced to verify that the correct code has been selected from the table and that a more specific site code does not exist.

See Section I.C.21. Factors influencing health status and contact with health services, Status, for information regarding Z15.0, codes for genetic susceptibility to cancer.

a. **Treatment directed at the malignancy**

If the treatment is directed at the malignancy, designate the malignancy as the principal diagnosis.

The only exception to this guideline is if a patient admission/encounter is solely for the administration of chemotherapy, immunotherapy or radiation therapy, assign the appropriate Z51.- code as the first-listed or principal diagnosis, and the diagnosis or problem for which the service is being performed as a secondary diagnosis.

b. **Treatment of secondary site**

When a patient is admitted because of a primary neoplasm with metastasis and treatment is directed toward the secondary site only, the secondary neoplasm is designated as the principal diagnosis even though the primary malignancy is still present.

c. **Coding and sequencing of complications**

Coding and sequencing of complications associated with the malignancies or with the therapy thereof are subject to the following guidelines:

1) **Anemia associated with malignancy**

When admission/encounter is for management of an anemia associated with the malignancy, and the treatment is only for anemia, the appropriate code for the malignancy is sequenced as the principal or first-listed diagnosis followed by the appropriate code for the anemia (such as code D63.0, Anemia in neoplastic disease).

2) **Anemia associated with chemotherapy, immunotherapy and radiation therapy**

When the admission/encounter is for management of an anemia associated with an adverse effect of the administration of chemotherapy or immunotherapy and the only treatment is for the anemia, the anemia code is sequenced first followed by the appropriate codes for the neoplasm and the adverse effect (T45.1X5, Adverse effect of antineoplastic and immunosuppressive drugs).

When the admission/encounter is for management of an anemia associated with an adverse effect of radiotherapy, the anemia code should be sequenced first, followed by the appropriate neoplasm code and code Y84.2, Radiological procedure and radiotherapy as the cause of abnormal reaction of the patient, or of later complication, without mention of misadventure at the time of the procedure.

3) **Management of dehydration due to the malignancy**

When the admission/encounter is for management of dehydration due to the malignancy and only the dehydration is being treated (intravenous rehydration), the dehydration is sequenced first, followed by the code(s) for the malignancy.

4) **Treatment of a complication resulting from a surgical procedure**

When the admission/encounter is for treatment of a complication resulting from a surgical procedure, designate the complication as the principal or first-listed diagnosis if treatment is directed at resolving the complication.

d. **Primary malignancy previously excised**

When a primary malignancy has been previously excised or eradicated from its site and there is no further treatment directed to that site and there is no evidence of any existing primary malignancy, a code from category Z85, Personal history of malignant neoplasm, should be used to indicate the former site of the malignancy. Any mention of extension, invasion, or metastasis to another site is coded as a secondary malignant neoplasm to that site. The secondary site may be the principal or first-listed with the Z85 code used as a secondary code.

e. **Admissions/Encounters involving chemotherapy, immunotherapy and radiation therapy**

1) **Episode of care involves surgical removal of neoplasm**

When an episode of care involves the surgical removal of a neoplasm, primary or secondary site, followed by adjunct chemotherapy or radiation treatment during the same episode of care, the code for the neoplasm should be assigned as principal or first-listed diagnosis.

2) Patient admission/encounter solely for administration of chemotherapy, immunotherapy and radiation therapy

If a patient admission/encounter is solely for the administration of chemotherapy, immunotherapy or radiation therapy assign code Z51.0, Encounter for antineoplastic radiation therapy, or Z51.11, Encounter for antineoplastic chemotherapy, or Z51.12, Encounter for antineoplastic immunotherapy as the first-listed or principal diagnosis. If a patient receives more than one of these therapies during the same admission more than one of these codes may be assigned, in any sequence.

The malignancy for which the therapy is being administered should be assigned as a secondary diagnosis.

3) Patient admitted for radiation therapy, chemotherapy or immunotherapy and develops complications

When a patient is admitted for the purpose of radiotherapy, immunotherapy or chemotherapy and develops complications such as uncontrolled nausea and vomiting or dehydration, the principal or first-listed diagnosis is Z51.0, Encounter for antineoplastic radiation therapy, or Z51.11, Encounter for antineoplastic chemotherapy, or Z51.12, Encounter for antineoplastic immunotherapy followed by any codes for the complications.

f. Admission/encounter to determine extent of malignancy

When the reason for admission/encounter is to determine the extent of the malignancy, or for a procedure such as paracentesis or thoracentesis, the primary malignancy or appropriate metastatic site is designated as the principal or first-listed diagnosis, even though chemotherapy or radiotherapy is administered.

g. Symptoms, signs, and abnormal findings listed in Chapter 18 associated with neoplasms

Symptoms, signs, and ill-defined conditions listed in Chapter 18 characteristic of, or associated with, an existing primary or secondary site malignancy cannot be used to replace the malignancy as principal or first-listed diagnosis, regardless of the number of admissions or encounters for treatment and care of the neoplasm.

See section I.C.21. Factors influencing health status and contact with health services, Encounter for prophylactic organ removal.

h. Admission/encounter for pain control/management

See Section I.C.6. for information on coding admission/encounter for pain control/management.

i. Malignancy in two or more noncontiguous sites

A patient may have more than one malignant tumor in the same organ. These tumors may represent different primaries or metastatic disease, depending on the site. Should the documentation be unclear, the provider should be queried as to the status of each tumor so that the correct codes can be assigned.

j. Disseminated malignant neoplasm, unspecified

Code C80.0, Disseminated malignant neoplasm, unspecified, is for use only in those cases where the patient has advanced metastatic disease and no known primary or secondary sites are specified. It should not be used in place of assigning codes for the primary site and all known secondary sites.

k. Malignant neoplasm without specification of site

Code C80.1, Malignant (primary) neoplasm, unspecified, equates to Cancer, unspecified. This code should only be used when no determination can be made as to the primary site of a malignancy. This code should rarely be used in the inpatient setting.

l. Sequencing of neoplasm codes

1) Encounter for treatment of primary malignancy

If the reason for the encounter is for treatment of a primary malignancy, assign the malignancy as the principal/first-listed diagnosis. The primary site is to be sequenced first, followed by any metastatic sites.

2) Encounter for treatment of secondary malignancy

When an encounter is for a primary malignancy with metastasis and treatment is directed toward the metastatic (secondary) site(s) only, the metastatic site(s) is designated as the principal/first-listed diagnosis. The primary malignancy is coded as an additional code.

3) Malignant neoplasm in a pregnant patient

When a pregnant woman has a malignant neoplasm, a code from subcategory O9A.1-, Malignant neoplasm complicating pregnancy, childbirth, and the puerperium, should be sequenced first, followed by the appropriate code from Chapter 2 to indicate the type of neoplasm.

4) Encounter for complication associated with a neoplasm

When an encounter is for management of a complication associated with a neoplasm, such as dehydration, and the treatment is only for the complication, the complication is coded first, followed by the appropriate code(s) for the neoplasm.

The exception to this guideline is anemia. When the admission/encounter is for management of an anemia associated with the malignancy, and the treatment is only for anemia, the appropriate code for the malignancy is sequenced as the principal or first-listed diagnosis followed by code D63.0, Anemia in neoplastic disease.

5) Complication from surgical procedure for treatment of a neoplasm

When an encounter is for treatment of a complication resulting from a surgical procedure performed for the treatment of the neoplasm, designate the complication as the principal/first-listed diagnosis. See guideline regarding the coding of a current malignancy versus personal history to determine if the code for the neoplasm should also be assigned.

6) Pathologic fracture due to a neoplasm

When an encounter is for a pathological fracture due to a neoplasm, and the focus of treatment is the fracture, a code from subcategory M84.5, Pathological fracture in neoplastic disease, should be sequenced first, followed by the code for the neoplasm.

If the focus of treatment is the neoplasm with an associated pathological fracture, the neoplasm code should be sequenced first, followed by a code from M84.5 for the pathological fracture.

m. Current malignancy versus personal history of malignancy

When a primary malignancy has been excised but further treatment, such as an additional surgery for the malignancy, radiation therapy or chemotherapy is directed to that site, the primary malignancy code should be used until treatment is completed.

When a primary malignancy has been previously excised or eradicated from its site, there is no further treatment (of the malignancy) directed to that site, and there is no evidence of any existing primary malignancy, a code from category Z85, Personal history of malignant neoplasm, should be used to indicate the former site of the malignancy.

See Section I.C.21. Factors influencing health status and contact with health services, History (of)

n. Leukemia, multiple myeloma, and malignant plasma cell neoplasms in remission versus personal history

The categories for leukemia, and category C90, Multiple myeloma and malignant plasma cell neoplasms, have codes indicating whether or not the leukemia has achieved remission. There are also codes Z85.6, Personal history of leukemia, and Z85.79, Personal history of other malignant neoplasms of lymphoid, hematopoietic and related tissues. If the documentation is unclear, as to whether the leukemia has achieved remission, the provider should be queried.

See Section I.C.21. Factors influencing health status and contact with health services, History (of)

o. Aftercare following surgery for neoplasm

See Section I.C.21. Factors influencing health status and contact with health services, Aftercare

p. Follow-up care for completed treatment of a malignancy

See Section I.C.21. Factors influencing health status and contact with health services, Follow-up

q. Prophylactic organ removal for prevention of malignancy

See Section I.C. 21, Factors influencing health status and contact with health services, Prophylactic organ removal

r. **Malignant neoplasm associated with transplanted organ**
A malignant neoplasm of a transplanted organ should be coded as a transplant complication. Assign first the appropriate code from category T86.-, Complications of transplanted organs and tissue, followed by code C80.2, Malignant neoplasm associated with transplanted organ. Use an additional code for the specific malignancy.

3. **Chapter 3: Disease of the blood and blood-forming organs and certain disorders involving the immune mechanism (D50-D89)**
Reserved for future guideline expansion

4. **Chapter 4: Endocrine, Nutritional, and Metabolic Diseases (E00-E89)**
   a. **Diabetes mellitus**
   The diabetes mellitus codes are combination codes that include the type of diabetes mellitus, the body system affected, and the complications affecting that body system. As many codes within a particular category as are necessary to describe all of the complications of the disease may be used. They should be sequenced based on the reason for a particular encounter. Assign as many codes from categories E08 – E13 as needed to identify all of the associated conditions that the patient has.

   1) **Type of diabetes**
   The age of a patient is not the sole determining factor, though most type 1 diabetics develop the condition before reaching puberty. For this reason type 1 diabetes mellitus is also referred to as juvenile diabetes.

   2) **Type of diabetes mellitus not documented**
   If the type of diabetes mellitus is not documented in the medical record the default is E11.-, Type 2 diabetes mellitus.

   3) **Diabetes mellitus and the use of insulin**
   If the documentation in a medical record does not indicate the type of diabetes but does indicate that the patient uses insulin, code E11, Type 2 diabetes mellitus, should be assigned. Code Z79.4, Long-term (current) use of insulin, should also be assigned to indicate that the patient uses insulin. Code Z79.4 should not be assigned if insulin is given temporarily to bring a type 2 patient's blood sugar under control during an encounter.

   4) **Diabetes mellitus in pregnancy and gestational diabetes**
   See Section I.C.15. Diabetes mellitus in pregnancy.

   See Section I.C.15. Gestational (pregnancy induced) diabetes

   5) **Complications due to insulin pump malfunction**
      (a) **Underdose of insulin due to insulin pump failure**
      An underdose of insulin due to an insulin pump failure should be assigned to a code from subcategory T85.6, Mechanical complication of other specified internal and external prosthetic devices, implants and grafts, that specifies the type of pump malfunction, as the principal or first-listed code, followed by code T38.3x6-, Underdosing of insulin and oral hypoglycemic [antidiabetic] drugs. Additional codes for the type of diabetes mellitus and any associated complications due to the underdosing should also be assigned.

      (b) **Overdose of insulin due to insulin pump failure**
      The principal or first-listed code for an encounter due to an insulin pump malfunction resulting in an overdose of insulin, should also be T85.6-, Mechanical complication of other specified internal and external prosthetic devices, implants and grafts, followed by code T38.3X1-, Poisoning by insulin and oral hypoglycemic [antidiabetic] drugs, accidental (unintentional).

   6) **Secondary diabetes mellitus**
   Codes under categories E08, Diabetes mellitus due to underlying condition, E09, Drug or chemical induced diabetes mellitus, and E13, Other specified diabetes mellitus, identify complications/manifestations associated with secondary diabetes mellitus. Secondary diabetes is always caused by another condition or event (e.g., cystic fibrosis, malignant neoplasm of pancreas, pancreatectomy, adverse effect of drug, or poisoning).

      (a) **Secondary diabetes mellitus and the use of insulin**
      For patients who routinely use insulin, code Z79.4, Long-term (current) use of insulin, should also be assigned. Code Z79.4 should not be assigned if insulin is given temporarily to bring a patient's blood sugar under control during an encounter.

      (b) **Assigning and sequencing secondary diabetes codes and its causes**
      The sequencing of the secondary diabetes codes in relationship to codes for the cause of the diabetes is based on the Tabular List instructions for categories E08, E09 and E13.

      (i) **Secondary diabetes mellitus due to pancreatectomy**
      For postpancreatectomy diabetes mellitus (lack of insulin due to the surgical removal of all or part of the pancreas), assign code E89.1, Postprocedural hypoinsulinemia. Assign a code from category E13 and a code from subcategory Z90.41-, Acquired absence of pancreas, as additional codes.

      (ii) **Secondary diabetes due to drugs**
      Secondary diabetes may be caused by an adverse effect of correctly administered medications, poisoning or sequela of poisoning.
      See section I.C.19.e for coding of adverse effects and poisoning, and section I.C.20 for external cause code reporting.

5. **Chapter 5: Mental, Behavioral and Neurodevelopmental disorders (F01 – F99)**
   a. **Pain disorders related to psychological factors**
   Assign code F45.41, for pain that is exclusively related to psychological disorders. As indicated by the Excludes 1 note under category G89, a code from category G89 should not be assigned with code F45.41.

   Code F45.42, Pain disorders with related psychological factors, should be used with a code from category G89, Pain, not elsewhere classified, if there is documentation of a psychological component for a patient with acute or chronic pain.
   See Section I.C.6. Pain

   b. **Mental and behavioral disorders due to psychoactive substance use**
   1) **In remission**
   Selection of codes for "in remission" for categories F10-F19, Mental and behavioral disorders due to psychoactive substance use (categories F10-F19 with -.21) requires the provider's clinical judgment. The appropriate codes for "in remission" are assigned only on the basis of provider documentation (as defined in the Official Guidelines for Coding and Reporting).

   2) **Psychoactive substance use, abuse and dependence**
   When the provider documentation refers to use, abuse and dependence of the same substance (e.g. alcohol, opioid, cannabis, etc.), only one code should be assigned to identify the pattern of use based on the following hierarchy:

   - If both use and abuse are documented, assign only the code for abuse
   - If both abuse and dependence are documented, assign only the code for dependence
   - If use, abuse and dependence are all documented, assign only the code for dependence
   - If both use and dependence are documented, assign only the code for dependence.

   3) **Psychoactive substance use**
   As with all other diagnoses, the codes for psychoactive substance use (F10.9-, F11.9-, F12.9-, F13.9-, F14.9-, F15.9-, F16.9-) should only be assigned based on provider documentation and when they meet the definition of a reportable diagnosis (see Section III, Reporting Additional Diagnoses). The codes are to be used only when the psychoactive substance use is associated with a mental or behavioral disorder, and such a relationship is documented by the provider.

6. **Chapter 6: Diseases of Nervous System (G00-G99)**
   a. **Dominant/nondominant side**
   Codes from category G81, Hemiplegia and hemiparesis, and subcategories, G83.1, Monoplegia of lower limb, G83.2, Monoplegia of upper limb, and G83.3, Monoplegia, unspecified, identify whether the dominant or nondominant side is affected. Should the affected side be documented, but not specified as dominant or nondominant, and the classification system does not indicate a default, code selection is as follows:

   - For ambidextrous patients, the default should be dominant.
   - If the left side is affected, the default is non-dominant.
   - If the right side is affected, the default is dominant.

   b. **Pain - Category G89**
   1) **General coding information**
   Codes in category G89, Pain, not elsewhere classified, may be used in conjunction with codes from other categories and chapters to provide more detail about acute or chronic pain and neoplasm-related pain, unless otherwise indicated below.

   If the pain is not specified as acute or chronic, post-thoracotomy, postprocedural, or neoplasm-related, do not assign codes from category G89.

   A code from category G89 should not be assigned if the underlying (definitive) diagnosis is known, unless the reason for the encounter is pain control/ management and not management of the underlying condition.

   When an admission or encounter is for a procedure aimed at treating the underlying condition (e.g., spinal fusion, kyphoplasty), a code for the underlying condition (e.g., vertebral fracture, spinal stenosis) should be assigned as the principal diagnosis. No code from category G89 should be assigned.

   (a) **Category G89 codes as principal or first-listed diagnosis**
   Category G89 codes are acceptable as principal diagnosis or the first-listed code:

   - When pain control or pain management is the reason for the admission/encounter (e.g., a patient with displaced intervertebral disc, nerve impingement and severe back pain presents for injection of steroid into the spinal canal). The underlying cause of the pain should be reported as an additional diagnosis, if known.

   - When a patient is admitted for the insertion of a neurostimulator for pain control, assign the appropriate pain code as the principal or first-listed diagnosis. When an admission or encounter is for a procedure aimed at treating the underlying condition and a neurostimulator is inserted for pain control during the same admission/encounter, a code for the underlying condition should be assigned as the principal diagnosis and the appropriate pain code should be assigned as a secondary diagnosis.

   (b) **Use of category G89 codes in conjunction with site specific pain codes**
   (i) **Assigning category G89 and site-specific pain codes**
   Codes from category G89 may be used in conjunction with codes that identify the site of pain (including codes from chapter 18) if the category G89 code provides additional information. For example, if the code describes the site of the pain, but does not fully describe whether the pain is acute or chronic, then both codes should be assigned.

   (ii) **Sequencing of category G89 codes with site-specific pain codes**
   The sequencing of category G89 codes with site-specific pain codes (including chapter 18 codes), is dependent on the circumstances of the encounter/admission as follows:

   - If the encounter is for pain control or pain management, assign the code from category G89 followed by the code identifying the specific site of pain (e.g., encounter for pain management for acute neck pain from trauma is assigned code G89.11, Acute pain due to trauma, followed by code M54.2, Cervicalgia, to identify the site of pain).

   - If the encounter is for any other reason except pain control or pain management, and a related definitive diagnosis has not been established (confirmed) by the provider, assign the code for the specific site of pain first, followed by the appropriate code from category G89.

   2) **Pain due to devices, implants and grafts**
   See Section I.C.19. Pain due to medical devices

   3) **Postoperative pain**
   The provider's documentation should be used to guide the coding of postoperative pain, as well as *Section III. Reporting Additional Diagnoses* and *Section IV. Diagnostic Coding and Reporting in the Outpatient Setting.*

   The default for post-thoracotomy and other postoperative pain not specified as acute or chronic is the code for the acute form.

   Routine or expected postoperative pain immediately after surgery should not be coded.

   (a) **Postoperative pain not associated with specific postoperative complication**
   Postoperative pain not associated with a specific postoperative complication is assigned to the appropriate postoperative pain code in category G89.

   (b) **Postoperative pain associated with specific postoperative complication**
   Postoperative pain associated with a specific postoperative complication (such as painful wire sutures) is assigned to the appropriate code(s) found in Chapter 19, Injury, poisoning, and certain other consequences of external causes. If appropriate, use additional code(s) from category G89 to identify acute or chronic pain (G89.18 or G89.28).

   4) **Chronic pain**
   Chronic pain is classified to subcategory G89.2. There is no time frame defining when pain becomes chronic pain. The provider's documentation should be used to guide use of these codes.

   5) **Neoplasm related pain**
   Code G89.3 is assigned to pain documented as being related, associated or due to cancer, primary or secondary malignancy, or tumor. This code is assigned regardless of whether the pain is acute or chronic.

   This code may be assigned as the principal or first-listed code when the stated reason for the admission/encounter is documented as pain control/pain management. The underlying neoplasm should be reported as an additional diagnosis.

   When the reason for the admission/encounter is management of the neoplasm and the pain associated with the neoplasm is also documented, code G89.3 may be assigned as an additional diagnosis. It is not necessary to assign an additional code for the site of the pain.

   See Section I.C.2 for instructions on the sequencing of neoplasms for all other stated reasons for the admission/encounter (except for pain control/pain management).

   6) **Chronic pain syndrome**
   Central pain syndrome (G89.0) and chronic pain syndrome (G89.4) are different than the term "chronic pain," and therefore codes should only be used when the provider has specifically documented this condition.

   See Section I.C.5. Pain disorders related to psychological factors

7. **Chapter 7: Diseases of Eye and Adnexa (H00-H59)**
   a. **Glaucoma**
   1) **Assigning glaucoma codes**
   Assign as many codes from category H40, Glaucoma, as needed to identify the type of glaucoma, the affected eye, and the glaucoma stage.

   2) **Bilateral glaucoma with same type and stage**
   When a patient has bilateral glaucoma and both eyes are documented as being the same type and stage, and there is a

code for bilateral glaucoma, report only the code for the type of glaucoma, bilateral, with the seventh character for the stage.

When a patient has bilateral glaucoma and both eyes are documented as being the same type and stage, and the classification does not provide a code for bilateral glaucoma (i.e. subcategories H40.10, H40.11 and H40.20) report only one code for the type of glaucoma with the appropriate seventh character for the stage.

3) Bilateral glaucoma stage with different types or stages
When a patient has bilateral glaucoma and each eye is documented as having a different type or stage, and the classification distinguishes laterality, assign the appropriate code for each eye rather than the code for bilateral glaucoma.

When a patient has bilateral glaucoma and each eye is documented as having a different type, and the classification does not distinguish laterality (i.e. subcategories H40.10, H40.11 and H40.20), assign one code for each type of glaucoma with the appropriate seventh character for the stage.

When a patient has bilateral glaucoma and each eye is documented as having the same type, but different stage, and the classification does not distinguish laterality (i.e. subcategories H40.10, H40.11 and H40.20), assign a code for the type of glaucoma for each eye with the seventh character for the specific glaucoma stage documented for each eye.

4) Patient admitted with glaucoma and stage evolves during the admission
If a patient is admitted with glaucoma and the stage progresses during the admission, assign the code for highest stage documented.

5) Indeterminate stage glaucoma
Assignment of the seventh character "4" for "indeterminate stage" should be based on the clinical documentation. The seventh character "4" is used for glaucomas whose stage cannot be clinically determined. This seventh character should not be confused with the seventh character "0", unspecified, which should be assigned when there is no documentation regarding the stage of the glaucoma.

8. Chapter 8: Diseases of Ear and Mastoid Process (H60-H95)
Reserved for future guideline expansion

9. Chapter 9: Diseases of Circulatory System (I00-I99)
a. Hypertension
1) Hypertension with heart disease
Heart conditions classified to I50.- or I51.4-I51.9, are assigned to, a code from category I11, Hypertensive heart disease, when a causal relationship is stated (due to hypertension) or implied (hypertensive). Use an additional code from category I50, Heart failure, to identify the type of heart failure in those patients with heart failure.

The same heart conditions (I50.-, I51.4-I51.9) with hypertension, but without a stated causal relationship, are coded separately. Sequence according to the circumstances of the admission/encounter.

2) Hypertensive chronic kidney disease
Assign codes from category I12, Hypertensive chronic kidney disease, when both hypertension and a condition classifiable to category N18, Chronic kidney disease (CKD), are present. Unlike hypertension with heart disease, ICD-10-CM presumes a cause-and-effect relationship and classifies chronic kidney disease with hypertension as hypertensive chronic kidney disease.

The appropriate code from category N18 should be used as a secondary code with a code from category I12 to identify the stage of chronic kidney disease.
See Section I.C.14. Chronic kidney disease.

If a patient has hypertensive chronic kidney disease and acute renal failure, an additional code for the acute renal failure is required.

3) Hypertensive heart and chronic kidney disease
Assign codes from combination category I13, Hypertensive heart and chronic kidney disease, when both hypertensive

kidney disease and hypertensive heart disease are stated in the diagnosis. Assume a relationship between the hypertension and the chronic kidney disease, whether or not the condition is so designated. If heart failure is present, assign an additional code from category I50 to identify the type of heart failure.

The appropriate code from category N18, Chronic kidney disease, should be used as a secondary code with a code from category I13 to identify the stage of chronic kidney disease.
See Section I.C.14. Chronic kidney disease.

The codes in category I13, Hypertensive heart and chronic kidney disease, are combination codes that include hypertension, heart disease and chronic kidney disease. The Includes note at I13 specifies that the conditions included at I11 and I12 are included together in I13. If a patient has hypertension, heart disease and chronic kidney disease then a code from I13 should be used, not individual codes for hypertension, heart disease and chronic kidney disease, or codes from I11 or I12.

For patients with both acute renal failure and chronic kidney disease an additional code for acute renal failure is required.

4) Hypertensive cerebrovascular disease
For hypertensive cerebrovascular disease, first assign the appropriate code from categories I60-I69, followed by the appropriate hypertension code.

5) Hypertensive retinopathy
Subcategory H35.0, Background retinopathy and retinal vascular changes, should be used with a code from category I10 – I15, Hypertensive disease to include the systemic hypertension. The sequencing is based on the reason for the encounter.

6) Hypertension, secondary
Secondary hypertension is due to an underlying condition. Two codes are required: one to identify the underlying etiology and one from category I15 to identify the hypertension. Sequencing of codes is determined by the reason for admission/encounter.

7) Hypertension, transient
Assign code R03.0, Elevated blood pressure reading without diagnosis of hypertension, unless patient has an established diagnosis of hypertension. Assign code O13.-, Gestational [pregnancy-induced] hypertension without significant proteinuria, or O14.-, Pre-eclampsia, for transient hypertension of pregnancy.

8) Hypertension, controlled
This diagnostic statement usually refers to an existing state of hypertension under control by therapy. Assign the appropriate code from categories I10-I15, Hypertensive diseases.

9) Hypertension, uncontrolled
Uncontrolled hypertension may refer to untreated hypertension or hypertension not responding to current therapeutic regimen. In either case, assign the appropriate code from categories I10-I15, Hypertensive diseases.

b. Atherosclerotic coronary artery disease and angina
ICD-10-CM has combination codes for atherosclerotic heart disease with angina pectoris. The subcategories for these codes are I25.11, Atherosclerotic heart disease of native coronary artery with angina pectoris and I25.7, Atherosclerosis of coronary artery bypass graft(s) and coronary artery of transplanted heart with angina pectoris.

When using one of these combination codes it is not necessary to use an additional code for angina pectoris. A causal relationship can be assumed in a patient with both atherosclerosis and angina pectoris, unless the documentation indicates the angina is due to something other than the atherosclerosis.

If a patient with coronary artery disease is admitted due to an acute myocardial infarction (AMI), the AMI should be sequenced before the coronary artery disease.
See Section I.C.9. Acute myocardial infarction (AMI)

c. Intraoperative and postprocedural cerebrovascular accident
Medical record documentation should clearly specify the cause-and-effect relationship between the medical intervention and the

cerebrovascular accident in order to assign a code for intraoperative or postprocedural cerebrovascular accident.

Proper code assignment depends on whether it was an infarction or hemorrhage and whether it occurred intraoperatively or postoperatively. If it was a cerebral hemorrhage, code assignment depends on the type of procedure performed.

d. Sequelae of cerebrovascular disease

1) Category I69, sequelae of cerebrovascular disease

Category I69 is used to indicate conditions classifiable to categories I60-I67 as the causes of sequela (neurologic deficits), themselves classified elsewhere. These "late effects" include neurologic deficits that persist after initial onset of conditions classifiable to categories I60-I67. The neurologic deficits caused by cerebrovascular disease may be present from the onset or may arise at any time after the onset of the condition classifiable to categories I60-I67.

Codes from category I69, Sequelae of cerebrovascular disease, that specify hemiplegia, hemiparesis and monoplegia identify whether the dominant or nondominant side is affected. Should the affected side be documented, but not specified as dominant or nondominant, and the classification system does not indicate a default, code selection is as follows:

- For ambidextrous patients, the default should be dominant.
- If the left side is affected, the default is non-dominant.
- If the right side is affected, the default is dominant.

2) Codes from category I69 with codes from I60-I67

Codes from category I69 may be assigned on a health care record with codes from I60-I67, if the patient has a current cerebrovascular disease and deficits from an old cerebrovascular disease.

3) Codes from category I69 and Personal history of transient ischemic attack (TIA) and cerebral infarction (Z86.73)

Codes from category I69 should not be assigned if the patient does not have neurologic deficits.

See Section I.C.21. 4. History (of) for use of personal history codes

e. Acute myocardial infarction (AMI)

1) ST elevation myocardial infarction (STEMI) and non ST elevation myocardial infarction (NSTEMI)

The ICD-10-CM codes for acute myocardial infarction (AMI) identify the site, such as anterolateral wall or true posterior wall. Subcategories I21.0-I21.2 and code I21.3 are used for ST elevation myocardial infarction (STEMI). Code I21.4, Non-ST elevation (NSTEMI) myocardial infarction, is used for non ST elevation myocardial infarction (NSTEMI) and nontransmural MIs.

If NSTEMI evolves to STEMI, assign the STEMI code. If STEMI converts to NSTEMI due to thrombolytic therapy, it is still coded as STEMI.

For encounters occurring while the myocardial infarction is equal to, or less than, four weeks old, including transfers to another acute setting or a postacute setting, and the patient requires continued care for the myocardial infarction, codes from category I21 may continue to be reported. For encounters after the 4 week time frame and the patient is still receiving care related to the myocardial infarction, the appropriate aftercare code should be assigned, rather than a code from category I21. For old or healed myocardial infarctions not requiring further care, code I25.2, Old myocardial infarction, may be assigned.

2) Acute myocardial infarction, unspecified

Code I21.3, ST elevation (STEMI) myocardial infarction of unspecified site, is the default for the unspecified term acute myocardial infarction. If only STEMI or transmural MI without the site is documented, query the provider as to the site, or assign code I21.3.

3) AMI documented as nontransmural or subendocardial but site provided

If an AMI is documented as nontransmural or subendocardial, but the site is provided, it is still coded as a subendocardial AMI.

See Section I.C.21.3 for information on coding status post administration of tPA in a different facility within the last 24 hrs.

4) Subsequent acute myocardial infarction

A code from category I22, Subsequent ST elevation (STEMI) and non ST elevation (NSTEMI) myocardial infarction, is to be used when a patient who has suffered an AMI has a new AMI within the 4 week time frame of the initial AMI. A code from category I22 must be used in conjunction with a code from category I21. The sequencing of the I22 and I21 codes depends on the circumstances of the encounter.

10. Chapter 10: Diseases of the Respiratory System (J00-J99)

a. Chronic Obstructive Pulmonary Disease [COPD] and Asthma

1) Acute exacerbation of chronic obstructive bronchitis and asthma

The codes in categories J44 and J45 distinguish between uncomplicated cases and those in acute exacerbation. An acute exacerbation is a worsening or a decompensation of a chronic condition. An acute exacerbation is not equivalent to an infection superimposed on a chronic condition, though an exacerbation may be triggered by an infection.

b. Acute Respiratory Failure

1) Acute respiratory failure as principal diagnosis

A code from subcategory J96.0, Acute respiratory failure, or subcategory J96.2, Acute and chronic respiratory failure, may be assigned as a principal diagnosis when it is the condition established after study to be chiefly responsible for occasioning the admission to the hospital, and the selection is supported by the Alphabetic Index and Tabular List. However, chapter-specific coding guidelines (such as obstetrics, poisoning, HIV, newborn) that provide sequencing direction take precedence.

2) Acute respiratory failure as secondary diagnosis

Respiratory failure may be listed as a secondary diagnosis if it occurs after admission, or if it is present on admission, but does not meet the definition of principal diagnosis.

3) Sequencing of acute respiratory failure and another acute condition

When a patient is admitted with respiratory failure and another acute condition, (e.g., myocardial infarction, cerebrovascular accident, aspiration pneumonia), the principal diagnosis will not be the same in every situation. This applies whether the other acute condition is a respiratory or nonrespiratory condition. Selection of the principal diagnosis will be dependent on the circumstances of admission. If both the respiratory failure and the other acute condition are equally responsible for occasioning the admission to the hospital, and there are no chapter-specific sequencing rules, the guideline regarding two or more diagnoses that equally meet the definition for principal diagnosis (Section II, C.) may be applied in these situations.

If the documentation is not clear as to whether acute respiratory failure and another condition are equally responsible for occasioning the admission, query the provider for clarification.

c. Influenza due to certain identified influenza viruses

Code only confirmed cases of influenza due to certain identified influenza viruses (category J09), and due to other identified influenza virus (category J10). This is an exception to the hospital inpatient guideline Section II, H. (Uncertain Diagnosis).

In this context, "confirmation" does not require documentation of positive laboratory testing specific for avian or other novel influenza A or other identified influenza virus. However, coding should be based on the provider's diagnostic statement that the patient has avian influenza, or other novel influenza A, for category J09, or has another particular identified strain of influenza, such as H1N1 or H3N2, but not identified as novel or variant, for category J10.

If the provider records "suspected" or "possible" or "probable" avian influenza, or novel influenza, or other identified influenza, then the appropriate influenza code from category J11, Influenza due to unidentified influenza virus, should be assigned. A code from category J09, Influenza due to certain identified influenza viruses, should not be assigned nor should a code from category J10, Influenza due to other identified influenza virus.

d. **Ventilator associated pneumonia**

1) **Documentation of ventilator associated pneumonia**

As with all procedural or postprocedural complications, code assignment is based on the provider's documentation of the relationship between the condition and the procedure.

Code J95.851, Ventilator associated pneumonia, should be assigned only when the provider has documented ventilator associated pneumonia (VAP). An additional code to identify the organism (e.g., Pseudomonas aeruginosa, code B96.5) should also be assigned. Do not assign an additional code from categories J12-J18 to identify the type of pneumonia.

Code J95.851 should not be assigned for cases where the patient has pneumonia and is on a mechanical ventilator and the provider has not specifically stated that the pneumonia is ventilator-associated pneumonia. If the documentation is unclear as to whether the patient has a pneumonia that is a complication attributable to the mechanical ventilator, query the provider.

2) **Ventilator associated pneumonia develops after admission**

A patient may be admitted with one type of pneumonia (e.g., code J13, Pneumonia due to Streptococcus pneu- monia) and subsequently develop VAP. In this instance, the principal diagnosis would be the appro- priate code from categories J12-J18 for the pneumonia diagnosed at the time of admission. Code J95.851, Ventilator assoc- iated pneumonia, would be assigned as an additional diagnosis when the provider has also documented the presence of ventilator associated pneumonia.

11. **Chapter 11: Diseases of the Digestive System (K00-K95)**

Reserved for future guideline expansion

12. **Chapter 12: Diseases of the Skin and Subcutaneous Tissue (L00-L99)**

a. **Pressure ulcer stage codes**

1) **Pressure ulcer stages**

Codes from category L89, Pressure ulcer, are combination codes that identify the site of the pressure ulcer as well as the stage of the ulcer.

The ICD-10-CM classifies pressure ulcer stages based on severity, which is designated by stages 1-4, unspecified stage and unstageable.

Assign as many codes from category L89 as needed to identify all the pressure ulcers the patient has, if applicable.

2) **Unstageable pressure ulcers**

Assignment of the code for unstageable pressure ulcer (L89.--0) should be based on the clinical documentation. These codes are used for pressure ulcers whose stage cannot be clinically determined (e.g., the ulcer is covered by eschar or has been treated with a skin or muscle graft) and pressure ulcers that are documented as deep tissue injury but not documented as due to trauma. This code should not be confused with the codes for unspecified stage (L89.--9). When there is no documentation regarding the stage of the pressure ulcer, assign the appropriate code for unspecified stage (L89.--9).

3) **Documented pressure ulcer stage**

Assignment of the pressure ulcer stage code should be guided by clinical documentation of the stage or documentation of the terms found in the Alphabetic Index. For clinical terms describing the stage that are not found in the Alphabetic Index, and there is no documentation of the stage, the provider should be queried.

4) **Patients admitted with pressure ulcers documented as healed**

No code is assigned if the documentation states that the pressure ulcer is completely healed.

5) **Patients admitted with pressure ulcers documented as healing**

Pressure ulcers described as healing should be assigned the appropriate pressure ulcer stage code based on the documentation in the medical record. If the documentation does not provide information about the stage of the healing pressure ulcer, assign the appropriate code for unspecified stage.

If the documentation is unclear as to whether the patient has a current (new) pressure ulcer or if the patient is being treated for a healing pressure ulcer, query the provider.

6) **Patient admitted with pressure ulcer evolving into another stage during the admission**

If a patient is admitted with a pressure ulcer at one stage and it progresses to a higher stage, assign the code for the highest stage reported for that site.

13. **Chapter 13: Diseases of the Musculoskeletal System and Connective Tissue (M00-M99)**

a. **Site and laterality**

Most of the codes within Chapter 13 have site and laterality designations. The site represents the bone, joint or the muscle involved. For some conditions where more than one bone, joint or muscle is usually involved, such as osteoarthritis, there is a "multiple sites" code available. For categories where no multiple site code is provided and more than one bone, joint or muscle is involved, multiple codes should be used to indicate the different sites involved.

1) **Bone versus joint**

For certain conditions, the bone may be affected at the upper or lower end, (e.g., avascular necrosis of bone, M87, Osteoporosis, M80, M81). Though the portion of the bone affected may be at the joint, the site designation will be the bone, not the joint.

b. **Acute traumatic versus chronic or recurrent musculoskeletal conditions**

Many musculoskeletal conditions are a result of previous injury or trauma to a site, or are recurrent conditions. Bone, joint or muscle conditions that are the result of a healed injury are usually found in chapter 13. Recurrent bone, joint or muscle conditions are also usually found in chapter 13. Any current, acute injury should be coded to the appropriate injury code from chapter 19. Chronic or recurrent conditions should generally be coded with a code from chapter 13. If it is difficult to determine from the documentation in the record which code is best to describe a condition, query the provider.

c. **Coding of Pathologic Fractures**

7th character A is for use as long as the patient is receiving active treatment for the fracture. Examples of active treatment are: surgical treatment, emergency department encounter, evaluation and continuing treatment by the same or a different physician. While the patient may be seen by a new or different provider over the course of treatment for a pathological fracture, assignment of the 7th character is based on whether the patient is undergoing active treatment and not whether the provider is seeing the patient for the first time.

7th character, D is to be used for encounters after the patient has completed active treatment. The other 7th characters, listed under each subcategory in the Tabular List, are to be used for subsequent encounters for treatment of problems associated with the healing, such as malunions, nonunions, and sequelae.

Care for complications of surgical treatment for fracture repairs during the healing or recovery phase should be coded with the appropriate complication codes.

See Section I.C.19. Coding of traumatic fractures.

d. **Osteoporosis**

Osteoporosis is a systemic condition, meaning that all bones of the musculoskeletal system are affected. Therefore, site is not a component of the codes under category M81, Osteoporosis without current pathological fracture. The site codes under category M80, Osteoporosis with current pathological fracture, identify the site of the fracture, not the osteoporosis.

1) **Osteoporosis without pathological fracture**

Category M81, Osteoporosis without current pathological fracture, is for use for patients with osteoporosis who do not currently have a pathologic fracture due to the osteoporosis, even if they have had a fracture in the past. For patients with a history of osteoporosis fractures, status code Z87.310, Personal history of (healed) osteoporosis fracture, should follow the code from M81.

    2) Osteoporosis with current pathological fracture
      Category M80, Osteoporosis with current pathological fracture, is for patients who have a current pathologic fracture at the time of an encounter. The codes under M80 identify the site of the fracture. A code from category M80, not a traumatic fracture code, should be used for any patient with known osteoporosis who suffers a fracture, even if the patient had a minor fall or trauma, if that fall or trauma would not usually break a normal, healthy bone.

14. Chapter 14: Diseases of Genitourinary System (N00-N99)
a. Chronic kidney disease
1) Stages of chronic kidney disease (CKD)
The ICD-10-CM classifies CKD based on severity. The severity of CKD is designated by stages 1-5. Stage 2, code N18.2, equates to mild CKD; stage 3, code N18.3, equates to moderate CKD; and stage 4, code N18.4, equates to severe CKD. Code N18.6, End stage renal disease (ESRD), is assigned when the provider has documented end-stage-renal disease (ESRD).

If both a stage of CKD and ESRD are documented, assign code N18.6 only.

2) Chronic kidney disease and kidney transplant status
Patients who have undergone kidney transplant may still have some form of chronic kidney disease (CKD) because the kidney transplant may not fully restore kidney function. Therefore, the presence of CKD alone does not constitute a transplant complication. Assign the appropriate N18 code for the patient's stage of CKD and code Z94.0, Kidney transplant status. If a transplant complication such as failure or rejection or other transplant complication is documented, see section I.C.19.g for information on coding complications of a kidney transplant. If the documentation is unclear as to whether the patient has a complication of the transplant, query the provider.

3) Chronic kidney disease with other conditions
Patients with CKD may also suffer from other serious conditions, most commonly diabetes mellitus and hypertension. The sequencing of the CKD code in relationship to codes for other contributing conditions is based on the conventions in the Tabular List.

See I.C.9. Hypertensive chronic kidney disease.

See I.C.19. Chronic kidney disease and kidney transplant complications.

15. Chapter 15: Pregnancy, Childbirth, and the Puerperium (O00-O9A)
a. General Rules for Obstetric Cases
1) Codes from chapter 15 and sequencing priority
Obstetric cases require codes from chapter 15, codes in the range O00-O9A, Pregnancy, Childbirth, and the Puerperium. Chapter 15 codes have sequencing priority over codes from other chapters. Additional codes from other chapters may be used in conjunction with chapter 15 codes to further specify conditions. Should the provider document that the pregnancy is incidental to the encounter, then code Z33.1, Pregnant state, incidental, should be used in place of any chapter 15 codes. It is the provider's responsibility to state that the condition being treated is not affecting the pregnancy.

2) Chapter 15 codes used only on the maternal record
Chapter 15 codes are to be used only on the maternal record, never on the record of the newborn.

3) Final character for trimester
The majority of codes in Chapter 15 have a final character indicating the trimester of pregnancy. The timeframes for the trimesters are indicated at the beginning of the chapter. If trimester is not a component of a code it is because the condition always occurs in a specific trimester, or the concept of trimester of pregnancy is not applicable. Certain codes have characters for only certain trimesters because the condition does not occur in all trimesters, but it may occur in more than just one.

Assignment of the final character for trimester should be based on the provider's documentation of the trimester (or number of weeks) for the current admission/encounter. This applies to the assignment of trimester for pre-existing conditions as well as

those that develop during or are due to the pregnancy. The provider's documentation of the number of weeks may be used to assign the appropriate code identifying the trimester.

Whenever delivery occurs during the current admission, and there is an "in childbirth" option for the obstetric complication being coded, the "in childbirth" code should be assigned.

4) Selection of trimester for inpatient admissions that encompass more than one trimesters
In instances when a patient is admitted to a hospital for complications of pregnancy during one trimester and remains in the hospital into a subsequent trimester, the trimester character for the antepartum complication code should be assigned on the basis of the trimester when the complication developed, not the trimester of the discharge. If the condition developed prior to the current admission/encounter or represents a pre-existing condition, the trimester character for the trimester at the time of the admission/encounter should be assigned.

5) Unspecified trimester
Each category that includes codes for trimester has a code for "unspecified trimester." The "unspecified trimester" code should rarely be used, such as when the documentation in the record is insufficient to determine the trimester and it is not possible to obtain clarification.

6) 7th character for fetus identification
Where applicable, a 7th character is to be assigned for certain categories (O31, O32, O33.3 - O33.6, O35, O36, O40, O41, O60.1, O60.2, O64, and O69) to identify the fetus for which the complication code applies.

Assign 7th character "0":
- For single gestations
- When the documentation in the record is insufficient to determine the fetus affected and it is not possible to obtain clarification.
- When it is not possible to clinically determine which fetus is affected.

b. Selection of OB principal or first-listed diagnosis
1) Routine outpatient prenatal visits
For routine outpatient prenatal visits when no complications are present, a code from category Z34, Encounter for supervision of normal pregnancy, should be used as the first-listed diagnosis. These codes should not be used in conjunction with chapter 15 codes.

2) Prenatal outpatient visits for high-risk patients
For routine prenatal outpatient visits for patients with high-risk pregnancies, a code from category O09, Supervision of high-risk pregnancy, should be used as the first-listed diagnosis. Secondary chapter 15 codes may be used in conjunction with these codes if appropriate.

3) Episodes when no delivery occurs
In episodes when no delivery occurs, the principal diagnosis should correspond to the principal complication of the pregnancy which necessitated the encounter. Should more than one complication exist, all of which are treated or monitored, any of the complications codes may be sequenced first.

4) When a delivery occurs
When a delivery occurs, the principal diagnosis should correspond to the main circumstances or complication of the delivery. In cases of cesarean delivery, the selection of the principal diagnosis should be the condition established after study that was responsible for the patient's admission. If the patient was admitted with a condition that resulted in the performance of a cesarean procedure, that condition should be selected as the principal diagnosis. If the reason for the admission/encounter was unrelated to the condition resulting in the cesarean delivery, the condition related to the reason for the admission/encounter should be selected as the principal diagnosis.

5) **Outcome of delivery**

A code from category Z37, Outcome of delivery, should be included on every maternal record when a delivery has occurred. These codes are not to be used on subsequent records or on the newborn record.

c. **Pre-existing conditions versus conditions due to the pregnancy**

Certain categories in Chapter 15 distinguish between conditions of the mother that existed prior to pregnancy (pre-existing) and those that are a direct result of pregnancy. When assigning codes from Chapter 15, it is important to assess if a condition was pre-existing prior to pregnancy or developed during or due to the pregnancy in order to assign the correct code.

Categories that do not distinguish between pre-existing and pregnancy-related conditions may be used for either. It is acceptable to use codes specifically for the puerperium with codes complicating pregnancy and childbirth if a condition arises postpartum during the delivery encounter.

d. **Pre-existing hypertension in pregnancy**

Category O10, Pre-existing hypertension complicating pregnancy, childbirth and the puerperium, includes codes for hypertensive heart and hypertensive chronic kidney disease. When assigning one of the O10 codes that includes hypertensive heart disease or hypertensive chronic kidney disease, it is necessary to add a secondary code from the appropriate hypertension category to specify the type of heart failure or chronic kidney disease.

See Section I.C.9. Hypertension.

e. **Fetal conditions affecting the management of the mother**

1) **Codes from categories O35 and O36**

Codes from categories O35, Maternal care for known or suspected fetal abnormality and damage, and O36, Maternal care for other fetal problems, are assigned only when the fetal condition is actually responsible for modifying the management of the mother, i.e., by requiring diagnostic studies, additional observation, special care, or termination of pregnancy. The fact that the fetal condition exists does not justify assigning a code from this series to the mother's record.

2) **In utero surgery**

In cases when surgery is performed on the fetus, a diagnosis code from category O35, Maternal care for known or suspected fetal abnormality and damage, should be assigned identifying the fetal condition. Assign the appropriate procedure code for the procedure performed.

No code from Chapter 16, the perinatal codes, should be used on the mother's record to identify fetal conditions. Surgery performed in utero on a fetus is still to be coded as an obstetric encounter.

f. **HIV Infection in pregnancy, childbirth and the puerperium**

During pregnancy, childbirth or the puerperium, a patient admitted because of an HIV-related illness should receive a principal diagnosis from subcategory O98.7-, Human immunodeficiency [HIV] disease complicating pregnancy, childbirth and the puerperium, followed by the code(s) for the HIV-related illness(es).

Patients with asymptomatic HIV infection status admitted during pregnancy, childbirth, or the puerperium should receive codes of O98.7- and Z21, Asymptomatic human immunodeficiency virus [HIV] infection status.

g. **Diabetes mellitus in pregnancy**

Diabetes mellitus is a significant complicating factor in pregnancy. Pregnant women who are diabetic should be assigned a code from category O24, Diabetes mellitus in pregnancy, childbirth, and the puerperium, first, followed by the appropriate diabetes code(s) (E08-E13) from Chapter 4.

h. **Long term use of insulin**

Code Z79.4, Long-term (current) use of insulin, should also be assigned if the diabetes mellitus is being treated with insulin.

i. **Gestational (pregnancy induced) diabetes**

Gestational (pregnancy induced) diabetes can occur during the second and third trimester of pregnancy in women who were not diabetic prior to pregnancy. Gestational diabetes can cause complications in the pregnancy similar to those of pre-existing

diabetes mellitus. It also puts the woman at greater risk of developing diabetes after the pregnancy. Codes for gestational diabetes are in subcategory O24.4, Gestational diabetes mellitus. No other code from category O24, Diabetes mellitus in pregnancy, childbirth, and the puerperium, should be used with a code from O24.4.

The codes under subcategory O24.4 include diet controlled and insulin controlled. If a patient with gestational diabetes is treated with both diet and insulin, only the code for insulin-controlled is required.

Code Z79.4, Long-term (current) use of insulin, should not be assigned with codes from subcategory O24.4.

An abnormal glucose tolerance in pregnancy is assigned a code from subcategory O99.81, Abnormal glucose complicating pregnancy, childbirth, and the puerperium.

j. **Sepsis and septic shock complicating abortion, pregnancy, childbirth and the puerperium**

When assigning a chapter 15 code for sepsis complicating abortion, pregnancy, childbirth, and the puerperium, a code for the specific type of infection should be assigned as an additional diagnosis. If severe sepsis is present, a code from subcategory R65.2, Severe sepsis, and code(s) for associated organ dysfunction(s) should also be assigned as additional diagnoses.

k. **Puerperal sepsis**

Code O85, Puerperal sepsis, should be assigned with a secondary code to identify the causal organism (e.g., for a bacterial infection, assign a code from category B95-B96, Bacterial infections in conditions classified elsewhere). A code from category A40, Streptococcal sepsis, or A41, Other sepsis, should not be used for puerperal sepsis. If applicable, use additional codes to identify severe sepsis (R65.2-) and any associated acute organ dysfunction.

l. **Alcohol and tobacco use during pregnancy, childbirth and the puerperium**

1) **Alcohol use during pregnancy, childbirth and the puerperium**

Codes under subcategory O99.31, Alcohol use complicating pregnancy, childbirth, and the puerperium, should be assigned for any pregnancy case when a mother uses alcohol during the pregnancy or postpartum. A secondary code from category F10, Alcohol related disorders, should also be assigned to identify manifestations of the alcohol use.

2) **Tobacco use during pregnancy, childbirth and the puerperium**

Codes under subcategory O99.33, Smoking (tobacco) complicating pregnancy, childbirth, and the puerperium, should be assigned for any pregnancy case when a mother uses any type of tobacco product during the pregnancy or postpartum. A secondary code from category F17, Nicotine dependence, or code Z72.0, Tobacco use, should also be assigned to identify the type of nicotine dependence.

m. **Poisoning, toxic effects, adverse effects and underdosing in a pregnant patient**

A code from subcategory O9A.2, Injury, poisoning and certain other consequences of external causes complicating pregnancy, childbirth, and the puerperium, should be sequenced first, followed by the appropriate injury, poisoning, toxic effect, adverse effect or underdosing code, and then the additional code(s) that specifies the condition caused by the poisoning, toxic effect, adverse effect or underdosing.

See Section I.C.19. Adverse effects, poisoning, underdosing and toxic effects.

n. **Normal delivery, code O80**

1) **Encounter for full term uncomplicated delivery**

Code O80 should be assigned when a woman is admitted for a full-term normal delivery and delivers a single, healthy infant without any complications antepartum, during the delivery, or postpartum during the delivery episode. Code O80 is always a principal diagnosis. It is not to be used if any other code from chapter 15 is needed to describe a current complication of the antenatal, delivery, or perinatal period. Additional codes from other chapters may be used with code O80 if they are not related to or are in any way complicating the pregnancy.

2) Uncomplicated delivery with resolved antepartum complication

Code O80 may be used if the patient had a complication at some point during the pregnancy, but the complication is not present at the time of the admission for delivery.

3) Outcome of delivery for O80

Z37.0, Single live birth, is the only outcome of delivery code appropriate for use with O80.

o. The peripartum and postpartum periods

1) Peripartum and postpartum periods

The postpartum period begins immediately after delivery and continues for six weeks following delivery. The peripartum period is defined as the last month of pregnancy to five months postpartum.

2) Peripartum and postpartum complication

A postpartum complication is any complication occurring within the six-week period.

3) Pregnancy-related complications after 6 week period

Chapter 15 codes may also be used to describe pregnancy-related complications after the peripartum or postpartum period if the provider documents that a condition is pregnancy related.

4) Admission for routine postpartum care following delivery outside hospital

When the mother delivers outside the hospital prior to admission and is admitted for routine postpartum care and no complications are noted, code Z39.0, Encounter for care and examination of mother immediately after delivery, should be assigned as the principal diagnosis.

5) Pregnancy associated cardiomyopathy

Pregnancy associated cardiomyopathy, code O90.3, is unique in that it may be diagnosed in the third trimester of pregnancy but may continue to progress months after delivery. For this reason, it is referred to as peripartum cardiomyopathy. Code O90.3 is only for use when the cardiomyopathy develops as a result of pregnancy in a woman who did not have pre-existing heart disease.

p. Code O94, Sequelae of complication of pregnancy, childbirth, and the puerperium

1) Code O94

Code O94, Sequelae of complication of pregnancy, childbirth, and the puerperium, is for use in those cases when an initial complication of a pregnancy develops a sequelae requiring care or treatment at a future date.

2) After the initial postpartum period

This code may be used at any time after the initial postpartum period.

3) Sequencing of code O94

This code, like all late effect codes, is to be sequenced following the code describing the sequelae of the complication.

q. *Termination of Pregnancy and Spontaneous abortions*

1) Abortion with Liveborn Fetus

When an attempted termination of pregnancy results in a liveborn fetus, assign code Z33.2, Encounter for elective termination of pregnancy and a code from category Z37, Outcome of Delivery.

2) Retained Products of Conception following an abortion

Subsequent encounters for retained products of conception following a spontaneous abortion or elective termination of pregnancy are assigned the appropriate code from category O03, Spontaneous abortion, or codes O07.4, Failed attempted termination of pregnancy without complication and Z33.2, Encounter for elective termination of pregnancy. This advice is appropriate even when the patient was discharged previously with a discharge diagnosis of complete abortion.

3) Complications leading to abortion

Codes from Chapter 15 may be used as additional codes to identify any documented complications of the pregnancy in conjunction with codes in categories in O07 and O08.

r. Abuse in a pregnant patient

For suspected or confirmed cases of abuse of a pregnant patient, a code(s) from subcategories O9A.3, Physical abuse complicating pregnancy, childbirth, and the puerperium, O9A.4, Sexual abuse complicating pregnancy, childbirth, and the puerperium, and O9A.5, Psychological abuse complicating pregnancy, childbirth, and the puerperium, should be sequenced first, followed by the appropriate codes (if applicable) to identify any associated current injury due to physical abuse, sexual abuse, and the perpetrator of abuse.

See Section I.C.19. Adult and child abuse, neglect and other maltreatment.

16. Chapter 16: Certain Conditions Originating in the Perinatal Period (P00- P96)

For coding and reporting purposes the perinatal period is defined as before birth through the 28th day following birth. The following guidelines are provided for reporting purposes

a. General Perinatal Rules

1) Use of Chapter 16 codes

Codes in this chapter are <u>never</u> for use on the maternal record. Codes from Chapter 15, the obstetric chapter, are never permitted on the newborn record. Chapter 16 codes may be used throughout the life of the patient if the condition is still present.

2) Principal diagnosis for birth record

When coding the birth episode in a newborn record, assign a code from category Z38, Liveborn infants according to place of birth and type of delivery, as the principal diagnosis. A code from category Z38 is assigned only once, to a newborn at the time of birth. If a newborn is transferred to another institution, a code from category Z38 should not be used at the receiving hospital.

A code from category Z38 is used only on the newborn record, not on the mother's record.

3) Use of codes from other chapters with codes from Chapter 16

Codes from other chapters may be used with codes from chapter 16 if the codes from the other chapters provide more specific detail. Codes for signs and symptoms may be assigned when a definitive diagnosis has not been established. If the reason for the encounter is a perinatal condition, the code from chapter 16 should be sequenced first.

4) Use of Chapter 16 codes after the perinatal period

Should a condition originate in the perinatal period, and continue throughout the life of the patient, the perinatal code should continue to be used regardless of the patient's age.

5) Birth process or community acquired conditions

If a newborn has a condition that may be either due to the birth process or community acquired and the documentation does not indicate which it is, the default is due to the birth process and the code from Chapter 16 should be used. If the condition is community-acquired, a code from Chapter 16 should not be assigned.

6) Code all clinically significant conditions

All clinically significant conditions noted on routine newborn examination should be coded. A condition is clinically significant if it requires:

- clinical evaluation; or
- therapeutic treatment; or
- diagnostic procedures; or
- extended length of hospital stay; or
- increased nursing care and/or monitoring; or
- has implications for future health care needs

Note: The perinatal guidelines listed above are the same as the general coding guidelines for "additional diagnoses", except for the final point regarding implications for future health care needs. Codes should be assigned for conditions that have been specified by the provider as having implications for future health care needs.

b. **Observation and Evaluation of Newborns for Suspected Conditions not Found**

Reserved for future expansion

c. **Coding Additional Perinatal Diagnoses**

1) **Assigning codes for conditions that require treatment**

Assign codes for conditions that require treatment or further investigation, prolong the length of stay, or require resource utilization.

2) **Codes for conditions specified as having implications for future health care needs**

Assign codes for conditions that have been specified by the provider as having implications for future health care needs.

Note: This guideline should not be used for adult patients.

d. **Prematurity and Fetal Growth Retardation**

Providers utilize different criteria in determining prematurity. A code for prematurity should not be assigned unless it is documented. Assignment of codes in categories P05, Disorders of newborn related to slow fetal growth and fetal malnutrition, and P07, Disorders of newborn related to short gestation and low birth weight, not elsewhere classified, should be based on the recorded birth weight and estimated gestational age. Codes from category P05 should not be assigned with codes from category P07.

When both birth weight and gestational age are available, two codes from category P07 should be assigned, with the code for birth weight sequenced before the code for gestational age.

e. **Low birth weight and immaturity status**

Codes from category P07, Disorders of newborn related to short gestation and low birth weight, not elsewhere classified, are for use for a child or adult who was premature or had a low birth weight as a newborn and this is affecting the patient's current health status.

See Section I.C.21. Factors influencing health status and contact with health services, Status.

f. **Bacterial Sepsis of Newborn**

Category P36, Bacterial sepsis of newborn, includes congenital sepsis. If a perinate is documented as having sepsis without documentation of congenital or community acquired, the default is congenital and a code from category P36 should be assigned. If the P36 code includes the causal organism, an additional code from category B95, Streptococcus, Staphylococcus, and Enterococcus as the cause of diseases classified elsewhere, or B96, Other bacterial agents as the cause of diseases classified elsewhere, should not be assigned. If the P36 code does not include the causal organism, assign an additional code from category B96. If applicable, use additional codes to identify severe sepsis (R65.2-) and any associated acute organ dysfunction.

g. **Stillbirth**

Code P95, Stillbirth, is only for use in institutions that maintain separate records for stillbirths. No other code should be used with P95. Code P95 should not be used on the mother's record.

17. **Chapter 17: Congenital malformations, deformations, and chromosomal abnormalities (Q00-Q99)**

Assign an appropriate code(s) from categories Q00-Q99, Congenital malformations, deformations, and chromosomal abnormalities when a malformation/deformation or chromosomal abnormality is documented. A malformation/deformation/or chromosomal abnormality may be the principal/first-listed diagnosis on a record or a secondary diagnosis.

When a malformation/deformation/or chromosomal abnormality does not have a unique code assignment, assign additional code(s) for any manifestations that may be present.

When the code assignment specifically identifies the malformation/deformation/or chromosomal abnormality, manifestations that are an inherent component of the anomaly should not be coded separately. Additional codes should be assigned for manifestations that are not an inherent component.

Codes from Chapter 17 may be used throughout the life of the patient. If a congenital malformation or deformity has been corrected, a personal history code should be used to identify the history of the malformation or deformity. Although present at birth, malformation/deformation/or chromosomal abnormality may not be identified until later in life. Whenever the condition is diagnosed by the physician, it is appropriate

to assign a code from codes Q00-Q99.For the birth admission, the appropriate code from category Z38, Liveborn infants, according to place of birth and type of delivery, should be sequenced as the principal diagnosis, followed by any congenital anomaly codes, Q00- Q99.

18. **Chapter 18: Symptoms, signs, and abnormal clinical and laboratory findings, not elsewhere classified (R00-R99)**

Chapter 18 includes symptoms, signs, abnormal results of clinical or other investigative procedures, and ill-defined conditions regarding which no diagnosis classifiable elsewhere is recorded. Signs and symptoms that point to a specific diagnosis have been assigned to a category in other chapters of the classification.

a. **Use of symptom codes**

Codes that describe symptoms and signs are acceptable for reporting purposes when a related definitive diagnosis has not been established (confirmed) by the provider.

b. **Use of a symptom code with a definitive diagnosis code**

Codes for signs and symptoms may be reported in addition to a related definitive diagnosis when the sign or symptom is not routinely associated with that diagnosis, such as the various signs and symptoms associated with complex syndromes. The definitive diagnosis code should be sequenced before the symptom code.

Signs or symptoms that are associated routinely with a disease process should not be assigned as additional codes, unless otherwise instructed by the classification.

c. **Combination codes that include symptoms**

ICD-10-CM contains a number of combination codes that identify both the definitive diagnosis and common symptoms of that diagnosis. When using one of these combination codes, an additional code should not be assigned for the symptom.

d. **Repeated falls**

Code R29.6, Repeated falls, is for use for encounters when a patient has recently fallen and the reason for the fall is being investigated.

Code Z91.81, History of falling, is for use when a patient has fallen in the past and is at risk for future falls. When appropriate, both codes R29.6 and Z91.81 may be assigned together.

e. **Coma scale**

The coma scale codes (R40.2-) can be used in conjunction with traumatic brain injury codes, acute cerebrovascular disease or sequelae of cerebrovascular disease codes. These codes are primarily for use by trauma registries, but they may be used in any setting where this information is collected. The coma scale codes should be sequenced after the diagnosis code(s).

These codes, one from each subcategory, are needed to complete the scale. The 7th character indicates when the scale was recorded. The 7th character should match for all three codes.

At a minimum, report the initial score documented on presentation at your facility. This may be a score from the emergency medicine technician (EMT) or in the emergency department. If desired, a facility may choose to capture multiple Glasgow coma scale scores.

Assign code R40.24, Glasgow coma scale, total score, when only the total score is documented in the medical record and not the individual score(s).

f. **Functional quadriplegia**

Functional quadriplegia (code R53.2) is the lack of ability to use one's limbs or to ambulate due to extreme debility. It is not associated with neurologic deficit or injury, and code R53.2 should not be used for cases of neurologic quadriplegia. It should only be assigned if functional quadriplegia is specifically documented in the medical record.

g. **SIRS due to non-infectious process**

The systemic inflammatory response syndrome (SIRS) can develop as a result of certain non-infectious disease processes, such as trauma, malignant neoplasm, or pancreatitis. When SIRS is documented with a noninfectious condition, and no subsequent infection is documented, the code for the underlying condition, such as an injury, should be assigned, followed by code R65.10, Systemic inflammatory response syndrome (SIRS) of non-infectious origin without acute organ dysfunction, or code R65.11, Systemic inflammatory response syndrome (SIRS) of non-infectious origin with acute organ dysfunction. If an associated acute organ dysfunction is documented, the appropriate code(s) for the specific type of organ dysfunction(s) should be assigned in addition to code R65.11. If acute organ dysfunction is documented, but it cannot be determined if the acute organ dysfunction is associated with SIRS or due to another condition (e.g., directly due to the trauma), the provider should be queried.

h. Death NOS
Code R99, Ill-defined and unknown cause of mortality, is only for use in the very limited circumstance when a patient who has already died is brought into an emergency department or other healthcare facility and is pronounced dead upon arrival. It does not represent the discharge disposition of death.

19. Chapter 19: Injury, poisoning, and certain other consequences of external causes (S00-T88)

a. Application of 7th Characters in Chapter 19
Most categories in chapter 19 have a 7th character requirement for each applicable code. Most categories in this chapter have three 7th character values (with the exception of fractures): A, initial encounter, D, subsequent encounter and S, sequela. Categories for traumatic fractures have additional 7th character values. While the patient may be seen by a new or different provider over the course of treatment for an injury, assignment of the 7th character is based on whether the patient is undergoing active treatment and not whether the provider is seeing the patient for the first time.

For complication codes, active treatment refers to treatment for the condition described by the code, even though it may be related to an earlier precipitating problem. For example, code T84.50XA, Infection and inflammatory reaction due to unspecified internal joint prosthesis, initial encounter, is used when active treatment is provided for the infection, even though the condition relates to the prosthetic device, implant or graft that was placed at a previous encounter.

7th character "A", initial encounter is used while the patient is receiving active treatment for the condition. Examples of active treatment are: surgical treatment, emergency department encounter, and evaluation and continuing treatment by the same or a different physician.

7th character "D" subsequent encounter is used for encounters after the patient has received active treatment of the condition and is receiving routine care for the condition during the healing or recovery phase. Examples of subsequent care are: cast change or removal, an x-ray to check healing status of fracture, removal of external or internal fixation device, medication adjustment, other aftercare and follow up visits following treatment of the injury or condition.

The aftercare Z codes should not be used for aftercare for conditions such as injuries or poisonings, where 7th characters are provided to identify subsequent care. For example, for aftercare of an injury, assign the acute injury code with the 7th character "D" (subsequent encounter).

7th character "S", sequela, is for use for complications or conditions that arise as a direct result of a condition, such as scar formation after a burn. The scars are sequelae of the burn. When using 7th character "S", it is necessary to use both the injury code that precipitated the sequela and the code for the sequela itself. The "S" is added only to the injury code, not the sequela code. The 7th character "S" identifies the injury responsible for the sequela. The specific type of sequela (e.g. scar) is sequenced first, followed by the injury code.

See Section I.B.10 Sequelae, (Late Effects)

b. Coding of injuries
When coding injuries, assign separate codes for each injury unless a combination code is provided, in which case the combination code is assigned. Code T07, Unspecified multiple injuries should not be assigned in the inpatient setting unless information for a more specific code is not available. Traumatic injury codes (S00-T14.9) are not to be used for normal, healing surgical wounds or to identify complications of surgical wounds.

The code for the most serious injury, as determined by the provider and the focus of treatment, is sequenced first.

1) Superficial injuries
Superficial injuries such as abrasions or contusions are not coded when associated with more severe injuries of the same site.

2) Primary injury with damage to nerves/blood vessels
When a primary injury results in minor damage to peripheral nerves or blood vessels, the primary injury is sequenced first with additional code(s) for injuries to nerves and spinal cord (such as category S04), and/or injury to blood vessels (such as category S15). When the primary injury is to the blood vessels or nerves, that injury should be sequenced first.

c. Coding of Traumatic Fractures
The principles of multiple coding of injuries should be followed in coding fractures. Fractures of specified sites are coded individually by site in accordance with both the provisions within categories S02, S12, S22, S32, S42, S49, S52, S59, S62, S72, S79, S82, S89, S92 and the level of detail furnished by medical record content.

A fracture not indicated as open or closed should be coded to closed. A fracture not indicated whether displaced or not displaced should be coded to displaced.

More specific guidelines are as follows:

1) Initial vs. Subsequent Encounter for Fractures
Traumatic fractures are coded using the appropriate 7th character for initial encounter (A, B, C) while the patient is receiving active treatment for the fracture. Examples of active treatment are: surgical treatment, emergency department encounter, and evaluation and continuing (ongoing) treatment by the same or different physician. The appropriate 7th character for initial encounter should also be assigned for a patient who delayed seeking treatment for the fracture or nonunion.

Fractures are coded using the appropriate 7th character for subsequent care for encounters after the patient has completed active treatment of the fracture and is receiving routine care for the fracture during the healing or recovery phase. Examples of fracture aftercare are: cast change or removal, an x-ray to check healing status of fracture, removal of external or internal fixation device, medication adjustment, and follow-up visits following fracture treatment.

Care for complications of surgical treatment for fracture repairs during the healing or recovery phase should be coded with the appropriate complication codes.

Care of complications of fractures, such as malunion and nonunion, should be reported with the appropriate 7th character for subsequent care with nonunion (K, M, N,) or subsequent care with malunion (P, Q, R).

Malunion/nonunion: The appropriate 7th character for initial encounter should also be assigned for a patient who delayed seeking treatment for the fracture or nonunion.

A code from category M80, not a traumatic fracture code, should be used for any patient with known osteoporosis who suffers a fracture, even if the patient had a minor fall or trauma, if that fall or trauma would not usually break a normal, healthy bone.

See Section I.C.13. Osteoporosis.

The aftercare Z codes should not be used for aftercare for traumatic fractures. For aftercare of a traumatic fracture, assign the acute fracture code with the appropriate 7th character.

2) Multiple fractures sequencing
Multiple fractures are sequenced in accordance with the severity of the fracture.

d. Coding of burns and corrosions
The ICD-10-CM makes a distinction between burns and corrosions. The burn codes are for thermal burns, except sunburns, that come from a heat source, such as a fire or hot appliance. The burn codes are also for burns resulting from electricity and radiation. Corrosions are burns due to chemicals. The guidelines are the same for burns and corrosions.

Current burns (T20-T25) are classified by depth, extent and by agent (X code). Burns are classified by depth as first degree (erythema), second degree (blistering), and third degree (full-thickness involvement). Burns of the eye and internal organs (T26-T28) are classified by site, but not by degree.

1) **Sequencing of burn and related condition codes**
Sequence first the code that reflects the highest degree of burn when more than one burn is present.

  a. When the reason for the admission or encounter is for treatment of external multiple burns, sequence first the code that reflects the burn of the highest degree.

  b. When a patient has both internal and external burns, the circumstances of admission govern the selection of the principal diagnosis or first-listed diagnosis.

  c. When a patient is admitted for burn injuries and other related conditions such as smoke inhalation and/or respiratory failure, the circumstances of admission govern the selection of the principal or first-listed diagnosis.

2) **Burns of the same local site**
Classify burns of the same local site (three-character category level, T20-T28) but of different degrees to the subcategory identifying the highest degree recorded in the diagnosis.

3) **Non-healing burns**
Non-healing burns are coded as acute burns.

Necrosis of burned skin should be coded as a non-healed burn.

4) **Infected burn**
For any documented infected burn site, use an additional code for the infection.

5) **Assign separate codes for each burn site**
When coding burns, assign separate codes for each burn site. Category T30, Burn and corrosion, body region unspecified is extremely vague and should rarely be used.

6) **Burns and corrosions classified according to extent of body surface involved**
Assign codes from category T31, Burns classified according to extent of body surface involved, or T32, Corrosions classified according to extent of body surface involved, when the site of the burn is not specified or when there is a need for additional data. It is advisable to use category T31 as additional coding when needed to provide data for evaluating burn mortality, such as that needed by burn units. It is also advisable to use category T31 as an additional code for reporting purposes when there is mention of a third-degree burn involving 20 percent or more of the body surface.

Categories T31 and T32 are based on the classic "rule of nines" in estimating body surface involved: head and neck are assigned nine percent, each arm nine percent, each leg 18 percent, the anterior trunk 18 percent, posterior trunk 18 percent, and genitalia one percent. Providers may change these percentage assignments where necessary to accommodate infants and children who have proportionately larger heads than adults, and patients who have large buttocks, thighs, or abdomen that involve burns.

7) **Encounters for treatment of sequela of burns**
Encounters for the treatment of the late effects of burns or corrosions (i.e., scars or joint contractures) should be coded with a burn or corrosion code with the 7th character "S" for sequela.

8) **Sequelae with a late effect code and current burn**
When appropriate, both a code for a current burn or corrosion with 7th character "A" or "D" and a burn or corrosion code with 7th character "S" may be assigned on the same record (when both a current burn and sequelae of an old burn exist). Burns and corrosions do not heal at the same rate and a current healing wound may still exist with sequela of a healed burn or corrosion.

    See Section I.B.10 Sequela (Late Effects)

9) **Use of an external cause code with burns and corrosions**
An external cause code should be used with burns and corrosions to identify the source and intent of the burn, as well as the place where it occurred.

e. **Adverse effects, poisoning, underdosing and toxic effects**
Codes in categories T36-T65 are combination codes that include the substance that was taken as well as the intent. No additional external cause code is required for poisonings, toxic effects, adverse effects and underdosing codes.

1) **Do not code directly from the Table of Drugs**
Do not code directly from the Table of Drugs and Chemicals. Always refer back to the Tabular List.

2) **Use as many codes as necessary to describe**
Use as many codes as necessary to describe completely all drugs, medicinal or biological substances.

3) **If the same code would describe the causative agent**
If the same code would describe the causative agent for more than one adverse reaction, poisoning, toxic effect or underdosing, assign the code only once.

4) **If two or more drugs, medicinal or biological substances**
If two or more drugs, medicinal or biological substances are reported, code each individually unless a combination code is listed in the Table of Drugs and Chemicals.

5) **The occurrence of drug toxicity is classified in ICD-10-CM as follows:**

  (a) **Adverse effect**
When coding an adverse effect of a drug that has been correctly prescribed and properly administered, assign the appropriate code for the nature of the adverse effect followed by the appropriate code for the adverse effect of the drug (T36-T50). The code for the drug should have a 5th or 6th character "5" (for example T36.0X5-) Examples of the nature of an adverse effect are tachycardia, delirium, gastrointestinal hemorrhaging, vomiting, hypokalemia, hepatitis, renal failure, or respiratory failure.

  (b) **Poisoning**
When coding a poisoning or reaction to the improper use of a medication (e.g., overdose, wrong substance given or taken in error, wrong route of administration), first assign the appropriate code from categories T36-T50. The poisoning codes have an associated intent as their 5th or 6th character (accidental, intentional self-harm, assault and undetermined. Use additional code(s) for all manifestations of poisonings.

If there is also a diagnosis of abuse or dependence of the substance, the abuse or dependence is assigned as an additional code.

Examples of poisoning include:

  (i) Error was made in drug prescription

      Errors made in drug prescription or in the administration of the drug by provider, nurse, patient, or other person.

  (ii) Overdose of a drug intentionally taken

      If an overdose of a drug was intentionally taken or administered and resulted in drug toxicity, it would be coded as a poisoning.

  (iii) Nonprescribed drug taken with correctly prescribed and properly administered drug

      If a nonprescribed drug or medicinal agent was taken in combination with a correctly prescribed and properly administered drug, any drug toxicity or other reaction resulting from the interaction of the two drugs would be classified as a poisoning.

  (iv) Interaction of drug(s) and alcohol

      When a reaction results from the interaction of a drug(s) and alcohol, this would be classified as poisoning.
      See Section I.C.4. if poisoning is the result of insulin pump malfunctions.

  (c) **Underdosing**
Underdosing refers to taking less of a medication than is prescribed by a provider or a manufacturer's instruction. For underdosing, assign the code from categories T36-T50 (fifth or sixth character "6").

Codes for underdosing should never be assigned as principal or first-listed codes. If a patient has a relapse or exacerbation of the medical condition for which the drug is prescribed because of the reduction in dose, then the medical condition itself should be coded.

Noncompliance (Z91.12-, Z91.13-) or complication of care (Y63.61, Y63.8-Y63.9) codes are to be used with an underdosing code to indicate intent, if known.

(d) Toxic effects

When a harmful substance is ingested or comes in contact with a person, this is classified as a toxic effect. The toxic effect codes are in categories T51-T65.

Toxic effect codes have an associated intent: accidental, intentional self-harm, assault and undetermined.

f. Adult and child abuse, neglect and other maltreatment

Sequence first the appropriate code from categories T74.- (Adult and child abuse, neglect and other maltreatment, confirmed) or T76.- (Adult and child abuse, neglect and other maltreatment, suspected) for abuse, neglect and other maltreatment, followed by any accompanying mental health or injury code(s).

If the documentation in the medical record states abuse or neglect it is coded as confirmed (T74.-). It is coded as suspected if it is documented as suspected (T76.-).

For cases of confirmed abuse or neglect an external cause code from the assault section (X92-Y08) should be added to identify the cause of any physical injuries. A perpetrator code (Y07) should be added when the perpetrator of the abuse is known. For suspected cases of abuse or neglect, do not report external cause or perpetrator code.

If a suspected case of abuse, neglect or mistreatment is ruled out during an encounter code Z04.71, Encounter for examination and observation following alleged physical adult abuse, ruled out, or code Z04.72, Encounter for examination and observation following alleged child physical abuse, ruled out, should be used, not a code from T76.

If a suspected case of alleged rape or sexual abuse is ruled out during an encounter code Z04.41, Encounter for examination and observation following alleged physical adult abuse, ruled out, or code Z04.42, Encounter for examination and observation following alleged rape or sexual abuse, ruled out, should be used, not a code from T76.

See Section I.C.15. Abuse in a pregnant patient.

g. Complications of care

1) General guidelines for complications of care

(a) Documentation of complications of care

See Section I.B.16. for information on documentation of complications of care.

2) Pain due to medical devices

Pain associated with devices, implants or grafts left in a surgical site (for example painful hip prosthesis) is assigned to the appropriate code(s) found in Chapter 19, Injury, poisoning, and certain other consequences of external causes. Specific codes for pain due to medical devices are found in the T code section of the ICD-10-CM. Use additional code(s) from category G89 to identify acute or chronic pain due to presence of the device, implant or graft (G89.18 or G89.28).

3) Transplant complications

(a) Transplant complications other than kidney

Codes under category T86, Complications of transplanted organs and tissues, are for use for both complications and rejection of transplanted organs. A transplant complication code is only assigned if the complication affects the function of the transplanted organ. Two codes are required to fully describe a transplant complication: the appropriate code from category T86 and a secondary code that identifies the complication.

Pre-existing conditions or conditions that develop after the transplant are not coded as complications unless they affect the function of the transplanted organs.

See I.C.21. for transplant organ removal status

See I.C.2. for malignant neoplasm associated with transplanted organ.

(b) Kidney transplant complications

Patients who have undergone kidney transplant may still have some form of chronic kidney disease (CKD) because the kidney transplant may not fully restore kidney function. Code T86.1- should be assigned for documented complications of a kidney transplant, such as transplant failure or rejection or other transplant complication. Code T86.1- should not be assigned for post kidney transplant patients who have chronic kidney (CKD) unless a transplant complication such as transplant failure or rejection is documented. If the documentation is unclear as to whether the patient has a complication of the transplant, query the provider.

Conditions that affect the function of the transplanted kidney, other than CKD, should be assigned a code from subcategory T86.1, Complications of transplanted organ, Kidney, and a secondary code that identifies the complication.

For patients with CKD following a kidney transplant, but who do not have a complication such as failure or rejection, *see section I.C.14. Chronic kidney disease and kidney transplant status.*

4) Complication codes that include the external cause

As with certain other T codes, some of the complications of care codes have the external cause included in the code. The code includes the nature of the complication as well as the type of procedure that caused the complication. No external cause code indicating the type of procedure is necessary for these codes.

5) Complications of care codes within the body system chapters

Intraoperative and postprocedural complication codes are found within the body system chapters with codes specific to the organs and structures of that body system. These codes should be sequenced first, followed by a code(s) for the specific complication, if applicable.

20. Chapter 20: External Causes of Morbidity (V00-Y99)

The external causes of morbidity codes should never be sequenced as the first- listed or principal diagnosis.

External cause codes are intended to provide data for injury research and evaluation of injury prevention strategies. These codes capture how the injury or health condition happened (cause), the intent (unintentional or accidental; or intentional, such as suicide or assault), the place where the event occurred the activity of the patient at the time of the event, and the person's status (e.g., civilian, military).

There is no national requirement for mandatory ICD-10-CM external cause code reporting. Unless a provider is subject to a state-based external cause code reporting mandate or these codes are required by a particular payer, reporting of ICD-10-CM codes in Chapter 20, External Causes of Morbidity, is not required. In the absence of a mandatory reporting requirement, providers are encouraged to voluntarily report external cause codes, as they provide valuable data for injury research and evaluation of injury prevention strategies.

a. General External Cause Coding Guidelines

1) Used with any code in the range of A00.0-T88.9, Z00-Z99

An external cause code may be used with any code in the range of A00.0-T88.9, Z00-Z99, classification that is a health condition due to an external cause. Though they are most applicable to injuries, they are also valid for use with such things as infections or diseases due to an external source, and other health conditions, such as a heart attack that occurs during strenuous physical activity.

2) External cause code used for length of treatment

Assign the external cause code, with the appropriate 7th character (initial encounter, subsequent encounter or sequela) for each encounter for which the injury or condition is being treated.

Most categories in chapter 20 have a 7th character requirement for each applicable code. Most categories in this chapter have three 7th character values: A, initial encounter, D, subsequent encounter and S, sequela. While the patient may be seen by a new or different provider over the course of treatment for an injury or condition, assignment of the 7th character for external cause should match the 7th character of the code assigned for the associated injury or condition for the encounter.

3) **Use the full range of external cause codes**
Use the full range of external cause codes to completely describe the cause, the intent, the place of occurrence, and if applicable, the activity of the patient at the time of the event, and the patient's status, for all injuries, and other health conditions due to an external cause.

4) **Assign as many external cause codes as necessary**
Assign as many external cause codes as necessary to fully explain each cause. If only one external code can be recorded, assign the code most related to the principal diagnosis.

5) **The selection of the appropriate external cause code**
The selection of the appropriate external cause code is guided by the Alphabetic Index of External Causes and by Inclusion and Exclusion notes in the Tabular List.

6) **External cause code can never be a principal diagnosis**
An external cause code can never be a principal (first-listed) diagnosis.

7) **Combination external cause codes**
Certain of the external cause codes are combination codes that identify sequential events that result in an injury, such as a fall which results in striking against an object. The injury may be due to either event or both. The combination external cause code used should correspond to the sequence of events regardless of which caused the most serious injury.

8) **No external cause code needed in certain circumstances**
No external cause code from Chapter 20 is needed if the external cause and intent are included in a code from another chapter (e.g. T36.0X1- Poisoning by penicillins, accidental (unintentional)).

b. **Place of Occurrence Guideline**
Codes from category Y92, Place of occurrence of the external cause, are secondary codes for use after other external cause codes to identify the location of the patient at the time of injury or other condition.

Generally, a place of occurrence code is assigned only once, at the initial encounter for treatment. However, in the rare instance that a new injury occurs during hospitalization, an additional place of occurrence code may be assigned. No 7th characters are used for Y92.

Do not use place of occurrence code Y92.9 if the place is not stated or is not applicable.

c. **Activity code**
Assign a code from category Y93, Activity code, to describe the activity of the patient at the time the injury or other health condition occurred.

An activity code is used only once, at the initial encounter for treatment. Only one code from Y93 should be recorded on a medical record. An activity code should be used in conjunction with a place of occurrence code, Y92.

The activity codes are not applicable to poisonings, adverse effects, misadventures or sequela.

Do not assign Y93.9, Unspecified activity, if the activity is not stated.

A code from category Y93 is appropriate for use with external cause and intent codes if identifying the activity provides additional information about the event.

d. **Place of occurrence, activity, and status codes used with other external cause code**
When applicable, place of occurrence, activity, and external cause status codes are sequenced after the main external cause code(s). Regardless of the number of external cause codes assigned, there should be only one place of occurrence code, one activity code, and one external cause status code assigned to an encounter.

e. **If the reporting format limits the number of external cause codes**
If the reporting format limits the number of external cause codes that can be used in reporting clinical data, report the code for the cause/intent most related to the principal diagnosis. If the format permits capture of additional external cause codes, the cause/intent, including medical misadventures, of the additional events should be reported rather than the codes for place, activity, or external status.

f. **Multiple external cause coding guidelines**
More than one external cause code is required to fully describe the external cause of an illness or injury. The assignment of external cause codes should be sequenced in the following priority:

If two or more events cause separate injuries, an external cause code should be assigned for each cause. The first-listed external cause code will be selected in the following order:

External codes for child and adult abuse take priority over all other external cause codes.

See Section I.C.19., Child and Adult abuse guidelines.

External cause codes for terrorism events take priority over all other external cause codes except child and adult abuse.

External cause codes for cataclysmic events take priority over all other external cause codes except child and adult abuse and terrorism.

External cause codes for transport accidents take priority over all other external cause codes except cataclysmic events, child and adult abuse and terrorism.

Activity and external cause status codes are assigned following all causal (intent) external cause codes.

The first-listed external cause code should correspond to the cause of the most serious diagnosis due to an assault, accident, or self-harm, following the order of hierarchy listed above.

g. **Child and adult abuse guideline**
Adult and child abuse, neglect and maltreatment are classified as assault. Any of the assault codes may be used to indicate the external cause of any injury resulting from the confirmed abuse.

For confirmed cases of abuse, neglect and maltreatment, when the perpetrator is known, a code from Y07, Perpetrator of maltreatment and neglect, should accompany any other assault codes.

See Section I.C.19. Adult and child abuse, neglect and other maltreatment

h. **Unknown or undetermined intent guideline**
If the intent (accident, self-harm, assault) of the cause of an injury or other condition is unknown or unspecified, code the intent as accidental intent. All transport accident categories assume accidental intent.

1) **Use of undetermined intent**
External cause codes for events of undetermined intent are only for use if the documentation in the record specifies that the intent cannot be determined.

i. **Sequelae (Late Effects) of External Cause Guidelines**

1) **Sequelae external cause codes**
Sequela are reported using the external cause code with the 7th character "S" for sequela. These codes should be used with any report of a late effect or sequela resulting from a previous injury.

See Section I.B.10 Sequela (Late Effects)

2) **Sequela external cause code with a related current injury**
A sequela external cause code should never be used with a related current nature of injury code.

3) **Use of sequela external cause codes for subsequent visits**
Use a late effect external cause code for subsequent visits when a late effect of the initial injury is being treated. Do not use a late effect external cause code for subsequent visits for follow-up care (e.g., to assess healing, to receive rehabilitative therapy) of the injury when no late effect of the injury has been documented.

j. **Terrorism guidelines**

1) **Cause of injury identified by the Federal Government (FBI) as terrorism**
When the cause of an injury is identified by the Federal Government (FBI) as terrorism, the first-listed external cause code should be a code from category Y38, Terrorism. The definition of terrorism employed by the FBI is found at the

inclusion note at the beginning of category Y38. Use additional code for place of occurrence (Y92.-). More than one Y38 code may be assigned if the injury is the result of more than one mechanism of terrorism.

2) Cause of an injury is suspected to be the result of terrorism
When the cause of an injury is suspected to be the result of terrorism a code from category Y38 should not be assigned. Suspected cases should be classified as assault.

3) Code Y38.9, terrorism, secondary effects
Assign code Y38.9, Terrorism, secondary effects, for conditions occurring subsequent to the terrorist event. This code should not be assigned for conditions that are due to the initial terrorist act.

It is acceptable to assign code Y38.9 with another code from Y38 if there is an injury due to the initial terrorist event and an injury that is a subsequent result of the terrorist event.

k. External cause status
A code from category Y99, External cause status, should be assigned whenever any other external cause code is assigned for an encounter, including an Activity code, except for the events noted below. Assign a code from category Y99, External cause status, to indicate the work status of the person at the time the event occurred. The status code indicates whether the event occurred during military activity, whether a non-military person was at work, whether an individual including a student or volunteer was involved in a non-work activity at the time of the causal event.

A code from Y99, External cause status, should be assigned, when applicable, with other external cause codes, such as transport accidents and falls. The external cause status codes are not applicable to poisonings, adverse effects, misadventures or late effects.

Do not assign a code from category Y99 if no other external cause codes (cause, activity) are applicable for the encounter.

An external cause status code is used only once, at the initial encounter for treatment. Only one code from Y99 should be recorded on a medical record.

Do not assign code Y99.9, Unspecified external cause status, if the status is not stated.

21. Chapter 21: Factors influencing health status and contact with health services (Z00-Z99)
Note: The chapter specific guidelines provide additional information about the use of Z codes for specified encounters.

a. Use of Z codes in any healthcare setting
Z codes are for use in any healthcare setting. Z codes may be used as either a first-listed (principal diagnosis code in the inpatient setting) or secondary code, depending on the circumstances of the encounter. Certain Z codes may only be used as first-listed or principal diagnosis.

b. Z Codes indicate a reason for an encounter
Z codes are not procedure codes. A corresponding procedure code must accompany a Z code to describe any procedure performed.

c. Categories of Z Codes
1) Contact/Exposure
Category Z20 indicates contact with, and suspected exposure to, communicable diseases. These codes are for patients who do not show any sign or symptom of a disease but are suspected to have been exposed to it by close personal contact with an infected individual or are in an area where a disease is epidemic.

Category Z77, Other contact with and (suspected) exposures hazardous to health, indicates contact with and suspected exposures hazardous to health.

Contact/exposure codes may be used as a first-listed code to explain an encounter for testing, or, more commonly, as a secondary code to identify a potential risk.

2) Inoculations and vaccinations
Code Z23 is for encounters for inoculations and vaccinations. It indicates that a patient is being seen to receive a prophylactic inoculation against a disease. Procedure codes are required to identify the actual administration of the injection and the type(s) of immunizations given. Code Z23 may be used as a secondary code if the inoculation is given as a routine part of preventive health care, such as a well-baby visit.

3) Status
Status codes indicate that a patient is either a carrier of a disease or has the sequelae or residual of a past disease or condition. This includes such things as the presence of prosthetic or mechanical devices resulting from past treatment. A status code is informative, because the status may affect the course of treatment and its outcome. A status code is distinct from a history code. The history code indicates that the patient no longer has the condition.

A status code should not be used with a diagnosis code from one of the body system chapters, if the diagnosis code includes the information provided by the status code. For example, code Z94.1, Heart transplant status, should not be used with a code from subcategory T86.2, Complications of heart transplant. The status code does not provide additional information. The complication code indicates that the patient is a heart transplant patient.

For encounters for weaning from a mechanical ventilator, assign a code from subcategory J96.1, Chronic respiratory failure, followed by code Z99.11, Dependence on respirator [ventilator] status.

The status Z codes/categories are:

Z14　Genetic carrier

　　　Genetic carrier status indicates that a person carries a gene, associated with a particular disease, which may be passed to offspring who may develop that disease. The person does not have the disease and is not at risk of developing the disease.

Z15　Genetic susceptibility to disease

　　　Genetic susceptibility indicates that a person has a gene that increases the risk of that person developing the disease.

　　　Codes from category Z15 should not be used as principal or first-listed codes. If the patient has the condition to which he/she is susceptible, and that condition is the reason for the encounter, the code for the current condition should be sequenced first. If the patient is being seen for follow-up after completed treatment for this condition, and the condition no longer exists, a follow-up code should be sequenced first, followed by the appropriate personal history and genetic susceptibility codes. If the purpose of the encounter is genetic counseling associated with procreative management, code Z31.5, Encounter for genetic counseling, should be assigned as the first-listed code, followed by a code from category Z15. Additional codes should be assigned for any applicable family or personal history.

Z16　Resistance to antimicrobial drugs

　　　This code indicates that a patient has a condition that is resistant to antimicrobial drug treatment. Sequence the infection code first.

Z17　Estrogen receptor status

Z18　Retained foreign body fragments

Z21　Asymptomatic HIV infection status

　　　This code indicates that a patient has tested positive for HIV but has manifested no signs or symptoms of the disease.

Z22　Carrier of infectious disease

　　　Carrier status indicates that a person harbors the specific organisms of a disease without manifest symptoms and is capable of transmitting the infection.

Z28.3　Underimmunization status

Z33.1　Pregnant state, incidental

　　　This code is a secondary code only for use when the pregnancy is in no way complicating the reason for visit. Otherwise, a code from the obstetric chapter is required.

Z66   Do not resuscitate

This code may be used when it is documented by the provider that a patient is on do not resuscitate status at any time during the stay.

Z67   Blood type

Z68   Body mass index (BMI)

Z74.Ø1 Bed confinement status

Z76.82 Awaiting organ transplant status

Z78   Other specified health status

Code Z78.1, Physical restraint status, may be used when it is documented by the provider that a patient has been put in restraints during the current encounter. Please note that this code should not be reported when it is documented by the provider that a patient is temporarily restrained during a procedure.

Z79   Long-term (current) drug therapy

Codes from this category indicate a patient's continuous use of a prescribed drug (including such things as aspirin therapy) for the long-term treatment of a condition or for prophylactic use. It is not for use for patients who have addictions to drugs. This subcategory is not for use of medications for detoxification or maintenance programs to prevent withdrawal symptoms in patients with drug dependence (e.g., methadone maintenance for opiate dependence). Assign the appropriate code for the drug dependence instead.

Assign a code from Z79 if the patient is receiving a medication for an extended period as a prophylactic measure (such as for the prevention of deep vein thrombosis) or as treatment of a chronic condition (such as arthritis) or a disease requiring a lengthy course of treatment (such as cancer). Do not assign a code from category Z79 for medication being administered for a brief period of time to treat an acute illness or injury (such as a course of antibiotics to treat acute bronchitis).

Z88   Allergy status to drugs, medicaments and biological substances

Except: Z88.9, Allergy status to unspecified drugs, medicaments and biological substances status

Z89   Acquired absence of limb

Z9Ø   Acquired absence of organs, not elsewhere classified

Z91.Ø- Allergy status, other than to drugs and biological substances

Z92.82 Status post administration of tPA (rtPA) in a different facility within the last 24 hours prior to admission to a current facility

Assign code Z92.82, Status post administration of tPA (rtPA) in a different facility within the last 24 hours prior to admission to current facility, as a secondary diagnosis when a patient is received by transfer into a facility and documentation indicates they were administered tissue plasminogen activator (tPA) within the last 24 hours prior to admission to the current facility.

This guideline applies even if the patient is still receiving the tPA at the time they are received into the current facility.

The appropriate code for the condition for which the tPA was administered (such as cerebrovascular disease or myocardial infarction) should be assigned first.

Code Z92.82 is only applicable to the receiving facility record and not to the transferring facility record.

Z93   Artificial opening status

Z94   Transplanted organ and tissue status

Z95   Presence of cardiac and vascular implants and grafts

Z96   Presence of other functional implants

Z97   Presence of other devices

Z98   Other postprocedural states

Assign code Z98.85, Transplanted organ removal status, to indicate that a transplanted organ has been previously removed. This code should not be assigned for the encounter in which the transplanted organ is removed. The complication necessitating removal of the transplant organ should be assigned for that encounter.

See section I.C19. for information on the coding of organ transplant complications.

Z99   Dependence on enabling machines and devices, not elsewhere classified

Note: Categories Z89-Z9Ø and Z93-Z99 are for use only if there are no complications or malfunctions of the organ or tissue replaced, the amputation site or the equipment on which the patient is dependent.

4)   **History (of)**

There are two types of history Z codes, personal and family. Personal history codes explain a patient's past medical condition that no longer exists and is not receiving any treatment, but that has the potential for recurrence, and therefore may require continued monitoring.

Family history codes are for use when a patient has a family member(s) who has had a particular disease that causes the patient to be at higher risk of also contracting the disease.

Personal history codes may be used in conjunction with follow-up codes and family history codes may be used in conjunction with screening codes to explain the need for a test or procedure. History codes are also acceptable on any medical record regardless of the reason for visit. A history of an illness, even if no longer present, is important information that may alter the type of treatment ordered.

The history Z code categories are:

Z8Ø   Family history of primary malignant neoplasm

Z81   Family history of mental and behavioral disorders

Z82   Family history of certain disabilities and chronic diseases (leading to disablement)

Z83   Family history of other specific disorders

Z84   Family history of other conditions

Z85   Personal history of malignant neoplasm

Z86   Personal history of certain other diseases

Z87   Personal history of other diseases and conditions

Z91.4- Personal history of psychological trauma, not elsewhere classified

Z91.5   Personal history of self-harm

Z91.8- Other specified personal risk factors, not elsewhere classified

Exception:

Z91.83, Wandering in diseases classified elsewhere

Z92   Personal history of medical treatment

Except: Z92.Ø, Personal history of contraception

Except: Z92.82, Status post administration of tPA (rtPA) in a different facility within the last 24 hours prior to admission to a current facility

5)   **Screening**

Screening is the testing for disease or disease precursors in seemingly well individuals so that early detection and treatment can be provided for those who test positive for the disease (e.g., screening mammogram).

The testing of a person to rule out or confirm a suspected diagnosis because the patient has some sign or symptom is a diagnostic examination, not a screening. In these cases, the sign or symptom is used to explain the reason for the test.

A screening code may be a first-listed code if the reason for the visit is specifically the screening exam. It may also be used as an additional code if the screening is done during an office visit for other health problems. A screening code is not necessary if the screening is inherent to a routine examination, such as a pap smear done during a routine pelvic examination.

Should a condition be discovered during the screening then the code for the condition may be assigned as an additional diagnosis.

The Z code indicates that a screening exam is planned. A procedure code is required to confirm that the screening was performed.

The screening Z codes/categories:

Z11   Encounter for screening for infectious and parasitic diseases

Z12   Encounter for screening for malignant neoplasms

Z13   Encounter for screening for other diseases and disorders

Except: Z13.9, Encounter for screening, unspecified

Z36   Encounter for antenatal screening for mother

6) Observation

There are two observation Z code categories. They are for use in very limited circumstances when a person is being observed for a suspected condition that is ruled out. The observation codes are not for use if an injury or illness or any signs or symptoms related to the suspected condition are present. In such cases the diagnosis/symptom code is used with the corresponding external cause code.

The observation codes are to be used as principal diagnosis only. Additional codes may be used in addition to the observation code but only if they are unrelated to the suspected condition being observed.

Codes from subcategory Z03.7, Encounter for suspected maternal and fetal conditions ruled out, may either be used as a first-listed or as an additional code assignment depending on the case. They are for use in very limited circumstances on a maternal record when an encounter is for a suspected maternal or fetal condition that is ruled out during that encounter (for example, a maternal or fetal condition may be suspected due to an abnormal test result). These codes should not be used when the condition is confirmed. In those cases, the confirmed condition should be coded. In addition, these codes are not for use if an illness or any signs or symptoms related to the suspected condition or problem are present. In such cases the diagnosis/symptom code is used.

Additional codes may be used in addition to the code from subcategory Z03.7, but only if they are unrelated to the suspected condition being evaluated.

Codes from subcategory Z03.7 may not be used for encounters for antenatal screening of mother. *See Section I.C.21.c.5, Screening.*

For encounters for suspected fetal condition that are inconclusive following testing and evaluation, assign the appropriate code from category O35, O36, O40 or O41.

The observation Z code categories:

Z03   Encounter for medical observation for suspected diseases and conditions ruled out

Z04   Encounter for examination and observation for other reasons

Except: Z04.9, Encounter for examination and observation for unspecified reason

7) Aftercare

Aftercare visit codes cover situations when the initial treatment of a disease has been performed and the patient requires continued care during the healing or recovery phase, or for the long-term consequences of the disease. The aftercare Z code should not be used if treatment is directed at a current, acute disease. The diagnosis code is to be used in these cases. Exceptions to this rule are codes Z51.0, Encounter for antineoplastic radiation therapy, and codes from subcategory Z51.1, Encounter for antineoplastic chemotherapy and immunotherapy. These codes are to be first-listed, followed by the diagnosis code when a patient's encounter is solely to receive radiation therapy, chemotherapy, or immunotherapy for the treatment of a neoplasm. If the reason for the encounter is more than one type of antineoplastic therapy, code Z51.0 and a code from subcategory Z51.1 may be assigned together, in

which case one of these codes would be reported as a secondary diagnosis.

The aftercare Z codes should also not be used for aftercare for injuries. For aftercare of an injury, assign the acute injury code with the appropriate 7th character (for subsequent encounter).

The aftercare codes are generally first-listed to explain the specific reason for the encounter. An aftercare code may be used as an additional code when some type of aftercare is provided in addition to the reason for admission and no diagnosis code is applicable. An example of this would be the closure of a colostomy during an encounter for treatment of another condition.

Aftercare codes should be used in conjunction with other aftercare codes or diagnosis codes to provide better detail on the specifics of an aftercare encounter visit, unless otherwise directed by the classification. Should a patient receive multiple types of antineoplastic therapy during the same encounter, code Z51.0, Encounter for antineoplastic radiation therapy, and codes from subcategory Z51.1, Encounter for antineoplastic chemotherapy and immunotherapy, may be used together on a record. The sequencing of multiple aftercare codes depends on the circumstances of the encounter.

Certain aftercare Z code categories need a secondary diagnosis code to describe the resolving condition or sequelae. For others, the condition is included in the code title.

Additional Z code aftercare category terms include fitting and adjustment, and attention to artificial openings.

Status Z codes may be used with aftercare Z codes to indicate the nature of the aftercare. For example code Z95.1, Presence of aortocoronary bypass graft, may be used with code Z48.812, Encounter for surgical aftercare following surgery on the circulatory system, to indicate the surgery for which the aftercare is being performed. A status code should not be used when the aftercare code indicates the type of status, such as using Z43.0, Encounter for attention to tracheostomy, with Z93.0, Tracheostomy status.

The aftercare Z category/codes:

Z42   Encounter for plastic and reconstructive surgery following medical procedure or healed injury

Z43   Encounter for attention to artificial openings

Z44   Encounter for fitting and adjustment of external prosthetic device

Z45   Encounter for adjustment and management of implanted device

Z46   Encounter for fitting and adjustment of other devices

Z47   Orthopedic aftercare

Z48   Encounter for other postprocedural aftercare

Z49   Encounter for care involving renal dialysis

Z51   Encounter for other aftercare

8) Follow-up

The follow-up codes are used to explain continuing surveillance following completed treatment of a disease, condition, or injury. They imply that the condition has been fully treated and no longer exists. They should not be confused with aftercare codes, or injury codes with a 7th character for subsequent encounter, that explain ongoing care of a healing condition or its sequelae. Follow-up codes may be used in conjunction with history codes to provide the full picture of the healed condition and its treatment. The follow-up code is sequenced first, followed by the history code.

A follow-up code may be used to explain multiple visits. Should a condition be found to have recurred on the follow-up visit, then the diagnosis code for the condition should be assigned in place of the follow-up code.

The follow-up Z code categories:

Z08   Encounter for follow-up examination after completed treatment for malignant neoplasm

Z09   Encounter for follow-up examination after completed treatment for conditions other than malignant neoplasm

Z39   Encounter for maternal postpartum care and examination

9) Donor

Codes in category Z52, Donors of organs and tissues, are used for living individuals who are donating blood or other body tissue. These codes are only for individuals donating for others, not for self-donations. They are not used to identify cadaveric donations.

10) Counseling

Counseling Z codes are used when a patient or family member receives assistance in the aftermath of an illness or injury, or when support is required in coping with family or social problems. They are not used in conjunction with a diagnosis code when the counseling component of care is considered integral to standard treatment.

The counseling Z codes/categories:

Z30.0-   Encounter for general counseling and advice on contraception

Z31.5   Encounter for genetic counseling

Z31.6-   Encounter for general counseling and advice on procreation

Z32.2   Encounter for childbirth instruction

Z32.3   Encounter for childcare instruction

Z69   Encounter for mental health services for victim and perpetrator of abuse

Z70   Counseling related to sexual attitude, behavior and orientation

Z71   Persons encountering health services for other counseling and medical advice, not elsewhere classified

Z76.81   Expectant mother prebirth pediatrician visit

11) Encounters for obstetrical and reproductive services

See Section I.C.15. Pregnancy, Childbirth, and the Puerperium, for further instruction on the use of these codes.

Z codes for pregnancy are for use in those circumstances when none of the problems or complications included in the codes from the Obstetrics chapter exist (a routine prenatal visit or postpartum care). Codes in category Z34, Encounter for supervision of normal pregnancy, are always first-listed and are not to be used with any other code from the OB chapter.

Codes in category Z3A, Weeks of gestation, may be assigned to provide additional information about the pregnancy. The date of the admission should be used to determine weeks of gestation for inpatient admissions that encompass more than one gestational week.

The outcome of delivery, category Z37, should be included on all maternal delivery records. It is always a secondary code.

Z codes for family planning (contraceptive) or procreative management and counseling should be included on an obstetric record either during the pregnancy or the postpartum stage, if applicable.

Z codes/categories for obstetrical and reproductive services:

Z30   Encounter for contraceptive management

Z31   Encounter for procreative management

Z32.2   Encounter for childbirth instruction

Z32.3   Encounter for childcare instruction

Z33   Pregnant state

Z34   Encounter for supervision of normal pregnancy

Z36   Encounter for antenatal screening of mother

Z3A   Weeks of gestation

Z37   Outcome of delivery

Z39   Encounter for maternal postpartum care and examination

Z76.81   Expectant mother prebirth pediatrician visit

12) Newborns and Infants

See Section I.C.16. Newborn (Perinatal) Guidelines, for further instruction on the use of these codes.

Newborn Z codes/categories:

Z76.1   Encounter for health supervision and care of foundling

Z00.1-   Encounter for routine child health examination

Z38   Liveborn infants according to place of birth and type of delivery

13) Routine and administrative examinations

The Z codes allow for the description of encounters for routine examinations, such as, a general check-up, or, examinations for administrative purposes, such as, a pre-employment physical. The codes are not to be used if the examination is for diagnosis of a suspected condition or for treatment purposes. In such cases the diagnosis code is used. During a routine exam, should a diagnosis or condition be discovered, it should be coded as an additional code. Pre-existing and chronic conditions and history codes may also be included as additional codes as long as the examination is for administrative purposes and not focused on any particular condition.

Some of the codes for routine health examinations distinguish between "with" and "without" abnormal findings. Code assignment depends on the information that is known at the time the encounter is being coded. For example, if no abnormal findings were found during the examination, but the encounter is being coded before test results are back, it is acceptable to assign the code for "without abnormal findings." When assigning a code for "with abnormal findings," additional code(s) should be assigned to identify the specific abnormal finding(s).

Pre-operative examination and pre-procedural laboratory examination Z codes are for use only in those situations when a patient is being cleared for a procedure or surgery and no treatment is given.

The Z codes/categories for routine and administrative examinations:

Z00   Encounter for general examination without complaint, suspected or reported diagnosis

Z01   Encounter for other special examination without complaint, suspected or reported diagnosis

Z02   Encounter for administrative examination

    Except: Z02.9, Encounter for administrative examinations, unspecified

Z32.0-   Encounter for pregnancy test

14) Miscellaneous Z codes

The miscellaneous Z codes capture a number of other health care encounters that do not fall into one of the other categories. Certain of these codes identify the reason for the encounter; others are for use as additional codes that provide useful information on circumstances that may affect a patient's care and treatment.

Prophylactic Organ Removal

For encounters specifically for prophylactic removal of an organ (such as prophylactic removal of breasts due to a genetic susceptibility to cancer or a family history of cancer), the principal or first-listed code should be a code from category Z40, Encounter for prophylactic surgery, followed by the appropriate codes to identify the associated risk factor (such as genetic susceptibility or family history).

If the patient has a malignancy of one site and is having prophylactic removal at another site to prevent either a new primary malignancy or metastatic disease, a code for the malignancy should also be assigned in addition to a code from subcategory Z40.0, Encounter for prophylactic surgery for risk factors related to malignant neoplasms. A Z40.0 code should not be assigned if the patient is having organ removal for treatment of a malignancy, such as the removal of the testes for the treatment of prostate cancer.

Miscellaneous Z codes/categories:

Z28   Immunization not carried out

Except: Z28.3, Underimmunization status

Z40   Encounter for prophylactic surgery

Z41   Encounter for procedures for purposes other than remedying health state

Except: Z41.9, Encounter for procedure for purposes other than remedying health state, unspecified

Z53   Persons encountering health services for specific procedures and treatment, not carried out

Z55   Problems related to education and literacy

Z56   Problems related to employment and unemployment

Z57   Occupational exposure to risk factors

Z58   Problems related to physical environment

Z59   Problems related to housing and economic circumstances

Z60   Problems related to social environment

Z62   Problems related to upbringing

Z63   Other problems related to primary support group, including family circumstances

Z64   Problems related to certain psychosocial circumstances

Z65   Problems related to other psychosocial circumstances

Z72   Problems related to lifestyle

Z73   Problems related to life management difficulty

Z74   Problems related to care provider dependency

Except: Z74.01, Bed confinement status

Z75   Problems related to medical facilities and other health care

Z76.0   Encounter for issue of repeat prescription

Z76.3   Healthy person accompanying sick person

Z76.4   Other boarder to healthcare facility

Z76.5   Malingerer [conscious simulation]

Z91.1-   Patient's noncompliance with medical treatment and regimen

Z91.83   Wandering in diseases classified elsewhere

Z91.89   Other specified personal risk factors, not elsewhere classified

15) Nonspecific Z codes

Certain Z codes are so non-specific, or potentially redundant with other codes in the classification, that there can be little justification for their use in the inpatient setting. Their use in the outpatient setting should be limited to those instances when there is no further documentation to permit more precise coding. Otherwise, any sign or symptom or any other reason for visit that is captured in another code should be used.

Nonspecific Z codes/categories:

Z02.9   Encounter for administrative examinations, unspecified

Z04.9   Encounter for examination and observation for unspecified reason

Z13.9   Encounter for screening, unspecified

Z41.9   Encounter for procedure for purposes other than remedying health state, unspecified

Z52.9   Donor of unspecified organ or tissue

Z86.59   Personal history of other mental and behavioral disorders

Z88.9   Allergy status to unspecified drugs, medicaments and biological substances status

Z92.0   Personal history of contraception

16) Z codes that may only be principal/first-listed diagnosis

The following Z codes/categories may only be reported as the principal/first-listed diagnosis, except when there are multiple encounters on the same day and the medical records for the encounters are combined:

Z00   Encounter for general examination without complaint, suspected or reported diagnosis

Except: Z00.6

Z01   Encounter for other special examination without complaint, suspected or reported diagnosis

Z02   Encounter for administrative examination

Z03   Encounter for medical observation for suspected diseases and conditions ruled out

Z04   Encounter for examination and observation for other reasons

Z33.2   Encounter for elective termination of pregnancy

Z31.81   Encounter for male factor infertility in female patient

Z31.82   Encounter for Rh incompatibility status

Z31.83   Encounter for assisted reproductive fertility procedure cycle

Z31.84   Encounter for fertility preservation procedure

Z34   Encounter for supervision of normal pregnancy

Z39   Encounter for maternal postpartum care and examination

Z38   Liveborn infants according to place of birth and type of delivery

Z42   Encounter for plastic and reconstructive surgery following medical procedure or healed injury

Z51.0   Encounter for antineoplastic radiation therapy

Z51.1-   Encounter for antineoplastic chemotherapy and immunotherapy

Z52   Donors of organs and tissues

Except: Z52.9, Donor of unspecified organ or tissue

Z76.1   Encounter for health supervision and care of foundling

Z76.2   Encounter for health supervision and care of other healthy infant and child

Z99.12   Encounter for respirator [ventilator] dependence during power failure

Section II. Selection of Principal Diagnosis

The circumstances of inpatient admission always govern the selection of principal diagnosis.

The principal diagnosis is defined in the Uniform Hospital Discharge Data Set (UHDDS) as "that condition established after study to be chiefly responsible for occasioning the admission of the patient to the hospital for care."

The UHDDS definitions are used by hospitals to report inpatient data elements in a standardized manner. These data elements and their definitions can be found in the July 31, 1985, Federal Register (Vol. 50, No, 147), pp. 31038-40.

Since that time the application of the UHDDS definitions has been expanded to include all non- outpatient settings (acute care, short term, long term care and psychiatric hospitals; home health agencies; rehab facilities; nursing homes, etc).

In determining principal diagnosis, coding conventions in the ICD-10-CM, the Tabular List and Alphabetic Index take precedence over these official coding guidelines.

(See Section I.A., Conventions for the ICD-10-CM)

The importance of consistent, complete documentation in the medical record cannot be overemphasized. Without such documentation the application of all coding guidelines is a difficult, if not impossible, task.

A. Codes for symptoms, signs, and ill-defined conditions

Codes for symptoms, signs, and ill-defined conditions from Chapter 18 are not to be used as principal diagnosis when a related definitive diagnosis has been established.

B. Two or more interrelated conditions, each potentially meeting the definition for principal diagnosis

When there are two or more interrelated conditions (such as diseases in the same ICD-10-CM chapter or manifestations characteristically associated with a certain disease) potentially meeting the definition of principal diagnosis, either condition may be sequenced first, unless the circumstances of the admission, the therapy provided, the Tabular List, or the Alphabetic Index indicate otherwise.

C. Two or more diagnoses that equally meet the definition for principal diagnosis

In the unusual instance when two or more diagnoses equally meet the criteria for principal diagnosis as determined by the circumstances of admission, diagnostic workup and/or therapy provided, and the Alphabetic Index, Tabular List, or another coding guidelines does not provide sequencing direction, any one of the diagnoses may be sequenced first.

D. Two or more comparative or contrasting conditions

In those rare instances when two or more contrasting or comparative diagnoses are documented as "either/or" (or similar terminology), they are coded as if the diagnoses were confirmed and the diagnoses are sequenced according to the circumstances of the admission. If no further determination can be made as to which diagnosis should be principal, either diagnosis may be sequenced first.

E. A symptom(s) followed by contrasting/comparative diagnoses

GUIDELINE HAS BEEN DELETED EFFECTIVE OCTOBER 1, 2014

F. Original treatment plan not carried out

Sequence as the principal diagnosis the condition, which after study occasioned the admission to the hospital, even though treatment may not have been carried out due to unforeseen circumstances.

G. Complications of surgery and other medical care

When the admission is for treatment of a complication resulting from surgery or other medical care, the complication code is sequenced as the principal diagnosis. If the complication is classified to the T80-T88 series and the code lacks the necessary specificity in describing the complication, an additional code for the specific complication should be assigned.

H. Uncertain diagnosis

If the diagnosis documented at the time of discharge is qualified as "probable", "suspected", "likely", "questionable", "possible", or "still to be ruled out", or other similar terms indicating uncertainty, code the condition as if it existed or was established. The bases for these guidelines are the diagnostic workup, arrangements for further workup or observation, and initial therapeutic approach that correspond most closely with the established diagnosis.

Note: This guideline is applicable only to inpatient admissions to short-term, acute, long-term care and psychiatric hospitals.

I. Admission from observation unit

1. **Admission Following Medical Observation**
   When a patient is admitted to an observation unit for a medical condition, which either worsens or does not improve, and is subsequently admitted as an inpatient of the same hospital for this same medical condition, the principal diagnosis would be the medical condition which led to the hospital admission.

2. **Admission Following Post-Operative Observation**
   When a patient is admitted to an observation unit to monitor a condition (or complication) that develops following outpatient surgery, and then is subsequently admitted as an inpatient of the same hospital, hospitals should apply the Uniform Hospital Discharge Data Set (UHDDS) definition of principal diagnosis as "that condition established after study to be chiefly responsible for occasioning the admission of the patient to the hospital for care."

J. Admission from outpatient surgery

When a patient receives surgery in the hospital's outpatient surgery department and is subsequently admitted for continuing inpatient care at the same hospital, the following guidelines should be followed in selecting the principal diagnosis for the inpatient admission:

- If the reason for the inpatient admission is a complication, assign the complication as the principal diagnosis.
- If no complication, or other condition, is documented as the reason for the inpatient admission, assign the reason for the outpatient surgery as the principal diagnosis.
- If the reason for the inpatient admission is another condition unrelated to the surgery, assign the unrelated condition as the principal diagnosis.

K. Admissions/Encounters for Rehabilitation

When the purpose for the admission/encounter is rehabilitation, sequence first the code for the condition for which the service is being performed. For example, for an admission/encounter for rehabilitation for right-sided dominant hemiplegia following a cerebrovascular infarction, report code I69.351, Hemiplegia and hemiparesis following cerebral infarction affecting right dominant side, as the first-listed or principal diagnosis.

If the condition for which the rehabilitation service is no longer present, report the appropriate aftercare code as the first-listed or principal diagnosis. For example, if a patient with severe degenerative osteoarthritis of the hip, underwent hip replacement and the current encounter/admission is for rehabilitation, report code Z47.1, Aftercare following joint replacement surgery, as the first-listed or principal diagnosis.

See Section I.C.21.c.7, Factors influencing health states and contact with health services, Aftercare.

Section III. Reporting Additional Diagnoses

GENERAL RULES FOR OTHER (ADDITIONAL) DIAGNOSES

For reporting purposes the definition for "other diagnoses" is interpreted as additional conditions that affect patient care in terms of requiring:

> clinical evaluation; or
>
> therapeutic treatment; or
>
> diagnostic procedures; or
>
> extended length of hospital stay; or
>
> increased nursing care and/or monitoring.

The UHDDS item #11-b defines Other Diagnoses as "all conditions that coexist at the time of admission, that develop subsequently, or that affect the treatment received and/or the length of stay. Diagnoses that relate to an earlier episode which have no bearing on the current hospital stay are to be excluded." UHDDS definitions apply to inpatients in acute care, short-term, long term care and psychiatric hospital setting. The UHDDS definitions are used by acute care short-term hospitals to report inpatient data elements in a standardized manner. These data elements and their definitions can be found in the July 31, 1985, Federal Register (Vol. 50, No, 147), pp. 31038-40.

Since that time the application of the UHDDS definitions has been expanded to include all non-outpatient settings (acute care, short term, long term care and psychiatric hospitals; home health agencies; rehab facilities; nursing homes, etc).

The following guidelines are to be applied in designating "other diagnoses" when neither the Alphabetic Index nor the Tabular List in ICD-10-CM provide direction. The listing of the diagnoses in the patient record is the responsibility of the attending provider.

A. **Previous conditions**
   If the provider has included a diagnosis in the final diagnostic statement, such as the discharge summary or the face sheet, it should ordinarily be coded. Some providers include in the diagnostic statement resolved conditions or diagnoses and status-post procedures from previous admission that have no bearing on the current stay. Such conditions are not to be reported and are coded only if required by hospital policy.

   However, history codes (categories Z80-Z87) may be used as secondary codes if the historical condition or family history has an impact on current care or influences treatment.

B. **Abnormal findings**
   Abnormal findings (laboratory, x-ray, pathologic, and other diagnostic results) are not coded and reported unless the provider indicates their clinical significance. If the findings are outside the normal range and the attending provider has ordered other tests to evaluate the condition or prescribed treatment, it is appropriate to ask the provider whether the abnormal finding should be added.

   Please note: This differs from the coding practices in the outpatient setting for coding encounters for diagnostic tests that have been interpreted by a provider.

C. **Uncertain Diagnosis**
   If the diagnosis documented at the time of discharge is qualified as "probable", "suspected", "likely", "questionable", "possible", or "still to be ruled out" or other similar terms indicating uncertainty, code the condition as if it existed or was established. The bases for these guidelines are the diagnostic workup, arrangements for further workup

or observation, and initial therapeutic approach that correspond most closely with the established diagnosis.

Note: This guideline is applicable only to inpatient admissions to short-term, acute, long-term care and psychiatric hospitals.

Section IV. Diagnostic Coding and Reporting Guidelines for Outpatient Services

These coding guidelines for outpatient diagnoses have been approved for use by hospitals/ providers in coding and reporting hospital-based outpatient services and provider-based office visits.

Information about the use of certain abbreviations, punctuation, symbols, and other conventions used in the ICD-10-CM Tabular List (code numbers and titles), can be found in Section IA of these guidelines, under "Conventions Used in the Tabular List." Section I.B. contains general guidelines that apply to the entire classification. Section I.C. contains chapter-specific guidelines that correspond to the chapters as they are arranged in the classification. Information about the correct sequence to use in finding a code is also described in Section I.

The terms encounter and visit are often used interchangeably in describing outpatient service contacts and, therefore, appear together in these guidelines without distinguishing one from the other.

Though the conventions and general guidelines apply to all settings, coding guidelines for outpatient and provider reporting of diagnoses will vary in a number of instances from those for inpatient diagnoses, recognizing that:

The Uniform Hospital Discharge Data Set (UHDDS) definition of principal diagnosis applies only to inpatients in acute, short-term, long-term care and psychiatric hospitals.

Coding guidelines for inconclusive diagnoses (probable, suspected, rule out, etc.) were developed for inpatient reporting and do not apply to outpatients.

A. Selection of first-listed condition

In the outpatient setting, the term first-listed diagnosis is used in lieu of principal diagnosis.

In determining the first-listed diagnosis the coding conventions of ICD-10-CM, as well as the general and disease specific guidelines take precedence over the outpatient guidelines.

Diagnoses often are not established at the time of the initial encounter/visit. It may take two or more visits before the diagnosis is confirmed.

The most critical rule involves beginning the search for the correct code assignment through the Alphabetic Index. Never begin searching initially in the Tabular List as this will lead to coding errors.

1. Outpatient surgery

When a patient presents for outpatient surgery (same day surgery), code the reason for the surgery as the first-listed diagnosis (reason for the encounter), even if the surgery is not performed due to a contraindication.

2. Observation stay

When a patient is admitted for observation for a medical condition, assign a code for the medical condition as the first-listed diagnosis.

When a patient presents for outpatient surgery and develops complications requiring admission to observation, code the reason for the surgery as the first reported diagnosis (reason for the encounter), followed by codes for the complications as secondary diagnoses.

B. Codes from A00.0 through T88.9, Z00-Z99

The appropriate code(s) from A00.0 through T88.9, Z00-Z99 must be used to identify diagnoses, symptoms, conditions, problems, complaints, or other reason(s) for the encounter/visit.

C. Accurate reporting of ICD-10-CM diagnosis codes

For accurate reporting of ICD-10-CM diagnosis codes, the documentation should describe the patient's condition, using terminology which includes specific diagnoses as well as symptoms, problems, or reasons for the encounter. There are ICD-10-CM codes to describe all of these.

D. Codes that describe symptoms and signs

Codes that describe symptoms and signs, as opposed to diagnoses, are acceptable for reporting purposes when a diagnosis has not been established (confirmed) by the provider. Chapter 18 of ICD-10-CM, Symptoms, Signs, and Abnormal Clinical and Laboratory Findings Not Elsewhere Classified (codes R00-R99) contain many, but not all codes for symptoms.

E. Encounters for circumstances other than a disease or injury

ICD-10-CM provides codes to deal with encounters for circumstances other than a disease or injury. The Factors Influencing Health Status and Contact with Health Services codes (Z00-Z99) are provided to deal with occasions when circumstances other than a disease or injury are recorded as diagnosis or problems.

See Section I.C.21. Factors influencing health status and contact with health services.

F. Level of Detail in Coding

1. ICD-10-CM codes with 3, 4, 5, 6 or 7 characters

ICD-10-CM is composed of codes with 3, 4, 5, 6 or 7 characters. Codes with three characters are included in ICD-10-CM as the heading of a category of codes that may be further subdivided by the use of fourth, fifth, sixth or seventh characters to provide greater specificity.

2. Use of full number of *characters* required for a code

A three-character code is to be used only if it is not further subdivided. A code is invalid if it has not been coded to the full number of characters required for that code, including the 7th character extension, if applicable.

G. ICD-10-CM code for the diagnosis, condition, problem, or other reason for encounter/visit

List first the ICD-10-CM code for the diagnosis, condition, problem, or other reason for encounter/visit shown in the medical record to be chiefly responsible for the services provided. List additional codes that describe any coexisting conditions. In some cases the first-listed diagnosis may be a symptom when a diagnosis has not been established (confirmed) by the physician.

H. Uncertain diagnosis

Do not code diagnoses documented as "probable", "suspected," "questionable," "rule out," or "working diagnosis" or other similar terms indicating uncertainty. Rather, code the condition(s) to the highest degree of certainty for that encounter/visit, such as symptoms, signs, abnormal test results, or other reason for the visit.

Please note: This differs from the coding practices used by short-term, acute care, long-term care and psychiatric hospitals.

I. Chronic diseases

Chronic diseases treated on an ongoing basis may be coded and reported as many times as the patient receives treatment and care for the condition(s)

J. Code all documented conditions that coexist

Code all documented conditions that coexist at the time of the encounter/visit, and require or affect patient care treatment or management. Do not code conditions that were previously treated and no longer exist. However, history codes (categories Z80-Z87) may be used as secondary codes if the historical condition or family history has an impact on current care or influences treatment.

K. Patients receiving diagnostic services only

For patients receiving diagnostic services only during an encounter/visit, sequence first the diagnosis, condition, problem, or other reason for encounter/visit shown in the medical record to be chiefly responsible for the outpatient services provided during the encounter/visit. Codes for other diagnoses (e.g., chronic conditions) may be sequenced as additional diagnoses.

For encounters for routine laboratory/radiology testing in the absence of any signs, symptoms, or associated diagnosis, assign Z01.89, Encounter for other specified special examinations. If routine testing is performed during the same encounter as a test to evaluate a sign, symptom, or diagnosis, it is appropriate to assign both the Z code and the code describing the reason for the non-routine test.

For outpatient encounters for diagnostic tests that have been interpreted by a physician, and the final report is available at the time of coding, code any confirmed or definitive diagnosis(es) documented in the interpretation. Do not code related signs and symptoms as additional diagnoses.

Please note: This differs from the coding practice in the hospital inpatient setting regarding abnormal findings on test results.

L. Patients receiving therapeutic services only

For patients receiving therapeutic services only during an encounter/visit, sequence first the diagnosis, condition, problem, or other reason for encounter/visit shown in the medical record to be chiefly responsible for the outpatient services provided during the encounter/visit. Codes for other diagnoses (e.g., chronic conditions) may be sequenced as additional diagnoses.

The only exception to this rule is that when the primary reason for the admission/encounter is chemotherapy or radiation therapy, the appropriate Z code for the service is listed first, and the diagnosis or problem for which the service is being performed listed second.

M. Patients receiving preoperative evaluations only

For patients receiving preoperative evaluations only, sequence first a code from subcategory Z01.81, Encounter for pre-procedural examinations, to describe the pre-op consultations. Assign a code for the condition to describe the reason for the surgery as an additional diagnosis. Code also any findings related to the pre-op evaluation.

N. Ambulatory surgery

For ambulatory surgery, code the diagnosis for which the surgery was performed. If the postoperative diagnosis is known to be different from the preoperative diagnosis at the time the diagnosis is confirmed, select the postoperative diagnosis for coding, since it is the most definitive.

O. Routine outpatient prenatal visits

See Section I.C.15. Routine outpatient prenatal visits.

P. Encounters for general medical examinations with abnormal findings

The subcategories for encounters for general medical examinations, Z00.0-, provide codes for with and without abnormal findings. Should a general medical examination result in an abnormal finding, the code for general medical examination with abnormal finding should be assigned as the first-listed diagnosis. A secondary code for the abnormal finding should also be coded.

Q. Encounters for routine health screenings

See Section I.C.21. Factors influencing health status and contact with health services, Screening

Appendix I. Present on Admission Reporting Guidelines

Introduction

These guidelines are to be used as a supplement to the *ICD-10-CM Official Guidelines for Coding and Reporting* to facilitate the assignment of the Present on Admission (POA) indicator for each diagnosis and external cause of injury code reported on claim forms (UB-04 and 837 Institutional).

These guidelines are not intended to replace any guidelines in the main body of the *ICD-10-CM Official Guidelines for Coding and Reporting*. The POA guidelines are not intended to provide guidance on when a condition should be coded, but rather, how to apply the POA indicator to the final set of diagnosis codes that have been assigned in accordance with Sections I, II, and III of the official coding guidelines. Subsequent to the assignment of the ICD-10-CM codes, the POA indicator should then be assigned to those conditions that have been coded.

As stated in the Introduction to the *ICD-10-CM Official Guidelines for Coding and Reporting*, a joint effort between the healthcare provider and the coder is essential to achieve complete and accurate documentation, code assignment, and reporting of diagnoses and procedures. The importance of consistent, complete documentation in the medical record cannot be overemphasized. Medical record documentation from any provider involved in the care and treatment of the patient may be used to support the determination of whether a condition was present on admission or not. In the context of the official coding guidelines, the term "provider" means a physician or any qualified healthcare practitioner who is legally accountable for establishing the patient's diagnosis.

These guidelines are not a substitute for the provider's clinical judgment as to the determination of whether a condition was/was not present on admission. The provider should be queried regarding issues related to the linking of signs/symptoms, timing of test results, and the timing of findings.

General Reporting Requirements

All claims involving inpatient admissions to general acute care hospitals or other facilities that are subject to a law or regulation mandating collection of present on admission information.

Present on admission is defined as present at the time the order for inpatient admission occurs -- conditions that develop during an outpatient encounter, including emergency department, observation, or outpatient surgery, are considered as present on admission.

POA indicator is assigned to principal and secondary diagnoses (as defined in Section II of the Official Guidelines for Coding and Reporting) and the external cause of injury codes.

Issues related to inconsistent, missing, conflicting or unclear documentation must still be resolved by the provider.

If a condition would not be coded and reported based on UHDDS definitions and current official coding guidelines, then the POA indicator would not be reported.

Reporting Options

Y –	Yes
N –	No
U –	Unknown
W –	Clinically undetermined
	Unreported/Not used (or "1" for Medicare usage) – (Exempt from POA reporting)

Reporting Definitions

Y –	present at the time of inpatient admission
N –	not present at the time of inpatient admission
U –	documentation is insufficient to determine if condition is present on admission
W –	provider is unable to clinically determine whether condition was present on admission or not

Timeframe for POA Identification and Documentation

There is no required timeframe as to when a provider (per the definition of "provider" used in these guidelines) must identify or document a condition to be present on admission. In some clinical situations, it may not be possible for a provider to make a definitive diagnosis (or a condition may not be recognized or reported by the patient) for a period of time after admission. In some cases it may be several days before the provider arrives at a definitive diagnosis. This does not mean that the condition was not present on admission. Determination of whether the condition was present on admission or not will be based on the applicable POA guideline as identified in this document, or on the provider's best clinical judgment.

If at the time of code assignment the documentation is unclear as to whether a condition was present on admission or not, it is appropriate to query the provider for clarification.

Assigning the POA Indicator

Condition is on the "Exempt from Reporting" list

Leave the "present on admission" field blank if the condition is on the list of ICD-10-CM codes for which this field is not applicable. This is the only circumstance in which the field may be left blank.

POA Explicitly Documented

Assign "Y" for any condition the provider explicitly documents as being present on admission.

Assign "N" for any condition the provider explicitly documents as not present at the time of admission.

Conditions diagnosed prior to inpatient admission

Assign "Y" for conditions that were diagnosed prior to admission (example: hypertension, diabetes mellitus, asthma).

Conditions diagnosed during the admission but clearly present before admission

Assign "Y" for conditions diagnosed during the admission that were clearly present but not diagnosed until after admission occurred.

Diagnoses subsequently confirmed after admission are considered present on admission if at the time of admission they are documented as suspected, possible, rule out, differential diagnosis, or constitute an underlying cause of a symptom that is present at the time of admission.

Condition develops during outpatient encounter prior to inpatient admission

Assign "Y" for any condition that develops during an outpatient encounter prior to a written order for inpatient admission.

Documentation does not indicate whether condition was present on admission

Assign "U" when the medical record documentation is unclear as to whether the condition was present on admission. "U" should not be routinely assigned and used only in very limited circumstances. Coders are encouraged to query the providers when the documentation is unclear.

Documentation states that it cannot be determined whether the condition was or was not present on admission

Assign "W" when the medical record documentation indicates that it cannot be clinically determined whether or not the condition was present on admission.

Chronic condition with acute exacerbation during the admission

If a single code identifies both the chronic condition and the acute exacerbation, see POA guidelines pertaining to combination codes.

If a single code only identifies the chronic condition and not the acute exacerbation (e.g., acute exacerbation of chronic leukemia), assign "Y."

Conditions documented as possible, probable, suspected, or rule out at the time of discharge

If the final diagnosis contains a possible, probable, suspected, or rule out diagnosis, and this diagnosis was based on signs, symptoms or clinical findings suspected at the time of inpatient admission, assign "Y."

If the final diagnosis contains a possible, probable, suspected, or rule out diagnosis, and this diagnosis was based on signs, symptoms or clinical findings that were not present on admission, assign "N".

Conditions documented as impending or threatened at the time of discharge

If the final diagnosis contains an impending or threatened diagnosis, and this diagnosis is based on symptoms or clinical findings that were present on admission, assign "Y".

If the final diagnosis contains an impending or threatened diagnosis, and this diagnosis is based on symptoms or clinical findings that were not present on admission, assign "N".

Acute and Chronic Conditions

Assign "Y" for acute conditions that are present at time of admission and N for acute conditions that are not present at time of admission.

Assign "Y" for chronic conditions, even though the condition may not be diagnosed until after admission.

If a single code identifies both an acute and chronic condition, see the POA guidelines for combination codes.

Combination Codes

Assign "N" if any part of the combination code was not present on admission (e.g., COPD with acute exacerbation and the exacerbation was not present on admission; gastric ulcer that does not start bleeding until after admission; asthma patient develops status asthmaticus after admission).

Assign "Y" if all parts of the combination code were present on admission (e.g., patient with acute prostatitis admitted with hematuria).

If the final diagnosis includes comparative or contrasting diagnoses, and both were present, or suspected, at the time of admission, assign "Y".

For infection codes that include the causal organism, assign "Y" if the infection (or signs of the infection) was present on admission, even though the culture results may not be known until after admission (e.g., patient is admitted with pneumonia and the provider documents pseudomonas as the causal organism a few days later).

Same Diagnosis Code for Two or More Conditions

When the same ICD-10-CM diagnosis code applies to two or more conditions during the same encounter (e.g. two separate conditions classified to the same ICD-10-CM diagnosis code):

Assign "Y" if all conditions represented by the single ICD-10-CM code were present on admission (e.g. bilateral unspecified age-related cataracts).

Assign "N" if any of the conditions represented by the single ICD-10-CM code was not present on admission (e.g. traumatic secondary and recurrent hemorrhage and seroma is assigned to a single code T79.2, but only one of the conditions was present on admission).

Obstetrical conditions

Whether or not the patient delivers during the current hospitalization does not affect assignment of the POA indicator. The determining factor for POA assignment is whether the pregnancy complication or obstetrical condition described by the code was present at the time of admission or not.

If the pregnancy complication or obstetrical condition was present on admission (e.g., patient admitted in preterm labor), assign "Y".

If the pregnancy complication or obstetrical condition was not present on admission (e.g., 2nd degree laceration during delivery, postpartum hemorrhage that occurred during current hospitalization, fetal distress develops after admission), assign "N".

If the obstetrical code includes more than one diagnosis and any of the diagnoses identified by the code were not present on admission assign "N". (e.g., Category O11, Pre-existing hypertension with pre-eclampsia).

Perinatal conditions

Newborns are not considered to be admitted until after birth. Therefore, any condition present at birth or that developed in utero is considered present at admission and should be assigned "Y". This includes conditions that occur during delivery (e.g., injury during delivery, meconium aspiration, exposure to streptococcus B in the vaginal canal).

Congenital conditions and anomalies

Assign "Y" for congenital conditions and anomalies except for categories Q00-Q99, Congenital anomalies, which are on the exempt list. Congenital conditions are always considered present on admission.

External cause of injury codes

Assign "Y" for any external cause code representing an external cause of morbidity that occurred prior to inpatient admission (e.g., patient fell out of bed at home, patient fell out of bed in emergency room prior to admission).

Assign "N" for any external cause code representing an external cause of morbidity that occurred during inpatient hospitalization (e.g., patient fell out of hospital bed during hospital stay, patient experienced an adverse reaction to a medication administered after inpatient admission).

Categories and Codes Exempt from Diagnosis Present on Admission Requirement

Note: "Diagnosis present on admission" for these code categories are exempt because they represent circumstances regarding the healthcare encounter or factors influencing health status that do not represent a current disease or injury or are always present on admission.

B90–B94	Sequelae of infectious and parasitic diseases
E64	Sequelae of malnutrition and other nutritional deficiencies
I25.2	Old myocardial infarction
I69	Sequelae of cerebrovascular disease
O09	Supervision of high risk pregnancy
O66.5	Attempted application of vacuum extractor and forceps
O80	Encounter for full-term uncomplicated delivery
O94	Sequelae of complication of pregnancy, childbirth, and the puerperium
P00	Newborn (suspected to be) affected by maternal conditions that may be unrelated to present pregnancy
Q00-Q99	Congenital malformations, deformations and chromosomal abnormalities

S00-T88.9	Injury, poisoning and certain other consequences of external causes with 7th character representing subsequent encounter or sequela
V00-V09	Pedestrian injured in transport accident
	Except:V00.81-, Accident with wheelchair (powered) V00.83-, Accident with motorized mobility scooter
V10-V19	Pedal cycle rider injured in transport accident
V20-V29	Motorcycle rider injured in transport accident
V30-V39	Occupant of three-wheeled motor vehicle injured in transport accident
V40-V49	Car occupant injured in transport accident
V50-V59	Occupant of pick-up truck or van injured in transport accident
V60-V69	Occupant of heavy transport vehicle injured in transport accident
V70-V79	Bus occupant injured in transport accident
V80-V89	Other land transport accidents
V90-V94	Water transport accidents
V95-V97	Air and space transport accidents
V98-V99	Other and unspecified transport accidents
W09	Fall on and from playground equipment
W14	Fall from tree
W15	Fall from cliff
W17.0	Fall into well
W17.1	Fall into storm drain or manhole
W18.01	Striking against sports equipment with subsequent fall
W21	Striking against or struck by sports equipment
W30	Contact with agricultural machinery
W31	Contact with other and unspecified machinery
W32-W34	Accidental handgun discharge and malfunction
W35-W40	Exposure to inanimate mechanical forces
W52	Crushed, pushed or stepped on by crowd or human stampede
W56	Contact with nonvenomous marine animal
W58	Contact with crocodile or alligator
W61	Contact with birds (domestic) (wild)
W62	Contact with nonvenomous amphibians
W89	Exposure to man-made visible and ultraviolet light
X02	Exposure to controlled fire in building or structure
X03	Exposure to controlled fire, not in building or structure
X04	Exposure to ignition of highly flammable material
X52	Prolonged stay in weightless environment
X71	Intentional self-harm by drowning and submersion
	Except: X71.0-, Intentional self-harm by drowning and submersion while in bath tub
X72	Intentional self-harm by handgun discharge
X73	Intentional self-harm by rifle, shotgun and larger firearm discharge
X74	Intentional self-harm by other and unspecified firearm and gun discharge
X75	Intentional self-harm by explosive material
X76	Intentional self-harm by smoke, fire and flames
X77	Intentional self-harm by steam, hot vapors and hot objects
X81	Intentional self-harm by jumping or lying in front of moving object
X82	Intentional self-harm by crashing of motor vehicle
X83	Intentional self-harm by other specified means
Y03	Assault by crashing of motor vehicle
Y07	Perpetrator of assault, maltreatment and neglect
Y08.8	Assault by strike by sports equipment
Y21	Drowning and submersion, undetermined intent
Y22	Handgun discharge, undetermined intent
Y23	Rifle, shotgun and larger firearm discharge, undetermined intent
Y24	Other and unspecified firearm discharge, undetermined intent
Y30	Falling, jumping or pushed from a high place, undetermined intent
Y32	Assault by crashing of motor vehicle, undetermined intent
Y36	Operations of war
Y37	Military operations
Y92	Place of occurrence of the external cause
Y93	Activity code
Y99	External cause status

Z00	Encounter for general examination without complaint, suspected or reported diagnosis
Z01	Encounter for other special examination without complaint, suspected or reported diagnosis
Z02	Encounter for administrative examination
Z03	Encounter for medical observation for suspected diseases and conditions ruled out
Z08	Encounter for follow-up examination following completed treatment for malignant neoplasm
Z09	Encounter for follow-up examination after completed treatment for conditions other than malignant neoplasm
Z11	Encounter for screening for infectious and parasitic diseases
Z11.8	Encounter for screening for other infectious and parasitic diseases
Z12	Encounter for screening for malignant neoplasms
Z13	Encounter for screening for other diseases and disorders
Z13.4	Encounter for screening for certain developmental disorders in childhood
Z13.5	Encounter for screening for eye and ear disorders
Z13.6	Encounter for screening for cardiovascular disorders
Z13.83	Encounter for screening for respiratory disorder NEC
Z13.89	Encounter for screening for other disorder
Z14	Genetic carrier
Z15	Genetic susceptibility to disease
Z17	Estrogen receptor status
Z18	Retained foreign body fragments
Z22	Carrier of infectious disease
Z23	Encounter for immunization
Z28	Immunization not carried out and underimmunization status
Z28.3	Underimmunization status
Z30	Encounter for contraceptive management
Z31	Encounter for procreative management
Z34	Encounter for supervision of normal pregnancy
Z36	Encounter for antenatal screening of mother
Z37	Outcome of delivery
Z38	Liveborn infants according to place of birth and type of delivery
Z39	Encounter for maternal postpartum care and examination
Z41	Encounter for procedures for purposes other than remedying health state
Z42	Encounter for plastic and reconstructive surgery following medical procedure or healed injury
Z43	Encounter for attention to artificial openings
Z44	Encounter for fitting and adjustment of external prosthetic device
Z45	Encounter for adjustment and management of implanted device
Z46	Encounter for fitting and adjustment of other devices
Z47.8	Encounter for other orthopedic aftercare
Z49	Encounter for care involving renal dialysis
Z51	Encounter for other aftercare
Z51.5	Encounter for palliative care
Z51.8	Encounter for other specified aftercare
Z52	Donors of organs and tissues
Z59	Problems related to housing and economic circumstances
Z63	Other problems related to primary support groupincluding family circumstances
Z65	Problems related to other psychosocial circumstances
Z65.8	Other specified problems related to psychosocial circumstances
Z67.1-Z67.9	Blood type
Z68	Body mass index (BMI)
Z72	Problems related to lifestyle
Z74.01	Bed confinement status
Z76	Persons encountering health services in other circumstances
Z77.110-Z77.128	Environmental pollution and hazards in the physical environment
Z78	Other specified health status
Z79	Long term (current) drug therapy
Z80	Family history of primary malignant neoplasm
Z81	Family history of mental and behavioral disorders
Z82	Family history of certain disabilities and chronic diseases (leading to disablement)
Z83	Family history of other specific disorders

Z84	Family history of other conditions	Z92	Personal history of medical treatment
Z85	Personal history of primary malignant neoplasm	Z93	Artificial opening status
Z86	Personal history of certain other diseases	Z94	Transplanted organ and tissue status
Z87	Personal history of other diseases and conditions	Z95	Presence of cardiac and vascular implants and grafts
Z87.828	Personal history of other (healed) physical injury and trauma	Z97	Presence of other devices
Z87.891	Personal history of nicotine dependence	Z98	Other postprocedural states
Z88	Allergy status to drugs, medicaments and biological substances	Z99	Dependence on enabling machines and devices, not elsewhere classified
Z89	Acquired absence of limb		
Z90.710	Acquired absence of both cervix and uterus		
Z91.0	Allergy status, other than to drugs and biological substances		
Z91.4	Personal history of psychological trauma, not elsewhere classified		
Z91.5	Personal history of self-harm		
Z91.8	Other specified risk factors, not elsewhere classified		

ICD-10-CM Index to Diseases and Injuries

A

Aarskog's syndrome Q87.1
Abandonment — *see* Maltreatment
Abasia (-astasia) (hysterical) F44.4
Abderhalden-Kaufmann-Lignac syndrome (cystinosis) E72.04
Abdomen, abdominal (*see also* condition)
  acute R10.0
  angina K55.1
  muscle deficiency syndrome Q79.4
Abdominalgia — *see* Pain, abdominal
Abduction contracture, hip or other joint — *see* Contraction, joint
Aberrant (congenital) (*see also* Malposition, congenital)
  adrenal gland Q89.1
  artery (peripheral) Q27.8
    basilar NEC Q28.1
    cerebral Q28.3
    coronary Q24.5
    digestive system Q27.8
    eye Q15.8
    lower limb Q27.8
    precerebral Q28.1
    pulmonary Q25.79
    renal Q27.2
    retina Q14.1
    specified site NEC Q27.8
    subclavian Q27.8
    upper limb Q27.8
    vertebral Q28.1
  breast Q83.8
  endocrine gland NEC Q89.2
  hepatic duct Q44.5
  pancreas Q45.3
  parathyroid gland Q89.2
  pituitary gland Q89.2
  sebaceous glands, mucous membrane, mouth, congenital Q38.6
  spleen Q89.09
  subclavian artery Q27.8
  thymus (gland) Q89.2
  thyroid gland Q89.2
  vein (peripheral) NEC Q27.8
    cerebral Q28.3
    digestive system Q27.8
    lower limb Q27.8
    precerebral Q28.1
    specified site NEC Q27.8
    upper limb Q27.8
Aberration
  distantial — *see* Disturbance, visual
  mental F99
Abetalipoproteinemia E78.6
Abiotrophy R68.89
Ablatio, ablation
  retinae — *see* Detachment, retina
Ablepharia, ablepharon Q10.3
Abnormal, abnormality, abnormalities (*see also* Anomaly)
  acid-base balance (mixed) E87.4
  albumin R77.0
  alphafetoprotein R77.2
  alveolar ridge K08.9
  anatomical relationship Q89.9
  apertures, congenital, diaphragm Q79.1
  auditory perception H93.29- ☑
    diplacusis — *see* Diplacusis
    hyperacusis — *see* Hyperacusis
    recruitment — *see* Recruitment, auditory
    threshold shift — *see* Shift, auditory threshold
  autosomes Q99.9
    fragile site Q95.5
  basal metabolic rate R94.8
  biosynthesis, testicular androgen E29.1
  bleeding time R79.1
  blood level (of)
    cobalt R79.0
    copper R79.0
    iron R79.0
    lithium R78.89

Abnormal, abnormality, abnormalities — *continued*
  blood level — *continued*
    magnesium R79.0
    mineral NEC R79.0
    zinc R79.0
  blood pressure
    elevated R03.0
    low reading (nonspecific) R03.1
  blood sugar R73.09
  blood-gas level R79.81
  bowel sounds R19.15
    absent R19.11
    hyperactive R19.12
  brain scan R94.02
  breathing R06.9
  caloric test R94.138
  cerebrospinal fluid R83.9
    cytology R83.6
    drug level R83.2
    enzyme level R83.0
    hormones R83.1
    immunology R83.4
    microbiology R83.5
    nonmedicinal level R83.3
    specified type NEC R83.8
  chemistry, blood R79.9
    C-reactive protein R79.82
    drugs — *see* Findings, abnormal, in blood
    gas level R79.81
    minerals R79.0
    pancytopenia D61.818
    PTT R79.1
    specified NEC R79.89
    toxins — *see* Findings, abnormal, in blood
  chest sounds (friction) (rales) R09.89
  chromosome, chromosomal Q99.9
    with more than three X chromosomes, female Q97.1
    analysis result R89.8
      bronchial washings R84.8
      cerebrospinal fluid R83.8
      cervix uteri NEC R87.89
      nasal secretions R84.8
      nipple discharge R89.8
      peritoneal fluid R85.89
      pleural fluid R84.8
      prostatic secretions R86.8
      saliva R85.89
      seminal fluid R86.8
      sputum R84.8
      synovial fluid R89.8
      throat scrapings R84.8
      vagina R87.89
      vulva R87.89
      wound secretions R89.8
    dicentric replacement Q93.2
    ring replacement Q93.2
    sex Q99.8
      female phenotype Q97.9
        specified NEC Q97.8
      male phenotype Q98.9
        specified NEC Q98.8
      structural male Q98.6
    specified NEC Q99.8
  clinical findings NEC R68.89
  coagulation D68.9
    newborn, transient P61.6
    profile R79.1
    time R79.1
  communication — *see* Fistula
  conjunctiva, vascular H11.41- ☑
  coronary artery Q24.5
  cortisol-binding globulin E27.8
  course, eustachian tube Q17.8
  creatinine clearance R94.4
  cytology
    anus R85.619
      atypical squamous cells cannot exclude high grade squamous intraepithelial lesion (ASC-H) R85.611
      atypical squamous cells of undetermined significance (ASC-US) R85.610

Abnormal, abnormality, abnormalities — *continued*
  cytology — *continued*
    anus — *continued*
      cytologic evidence of malignancy R85.614
      high grade squamous intraepithelial lesion (HGSIL) R85.613
      human papillomavirus (HPV) DNA test
        high risk positive R85.81
        low risk postive R85.82
      inadequate smear R85.615
      low grade squamous intraepithelial lesion (LGSIL) R85.612
      satisfactory anal smear but lacking transformation zone R85.616
      specified NEC R85.618
      unsatisfactory smear R85.615
    female genital organs — *see* Abnormal, Papanicolaou (smear)
  dark adaptation curve H53.61
  dentofacial NEC — *see* Anomaly, dentofacial
  development, developmental Q89.9
    central nervous system Q07.9
  diagnostic imaging
    abdomen, abdominal region NEC R93.5
    biliary tract R93.2
    breast R92.8
    central nervous system NEC R90.89
    cerebrovascular NEC R90.89
    coronary circulation R93.1
    digestive tract NEC R93.3
    gastrointestinal (tract) R93.3
    genitourinary organs R93.8
    head R93.0
    heart R93.1
    intrathoracic organ NEC R93.8
    limbs R93.6
    liver R93.2
    lung (field) R91.8
    musculoskeletal system NEC R93.7
    retroperitoneum R93.5
    site specified NEC R93.8
    skin and subcutaneous tissue R93.8
    skull R93.0
    urinary organs R93.4
  direction, teeth, fully erupted M26.30
  ear ossicles, acquired NEC H74.39- ☑
    ankylosis — *see* Ankylosis, ear ossicles
    discontinuity — *see* Discontinuity, ossicles, ear
    partial loss — *see* Loss, ossicles, ear (partial)
  Ebstein Q22.5
  echocardiogram R93.1
  echoencephalogram R90.81
  echogram — *see* Abnormal, diagnostic imaging
  electrocardiogram [ECG] [EKG] R94.31
  electroencephalogram [EEG] R94.01
  electrolyte — *see* Imbalance, electrolyte
  electromyogram [EMG] R94.131
  electro-oculogram [EOG] R94.110
  electrophysiological intracardiac studies R94.39
  electroretinogram [ERG] R94.111
  erythrocytes
    congenital, with perinatal jaundice D58.9
  feces (color) (contents) (mucus) R19.5
  finding — *see* Findings, abnormal, without diagnosis
  fluid
    amniotic — *see* Abnormal, specimen, specified
    cerebrospinal — *see* Abnormal, cerebrospinal fluid
    peritoneal — *see* Abnormal, specimen, digestive organs
    pleural — *see* Abnormal, specimen, respiratory organs
    synovial — *see* Abnormal, specimen, specified
    thorax (bronchial washings) (pleural fluid) — *see* Abnormal, specimen, respiratory organs
    vaginal — *see* Abnormal, specimen, female genital organs
  form
    teeth K00.2
    uterus — *see* Anomaly, uterus
  function studies
    auditory R94.120
    bladder R94.8

Abnormal, abnormality, abnormalities —
   continued
  function studies — *continued*
    brain R94.09
    cardiovascular R94.30
    ear R94.128
    endocrine NEC R94.7
    eye NEC R94.118
    kidney R94.4
    liver R94.5
    nervous system
      central NEC R94.09
      peripheral NEC R94.138
    pancreas R94.8
    placenta R94.8
    pulmonary R94.2
    special senses NEC R94.128
    spleen R94.8
    thyroid R94.6
    vestibular R94.121
  gait — *see* Gait
    hysterical F44.4
  gastrin secretion E16.4
  globulin R77.1
    cortisol-binding E27.8
    thyroid-binding E07.89
  glomerular, minor (*see also* N00-N07 with fourth
    character .0) N05.0
  glucagon secretion E16.3
  glucose tolerance (test) (non-fasting) R73.09
  gravitational (G) forces or states (effect of) T75.81 ☑
  hair (color) (shaft) L67.9
    specified NEC L67.8
  hard tissue formation in pulp (dental) K04.3
  head movement R25.0
  heart
    rate R00.9
      specified NEC R00.8
    shadow R93.1
    sounds NEC R01.2
  hemoglobin (disease) (*see also* Disease, hemoglobin)
    D58.2
    trait — *see* Trait, hemoglobin, abnormal
  histology NEC R89.7
  immunological findings R89.4
    in serum R76.9
      specified NEC R76.8
  increase in appetite R63.2
  involuntary movement — *see* Abnormal, movement,
    involuntary
  jaw closure M26.51
  karyotype R89.8
  kidney function test R94.4
  knee jerk R29.2
  leukocyte (cell) (differential) NEC D72.9
  liver
  loss of
    height R29.890
    weight R63.4
  mammogram NEC R92.8
    calcification (calculus) R92.1
    microcalcification R92.0
  Mantoux test R76.11
  movement (disorder) (*see also* Disorder, movement)
    head R25.0
    involuntary R25.9
      fasciculation R25.3
      of head R25.0
      spasm R25.2
      specified type NEC R25.8
      tremor R25.1
  myoglobin (Aberdeen) (Annapolis) R89.7
  neonatal screening P09
  oculomotor study R94.113
  palmar creases Q82.8
  Papanicolaou (smear)
    anus R85.619
      atypical squamous cells cannot exclude high
        grade squamous intraepithelial lesion
        (ASC-H) R85.611
      atypical squamous cells of undetermined signif-
        icance (ASC-US) R85.610
      cytologic evidence of malignancy R85.614
      high grade squamous intraepithelial lesion
        (HGSIL) R85.613
      human papillomavirus (HPV) DNA test
        high risk positive R85.81
        low risk postive R85.82

Abnormal, abnormality, abnormalities —
   continued
  Papanicolaou — *continued*
    anus — *continued*
      inadequate smear R85.615
      low grade squamous intraepithelial lesion
        (LGSIL) R85.612
      satisfactory anal smear but lacking transforma-
        tion zone R85.616
      specified NEC R85.618
      unsatisfactory smear R85.615
    bronchial washings R84.6
    cerebrospinal fluid R83.6
    cervix R87.619
      atypical squamous cells cannot exclude high
        grade squamous intraepithelial lesion
        (ASC-H) R87.611
      atypical squamous cells of undetermined signif-
        icance (ASC-US) R87.610
      cytologic evidence of malignancy R87.614
      high grade squamous intraepithelial lesion
        (HGSIL) R87.613
      inadequate smear R87.615
      low grade squamous intraepithelial lesion
        (LGSIL) R87.612
      non-atypical endometrial cells R87.618
      satisfactory cervical smear but lacking transfor-
        mation zone R87.616
      specified NEC R87.618
      thin preparaton R87.619
      unsatisfactory smear R87.615
    nasal secretions R84.6
    nipple discharge R89.6
    peritoneal fluid R85.69
    pleural fluid R84.6
    prostatic secretions R86.6
    saliva R85.69
    seminal fluid R86.6
    sites NEC R89.6
    sputum R84.6
    synovial fluid R89.6
    throat scrapings R84.6
    vagina R87.629
      atypical squamous cells cannot exclude high
        grade squamous intraepithelial lesion
        (ASC-H) R87.621
      atypical squamous cells of undetermined signif-
        icance (ASC-US) R87.620
      cytologic evidence of malignancy R87.624
      high grade squamous intraepithelial lesion
        (HGSIL) R87.623
      inadequate smear R87.625
      low grade squamous intraepithelial lesion
        (LGSIL) R87.622
      specified NEC R87.628
      thin preparation R87.629
      unsatisfactory smear R87.625
    vulva R87.69
    wound secretions R89.6
  partial thromboplastin time (PTT) R79.1
  pelvis (bony) — *see* Deformity, pelvis
  percussion, chest (tympany) R09.89
  periods (grossly) — *see* Menstruation
  phonocardiogram R94.39
  plantar reflex R29.2
  plasma
    protein R77.9
      specified NEC R77.8
    viscosity R70.1
  pleural (folds) Q34.0
  posture R29.3
  product of conception O02.9
    specified type NEC O02.89
  prothrombin time (PT) R79.1
  pulmonary
    artery, congenital Q25.79
    function, newborn P28.89
    test results R94.2
  pulsations in neck R00.2
  pupillary H21.56- ☑
    function (reaction) (reflex) — *see* Anomaly, pupil,
      function
  radiological examination — *see* Abnormal, diagnostic
    imaging
  red blood cell(s) (morphology) (volume) R71.8
  reflex — *see* Reflex
  renal function test R94.4
  response to nerve stimulation R94.130

Abnormal, abnormality, abnormalities —
   continued
  retinal correspondence H53.31
  retinal function study R94.111
  rhythm, heart (*see also* Arrhythmia)
  saliva — *see* Abnormal, specimen, digestive organs
  scan
    kidney R94.4
    liver R93.2
    thyroid R94.6
  secretion
    gastrin E16.4
    glucagon E16.3
  semen, seminal fluid — *see* Abnormal, specimen, male
    genital organs
  serum level (of)
    acid phosphatase R74.8
    alkaline phosphatase R74.8
    amylase R74.8
    enzymes R74.9
      specified NEC R74.8
    lipase R74.8
    triacylglycerol lipase R74.8
  shape
    gravid uterus — *see* Anomaly, uterus
  sinus venosus Q21.1
  size, tooth, teeth K00.2
  spacing, tooth, teeth, fully erupted M26.30
  specimen
    digestive organs (peritoneal fluid) (saliva) R85.9
      cytology R85.69
      drug level R85.2
      enzyme level R85.0
      histology R85.7
      hormones R85.1
      immunology R85.4
      microbiology R85.5
      nonmedicinal level R85.3
      specified type NEC R85.89
    female genital organs (secretions) (smears) R87.9
      cytology R87.69
        cervix R87.619
          human papillomavirus (HPV) DNA test
            high risk positive R87.810
            low risk positive R87.820
          inadequate (unsatisfactory) smear
            R87.615
          non-atypical endometrial cells R87.618
          specified NEC R87.618
        vagina R87.629
          human papillomavirus (HPV) DNA test
            high risk positive R87.811
            low risk positive R87.821
          inadequate (unsatisfactory) smear
            R87.625
        vulva R87.69
      drug level R87.2
      enzyme level R87.0
      histological R87.7
      hormones R87.1
      immunology R87.4
      microbiology R87.5
      nonmedicinal level R87.3
      specified type NEC R87.89
    male genital organs (prostatic secretions) (semen)
      R86.9
      cytology R86.6
      drug level R86.2
      enzyme level R86.0
      histological R86.7
      hormones R86.1
      immunology R86.4
      microbiology R86.5
      nonmedicinal level R86.3
      specified type NEC R86.8
    nipple discharge — *see* Abnormal, specimen,
      specified
    respiratory organs (bronchial washings) (nasal se-
      cretions) (pleural fluid) (sputum) R84.9
      cytology R84.6
      drug level R84.2
      enzyme level R84.0
      histology R84.7
      hormones R84.1
      immunology R84.4
      microbiology R84.5
      nonmedicinal level R84.3
      specified type NEC R84.8

Abnormal, abnormality, abnormalities — *continued*
  specimen — *continued*
    specified organ, system and tissue NOS R89.9
      cytology R89.6
      drug level R89.2
      enzyme level R89.0
      histology R89.7
      hormones R89.1
      immunology R89.4
      microbiology R89.5
      nonmedicinal level R89.3
      specified type NEC R89.8
    synovial fluid — *see* Abnormal, specimen, specified
    thorax (bronchial washings) (pleural fluids) — *see* Abnormal, specimen, respiratory organs
    vagina (secretion) (smear) R87.629
    vulva (secretion) (smear) R87.69
    wound secretion — *see* Abnormal, specimen, specified
  spermatozoa — *see* Abnormal, specimen, male genital organs
  sputum (amount) (color) (odor) R09.3
  stool (color) (contents) (mucus) R19.5
    bloody K92.1
    guaiac positive R19.5
  synchondrosis Q78.8
  thermography (*see also* Abnormal, diagnostic imaging) R93.8
  thyroid-binding globulin E07.89
  tooth, teeth (form) (size) K00.2
  toxicology (findings) R78.9
  transport protein E88.09
  tumor marker NEC R97.8
  ultrasound results — *see* Abnormal, diagnostic imaging
  umbilical cord complicating delivery O69.9 ☑
  urination NEC R39.19
  urine (constituents) R82.90
    bile R82.2
    cytological examination R82.8
    drugs R82.5
    fat R82.0
    glucose R81
    heavy metals R82.6
    hemoglobin R82.3
    histological examination R82.8
    ketones R82.4
    microbiological examination (culture) R82.7
    myoglobin R82.1
    positive culture R82.7
    protein — *see* Proteinuria
    specified substance NEC R82.99
      chromoabnormality NEC R82.91
    substances nonmedical R82.6
  uterine hemorrhage — *see* Hemorrhage, uterus
  vectorcardiogram R94.39
  visually evoked potential (VEP) R94.112
  white blood cells D72.9
    specified NEC D72.89
  X-ray examination — *see* Abnormal, diagnostic imaging
Abnormity (any organ or part) — *see* Anomaly
Abocclusion M26.29
  hemolytic disease (newborn) P55.1
  incompatibility reaction ABO — *see* Complication(s), transfusion, incompatibility reaction, ABO
Abolition, language R48.8
Aborter, habitual or recurrent — *see* Loss (of), pregnancy, recurrent
Abortion (complete) (spontaneous) O03.9
  with
    retained products of conception — *see* Abortion, incomplete
  attempted (elective) (failed) O07.4
    complicated by O07.30
      afibrinogenemia O07.1
      cardiac arrest O07.36
      chemical damage of pelvic organ(s) O07.34
      circulatory collapse O07.31
      cystitis O07.38
      defibrination syndrome O07.1
      electrolyte imbalance O07.33
      embolism (air) (amniotic fluid) (blood clot) (fat) (pulmonary) (septic) (soap) O07.2
      endometritis O07.0
      genital tract and pelvic infection O07.0
      hemolysis O07.1

Abortion — *continued*
  attempted — *continued*
    complicated by — *continued*
      hemorrhage (delayed) (excessive) O07.1
      infection
        genital tract or pelvic O07.0
        urinary tract tract O07.38
      intravascular coagulation O07.1
      laceration of pelvic organ(s) O07.34
      metabolic disorder O07.33
      oliguria O07.32
      oophoritis O07.0
      parametritis O07.0
      pelvic peritonitis O07.0
      perforation of pelvic organ(s) O07.34
      renal failure or shutdown O07.32
      salpingitis or salpingo-oophoritis O07.0
      sepsis O07.37
      shock O07.31
      specified condition NEC O07.39
      tubular necrosis (renal) O07.32
      uremia O07.32
      urinary tract infection O07.38
      venous complication NEC O07.35
        embolism (air) (amniotic fluid) (blood clot) (fat) (pulmonary) (septic) (soap) O07.2
  complicated (by) (following) O03.80
    afibrinogenemia O03.6
    cardiac arrest O03.86
    chemical damage of pelvic organ(s) O03.84
    circulatory collapse O03.81
    cystitis O03.88
    defibrination syndrome O03.6
    electrolyte imbalance O03.83
    embolism (air) (amniotic fluid) (blood clot) (fat) (pulmonary) (septic) (soap) O03.7
    endometritis O03.5
    genital tract and pelvic infection O03.5
    hemolysis O03.6
    hemorrhage (delayed) (excessive) O03.6
    infection
      genital tract or pelvic O03.5
      urinary tract O03.88
    intravascular coagulation O03.6
    laceration of pelvic organ(s) O03.84
    metabolic disorder O03.83
    oliguria O03.82
    oophoritis O03.5
    parametritis O03.5
    pelvic peritonitis O03.5
    perforation of pelvic organ(s) O03.84
    renal failure or shutdown O03.82
    salpingitis or salpingo-oophoritis O03.5
    sepsis O03.87
    shock O03.81
    specified condition NEC O03.89
    tubular necrosis (renal) O03.82
    uremia O03.82
    urinary tract infection O03.88
    venous complication NEC O03.85
      embolism (air) (amniotic fluid) (blood clot) (fat) (pulmonary) (septic) (soap) O03.7
  failed — *see* Abortion, attempted
  habitual or recurrent N96
    with current abortion — *see* categories O03-O06
    without current pregnancy N96
    care in current pregnancy O26.2- ☑
  incomplete (spontaneous) O03.4
    complicated (by) (following) O03.30
      afibrinogenemia O03.1
      cardiac arrest O03.36
      chemical damage of pelvic organ(s) O03.34
      circulatory collapse O03.31
      cystitis O03.38
      defibrination syndrome O03.1
      electrolyte imbalance O03.33
      embolism (air) (amniotic fluid) (blood clot) (fat) (pulmonary) (septic) (soap) O03.2
      endometritis O03.0
      genital tract and pelvic infection O03.0
      hemolysis O03.1
      hemorrhage (delayed) (excessive) O03.1
      infection
        genital tract or pelvic O03.0
        urinary tract O03.38
      intravascular coagulation O03.1
      laceration of pelvic organ(s) O03.34
      metabolic disorder O03.33

Abortion — *continued*
  incomplete — *continued*
    complicated — *continued*
      oliguria O03.32
      oophoritis O03.0
      parametritis O03.0
      pelvic peritonitis O03.0
      perforation of pelvic organ(s) O03.34
      renal failure or shutdown O03.32
      salpingitis or salpingo-oophoritis O03.0
      sepsis O03.37
      shock O03.31
      specified condition NEC O03.39
      tubular necrosis (renal) O03.32
      uremia O03.32
      urinary infection O03.38
      venous complication NEC O03.35
        embolism (air) (amniotic fluid) (blood clot) (fat) (pulmonary) (septic) (soap) O03.2
  induced (encounter for) Z33.2
    complicated by O04.80
      afibrinogenemia O04.6
      cardiac arrest O04.86
      chemical damage of pelvic organ(s) O04.84
      circulatory collapse O04.81
      cystitis O04.88
      defibrination syndrome O04.6
      electrolyte imbalance O04.83
      embolism (air) (amniotic fluid) (blood clot) (fat) (pulmonary) (septic) (soap) O04.7
      endometritis O04.5
      genital tract and pelvic infection O04.5
      hemolysis O04.6
      hemorrhage (delayed) (excessive) O04.6
      infection
        genital tract or pelvic O04.5
        urinary tract O04.88
      intravascular coagulation O04.6
      laceration of pelvic organ(s) O04.84
      metabolic disorder O04.83
      oliguria O04.82
      oophoritis O04.5
      parametritis O04.5
      pelvic peritonitis O04.5
      perforation of pelvic organ(s) O04.84
      renal failure or shutdown O04.82
      salpingitis or salpingo-oophoritis O04.5
      sepsis O04.87
      shock O04.81
      specified condition NEC O04.89
      tubular necrosis (renal) O04.82
      uremia O04.82
      urinary tract infection O04.88
      venous complication NEC O04.85
        embolism (air) (amniotic fluid) (blood clot) (fat) (pulmonary) (septic) (soap) O04.7
  missed O02.1
  spontaneous — *see* Abortion (complete) (spontaneous)
    threatened O20.0
  threatened (spontaneous) O20.0
  tubal O00.1
Abortus fever A23.1
Aboulomania F60.7
Abrami's disease D59.8
Abramov-Fiedler myocarditis (acute isolated myocarditis) I40.1
Abrasion T14.8
  abdomen, abdominal (wall) S30.811 ☑
  alveolar process S00.512 ☑
  ankle S90.51- ☑
  antecubital space — *see* Abrasion, elbow
  anus S30.817 ☑
  arm (upper) S40.81- ☑
  auditory canal — *see* Abrasion, ear
  auricle — *see* Abrasion, ear
  axilla — *see* Abrasion, arm
  back, lower S30.810 ☑
  breast S20.11- ☑
  brow S00.81 ☑
  buttock S30.810 ☑
  calf — *see* Abrasion, leg
  canthus — *see* Abrasion, eyelid
  cheek S00.81 ☑
    internal S00.512 ☑
  chest wall — *see* Abrasion, thorax
  chin S00.81 ☑
  clitoris S30.814 ☑

Abrasion — *continued*
- cornea S05.0- ☑
- costal region — *see* Abrasion, thorax
- dental K03.1
- digit(s)
  - foot — *see* Abrasion, toe
  - hand — *see* Abrasion, finger
- ear S00.41- ☑
- elbow S50.31- ☑
- epididymis S30.813 ☑
- epigastric region S30.811 ☑
- epiglottis S10.11 ☑
- esophagus (thoracic) S27.818 ☑
  - cervical S10.11 ☑
- eyebrow — *see* Abrasion, eyelid
- eyelid S00.21- ☑
- face S00.81 ☑
- finger(s) S60.41- ☑
  - index S60.41- ☑
  - little S60.41- ☑
  - middle S60.41- ☑
  - ring S60.41- ☑
- flank S30.811 ☑
- foot (except toe(s) alone) S90.81- ☑
  - toe — *see* Abrasion, toe
- forearm S50.81- ☑
  - elbow only — *see* Abrasion, elbow
- forehead S00.81 ☑
- genital organs, external
  - female S30.816 ☑
  - male S30.815 ☑
- groin S30.811 ☑
- gum S00.512 ☑
- hand S60.51- ☑
- head S00.91 ☑
  - ear — *see* Abrasion, ear
  - eyelid — *see* Abrasion, eyelid
  - lip S00.511 ☑
  - nose S00.31 ☑
  - oral cavity S00.512 ☑
  - scalp S00.01 ☑
  - specified site NEC S00.81 ☑
- heel — *see* Abrasion, foot
- hip S70.21- ☑
- inguinal region S30.811 ☑
- interscapular region S20.419 ☑
- jaw S00.81 ☑
- knee S80.21- ☑
- labium (majus) (minus) S30.814 ☑
- larynx S10.11 ☑
- leg (lower) S80.81- ☑
  - knee — *see* Abrasion, knee
  - upper — *see* Abrasion, thigh
- lip S00.511 ☑
- lower back S30.810 ☑
- lumbar region S30.810 ☑
- malar region S00.81 ☑
- mammary — *see* Abrasion, breast
- mastoid region S00.81 ☑
- mouth S00.512 ☑
- nail
  - finger — *see* Abrasion, finger
  - toe — *see* Abrasion, toe
- nape S10.81 ☑
- nasal S00.31 ☑
- neck S10.91 ☑
  - specified site NEC S10.81 ☑
  - throat S10.11 ☑
- nose S00.31 ☑
- occipital region S00.01 ☑
- oral cavity S00.512 ☑
- orbital region — *see* Abrasion, eyelid
- palate S00.512 ☑
- palm — *see* Abrasion, hand
- parietal region S00.01 ☑
- pelvis S30.810 ☑
- penis S30.812 ☑
- perineum
  - female S30.814 ☑
  - male S30.810 ☑
- periocular area — *see* Abrasion, eyelid
- phalanges
  - finger — *see* Abrasion, finger
  - toe — *see* Abrasion, toe
- pharynx S10.11 ☑
- pinna — *see* Abrasion, ear

Abrasion — *continued*
- popliteal space — *see* Abrasion, knee
- prepuce S30.812 ☑
- pubic region S30.810 ☑
- pudendum
  - female S30.816 ☑
  - male S30.815 ☑
- sacral region S30.810 ☑
- scalp S00.01 ☑
- scapular region — *see* Abrasion, shoulder
- scrotum S30.813 ☑
- shin — *see* Abrasion, leg
- shoulder S40.21- ☑
- skin NEC T14.8
- sternal region S20.319 ☑
- submaxillary region S00.81 ☑
- submental region S00.81 ☑
- subungual
  - finger(s) — *see* Abrasion, finger
  - toe(s) — *see* Abrasion, toe
- supraclavicular fossa S10.81 ☑
- supraorbital S00.81 ☑
- temple S00.81 ☑
- temporal region S00.81 ☑
- testis S30.813 ☑
- thigh S70.31- ☑
- thorax, thoracic (wall) S20.91 ☑
  - back S20.41- ☑
  - front S20.31- ☑
- throat S10.11 ☑
- thumb S60.31- ☑
- toe(s) (lesser) S90.416 ☑
  - great S90.41- ☑
- tongue S00.512 ☑
- tooth, teeth (dentifrice) (habitual) (hard tissues) (occupational) (ritual) (traditional) K03.1
- trachea S10.11 ☑
- tunica vaginalis S30.813 ☑
- tympanum, tympanic membrane — *see* Abrasion, ear
- uvula S00.512 ☑
- vagina S30.814 ☑
- vocal cords S10.11 ☑
- vulva S30.814 ☑
- wrist S60.81- ☑

Abrism — *see* Poisoning, food, noxious, plant

Abruptio placentae O45.9- ☑
- with
  - afibrinogenemia O45.01- ☑
  - coagulation defect O45.00- ☑
    - specified NEC O45.09- ☑
  - disseminated intravascular coagulation O45.02- ☑
  - hypofibrinogenemia O45.01- ☑
- specified NEC O45.8- ☑

Abruption, placenta — *see* Abruptio placentae

Abscess (connective tissue) (embolic) (fistulous) (infective) (metastatic) (multiple) (pernicious) (pyogenic) (septic) L02.91
- with
  - diverticular disease (intestine) K57.80
    - with bleeding K57.81
    - large intestine K57.20
      - with
        - bleeding K57.21
        - small intestine K57.40
          - with bleeding K57.41
    - small intestine K57.00
      - with
        - bleeding K57.01
        - large intestine K57.40
          - with bleeding K57.41
  - lymphangitis — *code by* site under Abscess
- abdomen, abdominal
  - cavity K65.1
  - wall L02.211
- abdominopelvic K65.1
- accessory sinus — *see* Sinusitis
- adrenal (capsule) (gland) E27.8
- alveolar K04.7
  - with sinus K04.6
- amebic A06.4
  - brain (and liver or lung abscess) A06.6
  - genitourinary tract A06.82
  - liver (without mention of brain or lung abscess) A06.4
  - lung (and liver) (without mention of brain abscess) A06.5
  - specified site NEC A06.89

Abscess — *continued*
- amebic — *continued*
  - spleen A06.89
- anerobic A48.0
- ankle — *see* Abscess, lower limb
- anorectal K61.2
- antecubital space — *see* Abscess, upper limb
- antrum (chronic) (Highmore) — *see* Sinusitis, maxillary
- anus K61.0
- apical (tooth) K04.7
  - with sinus (alveolar) K04.6
- appendix K35.3
- areola (acute) (chronic) (nonpuerperal) N61
  - puerperal, postpartum or gestational — *see* Infection, nipple
- arm (any part) — *see* Abscess, upper limb
- artery (wall) I77.89
- atheromatous I77.2
- auricle, ear — *see* Abscess, ear, external
- axilla (region) L02.41- ☑
  - lymph gland or node L04.2
- back (any part, except buttock) L02.212
- Bartholin's gland N75.1
  - with
    - abortion — *see* Abortion, by type complicated by, sepsis
    - ectopic or molar pregnancy O08.0
  - following ectopic or molar pregnancy O08.0
- Bezold's — *see* Mastoiditis, acute
- bilharziasis B65.1
- bladder (wall) — *see* Cystitis, specified type NEC
- bone (subperiosteal) (*see also* Osteomyelitis, specified type NEC)
  - accessory sinus (chronic) — *see* Sinusitis
  - chronic or old — *see* Osteomyelitis, chronic
  - jaw (lower) (upper) M27.2
  - mastoid — *see* Mastoiditis, acute, subperiosteal
  - petrous — *see* Petrositis
  - spinal (tuberculous) A18.01
    - nontuberculous — *see* Osteomyelitis, vertebra
- bowel K63.0
- brain (any part) (cystic) (otogenic) G06.0
  - amebic (with abscess of any other site) A06.6
  - gonococcal A54.82
  - pheomycotic (chromomycotic) B43.1
  - tuberculous A17.81
- breast (acute) (chronic) (nonpuerperal) N61
  - newborn P39.0
  - puerperal, postpartum, gestational — *see* Mastitis, obstetric, purulent
- broad ligament N73.2
  - acute N73.0
  - chronic N73.1
- Brodie's (localized) (chronic) M86.8X- ☑
- bronchi J98.09
- buccal cavity K12.2
- bulbourethral gland N34.0
- bursa M71.00
  - ankle M71.07- ☑
  - elbow M71.02- ☑
  - foot M71.07- ☑
  - hand M71.04- ☑
  - hip M71.05- ☑
  - knee M71.06- ☑
  - multiple sites M71.09
  - pharyngeal J39.1
  - shoulder M71.01- ☑
  - specified site NEC M71.08
  - wrist M71.03- ☑
- buttock L02.31
- canthus — *see* Blepharoconjunctivitis
- cartilage — *see* Disorder, cartilage, specified type NEC
- cecum K35.3
- cerebellum, cerebellar G06.0
  - sequelae G09
- cerebral (embolic) G06.0
  - sequelae G09
- cervical (meaning neck) L02.11
  - lymph gland or node L04.0
- cervix (stump) (uteri) — *see* Cervicitis
- cheek (external) L02.01
  - inner K12.2
- chest J86.9
  - with fistula J86.0
  - wall L02.213
- chin L02.01
- choroid — *see* Inflammation, chorioretinal

☑ Additional Character Required — Refer to the Tabular List for Character Selection   ▽ Subterms under main terms may continue to next column or page

Abscess — *continued*
- circumtonsillar J36
- cold (lung) (tuberculous) (*see also* Tuberculosis, abscess, lung)
  - articular — *see* Tuberculosis, joint
- colon (wall) K63.0
- colostomy K94.02
- conjunctiva — *see* Conjunctivitis, acute
- cornea H16.31- ☑
- corpus
  - cavernosum N48.21
  - luteum — *see* Oophoritis
- Cowper's gland N34.0
- cranium G06.0
- cul-de-sac (Douglas') (posterior) — *see* Peritonitis, pelvic, female
- cutaneous — *see* Abscess, by site
- dental K04.7
  - with sinus (alveolar) K04.6
- dentoalveolar K04.7
  - with sinus K04.6
- diaphragm, diaphragmatic K65.1
- Douglas' cul-de-sac or pouch — *see* Peritonitis, pelvic, female
- Dubois A50.59
- ear (middle) (*see also* Otitis, media, suppurative)
  - acute — *see* Otitis, media, suppurative, acute
  - external H60.0- ☑
- entamebic — *see* Abscess, amebic
- enterostomy K94.12
- epididymis N45.4
- epidural G06.2
  - brain G06.0
  - spinal cord G06.1
- epiglottis J38.7
- epiploon, epiploic K65.1
- erysipelatous — *see* Erysipelas
- esophagus K20.8
- ethmoid (bone) (chronic) (sinus) J32.2
- external auditory canal — *see* Abscess, ear, external
- extradural G06.2
  - brain G06.0
    - sequelae G09
  - spinal cord G06.1
- extraperitoneal K68.19
- eye — *see* Endophthalmitis, purulent
- eyelid H00.03- ☑
- face (any part, except ear, eye and nose) L02.01
- fallopian tube — *see* Salpingitis
- fascia M72.8
- fauces J39.1
- fecal K63.0
- femoral (region) — *see* Abscess, lower limb
- filaria, filarial — *see* Infestation, filarial
- finger (any) (*see also* Abscess, hand)
  - nail — *see* Cellulitis, finger
- foot L02.61- ☑
- forehead L02.01
- frontal sinus (chronic) J32.1
- gallbladder K81.0
- genital organ or tract
  - female (external) N76.4
  - male N49.9
    - multiple sites N49.8
    - specified NEC N49.8
- gestational mammary O91.11- ☑
- gestational subareolar O91.11- ☑
- gingival K05.21
- gland, glandular (lymph) (acute) — *see* Lymphadenitis, acute
- gluteal (region) L02.31
- gonorrheal — *see* Gonococcus
- groin L02.214
- gum K05.21
- hand L02.51- ☑
- head NEC L02.811
  - face (any part, except ear, eye and nose) L02.01
- heart — *see* Carditis
- heel — *see* Abscess, foot
- helminthic — *see* Infestation, helminth
- hepatic (cholangitic) (hematogenic) (lymphogenic) (pylephlebitic) K75.0
  - amebic A06.4
- hip (region) — *see* Abscess, lower limb
- ileocecal K35.3
- ileostomy (bud) K94.12

Abscess — *continued*
- iliac (region) L02.214
  - fossa K35.3
- infraclavicular (fossa) — *see* Abscess, upper limb
- inguinal (region) L02.214
  - lymph gland or node L04.1
- intestine, intestinal NEC K63.0
  - rectal K61.1
- intra-abdominal (*see also* Abscess, peritoneum) K65.1
  - postoperative T81.4 ☑
  - retroperitoneal K68.11
- intracranial G06.0
- intramammary — *see* Abscess, breast
- intraorbital — *see* Abscess, orbit
- intraperitoneal K65.1
- intrasphincteric (anus) K61.4
- intraspinal G06.1
- intratonsillar J36
- ischiorectal (fossa) K61.3
- jaw (bone) (lower) (upper) M27.2
- joint — *see* Arthritis, pyogenic or pyemic
  - spine (tuberculous) A18.01
    - nontuberculous — *see* Spondylopathy, infective
- kidney N15.1
  - with calculus N20.0
    - with hydronephrosis N13.6
  - puerperal (postpartum) O86.21
- knee (*see also* Abscess, lower limb)
  - joint M00.9
- labium (majus) (minus) N76.4
- lacrimal
  - caruncle — *see* Inflammation, lacrimal, passages, acute
  - gland — *see* Dacryoadenitis
  - passages (duct) (sac) — *see* Inflammation, lacrimal, passages, acute
- lacunar N34.0
- larynx J38.7
- lateral (alveolar) K04.7
  - with sinus K04.6
- leg (any part) — *see* Abscess, lower limb
- lens H27.8
- lingual K14.0
  - tonsil J36
- lip K13.0
- Littre's gland N34.0
- liver (cholangitic) (hematogenic) (lymphogenic) (pylephlebitic) (pyogenic) K75.0
  - amebic (due to Entamoeba histolytica) (dysenteric) (tropical) A06.4
    - with
      - brain abscess (and liver or lung abscess) A06.6
      - lung abscess A06.5
- loin (region) L02.211
- lower limb L02.41- ☑
- lumbar (tuberculous) A18.01
  - nontuberculous L02.212
- lung (miliary) (putrid) J85.2
  - with pneumonia J85.1
    - due to specified organism (*see* Pneumonia, in (due to))
  - amebic (with liver abscess) A06.5
    - with
      - brain abscess A06.6
      - pneumonia A06.5
- lymph, lymphatic, gland or node (acute) (*see also* Lymphadenitis, acute)
  - mesentery I88.0
- malar M27.2
- mammary gland — *see* Abscess, breast
- marginal, anus K61.0
- mastoid — *see* Mastoiditis, acute
- maxilla, maxillary M27.2
  - molar (tooth) K04.7
    - with sinus K04.6
  - premolar K04.7
  - sinus (chronic) J32.0
- mediastinum J85.3
- meibomian gland — *see* Hordeolum
- meninges G06.2
- mesentery, mesenteric K65.1
- mesosalpinx — *see* Salpingitis
- mons pubis L02.215
- mouth (floor) K12.2
- muscle — *see* Myositis, infective
- myocardium I40.0

Abscess — *continued*
- nabothian (follicle) — *see* Cervicitis
- nasal J32.9
- nasopharyngeal J39.1
- navel L02.216
  - newborn P38.9
    - with mild hemorrhage P38.1
    - without hemorrhage P38.9
- neck (region) L02.11
  - lymph gland or node L04.0
- nephritic — *see* Abscess, kidney
- nipple N61
  - associated with
    - lactation — *see* Pregnancy, complicated by, pregnancy — *see* Pregnancy, complicated by
- nose (external) (fossa) (septum) J34.0
  - sinus (chronic) — *see* Sinusitis
- omentum K65.1
- operative wound T81.4 ☑
- orbit, orbital — *see* Cellulitis, orbit
- otogenic G06.0
- ovary, ovarian (corpus luteum) — *see* Oophoritis
- oviduct — *see* Oophoritis
- palate (soft) K12.2
  - hard M27.2
- palmar (space) — *see* Abscess, hand
- pancreas (duct) — *see* Pancreatitis, acute
- parafrenal N48.21
- parametric, parametrium N73.2
  - acute N73.0
  - chronic N73.1
- paranephric N15.1
- parapancreatic — *see* Pancreatitis, acute
- parapharyngeal J39.0
- pararectal K61.1
- parasinus — *see* Sinusitis
- parauterine (*see also* Disease, pelvis, inflammatory) N73.2
- paravaginal — *see* Vaginitis
- parietal region (scalp) L02.811
- parodontal K05.21
- parotid (duct) (gland) K11.3
  - region K12.2
- pectoral (region) L02.213
- pelvis, pelvic
  - female — *see* Disease, pelvis, inflammatory
  - male, peritoneal K65.1
- penis N48.21
  - gonococcal (accessory gland) (periurethral) A54.1
- perianal K61.0
- periapical K04.7
  - with sinus (alveolar) K04.6
- periappendicular K35.3
- pericardial I30.1
- pericecal K35.3
- pericemental K05.21
- pericholecystic — *see* Cholecystitis, acute
- pericoronal K05.21
- peridental K05.21
- perimetric (*see also* Disease, pelvis, inflammatory) N73.2
- perinephric, perinephritic — *see* Abscess, kidney
- perineum, perineal (superficial) L02.215
  - urethra N34.0
- periodontal (parietal) K05.21
  - apical K04.7
- periosteum, periosteal (*see also* Osteomyelitis, specified type NEC)
  - with osteomyelitis (*see also* Osteomyelitis, specified type NEC)
    - acute — *see* Osteomyelitis, acute
    - chronic — *see* Osteomyelitis, chronic
- peripharyngeal J39.0
- peripleuritic J86.9
  - with fistula J86.0
- periprostatic N41.2
- perirectal K61.1
- perirenal (tissue) — *see* Abscess, kidney
- perisinuous (nose) — *see* Sinusitis
- peritoneum, peritoneal (perforated) (ruptured) K65.1
  - with appendicitis K35.3
  - pelvic
    - female — *see* Peritonitis, pelvic, female
    - male K65.1
  - postoperative T81.4 ☑
  - puerperal, postpartum, childbirth O85
  - tuberculous A18.31
- peritonsillar J36

Index

Abscess — *continued*
perityphlic K35.3
periureteral N28.89
periurethral N34.0
   gonococcal (accessory gland) (periurethral) A54.1
periuterine (*see also* Disease, pelvis, inflammatory)
   N73.2
perivesical — *see* Cystitis, specified type NEC
petrous bone — *see* Petrositis
phagedenic NOS L02.91
   chancroid A57
pharynx, pharyngeal (lateral) J39.1
pilonidal L05.01
pituitary (gland) E23.6
pleura J86.9
   with fistula J86.0
popliteal — *see* Abscess, lower limb
postcecal K35.3
postlaryngeal J38.7
postnasal J34.0
postoperative (any site) T81.4 ☑
   retroperitoneal K68.11
postpharyngeal J39.0
posttonsillar J36
post-typhoid A01.09
pouch of Douglas — *see* Peritonitis, pelvic, female
premammary — *see* Abscess, breast
prepatellar — *see* Abscess, lower limb
prostate N41.2
   gonococcal (acute) (chronic) A54.22
psoas muscle K68.12
puerperal — *code by* site under Puerperal, abscess
pulmonary — *see* Abscess, lung
pulp, pulpal (dental) K04.0
rectovaginal septum K63.0
rectovesical — *see* Cystitis, specified type NEC
rectum K61.1
renal — *see* Abscess, kidney
retina — *see* Inflammation, chorioretinal
retrobulbar — *see* Abscess, orbit
retrocecal K65.1
retrolaryngeal J38.7
retromammary — *see* Abscess, breast
retroperitoneal NEC K68.19
   postprocedural K68.11
retropharyngeal J39.0
retrouterine — *see* Peritonitis, pelvic, female
retrovesical — *see* Cystitis, specified type NEC
root, tooth K04.7
   with sinus (alveolar) K04.6
round ligament (*see also* Disease, pelvis, inflammatory)
   N73.2
rupture (spontaneous) NOS L02.91
sacrum (tuberculous) A18.01
   nontuberculous M46.28
salivary (duct) (gland) K11.3
scalp (any part) L02.811
scapular — *see* Osteomyelitis, specified type NEC
sclera — *see* Scleritis
scrofulous (tuberculous) A18.2
scrotum N49.2
seminal vesicle N49.0
septal, dental K04.7
   with sinus (alveolar) K04.6
serous — *see* Periostitis
shoulder (region) — *see* Abscess, upper limb
sigmoid K63.0
sinus (accessory) (chronic) (nasal) (*see also* Sinusitis)
   intracranial venous (any) G06.0
Skene's duct or gland N34.0
skin — *see* Abscess, by site
specified site NEC L02.818
spermatic cord N49.1
sphenoidal (sinus) (chronic) J32.3
spinal cord (any part) (staphylococcal) G06.1
   tuberculous A17.81
spine (column) (tuberculous) A18.01
   epidural G06.1
   nontuberculous — *see* Osteomyelitis, vertebra
spleen D73.3
   amebic A06.89
stitch T81.4 ☑
subarachnoid G06.2
   brain G06.0
   spinal cord G06.1
subareolar — *see* Abscess, breast
subcecal K35.3

Abscess — *continued*
subcutaneous (*see also* Abscess, by site)
   pheomycotic (chromomycotic) B43.2
subdiaphragmatic K65.1
subdural G06.2
   brain G06.0
     sequelae G09
   spinal cord G06.1
subgaleal L02.811
subhepatic K65.1
sublingual K12.2
   gland K11.3
submammary — *see* Abscess, breast
submandibular (region) (space) (triangle) K12.2
   gland K11.3
submaxillary (region) L02.01
   gland K11.3
submental L02.01
   gland K11.3
subperiosteal — *see* Osteomyelitis, specified type
   NEC
subphrenic K65.1
   postoperative T81.4 ☑
suburethral N34.0
sudoriparous L75.8
supraclavicular (fossa) — *see* Abscess, upper limb
suprapelvic, acute N73.0
suprarenal (capsule) (gland) E27.8
sweat gland L74.8
tear duct — *see* Inflammation, lacrimal, passages,
   acute
temple L02.01
temporal region L02.01
temporosphenoidal G06.0
tendon (sheath) M65.00
   ankle M65.07- ☑
   foot M65.07- ☑
   forearm M65.03- ☑
   hand M65.04- ☑
   lower leg M65.06- ☑
   pelvic region M65.05- ☑
   shoulder region M65.01- ☑
   specified site NEC M65.08
   thigh M65.05- ☑
   upper arm M65.02- ☑
testis N45.4
thigh — *see* Abscess, lower limb
thorax J86.9
   with fistula J86.0
throat J39.1
thumb (*see also* Abscess, hand)
   nail — *see* Cellulitis, finger
thymus (gland) E32.1
thyroid (gland) E06.0
toe (any) (*see also* Abscess, foot)
   nail — *see* Cellulitis, toe
tongue (staphylococcal) K14.0
tonsil(s) (lingual) J36
tonsillopharyngeal J36
tooth, teeth (root) K04.7
   with sinus (alveolar) K04.6
   supporting structures NEC K05.21
trachea J39.8
trunk L02.219
   abdominal wall L02.211
   back L02.212
   chest wall L02.213
   groin L02.214
   perineum L02.215
   umbilicus L02.216
tubal — *see* Salpingitis
tuberculous — *see* Tuberculosis, abscess
tubo-ovarian — *see* Salpingo-oophoritis
tunica vaginalis N49.1
umbilicus L02.216
upper
   limb L02.41- ☑
   respiratory J39.8
urethral (gland) N34.0
urinary N34.0
uterus, uterine (wall) (*see also* Endometritis)
   ligament (*see also* Disease, pelvis, inflammatory)
     N73.2
   neck — *see* Cervicitis
uvula K12.2
vagina (wall) — *see* Vaginitis
vaginorectal — *see* Vaginitis

Abscess — *continued*
vas deferens N49.1
vermiform appendix K35.3
vertebra (column) (tuberculous) A18.01
   nontuberculous — *see* Osteomyelitis, vertebra
vesical — *see* Cystitis, specified type NEC
vesico-uterine pouch — *see* Peritonitis, pelvic, female
vitreous (humor) — *see* Endophthalmitis, purulent
vocal cord J38.3
von Bezold's — *see* Mastoiditis, acute
vulva N76.4
vulvovaginal gland N75.1
web space — *see* Abscess, hand
wound T81.4 ☑
wrist — *see* Abscess, upper limb
Absence (of) (organ or part) (complete or partial)
adrenal (gland) (congenital) Q89.1
   acquired E89.6
albumin in blood E88.09
alimentary tract (congenital) Q45.8
   upper Q40.8
alveolar process (acquired) — *see* Anomaly, alveolar
ankle (acquired) Z89.44- ☑
anus (congenital) Q42.3
   with fistula Q42.2
aorta (congenital) Q25.4
appendix, congenital Q42.8
arm (acquired) Z89.20- ☑
   above elbow Z89.22- ☑
     congenital (with hand present) — *see* Agenesis,
       arm, with hand present
       and hand — *see* Agenesis, forearm, and
         hand
     below elbow Z89.21- ☑
       congenital (with hand present) — *see* Agenesis,
        arm, with hand present
       and hand — *see* Agenesis, forearm, and
         hand
   congenital — *see* Defect, reduction, upper limb
   shoulder (following explantation of shoulder joint
     prosthesis) (joint) (with or without presence
     of antibiotic-impregnated cement spacer)
     Z89.23- ☑
   congenital (with hand present) — *see* Agenesis,
     arm, with hand present
artery (congenital) (peripheral) Q27.8
   brain Q28.3
   coronary Q24.5
   pulmonary Q25.79
   specified NEC Q27.8
   umbilical Q27.0
atrial septum (congenital) Q21.1
auditory canal (congenital) (external) Q16.1
auricle (ear), congenital Q16.0
bile, biliary duct, congenital Q44.5
bladder (acquired) Z90.6
   congenital Q64.5
bowel sounds R19.11
brain Q00.0
   part of Q04.3
breast(s) (and nipple(s)) (acquired) Z90.1- ☑
   congenital Q83.8
broad ligament Q50.6
bronchus (congenital) Q32.4
canaliculus lacrimalis, congenital Q10.4
cerebellum (vermis) Q04.3
cervix (acquired) (with uterus) Z90.710
   with remaining uterus Z90.712
   congenital Q51.5
chin, congenital Q18.8
cilia (congenital) Q10.3
   acquired — *see* Madarosis
clitoris (congenital) Q52.6
coccyx, congenital Q76.49
cold sense R20.8
congenital
   lumen — *see* Atresia
   organ or site NEC — *see* Agenesis
   septum — *see* Imperfect, closure
corpus callosum Q04.0
cricoid cartilage, congenital Q31.8
diaphragm (with hernia), congenital Q79.1
digestive organ(s) or tract, congenital Q45.8
   acquired NEC Z90.49
   upper Q40.8
ductus arteriosus Q28.8
duodenum (acquired) Z90.49
   congenital Q41.0

Absence — *continued*
- ear, congenital Q16.9
  - acquired H93.8- ☑
  - auricle Q16.0
  - external Q16.0
  - inner Q16.5
  - lobe, lobule Q17.8
  - middle, except ossicles Q16.4
    - ossicles Q16.3
  - ossicles Q16.3
- ejaculatory duct (congenital) Q55.4
- endocrine gland (congenital) NEC Q89.2
  - acquired E89.89
- epididymis (congenital) Q55.4
  - acquired Z90.79
- epiglottis, congenital Q31.8
- esophagus (congenital) Q39.8
  - acquired (partial) Z90.49
- eustachian tube (congenital) Q16.2
- extremity (acquired) Z89.9
  - congenital Q73.0
  - knee (following explantation of knee joint prosthesis) (joint) (with or without presence of antibiotic-impregnated cement spacer) Z89.52- ☑
  - lower (above knee) Z89.619
    - below knee Z89.51-
  - upper — *see* Absence, arm
- eye (acquired) Z90.01
  - congenital Q11.1
  - muscle (congenital) Q10.3
- eyeball (acquired) Z90.01
- eyelid (fold) (congenital) Q10.3
  - acquired Z90.01
- face, specified part NEC Q18.8
- fallopian tube(s) (acquired) Z90.79
  - congenital Q50.6
- family member (causing problem in home) NEC (*see also* Disruption, family) Z63.32
- femur, congenital — *see* Defect, reduction, lower limb, longitudinal, femur
- fibrinogen (congenital) D68.2
  - acquired D65
- finger(s) (acquired) Z89.02- ☑
  - congenital — *see* Agenesis, hand
- foot (acquired) Z89.43- ☑
  - congenital — *see* Agenesis, foot
- forearm (acquired) — *see* Absence, arm, below elbow
- gallbladder (acquired) Z90.49
  - congenital Q44.0
- gamma globulin in blood D80.1
  - hereditary D80.0
- genital organs
  - acquired (female) (male) Z90.79
  - female, congenital Q52.8
    - external Q52.71
    - internal NEC Q52.8
  - male, congenital Q55.8
- genitourinary organs, congenital NEC
  - female Q52.8
  - male Q55.8
- globe (acquired) Z90.01
  - congenital Q11.1
- glottis, congenital Q31.8
- hand and wrist (acquired) Z89.11- ☑
  - congenital — *see* Agenesis, hand
- head, part (acquired) NEC Z90.09
- heat sense R20.8
- hip (following explantation of hip joint prosthesis) (joint) (with or without presence of antibiotic-impregnated cement spacer) Z89.62- ☑
- hymen (congenital) Q52.4
- ileum (acquired) Z90.49
  - congenital Q41.2
- immunoglobulin, isolated NEC D80.3
  - IgA D80.2
  - IgG D80.3
  - IgM D80.4
- incus (acquired) — *see* Loss, ossicles, ear
  - congenital Q16.3
- inner ear, congenital Q16.5
- intestine (acquired) (small) Z90.49
  - congenital Q41.9
    - specified NEC Q41.8
  - large Z90.49
    - congenital Q42.9
      - specified NEC Q42.8
- iris, congenital Q13.1

Absence — *continued*
- jejunum (acquired) Z90.49
  - congenital Q41.1
- joint
  - acquired
    - hip (following explantation of hip joint prosthesis) (with or without presence of antibiotic-impregnated cement spacer) Z89.62- ☑
    - knee (following explantation of knee joint prosthesis) (with or without presence of antibiotic-impregnated cement spacer) Z89.52- ☑
    - shoulder (following explantation of shoulder joint prosthesis) (with or without presence of antibiotic-impregnated cement spacer) Z89.23- ☑
  - congenital NEC Q74.8
- kidney(s) (acquired) Z90.5
  - congenital Q60.2
    - bilateral Q60.1
    - unilateral Q60.0
- knee (following explantation of knee joint prosthesis) (joint) (with or without presence of antibiotic-impregnated cement spacer) Z89.52- ☑
- labyrinth, membranous Q16.5
- larynx (congenital) Q31.8
  - acquired Z90.02
- leg (acquired) (above knee) Z89.61- ☑
  - below knee (acquired) Z89.51- ☑
  - congenital — *see* Defect, reduction, lower limb
- lens (acquired) (*see also* Aphakia)
  - congenital Q12.3
  - post cataract extraction Z98.4- ☑
- limb (acquired) — *see* Absence, extremity
- lip Q38.6
- liver (congenital) Q44.7
- lung (fissure) (lobe) (bilateral) (unilateral) (congenital) Q33.3
  - acquired (any part) Z90.2
- menstruation — *see* Amenorrhea
- muscle (congenital) (pectoral) Q79.8
  - ocular Q10.3
- neck, part Q18.8
- neutrophil — *see* Agranulocytosis
- nipple(s) (with breast(s)) (acquired) Z90.1- ☑
  - congenital Q83.2
- nose (congenital) Q30.1
  - acquired Z90.09
- organ
  - of Corti, congenital Q16.5
  - or site, congenital NEC Q89.8
    - acquired NEC Z90.89
- osseous meatus (ear) Q16.4
- ovary (acquired)
  - bilateral Z90.722
  - congenital
    - bilateral Q50.02
    - unilateral Q50.01
  - unilateral Z90.721
- oviduct (acquired)
  - bilateral Z90.722
  - congenital Q50.6
  - unilateral Z90.721
- pancreas (congenital) Q45.0
  - acquired Z90.410
    - complete Z90.410
    - partial Z90.411
    - total Z90.410
- parathyroid gland (acquired) E89.2
  - congenital Q89.2
- patella, congenital Q74.1
- penis (congenital) Q55.5
  - acquired Z90.79
- pericardium (congenital) Q24.8
- pituitary gland (congenital) Q89.2
  - acquired E89.3
- prostate (acquired) Z90.79
  - congenital Q55.4
- pulmonary valve Q22.0
- punctum lacrimale (congenital) Q10.4
- radius, congenital — *see* Defect, reduction, upper limb, longitudinal, radius
- rectum (congenital) Q42.1
  - with fistula Q42.0
  - acquired Z90.49
- respiratory organ NOS Q34.9

Absence — *continued*
- rib (acquired) Z90.89
  - congenital Q76.6
- sacrum, congenital Q76.49
- salivary gland(s), congenital Q38.4
- scrotum, congenital Q55.29
- seminal vesicles (congenital) Q55.4
  - acquired Z90.79
- septum
  - atrial (congenital) Q21.1
  - between aorta and pulmonary artery Q21.4
  - ventricular (congenital) Q20.4
- sex chromosome
  - female phenotype Q97.8
  - male phenotype Q98.8
- skull bone (congenital) Q75.8
  - with
    - anencephaly Q00.0
    - encephalocele — *see* Encephalocele
    - hydrocephalus Q03.9
      - with spina bifida — *see* Spina bifida, by site, with hydrocephalus
    - microcephaly Q02
- spermatic cord, congenital Q55.4
- spine, congenital Q76.49
- spleen (congenital) Q89.01
  - acquired Z90.81
- sternum, congenital Q76.7
- stomach (acquired) (partial) Z90.3
  - congenital Q40.2
- superior vena cava, congenital Q26.8
- teeth, tooth (congenital) K00.0
  - acquired (complete) K08.109
    - class I K08.101
    - class II K08.102
    - class III K08.103
    - class IV K08.104
    - due to
      - caries K08.139
        - class I K08.131
        - class II K08.132
        - class III K08.133
        - class IV K08.134
      - periodontal disease K08.129
        - class I K08.121
        - class II K08.122
        - class III K08.123
        - class IV K08.124
      - specified NEC K08.199
        - class I K08.191
        - class II K08.192
        - class III K08.193
        - class IV K08.194
      - trauma K08.119
        - class I K08.111
        - class II K08.112
        - class III K08.113
        - class IV K08.114
    - partial K08.409
      - class I K08.401
      - class II K08.402
      - class III K08.403
      - class IV K08.404
      - due to
        - caries K08.439
          - class I K08.431
          - class II K08.432
          - class III K08.433
          - class IV K08.434
        - periodontal disease K08.429
          - class I K08.421
          - class II K08.422
          - class III K08.423
          - class IV K08.424
        - specified NEC K08.499
          - class I K08.491
          - class II K08.492
          - class III K08.493
          - class IV K08.494
        - trauma K08.419
          - class I K08.411
          - class II K08.412
          - class III K08.413
          - class IV K08.414
- tendon (congenital) Q79.8
- testis (congenital) Q55.0
  - acquired Z90.79

Absence — *continued*
  thumb (acquired) Z89.01- ☑
    congenital — *see* Agenesis, hand
  thymus gland Q89.2
  thyroid (gland) (acquired) E89.0
    cartilage, congenital Q31.8
    congenital E03.1
  toe(s) (acquired) Z89.42- ☑
    with foot — *see* Absence, foot and ankle
    congenital — *see* Agenesis, foot
    great Z89.41- ☑
  tongue, congenital Q38.3
  trachea (cartilage), congenital Q32.1
  transverse aortic arch, congenital Q25.4
  tricuspid valve Q22.4
  umbilical artery, congenital Q27.0
  upper arm and forearm with hand present, congenital
      — *see* Agenesis, arm, with hand present
  ureter (congenital) Q62.4
    acquired Z90.6
  urethra, congenital Q64.5
  uterus (acquired) Z90.710
    with cervix Z90.710
    with remaining cervical stump Z90.711
    congenital Q51.0
  uvula, congenital Q38.5
  vagina, congenital Q52.0
  vas deferens (congenital) Q55.4
    acquired Z90.79
  vein (peripheral) congenital NEC Q27.8
    cerebral Q28.3
    digestive system Q27.8
    great Q26.8
    lower limb Q27.8
    portal Q26.5
    precerebral Q28.1
    specified site NEC Q27.8
    upper limb Q27.8
  vena cava (inferior) (superior), congenital Q26.8
  ventricular septum Q20.4
  vertebra, congenital Q76.49
  vulva, congenital Q52.71
  wrist (acquired) Z89.12- ☑
Absorbent system disease I87.8
Absorption
  carbohydrate, disturbance K90.4
  chemical — *see* Table of Drugs and Chemicals
    through placenta (newborn) P04.9
      environmental substance P04.6
      nutritional substance P04.5
      obstetric anesthetic or analgesic drug P04.0
  drug NEC — *see* Table of Drugs and Chemicals
    addictive
      through placenta (newborn) P04.49
        cocaine P04.41
    medicinal
      through placenta (newborn) P04.1
    through placenta (newborn) P04.1
      obstetric anesthetic or analgesic drug P04.0
  fat, disturbance K90.4
    pancreatic K90.3
  noxious substance — *see* Table of Drugs and Chemicals
  protein, disturbance K90.4
  starch, disturbance K90.4
  toxic substance — *see* Table of Drugs and Chemicals
  uremic — *see* Uremia
Abstinence symptoms, syndrome
  alcohol F10.239
    with delirium F10.231
  cocaine F14.23
  neonatal P96.1
  nicotine — *see* Dependence, drug, nicotine, with, withdrawal
  opioid F11.93
    with dependence F11.23
  psychoactive NEC F19.939
    with
      delirium F19.931
      dependence F19.239
        with
          delirium F19.231
          perceptual disturbance F19.232
        uncomplicated F19.230
      perceptual disturbance F19.932
    uncomplicated F19.930

Abstinence symptoms, syndrome — *continued*
  sedative F13.939
    with
      delirium F13.931
      dependence F13.239
        with
          delirium F13.231
          perceptual disturbance F13.232
        uncomplicated F13.230
      perceptual disturbance F13.932
    uncomplicated F13.930
  stimulant NEC F15.93
    with dependence F15.23
Abulia R68.89
Abulomania F60.7
Abuse
  adult — *see* Maltreatment, adult
    as reason for
      couple seeking advice (including offender) Z63.0
  alcohol (non-dependent) F10.10
    with
      anxiety disorder F10.180
      intoxication F10.129
        with delirium F10.121
        uncomplicated F10.120
      mood disorder F10.14
      other specified disorder F10.188
      psychosis F10.159
        delusions F10.150
        hallucinations F10.151
      sexual dysfunction F10.181
      sleep disorder F10.182
      unspecified disorder F10.19
    counseling and surveillance Z71.41
  amphetamine (or related substance) — *see* Abuse, drug, stimulant NEC
  analgesics (non-prescribed) (over the counter) F55.8
  antacids F55.0
  antidepressants — *see* Abuse, drug, psychoactive NEC
  anxiolytic — *see* Abuse, drug, sedative
  barbiturates — *see* Abuse, drug, sedative
  caffeine — *see* Abuse, drug, stimulant NEC
  cannabis, cannabinoids — *see* Abuse, drug, cannabis
  child — *see* Maltreatment, child
  cocaine — *see* Abuse, drug, cocaine
  drug NEC (non-dependent) F19.10
    with sleep disorder F19.182
    amphetamine type — *see* Abuse, drug, stimulant NEC
    analgesics (non-prescribed) (over the counter) F55.8
    antacids F55.0
    antidepressants — *see* Abuse, drug, psychoactive NEC
    anxiolytics — *see* Abuse, drug, sedative
    barbiturates — *see* Abuse, drug, sedative
    caffeine — *see* Abuse, drug, stimulant NEC
    cannabis F12.10
      with
        anxiety disorder F12.180
        intoxication F12.129
          with
            delirium F12.121
            perceptual disturbance F12.122
          uncomplicated F12.120
        other specified disorder F12.188
        psychosis F12.159
          delusions F12.150
          hallucinations F12.151
        unspecified disorder F12.19
    cocaine F14.10
      with
        anxiety disorder F14.180
        intoxication F14.129
          with
            delirium F14.121
            perceptual disturbance F14.122
          uncomplicated F14.120
        mood disorder F14.14
        other specified disorder F14.188
        psychosis F14.159
          delusions F14.150
          hallucinations F14.151
        sexual dysfunction F14.181
        sleep disorder F14.182
        unspecified disorder F14.19
    counseling and surveillance Z71.51

Abuse — *continued*
  drug — *continued*
    hallucinogen F16.10
      with
        anxiety disorder F16.180
        flashbacks F16.183
        intoxication F16.129
          with
            delirium F16.121
            perceptual disturbance F16.122
          uncomplicated F16.120
        mood disorder F16.14
        other specified disorder F16.188
        perception disorder, persisting F16.183
        psychosis F16.159
          delusions F16.150
          hallucinations F16.151
        unspecified disorder F16.19
    hashish — *see* Abuse, drug, cannabis
    herbal or folk remedies F55.1
    hormones F55.3
    hypnotics — *see* Abuse, drug, sedative
    inhalant F18.10
      with
        anxiety disorder F18.180
        dementia, persisting F18.17
        intoxication F18.129
          with delirium F18.121
          uncomplicated F18.120
        mood disorder F18.14
        other specified disorder F18.188
        psychosis F18.159
          delusions F18.150
          hallucinations F18.151
        unspecified disorder F18.19
    laxatives F55.2
    LSD — *see* Abuse, drug, hallucinogen
    marihuana — *see* Abuse, drug, cannabis
    morphine type (opioids) — *see* Abuse, drug, opioid
    opioid F11.10
      with
        intoxication F11.129
          with
            delirium F11.121
            perceptual disturbance F11.122
          uncomplicated F11.120
        mood disorder F11.14
        other specified disorder F11.188
        psychosis F11.159
          delusions F11.150
          hallucinations F11.151
        sexual dysfunction F11.181
        sleep disorder F11.182
        unspecified disorder F11.19
    PCP (phencyclidine) (or related substance) — *see* Abuse, drug, hallucinogen
    psychoactive NEC F19.10
      with
        amnestic disorder F19.16
        anxiety disorder F19.180
        dementia F19.17
        intoxication F19.129
          with
            delirium F19.121
            perceptual disturbance F19.122
          uncomplicated F19.120
        mood disorder F19.14
        other specified disorder F19.188
        psychosis F19.159
          delusions F19.150
          hallucinations F19.151
        sexual dysfunction F19.181
        sleep disorder F19.182
        unspecified disorder F19.19
    sedative, hypnotic or anxiolytic F13.10
      with
        anxiety disorder F13.180
        intoxication F13.129
          with delirium F13.121
          uncomplicated F13.120
        mood disorder F13.14
        other specified disorder F13.188
        psychosis F13.159
          delusions F13.150
          hallucinations F13.151
        sexual dysfunction F13.181
        sleep disorder F13.182
        unspecified disorder F13.19

Abuse — *continued*
  drug — *continued*
    solvent — *see* Abuse, drug, inhalant
    steroids F55.3
    stimulant NEC F15.10
      with
        anxiety disorder F15.180
        intoxication F15.129
          with
            delirium F15.121
            perceptual disturbance F15.122
          uncomplicated F15.120
        mood disorder F15.14
        other specified disorder F15.188
        psychosis F15.159
          delusions F15.150
          hallucinations F15.151
        sexual dysfunction F15.181
        sleep disorder F15.182
        unspecified disorder F15.19
    tranquilizers — *see* Abuse, drug, sedative
    vitamins F55.4
  hallucinogens — *see* Abuse, drug, hallucinogen
  hashish — *see* Abuse, drug, cannabis
  herbal or folk remedies F55.1
  hormones F55.3
  hypnotic — *see* Abuse, drug, sedative
  inhalant — *see* Abuse, drug, inhalant
  laxatives F55.2
  LSD — *see* Abuse, drug, hallucinogen
  marihuana — *see* Abuse, drug, cannabis
  morphine type (opioids) — *see* Abuse, drug, opioid
  non-psychoactive substance NEC F55.8
    antacids F55.0
    folk remedies F55.1
    herbal remedies F55.1
    hormones F55.3
    laxatives F55.2
    steroids F55.3
    vitamins F55.4
  opioids — *see* Abuse, drug, opioid
  PCP (phencyclidine) (or related substance) — *see* Abuse, drug, hallucinogen
  physical (adult) (child) — *see* Maltreatment
  psychoactive substance — *see* Abuse, drug, psychoactive NEC
  psychological (adult) (child) — *see* Maltreatment
  sedative — *see* Abuse, drug, sedative
  sexual — *see* Maltreatment
  solvent — *see* Abuse, drug, inhalant
  steroids F55.3
  vitamins F55.4
Acalculia R48.8
  developmental F81.2
Acanthamebiasis (with) B60.10
  conjunctiva B60.12
  keratoconjunctivitis B60.13
  meningoencephalitis B60.11
  other specified B60.19
Acanthocephaliasis B83.8
Acanthocheilonemiasis B74.4
Acanthocytosis E78.6
Acantholysis L11.9
Acanthosis (acquired) (nigricans) L83
  benign Q82.8
  congenital Q82.8
  seborrheic L82.1
    inflamed L82.0
  tongue K14.3
Acapnia E87.3
Acarbia E87.2
Acardia, acardius Q89.8
Acardiacus amorphus Q89.8
Acardiotrophia I51.4
Acariasis B88.0
  scabies B86
Acarodermatitis (urticarioides) B88.0
Acarophobia F40.218
Acatalasemia, acatalasia E80.3
Acathisia (drug induced) G25.71
Accelerated atrioventricular conduction I45.6
Accentuation of personality traits (type A) Z73.1
Accessory (congenital)
  adrenal gland Q89.1
  anus Q43.4
  appendix Q43.4
  atrioventricular conduction I45.6

Accessory — *continued*
  auditory ossicles Q16.3
  auricle (ear) Q17.0
  biliary duct or passage Q44.5
  bladder Q64.79
  blood vessels NEC Q27.9
    coronary Q24.5
  bone NEC Q79.8
  breast tissue, axilla Q83.1
  carpal bones Q74.0
  cecum Q43.4
  chromosome(s) NEC (nonsex) Q92.9
    with complex rearrangements NEC Q92.5
      seen only at prometaphase Q92.8
    13 — *see* Trisomy, 13
    18 — *see* Trisomy, 18
    21 — *see* Trisomy, 21
    partial Q92.9
    sex
      female phenotype Q97.8
  coronary artery Q24.5
  cusp(s), heart valve NEC Q24.8
    pulmonary Q22.3
  cystic duct Q44.5
  digit(s) Q69.9
  ear (auricle) (lobe) Q17.0
  endocrine gland NEC Q89.2
  eye muscle Q10.3
  eyelid Q10.3
  face bone(s) Q75.8
  fallopian tube (fimbria) (ostium) Q50.6
  finger(s) Q69.0
  foreskin N47.8
  frontonasal process Q75.8
  gallbladder Q44.1
  genital organ(s)
    female Q52.8
      external Q52.79
      internal NEC Q52.8
    male Q55.8
  genitourinary organs NEC Q89.8
    female Q52.8
    male Q55.8
  hallux Q69.2
  heart Q24.8
    valve NEC Q24.8
      pulmonary Q22.3
  hepatic ducts Q44.5
  hymen Q52.4
  intestine (large) (small) Q43.4
  kidney Q63.0
  lacrimal canal Q10.6
  leaflet, heart valve NEC Q24.8
  ligament, broad Q50.6
  liver Q44.7
    duct Q44.5
  lobule (ear) Q17.0
  lung (lobe) Q33.1
  muscle Q79.8
  navicular of carpus Q74.0
  nervous system, part NEC Q07.8
  nipple Q83.3
  nose Q30.8
  organ or site not listed — *see* Anomaly, by site
  ovary Q50.31
  oviduct Q50.6
  pancreas Q45.3
  parathyroid gland Q89.2
  parotid gland (and duct) Q38.4
  pituitary gland Q89.2
  preauricular appendage Q17.0
  prepuce N47.8
  renal arteries (multiple) Q27.2
  rib Q76.6
    cervical Q76.5
  roots (teeth) K00.2
  salivary gland Q38.4
  sesamoid bones Q74.8
    foot Q74.2
    hand Q74.0
  skin tags Q82.8
  spleen Q89.09
  sternum Q76.7
  submaxillary gland Q38.4
  tarsal bones Q74.2
  teeth, tooth K00.1
  tendon Q79.8
  thumb Q69.1

Accessory — *continued*
  thymus gland Q89.2
  thyroid gland Q89.2
  toes Q69.2
  tongue Q38.3
  tooth, teeth K00.1
  tragus Q17.0
  ureter Q62.5
  urethra Q64.79
  urinary organ or tract NEC Q64.8
  uterus Q51.2
  vagina Q52.10
  valve, heart NEC Q24.8
    pulmonary Q22.3
  vertebra Q76.49
  vocal cords Q31.8
  vulva Q52.79
Accident
  birth — *see* Birth, injury
  cardiac — *see* Infarct, myocardium
  cerebral I63.9
  cerebrovascular (embolic) (ischemic) (thrombotic) I63.9
    aborted I63.9
    hemorrhagic — *see* Hemorrhage, intracranial, intracerebral
    old (without sequelae) Z86.73
      with sequelae (of) — *see* Sequelae, infarction, cerebral
  coronary — *see* Infarct, myocardium
  craniovascular I63.9
  vascular, brain I63.9
Accidental — *see* condition
Accommodation (disorder) (*see also* condition)
  hysterical paralysis of F44.89
  insufficiency of H52.4
  paresis — *see* Paresis, of accommodation
  spasm — *see* Spasm, of accommodation
Accouchement — *see* Delivery
Accreta placenta O43.21- ☑
Accretio cordis (nonrheumatic) I31.0
Accretions, tooth, teeth K03.6
Acculturation difficulty Z60.3
Accumulation secretion, prostate N42.89
Acephalia, acephalism, acephalus, acephaly Q00.0
Acephalobrachia monster Q89.8
Acephalochirus monster Q89.8
Acephalogaster Q89.8
Acephalostomus monster Q89.8
Acephalothorax Q89.8
Acerophobia F40.298
Acetonemia R79.89
  in Type 1 diabetes E10.10
    with coma E10.11
Acetonuria R82.4
Achalasia (cardia) (esophagus) K22.0
  congenital Q39.5
  pylorus Q40.0
  sphincteral NEC K59.8
Ache(s) — *see* Pain
Acheilia Q38.6
Achilloburitis — *see* Tendinitis, Achilles
Achillodynia — *see* Tendinitis, Achilles
Achlorhydria, achlorhydric (neurogenic) K31.83
  anemia D50.8
  diarrhea K31.83
  psychogenic F45.8
  secondary to vagotomy K91.1
Achluophobia F40.228
Acholia K82.8
Acholuric jaundice (familial) (splenomegalic) (*see also* Spherocytosis)
  acquired D59.8
Achondrogenesis Q77.0
Achondroplasia (osteosclerosis congenita) Q77.4
Achroma, cutis L80
Achromat (ism), achromatopsia (acquired) (congenital) H53.51
Achromia, congenital — *see* Albinism
Achromia parasitica B36.0
Achylia gastrica K31.89
  psychogenic F45.8
Acid
  burn — *see* Corrosion
  deficiency
    amide nicotinic E52
    ascorbic E54
    folic E53.8

▽ Subterms under main terms may continue to next column or page   ☑ Additional Character Required — Refer to the Tabular List for Character Selection   9

Abuse — Acid

Acid — *continued*
  deficiency — *continued*
    nicotinic E52
    pantothenic E53.8
  intoxication E87.2
  peptic disease K30
  phosphatase deficiency E83.39
  stomach K30
    psychogenic F45.8
Acidemia E87.2
  argininosuccinic E72.22
  isovaleric E71.110
  metabolic (newborn) P19.9
    first noted before onset of labor P19.0
    first noted during labor P19.1
    noted at birth P19.2
  methylmalonic E71.120
  pipecolic E72.3
  propionic E71.121
Acidity, gastric (high) K30
  psychogenic F45.8
Acidocytopenia — *see* Agranulocytosis
Acidocytosis D72.1
Acidopenia — *see* Agranulocytosis
Acidosis (lactic) (respiratory) E87.2
  in Type 1 diabetes E10.10
    with coma E10.11
  kidney, tubular N25.89
  lactic E87.2
  metabolic NEC E87.2
    with respiratory acidosis E87.4
    late, of newborn P74.0
  mixed metabolic and respiratory, newborn P84
  newborn P84
  renal (hyperchloremic) (tubular) N25.89
  respiratory E87.2
    complicated by
      metabolic
        acidosis E87.4
        alkalosis E87.4
Aciduria
  argininosuccinic E72.22
  glutaric (type I) E72.3
    type II E71.313
    type III E71.5- ☑
  orotic (congenital) (hereditary) (pyrimidine deficiency)
    E79.8
    anemia D53.0
Acladiosis (skin) B36.0
Aclasis, diaphyseal Q78.6
Acleistocardia Q21.1
Aclusion — *see* Anomaly, dentofacial, malocclusion
Acne L70.9
  artificialis L70.8
  atrophica L70.2
  cachecticorum (Hebra) L70.8
  conglobata L70.1
  cystic L70.0
  decalvans L66.2
  excoriée des jeunes filles L70.5
  frontalis L70.2
  indurata L70.0
  infantile L70.4
  keloid L73.0
  lupoid L70.2
  necrotic, necrotica (miliaris) L70.2
  neonatal L70.4
  nodular L70.0
  occupational L70.8
  picker's L70.5
  pustular L70.0
  rodens L70.2
  rosacea L71.9
  specified NEC L70.8
  tropica L70.3
  varioliformis L70.2
  vulgaris L70.0
Acnitis (primary) A18.4
Acosta's disease T70.29 ☑
Acoustic — *see* condition
Acousticophobia F40.298
Acquired (*see also* condition)
  immunodeficiency syndrome (AIDS) B20
Acrania Q00.0
Acroangiodermatitis I78.9
Acroasphyxia, chronic I73.89
Acrobystitis N47.7
Acrocephalopolysyndactyly Q87.0

Acrocephalosyndactyly Q87.0
Acrocephaly Q75.0
Acrochondrohyperplasia — *see* Syndrome, Marfan's
Acrocyanosis I73.8 ☑
  newborn P28.2
    meaning transient blue hands and feet — *omit code*
Acrodermatitis L30.8
  atrophicans (chronica) L90.4
  continua (Hallopeau) L40.2
  enteropathica (hereditary) E83.2
  Hallopeau's L40.2
  infantile papular L44.4
  perstans L40.2
  pustulosa continua L40.2
  recalcitrant pustular L40.2
Acrodynia — *see* Poisoning, mercury
Acromegaly, acromegalia E22.0
Acromelalgia I73.81
Acromicria, acromikria Q79.8
Acronyx L60.0
Acropachy, thyroid — *see* Thyrotoxicosis
Acroparesthesia (simple) (vasomotor) I73.89
Acropathy, thyroid — *see* Thyrotoxicosis
Acrophobia F40.241
Acroposthitis N47.7
Acroscleriasis, acroscleroderma, acrosclerosis — *see* Sclerosis, systemic
Acrosphacelus I96
Acrospiroma, eccrine — *see* Neoplasm, skin, benign
Acrostealgia — *see* Osteochondropathy
Acrotrophodynia — *see* Immersion
ACTH ectopic syndrome E24.3
Actinic — *see* condition
Actinobacillosis, actinobacillus A28.8
  mallei A24.0
  muris A25.1
Actinomyces israelii (infection) — *see* Actinomycosis
Actinomycetoma (foot) B47.1
Actinomycosis, actinomycotic A42.9
  with pneumonia A42.0
  abdominal A42.1
  cervicofacial A42.2
  cutaneous A42.89
  gastrointestinal A42.1
  pulmonary A42.0
  sepsis A42.7
  specified site NEC A42.89
Actinoneuritis G62.82
Action, heart
  disorder I49.9
  irregular I49.9
    psychogenic F45.8
Activated protein C resistance D68.51
Active — *see* condition
Acute (*see also* condition)
  abdomen R10.0
  gallbladder — *see* Cholecystitis, acute
Acyanotic heart disease (congenital) Q24.9
Acystia Q64.5
Adair-Dighton syndrome (brittle bones and blue sclera, deafness) Q78.0
Adamantinoblastoma — *see* Ameloblastoma
Adamantinoma (*see also* Cyst, calcifying odontogenic)
  long bones C40.90
    lower limb C40.2- ☑
    upper limb C40.0- ☑
  malignant C41.1
    jaw (bone) (lower) C41.1
      upper C41.0
  tibial C40.2- ☑
Adamantoblastoma — *see* Ameloblastoma
Adams-Stokes (-Morgagni) disease or syndrome I45.9
Adaption reaction — *see* Disorder, adjustment
Addiction (*see also* Dependence) F19.20
  alcohol, alcoholic (ethyl) (methyl) (wood) (without remission) F10.20
    with remission F10.21
  drug — *see* Dependence, drug
  ethyl alcohol (without remission) F10.20
    with remission F10.21
  heroin — *see* Dependence, drug, opioid
  methyl alcohol (without remission) F10.20
    with remission F10.21
  methylated spirit (without remission) F10.20
    with remission F10.21

Addiction — *continued*
  morphine (-like substances) — *see* Dependence, drug, opioid
  nicotine — *see* Dependence, drug, nicotine
  opium and opioids — *see* Dependence, drug, opioid
  tobacco — *see* Dependence, drug, nicotine
Addison-Biermer anemia (pernicious) D51.0
Addisonian crisis E27.2
Addison's
  anemia (pernicious) D51.0
  disease (bronze) or syndrome E27.1
    tuberculous A18.7
  keloid L94.0
Addison-Schilder complex E71.528
Additional (*see also* Accessory)
  chromosome(s) Q99.8
    21 — *see* Trisomy, 21
    sex — *see* Abnormal, chromosome, sex
Adduction contracture, hip or other joint — *see* Contraction, joint
Adenitis (*see also* Lymphadenitis)
  acute, unspecified site L04.9
  axillary I88.9
    acute L04.2
    chronic or subacute I88.1
  Bartholin's gland N75.8
  bulbourethral gland — *see* Urethritis
  cervical I88.9
    acute L04.0
    chronic or subacute I88.1
  chancroid (Hemophilus ducreyi) A57
  chronic, unspecified site I88.1
  Cowper's gland — *see* Urethritis
  due to Pasteurella multocida (p. septica) A28.0
  epidemic, acute B27.09
  gangrenous L04.9
  gonorrheal NEC A54.89
  groin I88.9
    acute L04.1
    chronic or subacute I88.1
  infectious (acute) (epidemic) B27.09
  inguinal I88.9
    acute L04.1
    chronic or subacute I88.1
  lymph gland or node, except mesenteric I88.9
    acute — *see* Lymphadenitis, acute
    chronic or subacute I88.1
  mesenteric (acute) (chronic) (nonspecific) (subacute) I88.0
  parotid gland (suppurative) — *see* Sialoadenitis
  salivary gland (any) (suppurative) — *see* Sialoadenitis
  scrofulous (tuberculous) A18.2
  Skene's duct or gland — *see* Urethritis
  strumous, tuberculous A18.2
  subacute, unspecified site I88.1
  sublingual gland (suppurative) — *see* Sialoadenitis
  submandibular gland (suppurative) — *see* Sialoadenitis
  submaxillary gland (suppurative) — *see* Sialoadenitis
  tuberculous — *see* Tuberculosis, lymph gland
  urethral gland — *see* Urethritis
  Wharton's duct (suppurative) — *see* Sialoadenitis
Adenoacanthoma — *see* Neoplasm, malignant, by site
Adenoameloblastoma — *see* Cyst, calcifying odontogenic
Adenocarcinoid (tumor) — *see* Neoplasm, malignant, by site
Adenocarcinoma (*see also* Neoplasm, malignant, by site)
  acidophil
    specified site — *see* Neoplasm, malignant, by site
    unspecified site C75.1
  adrenal cortical C74.0- ☑
  alveolar — *see* Neoplasm, lung, malignant
  apocrine
    breast — *see* Neoplasm, breast, malignant
    in situ
      breast D05.8- ☑
      specified site NEC — *see* Neoplasm, skin, in situ
      unspecified site D04.9
    specified site NEC — *see* Neoplasm, skin, malignant
    unspecified site C44.99
  basal cell
    specified site — *see* Neoplasm, skin, malignant
    unspecified site C08.9
  basophil
    specified site — *see* Neoplasm, malignant, by site

☑ **Additional Character Required** — Refer to the Tabular List for Character Selection ▽ **Subterms under main terms may continue to next column or page**

Adenocarcinoma — *continued*
 basophil — *continued*
  unspecified site C75.1
 bile duct type C22.1
  liver C22.1
  specified site NEC — *see* Neoplasm, malignant, by
   site
  unspecified site C22.1
 bronchiolar — *see* Neoplasm, lung, malignant
 bronchioloalveolar — *see* Neoplasm, lung, malignant
 ceruminous C44.29- ☑
 cervix, in situ (*see also* Carcinoma, cervix uteri, in situ)
  D06.9
 chromophobe
  specified site — *see* Neoplasm, malignant, by site
  unspecified site C75.1
 diffuse type
  specified site — *see* Neoplasm, malignant, by site
  unspecified site C16.9
 duct
  infiltrating
   with Paget's disease — *see* Neoplasm, breast,
    malignant
   specified site — *see* Neoplasm, malignant, by
    site
   unspecified site (female) C50.91- ☑
    male C50.92- ☑
  specified site — *see* Neoplasm, malignant, by site
  unspecified site
   female C56.9
   male C61
 eosinophil
  specified site — *see* Neoplasm, malignant, by site
  unspecified site C75.1
 follicular
  with papillary C73
  moderately differentiated C73
  specified site — *see* Neoplasm, malignant, by site
  trabecular C73
  unspecified site C73
  well differentiated C73
 Hurthle cell C73
 in
  adenomatous
   polyposis coli C18.9
  infiltrating duct
   with Paget's disease — *see* Neoplasm, breast, ma-
    lignant
   specified site — *see* Neoplasm, by site, malignant
   unspecified site (female) C50.91- ☑
    male C50.92- ☑
 inflammatory
  specified site — *see* Neoplasm, by site, malignant
  unspecified site (female) C50.91- ☑
   male C50.92- ☑
 intestinal type
  specified site — *see* Neoplasm, by site, malignant
  unspecified site C16.9
 intracystic papillary
 intraductal
  breast D05.1- ☑
  noninfiltrating
   breast D05.1- ☑
   papillary
    with invasion
     specified site — *see* Neoplasm, by site,
      malignant
     unspecified site (female) C50.91- ☑
      male C50.92- ☑
    breast D05.1- ☑
    specified site NEC — *see* Neoplasm, in situ,
     by site
    unspecified site D05.1- ☑
   specified site NEC — *see* Neoplasm, in situ, by
    site
   unspecified site D05.1- ☑
  papillary
   with invasion
    specified site — *see* Neoplasm, malignant,
     by site
    unspecified site (female) C50.91- ☑
     male C50.92- ☑
   breast D05.1- ☑
   specified site — *see* Neoplasm, in situ, by site
   unspecified site D05.1- ☑
  specified site NEC — *see* Neoplasm, in situ, by site
  unspecified site D05.1- ☑

Adenocarcinoma — *continued*
 islet cell
  with exocrine, mixed
   specified site — *see* Neoplasm, malignant, by
    site
   unspecified site C25.9
  pancreas C25.4
  specified site NEC — *see* Neoplasm, malignant, by
   site
  unspecified site C25.4
 lobular
  in situ
   breast D05.0- ☑
   specified site NEC — *see* Neoplasm, in situ, by
    site
   unspecified site D05.0- ☑
  specified site — *see* Neoplasm, malignant, by site
  unspecified site (female) C50.91- ☑
   male C50.92- ☑
 mucoid (*see also* Neoplasm, malignant, by site)
  cell
   specified site — *see* Neoplasm, malignant, by
    site
   unspecified site C75.1
 nonencapsulated sclerosing C73
 papillary
  with follicular C73
  follicular variant C73
  intraductal (noninfiltrating)
   with invasion
    specified site — *see* Neoplasm, malignant,
     by site
    unspecified site (female) C50.91- ☑
     male C50.92- ☑
   breast D05.1- ☑
   specified site NEC — *see* Neoplasm, in situ, by
    site
   unspecified site D05.1- ☑
  serous
   specified site — *see* Neoplasm, malignant, by
    site
   unspecified site C56.9
 papillocystic
  specified site — *see* Neoplasm, malignant, by site
  unspecified site C56.9
 pseudomucinous
  specified site — *see* Neoplasm, malignant, by site
  unspecified site C56.9
 renal cell C64- ☑
 sebaceous — *see* Neoplasm, skin, malignant
 serous (*see also* Neoplasm, malignant, by site)
  papillary
   specified site — *see* Neoplasm, malignant, by
    site
   unspecified site C56.9
 sweat gland — *see* Neoplasm, skin, malignant
 water-clear cell C75.0
Adenocarcinoma-in-situ (*see also* Neoplasm, in situ, by
  site)
 breast D05.9- ☑
Adenofibroma
 clear cell — *see* Neoplasm, benign, by site
 endometrioid D27.9
  borderline malignancy D39.10
  malignant C56- ☑
 mucinous
  specified site — *see* Neoplasm, benign, by site
  unspecified site D27.9
 papillary
  specified site — *see* Neoplasm, benign, by site
  unspecified site D27.9
 prostate — *see* Enlargement, enlarged, prostate
 serous
  specified site — *see* Neoplasm, benign, by site
  unspecified site D27.9
 specified site — *see* Neoplasm, benign, by site
 unspecified site D27.9
Adenofibrosis
 breast — *see* Fibroadenosis, breast
 endometrioid N80.0
Adenoiditis (chronic) J35.02
 with tonsillitis J35.03
 acute J03.90
  recurrent J03.91
  specified organism NEC J03.80
   recurrent J03.81

Adenoiditis — *continued*
 acute — *continued*
  staphylococcal J03.80
   recurrent J03.81
  streptococcal J03.00
   recurrent J03.01
Adenoids — *see* condition
Adenolipoma — *see* Neoplasm, benign, by site
Adenolipomatosis, Launois-Bensaude E88.89
Adenolymphoma
 specified site — *see* Neoplasm, benign, by site
 unspecified site D11.9
Adenoma (*see also* Neoplasm, benign, by site)
 acidophil
  specified site — *see* Neoplasm, benign, by site
  unspecified site D35.2
 acidophil-basophil, mixed
  specified site — *see* Neoplasm, benign, by site
  unspecified site D35.2
 adrenal (cortical) D35.00
  clear cell D35.00
  compact cell D35.00
  glomerulosa cell D35.00
  heavily pigmented variant D35.00
  mixed cell D35.00
 alpha-cell
  pancreas D13.7
  specified site NEC — *see* Neoplasm, benign, by site
  unspecified site D13.7
 alveolar D14.30
 apocrine
  breast D24- ☑
  specified site NEC — *see* Neoplasm, skin, benign,
   by site
  unspecified site D23.9
 basal cell D11.9
 basophil
  specified site — *see* Neoplasm, benign, by site
  unspecified site D35.2
 basophil-acidophil, mixed
  specified site — *see* Neoplasm, benign, by site
  unspecified site D35.2
 beta-cell
  pancreas D13.7
  specified site NEC — *see* Neoplasm, benign, by site
  unspecified site D13.7
 bile duct D13.4
  common D13.5
  extrahepatic D13.5
  intrahepatic D13.4
  specified site NEC — *see* Neoplasm, benign, by site
  unspecified site D13.4
 black D35.00
 bronchial D38.1
  cylindroid type — *see* Neoplasm, lung, malignant
 ceruminous D23.2- ☑
 chief cell D35.1
 chromophobe
  specified site — *see* Neoplasm, benign, by site
  unspecified site D35.2
 colloid
  specified site — *see* Neoplasm, benign, by site
  unspecified site D34
 duct
 eccrine, papillary — *see* Neoplasm, skin, benign
 endocrine, multiple
  single specified site — *see* Neoplasm, uncertain
   behavior, by site
  two or more specified sites D44- ☑
  unspecified site D44.9
 endometrioid (*see also* Neoplasm, benign)
  borderline malignancy — *see* Neoplasm, uncertain
   behavior, by site
 eosinophil
  specified site — *see* Neoplasm, benign, by site
  unspecified site D35.2
 fetal
  specified site — *see* Neoplasm, benign, by site
  unspecified site D34
 follicular
  specified site — *see* Neoplasm, benign, by site
  unspecified site D34
 hepatocellular D13.4
 Hurthle cell D34
 islet cell
  pancreas D13.7
  specified site NEC — *see* Neoplasm, benign, by site
  unspecified site D13.7

Adenoma — *continued*
liver cell D13.4
macrofollicular
   specified site — *see* Neoplasm, benign, by site
   unspecified site D34
malignant, malignum — *see* Neoplasm, malignant,
      by site
microcystic
   pancreas D13.7
   specified site NEC — *see* Neoplasm, benign, by site
   unspecified site D13.7
microfollicular
   specified site — *see* Neoplasm, benign, by site
   unspecified site D34
mucoid cell
   specified site — *see* Neoplasm, benign, by site
   unspecified site D35.2
multiple endocrine
   single specified site — *see* Neoplasm, uncertain
      behavior, by site
   two or more specified sites D44- ☑
   unspecified site D44.9
nipple D24- ☑
papillary (*see also* Neoplasm, benign, by site)
   eccrine — *see* Neoplasm, skin, benign, by site
Pick's tubular
   specified site — *see* Neoplasm, benign, by site
   unspecified site
      female D27.9
      male D29.20
pleomorphic
   carcinoma in — *see* Neoplasm, salivary gland,
      malignant
      specified site — *see* Neoplasm, malignant, by
         site
      unspecified site C08.9
polypoid (*see also* Neoplasm, benign)
   adenocarcinoma in — *see* Neoplasm, malignant,
      by site
   adenocarcinoma in situ — *see* Neoplasm, in situ,
      by site
prostate — *see* Neoplasm, benign, prostate
rete cell D29.20
sebaceous — *see* Neoplasm, skin, benign
Sertoli cell
   specified site — *see* Neoplasm, benign, by site
   unspecified site
      female D27.9
      male D29.20
skin appendage — *see* Neoplasm, skin, benign
sudoriferous gland — *see* Neoplasm, skin, benign
sweat gland — *see* Neoplasm, skin, benign
testicular
   specified site — *see* Neoplasm, benign, by site
   unspecified site
      female D27.9
      male D29.20
tubular (*see also* Neoplasm, benign, by site)
   adenocarcinoma in — *see* Neoplasm, malignant,
      by site
   adenocarcinoma in situ — *see* Neoplasm, in situ,
      by site
   Pick's
      specified site — *see* Neoplasm, benign, by site
      unspecified site
         female D27.9
         male D29.20
tubulovillous (*see also* Neoplasm, benign, by site)
   adenocarcinoma in — *see* Neoplasm, malignant,
      by site
   adenocarcinoma in situ — *see* Neoplasm, in situ,
      by site
villous — *see* Neoplasm, uncertain behavior, by site
   adenocarcinoma in — *see* Neoplasm, malignant,
      by site
   adenocarcinoma in situ — *see* Neoplasm, in situ,
      by site
water-clear cell D35.1
Adenomatosis
endocrine (multiple) E31.20
   single specified site — *see* Neoplasm, uncertain
      behavior, by site
erosive of nipple D24- ☑
pluriendocrine — *see* Adenomatosis, endocrine
pulmonary D38.1
   malignant — *see* Neoplasm, lung, malignant
specified site — *see* Neoplasm, benign, by site

Adenomatosis — *continued*
unspecified site D12.6
Adenomatous
goiter (nontoxic) E04.9
   with hyperthyroidism — *see* Hyperthyroidism,
      with, goiter, nodular
   toxic — *see* Hyperthyroidism, with, goiter, nodular
Adenomyoma (*see also* Neoplasm, benign, by site)
prostate — *see* Enlarged, prostate
Adenomyometritis N80.0
Adenomyosis N80.0
Adenopathy (lymph gland) R59.9
generalized R59.1
inguinal R59.0
localized R59.0
mediastinal R59.0
mesentery R59.0
syphilitic (secondary) A51.49
tracheobronchial R59.0
   tuberculous A15.4
      primary (progressive) A15.7
tuberculous (*see also* Tuberculosis, lymph gland)
   tracheobronchial A15.4
      primary (progressive) A15.7
Adenosalpingitis — *see* Salpingitis
Adenosarcoma — *see* Neoplasm, malignant, by site
Adenosclerosis I88.8
Adenosis (sclerosing) breast — *see* Fibroadenosis, breast
Adenovirus, as cause of disease classified elsewhere
B97.0
Adentia (complete) (partial) — *see* Absence, teeth
Adherent (*see also* Adhesions)
labia (minora) N90.89
pericardium (nonrheumatic) I31.0
   rheumatic I09.2
placenta (with hemorrhage) O72.0
   without hemorrhage O73.0
prepuce, newborn N47.0
scar (skin) L90.5
tendon in scar L90.5
Adhesions, adhesive (postinfective) K66.0
with intestinal obstruction K56.5
abdominal (wall) — *see* Adhesions, peritoneum
appendix K38.8
bile duct (common) (hepatic) K83.8
bladder (sphincter) N32.89
bowel — *see* Adhesions, peritoneum
cardiac I31.0
   rheumatic I09.2
cecum — *see* Adhesions, peritoneum
cervicovaginal N88.1
   congenital Q52.8
   postpartal O90.89
      old N88.1
cervix N88.1
ciliary body NEC — *see* Adhesions, iris
clitoris N90.89
colon — *see* Adhesions, peritoneum
common duct K83.8
congenital (*see also* Anomaly, by site)
   fingers — *see* Syndactylism, complex, fingers
   omental, anomalous Q43.3
   peritoneal Q43.3
   tongue (to gum or roof of mouth) Q38.3
conjunctiva (acquired) H11.21- ☑
   congenital Q15.8
cystic duct K82.8
diaphragm — *see* Adhesions, peritoneum
due to foreign body — *see* Foreign body
duodenum — *see* Adhesions, peritoneum
ear
   middle H74.1- ☑
epididymis N50.8
epidural — *see* Adhesions, meninges
epiglottis J38.7
eyelid H02.59
female pelvis N73.6
gallbladder K82.8
globe H44.89
heart I31.0
   rheumatic I09.2
ileocecal (coil) — *see* Adhesions, peritoneum
ileum — *see* Adhesions, peritoneum
intestine (*see also* Adhesions, peritoneum)
   with obstruction K56.5
intra-abdominal — *see* Adhesions, peritoneum

Adhesions, adhesive — *continued*
iris H21.50- ☑
   anterior H21.51- ☑
   goniosynechiae H21.52- ☑
   posterior H21.54- ☑
   to corneal graft T85.89 ☑
joint — *see* Ankylosis
   knee M23.8X ☑
   temporomandibular M26.61
labium (majus) (minus), congenital Q52.5
liver — *see* Adhesions, peritoneum
lung J98.4
mediastinum J98.5
meninges (cerebral) (spinal) G96.12
   congenital Q07.8
   tuberculous (cerebral) (spinal) A17.0
mesenteric — *see* Adhesions, peritoneum
nasal (septum) (to turbinates) J34.89
ocular muscle — *see* Strabismus, mechanical
omentum — *see* Adhesions, peritoneum
ovary N73.6
   congenital (to cecum, kidney or omentum) Q50.39
paraovarian N73.6
pelvic (peritoneal)
   female N73.6
      postprocedural N99.4
   male — *see* Adhesions, peritoneum
   postpartal (old) N73.6
   tuberculous A18.17
penis to scrotum (congenital) Q55.8
periappendiceal (*see also* Adhesions, peritoneum)
pericardium (nonrheumatic) I31.0
   focal I31.8
   rheumatic I09.2
   tuberculous A18.84
pericholecystic K82.8
perigastric — *see* Adhesions, peritoneum
periovarian N73.6
periprostatic N42.89
perirectal — *see* Adhesions, peritoneum
perirenal N28.89
peritoneum, peritoneal (postinfective) (postprocedu-
      ral) K66.0
   with obstruction (intestinal) K56.5
   congenital Q43.3
   pelvic, female N73.6
      postprocedural N99.4
   postpartal, pelvic N73.6
   to uterus N73.6
peritubal N73.6
periureteral N28.89
periuterine N73.6
perivesical N32.89
perivesicular (seminal vesicle) N50.8
pleura, pleuritic J94.8
   tuberculous NEC A15.6
pleuropericardial J94.8
postoperative (gastrointestinal tract) K66.0
   with obstruction K91.3
   due to foreign body accidentally left in wound —
         see Foreign body, accidentally left during a
         procedure
   pelvic peritoneal N99.4
   urethra — *see* Stricture, urethra, postprocedural
   vagina N99.2
postpartal, old (vulva or perineum) N90.89
preputial, prepuce N47.5
pulmonary J98.4
pylorus — *see* Adhesions, peritoneum
sciatic nerve — *see* Lesion, nerve, sciatic
seminal vesicle N50.8
shoulder (joint) — *see* Capsulitis, adhesive
sigmoid flexure — *see* Adhesions, peritoneum
spermatic cord (acquired) N50.8
   congenital Q55.4
spinal canal G96.12
stomach — *see* Adhesions, peritoneum
subscapular — *see* Capsulitis, adhesive
temporomandibular M26.61
tendinitis (*see also* Tenosynovitis, specified type NEC)
   shoulder — *see* Capsulitis, adhesive
testis N44.8
tongue, congenital (to gum or roof of mouth) Q38.3
   acquired K14.8
trachea J39.8
tubo-ovarian N73.6
tunica vaginalis N44.8

Adhesions, adhesive — *continued*
  uterus N73.6
    internal N85.6
    to abdominal wall N73.6
  vagina (chronic) N89.5
    postoperative N99.2
  vitreomacular H43.82- ☑
  vitreous H43.89
  vulva N90.89
Adiaspiromycosis B48.8
Adie (-Holmes) **pupil or syndrome** — *see* Anomaly,
    pupil, function, tonic pupil
Adiponecrosis neonatorum P83.8
Adiposis (*see also* Obesity)
  cerebralis E23.6
  dolorosa E88.2
Adiposity (*see also* Obesity)
  heart — *see* Degeneration, myocardial
  localized E65
Adiposogenital dystrophy E23.6
Adjustment
  disorder — *see* Disorder, adjustment
  implanted device — *see* Encounter (for), adjustment
    (of)
  prosthesis, external — *see* Fitting
  reaction — *see* Disorder, adjustment
Administration of tPA (rtPA) in a different facility within
    the last 24 hours prior to admission to current facil-
    ity Z92.82
Admission (for) (*see also* Encounter (for))
  adjustment (of)
    artificial
      arm Z44.00- ☑
        complete Z44.01- ☑
        partial Z44.02- ☑
      eye Z44.2- ☑
      leg Z44.10- ☑
        complete Z44.11- ☑
        partial Z44.12- ☑
    brain neuropacemaker Z46.2
      implanted Z45.42
    breast
      implant Z45.81 ☑
      prosthesis (external) Z44.3 ☑
    colostomy belt Z46.89
    contact lenses Z46.0
    cystostomy device Z46.6
    dental prosthesis Z46.3
    device NEC
      abdominal Z46.89
      implanted Z45.89
        cardiac Z45.09
          defibrillator (with synchronous cardiace
              pacemaker) Z45.02
          pacemaker Z45.018
            pulse generator Z45.010
        hearing device Z45.328
          bone conduction Z45.320
          cochlear Z45.321
        infusion pump Z45.1
        nervous system Z45.49
          CSF drainage Z45.41
          hearing device — *see* Admission, adjust-
              ment, device, implanted, hearing
              device
          neuropacemaker Z45.42
          visual substitution Z45.31
        specified NEC Z45.89
        vascular access Z45.2
        visual substitution Z45.31
      nervous system Z46.2
        implanted — *see* Admission, adjustment,
            device, implanted, nervous system
      orthodontic Z46.4
      prosthetic Z44.9
        arm — *see* Admission, adjustment, artificial,
            arm
        breast Z44.3 ☑
        dental Z46.3
        eye Z44.2 ☑
        leg — *see* Admission, adjustment, artificial,
            leg
        specified type NEC Z44.8

Admission — *continued*
  adjustment — *continued*
    device — *continued*
      substitution
        auditory Z46.2
          implanted — *see* Admission, adjust-
              ment, device, implanted, hearing
              device
        nervous system Z46.2
          implanted — *see* Admission, adjust-
              ment, device, implanted, nervous
              system
        visual Z46.2
          implanted Z45.31
      urinary Z46.6
    hearing aid Z46.1
      implanted — *see* Admission, adjustment, de-
          vice, implanted, hearing device
    ileostomy device Z46.89
    intestinal appliance or device NEC Z46.89
    neuropacemaker (brain) (peripheral nerve) (spinal
        cord) Z46.2
      implanted Z45.42
    orthodontic device Z46.4
    orthopedic (brace) (cast) (device) (shoes) Z46.89
    pacemaker
      cardiac Z45.018
        pulse generator Z45.010
      nervous system Z46.2
        implanted Z45.42
    portacath (port-a-cath) Z45.2
    prosthesis Z44.9
      arm — *see* Admission, adjustment, artificial,
          arm
      breast Z44.3 ☑
      dental Z46.3
      eye Z44.2 ☑
      leg — *see* Admission, adjustment, artificial, leg
      specified NEC Z44.8
    spectacles Z46.0
  aftercare (*see also* Aftercare) Z51.89
    postpartum
      immediately after delivery Z39.0
      routine follow-up Z39.2
    radiation therapy (antineoplastic) Z51.0
  attention to artificial opening (of) Z43.9
    artificial vagina Z43.7
    colostomy Z43.3
    cystostomy Z43.5
    enterostomy Z43.4
    gastrostomy Z43.1
    ileostomy Z43.2
    jejunostomy Z43.4
    nephrostomy Z43.6
    specified site NEC Z43.8
      intestinal tract Z43.4
      urinary tract Z43.6
    tracheostomy Z43.0
    ureterostomy Z43.6
    urethrostomy Z43.6
  breast augmentation or reduction Z41.1
  breast reconstruction following mastectomy Z42.1
  change of
    dressing (nonsurgical) Z48.00
    neuropacemaker device (brain) (peripheral nerve)
        (spinal cord) Z46.2
      implanted Z45.42
    surgical dressing Z48.01
  circumcision, ritual or routine (in absence of diagnosis)
      Z41.2
  clinical research investigation (control) (normal com-
      parison) (participant) Z00.6
  contraceptive management Z30.9
  cosmetic surgery NEC Z41.1
  counseling (*see also* Counseling)
    dietary Z71.3
    HIV Z71.7
    human immunodeficiency virus Z71.7
    nonattending third party Z71.0
    procreative management NEC Z31.69
  delivery, full-term, uncomplicated O80
    cesarean, without indication O82
  dietary surveillance and counseling Z71.3
  ear piercing Z41.3
  examination at health care facility (adult) (*see also*
      Examination) Z00.00
    with abnormal findings Z00.01

Admission — *continued*
  examination at health care facility (*see also* Examina-
      tion) — *continued*
    clinical research investigation (control) (normal
        comparison) (participant) Z00.6
    dental Z01.20
      with abnormal findings Z01.21
    donor (potential) Z00.5
    ear Z01.10
      with abnormal findings NEC Z01.118
    eye Z01.00
      with abnormal findings Z01.01
    general, specified reason NEC Z00.8
    hearing Z01.10
      with abnormal findings NEC Z01.118
    postpartum checkup Z39.2
    psychiatric (general) Z00.8
      requested by authority Z04.6
    vision Z01.00
      with abnormal findings Z01.01
  fitting (of)
    artificial
      arm — *see* Admission, adjustment, artificial,
          arm
      eye Z44.2 ☑
      leg — *see* Admission, adjustment, artificial, leg
    brain neuropacemaker Z46.2
      implanted Z45.42
    breast prosthesis (external) Z44.3 ☑
    colostomy belt Z46.89
    contact lenses Z46.0
    cystostomy device Z46.6
    dental prosthesis Z46.3
    dentures Z46.3
    device NEC
      abdominal Z46.89
      nervous system Z46.2
        implanted — *see* Admission, adjustment,
            device, implanted, nervous system
      orthodontic Z46.4
      prosthetic Z44.9
        breast Z44.3 ☑
        dental Z46.3
        eye Z44.2 ☑
      substitution
        auditory Z46.2
          implanted — *see* Admission, adjust-
              ment, device, implanted, hearing
              device
        nervous system Z46.2
          implanted — *see* Admission, adjust-
              ment, device, implanted, nervous
              system
        visual Z46.2
          implanted Z45.31
    hearing aid Z46.1
    ileostomy device Z46.89
    intestinal appliance or device NEC Z46.89
    neuropacemaker (brain) (peripheral nerve) (spinal
        cord) Z46.2
      implanted Z45.42
    orthodontic device Z46.4
    orthopedic device (brace) (cast) (shoes) Z46.89
    prosthesis Z44.9
      arm — *see* Admission, adjustment, artificial,
          arm
      breast Z44.3 ☑
      dental Z46.3
      eye Z44.2 ☑
      leg — *see* Admission, adjustment, artificial, leg
      specified type NEC Z44.8
    spectacles Z46.0
  follow-up examination Z09
  intrauterine device management Z30.431
    initial prescription Z30.014
  mental health evaluation Z00.8
    requested by authority Z04.6
  observation — *see* Observation
  Papanicolaou smear, cervix Z12.4
    for suspected malignant neoplasm Z12.4
  plastic and reconstructive surgery following medical
      procedure or healed injury NEC Z42.8
  plastic surgery, cosmetic NEC Z41.1
  postpartum observation
    immediately after delivery Z39.0
    routine follow-up Z39.2
  poststerilization (for restoration) Z31.0
    aftercare Z31.42

Admission — continued
  procreative management Z31.9
  prophylactic (measure)
    organ removal Z40.00
      breast Z40.01
      ovary Z40.02
      specified organ NEC Z40.09
      testes Z40.09
    vaccination Z23
  psychiatric examination (general) Z00.8
    requested by authority Z04.6
  radiation therapy (antineoplastic) Z51.0
  reconstructive surgery following medical procedure
    or healed injury NEC Z42.8
  removal of
    cystostomy catheter Z43.5
    drains Z48.03
    dressing (nonsurgical) Z48.00
    intrauterine contraceptive device Z30.432
    neuropacemaker (brain) (peripheral nerve) (spinal
      cord) Z46.2
      implanted Z45.42
    staples Z48.02
    surgical dressing Z48.01
    sutures Z48.02
    ureteral stent Z46.6
  respirator [ventilator] use during power failure Z99.12
  restoration of organ continuity (poststerilization) Z31.0
    aftercare Z31.42
  sensitivity test (see also Test, skin)
    allergy NEC Z01.82
    Mantoux Z11.1
  tuboplasty following previous sterilization Z31.0
    aftercare Z31.42
  vasoplasty following previous sterilization Z31.0
    aftercare Z31.42
  vision examination Z01.00
    with abnormal findings Z01.01
  waiting period for admission to other facility Z75.1
Adnexitis (suppurative) — see Salpingo-oophoritis
Adolescent X-linked adrenoleukodystrophy E71.521
Adrenal (gland) — see condition
Adrenalism, tuberculous A18.7
Adrenalitis, adrenitis E27.8
  autoimmune E27.1
  meningococcal, hemorrhagic A39.1
Adrenarche, premature E27.0
Adrenocortical syndrome — see Cushing's, syndrome
Adrenogenital syndrome E25.9
  acquired E25.8
  congenital E25.0
  salt loss E25.0
Adrenogenitalism, congenital E25.0
Adrenoleukodystrophy E71.529
  neonatal E71.511
  X-linked E71.529
    Addison only phenotype E71.528
    Addison-Schilder E71.528
    adolescent E71.521
    adrenomyeloneuropathy E71.522
    childhood cerebral E71.520
    other specified E71.528
Adrenomyeloneuropathy E71.522
Adventitious bursa — see Bursopathy, specified type
  NEC
Adverse effect — see Table of Drugs and Chemicals,
  categories T36-T50, with 6th character 5
Advice — see Counseling
Adynamia (episodica) (hereditary) (periodic) G72.3
Aeration lung imperfect, newborn — see Atelectasis
Aerobullosis T70.3 ☑
Aerocele — see Embolism, air
Aerodermectasia
  subcutaneous (traumatic) T79.7 ☑
Aerodontalgia T70.29 ☑
Aeroembolism T70.3 ☑
Aerogenes capsulatus infection A48.0
Aero-otitis media T70.0 ☑
Aerophagy, aerophagia (psychogenic) F45.8
Aerophobia F40.228
Aerosinusitis T70.1 ☑
Aerotitis T70.0 ☑
Affection — see Disease
Afibrinogenemia (see also Defect, coagulation) D68.8
  acquired D65
  congenital D68.2
  following ectopic or molar pregnancy O08.1

Afibrinogenemia — continued
  in abortion — see Abortion, by type, complicated by,
    afibrinogenemia
  puerperal O72.3
African
  sleeping sickness B56.9
  tick fever A68.1
  trypanosomiasis B56.9
    gambian B56.0
    rhodesian B56.1
Aftercare (see also Care) Z51.89
  following surgery (for) (on)
    amputation Z47.81
    attention to
      drains Z48.03
      dressings (nonsurgical) Z48.00
        surgical Z48.01
      sutures Z48.02
    circulatory system Z48.812
    delayed (planned) wound closure Z48.1
    digestive system Z48.815
    explantation of joint prosthesis (staged procedure)
      hip Z47.32
      knee Z47.33
      shoulder Z47.31
    genitourinary system Z48.816
    joint replacement Z47.1
    neoplasm Z48.3
    nervous system Z48.811
    oral cavity Z48.814
    organ transplant
      bone marrow Z48.290
      heart Z48.21
      heart lung Z48.280
      kidney Z48.22
      liver Z48.23
      lung Z48.24
      multiple organs NEC Z48.288
      specified NEC Z48.298
    orthopedic NEC Z47.89
    planned wound closure Z48.1
    removal of internal fixation device Z47.2
    respiratory system Z48.813
    scoliosis Z47.82
    sense organs Z48.810
    skin and subcutaneous tissue Z48.817
    specified body system
      circulatory Z48.812
      digestive Z48.815
      genitourinary Z48.816
      nervous Z48.811
      oral cavity Z48.814
      respiratory Z48.813
      sense organs Z48.810
      skin and subcutaneous tissue Z48.817
      teeth Z48.814
    specified NEC Z48.89
    spinal Z48.89
    teeth Z48.814
  fracture — code to fracture with seventh character D
  involving
    removal of
      drains Z48.03
      dressings (nonsurgical) Z48.00
      staples Z48.02
      surgical dressings Z48.01
      sutures Z48.02
  neuropacemaker (brain) (peripheral nerve) (spinal
    cord) Z46.2
    implanted Z45.42
  orthopedic NEC Z47.89
  postprocedural — see Aftercare, following surgery
After-cataract — see Cataract, secondary
Agalactia (primary) O92.3
  elective, secondary or therapeutic O92.5
Agammaglobulinemia (acquired (secondary)) (nonfamilial) D80.1
  with
    immunoglobulin-bearing B-lymphocytes D80.1
    lymphopenia D81.9
  autosomal recessive (Swiss type) D80.0
  Bruton's X-linked D80.0
  common variable (CVAgamma) D80.1
  congenital sex-linked D80.0
  hereditary D80.0
  lymphopenic D81.9
  Swiss type (autosomal recessive) D80.0

Agammaglobulinemia — continued
  X-linked (with growth hormone deficiency)(Bruton)
    D80.0
Aganglionosis (bowel) (colon) Q43.1
Age (old) — see Senility
Agenesis
  adrenal (gland) Q89.1
  alimentary tract (complete) (partial) NEC Q45.8
    upper Q40.8
  anus, anal (canal) Q42.3
    with fistula Q42.2
  aorta Q25.4
  appendix Q42.8
  arm (complete) Q71.0- ☑
    with hand present Q71.1- ☑
  artery (peripheral) Q27.9
    brain Q28.3
    coronary Q24.5
    pulmonary Q25.79
    specified NEC Q27.8
    umbilical Q27.0
  auditory (canal) (external) Q16.1
  auricle (ear) Q16.0
  bile duct or passage Q44.5
  bladder Q64.5
  bone Q79.9
  brain Q00.0
    part of Q04.3
  breast (with nipple present) Q83.8
    with absent nipple Q83.0
  bronchus Q32.4
  canaliculus lacrimalis Q10.4
  carpus — see Agenesis, hand
  cartilage Q79.9
  cecum Q42.8
  cerebellum Q04.3
  cervix Q51.5
  chin Q18.8
  cilia Q10.3
  circulatory system, part NOS Q28.9
  clavicle Q74.0
  clitoris Q52.6
  coccyx Q76.49
  colon Q42.9
    specified NEC Q42.8
  corpus callosum Q04.0
  cricoid cartilage Q31.8
  diaphragm (with hernia) Q79.1
  digestive organ(s) or tract (complete) (partial) NEC
    Q45.8
    upper Q40.8
  ductus arteriosus Q28.8
  duodenum Q41.0
  ear Q16.9
    auricle Q16.0
    lobe Q17.8
  ejaculatory duct Q55.4
  endocrine (gland) NEC Q89.2
  epiglottis Q31.8
  esophagus Q39.8
  eustachian tube Q16.2
  eye Q11.1
    adnexa Q15.8
  eyelid (fold) Q10.3
  face
    bones NEC Q75.8
    specified part NEC Q18.8
  fallopian tube Q50.6
  femur — see Defect, reduction, lower limb, longitudi-
    nal, femur
  fibula — see Defect, reduction, lower limb, longitudi-
    nal, fibula
  finger (complete) (partial) — see Agenesis, hand
  foot (and toes) (complete) (partial) Q72.3- ☑
  forearm (with hand present) — see Agenesis, arm,
    with hand present
    and hand Q71.2- ☑
  gallbladder Q44.0
  gastric Q40.2
  genitalia, genital (organ(s))
    female Q52.8
      external Q52.71
      internal NEC Q52.8
    male Q55.8
  glottis Q31.8
  hair Q84.0
  hand (and fingers) (complete) (partial) Q71.3- ☑

☑ Additional Character Required — Refer to the Tabular List for Character Selection   ▽ Subterms under main terms may continue to next column or page

Agenesis — *continued*
- heart Q24.8
  - valve NEC Q24.8
    - pulmonary Q22.0
- hepatic Q44.7
- humerus — *see* Defect, reduction, upper limb
- hymen Q52.4
- ileum Q41.2
- incus Q16.3
- intestine (small) Q41.9
  - large Q42.9
    - specified NEC Q42.8
- iris (dilator fibers) Q13.1
- jaw M26.09
- jejunum Q41.1
- kidney(s) (partial) Q60.2
  - bilateral Q60.1
  - unilateral Q60.0
- labium (majus) (minus) Q52.71
- labyrinth, membranous Q16.5
- lacrimal apparatus Q10.4
- larynx Q31.8
- leg (complete) Q72.0- ☑
  - with foot present Q72.1- ☑
  - lower leg (with foot present) — *see* Agenesis, leg, with foot present
  - and foot Q72.2- ☑
- lens Q12.3
- limb (complete) Q73.0
  - lower — *see* Agenesis, leg
  - upper — *see* Agenesis, arm
- lip Q38.0
- liver Q44.7
- lung (fissure) (lobe) (bilateral) (unilateral) Q33.3
- mandible, maxilla M26.09
- metacarpus — *see* Agenesis, hand
- metatarsus — *see* Agenesis, foot
- muscle Q79.8
  - eyelid Q10.3
  - ocular Q15.8
- musculoskeletal system NEC Q79.8
- nail(s) Q84.3
- neck, part Q18.8
- nerve Q07.8
- nervous system, part NEC Q07.8
- nipple Q83.2
- nose Q30.1
- nuclear Q07.8
- organ
  - of Corti Q16.5
  - or site not listed — *see* Anomaly, by site
- osseous meatus (ear) Q16.1
- ovary
  - bilateral Q50.02
  - unilateral Q50.01
- oviduct Q50.6
- pancreas Q45.0
- parathyroid (gland) Q89.2
- parotid gland(s) Q38.4
- patella Q74.1
- pelvic girdle (complete) (partial) Q74.2
- penis Q55.5
- pericardium Q24.8
- pituitary (gland) Q89.2
- prostate Q55.4
- punctum lacrimale Q10.4
- radioulnar — *see* Defect, reduction, upper limb
- radius — *see* Defect, reduction, upper limb, longitudinal, radius
- rectum Q42.1
  - with fistula Q42.0
- renal Q60.2
  - bilateral Q60.1
  - unilateral Q60.0
- respiratory organ NEC Q34.8
- rib Q76.6
- roof of orbit Q75.8
- round ligament Q52.8
- sacrum Q76.49
- salivary gland Q38.4
- scapula Q74.0
- scrotum Q55.29
- seminal vesicles Q55.4
- septum
  - atrial Q21.1
  - between aorta and pulmonary artery Q21.4
  - ventricular Q20.4
- shoulder girdle (complete) (partial) Q74.0

Agenesis — *continued*
- skull (bone) Q75.8
  - with
    - anencephaly Q00.0
    - encephalocele — *see* Encephalocele
    - hydrocephalus Q03.9
      - with spina bifida — *see* Spina bifida, by site, with hydrocephalus
    - microcephaly Q02
- spermatic cord Q55.4
- spinal cord Q06.0
- spine Q76.49
- spleen Q89.01
- sternum Q76.7
- stomach Q40.2
- submaxillary gland(s) (congenital) Q38.4
- tarsus — *see* Agenesis, foot
- tendon Q79.8
- testicle Q55.0
- thymus (gland) Q89.2
- thyroid (gland) E03.1
  - cartilage Q31.8
- tibia — *see* Defect, reduction, lower limb, longitudinal, tibia
- tibiofibular — *see* Defect, reduction, lower limb, specified type NEC
- toe (and foot) (complete) (partial) — *see* Agenesis, foot
- tongue Q38.3
- trachea (cartilage) Q32.1
- ulna — *see* Defect, reduction, upper limb, longitudinal, ulna
- upper limb — *see* Agenesis, arm
- ureter Q62.4
- urethra Q64.5
- urinary tract NEC Q64.8
- uterus Q51.0
- uvula Q38.5
- vagina Q52.0
- vas deferens Q55.4
- vein(s) (peripheral) Q27.9
  - brain Q28.3
  - great NEC Q26.8
  - portal Q26.5
  - vena cava (inferior) (superior) Q26.8
- vermis of cerebellum Q04.3
- vertebra Q76.49
- vulva Q52.71

Ageusia R43.2
Agitated — *see* condition
Agitation R45.1
Aglossia (congenital) Q38.3
Aglossia-adactylia syndrome Q87.0
Aglycogenosis E74.00
Agnosia (body image) (other senses) (tactile) R48.1
- developmental F88
- verbal R48.1
  - auditory R48.1
    - developmental F80.2
  - developmental F80.2
- visual (object) R48.3

Agoraphobia F40.00
- with panic disorder F40.01
- without panic disorder F40.02

Agrammatism R48.8
Agranulocytopenia — *see* Agranulocytosis
Agranulocytosis (chronic) (cyclical) (genetic) (infantile) (periodic) (pernicious) (*see also* Neutropenia) D70.9
- congenital D70.0
- cytoreductive cancer chemotherapy sequela D70.1
- drug-induced D70.2
  - due to cytoreductive cancer chemotherapy D70.1
- due to infection D70.3
- secondary D70.4
  - drug-induced D70.2
    - due to cytoreductive cancer chemotherapy D70.1

Agraphia (absolute) R48.8
- with alexia R48.0
- developmental F81.81

Ague (dumb) — *see* Malaria
Agyria Q04.3
Ahumada-del Castillo syndrome E23.0
Aichmophobia F40.298
AIDS (related complex) B20
Ailment heart — *see* Disease, heart
Ailurophobia F40.218
Ainhum (disease) L94.6

AIPHI (acute idiopathic pulmonary hemorrhage in infants (over 28 days old)) R04.81
Air
- anterior mediastinum J98.2
- compressed, disease T70.3 ☑
- conditioner lung or pneumonitis J67.7
- embolism (artery) (cerebral) (any site) T79.0 ☑
  - with ectopic or molar pregnancy O08.2
  - due to implanted device NEC — *see* Complications, by site and type, specified NEC
  - following
    - abortion — *see* Abortion by type, complicated by, embolism
    - ectopic or molar pregnancy O08.2
  - infusion, therapeutic injection or transfusion T80.0 ☑
  - in pregnancy, childbirth or puerperium — *see* Embolism, obstetric
  - traumatic T79.0 ☑
- hunger, psychogenic F45.8
- rarefied, effects of — *see* Effect, adverse, high altitude
- sickness T75.3 ☑

Airplane sickness T75.3 ☑
Akathisia (drug-induced) (treatment-induced) G25.71
- neuroleptic induced (acute) G25.71
Akinesia R29.898
Akinetic mutism R41.89
Akureyri's disease G93.3
Alactasia, congenital E73.0
Alagille's syndrome Q44.7
Alastrim B03
Albers-Schönberg syndrome Q78.2
Albert's syndrome — *see* Tendinitis, Achilles
Albinism, albino E70.30
- with hematologic abnormality E70.339
  - Chédiak-Higashi syndrome E70.330
  - Hermansky-Pudlak syndrome E70.331
  - other specified E70.338
- I E70.320
- II E70.321
- ocular E70.319
  - autosomal recessive E70.311
  - other specified E70.318
  - X-linked E70.310
- oculocutaneous E70.329
  - other specified E70.328
  - tyrosinase (ty) negative E70.320
  - tyrosinase (ty) positive E70.321
- other specified E70.39
Albinismus E70.30
Albright (-McCune)(-Sternberg) syndrome Q78.1
Albuminous — *see* condition
Albuminuria, albuminuric (acute) (chronic) (subacute) (*see also* Proteinuria) R80.9
- complicating pregnancy — *see* Proteinuria, gestational
- with
  - gestational hypertension — *see* Pre-eclampsia
  - pre-existing hypertension — *see* Hypertension, complicating pregnancy, pre-existing, with, pre-eclampsia
- gestational — *see* Proteinuria, gestational
- with
  - gestational hypertension — *see* Pre-eclampsia
  - pre-existing hypertension — *see* Hypertension, complicating pregnancy, pre-existing, with, pre-eclampsia
- orthostatic R80.2
- postural R80.2
- pre-eclamptic — *see* Pre-eclampsia
- scarlatinal A38.8
Albuminurophobia F40.298
Alcaptonuria E70.29
Alcohol, alcoholic, alcohol-induced
- addiction (without remission) F10.20
  - with remission F10.21
- amnestic disorder, persisting F10.96
  - with dependence F10.26
- brain syndrome, chronic F10.97
  - with dependence F10.27
- cardiopathy I42.6
- counseling and surveillance Z71.41
  - family member Z71.42
- delirium (acute) (tremens) (withdrawal) F10.231
  - with intoxication F10.921
  - in
    - abuse F10.121
    - dependence F10.221

Alcohol, alcoholic, alcohol-induced — *continued*
dementia F10.97
  with dependence F10.27
deterioration F10.97
  with dependence F10.27
hallucinosis (acute) F10.951
  in
    abuse F10.151
    dependence F10.251
insanity F10.959
intoxication (acute) (without dependence) F10.129
  with
    delirium F10.121
    dependence F10.229
      with delirium F10.221
      uncomplicated F10.220
    uncomplicated F10.120
jealousy F10.988
Korsakoff's, Korsakov's, Korsakow's F10.26
liver K70.9
  acute — *see* Disease, liver, alcoholic, hepatitis
mania (acute) (chronic) F10.959
paranoia, paranoid (type) psychosis F10.950
pellagra E52
poisoning, accidental (acute) NEC — *see* Table of Drugs and Chemicals, alcohol, poisoning
psychosis — *see* Psychosis, alcoholic
withdrawal (without convulsions) F10.239
  with delirium F10.231
Alcoholism (chronic) (without remission) F10.20
with
  psychosis — *see* Psychosis, alcoholic
  remission F10.21
  Korsakov's F10.96
    with dependence F10.26
Alder (-Reilly) **anomaly or syndrome** (leukocyte granulation) D72.0
Aldosteronism E26.9
familial (type I) E26.02
glucocorticoid-remediable E26.02
primary (due to (bilateral) adrenal hyperplasia) E26.09
primary NEC E26.09
secondary E26.1
specified NEC E26.89
Aldosteronoma D44.10
Aldrich (-Wiskott) **syndrome** (eczema-thrombocytopenia) D82.0
Alektorophobia F40.218
Aleppo boil B55.1
Aleukemic — *see* condition
Aleukia
congenital D70.0
hemorrhagica D61.9
  congenital D61.09
splenica D73.1
Alexia R48.0
developmental F81.0
secondary to organic lesion R48.0
Algoneurodystrophy M89.00
ankle M89.07- ☑
foot M89.07- ☑
forearm M89.03- ☑
hand M89.04- ☑
lower leg M89.06- ☑
multiple sites M89.0- ☑
shoulder M89.01- ☑
specified site NEC M89.08
thigh M89.05- ☑
upper arm M89.02- ☑
Algophobia F40.298
Alienation, mental — *see* Psychosis
Alkalemia E87.3
Alkalosis E87.3
metabolic E87.3
  with respiratory acidosis E87.4
respiratory E87.3
Alkaptonuria E70.29
Allen-Masters syndrome N83.8
Allergy, allergic (reaction) (to) T78.40 ☑
air-borne substance NEC (rhinitis) J30.89
alveolitis (extrinsic) J67.9
  due to
    Aspergillus clavatus J67.4
    Cryptostroma corticale J67.6
    organisms (fungal, thermophilic actinomycete) growing in ventilation (air conditioning) systems J67.7

Allergy, allergic — *continued*
alveolitis — *continued*
  specified type NEC J67.8
anaphylactic reaction or shock T78.2 ☑
angioneurotic edema T78.3 ☑
animal (dander) (epidermal) (hair) (rhinitis) J30.81
bee sting (anaphylactic shock) — *see* Toxicity, venom, arthropod, bee
biological — *see* Allergy, drug
colitis K52.2
dander (animal) (rhinitis) J30.81
dandruff (rhinitis) J30.81
dental restorative material (existing) K08.55
dermatitis — *see* Dermatitis, contact, allergic
diathesis — *see* History, allergy
drug, medicament & biological (any) (external) (internal) T78.40 ☑
  correct substance properly administered — *see* Table of Drugs and Chemicals, by drug, adverse effect
  wrong substance given or taken NEC (by accident) — *see* Table of Drugs and Chemicals, by drug, poisoning
due to pollen J30.1
dust (house) (stock) (rhinitis) J30.89
  with asthma — *see* Asthma, allergic extrinsic
eczema — *see* Dermatitis, contact, allergic
epidermal (animal) (rhinitis) J30.81
feathers (rhinitis) J30.89
food (any) (ingested) NEC T78.1 ☑
  anaphylactic shock — *see* Shock, anaphylactic, due to food
  dermatitis — *see* Dermatitis, due to, food
  dietary counseling and surveillance Z71.3
  in contact with skin L23.6
  rhinitis J30.5
  status (without reaction) Z91.018
    eggs Z91.012
    milk products Z91.011
    peanuts Z91.010
    seafood Z91.013
    specified NEC Z91.018
gastrointestinal K52.2
grain J30.1
grass (hay fever) (pollen) J30.1
  asthma — *see* Asthma, allergic extrinsic
hair (animal) (rhinitis) J30.81
history (of) — *see* History, allergy
horse serum — *see* Allergy, serum
inhalant (rhinitis) J30.89
  pollen J30.1
kapok (rhinitis) J30.89
medicine — *see* Allergy, drug
milk protein K52.2
nasal, seasonal due to pollen J30.1
pneumonia J82
pollen (any) (hay fever) J30.1
  asthma — *see* Asthma, allergic extrinsic
primrose J30.1
primula J30.1
purpura D69.0
ragweed (hay fever) (pollen) J30.1
  asthma — *see* Asthma, allergic extrinsic
rose (pollen) J30.1
seasonal NEC J30.2
Senecio jacobae (pollen) J30.1
serum (*see also* Reaction, serum) T80.69 ☑
  anaphylactic shock T80.59 ☑
shock (anaphylactic) T78.2 ☑
  due to
    administration of blood and blood products T80.51 ☑
    adverse effect of correct medicinal substance properly administered T88.6 ☑
    immunization T80.52 ☑
    serum NEC T80.59 ☑
    vaccination T80.52 ☑
specific NEC T78.49 ☑
tree (any) (hay fever) (pollen) J30.1
  asthma — *see* Asthma, allergic extrinsic
upper respiratory J30.9
urticaria L50.0
vaccine — *see* Allergy, serum
wheat — *see* Allergy, food
Allescheriasis B48.2
Alligator skin disease Q80.9
Allocheiria, allochiria R20.8

Almeida's disease — *see* Paracoccidioidomycosis
Alopecia (hereditaria) (seborrheica) L65.9
androgenic L64.9
  drug-induced L64.0
  specified NEC L64.8
areata L63.9
  ophiasis L63.2
  specified NEC L63.8
  totalis L63.0
  universalis L63.1
cicatricial L66.9
  specified NEC L66.8
circumscripta L63.9
congenital, congenitalis Q84.0
due to cytotoxic drugs NEC L65.8
mucinosa L65.2
postinfective NEC L65.8
postpartum L65.0
premature L64.8
specific (syphilitic) A51.32
specified NEC L65.8
syphilitic (secondary) A51.32
totalis (capitis) L63.0
universalis (entire body) L63.1
X-ray L58.1
Alpers' disease G31.81
Alpine sickness T70.29 ☑
Alport syndrome Q87.81
ALTE (apparent life threatening event) **in newborn and infant** R68.13
Alteration (of), **Altered**
awareness, transient R40.4
mental status R41.82
pattern of family relationships affecting child Z62.898
sensation
  following
    cerebrovascular disease I69.998
      cerebral infarction I69.398
      intracerebral hemorrhage I69.198
      nontraumatic intracranial hemorrhage NEC I69.298
      specified disease NEC I69.898
      subarachnoid hemorrhage I69.098
Alternating — *see* condition
Altitude, high (effects) — *see* Effect, adverse, high altitude
Aluminosis (of lung) J63.0
Alveolitis
allergic (extrinsic) — *see* Pneumonitis, hypersensitivity
due to
  Aspergillus clavatus J67.4
  Cryptostroma corticale J67.6
fibrosing (cryptogenic) (idiopathic) J84.112
jaw M27.3
sicca dolorosa M27.3
Alveolus, alveolar — *see* condition
Alymphocytosis D72.810
thymic (with immunodeficiency) D82.1
Alymphoplasia, thymic D82.1
Alzheimer's disease or sclerosis — *see* Disease, Alzheimer's
Amastia (with nipple present) Q83.8
with absent nipple Q83.0
Amathophobia F40.228
Amaurosis (acquired) (congenital) (*see also* Blindness)
fugax G45.3
hysterical F44.6
Leber's congenital H35.50
uremic — *see* Uremia
Amaurotic idiocy (infantile) (juvenile) (late) E75.4
Amaxophobia F40.248
Ambiguous genitalia Q56.4
Amblyopia (congenital) (ex anopsia) (partial) (suppression) H53.00- ☑
anisometropic — *see* Amblyopia, refractive
deprivation H53.01- ☑
hysterical F44.6
nocturnal (*see also* Blindness, night)
  vitamin A deficiency E50.5
refractive H53.02- ☑
strabismic H53.03- ☑
tobacco H53.8
toxic NEC H53.8
uremic — *see* Uremia
Ameba, amebic (histolytica) (*see also* Amebiasis)
abscess (liver) A06.4

Amebiasis A06.9
- with abscess — *see* Abscess, amebic
- acute A06.0
- chronic (intestine) A06.1
  - with abscess — *see* Abscess, amebic
- cutaneous A06.7
- cutis A06.7
- cystitis A06.81
- genitourinary tract NEC A06.82
- hepatic — *see* Abscess, liver, amebic
- intestine A06.0
- nondysenteric colitis A06.2
- skin A06.7
- specified site NEC A06.89

Ameboma (of intestine) A06.3

Amelia Q73.0
- lower limb — *see* Agenesis, leg
- upper limb — *see* Agenesis, arm

Ameloblastoma (*see also* Cyst, calcifying odontogenic)
- long bones C40.9-
  - lower limb C40.2- ☑
  - upper limb C40.0- ☑
- malignant C41.1
  - jaw (bone) (lower) C41.1
    - upper C41.0
- tibial C40.2- ☑

Amelogenesis imperfecta K00.5
- nonhereditaria (segmentalis) K00.4

Amenorrhea N91.2
- hyperhormonal E28.8
- primary N91.0
- secondary N91.1

Amentia — *see* Disability, intellectual
- Meynert's (nonalcoholic) F04

American
- leishmaniasis B55.2
- mountain tick fever A93.2

Ametropia — *see* Disorder, refraction

Amianthosis J61

Amimia R48.8

Amino-acid disorder E72.9
- anemia D53.0

Aminoacidopathy E72.9

Aminoaciduria E72.9

Amnesia R41.3
- anterograde R41.1
- auditory R48.8
- dissociative F44.0
- hysterical F44.0
- postictal in epilepsy — *see* Epilepsy
- psychogenic F44.0
- retrograde R41.2
- transient global G45.4

Amnes(t)ic syndrome (post-traumatic) F04
- induced by
  - alcohol F10.96
    - with dependence F10.26
  - psychoactive NEC F19.96
    - with
      - abuse F19.16
      - dependence F19.26
  - sedative F13.96
    - with dependence F13.26

Amnion, amniotic — *see* condition

Amnionitis — *see* Pregnancy, complicated by

Amok F68.8

Amoral traits F60.89

Ampulla
- lower esophagus K22.8
- phrenic K22.8

Amputation (*see also* Absence, by site, acquired)
- neuroma (postoperative) (traumatic) — *see* Complications, amputation stump, neuroma
- stump (surgical)
  - abnormal, painful, or with complication (late) — *see* Complications, amputation stump
  - healed or old NOS Z89.9
- traumatic (complete) (partial)
  - arm (upper) (complete) S48.91- ☑
    - at
      - elbow S58.01- ☑
        - partial S58.02- ☑
      - shoulder joint (complete) S48.01- ☑
        - partial S48.02- ☑
    - between
      - elbow and wrist (complete) S58.11- ☑
        - partial S58.12- ☑

Amputation — *continued*
- traumatic — *continued*
  - arm — *continued*
    - between — *continued*
      - shoulder and elbow (complete) S48.11- ☑
        - partial S48.12- ☑
    - partial S48.92- ☑
  - breast (complete) S28.21- ☑
    - partial S28.22- ☑
  - clitoris (complete) S38.211
    - partial S38.212
  - ear (complete) S08.11- ☑
    - partial S08.12- ☑
  - finger (complete) (metacarpophalangeal)
    - S68.11- ☑
    - index S68.11- ☑
    - little S68.11- ☑
    - middle S68.11- ☑
    - partial S68.12- ☑
      - index S68.12- ☑
      - little S68.12- ☑
      - middle S68.12- ☑
      - ring S68.12- ☑
    - ring S68.11- ☑
    - thumb — *see* Amputation, traumatic, thumb
    - transphalangeal (complete) S68.61- ☑
      - index S68.61- ☑
      - little S68.61- ☑
      - middle S68.61- ☑
      - partial S68.62- ☑
        - index S68.62- ☑
        - little S68.62- ☑
        - middle S68.62- ☑
        - ring S68.62- ☑
      - ring S68.61- ☑
  - foot (complete) S98.91- ☑
    - at ankle level S98.01- ☑
      - partial S98.02- ☑
    - midfoot S98.31- ☑
      - partial S98.32- ☑
    - partial S98.92- ☑
  - forearm (complete) S58.91- ☑
    - at elbow level (complete) S58.01- ☑
      - partial S58.02- ☑
    - between elbow and wrist (complete) S58.11- ☑
      - partial S58.12- ☑
    - partial S58.92- ☑
  - genital organ(s) (external)
    - female (complete) S38.211 ☑
      - partial S38.212 ☑
    - male
      - penis (complete) S38.221 ☑
        - partial S38.222 ☑
      - scrotum (complete) S38.231 ☑
        - partial S38.232 ☑
      - testes (complete) S38.231 ☑
        - partial S38.232 ☑
  - hand (complete) (wrist level) S68.41- ☑
    - finger(s) alone — *see* Amputation, traumatic, finger
    - partial S68.42- ☑
    - thumb alone — *see* Amputation, traumatic, thumb
    - transmetacarpal (complete) S68.71- ☑
      - partial S68.72- ☑
  - head
    - ear — *see* Amputation, traumatic, ear
    - nose (partial) S08.812 ☑
      - complete S08.811 ☑
    - part S08.89
      - scalp S08.0 ☑
  - hip (and thigh) (complete) S78.91- ☑
    - at hip joint (complete) S78.01- ☑
      - partial S78.02- ☑
    - between hip and knee (complete) S78.11- ☑
      - partial S78.12- ☑
    - partial S78.92- ☑
  - labium (majus) (minus) (complete) S38.21- ☑
    - partial S38.21- ☑
  - leg (lower) S88.91- ☑
    - at knee level S88.01- ☑
      - partial S88.02- ☑
    - between knee and ankle S88.11- ☑
      - partial S88.12- ☑
    - partial S88.92- ☑

Amputation — *continued*
- traumatic — *continued*
  - nose (partial) S08.812 ☑
    - complete S08.811 ☑
  - penis (complete) S38.221 ☑
    - partial S38.222 ☑
  - scrotum (complete) S38.231 ☑
    - partial S38.232 ☑
  - shoulder — *see* Amputation, traumatic, arm
    - at shoulder joint — *see* Amputation, traumatic, arm, at shoulder joint
  - testes (complete) S38.231 ☑
    - partial S38.232 ☑
  - thigh — *see* Amputation, traumatic, hip
  - thorax, part of S28.1 ☑
    - breast — *see* Amputation, traumatic, breast
  - thumb (complete) (metacarpophalangeal)
    - S68.01- ☑
    - partial S68.02- ☑
    - transphalangeal (complete) S68.51- ☑
      - partial S68.52- ☑
  - toe (lesser) S98.13- ☑
    - great S98.11- ☑
      - partial S98.12- ☑
    - more than one S98.21- ☑
      - partial S98.22- ☑
    - partial S98.14- ☑
  - vulva (complete) S38.211 ☑
    - partial S38.212 ☑

Amputee (bilateral) (old) Z89.9

Amsterdam dwarfism Q87.1

Amusia R48.8
- developmental F80.89

Amyelencephalus, amyelencephaly Q00.0

Amyelia Q06.0

Amygdalitis — *see* Tonsillitis

Amygdalolith J35.8

Amyloid heart (disease) E85.4 [I43]

Amyloidosis (generalized) (primary) E85.9
- with lung involvement E85.4 [J99]
- familial E85.2
- genetic E85.2
- heart E85.4 [I43]
- hemodialysis-associated E85.3
- liver E85.4 [K77]
- localized E85.4
- neuropathic heredofamilial E85.1
- non-neuropathic heredofamilial E85.0
- organ limited E85.4
- Portuguese E85.1
- pulmonary E85.4 [J99]
- secondary systemic E85.3
- skin (lichen) (macular) E85.4 [L99]
- specified NEC E85.8
- subglottic E85.4 [J99]

Amylopectinosis (brancher enzyme deficiency) E74.03

Amylophagia — *see* Pica

Amyoplasia congenita Q79.8

Amyotonia M62.89
- congenita G70.2

Amyotrophia, amyotrophy, amyotrophic G71.8
- congenita Q79.8
- diabetic — *see* Diabetes, amyotrophy
- lateral sclerosis G12.21
- neuralgic G54.5
- spinal progressive G12.21

Anacidity, gastric K31.83
- psychogenic F45.8

Anaerosis of newborn P28.89

Analbuminemia E88.09

Analgesia — *see* Anesthesia

Analphalipoproteinemia E78.6

Anaphylactic
- purpura D69.0
- shock or reaction — *see* Shock, anaphylactic

Anaphylactoid shock or reaction — *see* Shock, anaphylactic

Anaphylactoid syndrome of pregnancy O88.01- ☑

Anaphylaxis — *see* Shock, anaphylactic

Anaplasia cervix (*see also* Dysplasia, cervix) N87.9

Anaplasmosis, human A77.49

Anarthria R47.1

Anasarca R60.1
- cardiac — *see* Failure, heart, congestive
- lung J18.2
- newborn P83.2
- nutritional E43

Anasarca — *continued*
pulmonary J18.2
renal N04.9
Anastomosis
aneurysmal — *see* Aneurysm
arteriovenous ruptured brain I60.8
intestinal K63.89
complicated NEC K91.89
involving urinary tract N99.89
retinal and choroidal vessels (congenital) Q14.8
Anatomical narrow angle H40.03- ☑
Ancylostoma, ancylostomiasis (braziliense) (caninum) (ceylanicum) (duodenale) B76.0
Necator americanus B76.1
Andersen's disease (glycogen storage) E74.09
Anderson-Fabry disease E75.21
Andes disease T70.29 ☑
Andrews' disease (bacterid) L08.89
Androblastoma
benign
specified site — *see* Neoplasm, benign, by site
unspecified site
female D27.9
male D29.20
malignant
specified site — *see* Neoplasm, malignant, by site
unspecified site
female C56.9
male C62.90
specified site — *see* Neoplasm, uncertain behavior, by site
tubular
with lipid storage
specified site — *see* Neoplasm, benign, by site
unspecified site
female D27.9
male D29.20
specified site — *see* Neoplasm, benign, by site
unspecified site
female D27.9
male D29.20
unspecified site
female D39.10
male D40.10
Androgen insensitivity syndrome (*see also* Syndrome, androgen insensitivity) E34.50
Androgen resistance syndrome (*see also* Syndrome, androgen insensitivity) E34.50
Android pelvis Q74.2
with disproportion (fetopelvic) O33.3 ☑
causing obstructed labor O65.3
Androphobia F40.290
Anectasis, pulmonary (newborn) — *see* Atelectasis
Anemia (essential) (general) (hemoglobin deficiency) (infantile) (primary) (profound) D64.9
with (due to) (in)
disorder of
anaerobic glycolysis D55.2
pentose phosphate pathway D55.1
koilonychia D50.9
achlorhydric D50.8
achrestic D53.1
Addison (-Biermer) (pernicious) D51.0
agranulocytic — *see* Agranulocytosis
amino-acid-deficiency D53.0
aplastic D61.9
congenital D61.09
drug-induced D61.1
due to
drugs D61.1
external agents NEC D61.2
infection D61.2
radiation D61.2
idiopathic D61.3
red cell (pure) D60.9
chronic D60.0
congenital D61.01
specified type NEC D60.8
transient D60.1
specified type NEC D61.89
toxic D61.2
aregenerative
congenital D61.09
asiderotic D50.9
atypical (primary) D64.9
Baghdad spring D55.0
Balantidium coli A07.0
Biermer's (pernicious) D51.0

Anemia — *continued*
blood loss (chronic) D50.0
acute D62
bothriocephalus B70.0 [D63.8]
brickmaker's B76.9 [D63.8]
cerebral I67.89
childhood D58.9
chlorotic D50.8
chronic
blood loss D50.0
hemolytic D58.9
idiopathic D59.9
simple D53.9
chronica congenita aregenerativa D61.09
combined system disease NEC D51.0 [G32.0]
due to dietary vitamin B12 deficiency D51.3 [G32.0]
complicating pregnancy, childbirth or puerperium — *see* Pregnancy, complicated by (management affected by), anemia
congenital P61.4
aplastic D61.09
due to isoimmunization NOS P55.9
dyserythropoietic, dyshematopoietic D64.4
following fetal blood loss P61.3
Heinz body D58.2
hereditary hemolytic NOS D58.9
pernicious D51.0
spherocytic D58.0
Cooley's (erythroblastic) D56.1
cytogenic D51.0
deficiency D53.9
6-PGD D55.1
2, 3 diphosphoglycurate mutase D55.2
2, 3 PG D55.2
6 phosphogluconate dehydrogenase D55.1
amino-acid D53.0
combined B12 and folate D53.1
enzyme D55.9
drug-induced (hemolytic) D59.2
glucose-6-phosphate dehydrogenase (G6PD) D55.0
glycolytic D55.2
nucleotide metabolism D55.3
related to hexose monophosphate (HMP) shunt pathway NEC D55.1
specified type NEC D55.8
erythrocytic glutathione D55.1
folate D52.9
dietary D52.0
drug-induced D52.1
folic acid D52.9
dietary D52.0
drug-induced D52.1
G SH D55.1
G6PD D55.0
GGS-R D55.1
glucose-6-phosphate dehydrogenase D55.0
glutathione reductase D55.1
glyceraldehyde phosphate dehydrogenase D55.2
hexokinase D55.2
iron D50.9
secondary to blood loss (chronic) D50.0
nutritional D53.9
with
poor iron absorption D50.8
specified deficiency NEC D53.8
phosphofructo-aldolase D55.2
phosphoglycerate kinase D55.2
PK D55.2
protein D53.0
pyruvate kinase D55.2
transcobalamin II D51.2
triose-phosphate isomerase D55.2
vitamin B12 NOS D51.9
dietary D51.3
due to
intrinsic factor deficiency D51.0
selective vitamin B12 malabsorption with proteinuria D51.1
pernicious D51.0
specified type NEC D51.8
Diamond-Blackfan (congenital hypoplastic) D61.01
dibothriocephalus B70.0 [D63.8]
dimorphic D53.1
diphasic D53.1
Diphyllobothrium (Dibothriocephalus) B70.0 [D63.8]
due to (in) (with)
antineoplastic chemotherapy D64.81

Anemia — *continued*
due to — *continued*
blood loss (chronic) D50.0
acute D62
chemotherapy, antineoplastic D64.81
chronic disease classified elsewhere NEC D63.8
chronic kidney disease D63.1
deficiency
amino-acid D53.0
copper D53.8
folate (folic acid) D52.9
dietary D52.0
drug-induced D52.1
molybdenum D53.8
protein D53.0
zinc D53.8
dietary vitamin B12 deficiency D51.3
disorder of
glutathione metabolism D55.1
nucleotide metabolism D55.3
drug — *see* Anemia, by type (*see also* Table of Drugs and Chemicals)
end stage renal disease D63.1
enzyme disorder D55.9
fetal blood loss P61.3
fish tapeworm (D.latum) infestation B70.0 [D63.8]
hemorrhage (chronic) D50.0
acute D62
impaired absorption D50.9
loss of blood (chronic) D50.0
acute D62
myxedema E03.9 [D63.8]
Necator americanus B76.1 [D63.8]
prematurity P61.2
selective vitamin B12 malabsorption with protein-uria D51.1
transcobalamin II deficiency D51.2
Dyke-Young type (secondary) (symptomatic) D59.1
dyserythropoietic (congenital) D64.4
dyshematopoietic (congenital) D64.4
Egyptian B76.9 [D63.8]
elliptocytosis — *see* Elliptocytosis
enzyme-deficiency, drug-induced D59.2
epidemic (*see also* Ancylostomiasis) B76.9 [D63.8]
erythroblastic
familial D56.1
newborn (*see also* Disease, hemolytic) P55.9
of childhood D56.1
erythrocytic glutathione deficiency D55.1
erythropoietin-resistant anemia (EPO resistant anemia) D63.1
Faber's (achlorhydric anemia) D50.9
factitious (self-induced blood letting) D50.0
familial erythroblastic D56.1
Fanconi's (congenital pancytopenia) D61.09
favism D55.0
fish tapeworm (D. latum) infestation B70.0 [D63.8]
folate (folic acid) deficiency D52.9
glucose-6-phosphate dehydrogenase (G6PD) deficiency D55.0
glutathione-reductase deficiency D55.1
goat's milk D52.0
granulocytic — *see* Agranulocytosis
Heinz body, congenital D58.2
hemolytic D58.9
acquired D59.9
with hemoglobinuria NEC D59.6
autoimmune NEC D59.1
infectious D59.4
specified type NEC D59.8
toxic D59.4
acute D59.9
due to enzyme deficiency specified type NEC D55.8
Lederer's D59.1
autoimmune D59.1
drug-induced D59.0
chronic D58.9
idiopathic D59.9
cold type (secondary) (symptomatic) D59.1
congenital (spherocytic) — *see* Spherocytosis
due to
cardiac conditions D59.4
drugs (nonautoimmune) D59.2
autoimmune D59.0
enzyme disorder D55.9
drug-induced D59.2

☑ **Additional Character Required — Refer to the Tabular List for Character Selection**   ⬙ **Subterms under main terms may continue to next column or page**

Anemia — *continued*
  hemolytic — *continued*
    due to — *continued*
      presence of shunt or other internal prosthetic
        device D59.4
     familial D58.9
     hereditary D58.9
      due to enzyme disorder D55.9
       specified type NEC D55.8
      specified type NEC D58.8
    idiopathic (chronic) D59.9
    mechanical D59.4
    microangiopathic D59.4
    nonautoimmune D59.4
     drug-induced D59.2
    nonspherocytic
     congenital or hereditary NEC D55.8
      glucose-6-phosphate dehydrogenase defi-
       ciency D55.0
      pyruvate kinase deficiency D55.2
      type
       I D55.1
       II D55.2
     type
      I D55.1
      II D55.2
    secondary D59.4
     autoimmune D59.1
    specified (hereditary) type NEC D58.8
    Stransky-Regala type (*see also* Hemoglobinopathy)
     D58.8
    symptomatic D59.4
     autoimmune D59.1
    toxic D59.4
    warm type (secondary) (symptomatic) D59.1
  hemorrhagic (chronic) D50.0
   acute D62
  Herrick's D57.1
  hexokinase deficiency D55.2
  hookworm B76.9 [D63.8]
  hypochromic (idiopathic) (microcytic) (normoblastic)
   D50.9
   due to blood loss (chronic) D50.0
    acute D62
   familial sex-linked D64.0
   pyridoxine-responsive D64.3
   sideroblastic, sex-linked D64.0
  hypoplasia, red blood cells D61.9
   congenital or familial D61.01
  hypoplastic (idiopathic) D61.9
   congenital or familial (of childhood) D61.01
  hypoproliferative (refractive) D61.9
  idiopathic D64.9
   aplastic D61.3
   hemolytic, chronic D59.9
  in (due to) (with)
   chronic kidney disease D63.1
   end stage renal disease D63.1
   failure, kidney (renal) D63.1
   neoplastic disease (*see also* Neoplasm) D63.0
  intertropical (*see also* Ancylostomiasis) D63.8
  iron deficiency D50.9
   secondary to blood loss (chronic) D50.0
    acute D62
   specified type NEC D50.8
  Joseph-Diamond-Blackfan (congenital hypoplastic)
   D61.01
  Lederer's (hemolytic) D59.1
  leukoerythroblastic D61.82
  macrocytic D53.9
   nutritional D52.0
   tropical D52.8
  malarial (*see also* Malaria) B54 [D63.8]
  malignant (progressive) D51.0
  malnutrition D53.9
  marsh (*see also* Malaria) B54 [D63.8]
  Mediterranean (with other hemoglobinopathy) D56.9
  megaloblastic D53.1
   combined B12 and folate deficiency D53.1
   hereditary D51.1
   nutritional D52.0
   orotic aciduria D53.0
   refractory D53.1
   specified type NEC D53.1
  megalocytic D53.1
  microcytic (hypochromic) D50.9
   due to blood loss (chronic) D50.0
    acute D62

Anemia — *continued*
  microcytic — *continued*
   familial D56.8
  microdrepanocytosis D57.40
  microelliptopoikilocytic (Rietti-Greppi- Micheli) D56.9
  miner's B76.9 [D63.8]
  myelodysplastic D46.9
  myelofibrosis D75.81
  myelogenous D64.89
  myelopathic D64.89
  myelophthisic D61.82
  myeloproliferative D47.Z9 (*following* D47.4)
  newborn P61.4
   due to
    ABO (antibodies, isoimmunization, maternal/fe-
     tal incompatibility) P55.1
    Rh (antibodies, isoimmunization, maternal/fetal
     incompatibility) P55.0
   following fetal blood loss P61.3
   posthemorrhagic (fetal) P61.3
  nonspherocytic hemolytic — *see* Anemia, hemolytic,
   nonspherocytic
  normocytic (infectional) D64.9
   due to blood loss (chronic) D50.0
    acute D62
   myelophthisic D61.82
  nutritional (deficiency) D53.9
   with
    poor iron absorption D50.8
    specified deficiency NEC D53.8
    megaloblastic D52.0
  of prematurity P61.2
  orotaciduric (congenital) (hereditary) D53.0
  osteosclerotic D64.89
  ovalocytosis (hereditary) — *see* Elliptocytosis
  paludal (*see also* Malaria) B54 [D63.8]
  pernicious (congenital) (malignant) (progressive) D51.0
  pleochromic D64.89
   of sprue D52.8
  posthemorrhagic (chronic) D50.0
   acute D62
   newborn P61.3
  postoperative (postprocedural)
   due to (acute) blood loss D62
    chronic blood loss D50.0
   specified NEC D64.9
  postpartum O90.81
  pressure D64.89
  progressive D64.9
   malignant D51.0
   pernicious D51.0
  protein-deficiency D53.0
  pseudoleukemica infantum D64.89
  pure red cell D60.9
   congenital D61.01
  pyridoxine-responsive D64.3
  pyruvate kinase deficiency D55.2
  refractory D46.4
   with
    excess of blasts D46.20
     1 (RAEB 1) D46.21
     2 (RAEB 2) D46.22
     in transformation (RAEB T) — *see* Leukemia,
      acute myeloblastic
    hemochromatosis D46.1
    sideroblasts (ring) (RARS) D46.1
   without ring sideroblasts, so stated D46.0
   without sideroblasts without excess of blasts D46.0
   megaloblastic D53.1
   sideroblastic D46.1
   sideropenic D50.9
  Rietti-Greppi-Micheli D56.9
  scorbutic D53.2
  secondary to
   blood loss (chronic) D50.0
    acute D62
   hemorrhage (chronic) D50.0
    acute D62
  semiplastic D61.89
  sickle-cell — *see* Disease, sickle-cell
  sideroblastic D64.3
   hereditary D64.0
   hypochromic, sex-linked D64.0
   pyridoxine-responsive NEC D64.3
   refractory D46.1
   secondary (due to)
    disease D64.1
    drugs and toxins D64.2

Anemia — *continued*
  sideroblastic — *continued*
   specified type NEC D64.3
  sideropenic (refractory) D50.9
   due to blood loss (chronic) D50.0
    acute D62
  simple chronic D53.9
  specified type NEC D64.89
  spherocytic (hereditary) — *see* Spherocytosis
  splenic D64.89
  splenomegalic D64.89
  stomatocytosis D58.8
  syphilitic (acquired) (late) A52.79 [D63.8]
  target cell D64.89
  thalassemia D56.9
  thrombocytopenic — *see* Thrombocytopenia
  toxic D61.2
  tropical B76.9 [D63.8]
   macrocytic D52.8
  tuberculous A18.89 [D63.8]
  vegan D51.3
  vitamin
   B6-responsive D64.3
   B12 deficiency (dietary) pernicious D51.0
  von Jaksch's D64.89
  Witts' (achlorhydric anemia) D50.8
Anemophobia F40.228
Anencephalus, anencephaly Q00.0
Anergasia — *see* Psychosis, organic
Anesthesia, anesthetic R20.0
  complication or reaction NEC (*see also* Complications,
   anesthesia) T88.59 ☑
   due to
    correct substance properly administered — *see*
     Table of Drugs and Chemicals, by drug,
     adverse effect
    overdose or wrong substance given — *see* Ta-
     ble of Drugs and Chemicals, by drug,
     poisoning
  cornea H18.81- ☑
  dissociative F44.6
  functional (hysterical) F44.6
  hyperesthetic, thalamic G89.0
  hysterical F44.6
  local skin lesion R20.0
  sexual (psychogenic) F52.1
  shock (due to) T88.2 ☑
  skin R20.0
  testicular N50.9
Anetoderma (maculosum) (of) L90.8
  Jadassohn-Pellizzari L90.2
  Schweniger-Buzzi L90.1
Aneurin deficiency E51.9
Aneurysm (anastomotic) (artery) (cirsoid) (diffuse) (false)
  (fusiform) (multiple) (saccular) I72.9
  abdominal (aorta) I71.4
   ruptured I71.3
   syphilitic A52.01
  aorta, aortic (nonsyphilitic) I71.9
   abdominal I71.4
    ruptured I71.3
   arch I71.2
    ruptured I71.1
   arteriosclerotic I71.9
    ruptured I71.8
   ascending I71.2
    ruptured I71.1
   congenital Q25.4
   descending I71.9
    abdominal I71.4
     ruptured I71.3
    ruptured I71.8
    thoracic I71.2
     ruptured I71.1
   ruptured I71.8
   sinus, congenital Q25.4
   syphilitic A52.01
   thoracic I71.2
    ruptured I71.1
   thoracoabdominal I71.6
    ruptured I71.5
   thorax, thoracic (arch) I71.2
    ruptured I71.1
   transverse I71.2
    ruptured I71.1
   valve (heart) (*see also* Endocarditis, aortic) I35.8

Aneurysm — *continued*
- arteriosclerotic I72.9
  - cerebral I67.1
    - ruptured — *see* Hemorrhage, intracranial, subarachnoid
  - arteriovenous (congenital) (*see also* Malformation, arteriovenous)
    - acquired I77.0
      - brain I67.1
      - coronary I25.41
      - pulmonary I28.0
    - brain Q28.2
      - ruptured I60.8
    - peripheral — *see* Malformation, arteriovenous, peripheral
    - precerebral vessels Q28.0
    - specified site NEC (*see also* Malformation, arteriovenous)
      - acquired I77.0
- basal — *see* Aneurysm, brain
- berry (congenital) (nonruptured) I67.1
  - ruptured I60.7
- brain I67.1
  - arteriosclerotic I67.1
    - ruptured — *see* Hemorrhage, intracranial, subarachnoid
  - arteriovenous (congenital) (nonruptured) Q28.2
    - acquired I67.1
      - ruptured I60.8
    - ruptured I60.8
  - berry (congenital) (nonruptured) I67.1
    - ruptured (*see also* Hemorrhage, intracranial, subarachnoid) I60.7
  - congenital Q28.3
    - ruptured I60.7
  - meninges I67.1
    - ruptured I60.8
  - miliary (congenital) (nonruptured) I67.1
    - ruptured (*see also* Hemorrhage, intracranial, subarachnoid) I60.7
  - mycotic I33.0
  - ruptured — *see* Hemorrhage, intracranial, subarachnoid
  - syphilitic (hemorrhage) A52.05
- cardiac (false) (*see also* Aneurysm, heart) I25.3
- carotid artery (common) (external) I72.0
  - internal (intracranial) I67.1
    - extracranial portion I72.0
    - ruptured into brain I60.0- ☑
  - syphilitic A52.09
    - intracranial A52.05
- cavernous sinus I67.1
  - arteriovenous (congenital) (nonruptured) Q28.3
    - ruptured I60.8
- celiac I72.8
- central nervous system, syphilitic A52.05
- cerebral — *see* Aneurysm, brain
- chest — *see* Aneurysm, thorax
- circle of Willis I67.1
  - congenital Q28.3
    - ruptured I60.6
  - ruptured I60.6
- common iliac artery I72.3
- congenital (peripheral) Q27.8
  - brain Q28.3
    - ruptured I60.7
  - coronary Q24.5
  - digestive system Q27.8
  - lower limb Q27.8
  - pulmonary Q25.79
  - retina Q14.1
  - specified site NEC Q27.8
  - upper limb Q27.8
- conjunctiva — *see* Abnormality, conjunctiva, vascular
- conus arteriosus — *see* Aneurysm, heart
- coronary (arteriosclerotic) (artery) I25.41
  - arteriovenous, congenital Q24.5
  - congenital Q24.5
  - ruptured — *see* Infarct, myocardium
  - syphilitic A52.06
  - vein I25.89
- cylindroid (aorta) I71.9
  - ruptured I71.8
  - syphilitic A52.01
- ductus arteriosus Q25.0
- endocardial, infective (any valve) I33.0
- femoral (artery) (ruptured) I72.4
- gastroduodenal I72.8

Aneurysm — *continued*
- gastroepiploic I72.8
- heart (wall) (chronic or with a stated duration of over 4 weeks) I25.3
  - valve — *see* Endocarditis
- hepatic I72.8
- iliac (common) (artery) (ruptured) I72.3
- infective I72.9
  - endocardial (any valve) I33.0
- innominate (nonsyphilitic) I72.8
  - syphilitic A52.09
- interauricular septum — *see* Aneurysm, heart
- interventricular septum — *see* Aneurysm, heart
- intrathoracic (nonsyphilitic) I71.2
  - ruptured I71.1
  - syphilitic A52.01
- lower limb I72.4
- lung (pulmonary artery) I28.1
- mediastinal (nonsyphilitic) I72.8
  - syphilitic A52.09
- miliary (congenital) I67.1
  - ruptured — *see* Hemorrhage, intracerebral, subarachnoid, intracranial
- mitral (heart) (valve) I34.8
- mural — *see* Aneurysm, heart
- mycotic I72.9
  - endocardial (any valve) I33.0
  - ruptured, brain — *see* Hemorrhage, intracerebral, subarachnoid
- myocardium — *see* Aneurysm, heart
- neck I72.0
- pancreaticoduodenal I72.8
- patent ductus arteriosus Q25.0
- peripheral NEC I72.8
  - congenital Q27.8
    - digestive system Q27.8
    - lower limb Q27.8
    - specified site NEC Q27.8
    - upper limb Q27.8
- popliteal (artery) (ruptured) I72.4
- precerebral, congenital (nonruptured) Q28.1
- pulmonary I28.1
  - arteriovenous Q25.72
    - acquired I28.0
  - syphilitic A52.09
  - valve (heart) — *see* Endocarditis, pulmonary
- racemose (peripheral) I72.9
  - congenital — *see* Aneurysm, congenital
- radial I72.1
- Rasmussen NEC A15.0
- renal (artery) I72.2
- retina (*see also* Disorder, retina, microaneurysms)
  - congenital Q14.1
  - diabetic — *see* Diabetes, microaneurysms, retinal
- sinus of Valsalva Q25.4
- specified NEC I72.8
- spinal (cord) I72.8
  - syphilitic (hemorrhage) A52.09
- splenic I72.8
- subclavian (artery) (ruptured) I72.8
  - syphilitic A52.09
- superior mesenteric I72.8
- syphilitic (aorta) A52.01
  - central nervous system A52.05
  - congenital (late) A50.54 [I79.0]
  - spine, spinal A52.09
- thoracoabdominal (aorta) I71.6
  - ruptured I71.5
  - syphilitic A52.01
- thorax, thoracic (aorta) (arch) (nonsyphilitic) I71.2
  - ruptured I71.1
  - syphilitic A52.01
- traumatic (complication) (early), specified site — *see* Injury, blood vessel
- tricuspid (heart) (valve) I07.8
- ulnar I72.1
- upper limb (ruptured) I72.1
- valve, valvular — *see* Endocarditis
- venous (*see also* Varix) I86.8
  - congenital Q27.8
    - digestive system Q27.8
    - lower limb Q27.8
    - specified site NEC Q27.8
    - upper limb Q27.8
- ventricle — *see* Aneurysm, heart
- visceral NEC I72.8

Angelman syndrome Q93.5
Anger R45.4

Angiectasis, angiectopia I99.8
Angiitis I77.6
- allergic granulomatous M30.1
- hypersensitivity M31.0
- necrotizing M31.9
  - specified NEC M31.8
- nervous system, granulomatous I67.7
Angina (attack) (cardiac) (chest) (heart) (pectoris) (syndrome) (vasomotor) I20.9
- with
  - atherosclerotic heart disease — *see* Arteriosclerosis, coronary (artery),
  - documented spasm I20.1
- abdominal K55.1
- accelerated — *see* Angina, unstable
- agranulocytic — *see* Agranulocytosis
- angiospastic — *see* Angina, with documented spasm
- aphthous B08.5
- crescendo — *see* Angina, unstable
- croupous J05.0
- cruris I73.9
- de novo effort — *see* Angina, unstable
- diphtheritic, membranous A36.0
- equivalent I20.8
- exudative, chronic J37.0
- following acute myocardial infarction I23.7
- gangrenous diphtheritic A36.0
- intestinal K55.1
- Ludovici K12.2
- Ludwig's K12.2
- malignant diphtheritic A36.0
- membranous J05.0
  - diphtheritic A36.0
  - Vincent's A69.1
- mesenteric K55.1
- monocytic — *see* Mononucleosis, infectious
- of effort — *see* Angina, specified NEC
- phlegmonous J36
  - diphtheritic A36.0
- post-infarctional I23.7
- pre-infarctional — *see* Angina, unstable
- Prinzmetal — *see* Angina, with documented spasm
- progressive — *see* Angina, unstable
- pseudomembranous A69.1
- pultaceous, diphtheritic A36.0
- spasm-induced — *see* Angina, with documented spasm
- specified NEC I20.8
- stable I20.9
- stenocardia — *see* Angina, specified NEC
- stridulous, diphtheritic A36.2
- tonsil J36
- trachealis J05.0
- unstable I20.0
- variant — *see* Angina, with documented spasm
- Vincent's A69.1
- worsening effort — *see* Angina, unstable
Angioblastoma — *see* Neoplasm, connective tissue, uncertain behavior
Angiocholecystitis — *see* Cholecystitis, acute
Angiocholitis (*see also* Cholecystitis, acute) K83.0
Angiodysgenesis spinalis G95.19
Angiodysplasia (cecum) (colon) K55.20
- with bleeding K55.21
- duodenum (and stomach) K31.819
  - with bleeding K31.811
- stomach (and duodenum) K31.819
  - with bleeding K31.811
Angioedema (allergic) (any site) (with urticaria) T78.3 ☑
- hereditary D84.1
Angioendothelioma — *see* Neoplasm, uncertain behavior, by site
- benign D18.00
  - intra-abdominal D18.03
  - intracranial D18.02
  - skin D18.01
  - specified site NEC D18.09
- bone — *see* Neoplasm, bone, malignant
- Ewing's — *see* Neoplasm, bone, malignant
Angioendotheliomatosis C85.8- ☑
Angiofibroma (*see also* Neoplasm, benign, by site)
- juvenile
  - specified site — *see* Neoplasm, benign, by site
  - unspecified site D10.6
Angiohemophilia (A) (B) D68.0
Angioid streaks (choroid) (macula) (retina) H35.33

Angiokeratoma — *see* Neoplasm, skin, benign
  corporis diffusum E75.21
Angioleiomyoma — *see* Neoplasm, connective tissue,
  benign
Angiolipoma (*see also* Lipoma)
  infiltrating — *see* Lipoma
Angioma (*see also* Hemangioma, by site)
  capillary I78.1
  hemorrhagicum hereditaria I78.0
  intra-abdominal D18.03
  intracranial D18.02
  malignant — *see* Neoplasm, connective tissue, malig-
    nant
  plexiform D18.00
    intra-abdominal D18.03
    intracranial D18.02
    skin D18.01
    specified site NEC D18.09
  senile I78.1
  serpiginosum L81.7
  skin D18.01
  specified site NEC D18.09
  spider I78.1
  stellate I78.1
  venous Q28.3
Angiomatosis Q82.8
  bacillary A79.89
  encephalotrigeminal Q85.8
  hemorrhagic familial I78.0
  hereditary familial I78.0
  liver K76.4
Angiomyolipoma — *see* Lipoma
Angiomyoliposarcoma — *see* Neoplasm, connective
  tissue, malignant
Angiomyoma — *see* Neoplasm, connective tissue, benign
Angiomyosarcoma — *see* Neoplasm, connective tissue,
  malignant
Angiomyxoma — *see* Neoplasm, connective tissue, uncertain behavior
Angioneurosis F45.8
Angioneurotic edema (allergic) (any site) (with urticaria)
  T78.3 ☑
  hereditary D84.1
Angiopathia, angiopathy I99.9
  cerebral I67.9
    amyloid E85.4 [I68.0]
  diabetic (peripheral) — *see* Diabetes, angiopathy
  peripheral I73.9
    diabetic — *see* Diabetes, angiopathy
    specified type NEC I73.89
  retinae syphilitica A52.05
  retinalis (juvenilis)
    diabetic — *see* Diabetes, retinopathy
    proliferative — *see* Retinopathy, proliferative
Angiosarcoma (*see also* Neoplasm, connective tissue,
  malignant)
  liver C22.3
Angiosclerosis — *see* Arteriosclerosis
Angiospasm (peripheral) (traumatic) (vessel) I73.9
  brachial plexus G54.0
  cerebral G45.9
  cervical plexus G54.2
  nerve
    arm — *see* Mononeuropathy, upper limb
      axillary G54.0
      median — *see* Lesion, nerve, median
      ulnar — *see* Lesion, nerve, ulnar
    axillary G54.0
    leg — *see* Mononeuropathy, lower limb
    median — *see* Lesion, nerve, median
    plantar — *see* Lesion, nerve, plantar
    ulnar — *see* Lesion, nerve, ulnar
Angiospastic disease or edema I73.9
Angiostrongyliasis
  due to
    Parastrongylus
      cantonensis B83.2
      costaricensis B81.3
  intestinal B81.3
Anguillulosis — *see* Strongyloidiasis
Angulation
  cecum — *see* Obstruction, intestine
  coccyx (acquired) (*see also* subcategory) M43.8 ☑
    congenital NEC Q76.49

Angulation — *continued*
  femur (acquired) (*see also* Deformity, limb, specified
    type NEC, thigh)
    congenital Q74.2
  intestine (large) (small) — *see* Obstruction, intestine
  sacrum (acquired) (*see also* subcategory) M43.8 ☑
    congenital NEC Q76.49
  sigmoid (flexure) — *see* Obstruction, intestine
  spine — *see* Dorsopathy, deforming, specified NEC
  tibia (acquired) (*see also* Deformity, limb, specified
    type NEC, lower leg)
    congenital Q74.2
  ureter N13.5
    with infection N13.6
  wrist (acquired) (*see also* Deformity, limb, specified
    type NEC, forearm)
    congenital Q74.0
Angulus infectiosus (lips) K13.0
Anhedonia R45.84
Anhidrosis L74.4
Anhydration, anhydremia E86.0
  with
    hypernatremia E87.0
    hyponatremia E87.1
Anhydremia E86.0
  with
    hypernatremia E87.0
    hyponatremia E87.1
Anidrosis L74.4
Aniridia (congenital) Q13.1
Anisakiasis (infection) (infestation) B81.0
Anisakis larvae infestation B81.0
Aniseikonia H52.32
Anisocoria (pupil) H57.02
  congenital Q13.2
Anisocytosis R71.8
Anisometropia (congenital) H52.31
Ankle — *see* condition
Ankyloblepharon (eyelid) (acquired) (*see also* Blepharophimosis)
  filiforme (adnatum) (congenital) Q10.3
  total Q10.3
Ankyloglossia Q38.1
Ankylosis (fibrous) (osseous) (joint) M24.60
  ankle M24.67- ☑
  arthrodesis status Z98.1
  cricoarytenoid (cartilage) (joint) (larynx) J38.7
  dental K03.5
  ear ossicles H74.31- ☑
  elbow M24.62- ☑
  foot M24.67- ☑
  hand M24.64- ☑
  hip M24.65- ☑
  incostapedial joint (infectional) — *see* Ankylosis, ear
    ossicles
  jaw (temporomandibular) M26.61
  knee M24.66- ☑
  lumbosacral (joint) M43.27
  postoperative (status) Z98.1
  produced by surgical fusion, status Z98.1
  sacro-iliac (joint) M43.28
  shoulder M24.61- ☑
  spine (joint) (*see also* Fusion, spine)
    spondylitic — *see* Spondylitis, ankylosing
  surgical Z98.1
  temporomandibular M26.61
  tooth, teeth (hard tissues) K03.5
  wrist M24.63- ☑
Ankylostoma — *see* Ancylostoma
Ankylostomiasis — *see* Ancylostomiasis
Ankylurethria — *see* Stricture, urethra
Annular (*see also* condition)
  detachment, cervix N88.8
  organ or site, congenital NEC — *see* Distortion
  pancreas (congenital) Q45.1
Anodontia (complete) (partial) (vera) K00.0
  acquired K08.10 ☑
Anomaly, anomalous (congenital) (unspecified type)
  Q89.9
  abdominal wall NEC Q79.59
  acoustic nerve Q07.8
  adrenal (gland) Q89.1
  Alder (-Reilly) (leukocyte granulation) D72.0
  alimentary tract Q45.9
    upper Q40.9

Anomaly, anomalous — *continued*
  alveolar M26.70
    hyperplasia M26.79
      mandibular M26.72
      maxillary M26.71
    hypoplasia M26.79
      mandibular M26.74
      maxillary M26.73
    ridge (process) M26.79
    specified NEC M26.79
  ankle (joint) Q74.2
  anus Q43.9
  aorta (arch) NEC Q25.4
    coarctation (preductal) (postductal) Q25.1
  aortic cusp or valve Q23.9
  appendix Q43.8
  apple peel syndrome Q41.1
  aqueduct of Sylvius Q03.0
    with spina bifida — *see* Spina bifida, with hydro-
      cephalus
  arm Q74.0
  arteriovenous NEC
    coronary Q24.5
    gastrointestinal Q27.33
      acquired — *see* Angiodysplasia
  artery (peripheral) Q27.9
    basilar NEC Q28.1
    cerebral Q28.3
    coronary Q24.5
    digestive system Q27.8
    eye Q15.8
    great Q25.9
      specified NEC Q25.8
    lower limb Q27.8
    peripheral Q27.9
      specified NEC Q27.8
    pulmonary NEC Q25.79
    renal Q27.2
    retina Q14.1
    specified site NEC Q27.8
    subclavian Q27.8
    umbilical Q27.0
    upper limb Q27.8
    vertebral NEC Q28.1
  aryteno-epiglottic folds Q31.8
  atrial
    bands or folds Q20.8
    septa Q21.1
  atrioventricular
    excitation I45.6
    septum Q21.0
  auditory canal Q17.8
  auricle
    ear Q17.8
      causing impairment of hearing Q16.9
    heart Q20.8
  Axenfeld's Q15.0
  back Q89.9
  band
    atrial Q20.8
    heart Q24.8
    ventricular Q24.8
  Bartholin's duct Q38.4
  biliary duct or passage Q44.5
  bladder Q64.70
    absence Q64.5
    diverticulum Q64.6
    exstrophy Q64.10
      cloacal Q64.12
      extroversion Q64.19
      specified type NEC Q64.19
      supravesical fissure Q64.11
    neck obstruction Q64.31
    specified type NEC Q64.79
  bone Q79.9
    arm Q74.0
    face Q75.9
    leg Q74.2
    pelvic girdle Q74.2
    shoulder girdle Q74.0
    skull Q75.9
      with
        anencephaly Q00.0
        encephalocele — *see* Encephalocele
        hydrocephalus Q03.9
          with spina bifida — *see* Spina bifida, by
            site, with hydrocephalus
        microcephaly Q02

Anomaly, anomalous — *continued*
- brain (multiple) Q04.9
  - vessel Q28.3
- breast Q83.9
- broad ligament Q50.6
- bronchus Q32.4
- bulbus cordis Q21.9
- bursa Q79.9
- canal of Nuck Q52.4
- canthus Q10.3
- capillary Q27.9
- cardiac Q24.9
  - chambers Q20.9
    - specified NEC Q20.8
  - septal closure Q21.9
    - specified NEC Q21.8
  - valve NEC Q24.8
    - pulmonary Q22.3
- cardiovascular system Q28.8
- carpus Q74.0
- caruncle, lacrimal Q10.6
- cascade stomach Q40.2
- cauda equina Q06.3
- cecum Q43.9
- cerebral Q04.9
  - vessels Q28.3
- cervix Q51.9
- Chédiak-Higashi (-Steinbrinck) (congenital gigantism of peroxidase granules) E70.330
- cheek Q18.9
- chest wall Q67.8
  - bones Q76.9
- chin Q18.9
- chordae tendineae Q24.8
- choroid Q14.3
  - plexus Q07.8
- chromosomes, chromosomal Q99.9
  - D (1) — *see* condition, chromosome 13
  - E (3) — *see* condition, chromosome 18
  - G — *see* condition, chromosome 21
  - sex
    - female phenotype Q97.8
    - gonadal dysgenesis (pure) Q99.1
    - Klinefelter's Q98.4
    - male phenotype Q98.9
    - Turner's Q96.9
  - specified NEC Q99.8
- cilia Q10.3
- circulatory system Q28.9
- clavicle Q74.0
- clitoris Q52.6
- coccyx Q76.49
- colon Q43.9
- common duct Q44.5
- communication
  - coronary artery Q24.5
  - left ventricle with right atrium Q21.0
- concha (ear) Q17.3
- connection
  - portal vein Q26.5
  - pulmonary venous Q26.4
    - partial Q26.3
    - total Q26.2
  - renal artery with kidney Q27.2
- cornea (shape) Q13.4
- coronary artery or vein Q24.5
- cranium — *see* Anomaly, skull
- cricoid cartilage Q31.8
- cystic duct Q44.5
- dental
  - alveolar — *see* Anomaly, alveolar
  - arch relationship M26.20
    - specified NEC M26.29
- dentofacial M26.9
  - alveolar — *see* Anomaly, alveolar
  - dental arch relationship M26.20
    - specified NEC M26.29
  - functional M26.50
    - specified NEC M26.59
  - jaw size M26.00
    - macrogenia M26.05
    - mandibular
      - hyperplasia M26.03
      - hypoplasia M26.04
    - maxillary
      - hyperplasia M26.01
      - hypoplasia M26.02
    - microgenia M26.06

Anomaly, anomalous — *continued*
- dentofacial — *continued*
  - jaw size — *continued*
    - specified type NEC M26.09
  - jaw-cranial base relationship M26.10
    - asymmetry M26.12
      - maxillary M26.11
    - specified type NEC M26.19
  - malocclusion M26.4
    - dental arch relationship NEC M26.29
    - jaw size — *see* Anomaly, dentofacial, jaw size
    - jaw-cranial base relationship — *see* Anomaly, dentofacial, jaw-cranial base relationship
  - specified type NEC M26.89
  - temporomandibular joint M26.60
    - adhesions M26.61
    - ankylosis M26.61
    - arthralgia M26.62
    - articular disc M26.63
    - specified type NEC M26.69
  - tooth position, fully erupted M26.30
    - specified NEC M26.39
- dermatoglyphic Q82.8
- diaphragm (apertures) NEC Q79.1
- digestive organ(s) or tract Q45.9
  - lower Q43.9
  - upper Q40.9
- distance, interarch (excessive) (inadequate) M26.25
- distribution, coronary artery Q24.5
- ductus
  - arteriosus Q25.0
  - botalli Q25.0
- duodenum Q43.9
- dura (brain) Q04.9
  - spinal cord Q06.9
- ear (external) Q17.9
  - causing impairment of hearing Q16.9
  - inner Q16.5
  - middle (causing impairment of hearing) Q16.4
    - ossicles Q16.3
- Ebstein's (heart) (tricuspid valve) Q22.5
- ectodermal Q82.9
- Eisenmenger's (ventricular septal defect) Q21.8
- ejaculatory duct Q55.4
- elbow Q74.0
- endocrine gland NEC Q89.2
- epididymis Q55.4
- epiglottis Q31.8
- esophagus Q39.9
- eustachian tube Q17.8
- eye Q15.9
  - anterior segment Q13.9
    - specified NEC Q13.89
  - posterior segment Q14.9
    - specified NEC Q14.8
  - ptosis (eyelid) Q10.0
  - specified NEC Q15.8
- eyebrow Q18.8
- eyelid Q10.3
  - ptosis Q10.0
- face Q18.9
  - bone(s) Q75.9
- fallopian tube Q50.6
- fascia Q79.9
- femur NEC Q74.2
- fibula NEC Q74.2
- finger Q74.0
- fixation, intestine Q43.3
- flexion (joint) NOS Q74.9
  - hip or thigh Q65.89
- foot NEC Q74.2
  - varus (congenital) Q66.3
- foramen
  - Botalli Q21.1
  - ovale Q21.1
- forearm Q74.0
- forehead Q75.8
- form, teeth K00.2
- fovea centralis Q14.1
- frontal bone — *see* Anomaly, skull
- gallbladder (position) (shape) (size) Q44.1
- Gartner's duct Q52.4
- gastrointestinal tract Q45.9
- genitalia, genital organ(s) or system
  - female Q52.9
    - external Q52.70
    - internal NOS Q52.9

Anomaly, anomalous — *continued*
- genitalia, genital organ(s) or system — *continued*
  - male Q55.9
    - hydrocele P83.5
    - specified NEC Q55.8
- genitourinary NEC
  - female Q52.9
  - male Q55.9
- Gerbode Q21.0
- glottis Q31.8
- granulation or granulocyte, genetic (constitutional) (leukocyte) D72.0
- gum Q38.6
- gyri Q07.9
- hair Q84.2
- hand Q74.0
- hard tissue formation in pulp K04.3
- head — *see* Anomaly, skull
- heart Q24.9
  - auricle Q20.8
  - bands or folds Q24.8
  - fibroelastosis cordis I42.4
  - obstructive NEC Q22.6
  - patent ductus arteriosus (Botalli) Q25.0
  - septum Q21.9
    - auricular Q21.1
    - interatrial Q21.1
    - interventricular Q21.0
      - with pulmonary stenosis or atresia, dextraposition of aorta and hypertrophy of right ventricle Q21.3
    - specified NEC Q21.8
    - ventricular Q21.0
      - with pulmonary stenosis or atresia, dextraposition of aorta and hypertrophy of right ventricle Q21.3
  - tetralogy of Fallot Q21.3
  - valve NEC Q24.8
    - aortic
      - bicuspid valve Q23.1
      - insufficiency Q23.1
      - stenosis Q23.0
        - subaortic Q24.4
    - mitral
      - insufficiency Q23.3
      - stenosis Q23.2
    - pulmonary Q22.3
      - atresia Q22.0
      - insufficiency Q22.2
      - stenosis Q22.1
        - infundibular Q24.3
        - subvalvular Q24.3
    - tricuspid
      - atresia Q22.4
      - stenosis Q22.4
  - ventricle Q20.8
- heel NEC Q74.2
- Hegglin's D72.0
- hemianencephaly Q00.0
- hemicephaly Q00.0
- hemicrania Q00.0
- hepatic duct Q44.5
- hip NEC Q74.2
- hourglass stomach Q40.2
- humerus Q74.0
- hydatid of Morgagni
  - female Q50.5
  - male (epididymal) Q55.4
    - testicular Q55.29
- hymen Q52.4
- hypersegmentation of neutrophils, hereditary D72.0
- hypophyseal Q89.2
- ileocecal (coil) (valve) Q43.9
- ileum Q43.9
- ilium NEC Q74.2
- integument Q84.9
  - specified NEC Q84.8
- interarch distance (excessive) (inadequate) M26.25
- intervertebral cartilage or disc Q76.49
- intestine (large) (small) Q43.9
  - with anomalous adhesions, fixation or malrotation Q43.3
- iris Q13.2
- ischium NEC Q74.2
- jaw — *see* Anomaly, dentofacial
  - alveolar — *see* Anomaly, alveolar
- jaw-cranial base relationship — *see* Anomaly, dentofacial, jaw-cranial base relationship

Anomaly, anomalous — *continued*
- jejunum Q43.8
- joint Q74.9
  - specified NEC Q74.8
- Jordan's D72.0
- kidney(s) (calyx) (pelvis) Q63.9
  - artery Q27.2
  - specified NEC Q63.8
- Klippel-Feil (brevicollis) Q76.1
- knee Q74.1
- labium (majus) (minus) Q52.70
- labyrinth, membranous Q16.5
- lacrimal apparatus or duct Q10.6
- larynx, laryngeal (muscle) Q31.9
  - web (bed) Q31.0
- lens Q12.9
- leukocytes, genetic D72.0
  - granulation (constitutional) D72.0
- lid (fold) Q10.3
- ligament Q79.9
  - broad Q50.6
  - round Q52.8
- limb Q74.9
  - lower NEC Q74.2
    - reduction deformity — *see* Defect, reduction, lower limb
  - upper Q74.0
- lip Q38.0
- liver Q44.7
  - duct Q44.5
- lower limb NEC Q74.2
- lumbosacral (joint) (region) Q76.49
  - kyphosis — *see* Kyphosis, congenital
  - lordosis — *see* Lordosis, congenital
- lung (fissure) (lobe) Q33.9
- mandible — *see* Anomaly, dentofacial
- maxilla — *see* Anomaly, dentofacial
- May (-Hegglin) D72.0
- meatus urinarius NEC Q64.79
- meningeal bands or folds Q07.9
  - constriction of Q07.8
    - spinal Q06.9
- meninges Q07.9
  - cerebral Q04.8
  - spinal Q06.9
- meningocele Q05.9
- mesentery Q45.9
- metacarpus Q74.0
- metatarsus NEC Q74.2
- middle ear Q16.4
  - ossicles Q16.3
- mitral (leaflets) (valve) Q23.9
  - insufficiency Q23.3
  - specified NEC Q23.8
  - stenosis Q23.2
- mouth Q38.6
- Müllerian (*see also* Anomaly, by site)
  - uterus NEC Q51.818
- multiple NEC Q89.7
- muscle Q79.9
  - eyelid Q10.3
- musculoskeletal system, except limbs Q79.9
- myocardium Q24.8
- nail Q84.6
- narrowness, eyelid Q10.3
- nasal sinus (wall) Q30.8
- neck (any part) Q18.9
- nerve Q07.9
  - acoustic Q07.8
  - optic Q07.8
- nervous system (central) Q07.9
- nipple Q83.9
- nose, nasal (bones) (cartilage) (septum) (sinus) Q30.9
  - specified NEC Q30.8
- ocular muscle Q15.8
- omphalomesenteric duct Q43.0
- opening, pulmonary veins Q26.4
- optic
  - disc Q14.2
  - nerve Q07.8
- opticociliary vessels Q13.2
- orbit (eye) Q10.7
- organ Q89.9
  - of Corti Q16.5
- origin
  - artery
    - innominate Q25.8
    - pulmonary Q25.79

Anomaly, anomalous — *continued*
- origin — *continued*
  - artery — *continued*
    - renal Q27.2
    - subclavian Q25.8
  - osseous meatus (ear) Q16.1
- ovary Q50.39
- oviduct Q50.6
- palate (hard) (soft) NEC Q38.5
- pancreas or pancreatic duct Q45.3
- papillary muscles Q24.8
- parathyroid gland Q89.2
- paraurethral ducts Q64.79
- parotid (gland) Q38.4
- patella Q74.1
- Pelger-Huët (hereditary hyposegmentation) D72.0
- pelvic girdle NEC Q74.2
- pelvis (bony) NEC Q74.2
  - rachitic E64.3
- penis (glans) Q55.69
- pericardium Q24.8
- peripheral vascular system Q27.9
- Peter's Q13.4
- pharynx Q38.8
- pigmentation L81.9
  - congenital Q82.8
- pituitary (gland) Q89.2
- pleural (folds) Q34.0
- portal vein Q26.5
  - connection Q26.5
- position, tooth, teeth, fully erupted M26.30
  - specified NEC M26.39
- precerebral vessel Q28.1
- prepuce Q55.69
- prostate Q55.4
- pulmonary Q33.9
  - artery NEC Q25.79
  - valve Q22.3
    - atresia Q22.0
    - insufficiency Q22.2
    - specified type NEC Q22.3
    - stenosis Q22.1
      - infundibular Q24.3
      - subvalvular Q24.3
  - venous connection Q26.4
    - partial Q26.3
    - total Q26.2
- pupil Q13.2
  - function H57.00
    - anisocoria H57.02
    - Argyll Robertson pupil H57.01
    - miosis H57.03
    - mydriasis H57.04
    - specified type NEC H57.09
    - tonic pupil H57.05- ☑
- pylorus Q40.3
- radius Q74.0
- rectum Q43.9
- reduction (extremity) (limb)
  - femur (longitudinal) — *see* Defect, reduction, lower limb, longitudinal, femur
  - fibula (longitudinal) — *see* Defect, reduction, lower limb, longitudinal, fibula
  - lower limb — *see* Defect, reduction, lower limb
  - radius (longitudinal) — *see* Defect, reduction, upper limb, longitudinal, radius
  - tibia (longitudinal) — *see* Defect, reduction, lower limb, longitudinal, tibia
  - ulna (longitudinal) — *see* Defect, reduction, upper limb, longitudinal, ulna
  - upper limb — *see* Defect, reduction, upper limb
- refraction — *see* Disorder, refraction
- renal Q63.9
  - artery Q27.2
  - pelvis Q63.9
    - specified NEC Q63.8
- respiratory system Q34.9
  - specified NEC Q34.8
- retina Q14.1
- rib Q76.6
  - cervical Q76.5
- Rieger's Q13.81
- rotation — *see* Malrotation
  - hip or thigh Q65.89
- round ligament Q52.8
- sacroiliac (joint) NEC Q74.2
- sacrum NEC Q76.49
  - kyphosis — *see* Kyphosis, congenital

Anomaly, anomalous — *continued*
- sacrum — *continued*
  - lordosis — *see* Lordosis, congenital
- saddle nose, syphilitic A50.57
- salivary duct or gland Q38.4
- scapula Q74.0
- scrotum — *see* Malformation, testis and scrotum
- sebaceous gland Q82.9
- seminal vesicles Q55.4
- sense organs NEC Q07.8
- sex chromosomes NEC (*see also* Anomaly, chromosomes)
  - female phenotype Q97.8
  - male phenotype Q98.9
- shoulder (girdle) (joint) Q74.9
- sigmoid (flexure) Q43.9
- simian crease Q82.8
- sinus of Valsalva Q25.4
- skeleton generalized Q78.9
- skin (appendage) Q82.9
- skull Q75.9
  - with
    - anencephaly Q00.0
    - encephalocele — *see* Encephalocele
    - hydrocephalus Q03.9
      - with spina bifida — *see* Spina bifida, by site, with hydrocephalus
    - microcephaly Q02
- specified organ or site NEC Q89.8
- spermatic cord Q55.4
- spine, spinal NEC Q76.49
  - column NEC Q76.49
    - kyphosis — *see* Kyphosis, congenital
    - lordosis — *see* Lordosis, congenital
  - cord Q06.9
  - nerve root Q07.8
- spleen Q89.09
  - agenesis Q89.01
- stenonian duct Q38.4
- sternum NEC Q76.7
- stomach Q40.3
- submaxillary gland Q38.4
- tarsus NEC Q74.2
- tendon Q79.9
- testis — *see* Malformation, testis and scrotum
- thigh NEC Q74.2
- thorax (wall) Q67.8
  - bony Q76.9
- throat Q38.8
- thumb Q74.0
- thymus gland Q89.2
- thyroid (gland) Q89.2
  - cartilage Q31.8
- tibia NEC Q74.2
  - saber A50.56
- toe Q74.2
- tongue Q38.3
- tooth, teeth K00.9
  - eruption K00.6
  - position, fully erupted M26.30
  - spacing, fully erupted M26.30
- trachea (cartilage) Q32.1
- tragus Q17.9
- tricuspid (leaflet) (valve) Q22.9
  - atresia or stenosis Q22.4
  - Ebstein's Q22.5
- Uhl's (hypoplasia of myocardium, right ventricle) Q24.8
- ulna Q74.0
- umbilical artery Q27.0
- union
  - cricoid cartilage and thyroid cartilage Q31.8
  - thyroid cartilage and hyoid bone Q31.8
  - trachea with larynx Q31.8
- upper limb Q74.0
- urachus Q64.4
- ureter Q62.8
  - obstructive NEC Q62.39
    - cecoureterocele Q62.32
    - orthotopic ureterocele Q62.31
- urethra Q64.70
  - absence Q64.5
  - double Q64.74
  - fistula to rectum Q64.73
  - obstructive Q64.39
    - stricture Q64.32
  - prolapse Q64.71
  - specified type NEC Q64.79
- urinary tract Q64.9

Anomaly, anomalous — *continued*
  uterus Q51.9
    with only one functioning horn Q51.4
  uvula Q38.5
  vagina Q52.4
  valleculae Q31.8
  valve (heart) NEC Q24.8
    coronary sinus Q24.5
    inferior vena cava Q24.8
    pulmonary Q22.3
    sinus coronario Q24.5
    venae cavae inferioris Q24.8
  vas deferens Q55.4
  vascular Q27.9
    brain Q28.3
    ring Q25.4
  vein(s) (peripheral) Q27.9
    brain Q28.3
    cerebral Q28.3
    coronary Q24.5
    developmental Q28.3
    great Q26.9
      specified NEC Q26.8
  vena cava (inferior) (superior) Q26.9
  venous — *see* Anomaly, vein(s)
  venous return Q26.8
  ventricular
    bands or folds Q24.8
    septa Q21.0
  vertebra Q76.49
    kyphosis — *see* Kyphosis, congenital
    lordosis — *see* Lordosis, congenital
  vesicourethral orifice Q64.79
  vessel(s) Q27.9
    optic papilla Q14.2
    precerebral Q28.1
  vitelline duct Q43.0
  vitreous body or humor Q14.0
  vulva Q52.70
  wrist (joint) Q74.0
Anomia R48.8
Anonychia (congenital) Q84.3
  acquired L60.8
Anophthalmos, anophthalmus (congenital) (globe)
    Q11.1
  acquired Z90.01
Anopia, anopsia H53.46- ☑
  quadrant H53.46- ☑
Anorchia, anorchism, anorchidism Q55.0
Anorexia R63.0
  hysterical F44.89
  nervosa F50.00
    atypical F50.9
    binge-eating type F50.2
      with purging F50.02
    restricting type F50.01
Anorgasmy, psychogenic (female) F52.31
  male F52.32
Anosmia R43.0
  hysterical F44.6
  postinfectional J39.8
Anosognosia R41.89
Anosteoplasia Q78.9
Anovulatory cycle N97.0
Anoxemia R09.02
  newborn P84
Anoxia (pathological) R09.02
  altitude T70.29 ☑
  cerebral G93.1
    complicating
      anesthesia (general) (local) or other sedation
        T88.59 ☑
        in labor and delivery O74.3
        in pregnancy O29.21- ☑
        postpartum, puerperal O89.2
      delivery (cesarean) (instrumental) O75.4
    during a procedure G97.81
    newborn P84
    resulting from a procedure G97.82
  due to
    drowning T75.1 ☑
    high altitude T70.29 ☑
  heart — *see* Insufficiency, coronary
  intrauterine P84
  myocardial — *see* Insufficiency, coronary
  newborn P84
  spinal cord G95.11

Anoxia — *continued*
  systemic (by suffocation) (low content in atmosphere)
    — *see* Asphyxia, traumatic
Anteflexion — *see* Anteversion
Antenatal
  care (normal pregnancy) Z34.90
  screening (encounter for) of mother Z36
Antepartum — *see* condition
Anterior — *see* condition
Antero-occlusion M26.220
Anteversion
  cervix — *see* Anteversion, uterus
  femur (neck), congenital Q65.89
  uterus, uterine (cervix) (postinfectional) (postpartal,
    old) N85.4
    congenital Q51.818
    in pregnancy or childbirth — *see* Pregnancy,
      complicated by
Anthophobia F40.228
Anthracosilicosis J60
Anthracosis (lung) (occupational) J60
  lingua K14.3
Anthrax A22.9
  with pneumonia A22.1
  cerebral A22.8
  colitis A22.2
  cutaneous A22.0
  gastrointestinal A22.2
  inhalation A22.1
  intestinal A22.2
  meningitis A22.8
  pulmonary A22.1
  respiratory A22.1
  sepsis A22.7
  specified manifestation NEC A22.8
Anthropoid pelvis Q74.2
  with disproportion (fetopelvic) O33.0
Anthropophobia F40.10
  generalized F40.11
Antibodies, maternal (blood group) — *see* Isoimmu-
    nization, affecting management of pregnancy
  anti-D — *see* Isoimmunization, affecting management
    of pregnancy, Rh
  newborn P55.0
Antibody
  anticardiolipin R76.0
    with
      hemorrhagic disorder D68.312
      hypercoagulable state D68.61
  antiphosphatidylglycerol R76.0
    with
      hemorrhagic disorder D68.312
      hypercoagulable state D68.61
  antiphosphatidylinositol R76.0
    with
      hemorrhagic disorder D68.312
      hypercoagulable state D68.61
  antiphosphatidylserine R76.0
    with
      hemorrhagic disorder D68.312
      hypercoagulable state D68.61
  antiphospholipid R76.0
    with
      hemorrhagic disorder D68.312
      hypercoagulable state D68.61
Anticardiolipin syndrome D68.61
Anticoagulant, circulating (intrinsic) (*see also* Disorder,
    hemorrhagic) D68.318
  drug-induced (extrinsic) (*see also* Disorder, hemorrhag-
    ic) D68.32
Antidiuretic hormone syndrome E22.2
Antimonial cholera — *see* Poisoning, antimony
Antiphospholipid
  antibody
    with hemorrhagic disorder D68.312
    syndrome D68.61
Antisocial personality F60.2
Antithrombinemia — *see* Circulating anticoagulants
Antithromboplastinemia D68.318
Antithromboplastinogenemia D68.318
Antitoxin complication or reaction — *see* Complica-
    tions, vaccination
Antlophobia F40.228
Antritis J32.0
  maxilla J32.0
    acute J01.00
      recurrent J01.01

Antritis — *continued*
  stomach K29.60
    with bleeding K29.61
Antrum, antral — *see* condition
Anuria R34
  calculous (impacted) (recurrent) (*see also* Calculus,
    urinary) N20.9
  following
    abortion — *see* Abortion by type complicated by,
      renal failure
    ectopic or molar pregnancy O08.4
  newborn P96.0
  postprocedural N99.0
  postrenal N13.8
  traumatic (following crushing) T79.5 ☑
Anus, anal — *see* condition
Anusitis K62.89
Anxiety F41.9
  depression F41.8
  episodic paroxysmal F41.0
  generalized F41.1
  hysteria F41.8
  neurosis F41.1
  panic type F41.0
  reaction F41.1
  separation, abnormal (of childhood) F93.0
  specified NEC F41.8
  state F41.1
Aorta, aortic — *see* condition
Aortectasia — *see* Ectasia, aorta
  with aneurysm — *see* Aneurysm, aorta
Aortitis (nonsyphilitic) (calcific) I77.6
  arteriosclerotic I70.0
  Doehle-Heller A52.02
  luetic A52.02
  rheumatic — *see* Endocarditis, acute, rheumatic
  specific (syphilitic) A52.02
  syphilitic A52.02
    congenital A50.54 [I79.1]
Apathetic thyroid storm — *see* Thyrotoxicosis
Apathy R45.3
Apeirophobia F40.228
Apepsia K30
  psychogenic F45.8
Aperistalsis, esophagus K22.0
Apertognathia M26.29
Apert's syndrome Q87.0
Aphagia R13.0
  psychogenic F50.9
Aphakia (acquired) (postoperative) H27.0- ☑
  congenital Q12.3
Aphasia (amnestic) (global) (nominal) (semantic) (syntac-
    tic) R47.01
  acquired, with epilepsy (Landau-Kleffner syndrome)
    — *see* Epilepsy, specified NEC
  auditory (developmental) F80.2
  developmental (receptive type) F80.2
    expressive type F80.1
    Wernicke's F80.2
  following
    cerebrovascular disease I69.920
      cerebral infarction I69.320
      intracerebral hemorrhage I69.120
      nontraumatic intracranial hemorrhage NEC
        I69.220
      specified disease NEC I69.820
      subarachnoid hemorrhage I69.020
  primary progressive G31.01 [F02.80]
    with behavioral disturbance G31.01 [F02.81]
  progressive isolated G31.01 [F02.80]
    with behavioral disturbance G31.01 [F02.81]
  sensory F80.2
  syphilis, tertiary A52.19
  Wernicke's (developmental) F80.2
Aphonia (organic) R49.1
  hysterical F44.4
  psychogenic F44.4
Aphthae, aphthous (*see also* condition)
  Bednar's K12.0
  cachectic K14.0
  epizootic B08.8
  fever B08.8
  oral (recurrent) K12.0
  stomatitis (major) (minor) K12.0
  thrush B37.0
  ulcer (oral) (recurrent) K12.0
    genital organ(s) NEC
      female N76.6

Aphthae, aphthous — *continued*
  ulcer — *continued*
    genital organ(s) — *continued*
      male N50.8
    larynx J38.7
Apical — *see* condition
Apiphobia F40.218
Aplasia (*see also* Agenesis)
  abdominal muscle syndrome Q79.4
  alveolar process (acquired) — *see* Anomaly, alveolar
    congenital Q38.6
  aorta (congenital) Q25.4
  axialis extracorticalis (congenita) E75.29
  bone marrow (myeloid) D61.9
    congenital D61.01
  brain Q00.0
    part of Q04.3
  bronchus Q32.4
  cementum K00.4
  cerebellum Q04.3
  cervix (congenital) Q51.5
  congenital pure red cell D61.01
  corpus callosum Q04.0
  cutis congenita Q84.8
  erythrocyte congenital D61.01
  extracortical axial E75.29
  eye Q11.1
  fovea centralis (congenital) Q14.1
  gallbladder, congenital Q44.0
  iris Q13.1
  labyrinth, membranous Q16.5
  limb (congenital) Q73.8
    lower — *see* Defect, reduction, lower limb
    upper — *see* Agenesis, arm
  lung, congenital (bilateral) (unilateral) Q33.3
  pancreas Q45.0
  parathyroid-thymic D82.1
  Pelizaeus-Merzbacher E75.29
  penis Q55.5
  prostate Q55.4
  red cell (with thymoma) D60.9
    acquired D60.9
      due to drugs D60.9
    adult D60.9
    chronic D60.0
    congenital D61.01
    constitutional D61.01
    due to drugs D60.9
    hereditary D61.01
    of infants D61.01
    primary D61.01
    pure D61.01
      due to drugs D60.9
    specified type NEC D60.8
    transient D60.1
  round ligament Q52.8
  skin Q84.8
  spermatic cord Q55.4
  spleen Q89.01
  testicle Q55.0
  thymic, with immunodeficiency D82.1
  thyroid (congenital) (with myxedema) E03.1
  uterus Q51.0
  ventral horn cell Q06.1
Apnea, apneic (of) (spells) R06.81
  newborn NEC P28.4
    obstructive P28.4
    sleep (central) (obstructive) (primary) P28.3
  prematurity P28.4
  sleep G47.30
    central (primary) G47.31
      in conditions classified elsewhere G47.37
    obstructive (adult) (pediatric) G47.33
    primary central G47.31
    specified NEC G47.39
Apneumatosis, newborn P28.0
Apocrine metaplasia (breast) — *see* Dysplasia, mammary, specified type NEC
Apophysitis (bone) (*see also* Osteochondropathy)
  calcaneus M92.8
  juvenile M92.9
Apoplectiform convulsions (cerebral ischemia) I67.82
Apoplexia, apoplexy, apoplectic
  adrenal A39.1
  heart (auricle) (ventricle) — *see* Infarct, myocardium
  heat T67.0 ☑
  hemorrhagic (stroke) — *see* Hemorrhage, intracranial

Apoplexia, apoplexy, apoplectic — *continued*
  meninges, hemorrhagic — *see* Hemorrhage, intracranial, subarachnoid
  uremic N18.9 [I68.8]
Appearance
  bizarre R46.1
  specified NEC R46.89
  very low level of personal hygiene R46.0
Appendage
  epididymal (organ of Morgagni) Q55.4
  intestine (epiploic) Q43.8
  preauricular Q17.0
  testicular (organ of Morgagni) Q55.29
Appendicitis (pneumococcal) (retrocecal) K37
  with
    perforation or rupture K35.2
    peritoneal abscess K35.3
    peritonitis NEC K35.3
      generalized (with perforation or rupture) K35.2
      localized (with perforation or rupture) K35.3
  acute (catarrhal) (fulminating) (gangrenous) (obstructive) (retrocecal) (suppurative) K35.80
    with
      peritoneal abscess K35.3
      peritonitis NEC K35.3
        generalized (with perforation or rupture) K35.2
        localized (with perforation or rupture) K35.3
    specified NEC K35.89
  amebic A06.89
  chronic (recurrent) K36
  exacerbation — *see* Appendicitis, acute
  gangrenous — *see* Appendicitis, acute
  healed (obliterative) K36
  interval K36
  neurogenic K36
  obstructive K36
  recurrent K36
  relapsing K36
  subacute (adhesive) K36
  subsiding K36
  suppurative — *see* Appendicitis, acute
  tuberculous A18.32
Appendicopathia oxyurica B80
Appendix, appendicular (*see also* condition)
  epididymis Q55.4
  Morgagni
    female Q50.5
    male (epididymal) Q55.4
    testicular Q55.29
  testis Q55.29
Appetite
  depraved — *see* Pica
  excessive R63.2
  lack or loss (*see also* Anorexia) R63.0
    nonorganic origin F50.8
    psychogenic F50.8
  perverted (hysterical) — *see* Pica
Apple peel syndrome Q41.1
Apprehension state F41.1
Apprehensiveness, abnormal F41.9
Approximal wear K03.0
Apraxia (classic) (ideational) (ideokinetic) (ideomotor) (motor) (verbal) R48.2
  following
    cerebrovascular disease I69.990
      cerebral infarction I69.390
      intracerebral hemorrhage I69.190
      nontraumatic intracranial hemorrhage NEC I69.290
      specified disease NEC I69.890
      subarachnoid hemorrhage I69.090
  oculomotor, congenital H51.8
Aptyalism K11.7
Apudoma — *see* Neoplasm, uncertain behavior, by site
Aqueous misdirection H40.83- ☑
Arabicum elephantiasis — *see* Infestation, filarial
Arachnitis — *see* Meningitis
Arachnodactyly — *see* Syndrome, Marfan's
Arachnoiditis (acute) (adhesive) (basal) (brain) (cerebrospinal) — *see* Meningitis
Arachnophobia F40.210
Arboencephalitis, Australian A83.4
Arborization block (heart) I45.5
ARC (AIDS-related complex) B20
Arches — *see* condition
Arcuate uterus Q51.810

Arcuatus uterus Q51.810
Arcus (cornea) senilis — *see* Degeneration, cornea, senile
Arc-welder's lung J63.4
Areflexia R29.2
Areola — *see* condition
Argentaffinoma (*see also* Neoplasm, uncertain behavior, by site)
  malignant — *see* Neoplasm, malignant, by site
  syndrome E34.0
Argininemia E72.21
Arginosuccinic aciduria E72.22
Argyll Robertson phenomenon, pupil or syndrome (syphilitic) A52.19
  atypical H57.09
  nonsyphilitic H57.09
Argyria, argyriasis
  conjunctival H11.13- ☑
  from drug or medicament — *see* Table of Drugs and Chemicals, by substance
Argyrosis, conjunctival H11.13- ☑
Arhinencephaly Q04.1
Ariboflavinosis E53.0
Arm — *see* condition
Arnold-Chiari disease, obstruction or syndrome (type II) Q07.00
  with
    hydrocephalus Q07.02
      with spina bifida Q07.03
    spina bifida Q07.01
      with hydrocephalus Q07.03
  type III — *see* Encephalocele
  type IV Q04.8
Aromatic amino-acid metabolism disorder E70.9
  specified NEC E70.8
Arousals, confusional G47.51
Arrest, arrested
  cardiac I46.9
    complicating
      abortion — *see* Abortion, by type, complicated by, cardiac arrest
      anesthesia (general) (local) or other sedation — *see* Table of Drugs and Chemicals, by drug
        in labor and delivery O74.2
        in pregnancy O29.11- ☑
        postpartum, puerperal O89.1
      delivery (cesarean) (instrumental) O75.4
    due to
      cardiac condition I46.2
      specified condition NEC I46.8
    intraoperative I97.71- ☑
    newborn P29.81
    postprocedural I97.12- ☑
      obstetric procedure O75.4
  cardiorespiratory — *see* Arrest, cardiac
  circulatory — *see* Arrest, cardiac
  deep transverse O64.0 ☑
  development or growth
    bone — *see* Disorder, bone, development or growth
    child R62.50
    tracheal rings Q32.1
  epiphyseal
    complete
      femur M89.15- ☑
      humerus M89.12- ☑
      tibia M89.16- ☑
      ulna M89.13- ☑
      forearm M89.13- ☑
        specified NEC M89.13- ☑
        ulna — *see* Arrest, epiphyseal, by type, ulna
      lower leg M89.16- ☑
        specified NEC M89.168
        tibia — *see* Arrest, epiphyseal, by type, tibia
    partial
      femur M89.15- ☑
      humerus M89.12- ☑
      tibia M89.16- ☑
      ulna M89.13- ☑
    specified NEC M89.18
  granulopoiesis — *see* Agranulocytosis
  growth plate — *see* Arrest, epiphyseal
  heart — *see* Arrest, cardiac
  legal, anxiety concerning Z65.3
  physeal — *see* Arrest, epiphyseal
  respiratory R09.2
    newborn P28.81

Arrest, arrested — continued
　sinus I45.5
　spermatogenesis (complete) — see Azoospermia
　　incomplete — see Oligospermia
　transverse (deep) O64.0 ☑
Arrhenoblastoma
　benign
　　specified site — see Neoplasm, benign, by site
　　unspecified site
　　　female D27.9
　　　male D29.20
　malignant
　　specified site — see Neoplasm, malignant, by site
　　unspecified site
　　　female C56.9
　　　male C62.90
　specified site — see Neoplasm, uncertain behavior,
　　by site
　unspecified site
　　female D39.10
　　male D40.10
Arrhythmia (auricle) (cardiac) (juvenile) (nodal) (reflex)
　　(sinus) (supraventricular) (transitory) (ventricle) I49.9
　block I45.9
　extrasystolic I49.49
　newborn
　　bradycardia P29.12
　　occurring before birth P03.819
　　　before onset of labor P03.810
　　　during labor P03.811
　　tachycardia P29.11
　psychogenic F45.8
　specified NEC I49.8
　vagal R55
　ventricular re-entry I47.0
Arrillaga-Ayerza syndrome (pulmonary sclerosis with
　　pulmonary hypertension) I27.0
Arsenical pigmentation L81.8
　from drug or medicament — see Table of Drugs and
　　Chemicals
Arsenism — see Poisoning, arsenic
Arterial — see condition
Arteriofibrosis — see Arteriosclerosis
Arteriolar sclerosis — see Arteriosclerosis
Arteriolith — see Arteriosclerosis
Arteriolitis I77.6
　necrotizing, kidney I77.5
　renal — see Hypertension, kidney
Arteriolosclerosis — see Arteriosclerosis
Arterionephrosclerosis — see Hypertension, kidney
Arteriopathy I77.9
Arteriosclerosis, arteriosclerotic (diffuse) (obliterans)
　　(of) (senile) (with calcification) I70.90
　aorta I70.0
　arteries of extremities — see Arteriosclerosis, extrem-
　　ities
　brain I67.2
　bypass graft
　　coronary — see Arteriosclerosis, coronary, bypass
　　　graft
　　extremities — see Arteriosclerosis, extremities,
　　　bypass graft
　cardiac — see Disease, heart, ischemic, atherosclerotic
　cardiopathy — see Disease, heart, ischemic,
　　atherosclerotic
　cardiorenal — see Hypertension, cardiorenal
　cardiovascular — see Disease, heart, ischemic,
　　atherosclerotic
　carotid (see also Occlusion, artery, carotid) I65.2- ☑
　central nervous system I67.2
　cerebral I67.2
　cerebrovascular I67.2
　coronary (artery) I25.10
　　bypass graft I25.810
　　　with
　　　　angina pectoris I25.709
　　　　　with documented spasm I25.701
　　　　　specified type NEC I25.708
　　　　　unstable I25.700
　　　　ischemic chest pain I25.709
　　　autologous artery I25.810
　　　　with
　　　　　angina pectoris I25.729
　　　　　　with documented spasm I25.721
　　　　　　specified type I25.728
　　　　　　unstable I25.720
　　　　　ischemic chest pain I25.729

Arteriosclerosis, arteriosclerotic — continued
　coronary — continued
　　bypass graft — continued
　　　autologous vein I25.810
　　　　with
　　　　　angina pectoris I25.719
　　　　　　with documented spasm I25.711
　　　　　　specified type I25.718
　　　　　　unstable I25.710
　　　　　ischemic chest pain I25.719
　　　nonautologous biological I25.810
　　　　with
　　　　　angina pectoris I25.739
　　　　　　with documented spasm I25.731
　　　　　　specified type I25.738
　　　　　　unstable I25.730
　　　　　ischemic chest pain I25.739
　　　specified type NEC I25.810
　　　　with
　　　　　angina pectoris I25.799
　　　　　　with documented spasm I25.791
　　　　　　specified type I25.798
　　　　　　unstable I25.790
　　　　　ischemic chest pain I25.799
　　due to
　　　calcified coronary lesion (severely) I25.84
　　　lipid rich plaque I25.83
　　native vessel
　　　with
　　　　angina pectoris I25.119
　　　　　with documented spasm I25.111
　　　　　specified type NEC I25.118
　　　　　unstable I25.110
　　　　ischemic chest pain I25.119
　　transplanted heart I25.811
　　　bypass graft I25.812
　　　　with
　　　　　angina pectoris I25.769
　　　　　　with documented spasm I25.761
　　　　　　specified type I25.768
　　　　　　unstable I25.760
　　　　　ischemic chest pain I25.769
　　　native coronary artery I25.811
　　　　with
　　　　　angina pectoris I25.759
　　　　　　with documented spasm I25.751
　　　　　　specified type I25.758
　　　　　　unstable I25.750
　　　　　ischemic chest pain I25.759
　extremities (native arteries) I70.209
　　bypass graft I70.309
　　　autologous vein graft I70.409
　　　　leg I70.409
　　　　　with
　　　　　　gangrene (and intermittent claudica-
　　　　　　　tion, rest pain and ulcer)
　　　　　　　I70.469
　　　　　　intermittent claudication I70.419
　　　　　　rest pain (and intermittent claudica-
　　　　　　　tion) I70.429
　　　　　　specified type NEC I70.493
　　　　　bilateral I70.403
　　　　　　with
　　　　　　　gangrene (and intermittent clau-
　　　　　　　　dication, rest pain and ul-
　　　　　　　　cer) I70.463
　　　　　　　intermittent claudication I70.463
　　　　　　　rest pain (and intermittent claudi-
　　　　　　　　cation) I70.423
　　　　　　　specified type NEC I70.493
　　　　　left I70.402
　　　　　　with
　　　　　　　gangrene (and intermittent clau-
　　　　　　　　dication, rest pain and ul-
　　　　　　　　cer) I70.462
　　　　　　　intermittent claudication I70.412
　　　　　　　rest pain (and intermittent claudi-
　　　　　　　　cation) I70.422
　　　　　　　ulceration (and intermittent
　　　　　　　　claudication and rest pain)
　　　　　　　　I70.449
　　　　　　　ankle I70.443
　　　　　　　calf I70.442
　　　　　　　foot site NEC I70.445
　　　　　　　heel I70.444
　　　　　　　lower leg NEC I70.448
　　　　　　　midfoot I70.444
　　　　　　　thigh I70.441
　　　　　　specified type NEC I70.492

Arteriosclerosis, arteriosclerotic — continued
　extremities — continued
　　bypass graft — continued
　　　autologous vein graft — continued
　　　　leg — continued
　　　　　right I70.401
　　　　　　with
　　　　　　　gangrene (and intermittent clau-
　　　　　　　　dication, rest pain and ul-
　　　　　　　　cer) I70.461
　　　　　　　intermittent claudication I70.411
　　　　　　　rest pain (and intermittent claudi-
　　　　　　　　cation) I70.421
　　　　　　　ulceration (and intermittent
　　　　　　　　claudication and rest pain)
　　　　　　　　I70.439
　　　　　　　ankle I70.433
　　　　　　　calf I70.432
　　　　　　　foot site NEC I70.435
　　　　　　　heel I70.434
　　　　　　　lower leg NEC I70.438
　　　　　　　midfoot I70.434
　　　　　　　thigh I70.431
　　　　　　specified type NEC I70.491
　　　　specified type NEC I70.499
　　　specified NEC I70.408
　　　　with
　　　　　gangrene (and intermittent claudica-
　　　　　　tion, rest pain and ulcer)
　　　　　　I70.468
　　　　　intermittent claudication I70.418
　　　　　rest pain (and intermittent claudica-
　　　　　　tion) I70.428
　　　　　ulceration (and intermittent claudica-
　　　　　　tion and rest pain) I70.45
　　　　　specified type NEC I70.498
　　　leg I70.309
　　　　with
　　　　　gangrene (and intermittent claudication,
　　　　　　rest pain and ulcer) I70.369
　　　　　intermittent claudication I70.319
　　　　　rest pain (and intermittent claudication)
　　　　　　I70.329
　　　　bilateral I70.303
　　　　　with
　　　　　　gangrene (and intermittent claudica-
　　　　　　　tion, rest pain and ulcer)
　　　　　　　I70.363
　　　　　　intermittent claudication I70.313
　　　　　　rest pain (and intermittent claudica-
　　　　　　　tion) I70.323
　　　　　　specified type NEC I70.393
　　　　left I70.302
　　　　　with
　　　　　　gangrene (and intermittent claudica-
　　　　　　　tion, rest pain and ulcer)
　　　　　　　I70.362
　　　　　　intermittent claudication I70.312
　　　　　　rest pain (and intermittent claudica-
　　　　　　　tion) I70.322
　　　　　　ulceration (and intermittent claudica-
　　　　　　　tion and rest pain) I70.349
　　　　　　ankle I70.343
　　　　　　calf I70.342
　　　　　　foot site NEC I70.345
　　　　　　heel I70.344
　　　　　　lower leg NEC I70.348
　　　　　　midfoot I70.344
　　　　　　thigh I70.341
　　　　　specified type NEC I70.392
　　　　right I70.301
　　　　　with
　　　　　　gangrene (and intermittent claudica-
　　　　　　　tion, rest pain and ulcer)
　　　　　　　I70.361
　　　　　　intermittent claudication I70.311
　　　　　　rest pain (and intermittent claudica-
　　　　　　　tion) I70.321
　　　　　　ulceration (and intermittent claudica-
　　　　　　　tion and rest pain I70.339
　　　　　　ankle I70.333
　　　　　　calf I70.332
　　　　　　foot site NEC I70.335
　　　　　　heel I70.334
　　　　　　lower leg NEC I70.338
　　　　　　midfoot I70.334
　　　　　　thigh I70.331
　　　　　specified type NEC I70.391

Arteriosclerosis, arteriosclerotic — *continued*
  extremities — *continued*
    bypass graft — *continued*
      leg — *continued*
        specified type NEC I70.399
      nonautologous biological graft I70.509
        leg I70.509
          with
            gangrene (and intermittent claudication, rest pain and ulcer) I70.569
            intermittent claudication I70.519
            rest pain (and intermittent claudication) I70.529
          bilateral I70.503
            with
              gangrene (and intermittent claudication, rest pain and ulcer) I70.563
              intermittent claudication I70.513
              rest pain (and intermittent claudication) I70.523
            specified type NEC I70.593
          left I70.502
            with
              gangrene (and intermittent claudication, rest pain and ulcer) I70.562
              intermittent claudication I70.512
              rest pain (and intermittent claudication) I70.522
              ulceration (and intermittent claudication and rest pain) I70.549
                ankle I70.543
                calf I70.542
                foot site NEC I70.545
                heel I70.544
                lower leg NEC I70.548
                midfoot I70.544
                thigh I70.541
            specified type NEC I70.592
          right I70.501
            with
              gangrene (and intermittent claudication, rest pain and ulcer) I70.561
              intermittent claudication I70.511
              rest pain (and intermittent claudication) I70.521
              ulceration (and intermittent claudication and rest pain) I70.539
                ankle I70.533
                calf I70.532
                foot site NEC I70.535
                heel I70.534
                lower leg NEC I70.538
                midfoot I70.534
                thigh I70.531
            specified type NEC I70.591
        specified type NEC I70.599
        specified NEC I70.508
          with
            gangrene (and intermittent claudication, rest pain and ulcer) I70.568
            intermittent claudication I70.518
            rest pain (and intermittent claudication) I70.528
            ulceration (and intermittent claudication and rest pain) I70.55
          specified type NEC I70.598
      nonbiological graft I70.609
        leg I70.609
          with
            gangrene (and intermittent claudication, rest pain and ulcer) I70.669
            intermittent claudication I70.619
            rest pain (and intermittent claudication) I70.629
          bilateral I70.603
            with
              gangrene (and intermittent claudication, rest pain and ulcer) I70.663
              intermittent claudication I70.613

Arteriosclerosis, arteriosclerotic — *continued*
  extremities — *continued*
    bypass graft — *continued*
      nonbiological graft — *continued*
        leg — *continued*
          bilateral — *continued*
            with — *continued*
              rest pain (and intermittent claudication) I70.623
              specified type NEC I70.693
          left I70.602
            with
              gangrene (and intermittent claudication, rest pain and ulcer) I70.662
              intermittent claudication I70.612
              rest pain (and intermittent claudication) I70.622
              ulceration (and intermittent claudication and rest pain) I70.649
                ankle I70.643
                calf I70.642
                foot site NEC I70.645
                heel I70.644
                lower leg NEC I70.648
                midfoot I70.644
                thigh I70.641
            specified type NEC I70.692
          right I70.601
            with
              gangrene (and intermittent claudication, rest pain and ulcer) I70.661
              intermittent claudication I70.611
              rest pain (and intermittent claudication) I70.621
              ulceration (and intermittent claudication and rest pain) I70.639
                ankle I70.633
                calf I70.632
                foot site NEC I70.635
                heel I70.634
                lower leg NEC I70.638
                midfoot I70.634
                thigh I70.631
            specified type NEC I70.691
          specified NEC I70.608
            with
              gangrene (and intermittent claudication, rest pain and ulcer) I70.668
              intermittent claudication I70.618
              rest pain (and intermittent claudication) I70.628
              ulceration (and intermittent claudication and rest pain) I70.65
            specified type NEC I70.698
      specified graft NEC I70.709
        leg I70.709
          with
            gangrene (and intermittent claudication, rest pain and ulcer) I70.769
            intermittent claudication I70.719
            rest pain (and intermittent claudication) I70.729
          bilateral I70.703
            with
              gangrene (and intermittent claudication, rest pain and ulcer) I70.763
              intermittent claudication I70.713
              rest pain (and intermittent claudication) I70.723
            specified type NEC I70.793
          left I70.702
            with
              gangrene (and intermittent claudication, rest pain and ulcer) I70.762
              intermittent claudication I70.712
              rest pain (and intermittent claudication) I70.722

Arteriosclerosis, arteriosclerotic — *continued*
  extremities — *continued*
    bypass graft — *continued*
      specified graft — *continued*
        leg — *continued*
          left — *continued*
            with — *continued*
              ulceration (and intermittent claudication and rest pain) I70.749
                ankle I70.743
                calf I70.742
                foot site NEC I70.745
                heel I70.744
                lower leg NEC I70.748
                midfoot I70.744
                thigh I70.741
            specified type NEC I70.792
          right I70.701
            with
              gangrene (and intermittent claudication, rest pain and ulcer) I70.761
              intermittent claudication I70.711
              rest pain (and intermittent claudication) I70.721
              ulceration (and intermittent claudication and rest pain) I70.739
                ankle I70.733
                calf I70.732
                foot site NEC I70.735
                heel I70.734
                lower leg NEC I70.738
                midfoot I70.734
                thigh I70.731
            specified type NEC I70.791
          specified type NEC I70.799
        specified NEC I70.708
          with
            gangrene (and intermittent claudication, rest pain and ulcer) I70.768
            intermittent claudication I70.718
            rest pain (and intermittent claudication) I70.728
            ulceration (and intermittent claudication and rest pain) I70.75
          specified type NEC I70.798
    specified NEC I70.308
      with
        gangrene (and intermittent claudication, rest pain and ulcer) I70.368
        intermittent claudication I70.318
        rest pain (and intermittent claudication) I70.328
        ulceration (and intermittent claudication and rest pain) I70.35
      specifiec type NEC I70.398
    leg I70.209
      with
        gangrene (and intermittent claudication, rest pain and ulcer) I70.269
        intermittent claudication I70.219
        rest pain (and intermittent claudication) I70.229
      bilateral I70.203
        with
          gangrene (and intermittent claudication, rest pain and ulcer) I70.263
          intermittent claudication I70.213
          rest pain (and intermittent claudication) I70.223
        specified type NEC I70.293
      left I70.202
        with
          gangrene (and intermittent claudication, rest pain and ulcer) I70.262
          intermittent claudication I70.212
          rest pain (and intermittent claudication) I70.222
          ulceration (and intermittent claudication and rest pain) I70.249
            ankle I70.243
            calf I70.242
            foot site NEC I70.245
            heel I70.244
            lower leg NEC I70.248

Arteriosclerosis, arteriosclerotic — *continued*
  extremities — *continued*
    leg — *continued*
      left — *continued*
        with — *continued*
          ulceration — *continued*
            midfoot I70.244
            thigh I70.241
          specified type NEC I70.292
       right I70.201
        with
          gangrene (and intermittent claudication, rest pain and ulcer) I70.261
          intermittent claudication I70.211
          rest pain (and intermittent claudication) I70.221
          ulceration (and intermittent claudication and rest pain) I70.239
            ankle I70.233
            calf I70.232
            foot site NEC I70.235
            heel I70.234
            lower leg NEC I70.238
            midfoot I70.234
            thigh I70.231
        specified type NEC I70.291
      specified site NEC I70.208
       with
        gangrene (and intermittent claudication, rest pain and ulcer) I70.268
        intermittent claudication I70.218
        rest pain (and intermittent claudication) I70.228
        ulceration (and intermittent claudication and rest pain) I70.25
      specified type NEC I70.298
  generalized I70.91
  heart (disease) — *see* Arteriosclerosis, coronary (artery),
  kidney — *see* Hypertension, kidney
  medial — *see* Arteriosclerosis, extremities
  mesenteric (artery) K55.1
  Mönckeberg's — *see* Arteriosclerosis, extremities
  myocarditis I51.4
  peripheral (of extremities) — *see* Arteriosclerosis, extremities
  pulmonary (idiopathic) I27.0
  renal (arterioles) (*see also* Hypertension, kidney)
    artery I70.1
  retina (vascular) I70.8 [H35.0-] ☑
  specified artery NEC I70.8
  spinal (cord) G95.19
  vertebral (artery) I67.2
Arteriospasm I73.9
Arteriovenous — *see* condition
Arteritis I77.6
  allergic M31.0
  aorta (nonsyphilitic) I77.6
    syphilitic A52.02
  aortic arch M31.4
  brachiocephalic M31.4
  brain I67.7
    syphilitic A52.04
  cerebral I67.7
    in systemic lupus erythematosus M32.19
    listerial A32.89
    syphilitic A52.04
    tuberculous A18.89
  coronary (artery) I25.89
    rheumatic I01.8
      chronic I09.89
    syphilitic A52.06
  cranial (left) (right), giant cell M31.6
  deformans — *see* Arteriosclerosis
  giant cell NEC M31.6
    with polymyalgia rheumatica M31.5
  necrosing or necrotizing M31.9
    specified NEC M31.8
  nodosa M30.0
  obliterans — *see* Arteriosclerosis
  pulmonary I28.8
  rheumatic — *see* Fever, rheumatic
  senile — *see* Arteriosclerosis
  suppurative I77.2
  syphilitic (general) A52.09
    brain A52.04
    coronary A52.06

Arteritis — *continued*
  syphilitic — *continued*
    spinal A52.09
  temporal, giant cell M31.6
  young female aortic arch syndrome M31.4
Artery, arterial (*see also* condition)
  abscess I77.89
  single umbilical Q27.0
Arthralgia (allergic) (*see also* Pain, joint)
  in caisson disease T70.3 ☑
  temporomandibular M26.62
Arthritis, arthritic (acute) (chronic) (nonpyogenic) (subacute) M19.90
  allergic — *see* Arthritis, specified form NEC
  ankylosing (crippling) (spine) (*see also* Spondylitis, ankylosing)
    sites other than spine — *see* Arthritis, specified form NEC
  atrophic — *see* Osteoarthritis
    spine — *see* Spondylitis, ankylosing
  back — *see* Spondylopathy, inflammatory
  blennorrhagic (gonococcal) A54.42
  Charcot's — *see* Arthropathy, neuropathic
    diabetic — *see* Diabetes, arthropathy, neuropathic
    syringomyelic G95.0
  chylous (filarial) (*see also* category M01) B74.9
  climacteric (any site) NEC — *see* Arthritis, specified form NEC
  crystal (-induced) — *see* Arthritis, in, crystals
  deformans — *see* Osteoarthritis
  degenerative — *see* Osteoarthritis
  due to or associated with
    acromegaly E22.0
    brucellosis — *see* Brucellosis
    caisson disease T70.3 ☑
    diabetes — *see* Diabetes, arthropathy
    dracontiasis (*see also* category M01) B72
    enteritis NEC
      regional — *see* Enteritis, regional
    erysipelas (*see also* category M01) A46
    erythema
      epidemic A25.1
      nodosum L52
    filariasis NOS B74.9
    glanders A24.0
    helminthiasis (*see also* category M01) B83.9
    hemophilia D66 [M36.2]
    Henoch- (Schönlein) purpura D69.0 [M36.4]
    human parvovirus (*see also* category M01) B97.6
    infectious disease NEC M01 ☑
    leprosy (see also category M01) (*see also* Leprosy) A30.9
    Lyme disease A69.23
    mycobacteria (*see also* category M01) A31.8
    parasitic disease NEC (*see also* category M01) B89
    paratyphoid fever (see also category M01) (*see also* Fever, paratyphoid) A01.4
    rat bite fever (*see also* category M01) A25.1
    regional enteritis — *see* Enteritis, regional
    respiratory disorder NOS J98.9
    serum sickness (*see also* Reaction, serum) T80.69 ☑
    syringomyelia G95.0
    typhoid fever A01.04
  epidemic erythema A25.1
  febrile — *see* Fever, rheumatic
  gonococcal A54.42
  gouty (acute) — *see* Gout, idiopathic
  in (due to)
    acromegaly (*see also* subcategory M14.8-) E22.0
    amyloidosis (*see also* subcategory M14.8-) E85.4
    bacterial disease (*see also* subcategory M01) A49.9
    Behçet's syndrome M35.2
    caisson disease (*see also* subcategory M14.8-) T70.3 ☑
    coliform bacilli (Escherichia coli) — *see* Arthritis, in, pyogenic organism NEC
    crystals M11.9
      dicalcium phosphate — *see* Arthritis, in, crystals, specified type NEC
      hydroxyapatite M11.0- ☑
      pyrophosphate — *see* Arthritis, in, crystals, specified type NEC
      specified type NEC M11.80
        ankle M11.87- ☑
        elbow M11.82- ☑
        foot joint M11.87- ☑
        hand joint M11.84- ☑

Arthritis, arthritic — *continued*
  in — *continued*
    crystals — *continued*
      specified type — *continued*
        hip M11.85- ☑
        knee M11.86- ☑
        multiple sites M11.8- ☑
        shoulder M11.81- ☑
        vertebrae M11.88
        wrist M11.83- ☑
    dermatoarthritis, lipoid E78.81
    dracontiasis (dracunculiasis) (*see also* category M01) B72
    endocrine disorder NEC (*see also* subcategory M14.8-) E34.9
    enteritis, infectious NEC (*see also* category M01) A09
      specified organism NEC (*see also* category M01) A08.8
    erythema
      multiforme (*see also* subcategory M14.8-) L51.9
      nodosum (*see also* subcategory M14.8-) L52
    gout — *see* Gout, idiopathic
    helminthiasis NEC (*see also* category M01) B83.9
    hemochromatosis (*see also* subcategory M14.8-) E83.118
    hemoglobinopathy NEC D58.2 [M36.3]
    hemophilia NEC D66 [M36.2]
    Hemophilus influenzae M00.8- ☑ [B96.3]
    Henoch (-Schönlein) purpura D69.0 [M36.4]
    hyperparathyroidism NEC (*see also* subcategory M14.8-) E21.3
    hypersensitivity reaction NEC T78.49 ☑ [M36.4]
    hypogammaglobulinemia (*see also* subcategory M14.8-) D80.1
    hypothyroidism NEC (*see also* subcategory M14.8-) E03.9
    infection — *see* Arthritis, pyogenic or pyemic
      spine — *see* Spondylopathy, infective
    infectious disease NEC M01 ☑
    leprosy (*see also* category M01) A30.9
    leukemia NEC C95.9- ☑ [M36.1]
    lipoid dermatoarthritis E78.81
    Lyme disease A69.23
    Mediterranean fever, familial (*see also* subcategory M14.8-) E85.0
    Meningococcus A39.83
    metabolic disorder NEC (*see also* subcategory M14.8-) E88.9
    multiple myelomatosis C90.0- ☑ [M36.1]
    mumps B26.85
    mycosis NEC (*see also* category M01) B49
    myelomatosis (multiple) C90.0- ☑ [M36.1]
    neurological disorder NEC G98.0
    ochronosis (*see also* subcategory M14.8-) E70.29
    O'nyong-nyong (*see also* category M01) A92.1
    parasitic disease NEC (*see also* category M01) B89
    paratyphoid fever (*see also* category M01) A01.4
    Pseudomonas — *see* Arthritis, pyogenic, bacterial NEC
    psoriasis L40.50
    pyogenic organism NEC — *see* Arthritis, pyogenic, bacterial NEC
    Reiter's disease — *see* Reiter's disease
    respiratory disorder NEC (*see also* subcategory M14.8-) J98.9
    reticulosis, malignant (*see also* subcategory M14.8-) C86.0
    rubella B06.82
    Salmonella (arizonae) (cholerae-suis) (enteritidis) (typhimurium) A02.23
    sarcoidosis D86.86
    specified bacteria NEC — *see* Arthritis, pyogenic, bacterial NEC
    sporotrichosis B42.82
    syringomyelia G95.0
    thalassemia NEC D56.9 [M36.3]
    tuberculosis — *see* Tuberculosis, arthritis
    typhoid fever A01.04
    urethritis, Reiter's — *see* Reiter's disease
    viral disease NEC (*see also* category M01) B34.9
  infectious or infective (*see also* Arthritis, pyogenic or pyemic)
    spine — *see* Spondylopathy, infective
  juvenile M08.90
    with systemic onset — *see* Still's disease
    ankle M08.97- ☑

Arthritis, arthritic — *continued*
　juvenile — *continued*
　　elbow M08.92- ☑
　　foot joint M08.97- ☑
　　hand joint M08.94- ☑
　　hip M08.95- ☑
　　knee M08.96- ☑
　　multiple site M08.99
　　pauciarticular M08.40
　　　ankle M08.47- ☑
　　　elbow M08.42- ☑
　　　foot joint M08.47- ☑
　　　hand joint M08.44- ☑
　　　hip M08.45- ☑
　　　knee M08.46- ☑
　　　shoulder M08.41- ☑
　　　vertebrae M08.48
　　　wrist M08.43- ☑
　　psoriatic L40.54
　　rheumatoid — *see* Arthritis, rheumatoid, juvenile
　　shoulder M08.91- ☑
　　specified type NEC M08.80
　　　ankle M08.87- ☑
　　　elbow M08.82- ☑
　　　foot joint M08.87- ☑
　　　hand joint M08.84- ☑
　　　hip M08.85- ☑
　　　knee M08.86- ☑
　　　multiple site M08.89
　　　shoulder M08.81- ☑
　　　specified joint NEC M08.88
　　　vertebrae M08.88
　　　wrist M08.83- ☑
　　wrist M08.93- ☑
　meaning osteoarthritis — *see* Osteoarthritis
　meningococcal A39.83
　menopausal (any site) NEC — *see* Arthritis, specified form NEC
　mutilans (psoriatic) L40.52
　mycotic NEC (*see also* category M01) B49
　neuropathic (Charcot) — *see* Arthropathy, neuropathic
　　diabetic — *see* Diabetes, arthropathy, neuropathic
　　nonsyphilitic NEC G98.0
　　syringomyelic G95.0
　ochronotic (*see also* subcategory M14.8-) E70.29
　palindromic (any site) — *see* Rheumatism, palindromic
　pneumococcal M00.10
　　ankle M00.17- ☑
　　elbow M00.12- ☑
　　foot joint — *see* Arthritis, pneumococcal, ankle
　　hand joint M00.14- ☑
　　hip M00.15- ☑
　　knee M00.16- ☑
　　multiple site M00.19
　　shoulder M00.11- ☑
　　vertebra M00.18
　　wrist M00.13- ☑
　postdysenteric — *see* Arthropathy, postdysenteric
　postmeningococcal A39.84
　postrheumatic, chronic — *see* Arthropathy, postrheumatic, chronic
　primary progressive (*see also* Arthritis, specified form NEC)
　　spine — *see* Spondylitis, ankylosing
　psoriatic L40.50
　purulent (any site except spine) — *see* Arthritis, pyogenic or pyemic
　　spine — *see* Spondylopathy, infective
　pyogenic or pyemic (any site except spine) M00.9
　　bacterial NEC M00.80
　　　ankle M00.87- ☑
　　　elbow M00.82- ☑
　　　foot joint — *see* Arthritis, pyogenic, bacterial NEC, ankle
　　　hand joint M00.84- ☑
　　　hip M00.85- ☑
　　　knee M00.86- ☑
　　　multiple site M00.89
　　　shoulder M00.81- ☑
　　　vertebra M00.88
　　　wrist M00.83- ☑
　　pneumococcal — *see* Arthritis, pneumococcal
　　spine — *see* Spondylopathy, infective
　　staphylococcal — *see* Arthritis, staphylococcal
　　streptococcal — *see* Arthritis, streptococcal NEC
　　　pneumococcal — *see* Arthritis, pneumococcal

Arthritis, arthritic — *continued*
　reactive — *see* Reiter's disease
　rheumatic (*see also* Arthritis, rheumatoid)
　　acute or subacute — *see* Fever, rheumatic
　rheumatoid M06.9
　　with
　　　carditis — *see* Rheumatoid, carditis
　　　endocarditis — *see* Rheumatoid, carditis
　　　heart involvement NEC — *see* Rheumatoid, carditis
　　　lung involvement — *see* Rheumatoid, lung
　　　myocarditis — *see* Rheumatoid, carditis
　　　myopathy — *see* Rheumatoid, myopathy
　　　pericarditis — *see* Rheumatoid, carditis
　　　polyneuropathy — *see* Rheumatoid, polyneuropathy
　　　rheumatoid factor — *see* Arthritis, rheumatoid, seropositive
　　　splenoadenomegaly and leukopenia — *see* Felty's syndrome
　　　vasculitis — *see* Rheumatoid, vasculitis
　　　visceral involvement NEC — *see* Rheumatoid, arthritis, with involvement of organs NEC
　　juvenile (with or without rheumatoid factor) M08.00
　　　ankle M08.07- ☑
　　　elbow M08.02- ☑
　　　foot joint M08.07- ☑
　　　hand joint M08.04- ☑
　　　hip M08.05- ☑
　　　knee M08.06- ☑
　　　multiple site M08.09
　　　shoulder M08.01- ☑
　　　vertebra M08.08
　　　wrist M08.03- ☑
　　seronegative M06.00
　　　ankle M06.07- ☑
　　　elbow M06.02- ☑
　　　foot joint M06.07- ☑
　　　hand joint M06.04- ☑
　　　hip M06.05- ☑
　　　knee M06.06- ☑
　　　multiple site M06.09
　　　shoulder M06.01- ☑
　　　vertebra M06.08
　　　wrist M06.03- ☑
　　seropositive M05.9
　　　without organ involvement M05.70
　　　　ankle M05.77- ☑
　　　　elbow M05.72- ☑
　　　　foot joint M05.77- ☑
　　　　hand joint M05.74- ☑
　　　　hip M05.75- ☑
　　　　knee M05.76- ☑
　　　　multiple sites M05.79
　　　　shoulder M05.71- ☑
　　　　vertebra — *see* Spondylitis, ankylosing
　　　　wrist M05.73- ☑
　　　specified NEC M05.80
　　　　ankle M05.87- ☑
　　　　elbow M05.82- ☑
　　　　foot joint M05.87- ☑
　　　　hand joint M05.84- ☑
　　　　hip M05.85- ☑
　　　　knee M05.86- ☑
　　　　multiple sites M05.89
　　　　shoulder M05.81- ☑
　　　　vertebra — *see* Spondylitis, ankylosing
　　　　wrist M05.83- ☑
　　specified type NEC M06.80
　　　ankle M06.87- ☑
　　　elbow M06.82- ☑
　　　foot joint M06.87- ☑
　　　hand joint M06.84- ☑
　　　hip M06.85- ☑
　　　knee M06.86- ☑
　　　multiple site M06.89
　　　shoulder M06.81- ☑
　　　vertebra M06.88
　　　wrist M06.83- ☑
　　spine — *see* Spondylitis, ankylosing
　rubella B06.82
　scorbutic (*see also* subcategory M14.8-) E54
　senile or senescent — *see* Osteoarthritis

Arthritis, arthritic — *continued*
　septic (any site except spine) — *see* Arthritis, pyogenic or pyemic
　　spine — *see* Spondylopathy, infective
　serum (nontherapeutic) (therapeutic) — *see* Arthropathy, postimmunization
　specified form NEC M13.80
　　ankle M13.87- ☑
　　elbow M13.82- ☑
　　foot joint M13.87- ☑
　　hand joint M13.84- ☑
　　hip M13.85- ☑
　　knee M13.86- ☑
　　multiple site M13.89
　　shoulder M13.81- ☑
　　specified joint NEC M13.88
　　wrist M13.83- ☑
　spine (*see also* Spondylopathy, inflammatory)
　　infectious or infective NEC — *see* Spondylopathy, infective
　　Marie-Strümpell — *see* Spondylitis, ankylosing
　　pyogenic — *see* Spondylopathy, infective
　　rheumatoid — *see* Spondylitis, ankylosing
　　traumatic (old) — *see* Spondylopathy, traumatic
　　tuberculous A18.01
　staphylococcal M00.00
　　ankle M00.07- ☑
　　elbow M00.02- ☑
　　foot joint — *see* Arthritis, staphylococcal, ankle
　　hand joint M00.04- ☑
　　hip M00.05- ☑
　　knee M00.06- ☑
　　multiple site M00.09
　　shoulder M00.01- ☑
　　vertebra M00.08
　　wrist M00.03- ☑
　streptococcal NEC M00.20
　　ankle M00.27- ☑
　　elbow M00.22- ☑
　　foot joint — *see* Arthritis, streptococcal, ankle
　　hand joint M00.24- ☑
　　hip M00.25- ☑
　　knee M00.26- ☑
　　multiple site M00.29
　　shoulder M00.21- ☑
　　vertebra M00.28
　　wrist M00.23- ☑
　suppurative — *see* Arthritis, pyogenic or pyemic
　syphilitic (late) A52.16
　　congenital A50.55 [M12.80]
　syphilitica deformans (Charcot) A52.16
　temporomandibular M26.69
　toxic of menopause (any site) — *see* Arthritis, specified form NEC
　transient — *see* Arthropathy, specified form NEC
　traumatic (chronic) — *see* Arthropathy, traumatic
　tuberculous A18.02
　　spine A18.01
　uratic — *see* Gout, idiopathic
　urethritica (Reiter's) — *see* Reiter's disease
　vertebral — *see* Spondylopathy, inflammatory
　villous (any site) — *see* Arthropathy, specified form NEC
Arthrocele — *see* Effusion, joint
Arthrodesis status Z98.1
Arthrodynia (*see also* Pain, joint)
Arthrodysplasia Q74.9
Arthrofibrosis, joint — *see* Ankylosis
Arthrogryposis (congenital) Q68.8
　multiplex congenita Q74.3
Arthrokatadysis M24.7
Arthropathy (*see also* Arthritis) M12.9
　Charcot's — *see* Arthropathy, neuropathic
　　diabetic — *see* Diabetes, arthropathy, neuropathic
　　syringomyelic G95.0
　cricoarytenoid J38.7
　crystal (-induced) — *see* Arthritis, in, crystals
　diabetic NEC — *see* Diabetes, arthropathy
　distal interphalangeal, psoriatic L40.51
　enteropathic M07.60
　　ankle M07.67- ☑
　　elbow M07.62- ☑
　　foot joint M07.67- ☑
　　hand joint M07.64- ☑
　　hip M07.65- ☑
　　knee M07.66- ☑

Arthropathy — *continued*
  enteropathic — *continued*
    multiple site M07.69
    shoulder M07.61- ☑
    vertebra M07.68
    wrist M07.63- ☑
  following intestinal bypass M02.00
    ankle M02.07- ☑
    elbow M02.02- ☑
    foot joint M02.07- ☑
    hand joint M02.04- ☑
    hip M02.05- ☑
    knee M02.06- ☑
    multiple site M02.09
    shoulder M02.01- ☑
    vertebra M02.08
    wrist M02.03- ☑
  gouty (*see also* Gout, idiopathic)
    in (due to)
      Lesch-Nyhan syndrome E79.1 [M14.8-] ☑
      sickle-cell disorders D57- ☑ [M14.8-] ☑
  hemophilic NEC D66 [M36.2]
    in (due to)
      hyperparathyroidism NEC E21.3 [M14.8-] ☑
      metabolic disease NOS E88.9 [M14.8-] ☑
  in (due to)
    acromegaly E22.0 [M14.8-] ☑
    amyloidosis E85.4 [M14.8-] ☑
    blood disorder NOS D75.9 [M36.3]
    diabetes — *see* Diabetes, arthropathy
    endocrine disease NOS E34.9 [M14.8-] ☑
    erythema
      multiforme L51.9 [M14.8-] ☑
      nodosum L52 [M14.8-] ☑
    hemochromatosis E83.118 [M14.8-] ☑
    hemoglobinopathy NEC D58.2 [M36.3]
    hemophilia NEC D66 [M36.2]
    Henoch-Schönlein purpura D69.0 [M36.4]
    hyperthyroidism E05.90 [M14.8-] ☑
    hypothyroidism E03.9 [M14.8-] ☑
    infective endocarditis I33.0 [M12.80]
    leukemia NEC C95.9- ☑ [M36.1]
    malignant histiocytosis C96.A [M36.1]
    metabolic disease NOS E88.9 [M14.8-] ☑
    multiple myeloma C90.0- ☑ [M36.1]
    neoplastic disease NOS (*see also* Neoplasm)
      D49.9 [M36.1]
    nutritional deficiency (*see also* subcategory
      M14.8-) E63.9
    psoriasis NOS L40.50
    sarcoidosis D86.86
    syphilis (late) A52.77
      congenital A50.55 [M12.80]
    thyrotoxicosis (*see also* subcategory M14.8-) E05.90
    ulcerative colitis K51.90 [M07.60]
    viral hepatitis (postinfectious) NEC B19.9 [M12.80]
    Whipple's disease (*see also* subcategory M14.8-)
      K90.81
  Jaccoud — *see* Arthropathy, postrheumatic, chronic
  juvenile — *see* Arthritis, juvenile
    psoriatic L40.54
  mutilans (psoriatic) L40.52
  neuropathic (Charcot) M14.60
    ankle M14.67- ☑
    diabetic — *see* Diabetes, arthropathy, neuropathic
    elbow M14.62- ☑
    foot joint M14.67- ☑
    hand joint M14.64- ☑
    hip M14.65- ☑
    knee M14.66- ☑
    multiple site M14.69
    nonsyphilitic NEC G98.0
    shoulder M14.61- ☑
    syringomyelic G95.0
    vertebra M14.68
    wrist M14.63- ☑
  osteopulmonary — *see* Osteoarthropathy, hyper-
    trophic, specified NEC
  postdysenteric M02.10
    ankle M02.17- ☑
    elbow M02.12- ☑
    foot joint M02.17- ☑
    hand joint M02.14- ☑
    hip M02.15- ☑
    knee M02.16- ☑
    multiple site M02.19
    shoulder M02.11- ☑

Arthropathy — *continued*
  postdysenteric — *continued*
    vertebra M02.18
    wrist M02.13- ☑
  postimmunization M02.20
    ankle M02.27- ☑
    elbow M02.22- ☑
    foot joint M02.27- ☑
    hand joint M02.24- ☑
    hip M02.25- ☑
    knee M02.26- ☑
    multiple site M02.29
    shoulder M02.21- ☑
    vertebra M02.28
    wrist M02.23- ☑
  postinfectious NEC B99 ☑ [M12.80]
    in (due to)
      enteritis due to Yersinia enterocolitica
        A04.6 [M12.80]
      syphilis A52.77
      viral hepatitis NEC B19.9 [M12.80]
  postrheumatic, chronic (Jaccoud) M12.00
    ankle M12.07- ☑
    elbow M12.02- ☑
    foot joint M12.07- ☑
    hand joint M12.04- ☑
    hip M12.05- ☑
    knee M12.06- ☑
    multiple site M12.09
    shoulder M12.01- ☑
    specified joint NEC M12.08
    vertebrae M12.08
    wrist M12.03- ☑
  psoriatic NEC L40.59
    interphalangeal, distal L40.51
  reactive M02.9
    in (due to)
      infective endocarditis I33.0 [M02.9]
    specified type NEC M02.80
      ankle M02.87- ☑
      elbow M02.82- ☑
      foot joint M02.87- ☑
      hand joint M02.84- ☑
      hip M02.85- ☑
      knee M02.86- ☑
      multiple site M02.89
      shoulder M02.81- ☑
      vertebra M02.88
      wrist M02.83- ☑
  specified form NEC M12.80
    ankle M12.87- ☑
    elbow M12.82- ☑
    foot joint M12.87- ☑
    hand joint M12.84- ☑
    hip M12.85- ☑
    knee M12.86- ☑
    multiple site M12.89
    shoulder M12.81- ☑
    specified joint NEC M12.88
    vertebrae M12.88
    wrist M12.83- ☑
  syringomyelic G95.0
  tabes dorsalis A52.16
  tabetic A52.16
  transient — *see* Arthropathy, specified form NEC
  traumatic M12.50
    ankle M12.57- ☑
    elbow M12.52- ☑
    foot joint M12.57- ☑
    hand joint M12.54- ☑
    hip M12.55- ☑
    knee M12.56- ☑
    multiple site M12.59
    shoulder M12.51- ☑
    specified joint NEC M12.58
    vertebrae M12.58
    wrist M12.53- ☑
Arthropyosis — *see* Arthritis, pyogenic or pyemic
Arthrosis (deformans) (degenerative) (localized) (*see also* Osteoarthritis) M19.90
  spine — *see* Spondylosis
Arthus' phenomenon or reaction T78.41 ☑
  due to
    drug — *see* Table of Drugs and Chemicals, by drug
Articular — *see* condition
Articulation, reverse (teeth) M26.24

Artificial
  insemination complication — *see* Complications, arti-
    ficial, fertilization
  opening status (functioning) (without complication)
    Z93.9
    anus (colostomy) Z93.3
    colostomy Z93.3
    cystostomy Z93.50
      appendico-vesicostomy Z93.52
      cutaneous Z93.51
      specified NEC Z93.59
    enterostomy Z93.4
    gastrostomy Z93.1
    ileostomy Z93.2
    intestinal tract NEC Z93.4
    jejunostomy Z93.4
    nephrostomy Z93.6
    specified site NEC Z93.8
    tracheostomy Z93.0
    ureterostomy Z93.6
    urethrostomy Z93.6
    urinary tract NEC Z93.6
    vagina Z93.8
  vagina status Z93.8
Arytenoid — *see* condition
Asbestosis (occupational) J61
Ascariasis B77.9
  with
    complications NEC B77.89
    intestinal complications B77.0
    pneumonia, pneumonitis B77.81
Ascaridosis, ascaridiasis — *see* Ascariasis
Ascaris (infection) (infestation) (lumbricoides) — *see* Ascariasis
Ascending — *see* condition
ASC-H (atypical squamous cells cannot exclude high grade squamous intraepithelial lesion on cytologic smear)
  anus R85.611
  cervix R87.611
  vagina R87.621
Aschoff's bodies — *see* Myocarditis, rheumatic
Ascites (abdominal) R18.8
  cardiac I50.9
  chylous (nonfilarial) I89.8
    filarial — *see* Infestation, filarial
  due to
    cirrhosis, alcoholic K70.31
    hepatitis
      alcoholic K70.11
      chronic active K71.51
    S. japonicum B65.2
  heart I50.9
  malignant R18.0
  pseudochylous R18.8
  syphilitic A52.74
  tuberculous A18.31
ASC-US (atypical squamous cells of undetermined significance on cytologic smear)
  anus R85.610
  cervix R87.610
  vagina R87.620
Aseptic — *see* condition
Asherman's syndrome N85.6
Asialia K11.7
Asiatic cholera — *see* Cholera
Asimultagnosia (simultanagnosia) R48.3
Askin's tumor — *see* Neoplasm, connective tissue, malignant
Asocial personality F60.2
Asomatognosia R41.4
Aspartylglucosaminuria E77.1
Asperger's disease or syndrome F84.5
Aspergilloma — *see* Aspergillosis
Aspergillosis (with pneumonia) B44.9
  bronchopulmonary, allergic B44.81
  disseminated B44.7
  generalized B44.7
  pulmonary NEC B44.1
    allergic B44.81
    invasive B44.0
  specified NEC B44.89
  tonsillar B44.2
Aspergillus (flavus) (fumigatus) (infection) (terreus) — *see* Aspergillosis
Aspermatogenesis — *see* Azoospermia
Aspermia (testis) — *see* Azoospermia

☑ **Additional Character Required — Refer to the Tabular List for Character Selection**   ▽ **Subterms under main terms may continue to next column or page**

Asphyxia, asphyxiation (by) R09.01
  antenatal P84
  birth P84
  bunny bag — see Asphyxia, due to, mechanical threat to breathing, trapped in bed clothes
  crushing S28.0 ☑
  drowning T75.1 ☑
  gas, fumes, or vapor — see Table of Drugs and Chemicals
  inhalation — see Inhalation
  intrauterine P84
  local I73.00
    with gangrene I73.01
  mucus (see also Foreign body, respiratory tract, causing asphyxia)
  newborn P84
  pathological R09.01
  postnatal P84
    mechanical — see Asphyxia, due to, mechanical threat to breathing
  prenatal P84
  reticularis R23.1
  strangulation — see Asphyxia, due to, mechanical threat to breathing
  submersion T75.1 ☑
  traumatic T71.9 ☑
    due to
      crushed chest S28.0 ☑
      foreign body (in) — see Foreign body, respiratory tract, causing asphyxia
      low oxygen content of ambient air T71.20 ☑
        due to
          being trapped in
            low oxygen environment T71.29 ☑
            in car trunk T71.221 ☑
              circumstances undetermined T71.224 ☑
              done with intent to harm by
                another person T71.223 ☑
                self T71.222 ☑
            in refrigerator T71.231 ☑
              circumstances undetermined T71.234 ☑
              done with intent to harm by
                another person T71.233 ☑
                self T71.232 ☑
      cave-in T71.21 ☑
      mechanical threat to breathing (accidental) T71.191 ☑
      circumstances undetermined T71.194 ☑
      done with intent to harm by
        another person T71.193 ☑
        self T71.192 ☑
      hanging T71.161 ☑
        circumstances undetermined T71.164 ☑
        done with intent to harm by
          another person T71.163 ☑
          self T71.162 ☑
      plastic bag T71.121 ☑
        circumstances undetermined T71.124 ☑
        done with intent to harm by
          another person T71.123 ☑
          self T71.122 ☑
      smothering
        in furniture T71.151 ☑
          circumstances undetermined T71.154 ☑
          done with intent to harm by
            another person T71.153 ☑
            self T71.152 ☑
        under
          another person's body T71.141 ☑
            circumstances undetermined T71.144 ☑
            done with intent to harm T71.143 ☑
          pillow T71.111 ☑
            circumstances undetermined T71.114 ☑
            done with intent to harm by
              another person T71.113 ☑
              self T71.112 ☑
      trapped in bed clothes T71.131 ☑
        circumstances undetermined T71.134 ☑
        done with intent to harm by
          another person T71.133 ☑
          self T71.132 ☑

Asphyxia, asphyxiation — continued
  vomiting, vomitus — see Foreign body, respiratory tract, causing asphyxia
Aspiration
  amniotic (clear) fluid (newborn) P24.10
    with
      pneumonia (pneumonitis) P24.11
      respiratory symptoms P24.11
  blood
    newborn (without respiratory symptoms) P24.20
      with
        pneumonia (pneumonitis) P24.21
        respiratory symptoms P24.21
    specified age NEC — see Foreign body, respiratory tract
  bronchitis J69.0
  food or foreign body (with asphyxiation) — see Asphyxia, food
  liquor (amnii) (newborn) P24.10
    with
      pneumonia (pneumonitis) P24.11
      respiratory symptoms P24.11
  meconium (newborn) (without respiratory symptoms) P24.00
    with
      pneumonitis (pneumonitis) P24.01
      respiratory symptoms P24.01
  milk (newborn) (without respiratory symptoms) P24.30
    with
      pneumonia (pneumonitis) P24.31
      respiratory symptoms P24.31
    specified age NEC — see Foreign body, respiratory tract
  mucus (see also Foreign body, by site, causing asphyxia)
    newborn P24.10
      with
        pneumonia (pneumonitis) P24.11
        respiratory symptoms P24.11
  neonatal P24.9
    specific NEC (without respiratory symptoms) P24.80
      with
        pneumonia (pneumonitis) P24.81
        respiratory symptoms P24.81
  newborn P24.9
    specific NEC (without respiratory symptoms) P24.80
      with
        pneumonia (pneumonitis) P24.81
        respiratory symptoms P24.81
  pneumonia J69.0
  pneumonitis J69.0
  syndrome of newborn — see Aspiration, by substance, with pneumonia
  vernix caseosa (newborn) P24.80
    with
      pneumonia (pneumonitis) P24.81
      respiratory symptoms P24.81
  vomitus (see also Foreign body, respiratory tract)
    newborn (without respiratory symptoms) P24.30
      with
        pneumonia (pneumonitis) P24.31
        respiratory symptoms P24.31
Asplenia (congenital) Q89.01
  postsurgical Z90.81
Assam fever B55.0
Assault, sexual — see Maltreatment
Assmann's focus NEC A15.0
Astasia (-abasia) (hysterical) F44.4
Asteatosis cutis L85.3
Astereognosia, astereognosis R48.1
Asterixis R27.8
  in liver disease K71.3
Asteroid hyalitis — see Deposit, crystalline
Asthenia, asthenic R53.1
  cardiac (see also Failure, heart) I50.9
    psychogenic F45.8
  cardiovascular (see also Failure, heart) I50.9
    psychogenic F45.8
  heart (see also Failure, heart) I50.9
    psychogenic F45.8
  hysterical F44.4
  myocardial (see also Failure, heart) I50.9
    psychogenic F45.8
  nervous F48.8
  neurocirculatory F45.8
  neurotic F48.8
  psychogenic F48.8
  psychoneurotic F48.8

Asthenia, asthenic — continued
  psychophysiologic F48.8
  reaction (psychophysiologic) F48.8
  senile R54
Asthenopia (see also Discomfort, visual)
  hysterical F44.6
  psychogenic F44.6
Asthenospermia — see Abnormal, specimen, male genital organs
Asthma, asthmatic (bronchial) (catarrh) (spasmodic) J45.909
  with
    chronic obstructive bronchitis J44.9
      with
        acute lower respiratory infection J44.0
        exacerbation (acute) J44.1
    chronic obstructive pulmonary disease J44.9
      with
        acute lower respiratory infection J44.0
        exacerbation (acute) J44.1
    exacerbation (acute) J45.901
    hay fever — see Asthma, allergic extrinsic
    rhinitis, allergic — see Asthma, allergic extrinsic
    status asthmaticus J45.902
  allergic extrinsic J45.909
    with
      exacerbation (acute) J45.901
      status asthmaticus J45.902
  atopic — see Asthma, allergic extrinsic
  cardiac — see Failure, ventricular, left
  cardiobronchial I50.1
  childhood J45.909
    with
      exacerbation (acute) J45.901
      status asthmaticus J45.902
  chronic obstructive J44.9
    with
      acute lower respiratory infection J44.0
      exacerbation (acute) J44.1
  collier's J60
  cough variant J45.991
  detergent J69.8
  due to
    detergent J69.8
    inhalation of fumes J68.3
  eosinophilic J82
  extrinsic, allergic — see Asthma, allergic extrinsic
  grinder's J62.8
  hay — see Asthma, allergic extrinsic
  heart I50.9
  idiosyncratic — see Asthma, nonallergic
  intermittent (mild) J45.20
    with
      exacerbation (acute) J45.21
      status asthmaticus J45.22
  intrinsic, nonallergic — see Asthma, nonallergic
  Kopp's E32.8
  late-onset J45.909
    with
      exacerbation (acute) J45.901
      status asthmaticus J45.902
  mild intermittent J45.20
    with
      exacerbation (acute) J45.21
      status asthmaticus J45.22
  mild persistent J45.30
    with
      exacerbation (acute) J45.31
      status asthmaticus J45.32
  Millar's (laryngismus stridulus) J38.5
  miner's J60
  mixed J45.909
    with
      exacerbation (acute) J45.901
      status asthmaticus J45.902
  moderate persistent J45.40
    with
      exacerbation (acute) J45.41
      status asthmaticus J45.42
  nervous — see Asthma, nonallergic
  nonallergic (intrinsic) J45.909
    with
      exacerbation (acute) J45.901
      status asthmaticus J45.902
  persistent
    mild J45.30
      with
        exacerbation (acute) J45.31

Asthma, asthmatic — *continued*
  persistent — *continued*
    mild — *continued*
      with — *continued*
        status asthmaticus J45.32
      moderate J45.40
        with
          exacerbation (acute) J45.41
          status asthmaticus J45.42
      severe J45.50
        with
          exacerbation (acute) J45.51
          status asthmaticus J45.52
    platinum J45.998
    pneumoconiotic NEC J64
    potter's J62.8
    predominantly allergic J45.909
    psychogenic F54
    pulmonary eosinophilic J82
    red cedar J67.8
    Rostan's I50.1
    sandblaster's J62.8
    sequoiosis J67.8
    severe persistent J45.50
      with
        exacerbation (acute) J45.51
        status asthmaticus J45.52
    specified NEC J45.998
    stonemason's J62.8
    thymic E32.8
    tuberculous — *see* Tuberculosis, pulmonary
    Wichmann's (laryngismus stridulus) J38.5
    wood J67.8
Astigmatism (compound) (congenital) H52.20- ☑
  irregular H52.21- ☑
  regular H52.22- ☑
Astraphobia F40.220
Astroblastoma
  specified site — *see* Neoplasm, malignant, by site
  unspecified site C71.9
Astrocytoma (cystic)
  anaplastic
    specified site — *see* Neoplasm, malignant, by site
    unspecified site C71.9
  fibrillary
    specified site — *see* Neoplasm, malignant, by site
    unspecified site C71.9
  fibrous
    specified site — *see* Neoplasm, malignant, by site
    unspecified site C71.9
  gemistocytic
    specified site — *see* Neoplasm, malignant, by site
    unspecified site C71.9
  juvenile
    specified site — *see* Neoplasm, malignant, by site
    unspecified site C71.9
  pilocytic
    specified site — *see* Neoplasm, malignant, by site
    unspecified site C71.9
  piloid
    specified site — *see* Neoplasm, malignant, by site
    unspecified site C71.9
  protoplasmic
    specified site — *see* Neoplasm, malignant, by site
    unspecified site C71.9
  specified site NEC — *see* Neoplasm, malignant, by site
  subependymal D43.2
    giant cell
      specified site — *see* Neoplasm, uncertain behavior, by site
      unspecified site D43.2
    specified site — *see* Neoplasm, uncertain behavior, by site
    unspecified site D43.2
  unspecified site C71.9
Astroglioma
  specified site — *see* Neoplasm, malignant, by site
  unspecified site C71.9
Asymbolia R48.8
Asymmetry (*see also* Distortion)
  between native and reconstructed breast N65.1
  face Q67.0
  jaw (lower) — *see* Anomaly, dentofacial, jaw-cranial base relationship, asymmetry
Asynergia, asynergy R27.8
  ventricular I51.89
Asystole (heart) — *see* Arrest, cardiac

At risk
  for falling Z91.81
Ataxia, ataxy, ataxic R27.0
  acute R27.8
  brain (hereditary) G11.9
  cerebellar (hereditary) G11.9
    with defective DNA repair G11.3
    alcoholic G31.2
    early-onset G11.1
    in
      alcoholism G31.2
      myxedema E03.9 [G13.2]
      neoplastic disease (*see also* Neoplasm) D49.9 [G13.1]
      specified disease NEC G32.81
    late-onset (Marie's) G11.2
  cerebral (hereditary) G11.9
  congenital nonprogressive G11.0
  family, familial — *see* Ataxia, hereditary
  following
    cerebrovascular disease I69.993
      cerebral infarction I69.393
      intracerebral hemorrhage I69.193
      nontraumatic intracranial hemorrhage NEC I69.293
      specified disease NEC I69.893
      subarachnoid hemorrhage I69.093
  Friedreich's (heredofamilial) (cerebellar) (spinal) G11.1
  gait R26.0
    hysterical F44.4
  general R27.8
  gluten M35.9 [G32.81]
    with celiac disease K90.0 [G32.81]
  hereditary G11.9
    with neuropathy G60.2
    cerebellar — *see* Ataxia, cerebellar
    spastic G11.4
    specified NEC G11.8
    spinal (Friedreich's) G11.1
  heredofamilial — *see* Ataxia, hereditary
  Hunt's G11.1
  hysterical F44.4
  locomotor (progressive) (syphilitic) (partial) (spastic) A52.11
    diabetic — *see* Diabetes, ataxia
  Marie's (cerebellar) (heredofamilial) (late-onset) G11.2
  nonorganic origin F44.4
  nonprogressive, congenital G11.0
  psychogenic F44.4
  Roussy-Lévy G60.0
  Sanger-Brown's (hereditary) G11.2
  spastic hereditary G11.4
  spinal
    hereditary (Friedreich's) G11.1
    progressive (syphilitic) A52.11
  spinocerebellar, X-linked recessive G11.1
  telangiectasia (Louis-Bar) G11.3
Ataxia-telangiectasia (Louis-Bar) G11.3
Atelectasis (massive) (partial) (pressure) (pulmonary) J98.11
  newborn P28.10
    due to resorption P28.11
    partial P28.19
    primary P28.0
    secondary P28.19
  primary (newborn) P28.0
  tuberculous — *see* Tuberculosis, pulmonary
Atelocardia Q24.9
Atelomyelia Q06.1
Atheroembolism
  of
    extremities
      lower I75.02- ☑
      upper I75.01- ☑
    kidney I75.81
    specified NEC I75.89
Atheroma, atheromatous (*see also* Arteriosclerosis) I70.90
  aorta, aortic I70.0
    valve (*see also* Endocarditis, aortic) I35.8
  aorto-iliac I70.0
  artery — *see* Arteriosclerosis
  basilar (artery) I67.2
  carotid (artery) (common) (internal) I67.2
  cerebral (arteries) I67.2
  coronary (artery) I25.10
    with angina pectoris — *see* Arteriosclerosis, coronary (artery),

Atheroma, atheromatous — *continued*
  degeneration — *see* Arteriosclerosis
  heart, cardiac — *see* Disease, heart, ischemic, atherosclerotic
  mitral (valve) I34.8
  myocardium, myocardial — *see* Disease, heart, ischemic, atherosclerotic
  pulmonary valve (heart) (*see also* Endocarditis, pulmonary) I37.8
  tricuspid (heart) (valve) I36.8
  valve, valvular — *see* Endocarditis
  vertebral (artery) I67.2
Atheromatosis — *see* Arteriosclerosis
Atherosclerosis (*see also* Arteriosclerosis)
  coronary
    artery I25.10
      with angina pectoris — *see* Arteriosclerosis, coronary (artery),
      due to
        calcified coronary lesion (severely) I25.84
        lipid rich plaque I25.83
    transplanted heart I25.811
      bypass graft I25.812
        with angina pectoris — *see* Arteriosclerosis, coronary (artery),
      native coronary artery I25.811
        with angina pectoris — *see* Arteriosclerosis, coronary (artery),
Athetosis (acquired) R25.8
  bilateral (congenital) G80.3
  congenital (bilateral) (double) G80.3
  double (congenital) G80.3
  unilateral R25.8
Athlete's
  foot B35.3
  heart I51.7
Athrepsia E41
Athyrea (acquired) (*see also* Hypothyroidism)
  congenital E03.1
Atonia, atony, atonic
  bladder (sphincter) (neurogenic) N31.2
  capillary I78.8
  cecum K59.8
    psychogenic F45.8
  colon — *see* Atony, intestine
  congenital P94.2
  esophagus K22.8
  intestine K59.8
    psychogenic F45.8
  stomach K31.89
    neurotic or psychogenic F45.8
  uterus (during labor) O62.2
    with hemorrhage (postpartum) O72.1
    postpartum (with hemorrhage) O72.1
      without hemorrhage O75.89
Atopy — *see* History, allergy
Atransferrinemia, congenital E88.09
Atresia, atretic
  alimentary organ or tract NEC Q45.8
    upper Q40.8
  ani, anus, anal (canal) Q42.3
    with fistula Q42.2
  aorta (arch) (ring) Q25.2
  aortic (orifice) (valve) Q23.0
    arch Q25.2
    congenital with hypoplasia of ascending aorta and defective development of left ventricle (with mitral stenosis) Q23.4
    in hypoplastic left heart syndrome Q23.4
  aqueduct of Sylvius Q03.0
    with spina bifida — *see* Spina bifida, with hydrocephalus
  artery NEC Q27.8
    cerebral Q28.3
    coronary Q24.5
    digestive system Q27.8
    eye Q15.8
    lower limb Q27.8
    pulmonary Q25.5
    specified site NEC Q27.8
    umbilical Q27.0
    upper limb Q27.8
  auditory canal (external) Q16.1
  bile duct (common) (congenital) (hepatic) Q44.2
    acquired — *see* Obstruction, bile duct
  bladder (neck) Q64.39
    obstruction Q64.31
  bronchus Q32.4

☑ **Additional Character Required** — Refer to the Tabular List for Character Selection   ▽ **Subterms under main terms may continue to next column or page**

Atresia, atretic — *continued*
  cecum Q42.8
  cervix (acquired) N88.2
    congenital Q51.828
    in pregnancy or childbirth — *see* Anomaly, cervix, in pregnancy or childbirth
      causing obstructed labor O65.5
  choana Q30.0
  colon Q42.9
    specified NEC Q42.8
  common duct Q44.2
  cricoid cartilage Q31.8
  cystic duct Q44.2
    acquired K82.8
      with obstruction K82.0
  digestive organs NEC Q45.8
  duodenum Q41.0
  ear canal Q16.1
  ejaculatory duct Q55.4
  epiglottis Q31.8
  esophagus Q39.0
    with tracheoesophageal fistula Q39.1
  eustachian tube Q17.8
  fallopian tube (congenital) Q50.6
    acquired N97.1
  follicular cyst N83.0
  foramen of
    Luschka Q03.1
      with spina bifida — *see* Spina bifida, with hydrocephalus
    Magendie Q03.1
      with spina bifida — *see* Spina bifida, with hydrocephalus
  gallbladder Q44.1
  genital organ
    external
      female Q52.79
      male Q55.8
    internal
      female Q52.8
      male Q55.8
  glottis Q31.8
  gullet Q39.0
    with tracheoesophageal fistula Q39.1
  heart valve NEC Q24.8
    pulmonary Q22.0
    tricuspid Q22.4
  hymen Q52.3
    acquired (postinfective) N89.6
  ileum Q41.2
  intestine (small) Q41.9
    large Q42.9
      specified NEC Q42.8
  iris, filtration angle Q15.0
  jejunum Q41.1
  lacrimal apparatus Q10.4
  larynx Q31.8
  meatus urinarius Q64.33
  mitral valve Q23.2
    in hypoplastic left heart syndrome Q23.4
  nares (anterior) (posterior) Q30.0
  nasopharynx Q34.8
  nose, nostril Q30.0
    acquired J34.89
  organ or site NEC Q89.8
  osseous meatus (ear) Q16.1
  oviduct (congenital) Q50.6
    acquired N97.1
  parotid duct Q38.4
    acquired K11.8
  pulmonary (artery) Q25.5
    valve Q22.0
  pulmonic Q22.0
  pupil Q13.2
  rectum Q42.1
    with fistula Q42.0
  salivary duct Q38.4
    acquired K11.8
  sublingual duct Q38.4
    acquired K11.8
  submandibular duct Q38.4
    acquired K11.8
  submaxillary duct Q38.4
    acquired K11.8
  thyroid cartilage Q31.8
  trachea Q32.1
  tricuspid valve Q22.4

Atresia, atretic — *continued*
  ureter Q62.10
    pelvic junction Q62.11
    vesical orifice Q62.12
  ureteropelvic junction Q62.11
  ureterovesical orifice Q62.12
  urethra (valvular) Q64.39
    stricture Q64.32
  urinary tract NEC Q64.8
  uterus Q51.818
    acquired N85.8
  vagina (congenital) Q52.4
    acquired (postinfectional) (senile) N89.5
  vas deferens Q55.3
  vascular NEC Q27.8
    cerebral Q28.3
    digestive system Q27.8
    lower limb Q27.8
    specified site NEC Q27.8
    upper limb Q27.8
  vein NEC Q27.8
    digestive system Q27.8
    great Q26.8
    lower limb Q27.8
    portal Q26.5
    pulmonary Q26.3
    specified site NEC Q27.8
    upper limb Q27.8
  vena cava (inferior) (superior) Q26.8
  vesicourethral orifice Q64.31
  vulva Q52.79
    acquired N90.5
Atrichia, atrichosis — *see* Alopecia
Atrophia (*see also* Atrophy)
  cutis senilis L90.8
    due to radiation L57.8
  gyrata of choroid and retina H31.23
  senilis R54
    dermatological L90.8
      due to radiation (nonionizing) (solar) L57.8
  unguium L60.3
    congenita Q84.6
Atrophie blanche (en plaque) (de Milian) L95.0
Atrophoderma, atrophodermia (of) L90.9
  diffusum (idiopathic) L90.4
  maculatum L90.8
    et striatum L90.8
      due to syphilis A52.79
    syphilitic A51.39
  neuriticum L90.8
  Pasini and Pierini L90.3
  pigmentosum Q82.1
  reticulatum symmetricum faciei L66.4
  senile L90.8
    due to radiation (nonionizing) (solar) L57.8
  vermiculata (cheeks) L66.4
Atrophy, atrophic (of)
  adrenal (capsule) (gland) E27.49
    primary (autoimmune) E27.1
  alveolar process or ridge (edentulous) K08.20
  anal sphincter (disuse) N81.84
  appendix K38.8
  arteriosclerotic — *see* Arteriosclerosis
  bile duct (common) (hepatic) K83.8
  bladder N32.89
    neurogenic N31.8
  blanche (en plaque) (of Milian) L95.0
  bone (senile) NEC (*see also* Disorder, bone, specified type NEC)
    due to
      tabes dorsalis (neurogenic) A52.11
  brain (cortex) (progressive) G31.9
    frontotemporal circumscribed G31.01 [F02.80]
      with behavioral disturbance G31.01 [F02.81]
    senile NEC G31.1
  breast N64.2
    obstetric — *see* Disorder, breast, specified type NEC
  buccal cavity K13.79
  cardiac — *see* Degeneration, myocardial
  cartilage (infectional) (joint) — *see* Disorder, cartilage, specified NEC
  cerebellar — *see* Atrophy, brain
  cerebral — *see* Atrophy, brain
  cervix (mucosa) (senile) (uteri) N88.8
    menopausal N95.8
  Charcot-Marie-Tooth G60.0

Atrophy, atrophic — *continued*
  choroid (central) (macular) (myopic) (retina) H31.10- ☑
    diffuse secondary H31.12- ☑
    gyrate H31.23
    senile H31.11- ☑
  ciliary body — *see* Atrophy, iris
  conjunctiva (senile) H11.89
  corpus cavernosum N48.89
  cortical — *see* Atrophy, brain
  cystic duct K82.8
  Déjérine-Thomas G23.8
  disuse NEC — *see* Atrophy, muscle
  Duchenne-Aran G12.21
  ear H93.8- ☑
  edentulous alveolar ridge K08.20
  endometrium (senile) N85.8
    cervix N88.8
  enteric K63.89
  epididymis N50.8
  eyeball — *see* Disorder, globe, degenerated condition, atrophy
  eyelid (senile) — *see* Disorder, eyelid, degenerative
  facial (skin) L90.9
  fallopian tube (senile) N83.32
    with ovary N83.33
  fascioscapulohumeral (Landouzy- Déjérine) G71.0
  fatty, thymus (gland) E32.8
  gallbladder K82.8
  gastric K29.40
    with bleeding K29.41
  gastrointestinal K63.89
  glandular I89.8
  globe H44.52- ☑
  gum K06.0
  hair L67.8
  heart (brown) — *see* Degeneration, myocardial
  hemifacial Q67.4
    Romberg G51.8
  infantile E41
    paralysis, acute — *see* Poliomyelitis, paralytic
  intestine K63.89
  iris (essential) (progressive) H21.26- ☑
    specified NEC H21.29
  kidney (senile) (terminal) (*see also* Sclerosis, renal) N26.1
    congenital or infantile Q60.5
      bilateral Q60.4
      unilateral Q60.3
    hydronephrotic — *see* Hydronephrosis
  lacrimal gland (primary) H04.14- ☑
    secondary H04.15- ☑
  Landouzy-Déjérine G71.0
  laryngitis, infective J37.0
  larynx J38.7
  Leber's optic (hereditary) H47.22
  lip K13.0
  liver (yellow) K72.90
    with coma K72.91
    acute, subacute K72.00
      with coma K72.01
    chronic K72.10
      with coma K72.11
  lung (senile) J98.4
  macular (dermatological) L90.8
    syphilitic, skin A51.39
      striated A52.79
  mandible (edentulous) K08.20
    minimal K08.21
    moderate K08.22
    severe K08.23
  maxilla K08.20
    minimal K08.24
    moderate K08.25
    severe K08.26
  muscle, muscular (diffuse) (general) (idiopathic) (primary) M62.50
    ankle M62.57- ☑
    Duchenne-Aran G12.21
    foot M62.57- ☑
    forearm M62.53- ☑
    hand M62.54- ☑
    infantile spinal G12.0
    lower leg M62.56- ☑
    multiple sites M62.59
    myelopathic — *see* Atrophy, muscle, spinal
    myotonic G71.11
    neuritic G58.9
    neuropathic (peroneal) (progressive) G60.0

Atrophy, atrophic — continued
  muscle, muscular — continued
    pelvic (disuse) N81.84
    peroneal G60.0
    progressive (bulbar) G12.21
      adult G12.1
      infantile (spinal) G12.0
      spinal G12.9
        adult G12.1
        infantile G12.0
    pseudohypertrophic G71.0
    shoulder region M62.51- ☑
    specified site NEC M62.58
    spinal G12.9
      adult form G12.1
      Aran-Duchenne G12.21
      childhood form, type II G12.1
      distal G12.1
      hereditary NEC G12.1
      infantile, type I (Werdnig-Hoffmann) G12.0
      juvenile form, type III (Kugelberg- Welander) G12.1
      progressive G12.21
      scapuloperoneal form G12.1
      specified NEC G12.8
    syphilitic A52.78
    thigh M62.55- ☑
    upper arm M62.52- ☑
  myocardium — see Degeneration, myocardial
  myometrium (senile) N85.8
    cervix N88.8
  myopathic NEC — see Atrophy, muscle
  myotonia G71.11
  nail L60.3
  nasopharynx J31.1
  nerve (see also Disorder, nerve)
    abducens — see Strabismus, paralytic, sixth nerve
    accessory G52.8
    acoustic or auditory H93.3 ☑
    cranial G52.9
      eighth (auditory) H93.3 ☑
      eleventh (accessory) G52.8
      fifth (trigeminal) G50.8
      first (olfactory) G52.0
      fourth (trochlear) — see Strabismus, paralytic, fourth nerve
      second (optic) H47.20
      sixth (abducens) — see Strabismus, paralytic, sixth nerve
      tenth (pneumogastric) (vagus) G52.2
      third (oculomotor) — see Strabismus, paralytic, third nerve
      twelfth (hypoglossal) G52.3
    hypoglossal G52.3
    oculomotor — see Strabismus, paralytic, third nerve
    olfactory G52.0
    optic (papillomacular bundle)
      syphilitic (late) A52.15
        congenital A50.44
    pneumogastric G52.2
    trigeminal G50.8
    trochlear — see Strabismus, paralytic, fourth nerve
    vagus (pneumogastric) G52.2
  neurogenic, bone, tabetic A52.11
  nutritional E41
  old age R54
  olivopontocerebellar G23.8
  optic (nerve) H47.20
    glaucomatous H47.23- ☑
    hereditary H47.22
    primary H47.21- ☑
    specified type NEC H47.29- ☑
    syphilitic (late) A52.15
      congenital A50.44
  orbit H05.31- ☑
  ovary (senile) N83.31
    with fallopian tube N83.33
  oviduct (senile) — see Atrophy, fallopian tube
  palsy, diffuse (progressive) G12.22
  pancreas (duct) (senile) K86.8
  parotid gland K11.0
  pelvic muscle N81.84
  penis N48.89
  pharynx J39.2
  pluriglandular E31.8
    autoimmune E31.0
  polyarthritis M15.9

Atrophy, atrophic — continued
  prostate N42.89
  pseudohypertrophic (muscle) G71.0
  renal (see also Sclerosis, renal) N26.1
  retina, retinal (postinfectional) H35.89
  rhinitis J31.0
  salivary gland K11.0
  scar L90.5
  sclerosis, lobar (of brain) G31.09 [F02.80]
    with behavioral disturbance G31.09 [F02.81]
  scrotum N50.8
  seminal vesicle N50.8
  senile R54
    due to radiation (nonionizing) (solar) L57.8
  skin (patches) (spots) L90.9
    degenerative (senile) L90.8
    due to radiation (nonionizing) (solar) L57.8
    senile L90.8
  spermatic cord N50.8
  spinal (acute) (cord) G95.89
    muscular — see Atrophy, muscle, spinal
    paralysis G12.20
      acute — see Poliomyelitis, paralytic
      meaning progressive muscular atrophy G12.21
  spine (column) — see Spondylopathy, specified NEC
  spleen (senile) D73.0
  stomach K29.40
    with bleeding K29.41
  striate (skin) L90.6
    syphilitic A52.79
  subcutaneous L90.9
  sublingual gland K11.0
  submandibular gland K11.0
  submaxillary gland K11.0
  Sudeck's — see Algoneurodystrophy
  suprarenal (capsule) (gland) E27.49
    primary E27.1
  systemic affecting central nervous system in
      myxedema E03.9 [G13.2]
      neoplastic disease (see also Neoplasm) D49.9 [G13.1]
      specified disease NEC G13.8
  tarso-orbital fascia, congenital Q10.3
  testis N50.0
  thenar, partial — see Syndrome, carpal tunnel
  thymus (fatty) E32.8
  thyroid (gland) (acquired) E03.4
    with cretinism E03.1
    congenital (with myxedema) E03.1
  tongue (senile) K14.8
    papillae K14.4
  trachea J39.8
  tunica vaginalis N50.8
  turbinate J34.89
  tympanic membrane (nonflaccid) H73.82- ☑
    flaccid H73.81- ☑
  upper respiratory tract J39.8
  uterus, uterine (senile) N85.8
    cervix N88.8
    due to radiation (intended effect) N85.8
      adverse effect or misadventure N99.89
  vagina (senile) N95.2
  vas deferens N50.8
  vascular I99.8
  vertebra (senile) — see Spondylopathy, specified NEC
  vulva (senile) N90.5
  Werdnig-Hoffmann G12.0
  yellow — see Failure, hepatic

Attack, attacks
  with alteration of consciousness (with automatisms) — see Epilepsy, localization-related, symptomatic, with complex partial seizures
  without alteration of consciousness — see Epilepsy, localization-related, symptomatic, with simple partial seizures
  Adams-Stokes I45.9
  akinetic — see Epilepsy, generalized, specified NEC
  angina — see Angina
  atonic — see Epilepsy, generalized, specified NEC
  benign shuddering G25.83
  cataleptic — see Catalepsy
  coronary — see Infarct, myocardium
  cyanotic, newborn P28.2
  drop NEC R55
  epileptic — see Epilepsy
  heart — see Infarct, myocardium
  hysterical F44.9

Attack, attacks — continued
  jacksonian — see Epilepsy, localization-related, symptomatic, with simple partial seizures
  myocardium, myocardial — see Infarct, myocardium
  myoclonic — see Epilepsy, generalized, specified NEC
  panic F41.0
  psychomotor — see Epilepsy, localization-related, symptomatic, with complex partial seizures
  salaam — see Epilepsy, spasms
  schizophreniform, brief F23
  shuddering, benign G25.83
  Stokes-Adams I45.9
  syncope R55
  transient ischemic (TIA) G45.9
    specified NEC G45.8
  unconsciousness R55
    hysterical F44.89
  vasomotor R55
  vasovagal (paroxysmal) (idiopathic) R55

Attention (to)
  artificial
    opening (of) Z43.9
      digestive tract NEC Z43.4
        colon Z43.3
        ilium Z43.2
        stomach Z43.1
      specified NEC Z43.8
      trachea Z43.0
      urinary tract NEC Z43.6
        cystostomy Z43.5
        nephrostomy Z43.6
        ureterostomy Z43.6
        urethrostomy Z43.6
    vagina Z43.7
  colostomy Z43.3
  cystostomy Z43.5
  deficit disorder or syndrome F98.8
    with hyperactivity — see Disorder, attention-deficit hyperactivity
  gastrostomy Z43.1
  ileostomy Z43.2
  jejunostomy Z43.4
  nephrostomy Z43.6
  surgical dressings Z48.01
  sutures Z48.02
  tracheostomy Z43.0
  ureterostomy Z43.6
  urethrostomy Z43.6

Attrition
  gum K06.0
  tooth, teeth (excessive) (hard tissues) K03.0

Atypical, atypism (see also condition)
  cells (on cytolgocial smear) (endocervical) (endometrial) (glandular)
    cervix R87.619
    vagina R87.629
  cervical N87.9
  endometrium N85.9
    hyperplasia N85.00
  parenting situation Z62.9

Auditory — see condition

Aujeszky's disease B33.8

Aurantiasis, cutis E67.1

Auricle, auricular (see also condition)
  cervical Q18.2

Auriculotemporal syndrome G50.8

Austin Flint murmur (aortic insufficiency) I35.1

Australian
  Q fever A78
  X disease A83.4

Autism, autistic (childhood) (infantile) F84.0
  atypical F84.9

Autodigestion R68.89

Autoerythrocyte sensitization (syndrome) D69.2

Autographism L50.3

Autoimmune
  disease (systemic) M35.9
  inhibitors to clotting factors D68.311
  lymphoproliferative syndrome [ALPS] D89.82
  thyroiditis E06.3

Autointoxication R68.89

Automatism G93.89
  with temporal sclerosis G93.81
  epileptic — see Epilepsy, localization-related, symptomatic, with complex partial seizures
  paroxysmal, idiopathic — see Epilepsy, localization-related, symptomatic, with complex partial seizures

☑ Additional Character Required — Refer to the Tabular List for Character Selection   ▼ Subterms under main terms may continue to next column or page

Autonomic, autonomous
  bladder (neurogenic) N31.2
  hysteria seizure F44.5
Autosensitivity, erythrocyte D69.2
Autosensitization, cutaneous L30.2
Autosome — see condition by chromosome involved
Autotopagnosia R48.1
Autotoxemia R68.89
Autumn — see condition
Avellis' syndrome G46.8
Aversion
  oral R63.3
    newborn P92.- ☑
    nonorganic origin F98.2 ☑
  sexual F52.1
Aviator's
  disease or sickness — see Effect, adverse, high altitude
  ear T70.0 ☑
Avitaminosis (multiple) (see also Deficiency, vitamin)
    E56.9
  B E53.9
    with
      beriberi E51.11
      pellagra E52
  B2 E53.0
  B6 E53.1
  B12 E53.8
  D E55.9
    with rickets E55.0
  G E53.0
  K E56.1
  nicotinic acid E52
AVNRT (atrioventricular nodal re-entrant tachycardia)
    I47.1
AVRT (atrioventricular nodal re-entrant tachycardia) I47.1
Avulsion (traumatic)
  blood vessel — see Injury, blood vessel
  bone — see Fracture, by site
  cartilage (see also Dislocation, by site)
    symphyseal (inner), complicating delivery O71.6
  external site other than limb — see Wound, open, by
    site
  eye S05.7- ☑
  head (intracranial)
    external site NEC S08.89 ☑
    scalp S08.0 ☑
  internal organ or site — see Injury, by site
  joint (see also Dislocation, by site)
    capsule — see Sprain, by site
  kidney S37.06- ☑
  ligament — see Sprain, by site
  limb (see also Amputation, traumatic, by site)
    skin and subcutaneous tissue — see Wound, open,
      by site
  muscle — see Injury, muscle
  nerve (root) — see Injury, nerve
  scalp S08.0 ☑
  skin and subcutaneous tissue — see Wound, open, by
    site
  spleen S36.032 ☑
  symphyseal cartilage (inner), complicating delivery
    O71.6
  tendon — see Injury, muscle
  tooth S03.2 ☑
Awareness of heart beat R00.2
Axenfeld's
  anomaly or syndrome Q15.0
  degeneration (calcareous) Q13.4
Axilla, axillary (see also condition)
  breast Q83.1
Axonotmesis — see Injury, nerve
Ayerza's disease or syndrome (pulmonary artery scle-
    rosis with pulmonary hypertension) I27.0
Azoospermia (organic) N46.01
  due to
    drug therapy N46.021
    efferent duct obstruction N46.023
    infection N46.022
    radiation N46.024
    specified cause NEC N46.029
    systemic disease N46.025
Azotemia R79.89
  meaning uremia N19
Aztec ear Q17.3
Azygos
  continuation inferior vena cava Q26.8
  lobe (lung) Q33.1

B

Baastrup's disease — see Kissing spine
Babesiosis B60.0
Babington's disease (familial hemorrhagic telangiecta-
    sia) I78.0
Babinski's syndrome A52.79
Baby
  crying constantly R68.11
  floppy (syndrome) P94.2
Bacillary — see condition
Bacilluria N39.0
Bacillus (see also Infection, bacillus)
  abortus infection A23.1
  anthracis infection A22.9
  coli infection (see also Escherichia coli) B96.20
  Flexner's A03.1
  mallei infection A24.0
  Shiga's A03.0
  suipestifer infection — see Infection, salmonella
Back — see condition
Backache (postural) M54.9
  sacroiliac M53.3
  specified NEC M54.89
Backflow — see Reflux
Backward reading (dyslexia) F81.0
Bacteremia R78.81
  with sepsis — see Sepsis
Bactericholia — see Cholecystitis, acute
Bacterid, bacteride (pustular) L40.3
Bacterium, bacteria, bacterial
  agent NEC, as cause of disease classified elsewhere
    B96.89
  in blood — see Bacteremia
  in urine — see Bacteriuria
Bacteriuria, bacteruria N39.0
  asymptomatic N39.0
Bacteroides
  fragilis, as cause of disease classified elsewhere B96.6
Bad
  heart — see Disease, heart
  trip
    due to drug abuse — see Abuse, drug, hallucino-
      gen
    due to drug dependence — see Dependence, drug,
      hallucinogen
Baelz's disease (cheilitis glandularis apostematosa) K13.0
Baerensprung's disease (eczema marginatum) B35.6
Bagasse disease or pneumonitis J67.1
Bagassosis J67.1
Baker's cyst — see Cyst, Baker's
Bakwin-Krida syndrome (craniometaphyseal dysplasia)
    Q78.5
Balancing side interference M26.56
Balanitis (circinata) (erosiva) (gangrenosa) (phagedenic)
    (vulgaris) N48.1
  amebic A06.82
  candidal B37.42
  due to Haemophilus ducreyi A57
  gonococcal (acute) (chronic) A54.09
  xerotica obliterans N48.0
Balanoposthitis N47.6
  gonococcal (acute) (chronic) A54.09
  ulcerative (specific) A63.8
Balanorrhagia — see Balanitis
Balantidiasis, balantidiosis A07.0
Bald tongue K14.4
Baldness (see also Alopecia)
  male-pattern — see Alopecia, androgenic
Balkan grippe A78
Balloon disease — see Effect, adverse, high altitude
Balo's disease (concentric sclerosis) G37.5
Bamberger-Marie disease — see Osteoarthropathy,
    hypertrophic, specified type NEC
Bancroft's filariasis B74.0
Band(s)
  adhesive — see Adhesions, peritoneum
  anomalous or congenital (see also Anomaly, by site)
    heart (atrial) (ventricular) Q24.8
    intestine Q43.3
    omentum Q43.3
  cervix N88.1
  constricting, congenital Q79.8
  gallbladder (congenital) Q44.1
  intestinal (adhesive) — see Adhesions, peritoneum

Band(s) — continued
  obstructive
    intestine K56.5
    peritoneum K56.5
  periappendiceal, congenital Q43.3
  peritoneal (adhesive) — see Adhesions, peritoneum
  uterus N73.6
    internal N85.6
  vagina N89.5
Bandemia D72.825
Bandl's ring (contraction), complicating delivery O62.4
Bangkok hemorrhagic fever A91
Bang's disease (brucella abortus) A23.1
Bankruptcy, anxiety concerning Z59.8
Bannister's disease T78.3 ☑
  hereditary D84.1
Banti's disease or syndrome (with cirrhosis) (with portal
    hypertension) K76.6
Bar, median, prostate — see Enlargement, enlarged,
    prostate
Barcoo disease or rot — see Ulcer, skin
Barlow's disease E54
Barodontalgia T70.29 ☑
Baron Münchausen syndrome — see Disorder, facti-
    tious
Barosinusitis T70.1 ☑
Barotitis T70.0 ☑
Barotrauma T70.29 ☑
  odontalgia T70.29 ☑
  otitic T70.0 ☑
  sinus T70.1 ☑
Barraquer (-Simons) **disease or syndrome** (progressive
    lipodystrophy) E88.1
Barré-Guillain disease or syndrome G61.0
Barrel chest M95.4
Barré-Liéou syndrome (posterior cervical sympathetic)
    M53.0
Barrett's
  disease — see Barrett's, esophagus
  esophagus K22.70
    with dysplasia K22.719
      high grade K22.711
      low grade K22.710
    without dysplasia K22.70
  syndrome — see Barrett's, esophagus
  ulcer K22.10
    with bleeding K22.11
    without bleeding K22.10
Bársony (-Polgár) (-Teschendorf) **syndrome** (corkscrew
    esophagus) K22.4
Barth syndrome E78.71
Bartholinitis (suppurating) N75.8
  gonococcal (acute) (chronic) (with abscess) A54.1
Bartonellosis A44.9
  cutaneous A44.1
  mucocutaneous A44.1
  specified NEC A44.8
  systemic A44.0
Barton's fracture S52.56- ☑
Bartter's syndrome E26.81
Basal — see condition
Basan's (hidrotic) ectodermal dysplasia Q82.4
Baseball finger — see Dislocation, finger
Basedow's disease (exophthalmic goiter) — see Hyper-
    thyroidism, with, goiter
Basic — see condition
Basilar — see condition
Bason's (hidrotic) ectodermal dysplasia Q82.4
Basopenia — see Agranulocytosis
Basophilia D72.824
Basophilism (cortico-adrenal) (Cushing's) (pituitary)
    E24.0
Bassen-Kornzweig disease or syndrome E78.6
Bat ear Q17.5
Bateman's
  disease B08.1
  purpura (senile) D69.2
Bathing cramp T75.1 ☑
Bathophobia F40.248
Batten (-Mayou) **disease** E75.4
  retina E75.4 [H36]
Batten-Steinert syndrome G71.11
Battered — see Maltreatment
Battey Mycobacterium infection A31.0
Battle exhaustion F43.0
Battledore placenta O43.19- ☑

Index   Autonomic, autonomous — Battledore placenta

☞ **Subterms under main terms may continue to next column or page**   ☑ **Additional Character Required — Refer to the Tabular List for Character Selection**

Baumgarten-Cruveilhier cirrhosis, disease or syndrome K74.69
Bauxite fibrosis (of lung) J63.1
Bayle's disease (general paresis) A52.17
Bazin's disease (primary) (tuberculous) A18.4
Beach ear — *see* Swimmer's, ear
Beaded hair (congenital) Q84.1
Béal conjunctivitis or syndrome B30.2
Beard's disease (neurasthenia) F48.8
Beat(s)
  atrial, premature I49.1
  ectopic I49.49
  elbow — *see* Bursitis, elbow
  escaped, heart I49.49
  hand — *see* Bursitis, hand
  knee — *see* Bursitis, knee
  premature I49.40
    atrial I49.1
    auricular I49.1
    supraventricular I49.1
Beau's
  disease or syndrome — *see* Degeneration, myocardial
  lines (transverse furrows on fingernails) L60.4
Bechterev's syndrome — *see* Spondylitis, ankylosing
Becker's
  cardiomyopathy I42.8
  disease
    idiopathic mural endomyocardial disease I42.3
    myotonia congenita, recessive form G71.12
  dystrophy G71.0
  pigmented hairy nevus D22.5
Beck's syndrome (anterior spinal artery occlusion) I65.8
Beckwith-Wiedemann syndrome Q87.3
Bed confinement status Z74.01
Bed sore — *see* Ulcer, pressure, by site
Bedbug bite(s) — *see* Bite(s), by site, superficial, insect
Bedclothes, asphyxiation or suffocation by — *see* Asphyxia, traumatic, due to, mechanical, trapped
Bednar's
  aphthae K12.0
  tumor — *see* Neoplasm, malignant, by site
Bedridden Z74.01
Bedsore — *see* Ulcer, pressure, by site
Bedwetting — *see* Enuresis
Bee sting (with allergic or anaphylactic shock) — *see* Toxicity, venom, arthropod, bee
Beer drinker's heart (disease) I42.6
Begbie's disease (exophthalmic goiter) — *see* Hyperthyroidism, with, goiter
Behavior
  antisocial
    adult Z72.811
    child or adolescent Z72.810
  disorder, disturbance — *see* Disorder, conduct
  disruptive — *see* Disorder, conduct
  drug seeking Z72.89
  inexplicable R46.2
  marked evasiveness R46.5
  obsessive-compulsive R46.81
  overactivity R46.3
  poor responsiveness R46.4
  self-damaging (life-style) Z72.89
  sleep-incompatible Z72.821
  slowness R46.4
  specified NEC R46.89
  strange (and inexplicable) R46.2
  suspiciousness R46.5
  type A pattern Z73.1
  undue concern or preoccupation with stressful events R46.6
  verbosity and circumstantial detail obscuring reason for contact R46.7
Behçet's disease or syndrome M35.2
Behr's disease — *see* Degeneration, macula
Beigel's disease or morbus (white piedra) B36.2
Bejel A65
Bekhterev's syndrome — *see* Spondylitis, ankylosing
Belching — *see* Eructation
Bell's
  mania F30.8
  palsy, paralysis G51.0
    infant or newborn P11.3
  spasm G51.3
Bence Jones albuminuria or proteinuria NEC R80.3
Bends T70.3 ☑
Benedikt's paralysis or syndrome G46.3

Benign (*see also* condition)
  prostatic hyperplasia — *see* Hyperplasia, prostate
Bennett's fracture (displaced) S62.21- ☑
Benson's disease — *see* Deposit, crystalline
Bent
  back (hysterical) F44.4
  nose M95.0
    congenital Q67.4
Bereavement (uncomplicated) Z63.4
Bergeron's disease (hysterical chorea) F44.4
Berger's disease — *see* Nephropathy, IgA
Beriberi (dry) E51.11
  heart (disease) E51.12
  polyneuropathy E51.11
  wet E51.12
    involving circulatory system E51.11
Berlin's disease or edema (traumatic) S05.8X- ☑
Berlock (berloque) **dermatitis** L56.2
Bernard-Horner syndrome G90.2
Bernard-Soulier disease or thrombopathia D69.1
Bernhardt (-Roth) **disease** — *see* Mononeuropathy, lower limb, meralgia paresthetica
Bernheim's syndrome — *see* Failure, heart, congestive
Bertielliasis B71.8
Berylliosis (lung) J63.2
Besnier-Boeck (-Schaumann) **disease** — *see* Sarcoidosis
Besnier's
  lupus pernio D86.3
  prurigo L20.0
Bestiality F65.89
Best's disease H35.50
Betalipoproteinemia, broad or floating E78.2
Beta-mercaptolactate-cysteine disulfiduria E72.09
Betting and gambling Z72.6
  pathological (compulsive) F63.0
Bezoar T18.9 ☑
  intestine T18.3 ☑
  stomach T18.2 ☑
Bezold's abscess — *see* Mastoiditis, acute
Bianchi's syndrome R48.8
Bicornate or bicornis uterus Q51.3
  in pregnancy or childbirth O34.59- ☑
    causing obstructed labor O65.5
Bicuspid aortic valve Q23.1
Biedl-Bardet syndrome Q87.89
Bielschowsky (-Jansky) **disease** E75.4
Biermer's (pernicious) **anemia or disease** D51.0
Biett's disease L93.0
Bifid (congenital)
  apex, heart Q24.8
  clitoris Q52.6
  kidney Q63.8
  nose Q30.2
  patella Q74.1
  scrotum Q55.29
  toe NEC Q74.2
  tongue Q38.3
  ureter Q62.8
  uterus Q51.3
  uvula Q35.7
Biforis uterus (suprasimplex) Q51.3
Bifurcation (congenital)
  gallbladder Q44.1
  kidney pelvis Q63.8
  renal pelvis Q63.8
  rib Q76.6
  tongue, congenital Q38.3
  trachea Q32.1
  ureter Q62.8
  urethra Q64.74
  vertebra Q76.49
Big spleen syndrome D73.1
Bigeminal pulse R00.8
Bilateral — *see* condition
Bile
  duct — *see* condition
  pigments in urine R82.2
Bilharziasis (*see also* Schistosomiasis)
  chyluria B65.0
  cutaneous B65.3
  galacturia B65.0
  hematochyluria B65.0
  intestinal B65.1
  lipemia B65.9
  lipuria B65.0
  oriental B65.2
  piarhemia B65.9

Bilharziasis — *continued*
  pulmonary NOS B65.9 [J99]
    pneumonia B65.9 [J17]
  tropical hematuria B65.0
  vesical B65.0
Biliary — *see* condition
Bilirubin metabolism disorder E80.7
  specified NEC E80.6
Bilirubinemia, familial nonhemolytic E80.4
Bilirubinuria R82.2
Biliuria R82.2
Bilocular stomach K31.2
Binswanger's disease I67.3
Biparta, bipartite
  carpal scaphoid Q74.0
  patella Q74.1
  vagina Q52.10
Bird
  face Q75.8
  fancier's disease or lung J67.2
Birth
  complications in mother — *see* Delivery, complicated
  compression during NOS P15.9
  defect — *see* Anomaly
  immature (less than 37 completed weeks) — *see* Preterm, newborn
    extremely (less than 28 completed weeks) — *see* Immaturity, extreme
  inattention, at or after — *see* Maltreatment, child, neglect
  injury NOS P15.9
    basal ganglia P11.1
    brachial plexus NEC P14.3
    brain (compression) (pressure) P11.2
    central nervous system NOS P11.9
    cerebellum P11.1
    cerebral hemorrhage P10.1
    external genitalia P15.5
    eye P15.3
    face P15.4
    fracture
      bone P13.9
        specified NEC P13.8
      clavicle P13.4
      femur P13.2
      humerus P13.3
      long bone, except femur P13.3
      radius and ulna P13.3
      skull P13.0
      spine P11.5
      tibia and fibula P13.3
    intracranial P11.2
      laceration or hemorrhage P10.9
        specified NEC P10.8
    intraventricular hemorrhage P10.2
    laceration
      brain P10.1
      by scalpel P15.8
      peripheral nerve P14.9
    liver P15.0
    meninges
      brain P11.1
      spinal cord P11.5
    nerve
      brachial plexus P14.3
      cranial NEC (except facial) P11.4
      facial P11.3
      peripheral P14.9
      phrenic (paralysis) P14.2
    paralysis
      facial nerve P11.3
      spinal P11.5
    penis P15.5
    rupture
      spinal cord P11.5
    scalp P12.9
    scalpel wound P15.8
    scrotum P15.5
    skull NEC P13.1
      fracture P13.0
    specified type NEC P15.8
    spinal cord P11.5
    spine P11.5
    spleen P15.1
    sternomastoid (hematoma) P15.2
    subarachnoid hemorrhage P10.3
    subcutaneous fat necrosis P15.6
    subdural hemorrhage P10.0

Birth — *continued*
  injury — *continued*
    tentorial tear P10.4
    testes P15.5
    vulva P15.5
  lack of care, at or after — *see* Maltreatment, child, neglect
  neglect, at or after — *see* Maltreatment, child, neglect
  palsy or paralysis, newborn, NOS (birth injury) P14.9
  premature (infant) — *see* Preterm, newborn
  shock, newborn P96.89
  trauma — *see* Birth, injury
  weight
    4000 grams to 4499 grams P08.1
    4500 grams or more P08.0
    low (2499 grams or less) — *see* Low, birthweight
      extremely (999 grams or less) — *see* Low, birthweight, extreme
Birthmark Q82.5
Birt-Hogg-Dube syndrome Q87.89
Bisalbuminemia E88.09
Biskra's button B55.1
Bite(s) (animal) (human)
  abdomen, abdominal
    wall S31.159 ☑
      with penetration into peritoneal cavity S31.659 ☑
      epigastric region S31.152 ☑
        with penetration into peritoneal cavity S31.652 ☑
      left
        lower quadrant S31.154 ☑
          with penetration into peritoneal cavity S31.654 ☑
        upper quadrant S31.151 ☑
          with penetration into peritoneal cavity S31.651 ☑
      periumbilic region S31.155 ☑
        with penetration into peritoneal cavity S31.655 ☑
      right
        lower quadrant S31.153 ☑
          with penetration into peritoneal cavity S31.653 ☑
        upper quadrant S31.150 ☑
          with penetration into peritoneal cavity S31.650 ☑
      superficial NEC S30.871 ☑
        insect S30.861 ☑
  alveolar (process) — *see* Bite, oral cavity
  amphibian (venomous) — *see* Venom, bite, amphibian
  animal (*see also* Bite, by site)
    venomous — *see* Venom
  ankle S91.05- ☑
    superficial NEC S90.57- ☑
      insect S90.56- ☑
  antecubital space — *see* Bite, elbow
  anus S31.835 ☑
    superficial NEC S30.877 ☑
      insect S30.867 ☑
  arm (upper) S41.15- ☑
    lower — *see* Bite, forearm
    superficial NEC S40.87- ☑
      insect S40.86- ☑
  arthropod NEC — *see* Venom, bite, arthropod
  auditory canal (external) (meatus) — *see* Bite, ear
  auricle, ear — *see* Bite, ear
  axilla — *see* Bite, arm
  back (*see also* Bite, thorax, back)
    lower S31.050 ☑
      with penetration into retroperitoneal space S31.051 ☑
      superficial NEC S30.870 ☑
        insect S30.860 ☑
  bedbug — *see* Bite(s), by site, superficial, insect
  breast S21.05- ☑
    superficial NEC S20.17- ☑
      insect S20.16- ☑
  brow — *see* Bite, head, specified site NEC
  buttock S31.805 ☑
    left S31.825 ☑
    right S31.815 ☑
    superficial NEC S30.870 ☑
      insect S30.860 ☑
  calf — *see* Bite, leg
  canaliculus lacrimalis — *see* Bite, eyelid

Bite(s) — *continued*
  canthus, eye — *see* Bite, eyelid
  centipede — *see* Toxicity, venom, arthropod, centipede
  cheek (external) S01.45- ☑
    internal — *see* Bite, oral cavity
    superficial NEC S00.87 ☑
      insect S00.86 ☑
  chest wall — *see* Bite, thorax
  chigger B88.0
  chin — *see* Bite, head, specified site NEC
  clitoris — *see* Bite, vulva
  costal region — *see* Bite, thorax
  digit(s)
    hand — *see* Bite, finger
    toe — *see* Bite, toe
  ear (canal) (external) S01.35- ☑
    superficial NEC S00.47- ☑
      insect S00.46- ☑
  elbow S51.05- ☑
    superficial NEC S50.37- ☑
      insect S50.36- ☑
  epididymis — *see* Bite, testis
  epigastric region — *see* Bite, abdomen
  epiglottis — *see* Bite, neck, specified site NEC
  esophagus, cervical S11.25 ☑
    superficial NEC S10.17 ☑
      insect S10.16 ☑
  eyebrow — *see* Bite, eyelid
  eyelid S01.15- ☑
    superficial NEC S00.27- ☑
      insect S00.26- ☑
  face NEC — *see* Bite, head, specified site NEC
  finger(s) S61.259 ☑
    with
      damage to nail S61.359 ☑
    index S61.258 ☑
      with
        damage to nail S61.358 ☑
      left S61.251 ☑
        with
          damage to nail S61.351 ☑
      right S61.250 ☑
        with
          damage to nail S61.350 ☑
      superficial NEC S60.478 ☑
        insect S60.46- ☑
    little S61.25- ☑
      with
        damage to nail S61.35- ☑
      superficial NEC S60.47- ☑
        insect S60.46- ☑
    middle S61.25- ☑
      with
        damage to nail S61.35- ☑
      superficial NEC S60.47- ☑
        insect S60.46- ☑
    ring S61.25- ☑
      with
        damage to nail S61.35- ☑
      superficial NEC S60.47- ☑
        insect S60.46- ☑
    superficial NEC S60.479 ☑
      insect S60.469 ☑
    thumb — *see* Bite, thumb
  flank — *see* Bite, abdomen, wall
  flea — *see* Bite, by site, superficial, insect
  foot (except toe(s) alone) S91.35- ☑
    superficial NEC S90.87- ☑
      insect S90.86- ☑
    toe — *see* Bite, toe
  forearm S51.85- ☑
    elbow only — *see* Bite, elbow
    superficial NEC S50.87- ☑
      insect S50.86- ☑
  forehead — *see* Bite, head, specified site NEC
  genital organs, external
    female S31.552 ☑
      superficial NEC S30.876 ☑
        insect S30.866 ☑
      vagina and vulva — *see* Bite, vulva
    male S31.551 ☑
      penis — *see* Bite, penis
      scrotum — *see* Bite, scrotum
      superficial NEC S30.875 ☑
        insect S30.865 ☑

Bite(s) — *continued*
  genital organs, external — *continued*
    male — *continued*
      testes — *see* Bite, testis
  groin — *see* Bite, abdomen, wall
  gum — *see* Bite, oral cavity
  hand S61.45- ☑
    finger — *see* Bite, finger
    superficial NEC S60.57- ☑
      insect S60.56- ☑
    thumb — *see* Bite, thumb
  head S01.95- ☑
    cheek — *see* Bite, cheek
    ear — *see* Bite, ear
    eyelid — *see* Bite, eyelid
    lip — *see* Bite, lip
    nose — *see* Bite, nose
    oral cavity — *see* Bite, oral cavity
    scalp — *see* Bite, scalp
    specified site NEC S01.85 ☑
      superficial NEC S00.87 ☑
        insect S00.86 ☑
    superficial NEC S00.97 ☑
      insect S00.96 ☑
    temporomandibular area — *see* Bite, cheek
  heel — *see* Bite, foot
  hip S71.05- ☑
    superficial NEC S70.27- ☑
      insect S70.26- ☑
  hymen S31.45 ☑
  hypochondrium — *see* Bite, abdomen, wall
  hypogastric region — *see* Bite, abdomen, wall
  inguinal region — *see* Bite, abdomen, wall
  insect — *see* Bite, by site, superficial, insect
  instep — *see* Bite, foot
  interscapular region — *see* Bite, thorax, back
  jaw — *see* Bite, head, specified site NEC
  knee S81.05- ☑
    superficial NEC S80.27- ☑
      insect S80.26- ☑
  labium (majus) (minus) — *see* Bite, vulva
  lacrimal duct — *see* Bite, eyelid
  larynx S11.015 ☑
    superficial NEC S10.17 ☑
      insect S10.16 ☑
  leg (lower) S81.85- ☑
    ankle — *see* Bite, ankle
    foot — *see* Bite, foot
    knee — *see* Bite, knee
    superficial NEC S80.87- ☑
      insect S80.86- ☑
    toe — *see* Bite, toe
    upper — *see* Bite, thigh
  lip S01.551 ☑
    superficial NEC S00.571 ☑
      insect S00.561 ☑
  lizard (venomous) — *see* Venom, bite, reptile
  loin — *see* Bite, abdomen, wall
  lower back — *see* Bite, back, lower
  lumbar region — *see* Bite, back, lower
  malar region — *see* Bite, head, specified site NEC
  mammary — *see* Bite, breast
  marine animals (venomous) — *see* Toxicity, venom, marine animal
  mastoid region — *see* Bite, head, specified site NEC
  mouth — *see* Bite, oral cavity
  nail
    finger — *see* Bite, finger
    toe — *see* Bite, toe
  nape — *see* Bite, neck, specified site NEC
  nasal (septum) (sinus) — *see* Bite, nose
  nasopharynx — *see* Bite, head, specified site NEC
  neck S11.95 ☑
    involving
      cervical esophagus — *see* Bite, esophagus, cervical
      larynx — *see* Bite, larynx
      pharynx — *see* Bite, pharynx
      thyroid gland S11.15 ☑
      trachea — *see* Bite, trachea
    specified site NEC S11.85 ☑
      superficial NEC S10.87 ☑
        insect S10.86 ☑
    superficial NEC S10.97 ☑
      insect S10.96 ☑

Index

Bite(s) — *continued*
- neck — *continued*
  - throat S11.85 ☑
    - superficial NEC S10.17 ☑
      - insect S10.16 ☑
- nose (septum) (sinus) S01.25 ☑
  - superficial NEC S00.37 ☑
    - insect S00.36 ☑
- occipital region — *see* Bite, scalp
- oral cavity S01.552 ☑
  - superficial NEC S00.572 ☑
    - insect S00.562 ☑
- orbital region — *see* Bite, eyelid
- palate — *see* Bite, oral cavity
- palm — *see* Bite, hand
- parietal region — *see* Bite, scalp
- pelvis S31.050 ☑
  - with penetration into retroperitoneal space S31.051 ☑
  - superficial NEC S30.870 ☑
    - insect S30.860 ☑
- penis S31.25 ☑
  - superficial NEC S30.872 ☑
    - insect S30.862 ☑
- perineum
  - female — *see* Bite, vulva
  - male — *see* Bite, pelvis
- periocular area (with or without lacrimal passages) — *see* Bite, eyelid
- phalanges
  - finger — *see* Bite, finger
  - toe — *see* Bite, toe
- pharynx S11.25 ☑
  - superficial NEC S10.17 ☑
    - insect S10.16 ☑
- pinna — *see* Bite, ear
- poisonous — *see* Venom
- popliteal space — *see* Bite, knee
- prepuce — *see* Bite, penis
- pubic region — *see* Bite, abdomen, wall
- rectovaginal septum — *see* Bite, vulva
- red bug B88.0
- reptile NEC (*see also* Venom, bite, reptile)
  - nonvenomous — *see* Bite, by site
  - snake — *see* Venom, bite, snake
- sacral region — *see* Bite, back, lower
- sacroiliac region — *see* Bite, back, lower
- salivary gland — *see* Bite, oral cavity
- scalp S01.05 ☑
  - superficial NEC S00.07 ☑
    - insect S00.06 ☑
- scapular region — *see* Bite, shoulder
- scrotum S31.35 ☑
  - superficial NEC S30.873 ☑
    - insect S30.863 ☑
- sea-snake (venomous) — *see* Toxicity, venom, snake, sea snake
- shin — *see* Bite, leg
- shoulder S41.05- ☑
  - superficial NEC S40.27- ☑
    - insect S40.26- ☑
- snake (*see also* Venom, bite, snake)
  - nonvenomous — *see* Bite, by site
- spermatic cord — *see* Bite, testis
- spider (venomous) — *see* Toxicity, venom, spider
  - nonvenomous — *see* Bite, by site, superficial, insect
- sternal region — *see* Bite, thorax, front
- submaxillary region — *see* Bite, head, specified site NEC
- submental region — *see* Bite, head, specified site NEC
- subungual
  - finger(s) — *see* Bite, finger
  - toe — *see* Bite, toe
- superficial — *see* Bite, by site, superficial
- supraclavicular fossa S11.85 ☑
- supraorbital — *see* Bite, head, specified site NEC
- temple, temporal region — *see* Bite, head, specified site NEC
- temporomandibular area — *see* Bite, cheek
- testis S31.35 ☑
  - superficial NEC S30.873 ☑
    - insect S30.863 ☑
- thigh S71.15- ☑
  - superficial NEC S70.37- ☑
    - insect S70.36- ☑

Bite(s) — *continued*
- thorax, thoracic (wall) S21.95 ☑
  - back S21.25- ☑
    - with penetration into thoracic cavity S21.45- ☑
  - breast — *see* Bite, breast
  - front S21.15- ☑
    - with penetration into thoracic cavity S21.35- ☑
  - superficial NEC S20.97 ☑
    - back S20.47- ☑
    - front S20.37- ☑
    - insect S20.96 ☑
      - back S20.46- ☑
      - front S20.36- ☑
- throat — *see* Bite, neck, throat
- thumb S61.05- ☑
  - with damage to nail S61.15- ☑
  - superficial NEC S60.37- ☑
    - insect S60.36- ☑
- thyroid S11.15 ☑
  - superficial NEC S10.87 ☑
    - insect S10.86 ☑
- toe(s) S91.15- ☑
  - with damage to nail S91.25- ☑
  - great S91.15- ☑
    - with damage to nail S91.25- ☑
  - lesser S91.15- ☑
    - with damage to nail S91.25- ☑
  - superficial NEC S90.47- ☑
    - great S90.4/- ☑
    - insect S90.46- ☑
      - great S90.46- ☑
- tongue S01.552 ☑
- trachea S11.025 ☑
  - superficial NEC S10.17 ☑
    - insect S10.16 ☑
- tunica vaginalis — *see* Bite, testis
- tympanum, tympanic membrane — *see* Bite, ear
- umbilical region S31.155 ☑
- uvula — *see* Bite, oral cavity
- vagina — *see* Bite, vulva
- venomous — *see* Venom
- vocal cords S11.035 ☑
  - superficial NEC S10.17 ☑
    - insect S10.16 ☑
- vulva S31.45 ☑
  - superficial NEC S30.874 ☑
    - insect S30.864 ☑
- wrist S61.55- ☑
  - superficial NEC S60.87- ☑
    - insect S60.86- ☑

Biting, cheek or lip K13.1
Biventricular failure (heart) I50.9
Björck (-Thorson) **syndrome** (malignant carcinoid) E34.0
Black
- death A20.9
- eye S00.1- ☑
- hairy tongue K14.3
- heel (foot) S90.3- ☑
- lung (disease) J60
- palm (hand) S60.22- ☑

Blackfan-Diamond anemia or syndrome (congenital hypoplastic anemia) D61.01
Blackhead L70.0
Blackout R55
Bladder — *see* condition
Blast (air) (hydraulic) (immersion) (underwater)
- blindness S05.8X- ☑
- injury
  - abdomen or thorax — *see* Injury, by site
  - ear (acoustic nerve trauma) — *see* Injury, nerve, acoustic, specified type NEC
- syndrome NEC T70.8 ☑
Blastoma — *see* Neoplasm, malignant, by site
- pulmonary — *see* Neoplasm, lung, malignant
Blastomycosis, blastomycotic B40.9
- Brazilian — *see* Paracoccidioidomycosis
- cutaneous B40.3
- disseminated B40.7
- European — *see* Cryptococcosis
- generalized B40.7
- keloidal B48.0
- North American B40.9

Blastomycosis, blastomycotic — *continued*
- primary pulmonary B40.0
- pulmonary B40.2
  - acute B40.0
  - chronic B40.1
- skin B40.3
- South American — *see* Paracoccidioidomycosis
- specified NEC B40.89
Bleb(s) R23.8
- emphysematous (lung) (solitary) J43.9
- endophthalmitis H59.43
- filtering (vitreous), after glaucoma surgery Z98.83
- inflamed (infected), postprocedural H59.40
  - stage 1 H59.41
  - stage 2 H59.42
  - stage 3 H59.43
- lung (ruptured) J43.9
  - congenital — *see* Atelectasis
  - newborn P25.8
- subpleural (emphysematous) J43.9
Blebitis, postprocedural H59.40
- stage 1 H59.41
- stage 2 H59.42
- stage 3 H59.43
Bleeder (familial) (hereditary) — *see* Hemophilia
Bleeding (*see also* Hemorrhage)
- anal K62.5
- anovulatory N97.0
- atonic, following delivery O72.1
- capillary I78.8
  - puerperal O72.2
- contact (postcoital) N93.0
- due to uterine subinvolution N85.3
- ear — *see* Otorrhagia
- excessive, associated with menopausal onset N92.4
- familial — *see* Defect, coagulation
- following intercourse N93.0
- gastrointestinal K92.2
- hemorrhoids — *see* Hemorrhoids
- intermenstrual (regular) N92.3
  - irregular N92.1
- intraoperative — *see* Complication, intraoperative, hemorrhage
- irregular N92.6
- menopausal N92.4
- newborn, intraventricular — *see* Newborn, affected by, hemorrhage, intraventricular
- nipple N64.59
- nose R04.0
- ovulation N92.3
- postclimacteric N95.0
- postcoital N93.0
- postmenopausal N95.0
- postoperative — *see* Complication, postprocedural, hemorrhage
- preclimacteric N92.4
- puberty (excessive, with onset of menstrual periods) N92.2
- rectum, rectal K62.5
  - newborn P54.2
- tendencies — *see* Defect, coagulation
- throat R04.1
- tooth socket (post-extraction) K91.840
- umbilical stump P51.9
- uterus, uterine NEC N93.9
  - climacteric N92.4
  - dysfunctional of functional N93.8
  - menopausal N92.4
  - preclimacteric or premenopausal N92.4
  - unrelated to menstrual cycle N93.9
- vagina, vaginal (abnormal) N93.9
  - dysfunctional or functional N93.8
  - newborn P54.6
- vicarious N94.89
Blennorrhagia, blennorrhagic — *see* Gonorrhea
Blennorrhea (acute) (chronic) (*see also* Gonorrhea)
- inclusion (neonatal) (newborn) P39.1
- lower genitourinary tract (gonococcal) A54.00
- neonatorum (gonococcal ophthalmia) A54.31
Blepharelosis — *see* Entropion
Blepharitis (angularis) (ciliaris) (eyelid) (marginal) (nonulcerative) H01.009
- herpes zoster B02.39
- left H01.006
  - lower H01.005
  - upper H01.004
- right H01.003
  - lower H01.002

Bite — Blepharitis

Blepharitis — *continued*
  right — *continued*
    upper H01.001
    squamous H01.029
      left H01.026
        lower H01.025
        upper H01.024
      right H01.023
        lower H01.022
        upper H01.021
    ulcerative H01.019
      left H01.016
        lower H01.015
        upper H01.014
      right H01.013
        lower H01.012
        upper H01.011
Blepharochalasis H02.30
  congenital Q10.0
  left H02.36
    lower H02.35
    upper H02.34
  right H02.33
    lower H02.32
    upper H02.31
Blepharoclonus H02.59
Blepharoconjunctivitis H10.50- ☑
  angular H10.52- ☑
  contact H10.53- ☑
  ligneous H10.51- ☑
Blepharophimosis (eyelid) H02.529
  congenital Q10.3
  left H02.526
    lower H02.525
    upper H02.524
  right H02.523
    lower H02.522
    upper H02.521
Blepharoptosis H02.40- ☑
  congenital Q10.0
  mechanical H02.41- ☑
  myogenic H02.42- ☑
  neurogenic H02.43- ☑
  paralytic H02.43- ☑
Blepharopyorrhea, gonococcal A54.39
Blepharospasm G24.5
  drug induced G24.01
Blighted ovum O02.0
Blind (*see also* Blindness)
  bronchus (congenital) Q32.4
  loop syndrome K90.2
    congenital Q43.8
  sac, fallopian tube (congenital) Q50.6
  spot, enlarged — *see* Defect, visual field, localized, scotoma, blind spot area
  tract or tube, congenital NEC — *see* Atresia, by site
Blindness (acquired) (congenital) (both eyes) H54.0
  blast S05.8X- ☑
  color — *see* Deficiency, color vision
  concussion S05.8X- ☑
  cortical H47.619
    left brain H47.612
    right brain H47.611
  day H53.11
  due to injury (current episode) S05.9- ☑
    sequelae — *code to* injury with seventh character S
  eclipse (total) — *see* Retinopathy, solar
  emotional (hysterical) F44.6
  face H53.16
  hysterical F44.6
  legal (both eyes) (USA definition) H54.8
  mind R48.8
  night H53.60
    abnormal dark adaptation curve H53.61
    acquired H53.62
    congenital H53.63
    specified type NEC H53.69
    vitamin A deficiency E50.5
  one eye (other eye normal) H54.40
    left (normal vision on right) H54.42
      low vision on right H54.12
    low vision, other eye H54.10
    right (normal vision on left) H54.41
      low vision on left H54.11
  psychic R48.8
  river B73.01
  snow — *see* Photokeratitis

Blindness — *continued*
  sun, solar — *see* Retinopathy, solar
  transient — *see* Disturbance, vision, subjective, loss, transient
  traumatic (current episode) S05.9- ☑
  word (developmental) F81.0
    acquired R48.0
    secondary to organic lesion R48.0
Blister (nonthermal)
  abdominal wall S30.821 ☑
  alveolar process S00.522 ☑
  ankle S90.52- ☑
  antecubital space — *see* Blister, elbow
  anus S30.827 ☑
  arm (upper) S40.82- ☑
  auditory canal — *see* Blister, ear
  auricle — *see* Blister, ear
  axilla — *see* Blister, arm
  back, lower S30.820 ☑
  beetle dermatitis L24.89
  breast S20.12- ☑
  brow S00.82 ☑
  calf — *see* Blister, leg
  canthus — *see* Blister, eyelid
  cheek S00.82 ☑
    internal S00.522 ☑
  chest wall — *see* Blister, thorax
  chin S00.82 ☑
  costal region — *see* Blister, thorax
  digit(s)
    foot — *see* Blister, toe
    hand — *see* Blister, finger
  due to burn — *see* Burn, by site, second degree
  ear S00.42- ☑
  elbow S50.32- ☑
  epiglottis S10.12 ☑
  esophagus, cervical S10.12 ☑
  eyebrow — *see* Blister, eyelid
  eyelid S00.22- ☑
  face S00.82 ☑
  fever B00.1
  finger(s) S60.429 ☑
    index S60.42- ☑
    little S60.42- ☑
    middle S60.42- ☑
    ring S60.42- ☑
  foot (except toe(s) alone) S90.82- ☑
    toe — *see* Blister, toe
  forearm S50.82- ☑
    elbow only — *see* Blister, elbow
  forehead S00.82 ☑
  fracture — *omit code*
  genital organ
    female S30.826 ☑
    male S30.825 ☑
  gum S00.522 ☑
  hand S60.52- ☑
  head S00.92 ☑
    ear — *see* Blister, ear
    eyelid — *see* Blister, eyelid
    lip S00.521 ☑
    nose S00.32 ☑
    oral cavity S00.522 ☑
    scalp S00.02 ☑
    specified site NEC S00.82 ☑
  heel — *see* Blister, foot
  hip S70.22- ☑
  interscapular region S20.429 ☑
  jaw S00.82 ☑
  knee S80.22- ☑
  larynx S10.12 ☑
  leg (lower) S80.82- ☑
    knee — *see* Blister, knee
    upper — *see* Blister, thigh
  lip S00.521 ☑
  malar region S00.82 ☑
  mammary — *see* Blister, breast
  mastoid region S00.82 ☑
  mouth S00.522 ☑
  multiple, skin, nontraumatic R23.8
  nail
    finger — *see* Blister, finger
    toe — *see* Blister, toe
  nasal S00.32 ☑
  neck S10.92 ☑
    specified site NEC S10.82 ☑

Blister — *continued*
  neck — *continued*
    throat S10.12 ☑
  nose S00.32 ☑
  occipital region S00.02 ☑
  oral cavity S00.522 ☑
  orbital region — *see* Blister, eyelid
  palate S00.522 ☑
  palm — *see* Blister, hand
  parietal region S00.02 ☑
  pelvis S30.820 ☑
  penis S30.822 ☑
  periocular area — *see* Blister, eyelid
  phalanges
    finger — *see* Blister, finger
    toe — *see* Blister, toe
  pharynx S10.12 ☑
  pinna — *see* Blister, ear
  popliteal space — *see* Blister, knee
  scalp S00.02 ☑
  scapular region — *see* Blister, shoulder
  scrotum S30.823 ☑
  shin — *see* Blister, leg
  shoulder S40.22- ☑
  sternal region S20.329 ☑
  submaxillary region S00.82 ☑
  submental region S00.82 ☑
  subungual
    finger(s) — *see* Blister, finger
    toe(s) — *see* Blister, toe
  supraclavicular fossa S10.82 ☑
  supraorbital S00.82 ☑
  temple S00.82 ☑
  temporal region S00.82 ☑
  testis S30.823 ☑
  thermal — *see* Burn, second degree, by site
  thigh S70.32- ☑
  thorax, thoracic (wall) S20.92 ☑
    back S20.42- ☑
    front S20.32- ☑
  throat S10.12 ☑
  thumb S60.32- ☑
  toe(s) S90.42- ☑
    great S90.42- ☑
  tongue S00.522 ☑
  trachea S10.12 ☑
  tympanum, tympanic membrane — *see* Blister, ear
  upper arm — *see* Blister, arm (upper)
  uvula S00.522 ☑
  vagina S30.824 ☑
  vocal cords S10.12 ☑
  vulva S30.824 ☑
  wrist S60.82- ☑
Bloating R14.0
Bloch-Sulzberger disease or syndrome Q82.3
Block, blocked
  alveolocapillary J84.10
  arborization (heart) I45.5
  arrhythmic I45.9
  atrioventricular (incomplete) (partial) I44.30
    with atrioventricular dissociation I44.2
    complete I44.2
      congenital Q24.6
    congenital Q24.6
    first degree I44.0
    second degree (types I and II) I44.1
    specified NEC I44.39
    third degree I44.2
    types I and II I44.1
  auriculoventricular — *see* Block, atrioventricular
  bifascicular (cardiac) I45.2
  bundle-branch (complete) (false) (incomplete) I45.4
    bilateral I45.2
    left I44.7
      with right bundle branch block I45.2
      hemiblock I44.60
        anterior I44.4
        posterior I44.5
      incomplete I44.7
        with right bundle branch block I45.2
    right I45.10
      with
        left bundle branch block I45.2
        left fascicular block I45.2
      specified NEC I45.19
    Wilson's type I45.19
  cardiac I45.9

Index

Block, blocked — Brachycephaly

Block, blocked — continued
  conduction I45.9
    complete I44.2
  fascicular (left) I44.60
    anterior I44.4
    posterior I44.5
    right I45.0
    specified NEC I44.69
  foramen Magendie (acquired) G91.1
    congenital Q03.1
      with spina bifida — see Spina bifida, by site,
        with hydrocephalus
  heart I45.9
    bundle branch I45.4
      bilateral I45.2
    complete (atrioventricular) I44.2
    congenital Q24.6
    first degree (atrioventricular) I44.0
    second degree (atrioventricular) I44.1
    specified type NEC I45.5
    third degree (atrioventricular) I44.2
  hepatic vein I82.0
  intraventricular (nonspecific) I45.4
    bundle branch
      bilateral I45.2
  kidney N28.9
    postcystoscopic or postprocedural N99.0
  Mobitz (types I and II) I44.1
  myocardial — see Block, heart
  nodal I45.5
  organ or site, congenital NEC — see Atresia, by site
  portal (vein) I81
  second degree (types I and II) I44.1
  sinoatrial I45.5
  sinoauricular I45.5
  third degree I44.2
  trifascicular I45.3
  tubal N97.1
  vein NOS I82.90
  Wenckebach (types I and II) I44.1
Blockage — see Obstruction
Blocq's disease F44.4
Blood
  constituents, abnormal R78.9
  disease D75.9
  donor — see Donor, blood
  dyscrasia D75.9
    with
      abortion — see Abortion, by type, complicated
        by, hemorrhage
      ectopic pregnancy O08.1
      molar pregnancy O08.1
    following ectopic or molar pregnancy O08.1
    newborn P61.9
    puerperal, postpartum O72.3
  flukes NEC — see Schistosomiasis
  in
    feces K92.1
      occult R19.5
    urine — see Hematuria
  mole O02.0
  occult in feces R19.5
  pressure
    decreased, due to shock following injury T79.4 ☑
    examination only Z01.30
    fluctuating I99.8
    high — see Hypertension
      borderline R03.0
      incidental reading, without diagnosis of hyper-
        tension R03.0
    low (see also Hypotension)
      incidental reading, without diagnosis of hy-
        potension R03.1
  spitting — see Hemoptysis
  staining cornea — see Pigmentation, cornea, stromal
  transfusion
    reaction or complication — see Complications,
      transfusion
  type
    A (Rh positive) Z67.10
      Rh negative Z67.11
    AB (Rh positive) Z67.30
      Rh negative Z67.31
    B (Rh positive) Z67.20
      Rh negative Z67.21
    O (Rh positive) Z67.40
      Rh negative Z67.41
    Rh (positive) Z67.90

Blood — continued
  type — continued
    Rh (positive) Z67.90
      negative Z67.91
  vessel rupture — see Hemorrhage
  vomiting — see Hematemesis
Blood-forming organs, disease D75.9
Bloodgood's disease — see Mastopathy, cystic
Bloom (-Machacek)(-Torre) **syndrome** Q82.8
Blount's disease or osteochondrosis — see Osteochon-
    drosis, juvenile, tibia
Blue
  baby Q24.9
  diaper syndrome E72.09
  dome cyst (breast) — see Cyst, breast
  dot cataract Q12.0
  nevus D22.9
  sclera Q13.5
    with fragility of bone and deafness Q78.0
  toe syndrome I75.02- ☑
Blueness — see Cyanosis
Blues, postpartal O90.6
  baby O90.6
Blurring, visual H53.8
Blushing (abnormal) (excessive) R23.2
BMI — see Body, mass index
Boarder, hospital NEC Z76.4
  accompanying sick person Z76.3
  healthy infant or child Z76.2
    foundling Z76.1
Bockhart's impetigo L01.02
Bodechtel-Guttman disease (subacute sclerosing pan-
    nencephalitis) A81.1
Boder-Sedgwick syndrome (ataxia-telangiectasia)
    G11.3
Body, bodies
  Aschoff's — see Myocarditis, rheumatic
  asteroid, vitreous — see Deposit, crystalline
  cytoid (retina) — see Occlusion, artery, retina
  drusen (degenerative) (macula) (retinal) (see also De-
    generation, macula, drusen)
    optic disc — see Drusen, optic disc
  foreign — see Foreign body
  loose
    joint, except knee — see Loose, body, joint
      knee M23.4- ☑
    sheath, tendon — see Disorder, tendon, specified
      type NEC
  mass index (BMI)
    adult
      19 or less Z68.1
      20.0-20.9 Z68.20
      21.0-21.9 Z68.21
      22.0-22.9 Z68.22
      23.0-23.9 Z68.23
      24.0-24.9 Z68.24
      25.0-25.9 Z68.25
      26.0-26.9 Z68.26
      27.0-27.9 Z68.27
      28.0-28.9 Z68.28
      29.0-29.9 Z68.29
      30.0-30.9 Z68.30
      31.0-31.9 Z68.31
      32.0-32.9 Z68.32
      33.0-33.9 Z68.33
      34.0-34.9 Z68.34
      35.0-35.9 Z68.35
      36.0-36.9 Z68.36
      37.0-37.9 Z68.37
      38.0-38.9 Z68.38
      39.0-39.9 Z68.39
      40.0-44.9 Z68.41
      45.0-49.9 Z68.42
      50.0-59.9 Z68.43
      60.0-69.9 Z68.44
      70 and over Z68.45
    pediatric
      5th percentile to less than 85th percentile for
        age Z68.52
      85th percentile to less than 95th percentile for
        age Z68.53
      less than fifth percentile for age Z68.51
      greater than or equal to ninety-fifth percentile
        for age Z68.54
  Mooser's A75.2
  rice (see also Loose, body, joint)
    knee M23.4- ☑
  rocking F98.4

Boeck's
  disease or sarcoid — see Sarcoidosis
  lupoid (miliary) D86.3
Boerhaave's syndrome (spontaneous esophageal rup-
    ture) K22.3
Boggy
  cervix N88.8
  uterus N85.8
Boil (see also Furuncle, by site)
  Aleppo B55.1
  Baghdad B55.1
  Delhi B55.1
  lacrimal
    gland — see Dacryoadenitis
    passages (duct) (sac) — see Inflammation, lacrimal,
      passages, acute
  Natal B55.1
  orbit, orbital — see Abscess, orbit
  tropical B55.1
Bold hives — see Urticaria
Bombé, iris — see Membrane, pupillary
Bone — see condition
Bonnevie-Ullrich syndrome Q87.1
Bonnier's syndrome H81.8 ☑
Bonvale dam fever T73.3 ☑
Bony block of joint — see Ankylosis
BOOP (bronchiolitis obliterans organized pneumonia)
    J84.89
Borderline
  diabetes mellitus R73.09
  hypertension R03.0
  osteopenia M85.8- ☑
  pelvis, with obstruction during labor O65.1
  personality F60.3
Borna disease A83.9
Bornholm disease B33.0
Boston exanthem A88.0
Botalli, ductus (patent) (persistent) Q25.0
Bothriocephalus latus infestation B70.0
Botulism (foodborne intoxication) A05.1
  infant A48.51
  non-foodborne A48.52
  wound A48.52
Bouba — see Yaws
Bouchard's nodes (with arthropathy) M15.2
Bouffée délirante F23
Bouillaud's disease or syndrome (rheumatic heart
    disease) I01.9
Bourneville's disease Q85.1
Boutonniere deformity (finger) — see Deformity, finger,
    boutonniere
Bouveret (-Hoffmann) **syndrome** (paroxysmal tachycar-
    dia) I47.9
Bovine heart — see Hypertrophy, cardiac
Bowel — see condition
Bowen's
  dermatosis (precancerous) — see Neoplasm, skin, in
    situ
  disease — see Neoplasm, skin, in situ
  epithelioma — see Neoplasm, skin, in situ
  type
    epidermoid carcinoma-in-situ — see Neoplasm,
      skin, in situ
    intraepidermal squamous cell carcinoma — see
      Neoplasm, skin, in situ
Bowing
  femur (see also Deformity, limb, specified type NEC,
    thigh)
    congenital Q68.3
  fibula (see also Deformity, limb, specified type NEC,
    lower leg)
    congenital Q68.4
  forearm — see Deformity, limb, specified type NEC,
    forearm
  leg(s), long bones, congenital Q68.5
  radius (see also Deformity, limb, specified type NEC,
    forearm)
  tibia (see also Deformity, limb, specified type NEC,
    lower leg)
    congenital Q68.4
Bowleg(s) (acquired) M21.16- ☑
  congenital Q68.5
  rachitic E64.3
Boyd's dysentery A03.2
Brachial — see condition
Brachycardia R00.1
Brachycephaly Q75.0

Bradley's disease A08.19
Bradyarrhythmia, cardiac I49.8
Bradycardia (sinoatrial) (sinus) (vagal) R00.1
  neonatal P29.12
  reflex G90.09
  tachycardia syndrome I49.5
Bradykinesia R25.8
Bradypnea R06.89
Bradytachycardia I49.5
Brailsford's disease or osteochondrosis — see Osteo-
  chondrosis, juvenile, radius
Brain (see also condition)
  death G93.82
  syndrome — see Syndrome, brain
Branched-chain amino-acid disorder E71.2
Branchial — see condition
  cartilage, congenital Q18.2
Branchiogenic remnant (in neck) Q18.0
Brandt's syndrome (acrodermatitis enteropathica) E83.2
Brash (water) R12
Bravais-jacksonian epilepsy — see Epilepsy, localiza-
  tion-related, symptomatic, with simple partial
  seizures
Braxton Hicks contractions — see False, labor
Brazilian leishmaniasis B55.2
BRBPR K62.5
Break, retina (without detachment) H33.30- ☑
  with retinal detachment — see Detachment, retina
  horseshoe tear H33.31- ☑
  multiple H33.33- ☑
  round hole H33.32- ☑
Breakdown
  device, graft or implant (see also Complications, by
    site and type, mechanical) T85.618 ☑
    arterial graft NEC — see Complication, cardiovas-
      cular device, mechanical, vascular
    breast (implant) T85.41 ☑
    catheter NEC T85.618 ☑
      cystostomy T83.010 ☑
      dialysis (renal) T82.41 ☑
        intraperitoneal T85.611 ☑
      infusion NEC T82.514 ☑
        spinal (epidural) (subdural) T85.610 ☑
      urinary (indwelling) T83.018 ☑
    electronic (electrode) (pulse generator) (stimulator)
      bone T84.310 ☑
      cardiac T82.119 ☑
        electrode T82.110 ☑
        pulse generator T82.111 ☑
        specified type NEC T82.118 ☑
      nervous system — see Complication, prosthetic
        device, mechanical, electronic nervous
        system stimulator
      urinary — see Complication, genitourinary,
        device, urinary, mechanical
    fixation, internal (orthopedic) NEC — see Compli-
      cation, fixation device, mechanical
    gastrointestinal — see Complications, prosthetic
      device, mechanical, gastrointestinal device
    genital NEC T83.418 ☑
      intrauterine contraceptive device T83.31 ☑
      penile prosthesis T83.410 ☑
    heart NEC — see Complication, cardiovascular de-
      vice, mechanical
    joint prosthesis — see Complications..., joint pros-
      thesis,internal, mechanical, by site
    ocular NEC — see Complications, prosthetic device,
      mechanical, ocular device
    orthopedic NEC — see Complication, orthopedic,
      device, mechanical
    specified NEC T85.618 ☑
    sutures, permanent T85.612 ☑
      used in bone repair — see Complications, fixa-
        tion device, internal (orthopedic), me-
        chanical
    urinary NEC (see also Complication, genitourinary,
      device, urinary, mechanical)
      graft T83.21 ☑
    vascular NEC — see Complication, cardiovascular
      device, mechanical
    ventricular intracranial shunt T85.01 ☑
  nervous F48.8
  perineum O90.1
  respirator J95.850
    specified NEC J95.859
  ventilator

Breakdown — continued
  ventilator J95.850
    specified NEC J95.859
Breast (see also condition)
  buds E30.1
    in newborn P96.89
  dense R92.2
  nodule N63
Breath
  foul R19.6
  holder, child R06.89
  holding spell R06.89
  shortness R06.02
Breathing
  labored — see Hyperventilation
  mouth R06.5
    causing malocclusion M26.5 ☑
  periodic R06.3
    high altitude G47.32
Breathlessness R06.81
Breda's disease — see Yaws
Breech presentation (mother) O32.1 ☑
  causing obstructed labor O64.1 ☑
  footling O32.8 ☑
    causing obstructed labor O64.8 ☑
  incomplete O32.8 ☑
    causing obstructed labor O64.8 ☑
Breisky's disease N90.4
Brennemann's syndrome I88.0
Brenner
  tumor (benign) D27.9
    borderline malignancy D39.1- ☑
    malignant C56 ☑
    proliferating D39.1- ☑
Bretonneau's disease or angina A36.0
Breus' mole O02.0
Brevicollis Q76.49
Brickmakers' anemia B76.9 [D63.8]
Bridge, myocardial Q24.5
Bright red blood per rectum (BRBPR) K62.5
Bright's disease (see also Nephritis)
  arteriosclerotic — see Hypertension, kidney
Brill (-Zinsser) **disease** (recrudescent typhus) A75.1
  flea-borne A75.2
  louse-borne A75.1
Brill-Symmers' disease C82.90
Brion-Kayser disease — see Fever, parathyroid
Briquet's disorder or syndrome F45.0
Brissaud's
  infantilism or dwarfism E23.0
  motor-verbal tic F95.2
Brittle
  bones disease Q78.0
  nails L60.3
    congenital Q84.6
Broad (see also condition)
  beta disease E78.2
  ligament laceration syndrome N83.8
Broad- or floating-betalipoproteinemia E78.2
Brock's syndrome (atelectasis due to enlarged lymph
  nodes) J98.19
Brocq-Duhring disease (dermatitis herpetiformis) L13.0
Brodie's abscess or disease M86.8X- ☑
Broken
  arches (see also Deformity, limb, flat foot)
  arm (meaning upper limb) — see Fracture, arm
  back — see Fracture, vertebra
  bone — see Fracture
  implant or internal device — see Complications, by
    site and type, mechanical
  leg (meaning lower limb) — see Fracture, leg
  nose S02.2 ☑
  tooth, teeth — see Fracture, tooth
Bromhidrosis, bromidrosis L75.0
Bromidism, bromism G92
  chronic (dependence) F13.20
  due to
    correct substance properly administered — see
      Table of Drugs and Chemicals, by drug, ad-
      verse effect
    overdose or wrong substance given or taken —
      see Table of Drugs and Chemicals, by drug,
      poisoning
Bromidrosiphobia F40.298
Bronchi, bronchial — see condition
Bronchiectasis (cylindrical) (diffuse) (fusiform) (localized)
  (saccular) J47.9

Bronchiectasis — continued
  with
    acute
      bronchitis J47.0
      lower respiratory infection J47.0
    exacerbation (acute) J47.1
  congenital Q33.4
  tuberculous NEC — see Tuberculosis, pulmonary
Bronchiolectasis — see Bronchiectasis
Bronchiolitis (acute) (infective) (subacute) J21.9
  with
    bronchospasm or obstruction J21.9
    influenza, flu or grippe — see Influenza, with, res-
      piratory manifestations NEC
  chemical (chronic) J68.4
    acute J68.0
  chronic (fibrosing) (obliterative) J44.9
  due to
    external agent — see Bronchitis, acute, due to
    human metapneumovirus J21.1
    respiratory syncytial virus J21.0
    specified organism NEC J21.8
  fibrosa obliterans J44.9
  influenzal — see Influenza, with, respiratory manifes-
    tations NEC
  obliterans J42
    with organizing pneumonia (BOOP) J84.89
  obliterative (chronic) (subacute) J44.9
    due to chemicals, gases, fumes or vapors (inhala-
      tion) J68.4
    due to fumes or vapors J68.4
  respiratory, interstitial lung disease J84.115
Bronchitis (diffuse) (fibrinous) (hypostatic) (infective)
  (membranous) J40
  with
    influenza, flu or grippe — see Influenza, with, res-
      piratory manifestations NEC
    obstruction (airway) (lung) J44.9
    tracheitis (I5 years of age and above) J40
      acute or subacute J20.9
      chronic J42
      under I5 years of age J20.9
  acute or subacute (with bronchospasm or obstruction)
    J20.9
    with
      bronchiectasis J47.0
      chronic obstructive pulmonary disease J44.0
    chemical (due to gases, fumes or vapors) J68.0
    due to
      fumes or vapors J68.0
      Haemophilus influenzae J20.1
      Mycoplasma pneumoniae J20.0
      radiation J70.0
      specified organism NEC J20.8
      Streptococcus J20.2
      virus
        coxsackie J20.3
        echovirus J20.7
        parainfluenzae J20.4
        respiratory syncytial J20.5
        rhinovirus J20.6
    viral NEC J20.8
  allergic (acute) J45.909
    with
      exacerbation (acute) J45.901
      status asthmaticus J45.902
  arachidic T17.528 ☑
  aspiration (due to fumes or vapors) J68.0
  asthmatic J45.9 ☑
    chronic J44.9
      with
        acute lower respiratory infection J44.0
        exacerbation (acute) J44.1
  capillary — see Pneumonia, broncho
  caseous (tuberculous) A15.5
  Castellani's A69.8
  catarrhal (I5 years of age and above) J40
    acute — see Bronchitis, acute
    chronic J41.0
    under I5 years of age J20.9
  chemical (acute) (subacute) J68.0
    chronic J68.4
    due to fumes or vapors J68.0
      chronic J68.4
  chronic J42
    with
      airways obstruction J44.9
      tracheitis (chronic) J42

Bronchitis — *continued*
  chronic — *continued*
    asthmatic (obstructive) J44.9
    catarrhal J41.Ø
    chemical (due to fumes or vapors) J68.4
    due to
      chemicals, gases, fumes or vapors (inhalation)
        J68.4
      radiation J7Ø.1
      tobacco smoking J41.Ø
    emphysematous J44.9
    mucopurulent J41.1
    non-obstructive J41.Ø
    obliterans J44.9
    obstructive J44.9
    purulent J41.1
    simple J41.Ø
  croupous — *see* Bronchitis, acute
  due to gases, fumes or vapors (chemical) J68.Ø
  emphysematous (obstructive) J44.9
  exudative — *see* Bronchitis, acute
  fetid J41.1
  grippal — *see* Influenza, with, respiratory manifestations NEC
  in those under l5 years age — *see* Bronchitis, acute
    chronic — *see* Bronchitis, chronic
  influenzal — *see* Influenza, with, respiratory manifestations NEC
  mixed simple and mucopurulent J41.8
  moulder's J62.8
  mucopurulent (chronic) (recurrent) J41.1
    acute or subacute J2Ø.9
    simple (mixed) J41.8
  obliterans (chronic) J44.9
  obstructive (chronic) (diffuse) J44.9
  pituitous J41.1
  pneumococcal, acute or subacute J2Ø.2
  pseudomembranous, acute or subacute — *see* Bronchitis, acute
  purulent (chronic) (recurrent) J41.1
    acute or subacute — *see* Bronchitis, acute
  putrid J41.1
  senile (chronic) J42
  simple and mucopurulent (mixed) J41.8
  smokers' J41.Ø
  spirochetal NEC A69.8
  subacute — *see* Bronchitis, acute
  suppurative (chronic) J41.1
    acute or subacute — *see* Bronchitis, acute
  tuberculous A15.5
  under l5 years of age — *see* Bronchitis, acute
    chronic — *see* Bronchitis, chronic
  viral NEC, acute or subacute (*see also* Bronchitis, acute) J2Ø.8
Bronchoalveolitis J18.Ø
Bronchoaspergillosis B44.1
Bronchocele meaning goiter EØ4.Ø
Broncholithiasis J98.Ø9
  tuberculous NEC A15.5
Bronchomalacia J98.Ø9
  congenital Q32.2
Bronchomycosis NOS B49 [J99]
  candidal B37.1
Bronchopleuropneumonia — *see* Pneumonia, broncho
Bronchopneumonia — *see* Pneumonia, broncho
Bronchopneumonitis — *see* Pneumonia, broncho
Bronchopulmonary — *see* condition
Bronchopulmonitis — *see* Pneumonia, broncho
Bronchorrhagia (see Hemoptysis)
Bronchorrhea J98.Ø9
  acute J2Ø.9
  chronic (infective) (purulent) J42
Bronchospasm (acute) J98.Ø1
  with
    bronchiolitis, acute J21.9
    bronchitis, acute (conditions in J2Ø) — *see* Bronchitis, acute
  due to external agent — *see* condition, respiratory, acute, due to
  exercise induced J45.99Ø
Bronchospirochetosis A69.8
  Castellani A69.8
Bronchostenosis J98.Ø9
Bronchus — *see* condition
Brontophobia F4Ø.22Ø
Bronze baby syndrome P83.8
Brooke's tumor — *see* Neoplasm, skin, benign

Brown enamel of teeth (hereditary) KØØ.5
Brown's sheath syndrome H5Ø.61- ✓
Brown-Séquard disease, paralysis or syndrome G83.81
Bruce sepsis A23.Ø
Brucellosis (infection) A23.9
  abortus A23.1
  canis A23.3
  dermatitis A23.9
  melitensis A23.Ø
  mixed A23.8
  sepsis A23.9
    melitensis A23.Ø
    specified NEC A23.8
  suis A23.2
Bruck-de Lange disease Q87.1
Bruck's disease — *see* Deformity, limb
Brugsch's syndrome Q82.8
Bruise (skin surface intact) (*see also* Contusion)
  with
    open wound — *see* Wound, open
  internal organ — *see* Injury, by site
  newborn P54.5
  scalp, due to birth injury, newborn P12.3
  umbilical cord O69.5 ✓
Bruit (arterial) RØ9.89
  cardiac RØ1.1
Brush burn — *see* Abrasion, by site
Bruton's X-linked agammaglobulinemia D8Ø.Ø
Bruxism
  psychogenic F45.8
  sleep related G47.63
Bubbly lung syndrome P27.Ø
Bubo I88.8
  blennorrhagic (gonococcal) A54.89
  chancroidal A57
  climatic A55
  due to Haemophilus ducreyi A57
  gonococcal A54.89
  indolent (nonspecific) I88.8
  inguinal (nonspecific) I88.8
    chancroidal A57
    climatic A55
    due to H. ducreyi A57
    infective I88.8
  scrofulous (tuberculous) A18.2
  soft chancre A57
  suppurating — *see* Lymphadenitis, acute
  syphilitic (primary) A51.Ø
    congenital A5Ø.Ø7
  tropical A55
  virulent (chancroidal) A57
Bubonic plague A2Ø.Ø
Bubonocele — *see* Hernia, inguinal
Buccal — *see* condition
Buchanan's disease or osteochondrosis M91.Ø
Buchem's syndrome (hyperostosis corticalis) M85.2
Bucket-handle fracture or tear (semilunar cartilage) — *see* Tear, meniscus
Budd-Chiari syndrome (hepatic vein thrombosis) I82.Ø
Budgerigar fancier's disease or lung J67.2
Buds
  breast E3Ø.1
    in newborn P96.89
Buerger's disease (thromboangiitis obliterans) I73.1
Bulbar — *see* condition
Bulbus cordis (left ventricle) (persistent) Q21.8
Bulimia (nervosa) F5Ø.2
  atypical F5Ø.9
  normal weight F5Ø.9
Bulky
  stools R19.5
  uterus N85.2
Bulla (e) R23.8
  lung (emphysematous) (solitary) J43.9
    newborn P25.8
Bullet wound (*see also* Wound, open)
  fracture — *code as* Fracture, by site
  internal organ — *see* Injury, by site
Bundle
  branch block (complete) (false) (incomplete) — *see* Block, bundle-branch
  of His — *see* condition
Bunion — *see* Deformity, toe, hallux valgus
Buphthalmia, buphthalmos (congenital) Q15.Ø
Burdwan fever B55.Ø
Bürger-Grütz disease or syndrome E78.3

Buried
  penis (congenital) Q55.64
    acquired N48.83
  roots KØ8.3
Burke's syndrome K86.8
Burkitt
  cell leukemia C91.Ø- ✓
  lymphoma (malignant) C83.7- ✓
    small noncleaved, diffuse C83.7- ✓
    spleen C83.77
    undifferentiated C83.7- ✓
  tumor C83.7- ✓
  type
    acute lymphoblastic leukemia C91.Ø- ✓
    undifferentiated C83.7- ✓
Burn (electricity) (flame) (hot gas, liquid or hot object) (radiation) (steam) (thermal) T3Ø.Ø
  abdomen, abdominal (muscle) (wall) T21.Ø2 ✓
    first degree T21.12 ✓
    second degree T21.22 ✓
    third degree T21.32 ✓
  above elbow T22.Ø39 ✓
    first degree T22.139 ✓
    left T22.Ø32 ✓
      first degree T22.132 ✓
      second degree T22.232 ✓
      third degree T22.332 ✓
    right T22.Ø31 ✓
      first degree T22.131 ✓
      second degree T22.231 ✓
      third degree T22.331 ✓
    second degree T22.239 ✓
    third degree T22.339 ✓
  acid (caustic) (external) (internal) — *see* Corrosion, by site
  alimentary tract NEC T28.2 ✓
    esophagus T28.1 ✓
    mouth T28.Ø ✓
    pharynx T28.Ø ✓
  alkaline (caustic) (external) (internal) — *see* Corrosion, by site
  ankle T25.Ø19 ✓
    first degree T25.119 ✓
    left T25.Ø12 ✓
      first degree T25.112 ✓
      second degree T25.212 ✓
      third degree T25.312 ✓
    multiple with foot — *see* Burn, lower, limb, multiple, ankle and foot
    right T25.Ø11 ✓
      first degree T25.111 ✓
      second degree T25.211 ✓
      third degree T25.311 ✓
    second degree T25.219 ✓
    third degree T25.319 ✓
  anus — *see* Burn, buttock
  arm (lower) (upper) — *see* Burn, upper, limb
  axilla T22.Ø49 ✓
    first degree T22.149 ✓
    left T22.Ø42 ✓
      first degree T22.142 ✓
      second degree T22.242 ✓
      third degree T22.342 ✓
    right T22.Ø41 ✓
      first degree T22.141 ✓
      second degree T22.241 ✓
      third degree T22.341 ✓
    second degree T22.249 ✓
    third degree T22.349 ✓
  back (lower) T21.Ø4 ✓
    first degree T21.14 ✓
    second degree T21.24 ✓
    third degree T21.34 ✓
    upper T21.Ø3 ✓
      first degree T21.13 ✓
      second degree T21.23 ✓
      third degree T21.33 ✓
  blisters — *code as* Burn, second degree, by site
  breast(s) — *see* Burn, chest wall
  buttock(s) T21.Ø5 ✓
    first degree T21.15 ✓
    second degree T21.25 ✓
    third degree T21.35 ✓
  calf T24.Ø39 ✓
    first degree T24.139 ✓

Burn — *continued*
  calf — *continued*
    left T24.032 ☑
      first degree T24.132 ☑
      second degree T24.232 ☑
      third degree T24.332 ☑
    right T24.031 ☑
      first degree T24.131 ☑
      second degree T24.231 ☑
      third degree T24.331 ☑
    second degree T24.239 ☑
    third degree T24.339 ☑
  canthus (eye) — *see* Burn, eyelid
  caustic acid or alkaline — *see* Corrosion, by site
  cervix T28.3 ☑
  cheek T20.06 ☑
    first degree T20.16 ☑
    second degree T20.26 ☑
    third degree T20.36 ☑
  chemical (acids) (alkalines) (caustics) (external) (internal) — *see* Corrosion, by site
  chest wall T21.01 ☑
    first degree T21.11 ☑
    second degree T21.21 ☑
    third degree T21.31 ☑
  chin T20.03 ☑
    first degree T20.13 ☑
    second degree T20.23 ☑
    third degree T20.33 ☑
  colon T28.2 ☑
  conjunctiva (and cornea) — *see* Burn, cornea
  cornea (and conjunctiva) T26.1- ☑
    chemical — *see* Corrosion, cornea
  corrosion (external) (internal) — *see* Corrosion, by site
  deep necrosis of underlying tissue — *code as* Burn, third degree, by site
  dorsum of hand T23.069 ☑
    first degree T23.169 ☑
    left T23.062 ☑
      first degree T23.162 ☑
      second degree T23.262 ☑
      third degree T23.362 ☑
    right T23.061 ☑
      first degree T23.161 ☑
      second degree T23.261 ☑
      third degree T23.361 ☑
    second degree T23.269 ☑
    third degree T23.369 ☑
  due to ingested chemical agent — *see* Corrosion, by site
  ear (auricle) (external) (canal) T20.01 ☑
    first degree T20.11 ☑
    second degree T20.21 ☑
    third degree T20.31 ☑
  elbow T22.029 ☑
    first degree T22.129 ☑
    left T22.022 ☑
      first degree T22.122 ☑
      second degree T22.222 ☑
      third degree T22.322 ☑
    right T22.021 ☑
      first degree T22.121 ☑
      second degree T22.221 ☑
      third degree T22.321 ☑
    second degree T22.229 ☑
    third degree T22.329 ☑
  epidermal loss — *code as* Burn, second degree, by site
  erythema, erythematous — *code as* Burn, first degree, by site
  esophagus T28.1 ☑
  extent (percentage of body surface)
    less than 10 percent T31.0
    10-19 percent T31.10
      with 0-9 percent third degree burns T31.10
      with 10-19 percent third degree burns T31.11
    20-29 percent T31.20
      with 0-9 percent third degree burns T31.20
      with 10-19 percent third degree burns T31.21
      with 20-29 percent third degree burns T31.22
    30-39 percent T31.30
      with 0-9 percent third degree burns T31.30
      with 10-19 percent third degree burns T31.31
      with 20-29 percent third degree burns T31.32
      with 30-39 percent third degree burns T31.33
    40-49 percent T31.40
      with 0-9 percent third degree burns T31.40

Burn — *continued*
  extent — *continued*
    40-49 percent — *continued*
      with 10-19 percent third degree burns T31.41
      with 20-29 percent third degree burns T31.42
      with 30-39 percent third degree burns T31.43
      with 40-49 percent third degree burns T31.44
    50-59 percent T31.50
      with 0-9 percent third degree burns T31.50
      with 10-19 percent third degree burns T31.51
      with 20-29 percent third degree burns T31.52
      with 30-39 percent third degree burns T31.53
      with 40-49 percent third degree burns T31.54
      with 50-59 percent third degree burns T31.55
    60-69 percent T31.60
      with 0-9 percent third degree burns T31.60
      with 10-19 percent third degree burns T31.61
      with 20-29 percent third degree burns T31.62
      with 30-39 percent third degree burns T31.63
      with 40-49 percent third degree burns T31.64
      with 50-59 percent third degree burns T31.65
      with 60-69 percent third degree burns T31.66
    70-79 percent T31.70
      with 0-9 percent third degree burns T31.70
      with 10-19 percent third degree burns T31.71
      with 20-29 percent third degree burns T31.72
      with 30-39 percent third degree burns T31.73
      with 40-49 percent third degree burns T31.74
      with 50-59 percent third degree burns T31.75
      with 60-69 percent third degree burns T31.76
      with 70-79 percent third degree burns T31.77
    80-89 percent T31.80
      with 0-9 percent third degree burns T31.80
      with 10-19 percent third degree burns T31.81
      with 20-29 percent third degree burns T31.82
      with 30-39 percent third degree burns T31.83
      with 40-49 percent third degree burns T31.84
      with 50-59 percent third degree burns T31.85
      with 60-69 percent third degree burns T31.86
      with 70-79 percent third degree burns T31.87
      with 80-89 percent third degree burns T31.88
    90 percent or more T31.90
      with 0-9 percent third degree burns T31.90
      with 10-19 percent third degree burns T31.91
      with 20-29 percent third degree burns T31.92
      with 30-39 percent third degree burns T31.93
      with 40-49 percent third degree burns T31.94
      with 50-59 percent third degree burns T31.95
      with 60-69 percent third degree burns T31.96
      with 70-79 percent third degree burns T31.97
      with 80-89 percent third degree burns T31.98
      with 90 percent or more third degree burns T31.99
  extremity — *see* Burn, limb
  eye(s) and adnexa T26.4- ☑
    with resulting rupture and destruction of eyeball T26.2- ☑
    conjunctival sac — *see* Burn, cornea
    cornea — *see* Burn, cornea
    lid — *see* Burn, eyelid
    periocular area — *see* Burn, eyelid
    specified site NEC T26.3- ☑
  eyeball — *see* Burn, eye
  eyelid(s) T26.0- ☑
    chemical — *see* Corrosion, eyelid
  face — *see* Burn, head
  finger T23.029 ☑
    first degree T23.129 ☑
    left T23.022 ☑
      first degree T23.122 ☑
      second degree T23.222 ☑
      third degree T23.322 ☑
    multiple sites (without thumb) T23.039 ☑
      with thumb T23.049 ☑
        first degree T23.149 ☑
        left T23.042 ☑
          first degree T23.142 ☑
          second degree T23.242 ☑
          third degree T23.342 ☑
        right T23.041 ☑
          first degree T23.141 ☑
          second degree T23.241 ☑
          third degree T23.341 ☑
        second degree T23.249 ☑
        third degree T23.349 ☑
      first degree T23.139 ☑

Burn — *continued*
  finger — *continued*
    multiple sites — *continued*
      left T23.032 ☑
        first degree T23.132 ☑
        second degree T23.232 ☑
        third degree T23.332 ☑
      right T23.031 ☑
        first degree T23.131 ☑
        second degree T23.231 ☑
        third degree T23.331 ☑
      second degree T23.239 ☑
      third degree T23.339 ☑
    right T23.021 ☑
      first degree T23.121 ☑
      second degree T23.221 ☑
      third degree T23.321 ☑
    second degree T23.229 ☑
    third degree T23.329 ☑
  flank — *see* Burn, abdominal wall
  foot T25.029 ☑
    first degree T25.129 ☑
    left T25.022 ☑
      first degree T25.122 ☑
      second degree T25.222 ☑
      third degree T25.322 ☑
    multiple with ankle — *see* Burn, lower, limb, multiple, ankle and foot
    right T25.021 ☑
      first degree T25.121 ☑
      second degree T25.221 ☑
      third degree T25.321 ☑
    second degree T25.229 ☑
    third degree T25.329 ☑
  forearm T22.019 ☑
    first degree T22.119 ☑
    left T22.012 ☑
      first degree T22.112 ☑
      second degree T22.212 ☑
      third degree T22.312 ☑
    right T22.011 ☑
      first degree T22.111 ☑
      second degree T22.211 ☑
      third degree T22.311 ☑
    second degree T22.219 ☑
    third degree T22.319 ☑
  forehead T20.06 ☑
    first degree T20.16 ☑
    second degree T20.26 ☑
    third degree T20.36 ☑
  fourth degree — *code as* Burn, third degree, by site
  friction — *see* Burn, by site
  from swallowing caustic or corrosive substance NEC — *see* Corrosion, by site
  full thickness skin loss — *code as* Burn, third degree, by site
  gastrointestinal tract NEC T28.2 ☑
    from swallowing caustic or corrosive substance T28.7 ☑
  genital organs
    external
      female T21.07 ☑
        first degree T21.17 ☑
        second degree T21.27 ☑
        third degree T21.37 ☑
      male T21.06 ☑
        first degree T21.16 ☑
        second degree T21.26 ☑
        third degree T21.36 ☑
    internal T28.3 ☑
      from caustic or corrosive substance T28.8 ☑
  groin — *see* Burn, abdominal wall
  hand(s) T23.009 ☑
    back — *see* Burn, dorsum of hand
    finger — *see* Burn, finger
    first degree T23.109 ☑
    left T23.002 ☑
      first degree T23.102 ☑
      second degree T23.202 ☑
      third degree T23.302 ☑
    multiple sites with wrist T23.099 ☑
      first degree T23.199 ☑
      left T23.092 ☑
        first degree T23.192 ☑
        second degree T23.292 ☑
        third degree T23.392 ☑

▽ Subterms under main terms may continue to next column or page   ☑ Additional Character Required — Refer to the Tabular List for Character Selection   43

Burn — Burn

Burn — continued
  hand(s) — continued
    multiple sites with wrist — continued
      right T23.091 ☑
        first degree T23.191 ☑
        second degree T23.291 ☑
        third degree T23.391 ☑
      second degree T23.299 ☑
      third degree T23.399 ☑
    palm — see Burn, palm
    right T23.001 ☑
      first degree T23.101 ☑
      second degree T23.201 ☑
      third degree T23.301 ☑
    second degree T23.209 ☑
    third degree T23.309 ☑
    thumb — see Burn, thumb
  head (and face) (and neck) T20.00 ☑
    cheek — see Burn, cheek
    chin — see Burn, chin
    ear — see Burn, ear
    eye(s) only — see Burn, eye
    first degree T20.10 ☑
    forehead — see Burn, forehead
    lip — see Burn, lip
    multiple sites T20.09 ☑
      first degree T20.19 ☑
      second degree T20.29 ☑
      third degree T20.39 ☑
    neck — see Burn, neck
    nose — see Burn, nose
    scalp — see Burn, scalp
    second degree T20.20 ☑
    third degree T20.30 ☑
  hip(s) — see Burn, lower, limb
  inhalation — see Burn, respiratory tract
    caustic or corrosive substance (fumes) — see Corrosion, respiratory tract
  internal organ(s) T28.40 ☑
    alimentary tract T28.2 ☑
      esophagus T28.1 ☑
    eardrum T28.41 ☑
    esophagus T28.1 ☑
    from caustic or corrosive substance (swallowing) NEC — see Corrosion, by site
    genitourinary T28.3 ☑
    mouth T28.0 ☑
    pharynx T28.0 ☑
    respiratory tract — see Burn, respiratory tract
    specified organ NEC T28.49 ☑
  interscapular region — see Burn, back, upper
  intestine (large) (small) T28.2 ☑
  knee T24.029 ☑
    first degree T24.129 ☑
    left T24.022 ☑
      first degree T24.122 ☑
      second degree T24.222 ☑
      third degree T24.322 ☑
    right T24.021 ☑
      first degree T24.121 ☑
      second degree T24.221 ☑
      third degree T24.321 ☑
    second degree T24.229 ☑
    third degree T24.329 ☑
  labium (majus) (minus) — see Burn, genital organs, external, female
  lacrimal apparatus, duct, gland or sac — see Burn, eye, specified site NEC
  larynx T27.0 ☑
    with lung T27.1 ☑
  leg(s) (lower) (upper) — see Burn, lower, limb
  lightning — see Burn, by site
  limb(s)
    lower (except ankle or foot alone) — see Burn, lower, limb
    upper — see Burn, upper limb
  lip(s) T20.02 ☑
    first degree T20.12 ☑
    second degree T20.22 ☑
    third degree T20.32 ☑
  lower
    back — see Burn, back
    limb T24.009 ☑
      ankle — see Burn, ankle
      calf — see Burn, calf
      first degree T24.109 ☑

Burn — continued
  lower — continued
    limb — continued
      foot — see Burn, foot
      hip — see Burn, thigh
      knee — see Burn, knee
      left T24.002 ☑
        first degree T24.102 ☑
        second degree T24.202 ☑
        third degree T24.302 ☑
      multiple sites, except ankle and foot T24.099 ☑
        ankle and foot T25.099 ☑
          first degree T25.199 ☑
          left T25.092 ☑
            first degree T25.192 ☑
            second degree T25.292 ☑
            third degree T25.392 ☑
          right T25.091 ☑
            first degree T25.191 ☑
            second degree T25.291 ☑
            third degree T25.391 ☑
          second degree T25.299 ☑
          third degree T25.399 ☑
        first degree T24.199 ☑
        left T24.092 ☑
          first degree T24.192 ☑
          second degree T24.292 ☑
          third degree T24.392 ☑
        right T24.091 ☑
          first degree T24.191 ☑
          second degree T24.291 ☑
          third degree T24.391 ☑
        second degree T24.299 ☑
        third degree T24.399 ☑
      right T24.001 ☑
        first degree T24.101 ☑
        second degree T24.201 ☑
        third degree T24.301 ☑
      second degree T24.209 ☑
      thigh — see Burn, thigh
      third degree T24.309 ☑
      toe — see Burn, toe
  lung (with larynx and trachea) T27.1 ☑
  mouth T28.0 ☑
  neck T20.07 ☑
    first degree T20.17 ☑
    second degree T20.27 ☑
    third degree T20.37 ☑
  nose (septum) T20.04 ☑
    first degree T20.14 ☑
    second degree T20.24 ☑
    third degree T20.34 ☑
  ocular adnexa — see Burn, eye
  orbit region — see Burn, eyelid
  palm T23.059 ☑
    first degree T23.159 ☑
    left T23.052 ☑
      first degree T23.152 ☑
      second degree T23.252 ☑
      third degree T23.352 ☑
    right T23.051 ☑
      first degree T23.151 ☑
      second degree T23.251 ☑
      third degree T23.351 ☑
    second degree T23.259 ☑
    third degree T23.359 ☑
  partial thickness — code as Burn, unspecified degree, by site
  pelvis — see Burn, trunk
  penis — see Burn, genital organs, external, male
  perineum
    female — see Burn, genital organs, external, female
    male — see Burn, genital organs, external, male
  periocular area — see Burn, eyelid
  pharynx T28.0 ☑
  rectum T28.2 ☑
  respiratory tract T27.3 ☑
    larynx — see Burn, larynx
    specified part NEC T27.2 ☑
    trachea — see Burn, trachea
  sac, lacrimal — see Burn, eye, specified site NEC
  scalp T20.05 ☑
    first degree T20.15 ☑
    second degree T20.25 ☑
    third degree T20.35 ☑

Burn — continued
  scapular region T22.069 ☑
    first degree T22.169 ☑
    left T22.062 ☑
      first degree T22.162 ☑
      second degree T22.262 ☑
      third degree T22.362 ☑
    right T22.061 ☑
      first degree T22.161 ☑
      second degree T22.261 ☑
      third degree T22.361 ☑
    second degree T22.269 ☑
    third degree T22.369 ☑
  sclera — see Burn, eye, specified site NEC
  scrotum — see Burn, genital organs, external, male
  shoulder T22.059 ☑
    first degree T22.159 ☑
    left T22.052 ☑
      first degree T22.152 ☑
      second degree T22.252 ☑
      third degree T22.352 ☑
    right T22.051 ☑
      first degree T22.151 ☑
      second degree T22.251 ☑
      third degree T22.351 ☑
    second degree T22.259 ☑
    third degree T22.359 ☑
  stomach T28.2 ☑
  temple — see Burn, head
  testis — see Burn, genital organs, external, male
  thigh T24.019 ☑
    first degree T24.119 ☑
    left T24.012 ☑
      first degree T24.112 ☑
      second degree T24.212 ☑
      third degree T24.312 ☑
    right T24.011 ☑
      first degree T24.111 ☑
      second degree T24.211 ☑
      third degree T24.311 ☑
    second degree T24.219 ☑
    third degree T24.319 ☑
  thorax (external) — see Burn, trunk
  throat (meaning pharynx) T28.0 ☑
  thumb(s) T23.019 ☑
    first degree T23.119 ☑
    left T23.012 ☑
      first degree T23.112 ☑
      second degree T23.212 ☑
      third degree T23.312 ☑
    multiple sites with fingers T23.049 ☑
      first degree T23.149 ☑
      left T23.042 ☑
        first degree T23.142 ☑
        second degree T23.242 ☑
        third degree T23.342 ☑
      right T23.041 ☑
        first degree T23.141 ☑
        second degree T23.241 ☑
        third degree T23.341 ☑
      second degree T23.249 ☑
      third degree T23.349 ☑
    right T23.011 ☑
      first degree T23.111 ☑
      second degree T23.211 ☑
      third degree T23.311 ☑
    second degree T23.219 ☑
    third degree T23.319 ☑
  toe T25.039 ☑
    first degree T25.139 ☑
    left T25.032 ☑
      first degree T25.132 ☑
      second degree T25.232 ☑
      third degree T25.332 ☑
    right T25.031 ☑
      first degree T25.131 ☑
      second degree T25.231 ☑
      third degree T25.331 ☑
    second degree T25.239 ☑
    third degree T25.339 ☑
  tongue T28.0 ☑
  tonsil(s) T28.0 ☑
  trachea T27.0 ☑
    with lung T27.1 ☑

☑ Additional Character Required — Refer to the Tabular List for Character Selection   ▽ Subterms under main terms may continue to next column or page

Burn — *continued*
  trunk T21.00 ☑
    abdominal wall — *see* Burn, abdominal wall
    anus — *see* Burn, buttock
    axilla — *see* Burn, upper limb
    back — *see* Burn, back
    breast — *see* Burn, chest wall
    buttock — *see* Burn, buttock
    chest wall — *see* Burn, chest wall
    first degree T21.10 ☑
    flank — *see* Burn, abdominal wall
    genital
      female — *see* Burn, genital organs, external, female
      male — *see* Burn, genital organs, external, male
    groin — *see* Burn, abdominal wall
    interscapular region — *see* Burn, back, upper
    labia — *see* Burn, genital organs, external, female
    lower back — *see* Burn, back
    penis — *see* Burn, genital organs, external, male
    perineum
      female — *see* Burn, genital organs, external, female
      male — *see* Burn, genital organs, external, male
    scapula region — *see* Burn, scapular region
    scrotum — *see* Burn, genital organs, external, male
    second degree T21.20 ☑
    specified site NEC T21.09 ☑
      first degree T21.19 ☑
      second degree T21.29 ☑
      third degree T21.39 ☑
    testes — *see* Burn, genital organs, external, male
    third degree T21.30 ☑
    upper back — *see* Burn, back, upper
    vulva — *see* Burn, genital organs, external, female
  unspecified site with extent of body surface involved
    specified
      less than 10 per cent T31.0
      10-19 per cent (0-9 percent third degree) T31.10
        with 10-19 percent third degree T31.11
      20-29 per cent (0-9 percent third degree) T31.20
        with
          10-19 percent third degree T31.21
          20-29 percent third degree T31.22
      30-39 per cent (0-9 percent third degree) T31.30
        with
          10-19 percent third degree T31.31
          20-29 percent third degree T31.32
          30-39 percent third degree T31.33
      40-49 per cent (0-9 percent third degree) T31.40
        with
          10-19 percent third degree T31.41
          20-29 percent third degree T31.42
          30-39 percent third degree T31.43
          40-49 percent third degree T31.44
      50-59 per cent (0-9 percent third degree) T31.50
        with
          10-19 percent third degree T31.51
          20-29 percent third degree T31.52
          30-39 percent third degree T31.53
          40-49 percent third degree T31.54
          50-59 percent third degree T31.55
      60-69 per cent (0-9 percent third degree) T31.60
        with
          10-19 percent third degree T31.61
          20-29 percent third degree T31.62
          30-39 percent third degree T31.63
          40-49 percent third degree T31.64
          50-59 percent third degree T31.65
          60-69 percent third degree T31.66
      70-79 per cent (0-9 percent third degree) T31.70
        with
          10-19 percent third degree T31.71
          20-29 percent third degree T31.72
          30-39 percent third degree T31.73
          40-49 percent third degree T31.74
          50-59 percent third degree T31.75
          60-69 percent third degree T31.76
          70-79 percent third degree T31.77
      80-89 per cent (0-9 percent third degree) T31.80
        with
          10-19 percent third degree T31.81
          20-29 percent third degree T31.82
          30-39 percent third degree T31.83
          40-49 percent third degree T31.84
          50-59 percent third degree T31.85
          60-69 percent third degree T31.86
          70-79 percent third degree T31.87

Burn — *continued*
  unspecified site with extent of body surface involved
    specified — *continued*
      80-89 per cent — *continued*
        with — *continued*
          80-89 percent third degree T31.88
      90 per cent or more (0-9 percent third degree) T31.90
        with
          10-19 percent third degree T31.91
          20-29 percent third degree T31.92
          30-39 percent third degree T31.93
          40-49 percent third degree T31.94
          50-59 percent third degree T31.95
          60-69 percent third degree T31.96
          70-79 percent third degree T31.97
          80-89 percent third degree T31.98
          90-99 percent third degree T31.99
  upper limb T22.00 ☑
    above elbow — *see* Burn, above elbow
    axilla — *see* Burn, axilla
    elbow — *see* Burn, elbow
    first degree T22.10 ☑
    forearm — *see* Burn, forearm
    hand — *see* Burn, hand
    interscapular region — *see* Burn, back, upper
    multiple sites T22.099 ☑
      first degree T22.199 ☑
      left T22.092 ☑
        first degree T22.192 ☑
        second degree T22.292 ☑
        third degree T22.392 ☑
      right T22.091 ☑
        first degree T22.191 ☑
        second degree T22.291 ☑
        third degree T22.391 ☑
      second degree T22.299 ☑
      third degree T22.399 ☑
    scapular region — *see* Burn, scapular region
    second degree T22.20 ☑
    shoulder — *see* Burn, shoulder
    third degree T22.30 ☑
    wrist — *see* Burn, wrist
  uterus T28.3
  vagina T28.3
  vulva — *see* Burn, genital organs, external, female
  wrist T23.079 ☑
    first degree T23.179 ☑
    left T23.072 ☑
      first degree T23.172 ☑
      second degree T23.272 ☑
      third degree T23.372 ☑
    multiple sites with hand T23.099 ☑
      first degree T23.199 ☑
      left T23.092 ☑
        first degree T23.192 ☑
        second degree T23.292 ☑
        third degree T23.392 ☑
      right T23.091 ☑
        first degree T23.191 ☑
        second degree T23.291 ☑
        third degree T23.391 ☑
      second degree T23.299 ☑
      third degree T23.399 ☑
    right T23.071 ☑
      first degree T23.171 ☑
      second degree T23.271 ☑
      third degree T23.371 ☑
    second degree T23.279 ☑
    third degree T23.379 ☑
Burnett's syndrome E83.52
Burning
  feet syndrome E53.9
  sensation R20.8
  tongue K14.6
Burn-out (state) Z73.0
Burns' disease or osteochondrosis — *see* Osteochondrosis, juvenile, ulna
Bursa — *see* condition
Bursitis M71.9
  Achilles — *see* Tendinitis, Achilles
  adhesive — *see* Bursitis, specified NEC
  ankle — *see* Enthesopathy, lower limb, ankle, specified type NEC
  calcaneal — *see* Enthesopathy, foot, specified type NEC

Bursitis — *continued*
  collateral ligament, tibial — *see* Bursitis, tibial collateral
  due to use, overuse, pressure (*see also* Disorder, soft tissue, due to use, specified type NEC)
    specified NEC — *see* Disorder, soft tissue, due to use, specified NEC
  Duplay's M75.0
  elbow NEC M70.3- ☑
    olecranon M70.2- ☑
  finger — *see* Disorder, soft tissue, due to use, specified type NEC, hand
  foot — *see* Enthesopathy, foot, specified type NEC
  gonococcal A54.49
  gouty — *see* Gout, idiopathic
  hand M70.1- ☑
  hip NEC M70.7- ☑
    trochanteric M70.6- ☑
  infective NEC M71.10
    abscess — *see* Abscess, bursa
    ankle M71.17- ☑
    elbow M71.12- ☑
    foot M71.17- ☑
    hand M71.14- ☑
    hip M71.15- ☑
    knee M71.16- ☑
    multiple sites M71.19
    shoulder M71.11- ☑
    specified site NEC M71.18
    wrist M71.13- ☑
  ischial — *see* Bursitis, hip
  knee NEC M70.5- ☑
    prepatellar M70.4- ☑
  occupational NEC (*see also* Disorder, soft tissue, due to, use)
  olecranon — *see* Bursitis, elbow, olecranon
  pharyngeal J39.1
  popliteal — *see* Bursitis, knee
  prepatellar M70.4- ☑
  radiohumeral M77.8
  rheumatoid M06.20
    ankle M06.27- ☑
    elbow M06.22- ☑
    foot joint M06.27- ☑
    hand joint M06.24- ☑
    hip M06.25- ☑
    knee M06.26- ☑
    multiple site M06.29
    shoulder M06.21- ☑
    vertebra M06.28
    wrist M06.23- ☑
  scapulohumeral — *see* Bursitis, shoulder
  semimembranous muscle (knee) — *see* Bursitis, knee
  shoulder M75.5- ☑
    adhesive — *see* Capsulitis, adhesive
  specified NEC M71.50
    ankle M71.57- ☑
    due to use, overuse or pressure — *see* Disorder, soft tissue, due to, use
    elbow M71.52- ☑
    foot M71.57- ☑
    hand M71.54- ☑
    hip M71.55- ☑
    knee M71.56- ☑
    shoulder — *see* Bursitis, shoulder
    specified site NEC M71.58
    tibial collateral M76.4- ☑
    wrist M71.53- ☑
  subacromial — *see* Bursitis, shoulder
  subcoracoid — *see* Bursitis, shoulder
  subdeltoid — *see* Bursitis, shoulder
  syphilitic A52.78
  Thornwaldt, Tornwaldt J39.2
  tibial collateral — *see* Bursitis, tibial collateral
  toe — *see* Enthesopathy, foot, specified type NEC
  trochanteric (area) — *see* Bursitis, hip, trochanteric
  wrist — *see* Bursitis, hand
Bursopathy M71.9
  specified type NEC M71.80
    ankle M71.87- ☑
    elbow M71.82- ☑
    foot M71.87- ☑
    hand M71.84- ☑
    hip M71.85- ☑
    knee M71.86- ☑
    multiple sites M71.89
    shoulder M71.81- ☑

Bursopathy — continued
  specified type — continued
    specified site NEC M71.88
    wrist M71.83-☑
Burst stitches or sutures (complication of surgery)
    T81.31 ☑
  external operation wound T81.31 ☑
  internal operation wound T81.32 ☑
Buruli ulcer A31.1
Bury's disease L95.1
Buschke's
  disease B45.3
  scleredema — see Sclerosis, systemic
Busse-Buschke disease B45.3
Buttock — see condition
Button
  Biskra B55.1
  Delhi B55.1
  oriental B55.1
Buttonhole deformity (finger) — see Deformity, finger, boutonniere
Bwamba fever A92.8
Byssinosis J66.0
Bywaters' syndrome T79.5 ☑

C

Cachexia R64
  cancerous R64
  cardiac — see Disease, heart
  dehydration E86.0
    with
      hypernatremia E87.0
      hyponatremia E87.1
    due to malnutrition R64
  exophthalmic — see Hyperthyroidism
  heart — see Disease, heart
  hypophyseal E23.0
  hypopituitary E23.0
  lead — see Poisoning, lead
  malignant R64
  marsh — see Malaria
  nervous F48.8
  old age R54
  paludal — see Malaria
  pituitary E23.0
  renal N28.9
  saturnine — see Poisoning, lead
  senile R54
  Simmonds' E23.0
  splenica D73.0
  strumipriva E03.4
  tuberculous NEC — see Tuberculosis
Café, au lait spots L81.3
Caffey's syndrome Q78.8
Caisson disease T70.3 ☑
Cake kidney Q63.1
Caked breast (puerperal, postpartum) O92.79
Calabar swelling B74.3
Calcaneal spur — see Spur, bone, calcaneal
Calcaneo-apophysitis M92.8
Calcareous — see condition
Calcicosis J62.8
Calciferol (vitamin D) deficiency E55.9
  with rickets E55.0
Calcification
  adrenal (capsule) (gland) E27.49
    tuberculous E35 [B90.8]
  aorta I70.0
  artery (annular) — see Arteriosclerosis
  auricle (ear) — see Disorder, pinna, specified type NEC
  basal ganglia G23.8
  bladder N32.89
    due to Schistosoma hematobium B65.0
  brain (cortex) — see Calcification, cerebral
  bronchus J98.09
  bursa M71.40
    ankle M71.47-☑
    elbow M71.42-☑
    foot M71.47-☑
    hand M71.44-☑
    hip M71.45-☑
    knee M71.46-☑
    multiple sites M71.49
    shoulder M75.3-☑
    specified site NEC M71.48
    wrist M71.43-☑

Calcification — continued
  cardiac — see Degeneration, myocardial
  cerebral (cortex) G93.89
    artery I67.2
  cervix (uteri) N88.8
  choroid plexus G93.89
  conjunctiva — see Concretion, conjunctiva
  corpora cavernosa (penis) N48.89
  cortex (brain) — see Calcification, cerebral
  dental pulp (nodular) K04.2
  dentinal papilla K00.4
  fallopian tube N83.8
  falx cerebri G96.19
  gallbladder K82.8
  general E83.59
  heart (see also Degeneration, myocardial)
    valve — see Endocarditis
  idiopathic infantile arterial (IIAC) Q28.8
  intervertebral cartilage or disc (postinfective) — see Disorder, disc, specified NEC
  intracranial — see Calcification, cerebral
  joint — see Disorder, joint, specified type NEC
  kidney N28.89
    tuberculous N29 [B90.1]
  larynx (senile) J38.7
  lens — see Cataract, specified NEC
  lung (active) (postinfectional) J98.4
    tuberculous B90.9
  lymph gland or node (postinfectional) I89.8
    tuberculous (see also Tuberculosis, lymph gland) B90.8
  mammographic R92.1
  massive (paraplegic) — see Myositis, ossificans, in, quadriplegia
  medial — see Arteriosclerosis, extremities
  meninges (cerebral) (spinal) G96.19
  metastatic E83.59
  Mönckeberg's — see Arteriosclerosis, extremities
  muscle M61.9
    due to burns — see Myositis, ossificans, in, burns
    paralytic — see Myositis, ossificans, in, quadriplegia
    specified type NEC M61.40
      ankle M61.47-☑
      foot M61.47-☑
      forearm M61.43-☑
      hand M61.44-☑
      lower leg M61.46-☑
      multiple sites M61.49
      pelvic region M61.45-☑
      shoulder region M61.41-☑
      specified site NEC M61.48
      thigh M61.45-☑
      upper arm M61.42-☑
  myocardium, myocardial — see Degeneration, myocardial
  ovary N83.8
  pancreas K86.8
  penis N48.89
  periarticular — see Disorder, joint, specified type NEC
  pericardium (see also Pericarditis) I31.1
  pineal gland E34.8
  pleura J94.8
    postinfectional J94.8
    tuberculous NEC B90.9
  pulpal (dental) (nodular) K04.2
  sclera H15.89
  spleen D73.89
  subcutaneous L94.2
  suprarenal (capsule) (gland) E27.49
  tendon (sheath) (see also Tenosynovitis, specified type NEC)
    with bursitis, synovitis or tenosynovitis — see Tendinitis, calcific
  trachea J39.8
  ureter N28.89
  uterus N85.8
  vitreous — see Deposit, crystalline
Calcified — see Calcification
Calcinosis (interstitial) (tumoral) (universalis) E83.59
  with Raynaud's phenomenon, esophageal dysfunction, sclerodactyly, telangiectasia (CREST syndrome) M34.1
  circumscripta (skin) L94.2
  cutis L94.2
Calciphylaxis (see also Calcification, by site) E83.59
Calcium
  deposits — see Calcification, by site

Calcium — continued
  metabolism disorder E83.50
  salts or soaps in vitreous — see Deposit, crystalline
Calciuria R82.99
Calculi — see Calculus
Calculosis, intrahepatic — see Calculus, bile duct
Calculus, calculi, calculous
  ampulla of Vater — see Calculus, bile duct
  anuria (impacted) (recurrent) (see also Calculus, urinary) N20.9
  appendix K38.1
  bile duct (common) (hepatic) K80.50
    duct
      calculus of gallbladder — see Calculus, gallbladder and bile duct
      cholangitis K80.30
        with
          cholecystitis — see Calculus, bile duct, with cholecystitis
          obstruction K80.31
        acute K80.32
          with
            chronic cholangitis K80.36
              with obstruction K80.37
            obstruction K80.33
        chronic K80.34
          with
            acute cholangitis K80.36
              with obstruction K80.37
            obstruction K80.35
      cholecystitis (with cholangitis) K80.40
        with obstruction K80.41
        acute K80.42
          with
            chronic cholecystitis K80.46
              with obstruction K80.47
            obstruction K80.43
        chronic K80.44
          with
            acute cholecystitis K80.46
              with obstruction K80.47
            obstruction K80.45
      obstruction K80.51
  biliary (see also Calculus, gallbladder)
    specified NEC K80.80
      with obstruction K80.81
  bilirubin, multiple — see Calculus, gallbladder
  bladder (encysted) (impacted) (urinary) (diverticulum) N21.0
  bronchus J98.09
  calyx (kidney) (renal) — see Calculus, kidney
  cholesterol (pure) (solitary) — see Calculus, gallbladder
  common duct (bile) — see Calculus, bile duct
  conjunctiva — see Concretion, conjunctiva
  cystic N21.0
    duct — see Calculus, gallbladder
  dental (subgingival) (supragingival) K03.6
  diverticulum
    bladder N21.0
    kidney N20.0
  epididymis N50.8
  gallbladder K80.20
    with
      bile duct calculus — see Calculus, gallbladder and bile duct
      cholecystitis K80.10
        with obstruction K80.11
        acute K80.00
          with
            chronic cholecystitis K80.12
              with obstruction K80.13
            obstruction K80.01
        chronic K80.10
          with
            acute cholecystitis K80.12
              with obstruction K80.13
            obstruction K80.11
      specified NEC K80.18
        with obstruction K80.19
    obstruction K80.21
  gallbladder and bile duct K80.70
    with
      cholecystitis K80.60
        with obstruction K80.61
        acute K80.62
          with
            chronic cholecystitis K80.66
              with obstruction K80.67

Calculus, calculi, calculous — *continued*
gallbladder and bile duct — *continued*
with — *continued*
cholecystitis — *continued*
acute — *continued*
with — *continued*
obstruction K80.63
chronic K80.64
with
acute cholecystitis K80.66
with obstruction K80.67
obstruction K80.65
obstruction K80.71
hepatic (duct) — *see* Calculus, bile duct
ileal conduit N21.8
intestinal (impaction) (obstruction) K56.49
kidney (impacted) (multiple) (pelvis) (recurrent)
(staghorn) N20.0
with calculus, ureter N20.2
congenital Q63.8
lacrimal passages — *see* Dacryolith
liver (impacted) — *see* Calculus, bile duct
lung J98.4
mammographic R92.1
nephritic (impacted) (recurrent) — *see* Calculus, kidney
nose J34.89
pancreas (duct) K86.8
parotid duct or gland K11.5
pelvis, encysted — *see* Calculus, kidney
prostate N42.0
pulmonary J98.4
pyelitis (impacted) (recurrent) N20.0
with hydronephrosis N13.2
pyelonephritis (impacted) (recurrent) N20 ☑
with hydronephrosis N13.2
renal (impacted) (recurrent) — *see* Calculus, kidney
salivary (duct) (gland) K11.5
seminal vesicle N50.8
staghorn — *see* Calculus, kidney
Stensen's duct K11.5
stomach K31.89
sublingual duct or gland K11.5
congenital Q38.4
submandibular duct, gland or region K11.5
submaxillary duct, gland or region K11.5
suburethral N21.8
tonsil J35.8
tooth, teeth (subgingival) (supragingival) K03.6
tunica vaginalis N50.8
ureter (impacted) (recurrent) N20.1
with calculus, kidney N20.2
with hydronephrosis N13.2
with infection N13.6
urethra (impacted) N21.1
urinary (duct) (impacted) (passage) (tract) N20.9
with hydronephrosis N13.2
with infection N13.6
in (due to)
lower N21.9
specified NEC N21.8
vagina N89.8
vesical (impacted) N21.0
Wharton's duct K11.5
xanthine E79.8 [N22]
Calicectasis N28.89
Caliectasis N28.89
California
disease B38.9
encephalitis A83.5
Caligo cornea — *see* Opacity, cornea, central
Callositas, callosity (infected) L84
Callus (infected) L84
bone — *see* Osteophyte
excessive, following fracture — *code as* Sequelae of fracture
Calorie deficiency or malnutrition (*see also* Malnutrition) E46
Calvé-Perthes disease — *see* Legg-Calvé-Perthes disease
Calvé's disease — *see* Osteochondrosis, juvenile, spine
Calvities — *see* Alopecia, androgenic
Cameroon fever — *see* Malaria
Camptocormia (hysterical) F44.4
Camurati-Engelmann syndrome Q78.3
Canal (*see also* condition)
atrioventricular common Q21.2
Canaliculitis (lacrimal) (acute) (subacute) H04.33- ☑
Actinomyces A42.89

Canaliculitis — *continued*
chronic H04.42- ☑
Canavan's disease E75.29
Canceled procedure (surgical) Z53.9
because of
contraindication Z53.09
smoking Z53.01
left against medical advice (AMA) Z53.21
patient's decision Z53.20
for reasons of belief or group pressure Z53.1
specified reason NEC Z53.29
specified reason NEC Z53.8
Cancer (*see also* Neoplasm, by site, malignant)
bile duct type liver C22.1
blood — *see* Leukemia
breast (*see also* Neoplasm, breast, malignant)
C50.91- ☑
hepatocellular C22.0
lung (*see also* Neoplasm, lung, malignant) C34.90
ovarian (*see also* Neoplasm ovary, malignant) C56.9
unspecified site (primary) C80.1
Cancer (o)**phobia** F45.29
Cancerous — *see* Neoplasm, malignant, by site
Cancrum oris A69.0
Candidiasis, candidal B37.9
balanitis B37.42
bronchitis B37.1
cheilitis B37.83
congenital P37.5
cystitis B37.41
disseminated B37.7
endocarditis B37.6
enteritis B37.82
esophagitis B37.81
intertrigo B37.2
lung B37.1
meningitis B37.5
mouth B37.0
nails B37.2
neonatal P37.5
onychia B37.2
oral B37.0
osteomyelitis B37.89
otitis externa B37.84
paronychia B37.2
perionyxis B37.2
pneumonia B37.1
proctitis B37.82
pulmonary B37.1
pyelonephritis B37.49
sepsis B37.7
skin B37.2
specified site NEC B37.89
stomatitis B37.0
systemic B37.7
urethritis B37.41
urogenital site NEC B37.49
vagina B37.3
vulva B37.3
vulvovaginitis B37.3
Candidid L30.2
Candidosis — *see* Candidiasis
Candiru infection or infestation B88.8
Canities (premature) L67.1
congenital Q84.2
Canker (mouth) (sore) K12.0
rash A38.9
Cannabinosis J66.2
Canton fever A75.9
Cantrell's syndrome Q87.89
Capillariasis (intestinal) B81.1
hepatic B83.8
Capillary — *see* condition
Caplan's syndrome — *see* Rheumatoid, lung
Capsule — *see* condition
Capsulitis (joint) (*see also* Enthesopathy)
adhesive (shoulder) M75.0- ☑
hepatic K65.8
labyrinthine — *see* Otosclerosis, specified NEC
thyroid E06.9
Caput
crepitus Q75.8
medusae I86.8
succedaneum P12.81
Car sickness T75.3 ☑
Carapata (disease) A68.0
Carate — *see* Pinta

Carbon lung J60
Carbuncle L02.93
abdominal wall L02.231
anus K61.0
auditory canal, external — *see* Abscess, ear, external
auricle ear — *see* Abscess, ear, external
axilla L02.43- ☑
back (any part) L02.232
breast N61
buttock L02.33
cheek (external) L02.03
chest wall L02.233
chin L02.03
corpus cavernosum N48.21
ear (any part) (external) (middle) — *see* Abscess, ear, external
external auditory canal — *see* Abscess, ear, external
eyelid — *see* Abscess, eyelid
face NEC L02.03
femoral (region) — *see* Carbuncle, lower limb
finger — *see* Carbuncle, hand
flank L02.231
foot L02.63- ☑
forehead L02.03
genital — *see* Abscess, genital
gluteal (region) L02.33
groin L02.234
hand L02.53- ☑
head NEC L02.831
heel — *see* Carbuncle, foot
hip — *see* Carbuncle, lower limb
kidney — *see* Abscess, kidney
knee — *see* Carbuncle, lower limb
labium (majus) (minus) N76.4
lacrimal
gland — *see* Dacryoadenitis
passages (duct) (sac) — *see* Inflammation, lacrimal, passages, acute
leg — *see* Carbuncle, lower limb
lower limb L02.43- ☑
malignant A22.0
navel L02.236
neck L02.13
nose (external) (septum) J34.0
orbit, orbital — *see* Abscess, orbit
palmar (space) — *see* Carbuncle, hand
partes posteriores L02.33
pectoral region L02.233
penis N48.21
perineum L02.235
pinna — *see* Abscess, ear, external
popliteal — *see* Carbuncle, lower limb
scalp L02.831
seminal vesicle N49.0
shoulder — *see* Carbuncle, upper limb
specified site NEC L02.838
temple (region) L02.03
thumb — *see* Carbuncle, hand
toe — *see* Carbuncle, foot
trunk L02.239
abdominal wall L02.231
back L02.232
chest wall L02.233
groin L02.234
perineum L02.235
umbilicus L02.236
umbilicus L02.236
upper limb L02.43- ☑
urethra N34.0
vulva N76.4
Carbunculus — *see* Carbuncle
Carcinoid (tumor) — *see* Tumor, carcinoid
Carcinoidosis E34.0
Carcinoma (malignant) (*see also* Neoplasm, by site, malignant)
acidophil
specified site — *see* Neoplasm, malignant, by site
unspecified site C75.1
acidophil-basophil, mixed
specified site — *see* Neoplasm, malignant, by site
unspecified site C75.1
adnexal (skin) — *see* Neoplasm, skin, malignant
adrenal cortical C74.0- ☑
alveolar — *see* Neoplasm, lung, malignant
cell — *see* Neoplasm, lung, malignant
ameloblastic C41.1
upper jaw (bone) C41.0

Carcinoma — *continued*
  apocrine
    breast — *see* Neoplasm, breast, malignant
    specified site NEC — *see* Neoplasm, skin, malignant
    unspecified site C44.99
  basal cell (pigmented) (*see also* Neoplasm, skin, malignant) C44.91
    fibro-epithelial — *see* Neoplasm, skin, malignant
    morphea — *see* Neoplasm, skin, malignant
    multicentric — *see* Neoplasm, skin, malignant
  basaloid
  basal-squamous cell, mixed — *see* Neoplasm, skin, malignant
  basophil
    specified site — *see* Neoplasm, malignant, by site
    unspecified site C75.1
  basophil-acidophil, mixed
    specified site — *see* Neoplasm, malignant, by site
    unspecified site C75.1
  basosquamous — *see* Neoplasm, skin, malignant
  bile duct
    with hepatocellular, mixed C22.0
    liver C22.1
    specified site NEC — *see* Neoplasm, malignant, by site
    unspecified site C22.1
  branchial or branchiogenic C10.4
  bronchial or bronchogenic — *see* Neoplasm, lung, malignant
  bronchiolar — *see* Neoplasm, lung, malignant
  bronchioloalveolar — *see* Neoplasm, lung, malignant
  C cell
    specified site — *see* Neoplasm, malignant, by site
    unspecified site C73
  ceruminous C44.29- ☑
  cervix uteri
    in situ D06.9
      endocervix D06.0
      exocervix D06.1
      specified site NEC D06.7
  chorionic
    specified site — *see* Neoplasm, malignant, by site
    unspecified site
      female C58
      male C62.90
  chromophobe
    specified site — *see* Neoplasm, malignant, by site
    unspecified site C75.1
  cloacogenic
    specified site — *see* Neoplasm, malignant, by site
    unspecified site C21.2
  diffuse type
    specified site — *see* Neoplasm, malignant, by site
    unspecified site C16.9
  duct (cell)
    with Paget's disease — *see* Neoplasm, breast, malignant
    infiltrating
      with lobular carcinoma (in situ)
        specified site — *see* Neoplasm, malignant, by site
        unspecified site (female) C50.91- ☑
          male C50.92- ☑
      specified site — *see* Neoplasm, malignant, by site
      unspecified site (female) C50.91- ☑
        male C50.92- ☑
  ductal
    with lobular
      specified site — *see* Neoplasm, malignant, by site
      unspecified site (female) C50.91- ☑
        male C50.92- ☑
    ductular, infiltrating
      specified site — *see* Neoplasm, malignant, by site
      unspecified site (female) C50.91- ☑
        male C50.92- ☑
  embryonal
    liver C22.7
  endometrioid
    specified site — *see* Neoplasm, malignant, by site
    unspecified site
      female C56.9
      male C61
  eosinophil
    specified site — *see* Neoplasm, malignant, by site
    unspecified site C75.1

Carcinoma — *continued*
  epidermoid (*see also* Neoplasm, skin, malignant)
    in situ, Bowen's type — *see* Neoplasm, skin, in situ
  fibroepithelial, basal cell — *see* Neoplasm, skin, malignant
  follicular
    with papillary (mixed) C73
    moderately differentiated C73
    pure follicle C73
    specified site — *see* Neoplasm, malignant, by site
    trabecular C73
    unspecified site C73
    well differentiated C73
  generalized, with unspecified primary site C80.0
  glycogen-rich — *see* Neoplasm, breast, malignant
  granulosa cell C56- ☑
  hepatic cell C22.0
  hepatocellular C22.0
    with bile duct, mixed C22.0
    fibrolamellar C22.0
  hepatocholangiolitic C22.0
  Hurthle cell C73
  in
    adenomatous
      polyposis coli C18.9
    pleomorphic adenoma — *see* Neoplasm, salivary glands, malignant
    situ — *see* Carcinoma-in-situ
  infiltrating
    duct
      with lobular
        specified site — *see* Neoplasm, malignant, by site
        unspecified site (female) C50.91- ☑
          male C50.92- ☑
      with Paget's disease — *see* Neoplasm, breast, malignant
      specified site — *see* Neoplasm, malignant
      unspecified site (female) C50.91- ☑
        male C50.92- ☑
    ductular
      specified site — *see* Neoplasm, malignant
      unspecified site (female) C50.91- ☑
        male C50.92- ☑
    lobular
      specified site — *see* Neoplasm, malignant
      unspecified site (female) C50.91- ☑
        male C50.92- ☑
  inflammatory
    specified site — *see* Neoplasm, malignant
    unspecified site (female) C50.91- ☑
      male C50.92- ☑
  intestinal type
    specified site — *see* Neoplasm, malignant, by site
    unspecified site C16.9
  intracystic
    noninfiltrating — *see* Neoplasm, in situ, by site
  intraductal (noninfiltrating)
    with Paget's disease — *see* Neoplasm, breast, malignant
    breast D05.1- ☑
    papillary
      with invasion
        specified site — *see* Neoplasm, malignant, by site
        unspecified site (female) C50.91- ☑
          male C50.92- ☑
      breast D05.1- ☑
      specified site NEC — *see* Neoplasm, in situ, by site
      unspecified site (female) D05.1- ☑
    specified site NEC — *see* Neoplasm, in situ, by site
    unspecified site (female) D05.1- ☑
  intraepidermal — *see* Neoplasm, in situ
    squamous cell, Bowen's type — *see* Neoplasm, skin, in situ
  intraepithelial — *see* Neoplasm, in situ, by site
    squamous cell — *see* Neoplasm, in situ, by site
  intraosseous C41.1
    upper jaw (bone) C41.0
  islet cell
    with exocrine, mixed
      specified site — *see* Neoplasm, malignant, by site
      unspecified site C25.9
    pancreas C25.4

Carcinoma — *continued*
  islet cell — *continued*
    specified site NEC — *see* Neoplasm, malignant, by site
    unspecified site C25.4
  juvenile, breast — *see* Neoplasm, breast, malignant
  large cell
    small cell
      specified site — *see* Neoplasm, malignant, by site
      unspecified site C34.90
  Leydig cell (testis)
    specified site — *see* Neoplasm, malignant, by site
    unspecified site
      female C56.9
      male C62.90
  lipid-rich (female) C50.91- ☑
    male C50.92- ☑
  liver cell C22.0
  liver NEC C22.7
  lobular (infiltrating)
    with intraductal
      specified site — *see* Neoplasm, malignant, by site
      unspecified site (female) C50.91- ☑
        male C50.92- ☑
    noninfiltrating
      breast D05.0- ☑
      specified site NEC — *see* Neoplasm, in situ, by site
      unspecified site D05.0- ☑
    specified site — *see* Neoplasm, malignant, by site
    unspecified site (female) C50.91- ☑
      male C50.92- ☑
  medullary
    with
      amyloid stroma
        specified site — *see* Neoplasm, malignant, by site
        unspecified site C73
      lymphoid stroma
        specified site — *see* Neoplasm, malignant, by site
        unspecified site (female) C50.91- ☑
          male C50.92- ☑
  Merkel cell C4A.9 (*following* C43)
    anal margin C4A.51 (*following* C43)
    anal skin C4A.51 (*following* C43)
    canthus C4A.1- ☑ (*following* C43)
    ear and external auricular canal C4A.2- ☑ (*following* C43)
    external auricular canal C4A.2- ☑ (*following* C43)
    eyelid, including canthus C4A.1- ☑ (*following* C43)
    face C4A.30 (*following* C43)
      specified NEC C4A.39 (*following* C43)
    hip C4A.7- ☑ (*following* C43)
    lip C4A.0 (*following* C43)
    lower limb, including hip C4A.7- ☑ (*following* C43)
    neck C4A.4 (*following* C43)
    nodal presentation C7B.1 (*following* C75)
    nose C4A.31 (*following* C43)
    overlapping sites C4A.8 (*following* C43)
    perianal skin C4A.51 (*following* C43)
    scalp C4A.4 (*following* C43)
    secondary C7B.1 (*following* C75)
    shoulder C4A.6- ☑ (*following* C43)
    skin of breast C4A.52 (*following* C43)
    trunk NEC C4A.59 (*following* C43)
    upper limb, including shoulder C4A.6- ☑ (*following* C43)
    visceral metastatic C7B.1 (*following* C75)
  metastatic — *see* Neoplasm, secondary, by site
  metatypical — *see* Neoplasm, skin, malignant
  morphea, basal cell — *see* Neoplasm, skin, malignant
  mucoid
    cell
      specified site — *see* Neoplasm, malignant, by site
      unspecified site C75.1
  neuroendocrine (*see also* Tumor, neuroendocrine)
    high grade, any site C7A.1 (*following* C75)
    poorly differentiated, any site C7A.1 (*following* C75)
  nonencapsulated sclerosing C73
  noninfiltrating
    intracystic — *see* Neoplasm, in situ, by site
    intraductal
      breast D05.1- ☑

☑ **Additional Character Required — Refer to the Tabular List for Character Selection**   ◤ᴱᴸ **Subterms under main terms may continue to next column or page**

Carcinoma — *continued*
  noninfiltrating — *continued*
    intraductal — *continued*
      papillary
        breast D05.1- ☑
        specified site NEC — *see* Neoplasm, in situ, by site
        unspecified site D05.1- ☑
      specified site — *see* Neoplasm, in situ, by site
      unspecified site D05.1- ☑
      lobular
        breast D05.0- ☑
        specified site NEC — *see* Neoplasm, in situ, by site
        unspecified site (female) D05.0- ☑
  oat cell
    specified site — *see* Neoplasm, malignant, by site
    unspecified site C34.90
  odontogenic C41.1
    upper jaw (bone) C41.0
  papillary
    with follicular (mixed) C73
    follicular variant C73
    intraductal (noninfiltrating)
      with invasion
        specified site — *see* Neoplasm, malignant, by site
        unspecified site (female) C50.91- ☑
          male C50.92- ☑
      breast D05.1- ☑
      specified site NEC — *see* Neoplasm, in situ, by site
      unspecified site D05.1- ☑
    serous
      specified site — *see* Neoplasm, malignant, by site
    surface
      specified site — *see* Neoplasm, malignant, by site
      unspecified site C56.9
    unspecified site C56.9
  papillocystic
    specified site — *see* Neoplasm, malignant, by site
    unspecified site C56.9
  parafollicular cell
    specified site — *see* Neoplasm, malignant, by site
    unspecified site C73
  pilomatrix — *see* Neoplasm, skin, malignant
  pseudomucinous
    specified site — *see* Neoplasm, malignant, by site
    unspecified site C56.9
  renal cell C64- ☑
  Schmincke — *see* Neoplasm, nasopharynx, malignant
  Schneiderian
    specified site — *see* Neoplasm, malignant, by site
    unspecified site C30.0
  sebaceous — *see* Neoplasm, skin, malignant
  secondary (*see also* Neoplasm, secondary, by site)
    Merkel cell C7B.1 (*following* C75)
  secretory, breast — *see* Neoplasm, breast, malignant
  serous
    papillary
      specified site — *see* Neoplasm, malignant, by site
      unspecified site C56.9
    surface, papillary
      specified site — *see* Neoplasm, malignant, by site
      unspecified site C56.9
  Sertoli cell
    specified site — *see* Neoplasm, malignant, by site
    unspecified site C62.90
      female C56.9
      male C62.90
  skin appendage — *see* Neoplasm, skin, malignant
  small cell
    fusiform cell
      specified site — *see* Neoplasm, malignant, by site
      unspecified site C34.90
    intermediate cell
      specified site — *see* Neoplasm, malignant, by site
      unspecified site C34.90
    large cell
      specified site — *see* Neoplasm, malignant, by site

Carcinoma — *continued*
  small cell — *continued*
    large cell — *continued*
      unspecified site C34.90
    solid
      with amyloid stroma
        specified site — *see* Neoplasm, malignant, by site
        unspecified site C73
    microinvasive
      specified site — *see* Neoplasm, malignant, by site
      unspecified site C53.9
  sweat gland — *see* Neoplasm, skin, malignant
  theca cell C56.- ☑
  thymic C37
  unspecified site (primary) C80.1
  water-clear cell C75.0
Carcinoma-in-situ (*see also* Neoplasm, in situ, by site)
  breast NOS D05.9- ☑
    specified type NEC D05.8- ☑
  epidermoid (*see also* Neoplasm, in situ, by site)
    with questionable stromal invasion
      cervix D06.9
      specified site NEC — *see* Neoplasm, in situ, by site
      unspecified site D06.9
    Bowen's type — *see* Neoplasm, skin, in situ
  intraductal
    breast D05.1- ☑
    specified site NEC — *see* Neoplasm, in situ, by site
    unspecified site D05.1- ☑
  lobular
    with
      infiltrating duct
        breast (female) C50.91- ☑
          male C50.92- ☑
        specified site NEC — *see* Neoplasm, malignant
        unspecified site (female) C50.91- ☑
          male C50.92- ☑
      intraductal
        breast D05.8- ☑
        specified site NEC — *see* Neoplasm, in situ, by site
        unspecified site (female) D05.8- ☑
    breast D05.0- ☑
    specified site NEC — *see* Neoplasm, in situ, by site
    unspecified site D05.0- ☑
  squamous cell (*see also* Neoplasm, in situ, by site)
    with questionable stromal invasion
      cervix D06.9
      specified site NEC — *see* Neoplasm, in situ, by site
      unspecified site D06.9
Carcinomaphobia F45.29
Carcinomatosis C80.0
  peritonei C78.6
  unspecified site (primary) (secondary) C80.0
Carcinosarcoma — *see* Neoplasm, malignant, by site
  embryonal — *see* Neoplasm, malignant, by site
Cardia, cardial — *see* condition
Cardiac (*see also* condition)
  death, sudden — *see* Arrest, cardiac
  pacemaker
    in situ Z95.0
    management or adjustment Z45.018
  tamponade I31.4
Cardialgia — *see* Pain, precordial
Cardiectasis — *see* Hypertrophy, cardiac
Cardiochalasia K21.9
Cardiomalacia I51.5
Cardiomegalia glycogenica diffusa E74.02 [I43]
Cardiomegaly (*see also* Hypertrophy, cardiac)
  congenital Q24.8
  glycogen E74.02 [I43]
  idiopathic I51.7
Cardiomyoliposis I51.5
Cardiomyopathy (familial) (idiopathic) I42.9
  alcoholic I42.6
  amyloid E85.4 [I43]
  arteriosclerotic — *see* Disease, heart, ischemic, atherosclerotic
  beriberi E51.12
  cobalt-beer I42.6
  congenital I42.4
  congestive I42.0

Cardiomyopathy — *continued*
  constrictive NOS I42.5
  dilated I42.0
  due to
    alcohol I42.6
    beriberi E51.12
    cardiac glycogenosis E74.02 [I43]
    drugs I42.7
    external agents NEC I42.7
    Friedreich's ataxia G11.1
    myotonia atrophica G71.11 [I43]
    progressive muscular dystrophy G71.0
  glycogen storage E74.02 [I43]
  hypertensive — *see* Hypertension, heart
  hypertrophic (nonobstructive) I42.2
    obstructive I42.1
      congenital Q24.8
  in
    Chagas' disease (chronic) B57.2
      acute B57.0
    sarcoidosis D86.85
  ischemic I25.5
  metabolic E88.9 [I43]
    thyrotoxic E05.90 [I43]
      with thyroid storm E05.91 [I43]
  newborn I42.8
    congenital I42.4
  nutritional E63.9 [I43]
    beriberi E51.12
  obscure of Africa I42.8
  peripartum O90.3
  postpartum O90.3
  restrictive NEC I42.5
  rheumatic I09.0
  secondary I42.9
  stress induced I51.81
  takotsubo I51.81
  thyrotoxic E05.90 [I43]
    with thyroid storm E05.91 [I43]
  toxic NEC I42.7
  tuberculous A18.84
  viral B33.24
Cardionephritis — *see* Hypertension, cardiorenal
Cardionephropathy — *see* Hypertension, cardiorenal
Cardionephrosis — *see* Hypertension, cardiorenal
Cardiopathia nigra I27.0
Cardiopathy (*see also* Disease, heart) I51.9
  idiopathic I42.9
  mucopolysaccharidosis E76.3 [I52]
Cardiopericarditis — *see* Pericarditis
Cardiophobia F45.29
Cardiorenal — *see* condition
Cardiorrhexis — *see* Infarct, myocardium
Cardiosclerosis — *see* Disease, heart, ischemic, atherosclerotic
Cardiosis — *see* Disease, heart
Cardiospasm (esophagus) (reflex) (stomach) K22.0
  congenital Q39.5
    with megaesophagus Q39.5
Cardiostenosis — *see* Disease, heart
Cardiosymphysis I31.0
Cardiovascular — *see* condition
Carditis (acute) (bacterial) (chronic) (subacute) I51.89
  meningococcal A39.50
  rheumatic — *see* Disease, heart, rheumatic
  rheumatoid — *see* Rheumatoid, carditis
  viral B33.20
Care (of) (for) (following)
  child (routine) Z76.2
  family member (handicapped) (sick)
    creating problem for family Z63.6
    provided away from home for holiday relief Z75.5
    unavailable, due to
      absence (person rendering care) (sufferer) Z74.2
      inability (any reason) of person rendering care Z74.2
  foundling Z76.1
  holiday relief Z75.5
  improper — *see* Maltreatment
  lack of (at or after birth) (infant) — *see* Maltreatment, child, neglect
  lactating mother Z39.1
  palliative Z51.5
  postpartum
    immediately after delivery Z39.0
    routine follow-up Z39.2
  respite Z75.5

Care — *continued*
  unavailable, due to
    absence of person rendering care Z74.2
    inability (any reason) of person rendering care
      Z74.2
  well-baby Z76.2
Caries
  bone NEC A18.03
  dental K02.9
    arrested (coronal) (root) K02.3
    chewing surface
      limited to enamel K02.51
      penetrating into dentin K02.52
      penetrating into pulp K02.53
    coronal surface
      chewing surface
        limited to enamel K02.51
        penetrating into dentin K02.52
        penetrating into pulp K02.53
      pit and fissure surface
        limited to enamel K02.51
        penetrating into dentin K02.52
        penetrating into pulp K02.53
      smooth surface
        limited to enamel K02.61
        penetrating into dentin K02.62
        penetrating into pulp K02.63
    pit and fissure surface
      limited to enamel K02.51
      penetrating into dentin K02.52
      penetrating into pulp K02.53
    root K02.7
    smooth surface
      limited to enamel K02.61
      penetrating into dentin K02.62
      penetrating into pulp K02.63
  external meatus — *see* Disorder, ear, external, specified type NEC
  hip (tuberculous) A18.02
  initial (tooth)
    chewing surface K02.51
    pit and fissure surface K02.51
    smooth surface K02.61
  knee (tuberculous) A18.02
  labyrinth H83.8 ☑
  limb NEC (tuberculous) A18.03
  mastoid process (chronic) — *see* Mastoiditis, chronic tuberculous A18.03
  middle ear H74.8 ☑
  nose (tuberculous) A18.03
  orbit (tuberculous) A18.03
  ossicles, ear — *see* Abnormal, ear ossicles
  petrous bone — *see* Petrositis
  root (dental) (tooth) K02.7
  sacrum (tuberculous) A18.01
  spine, spinal (column) (tuberculous) A18.01
  syphilitic A52.77
    congenital (early) A50.02 [M90.80]
  tooth, teeth — *see* Caries, dental
  tuberculous A18.03
  vertebra (column) (tuberculous) A18.01
Carious teeth — *see* Caries, dental
Carneous mole O02.0
Carnitine insufficiency E71.40
Carotid body or sinus syndrome G90.01
Carotidynia G90.01
Carotinemia (dietary) E67.1
Carotinosis (cutis) (skin) E67.1
Carpal tunnel syndrome — *see* Syndrome, carpal tunnel
Carpenter's syndrome Q87.0
Carpopedal spasm — *see* Tetany
Carr-Barr-Plunkett syndrome Q97.1
Carrier (suspected) of
  amebiasis Z22.1
  bacterial disease NEC Z22.39
    diphtheria Z22.2
    intestinal infectious NEC Z22.1
      typhoid Z22.0
    meningococcal Z22.31
    sexually transmitted Z22.4
    specified NEC Z22.39
    staphylococcal (Methicillin susceptible) Z22.321
      Methicillin resistant Z22.322
    streptococcal Z22.338
      group B Z22.330
    typhoid Z22.0
  cholera Z22.1
  diphtheria Z22.2

Carrier of — *continued*
  gastrointestinal pathogens NEC Z22.1
  genetic Z14.8
    cystic fibrosis Z14.1
    hemophilia A (asymptomatic) Z14.01
      symptomatic Z14.02
  gonorrhea Z22.4
  HAA (hepatitis Australian-antigen) Z22.59
  HB (c)(s)-AG Z22.51
  hepatitis (viral) Z22.50
    Australia-antigen (HAA) Z22.59
    B surface antigen (HBsAg) Z22.51
      with acute delta- (super)infection B17.0
    C Z22.52
    specified NEC Z22.59
  human T-cell lymphotropic virus type-1 (HTLV-1) infection Z22.6
  infectious organism Z22.9
    specified NEC Z22.8
  meningococci Z22.31
  Salmonella typhosa Z22.0
  serum hepatitis — *see* Carrier, hepatitis
  staphylococci (Methicillin susceptible) Z22.321
    Methicillin resistant Z22.322
  streptococci Z22.338
    group B Z22.330
  syphilis Z22.4
  typhoid Z22.0
  venereal disease NEC Z22.4
Carrion's disease A44.0
Carter's relapsing fever (Asiatic) A68.1
Cartilage — *see* condition
Caruncle (inflamed)
  conjunctiva (acute) — *see* Conjunctivitis, acute
  labium (majus) (minus) N90.89
  lacrimal — *see* Inflammation, lacrimal, passages
  myrtiform N89.8
  urethral (benign) N36.2
Cascade stomach K31.2
Caseation lymphatic gland (tuberculous) A18.2
Cassidy (-Scholte) syndrome (malignant carcinoid) E34.0
Castellani's disease A69.8
Castration, traumatic, male S38.231 ☑
Casts in urine R82.99
Cat
  cry syndrome Q93.4
  ear Q17.3
  eye syndrome Q92.8
Catabolism, senile R54
Catalepsy (hysterical) F44.2
  schizophrenic F20.2
Cataplexy (idiopathic) — *see* Narcolepsy
Cataract (cortical) (immature) (incipient) H26.9
  with
    neovascularization — *see* Cataract, complicated
  age-related — *see* Cataract, senile
  anterior
    and posterior axial embryonal Q12.0
    pyramidal Q12.0
  associated with
    galactosemia E74.21 [H28]
    myotonic disorders G71.19 [H28]
  blue Q12.0
  central Q12.0
  cerulean Q12.0
  complicated H26.20
    with
      neovascularization H26.21- ☑
      ocular disorder H26.22- ☑
    glaucomatous flecks H26.23- ☑
  congenital Q12.0
  coraliform Q12.0
  coronary Q12.0
  crystalline Q12.0
  diabetic — *see* Diabetes, cataract
  drug-induced H26.3- ☑
  due to
    ocular disorder — *see* Cataract, complicated
    radiation H26.8
  electric H26.8
  extraction status Z98.4- ☑
  glass-blower's H26.8
  heat ray H26.8
  heterochromic — *see* Cataract, complicated
  hypermature — *see* Cataract, senile, morgagnian type
  in (due to)
    chronic iridocyclitis — *see* Cataract, complicated

Cataract — *continued*
  in — *continued*
    diabetes — *see* Diabetes, cataract
    endocrine disease E34.9 [H28]
    eye disease — *see* Cataract, complicated
    hypoparathyroidism E20.9 [H28]
    malnutrition-dehydration E46 [H28]
    metabolic disease E88.9 [H28]
    myotonic disorders G71.19 [H28]
    nutritional disease E63.9 [H28]
  infantile — *see* Cataract, presenile
  irradiational — *see* Cataract, specified NEC
  juvenile — *see* Cataract, presenile
  malnutrition-dehydration E46 [H28]
  morgagnian — *see* Cataract, senile, morgagnian type
  myotonic G71.19 [H28]
  myxedema E03.9 [H28]
  nuclear
    embryonal Q12.0
    sclerosis — *see* Cataract, senile, nuclear
  presenile H26.00- ☑
    combined forms H26.06- ☑
    cortical H26.01- ☑
    lamellar — *see* Cataract, presenile, cortical
    nuclear H26.03- ☑
    specified NEC H26.09
    subcapsular polar (anterior) H26.04- ☑
      posterior H26.05- ☑
    zonular — *see* Cataract, presenile, cortical
  secondary H26.40
    Soemmering's ring H26.41- ☑
    specified NEC H26.49- ☑
    to eye disease — *see* Cataract, complicated
  senile H25.9
    brunescens — *see* Cataract, senile, nuclear
    combined forms H25.81- ☑
    coronary — *see* Cataract, senile, incipient
    cortical H25.01- ☑
    hypermature — *see* Cataract, senile, morgagnian type
    incipient (mature) (total) H25.09- ☑
      cortical — *see* Cataract, senile, cortical
      subcapsular — *see* Cataract, senile, subcapsular
    morgagnian type (hypermature) H25.2- ☑
    nuclear (sclerosis) H25.1- ☑
    polar subcapsular (anterior) (posterior) — *see* Cataract, senile, incipient
    punctate — *see* Cataract, senile, incipient
    specified NEC H25.89
    subcapsular polar (anterior) H25.03- ☑
      posterior H25.04- ☑
  snowflake — *see* Diabetes, cataract
  specified NEC H26.8
  toxic — *see* Cataract, drug-induced
  traumatic H26.10- ☑
    localized H26.11- ☑
    partially resolved H26.12- ☑
    total H26.13- ☑
  zonular (perinuclear) Q12.0
Cataracta (*see also* Cataract)
  brunescens — *see* Cataract, senile, nuclear
  centralis pulverulenta Q12.0
  cerulea Q12.0
  complicata — *see* Cataract, complicated
  congenita Q12.0
  coralliformis Q12.0
  coronaria Q12.0
  diabetic — *see* Diabetes, cataract
  membranacea
    accreta — *see* Cataract, secondary
    congenita Q12.0
  nigra — *see* Cataract, senile, nuclear
  sunflower — *see* Cataract, complicated
Catarrh, catarrhal (acute) (febrile) (infectious) (inflammation) (*see also* condition) J00
  bronchial — *see* Bronchitis
  chest — *see* Bronchitis
  chronic J31.0
  due to congenital syphilis A50.03
  enteric — *see* Enteritis
  eustachian H68.009
  fauces — *see* Pharyngitis
  gastrointestinal — *see* Enteritis
  gingivitis K05.00
    nonplaque induced K05.01
    plaque induced K05.00
  hay — *see* Fever, hay

Catarrh, catarrhal — *continued*
  intestinal — *see* Enteritis
  larynx, chronic J37.0
  liver B15.9
    with hepatic coma B15.0
  lung — *see* Bronchitis
  middle ear, chronic — *see* Otitis, media, nonsuppurative, chronic, serous
  mouth K12.1
  nasal (chronic) — *see* Rhinitis
  nasobronchial J31.1
  nasopharyngeal (chronic) J31.1
    acute J00
  pulmonary — *see* Bronchitis
  spring (eye) (vernal) — *see* Conjunctivitis, acute, atopic
  summer (hay) — *see* Fever, hay
  throat J31.2
  tubotympanal (*see also* Otitis, media, nonsuppurative)
    chronic — *see* Otitis, media, nonsuppurative, chronic, serous
Catatonia (schizophrenic) F20.2
Catatonic
  disorder due to known physiologic condition F06.1
  schizophrenia F20.2
  stupor R40.1
Cat-scratch (*see also* Abrasion)
  disease or fever A28.1
Cauda equina — *see* condition
Cauliflower ear M95.1- ☑
Causalgia (upper limb) G56.4- ☑
  lower limb G57.7- ☑
Cause
  external, general effects T75.89 ☑
Caustic burn — *see* Corrosion, by site
Cavare's disease (familial periodic paralysis) G72.3
Cave-in, injury
  crushing (severe) — *see* Crush
  suffocation — *see* Asphyxia, traumatic, due to low oxygen, due to cave-in
Cavernitis (penis) N48.29
Cavernositis N48.29
Cavernous — *see* condition
Cavitation of lung (*see also* Tuberculosis, pulmonary)
  nontuberculous J98.4
Cavities, dental — *see* Caries, dental
Cavity
  lung — *see* Cavitation of lung
  optic papilla Q14.2
  pulmonary — *see* Cavitation of lung
Cavovarus foot, congenital Q66.1
Cavus foot (congenital) Q66.7
  acquired — *see* Deformity, limb, foot, specified NEC
Cazenave's disease L10.2
Cecitis K52.9
  with perforation, peritonitis, or rupture K65.8
Cecum — *see* condition
Celiac
  artery compression syndrome I77.4
  disease K90.0
  infantilism K90.0
Cell(s), **cellular** (*see also* condition)
  in urine R82.99
Cellulitis (diffuse) (phlegmonous) (septic) (suppurative) L03.90
  abdominal wall L03.311
  anaerobic A48.0
  ankle — *see* Cellulitis, lower limb
  anus K61.0
  arm — *see* Cellulitis, upper limb
  auricle (ear) — *see* Cellulitis, ear
  axilla L03.11- ☑
  back (any part) L03.312
  broad ligament
    acute N73.0
  buttock L03.317
  cervical (meaning neck) L03.221
  cervix (uteri) — *see* Cervicitis
  cheek (external) L03.211
    internal K12.2
  chest wall L03.313
  chronic L03.90
  clostridial A48.0
  corpus cavernosum N48.22
  digit
    finger — *see* Cellulitis, finger
    toe — *see* Cellulitis, toe

Cellulitis — *continued*
  Douglas' cul-de-sac or pouch
    acute N73.0
  drainage site (following operation) T81.4 ☑
  ear (external) H60.1- ☑
  eosinophilic (granulomatous) L98.3
  erysipelatous — *see* Erysipelas
  external auditory canal — *see* Cellulitis, ear
  eyelid — *see* Abscess, eyelid
  face NEC L03.211
  finger (intrathecal) (periosteal) (subcutaneous) (subcuticular) L03.01- ☑
  foot — *see* Cellulitis, lower limb
  gangrenous — *see* Gangrene
  genital organ NEC
    female (external) N76.4
    male N49.9
      multiple sites N49.8
      specified NEC N49.8
  gluteal (region) L03.317
  gonococcal A54.89
  groin L03.314
  hand — *see* Cellulitis, upper limb
  head NEC L03.811
    face (any part, except ear, eye and nose) L03.211
  heel — *see* Cellulitis, lower limb
  hip — *see* Cellulitis, lower limb
  jaw (region) L03.211
  knee — *see* Cellulitis, lower limb
  labium (majus) (minus) — *see* Vulvitis
  lacrimal passages — *see* Inflammation, lacrimal, passages
  larynx J38.7
  leg — *see* Cellulitis, lower limb
  lip K13.0
  lower limb L03.11- ☑
    toe — *see* Cellulitis, toe
  mouth (floor) K12.2
  multiple sites, so stated L03.90
  nasopharynx J39.1
  navel L03.316
    newborn P38.9
      with mild hemorrhage P38.1
      without hemorrhage P38.9
  neck (region) L03.221
  nose (septum) (external) J34.0
  orbit, orbital H05.01- ☑
  palate (soft) K12.2
  pectoral (region) L03.313
  pelvis, pelvic (chronic)
    female (*see also* Disease, pelvis, inflammatory) N73.2
      acute N73.0
    following ectopic or molar pregnancy O08.0
    male K65.0
  penis N48.22
  perineal, perineum L03.315
  perirectal K61.1
  peritonsillar J36
  periurethral N34.0
  periuterine (*see also* Disease, pelvis, inflammatory) N73.2
    acute N73.0
  pharynx J39.1
  rectum K61.1
  retroperitoneal K68.9
  round ligament
    acute N73.0
  scalp (any part) L03.811
  scrotum N49.2
  seminal vesicle N49.0
  shoulder — *see* Cellulitis, upper limb
  specified site NEC L03.818
  submandibular (region) (space) (triangle) K12.2
    gland K11.3
  submaxillary (region) K12.2
    gland K11.3
  thigh — *see* Cellulitis, lower limb
  thumb (intrathecal) (periosteal) (subcutaneous) (subcuticular) — *see* Cellulitis, finger
  toe (intrathecal) (periosteal) (subcutaneous) (subcuticular) L03.03- ☑
  tonsil J36
  trunk L03.319
    abdominal wall L03.311
    back (any part) L03.312
    buttock L03.317
    chest wall L03.313

Cellulitis — *continued*
  trunk — *continued*
    groin L03.314
    perineal, perineum L03.315
    umbilicus L03.316
  tuberculous (primary) A18.4
  umbilicus L03.316
  upper limb L03.11- ☑
    axilla — *see* Cellulitis, axilla
    finger — *see* Cellulitis, finger
    thumb — *see* Cellulitis, finger
  vaccinal T88.0 ☑
  vocal cord J38.3
  vulva — *see* Vulvitis
  wrist — *see* Cellulitis, upper limb
Cementoblastoma, benign — *see* Cyst, calcifying odontogenic
Cementoma — *see* Cyst, calcifying odontogenic
Cementoperiostitis — *see* Periodontitis
Cementosis K03.4
Central auditory processing disorder H93.25
Central pain syndrome G89.0
Cephalematocele, cephal (o)hematocele
  newborn P52.8
    birth injury P10.8
  traumatic — *see* Hematoma, brain
Cephalematoma, cephalhematoma (calcified)
  newborn (birth injury) P12.0
  traumatic — *see* Hematoma, brain
Cephalgia, cephalalgia (*see also* Headache)
  histamine G44.009
    intractable G44.001
    not intractable G44.009
  trigeminal autonomic (TAC) NEC G44.099
    intractable G44.091
    not intractable G44.099
Cephalic — *see* condition
Cephalitis — *see* Encephalitis
Cephalocele — *see* Encephalocele
Cephalomenia N94.89
Cephalopelvic — *see* condition
Cerclage (with cervical incompetence) in pregnancy — *see* Incompetence, cervix, in pregnancy
Cerebellitis — *see* Encephalitis
Cerebellum, cerebellar — *see* condition
Cerebral — *see* condition
Cerebritis — *see* Encephalitis
Cerebro-hepato-renal syndrome Q87.89
Cerebromalacia — *see* Softening, brain
  sequelae of cerebrovascular disease I69.398
Cerebroside lipidosis E75.22
Cerebrospasticity (congenital) G80.1
Cerebrospinal — *see* condition
Cerebrum — *see* condition
Ceroid-lipofuscinosis, neuronal E75.4
Cerumen (accumulation) (impacted) H61.2- ☑
Cervical (*see also* condition)
  auricle Q18.2
  dysplasia in pregnancy — *see* Abnormal, cervix, in pregnancy or childbirth
  erosion in pregnancy — *see* Abnormal, cervix, in pregnancy or childbirth
  fibrosis in pregnancy — *see* Abnormal, cervix, in pregnancy or childbirth
  fusion syndrome Q76.1
  rib Q76.5
  shortening (complicating pregnancy) O26.87- ☑
Cervicalgia M54.2
Cervicitis (acute) (chronic) (nonvenereal) (senile (atrophic)) (subacute) (with ulceration) N72
  with
    abortion — *see* Abortion, by type complicated by genital tract and pelvic infection
    ectopic pregnancy O08.0
    molar pregnancy O08.0
  chlamydial A56.09
  gonococcal A54.03
  herpesviral A60.03
  puerperal (postpartum) O86.11
  syphilitic A52.76
  trichomonal A59.09
  tuberculous A18.16
Cervicocolpitis (emphysematosa) (*see also* Cervicitis) N72
Cervix — *see* condition
Cesarean delivery, previous, affecting management of pregnancy O34.21

Céstan (-Chenais) paralysis or syndrome G46.3
Céstan-Raymond syndrome I65.8
Cestode infestation B71.9
　specified type NEC B71.8
Cestodiasis B71.9
Chabert's disease A22.9
Chacaleh E53.8
Chafing L30.4
Chagas' (-Mazza) disease (chronic) B57.2
　with
　　cardiovascular involvement NEC B57.2
　　digestive system involvement B57.30
　　　megacolon B57.32
　　　megaesophagus B57.31
　　　other specified B57.39
　　megacolon B57.32
　　megaesophagus B57.31
　　myocarditis B57.2
　　nervous system involvement B57.40
　　　meningitis B57.41
　　　meningoencephalitis B57.42
　　　other specified B57.49
　　specified organ involvement NEC B57.5
　acute (with) B57.1
　　cardiovascular NEC B57.0
　　myocarditis B57.0
Chagres fever B50.9
Chairridden Z74.09
Chalasia (cardiac sphincter) K21.9
Chalazion H00.19
　left H00.16
　　lower H00.15
　　upper H00.14
　right H00.13
　　lower H00.12
　　upper H00.11
Chalcosis (see also Disorder, globe, degenerative, chalcosis)
　cornea — see Deposit, cornea
　crystalline lens — see Cataract, complicated
　retina H35.89
Chalicosis (pulmonum) J62.8
Chancre (any genital site) (hard) (hunterian) (mixed) (primary) (seronegative) (seropositive) (syphilitic) A51.0
　congenital A50.07
　conjunctiva NEC A51.2
　Ducrey's A57
　extragenital A51.2
　eyelid A51.2
　lip A51.2
　nipple A51.2
　Nisbet's A57
　of
　　carate A67.0
　　pinta A67.0
　　yaws A66.0
　palate, soft A51.2
　phagedenic A57
　simple A57
　soft A57
　　bubo A57
　　palate A51.2
　urethra A51.0
　yaws A66.0
Chancroid (anus) (genital) (penis) (perineum) (rectum) (urethra) (vulva) A57
Chandler's disease (osteochondritis dissecans, hip) — see Osteochondritis, dissecans, hip
Change(s) (in) (of) (see also Removal)
　arteriosclerotic — see Arteriosclerosis
　bone (see also Disorder, bone)
　　diabetic — see Diabetes, bone change
　bowel habit R19.4
　cardiorenal (vascular) — see Hypertension, cardiorenal
　cardiovascular — see Disease, cardiovascular
　circulatory I99.9
　cognitive (mild) (organic) R41.89
　color, tooth, teeth
　　during formation K00.8
　　posteruptive K03.7
　contraceptive device Z30.433
　corneal membrane H18.30
　　Bowman's membrane fold or rupture H18.31- ☑
　　Descemet's membrane
　　　fold H18.32- ☑
　　　rupture H18.33- ☑
　coronary — see Disease, heart, ischemic

Change(s) — continued
　degenerative, spine or vertebra — see Spondylosis
　dental pulp, regressive K04.2
　dressing (nonsurgical) Z48.00
　　surgical Z48.01
　heart — see Disease, heart
　hip joint — see Derangement, joint, hip
　hyperplastic larynx J38.7
　hypertrophic
　　nasal sinus J34.89
　　turbinate, nasal J34.3
　　upper respiratory tract J39.8
　indwelling catheter Z46.6
　inflammatory (see also Inflammation)
　　sacroiliac M46.1
　job, anxiety concerning Z56.1
　joint — see Derangement, joint
　life — see Menopause
　mental status R41.82
　minimal (glomerular) (see also N00–N07 with fourth character .0) N05.0
　myocardium, myocardial — see Degeneration, myocardial
　of life — see Menopause
　pacemaker Z45.018
　　pulse generator Z45.010
　personality (enduring) F68.8
　　due to (secondary to)
　　　general medical condition F07.0
　　secondary (nonspecific) F60.89
　regressive, dental pulp K04.2
　renal — see Disease, renal
　retina H35.9
　　myopic I I44.2- ☑
　sacroiliac joint M53.3
　senile (see also condition) R54
　sensory R20.8
　skin R23.9
　　acute, due to ultraviolet radiation L56.9
　　　specified NEC L56.8
　　chronic, due to nonionizing radiation L57.9
　　　specified NEC L57.8
　　cyanosis R23.0
　　flushing R23.2
　　pallor R23.1
　　petechiae R23.3
　　specified change NEC R23.8
　　swelling — see Mass, localized
　　texture R23.4
　trophic
　　arm — see Mononeuropathy, upper limb
　　leg — see Mononeuropathy, lower limb
　vascular I99.9
　vasomotor I73.9
　voice R49.9
　　psychogenic F44.4
　　specified NEC R49.8
Changing sleep-work schedule, affecting sleep G47.26
Changuinola fever A93.1
Chapping skin T69.8 ☑
Charcot-Marie-Tooth disease, paralysis or syndrome G60.0
Charcot's
　arthropathy — see Arthropathy, neuropathic
　cirrhosis K74.3
　disease (tabetic arthropathy) A52.16
　joint (disease) (tabetic) A52.16
　　diabetic — see Diabetes, with, arthropathy
　　syringomyelic G95.0
　syndrome (intermittent claudication) I73.9
CHARGE association Q89.8
Charley-horse (quadriceps) M62.831
　traumatic (quadriceps) S76.11- ☑
Charlouis' disease — see Yaws
Cheadle's disease E54
Checking (of)
　cardiac pacemaker (battery) (electrode(s)) Z45.018
　　pulse generator Z45.010
　intrauterine contraceptive device Z30.431
Check-up — see Examination
Chédiak-Higashi (-Steinbrinck) **syndrome** (congenital gigantism of peroxidase granules) E70.330
Cheek — see condition
Cheese itch B88.0
Cheese-washer's lung J67.8
Cheese-worker's lung J67.8

Cheilitis (acute) (angular) (catarrhal) (chronic) (exfoliative) (gangrenous) (glandular) (infectional) (suppurative) (ulcerative) (vesicular) K13.0
　actinic (due to sun) L56.8
　　other than from sun L59.8
　candidal B37.83
Cheilodynia K13.0
Cheiloschisis — see Cleft, lip
Cheilosis (angular) K13.0
　with pellagra E52
　due to
　　vitamin B2 (riboflavin) deficiency E53.0
Cheiromegaly M79.89
Cheiropompholyx L30.1
Cheloid — see Keloid
Chemical burn — see Corrosion, by site
Chemodectoma — see Paraganglioma, nonchromaffin
Chemosis, conjunctiva — see Edema, conjunctiva
Chemotherapy (session) (for)
　cancer Z51.11
　neoplasm Z51.11
Cherubism M27.8
Chest — see condition
Cheyne-Stokes breathing (respiration) R06.3
Chiari's
　disease or syndrome (hepatic vein thrombosis) I82.0
　malformation
　　type I G93.5
　　type II — see Spina bifida
　net Q24.8
Chicago disease B40.9
Chickenpox — see Varicella
Chiclero ulcer or sore B55.1
Chigger (infestation) B88.0
Chignon (disease) B36.8
　newborn (from vacuum extraction) (birth injury) P12.1
Chilaiditi's syndrome (subphrenic displacement, colon) Q43.3
Chilblain(s) (lupus) T69.1 ☑
Child
　custody dispute Z65.3
Childbirth — see Delivery
Childhood
　cerebral X-linked adrenoleukodystrophy E71.520
　period of rapid growth Z00.2
Chill(s) R68.83
　with fever R50.9
　without fever R68.83
　congestive in malarial regions B54
Chilomastigiasis A07.8
Chimera 46,XX/46,XY Q99.0
Chin — see condition
Chinese dysentery A03.9
Chionophobia F40.228
Chitral fever A93.1
Chlamydia, chlamydial A74.9
　cervicitis A56.09
　conjunctivitis A74.0
　cystitis A56.01
　endometritis A56.11
　epididymitis A56.19
　female
　　pelvic inflammatory disease A56.11
　　pelviperitonitis A56.11
　orchitis A56.19
　peritonitis A74.81
　pharyngitis A56.4
　proctitis A56.3
　psittaci (infection) A70
　salpingitis A56.11
　sexually-transmitted infection NEC A56.8
　specified NEC A74.89
　urethritis A56.01
　vulvovaginitis A56.02
Chlamydiosis — see Chlamydia
Chloasma (skin) (idiopathic) (symptomatic) L81.1
　eyelid H02.719
　　hyperthyroid E05.90 [H02.719]
　　　with thyroid storm E05.91 [H02.719]
　　left H02.716
　　　lower H02.715
　　　upper H02.714
　　right H02.713
　　　lower H02.712
　　　upper H02.711
Chloroma C92.3- ☑

☑ Additional Character Required — Refer to the Tabular List for Character Selection　　　▽ Subterms under main terms may continue to next column or page

Chlorosis D50.9
  Egyptian B76.9 [D63.8]
  miner's B76.9 [D63.8]
Chlorotic anemia D50.8
Chocolate cyst (ovary) N80.1
Choked
  disc or disk — *see* Papilledema
  on food, phlegm, or vomitus NOS — *see* Foreign body, by site
  while vomiting NOS — *see* Foreign body, by site
Chokes (resulting from bends) T70.3 ☑
Choking sensation R09.89
Cholangiectasis K83.8
Cholangiocarcinoma
  with hepatocellular carcinoma, combined C22.0
  liver C22.1
  specified site NEC — *see* Neoplasm, malignant, by site
  unspecified site C22.1
Cholangiohepatitis K83.8
  due to fluke infestation B66.1
Cholangiohepatoma C22.0
Cholangiolitis (acute) (chronic) (extrahepatic) (gangrenous) (intrahepatic) K83.0
  paratyphoidal — *see* Fever, paratyphoid
  typhoidal A01.09
Cholangioma D13.4
  malignant — *see* Cholangiocarcinoma
Cholangitis (ascending) (primary) (recurrent) (sclerosing) (secondary) (stenosing) (suppurative) K83.0
  with calculus, bile duct — *see* Calculus, bile duct, with cholangitis
  chronic nonsuppurative destructive K74.3
Cholecystectasia K82.8
Cholecystitis K81.9
  with
    calculus, stones in
      bile duct (common) (hepatic) — *see* Calculus, bile duct, with cholecystitis
      cystic duct — *see* Calculus, gallbladder, with cholecystitis
      gallbladder — *see* Calculus, gallbladder, with cholecystitis
      choledocholithiasis — *see* Calculus, bile duct, with cholecystitis
      cholelithiasis — *see* Calculus, gallbladder, with cholecystitis
  acute (emphysematous) (gangrenous) (suppurative) K81.0
    with
      calculus, stones in
        cystic duct — *see* Calculus, gallbladder, with cholecystitis, acute
        gallbladder — *see* Calculus, gallbladder, with cholecystitis, acute
        choledocholithiasis — *see* Calculus, bile duct, with cholecystitis, acute
        cholelithiasis — *see* Calculus, gallbladder, with cholecystitis, acute
      chronic cholecystitis K81.2
        with gallbladder calculus K80.12
          with obstruction K80.13
  chronic K81.1
    with acute cholecystitis K81.2
      with gallbladder calculus K80.12
        with obstruction K80.13
  emphysematous (acute) — *see* Cholecystitis, acute
  gangrenous — *see* Cholecystitis, acute
  paratyphoidal, current A01.4
  suppurative — *see* Cholecystitis, acute
  typhoidal A01.09
Cholecystolithiasis — *see* Calculus, gallbladder
Choledochitis (suppurative) K83.0
Choledocholith — *see* Calculus, bile duct
Choledocholithiasis (common duct) (hepatic duct) — *see* Calculus, bile duct
  cystic — *see* Calculus, gallbladder
  typhoidal A01.09
Cholelithiasis (cystic duct) (gallbladder) (impacted) (multiple) — *see* Calculus, gallbladder
  bile duct (common) (hepatic) — *see* Calculus, bile duct
  hepatic duct — *see* Calculus, bile duct
  specified NEC K80.80
    with obstruction K80.81
Cholemia (*see also* Jaundice)
  familial (simple) (congenital) E80.4
  Gilbert's E80.4
Choleperitoneum, choleperitonitis K65.3

Cholera (Asiatic) (epidemic) (malignant) A00.9
  antimonial — *see* Poisoning, antimony
  classical A00.0
  due to Vibrio cholerae 01 A00.9
    biovar cholerae A00.0
    biovar eltor A00.1
    el tor A00.1
  el tor A00.1
Cholerine — *see* Cholera
Cholestasis NEC K83.1
  with hepatocyte injury K71.0
  due to total parenteral nutrition (TPN) K76.89
  pure K71.0
Cholesteatoma (ear) (middle) (with reaction) H71.9-☑
  attic H71.0-☑
  external ear (canal) H60.4-☑
  mastoid H71.2-☑
  postmastoidectomy cavity (recurrent) — *see* Complications, postmastoidectomy, recurrent cholesteatoma
  recurrent (postmastoidectomy) — *see* Complications, postmastoidectomy, recurrent cholesteatoma
  tympanum H71.1-☑
Cholesteatosis, diffuse H71.3-☑
Cholesteremia E78.0
Cholesterin in vitreous — *see* Deposit, crystalline
Cholesterol
  deposit
    retina H35.89
    vitreous — *see* Deposit, crystalline
  elevated (high) E78.0
    with elevated (high) triglycerides E78.2
    screening for Z13.220
  imbibition of gallbladder K82.4
Cholesterolemia (essential) (familial) (hereditary) (pure) E78.0
Cholesterolosis, cholesterosis (gallbladder) K82.4
  cerebrotendinous E75.5
Cholocolic fistula K82.3
Choluria R82.2
Chondritis M94.8X9
  aurical H61.03-☑
  costal (Tietze's) M94.0
  external ear H61.03-☑
  patella, posttraumatic — *see* Chondromalacia, patella
  pinna H61.03-☑
  purulent M94.8X-☑
  tuberculous NEC A18.02
    intervertebral A18.01
Chondroblastoma (*see also* Neoplasm, bone, benign)
  malignant — *see* Neoplasm, bone, malignant
Chondrocalcinosis M11.20
  ankle M11.27-☑
  elbow M11.22-☑
  familial M11.10
    ankle M11.17-☑
    elbow M11.12-☑
    foot joint M11.17-☑
    hand joint M11.14-☑
    hip M11.15-☑
    knee M11.16-☑
    multiple site M11.19
    shoulder M11.11-☑
    vertebrae M11.18
    wrist M11.13-☑
  foot joint M11.27-☑
  hand joint M11.24-☑
  hip M11.25-☑
  knee M11.26-☑
  multiple site M11.29
  shoulder M11.21-☑
  specified type NEC M11.20
    ankle M11.27-☑
    elbow M11.22-☑
    foot joint M11.27-☑
    hand joint M11.24-☑
    hip M11.25-☑
    knee M11.26-☑
    multiple site M11.29
    shoulder M11.21-☑
    vertebrae M11.28
    wrist M11.23-☑
  vertebrae M11.28
  wrist M11.23-☑
Chondrodermatitis nodularis helicis or anthelicis — *see* Perichondritis, ear

Chondrodysplasia Q78.9
  with hemangioma Q78.4
  calcificans congenita Q77.3
  fetalis Q77.4
  metaphyseal (Jansen's) (McKusick's) (Schmid's) Q78.5
  punctata Q77.3
Chondrodystrophy, chondrodystrophia (familial) (fetalis) (hypoplastic) Q78.9
  calcificans congenita Q77.3
  myotonic (congenital) G71.13
  punctata Q77.3
Chondroectodermal dysplasia Q77.6
Chondrogenesis imperfecta Q77.4
Chondrolysis M94.35-☑
Chondroma (*see also* Neoplasm, cartilage, benign)
  juxtacortical — *see* Neoplasm, bone, benign
  periosteal — *see* Neoplasm, bone, benign
Chondromalacia (systemic) M94.20
  acromioclavicular joint M94.21-☑
  ankle M94.27-☑
  elbow M94.22-☑
  foot joint M94.27-☑
  glenohumeral joint M94.21-☑
  hand joint M94.24-☑
  hip M94.25-☑
  knee M94.26-☑
    patella M22.4-☑
  multiple sites M94.29
  patella M22.4-☑
  rib M94.28
  sacroiliac joint M94.259
  shoulder M94.21-☑
  sternoclavicular joint M94.21-☑
  vertebral joint M94.28
  wrist M94.23-☑
Chondromatosis (*see also* Neoplasm, cartilage, uncertain behavior)
  internal M94.8X9
Chondromyxosarcoma — *see* Neoplasm, cartilage, malignant
Chondro-osteodysplasia (Morquio-Brailsford type) E76.219
Chondro-osteodystrophy E76.29
Chondro-osteoma — *see* Neoplasm, bone, benign
Chondropathia tuberosa M94.0
Chondrosarcoma — *see* Neoplasm, cartilage, malignant
  juxtacortical — *see* Neoplasm, bone, malignant
  mesenchymal — *see* Neoplasm, connective tissue, malignant
  myxoid — *see* Neoplasm, cartilage, malignant
Chordee (nonvenereal) N48.89
  congenital Q54.4
  gonococcal A54.09
Chorditis (fibrinous) (nodosa) (tuberosa) J38.2
Chordoma — *see* Neoplasm, vertebral (column), malignant
Chorea (chronic) (gravis) (posthemiplegic) (senile) (spasmodic) G25.5
  with
    heart involvement I02.0
      active or acute (conditions in I01-) I02.0
        rheumatic I02.9
          with valvular disorder I02.0
      rheumatic heart disease (chronic) (inactive)(quiescent) — *code to* rheumatic heart condition involved
  drug-induced G25.4
  habit F95.8
  hereditary G10
  Huntington's G10
  hysterical F44.4
  minor I02.9
    with heart involvement I02.0
  progressive G25.5
    hereditary G10
  rheumatic (chronic) I02.9
    with heart involvement I02.0
  Sydenham's I02.9
    with heart involvement — *see* Chorea, with rheumatic heart disease
  nonrheumatic G25.5
Choreoathetosis (paroxysmal) G25.5
Chorioadenoma (destruens) D39.2
Chorioamnionitis O41.12-☑
Chorioangioma D26.7

Index

Choriocarcinoma — Claudicatio venosa intermittens

Choriocarcinoma — see Neoplasm, malignant, by site
  combined with
    embryonal carcinoma — see Neoplasm, malignant,
      by site
    other germ cell elements — see Neoplasm, malig-
      nant, by site
    teratoma — see Neoplasm, malignant, by site
  specified site — see Neoplasm, malignant, by site
  unspecified site
    female C58
    male C62.90
Chorioencephalitis (acute) (lymphocytic) (serous) A87.2
Chorioepithelioma — see Choriocarcinoma
Choriomeningitis (acute) (lymphocytic) (serous) A87.2
Chorionepithelioma — see Choriocarcinoma
Chorioretinitis (see also Inflammation, chorioretinal)
  disseminated (see also Inflammation, chorioretinal,
    disseminated)
    in neurosyphilis A52.19
  Egyptian B76.9 [D63.8]
  focal (see also Inflammation, chorioretinal, focal)
  histoplasmic B39.9 [H32]
  in (due to)
    histoplasmosis B39.9 [H32]
    syphilis (secondary) A51.43
      late A52.71
    toxoplasmosis (acquired) B58.01
      congenital (active) P37.1 [H32]
    tuberculosis A18.53
  juxtapapillary, juxtapapillaris — see Inflammation,
    chorioretinal, focal, juxtapapillary
  leprous A30.9 [H32]
  miner's B76.9 [D63.8]
  progressive myopia (degeneration) H44.2- ☑
  syphilitic (secondary) A51.43
    congenital (early) A50.01 [H32]
      late A50.32
    late A52.71
  tuberculous A18.53
Chorioretinopathy, central serous H35.71- ☑
Choroid — see condition
Choroideremia H31.21
Choroiditis — see Chorioretinitis
Choroidopathy — see Disorder, choroid
Choroidoretinitis — see Chorioretinitis
Choroidoretinopathy, central serous — see Chori-
  oretinopathy, central serous
Christian-Weber disease M35.6
Christmas disease D67
Chromaffinoma (see also Neoplasm, benign, by site)
  malignant — see Neoplasm, malignant, by site
Chromatopsia — see Deficiency, color vision
Chromhidrosis, chromidrosis L75.1
Chromoblastomycosis — see Chromomycosis
Chromoconversion R82.91
Chromomycosis B43.9
  brain abscess B43.1
  cerebral B43.1
  cutaneous B43.0
  skin B43.0
  specified NEC B43.8
  subcutaneous abscess or cyst B43.2
Chromophytosis B36.0
Chromosome — see Anomaly, by chromosome involved
  D (1) — see Anomaly, chromosome 13
  E (3) — see Anomaly, chromosome 18
  G — see Anomaly, chromosome 21
Chromotrichomycosis B36.8
Chronic — see condition
  fracture — see Fracture, pathological
Churg-Strauss syndrome M30.1
Chyle cyst, mesentery I89.8
Chylocele (nonfilarial) I89.8
  filarial (see also Infestation, filarial) B74.9 [N51]
  tunica vaginalis N50.8
    filarial (see also Infestation, filarial) B74.9 [N51]
Chylomicronemia (fasting) (with hyperprebetalipopro-
  teinemia) E78.3
Chylopericardium I31.3
  acute I30.9
Chylothorax (nonfilarial) I89.8
  filarial (see also Infestation, filarial) B74.9 [J91.8]
Chylous — see condition
Chyluria (nonfilarial) R82.0
  due to
    bilharziasis B65.0

Chyluria — continued
  due to — continued
    Brugia (malayi) B74.1
      timori B74.2
    schistosomiasis (bilharziasis) B65.0
    Wuchereria (bancrofti) B74.0
  filarial — see Infestation, filarial
Cicatricial (deformity) — see Cicatrix
Cicatrix (adherent) (contracted) (painful) (vicious) (see
  also Scar) L90.5
  adenoid (and tonsil) J35.8
  alveolar process M26.79
  anus K62.89
  auricle — see Disorder, pinna, specified type NEC
  bile duct (common) (hepatic) K83.8
  bladder N32.89
  bone — see Disorder, bone, specified type NEC
  brain G93.89
  cervix (postoperative) (postpartal) N88.1
  common duct K83.8
  cornea H17.9
    tuberculous A18.59
  duodenum (bulb), obstructive K31.5
  esophagus K22.2
  eyelid — see Disorder, eyelid function
  hypopharynx J39.2
  lacrimal passages — see Obstruction, lacrimal
  larynx J38.7
  lung J98.4
  middle ear H74.8 ☑
  mouth K13.79
  muscle M62.89
    with contracture — see Contraction, muscle NEC
  nasopharynx J39.2
  palate (soft) K13.79
  penis N48.89
  pharynx J39.2
  prostate N42.89
  rectum K62.89
  retina — see Scar, chorioretinal
  semilunar cartilage — see Derangement, meniscus
  seminal vesicle N50.8
  skin L90.5
    infected L08.89
    postinfective L90.5
    tuberculous B90.8
  specified site NEC L90.5
  throat J39.2
  tongue K14.8
  tonsil (and adenoid) J35.8
  trachea J39.8
  tuberculous NEC B90.9
  urethra N36.8
  uterus N85.8
  vagina N89.8
    postoperative N99.2
  vocal cord J38.3
  wrist, constricting (annular) L90.5
CIDP (chronic inflammatory demyelinating polyneuropathy) G61.81
CIN — see Neoplasia, intraepithelial, cervix
Cinchonism — see Deafness, ototoxic
  correct substance properly administered — see Table
    of Drugs and Chemicals, by drug, adverse effect
  overdose or wrong substance given or taken — see
    Table of Drugs and Chemicals, by drug, poison-
    ing
Circle of Willis — see condition
Circular — see condition
Circulating anticoagulants (see also Disorder, hemorrhagic) D68.318
  due to drugs (see also Disorder, hemorrhagic) D68.32
  following childbirth O72.3
Circulation
  collateral, any site I99.8
  defective (lower extremity) I99.8
    congenital Q28.9
  embryonic Q28.9
  failure (peripheral) R57.9
    newborn P29.89
  fetal, persistent P29.3
  heart, incomplete Q28.9
Circulatory system — see condition
Circulus senilis (cornea) — see Degeneration, cornea,
  senile
Circumcision (in absence of medical indication) (ritual)
  (routine) Z41.2
Circumscribed — see condition

Circumvallate placenta O43.11- ☑
Cirrhosis, cirrhotic (hepatic) (liver) K74.60
  alcoholic K70.30
    with ascites K70.31
  atrophic — see Cirrhosis, liver
  Baumgarten-Cruveilhier K74.69
  biliary (cholangiolitic) (cholangitic) (hypertrophic)
    (obstructive) (pericholangiolitic) K74.5
    due to
      Clonorchiasis B66.1
      flukes B66.3
    primary K74.3
    secondary K74.4
  cardiac (of liver) K76.1
  Charcot's K74.3
  cholangiolitic, cholangitic, cholostatic (primary) K74.3
  congestive K76.1
  Cruveilhier-Baumgarten K74.69
  cryptogenic (liver) K74.69
  due to
    hepatolenticular degeneration E83.01
    Wilson's disease E83.01
    xanthomatosis E78.2
  fatty K76.0
    alcoholic K70.0
  Hanot's (hypertrophic) K74.3
  hepatic — see Cirrhosis, liver
  hypertrophic K74.3
  Indian childhood K74.69
  kidney — see Sclerosis, renal
  Laennec's K70.30
    with ascites K70.31
    alcoholic K70.30
      with ascites K70.31
    nonalcoholic K74.69
  liver K74.60
    alcoholic K70.30
      with ascites K70.31
      fatty K70.0
    congenital P78.81
    syphilitic A52.74
  lung (chronic) J84.10
  macronodular K74.69
    alcoholic K70.30
      with ascites K70.31
  micronodular K74.69
    alcoholic K70.30
      with ascites K70.31
  mixed type K74.69
  monolobular K74.3
  nephritis — see Sclerosis, renal
  nutritional K74.69
    alcoholic K70.30
      with ascites K70.31
  obstructive — see Cirrhosis, biliary
  ovarian N83.8
  pancreas (duct) K86.8
  pigmentary E83.110
  portal K74.69
    alcoholic K70.30
      with ascites K70.31
  postnecrotic K74.69
    alcoholic K70.30
      with ascites K70.31
  pulmonary J84.10
  renal — see Sclerosis, renal
  spleen D73.2
  stasis K76.1
  Todd's K74.3
  unilobar K74.3
  xanthomatous (biliary) K74.5
    due to xanthomatosis (familial) (metabolic) (prima-
      ry) E78.2
Cistern, subarachnoid R93.0
Citrullinemia E72.23
Citrullinuria E72.23
Civatte's disease or poikiloderma L57.3
Clam digger's itch B65.3
Clammy skin R23.1
Clap — see Gonorrhea
Clarke-Hadfield syndrome (pancreatic infantilism)
  K86.8
Clark's paralysis G80.9
Clastothrix L67.8
Claude Bernard-Horner syndrome G90.2
  traumatic — see Injury, nerve, cervical sympathetic
Claude's disease or syndrome G46.3
Claudicatio venosa intermittens I87.8

Claudication, intermittent I73.9
  cerebral (artery) G45.9
  spinal cord (arteriosclerotic) G95.19
    syphilitic A52.09
  venous (axillary) I87.8
Claustrophobia F40.240
Clavus (infected) L84
Clawfoot (congenital) Q66.89
  acquired — *see* Deformity, limb, clawfoot
Clawhand (acquired) (*see also* Deformity, limb, clawhand)
  congenital Q68.1
Clawtoe (congenital) Q66.89
  acquired — *see* Deformity, toe, specified NEC
Clay eating — *see* Pica
Cleansing of artificial opening — *see* Attention to, artificial, opening
Cleft (congenital) (*see also* Imperfect, closure)
  alveolar process M26.79
  branchial (cyst) (persistent) Q18.2
  cricoid cartilage, posterior Q31.8
  lip (unilateral) Q36.9
    with cleft palate Q37.9
      hard Q37.1
        with soft Q37.5
      soft Q37.3
        with hard Q37.5
      bilateral Q36.0
        with cleft palate Q37.8
          hard Q37.0
            with soft Q37.4
          soft Q37.2
            with hard Q37.4
    median Q36.1
  nose Q30.2
  palate Q35.9
    with cleft lip (unilateral) Q37.9
      bilateral Q37.8
    hard Q35.1
      with
        cleft lip (unilateral) Q37.1
          bilateral Q37.0
        soft Q35.5
          with cleft lip (unilateral) Q37.5
            bilateral Q37.4
    medial Q35.5
    soft Q35.3
      with
        cleft lip (unilateral) Q37.3
          bilateral Q37.2
        hard Q35.5
          with cleft lip (unilateral) Q37.5
            bilateral Q37.4
  penis Q55.69
  scrotum Q55.29
  thyroid cartilage Q31.8
  uvula Q35.7
Cleidocranial dysostosis Q74.0
Cleptomania F63.2
Clicking hip (newborn) R29.4
Climacteric (female) (*see also* Menopause)
  arthritis (any site) NEC — *see* Arthritis, specified form NEC
  depression (single episode) F32.8
  male (symptoms) (syndrome) NEC N50.8
  paranoid state F22
  polyarthritis NEC — *see* Arthritis, specified form NEC
  symptoms (female) N95.1
Clinical research investigation (clinical trial) (control subject) (normal comparison) (participant) Z00.6
Clitoris — *see* condition
Cloaca (persistent) Q43.7
Clonorchiasis, clonorchis infection (liver) B66.1
Clonus R25.8
Closed bite M26.29
Clostridium (C.) **perfringens, as cause of disease classified elsewhere** B96.7
Closure
  congenital, nose Q30.0
  cranial sutures, premature Q75.0
  defective or imperfect NEC — *see* Imperfect, closure
  fistula, delayed — *see* Fistula
  foramen ovale, imperfect Q21.1
  hymen N89.6
  interauricular septum, defective Q21.1
  interventricular septum, defective Q21.0
  lacrimal duct (*see also* Stenosis, lacrimal, duct)
    congenital Q10.5

Closure — *continued*
  nose (congenital) Q30.0
    acquired M95.0
  of artificial opening — *see* Attention to, artificial, opening
  vagina N89.5
  valve — *see* Endocarditis
  vulva N90.5
Clot (blood) (*see also* Embolism)
  artery (obstruction) (occlusion) — *see* Embolism
  bladder N32.89
  brain (intradural or extradural) — *see* Occlusion, artery, cerebral
  circulation I74.9
  heart (*see also* Infarct, myocardium)
    not resulting in infarction I24.0
  vein — *see* Thrombosis
Clouded state R40.1
  epileptic — *see* Epilepsy, specified NEC
  paroxysmal — *see* Epilepsy, specified NEC
Cloudy antrum, antra J32.0
Clouston's (hidrotic) **ectodermal dysplasia** Q82.4
Clubbed nail pachydermoperiostosis M89.40 [L62]
Clubbing of finger(s) (nails) R68.3
Clubfinger R68.3
  congenital Q68.1
Clubfoot (congenital) Q66.89
  acquired — *see* Deformity, limb, clubfoot
  equinovarus Q66.0
  paralytic — *see* Deformity, limb, clubfoot
Clubhand (congenital) (radial) Q71.4- ☑
  acquired — *see* Deformity, limb, clubhand
Clubnail R68.3
  congenital Q84.6
Clump, kidney Q63.1
Clumsiness, clumsy child syndrome F82
Cluttering F80.81
Clutton's joints A50.51 [M12.80]
Coagulation, intravascular (diffuse) (disseminated) (*see also* Defibrination syndrome)
  complicating abortion — *see* Abortion, by type, complicated by, intravascular coagulation
  following ectopic or molar pregnancy O08.1
Coagulopathy (*see also* Defect, coagulation)
  consumption D65
  intravascular D65
    newborn P60
Coalition
  calcaneo-scaphoid Q66.89
  tarsal Q66.89
Coalminer's
  elbow — *see* Bursitis, elbow, olecranon
  lung or pneumoconiosis J60
Coalworker's lung or pneumoconiosis J60
Coarctation
  aorta (preductal) (postductal) Q25.1
  pulmonary artery Q25.71
Coated tongue K14.3
Coats' disease (exudative retinopathy) — *see* Retinopathy, exudative
Cocainism — *see* Dependence, drug, cocaine
Coccidioidomycosis B38.9
  cutaneous B38.3
  disseminated B38.7
  generalized B38.7
  meninges B38.4
  prostate B38.81
  pulmonary B38.2
    acute B38.0
    chronic B38.1
  skin B38.3
  specified NEC B38.89
Coccidioidosis — *see* Coccidioidomycosis
Coccidiosis (intestinal) A07.3
Coccydynia, coccygodynia M53.3
Coccyx — *see* condition
Cochin-China diarrhea K90.1
Cockayne's syndrome Q87.1
Cocked up toe — *see* Deformity, toe, specified NEC
Cock's peculiar tumor L72.3
Codman's tumor — *see* Neoplasm, bone, benign
Coenurosis B71.8
Coffee-worker's lung J67.8
Cogan's syndrome H16.32- ☑
  oculomotor apraxia H51.8
Coitus, painful (female) N94.1
  male N53.12

Coitus, painful — *continued*
  psychogenic F52.6
Cold J00
  with influenza, flu, or grippe — *see* Influenza, with, respiratory manifestations NEC
  agglutinin disease or hemoglobinuria (chronic) D59.1
  bronchial — *see* Bronchitis
  chest — *see* Bronchitis
  common (head) J00
  effects of T69.9 ☑
    specified effect NEC T69.8 ☑
  excessive, effects of T69.9 ☑
    specified effect NEC T69.8 ☑
  exhaustion from T69.8 ☑
  exposure to T69.9 ☑
    specified effect NEC T69.8 ☑
  head J00
  injury syndrome (newborn) P80.0
  on lung — *see* Bronchitis
  rose J30.1
  sensitivity, auto-immune D59.1
  virus J00
Coldsore B00.1
Colibacillosis A49.8
  as the cause of other disease (*see also* Escherichia coli) B96.20
  generalized A41.50
Colic (bilious) (infantile) (intestinal) (recurrent) (spasmodic) R10.83
  abdomen R10.83
    psychogenic F45.8
  appendix, appendicular K38.8
  bile duct — *see* Calculus, bile duct
  biliary — *see* Calculus, bile duct
  common duct — *see* Calculus, bile duct
  cystic duct — *see* Calculus, gallbladder
  Devonshire NEC — *see* Poisoning, lead
  gallbladder — *see* Calculus, gallbladder
  gallstone — *see* Calculus, gallbladder
    gallbladder or cystic duct — *see* Calculus, gallbladder
  hepatic (duct) — *see* Calculus, bile duct
  hysterical F45.8
  kidney N23
  lead NEC — *see* Poisoning, lead
  mucous K58.9
    with diarrhea K58.0
    psychogenic F54
  nephritic N23
  painter's NEC — *see* Poisoning, lead
  pancreas K86.8
  psychogenic F45.8
  renal N23
  saturnine NEC — *see* Poisoning, lead
  ureter N23
  urethral N36.8
    due to calculus N21.1
  uterus NEC N94.89
    menstrual — *see* Dysmenorrhea
  worm NOS B83.9
Colicystitis — *see* Cystitis
Colitis (acute) (catarrhal) (chronic) (noninfective) (hemorrhagic) (*see also* Enteritis) K52.9
  allergic K52.2
  amebic (acute) (*see also* Amebiasis) A06.0
    nondysenteric A06.2
  anthrax A22.2
  bacillary — *see* Infection, Shigella
  balantidial A07.0
  Clostridium difficile A04.7
  coccidial A07.3
  collagenous K52.89
  cystica superficialis K52.89
  dietary counseling and surveillance (for) Z71.3
  dietetic K52.2
  drug-induced K52.1
  due to radiation K52.0
  eosinophilic K52.82
  food hypersensitivity K52.2
  giardial A07.1
  granulomatous — *see* Enteritis, regional, large intestine
  infectious — *see* Enteritis, infectious
  ischemic K55.9
    acute (fulminant) (subacute) K55.0
    chronic K55.1
    due to mesenteric artery insufficiency K55.1

Colitis — *continued*
 ischemic — *continued*
  fulminant (acute) K55.0
 left sided K51.50
  with
   abscess K51.514
   complication K51.519
    specified NEC K51.518
   fistula K51.513
   obstruction K51.512
   rectal bleeding K51.511
 lymphocytic K52.89
 membranous
  psychogenic F54
 microscopic (collagenous) (lymphocytic) K52.89
 mucous — *see* Syndrome, irritable, bowel
  psychogenic F54
 noninfective K52.9
  specified NEC K52.89
 polyposa — *see* Polyp, colon, inflammatory
 protozoal A07.9
 pseudomembranous A04.7
 pseudomucinous — *see* Syndrome, irritable, bowel
 regional — *see* Enteritis, regional, large intestine
 segmental — *see* Enteritis, regional, large intestine
 septic — *see* Enteritis, infectious
 spastic K58.9
  with diarrhea K58.0
  psychogenic F54
 staphylococcal A04.8
  foodborne A05.0
 subacute ischemic K55.0
 thromboulcerative K55.0
 toxic NEC K52.1
  due to Clostridium difficile A04.7
 transmural — *see* Enteritis, regional, large intestine
 trichomonal A07.8
 tuberculous (ulcerative) A18.32
 ulcerative (chronic) K51.90
  with
   complication K51.919
    abscess K51.914
    fistula K51.913
    obstruction K51.912
    rectal bleeding K51.911
    specified complication NEC K51.918
  enterocolitis — *see* Enterocolitis, ulcerative
  ileocolitis — *see* Ileocolitis, ulcerative
  mucosal proctocolitis — *see* Proctocolitis, mucosal
  proctitis — *see* Proctitis, ulcerative
  pseudopolyposis — *see* Polyp, colon, inflammatory
  psychogenic F54
  rectosigmoiditis — *see* Rectosigmoiditis, ulcerative
  specified type NEC K51.80
   with
    complication K51.819
     abscess K51.814
     fistula K51.813
     obstruction K51.812
     rectal bleeding K51.811
     specified complication NEC K51.818

Collagenosis, collagen disease (nonvascular) (vascular) M35.9
 cardiovascular I42.8
 reactive perforating L87.1
 specified NEC M35.8
Collapse R55
 adrenal E27.2
 cardiorespiratory R57.0
 cardiovascular R57.0
  newborn P29.89
 circulatory (peripheral) R57.9
  during or after labor and delivery O75.1
  following ectopic or molar pregnancy O08.3
  newborn P29.89
 during or
  after labor and delivery O75.1
  resulting from a procedure, not elsewhere classified T81.10 ☑
 external ear canal — *see* Stenosis, external ear canal
 general R55
 heart — *see* Disease, heart
 heat T67.1 ☑
 hysterical F44.89
 labyrinth, membranous (congenital) Q16.5

Collapse — *continued*
 lung (*see also* Atelectasis) J98.19
  pressure due to anesthesia (general) (local) or other sedation T88.2 ☑
   during labor and delivery O74.1
   in pregnancy O29.02- ☑
   postpartum, puerperal O89.09
 myocardial — *see* Disease, heart
 nervous F48.8
 neurocirculatory F45.8
 nose M95.0
 postoperative T81.10 ☑
 pulmonary (*see also* Atelectasis) J98.19
  newborn — *see* Atelectasis
 trachea J39.8
 tracheobronchial J98.09
 valvular — *see* Endocarditis
 vascular (peripheral) R57.9
  during or after labor and delivery O75.1
  following ectopic or molar pregnancy O08.3
  newborn P29.89
 vertebra M48.50- ☑
  cervical region M48.52- ☑
  cervicothoracic region M48.53- ☑
  in (due to)
   metastasis — *see* Collapse, vertebra, in, specified disease NEC
   osteoporosis (*see also* Osteoporosis) M80.88 ☑
    cervical region M80.88 ☑
    cervicothoracic region M80.88 ☑
    lumbar region M80.88 ☑
    lumbosacral region M80.88 ☑
    multiple sites M80.88 ☑
    occipito-atlanto-axial region M80.88 ☑
    sacrococcygeal region M80.88 ☑
    thoracic region M80.88 ☑
    thoracolumbar region M80.88 ☑
   specified disease NEC M48.50- ☑
    cervical region M48.52- ☑
    cervicothoracic region M48.53- ☑
    lumbar region M48.56- ☑
    lumbosacral region M48.57- ☑
    occipito-atlanto-axial region M48.51- ☑
    sacrococcygeal region M48.58- ☑
    thoracic region M48.54- ☑
    thoracolumbar region M48.55- ☑
  lumbar region M48.56- ☑
  lumbosacral region M48.57- ☑
  occipito-atlanto-axial region M48.51- ☑
  sacrococcygeal region M48.58- ☑
  thoracic region M48.54- ☑
  thoracolumbar region M48.55- ☑
Collateral (*see also* condition)
 circulation (venous) I87.8
 dilation, veins I87.8
Colles' fracture S52.53- ☑
Collet (-Sicard) syndrome G52.7
Collier's asthma or lung J60
Collodion baby Q80.2
Colloid nodule (of thyroid) (cystic) E04.1
Coloboma (iris) Q13.0
 eyelid Q10.3
 fundus Q14.8
 lens Q12.2
 optic disc (congenital) Q14.2
  acquired H47.31- ☑
Coloenteritis — *see* Enteritis
Colon — *see* condition
Colonization
 MRSA (Methicillin resistant Staphylococcus aureus) Z22.322
 MSSA (Methicillin susceptible Staphylococcus aureus) Z22.321
 status — *see* Carrier (suspected) of
Coloptosis K63.4
Color blindness — *see* Deficiency, color vision
Colostomy
 attention to Z43.3
 fitting or adjustment Z46.89
 malfunctioning K94.03
 status Z93.3
Colpitis (acute) — *see* Vaginitis
Colpocele N81.5
Colpocystitis — *see* Vaginitis
Colpospasm N94.2
Column, spinal, vertebral — *see* condition

Coma R40.20
 with
  motor response (none) R40.231 ☑
   abnormal R40.233 ☑
   extension R40.232 ☑
   flexion withdrawal R40.234 ☑
   localizes pain R40.235 ☑
   obeys commands R40.236 ☑
  opening of eyes (never) R40.211 ☑
   in response to
    pain R40.212 ☑
    sound R40.213 ☑
   spontaneous R40.214 ☑
  verbal response (none) R40.221 ☑
   confused conversation R40.224 ☑
   inappropriate words R40.223 ☑
   incomprehensible words R40.222 ☑
   oriented R40.225 ☑
 eclamptic — *see* Eclampsia
 epileptic — *see* Epilepsy
 Glasgow, scale score — *see* Glasgow coma scale
 hepatic — *see* Failure, hepatic, by type, with coma
 hyperglycemic (diabetic) — *see* Diabetes, coma
 hyperosmolar (diabetic) — *see* Diabetes, coma
 hypoglycemic (diabetic) — *see* Diabetes, coma, hypoglycemic
  nondiabetic E15
 in diabetes — *see* Diabetes, coma
 insulin-induced — *see* Coma, hypoglycemic
 myxedematous E03.5
 newborn P91.5
 persistent vegetative state R40.3
 specified NEC, without documented Glasgow coma scale score, or with partial Glasgow coma scale score reported R40.244
Comatose — *see* Coma
Combat fatigue F43.0
Combined — *see* condition
Comedo, comedones (giant) L70.0
Comedocarcinoma (*see also* Neoplasm, breast, malignant)
 noninfiltrating
  breast D05.8- ☑
  specified site — *see* Neoplasm, in situ, by site
  unspecified site D05.8- ☑
Comedomastitis — *see* Ectasia, mammary duct
Comminuted fracture — *code as* Fracture, closed
Common
 arterial trunk Q20.0
 atrioventricular canal Q21.2
 atrium Q21.1
 cold (head) J00
 truncus (arteriosus) Q20.0
 variable immunodeficiency — *see* Immunodeficiency, common variable
 ventricle Q20.4
Commotio, commotion (current)
 brain — *see* Injury, intracranial, concussion
 cerebri — *see* Injury, intracranial, concussion
 retinae S05.8X- ☑
 spinal cord — *see* Injury, spinal cord, by region
 spinalis — *see* Injury, spinal cord, by region
Communication
 between
  base of aorta and pulmonary artery Q21.4
  left ventricle and right atrium Q20.5
  pericardial sac and pleural sac Q34.8
  pulmonary artery and pulmonary vein, congenital Q25.72
 congenital between uterus and digestive or urinary tract Q51.7
Compartment syndrome (deep) (posterior) (traumatic) T79.A0 ☑ (*following* T79.7)
 abdomen T79.A3 ☑ (*following* T79.7)
 lower extremity (hip, buttock, thigh, leg, foot, toes) T79.A2 ☑ (*following* T79.7)
 nontraumatic
  abdomen M79.A3 (*following* M79.7)
  lower extremity (hip, buttock, thigh, leg, foot, toes) M79.A2- ☑ (*following* M79.7)
  specified site NEC M79.A9 (*following* M79.7)
  upper extremity (shoulder, arm, forearm, wrist, hand, fingers) M79.A1- ☑ (*following* M79.7)
 specified site NEC T79.A9 ☑ (*following* T79.7)
 upper extremity (shoulder, arm, forearm, wrist, hand, fingers) T79.A1- ☑ (*following* T79.7)

Compensation
  failure — *see* Disease, heart
  neurosis, psychoneurosis — *see* Disorder, factitious
Complaint (*see also* Disease)
  bowel, functional K59.9
    psychogenic F45.8
  intestine, functional K59.9
    psychogenic F45.8
  kidney — *see* Disease, renal
  miners' J60
Complete — *see* condition
Complex
  Addison-Schilder E71.528
  cardiorenal — *see* Hypertension, cardiorenal
  Costen's M26.69
  disseminated mycobacterium avium- intracellulare (DMAC) A31.2
  Eisenmenger's (ventricular septal defect) I27.89
  hypersexual F52.8
  jumped process, spine — *see* Dislocation, vertebra
  primary, tuberculous A15.7
  Schilder-Addison E71.528
  subluxation (vertebral) M99.19
    abdomen M99.19
    acromioclavicular M99.17
    cervical region M99.11
    cervicothoracic M99.11
    costochondral M99.18
    costovertebral M99.18
    head region M99.10
    hip M99.15
    lower extremity M99.16
    lumbar region M99.13
    lumbosacral M99.13
    occipitocervical M99.10
    pelvic region M99.15
    pubic M99.15
    rib cage M99.18
    sacral region M99.14
    sacrococcygeal M99.14
    sacroiliac M99.14
    specified NEC M99.19
    sternochondral M99.18
    sternoclavicular M99.17
    thoracic region M99.12
    thoracolumbar M99.12
    upper extremity M99.17
  Taussig-Bing (transposition, aorta and overriding pulmonary artery) Q20.1
Complication(s) (from) (of)
  accidental puncture or laceration during a procedure (of) — *see* Complications, intraoperative (intraprocedural), puncture or laceration
  amputation stump (surgical) (late) NEC T87.9
    dehiscence T87.81
    infection or inflammation T87.40
      lower limb T87.4- ☑
      upper limb T87.4- ☑
    necrosis T87.50
      lower limb T87.5- ☑
      upper limb T87.5- ☑
    neuroma T87.30
      lower limb T87.3- ☑
      upper limb T87.3- ☑
    specified type NEC T87.89
  anastomosis (and bypass) (*see also* Complications, prosthetic device or implant)
    intestinal (internal) NEC K91.89
      involving urinary tract N99.89
    urinary tract (involving intestinal tract) N99.89
    vascular — *see* Complications, cardiovascular device or implant
  anesthesia, anesthetic (*see also* Anesthesia, complication) T88.59 ☑
    brain, postpartum, puerperal O89.2
    cardiac
      in
        labor and delivery O74.2
        pregnancy O29.19- ☑
      postpartum, puerperal O89.1
    central nervous system
      in
        labor and delivery O74.3
        pregnancy O29.29- ☑
      postpartum, puerperal O89.2
    difficult or failed intubation T88.4 ☑
      in pregnancy O29.6- ☑

Complication(s) — *continued*
  anesthesia, anesthetic (*see also* Anesthesia, complication) — *continued*
    failed sedation (conscious) (moderate) during procedure T88.52 ☑
    hyperthermia, malignant T88.3 ☑
    hypothermia T88.51 ☑
    intubation failure T88.4 ☑
    malignant hyperthermia T88.3 ☑
    pulmonary
      in
        labor and delivery O74.1
        pregnancy NEC O29.09- ☑
      postpartum, puerperal O89.09
    shock T88.2 ☑
    spinal and epidural
      in
        labor and delivery NEC O74.6
          headache O74.5
        pregnancy NEC O29.5X- ☑
      postpartum, puerperal NEC O89.5
        headache O89.4
  anti-reflux device — *see* Complications, esophageal anti-reflux device
  aortic (bifurcation) graft — *see* Complications, graft, vascular
  aortocoronary (bypass) graft — *see* Complications, coronary artery (bypass) graft
  aortofemoral (bypass) graft — *see* Complications, extremity artery (bypass) graft
  arteriovenous
    fistula, surgically created T82.9 ☑
      embolism T82.818 ☑
      fibrosis T82.828 ☑
      hemorrhage T82.838 ☑
      infection or inflammation T82.7 ☑
      mechanical
        breakdown T82.510 ☑
        displacement T82.520 ☑
        leakage T82.530 ☑
        malposition T82.520 ☑
        obstruction T82.590 ☑
        perforation T82.590 ☑
        protrusion T82.590 ☑
      pain T82.848 ☑
      specified type NEC T82.898 ☑
      stenosis T82.858 ☑
      thrombosis T82.868 ☑
    shunt, surgically created T82.9 ☑
      embolism T82.818 ☑
      fibrosis T82.828 ☑
      hemorrhage T82.838 ☑
      infection or inflammation T82.7 ☑
      mechanical
        breakdown T82.511 ☑
        displacement T82.521 ☑
        leakage T82.531 ☑
        malposition T82.521 ☑
        obstruction T82.591 ☑
        perforation T82.591 ☑
        protrusion T82.591 ☑
      pain T82.848 ☑
      specified type NEC T82.898 ☑
      stenosis T82.858 ☑
      thrombosis T82.868 ☑
  arthroplasty — *see* Complications, joint prosthesis
  artificial
    fertilization or insemination N98.9
      attempted introduction (of)
        embryo in embryo transfer N98.3
        ovum following in vitro fertilization N98.2
      hyperstimulation of ovaries N98.1
      infection N98.0
      specified NEC N98.8
    heart T82.9 ☑
      embolism T82.817 ☑
      fibrosis T82.827 ☑
      hemorrhage T82.837 ☑
      infection or inflammation T82.7 ☑
      mechanical
        breakdown T82.512 ☑
        displacement T82.522 ☑
        leakage T82.532 ☑
        malposition T82.522 ☑
        obstruction T82.592 ☑
        perforation T82.592 ☑

Complication(s) — *continued*
  artificial — *continued*
    heart — *continued*
      mechanical — *continued*
        protrusion T82.592 ☑
      pain T82.847 ☑
      specified type NEC T82.897 ☑
      stenosis T82.857 ☑
      thrombosis T82.867 ☑
    opening
      cecostomy — *see* Complications, colostomy
      colostomy — *see* Complications, colostomy
      cystostomy — *see* Complications, cystostomy
      enterostomy — *see* Complications, enterostomy
      gastrostomy — *see* Complications, gastrostomy
      ileostomy — *see* Complications, enterostomy
      jejunostomy — *see* Complications, enterostomy
      nephrostomy — *see* Complications, stoma, urinary tract
      tracheostomy — *see* Complications, tracheostomy
      ureterostomy — *see* Complications, stoma, urinary tract
      urethrostomy — *see* Complications, stoma, urinary tract
  balloon implant or device
    gastrointestinal T85.9 ☑
      embolism T85.81 ☑
      fibrosis T85.82 ☑
      hemorrhage T85.83 ☑
      infection and inflammation T85.79 ☑
      pain T85.84 ☑
      specified type NEC T85.89 ☑
      stenosis T85.85 ☑
      thrombosis T85.86 ☑
    vascular (counterpulsation) T82.9 ☑
      embolism T82.818 ☑
      fibrosis T82.828 ☑
      hemorrhage T82.838 ☑
      infection or inflammation T82.7 ☑
      mechanical
        breakdown T82.513 ☑
        displacement T82.523 ☑
        leakage T82.533 ☑
        malposition T82.523 ☑
        obstruction T82.593 ☑
        perforation T82.593 ☑
        protrusion T82.593 ☑
      pain T82.848 ☑
      specified type NEC T82.898 ☑
      stenosis T82.858 ☑
      thrombosis T82.868 ☑
  bariatric procedure
    gastric band procedure K95.09
      infection K95.01
    specified procedure NEC K95.89
      infection K95.81
  bile duct implant (prosthetic) T85.9 ☑
    embolism T85.81 ☑
    fibrosis T85.82 ☑
    hemorrhage T85.83 ☑
    infection and inflammation T85.79 ☑
    mechanical
      breakdown T85.510 ☑
      displacement T85.520 ☑
      malfunction T85.510 ☑
      malposition T85.520 ☑
      obstruction T85.590 ☑
      perforation T85.590 ☑
      protrusion T85.590 ☑
      specified NEC T85.590 ☑
    pain T85.84 ☑
    specified type NEC T85.89 ☑
    stenosis T85.85 ☑
    thrombosis T85.86 ☑
  bladder device (auxiliary) — *see* Complications, genitourinary, device or implant, urinary system
  bleeding (postoperative) — *see* Complication, postoperative, hemorrhage
    intraoperative — *see* Complication, intraoperative, hemorrhage
  blood vessel graft — *see* Complications, graft, vascular
  bone
    device NEC T84.9 ☑
      embolism T84.81 ☑

☂ Subterms under main terms may continue to next column or page

Complication(s) — *continued*
- bone — *continued*
  - device — *continued*
    - fibrosis T84.82 ☑
    - hemorrhage T84.83 ☑
    - infection or inflammation T84.7 ☑
    - mechanical
      - breakdown T84.318 ☑
      - displacement T84.328 ☑
      - malposition T84.328 ☑
      - obstruction T84.398 ☑
      - perforation T84.398 ☑
      - protrusion T84.398 ☑
    - pain T84.84 ☑
    - specified type NEC T84.89 ☑
    - stenosis T84.85 ☑
    - thrombosis T84.86 ☑
  - graft — *see* Complications, graft, bone
  - growth stimulator (electrode) — *see* Complications, electronic stimulator device, bone
  - marrow transplant — *see* Complications, transplant, bone, marrow
- brain neurostimulator (electrode) — *see* Complications, electronic stimulator device, brain
- breast implant (prosthetic) T85.9 ☑
  - capsular contracture T85.44 ☑
  - embolism T85.81 ☑
  - fibrosis T85.82 ☑
  - hemorrhage T85.83 ☑
  - infection and inflammation T85.79 ☑
  - mechanical
    - breakdown T85.41 ☑
    - displacement T85.42 ☑
    - leakage T85.43 ☑
    - malposition T85.42 ☑
    - obstruction T85.49 ☑
    - perforation T85.49 ☑
    - protrusion T85.49 ☑
    - specified NEC T85.49 ☑
  - pain T85.84 ☑
  - specified type NEC T85.89 ☑
  - stenosis T85.85 ☑
  - thrombosis T85.86 ☑
- bypass (*see also* Complications, prosthetic device or implant)
  - aortocoronary — *see* Complications, coronary artery (bypass) graft
  - arterial (*see also* Complications, graft, vascular)
    - extremity — *see* Complications, extremity artery (bypass) graft
- cardiac (*see also* Disease, heart)
  - device, implant or graft T82.9 ☑
    - embolism T82.817 ☑
    - fibrosis T82.827 ☑
    - hemorrhage T82.837 ☑
    - infection or inflammation T82.7 ☑
      - valve prosthesis T82.6 ☑
    - mechanical
      - breakdown T82.519 ☑
        - specified device NEC T82.518 ☑
      - displacement T82.529 ☑
        - specified device NEC T82.528 ☑
      - leakage T82.539 ☑
        - specified device NEC T82.538 ☑
      - malposition T82.529 ☑
        - specified device NEC T82.528 ☑
      - obstruction T82.599 ☑
        - specified device NEC T82.598 ☑
      - perforation T82.599 ☑
        - specified device NEC T82.598 ☑
      - protrusion T82.599 ☑
        - specified device NEC T82.598 ☑
    - pain T82.847 ☑
    - specified type NEC T82.897 ☑
    - stenosis T82.857 ☑
    - thrombosis T82.867 ☑
- cardiovascular device, graft or implant T82.9 ☑
  - aortic graft — *see* Complications, graft, vascular
  - arteriovenous
    - fistula, artificial — *see* Complication, arteriovenous, fistula, surgically created
    - shunt — *see* Complication, arteriovenous, shunt, surgically created
  - artificial heart — *see* Complication, artificial, heart
  - balloon (counterpulsation) device — *see* Complication, balloon implant, vascular

Complication(s) — *continued*
- cardiovascular device, graft or implant — *continued*
  - carotid artery graft — *see* Complications, graft, vascular
  - coronary bypass graft — *see* Complications, coronary artery (bypass) graft
  - dialysis catheter (vascular) — *see* Complication, catheter, dialysis
  - electronic T82.9 ☑
    - electrode T82.9 ☑
      - embolism T82.817 ☑
      - fibrosis T82.827 ☑
      - hemorrhage T82.837 ☑
      - infection T82.7 ☑
      - mechanical
        - breakdown T82.110 ☑
        - displacement T82.120 ☑
        - leakage T82.190 ☑
        - obstruction T82.190 ☑
        - perforation T82.190 ☑
        - protrusion T82.190 ☑
        - specified type NEC T82.190 ☑
      - pain T82.847 ☑
      - specified NEC T82.897 ☑
      - stenosis T82.857 ☑
      - thrombosis T82.867 ☑
    - embolism T82.817 ☑
    - fibrosis T82.827 ☑
    - hemorrhage T82.837 ☑
    - infection T82.7 ☑
    - mechanical
      - breakdown T82.119 ☑
      - displacement T82.129 ☑
      - leakage T82.199 ☑
      - obstruction T82.199 ☑
      - perforation T82.199 ☑
      - protrusion T82.199 ☑
      - specified type NEC T82.199 ☑
    - pain T82.847 ☑
    - pulse generator T82.9 ☑
      - embolism T82.817 ☑
      - fibrosis T82.827 ☑
      - hemorrhage T82.837 ☑
      - infection T82.7 ☑
      - mechanical
        - breakdown T82.111 ☑
        - displacement T82.121 ☑
        - leakage T82.191 ☑
        - obstruction T82.191 ☑
        - perforation T82.191 ☑
        - protrusion T82.191 ☑
        - specified type NEC T82.191 ☑
      - pain T82.847 ☑
      - specified NEC T82.897 ☑
      - stenosis T82.857 ☑
      - thrombosis T82.867 ☑
    - specified condition NEC T82.897 ☑
    - specified device NEC T82.9 ☑
      - embolism T82.817 ☑
      - fibrosis T82.827 ☑
      - hemorrhage T82.837 ☑
      - infection T82.7 ☑
      - mechanical
        - breakdown T82.118 ☑
        - displacement T82.128 ☑
        - leakage T82.198 ☑
        - obstruction T82.198 ☑
        - perforation T82.198 ☑
        - protrusion T82.198 ☑
        - specified type NEC T82.198 ☑
      - pain T82.847 ☑
      - specified NEC T82.897 ☑
      - stenosis T82.857 ☑
      - thrombosis T82.867 ☑
    - stenosis T82.857 ☑
    - thrombosis T82.867 ☑
  - extremity artery graft — *see* Complication, extremity artery (bypass) graft
  - femoral artery graft — *see* Complication, extremity artery (bypass) graft
  - heart
    - transplant — *see* Complication, transplant, heart
    - valve — *see* Complication, prosthetic device, heart valve

Complication(s) — *continued*
- cardiovascular device, graft or implant — *continued*
  - heart — *continued*
    - valve — *see* Complication, prosthetic device, heart valve — *continued*
      - graft — *see* Complication, heart, valve, graft
    - heart-lung transplant — *see* Complication, transplant, heart, with lung
    - infection or inflammation T82.7 ☑
    - umbrella device — *see* Complication, umbrella device, vascular
    - vascular graft (or anastomosis) — *see* Complication, graft, vascular
  - carotid artery (bypass) graft — *see* Complications, graft, vascular
  - catheter (device) NEC (*see also* Complications, prosthetic device or implant)
    - cystostomy T83.9 ☑
      - embolism T83.81 ☑
      - fibrosis T83.82 ☑
      - hemorrhage T83.83 ☑
      - infection and inflammation T83.59 ☑
      - mechanical
        - breakdown T83.010 ☑
        - displacement T83.020 ☑
        - leakage T83.030 ☑
        - malposition T83.020 ☑
        - obstruction T83.090 ☑
        - perforation T83.090 ☑
        - protrusion T83.090 ☑
        - specified NEC T83.090 ☑
      - pain T83.84 ☑
      - specified type NEC T83.89 ☑
      - stenosis T83.85 ☑
      - thrombosis T83.86 ☑
    - dialysis (vascular) T82.9 ☑
      - embolism T82.818 ☑
      - fibrosis T82.828 ☑
      - hemorrhage T82.838 ☑
      - infection and inflammation T82.7 ☑
      - intraperitoneal — *see* Complications, catheter, intraperitoneal
      - mechanical
        - breakdown T82.41 ☑
        - displacement T82.42 ☑
        - leakage T82.43 ☑
        - malposition T82.42 ☑
        - obstruction T82.49 ☑
        - perforation T82.49 ☑
        - protrusion T82.49 ☑
      - pain T82.848 ☑
      - specified type NEC T82.898 ☑
      - stenosis T82.858 ☑
      - thrombosis T82.868 ☑
    - epidural infusion T85.9 ☑
      - embolism T85.81 ☑
      - fibrosis T85.82 ☑
      - hemorrhage T85.83 ☑
      - infection and inflammation T85.79 ☑
      - mechanical
        - breakdown T85.610 ☑
        - displacement T85.620 ☑
        - leakage T85.630 ☑
        - malfunction T85.610 ☑
        - malposition T85.620 ☑
        - obstruction T85.690 ☑
        - perforation T85.690 ☑
        - protrusion T85.690 ☑
        - specified NEC T85.690 ☑
      - pain T85.84 ☑
      - specified type NEC T85.89 ☑
      - stenosis T85.85 ☑
      - thrombosis T85.86 ☑
    - intraperitoneal dialysis T85.9 ☑
      - embolism T85.81 ☑
      - fibrosis T85.82 ☑
      - hemorrhage T85.83 ☑
      - infection and inflammation T85.71 ☑
      - mechanical
        - breakdown T85.611 ☑
        - displacement T85.621 ☑
        - leakage T85.631 ☑
        - malfunction T85.611 ☑
        - malposition T85.621 ☑
        - obstruction T85.691 ☑

☑ Additional Character Required — Refer to the Tabular List for Character Selection   ▽ Subterms under main terms may continue to next column or page

Complication(s) — *continued*
catheter (*see also* Complications, prosthetic device or implant) — *continued*
  intraperitoneal dialysis — *continued*
    mechanical — *continued*
      perforation T85.691 ☑
      protrusion T85.691 ☑
      specified NEC T85.691 ☑
    pain T85.84 ☑
    specified type NEC T85.89 ☑
    stenosis T85.85 ☑
    thrombosis T85.86 ☑
  intravenous infusion T82.9 ☑
    embolism T82.818 ☑
    fibrosis T82.828 ☑
    hemorrhage T82.838 ☑
    infection or inflammation T82.7 ☑
    mechanical
      breakdown T82.514 ☑
      displacement T82.524 ☑
      leakage T82.534 ☑
      malposition T82.524 ☑
      obstruction T82.594 ☑
      perforation T82.594 ☑
      protrusion T82.594 ☑
    pain T82.848 ☑
    specified type NEC T82.898 ☑
    stenosis T82.858 ☑
    thrombosis T82.868 ☑
  subdural infusion T85.9 ☑
    embolism T85.81 ☑
    fibrosis T85.82 ☑
    hemorrhage T85.83 ☑
    infection and inflammation T85.79 ☑
    mechanical
      breakdown T85.610 ☑
      displacement T85.620 ☑
      leakage T85.630 ☑
      malfunction T85.610 ☑
      malposition T85.620 ☑
      obstruction T85.690 ☑
      perforation T85.690 ☑
      protrusion T85.690 ☑
      specified NEC T85.690 ☑
    pain T85.84 ☑
    specified type NEC T85.89 ☑
    stenosis T85.85 ☑
    thrombosis T85.86 ☑
  urethral, indwelling T83.9 ☑
    displacement T83.028 ☑
    embolism T83.81 ☑
    fibrosis T83.82 ☑
    hemorrhage T83.83 ☑
    infection and inflammation T83.51 ☑
    leakage T83.038 ☑
    malposition T83.028 ☑
    mechanical
      breakdown T83.018 ☑
    obstruction (mechanical) T83.098 ☑
    pain T83.84 ☑
    perforation T83.098 ☑
    protrusion T83.098 ☑
    specified type NEC T83.098 ☑
    stenosis T83.85 ☑
    thrombosis T83.86 ☑
  urinary (indwelling) — *see* Complications, catheter, urethral, indwelling
cecostomy (stoma) — *see* Complications, colostomy
cesarean delivery wound NEC O90.89
  disruption O90.0
  hematoma O90.2
  infection (following delivery) O86.0
chemotherapy (antineoplastic) NEC T88.7 ☑
chin implant (prosthetic) — *see* Complication, prosthetic device or implant, specified NEC
circulatory system I99.8
  intraoperative I97.88
  postprocedural I97.89
    following cardiac surgery I97.19- ☑
      postcardiotomy syndrome I97.0
    hypertension I97.3
    lymphedema after mastectomy I97.2
    postcardiotomy syndrome I97.0
    specified NEC I97.89
colostomy (stoma) K94.00
  hemorrhage K94.01

Complication(s) — *continued*
colostomy — *continued*
  infection K94.02
  malfunction K94.03
  mechanical K94.03
  specified complication NEC K94.09
contraceptive device, intrauterine — *see* Complications, intrauterine, contraceptive device
cord (umbilical) — *see* Complications, umbilical cord
corneal graft — *see* Complications, graft, cornea
coronary artery (bypass) graft T82.9
  atherosclerosis — *see* Arteriosclerosis, coronary (artery),
  embolism T82.818 ☑
  fibrosis T82.828 ☑
  hemorrhage T82.838 ☑
  infection and inflammation T82.7 ☑
  mechanical
    breakdown T82.211 ☑
    displacement T82.212 ☑
    leakage T82.213 ☑
    malposition T82.212 ☑
    obstruction T82.218 ☑
    perforation T82.218 ☑
    protrusion T82.218 ☑
    specified NEC T82.218 ☑
  pain T82.848 ☑
  specified type NEC T82.897 ☑
  stenosis T82.858 ☑
  thrombosis T82.868 ☑
counterpulsation device (balloon), intra-aortic — *see* Complications, balloon implant, vascular
cystostomy (stoma) N99.518
  catheter — *see* Complications, catheter, cystostomy
  hemorrhage N99.510
  infection N99.511
  malfunction N99.512
  specified type NEC N99.518
delivery (*see also* Complications, obstetric) O75.9
  procedure (instrumental) (manual) (surgical) O75.4
  specified NEC O75.89
dialysis (peritoneal) (renal) (*see also* Complications, infusion)
  catheter (vascular) — *see* Complication, catheter, dialysis
    peritoneal, intraperitoneal — *see* Complications, catheter, intraperitoneal
dorsal column (spinal) neurostimulator — *see* Complications, electronic stimulator device, spinal cord
drug NEC T88.7 ☑
ear procedure (*see also* Disorder, ear)
  intraoperative H95.88
    hematoma — *see* Complications, intraoperative, hemorrhage (hematoma) (of), ear
    hemorrhage — *see* Complications, intraoperative, hemorrhage (hematoma) (of), ear
    laceration — *see* Complications, intraoperative, puncture or laceration..., ear
    specified NEC H95.88
  postoperative H95.89
    external ear canal stenosis H95.81- ☑
    hematoma — *see* Complications, postprocedural, hemorrhage (hematoma) (of), ear
    hemorrhage — *see* Complications, postprocedural, hemorrhage (hematoma) (of), ear
    postmastoidectomy — *see* Complications, postmastoidectomy
    specified NEC H95.89
ectopic pregnancy O08.9
  damage to pelvic organs O08.6
  embolism O08.2
  genital infection O08.0
  hemorrhage (delayed) (excessive) O08.1
  metabolic disorder O08.5
  renal failure O08.4
  shock O08.3
  specified type NEC O08.0
  venous complication NEC O08.7
electronic stimulator device
  bladder (urinary) — *see* Complications, electronic stimulator device, urinary
  bone T84.9 ☑
    breakdown T84.310 ☑
    displacement T84.320 ☑
    embolism T84.81 ☑
    fibrosis T84.82 ☑

Complication(s) — *continued*
electronic stimulator device — *continued*
  bone — *continued*
    hemorrhage T84.83 ☑
    infection or inflammation T84.7 ☑
    malfunction T84.310 ☑
    malposition T84.320 ☑
    mechanical NEC T84.390 ☑
    obstruction T84.390 ☑
    pain T84.84 ☑
    perforation T84.390 ☑
    protrusion T84.390 ☑
    specified type NEC T84.89 ☑
    stenosis T84.85 ☑
    thrombosis T84.86 ☑
  brain T85.9 ☑
    embolism T85.81 ☑
    fibrosis T85.82 ☑
    hemorrhage T85.83 ☑
    infection and inflammation T85.79 ☑
    mechanical
      breakdown T85.110 ☑
      displacement T85.120 ☑
      leakage T85.190 ☑
      malposition T85.120 ☑
      obstruction T85.190 ☑
      perforation T85.190 ☑
      protrusion T85.190 ☑
      specified NEC T85.190 ☑
    pain T85.84 ☑
    specified type NEC T85.89 ☑
    stenosis T85.85 ☑
    thrombosis T85.86 ☑
  cardiac (defibrillator) (pacemaker) — *see* Complications, cardiovascular device or implant, electronic
  muscle T84.9 ☑
    breakdown T84.418 ☑
    displacement T84.428 ☑
    embolism T84.81 ☑
    fibrosis T84.82 ☑
    hemorrhage T84.83 ☑
    infection or inflammation T84.7 ☑
    mechanical NEC T84.498 ☑
    pain T84.84 ☑
    specified type NEC T84.89 ☑
    stenosis T84.85 ☑
    thrombosis T84.86 ☑
  nervous system T85.9 ☑
    brain — *see* Complications, electronic stimulator device, brain
    embolism T85.81 ☑
    fibrosis T85.82 ☑
    hemorrhage T85.83 ☑
    infection and inflammation T85.79 ☑
    mechanical
      breakdown T85.118 ☑
      displacement T85.128 ☑
      leakage T85.199 ☑
      malposition T85.128 ☑
      obstruction T85.199 ☑
      perforation T85.199 ☑
      protrusion T85.199 ☑
      specified NEC T85.199 ☑
    pain T85.84 ☑
    peripheral nerve — *see* Complications, electronic stimulator device, peripheral nerve
    specified type NEC T85.89 ☑
    spinal cord — *see* Complications, electronic stimulator device, spinal cord
    stenosis T85.85 ☑
    thrombosis T85.86 ☑
  peripheral nerve T85.9 ☑
    embolism T85.81 ☑
    fibrosis T85.82 ☑
    hemorrhage T85.83 ☑
    infection and inflammation T85.79 ☑
    mechanical
      breakdown T85.111 ☑
      displacement T85.121 ☑
      leakage T85.191 ☑
      malposition T85.121 ☑
      obstruction T85.191 ☑
      perforation T85.191 ☑
      protrusion T85.191 ☑
      specified NEC T85.191 ☑

Complication(s) — *continued*
electronic stimulator device — *continued*
  peripheral nerve — *continued*
    pain T85.84 ☑
    specified type NEC T85.89 ☑
    stenosis T85.85 ☑
    thrombosis T85.86 ☑
  spinal cord T85.9 ☑
    embolism T85.81 ☑
    fibrosis T85.82 ☑
    hemorrhage T85.83 ☑
    infection and inflammation T85.79 ☑
    mechanical
      breakdown T85.112 ☑
      displacement T85.122 ☑
      leakage T85.192 ☑
      malposition T85.122 ☑
      obstruction T85.192 ☑
      perforation T85.192 ☑
      protrusion T85.192 ☑
      specified NEC T85.192 ☑
    pain T85.84 ☑
    specified type NEC T85.89 ☑
    stenosis T85.85 ☑
    thrombosis T85.86 ☑
  urinary T83.9 ☑
    embolism T83.81 ☑
    fibrosis T83.82 ☑
    hemorrhage T83.83 ☑
    infection and inflammation T83.59 ☑
    mechanical
      breakdown T83.110 ☑
      displacement T83.120 ☑
      malposition T83.120 ☑
      perforation T83.190 ☑
      protrusion T83.190 ☑
      specified NEC T83.190 ☑
    pain T83.84 ☑
    specified type NEC T83.89 ☑
    stenosis T83.85 ☑
    thrombosis T83.86 ☑
electroshock therapy T88.9 ☑
  specified NEC T88.8 ☑
endocrine E34.9
  postprocedural
    adrenal hypofunction E89.6
    hypoinsulinemia E89.1
    hypoparathyroidism E89.2
    hypopituitarism E89.3
    hypothyroidism E89.0
    ovarian failure E89.40
      asymptomatic E89.40
      symptomatic E89.41
    specified NEC E89.89
    testicular hypofunction E89.5
endodontic treatment NEC M27.59
enterostomy (stoma) K94.10
  hemorrhage K94.11
  infection K94.12
  malfunction K94.13
  mechanical K94.13
  specified complication NEC K94.19
episiotomy, disruption O90.1
esophageal anti-reflux device T85.9 ☑
  embolism T85.81 ☑
  fibrosis T85.82 ☑
  hemorrhage T85.83 ☑
  infection and inflammation T85.79 ☑
  mechanical
    breakdown T85.511 ☑
    displacement T85.521 ☑
    malfunction T85.511 ☑
    malposition T85.521 ☑
    obstruction T85.591 ☑
    perforation T85.591 ☑
    protrusion T85.591 ☑
    specified NEC T85.591 ☑
  pain T85.84 ☑
  specified type NEC T85.89 ☑
  stenosis T85.85 ☑
  thrombosis T85.86 ☑
esophagostomy K94.30
  hemorrhage K94.31
  infection K94.32
  malfunction K94.33
  mechanical K94.33

Complication(s) — *continued*
esophagostomy — *continued*
  specified complication NEC K94.39
extracorporeal circulation T80.90 ☑
extremity artery (bypass) graft T82.9 ☑
  arteriosclerosis — *see* Arteriosclerosis, extremities,
    bypass graft
  embolism T82.818 ☑
  fibrosis T82.828 ☑
  hemorrhage T82.838 ☑
  infection and inflammation T82.7 ☑
  mechanical
    breakdown T82.318 ☑
      femoral artery T82.312 ☑
    displacement T82.328 ☑
      femoral artery T82.322 ☑
    leakage T82.338 ☑
      femoral artery T82.332 ☑
    malposition T82.328 ☑
      femoral artery T82.322 ☑
    obstruction T82.398 ☑
      femoral artery T82.392 ☑
    perforation T82.398 ☑
      femoral artery T82.392 ☑
    protrusion T82.398 ☑
      femoral artery T82.392 ☑
  pain T82.848 ☑
  specified type NEC T82.898 ☑
  stenosis T82.858 ☑
  thrombosis T82.868 ☑
eye H57.9
  corneal graft — *see* Complications, graft, cornea
  implant (prosthetic) T85.9 ☑
    embolism T85.81 ☑
    fibrosis T85.82 ☑
    hemorrhage T85.83 ☑
    infection and inflammation T85.79 ☑
    mechanical
      breakdown T85.318 ☑
      displacement T85.328 ☑
      leakage T85.398 ☑
      malposition T85.328 ☑
      obstruction T85.398 ☑
      perforation T85.398 ☑
      protrusion T85.398 ☑
      specified NEC T85.398 ☑
    pain T85.84 ☑
    specified type NEC T85.89 ☑
    stenosis T85.85 ☑
    thrombosis T85.86 ☑
  intraocular lens — *see* Complications, intraocular
    lens
  orbital prosthesis — *see* Complications, orbital
    prosthesis
female genital N94.9
  device, implant or graft NEC — *see* Complications,
    genitourinary, device or implant, genital tract
femoral artery (bypass) graft — *see* Complication, extremity artery (bypass) graft
fixation device, internal (orthopedic) T84.9 ☑
  infection and inflammation T84.60 ☑
    arm T84.61- ☑
      humerus T84.61- ☑
      radius T84.61- ☑
      ulna T84.61- ☑
    leg T84.629 ☑
      femur T84.62- ☑
      fibula T84.62- ☑
      tibia T84.62- ☑
    specified site NEC T84.89 ☑
    spine T84.63 ☑
  mechanical
    breakdown
      limb T84.119 ☑
        carpal T84.210 ☑
        femur T84.11- ☑
        fibula T84.11- ☑
        humerus T84.11- ☑
        metacarpal T84.210 ☑
        metatarsal T84.213 ☑
        phalanx
          foot T84.213 ☑
          hand T84.210 ☑
        radius T84.11- ☑
        tarsal T84.213 ☑
        tibia T84.11- ☑

Complication(s) — *continued*
fixation device, internal — *continued*
  mechanical — *continued*
    breakdown — *continued*
      limb — *continued*
        ulna T84.11- ☑
        specified bone NEC T84.218 ☑
      spine T84.216 ☑
    displacement
      limb T84.129 ☑
        carpal T84.220 ☑
        femur T84.12- ☑
        fibula T84.12- ☑
        humerus T84.12- ☑
        metacarpal T84.220 ☑
        metatarsal T84.223 ☑
        phalanx
          foot T84.223 ☑
          hand T84.220 ☑
        radius T84.12- ☑
        tarsal T84.223 ☑
        tibia T84.12- ☑
        ulna T84.12- ☑
      specified bone NEC T84.228 ☑
      spine T84.226 ☑
    malposition — *see* Complications, fixation device, internal, mechanical, displacement
    obstruction — *see* Complications, fixation device, internal, mechanical, specified type NEC
    perforation — *see* Complications, fixation device, internal, mechanical, specified type NEC
    protrusion — *see* Complications, fixation device, internal, mechanical, specified type NEC
    specified type NEC
      limb T84.199 ☑
        carpal T84.290 ☑
        femur T84.19- ☑
        fibula T84.19- ☑
        humerus T84.19- ☑
        metacarpal T84.290 ☑
        metatarsal T84.293 ☑
        phalanx
          foot T84.293 ☑
          hand T84.290 ☑
        radius T84.19- ☑
        tarsal T84.293 ☑
        tibia T84.19- ☑
        ulna T84.19- ☑
      specified bone NEC T84.298 ☑
      vertebra T84.296 ☑
  specified type NEC T84.89 ☑
    embolism T84.81 ☑
    fibrosis T84.82 ☑
    hemorrhage T84.83 ☑
    pain T84.84 ☑
    specified complication NEC T84.89 ☑
    stenosis T84.85 ☑
    thrombosis T84.86 ☑
following
  acute myocardial infarction NEC I23.8
    aneurysm (false) (of cardiac wall) (of heart wall) (ruptured) I23.3
    angina I23.7
    atrial
      septal defect I23.1
      thrombosis I23.6
    cardiac wall rupture I23.3
    chordae tendinae rupture I23.4
    defect
      septal
        atrial (heart) I23.1
        ventricular (heart) I23.2
    hemopericardium I23.0
    papillary muscle rupture I23.5
    rupture
      cardiac wall I23.3
        with hemopericardium I23.0
      chordae tendineae I23.4
      papillary muscle I23.5
    specified NEC I23.8
    thrombosis
      atrium I23.6
      auricular appendage I23.6
      ventricle (heart) I23.6

☑ **Additional Character Required — Refer to the Tabular List for Character Selection**   ▽ **Subterms under main terms may continue to next column or page**

Complication(s) — *continued*
  following — *continued*
    acute myocardial infarction — *continued*
      ventricular
        septal defect I23.2
        thrombosis I23.6
    ectopic or molar pregnancy O08.9
      cardiac arrest O08.81
      sepsis O08.82
      specified type NEC O08.89
      urinary tract infection O08.83
    termination of pregnancy — *see* Abortion
  gastrointestinal K92.9
    bile duct prosthesis — *see* Complications, bile duct implant
    esophageal anti-reflux device — *see* Complications, esophageal anti-reflux device
    postoperative
      colostomy — *see* Complications, colostomy
      dumping syndrome K91.1
      enterostomy — *see* Complications, enterostomy
      gastrostomy — *see* Complications, gastrostomy
      malabsorption NEC K91.2
      obstruction K91.3
      postcholecystectomy syndrome K91.5
      specified NEC K91.89
      vomiting after GI surgery K91.0
    prosthetic device or implant
      bile duct prosthesis — *see* Complications, bile duct implant
      esophageal anti-reflux device — *see* Complications, esophageal anti-reflux device
      specified type NEC
        embolism T85.81 ☑
        fibrosis T85.82 ☑
        hemorrhage T85.83 ☑
        mechanical
          breakdown T85.518 ☑
          displacement T85.528 ☑
          malfunction T85.518 ☑
          malposition T85.528 ☑
          obstruction T85.598 ☑
          perforation T85.598 ☑
          protrusion T85.598 ☑
          specified NEC T85.598 ☑
        pain T85.84 ☑
        specified complication NEC T85.89 ☑
        stenosis T85.85 ☑
        thrombosis T85.86 ☑
  gastrostomy (stoma) K94.20
    hemorrhage K94.21
    infection K94.22
    malfunction K94.23
    mechanical K94.23
    specified complication NEC K94.29
  genitourinary
    device or implant T83.9 ☑
      genital tract T83.9 ☑
        infection or inflammation T83.6 ☑
        intrauterine contraceptive device — *see* Complications, intrauterine, contraceptive device
        mechanical — *see* Complications, by device, mechanical
        mesh — *see* Complications, mesh
        penile prosthesis — *see* Complications, prosthetic device, penile
        specified type NEC T83.89 ☑
          embolism T83.81 ☑
          fibrosis T83.82 ☑
          hemorrhage T83.83 ☑
          pain T83.84 ☑
          specified complication NEC T83.89 ☑
          stenosis T83.85 ☑
          thrombosis T83.86 ☑
        vaginal mesh — *see* Complications, mesh
      urinary system T83.9 ☑
        cystostomy catheter — *see* Complication, catheter, cystostomy
        electronic stimulator — *see* Complications, electronic stimulator device, urinary
        indwelling urethral catheter — *see* Complications, catheter, urethral, indwelling
        infection or inflammation T83.59 ☑
          indwelling urinary catheter T83.51 ☑

Complication(s) — *continued*
  genitourinary — *continued*
    device or implant — *continued*
      urinary system — *continued*
        kidney transplant — *see* Complication, transplant, kidney
        organ graft — *see* Complication, graft, urinary organ
        specified type NEC T83.89 ☑
          embolism T83.81 ☑
          fibrosis T83.82 ☑
          hemorrhage T83.83 ☑
          mechanical T83.198 ☑
            breakdown T83.118 ☑
            displacement T83.128 ☑
            malfunction T83.118 ☑
            malposition T83.128 ☑
            obstruction T83.198 ☑
            perforation T83.198 ☑
            protrusion T83.198 ☑
            specified NEC T83.198 ☑
          pain T83.84 ☑
          specified complication NEC T83.89 ☑
          stenosis T83.85 ☑
          thrombosis T83.86 ☑
        sphincter implant — *see* Complications, implant, urinary sphincter
    postprocedural
      pelvic peritoneal adhesions N99.4
      renal failure N99.0
      specified NEC N99.89
      stoma — *see* Complications, stoma, urinary tract
      urethral stricture — *see* Stricture, urethra, postprocedural
      vaginal
        adhesions N99.2
        vault prolapse N99.3
  graft (bypass) (patch) (*see also* Complications, prosthetic device or implant)
    aorta — *see* Complications, graft, vascular
    arterial — *see* Complication, graft, vascular
    bone T86.839
      failure T86.831
      infection T86.832
      mechanical T84.318 ☑
        breakdown T84.318 ☑
        displacement T84.328 ☑
        protrusion T84.398 ☑
        specified type NEC T84.398 ☑
      rejection T86.830
      specified type NEC T86.838
    carotid artery — *see* Complications, graft, vascular
    cornea T86.849
      failure T86.841
      infection T86.842
      mechanical T85.398 ☑
        breakdown T85.318 ☑
        displacement T85.328 ☑
        protrusion T85.398 ☑
        specified type NEC T85.398 ☑
      rejection T86.840
      retroprosthetic membrane T85.398 ☑
      specified type NEC T86.848
    femoral artery (bypass) — *see* Complication, extremity artery (bypass) graft
    genital organ or tract — *see* Complications, genitourinary, device or implant, genital tract
    muscle T84.9 ☑
      breakdown T84.410 ☑
      displacement T84.420 ☑
      embolism T84.81 ☑
      fibrosis T84.82 ☑
      hemorrhage T84.83 ☑
      infection and inflammation T84.7 ☑
      mechanical NEC T84.490 ☑
      pain T84.84 ☑
      specified type NEC T84.89 ☑
      stenosis T84.85 ☑
      thrombosis T84.86 ☑
    nerve — *see* Complication, prosthetic device or implant, specified NEC
    skin — *see* Complications, prosthetic device or implant, skin graft
    tendon T84.9 ☑
      breakdown T84.410 ☑

Complication(s) — *continued*
  graft (*see also* Complications, prosthetic device or implant) — *continued*
    tendon — *continued*
      displacement T84.420 ☑
      embolism T84.81 ☑
      fibrosis T84.82 ☑
      hemorrhage T84.83 ☑
      infection and inflammation T84.7 ☑
      mechanical NEC T84.490 ☑
      pain T84.84 ☑
      specified type NEC T84.89 ☑
      stenosis T84.85 ☑
      thrombosis T84.86 ☑
    urinary organ T83.9 ☑
      embolism T83.81 ☑
      fibrosis T83.82 ☑
      hemorrhage T83.83 ☑
      infection and inflammation T83.59 ☑
        indwelling urinary catheter T83.51 ☑
      mechanical
        breakdown T83.21 ☑
        displacement T83.22 ☑
        leakage T83.23 ☑
        malposition T83.22 ☑
        obstruction T83.29 ☑
        perforation T83.29 ☑
        protrusion T83.29 ☑
        specified NEC T83.29 ☑
      pain T83.84 ☑
      specified type NEC T83.89 ☑
      stenosis T83.85 ☑
      thrombosis T83.86 ☑
    vascular T82.9 ☑
      embolism T82.818 ☑
      femoral artery — *see* Complication, extremity artery (bypass) graft
      fibrosis T82.828 ☑
      hemorrhage T82.838 ☑
      mechanical
        breakdown T82.319 ☑
          aorta (bifurcation) T82.310 ☑
          carotid artery T82.311 ☑
          specified vessel NEC T82.318 ☑
        displacement T82.329 ☑
          aorta (bifurcation) T82.320 ☑
          carotid artery T82.321 ☑
          specified vessel NEC T82.328 ☑
        leakage T82.339 ☑
          aorta (bifurcation) T82.330 ☑
          carotid artery T82.331 ☑
          specified vessel NEC T82.338 ☑
        malposition T82.329 ☑
          aorta (bifurcation) T82.320 ☑
          carotid artery T82.321 ☑
          specified vessel NEC T82.328 ☑
        obstruction T82.399 ☑
          aorta (bifurcation) T82.390 ☑
          carotid artery T82.391 ☑
          specified vessel NEC T82.398 ☑
        perforation T82.399 ☑
          aorta (bifurcation) T82.390 ☑
          carotid artery T82.391 ☑
          specified vessel NEC T82.398 ☑
        protrusion T82.399 ☑
          aorta (bifurcation) T82.390 ☑
          carotid artery T82.391 ☑
          specified vessel NEC T82.398 ☑
      pain T82.848 ☑
      specified complication NEC T82.898 ☑
      stenosis T82.858 ☑
      thrombosis T82.868 ☑
  heart I51.9
    assist device
      infection and inflammation T82.7 ☑
    following acute myocardial infarction — *see* Complications, following, acute myocardial infarction
    postoperative — *see* Complications, circulatory system
    transplant — *see* Complication, transplant, heart and lung(s) — *see* Complications, transplant, heart, with lung
    valve
      graft (biological) T82.9 ☑
        embolism T82.817 ☑

Complication(s) — *continued*
- heart — *continued*
  - valve — *continued*
    - graft — *continued*
      - fibrosis T82.827 ☑
      - hemorrhage T82.837 ☑
      - infection and inflammation T82.7 ☑
      - mechanical T82.228 ☑
        - breakdown T82.221 ☑
        - displacement T82.222 ☑
        - leakage T82.223 ☑
        - malposition T82.222 ☑
        - obstruction T82.228 ☑
        - perforation T82.228 ☑
        - protrusion T82.228 ☑
      - pain T82.847 ☑
      - specified type NEC T82.897 ☑
      - stenosis T82.857 ☑
      - thrombosis T82.867 ☑
    - prosthesis T82.9 ☑
      - embolism T82.817 ☑
      - fibrosis T82.827 ☑
      - hemorrhage T82.837 ☑
      - infection or inflammation T82.6 ☑
      - mechanical T82.09 ☑
        - breakdown T82.01 ☑
        - displacement T82.02 ☑
        - leakage T82.03 ☑
        - malposition T82.02 ☑
        - obstruction T82.09 ☑
        - perforation T82.09 ☑
        - protrusion T82.09 ☑
      - pain T82.847 ☑
      - specified type NEC T82.897 ☑
        - mechanical T82.09 ☑
      - stenosis T82.857 ☑
      - thrombosis T82.867 ☑
- hematoma
  - intraoperative — *see* Complication, intraoperative, hemorrhage
  - postprocedural — *see* Complication, postprocedural, hemorrhage
- hemodialysis — *see* Complications, dialysis
- hemorrhage
  - intraoperative — *see* Complication, intraoperative, hemorrhage
  - postprocedural — *see* Complication, postprocedural, hemorrhage
- ileostomy (stoma) — *see* Complications, enterostomy
- immunization (procedure) — *see* Complications, vaccination
- implant (*see also* Complications, by site and type)
  - urinary sphincter T83.9 ☑
    - embolism T83.81 ☑
    - fibrosis T83.82 ☑
    - hemorrhage T83.83 ☑
    - infection and inflammation T83.59 ☑
    - mechanical
      - breakdown T83.111 ☑
      - displacement T83.121 ☑
      - leakage T83.191 ☑
      - malposition T83.121 ☑
      - obstruction T83.191 ☑
      - perforation T83.191 ☑
      - protrusion T83.191 ☑
      - specified NEC T83.191 ☑
    - pain T83.84 ☑
    - specified type NEC T83.89 ☑
    - stenosis T83.85 ☑
    - thrombosis T83.86 ☑
- infusion (procedure) T80.90 ☑
  - air embolism T80.0 ☑
  - blood — *see* Complications, transfusion
  - catheter — *see* Complications, catheter
  - infection T80.29 ☑
  - pump — *see* Complications, cardiovascular, device or implant
  - sepsis T80.29 ☑
  - serum reaction (*see also* Reaction, serum) T80.69 ☑
    - anaphylactic shock (*see also* Shock, anaphylactic) T80.59 ☑
  - specified type NEC T80.89 ☑
- inhalation therapy NEC T81.81 ☑
- injection (procedure) T80.90 ☑
  - drug reaction — *see* Reaction, drug
  - infection T80.29 ☑

Complication(s) — *continued*
- injection — *continued*
  - sepsis T80.29 ☑
  - serum (prophylactic) (therapeutic) — *see* Complications, vaccination
  - specified type NEC T80.89 ☑
  - vaccine (any) — *see* Complications, vaccination
- inoculation (any) — *see* Complications, vaccination
- insulin pump
  - infection and inflammation T85.72 ☑
  - mechanical
    - breakdown T85.614 ☑
    - displacement T85.624 ☑
    - leakage T85.633 ☑
    - malposition T85.624 ☑
    - obstruction T85.694 ☑
    - perforation T85.694 ☑
    - protrusion T85.694 ☑
    - specified NEC T85.694 ☑
- intestinal pouch NEC K91.858
- intraocular lens (prosthetic) T85.9 ☑
  - embolism T85.81 ☑
  - fibrosis T85.82 ☑
  - hemorrhage T85.83 ☑
  - infection and inflammation T85.79 ☑
  - mechanical
    - breakdown T85.21 ☑
    - displacement T85.22 ☑
    - malposition T85.22 ☑
    - obstruction T85.29 ☑
    - perforation T85.29 ☑
    - protrusion T85.29 ☑
    - specified NEC T85.29 ☑
  - pain T85.84 ☑
  - specified type NEC T85.89 ☑
  - stenosis T85.85 ☑
  - thrombosis T85.86 ☑
- intraoperative (intraprocedural)
  - cardiac arrest
    - during cardiac surgery I97.710
    - during other surgery I97.711
  - cardiac functional disturbance NEC
    - during cardiac surgery I97.790
    - during other surgery I97.791
  - hemorrhage (hematoma) (of)
    - circulatory system organ or structure
      - during cardiac bypass I97.411
      - during cardiac catheterization I97.410
      - during other circulatory system procedure I97.418
      - during other procedure I97.42
    - digestive system organ
      - during procedure on digestive system K91.61
      - during procedure on other organ K91.62
    - ear
      - during procedure on ear and mastoid process H95.21
      - during procedure on other organ H95.22
    - endocrine system organ or structure
      - during procedure on endocrine system organ or structure E36.01
      - during procedure on other organ E36.02
    - eye and adnexa
      - during ophthalmic procedure H59.11- ☑
      - during other procedure H59.12- ☑
    - genitourinary organ or structure
      - during procedure on genitourinary organ or structure N99.61
      - during procedure on other organ N99.62
    - mastoid process
      - during procedure on ear and mastoid process H95.21
      - during procedure on other organ H95.22
    - musculoskeletal structure
      - during musculoskeletal surgery M96.810
      - during non-orthopedic surgery M96.811
      - during orthopedic surgery M96.810
    - nervous system
      - during a nervous system procedure G97.31
      - during other procedure G97.32
    - respiratory system
      - during other procedure J95.62
      - during procedure on respiratory system organ or structure J95.61
    - skin and subcutaneous tissue
      - during a dermatologic procedure L76.01

Complication(s) — *continued*
- intraoperative — *continued*
  - hemorrhage — *continued*
    - skin and subcutaneous tissue — *continued*
      - during a procedure on other organ L76.02
    - spleen
      - during a procedure on other organ D78.02
      - during a procedure on the spleen D78.01
  - puncture or laceration (accidental) (unintentional) (of)
    - brain
      - during a nervous system procedure G97.48
      - during other procedure G97.49
    - circulatory system organ or structure
      - during circulatory system procedure I97.51
      - during other procedure I97.52
    - digestive system
      - during procedure on digestive system K91.71
      - during procedure on other organ K91.72
    - ear
      - during procedure on ear and mastoid process H95.31
      - during procedure on other organ H95.32
    - endocrine system organ or structure
      - during procedure on endocrine system organ or structure E36.11
      - during procedure on other organ E36.12
    - eye and adnexa
      - during ophthalmic procedure H59.21- ☑
      - during other procedure H59.22- ☑
    - genitourinary organ or structure
      - during procedure on genitourinary organ or structure N99.71
      - during procedure on other organ N99.72
    - mastoid process
      - during procedure on ear and mastoid process H95.31
      - during procedure on other organ H95.32
    - musculoskeletal structure
      - during musculoskeletal surgery M96.820
      - during non-orthopedic surgery M96.821
      - during orthopedic surgery M96.820
    - nervous system
      - during a nervous system procedure G97.48
      - during other procedure G97.49
    - respiratory system
      - during other procedure J95.72
      - during procedure on respiratory system organ or structure J95.71
    - skin and subcutaneous tissue
      - during a dermatologic procedure L76.11
      - during a procedure on other organ L76.12
    - spleen
      - during a procedure on other organ D78.12
      - during a procedure on the spleen D78.11
  - specified NEC
    - circulatory system I97.88
    - digestive system K91.81
    - ear H95.88
    - endocrine system E36.8
    - eye and adnexa H59.88
    - genitourinary system N99.81
    - mastoid process H95.88
    - musculoskeletal structure M96.89
    - nervous system G97.81
    - respiratory system J95.88
    - skin and subcutaneous tissue L76.81
    - spleen D78.81
- intraperitoneal catheter (dialysis) (infusion) — *see* Complications, catheter, intraperitoneal
- intrauterine
  - contraceptive device
    - embolism T83.81 ☑
    - fibrosis T83.82 ☑
    - hemorrhage T83.83 ☑
    - infection and inflammation T83.6 ☑
    - mechanical
      - breakdown T83.31 ☑
      - displacement T83.32 ☑
      - malposition T83.32 ☑
      - obstruction T83.39 ☑
      - perforation T83.39 ☑
      - protrusion T83.39 ☑
      - specified NEC T83.39 ☑
    - pain T83.84 ☑
    - specified type NEC T83.89 ☑
    - stenosis T83.85 ☑

  ☑ **Additional Character Required — Refer to the Tabular List for Character Selection**   🜊 **Subterms under main terms may continue to next column or page**

Complication(s) — *continued*
  intrauterine — *continued*
    contraceptive device — *continued*
      thrombosis T83.86 ☑
      procedure (fetal), to newborn P96.5
  jejunostomy (stoma) — *see* Complications, enterostomy
  joint prosthesis, internal T84.9 ☑
    breakage (fracture) T84.01- ☑
    dislocation T84.02- ☑
    fracture T84.01- ☑
    infection or inflammation T84.50 ☑
      hip T84.5- ☑
      knee T84.5- ☑
      specified joint NEC T84.59 ☑
    instability T84.02- ☑
    malposition — *see* Complications, joint prosthesis, mechanical, displacement
    mechanical
      breakage, broken T84.01- ☑
      dislocation T84.02- ☑
      fracture T84.01- ☑
      instability T84.02- ☑
      leakage — *see* Complications, joint prosthesis, mechanical, specified NEC
      loosening T84.039 ☑
        hip T84.03- ☑
        knee T84.03- ☑
        specified joint NEC T84.038 ☑
      obstruction — *see* Complications, joint prosthesis, mechanical, specified NEC
      perforation — *see* Complications, joint prosthesis, mechanical, specified NEC
      periprosthetic
        fracture T84.049 ☑
          hip T84.04- ☑
          knee T84.04- ☑
          other specified joint T84.048 ☑
        osteolysis T84.059 ☑
          hip T84.05- ☑
          knee T84.05- ☑
          other specified joint T84.058 ☑
      protrusion — *see* Complications, joint prosthesis, mechanical, specified NEC
      specified complication NEC T84.099 ☑
        hip T84.09- ☑
        knee T84.09- ☑
        other specified joint T84.098 ☑
      subluxation T84.02- ☑
      wear of articular bearing surface T84.069 ☑
        hip T84.06- ☑
        knee T84.06- ☑
        other specified joint T84.068 ☑
    specified joint NEC T84.89 ☑
      embolism T84.81 ☑
      fibrosis T84.82 ☑
      hemorrhage T84.83 ☑
      pain T84.84 ☑
      specified complication NEC T84.89 ☑
      stenosis T84.85 ☑
      thrombosis T84.86 ☑
    subluxation T84.02- ☑
  kidney transplant — *see* Complications, transplant, kidney
  labor O75.9
    specified NEC O75.89
  liver transplant (immune or nonimmune) — *see* Complications, transplant, liver
  lumbar puncture G97.1
    cerebrospinal fluid leak G97.0
    headache or reaction G97.1
  lung transplant — *see* Complications, transplant, lung and heart — *see* Complications, transplant, lung, with heart
  male genital N50.9
    device, implant or graft — *see* Complications, genitourinary, device or implant, genital tract
    postprocedural or postoperative — *see* Complications, genitourinary, postprocedural
    specified NEC N99.89
  mastoid (process) procedure
    intraoperative H95.88
      hematoma — *see* Complications, intraoperative, hemorrhage (hematoma) (of), mastoid process

Complication(s) — *continued*
  mastoid procedure — *continued*
    intraoperative — *continued*
      hemorrhage — *see* Complications, intraoperative, hemorrhage (hematoma) (of), mastoid process
      laceration — *see* Complications, intraoperative, puncture or laceration, mastoid process
      specified NEC H95.88
    postmastoidectomy — *see* Complications, postmastoidectomy
    postoperative H95.89
      external ear canal stenosis H95.81 ☑
      hematoma — *see* Complications, postprocedural, hemorrhage (hematoma) (of), mastoid process
      hemorrhage — *see* Complications, postprocedural, hemorrhage (hematoma) (of), mastoid process
      postmastoidectomy — *see* Complications, postmastoidectomy
      specified NEC H95.89
  mastoidectomy cavity — *see* Complications, postmastoidectomy
  mechanical — *see* Complications, by site and type, mechanical
  medical procedures (*see also* Complication(s), intraoperative) T88.9 ☑
  metabolic E88.9
    postoperative E89.89
      specified NEC E89.89
  molar pregnancy NOS O08.9
    damage to pelvic organs O08.6
    embolism O08.2
    genital infection O08.0
    hemorrhage (delayed) (excessive) O08.1
    metabolic disorder O08.5
    renal failure O08.4
    shock O08.3
    specified type NEC O08.0
    venous complication NEC O08.7
  musculoskeletal system (*see also* Complication, intraoperative (intraprocedural), by site)
    device, implant or graft NEC — *see* Complications, orthopedic, device or implant
    internal fixation (nail) (plate) (rod) — *see* Complications, fixation device, internal
    joint prosthesis — *see* Complications, joint prosthesis
    post radiation M96.89
      kyphosis M96.3
      scoliosis M96.5
      specified complication NEC M96.89
    postoperative (postprocedural) M96.89
      with osteoporosis — *see* Osteoporosis
      fracture following insertion of device — *see* Fracture, following insertion of orthopedic implant, joint prosthesis or bone plate
      joint instability after prosthesis removal M96.89
      lordosis M96.4
      postlaminectomy syndrome NEC M96.1
        kyphosis M96.3
      pseudarthrosis M96.0
      specified complication NEC M96.89
  nephrostomy (stoma) — *see* Complications, stoma, urinary tract, external NEC
  nervous system G98.8
    central G96.9
    device, implant or graft (*see also* Complication, prosthetic device or implant, specified NEC)
      electronic stimulator (electrode(s)) — *see* Complications, electronic stimulator device
      ventricular shunt — *see* Complications, ventricular shunt
    electronic stimulator (electrode(s)) — *see* Complications, electronic stimulator device
    postprocedural G97.82
      intracranial hypotension G97.2
      specified NEC G97.82
      spinal fluid leak G97.0
  newborn, due to intrauterine (fetal) procedure P96.5
  nonabsorbable (permanent) sutures — *see* Complication, sutures, permanent
  obstetric O75.9
    procedure (instrumental) (manual) (surgical)
      specified NEC O75.4
    specified NEC O75.89

Complication(s) — *continued*
  obstetric — *continued*
    surgical wound NEC O90.89
      hematoma O90.2
      infection O86.0
    ocular lens implant — *see* Complications, intraocular lens
  ophthalmologic
    postprocedural bleb — *see* Blebitis
  orbital prosthesis T85.9 ☑
    embolism T85.81 ☑
    fibrosis T85.82 ☑
    hemorrhage T85.83 ☑
    infection and inflammation T85.79 ☑
    mechanical
      breakdown T85.31- ☑
      displacement T85.32- ☑
      malposition T85.32- ☑
      obstruction T85.39- ☑
      perforation T85.39- ☑
      protrusion T85.39- ☑
      specified NEC T85.39- ☑
    pain T85.84 ☑
    specified type NEC T85.89 ☑
    stenosis T85.85 ☑
    thrombosis T85.86 ☑
  organ or tissue transplant (partial) (total) — *see* Complications, transplant
  orthopedic (*see also* Disorder, soft tissue)
    device or implant T84.9 ☑
      bone
        device or implant — *see* Complication, bone, device NEC
        graft — *see* Complication, graft, bone
      breakdown T84.418 ☑
      displacement T84.428 ☑
      electronic bone stimulator — *see* Complications, electronic stimulator device, bone
      embolism T84.81 ☑
      fibrosis T84.82 ☑
      fixation device — *see* Complication, fixation device, internal
      hemorrhage T84.83 ☑
      infection or inflammation T84.7 ☑
      joint prosthesis — *see* Complication, joint prosthesis, internal
      malfunction T84.418 ☑
      malposition T84.428 ☑
      mechanical NEC T84.498 ☑
      muscle graft — *see* Complications, graft, muscle
      obstruction T84.498 ☑
      pain T84.84 ☑
      perforation T84.498 ☑
      protrusion T84.498 ☑
      specified complication NEC T84.89 ☑
      stenosis T84.85 ☑
      tendon graft — *see* Complications, graft, tendon
      thrombosis T84.86 ☑
    fracture (following insertion of device) — *see* Fracture, following insertion of orthopedic implant, joint prosthesis or bone plate
    postprocedural M96.89
      fracture — *see* Fracture, following insertion of orthopedic implant, joint prosthesis or bone plate
      postlaminectomy syndrome NEC M96.1
        kyphosis M96.3
        lordosis M96.4
      postradiation
        kyphosis M96.2
        scoliosis M96.5
      pseudarthrosis post-fusion M96.0
      specified type NEC M96.89
  pacemaker (cardiac) — *see* Complications, cardiovascular device or implant, electronic
  pancreas transplant — *see* Complications, transplant, pancreas
  penile prosthesis (implant) — *see* Complications, prosthetic device, penile
  perfusion NEC T80.90 ☑
  perineal repair (obstetrical) NEC O90.89
    disruption O90.1
    hematoma O90.2
    infection (following delivery) O86.0
  phototherapy T88.9 ☑
    specified NEC T88.8 ☑

Complication(s) — *continued*
postmastoidectomy NEC H95.19- ☑
cyst, mucosal H95.13- ☑
granulation H95.12- ☑
inflammation, chronic H95.11- ☑
recurrent cholesteatoma H95.0- ☑
postoperative — *see* Complications, postprocedural
circulatory — *see* Complications, circulatory system
ear — *see* Complications, ear
endocrine — *see* Complications, endocrine
eye — *see* Complications, eye
lumbar puncture G97.1
cerebrospinal fluid leak G97.0
nervous system (central) (peripheral) — *see* Complications, nervous system
respiratory system — *see* Complications, respiratory system
postprocedural (*see also* Complications, surgical procedure)
cardiac arrest
following cardiac surgery I97.120
following other surgery I97.121
cardiac functional disturbance NEC
following cardiac surgery I97.190
following other surgery I97.191
cardiac insufficiency
following cardiac surgery I97.110
following other surgery I97.111
chorioretinal scars following retinal surgery H59.81- ☑
following cataract surgery
cataract (lens) fragments H59.02- ☑
cystoid macular edema H59.03- ☑
specified NEC H59.09- ☑
vitreous (touch) syndrome H59.01- ☑
heart failure
following cardiac surgery I97.130
following other surgery I97.131
hemorrhage (hematoma) (of)
circulatory system organ or structure
following a cardiac bypass I97.611
following a cardiac catheterization I97.610
following other circulatory system procedure I97.618
following other procedure I97.62
digestive system
following procedure on digestive system K91.840
following procedure on other organ K91.841
ear
following other procedure H95.42
following procedure on ear and mastoid process H95.41
endocrine system
following endocrine system procedure E89.810
following other procedure E89.811
eye and adnexa
following ophthalmic procedure H59.31- ☑
following other procedure H59.32- ☑
genitourinary organ or structure
following procedure on genitourinary organ or structure N99.820
following procedure on other organ N99.821
mastoid process
following other procedure H95.42
following procedure on ear and mastoid process H95.41
musculoskeletal structure
following musculoskeletal surgery M96.830
following non-orthopedic surgery M96.831
following orthopedic surgery M96.830
nervous system
following a nervous system procedure G97.51
following other procedure G97.52
respiratory system
following a respiratory system procedure J95.830
following other procedure J95.831
skin and subcutaneous tissue
following a dermatologic procedure L76.21
following a procedure on other organ L76.22
spleen
following procedure on other organ D78.22
following procedure on the spleen D78.21

Complication(s) — *continued*
postprocedural (*see also* Complications, surgical procedure) — *continued*
specified NEC
circulatory system I97.89
digestive K91.89
ear H95.89
endocrine E89.89
eye and adnexa H59.89
genitourinary N99.89
mastoid process H95.89
metabolic E89.89
musculoskeletal structure M96.89
nervous system G97.82
respiratory system J95.89
skin and subcutaneous tissue L76.82
spleen D78.89
pregnancy NEC — *see* Pregnancy, complicated by
prosthetic device or implant T85.9
bile duct — *see* Complications, bile duct implant
breast — *see* Complications, breast implant
cardiac and vascular NEC — *see* Complications, cardiovascular device or implant
corneal transplant — *see* Complications, graft, cornea
electronic nervous system stimulator — *see* Complications, electronic stimulator device
epidural infusion catheter — *see* Complications, catheter, epidural
esophageal anti-reflux device — *see* Complications, esophageal anti-reflux device
genital organ or tract — *see* Complications, genitourinary, device or implant, genital tract
heart valve — *see* Complications, heart, valve, prosthesis
infection or inflammation T85.79 ☑
intestine transplant T86.892
liver transplant T86.43
lung transplant T86.812
pancreas transplant T86.892
skin graft T86.822
intraocular lens — *see* Complications, intraocular lens
intraperitoneal (dialysis) catheter — *see* Complications, catheter, intraperitoneal
joint — *see* Complications, joint prosthesis, internal
mechanical NEC T85.698 ☑
dialysis catheter (vascular) (*see also* Complication, catheter, dialysis, mechanical)
peritoneal — *see* Complication, catheter, intraperitoneal, mechanical
gastrointestinal device T85.598 ☑
ocular device T85.398 ☑
subdural (infusion) catheter T85.690 ☑
suture, permanent T85.692 ☑
that for bone repair — *see* Complications, fixation device, internal (orthopedic), mechanical
ventricular shunt
breakdown T85.01 ☑
displacement T85.02 ☑
leakage T85.03 ☑
malposition T85.02 ☑
obstruction T85.09 ☑
perforation T85.09 ☑
protrusion T85.09 ☑
specified NEC T85.09 ☑
mesh
erosion (to surrounding organ or tissue) T83.718 ☑
vaginal (into pelvic floor muscles) T83.711 ☑
exposure (into surrounding organ or tissue) T83.728 ☑
vaginal (into vagina) (through vaginal wall) T83.721 ☑
orbital — *see* Complications, orbital prosthesis
penile T83.9 ☑
embolism T83.81 ☑
fibrosis T83.82 ☑
hemorrhage T83.83 ☑
infection and inflammation T83.6 ☑
mechanical
breakdown T83.410 ☑
displacement T83.420 ☑
leakage T83.490 ☑
malposition T83.420 ☑

Complication(s) — *continued*
prosthetic device or implant — *continued*
penile — *continued*
mechanical — *continued*
obstruction T83.490 ☑
perforation T83.490 ☑
protrusion T83.490 ☑
specified NEC T83.490 ☑
pain T83.84 ☑
specified type NEC T83.89 ☑
stenosis T83.85 ☑
thrombosis T83.86 ☑
prosthetic materials NEC
erosion (to surrounding organ or tissue) T83.718 ☑
vaginal (into pelvic floor muscles) T83.711 ☑
exposure (into surrounding organ or tissue) T83.728 ☑
vaginal (into vagina) (through vaginal wall) T83.721 ☑
skin graft T86.829
artificial skin or decellularized allodermis
embolism T85.81 ☑
fibrosis T85.82 ☑
hemorrhage T85.83 ☑
infection and inflammation T85.79 ☑
mechanical
breakdown T85.613 ☑
displacement T85.623 ☑
malfunction T85.613 ☑
malposition T85.623 ☑
obstruction T85.693 ☑
perforation T85.693 ☑
protrusion T85.693 ☑
specified NEC T85.693 ☑
pain T85.84 ☑
specified type NEC T85.89 ☑
stenosis T85.85 ☑
thrombosis T85.86 ☑
failure T86.821
infection T86.822
rejection T86.820
specified NEC T86.828
specified NEC T85.9 ☑
embolism T85.81 ☑
fibrosis T85.82 ☑
hemorrhage T85.83 ☑
infection and inflammation T85.79 ☑
mechanical
breakdown T85.618 ☑
displacement T85.628 ☑
leakage T85.638 ☑
malfunction T85.618 ☑
malposition T85.628 ☑
obstruction T85.698 ☑
perforation T85.698 ☑
protrusion T85.698 ☑
specified NEC T85.698 ☑
pain T85.84 ☑
specified type NEC T85.89 ☑
stenosis T85.85 ☑
thrombosis T85.86 ☑
subdural infusion catheter — *see* Complications, catheter, subdural
sutures — *see* Complications, sutures
urinary organ or tract NEC — *see* Complications, genitourinary, device or implant, urinary system
vascular — *see* Complications, cardiovascular device or implant
ventricular shunt — *see* Complications, ventricular shunt (device)
puerperium — *see* Puerperal
puncture, spinal G97.1
cerebrospinal fluid leak G97.0
headache or reaction G97.1
pyelogram N99.89
radiation
kyphosis M96.2
scoliosis M96.5
reattached
extremity (infection) (rejection)
lower T87.1X- ☑
upper T87.0X- ☑
specified body part NEC T87.2

☑ **Additional Character Required** — Refer to the Tabular List for Character Selection   Subterms under main terms may continue to next column or page

Complication(s) — *continued*
reconstructed breast
  asymmetry between native and reconstructed
    breast N65.1
  deformity N65.0
  disproportion between native and reconstructed
    breast N65.1
  excess tissue N65.0
  misshappen N65.0
reimplant NEC (*see also* Complications, prosthetic device or implant)
  limb (infection) (rejection) — *see* Complications,
    reattached, extremity
  organ (partial) (total) — *see* Complications, trans-
    plant
  prosthetic device NEC — *see* Complications, pros-
    thetic device
renal N28.9
  allograft — *see* Complications, transplant, kidney
  dialysis — *see* Complications, dialysis
respirator
  mechanical J95.850
    specified NEC J95.859
respiratory system J98.9
  device, implant or graft — *see* Complication,
    prosthetic device or implant, specified NEC
  lung transplant — *see* Complications, prosthetic
    device or implant, lung transplant
  postoperative J95.89
    air leak J95.812
    Mendelson's syndrome (chemical pneumonitis)
      J95.4
    pneumothorax J95.811
    pulmonary insufficiency (acute) (after nontho-
      racic surgery) J95.2
      chronic J95.3
      following thoracic surgery J95.1
    respiratory failure (acute) J95.821
      acute and chronic J95.822
    specified NEC J95.89
    subglottic stenosis J95.5
    tracheostomy complication — *see* Complica-
      tions, tracheostomy
  therapy T81.89 ☑
sedation during labor and delivery O74.9
  cardiac O74.2
  central nervous system O74.3
  pulmonary NEC O74.1
shunt (*see also* Complications, prosthetic device or
  implant)
  arteriovenous — *see* Complications, arteriovenous,
    shunt
  ventricular (communicating) — *see* Complications,
    ventricular shunt
skin
  graft T86.829
    failure T86.821
    infection T86.822
    rejection T86.820
    specified type NEC T86.828
spinal
  anesthesia — *see* Complications, anesthesia, spinal
  catheter (epidural) (subdural) — *see* Complications,
    catheter
  puncture or tap G97.1
    cerebrospinal fluid leak G97.0
    headache or reaction G97.1
stent
  bile duct — *see* Complications, bile duct prosthesis
  urinary T83.9 ☑
    embolism T83.81 ☑
    fibrosis T83.82 ☑
    hemorrhage T83.83 ☑
    infection and inflammation T83.59 ☑
    mechanical
      breakdown T83.112 ☑
      displacement T83.122 ☑
      leakage T83.192 ☑
      malposition T83.122 ☑
      obstruction T83.192 ☑
      perforation T83.192 ☑
      protrusion T83.192 ☑
      specified NEC T83.192 ☑
    pain T83.84 ☑
    specified type NEC T83.89 ☑
    stenosis T83.85 ☑
    thrombosis T83.86 ☑

Complication(s) — *continued*
stoma
  digestive tract
    colostomy — *see* Complications, colostomy
    enterostomy — *see* Complications, enterosto-
      my
    esophagostomy — *see* Complications,
      esophagostomy
    gastrostomy — *see* Complications, gastrostomy
  urinary tract N99.538
    cystostomy — *see* Complications, cystostomy
    external NOS N99.528
      hemorrhage N99.520
      infection N99.521
      malfunction N99.522
      specified type NEC N99.528
    hemorrhage N99.530
    infection N99.531
    malfunction N99.532
    specified type NEC N99.538
stomach banding — *see* Complication(s), bariatric
  procedure
stomach stapling — *see* Complication(s), bariatric
  procedure
surgical material, nonabsorbable — *see* Complication,
  suture, permanent
surgical procedure (on) T81.9 ☑
  amputation stump (late) — *see* Complications,
    amputation stump
  cardiac — *see* Complications, circulatory system
  cholesteatoma, recurrent — *see* Complications,
    postmastoidectomy, recurrent
    cholesteatoma
  circulatory (early) — *see* Complications, circulatory
    system
  digestive system — *see* Complications, gastroin-
    testinal
  dumping syndrome (postgastrectomy) K91.1
  ear — *see* Complications, ear
  elephantiasis or lymphedema I97.89
    postmastectomy I97.2
  emphysema (surgical) T81.82 ☑
  endocrine — *see* Complications, endocrine
  eye — *see* Complications, eye
  fistula (persistent postoperative) T81.83 ☑
  foreign body inadvertently left in wound (sponge)
    (suture) (swab) — *see* Foreign body, acciden-
    tally left during a procedure
  gastrointestinal — *see* Complications, gastrointesti-
    nal
  genitourinary NEC N99.89
  hematoma
    intraoperative — *see* Complication, intraopera-
      tive, hemorrhage
    postprocedural — *see* Complication, postpro-
      cedural, hemorrhage
  hemorrhage
    intraoperative — *see* Complication, intraopera-
      tive, hemorrhage
    postprocedural — *see* Complication, postpro-
      cedural, hemorrhage
  hepatic failure K91.82
  hyperglycemia (postpancreatectomy) E89.1
  hypoinsulinemia (postpancreatectomy) E89.1
  hypoparathyroidism (postparathyroidectomy)
    E89.2
  hypopituitarism (posthypophysectomy) E89.3
  hypothyroidism (post-thyroidectomy) E89.0
  intestinal obstruction K91.3
  intracranial hypotension following ventricular
    shunting (ventriculostomy) G97.2
  lymphedema I97.89
    postmastectomy I97.2
  malabsorption (postsurgical) NEC K91.2
    osteoporosis — *see* Osteoporosis, postsurgical
      malabsorption
  mastoidectomy cavity NEC — *see* Complications,
    postmastoidectomy
  metabolic E89.89
    specified NEC E89.89
  musculoskeletal — *see* Complications, muscu-
    loskeletal system
  nervous system (central) (peripheral) — *see* Com-
    plications, nervous system
  ovarian failure E89.40
    asymptomatic E89.40
    symptomatic E89.41

Complication(s) — *continued*
surgical procedure — *continued*
  peripheral vascular — *see* Complications, surgical
    procedure, vascular
  postcardiotomy syndrome I97.0
  postcholecystectomy syndrome K91.5
  postcommissurotomy syndrome I97.0
  postgastrectomy dumping syndrome K91.1
  postlaminectomy syndrome NEC M96.1
    kyphosis M96.3
  postmastectomy lymphedema syndrome I97.2
  postmastoidectomy cholesteatoma — *see* Compli-
    cations, postmastoidectomy, recurrent
    cholesteatoma
  postvagotomy syndrome K91.1
  postvalvulotomy syndrome I97.0
  pulmonary insufficiency (acute) J95.2
    chronic J95.3
    following thoracic surgery J95.1
  reattached body part — *see* Complications, reat-
    tached
  respiratory — *see* Complications, respiratory sys-
    tem
  shock (hypovolemic) T81.19 ☑
  spleen (postoperative) D78.89
    intraoperative D78.81
  stitch abscess T81.4 ☑
  subglottic stenosis (postsurgical) J95.5
  testicular hypofunction E89.5
  transplant — *see* Complications, organ or tissue
    transplant
  urinary NEC N99.89
  vaginal vault prolapse (posthysterectomy) N99.3
  vascular (peripheral)
    artery T81.719 ☑
      mesenteric T81.710 ☑
      renal T81.711 ☑
      specified NEC T81.718 ☑
    vein T81.72 ☑
  wound infection T81.4 ☑
suture, permanent (wire) NEC T85.9 ☑
  with repair of bone — *see* Complications, fixation
    device, internal
  embolism T85.81 ☑
  fibrosis T85.82 ☑
  hemorrhage T85.83 ☑
  infection and inflammation T85.79 ☑
  mechanical
    breakdown T85.612 ☑
    displacement T85.622 ☑
    malfunction T85.612 ☑
    malposition T85.622 ☑
    obstruction T85.692 ☑
    perforation T85.692 ☑
    protrusion T85.692 ☑
    specified NEC T85.692 ☑
  pain T85.84 ☑
  specified type NEC T85.89 ☑
  stenosis T85.85 ☑
  thrombosis T85.86 ☑
tracheostomy J95.00
  granuloma J95.09
  hemorrhage J95.01
  infection J95.02
  malfunction J95.03
  mechanical J95.03
  obstruction J95.03
  specified type NEC J95.09
  tracheo-esophageal fistula J95.04
transfusion (blood) (lymphocytes) (plasma) T80.92 ☑
  air emblism T80.0 ☑
  circulatory overload E87.71
  febrile nonhemolytic transfusion reaction R50.84
  hemochromatosis E83.111
  hemolysis T80.89 ☑
  hemolytic reaction (antigen unspecified)
    T80.919 ☑
  incompatibility reaction (antigen unspecified)
    T80.919 ☑
    ABO T80.30 ☑
      delayed serologic (DSTR) T80.39 ☑
      hemolytic transfusion reaction (HTR) (un-
        specified time after transfusion)
        T80.319 ☑
        acute (AHTR) (less than 24 hours after
          transfusion) T80.310 ☑

Complication(s) — *continued*
transfusion — *continued*
incompatibility reaction — *continued*
ABO — *continued*
hemolytic transfusion reaction — *continued*
delayed (DHTR) (24 hours or more after transfusion) T80.311 ☑
specified NEC T80.39 ☑
acute (antigen unspecified) T80.910 ☑
delayed (antigen unspecified) T80.911 ☑
delayed serologic (DSTR) T80.89 ☑
non-ABO (minor antigens (Duffy) (Kell) (Kidd) (Lewis) (M) (N) (P) (S)) T80.A0 ☑ (*following* T80.4)
delayed serologic (DSTR) T80.A9 ☑ (*following* T80.4)
hemolytic transfusion reaction (HTR) (unspecified time after transfusion) T80.A19 ☑ (*following* T80.4)
acute (AHTR) (less than 24 hours after transfusion) T80.A10 ☑ (*following* T80.4)
delayed (DHTR) (24 hours or more after transfusion) T80.A11 ☑ (*following* T80.4)
specified NEC T80.A9 ☑ (*following* T80.4)
Rh (antigens (C) (c) (D) (E) (e)) (factor) T80.40 ☑
delayed serologic (DSTR) T80.49 ☑
hemolytic transfusion reaction (HTR) (unspecified time after transfusion) T80.419 ☑
acute (AHTR) (less than 24 hours after transfusion) T80.410 ☑
delayed (DHTR) (24 hours or more after transfusion) T80.411 ☑
specified NEC T80.49 ☑
infection T80.29 ☑
reaction NEC T80.89 ☑
sepsis T80.29 ☑
shock T80.89 ☑
transplant T86.90
bone T86.839
failure T86.831
infection T86.832
rejection T86.830
specified type NEC T86.838
bone marrow T86.00
failure T86.02
infection T86.03
rejection T86.01
specified type NEC T86.09
cornea T86.849
failure T86.841
infection T86.842
rejection T86.840
specified type NEC T86.848
failure T86.92
heart T86.20
with lung T86.30
cardiac allograft vasculopathy T86.290
failure T86.32
infection T86.33
rejection T86.31
specified type NEC T86.39
failure T86.22
infection T86.23
rejection T86.21
specified type NEC T86.298
infection T86.93
intestine T86.859
failure T86.851
infection T86.852
rejection T86.850
specified type NEC T86.858
kidney T86.10
failure T86.12
infection T86.13
rejection T86.11
specified type NEC T86.19
liver T86.40
failure T86.42
infection T86.43
rejection T86.41
specified type NEC T86.49
lung T86.819
with heart T86.30
failure T86.32

Complication(s) — *continued*
transplant — *continued*
lung — *continued*
with heart — *continued*
infection T86.33
rejection T86.31
specified type NEC T86.39
failure T86.811
infection T86.812
rejection T86.810
specified type NEC T86.818
malignant neoplasm C80.2
pancreas T86.899
failure T86.891
infection T86.892
rejection T86.890
specified type NEC T86.898
peripheral blood stem cells T86.5
post-transplant lymphoproliferative disorder (PTLD) D47.Z1 (*following* D47.1)
rejection T86.91
skin T86.829
failure T86.821
infection T86.822
rejection T86.820
specified type NEC T86.828
specified
tissue T86.899
failure T86.891
infection T86.892
rejection T86.890
specified type NEC T86.898
type NEC T86.99
stem cell (from peripheral blood) (from umbilical cord) T86.5
umbilical cord stem cells T86.5
trauma (early) T79.9 ☑
specified NEC T79.8 ☑
ultrasound therapy NEC T88.9 ☑
umbilical cord NEC
complicating delivery O69.9 ☑
specified NEC O69.89 ☑
umbrella device, vascular T82.9 ☑
embolism T82.818 ☑
fibrosis T82.828 ☑
hemorrhage T82.838 ☑
infection or inflammation T82.7 ☑
mechanical
breakdown T82.515 ☑
displacement T82.525 ☑
leakage T82.535 ☑
malposition T82.525 ☑
obstruction T82.595 ☑
perforation T82.595 ☑
protrusion T82.595 ☑
pain T82.848 ☑
specified type NEC T82.898 ☑
stenosis T82.858 ☑
thrombosis T82.868 ☑
urethral catheter — *see* Complications, catheter, urethral, indwelling
vaccination T88.1 ☑
anaphylaxis NEC T80.52 ☑
arthropathy — *see* Arthropathy, postimmunization
cellulitis T88.0 ☑
encephalitis or encephalomyelitis G04.02
infection (general) (local) NEC T88.0 ☑
meningitis G03.8
myelitis G04.89
protein sickness T80.62 ☑
rash T88.1 ☑
reaction (allergic) T88.1 ☑
serum T80.62 ☑
sepsis T88.0 ☑
serum intoxication, sickness, rash, or other serum reaction NEC T80.62 ☑
anaphylactic shock T80.52 ☑
shock (allergic) (anaphylactic) T80.52 ☑
vaccinia (generalized) (localized) T88.1 ☑
vas deferens device or implant — *see* Complications, genitourinary, device or implant, genital tract
vascular I99.9
device or implant T82.9 ☑
embolism T82.818 ☑
fibrosis T82.828 ☑
hemorrhage T82.838 ☑
infection or inflammation T82.7 ☑

Complication(s) — *continued*
vascular — *continued*
device or implant — *continued*
mechanical
breakdown T82.519 ☑
specified device NEC T82.518 ☑
displacement T82.529 ☑
specified device NEC T82.528 ☑
leakage T82.539 ☑
specified device NEC T82.538 ☑
malposition T82.529 ☑
specified device NEC T82.528 ☑
obstruction T82.599 ☑
specified device NEC T82.598 ☑
perforation T82.599 ☑
specified device NEC T82.598 ☑
protrusion T82.599 ☑
specified device NEC T82.598 ☑
pain T82.848 ☑
specified type NEC T82.898 ☑
stenosis T82.858 ☑
thrombosis T82.868 ☑
dialysis catheter — *see* Complication, catheter, dialysis
following infusion, therapeutic injection or transfusion T80.1 ☑
graft T82.9 ☑
embolism T82.818 ☑
fibrosis T82.828 ☑
hemorrhage T82.838 ☑
mechanical
breakdown T82.319 ☑
aorta (bifurcation) T82.310 ☑
carotid artery T82.311 ☑
specified vessel NEC T82.318 ☑
displacement T82.329 ☑
aorta (bifurcation) T82.320 ☑
carotid artery T82.321 ☑
specified vessel NEC T82.328 ☑
leakage T82.339 ☑
aorta (bifurcation) T82.330 ☑
carotid artery T82.331 ☑
specified vessel NEC T82.338 ☑
malposition T82.329 ☑
aorta (bifurcation) T82.320 ☑
carotid artery T82.321 ☑
specified vessel NEC T82.328 ☑
obstruction T82.399 ☑
aorta (bifurcation) T82.390 ☑
carotid artery T82.391 ☑
specified vessel NEC T82.398 ☑
perforation T82.399 ☑
aorta (bifurcation) T82.390 ☑
carotid artery T82.391 ☑
specified vessel NEC T82.398 ☑
protrusion T82.399 ☑
aorta (bifurcation) T82.390 ☑
carotid artery T82.391 ☑
specified vessel NEC T82.398 ☑
pain T82.848 ☑
specified complication NEC T82.898 ☑
stenosis T82.858 ☑
thrombosis T82.868 ☑
postoperative — *see* Complications, postoperative, circulatory
vena cava device (filter) (sieve) (umbrella) — *see* Complications, umbrella device, vascular
ventilation therapy NEC T81.81 ☑
ventilator
mechanical J95.850
specified NEC J95.859
ventricular (communicating) shunt (device) T85.9 ☑
embolism T85.81 ☑
fibrosis T85.82 ☑
hemorrhage T85.83 ☑
infection and inflammation T85.79 ☑
mechanical
breakdown T85.01 ☑
displacement T85.02 ☑
leakage T85.03 ☑
malposition T85.02 ☑
obstruction T85.09 ☑
perforation T85.09 ☑
protrusion T85.09 ☑
specified NEC T85.09 ☑
pain T85.84 ☑

Complication(s) — *continued*
  ventricular shunt — *continued*
    specified type NEC T85.89 ☑
    stenosis T85.85 ☑
    thrombosis T85.86 ☑
  wire suture, permanent (implanted) — *see* Complications, suture, permanent
Compressed air disease T70.3 ☑
Compression
  with injury — *code by* Nature of injury
  artery I77.1
    celiac, syndrome I77.4
  brachial plexus G54.0
  brain (stem) G93.5
    due to
      contusion (diffuse) — *see* Injury, intracranial, diffuse
        focal — *see* Injury, intracranial, focal
      injury NEC — *see* Injury, intracranial, diffuse
      traumatic — *see* Injury, intracranial, diffuse
  bronchus J98.09
  cauda equina G83.4
  celiac (artery) (axis) I77.4
  cerebral — *see* Compression, brain
  cervical plexus G54.2
  cord
    spinal — *see* Compression, spinal
    umbilical — *see* Compression, umbilical cord
  cranial nerve G52.9
    eighth H93.3 ☑
    eleventh G52.8
    fifth G50.8
    first G52.0
    fourth — *see* Strabismus, paralytic, fourth nerve
    ninth G52.1
    second — *see* Disorder, nerve, optic
    seventh G52.8
    sixth — *see* Strabismus, paralytic, sixth nerve
    tenth G52.2
    third — *see* Strabismus, paralytic, third nerve
    twelfth G52.3
  diver's squeeze T70.3 ☑
  during birth (newborn) P15.9
  esophagus K22.2
  eustachian tube — *see* Obstruction, eustachian tube, cartilaginous
  facies Q67.1
  fracture — *see* Fracture
  heart — *see* Disease, heart
  intestine — *see* Obstruction, intestine
  laryngeal nerve, recurrent G52.2
    with paralysis of vocal cords and larynx J38.00
      bilateral J38.02
      unilateral J38.01
  lumbosacral plexus G54.1
  lung J98.4
  lymphatic vessel I89.0
  medulla — *see* Compression, brain
  nerve (*see also* Disorder, nerve) G58.9
    arm NEC — *see* Mononeuropathy, upper limb
    axillary G54.0
    cranial — *see* Compression, cranial nerve
    leg NEC — *see* Mononeuropathy, lower limb
    median (in carpal tunnel) — *see* Syndrome, carpal tunnel
    optic — *see* Disorder, nerve, optic
    plantar — *see* Lesion, nerve, plantar
    posterior tibial (in tarsal tunnel) — *see* Syndrome, tarsal tunnel
    root or plexus NOS (in) G54.9
      intervertebral disc disorder NEC — *see* Disorder, disc, with, radiculopathy
        with myelopathy — *see* Disorder, disc, with, myelopathy
      neoplastic disease (*see also* Neoplasm) D49.9 [G55]
      spondylosis — *see* Spondylosis, with radiculopathy
    sciatic (acute) — *see* Lesion, nerve, sciatic
    sympathetic G90.8
    traumatic — *see* Injury, nerve
    ulnar — *see* Lesion, nerve, ulnar
    upper extremity NEC — *see* Mononeuropathy, upper limb
  spinal (cord) G95.20
    by displacement of intervertebral disc NEC (*see also* Disorder, disc, with, myelopathy)

Compression — *continued*
  spinal — *continued*
    nerve root NOS G54.9
      due to displacement of intervertebral disc NEC — *see* Disorder, disc, with, radiculopathy
        with myelopathy — *see* Disorder, disc, with, myelopathy
    specified NEC G95.29
    spondylogenic (cervical) (lumbar, lumbosacral) (thoracic) — *see* Spondylosis, with myelopathy NEC
      anterior — *see* Syndrome, anterior, spinal artery, compression
    traumatic — *see* Injury, spinal cord, by region
  subcostal nerve (syndrome) — *see* Mononeuropathy, upper limb, specified NEC
  sympathetic nerve NEC G90.8
  syndrome T79.5 ☑
  trachea J39.8
  ulnar nerve (by scar tissue) — *see* Lesion, nerve, ulnar
  umbilical cord
    complicating delivery O69.2 ☑
      cord around neck O69.1 ☑
      prolapse O69.0 ☑
      specified NEC O69.2 ☑
  ureter N13.5
  vein I87.1
  vena cava (inferior) (superior) I87.1
Compulsion, compulsive
  gambling F63.0
  neurosis F42
  personality F60.5
  states F42
  swearing F42
    in Gilles de la Tourette's syndrome F95.2
  tics and spasms F95.9
Concato's disease (pericardial polyserositis) A19.9
  nontubercular I31.1
  pleural — *see* Pleurisy, with effusion
Concavity chest wall M95.4
Concealed penis Q55.69
Concern (normal) **about sick person in family** Z63.6
Concrescence (teeth) K00.2
Concretio cordis I31.1
  rheumatic I09.2
Concretion (*see also* Calculus)
  appendicular K38.1
  canaliculus — *see* Dacryolith
  clitoris N90.89
  conjunctiva H11.12- ☑
  eyelid — *see* Disorder, eyelid, specified type NEC
  lacrimal passages — *see* Dacryolith
  prepuce (male) N47.8
  salivary gland (any) K11.5
  seminal vesicle N50.8
  tonsil J35.8
Concussion (brain) (cerebral) (current) S06.0X- ☑
  blast (air) (hydraulic) (immersion) (underwater)
    abdomen or thorax — *see* Injury, blast, by site
    ear with acoustic nerve injury — *see* Injury, nerve, acoustic, specified type NEC
  cauda equina S34.3 ☑
  conus medullaris S34.02 ☑
  ocular S05.8X- ☑
  spinal (cord)
    cervical S14.0 ☑
    lumbar S34.01 ☑
    sacral S34.02 ☑
    thoracic S24.0 ☑
  syndrome F07.81
Condition — *see* Disease
Conditions arising in the perinatal period — *see* Newborn, affected by
Conduct disorder — *see* Disorder, conduct
Condyloma A63.0
  acuminatum A63.0
  gonorrheal A54.09
  latum A51.31
  syphilitic A51.31
    congenital A50.07
  venereal, syphilitic A51.31
Conflagration (*see also* Burn)
  asphyxia (by inhalation of gases, fumes or vapors) (*see also* Table of Drugs and Chemicals) T59.9- ☑
Conflict (with) (*see also* Discord)
  family Z73.9

Conflict — *continued*
  marital Z63.0
    involving divorce or estrangement Z63.5
  parent-child Z62.820
    parent-adopted child Z62.821
    parent-biological child Z62.820
    parent-foster child Z62.822
  social role NEC Z73.5
Confluent — *see* condition
Confusion, confused R41.0
  epileptic F05
  mental state (psychogenic) F44.89
  psychogenic F44.89
  reactive (from emotional stress, psychological trauma) F44.89
Confusional arousals G47.51
Congelation T69.9 ☑
Congenital (*see also* condition)
  aortic septum Q25.4
  intrinsic factor deficiency D51.0
  malformation — *see* Anomaly
Congestion, congestive
  bladder N32.89
  bowel K63.89
  brain G93.89
  breast N64.59
  bronchial J98.09
  catarrhal J31.0
  chest R09.89
  chill, malarial — *see* Malaria
  circulatory NEC I99.8
  duodenum K31.89
  eye — *see* Hyperemia, conjunctiva
  facial, due to birth injury P15.4
  general R68.89
  glottis J37.0
  heart — *see* Failure, heart, congestive
  hepatic K76.1
  hypostatic (lung) — *see* Edema, lung
  intestine K63.89
  kidney N28.89
  labyrinth H83.8 ☑
  larynx J37.0
  liver K76.1
  lung R09.89
    active or acute — *see* Pneumonia
  malaria, malarial — *see* Malaria
  nasal R09.81
  nose R09.81
  orbit, orbital (*see also* Exophthalmos)
    inflammatory (chronic) — *see* Inflammation, orbit
  ovary N83.8
  pancreas K86.8
  pelvic, female N94.89
  pleural J94.8
  prostate (active) N42.1
  pulmonary — *see* Congestion, lung
  renal N28.89
  retina H35.81
  seminal vesicle N50.1
  spinal cord G95.19
  spleen (chronic) D73.2
  stomach K31.89
  trachea — *see* Tracheitis
  urethra N36.8
  uterus N85.8
    with subinvolution N85.3
  venous (passive) I87.8
  viscera R68.89
Congestive — *see* Congestion
Conical
  cervix (hypertrophic elongation) N88.4
  cornea — *see* Keratoconus
  teeth K00.2
Conjoined twins Q89.4
Conjugal maladjustment Z63.0
  involving divorce or estrangement Z63.5
Conjunctiva — *see* condition
Conjunctivitis (staphylococcal) (streptococcal) NOS H10.9
  Acanthamoeba B60.12
  acute H10.3- ☑
    atopic H10.1- ☑
    chemical (*see also* Corrosion, cornea) H10.21- ☑
    mucopurulent H10.02- ☑
      follicular H10.01- ☑
    pseudomembranous H10.22- ☑

Conjunctivitis — Constriction

Conjunctivitis — *continued*
  acute — *continued*
    serous except viral H10.23- ☑
      viral — *see* Conjunctivitis, viral
    toxic H10.21- ☑
  adenoviral (acute) (follicular) B30.1
  allergic (acute) — *see* Conjunctivitis, acute, atopic
    chronic H10.45
      vernal H10.44
  anaphylactic — *see* Conjunctivitis, acute, atopic
  Apollo B30.3
  atopic (acute) — *see* Conjunctivitis, acute, atopic
  Béal's B30.2
  blennorrhagic (gonococcal) (neonatorum) A54.31
  chemical (acute) (*see also* Corrosion, cornea)
    H10.21- ☑
  chlamydial A74.0
    due to trachoma A71.1
    neonatal P39.1
  chronic (nodosa) (petrificans) (phlyctenular) H10.40- ☑
    allergic H10.45
      vernal H10.44
    follicular H10.43- ☑
    giant papillary H10.41- ☑
    simple H10.42- ☑
    vernal H10.44
  coxsackievirus 24 B30.3
  diphtheritic A36.86
  due to
    dust — *see* Conjunctivitis, acute, atopic
    filariasis B74.9
    mucocutaneous leishmaniasis B55.2
  enterovirus type 70 (hemorrhagic) B30.3
  epidemic (viral) B30.9
    hemorrhagic B30.3
  gonococcal (neonatorum) A54.31
  granular (trachomatous) A71.1
    sequelae (late effect) B94.0
  hemorrhagic (acute) (epidemic) B30.3
  herpes zoster B02.31
  in (due to)
    Acanthamoeba B60.12
    adenovirus (acute) (follicular) B30.1
    Chlamydia A74.0
    coxsackievirus 24 B30.3
    diphtheria A36.86
    enterovirus type 70 (hemorrhagic) B30.3
    filariasis B74.9
    gonococci A54.31
    herpes (simplex) virus B00.53
      zoster B02.31
    infectious disease NEC B99 ☑
    meningococci A39.89
    mucocutaneous leishmaniasis B55.2
    rosacea L71.9
    syphilis (late) A52.71
    zoster B02.31
  inclusion A74.0
  infantile P39.1
    gonococcal A54.31
  Koch-Weeks' — *see* Conjunctivitis, acute, mucopurulent
  light — *see* Conjunctivitis, acute, atopic
  ligneous — *see* Blepharoconjunctivitis, ligneous
  meningococcal A39.89
  mucopurulent — *see* Conjunctivitis, acute, mucopurulent
  neonatal P39.1
    gonococcal A54.31
  Newcastle B30.8
  of Béal B30.2
  parasitic
    filariasis B74.9
    mucocutaneous leishmaniasis B55.2
  Parinaud's H10.89
  petrificans H10.89
  rosacea L71.9
  specified NEC H10.89
  swimming-pool B30.1
  trachomatous A71.1
    acute A71.0
    sequelae (late effect) B94.0
  traumatic NEC H10.89
  tuberculous A18.59
  tularemic A21.1
  tularensis A21.1

Conjunctivitis — *continued*
  viral B30.9
    due to
      adenovirus B30.1
      enterovirus B30.3
    specified NEC B30.8
Conjunctivochalasis H11.82- ☑
Connective tissue — *see* condition
Conn's syndrome E26.01
Conradi (-Hunermann) **disease** Q77.3
Consanguinity Z84.3
  counseling Z71.89
Conscious simulation (of illness) Z76.5
Consecutive — *see* condition
Consolidation lung (base) — *see* Pneumonia, lobar
Constipation (atonic) (neurogenic) (simple) (spastic) K59.00
  drug-induced — *see* Table of Drugs and Chemicals
  outlet dysfunction K59.02
  psychogenic F45.8
  slow transit K59.01
  specified NEC K59.09
Constitutional (*see also* condition)
  substandard F60.7
Constitutionally substandard F60.7
Constriction (*see also* Stricture)
  auditory canal — *see* Stenosis, external ear canal
  bronchial J98.09
  duodenum K31.5
  esophagus K22.2
  external
    abdomen, abdominal (wall) S30.841 ☑
    alveolar process S00.542 ☑
    ankle S90.54- ☑
    antecubital space — *see* Constriction, external, forearm
    arm (upper) S40.84- ☑
    auricle — *see* Constriction, external, ear
    axilla — *see* Constriction, external, arm
    back, lower S30.840 ☑
    breast S20.14- ☑
    brow S00.84 ☑
    buttock S30.840 ☑
    calf — *see* Constriction, external, leg
    canthus — *see* Constriction, external, eyelid
    cheek S00.84 ☑
      internal S00.542 ☑
    chest wall — *see* Constriction, external, thorax
    chin S00.84 ☑
    clitoris S30.844 ☑
    costal region — *see* Constriction, external, thorax
    digit(s)
      foot — *see* Constriction, external, toe
      hand — *see* Constriction, external, finger
    ear S00.44- ☑
    elbow S50.34- ☑
    epididymis S30.843 ☑
    epigastric region S30.841 ☑
    esophagus, cervical S10.14 ☑
    eyebrow — *see* Constriction, external, eyelid
    eyelid S00.24- ☑
    face S00.84 ☑
    finger(s) S60.44- ☑
      index S60.44- ☑
      little S60.44- ☑
      middle S60.44- ☑
      ring S60.44- ☑
    flank S30.841 ☑
    foot (except toe(s) alone) S90.84- ☑
      toe — *see* Constriction, external, toe
    forearm S50.84- ☑
      elbow only — *see* Constriction, external, elbow
    forehead S00.84 ☑
    genital organs, external
      female S30.846 ☑
      male S30.845 ☑
    groin S30.841 ☑
    gum S00.542 ☑
    hand S60.54- ☑
    head S00.94 ☑
      ear — *see* Constriction, external, ear
      eyelid — *see* Constriction, external, eyelid
      lip S00.541 ☑
      nose S00.34 ☑
      oral cavity S00.542 ☑
      scalp S00.04 ☑

Constriction — *continued*
  external — *continued*
    head — *continued*
      specified site NEC S00.84 ☑
    heel — *see* Constriction, external, foot
    hip S70.24- ☑
    inguinal region S30.841 ☑
    interscapular region S20.449 ☑
    jaw S00.84 ☑
    knee S80.24- ☑
    labium (majus) (minus) S30.844 ☑
    larynx S10.14 ☑
    leg (lower) S80.84- ☑
      knee — *see* Constriction, external, knee
      upper — *see* Constriction, external, thigh
    lip S00.541 ☑
    lower back S30.840 ☑
    lumbar region S30.840 ☑
    malar region S00.84 ☑
    mammary — *see* Constriction, external, breast
    mastoid region S00.84 ☑
    mouth S00.542 ☑
    nail
      finger — *see* Constriction, external, finger
      toe — *see* Constriction, external, toe
    nasal S00.34 ☑
    neck S10.94 ☑
      specified site NEC S10.84 ☑
      throat S10.14 ☑
    nose S00.34 ☑
    occipital region S00.04 ☑
    oral cavity S00.542 ☑
    orbital region — *see* Constriction, external, eyelid
    palate S00.542 ☑
    palm — *see* Constriction, external, hand
    parietal region S00.04 ☑
    pelvis S30.840 ☑
    penis S30.842 ☑
    perineum
      female S30.844 ☑
      male S30.840 ☑
    periocular area — *see* Constriction, external, eyelid
    phalanges
      finger — *see* Constriction, external, finger
      toe — *see* Constriction, external, toe
    pharynx S10.14 ☑
    pinna — *see* Constriction, external, ear
    popliteal space — *see* Constriction, external, knee
    prepuce S30.842 ☑
    pubic region S30.840 ☑
    pudendum
      female S30.846 ☑
      male S30.845 ☑
    sacral region S30.840 ☑
    scalp S00.04 ☑
    scapular region — *see* Constriction, external, shoulder
    scrotum S30.843 ☑
    shin — *see* Constriction, external, leg
    shoulder S40.24- ☑
    sternal region S20.349 ☑
    submaxillary region S00.84 ☑
    submental region S00.84 ☑
    subungual
      finger(s) — *see* Constriction, external, finger
      toe(s) — *see* Constriction, external, toe
    supraclavicular fossa S10.84 ☑
    supraorbital S00.84 ☑
    temple S00.84 ☑
    temporal region S00.84 ☑
    testis S30.843 ☑
    thigh S70.34- ☑
    thorax, thoracic (wall) S20.94 ☑
      back S20.44- ☑
      front S20.34- ☑
    throat S10.14 ☑
    thumb S60.34- ☑
    toe(s) (lesser) S90.44- ☑
      great S90.44- ☑
    tongue S00.542 ☑
    trachea S10.14 ☑
    tunica vaginalis S30.843 ☑
    uvula S00.542 ☑
    vagina S30.844 ☑
    vulva S30.844 ☑
    wrist S60.84- ☑

☑ **Additional Character Required** — Refer to the Tabular List for Character Selection   ▽ **Subterms under main terms may continue to next column or page**

Constriction — *continued*
    gallbladder — *see* Obstruction, gallbladder
    intestine — *see* Obstruction, intestine
    larynx J38.6
        congenital Q31.8
            specified NEC Q31.8
            subglottic Q31.1
    organ or site, congenital NEC — *see* Atresia, by site
    prepuce (acquired) (congenital) N47.1
    pylorus (adult hypertrophic) K31.1
        congenital or infantile Q40.0
            newborn Q40.0
    ring dystocia (uterus) O62.4
    spastic (*see also* Spasm)
        ureter N13.5
    ureter N13.5
        with infection N13.6
    urethra — *see* Stricture, urethra
    visual field (peripheral) (functional) — *see* Defect, visual field
Constrictive — *see* condition
Consultation
    without complaint or sickness Z71.9
        feared complaint unfounded Z71.1
        specified reason NEC Z71.89
    medical — *see* Counseling, medical
    religious Z71.81
    specified reason NEC Z71.89
    spiritual Z71.81
Consumption — *see* Tuberculosis
Contact (with) (*see also* Exposure (to))
    acariasis Z20.7
    AIDS virus Z20.6
    air pollution Z77.110
    algae and algae toxins Z77.121
    algae bloom Z77.121
    anthrax Z20.810
    aromatic amines Z77.020
    aromatic (hazardous) compounds NEC Z77.028
    aromatic dyes NOS Z77.028
    arsenic Z77.010
    asbestos Z77.090
    bacterial disease NEC Z20.818
    benzene Z77.021
    blue-green algae bloom Z77.121
    body fluids (potentially hazardous) Z77.21
    brown tide Z77.121
    chemicals (chiefly nonmedicinal) (hazardous) NEC Z77.098
    cholera Z20.09
    chromium compounds Z77.018
    communicable disease Z20.9
        bacterial NEC Z20.818
        specified NEC Z20.89
        viral NEC Z20.828
    cyanobacteria bloom Z77.121
    dyes Z77.098
    Escherichia coli (E. coli) Z20.01
    fiberglass — *see* Table of Drugs and Chemicals, fiberglass
    German measles Z20.4
    gonorrhea Z20.2
    hazardous metals NEC Z77.018
    hazardous substances NEC Z77.29
    hazards in the physical environment NEC Z77.128
    hazards to health NEC Z77.9
    HIV Z20.6
    HTLV-III/LAV Z20.6
    human immunodeficiency virus (HIV) Z20.6
    infection Z20.9
        specified NEC Z20.89
    infestation (parasitic) NEC Z20.7
    intestinal infectious disease NEC Z20.09
        Escherichia coli (E. coli) Z20.01
    lead Z77.011
    meningococcus Z20.811
    mold (toxic) Z77.120
    nickel dust Z77.018
    noise Z77.122
    parasitic disease Z20.7
    pediculosis Z20.7
    pfiesteria piscicida Z77.121
    poliomyelitis Z20.89
    pollution
        air Z77.110
        environmental NEC Z77.118
        soil Z77.112
        water Z77.111

Contact — *continued*
    polycyclic aromatic hydrocarbons Z77.028
    rabies Z20.3
    radiation, naturally occurring NEC Z77.123
    radon Z77.123
    red tide (Florida) Z77.121
    rubella Z20.4
    sexually-transmitted disease Z20.2
    smallpox (laboratory) Z20.89
    syphilis Z20.2
    tuberculosis Z20.1
    uranium Z77.012
    varicella Z20.820
    venereal disease Z20.2
    viral disease NEC Z20.828
    viral hepatitis Z20.5
    water pollution Z77.111
Contamination, food — *see* Intoxication, foodborne
Contraception, contraceptive
    advice Z30.09
    counseling Z30.09
    device (intrauterine) (in situ) Z97.5
        causing menorrhagia T83.83 ☑
        checking Z30.431
        complications — *see* Complications, intrauterine, contraceptive device
        in place Z97.5
        initial prescription Z30.014
        reinsertion Z30.433
        removal Z30.432
        replacement Z30.433
    emergency (postcoital) Z30.012
    initial prescription Z30.019
        injectable Z30.013
        intrauterine device Z30.014
        pills Z30.011
        postcoital (emergency) Z30.012
        specified type NEC Z30.018
        subdermal implantable Z30.019
    maintenance Z30.40
        examination Z30.8
        injectable Z30.42
        intrauterine device Z30.431
        pills Z30.41
        specified type NEC Z30.49
        subdermal implantable Z30.49
    management Z30.9
        specified NEC Z30.8
    postcoital (emergency) Z30.012
    prescription Z30.019
        repeat Z30.40
    sterilization Z30.2
    surveillance (drug) — *see* Contraception, maintenance
Contraction(s), contracture, contracted
    Achilles tendon (*see also* Short, tendon, Achilles)
        congenital Q66.89
    amputation stump (surgical) (flexion) (late) (next proximal joint) T87.89
    anus K59.8
    bile duct (common) (hepatic) K83.8
    bladder N32.89
        neck or sphincter N32.0
    bowel, cecum, colon or intestine, any part — *see* Obstruction, intestine
    Braxton Hicks — *see* False, labor
    breast implant, capsular T85.44 ☑
    bronchial J98.09
    burn (old) — *see* Cicatrix
    cervix — *see* Stricture, cervix
    cicatricial — *see* Cicatrix
    conjunctiva, trachomatous, active A71.1
        sequelae (late effect) B94.0
    Dupuytren's M72.0
    eyelid — *see* Disorder, eyelid function
    fascia (lata) (postural) M72.8
        Dupuytren's M72.0
        palmar M72.0
        plantar M72.2
    finger NEC (*see also* Deformity, finger)
        congenital Q68.1
        joint — *see* Contraction, joint, hand
    flaccid — *see* Contraction, paralytic
    gallbladder K82.0
    heart valve — *see* Endocarditis
    hip — *see* Contraction, joint, hip
    hourglass
        bladder N32.89
            congenital Q64.79

Contraction(s), contracture, contracted — *continued*
    hourglass — *continued*
        gallbladder K82.0
            congenital Q44.1
        stomach K31.89
            congenital Q40.2
            psychogenic F45.8
        uterus (complicating delivery) O62.4
    hysterical F44.4
    internal os — *see* Stricture, cervix
    joint (abduction) (acquired) (adduction) (flexion) (rotation) M24.50
        ankle M24.57- ☑
        congenital NEC Q68.8
            hip Q65.89
        elbow M24.52- ☑
        foot joint M24.57- ☑
        hand joint M24.54- ☑
        hip M24.55- ☑
            congenital Q65.89
        hysterical F44.4
        knee M24.56- ☑
        shoulder M24.51- ☑
        wrist M24.53- ☑
    kidney (granular) (secondary) N26.9
        congenital Q63.8
        hydronephritic — *see* Hydronephrosis Page N26.2
        pyelonephritic — *see* Pyelitis, chronic
        tuberculous A18.11
    ligament (*see also* Disorder, ligament)
        congenital Q79.8
    muscle (postinfective) (postural) NEC M62.40
        with contracture of joint — *see* Contraction, joint
        ankle M62.47- ☑
        congenital Q79.8
            sternocleidomastoid Q68.0
        extraocular — *see* Strabismus
        eye (extrinsic) — *see* Strabismus
        foot M62.47- ☑
        forearm M62.43- ☑
        hand M62.44- ☑
        hysterical F44.4
        ischemic (Volkmann's) T79.6 ☑
        lower leg M62.46- ☑
        multiple sites M62.49
        pelvic region M62.45- ☑
        posttraumatic — *see* Strabismus, paralytic
        psychogenic F45.8
            conversion reaction F44.4
        shoulder region M62.41- ☑
        specified site NEC M62.48
        thigh M62.45- ☑
        upper arm M62.42- ☑
    neck — *see* Torticollis
    ocular muscle — *see* Strabismus
    organ or site, congenital NEC — *see* Atresia, by site
    outlet (pelvis) — *see* Contraction, pelvis
    palmar fascia M72.0
    paralytic
        joint — *see* Contraction, joint
        muscle (*see also* Contraction, muscle NEC)
            ocular — *see* Strabismus, paralytic
    pelvis (acquired) (general) M95.5
        with disproportion (fetopelvic) O33.1
            causing obstructed labor O65.1
            inlet O33.2
            mid-cavity O33.3 ☑
            outlet O33.3 ☑
    plantar fascia M72.2
    premature
        atrium I49.1
        auriculoventricular I49.49
        heart I49.49
        junctional I49.2
        supraventricular I49.1
        ventricular I49.3
    prostate N42.89
    pylorus NEC (*see also* Pylorospasm)
        psychogenic F45.8
    rectum, rectal (sphincter) K59.8
    ring (Bandl's) (complicating delivery) O62.4
    scar — *see* Cicatrix
    spine — *see* Dorsopathy, deforming
    sternocleidomastoid (muscle), congenital Q68.0

Contraction(s), contracture, contracted — *continued*
- stomach K31.89
  - hourglass K31.89
    - congenital Q40.2
    - psychogenic F45.8
  - psychogenic F45.8
- tendon (sheath) M62.40
  - with contracture of joint — *see* Contraction, joint
  - Achilles — *see* Short, tendon, Achilles
  - ankle M62.47- ☑
    - Achilles — *see* Short, tendon, Achilles
  - foot M62.47- ☑
  - forearm M62.43- ☑
  - hand M62.44- ☑
  - lower leg M62.46- ☑
  - multiple sites M62.49
  - neck M62.48
  - pelvic region M62.45- ☑
  - shoulder region M62.41- ☑
  - specified site NEC M62.48
  - thigh M62.45- ☑
  - thorax M62.48
  - trunk M62.48
  - upper arm M62.42- ☑
- toe — *see* Deformity, toe, specified NEC
- ureterovesical orifice (postinfectional) N13.5
  - with infection N13.6
- urethra (*see also* Stricture, urethra)
  - orifice N32.0
- uterus N85.8
  - abnormal NEC O62.9
  - clonic (complicating delivery) O62.4
  - dyscoordinate (complicating delivery) O62.4
  - hourglass (complicating delivery) O62.4
  - hypertonic O62.4
  - hypotonic NEC O62.2
  - inadequate
    - primary O62.0
    - secondary O62.1
  - incoordinate (complicating delivery) O62.4
  - poor O62.2
  - tetanic (complicating delivery) O62.4
- vagina (outlet) N89.5
- vesical N32.89
  - neck or urethral orifice N32.0
- visual field — *see* Defect, visual field, generalized
- Volkmann's (ischemic) T79.6 ☑

Contusion (skin surface intact) T14.8
- abdomen, abdominal (muscle) (wall) S30.1 ☑
- adnexa, eye NEC S05.8X- ☑
- adrenal gland S37.812 ☑
- alveolar process S00.532 ☑
- ankle S90.0- ☑
- antecubital space — *see* Contusion, forearm
- anus S30.3 ☑
- arm (upper) S40.02- ☑
  - lower (with elbow) — *see* Contusion, forearm
- auditory canal — *see* Contusion, ear
- auricle — *see* Contusion, ear
- axilla — *see* Contusion, arm, upper
- back (*see also* Contusion, thorax, back)
  - lower S30.0 ☑
- bile duct S36.13 ☑
- bladder S37.22 ☑
- bone NEC T14.8
- brain (diffuse) — *see* Injury, intracranial, diffuse
  - focal — *see* Injury, intracranial, focal
- brainstem S06.38- ☑
- breast S20.0- ☑
- broad ligament S37.892 ☑
- brow S00.83 ☑
- buttock S30.0 ☑
- canthus, eye S00.1- ☑
- cauda equina S34.3 ☑
- cerebellar, traumatic S06.37- ☑
- cerebral S06.33- ☑
  - left side S06.32- ☑
  - right side S06.31- ☑
- cheek S00.83 ☑
  - internal S00.532 ☑
- chest (wall) — *see* Contusion, thorax
- chin S00.83 ☑
- clitoris S30.23 ☑
- colon — *see* Injury, intestine, large, contusion
- common bile duct S36.13 ☑

Contusion — *continued*
- conjunctiva S05.1- ☑
  - with foreign body (in conjunctival sac) — *see* Foreign body, conjunctival sac
- conus medullaris (spine) S34.139 ☑
- cornea — *see* Contusion, eyeball
  - with foreign body — *see* Foreign body, cornea
- corpus cavernosum S30.21 ☑
- cortex (brain) (cerebral) — *see* Injury, intracranial, diffuse
  - focal — *see* Injury, intracranial, focal
- costal region — *see* Contusion, thorax
- cystic duct S36.13 ☑
- diaphragm S27.802 ☑
- duodenum S36.420 ☑
- ear S00.43- ☑
- elbow S50.0- ☑
  - with forearm — *see* Contusion, forearm
- epididymis S30.22 ☑
- epigastric region S30.1 ☑
- epiglottis S10.0 ☑
- esophagus (thoracic) S27.812 ☑
  - cervical S10.0 ☑
- eyeball S05.1- ☑
- eyebrow S00.1- ☑
- eyelid (and periocular area) S00.1- ☑
- face NEC S00.83 ☑
- fallopian tube S37.529 ☑
  - bilateral S37.522 ☑
  - unilateral S37.521 ☑
- femoral triangle S30.1 ☑
- finger(s) S60.00 ☑
  - with damage to nail (matrix) S60.10 ☑
  - index S60.02- ☑
    - with damage to nail S60.12- ☑
  - little S60.05- ☑
    - with damage to nail S60.15- ☑
  - middle S60.03- ☑
    - with damage to nail S60.13- ☑
  - ring S60.04- ☑
    - with damage to nail S60.14- ☑
  - thumb — *see* Contusion, thumb
- flank S30.1 ☑
- foot (except toe(s) alone) S90.3- ☑
  - toe — *see* Contusion, toe
- forearm S50.1- ☑
  - elbow only — *see* Contusion, elbow
- forehead S00.83 ☑
- gallbladder S36.122 ☑
- genital organs, external
  - female S30.202 ☑
  - male S30.201 ☑
- globe (eye) — *see* Contusion, eyeball
- groin S30.1 ☑
- gum S00.532 ☑
- hand S60.22- ☑
  - finger(s) — *see* Contusion, finger
  - wrist — *see* Contusion, wrist
- head S00.93 ☑
  - ear — *see* Contusion, ear
  - eyelid — *see* Contusion, eyelid
  - lip S00.531 ☑
  - nose S00.33 ☑
  - oral cavity S00.532 ☑
  - scalp S00.03 ☑
  - specified part NEC S00.83 ☑
- heel — *see* Contusion, foot
- hepatic duct S36.13 ☑
- hip S70.0- ☑
- ileum S36.428 ☑
- iliac region S30.1 ☑
- inguinal region S30.1 ☑
- interscapular region S20.229 ☑
- intra-abdominal organ S36.92 ☑
  - colon — *see* Injury, intestine, large, contusion
  - liver S36.112 ☑
  - pancreas — *see* Contusion, pancreas
  - rectum S36.62 ☑
  - small intestine — *see* Injury, intestine, small, contusion
  - specified organ NEC S36.892 ☑
  - spleen — *see* Contusion, spleen
  - stomach S36.32 ☑
- iris (eye) — *see* Contusion, eyeball
- jaw S00.83 ☑
- jejunum S36.428 ☑

Contusion — *continued*
- kidney S37.01- ☑
  - major (greater than 2 cm) S37.02- ☑
  - minor (less than 2 cm) S37.01- ☑
- knee S80.0- ☑
- labium (majus) (minus) S30.23 ☑
- lacrimal apparatus, gland or sac S05.8X- ☑
- larynx S10.0 ☑
- leg (lower) S80.1- ☑
  - knee — *see* Contusion, knee
- lens — *see* Contusion, eyeball
- lip S00.531 ☑
- liver S36.112 ☑
- lower back S30.0 ☑
- lumbar region S30.0 ☑
- lung S27.329 ☑
  - bilateral S27.322 ☑
  - unilateral S27.321 ☑
- malar region S00.83 ☑
- mastoid region S00.83 ☑
- membrane, brain — *see* Injury, intracranial, diffuse
  - focal — *see* Injury, intracranial, focal
- mesentery S36.892 ☑
- mesosalpinx S37.892 ☑
- mouth S00.532 ☑
- muscle — *see* Contusion, by site
- nail
  - finger — *see* Contusion, finger, with damage to nail
  - toe — *see* Contusion, toe, with damage to nail
- nasal S00.33 ☑
- neck S10.93 ☑
  - specified site NEC S10.83 ☑
  - throat S10.0 ☑
- nerve — *see* Injury, nerve
- newborn P54.5
- nose S00.33 ☑
- occipital
  - lobe (brain) — *see* Injury, intracranial, diffuse
  - focal — *see* Injury, intracranial, focal
  - region (scalp) S00.03 ☑
- orbit (region) (tissues) S05.1- ☑
- ovary S37.429 ☑
  - bilateral S37.422 ☑
  - unilateral S37.421 ☑
- palate S00.532 ☑
- pancreas S36.229 ☑
  - body S36.221 ☑
  - head S36.220 ☑
  - tail S36.222 ☑
- parietal
  - lobe (brain) — *see* Injury, intracranial, diffuse
  - focal — *see* Injury, intracranial, focal
  - region (scalp) S00.03 ☑
- pelvic organ S37.92 ☑
  - adrenal gland S37.812 ☑
  - bladder S37.22 ☑
  - fallopian tube — *see* Contusion, fallopian tube
  - kidney — *see* Contusion, kidney
  - ovary — *see* Contusion, ovary
  - prostate S37.822 ☑
  - specified organ NEC S37.892 ☑
  - ureter S37.12 ☑
  - urethra S37.32 ☑
  - uterus S37.62 ☑
- pelvis S30.0 ☑
- penis S30.21 ☑
- perineum
  - female S30.23 ☑
  - male S30.0 ☑
- periocular area S00.1- ☑
- peritoneum S36.81 ☑
- periurethral tissue — *see* Contusion, urethra
- pharynx S10.0 ☑
- pinna — *see* Contusion, ear
- popliteal space — *see* Contusion, knee
- prepuce S30.21 ☑
- prostate S37.822 ☑
- pubic region S30.1 ☑
- pudendum
  - female S30.202 ☑
  - male S30.201 ☑
- quadriceps femoris — *see* Contusion, thigh
- rectum S36.62 ☑
- retroperitoneum S36.892 ☑
- round ligament S37.892 ☑

☑ **Additional Character Required — Refer to the Tabular List for Character Selection**   ▽ **Subterms under main terms may continue to next column or page**

Index

Contusion — *continued*
  sacral region S30.0 ☑
  scalp S00.03 ☑
    due to birth injury P12.3
  scapular region — *see* Contusion, shoulder
  sclera — *see* Contusion, eyeball
  scrotum S30.22 ☑
  seminal vesicle S37.892 ☑
  shoulder S40.01- ☑
  skin NEC T14.8
  small intestine — *see* Injury, intestine, small, contusion
  spermatic cord S30.22 ☑
  spinal cord — *see* Injury, spinal cord, by region
    cauda equina S34.3 ☑
    conus medullaris S34.139 ☑
  spleen S36.029 ☑
    major S36.021 ☑
    minor S36.020 ☑
  sternal region S20.219 ☑
  stomach S36.32 ☑
  subconjunctival S05.1- ☑
  subcutaneous NEC T14.8
  submaxillary region S00.83 ☑
  submental region S00.83 ☑
  subperiosteal NEC T14.8
  subungual
    finger — *see* Contusion, finger, with damage to nail
    toe — *see* Contusion, toe, with damage to nail
  supraclavicular fossa S10.83 ☑
  supraorbital S00.83 ☑
  suprarenal gland S37.812 ☑
  temple (region) S00.83 ☑
  temporal
    lobe (brain) — *see* Injury, intracranial, diffuse
    focal — *see* Injury, intracranial, focal
    region S00.83 ☑
  testis S30.22 ☑
  thigh S70.1- ☑
  thorax (wall) S20.20 ☑
    back S20.22- ☑
    front S20.21- ☑
  throat S10.0 ☑
  thumb S60.01- ☑
    with damage to nail S60.11- ☑
  toe(s) (lesser) S90.12- ☑
    with damage to nail S90.22- ☑
    great S90.11- ☑
      with damage to nail S90.21- ☑
      specified type NEC S90.221 ☑
  tongue S00.532 ☑
  trachea (cervical) S10.0 ☑
    thoracic S27.52 ☑
  tunica vaginalis S30.22 ☑
  tympanum, tympanic membrane — *see* Contusion, ear
  ureter S37.12 ☑
  urethra S37.32 ☑
  urinary organ NEC S37.892 ☑
  uterus S37.62 ☑
  uvula S00.532 ☑
  vagina S30.23 ☑
  vas deferens S37.892 ☑
  vesical S37.22 ☑
  vocal cord(s) S10.0 ☑
  vulva S30.23 ☑
  wrist S60.21- ☑
Conus (congenital) (any type) Q14.8
  cornea — *see* Keratoconus
  medullaris syndrome G95.81
Conversion hysteria, neurosis or reaction F44.9
Converter, tuberculosis (test reaction) R76.11
Conviction (legal), **anxiety concerning** Z65.0
  with imprisonment Z65.1
Convulsions (idiopathic) (*see also* Seizure(s)) R56.9
  apoplectiform (cerebral ischemia) I67.82
  benign neonatal (familial) — *see* Epilepsy, generalized, idiopathic
  dissociative F44.5
  epileptic — *see* Epilepsy
  epileptiform, epileptoid — *see* Seizure, epileptiform
  ether (anesthetic) — *see* Table of Drugs and Chemicals, by drug
  febrile R56.00
    with status epilepticus G40.901

Convulsions — *continued*
  febrile — *continued*
    complex R56.01
      with status epilepticus G40.901
    simple R56.00
  hysterical F44.5
  infantile P90
    epilepsy — *see* Epilepsy
  jacksonian — *see* Epilepsy, localization-related, symptomatic, with simple partial seizures
  myoclonic G25.3
  neonatal, benign (familial) — *see* Epilepsy, generalized, idiopathic
  newborn P90
  obstetrical (nephritic) (uremic) — *see* Eclampsia
  paretic A52.17
  post traumatic R56.1
  psychomotor — *see* Epilepsy, localization-related, symptomatic, with complex partial seizures
  recurrent R56.9
  reflex R25.8
  scarlatinal A38.8
  tetanus, tetanic — *see* Tetanus
  thymic E32.8
Convulsive (*see also* Convulsions)
Cooley's anemia D56.1
Coolie itch B76.9
Cooper's
  disease — *see* Mastopathy, cystic
  hernia — *see* Hernia, abdomen, specified site NEC
Copra itch B88.0
Coprophagy F50.8
Coprophobia F40.298
Coproporphyria, hereditary E80.29
Cor
  biloculare Q20.8
  bovis, bovinum — *see* Hypertrophy, cardiac
  pulmonale (chronic) I27.81
    acute I26.09
  triatriatum, triatrium Q24.2
  triloculare Q20.8
    biatrium Q20.4
    biventriculare Q21.1
Corbus' disease (gangrenous balanitis) N48.1
Cord (*see also* condition)
  around neck (tightly) (with compression)
    complicating delivery O69.1 ☑
  bladder G95.89
    tabetic A52.19
Cordis ectopia Q24.8
Corditis (spermatic) N49.1
Corectopia Q13.2
Cori's disease (glycogen storage) E74.03
Corkhandler's disease or lung J67.3
Corkscrew esophagus K22.4
Corkworker's disease or lung J67.3
Corn (infected) L84
Cornea (*see also* condition)
  donor Z52.5
  plana Q13.4
Cornelia de Lange syndrome Q87.1
Cornu cutaneum L85.8
Cornual gestation or pregnancy O00.8
Coronary (artery) — *see* condition
Coronavirus, as cause of disease classified elsewhere B97.29
  SARS-associated B97.21
Corpora (*see also* condition)
  amylacea, prostate N42.89
  cavernosa — *see* condition
Corpulence — *see* Obesity
Corpus — *see* condition
Corrected transposition Q20.5
Corrosion (injury) (acid) (caustic) (chemical) (lime) (external) (internal) T30.4
  abdomen, abdominal (muscle) (wall) T21.42 ☑
    first degree T21.52 ☑
    second degree T21.62 ☑
    third degree T21.72 ☑
  above elbow T22.439 ☑
    first degree T22.539 ☑
    left T22.432 ☑
      first degree T22.532 ☑
      second degree T22.632 ☑
      third degree T22.732 ☑
    right T22.431 ☑
      first degree T22.531 ☑

Corrosion — *continued*
  above elbow — *continued*
    right — *continued*
      second degree T22.631 ☑
      third degree T22.731 ☑
    second degree T22.639 ☑
    third degree T22.739 ☑
  alimentary tract NEC T28.7
  ankle T25.419 ☑
    first degree T25.519 ☑
    left T25.412 ☑
      first degree T25.512 ☑
      second degree T25.612 ☑
      third degree T25.712 ☑
    multiple with foot — *see* Corrosion, lower, limb, multiple, ankle and foot
    right T25.411 ☑
      first degree T25.511 ☑
      second degree T25.611 ☑
      third degree T25.711 ☑
    second degree T25.619 ☑
    third degree T25.719 ☑
  anus — *see* Corrosion, buttock
  arm(s) (meaning upper limb(s)) — *see* Corrosion, upper limb
  axilla T22.449 ☑
    first degree T22.549 ☑
    left T22.442 ☑
      first degree T22.542 ☑
      second degree T22.642 ☑
      third degree T22.742 ☑
    right T22.441 ☑
      first degree T22.541 ☑
      second degree T22.641 ☑
      third degree T22.741 ☑
    second degree T22.649 ☑
    third degree T22.749 ☑
  back (lower) T21.44 ☑
    first degree T21.54 ☑
    second degree T21.64 ☑
    third degree T21.74 ☑
    upper T21.43 ☑
      first degree T21.53 ☑
      second degree T21.63 ☑
      third degree T21.73 ☑
  blisters — *code as* Corrosion, second degree, by site
  breast(s) — *see* Corrosion, chest wall
  buttock(s) T21.45 ☑
    first degree T21.55 ☑
    second degree T21.65 ☑
    third degree T21.75 ☑
  calf T24.439 ☑
    first degree T24.539 ☑
    left T24.432 ☑
      first degree T24.532 ☑
      second degree T24.632 ☑
      third degree T24.732 ☑
    right T24.431 ☑
      first degree T24.531 ☑
      second degree T24.631 ☑
      third degree T24.731 ☑
    second degree T24.639 ☑
    third degree T24.739 ☑
  canthus (eye) — *see* Corrosion, eyelid
  cervix T28.8 ☑
  cheek T20.46 ☑
    first degree T20.56 ☑
    second degree T20.66 ☑
    third degree T20.76 ☑
  chest wall T21.41 ☑
    first degree T21.51 ☑
    second degree T21.61 ☑
    third degree T21.71 ☑
  chin T20.43 ☑
    first degree T20.53 ☑
    second degree T20.63 ☑
    third degree T20.73 ☑
  colon T28.7 ☑
  conjunctiva (and cornea) — *see* Corrosion, cornea
  cornea (and conjunctiva) T26.6- ☑
  deep necrosis of underlying tissue — *code as* Corrosion, third degree, by site
  dorsum of hand T23.469 ☑
    first degree T23.569 ☑

Corrosion — *continued*
dorsum of hand — *continued*
  left T23.462 ☑
    first degree T23.562 ☑
    second degree T23.662 ☑
    third degree T23.762 ☑
  right T23.461 ☑
    first degree T23.561 ☑
    second degree T23.661 ☑
    third degree T23.761 ☑
  second degree T23.669 ☑
  third degree T23.769 ☑
ear (auricle) (external) (canal) T20.41 ☑
  drum T28.91 ☑
  first degree T20.51 ☑
  second degree T20.61 ☑
  third degree T20.71 ☑
elbow T22.429 ☑
  first degree T22.529 ☑
  left T22.422 ☑
    first degree T22.522 ☑
    second degree T22.622 ☑
    third degree T22.722 ☑
  right T22.421 ☑
    first degree T22.521 ☑
    second degree T22.621 ☑
    third degree T22.721 ☑
  second degree T22.629 ☑
  third degree T22.729 ☑
entire body — *see* Corrosion, multiple body regions
epidermal loss — *code as* Corrosion, second degree, by site
epiglottis T27.4 ☑
erythema, erythematous — *code as* Corrosion, first degree, by site
esophagus T28.6 ☑
extent (percentage of body surface)
  less than 10 per cent T32.0
  10-19 per cent (0-9 percent third degree) T32.10
    with 10-19 percent third degree T32.11
  20-29 per cent (0-9 percent third degree) T32.20
    with
      10-19 percent third degree T32.21
      20-29 percent third degree T32.22
  30-39 per cent (0-9 percent third degree) T32.30
    with
      10-19 percent third degree T32.31
      20-29 percent third degree T32.32
      30-39 percent third degree T32.33
  40-49 per cent (0-9 percent third degree) T32.40
    with
      10-19 percent third degree T32.41
      20-29 percent third degree T32.42
      30-39 percent third degree T32.43
      40-49 percent third degree T32.44
  50-59 per cent (0-9 percent third degree) T32.50
    with
      10-19 percent third degree T32.51
      20-29 percent third degree T32.52
      30-39 percent third degree T32.53
      40-49 percent third degree T32.54
      50-59 percent third degree T32.55
  60-69 per cent (0-9 percent third degree) T32.60
    with
      10-19 percent third degree T32.61
      20-29 percent third degree T32.62
      30-39 percent third degree T32.63
      40-49 percent third degree T32.64
      50-59 percent third degree T32.65
      60-69 percent third degree T32.66
  70-79 per cent (0-9 percent third degree) T32.70
    with
      10-19 percent third degree T32.71
      20-29 percent third degree T32.72
      30-39 percent third degree T32.73
      40-49 percent third degree T32.74
      50-59 percent third degree T32.75
      60-69 percent third degree T32.76
      70-79 percent third degree T32.77
  80-89 per cent (0-9 percent third degree) T32.80
    with
      10-19 percent third degree T32.81
      20-29 percent third degree T32.82
      30-39 percent third degree T32.83
      40-49 percent third degree T32.84
      50-59 percent third degree T32.85
      60-69 percent third degree T32.86

Corrosion — *continued*
extent — *continued*
  80-89 per cent — *continued*
    with — *continued*
      70-79 percent third degree T32.87
      80-89 percent third degree T32.88
  90 per cent or more (0-9 percent third degree) T32.90
    with
      10-19 percent third degree T32.91
      20-29 percent third degree T32.92
      30-39 percent third degree T32.93
      40-49 percent third degree T32.94
      50-59 percent third degree T32.95
      60-69 percent third degree T32.96
      70-79 percent third degree T32.97
      80-89 percent third degree T32.98
      90-99 percent third degree T32.99
extremity — *see* Corrosion, limb
eye(s) and adnexa T26.9- ☑
  with resulting rupture and destruction of eyeball T26.7- ☑
  conjunctival sac — *see* Corrosion, cornea
  cornea — *see* Corrosion, cornea
  lid — *see* Corrosion, eyelid
  periocular area — *see* Corrosion eyelid
  specified site NEC T26.8- ☑
eyeball — *see* Corrosion, eye
eyelid(s) T26.5- ☑
face — *see* Corrosion, head
finger T23.429 ☑
  first degree T23.529 ☑
  left T23.422 ☑
    first degree T23.522 ☑
    second degree T23.622 ☑
    third degree T23.722 ☑
  multiple sites (without thumb) T23.439 ☑
    with thumb T23.449 ☑
      first degree T23.549 ☑
      left T23.442 ☑
        first degree T23.542 ☑
        second degree T23.642 ☑
        third degree T23.742 ☑
      right T23.441 ☑
        first degree T23.541 ☑
        second degree T23.641 ☑
        third degree T23.741 ☑
      second degree T23.649 ☑
      third degree T23.749 ☑
  first degree T23.539 ☑
  left T23.432 ☑
    first degree T23.532 ☑
    second degree T23.632 ☑
    third degree T23.732 ☑
  right T23.431 ☑
    first degree T23.531 ☑
    second degree T23.631 ☑
    third degree T23.731 ☑
  second degree T23.639 ☑
  third degree T23.739 ☑
  right T23.421 ☑
    first degree T23.521 ☑
    second degree T23.621 ☑
    third degree T23.721 ☑
  second degree T23.629 ☑
  third degree T23.729 ☑
flank — *see* Corrosion, abdomen
foot T25.429 ☑
  first degree T25.529 ☑
  left T25.422 ☑
    first degree T25.522 ☑
    second degree T25.622 ☑
    third degree T25.722 ☑
  multiple with ankle — *see* Corrosion, lower, limb, multiple, ankle and foot
  right T25.421 ☑
    first degree T25.521 ☑
    second degree T25.621 ☑
    third degree T25.721 ☑
  second degree T25.629 ☑
  third degree T25.729 ☑
forearm T22.419 ☑
  first degree T22.519 ☑
  left T22.412 ☑
    first degree T22.512 ☑
    second degree T22.612 ☑

Corrosion — *continued*
forearm — *continued*
  left — *continued*
    third degree T22.712 ☑
  right T22.411 ☑
    first degree T22.511 ☑
    second degree T22.611 ☑
    third degree T22.711 ☑
  second degree T22.619 ☑
  third degree T22.719 ☑
forehead T20.46 ☑
  first degree T20.56 ☑
  second degree T20.66 ☑
  third degree T20.76 ☑
fourth degree — *code as* Corrosion, third degree, by site
full thickness skin loss — *code as* Corrosion, third degree, by site
gastrointestinal tract NEC T28.7 ☑
genital organs
  external
    female T21.47 ☑
      first degree T21.57 ☑
      second degree T21.67 ☑
      third degree T21.77 ☑
    male T21.46 ☑
      first degree T21.56 ☑
      second degree T21.66 ☑
      third degree T21.76 ☑
  internal T28.8 ☑
groin — *see* Corrosion, abdominal wall
hand(s) T23.409 ☑
  back — *see* Corrosion, dorsum of hand
  finger — *see* Corrosion, finger
  first degree T23.509 ☑
  left T23.402 ☑
    first degree T23.502 ☑
    second degree T23.602 ☑
    third degree T23.702 ☑
  multiple sites with wrist T23.499 ☑
    first degree T23.599 ☑
    left T23.492 ☑
      first degree T23.592 ☑
      second degree T23.692 ☑
      third degree T23.792 ☑
    right T23.491 ☑
      first degree T23.591 ☑
      second degree T23.691 ☑
      third degree T23.791 ☑
    second degree T23.699 ☑
    third degree T23.799 ☑
  palm — *see* Corrosion, palm
  right T23.401 ☑
    first degree T23.501 ☑
    second degree T23.601 ☑
    third degree T23.701 ☑
  second degree T23.609 ☑
  third degree T23.709 ☑
  thumb — *see* Corrosion, thumb
head (and face) (and neck) T20.40 ☑
  cheek — *see* Corrosion, cheek
  chin — *see* Corrosion, chin
  ear — *see* Corrosion, ear
  eye(s) only — *see* Corrosion, eye
  first degree T20.50 ☑
  forehead — *see* Corrosion, forehead
  lip — *see* Corrosion, lip
  multiple sites T20.49 ☑
    first degree T20.59 ☑
    second degree T20.69 ☑
    third degree T20.79 ☑
  neck — *see* Corrosion, neck
  nose — *see* Corrosion, nose
  scalp — *see* Corrosion, scalp
  second degree T20.60 ☑
  third degree T20.70 ☑
hip(s) — *see* Corrosion, lower, limb
inhalation — *see* Corrosion, respiratory tract
internal organ(s) (*see also* Corrosion, by site) T28.90 ☑
  alimentary tract T28.7 ☑
    esophagus T28.6 ☑
  esophagus T28.6 ☑
  genitourinary T28.8 ☑
  mouth T28.5 ☑
  pharynx T28.5 ☑
  specified organ NEC T28.99 ☑

Corrosion — *continued*
  interscapular region — *see* Corrosion, back, upper
  intestine (large) (small) T28.7 ☑
  knee T24.429 ☑
    first degree T24.529 ☑
    left T24.422 ☑
      first degree T24.522 ☑
      second degree T24.622 ☑
      third degree T24.722 ☑
    right T24.421 ☑
      first degree T24.521 ☑
      second degree T24.621 ☑
      third degree T24.721 ☑
    second degree T24.629 ☑
    third degree T24.729 ☑
  labium (majus) (minus) — *see* Corrosion, genital organs, external, female
  lacrimal apparatus, duct, gland or sac — *see* Corrosion, eye, specified site NEC
  larynx T27.4 ☑
    with lung T27.5 ☑
  leg(s) (meaning lower limb(s)) — *see* Corrosion, lower limb
  limb(s)
    lower — *see* Corrosion, lower, limb
    upper — *see* Corrosion, upper limb
  lip(s) T20.42 ☑
    first degree T20.52 ☑
    second degree T20.62 ☑
    third degree T20.72 ☑
  lower
    back — *see* Corrosion, back
    limb T24.409 ☑
      ankle — *see* Corrosion, ankle
      calf — *see* Corrosion, calf
      first degree T24.509 ☑
      foot — *see* Corrosion, foot
      hip — *see* Corrosion, thigh
      knee — *see* Corrosion, knee
      left T24.402 ☑
        first degree T24.502 ☑
        second degree T24.602 ☑
        third degree T24.702 ☑
      multiple sites, except ankle and foot T24.499 ☑
        ankle and foot T25.499 ☑
          first degree T25.599 ☑
          left T25.492 ☑
            first degree T25.592 ☑
            second degree T25.692 ☑
            third degree T25.792 ☑
          right T25.491 ☑
            first degree T25.591 ☑
            second degree T25.691 ☑
            third degree T25.791 ☑
          second degree T25.699 ☑
          third degree T25.799 ☑
        first degree T24.599 ☑
        left T24.492 ☑
          first degree T24.592 ☑
          second degree T24.692 ☑
          third degree T24.792 ☑
        right T24.491 ☑
          first degree T24.591 ☑
          second degree T24.691 ☑
          third degree T24.791 ☑
        second degree T24.699 ☑
        third degree T24.799 ☑
      right T24.401 ☑
        first degree T24.501 ☑
        second degree T24.601 ☑
        third degree T24.701 ☑
      second degree T24.609 ☑
      thigh — *see* Corrosion, thigh
      third degree T24.709 ☑
  lung (with larynx and trachea) T27.5 ☑
  mouth T28.5 ☑
  neck T20.47 ☑
    first degree T20.57 ☑
    second degree T20.67 ☑
    third degree T20.77 ☑
  nose (septum) T20.44 ☑
    first degree T20.54 ☑
    second degree T20.64 ☑
    third degree T20.74 ☑
  ocular adnexa — *see* Corrosion, eye
  orbit region — *see* Corrosion, eyelid

Corrosion — *continued*
  palm T23.459 ☑
    first degree T23.559 ☑
    left T23.452 ☑
      first degree T23.552 ☑
      second degree T23.652 ☑
      third degree T23.752 ☑
    right T23.451 ☑
      first degree T23.551 ☑
      second degree T23.651 ☑
      third degree T23.751 ☑
    second degree T23.659 ☑
    third degree T23.759 ☑
  partial thickness — *code as* Corrosion, unspecified degree, by site
  pelvis — *see* Corrosion, trunk
  penis — *see* Corrosion, genital organs, external, male
  perineum
    female — *see* Corrosion, genital organs, external, female
    male — *see* Corrosion, genital organs, external, male
  periocular area — *see* Corrosion, eyelid
  pharynx T28.5 ☑
  rectum T28.7 ☑
  respiratory tract T27.7 ☑
    larynx — *see* Corrosion, larynx
    specified part NEC T27.6 ☑
    trachea — *see* Corrosion, larynx
  sac, lacrimal — *see* Corrosion, eye, specified site NEC
  scalp T20.45 ☑
    first degree T20.55 ☑
    second degree T20.65 ☑
    third degree T20.75 ☑
  scapular region T22.469 ☑
    first degree T22.569 ☑
    left T22.462 ☑
      first degree T22.562 ☑
      second degree T22.662 ☑
      third degree T22.762 ☑
    right T22.461 ☑
      first degree T22.561 ☑
      second degree T22.661 ☑
      third degree T22.761 ☑
    second degree T22.669 ☑
    third degree T22.769 ☑
  sclera — *see* Corrosion, eye, specified site NEC
  scrotum — *see* Corrosion, genital organs, external, male
  shoulder T22.459 ☑
    first degree T22.559 ☑
    left T22.452 ☑
      first degree T22.552 ☑
      second degree T22.652 ☑
      third degree T22.752 ☑
    right T22.451 ☑
      first degree T22.551 ☑
      second degree T22.651 ☑
      third degree T22.751 ☑
    second degree T22.659 ☑
    third degree T22.759 ☑
  stomach T28.7 ☑
  temple — *see* Corrosion, head
  testis — *see* Corrosion, genital organs, external, male
  thigh T24.419 ☑
    first degree T24.519 ☑
    left T24.412 ☑
      first degree T24.512 ☑
      second degree T24.612 ☑
      third degree T24.712 ☑
    right T24.411 ☑
      first degree T24.511 ☑
      second degree T24.611 ☑
      third degree T24.711 ☑
    second degree T24.619 ☑
    third degree T24.719 ☑
  thorax (external) — *see* Corrosion, trunk
  throat (meaning pharynx) T28.5 ☑
  thumb(s) T23.419 ☑
    first degree T23.519 ☑
    left T23.412 ☑
      first degree T23.512 ☑
      second degree T23.612 ☑
      third degree T23.712 ☑

Corrosion — *continued*
  thumb(s) — *continued*
    multiple sites with fingers T23.449 ☑
      first degree T23.549 ☑
      left T23.442 ☑
        first degree T23.542 ☑
        second degree T23.642 ☑
        third degree T23.742 ☑
      right T23.441 ☑
        first degree T23.541 ☑
        second degree T23.641 ☑
        third degree T23.741 ☑
      second degree T23.649 ☑
      third degree T23.749 ☑
    right T23.411 ☑
      first degree T23.511 ☑
      second degree T23.611 ☑
      third degree T23.711 ☑
    second degree T23.619 ☑
    third degree T23.719 ☑
  toe T25.439 ☑
    first degree T25.539 ☑
    left T25.432 ☑
      first degree T25.532 ☑
      second degree T25.632 ☑
      third degree T25.732 ☑
    right T25.431 ☑
      first degree T25.531 ☑
      second degree T25.631 ☑
      third degree T25.731 ☑
    second degree T25.639 ☑
    third degree T25.739 ☑
  tongue T28.5 ☑
  tonsil(s) T28.5 ☑
  total body — *see* Corrosion, multiple body regions
  trachea T27.4 ☑
    with lung T27.5 ☑
  trunk T21.40 ☑
    abdominal wall — *see* Corrosion, abdominal wall
    anus — *see* Corrosion, buttock
    axilla — *see* Corrosion, upper limb
    back — *see* Corrosion, back
    breast — *see* Corrosion, chest wall
    buttock — *see* Corrosion, buttock
    chest wall — *see* Corrosion, chest wall
    first degree T21.50 ☑
    flank — *see* Corrosion, abdominal wall
    genital
      female — *see* Corrosion, genital organs, external, female
      male — *see* Corrosion, genital organs, external, male
    groin — *see* Corrosion, abdominal wall
    interscapular region — *see* Corrosion, back, upper
    labia — *see* Corrosion, genital organs, external, female
    lower back — *see* Corrosion, back
    penis — *see* Corrosion, genital organs, external, male
    perineum
      female — *see* Corrosion, genital organs, external, female
      male — *see* Corrosion, genital organs, external, male
    scapular region — *see* Corrosion, upper limb
    scrotum — *see* Corrosion, genital organs, external, male
    second degree T21.60 ☑
    shoulder — *see* Corrosion, upper limb
    specified site NEC T21.49 ☑
      first degree T21.59 ☑
      second degree T21.69 ☑
      third degree T21.79 ☑
    testes — *see* Corrosion, genital organs, external, male
    third degree T21.70 ☑
    upper back — *see* Corrosion, back, upper
    vagina T28.8 ☑
    vulva — *see* Corrosion, genital organs, external, female
  unspecified site with extent of body surface involved
    specified
      less than 10 per cent T32.0
      10-19 per cent (0-9 percent third degree) T32.10
        with 10-19 percent third degree T32.11

Corrosion — *continued*
unspecified site with extent of body surface involved
specified — *continued*
20-29 per cent (0-9 percent third degree) T32.20
with
10-19 percent third degree T32.21
20-29 percent third degree T32.22
30-39 per cent (0-9 percent third degree) T32.30
with
10-19 percent third degree T32.31
20-29 percent third degree T32.32
30-39 percent third degree T32.33
40-49 per cent (0-9 percent third degree) T32.40
with
10-19 percent third degree T32.41
20-29 percent third degree T32.42
30-39 percent third degree T32.43
40-49 percent third degree T32.44
50-59 per cent (0-9 percent third degree) T32.50
with
10-19 percent third degree T32.51
20-29 percent third degree T32.52
30-39 percent third degree T32.53
40-49 percent third degree T32.54
50-59 percent third degree T32.55
60-69 per cent (0-9 percent third degree) T32.60
with
10-19 percent third degree T32.61
20-29 percent third degree T32.62
30-39 percent third degree T32.63
40-49 percent third degree T32.64
50-59 percent third degree T32.65
60-69 percent third degree T32.66
70-79 per cent (0-9 percent third degree) T32.70
with
10-19 percent third degree T32.71
20-29 percent third degree T32.72
30-39 percent third degree T32.73
40-49 percent third degree T32.74
50-59 percent third degree T32.75
60-69 percent third degree T32.76
70-79 percent third degree T32.77
80-89 per cent (0-9 percent third degree) T32.80
with
10-19 percent third degree T32.81
20-29 percent third degree T32.82
30-39 percent third degree T32.83
40-49 percent third degree T32.84
50-59 percent third degree T32.85
60-69 percent third degree T32.86
70-79 percent third degree T32.87
80-89 percent third degree T32.88
90 per cent or more (0-9 percent third degree) T32.90
with
10-19 percent third degree T32.91
20-29 percent third degree T32.92
30-39 percent third degree T32.93
40-49 percent third degree T32.94
50-59 percent third degree T32.95
60-69 percent third degree T32.96
70-79 percent third degree T32.97
80-89 percent third degree T32.98
90-99 percent third degree T32.99
upper limb (axilla) (scapular region) T22.40 ☑
above elbow — *see* Corrosion, above elbow
axilla — *see* Corrosion, axilla
elbow — *see* Corrosion, elbow
first degree T22.50 ☑
forearm — *see* Corrosion, forearm
hand — *see* Corrosion, hand
interscapular region — *see* Corrosion, back, upper
multiple sites T22.499 ☑
first degree T22.599 ☑
left T22.492 ☑
first degree T22.592 ☑
second degree T22.692 ☑
third degree T22.792 ☑
right T22.491 ☑
first degree T22.591 ☑
second degree T22.691 ☑
third degree T22.791 ☑
second degree T22.699 ☑
third degree T22.799 ☑
scapular region — *see* Corrosion, scapular region
second degree T22.60 ☑
shoulder — *see* Corrosion, shoulder
third degree T22.70 ☑

Corrosion — *continued*
upper limb — *continued*
wrist — *see* Corrosion, hand
uterus T28.8 ☑
vagina T28.8 ☑
vulva — *see* Corrosion, genital organs, external, female
wrist T23.479 ☑
first degree T23.579 ☑
left T23.472 ☑
first degree T23.572 ☑
second degree T23.672 ☑
third degree T23.772 ☑
multiple sites with hand T23.499 ☑
first degree T23.599 ☑
left T23.492 ☑
first degree T23.592 ☑
second degree T23.692 ☑
third degree T23.792 ☑
right T23.491 ☑
first degree T23.591 ☑
second degree T23.691 ☑
third degree T23.791 ☑
second degree T23.699 ☑
third degree T23.799 ☑
right T23.471 ☑
first degree T23.571 ☑
second degree T23.671 ☑
third degree T23.771 ☑
second degree T23.679 ☑
third degree T23.779 ☑
Corrosive burn — *see* Corrosion
Corsican fever — *see* Malaria
Cortical — *see* condition
Cortico-adrenal — *see* condition
Coryza (acute) J00
with grippe or influenza — *see* Influenza, with, respiratory manifestations NEC
syphilitic
congenital (chronic) A50.05
Costen's syndrome or complex M26.69
Costiveness — *see* Constipation
Costochondritis M94.0
Cot death R99
Cotard's syndrome F22
Cotia virus B08.8
Cotton wool spots (retinal) H35.81
Cotungo's disease — *see* Sciatica
Cough (affected) (chronic) (epidemic) (nervous) R05
with hemorrhage — *see* Hemoptysis
bronchial R05
with grippe or influenza — *see* Influenza, with, respiratory manifestations NEC
functional F45.8
hysterical F45.8
laryngeal, spasmodic R05
psychogenic F45.8
smokers' J41.0
tea taster's B49
Counseling (for) Z71.9
abuse NEC
perpetrator Z69.82
victim Z69.81
alcohol abuser Z71.41
family Z71.42
child abuse
nonparental
perpetrator Z69.021
victim Z69.020
parental
perpetrator Z69.011
victim Z69.010
consanguinity Z71.89
contraceptive Z30.09
dietary Z71.3
drug abuser Z71.51
family member Z71.52
family Z71.89
fertility preservation (prior to cancer therapy) (prior to removal of gonads) Z31.62
for non-attending third party Z71.0
related to sexual behavior or orientation Z70.2
genetic NEC Z31.5
health (advice) (education) (instruction) — *see* Counseling, medical
human immunodeficiency virus (HIV) Z71.7
impotence Z70.1
insulin pump use Z46.81

Counseling — *continued*
medical (for) Z71.9
boarding school resident Z59.3
consanguinity Z71.89
feared complaint and no disease found Z71.1
human immunodeficiency virus (HIV) Z71.7
institutional resident Z59.3
on behalf of another Z71.0
related to sexual behavior or orientation Z70.2
person living alone Z60.2
specified reason NEC Z71.89
natural family planning
procreative Z31.61
to avoid pregnancy Z30.02
perpetrator (of)
abuse NEC Z69.82
child abuse
non-parental Z69.021
parental Z69.011
rape NEC Z69.82
spousal abuse Z69.12
procreative NEC Z31.69
fertility preservation (prior to cancer therapy) (prior to removal of gonads) Z31.62
using natural family planning Z31.61
promiscuity Z70.1
rape victim Z69.81
religious Z71.81
sex, sexual (related to) Z70.9
attitude(s) Z70.0
behavior or orientation Z70.1
combined concerns Z70.3
non-responsiveness Z70.1
on behalf of third party Z70.2
specified reason NEC Z70.8
specified reason NEC Z71.89
spiritual Z71.81
spousal abuse (perpetrator) Z69.12
victim Z69.11
substance abuse Z71.89
alcohol Z71.41
drug Z71.51
tobacco Z71.6
tobacco use Z71.6
use (of)
insulin pump Z46.81
victim (of)
abuse Z69.81
child abuse
by parent Z69.010
non-parental Z69.020
rape NEC Z69.81
Coupled rhythm R00.8
Couvelaire syndrome or uterus (complicating delivery) O45.8X- ☑
Cowperitis — *see* Urethritis
Cowper's gland — *see* condition
Cowpox B08.010
due to vaccination T88.1 ☑
Coxa
magna M91.4- ☑
plana M91.2- ☑
valga (acquired) (*see also* Deformity, limb, specified type NEC, thigh)
congenital Q65.81
sequelae (late effect) of rickets E64.3
vara (acquired) (*see also* Deformity, limb, specified type NEC, thigh)
congenital Q65.82
sequelae (late effect) of rickets E64.3
Coxalgia, coxalgic (nontuberculous) (*see also* Pain, joint, hip)
tuberculous A18.02
Coxitis — *see* Monoarthritis, hip
Coxsackie (virus) (infection) B34.1
as cause of disease classified elsewhere B97.11
carditis B33.20
central nervous system NEC A88.8
endocarditis B33.21
enteritis A08.39
meningitis (aseptic) A87.0
myocarditis B33.22
pericarditis B33.23
pharyngitis B08.5
pleurodynia B33.0
specific disease NEC B33.8
Crabs, meaning pubic lice B85.3
Crack baby P04.41

74

☑ Additional Character Required — Refer to the Tabular List for Character Selection   ▽ Subterms under main terms may continue to next column or page

Corrosion — Crack baby

Cracked nipple N64.0
  associated with
    lactation O92.13
    pregnancy O92.11- ☑
    puerperium O92.12
Cracked tooth K03.81
Cradle cap L21.0
Craft neurosis F48.8
Cramp(s) R25.2
  abdominal — see Pain, abdominal
  bathing T75.1 ☑
  colic R10.83
    psychogenic F45.8
  due to immersion T75.1 ☑
  fireman T67.2 ☑
  heat T67.2 ☑
  immersion T75.1 ☑
  intestinal — see Pain, abdominal
    psychogenic F45.8
  leg, sleep related G47.62
  limb (lower) (upper) NEC R25.2
    sleep related G47.62
  linotypist's F48.8
    organic G25.89
  muscle (limb) (general) R25.2
    due to immersion T75.1 ☑
    psychogenic F45.8
  occupational (hand) F48.8
    organic G25.89
  salt-depletion E87.1
  sleep related, leg G47.62
  stoker's T67.2 ☑
  swimmer's T75.1 ☑
  telegrapher's F48.8
    organic G25.89
  typist's F48.8
    organic G25.89
  uterus N94.89
    menstrual — see Dysmenorrhea
  writer's F48.8
    organic G25.89
Cranial — see condition
Craniocleidodysostosis Q74.0
Craniofenestria (skull) Q75.8
Craniolacunia (skull) Q75.8
Craniopagus Q89.4
Craniopathy, metabolic M85.2
Craniopharyngeal — see condition
Craniopharyngioma D44.4
Craniorachischisis (totalis) Q00.1
Cranioschisis Q75.8
Craniostenosis Q75.0
Craniosynostosis Q75.0
Craniotabes (cause unknown) M83.8
  neonatal P96.3
  rachitic E64.3
  syphilitic A50.56
Cranium — see condition
Craw-craw — see Onchocerciasis
Creaking joint — see Derangement, joint, specified type
    NEC
Creeping
  eruption B76.9
  palsy or paralysis G12.22
Crenated tongue K14.8
Creotoxism A05.9
Crepitus
  caput Q75.8
  joint — see Derangement, joint, specified type NEC
Crescent or conus choroid, congenital Q14.3
CREST syndrome M34.1
Cretin, cretinism (congenital) (endemic) (nongoitrous)
    (sporadic) E00.9
  pelvis
    with disproportion (fetopelvic) O33.0
      causing obstructed labor O65.0
  type
    hypothyroid E00.1
    mixed E00.2
    myxedematous E00.1
    neurological E00.0
Creutzfeldt-Jakob disease or syndrome (with demen-
    tia) A81.00
  familial A81.09
  iatrogenic A81.09
  specified NEC A81.09
  sporadic A81.09

Creutzfeldt-Jakob disease or syndrome —
    continued
    variant (vCJD) A81.01
Crib death R99
Cribriform hymen Q52.3
Cri-du-chat syndrome Q93.4
Crigler-Najjar disease or syndrome E80.5
Crime, victim of Z65.4
Crimean hemorrhagic fever A98.0
Criminalism F60.2
Crisis
  abdomen R10.0
  acute reaction F43.0
  addisonian E27.2
  adrenal (cortical) E27.2
  celiac K90.0
  Dietl's N13.8
  emotional (see also Disorder, adjustment)
    acute reaction to stress F43.0
    specific to childhood and adolescence F93.8
  glaucomatocyclitic — see Glaucoma, secondary, in-
      flammation
  heart — see Failure, heart
  nitritoid I95.2
    correct substance properly administered — see
        Table of Drugs and Chemicals, by drug, ad-
        verse effect
    overdose or wrong substance given or taken —
        see Table of Drugs and Chemicals, by drug,
        poisoning
  oculogyric H51.8
    psychogenic F45.8
  Pel's (tabetic) A52.11
  psychosexual identity F64.2
  renal N28.0
  sickle-cell D57.00
    with
      acute chest syndrome D57.01
      splenic sequestration D57.02
  state (acute reaction) F43.0
  tabetic A52.11
  thyroid — see Thyrotoxicosis with thyroid storm
  thyrotoxic — see Thyrotoxicosis with thyroid storm
Crocq's disease (acrocyanosis) I73.89
Crohn's disease — see Enteritis, regional
Crooked septum, nasal J34.2
Cross syndrome E70.328
Crossbite (anterior) (posterior) M26.24
Cross-eye — see Strabismus, convergent concomitant
Croup, croupous (catarrhal) (infectious) (inflammatory)
    (nondiphtheritic) J05.0
  bronchial J20.9
  diphtheritic A36.2
  false J38.5
  spasmodic J38.5
    diphtheritic A36.2
  stridulous J38.5
    diphtheritic A36.2
Crouzon's disease Q75.1
Crowding, tooth, teeth, fully erupted M26.31
CRST syndrome M34.1
Cruchet's disease A85.8
Cruelty in children (see also Disorder, conduct)
Crural ulcer — see Ulcer, lower limb
Crush, crushed, crushing T14.8
  abdomen S38.1 ☑
  ankle S97.0- ☑
  arm (upper) (and shoulder) S47.- ☑
  axilla — see Crush, arm
  back, lower S38.1 ☑
  buttock S38.1 ☑
  cheek S07.0 ☑
  chest S28.0 ☑
  cranium S07.1 ☑
  ear S07.0 ☑
  elbow S57.0- ☑
  extremity
    lower
      ankle — see Crush, ankle
      below knee — see Crush, leg
      foot — see Crush, foot
      hip — see Crush, hip
      knee — see Crush, knee
      thigh — see Crush, thigh
      toe — see Crush, toe
    upper
      below elbow S67.9- ☑

Crush, crushed, crushing — continued
  extremity — continued
    upper — continued
      elbow — see Crush, elbow
      finger — see Crush, finger
      forearm — see Crush, forearm
      hand — see Crush, hand
      thumb — see Crush, thumb
      upper arm — see Crush, arm
      wrist — see Crush, wrist
  face S07.0 ☑
  finger(s) S67.1- ☑
    with hand (and wrist) — see Crush, hand, specified
        site NEC
    index S67.19- ☑
    little S67.19- ☑
    middle S67.19- ☑
    ring S67.19- ☑
    thumb — see Crush, thumb
  foot S97.8- ☑
    toe — see Crush, toe
  forearm S57.8- ☑
  genitalia, external
    female S38.002 ☑
      vagina S38.03 ☑
      vulva S38.03 ☑
    male S38.001 ☑
      penis S38.01 ☑
      scrotum S38.02 ☑
      testis S38.02 ☑
  hand (except fingers alone) S67.2- ☑
    with wrist S67.4- ☑
  head S07.9 ☑
    specified NEC S07.8 ☑
  heel — see Crush, foot
  hip S77.0- ☑
    with thigh S77.2- ☑
  internal organ (abdomen, chest, or pelvis) NEC T14.8
  knee S87.0- ☑
  labium (majus) (minus) S38.03 ☑
  larynx S17.0 ☑
  leg (lower) S87.8- ☑
    knee — see Crush, knee
  lip S07.0 ☑
  lower
    back S38.1 ☑
    leg — see Crush, leg
  neck S17.9 ☑
  nerve — see Injury, nerve
  nose S07.0 ☑
  pelvis S38.1 ☑
  penis S38.01 ☑
  scalp S07.8 ☑
  scapular region — see Crush, arm
  scrotum S38.02 ☑
  severe, unspecified site T14.8
  shoulder (and upper arm) — see Crush, arm
  skull S07.1 ☑
  syndrome (complication of trauma) T79.5 ☑
  testis S38.02 ☑
  thigh S77.1- ☑
    with hip S77.2- ☑
  throat S17.8 ☑
  thumb S67.0- ☑
    with hand (and wrist) — see Crush, hand, specified
        site NEC
  toe(s) S97.10- ☑
    great S97.11- ☑
    lesser S97.12- ☑
  trachea S17.0 ☑
  vagina S38.03 ☑
  vulva S38.03 ☑
  wrist S67.3- ☑
    with hand S67.4- ☑
Crusta lactea L21.0
Crusts R23.4
Crutch paralysis — see Injury, brachial plexus
**Cruveilhier-Baumgarten cirrhosis, disease or syn-
    drome** K74.69
Cruveilhier's atrophy or disease G12.8
Crying (constant) (continuous) (excessive)
  child, adolescent or adult R45.83
  infant (baby) (newborn) R68.11
Cryofibrinogenemia D89.2
Cryoglobulinemia (essential) (idiopathic) (mixed) (pri-
    mary) (purpura) (secondary) (vasculitis) D89.1

Cryoglobulinemia — *continued*
  with lung involvement D89.1 [J99]
Cryptitis (anal) (rectal) K62.89
Cryptococcosis, cryptococcus (infection) (neoformans) B45.9
  bone B45.3
  cerebral B45.0
  cutaneous B45.2
  disseminated B45.7
  generalized B45.7
  meningitis B45.1
  meningocerebralis B45.1
  osseous B45.3
  pulmonary B45.0
  skin B45.2
  specified NEC B45.8
Cryptopapillitis (anus) K62.89
Cryptophthalmos Q11.2
  syndrome Q87.0
Cryptorchid, cryptorchism, cryptorchidism Q53.9
  bilateral Q53.20
    abdominal Q53.21
    perineal Q53.22
  unilateral Q53.10
    abdominal Q53.11
    perineal Q53.12
Cryptosporidiosis A07.2
  hepatobiliary B88.8
  respiratory B88.8
Cryptostromosis J67.6
Crystalluria R82.99
Cubitus
  congenital Q68.8
  valgus (acquired) M21.0- ☑
    congenital Q68.8
    sequelae (late effect) of rickets E64.3
  varus (acquired) M21.1- ☑
    congenital Q68.8
    sequelae (late effect) of rickets E64.3
Cultural deprivation or shock Z60.3
Curling esophagus K22.4
Curling's ulcer — *see* Ulcer, peptic, acute
Curschmann (-Batten) (-Steinert) **disease or syndrome** G71.11
Curse, Ondine's — *see* Apnea, sleep
Curvature
  organ or site, congenital NEC — *see* Distortion
  penis (lateral) Q55.61
  Pott's (spinal) A18.01
  radius, idiopathic, progressive (congenital) Q74.0
  spine (acquired) (angular) (idiopathic) (incorrect) (postural) — *see* Dorsopathy, deforming
    congenital Q67.5
    due to or associated with
      Charcot-Marie-Tooth disease (*see also* subcategory M49.8) G60.0
      osteitis
        deformans M88.88
        fibrosa cystica (*see also* subcategory M49.8) E21.0
      tuberculosis (Pott's curvature) A18.01
    sequelae (late effect) of rickets E64.3
    tuberculous A18.01
Cushingoid due to steroid therapy E24.2
  correct substance properly administered — *see* Table of Drugs and Chemicals, by drug, adverse effect
  overdose or wrong substance given or taken — *see* Table of Drugs and Chemicals, by drug, poisoning
Cushing's
  syndrome or disease E24.9
    drug-induced E24.2
    iatrogenic E24.2
    pituitary-dependent E24.0
    specified NEC E24.8
  ulcer — *see* Ulcer, peptic, acute
Cusp, Carabelli — *omit code*
Cut (external) (*see also* Laceration)
  muscle — *see* Injury, muscle
Cutaneous (*see also* condition)
  hemorrhage R23.3
  larva migrans B76.9
Cutis (*see also* condition)
  hyperelastica Q82.8
    acquired L57.4
  laxa (hyperelastica) — *see* Dermatolysis
  marmorata R23.8

Cutis — *continued*
  osteosis L94.2
  pendula — *see* Dermatolysis
  rhomboidalis nuchae L57.2
  verticis gyrata Q82.8
    acquired L91.8
Cyanosis R23.0
  due to
    patent foramen botalli Q21.1
    persistent foramen ovale Q21.1
  enterogenous D74.8
  paroxysmal digital — *see* Raynaud's disease
    with gangrene I73.01
  retina, retinal H35.89
Cyanotic heart disease I24.9
  congenital Q24.9
Cycle
  anovulatory N97.0
  menstrual, irregular N92.6
Cyclencephaly Q04.9
Cyclical vomiting (*see also* Vomiting, cyclical) G43.A0
  (*following* G43.7)
  psychogenic F50.8
Cyclitis (*see also* Iridocyclitis) H20.9
  chronic — *see* Iridocyclitis, chronic
  Fuchs' heterochromic H20.81- ☑
  granulomatous — *see* Iridocyclitis, chronic
  lens-induced — *see* Iridocyclitis, lens-induced
  posterior H30.2- ☑
Cycloid personality F34.0
Cyclophoria H50.54
Cyclopia, cyclops Q87.0
Cyclopism Q87.0
Cyclosporiasis A07.4
Cyclothymia F34.0
Cyclothymic personality F34.0
Cyclotropia H50.41- ☑
Cylindroma (*see also* Neoplasm, malignant, by site)
  eccrine dermal — *see* Neoplasm, skin, benign
  skin — *see* Neoplasm, skin, benign
Cylindruria R82.99
Cynanche
  diphtheritic A36.2
  tonsillaris J36
Cynophobia F40.218
Cynorexia R63.2
Cyphosis — *see* Kyphosis
Cyprus fever — *see* Brucellosis
Cyst (colloid) (mucous) (simple) (retention)
  adenoid (infected) J35.8
  adrenal gland E27.8
    congenital Q89.1
  air, lung J98.4
  allantoic Q64.4
  alveolar process (jaw bone) M27.40
  amnion, amniotic O41.8X- ☑
  anterior
    chamber (eye) — *see* Cyst, iris
    nasopalatine K09.1
  antrum J34.1
  anus K62.89
  apical (tooth) (periodontal) K04.8
  appendix K38.8
  arachnoid, brain (acquired) G93.0
    congenital Q04.6
  arytenoid J38.7
  Baker's M71.2- ☑
    ruptured M66.0
    tuberculous A18.02
  Bartholin's gland N75.0
  bile duct (common) (hepatic) K83.5
  bladder (multiple) (trigone) N32.89
  blue dome (breast) — *see* Cyst, breast
  bone (local) NEC M85.60
    aneurysmal M85.50
      ankle M85.57- ☑
      foot M85.57- ☑
      forearm M85.53- ☑
      hand M85.54- ☑
      jaw M27.49
      lower leg M85.56- ☑
      multiple site M85.59
      neck M85.58
      rib M85.58
      shoulder M85.51- ☑
      skull M85.58
      specified site NEC M85.58

Cyst — *continued*
  bone — *continued*
    aneurysmal — *continued*
      thigh M85.55- ☑
      toe M85.57- ☑
      upper arm M85.52- ☑
      vertebra M85.58
    solitary M85.40
      ankle M85.47- ☑
      fibula M85.46- ☑
      foot M85.47- ☑
      hand M85.44- ☑
      humerus M85.42- ☑
      jaw M27.49
      neck M85.48
      pelvis M85.45- ☑
      radius M85.43- ☑
      rib M85.48
      shoulder M85.41- ☑
      skull M85.48
      specified site NEC M85.48
      tibia M85.46- ☑
      toe M85.47- ☑
      ulna M85.43- ☑
      vertebra M85.48
    specified type NEC M85.60
      ankle M85.67- ☑
      foot M85.67- ☑
      forearm M85.63- ☑
      hand M85.64- ☑
      jaw M27.40
        developmental (nonodontogenic) K09.1
        odontogenic K09.0
        latent M27.0
      lower leg M85.66- ☑
      multiple site M85.69
      neck M85.68
      rib M85.68
      shoulder M85.61- ☑
      skull M85.68
      specified site NEC M85.68
      thigh M85.65- ☑
      toe M85.67- ☑
      upper arm M85.62- ☑
      vertebra M85.68
  brain (acquired) G93.0
    congenital Q04.6
    hydatid B67.99 [G94]
    third ventricle (colloid), congenital Q04.6
  branchial (cleft) Q18.0
  branchiogenic Q18.0
  breast (benign) (blue dome) (pedunculated) (solitary) N60.0- ☑
    involution — *see* Dysplasia, mammary, specified type NEC
    sebaceous — *see* Dysplasia, mammary, specified type NEC
  broad ligament (benign) N83.8
  bronchogenic (mediastinal) (sequestration) J98.4
    congenital Q33.0
  buccal K09.8
  bulbourethral gland N36.8
  bursa, bursal NEC M71.30
    with rupture — *see* Rupture, synovium
    ankle M71.37- ☑
    elbow M71.32- ☑
    foot M71.37- ☑
    hand M71.34- ☑
    hip M71.35- ☑
    multiple sites M71.39
    pharyngeal J39.2
    popliteal space — *see* Cyst, Baker's
    shoulder M71.31- ☑
    specified site NEC M71.38
    wrist M71.33- ☑
  calcifying odontogenic D16.5
    upper jaw (bone) (maxilla) D16.4
  canal of Nuck (female) N94.89
    congenital Q52.4
  canthus — *see* Cyst, conjunctiva
  carcinomatous — *see* Neoplasm, malignant, by site
  cauda equina G95.89
  cavum septi pellucidi — *see* Cyst, brain
  celomic (pericardium) Q24.8
  cerebellopontine (angle) — *see* Cyst, brain
  cerebellum — *see* Cyst, brain
  cerebral — *see* Cyst, brain

Cyst — *continued*
- cervical lateral Q18.1
- cervix NEC N88.8
  - embryonic Q51.6
  - nabothian N88.8
- chiasmal optic NEC — *see* Disorder, optic, chiasm
- chocolate (ovary) N80.1
- choledochus, congenital Q44.4
- chorion O41.8X- ☑
- choroid plexus G93.0
- ciliary body — *see* Cyst, iris
- clitoris N90.7
- colon K63.89
- common (bile) duct K83.5
- congenital NEC Q89.8
  - adrenal gland Q89.1
  - epiglottis Q31.8
  - esophagus Q39.8
  - fallopian tube Q50.4
  - kidney Q61.00
    - more than one (multiple) Q61.02
      - specified as polycystic Q61.3
        - adult type Q61.2
        - infantile type NEC Q61.19
          - collecting duct dilation Q61.11
    - solitary Q61.01
  - larynx Q31.8
  - liver Q44.6
  - lung Q33.0
  - mediastinum Q34.1
  - ovary Q50.1
  - oviduct Q50.4
  - periurethral (tissue) Q64.79
  - prepuce Q55.69
  - salivary gland (any) Q38.4
  - sublingual Q38.6
  - submaxillary gland Q38.6
  - thymus (gland) Q89.2
  - tongue Q38.3
  - ureterovesical orifice Q62.8
  - vulva Q52.79
- conjunctiva H11.44- ☑
- cornea H18.89- ☑
- corpora quadrigemina G93.0
- corpus
  - albicans N83.29
  - luteum (hemorrhagic) (ruptured) N83.1
- Cowper's gland (benign) (infected) N36.8
- cranial meninges G93.0
- craniobuccal pouch E23.6
- craniopharyngeal pouch E23.6
- cystic duct K82.8
- Cysticercus — *see* Cysticercosis
- Dandy-Walker Q03.1
  - with spina bifida — *see* Spina bifida
- dental (root) K04.8
  - developmental K09.0
  - eruption K09.0
  - primordial K09.0
- dentigerous (mandible) (maxilla) K09.0
- dermoid — *see* Neoplasm, benign, by site
  - with malignant transformation C56.- ☑
  - implantation
    - external area or site (skin) NEC L72.0
    - iris — *see* Cyst, iris, implantation
    - vagina N89.8
    - vulva N90.7
  - mouth K09.8
  - oral soft tissue K09.8
  - sacrococcygeal — *see* Cyst, pilonidal
- developmental K09.1
  - odontogenic K09.0
  - oral region (nonodontogenic) K09.1
  - ovary, ovarian Q50.1
- dura (cerebral) G93.0
  - spinal G96.19
- ear (external) Q18.1
- echinococcal — *see* Echinococcus
- embryonic
  - cervix uteri Q51.6
  - fallopian tube Q50.4
  - vagina Q51.6
- endometrium, endometrial (uterus) N85.8
  - ectopic — *see* Endometriosis
- enterogenous Q43.8
- epidermal, epidermoid (inclusion) (*see also* Cyst, skin) L72.0
  - mouth K09.8

Cyst — *continued*
- epidermal, epidermoid (*see also* Cyst, skin) — *continued*
  - oral soft tissue K09.8
- epididymis N50.3
- epiglottis J38.7
- epiphysis cerebri E34.8
- epithelial (inclusion) L72.0
- epoophoron Q50.5
- eruption K09.0
- esophagus K22.8
- ethmoid sinus J34.1
- external female genital organs NEC N90.7
- eyelid (sebaceous) H02.829
  - infected — *see* Hordeolum
  - left H02.826
    - lower H02.825
    - upper H02.824
  - right H02.823
    - lower H02.822
    - upper H02.821
- eye NEC H57.8
  - congenital Q15.8
- fallopian tube N83.8
  - congenital Q50.4
- fimbrial (twisted) Q50.4
- fissural (oral region) K09.1
- follicle (graafian) (hemorrhagic) N83.0
  - nabothian N88.8
- follicular (atretic) (hemorrhagic) (ovarian) N83.0
  - dentigerous K09.0
  - odontogenic K09.0
  - skin L72.9
    - specified NEC L72.8
- frontal sinus J34.1
- gallbladder K82.8
- ganglion — *see* Ganglion
- Gartner's duct Q52.4
- gingiva K09.0
- gland of Moll — *see* Cyst, eyelid
- globulomaxillary K09.1
- graafian follicle (hemorrhagic) N83.0
- granulosal lutein (hemorrhagic) N83.1
- hemangiomatous D18.00
  - intra-abdominal D18.03
  - intracranial D18.02
  - skin D18.01
  - specified site NEC D18.09
- hydatid (*see also* Echinococcus) B67.90
  - brain B67.99 [G94]
  - liver (*see also* Cyst, liver, hydatid) B67.8
  - lung NEC B67.99 [J99]
  - Morgagni
    - female Q50.5
    - male (epididymal) Q55.4
      - testicular Q55.29
  - specified site NEC B67.99
- hymen N89.8
  - embryonic Q52.4
- hypopharynx J39.2
- hypophysis, hypophyseal (duct) (recurrent) E23.6
  - cerebri E23.6
- implantation (dermoid)
  - external area or site (skin) NEC L72.0
  - iris — *see* Cyst, iris, implantation
  - vagina N89.8
  - vulva N90.7
- incisive canal K09.1
- inclusion (epidermal) (epithelial) (epidermoid) (squamous) L72.0
  - not of skin — *code under* Cyst, by site
- intestine (large) (small) K63.89
- intracranial — *see* Cyst, brain
- intraligamentous (*see also* Disorder, ligament)
  - knee — *see* Derangement, knee
- intrasellar E23.6
- iris H21.309
  - exudative H21.31- ☑
  - idiopathic H21.30- ☑
  - implantation H21.32- ☑
  - parasitic H21.33- ☑
  - pars plana (primary) H21.34- ☑
    - exudative H21.35- ☑
- jaw (bone) M27.40
  - aneurysmal M27.49
  - developmental (odontogenic) K09.0
  - fissural K09.1
  - hemorrhagic M27.49

Cyst — *continued*
- jaw — *continued*
  - traumatic M27.49
- joint NEC — *see* Disorder, joint, specified type NEC
- kidney (acquired) N28.1
  - calyceal — *see* Hydronephrosis
  - congenital Q61.00
    - more than one (multiple) Q61.02
      - specified as polycystic Q61.3
        - adult type (autosomal dominant) Q61.2
        - infantile type (autosomal recessive) NEC Q61.19
          - collecting duct dilation Q61.11
  - pyelogenic — *see* Hydronephrosis
  - simple N28.1
  - solitary (single) Q61.01
    - acquired N28.1
- labium (majus) (minus) N90.7
  - sebaceous N90.7
- lacrimal (*see also* Disorder, lacrimal system, specified NEC)
  - gland H04.13- ☑
  - passages or sac — *see* Disorder, lacrimal system, specified NEC
- larynx J38.7
- lateral periodontal K09.0
- lens H27.8
  - congenital Q12.8
- lip (gland) K13.0
- liver (idiopathic) (simple) K76.89
  - congenital Q44.6
  - hydatid B67.8
    - granulosus B67.0
    - multilocularis B67.5
- lung J98.4
  - congenital Q33.0
  - giant bullous J43.9
- lutein N83.1
- lymphangiomatous D18.1
- lymphoepithelial, oral soft tissue K09.8
- macula — *see* Degeneration, macula, hole
- malignant — *see* Neoplasm, malignant, by site
- mammary gland — *see* Cyst, breast
- mandible M27.40
  - dentigerous K09.0
  - radicular K04.8
- maxilla M27.40
  - dentigerous K09.0
  - radicular K04.8
- medial, face and neck Q18.8
- median
  - anterior maxillary K09.1
  - palatal K09.1
- mediastinum, congenital Q34.1
- meibomian (gland) — *see* Chalazion
  - infected — *see* Hordeolum
- membrane, brain G93.0
- meninges (cerebral) G93.0
  - spinal G96.19
- meniscus, knee — *see* Derangement, knee, meniscus, cystic
- mesentery, mesenteric K66.8
  - chyle I89.8
- mesonephric duct
  - female Q50.5
  - male Q55.4
- milk N64.89
- Morgagni (hydatid)
  - female Q50.5
  - male (epididymal) Q55.4
    - testicular Q55.29
- mouth K09.8
- Müllerian duct Q50.4
  - appendix testis Q55.29
  - cervix Q51.6
  - fallopian tube Q50.4
  - female Q50.4
  - male Q55.29
  - prostatic utricle Q55.4
  - vagina (embryonal) Q52.4
- multilocular (ovary) D39.10
  - benign — *see* Neoplasm, benign, by site
- myometrium N85.8
- nabothian (follicle) (ruptured) N88.8
- nasoalveolar K09.1
- nasolabial K09.1
- nasopalatine (anterior) (duct) K09.1
- nasopharynx J39.2

▽ **Subterms under main terms may continue to next column or page**   ☑ **Additional Character Required — Refer to the Tabular List for Character Selection**   **77**

Cyst—Cyst

Cyst — *continued*

neoplastic — *see* Neoplasm, uncertain behavior, by site
benign — *see* Neoplasm, benign, by site
nervous system NEC G96.8
neuroenteric (congenital) Q06.8
nipple — *see* Cyst, breast
nose (turbinates) J34.1
sinus J34.1
odontogenic, developmental K09.0
omentum (lesser) K66.8
congenital Q45.8
ora serrata — *see* Cyst, retina, ora serrata
oral
region K09.9
developmental (nonodontogenic) K09.1
specified NEC K09.8
soft tissue K09.9
specified NEC K09.8
orbit H05.81- ☑
ovary, ovarian (twisted) N83.20
adherent N83.20
chocolate N80.1
corpus
albicans N83.29
luteum (hemorrhagic) N83.1
dermoid D27.9
developmental Q50.1
due to failure of involution NEC N83.20
endometrial N80.1
follicular (graafian) (hemorrhagic) N83.0
hemorrhagic N83.20
in pregnancy or childbirth O34.8- ☑
with obstructed labor O65.5
multilocular D39.10
pseudomucinous D27.9
retention N83.29
serous N83.20
specified NEC N83.29
theca lutein (hemorrhagic) N83.1
tuberculous A18.18
oviduct N83.8
palate (median) (fissural) K09.1
palatine papilla (jaw) K09.1
pancreas, pancreatic (hemorrhagic) (true) K86.2
congenital Q45.2
false K86.3
paralabral
hip M24.85- ☑
shoulder S43.43- ☑
paramesonephric duct Q50.4
female Q50.4
male Q55.29
paranephric N28.1
paraphysis, cerebri, congenital Q04.6
parasitic B89
parathyroid (gland) E21.4
paratubal N83.8
paraurethral duct N36.8
paroophoron Q50.5
parotid gland K11.6
parovarian Q50.5
pelvis, female N94.89
in pregnancy or childbirth O34.8- ☑
causing obstructed labor O65.5
penis (sebaceous) N48.89
periapical K04.8
pericardial (congenital) Q24.8
acquired (secondary) I31.8
pericoronal K09.0
periodontal K04.8
lateral K09.0
peripelvic (lymphatic) N28.1
peritoneum K66.8
chylous I89.8
periventricular, acquired, newborn P91.1
pharynx (wall) J39.2
pilar L72.11
pilonidal (infected) (rectum) L05.91
with abscess L05.01
malignant C44.59- ☑
pituitary (duct) (gland) E23.6
placenta O43.19- ☑
pleura J94.8
popliteal — *see* Cyst, Baker's
porencephalic Q04.6
acquired G93.0
postanal (infected) — *see* Cyst, pilonidal

Cyst — *continued*

postmastoidectomy cavity (mucosal) — *see* Complications, postmastoidectomy, cyst
preauricular Q18.1
prepuce N47.4
congenital Q55.69
primordial (jaw) K09.0
prostate N42.83
pseudomucinous (ovary) D27.9
pupillary, miotic H21.27- ☑
radicular (residual) K04.8
radiculodental K04.8
ranular K11.8
Rathke's pouch E23.6
rectum (epithelium) (mucous) K62.89
renal — *see* Cyst, kidney
residual (radicular) K04.8
retention (ovary) N83.29
salivary gland K11.6
retina H33.19- ☑
ora serrata H33.11- ☑
parasitic H33.12- ☑
retroperitoneal K68.9
sacrococcygeal (dermoid) — *see* Cyst, pilonidal
salivary gland or duct (mucous extravasation or retention) K11.6
Sampson's N80.1
sclera H15.89
scrotum L72.9
sebaceous L72.3
sebaceous (duct) (gland) L72.3
breast — *see* Dysplasia, mammary, specified type NEC
eyelid — *see* Cyst, eyelid
genital organ NEC
female N94.89
male N50.8
scrotum L72.3
semilunar cartilage (knee) (multiple) — *see* Derangement, knee, meniscus, cystic
seminal vesicle N50.8
serous (ovary) N83.20
sinus (accessory) (nasal) J34.1
Skene's gland N36.8
skin L72.9
breast — *see* Dysplasia, mammary, specified type NEC
epidermal, epidermoid L72.0
epithelial L72.0
eyelid — *see* Cyst, eyelid
genital organ NEC
female N90.7
male N50.8
inclusion L72.0
scrotum L72.9
sebaceous L72.3
sweat gland or duct L74.8
solitary
bone — *see* Cyst, bone, solitary
jaw M27.40
kidney N28.1
spermatic cord N50.8
sphenoid sinus J34.1
spinal meninges G96.19
spleen NEC D73.4
congenital Q89.09
hydatid (*see also* Echinococcus) B67.99 [D77]
Stafne's M27.0
subarachnoid intrasellar R93.0
subcutaneous, pheomycotic (chromomycotic) B43.2
subdural (cerebral) G93.0
spinal cord G96.19
sublingual gland K11.6
submandibular gland K11.6
submaxillary gland K11.6
suburethral N36.8
suprarenal gland E27.8
suprasellar — *see* Cyst, brain
sweat gland or duct L74.8
synovial (*see also* Cyst, bursa)
ruptured — *see* Rupture, synovium
tarsal — *see* Chalazion
tendon (sheath) — *see* Disorder, tendon, specified type NEC
testis N44.2
tunica albuginea N44.1
theca lutein (ovary) N83.1
Thornwaldt's J39.2

Cyst — *continued*

thymus (gland) E32.8
thyroglossal duct (infected) (persistent) Q89.2
thyroid (gland) E04.1
thyrolingual duct (infected) (persistent) Q89.2
tongue K14.8
tonsil J35.8
tooth — *see* Cyst, dental
Tornwaldt's J39.2
trichilemmal (proliferating) L72.12
trichodermal L72.12
tubal (fallopian) N83.8
inflammatory — *see* Salpingitis, chronic
tubo-ovarian N83.8
inflammatory N70.13
tunica
albuginea testis N44.1
vaginalis N50.8
turbinate (nose) J34.1
Tyson's gland N48.89
urachus, congenital Q64.4
ureter N28.89
ureterovesical orifice N28.89
urethra, urethral (gland) N36.8
uterine ligament N83.8
uterus (body) (corpus) (recurrent) N85.8
embryonic Q51.818
cervix Q51.6
vagina, vaginal (implantation) (inclusion) (squamous cell) (wall) N89.8
embryonic Q52.4
vallecula, vallecular (epiglottis) J38.7
vesical (orifice) N32.89
vitreous body H43.89
vulva (implantation) (inclusion) N90.7
congenital Q52.79
sebaceous gland N90.7
vulvovaginal gland N90.7
wolffian
female Q50.5
male Q55.4

Cystadenocarcinoma — *see* Neoplasm, malignant, by site
bile duct C22.1
endometrioid — *see* Neoplasm, malignant, by site
specified site — *see* Neoplasm, malignant, by site
unspecified site
female C56.9
male C61
mucinous
papillary
specified site — *see* Neoplasm, malignant, by site
unspecified site C56.9
specified site — *see* Neoplasm, malignant, by site
unspecified site C56.9
papillary
mucinous
specified site — *see* Neoplasm, malignant, by site
unspecified site C56.9
pseudomucinous
specified site — *see* Neoplasm, malignant, by site
unspecified site C56.9
serous
specified site — *see* Neoplasm, malignant, by site
unspecified site C56.9
specified site — *see* Neoplasm, malignant, by site
unspecified site C56.9
pseudomucinous
papillary
specified site — *see* Neoplasm, malignant, by site
unspecified site C56.9
specified site — *see* Neoplasm, malignant, by site
unspecified site C56.9
serous
papillary
specified site — *see* Neoplasm, malignant, by site
unspecified site C56.9
specified site — *see* Neoplasm, malignant, by site
unspecified site C56.9

Cystadenofibroma
clear cell — *see* Neoplasm, benign, by site
endometrioid D27.9

☑ Additional Character Required — Refer to the Tabular List for Character Selection

Subterms under main terms may continue to next column or page

Cystadenofibroma — *continued*
  endometrioid D27.9
    borderline malignancy D39.1- ☑
    malignant C56.- ☑
  mucinous
    specified site — *see* Neoplasm, benign, by site
    unspecified site D27.9
  serous
    specified site — *see* Neoplasm, benign, by site
    unspecified site D27.9
  specified site — *see* Neoplasm, benign, by site
  unspecified site D27.9
Cystadenoma (*see also* Neoplasm, benign, by site)
  bile duct D13.4
  endometrioid — *see* Neoplasm, benign, by site
    borderline malignancy — *see* Neoplasm, uncertain behavior, by site
  malignant — *see* Neoplasm, malignant, by site
  mucinous
    borderline malignancy
      ovary C56.- ☑
      specified site NEC — *see* Neoplasm, uncertain behavior, by site
      unspecified site C56.9
    papillary
      borderline malignancy
        ovary C56.- ☑
        specified site NEC — *see* Neoplasm, uncertain behavior, by site
        unspecified site C56.9
      specified site — *see* Neoplasm, benign, by site
      unspecified site D27.9
    specified site — *see* Neoplasm, benign, by site
    unspecified site D27.9
  papillary
    borderline malignancy
      ovary C56.- ☑
      specified site NEC — *see* Neoplasm, uncertain behavior, by site
      unspecified site C56.9
    lymphomatosum
      specified site — *see* Neoplasm, benign, by site
      unspecified site D11.9
    mucinous
      borderline malignancy
        ovary C56.- ☑
        specified site NEC — *see* Neoplasm, uncertain behavior, by site
        unspecified site C56.9
      specified site — *see* Neoplasm, benign, by site
      unspecified site D27.9
    pseudomucinous
      borderline malignancy
        ovary C56.- ☑
        specified site NEC — *see* Neoplasm, uncertain behavior, by site
        unspecified site C56.9
      specified site — *see* Neoplasm, benign, by site
      unspecified site D27.9
    serous
      borderline malignancy
        ovary C56.- ☑
        specified site NEC — *see* Neoplasm, uncertain behavior, by site
        unspecified site C56.9
      specified site — *see* Neoplasm, benign, by site
      unspecified site D27.9
    pseudomucinous
      borderline malignancy
        ovary C56.- ☑
        specified site NEC — *see* Neoplasm, uncertain behavior, by site
        unspecified site C56.9
      papillary
        borderline malignancy
          ovary C56.- ☑
          specified site NEC — *see* Neoplasm, uncertain behavior, by site
          unspecified site C56.9
        specified site — *see* Neoplasm, benign, by site
        unspecified site D27.9
      specified site — *see* Neoplasm, benign, by site

Cystadenoma — *continued*
  pseudomucinous — *continued*
    unspecified site D27.9
  serous
    borderline malignancy
      ovary C56.- ☑
      specified site NEC — *see* Neoplasm, uncertain behavior, by site
      unspecified site C56.9
    papillary
      borderline malignancy
        ovary C56.- ☑
        specified site NEC — *see* Neoplasm, uncertain behavior, by site
        unspecified site C56.9
      specified site — *see* Neoplasm, benign, by site
      unspecified site D27.9
    specified site — *see* Neoplasm, benign, by site
    unspecified site D27.9
Cystathionine synthase deficiency E72.11
Cystathioninemia E72.19
Cystathioninuria E72.19
Cystic (*see also* condition)
  breast (chronic) — *see* Mastopathy, cystic
  corpora lutea (hemorrhagic) N83.1
  duct — *see* condition
  eyeball (congenital) Q11.0
  fibrosis — *see* Fibrosis, cystic
  kidney (congenital) Q61.9
    adult type Q61.2
    infantile type NEC Q61.19
      collecting duct dilatation Q61.11
    medullary Q61.5
  liver, congenital Q44.6
  lung disease J98.4
    congenital Q33.0
  mastitis, chronic — *see* Mastopathy, cystic
  medullary, kidney Q61.5
  meniscus — *see* Derangement, knee, meniscus, cystic
  ovary N83.20
Cysticercosis, cysticerciasis B69.9
  with
    epileptiform fits B69.0
    myositis B69.81
  brain B69.0
  central nervous system B69.0
  cerebral B69.0
  ocular B69.1
  specified NEC B69.89
Cysticercus cellulose infestation — *see* Cysticercosis
Cystinosis (malignant) E72.04
Cystinuria E72.01
Cystitis (exudative) (hemorrhagic) (septic) (suppurative) N30.90
  with
    fibrosis — *see* Cystitis, chronic, interstitial
    hematuria N30.91
    leukoplakia — *see* Cystitis, chronic, interstitial
    malakoplakia — *see* Cystitis, chronic, interstitial
    metaplasia — *see* Cystitis, chronic, interstitial
    prostatitis N41.3
  acute N30.00
    with hematuria N30.01
    of trigone N30.30
      with hematuria N30.31
  allergic — *see* Cystitis, specified type NEC
  amebic A06.81
  bilharzial B65.9 [N33]
  blennorrhagic (gonococcal) A54.01
  bullous — *see* Cystitis, specified type NEC
  calculous N21.0
  chlamydial A56.01
  chronic N30.20
    with hematuria N30.21
    interstitial N30.10
      with hematuria N30.11
    of trigone N30.30
      with hematuria N30.31
    specified NEC N30.20
      with hematuria N30.21
  cystic (a) — *see* Cystitis, specified type NEC
  diphtheritic A36.85
  echinococcal
    granulosus B67.39

Cystitis — *continued*
  echinococcal — *continued*
    multilocularis B67.69
  emphysematous — *see* Cystitis, specified type NEC
  encysted — *see* Cystitis, specified type NEC
  eosinophilic — *see* Cystitis, specified type NEC
  follicular — *see* Cystitis, of trigone
  gangrenous — *see* Cystitis, specified type NEC
  glandularis — *see* Cystitis, specified type NEC
  gonococcal A54.01
  incrusted — *see* Cystitis, specified type NEC
  interstitial (chronic) — *see* Cystitis, chronic, interstitial
  irradiation N30.40
    with hematuria N30.41
  irritation — *see* Cystitis, specified type NEC
  malignant — *see* Cystitis, specified type NEC
  of trigone N30.30
    with hematuria N30.31
  panmural — *see* Cystitis, chronic, interstitial
  polyposa — *see* Cystitis, specified type NEC
  prostatic N41.3
  puerperal (postpartum) O86.22
  radiation — *see* Cystitis, irradiation
  specified type NEC N30.80
    with hematuria N30.81
  subacute — *see* Cystitis, chronic
  submucous — *see* Cystitis, chronic, interstitial
  syphilitic (late) A52.76
  trichomonal A59.03
  tuberculous A18.12
  ulcerative — *see* Cystitis, chronic, interstitial
Cystocele (-urethrocele)
  female N81.10
    with prolapse of uterus — *see* Prolapse, uterus
    lateral N81.12
    midline N81.11
    paravaginal N81.12
  in pregnancy or childbirth O34.8- ☑
    causing obstructed labor O65.5
  male N32.89
Cystolithiasis N21.0
Cystoma (*see also* Neoplasm, benign, by site)
  endometrial, ovary N80.1
  mucinous
    specified site — *see* Neoplasm, benign, by site
    unspecified site D27.9
  serous
    specified site — *see* Neoplasm, benign, by site
    unspecified site D27.9
  simple (ovary) N83.29
Cystoplegia N31.2
Cystoptosis N32.89
Cystopyelitis — *see* Pyelonephritis
Cystorrhagia N32.89
Cystosarcoma phyllodes D48.6- ☑
  benign D24- ☑
  malignant — *see* Neoplasm, breast, malignant
Cystostomy
  attention to Z43.5
  complication — *see* Complications, cystostomy
  status Z93.50
    appendico-vesicostomy Z93.52
    cutaneous Z93.51
    specified NEC Z93.59
Cystourethritis — *see* Urethritis
Cystourethrocele (*see also* Cystocele)
  female N81.10
    with uterine prolapse — *see* Prolapse, uterus
    lateral N81.12
    midline N81.11
    paravaginal N81.12
  male N32.89
Cytomegalic inclusion disease
  congenital P35.1
Cytomegalovirus infection B25.9
Cytomycosis (reticuloendothelial) B39.4
Cytopenia D75.9
  refractory
    with multilineage dysplasia D46.A (*following* D46.2)
    and ring sideroblasts (RCMD RS) D46.B (*following* D46.2)
Czerny's disease (periodic hydrarthrosis of the knee) — *see* Effusion, joint, knee

D

Da Costa's syndrome F45.8
Daae (-Finsen) **disease** (epidemic pleurodynia) B33.0
Dabney's grip B33.0
Dacryoadenitis, dacryadenitis H04.00- ☑
  acute H04.01- ☑
  chronic H04.02- ☑
Dacryocystitis H04.30- ☑
  acute H04.32- ☑
  chronic H04.41- ☑
  neonatal P39.1
  phlegmonous H04.31- ☑
  syphilitic A52.71
    congenital (early) A50.01
  trachomatous, active A71.1
    sequelae (late effect) B94.0
Dacryocystoblenorrhea — *see* Inflammation, lacrimal, passages, chronic
Dacryocystocele — *see* Disorder, lacrimal system, changes
Dacryolith, dacryolithiasis H04.51- ☑
Dacryoma — *see* Disorder, lacrimal system, changes
Dacryopericystitis — *see* Dacryocystitis
Dacryops H04.11- ☑
Dacryostenosis (*see also* Stenosis, lacrimal)
  congenital Q10.5
Dactylitis
  bone — *see* Osteomyelitis
  sickle-cell D57.00
    Hb C D57.219
    Hb SS D57.00
    specified NEC D57.819
  skin L08.9
  syphilitic A52.77
  tuberculous A18.03
Dactylolysis spontanea (ainhum) L94.6
Dactylosymphysis Q70.9
  fingers — *see* Syndactylism, complex, fingers
  toes — *see* Syndactylism, complex, toes
Damage
  arteriosclerotic — *see* Arteriosclerosis
  brain (nontraumatic) G93.9
    anoxic, hypoxic G93.1
      resulting from a procedure G97.82
    child NEC G80.9
    due to birth injury P11.2
  cardiorenal (vascular) — *see* Hypertension, cardiorenal
  cerebral NEC — *see* Damage, brain
  coccyx, complicating delivery O71.6
  coronary — *see* Disease, heart, ischemic
  eye, birth injury P15.3
  liver (nontraumatic) K76.9
    alcoholic K70.9
    due to drugs — *see* Disease, liver, toxic
    toxic — *see* Disease, liver, toxic
  medication T88.7 ☑
  pelvic
    joint or ligament, during delivery O71.6
    organ NEC
      during delivery O71.5
      following ectopic or molar pregnancy O08.6
  renal — *see* Disease, renal
  subendocardium, subendocardial — *see* Degeneration, myocardial
  vascular I99.9
Dana-Putnam syndrome (subacute combined sclerosis with pernicious anemia) — *see* Degeneration, combined
Danbolt (-Cross) **syndrome** (acrodermatitis enteropathica) E83.2
Dandruff L21.0
Dandy-Walker syndrome Q03.1
  with spina bifida — *see* Spina bifida
Danlos' syndrome Q79.6
Darier (-White) **disease** (congenital) Q82.8
  meaning erythema annulare centrifugum L53.1
Darier-Roussy sarcoid D86.3
Darling's disease or histoplasmosis B39.4
Darwin's tubercle Q17.8

Dawson's (inclusion body) **encephalitis** A81.1
De Beurmann (-Gougerot) **disease** B42.1
De la Tourette's syndrome F95.2
De Lange's syndrome Q87.1
De Morgan's spots (senile angiomas) I78.1
De Quervain's
  disease (tendon sheath) M65.4
  syndrome E34.51
  thyroiditis (subacute granulomatous thyroiditis) E06.1
De Toni-Fanconi (-Debré) **syndrome** E72.09
  with cystinosis E72.04
Dead
  fetus, retained (mother) O36.4 ☑
    early pregnancy O02.1
  labyrinth H83.2 ☑
  ovum, retained O02.0
Deaf nonspeaking NEC H91.3
Deafmutism (acquired) (congenital) NEC H91.3
  hysterical F44.6
  syphilitic, congenital (*see also* subcategory) H94.8
    A50.09
Deafness (acquired) (complete) (hereditary) (partial) H91.9-
  with blue sclera and fragility of bone Q78.0
  auditory fatigue — *see* Deafness, specified type NEC
  aviation T70.0 ☑
    nerve injury — *see* Injury, nerve, acoustic, specified type NEC
  boilermaker's H83.3 ☑
  central — *see* Deafness, sensorineural
  conductive H90.2
    and sensorineural, mixed H90.8
      bilateral H90.6
    bilateral H90.0
    unilateral H90.1- ☑
  congenital H90.5
    with blue sclera and fragility of bone Q78.0
  due to toxic agents — *see* Deafness, ototoxic
  emotional (hysterical) F44.6
  functional (hysterical) F44.6
  high frequency H91.9- ☑
  hysterical F44.6
  low frequency H91.9- ☑
  mental R48.8
  mixed conductive and sensorineural H90.8
    bilateral H90.6
    unilateral H90.7- ☑
  nerve — *see* Deafness, sensorineural
  neural — *see* Deafness, sensorineural
  noise-induced (*see also* subcategory) H83.3 ☑
    nerve injury — *see* Injury, nerve, acoustic, specified type NEC
  nonspeaking H91.3
  ototoxic H91.0 ☑
  perceptive — *see* Deafness, sensorineural
  psychogenic (hysterical) F44.6
  sensorineural H90.5
    and conductive, mixed H90.8
      bilateral H90.6
    bilateral H90.3
    unilateral H90.4- ☑
  sensory — *see* Deafness, sensorineural
  specified type NEC H91.8 ☑
  sudden (idiopathic) H91.2- ☑
  syphilitic A52.15
  transient ischemic H93.01- ☑
  traumatic — *see* Injury, nerve, acoustic, specified type NEC
  word (developmental) H93.25
Death (cause unknown) (of) (unexplained) (unspecified cause) R99
  brain G93.82
  cardiac (sudden) (with successful resuscitation) — *code to* underlying disease
    family history of Z82.41
    personal history of Z86.74
  family member (assumed) Z63.4
Debility (chronic) (general) (nervous) R53.81
  congenital or neonatal NOS P96.9
  nervous R53.81
  old age R54
  senile R54

Débove's disease (splenomegaly) R16.1
Decalcification
  bone — *see* Osteoporosis
  teeth K03.89
Decapsulation, kidney N28.89
Decay
  dental — *see* Caries, dental
  senile R54
  tooth, teeth — *see* Caries, dental
Deciduitis (acute)
  following ectopic or molar pregnancy O08.0
Decline (general) — *see* Debility
  cognitive, age-associated R41.81
Decompensation
  cardiac (acute) (chronic) — *see* Disease, heart
  cardiovascular — *see* Disease, cardiovascular
  heart — *see* Disease, heart
  hepatic — *see* Failure, hepatic
  myocardial (acute) (chronic) — *see* Disease, heart
  respiratory J98.8
Decompression sickness T70.3 ☑
Decrease (d)
  absolute neutrophile count — *see* Neutropenia
  blood
    platelets — *see* Thrombocytopenia
    pressure R03.1
      due to shock following
        injury T79.4 ☑
        operation T81.19 ☑
  estrogen E28.39
    postablative E89.40
      asymptomatic E89.40
      symptomatic E89.41
  fragility of erythrocytes D58.8
  function
    lipase (pancreatic) K90.3
    ovary in hypopituitarism E23.0
    parenchyma of pancreas K86.8
    pituitary (gland) (anterior) (lobe) E23.0
      posterior (lobe) E23.0
  functional activity R68.89
  glucose R73.09
  hematocrit R71.0
  hemoglobin R71.0
  leukocytes D72.819
    specified NEC D72.818
  libido R68.82
  lymphocytes D72.810
  platelets D69.6
  respiration, due to shock following injury T79.4 ☑
  sexual desire R68.82
  tear secretion NEC — *see* Syndrome, dry eye
  tolerance
    fat K90.4
    glucose R73.09
    pancreatic K90.3
    salt and water E87.8
  vision NEC H54.7
  white blood cell count D72.819
    specified NEC D72.818
Decubitus (ulcer) — *see* Ulcer, pressure, by site
  cervix N86
Deepening acetabulum — *see* Derangement, joint, specified type NEC, hip
Defect, defective Q89.9
  3-beta-hydroxysteroid dehydrogenase E25.0
  11-hydroxylase E25.0
  21-hydroxylase E25.0
  abdominal wall, congenital Q79.59
  antibody immunodeficiency D80.9
  aorticopulmonary septum Q21.4
  atrial septal (ostium secundum type) Q21.1
    following acute myocardial infarction (current complication) I23.1
    ostium primum type Q21.2
  atrioventricular
    canal Q21.2
    septum Q21.2
  auricular septal Q21.1
  bilirubin excretion NEC E80.6
  biosynthesis, androgen (testicular) E29.1
  bulbar septum Q21.0

80

☑ Additional Character Required — Refer to the Tabular List for Character Selection   ▽ Subterms under main terms may continue to next column or page

Defect, defective — *continued*
- catalase E80.3
- cell membrane receptor complex (CR3) D71
- circulation I99.9
  - congenital Q28.9
  - newborn Q28.9
- coagulation (factor) (*see also* Deficiency, factor) D68.9
  - with
    - ectopic pregnancy O08.1
    - molar pregnancy O08.1
  - acquired D68.4
  - antepartum with hemorrhage — *see* Hemorrhage, antepartum, with coagulation defect
  - due to
    - liver disease D68.4
    - vitamin K deficiency D68.4
  - hereditary NEC D68.2
  - intrapartum O67.0
  - newborn, transient P61.6
  - postpartum O72.3
  - specified type NEC D68.8
- complement system D84.1
- conduction (heart) I45.9
  - bone — *see* Deafness, conductive
- congenital, organ or site not listed — *see* Anomaly, by site
- coronary sinus Q21.1
- cushion, endocardial Q21.2
- degradation, glycoprotein E77.1
- dental bridge, crown, fillings — *see* Defect, dental restoration
- dental restoration K08.50
  - specified NEC K08.59
- dentin (hereditary) K00.5
- Descemet's membrane, congenital Q13.89
- developmental (*see also* Anomaly)
  - cauda equina Q06.3
- diaphragm
  - with elevation, eventration or hernia — *see* Hernia, diaphragm
  - congenital Q79.1
    - with hernia Q79.0
    - gross (with hernia) Q79.0
- ectodermal, congenital Q82.9
- Eisenmenger's Q21.8
- enzyme
  - catalase E80.3
  - peroxidase E80.3
- esophagus, congenital Q39.9
- extensor retinaculum M62.89
- fibrin polymerization D68.2
- filling
  - bladder R93.4
  - kidney R93.4
  - stomach R93.3
  - ureter R93.4
- Gerbode Q21.0
- glycoprotein degradation E77.1
- Hageman (factor) D68.2
- hearing — *see* Deafness
- high grade F70
- interatrial septal Q21.1
- interauricular septal Q21.1
- interventricular septal Q21.0
  - with dextroposition of aorta, pulmonary stenosis and hypertrophy of right ventricle Q21.3
  - in tetralogy of Fallot Q21.3
- learning (specific) — *see* Disorder, learning
- lymphocyte function antigen-1 (LFA-1) D84.0
- lysosomal enzyme, post-translational modification E77.0
- major osseous M89.70
  - ankle M89.77- ☑
  - carpus M89.74- ☑
  - clavicle M89.71- ☑
  - femur M89.75- ☑
  - fibula M89.76- ☑
  - fingers M89.74- ☑
  - foot M89.77- ☑
  - forearm M89.73- ☑
  - hand M89.74- ☑
  - humerus M89.72- ☑
  - lower leg M89.76- ☑
  - metacarpus M89.74- ☑
  - metatarsus M89.77- ☑
  - multiple sites M89.79
  - pelvic region M89.75- ☑
  - pelvis M89.75- ☑

Defect, defective — *continued*
- major osseous — *continued*
  - radius M89.73- ☑
  - scapula M89.71- ☑
  - shoulder region M89.71- ☑
  - specified NEC M89.78
  - tarsus M89.77- ☑
  - thigh M89.75- ☑
  - tibia M89.76- ☑
  - toes M89.77- ☑
  - ulna M89.73- ☑
- mental — *see* Disability, intellectual
- modification, lysosomal enzymes, post-translational E77.0
- obstructive, congenital
  - renal pelvis Q62.39
  - ureter Q62.39
    - atresia — *see* Atresia, ureter
    - cecoureterocele Q62.32
    - megaureter Q62.2
    - orthotopic ureterocele Q62.31
- osseous, major M89.70
  - ankle M89.77- ☑
  - carpus M89.74- ☑
  - clavicle M89.71- ☑
  - femur M89.75- ☑
  - fibula M89.76- ☑
  - fingers M89.74- ☑
  - foot M89.77- ☑
  - forearm M89.73- ☑
  - hand M89.74- ☑
  - humerus M89.72- ☑
  - lower leg M89.76- ☑
  - metacarpus M89.74- ☑
  - metatarsus M89.77- ☑
  - multiple sites M89.9
  - pelvic region M89.75- ☑
  - pelvis M89.75- ☑
  - radius M89.73- ☑
  - scapula M89.71- ☑
  - shoulder region M89.71- ☑
  - specified NEC M89.78
  - tarsus M89.77- ☑
  - thigh M89.75- ☑
  - tibia M89.76- ☑
  - toes M89.77- ☑
  - ulna M89.73- ☑
- osteochondral NEC (*see also* Deformity) M95.8
- ostium
  - primum Q21.2
  - secundum Q21.1
- peroxidase E80.3
- placental blood supply — *see* Insufficiency, placental
- platelets, qualitative D69.1
  - constitutional D68.0
- postural NEC, spine — *see* Dorsopathy, deforming
- reduction
  - limb Q73.8
    - lower Q72.9- ☑
      - absence — *see* Agenesis, leg
        - foot — *see* Agenesis, foot
      - longitudinal
        - femur Q72.4- ☑
        - fibula Q72.6- ☑
        - tibia Q72.5- ☑
      - specified type NEC Q72.89- ☑
      - split foot Q72.7- ☑
    - upper Q71.9- ☑
      - absence — *see* Agenesis, arm
        - forearm — *see* Agenesis, forearm
        - hand — *see* Agenesis, hand
      - lobster-claw hand Q71.6- ☑
      - longitudinal
        - radius Q71.4- ☑
        - ulna Q71.5- ☑
      - specified type NEC Q71.89- ☑
- renal pelvis Q63.8
  - obstructive Q62.39
- respiratory system, congenital Q34.9
- restoration, dental K08.50
  - specified NEC K08.59
- retinal nerve bundle fibers H35.89
- septal (heart) NOS Q21.9
  - acquired (atrial) (auricular) (ventricular) (old) I51.0

Defect, defective — *continued*
- septal — *continued*
  - atrial Q21.1
    - concurrent with acute myocardial infarction — *see* Infarct, myocardium
    - following acute myocardial infarction (current complication) I23.1
    - ventricular (*see also* Defect, ventricular septal) Q21.0
  - sinus venosus Q21.1
- speech R47.9
  - developmental F80.9
  - specified NEC R47.89
- Taussig-Bing (aortic transposition and overriding pulmonary artery) Q20.1
- teeth, wedge K03.1
- vascular (local) I99.9
  - congenital Q27.9
- ventricular septal Q21.0
  - concurrent with acute myocardial infarction — *see* Infarct, myocardium
  - following acute myocardial infarction (current complication) I23.2
  - in tetralogy of Fallot Q21.3
- vision NEC H54.7
- visual field H53.40
  - bilateral
    - heteronymous H53.47
    - homonymous H53.46- ☑
  - generalized contraction H53.48- ☑
  - localized
    - arcuate H53.43- ☑
    - scotoma (central area) H53.41- ☑
      - blind spot area H53.42- ☑
    - sector H53.43- ☑
    - specified type NEC H53.45- ☑
- voice R49.9
  - specified NEC R49.8
- wedge, tooth, teeth (abrasion) K03.1

Deferentitis N49.1
- gonorrheal (acute) (chronic) A54.23

Defibrination (syndrome) D65
- antepartum — *see* Hemorrhage, antepartum, with coagulation defect, disseminated intravascular coagulation
- following ectopic or molar pregnancy O08.1
- intrapartum O67.0
- newborn P60
- postpartum O72.3

Deficiency, deficient
- 3-beta hydroxysteroid dehydrogenase E25.0
- 5-alpha reductase (with male pseudohermaphroditism) E29.1
- 11-hydroxylase E25.0
- 21-hydroxylase E25.0
- abdominal muscle syndrome Q79.4
- AC globulin (congenital) (hereditary) D68.2
  - acquired D68.4
- accelerator globulin (Ac G) (blood) D68.2
- acid phosphatase E83.39
- activating factor (blood) D68.2
- adenosine deaminase (ADA) D81.3
- aldolase (hereditary) E74.19
- alpha-1-antitrypsin E88.01
- amino-acids E72.9
- anemia — *see* Anemia
- aneurin E51.9
- antibody with
  - hyperimmunoglobulinemia D80.6
  - near-normal immunoglobins D80.6
- antidiuretic hormone E23.2
- anti-hemophilic
  - factor (A) D66
    - B D67
    - C D68.1
  - globulin (AHG) NEC D66
- antithrombin (antithrombin III) D68.59
- ascorbic acid E54
- attention (disorder) (syndrome) F98.8
  - with hyperactivity — *see* Disorder, attention-deficit hyperactivity
- autoprothrombin
  - C D68.2
  - I D68.2
  - II D67
- beta-glucuronidase E76.29
- biotin E53.8
- biotin-dependent carboxylase D81.819

Deficiency, deficient — *continued*
 biotinidase D81.810
 brancher enzyme (amylopectinosis) E74.03
 C1 esterase inhibitor (C1-INH) D84.1
 calciferol E55.9
  with
    adult osteomalacia M83.8
    rickets — *see* Rickets
 calcium (dietary) E58
 calorie, severe E43
  with marasmus E41
    and kwashiorkor E42
 cardiac — *see* Insufficiency, myocardial
 carnitine E71.40
  due to
    hemodialysis E71.43
    inborn errors of metabolism E71.42
    Valproic acid therapy E71.43
  iatrogenic E71.43
  muscle palmityltransferase E71.314
  primary E71.41
  secondary E71.448
 carotene E50.9
 central nervous system G96.8
 ceruloplasmin (Wilson) E83.01
 choline E53.8
 Christmas factor D67
 chromium E61.4
 clotting (blood) (*see also* Deficiency, coagulation factor) D68.9
 clotting factor NEC (hereditary) (*see also* Deficiency, factor) D68.2
 coagulation NOS D68.9
  with
    ectopic pregnancy O08.1
    molar pregnancy O08.1
  acquired (any) D68.4
  antepartum hemorrhage — *see* Hemorrhage, antepartum, with coagulation defect
  clotting factor NEC (*see also* Deficiency, factor) D68.2
  due to
    hyperprothrombinemia D68.4
    liver disease D68.4
    vitamin K deficiency D68.4
  newborn, transient P61.6
  postpartum O72.3
  specified NEC D68.8
 cognitive F09
 color vision H53.50
  achromatopsia H53.51
  acquired H53.52
  deuteranomaly H53.53
  protanomaly H53.54
  specified type NEC H53.59
  tritanomaly H53.55
 combined glucocorticoid and mineralocorticoid E27.49
 contact factor D68.2
 copper (nutritional) E61.0
 corticoadrenal E27.40
  primary E27.1
 craniofacial axis Q75.0
 cyanocobalamin E53.8
 debrancher enzyme (limit dextrinosis) E74.03
 dehydrogenase
  long chain/very long chain acyl CoA E71.310
  medium chain acyl CoA E71.311
  short chain acyl CoA E71.312
 diet E63.9
 dihydropyrimidine dehydrogenase (DPD) E88.89
 disaccharidase E73.9
 edema — *see* Malnutrition, severe
 endocrine E34.9
 energy-supply — *see* Malnutrition
 enzymes, circulating NEC E88.09
 ergosterol E55.9
  with
    adult osteomalacia M83.8
    rickets — *see* Rickets
 essential fatty acid (EFA) E63.0
 factor (*see also* Deficiency, coagulation)
  Hageman D68.2
  I (congenital) (hereditary) D68.2
  II (congenital) (hereditary) D68.2
  IX (congenital) (functional) (hereditary) (with functional defect) D67
  multiple (congenital) D68.8
    acquired D68.4

Deficiency, deficient — *continued*
 factor (*see also* Deficiency, coagulation) — *continued*
  V (congenital) (hereditary) D68.2
  VII (congenital) (hereditary) D68.2
  VIII (congenital) (functional) (hereditary) (with functional defect) D66
    with vascular defect D68.0
  X (congenital) (hereditary) D68.2
  XI (congenital) (hereditary) D68.1
  XII (congenital) (hereditary) D68.2
  XIII (congenital) (hereditary) D68.2
 femoral, proximal focal (congenital) — *see* Defect, reduction, lower limb, longitudinal, femur
 fibrinase D68.2
 fibrinogen (congenital) (hereditary) D68.2
  acquired D65
 fibrin-stabilizing factor (congenital) (hereditary) D68.2
  acquired D68.4
 folate E53.8
 folic acid E53.8
 foreskin N47.3
 fructokinase E74.11
 fructose 1,6-diphosphatase E74.19
 fructose-1-phosphate aldolase E74.19
 galactokinase E74.29
 galactose-1-phosphate uridyl transferase E74.29
 gammaglobulin in blood D80.1
  hereditary D80.0
 glass factor D68.2
 glucocorticoid E27.49
  mineralocorticoid E27.49
 glucose-6-phosphatase E74.01
 glucose-6-phosphate dehydrogenase anemia D55.0
 glucuronyl transferase E80.5
 glycogen synthetase E74.09
 gonadotropin (isolated) E23.0
 growth hormone (idiopathic) (isolated) E23.0
 Hageman factor D68.2
 hemoglobin D64.9
 hepatophosphorylase E74.09
 homogentisate 1,2-dioxygenase E70.29
 hormone
  anterior pituitary (partial) NEC E23.0
    growth E23.0
  growth (isolated) E23.0
  pituitary E23.0
  testicular E29.1
 hypoxanthine- (guanine)-phosphoribosyltransferase (HG- PRT) (total H-PRT) E79.1
 immunity D84.9
  cell-mediated D84.8
    with thrombocytopenia and eczema D82.0
  combined D81.9
  humoral D80.9
  IgA (secretory) D80.2
  IgG D80.3
  IgM D80.4
 immuno — *see* Immunodeficiency
 immunoglobulin, selective
  A (IgA) D80.2
  G (IgG) (subclasses) D80.3
  M (IgM) D80.4
 inositol (B complex) E53.8
 intrinsic
  factor (congenital) D51.0
  sphincter N36.42
    with urethral hypermobility N36.43
 iodine E61.8
  congenital syndrome — *see* Syndrome, iodine-deficiency, congenital
 iron E61.1
  anemia D50.9
 kalium E87.6
 kappa-light chain D80.8
 labile factor (congenital) (hereditary) D68.2
  acquired D68.4
 lacrimal fluid (acquired) (*see also* Syndrome, dry eye)
  congenital Q10.6
 lactase
  congenital E73.0
  secondary E73.1
 Laki-Lorand factor D68.2
 lecithin cholesterol acyltransferase E78.6
 lipocaic K86.8
 lipoprotein (familial) (high density) E78.6
 liver phosphorylase E74.09
 lysosomal alpha-1, 4 glucosidase E74.02

Deficiency, deficient — *continued*
 magnesium E61.2
 major histocompatibility complex
  class I D81.6
  class II D81.7
 manganese E61.3
 menadione (vitamin K) E56.1
  newborn P53
 mental (familial) (hereditary) — *see* Disability, intellectual
 methylenetetrahydrofolate reductase (MTHFR) E72.12
 mineralocorticoid E27.49
  with glucocorticoid E27.49
 mineral NEC E61.8
 molybdenum (nutritional) E61.5
 moral F60.2
 multiple nutrient elements E61.7
 muscle
  carnitine (palmityltransferase) E71.314
  phosphofructokinase E74.09
 myoadenylate deaminase E79.2
 myocardial — *see* Insufficiency, myocardial
 myophosphorylase E74.04
 NADH diaphorase or reductase (congenital) D74.0
 NADH-methemoglobin reductase (congenital) D74.0
 natrium E87.1
 niacin (amide) (-tryptophan) E52
 nicotinamide E52
 nicotinic acid E52
 number of teeth — *see* Anodontia
 nutrient element E61.9
  multiple E61.7
  specified NEC E61.8
 nutrition, nutritional E63.9
  sequelae — *see* Sequelae, nutritional deficiency
  specified NEC E63.8
 ornithine transcarbamylase E72.4
 ovarian E28.39
 oxygen — *see* Anoxia
 pantothenic acid E53.8
 parathyroid (gland) E20.9
 perineum (female) N81.89
 phenylalanine hydroxylase E70.1
 phosphoenolpyruvate carboxykinase E74.4
 phosphofructokinase E74.19
 phosphomannomutase E74.8
 phosphomannose isomerase E74.8
 phosphomannosyl mutase E74.8
 phosphorylase kinase, liver E74.09
 pituitary hormone (isolated) E23.0
 plasma thromboplastin
  antecedent (PTA) D68.1
  component (PTC) D67
 platelet NEC D69.1
  constitutional D68.0
 polyglandular E31.8
  autoimmune E31.0
 potassium (K) E87.6
 prepuce N47.3
 proaccelerin (congenital) (hereditary) D68.2
  acquired D68.4
 proconvertin factor (congenital) (hereditary) D68.2
  acquired D68.4
 protein (*see also* Malnutrition) E46
  anemia D53.0
  C D68.59
  S D68.59
 prothrombin (congenital) (hereditary) D68.2
  acquired D68.4
 Prower factor D68.2
 pseudocholinesterase E88.09
 PTA (plasma thromboplastin antecedent) D68.1
 PTC (plasma thromboplastin component) D67
 purine nucleoside phosphorylase (PNP) D81.5
 pyracin (alpha) (beta) E53.1
 pyridoxal E53.1
 pyridoxamine E53.1
 pyridoxine (derivatives) E53.1
 pyruvate
  carboxylase E74.4
  dehydrogenase E74.4
 riboflavin (vitamin B2) E53.0
 salt E87.1
 secretion
  ovary E28.39
  salivary gland (any) K11.7
  urine R34
 selenium (dietary) E59

☑ **Additional Character Required — Refer to the Tabular List for Character Selection**   ▽ Subterms under main terms may continue to next column or page

Deficiency, deficient — *continued*
serum antitrypsin, familial E88.01
short stature homeobox gene (SHOX)
  with
    dyschondrosteosis Q78.8
    short stature (idiopathic) E34.3
    Turner's syndrome Q96.9
sodium (Na) E87.1
SPCA (factor VII) D68.2
sphincter, intrinsic N36.42
  with urethral hypermobility N36.43
stable factor (congenital) (hereditary) D68.2
  acquired D68.4
Stuart-Prower (factor X) D68.2
sucrase E74.39
sulfatase E75.29
sulfite oxidase E72.19
thiamin, thiaminic (chloride) E51.9
  beriberi (dry) E51.11
    wet E51.12
thrombokinase D68.2
  newborn P53
thyroid (gland) — *see* Hypothyroidism
tocopherol E56.0
tooth bud K00.0
transcobalamine II (anemia) D51.2
vanadium E61.6
vascular I99.9
vasopressin E23.2
viosterol — *see* Deficiency, calciferol
vitamin (multiple) NOS E56.9
  A E50.9
    with
      Bitot's spot (corneal) E50.1
      follicular keratosis E50.8
      keratomalacia E50.4
      manifestations NEC E50.8
      night blindness E50.5
      scar of cornea, xerophthalmic E50.6
      xeroderma E50.8
      xerophthalmia E50.7
      xerosis
        conjunctival E50.0
          and Bitot's spot E50.1
        cornea E50.2
          and ulceration E50.3
    sequelae E64.1
  B (complex) NOS E53.9
    with
      beriberi (dry) E51.11
        wet E51.12
      pellagra E52
  B1 NOS E51.9
    beriberi (dry) E51.11
      with circulatory system manifestations
        E51.11
      wet E51.12
  B2 (riboflavin) E53.0
  B6 E53.1
  B12 E53.8
  C E54
    sequelae E64.2
  D E55.9
    with
      adult osteomalacia M83.8
      rickets — *see* Rickets
    25-hydroxylase E83.32
  E E56.0
  folic acid E53.8
  G E53.0
  group B E53.9
    specified NEC E53.8
  H (biotin) E53.8
  K E56.1
    of newborn P53
  nicotinic E52
  P E56.8
  PP (pellagra-preventing) E52
  specified NEC E56.8
  thiamin E51.9
    beriberi — *see* Beriberi
zinc, dietary E60
Deficit (*see also* Deficiency)
  attention and concentration R41.840
    disorder — *see* Attention, deficit
  cognitive communication R41.841

Deficit — *continued*
  cognitive NEC R41.89
    following
      cerebral infarction I69.31
      cerebrovascular disease I69.91
        specified disease NEC I69.81
      intracerebral hemorrhage I69.11
      nontraumatic intracranial hemorrhage NEC
        I69.21
      subarachnoid hemorrhage I69.01
  concentration R41.840
  executive function R41.844
  frontal lobe R41.844
  neurologic NEC R29.818
    ischemic
      reversible (RIND) I63.9
        prolonged (PRIND) I63.9
  oxygen R09.02
  prolonged reversible ischemic neurologic (PRIND) I63.9
  psychomotor R41.843
  visuospatial R41.842
Deflection
  radius — *see* Deformity, limb, specified type NEC,
    forearm
  septum (acquired) (nasal) (nose) J34.2
  spine — *see* Curvature, spine
  turbinate (nose) J34.2
Defluvium
  capillorum — *see* Alopecia
  ciliorum — *see* Madarosis
  unguium L60.8
Deformity Q89.9
  abdomen, congenital Q89.9
  abdominal wall
    acquired M95.8
    congenital Q79.59
  acquired (unspecified site) M95.9
  adrenal gland Q89.1
  alimentary tract, congenital Q45.9
    upper Q40.9
  ankle (joint) (acquired) (*see also* Deformity, limb, lower
    leg)
    abduction — *see* Contraction, joint, ankle
    congenital Q68.8
    contraction — *see* Contraction, joint, ankle
    specified type NEC — *see* Deformity, limb, foot,
      specified NEC
  anus (acquired) K62.89
    congenital Q43.9
  aorta (arch) (congenital) Q25.4
    acquired I77.89
  aortic
    arch, acquired I77.89
    cusp or valve (congenital) Q23.8
      acquired (*see also* Endocarditis, aortic) I35.8
  arm (acquired) (upper) (*see also* Deformity, limb, upper
    arm)
    congenital Q68.8
    forearm — *see* Deformity, limb, forearm
  artery (congenital) (peripheral) NOS Q27.9
    acquired I77.89
    coronary (acquired) I25.9
      congenital Q24.5
    umbilical Q27.0
  atrial septal Q21.1
  auditory canal (external) (congenital) (*see also* Malfor-
    mation, ear, external)
    acquired — *see* Disorder, ear, external, specified
      type NEC
  auricle
    ear (congenital) (*see also* Malformation, ear, exter-
      nal)
      acquired — *see* Disorder, pinna, deformity
  back — *see* Dorsopathy, deforming
  bile duct (common) (congenital) (hepatic) Q44.5
    acquired K83.8
  biliary duct or passage (congenital) Q44.5
    acquired K83.8
  bladder (neck) (trigone) (sphincter) (acquired) N32.89
    congenital Q64.79
  bone (acquired) NOS M95.9
    congenital Q79.9
    turbinate M95.0
  brain (congenital) Q04.9
    acquired G93.89
    reduction Q04.3
  breast (acquired) N64.89
    congenital Q83.9

Deformity — *continued*
  breast — *continued*
    reconstructed N65.0
  bronchus (congenital) Q32.4
    acquired NEC J98.09
  bursa, congenital Q79.9
  canaliculi (lacrimalis) (acquired) (*see also* Disorder,
    lacrimal system, changes)
    congenital Q10.6
  canthus, acquired — *see* Disorder, eyelid, specified
    type NEC
  capillary (acquired) I78.8
  cardiovascular system, congenital Q28.9
  caruncle, lacrimal (acquired) (*see also* Disorder,
    lacrimal system, changes)
    congenital Q10.6
  cascade, stomach K31.2
  cecum (congenital) Q43.9
    acquired K63.89
  cerebral, acquired G93.89
    congenital Q04.9
  cervix (uterus) (acquired) NEC N88.8
    congenital Q51.9
  cheek (acquired) M95.2
    congenital Q18.9
  chest (acquired) (wall) M95.4
    congenital Q67.8
    sequelae (late effect) of rickets E64.3
  chin (acquired) M95.2
    congenital Q18.9
  choroid (congenital) Q14.3
    acquired H31.8
    plexus Q07.8
      acquired G96.19
  cicatricial — *see* Cicatrix
  cilia, acquired — *see* Disorder, eyelid, specified type
    NEC
  clavicle (acquired) M95.8
    congenital Q68.8
  clitoris (congenital) Q52.6
    acquired N90.89
  clubfoot — *see* Clubfoot
  coccyx (acquired) — *see* subcategory M43.8 ☑
  colon (congenital) Q43.9
    acquired K63.89
  concha (ear), congenital (*see also* Malformation, ear,
    external)
    acquired — *see* Disorder, pinna, deformity
  cornea (acquired) H18.70
    congenital Q13.4
    descemetocele — *see* Descemetocele
    ectasia — *see* Ectasia, cornea
    specified NEC H18.79- ☑
    staphyloma — *see* Staphyloma, cornea
  coronary artery (acquired) I25.9
    congenital Q24.5
  cranium (acquired) — *see* Deformity, skull
  cricoid cartilage (congenital) Q31.8
    acquired J38.7
  cystic duct (congenital) Q44.5
    acquired K82.8
  Dandy-Walker Q03.1
    with spina bifida — *see* Spina bifida
  diaphragm (congenital) Q79.1
    acquired J98.6
  digestive organ NOS Q45.9
  ductus arteriosus Q25.0
  duodenal bulb K31.89
  duodenum (congenital) Q43.9
    acquired K31.89
  dura — *see* Deformity, meninges
  ear (acquired) (*see also* Disorder, pinna, deformity)
    congenital Q17.9
      congenital (external) Q17.9
        internal Q16.5
        middle Q16.4
          ossicles Q16.3
        ossicles Q16.3
  ectodermal (congenital) NEC Q84.9
  ejaculatory duct (congenital) Q55.4
    acquired N50.8
  elbow (joint) (acquired) (*see also* Deformity, limb, up-
    per arm)
    congenital Q68.8
    contraction — *see* Contraction, joint, elbow
  endocrine gland NEC Q89.2
  epididymis (congenital) Q55.4
    acquired N50.8

▽ **Subterms under main terms may continue to next column or page**   ☑ **Additional Character Required** — **Refer to the Tabular List for Character Selection**   **83**

Deficiency, deficient — Deformity

Deformity — *continued*
  epiglottis(congenital) Q31.8
    acquired J38.7
  esophagus (congenital) Q39.9
    acquired K22.8
  eustachian tube (congenital) NEC Q17.8
  eye, congenital Q15.9
  eyebrow (congenital) Q18.8
  eyelid (acquired) (*see also* Disorder, eyelid,
     specified type NEC)
    congenital Q10.3
  face (acquired) M95.2
    congenital Q18.9
  fallopian tube, acquired N83.8
  femur (acquired) — *see* Deformity, limb, specified type
     NEC, thigh
  fetal
    with fetopelvic disproportion O33.7
    causing obstructed labor O66.3
  finger (acquired) M20.00- ☑
    boutonniere M20.02- ☑
    congenital Q68.1
    flexion contracture — *see* Contraction, joint, hand
    mallet finger M20.01- ☑
    specified NEC M20.09- ☑
    swan-neck M20.03- ☑
  flexion (joint) (acquired) (*see also* Deformity, limb,
     flexion) M21.20
    congenital NOS Q74.9
     hip Q65.89
  foot (acquired) (*see also* Deformity, limb, lower leg)
    cavovarus (congenital) Q66.1
    congenital NOS Q66.9
     specified type NEC Q66.89
    specified type NEC — *see* Deformity, limb, foot,
      specified NEC
    valgus (congenital) Q66.6
     acquired — *see* Deformity, valgus, ankle
    varus (congenital) NEC Q66.3
     acquired — *see* Deformity, varus, ankle
  forearm (acquired) (*see also* Deformity, limb, forearm)
    congenital Q68.8
  forehead (acquired) M95.2
    congenital Q75.8
  frontal bone (acquired) M95.2
    congenital Q75.8
  gallbladder (congenital) Q44.1
    acquired K82.8
  gastrointestinal tract (congenital) NOS Q45.9
    acquired K63.89
  genitalia, genital organ(s) or system NEC
    female (congenital) Q52.9
     acquired N94.89
     external Q52.70
    male (congenital) Q55.9
     acquired N50.8
  globe (eye) (congenital) Q15.8
    acquired H44.89
  gum, acquired NEC K06.8
  hand (acquired) — *see* Deformity, limb, hand
    congenital Q68.1
  head (acquired) M95.2
    congenital Q75.8
  heart (congenital) Q24.9
    septum Q21.9
     auricular Q21.1
     ventricular Q21.0
    valve (congenital) NEC Q24.8
     acquired — *see* Endocarditis
  heel (acquired) — *see* Deformity, foot
  hepatic duct (congenital) Q44.5
    acquired K83.8
  hip (joint) (acquired) (*see also* Deformity, limb, thigh)
    congenital Q65.9
    due to (previous) juvenile osteochondrosis — *see*
     Coxa, plana
    flexion — *see* Contraction, joint, hip
  hourglass — *see* Contraction, hourglass
  humerus (acquired) M21.82- ☑
    congenital Q74.0
  hypophyseal (congenital) Q89.2
  ileocecal (coil) (valve) (acquired) K63.89
    congenital Q43.9
  ileum (congenital) Q43.9
    acquired K63.89
  ilium (acquired) M95.5
    congenital Q74.2
  integument (congenital) Q84.9

Deformity — *continued*
  intervertebral cartilage or disc (acquired) — *see* Disor-
    der, disc, specified NEC
  intestine (large) (small) (congenital) NOS Q43.9
    acquired K63.89
  intrinsic minus or plus (hand) — *see* Deformity, limb,
    specified type NEC, forearm
  iris (acquired) H21.89
    congenital Q13.2
  ischium (acquired) M95.5
    congenital Q74.2
  jaw (acquired) (congenital) M26.9
  joint (acquired) NEC M21.90
    congenital Q68.8
    elbow M21.92- ☑
    hand M21.94- ☑
    hip M21.95- ☑
    knee M21.96- ☑
    shoulder M21.92- ☑
    wrist M21.93- ☑
  kidney(s) (calyx) (pelvis) (congenital) Q63.9
    acquired N28.89
    artery (congenital) Q27.2
     acquired I77.89
  Klippel-Feil (brevicollis) Q76.1
  knee (acquired) NEC (*see also* Deformity, limb, lower
    leg)
    congenital Q68.2
  labium (majus) (minus) (congenital) Q52.79
    acquired N90.89
  lacrimal passages or duct (congenital) NEC Q10.6
    acquired — *see* Disorder, lacrimal system, changes
  larynx (muscle) (congenital) Q31.8
    acquired J38.7
    web (glottic) Q31.0
  leg (upper) (acquired) NEC (*see also* Deformity, limb,
    thigh)
    congenital Q68.8
    lower leg — *see* Deformity, limb, lower leg
  lens (acquired) H27.8
    congenital Q12.9
  lid (fold) (acquired) (*see also* Disorder, eyelid, specified
    type NEC)
    congenital Q10.3
  ligament (acquired) — *see* Disorder, ligament
    congenital Q79.9
  limb (acquired) M21.90
    clawfoot M21.53- ☑
    clawhand M21.51- ☑
    clubfoot M21.54- ☑
    clubhand M21.52- ☑
    congenital, except reduction deformity Q74.9
    flat foot M21.4- ☑
    flexion M21.20
     ankle M21.27- ☑
     elbow M21.22- ☑
     finger M21.24- ☑
     hip M21.25- ☑
     knee M21.26- ☑
     shoulder M21.21- ☑
     toe M21.27- ☑
     wrist M21.23- ☑
    foot
     claw — *see* Deformity, limb, clawfoot
     club — *see* Deformity, limb, clubfoot
     drop M21.37- ☑
     flat — *see* Deformity, limb, flat foot
     specified NEC M21.6X- ☑
    forearm M21.93- ☑
    hand M21.94- ☑
    lower leg M21.96- ☑
    specified type NEC M21.80
     forearm M21.83- ☑
     lower leg M21.86- ☑
     thigh M21.85- ☑
     upper arm M21.82- ☑
    thigh M21.95- ☑
    unequal length M21.70
     short site is
      femur M21.75- ☑
      fibula M21.76- ☑
      humerus M21.72- ☑
      radius M21.73- ☑
      tibia M21.76- ☑
      ulna M21.73- ☑
    upper arm M21.92- ☑
    valgus — *see* Deformity, valgus

Deformity — *continued*
  limb — *continued*
    varus — *see* Deformity, varus
     wrist drop M21.33- ☑
  lip (acquired) NEC K13.0
    congenital Q38.0
  liver (congenital) Q44.7
    acquired K76.89
  lumbosacral (congenital) (joint) (region) Q76.49
    acquired — *see* subcategory M43.8 ☑
    kyphosis — *see* Kyphosis, congenital
    lordosis — *see* Lordosis, congenital
  lung (congenital) Q33.9
    acquired J98.4
  lymphatic system, congenital Q89.9
  Madelung's (radius) Q74.0
  mandible (acquired) (congenital) M26.9
  maxilla (acquired) (congenital) M26.9
  meninges or membrane (congenital) Q07.9
    cerebral Q04.8
     acquired G96.19
    spinal cord (congenital) G96.19
     acquired G96.19
  metacarpus (acquired) — *see* Deformity, limb, forearm
    congenital Q74.0
  metatarsus (acquired) — *see* Deformity, foot
    congenital Q66.9
  middle ear (congenital) Q16.4
    ossicles Q16.3
  mitral (leaflets) (valve) I05.8
    parachute Q23.2
    stenosis, congenital Q23.2
  mouth (acquired) K13.79
    congenital Q38.6
  multiple, congenital NEC Q89.7
  muscle (acquired) M62.89
    congenital Q79.9
     sternocleidomastoid Q68.0
  musculoskeletal system (acquired) M95.9
    congenital Q79.9
    specified NEC M95.8
  nail (acquired) L60.8
    congenital Q84.6
  nasal — *see* Deformity, nose
  neck (acquired) M95.3
    congenital Q18.9
     sternocleidomastoid Q68.0
  nervous system (congenital) Q07.9
  nipple (congenital) Q83.9
    acquired N64.89
  nose (acquired) (cartilage) M95.0
    bone (turbinate) M95.0
    congenital Q30.9
     bent or squashed Q67.4
    saddle M95.0
     syphilitic A50.57
    septum (acquired) J34.2
     congenital Q30.8
    sinus (wall) (congenital) Q30.8
     acquired M95.0
    syphilitic (congenital) A50.57
     late A52.73
  ocular muscle (congenital) Q10.3
    acquired — *see* Strabismus, mechanical
  opticociliary vessels (congenital) Q13.2
  orbit (eye) (acquired) H05.30
    atrophy — *see* Atrophy, orbit
    congenital Q10.7
    due to
     bone disease NEC H05.32- ☑
     trauma or surgery H05.33- ☑
    enlargement — *see* Enlargement, orbit
    exostosis — *see* Exostosis, orbit
  organ of Corti (congenital) Q16.5
  ovary (congenital) Q50.39
    acquired N83.8
  oviduct, acquired N83.8
  palate (congenital) Q38.5
    acquired M27.8
    cleft (congenital) — *see* Cleft, palate
  pancreas (congenital) Q45.3
    acquired K86.8
  parathyroid (gland) Q89.2
  parotid (gland) (congenital) Q38.4
    acquired K11.8
  patella (acquired) — *see* Disorder, patella, specified
    NEC

  ☑ **Additional Character Required — Refer to the Tabular List for Character Selection**   ▽ **Subterms under main terms may continue to next column or page**

Deformity — *continued*
  pelvis, pelvic (acquired) (bony) M95.5
    with disproportion (fetopelvic) O33.0
      causing obstructed labor O65.0
    congenital Q74.2
    rachitic sequelae (late effect) E64.3
  penis (glans) (congenital) Q55.69
    acquired N48.89
  pericardium (congenital) Q24.8
    acquired — *see* Pericarditis
  pharynx (congenital) Q38.8
    acquired J39.2
  pinna, acquired (*see also* Disorder, pinna, deformity)
    congenital Q17.9
  pituitary (congenital) Q89.2
  posture — *see* Dorsopathy, deforming
  prepuce (congenital) Q55.69
    acquired N47.8
  prostate (congenital) Q55.4
    acquired N42.89
  pupil (congenital) Q13.2
    acquired — *see* Abnormality, pupillary
  pylorus (congenital) Q40.3
    acquired K31.89
  rachitic (acquired), old or healed E64.3
  radius (acquired) (*see also* Deformity, limb, forearm)
    congenital Q68.8
  rectum (congenital) Q43.9
    acquired K62.89
  reduction (extremity) (limb), congenital (*see also* condition and site) Q73.8
    brain Q04.3
    lower — *see* Defect, reduction, lower limb
    upper — *see* Defect, reduction, upper limb
  renal — *see* Deformity, kidney
  respiratory system (congenital) Q34.9
  rib (acquired) M95.4
    congenital Q76.6
      cervical Q76.5
  rotation (joint) (acquired) — *see* Deformity, limb, specified site NEC
    congenital Q74.9
    hip — *see* Deformity, limb, specified type NEC, thigh
      congenital Q65.89
  sacroiliac joint (congenital) — *see* subcategory Q74.2
    acquired — *see* subcategory M43.8 ☑
  sacrum (acquired) — *see* subcategory M43.8 ☑
  saddle
    back — *see* Lordosis
    nose M95.0
      syphilitic A50.57
  salivary gland or duct (congenital) Q38.4
    acquired K11.8
  scapula (acquired) M95.8
    congenital Q68.8
  scrotum (congenital) (*see also* Malformation, testis and scrotum)
    acquired N50.8
  seminal vesicles (congenital) Q55.4
    acquired N50.8
  septum, nasal (acquired) J34.2
  shoulder (joint) (acquired) — *see* Deformity, limb, upper arm
    congenital Q74.0
    contraction — *see* Contraction, joint, shoulder
  sigmoid (flexure) (congenital) Q43.9
    acquired K63.89
  skin (congenital) Q82.9
  skull (acquired) M95.2
    congenital Q75.8
      with
        anencephaly Q00.0
        encephalocele — *see* Encephalocele
        hydrocephalus Q03.9
          with spina bifida — *see* Spina bifida, by site, with hydrocephalus
        microcephaly Q02
  soft parts, organs or tissues (of pelvis)
    in pregnancy or childbirth NEC O34.8- ☑
      causing obstructed labor O65.5
  spermatic cord (congenital) Q55.4
    acquired N50.8
    torsion — *see* Torsion, spermatic cord
  spinal — *see* Dorsopathy, deforming
    column (acquired) — *see* Dorsopathy, deforming
    congenital Q67.5

Deformity — *continued*
  spinal — *see* Dorsopathy, deforming — *continued*
    cord (congenital) Q06.9
      acquired G95.89
    nerve root (congenital) Q07.9
  spine (acquired) (*see also* Dorsopathy, deforming)
    congenital Q67.5
    rachitic E64.3
    specified NEC — *see* Dorsopathy, deforming, specified NEC
  spleen
    acquired D73.89
    congenital Q89.09
  Sprengel's (congenital) Q74.0
  sternocleidomastoid (muscle), congenital Q68.0
  sternum (acquired) M95.4
    congenital NEC Q76.7
  stomach (congenital) Q40.3
    acquired K31.89
  submandibular gland (congenital) Q38.4
  submaxillary gland (congenital) Q38.4
    acquired K11.8
  talipes — *see* Talipes
  testis (congenital) (*see also* Malformation, testis and scrotum)
    acquired N44.8
      torsion — *see* Torsion, testis
  thigh (acquired) (*see also* Deformity, limb, thigh)
    congenital NEC Q68.8
  thorax (acquired) (wall) M95.4
    congenital Q67.8
    sequelae of rickets E64.3
  thumb (acquired) (*see also* Deformity, finger)
    congenital NEC Q68.1
  thymus (tissue) (congenital) Q89.2
  thyroid (gland) (congenital) Q89.2
    cartilage Q31.8
      acquired J38.7
  tibia (acquired) (*see also* Deformity, limb, specified type NEC, lower leg)
    congenital NEC Q68.8
    saber (syphilitic) A50.56
  toe (acquired) M20.6- ☑
    congenital Q66.9
    hallux rigidus M20.2- ☑
    hallux valgus M20.1- ☑
    hallux varus M20.3- ☑
    hammer toe M20.4- ☑
    specified NEC M20.5X- ☑
  tongue (congenital) Q38.3
    acquired K14.8
  tooth, teeth K00.2
  trachea (rings) (congenital) Q32.1
    acquired J39.8
  transverse aortic arch (congenital) Q25.4
  tricuspid (leaflets) (valve) I07.8
    atresia or stenosis Q22.4
    Ebstein's Q22.5
  trunk (acquired) M95.8
    congenital Q89.9
  ulna (acquired) (*see also* Deformity, limb, forearm)
    congenital NEC Q68.8
  urachus, congenital Q64.4
  ureter (opening) (congenital) Q62.8
    acquired N28.89
  urethra (congenital) Q64.79
    acquired N36.8
  urinary tract (congenital) Q64.9
    urachus Q64.4
  uterus (congenital) Q51.9
    acquired N85.8
  uvula (congenital) Q38.5
  vagina (acquired) N89.8
    congenital Q52.4
  valgus NEC M21.00
    ankle M21.07- ☑
    elbow M21.02- ☑
    hip M21.05- ☑
    knee M21.06- ☑
  valve, valvular (congenital) (heart) Q24.8
    acquired — *see* Endocarditis
  varus NEC M21.10
    ankle M21.17- ☑
    elbow M21.12- ☑
    hip M21.15 ☑
    knee M21.16- ☑
    tibia — *see* Osteochondrosis, juvenile, tibia

Deformity — *continued*
  vas deferens (congenital) Q55.4
    acquired N50.8
  vein (congenital) Q27.9
    great Q26.9
  vertebra — *see* Dorsopathy, deforming
  vertical talus (congenital) Q66.80
    left foot Q66.82
    right foot Q66.81
  vesicourethral orifice (acquired) N32.89
    congenital NEC Q64.79
  vessels of optic papilla (congenital) Q14.2
  visual field (contraction) — *see* Defect, visual field
  vitreous body, acquired H43.89
  vulva (congenital) Q52.79
    acquired N90.89
  wrist (joint) (acquired) (*see also* Deformity, limb, forearm)
    congenital Q68.8
    contraction — *see* Contraction, joint, wrist

Degeneration, degenerative
  adrenal (capsule) (fatty) (gland) (hyaline) (infectional) E27.8
  amyloid (*see also* Amyloidosis) E85.9
  anterior cornua, spinal cord G12.29
  anterior labral S43.49- ☑
  aorta, aortic I70.0
    fatty I77.89
  aortic valve (heart) — *see* Endocarditis, aortic
  arteriovascular — *see* Arteriosclerosis
  artery, arterial (atheromatous) (calcareous) (*see also* Arteriosclerosis)
    cerebral, amyloid E85.4 [I68.0]
    medial — *see* Arteriosclerosis, extremities
  articular cartilage NEC — *see* Derangement, joint, articular cartilage, by site
  atheromatous — *see* Arteriosclerosis
  basal nuclei or ganglia G23.9
    specified NEC G23.8
  bone NEC — *see* Disorder, bone, specified type NEC
  brachial plexus G54.0
  brain (cortical) (progressive) G31.9
    alcoholic G31.2
    arteriosclerotic I67.2
    childhood G31.9
      specified NEC G31.89
    cystic G31.89
      congenital Q04.6
    in
      alcoholism G31.2
      beriberi E51.2
      cerebrovascular disease I67.9
      congenital hydrocephalus Q03.9
        with spina bifida (*see also* Spina bifida)
      Fabry-Anderson disease E75.21
      Gaucher's disease E75.22
      Hunter's syndrome E76.1
      lipidosis
        cerebral E75.4
        generalized E75.6
      mucopolysaccharidosis — *see* Mucopolysaccharidosis
      myxedema E03.9 [G32.89]
      neoplastic disease (*see also* Neoplasm) D49.6 [G32.89]
      Niemann-Pick disease E75.249 [G32.89]
      sphingolipidosis E75.3 [G32.89]
      vitamin B12 deficiency E53.8 [G32.89]
    senile NEC G31.1
  breast N64.89
  Bruch's membrane — *see* Degeneration, choroid
  capillaries (fatty) I78.8
    amyloid E85.8 [I79.8]
  cardiac (*see also* Degeneration, myocardial)
    valve, valvular — *see* Endocarditis
  cardiorenal — *see* Hypertension, cardiorenal
  cardiovascular (*see also* Disease, cardiovascular)
    renal — *see* Hypertension, cardiorenal
  cerebellar NOS G31.9
    alcoholic G31.2
    primary (hereditary) (sporadic) G11.9
  cerebral — *see* Degeneration, brain
  cerebrovascular I67.9
    due to hypertension I67.4
  cervical plexus G54.2
  cervix N88.8
    due to radiation (intended effect) N88.8
      adverse effect or misadventure N99.89

Degeneration, degenerative — *continued*
  chamber angle H21.21- ☑
  changes, spine or vertebra — *see* Spondylosis
  chorioretinal (*see also* Degeneration, choroid)
    hereditary H31.20
  choroid (colloid) (drusen) H31.10- ☑
    atrophy — *see* Atrophy, choroidal
    hereditary — *see* Dystrophy, choroidal, hereditary
  ciliary body H21.22- ☑
  cochlear — *see* subcategory H83.8 ☑
  combined (spinal cord) (subacute) E53.8 [G32.0]
    with anemia (pernicious) D51.0 [G32.0]
      due to dietary vitamin B12 deficiency
        D51.3 [G32.0]
    in (due to)
      vitamin B12 deficiency E53.8 [G32.0]
        anemia D51.9 [G32.0]
  conjunctiva H11.10
    concretions — *see* Concretion, conjunctiva
    deposits — *see* Deposit, conjunctiva
    pigmentations — *see* Pigmentation, conjunctiva
    pinguecula — *see* Pinguecula
    xerosis — *see* Xerosis, conjunctiva
  cornea H18.40
    calcerous H18.43
      band keratopathy H18.42- ☑
    familial, hereditary — *see* Dystrophy, cornea
    hyaline (of old scars) H18.49
    keratomalacia — *see* Keratomalacia
    nodular H18.45- ☑
    peripheral H18.46- ☑
    senile H18.41- ☑
    specified type NEC H18.49
  cortical (cerebellar) (parenchymatous) G31.89
    alcoholic G31.2
    diffuse, due to arteriopathy I67.2
  corticobasal G31.85
  cutis L98.8
    amyloid E85.4 [L99]
  dental pulp K04.2
  disc disease — *see* Degeneration, intervertebral disc
    NEC
  dorsolateral (spinal cord) — *see* Degeneration, combined
  extrapyramidal G25.9
  eye, macular (*see also* Degeneration, macula)
    congenital or hereditary — *see* Dystrophy, retina
  facet joints — *see* Spondylosis
  fatty
    liver NEC K76.0
      alcoholic K70.0
  grey matter (brain) (Alpers') G31.81
  heart (*see also* Degeneration, myocardial)
    amyloid E85.4 [I43]
    atheromatous — *see* Disease, heart, ischemic, atherosclerotic
    ischemic — *see* Disease, heart, ischemic
  hepatolenticular (Wilson's) E83.01
  hepatorenal K76.7
  hyaline (diffuse) (generalized)
    localized — *see* Degeneration, by site
  infrapatellar fat pad M79.4
  intervertebral disc NOS
    with
      myelopathy — *see* Disorder, disc, with, myelopathy
      radiculitis or radiculopathy — *see* Disorder, disc, with, radiculopathy
    cervical, cervicothoracic — *see* Disorder, disc, cervical, degeneration
      with
        myelopathy — *see* Disorder, disc, cervical, with myelopathy
        neuritis, radiculitis or radiculopathy — *see* Disorder, disc, cervical, with neuritis
    lumbar region M51.36
      with
        myelopathy M51.06
        neuritis, radiculitis, radiculopathy or sciatica M51.16
    lumbosacral region M51.37
      with
        neuritis, radiculitis, radiculopathy or sciatica M51.17
    sacrococcygeal region M53.3

Degeneration, degenerative — *continued*
  intervertebral disc — *continued*
    thoracic region M51.34
      with
        myelopathy M51.04
        neuritis, radiculitis, radiculopathy M51.14
    thoracolumbar region M51.35
      with
        myelopathy M51.05
        neuritis, radiculitis, radiculopathy M51.15
  intestine, amyloid E85.4
  iris (pigmentary) H21.23- ☑
  ischemic — *see* Ischemia
  joint disease — *see* Osteoarthritis
  kidney N28.89
    amyloid E85.4 [N29]
    cystic, congenital Q61.9
    fatty N28.89
    polycystic Q61.3
      adult type (autosomal dominant) Q61.2
      infantile type (autosomal recessive) NEC Q61.19
        collecting duct dilatation Q61.11
  Kuhnt-Junius (*see also* Degeneration, macula) H35.32
  lens — *see* Cataract
  lenticular (familial) (progressive) (Wilson's) (with cirrhosis of liver) E83.01
  liver (diffuse) NEC K76.89
    amyloid E85.4 [K77]
    cystic K76.89
      congenital Q44.6
    fatty NEC K76.0
      alcoholic K70.0
    hypertrophic K76.89
    parenchymatous, acute or subacute K72.00
      with coma K72.01
    pigmentary K76.89
    toxic (acute) K71.9
  lung J98.4
  lymph gland I89.8
    hyaline I89.8
  macula, macular (acquired) (age-related) (senile) H35.30
    angioid streaks H35.33
    atrophic age-related H35.31
    congenital or hereditary — *see* Dystrophy, retina
    cystoid H35.35- ☑
    drusen H35.36- ☑
    exudative H35.32
    hole H35.34- ☑
    nonexudative H35.31
    puckering H35.37- ☑
    toxic H35.38- ☑
  membranous labyrinth, congenital (causing impairment of hearing) Q16.5
  meniscus — *see* Derangement, meniscus
  mitral — *see* Insufficiency, mitral
  Mönckeberg's — *see* Arteriosclerosis, extremities
  motor centers, senile G31.1
  multi-system G90.3
  mural — *see* Degeneration, myocardial
  muscle (fatty) (fibrous) (hyaline) (progressive) M62.89
    heart — *see* Degeneration, myocardial
  myelin, central nervous system G37.9
  myocardial, myocardium (fatty) (hyaline) (senile) I51.5
    with rheumatic fever (conditions in I00) I09.0
      active, acute or subacute I01.2
        with chorea I02.0
      inactive or quiescent (with chorea) I09.0
    hypertensive — *see* Hypertension, heart
    rheumatic — *see* Degeneration, myocardial, with rheumatic fever
    syphilitic A52.06
  nasal sinus (mucosa) J32.9
    frontal J32.1
    maxillary J32.0
  nerve — *see* Disorder, nerve
  nervous system G31.9
    alcoholic G31.2
    amyloid E85.4 [G99.8]
    autonomic G90.9
    fatty G31.89
    specified NEC G31.89
  nipple N64.89
  olivopontocerebellar (hereditary) (familial) G23.8
  osseous labyrinth — *see* subcategory H83.8 ☑
  ovary N83.8
    cystic N83.20
    microcystic N83.20

Degeneration, degenerative — *continued*
  pallidal pigmentary (progressive) G23.0
  pancreas K86.8
    tuberculous A18.83
  penis N48.89
  pigmentary (diffuse) (general)
    localized — *see* Degeneration, by site
    pallidal (progressive) G23.0
  pineal gland E34.8
  pituitary (gland) E23.6
  popliteal fat pad M79.4
  posterolateral (spinal cord) — *see* Degeneration, combined
  pulmonary valve (heart) I37.8
  pulp (tooth) K04.2
  pupillary margin H21.24- ☑
  renal — *see* Degeneration, kidney
  retina H35.9
    hereditary (cerebroretinal) (congenital) (juvenile) (macula) (peripheral) (pigmentary) — *see* Dystrophy, retina
    Kuhnt-Junius (*see also* Degeneration, macula) H35.32
    macula (cystic) (exudative) (hole) (nonexudative) (pseudohole) (senile) (toxic) — *see* Degeneration, macula
    peripheral H35.40
      lattice H35.41- ☑
      microcystoid H35.42- ☑
      paving stone H35.43- ☑
      secondary
        pigmentary H35.45- ☑
        vitreoretinal H35.46- ☑
      senile reticular H35.44- ☑
    pigmentary (primary) (*see also* Dystrophy, retina)
      secondary — *see* Degeneration, retina, peripheral, secondary
    posterior pole — *see* Degeneration, macula
  saccule, congenital (causing impairment of hearing) Q16.5
  senile R54
    brain G31.1
    cardiac, heart or myocardium — *see* Degeneration, myocardial
    motor centers G31.1
    vascular — *see* Arteriosclerosis
  sinus (cystic) (*see also* Sinusitis)
    polypoid J33.1
  skin L98.8
    amyloid E85.4 [L99]
    colloid L98.8
  spinal (cord) G31.89
    amyloid E85.4 [G32.89]
    combined (subacute) — *see* Degeneration, combined
    dorsolateral — *see* Degeneration, combined
    familial NEC G31.89
    fatty G31.89
    funicular — *see* Degeneration, combined
    posterolateral — *see* Degeneration, combined
    subacute combined — *see* Degeneration, combined
    tuberculous A17.81
  spleen D73.0
    amyloid E85.4 [D77]
  stomach K31.89
  striatonigral G23.2
  suprarenal (capsule) (gland) E27.8
  synovial membrane (pulpy) — *see* Disorder, synovium, specified type NEC
  tapetoretinal — *see* Dystrophy, retina
  thymus (gland) E32.8
    fatty E32.8
  thyroid (gland) E07.89
  tricuspid (heart) (valve) I07.9
  tuberculous NEC — *see* Tuberculosis
  turbinate J34.89
  uterus (cystic) N85.8
  vascular (senile) — *see* Arteriosclerosis
    hypertensive — *see* Hypertension
  vitreoretinal, secondary — *see* Degeneration, retina, peripheral, secondary, vitreoretinal
  vitreous (body) H43.81- ☑
  Wallerian — *see* Disorder, nerve
  Wilson's hepatolenticular E83.01

Deglutition
  paralysis R13.0
    hysterical F44.4
  pneumonia J69.0
Degos' disease I77.89
Dehiscence (of)
  amputation stump T87.81
  cesarean wound O90.0
  closure of
    cornea T81.31 ☑
    craniotomy T81.32 ☑
    fascia (muscular) (superficial) T81.32 ☑
    internal organ or tissue T81.32 ☑
    laceration (external) (internal) T81.33 ☑
    ligament T81.32 ☑
    mucosa T81.31 ☑
    muscle or muscle flap T81.32 ☑
    ribs or rib cage T81.32 ☑
    skin and subcutaneous tissue (full-thickness) (su-
      perficial) T81.31 ☑
    skull T81.32 ☑
    sternum (sternotomy) T81.32 ☑
    tendon T81.32 ☑
    traumatic laceration (external) (internal) T81.33 ☑
  episiotomy O90.1
  operation wound NEC T81.31 ☑
    external operation wound (superficial) T81.31 ☑
    internal operation wound (deep) T81.32 ☑
  perineal wound (postpartum) O90.1
  traumatic injury wound repair T81.33 ☑
  wound T81.30 ☑
    traumatic repair T81.33 ☑
Dehydration E86.0
  hypertonic E87.0
  hypotonic E87.1
  newborn P74.1
Déjérine-Roussy syndrome G89.0
Déjérine-Sottas disease or neuropathy (hypertrophic)
  G60.0
Déjérine-Thomas atrophy G23.8
Delay, delayed
  any plane in pelvis
    complicating delivery O66.9
  birth or delivery NOS O63.9
  closure, ductus arteriosus (Botalli) P29.3
  coagulation — see Defect, coagulation
  conduction (cardiac) (ventricular) I45.9
  delivery, second twin, triplet, etc O63.2
  development R62.50
    global F88
    intellectual (specific) F81.9
    language F80.9
      due to hearing loss F80.4
    learning F81.9
    pervasive F84.9
    physiological R62.50
      specified stage NEC R62.0
    reading F81.0
    sexual E30.0
    speech F80.9
      due to hearing loss F80.4
    spelling F81.81
  gastric emptying K30
  menarche E30.0
  menstruation (cause unknown) N91.0
  milestone R62.0
  passage of meconium (newborn) P76.0
  primary respiration P28.9
  puberty (constitutional) E30.0
  separation of umbilical cord P96.82
  sexual maturation, female E30.0
  sleep phase syndrome G47.21
  union, fracture — see Fracture, by site
  vaccination Z28.9
Deletion(s)
  autosome Q93.9
    identified by fluorescence in situ hybridization
      (FISH) Q93.89
    identified by in situ hybridization (ISH) Q93.89
  chromosome
    with complex rearrangements NEC Q93.7
    part of NEC Q93.5
    seen only at prometaphase Q93.89
    short arm
      22q11.2 Q93.81
      4 Q93.3
      5p Q93.4

Deletion(s) — continued
  chromosome — continued
    specified NEC Q93.89
  long arm chromosome 18 or 21 Q93.89
    with complex rearrangements NEC Q93.7
  microdeletions NEC Q93.88
Delhi boil or button B55.1
Delinquency (juvenile) (neurotic) F91.8
  group Z72.810
Delinquent immunization status Z28.3
Delirium, delirious (acute or subacute) (not alcohol- or
  drug-induced) (with dementia) R41.0
  alcoholic (acute) (tremens) (withdrawal) F10.921
    with intoxication F10.921
      in
        abuse F10.121
        dependence F10.221
  due to (secondary to)
    alcohol
      intoxication F10.921
        in
          abuse F10.121
          dependence F10.221
      withdrawal F10.231
    amphetamine intoxication F15.921
      in
        abuse F15.121
        dependence F15.221
    anxiolytic
      intoxication F13.921
        in
          abuse F13.121
          dependence F13.221
      withdrawal F13.231
    cannabis intoxication (acute) F12.921
      in
        abuse F12.121
        dependence F12.221
    cocaine intoxication (acute) F14.921
      in
        abuse F14.121
        dependence F14.221
    general medical condition F05
    hallucinogen intoxication F16.921
      in
        abuse F16.121
        dependence F16.221
    hypnotic
      intoxication F13.921
        in
          abuse F13.121
          dependence F13.221
      withdrawal F13.231
    inhalant intoxication (acute) F18.921
      in
        abuse F18.121
        dependence F18.221
    multiple etiologies F05
    opioid intoxication (acute) F11.921
      in
        abuse F11.121
        dependence F11.221
    phencyclidine intoxication (acute) F16.921
      in
        abuse F16.121
        dependence F16.221
    psychoactive substance NEC intoxication (acute)
      F19.921
      in
        abuse F19.121
        dependence F19.221
    sedative
      intoxication F13.921
        in
          abuse F13.121
          dependence F13.221
      withdrawal F13.231
    unknown etiology F05
  exhaustion F43.0
  hysterical F44.89
  postprocedural (postoperative) F05
  puerperal F05
  thyroid — see Thyrotoxicosis with thyroid storm
  traumatic — see Injury, intracranial
  tremens (alcohol-induced) F10.231
    sedative-induced F13.231
Delivery (childbirth) (labor)
  arrested active phase O62.1

Delivery — continued
  cesarean (for)
    without indication O82
    abnormal
      pelvis (bony) (deformity) (major) NEC with dis-
        proportion (fetopelvic) O33.0
        with obstructed labor O65.0
      presentation or position O32.9 ☑
    abruptio placentae (see also Abruptio placentae)
      O45.9- ☑
    acromion presentation O32.2 ☑
    atony, uterus O62.2
    breech presentation O32.1 ☑
      incomplete O32.8 ☑
    brow presentation O32.3 ☑
    cephalopelvic disproportion O33.9
    cerclage O34.3- ☑
    chin presentation O32.3 ☑
    cicatrix of cervix O34.4- ☑
    contracted pelvis (general)
      inlet O33.2
      outlet O33.3
    cord presentation or prolapse O69.0 ☑
    cystocele O34.8- ☑
    deformity (acquired) (congenital)
      pelvic organs or tissues NEC O34.8- ☑
      pelvis (bony) NEC O33.0
    disproportion NOS O33.9
    eclampsia — see Eclampsia
    face presentation O32.3 ☑
    failed
      forceps O66.5
      induction of labor O61.9
        instrumental O61.1
        mechanical O61.1
        medical O61.0
        specified NEC O61.8
        surgical O61.1
      trial of labor NOS O66.40
        following previous cesarean delivery O66.41
      vacuum extraction O66.5
      ventouse O66.5
    fetal-maternal hemorrhage O43.01- ☑
    hemorrhage (intrapartum) O67.9
      with coagulation defect O67.0
      specified cause NEC O67.8
    high head at term O32.4 ☑
    hydrocephalic fetus O33.6 ☑
    incarceration of uterus O34.51- ☑
    incoordinate uterine action O62.4
    increased size, fetus O33.5 ☑
    inertia, uterus O62.2
      primary O62.0
      secondary O62.1
    lateroversion, uterus O34.59- ☑
    mal lie O32.9 ☑
    malposition
      fetus O32.9 ☑
      pelvic organs or tissues NEC O34.8- ☑
      uterus NEC O34.59- ☑
    malpresentation NOS O32.9 ☑
    oblique presentation O32.2 ☑
    occurring after 37 completed weeks of gestation
      but before 39 completed weeks gestation
      due to (spontaneous) onset of labor O75.82
    oversize fetus O33.5 ☑
    pelvic tumor NEC O34.8- ☑
    placenta previa O44.1- ☑
      without hemorrhage O44.0- ☑
    placental insufficiency O36.51- ☑
    planned, occurring after 37 completed weeks of
      gestation but before 39 completed weeks
      gestation due to (spontaneous) onset of la-
      bor O75.82
    polyp, cervix O34.4- ☑
      causing obstructed labor O65.5
    poor dilatation, cervix O62.0
    pre-eclampsia O14.9- ☑
      mild O14.0- ☑
      moderate O14.0- ☑
      severe
        with hemolysis, elevated liver enzymes and
          low platelet count (HELLP) O14.2- ☑
    previous
      cesarean delivery O34.21
      surgery (to)
        cervix O34.4- ☑

Delivery — *continued*
  cesarean — *continued*
    previous — *continued*
      surgery — *continued*
        gynecological NEC O34.8- ☑
        rectum O34.7- ☑
        uterus O34.29
        vagina O34.6- ☑
    prolapse
      arm or hand O32.2 ☑
      uterus O34.52- ☑
    prolonged labor NOS O63.9
    rectocele O34.8- ☑
    retroversion
      uterus O34.53- ☑
    rigid
      cervix O34.4- ☑
      pelvic floor O34.8- ☑
      perineum O34.7- ☑
      vagina O34.6 ☑
      vulva O34.7- ☑
    sacculation, pregnant uterus O34.59- ☑
    scar(s)
      cervix O34.4- ☑
      cesarean delivery O34.21
      uterus O34.29
    Shirodkar suture in situ O34.3- ☑
    shoulder presentation O32.2 ☑
    stenosis or stricture, cervix O34.4- ☑
    streptococcus B carrier state O99.824
    transverse presentation or lie O32.2 ☑
    tumor, pelvic organs or tissues NEC O34.8- ☑
      cervix O34.4- ☑
    umbilical cord presentation or prolapse O69.0 ☑
  completely normal case O80
  complicated O75.9
    by
      abnormal, abnormality (of)
        forces of labor O62.9
          specified type NEC O62.8
        glucose O99.814
        uterine contractions NOS O62.9
      abruptio placentae (*see also* Abruptio placentae) O45.9- ☑
      abuse
        physical O9A.32 (*following* O99)
        psychological O9A.52 (*following* O99)
        sexual O9A.42 (*following* O99)
      adherent placenta O72.0
        without hemorrhage O73.0
      alcohol use O99.314
      anemia (pre-existing) O99.02
      anesthetic death O74.8
      annular detachment of cervix O71.3
      atony, uterus O62.2
      attempted vacuum extraction and forceps O66.5
      Bandl's ring O62.4
      bariatric surgery status O99.844
      biliary tract disorder O26.62
      bleeding — *see* Delivery, complicated by, hemorrhage
      blood disorder NEC O99.12
      cervical dystocia (hypotonic) O62.2
        primary O62.0
        secondary O62.1
      circulatory system disorder O99.42
      compression of cord (umbilical) NEC O69.2 ☑
      condition NEC O99.89
      contraction, contracted ring O62.4
      cord (umbilical)
        around neck
          with compression O69.1 ☑
          without compression O69.81 ☑
        bruising O69.5 ☑
        complication O69.9 ☑
          specified NEC O69.89 ☑
        compression NEC O69.2 ☑
        entanglement O69.2 ☑
          without compression O69.82 ☑
        hematoma O69.5 ☑
        presentation O69.0 ☑
        prolapse O69.0 ☑
        short O69.3 ☑
        thrombosis (vessels) O69.5 ☑
        vascular lesion O69.5 ☑
      Couvelaire uterus O45.8X- ☑

Delivery — *continued*
  complicated — *continued*
    by — *continued*
      damage to (injury to) NEC
        perineum O71.82
        periurethral tissue O71.82
        vulva O71.82
      delay following rupture of membranes (spontaneous) — *see* Pregnancy, complicated by, premature rupture of membranes
      depressed fetal heart tones O76
      diabetes O24.92
        gestational O24.429
          diet controlled O24.420
          insulin controlled O24.424
        pre-existing O24.32
          specified NEC O24.82
          type 1 O24.02
          type 2 O24.12
      diastasis recti (abdominis) O71.89
      dilatation
        bladder O66.8
        cervix incomplete, poor or slow O62.0
      disease NEC O99.89
      disruptio uteri — *see* Delivery, complicated by, rupture, uterus
      drug use O99.324
      dysfunction, uterus NOS O62.9
        hypertonic O62.4
        hypotonic O62.2
          primary O62.0
          secondary O62.1
        incoordinate O62.4
      eclampsia O15.1
      embolism (pulmonary) — *see* Embolism, obstetric
      endocrine, nutritional or metabolic disease NEC O99.284
      failed
        attempted vaginal birth after previous cesarean delivery O66.41
        induction of labor O61.9
          instrumental O61.1
          mechanical O61.1
          medical O61.0
          specified NEC O61.8
          surgical O61.1
        trial of labor O66.40
      female genital mutilation O65.5
      fetal
        abnormal acid-base balance O68
        acidemia O68
        acidosis O68
        alkalosis O68
        death, early O02.1
        deformity O66.3
        heart rate or rhythm (abnormal) (non-reassuring) O76
        hypoxia O77.8
        stress O77.9
          due to drug administration O77.1
          electrocardiographic evidence of O77.8
          specified NEC O77.8
          ultrasound evidence of O77.8
      fever during labor O75.2
      gastric banding status O99.844
      gastric bypass status O99.844
      gastrointestinal disease NEC O99.62
      gestational diabetes O24.429
        diet controlled O24.420
        insulin (and diet) controlled O24.424
      gonorrhea O98.22
      hematoma O71.7
        ischial spine O71.7
        pelvic O71.7
        vagina O71.7
        vulva or perineum O71.7
      hemorrhage (uterine) O67.9
        associated with
          afibrinogenemia O67.0
          coagulation defect O67.0
          hyperfibrinolysis O67.0
          hypofibrinogenemia O67.0
        due to
          low-lying placenta O44.1- ☑
          placenta previa O44.1- ☑

Delivery — *continued*
  complicated — *continued*
    by — *continued*
      hemorrhage — *continued*
        due to — *continued*
          premature separation of placenta (normally implanted) (*see also* Abruptio placentae) O45.9- ☑
          retained placenta O72.0
          uterine leiomyoma O67.8
        placenta NEC O67.8
        postpartum NEC (atonic) (immediate) O72.1
          with retained or trapped placenta O72.0
          delayed O72.2
          secondary O72.2
          third stage O72.0
      hourglass contraction, uterus O62.4
      hypertension, hypertensive (pre-existing) — *see* Hypertension, complicated by, childbirth (labor)
      hypotension O26.5- ☑
      incomplete dilatation (cervix) O62.0
      incoordinate uterus contractions O62.4
      inertia, uterus O62.2
        during latent phase of labor O62.0
        primary O62.0
        secondary O62.1
      infection (maternal) O98.92
        carrier state NEC O99.834
        gonorrhea O98.22
        human immunodeficiency virus (HIV) O98.72
        sexually transmitted NEC O98.32
        specified NEC O98.82
        syphilis O98.12
        tuberculosis O98.02
        viral hepatitis O98.42
        viral NEC O98.52
      injury (to mother) (*see also* Delivery, complicated, by, damage to) O71.9
        nonobstetric O9A.22 (*following* O99)
          caused by abuse — *see* Delivery, complicated by, abuse
      intrauterine fetal death, early O02.1
      inversion, uterus O71.2
      laceration (perineal) O70.9
        anus (sphincter) O70.4
          with third degree laceration O70.2
            with mucosa O70.3
          without third degree laceration O70.4
        bladder (urinary) O71.5
        bowel O71.5
        cervix (uteri) O71.3
        fourchette O70.0
        hymen O70.0
        labia O70.0
        pelvic
          floor O70.1
          organ NEC O71.5
        perineum, perineal O70.9
          first degree O70.0
          fourth degree O70.3
          muscles O70.1
          second degree O70.1
          skin O70.0
          slight O70.0
          third degree O70.2
        peritoneum (pelvic) O71.5
        rectovaginal (septum) (without perineal laceration) O71.4
          with perineum O70.2
            with anal or rectal mucosa O70.3
        specified NEC O71.89
        sphincter ani — *see* Delivery, complicated, by, laceration, anus (sphincter)
        urethra O71.5
        uterus O71.81
          before labor O71.81
        vagina, vaginal (deep) (high) (without perineal laceration) O71.4
          with perineum O70.0
          muscles, with perineum O70.1
        vulva O70.0
      liver disorder O26.62
      malignancy O9A.12 (*following* O99)
      malnutrition O25.2

☑ **Additional Character Required** — Refer to the Tabular List for Character Selection   ▽ **Subterms under main terms may continue to next column or page**

Delivery — *continued*
  complicated — *continued*
    by — *continued*
      malposition, malpresentation
        without obstruction (*see also* Delivery,
              complicated by, obstruction) O32.9 ☑
          breech O32.1 ☑
          compound O32.6 ☑
          face (brow) (chin) O32.3 ☑
          footling O32.8 ☑
          high head O32.4 ☑
          oblique O32.2 ☑
          specified NEC O32.8 ☑
          transverse O32.2 ☑
          unstable lie O32.0 ☑
        placenta (with hemorrhage) O44.1- ☑
          without hemorrhage O44.0- ☑
        uterus or cervix O65.5
      meconium in amniotic fluid O77.0
      mental disorder NEC O99.344
      metrorrhexis — *see* Delivery, complicated by,
          rupture, uterus
      nervous system disorder O99.354
      obesity (pre-existing) O99.214
      obesity surgery status O99.844
      obstetric trauma O71.9
        specified NEC O71.89
      obstructed labor
        due to
          breech (complete) (frank) presentation
              O64.1 ☑
            incomplete O64.8 ☑
          brow presenation O64.3 ☑
          buttock presentation O64.1 ☑
          chin presentation O64.2 ☑
          compound presentation O64.5 ☑
          contracted pelvis O65.1
          deep transverse arrest O64.0 ☑
          deformed pelvis O65.0
          dystocia (fetal) O66.9
            due to
              conjoined twins O66.3
              fetal
                abnormality NEC O66.3
                ascites O66.3
                hydrops O66.3
                meningomyelocele O66.3
                sacral teratoma O66.3
                tumor O66.3
              hydrocephalic fetus O66.3
              shoulder O66.0
          face presentation O64.2 ☑
          fetopelvic disproportion O65.4
          footling presentation O64.8 ☑
          impacted shoulders O66.0
          incomplete rotation of fetal head
              O64.0 ☑
          large fetus O66.2
          locked twins O66.1
          malposition O64.9 ☑
            specified NEC O64.8 ☑
          malpresentation O64.9 ☑
            specified NEC O64.8 ☑
          multiple fetuses NEC O66.6
          pelvic
            abnormality (maternal) O65.9
              organ O65.5
                specified NEC O65.8
            contraction
              inlet O65.2
              mid-cavity O65.3
              outlet O65.3
          persistent (position)
            occipitoiliac O64.0 ☑
            occipitoposterior O64.0 ☑
            occipitosacral O64.0 ☑
            occipitotransverse O64.0 ☑
          prolapsed arm O64.4 ☑
          shoulder presentation O64.4 ☑
        specified NEC O66.8
      pathological retraction ring, uterus O62.4
      penetration, pregnant uterus by instrument
          O71.1
      perforation — *see* Delivery, complicated by,
          laceration

Delivery — *continued*
  complicated — *continued*
    by — *continued*
      placenta, placental
        ablatio (*see also* Abruptio placentae)
            O45.9- ☑
        abnormality O43.9- ☑
          specified NEC O43.89- ☑
        abruptio (*see also* Abruptio placentae)
            O45.9- ☑
        accreta O43.21- ☑
        adherent (with hemorrhage) O72.0
          without hemorrhage O73.0
        detachment (premature) (*see also* Abruptio
            placentae) O45.9- ☑
        disorder O43.9- ☑
          specified NEC O43.89- ☑
        hemorrhage NEC O67.8
        increta O43.22- ☑
        low (implantation) O44.1- ☑
          without hemorrhage O44.0- ☑
        malformation O43.10- ☑
        malposition O44.1- ☑
          without hemorrhage O44.0- ☑
        percreta O43.23- ☑
        previa (central) (lateral) (low) (marginal)
            (partial) (total) O44.1- ☑
          without hemorrhage O44.0- ☑
        retained (with hemorrhage) O72.0
          without hemorrhage O73.0
        separation (premature) O45.9- ☑
          specified NEC O45.8X- ☑
        vicious insertion O44.1- ☑
      precipitate labor O62.3
      premature rupture, membranes (*see also* Preg-
          nancy, complicated by, premature rup-
          ture of membranes) O42.90
      prolapse
        arm or hand O32.2 ☑
        cord (umbilical) O69.0 ☑
        foot or leg O32.8 ☑
        uterus O34.52- ☑
      prolonged labor O63.9
        first stage O63.0
        second stage O63.1
      protozoal disease (maternal) O98.62
      respiratory disease NEC O99.52
      retained membranes or portions of placenta
          O72.2
        without hemorrhage O73.1
      retarded birth O63.9
      retention of secundines (with hemorrhage)
          O72.0
        without hemorrhage O73.0
        partial O72.2
          without hemorrhage O73.1
      rupture
        bladder (urinary) O71.5
        cervix O71.3
        pelvic organ NEC O71.5
        urethra O71.5
        uterus (during or after labor) O71.1
          before labor O71.0- ☑
      separation, pubic bone (symphysis pubis) O71.6
      shock O75.1
      shoulder presentation O64.4 ☑
      skin disorder NEC O99.72
      spasm, cervix O62.4
      stenosis or stricture, cervix O65.5
      streptococcus B carrier state O99.824
      subluxation of symphysis (pubis) O26.72
      syphilis (maternal) O98.12
      tear — *see* Delivery, complicated by, laceration
      tetanic uterus O62.4
      trauma (obstetrical) (*see also* Delivery, compli-
          cated, by, damage to) O71.9
        non-obstetric O9A.22 (*following* O99)
          periurethral O71.82
          specified NEC O71.89
      tuberculosis (maternal) O98.02
      tumor, pelvic organs or tissues NEC O65.5
      umbilical cord around neck
        with compression O69.1 ☑
        without compression O69.81 ☑
      uterine inertia O62.2
        during latent phase of labor O62.0
        primary O62.0

Delivery — *continued*
  complicated — *continued*
    by — *continued*
      uterine inertia — *continued*
        secondary O62.1
        vasa previa O69.4 ☑
        velamentous insertion of cord O43.12- ☑
      specified complication NEC O75.89
  delayed NOS O63.9
    following rupture of membranes
      artificial O75.5
    second twin, triplet, etc. O63.2
  forceps, low following failed vacuum extraction O66.5
  missed (at or near term) O36.4 ☑
  normal O80
  obstructed — *see* Delivery, complicated by, obstruc-
      tion
  precipitate O62.3
  preterm (*see also* Pregnancy, complicated by, preterm
      labor) O60.10 ☑
  spontaneous O80
  term pregnancy NOS O80
  uncomplicated O80
  vaginal, following previous cesarean delivery O34.21
Delusions (paranoid) — *see* Disorder, delusional
Dementia (degenerative (primary)) (old age) (persisting)
    F03.90
  with
    aggressive behavior F03.91
    behavioral disturbance F03.91
    combative behavior F03.91
    Lewy bodies G31.83 [F02.80]
      with behavioral disturbance G31.83 [F02.81]
    Parkinsonism G31.83 [F02.80]
      with behavioral disturbance G31.83 [F02.81]
    Parkinson's disease G20 [F02.80]
      with behavioral disturbance G20 [F02.81]
    violent behavior F03.91
  alcoholic F10.97
    with dependence F10.27
  Alzheimer's type — *see* Disease, Alzheimer's
  arteriosclerotic — *see* Dementia, vascular
  atypical, Alzheimer's type — *see* Disease, Alzheimer's,
      specified NEC
  congenital — *see* Disability, intellectual
  frontal (lobe) G31.09 [F02.80]
    with behavioral disturbance G31.09 [F02.81]
  frontotemporal G31.09 [F02.80]
    with behavioral disturbance G31.09 [F02.81]
    specified NEC G31.09 [F02.80]
      with behavioral disturbance G31.09 [F02.81]
  in (due to)
    with behavioral disturbance G31.83 [F02.81]
    alcohol F10.97
      with dependence F10.27
    Alzheimer's disease — *see* Disease, Alzheimer's
    arteriosclerotic brain disease — *see* Dementia,
        vascular
    cerebral lipidoses E75.- ☑ [F02.80]
      with behavioral disturbance E75.- ☑ [F02.81]
    Creutzfeldt-Jakob disease (*see also* Creutzfeldt-
        Jakob disease or syndrome (with dementia))
        A81.00
    epilepsy G40.- ☑ [F02.80]
      with behavioral disturbance G40.- ☑ [F02.81]
    hepatolenticular degeneration E83.01 [F02.80]
      with behavioral disturbance E83.01 [F02.81]
    human immunodeficiency virus (HIV) disease
        B20 [F02.80]
      with behavioral disturbance B20 [F02.81]
    Huntington's disease or chorea G10
    hypercalcemia E83.52 [F02.80]
      with behavioral disturbance E83.52 [F02.81]
    hypothyroidism, acquired E03.9 [F02.80]
      with behavioral disturbance E03.9 [F02.81]
      due to iodine deficiency E01.8 [F02.80]
        with behavioral disturbance E01.8 [F02.81]
    inhalants F18.97
      with dependence F18.27
    multiple
      etiologies F03 ☑
      sclerosis G35 [F02.80]
        with behavioral disturbance G35 [F02.81]
      neurosyphilis A52.17 [F02.80]
        with behavioral disturbance A52.17 [F02.81]
      juvenile A50.49 [F02.80]
        with behavioral disturbance A50.49 [F02.81]

Index

Delivery — Dementia

Dementia — *continued*
  in — *continued*
    niacin deficiency E52 [F02.80]
      with behavioral disturbance E52 [F02.81]
    paralysis agitans G20 [F02.80]
      with behavioral disturbance G20 [F02.81]
    Parkinson's disease G20 [F02.80]
    pellagra E52 [F02.80]
      with behavioral disturbance E52 [F02.81]
    Pick's G31.01 [F02.80]
      with behavioral disturbance G31.01 [F02.81]
    polyarteritis nodosa M30.0 [F02.80]
      with behavioral disturbance M30.0 [F02.81]
    psychoactive drug F19.97
      with dependence F19.27
      inhalants F18.97
        with dependence F18.27
      sedatives, hypnotics or anxiolytics F13.97
        with dependence F13.27
    sedatives, hypnotics or anxiolytics F13.97
      with dependence F13.27
    systemic lupus erythematosus M32.- ☑ [F02.80]
      with behavioral disturbance M32.- ☑ [F02.81]
    trypanosomiasis
      African B56.9 [F02.80]
        with behavioral disturbance B56.9 [F02.81]
    unknown etiology F03 ☑
    vitamin B12 deficiency E53.8 [F02.80]
      with behavioral disturbance E53.8 [F02.81]
    volatile solvents F18.97
      with dependence F18.27
  infantile, infantilis F84.3
  Lewy body G31.83 [F02.80]
    with behavioral disturbance G31.83 [F02.81]
  multi-Infarct — *see* Dementia, vascular
  paralytica, paralytic (syphilitic) A52.17 [F02.80]
    with behavioral disturbance A52.17 [F02.81]
    juvenilis A50.45
  paretic A52.17
  praecox — *see* Schizophrenia
  presenile F03 ☑
    Alzheimer's type — *see* Disease, Alzheimer's, early onset
  primary degenerative F03 ☑
  progressive, syphilitic A52.17
  senile F03 ☑
    with acute confusional state F05
    Alzheimer's type — *see* Disease, Alzheimer's, late onset
    depressed or paranoid type F03 ☑
  vascular (acute onset) (mixed) (multi-infarct) (subcortical) F01.50
    with behavioral disturbance F01.51
Demineralization, bone — *see* Osteoporosis
Demodex folliculorum (infestation) B88.0
Demophobia F40.248
Demoralization R45.3
Demyelination, demyelinization
  central nervous system G37.9
    specified NEC G37.8
  corpus callosum (central) G37.1
  disseminated, acute G36.9
    specified NEC G36.8
  global G35
  in optic neuritis G36.0
Dengue (classical) (fever) A90
  hemorrhagic A91
  sandfly A93.1
Dennie-Marfan syphilitic syndrome A50.45
Dens evaginatus, in dente or invaginatus K00.2
Dense breasts R92.2
Density
  increased, bone (disseminated) (generalized) (spotted) — *see* Disorder, bone, density and structure, specified type NEC
  lung (nodular) J98.4
Dental (*see also* condition)
  examination Z01.20
    with abnormal findings Z01.21
  restoration
    aesthetically inadequate or displeasing K08.56
    defective K08.50
      specified NEC K08.59
    failure of marginal integrity K08.51
    failure of periodontal anatomical integrity K08.54
Dentia praecox K00.6
Denticles (pulp) K04.2
Dentigerous cyst K09.0

Dentin
  irregular (in pulp) K04.3
  opalescent K00.5
  secondary (in pulp) K04.3
  sensitive K03.89
Dentinogenesis imperfecta K00.5
Dentinoma — *see* Cyst, calcifying odontogenic
Dentition (syndrome) K00.7
  delayed K00.6
  difficult K00.7
  precocious K00.6
  premature K00.6
  retarded K00.6
Dependence (on) (syndrome) F19.20
  with remission F19.21
  alcohol (ethyl) (methyl) (without remission) F10.20
    with
      amnestic disorder, persisting F10.26
      anxiety disorder F10.280
      dementia, persisting F10.27
      intoxication F10.229
        with delirium F10.221
        uncomplicated F10.220
      mood disorder F10.24
      psychotic disorder F10.259
        with
          delusions F10.250
          hallucinations F10.251
      remission F10.21
      sexual dysfunction F10.281
      sleep disorder F10.282
      specified disorder NEC F10.288
      withdrawal F10.239
        with
          delirium F10.231
          perceptual disturbance F10.232
        uncomplicated F10.230
    counseling and surveillance Z71.41
  amobarbital — *see* Dependence, drug, sedative
  amphetamine(s) (type) — *see* Dependence, drug, stimulant NEC
  amytal (sodium) — *see* Dependence, drug, sedative
  analgesic NEC F55.8
  anesthetic (agent) (gas) (general) (local) NEC — *see* Dependence, drug, psychoactive NEC
  anxiolytic NEC — *see* Dependence, drug, sedative
  barbital(s) — *see* Dependence, drug, sedative
  barbiturate(s) (compounds) (drugs classifiable to T42) — *see* Dependence, drug, sedative
  benzedrine — *see* Dependence, drug, stimulant NEC
  bhang — *see* Dependence, drug, cannabis
  bromide(s) NEC — *see* Dependence, drug, sedative
  caffeine — *see* Dependence, drug, stimulant NEC
  cannabis (sativa) (indica) (resin) (derivatives) (type) — *see* Dependence, drug, cannabis
  chloral (betaine) (hydrate) — *see* Dependence, drug, sedative
  chlordiazepoxide — *see* Dependence, drug, sedative
  coca (leaf) (derivatives) — *see* Dependence, drug, cocaine
  cocaine — *see* Dependence, drug, cocaine
  codeine — *see* Dependence, drug, opioid
  combinations of drugs F19.20
  dagga — *see* Dependence, drug, cannabis
  demerol — *see* Dependence, drug, opioid
  dexamphetamine — *see* Dependence, drug, stimulant NEC
  dexedrine — *see* Dependence, drug, stimulant NEC
  dextromethorphan — *see* Dependence, drug, opioid
  dextromoramide — *see* Dependence, drug, opioid
  dextro-nor-pseudo-ephedrine — *see* Dependence, drug, stimulant NEC
  dextrorphan — *see* Dependence, drug, opioid
  diazepam — *see* Dependence, drug, sedative
  dilaudid — *see* Dependence, drug, opioid
  D-lysergic acid diethylamide — *see* Dependence, drug, hallucinogen
  drug NEC F19.20
    with sleep disorder F19.282
    cannabis F12.20
      with
        anxiety disorder F12.280
        intoxication F12.229
          with
            delirium F12.221
            perceptual disturbance F12.222
          uncomplicated F12.220

Dependence — *continued*
  drug — *continued*
    cannabis — *continued*
      with — *continued*
        other specified disorder F12.288
        psychosis F12.259
          delusions F12.250
          hallucinations F12.251
        unspecified disorder F12.29
      in remission F12.21
    cocaine F14.20
      with
        anxiety disorder F14.280
        intoxication F14.229
          with
            delirium F14.221
            perceptual disturbance F14.222
          uncomplicated F14.220
        mood disorder F14.24
        other specified disorder F14.288
        psychosis F14.259
          delusions F14.250
          hallucinations F14.251
        sexual dysfunction F14.281
        sleep disorder F14.282
        unspecified disorder F14.29
        withdrawal F14.23
      in remission F14.21
      withdrawal symptoms in newborn P96.1
    counseling and surveillance Z71.51
    hallucinogen F16.20
      with
        anxiety disorder F16.280
        flashbacks F16.283
        intoxication F16.229
          with delirium F16.221
          uncomplicated F16.220
        mood disorder F16.24
        other specified disorder F16.288
        perception disorder, persisting F16.283
        psychosis F16.259
          delusions F16.250
          hallucinations F16.251
        unspecified disorder F16.29
      in remission F16.21
    in remission F19.21
    inhalant F18.20
      with
        anxiety disorder F18.280
        dementia, persisting F18.27
        intoxication F18.229
          with delirium F18.221
          uncomplicated F18.220
        mood disorder F18.24
        other specified disorder F18.288
        psychosis F18.259
          delusions F18.250
          hallucinations F18.251
        unspecified disorder F18.29
      in remission F18.21
    nicotine F17.200
      with disorder F17.209
        remission F17.201
        specified disorder NEC F17.208
        withdrawal F17.203
      chewing tobacco F17.220
        with disorder F17.229
          remission F17.221
          specified disorder NEC F17.228
          withdrawal F17.223
      cigarettes F17.210
        with disorder F17.219
          remission F17.211
          specified disorder NEC F17.218
          withdrawal F17.213
      specified product NEC F17.290
        with disorder F17.299
          remission F17.291
          specified disorder NEC F17.298
          withdrawal F17.293
    opioid F11.20
      with
        intoxication F11.229
          with
            delirium F11.221
            perceptual disturbance F11.222
          uncomplicated F11.220
        mood disorder F11.24

Dependence — *continued*
　drug — *continued*
　　opioid — *continued*
　　　with — *continued*
　　　　other specified disorder F11.288
　　　　psychosis F11.259
　　　　　delusions F11.250
　　　　　hallucinations F11.251
　　　　sexual dysfunction F11.281
　　　　sleep disorder F11.282
　　　　unspecified disorder F11.29
　　　　withdrawal F11.23
　　　in remission F11.21
　　psychoactive NEC F19.20
　　　with
　　　　amnestic disorder F19.26
　　　　anxiety disorder F19.280
　　　　dementia F19.27
　　　　intoxication F19.229
　　　　　with
　　　　　　delirium F19.221
　　　　　　perceptual disturbance F19.222
　　　　　uncomplicated F19.220
　　　　mood disorder F19.24
　　　　other specified disorder F19.288
　　　　psychosis F19.259
　　　　　delusions F19.250
　　　　　hallucinations F19.251
　　　　sexual dysfunction F19.281
　　　　sleep disorder F19.282
　　　　unspecified disorder F19.29
　　　　withdrawal F19.239
　　　　　with
　　　　　　delirium F19.231
　　　　　　perceptual disturbance F19.232
　　　　　uncomplicated F19.230
　　sedative, hypnotic or anxiolytic F13.20
　　　with
　　　　amnestic disorder F13.26
　　　　anxiety disorder F13.280
　　　　dementia, persisting F13.27
　　　　intoxication F13.229
　　　　　with delirium F13.221
　　　　　uncomplicated F13.220
　　　　mood disorder F13.24
　　　　other specified disorder F13.288
　　　　psychosis F13.259
　　　　　delusions F13.250
　　　　　hallucinations F13.251
　　　　sexual dysfunction F13.281
　　　　sleep disorder F13.282
　　　　unspecified disorder F13.29
　　　　withdrawal F13.239
　　　　　with
　　　　　　delirium F13.231
　　　　　　perceptual disturbance F13.232
　　　　　uncomplicated F13.230
　　　in remission F13.21
　　stimulant NEC F15.20
　　　with
　　　　anxiety disorder F15.280
　　　　intoxication F15.229
　　　　　with
　　　　　　delirium F15.221
　　　　　　perceptual disturbance F15.222
　　　　　uncomplicated F15.220
　　　　mood disorder F15.24
　　　　other specified disorder F15.288
　　　　psychosis F15.259
　　　　　delusions F15.250
　　　　　hallucinations F15.251
　　　　sexual dysfunction F15.281
　　　　sleep disorder F15.282
　　　　unspecified disorder F15.29
　　　　withdrawal F15.23
　　　in remission F15.21
　ethyl
　　alcohol (without remission) F10.20
　　　with remission F10.21
　　bromide — *see* Dependence, drug, sedative
　　carbamate F19.20
　　chloride F19.20
　　morphine — *see* Dependence, drug, opioid
　ganja — *see* Dependence, drug, cannabis
　glue (airplane) (sniffing) — *see* Dependence, drug, inhalant
　glutethimide — *see* Dependence, drug, sedative

Dependence — *continued*
　hallucinogenics — *see* Dependence, drug, hallucinogen
　hashish — *see* Dependence, drug, cannabis
　hemp — *see* Dependence, drug, cannabis
　heroin (salt) (any) — *see* Dependence, drug, opioid
　hypnotic NEC — *see* Dependence, drug, sedative
　Indian hemp — *see* Dependence, drug, cannabis
　inhalants — *see* Dependence, drug, inhalant
　khat — *see* Dependence, drug, stimulant NEC
　laudanum — *see* Dependence, drug, opioid
　LSD (-25) (derivatives) — *see* Dependence, drug, hallucinogen
　luminal — *see* Dependence, drug, sedative
　lysergic acid — *see* Dependence, drug, hallucinogen
　maconha — *see* Dependence, drug, cannabis
　marihuana — *see* Dependence, drug, cannabis
　meprobamate — *see* Dependence, drug, sedative
　mescaline — *see* Dependence, drug, hallucinogen
　methadone — *see* Dependence, drug, opioid
　methamphetamine(s) — *see* Dependence, drug, stimulant NEC
　methaqualone — *see* Dependence, drug, sedative
　methyl
　　alcohol (without remission) F10.20
　　　with remission F10.21
　　bromide — *see* Dependence, drug, sedative
　　morphine — *see* Dependence, drug, opioid
　　phenidate — *see* Dependence, drug, stimulant NEC
　　sulfonal — *see* Dependence, drug, sedative
　morphine (sulfate) (sulfite) (type) — *see* Dependence, drug, opioid
　narcotic (drug) NEC — *see* Dependence, drug, opioid
　nembutal — *see* Dependence, drug, sedative
　neraval — *see* Dependence, drug, sedative
　neravan — *see* Dependence, drug, sedative
　neurobarb — *see* Dependence, drug, sedative
　nicotine — *see* Dependence, drug, nicotine
　nitrous oxide F19.20
　nonbarbiturate sedatives and tranquilizers with similar effect — *see* Dependence, drug, sedative
　on
　　artificial heart (fully implantable) (mechanical) Z95.812
　　aspirator Z99.0
　　care provider (because of) Z74.9
　　　impaired mobility Z74.09
　　　need for
　　　　assistance with personal care Z74.1
　　　　continuous supervision Z74.3
　　　no other household member able to render care Z74.2
　　　specified reason NEC Z74.8
　　machine Z99.89
　　　enabling NEC Z99.89
　　　specified type NEC Z99.89
　　renal dialysis (hemodialysis) (peritoneal) Z99.2
　　respirator Z99.11
　　ventilator Z99.11
　　wheelchair Z99.3
　opiate — *see* Dependence, drug, opioid
　opioids — *see* Dependence, drug, opioid
　opium (alkaloids) (derivatives) (tincture) — *see* Dependence, drug, opioid
　oxygen (long-term) (supplemental) Z99.81
　paraldehyde — *see* Dependence, drug, sedative
　paregoric — *see* Dependence, drug, opioid
　PCP (phencyclidine) (*see also* Abuse, drug, hallucinogen) F16.20
　pentobarbital — *see* Dependence, drug, sedative
　pentobarbitone (sodium) — *see* Dependence, drug, sedative
　pentothal — *see* Dependence, drug, sedative
　peyote — *see* Dependence, drug, hallucinogen
　phencyclidine (PCP) (and related substances) (*see also* Abuse, drug, hallucinogen) F16.20
　phenmetrazine — *see* Dependence, drug, stimulant NEC
　phenobarbital — *see* Dependence, drug, sedative
　polysubstance F19.20
　psilocibin, psilocin, psilocyn, psilocyline — *see* Dependence, drug, hallucinogen
　psychostimulant NEC — *see* Dependence, drug, stimulant NEC
　secobarbital — *see* Dependence, drug, sedative
　seconal — *see* Dependence, drug, sedative

Dependence — *continued*
　sedative NEC — *see* Dependence, drug, sedative
　specified drug NEC — *see* Dependence, drug
　stimulant NEC — *see* Dependence, drug, stimulant NEC
　substance NEC — *see* Dependence, drug
　supplemental oxygen Z99.81
　tobacco — *see* Dependence, drug, nicotine
　　counseling and surveillance Z71.6
　tranquilizer NEC — *see* Dependence, drug, sedative
　vitamin B6 E53.1
　volatile solvents — *see* Dependence, drug, inhalant
Dependency
　care-provider Z74.9
　passive F60.7
　reactions (persistent) F60.7
Depersonalization (in neurotic state) (neurotic) (syndrome) F48.1
Depletion
　extracellular fluid E86.9
　plasma E86.1
　potassium E87.6
　　nephropathy N25.89
　salt or sodium E87.1
　　causing heat exhaustion or prostration T67.4 ☑
　　nephropathy N28.9
　volume NOS E86.9
Deployment (current) (military) status Z56.82
　in theater or in support of military war, peacekeeping and humanitarian operations Z56.82
　personal history of Z91.82
　　military war, peacekeeping and humanitarian deployment (current or past conflict) Z91.82
　returned from Z91.82
Depolarization, premature I49.40
　atrial I49.1
　junctional I49.2
　specified NEC I49.49
　ventricular I49.3
Deposit
　bone in Boeck's sarcoid D86.89
　calcareous, calcium — *see* Calcification
　cholesterol
　　retina H35.89
　　vitreous (body) (humor) — *see* Deposit, crystalline
　conjunctiva H11.11- ☑
　cornea H18.00- ☑
　　argentous H18.02- ☑
　　due to metabolic disorder H18.03- ☑
　　Kayser-Fleischer ring H18.04- ☑
　　pigmentation — *see* Pigmentation, cornea
　crystalline, vitreous (body) (humor) H43.2- ☑
　hemosiderin in old scars of cornea — *see* Pigmentation, cornea, stromal
　metallic in lens — *see* Cataract, specified NEC
　skin R23.8
　tooth, teeth (betel) (black) (green) (materia alba) (orange) (tobacco) K03.6
　urate, kidney — *see* Calculus, kidney
Depraved appetite — *see* Pica
Depressed
　HDL cholesterol E78.6
Depression (acute) (mental) F32.9
　agitated (single episode) F32.2
　anaclitic — *see* Disorder, adjustment
　anxiety F41.8
　　persistent F34.1
　arches (*see also* Deformity, limb, flat foot)
　atypical (single episode) F32.8
　basal metabolic rate R94.8
　bone marrow D75.89
　central nervous system R09.2
　cerebral R29.818
　　newborn P91.4
　cerebrovascular I67.9
　chest wall M95.4
　climacteric (single episode) F32.8
　endogenous (without psychotic symptoms) F33.2
　　with psychotic symptoms F33.3
　functional activity R68.89
　hysterical F44.89
　involutional (single episode) F32.8
　major F32.9
　　with psychotic symptoms F32.3
　　recurrent — *see* Disorder, depressive, recurrent
　manic-depressive — *see* Disorder, depressive, recurrent

Subterms under main terms may continue to next column or page　　☑ **Additional Character Required** — Refer to the Tabular List for Character Selection　　**91**

Dependence — Depression

Depression — *continued*
  masked (single episode) F32.8
  medullary G93.89
  menopausal (single episode) F32.8
  metatarsus — *see* Depression, arches
  monopolar F33.9
  nervous F34.1
  neurotic F34.1
  nose M95.0
  postnatal F53
  postpartum F53
  post-psychotic of schizophrenia F32.8
  post-schizophrenic F32.8
  psychogenic (reactive) (single episode) F32.9
  psychoneurotic F34.1
  psychotic (single episode) F32.3
    recurrent F33.3
  reactive (psychogenic) (single episode) F32.9
    psychotic (single episode) F32.3
  recurrent — *see* Disorder, depressive, recurrent
  respiratory center G93.89
  seasonal — *see* Disorder, depressive, recurrent
  senile F03 ☑
  severe, single episode F32.2
  situational F43.21
  skull Q67.4
  specified NEC (single episode) F32.8
  sternum M95.4
  visual field — *see* Defect, visual field
  vital (recurrent) (without psychotic symptoms) F33.2
    with psychotic symptoms F33.3
    single episode F32.2

Deprivation
  cultural Z60.3
  effects NOS T73.9 ☑
    specified NEC T73.8 ☑
  emotional NEC Z65.8
    affecting infant or child — *see* Maltreatment, child, psychological
  food T73.0 ☑
  protein — *see* Malnutrition
  sleep Z72.820
  social Z60.4
    affecting infant or child — *see* Maltreatment, child, psychological
  specified NEC T73.8 ☑
  vitamins — *see* Deficiency, vitamin
  water T73.1 ☑

Derangement
  ankle (internal) — *see* Derangement, joint, ankle
  cartilage (articular) NEC — *see* Derangement, joint, articular cartilage, by site
    recurrent — *see* Dislocation, recurrent
  cruciate ligament, anterior, current injury — *see* Sprain, knee, cruciate, anterior
  elbow (internal) — *see* Derangement, joint, elbow
  hip (joint) (internal) (old) — *see* Derangement, joint, hip
  joint (internal) M24.9
    ankylosis — *see* Ankylosis
    articular cartilage M24.10
      ankle M24.17- ☑
      elbow M24.12- ☑
      foot M24.17- ☑
      hand M24.14- ☑
      hip M24.15- ☑
      knee NEC M23.9- ☑
      loose body — *see* Loose, body
      shoulder M24.11- ☑
      wrist M24.13- ☑
    contracture — *see* Contraction, joint
    current injury (*see also* Dislocation)
      knee, meniscus or cartilage — *see* Tear, meniscus
    dislocation
      pathological — *see* Dislocation, pathological
      recurrent — *see* Dislocation, recurrent
    knee — *see* Derangement, knee
    ligament — *see* Disorder, ligament
    loose body — *see* Loose, body
    recurrent — *see* Dislocation, recurrent
    specified type NEC M24.80
      ankle M24.87- ☑
      elbow M24.82- ☑
      foot joint M24.87- ☑
      hand joint M24.84- ☑
      hip M24.85- ☑

Derangement — *continued*
  joint — *continued*
    specified type — *continued*
      shoulder M24.81- ☑
      wrist M24.83- ☑
    temporomandibular M26.69
  knee (recurrent) M23.9- ☑
    ligament disruption, spontaneous M23.60- ☑
      anterior cruciate M23.61- ☑
      capsular M23.67- ☑
      instability, chronic M23.5- ☑
      lateral collateral M23.64- ☑
      medial collateral M23.63- ☑
      posterior cruciate M23.62- ☑
    loose body M23.4- ☑
    meniscus M23.30- ☑
      cystic M23.00- ☑
        lateral M23.002
          anterior horn M23.04- ☑
          posterior horn M23.05 ☑
          specified NEC M23.06- ☑
        medial M23.005
          anterior horn M23.01- ☑
          posterior horn M23.02- ☑
          specified NEC M23.03- ☑
      degenerate — *see* Derangement, knee, meniscus, specified NEC
      detached — *see* Derangement, knee, meniscus, specified NEC
      due to old tear or injury M23.20- ☑
        lateral M23.20- ☑
          anterior horn M23.24- ☑
          posterior horn M23.25- ☑
          specified NEC M23.26- ☑
        medial M23.20- ☑
          anterior horn M23.21- ☑
          posterior horn M23.22- ☑
          specified NEC M23.23- ☑
      retained — *see* Derangement, knee, meniscus, specified NEC
      specified NEC M23.30- ☑
        lateral M23.30- ☑
          anterior horn M23.34- ☑
          posterior horn M23.35- ☑
          specified NEC M23.36- ☑
        medial M23.30- ☑
          anterior horn M23.31- ☑
          posterior horn M23.32- ☑
          specified NEC M23.33- ☑
      old M23.8X- ☑
      specified NEC — *see* subcategory M23.8 ☑
  low back NEC — *see* Dorsopathy, specified NEC
  meniscus — *see* Derangement, knee, meniscus
  mental — *see* Psychosis
  patella, specified NEC — *see* Disorder, patella, derangement NEC
  semilunar cartilage (knee) — *see* Derangement, knee, meniscus, specified NEC
  shoulder (internal) — *see* Derangement, joint, shoulder

Dercum's disease E88.2
Derealization (neurotic) F48.1
Dermal — *see* condition
Dermaphytid — *see* Dermatophytosis
Dermatitis (eczematous) L30.9
  ab igne L59.0
  acarine B88.0
  actinic (due to sun) L57.8
    other than from sun L59.8
  allergic — *see* Dermatitis, contact, allergic
  ambustionis, due to burn or scald — *see* Burn
  amebic A06.7
  ammonia L22
  arsenical (ingested) L27.8
  artefacta L98.1
    psychogenic F54
  atopic L20.9
    psychogenic F54
    specified NEC L20.89
  autoimmune progesterone L30.8
  berlock, berloque L56.2
  blastomycotic B40.3
  blister beetle L24.89
  bullous, bullosa L13.9
    mucosynechial, atrophic L12.1
    seasonal L30.8

Dermatitis — *continued*
  bullous, bullosa — *continued*
    specified NEC L13.8
  calorica L59.0
    due to burn or scald — *see* Burn
  caterpillar L24.89
  cercarial B65.3
  combustionis L59.0
    due to burn or scald — *see* Burn
  congelationis T69.1 ☑
  contact (occupational) L25.9
    allergic L23.9
      due to
        adhesives L23.1
        cement L23.5
        chemical products NEC L23.5
        chromium L23.0
        cosmetics L23.2
        dander (cat) (dog) L23.81
        drugs in contact with skin L23.3
        dyes L23.4
        food in contact with skin L23.6
        hair (cat) (dog) L23.81
        insecticide L23.5
        metals L23.0
        nickel L23.0
        plants, non-food L23.7
        plastic L23.5
        rubber L23.5
        specified agent NEC L23.89
    due to
      cement L25.3
      chemical products NEC L25.3
      cosmetics L25.0
      dander (cat) (dog) L23.81
      drugs in contact with skin L25.1
      dyes L25.2
      food in contact with skin L25.4
      hair (cat) (dog) L23.81
      plants, non-food L25.5
      specified agent NEC L25.8
    irritant L24.9
      due to
        cement L25.3
        chemical products NEC L24.5
        cosmetics L24.3
        detergents L24.0
        drugs in contact with skin L24.4
        food in contact with skin L24.6
        oils and greases L24.1
        plants, non-food L24.7
        solvents L24.2
        specified agent NEC L24.89
  contusiformis L52
  diabetic — *see* E08-E13 with .620
  diaper L22
  diphtheritica A36.3
  dry skin L85.3
  due to
    acetone (contact) (irritant) L24.2
    acids (contact) (irritant) L24.5
    adhesive(s) (allergic) (contact) (plaster) L23.1
      irritant L24.5
    alcohol (irritant) (skin contact) (substances in category T51) L24.2
      taken internally L27.8
    alkalis (contact) (irritant) L24.5
    arsenic (ingested) L27.8
    carbon disulfide (contact) (irritant) L24.2
    caustics (contact) (irritant) L24.5
    cement (contact) L25.3
    cereal (ingested) L27.2
    chemical(s) NEC L25.3
      taken internally L27.8
    chlorocompounds L24.2
    chromium (contact) (irritant) L24.81
    coffee (ingested) L27.2
    cold weather L30.8
    cosmetics (contact) L25.0
      allergic L23.2
      irritant L24.3
    cyclohexanes L24.2
    dander (cat) (dog) L23.81
    Demodex species B88.0
    Dermanyssus gallinae B88.0
    detergents (contact) (irritant) L24.0
    dichromate L24.81

92

☑ **Additional Character Required** — Refer to the Tabular List for Character Selection   ▽ **Subterms under main terms may continue to next column or page**

Dermatitis — *continued*
due to — *continued*
drugs and medicaments (generalized) (internal use) L27.0
external — *see* Dermatitis, due to, drugs, in contact with skin
in contact with skin L25.1
allergic L23.3
irritant L24.4
localized skin eruption L27.1
specified substance — *see* Table of Drugs and Chemicals
dyes (contact) L25.2
allergic L23.4
irritant L24.89
epidermophytosis — *see* Dermatophytosis
esters L24.2
external irritant NEC L24.9
fish (ingested) L27.2
flour (ingested) L27.2
food (ingested) L27.2
in contact with skin L25.4
fruit (ingested) L27.2
furs (allergic) (contact) L23.81
glues — *see* Dermatitis, due to, adhesives
glycols L24.2
greases NEC (contact) (irritant) L24.1
hair (cat) (dog) L23.81
hot
objects and materials — *see* Burn
weather or places L59.0
hydrocarbons L24.2
infrared rays L59.8
ingestion, ingested substance L27.9
chemical NEC L27.8
drugs and medicaments — *see* Dermatitis, due to, drugs
food L27.2
specified NEC L27.8
insecticide in contact with skin L24.5
internal agent L27.9
drugs and medicaments (generalized) — *see* Dermatitis, due to, drugs
food L27.2
irradiation — *see* Dermatitis, due to, radioactive substance
ketones L24.2
lacquer tree (allergic) (contact) L23.7
light (sun) NEC L57.8
acute L56.8
other L59.8
Liponyssoides sanguineus B88.0
low temperature L30.8
meat (ingested) L27.2
metals, metal salts (contact) (irritant) L24.81
milk (ingested) L27.2
nickel (contact) (irritant) L24.81
nylon (contact) (irritant) L24.5
oils NEC (contact) (irritant) L24.1
paint solvent (contact) (irritant) L24.2
petroleum products (contact) (irritant) (substances in T52.0) L24.2
plants NEC (contact) L25.5
allergic L23.7
irritant L24.7
plasters (adhesive) (any) (allergic) (contact) L23.1
irritant L24.5
plastic (contact) L25.3
preservatives (contact) — *see* Dermatitis, due to, chemical, in contact with skin
primrose (allergic) (contact) L23.7
primula (allergic) (contact) L23.7
radiation L59.8
nonionizing (chronic exposure) L57.8
sun NEC L57.8
acute L56.8
radioactive substance L58.9
acute L58.0
chronic L58.1
radium L58.9
acute L58.0
chronic L58.1
ragweed (allergic) (contact) L23.7
Rhus (allergic) (contact) (diversiloba) (radicans) (toxicodendron) (venenata) (verniciflua) L23.7
rubber (contact) L24.5
Senecio jacobaea (allergic) (contact) L23.7

Dermatitis — *continued*
due to — *continued*
solvents (contact) (irritant) (substances in category T52) L24.2
specified agent NEC (contact) L25.8
allergic L23.89
irritant L24.89
sunshine NEC L57.8
acute L56.8
tetrachlorethylene (contact) (irritant) L24.2
toluene (contact) (irritant) L24.2
turpentine (contact) L24.2
ultraviolet rays (sun NEC) (chronic exposure) L57.8
acute L56.8
vaccine or vaccination L27.0
specified substance — *see* Table of Drugs and Chemicals
varicose veins — *see* Varix, leg, with, inflammation
X-rays L58.9
acute L58.0
chronic L58.1
dyshidrotic L30.1
dysmenorrheica N94.6
escharotica — *see* Burn
exfoliative, exfoliativa (generalized) L26
neonatorum L00
eyelid (*see also* Dermatosis, eyelid)
allergic H01.119
left H01.116
lower H01.115
upper H01.114
right H01.113
lower H01.112
upper H01.111
contact — *see* Dermatitis, eyelid, allergic
due to
Demodex species B88.0
herpes (zoster) B02.39
simplex B00.59
eczematous H01.139
left H01.136
lower H01.135
upper H01.134
right H01.133
lower H01.132
upper H01.131
facta, factitia, factitial L98.1
psychogenic F54
flexural NEC L20.82
friction L30.4
fungus B36.9
specified type NEC B36.8
gangrenosa, gangrenous infantum L08.0
harvest mite B88.0
heat L59.0
herpesviral, vesicular (ear) (lip) B00.1
herpetiformis (bullous) (erythematous) (pustular) (vesicular) L13.0
juvenile L12.2
senile L12.0
hiemalis L30.8
hypostatic, hypostatica — *see* Varix, leg, with, inflammation
infectious eczematoid L30.3
infective L30.3
irritant — *see* Dermatitis, contact, irritant
Jacquet's (diaper dermatitis) L22
Leptus B88.0
lichenified NEC L28.0
medicamentosa (generalized) (internal use) — *see* Dermatitis, due to drugs
mite B88.0
multiformis L13.0
juvenile L12.2
napkin L22
neurotica L13.0
nummular L30.0
papillaris capillitii L73.0
pellagrous E52
perioral L71.0
photocontact L56.2
polymorpha dolorosa L13.0
pruriginosa L13.0
pruritic NEC L30.8
psychogenic F54
purulent L08.0
pustular
contagious B08.02

Dermatitis — *continued*
pustular — *continued*
subcorneal L13.1
pyococcal L08.0
pyogenica L08.0
repens L40.2
Ritter's (exfoliativa) L00
Schamberg's L81.7
schistosome B65.3
seasonal bullous L30.8
seborrheic L21.9
infantile L21.1
specified NEC L21.8
sensitization NOS L23.9
septic L08.0
solare L57.8
specified NEC L30.8
stasis I87.2
with varicose ulcer — *see* Varix, leg, with ulcer, with inflammation
due to postthrombotic syndrome — *see* Syndrome, postthrombotic
suppurative L08.0
traumatic NEC L30.4
trophoneurotica L13.0
ultraviolet (sun) (chronic exposure) L57.8
acute L56.8
varicose — *see* Varix, leg, with, inflammation
vegetans L10.1
verrucosa B43.0
vesicular, herpesviral B00.1
Dermatoarthritis, lipoid E78.81
Dermatochalasis, eyelid H02.839
left H02.836
lower H02.835
upper H02.834
right H02.833
lower H02.832
upper H02.831
Dermatofibroma (lenticulare) — *see* Neoplasm, skin, benign
protuberans — *see* Neoplasm, skin, uncertain behavior
Dermatofibrosarcoma (pigmented) (protuberans) — *see* Neoplasm, skin, malignant
Dermatographia L50.3
Dermatolysis (exfoliativa) (congenital) Q82.8
acquired L57.4
eyelids — *see* Blepharochalasis
palpebrarum — *see* Blepharochalasis
senile L57.4
Dermatomegaly NEC Q82.8
Dermatomucosomyositis M33.10
with
myopathy M33.12
respiratory involvement M33.11
specified organ involvement NEC M33.19
Dermatomycosis B36.9
furfuracea B36.0
specified type NEC B36.8
Dermatomyositis (acute) (chronic) (*see also* Dermatopolymyositis)
in (due to) neoplastic disease (*see also* Neoplasm) D49.9 [M36.0]
Dermatoneuritis of children — *see* Poisoning, mercury
Dermatophilosis A48.8
Dermatophytid L30.2
Dermatophytide — *see* Dermatophytosis
Dermatophytosis (epidermophyton) (infection) (Microsporum) (tinea) (Trichophyton) B35.9
beard B35.0
body B35.4
capitis B35.0
corporis B35.4
deep-seated B35.8
disseminated B35.8
foot B35.3
granulomatous B35.8
groin B35.6
hand B35.2
nail B35.1
perianal (area) B35.6
scalp B35.0
specified NEC B35.8
Dermatopolymyositis M33.90
with
myopathy M33.92
respiratory involvement M33.91
specified organ involvement NEC M33.99

Dermatopolymyositis — *continued*
in neoplastic disease (*see also* Neoplasm)
D49.9 [M36.0]
juvenile M33.00
with
myopathy M33.02
respiratory involvement M33.01
specified organ involvement NEC M33.09
specified NEC M33.10
myopathy M33.12
respiratory involvement M33.11
specified organ involvement NEC M33.19
Dermatopolyneuritis — *see* Poisoning, mercury
Dermatorrhexis Q79.6
acquired L57.4
Dermatosclerosis (*see also* Scleroderma)
localized L94.0
Dermatosis L98.9
Andrews' L08.89
Bowen's — *see* Neoplasm, skin, in situ
bullous L13.9
specified NEC L13.8
exfoliativa L26
eyelid (noninfectious)
dermatitis — *see* Dermatitis, eyelid
discoid lupus erythematosus — *see* Lupus, erythematosus, eyelid
xeroderma — *see* Xeroderma, acquired, eyelid
factitial L98.1
febrile neutrophilic L98.2
gonococcal A54.89
herpetiformis L13.0
juvenile L12.2
linear IgA L13.8
menstrual NEC L98.8
neutrophilic, febrile L98.2
occupational — *see* Dermatitis, contact
papulosa nigra L82.1
pigmentary L81.9
progressive L81.7
Schamberg's L81.7
psychogenic F54
purpuric, pigmented L81.7
pustular, subcorneal L13.1
transient acantholytic L11.1
Dermographia, dermographism L50.3
Dermoid (cyst) (*see also* Neoplasm, benign, by site)
with malignant transformation C56- ☑
due to radiation (nonionizing) L57.8
Dermopathy
infiltrative with thyrotoxicosis — *see* Thyrotoxicosis
nephrogenic fibrosing L90.8
Dermophytosis — *see* Dermatophytosis
Descemetocele H18.73- ☑
Descemet's membrane — *see* condition
Descending — *see* condition
Descensus uteri — *see* Prolapse, uterus
Desert
rheumatism B38.0
sore — *see* Ulcer, skin
Desertion (newborn) — *see* Maltreatment
Desmoid (extra-abdominal) (tumor) — *see* Neoplasm, connective tissue, uncertain behavior
abdominal D48.1
Despondency F32.9
Desquamation, skin R23.4
Destruction, destructive (*see also* Damage)
articular facet (*see also* Derangement, joint, specified type NEC)
knee M23.8X- ☑
vertebra — *see* Spondylosis
bone (*see also* Disorder, bone, specified type NEC)
syphilitic A52.77
joint (*see also* Derangement, joint, specified type NEC)
sacroiliac M53.3
rectal sphincter K62.89
septum (nasal) J34.89
tuberculous NEC — *see* Tuberculosis
tympanum, tympanic membrane (nontraumatic) — *see* Disorder, tympanic membrane, specified NEC
vertebral disc — *see* Degeneration, intervertebral disc
Destructiveness (*see also* Disorder, conduct)
adjustment reaction — *see* Disorder, adjustment
Desultory labor O62.2
Detachment
cartilage — *see* Sprain

Detachment — *continued*
cervix, annular N88.8
complicating delivery O71.3
choroid (old) (postinfectional) (simple) (spontaneous)
H31.40- ☑
hemorrhagic H31.41- ☑
serous H31.42- ☑
ligament — *see* Sprain
meniscus (knee) (*see also* Derangement, knee, meniscus, specified NEC)
current injury — *see* Tear, meniscus
due to old tear or injury — *see* Derangement, knee, meniscus, due to old tear
retina (without retinal break) (serous) H33.2- ☑
with retinal:
break H33.00- ☑
giant H33.03- ☑
multiple H33.02- ☑
single H33.01- ☑
dialysis H33.04- ☑
pigment epithelium — *see* Degeneration, retina, separation of layers, pigment epithelium detachment
rhegmatogenous — *see* Detachment, retina, with retinal, break
specified NEC H33.8
total H33.05- ☑
traction H33.4- ☑
vitreous (body) H43.81 ☑
Detergent asthma J69.8
Deterioration
epileptic F06.8
general physical R53.81
heart, cardiac — *see* Degeneration, myocardial
mental — *see* Psychosis
myocardial, myocardium — *see* Degeneration, myocardial
senile (simple) R54
Deuteranomaly (anomalous trichromat) H53.53
Deuteranopia (complete) (incomplete) H53.53
Development
abnormal, bone Q79.9
arrested R62.50
bone — *see* Arrest, development or growth, bone
child R62.50
due to malnutrition E45
defective, congenital (*see also* Anomaly, by site)
cauda equina Q06.3
left ventricle Q24.8
in hypoplastic left heart syndrome Q23.4
valve Q24.8
pulmonary Q22.3
delayed (*see also* Delay, development) R62.50
arithmetical skills F81.2
language (skills) (expressive) F80.1
learning skill F81.9
mixed skills F88
motor coordination F82
reading F81.0
specified learning skill NEC F81.89
speech F80.9
spelling F81.81
written expression F81.81
imperfect, congenital (*see also* Anomaly, by site)
heart Q24.9
lungs Q33.6
incomplete
bronchial tree Q32.4
organ or site not listed — *see* Hypoplasia, by site
respiratory system Q34.9
sexual, precocious NEC E30.1
tardy, mental (*see also* Disability, intellectual) F79
Developmental — *see* condition
testing, child — *see* Examination, child
Devergie's disease (pityriasis rubra pilaris) L44.0
Deviation (in)
conjugate palsy (eye) (spastic) H51.0
esophagus (acquired) K22.8
eye, skew H51.8
midline (jaw) (teeth) (dental arch) M26.29
specified site NEC — *see* Malposition
nasal septum J34.2
congenital Q67.4
opening and closing of the mandible M26.53
organ or site, congenital NEC — *see* Malposition, congenital
septum

Deviation — *continued*
septum (nasal) (acquired) J34.2
congenital Q67.4
sexual F65.9
bestiality F65.89
erotomania F52.8
exhibitionism F65.2
fetishism, fetishistic F65.0
transvestism F65.1
frotteurism F65.81
masochism F65.51
multiple F65.89
necrophilia F65.89
nymphomania F52.8
pederosis F65.4
pedophilia F65.4
sadism, sadomasochism F65.52
satyriasis F52.8
specified type NEC F65.89
transvestism F64.1
voyeurism F65.3
teeth, midline M26.29
trachea J39.8
ureter, congenital Q62.61
Device
cerebral ventricle (communicating) in situ Z98.2
contraceptive — *see* Contraceptive, device
drainage, cerebrospinal fluid, in situ Z98.2
Devic's disease G36.0
Devil's
grip B33.0
pinches (purpura simplex) D69.2
Devitalized tooth K04.99
Devonshire colic — *see* Poisoning, lead
Dextraposition, aorta Q20.3
in tetralogy of Fallot Q21.3
Dextrinosis, limit (debrancher enzyme deficiency)
E74.03
Dextrocardia (true) Q24.0
with
complete transposition of viscera Q89.3
situs inversus Q89.3
Dextrotransposition, aorta Q20.3
d-glycericacidemia E72.59
Dhat syndrome F48.8
Dhobi itch B35.6
Di George's syndrome D82.1
Di Guglielmo's disease C94.0- ☑
Diabetes, diabetic (mellitus) (sugar) E11.9
with
amyotrophy E11.44
arthropathy NEC E11.618
autonomic (poly)neuropathy E11.43
cataract E11.36
Charcot's joints E11.610
chronic kidney disease E11.22
circulatory complication NEC E11.59
complication E11.8
specified NEC E11.69
dermatitis E11.620
foot ulcer E11.621
gangrene E11.52
gastroparesis E11.43
glomerulonephrosis, intracapillary E11.21
glomerulosclerosis, intercapillary E11.21
hyperglycemia E11.65
hyperosmolarity E11.00
with coma E11.01
hypoglycemia E11.649
with coma E11.641
kidney complications NEC E11.29
Kimmelstiel-Wilson disease E11.21
loss of protective sensation (LOPS) — *see* Diabetes, by type, with neuropathy
mononeuropathy E11.41
myasthenia E11.44
necrobiosis lipoidica E11.620
nephropathy E11.21
neuralgia E11.42
neurologic complication NEC E11.49
neuropathic arthropathy E11.610
neuropathy E11.40
ophthalmic complication NEC E11.39
oral complication NEC E11.638
periodontal disease E11.630
peripheral angiopathy E11.51
with gangrene E11.52
polyneuropathy E11.42

☑ **Additional Character Required** — Refer to the Tabular List for Character Selection ⓇUL **Subterms under main terms may continue to next column or page**

Diabetes, diabetic — *continued*
  with — *continued*
    renal complication NEC E11.29
    renal tubular degeneration E11.29
    retinopathy E11.319
      with macular edema E11.311
      nonproliferative E11.329
        with macular edema E11.321
        mild E11.329
          with macular edema E11.321
        moderate E11.339
          with macular edema E11.331
        severe E11.349
          with macular edema E11.341
      proliferative E11.359
        with macular edema E11.351
    skin complication NEC E11.628
    skin ulcer NEC E11.622
  bronzed E83.110
  complicating pregnancy — *see* Pregnancy, complicated by, diabetes
  dietary counseling and surveillance Z71.3
  due to drug or chemical E09.9
    with
      amyotrophy E09.44
      arthropathy NEC E09.618
      autonomic (poly)neuropathy E09.43
      cataract E09.36
      Charcot's joints E09.610
      chronic kidney disease E09.22
      circulatory complication NEC E09.59
      complication E09.8
        specified NEC E09.69
      dermatitis E09.620
      foot ulcer E09.621
      gangrene E09.52
      gastroparesis E09.43
      glomerulonephrosis, intracapillary E09.21
      glomerulosclerosis, intercapillary E09.21
      hyperglycemia E09.65
      hyperosmolarity E09.00
        with coma E09.01
      hypoglycemia E09.649
        with coma E09.641
      ketoacidosis E09.10
        with coma E09.11
      kidney complications NEC E09.29
      Kimmelstiel-Wilson disease E09.21
      mononeuropathy E09.41
      myasthenia E09.44
      necrobiosis lipoidica E09.620
      nephropathy E09.21
      neuralgia E09.42
      neurologic complication NEC E09.49
      neuropathic arthropathy E09.610
      neuropathy E09.40
      ophthalmic complication NEC E09.39
      oral complication NEC E09.638
      periodontal disease E09.630
      peripheral angiopathy E09.51
        with gangrene E09.52
      polyneuropathy E09.42
      renal complication NEC E09.29
      renal tubular degeneration E09.29
      retinopathy E09.319
        with macular edema E09.311
        nonproliferative E09.329
          with macular edema E09.321
          mild E09.329
            with macular edema E09.321
          moderate E09.339
            with macular edema E09.331
          severe E09.349
            with macular edema E09.341
        proliferative E09.359
          with macular edema E09.351
      skin complication NEC E09.628
      skin ulcer NEC E09.622
  due to underlying condition E08.9
    with
      amyotrophy E08.44
      arthropathy NEC E08.618
      autonomic (poly)neuropathy E08.43
      cataract E08.36
      Charcot's joints E08.610
      chronic kidney disease E08.22
      circulatory complication NEC E08.59

Diabetes, diabetic — *continued*
  due to underlying condition — *continued*
    with — *continued*
      complication E08.8
        specified NEC E08.69
      dermatitis E08.620
      foot ulcer E08.621
      gangrene E08.52
      gastroparesis E08.43
      glomerulonephrosis, intracapillary E08.21
      glomerulosclerosis, intercapillary E08.21
      hyperglycemia E08.65
      hyperosmolarity E08.00
        with coma E08.01
      hypoglycemia E08.649
        with coma E08.641
      ketoacidosis E08.10
        with coma E08.11
      kidney complications NEC E08.29
      Kimmelstiel-Wilson disease E08.21
      mononeuropathy E08.41
      myasthenia E08.44
      necrobiosis lipoidica E08.620
      nephropathy E08.21
      neuralgia E08.42
      neurologic complication NEC E08.49
      neuropathic arthropathy E08.610
      neuropathy E08.40
      ophthalmic complication NEC E08.39
      oral complication NEC E08.638
      periodontal disease E08.630
      peripheral angiopathy E08.51
        with gangrene E08.52
      polyneuropathy E08.42
      renal complication NEC E08.29
      renal tubular degeneration E08.29
      retinopathy E08.319
        with macular edema E08.311
        nonproliferative E08.329
          with macular edema E08.321
          mild E08.329
            with macular edema E08.321
          moderate E08.339
            with macular edema E08.331
          severe E08.349
            with macular edema E08.341
        proliferative E08.359
          with macular edema E08.351
      skin complication NEC E08.628
      skin ulcer NEC E08.622
  gestational (in pregnancy) O24.419
    affecting newborn P70.0
    diet controlled O24.410
    in childbirth O24.429
      diet controlled O24.420
      insulin (and diet) controlled O24.424
    insulin (and diet) controlled O24.414
    puerperal O24.439
      diet controlled O24.430
      insulin (and diet) controlled O24.434
  hepatogenous E13.9
  inadequately controlled — *code to* Diabetes, by type, with hyperglycemia
  insipidus E23.2
    nephrogenic N25.1
    pituitary E23.2
    vasopressin resistant N25.1
  insulin dependent — *code to* type of diabetes
  juvenile-onset — *see* Diabetes, type 1
  ketosis-prone — *see* Diabetes, type 1
  latent R73.09
  neonatal (transient) P70.2
  non-insulin dependent — *code to* type of diabetes
  out of control — *code to* Diabetes, by type, with hyperglycemia
  phosphate E83.39
  poorly controlled — *code to* Diabetes, by type, with hyperglycemia
  postpancreatectomy — *see* Diabetes, specified type NEC
  postprocedural — *see* Diabetes, specified type NEC
  secondary diabetes mellitus NEC — *see* Diabetes, specified type NEC
  specified type NEC E13.9
    with
      amyotrophy E13.44
      arthropathy NEC E13.618
      autonomic (poly)neuropathy E13.43

Diabetes, diabetic — *continued*
  specified type — *continued*
    with — *continued*
      cataract E13.36
      Charcot's joints E13.610
      chronic kidney disease E13.22
      circulatory complication NEC E13.59
      complication E13.8
        specified NEC E13.69
      dermatitis E13.620
      foot ulcer E13.621
      gangrene E13.52
      gastroparesis E13.43
      glomerulonephrosis, intracapillary E13.21
      glomerulosclerosis, intercapillary E13.21
      hyperglycemia E13.65
      hyperosmolarity E13.00
        with coma E13.01
      hypoglycemia E13.649
        with coma E13.641
      ketoacidosis E13.10
        with coma E13.11
      kidney complications NEC E13.29
      Kimmelstiel-Wilson disease E13.21
      mononeuropathy E13.41
      myasthenia E13.44
      necrobiosis lipoidica E13.620
      nephropathy E13.21
      neuralgia E13.42
      neurologic complication NEC E13.49
      neuropathic arthropathy E13.610
      neuropathy E13.40
      ophthalmic complication NEC E13.39
      oral complication NEC E13.638
      periodontal disease E13.630
      peripheral angiopathy E13.51
        with gangrene E13.52
      polyneuropathy E13.42
      renal complication NEC E13.29
      renal tubular degeneration E13.29
      retinopathy E13.319
        with macular edema E13.311
        nonproliferative E13.329
          with macular edema E13.321
          mild E13.329
            with macular edema E13.321
          moderate E13.339
            with macular edema E13.331
          severe E13.349
            with macular edema E13.341
        proliferative E13.359
          with macular edema E13.351
    skin complication NEC E13.628
    skin ulcer NEC E13.622
  steroid-induced — *see* Diabetes, due to, drug or chemical
  type 1 E10.9
    with
      amyotrophy E10.44
      arthropathy NEC E10.618
      autonomic (poly)neuropathy E10.43
      cataract E10.36
      Charcot's joints E10.610
      chronic kidney disease E10.22
      circulatory complication NEC E10.59
      complication E10.8
        specified NEC E10.69
      dermatitis E10.620
      foot ulcer E10.621
      gangrene E10.52
      gastroparesis E10.43
      glomerulonephrosis, intracapillary E10.21
      glomerulosclerosis, intercapillary E10.21
      hyperglycemia E10.65
      hypoglycemia E10.649
        with coma E10.641
      ketoacidosis E10.10
        with coma E10.11
      kidney complications NEC E10.29
      Kimmelstiel-Wilson disease E10.21
      mononeuropathy E10.41
      myasthenia E10.44
      necrobiosis lipoidica E10.620
      nephropathy E10.21
      neuralgia E10.42
      neurologic complication NEC E10.49
      neuropathic arthropathy E10.610
      neuropathy E10.40

Diabetes, diabetic — *continued*
- type 1 — *continued*
  - with — *continued*
    - ophthalmic complication NEC E10.39
    - oral complication NEC E10.638
    - periodontal disease E10.630
    - peripheral angiopathy E10.51
      - with gangrene E10.52
    - polyneuropathy E10.42
    - renal complication NEC E10.29
    - renal tubular degeneration E10.29
    - retinopathy E10.319
      - with macular edema E10.311
      - nonproliferative E10.329
        - with macular edema E10.321
        - mild E10.329
          - with macular edema E10.321
        - moderate E10.339
          - with macular edema E10.331
        - severe E10.349
          - with macular edema E10.341
      - proliferative E10.359
        - with macular edema E10.351
    - skin complication NEC E10.628
    - skin ulcer NEC E10.622
- type 2 E11.9
  - with
    - amyotrophy E11.44
    - arthropathy NEC E11.618
    - autonomic (poly)neuropathy E11.43
    - cataract E11.36
    - Charcot's joints E11.610
    - chronic kidney disease E11.22
    - circulatory complication NEC E11.59
    - complication E11.8
      - specified NEC E11.69
    - dermatitis E11.620
    - foot ulcer E11.621
    - gangrene E11.52
    - gastroparesis E11.43
    - glomerulonephrosis, intracapillary E11.21
    - glomerulosclerosis, intercapillary E11.21
    - hyperglycemia E11.65
    - hyperosmolarity E11.00
      - with coma E11.01
    - hypoglycemia E11.649
      - with coma E11.641
    - kidney complications NEC E11.29
    - Kimmelstiel-Wilson disease E11.21
    - mononeuropathy E11.41
    - myasthenia E11.44
    - necrobiosis lipoidica E11.620
    - nephropathy E11.21
    - neuralgia E11.42
    - neurologic complication NEC E11.49
    - neuropathic arthropathy E11.610
    - neuropathy E11.40
    - ophthalmic complication NEC E11.39
    - oral complication NEC E11.638
    - periodontal disease E11.630
    - peripheral angiopathy E11.51
      - with gangrene E11.52
    - polyneuropathy E11.42
    - renal complication NEC E11.29
    - renal tubular degeneration E11.29
    - retinopathy E11.319
      - with macular edema E11.311
      - nonproliferative E11.329
        - with macular edema E11.321
        - mild E11.329
          - with macular edema E11.321
        - moderate E11.339
          - with macular edema E11.331
        - severe E11.349
          - with macular edema E11.341
      - proliferative E11.359
        - with macular edema E11.351
    - skin complication NEC E11.628
    - skin ulcer NEC E11.622

Diacyclothrombopathia D69.1
Diagnosis deferred R69
Dialysis (intermittent) (treatment)
- noncompliance (with) Z91.15
- renal (hemodialysis) (peritoneal), status Z99.2
- retina, retinal — *see* Detachment, retina, with retinal, dialysis

Diamond-Blackfan anemia (congenital hypoplastic) D61.01

Diamond-Gardener syndrome (autoerythrocyte sensitization) D69.2
Diaper rash L22
Diaphoresis (excessive) R61
Diaphragm — *see* condition
Diaphragmalgia R07.1
Diaphragmatitis, diaphragmitis J98.6
Diaphysial aclasis Q78.6
Diaphysitis — *see* Osteomyelitis, specified type NEC
Diarrhea, diarrheal (disease) (infantile) (inflammatory) R19.7
- achlorhydric K31.83
- allergic K52.2
- amebic (*see also* Amebiasis) A06.0
  - with abscess — *see* Abscess, amebic
  - acute A06.0
  - chronic A06.1
  - nondysenteric A06.2
- bacillary — *see* Dysentery, bacillary
- balantidial A07.0
- cachectic NEC K52.89
- Chilomastix A07.8
- choleriformis A00.1
- chronic (noninfectious) K52.9
- coccidial A07.3
- Cochin-China K90.1
  - strongyloidiasis B78.0
- Dientamoeba A07.8
- dietetic K52.2
- drug-induced K52.1
- due to
  - bacteria A04.9
    - specified NEC A04.8
  - Campylobacter A04.5
  - Capillaria philippinensis B81.1
  - Clostridium difficile A04.7
  - Clostridium perfringens (C) (F) A04.8
  - Cryptosporidium A07.2
  - drugs K52.1
  - Escherichia coli A04.4
    - enteroaggregative A04.4
    - enterohemorrhagic A04.3
    - enteroinvasive A04.2
    - enteropathogenic A04.0
    - enterotoxigenic A04.1
    - specified NEC A04.4
  - food hypersensitivity K52.2
  - Necator americanus B76.1
  - S. japonicum B65.2
  - specified organism NEC A08.8
    - bacterial A04.8
    - viral A08.39
  - Staphylococcus A04.8
  - Trichuris trichiuria B79
  - virus — *see* Enteritis, viral
  - Yersinia enterocolitica A04.6
- dysenteric A09
- endemic A09
- epidemic A09
- flagellate A07.9
- Flexner's (ulcerative) A03.1
- functional K59.1
  - following gastrointestinal surgery K91.89
  - psychogenic F45.8
- Giardia lamblia A07.1
- giardial A07.1
- hill K90.1
- infectious A09
- malarial — *see* Malaria
- mite B88.0
- mycotic NEC B49
- neonatal (noninfectious) P78.3
- nervous F45.8
- neurogenic K59.1
- noninfectious K52.9
- postgastrectomy K91.1
- postvagotomy K91.1
- protozoal A07.9
  - specified NEC A07.8
- psychogenic F45.8
- specified
  - bacterium NEC A04.8
  - virus NEC A08.39
- strongyloidiasis B78.0
- toxic K52.1
- trichomonal A07.8
- tropical K90.1
- tuberculous A18.32

Diarrhea, diarrheal — *continued*
- viral — *see* Enteritis, viral
Diastasis
- cranial bones M84.88
  - congenital NEC Q75.8
- joint (traumatic) — *see* Dislocation
- muscle M62.00
  - ankle M62.07- ☑
  - congenital Q79.8
  - foot M62.07- ☑
  - forearm M62.03- ☑
  - hand M62.04- ☑
  - lower leg M62.06- ☑
  - pelvic region M62.05- ☑
  - shoulder region M62.01- ☑
  - specified site NEC M62.08
  - thigh M62.05- ☑
  - upper arm M62.02- ☑
- recti (abdomen)
  - complicating delivery O71.89
  - congenital Q79.59
Diastema, tooth, teeth, fully erupted M26.32
Diastematomyelia Q06.2
Diataxia, cerebral G80.4
Diathesis
- allergic — *see* History, allergy
- bleeding (familial) D69.9
- cystine (familial) E72.00
- gouty — *see* Gout
- hemorrhagic (familial) D69.9
  - newborn NEC P53
- spasmophilic R29.0
Diaz's disease or osteochondrosis (juvenile) (talus) — *see* Osteochondrosis, juvenile, tarsus
Dibothriocephalus, dibothriocephaliasis (latus) (infection) (infestation) B70.0
- larval B70.1
Dicephalus, dicephaly Q89.4
Dichotomy, teeth K00.2
Dichromat, dichromatopsia (congenital) — *see* Deficiency, color vision
Dichuchwa A65
Dicroceliasis B66.2
Didelphia, didelphys — *see* Double uterus
Didymytis N45.1
- with orchitis N45.3
Dietary
- inadequacy or deficiency E63.9
- surveillance and counseling Z71.3
Dietl's crisis N13.8
Dieulafoy lesion (hemorrhagic)
- duodenum K31.82
- esophagus K22.8
- intestine (colon) K63.81
- stomach K31.82
Difficult, difficulty (in)
- acculturation Z60.3
- feeding R63.3
  - newborn P92.9
    - breast P92.5
    - specified NEC P92.8
  - nonorganic (infant or child) F98.29
- intubation, in anesthesia T88.4 ☑
- mechanical, gastroduodenal stoma K91.89
  - causing obstruction K91.3
- reading (developmental) F81.0
  - secondary to emotional disorders F93.9
- spelling (specific) F81.81
  - with reading disorder F81.89
  - due to inadequate teaching Z55.8
- swallowing — *see* Dysphagia
- walking R26.2
- work
  - conditions NEC Z56.5
  - schedule Z56.3
Diffuse — *see* condition
Digestive — *see* condition
Dihydropyrimidine dehydrogenase disease (DPD) E88.89
Diktyoma — *see* Neoplasm, malignant, by site
Dilaceration, tooth K00.4
Dilatation
- anus K59.8
  - venule — *see* Hemorrhoids
- aorta (focal) (general) — *see* Ectasia, aorta
  - with aneurysm — *see* Aneurysm, aorta
- artery — *see* Aneurysm

Dilatation — *continued*
bladder (sphincter) N32.89
  congenital Q64.79
blood vessel I99.8
bronchial J47.9
  with
    exacerbation (acute) J47.1
    lower respiratory infection J47.0
calyx (due to obstruction) — *see* Hydronephrosis
capillaries I78.8
cardiac (acute) (chronic) (*see also* Hypertrophy, cardiac)
  congenital Q24.8
    valve NEC Q24.8
      pulmonary Q22.3
  valve — *see* Endocarditis
cavum septi pellucidi Q06.8
cervix (uteri) (*see also* Incompetency, cervix)
  incomplete, poor, slow complicating delivery O62.0
colon K59.3
  congenital Q43.1
  psychogenic F45.8
common duct (acquired) K83.8
  congenital Q44.5
cystic duct (acquired) K82.8
  congenital Q44.5
duct, mammary — *see* Ectasia, mammary duct
duodenum K59.8
esophagus K22.8
  congenital Q39.5
  due to achalasia K22.0
eustachian tube, congenital Q17.8
gallbladder K82.8
gastric — *see* Dilatation, stomach
heart (acute) (chronic) (*see also* Hypertrophy, cardiac)
  congenital Q24.8
  valve — *see* Endocarditis
ileum K59.8
  psychogenic F45.8
jejunum K59.8
  psychogenic F45.8
kidney (calyx) (collecting structures) (cystic)
  (parenchyma) (pelvis) (idiopathic) N28.89
lacrimal passages or duct — *see* Disorder, lacrimal
  system, changes
lymphatic vessel I89.0
mammary duct — *see* Ectasia, mammary duct
Meckel's diverticulum (congenital) Q43.0
  malignant — *see* Table of Neoplasms, small intes-
    tine, malignant
myocardium (acute) (chronic) — *see* Hypertrophy,
  cardiac
organ or site, congenital NEC — *see* Distortion
pancreatic duct K86.8
pericardium — *see* Pericarditis
pharynx J39.2
prostate N42.89
pulmonary
  artery (idiopathic) I28.8
  valve, congenital Q22.3
pupil H57.04
rectum K59.3
saccule, congenital Q16.5
salivary gland (duct) K11.8
sphincter ani K62.89
stomach K31.89
  acute K31.0
  psychogenic F45.8
submaxillary duct K11.8
trachea, congenital Q32.1
ureter (idiopathic) N28.82
  congenital Q62.2
  due to obstruction N13.4
urethra (acquired) N36.8
vasomotor I73.9
vein I86.8
ventricular, ventricle (acute) (chronic) (*see also* Hypertrophy, cardiac)
  cerebral, congenital Q04.8
venule NEC I86.8
vesical orifice N32.89
Dilated, dilation — *see* Dilatation
Diminished, diminution
hearing (acuity) — *see* Deafness
sense or sensation (cold) (heat) (tactile) (vibratory)
  R20.8
vision NEC H54.7
vital capacity R94.2
Diminuta taenia B71.0

Dimitri-Sturge-Weber disease Q85.8
Dimple
parasacral, pilonidal or postanal — *see* Cyst, pilonidal
Dioctophyme renalis (infection) (infestation) B83.8
Dipetalonemiasis B74.4
Diphallus Q55.69
Diphtheria, diphtheritic (gangrenous) (hemorrhagic)
  A36.9
carrier (suspected) Z22.2
cutaneous A36.3
faucial A36.0
infection of wound A36.3
laryngeal A36.2
myocarditis A36.81
nasal, anterior A36.89
nasopharyngeal A36.1
neurological complication A36.89
pharyngeal A36.0
specified site NEC A36.89
tonsillar A36.0
Diphyllobothriasis (intestine) B70.0
larval B70.1
Diplacusis H93.22- ☑
Diplegia (upper limbs) G83.0
congenital (cerebral) G80.8
facial G51.0
lower limbs G82.20
spastic G80.1
Diplococcus, diplococcal — *see* condition
Diplopia H53.2
Dipsomania F10.20
  with
    psychosis — *see* Psychosis, alcoholic
    remission F10.21
Dipylidiasis B71.1
Direction, teeth, abnormal, fully erupted M26.30
Dirofilariasis B74.8
Dirt-eating child F98.3
Disability, disabilities
heart — *see* Disease, heart
intellectual F79
  with
    autistic features F84.9
  mild (I.Q. 50-69) F70
  moderate (I.Q. 35-49) F71
  profound (I.Q. under 20) F73
  severe (I.Q. 20-34) F72
  specified level NEC F78
knowledge acquisition F81.9
learning F81.9
limiting activities Z73.6
spelling, specific F81.81
Disappearance of family member Z63.4
Disarticulation — *see* Amputation
meaning traumatic amputation — *see* Amputation,
  traumatic
Discharge (from)
abnormal finding in — *see* Abnormal, specimen
breast (female) (male) N64.52
diencephalic autonomic idiopathic — *see* Epilepsy,
  specified NEC
ear (*see also* Otorrhea)
  blood — *see* Otorrhagia
excessive urine R35.8
nipple N64.52
penile R36.9
postnasal R09.82
prison, anxiety concerning Z65.2
urethral R36.9
  without blood R36.0
  hematospermia R36.1
vaginal N89.8
Discitis, diskitis M46.40
cervical region M46.42
cervicothoracic region M46.43
lumbar region M46.46
lumbosacral region M46.47
multiple sites M46.49
occipito-atlanto-axial region M46.41
pyogenic — *see* Infection, intervertebral disc, pyogenic
sacrococcygeal region M46.48
thoracic region M46.44
thoracolumbar region M46.45
Discoid
meniscus (congenital) Q68.6
semilunar cartilage (congenital) — *see* Derangement,
  knee, meniscus, specified NEC

Discoloration
nails L60.8
teeth (posteruptive) K03.7
  during formation K00.8
Discomfort
chest R07.89
visual H53.14- ☑
Discontinuity, ossicles, ear H74.2- ☑
Discord (with)
boss Z56.4
classmates Z55.4
counselor Z64.4
employer Z56.4
family Z63.8
fellow employees Z56.4
in-laws Z63.1
landlord Z59.2
lodgers Z59.2
neighbors Z59.2
probation officer Z64.4
social worker Z64.4
teachers Z55.4
workmates Z56.4
Discordant connection
atrioventricular (congenital) Q20.5
ventriculoarterial Q20.3
Discrepancy
centric occlusion maximum intercuspation M26.55
leg length (acquired) — *see* Deformity, limb, unequal
  length
  congenital — *see* Defect, reduction, lower limb
uterine size date O26.84- ☑
Discrimination
ethnic Z60.5
political Z60.5
racial Z60.5
religious Z60.5
sex Z60.5
Disease, diseased (*see also* Syndrome)
absorbent system I87.8
acid-peptic K30
Acosta's T70.29 ☑
Adams-Stokes (-Morgagni) (syncope with heart block)
  I45.9
Addison's anemia (pernicious) D51.0
adenoids (and tonsils) J35.9
adrenal (capsule) (cortex) (gland) (medullary) E27.9
  hyperfunction E27.0
  specified NEC E27.8
ainhum L94.6
airway
  obstructive, chronic J44.9
    due to
      cotton dust J66.0
      specific organic dusts NEC J66.8
  reactive — *see* Asthma
akamushi (scrub typhus) A75.3
Albers-Schönberg (marble bones) Q78.2
Albert's — *see* Tendinitis, Achilles
alimentary canal K63.9
alligator-skin Q80.9
  acquired L85.0
alpha heavy chain C88.3
alpine T70.29 ☑
altitude T70.20 ☑
alveolar ridge
  edentulous K06.9
    specified NEC K06.8
alveoli, teeth K08.9
Alzheimer's G30.9 [F02.80]
  with behavioral disturbance G30.9 [F02.81]
  early onset G30.0 [F02.80]
    with behavioral disturbance G30.0 [F02.81]
  late onset G30.1 [F02.80]
    with behavioral disturbance G30.1 [F02.81]
  specified NEC G30.8 [F02.80]
    with behavioral disturbance G30.8 [F02.81]
amyloid — *see* Amyloidosis
Andersen's (glycogenosis IV) E74.09
Andes T70.29 ☑
Andrews' (bacterid) L08.89
angiospastic I73.9
  cerebral G45.9
  vein I87.8
anterior
  chamber H21.9
  horn cell G12.29

Disease, diseased — *continued*
antiglomerular basement membrane (anti- GBM) anti-
    body M31.0
    tubulo-interstitial nephritis N12
antral — *see* Sinusitis, maxillary
anus K62.9
    specified NEC K62.89
aorta (nonsyphilitic) I77.9
    syphilitic NEC A52.02
aortic (heart) (valve) I35.9
    rheumatic I06.9
Apollo B30.3
aponeuroses — *see* Enthesopathy
appendix K38.9
    specified NEC K38.8
aqueous (chamber) H21.9
Arnold-Chiari — *see* Arnold-Chiari disease
arterial I77.9
    occlusive — *see* Occlusion, by site
        due to stricture or stenosis I77.1
arteriocardiorenal — *see* Hypertension, cardiorenal
arteriolar (generalized) (obliterative) I77.9
arteriorenal — *see* Hypertension, kidney
arteriosclerotic (*see also* Arteriosclerosis)
    cardiovascular — *see* Disease, heart, ischemic,
        atherosclerotic
    coronary (artery) — *see* Disease, heart, ischemic,
        atherosclerotic
    heart — *see* Disease, heart, ischemic, atherosclerot-
        ic
artery I77.9
    cerebral I67.9
    coronary I25.10
        with angina pectoris — *see* Arteriosclerosis,
            coronary (artery)
arthropod-borne NOS (viral) A94
    specified type NEC A93.8
atticoantral, chronic H66.20
    left H66.22
        with right H66.23
    right H66.21
        with left H66.23
auditory canal — *see* Disorder, ear, external
auricle, ear NEC — *see* Disorder, pinna
Australian X A83.4
autoimmune (systemic) NOS M35.9
    hemolytic (cold type) (warm type) D59.1
        drug-induced D59.0
    thyroid E06.3
aviator's — *see* Effect, adverse, high altitude
Ayala's Q78.5
Ayerza's (pulmonary artery sclerosis with pulmonary
    hypertension) I27.0
Babington's (familial hemorrhagic telangiectasia) I78.0
bacterial A49.9
    specified NEC A48.8
    zoonotic A28.9
        specified type NEC A28.8
Baelz's (cheilitis glandularis apostematosa) K13.0
bagasse J67.1
balloon — *see* Effect, adverse, high altitude
Bang's (brucella abortus) A23.1
Bannister's T78.3 ☑
barometer makers' — *see* Poisoning, mercury
Barraquer (-Simons') (progressive lipodystrophy) E88.1
Barrett's — *see* Barrett's, esophagus
Bartholin's gland N75.9
basal ganglia G25.9
    degenerative G23.9
        specified NEC G23.8
    specified NEC G25.89
Basedow's (exophthalmic goiter) — *see* Hyperthy-
    roidism, with, goiter (diffuse)
Bateman's B08.1
Batten-Steinert G71.11
Battey A31.0
Beard's (neurasthenia) F48.8
Becker
    idiopathic mural endomyocardial I42.3
    myotonia congenita G71.12
Begbie's (exophthalmic goiter) — *see* Hyperthy-
    roidism, with, goiter (diffuse)
behavioral, organic F07.9
Beigel's (white piedra) B36.2
Benson's — *see* Deposit, crystalline
Bernard-Soulier (thrombopathy) D69.1
Bernhardt (-Roth) — *see* Mononeuropathy, lower limb,
    meralgia paresthetica

Disease, diseased — *continued*
Biermer's (pernicious anemia) D51.0
bile duct (common) (hepatic) K83.9
    with calculus, stones — *see* Calculus, bile duct
    specified NEC K83.8
biliary (tract) K83.9
    specified NEC K83.8
Billroth's — *see* Spina bifida
bird fancier's J67.2
black lung J60
bladder N32.9
    in (due to)
        schistosomiasis (bilharziasis) B65.0 [N33]
    specified NEC N32.89
bleeder's D66
blood D75.9
    forming organs D75.9
    vessel I99.9
Bloodgood's — *see* Mastopathy, cystic
Bodechtel-Guttmann (subacute sclerosing panen-
    cephalitis) A81.1
bone (*see also* Disorder, bone)
    aluminum M83.4
    fibrocystic NEC
        jaw M27.49
bone-marrow D75.9
Borna A83.9
Bornholm (epidemic pleurodynia) B33.0
Bouchard's (myopathic dilatation of the stomach)
    K31.0
Bouillaud's (rheumatic heart disease) I01.9
Bourneville (-Brissaud) (tuberous sclerosis) Q85.1
Bouveret (-Hoffmann) (paroxysmal tachycardia) I47.9
bowel K63.9
    functional K59.9
        psychogenic F45.8
brain G93.9
    arterial, artery I67.9
    arteriosclerotic I67.2
    congenital Q04.9
    degenerative — *see* Degeneration, brain
    inflammatory — *see* Encephalitis
    organic G93.9
        arteriosclerotic I67.2
    parasitic NEC B71.9 [G94]
    senile NEC G31.1
    specified NEC G93.89
breast (*see also* Disorder, breast) N64.9
    cystic (chronic) — *see* Mastopathy, cystic
    fibrocystic — *see* Mastopathy, cystic
    Paget's
        female, unspecified side C50.91- ☑
        male, unspecified side C50.92- ☑
    specified NEC N64.89
Breda's — *see* Yaws
Bretonneau's (diphtheritic malignant angina) A36.0
Bright's — *see* Nephritis
    arteriosclerotic — *see* Hypertension, kidney
Brill's (recrudescent typhus) A75.1
Brill-Zinsser (recrudescent typhus) A75.1
Brion-Kayser — *see* Fever, paratyphoid
broad
    beta E78.2
    ligament (noninflammatory) N83.9
        inflammatory — *see* Disease, pelvis, inflamma-
            tory
        specified NEC N83.8
Brocq-Duhring (dermatitis herpetiformis) L13.0
Brocq's
    meaning
        dermatitis herpetiformis L13.0
        prurigo L28.2
bronchopulmonary J98.4
bronchus NEC J98.09
bronze Addison's E27.1
    tuberculous A18.7
budgerigar fancier's J67.2
Buerger's (thromboangiitis obliterans) I73.1
bullous L13.9
    chronic of childhood L12.2
    specified NEC L13.8
Bürger-Grütz (essential familial hyperlipemia) E78.3
bursa — *see* Bursopathy
caisson T70.3 ☑
California — *see* Coccidioidomycosis
capillaries I78.9
    specified NEC I78.8
Carapata A68.0

Disease, diseased — *continued*
cardiac — *see* Disease, heart
cardiopulmonary, chronic I27.9
cardiorenal (hepatic) (hypertensive) (vascular) — *see*
    Hypertension, cardiorenal
cardiovascular (atherosclerotic) I25.10
    with angina pectoris — *see* Arteriosclerosis, coro-
        nary (artery),
    congenital Q28.9
    hypertensive — *see* Hypertension, heart
    newborn P29.9
        specified NEC P29.89
    renal (hypertensive) — *see* Hypertension, cardiore-
        nal
    syphilitic (asymptomatic) A52.00
cartilage — *see* Disorder, cartilage
Castellani's A69.8
cat-scratch A28.1
Cavare's (familial periodic paralysis) G72.3
cecum K63.9
celiac (adult) (infantile) K90.0
cellular tissue L98.9
central core G71.2
cerebellar, cerebellum — *see* Disease, brain
cerebral (*see also* Disease, brain)
    degenerative — *see* Degeneration, brain
cerebrospinal G96.9
cerebrovascular I67.9
    acute I67.89
        embolic I63.4- ☑
        thrombotic I63.3- ☑
    arteriosclerotic I67.2
    specified NEC I67.89
cervix (uteri) (noninflammatory) N88.9
    inflammatory — *see* Cervicitis
    specified NEC N88.8
Chabert's A22.9
Chandler's (osteochondritis dissecans, hip) — *see* Os-
    teochondritis, dissecans, hip
Charlouis — *see* Yaws
Chédiak-Steinbrinck (-Higashi) (congenital gigantism
    of peroxidase granules) E70.330
chest J98.9
Chiari's (hepatic vein thrombosis) I82.0
Chicago B40.9
Chignon B36.8
chigo, chigoe B88.1
childhood granulomatous D71
Chinese liver fluke B66.1
chlamydial A74.9
    specified NEC A74.89
cholecystic K82.9
choroid H31.9
    specified NEC H31.8
Christmas D67
chronic bullous of childhood L12.2
chylomicron retention E78.3
ciliary body H21.9
    specified NEC H21.89
circulatory (system) NEC I99.8
    newborn P29.9
    syphilitic A52.00
        congenital A50.54
coagulation factor deficiency (congenital) — *see* De-
    fect, coagulation
coccidioidal — *see* Coccidioidomycosis
cold
    agglutinin or hemoglobinuria D59.1
        paroxysmal D59.6
    hemagglutinin (chronic) D59.1
collagen NOS (nonvascular) (vascular) M35.9
    specified NEC M35.8
colon K63.9
    functional K59.9
        congenital Q43.2
    ischemic K55.0
combined system — *see* Degeneration, combined
compressed air T70.3 ☑
Concato's (pericardial polyserositis) A19.9
    nontubercular I31.1
    pleural — *see* Pleurisy, with effusion
conjunctiva H11.9
    chlamydial A74.0
    specified NEC H11.89
    viral B30.9
        specified NEC B30.8

☑ **Additional Character Required — Refer to the Tabular List for Character Selection**

▽ **Subterms under main terms may continue to next column or page**

Disease, diseased — *continued*
connective tissue, systemic (diffuse) M35.9
  in(due to)
    hypogammaglobulinemia D8Ø.1 [M36.8]
    ochronosis E7Ø.29 [M36.8]
  specified NEC M35.8
Conor and Bruch's (boutonneuse fever) A77.1
Cooper's — *see* Mastopathy, cystic
Cori's (glycogenosis III) E74.Ø3
corkhandler's or corkworker's J67.3
cornea H18.9
  specified NEC H18.89- ☑
coronary (artery) — *see* Disease, heart, ischemic,
    atherosclerotic
  congenital Q24.5
  ostial, syphilitic (aortic) (mitral) (pulmonary) A52.Ø3
corpus cavernosum N48.9
  specified NEC N48.89
Cotugno's — *see* Sciatica
coxsackie (virus) NEC B34.1
cranial nerve NOS G52.9
Creutzfeldt-Jakob — *see* Creutzfeldt-Jakob disease or
    syndrome
Crocq's (acrocyanosis) I73.89
Crohn's — *see* Enteritis, regional
Curschmann G71.11
cystic
  breast (chronic) — *see* Mastopathy, cystic
  kidney, congenital Q61.9
  liver, congenital Q44.6
  lung J98.4
    congenital Q33.Ø
cytomegalic inclusion (generalized) B25.9
  with pneumonia B25.Ø
  congenital P35.1
cytomegaloviral B25.9
  specified NEC B25.8
Czerny's (periodic hydrarthrosis of the knee) — *see*
    Effusion, joint, knee
Daae (-Finsen) (epidemic pleurodynia) B33.Ø
Darling's — *see* Histoplasmosis capsulati
de Quervain's (tendon sheath) M65.4
  thyroid (subacute granulomatous thyroiditis) E06.1
Débove's (splenomegaly) R16.1
deer fly — *see* Tularemia
Degos' I77.89
demyelinating, demyelinizating (nervous system)
    G37.9
  multiple sclerosis G35
  specified NEC G37.8
dense deposit (*see also* NØØ-NØ7 with fourth character
    .6) NØ5.6
deposition, hydroxyapatite — *see* Disease, hydroxya-
    patite deposition
Devergie's (pityriasis rubra pilaris) L44.Ø
Devic's G36.Ø
diaphorase deficiency D74.Ø
diaphragm J98.6
diarrheal, infectious NEC AØ9
digestive system K92.9
  specified NEC K92.89
disc, degenerative — *see* Degeneration, intervertebral
    disc
discogenic (*see also* Displacement, intervertebral disc
    NEC)
  with myelopathy — *see* Disorder, disc, with,
    myelopathy
diverticular — *see* Diverticula
Dubois (thymus) A5Ø.59 [E35]
Duchenne-Griesinger G71.Ø
Duchenne's
  muscular dystrophy G71.Ø
  pseudohypertrophy, muscles G71.Ø
ductless glands E34.9
Duhring's (dermatitis herpetiformis) L13.Ø
duodenum K31.9
  specified NEC K31.89
Dupré's (meningism) R29.1
Dupuytren's (muscle contracture) M72.Ø
Durand-Nicholas-Favre (climatic bubo) A55
Duroziez's (congenital mitral stenosis) Q23.2
ear — *see* Disorder, ear
Eberth's — *see* Fever, typhoid
Ebola (virus) A98.4
Ebstein's heart Q22.5
Echinococcus — *see* Echinococcus
echovirus NEC B34.1
Eddowes' (brittle bones and blue sclera) Q78.Ø

Disease, diseased — *continued*
edentulous (alveolar) ridge KØ6.9
  specified NEC KØ6.8
Edsall's T67.2 ☑
Eichstedt's (pityriasis versicolor) B36.Ø
Ellis-van Creveld (chondroectodermal dysplasia) Q77.6
end stage renal (ESRD) N18.6
  due to hypertension I12.Ø
endocrine glands or system NEC E34.9
endomyocardial (eosinophilic) I42.3
English (rickets) E55.Ø
enteroviral, enterovirus NEC B34.1
  central nervous system NEC A88.8
epidemic B99.9
  specified NEC B99.8
epididymis N5Ø.9
Erb (-Landouzy) G71.Ø
Erdheim-Chester (ECD) E88.89
esophagus K22.9
  functional K22.4
  psychogenic F45.8
  specified NEC K22.8
Eulenburg's (congenital paramyotonia) G71.19
eustachian tube — *see* Disorder, eustachian tube
external
  auditory canal — *see* Disorder, ear, external
  ear — *see* Disorder, ear, external
extrapyramidal G25.9
  specified NEC G25.89
eye H57.9
  anterior chamber H21.9
  inflammatory NEC H57.8
  muscle (external) — *see* Strabismus
  specified NEC H57.8
  syphilitic — *see* Oculopathy, syphilitic
eyeball H44.9
  specified NEC H44.89
eyelid — *see* Disorder, eyelid
  specified NEC — *see* Disorder, eyelid, specified type
    NEC
eyeworm of Africa B74.3
facial nerve (seventh) G51.9
  newborn (birth injury) P11.3
Fahr (of brain) G23.8
Fahr Volhard (of kidney) I12.- ☑
fallopian tube (noninflammatory) N83.9
  inflammatory — *see* Salpingo-oophoritis
  specified NEC N83.8
familial periodic paralysis G72.3
Fanconi's (congenital pancytopenia) D61.Ø9
fascia NEC (*see also* Disorder, muscle)
  inflammatory — *see* Myositis
  specified NEC M62.89
Fauchard's (periodontitis) — *see* Periodontitis
Favre-Durand-Nicolas (climatic bubo) A55
Fede's K14.Ø
Feer's — *see* Poisoning, mercury
female pelvic inflammatory (*see also* Disease, pelvis,
    inflammatory) N73.9
  syphilitic (secondary) A51.42
  tuberculous A18.17
Fernels' (aortic aneurysm) I71.9
fibrocaseous of lung — *see* Tuberculosis, pulmonary
fibrocystic — *see* Fibrocystic disease
Fiedler's (leptospiral jaundice) A27.Ø
fifth BØ8.3
file-cutter's — *see* Poisoning, lead
fish-skin Q8Ø.9
  acquired L85.Ø
Flajani (-Basedow) (exophthalmic goiter) — *see* Hyper-
    thyroidism, with, goiter (diffuse)
flax-dresser's J66.1
fluke — *see* Infestation, fluke
foot and mouth BØ8.8
foot process NØ4.9
Forbes' (glycogenosis III) E74.Ø3
Fordyce-Fox (apocrine miliaria) L75.2
Fordyce's (ectopic sebaceous glands) (mouth) Q38.6
Forestier's (rhizomelic pseudopolyarthritis) M35.3
  meaning ankylosing hyperostosis — *see* Hyperos-
    tosis, ankylosing
Fothergill's
  neuralgia — *see* Neuralgia, trigeminal
  scarlatina anginosa A38.9
Fournier (gangrene) N49.3
  female N76.89
fourth BØ8.8
Fox (-Fordyce) (apocrine miliaria) L75.2

Disease, diseased — *continued*
Francis' — *see* Tularemia
Franklin C88.2
Frei's (climatic bubo) A55
Friedreich's
  combined systemic or ataxia G11.1
  myoclonia G25.3
frontal sinus — *see* Sinusitis, frontal
fungus NEC B49
Gaisböck's (polycythemia hypertonica) D75.1
gallbladder K82.9
  calculus — *see* Calculus, gallbladder
  cholecystitis — *see* Cholecystitis
  cholesterolosis K82.4
  fistula — *see* Fistula, gallbladder
  hydrops K82.1
  obstruction — *see* Obstruction, gallbladder
  perforation K82.2
  specified NEC K82.8
gamma heavy chain C88.2
Gamna's (siderotic splenomegaly) D73.2
Gamstorp's (adynamia episodica hereditaria) G72.3
Gandy-Nanta (siderotic splenomegaly) D73.2
ganister J62.8
gastric — *see* Disease, stomach
gastroesophageal reflux (GERD) K21.9
  with esophagitis K21.Ø
gastrointestinal (tract) K92.9
  amyloid E85.4
  functional K59.9
    psychogenic F45.8
  specified NEC K92.89
Gee (-Herter) (-Heubner) (-Thaysen) (nontropical sprue)
    K9Ø.Ø
genital organs
  female N94.9
  male N5Ø.9
Gerhardt's (erythromelalgia) I73.81
Gibert's (pityriasis rosea) L42
Gierke's (glycogenosis I) E74.Ø1
Gilles de la Tourette's (motor-verbal tic) F95.2
gingiva KØ6.9
  specified NEC KØ6.8
gland (lymph) I89.9
Glanzmann's (hereditary hemorrhagic thrombasthenia)
    D69.1
glass-blower's (cataract) — *see* Cataract, specified NEC
  salivary gland hypertrophy K11.1
Glisson's — *see* Rickets
globe H44.9
  specified NEC H44.89
glomerular (*see also* Glomerulonephritis)
  with edema — *see* Nephrosis
  acute — *see* Nephritis, acute
  chronic — *see* Nephritis, chronic
  minimal change NØ5.Ø
  rapidly progressive NØ1.9
glycogen storage E74.ØØ
  Andersen's E74.Ø9
  Cori's E74.Ø3
  Forbes' E74.Ø3
  generalized E74.ØØ
  glucose-6-phosphatase deficiency E74.Ø1
  heart E74.Ø2 [I43]
  hepatorenal E74.Ø9
  Hers' E74.Ø9
  liver and kidney E74.Ø9
  McArdle's E74.Ø4
  muscle phosphofructokinase E74.Ø9
  myocardium E74.Ø2 [I43]
  Pompe's E74.Ø2
  Tauri's E74.Ø9
  type Ø E74.Ø9
  type I E74.Ø1
  type II E74.Ø2
  type III E74.Ø3
  type IV E74.Ø9
  type V E74.Ø4
  type VI-XI E74.Ø9
  Von Gierke's E74.Ø1
Goldstein's (familial hemorrhagic telangiectasia) I78.Ø
gonococcal NOS A54.9
graft-versus-host (GVH) D89.813
  acute D89.81Ø
  acute on chronic D89.812
  chronic D89.811
grainhandler's J67.8
granulomatous (childhood) (chronic) D71

Disease, diseased — *continued*
Graves' (exophthalmic goiter) — *see* Hyperthyroidism,
    with, goiter (diffuse)
Griesinger's — *see* Ancylostomiasis
Grisel's M43.6
Gruby's (tinea tonsurans) B35.0
Guillain-Barré G61.0
Guinon's (motor-verbal tic) F95.2
gum K06.9
gynecological N94.9
H (Hartnup's) E72.02
Haff — *see* Poisoning, mercury
Hageman (congenital factor XII deficiency) D68.2
hair (color) (shaft) L67.9
    follicles L73.9
        specified NEC L73.8
Hamman's (spontaneous mediastinal emphysema)
    J98.2
hand, foot and mouth B08.4
Hansen's — *see* Leprosy
Hantavirus, with pulmonary manifestations B33.4
    with renal manifestations A98.5
Harada's H30.81- ☑
Hartnup (pellagra-cerebellar ataxia-renal
    aminoaciduria) E72.02
Hart's (pellagra-cerebellar ataxia-renal aminoaciduria)
    E72.02
Hashimoto's (struma lymphomatosa) E06.3
Hb — *see* Disease, hemoglobin
heart (organic) I51.9
    with
        pulmonary edema (acute) (*see also* Failure,
            ventricular, left) I50.1
        rheumatic fever (conditions in I00)
            active I01.9
                with chorea I02.0
                specified NEC I01.8
            inactive or quiescent (with chorea) I09.9
            specified NEC I09.89
    amyloid E85.4 [I43]
    aortic (valve) I35.9
    arteriosclerotic or sclerotic (senile) — *see* Disease,
        heart, ischemic, atherosclerotic
    artery, arterial — *see* Disease, heart, ischemic,
        atherosclerotic
    beer drinkers' I42.6
    beriberi (wet) E51.12
    black I27.0
    congenital Q24.9
        cyanotic Q24.9
        specified NEC Q24.8
    coronary — *see* Disease, heart, ischemic
    cryptogenic I51.9
    fibroid — *see* Myocarditis
    functional I51.89
        psychogenic F45.8
    glycogen storage E74.02 [I43]
    gonococcal A54.83
    hypertensive — *see* Hypertension, heart
    hyperthyroid (*see also* Hyperthyroidism)
        E05.90 [I43]
        with thyroid storm E05.91 [I43]
    ischemic (chronic or with a stated duration of over
        4 weeks) I25.9
        atherosclerotic (of) I25.10
            with angina pectoris — *see* Arteriosclerosis,
                coronary (artery)
            coronary artery bypass graft — *see* Arte-
                riosclerosis, coronary (artery),
                cardiomyopathy I25.5
        diagnosed on ECG or other special investiga-
            tion, but currently presenting no symp-
            toms I25.6
        silent I25.6
        specified form NEC I25.89
    kyphoscoliotic I27.1
    meningococcal A39.50
        endocarditis A39.51
        myocarditis A39.52
        pericarditis A39.53
    mitral I05.9
        specified NEC I05.8
    muscular — *see* Degeneration, myocardial
    psychogenic (functional) F45.8
    pulmonary (chronic) I27.9
        in schistosomiasis B65.9 [I52]
        specified NEC I27.89

Disease, diseased — *continued*
heart — *continued*
    rheumatic (chronic) (inactive) (old) (quiescent)
        (with chorea) I09.9
        active or acute I01.9
            with chorea (acute) (rheumatic) (Syden-
                ham's) I02.0
        specified NEC I09.89
    senile — *see* Myocarditis
    syphilitic A52.06
        aortic A52.03
            aneurysm A52.01
        congenital A50.54 [I52]
    thyrotoxic (*see also* Thyrotoxicosis) E05.90 [I43]
        with thyroid storm E05.91 [I43]
    valve, valvular (obstructive) (regurgitant) (*see also*
        Endocarditis)
        congenital NEC Q24.8
            pulmonary Q22.3
    vascular — *see* Disease, cardiovascular
heavy chain NEC C88.2
    alpha C88.3
    gamma C88.2
    mu C88.2
Hebra's
    pityriasis
        maculata et circinata L42
        rubra pilaris L44.0
    prurigo L28.2
hematopoietic organs D75.9
hemoglobin or Hb
    abnormal (mixed) NEC D58.2
        with thalassemia D56.9
    AS genotype D57.3
    Bart's D56.0
    C (Hb-C) D58.2
        with other abnormal hemoglobin NEC D58.2
        elliptocytosis D58.1
        Hb-S D57.2- ☑
        sickle-cell D57.2- ☑
        thalassemia D56.8
    Constant Spring D58.2
    D (Hb-D) D58.2
    E (Hb-E) D58.2
    E-beta thalassemia D56.5
    elliptocytosis D58.1
    H (Hb-H) (thalassemia) D56.0
        with other abnormal hemoglobin NEC D56.9
        Constant Spring D56.0
    I thalassemia D56.9
    M D74.0
    S or SS D57.1
    SC D57.2- ☑
    SD D57.8- ☑
    SE D57.8- ☑
    spherocytosis D58.0
    unstable, hemolytic D58.2
hemolytic (newborn) P55.9
    autoimmune (cold type) (warm type) D59.1
    drug-induced D59.0
    due to or with
        incompatibility
            ABO (blood group) P55.1
            blood (group) (Duffy) (K(ell)) (Kidd) (Lewis)
                (M) (S) NEC P55.8
            Rh (blood group) (factor) P55.0
        Rh negative mother P55.0
    specified type NEC P55.8
    unstable hemoglobin D58.2
hemorrhagic D69.9
    newborn P53
Henoch (-Schönlein) (purpura nervosa) D69.0
hepatic — *see* Disease, liver
hepatolenticular E83.01
heredodegenerative NEC
    spinal cord G95.89
herpesviral, disseminated B00.7
Hers' (glycogenosis VI) E74.09
Herter (-Gee) (-Heubner) (nontropical sprue) K90.0
Heubner-Herter (nontropical sprue) K90.0
high fetal gene or hemoglobin thalassemia D56.9
Hildenbrand's — *see* Typhus
hip (joint) M25.9
    congenital Q65.89
    suppurative M00.9
    tuberculous A18.02
His (-Werner) (trench fever) A79.0

Disease, diseased — *continued*
Hodgson's I71.2
    ruptured I71.1
Holla — *see* Spherocytosis
hookworm B76.9
    specified NEC B76.8
host-versus-graft D89.813
    acute D89.810
    acute on chronic D89.812
    chronic D89.811
human immunodeficiency virus (HIV) B20
Huntington's G10
Hutchinson's (cheiropompholyx) — *see* Hutchinson's
    disease
hyaline (diffuse) (generalized)
    membrane (lung) (newborn) P22.0
        adult J80
hydatid — *see* Echinococcus
hydroxyapatite deposition M11.00
    ankle M11.07- ☑
    elbow M11.02- ☑
    foot joint M11.07- ☑
    hand joint M11.04- ☑
    hip M11.05- ☑
    knee M11.06- ☑
    multiple site M11.09
    shoulder M11.01- ☑
    vertebra M11.08
    wrist M11.03- ☑
hyperkinetic — *see* Hyperkinesia
hypertensive — *see* Hypertension
hypophysis E23.7
Iceland G93.3
I-cell E77.0
immune D89.9
immunoproliferative (malignant) C88.9
    small intestinal C88.3
    specified NEC C88.8
inclusion B25.9
    salivary gland B25.9
infectious, infective B99.9
    congenital P37.9
        specified NEC P37.8
        viral P35.9
            specified type NEC P35.8
    specified NEC B99.8
inflammatory
    penis N48.29
        abscess N48.21
        cellulitis N48.22
    prepuce N47.7
        balanoposthitis N47.6
    tubo-ovarian — *see* Salpingo-oophoritis
intervertebral disc (*see also* Disorder, disc)
    with myelopathy — *see* Disorder, disc, with,
        myelopathy
    cervical, cervicothoracic — *see* Disorder, disc, cer-
        vical
        with
            myelopathy — *see* Disorder, disc, cervical,
                with myelopathy
            neuritis, radiculitis or radiculopathy — *see*
                Disorder, disc, cervical, with neuritis
            specified NEC — *see* Disorder, disc, cervical,
                specified type NEC
    lumbar (with)
        myelopathy M51.06
        neuritis, radiculitis, radiculopathy or sciatica
            M51.16
        specified NEC M51.86
    lumbosacral (with)
        neuritis, radiculitis, radiculopathy or sciatica
            M51.17
        specified NEC M51.87
    specified NEC — *see* Disorder, disc, specified NEC
    thoracic (with)
        myelopathy M51.04
        neuritis, radiculitis or radiculopathy M51.14
        specified NEC M51.84
    thoracolumbar (with)
        myelopathy M51.05
        neuritis, radiculitis or radiculopathy M51.15
        specified NEC M51.85
intestine K63.9
    functional K59.9
        psychogenic F45.8
        specified NEC K59.8
    organic K63.9

100

☑ **Additional Character Required** — **Refer to the Tabular List for Character Selection**   ▽ **Subterms under main terms may continue to next column or page**

Disease, diseased — *continued*
  intestine — *continued*
    protozoal A07.9
    specified NEC K63.89
  iris H21.9
    specified NEC H21.89
  iron metabolism or storage E83.10
  island (scrub typhus) A75.3
  itai-itai — *see* Poisoning, cadmium
  Jakob-Creutzfeldt — *see* Creutzfeldt-Jakob disease or
      syndrome
  jaw M27.9
    fibrocystic M27.49
    specified NEC M27.8
  jigger B88.1
  joint (*see also* Disorder, joint)
    Charcot's — *see* Arthropathy, neuropathic (Char-
        cot)
    degenerative — *see* Osteoarthritis
      multiple M15.9
      spine — *see* Spondylosis
    hypertrophic — *see* Osteoarthritis
    sacroiliac M53.3
    specified NEC — *see* Disorder, joint, specified type
        NEC
    spine NEC — *see* Dorsopathy
    suppurative — *see* Arthritis, pyogenic or pyemic
  Jourdain's (acute gingivitis) K05.00
    nonplaque induced K05.01
    plaque induced K05.00
  Kaschin-Beck (endemic polyarthritis) M12.10
    ankle M12.17- ✓
    elbow M12.12- ✓
    foot joint M12.17- ✓
    hand joint M12.14- ✓
    hip M12.15- ✓
    knee M12.16- ✓
    multiple site M12.19
    shoulder M12.11- ✓
    vertebra M12.18
    wrist M12.13- ✓
  Katayama B65.2
  Kedani (scrub typhus) A75.3
  Keshan E59
  kidney (functional) (pelvis) N28.9
    chronic N18.9
      hypertensive — *see* Hypertension, kidney
      stage 1 N18.1
      stage 2 (mild) N18.2
      stage 3 (moderate) N18.3
      stage 4 (severe) N18.4
      stage 5 N18.5
    complicating pregnancy — *see* Pregnancy, compli-
        cated by, renal disease
    cystic (congenital) Q61.9
    fibrocystic (congenital) Q61.8
    hypertensive — *see* Hypertension, kidney
    in (due to)
      schistosomiasis (bilharziasis) B65.9 [N29]
    multicystic Q61.4
    polycystic Q61.3
      adult type Q61.2
      childhood type NEC Q61.19
        collecting duct dilatation Q61.11
  Kimmelstiel (-Wilson) (intercapillary polycystic (con-
      genital) glomerulosclerosis) — *see* E08-E13 with
      .21
  Kinnier Wilson's (hepatolenticular degeneration)
      E83.01
  kissing — *see* Mononucleosis, infectious
  Klebs' (*see also* Glomerulonephritis) N05- ✓
  Klippel-Feil (brevicollis) Q76.1
  Köhler-Pellegrini-Stieda (calcification, knee joint) —
      see Bursitis, tibial collateral
  Kok Q89.8
  König's (osteochondritis dissecans) — *see* Osteochon-
      dritis, dissecans
  Korsakoff's (nonalcoholic) F04
    alcoholic F10.96
      with dependence F10.26
  Kostmann's (infantile genetic agranulocytosis) D70.0
  kuru A81.81
  Kyasanur Forest A98.2
  labyrinth, ear — *see* Disorder, ear, inner
  lacrimal system — *see* Disorder, lacrimal system
  Lafora's — *see* Epilepsy, generalized, idiopathic
  Lancereaux-Mathieu (leptospiral jaundice) A27.0
  Landry's G61.0

Disease, diseased — *continued*
  Larrey-Weil (leptospiral jaundice) A27.0
  larynx J38.7
  legionnaires' A48.1
    nonpneumonic A48.2
  Lenegre's I44.2
  lens H27.9
    specified NEC H27.8
  Lev's (acquired complete heart block) I44.2
  Lewy body (dementia) G31.83 [F02.80]
    with behavioral disturbance G31.83 [F02.81]
  Lichtheim's (subacute combined sclerosis with perni-
      cious anemia) D51.0
  Lightwood's (renal tubular acidosis) N25.89
  Lignac's (cystinosis) E72.04
  lip K13.0
  lipid-storage E75.6
    specified NEC E75.5
  Lipschütz's N76.6
  liver (chronic) (organic) K76.9
    alcoholic (chronic) K70.9
      acute — *see* Disease, liver, alcoholic, hepatitis
      cirrhosis K70.30
        with ascites K70.31
      failure K70.40
        with coma K70.41
      fatty liver K70.0
      fibrosis K70.2
      hepatitis K70.10
        with ascites K70.11
      sclerosis K70.2
    cystic, congenital Q44.6
    drug-induced (idiosyncratic) (toxic) (predictable)
        (unpredictable) — *see* Disease, liver, toxic
    end stage K72.90
      due to hepatitis — *see* Hepatitis
    fatty, nonalcoholic (NAFLD) K76.0
      alcoholic K70.0
    fibrocystic (congenital) Q44.6
    fluke
      Chinese B66.1
      oriental B66.1
      sheep B66.3
    glycogen storage E74.09 [K77]
    in (due to)
      schistosomiasis (bilharziasis) B65.9 [K77]
    inflammatory K75.9
      alcoholic K70.1 ✓
      specified NEC K75.89
    polycystic (congenital) Q44.6
    toxic K71.9
      with
        cholestasis K71.0
        cirrhosis (liver) K71.7
        fibrosis (liver) K71.7
        focal nodular hyperplasia K71.8
        hepatic granuloma K71.8
        hepatic necrosis K71.10
          with coma K71.11
        hepatitis NEC K71.6
          acute K71.2
          chronic
            active K71.50
              with ascites K71.51
            lobular K71.4
            persistent K71.3
          lupoid K71.50
            with ascites K71.51
        peliosis hepatis K71.8
        veno-occlusive disease (VOD) of liver K71.8
      veno-occlusive K76.5
  Lobo's (keloid blastomycosis) B48.0
  Lobstein's (brittle bones and blue sclera) Q78.0
  Ludwig's (submaxillary cellulitis) K12.2
  lumbosacral region M53.87
  lung J98.4
    black J60
    congenital Q33.9
    cystic J98.4
      congenital Q33.0
    fibroid (chronic) — *see* Fibrosis, lung
    fluke B66.4
      oriental B66.4
    in
      amyloidosis E85.4 [J99]
      sarcoidosis D86.0
      Sjögren's syndrome M35.02

Disease, diseased — *continued*
  lung — *continued*
    in — *continued*
      systemic
        lupus erythematosus M32.13
        sclerosis M34.81
    interstitial J84.9
      of childhood, specified NEC J84.848
      respiratory bronchiolitis J84.115
      specified NEC J84.89
    obstructive (chronic) J44.9
      with
        acute
          bronchitis J44.0
          exacerbation NEC J44.1
          lower respiratory infection J44.0
        alveolitis, allergic J67.9
        asthma J44.9
        bronchiectasis J47.9
          with
            exacerbation (acute) J47.1
            lower respiratory infection J47.0
        bronchitis J44.9
          with
            exacerbation (acute) J44.1
            lower respiratory infection J44.0
        emphysema J44.9
        hypersensitivity pneumonitis J67.9
      decompensated J44.1
        with
          exacerbation (acute) J44.1
    polycystic J98.4
      congenital Q33.0
    rheumatoid (diffuse) (interstitial) — *see* Rheuma-
        toid, lung
  Lutembacher's (atrial septal defect with mitral stenosis)
      Q21.1
  Lyme A69.20
  lymphatic (gland) (system) (channel) (vessel) I89.9
  lymphoproliferative D47.9
    specified NEC D47.Z9 (*following* D47.4)
    T-gamma D47.Z9 (*following* D47.4)
    X-linked D82.3
  Magitot's M27.2
  malarial — *see* Malaria
  malignant (*see also* Neoplasm, malignant, by site)
  Manson's B65.1
  maple bark J67.6
  maple-syrup-urine E71.0
  Marburg (virus) A98.3
  Marion's (bladder neck obstruction) N32.0
  Marsh's (exophthalmic goiter) — *see* Hyperthyroidism,
      with, goiter (diffuse)
  mastoid (process) — *see* Disorder, ear, middle
  Mathieu's (leptospiral jaundice) A27.0
  Maxcy's A75.2
  McArdle (-Schmid-Pearson) (glycogenosis V) E74.04
  mediastinum J98.5
  medullary center (idiopathic) (respiratory) G93.89
  Meige's (chronic hereditary edema) Q82.0
  meningococcal — *see* Infection, meningococcal
  mental F99
    organic F09
  mesenchymal M35.9
  mesenteric embolic K55.0
  metabolic, metabolism E88.9
    bilirubin E80.7
  metal-polisher's J62.8
  metastatic (*see also* Neoplasm, secondary, by site)
      C79.9
  microvascular - code to condition
  microvillus
    atrophy Q43.8
    inclusion (MVD) Q43.8
  middle ear — *see* Disorder, ear, middle
  Mikulicz' (dryness of mouth, absent or decreased
      lacrimation) K11.8
  Milroy's (chronic hereditary edema) Q82.0
  Minamata — *see* Poisoning, mercury
  minicore G71.2
  Minor's G95.19
  Minot's (hemorrhagic disease, newborn) P53
  Minot-von Willebrand-Jürgens (angiohemophilia)
      D68.0
  Mitchell's (erythromelalgia) I73.81
  mitral (valve) I05.9
    nonrheumatic I34.9
  mixed connective tissue M35.1

Disease, diseased — *continued*
moldy hay J67.0
Monge's T70.29 ☑
Morgagni-Adams-Stokes (syncope with heart block) I45.9
Morgagni's (syndrome) (hyperostosis frontalis interna) M85.2
Morton's (with metatarsalgia) — *see* Lesion, nerve, plantar
Morvan's G60.8
motor neuron (bulbar) (familial) (mixed type) (spinal) G12.20
amyotrophic lateral sclerosis G12.21
progressive bulbar palsy G12.22
specified NEC G12.29
moyamoya I67.5
mu heavy chain disease C88.2
multicore G71.2
muscle (*see also* Disorder, muscle)
inflammatory *see* Myositis
ocular (external) — *see* Strabismus
musculoskeletal system, soft tissue — *see also* Disorder, soft tissue
specified NEC — *see* Disorder, soft tissue, specified type NEC
mushroom workers' J67.5
mycotic B49
myelodysplastic, not classified C94.6
myeloproliferative, not classified C94.6
chronic D47.1
myocardium, myocardial (*see also* Degeneration, myocardial) I51.5
primary (idiopathic) I42.9
myoneural G70.9
Naegeli's D69.1
nails L60.9
specified NEC L60.8
Nairobi (sheep virus) A93.8
nasal J34.9
nemaline body G71.2
nerve — *see* Disorder, nerve
nervous system G98.8
autonomic G90.9
central G96.9
specified NEC G96.8
congenital Q07.9
parasympathetic G90.9
specified NEC G98.8
sympathetic G90.9
vegetative G90.9
neuromuscular system G70.9
Newcastle B30.8
Nicolas (-Durand)-Favre (climatic bubo) A55
nipple N64.9
Paget's C50.01- ☑
female C50.01- ☑
male C50.02- ☑
Nishimoto (-Takeuchi) I67.5
nonarthropod-borne NOS (viral) B34.9
enterovirus NEC B34.1
nonautoimmune hemolytic D59.4
drug-induced D59.2
Nonne-Milroy-Meige (chronic hereditary edema) Q82.0
nose J34.9
nucleus pulposus — *see* Disorder, disc
nutritional E63.9
oast-house-urine E72.19
ocular
herpesviral B00.50
zoster B02.30
obliterative vascular I77.1
Ohara's — *see* Tularemia
Opitz's (congestive splenomegaly) D73.2
Oppenheim-Urbach (necrobiosis lipoidica diabeticorum) — *see* E08-E13 with .620
optic nerve NEC — *see* Disorder, nerve, optic
orbit — *see* Disorder, orbit
Oriental liver fluke B66.1
Oriental lung fluke B66.4
Ormond's N13.5
Oropouche virus A93.0
Osler-Rendu (familial hemorrhagic telangiectasia) I78.0
osteofibrocystic E21.0
Otto's M24.7
outer ear — *see* Disorder, ear, external
ovary (noninflammatory) N83.9
cystic N83.20
inflammatory — *see* Salpingo-oophoritis

Disease, diseased — *continued*
ovary — *continued*
polycystic E28.2
specified NEC N83.8
Owren's (congenital) — *see* Defect, coagulation
pancreas K86.9
cystic K86.2
fibrocystic E84.9
specified NEC K86.8
panvalvular I08.9
specified NEC I08.8
parametrium (noninflammatory) N83.9
parasitic B89
cerebral NEC B71.9 [G94]
intestinal NOS B82.9
mouth B37.0
skin NOS B88.9
specified type — *see* Infestation
tongue B37.0
parathyroid (gland) E21.5
specified NEC E21.4
Parkinson's G20
parodontal K05.6
Parrot's (syphilitic osteochondritis) A50.02
Parry's (exophthalmic goiter) — *see* Hyperthyroidism, with, goiter (diffuse)
Parson's (exophthalmic goiter) — *see* Hyperthyroidism, with, goiter (diffuse)
Paxton's (white piedra) B36.2
pearl-worker's — *see* Osteomyelitis, specified type NEC
Pellegrini-Stieda (calcification, knee joint) — *see* Bursitis, tibial collateral
pelvis, pelvic
female NOS N94.9
specified NEC N94.89
gonococcal (acute) (chronic) A54.24
inflammatory (female) N73.9
acute N73.0
chronic N73.1
specified NEC N73.8
syphilitic (secondary) A51.42
late A52.76
tuberculous A18.17
organ, female N94.9
peritoneum, female NEC N94.89
penis N48.9
inflammatory N48.29
abscess N48.21
cellulitis N48.22
specified NEC N48.89
periapical tissues NOS K04.90
periodontal K05.6
specified NEC K05.5
periosteum — *see* Disorder, bone, specified type NEC
peripheral
arterial I73.9
autonomic nervous system G90.9
nerves — *see* Polyneuropathy
vascular NOS I73.9
peritoneum K66.9
pelvic, female NEC N94.89
specified NEC K66.8
persistent mucosal (middle ear) H66.20
left H66.22
with right H66.23
right H66.21
with left H66.23
Petit's — *see* Hernia, abdomen, specified site NEC
pharynx J39.2
specified NEC J39.2
Phocas' — *see* Mastopathy, cystic
photochromogenic (acid-fast bacilli) (pulmonary) A31.0
nonpulmonary A31.9
Pick's G31.01 [F02.80]
with behavioral disturbance G31.01 [F02.81]
pigeon fancier's J67.2
pineal gland E34.8
pink — *see* Poisoning, mercury
Pinkus' (lichen nitidus) L44.1
pinworm B80
Piry virus A93.8
pituitary (gland) E23.7
pituitary-snuff-taker's J67.8
pleura (cavity) J94.9
specified NEC J94.8
pneumatic drill (hammer) T75.21 ☑

Disease, diseased — *continued*
Pollitzer's (hidradenitis suppurativa) L73.2
polycystic
kidney or renal Q61.3
adult type Q61.2
childhood type NEC Q61.19
collecting duct dilatation Q61.11
liver or hepatic Q44.6
lung or pulmonary J98.4
congenital Q33.0
ovary, ovaries E28.2
spleen Q89.09
polyethylene T84.05- ☑
Pompe's (glycogenosis II) E74.02
Posadas-Wernicke B38.9
Potain's (pulmonary edema) — *see* Edema, lung
prepuce N47.8
inflammatory N47.7
balanoposthitis N47.6
Pringle's (tuberous sclerosis) Q85.1
prion, central nervous system A81.9
specified NEC A81.89
prostate N42.9 (congenital) Q61.3
specified NEC N42.89
protozoal B64
acanthamebiasis — *see* Acanthamebiasis
African trypanosomiasis — *see* African trypanosomiasis
babesiosis B60.0
Chagas disease — *see* Chagas disease
intestine, intestinal A07.9
leishmaniasis — *see* Leishmaniasis
malaria — *see* Malaria
naegleriasis B60.2
pneumocystosis B59
specified organism NEC B60.8
toxoplasmosis — *see* Toxoplasmosis
pseudo-Hurler's E77.0
psychiatric F99
psychotic — *see* Psychosis
Puente's (simple glandular cheilitis) K13.0
puerperal (*see also* Puerperal) O90.89
pulmonary (*see also* Disease, lung)
artery I28.9
chronic obstructive J44.9
with
acute bronchitis J44.0
exacerbation (acute) J44.1
lower respiratory infection (acute) J44.0
decompensated J44.1
with
exacerbation (acute) J44.1
heart I27.9
specified NEC I27.89
hypertensive (vascular) I27.0
valve I37.9
rheumatic I09.89
pulp (dental) NOS K04.90
pulseless M31.4
Putnam's (subacute combined sclerosis with pernicious anemia) D51.0
Pyle (-Cohn) (craniometaphyseal dysplasia) Q78.5
ragpicker's or ragsorter's A22.1
Raynaud's — *see* Raynaud's disease
reactive airway — *see* Asthma
Reclus' (cystic) — *see* Mastopathy, cystic
rectum K62.9
specified NEC K62.89
Refsum's (heredopathia atactica polyneuritiformis) G60.1
renal (functional) (pelvis) (*see also* Disease, kidney) N28.9
with
edema — *see* Nephrosis
glomerular lesion — *see* Glomerulonephritis
with edema — *see* Nephrosis
interstitial nephritis N12
acute N28.9
chronic (*see also* Disease, kidney, chronic) N18.9
cystic, congenital Q61.9
diabetic — *see* E08-E13 with .22
end-stage (failure) N18.6
due to hypertension I12.0
fibrocystic (congenital) Q61.8
hypertensive — *see* Hypertension, kidney
lupus M32.14
phosphate-losing (tubular) N25.0

Disease, diseased — *continued*
  renal (*see also* Disease, kidney) — *continued*
    polycystic (congenital) Q61.3
      adult type Q61.2
      childhood type NEC Q61.19
        collecting duct dilatation Q61.11
    rapidly progressive N01.9
    subacute N01.9
  Rendu-Osler-Weber (familial hemorrhagic telangiectasia) I78.0
  renovascular (arteriosclerotic) — *see* Hypertension, kidney
  respiratory (tract) J98.9
    acute or subacute NOS J06.9
      due to
        chemicals, gases, fumes or vapors (inhalation) J68.3
        external agent J70.9
          specified NEC J70.8
        radiation J70.0
        smoke inhalation J70.5
      noninfectious J39.8
    chronic NOS J98.9
      due to
        chemicals, gases, fumes or vapors J68.4
        external agent J70.9
          specified NEC J70.8
        radiation J70.1
    newborn P27.9
      specified NEC P27.8
    due to
      chemicals, gases, fumes or vapors J68.9
        acute or subacute NEC J68.3
        chronic J68.4
      external agent J70.9
        specified NEC J70.8
    newborn P28.9
      specified type NEC P28.89
    upper J39.9
      acute or subacute J06.9
      noninfectious NEC J39.8
      specified NEC J39.8
      streptococcal J06.9
  retina, retinal H35.9
    Batten's or Batten-Mayou E75.4 [H36]
    specified NEC H35.89
  rheumatoid — *see* Arthritis, rheumatoid
  rickettsial NOS A79.9
    specified type NEC A79.89
  Riga (-Fede) (cachectic aphthae) K14.0
  Riggs' (compound periodontitis) — *see* Periodontitis
  Ritter's L00
  Rivalta's (cervicofacial actinomycosis) A42.2
  Robles' (onchocerciasis) B73.01
  Roger's (congenital interventricular septal defect) Q21.0
  Rosenthal's (factor XI deficiency) D68.1
  Ross River B33.1
  Rossbach's (hyperchlorhydria) K30
  Rotes Quérol — *see* Hyperostosis, ankylosing
  Roth (-Bernhardt) — *see* Mononeuropathy, lower limb, meralgia paresthetica
  Runeberg's (progressive pernicious anemia) D51.0
  sacroiliac NEC M53.3
  salivary gland or duct K11.9
    inclusion B25.9
    specified NEC K11.8
    virus B25.9
  sandworm B76.9
  Schimmelbusch's — *see* Mastopathy, cystic
  Schmorl's — *see* Schmorl's disease or nodes
  Schönlein (-Henoch) (purpura rheumatica) D69.0
  Schottmüller's — *see* Fever, paratyphoid
  Schultz's (agranulocytosis) — *see* Agranulocytosis
  Schwalbe-Ziehen-Oppenheim G24.1
  Schwartz-Jampel G71.13
  sclera H15.9
    specified NEC H15.89
  scrofulous (tuberculous) A18.2
  scrotum N50.9
  sebaceous glands L73.9
  semilunar cartilage, cystic (*see also* Derangement, knee, meniscus, cystic)
  seminal vesicle N50.9
  serum NEC (*see also* Reaction, serum) T80.69 ☑
  sexually transmitted A64
    anogenital
      herpesviral infection — *see* Herpes, anogenital

Disease, diseased — *continued*
  sexually transmitted — *continued*
    anogenital — *continued*
      warts A63.0
    chancroid A57
    chlamydial infection — *see* Chlamydia
    gonorrhea — *see* Gonorrhea
    granuloma inguinale A58
    specified organism NEC A63.8
    syphilis — *see* Syphilis
    trichomoniasis — *see* Trichomoniasis
  Sézary C84.1- ☑
  shimamushi (scrub typhus) A75.3
  shipyard B30.0
  sickle-cell D57.1
    with crisis (vasoocclusive pain) D57.00
      with
        acute chest syndrome D57.01
        splenic sequestration D57.02
    elliptocytosis D57.8- ☑
    Hb-C D57.20
      with crisis (vasoocclusive pain) D57.219
        with
          acute chest syndrome D57.211
          splenic sequestration D57.212
      without crisis D57.20
    Hb-SD D57.80
      with crisis D57.819
        with
          acute chest syndrome D57.811
          splenic sequestration D57.812
    Hb-SE D57.80
      with crisis D57.819
        with
          acute chest syndrome D57.811
          splenic sequestration D57.812
    specified NEC D57.80
      with crisis D57.819
        with
          acute chest syndrome D57.811
          splenic sequestration D57.812
    spherocytosis D57.80
      with crisis D57.819
        with
          acute chest syndrome D57.811
          splenic sequestration D57.812
    thalassemia D57.40
      with crisis (vasoocclusive pain) D57.419
        with
          acute chest syndrome D57.411
          splenic sequestration D57.412
      without crisis D57.40
  silo-filler's J68.8
    bronchitis J68.0
    pneumonitis J68.0
    pulmonary edema J68.1
  simian B B00.4
  Simons' (progressive lipodystrophy) E88.1
  sin nombre virus B33.4
  sinus — *see* Sinusitis
  Sirkari's B55.0
  sixth B08.20
    due to human herpesvirus 6 B08.21
    due to human herpesvirus 7 B08.22
  skin L98.9
    due to metabolic disorder NEC E88.9 [L99]
    specified NEC L98.8
  slim (HIV) B20
  small vessel I73.9
  Sneddon-Wilkinson (subcorneal pustular dermatosis) L13.1
  South African creeping B88.0
  spinal (cord) G95.9
    congenital Q06.9
    specified NEC G95.89
  spine (*see also* Spondylopathy)
    joint — *see* Dorsopathy
    tuberculous A18.01
  spinocerebellar (hereditary) G11.9
    specified NEC G11.8
  spleen D73.9
    amyloid E85.4 [D77]
    organic D73.9
    polycystic Q89.09
    postinfectional D73.89
  sponge-diver's — *see* Toxicity, venom, marine animal, sea anemone
  Startle Q89.8

Disease, diseased — *continued*
  Steinert's G71.11
  Sticker's (erythema infectiosum) B08.3
  Stieda's (calcification, knee joint) — *see* Bursitis, tibial collateral
  Stokes' (exophthalmic goiter) — *see* Hyperthyroidism, with, goiter (diffuse)
  Stokes-Adams (syncope with heart block) I45.9
  stomach K31.9
    functional, psychogenic F45.8
    specified NEC K31.89
  stonemason's J62.8
  storage
    glycogen — *see* Disease, glycogen storage
    mucopolysaccharide — *see* Mucopolysaccharidosis
  striatopallidal system NEC G25.89
  Stuart-Prower (congenital factor X deficiency) D68.2
  Stuart's (congenital factor X deficiency) D68.2
  subcutaneous tissue — *see* Disease, skin
  supporting structures of teeth K08.9
    specified NEC K08.8
  suprarenal (capsule) (gland) E27.9
    hyperfunction E27.0
    specified NEC E27.8
  sweat glands L74.9
    specified NEC L74.8
  Sweeley-Klionsky E75.21
  Swift (-Feer) — *see* Poisoning, mercury
  swimming-pool granuloma A31.1
  Sylvest's (epidemic pleurodynia) B33.0
  sympathetic nervous system G90.9
  synovium — *see* Disorder, synovium
  syphilitic — *see* Syphilis
  systemic tissue mast cell C96.2
  tanapox (virus) B08.71
  Tangier E78.6
  Tarral-Besnier (pityriasis rubra pilaris) L44.0
  Tauri's E74.09
  tear duct — *see* Disorder, lacrimal system
  tendon, tendinous (*see also* Disorder, tendon)
    nodular — *see* Trigger finger
  terminal vessel I73.9
  testis N50.9
  thalassemia Hb-S — *see* Disease, sickle-cell, thalassemia
  Thaysen-Gee (nontropical sprue) K90.0
  Thomsen G71.12
  throat J39.2
    septic J02.0
  thromboembolic — *see* Embolism
  thymus (gland) E32.9
    specified NEC E32.8
  thyroid (gland) E07.9
    heart (*see also* Hyperthyroidism) E05.90 [I43]
      with thyroid storm E05.91 [I43]
    specified NEC E07.89
  Tietze's M94.0
  tongue K14.9
    specified NEC K14.8
  tonsils, tonsillar (and adenoids) J35.9
  tooth, teeth K08.9
    hard tissues K03.9
      specified NEC K03.89
    pulp NEC K04.99
    specified NEC K08.8
  Tourette's F95.2
  trachea NEC J39.8
  tricuspid I07.9
    nonrheumatic I36.9
  triglyceride-storage E75.5
  trophoblastic — *see* Mole, hydatidiform
  tsutsugamushi A75.3
  tube (fallopian) (noninflammatory) N83.9
    inflammatory — *see* Salpingitis
    specified NEC N83.8
  tuberculous NEC — *see* Tuberculosis
  tubo-ovarian (noninflammatory) N83.9
    inflammatory — *see* Salpingo-oophoritis
    specified NEC N83.8
  tubotympanic, chronic — *see* Otitis, media, suppurative, chronic, tubotympanic
  tubulo-interstitial N15.9
    specified NEC N15.8
  tympanum — *see* Disorder, tympanic membrane
  Uhl's Q24.8
  Underwood's (sclerema neonatorum) P83.0
  Unverricht (-Lundborg) — *see* Epilepsy, generalized, idiopathic

Disease, diseased — *continued*
- Urbach-Oppenheim (necrobiosis lipoidica diabeticorum) — *see* E08-E13 with .620
- ureter N28.9
  - in (due to)
    - schistosomiasis (bilharziasis) B65.0 [N29]
- urethra N36.9
  - specified NEC N36.8
- urinary (tract) N39.9
  - bladder N32.9
    - specified NEC N32.89
  - specified NEC N39.8
- uterus (noninflammatory) N85.9
  - infective — *see* Endometritis
  - inflammatory — *see* Endometritis
  - specified NEC N85.8
- uveal tract (anterior) H21.9
  - posterior H31.9
- vagabond's B85.1
- vagina, vaginal (noninflammatory) N89.9
  - inflammatory NEC N76.89
  - specified NEC N89.8
- valve, valvular I38
  - multiple I08.9
    - specified NEC I08.8
- van Creveld-von Gierke (glycogenosis I) E74.01
- vas deferens N50.9
- vascular I99.9
  - arteriosclerotic — *see* Arteriosclerosis
  - ciliary body NEC — *see* Disorder, iris, vascular
  - hypertensive — *see* Hypertension
  - iris NEC — *see* Disorder, iris, vascular
  - obliterative I77.1
    - peripheral I73.9
  - occlusive I99.8
  - peripheral (occlusive) I73.9
    - in diabetes mellitus — *see* E08-E13 with .51
- vasomotor I73.9
- vasospastic I73.9
- vein I87.9
- venereal (*see also* Disease, sexually transmitted) A64
  - chlamydial NEC A56.8
    - anus A56.3
    - genitourinary NOS A56.2
    - pharynx A56.4
    - rectum A56.3
  - fifth A55
  - sixth A55
  - specified nature or type NEC A63.8
- vertebra, vertebral (*see also* Spondylopathy)
  - disc — *see* Disorder, disc
- vibration — *see* Vibration, adverse effects
- viral, virus (*see also* Disease, by type of virus) B34.9
  - arbovirus NOS A94
  - arthropod-borne NOS A94
  - congenital P35.9
    - specified NEC P35.8
  - Hanta (with renal manifestations) (Dobrava) (Puumala) (Seoul) A98.5
    - with pulmonary manifestations (Andes) (Bayou) (Bermejo) (Black Creek Canal) (Choclo) (Juquitiba) (Laguna negra) (Lechiguanas) (New York) (Oran) (Sin nombre) B33.4
  - Hantaan (Korean hemorrhagic fever) A98.5
  - human immunodeficiency (HIV) B20
  - Kunjin A83.4
  - nonarthropod-borne NOS B34.9
  - Powassan A84.8
  - Rocio (encephalitis) A83.6
  - Sin nombre (Hantavirus) (cardio)-pulmonary syndrome) B33.4
  - Tahyna B33.8
  - vesicular stomatitis A93.8
- vitreous H43.9
  - specified NEC H43.89
- vocal cord J38.3
- Volkmann's, acquired T79.6 ☑
- von Eulenburg's (congenital paramyotonia) G71.19
- von Gierke's (glycogenosis I) E74.01
- von Graefe's — *see* Strabismus, paralytic, ophthalmoplegia, progressive
- von Willebrand (-Jürgens) (angiohemophilia) D68.0
- Vrolik's (osteogenesis imperfecta) Q78.0
- vulva (noninflammatory) N90.9
  - inflammatory NEC N76.89
  - specified NEC N90.89
- Wallgren's (obstruction of splenic vein with collateral circulation) I87.8

Disease, diseased — *continued*
- Wassilieff's (leptospiral jaundice) A27.0
- wasting NEC R64
  - due to malnutrition E41
- Waterhouse-Friderichsen A39.1
- Wegner's (syphilitic osteochondritis) A50.02
- Weil's (leptospiral jaundice of lung) A27.0
- Weir Mitchell's (erythromelalgia) I73.81
- Werdnig-Hoffmann G12.0
- Wermer's E31.21
- Werner-His (trench fever) A79.0
- Werner-Schultz (neutropenic splenomegaly) D73.81
- Wernicke-Posadas B38.9
- whipworm B79
- white blood cells D72.9
  - specified NEC D72.89
- white matter R90.82
- white-spot, meaning lichen sclerosus et atrophicus L90.0
  - penis N48.0
  - vulva N90.4
- Wilkie's K55.1
- Wilkinson-Sneddon (subcorneal pustular dermatosis) L13.1
- Willis' — *see* Diabetes
- Wilson's (hepatolenticular degeneration) E83.01
- woolsorter's A22.1
- yaba monkey tumor B08.72
- yaba pox (virus) B08.72
- zoonotic, bacterial A28.9
  - specified type NEC A28.8

Disfigurement (due to scar) L90.5

Disgerminoma — *see* Dysgerminoma

DISH (diffuse idiopathic skeletal hyperostosis) — *see* Hyperostosis, ankylosing

Disinsertion, retina — *see* Detachment, retina

Dislocatable hip, congenital Q65.6

Dislocation (articular)
- with fracture — *see* Fracture
- acromioclavicular (joint) S43.10- ☑
  - with displacement
    - 100%-200% S43.12- ☑
    - more than 200% S43.13- ☑
  - inferior S43.14- ☑
  - posterior S43.15- ☑
- ankle S93.0- ☑
- astragalus — *see* Dislocation, ankle
- atlantoaxial S13.121 ☑
- atlantooccipital S13.111 ☑
- atloidooccipital S13.111 ☑
- breast bone S23.29 ☑
- capsule, joint — *code by* site under Dislocation
- carpal (bone) — *see* Dislocation, wrist
- carpometacarpal (joint) NEC S63.05- ☑
  - thumb S63.04- ☑
- cartilage (joint) — *code by* site under Dislocation
- cervical spine (vertebra) — *see* Dislocation, vertebra, cervical
- chronic — *see* Dislocation, recurrent
- clavicle — *see* Dislocation, acromioclavicular joint
- coccyx S33.2 ☑
- congenital NEC Q68.8
- coracoid — *see* Dislocation, shoulder
- costal cartilage S23.29 ☑
- costochondral S23.29 ☑
- cricoarytenoid articulation S13.29 ☑
- cricothyroid articulation S13.29 ☑
- dorsal vertebra — *see* Dislocation, vertebra, thoracic
- ear ossicle — *see* Discontinuity, ossicles, ear
- elbow S53.10- ☑
  - congenital Q68.8
  - pathological — *see* Dislocation, pathological NEC, elbow
  - radial head alone — *see* Dislocation, radial head
  - recurrent — *see* Dislocation, recurrent, elbow
  - traumatic S53.10- ☑
    - anterior S53.11- ☑
    - lateral S53.14- ☑
    - medial S53.13- ☑
    - posterior S53.12- ☑
    - specified type NEC S53.19- ☑
- eye, nontraumatic — *see* Luxation, globe
- eyeball, nontraumatic — *see* Luxation, globe
- femur
  - distal end — *see* Dislocation, knee
  - proximal end — *see* Dislocation, hip

Dislocation — *continued*
- fibula
  - distal end — *see* Dislocation, ankle
  - proximal end — *see* Dislocation, knee
- finger S63.25- ☑
  - index S63.25- ☑
  - interphalangeal S63.27- ☑
    - distal S63.29- ☑
      - index S63.29- ☑
      - little S63.29- ☑
      - middle S63.29- ☑
      - ring S63.29- ☑
    - index S63.27- ☑
    - little S63.27- ☑
    - middle S63.27- ☑
    - proximal S63.28- ☑
      - index S63.28- ☑
      - little S63.28- ☑
      - middle S63.28- ☑
      - ring S63.28- ☑
    - ring S63.27- ☑
  - little S63.25- ☑
  - metacarpophalangeal S63.26- ☑
    - index S63.26- ☑
    - little S63.26- ☑
    - middle S63.26- ☑
    - ring S63.26- ☑
  - middle S63.25- ☑
  - recurrent — *see* Dislocation, recurrent, finger
  - ring S63.25- ☑
  - thumb — *see* Dislocation, thumb
- foot S93.30- ☑
  - recurrent — *see* Dislocation, recurrent, foot
  - specified site NEC S93.33- ☑
  - tarsal joint S93.31- ☑
  - tarsometatarsal joint S93.32- ☑
  - toe — *see* Dislocation, toe
- fracture — *see* Fracture
- glenohumeral (joint) — *see* Dislocation, shoulder
- glenoid — *see* Dislocation, shoulder
- habitual — *see* Dislocation, recurrent
- hip S73.00- ☑
  - anterior S73.03- ☑
    - obturator S73.02- ☑
  - central S73.04- ☑
  - congenital (total) Q65.2
    - bilateral Q65.1
    - partial Q65.5
      - bilateral Q65.4
      - unilateral Q65.3- ☑
    - unilateral Q65.0- ☑
  - developmental M24.85- ☑
  - pathological — *see* Dislocation, pathological NEC, hip
  - posterior S73.01- ☑
  - recurrent — *see* Dislocation, recurrent, hip
- humerus, proximal end — *see* Dislocation, shoulder
- incomplete — *see* Subluxation, by site
- incus — *see* Discontinuity, ossicles, ear
- infracoracoid — *see* Dislocation, shoulder
- innominate (pubic junction) (sacral junction) S33.39 ☑
  - acetabulum — *see* Dislocation, hip
- interphalangeal (joint(s))
  - finger S63.279 ☑
    - distal S63.29- ☑
      - index S63.29- ☑
      - little S63.29- ☑
      - middle S63.29- ☑
      - ring S63.29- ☑
    - index S63.27- ☑
    - little S63.27- ☑
    - middle S63.27- ☑
    - proximal S63.28- ☑
      - index S63.28- ☑
      - little S63.28- ☑
      - middle S63.28- ☑
      - ring S63.28- ☑
    - ring S63.27- ☑
  - foot or toe — *see* Dislocation, toe
  - thumb S63.12- ☑
    - distal joint S63.14- ☑
    - proximal joint S63.13- ☑
- jaw (cartilage) (meniscus) S03.0 ☑
- joint prosthesis — *see* Complications, joint prosthesis, mechanical, displacement, by site
- knee S83.106 ☑

Dislocation — *continued*
- knee S83.106 ☑
  - cap — *see* Dislocation, patella
  - congenital Q68.2
  - old M23.8X- ☑
  - patella — *see* Dislocation, patella
  - pathological — *see* Dislocation, pathological NEC, knee
  - proximal tibia
    - anteriorly S83.11- ☑
    - laterally S83.14- ☑
    - medially S83.13- ☑
    - posteriorly S83.12- ☑
  - recurrent (*see also* Derangement, knee, specified NEC)
  - specified type NEC S83.19- ☑
- lacrimal gland H04.16- ☑
- lens (complete) H27.10
  - anterior H27.12- ☑
  - congenital Q12.1
  - ocular implant — *see* Complications, intraocular lens
  - partial H27.11- ☑
  - posterior H27.13- ☑
  - traumatic S05.8X- ☑
- ligament — *code by* site under Dislocation
- lumbar (vertebra) — *see* Dislocation, vertebra, lumbar
- lumbosacral (vertebra) (*see also* Dislocation, vertebra, lumbar)
  - congenital Q76.49
- mandible S03.0 ☑
- meniscus (knee) — *see* Tear, meniscus
  - other sites - code by site under Dislocation
- metacarpal (bone)
  - distal end — *see* Dislocation, finger
  - proximal end S63.06- ☑
- metacarpophalangeal (joint)
  - finger S63.26- ☑
    - index S63.26- ☑
    - little S63.26- ☑
    - middle S63.26- ☑
    - ring S63.26- ☑
  - thumb S63.11- ☑
- metatarsal (bone) — *see* Dislocation, foot
- metatarsophalangeal (joint(s)) — *see* Dislocation, toe
- midcarpal (joint) S63.03- ☑
- midtarsal (joint) — *see* Dislocation, foot
- neck S13.20 ☑
  - specified site NEC S13.29 ☑
  - vertebra — *see* Dislocation, vertebra, cervical
- nose (septal cartilage) S03.1 ☑
- occipitoatloid S13.111 ☑
- old — *see* Derangement, joint, specified type NEC
- ossicles, ear — *see* Discontinuity, ossicles, ear
- partial — *see* Subluxation, by site
- patella S83.006 ☑
  - congenital Q74.1
  - lateral S83.01- ☑
  - recurrent (nontraumatic) M22.0- ☑
    - incomplete M22.1- ☑
  - specified type NEC S83.09- ☑
- pathological NEC M24.30
  - ankle M24.37- ☑
  - elbow M24.32- ☑
  - foot joint M24.37- ☑
  - hand joint M24.34- ☑
  - hip M24.35- ☑
  - knee M24.36- ☑
  - lumbosacral joint — *see* subcategory M53.2
  - pelvic region — *see* Dislocation, pathological, hip
  - sacroiliac — *see* subcategory M53.2
  - shoulder M24.31- ☑
  - wrist M24.33- ☑
- pelvis NEC S33.30 ☑
  - specified NEC S33.39 ☑
- phalanx
  - finger or hand — *see* Dislocation, finger
  - foot or toe — *see* Dislocation, toe
- prosthesis, internal — *see* Complications, prosthetic device, by site, mechanical
- radial head S53.006 ☑
  - anterior S53.01- ☑
  - posterior S53.02- ☑
  - specified type NEC S53.09- ☑
- radiocarpal (joint) S63.02- ☑
- radiohumeral (joint) — *see* Dislocation, radial head

Dislocation — *continued*
- radioulnar (joint)
  - distal S63.01- ☑
  - proximal — *see* Dislocation, elbow
- radius
  - distal end — *see* Dislocation, wrist
  - proximal end — *see* Dislocation, radial head
- recurrent M24.40
  - ankle M24.47- ☑
  - elbow M24.42- ☑
  - finger M24.44- ☑
  - foot joint M24.47- ☑
  - hand joint M24.44- ☑
  - hip M24.45- ☑
  - knee M24.46- ☑
    - patella — *see* Dislocation, patella, recurrent
  - patella — *see* Dislocation, patella, recurrent
  - sacroiliac — *see* subcategory M53.2
  - shoulder M24.41- ☑
  - toe M24.47- ☑
  - vertebra (*see also* subcategory) M43.5 ☑
    - atlantoaxial M43.4
      - with myelopathy M43.3
  - wrist M24.43- ☑
- rib (cartilage) S23.29 ☑
- sacrococcygeal S33.2 ☑
- sacroiliac (joint) (ligament) S33.2 ☑
  - congenital Q74.2
  - recurrent — *see* subcategory M53.2
- sacrum S33.2 ☑
- scaphoid (bone) (hand) (wrist) — *see* Dislocation, wrist
  - foot — *see* Dislocation, foot
- scapula — *see* Dislocation, shoulder, girdle, scapula
- semilunar cartilage, knee — *see* Tear, meniscus
- septal cartilage (nose) S03.1 ☑
- septum (nasal) (old) J34.2
- sesamoid bone — *code by* site under Dislocation
- shoulder (blade) (ligament) (joint) (traumatic) S43.006 ☑
  - acromioclavicular — *see* Dislocation, acromioclavicular
  - chronic — *see* Dislocation, recurrent, shoulder
  - congenital Q68.8
  - girdle S43.30- ☑
    - scapula S43.31- ☑
    - specified site NEC S43.39- ☑
  - humerus S43.00- ☑
    - anterior S43.01- ☑
    - inferior S43.03- ☑
    - posterior S43.02- ☑
  - pathological — *see* Dislocation, pathological NEC, shoulder
  - recurrent — *see* Dislocation, recurrent, shoulder
  - specified type NEC S43.08- ☑
- spine
  - cervical — *see* Dislocation, vertebra, cervical
  - congenital Q76.49
  - due to birth trauma P11.5
  - lumbar — *see* Dislocation, vertebra, lumbar
  - thoracic — *see* Dislocation, vertebra, thoracic
- spontaneous — *see* Dislocation, pathological
- sternoclavicular (joint) S43.206 ☑
  - anterior S43.21- ☑
  - posterior S43.22- ☑
- sternum S23.29 ☑
- subglenoid — *see* Dislocation, shoulder
- symphysis pubis S33.4 ☑
- talus — *see* Dislocation, ankle
- tarsal (bone(s)) (joint(s)) — *see* Dislocation, foot
- tarsometatarsal (joint(s)) — *see* Dislocation, foot
- temporomandibular (joint) S03.0 ☑
- thigh, proximal end — *see* Dislocation, hip
- thorax S23.20 ☑
  - specified site NEC S23.29 ☑
  - vertebra — *see* Dislocation, vertebra
- thumb S63.10- ☑
  - interphalangeal joint — *see* Dislocation, interphalangeal (joint), thumb
  - metacarpophalangeal joint — *see* Dislocation, metacarpophalangeal (joint), thumb
- thyroid cartilage S13.29 ☑
- tibia
  - distal end — *see* Dislocation, ankle
  - proximal end — *see* Dislocation, knee
- tibiofibular (joint)
  - distal — *see* Dislocation, ankle

Dislocation — *continued*
- tibiofibular — *continued*
  - superior — *see* Dislocation, knee
- toe(s) S93.106 ☑
  - great S93.10- ☑
    - interphalangeal joint S93.11- ☑
    - metatarsophalangeal joint S93.12- ☑
  - interphalangeal joint S93.119 ☑
  - lesser S93.106 ☑
    - interphalangeal joint S93.11- ☑
    - metatarsophalangeal joint S93.12- ☑
  - metatarsophalangeal joint S93.12- ☑
- tooth S03.2 ☑
- trachea S23.29 ☑
- ulna
  - distal end S63.07- ☑
  - proximal end — *see* Dislocation, elbow
- ulnohumeral (joint) — *see* Dislocation, elbow
- vertebra (articular process) (body) (traumatic)
  - cervical S13.101 ☑
    - atlantoaxial joint S13.121 ☑
    - atlantooccipital joint S13.111 ☑
    - atloidooccipital joint S13.111 ☑
    - joint between
      - C0 and C1 S13.111 ☑
      - C1 and C2 S13.121 ☑
      - C2 and C3 S13.131 ☑
      - C3 and C4 S13.141 ☑
      - C4 and C5 S13.151 ☑
      - C5 and C6 S13.161 ☑
      - C6 and C7 S13.171 ☑
      - C7 and T1 S13.181 ☑
    - occipitoatloid joint S13.111 ☑
  - congenital Q76.49
  - lumbar S33.101 ☑
    - joint between
      - L1 and L2 S33.111 ☑
      - L2 and L3 S33.121 ☑
      - L3 and L4 S33.131 ☑
      - L4 and L5 S33.141 ☑
  - nontraumatic — *see* Displacement, intervertebral disc
  - partial — *see* Subluxation, by site
  - recurrent NEC — *see* subcategory M43.5
  - thoracic S23.101 ☑
    - joint between
      - T1 and T2 S23.111 ☑
      - T2 and T3 S23.121 ☑
      - T3 and T4 S23.123 ☑
      - T4 and T5 S23.131 ☑
      - T5 and T6 S23.133 ☑
      - T6 and T7 S23.141 ☑
      - T7 and T8 S23.143 ☑
      - T8 and T9 S23.151 ☑
      - T9 and T10 S23.153 ☑
      - T10 and T11 S23.161 ☑
      - T11 and T12 S23.163 ☑
      - T12 and L1 S23.171 ☑
- wrist (carpal bone) S63.006 ☑
  - carpometacarpal joint — *see* Dislocation, carpometacarpal (joint)
  - distal radioulnar joint — *see* Dislocation, radioulnar (joint), distal
  - metacarpal bone, proximal — *see* Dislocation, metacarpal (bone), proximal end
  - midcarpal — *see* Dislocation, midcarpal (joint)
  - radiocarpal joint — *see* Dislocation, radiocarpal (joint)
  - recurrent — *see* Dislocation, recurrent, wrist
  - specified site NEC S63.09- ☑
  - ulna — *see* Dislocation, ulna, distal end
- xiphoid cartilage S23.29 ☑

Disorder (of) (*see also* Disease)
- acantholytic L11.9
  - specified NEC L11.8
- acute
  - psychotic — *see* Psychosis, acute
  - stress F43.0
- adjustment (grief) F43.20
  - with
    - anxiety F43.22
      - with depressed mood F43.23
    - conduct disturbance F43.24
      - with emotional disturbance F43.25
    - depressed mood F43.21
      - with anxiety F43.23

Disorder — *continued*
  adjustment — *continued*
    with — *continued*
      other specified symptom F43.29
  adrenal (capsule) (gland) (medullary) E27.9
    specified NEC E27.8
  adrenogenital E25.9
    drug-induced E25.8
    iatrogenic E25.8
    idiopathic E25.8
  adult personality (and behavior) F69
    specified NEC F68.8
  affective (mood) — *see* Disorder, mood
  aggressive, unsocialized F91.1
  alcohol-related F10.99
    with
      amnestic disorder, persisting F10.96
      anxiety disorder F10.980
      dementia, persisting F10.97
      intoxication F10.929
        with delirium F10.921
        uncomplicated F10.920
      mood disorder F10.94
      other specified F10.988
      psychotic disorder F10.959
        with
          delusions F10.950
          hallucinations F10.951
      sexual dysfunction F10.981
      sleep disorder F10.982
  allergic — *see* Allergy
  alveolar NEC J84.09
  amino-acid
    cystathioninuria E72.19
    cystinosis E72.04
    cystinuria E72.01
    glycinuria E72.09
    homocystinuria E72.11
    metabolism — *see* Disturbance, metabolism,
      amino-acid
    specified NEC E72.8
    neonatal, transitory P74.8
    renal transport NEC E72.09
    transport NEC E72.09
  amnesic, amnestic
    alcohol-induced F10.96
      with dependence F10.26
    due to (secondary to) general medical condition
      F04
    psychoactive NEC-induced F19.96
      with
        abuse F19.16
        dependence F19.26
    sedative, hypnotic or anxiolytic-induced F13.96
      with dependence F13.26
  anaerobic glycolysis with anemia D55.2
  anxiety F41.9
    due to (secondary to)
      alcohol F10.980
      amphetamine F15.980
        in
          abuse F15.180
          dependence F15.280
      anxiolytic F13.980
        in
          abuse F13.180
          dependence F13.280
      caffeine F15.980
        in
          abuse F15.180
          dependence F15.280
      cannabis F12.980
        in
          abuse F12.180
          dependence F12.280
      cocaine F14.980
        in
          abuse F14.180
          dependence F14.180
      general medical condition F06.4
      hallucinogen F16.980
        in
          abuse F16.180
          dependence F16.280
      hypnotic F13.980
        in
          abuse F13.180
          dependence F13.280

Disorder — *continued*
  anxiety — *continued*
    due to — *continued*
      inhalant F18.980
        in
          abuse F18.180
          dependence F18.280
      phencyclidine F16.980
        in
          abuse F16.180
          dependence F16.280
      psychoactive substance NEC F19.980
        in
          abuse F19.180
          dependence F19.280
      sedative F13.980
        in
          abuse F13.180
          dependence F13.280
      volatile solvents F18.980
        in
          abuse F18.180
          dependence F18.280
    generalized F41.1
    mixed
      with depression (mild) F41.8
      specified NEC F41.3
    organic F06.4
    phobic F40.9
      of childhood F40.8
    specified NEC F41.8
  aortic valve — *see* Endocarditis, aortic
  aromatic amino-acid metabolism E70.9
    specified NEC E70.8
  arteriole NEC I77.89
  artery NEC I77.89
  articulation — *see* Disorder, joint
  attachment (childhood)
    disinhibited F94.2
    reactive F94.1
  attention-deficit hyperactivity (adolescent) (adult)
    (child) F90.9
    combined type F90.2
    hyperactive type F90.1
    inattentive type F90.0
    specified type NEC F90.8
  attention-deficit without hyperactivity (adolescent)
    (adult) (child) F90.0
  auditory processing (central) H93.25
  autistic F84.0
  autonomic nervous system G90.9
    specified NEC G90.8
  avoidant, child or adolescent F40.10
  balance
    acid-base E87.8
      mixed E87.4
    electrolyte E87.8
    fluid NEC E87.8
  behavioral (disruptive) — *see* Disorder, conduct
  beta-amino-acid metabolism E72.8
  bile acid and cholesterol metabolism E78.70
    Barth syndrome E78.71
    other specified E78.79
    Smith-Lemli-Opitz syndrome E78.72
  bilirubin excretion E80.6
  binocular
    movement H51.9
      convergence
        excess H51.12
        insufficiency H51.11
      internuclear ophthalmoplegia — *see* Ophthal-
        moplegia, internuclear
      palsy of conjugate gaze H51.0
      specified type NEC H51.8
    vision NEC — *see* Disorder, vision, binocular
  bipolar (I) F31.9
    current episode
      depressed F31.9
        with psychotic features F31.5
        without psychotic features F31.30
          mild F31.31
          moderate F31.32
          severe (without psychotic features) F31.4
            with psychotic features F31.5
      hypomanic F31.0
      manic F31.9
        with psychotic features F31.2

Disorder — *continued*
  bipolar — *continued*
    current episode — *continued*
      manic — *continued*
        without psychotic features F31.10
          mild F31.11
          moderate F31.12
          severe (without psychotic features)
            F31.13
          with psychotic features F31.2
      mixed F31.60
        mild F31.61
        moderate F31.62
        severe (without psychotic features) F31.63
          with psychotic features F31.64
      severe depression (without psychotic features)
        F31.4
        with psychotic features F31.5
    in remission (currently) F31.70
      in full remission
        most recent episode
          depressed F31.76
          hypomanic F31.72
          manic F31.74
          mixed F31.78
      in partial remission
        most recent episode
          depressed F31.75
          hypomanic F31.71
          manic F31.73
          mixed F31.77
    organic F06.30
    single manic episode F30.9
      mild F30.11
      moderate F30.12
      severe (without psychotic symptoms) F30.13
        with psychotic symptoms F30.2
    specified NEC F31.89
  bipolar II F31.81
  bladder N32.9
    functional NEC N31.9
    in schistosomiasis B65.0 [N33]
    specified NEC N32.89
  bleeding D68.9
  blood D75.9
    in congenital early syphilis A50.09 [D77]
  body dysmorphic F45.22
  bone M89.9
    continuity M84.9
      specified type NEC M84.80
        ankle M84.87- ☑
        fibula M84.86- ☑
        foot M84.87- ☑
        hand M84.84- ☑
        humerus M84.82- ☑
        neck M84.88
        pelvis M84.859
        radius M84.83- ☑
        rib M84.88
        shoulder M84.81- ☑
        skull M84.88
        thigh M84.85- ☑
        tibia M84.86- ☑
        ulna M84.83- ☑
        vertebra M84.88
    density and structure M85.9
      cyst (*see also* Cyst, bone, specified type NEC)
        aneurysmal — *see* Cyst, bone, aneurysmal
        solitary — *see* Cyst, bone, solitary
      diffuse idiopathic skeletal hyperostosis — *see*
        Hyperostosis, ankylosing
      fibrous dysplasia (monostotic) — *see* Dysplasia,
        fibrous, bone
      fluorosis — *see* Fluorosis, skeletal
      hyperostosis of skull M85.2
      osteitis condensans — *see* Osteitis, condensans
      specified type NEC M85.8- ☑
        ankle M85.87- ☑
        foot M85.87- ☑
        forearm M85.83- ☑
        hand M85.84- ☑
        lower leg M85.86- ☑
        multiple sites M85.89
        neck M85.88
        rib M85.88
        shoulder M85.81- ☑
        skull M85.88
        thigh M85.85- ☑

☑ **Additional Character Required** — Refer to the Tabular List for Character Selection   ▽ **Subterms under main terms may continue to next column or page**

Disorder — continued
　bone — continued
　　density and structure — continued
　　　specified type — continued
　　　　upper arm M85.82- ☑
　　　　vertebra M85.88
　　development and growth NEC M89.20
　　　carpus M89.24- ☑
　　　clavicle M89.21- ☑
　　　femur M89.25- ☑
　　　fibula M89.26- ☑
　　　finger M89.24- ☑
　　　humerus M89.22- ☑
　　　ilium M89.259
　　　ischium M89.259
　　　metacarpus M89.24- ☑
　　　metatarsus M89.27- ☑
　　　multiple sites M89.29
　　　neck M89.28
　　　radius M89.23- ☑
　　　rib M89.28
　　　scapula M89.21- ☑
　　　skull M89.28
　　　tarsus M89.27- ☑
　　　tibia M89.26- ☑
　　　toe M89.27- ☑
　　　ulna M89.23- ☑
　　　vertebra M89.28
　　　specified type NEC M89.8X- ☑
　brachial plexus G54.0
　branched-chain amino-acid metabolism E71.2
　　specified NEC E71.19
　breast N64.9
　　agalactia — see Agalactia
　　associated with
　　　lactation O92.70
　　　　specified NEC O92.79
　　　pregnancy O92.20
　　　　specified NEC O92.29
　　　puerperium O92.20
　　　　specified NEC O92.29
　　cracked nipple — see Cracked nipple
　　galactorrhea — see Galactorrhea
　　hypogalactia O92.4
　　lactation disorder NEC O92.79
　　mastitis — see Mastitis
　　nipple infection — see Infection, nipple
　　retracted nipple — see Retraction, nipple
　　specified type NEC N64.89
　Briquet's F45.0
　bullous, in diseases classified elsewhere L14
　cannabis use
　　due to drug abuse — see Abuse, drug, cannabis
　　due to drug dependence — see Dependence, drug,
　　　cannabis
　carbohydrate
　　absorption, intestinal NEC E74.39
　　metabolism (congenital) E74.9
　　　specified NEC E74.8
　cardiac, functional I51.89
　carnitine metabolism E71.40
　cartilage M94.9
　　articular NEC — see Derangement, joint, articular
　　　cartilage
　　chondrocalcinosis — see Chondrocalcinosis
　　specified type NEC M94.8X- ☑
　　　articular — see Derangement, joint, articular
　　　　cartilage
　　　multiple sites M94.8X0
　catatonic
　　due to (secondary to) known physiological condi-
　　　tion F06.1
　　organic F06.1
　central auditory processing H93.25
　cervical
　　region NEC M53.82
　　root (nerve) NEC G54.2
　character NOS F60.9
　childhood disintegrative NEC F84.3
　cholesterol and bile acid metabolism E78.70
　　Barth syndrome E78.71
　　other specified E78.79
　　Smith-Lemli-Opitz syndrome E78.72
　choroid H31.9
　　atrophy — see Atrophy, choroid
　　degeneration — see Degeneration, choroid
　　detachment — see Detachment, choroid

Disorder — continued
　choroid — continued
　　dystrophy — see Dystrophy, choroid
　　hemorrhage — see Hemorrhage, choroid
　　rupture — see Rupture, choroid
　　scar — see Scar, chorioretinal
　　solar retinopathy — see Retinopathy, solar
　　specified type NEC H31.8
　ciliary body — see Disorder, iris
　　degeneration — see Degeneration, ciliary body
　coagulation (factor) (see also Defect, coagulation)
　　D68.9
　　newborn, transient P61.6
　coccyx NEC M53.3
　cognitive F09
　　due to (secondary to) general medical condition
　　　F09
　　persisting R41.89
　　　due to
　　　　alcohol F10.97
　　　　　with dependence F10.27
　　　　anxiolytics F13.97
　　　　　with dependence F13.27
　　　　hypnotics F13.97
　　　　　with dependence F13.27
　　　　sedatives F13.97
　　　　　with dependence F13.27
　　　　specified substance NEC F19.97
　　　　　with
　　　　　　abuse F19.17
　　　　　　dependence F19.27
　communication F80.9
　conduct (childhood) F91.9
　　adjustment reaction — see Disorder, adjustment
　　adolescent onset type F91.2
　　childhood onset type F91.1
　　compulsive F63.9
　　confined to family context F91.0
　　depressive F91.8
　　group type F91.2
　　hyperkinetic — see Disorder, attention-deficit hy-
　　　peractivity
　　oppositional defiance F91.3
　　socialized F91.2
　　solitary aggressive type F91.1
　　specified NEC F91.8
　　unsocialized (aggressive) F91.1
　conduction, heart I45.9
　congenital glycosylation (CDG) E74.8
　conjunctiva H11.9
　　infection — see Conjunctivitis
　connective tissue, localized L94.9
　　specified NEC L94.8
　conversion — see Disorder, dissociative
　convulsive (secondary) — see Convulsions
　cornea H18.9
　　deformity — see Deformity, cornea
　　degeneration — see Degeneration, cornea
　　deposits — see Deposit, cornea
　　due to contact lens H18.82- ☑
　　　specified as edema — see Edema, cornea
　　edema — see Edema, cornea
　　keratitis — see Keratitis
　　keratoconjunctivitis — see Keratoconjunctivitis
　　membrane change — see Change, corneal mem-
　　　brane
　　neovascularization — see Neovascularization,
　　　cornea
　　scar — see Opacity, cornea
　　specified type NEC H18.89- ☑
　　ulcer — see Ulcer, cornea
　corpus cavernosum N48.9
　cranial nerve — see Disorder, nerve, cranial
　cyclothymic F34.0
　defiant oppositional F91.3
　delusional (persistent) (systematized) F22
　　induced F24
　depersonalization F48.1
　depressive F32.9
　　major F32.9
　　　with psychotic symptoms F32.3
　　　in remission (full) F32.5
　　　　partial F32.4
　　　recurrent F33.9
　　　single episode F32.9
　　　　mild F32.0
　　　　moderate F32.1

Disorder — continued
　depressive — continued
　　major — continued
　　　single episode — continued
　　　　severe (without psychotic symptoms) F32.2
　　　　　with psychotic symptoms F32.3
　　　organic F06.31
　　　recurrent F33.9
　　　　current episode
　　　　　mild F33.0
　　　　　moderate F33.1
　　　　　severe (without psychotic symptoms) F33.2
　　　　　　with psychotic symptoms F33.3
　　　　in remission F33.40
　　　　　full F33.42
　　　　　partial F33.41
　　　　specified NEC F33.8
　　　single episode — see Episode, depressive
　developmental F89
　　arithmetical skills F81.2
　　coordination (motor) F82
　　expressive writing F81.81
　　language F80.9
　　　expressive F80.1
　　　mixed receptive and expressive F80.2
　　　receptive type F80.2
　　　specified NEC F80.89
　　learning F81.9
　　　arithmetical F81.2
　　　reading F81.0
　　mixed F88
　　motor coordination or function F82
　　pervasive F84.9
　　　specified NEC F84.8
　　phonological F80.0
　　reading F81.0
　　scholastic skills (see also Disorder, learning)
　　　mixed F81.89
　　specified NEC F88
　　speech F80.9
　　　articulation F80.0
　　　specified NEC F80.89
　　written expression F81.81
　diaphragm J98.6
　digestive (system) K92.9
　　newborn P78.9
　　　specified NEC P78.89
　　postprocedural — see Complication, gastrointesti-
　　　nal
　　psychogenic F45.8
　disc (intervertebral) M51.9
　　with
　　　myelopathy
　　　　cervical region M50.00
　　　　cervicothoracic region M50.03
　　　　high cervical region M50.01
　　　　lumbar region M51.06
　　　　mid-cervical region M50.02
　　　　sacrococcygeal region M53.3
　　　　thoracic region M51.04
　　　　thoracolumbar region M51.05
　　　radiculopathy
　　　　cervical region M50.10
　　　　cervicothoracic region M50.13
　　　　high cervical region M50.11
　　　　lumbar region M51.16
　　　　lumbosacral region M51.17
　　　　mid-cervical region M50.12
　　　　sacrococcygeal region M53.3
　　　　thoracic region M51.14
　　　　thoracolumbar region M51.15
　　cervical M50.90
　　　with
　　　　myelopathy M50.00
　　　　　C2-C3 M50.01
　　　　　C3-C4 M50.01
　　　　　C4-C5 M50.02
　　　　　C5-C6 M50.02
　　　　　C6-C7 M50.02
　　　　　C7-T1 M50.03
　　　　　cervicothoracic region M50.03
　　　　　high cervical region M50.01
　　　　　mid-cervical region M50.02
　　　　neuritis, radiculitis or radiculopathy M50.10
　　　　　C2-C3 M50.11
　　　　　C3-C4 M50.11
　　　　　C4-C5 M50.12
　　　　　C5-C6 M50.12

Disorder — *continued*
  disc — *continued*
    cervical — *continued*
      with — *continued*
        neuritis, radiculitis or radiculopathy — *continued*
          C6-C7 M50.12
          C7-T1 M50.13
          cervicothoracic region M50.13
          high cervical region M50.11
          mid-cervical region M50.12
        C2-C3 M50.91
        C3-C4 M50.91
        C4-C5 M50.92
        C5-C6 M50.92
        C6-C7 M50.92
        C7-T1 M50.93
        cervicothoracic region M50.93
        degeneration M50.30
          C2-C3 M50.31
          C3-C4 M50.31
          C4-C5 M50.32
          C5-C6 M50.32
          C6-C7 M50.32
          C7-T1 M50.33
          cervicothoracic region M50.33
          high cervical region M50.31
          mid-cervical region M50.32
        displacement M50.20
          C2-C3 M50.21
          C3-C4 M50.21
          C4-C5 M50.22
          C5-C6 M50.22
          C6-C7 M50.22
          C7-T1 M50.23
          cervicothoracic region M50.23
          high cervical region M50.21
          mid-cervical region M50.22
        high cervical region M50.91
        mid-cervical region M50.92
        specified type NEC M50.80
          C2-C3 M50.81
          C3-C4 M50.81
          C4-C5 M50.82
          C5-C6 M50.82
          C6-C7 M50.82
          C7-T1 M50.83
          cervicothoracic region M50.83
          high cervical region M50.81
          mid-cervical region M50.82
    specified NEC
      lumbar region M51.86
      lumbosacral region M51.87
      sacrococcygeal region M53.3
      thoracic region M51.84
      thoracolumbar region M51.85
  disinhibited attachment (childhood) F94.2
  disintegrative, childhood NEC F84.3
  disruptive behavior F98.9
  dissocial personality F60.2
  dissociative F44.9
    affecting
      motor function F44.4
        and sensation F44.7
      sensation F44.6
        and motor function F44.7
    brief reactive F43.0
    due to (secondary to) general medical condition F06.8
    mixed F44.7
    organic F06.8
    other specified NEC F44.89
  double heterozygous sickling — *see* Disease, sickle-cell
  dream anxiety F51.5
  drug induced hemorrhagic D68.32
  drug related F19.99
    abuse — *see* Abuse, drug
    dependence — *see* Dependence, drug
  dysmorphic body F45.1
  dysthymic F34.1
  ear H93.9- ☑
    bleeding — *see* Otorrhagia
    deafness — *see* Deafness
    degenerative H93.09- ☑
    discharge — *see* Otorrhea

Disorder — *continued*
  ear — *continued*
    external H61.9- ☑
      auditory canal stenosis — *see* Stenosis, external ear canal
      exostosis — *see* Exostosis, external ear canal
      impacted cerumen — *see* Impaction, cerumen
      otitis — *see* Otitis, externa
      perichondritis — *see* Perichondritis, ear
      pinna — *see* Disorder, pinna
      specified type NEC H61.89- ☑
    inner H83.9- ☑
      vestibular dysfunction — *see* Disorder, vestibular function
    middle H74.9- ☑
      adhesive H74.1- ☑
      ossicle — *see* Abnormal, ear ossicles
      polyp — *see* Polyp, ear (middle)
      specified NEC, in diseases classified elsewhere H75.8- ☑
    postprocedural — *see* Complications, ear, procedure
    specified NEC, in diseases classified elsewhere H94.8- ☑
  eating (adult) (psychogenic) F50.9
    anorexia — *see* Anorexia
    bulimia F50.2
    child F98.29
      pica F98.3
      rumination disorder F98.21
    pica F50.8
      childhood F98.3
  electrolyte (balance) NEC E87.8
    with
      abortion — *see* Abortion by type complicated by specified condition NEC
      ectopic pregnancy O08.5
      molar pregnancy O08.5
    acidosis (metabolic) (respiratory) E87.2
    alkalosis (metabolic) (respiratory) E87.3
  elimination, transepidermal L87.9
    specified NEC L87.8
  emotional (persistent) F34.9
    of childhood F93.9
      specified NEC F93.8
  endocrine E34.9
    postprocedural E89.89
    specified NEC E89.89
  erectile (male) (organic) (*see also* Dysfunction, sexual, male, erectile) N52.9
    nonorganic F52.21
  erythematous — *see* Erythema
  esophagus K22.9
    functional K22.4
    psychogenic F45.8
  eustachian tube H69.9- ☑
    infection — *see* Salpingitis, eustachian
    obstruction — *see* Obstruction, eustachian tube
    patulous — *see* Patulous, eustachian tube
    specified NEC H69.8- ☑
  extrapyramidal G25.9
    in deseases classified elsewhere — *see* category G26
    specified type NEC G25.89
  eye H57.9
    postprocedural — *see* Complication, postprocedural, eye
  eyelid H02.9
    cyst — *see* Cyst, eyelid
    degenerative H02.70
      chloasma — *see* Chloasma, eyelid
      madarosis — *see* Madarosis
      specified type NEC H02.79
      vitiligo — *see* Vitiligo, eyelid
      xanthelasma — *see* Xanthelasma
    dermatochalasis — *see* Dermatochalasis
    edema — *see* Edema, eyelid
    elephantiasis — *see* Elephantiasis, eyelid
    foreign body, retained — *see* Foreign body, retained, eyelid
    function H02.59
      abnormal innervation syndrome — *see* Syndrome, abnormal innervation
      blepharochalasis — *see* Blepharochalasis
      blepharoclonus — *see* Blepharoclonus
      blepharophimosis — *see* Blepharophimosis
      blepharoptosis — *see* Blepharoptosis

Disorder — *continued*
  eyelid — *continued*
    function — *continued*
      lagophthalmos — *see* Lagophthalmos
      lid retraction — *see* Retraction, lid
    hypertrichosis — *see* Hypertrichosis, eyelid
    specified type NEC H02.89
    vascular H02.879
      left H02.876
        lower H02.875
        upper H02.874
      right H02.873
        lower H02.872
        upper H02.871
  factitious F68.10
    with predominantly
      physical symptoms F68.12
        with psychological symptoms F68.13
      psychological symptoms F68.11
        with physical symptoms F68.13
  factor, coagulation — *see* Defect, coagulation
  fatty acid
    metabolism E71.30
      specified NEC E71.39
    oxidation
      LCAD E71.310
      MCAD E71.311
      SCAD E71.312
      specified deficiency NEC E71.318
  feeding (infant or child) (*see also* Disorder, eating) R63.3
  feigned (with obvious motivation) Z76.5
    without obvious motivation — *see* Disorder, factitious
  female
    hypoactive sexual desire F52.0
    orgasmic F52.31
    sexual arousal F52.22
  fibroblastic M72.9
    specified NEC M72.8
  fluency
    adult onset F98.5
    childhood onset F80.81
    following
      cerebral infarction I69.323
      cerebrovascular disease I69.923
        specified disease NEC I69.823
      intracerebral hemorrhage I69.123
      nontraumatic intracranial hemorrhage NEC I69.223
      subarachnoid hemorrhage I69.023
    in conditions classified elsewhere R47.82
  fluid balance E87.8
  follicular (skin) L73.9
    specified NEC L73.8
  fructose metabolism E74.10
    essential fructosuria E74.11
    fructokinase deficiency E74.11
    fructose-1, 6-diphosphatase deficiency E74.19
    hereditary fructose intolerance E74.12
    other specified E74.19
  functional polymorphonuclear neutrophils D71
  gallbladder, biliary tract and pancreas in diseases classified elsewhere K87
  gamma-glutamyl cycle E72.8
  gastric (functional) K31.9
    motility K30
    psychogenic F45.8
    secretion K30
  gastrointestinal (functional) NOS K92.9
    newborn P78.9
    psychogenic F45.8
  gender-identity or -role F64.9
    childhood F64.2
    effect on relationship F66
    of adolescence or adulthood (nontranssexual) F64.1
    specified NEC F64.8
    uncertainty F66
  genitourinary system
    female N94.9
    male N50.9
    psychogenic F45.8
  globe H44.9
    degenerated condition H44.50
      absolute glaucoma H44.51- ☑
      atrophy H44.52- ☑
      leucocoria H44.53- ☑
    degenerative H44.30

Index

Disorder — *continued*
  globe — *continued*
    degenerative H44.30
      chalcosis H44.31- ☑
      myopia H44.2- ☑
      siderosis H44.32- ☑
      specified type NEC H44.39- ☑
    endophthalmitis — *see* Endophthalmitis
    foreign body, retained — *see* Foreign body, intraoc-
        ular, old, retained
    hemophthalmos — *see* Hemophthalmos
    hypotony H44.40
      due to
        ocular fistula H44.42- ☑
        specified disorder NEC H44.43- ☑
      flat anterior chamber H44.41- ☑
      primary H44.44- ☑
    luxation — *see* Luxation, globe
    specified type NEC H44.89
  glomerular (in) N05.9
    amyloidosis E85.4 [N08]
    cryoglobulinemia D89.1 [N08]
    disseminated intravascular coagulation D65 [N08]
    Fabry's disease E75.21 [N08]
    familial lecithin cholesterol acyltransferase deficien-
        cy E78.6 [N08]
    Goodpasture's syndrome M31.0
    hemolytic-uremic syndrome D59.3
    Henoch (-Schönlein) purpura D69.0 [N08]
    malariae malaria B52.0
    microscopic polyangiitis M31.7 [N08]
    multiple myeloma C90.0- ☑ [N08]
    mumps B26.83
    schistosomiasis B65.9 [N08]
    sepsis NEC A41.- ☑ [N08]
      streptococcal A40.- ☑ [N08]
    sickle-cell disorders D57.- ☑ [N08]
    strongyloidiasis B78.9 [N08]
    subacute bacterial endocarditis I33.0 [N08]
    syphilis A52.75
    systemic lupus erythematosus M32.14
    thrombotic thrombocytopenic purpura
        M31.1 [N08]
    Waldenström macroglobulinemia C88.0 [N08]
    Wegener's granulomatosis M31.31
  gluconeogenesis E74.4
  glucosaminoglycan metabolism — *see* Disorder,
      metabolism, glucosaminoglycan
  glycine metabolism E72.50
    d-glycericacidemia E72.59
    hyperhydroxyprolinemia E72.59
    hyperoxaluria E72.53
    hyperprolinemia E72.59
    non-ketotic hyperglycinemia E72.51
    oxalosis E72.53
    oxaluria E72.53
    sarcosinemia E72.59
    trimethylaminuria E72.52
  glycoprotein metabolism E77.9
    specified NEC E77.8
  habit (and impulse) F63.9
    involving sexual behavior NEC F65.9
    specified NEC F63.89
  heart action I49.9
  hematological D75.9
    newborn (transient) P61.9
      specified NEC P61.8
  hematopoietic organs D75.9
  hemorrhagic NEC D69.9
    drug-induced D68.32
    due to
      extrinsic circulating anticoagulants D68.32
      increase in
        anti-IIa D68.32
        anti-Xa D68.32
      intrinsic
        circulating anticoagulants D68.318
        increase in
          anti-IXa D68.318
          antithrombin D68.318
          anti-VIIIa D68.318
          anti-XIa D68.318
    following childbirth O72.3
  hemostasis — *see* Defect, coagulation
  histidine metabolism E70.40
    histidinemia E70.41
    other specified E70.49

Disorder — *continued*
  hyperkinetic — *see* Disorder, attention-deficit hyper-
      activity
  hyperleucine-isoleucinemia E71.19
  hypervalinemia E71.19
  hypoactive sexual desire F52.0
  hypochondriacal F45.20
    body dysmorphic F45.22
    neurosis F45.21
    other specified F45.29
  identity
    dissociative F44.81
    of childhood F93.8
  immune mechanism (immunity) D89.9
    specified type NEC D89.89
  impaired renal tubular function N25.9
    specified NEC N25.89
  impulse (control) F63.9
  inflammatory
    pelvic, in diseases classified elsewhere — *see* cate-
        gory N74
    penis N48.29
      abscess N48.21
      cellulitis N48.22
  integument, newborn P83.9
    specified NEC P83.8
  intermittent explosive F63.81
  internal secretion pancreas — *see* Increased, secretion,
      pancreas, endocrine
  intestine, intestinal
    carbohydrate absorption NEC E74.39
      postoperative K91.2
    functional NEC K59.9
      postoperative K91.89
    psychogenic F45.8
    vascular K55.9
      chronic K55.1
      specified NEC K55.8
  intraoperative (intraprocedural) — *see* Complications,
      intraoperative
  involuntary emotional expression (IEED) F07.89
  iris H21.9
    adhesions — *see* Adhesions, iris
    atrophy — *see* Atrophy, iris
    chamber angle recession — *see* Recession, cham-
        ber angle
    cyst — *see* Cyst, iris
    degeneration — *see* Degeneration, iris
    in diseases classified elsewhere H22
    iridodialysis — *see* Iridodialysis
    iridoschisis — *see* Iridoschisis
    miotic pupillary cyst — *see* Cyst, pupillary
    pupillary
      abnormality — *see* Abnormality, pupillary
      membrane — *see* Membrane, pupillary
    specified type NEC H21.89
    vascular NEC H21.1X- ☑
  iron metabolism E83.10
    specified NEC E83.19
  isovaleric acidemia E71.110
  jaw, developmental M27.0
    temporomandibular — *see* Anomaly, dentofacial,
        temporomandibular joint
  joint M25.9
    derangement — *see* Derangement, joint
    effusion — *see* Effusion, joint
    fistula — *see* Fistula, joint
    hemarthrosis — *see* Hemarthrosis
    instability — *see* Instability, joint
    osteophyte — *see* Osteophyte
    pain — *see* Pain, joint
    psychogenic F45.8
    specified type NEC M25.80
      ankle M25.87- ☑
      elbow M25.82- ☑
      foot joint M25.87- ☑
      hand joint M25.84- ☑
      hip M25.85- ☑
      knee M25.86- ☑
      shoulder M25.81- ☑
      wrist M25.83- ☑
    stiffness — *see* Stiffness, joint
  ketone metabolism E71.32
  kidney N28.9
    functional (tubular) N25.9
    in
      schistosomiasis B65.9 [N29]

Disorder — *continued*
  kidney — *continued*
    tubular function N25.9
      specified NEC N25.89
  lacrimal system H04.9
    changes H04.69
      fistula — *see* Fistula, lacrimal
    gland H04.19
      atrophy — *see* Atrophy, lacrimal gland
      cyst — *see* Cyst, lacrimal, gland
      dacryops — *see* Dacryops
      dislocation — *see* Dislocation, lacrimal gland
      dry eye syndrome — *see* Syndrome, dry eye
      infection — *see* Dacryoadenitis
      granuloma — *see* Granuloma, lacrimal
      inflammation — *see* Inflammation, lacrimal
      obstruction — *see* Obstruction, lacrimal
      specified NEC H04.89
  lactation NEC O92.79
  language (developmental) F80.9
    expressive F80.1
    mixed receptive and expressive F80.2
    receptive F80.2
  late luteal phase dysphoric N94.89
  learning (specific) F81.9
    acalculia R48.8
    alexia R48.0
    mathematics F81.2
    reading F81.0
    specified NEC F81.89
    spelling F81.81
    written expression F81.81
  lens H27.9
    aphakia — *see* Aphakia
    cataract — *see* Cataract
    dislocation — *see* Dislocation, lens
    specified type NEC H27.8
  ligament M24.20
    ankle M24.27- ☑
    attachment, spine — *see* Enthesopathy, spinal
    elbow M24.22- ☑
    foot joint M24.27- ☑
    hand joint M24.24- ☑
    hip M24.25- ☑
    knee — *see* Derangement, knee, specified NEC
    shoulder M24.21- ☑
    vertebra M24.28
    wrist M24.23- ☑
  ligamentous attachments (*see also* Enthesopathy)
    spine — *see* Enthesopathy, spinal
  lipid
    metabolism, congenital E78.9
    storage E75.6
      specified NEC E75.5
  lipoprotein
    deficiency (familial) E78.6
    metabolism E78.9
      specified NEC E78.89
  liver K76.9
    malarial B54 [K77]
  low back (*see also* Dorsopathy, specified NEC)
  lumbosacral
    plexus G54.1
    root (nerve) NEC G54.4
  lung, interstitial, drug-induced J70.4
    acute J70.2
    chronic J70.3
  lymphoproliferative, post-transplant (PTLD) D47.Z1
      (*following* D47.4)
  lysine and hydroxylysine metabolism E72.3
  male
    erectile (organic) (*see also* Dysfunction, sexual,
        male, erectile) N52.9
      nonorganic F52.21
    hypoactive sexual desire F52.0
    orgasmic F52.32
  manic F30.9
    organic F06.33
  mastoid (*see also* Disorder, ear, middle)
    postprocedural — *see* Complications, ear, proce-
        dure
  meniscus — *see* Derangement, knee, meniscus
  menopausal N95.9
    specified NEC N95.8
  menstrual N92.6
    psychogenic F45.8
    specified NEC N92.5

Disorder — Disorder

Disorder — *continued*
  mental (or behavioral) (nonpsychotic) F99
    due to (secondary to)
      amphetamine
        due to drug abuse — *see* Abuse, drug, stimulant
        due to drug dependence — *see* Dependence, drug, stimulant
      brain disease, damage and dysfunction F09
      caffeine use
        due to drug abuse — *see* Abuse, drug, stimulant
        due to drug dependence — *see* Dependence, drug, stimulant
      cannabis use
        due to drug abuse — *see* Abuse, drug, cannabis
        due to drug dependence — *see* Dependence, drug, cannabis
      general medical condition F09
      sedative or hypnotic use
        due to drug abuse — *see* Abuse, drug, sedative
        due to drug dependence — *see* Dependence, drug, sedative
      tobacco (nicotine) use — *see* Dependence, drug, nicotine
    following organic brain damage F07.9
      frontal lobe syndrome F07.0
      personality change F07.0
      postconcussional syndrome F07.81
      specified NEC F07.89
    infancy, childhood or adolescence F98.9
    neurotic — *see* Neurosis
    organic or symptomatic F09
    presenile, psychotic F03 ☑
    problem NEC
    psychoneurotic — *see* Neurosis
    psychotic — *see* Psychosis
    puerperal F53
    senile, psychotic NEC F03 ☑
  metabolic, amino acid, transitory, newborn P74.8
  metabolism NOS E88.9
    amino-acid E72.9
      aromatic E70.9
        albinism — *see* Albinism
        histidine E70.40
          histidinemia E70.41
          other specified E70.49
        hyperphenylalaninemia E70.1
          classical phenylketonuria E70.0
        other specified E70.8
        tryptophan E70.5
        tyrosine E70.20
          hypertyrosinemia E70.21
          other specified E70.29
      branched chain E71.2
        3-methylglutaconic aciduria E71.111
        hyperleucine-isoleucinemia E71.19
        hypervalinemia E71.19
        isovaleric acidemia E71.110
        maple syrup urine disease E71.0
        methylmalonic acidemia E71.120
        organic aciduria NEC E71.118
        other specified E71.19
        proprionate NEC E71.128
        proprionic acidemia E71.121
      glycine E72.50
        d-glycericacidemia E72.59
        hyperhydroxyprolinemia E72.59
        hyperoxaluria E72.53
        hyperprolinemia E72.59
        non-ketotic hyperglycinemia E72.51
        other specified E72.59
        sarcosinemia E72.59
        trimethylaminuria E72.52
      hydroxylysine E72.3
      lysine E72.3
      ornithine E72.4
      other specified E72.8
        beta-amino acid E72.8
        gamma-glutamyl cycle E72.8
      straight-chain E72.8
      sulfur-bearing E72.10
        homocystinuria E72.11
        methylenetetrahydrofolate reductase deficiency E72.12
        other specified E72.19

Disorder — *continued*
  metabolism — *continued*
    bile acid and cholesterol metabolism E78.70
    bilirubin E80.7
      specified NEC E80.6
    calcium E83.50
      hypercalcemia E83.52
      hypocalcemia E83.51
      other specified E83.59
    carbohydrate E74.9
      specified NEC E74.8
    cholesterol and bile acid metabolism E78.70
    congenital E88.9
    copper E83.00
      specified type NEC E83.09
      Wilson's disease E83.01
    cystinuria E72.01
    fructose E74.10
    galactose E74.20
    glucosaminoglycan E76.9
      mucopolysaccharidosis — *see* Mucopolysaccharidosis
      specified NEC E76.8
    glutamine E72.8
    glycine E72.50
    glycogen storage (hepatorenal) E74.09
    glycoprotein E77.9
      specified NEC E77.8
    glycosaminoglycan E76.9
      specified NEC E76.8
    in labor and delivery O75.89
    iron E83.10
    isoleucine E71.19
    leucine E71.19
    lipoid E78.9
    lipoprotein E78.9
      specified NEC E78.89
    magnesium E83.40
      hypermagnesemia E83.41
      hypomagnesemia E83.42
      other specified E83.49
    mineral E83.9
      specified NEC E83.89
    mitochondrial E88.40
      MELAS syndrome E88.41
      MERRF syndrome (myoclonic epilepsy associated with ragged-red fibers) E88.42
      other specified E88.49
    ornithine E72.4
    phosphatases E83.30
    phosphorus E83.30
      acid phosphatase deficiency E83.39
      hypophosphatasia E83.39
      hypophosphatemia E83.39
        familial E83.31
      other specified E83.39
      pseudovitamin D deficiency E83.32
    plasma protein NEC E88.09
    porphyrin — *see* Porphyria
    postprocedural E89.89
      specified NEC E89.89
    purine E79.9
      specified NEC E79.8
    pyrimidine E79.9
      specified NEC E79.8
    pyruvate E74.4
    serine E72.8
    sodium E87.8
    specified NEC E88.89
    threonine E72.8
    valine E71.19
    zinc E83.2
  methylmalonic acidemia E71.120
  micturition NEC R39.19
    feeling of incomplete emptying R39.14
    hesitancy R39.11
    poor stream R39.12
    psychogenic F45.8
    split stream R39.13
    straining R39.16
    urgency R39.15
  mitochondrial metabolism E88.40
  mitral (valve) — *see* Endocarditis, mitral
  mixed
    anxiety and depressive F41.8
    of scholastic skills (developmental) F81.89
    receptive expressive language F80.2

Disorder — *continued*
  mood F39
    bipolar — *see* Disorder, bipolar
    depressive — *see* Disorder, depressive
    due to (secondary to)
      alcohol F10.94
      amphetamine F15.94
        in
          abuse F15.14
          dependence F15.24
      anxiolytic F13.94
        in
          abuse F13.14
          dependence F13.24
      cocaine F14.94
        in
          abuse F14.14
          dependence F14.24
      general medical condition F06.30
      hallucinogen F16.94
        in
          abuse F16.14
          dependence F16.24
      hypnotic F13.94
        in
          abuse F13.14
          dependence F13.24
      inhalant F18.94
        in
          abuse F18.14
          dependence F18.24
      opioid F11.94
        in
          abuse F11.14
          dependence F11.24
      phencyclidine (PCP) F16.94
        in
          abuse F16.14
          dependence F16.24
      physiological condition F06.30
        with
          depressive features F06.31
          major depressive-like episode F06.32
          manic features F06.33
          mixed features F06.34
      psychoactive substance NEC F19.94
        in
          abuse F19.14
          dependence F19.24
      sedative F13.94
        in
          abuse F13.14
          dependence F13.24
      volatile solvents F18.94
        in
          abuse F18.14
          dependence F18.24
    manic episode F30.9
      with psychotic symptoms F30.2
      without psychotic symptoms F30.10
        mild F30.11
        moderate F30.12
        severe F30.13
      in remission (full) F30.4
        partial F30.3
      specified type NEC F30.8
    organic F06.30
      right hemisphere F07.89
    persistent F34.9
      cyclothymia F34.0
      dysthymia F34.1
      specified type NEC F34.8
    recurrent F39
    right hemisphere organic F07.89
  movement G25.9
    drug-induced G25.70
      akathisia G25.71
      specified NEC G25.79
    hysterical F44.4
    in diseases classified elsewhere — *see* category G26
    periodic limb G47.61
      sleep related G47.61
    sleep related NEC G47.69
    specified NEC G25.89
    stereotyped F98.4
    treatment-induced G25.9
  multiple personality F44.81

☑ **Additional Character Required** — Refer to the Tabular List for Character Selection   ▽ **Subterms under main terms may continue to next column or page**

Disorder — *continued*
  muscle M62.9
    attachment, spine — *see* Enthesopathy, spinal
    in trichinellosis — *see* Trichinellosis, with muscle
      disorder
    psychogenic F45.8
    specified type NEC M62.89
    tone, newborn P94.9
      specified NEC P94.8
  muscular
    attachments (*see also* Enthesopathy)
      spine — *see* Enthesopathy, spinal
    urethra N36.44
  musculoskeletal system, soft tissue — *see* Disorder,
    soft tissue
    postprocedural M96.89
    psychogenic F45.8
  myoneural G70.9
    due to lead G70.1
    specified NEC G70.89
    toxic G70.1
  myotonic NEC G71.19
  nail, in diseases classified elsewhere L62
  neck region NEC — *see* Dorsopathy, specified NEC
  nerve G58.9
    abducent NEC — *see* Strabismus, paralytic, sixth
      nerve
    accessory G52.8
    acoustic — *see* subcategory H93.3 ☑
    auditory — *see* subcategory H93.3 ☑
    auriculotemporal G50.8
    axillary G54.0
    cerebral — *see* Disorder, nerve, cranial
    cranial G52.9
      eighth — *see* subcategory H93.3 ☑
      eleventh G52.8
      fifth G50.9
      first G52.0
      fourth NEC — *see* Strabismus, paralytic, fourth
        nerve
      multiple G52.7
      ninth G52.1
      second NEC — *see* Disorder, nerve, optic
      seventh NEC G51.8
      sixth NEC — *see* Strabismus, paralytic, sixth
        nerve
      specified NEC G52.8
      tenth G52.2
      third NEC — *see* Strabismus, paralytic, third
        nerve
      twelfth G52.3
    entrapment — *see* Neuropathy, entrapment
    facial G51.9
      specified NEC G51.8
    femoral — *see* Lesion, nerve, femoral
    glossopharyngeal NEC G52.1
    hypoglossal G52.3
    intercostal G58.0
    lateral
      cutaneous of thigh — *see* Mononeuropathy,
        lower limb, meralgia paresthetica
      popliteal — *see* Lesion, nerve, popliteal
    lower limb — *see* Mononeuropathy, lower limb
    medial popliteal — *see* Lesion, nerve, popliteal,
      medial
    median NEC — *see* Lesion, nerve, median
    multiple G58.7
    oculomotor NEC — *see* Strabismus, paralytic, third
      nerve
    olfactory G52.0
    optic NEC H47.09- ☑
      hemorrhage into sheath — *see* Hemorrhage,
        optic nerve
      ischemic H47.01- ☑
    peroneal — *see* Lesion, nerve, popliteal
    phrenic G58.8
    plantar — *see* Lesion, nerve, plantar
    pneumogastric G52.2
    posterior tibial — *see* Syndrome, tarsal tunnel
    radial — *see* Lesion, nerve, radial
    recurrent laryngeal G52.2
    root G54.9
      cervical G54.2
      lumbosacral G54.1
      specified NEC G54.8
      thoracic G54.3
    sciatic NEC — *see* Lesion, nerve, sciatic

Disorder — *continued*
  nerve — *continued*
    specified NEC G58.8
      lower limb — *see* Mononeuropathy, lower limb,
        specified NEC
      upper limb — *see* Mononeuropathy, upper
        limb, specified NEC
    sympathetic G90.9
    tibial — *see* Lesion, nerve, popliteal, medial
    trigeminal G50.9
      specified NEC G50.8
    trochlear NEC — *see* Strabismus, paralytic, fourth
      nerve
    ulnar — *see* Lesion, nerve, ulnar
    upper limb — *see* Mononeuropathy, upper limb
    vagus G52.2
  nervous system G98.8
    autonomic (peripheral) G90.9
      specified NEC G90.8
    central G96.9
      specified NEC G96.8
    parasympathetic G90.9
    specified NEC G98.8
    sympathetic G90.9
    vegetative G90.9
  neurohypophysis NEC E23.3
  neurological NEC R29.818
  neuromuscular G70.9
    hereditary NEC G71.9
    specified NEC G70.89
    toxic G70.1
  neurotic F48.9
    specified NEC F48.8
  neutrophil, polymorphonuclear D71
  nicotine use — *see* Dependence, drug, nicotine
  nightmare F51.5
  nose J34.9
    specified NEC J34.89
  obsessive-compulsive F42
  odontogenesis NOS K00.9
  opioid use
    with
      opioid-induced psychotic disorder F11.959
        with
          delusions F11.950
          hallucinations F11.951
    due to drug abuse — *see* Abuse, drug, opioid
    due to drug dependence — *see* Dependence, drug,
      opioid
  oppositional defiant F91.3
  optic
    chiasm H47.49
      due to
        inflammatory disorder H47.41
        neoplasm H47.42
        vascular disorder H47.43
    disc H47.39- ☑
      coloboma — *see* Coloboma, optic disc
      drusen — *see* Drusen, optic disc
      pseudopapilledema — *see* Pseudopapilledema
    radiations — *see* Disorder, visual, pathway
    tracts — *see* Disorder, visual, pathway
  orbit H05.9
    cyst — *see* Cyst, orbit
    deformity — *see* Deformity, orbit
    edema — *see* Edema, orbit
    enophthalmos — *see* Enophthalmos
    exophthalmos — *see* Exophthalmos
    hemorrhage — *see* Hemorrhage, orbit
    inflammation — *see* Inflammation, orbit
    myopathy — *see* Myopathy, extraocular muscles
    retained foreign body — *see* Foreign body, orbit,
      old
    specified type NEC H05.89
  organic
    anxiety F06.4
    catatonic F06.1
    delusional F06.2
    dissociative F06.8
    emotionally labile (asthenic) F06.8
    mood (affective) F06.30
    schizophrenia-like F06.2
  orgasmic (female) F52.31
    male F52.32
  ornithine metabolism E72.4
  overanxious F41.1
    of childhood F93.8

Disorder — *continued*
  pain
    with related psychological factors F45.42
    exclusively related to psychological factors F45.41
  pancreatic internal secretion E16.9
    specified NEC E16.8
  panic F41.0
    with agoraphobia F40.01
  papulosquamous L44.9
    in diseases classified elsewhere L45
    specified NEC L44.8
  paranoid F22
    induced F24
    shared F24
  parathyroid (gland) E21.5
    specified NEC E21.4
  parietoalveolar NEC J84.09
  paroxysmal, mixed R56.9
  patella M22.9- ☑
    chondromalacia — *see* Chondromalacia, patella
    derangement NEC M22.3X- ☑
    recurrent
      dislocation — *see* Dislocation, patella, recurrent
      subluxation — *see* Dislocation, patella, recur-
        rent, incomplete
    specified NEC M22.8X- ☑
  patellofemoral M22.2X- ☑
  pentose phosphate pathway with anemia D55.1
  perception, due to hallucinogens F16.983
    in
      abuse F16.183
      dependence F16.283
  peripheral nervous system NEC G64
  peroxisomal E71.50
    biogenesis
      neonatal adrenoleukodystrophy E71.511
      specified disorder NEC E71.518
      Zellweger syndrome E71.510
    rhizomelic chondrodysplasia punctata E71.540
    specified form NEC E71.548
      group 1 E71.518
      group 2 E71.53
      group 3 E71.542
    X-linked adrenoleukodystrophy E71.529
      adolescent E71.521
      adrenomyeloneuropathy E71.522
      childhood E71.520
      specified form NEC E71.528
    Zellweger-like syndrome E71.541
  persistent
    (somatoform) pain F45.41
    affective (mood) F34.9
  personality (*see also* Personality) F60.9
    affective F34.0
    aggressive F60.3
    amoral F60.2
    anankastic F60.5
    antisocial F60.2
    anxious F60.6
    asocial F60.2
    asthenic F60.7
    avoidant F60.6
    borderline F60.3
    change (secondary) due to general medical condi-
      tion F07.0
    compulsive F60.5
    cyclothymic F34.0
    dependent (passive) F60.7
    depressive F34.1
    dissocial F60.2
    emotional instability F60.3
    expansive paranoid F60.0
    explosive F60.3
    following organic brain damage F07.9
    histrionic F60.4
    hyperthymic F34.0
    hypothymic F34.1
    hysterical F60.4
    immature F60.89
    inadequate F60.7
    labile F60.3
    mixed (nonspecific) F60.89
    moral deficiency F60.2
    narcissistic F60.81
    negativistic F60.89
    obsessional F60.5
    obsessive (-compulsive) F60.5
    organic F07.9

Disorder — *continued*
  personality (*see also* Personality) — *continued*
    overconscientious F60.5
    paranoid F60.0
    passive (-dependent) F60.7
    passive-aggressive F60.89
    pathological NEC F60.9
    pseudosocial F60.2
    psychopathic F60.2
    schizoid F60.1
    schizotypal F21
    self-defeating F60.7
    specified NEC F60.89
    type A F60.5
    unstable (emotional) F60.3
  pervasive, developmental F84.9
  phobic anxiety, childhood F40.8
  phosphate-losing tubular N25.0
  pigmentation L81.9
    choroid, congenital Q14.3
    diminished melanin formation L81.6
    iron L81.8
    specified NEC L81.8
  pinna (noninfective) H61.10- ☑
    deformity, acquired H61.11- ☑
    hematoma H61.12- ☑
    perichondritis — *see* Perichondritis, ear
    specified type NEC H61.19- ☑
  pituitary gland E23.7
    iatrogenic (postprocedural) E89.3
    specified NEC E23.6
  platelets D69.1
  plexus G54.9
    specified NEC G54.8
  polymorphonuclear neutrophils D71
  porphyrin metabolism — *see* Porphyria
  postconcussional F07.81
  posthallucinogen perception F16.983
    in
      abuse F16.183
      dependence F16.283
  postmenopausal N95.9
    specified NEC N95.8
  postprocedural (postoperative) — *see* Complications, postprocedural
  post-transplant lymphoproliferative D47.Z1 (*following* D47.4)
  post-traumatic stress (PTSD) F43.10
    acute F43.11
    chronic F43.12
  premenstrual dysphoric (PMDD) N94.3
  prepuce N47.8
  propionic acidemia E71.121
  prostate N42.9
    specified NEC N42.89
  psychogenic NOS (*see also* condition) F45.9
    anxiety F41.8
    appetite F50.9
    asthenic F48.8
    cardiovascular (system) F45.8
    compulsive F42
    cutaneous F54
    depressive F32.9
    digestive (system) F45.8
    dysmenorrheic F45.8
    dyspneic F45.8
    endocrine (system) F54
    eye NEC F45.8
    feeding — *see* Disorder, eating
    functional NEC F45.8
    gastric F45.8
    gastrointestinal (system) F45.8
    genitourinary (system) F45.8
    heart (function) (rhythm) F45.8
    hyperventilatory F45.8
    hypochondriacal — *see* Disorder, hypochondriacal
    intestinal F45.8
    joint F45.8
    learning F81.9
    limb F45.8
    lymphatic (system) F45.8
    menstrual F45.8
    micturition F45.8
    monoplegic NEC F44.4
    motor F44.4
    muscle F45.8
    musculoskeletal F45.8
    neurocirculatory F45.8

Disorder — *continued*
  psychogenic (*see also* condition) — *continued*
    obsessive F42
    occupational F48.8
    organ or part of body NEC F45.8
    paralytic NEC F44.4
    phobic F40.9
    physical NEC F45.8
    rectal F45.8
    respiratory (system) F45.8
    rheumatic F45.8
    sexual (function) F52.9
    skin (allergic) (eczematous) F54
    sleep F51.9
    specified part of body NEC F45.8
    stomach F45.8
  psychological F99
    associated with
      disease classified elsewhere F54
      sexual
        development F66
        relationship F66
      uncertainty about gender identity F66
  psychomotor NEC F44.4
    hysterical F44.4
  psychoneurotic (*see also* Neurosis)
    mixed NEC F48.8
  psychophysiologic — *see* Disorder, somatoform
  psychosexual F65.9
    development F66
    identity of childhood F64.2
  psychosomatic NOS — *see* Disorder, somatoform
    multiple F45.0
    undifferentiated F45.1
  psychotic — *see* Psychosis
    transient (acute) F23
  puberty E30.9
    specified NEC E30.8
  pulmonary (valve) — *see* Endocarditis, pulmonary
  purine metabolism E79.9
  pyrimidine metabolism E79.9
  pyruvate metabolism E74.4
  reactive attachment (childhood) F94.1
  reading R48.0
    developmental (specific) F81.0
  receptive language F80.2
  receptor, hormonal, peripheral (*see also* Syndrome, androgen insensitivity) E34.50
  recurrent brief depressive F33.8
  reflex R29.2
  refraction H52.7
    aniseikonia H52.32
    anisometropia H52.31
    astigmatism — *see* Astigmatism
    hypermetropia — *see* Hypermetropia
    myopia — *see* Myopia
    presbyopia H52.4
    specified NEC H52.6
  relationship F68.8
    due to sexual orientation F66
  REM sleep behavior G47.52
  renal function, impaired (tubular) N25.9
  resonance R49.9
    specified NEC R49.8
  respiratory function, impaired (*see also* Failure, respiration)
    postprocedural — *see* Complication, postoperative, respiratory system
    psychogenic F45.8
  retina H35.9
    angioid streaks H35.33
    changes in vascular appearance H35.01- ☑
    degeneration — *see* Degeneration, retina
    dystrophy (hereditary) — *see* Dystrophy, retina
    edema H35.81
    hemorrhage — *see* Hemorrhage, retina
    ischemia H35.82
    macular degeneration — *see* Degeneration, macula
    microaneurysms H35.04- ☑
    microvascular abnormality NEC H35.09
    neovascularization — *see* Neovascularization, retina
    retinopathy — *see* Retinopathy
    separation of layers H35.70
      central serous chorioretinopathy H35.71- ☑
      pigment epithelium detachment (serous) H35.72- ☑
        hemorrhagic H35.73- ☑

Disorder — *continued*
  retina — *continued*
    specified type NEC H35.89
    telangiectasis — *see* Telangiectasis, retina
    vasculitis — *see* Vasculitis, retina
  retroperitoneal K68.9
  right hemisphere organic affective F07.89
  rumination (infant or child) F98.21
  sacrum, sacrococcygeal NEC M53.3
  schizoaffective F25.9
    bipolar type F25.0
    depressive type F25.1
    manic type F25.0
    mixed type F25.0
    specified NEC F25.8
  schizoid of childhood F84.5
  schizophreniform F20.81
    brief F23
  schizotypal (personality) F21
  secretion, thyrocalcitonin E07.0
  seizure (*see also* Epilepsy) G40.909
    intractable G40.919
      with status epilepticus G40.911
  semantic pragmatic F80.89
    with autism F84.0
  sense of smell R43.1
    psychogenic F45.8
  separation anxiety, of childhood F93.0
  sexual
    arousal, female F52.22
    aversion F52.1
    function, psychogenic F52.9
    maturation F66
    nonorganic F52.9
    preference (*see also* Deviation, sexual) F65.9
      fetishistic transvestism F65.1
    relationship F66
  shyness, of childhood and adolescence F40.10
  sibling rivalry F93.8
  sickle-cell (sickling) (homozygous) — *see* Disease, sickle-cell
    heterozygous D57.3
    specified type NEC D57.8- ☑
    trait D57.3
  sinus (nasal) J34.9
    specified NEC J34.89
  skin L98.9
    atrophic L90.9
      specified NEC L90.8
    granulomatous L92.9
      specified NEC L92.8
    hypertrophic L91.9
      specified NEC L91.8
    infiltrative NEC L98.6
    newborn P83.9
      specified NEC P83.8
    psychogenic (allergic) (eczematous) F54
  sleep G47.9
    breathing-related — *see* Apnea, sleep
    circadian rhythm G47.20
      advance sleep phase type G47.22
      delayed sleep phase type G47.21
      due to
        alcohol
          abuse F10.182
          dependence F10.282
          use F10.982
        amphetamines
          abuse F15.182
          dependence F15.282
          use F15.982
        caffeine
          abuse F15.182
          dependence F15.282
          use F15.982
        cocaine
          abuse F14.182
          dependence F14.282
          use F14.982
        drug NEC
          abuse F19.182
          dependence F19.282
          use F19.982
        opioid
          abuse F11.182
          dependence F11.282
          use F11.982

Disorder — *continued*
  sleep — *continued*
    circadian rhythm — *continued*
      due to — *continued*
        psychoactive substance NEC
          abuse F19.182
          dependence F19.282
          use F19.982
        sedative, hypnotic, or anxiolytic
          abuse F13.182
          dependence F13.282
          use F13.982
        stimulant NEC
          abuse F15.182
          dependence F15.282
          use F15.982
      free running type G47.24
      in conditions classified elsewhere G47.27
      irregular sleep wake type G47.23
      jet lag type G47.25
      shift work type G47.26
      specified NEC G47.29
    due to
      alcohol
        abuse F10.182
        dependence F10.282
        use F10.982
      amphetamine
        abuse F15.182
        dependence F15.282
        use F15.982
      anxiolytic
        abuse F13.182
        dependence F13.282
        use F13.982
      caffeine
        abuse F15.182
        dependence F15.282
        use F15.982
      cocaine
        abuse F14.182
        dependence F14.282
        use F14.982
      drug NEC
        abuse F19.182
        dependence F19.282
        use F19.982
      hypnotic
        abuse F13.182
        dependence F13.282
        use F13.982
      opioid
        abuse F11.182
        dependence F11.282
        use F11.982
      psychoactive substance NEC
        abuse F19.182
        dependence F19.282
        use F19.982
      sedative
        abuse F13.182
        dependence F13.282
        use F13.982
      stimulant NEC
        abuse F15.182
        dependence F15.282
        use F15.982
    emotional F51.9
    excessive somnolence — *see* Hypersomnia
    hypersomnia type — *see* Hypersomnia
    initiating or maintaining — *see* Insomnia
    nightmares F51.5
    nonorganic F51.9
      specified NEC F51.8
    parasomnia type G47.50
    specified NEC G47.8
    terrors F51.4
    walking F51.3
  sleep-wake pattern or schedule — *see* Disorder, sleep, circadian rhythm
  social
    anxiety of childhood F40.10
    functioning in childhood F94.9
      specified NEC F94.8
  soft tissue M79.9
    ankle M79.9
    due to use, overuse and pressure M70.90
      ankle M70.97- ☑

Disorder — *continued*
  soft tissue — *continued*
    due to use, overuse and pressure — *continued*
      bursitis — *see* Bursitis
      foot M70.97- ☑
      forearm M70.93- ☑
      hand M70.94- ☑
      lower leg M70.96- ☑
      multiple sites M70.99
      pelvic region M70.95- ☑
      shoulder region M70.91- ☑
      specified site NEC M70.98
      specified type NEC M70.80
        ankle M70.87- ☑
        foot M70.87- ☑
        forearm M70.83- ☑
        hand M70.84- ☑
        lower leg M70.86- ☑
        multiple sites M70.89
        pelvic region M70.85- ☑
        shoulder region M70.81- ☑
        specified site NEC M70.88
        thigh M70.85- ☑
        upper arm M70.82- ☑
      thigh M70.95- ☑
      upper arm M70.92- ☑
    foot M79.9
    forearm M79.9
    hand M79.9
    lower leg M79.9
    multiple sites M79.9
    occupational — *see* Disorder, soft tissue, due to use, overuse and pressure
    pelvic region M79.9
    shoulder region M79.9
    specified type NEC M79.89
    thigh M79.9
    upper arm M79.9
  somatization F45.0
  somatoform F45.9
    pain (persistent) F45.41
    somatization (multiple) (long-lasting) F45.0
    specified NEC F45.8
    undifferentiated F45.1
  somnolence, excessive — *see* Hypersomnia
  specific
    arithmetical F81.2
    developmental, of motor F82
    reading F81.0
    speech and language F80.9
    spelling F81.81
    written expression F81.81
  speech R47.9
    articulation (functional) (specific) F80.0
    developmental F80.9
    specified NEC R47.89
  spelling (specific) F81.81
  spine (*see also* Dorsopathy)
    ligamentous or muscular attachments, peripheral — *see* Enthesopathy, spinal
    specified NEC — *see* Dorsopathy, specified NEC
  stereotyped, habit or movement F98.4
  stomach (functional) — *see* Disorder, gastric
  stress F43.9
    post-traumatic F43.10
      acute F43.11
      chronic F43.12
  sulfur-bearing amino-acid metabolism E72.10
  sweat gland (eccrine) L74.9
    apocrine L75.9
      specified NEC L75.8
    specified NEC L74.8
  synovium M67.90
    acromioclavicular M67.91- ☑
    ankle M67.97- ☑
    elbow M67.92- ☑
    foot M67.97- ☑
    forearm M67.93- ☑
    hand M67.94- ☑
    hip M67.95- ☑
    knee M67.96- ☑
    multiple sites M67.99
    rupture — *see* Rupture, synovium
    shoulder M67.91- ☑
    specified type NEC M67.80
      acromioclavicular M67.81- ☑
      ankle M67.87- ☑

Disorder — *continued*
  synovium — *continued*
    specified type — *continued*
      elbow M67.82- ☑
      foot M67.87- ☑
      hand M67.84- ☑
      hip M67.85- ☑
      knee M67.86- ☑
      multiple sites M67.89
      wrist M67.83- ☑
    synovitis — *see* Synovitis
    upper arm M67.92- ☑
    wrist M67.93- ☑
  temperature regulation, newborn P81.9
    specified NEC P81.8
  temporomandibular joint — *see* Anomaly, dentofacial, temporomandibular joint
  tendon M67.90
    acromioclavicular M67.91- ☑
    ankle M67.97- ☑
    contracture — *see* Contracture, tendon
    elbow M67.92- ☑
    foot M67.97- ☑
    forearm M67.93- ☑
    hand M67.94- ☑
    hip M67.95- ☑
    knee M67.96- ☑
    multiple sites M67.99
    rupture — *see* Rupture, tendon
    shoulder M67.91- ☑
    specified type NEC M67.80
      acromioclavicular M67.81- ☑
      ankle M67.87- ☑
      elbow M67.82- ☑
      foot M67.87- ☑
      hand M67.84- ☑
      hip M67.85- ☑
      knee M67.86- ☑
      multiple sites M67.89
      trunk M67.88
      wrist M67.83- ☑
    synovitis — *see* Synovitis
    tendinitis — *see* Tendinitis
    tenosynovitis — *see* Tenosynovitis
    trunk M67.98
    upper arm M67.92- ☑
    wrist M67.93- ☑
  thoracic root (nerve) NEC G54.3
  thyrocalcitonin hypersecretion E07.0
  thyroid (gland) E07.9
    function NEC, neonatal, transitory P72.2
    iodine-deficiency related E01.8
    specified NEC E07.89
  tic — *see* Tic
  tooth K08.9
    development K00.9
      specified NEC K00.8
    eruption K00.6
  Tourette's F95.2
  trance and possession F44.89
  tricuspid (valve) — *see* Endocarditis, tricuspid
  tryptophan metabolism E70.5
  tubular, phosphate-losing N25.0
  tubulo-interstitial (in)
    brucellosis A23.9 [N16]
    cystinosis E72.04
    diphtheria A36.84
    glycogen storage disease E74.00 [N16]
    leukemia NEC C95.9- ☑ [N16]
    lymphoma NEC C85.9- ☑ [N16]
    mixed cryoglobulinemia D89.1 [N16]
    multiple myeloma C90.0- ☑ [N16]
    Salmonella infection A02.25
    sarcoidosis D86.84
    sepsis A41.9 [N16]
      streptococcal A40.9 [N16]
    systemic lupus erythematosus M32.15
    toxoplasmosis B58.83
    transplant rejection T86.91 [N16]
    Wilson's disease E83.01 [N16]
  tubulo-renal function, impaired N25.9
    specified NEC N25.89
  tympanic membrane H73.9- ☑
    atrophy — *see* Atrophy, tympanic membrane
    infection — *see* Myringitis
    perforation — *see* Perforation, tympanum
    specified NEC H73.89- ☑

Index

Disorder — Disorder

Disorder — *continued*
  unsocialized aggressive F91.1
  urea cycle metabolism E72.20
    argininemia E72.21
    arginosuccinic aciduria E72.22
    citrullinemia E72.23
    ornithine transcarbamylase deficiency E72.4
    other specified E72.29
  ureter (in) N28.9
    schistosomiasis B65.0 [N29]
    tuberculosis A18.11
  urethra N36.9
    specified NEC N36.8
  urinary system N39.9
    specified NEC N39.8
  valve, heart
    aortic — *see* Endocarditis, aortic
    mitral — *see* Endocarditis, mitral
    pulmonary — *see* Endocarditis, pulmonary
    rheumatic
      aortic — *see* Endocarditis, aortic, rheumatic
      mitral — *see* Endocarditis, mitral
      pulmonary — *see* Endocarditis, pulmonary, rheumatic
      tricuspid — *see* Endocarditis, tricuspid
    tricuspid — *see* Endocarditis, tricuspid
  vestibular function H81.9-
    specified NEC — *see* subcategory H81.8 ☑
      in diseases classified elsewhere H82.- ☑
    vertigo — *see* Vertigo
  vision, binocular H53.30
    abnormal retinal correspondence H53.31
    diplopia H53.2
    fusion with defective stereopsis H53.32
    simultaneous perception H53.33
    suppression H53.34
  visual
    cortex
      blindness H47.619
        left brain H47.612
        right brain H47.611
      due to
        inflammatory disorder H47.629
          left brain H47.622
          right brain H47.621
        neoplasm H47.639
          left brain H47.632
          right brain H47.631
        vascular disorder H47.649
          left brain H47.642
          right brain H47.641
    pathway H47.9
      due to
        inflammatory disorder H47.51- ☑
        neoplasm H47.52- ☑
        vascular disorder H47.53- ☑
    optic chiasm — *see* Disorder, optic, chiasm
  vitreous body H43.9
    crystalline deposits — *see* Deposit, crystalline
    degeneration — *see* Degeneration, vitreous
    hemorrhage — *see* Hemorrhage, vitreous
    opacities — *see* Opacity, vitreous
    prolapse — *see* Prolapse, vitreous
    specified type NEC H43.89
  voice R49.9
    specified type NEC R49.8
  volatile solvent use
    due to drug abuse — *see* Abuse, drug, inhalant
    due to drug dependence — *see* Dependence, drug, inhalant
  white blood cells D72.9
    specified NEC D72.89
  withdrawing, child or adolescent F40.10
Disorientation R41.0
Displacement, displaced
  acquired traumatic of bone, cartilage, joint, tendon NEC — *see* Dislocation
  adrenal gland (congenital) Q89.1
  appendix, retrocecal (congenital) Q43.8
  auricle (congenital) Q17.4
  bladder (acquired) N32.89
    congenital Q64.19
  brachial plexus (congenital) Q07.8
  brain stem, caudal (congenital) Q04.8
  canaliculus (lacrimalis), congenital Q10.6
  cardia through esophageal hiatus (congenital) Q40.1
  cerebellum, caudal (congenital) Q04.8
  cervix — *see* Malposition, uterus

Displacement, displaced — *continued*
  colon (congenital) Q43.3
  device, implant or graft (*see also* Complications, by site and type, mechanical) T85.628 ☑
    arterial graft NEC — *see* Complication, cardiovascular device, mechanical, vascular
    breast (implant) T85.42 ☑
    catheter NEC T85.628 ☑
      dialysis (renal) T82.42 ☑
        intraperitoneal T85.621 ☑
      infusion NEC T82.524 ☑
        spinal (epidural) (subdural) T85.620 ☑ ☑
      urinary (indwelling) T83.028 ☑
        cystostomy T83.020 ☑
    electronic (electrode) (pulse generator) (stimulator) — *see* Complication, electronic stimulator
    fixation, internal (orthopedic) NEC — *see* Complication, fixation device, mechanical
    gastrointestinal — *see* Complications, prosthetic device, mechanical, gastrointestinal device
    genital NEC T83.428 ☑
      intrauterine contraceptive device T83.32 ☑
      penile prosthesis T83.420 ☑
    heart NEC — *see* Complication, cardiovascular device, mechanical
    joint prosthesis — *see* Complications, joint prosthesis, mechanical
    ocular — *see* Complications, prosthetic device, mechanical, ocular device
    orthopedic NEC — *see* Complication, orthopedic, device or graft, mechanical
    specified NEC T85.628 ☑
    urinary NEC (*see also* Complication, genitourinary, device, urinary, mechanical)
      graft T83.22 ☑
    vascular NEC — *see* Complication, cardiovascular device, mechanical
    ventricular intracranial shunt T85.02 ☑
  electronic stimulator
    bone T84.320 ☑
    cardiac — *see* Complications, cardiac device, electronic
    nervous system — *see* Complication, prosthetic device, mechanical, electronic nervous system stimulator
    urinary — *see* Complications, electronic stimulator, urinary
  esophageal mucosa into cardia of stomach, congenital Q39.8
  esophagus (acquired) K22.8
    congenital Q39.8
  eyeball (acquired) (lateral) (old) — *see* Displacement, globe
    congenital Q15.8
    current — *see* Avulsion, eye
  fallopian tube (acquired) N83.4
    congenital Q50.6
    opening (congenital) Q50.6
  gallbladder (congenital) Q44.1
  gastric mucosa (congenital) Q40.2
  globe (acquired) (old) (lateral) H05.21- ☑
    current — *see* Avulsion, eye
  heart (congenital) Q24.8
    acquired I51.89
  hymen (upward) (congenital) Q52.4
  intervertebral disc NEC
    with myelopathy — *see* Disorder, disc, with, myelopathy
    cervical, cervicothoracic (with) M50.20
      myelopathy — *see* Disorder, disc, cervical, with myelopathy
      neuritis, radiculitis or radiculopathy — *see* Disorder, disc, cervical, with neuritis
    due to trauma — *see* Dislocation, vertebra
    lumbar region M51.26
      with
        myelopathy M51.06
        neuritis, radiculitis, radiculopathy or sciatica M51.16
    lumbosacral region M51.27
      with
        neuritis, radiculitis, radiculopathy or sciatica M51.17
    sacrococcygeal region M53.3
    thoracic region M51.24
      with
        myelopathy M51.04

Displacement, displaced — *continued*
  intervertebral disc — *continued*
    thoracic region — *continued*
      with — *continued*
        neuritis, radiculitis, radiculopathy M51.14
    thoracolumbar region M51.25
      with
        myelopathy M51.05
        neuritis, radiculitis, radiculopathy M51.15
  intrauterine device T83.32 ☑
  kidney (acquired) N28.83
    congenital Q63.2
  lachrymal, lacrimal apparatus or duct (congenital) Q10.6
  lens, congenital Q12.1
  macula (congenital) Q14.1
  Meckel's diverticulum Q43.0
    malignant — *see* Table of Neoplasms, small intestine, malignant
  nail (congenital) Q84.6
    acquired L60.8
  opening of Wharton's duct in mouth Q38.4
  organ or site, congenital NEC — *see* Malposition, congenital
  ovary (acquired) N83.4
    congenital Q50.39
    free in peritoneal cavity (congenital) Q50.39
    into hernial sac N83.4
  oviduct (acquired) N83.4
    congenital Q50.6
  parathyroid (gland) E21.4
  parotid gland (congenital) Q38.4
  punctum lacrimale (congenital) Q10.6
  sacro-iliac (joint) (congenital) Q74.2
    current injury S33.2 ☑
    old — *see* subcategory M53.2 ☑
  salivary gland (any) (congenital) Q38.4
  spleen (congenital) Q89.09
  stomach, congenital Q40.2
  sublingual duct Q38.4
  tongue (downward) (congenital) Q38.3
  tooth, teeth, fully erupted M26.30
    horizontal M26.33
    vertical M26.34
  trachea (congenital) Q32.1
  ureter or ureteric opening or orifice (congenital) Q62.62
  uterine opening of oviducts or fallopian tubes Q50.6
  uterus, uterine — *see* Malposition, uterus
  ventricular septum Q21.0
    with rudimentary ventricle Q20.4
Disproportion
  between native and reconstructed breast N65.1
  fiber-type G71.2
Disruptio uteri — *see* Rupture, uterus
Disruption (of)
  ciliary body NEC H21.89
  closure of
    cornea T81.31 ☑
    craniotomy T81.32 ☑
    fascia (muscular) (superficial) T81.32 ☑
    internal organ or tissue T81.32 ☑
    laceration (external) (internal) T81.33 ☑
    ligament T81.32 ☑
    mucosa T81.31 ☑
    muscle or muscle flap T81.32 ☑
    ribs or rib cage T81.32 ☑
    skin and subcutaneous tissue (full-thickness) (superficial) T81.31 ☑
    skull T81.32 ☑
    sternum (sternotomy) T81.32 ☑
    tendon T81.32 ☑
    traumatic laceration (external) (internal) T81.33 ☑
  family Z63.8
    due to
      absence of family member due to military deployment Z63.31
      absence of family member NEC Z63.32
      alcoholism and drug addiction in family Z63.72
      bereavement Z63.4
      death (assumed) or disappearance of family member Z63.4
      divorce or separation Z63.5
      drug addiction in family Z63.72
      return of family member from military deployment (current or past conflict) Z63.71
      stressful life events NEC Z63.79
  iris NEC H21.89

☑ **Additional Character Required** — **Refer to the Tabular List for Character Selection**   🔺 **Subterms under main terms may continue to next column or page**

Disruption — *continued*
  ligament(s) (*see also* Sprain)
    knee
      current injury — *see* Dislocation, knee
      old (chronic) — *see* Derangement, knee, insta-
        bility
      spontaneous NEC — *see* Derangement, knee,
        disruption ligament
  ossicular chain — *see* Discontinuity, ossicles, ear
  pelvic ring (stable) S32.810 ☑
    unstable S32.811 ☑
  traumatic injury wound repair T81.33 ☑
  wound T81.30 ☑
    episiotomy O90.1
    operation T81.31 ☑
      cesarean O90.0
      external operation wound (superficial)
        T81.31 ☑
      internal operation wound (deep) T81.32 ☑
    perineal (obstetric) O90.1
    traumatic injury repair T81.33 ☑

Dissatisfaction with
  employment Z56.9
  school environment Z55.4
Dissecting — *see* condition
Dissection
  aorta I71.00
    abdominal I71.02
    thoracic I71.01
    thoracoabdominal I71.03
  artery
    carotid I77.71
    cerebral (nonruptured) I67.0
      ruptured — *see* Hemorrhage, intracranial,
        subarachnoid
    coronary I25.42
    iliac I77.72
    renal I77.73
    specified NEC I77.79
    vertebral I77.74
  traumatic — *see* Wound, open, by site
  vascular I99.8
  wound — *see* Wound, open
Disseminated — *see* condition
Dissociation
  auriculoventricular or atrioventricular (AV) (any de-
    gree) (isorhythmic) I45.89
    with heart block I44.2
  interference I45.89
Dissociative reaction, state F44.9
Dissolution, vertebra — *see* Osteoporosis
Distension, distention
  abdomen R14.0
  bladder N32.89
  cecum K63.89
  colon K63.89
  gallbladder K82.8
  intestine K63.89
  kidney N28.89
  liver K76.89
  seminal vesicle N50.8
  stomach K31.89
    acute K31.0
    psychogenic F45.8
  ureter — *see* Dilatation, ureter
  uterus N85.8
Distoma hepaticum infestation B66.3
Distomiasis B66.9
  bile passages B66.3
  hemic B65.9
  hepatic B66.3
    due to Clonorchis sinensis B66.1
  intestinal B66.5
  liver B66.3
    due to Clonorchis sinensis B66.1
  lung B66.4
  pulmonary B66.4
Distomolar (fourth molar) K00.1
Disto-occlusion (Division I) (Division II) M26.212
Distortion(s) (congenital)
  adrenal (gland) Q89.1
  arm NEC Q68.8
  bile duct or passage Q44.5
  bladder Q64.79
  brain Q04.9
  cervix (uteri) Q51.9
  chest (wall) Q67.8

Distortion(s) — *continued*
  chest (wall) Q67.8
    bones Q76.8
  clavicle Q74.0
  clitoris Q52.6
  coccyx Q76.49
  common duct Q44.5
  coronary Q24.5
  cystic duct Q44.5
  ear (auricle) (external) Q17.3
    inner Q16.5
    middle Q16.4
      ossicles Q16.3
  endocrine NEC Q89.2
  eustachian tube Q17.8
  eye (adnexa) Q15.8
  face bone(s) NEC Q75.8
  fallopian tube Q50.6
  femur NEC Q68.8
  fibula NEC Q68.8
  finger(s) Q68.1
  foot Q66.9
  genitalia, genital organ(s)
    female Q52.8
      external Q52.79
      internal NEC Q52.8
  gyri Q04.8
  hand bone(s) Q68.1
  heart (auricle) (ventricle) Q24.8
    valve (cusp) Q24.8
  hepatic duct Q44.5
  humerus NEC Q68.8
  hymen Q52.4
  intrafamilial communications Z63.8
  jaw NEC M26.89
  labium (majus) (minus) Q52.79
  leg NEC Q68.8
  lens Q12.8
  liver Q44.7
  lumbar spine Q76.49
    with disproportion O33.8
      causing obstructed labor O65.0
  lumbosacral (joint) (region) Q76.49
    kyphosis — *see* Kyphosis, congenital
    lordosis — *see* Lordosis, congenital
  nerve Q07.8
  nose Q30.8
  organ
    of Corti Q16.5
    or site not listed — *see* Anomaly, by site
  ossicles, ear Q16.3
  oviduct Q50.6
  pancreas Q45.3
  parathyroid (gland) Q89.2
  pituitary (gland) Q89.2
  radius NEC Q68.8
  sacroiliac joint Q74.2
  sacrum Q76.49
  scapula Q74.0
  shoulder girdle Q74.0
  skull bone(s) NEC Q75.8
    with
      anencephalus Q00.0
      encephalocele — *see* Encephalocele
      hydrocephalus Q03.9
        with spina bifida — *see* Spina bifida, with
          hydrocephalus
      microcephaly Q02
  spinal cord Q06.8
  spine Q76.49
    kyphosis — *see* Kyphosis, congenital
    lordosis — *see* Lordosis, congenital
  spleen Q89.09
  sternum NEC Q76.7
  thorax (wall) Q67.8
    bony Q76.8
  thymus (gland) Q89.2
  thyroid (gland) Q89.2
  tibia NEC Q68.8
  toe(s) Q66.9
  tongue Q38.3
  trachea (cartilage) Q32.1
  ulna NEC Q68.8
  ureter Q62.8
  urethra Q64.79
    causing obstruction Q64.39
  uterus Q51.9
  vagina Q52.4

Distortion(s) — *continued*
  vertebra Q76.49
    kyphosis — *see* Kyphosis, congenital
    lordosis — *see* Lordosis, congenital
  visual (*see also* Disturbance, vision)
    shape and size H53.15
  vulva Q52.79
  wrist (bones) (joint) Q68.8
Distress
  abdomen — *see* Pain, abdominal
  acute respiratory (adult) (child) J80
  epigastric R10.13
  fetal P84
    complicating pregnancy — *see* Stress, fetal
  gastrointestinal (functional) K30
    psychogenic F45.8
  intestinal (functional) NOS K59.9
    psychogenic F45.8
  maternal, during labor and delivery O75.0
  respiratory R06.00
    adult J80
    child J80
    newborn P22.9
      specified NEC P22.8
    orthopnea R06.01
    psychogenic F45.8
    shortness of breath R06.02
    specified type NEC R06.09
Distribution vessel, atypical Q27.9
  coronary artery Q24.5
  precerebral Q28.1
Districhiasis L68.8
Disturbance(s) (*see also* Disease)
  absorption K90.9
    calcium E58
    carbohydrate K90.4
    fat K90.4
      pancreatic K90.3
    protein K90.4
    starch K90.4
    vitamin — *see* Deficiency, vitamin
  acid-base equilibrium E87.8
    mixed E87.4
  activity and attention (with hyperkinesis) — *see* Disor-
    der, attention-deficit hyperactivity
  amino acid transport E72.00
  assimilation, food K90.9
  auditory nerve, except deafness — *see* subcategory
    H93.3 ☑
  behavior — *see* Disorder, conduct
  blood clotting (mechanism) (*see also* Defect, coagula-
    tion) D68.9
  cerebral
    nerve — *see* Disorder, nerve, cranial
    status, newborn P91.9
      specified NEC P91.8
  circulatory I99.9
  conduct (*see also* Disorder, conduct) F91.9
    adjustment reaction — *see* Disorder, adjustment
    compulsive F63.9
    disruptive F91.9
    hyperkinetic — *see* Disorder, attention-deficit hy-
      peractivity
    socialized F91.2
    specified NEC F91.8
    unsocialized F91.1
  coordination R27.8
  cranial nerve — *see* Disorder, nerve, cranial
  deep sensibility — *see* Disturbance, sensation
  digestive K30
    psychogenic F45.8
  electrolyte (*see also* Imbalance, electrolyte)
    newborn, transitory P74.4
      hyperammonemia P74.6
      potassium balance P74.3
      sodium balance P74.2
      specified type NEC P74.4
  emotions specific to childhood and adolescence F93.9
    with
      anxiety and fearfulness NEC F93.8
      elective mutism F94.0
      oppositional disorder F91.3
      sensitivity (withdrawal) F40.10
      shyness F40.10
      social withdrawal F40.10
    involving relationship problems F93.8
    mixed F93.8
    specified NEC F93.8

Disturbance(s) — *continued*
  endocrine (gland) E34.9
    neonatal, transitory P72.9
      specified NEC P72.8
  equilibrium R42
  fructose metabolism E74.10
  gait — *see* Gait
    hysterical F44.4
    psychogenic F44.4
  gastrointestinal (functional) K30
    psychogenic F45.8
  habit, child F98.9
  hearing, except deafness and tinnitus — *see* Abnormal, auditory perception
  heart, functional (conditions in I44-I50)
    due to presence of (cardiac) prosthesis I97.19- ☑
    postoperative I97.89
      cardiac surgery I97.19- ☑
  hormones E34.9
  innervation uterus (parasympathetic) (sympathetic) N85.8
  keratinization NEC
    gingiva K05.10
      nonplaque induced K05.11
      plaque induced K05.10
    lip K13.0
    oral (mucosa) (soft tissue) K13.29
    tongue K13.29
  learning (specific) — *see* Disorder, learning
  memory — *see* Amnesia
    mild, following organic brain damage F06.8
  mental F99
    associated with diseases classified elsewhere F54
  metabolism E88.9
    with
      abortion — *see* Abortion, by type with other specified complication
      ectopic pregnancy O08.5
      molar pregnancy O08.5
    amino-acid E72.9
      aromatic E70.9
      branched-chain E71.2
      straight-chain E72.8
      sulfur-bearing E72.10
    ammonia E72.20
    arginine E72.21
    arginosuccinic acid E72.22
    carbohydrate E74.9
    cholesterol E78.9
    citrulline E72.23
    cystathionine E72.19
    general E88.9
    glutamine E72.8
    histidine E70.40
    homocystine E72.19
    hydroxylysine E72.3
    in labor or delivery O75.89
    iron E83.10
    lipoid E78.9
    lysine E72.3
    methionine E72.19
    neonatal, transitory P74.9
      calcium and magnesium P71.9
        specified type NEC P71.8
      carbohydrate metabolism P70.9
        specified type NEC P70.8
      specified NEC P74.8
    ornithine E72.4
    phosphate E83.39
    sodium NEC E87.8
    threonine E72.8
    tryptophan E70.5
    tyrosine E70.20
    urea cycle E72.20
  motor R29.2
  nervous, functional R45.0
  neuromuscular mechanism (eye), due to syphilis A52.15
  nutritional E63.9
    nail L60.3
  ocular motion H51.9
    psychogenic F45.8
  oculogyric H51.8
    psychogenic F45.8
  oculomotor H51.9
    psychogenic F45.8
  olfactory nerve R43.1
  optic nerve NEC — *see* Disorder, nerve, optic

Disturbance(s) — *continued*
  oral epithelium, including tongue NEC K13.29
  perceptual due to
    alcohol withdrawal F10.232
    amphetamine intoxication F15.922
      in
        abuse F15.122
        dependence F15.222
    anxiolytic withdrawal F13.232
    cannabis intoxication (acute) F12.922
      in
        abuse F12.122
        dependence F12.222
    cocaine intoxication (acute) F14.922
      in
        abuse F14.122
        dependence F14.222
    hypnotic withdrawal F13.232
    opioid intoxication (acute) F11.922
      in
        abuse F11.122
        dependence F11.222
    phencyclidine intoxication (acute) F19.922
      in
        abuse F19.122
        dependence F19.222
    sedative withdrawal F13.232
  personality (pattern) (trait) (*see also* Disorder, personality) F60.9
    following organic brain damage F07.9
  polyglandular E31.9
    specified NEC E31.8
  potassium balance, newborn P74.3
  psychogenic F45.9
  psychomotor F44.4
  psychophysical visual H53.16
  pupillary — *see* Anomaly, pupil, function
  reflex R29.2
  rhythm, heart I49.9
  salivary secretion K11.7
  sensation (cold) (heat) (localization) (tactile discrimination) (texture) (vibratory) NEC R20.9
    hysterical F44.6
    skin R20.9
      anesthesia R20.0
      hyperesthesia R20.3
      hypoesthesia R20.1
      paresthesia R20.2
      specified type NEC R20.8
    smell R43.9
      and taste (mixed) R43.8
      anosmia R43.0
      parosmia R43.1
      specified NEC R43.8
    taste R43.9
      and smell (mixed) R43.8
      parageusia R43.2
      specified NEC R43.8
  sensory — *see* Disturbance, sensation
  situational (transient) (*see also* Disorder, adjustment)
    acute F43.0
  sleep G47.9
    nonorganic origin F51.9
  smell — *see* Disturbance, sensation, smell
  sociopathic F60.2
  sodium balance, newborn P74.2
  speech R47.9
    developmental F80.9
    specified NEC R47.89
  stomach (functional) K31.9
  sympathetic (nerve) G90.9
  taste — *see* Disturbance, sensation, taste
  temperature
    regulation, newborn P81.9
      specified NEC P81.8
    sense R20.8
      hysterical F44.6
  tooth
    eruption K00.6
    formation K00.4
    structure, hereditary NEC K00.5
  touch — *see* Disturbance, sensation
  vascular I99.9
    arteriosclerotic — *see* Arteriosclerosis
  vasomotor I73.9
  vasospastic I73.9
  vision, visual H53.9

Disturbance(s) — *continued*
  vision, visual — *continued*
    following
      cerebral infarction I69.398
      cerebrovascular disease I69.998
        specified NEC I69.898
      intracerebral hemorrhage I69.198
      nontraumatic intracranial hemorrhage NEC I69.298
      specified disease NEC I69.898
      subarachnoid hemorrhage I69.098
    psychophysical H53.16
    specified NEC H53.8
    subjective H53.10
      day blindness H53.11
      discomfort H53.14- ☑
      distortions of shape and size H53.15
      loss
        sudden H53.13- ☑
        transient H53.12- ☑
      specified type NEC H53.19
  voice R49.9
    psychogenic F44.4
    specified NEC R49.8
Diuresis R35.8
Diver's palsy, paralysis or squeeze T70.3 ☑
Diverticulitis (acute) K57.92
  bladder — *see* Cystitis
  ileum — *see* Diverticulitis, intestine, small
  intestine K57.92
    with
      abscess, perforation or peritonitis K57.80
        with bleeding K57.81
      bleeding K57.93
    congenital Q43.8
    large K57.32
      with
        abscess, perforation or peritonitis K57.20
          with bleeding K57.21
        bleeding K57.33
        small intestine K57.52
          with
            abscess, perforation or peritonitis K57.40
              with bleeding K57.41
            bleeding K57.53
    small K57.12
      with
        abscess, perforation or peritonitis K57.00
          with bleeding K57.01
        bleeding K57.13
        large intestine K57.52
          with
            abscess, perforation or peritonitis K57.40
              with bleeding K57.41
            bleeding K57.53
Diverticulosis K57.90
  with bleeding K57.91
  large intestine K57.30
    with
      bleeding K57.31
      small intestine K57.50
        with bleeding K57.51
  small intestine K57.10
    with
      bleeding K57.11
      large intestine K57.50
        with bleeding K57.51
Diverticulum, diverticula (multiple) K57.90
  appendix (noninflammatory) K38.2
  bladder (sphincter) N32.3
    congenital Q64.6
  bronchus (congenital) Q32.4
    acquired J98.09
  calyx, calyceal (kidney) N28.89
  cardia (stomach) K31.4
  cecum — *see* Diverticulosis, intestine, large
    congenital Q43.8
  colon — *see* Diverticulosis, intestine, large
    congenital Q43.8
  duodenum — *see* Diverticulosis, intestine, small
    congenital Q43.8
  epiphrenic (esophagus) K22.5
  esophagus (congenital) Q39.6
    acquired (epiphrenic) (pulsion) (traction) K22.5
  eustachian tube — *see* Disorder, eustachian tube, specified NEC

Diverticulum, diverticula — *continued*
　fallopian tube N83.8
　gastric K31.4
　heart (congenital) Q24.8
　ileum — *see* Diverticulosis, intestine, small
　jejunum — *see* Diverticulosis, intestine, small
　kidney (pelvis) (calyces) N28.89
　　with calculus — *see* Calculus, kidney
　Meckel's (displaced) (hypertrophic) Q43.0
　　malignant — *see* Table of Neoplasms, small intestine, malignant
　midthoracic K22.5
　organ or site, congenital NEC — *see* Distortion
　pericardium (congenital) (cyst) Q24.8
　　acquired I31.8
　pharyngoesophageal (congenital) Q39.6
　　acquired K22.5
　pharynx (congenital) Q38.7
　rectosigmoid — *see* Diverticulosis, intestine, large
　　congenital Q43.8
　rectum — *see* Diverticulosis, intestine, large
　Rokitansky's K22.5
　seminal vesicle N50.8
　sigmoid — *see* Diverticulosis, intestine, large
　　congenital Q43.8
　stomach (acquired) K31.4
　　congenital Q40.2
　trachea (acquired) J39.8
　ureter (acquired) N28.89
　　congenital Q62.8
　ureterovesical orifice N28.89
　urethra (acquired) N36.1
　　congenital Q64.79
　ventricle, left (congenital) Q24.8
　vesical N32.3
　　congenital Q64.6
　Zenker's (esophagus) K22.5
Division
　cervix uteri (acquired) N88.8
　glans penis Q55.69
　labia minora (congenital) Q52.79
　ligament (partial or complete) (current) (*see also* Sprain)
　　with open wound — *see* Wound, open
　muscle (partial or complete) (current) (*see also* Injury, muscle)
　　with open wound — *see* Wound, open
　nerve (traumatic) — *see* Injury, nerve
　spinal cord — *see* Injury, spinal cord, by region
　vein I87.8
Divorce, causing family disruption Z63.5
Dix-Hallpike neurolabyrinthitis — *see* Neuronitis, vestibular
Dizziness R42
　hysterical F44.89
　psychogenic F45.8
DMAC (disseminated mycobacterium avium- intracellulare complex) A31.2
DNR (do not resuscitate) Z66
Doan-Wiseman syndrome (primary splenic neutropenia) — *see* Agranulocytosis
Doehle-Heller aortitis A52.02
Dog bite — *see* Bite
Dohle body panmyelopathic syndrome D72.0
Dolichocephaly Q67.2
Dolichocolon Q43.8
Dolichostenomelia — *see* Syndrome, Marfan's
Donohue's syndrome E34.8
Donor (organ or tissue) Z52.9
　blood (whole) Z52.000
　　autologous Z52.010
　　specified component (lymphocytes) (platelets) NEC Z52.008
　　　autologous Z52.018
　　　specified donor NEC Z52.098
　　specified donor NEC Z52.090
　　stem cells Z52.001
　　　autologous Z52.011
　　　specified donor NEC Z52.091
　bone Z52.20
　　autologous Z52.21
　　marrow Z52.3
　　specified type NEC Z52.29
　cornea Z52.5
　egg (Oocyte) Z52.819
　　age 35 and over Z52.812
　　　anonymous recipient Z52.812
　　　designated recipient Z52.813

Donor — *continued*
　egg — *continued*
　　under age 35 Z52.810
　　　anonymous recipient Z52.810
　　　designated recipient Z52.811
　kidney Z52.4
　liver Z52.6
　lung Z52.89
　lymphocyte — *see* Donor, blood, specified components NEC
　Oocyte — *see* Donor, egg
　platelets Z52.008
　potential, examination of Z00.5
　semen Z52.89
　skin Z52.10
　　autologous Z52.11
　　specified type NEC Z52.19
　specified organ or tissue NEC Z52.89
　sperm Z52.89
Donovanosis A58
Dorsalgia M54.9
　psychogenic F45.41
　specified NEC M54.89
Dorsopathy M53.9
　deforming M43.9
　　specified NEC — *see* subcategory M43.8 ☑
　specified NEC M53.80
　　cervical region M53.82
　　cervicothoracic region M53.83
　　lumbar region M53.86
　　lumbosacral region M53.87
　　occipito-atlanto-axial region M53.81
　　sacrococcygeal region M53.88
　　thoracic region M53.84
　　thoracolumbar region M53.85
Double
　albumin E88.09
　aortic arch Q25.4
　auditory canal Q17.8
　auricle (heart) Q20.8
　bladder Q64.79
　cervix Q51.820
　　with doubling of uterus (and vagina) Q51.10
　　　with obstruction Q51.11
　inlet ventricle Q20.4
　kidney with double pelvis (renal) Q63.0
　meatus urinarius Q64.75
　monster Q89.4
　outlet
　　left ventricle Q20.2
　　right ventricle Q20.1
　pelvis (renal) with double ureter Q62.5
　tongue Q38.3
　ureter (one or both sides) Q62.5
　　with double pelvis (renal) Q62.5
　urethra Q64.74
　urinary meatus Q64.75
　uterus Q51.2
　　with
　　　doubling of cervix (and vagina) Q51.10
　　　　with obstruction Q51.11
　　in pregnancy or childbirth O34.59- ☑
　　　causing obstructed labor O65.5
　vagina Q52.10
　　with doubling of uterus (and cervix) Q51.10
　　　with obstruction Q51.11
　vision H53.2
　vulva Q52.79
Douglas' pouch, cul-de-sac — *see* condition
Down syndrome Q90.9
　meiotic nondisjunction Q90.0
　mitotic nondisjunction Q90.1
　mosaicism Q90.1
　translocation Q90.2
DPD (dihydropyrimidine dehydrogenase deficiency) E88.89
Dracontiasis B72
Dracunculiasis, dracunculosis B72
Dream state, hysterical F44.89
Drepanocytic anemia — *see* Disease, sickle-cell
Dresbach's syndrome (elliptocytosis) D58.1
Dreschlera (hawaiiensis) (infection) B43.8
Dressler's syndrome I24.1
Drift, ulnar — *see* Deformity, limb, specified type NEC, forearm

Drinking (alcohol)
　excessive, to excess NEC (without dependence) F10.10
　　habitual (continual) (without remission) F10.20
　　　with remission F10.21
Drip, postnasal (chronic) R09.82
　due to
　　allergic rhinitis — *see* Rhinitis, allergic
　　common cold J00
　　gastroesophageal reflux — *see* Reflux, gastroesophageal
　　nasopharyngitis — *see* Nasopharyngitis
　　other known condition — *code to* condition
　　sinusitis — *see* Sinusitis
Droop
　facial R29.810
　　cerebrovascular disease I69.992
　　　cerebral infarction I69.392
　　　intracerebral hemorrhage I69.192
　　　nontraumatic intracranial hemorrhage NEC I69.292
　　　specified disease NEC I69.892
　　　subarachnoid hemorrhage I69.092
Drop (in)
　attack NEC R55
　finger — *see* Deformity, finger
　foot — *see* Deformity, limb, foot, drop
　hematocrit (precipitous) R71.0
　hemoglobin R71.0
　toe — *see* Deformity, toe, specified NEC
　wrist — *see* Deformity, limb, wrist drop
Dropped heart beats I45.9
Dropsy, dropsical (*see also* Hydrops)
　abdomen R18.8
　brain — *see* Hydrocephalus
　cardiac, heart — *see* Failure, heart, congestive
　gangrenous — *see* Gangrene
　heart — *see* Failure, heart, congestive
　kidney — *see* Nephrosis
　lung — *see* Edema, lung
　newborn due to isoimmunization P56.0
　pericardium — *see* Pericarditis
Drowned, drowning (near) T75.1 ☑
Drowsiness R40.0
Drug
　abuse counseling and surveillance Z71.51
　addiction — *see* Dependence
　dependence — *see* Dependence
　habit — *see* Dependence
　harmful use — *see* Abuse, drug
　induced fever R50.2
　overdose — *see* Table of Drugs and Chemicals, by drug, poisoning
　poisoning — *see* Table of Drugs and Chemicals, by drug, poisoning
　resistant organism infection (*see also* Resistant, organism, to, drug) Z16.30
　therapy
　　long term (current) (prophylactic) — *see* Therapy, drug long-term (current) (prophylactic)
　　short term — *omit code*
　wrong substance given or taken in error — *see* Table of Drugs and Chemicals, by drug, poisoning
Drunkenness (without dependence) F10.129
　acute in alcoholism F10.229
　chronic (without remission) F10.20
　　with remission F10.21
　pathological (without dependence) F10.129
　　with dependence F10.229
　sleep F51.9
Drusen
　macula (degenerative) (retina) — *see* Degeneration, macula, drusen
　optic disc H47.32- ☑
Dry, dryness (*see also* condition)
　larynx J38.7
　mouth R68.2
　　due to dehydration E86.0
　nose J34.89
　socket (teeth) M27.3
　throat J39.2
DSAP L56.5
Duane's syndrome H50.81- ☑
Dubin-Johnson disease or syndrome E80.6
Dubois' disease (thymus gland) A50.59 [E35]
Dubowitz' syndrome Q87.1
Duchenne-Aran muscular atrophy G12.21
Duchenne-Griesinger disease G71.0

Duchenne's
disease or syndrome
motor neuron disease G12.22
muscular dystrophy G71.0
locomotor ataxia (syphilitic) A52.11
paralysis
birth injury P14.0
due to or associated with
motor neuron disease G12.22
muscular dystrophy G71.0
Ducrey's chancre A57
Duct, ductus — *see* condition
Duhring's disease (dermatitis herpetiformis) L13.0
Dullness, cardiac (decreased) (increased) R01.2
Dumb ague — *see* Malaria
Dumbness — *see* Aphasia
Dumdum fever B55.0
Dumping syndrome (postgastrectomy) K91.1
Duodenitis (nonspecific) (peptic) K29.80
with bleeding K29.81
Duodenocholangitis — *see* Cholangitis
Duodenum, duodenal — *see* condition
Duplay's bursitis or periarthritis — *see* Tendinitis, calcific, shoulder
Duplication, duplex (*see also* Accessory)
alimentary tract Q45.8
anus Q43.4
appendix (and cecum) Q43.4
biliary duct (any) Q44.5
bladder Q64.79
cecum (and appendix) Q43.4
cervix Q51.820
chromosome NEC
with complex rearrangements NEC Q92.5
seen only at prometaphase Q92.8
cystic duct Q44.5
digestive organs Q45.8
esophagus Q39.8
frontonasal process Q75.8
intestine (large) (small) Q43.4
kidney Q63.0
liver Q44.7
pancreas Q45.3
penis Q55.69
respiratory organs NEC Q34.8
salivary duct Q38.4
spinal cord (incomplete) Q06.2
stomach Q40.2
Dupré's disease (meningism) R29.1
Dupuytren's contraction or disease M72.0
Durand-Nicolas-Favre disease A55
Durotomy (inadvertent) (incidental) G97.41
Duroziez's disease (congenital mitral stenosis) Q23.2
Dutton's relapsing fever (West African) A68.1
Dwarfism E34.3
achondroplastic Q77.4
congenital E34.3
constitutional E34.3
hypochondroplastic Q77.4
hypophyseal E23.0
infantile E34.3
Laron-type E34.3
Lorain (-Levi) type E23.0
metatropic Q77.8
nephrotic-glycosuric (with hypophosphatemic rickets) E72.09
nutritional E45
pancreatic K86.8
pituitary E23.0
renal N25.0
thanatophoric Q77.1
Dyke-Young anemia (secondary) (symptomatic) D59.1
Dysacusis — *see* Abnormal, auditory perception
Dysadrenocortism E27.9
hyperfunction E27.0
Dysarthria R47.1
following
cerebral infarction I69.322
cerebrovascular disease I69.922
specified disease NEC I69.822
intracerebral hemorrhage I69.122
nontraumatic intracranial hemorrhage NEC I69.222
subarachnoid hemorrhage I69.022
Dysautonomia (familial) G90.1
Dysbarism T70.3 ☑
Dysbasia R26.2
angiosclerotica intermittens I73.9
hysterical F44.4

Dysbasia — *continued*
lordotica (progressiva) G24.1
nonorganic origin F44.4
psychogenic F44.4
Dysbetalipoproteinemia (familial) E78.2
Dyscalculia R48.8
developmental F81.2
Dyschezia K59.00
Dyschondroplasia (with hemangiomata) Q78.4
Dyschromia (skin) L81.9
Dyscollagenosis M35.9
Dyscranio-pygo-phalangy Q87.0
Dyscrasia
blood (with) D75.9
antepartum hemorrhage — *see* Hemorrhage, antepartum, with coagulation defect
intrapartum hemorrhage O67.0
newborn P61.9
specified type NEC P61.8
puerperal, postpartum O72.3
polyglandular, pluriglandular E31.9
Dysendocrinism E34.9
Dysentery, dysenteric (catarrhal) (diarrhea) (epidemic) (hemorrhagic) (infectious) (sporadic) (tropical) A09
abscess, liver A06.4
amebic (*see also* Amebiasis) A06.0
with abscess — *see* Abscess, amebic
acute A06.0
chronic A06.1
arthritis (*see also* category M01) A09
bacillary (*see also* category M01) A03.9
bacillary A03.9
arthritis (*see also* category M01) A03.9
Boyd A03.2
Flexner A03.1
Schmitz (-Stutzer) A03.0
Shiga (-Kruse) A03.0
Shigella A03.9
boydii A03.2
dysenteriae A03.0
flexneri A03.1
group A A03.0
group B A03.1
group C A03.2
group D A03.3
sonnei A03.3
specified type NEC A03.8
Sonne A03.3
specified type NEC A03.8
balantidial A07.0
Balantidium coli A07.0
Boyd's A03.2
candidal B37.82
Chilomastix A07.8
Chinese A03.9
coccidial A07.3
Dientamoeba (fragilis) A07.8
Embadomonas A07.8
Entamoeba, entamebic — *see* Dysentery, amebic
Flexner-Boyd A03.2
Flexner's A03.1
Giardia lamblia A07.1
Hiss-Russell A03.1
Lamblia A07.1
leishmanial B55.0
malarial — *see* Malaria
metazoal B82.0
monilial B37.82
protozoal A07.9
Salmonella A02.0
schistosomal B65.1
Schmitz (-Stutzer) A03.0
Shiga (-Kruse) A03.0
Shigella NOS — *see* Dysentery, bacillary
Sonne A03.3
strongyloidiasis B78.0
trichomonal A07.8
viral (*see also* Enteritis, viral) A08.4
Dysequilibrium R42
Dysesthesia R20.8
hysterical F44.6
Dysfibrinogenemia (congenital) D68.2
Dysfunction
adrenal E27.9
hyperfunction E27.0
autonomic
due to alcohol G31.2
somatoform F45.8

Dysfunction — *continued*
bladder N31.9
neurogenic NOS — *see* Dysfunction, bladder, neuromuscular
neuromuscular NOS N31.9
atonic (motor) (sensory) N31.2
autonomous N31.2
flaccid N31.2
nonreflex N31.2
reflex N31.1
specified NEC N31.8
uninhibited N31.0
bleeding, uterus N93.8
cerebral G93.89
colon K59.9
psychogenic F45.8
colostomy K94.03
cystic duct K82.8
cystostomy (stoma) — *see* Complications, cystostomy
ejaculatory N53.19
anejaculatory orgasm N53.13
painful N53.12
premature F52.4
retarded N53.11
endocrine NOS E34.9
endometrium N85.8
enterostomy K94.13
gallbladder K82.8
gastrostomy (stoma) K94.23
gland, glandular NOS E34.9
heart I51.89
hemoglobin D75.89
hepatic K76.89
hypophysis E23.7
hypothalamic NEC E23.3
ileostomy (stoma) K94.13
jejunostomy (stoma) K94.13
kidney — *see* Disease, renal
labyrinthine — *see* subcategory H83.2 ☑
left ventricular, following sudden emotional stress I51.81
liver K76.89
male — *see* Dysfunction, sexual, male
orgasmic (female) F52.31
male F52.32
ovary E28.9
specified NEC E28.8
papillary muscle I51.89
parathyroid E21.4
physiological NEC R68.89
psychogenic F59
pineal gland E34.8
pituitary (gland) E23.3
platelets D69.1
polyglandular E31.9
specified NEC E31.8
psychophysiologic F59
psychosexual F52.9
with
dyspareunia F52.6
premature ejaculation F52.4
vaginismus F52.5
pylorus K31.9
rectum K59.9
psychogenic F45.8
reflex (sympathetic) — *see* Syndrome, pain, complex regional I
segmental — *see* Dysfunction, somatic
senile R54
sexual (due to) R37
alcohol F10.981
amphetamine F15.981
in
abuse F15.181
dependence F15.281
anxiolytic F13.981
in
abuse F13.181
dependence F13.281
cocaine F14.981
in
abuse F14.181
dependence F14.281
excessive sexual drive F52.8
failure of genital response (male) F52.21
female F52.22
female N94.9
aversion F52.1

Dysfunction — *continued*
  sexual — *continued*
    female — *continued*
      dyspareunia N94.1
        psychogenic F52.6
      frigidity F52.22
      nymphomania F52.8
      orgasmic F52.31
      psychogenic F52.9
        aversion F52.1
        dyspareunia F52.6
        frigidity F52.22
        nymphomania F52.8
        orgasmic F52.31
        vaginismus F52.5
      vaginismus N94.2
        psychogenic F52.5
    hypnotic F13.981
      in
        abuse F13.181
        dependence F13.281
    inhibited orgasm (female) F52.31
      male F52.32
    lack
      of sexual enjoyment F52.1
      or loss of sexual desire F52.0
    male N53.9
      anejaculatory orgasm N53.13
      ejaculatory N53.19
        painful N53.12
        premature F52.4
        retarded N53.11
      erectile N52.9
        drug induced N52.2
        due to
          disease classified elsewhere N52.1
          drug N52.2
        postoperative (postprocedural) N52.39
          following
            prostatectomy N52.34
              radical N52.31
            radical cystectomy N52.32
            urethral surgery N52.33
        psychogenic F52.21
        specified cause NEC N52.8
        vasculogenic
          arterial insufficiency N52.01
            with corporo-venous occlusive N52.03
          corporo-venous occlusive N52.02
            with arterial insufficiency N52.03
      impotence — *see* Dysfunction, sexual, male, erectile
      psychogenic F52.9
        aversion F52.1
        erectile F52.21
        orgasmic F52.32
        premature ejaculation F52.4
        satyriasis F52.8
        specified type NEC F52.8
      specified type NEC N53.8
    nonorganic F52.9
      specified NEC F52.8
    opioid F11.981
      in
        abuse F11.181
        dependence F11.281
    orgasmic dysfunction (female) F52.31
      male F52.32
    premature ejaculation F52.4
    psychoactive substances NEC F19.981
      in
        abuse F19.181
        dependence F19.281
    psychogenic F52.9
    sedative F13.981
      in
        abuse F13.181
        dependence F13.281
    sexual aversion F52.1
    vaginismus (nonorganic) (psychogenic) F52.5
  sinoatrial node I49.5
  somatic M99.09
    abdomen M99.09
    acromioclavicular M99.07
    cervical region M99.01
    cervicothoracic M99.01
    costochondral M99.08

Dysfunction — *continued*
  somatic — *continued*
    costovertebral M99.08
    head region M99.00
    hip M99.05
    lower extremity M99.06
    lumbar region M99.03
    lumbosacral M99.03
    occipitocervical M99.00
    pelvic region M99.05
    pubic M99.05
    rib cage M99.08
    sacral region M99.04
    sacrococcygeal M99.04
    sacroiliac M99.04
    specified NEC M99.09
    sternochondral M99.08
    sternoclavicular M99.07
    thoracic region M99.02
    thoracolumbar M99.02
    upper extremity M99.07
  somatoform autonomic F45.8
  stomach K31.89
    psychogenic F45.8
  suprarenal E27.9
    hyperfunction E27.0
  symbolic R48.9
    specified type NEC R48.8
  temporomandibular (joint) M26.69
    joint-pain syndrome M26.62
  testicular (endocrine) E29.9
    specified NEC E29.8
  thymus E32.9
  thyroid E07.9
  ureterostomy (stoma) — *see* Complications, stoma, urinary tract
  urethrostomy (stoma) — *see* Complications, stoma, urinary tract
  uterus, complicating delivery O62.9
    hypertonic O62.4
    hypotonic O62.2
      primary O62.0
      secondary O62.1
  ventricular I51.9
    with congestive heart failure I50.9
    left, reversible, following sudden emotional stress I51.81

Dysgenesis
  gonadal (due to chromosomal anomaly) Q96.9
    pure Q99.1
  renal Q60.5
    bilateral Q60.4
    unilateral Q60.3
  reticular D72.0
  tidal platelet D69.3

Dysgerminoma
  specified site — *see* Neoplasm, malignant, by site
  unspecified site
    female C56.9
    male C62.90

Dysgeusia R43.2
Dysgraphia R27.8
Dyshidrosis, dysidrosis L30.1
Dyskaryotic cervical smear R87.619
Dyskeratosis L85.8
  cervix — *see* Dysplasia, cervix
  congenital Q82.8
  uterus NEC N85.8
Dyskinesia G24.9
  biliary (cystic duct or gallbladder) K82.8
  drug induced
    orofacial G24.01
  esophagus K22.4
  hysterical F44.4
  intestinal K59.8
  nonorganic origin F44.4
  orofacial (idiopathic) G24.4
    drug induced G24.01
  psychogenic F44.4
  subacute, drug induced G24.01
  tardive G24.01
    neuroleptic induced G24.01
  trachea J39.8
  tracheobronchial J98.09
Dyslalia (developmental) F80.0
Dyslexia R48.0
  developmental F81.0

Dyslipidemia E78.5
  depressed HDL cholesterol E78.6
  elevated fasting triglycerides E78.1
Dysmaturity (*see also* Light for dates)
  pulmonary (newborn) (Wilson-Mikity) P27.0
Dysmenorrhea (essential) (exfoliative) N94.6
  congestive (syndrome) N94.6
  primary N94.4
  psychogenic F45.8
  secondary N94.5
Dysmetabolic syndrome X E88.81
Dysmetria R27.8
Dysmorphism (due to)
  alcohol Q86.0
  exogenous cause NEC Q86.8
  hydantoin Q86.1
  warfarin Q86.2
Dysmorphophobia (nondelusional) F45.22
  delusional F22
Dysnomia R47.01
Dysorexia R63.0
  psychogenic F50.8
Dysostosis
  cleidocranial, cleidocranialis Q74.0
  craniofacial Q75.1
  Fairbank's (idiopathic familial generalized osteophytosis) Q78.9
  mandibulofacial (incomplete) Q75.4
  multiplex E76.01
  oculomandibular Q75.5
Dyspareunia (female) N94.1
  male N53.12
  nonorganic F52.6
  psychogenic F52.6
  secondary N94.1
Dyspepsia R10.13
  atonic K30
  functional (allergic) (congenital) (gastrointestinal) (occupational) (reflex) K30
  intestinal K59.8
  nervous F45.8
  neurotic F45.8
  psychogenic F45.8
Dysphagia R13.10
  cervical R13.19
  following
    cerebral infarction I69.391
    cerebrovascular disease I69.991
      specified NEC I69.891
    intracerebral hemorrhage I69.191
    nontraumatic intracranial hemorrhage NEC I69.291
    specified disease NEC I69.891
    subarachnoid hemorrhage I69.091
  functional (hysterical) F45.8
  hysterical F45.8
  nervous (hysterical) F45.8
  neurogenic R13.19
  oral phase R13.11
  oropharyngeal phase R13.12
  pharyneal phase R13.13
  pharyngoesophageal phase R13.14
  psychogenic F45.8
  sideropenic D50.1
  spastica K22.4
  specified NEC R13.19
Dysphagocytosis, congenital D71
Dysphasia R47.02
  developmental
    expressive type F80.1
    receptive type F80.2
  following
    cerebrovascular disease I69.921
      cerebral infarction I69.321
      intracerebral hemorrhage I69.121
      nontraumatic intracranial hemorrhage NEC I69.221
      specified disease NEC I69.821
      subarachnoid hemorrhage I69.021
Dysphonia R49.0
  functional F44.4
  hysterical F44.4
  psychogenic F44.4
  spastica J38.3
Dysphoria, postpartal O90.6
Dyspituitarism E23.3
Dysplasia (*see also* Anomaly)
  acetabular, congenital Q65.89
  alveolar capillary, with vein misalignment J84.843

Dysplasia — *continued*
  anus (histologically confirmed) (mild) (moderate)
      K62.82
    severe D01.3
  arrhythmogenic right ventricular I42.8
  arterial, fibromuscular I77.3
  asphyxiating thoracic (congenital) Q77.2
  brain Q07.9
  bronchopulmonary, perinatal P27.1
  cervix (uteri) N87.9
    mild N87.0
    moderate N87.1
    severe D06.9
  chondroectodermal Q77.6
  colon D12.6
  craniometaphyseal Q78.5
  dentinal K00.5
  diaphyseal, progressive Q78.3
  dystrophic Q77.5
  ectodermal (anhidrotic) (congenital) (hereditary) Q02.4
    hydrotic Q82.8
  epithelial, uterine cervix — *see* Dysplasia, cervix
  eye (congenital) Q11.2
  fibrous
    bone NEC (monostotic) M85.00
      ankle M85.07- ☑
      foot M85.07- ☑
      forearm M85.03- ☑
      hand M85.04- ☑
      lower leg M85.06- ☑
      multiple site M85.09
      neck M85.08
      rib M85.08
      shoulder M85.01- ☑
      skull M85.08
      specified site NEC M85.08
      thigh M85.05- ☑
      toe M85.07- ☑
      upper arm M85.02- ☑
      vertebra M85.08
    diaphyseal, progressive Q78.3
    jaw M27.8
    polyostotic Q78.1
  florid osseous (*see also* Cyst, calcifying odontogenic)
  high grade, focal D12.6
  hip, congenital Q65.89
  joint, congenital Q74.8
  kidney Q61.4
    multicystic Q61.4
  leg Q74.2
  lung, congenital (not associated with short gestation)
      Q33.6
  mammary (gland) (benign) N60.9- ☑
    cyst (solitary) — *see* Cyst, breast
    cystic — *see* Mastopathy, cystic
    duct ectasia — *see* Ectasia, mammary duct
    fibroadenosis — *see* Fibroadenosis, breast
    fibrosclerosis — *see* Fibrosclerosis, breast
    specified type NEC N60.8- ☑
  metaphyseal (Jansen's) (McKusick's) (Schmid's) Q78.5
  muscle Q79.8
  oculodentodigital Q87.0
  periapical (cemental) (cemento-osseous) — *see* Cyst,
      calcifying odontogenic
  periosteum — *see* Disorder, bone, specified type NEC
  polyostotic fibrous Q78.1
  prostate (*see also* Neoplasia, intraepithelial, prostate)
      N42.3
    severe D07.5
  renal Q61.4
    multicystic Q61.4
  retinal, congenital Q14.1
  right ventricular, arrhythmogenic I42.8
  septo-optic Q04.4
  skin L98.8
  spinal cord Q06.1
  spondyloepiphyseal Q77.7
  thymic, with immunodeficiency D82.1
  vagina N89.3
    mild N89.0
    moderate N89.1
    severe NEC D07.2
  vulva N90.3
    mild N90.0
    moderate N90.1
    severe NEC D07.1

Dyspnea (nocturnal) (paroxysmal) R06.00
  asthmatic (bronchial) J45.909
    with
      bronchitis J45.909
        with
          exacerbation (acute) J45.901
          status asthmaticus J45.902
        chronic J44.9
      exacerbation (acute) J45.901
      status asthmaticus J45.902
  cardiac — *see* Failure, ventricular, left
  cardiac — *see* Failure, ventricular, left
  functional F45.8
  hyperventilation R06.4
  hysterical F45.8
  newborn P28.89
  orthopnea R06.01
  psychogenic F45.8
  shortness of breath R06.02
  specified type NEC R06.09
Dyspraxia R27.8
  developmental (syndrome) F82
Dysproteinemia E88.09
Dysreflexia, autonomic G90.4
Dysrhythmia
  cardiac I49.9
    newborn
      bradycardia P29.12
        occurring before birth P03.819
          before onset of labor P03.810
          during labor P03.811
      tachycardia P29.11
    postoperative I97.89
  cerebral or cortical — *see* Epilepsy
Dyssomnia — *see* Disorder, sleep
Dyssynergia
  biliary K83.8
  bladder sphincter N36.44
  cerebellaris myoclonica (Hunt's ataxia) G11.1
Dysthymia F34.1
Dysthyroidism E07.9
Dystocia O66.9
  affecting newborn P03.1
  cervical (hypotonic) O62.2
    affecting newborn P03.6
    primary O62.0
    secondary O62.1
  contraction ring O62.4
  fetal O66.9
    abnormality NEC O66.3
    conjoined twins O66.3
    oversize O66.2
  maternal O66.9
  positional O64.9 ☑
  shoulder (girdle) O66.0
    causing obstructed labor O66.0
  uterine NEC O62.4
Dystonia G24.9
  deformans progressiva G24.1
  drug induced NEC G24.09
    acute G24.02
    specified NEC G24.09
  familial G24.1
  idiopathic G24.1
    familial G24.1
    nonfamilial G24.2
    orofacial G24.4
  lenticularis G24.8
  musculorum deformans G24.1
  neuroleptic induced (acute) G24.02
  orofacial (idiopathic) G24.4
  oromandibular G24.4
    due to drug G24.01
  specified NEC G24.8
  torsion (familial) (idiopathic) G24.1
    acquired G24.8
    genetic G24.1
    symptomatic (nonfamilial) G24.2
Dystonic movements R25.8
Dystrophy, dystrophia
  adiposogenital E23.6
  Becker's type G71.0
  cervical sympathetic G90.2
  choroid (hereditary) H31.20
    central areolar H31.22
    choroideremia H31.21
    gyrate atrophy H31.23
    specified type NEC H31.29

Dystrophy, dystrophia — *continued*
  cornea (hereditary) H18.50
    endothelial H18.51
    epithelial H18.52
    granular H18.53
    lattice H18.54
    macular H18.55
    specified type NEC H18.59
  Duchenne's type G71.0
  due to malnutrition E45
  Erb's G71.0
  Fuchs' H18.51
  Gower's muscular G71.0
  hair L67.8
  infantile neuraxonal G31.89
  Landouzy-Déjérine G71.0
  Leyden-Möbius G71.0
  muscular G71.0
    benign (Becker type) G71.0
    congenital (hereditary) (progressive) (with specific
        morphological abnormalities of the muscle
        fiber) G71.0
      myotonic G71.11
    distal G71.0
    Duchenne type G71.0
    Emery-Dreifuss G71.0
    Erb type G71.0
    facioscapulohumeral G71.0
    Gower's G71.0
    hereditary (progressive) G71.0
    Landouzy-Déjérine type G71.0
    limb-girdle G71.0
    myotonic G71.11
    progressive (hereditary) G71.0
      Charcot-Marie (-Tooth) type G60.0
    pseudohypertrophic (infantile) G71.0
    severe (Duchenne type) G71.0
  myocardium, myocardial — *see* Degeneration, myocar-
      dial
  nail L60.3
    congenital Q84.6
  nutritional E45
  ocular G71.0
  oculocerebrorenal E72.03
  oculopharyngeal G71.0
  ovarian N83.8
  polyglandular E31.8
  reflex (neuromuscular) (sympathetic) — *see* Syndrome,
      pain, complex regional I
  retinal (hereditary) H35.50
    in
      lipid storage disorders E75.6 [H36]
      systemic lipidoses E75.6 [H36]
    involving
      pigment epithelium H35.54
      sensory area H35.53
    pigmentary H35.52
    vitreoretinal H35.51
  Salzmann's nodular — *see* Degeneration, cornea,
      nodular
  scapuloperoneal G71.0
  skin NEC L98.8
  sympathetic (reflex) — *see* Syndrome, pain, complex
      regional I
    cervical G90.2
  tapetoretinal H35.54
  thoracic, asphyxiating Q77.2
  unguium L60.3
    congenital Q84.6
  vitreoretinal H35.51
  vulva N90.4
  yellow (liver) — *see* Failure, hepatic
Dysuria R30.0
  psychogenic F45.8

E

Eales' disease H35.06- ☑
Ear (*see also* condition)
  piercing Z41.3
  tropical B36.8
  wax (impacted) H61.20
    left H61.22
      with right H61.23
    right H61.21
      with left H61.23
Earache — *see* subcategory H92.0 ☑
Early satiety R68.81

☑ **Additional Character Required** — Refer to the Tabular List for Character Selection   ▽ **Subterms under main terms may continue to next column or page**

Eaton-Lambert syndrome — *see* Syndrome, Lambert-Eaton
Eberth's disease (typhoid fever) A01.00
Ebola virus disease A98.4
Ebstein's anomaly or syndrome (heart) Q22.5
Eccentro-osteochondrodysplasia E76.29
Ecchondroma — *see* Neoplasm, bone, benign
Ecchondrosis D48.0
Ecchymosis R58
  conjunctiva — *see* Hemorrhage, conjunctiva
  eye (traumatic) — *see* Contusion, eyeball
  eyelid (traumatic) — *see* Contusion, eyelid
  newborn P54.5
  spontaneous R23.3
  traumatic — *see* Contusion
Echinococciasis — *see* Echinococcus
Echinococcosis — *see* Echinococcus
Echinococcus (infection) B67.90
  granulosus B67.4
    bone B67.2
    liver B67.0
    lung B67.1
    multiple sites B67.32
    specified site NEC B67.39
    thyroid B67.31 [E35]
  liver NOS B67.8
    granulosus B67.0
    multilocularis B67.5
  lung NEC B67.99
    granulosus B67.1
    multilocularis B67.69
  multilocularis B67.7
    liver B67.5
    multiple sites B67.61
    specified site NEC B67.69
  specified site NEC B67.99
    granulosus B67.39
    multilocularis B67.69
  thyroid NEC B67.99
    granulosus B67.31 [E35]
    multilocularis B67.69 [E35]
Echinorhynchiasis B83.8
Echinostomiasis B66.8
Echolalia R48.8
Echovirus, as cause of disease classified elsewhere B97.12
Eclampsia, eclamptic (coma) (convulsions) (delirium) (with hypertension) NEC O15.9
  during labor and delivery O15.1
  postpartum O15.2
  pregnancy O15.0- ☑
  puerperal O15.2
Economic circumstances affecting care Z59.9
Economo's disease A85.8
Ectasia, ectasis
  annuloaortic I35.8
  aorta I77.819
    with aneurysm — *see* Aneurysm, aorta
    abdominal I77.811
    thoracic I77.810
    thoracoabdominal I77.812
  breast — *see* Ectasia, mammary duct
  capillary I78.8
  cornea H18.71- ☑
  gastric antral vascular (GAVE) K31.819
    with hemorrhage K31.811
    without hemorrhage K31.819
  mammary duct N60.4- ☑
  salivary gland (duct) K11.8
  sclera — *see* Sclerectasia
Ecthyma L08.0
  contagiosum B08.02
  gangrenosum L08.0
  infectiosum B08.02
Ectocardia Q24.8
Ectodermal dysplasia (anhidrotic) Q82.4
Ectodermosis erosiva pluriorificialis L51.1
Ectopic, ectopia (congenital)
  abdominal viscera Q45.8
    due to defect in anterior abdominal wall Q79.59
  ACTH syndrome E24.3
  adrenal gland Q89.1
  anus Q43.5
  atrial beats I49.1
  beats I49.49
    atrial I49.1
    ventricular I49.3

Ectopic, ectopia — *continued*
  bladder Q64.10
  bone and cartilage in lung Q33.5
  brain Q04.8
  breast tissue Q83.8
  cardiac Q24.8
  cerebral Q04.8
  cordis Q24.8
  endometrium — *see* Endometriosis
  gastric mucosa Q40.2
  gestation — *see* Pregnancy, by site
  heart Q24.8
  hormone secretion NEC E34.2
  kidney (crossed) (pelvis) Q63.2
  lens, lentis Q12.1
  mole — *see* Pregnancy, by site
  organ or site NEC — *see* Malposition, congenital
  pancreas Q45.3
  pregnancy — *see* Pregnancy, ectopic
  pupil — *see* Abnormality, pupillary
  renal Q63.2
  sebaceous glands of mouth Q38.6
  spleen Q89.09
  testis Q53.00
    bilateral Q53.02
    unilateral Q53.01
  thyroid Q89.2
  tissue in lung Q33.5
  ureter Q62.63
  ventricular beats I49.3
  vesicae Q64.10
Ectromelia Q73.8
  lower limb — *see* Defect, reduction, limb, lower, specified type NEC
  upper limb — *see* Defect, reduction, limb, upper, specified type NEC
Ectropion H02.109
  cervix N86
    with cervicitis N72
  congenital Q10.1
  eyelid (paralytic) H02.109
    cicatricial H02.119
      left H02.116
        lower H02.115
        upper H02.114
      right H02.113
        lower H02.112
        upper H02.111
    congenital Q10.1
    left H02.106
      lower H02.105
      upper H02.104
    mechanical H02.129
      left H02.126
        lower H02.125
        upper H02.124
      right H02.123
        lower H02.122
        upper H02.121
    right H02.103
      lower H02.102
      upper H02.101
    senile H02.139
      left H02.136
        lower H02.135
        upper H02.134
      right H02.133
        lower H02.132
        upper H02.131
    spastic H02.149
      left H02.146
        lower H02.145
        upper H02.144
      right H02.143
        lower H02.142
        upper H02.141
  iris H21.89
  lip (acquired) K13.0
    congenital Q38.0
  urethra N36.8
  uvea H21.89
Eczema (acute) (chronic) (erythematous) (fissum) (rubrum) (squamous) (*see also* Dermatitis) L30.9
  contact — *see* Dermatitis, contact
  dyshydrotic L30.1
  external ear — *see* Otitis, externa, acute, eczematoid
  flexural L20.82
  herpeticum B00.0

Eczema — *continued*
  hypertrophicum L28.0
  hypostatic — *see* Varix, leg, with, inflammation
  impetiginous L01.1
  infantile (due to any substance) L20.83
    intertriginous L21.1
    seborrheic L21.1
  intertriginous NEC L30.4
    infantile L21.1
  intrinsic (allergic) L20.84
  lichenified NEC L28.0
  marginatum (hebrae) B35.6
  pustular L30.3
  stasis — *see* Varix, leg, with, inflammation
  vaccination, vaccinatum T88.1 ☑
  varicose — *see* Varix, leg, with, inflammation
Eczematid L30.2
Eddowes (-Spurway) **syndrome** Q78.0
Edema, edematous (infectious) (pitting) (toxic) R60.9
  with nephritis — *see* Nephrosis
  allergic T78.3 ☑
  amputation stump (surgical) (sequelae) (late effect)) T87.89
  angioneurotic (allergic) (any site) (with urticaria) T78.3 ☑
    hereditary D84.1
  angiospastic I73.9
  Berlin's (traumatic) S05.8X- ☑
  brain (cytotoxic) (vasogenic) G93.6
    due to birth injury P11.0
    newborn (anoxia or hypoxia) P52.4
      birth injury P11.0
    traumatic — *see* Injury, intracranial, cerebral edema
  cardiac — *see* Failure, heart, congestive
  cardiovascular — *see* Failure, heart, congestive
  cerebral — *see* Edema, brain
  cerebrospinal — *see* Edema, brain
  cervix (uteri) (acute) N88.8
    puerperal, postpartum O90.89
  chronic hereditary Q82.0
  circumscribed, acute T78.3 ☑
    hereditary D84.1
  conjunctiva H11.42- ☑
  cornea H18.2- ☑
    idiopathic H18.22- ☑
    secondary H18.23- ☑
      due to contact lens H18.21- ☑
  due to
    lymphatic obstruction I89.0
    salt retention E87.0
  epiglottis — *see* Edema, glottis
  essential, acute T78.3 ☑
    hereditary D84.1
  extremities, lower — *see* Edema, legs
  eyelid NEC H02.849
    left H02.846
      lower H02.845
      upper H02.844
    right H02.843
      lower H02.842
      upper H02.841
  familial, hereditary Q82.0
  famine — *see* Malnutrition, severe
  generalized R60.1
  glottis, glottic, glottidis (obstructive) (passive) J38.4
    allergic T78.3 ☑
      hereditary D84.1
  heart — *see* Failure, heart, congestive
  heat T67.7 ☑
  hereditary Q82.0
  inanition — *see* Malnutrition, severe
  intracranial G93.6
  iris H21.89
  joint — *see* Effusion, joint
  larynx — *see* Edema, glottis
  legs R60.0
    due to venous obstruction I87.1
    hereditary Q82.0
  localized R60.0
    due to venous obstruction I87.1
  lower limbs — *see* Edema, legs
  lung J81.1
    with heart condition or failure — *see* Failure, ventricular, left
    acute J81.0
    chemical (acute) J68.1
      chronic J68.1

Edema, edematous — *continued*
  lung — *continued*
    chronic J81.1
      due to
        chemicals, gases, fumes or vapors (inhalation) J68.1
        external agent J70.9
          specified NEC J70.8
        radiation J70.1
    due to
      chemicals, fumes or vapors (inhalation) J68.1
      external agent J70.9
        specified NEC J70.8
      high altitude T70.29 ☑
      near drowning T75.1 ☑
      radiation J70.0
    meaning failure, left ventricle I50.1
  lymphatic I89.0
    due to mastectomy I97.2
  macula H35.81
    cystoid, following cataract surgery — *see* Complications, postprocedural, following cataract surgery
    diabetic — *see* Diabetes, by type, with, retinopathy, with macular edema
  malignant — *see* Gangrene, gas
  Milroy's Q82.0
  nasopharynx J39.2
  newborn P83.30
    hydrops fetalis — *see* Hydrops, fetalis
    specified NEC P83.39
  nutritional (*see also* Malnutrition, severe)
    with dyspigmentation, skin and hair E40
  optic disc or nerve — *see* Papilledema
  orbit H05.22- ☑
  pancreas K86.8
  papilla, optic — *see* Papilledema
  penis N48.89
  periodic T78.3 ☑
    hereditary D84.1
  pharynx J39.2
  pulmonary — *see* Edema, lung
  Quincke's T78.3 ☑
    hereditary D84.1
  renal — *see* Nephrosis
  retina H35.81
    diabetic — *see* Diabetes, by type, with, retinopathy, with macular edema
  salt E87.0
  scrotum N50.8
  seminal vesicle N50.8
  spermatic cord N50.8
  spinal (cord) (vascular) (nontraumatic) G95.19
  starvation — *see* Malnutrition, severe
  stasis — *see* Hypertension, venous, (chronic)
  subglottic — *see* Edema, glottis
  supraglottic — *see* Edema, glottis
  testis N44.8
  tunica vaginalis N50.8
  vas deferens N50.8
  vulva (acute) N90.89
Edentulism — *see* Absence, teeth, acquired
Edsall's disease T67.2 ☑
Educational handicap Z55.9
  specified NEC Z55.8
Edward's syndrome — *see* Trisomy, 18
Effect(s) (of) (from) — *see* Effect, adverse NEC
Effect, adverse
  abnormal gravitational (G) forces or states T75.81 ☑
  abuse — *see* Maltreatment
  air pressure T70.9 ☑
    specified NEC T70.8 ☑
  altitude (high) — *see* Effect, adverse, high altitude
  anesthesia (*see also* Anesthesia) T88.59 ☑
    in labor and delivery O74.9
    in pregnancy NEC O29.3- ☑
    local, toxic
      in labor and delivery O74.4
      postpartum, puerperal O89.3
    postpartum, puerperal O89.9
    specified NEC T88.59 ☑
      in labor and delivery O74.8
      postpartum, puerperal O89.8
    spinal and epidural T88.59 ☑
      headache T88.59 ☑
        in labor and delivery O74.5
          postpartum, puerperal O89.4

Effect, adverse — *continued*
  anesthesia (*see also* Anesthesia) — *continued*
    spinal and epidural — *continued*
      specified NEC
        in labor and delivery O74.6
        postpartum, puerperal O89.5
  antitoxin — *see* Complications, vaccination
  atmospheric pressure T70.9 ☑
    due to explosion T70.8 ☑
    high T70.3 ☑
    low — *see* Effect, adverse, high altitude
    specified effect NEC T70.8 ☑
  biological, correct substance properly administered — *see* Effect, adverse, drug
  blood (derivatives) (serum) (transfusion) — *see* Complications, transfusion
  chemical substance — *see* Table of Drugs and Chemicals
  cold (temperature) (weather) T69.9 ☑
    chilblains I69.1 ☑
    frostbite — *see* Frostbite
    specified effect NEC T69.8 ☑
  drugs and medicaments T88.7 ☑
    specified drug — *see* Table of Drugs and Chemicals, by drug, adverse effect
    specified effect — *code to* condition
  electric current, electricity (shock) T75.4 ☑
    burn — *see* Burn
  exertion (excessive) T73.3 ☑
  exposure — *see* Exposure
  external cause NEC T75.89 ☑
  foodstuffs T78.1 ☑
    allergic reaction — *see* Allergy, food
      causing anaphylaxis — *see* Shock, anaphylactic, due to food
    noxious — *see* Poisoning, food, noxious
  gases, fumes, or vapors T59.9- ☑
    specified agent — *see* Table of Drugs and Chemicals
  glue (airplane) sniffing
    due to drug abuse — *see* Abuse, drug, inhalant
    due to drug dependence — *see* Dependence, drug, inhalant
  heat — *see* Heat
  high altitude NEC T70.29 ☑
    anoxia T70.29 ☑
    on
      ears T70.0 ☑
      sinuses T70.1 ☑
    polycythemia D75.1
  high pressure fluids T70.4 ☑
  hot weather — *see* Heat
  hunger T73.0 ☑
  immersion, foot — *see* Immersion
  immunization — *see* Complications, vaccination
  immunological agents — *see* Complications, vaccination
  infrared (radiation) (rays) NOS T66 ☑
    dermatitis or eczema L59.8
  infusion — *see* Complications, infusion
  lack of care of infants — *see* Maltreatment, child
  lightning — *see* Lightning
  medical care T88.9 ☑
    specified NEC T88.8 ☑
  medicinal substance, correct, properly administered — *see* Effect, adverse, drug
  motion T75.3 ☑
  noise, on inner ear — *see* subcategory H83.3 ☑
  overheated places — *see* Heat
  psychosocial, of work environment Z56.5
  radiation (diagnostic) (infrared) (natural source) (therapeutic) (ultraviolet) (X-ray) NOS T66 ☑
    dermatitis or eczema — *see* Dermatitis, due to, radiation
    fibrosis of lung J70.1
    pneumonitis J70.0
    pulmonary manifestations
      acute J70.0
      chronic J70.1
    skin L59.9
  radioactive substance NOS
    dermatitis or eczema — *see* Radiodermatitis
  reduced temperature T69.9 ☑
    immersion foot or hand — *see* Immersion
    specified effect NEC T69.8 ☑
  serum NEC (*see also* Reaction, serum) T80.69 ☑

Effect, adverse — *continued*
  specified NEC T78.8 ☑
    external cause NEC T75.89 ☑
  strangulation — *see* Asphyxia, traumatic
  submersion T75.1 ☑
  thirst T73.1 ☑
  toxic — *see* Toxicity
  transfusion — *see* Complications, transfusion
  ultraviolet (radiation) (rays) NOS T66 ☑
    burn — *see* Burn
    dermatitis or eczema — *see* Dermatitis, due to, ultraviolet rays
      acute L56.8
  vaccine (any) — *see* Complications, vaccination
  vibration — *see* Vibration, adverse effects
  water pressure NEC T70.9 ☑
    specified NEC T70.8 ☑
  weightlessness T75.82 ☑
  whole blood — *see* Complications, transfusion
  work environment Z56.5
Effects, late — *see* Sequelae
Effluvium
  anagen L65.1
  telogen L65.0
Effort syndrome (psychogenic) F45.8
Effusion
  amniotic fluid — *see* Pregnancy, complicated by, prematue rupture of membranes
  brain (serous) G93.6
  bronchial — *see* Bronchitis
  cerebral G93.6
  cerebrospinal (*see also* Meningitis)
    vessel G93.6
  chest — *see* Effusion, pleura
  chylous, chyliform (pleura) J94.0
  intracranial G93.6
  joint M25.40
    ankle M25.47- ☑
    elbow M25.42- ☑
    foot joint M25.47- ☑
    hand joint M25.44- ☑
    hip M25.45- ☑
    knee M25.46- ☑
    shoulder M25.41- ☑
    specified joint NEC M25.48
    wrist M25.43- ☑
  malignant pleural J91.0
  meninges — *see* Meningitis
  pericardium, pericardial (noninflammatory) I31.3
    acute — *see* Pericarditis, acute
  peritoneal (chronic) R18.8
  pleura, pleurisy, pleuritic, pleuropericardial J90
    chylous, chyliform J94.0
    due to systemic lupus erythematosis M32.13
    influenzal — *see* Influenza, with, respiratory manifestations NEC
    malignant J91.0
    newborn P28.89
    tuberculous NEC A15.6
      primary (progressive) A15.7
  spinal — *see* Meningitis
  thorax, thoracic — *see* Effusion, pleura
Egg shell nails L60.3
  congenital Q84.6
Egyptian splenomegaly B65.1
Ehlers-Danlos syndrome Q79.6
Ehrlichiosis A77.40
  due to
    E. chafeensis A77.41
    E. sennetsu A79.81
    specified organism NEC A77.49
Eichstedt's disease B36.0
Eisenmenger's
  complex or syndrome I27.89
  defect Q21.8
Ejaculation
  painful N53.12
  premature F52.4
  retarded N53.11
  retrograde N53.14
  semen, painful N53.12
    psychogenic F52.6
Ekbom's syndrome (restless legs) G25.81
Ekman's syndrome (brittle bones and blue sclera) Q78.0
Elastic skin Q82.8
  acquired L57.4

Elastofibroma — *see* Neoplasm, connective tissue, benign
Elastoma (juvenile) Q82.8
  Miescher's L87.2
Elastomyofibrosis I42.4
Elastosis
  actinic, solar L57.8
  atrophicans (senile) L57.4
  perforans serpiginosa L87.2
  senilis L57.4
Elbow — *see* condition
Electric current, electricity, effects (concussion) (fatal) (nonfatal) (shock) T75.4 ☑
  burn — *see* Burn
Electric feet syndrome E53.8
Electrocution T75.4 ☑
  from electroshock gun (taser) T75.4 ☑
Electrolyte imbalance E87.8
  with
    abortion — *see* Abortion by type, complicated by, electrolyte imbalance
    ectopic pregnancy O08.5
    molar pregnancy O08.5
Elephantiasis (nonfilarial) I89.0
  arabicum — *see* Infestation, filarial
  bancroftian B74.0
  congenital (any site) (hereditary) Q82.0
  due to
    Brugia (malayi) B74.1
      timori B74.2
    mastectomy I97.2
    Wuchereria (bancrofti) B74.0
  eyelid H02.859
    left H02.856
      lower H02.855
      upper H02.854
    right H02.853
      lower H02.852
      upper H02.851
  filarial, filariensis — *see* Infestation, filarial
  glandular I89.0
  graecorum A30.9
  lymphangiectatic I89.0
  lymphatic vessel I89.0
    due to mastectomy I97.2
  scrotum (nonfilarial) I89.0
  streptococcal I89.0
  surgical I97.89
    postmastectomy I97.2
  telangiectodes I89.0
  vulva (nonfilarial) N90.89
Elevated, elevation
  antibody titer R76.0
  basal metabolic rate R94.8
  blood pressure (*see also* Hypertension)
    reading (incidental) (isolated) (nonspecific), no diagnosis of hypertension R03.0
  blood sugar R73.9
  body temperature (of unknown origin) R50.9
  cancer antigen 125 [CA 125] R97.1
  carcinoembryonic antigen [CEA] R97.0
  cholesterol E78.0
    with high triglycerides E78.2
  conjugate, eye H51.0
  C-reactive protein (CRP) R79.82
  diaphragm, congenital Q79.1
  erythrocyte sedimentation rate R70.0
  fasting glucose R73.01
  fasting triglycerides E78.1
  finding on laboratory examination — *see* Findings, abnormal, inconclusive, without diagnosis, by type of exam
  GFR (glomerular filtration rate) — *see* Findings, abnormal, inconclusive, without diagnosis, by type of exam
  glucose tolerance (oral) R73.02
  immunoglobulin level R76.8
  indoleacetic acid R82.5
  lactic acid dehydrogenase (LDH) level R74.0
  leukocytes D72.829
  lipoprotein a level E78.8 ☑
  liver function
    study R94.5
    test R79.89
      alkaline phosphatase R74.8
      aminotransferase R74.0
      bilirubin R17
      hepatic enzyme R74.8

Elevated, elevation — *continued*
  liver function — *continued*
    test — *continued*
      lactate dehydrogenase R74.0
  lymphocytes D72.820
  prostate specific antigen [PSA] R97.2
  Rh titer — *see* Complication(s), transfusion, incompatibility reaction, Rh (factor)
  scapula, congenital Q74.0
  sedimentation rate R70.0
  SGOT R74.0
  SGPT R74.0
  transaminase level R74.0
  triglycerides E78.1
    with high cholesterol E78.2
  tumor associated antigens [TAA] NEC R97.8
  tumor specific antigens [TSA] NEC R97.8
  urine level of
    17-ketosteroids R82.5
    catecholamine R82.5
    indoleacetic acid R82.5
    steroids R82.5
    vanillylmandelic acid (VMA) R82.5
  venous pressure I87.8
  white blood cell count D72.829
    specified NEC D72.828
Elliptocytosis (congenital) (hereditary) D58.1
  Hb C (disease) D58.1
  hemoglobin disease D58.1
  sickle-cell (disease) D57.8- ☑
    trait D57.3
Ellison-Zollinger syndrome E16.4
Ellis-van Creveld syndrome (chondroectodermal dysplasia) Q77.6
Elongated, elongation (congenital) (*see also* Distortion)
  bone Q79.9
  cervix (uteri) Q51.828
    acquired N88.4
    hypertrophic N88.4
  colon Q43.8
  common bile duct Q44.5
  cystic duct Q44.5
  frenulum, penis Q55.69
  labia minora (acquired) N90.6
  ligamentum patellae Q74.1
  petiolus (epiglottidis) Q31.8
  tooth, teeth K00.2
  uvula Q38.6
Eltor cholera A00.1
Emaciation (due to malnutrition) E41
Embadomoniasis A07.8
Embedded tooth, teeth K01.0
  root only K08.3
Embolic — *see* condition
Embolism (multiple) (paradoxical) I74.9
  air (any site) (traumatic) T79.0 ☑
    following
      abortion — *see* Abortion by type complicated by embolism
      ectopic pregnancy O08.2
    infusion, therapeutic injection or transfusion T80.0 ☑
    molar pregnancy O08.2
    procedure NEC
      artery T81.719 ☑
        mesenteric T81.710 ☑
        renal T81.711 ☑
        specified NEC T81.718 ☑
      vein T81.72 ☑
  in pregnancy, childbirth or puerperium — *see* Embolism, obstetric
  amniotic fluid (pulmonary) (*see also* Embolism, obstetric)
    following
      abortion — *see* Abortion by type complicated by embolism
      ectopic pregnancy O08.2
      molar pregnancy O08.2
  aorta, aortic I74.10
    abdominal I74.09
      saddle I74.01
    bifurcation I74.09
    saddle I74.01
    thoracic I74.11
  artery I74.9
    auditory, internal I65.8
    basilar — *see* Occlusion, artery, basilar

Embolism — *continued*
  artery — *continued*
    carotid (common) (internal) — *see* Occlusion, artery, carotid
    cerebellar (anterior inferior) (posterior inferior) (superior) I66.3
    cerebral — *see* Occlusion, artery, cerebral
    choroidal (anterior) I66.8
    communicating posterior I66.8
    coronary (*see also* Infarct, myocardium)
      not resulting in infarction I24.0
    extremity I74.4
      lower I74.3
      upper I74.2
    hypophyseal I66.8
    iliac I74.5
    limb I74.4
      lower I74.3
      upper I74.2
    mesenteric (with gangrene) K55.0
    ophthalmic — *see* Occlusion, artery, retina
    peripheral I74.4
    pontine I66.8
    precerebral — *see* Occlusion, artery, precerebral
    pulmonary — *see* Embolism, pulmonary
    renal N28.0
    retinal — *see* Occlusion, artery, retina
    septic I76
    specified NEC I74.8
    vertebral — *see* Occlusion, artery, vertebral
  basilar (artery) I65.1
  blood clot
    following
      abortion — *see* Abortion by type complicated by embolism
      ectopic or molar pregnancy O08.2
    in pregnancy, childbirth or puerperium — *see* Embolism, obstetric
  brain (*see also* Occlusion, artery, cerebral)
    following
      abortion — *see* Abortion by type complicated by embolism
      ectopic or molar pregnancy O08.2
    puerperal, postpartum, childbirth — *see* Embolism, obstetric
  capillary I78.8
  cardiac (*see also* Infarct, myocardium)
    not resulting in infarction I24.0
  carotid (artery) (common) (internal) — *see* Occlusion, artery, carotid
  cavernous sinus (venous) — *see* Embolism, intracranial venous sinus
  cerebral — *see* Occlusion, artery, cerebral
  cholesterol — *see* Atheroembolism
  coronary (artery or vein) (systemic) — *see* Occlusion, coronary
  due to device, implant or graft (*see also* Complications, by site and type, specified NEC)
    arterial graft NEC T82.818 ☑
    breast (implant) T85.81 ☑
    catheter NEC T85.81 ☑
      dialysis (renal) T82.818 ☑
        intraperitoneal T85.81 ☑
      infusion NEC T82.818 ☑
        spinal (epidural) (subdural) T85.81 ☑
      urinary (indwelling) T83.81 ☑
    electronic (electrode) (pulse generator) (stimulator)
      bone T84.81 ☑
      cardiac T82.817 ☑
      nervous system (brain) (peripheral nerve) (spinal) T85.81 ☑
      urinary T83.81 ☑
    fixation, internal (orthopedic) NEC T84.81 ☑
    gastrointestinal (bile duct) (esophagus) T85.81 ☑
    genital NEC T83.81 ☑
    heart (graft) (valve) T82.817 ☑
    joint prosthesis T84.81 ☑
    ocular (corneal graft) (orbital implant) T85.81 ☑
    orthopedic (bone graft) NEC T86.838
    specified NEC T85.81 ☑
    urinary (graft) NEC T83.81 ☑
    vascular NEC T82.818 ☑
    ventricular intracranial shunt T85.81 ☑
  extremities
    lower — *see* Embolism, vein, lower extremity
      arterial I74.3
    upper I74.2

Index

Embolism — Empyema

Embolism — *continued*
eye H34.9
fat (cerebral) (pulmonary) (systemic) T79.1 ☑
    complicating delivery — *see* Embolism, obstetric
    following
        abortion — *see* Abortion by type complicated
            by embolism
        ectopic or molar pregnancy O08.2
following
    abortion — *see* Abortion by type complicated by
        embolism
    ectopic or molar pregnancy O08.2
    infusion, therapeutic injection or transfusion
        air T80.0 ☑
heart (fatty) (*see also* Infarct, myocardium)
    not resulting in infarction I24.0
hepatic (vein) I82.0
in pregnancy, childbirth or puerperium — *see* Embolism, obstetric
intestine (artery) (vein) (with gangrene) K55.0
intracranial (*see also* Occlusion, artery, cerebral)
    venous sinus (any) G08
        nonpyogenic I67.6
intraspinal venous sinuses or veins G08
    nonpyogenic G95.19
kidney (artery) N28.0
lateral sinus (venous) — *see* Embolism, intracranial,
    venous sinus
leg — *see* Embolism, vein, lower extremity
    arterial I74.3
longitudinal sinus (venous) — *see* Embolism, intracranial, venous sinus
lung (massive) — *see* Embolism, pulmonary
meninges I66.8
mesenteric (artery) (vein) (with gangrene) K55.0
obstetric (in) (pulmonary)
    childbirth O88.82
        air O88.02
        amniotic fluid O88.12
        blood clot O88.22
        fat O88.82
        pyemic O88.32
        septic O88.32
        specified type NEC O88.82
    pregnancy O88.81- ☑
        air O88.01- ☑
        amniotic fluid O88.11- ☑
        blood clot O88.21- ☑
        fat O88.81- ☑
        pyemic O88.31- ☑
        septic O88.31- ☑
        specified type NEC O88.81- ☑
    puerperal O88.83
        air O88.03
        amniotic fluid O88.13
        blood clot O88.23
        fat O88.83
        pyemic O88.33
        septic O88.33
        specified type NEC O88.83
ophthalmic — *see* Occlusion, artery, retina
penis N48.81
peripheral artery NOS I74.4
pituitary E23.6
popliteal (artery) I74.3
portal (vein) I81
postoperative, postprocedural
    artery T81.719 ☑
        mesenteric T81.710 ☑
        renal T81.711 ☑
        specified NEC T81.718 ☑
    vein T81.72 ☑
precerebral artery — *see* Occlusion, artery, precerebral
puerperal — *see* Embolism, obstetric
pulmonary (acute) (artery) (vein) I26.99
    with acute cor pulmonale I26.09
    chronic I27.82
    following
        abortion — *see* Abortion by type complicated
            by embolism
        ectopic or molar pregnancy O08.2
    healed or old Z86.711
    in pregnancy, childbirth or puerperium — *see*
        Embolism, obstetric
    personal history of Z86.711
    saddle I26.92
        with acute cor pulmonale I26.02

Embolism — *continued*
pulmonary — *continued*
    septic I26.90
        with acute cor pulmonale I26.01
    pyemic (multiple) I76
        following
            abortion — *see* Abortion by type complicated
                by embolism
            ectopic or molar pregnancy O08.2
        Hemophilus influenzae A41.3
        pneumococcal A40.3
            with pneumonia J13
        puerperal, postpartum, childbirth (any organism)
            — *see* Embolism, obstetric
        specified organism NEC A41.89
        staphylococcal A41.2
        streptococcal A40.9
    renal (artery) N28.0
        vein I82.3
    retina, retinal — *see* Occlusion, artery, retina
    saddle
        abdominal aorta I74.01
        pulmonary artery I26.92
            with acute cor pulmonale I26.02
    septic (arterial) I76
        complicating abortion — *see* Abortion, by type,
            complicated by, embolism
    sinus — *see* Embolism, intracranial, venous sinus
    soap complicating abortion — *see* Abortion, by type,
        complicated by, embolism
    spinal cord G95.19
        pyogenic origin G06.1
    spleen, splenic (artery) I74.8
    upper extremity I74.2
    vein (acute) I82.90
        antecubital I82.61- ☑
            chronic I82.71- ☑
        axillary I82.A1- ☑ (*following* I82.7)
            chronic I82.A2- ☑ (*following* I82.7)
        basilic I82.61- ☑
            chronic I82.71- ☑
        brachial I82.62- ☑
            chronic I82.72- ☑
        brachiocephalic (innominate) I82.290
            chronic I82.291
        cephalic I82.61- ☑
            chronic I82.71- ☑
        chronic I82.91
        deep (DVT) I82.40- ☑
            calf I82.4Z- ☑
                chronic I82.5Z- ☑
            lower leg I82.4Z- ☑
                chronic I82.5Z- ☑
            thigh I82.4Y- ☑
                chronic I82.5Y- ☑
            upper leg I82.4Y ☑
                chronic I82.5Y-
        femoral I82.41- ☑
            chronic I82.51- ☑
        iliac (iliofemoral) I82.42- ☑
            chronic I82.52- ☑
        innominate I82.290
            chronic I82.291
        internal jugular I82.C1- ☑ (*following* I82.7)
            chronic I82.C2- ☑ (*following* I82.7)
        lower extremity
            deep I82.40- ☑
                chronic I82.50- ☑
                specified NEC I82.49- ☑
                    chronic NEC I82.59- ☑
            distal
                deep I82.4Z- ☑
            proximal
                deep I82.4Y- ☑
                    chronic I82.5Y- ☑
            superficial I82.81- ☑
        popliteal I82.43- ☑
            chronic I82.53- ☑
        radial I82.62- ☑
            chronic I82.72- ☑
        renal I82.3
        saphenous (greater) (lesser) I82.81- ☑
        specified NEC I82.890
            chronic NEC I82.891
        subclavian I82.B1- ☑ (*following* I82.7)
            chronic I82.B2- ☑ (*following* I82.7)

Embolism — *continued*
vein — *continued*
    thoracic NEC I82.290
        chronic I82.291
    tibial I82.44- ☑
        chronic I82.54- ☑
    ulnar I82.62- ☑
        chronic I82.72- ☑
    upper extremity I82.60- ☑
        chronic I82.70- ☑
        deep I82.62- ☑
            chronic I82.72- ☑
        superficial I82.61- ☑
            chronic I82.71- ☑
    vena cava
        inferior (acute) I82.220
            chronic I82.221
        superior (acute) I82.210
            chronic I82.211
    venous sinus G08
    vessels of brain — *see* Occlusion, artery, cerebral
Embolus — *see* Embolism
Embryoma (*see also* Neoplasm, uncertain behavior, by
        site)
    benign — *see* Neoplasm, benign, by site
    kidney C64.- ☑
    liver C22.0
    malignant (*see also* Neoplasm, malignant, by site)
        kidney C64.- ☑
        liver C22.0
        testis C62.9- ☑
            descended (scrotal) C62.1- ☑
            undescended C62.0- ☑
    testis C62.9- ☑
        descended (scrotal) C62.1- ☑
        undescended C62.0- ☑
Embryonic
    circulation Q28.9
    heart Q28.9
    vas deferens Q55.4
Embryopathia NOS Q89.9
Embryotoxon Q13.4
Emesis — *see* Vomiting
Emotional lability R45.86
Emotionality, pathological F60.3
Emotogenic disease — *see* Disorder, psychogenic
Emphysema (atrophic) (bullous) (chronic) (interlobular)
        (lung) (obstructive) (pulmonary) (senile) (vesicular)
        J43.9
    cellular tissue (traumatic) T79.7 ☑
        surgical T81.82 ☑
    centrilobular J43.2
    compensatory J98.3
    congenital (interstitial) P25.0
    conjunctiva H11.89
    connective tissue (traumatic) T79.7 ☑
        surgical T81.82 ☑
    due to chemicals, gases, fumes or vapors J68.4
    eyelid(s) — *see* Disorder, eyelid, specified type NEC
        surgical T81.82 ☑
        traumatic T79.7 ☑
    interstitial J98.2
        congenital P25.0
        perinatal period P25.0
    laminated tissue T79.7 ☑
        surgical T81.82 ☑
    mediastinal J98.2
        newborn P25.2
    orbit, orbital — *see* Disorder, orbit, specified type NEC
    panacinar J43.1
    panlobular J43.1
    specified NEC J43.8
    subcutaneous (traumatic) T79.7 ☑
        nontraumatic J98.2
        postprocedural T81.82 ☑
        surgical T81.82 ☑
    surgical T81.82 ☑
    thymus (gland) (congenital) E32.8
    traumatic (subcutaneous) T79.7 ☑
    unilateral J43.0
Empty nest syndrome Z60.0
Empyema (acute) (chest) (double) (pleura) (supradi-
        aphragmatic) (thorax) J86.9
    with fistula J86.0
    accessory sinus (chronic) — *see* Sinusitis
    antrum (chronic) — *see* Sinusitis, maxillary
    brain (any part) — *see* Abscess, brain

Empyema — *continued*
  ethmoidal (chronic) (sinus) — *see* Sinusitis, ethmoidal
  extradural — *see* Abscess, extradural
  frontal (chronic) (sinus) — *see* Sinusitis, frontal
  gallbladder K81.0
  mastoid (process) (acute) — *see* Mastoiditis, acute
  maxilla, maxillary M27.2
    sinus (chronic) — *see* Sinusitis, maxillary
  nasal sinus (chronic) — *see* Sinusitis
  sinus (accessory) (chronic) (nasal) — *see* Sinusitis
  sphenoidal (sinus) (chronic) — *see* Sinusitis, sphe-
      noidal
  subarachnoid — *see* Abscess, extradural
  subdural — *see* Abscess, subdural
  tuberculous A15.6
  ureter — *see* Ureteritis
  ventricular — *see* Abscess, brain
En coup de sabre lesion L94.1
Enamel pearls K00.2
Enameloma K00.2
Enanthema, viral B09
Encephalitis (chronic) (hemorrhagic) (idiopathic)
      (nonepidemic) (spurious) (subacute) G04.90
  acute (*see also* Encephalitis, viral) A86
    disseminated G04.00
      infectious G04.01
      noninfectious G04.81
      postimmunization (postvaccination) G04.02
      postinfectious G04.01
    inclusion body A85.8
    necrotizing hemorrhagic G04.30
      postimmunization G04.32
      postinfectious G04.31
      specified NEC G04.39
  arboviral, arbovirus NEC A85.2
  arthropod-borne NEC (viral) A85.2
  Australian A83.4
  California (virus) A83.5
  Central European (tick-borne) A84.1
  Czechoslovakian A84.1
  Dawson's (inclusion body) A81.1
  diffuse sclerosing A81.1
  disseminated, acute G04.00
  due to
    cat scratch disease A28.1
    human immunodeficiency virus (HIV) disease
        B20 [G05.3]
    malaria — *see* Malaria
    rickettsiosis — *see* Rickettsiosis
    smallpox inoculation G04.02
    typhus — *see* Typhus
  Eastern equine A83.2
  endemic (viral) A86
  epidemic NEC (viral) A86
  equine (acute) (infectious) (viral) A83.9
    Eastern A83.2
    Venezuelan A92.2
    Western A83.1
  Far Eastern (tick-borne) A84.0
  following vaccination or other immunization proce-
      dure G04.02
  herpes zoster B02.0
  herpesviral B00.4
    due to herpesvirus 6 B10.01
    due to herpesvirus 7 B10.09
    specified NEC B10.09
  Ilheus (virus) A83.8
  in (due to)
    actinomycosis A42.82
    adenovirus A85.1
    African trypanosomiasis B56.9 [G05.3]
    Chagas' disease (chronic) B57.42
    cytomegalovirus B25.8
    enterovirus A85.0
    herpes (simplex) virus B00.4
      due to herpesvirus 6 B10.01
      due to herpesvirus 7 B10.09
      specified NEC B10.09
    infectious disease NEC B99 ☑ [G05.3]
    influenza — *see* Influenza, with, encephalopathy
    listeriosis A32.12
    measles B05.0
    mumps B26.2
    naegleriasis B60.2
    parasitic disease NEC B89 [G05.3]
    poliovirus A80.9 [G05.3]
    rubella B06.01

Encephalitis — *continued*
  in — *continued*
    syphilis
      congenital A50.42
      late A52.14
    systemic lupus erythematosus M32.19
    toxoplasmosis (acquired) B58.2
      congenital P37.1
    tuberculosis A17.82
    zoster B02.0
  inclusion body A81.1
  infectious (acute) (virus) NEC A86
  Japanese (B type) A83.0
  La Crosse A83.5
  lead — *see* Poisoning, lead
  lethargica (acute) (infectious) A85.8
  louping ill A84.8
  lupus erythematosus, systemic M32.19
  lymphatica A87.2
  Mengo A85.8
  meningococcal A39.81
  Murray Valley A83.4
  otitic NEC H66.40 [G05.3]
  parasitic NOS B71.9
  periaxial G37.0
  periaxialis (concentrica) (diffuse) G37.5
  postchickenpox B01.11
  postexanthematous NEC B09
  postimmunization G04.02
  postinfectious NEC G04.01
  postmeasles B05.0
  postvaccinal G04.02
  postvaricella B01.11
  postviral NEC A86
  Powassan A84.8
  Rasmussen G04.81
  Rio Bravo A85.8
  Russian
    autumnal A83.0
    spring-summer (taiga) A84.0
  saturnine — *see* Poisoning, lead
  specified NEC G04.81
  St. Louis A83.3
  subacute sclerosing A81.1
  summer A83.0
  suppurative G04.81
  tick-borne A84.9
  Torula, torular (cryptococcal) B45.1
  toxic NEC G92
  trichinosis B75 [G05.3]
  type
    B A83.0
    C A83.3
  van Bogaert's A81.1
  Venezuelan equine A92.2
  Vienna A85.8
  viral, virus A86
    arthropod-borne NEC A85.2
      mosquito-borne A83.9
        Australian X disease A83.4
        California virus A83.5
        Eastern equine A83.2
        Japanese (B type) A83.0
        Murray Valley A83.4
        specified NEC A83.8
        St. Louis A83.3
        type B A83.0
        type C A83.3
        Western equine A83.1
      tick-borne A84.9
        biundulant A84.1
        central European A84.1
        Czechoslovakian A84.1
        diphasic meningoencephalitis A84.1
        Far Eastern A84.0
        Russian spring-summer (taiga) A84.0
        specified NEC A84.8
      specified type NEC A85.8
    Western equine A83.1
Encephalocele Q01.9
  frontal Q01.0
  nasofrontal Q01.1
  occipital Q01.2
  specified NEC Q01.8
Encephalocystocele — *see* Encephalocele
Encephaloduroarteriomyosynangiosis (EDAMS) I67.5
Encephalomalacia (brain) (cerebellar) (cerebral) — *see*
    Softening, brain

Encephalomeningitis — *see* Meningoencephalitis
Encephalomeningocele — *see* Encephalocele
Encephalomeningomyelitis — *see* Meningoencephali-
    tis
Encephalomyelitis (*see also* Encephalitis) G04.90
  acute disseminated G04.00
    infectious G04.01
    noninfectious G04.81
    postimmunization G04.02
    postinfectious G04.01
  acute necrotizing hemorrhagic G04.30
    postimmunization G04.32
    postinfectious G04.31
    specified NEC G04.39
  benign myalgic G93.3
  equine A83.9
    Eastern A83.2
    Venezuelan A92.2
    Western A83.1
  in diseases classified elsewhere G05.3
  myalgic, benign G93.3
  postchickenpox B01.11
  postinfectious NEC G04.01
  postmeasles B05.0
  postvaccinal G04.02
  postvaricella B01.11
  rubella B06.01
  specified NEC G04.81
  Venezuelan equine A92.2
Encephalomyelocele — *see* Encephalocele
Encephalomyelomeningitis — *see* Meningoencephali-
    tis
Encephalomyelopathy G96.9
Encephalomyeloradiculitis (acute) G61.0
Encephalomyeloradiculoneuritis (acute) (Guillain-
    Barré) G61.0
Encephalomyeloradiculopathy G96.9
Encephalopathia hyperbilirubinemica, newborn
    P57.9
  due to isoimmunization (conditions in P55) P57.0
Encephalopathy (acute) G93.40
  acute necrotizing hemorrhagic G04.30
    postimmunization G04.32
    postinfectious G04.31
    specified NEC G04.39
  alcoholic G31.2
  anoxic — *see* Damage, brain, anoxic
  arteriosclerotic I67.2
  centrolobar progressive (Schilder) G37.0
  congenital Q07.9
  degenerative, in specified disease NEC G32.89
  demyelinating callosal G37.1
  due to
    drugs (*see also* Table of Drugs and Chemicals) G92
  hepatic — *see* Failure, hepatic
  hyperbilirubinemic, newborn P57.9
    due to isoimmunization (conditions in P55) P57.0
  hypertensive I67.4
  hypoglycemic E16.2
  hypoxic — *see* Damage, brain, anoxic
  hypoxic ischemic P91.60
    mild P91.61
    moderate P91.62
    severe P91.63
  in (due to) (with)
    birth injury P11.1
    hyperinsulinism E16.1 [G94]
    influenza — *see* Influenza, with, encephalopathy
    lack of vitamin (*see also* Deficiency, vitamin)
        E56.9 [G32.89]
    neoplastic disease (*see also* Neoplasm)
        D49.9 [G13.1]
    serum (*see also* Reaction, serum) T80.69 ☑
    syphilis A52.17
    trauma (postconcussional) F07.81
      current injury — *see* Injury, intracranial
    vaccination G04.02
  lead — *see* Poisoning, lead
  metabolic G93.41
    drug induced G92
    toxic G92
  myoclonic, early, symptomatic — *see* Epilepsy, gener-
      alized, specified NEC
  necrotizing, subacute (Leigh) G31.82
  pellagrous E52 [G32.89]
  portosystemic — *see* Failure, hepatic
  postcontusional F07.81
    current injury — *see* Injury, intracranial, diffuse

Index

Empyema — Encephalopathy

Encephalopathy — continued
  posthypoglycemic (coma) E16.1 [G94]
  postradiation G93.89
  saturnine — see Poisoning, lead
  septic G93.41
  specified NEC G93.49
  spongioform, subacute (viral) A81.09
  toxic G92
    metabolic G92
  traumatic (postconcussional) F07.81
    current injury — see Injury, intracranial
  vitamin B deficiency NEC E53.9 [G32.89]
    vitamin B1 E51.2
  Wernicke's E51.2
Encephalorrhagia — see Hemorrhage, intracranial, intracerebral
Encephalosis, posttraumatic F07.81
Enchondroma (see also Neoplasm, bone, benign)
Enchondromatosis (cartilaginous) (multiple) Q78.4
Encopresis R15.9
  functional F98.1
  nonorganic origin F98.1
  psychogenic F98.1
Encounter (with health service) (for) Z76.89
  adjustment and management (of)
    breast implant Z45.81 ☑
    implanted device NEC Z45.89
    myringotomy device (stent) (tube) Z45.82
  administrative purpose only Z02.9
    examination for
      adoption Z02.82
      armed forces Z02.3
      disability determination Z02.71
      driving license Z02.4
      employment Z02.1
      insurance Z02.6
      medical certificate NEC Z02.79
      paternity testing Z02.81
      residential institution admission Z02.2
      school admission Z02.0
      sports Z02.5
      specified reason NEC Z02.89
  aftercare — see Aftercare
  antenatal screening Z36
  assisted reproductive fertility procedure cycle Z31.83
  blood typing Z01.83
    Rh typing Z01.83
  breast augmentation or reduction Z41.1
  breast implant exchange (different material) (different size) Z45.81 ☑
  breast reconstruction following mastectomy Z42.1
  check-up — see Examination
  chemotherapy for neoplasm Z51.11
  colonoscopy, screening Z12.11
  counseling — see Counseling
  delivery, full-term, uncomplicated O80
    cesarean, without indication O82
  ear piercing Z41.3
  examination — see Examination
  expectant parent(s) (adoptive) pre-birth pediatrician visit Z76.81
  fertility preservation procedure (prior to cancer therapy) (prior to removal of gonads) Z31.84
  fitting (of) — see Fitting (and adjustment) (of)
  genetic
    counseling Z31.5
    testing — see Test, genetic
  hearing conservation and treatment Z01.12
  immunotherapy for neoplasm Z51.12
  in vitro fertilization cycle Z31.83
  instruction (in)
    child care (postpartal) (prenatal) Z32.3
    childbirth Z32.2
    natural family planning
      procreative Z31.61
      to avoid pregnancy Z30.02
  insulin pump titration Z46.81
  joint prosthesis insertion following prior explantation of joint prosthesis (staged procedure)
    hip Z47.32
    knee Z47.33
    shoulder Z47.31
  laboratory (as part of a general medical examination) Z00.00
    with abnormal findings Z00.01
  mental health services (for)
    abuse NEC
      perpetrator Z69.82

Encounter — continued
  mental health services — continued
    abuse — continued
      victim Z69.81
    child abuse
      nonparental
        perpetrator Z69.021
        victim Z69.020
      parental
        perpetrator Z69.011
        victim Z69.010
    spousal or partner abuse
      perpetrator Z69.12
      victim Z69.11
  observation (for) (ruled out)
    exposure to (suspected)
      anthrax Z03.810
      biological agent NEC Z03.818
  pediatrician visit, by expectant parent(s) (adoptive) Z76.01
  plastic and reconstructive surgery following medical procedure or healed injury NEC Z42.8
  pregnancy
    supervision of — see Pregnancy, supervision of
    test Z32.00
      result negative Z32.02
      result positive Z32.01
  radiation therapy (antineoplastic) Z51.0
  radiological (as part of a general medical examination) Z00.00
    with abnormal findings Z00.01
  reconstructive surgery following medical procedure or healed injury NEC Z42.8
  removal (of) (see also Removal)
    artificial
      arm Z44.00- ☑
        complete Z44.01- ☑
        partial Z44.02- ☑
      eye Z44.2- ☑
      leg Z44.10- ☑
        complete Z44.11- ☑
        partial Z44.12- ☑
    breast implant Z45.81 ☑
      tissue expander (without synchronous insertion of permanent implant) Z45.81 ☑
    device Z46.9
      specified NEC Z46.89
    external
      fixation device — code to fracture with seventh character D
      prosthesis, prosthetic device Z44.9
        breast Z44.3- ☑
        specified NEC Z44.8
    implanted device NEC Z45.89
    insulin pump Z46.81
    internal fixation device Z47.2
    myringotomy device (stent) (tube) Z45.82
    nervous system device NEC Z46.2
      brain neuropacemaker Z46.2
      visual substitution device Z46.2
        implanted Z45.31
    non-vascular catheter Z46.82
    orthodontic device Z46.4
    stent
      ureteral Z46.6
    urinary device Z46.6
  repeat cervical smear to confirm findings of recent normal smear following initial abnormal smear Z01.42
  respirator [ventilator] use during power failure Z99.12
  Rh typing Z01.83
  screening — see Screening
  specified NEC Z76.89
  sterilization Z30.2
  suspected condition, ruled out
    amniotic cavity and membrane Z03.71
    cervical shortening Z03.75
    fetal anomaly Z03.73
    fetal growth Z03.74
    maternal and fetal conditions NEC Z03.79
    oligohydramnios Z03.71
    placental problem Z03.72
    polyhydramnios Z03.71
  suspected exposure (to), ruled out
    anthrax Z03.810
    biological agents NEC Z03.818
  termination of pregnancy, elective Z33.2
  testing — see Test

Encounter — continued
  therapeutic drug level monitoring Z51.81
  titration, insulin pump Z46.81
  to determine fetal viability of pregnancy O36.80 ☑
  training
    insulin pump Z46.81
  X-ray of chest (as part of a general medical examination) Z00.00
    with abnormal findings Z00.01
Encystment — see Cyst
Endarteritis (bacterial, subacute) (infective) I77.6
  brain I67.7
  cerebral or cerebrospinal I67.7
  deformans — see Arteriosclerosis
  embolic — see Embolism
  obliterans (see also Arteriosclerosis)
    pulmonary I28.8
  pulmonary I28.8
  retina — see Vasculitis, retina
  senile — see Arteriosclerosis
  syphilitic A52.09
    brain or cerebral A52.04
    congenital A50.54 [I79.8]
  tuberculous A18.89
Endemic — see condition
Endocarditis (chronic) (marantic) (nonbacterial) (thrombotic) (valvular) I38
  with rheumatic fever (conditions in I00)
    active — see Endocarditis, acute, rheumatic
    inactive or quiescent (with chorea) I09.1
  acute or subacute I33.9
    infective I33.0
    rheumatic (aortic) (mitral) (pulmonary) (tricuspid) I01.1
      with chorea (acute) (rheumatic) (Sydenham's) I02.0
  aortic (heart) (nonrheumatic) (valve) I35.8
    with
      mitral disease I08.0
        with tricuspid (valve) disease I08.3
        active or acute I01.1
          with chorea (acute) (rheumatic) (Sydenham's) I02.0
      rheumatic fever (conditions in I00)
        active — see Endocarditis, acute, rheumatic
        inactive or quiescent (with chorea) I06.9
      tricuspid (valve) disease I08.2
        with mitral (valve) disease I08.3
    acute or subacute I33.9
    arteriosclerotic I35.8
    rheumatic I06.9
      with mitral disease I08.0
        with tricuspid (valve) disease I08.3
        active or acute I01.1
          with chorea (acute) (rheumatic) (Sydenham's) I02.0
      active or acute I01.1
        with chorea (acute) (rheumatic) (Sydenham's) I02.0
      specified NEC I06.8
    specified cause NEC I35.8
    syphilitic A52.03
  arteriosclerotic I38
  atypical verrucous (Libman-Sacks) M32.11
  bacterial (acute) (any valve) (subacute) I33.0
  candidal B37.6
  congenital Q24.8
  constrictive I33.0
  Coxiella burnetii A78 [I39]
  Coxsackie B33.21
  due to
    prosthetic cardiac valve T82.6 ☑
    Q fever A78 [I39]
    Serratia marcescens I33.0
    typhoid (fever) A01.02
  gonococcal A54.83
  infectious or infective (acute) (any valve) (subacute) I33.0
  lenta (acute) (any valve) (subacute) I33.0
  Libman-Sacks M32.11
  listerial A32.82
  Löffler's I42.3
  malignant (acute) (any valve) (subacute) I33.0
  meningococcal A39.51
  mitral (chronic) (double) (fibroid) (heart) (inactive) (valve) (with chorea) I05.9
    with
      aortic (valve) disease I08.0

☑ Additional Character Required — Refer to the Tabular List for Character Selection   ▽ Subterms under main terms may continue to next column or page

Endocarditis — *continued*
  mitral — *continued*
    with — *continued*
      aortic disease — *continued*
        with tricuspid (valve) disease I08.3
          active or acute I01.1
            with chorea (acute) (rheumatic) (Sydenham's) I02.0
          rheumatic fever (conditions in I00)
            active — *see* Endocarditis, acute, rheumatic
            inactive or quiescent (with chorea) I05.9
        tricuspid (valve) disease I08.1
          with aortic (valve) disease I08.3
      active or acute I01.1
        with chorea (acute) (rheumatic) (Sydenham's) I02.0
      bacterial I33.0
    arteriosclerotic I34.8
    nonrheumatic I34.8
      acute or subacute I33.9
    specified NEC I05.8
  monilial B37.6
  multiple valves I08.9
    specified disorders I08.8
  mycotic (acute) (any valve) (subacute) I33.0
  pneumococcal (acute) (any valve) (subacute) I33.0
  pulmonary (chronic) (heart) (valve) I37.8
    with rheumatic fever (conditions in I00)
      active — *see* Endocarditis, acute, rheumatic
      inactive or quiescent (with chorea) I09.89
        with aortic, mitral or tricuspid disease I08.8
    acute or subacute I33.9
      rheumatic I01.1
        with chorea (acute) (rheumatic) (Sydenham's) I02.0
    arteriosclerotic I37.8
    congenital Q22.2
    rheumatic (chronic) (inactive) (with chorea) I09.89
      active or acute I01.1
        with chorea (acute) (rheumatic) (Sydenham's) I02.0
    syphilitic A52.03
  purulent (acute) (any valve) (subacute) I33.0
  Q fever A78 [I39]
  rheumatic (chronic) (inactive) (with chorea) I09.1
    active or acute (aortic) (mitral) (pulmonary) (tricuspid) I01.1
      with chorea (acute) (rheumatic) (Sydenham's) I02.0
  rheumatoid — *see* Rheumatoid, carditis
  septic (acute) (any valve) (subacute) I33.0
  streptococcal (acute) (any valve) (subacute) I33.0
  subacute — *see* Endocarditis, acute
  suppurative (acute) (any valve) (subacute) I33.0
  syphilitic A52.03
  toxic I33.9
  tricuspid (chronic) (heart) (inactive) (rheumatic) (valve) (with chorea) I07.9
    with
      aortic (valve) disease I08.2
        mitral (valve) disease I08.3
      mitral (valve) disease I08.1
        aortic (valve) disease I08.3
      rheumatic fever (conditions in I00)
        active — *see* Endocarditis, acute, rheumatic
        inactive or quiescent (with chorea) I07.8
    active or acute I01.1
      with chorea (acute) (rheumatic) (Sydenham's) I02.0
    arteriosclerotic I36.8
    nonrheumatic I36.8
      acute or subacute I33.9
    specified cause, except rheumatic I36.8
  tuberculous — *see* Tuberculosis, endocarditis
  typhoid A01.02
  ulcerative (acute) (any valve) (subacute) I33.0
  vegetative (acute) (any valve) (subacute) I33.0
  verrucous (atypical) (nonbacterial) (nonrheumatic) M32.11
Endocardium, endocardial (*see also* condition)
  cushion defect Q21.2
Endocervicitis (*see also* Cervicitis)
  due to intrauterine (contraceptive) device T83.6 ☑
  hyperplastic N72
Endocrine — *see* condition
Endocrinopathy, pluriglandular E31.9
Endodontic
  overfill M27.52

Endodontic — *continued*
  underfill M27.53
Endodontitis K04.0
Endomastoiditis — *see* Mastoiditis
Endometrioma N80.9
Endometriosis N80.9
  appendix N80.5
  bladder N80.8
  bowel N80.5
  broad ligament N80.3
  cervix N80.0
  colon N80.5
  cul-de-sac (Douglas') N80.3
  exocervix N80.0
  fallopian tube N80.2
  female genital organ NEC N80.8
  gallbladder N80.8
  in scar of skin N80.6
  internal N80.0
  intestine N80.5
  lung N80.8
  myometrium N80.0
  ovary N80.1
  parametrium N80.3
  pelvic peritoneum N80.3
  peritoneal (pelvic) N80.3
  rectovaginal septum N80.4
  rectum N80.5
  round ligament N80.3
  skin (scar) N80.6
  specified site NEC N80.8
  stromal D39.0
  umbilicus N80.8
  uterus (internal) N80.0
  vagina N80.4
  vulva N80.8
Endometritis (decidual) (nonspecific) (purulent) (senile) (atrophic) (suppurative) N71.9
  with ectopic pregnancy O08.0
  acute N71.0
  blenorrhagic (gonococcal) (acute) (chronic) A54.24
  cervix, cervical (with erosion or ectropion) (*see also* Cervicitis)
    hyperplastic N72
  chlamydial A56.11
  chronic N71.1
  following
    abortion — *see* Abortion by type complicated by genital infection
    ectopic or molar pregnancy O08.0
  gonococcal, gonorrheal (acute) (chronic) A54.24
  hyperplastic (*see also* Hyperplasia, endometrial) N85.00
    cervix N72
  puerperal, postpartum, childbirth O86.12
  subacute N71.0
  tuberculous A18.17
Endometrium — *see* condition
Endomyocardiopathy, South African I42.3
Endomyocarditis — *see* Endocarditis
Endomyofibrosis I42.3
Endomyometritis — *see* Endometritis
Endopericarditis — *see* Endocarditis
Endoperineuritis — *see* Disorder, nerve
Endophlebitis — *see* Phlebitis
Endophthalmia — *see* Endophthalmitis, purulent
Endophthalmitis (acute) (infective) (metastatic) (subacute) H44.009
  bleb associated (*see also* Bleb, inflamed (infected), postprocedural H59.4 ☑
  gonorrheal A54.39
  in (due to)
    cysticercosis B69.1
    onchocerciasis B73.01
    toxocariasis B83.0
  panuveitis — *see* Panuveitis
  parasitic H44.12- ☑
  purulent H44.00- ☑
    panophthalmitis — *see* Panophthalmitis
    vitreous abscess H44.02- ☑
  specified NEC H44.19
  sympathetic — *see* Uveitis, sympathetic
Endosalpingioma D28.2
Endosalpingiosis N94.89
Endosteitis — *see* Osteomyelitis
Endothelioma, bone — *see* Neoplasm, bone, malignant
Endotheliosis (hemorrhagic infectional) D69.8
Endotoxemia — code to condition

Endotrachelitis — *see* Cervicitis
Engelmann (-Camurati) **syndrome** Q78.3
English disease — *see* Rickets
Engman's disease L30.3
Engorgement
  breast N64.59
    newborn P83.4
    puerperal, postpartum O92.79
  lung (passive) — *see* Edema, lung
  pulmonary (passive) — *see* Edema, lung
  stomach K31.89
  venous, retina — *see* Occlusion, retina, vein, engorgement
Enlargement, enlarged (*see also* Hypertrophy)
  adenoids J35.2
    with tonsils J35.3
  alveolar ridge K08.8
    congenital — *see* Anomaly, alveolar
  apertures of diaphragm (congenital) Q79.1
  gingival K06.1
  heart, cardiac — *see* Hypertrophy, cardiac
  lacrimal gland, chronic H04.03- ☑
  liver — *see* Hypertrophy, liver
  lymph gland or node R59.9
    generalized R59.1
    localized R59.0
  orbit H05.34- ☑
  organ or site, congenital NEC — *see* Anomaly, by site
  parathyroid (gland) E21.0
  pituitary fossa R93.0
  prostate N40.0
    with lower urinary tract symptoms (LUTS) N40.1
    without lower urinary tract symtpoms (LUTS) N40.0
  sella turcica R93.0
  spleen — *see* Splenomegaly
  thymus (gland) (congenital) E32.0
  thyroid (gland) — *see* Goiter
  tongue K14.8
  tonsils J35.1
    with adenoids J35.3
  uterus N85.2
Enophthalmos H05.40- ☑
  due to
    orbital tissue atrophy H05.41- ☑
    trauma or surgery H05.42- ☑
Enostosis M27.8
Entamebic, entamebiasis — *see* Amebiasis
Entanglement
  umbilical cord(s) O69.2 ☑
    with compression O69.2 ☑
      without compression O69.82 ☑
    around neck (with compression) O69.1 ☑
      without compression O69.81 ☑
    of twins in monoamniotic sac O69.2 ☑
Enteralgia — *see* Pain, abdominal
Enteric — *see* condition
Enteritis (acute) (diarrheal) (hemorrhagic) (noninfective) (septic) K52.9
  adenovirus A08.2
  aertrycke infection A02.0
  allergic K52.2
  amebic (acute) A06.0
    with abscess — *see* Abscess, amebic
    chronic A06.1
      with abscess — *see* Abscess, amebic
      nondysenteric A06.2
    nondysenteric A06.2
  astrovirus A08.32
  bacillary NOS A03.9
  bacterial A04.9
    specified NEC A04.8
  calicivirus A08.31
  candidal B37.82
  Chilomastix A07.8
  choleriformis A00.1
  chronic (noninfectious) K52.9
    ulcerative — *see* Colitis, ulcerative
  cicatrizing (chronic) — *see* Enteritis, regional, small intestine
  Clostridium
    botulinum (food poisoning) A05.1
    difficile A04.7
  coccidial A07.3
  coxsackie virus A08.39
  dietetic K52.2
  drug-induced K52.1

Endocarditis — Enteritis

Subterms under main terms may continue to next column or page   ☑ Additional Character Required — Refer to the Tabular List for Character Selection   127

Enteritis — continued
  due to
    astrovirus A08.32
    calicivirus A08.31
    coxsackie virus A08.39
    drugs K52.1
    echovirus A08.39
    enterovirus NEC A08.39
    food hypersensitivity K52.2
    infectious organism (bacterial) (viral) — see Enteritis, infectious
    torovirus A08.39
    Yersinia enterocolitica A04.6
  echovirus A08.39
  eltor A00.1
  enterovirus NEC A08.39
  eosinophilic K52.81
  epidemic (infectious) A09
  fulminant K55.0
  gangrenous — see Enteritis, infectious
  giardial A07.1
  infectious NOS A09
    due to
      adenovirus A08.2
      Aerobacter aerogenes A04.8
      Arizona (bacillus) A02.0
      bacteria NOS A04.9
        specified NEC A04.8
      Campylobacter A04.5
      Clostridium difficile A04.7
      Clostridium perfringens A04.8
      Enterobacter aerogenes A04.8
      enterovirus A08.39
      Escherichia coli A04.4
        enteroaggregative A04.4
        enterohemorrhagic A04.3
        enteroinvasive A04.2
        enteropathogenic A04.0
        enterotoxigenic A04.1
        specified NEC A04.4
      specified
        bacteria NEC A04.8
        virus NEC A08.39
      Staphylococcus A04.8
      virus NEC A08.4
        specified type NEC A08.39
      Yersinia enterocolitica A04.6
    specified organism NEC A08.8
  influenzal — see Influenza, with, digestive manifestations
  ischemic K55.9
    acute K55.0
    chronic K55.1
  microsporidial A07.8
  mucomembranous, myxomembranous — see Syndrome, irritable bowel
  mucous — see Syndrome, irritable bowel
  necroticans A05.2
  necrotizing of newborn — see Enterocolitis, necrotizing, in newborn
  neurogenic — see Syndrome, irritable bowel
  newborn necrotizing — see Enterocolitis, necrotizing, in newborn
  noninfectious K52.9
  norovirus A08.11
  parasitic NEC B82.9
  paratyphoid (fever) — see Fever, paratyphoid
  protozoal A07.9
    specified NEC A07.8
  radiation K52.0
  regional (of) K50.90
    with
      complication K50.919
        abscess K50.914
        fistula K50.913
        intestinal obstruction K50.912
        rectal bleeding K50.911
        specified complication NEC K50.918
    colon — see Enteritis, regional, large intestine
    duodenum — see Enteritis, regional, small intestine
    ileum — see Enteritis, regional, small intestine
    jejunum — see Enteritis, regional, small intestine
    large bowel — see Enteritis, regional, large intestine
    large intestine (colon) (rectum) K50.10
      with
        complication K50.119
          abscess K50.114

Enteritis — continued
  regional — continued
    large intestine — continued
      with — continued
        complication — continued
          fistula K50.113
          intestinal obstruction K50.112
          rectal bleeding K50.111
          small intestine (duodenum) (ileum) (jejunum) involvement K50.80
            with
              complication K50.819
                abscess K50.814
                fistula K50.813
                intestinal obstruction K50.812
                rectal bleeding K50.811
                specified complication NEC K50.818
          specified complication NEC K50.118
    rectum — see Enteritis, regional, large intestine
    small intestine (duodenum) (ileum) (jejunum) K50.00
      with
        complication K50.019
          abscess K50.014
          fistula K50.013
          intestinal obstruction K50.012
          large intestine (colon) (rectum) involvement K50.80
            with
              complication K50.819
                abscess K50.814
                fistula K50.813
                intestinal obstruction K50.812
                rectal bleeding K50.811
                specified complication NEC K50.818
          rectal bleeding K50.011
          specified complication NEC K50.018
  rotaviral A08.0
  Salmonella, salmonellosis (arizonae) (cholerae-suis) (enteritidis) (typhimurium) A02.0
  segmental — see Enteritis, regional
  septic A09
  Shigella — see Infection, Shigella
  small round structured NEC A08.19
  spasmodic, spastic — see Syndrome, irritable bowel
  staphylococcal A04.8
    due to food A05.0
  torovirus A08.39
  toxic NEC K52.1
    due to Clostridium difficile A04.7
  trichomonal A07.8
  tuberculous A18.32
  typhosa A01.00
  ulcerative (chronic) — see Colitis, ulcerative
  viral A08.4
    adenovirus A08.2
    enterovirus A08.39
    Rotavirus A08.0
    small round structured NEC A08.19
    specified NEC A08.39
    virus specified NEC A08.39

Enterobiasis B80
Enterobius vermicularis (infection) (infestation) B80
Enterocele (see also Hernia, abdomen)
  pelvic, pelvis (acquired) (congenital) N81.5
  vagina, vaginal (acquired) (congenital) NEC N81.5
Enterocolitis (see also Enteritis) K52.9
  due to Clostridium difficile A04.7
  fulminant ischemic K55.0
  granulomatous — see Enteritis, regional
  hemorrhagic (acute) K55.0
    chronic K55.1
  infectious NEC A09
  ischemic K55.9
  necrotizing
    due to Clostridium difficile A04.7
    in newborn P77.9
      stage 1 (without pneumatosis, without perforation) P77.1
      stage 2 (with pneumatosis, without perforation) P77.2
      stage 3 (with pneumatosis, with perforation) P77.3
  noninfectious K52.9
  newborn — see Enterocolitis, necrotizing, in newborn

Enterocolitis — continued
  pseudomembranous (newborn) A04.7
  radiation K52.0
    newborn — see Enterocolitis, necrotizing, in newborn
  ulcerative (chronic) — see Pancolitis, ulcerative (chronic)
Enterogastritis — see Enteritis
Enteropathy K63.9
  gluten-sensitive K90.0
  hemorrhagic, terminal K55.0
  protein-losing K90.4
Enteroperitonitis — see Peritonitis
Enteroptosis K63.4
Enterorrhagia K92.2
Enterospasm (see also Syndrome, irritable, bowel)
  psychogenic F45.8
Enterostenosis (see also Obstruction, intestine) K56.69
Enterostomy
  complication — see Complication, enterostomy
  status Z93.4
Enterovirus, as cause of disease classified elsewhere B97.10
  coxsackievirus B97.11
  echovirus B97.12
  other specified B97.19
Enthesopathy (peripheral) M77.9
  Achilles tendinitis — see Tendinitis, Achilles
  ankle and tarsus M77.9
    specified type NEC — see Enthesopathy, foot, specified type NEC
  anterior tibial syndrome M76.81- ☑
  calcaneal spur — see Spur, bone, calcaneal
  elbow region M77.8
    lateral epicondylitis — see Epicondylitis, lateral
    medial epicondylitis — see Epicondylitis, medial
  foot NEC M77.9
    metatarsalgia — see Metatarsalgia
    specified type NEC M77.5- ☑
  forearm M77.9
  gluteal tendinitis — see Tendinitis, gluteal
  hand M77.9
  hip — see Enthesopathy, lower limb, specified type NEC
  iliac crest spur — see Spur, bone, iliac crest
  iliotibial band syndrome — see Syndrome, iliotibial band
  knee — see Enthesopathy, lower limb, lower leg, specified type NEC
  lateral epicondylitis — see Epicondylitis, lateral
  lower limb (excluding foot) M76.9
    Achilles tendinitis — see Tendinitis, Achilles
    anterior tibial syndrome M76.81- ☑
    gluteal tendinitis — see Tendinitis, gluteal
    iliac crest spur — see Spur, bone, iliac crest
    iliotibial band syndrome — see Syndrome, iliotibial band
    patellar tendinitis — see Tendinitis, patellar
    pelvic region — see Enthesopathy, lower limb, specified type NEC
    peroneal tendinitis — see Tendinitis, peroneal
    posterior tibial syndrome M76.82- ☑
    psoas tendinitis — see Tendinitis, psoas
    shoulder M77.9
    specified type NEC M76.89- ☑
    tibial collateral bursitis — see Bursitis, tibial collateral
  medial epicondylitis — see Epicondylitis, medial
  metatarsalgia — see Metatarsalgia
  multiple sites M77.9
  patellar tendinitis — see Tendinitis, patellar
  pelvis M77.9
  periarthritis of wrist — see Periarthritis, wrist
  peroneal tendinitis — see Tendinitis, peroneal
  posterior tibial syndrome M76.82- ☑
  psoas tendinitis — see Tendinitis, psoas
  shoulder region — see Lesion, shoulder
  specified site NEC M77.9
  specified type NEC M77.8
  spinal M46.00
    cervical region M46.02
    cervicothoracic region M46.03
    lumbar region M46.06
    lumbosacral region M46.07
    multiple sites M46.09
    occipito-atlanto-axial region M46.01
    sacrococcygeal region M46.08

Enthesopathy — *continued*
  spinal — *continued*
    thoracic region M46.04
    thoracolumbar region M46.05
  tibial collateral bursitis — *see* Bursitis, tibial collateral
  upper arm M77.9
  wrist and carpus NEC M77.8
    calcaneal spur — *see* Spur, bone, calcaneal
    periarthritis of wrist — *see* Periarthritis, wrist
Entomophobia F40.218
Entomophthoromycosis B46.8
Entrance, air into vein — *see* Embolism, air
Entrapment, nerve — *see* Neuropathy, entrapment
Entropion (eyelid) (paralytic) H02.009
  cicatricial H02.019
    left H02.016
      lower H02.015
      upper H02.014
    right H02.013
      lower H02.012
      upper H02.011
  congenital Q10.2
  left H02.006
    lower H02.005
    upper H02.004
  mechanical H02.029
    left H02.026
      lower H02.025
      upper H02.024
    right H02.023
      lower H02.022
      upper H02.021
  right H02.003
    lower H02.002
    upper H02.001
  senile H02.039
    left H02.036
      lower H02.035
      upper H02.034
    right H02.033
      lower H02.032
      upper H02.031
  spastic H02.049
    left H02.046
      lower H02.045
      upper H02.044
    right H02.043
      lower H02.042
      upper H02.041
Enucleated eye (traumatic, current) S05.7- ☑
Enuresis R32
  functional F98.0
  habit disturbance F98.0
  nocturnal N39.44
    psychogenic F98.0
  nonorganic origin F98.0
  psychogenic F98.0
Eosinopenia — *see* Agranulocytosis
Eosinophilia (allergic) (hereditary) (idiopathic) (secondary) D72.1
  with
    angiolymphoid hyperplasia (ALHE) D18.01
  infiltrative J82
  Löffler's J82
  peritoneal — *see* Peritonitis, eosinophilic
  pulmonary NEC J82
  tropical (pulmonary) J82
Eosinophilia-myalgia syndrome M35.8
Ependymitis (acute) (cerebral) (chronic) (granular) — *see* Encephalomyelitis
Ependymoblastoma
  specified site — *see* Neoplasm, malignant, by site
  unspecified site C71.9
Ependymoma (epithelial) (malignant)
  anaplastic
    specified site — *see* Neoplasm, malignant, by site
    unspecified site C71.9
  benign
    specified site — *see* Neoplasm, benign, by site
    unspecified site D33.2
  myxopapillary D43.2
    specified site — *see* Neoplasm, uncertain behavior, by site
    unspecified site D43.2
  papillary D43.2
    specified site — *see* Neoplasm, uncertain behavior, by site
    unspecified site D43.2

Ependymoma — *continued*
  specified site — *see* Neoplasm, malignant, by site
  unspecified site C71.9
Ependymopathy G93.89
Ephelis, ephelides L81.2
Epiblepharon (congenital) Q10.3
Epicanthus, epicanthic fold (eyelid) (congenital) Q10.3
Epicondylitis (elbow)
  lateral M77.1- ☑
  medial M77.0- ☑
Epicystitis — *see* Cystitis
Epidemic — *see* condition
Epidermidalization, cervix — *see* Dysplasia, cervix
Epidermis, epidermal — *see* condition
Epidermodysplasia verruciformis B07.8
Epidermolysis
  bullosa (congenital) Q81.9
    acquired L12.30
      drug-induced L12.31
      specified cause NEC L12.35
    dystrophica Q81.2
    letalis Q81.1
    simplex Q81.0
    specified NEC Q81.8
  necroticans combustiformis L51.2
    due to drug — *see* Table of Drugs and Chemicals, by drug
Epidermophytid — *see* Dermatophytosis
Epidermophytosis (infected) — *see* Dermatophytosis
Epididymis — *see* condition
Epididymitis (acute) (nonvenereal) (recurrent) (residual) N45.1
  with orchitis N45.3
  blennorrhagic (gonococcal) A54.23
  caseous (tuberculous) A18.15
  chlamydial A56.19
  filarial (*see also* Infestation, filarial) B74.9 [N51]
  gonococcal A54.23
  syphilitic A52.76
  tuberculous A18.15
Epididymo-orchitis (*see also* Epididymitis) N45.3
Epidural — *see* condition
Epigastrium, epigastric — *see* condition
Epigastrocele — *see* Hernia, ventral
Epiglottis — *see* condition
Epiglottitis, epiglottiditis (acute) J05.10
  with obstruction J05.11
  chronic J37.0
Epignathus Q89.4
Epilepsia partialis continua (*see also* Kozhevnikof's epilepsy) G40.1- ☑
Epilepsy, epileptic, epilepsia (attack) (cerebral) (convulsion) (fit) (seizure) G40.909

> *Note: the following terms are to be considered equivalent to intractable: pharmacoresistant (pharmacologically resistant), treatment resistant, refractory (medically) and poorly controlled*

  with
    complex partial seizures — *see* Epilepsy, localization-related, symptomatic, with complex partial seizures
    grand mal seizures on awakening — *see* Epilepsy, generalized, specified NEC
    myoclonic absences — *see* Epilepsy, generalized, specified NEC
    myoclonic-astatic seizures — *see* Epilepsy, generalized, specified NEC
    simple partial seizures — *see* Epilepsy, localization-related, symptomatic, with simple partial seizures
  akinetic — *see* Epilepsy, generalized, specified NEC
  benign childhood with centrotemporal EEG spikes — *see* Epilepsy, localization-related, idiopathic
  benign myoclonic in infancy G40.80- ☑
  Bravais-jacksonian — *see* Epilepsy, localization-related, symptomatic, with simple partial seizures
  childhood
    with occipital EEG paroxysms — *see* Epilepsy, localization-related, idiopathic
    absence G40.A09 (*following* G40.3)
      intractable G40.A19 (*following* G40.3)
        with status epilepticus G40.A11 (*following* G40.3)
        without status epilepticus G40.A19 (*following* G40.3)

Epilepsy, epileptic, epilepsia — *continued*
  childhood — *continued*
    absence — *continued*
      not intractable G40.A09 (*following* G40.3)
        with status epilepticus G40.A01 (*following* G40.3)
        without status epilepticus G40.A09 (*following* G40.3)
  climacteric — *see* Epilepsy, specified NEC
  cysticercosis B69.0
  deterioration (mental) F06.8
  due to syphilis A52.19
  focal — *see* Epilepsy, localization-related, symptomatic, with simple partial seizures
  generalized
    idiopathic G40.309
      intractable G40.319
        with status epilepticus G40.311
        without status epilepticus G40.319
      not intractable G40.309
        with status epilepticus G40.301
        without status epilepticus G40.309
    specified NEC G40.409
      intractable G40.419
        with status epilepticus G40.411
        without status epilepticus G40.419
      not intractable G40.409
        with status epilepticus G40.401
        without status epilepticus G40.409
  impulsive petit mal — *see* Epilepsy, juvenile myoclonic
  intractable G40.919
    with status epilepticus G40.911
    without status epilepticus G40.919
  juvenile absence G40.A09 (*following* G40.3)
    intractable G40.A19 (*following* G40.3)
      with status epilepticus G40.A11 (*following* G40.3)
      without status epilepticus G40.A19 (*following* G40.3)
    not intractable G40.A09 (*following* G40.3)
      with status epilepticus G40.A01 (*following* G40.3)
      without status epilepticus G40.A09 (*following* G40.3)
  juvenile myoclonic G40.B09 (*following* G40.3)
    intractable G40.B19 (*following* G40.3)
      with status epilepticus G40.B11 (*following* G40.3)
      without status epilepticus G40.B19 (*following* G40.3)
    not intractable G40.B09 (*following* G40.3)
      with status epilepticus G40.B01 (*following* G40.3)
      without status epilepticus G40.B09 (*following* G40.3)
  localization-related (focal) (partial)
    idiopathic G40.009
      with seizures of localized onset G40.009
        intractable G40.019
          with status epilepticus G40.011
          without status epilepticus G40.019
        not intractable G40.009
          with status epilepticus G40.001
          without status epilepticus G40.009
    symptomatic
      with complex partial seizures G40.209
        intractable G40.219
          with status epilepticus G40.211
          without status epilepticus G40.219
        not intractable G40.209
          with status epilepticus G40.201
          without status epilepticus G40.209
      with simple partial seizures G40.109
        intractable G40.119
          with status epilepticus G40.111
          without status epilepticus G40.119
        not intractable G40.109
          with status epilepticus G40.101
          without status epilepticus G40.109
  myoclonus, myoclonic (progressive) — *see* Epilepsy, generalized, specified NEC
  not intractable G40.909
    with status epilepticus G40.901
    without status epilepticus G40.909
  on awakening — *see* Epilepsy, generalized, specified NEC
  parasitic NOS B71.9 [G94]

Epilepsy, epileptic, epilepsia — *continued*
partialis continua (*see also* Kozhevnikof's epilepsy)
G40.1- ☑
peripheral — *see* Epilepsy, specified NEC
procursiva — *see* Epilepsy, localization-related,
symptomatic, with simple partial seizures
progressive (familial) myoclonic — *see* Epilepsy, generalized, idiopathic
reflex — *see* Epilepsy, specified NEC
related to
alcohol G40.509
not intractable G40.509
with status epilepticus G40.501
without status epilepticus G40.509
drugs G40.509
not intractable G40.509
with status epilepticus G40.501
without status epilepticus G40.509
external causes G40.509
not intractable G40.509
with status epilepticus G40.501
without status epilepticus G40.509
hormonal changes G40.509
not intractable G40.509
with status epilepticus G40.501
without status epilepticus G40.509
sleep deprivation G40.509
not intractable G40.509
with status epilepticus G40.501
without status epilepticus G40.509
stress G40.509
not intractable G40.509
with status epilepticus G40.501
without status epilepticus G40.509
somatomotor — *see* Epilepsy, localization-related,
symptomatic, with simple partial seizures
somatosensory — *see* Epilepsy, localization-related,
symptomatic, with simple partial seizures
spasms G40.822
intractable G40.824
with status epilepticus G40.823
without status epilepticus G40.824
not intractable G40.822
with status epilepticus G40.821
without status epilepticus G40.822
specified NEC G40.802
intractable G40.804
with status epilepticus G40.803
without status epilepticus G40.804
not intractable G40.802
with status epilepticus G40.801
without status epilepticus G40.802
syndromes
generalized
idiopathic G40.309
intractable G40.319
with status epilepticus G40.311
without status epilepticus G40.319
not intractable G40.309
with status epilepticus G40.301
without status epilepticus G40.309
specified NEC G40.409
intractable G40.419
with status epilepticus G40.411
without status epilepticus G40.419
not intractable G40.409
with status epilepticus G40.401
without status epilepticus G40.409
localization-related (focal) (partial)
idiopathic G40.009
with seizures of localized onset G40.009
intractable G40.019
with status epilepticus G40.011
without status epilepticus G40.019
not intractable G40.009
with status epilepticus G40.001
without status epilepticus G40.009
symptomatic
with complex partial seizures G40.209
intractable G40.219
with status epilepticus G40.211
without status epilepticus G40.219
not intractable G40.209
with status epilepticus G40.201
without status epilepticus G40.209
with simple partial seizures G40.109
intractable G40.119
with status epilepticus G40.111

Epilepsy, epileptic, epilepsia — *continued*
syndromes — *continued*
localization-related — *continued*
symptomatic — *continued*
with simple partial seizures — *continued*
intractable — *continued*
without status epilepticus G40.119
not intractable G40.109
with status epilepticus G40.101
without status epilepticus G40.109
specified NEC G40.802
intractable G40.804
with status epilepticus G40.803
without status epilepticus G40.804
not intractable G40.802
with status epilepticus G40.801
without status epilepticus G40.802
tonic (-clonic) — *see* Epilepsy, generalized, specified
NEC
twilight F05
uncinate (gyrus) — *see* Epilepsy, localization-related,
symptomatic, with complex partial seizures
Unverricht (-Lundborg) (familial myoclonic) — *see*
Epilepsy, generalized, idiopathic
visceral — *see* Epilepsy, specified NEC
visual — *see* Epilepsy, specified NEC
Epiloia Q85.1
Epimenorrhea N92.0
Epipharyngitis — *see* Nasopharyngitis
Epiphora H04.20- ☑
due to
excess lacrimation H04.21- ☑
insufficient drainage H04.22- ☑
Epiphyseal arrest — *see* Arrest, epiphyseal
Epiphyseolysis, epiphysiolysis — *see* Osteochondropathy
Epiphysitis (*see also* Osteochondropathy)
juvenile M92.9
syphilitic (congenital) A50.02
Epiplocele — *see* Hernia, abdomen
Epiploitis — *see* Peritonitis
Epiplosarcomphalocele — *see* Hernia, umbilicus
Episcleritis (suppurative) H15.10- ☑
in (due to)
syphilis A52.71
tuberculosis A18.51
nodular H15.12- ☑
periodica fugax H15.11- ☑
angioneurotic — *see* Edema, angioneurotic
syphilitic (late) A52.71
tuberculous A18.51
Episode
affective, mixed F39
depersonalization (in neurotic state) F48.1
depressive F32.9
major F32.9
mild F32.0
moderate F32.1
severe (without psychotic symptoms) F32.2
with psychotic symptoms F32.3
recurrent F33.9
brief F33.8
specified NEC F32.8
hypomanic F30.8
manic F30.9
with
psychotic symptoms F30.2
remission (full) F30.4
partial F30.3
without psychotic symptoms F30.10
mild F30.11
moderate F30.12
severe (without psychotic symptoms) F30.13
with psychotic symptoms F30.2
other specified F30.8
recurrent F31.89
psychotic F23
organic F06.8
schizophrenic (acute) NEC, brief F23
Epispadias (female) (male) Q64.0
Episplenitis D73.89
Epistaxis (multiple) R04.0
hereditary I78.0
vicarious menstruation N94.89
Epithelioma (malignant) (*see also* Neoplasm, malignant,
by site)
adenoides cysticum — *see* Neoplasm, skin, benign
basal cell — *see* Neoplasm, skin, malignant

Epithelioma — *continued*
benign — *see* Neoplasm, benign, by site
Bowen's — *see* Neoplasm, skin, in situ
calcifying, of Malherbe — *see* Neoplasm, skin, benign
external site — *see* Neoplasm, skin, malignant
intraepidermal, Jadassohn — *see* Neoplasm, skin, be-
nign
squamous cell — *see* Neoplasm, malignant, by site
Epitheliomatosis pigmented Q82.1
Epitheliopathy, multifocal placoid pigment
H30.14- ☑
Epithelium, epithelial — *see* condition
Epituberculosis (with atelectasis) (allergic) A15.7
Eponychia Q84.6
Epstein's
nephrosis or syndrome — *see* Nephrosis
pearl K09.8
Epulis (gingiva) (fibrous) (giant cell) K06.8
Equinia A24.0
Equinovarus (congenital) (talipes) Q66.0
acquired — *see* Deformity, limb, clubfoot
Equivalent
convulsive (abdominal) — *see* Epilepsy, specified NEC
epileptic (psychic) — *see* Epilepsy, localization-related,
symptomatic, with complex partial seizures
Erb (-Duchenne) **paralysis** (birth injury) (newborn) P14.0
Erb-Goldflam disease or syndrome G70.00
with exacerbation (acute) G70.01
in crisis G70.01
Erb's
disease G71.0
palsy, paralysis (brachial) (birth) (newborn) P14.0
spinal (spastic) syphilitic A52.17
pseudohypertrophic muscular dystrophy G71.0
Erdheim's syndrome (acromegalic macrospondylitis)
E22.0
Erection, painful (persistent) — *see* Priapism
Ergosterol deficiency (vitamin D) E55.9
with
adult osteomalacia M83.8
rickets — *see* Rickets
Ergotism (*see also* Poisoning, food, noxious, plant)
from ergot used as drug (migraine therapy) — *see*
Table of Drugs and Chemicals
Erosio interdigitalis blastomycetica B37.2
Erosion
artery I77.2
without rupture I77.89
bone — *see* Disorder, bone, density and structure,
specified NEC
bronchus J98.09
cartilage (joint) — *see* Disorder, cartilage, specified
type NEC
cervix (uteri) (acquired) (chronic) (congenital) N86
with cervicitis N72
cornea (nontraumatic) — *see* Ulcer, cornea
recurrent H18.83- ☑
traumatic — *see* Abrasion, cornea
dental (idiopathic) (occupational) (due to diet, drugs
or vomiting) K03.2
duodenum, postpyloric — *see* Ulcer, duodenum
esophagus K22.10
with bleeding K22.11
gastric — *see* Ulcer, stomach
gastrojejunal — *see* Ulcer, gastrojejunal
implanted mesh — *see* Complications, mesh
intestine K63.3
lymphatic vessel I89.8
pylorus, pyloric (ulcer) — *see* Ulcer, stomach
spine, aneurysmal A52.09
stomach — *see* Ulcer, stomach
teeth (idiopathic) (occupational) (due to diet, drugs
or vomiting) K03.2
urethra N36.8
uterus N85.8
Erotomania F52.8
Error
metabolism, inborn — *see* Disorder, metabolism
refractive — *see* Disorder, refraction
Eructation R14.2
nervous or psychogenic F45.8
Eruption
creeping B76.9
drug (generalized) (taken internally) L27.0
fixed L27.1
in contact with skin — *see* Dermatitis, due to drugs
localized L27.1

☑ **Additional Character Required** — **Refer to the Tabular List for Character Selection**   ▽ **Subterms under main terms may continue to next column or page**

Eruption — *continued*
  Hutchinson, summer L56.4
  Kaposi's varicelliform B00.0
  napkin L22
  polymorphous light (sun) L56.4
  recalcitrant pustular L13.8
  ringed R23.8
  skin (nonspecific) R21
    creeping (meaning hookworm) B76.9
    due to inoculation/vaccination (generalized) (*see also* Dermatitis, due to, vaccine) L27.0
      localized L27.1
    erysipeloid A26.0
    feigned L98.1
    Kaposi's varicelliform B00.0
    lichenoid L28.0
    meaning dermatitis — *see* Dermatitis
    toxic NEC L53.0
  tooth, teeth, abnormal (incomplete) (late) (premature) (sequence) K00.6
  vesicular R23.8
Erysipelas (gangrenous) (infantile) (newborn) (phlegmonous) (suppurative) A46
  external ear A46 [H62.40]
  puerperal, postpartum O86.89
Erysipeloid A26.9
  cutaneous (Rosenbach's) A26.0
  disseminated A26.8
  sepsis A26.7
  specified NEC A26.8
Erythema, erythematous (infectional) (inflammation) L53.9
  ab igne L59.0
  annulare (centrifugum) (rheumaticum) L53.1
  arthriticum epidemicum A25.1
  brucellum — *see* Brucellosis
  chronic figurate NEC L53.3
  chronicum migrans (Borrelia burgdorferi) A69.20
  diaper L22
  due to
    chemical NEC L53.0
      in contact with skin L24.5
    drug (internal use) — *see* Dermatitis, due to, drugs
  elevatum diutinum L95.1
  endemic E52
  epidemic, arthritic A25.1
  figuratum perstans L53.3
  gluteal L22
  heat — *code by site under* Burn, first degree
  ichthyosiforme congenitum bullous Q80.3
  in diseases classified elsewhere L54
  induratum (nontuberculous) L52
    tuberculous A18.4
  infectiosum B08.3
  intertrigo L30.4
  iris L51.9
  marginatum L53.2
    in (due to) acute rheumatic fever I00
  medicamentosum — *see* Dermatitis, due to, drugs
  migrans A26.0
    chronicum A69.20
    tongue K14.1
  multiforme (major) (minor) L51.9
    bullous, bullosum L51.1
    conjunctiva L51.1
    nonbullous L51.0
    pemphigoides L12.0
    specified NEC L51.8
  napkin L22
  neonatorum P83.8
    toxic P83.1
  nodosum L52
    tuberculous A18.4
  palmar L53.8
  pernio T69.1 ☑
  rash, newborn P83.8
  scarlatiniform (recurrent) (exfoliative) L53.8
  solare L55.0
  specified NEC L53.8
  toxic, toxicum NEC L53.0
    newborn P83.1
  tuberculous (primary) A18.4
Erythematous, erythematosus — *see* condition
Erythermalgia (primary) I73.81
Erythralgia I73.81
Erythrasma L08.1
Erythredema (polyneuropathy) — *see* Poisoning, mercury

Erythremia (acute) C94.0- ☑
  chronic D45
  secondary D75.1
Erythroblastopenia (*see also* Aplasia, red cell) D60.9
  congenital D61.01
Erythroblastophthisis D61.09
Erythroblastosis (fetalis) (newborn) P55.9
  due to
    ABO (antibodies) (incompatibility) (isoimmunization) P55.1
    Rh (antibodies) (incompatibility) (isoimmunization) P55.0
Erythrocyanosis (crurum) I73.89
Erythrocythemia — *see* Erythremia
Erythrocytosis (megalosplenic) (secondary) D75.1
  familial D75.0
  oval, hereditary — *see* Elliptocytosis
  secondary D75.1
  stress D75.1
Erythroderma (secondary) (*see also* Erythema) L53.9
  bullous ichthyosiform, congenital Q80.3
  desquamativum L21.1
  ichthyosiform, congenital (bullous) Q80.3
  neonatorum P83.8
  psoriaticum L40.8
Erythrodysesthesia, palmar plantar (PPE) L27.1
Erythrogenesis imperfecta D61.09
Erythroleukemia C94.0- ☑
Erythromelalgia I73.81
Erythrophagocytosis D75.89
Erythrophobia F40.298
Erythroplakia, oral epithelium, and tongue K13.29
Erythroplasia (Queyrat) D07.4
  specified site — *see* Neoplasm, skin, in situ
  unspecified site D07.4
Escherichia coli (E. coli), **as cause of disease classified elsewhere** B96.20
  non-O157 Shiga toxin-producing (with known O group) B96.22
  non-Shiga toxin-producing B96.29
  O157 B96.21
  O157 with confirmation of Shiga toxin when H antigen is unknown, or is not H7 B96.21
  O157:H- (nonmotile) with confirmation of Shiga toxin B96.21
  O157:H7 with or without confirmation of Shiga toxin-production B96.21
    specified NEC B96.22
  Shiga toxin-producing (with unspecified O group) (STEC) B96.23
  specified NEC B96.29
Esophagismus K22.4
Esophagitis (acute) (alkaline) (chemical) (chronic) (infectional) (necrotic) (peptic) (postoperative) K20.9
  candidal B37.81
  due to gastrointestinal reflux disease K21.0
  eosinophilic K20.0
  reflux K21.0
  specified NEC K20.8
  tuberculous A18.83
  ulcerative K22.10
    with bleeding K22.11
Esophagocele K22.5
Esophagomalacia K22.8
Esophagospasm K22.4
Esophagostenosis K22.2
Esophagostomiasis B81.8
Esophagotracheal — *see* condition
Esophagus — *see* condition
Esophoria H50.51
  convergence, excess H51.12
  divergence, insufficiency H51.8
Esotropia — *see* Strabismus, convergent concomitant
Espundia B55.2
Essential — *see* condition
Esthesioneuroblastoma C30.0
Esthesioneurocytoma C30.0
Esthesioneuroepithelioma C30.0
Esthiomene A55
Estivo-autumnal malaria (fever) B50.9
Estrangement (marital) Z63.5
  parent-child NEC Z62.890
Estriasis — *see* Myiasis
Ethanolism — *see* Alcoholism
Etherism — *see* Dependence, drug, inhalant
Ethmoid, ethmoidal — *see* condition

Ethmoiditis (chronic) (nonpurulent) (purulent) (*see also* Sinusitis, ethmoidal)
  influenzal — *see* Influenza, with, respiratory manifestations NEC
  Woakes' J33.1
Ethylism — *see* Alcoholism
Eulenburg's disease (congenital paramyotonia) G71.19
Eumycetoma B47.0
Eunuchoidism E29.1
  hypogonadotropic E23.0
European blastomycosis — *see* Cryptococcosis
Eustachian — *see* condition
Evaluation (for) (of)
  development state
    adolescent Z00.3
    period of
      delayed growth in childhood Z00.70
        with abnormal findings Z00.71
      rapid growth in childhood Z00.2
    puberty Z00.3
  growth and developmental state (period of rapid growth) Z00.2
  delayed growth Z00.70
    with abnormal findings Z00.71
  mental health (status) Z00.8
    requested by authority Z04.6
  period of
    delayed growth in childhood Z00.70
      with abnormal findings Z00.71
    rapid growth in childhood Z00.2
  suspected condition — *see* Observation
Evans syndrome D69.41
Event, apparent life threatening in newborn and infant (ALTE) R68.13
Eventration (*see also* Hernia, ventral)
  colon into chest — *see* Hernia, diaphragm
  diaphragm (congenital) Q79.1
Eversion
  bladder N32.89
  cervix (uteri) N86
    with cervicitis N72
  foot NEC (*see also* Deformity, valgus, ankle)
    congenital Q66.6
  punctum lacrimale (postinfectional) (senile) H04.52- ☑
  ureter (meatus) N28.89
  urethra (meatus) N36.8
  uterus N81.4
Evidence
  cytologic
    of malignancy on anal smear R85.614
    of malignancy on cervical smear R87.614
    of malignancy on vaginal smear R87.624
Evisceration
  birth injury P15.8
  traumatic NEC
    eye — *see* Enucleated eye
Evulsion — *see* Avulsion
Ewing's sarcoma or tumor — *see* Neoplasm, bone, malignant
Examination (for) (following) (general) (of) (routine) Z00.00
  with abnormal findings Z00.01
  abuse, physical (alleged), ruled out
    adult Z04.71
    child Z04.72
  adolescent (development state) Z00.3
  alleged rape or sexual assault (victim), ruled out
    adult Z04.41
    child Z04.42
  allergy Z01.82
  annual (adult) (periodic) (physical) Z00.00
    with abnormal findings Z00.01
    gynecological Z01.419
      with abnormal findings Z01.411
  antibody response Z01.84
  blood — *see* Examination, laboratory
  blood pressure Z01.30
    with abnormal findings Z01.31
  cancer staging — *see* Neoplasm, malignant, by site
  cervical Papanicolaou smear Z12.4
    as part of routine gynecological examination Z01.419
      with abnormal findings Z01.411
  child (over 28 days old) Z00.129
    with abnormal findings Z00.121
    under 28 days old — *see* Newborn, examination
  clinical research control or normal comparison (control) (participant) Z00.6

Examination — *continued*
contraceptive (drug) maintenance (routine) Z30.8
  device (intrauterine) Z30.431
dental Z01.20
  with abnormal findings Z01.21
developmental — *see* Examination, child
donor (potential) Z00.5
ear Z01.10
  with abnormal findings NEC Z01.118
eye Z01.00
  with abnormal findings Z01.01
following
  accident NEC Z04.3
    transport Z04.1
    work Z04.2
  assault, alleged, ruled out
    adult Z04.71
    child Z04.72
  motor vehicle accident Z04.1
  treatment (for) Z09
    combined NEC Z09
      fracture Z09
      malignant neoplasm Z08
    malignant neoplasm Z08
    mental disorder Z09
    specified condition NEC Z09
follow-up (routine) (following) Z09
  chemotherapy NEC Z09
    malignant neoplasm Z08
  fracture Z09
  malignant neoplasm Z08
  postpartum Z39.2
  psychotherapy Z09
  radiotherapy NEC Z09
    malignant neoplasm Z08
  surgery NEC Z09
    malignant neoplasm Z08
gynecological Z01.419
  with abnormal findings Z01.411
  for contraceptive maintenance Z30.8
health — *see* Examination, medical
hearing Z01.10
  with abnormal findings NEC Z01.118
  following failed hearing screening Z01.110
immunity status testing Z01.84
laboratory (as part of a general medical examination)
  Z00.00
  with abnormal findings Z00.01
  preprocedural Z01.812
lactating mother Z39.1
medical (adult) (for) (of) Z00.00
  with abnormal findings Z00.01
  administrative purpose only Z02.9
    specified NEC Z02.89
  admission to
    armed forces Z02.3
    old age home Z02.2
    prison Z02.89
    residential institution Z02.2
    school Z02.0
      following illness or medical treatment Z02.0
    summer camp Z02.89
  adoption Z02.82
  blood alcohol or drug level Z02.83
  camp (summer) Z02.89
  clinical research, normal subject (control) (participant) Z00.6
  control subject in clinical research (normal comparison) (participant) Z00.6
  donor (potential) Z00.5
  driving license Z02.4
  general (adult) Z00.00
    with abnormal findings Z00.01
  immigration Z02.89
  insurance purposes Z02.6
  marriage Z02.89
  medicolegal reasons NEC Z04.8
  naturalization Z02.89
  participation in sport Z02.5
  paternity testing Z02.81
  population survey Z00.8
  pre-employment Z02.1
  pre-operative — *see* Examination, pre-procedural
  pre-procedural
    cardiovascular Z01.810
    respiratory Z01.811
    specified NEC Z01.818

Examination — *continued*
medical — *continued*
  preschool children
    for admission to school Z02.0
  prisoners
    for entrance into prison Z02.89
  recruitment for armed forces Z02.3
  specified NEC Z00.8
  sport competition Z02.5
medicolegal reason NEC Z04.8
newborn — *see* Newborn, examination
pelvic (annual) (periodic) Z01.419
  with abnormal findings Z01.411
period of rapid growth in childhood Z00.2
periodic (adult) (annual) (routine) Z00.00
  with abnormal findings Z00.01
physical (adult) (*see also* Examination, medical) Z00.00
  sports Z02.5
postpartum
  immediately after delivery Z39.0
  routine follow-up Z39.2
pre-chemotherapy (antineoplastic) Z01.818
prenatal (normal pregnancy) (*see also* Pregnancy, normal) Z34.9- ☑
pre-procedural (pre-operative)
  cardiovascular Z01.810
  laboratory Z01.812
  respiratory Z01.811
  specified NEC Z01.818
prior to chemotherapy (antineoplastic) Z01.818
psychiatric NEC Z00.8
  follow-up not needing further care Z09
  requested by authority Z04.6
radiological (as part of a general medical examination) Z00.00
  with abnormal findings Z00.01
repeat cervical smear to confirm findings of recent normal smear following initial abnormal smear Z01.42
skin (hypersensitivity) Z01.82
special (*see also* Examination, by type) Z01.89
  specified type NEC Z01.89
specified type or reason NEC Z04.8
teeth Z01.20
  with abnormal findings Z01.21
urine — *see* Examination, laboratory
vision Z01.00
  with abnormal findings Z01.01

Exanthem, exanthema (*see also* Rash)
with enteroviral vesicular stomatitis B08.4
Boston A88.0
epidemic with meningitis A88.0 [G02]
subitum B08.20
  due to human herpesvirus 6 B08.21
  due to human herpesvirus 7 B08.22
viral, virus B09
  specified type NEC B08.8

Excess, excessive, excessively
alcohol level in blood R78.0
androgen (ovarian) E28.1
attrition, tooth, teeth K03.0
carotene, carotin (dietary) E67.1
cold, effects of T69.9 ☑
  specified effect NEC T69.8 ☑
convergence H51.12
crying
  in child, adolescent, or adult R45.83
  in infant R68.11
development, breast N62
divergence H51.8
drinking (alcohol) NEC (without dependence) F10.10
  habitual (continual) (without remission) F10.20
eating R63.2
estrogen E28.0
fat (*see also* Obesity)
  in heart — *see* Degeneration, myocardial
  localized E65
foreskin N47.8
gas R14.0
glucagon E16.3
heat — *see* Heat
intermaxillary vertical dimension of fully erupted teeth M26.37
interocclusal distance of fully erupted teeth M26.37
kalium E87.5
large
  colon K59.3
    congenital Q43.8

Excess, excessive, excessively — *continued*
large — *continued*
  infant P08.0
  organ or site, congenital NEC — *see* Anomaly, by site
long
  organ or site, congenital NEC — *see* Anomaly, by site
menstruation (with regular cycle) N92.0
  with irregular cycle N92.1
napping Z72.821
natrium E87.0
number of teeth K00.1
nutrient (dietary) NEC R63.2
potassium (K) E87.5
salivation K11.7
secretion (*see also* Hypersecretion)
  milk O92.6
  sputum R09.3
  sweat R61
sexual drive F52.8
short
  organ or site, congenital NEC — *see* Anomaly, by site
  umbilical cord in labor or delivery O69.3 ☑
skin, eyelid (acquired) — *see* Blepharochalasis
  congenital Q10.3
sodium (Na) E87.0
spacing of fully erupted teeth M26.32
sputum R09.3
sweating R61
thirst R63.1
  due to deprivation of water T73.1 ☑
tuberosity of jaw M26.07
vitamin
  A (dietary) E67.0
    administered as drug (prolonged intake) — *see* Table of Drugs and Chemicals, vitamins, adverse effect
    overdose or wrong substance given or taken — *see* Table of Drugs and Chemicals, vitamins, poisoning
  D (dietary) E67.3
    administered as drug (prolonged intake) — *see* Table of Drugs and Chemicals, vitamins, adverse effect
    overdose or wrong substance given or taken — *see* Table of Drugs and Chemicals, vitamins, poisoning
weight
  gain R63.5
  loss R63.4

Excitability, abnormal, under minor stress (personality disorder) F60.3

Excitation
anomalous atrioventricular I45.6
psychogenic F30.8
reactive (from emotional stress, psychological trauma) F30.8

Excitement
hypomanic F30.8
manic F30.9
mental, reactive (from emotional stress, psychological trauma) F30.8
state, reactive (from emotional stress, psychological trauma) F30.8

Excoriation (traumatic) (*see also* Abrasion)
neurotic L98.1

Exfoliation
due to erythematous conditions according to extent of body surface involved L49.0
  less than 10 percent of body surface L49.0
  10-19 percent of body surface L49.1
  20-29 percent of body surface L49.2
  30-39 percent of body surface L49.3
  40-49 percent of body surface L49.4
  50-59 percent of body surface L49.5
  60-69 percent of body surface L49.6
  70-79 percent of body surface L49.7
  80-89 percent of body surface L49.8
  90-99 percent of body surface L49.9
teeth, due to systemic causes K08.0

Exfoliative — *see* condition

Exhaustion, exhaustive (physical NEC) R53.83
battle F43.0
cardiac — *see* Failure, heart
delirium F43.0

☑ **Additional Character Required — Refer to the Tabular List for Character Selection**
🔻 Subterms under main terms may continue to next column or page

Exhaustion, exhaustive — *continued*
  due to
        cold T69.8 ☑
        excessive exertion T73.3 ☑
        exposure T73.2 ☑
        neurasthenia F48.8
  heart — *see* Failure, heart
  heat (*see also* Heat, exhaustion) T67.5 ☑
        due to
              salt depletion T67.4 ☑
              water depletion T67.3 ☑
  maternal, complicating delivery O75.81
  mental F48.8
  myocardium, myocardial — *see* Failure, heart
  nervous F48.8
  old age R54
  psychogenic F48.8
  psychosis F43.0
  senile R54
  vital NEC Z73.0
Exhibitionism F65.2
Exocervicitis — *see* Cervicitis
Exomphalos Q79.2
  meaning hernia — *see* Hernia, umbilicus
Exophoria H50.52
  convergence, insufficiency H51.11
  divergence, excess H51.8
Exophthalmos H05.2- ☑
  congenital Q15.8
  constant NEC H05.24- ☑
  displacement, globe — *see* Displacement, globe
  due to thyrotoxicosis (hyperthyroidism) — *see* Hyperthyroidism, with, goiter (diffuse)
  dysthyroid — *see* Hyperthyroidism, with, goiter (diffuse)
  goiter — *see* Hyperthyroidism, with, goiter (diffuse)
  intermittent NEC H05.25- ☑
  malignant — *see* Hyperthyroidism, with, goiter (diffuse)
  orbital
        edema — *see* Edema, orbit
        hemorrhage — *see* Hemorrhage, orbit
  pulsating NEC H05.26- ☑
  thyrotoxic, thyrotropic — *see* Hyperthyroidism, with, goiter (diffuse)
Exostosis (*see also* Disorder, bone)
  cartilaginous — *see* Neoplasm, bone, benign
  congenital (multiple) Q78.6
  external ear canal H61.81- ☑
  gonococcal A54.49
  jaw (bone) M27.8
  multiple, congenital Q78.6
  orbit H05.35- ☑
  osteocartilaginous — *see* Neoplasm, bone, benign
  syphilitic A52.77
Exotropia — *see* Strabismus, divergent concomitant
Explanation of
  investigation finding Z71.2
  medication Z71.89
Exposure (to) (*see also* Contact, with) T75.89 ☑
  acariasis Z20.7
  AIDS virus Z20.6
  air pollution Z77.110
  algae and algae toxins Z77.121
  algae bloom Z77.121
  anthrax Z20.810
  aromatic amines Z77.020
  aromatic (hazardous) compounds NEC Z77.028
  aromatic dyes NOS Z77.028
  arsenic Z77.010
  asbestos Z77.090
  bacterial disease NEC Z20.818
  benzene Z77.021
  blue-green algae bloom Z77.121
  body fluids (potentially hazardous) Z77.21
  brown tide Z77.121
  chemicals (chiefly nonmedicinal) (hazardous) NEC Z77.098
  cholera Z20.09
  chromium compounds Z77.018
  cold, effects of T69.9 ☑
        specified effect NEC T69.8 ☑
  communicable disease Z20.9
        bacterial NEC Z20.818
        specified NEC Z20.89
        viral NEC Z20.828
  cyanobacteria bloom Z77.121

Exposure — *continued*
  disaster Z65.5
  discrimination Z60.5
  dyes Z77.098
  effects of T73.9 ☑
  environmental tobacco smoke (acute) (chronic) Z77.22
  Escherichia coli (E. coli) Z20.01
  exhaustion due to T73.2 ☑
  fiberglass — *see* Table of Drugs and Chemicals, fiberglass
  German measles Z20.4
  gonorrhea Z20.2
  hazardous metals NEC Z77.018
  hazardous substances NEC Z77.29
  hazards in the physical environment NEC Z77.128
  hazards to health NEC Z77.9
  human immunodeficiency virus (HIV) Z20.6
  human T-lymphotropic virus type-1 (HTLV-1) Z20.89
  implanted
        mesh — *see* Complications, mesh
        prosthetic materials NEC — *see* Complications, prosthetic materials NEC
  infestation (parasitic) NEC Z20.7
  intestinal infectious disease NEC Z20.09
        Escherichia coli (E. coli) Z20.01
  lead Z77.011
  meningococcus Z20.811
  mold (toxic) Z77.120
  nickel dust Z77.018
  noise Z77.122
  occupational
        air contaminants NEC Z57.39
        dust Z57.2
        environmental tobacco smoke Z57.31
        extreme temperature Z57.6
        noise Z57.0
        radiation Z57.1
        risk factors Z57.9
              specified NEC Z57.8
        toxic agents (gases) (liquids) (solids) (vapors) in agriculture Z57.4
        toxic agents (gases) (liquids) (solids) (vapors) in industry NEC Z57.5
        vibration Z57.7
  parasitic disease NEC Z20.7
  pediculosis Z20.7
  persecution Z60.5
  pfiesteria piscicida Z77.121
  poliomyelitis Z20.89
  pollution
        air Z77.110
        environmental NEC Z77.118
        soil Z77.112
        water Z77.111
  polycyclic aromatic hydrocarbons Z77.028
  prenatal (drugs) (toxic chemicals) — *see* Newborn, affected by (suspected to be), noxious substances transmitted via placenta or breast milk
  rabies Z20.3
  radiation, naturally occurring NEC Z77.123
  radon Z77.123
  red tide (Florida) Z77.121
  rubella Z20.4
  second hand tobacco smoke (acute) (chronic) Z77.22
        in the perinatal period P96.81
  sexually-transmitted disease Z20.2
  smallpox (laboratory) Z20.89
  syphilis Z20.2
  terrorism Z65.4
  torture Z65.4
  tuberculosis Z20.1
  uranium Z77.012
  varicella Z20.820
  venereal disease Z20.2
  viral disease NEC Z20.828
  war Z65.5
  water pollution Z77.111
Exsanguination — *see* Hemorrhage
Exstrophy
  abdominal contents Q45.8
  bladder Q64.10
        cloacal Q64.12
        specified type NEC Q64.19
        supravesical fissure Q64.11
Extensive — *see* condition
Extra (*see also* Accessory)
  marker chromosomes (normal individual) Q92.61
        in abnormal individual Q92.62

Extra — *continued*
  rib Q76.6
        cervical Q76.5
Extrasystoles (supraventricular) I49.49
  atrial I49.1
  auricular I49.1
  junctional I49.2
  ventricular I49.3
Extrauterine gestation or pregnancy — *see* Pregnancy, by site
Extravasation
  blood R58
  chyle into mesentery I89.8
  pelvicalyceal N13.8
  pyelosinus N13.8
  urine (from ureter) R39.0
  vesicant agent
        antineoplastic chemotherapy T80.810 ☑
        other agent NEC T80.818 ☑
Extremity — *see* condition, limb
Extrophy — *see* Exstrophy
Extroversion
  bladder Q64.19
  uterus N81.4
        complicating delivery O71.2
        postpartal (old) N81.4
Extruded tooth (teeth) M26.34
Extrusion
  breast implant (prosthetic) T85.42 ☑
  eye implant (globe) (ball) T85.328 ☑
  intervertebral disc — *see* Displacement, intervertebral disc
  ocular lens implant (prosthetic) — *see* Complications, intraocular lens
  vitreous — *see* Prolapse, vitreous
Exudate
  pleural — *see* Effusion, pleura
  retina H35.89
Exudative — *see* condition
Eye, eyeball, eyelid — *see* condition
Eyestrain — *see* Disturbance, vision, subjective
Eyeworm disease of Africa B74.3

F

Faber's syndrome (achlorhydric anemia) D50.9
Fabry (-Anderson) **disease** E75.21
Faciocephalalgia, autonomic (*see also* Neuropathy, peripheral, autonomic) G90.09
Factor(s)
  psychic, associated with diseases classified elsewhere F54
  psychological
        affecting physical conditions F54
        or behavioral
              affecting general medical condition F54
              associated with disorders or diseases classified elsewhere F54
Fahr disease (of brain) G23.8
Fahr Volhard disease (of kidney) I12.- ☑
Failure, failed
  abortion — *see* Abortion, attempted
  aortic (valve) I35.8
        rheumatic I06.8
  attempted abortion — *see* Abortion, attempted
  biventricular I50.9
  bone marrow — *see* Anemia, aplastic
  cardiac — *see* Failure, heart
  cardiorenal (chronic) I50.9
        hypertensive I13.2
  cardiorespiratory (*see also* Failure, heart) R09.2
  cardiovascular (chronic) — *see* Failure, heart
  cerebrovascular I67.9
  cervical dilatation in labor O62.0
  circulation, circulatory (peripheral) R57.9
        newborn P29.89
  compensation — *see* Disease, heart
  compliance with medical treatment or regimen — *see* Noncompliance
  congestive — *see* Failure, heart, congestive
  dental implant (endosseous) M27.69
        due to
              failure of dental prosthesis M27.63
              lack of attached gingiva M27.62
              occlusal trauma (poor prosthetic design) M27.62
              parafunctional habits M27.62

Failure, failed — *continued*
dental implant — *continued*
  due to — *continued*
    periodontal infection (peri-implantitis) M27.62
    poor oral hygiene M27.62
    osseointegration M27.61
      due to
        complications of systemic disease M27.61
        poor bone quality M27.61
      iatrogenic M27.61
    post-osseointegration
      biological M27.62
        due to complications of systemic disease M27.62
      iatrogenic M27.62
      mechanical M27.63
    pre-integration M27.61
    pre-osseointegration M27.61
    specified NEC M27.69
descent of head (at term) of pregnancy (mother) O32.4 ☑
endosseous dental implant — *see* Failure, dental implant
engagement of head (term of pregnancy) (mother) O32.4 ☑
erection (penile) (*see also* Dysfunction, sexual, male, erectile) N52.9
  nonorganic F52.21
examination(s), anxiety concerning Z55.2
expansion terminal respiratory units (newborn) (primary) P28.0
forceps NOS (with subsequent cesarean delivery) O66.5
gain weight (child over 28 days old) R62.51
  adult R62.7
  newborn P92.6
genital response (male) F52.21
  female F52.22
heart (acute) (senile) (sudden) I50.9
  with
    acute pulmonary edema — *see* Failure, ventricular, left
    decompensation — *see* Failure, heart, congestive
    dilatation — *see* Disease, heart
  arteriosclerotic I70.90
  biventricular I50.9
  combined left-right sided I50.9
  compensated I50.9
  complicating
    anesthesia (general) (local) or other sedation
      in labor and delivery O74.2
      in pregnancy O29.12- ☑
      postpartum, puerperal O89.1
    delivery (cesarean) (instrumental) O75.4
  congestive (compensated) (decompensated) I50.9
    with rheumatic fever (conditions in I00)
      active I01.8
      inactive or quiescent (with chorea) I09.81
    newborn P29.0
    rheumatic (chronic) (inactive) (with chorea) I09.81
      active or acute I01.8
        with chorea I02.0
  decompensated I50.9
  degenerative — *see* Degeneration, myocardial
  diastolic (congestive) I50.30
    acute (congestive) I50.31
      and (on) chronic (congestive) I50.33
    chronic (congestive) I50.32
      and (on) acute (congestive) I50.33
    combined with systolic (congestive) I50.40
      acute (congestive) I50.41
        and (on) chronic (congestive) I50.43
      chronic (congestive) I50.42
        and (on) acute (congestive) I50.43
  due to presence of cardiac prosthesis I97.13- ☑
  following cardiac surgery I97.13- ☑
  high output NOS I50.9
  hypertensive — *see* Hypertension, heart
  left (ventricular) — *see* Failure, ventricular, left
  low output (syndrome) NOS I50.9
  newborn P29.0
  organic — *see* Disease, heart
  peripartum O90.3
  postprocedural I97.13- ☑
  rheumatic (chronic) (inactive) I09.9
  right (ventricular) (secondary to left heart failure) — *see* Failure, heart, congestive

Failure, failed — *continued*
heart — *continued*
  systolic (congestive) I50.20
    acute (congestive) I50.21
      and (on) chronic (congestive) I50.23
    chronic (congestive) I50.22
      and (on) acute (congestive) I50.23
    combined with diastolic (congestive) I50.40
      acute (congestive) I50.41
        and (on) chronic (congestive) I50.43
      chronic (congestive) I50.42
        and (on) acute (congestive) I50.43
  thyrotoxic (*see also* Thyrotoxicosis) E05.90 [I43]
    with thyroid storm E05.91 [I43]
  valvular — *see* Endocarditis
hepatic K72.90
  with coma K72.91
  acute or subacute K72.00
    with coma K72.01
    due to drugs K71.10
      with coma K71.11
  alcoholic (acute) (chronic) (subacute) K70.40
    with coma K70.41
  chronic K72.10
    with coma K72.11
    due to drugs (acute) (subacute) (chronic) K71.10
      with coma K71.11
  due to drugs (acute) (subacute) (chronic) K71.10
    with coma K71.11
  postprocedural K91.82
hepatorenal K76.7
induction (of labor) O61.9
  abortion — *see* Abortion, attempted
  by
    oxytocic drugs O61.0
    prostaglandins O61.0
  instrumental O61.1
  mechanical O61.1
  medical O61.0
  specified NEC O61.8
  surgical O61.1
intubation during anesthesia T88.4 ☑
  in pregnancy O29.6- ☑
  labor and delivery O74.7
  postpartum, puerperal O89.6
involution, thymus (gland) E32.0
kidney (*see also* Disease, kidney, chronic) N19
  acute (*see also* Failure, renal, acute) N17.9
lactation (complete) O92.3
  partial O92.4
Leydig's cell, adult E29.1
liver — *see* Failure, hepatic
menstruation at puberty N91.0
mitral I05.8
myocardial, myocardium (*see also* Failure, heart) I50.9
  chronic (*see also* Failure, heart, congestive) I50.9
  congestive (*see also* Failure, heart, congestive) I50.9
orgasm (female) (psychogenic) F52.31
  male F52.32
ovarian (primary) E28.39
  iatrogenic E89.40
    asymptomatic E89.40
    symptomatic E89.41
  postprocedural (postablative) (postirradiation) (postsurgical) E89.40
    asymptomatic E89.40
    symptomatic E89.41
ovulation causing infertility N97.0
polyglandular, autoimmune E31.0
prosthetic joint implant — *see* Complications, joint prosthesis, mechanical, breakdown, by site
renal N19
  with
    tubular necrosis (acute) N17.0
  acute N17.9
    with
      cortical necrosis N17.1
      medullary necrosis N17.2
      tubular necrosis N17.0
    specified NEC N17.8
  chronic N18.9
    hypertensive — *see* Hypertension, kidney
  congenital P96.0
  end stage (chronic) N18.6
    due to hypertension I12.0
  following
    abortion — *see* Abortion by type complicated by specified condition NEC

Failure, failed — *continued*
renal — *continued*
  following — *continued*
    crushing T79.5 ☑
    ectopic or molar pregnancy O08.4
    labor and delivery (acute) O90.4
  hypertensive — *see* Hypertension, kidney
  postprocedural N99.0
respiration, respiratory J96.90
  with
    hypercapnia J96.92
    hypoxia J96.91
  acute J96.00
    with
      hypercapnia J96.02
      hypoxia J96.01
  acute and (on) chronic J96.20
    with
      hypercapnia J96.22
      hypoxia J96.21
  center G93.89
  chronic J96.10
    with
      hypercapnia J96.12
      hypoxia J96.11
  newborn P28.5
  postprocedural (acute) J95.821
    acute and chronic J95.822
rotation
  cecum Q43.3
  colon Q43.3
  intestine Q43.3
  kidney Q63.2
sedation (conscious) (moderate) during procedure T88.52 ☑
  history of Z92.83
segmentation (*see also* Fusion)
  fingers — *see* Syndactylism, complex, fingers
  vertebra Q76.49
    with scoliosis Q76.3
seminiferous tubule, adult E29.1
senile (general) R54
sexual arousal (male) F52.21
  female F52.22
testicular endocrine function E29.1
to thrive (child over 28 days old) R62.51
  adult R62.7
  newborn P92.6
transplant T86.92
  bone T86.831
    marrow T86.02
  cornea T86.841
  heart T86.22
    with lung(s) T86.32
  intestine T86.851
  kidney T86.12
  liver T86.42
  lung(s) T86.811
    with heart T86.32
  pancreas T86.891
  skin (allograft) (autograft) T86.821
  specified organ or tissue NEC T86.891
  stem cell (peripheral blood) (umbilical cord) T86.5
trial of labor (with subsequent cesarean delivery) O66.40
  following previous cesarean delivery O66.41
tubal ligation N99.89
urinary — *see* Disease, kidney, chronic
vacuum extraction NOS (with subsequent cesarean delivery) O66.5
vasectomy N99.89
ventouse NOS (with subsequent cesarean delivery) O66.5
ventricular (*see also* Failure, heart) I50.9
  left I50.1
    with rheumatic fever (conditions in I00)
      active I01.8
        with chorea I02.0
      inactive or quiescent (with chorea) I09.81
    rheumatic (chronic) (inactive) (with chorea) I09.81
      active or acute I01.8
        with chorea I02.0
  right (*see also* Failure, heart, congestive) I50.9
vital centers, newborn P91.8
Fainting (fit) R55
Fallen arches — *see* Deformity, limb, flat foot

☑ Additional Character Required — Refer to the Tabular List for Character Selection   Subterms under main terms may continue to next column or page

Falling, falls (repeated) R29.6
　any organ or part — see Prolapse
Fallopian
　insufflation Z31.41
　tube — see condition
Fallot's
　pentalogy Q21.8
　tetrad or tetralogy Q21.3
　triad or trilogy Q22.3
False (see also condition)
　croup J38.5
　joint — see Nonunion, fracture
　labor (pains) O47.9
　　at or after 37 completed weeks of gestation O47.1
　　before 37 completed weeks of gestation O47.0- ☑
　passage, urethra (prostatic) N36.5
　pregnancy F45.8
Family, familial (see also condition)
　disruption Z63.8
　　involving divorce or separation Z63.5
　Li-Fraumeni (syndrome) Z15.01
　planning advice Z30.09
　problem Z63.9
　　specified NEC Z63.8
　retinoblastoma C69.2- ☑
Famine (effects of) T73.0 ☑
　edema — see Malnutrition, severe
Fanconi (-de Toni)(-Debré) **syndrome** E72.09
　with cystinosis E72.04
Fanconi's anemia (congenital pancytopenia) D61.09
Farber's disease or syndrome E75.29
Farcy A24.0
Farmer's
　lung J67.0
　skin L57.8
Farsightedness — see Hypermetropia
Fascia — see condition
Fasciculation R25.3
Fasciitis M72.9
　diffuse (eosinophilic) M35.4
　infective M72.8
　　necrotizing M72.6
　necrotizing M72.6
　nodular M72.4
　perirenal (with ureteral obstruction) N13.5
　　with infection N13.6
　plantar M72.2
　specified NEC M72.8
　traumatic (old) M72.8
　　current — code by site under Sprain
Fascioliasis B66.3
Fasciolopsis, fasciolopsiasis (intestinal) B66.5
Fascioscapulohumeral myopathy G71.0
Fast pulse R00.0
Fat
　embolism — see Embolism, fat
　excessive (see also Obesity)
　　in heart — see Degeneration, myocardial
　in stool R19.5
　localized (pad) E65
　　heart — see Degeneration, myocardial
　　knee M79.4
　　retropatellar M79.4
　necrosis
　　breast N64.1
　　mesentery K65.4
　　omentum K65.4
　pad E65
　　knee M79.4
Fatigue R53.83
　auditory deafness — see Deafness
　chronic R53.82
　combat F43.0
　general R53.83
　　psychogenic F48.8
　heat (transient) T67.6 ☑
　muscle M62.89
　myocardium — see Failure, heart
　neoplasm-related R53.0
　nervous, neurosis F48.8
　operational F48.8
　psychogenic (general) F48.8
　senile R54
　voice R49.8
Fatness — see Obesity
Fatty (see also condition)
　apron E65

Fatty — continued
　degeneration — see Degeneration, fatty
　heart (enlarged) — see Degeneration, myocardial
　liver NEC K76.0
　　alcoholic K70.0
　　nonalcoholic K76.0
　necrosis — see Degeneration, fatty
Fauces — see condition
Fauchard's disease (periodontitis) — see Periodontitis
Faucitis J02.9
Favism (anemia) D55.0
Favus — see Dermatophytosis
Fazio-Londe disease or syndrome G12.1
Fear complex or reaction F40.9
Fear of — see Phobia
Feared complaint unfounded Z71.1
Febris, febrile (see also Fever)
　flava (see also Fever, yellow) A95.9
　melitensis A23.0
　pestis — see Plague
　recurrens — see Fever, relapsing
　rubra A38.9
Fecal
　incontinence R15.9
　smearing R15.1
　soiling R15.1
　urgency R15.2
Fecalith (impaction) K56.41
　appendix K38.1
　congenital P76.8
Fede's disease K14.0
Feeble rapid pulse due to shock following injury
　T79.4 ☑
Feeble-minded F70
Feeding
　difficulties R63.3
　problem R63.3
　　newborn P92.9
　　　specified NEC P92.8
　　nonorganic (adult) — see Disorder, eating
Feeling (of)
　foreign body in throat R09.89
Feer's disease — see Poisoning, mercury
Feet — see condition
Feigned illness Z76.5
Feil-Klippel syndrome (brevicollis) Q76.1
Feinmesser's (hidrotic) **ectodermal dysplasia** Q82.4
Felinophobia F40.218
Felon (see also Cellulitis, digit)
　with lymphangitis — see Lymphangitis, acute, digit
Felty's syndrome M05.00
　ankle M05.07- ☑
　elbow M05.02- ☑
　foot joint M05.07- ☑
　hand joint M05.04- ☑
　hip M05.05- ☑
　knee M05.06- ☑
　multiple site M05.09
　shoulder M05.01- ☑
　vertebra — see Spondylitis, ankylosing
　wrist M05.03- ☑
Female genital cutting status — see Female genital
　mutilation status (FGM)
Female genital mutilation status (FGM) N90.810
　specified NEC N90.818
　type I (clitorectomy status) N90.811
　type II (clitorectomy with excision of labia minora status) N90.812
　type III (infibulation status) N90.813
　type IV N90.818
Femur, femoral — see condition
Fenestration, fenestrated (see also Imperfect, closure)
　aortico-pulmonary Q21.4
　cusps, heart valve NEC Q24.8
　　pulmonary Q22.3
　pulmonic cusps Q22.3
Fernell's disease (aortic aneurysm) I71.9
Fertile eunuch syndrome E23.0
Fetid
　breath R19.6
　sweat L75.0
Fetishism F65.0
　transvestic F65.1
Fetus, fetal (see also condition)
　alcohol syndrome (dysmorphic) Q86.0
　compressus O31.0- ☑
　hydantoin syndrome Q86.1

Fetus, fetal — continued
　lung tissue P28.0
　papyraceous O31.0- ☑
Fever (inanition) (of unknown origin) (persistent) (with chills) (with rigor) R50.9
　abortus A23.1
　Aden (dengue) A90
　African tick-borne A68.1
　American
　　mountain (tick) A93.2
　　spotted A77.0
　aphthous B08.8
　arbovirus, arboviral A94
　　hemorrhagic A94
　　specified NEC A93.8
　Argentinian hemorrhagic A96.0
　Assam B55.0
　Australian Q A78
　Bangkok hemorrhagic A91
　Barmah forest A92.8
　Bartonella A44.0
　bilious, hemoglobinuric B50.8
　blackwater B50.8
　blister B00.1
　Bolivian hemorrhagic A96.1
　Bonvale dam T73.3 ☑
　boutonneuse A77.1
　brain — see Encephalitis
　Brazilian purpuric A48.4
　breakbone A90
　Bullis A77.0
　Bunyamwera A92.8
　Burdwan B55.0
　Bwamba A92.8
　Cameroon — see Malaria
　Canton A75.9
　catarrhal (acute) J00
　　chronic J31.0
　cat-scratch A28.1
　Central Asian hemorrhagic A98.0
　cerebral — see Encephalitis
　cerebrospinal meningococcal A39.0
　Chagres B50.9
　Chandipura A92.8
　Changuinola A93.1
　Charcot's (biliary) (hepatic) (intermittent) — see Calculus, bile duct
　Chikungunya (viral) (hemorrhagic) A92.0
　Chitral A93.1
　Colombo — see Fever, paratyphoid
　Colorado tick (virus) A93.2
　congestive (remittent) — see Malaria
　Congo virus A98.0
　continued malarial B50.9
　Corsican — see Malaria
　Crimean-Congo hemorrhagic A98.0
　Cyprus — see Brucellosis
　dandy A90
　deer fly — see Tularemia
　dengue (virus) A90
　　hemorrhagic A91
　　sandfly A93.1
　desert B38.0
　drug induced R50.2
　due to
　　conditions classified elsewhere R50.81
　　heat T67.0 ☑
　enteric A01.00
　enteroviral exanthematous (Boston exanthem) A88.0
　ephemeral (of unknown origin) R50.9
　epidemic hemorrhagic A98.5
　erysipelatous — see Erysipelas
　estivo-autumnal (malarial) B50.9
　famine A75.0
　five day A79.0
　following delivery O86.4
　Fort Bragg A27.89
　gastroenteric A01.00
　gastromalarial — see Malaria
　Gibraltar — see Brucellosis
　glandular — see Mononucleosis, infectious
　Guama (viral) A92.8
　Haverhill A25.1
　hay (allergic) J30.1
　　with asthma (bronchial) J45.909
　　　with
　　　　exacerbation (acute) J45.901
　　　　status asthmaticus J45.902

Fever — *continued*
  hay — *continued*
    due to
      allergen other than pollen J30.89
      pollen, any plant or tree J30.1
  heat (effects) T67.0 ☑
  hematuric, bilious B50.8
  hemoglobinuric (malarial) (bilious) B50.8
  hemorrhagic (arthropod-borne) NOS A94
    with renal syndrome A98.5
    arenaviral A96.9
      specified NEC A96.8
    Argentinian A96.0
    Bangkok A91
    Bolivian A96.1
    Central Asian A98.0
    Chikungunya A92.0
    Crimean-Congo A98.0
    dengue (virus) A91
    epidemic A98.5
    Junin (virus) A96.0
    Korean A98.5
    Kyasanur forest A98.2
    Machupo (virus) A96.1
    mite-borne A93.8
    mosquito-borne A92.8
    Omsk A98.1
    Philippine A91
    Russian A98.5
    Singapore A91
    Southeast Asia A91
    Thailand A91
    tick-borne NEC A93.8
    viral A99
      specified NEC A98.8
  hepatic — *see* Cholecystitis
  herpetic — *see* Herpes
  icterohemorrhagic A27.0
  Indiana A93.8
  infective B99.9
    specified NEC B99.8
  intermittent (bilious) (*see also* Malaria)
    of unknown origin R50.9
    pernicious B50.9
  iodide R50.2
  Japanese river A75.3
  jungle (*see also* Malaria)
    yellow A95.0
  Junin (virus) hemorrhagic A96.0
  Katayama B65.2
  kedani A75.3
  Kenya (tick) A77.1
  Kew Garden A79.1
  Korean hemorrhagic A98.5
  Lassa A96.2
  Lone Star A77.0
  Machupo (virus) hemorrhagic A96.1
  malaria, malarial — *see* Malaria
  Malta A23.9
  Marseilles A77.1
  marsh — *see* Malaria
  Mayaro (viral) A92.8
  Mediterranean (*see also* Brucellosis) A23.9
    familial E85.0
    tick A77.1
  meningeal — *see* Meningitis
  Meuse A79.0
  Mexican A75.2
  mianeh A68.1
  miasmatic — *see* Malaria
  mosquito-borne (viral) A92.9
    hemorrhagic A92.8
  mountain (*see also* Brucellosis)
    meaning Rocky Mountain spotted fever A77.0
    tick (American) (Colorado) (viral) A93.2
  Mucambo (viral) A92.8
  mud A27.9
  Neapolitan — *see* Brucellosis
  neutropenic D70.9
  newborn P81.9
    environmental P81.0
  Nine-Mile A78
  non-exanthematous tick A93.2
  North Asian tick-borne A77.2
  Omsk hemorrhagic A98.1
  O'nyong-nyong (viral) A92.1
  Oropouche (viral) A93.0
  Oroya A44.0

Fever — *continued*
  paludal — *see* Malaria
  Panama (malarial) B50.9
  Pappataci A93.1
  paratyphoid A01.4
    A A01.1
    B A01.2
    C A01.3
  parrot A70
  periodic (Mediterranean) E85.0
  persistent (of unknown origin) R50.9
  petechial A39.0
  pharyngoconjunctival B30.2
  Philippine hemorrhagic A91
  phlebotomus A93.1
  Piry (virus) A93.8
  Pixuna (viral) A92.8
  Plasmodium ovale B53.0
  polioviral (nonparalytic) A80.4
  Pontiac A48.2
  postimmunization R50.83
  postoperative R50.82
    due to infection T81.4 ☑
  posttransfusion R50.84
  postvaccination R50.83
  presenting with conditions classified elsewhere R50.81
  pretibial A27.89
  puerperal O86.4
  Q A78
  quadrilateral A78
  quartan (malaria) B52.9
  Queensland (coastal) (tick) A77.3
  quintan A79.0
  rabbit — *see* Tularemia
  rat-bite A25.9
    due to
      Spirillum A25.0
      Streptobacillus moniliformis A25.1
  recurrent — *see* Fever, relapsing
  relapsing (Borrelia) A68.9
    Carter's (Asiatic) A68.1
    Dutton's (West African) A68.1
    Koch's A68.9
    louse-borne A68.0
    Novy's
      louse-borne A68.0
      tick-borne A68.1
    Obermeyer's (European) A68.0
    tick-borne A68.1
  remittent (bilious) (congestive) (gastric) — *see* Malaria
  rheumatic (active) (acute) (chronic) (subacute) I00
    with central nervous system involvement I02.9
    active with heart involvement — *see* category
      I01 ☑
    inactive or quiescent with
      cardiac hypertrophy I09.89
      carditis I09.9
      endocarditis I09.1
        aortic (valve) I06.9
          with mitral (valve) disease I08.0
        mitral (valve) I05.9
          with aortic (valve) disease I08.0
        pulmonary (valve) I09.89
        tricuspid (valve) I07.8
      heart disease NEC I09.89
      heart failure (congestive) (conditions in I50.9) I09.81
      left ventricular failure (conditions in I50.1) I09.81
      myocarditis, myocardial degeneration (conditions in I51.4) I09.0
      pancarditis I09.9
      pericarditis I09.2
  Rift Valley (viral) A92.4
  Rocky Mountain spotted A77.0
  rose J30.1
  Ross River B33.1
  Russian hemorrhagic A98.5
  San Joaquin (Valley) B38.0
  sandfly A93.1
  Sao Paulo A77.0
  scarlet A38.9
  seven day (leptospirosis) (autumnal) (Japanese) A27.89
    dengue A90
  shin-bone A79.0
  Singapore hemorrhagic A91
  solar A90
  Songo A98.5

Fever — *continued*
  sore B00.1
  South African tick-bite A68.1
  Southeast Asia hemorrhagic A91
  spinal — *see* Meningitis
  spirillary A25.0
  splenic — *see* Anthrax
  spotted A77.9
    American A77.0
    Brazilian A77.0
    cerebrospinal meningitis A39.0
    Colombian A77.0
    due to Rickettsia
      australis A77.3
      conorii A77.1
      rickettsii A77.0
      sibirica A77.2
      specified type NEC A77.8
    Ehrlichiosis A77.40
      due to
        E. chafeensis A77.41
        specified organism NEC A77.49
    Rocky Mountain A77.0
  steroid R50.2
  streptobacillary A25.1
  subtertian B50.9
  Sumatran mite A75.3
  sun A90
  swamp A27.9
  swine A02.8
  sylvatic, yellow A95.0
  Tahyna B33.8
  tertian — *see* Malaria, tertian
  Thailand hemorrhagic A91
  thermic T67.0 ☑
  three-day A93.1
  tick
    American mountain A93.2
    Colorado A93.2
    Kemerovo A93.8
    Mediterranean A77.1
    mountain A93.2
    nonexanthematous A93.2
    Quaranfil A93.8
  tick-bite NEC A93.8
  tick-borne (hemorrhagic) NEC A93.8
  trench A79.0
  tsutsugamushi A75.3
  typhogastric A01.00
  typhoid (abortive) (hemorrhagic) (intermittent) (malignant) A01.00
    complicated by
      arthritis A01.04
      heart involvement A01.02
      meningitis A01.01
      osteomyelitis A01.05
      pneumonia A01.03
      specified NEC A01.09
  typhomalarial — *see* Malaria
  typhus — *see* Typhus (fever)
  undulant — *see* Brucellosis
  unknown origin R50.9
  uveoparotid D86.89
  valley B38.0
  Venezuelan equine A92.2
  vesicular stomatitis A93.8
  viral hemorrhagic — *see* Fever, hemorrhagic, by type of virus
  Volhynian A79.0
  Wesselsbron (viral) A92.8
  West
    African B50.8
    Nile (viral) A92.30
      with
        complications NEC A92.39
        cranial nerve disorders A92.32
        encephalitis A92.31
        encephalomyelitis A92.31
        neurologic manifestation NEC A92.32
        optic neuritis A92.32
        polyradiculitis A92.32
  Whitmore's — *see* Melioidosis
  Wolhynian A79.0
  worm B83.9
  yellow A95.9
    jungle A95.0
    sylvatic A95.0
    urban A95.1

Fever — *continued*
  Zika (viral) A92.8
Fibrillation
  atrial or auricular (established) I48.91
    chronic I48.2
    paroxysmal I48.0
    permanent I48.2
    persistent I48.1
  cardiac I49.8
  heart I49.8
  muscular M62.89
  ventricular I49.01
Fibrin
  ball or bodies, pleural (sac) J94.1
  chamber, anterior (eye) (gelatinous exudate) — *see*
    Iridocyclitis, acute
Fibrinogenolysis — *see* Fibrinolysis
Fibrinogenopenia D68.8
  acquired D65
  congenital D68.2
Fibrinolysis (hemorrhagic) (acquired) D65
  antepartum hemorrhage — *see* Hemorrhage, antepartum, with coagulation defect
  following
    abortion — *see* Abortion by type complicated by hemorrhage
    ectopic or molar pregnancy O08.1
  intrapartum O67.0
  newborn, transient P60
  postpartum O72.3
Fibrinopenia (hereditary) D68.2
  acquired D68.4
Fibrinopurulent — *see* condition
Fibrinous — *see* condition
Fibroadenoma
  cellular intracanalicular D24- ☑
  giant D24- ☑
  intracanalicular
    cellular D24- ☑
    giant D24- ☑
    specified site — *see* Neoplasm, benign, by site
    unspecified site D24- ☑
  juvenile D24- ☑
  pericanalicular
    specified site — *see* Neoplasm, benign, by site
    unspecified site D24- ☑
  phyllodes D24- ☑
  prostate D29.1
  specified site NEC — *see* Neoplasm, benign, by site
  unspecified site D24- ☑
Fibroadenosis, breast (chronic) (cystic) (diffuse) (periodic) (segmental) N60.2- ☑
Fibroangioma (*see also* Neoplasm, benign, by site)
  juvenile
    specified site — *see* Neoplasm, benign, by site
    unspecified site D10.6
Fibrochondrosarcoma — *see* Neoplasm, cartilage, malignant
Fibrocystic
  disease (*see also* Fibrosis, cystic)
    breast — *see* Mastopathy, cystic
    jaw M27.49
    kidney (congenital) Q61.8
    liver Q44.6
    pancreas E84.9
  kidney (congenital) Q61.8
Fibrodysplasia ossificans progressiva — *see* Myositis, ossificans, progressiva
Fibroelastosis (cordis) (endocardial) (endomyocardial) I42.4
Fibroid (tumor) (*see also* Neoplasm, connective tissue, benign)
  disease, lung (chronic) — *see* Fibrosis, lung
  heart (disease) — *see* Myocarditis
  in pregnancy or childbirth O34.1- ☑
    causing obstructed labor O65.5
  induration, lung (chronic) — *see* Fibrosis, lung
  lung — *see* Fibrosis, lung
  pneumonia (chronic) — *see* Fibrosis, lung
  uterus D25.9
Fibrolipoma — *see* Lipoma
Fibroliposarcoma — *see* Neoplasm, connective tissue, malignant
Fibroma (*see also* Neoplasm, connective tissue, benign)
  ameloblastic — *see* Cyst, calcifying odontogenic
  bone (nonossifying) — *see* Disorder, bone, specified type NEC

Fibroma — *continued*
  bone — *see* Disorder, bone, specified type — *continued*
    ossifying — *see* Neoplasm, bone, benign
  cementifying — *see* Neoplasm, bone, benign
  chondromyxoid — *see* Neoplasm, bone, benign
  desmoplastic — *see* Neoplasm, connective tissue, uncertain behavior
  durum — *see* Neoplasm, connective tissue, benign
  fascial — *see* Neoplasm, connective tissue, benign
  invasive — *see* Neoplasm, connective tissue, uncertain behavior
  molle — *see* Lipoma
  myxoid — *see* Neoplasm, connective tissue, benign
  nasopharynx, nasopharyngeal (juvenile) D10.6
  nonosteogenic (nonossifying) — *see* Dysplasia, fibrous
  odontogenic (central) — *see* Cyst, calcifying odontogenic
  ossifying — *see* Neoplasm, bone, benign
  periosteal — *see* Neoplasm, bone, benign
  soft — *see* Lipoma
Fibromatosis M72.9
  abdominal — *see* Neoplasm, connective tissue, uncertain behavior
  aggressive — *see* Neoplasm, connective tissue, uncertain behavior
  congenital generalized — *see* Neoplasm, connective tissue, uncertain behavior
  Dupuytren's M72.0
  gingival K06.1
  palmar (fascial) M72.0
  plantar (fascial) M72.2
  pseudosarcomatous (proliferative) (subcutaneous) M72.4
  retroperitoneal D48.3
  specified NEC M72.8
Fibromyalgia M79.7
Fibromyoma (*see also* Neoplasm, connective tissue, benign)
  uterus (corpus) (*see also* Leiomyoma, uterus)
    in pregnancy or childbirth — *see* Fibroid, in pregnancy or childbirth
    causing obstructed labor O65.5
Fibromyositis M79.7
Fibromyxolipoma D17.9
Fibromyxoma — *see* Neoplasm, connective tissue, benign
Fibromyxosarcoma — *see* Neoplasm, connective tissue, malignant
Fibro-odontoma, ameloblastic — *see* Cyst, calcifying odontogenic
Fibro-osteoma — *see* Neoplasm, bone, benign
Fibroplasia, retrolental H35.17- ☑
Fibropurulent — *see* condition
Fibrosarcoma (*see also* Neoplasm, connective tissue, malignant)
  ameloblastic C41.1
    upper jaw (bone) C41.0
  congenital — *see* Neoplasm, connective tissue, malignant
  fascial — *see* Neoplasm, connective tissue, malignant
  infantile — *see* Neoplasm, connective tissue, malignant
  odontogenic C41.1
    upper jaw (bone) C41.0
  periosteal — *see* Neoplasm, bone, malignant
Fibrosclerosis
  breast N60.3- ☑
  multifocal M35.5
  penis (corpora cavernosa) N48.6
Fibrosis, fibrotic
  adrenal (gland) E27.8
  amnion O41.8X- ☑
  anal papillae K62.89
  arteriocapillary — *see* Arteriosclerosis
  bladder N32.89
    interstitial — *see* Cystitis, chronic, interstitial
    localized submucosal — *see* Cystitis, chronic, interstitial
    panmural — *see* Cystitis, chronic, interstitial
  breast — *see* Fibrosclerosis, breast
  capillary (*see also* Arteriosclerosis) I70.90
    lung (chronic) — *see* Fibrosis, lung
  cardiac — *see* Myocarditis
  cervix N88.8
  chorion O41.8X- ☑
  corpus cavernosum (sclerosing) N48.6

Fibrosis, fibrotic — *continued*
  cystic (of pancreas) E84.9
    with
      distal intestinal obstruction syndrome E84.19
      fecal impaction E84.19
      intestinal manifestations NEC E84.19
      pulmonary manifestations E84.0
      specified manifestations NEC E84.8
  due to device, implant or graft (*see also* Complications, by site and type, specified NEC) T85.82 ☑
    arterial graft NEC T82.828 ☑
    breast (implant) T85.82 ☑
    catheter NEC T85.82 ☑
      dialysis (renal) T82.828 ☑
        intraperitoneal T85.82 ☑
      infusion NEC T82.828 ☑
        spinal (epidural) (subdural) T85.82 ☑
      urinary (indwelling) T83.82 ☑
    electronic (electrode) (pulse generator) (stimulator)
      bone T84.82 ☑
      cardiac T82.827 ☑
      nervous system (brain) (peripheral nerve) (spinal) T85.82 ☑
      urinary T83.82 ☑
    fixation, internal (orthopedic) NEC T84.82 ☑
    gastrointestinal (bile duct) (esophagus) T85.82 ☑
    genital NEC T83.82 ☑
    heart NEC T82.827 ☑
    joint prosthesis T84.82 ☑
    ocular (corneal graft) (orbital implant) NEC T85.82 ☑
    orthopedic NEC T84.82 ☑
    specified NEC T85.82 ☑
    urinary NEC T83.82 ☑
    vascular NEC T82.828 ☑
    ventricular intracranial shunt T85.82 ☑
  ejaculatory duct N50.8
  endocardium — *see* Endocarditis
  endomyocardial (tropical) I42.3
  epididymis N50.8
  eye muscle — *see* Strabismus, mechanical
  heart — *see* Myocarditis
  hepatic — *see* Fibrosis, liver
  hepatolienal (portal hypertension) K76.6
  hepatosplenic (portal hypertension) K76.6
  infrapatellar fat pad M79.4
  intrascrotal N50.8
  kidney N26.9
  liver K74.0
    with sclerosis K74.2
    alcoholic K70.2
  lung (atrophic) (chronic) (confluent) (massive) (perialveolar) (peribronchial) J84.10
    with
      anthracosilicosis J60
      anthracosis J60
      asbestosis J61
      bagassosis J67.1
      bauxite J63.1
      berylliosis J63.2
      byssinosis J66.0
      calcicosis J62.8
      chalicosis J62.8
      dust reticulation J64
      farmer's lung J67.0
      ganister disease J62.8
      graphite J63.3
      pneumoconiosis NOS J64
      siderosis J63.4
      silicosis J62.8
    capillary J84.10
    congenital P27.8
    diffuse (idiopathic) J84.10
      chemicals, gases, fumes or vapors (inhalation) J68.4
      interstitial J84.10
        acute J84.114
      talc J62.0
    following radiation J70.1
    idiopathic J84.112
    postinflammatory J84.10
    silicotic J62.8
    tuberculous — *see* Tuberculosis, pulmonary
  lymphatic gland I89.8
  median bar — *see* Hyperplasia, prostate
  mediastinum (idiopathic) J98.5
  meninges G96.19

Fibrosis, fibrotic — *continued*
myocardium, myocardial — *see* Myocarditis
ovary N83.8
oviduct N83.8
pancreas K86.8
penis NEC N48.6
pericardium I31.0
perineum, in pregnancy or childbirth O34.7- ☑
causing obstructed labor O65.5
pleura J94.1
popliteal fat pad M79.4
prostate (chronic) — *see* Hyperplasia, prostate
pulmonary (*see also* Fibrosis, lung) J84.10
congenital P27.8
idiopathic J84.112
rectal sphincter K62.89
retroperitoneal, idiopathic (with ureteral obstruction) N13.5
with infection N13.6
sclerosing mesenteric (idiopathic) K65.4
scrotum N50.8
seminal vesicle N50.8
senile R54
skin L90.5
spermatic cord N50.8
spleen D73.89
in schistosomiasis (bilharziasis) B65.9 [D77]
subepidermal nodular — *see* Neoplasm, skin, benign
submucous (oral) (tongue) K13.5
testis N44.8
chronic, due to syphilis A52.76
thymus (gland) E32.8
tongue, submucous K13.5
tunica vaginalis N50.8
uterus (non-neoplastic) N85.8
vagina N89.8
valve, heart — *see* Endocarditis
vas deferens N50.8
vein I87.8
Fibrositis (periarticular) M79.7
nodular, chronic (Jaccoud's) (rheumatoid) — *see* Arthropathy, postrheumatic, chronic
Fibrothorax J94.1
Fibrotic — *see* Fibrosis
Fibrous — *see* condition
Fibroxanthoma (*see also* Neoplasm, connective tissue, benign)
atypical — *see* Neoplasm, connective tissue, uncertain behavior
malignant — *see* Neoplasm, connective tissue, malignant
Fibroxanthosarcoma — *see* Neoplasm, connective tissue, malignant
Fiedler's
disease (icterohemorrhagic leptospirosis) A27.0
myocarditis (acute) I40.1
Fifth disease B08.3
venereal A55
Filaria, filarial, filariasis — *see* Infestation, filarial
Filatov's disease — *see* Mononucleosis, infectious
File-cutter's disease — *see* Poisoning, lead
Filling defect
biliary tract R93.2
bladder R93.4
duodenum R93.3
gallbladder R93.2
gastrointestinal tract R93.3
intestine R93.3
kidney R93.4
stomach R93.3
ureter R93.4
Fimbrial cyst Q50.4
Financial problem affecting care NOS Z59.9
bankruptcy Z59.8
foreclosure on loan Z59.8
Findings, abnormal, inconclusive, without diagnosis (*see also* Abnormal)
17-ketosteroids, elevated R82.5
acetonuria R82.4
alcohol in blood R78.0
anisocytosis R71.8
antenatal screening of mother O28.9
biochemical O28.1
chromosomal O28.5
cytological O28.2
genetic O28.5
hematological O28.0
radiological O28.4

Findings, abnormal, inconclusive, without diagnosis — *continued*
antenatal screening of mother — *continued*
specified NEC O28.8
ultrasonic O28.3
antibody titer, elevated R76.0
anticardiolipin antibody R76.0
antiphosphatidylglycerol antibody R76.0
antiphosphatidylinositol antibody R76.0
antiphosphatidylserine antibody R76.0
antiphospholipid antibody R76.0
bacteriuria N39.0
bicarbonate E87.8
bile in urine R82.2
blood sugar R73.09
high R73.9
low (transient) E16.2
body fluid or substance, specified NEC R88.8
casts, urine R82.99
catecholamines R82.5
cells, urine R82.99
chloride E87.8
cholesterol E78.9
high E78.0
with high triglycerides E78.2
chyluria R82.0
cloudy
dialysis effluent R88.0
urine R82.90
creatinine clearance R94.4
crystals, urine R82.99
culture
blood R78.81
positive — *see* Positive, culture
echocardiogram R93.1
electrolyte level, urinary R82.99
function study NEC R94.8
bladder R94.8
endocrine NEC R94.7
thyroid R94.6
kidney R94.4
liver R94.5
pancreas R94.8
placenta R94.8
pulmonary R94.2
spleen R94.8
gallbladder, nonvisualization R93.2
glucose (tolerance test) (non-fasting) R73.09
glycosuria R81
heart
shadow R93.1
sounds R01.2
hematinuria R82.3
hematocrit drop (precipitous) R71.0
hemoglobinuria R82.3
human papillomavirus (HPV) DNA test positive
cervix
high risk R87.810
low risk R87.820
vagina
high risk R87.811
low risk R87.821
in blood (of substance not normally found in blood) R78.9
addictive drug NEC R78.4
alcohol (excessive level) R78.0
cocaine R78.2
hallucinogen R78.3
heavy metals (abnormal level) R78.79
lead R78.71
lithium (abnormal level) R78.89
opiate drug R78.1
psychotropic drug R78.5
specified substance NEC R78.89
steroid agent R78.6
indoleacetic acid, elevated R82.5
ketonuria R82.4
lactic acid dehydrogenase (LDH) R74.0
liver function test R79.89
mammogram NEC R92.8
calcification (calculus) R92.1
inconclusive result (due to dense breasts) R92.2
microcalcification R92.0
mediastinal shift R93.8
melanin, urine R82.99
myoglobinuria R82.1
neonatal screening P09
nonvisualization of gallbladder R93.2

Findings, abnormal, inconclusive, without diagnosis — *continued*
odor of urine NOS R82.90
Papanicolaou cervix R87.619
non-atypical endometrial cells R87.618
pneumoencephalogram R93.0
poikilocytosis R71.8
potassium (deficiency) E87.6
excess E87.5
PPD R76.11
radiologic (X-ray) R93.8
abdomen R93.5
biliary tract R93.2
breast R92.8
gastrointestinal tract R93.3
genitourinary organs R93.8
head R93.0
inconclusive due to excess body fat of patient R93.9
intrathoracic organs NEC R93.1
placenta R93.8
retroperitoneum R93.5
skin R93.8
skull R93.0
subcutaneous tissue R93.8
red blood cell (count) (morphology) (sickling) (volume) R71.8
scan NEC R94.8
bladder R94.8
bone R94.8
kidney R94.4
liver R93.2
lung R94.2
pancreas R94.8
placental R94.8
spleen R94.8
thyroid R94.6
sedimentation rate, elevated R70.0
SGOT R74.0
SGPT R74.0
sodium (deficiency) E87.1
excess E87.0
specified body fluid NEC R88.8
stress test R94.39
thyroid (function) (metabolic rate) (scan) (uptake) R94.6
transaminase (level) R74.0
triglycerides E78.9
high E78.1
with high cholesterol E78.2
tuberculin skin test (without active tuberculosis) R76.11
urine R82.90
acetone R82.4
bacteria N39.0
bile R82.2
casts or cells R82.99
chyle R82.0
culture positive R82.7
glucose R81
hemoglobin R82.3
ketone R82.4
sugar R81
vanillylmandelic acid (VMA), elevated R82.5
vectorcardiogram (VCG) R94.39
ventriculogram R93.0
white blood cell (count) (differential) (morphology) D72.9
xerography R92.8
Finger — *see* condition
Fire, Saint Anthony's — *see* Erysipelas
Fire-setting
pathological (compulsive) F63.1
Fish hook stomach K31.89
Fishmeal-worker's lung J67.8
Fissure, fissured
anus, anal K60.2
acute K60.0
chronic K60.1
congenital Q43.8
ear, lobule, congenital Q17.8
epiglottis (congenital) Q31.8
larynx J38.7
congenital Q31.8
lip K13.0
congenital — *see* Cleft, lip
nipple N64.0
associated with
lactation O92.13

☑ **Additional Character Required** — **Refer to the Tabular List for Character Selection**

⌖ **Subterms under main terms may continue to next column or page**

Fissure, fissured — *continued*
  nipple — *continued*
    associated with — *continued*
      pregnancy O92.11- ☑
      puerperium O92.12
  nose Q30.2
  palate (congenital) — *see* Cleft, palate
  skin R23.4
  spine (congenital) (*see also* Spina bifida)
    with hydrocephalus — *see* Spina bifida, by site,
      with hydrocephalus
  tongue (acquired) K14.5
    congenital Q38.3
Fistula (cutaneous) L98.8
  abdomen (wall) K63.2
    bladder N32.2
    intestine NEC K63.2
    ureter N28.89
    uterus N82.5
  abdominorectal K63.2
  abdominosigmoidal K63.2
  abdominothoracic J86.0
  abdominouterine N82.5
    congenital Q51.7
  abdominovesical N32.2
  accessory sinuses — *see* Sinusitis
  actinomycotic — *see* Actinomycosis
  alveolar antrum — *see* Sinusitis, maxillary
  alveolar process K04.6
  anorectal K60.5
  antrobuccal — *see* Sinusitis, maxillary
  antrum — *see* Sinusitis, maxillary
  anus, anal (recurrent) (infectional) K60.3
    congenital Q43.6
      with absence, atresia and stenosis Q42.2
    tuberculous A18.32
  aorta-duodenal I77.2
  appendix, appendicular K38.3
  arteriovenous (acquired) (nonruptured) I77.0
    brain I67.1
      congenital Q28.2
        ruptured I60.8
      ruptured I60.8
    cerebral — *see* Fistula, arteriovenous, brain
    congenital (peripheral) (*see also* Malformation, ar-
      teriovenous)
      brain Q28.2
        ruptured I60.8
      coronary Q24.5
      pulmonary Q25.72
    coronary I25.41
      congenital Q24.5
    pulmonary I28.0
      congenital Q25.72
    surgically created (for dialysis) Z99.2
      complication — *see* Complication, arteriove-
        nous, fistula, surgically created
    traumatic — *see* Injury, blood vessel
  artery I77.2
  aural (mastoid) — *see* Mastoiditis, chronic
  auricle (*see also* Disorder, pinna, specified type NEC)
    congenital Q18.1
  Bartholin's gland N82.8
  bile duct (common) (hepatic) K83.3
    with calculus, stones — *see* Calculus, bile duct
  biliary (tract) — *see* Fistula, bile duct
  bladder (sphincter) NEC (*see also* Fistula, vesico-) N32.2
    into seminal vesicle N32.2
  bone (*see also* Disorder, bone, specified type NEC)
    with osteomyelitis, chronic — *see* Osteomyelitis,
      chronic, with draining sinus
  brain G93.89
    arteriovenous (acquired) I67.1
      congenital Q28.2
  branchial (cleft) Q18.0
  branchiogenous Q18.0
  breast N61
    puerperal, postpartum or gestational, due to mas-
      titis (purulent) — *see* Mastitis, obstetric, pu-
      rulent
  bronchial J86.0
  bronchocutaneous, bronchomediastinal, bronchopleu-
    ral, bronchopleuromediastinal (infective) J86.0
    tuberculous NEC A15.5
  bronchoesophageal J86.0
    congenital Q39.2
      with atresia of esophagus Q39.1
  bronchovisceral J86.0

Fistula — *continued*
  buccal cavity (infective) K12.2
  cecosigmoidal K63.2
  cecum K63.2
  cerebrospinal (fluid) G96.0
  cervical, lateral Q18.1
  cervicoaural Q18.1
  cervicosigmoidal N82.4
  cervicovesical N82.1
  cervix N82.8
  chest (wall) J86.0
  cholecystenteric — *see* Fistula, gallbladder
  cholecystocolic — *see* Fistula, gallbladder
  cholecystocolonic — *see* Fistula, gallbladder
  cholecystoduodenal — *see* Fistula, gallbladder
  cholecystogastric — *see* Fistula, gallbladder
  cholecystointestinal — *see* Fistula, gallbladder
  choledochoduodenal — *see* Fistula, bile duct
  cholocolic K82.3
  coccyx — *see* Sinus, pilonidal
  colon K63.2
  colostomy K94.09
  common duct — *see* Fistula, bile duct
  congenital, site not listed — *see* Anomaly, by site
  coronary, arteriovenous I25.41
    congenital Q24.5
  costal region J86.0
  cul-de-sac, Douglas' N82.8
  cystic duct (*see also* Fistula, gallbladder)
    congenital Q44.5
  dental K04.6
  diaphragm J86.0
  duodenum K31.6
  ear (external) (canal) — *see* Disorder, ear, external,
    specified type NEC
  enterocolic K63.2
  enterocutaneous K63.2
  enterouterine N82.4
    congenital Q51.7
  enterovaginal N82.4
    congenital Q52.2
    large intestine N82.3
    small intestine N82.2
  enterovesical N32.1
  epididymis N50.8
    tuberculous A18.15
  esophagobronchial J86.0
    congenital Q39.2
      with atresia of esophagus Q39.1
  esophagocutaneous K22.8
  esophagopleural-cutaneous J86.0
  esophagotracheal J86.0
    congenital Q39.2
      with atresia of esophagus Q39.1
  esophagus K22.8
    congenital Q39.2
      with atresia of esophagus Q39.1
  ethmoid — *see* Sinusitis, ethmoidal
  eyeball (cornea) (sclera) — *see* Disorder, globe, hy-
    potony
  eyelid H01.8
  fallopian tube, external N82.5
  fecal K63.2
    congenital Q43.6
  from periapical abscess K04.6
  frontal sinus — *see* Sinusitis, frontal
  gallbladder K82.3
    with calculus, cholelithiasis, stones — *see* Calculus,
      gallbladder
  gastric K31.6
  gastrocolic K31.6
    congenital Q40.2
    tuberculous A18.32
  gastroenterocolic K31.6
  gastroesophageal K31.6
  gastrojejunal K31.6
  gastrojejunocolic K31.6
  genital tract (female) N82.9
    specified NEC N82.8
    to intestine NEC N82.4
    to skin N82.5
  hepatic artery-portal vein, congenital Q26.6
  hepatopleural J86.0
  hepatopulmonary J86.0
  ileorectal or ileosigmoidal K63.2
  ileovaginal N82.2
  ileovesical N32.1
  ileum K63.2

Fistula — *continued*
  in ano K60.3
    tuberculous A18.32
  inner ear (labyrinth) — *see* subcategory H83.1 ☑
  intestine NEC K63.2
  intestinocolonic (abdominal) K63.2
  intestinoureteral N28.89
  intestinouterine N82.4
  intestinovaginal N82.4
    large intestine N82.3
    small intestine N82.2
  intestinovesical N32.1
  ischiorectal (fossa) K61.3
  jejunum K63.2
  joint M25.10
    ankle M25.17- ☑
    elbow M25.12- ☑
    foot joint M25.17- ☑
    hand joint M25.14- ☑
    hip M25.15- ☑
    knee M25.16- ☑
    shoulder M25.11- ☑
    specified joint NEC M25.18
    tuberculous — *see* Tuberculosis, joint
    vertebrae M25.18
    wrist M25.13- ☑
  kidney N28.89
  labium (majus) (minus) N82.8
  labyrinth — *see* subcategory H83.1 ☑
  lacrimal (gland) (sac) H04.61- ☑
  lacrimonasal duct — *see* Fistula, lacrimal
  laryngotracheal, congenital Q34.8
  larynx J38.7
  lip K13.0
    congenital Q38.0
  lumbar, tuberculous A18.01
  lung J86.0
  lymphatic I89.8
  mammary (gland) N61
  mastoid (process) (region) — *see* Mastoiditis, chronic
  maxillary J32.0
  medial, face and neck Q18.8
  mediastinal J86.0
  mediastinobronchial J86.0
  mediastinocutaneous J86.0
  middle ear — *see* subcategory H74.8 ☑
  mouth K12.2
  nasal J34.89
    sinus — *see* Sinusitis
  nasopharynx J39.2
  nipple N64.0
  nose J34.89
  oral (cutaneous) K12.2
    maxillary J32.0
    nasal (with cleft palate) — *see* Cleft, palate
  orbit, orbital — *see* Disorder, orbit, specified type NEC
  oroantral J32.0
  oviduct, external N82.5
  palate (hard) M27.8
  pancreatic K86.8
  pancreaticoduodenal K86.8
  parotid (gland) K11.4
    region K12.2
  penis N48.89
  perianal K60.3
  pericardium (pleura) (sac) — *see* Pericarditis
  pericecal K63.2
  perineorectal K60.4
  perineosigmoidal K63.2
  perineum, perineal (with urethral involvement) NEC
    N36.0
    tuberculous A18.13
    ureter N28.89
  perirectal K60.4
    tuberculous A18.32
  peritoneum K65.9
  pharyngoesophageal J39.2
  pharynx J39.2
    branchial cleft (congenital) Q18.0
  pilonidal (infected) (rectum) — *see* Sinus, pilonidal
  pleura, pleural, pleurocutaneous, pleuroperitoneal
    J86.0
    tuberculous NEC A15.6
  pleuropericardial I31.8
  portal vein-hepatic artery, congenital Q26.6
  postauricular H70.81- ☑
  postoperative, persistent T81.83 ☑
    specified site — *see* Fistula, by site

Fistula — *continued*
  preauricular (congenital) Q18.1
  prostate N42.89
  pulmonary J86.0
    arteriovenous I28.0
      congenital Q25.72
    tuberculous — *see* Tuberculosis, pulmonary
  pulmonoperitoneal J86.0
  rectolabial N82.4
  rectosigmoid (intercommunicating) K63.2
  rectoureteral N28.89
  rectourethral N36.0
    congenital Q64.73
  rectouterine N82.4
    congenital Q51.7
  rectovaginal N82.3
    congenital Q52.2
    tuberculous A18.18
  rectovesical N32.1
    congenital Q64.79
  rectovesicovaginal N82.3
  rectovulval N82.4
    congenital Q52.79
  rectum (to skin) K60.4
    congenital Q43.6
      with absence, atresia and stenosis Q42.0
    tuberculous A18.32
  renal N28.89
  retroauricular — *see* Fistula, postauricular
  salivary duct or gland (any) K11.4
    congenital Q38.4
  scrotum (urinary) N50.8
    tuberculous A18.15
  semicircular canals — *see* subcategory H83.1 ☑
  sigmoid K63.2
    to bladder N32.1
  sinus — *see* Sinusitis
  skin L98.8
    to genital tract (female) N82.5
  splenocolic D73.89
  stercoral K63.2
  stomach K31.6
  sublingual gland K11.4
  submandibular gland K11.4
  submaxillary (gland) K11.4
    region K12.2
  thoracic J86.0
    duct I89.8
  thoracoabdominal J86.0
  thoracogastric J86.0
  thoracointestinal J86.0
  thorax J86.0
  thyroglossal duct Q89.2
  thyroid E07.89
  trachea, congenital (external) (internal) Q32.1
  tracheoesophageal J86.0
    congenital Q39.2
      with atresia of esophagus Q39.1
    following tracheostomy J95.04
  traumatic arteriovenous — *see* Injury, blood vessel,
    by site
  tuberculous — *code by* site under Tuberculosis
  typhoid A01.09
  umbilicourinary Q64.8
  urachus, congenital Q64.4
  ureter (persistent) N28.89
  ureteroabdominal N28.89
  ureterorectal N28.89
  ureterosigmoido-abdominal N28.89
  ureterovaginal N82.1
  ureterovesical N32.2
  urethra N36.0
    congenital Q64.79
    tuberculous A18.13
  urethroperineal N36.0
  urethroperineovesical N32.2
  urethrorectal N36.0
    congenital Q64.73
  urethroscrotal N50.8
  urethrovaginal N82.1
  urethrovesical N32.2
  urinary (tract) (persistent) (recurrent) N36.0
  uteroabdominal N82.5
    congenital Q51.7
  uteroenteric, uterointestinal N82.4
    congenital Q51.7
  uterorectal N82.4
    congenital Q51.7

Fistula — *continued*
  uteroureteric N82.1
  uterourethral Q51.7
  uterovaginal N82.8
  uterovesical N82.1
    congenital Q51.7
  uterus N82.8
  vagina (postpartal) (wall) N82.8
  vaginocutaneous (postpartal) N82.5
  vaginointestinal NEC N82.4
    large intestine N82.3
    small intestine N82.2
  vaginoperineal N82.5
  vasocutaneous, congenital Q55.7
  vesical NEC N32.2
  vesicoabdominal N32.2
  vesicocervicovaginal N82.1
  vesicocolic N32.1
  vesicocutaneous N32.2
  vesicoenteric N32.1
  vesicointestinal N32.1
  vesicometrorectal N82.4
  vesicoperineal N32.2
  vesicorectal N32.1
    congenital Q64.79
  vesicosigmoidal N32.1
  vesicosigmoidovaginal N82.3
  vesicoureteral N32.2
  vesicoureterovaginal N82.1
  vesicourethral N32.2
  vesicourethrorectal N32.1
  vesicouterine N82.1
    congenital Q51.7
  vesicovaginal N82.0
  vulvorectal N82.4
    congenital Q52.79
Fit R56.9
  epileptic — *see* Epilepsy
  fainting R55
  hysterical F44.5
  newborn P90
Fitting (and adjustment) (of)
  artificial
    arm — *see* Admission, adjustment, artificial, arm
    breast Z44.3 ☑
    eye Z44.2 ☑
    leg — *see* Admission, adjustment, artificial, leg
  automatic implantable cardiac defibrillator (with synchronous cardiac pacemaker) Z45.02
  brain neuropacemaker Z46.2
    implanted Z45.42
  cardiac defibrillator — *see* Fitting (and adjustment) (of), automatic implantable cardiac defibrillator
  catheter, non-vascular Z46.82
  colostomy belt Z46.89
  contact lenses Z46.0
  cystostomy device Z46.6
  defibrillator, cardiac — *see* Fitting (and adjustment) (of), automatic implantable cardiac defibrillator
  dentures Z46.3
  device NOS Z46.9
    abdominal Z46.89
    gastrointestinal NEC Z46.59
    implanted NEC Z45.89
    nervous system Z46.2
      implanted — *see* Admission, adjustment, device, implanted, nervous system
    orthodontic Z46.4
    orthoptic Z46.0
    orthotic Z46.89
    prosthetic (external) Z44.9
      breast Z44.3 ☑
      dental Z46.3
      eye Z44.2 ☑
      specified NEC Z44.8
    specified NEC Z46.89
    substitution
      auditory Z46.2
        implanted — *see* Admission, adjustment, device, implanted, hearing device
      nervous system Z46.2
        implanted — *see* Admission, adjustment, device, implanted, nervous system
      visual Z46.2
        implanted Z45.31
    urinary Z46.6
  gastric lap band Z46.51
  gastrointestinal appliance NEC Z46.59

Fitting — *continued*
  glasses (reading) Z46.0
  hearing aid Z46.1
  ileostomy device Z46.89
  insulin pump Z46.81
  intestinal appliance NEC Z46.89
  myringotomy device (stent) (tube) Z45.82
  neuropacemaker Z46.2
    implanted Z45.42
  non-vascular catheter Z46.82
  orthodontic device Z46.4
  orthopedic device (brace) (cast) (corset) (shoes) Z46.89
  pacemaker (cardiac) Z45.018
    nervous system (brain) (peripheral nerve) (spinal cord) Z46.2
      implanted Z45.42
    pulse generator Z45.010
  portacath (port-a-cath) Z45.2
  prosthesis (external) Z44.9
    arm — *see* Admission, adjustment, artificial, arm
    breast Z44.3 ☑
    dental Z46.3
    eye Z44.2 ☑
    leg — *see* Admission, adjustment, artificial, leg
    specified NEC Z44.8
  spectacles Z46.0
  wheelchair Z46.89
Fitzhugh-Curtis syndrome
  due to
    Chlamydia trachomatis A74.81
    Neisseria gonorrhorea (gonococcal peritonitis) A54.85
Fitz's syndrome (acute hemorrhagic pancreatitis) K85.8
Fixation
  joint — *see* Ankylosis
  larynx J38.7
  stapes — *see* Ankylosis, ear ossicles
    deafness — *see* Deafness, conductive
  uterus (acquired) — *see* Malposition, uterus
  vocal cord J38.3
Flabby ridge K06.8
Flaccid (*see also* condition)
  palate, congenital Q38.5
Flail
  chest S22.5 ☑
    newborn (birth injury) P13.8
  joint (paralytic) M25.20
    ankle M25.27- ☑
    elbow M25.22- ☑
    foot joint M25.27- ☑
    hand joint M25.24- ☑
    hip M25.25- ☑
    knee M25.26- ☑
    shoulder M25.21- ☑
    specified joint NEC M25.28
    wrist M25.23- ☑
Flajani's disease — *see* Hyperthyroidism, with, goiter (diffuse)
Flap, liver K71.3
Flashbacks (residual to hallucinogen use) F16.283
Flat
  chamber (eye) — *see* Disorder, globe, hypotony, flat anterior chamber
  chest, congenital Q67.8
  foot (acquired) (fixed type) (painful) (postural) (*see also* Deformity, limb, flat foot)
    congenital (rigid) (spastic (everted)) Q66.5- ☑
    rachitic sequelae (late effect) E64.3
  organ or site, congenital NEC — *see* Anomaly, by site
  pelvis M95.5
    with disproportion (fetopelvic) O33.0
      causing obstructed labor O65.0
    congenital Q74.2
Flatau-Schilder disease G37.0
Flatback syndrome M40.30
  lumbar region M40.36
  lumbosacral region M40.37
  thoracolumbar region M40.35
Flattening
  head, femur M89.8X5
  hip — *see* Coxa, plana
  lip (congenital) Q18.8
  nose (congenital) Q67.4
    acquired M95.0
Flatulence R14.3
  psychogenic F45.8
Flatus R14.3

Flatus — *continued*
  vaginalis N89.8
Flax-dresser's disease J66.1
Flea bite — *see* Injury, bite, by site, superficial, insect
Flecks, glaucomatous (subcapsular) — *see* Cataract, complicated
Fleischer (-Kayser) **ring** (cornea) H18.04- ☑
Fleshy mole O02.0
Flexibilitas cerea — *see* Catalepsy
Flexion
  amputation stump (surgical) T87.89
  cervix — *see* Malposition, uterus
  contracture, joint — *see* Contraction, joint
  deformity, joint (*see also* Deformity, limb, flexion) M21.20
    hip, congenital Q65.89
  uterus (*see also* Malposition, uterus)
    lateral — *see* Lateroversion, uterus
Flexner-Boyd dysentery A03.2
Flexner's dysentery A03.1
Flexure — *see* Flexion
Flint murmur (aortic insufficiency) I35.1
Floater, vitreous — *see* Opacity, vitreous
Floating
  cartilage (joint) (*see also* Loose, body, joint)
    knee — *see* Derangement, knee, loose body
  gallbladder, congenital Q44.1
  kidney N28.89
    congenital Q63.8
  spleen D73.89
Flooding N92.0
Floor — *see* condition
Floppy
  baby syndrome (nonspecific) P94.2
  iris syndrome (intraoperative) (IFIS) H21.81
  nonrheumatic mitral valve syndrome I34.1
Flu (*see also* Influenza)
  avian (*see also* Influenza, due to, identified novel influenza A virus) J09.X2
  bird (*see also* Influenza, due to, identified novel influenza A virus) J09.X2
  intestinal NEC A08.4
  swine (viruses that normally cause infections in pigs) (*see also* Influenza, due to, identified novel influenza A virus) J09.X2
Fluctuating blood pressure I99.8
Fluid
  abdomen R18.8
  chest J94.8
  heart — *see* Failure, heart, congestive
  joint — *see* Effusion, joint
  loss (acute) E86.9
    with
      hypernatremia E87.0
      hyponatremia E87.1
  lung — *see* Edema, lung
  overload E87.70
    specified NEC E87.79
  peritoneal cavity R18.8
  pleural cavity J94.8
  retention R60.9
Flukes NEC (*see also* Infestation, fluke)
  blood NEC — *see* Schistosomiasis
  liver B66.3
Fluor (vaginalis) N89.8
  trichomonal or due to Trichomonas (vaginalis) A59.00
Fluorosis
  dental K00.3
  skeletal M85.10
    ankle M85.17- ☑
    foot M85.17- ☑
    forearm M85.13- ☑
    hand M85.14- ☑
    lower leg M85.16- ☑
    multiple site M85.19
    neck M85.18
    rib M85.18
    shoulder M85.11- ☑
    skull M85.18
    specified site NEC M85.18
    thigh M85.15- ☑
    toe M85.17- ☑
    upper arm M85.12- ☑
    vertebra M85.18
Flush syndrome E34.0
Flushing R23.2
  menopausal N95.1

Flutter
  atrial or auricular I48.92
    atypical I48.4
    type I I48.3
    type II I48.4
    typical I48.3
  heart I49.8
    atrial or auricular I48.92
      atypical I48.4
      type I I48.3
      type II I48.4
      typical I48.3
    ventricular I49.02
  ventricular I49.02
FNHTR (febrile nonhemolytic transfusion reaction) R50.84
Fochier's abscess — *code by* site under Abscess
Focus, Assmann's — *see* Tuberculosis, pulmonary
Fogo selvagem L10.3
Foix-Alajouanine syndrome G95.19
Fold, folds (anomalous) (*see also* Anomaly, by site)
  Descemet's membrane — *see* Change, corneal membrane, Descemet's, fold
  epicanthic Q10.3
  heart Q24.8
Folie à deux F24
Follicle
  cervix (nabothian) (ruptured) N88.8
  graafian, ruptured, with hemorrhage N83.0
  nabothian N88.8
Follicular — *see* condition
Folliculitis (superficial) L73.9
  abscedens et suffodiens L66.3
  cyst N83.0
  decalvans L66.2
  deep — *see* Furuncle, by site
  gonococcal (acute) (chronic) A54.01
  keloid, keloidalis L73.0
  pustular L01.02
  ulerythematosa reticulata L66.4
Folliculome lipidique
  specified site — *see* Neoplasm, benign, by site
  unspecified site
    female D27.9
    male D29.20
Følling's disease E70.0
Follow-up — *see* Examination, follow-up
Fong's syndrome (hereditary osteo-onychodysplasia) Q78.5
Food
  allergy L27.2
  asphyxia (from aspiration or inhalation) — *see* Foreign body, by site
  choked on — *see* Foreign body, by site
  deprivation T73.0 ☑
    specified kind of food NEC E63.8
  intoxication — *see* Poisoning, food
  lack of T73.0 ☑
  poisoning — *see* Poisoning, food
  rejection NEC — *see* Disorder, eating
  strangulation or suffocation — *see* Foreign body, by site
  toxemia — *see* Poisoning, food
Foot — *see* condition
Foramen ovale (nonclosure) (patent) (persistent) Q21.1
Forbes' glycogen storage disease E74.03
Fordyce-Fox disease L75.2
Fordyce's disease (mouth) Q38.6
Forearm — *see* condition
Foreign body
  with
    laceration — *see* Laceration, by site, with foreign body
    puncture wound — *see* Puncture, by site, with foreign body
  accidentally left following a procedure T81.509 ☑
    aspiration T81.506 ☑
      resulting in
        adhesions T81.516 ☑
        obstruction T81.526 ☑
        perforation T81.536 ☑
        specified complication NEC T81.596 ☑
    cardiac catheterization T81.505 ☑
      resulting in
        acute reaction T81.60 ☑
          aseptic peritonitis T81.61 ☑
          specified NEC T81.69 ☑
        adhesions T81.515 ☑

Foreign body — *continued*
  accidentally left following a procedure — *continued*
    cardiac catheterization — *continued*
      resulting in — *continued*
        obstruction T81.525 ☑
        perforation T81.535 ☑
        specified complication NEC T81.595 ☑
    causing
      acute reaction T81.60 ☑
        aseptic peritonitis T81.61 ☑
        specified complication NEC T81.69 ☑
      adhesions T81.519 ☑
      aseptic peritonitis T81.61 ☑
      obstruction T81.529 ☑
      perforation T81.539 ☑
      specified complication NEC T81.599 ☑
    endoscopy T81.504 ☑
      resulting in
        adhesions T81.514 ☑
        obstruction T81.524 ☑
        perforation T81.534 ☑
        specified complication NEC T81.594 ☑
    immunization T81.503 ☑
      resulting in
        adhesions T81.513 ☑
        obstruction T81.523 ☑
        perforation T81.533 ☑
        specified complication NEC T81.593 ☑
    infusion T81.501 ☑
      resulting in
        adhesions T81.511 ☑
        obstruction T81.521 ☑
        perforation T81.531 ☑
        specified complication NEC T81.591 ☑
    injection T81.503 ☑
      resulting in
        adhesions T81.513 ☑
        obstruction T81.523 ☑
        perforation T81.533 ☑
        specified complication NEC T81.593 ☑
    kidney dialysis T81.502 ☑
      resulting in
        adhesions T81.512 ☑
        obstruction T81.522 ☑
        perforation T81.532 ☑
        specified complication NEC T81.592 ☑
    packing removal T81.507 ☑
      resulting in
        acute reaction T81.60 ☑
          aseptic peritonitis T81.61 ☑
          specified NEC T81.69 ☑
        adhesions T81.517 ☑
        obstruction T81.527 ☑
        perforation T81.537 ☑
        specified complication NEC T81.597 ☑
    puncture T81.506 ☑
      resulting in
        adhesions T81.516 ☑
        obstruction T81.526 ☑
        perforation T81.536 ☑
        specified complication NEC T81.596 ☑
    specified procedure NEC T81.508 ☑
      resulting in
        acute reaction T81.60 ☑
          aseptic peritonitis T81.61 ☑
          specified NEC T81.69 ☑
        adhesions T81.518 ☑
        obstruction T81.528 ☑
        perforation T81.538 ☑
        specified complication NEC T81.598 ☑
    surgical operation T81.500 ☑
      resulting in
        acute reaction T81.60 ☑
          aseptic peritonitis T81.61 ☑
          specified NEC T81.69 ☑
        adhesions T81.510 ☑
        obstruction T81.520 ☑
        perforation T81.530 ☑
        specified complication NEC T81.590 ☑
    transfusion T81.501 ☑
      resulting in
        adhesions T81.511 ☑
        obstruction T81.521 ☑
        perforation T81.531 ☑
        specified complication NEC T81.591 ☑

Foreign body — *continued*
  alimentary tract T18.9 ☑
    anus T18.5 ☑
    colon T18.4 ☑
    esophagus — *see* Foreign body, esophagus
    mouth T18.0 ☑
    multiple sites T18.8 ☑
    rectosigmoid (junction) T18.5 ☑
    rectum T18.5 ☑
    small intestine T18.3 ☑
    specified site NEC T18.8 ☑
    stomach T18.2 ☑
  anterior chamber (eye) S05.5- ☑
  auditory canal — *see* Foreign body, entering through orifice, ear
  bronchus T17.508 ☑
    causing
      asphyxiation T17.500 ☑
        food (bone) (seed) T17.520 ☑
        gastric contents (vomitus) T17.510 ☑
        specified type NEC T17.590 ☑
      injury NEC T17.508 ☑
        food (bone) (seed) T17.528 ☑
        gastric contents (vomitus) T17.518 ☑
        specified type NEC T17.598 ☑
  canthus — *see* Foreign body, conjunctival sac
  ciliary body (eye) S05.5- ☑
  conjunctival sac T15.1- ☑
  cornea T15.0- ☑
  entering through orifice
    accessory sinus T17.0 ☑
    alimentary canal T18.9 ☑
      multiple parts T18.8 ☑
      specified part NEC T18.8 ☑
    alveolar process T18.0 ☑
    antrum (Highmore's) T17.0 ☑
    anus T18.5 ☑
    appendix T18.4 ☑
    auditory canal — *see* Foreign body, entering through orifice, ear
    auricle — *see* Foreign body, entering through orifice, ear
    bladder T19.1 ☑
    bronchioles — *see* Foreign body, respiratory tract, specified site NEC
    bronchus (main) — *see* Foreign body, bronchus
    buccal cavity T18.0 ☑
    canthus (inner) — *see* Foreign body, conjunctival sac
    cecum T18.4 ☑
    cervix (canal) (uteri) T19.3 ☑
    colon T18.4 ☑
    conjunctival sac — *see* Foreign body, conjunctival sac
    cornea — *see* Foreign body, cornea
    digestive organ or tract NOS T18.9 ☑
      multiple parts T18.8 ☑
      specified part NEC T18.8 ☑
    duodenum T18.3 ☑
    ear (external) T16.- ☑
    esophagus — *see* Foreign body, esophagus
    eye (external) NOS T15.9- ☑
      conjunctival sac — *see* Foreign body, conjunctival sac
      cornea — *see* Foreign body, cornea
      specified part NEC T15.8- ☑
    eyeball (*see also* Foreign body, entering through orifice, eye, specified part NEC)
      with penetrating wound — *see* Puncture, eyeball
    eyelid (*see also* Foreign body, conjunctival sac) with
      laceration — *see* Laceration, eyelid, with foreign body
      puncture — *see* Puncture, eyelid, with foreign body
      superficial injury — *see* Foreign body, superficial, eyelid
    gastrointestinal tract T18.9 ☑
      multiple parts T18.8 ☑
      specified part NEC T18.8 ☑
    genitourinary tract T19.9 ☑
      multiple parts T19.8 ☑
      specified part NEC T19.8 ☑
    globe — *see* Foreign body, entering through orifice, eyeball

Foreign body — *continued*
  entering through orifice — *continued*
    gum T18.0 ☑
    Highmore's antrum T17.0 ☑
    hypopharynx — *see* Foreign body, pharynx
    ileum T18.3 ☑
    intestine (small) T18.3 ☑
      large T18.4 ☑
    lacrimal apparatus (punctum) — *see* Foreign body, entering through orifice, eye, specified part NEC
    large intestine T18.4 ☑
    larynx — *see* Foreign body, larynx
    lung — *see* Foreign body, respiratory tract, specified site NEC
    maxillary sinus T17.0 ☑
    mouth T18.0 ☑
    nasal sinus T17.0 ☑
    nasopharynx — *see* Foreign body, pharynx
    nose (passage) T17.1 ☑
    nostril T17.1 ☑
    oral cavity T18.0 ☑
    palate T18.0 ☑
    penis T19.4 ☑
    pharynx — *see* Foreign body, pharynx
    piriform sinus — *see* Foreign body, pharynx
    rectosigmoid (junction) T18.5 ☑
    rectum T18.5 ☑
    respiratory tract — *see* Foreign body, respiratory tract
    sinus (accessory) (frontal) (maxillary) (nasal) T17.0 ☑
      piriform — *see* Foreign body, pharynx
    small intestine T18.3 ☑
    stomach T18.2 ☑
    suffocation by — *see* Foreign body, by site
    tear ducts or glands — *see* Foreign body, entering through orifice, eye, specified part NEC
    throat — *see* Foreign body, pharynx
    tongue T18.0 ☑
    tonsil, tonsillar (fossa) — *see* Foreign body, pharynx
    trachea — *see* Foreign body, trachea
    ureter T19.8 ☑
    urethra T19.0 ☑
    uterus (any part) T19.3 ☑
    vagina T19.2 ☑
    vulva T19.2 ☑
  esophagus T18.108 ☑
    causing
      injury NEC T18.108 ☑
        food (bone) (seed) T18.128 ☑
        gastric contents (vomitus) T18.118 ☑
        specified type NEC T18.198 ☑
      tracheal compression T18.100 ☑
        food (bone) (seed) T18.120 ☑
        gastric contents (vomitus) T18.110 ☑
        specified type NEC T18.190 ☑
  felling of, in throat R09.89
  fragment — *see* Retained, foreign body fragments (type of)
  genitourinary tract T19.9 ☑
    bladder T19.1 ☑
    multiple parts T19.8 ☑
    penis T19.4 ☑
    specified site NEC T19.8 ☑
    urethra T19.0 ☑
    uterus T19.3 ☑
      IUD Z97.5
    vagina T19.2 ☑
      contraceptive device Z97.5
    vulva T19.2 ☑
  granuloma (old) (soft tissue) (*see also* Granuloma, foreign body)
    skin L92.3
  in
    laceration — *see* Laceration, by site, with foreign body
    puncture wound — *see* Puncture, by site, with foreign body
    soft tissue (residual) M79.5
  inadvertently left in operation wound — *see* Foreign body, accidentally left during a procedure
  ingestion, ingested NOS T18.9 ☑
  inhalation or inspiration — *see* Foreign body, by site
  internal organ, not entering through a natural orifice — code as specific injury with foreign body

Foreign body — *continued*
  intraocular S05.5- ☑
    old, retained (nonmagnetic) H44.70- ☑
      anterior chamber H44.71- ☑
      ciliary body H44.72- ☑
      iris H44.72- ☑
      lens H44.73- ☑
      magnetic H44.60- ☑
        anterior chamber H44.61- ☑
        ciliary body H44.62- ☑
        iris H44.62- ☑
        lens H44.63- ☑
        posterior wall H44.64- ☑
        specified site NEC H44.69- ☑
        vitreous body H44.65- ☑
      posterior wall H44.74- ☑
      specified site NEC H44.79- ☑
      vitreous body H44.75- ☑
  iris — *see* Foreign body, intraocular
  lacrimal punctum — *see* Foreign body, entering through orifice, eye, specified part NEC
  larynx T17.308 ☑
    causing
      asphyxiation T17.300 ☑
        food (bone) (seed) T17.320 ☑
        gastric contents (vomitus) T17.310 ☑
        specified type NEC T17.390 ☑
      injury NEC T17.308 ☑
        food (bone) (seed) T17.328 ☑
        gastric contents (vomitus) T17.318 ☑
        specified type NEC T17.398 ☑
  lens — *see* Foreign body, intraocular
  ocular muscle S05.4- ☑
    old, retained — *see* Foreign body, orbit, old
  old or residual
    soft tissue (residual) M79.5
  operation wound, left accidentally — *see* Foreign body, accidentally left during a procedure
  orbit S05.4- ☑
    old, retained H05.5- ☑
  pharynx T17.208 ☑
    causing
      asphyxiation T17.200 ☑
        food (bone) (seed) T17.220 ☑
        gastric contents (vomitus) T17.210 ☑
        specified type NEC T17.290 ☑
      injury NEC T17.208 ☑
        food (bone) (seed) T17.228 ☑
        gastric contents (vomitus) T17.218 ☑
        specified type NEC T17.298 ☑
  respiratory tract T17.908 ☑
    bronchioles — *see* Foreign body, respiratory tract, specified site NEC
    bronchus — *see* Foreign body, bronchus
    causing
      asphyxiation T17.900 ☑
        food (bone) (seed) T17.920 ☑
        gastric contents (vomitus) T17.910 ☑
        specified type NEC T17.990 ☑
      injury NEC T17.908 ☑
        food (bone) (seed) T17.928 ☑
        gastric contents (vomitus) T17.918 ☑
        specified type NEC T17.998 ☑
    larynx — *see* Foreign body, larynx
    lung — *see* Foreign body, respiratory tract, specified site NEC
    multiple parts — *see* Foreign body, respiratory tract, specified site NEC
    nasal sinus T17.0 ☑
    nasopharynx — *see* Foreign body, pharynx
    nose T17.1 ☑
    nostril T17.1 ☑
    pharynx — *see* Foreign body, pharynx
    specified site NEC T17.808 ☑
      causing
        asphyxiation T17.800 ☑
          food (bone) (seed) T17.820 ☑
          gastric contents (vomitus) T17.810 ☑
          specified type NEC T17.890 ☑
        injury NEC T17.808 ☑
          food (bone) (seed) T17.828 ☑
          gastric contents (vomitus) T17.818 ☑
          specified type NEC T17.898 ☑
  throat — *see* Foreign body, pharynx
  trachea — *see* Foreign body, trachea

Foreign body — *continued*
retained (old) (nonmagnetic) (in)
anterior chamber (eye) — *see* Foreign body, intraocular, old, retained, anterior chamber
magnetic — *see* Foreign body, intraocular, old, retained, magnetic, anterior chamber
ciliary body — *see* Foreign body, intraocular, old, retained, ciliary body
magnetic — *see* Foreign body, intraocular, old, retained, magnetic, ciliary body
eyelid H02.819
left H02.816
lower H02.815
upper H02.814
right H02.813
lower H02.812
upper H02.811
fragments — *see* Retained, foreign body fragments (type of)
globe — *see* Foreign body, intraocular, old, retained
magnetic — *see* Foreign body, intraocular, old, retained, magnetic
intraocular — *see* Foreign body, intraocular, old, retained
magnetic — *see* Foreign body, intraocular, old, retained, magnetic
iris — *see* Foreign body, intraocular, old, retained, iris
magnetic — *see* Foreign body, intraocular, old, retained, magnetic, iris
lens — *see* Foreign body, intraocular, old, retained, lens
magnetic — *see* Foreign body, intraocular, old, retained, magnetic, lens
muscle — *see* Foreign body, retained, soft tissue
orbit — *see* Foreign body, orbit, old
posterior wall of globe — *see* Foreign body, intraocular, old, retained, posterior wall
magnetic — *see* Foreign body, intraocular, old, retained, magnetic, posterior wall
retrobulbar — *see* Foreign body, orbit, old, retrobulbar
soft tissue M79.5
vitreous — *see* Foreign body, intraocular, old, retained, vitreous body
magnetic — *see* Foreign body, intraocular, old, retained, magnetic, vitreous body
retina S05.5- ☑
superficial, without open wound
abdomen, abdominal (wall) S30.851 ☑
alveolar process S00.552 ☑
ankle S90.55- ☑
antecubital space — *see* Foreign body, superficial, forearm
anus S30.857 ☑
arm (upper) S40.85- ☑
auditory canal — *see* Foreign body, superficial, ear
auricle — *see* Foreign body, superficial, ear
axilla — *see* Foreign body, superficial, arm
back, lower S30.850 ☑
breast S20.15- ☑
brow S00.85 ☑
buttock S30.850 ☑
calf — *see* Foreign body, superficial, leg
canthus — *see* Foreign body, superficial, eyelid
cheek S00.85 ☑
internal S00.552 ☑
chest wall — *see* Foreign body, superficial, thorax
chin S00.85 ☑
clitoris S30.854 ☑
costal region — *see* Foreign body, superficial, thorax
digit(s)
foot — *see* Foreign body, superficial, toe
hand — *see* Foreign body, superficial, finger
ear S00.45- ☑
elbow S50.35- ☑
epididymis S30.853 ☑
epigastric region S30.851 ☑
epiglottis S10.15 ☑
esophagus, cervical S10.15 ☑
eyebrow — *see* Foreign body, superficial, eyelid
eyelid S00.25- ☑
face S00.85 ☑
finger(s) S60.459 ☑
index S60.45- ☑

Foreign body — *continued*
superficial, without open wound — *continued*
finger(s) — *continued*
little S60.45- ☑
middle S60.45- ☑
ring S60.45- ☑
flank S30.851 ☑
foot (except toe(s) alone) S90.85- ☑
toe — *see* Foreign body, superficial, toe
forearm S50.85- ☑
elbow only — *see* Foreign body, superficial, elbow
forehead S00.85 ☑
genital organs, external
female S30.856 ☑
male S30.855 ☑
groin S30.851 ☑
gum S00.552 ☑
hand S60.55- ☑
head S00.95 ☑
ear — *see* Foreign body, superficial, ear
eyelid — *see* Foreign body, superficial, eyelid
lip S00.551 ☑
nose S00.35 ☑
oral cavity S00.552 ☑
scalp S00.05 ☑
specified site NEC S00.85 ☑
heel — *see* Foreign body, superficial, foot
hip S70.25- ☑
inguinal region S30.851 ☑
interscapular region S20.459 ☑
jaw S00.85 ☑
knee S80.25- ☑
labium (majus) (minus) S30.854 ☑
larynx S10.15 ☑
leg (lower) S80.85- ☑
knee — *see* Foreign body, superficial, knee
upper — *see* Foreign body, superficial, thigh
lip S00.551 ☑
lower back S30.850 ☑
lumbar region S30.850 ☑
malar region S00.85 ☑
mammary — *see* Foreign body, superficial, breast
mastoid region S00.85 ☑
mouth S00.552 ☑
nail
finger — *see* Foreign body, superficial, finger
toe — *see* Foreign body, superficial, toe
nape S10.85 ☑
nasal S00.35 ☑
neck S10.95 ☑
specified site NEC S10.85 ☑
throat S10.15 ☑
nose S00.35 ☑
occipital region S00.05 ☑
oral cavity S00.552 ☑
orbital region — *see* Foreign body, superficial, eyelid
palate S00.552 ☑
palm — *see* Foreign body, superficial, hand
parietal region S00.05 ☑
pelvis S30.850 ☑
penis S30.852 ☑
perineum
female S30.854 ☑
male S30.850 ☑
periocular area — *see* Foreign body, superficial, eyelid
phalanges
finger — *see* Foreign body, superficial, finger
toe — *see* Foreign body, superficial, toe
pharynx S10.15 ☑
pinna — *see* Foreign body, superficial, ear
popliteal space — *see* Foreign body, superficial, knee
prepuce S30.852 ☑
pubic region S30.850 ☑
pudendum
female S30.856 ☑
male S30.855 ☑
sacral region S30.850 ☑
scalp S00.05 ☑
scapular region — *see* Foreign body, superficial, shoulder
scrotum S30.853 ☑
shin — *see* Foreign body, superficial, leg

Foreign body — *continued*
superficial, without open wound — *continued*
shoulder S40.25- ☑
sternal region S20.359 ☑
submaxillary region S00.85 ☑
submental region S00.85 ☑
subungual
finger(s) — *see* Foreign body, superficial, finger
toe(s) — *see* Foreign body, superficial, toe
supraclavicular fossa S10.85 ☑
supraorbital S00.85 ☑
temple S00.85 ☑
temporal region S00.85 ☑
testis S30.853 ☑
thigh S70.35- ☑
thorax, thoracic (wall) S20.95 ☑
back S20.45- ☑
front S20.35- ☑
throat S10.15 ☑
thumb S60.35- ☑
toe(s) (lesser) S90.456 ☑
great S90.45- ☑
tongue S00.552 ☑
trachea S10.15 ☑
tunica vaginalis S30.853 ☑
tympanum, tympanic membrane — *see* Foreign body, superficial, ear
uvula S00.552 ☑
vagina S30.854 ☑
vocal cords S10.15 ☑
vulva S30.854 ☑
wrist S60.85- ☑
swallowed T18.9 ☑
trachea T17.408 ☑
causing
asphyxiation T17.400 ☑
food (bone) (seed) T17.420 ☑
gastric contents (vomitus) T17.410 ☑
specified type NEC T17.490 ☑
injury NEC T17.408 ☑
food (bone) (seed) T17.428 ☑
gastric contents (vomitus) T17.418 ☑
specified type NEC T17.498 ☑
type of fragment — *see* Retained, foreign body fragments (type of)
vitreous (humor) S05.5- ☑
Forestier's disease (rhizomelic pseudopolyarthritis) M35.3
meaning ankylosing hyperostosis — *see* Hyperostosis, ankylosing
Formation
hyalin in cornea — *see* Degeneration, cornea
sequestrum in bone (due to infection) — *see* Osteomyelitis, chronic
valve
colon, congenital Q43.8
ureter (congenital) Q62.39
Formication R20.2
Fort Bragg fever A27.89
Fossa (*see also* condition)
pyriform — *see* condition
Foster-Kennedy syndrome H47.14- ☑
Fothergill's
disease (trigeminal neuralgia) (*see also* Neuralgia, trigeminal)
scarlatina anginosa A38.9
Foul breath R19.6
Foundling Z76.1
Fournier disease or gangrene N49.3
female N76.89
Fourth
cranial nerve — *see* condition
molar K00.1
Foville's (peduncular) **disease or syndrome** G46.3
Fox (-Fordyce) disease (apocrine miliaria) L75.2
Fracture, burst — *see* Fracture, traumatic, by site
Fracture, chronic — *see* Fracture, pathological
Fracture, insufficiency — *see* Fracture, pathologic, by site
Fracture, pathological (pathologic) (*see also* Fracture, traumatic) M84.40 ☑
ankle M84.47- ☑
carpus M84.44- ☑
clavicle M84.41- ☑
dental implant M27.63

Fracture, pathological — *continued*
dental restorative material K08.539
   with loss of material K08.531
   without loss of material K08.530
  due to
    neoplastic disease NEC (*see also* Neoplasm)
      M84.50 ✓
     ankle M84.57- ✓
     carpus M84.54- ✓
     clavicle M84.51- ✓
     femur M84.55- ✓
     fibula M84.56- ✓
     finger M84.54- ✓
     hip M84.559 ✓
     humerus M84.52- ✓
     ilium M84.550 ✓
     ischium M84.550 ✓
     metacarpus M84.54- ✓
     metatarsus M84.57- ✓
     neck M84.58 ✓
     pelvis M84.550 ✓
     radius M84.53- ✓
     rib M84.58 ✓
     scapula M84.51- ✓
     skull M84.58 ✓
     specified site NEC M84.58 ✓
     tarsus M84.57- ✓
     tibia M84.56- ✓
     toe M84.57- ✓
     ulna M84.53- ✓
     vertebra M84.58 ✓
    osteoporosis M80.80 ✓
     disuse — *see* Osteoporosis, specified type NEC, with pathological fracture
     drug-induced — *see* Osteoporosis, drug induced, with pathological fracture
     idiopathic — *see* Osteoporosis, specified type NEC, with pathological fracture
     postmenopausal — *see* Osteoporosis, postmenopausal, with pathological fracture
     postoophorectomy — *see* Osteoporosis, postoophorectomy, with pathological fracture
     postsurgical malabsorption — *see* Osteoporosis, specified type NEC, with pathological fracture
     specified cause NEC — *see* Osteoporosis, specified type NEC, with pathological fracture
    specified disease NEC M84.60 ✓
     ankle M84.67- ✓
     carpus M84.64- ✓
     clavicle M84.61- ✓
     femur M84.65- ✓
     fibula M84.66- ✓
     finger M84.64- ✓
     hip M84.65- ✓
     humerus M84.62- ✓
     ilium M84.650 ✓
     ischium M84.650 ✓
     metacarpus M84.64- ✓
     metatarsus M84.67- ✓
     neck M84.68 ✓
     radius M84.63- ✓
     rib M84.68 ✓
     scapula M84.61- ✓
     skull M84.68 ✓
     tarsus M84.67- ✓
     tibia M84.66- ✓
     toe M84.67- ✓
     ulna M84.63- ✓
     vertebra M84.68 ✓
femur M84.45- ✓
fibula M84.46- ✓
finger M84.44- ✓
hip M84.459 ✓
humerus M84.42- ✓
ilium M84.454 ✓
ischium M84.454 ✓
joint prosthesis — *see* Complications, joint prosthesis, mechanical, breakdown, by site
  periprosthetic — *see* Complications, joint prosthesis, mechanical, periprosthesis, fracture, by site
metacarpus M84.44- ✓
metatarsus M84.47- ✓
neck M84.48 ✓

Fracture, pathological — *continued*
pelvis M84.454 ✓
radius M84.43- ✓
restorative material (dental) K08.539
  with loss of material K08.531
  without loss of material K08.530
rib M84.48 ✓
scapula M84.41- ✓
skull M84.48 ✓
tarsus M84.47- ✓
tibia M84.46- ✓
toe M84.47- ✓
ulna M84.43- ✓
vertebra M84.48 ✓
Fracture, traumatic (abduction) (adduction) (separation)
  (*see also* Fracture, pathological) T14.8
acetabulum S32.40- ✓
  column
    anterior (displaced) (iliopubic) S32.43- ✓
     nondisplaced S32.436 ✓
    posterior (displaced) (ilioischial) S32.443 ✓
     nondisplaced S32.44- ✓
    dome (displaced) S32.48- ✓
    nondisplaced S32.48 ✓
    specified NEC S32.49- ✓
    transverse (displaced) S32.45- ✓
     with associated posterior wall fracture (displaced) S32.46- ✓
      nondisplaced S32.46- ✓
     nondisplaced S32.45- ✓
    wall
     anterior (displaced) S32.41- ✓
      nondisplaced S32.41- ✓
     medial (displaced) S32.47- ✓
      nondisplaced S32.47- ✓
     posterior (displaced) S32.42- ✓
      with associated transverse fracture (displaced) S32.46- ✓
       nondisplaced S32.46- ✓
      nondisplaced S32.42- ✓
acromion — *see* Fracture, scapula, acromial process
ankle S82.899 ✓
  bimalleolar (displaced) S82.84- ✓
   nondisplaced S82.84- ✓
  lateral malleolus only (displaced) S82.6- ✓
   nondisplaced S82.6- ✓
  medial malleolus (displaced) S82.5- ✓
   associated with Maisonneuve's fracture — *see* Fracture, Maisonneuve's
   nondisplaced S82.5- ✓
  talus — *see* Fracture, tarsal, talus
  trimalleolar (displaced) S82.85- ✓
   nondisplaced S82.85- ✓
arm (upper) (*see also* Fracture, humerus, shaft)
  humerus — *see* Fracture, humerus
  radius — *see* Fracture, radius
  ulna — *see* Fracture, ulna
astragalus — *see* Fracture, tarsal, talus
atlas — *see* Fracture, neck, cervical vertebra, first
axis — *see* Fracture, neck, cervical vertebra, second
back — *see* Fracture, vertebra
Barton's — *see* Barton's fracture
base of skull — *see* Fracture, skull, base
basicervical (basal) (femoral) S72.0 ✓
Bennett's — *see* Bennett's fracture
bimalleolar — *see* Fracture, ankle, bimalleolar
blow-out S02.3 ✓
bone NEC T14.8
  birth injury P13.9
  following insertion of orthopedic implant, joint prosthesis or bone plate — *see* Fracture, following insertion of orthopedic implant, joint prosthesis or bone plate
  in (due to) neoplastic disease NEC — *see* Fracture, pathological, due to, neoplastic disease
  pathological (cause unknown) — *see* Fracture, pathological
breast bone — *see* Fracture, sternum
bucket handle (semilunar cartilage) — *see* Tear, meniscus
burst — *see* Fracture, traumatic, by site
calcaneus — *see* Fracture, tarsal, calcaneus
carpal bone(s) S62.10- ✓
  capitate (displaced) S62.13- ✓
   nondisplaced S62.13- ✓
  cuneiform — *see* Fracture, carpal bone, triquetrum

Fracture, traumatic — *continued*
carpal bone(s) — *continued*
  hamate (body) (displaced) S62.143 ✓
   hook process (displaced) S62.15- ✓
    nondisplaced S62.15- ✓
   nondisplaced S62.14- ✓
  larger multangular — *see* Fracture, carpal bones, trapezium
  lunate (displaced) S62.12- ✓
   nondisplaced S62.12- ✓
  navicular S62.00- ✓
   distal pole (displaced) S62.01- ✓
    nondisplaced S62.01- ✓
   middle third (displaced) S62.02- ✓
    nondisplaced S62.02- ✓
   proximal third (displaced) S62.03- ✓
    nondisplaced S62.03- ✓
   volar tuberosity — *see* Fracture, carpal bones, navicular, distal pole
  os magnum — *see* Fracture, carpal bones, capitate
  pisiform (displaced) S62.16- ✓
   nondisplaced S62.16- ✓
  semilunar — *see* Fracture, carpal bones, lunate
  smaller multangular — *see* Fracture, carpal bones, trapezoid
  trapezium (displaced) S62.17- ✓
   nondisplaced S62.17- ✓
  trapezoid (displaced) S62.18- ✓
   nondisplaced S62.18- ✓
  triquetrum (displaced) S62.11- ✓
   nondisplaced S62.11- ✓
  unciform — *see* Fracture, carpal bones, hamate
cervical — *see* Fracture, vertebra, cervical
clavicle S42.00- ✓
  acromial end (displaced) S42.03- ✓
   nondisplaced S42.03- ✓
  birth injury P13.4
  lateral end — *see* Fracture, clavicle, acromial end
  shaft (displaced) S42.02- ✓
   nondisplaced S42.02- ✓
  sternal end (anterior) (displaced) S42.01- ✓
   nondisplaced S42.01- ✓
   posterior S42.01- ✓
coccyx S32.2 ✓
collapsed — *see* Collapse, vertebra
collar bone — *see* Fracture, clavicle
Colles' — *see* Colles' fracture
compression, not due to trauma — *see* Collapse, vertebra
coronoid process — *see* Fracture, ulna, upper end, coronoid process
corpus cavernosum penis S39.840 ✓
costochondral cartilage S23.41 ✓
costochondral, costosternal junction — *see* Fracture, rib
cranium — *see* Fracture, skull
cricoid cartilage S12.8 ✓
cuboid (ankle) — *see* Fracture, tarsal, cuboid
cuneiform
  foot — *see* Fracture, tarsal, cuneiform
  wrist — *see* Fracture, carpal, triquetrum
delayed union — *see* Delay, union, fracture
dental restorative material K08.539
  with loss of material K08.531
  without loss of material K08.530
due to
  birth injury — *see* Birth, injury, fracture
  osteoporosis — *see* Osteoporosis, with fracture
Dupuytren's — *see* Fracture, ankle, lateral malleolus
elbow S42.40- ✓
ethmoid (bone) (sinus) — *see* Fracture, skull, base
face bone S02.92 ✓
fatigue (*see also* Fracture, stress)
  vertebra M48.40 ✓
   cervical region M48.42 ✓
   cervicothoracic region M48.43 ✓
   lumbar region M48.46 ✓
   lumbosacral region M48.47 ✓
   occipito-atlanto-axial region M48.41 ✓
   sacrococcygeal region M48.48 ✓
   thoracic region M48.44 ✓
   thoracolumbar region M48.45 ✓
femur, femoral S72.9- ✓
  basicervical (basal) S72.0 ✓
  birth injury P13.2
  capital epiphyseal S79.01- ✓

Fracture, traumatic — *continued*
  femur, femoral — *continued*
    condyles, epicondyles — *see* Fracture, femur, lower end
    distal end — *see* Fracture, femur, lower end
    epiphysis
      head — *see* Fracture, femur, upper end, epiphysis
      lower — *see* Fracture, femur, lower end, epiphysis
      upper — *see* Fracture, femur, upper end, epiphysis
    following insertion of implant, prosthesis or plate M96.66- ☑
    head — *see* Fracture, femur, upper end, head
    intertrochanteric — *see* Fracture, femur, trochanteric
    intratrochanteric — *see* Fracture, femur, trochanteric
    lower end S72.40- ☑
      condyle (displaced) S72.41- ☑
        lateral (displaced) S72.42- ☑
          nondisplaced S72.42- ☑
        medial (displaced) S72.43- ☑
          nondisplaced S72.43- ☑
        nondisplaced S72.41- ☑
      epiphysis (displaced) S72.44- ☑
        nondisplaced S72.44- ☑
      physeal S79.10- ☑
        Salter-Harris
          Type I S79.11- ☑
          Type II S79.12- ☑
          Type III S79.13- ☑
          Type IV S79.14- ☑
        specified NEC S79.19- ☑
      specified NEC S72.49- ☑
      supracondylar (displaced) S72.45- ☑
        with intracondylar extension (displaced) S72.46- ☑
          nondisplaced S72.46- ☑
        nondisplaced S72.45- ☑
      torus S72.47- ☑
    neck — *see* Fracture, femur, upper end, neck
    pertrochanteric — *see* Fracture, femur, trochanteric
    shaft (lower third) (middle third) (upper third) S72.30- ☑
      comminuted (displaced) S72.35- ☑
        nondisplaced S72.35- ☑
      oblique (displaced) S72.33- ☑
        nondisplaced S72.33- ☑
      segmental (displaced) S72.36- ☑
        nondisplaced S72.36- ☑
      specified NEC S72.39- ☑
      spiral (displaced) S72.34- ☑
        nondisplaced S72.34- ☑
      transverse (displaced) S72.32- ☑
        nondisplaced S72.32- ☑
    specified site NEC — *see* subcategory S72.8 ☑
    subcapital (displaced) S72.01- ☑
    subtrochanteric (region) (section) (displaced) S72.2- ☑
      nondisplaced S72.2- ☑
    transcervical — *see* Fracture, femur, upper end, neck
    transtrochanteric — *see* Fracture, femur, trochanteric
    trochanteric S72.10- ☑
      apophyseal (displaced) S72.13- ☑
        nondisplaced S72.13- ☑
      greater trochanter (displaced) S72.11- ☑
        nondisplaced S72.11- ☑
      intertrochanteric (displaced) S72.14- ☑
        nondisplaced S72.14- ☑
      lesser trochanter (displaced) S72.12- ☑
        nondisplaced S72.12- ☑
    upper end S72.00- ☑
      apophyseal (displaced) S72.13- ☑
        nondisplaced S72.13- ☑
      cervicotrochanteric — *see* Fracture, femur, upper end, neck, base
      epiphysis (displaced) S72.02- ☑
        nondisplaced S72.02- ☑
      head S72.05- ☑
        articular (displaced) S72.06- ☑
          nondisplaced S72.06- ☑

Fracture, traumatic — *continued*
  femur, femoral — *continued*
    upper end — *continued*
      head — *continued*
        specified NEC S72.09- ☑
      intertrochanteric (displaced) S72.14- ☑
        nondisplaced S72.14- ☑
      intracapsular S72.01- ☑
      midcervical (displaced) S72.03- ☑
        nondisplaced S72.03- ☑
      neck S72.00- ☑
        base (displaced) S72.04- ☑
          nondisplaced S72.04- ☑
        specified NEC S72.09- ☑
      pertrochanteric — *see* Fracture, femur, upper end, trochanteric
      physeal S79.00- ☑
        Salter-Harris type I S79.01- ☑
        specified NEC S79.09- ☑
      subcapital (displaced) S72.01- ☑
      subtrochanteric (displaced) S72.2- ☑
        nondisplaced S72.2- ☑
      transcervical — *see* Fracture, femur, upper end, midcervical
      trochanteric S72.10- ☑
        greater (displaced) S72.11- ☑
          nondisplaced S72.11- ☑
        lesser (displaced) S72.12- ☑
          nondisplaced S72.12- ☑
  fibula (shaft) (styloid) S82.40- ☑
    comminuted (displaced) S82.45- ☑
      nondisplaced S82.45- ☑
    following insertion of implant, prosthesis or plate M96.67- ☑
    involving ankle or malleolus — *see* Fracture, fibula, lateral malleolus
    lateral malleolus (displaced) S82.6- ☑
      nondisplaced S82.6- ☑
    lower end
      physeal S89.30- ☑
        Salter-Harris
          Type I S89.31- ☑
          Type II S89.32- ☑
        specified NEC S89.39- ☑
      specified NEC S82.83- ☑
      torus S82.82- ☑
    oblique (displaced) S82.43- ☑
      nondisplaced S82.43- ☑
    segmental (displaced) S82.46- ☑
      nondisplaced S82.46- ☑
    specified NEC S82.49- ☑
    spiral (displaced) S82.44- ☑
      nondisplaced S82.44- ☑
    transverse (displaced) S82.42- ☑
      nondisplaced S82.42- ☑
    upper end
      physeal S89.20- ☑
        Salter-Harris
          Type I S89.21- ☑
          Type II S89.22- ☑
        specified NEC S89.29- ☑
      specified NEC S82.83- ☑
      torus S82.81- ☑
  finger (except thumb) S62.60- ☑
    distal phalanx (displaced) S62.63- ☑
      nondisplaced S62.66- ☑
    index S62.60- ☑
      distal phalanx (displaced) S62.63- ☑
        nondisplaced S62.66- ☑
      medial phalanx (displaced) S62.62- ☑
        nondisplaced S62.65- ☑
      proximal phalanx (displaced) S62.61- ☑
        nondisplaced S62.64- ☑
    little S62.60- ☑
      distal phalanx (displaced) S62.63- ☑
        nondisplaced S62.66- ☑
      medial phalanx (displaced) S62.62- ☑
        nondisplaced S62.65- ☑
      proximal phalanx (displaced) S62.61- ☑
        nondisplaced S62.64- ☑
      medial phalanx (displaced) S62.62- ☑
        nondisplaced S62.65- ☑
    middle S62.60- ☑
      distal phalanx (displaced) S62.63- ☑
        nondisplaced S62.66- ☑

Fracture, traumatic — *continued*
  finger — *continued*
    middle — *continued*
      medial phalanx (displaced) S62.62- ☑
        nondisplaced S62.65- ☑
      proximal phalanx (displaced) S62.61- ☑
        nondisplaced S62.64- ☑
    proximal phalanx (displaced) S62.61- ☑
      nondisplaced S62.64- ☑
    ring S62.60- ☑
      distal phalanx (displaced) S62.63- ☑
        nondisplaced S62.66- ☑
      medial phalanx (displaced) S62.62- ☑
        nondisplaced S62.65- ☑
      proximal phalanx (displaced) S62.61- ☑
        nondisplaced S62.64- ☑
    thumb — *see* Fracture, thumb
  following insertion (intraoperative) (postoperative) of orthopedic implant, joint prosthesis or bone plate M96.69
    femur M96.66- ☑
    fibula M96.67- ☑
    humerus M96.62- ☑
    pelvis M96.65
    radius M96.63- ☑
    specified bone NEC M96.69
    tibia M96.67- ☑
    ulna M96.63- ☑
  foot S92.90- ☑
    astragalus — *see* Fracture, tarsal, talus
    calcaneus — *see* Fracture, tarsal, calcaneus
    cuboid — *see* Fracture, tarsal, cuboid
    cuneiform — *see* Fracture, tarsal, cuneiform
    metatarsal — *see* Fracture, metatarsal
    navicular — *see* Fracture, tarsal, navicular
    talus — *see* Fracture, tarsal, talus
    tarsal — *see* Fracture, tarsal
    toe — *see* Fracture, toe
  forearm S52.9- ☑
    radius — *see* Fracture, radius
    ulna — *see* Fracture, ulna
  fossa (anterior) (middle) (posterior) S02.19 ☑
  frontal (bone) (skull) S02.0 ☑
    sinus S02.19 ☑
  glenoid (cavity) (scapula) — *see* Fracture, scapula, glenoid cavity
  greenstick — *see* Fracture, by site
  hallux — *see* Fracture, toe, great
  hand S62.9- ☑
    carpal — *see* Fracture, carpal bone
    finger (except thumb) — *see* Fracture, finger
    metacarpal — *see* Fracture, metacarpal
    navicular (scaphoid) (hand) — *see* Fracture, carpal bone, navicular
    thumb — *see* Fracture, thumb
  healed or old
    with complications — *code by* Nature of the complication
  heel bone — *see* Fracture, tarsal, calcaneus
  Hill-Sachs S42.29- ☑
  hip — *see* Fracture, femur, neck
  humerus S42.30- ☑
    anatomical neck — *see* Fracture, humerus, upper end
    articular process — *see* Fracture, humerus, lower end
    capitellum — *see* Fracture, humerus, lower end, condyle, lateral
    distal end — *see* Fracture, humerus, lower end
    epiphysis
      lower — *see* Fracture, humerus, lower end, physeal
      upper — *see* Fracture, humerus, upper end, physeal
    external condyle — *see* Fracture, humerus, lower end, condyle, lateral
    following insertion of implant, prosthesis or plate M96.62- ☑
    great tuberosity — *see* Fracture, humerus, upper end, greater tuberosity
    intercondylar — *see* Fracture, humerus, lower end
    internal epicondyle — *see* Fracture, humerus, lower end, epicondyle, medial
    lesser tuberosity — *see* Fracture, humerus, upper end, lesser tuberosity

Fracture, traumatic — *continued*
humerus — *continued*
lower end S42.40- ☑
condyle
lateral (displaced) S42.45- ☑
nondisplaced S42.45- ☑
medial (displaced) S42.46- ☑
nondisplaced S42.46- ☑
epicondyle
lateral (displaced) S42.43- ☑
nondisplaced S42.43- ☑
medial (displaced) S42.44- ☑
incarcerated S42.44- ☑
nondisplaced S42.44- ☑
physeal S49.10- ☑
Salter-Harris
Type I S49.11- ☑
Type II S49.12- ☑
Type III S49.13- ☑
Type IV S49.14- ☑
specified NEC S49.19- ☑
specified NEC (displaced) S42.49- ☑
nondisplaced S42.49- ☑
supracondylar (simple) (displaced) S42.41- ☑
comminuted (displaced) S42.42- ☑
nondisplaced S42.42- ☑
nondisplaced S42.41- ☑
torus S42.48- ☑
transcondylar (displaced) S42.47- ☑
nondisplaced S42.47- ☑
proximal end — *see* Fracture, humerus, upper end
shaft S42.30- ☑
comminuted (displaced) S42.35- ☑
nondisplaced S42.35- ☑
greenstick S42.31- ☑
oblique (displaced) S42.33- ☑
nondisplaced S42.33- ☑
segmental (displaced) S42.36- ☑
nondisplaced S42.36- ☑
specified NEC S42.39- ☑
spiral (displaced) S42.34- ☑
nondisplaced S42.34- ☑
transverse (displaced) S42.32- ☑
nondisplaced S42.32- ☑
supracondylar — *see* Fracture, humerus, lower end
surgical neck — *see* Fracture, humerus, upper end, surgical neck
trochlea — *see* Fracture, humerus, lower end, condyle, medial
tuberosity — *see* Fracture, humerus, upper end
upper end S42.20- ☑
anatomical neck — *see* Fracture, humerus, upper end, specified NEC
articular head — *see* Fracture, humerus, upper end, specified NEC
epiphysis — *see* Fracture, humerus, upper end, physeal
greater tuberosity (displaced) S42.25- ☑
nondisplaced S42.25- ☑
lesser tuberosity (displaced) S42.26- ☑
nondisplaced S42.26- ☑
physeal S49.00- ☑
Salter-Harris
Type I S49.01- ☑
Type II S49.02- ☑
Type III S49.03- ☑
Type IV S49.04- ☑
specified NEC S49.09- ☑
specified NEC (displaced) S42.29- ☑
nondisplaced S42.29- ☑
surgical neck (displaced) S42.21- ☑
four-part S42.24- ☑
nondisplaced S42.21- ☑
three-part S42.23- ☑
two-part (displaced) S42.22- ☑
nondisplaced S42.22- ☑
torus S42.27- ☑
transepiphyseal — *see* Fracture, humerus, upper end, physeal
hyoid bone S12.8 ☑
ilium S32.30- ☑
with disruption of pelvic ring — *see* Disruption, pelvic ring
avulsion (displaced) S32.31- ☑
nondisplaced S32.31- ☑
specified NEC S32.39- ☑

Fracture, traumatic — *continued*
impaction, impacted — *code as* Fracture, by site
innominate bone — *see* Fracture, ilium
instep — *see* Fracture, foot
ischium S32.60- ☑
with disruption of pelvic ring — *see* Disruption, pelvic ring
avulsion (displaced) S32.61- ☑
nondisplaced S32.61- ☑
specified NEC S32.69- ☑
jaw (bone) (lower) — *see* Fracture, mandible
upper — *see* Fracture, maxilla
joint prosthesis — *see* Complications, joint prosthesis, mechanical, breakdown, by site
periprosthetic — *see* Complications, joint prosthesis, mechanical, periprosthesis, fracture, by site
knee cap — *see* Fracture, patella
larynx S12.8 ☑
late effects — *see* Sequelae, fracture
leg (lower) S82.9- ☑
ankle — *see* Fracture, ankle
femur — *see* Fracture, femur
fibula — *see* Fracture, fibula
malleolus — *see* Fracture, ankle
patella — *see* Fracture, patella
specified site NEC S82.89- ☑
tibia — *see* Fracture, tibia
lumbar spine — *see* Fracture, vertebra, lumbar
lumbosacral spine S32.9 ☑
Maisonneuve's (displaced) S82.86- ☑
nondisplaced S82.86- ☑
malar bone (*see also* Fracture, maxilla) S02.400 ☑
malleolus — *see* Fracture, ankle
malunion — *see* Fracture, by site
mandible (lower jaw (bone)) S02.609 ☑
alveolus S02.67 ☑
angle (of jaw) S02.65 ☑
body, unspecified S02.600 ☑
condylar process S02.61 ☑
coronoid process S02.63 ☑
ramus, unspecified S02.64 ☑
specified site NEC S02.69 ☑
subcondylar process S02.62 ☑
symphysis S02.66 ☑
manubrium (sterni) S22.21 ☑
dissociation from sternum S22.23 ☑
march — *see* Fracture, traumatic, stress, by site
maxilla, maxillary (bone) (sinus) (superior) (upper jaw) S02.401 ☑
alveolus S02.42 ☑
inferior — *see* Fracture, mandible
LeFort I S02.411 ☑
LeFort II S02.412 ☑
LeFort III S02.413 ☑
metacarpal S62.309 ☑
base (displaced) S62.319 ☑
nondisplaced S62.349 ☑
fifth S62.30- ☑
base (displaced) S62.31- ☑
nondisplaced S62.34- ☑
neck (displaced) S62.33- ☑
nondisplaced S62.36- ☑
shaft (displaced) S62.32- ☑
nondisplaced S62.35- ☑
specified NEC S62.398 ☑
first S62.20- ☑
base NEC (displaced) S62.23- ☑
nondisplaced S62.23- ☑
Bennett's — *see* Bennett's fracture
neck (displaced) S62.25- ☑
nondisplaced S62.25- ☑
shaft (displaced) S62.24- ☑
nondisplaced S62.24- ☑
specified NEC S62.29- ☑
fourth S62.30- ☑
base (displaced) S62.31- ☑
nondisplaced S62.34- ☑
neck (displaced) S62.33- ☑
nondisplaced S62.36- ☑
shaft (displaced) S62.32- ☑
nondisplaced S62.35- ☑
specified NEC S62.39- ☑
neck (displaced) S62.33- ☑
nondisplaced S62.36- ☑
Rolando's — *see* Rolando's fracture

Fracture, traumatic — *continued*
metacarpal — *continued*
second S62.30- ☑
base (displaced) S62.31- ☑
nondisplaced S62.34- ☑
neck (displaced) S62.33- ☑
nondisplaced S62.36- ☑
shaft (displaced) S62.32- ☑
nondisplaced S62.35- ☑
specified NEC S62.39- ☑
shaft (displaced) S62.32- ☑
nondisplaced S62.35- ☑
specified NEC S62.399 ☑
third S62.30- ☑
base (displaced) S62.31- ☑
nondisplaced S62.34- ☑
neck (displaced) S62.33- ☑
nondisplaced S62.36- ☑
shaft (displaced) S62.32- ☑
nondisplaced S62.35- ☑
specified NEC S62.39- ☑
metastatic — *see* Fracture, pathological, due to, neoplastic disease (*see also* Neoplasm)
metatarsal bone S92.30- ☑
fifth (displaced) S92.35- ☑
nondisplaced S92.35- ☑
first (displaced) S92.31- ☑
nondisplaced S92.31- ☑
fourth (displaced) S92.34- ☑
nondisplaced S92.34- ☑
second (displaced) S92.32- ☑
nondisplaced S92.32- ☑
third (displaced) S92.33- ☑
nondisplaced S92.33- ☑
Monteggia's — *see* Monteggia's fracture
multiple
hand (and wrist) NEC — *see* Fracture, by site
ribs — *see* Fracture, rib, multiple
nasal (bone(s)) S02.2 ☑
navicular (scaphoid) (foot) (*see also* Fracture, tarsal, navicular)
hand — *see* Fracture, carpal, navicular
neck S12.9 ☑
cervical vertebra S12.9 ☑
fifth (displaced) S12.400 ☑
nondisplaced S12.401 ☑
specified type NEC (displaced) S12.490 ☑
nondisplaced S12.491 ☑
first (displaced) S12.000 ☑
burst (stable) S12.01 ☑
unstable S12.02 ☑
lateral mass (displaced) S12.040 ☑
nondisplaced S12.041 ☑
nondisplaced S12.001 ☑
posterior arch (displaced) S12.030 ☑
nondisplaced S12.031 ☑
specified type NEC (displaced) S12.090 ☑
nondisplaced S12.091 ☑
fourth (displaced) S12.300 ☑
nondisplaced S12.301 ☑
specified type NEC (displaced) S12.390 ☑
nondisplaced S12.391 ☑
second (displaced) S12.100 ☑
dens (anterior) (displaced) (type II) S12.110 ☑
nondisplaced S12.112 ☑
posterior S12.111 ☑
specified type NEC (displaced) S12.120 ☑
nondisplaced S12.121 ☑
nondisplaced S12.101 ☑
specified type NEC (displaced) S12.190 ☑
nondisplaced S12.191 ☑
seventh (displaced) S12.600 ☑
nondisplaced S12.601 ☑
specified type NEC (displaced) S12.690 ☑
displaced S12.691 ☑
sixth (displaced) S12.500 ☑
nondisplaced S12.501 ☑
specified type NEC (displaced) S12.590 ☑
displaced S12.591 ☑
third (displaced) S12.200 ☑
nondisplaced S12.201 ☑
specified type NEC (displaced) S12.290 ☑
displaced S12.291 ☑

☑ Additional Character Required — Refer to the Tabular List for Character Selection   ▽ Subterms under main terms may continue to next column or page

Fracture, traumatic — *continued*
- neck — *continued*
  - hyoid bone S12.8 ☑
  - larynx S12.8 ☑
  - specified site NEC S12.8 ☑
  - thyroid cartilage S12.8 ☑
  - trachea S12.8 ☑
- neoplastic NEC — *see* Fracture, pathological, due to, neoplastic disease
- neural arch — *see* Fracture, vertebra
- newborn — *see* Birth, injury, fracture
- nontraumatic — *see* Fracture, pathological
- nonunion — *see* Nonunion, fracture
- nose, nasal (bone) (septum) S02.2 ☑
- occiput — *see* Fracture, skull, base, occiput
- odontoid process — *see* Fracture, neck, cervical vertebra, second
- olecranon (process) (ulna) — *see* Fracture, ulna, upper end, olecranon process
- orbit, orbital (bone) (region) S02.8 ☑
  - floor (blow-out) S02.3 ☑
  - roof S02.19 ☑
- os
  - calcis — *see* Fracture, tarsal, calcaneus
  - magnum — *see* Fracture, carpal, capitate
  - pubis — *see* Fracture, pubis
- palate S02.8 ☑
- parietal bone (skull) S02.0 ☑
- patella S82.00- ☑
  - comminuted (displaced) S82.04- ☑
    - nondisplaced S82.04- ☑
  - longitudinal (displaced) S82.02- ☑
    - nondisplaced S82.02- ☑
  - osteochondral (displaced) S82.01- ☑
    - nondisplaced S82.01- ☑
  - specified NEC S82.09- ☑
  - transverse (displaced) S82.03- ☑
    - nondisplaced S82.03- ☑
- pedicle (of vertebral arch) — *see* Fracture, vertebra
- pelvis, pelvic (bone) S32.9 ☑
  - acetabulum — *see* Fracture, acetabulum
  - circle — *see* Disruption, pelvic ring
  - following insertion of implant, prosthesis or plate M96.65
  - ilium — *see* Fracture, ilium
  - ischium — *see* Fracture, ischium
  - multiple
    - with disruption of pelvic ring (circle) — *see* Disruption, pelvic ring
    - without disruption of pelvic ring (circle) S32.82 ☑
  - pubis — *see* Fracture, pubis
  - sacrum — *see* Fracture, sacrum
  - specified site NEC S32.89 ☑
- phalanx
  - foot — *see* Fracture, toe
  - hand — *see* Fracture, finger
- pisiform — *see* Fracture, carpal, pisiform
- pond — *see* Fracture, skull
- prosthetic device, internal — *see* Complications, prosthetic device, by site, mechanical
- pubis S32.50- ☑
  - with disruption of pelvic ring — *see* Disruption, pelvic ring
  - specified site NEC S32.59- ☑
  - superior rim S32.51- ☑
- radius S52.9- ☑
  - distal end — *see* Fracture, radius, lower end
  - following insertion of implant, prosthesis or plate M96.63- ☑
  - head — *see* Fracture, radius, upper end, head
  - lower end S52.50- ☑
    - Barton's — *see* Barton's fracture
    - Colles' — *see* Colles' fracture
    - extraarticular NEC S52.55- ☑
    - intraarticular NEC S52.57- ☑
    - physeal S59.20- ☑
      - Salter-Harris
        - Type I S59.21- ☑
        - Type II S59.22- ☑
        - Type III S59.23- ☑
        - Type IV S59.24- ☑
      - specified NEC S59.29- ☑
    - Smith's — *see* Smith's fracture
    - specified NEC S52.59- ☑

Fracture, traumatic — *continued*
- radius — *continued*
  - lower end — *continued*
    - styloid process (displaced) S52.51- ☑
      - nondisplaced S52.51- ☑
    - torus S52.52- ☑
  - neck — *see* Fracture, radius, upper end
  - proximal end — *see* Fracture, radius, upper end
  - shaft S52.30- ☑
    - bent bone S52.38- ☑
    - comminuted (displaced) S52.35- ☑
      - nondisplaced S52.35- ☑
    - Galeazzi's — *see* Galeazzi's fracture
    - greenstick S52.31- ☑
    - oblique (displaced) S52.33- ☑
      - nondisplaced S52.33- ☑
    - segmental (displaced) S52.36- ☑
      - nondisplaced S52.36- ☑
    - specified NEC S52.39- ☑
    - spiral (displaced) S52.34- ☑
      - nondisplaced S52.34- ☑
    - transverse (displaced) S52.32- ☑
      - nondisplaced S52.32- ☑
  - upper end S52.10- ☑
    - head (displaced) S52.12- ☑
      - nondisplaced S52.12- ☑
    - neck (displaced) S52.13- ☑
      - nondisplaced S52.13- ☑
    - physeal S59.10- ☑
      - Salter-Harris
        - Type I S59.11- ☑
        - Type II S59.12- ☑
        - Type III S59.13- ☑
        - Type IV S59.14- ☑
      - specified NEC S59.19- ☑
    - specified NEC S52.18- ☑
    - torus S52.11- ☑
- ramus
  - inferior or superior, pubis — *see* Fracture, pubis
  - mandible — *see* Fracture, mandible
- restorative material (dental) K08.539
  - with loss of material K08.531
  - without loss of material K08.530
- rib S22.3- ☑
  - with flail chest — *see* Flail, chest
  - multiple S22.4- ☑
    - with flail chest — *see* Flail, chest
- root, tooth — *see* Fracture, tooth
- sacrum S32.10 ☑
  - specified NEC S32.19 ☑
  - Type
    - 1 S32.14 ☑
    - 2 S32.15 ☑
    - 3 S32.16 ☑
    - 4 S32.17 ☑
  - Zone
    - I S32.119 ☑
      - displaced (minimally) S32.111 ☑
        - severely S32.112 ☑
      - nondisplaced S32.110 ☑
    - II S32.129 ☑
      - displaced (minimally) S32.121 ☑
        - severely S32.122 ☑
      - nondisplaced S32.120 ☑
    - III S32.139 ☑
      - displaced (minimally) S32.131 ☑
        - severely S32.132 ☑
      - nondisplaced S32.130 ☑
- scaphoid (hand) (*see also* Fracture, carpal, navicular)
  - foot — *see* Fracture, tarsal, navicular
- scapula S42.10- ☑
  - acromial process (displaced) S42.12- ☑
    - nondisplaced S42.12- ☑
  - body (displaced) S42.11- ☑
    - nondisplaced S42.11- ☑
  - coracoid process (displaced) S42.13- ☑
    - nondisplaced S42.13- ☑
  - glenoid cavity (displaced) S42.14- ☑
    - nondisplaced S42.14- ☑
  - neck (displaced) S42.15- ☑
    - nondisplaced S42.15- ☑
  - specified NEC S42.19- ☑
- semilunar bone, wrist — *see* Fracture, carpal, lunate
- sequelae — *see* Sequelae, fracture
- sesamoid bone
  - hand — *see* Fracture, carpal

Fracture, traumatic — *continued*
- sesamoid bone — *continued*
  - other — *code by* site under Fracture
- shepherd's — *see* Fracture, tarsal, talus
- shoulder (girdle) S42.9- ☑
  - blade — *see* Fracture, scapula
  - sinus (ethmoid) (frontal) S02.19 ☑
- skull S02.91 ☑
  - base S02.10 ☑
    - occiput S02.119 ☑
      - condyle S02.113 ☑
        - type I S02.110 ☑
        - type II S02.111 ☑
        - type III S02.112 ☑
      - specified NEC S02.118 ☑
    - specified NEC S02.19 ☑
  - birth injury P13.0
  - frontal bone S02.0 ☑
  - parietal bone S02.0 ☑
  - specified site NEC S02.8 ☑
  - temporal bone S02.19 ☑
  - vault S02.0 ☑
- Smith's — *see* Smith's fracture
- sphenoid (bone) (sinus) S02.19 ☑
- spine — *see* Fracture, vertebra
- spinous process — *see* Fracture, vertebra
- spontaneous (cause unknown) — *see* Fracture, pathological
- stave (of thumb) — *see* Fracture, metacarpal, first
- sternum S22.20 ☑
  - with flail chest — *see* Flail, chest
  - body S22.22 ☑
  - manubrium S22.21 ☑
  - xiphoid (process) S22.24 ☑
- stress M84.30 ☑
  - ankle M84.37- ☑
  - carpus M84.34- ☑
  - clavicle M84.31- ☑
  - femoral neck M84.359 ☑
  - femur M84.35- ☑
  - fibula M84.36- ☑
  - finger M84.34- ☑
  - hip M84.359 ☑
  - humerus M84.32- ☑
  - ilium M84.350 ☑
  - ischium M84.350 ☑
  - metacarpus M84.34- ☑
  - metatarsus M84.37- ☑
  - neck — *see* Fracture, fatigue, vertebra
  - pelvis M84.350 ☑
  - radius M84.33- ☑
  - rib M84.38 ☑
  - scapula M84.31- ☑
  - skull M84.38 ☑
  - tarsus M84.37- ☑
  - tibia M84.36- ☑
  - toe M84.37- ☑
  - ulna M84.33- ☑
  - vertebra — *see* Fracture, fatigue, vertebra
- supracondylar, elbow — *see* Fracture, humerus, lower end, supracondylar
- symphysis pubis — *see* Fracture, pubis
- talus (ankle bone) — *see* Fracture, tarsal, talus
- tarsal bone(s) S92.20- ☑
  - astragalus — *see* Fracture, tarsal, talus
  - calcaneus S92.00- ☑
    - anterior process (displaced) S92.02- ☑
      - nondisplaced S92.02- ☑
    - body (displaced) S92.01- ☑
      - nondisplaced S92.01- ☑
    - extraarticular NEC (displaced) S92.05- ☑
      - nondisplaced S92.05- ☑
    - intraarticular (displaced) S92.06- ☑
      - nondisplaced S92.06- ☑
    - tuberosity (displaced) S92.04- ☑
      - avulsion (displaced) S92.03- ☑
        - nondisplaced S92.03- ☑
      - nondisplaced S92.04- ☑
  - cuboid (displaced) S92.21- ☑
    - nondisplaced S92.21- ☑
  - cuneiform
    - intermediate (displaced) S92.23- ☑
      - nondisplaced S92.23- ☑
    - lateral (displaced) S92.22- ☑
      - nondisplaced S92.22- ☑

Fracture, traumatic — *continued*
  tarsal bone(s) — *continued*
    cuneiform — *continued*
      medial (displaced) S92.24- ☑
        nondisplaced S92.24- ☑
    navicular (displaced) S92.25- ☑
      nondisplaced S92.25- ☑
    scaphoid — *see* Fracture, tarsal, navicular
    talus S92.10- ☑
      avulsion (displaced) S92.15- ☑
        nondisplaced S92.15- ☑
      body (displaced) S92.12- ☑
        nondisplaced S92.12- ☑
      dome (displaced) S92.14- ☑
        nondisplaced S92.14- ☑
      head (displaced) S92.12- ☑
        nondisplaced S92.12- ☑
      lateral process (displaced) S92.14- ☑
        nondisplaced S92.14- ☑
      neck (displaced) S92.11- ☑
        nondisplaced S92.11- ☑
      posterior process (displaced) S92.13- ☑
        nondisplaced S92.13- ☑
      specified NEC S92.19- ☑
  temporal bone (styloid) S02.19 ☑
  thorax (bony) S22.9 ☑
    with flail chest — *see* Flail, chest
    rib S22.3- ☑
      multiple S22.4- ☑
        with flail chest — *see* Flail, chest
    sternum S22.20 ☑
      body S22.22 ☑
      manubrium S22.21 ☑
      xiphoid process S22.24 ☑
    vertebra (displaced) S22.009 ☑
      burst (stable) S22.001 ☑
        unstable S22.002 ☑
      eighth S22.069 ☑
        burst (stable) S22.061 ☑
          unstable S22.062 ☑
        specified type NEC S22.068 ☑
        wedge compression S22.060 ☑
      eleventh S22.089 ☑
        burst (stable) S22.081 ☑
          unstable S22.082 ☑
        specified type NEC S22.088 ☑
        wedge compression S22.080 ☑
      fifth S22.059 ☑
        burst (stable) S22.051 ☑
          unstable S22.052 ☑
        specified type NEC S22.058 ☑
        wedge compression S22.050 ☑
      first S22.019 ☑
        burst (stable) S22.011 ☑
          unstable S22.012 ☑
        specified type NEC S22.018 ☑
        wedge compression S22.010 ☑
      fourth S22.049 ☑
        burst (stable) S22.041 ☑
          unstable S22.042 ☑
        specified type NEC S22.048 ☑
        wedge compression S22.040 ☑
      ninth S22.079 ☑
        burst (stable) S22.071 ☑
          unstable S22.072 ☑
        specified type NEC S22.078 ☑
        wedge compression S22.070 ☑
      nondisplaced S22.001 ☑
      second S22.029 ☑
        burst (stable) S22.021 ☑
          unstable S22.022 ☑
        specified type NEC S22.028 ☑
        wedge compression S22.020 ☑
      seventh S22.069 ☑
        burst (stable) S22.061 ☑
          unstable S22.062 ☑
        specified type NEC S22.068 ☑
        wedge compression S22.060 ☑
      sixth S22.059 ☑
        burst (stable) S22.051 ☑
          unstable S22.052 ☑
        specified type NEC S22.058 ☑
        wedge compression S22.050 ☑
      specified type NEC S22.008 ☑

Fracture, traumatic — *continued*
  thorax — *continued*
    vertebra — *continued*
      tenth S22.079 ☑
        burst (stable) S22.071 ☑
          unstable S22.072 ☑
        specified type NEC S22.078 ☑
        wedge compression S22.070 ☑
      third S22.039 ☑
        burst (stable) S22.031 ☑
          unstable S22.032 ☑
        specified type NEC S22.038 ☑
        wedge compression S22.030 ☑
      twelfth S22.089 ☑
        burst (stable) S22.081 ☑
          unstable S22.082 ☑
        specified type NEC S22.088 ☑
        wedge compression S22.080 ☑
      wedge compression S22.000 ☑
    thumb S62.50- ☑
      distal phalanx (displaced) S62.52- ☑
        nondisplaced S62.52- ☑
      proximal phalanx (displaced) S62.51- ☑
        nondisplaced S62.51- ☑
    thyroid cartilage S12.8 ☑
    tibia (shaft) S82.20- ☑
      comminuted (displaced) S82.25- ☑
        nondisplaced S82.25- ☑
      condyles — *see* Fracture, tibia, upper end
      distal end — *see* Fracture, tibia, lower end
      epiphysis
        lower — *see* Fracture, tibia, lower end
        upper — *see* Fracture, tibia, upper end
      following insertion of implant, prosthesis or plate
        M96.67- ☑
      head (involving knee joint) — *see* Fracture, tibia,
        upper end
      intercondyloid eminence — *see* Fracture, tibia,
        upper end
      involving ankle or malleolus — *see* Fracture, ankle,
        medial malleolus
      lower end S82.30- ☑
        physeal S89.10- ☑
          Salter-Harris
            Type I S89.11- ☑
            Type II S89.12- ☑
            Type III S89.13- ☑
            Type IV S89.14- ☑
          specified NEC S89.19- ☑
        pilon (displaced) S82.87- ☑
          nondisplaced S82.87- ☑
        specified NEC S82.39- ☑
        torus S82.31- ☑
      malleolus — *see* Fracture, ankle, medial malleolus
      oblique (displaced) S82.23- ☑
        nondisplaced S82.23- ☑
      pilon — *see* Fracture, tibia, lower end, pilon
      proximal end — *see* Fracture, tibia, upper end
      segmental (displaced) S82.26- ☑
        nondisplaced S82.26- ☑
      specified NEC S82.29- ☑
      spine — *see* Fracture, upper end, spine
      spiral (displaced) S82.24- ☑
        nondisplaced S82.24- ☑
      transverse (displaced) S82.22- ☑
        nondisplaced S82.22- ☑
      tuberosity — *see* Fracture, tibia, upper end,
        tuberosity
      upper end S82.10- ☑
        bicondylar (displaced) S82.14- ☑
          nondisplaced S82.14- ☑
        lateral condyle (displaced) S82.12- ☑
          nondisplaced S82.12- ☑
        medial condyle (displaced) S82.13- ☑
          nondisplaced S82.13- ☑
        physeal S89.00- ☑
          Salter-Harris
            Type I S89.01- ☑
            Type II S89.02- ☑
            Type III S89.03- ☑
            Type IV S89.04- ☑
          specified NEC S89.09- ☑
        plateau — *see* Fracture, tibia, upper end, bi-
          condylar
        specified NEC S82.19- ☑
        spine

Fracture, traumatic — *continued*
  tibia — *continued*
    upper end — *continued*
      spine (displaced) S82.11- ☑
        nondisplaced S82.11- ☑
      torus S82.16- ☑
      tuberosity (displaced) S82.15- ☑
        nondisplaced S82.15- ☑
  toe S92.91- ☑
    great (displaced) S92.40- ☑
      distal phalanx (displaced) S92.42- ☑
        nondisplaced S92.42- ☑
      nondisplaced S92.40- ☑
      proximal phalanx (displaced) S92.41- ☑
        nondisplaced S92.41- ☑
      specified NEC S92.49- ☑
    lesser (displaced) S92.50- ☑
      distal phalanx (displaced) S92.53- ☑
        nondisplaced S92.53- ☑
      medial phalanx (displaced) S92.52- ☑
        nondisplaced S92.52- ☑
      nondisplaced S92.50- ☑
      proximal phalanx (displaced) S92.51- ☑
        nondisplaced S92.51- ☑
      specified NEC S92.59- ☑
  tooth (root) S02.5 ☑
  trachea (cartilage) S12.8 ☑
  transverse process — *see* Fracture, vertebra
  trapezium or trapezoid bone — *see* Fracture, carpal
  trimalleolar — *see* Fracture, ankle, trimalleolar
  triquetrum (cuneiform of carpus) — *see* Fracture,
    carpal, triquetrum
  trochanter — *see* Fracture, femur, trochanteric
  tuberosity (external) — *code by* site under Fracture
  ulna (shaft) S52.20- ☑
    bent bone S52.28- ☑
    coronoid process — *see* Fracture, ulna, upper end,
      coronoid process
    distal end — *see* Fracture, ulna, lower end
    following insertion of implant, prosthesis or plate
      M96.63- ☑
    head S52.00- ☑
    lower end S52.60- ☑
      physeal S59.00- ☑
        Salter-Harris
          Type I S59.01- ☑
          Type II S59.02- ☑
          Type III S59.03- ☑
          Type IV S59.04- ☑
        specified NEC S59.09- ☑
      specified NEC S52.69- ☑
      styloid process (displaced) S52.61- ☑
        nondisplaced S52.61- ☑
      torus S52.62- ☑
    proximal end — *see* Fracture, ulna, upper end
    shaft S52.20- ☑
      comminuted (displaced) S52.25- ☑
        nondisplaced S52.25- ☑
      greenstick S52.21- ☑
      Monteggia's — *see* Monteggia's fracture
      oblique (displaced) S52.23- ☑
        nondisplaced S52.23- ☑
      segmental (displaced) S52.26- ☑
        nondisplaced S52.26- ☑
      specified NEC S52.29- ☑
      spiral (displaced) S52.24- ☑
        nondisplaced S52.24- ☑
      transverse (displaced) S52.22- ☑
        nondisplaced S52.22- ☑
    upper end S52.00- ☑
      coronoid process (displaced) S52.04- ☑
        nondisplaced S52.04- ☑
      olecranon process (displaced) S52.02- ☑
        with intraarticular extension S52.03- ☑
        nondisplaced S52.02- ☑
          with intraarticular extension S52.03- ☑
      specified NEC S52.09- ☑
      torus S52.01- ☑
  unciform — *see* Fracture, carpal, hamate
  vault of skull S02.0 ☑
  vertebra, vertebral (arch) (body) (column) (neural arch)
    (pedicle) (spinous process) (transverse process)
    atlas — *see* Fracture, neck, cervical vertebra, first
    axis — *see* Fracture, neck, cervical vertebra, second

Fracture, traumatic — *continued*
  vertebra, vertebral — *continued*
    cervical (teardrop) S12.9 ☑
      axis — *see* Fracture, neck, cervical vertebra, second
      first (atlas) — *see* Fracture, neck, cervical vertebra, first
      second (axis) — *see* Fracture, neck, cervical vertebra, second
    chronic M84.48 ☑
    coccyx S32.2 ☑
    dorsal — *see* Fracture, thorax, vertebra
    lumbar S32.009 ☑
      burst (stable) S32.001 ☑
        unstable S32.002 ☑
      fifth S32.059 ☑
        burst (stable) S32.051 ☑
          unstable S32.052 ☑
        specified type NEC S32.058 ☑
        wedge compression S32.050 ☑
      first S32.019 ☑
        burst (stable) S32.011 ☑
          unstable S32.012 ☑
        specified type NEC S32.018 ☑
        wedge compression S32.010 ☑
      fourth S32.049 ☑
        burst (stable) S32.041 ☑
          unstable S32.042 ☑
        specified type NEC S32.048 ☑
        wedge compression S32.040 ☑
      second S32.029 ☑
        burst (stable) S32.021 ☑
          unstable S32.022 ☑
        specified type NEC S32.028 ☑
        wedge compression S32.020 ☑
      specified type NEC S32.008 ☑
      third S32.039 ☑
        burst (stable) S32.031 ☑
          unstable S32.032 ☑
        specified type NEC S32.038 ☑
        wedge compression S32.030 ☑
      wedge compression S32.000 ☑
    metastatic — *see* Collapse, vertebra, in, specified disease NEC (*see also* Neoplasm)
    newborn (birth injury) P11.5
    sacrum S32.10 ☑
      specified NEC S32.19 ☑
      Type
        1 S32.14 ☑
        2 S32.15 ☑
        3 S32.16 ☑
        4 S32.17 ☑
      Zone
        I S32.119 ☑
          displaced (minimally) S32.111 ☑
            severely S32.112 ☑
          nondisplaced S32.110 ☑
        II S32.129 ☑
          displaced (minimally) S32.121 ☑
            severely S32.122 ☑
          nondisplaced S32.120 ☑
        III S32.139 ☑
          displaced (minimally) S32.131 ☑
            severely S32.132 ☑
          nondisplaced S32.130 ☑
    thoracic — *see* Fracture, thorax, vertebra
  vertex S02.0 ☑
  vomer (bone) S02.2 ☑
  wrist S62.10- ☑
    carpal — *see* Fracture, carpal bone
    navicular (scaphoid) (hand) — *see* Fracture, carpal, navicular
  xiphisternum, xiphoid (process) S22.24 ☑
  zygoma S02.402 ☑
Fragile, fragility
  autosomal site Q95.5
  bone, congenital (with blue sclera) Q78.0
  capillary (hereditary) D69.8
  hair L67.8
  nails L60.3
  non-sex chromosome site Q95.5
  X chromosome Q99.2
Fragilitas
  crinium L67.8
  ossium (with blue sclerae) (hereditary) Q78.0
  unguium L60.3

Fragilitas — *continued*
  unguium L60.3
    congenital Q84.6
Fragments, cataract (lens), **following cataract surgery** H59.02- ☑
  retained foreign body — *see* Retained, foreign body fragments (type of)
Frailty (frail) R54
  mental R41.81
Frambesia, frambesial (tropica) (*see also* Yaws)
  initial lesion or ulcer A66.0
  primary A66.0
Frambeside
  gummatous A66.4
  of early yaws A66.2
Frambesioma A66.1
Franceschetti-Klein (-Wildervanck) **disease or syndrome** Q75.4
Francis' disease — *see* Tularemia
Franklin disease C88.2
Frank's essential thrombocytopenia D69.3
Fraser's syndrome Q87.0
Freckle(s) L81.2
  malignant melanoma in — *see* Melanoma
  melanotic (Hutchinson's) — *see* Melanoma, in situ
  retinal D49.81
Frederickson's hyperlipoproteinemia, type
  I and V E78.3
  IIA E78.0
  IIB and III E78.2
  IV E78.1
Freeman Sheldon syndrome Q87.0
Freezing (*see also* Effect, adverse, cold) T69.9 ☑
Freiberg's disease (infraction of metatarsal head or osteochondrosis) — *see* Osteochondrosis, juvenile, metatarsus
Frei's disease A55
Fremitus, friction, cardiac R01.2
Frenum, frenulum
  external os Q51.828
  tongue (shortening) (congenital) Q38.1
Frequency micturition (nocturnal) R35.0
  psychogenic F45.8
Frey's syndrome
  auriculotemporal G50.8
  hyperhidrosis L74.52
Friction
  burn — *see* Burn, by site
  fremitus, cardiac R01.2
  precordial R01.2
  sounds, chest R09.89
Friderichsen-Waterhouse syndrome or disease A39.1
Friedländer's B (bacillus) **NEC** (*see also* condition) A49.8
Friedreich's
  ataxia G11.1
  combined systemic disease G11.1
  facial hemihypertrophy Q67.4
  sclerosis (cerebellum) (spinal cord) G11.1
Frigidity F52.22
Fröhlich's syndrome E23.6
Frontal (*see also* condition)
  lobe syndrome F07.0
Frostbite (superficial) T33.90 ☑
  with
    partial thickness skin loss — *see* Frostbite (superficial), by site
    tissue necrosis T34.90 ☑
  abdominal wall T33.3 ☑
    with tissue necrosis T34.3 ☑
  ankle T33.81- ☑
    with tissue necrosis T34.81- ☑
  arm T33.4- ☑
    with tissue necrosis T34.4- ☑
    finger(s) — *see* Frostbite, finger
    hand — *see* Frostbite, hand
    wrist — *see* Frostbite, wrist
  ear T33.01- ☑
    with tissue necrosis T34.01- ☑
  face T33.09 ☑
    with tissue necrosis T34.09 ☑
  finger T33.53- ☑
    with tissue necrosis T34.53- ☑
  foot T33.82- ☑
    with tissue necrosis T34.82- ☑
  hand T33.52- ☑
    with tissue necrosis T34.52- ☑

Frostbite — *continued*
  head T33.09 ☑
    with tissue necrosis T34.09 ☑
    ear — *see* Frostbite, ear
    nose — *see* Frostbite, nose
  hip (and thigh) T33.6- ☑
    with tissue necrosis T34.6- ☑
  knee T33.7- ☑
    with tissue necrosis T34.7- ☑
  leg T33.9- ☑
    with tissue necrosis T34.9- ☑
    ankle — *see* Frostbite, ankle
    foot — *see* Frostbite, foot
    knee — *see* Frostbite, knee
    lower T33.7- ☑
      with tissue necrosis T34.7- ☑
    thigh — *see* Frostbite, hip
    toe — *see* Frostbite, toe
  limb
    lower T33.99 ☑
      with tissue necrosis T34.99 ☑
    upper — *see* Frostbite, arm
  neck T33.1 ☑
    with tissue necrosis T34.1 ☑
  nose T33.02 ☑
    with tissue necrosis T34.02 ☑
  pelvis T33.3 ☑
    with tissue necrosis T34.3 ☑
  specified site NEC T33.99 ☑
    with tissue necrosis T34.99 ☑
  thigh — *see* Frostbite, hip
  thorax T33.2 ☑
    with tissue necrosis T34.2 ☑
  toes T33.83- ☑
    with tissue necrosis T34.83- ☑
  trunk T33.99 ☑
    with tissue necrosis T34.99 ☑
  wrist T33.51- ☑
    with tissue necrosis T34.51- ☑
Frotteurism F65.81
Frozen (*see also* Effect, adverse, cold) T69.9 ☑
  pelvis (female) N94.89
    male K66.8
  shoulder — *see* Capsulitis, adhesive
Fructokinase deficiency E74.11
Fructose 1,6 diphosphatase deficiency E74.19
Fructosemia (benign) (essential) E74.12
Fructosuria (benign) (essential) E74.11
Fuchs'
  black spot (myopic) H44.2- ☑
  dystrophy (corneal endothelium) H18.51
  heterochromic cyclitis — *see* Cyclitis, Fuchs' heterochromic
Fucosidosis E77.1
Fugue R68.89
  dissociative F44.1
  hysterical (dissociative) F44.1
  postictal in epilepsy — *see* Epilepsy
  reaction to exceptional stress (transient) F43.0
Fulminant, fulminating — *see* condition
Functional (*see also* condition)
  bleeding (uterus) N93.8
Functioning, intellectual, borderline R41.83
Fundus — *see* condition
Fungemia NOS B49
Fungus, fungous
  cerebral G93.89
  disease NOS B49
  infection — *see* Infection, fungus
Funiculitis (acute) (chronic) (endemic) N49.1
  gonococcal (acute) (chronic) A54.23
  tuberculous A18.15
Funnel
  breast (acquired) M95.4
    congenital Q67.6
    sequelae (late effect) of rickets E64.3
  chest (acquired) M95.4
    congenital Q67.6
    sequelae (late effect) of rickets E64.3
  pelvis (acquired) M95.5
    with disproportion (fetopelvic) O33.3 ☑
      causing obstructed labor O65.3
    congenital Q74.2
FUO (fever of unknown origin) R50.9
Furfur L21.0
  microsporon B36.0

Furrier's lung J67.8
Furrowed K14.5
  nail(s) (transverse) L60.4
    congenital Q84.6
  tongue K14.5
    congenital Q38.3
Furuncle L02.92
  abdominal wall L02.221
  ankle — *see* Furuncle, lower limb
  antecubital space — *see* Furuncle, upper limb
  anus K61.0
  arm — *see* Furuncle, upper limb
  auditory canal, external — *see* Abscess, ear, external
  auricle (ear) — *see* Abscess, ear, external
  axilla (region) L02.42- ☑
  back (any part) L02.222
  breast N61
  buttock L02.32
  cheek (external) L02.02
  chest wall L02.223
  chin L02.02
  corpus cavernosum N48.21
  ear, external — *see* Abscess, ear, external
  external auditory canal — *see* Abscess, ear, external
  eyelid — *see* Abscess, eyelid
  face L02.02
  femoral (region) — *see* Furuncle, lower limb
  finger — *see* Furuncle, hand
  flank L02.221
  foot L02.62- ☑
  forehead L02.02
  gluteal (region) L02.32
  groin L02.224
  hand L02.52- ☑
  head L02.821
    face L02.02
  hip — *see* Furuncle, lower limb
  kidney — *see* Abscess, kidney
  knee — *see* Furuncle, lower limb
  labium (majus) (minus) N76.4
  lacrimal
    gland — *see* Dacryoadenitis
    passages (duct) (sac) — *see* Inflammation, lacrimal, passages, acute
  leg (any part) — *see* Furuncle, lower limb
  lower limb L02.42- ☑
  malignant A22.0
  mouth K12.2
  navel L02.226

Furuncle — *continued*
  neck L02.12
  nose J34.0
  orbit, orbital — *see* Abscess, orbit
  palmar (space) — *see* Furuncle, hand
  partes posteriores L02.32
  pectoral region L02.223
  penis N48.21
  perineum L02.225
  pinna — *see* Abscess, ear, external
  popliteal — *see* Furuncle, lower limb
  prepatellar — *see* Furuncle, lower limb
  scalp L02.821
  seminal vesicle N49.0
  shoulder — *see* Furuncle, upper limb
  specified site NEC L02.828
  submandibular K12.2
  temple (region) L02.02
  thumb — *see* Furuncle, hand
  toe — *see* Furuncle, foot
  trunk L02.229
    abdominal wall L02.221
    back L02.222
    chest wall L02.223
    groin L02.224
    perineum L02.225
    umbilicus L02.226
  umbilicus L02.226
  upper limb L02.42- ☑
  vulva N76.4
Furunculosis — *see* Furuncle
Fused — *see* Fusion, fused
Fusion, fused (congenital)
  astragaloscaphoid Q74.2
  atria Q21.1
  auditory canal Q16.1
  auricles, heart Q21.1
  binocular with defective stereopsis H53.32
  bone Q79.8
  cervical spine M43.22
  choanal Q30.0
  commissure, mitral valve Q23.2
  cusps, heart valve NEC Q24.8
    mitral Q23.2
    pulmonary Q22.1
    tricuspid Q22.4
  ear ossicles Q16.3
  fingers Q70.0 ☑
  hymen Q52.3

Fusion, fused — *continued*
  joint (acquired) (*see also* Ankylosis)
    congenital Q74.8
  kidneys (incomplete) Q63.1
  labium (majus) (minus) Q52.5
  larynx and trachea Q34.8
  limb, congenital Q74.8
    lower Q74.2
    upper Q74.0
  lobes, lung Q33.8
  lumbosacral (acquired) M43.27
    arthrodesis status Z98.1
    congenital Q76.49
    postprocedural status Z98.1
  nares, nose, nasal, nostril(s) Q30.0
  organ or site not listed — *see* Anomaly, by site
  ossicles Q79.9
    auditory Q16.3
  pulmonic cusps Q22.1
  ribs Q76.6
  sacroiliac (joint) (acquired) M43.28
    arthrodesis status Z98.1
    congenital Q74.2
    postprocedural status Z98.1
  spine (acquired) NEC M43.20
    arthrodesis status Z98.1
    cervical region M43.22
    cervicothoracic region M43.23
    congenital Q76.49
    lumbar M43.26
    lumbosacral region M43.27
    occipito-atlanto-axial region M43.21
    postoperative status Z98.1
    sacrococcygeal region M43.28
    thoracic region M43.24
    thoracolumbar region M43.25
  sublingual duct with submaxillary duct at opening in mouth Q38.4
  testes Q55.1
  toes Q70.2- ☑
  tooth, teeth K00.2
  trachea and esophagus Q39.8
  twins Q89.4
  vagina Q52.4
  ventricles, heart Q21.0
  vertebra (arch) — *see* Fusion, spine
  vulva Q52.5
Fusospirillosis (mouth) (tongue) (tonsil) A69.1
Fussy baby R68.12

G

Gain in weight (abnormal) (excessive) (*see also* Weight, gain)
Gaisböck's disease (polycythemia hypertonica) D75.1
Gait abnormality R26.9
  ataxic R26.0
  falling R29.6
  hysterical (ataxic) (staggering) F44.4
  paralytic R26.1
  spastic R26.1
  specified type NEC R26.89
  staggering R26.0
  unsteadiness R26.81
  walking difficulty NEC R26.2
Galactocele (breast) N64.89
  puerperal, postpartum O92.79
Galactokinase deficiency E74.29
Galactophoritis N61
  gestational, puerperal, postpartum O91.2- ☑
Galactorrhea O92.6
  not associated with childbirth N64.3
Galactosemia (classic) (congenital) E74.21
Galactosuria E74.29
Galacturia R82.0
  schistosomiasis (bilharziasis) B65.0
Galeazzi's fracture S52.37- ☑
Galen's vein — *see* condition
Gall duct — *see* condition
Gallbladder (*see also* condition)
  acute K81.0
Gallop rhythm R00.8
Gallstone (colic) (cystic duct) (gallbladder) (impacted) (multiple) (*see also* Calculus, gallbladder)
  with
    cholecystitis — *see* Calculus, gallbladder, with cholecystitis
  bile duct (common) (hepatic) — *see* Calculus, bile duct
  causing intestinal obstruction K56.3
  specified NEC K80.80
    with obstruction K80.81
Gambling Z72.6
  pathological (compulsive) F63.0
Gammopathy (of undetermined significance [MGUS]) D47.2
  associated with lymphoplasmacytic dyscrasia D47.2
  monoclonal D47.2
  polyclonal D89.0
Gamna's disease (siderotic splenomegaly) D73.1
Gamophobia F40.298
Gampsodactylia (congenital) Q66.7
Gamstorp's disease (adynamia episodica hereditaria) G72.3
Gandy-Nanta disease (siderotic splenomegaly) D73.1
Gang
  membership offenses Z72.810
Gangliocytoma D36.10
Ganglioglioma — *see* Neoplasm, uncertain behavior, by site
Ganglion (compound) (diffuse) (joint) (tendon (sheath)) M67.40
  ankle M67.47- ☑
  foot M67.47- ☑
  forearm M67.43- ☑
  hand M67.44- ☑
  lower leg M67.46- ☑
  multiple sites M67.49
  of yaws (early) (late) A66.6
  pelvic region M67.45- ☑
  periosteal — *see* Periostitis
  shoulder region M67.41- ☑
  specified site NEC M67.48
  thigh region M67.45- ☑
  tuberculous A18.09
  upper arm M67.42- ☑
  wrist M67.43- ☑
Ganglioneuroblastoma — *see* Neoplasm, nerve, malignant

Ganglioneuroma D36.10
  malignant — *see* Neoplasm, nerve, malignant
Ganglioneuromatosis D36.10
Ganglionitis
  fifth nerve — *see* Neuralgia, trigeminal
  gasserian (postherpetic) (postzoster) B02.21
  geniculate G51.1
    newborn (birth injury) P11.3
    postherpetic, postzoster B02.21
  herpes zoster B02.21
  postherpetic geniculate B02.21
Gangliosidosis E75.10
  GM1 E75.19
  GM2 E75.00
    other specified E75.09
    Sandhoff disease E75.01
    Tay-Sachs disease E75.02
  GM3 E75.19
  mucolipidosis IV E75.11
Gangosa A66.5
Gangrene, gangrenous (connective tissue) (dropsical) (dry) (moist) (skin) (ulcer) (*see also* Necrosis) I96
  with diabetes (mellitus) — *see* Diabetes, gangrene
  abdomen (wall) I96
  alveolar M27.3
  appendix K35.80
    with
      perforation or rupture K35.2
      peritoneal abscess K35.3
      peritonitis NEC K35.3
        generalized (with perforation or rupture) K35.2
        localized (with perforation or rupture) K35.3
  arteriosclerotic (general) (senile) — *see* Arteriosclerosis, extremities, with, gangrene
  auricle I96
  Bacillus welchii A48.0
  bladder (infectious) — *see* Cystitis, specified type NEC
  bowel, cecum, or colon — *see* Gangrene, intestine
  Clostridium perfringens or welchii A48.0
  cornea H18.89- ☑
  corpora cavernosa N48.29
    noninfective N48.89
  cutaneous, spreading I96
  decubital — *see* Ulcer, pressure, by site
  diabetic (any site) — *see* Diabetes, gangrene
  emphysematous — *see* Gangrene, gas
  epidemic — *see* Poisoning, food, noxious, plant
  epididymis (infectional) N45.1
  erysipelas — *see* Erysipelas
  extremity (lower) (upper) I96
  Fournier N49.3
    female N76.89
  fusospirochetal A69.0
  gallbladder — *see* Cholecystitis, acute
  gas (bacillus) A48.0
    following
      abortion — *see* Abortion by type complicated by infection
      ectopic or molar pregnancy O08.0
  glossitis K14.0
  hernia — *see* Hernia, by site, with gangrene
  intestine, intestinal (hemorrhagic) (massive) K55.0
    with
      mesenteric embolism K55.0
      obstruction — *see* Obstruction, intestine
  laryngitis J04.0
  limb (lower) (upper) I96
  lung J85.0
    spirochetal A69.8
  lymphangitis I89.1
  Meleney's (synergistic) — *see* Ulcer, skin
  mesentery K55.0
    with
      embolism K55.0
      intestinal obstruction — *see* Obstruction, intestine
  mouth A69.0
  ovary — *see* Oophoritis
  pancreas K85.9
  penis N48.29
    noninfective N48.89

Gangrene, gangrenous — *continued*
  perineum I96
  pharynx (*see also* Pharyngitis)
    Vincent's A69.1
  presenile I73.1
  progressive synergistic — *see* Ulcer, skin
  pulmonary J85.0
  pulpal (dental) K04.1
  quinsy J36
  Raynaud's (symmetric gangrene) I73.01
  retropharyngeal J39.2
  scrotum N49.3
    noninfective N50.8
  senile (atherosclerotic) — *see* Arteriosclerosis, extremities, with, gangrene
  spermatic cord N49.1
    noninfective N50.8
  spine I96
  spirochetal NEC A69.8
  spreading cutaneous I96
  stomatitis A69.0
  symmetrical I73.01
  testis (infectional) N45.2
    noninfective N44.8
  throat (*see also* Pharyngitis)
    diphtheritic A36.0
    Vincent's A69.1
  thyroid (gland) E07.89
  tooth (pulp) K04.1
  tuberculous NEC — *see* Tuberculosis
  tunica vaginalis N49.1
    noninfective N50.8
  umbilicus I96
  uterus — *see* Endometritis
  uvulitis K12.2
  vas deferens N49.1
    noninfective N50.8
  vulva N76.89
Ganister disease J62.8
Ganser's syndrome (hysterical) F44.89
Gardner-Diamond syndrome (autoerythrocyte sensitization) D69.2
Gargoylism E76.01
Garré's disease, osteitis (sclerosing), osteomyelitis — *see* Osteomyelitis, specified type NEC
Garrod's pad, knuckle M72.1
Gartner's duct
  cyst Q52.4
  persistent Q50.6
Gas R14.3
  asphyxiation, inhalation, poisoning, suffocation NEC — *see* Table of Drugs and Chemicals
  excessive R14.0
  gangrene A48.0
    following
      abortion — *see* Abortion by type complicated by infection
      ectopic or molar pregnancy O08.0
  on stomach R14.0
  pains R14.1
Gastralgia (*see also* Pain, abdominal)
Gastrectasis K31.0
  psychogenic F45.8
Gastric — *see* condition
Gastrinoma
  malignant
    pancreas C25.4
    specified site NEC — *see* Neoplasm, malignant, by site
    unspecified site C25.4
  specified site — *see* Neoplasm, uncertain behavior
  unspecified site D37.9
Gastritis (simple) K29.70
  with bleeding K29.71
  acute (erosive) K29.00
    with bleeding K29.01
  alcoholic K29.20
    with bleeding K29.21
  allergic K29.60
    with bleeding K29.61
  atrophic (chronic) K29.40
    with bleeding K29.41

Gastritis — *continued*
  chronic (antral) (fundal) K29.50
    with bleeding K29.51
    atrophic K29.40
      with bleeding K29.41
    superficial K29.30
      with bleeding K29.31
  dietary counseling and surveillance Z71.3
  due to diet deficiency E63.9
  eosinophilic K52.81
  giant hypertrophic K29.60
    with bleeding K29.61
  granulomatous K29.60
    with bleeding K29.61
  hypertrophic (mucosa) K29.60
    with bleeding K29.61
  nervous F54
  spastic K29.60
    with bleeding K29.61
  specified NEC K29.60
    with bleeding K29.61
  superficial chronic K29.30
    with bleeding K29.31
  tuberculous A18.83
  viral NEC A08.4
Gastrocarcinoma — *see* Neoplasm, malignant, stomach
Gastrocolic — *see* condition
Gastrodisciasis, gastrodiscoidiasis B66.8
Gastroduodenitis K29.90
  with bleeding K29.91
  virus, viral A08.4
    specified type NEC A08.39
Gastrodynia — *see* Pain, abdominal
Gastroenteritis (acute) (chronic) (noninfectious) (*see also* Enteritis) K52.9
  allergic K52.2
  dietetic K52.2
  drug-induced K52.1
  due to
    Cryptosporidium A07.2
    drugs K52.1
    food poisoning — *see* Intoxication, foodborne
    radiation K52.0
  eosinophilic K52.81
  epidemic (infectious) A09
  food hypersensitivity K52.2
  infectious — *see* Enteritis, infectious
  influenzal — *see* Influenza, with gastroenteritis
  noninfectious K52.9
    specified NEC K52.89
  rotaviral A08.0
  Salmonella A02.0
  toxic K52.1
  viral NEC A08.4
    acute infectious A08.39
      type Norwalk A08.11
    infantile (acute) A08.39
    Norwalk agent A08.11
    rotaviral A08.0
    severe of infants A08.39
    specified type NEC A08.39
Gastroenteropathy (*see also* Gastroenteritis) K52.9
  acute, due to Norovirus A08.11
  acute, due to Norwalk agent A08.11
  infectious A09
Gastroenteroptosis K63.4
Gastroesophageal laceration- hemorrhage syndrome K22.6
Gastrointestinal — *see* condition
Gastrojejunal — *see* condition
Gastrojejunitis (*see also* Enteritis) K52.9
Gastrojejunocolic — *see* condition
Gastroliths K31.89
Gastromalacia K31.89
Gastroparalysis K31.84
  diabetic — *see* Diabetes, gastroparalysis
Gastroparesis K31.84
  diabetic — *see* Diabetes, by type, with gastroparesis
Gastropathy K31.9
  congestive portal K31.89
  erythematous K29.70
  exudative K90.89
  portal hypertensive K31.89
Gastroptosis K31.89
Gastrorrhagia K92.2
  psychogenic F45.8
Gastroschisis (congenital) Q79.3

Gastrospasm (neurogenic) (reflex) K31.89
  neurotic F45.8
  psychogenic F45.8
Gastrostaxis — *see* Gastritis, with bleeding
Gastrostenosis K31.89
Gastrostomy
  attention to Z43.1
  status Z93.1
Gastrosuccorrhea (continuous) (intermittent) K31.89
  neurotic F45.8
  psychogenic F45.8
Gatophobia F40.218
Gaucher's disease or splenomegaly (adult) (infantile) E75.22
Gee (-Herter)(-Thaysen) **disease** (nontropical sprue) K90.0
Gélineau's syndrome G47.419
  with cataplexy G47.411
Gemistocytoma
  specified site — *see* Neoplasm, malignant, by site
  unspecified site C71.9
General, generalized — *see* condition
Genetic
  carrier (status)
    cystic fibrosis Z14.1
    hemophilia A (asymptomatic) Z14.01
      symptomatic Z14.02
    specified NEC Z14.8
  susceptibility to disease NEC Z15.89
    malignant neoplasm Z15.09
      breast Z15.01
      endometrium Z15.04
      ovary Z15.02
      prostate Z15.03
      specified NEC Z15.09
    multiple endocrine neoplasia Z15.81
Genital — *see* condition
Genito-anorectal syndrome A55
Genitourinary system — *see* condition
Genu
  congenital Q74.1
  extrorsum (acquired) (*see also* Deformity, varus, knee)
    congenital Q74.1
    sequelae (late effect) of rickets E64.3
  introrsum (acquired) (*see also* Deformity, valgus, knee)
    congenital Q74.1
    sequelae (late effect) of rickets E64.3
  rachitic (old) E64.3
  recurvatum (acquired) (*see also* Deformity, limb, specified type NEC, lower leg)
    congenital Q68.2
    sequelae (late effect) of rickets E64.3
  valgum (acquired) (knock-knee) M21.06- ☑
    congenital Q74.1
    sequelae (late effect) of rickets E64.3
  varum (acquired) (bowleg) M21.16- ☑
    congenital Q74.1
    sequelae (late effect) of rickets E64.3
Geographic tongue K14.1
Geophagia — *see* Pica
Geotrichosis B48.3
  stomatitis B48.3
Gephyrophobia F40.242
Gerbode defect Q21.0
GERD (gastroesophageal reflux disease) K21.9
Gerhardt's
  disease (erythromelalgia) I73.81
  syndrome (vocal cord paralysis) J38.00
    bilateral J38.02
    unilateral J38.01
German measles (*see also* Rubella)
  exposure to Z20.4
Germinoblastoma (diffuse) C85.9- ☑
  follicular C82.9- ☑
Germinoma — *see* Neoplasm, malignant, by site
Gerontoxon — *see* Degeneration, cornea, senile
Gerstmann's syndrome R48.8
  developmental F81.2
Gerstmann-Sträussler-Scheinker syndrome (GSS) A81.82
Gestation (period) (*see also* Pregnancy)
  ectopic — *see* Pregnancy, by site
  multiple O30.9- ☑
    greater than quadruplets — *see* Pregnancy, multiple (gestation), specified NEC
    specified NEC — *see* Pregnancy, multiple (gestation), specified NEC

Gestational
  mammary abscess O91.11- ☑
  purulent mastitis O91.11- ☑
  subareolar abscess O91.11- ☑
Ghon tubercle, primary infection A15.7
Ghost
  teeth K00.4
  vessels (cornea) H16.41- ☑
Ghoul hand A66.3
Gianotti-Crosti disease L44.4
Giant
  cell
    epulis K06.8
    peripheral granuloma K06.8
  esophagus, congenital Q39.5
  kidney, congenital Q63.3
  urticaria T78.3 ☑
    hereditary D84.1
Giardiasis A07.1
Gibert's disease or pityriasis L42
Giddiness R42
  hysterical F44.89
  psychogenic F45.8
Gierke's disease (glycogenosis I) E74.01
Gigantism (cerebral) (hypophyseal) (pituitary) E22.0
  constitutional E34.4
Gilbert's disease or syndrome E80.4
Gilchrist's disease B40.9
Gilford-Hutchinson disease E34.8
Gilles de la Tourette's disease or syndrome (motor-verbal tic) F95.2
Gingivitis K05.10
  acute (catarrhal) K05.00
    necrotizing A69.1
    nonplaque induced K05.01
    plaque induced K05.00
  chronic (desquamative) (hyperplastic) (simple marginal) (ulcerative) K05.10
    nonplaque induced K05.11
    plaque induced K05.10
  expulsiva — *see* Periodontitis
  necrotizing ulcerative (acute) A69.1
  pellagrous E52
    acute necrotizing A69.1
  Vincent's A69.1
Gingivoglossitis K14.0
Gingivopericementitis — *see* Periodontitis
Gingivosis — *see* Gingivitis, chronic
Gingivostomatitis K05.10
  herpesviral B00.2
  necrotizing ulcerative (acute) A69.1
Gland, glandular — *see* condition
Glanders A24.0
Glanzmann (-Naegeli) **disease or thrombasthenia** D69.1
Glasgow coma scale
  total score
    3-8 R40.243
    9-12 R40.242
    13-15 R40.241
Glass-blower's disease (cataract) — *see* Cataract, specified NEC
Glaucoma H40.9
  with
    increased episcleral venous pressure H40.81- ☑
    pseudoexfoliation of lens — *see* Glaucoma, open angle, primary, capsular
  absolute H44.51- ☑
  angle-closure (primary) H40.20- ☑
    acute (attack) (crisis) H40.21- ☑
    chronic H40.22- ☑
    intermittent H40.23- ☑
    residual stage H40.24- ☑
  borderline H40.00- ☑
  capsular (with pseudoexfoliation of lens) — *see* Glaucoma, open angle, primary, capsular
  childhood Q15.0
  closed angle — *see* Glaucoma, angle-closure
  congenital Q15.0
  corticosteroid-induced — *see* Glaucoma, secondary, drugs
  hypersecretion H40.82- ☑
  in (due to)
    amyloidosis E85.4 [H42]
    aniridia Q13.1 [H42]
    concussion of globe — *see* Glaucoma, secondary, trauma

Glaucoma — *continued*
  in — *continued*
    dislocation of lens — *see* Glaucoma, secondary
    disorder of lens NEC — *see* Glaucoma, secondary
    drugs — *see* Glaucoma, secondary, drugs
    endocrine disease NOS E34.9 [H42]
    eye
      inflammation — *see* Glaucoma, secondary, in-
        flammation
      trauma — *see* Glaucoma, secondary, trauma
    hypermature cataract — *see* Glaucoma, secondary
    iridocyclitis — *see* Glaucoma, secondary, inflamma-
      tion
    lens disorder — *see* Glaucoma, secondary
    Lowe's syndrome E72.03 [H42]
    metabolic disease NOS E88.9 [H42]
    ocular disorders NEC — *see* Glaucoma, secondary
    onchocerciasis B73.02
    pupillary block — *see* Glaucoma, secondary
    retinal vein occlusion — *see* Glaucoma, secondary
    Rieger's anomaly Q13.81 [H42]
    rubeosis of iris — *see* Glaucoma, secondary
    tumor of globe — *see* Glaucoma, secondary
  infantile Q15.0
  low tension — *see* Glaucoma, open angle, primary,
    low-tension
  malignant H40.83- ☑
  narrow angle — *see* Glaucoma, angle-closure
  newborn Q15.0
  noncongestive (chronic) — *see* Glaucoma, open angle
  nonobstructive — *see* Glaucoma, open angle
  obstructive (*see also* Glaucoma, angle-closure)
    due to lens changes — *see* Glaucoma, secondary
  open angle H40.10- ☑
    primary H40.11- ☑
      capsular (with pseudoexfoliation of lens)
        H40.14- ☑
      low-tension H40.12- ☑
      pigmentary H40.13- ☑
      residual stage H40.15- ☑
  phacolytic — *see* Glaucoma, secondary
  pigmentary — *see* Glaucoma, open angle, primary,
    pigmentary
  postinfectious — *see* Glaucoma, secondary, inflamma-
    tion
  secondary (to) H40.5- ☑
    drugs H40.6- ☑
    inflammation H40.4- ☑
    trauma H40.3- ☑
  simple (chronic) H40.11 ☑
  simplex H40.11 ☑
  specified type NEC H40.89
  suspect H40.00- ☑
  syphilitic A52.71
  traumatic (*see also* Glaucoma, secondary, trauma)
    newborn (birth injury) P15.3
  tuberculous A18.59
Glaucomatous flecks (subcapsular) — *see* Cataract,
  complicated
Glazed tongue K14.4
Gleet (gonococcal) A54.01
Glénard's disease K63.4
Glioblastoma (multiforme)
  with sarcomatous component
    specified site — *see* Neoplasm, malignant, by site
    unspecified site C71.9
  giant cell
    specified site — *see* Neoplasm, malignant, by site
    unspecified site C71.9
  specified site — *see* Neoplasm, malignant, by site
  unspecified site C71.9
Glioma (malignant)
  astrocytic
    specified site — *see* Neoplasm, malignant, by site
    unspecified site C71.9
  mixed
    specified site — *see* Neoplasm, malignant, by site
    unspecified site C71.9
  nose Q30.8
  specified site NEC — *see* Neoplasm, malignant, by site
  subependymal D43.2
    specified site — *see* Neoplasm, uncertain behavior,
      by site
    unspecified site D43.2
  unspecified site C71.9
Gliomatosis cerebri C71.0

Glioneuroma — *see* Neoplasm, uncertain behavior, by
  site
Gliosarcoma
  specified site — *see* Neoplasm, malignant, by site
  unspecified site C71.9
Gliosis (cerebral) G93.89
  spinal G95.89
Glisson's disease — *see* Rickets
Globinuria R82.3
Globus (hystericus) F45.8
Glomangioma D18.00
  intra-abdominal D18.03
  intracranial D18.02
  skin D18.01
  specified site NEC D18.09
Glomangiomyoma D18.00
  intra-abdominal D18.03
  intracranial D18.02
  skin D18.01
  specified site NEC D18.09
Glomangiosarcoma — *see* Neoplasm, connective tissue,
  malignant
Glomerular
  disease in syphilis A52.75
  nephritis — *see* Glomerulonephritis
Glomerulitis — *see* Glomerulonephritis
Glomerulonephritis (*see also* Nephritis) N05.9
  with
    edema — *see* Nephrosis
    minimal change N05.0
    minor glomerular abnormality N05.0
  acute N00.9
  chronic N03.9
  crescentic (diffuse) NEC (*see also* N00-N07 with fourth
    character .7) N05.7
  dense deposit (*see also* N00-N07 with fourth character
    .6) N05.6
  diffuse
    crescentic (*see also* N00-N07 with fourth character
      .7) N05.7
    endocapillary proliferative (*see also* N00-N07 with
      fourth character .4) N05.4
    membranous (*see also* N00-N07 with fourth char-
      acter .2) N05.2
    mesangial proliferative (*see also* N00-N07 with
      fourth character .3) N05.3
    mesangiocapillary (*see also* N00-N07 with fourth
      character .5) N05.5
    sclerosing N05.8
  endocapillary proliferative (diffuse) NEC (*see also* N00-
    N07 with fourth character .4) N05.4
  extracapillary NEC (*see also* N00-N07 with fourth
    character .7) N05.7
  focal (and segmental) (*see also* N00-N07 with fourth
    character .1) N05.1
  hypocomplementemic — *see* Glomerulonephritis,
    membranoproliferative
  IgA — *see* Nephropathy, IgA
  immune complex (circulating) NEC N05.8
  in (due to)
    amyloidosis E85.4 [N08]
    bilharziasis B65.9 [N08]
    cryoglobulinemia D89.1 [N08]
    defibrination syndrome D65 [N08]
    diabetes mellitus — *see* Diabetes, glomeruloscle-
      rosis
    disseminated intravascular coagulation D65 [N08]
    Fabry (-Anderson) disease E75.21 [N08]
    Goodpasture's syndrome M31.0
    hemolytic-uremic syndrome D59.3
    Henoch (-Schönlein) purpura D69.0 [N08]
    lecithin cholesterol acyltransferase deficiency
      E78.6 [N08]
    microscopic polyangiitis M31.7 [N08]
    multiple myeloma C90.0- ☑ [N08]
    Plasmodium malariae B52.0
    schistosomiasis B65.9 [N08]
    sepsis A41.9 [N08]
      streptococcal A40- ☑ [N08]
    sickle-cell disorders D57.- ☑ [N08]
    strongyloidiasis B78.9 [N08]
    subacute bacterial endocarditis I33.0 [N08]
    syphilis (late) congenital A50.59 [N08]
    systemic lupus erythematosus M32.14
    thrombotic thrombocytopenic purpura
      M31.1 [N08]
    typhoid fever A01.09
    Waldenström macroglobulinemia C88.0 [N08]

Glomerulonephritis — *continued*
  in — *continued*
    Wegener's granulomatosis M31.31
  latent or quiescent N03.9
  lobular, lobulonodular — *see* Glomerulonephritis,
    membranoproliferative
  membranoproliferative (diffuse)(type 1 or 3) (*see also*
    N00-N07 with fourth character .5) N05.5
    dense deposit (type 2) NEC (*see also* N00-N07 with
      fourth character .6) N05.6
  membranous (diffuse) NEC (*see also* N00-N07 with
    fourth character .2) N05.2
  mesangial
    IgA/IgG — *see* Nephropathy, IgA
    proliferative (diffuse) NEC (*see also* N00-N07 with
      fourth character .3) N05.3
  mesangiocapillary (diffuse) NEC (*see also* N00-N07
    with fourth character .5) N05.5
  necrotic, necrotizing NEC (*see also* N00- N07 with
    fourth character .8) N05.8
  nodular — *see* Glomerulonephritis, membranoprolif-
    erative
  poststreptococcal NEC N05.9
    acute N00.9
    chronic N03.9
    rapidly progressive N01.9
  proliferative NEC (*see also* N00-N07 with fourth char-
    acter .8) N05.8
    diffuse (lupus) M32.14
  rapidly progressive N01.9
  sclerosing, diffuse N05.8
  specified pathology NEC (*see also* N00- N07 with fourth
    character .8) N05.8
  subacute N01.9
Glomerulopathy — *see* Glomerulonephritis
Glomerulosclerosis (*see also* Sclerosis, renal)
  intercapillary (nodular) (with diabetes) — *see* Diabetes,
    glomerulosclerosis
  intracapillary — *see* Diabetes, glomerulosclerosis
Glossagra K14.6
Glossalgia K14.6
Glossitis (chronic superficial) (gangrenous) (Moeller's)
  K14.0
  areata exfoliativa K14.1
  atrophic K14.4
  benign migratory K14.1
  cortical superficial, sclerotic K14.0
  Hunter's D51.0
  interstitial, sclerous K14.0
  median rhomboid K14.2
  pellagrous E52
  superficial, chronic K14.0
Glossocele K14.8
Glossodynia K14.6
  exfoliativa K14.4
Glossoncus K14.8
Glossopathy K14.9
Glossophytia K14.3
Glossoplegia K14.8
Glossoptosis K14.8
Glossopyrosis K14.6
Glossotrichia K14.3
Glossy skin L90.8
Glottis — *see* condition
Glottitis (*see also* Laryngitis) J04.0
Glucagonoma
  pancreas
    benign D13.7
    malignant C25.4
    uncertain behavior D37.8
  specified site NEC
    benign — *see* Neoplasm, benign, by site
    malignant — *see* Neoplasm, malignant, by site
    uncertain behavior — *see* Neoplasm, uncertain
      behavior, by site
  unspecified site
    benign D13.7
    malignant C25.4
    uncertain behavior D37.8
Glucoglycinuria E72.51
Glucose-galactose malabsorption E74.39
Glue
  ear — *see* Otitis, media, nonsuppurative, chronic,
    mucoid
  sniffing (airplane) — *see* Abuse, drug, inhalant
    dependence — *see* Dependence, drug, inhalant
Glutaric aciduria E72.3

Glycinemia E72.51
Glycinuria (renal) (with ketosis) E72.09
Glycogen
    infiltration — see Disease, glycogen storage
    storage disease — see Disease, glycogen storage
Glycogenosis (diffuse) (generalized) (see also Disease, glycogen storage)
    cardiac E74.02 [I43]
    diabetic, secondary — see Diabetes, glycogenosis, secondary
    pulmonary interstitial J84.842
Glycopenia E16.2
Glycosuria R81
    renal E74.8
Gnathostoma spinigerum (infection) (infestation), **gnathostomiasis** (wandering swelling) B83.1
Goiter (plunging) (substernal) E04.9
    with
        hyperthyroidism (recurrent) — see Hyperthyroidism, with, goiter
        thyrotoxicosis — see Hyperthyroidism, with, goiter
    adenomatous — see Goiter, nodular
    cancerous C73
    congenital (nontoxic) E03.0
        diffuse E03.0
        parenchymatous E03.0
        transitory, with normal functioning P72.0
    cystic E04.2
        due to iodine-deficiency E01.1
    due to
        enzyme defect in synthesis of thyroid hormone E07.1
        iodine-deficiency (endemic) E01.2
    dyshormonogenetic (familial) E07.1
    endemic (iodine-deficiency) E01.2
        diffuse E01.0
        multinodular E01.1
    exophthalmic — see Hyperthyroidism, with, goiter
    iodine-deficiency (endemic) E01.2
        diffuse E01.0
        multinodular E01.1
        nodular E01.1
    lingual Q89.2
    lymphadenoid E06.3
    malignant C73
    multinodular (cystic) (nontoxic) E04.2
        toxic or with hyperthyroidism E05.20
            with thyroid storm E05.21
    neonatal NEC P72.0
    nodular (nontoxic) (due to) E04.9
        with
            hyperthyroidism E05.20
                with thyroid storm E05.21
            thyrotoxicosis E05.20
                with thyroid storm E05.21
        endemic E01.1
        iodine-deficiency E01.1
        sporadic E04.9
        toxic E05.20
            with thyroid storm E05.21
    nontoxic E04.9
        diffuse (colloid) E04.0
        multinodular E04.2
        simple E04.0
        specified NEC E04.8
        uninodular E04.1
    simple E04.0
    toxic — see Hyperthyroidism, with, goiter
    uninodular (nontoxic) E04.1
        toxic or with hyperthyroidism E05.10
            with thyroid storm E05.11
Goiter-deafness syndrome E07.1
Goldberg syndrome Q89.8
Goldberg-Maxwell syndrome E34.51
Goldblatt's hypertension or kidney I70.1
Goldenhar (-Gorlin) **syndrome** Q87.0
Goldflam-Erb disease or syndrome G70.00
    with exacerbation (acute) G70.01
    in crisis G70.01
Goldscheider's disease Q81.8
Goldstein's disease (familial hemorrhagic telangiectasia) I78.0
Golfer's elbow — see Epicondylitis, medial
Gonadoblastoma
    specified site — see Neoplasm, uncertain behavior, by site
    unspecified site
        female D39.10

Gonadoblastoma — continued
    unspecified site — continued
        male D40.10
Gonecystitis — see Vesiculitis
Gongylonemiasis B83.8
Goniosynechiae — see Adhesions, iris, goniosynechiae
Gonococcemia A54.86
Gonococcus, gonococcal (disease) (infection) (see also condition) A54.9
    anus A54.6
    bursa, bursitis A54.49
    conjunctiva, conjunctivitis (neonatorum) A54.31
    endocardium A54.83
    eye A54.30
        conjunctivitis A54.31
        iridocyclitis A54.32
        keratitis A54.33
        newborn A54.31
        other specified A54.39
    fallopian tubes (acute) (chronic) A54.24
    genitourinary (organ) (system) (tract) (acute)
        lower A54.00
            with abscess (accessory gland) (periurethral) A54.1
        upper (see also condition) A54.29
    heart A54.83
    iridocyclitis A54.32
    joint A54.42
    lymphatic (gland) (node) A54.89
    meninges, meningitis A54.81
    musculoskeletal A54.40
        arthritis A54.42
        osteomyelitis A54.43
        other specified A54.49
        spondylopathy A54.41
    pelviperitonitis A54.24
    pelvis (acute) (chronic) A54.24
    pharynx A54.5
    proctitis A54.6
    pyosalpinx (acute) (chronic) A54.24
    rectum A54.6
    skin A54.89
    specified site NEC A54.89
    tendon sheath A54.49
    throat A54.5
    urethra (acute) (chronic) A54.01
        with abscess (accessory gland) (periurethral) A54.1
    vulva (acute) (chronic) A54.02
Gonocytoma
    specified site — see Neoplasm, uncertain behavior, by site
    unspecified site
        female D39.10
        male D40.10
Gonorrhea (acute) (chronic) A54.9
    Bartholin's gland (acute) (chronic) (purulent) A54.02
        with abscess (accessory gland) (periurethral) A54.1
    bladder A54.01
    cervix A54.03
    conjunctiva, conjunctivitis (neonatorum) A54.31
    contact Z20.2
    Cowper's gland (with abscess) A54.1
    exposure to Z20.2
    fallopian tube (acute) (chronic) A54.24
    kidney (acute) (chronic) A54.21
    lower genitourinary tract A54.00
        with abscess (accessory gland) (periurethral) A54.1
    ovary (acute) (chronic) A54.24
    pelvis (acute) (chronic) A54.24
        female pelvic inflammatory disease A54.24
    penis A54.09
    prostate (acute) (chronic) A54.22
    seminal vesicle (acute) (chronic) A54.23
    specified site not listed (see also Gonococcus) A54.89
    spermatic cord (acute) (chronic) A54.23
    urethra A54.01
        with abscess (accessory gland) (periurethral) A54.1
    vagina A54.02
    vas deferens (acute) (chronic) A54.23
    vulva A54.02
Goodall's disease A08.19
Goodpasture's syndrome M31.0
Gopalan's syndrome (burning feet) E53.0
Gorlin-Chaudry-Moss syndrome Q87.0
Gottron's papules L94.4
Gougerot-Blum syndrome (pigmented purpuric lichenoid dermatitis) L81.7

Gougerot-Carteaud disease or syndrome (confluent reticulate papillomatosis) L83
Gougerot's syndrome (trisymptomatic) L81.7
Gouley's syndrome (constrictive pericarditis) I31.1
Goundou A66.6
Gout, chronic (see also Gout, gouty) M1A.9 ☑ (following M08)
    drug-induced M1A.20 ☑ (following M08)
        ankle M1A.27- ☑ (following M08)
        elbow M1A.22- ☑ (following M08)
        foot joint M1A.27- ☑ (following M08)
        hand joint M1A.24- ☑ (following M08)
        hip M1A.25- ☑ (following M08)
        knee M1A.26- ☑ (following M08)
        multiple site M1A.29- ☑ (following M08)
        shoulder M1A.21- ☑ (following M08)
        vertebrae M1A.28 ☑ (following M08)
        wrist M1A.23- ☑ (following M08)
    idiopathic M1A.00 ☑ (following M08)
        ankle M1A.07- ☑ (following M08)
        elbow M1A.02- ☑ (following M08)
        foot joint M1A.07- ☑ (following M08)
        hand joint M1A.04- ☑ (following M08)
        hip M1A.05- ☑ (following M08)
        knee M1A.06- ☑ (following M08)
        multiple site M1A.09 ☑ (following M08)
        shoulder M1A.01- ☑ (following M08)
        vertebrae M1A.08 ☑ (following M08)
        wrist M1A.03- ☑ (following M08)
    in (due to) renal impairment M1A.30 ☑ (following M08)
        ankle M1A.37- ☑ (following M08)
        elbow M1A.32- ☑ (following M08)
        foot joint M1A.37- ☑ (following M08)
        hand joint M1A.34- ☑ (following M08)
        hip M1A.35- ☑ (following M08)
        knee M1A.36- ☑ (following M08)
        multiple site M1A.39 ☑ (following M08)
        shoulder M1A.31- ☑ (following M08)
        vertebrae M1A.38 ☑ (following M08)
        wrist M1A.33- ☑ (following M08)
    lead-induced M1A.10 ☑ (following M08)
        ankle M1A.17- ☑ (following M08)
        elbow M1A.12- ☑ (following M08)
        foot joint M1A.17- ☑ (following M08)
        hand joint M1A.14- ☑ (following M08)
        hip M1A.15- ☑ (following M08)
        knee M1A.16- ☑ (following M08)
        multiple site M1A.19 ☑ (following M08)
        shoulder M1A.11- ☑ (following M08)
        vertebrae M1A.18 ☑ (following M08)
        wrist M1A.13- ☑ (following M08)
    primary — see Gout, chronic, idiopathic
    saturnine — see Gout, chronic, lead-induced
    secondary NEC M1A.40 ☑ (following M08)
        ankle M1A.47- ☑ (following M08)
        elbow M1A.42- ☑ (following M08)
        foot joint M1A.47- ☑ (following M08)
        hand joint M1A.44- ☑ (following M08)
        hip M1A.45- ☑ (following M08)
        knee M1A.46- ☑ (following M08)
        multiple site M1A.49 ☑ (following M08)
        shoulder M1A.41- ☑ (following M08)
        vertebrae M1A.48 ☑ (following M08)
        wrist M1A.43- ☑ (following M08)
    syphilitic (see also subcategory M14.8-) A52.77
    tophi M1A.9 ☑ (following M08)
Gout, gouty (acute) (attack) (flare) (see also Gout, chronic) M10.9
    drug-induced M10.20
        ankle M10.27- ☑
        elbow M10.22- ☑
        foot joint M10.27- ☑
        hand joint M10.24- ☑
        hip M10.25- ☑
        knee M10.26- ☑
        multiple site M10.29
        shoulder M10.21- ☑
        vertebrae M10.28
        wrist M10.23- ☑
    idiopathic M10.00
        ankle M10.07- ☑
        elbow M10.02- ☑
        foot joint M10.07- ☑
        hand joint M10.04- ☑
        hip M10.05- ☑

Gout, gouty — *continued*
  idiopathic — *continued*
    knee M10.06- ☑
    multiple site M10.09
    shoulder M10.01- ☑
    vertebrae M10.08
    wrist M10.03- ☑
  in (due to) renal impairment M10.30
    ankle M10.37- ☑
    elbow M10.32- ☑
    foot joint M10.37- ☑
    hand joint M10.34- ☑
    hip M10.35- ☑
    knee M10.36- ☑
    multiple site M10.39
    shoulder M10.31- ☑
    vertebrae M10.38
    wrist M10.33- ☑
  lead-induced M10.10
    ankle M10.17- ☑
    elbow M10.12- ☑
    foot joint M10.17- ☑
    hand joint M10.14- ☑
    hip M10.15- ☑
    knee M10.16- ☑
    multiple site M10.19
    shoulder M10.11- ☑
    vertebrae M10.18
    wrist M10.13- ☑
  primary — *see* Gout, idiopathic
  saturnine — *see* Gout, lead-induced
  secondary NEC M10.40
    ankle M10.47- ☑
    elbow M10.42- ☑
    foot joint M10.47- ☑
    hand joint M10.44- ☑
    hip M10.45- ☑
    knee M10.46- ☑
    multiple site M10.49
    shoulder M10.41- ☑
    vertebrae M10.48
    wrist M10.43- ☑
  syphilitic (*see also* subcategory M14.8-) A52.77
  tophi — *see* Gout, chronic
Gower's
  muscular dystrophy G71.0
  syndrome (vasovagal attack) R55
Gradenigo's syndrome — *see* Otitis, media, suppurative, acute
Graefe's disease — *see* Strabismus, paralytic, ophthalmoplegia, progressive
Graft-versus-host disease D89.813
  acute D89.810
  acute on chronic D89.812
  chronic D89.811
Grain mite (itch) B88.0
Grainhandler's disease or lung J67.8
Grand mal — *see* Epilepsy, generalized, specified NEC
Grand multipara status only (not pregnant) Z64.1
  pregnant — *see* Pregnancy, complicated by, grand multiparity
Granite worker's lung J62.8
Granular (*see also* condition)
  inflammation, pharynx J31.2
  kidney (contracting) — *see* Sclerosis, renal
  liver K74.69
Granulation tissue (abnormal) (excessive) L92.9
  postmastoidectomy cavity — *see* Complications, postmastoidectomy, granulation
Granulocytopenia (primary) (malignant) — *see* Agranulocytosis
Granuloma L92.9
  abdomen K66.8
    from residual foreign body L92.3
    pyogenicum L98.0
  actinic L57.5
  annulare (perforating) L92.0
  apical K04.5
  aural — *see* Otitis, externa, specified NEC
  beryllium (skin) L92.3
  bone
    eosinophilic C96.6
    from residual foreign body — *see* Osteomyelitis, specified type NEC
    lung C96.6
  brain (any site) G06.0
    schistosomiasis B65.9 [G07]

Granuloma — *continued*
  canaliculus lacrimalis — *see* Granuloma, lacrimal
  candidal (cutaneous) B37.2
  cerebral (any site) G06.0
  coccidioidal (primary) (progressive) B38.7
    lung B38.1
    meninges B38.4
  colon K63.89
  conjunctiva H11.22- ☑
  dental K04.5
  ear, middle — *see* Cholesteatoma
  eosinophilic C96.6
    bone C96.6
    lung C96.6
    oral mucosa K13.4
    skin L92.2
  eyelid H01.8
  facial (e) L92.2
  foreign body (in soft tissue) NEC M60.20
    ankle M60.27- ☑
    foot M60.27- ☑
    forearm M60.23- ☑
    hand M60.24- ☑
    in operation wound — *see* Foreign body, accidentally left during a procedure
    lower leg M60.26- ☑
    pelvic region M60.25- ☑
    shoulder region M60.21- ☑
    skin L92.3
    specified site NEC M60.28
    subcutaneous tissue L92.3
    thigh M60.25- ☑
    upper arm M60.22- ☑
  gangraenescens M31.2
  genito-inguinale A58
  giant cell (central) (reparative) (jaw) M27.1
    gingiva (peripheral) K06.8
  gland (lymph) I88.8
  hepatic NEC K75.3
    in (due to)
      berylliosis J63.2 [K77]
      sarcoidosis D86.89
  Hodgkin C81.9 ☑
  ileum K63.89
  infectious B99.9
    specified NEC B99.8
  inguinale (Donovan) (venereal) A58
  intestine NEC K63.89
  intracranial (any site) G06.0
  intraspinal (any part) G06.1
  iridocyclitis — *see* Iridocyclitis, chronic
  jaw (bone) (central) M27.1
    reparative giant cell M27.1
  kidney (*see also* Infection, kidney) N15.8
  lacrimal H04.81- ☑
  larynx J38.7
  lethal midline (faciale(e)) M31.2
  liver NEC — *see* Granuloma, hepatic
  lung (infectious) (*see also* Fibrosis, lung)
    coccidioidal B38.1
    eosinophilic C96.6
  Majocchi's B35.8
  malignant (facial(e)) M31.2
  mandible (central) M27.1
  midline (lethal) M31.2
  monilial (cutaneous) B37.2
  nasal sinus — *see* Sinusitis
  operation wound T81.89 ☑
    foreign body — *see* Foreign body, accidentally left during a procedure
    stitch T81.89 ☑
    talc — *see* Foreign body, accidentally left during a procedure
  oral mucosa K13.4
  orbit, orbital H05.11- ☑
  paracoccidioidal B41.8
  penis, venereal A58
  periapical K04.5
  peritoneum K66.8
    due to ova of helminths NOS (*see also* Helminthiasis) B83.9 [K67]
  postmastoidectomy cavity — *see* Complications, postmastoidectomy, recurrent cholesteatoma
  prostate N42.89
  pudendi (ulcerating) A58
  pulp, internal (tooth) K03.3
  pyogenic, pyogenicum (of) (skin) L98.0
    gingiva K06.8

Granuloma — *continued*
  pyogenic, pyogenicum — *continued*
    maxillary alveolar ridge K04.5
    oral mucosa K13.4
  rectum K62.89
  reticulohistiocytic D76.3
  rubrum nasi L74.8
  Schistosoma — *see* Schistosomiasis
  septic (skin) L98.0
  silica (skin) L92.3
  sinus (accessory) (infective) (nasal) — *see* Sinusitis
  skin L92.9
    from residual foreign body L92.3
    pyogenicum L98.0
  spine
    syphilitic (epidural) A52.19
    tuberculous A18.01
  stitch (postoperative) T81.89 ☑
  suppurative (skin) L98.0
  swimming pool A31.1
  talc (*see also* Granuloma, foreign body)
    in operation wound — *see* Foreign body, accidentally left during a procedure
  telangiectaticum (skin) L98.0
  tracheostomy J95.09
  trichophyticum B35.8
  tropicum A66.4
  umbilicus L92.9
  urethra N36.8
  uveitis — *see* Iridocyclitis, chronic
  vagina A58
  venereum A58
  vocal cord J38.3
Granulomatosis L92.9
  lymphoid C83.8- ☑
  miliary (listerial) A32.89
  necrotizing, respiratory M31.30
  progressive septic D71
  specified NEC L92.8
  Wegener's M31.30
    with renal involvement M31.31
Granulomatous tissue (abnormal) (excessive) L92.9
Granulosis rubra nasi L74.8
Graphite fibrosis (of lung) J63.3
Graphospasm F48.8
  organic G25.89
Grating scapula M89.8X1
Gravel (urinary) — *see* Calculus, urinary
Graves' disease — *see* Hyperthyroidism, with, goiter
Gravis — *see* condition
Grawitz tumor C64.- ☑
Gray syndrome (newborn) P93.0
Grayness, hair (premature) L67.1
  congenital Q84.2
Green sickness D50.8
Greenfield's disease
  meaning
    concentric sclerosis (encephalitis periaxialis concentrica) G37.5
    metachromatic leukodystrophy E75.25
Greenstick fracture — *code as* Fracture, by site
Grey syndrome (newborn) P93.0
Grief F43.21
  prolonged F43.29
  reaction (*see also* Disorder, adjustment) F43.20
Griesinger's disease B76.9
Grinder's lung or pneumoconiosis J62.8
Grinding, teeth
  psychogenic F45.8
  sleep related G47.63
Grip
  Dabney's B33.0
  devil's B33.0
Grippe, grippal (*see also* Influenza)
  Balkan A78
  summer, of Italy A93.1
Grisel's disease M43.6
Groin — *see* condition
Grooved tongue K14.5
Ground itch B76.9
Grover's disease or syndrome L11.1
Growing pains, children R29.898
Growth (fungoid) (neoplastic) (new) (*see also* Neoplasm)
  adenoid (vegetative) J35.8
  benign — *see* Neoplasm, benign, by site
  malignant — *see* Neoplasm, malignant, by site
  rapid, childhood Z00.2

Growth — *continued*
　secondary — *see* Neoplasm, secondary, by site
Gruby's disease B35.0
Gubler-Millard paralysis or syndrome G46.3
Guerin-Stern syndrome Q74.3
Guidance, insufficient anterior (occlusal) M26.54
Guillain-Barré disease or syndrome G61.0
　sequelae G65.0
Guinea worms (infection) (infestation) B72
Guinon's disease (motor-verbal tic) F95.2
Gull's disease E03.4
Gum — *see* condition
Gumboil K04.7
　with sinus K04.6
Gumma (syphilitic) A52.79
　artery A52.09
　　cerebral A52.04
　bone A52.77
　　of yaws (late) A66.6
　brain A52.19
　cauda equina A52.19
　central nervous system A52.3
　ciliary body A52.71
　congenital A50.59
　eyelid A52.71
　heart A52.06
　intracranial A52.19
　iris A52.71
　kidney A52.75
　larynx A52.73
　leptomeninges A52.19
　liver A52.74
　meninges A52.19
　myocardium A52.06
　nasopharynx A52.73
　neurosyphilitic A52.3
　nose A52.73
　orbit A52.71
　palate (soft) A52.79
　penis A52.76
　pericardium A52.06
　pharynx A52.73
　pituitary A52.79
　scrofulous (tuberculous) A18.4
　skin A52.79
　specified site NEC A52.79
　spinal cord A52.19
　tongue A52.79
　tonsil A52.73
　trachea A52.73
　tuberculous A18.4
　ulcerative due to yaws A66.4
　ureter A52.75
　yaws A66.4
　　bone A66.6
Gunn's syndrome Q07.8
Gunshot wound (*see also* Wound, open)
　fracture — *code as* Fracture, by site
　internal organs — *see* Injury, by site
Gynandrism Q56.0
Gynandroblastoma
　specified site — *see* Neoplasm, uncertain behavior,
　　by site
　unspecified site
　　female D39.10
　　male D40.10
Gynecological examination (periodic) (routine) Z01.419
　with abnormal findings Z01.411
Gynecomastia N62
Gynephobia F40.291
Gyrate scalp Q82.8

H

H (Hartnup's) **disease** E72.02
Haas' disease or osteochondrosis (juvenile) (head of
　humerus) — *see* Osteochondrosis, juvenile,
　humerus
Habit, habituation
　bad sleep Z72.821
　chorea F95.8
　disturbance, child F98.9
　drug — *see* Dependence, drug
　irregular sleep Z72.821
　laxative F55.2
　spasm — *see* Tic
　tic — *see* Tic

Haemophilus (H.) **influenzae, as cause of disease
　classified elsewhere** B96.3
Haff disease — *see* Poisoning, mercury
Hageman's factor defect, deficiency or disease D68.2
Haglund's disease or osteochondrosis (juvenile) (os
　tibiale externum) — *see* Osteochondrosis, juvenile,
　tarsus
Hailey-Hailey disease Q82.8
Hair (*see also* condition)
　plucking F63.3
　　in stereotyped movement disorder F98.4
　tourniquet syndrome (*see also* Constriction, external,
　　by site)
　　finger S60.44- ☑
　　penis S30.842 ☑
　　thumb S60.34- ☑
　　toe S90.44- ☑
Hairball in stomach T18.2 ☑
Hair-pulling, pathological (compulsive) F63.3
Hairy black tongue K14.3
Half vertebra Q76.49
Halitosis R19.6
Hallerman-Streiff syndrome Q87.0
Hallervorden-Spatz disease G23.0
Hallopeau's acrodermatitis or disease L40.2
Hallucination R44.3
　auditory R44.0
　gustatory R44.2
　olfactory R44.2
　specified NEC R44.2
　tactile R44.2
　visual R44.1
Hallucinosis (chronic) F28
　alcoholic (acute) F10.951
　　in
　　　abuse F10.151
　　　dependence F10.251
　drug-induced F19.951
　　cannabis F12.951
　　cocaine F14.951
　　hallucinogen F16.151
　　in
　　　abuse F19.151
　　　　cannabis F12.151
　　　　cocaine F14.151
　　　　hallucinogen F16.151
　　　　inhalant F18.151
　　　　opioid F11.151
　　　　sedative, anxiolytic or hypnotic F13.151
　　　　stimulant NEC F15.151
　　　dependence F19.251
　　　　cannabis F12.251
　　　　cocaine F14.251
　　　　hallucinogen F16.251
　　　　inhalant F18.251
　　　　opioid F11.251
　　　　sedative, anxiolytic or hypnotic F13.251
　　　　stimulant NEC F15.251
　　inhalant F18.951
　　opioid F11.951
　　sedative, anxiolytic or hypnotic F13.951
　　stimulant NEC F15.951
　organic F06.0
Hallux
　deformity (acquired) NEC M20.5X- ☑
　limitus M20.5X- ☑
　malleus (acquired) NEC M20.3- ☑
　rigidus (acquired) M20.2- ☑
　　congenital Q74.2
　　sequelae (late effect) of rickets E64.3
　valgus (acquired) M20.1- ☑
　　congenital Q66.6
　varus (acquired) M20.3- ☑
　　congenital Q66.3
Halo, visual H53.19
Hamartoma, hamartoblastoma Q85.9
　epithelial (gingival), odontogenic, central or peripheral
　　— *see* Cyst, calcifying odontogenic
Hamartosis Q85.9
Hamman-Rich syndrome J84.114
Hammer toe (acquired) NEC (*see also* Deformity, toe,
　hammer toe)
　congenital Q66.89
　sequelae (late effect) of rickets E64.3
Hand — *see* condition
Hand-foot syndrome L27.1

Handicap, handicapped
　educational Z55.9
　　specified NEC Z55.8
Hand-Schüller-Christian disease or syndrome C96.5
Hanging (asphyxia) (strangulation) (suffocation) — *see*
　Asphyxia, traumatic, due to mechanical threat
Hangnail (*see also* Cellulitis, digit)
　with lymphangitis — *see* Lymphangitis, acute, digit
Hangover (alcohol) F10.129
Hanhart's syndrome Q87.0
Hanot-Chauffard (-Troisier) **syndrome** E83.19
Hanot's cirrhosis or disease K74.3
Hansen's disease — *see* Leprosy
Hantaan virus disease (Korean hemorrhagic fever) A98.5
Hantavirus disease (with renal manifestations) (Dobra-
　va) (Puumala) (Seoul) A98.5
　with pulmonary manifestations (Andes) (Bayou)
　　(Bermejo) (Black Creek Canal) (Choclo) (Juquiti-
　　ba) (Laguna negra) (Lechiguanas) (New York)
　　(Oran) (Sin nombre) B33.4
Happy puppet syndrome Q93.5
Harada's disease or syndrome H30.81- ☑
Hardening
　artery — *see* Arteriosclerosis
　brain G93.89
Harelip (complete) (incomplete) — *see* Cleft, lip
Harlequin (newborn) Q80.4
Harley's disease D59.6
Harmful use (of)
　alcohol F10.10
　anxiolytics — *see* Abuse, drug, sedative
　cannabinoids — *see* Abuse, drug, cannabis
　cocaine — *see* Abuse, drug, cocaine
　drug — *see* Abuse, drug
　hallucinogens — *see* Abuse, drug, hallucinogen
　hypnotics — *see* Abuse, drug, sedative
　opioids — *see* Abuse, drug, opioid
　PCP (phencyclidine) — *see* Abuse, drug, hallucinogen
　sedatives — *see* Abuse, drug, sedative
　stimulants NEC — *see* Abuse, drug, stimulant
Harris' lines — *see* Arrest, epiphyseal
Hartnup's disease E72.02
Harvester's lung J67.0
Harvesting ovum for in vitro fertilization Z31.83
Hashimoto's disease or thyroiditis E06.3
Hashitoxicosis (transient) E06.3
Hassal-Henle bodies or warts (cornea) H18.49
Haut mal — *see* Epilepsy, generalized, specified NEC
Haverhill fever A25.1
Hay fever (*see also* Fever, hay) J30.1
Hayem-Widal syndrome D59.8
Haygarth's nodes M15.8
Haymaker's lung J67.0
Hb (abnormal)
　Bart's disease D56.0
　disease — *see* Disease, hemoglobin
　trait — *see* Trait
Head — *see* condition
Headache R51
　allergic NEC G44.89
　associated with sexual activity G44.82
　chronic daily R51
　cluster G44.009
　　chronic G44.029
　　　intractable G44.021
　　　not intractable G44.029
　　episodic G44.019
　　　intractable G44.011
　　　not intractable G44.019
　　intractable G44.001
　　not intractable G44.009
　cough (primary) G44.83
　daily chronic R51
　drug-induced NEC G44.40
　　intractable G44.41
　　not intractable G44.40
　exertional (primary) G44.84
　histamine G44.009
　　intractable G44.001
　　not intractable G44.009
　hypnic G44.81
　lumbar puncture G97.1
　medication overuse G44.40
　　intractable G44.41
　　not intractable G44.40
　menstrual — *see* Migraine, menstrual
　migraine (type) (*see also* Migraine) G43.909

　☑ **Additional Character Required** — **Refer to the Tabular List for Character Selection**　🔻 **Subterms under main terms may continue to next column or page**

Headache — *continued*
  nasal septum R51
  neuralgiform, short lasting unilateral, with conjunctival
      injection and tearing (SUNCT) G44.059
    intractable G44.051
    not intractable G44.059
  new daily persistent (NDPH) G44.52
  orgasmic G44.82
  periodic syndromes in adults and children G43.C0
      (*following* G43.7)
    with refractory migraine G43.C1 (*following* G43.7)
    without refractory migraine G43.C0 (*following*
        G43.7)
    intractable G43.C1 (*following* G43.7)
    not intractable G43.C0 (*following* G43.7)
  postspinal puncture G97.1
  post-traumatic G44.309
    acute G44.319
      intractable G44.311
      not intractable G44.319
    chronic G44.329
      intractable G44.321
      not intractable G44.329
    intractable G44.301
    not intractable G44.309
  pre-menstrual — *see* Migraine, menstrual
  preorgasmic G44.82
  primary
    cough G44.83
    exertional G44.84
    stabbing G44.85
    thunderclap G44.53
  rebound G44.40
    intractable G44.41
    not intractable G44.40
  short lasting unilateral neuralgiform, with conjunctival
      injection and tearing (SUNCT) G44.059
    intractable G44.051
    not intractable G44.059
  specified syndrome NEC G44.89
  spinal and epidural anesthesia - induced T88.59 ☑
    in labor and delivery O74.5
    in pregnancy O29.4- ☑
    postpartum, puerperal O89.4
  spinal fluid loss (from puncture) G97.1
  stabbing (primary) G44.85
  tension (-type) G44.209
    chronic G44.229
      intractable G44.221
      not intractable G44.229
    episodic G44.219
      intractable G44.211
      not intractable G44.219
    intractable G44.201
    not intractable G44.209
  thunderclap (primary) G44.53
  vascular NEC G44.1
Healthy
  infant
    accompanying sick mother Z76.3
    receiving care Z76.2
  person accompanying sick person Z76.3
Hearing examination Z01.10
  with abnormal findings NEC Z01.118
  following failed hearing screening Z01.110
  for hearing conservation and treatment Z01.12
Heart — *see* condition
Heart beat
  abnormality R00.9
    specified NEC R00.8
  awareness R00.2
  rapid R00.0
  slow R00.1
Heartburn R12
  psychogenic F45.8
Heat (effects) T67.9 ☑
  apoplexy T67.0 ☑
  burn (*see also* Burn) L55.9
  collapse T67.1 ☑
  cramps T67.2 ☑
  dermatitis or eczema L59.0
  edema T67.7 ☑
  erythema — *code by site under* Burn, first degree
  excessive T67.9 ☑
    specified effect NEC T67.8 ☑
  exhaustion T67.5 ☑
    anhydrotic T67.3 ☑

Heat — *continued*
  exhaustion — *continued*
    due to
      salt (and water) depletion T67.4 ☑
      water depletion T67.3 ☑
        with salt depletion T67.4 ☑
  fatigue (transient) T67.6 ☑
  fever T67.0 ☑
  hyperpyrexia T67.0 ☑
  prickly L74.0
  prostration — *see* Heat, exhaustion
  pyrexia T67.0 ☑
  rash L74.0
  specified effect NEC T67.8 ☑
  stroke T67.0 ☑
  sunburn — *see* Sunburn
  syncope T67.1 ☑
Heavy-for-dates NEC (infant) (4000g to 4499g) P08.1
  exceptionally (4500g or more) P08.0
Hebephrenia, hebephrenic (schizophrenia) F20.1
Heberden's disease or nodes (with arthropathy) M15.1
Hebra's
  pityriasis L26
  prurigo L28.2
Heel — *see* condition
Heerfordt's disease D86.89
Hegglin's anomaly or syndrome D72.0
Heilmeyer-Schoner disease D45
Heine-Medin disease A80.9
Heinz body anemia, congenital D58.2
Heliophobia F40.228
Heller's disease or syndrome F84.3
HELLP syndrome (hemolysis, elevated liver enzymes
    and low platelet count) O14.2- ☑
Helminthiasis (*see also* Infestation, helminth)
  Ancylostoma B76.0
  intestinal B82.0
    mixed types (types classifiable to more than one
        of the titles B65.0-B81.3 and B81.8) B81.4
    specified type NEC B81.8
  mixed types (intestinal) (types classifiable to more
      than one of the titles B65.0-B81.3 and B81.8)
      B81.4
  Necator (americanus) B76.1
  specified type NEC B83.8
Heloma L84
Hemangioblastoma — *see* Neoplasm, connective tissue,
    uncertain behavior
  malignant — *see* Neoplasm, connective tissue, malig-
    nant
Hemangioendothelioma (*see also* Neoplasm, uncertain
    behavior, by site)
  benign D18.00
    intra-abdominal D18.03
    intracranial D18.02
    skin D18.01
    specified site NEC D18.09
  bone (diffuse) — *see* Neoplasm, bone, malignant
  epithelioid (*see also* Neoplasm, uncertain behavior,
      by site)
    malignant — *see* Neoplasm, malignant, by site
  malignant — *see* Neoplasm, connective tissue, malig-
    nant
Hemangiofibroma — *see* Neoplasm, benign, by site
Hemangiolipoma — *see* Lipoma
Hemangioma D18.00
  arteriovenous D18.00
    intra-abdominal D18.03
    intracranial D18.02
    skin D18.01
    specified site NEC D18.09
  capillary D18.00
    intra-abdominal D18.03
    intracranial D18.02
    skin D18.01
    specified site NEC D18.09
  cavernous D18.00
    intra-abdominal D18.03
    intracranial D18.02
    skin D18.01
    specified site NEC D18.09
  epithelioid D18.00
    intra-abdominal D18.03
    intracranial D18.02
    skin D18.01
    specified site NEC D18.09

Hemangioma — *continued*
  histiocytoid D18.00
    intra-abdominal D18.03
    intracranial D18.02
    skin D18.01
    specified site NEC D18.09
  infantile D18.00
    intra-abdominal D18.03
    intracranial D18.02
    skin D18.01
    specified site NEC D18.09
  intra-abdominal D18.03
  intracranial D18.02
  intramuscular D18.00
    intra-abdominal D18.03
    intracranial D18.02
    skin D18.01
    specified site NEC D18.09
  juvenile D18.00
  malignant — *see* Neoplasm, connective tissue, malig-
    nant
  plexiform D18.00
    intra-abdominal D18.03
    intracranial D18.02
    skin D18.01
    specified site NEC D18.09
  racemose D18.00
    intra-abdominal D18.03
    intracranial D18.02
    skin D18.01
    specified site NEC D18.09
  sclerosing — *see* Neoplasm, skin, benign
  simplex D18.00
    intra-abdominal D18.03
    intracranial D18.02
    skin D18.01
    specified site NEC D18.09
  skin D18.01
  specified site NEC D18.09
  venous D18.00
    intra-abdominal D18.03
    intracranial D18.02
    skin D18.01
    specified site NEC D18.09
  verrucous keratotic D18.00
    intra-abdominal D18.03
    intracranial D18.02
    skin D18.01
    specified site NEC D18.09
Hemangiomatosis (systemic) I78.8
  involving single site — *see* Hemangioma
Hemangiopericytoma (*see also* Neoplasm, connective
    tissue, uncertain behavior)
  benign — *see* Neoplasm, connective tissue, benign
  malignant — *see* Neoplasm, connective tissue, malig-
    nant
Hemangiosarcoma — *see* Neoplasm, connective tissue,
    malignant
Hemarthrosis (nontraumatic) M25.00
  ankle M25.07- ☑
  elbow M25.02- ☑
  foot joint M25.07- ☑
  hand joint M25.04- ☑
  hip M25.05- ☑
  in hemophilic arthropathy — *see* Arthropathy,
      hemophilic
  knee M25.06- ☑
  shoulder M25.01- ☑
  specified joint NEC M25.08
  traumatic — *see* Sprain, by site
  vertebrae M25.08
  wrist M25.03- ☑
Hematemesis K92.0
  with ulcer — *code by site under* Ulcer, with hemor-
      rhage K27.4
  newborn, neonatal P54.0
    due to swallowed maternal blood P78.2
Hematidrosis L74.8
Hematinuria (*see also* Hemoglobinuria)
  malarial B50.8
Hematobilia K83.8
Hematocele
  female NEC N94.89
    with ectopic pregnancy O00.9
    ovary N83.8
  male N50.1
Hematochezia (*see also* Melena) K92.1

Hematochyluria (see also Infestation, filarial)
schistosomiasis (bilharziasis) B65.0
Hematocolpos (with hematometra or hematosalpinx)
N89.7
Hematocornea — see Pigmentation, cornea, stromal
Hematogenous — see condition
Hematoma (traumatic) (skin surface intact) (see also
Contusion)
with
injury of internal organs — see Injury, by site
open wound — see Wound, open
amputation stump (surgical) (late) T87.89
aorta, dissecting I71.00
abdominal I71.02
thoracic I71.01
thoracoabdominal I71.03
aortic intramural — see Dissection, aorta
arterial (complicating trauma) — see Injury, blood
vessel, by site
auricle — see Contusion, ear
nontraumatic — see Disorder, pinna, hematoma
birth injury NEC P15.8
brain (traumatic)
with
cerebral laceration or contusion (diffuse) — see
Injury, intracranial, diffuse
focal — see Injury, intracranial, focal
cerebellar, traumatic S06.37- ☑
intracerebral, traumatic — see Injury, intracranial,
intracerebral hemorrhage
newborn NEC P52.4
birth injury P10.1
nontraumatic — see Hemorrhage, intracranial
subarachnoid, arachnoid, traumatic — see Injury,
intracranial, subarachnoid hemorrhage
subdural, traumatic — see Injury, intracranial,
subdural hemorrhage
breast (nontraumatic) N64.89
broad ligament (nontraumatic) N83.7
traumatic S37.892 ☑
cerebellar, traumatic S06.37- ☑
cerebral — see Hematoma, brain
cerebrum S06.36- ☑
left S06.35- ☑
right S06.34- ☑
cesarean delivery wound O90.2
complicating delivery (perineal) (pelvic) (vagina) (vulva) O71.7
corpus cavernosum (nontraumatic) N48.89
epididymis (nontraumatic) N50.1
epidural (traumatic) — see Injury, intracranial, epidural
hemorrhage
spinal — see Injury, spinal cord, by region
episiotomy O90.2
face, birth injury P15.4
genital organ NEC (nontraumatic)
female (nonobstetric) N94.89
traumatic S30.202 ☑
male N50.1
traumatic S30.201 ☑
internal organs — see Injury, by site
intracerebral, traumatic — see Injury, intracranial, intracerebral hemorrhage
intraoperative — see Complications, intraoperative,
hemorrhage
labia (nontraumatic) (nonobstetric) N90.89
liver (subcapsular) (nontraumatic) K76.89
birth injury P15.0
mediastinum — see Injury, intrathoracic
mesosalpinx (nontraumatic) N83.7
traumatic S37.898 ☑
muscle — code by site under Contusion
nontraumatic
muscle M79.81
soft tissue M79.81
obstetrical surgical wound O90.2
orbit, orbital (nontraumatic) (see also Hemorrhage,
orbit)
traumatic — see Contusion, orbit
pelvis (female) (nontraumatic) (nonobstetric) N94.89
obstetric O71.7
traumatic — see Injury, by site
penis (nontraumatic) N48.89
birth injury P15.5
perianal (nontraumatic) K64.5
perineal S30.23 ☑
complicating delivery O71.7

Hematoma — continued
perirenal — see Injury, kidney
pinna — see Contusion, ear
nontraumatic — see Disorder, pinna, hematoma
placenta O43.89- ☑
postoperative (postprocedural) — see Complication,
postprocedural, hemorrhage
retroperitoneal (nontraumatic) K66.1
traumatic S36.892 ☑
scrotum, superficial S30.22 ☑
birth injury P15.5
seminal vesicle (nontraumatic) N50.1
traumatic S37.892 ☑
spermatic cord (traumatic) S37.892 ☑
nontraumatic N50.1
spinal (cord) (meninges) (see also Injury, spinal cord,
by region)
newborn (birth injury) P11.5
spleen D73.5
intraoperative — see Complications, intraoperative,
hemorrhage, spleen
postprocedural (postoperative) — see Complications, postprocedural, hemorrhage, spleen
sternocleidomastoid, birth injury P15.2
sternomastoid, birth injury P15.2
subarachnoid (traumatic) — see Injury, intracranial,
subarachnoid hemorrhage
newborn (nontraumatic) P52.5
due to birth injury P10.3
nontraumatic — see Hemorrhage, intracranial,
subarachnoid
subdural (traumatic) — see Injury, intracranial, subdural hemorrhage
newborn (localized) P52.8
birth injury P10.0
nontraumatic — see Hemorrhage, intracranial,
subdural
superficial, newborn P54.5
testis (nontraumatic) N50.1
birth injury P15.5
tunica vaginalis (nontraumatic) N50.1
umbilical cord, complicating delivery O69.5 ☑
uterine ligament (broad) (nontraumatic) N83.7
traumatic S37.892 ☑
vagina (ruptured) (nontraumatic) N89.8
complicating delivery O71.7
vas deferens (nontraumatic) N50.1
traumatic S37.892 ☑
vitreous — see Hemorrhage, vitreous
vulva (nontraumatic) (nonobstetric) N90.89
complicating delivery O71.7
newborn (birth injury) P15.5
Hematometra N85.7
with hematocolpos N89.7
Hematomyelia (central) G95.19
newborn (birth injury) P11.5
traumatic T14.8
Hematomyelitis G04.90
Hematoperitoneum — see Hemoperitoneum
Hematophobia F40.230
Hematopneumothorax (see Hemothorax)
Hematopoiesis, cyclic D70.4
Hematoporphyria — see Porphyria
Hematorachis, hematorrhachis G95.19
newborn (birth injury) P11.5
Hematosalpinx N83.6
with
hematocolpos N89.7
hematometra N85.7
with hematocolpos N89.7
infectional — see Salpingitis
Hematospermia R36.1
Hematothorax (see Hemothorax)
Hematuria R31.9
benign (familial) (of childhood) (see also Hematuria,
idiopathic)
essential microscopic R31.1
due to sulphonamide, sulfonamide — see Table of
Drugs and Chemicals, by drug
endemic (see also Schistosomiasis) B65.0
gross R31.0
idiopathic N02.9
with glomerular lesion
crescentic (diffuse) glomerulonephritis N02.7
dense deposit disease N02.6
endocapillary proliferative glomerulonephritis
N02.4

Hematuria — continued
idiopathic — continued
with glomerular lesion — continued
focal and segmental hyalinosis or sclerosis
N02.1
membranoproliferative (diffuse) N02.5
membranous (diffuse) N02.2
mesangial proliferative (diffuse) N02.3
mesangiocapillary (diffuse) N02.5
minor abnormality N02.0
proliferative NEC N02.8
specified pathology NEC N02.8
intermittent — see Hematuria, idiopathic
malarial B50.8
microscopic NEC R31.2
benign essential R31.1
paroxysmal (see also Hematuria, idiopathic)
nocturnal D59.5
persistent — see Hematuria, idiopathic
recurrent — see Hematuria, idiopathic
tropical (see also Schistosomiasis) B65.0
tuberculous A18.13
Hemeralopia (day blindness) H53.11
vitamin A deficiency E50.5
Hemi-akinesia R41.4
Hemianalgesia R20.0
Hemianencephaly Q00.0
Hemianesthesia R20.0
Hemianopia, hemianopsia (heteronymous) H53.47
homonymous H53.46- ☑
syphilitic A52.71
Hemiathetosis R25.8
Hemiatrophy R68.89
cerebellar G31.9
face, facial, progressive (Romberg) G51.8
tongue K14.8
Hemiballism (us) G25.5
Hemicardia Q24.8
Hemicephalus, hemicephaly Q00.0
Hemichorea G25.5
Hemicolitis, left — see Colitis, left sided
Hemicrania
congenital malformation Q00.0
continua G44.51
meaning migraine (see also Migraine) G43.909
paroxysmal G44.039
chronic G44.049
intractable G44.041
not intractable G44.049
episodic G44.039
intractable G44.031
not intractable G44.039
intractable G44.031
not intractable G44.039
Hemidystrophy — see Hemiatrophy
Hemiectromelia Q73.8
Hemihypalgesia R20.8
Hemihypesthesia R20.1
Hemi-inattention R41.4
Hemimelia Q73.8
lower limb — see Defect, reduction, lower limb, specified type NEC
upper limb — see Defect, reduction, upper limb,
specified type NEC
Hemiparalysis — see Hemiplegia
Hemiparesis — see Hemiplegia
Hemiparesthesia R20.2
Hemiparkinsonism G20
Hemiplegia G81.9- ☑
alternans facialis G83.89
ascending NEC G81.90
spinal G95.89
congenital (cerebral) G80.8
spastic G80.2
embolic (current episode) I63.4- ☑
flaccid G81.0- ☑
following
cerebrovascular disease I69.959
cerebral infarction I69.35- ☑
intracerebral hemorrhage I69.15- ☑
nontraumatic intracranial hemorrhage NEC
I69.25- ☑
specified disease NEC I69.85- ☑
stroke NOS I69.35- ☑
subarachnoid hemorrhage I69.05- ☑
hysterical F44.4

Hemiplegia — continued
  newborn NEC P91.8
    birth injury P11.9
  spastic G81.1- ☑
    congenital G80.2
  thrombotic (current episode) I63.3 ☑
Hemisection, spinal cord — see Injury, spinal cord, by
      region
Hemispasm (facial) R25.2
Hemisporosis B48.8
Hemitremor R25.1
Hemivertebra Q76.49
  failure of segmentation with scoliosis Q76.3
  fusion with scoliosis Q76.3
Hemochromatosis E83.119
  with refractory anemia D46.1
  due to repeated red blood cell transfusion E83.111
  hereditary (primary) E83.110
  primary E83.110
  specified NEC E83.118
Hemoglobin (see also condition)
  abnormal (disease) — see Disease, hemoglobin
  AS genotype D57.3
  Constant Spring D58.2
  E-beta thalassemia D56.5
  fetal, hereditary persistence (HPFH) D56.4
  H Constant Spring D56.0
  low NOS D64.9
  S (Hb S), heterozygous D57.3
Hemoglobinemia D59.9
  due to blood transfusion T80.89 ☑
  paroxysmal D59.6
    nocturnal D59.5
Hemoglobinopathy (mixed) D58.2
  with thalassemia D56.8
  sickle-cell D57.1
    with thalassemia D57.40
      with crisis (vasoocclusive pain) D57.419
        with
          acute chest syndrome D57.411
          splenic sequestration D57.412
      without crisis D57.40
Hemoglobinuria R82.3
  with anemia, hemolytic, acquired (chronic) NEC D59.6
  cold (agglutinin) (paroxysmal) (with Raynaud's syn-
      drome) D59.6
  due to exertion or hemolysis NEC D59.6
  intermittent D59.6
  malarial B50.8
  march D59.6
  nocturnal (paroxysmal) D59.5
  paroxysmal (cold) D59.6
    nocturnal D59.5
Hemolymphangioma D18.1
Hemolysis
  intravascular
    with
      abortion — see Abortion, by type, complicated
          by, hemorrhage
      ectopic or molar pregnancy O08.1
      hemorrhage
        antepartum — see Hemorrhage, antepar-
            tum, with coagulation defect
        intrapartum (see also Hemorrhage, compli-
            cating, delivery) O67.0
      postpartum O72.3
  neonatal (excessive) P58.9
    specified NEC P58.8
Hemolytic — see condition
Hemopericardium I31.2
  following acute myocardial infarction (current compli-
      cation) I23.0
  newborn P54.8
  traumatic — see Injury, heart, with hemopericardium
Hemoperitoneum K66.1
  infectional K65.9
  traumatic S36.899 ☑
    with open wound — see Wound, open, with pene-
        tration into peritoneal cavity
Hemophilia (classical) (familial) (hereditary) D66
  A D66
  acquired D68.311
  autoimmune D68.311
  B D67
  C D68.1
  calcipriva (see also Defect, coagulation) D68.4
  nonfamilial (see also Defect, coagulation) D68.4
  secondary D68.311

Hemophilia — continued
  vascular D68.0
Hemophthalmos H44.81- ☑
Hemopneumothorax (see also Hemothorax)
  traumatic S27.2 ☑
Hemoptysis R04.2
  newborn P26.9
  tuberculous — see Tuberculosis, pulmonary
Hemorrhage, hemorrhagic (concealed) R58
  abdomen R58
  accidental antepartum — see Hemorrhage, antepar-
      tum
  acute idiopathic pulmonary, in infants R04.81
  adenoid J35.8
  adrenal (capsule) (gland) E27.49
    medulla E27.8
    newborn P54.4
  after delivery — see Hemorrhage, postpartum
  alveolar
    lung, newborn P26.8
    process K08.8
  alveolus K08.8
  amputation stump (surgical) T87.89
  anemia (chronic) D50.0
    acute D62
  antepartum (with) O46.90
    with coagulation defect O46.00- ☑
      afibrinogenemia O46.01- ☑
      disseminated intravascular coagulation
          O46.02- ☑
      hypofibrinogenemia O46.01- ☑
      specified defect NEC O46.09- ☑
    before 20 weeks gestation O20.9
      specified type NEC O20.8
      threatened abortion O20.0
    due to
      abruptio placenta (see also Abruptio placentae)
          O45.9- ☑
      leiomyoma, uterus — see Hemorrhage, antepar-
          tum, specified cause NEC
      placenta previa O44.1- ☑
    specified cause NEC — see subcategory O46.8X- ☑
  anus (sphincter) K62.5
  apoplexy (stroke) — see Hemorrhage, intracranial, in-
      tracerebral
  arachnoid — see Hemorrhage, intracranial, subarach-
      noid
  artery R58
    brain — see Hemorrhage, intracranial, intracerebral
  basilar (ganglion) I61.0
  bladder N32.89
  bowel K92.2
    newborn P54.3
  brain (miliary) (nontraumatic) — see Hemorrhage, in-
      tracranial, intracerebral
    due to
      birth injury P10.1
      syphilis A52.05
    epidural or extradural (traumatic) — see Injury,
        intracranial, epidural hemorrhage
    newborn P52.4
      birth injury P10.1
    subarachnoid — see Hemorrhage, intracranial,
        subarachnoid
    subdural — see Hemorrhage, intracranial, subdural
  brainstem (nontraumatic) I61.3
    traumatic S06.38- ☑
  breast N64.59
  bronchial tube — see Hemorrhage, lung
  bronchopulmonary — see Hemorrhage, lung
  bronchus — see Hemorrhage, lung
  bulbar I61.5
  capillary I78.85
    primary D69.8
  cecum K92.2
  cerebellar, cerebellum (nontraumatic) I61.4
    newborn P52.6
    traumatic S06.37- ☑
  cerebral, cerebrum (see also Hemorrhage, intracranial,
      intracerebral)
    lobe I61.1
    newborn (anoxic) P52.4
      birth injury P10.1
  cerebromeningeal I61.8
  cerebrospinal — see Hemorrhage, intracranial, intrac-
      erebral
  cervix (uteri) (stump) NEC N88.8

Hemorrhage, hemorrhagic — continued
  chamber, anterior (eye) — see Hyphema
  childbirth — see Hemorrhage, complicating, delivery
  choroid H31.30- ☑
    expulsive H31.31- ☑
  ciliary body — see Hyphema
  cochlea — see subcategory H83.8 ☑
  colon K92.2
  complicating
    abortion — see Abortion, by type, complicated by,
        hemorrhage
    delivery O67.9
      associated with coagulation defect (afibrinogen-
          emia) (DIC) (hyperfibrinolysis) O67.0
      specified cause NEC O67.8
      surgical procedure — see Hemorrhage, intraoper-
          ative
  conjunctiva H11.3- ☑
    newborn P54.8
  cord, newborn (stump) P51.9
  corpus luteum (ruptured) cyst N83.1
  cortical (brain) I61.1
  cranial — see Hemorrhage, intracranial
  cutaneous R23.3
    due to autosensitivity, erythrocyte D69.2
    newborn P54.5
  delayed
    following ectopic or molar pregnancy O08.1
    postpartum O72.2
  diathesis (familial) D69.9
  disease D69.9
    newborn P53
    specified type NEC D69.8
  due to or associated with
    afibrinogenemia or other coagulation defect
        (conditions in categories D65- D69)
      antepartum — see Hemorrhage, antepartum,
          with coagulation defect
      intrapartum O67.0
    dental implant M27.61
    device, implant or graft (see also Complications,
        by site and type, specified NEC) T85.83 ☑
      arterial graft NEC T82.838 ☑
      breast T85.83 ☑
      catheter NEC T85.83 ☑
        dialysis (renal) T82.838 ☑
          intraperitoneal T85.83 ☑
        infusion NEC T82.838 ☑
          spinal (epidural) (subdural) T85.83 ☑
        urinary (indwelling) T83.83 ☑
      electronic (electrode) (pulse generator) (stimu-
          lator)
        bone T84.83 ☑
        cardiac T82.837 ☑
        nervous system (brain) (peripheral nerve)
            (spinal) T85.83 ☑
        urinary T83.83 ☑
      fixation, internal (orthopedic) NEC T84.83 ☑
      gastrointestinal (bile duct) (esophagus)
          T85.83 ☑
      genital NEC T83.83 ☑
      heart NEC T82.837 ☑
      joint prosthesis T84.83 ☑
      ocular (corneal graft) (orbital implant) NEC
          T85.83 ☑
      orthopedic NEC T84.83 ☑
        bone graft T86.838
      specified NEC T85.83 ☑
      urinary NEC T83.83 ☑
      vascular NEC T82.838 ☑
      ventricular intracranial shunt T85.83 ☑
  duodenum, duodenal K92.2
    ulcer — see Ulcer, duodenum, with hemorrhage
  dura mater — see Hemorrhage, intracranial, subdural
  endotracheal — see Hemorrhage, lung
  epicranial subaponeurotic (massive), birth injury P12.2
  epidural (traumatic) (see also Injury, intracranial,
      epidural hemorrhage)
    nontraumatic I62.1
  esophagus K22.8
    varix I85.01
      secondary I85.11
  excessive, following ectopic gestation (subsequent
      episode) O08.1
  extradural (traumatic) — see Injury, intracranial,
      epidural hemorrhage
    birth injury P10.8

Hemorrhage, hemorrhagic — *continued*
  extradural — *see* Injury, intracranial, epidural hemor-
    rhage — *continued*
      newborn (anoxic) (nontraumatic) P52.8
      nontraumatic I62.1
  eye NEC H57.8
    fundus — *see* Hemorrhage, retina
    lid — *see* Disorder, eyelid, specified type NEC
  fallopian tube N83.6
  fibrinogenolysis — *see* Fibrinolysis
  fibrinolytic (acquired) — *see* Fibrinolysis
  from
    ear (nontraumatic) — *see* Otorrhagia
    tracheostomy stoma J95.01
  fundus, eye — *see* Hemorrhage, retina
  funis — *see* Hemorrhage, umbilicus, cord
  gastric — *see* Hemorrhage, stomach
  gastroenteric K92.2
    newborn P54.3
  gastrointestinal (tract) K92.2
    newborn P54.3
  genital organ, male N50.1
  genitourinary (tract) NOS R31.9
  gingiva K06.8
  globe (eye) — *see* Hemophthalmos
  graafian follicle cyst (ruptured) N83.0
  gum K06.8
  heart I51.89
  hypopharyngeal (throat) R04.1
  intermenstrual (regular) N92.3
    irregular N92.1
  internal (organs) NEC R58
    capsule I61.0
    ear — *see* subcategory H83.8 ☑
    newborn P54.8
  intestine K92.2
    newborn P54.3
  intra-abdominal R58
  intra-alveolar (lung), newborn P26.8
  intracerebral (nontraumatic) — *see* Hemorrhage, in-
    tracranial, intracerebral
  intracranial (nontraumatic) I62.9
    birth injury P10.9
    epidural, nontraumatic I62.1
    extradural, nontraumatic I62.1
    intracerebral (nontraumatic) (in) I61.9
      brain stem I61.3
      cerebellum I61.4
      hemisphere I61.2
        cortical (superficial) I61.1
        subcortical (deep) I61.0
      intraoperative
        during a nervous system procedure G97.31
        during other procedure G97.32
      intraventricular I61.5
      multiple localized I61.6
      newborn P52.4
        birth injury P10.1
      postprocedural
        following a nervous system procedure
          G97.51
        following other procedure G97.52
      specified NEC I61.8
      superficial I61.1
      traumatic (diffuse) — *see* Injury, intracranial,
        diffuse
        focal — *see* Injury, intracranial, focal
    newborn P52.9
      specified NEC P52.8
    subarachnoid (nontraumatic) (from) I60.9
      intracranial (cerebral) artery I60.7
        anterior communicating I60.2- ☑
        basilar I60.4
        carotid siphon and bifurcation I60.0- ☑
        communicating I60.7
          anterior I60.2- ☑
          posterior I60.3- ☑
        middle cerebral I60.1- ☑
        posterior communicating I60.3- ☑
        specified artery NEC I60.6
        vertebral I60.5- ☑
      newborn P52.5
        birth injury P10.3
      specified NEC I60.8
      traumatic S06.6X- ☑
    subdural (nontraumatic) I62.00
      acute I62.01
      birth injury P10.0

Hemorrhage, hemorrhagic — *continued*
  intracranial — *continued*
    subdural — *continued*
      chronic I62.03
      newborn (anoxic) (hypoxic) P52.8
        birth injury P10.0
      spinal G95.19
      subacute I62.02
      traumatic — *see* Injury, intracranial, subdural
        hemorrhage
    traumatic — *see* Injury, intracranial, focal brain in-
      jury
  intramedullary NEC G95.19
  intraocular — *see* Hemophthalmos
  intraoperative, intraprocedural — *see* Complication,
    hemorrhage (hematoma), intraoperative (in-
    traprocedural), by site
  intrapartum — *see* Hemorrhage, complicating, deliv-
    ery
  intrapelvic
    female N94.89
    male K66.1
  intraperitoneal K66.1
  intrapontine I61.3
  intraprocedural — *see* Complication, hemorrhage
    (hematoma), intraoperative (intraprocedural),
    by site
  intrauterine N85.7
    complicating delivery (*see also* Hemorrhage, com-
      plicating, delivery) O67.9
    postpartum — *see* Hemorrhage, postpartum
  intraventricular I61.5
    newborn (nontraumatic) (*see also* Newborn, affect-
      ed by, hemorrhage) P52.3
      due to birth injury P10.2
      grade
        1 P52.0
        2 P52.1
        3 P52.21
        4 P52.22
  intravesical N32.89
  iris (postinfectional) (postinflammatory) (toxic) — *see*
    Hyphema
  joint (nontraumatic) — *see* Hemarthrosis
  kidney N28.89
  knee (joint) (nontraumatic) — *see* Hemarthrosis, knee
  labyrinth — *see* subcategory H83.8 ☑
  lenticular striate artery I61.0
  ligature, vessel — *see* Hemorrhage, postoperative
  liver K76.89
  lung R04.89
    newborn P26.9
      massive P26.1
      specified NEC P26.8
    tuberculous — *see* Tuberculosis, pulmonary
  massive umbilical, newborn P51.0
  mediastinum — *see* Hemorrhage, lung
  medulla I61.3
  membrane (brain) I60.8
    spinal cord — *see* Hemorrhage, spinal cord
  meninges, meningeal (brain) (middle) I60.8
    spinal cord — *see* Hemorrhage, spinal cord
  mesentery K66.1
  metritis — *see* Endometritis
  mouth K13.79
  mucous membrane NEC R58
    newborn P54.8
  muscle M62.89
  nail (subungual) L60.8
  nasal turbinate R04.0
    newborn P54.8
  navel, newborn P51.9
  newborn P54.9
    specified NEC P54.8
  nipple N64.59
  nose R04.0
    newborn P54.8
  omentum K66.1
  optic nerve (sheath) H47.02- ☑
  orbit, orbital H05.23- ☑
  ovary NEC N83.8
  oviduct N83.6
  pancreas K86.8
  parathyroid (gland) (spontaneous) E21.4
  parturition — *see* Hemorrhage, complicating, delivery
  penis N48.89
  pericardium, pericarditis I31.2
  peritoneum, peritoneal K66.1

Hemorrhage, hemorrhagic — *continued*
  peritonsillar tissue J35.8
    due to infection J36
  petechial R23.3
    due to autosensitivity, erythrocyte D69.2
  pituitary (gland) E23.6
  pleura — *see* Hemorrhage, lung
  polioencephalitis, superior E51.2
  polymyositis — *see* Polymyositis
  pons, pontine I61.3
  posterior fossa (nontraumatic) I61.8
    newborn P52.6
  postmenopausal N95.0
  postnasal R04.0
  postoperative — *see* Complications, postprocedural,
    hemorrhage, by site
  postpartum NEC (following delivery of placenta) O72.1
    delayed or secondary O72.2
    retained placenta O72.0
    third stage O72.0
  pregnancy — *see* Hemorrhage, antepartum
  preretinal — *see* Hemorrhage, retina
  prostate N42.1
  puerperal — *see* Hemorrhage, postpartum
    delayed or secondary O72.2
  pulmonary R04.89
    newborn P26.9
      massive P26.1
      specified NEC P26.8
    tuberculous — *see* Tuberculosis, pulmonary
  purpura (primary) D69.3
  rectum (sphincter) K62.5
    newborn P54.2
  recurring, following initial hemorrhage at time of injury
    T79.2 ☑
  renal N28.89
  respiratory passage or tract R04.9
    specified NEC R04.89
  retina, retinal (vessels) H35.6- ☑
    diabetic — *see* Diabetes, retinal, hemorrhage
  retroperitoneal R58
  scalp R58
  scrotum N50.1
  secondary (nontraumatic) R58
    following initial hemorrhage at time of injury
      T79.2 ☑
  seminal vesicle N50.1
  skin R23.3
    newborn P54.5
  slipped umbilical ligature P51.8
  spermatic cord N50.1
  spinal (cord) G95.19
    newborn (birth injury) P11.5
  spleen D73.5
    intraoperative — *see* Complications, intraoperative,
      hemorrhage, spleen
    postprocedural — *see* Complications, postproce-
      dural, hemorrhage, spleen
  stomach K92.2
    newborn P54.3
    ulcer — *see* Ulcer, stomach, with hemorrhage
  subarachnoid (nontraumatic) — *see* Hemorrhage, in-
    tracranial, subarachnoid
  subconjunctival (*see also* Hemorrhage, conjunctiva)
    birth injury P15.3
  subcortical (brain) I61.0
  subcutaneous R23.3
  subdiaphragmatic R58
  subdural (acute) (nontraumatic) — *see* Hemorrhage,
    intracranial, subdural
  subependymal
    newborn P52.0
      with intraventricular extension P52.1
        and intracerebral extension P52.22
  subgaleal P12.1
  subhyaloid — *see* Hemorrhage, retina
  subperiosteal — *see* Disorder, bone, specified type
    NEC
  subretinal — *see* Hemorrhage, retina
  subtentorial — *see* Hemorrhage, intracranial, subdural
  subungual L60.8
  suprarenal (capsule) (gland) E27.49
    newborn P54.4
  tentorium (traumatic) NEC — *see* Hemorrhage, brain
    newborn (birth injury) P10.4
  testis N50.1
  third stage (postpartum) O72.0
  thorax — *see* Hemorrhage, lung

☑ **Additional Character Required — Refer to the Tabular List for Character Selection**   ▽ Subterms under main terms may continue to next column or page

Hemorrhage, hemorrhagic — *continued*
　throat R04.1
　thymus (gland) E32.8
　thyroid (cyst) (gland) E07.89
　tongue K14.8
　tonsil J35.8
　trachea — *see* Hemorrhage, lung
　tracheobronchial R04.89
　　newborn P26.0
　traumatic — *code to* specific injury
　　cerebellar — *see* Hemorrhage, brain
　　intracranial — *see* Hemorrhage, brain
　　recurring or secondary (following initial hemor-
　　　rhage at time of injury) T79.2 ☑
　tuberculous NEC (*see also* Tuberculosis, pulmonary)
　　A15.0
　tunica vaginalis N50.1
　ulcer — *code by* site under Ulcer, with hemorrhage
　　K27.4
　umbilicus, umbilical
　　cord
　　　after birth, newborn P51.9
　　　complicating delivery O69.5 ☑
　　newborn P51.9
　　　massive P51.0
　　　slipped ligature P51.8
　　　stump P51.9
　urethra (idiopathic) N36.8
　uterus, uterine (abnormal) N93.9
　　climacteric N92.4
　　complicating delivery — *see* Hemorrhage, compli-
　　　cating, delivery
　　dysfunctional or functional N93.8
　　intermenstrual (regular) N92.3
　　　irregular N92.1
　　postmenopausal N95.0
　　postpartum — *see* Hemorrhage, postpartum
　　preclimacteric or premenopausal N92.4
　　prepubertal N93.8
　　pubertal N92.2
　vagina (abnormal) N93.9
　　newborn P54.6
　vas deferens N50.1
　vasa previa O69.4 ☑
　ventricular I61.5
　vesical N32.89
　viscera NEC R58
　　newborn P54.8
　vitreous (humor) (intraocular) H43.1- ☑
　vulva N90.89
Hemorrhoids (bleeding) (without mention of degree)
　K64.9
　1st degree (grade/stage I) (without prolapse outside
　　of anal canal) K64.0
　2nd degree (grade/stage II) (that prolapse with
　　straining but retract spontaneously) K64.1
　3rd degree (grade/stage III) (that prolapse with
　　straining and require manual replacement back
　　inside anal canal) K64.2
　4th degree (grade/stage IV) (with prolapsed tissue that
　　cannot be manually replaced) K64.3
　complicating
　　pregnancy O22.4 ☑
　　puerperium O87.2
　external K64.4
　　with
　　　thrombosis K64.5
　internal (without mention of degree) K64.8
　prolapsed K64.8
　skin tags
　　anus K64.4
　　residual K64.4
　specified NEC K64.8
　strangulated (*see also* Hemorrhoids, by degree) K64.8
　thrombosed (*see also* Hemorrhoids, by degree) K64.5
　ulcerated (*see also* Hemorrhoids, by degree) K64.8
Hemosalpinx N83.6
　with
　　hematocolpos N89.7
　　hematometra N85.7
　　　with hematocolpos N89.7
Hemosiderosis (dietary) E83.19
　pulmonary, idiopathic E83.1- ☑ [J84.03]
　transfusion T80.89 ☑
Hemothorax (bacterial) (nontuberculous) J94.2
　newborn P54.8
　traumatic S27.1 ☑
　　with pneumothorax S27.2 ☑

Hemothorax — *continued*
　tuberculous NEC A15.6
Henoch (-Schönlein) **disease or syndrome** (purpura)
　D69.0
Henpue, henpuye A66.6
Hepar lobatum (syphilitic) A52.74
Hepatalgia K76.89
Hepatitis K75.9
　acute B17.9
　　with coma K72.01
　　with hepatic failure — *see* Failure, hepatic
　　alcoholic — *see* Hepatitis, alcoholic
　　infectious B15.9
　　　with hepatic coma B15.0
　　viral B17.9
　alcoholic (acute) (chronic) K70.10
　　with ascites K70.11
　amebic — *see* Abscess, liver, amebic
　anicteric, (viral) — *see* Hepatitis, viral
　antigen-associated (HAA) — *see* Hepatitis, B
　Australia-antigen (positive) — *see* Hepatitis, B
　autoimmune K75.4
　B B19.10
　　with hepatic coma B19.11
　　acute B16.9
　　　with
　　　　delta-agent (coinfection) (without hepatic
　　　　　coma) B16.1
　　　　　with hepatic coma B16.0
　　　　hepatic coma (without delta-agent coinfec-
　　　　　tion) B16.2
　　chronic B18.1
　　　with delta-agent B18.0
　bacterial NEC K75.89
　C (viral) B19.20
　　with hepatic coma B19.21
　　acute B17.10
　　　with hepatic coma B17.11
　　chronic B18.2
　catarrhal (acute) B15.9
　　with hepatic coma B15.0
　cholangiolitic K75.89
　cholestatic K75.89
　chronic K73.9
　　active NEC K73.2
　　lobular NEC K73.1
　　persistent NEC K73.0
　　specified NEC K73.8
　cytomegaloviral B25.1
　due to ethanol (acute) (chronic) — *see* Hepatitis, alco-
　　holic
　epidemic B15.9
　　with hepatic coma B15.0
　fulminant NEC (viral) — *see* Hepatitis, viral
　granulomatous NEC K75.3
　herpesviral B00.81
　history of
　　B Z86.19
　　C Z86.19
　homologous serum — *see* Hepatitis, viral, type B
　in (due to)
　　mumps B26.81
　　toxoplasmosis (acquired) B58.1
　　　congenital (active) P37.1 [K77]
　infectious, infective (acute) (chronic) (subacute) B15.9
　　with hepatic coma B15.0
　inoculation — *see* Hepatitis, viral, type B
　interstitial (chronic) K74.69
　lupoid NEC K75.4
　malignant NEC (with hepatic failure) K72.90
　　with coma K72.91
　neonatal (idiopathic) (toxic) P59.29
　neonatal giant cell P59.29
　newborn P59.29
　postimmunization — *see* Hepatitis, viral, type B
　post-transfusion — *see* Hepatitis, viral, type B
　reactive, nonspecific K75.2
　serum — *see* Hepatitis, viral, type B
　specified type NEC
　　with hepatic failure — *see* Failure, hepatic
　syphilitic (late) A52.74
　　congenital (early) A50.08 [K77]
　　　late A50.59 [K77]
　　secondary A51.45
　toxic (*see also* Disease, liver, toxic) K71.6
　tuberculous A18.83
　viral, virus B19.9
　　with hepatic coma B19.0

Hepatitis — *continued*
　viral, virus — *continued*
　　acute B17.9
　　chronic B18.9
　　　specified NEC B18.8
　　　type
　　　　B B18.1
　　　　　with delta-agent B18.0
　　　　C B18.2
　　congenital P35.3
　　coxsackie B33.8 [K77]
　　cytomegalic inclusion B25.1
　　in remission, any type — *code to* Hepatitis, chronic,
　　　by type
　　non-A, non-B B17.8
　　specified type NEC (with or without coma) B17.8
　　type
　　　A B15.9
　　　　with hepatic coma B15.0
　　　B B19.10
　　　　with hepatic coma B19.11
　　　　acute B16.9
　　　　　with
　　　　　　delta-agent (coinfection) (without
　　　　　　　hepatic coma) B16.1
　　　　　　　with hepatic coma B16.0
　　　　　　hepatic coma (without delta-agent
　　　　　　　coinfection) B16.2
　　　　chronic B18.1
　　　　　with delta-agent B18.0
　　　C B19.20
　　　　with hepatic coma B19.21
　　　　acute B17.10
　　　　　with hepatic coma B17.11
　　　　chronic B18.2
　　　E B17.2
　　non-A, non-B B17.8
Hepatization lung (acute) — *see* Pneumonia, lobar
Hepatoblastoma C22.2
Hepatocarcinoma C22.0
Hepatocholangiocarcinoma C22.0
Hepatocholangioma, benign D13.4
Hepatocholangitis K75.89
Hepatolenticular degeneration E83.01
Hepatoma (malignant) C22.0
　benign D13.4
　embryonal C22.0
Hepatomegaly (*see also* Hypertrophy, liver)
　with splenomegaly R16.2
　congenital Q44.7
　in mononucleosis
　　gammaherpesviral B27.09
　　infectious specified NEC B27.89
Hepatoptosis K76.89
Hepatorenal syndrome following labor and delivery
　O90.4
Hepatosis K76.89
Hepatosplenomegaly R16.2
　hyperlipemic (Bürger-Grütz type) E78.3 [K77]
Hereditary — *see* condition
Heredodegeneration, macular — *see* Dystrophy, retina
Heredopathia atactica polyneuritiformis G60.1
Heredosyphilis — *see* Syphilis, congenital
Herlitz' syndrome Q81.1
Hermansky-Pudlak syndrome E70.331
Hermaphrodite, hermaphroditism (true) Q56.0
　46,XX with streak gonads Q99.1
　46,XX/46,XY Q99.0
　46,XY with streak gonads Q99.1
　chimera 46,XX/46,XY Q99.0
Hernia, hernial (acquired) (recurrent) K46.9
　with
　　gangrene — *see* Hernia, by site, with, gangrene
　　incarceration — *see* Hernia, by site, with, obstruc-
　　　tion
　　irreducible — *see* Hernia, by site, with, obstruction
　　obstruction — *see* Hernia, by site, with, obstruction
　　strangulation — *see* Hernia, by site, with, obstruc-
　　　tion
　abdomen, abdominal K46.9
　　with
　　　gangrene (and obstruction) K46.1
　　　obstruction K46.0
　femoral — *see* Hernia, femoral
　incisional — *see* Hernia, incisional
　inguinal — *see* Hernia, inguinal
　specified site NEC K45.8

Hernia, hernial — *continued*
  abdomen, abdominal — *continued*
    specified site — *continued*
      with
        gangrene (and obstruction) K45.1
        obstruction K45.0
    umbilical — *see* Hernia, umbilical
    wall — *see* Hernia, ventral
  appendix — *see* Hernia, abdomen
  bladder (mucosa) (sphincter)
    congenital (female) (male) Q79.51
    female — *see* Cystocele
    male N32.89
  brain, congenital — *see* Encephalocele
  cartilage, vertebra — *see* Displacement, intervertebral disc
  cerebral, congenital (*see also* Encephalocele)
    endaural Q01.8
  ciliary body (traumatic) S05.2- ☑
  colon — *see* Hernia, abdomen
  Cooper's — *see* Hernia, abdomen, specified site NEC
  crural — *see* Hernia, femoral
  diaphragm, diaphragmatic K44.9
    with
      gangrene (and obstruction) K44.1
      obstruction K44.0
    congenital Q79.0
  direct (inguinal) — *see* Hernia, inguinal
  diverticulum, intestine — *see* Hernia, abdomen
  double (inguinal) — *see* Hernia, inguinal, bilateral
  due to adhesions (with obstruction) K56.5
  epigastric (*see also* Hernia, ventral) K43.9
  esophageal hiatus — *see* Hernia, hiatal
  external (inguinal) — *see* Hernia, inguinal
  fallopian tube N83.4
  fascia M62.89
  femoral K41.90
    with
      gangrene (and obstruction) K41.40
        not specified as recurrent K41.40
        recurrent K41.41
      obstruction K41.30
        not specified as recurrent K41.30
        recurrent K41.31
    bilateral K41.20
      with
        gangrene (and obstruction) K41.10
          not specified as recurrent K41.10
          recurrent K41.11
        obstruction K41.00
          not specified as recurrent K41.00
          recurrent K41.01
      not specified as recurrent K41.20
      recurrent K41.21
    not specified as recurrent K41.90
    recurrent K41.91
    unilateral K41.90
      with
        gangrene (and obstruction) K41.40
          not specified as recurrent K41.40
          recurrent K41.41
        obstruction K41.30
          not specified as recurrent K41.30
          recurrent K41.31
      not specified as recurrent K41.90
      recurrent K41.91
  foramen magnum G93.5
    congenital Q01.8
  funicular (umbilical) (*see also* Hernia, umbilicus)
    spermatic (cord) — *see* Hernia, inguinal
  gastrointestinal tract — *see* Hernia, abdomen
  Hesselbach's — *see* Hernia, femoral, specified site NEC
  hiatal (esophageal) (sliding) K44.9
    with
      gangrene (and obstruction) K44.1
      obstruction K44.0
    congenital Q40.1
  hypogastric — *see* Hernia, ventral
  incarcerated (*see also* Hernia, by site, with obstruction)
    with gangrene — *see* Hernia, by site, with gangrene
  incisional K43.2
    with
      gangrene (and obstruction) K43.1
      obstruction K43.0
  indirect (inguinal) — *see* Hernia, inguinal
  inguinal (direct) (external) (funicular) (indirect) (internal) (oblique) (scrotal) (sliding) K40.90

Hernia, hernial — *continued*
  inguinal — *continued*
    with
      gangrene (and obstruction) K40.40
        not specified as recurrent K40.40
        recurrent K40.41
      obstruction K40.30
        not specified as recurrent K40.30
        recurrent K40.31
    bilateral K40.20
      with
        gangrene (and obstruction) K40.10
          not specified as recurrent K40.10
          recurrent K40.11
        obstruction K40.00
          not specified as recurrent K40.00
          recurrent K40.01
      not specified as recurrent K40.20
      recurrent K40.21
    not specified as recurrent K40.90
    recurrent K40.91
    unilateral K40.90
      with
        gangrene (and obstruction) K40.40
          not specified as recurrent K40.40
          recurrent K40.41
        obstruction K40.30
          not specified as recurrent K40.30
          recurrent K40.31
      not specified as recurrent K40.90
      recurrent K40.91
  internal (*see also* Hernia, abdomen)
    inguinal — *see* Hernia, inguinal
  interstitial — *see* Hernia, abdomen
  intervertebral cartilage or disc — *see* Displacement, intervertebral disc
  intestine, intestinal — *see* Hernia, by site
  intra-abdominal — *see* Hernia, abdomen
  iris (traumatic) S05.2- ☑
  irreducible (*see also* Hernia, by site, with obstruction)
    with gangrene — *see* Hernia, by site, with gangrene
  ischiatic — *see* Hernia, abdomen, specified site NEC
  ischiorectal — *see* Hernia, abdomen, specified site NEC
  lens (traumatic) S05.2- ☑
  linea (alba) (semilunaris) — *see* Hernia, ventral
  Littre's — *see* Hernia, abdomen
  lumbar — *see* Hernia, abdomen, specified site NEC
  lung (subcutaneous) J98.4
  mediastinum J98.5
  mesenteric (internal) — *see* Hernia, abdomen
  midline — *see* Hernia, ventral
  muscle (sheath) M62.89
  nucleus pulposus — *see* Displacement, intervertebral disc
  oblique (inguinal) — *see* Hernia, inguinal
  obstructive (*see also* Hernia, by site, with obstruction)
    with gangrene — *see* Hernia, by site, with gangrene
  obturator — *see* Hernia, abdomen, specified site NEC
  omental — *see* Hernia, abdomen
  ovary N83.4
  oviduct N83.4
  paraesophageal (*see also* Hernia, diaphragm)
    congenital Q40.1
  parastomal K43.5
    with
      gangrene (and obstruction) K43.4
      obstruction K43.3
  paraumbilical — *see* Hernia, umbilicus
  perineal — *see* Hernia, abdomen, specified site NEC
  Petit's — *see* Hernia, abdomen, specified site NEC
  postoperative — *see* Hernia, incisional
  pregnant uterus — *see* Abnormal, uterus in pregnancy or childbirth
  prevesical N32.89
  properitoneal — *see* Hernia, abdomen, specified site NEC
  pudendal — *see* Hernia, abdomen, specified site NEC
  rectovaginal N81.6
  retroperitoneal — *see* Hernia, abdomen, specified site NEC
  Richter's — *see* Hernia, abdomen, with obstruction
  Rieux's, Riex's — *see* Hernia, abdomen, specified site NEC

Hernia, hernial — *continued*
  sac condition (adhesion) (dropsy) (inflammation) (laceration) (suppuration) — *code by site under* Hernia
  sciatic — *see* Hernia, abdomen, specified site NEC
  scrotum, scrotal — *see* Hernia, inguinal
  sliding (inguinal) (*see also* Hernia, inguinal)
    hiatus — *see* Hernia, hiatal
  spigelian — *see* Hernia, ventral
  spinal — *see* Spina bifida
  strangulated (*see also* Hernia, by site, with obstruction)
    with gangrene — *see* Hernia, by site, with gangrene
  subxiphoid — *see* Hernia, ventral
  supra-umbilicus — *see* Hernia, ventral
  tendon — *see* Disorder, tendon, specified type NEC
  Treitz's (fossa) — *see* Hernia, abdomen, specified site NEC
  tunica vaginalis Q55.29
  umbilicus, umbilical K42.9
    with
      gangrene (and obstruction) K42.1
      obstruction K42.0
  ureter N28.89
  urethra, congenital Q64.79
  urinary meatus, congenital Q64.79
  uterus N81.4
    pregnant — *see* Abnormal, uterus in pregnancy or childbirth
  vaginal (anterior) (wall) — *see* Cystocele
  Velpeau's — *see* Hernia, femoral
  ventral K43.9
    with
      gangrene (and obstruction) K43.7
      obstruction K43.6
    incisional K43.2
      with
        gangrene (and obstruction) K43.1
        obstruction K43.0
    recurrent — *see* Hernia, incisional
    specified NEC K43.9
      with
        gangrene (and obstruction) K43.7
        obstruction K43.6
  vesical
    congenital (female) (male) Q79.51
    female — *see* Cystocele
    male N32.89
  vitreous (into wound) S05.2- ☑
    into anterior chamber — *see* Prolapse, vitreous
Herniation (*see also* Hernia)
  brain (stem) G93.5
  cerebral G93.5
  mediastinum J98.5
  nucleus pulposus — *see* Displacement, intervertebral disc
Herpangina B08.5
Herpes, herpesvirus, herpetic B00.9
  anogenital A60.9
    perianal skin A60.1
    rectum A60.1
    urogenital tract A60.00
      cervix A60.03
      male genital organ NEC A60.02
      penis A60.01
      specified site NEC A60.09
      vagina A60.04
      vulva A60.04
  blepharitis (zoster) B02.39
    simplex B00.59
  circinatus B35.4
    bullosus L12.0
  conjunctivitis (simplex) B00.53
    zoster B02.31
  cornea B02.33
  encephalitis B00.4
    due to herpesvirus 6 B10.01
    due to herpesvirus 7 B10.09
    specified NEC B10.09
  eye (zoster) B02.30
    simplex B00.50
  eyelid (zoster) B02.39
    simplex B00.59
  facialis B00.1
  febrilis B00.1
  geniculate ganglionitis B02.21
  genital, genitalis A60.00
    female A60.09

☑ **Additional Character Required** — Refer to the Tabular List for Character Selection   ▽ **Subterms under main terms may continue to next column or page**

Herpes, herpesvirus, herpetic — *continued*
  genital, genitalis — *continued*
    male A60.02
  gestational, gestationis O26.4- ☑
  gingivostomatitis B00.2
  human B00.9
    1 — *see* Herpes, simplex
    2 — *see* Herpes, simplex
    3 — *see* Varicella
    4 — *see* Mononucleosis, Epstein-Barr (virus)
    5 — *see* Disease, cytomegalic inclusion (generalized)
    6
      encephalitis B10.01
      specified NEC B10.81
    7
      encephalitis B10.09
      specified NEC B10.82
    8 B10.89
  infection NEC B10.89
    Kaposi's sarcoma associated B10.89
  iridocyclitis (simplex) B00.51
    zoster B02.32
  iris (vesicular erythema multiforme) L51.9
  iritis (simplex) B00.51
  Kaposi's sarcoma associated B10.89
  keratitis (simplex) (dendritic) (disciform) (interstitial) B00.52
    zoster (interstitial) B02.33
  keratoconjunctivitis (simplex) B00.52
    zoster B02.33
  labialis B00.1
  lip B00.1
  meningitis (simplex) B00.3
    zoster B02.1
  ophthalmicus (zoster) NEC B02.30
    simplex B00.50
  penis A60.01
  perianal skin A60.1
  pharyngitis, pharyngotonsillitis B00.2
  rectum A60.1
  scrotum A60.02
  sepsis B00.7
  simplex B00.9
    complicated NEC B00.89
    congenital P35.2
    conjunctivitis B00.53
    external ear B00.1
    eyelid B00.59
    hepatitis B00.81
    keratitis (interstitial) B00.52
    myleitis B00.82
    specified complication NEC B00.89
    visceral B00.89
  stomatitis B00.2
  tonsurans B35.0
  visceral B00.89
  vulva A60.04
  whitlow B00.89
  zoster (see also condition) B02.9
    auricularis B02.21
    complicated NEC B02.8
    conjunctivitis B02.31
    disseminated B02.7
    encephalitis B02.0
    eye (lid) B02.39
    geniculate ganglionitis B02.21
    keratitis (interstitial) B02.33
    meningitis B02.1
    myelitis B02.24
    neuritis, neuralgia B02.29
    ophthalmicus NEC B02.30
    oticus B02.21
    polyneuropathy B02.23
    specified complication NEC B02.8
    trigeminal neuralgia B02.22
Herpesvirus (human) — *see* Herpes
Herpetophobia F40.218
Herrick's anemia — *see* Disease, sickle-cell
Hers' disease E74.09
Herter-Gee syndrome K90.0
Herxheimer's reaction R68.89
Hesitancy
  of micturition R39.11
  urinary R39.11
Hesselbach's hernia — *see* Hernia, femoral, specified site NEC

Heterochromia (congenital) Q13.2
  cataract — *see* Cataract, complicated
  cyclitis (Fuchs) — *see* Cyclitis, Fuchs' heterochromic
  hair L67.1
  iritis — *see* Cyclitis, Fuchs' heterochromic
  retained metallic foreign body (nonmagnetic) — *see* Foreign body, intraocular, old, retained
    magnetic — *see* Foreign body, intraocular, old, retained, magnetic
  uveitis — *see* Cyclitis, Fuchs' heterochromic
Heterophoria — *see* Strabismus, heterophoria
Heterophyes, heterophyiasis (small intestine) B66.8
Heterotopia, heterotopic (see also Malposition, congenital)
  cerebralis Q04.8
Heterotropia — *see* Strabismus
Heubner-Herter disease K90.0
Hexadactylism Q69.9
HGSIL (cytology finding) (high grade squamous intraepithelial lesion on cytologic smear) (Pap smear finding)
  anus R85.613
  cervix R87.613
    biopsy (histology) finding — *code to* CIN II or CIN III
  vagina R87.623
    biopsy (histology) finding — *code to* VAIN II or VAIN III
Hibernoma — *see* Lipoma
Hiccup, hiccough R06.6
  epidemic B33.0
  psychogenic F45.8
Hidden penis (congenital) Q55.64
  acquired N48.83
Hidradenitis (axillaris) (suppurative) L73.2
Hidradenoma (nodular) (see also Neoplasm, skin, benign)
  clear cell — *see* Neoplasm, skin, benign
  papillary — *see* Neoplasm, skin, benign
Hidrocystoma — *see* Neoplasm, skin, benign
High
  altitude effects T70.20 ☑
    anoxia T70.29 ☑
    on
      ears T70.0 ☑
      sinuses T70.1 ☑
    polycythemia D75.1
  arch
    foot Q66.7
    palate, congenital Q38.5
  arterial tension — *see* Hypertension
  basal metabolic rate R94.8
  blood pressure (see also Hypertension)
    borderline R03.0
    reading (incidental) (isolated) (nonspecific), without diagnosis of hypertension R03.0
  cholesterol E78.0
    with high triglycerides E78.2
  diaphragm (congenital) Q79.1
  expressed emotional level within family Z63.8
  head at term O32.4 ☑
  palate, congenital Q38.5
  risk
    infant NEC Z76.2
    sexual behavior (heterosexual) Z72.51
      bisexual Z72.53
      homosexual Z72.52
  temperature (of unknown origin) R50.9
  thoracic rib Q76.6
  triglycerides E78.1
    with high cholesterol E78.2
Hildenbrand's disease A75.0
Hilum — *see* condition
Hip — *see* condition
Hippel's disease Q85.8
Hippophobia F40.218
Hippus H57.09
Hirschsprung's disease or megacolon Q43.1
Hirsutism, hirsuties L68.0
Hirudiniasis
  external B88.3
  internal B83.4
Hiss-Russell dysentery A03.1
Histidinemia, histidinuria E70.41
Histiocytoma (see also Neoplasm, skin, benign)
  fibrous (see also Neoplasm, skin, benign)
    atypical — *see* Neoplasm, connective tissue, uncertain behavior

Histiocytoma — *continued*
  fibrous (see also Neoplasm, skin, benign) — *continued*
    malignant — *see* Neoplasm, connective tissue, malignant
Histiocytosis D76.3
  acute differentiated progressive C96.0
  Langerhans' cell NEC C96.6
    multifocal X
      multisystemic (disseminated) C96.0
      unisystemic C96.5
    pulmonary, adult (adult PLCH) J84.82
    unifocal (X) C96.6
  lipid, lipoid D76.3
    essential E75.29
  malignant C96.A (*following* C96.6)
  mononuclear phagocytes NEC D76.1
    Langerhans' cells C96.6
  non-Langerhans cell D76.3
  polyostotic sclerosing D76.3
  sinus, with massive lymphadenopathy D76.3
  syndrome NEC D76.3
  X NEC C96.6
    acute (progressive) C96.0
    chronic C96.6
    multifocal C96.5
    multisystemic C96.0
    unifocal C96.6
Histoplasmosis B39.9
  with pneumonia NEC B39.2
  African B39.5
  American — *see* Histoplasmosis, capsulati
  capsulati B39.4
    disseminated B39.3
    generalized B39.3
    pulmonary B39.2
      acute B39.0
      chronic B39.1
  Darling's B39.4
  duboisii B39.5
  lung NEC B39.2
History
  family (of) (see also History, personal (of))
    alcohol abuse Z81.1
    allergy NEC Z84.89
    anemia Z83.2
    arthritis Z82.61
    asthma Z82.5
    blindness Z82.1
    cardiac death (sudden) Z82.41
    carrier of genetic disease Z84.81
    chromosomal anomaly Z82.79
    chronic
      disabling disease NEC Z82.8
      lower respiratory disease Z82.5
    colonic polyps Z83.71
    congenital malformations and deformations Z82.79
      polycystic kidney Z82.71
    consanguinity Z84.3
    deafness Z82.2
    diabetes mellitus Z83.3
    disability NEC Z82.8
    disease or disorder (of)
      allergic NEC Z84.89
      behavioral NEC Z81.8
      blood and blood-forming organs Z83.2
      cardiovascular NEC Z82.49
      chronic disabling NEC Z82.8
      digestive Z83.79
      ear NEC Z83.52
      endocrine NEC Z83.49
      eye NEC Z83.518
        glaucoma Z83.511
      genitourinary NEC Z84.2
      glaucoma Z83.511
      hematological Z83.2
      immune mechanism Z83.2
      infectious NEC Z83.1
      ischemic heart Z82.49
      kidney Z84.1
      mental NEC Z81.8
      metabolic Z83.49
      musculoskeletal NEC Z82.69
      neurological NEC Z82.0
      nutritional Z83.49
      parasitic NEC Z83.1
      psychiatric NEC Z81.8
      respiratory NEC Z83.6

History — *continued*
  family (*see also* History, personal) — *continued*
    disease or disorder — *continued*
      skin and subcutaneous tissue NEC Z84.0
      specified NEC Z84.89
    drug abuse NEC Z81.3
    epilepsy Z82.0
    genetic disease carrier Z84.81
    glaucoma Z83.511
    hearing loss Z82.2
    human immunodeficiency virus (HIV) infection Z83.0
    Huntington's chorea Z82.0
    intellectual disability Z81.0
    leukemia Z80.6
    malignant neoplasm (of) NOS Z80.9
      bladder Z80.52
      breast Z80.3
      bronchus Z80.1
      digestive organ Z80.0
      gastrointestinal tract Z80.0
      genital organ Z80.49
        ovary Z80.41
        prostate Z80.42
        specified organ NEC Z80.49
        testis Z80.43
      hematopoietic NEC Z80.7
      intrathoracic organ NEC Z80.2
      kidney Z80.51
      lung Z80.1
      lymphatic NEC Z80.7
      ovary Z80.41
      prostate Z80.42
      respiratory organ NEC Z80.2
      specified site NEC Z80.8
      testis Z80.43
      trachea Z80.1
      urinary organ or tract Z80.59
        bladder Z80.52
        kidney Z80.51
    mental
      disorder NEC Z81.8
    multiple endocrine neoplasia (MEN) syndrome Z83.41
    osteoporosis Z82.62
    polycystic kidney Z82.71
    polyps (colon) Z83.71
    psychiatric disorder Z81.8
    psychoactive substance abuse NEC Z81.3
    respiratory condition NEC Z83.6
      asthma and other lower respiratory conditions Z82.5
    self-harmful behavior Z81.8
    skin condition Z84.0
    specified condition NEC Z84.89
    stroke (cerebrovascular) Z82.3
    substance abuse NEC Z81.4
      alcohol Z81.1
      drug NEC Z81.3
      psychoactive NEC Z81.3
      tobacco Z81.2
    sudden cardiac death Z82.41
    tobacco abuse Z81.2
    violence, violent behavior Z81.8
    visual loss Z82.1
  personal (of) (*see also* History, family (of))
    abuse
      adult Z91.419
        physical and sexual Z91.410
        psychological Z91.411
      childhood Z62.819
        physical Z62.810
        psychological Z62.811
        sexual Z62.810
    alcohol dependence F10.21
    allergy (to) Z88.9
      analgesic agent NEC Z88.6
      anesthetic Z88.4
      antibiotic agent NEC Z88.1
      anti-infective agent NEC Z88.3
      contrast media Z91.041
      drugs, medicaments and biological substances Z88.9
        specified NEC Z88.8
      food Z91.018
        additives Z91.02
        eggs Z91.012
        milk products Z91.011

History — *continued*
  personal (*see also* History, family) — *continued*
    allergy — *continued*
      food — *continued*
        peanuts Z91.010
        seafood Z91.013
        specified food NEC Z91.018
      insect Z91.038
        bee Z91.030
      latex Z91.040
      medicinal agents Z88.9
        specified NEC Z88.8
      narcotic agent NEC Z88.5
      nonmedicinal agents Z91.048
      penicillin Z88.0
      serum Z88.7
      specified NEC Z91.09
      sulfonamides Z88.2
      vaccine Z88.7
    anaphylactic shock Z87.892
    anaphylaxis Z87.892
    behavioral disorders Z86.59
    benign carcinoid tumor Z86.012
    benign neoplasm Z86.018
      brain Z86.011
      carcinoid Z86.012
      colonic polyps Z86.010
    brain injury (traumatic) Z87.820
    breast implant removal Z98.86
    calculi, renal Z87.442
    cancer — *see* History, personal (of), malignant neoplasm (of)
    cardiac arrest (death), successfully resuscitated Z86.74
    cerebral infarction without residual deficit Z86.73
    cervical dysplasia Z87.410
    chemotherapy for neoplastic condition Z92.21
    childhood abuse — *see* History, personal (of), abuse
    cleft lip (corrected) Z87.730
    cleft palate (corrected) Z87.730
    collapsed vertebra (healed) Z87.311
      due to osteoporosis Z87.310
    combat and operational stress reaction Z86.51
    congenital malformation (corrected) Z87.798
      circulatory system (corrected) Z87.74
      digestive system (corrected) NEC Z87.738
      ear (corrected) Z87.720
      eye (corrected) Z87.721
      face and neck (corrected) Z87.790
      genitourinary system (corrected) NEC Z87.718
      heart (corrected) Z87.74
      integument (corrected) Z87.76
      limb(s) (corrected) Z87.76
      musculoskeletal system (corrected) Z87.76
      neck (corrected) Z87.790
      nervous system (corrected) NEC Z87.728
      respiratory system (corrected) Z87.75
      sense organs (corrected) NEC Z87.728
      specified NEC Z87.798
    contraception Z92.0
    deployment (military) Z91.82
    diabetic foot ulcer Z86.31
    disease or disorder (of) Z87.898
      anaphylaxis Z87.892
      blood and blood-forming organs Z86.2
      circulatory system Z86.79
        specified condition NEC Z86.79
      connective tissue Z87.39
      digestive system Z87.19
        colonic polyp Z86.010
        peptic ulcer disease Z87.11
        specified condition NEC Z87.19
      ear Z86.69
      endocrine Z86.39
        diabetic foot ulcer Z86.31
        gestational diabetes Z86.32
        specified type NEC Z86.39
      eye Z86.69
      genital (track) system NEC
        female Z87.42
        male Z87.438
      hematological Z86.2
      Hodgkin Z85.71
      immune mechanism Z86.2
      infectious Z86.19
        malaria Z86.13

History — *continued*
  personal (*see also* History, family) — *continued*
    disease or disorder — *continued*
      infectious — *continued*
        Methicillin resistant Staphylococcus aureus (MRSA) Z86.14
        poliomyelitis Z86.12
        specified NEC Z86.19
        tuberculosis Z86.11
      mental NEC Z86.59
      metabolic Z86.39
        diabetic foot ulcer Z86.31
        gestational diabetes Z86.32
        specified type NEC Z86.39
      musculoskeletal NEC Z87.39
      nervous system Z86.69
      nutritional Z86.39
      parasitic Z86.19
      respiratory system NEC Z87.09
      sense organs Z86.69
      skin Z87.2
      specified site or type NEC Z87.898
      subcutaneous tissue Z87.2
      trophoblastic Z87.59
      urinary system NEC Z87.448
    drug dependence — *see* Dependence, drug, by type, in remission
    drug therapy
      antineoplastic chemotherapy Z92.21
      estrogen Z92.23
      immunosupression Z92.25
      inhaled steroids Z92.240
      monoclonal drug Z92.22
      specified NEC Z92.29
      steroid Z92.241
      systemic steroids Z92.241
    dysplasia
      cervical Z87.410
      prostatic Z87.430
      vaginal Z87.411
      vulvar Z87.412
    embolism (venous) Z86.718
      pulmonary Z86.711
    encephalitis Z86.61
    estrogen therapy Z92.23
    extracorporeal membrane oxygenation (ECMO) Z92.81
    failed conscious sedation Z92.83
    failed moderate sedation Z92.83
    fall, falling Z91.81
    fracture (healed)
      fatigue Z87.312
      fragility Z87.310
      osteoporosis Z87.310
      pathological NEC Z87.311
      stress Z87.312
      traumatic Z87.81
    gestational diabetes Z86.32
    hepatitis
      B Z86.19
      C Z86.19
    Hodgkin disease Z85.71
    hyperthermia, malignant Z88.4
    hypospadias (corrected) Z87.710
    hysterectomy Z90.710
    immunosupression therapy Z92.25
    in situ neoplasm
      breast Z86.000
      cervix uteri Z86.001
      specified NEC Z86.008
    in utero procedure during pregnancy Z98.870
    in utero procedure while a fetus Z98.871
    infection NEC Z86.19
      central nervous system Z86.61
      Methicillin resistant Staphylococcus aureus (MRSA) Z86.14
      urinary (recurrent) (tract) Z87.440
    injury NEC Z87.828
    irradiation Z92.3
    kidney stones Z87.442
    leukemia Z85.6
    lymphoma (non-Hodgkin) Z85.72
    malignant melanoma (skin) Z85.820
    malignant neoplasm (of) Z85.9
      accessory sinuses Z85.22
      anus NEC Z85.048
        carcinoid Z85.040
      bladder Z85.51

History — *continued*
personal (*see also* History, family) — *continued*
  malignant neoplasm — *continued*
    bone Z85.830
    brain Z85.841
    breast Z85.3
    bronchus NEC Z85.118
      carcinoid Z85.110
    carcinoid — *see* History, personal (of), malig-
      nant neoplasm, by site, carcinioid
    cervix Z85.41
    colon NEC Z85.038
      carcinoid Z85.030
    digestive organ Z85.00
      specified NEC Z85.09
    endocrine gland NEC Z85.858
    epididymis Z85.48
    esophagus Z85.01
    eye Z85.840
    gastrointestinal tract — *see* History, malignant
      neoplasm, digestive organ
    genital organ
      female Z85.40
        specified NEC Z85.44
      male Z85.45
        specified NEC Z85.49
    hematopoietic Z85.79
    intrathoracic organ Z85.20
    kidney NEC Z85.528
      carcinoid Z85.520
    large intestine NEC Z85.038
      carcinoid Z85.030
    larynx Z85.21
    liver Z85.05
    lung NEC Z85.118
      carcinoid Z85.110
    mediastinum Z85.29
    Merkel cell Z85.821
    middle ear Z85.22
    nasal cavities Z85.22
    nervous system NEC Z85.848
    oral cavity Z85.819
      specified site NEC Z85.818
    ovary Z85.43
    pancreas Z85.07
    pelvis Z85.53
    pharynx Z85.819
      specified site NEC Z85.818
    pleura Z85.29
    prostate Z85.46
    rectosigmoid junction NEC Z85.048
      carcinoid Z85.040
    rectum NEC Z85.048
      carcinoid Z85.040
    respiratory organ Z85.20
    sinuses, accessory Z85.22
    skin NEC Z85.828
      melanoma Z85.820
      Merkel cell Z85.821
    small intestine NEC Z85.068
      carcinoid Z85.060
    soft tissue Z85.831
    specified site NEC Z85.89
    stomach NEC Z85.028
      carcinoid Z85.020
    testis Z85.47
    thymus NEC Z85.238
      carcinoid Z85.230
    thyroid Z85.850
    tongue Z85.810
    trachea Z85.12
    urinary organ or tract Z85.50
      specified NEC Z85.59
    uterus Z85.42
  maltreatment Z91.89
  medical treatment NEC Z92.89
  melanoma (malignant) (skin) Z85.820
  meningitis Z86.61
  mental disorder Z86.59
  Merkel cell carcinoma (skin) Z85.821
  Methicillin resistant Staphylococcus aureus (MRSA)
    Z86.14
  military deployment Z91.82
  military war, peacekeeping and humanitarian de-
    ployment (current or past conflict) Z91.82
  myocardial infarction (old) I25.2
  neglect (in)
    adult Z91.412

History — *continued*
personal (*see also* History, family) — *continued*
  neglect — *continued*
    childhood Z62.812
  neoplasm
    benign Z86.018
      brain Z86.011
      colon polyp Z86.010
    in situ
      breast Z86.000
      cervix uteri Z86.001
      specified NEC Z86.008
    malignant — *see* History of, malignant neo-
      plasm
    uncertain behavior Z86.03
  nephrotic syndrome Z87.441
  nicotine dependence Z87.891
  noncompliance with medical treatment or regimen
    — *see* Noncompliance
  nutritional deficiency Z86.39
  obstetric complications Z87.59
    childbirth Z87.59
    pregnancy Z87.59
    pre-term labor Z87.51
    puerperium Z87.59
  osteoporosis fractures Z87.31 ☑
  parasuicide (attempt) Z91.5
  physical trauma NEC Z87.828
    self-harm or suicide attempt Z91.5
  pneumonia (recurrent) Z87.01
  poisoning NEC Z91.89
    self-harm or suicide attempt Z91.5
  poor personal hygiene Z91.89
  preterm labor Z87.51
  procedure during pregnancy Z98.870
  procedure while a fetus Z98.871
  prolonged reversible ischemic neurologic deficit
    (PRIND) Z86.73
  prostatic dysplasia Z87.430
  psychological
    abuse
      adult Z91.411
      child Z62.811
    trauma, specified NEC Z91.49
  radiation therapy Z92.3
  removal
    implant
      breast Z98.86
  renal calculi Z87.442
  respiratory condition NEC Z87.09
  retained foreign body fully removed Z87.821
  risk factors NEC Z91.89
  self-harm Z91.5
  self-poisoning attempt Z91.5
  sex reassignment Z87.890
  sleep-wake cycle problem Z72.821
  specified NEC Z87.898
  steroid therapy (systemic) Z92.241
    inhaled Z92.240
  stroke without residual deficits Z86.73
  substance abuse NEC F10-F19 with fifth character
    1
  sudden cardiac arrest Z86.74
  sudden cardiac death successfully resuscitated
    Z86.74
  suicide attempt Z91.5
  surgery NEC Z98.89
    sex reassignment Z87.890
    transplant — *see* Transplant
  thrombophlebitis Z86.72
  thrombosis (venous) Z86.718
    pulmonary Z86.711
  tobacco dependence Z87.891
  transient ischemic attack (TIA) without residual
    deficits Z86.73
  trauma (physical) NEC Z87.828
    psychological NEC Z91.49
    self-harm Z91.5
  traumatic brain injury Z87.820
  unhealthy sleep-wake cycle Z72.821
  urinary calculi Z87.442
  urinary (recurrent) (tract) infection(s) Z87.440
  vaginal dysplasia Z87.411
  venous thrombosis or embolism Z86.718
    pulmonary Z86.711
  vulvar dysplasia Z87.412
His-Werner disease A79.0

HIV (*see also* Human, immunodeficiency virus) B20
  laboratory evidence (nonconclusive) R75
  nonconclusive test (in infants) R75
  positive, seropositive Z21
Hives (bold) — *see* Urticaria
Hoarseness R49.0
Hobo Z59.0
Hodgkin disease — *see* Lymphoma, Hodgkin
Hodgson's disease I71.2
  ruptured I71.1
Hoffa-Kastert disease E88.89
Hoffa's disease E88.89
Hoffmann-Bouveret syndrome I47.9
Hoffmann's syndrome E03.9 [G73.7]
Hole (round)
  macula H35.34- ☑
  retina (without detachment) — *see* Break, retina,
    round hole
    with detachment — *see* Detachment, retina, with
      retinal, break
Holiday relief care Z75.5
Hollenhorst's plaque — *see* Occlusion, artery, retina
Hollow foot (congenital) Q66.7
  acquired — *see* Deformity, limb, foot, specified NEC
Holoprosencephaly Q04.2
Holt-Oram syndrome Q87.2
Homelessness Z59.0
Homesickness — *see* Disorder, adjustment
Homocystinemia, homocystinuria E72.11
Homogentisate 1,2-dioxygenase deficiency E70.29
Homologous serum hepatitis (prophylactic) (therapeu-
  tic) — *see* Hepatitis, viral, type B
Honeycomb lung J98.4
  congenital Q33.0
Hooded
  clitoris Q52.6
  penis Q55.69
Hookworm (anemia) (disease) (infection) (infestation)
  B76.9
  specified NEC B76.8
Hordeolum (eyelid) (externum) (recurrent) H00.019
  internum H00.029
    left H00.026
      lower H00.025
      upper H00.024
    right H00.023
      lower H00.022
      upper H00.021
  left H00.016
    lower H00.015
    upper H00.014
  right H00.013
    lower H00.012
    upper H00.011
Horn
  cutaneous L85.8
  nail L60.2
    congenital Q84.6
Horner (-Claude Bernard) **syndrome** G90.2
  traumatic — *see* Injury, nerve, cervical sympathetic
Horseshoe kidney (congenital) Q63.1
Horton's headache or neuralgia G44.099
  intractable G44.091
  not intractable G44.099
Hospital hopper syndrome — *see* Disorder, factitious
Hospitalism in children — *see* Disorder, adjustment
Hostility R45.5
  towards child Z62.3
Hot flashes
  menopausal N95.1
Hourglass (contracture) (*see also* Contraction, hourglass)
  stomach K31.89
    congenital Q40.2
    stricture K31.2
Household, housing circumstance affecting care
  Z59.9
  specified NEC Z59.8
Housemaid's knee — *see* Bursitis, prepatellar
Hudson (-Stähli) **line** (cornea) — *see* Pigmentation,
  cornea, anterior
Human
  bite (open wound) (*see also* Bite)
    intact skin surface — *see* Bite, superficial
  herpesvirus — *see* Herpes
  immunodeficiency virus (HIV) disease (infection) B20
    asymptomatic status Z21
    contact Z20.6

Human — *continued*
  immunodeficiency virus disease — *continued*
    counseling Z71.7
    dementia B20 [F02.80]
      with behavioral disturbance B20 [F02.81]
    exposure to Z20.6
    laboratory evidence R75
    type-2 (HIV 2) as cause of disease classified else-
      where B97.35
  papillomavirus (HPV)
    DNA test positive
      high risk
        cervix R87.810
        vagina R87.811
      low risk
        cervix R87.820
        vagina R87.821
    screening for Z11.51
  T-cell lymphotropic virus
    type-1 (HTLV-I) infection B33.3
      as cause of disease classified elsewhere B97.33
      carrier Z22.6
    type-2 (HTLV-II) as cause of disease classified else-
      where B97.34
Humidifier lung or pneumonitis J67.7
Humiliation (experience) **in childhood** Z62.898
Humpback (acquired) — *see* Kyphosis
Hunchback (acquired) — *see* Kyphosis
Hunger T73.0 ☑
  air, psychogenic F45.8
Hungry bone syndrome E83.81
Hunner's ulcer — *see* Cystitis, chronic, interstitial
Hunter's
  glossitis D51.0
  syndrome E76.1
Huntington's disease or chorea G10
  with dementia G10 [F02.80]
    with behavioral disturbance G10 [F02.81]
Hunt's
  disease or syndrome (herpetic geniculate ganglionitis)
    B02.21
    dyssynergia cerebellaris myoclonica G11.1
  neuralgia B02.21
Hurler (-Scheie) **disease or syndrome** E76.02
Hurst's disease G36.1
Hurthle cell
  adenocarcinoma C73
  adenoma D34
  carcinoma C73
  tumor D34
Hutchinson-Boeck disease or syndrome — *see* Sarcoidosis
Hutchinson-Gilford disease or syndrome E34.8
Hutchinson's
  disease, meaning
    angioma serpiginosum L81.7
    pompholyx (cheiropompholyx) L30.1
    prurigo estivalis L56.4
    summer eruption or summer prurigo L56.4
  melanotic freckle — *see* Melanoma, in situ
    malignant melanoma in — *see* Melanoma
  teeth or incisors (congenital syphilis) A50.52
  triad (congenital syphilis) A50.53
Hyalin plaque, sclera, senile H15.89
Hyaline membrane (disease) (lung) (pulmonary) (newborn) P22.0
Hyalinosis
  cutis (et mucosae) E78.89
  focal and segmental (glomerular) (*see also* N00-N07
    with fourth character .1) N05.1
Hyalitis, hyalosis, asteroid (*see also* Deposit, crystalline)
  syphilitic (late) A52.71
Hydatid
  cyst or tumor — *see* Echinococcus
  mole — *see* Hydatidiform mole
  Morgagni
    female Q50.5
    male (epididymal) Q55.4
      testicular Q55.29
Hydatidiform mole (benign) (complicating pregnancy)
  (delivered) (undelivered) O01.9
  classical O01.0
  complete O01.0
  incomplete O01.1
  invasive D39.2
  malignant D39.2
  partial O01.1
Hydatidosis — *see* Echinococcus

Hydradenitis (axillaris) (suppurative) L73.2
Hydradenoma — *see* Hidradenoma
Hydramnios O40.- ☑
Hydrancephaly, hydranencephaly Q04.3
  with spina bifida — *see* Spina bifida, with hydro-
    cephalus
Hydrargyrism NEC — *see* Poisoning, mercury
Hydrarthrosis (*see also* Effusion, joint)
  gonococcal A54.42
  intermittent M12.40
    ankle M12.47- ☑
    elbow M12.42- ☑
    foot joint M12.47- ☑
    hand joint M12.44- ☑
    hip M12.45- ☑
    knee M12.46- ☑
    multiple site M12.49
    shoulder M12.41- ☑
    specified joint NEC M12.48
    wrist M12.43- ☑
  of yaws (early) (late) (*see also* subcategory M14.8-)
    A66.6
  syphilitic (late) A52.77
  congenital A50.55 [M12.80]
Hydremia D64.89
Hydrencephalocele (congenital) — *see* Encephalocele
Hydrencephalomeningocele (congenital) — *see* Encephalocele
Hydroa R23.8
  aestivale L56.4
  vacciniforme L56.4
Hydroadenitis (axillaris) (suppurative) L73.2
Hydrocalycosis — *see* Hydronephrosis
Hydrocele (spermatic cord) (testis) (tunica vaginalis)
  N43.3
  canal of Nuck N94.89
  communicating N43.2
    congenital P83.5
  congenital P83.5
  encysted N43.0
  female NEC N94.89
  infected N43.1
  newborn P83.5
  round ligament N94.89
  specified NEC N43.2
  spinalis — *see* Spina bifida
  vulva N90.89
Hydrocephalus (acquired) (external) (internal) (malignant) (recurrent) G91.9
  aqueduct Sylvius stricture Q03.0
  causing disproportion O33.6 ☑
    with obstructed labor O66.3
  communicating G91.0
  congenital (external) (internal) Q03.9
    with spina bifida Q05.4
      cervical Q05.0
      dorsal Q05.1
      lumbar Q05.2
      lumbosacral Q05.2
      sacral Q05.3
      thoracic Q05.1
      thoracolumbar Q05.1
    specified NEC Q03.8
  due to toxoplasmosis (congenital) P37.1
  foramen Magendie block (acquired) G91.1
    congenital (*see also* Hydrocephalus, congenital)
      Q03.1
  in (due to)
    infectious disease NEC B89 [G91.4]
    neoplastic disease NEC (*see also* Neoplasm) G91.4
    parasitic disease B89 [G91.4]
  newborn Q03.9
    with spina bifida — *see* Spina bifida, with hydro-
      cephalus
  noncommunicating G91.1
  normal pressure G91.2
    secondary G91.0
  obstructive G91.1
  otitic G93.2
  post-traumatic NEC G91.3
  secondary G91.4
    post-traumatic G91.3
  specified NEC G91.8
  syphilitic, congenital A50.49
Hydrocolpos (congenital) N89.8
Hydrocystoma — *see* Neoplasm, skin, benign
Hydroencephalocele (congenital) — *see* Encephalocele

Hydroencephalomeningocele (congenital) — *see* En-
  cephalocele
Hydrohematopneumothorax — *see* Hemothorax
Hydromeningitis — *see* Meningitis
Hydromeningocele (spinal) (*see also* Spina bifida)
  cranial — *see* Encephalocele
Hydrometra N85.8
Hydrometrocolpos N89.8
Hydromicrocephaly Q02
Hydromphalos (since birth) Q45.8
Hydromyelia Q06.4
Hydromyelocele — *see* Spina bifida
Hydronephrosis (atrophic) (early) (functionless) (inter-
  mittent) (primary) (secondary) NEC N13.30
  with
    infection N13.6
    obstruction (by) (of)
      renal calculus N13.2
        with infection N13.6
      ureteral NEC N13.1
        with infection N13.6
        calculus N13.2
          with infection N13.6
      ureteropelvic junction (congenital) Q62.0
        with infection N13.6
    ureteral stricture NEC N13.1
      with infection N13.6
  congenital Q62.0
  specified type NEC N13.39
  tuberculous A18.11
Hydropericarditis — *see* Pericarditis
Hydropericardium — *see* Pericarditis
Hydroperitoneum R18.8
Hydrophobia — *see* Rabies
Hydrophthalmos Q15.0
Hydropneumohemothorax — *see* Hemothorax
Hydropneumopericarditis — *see* Pericarditis
Hydropneumopericardium — *see* Pericarditis
Hydropneumothorax J94.8
  traumatic — *see* Injury, intrathoracic, lung
  tuberculous NEC A15.6
Hydrops R60.9
  abdominis R18.8
  articulorum intermittens — *see* Hydrarthrosis, inter-
    mittent
  cardiac — *see* Failure, heart, congestive
  causing obstructed labor (mother) O66.3
  endolymphatic H81.0- ☑
  fetal — *see* Pregnancy, complicated by, hydrops, fetalis
  fetalis P83.2
    due to
      ABO isoimmunization P56.0
      alpha thalassemia D56.0
      hemolytic disease P56.90
        specified NEC P56.99
      isoimmunization (ABO) (Rh) P56.0
      other specified nonhemolytic disease NEC P83.2
      Rh incompatibility P56.0
    during pregnancy — *see* Pregnancy, complicated
      by, hydrops, fetalis
  gallbladder K82.1
  joint — *see* Effusion, joint
  labyrinth H81.0- ☑
  newborn (idiopathic) P83.2
    due to
      ABO isoimmunization P56.0
      alpha thalassemia D56.0
      hemolytic disease P56.90
        specified NEC P56.99
      isoimmunization (ABO) (Rh) P56.0
      Rh incompatibility P56.0
  nutritional — *see* Malnutrition, severe
  pericardium — *see* Pericarditis
  pleura — *see* Hydrothorax
  spermatic cord — *see* Hydrocele
Hydropyonephrosis N13.6
Hydrorachis Q06.4
Hydrorrhea (nasal) J34.89
  pregnancy — *see* Rupture, membranes, premature
Hydrosadenitis (axillaris) (suppurative) L73.2
Hydrosalpinx (fallopian tube) (follicularis) N70.11
Hydrothorax (double) (pleura) J94.8
  chylous (nonfilarial) I89.8
    filarial (*see also* Infestation, filarial) B74.9 [J91.8]
  traumatic — *see* Injury, intrathoracic
  tuberculous NEC (non primary) A15.6

Hydroureter (*see also* Hydronephrosis) N13.4
  with infection N13.6
  congenital Q62.39
Hydroureteronephrosis — *see* Hydronephrosis
Hydrourethra N36.8
Hydroxykynureninuria E70.8
Hydroxylysinemia E72.3
Hydroxyprolinemia E72.59
Hygiene, sleep
  abuse Z72.821
  inadequate Z72.821
  poor Z72.821
Hygroma (congenital) (cystic) D18.1
  praepatellare, prepatellar — *see* Bursitis, prepatellar
Hymen — *see* condition
Hymenolepis, hymenolepiasis (diminuta) (infection)
  (infestation) (nana) B71.0
Hypalgesia R20.8
Hyperacidity (gastric) K31.89
  psychogenic F45.8
Hyperactive, hyperactivity F90.9
  basal cell, uterine cervix — *see* Dysplasia, cervix
  bowel sounds R19.12
  cervix epithelial (basal) — *see* Dysplasia, cervix
  child F90.9
    attention deficit — *see* Disorder, attention-deficit
      hyperactivity
  detrusor muscle N32.81
  gastrointestinal K31.89
    psychogenic F45.8
  nasal mucous membrane J34.3
  stomach K31.89
  thyroid (gland) — *see* Hyperthyroidism
Hyperacusis H93.23- ☑
Hyperadrenalism E27.5
Hyperadrenocorticism E24.9
  congenital E25.0
  iatrogenic E24.2
    correct substance properly administered — *see*
      Table of Drugs and Chemicals, by drug, ad-
      verse effect
    overdose or wrong substance given or taken —
      see Table of Drugs and Chemicals, by drug,
      poisoning
  not associated with Cushing's syndrome E27.0
  pituitary-dependent E24.0
Hyperaldosteronism E26.9
  familial (type I) E26.02
  glucocorticoid-remediable E26.02
  primary (due to (bilateral) adrenal hyperplasia) E26.09
  primary NEC E26.09
  secondary E26.1
  specified NEC E26.89
Hyperalgesia R20.8
Hyperalimentation R63.2
  carotene, carotin E67.1
  specified NEC E67.8
  vitamin
    A E67.0
    D E67.3
Hyperaminoaciduria
  arginine E72.21
  cystine E72.01
  lysine E72.3
  ornithine E72.4
Hyperammonemia (congenital) E72.20
Hyperazotemia — *see* Uremia
Hyperbetalipoproteinemia (familial) E78.0
  with prebetalipoproteinemia E78.2
Hyperbilirubinemia
  constitutional E80.6
  familial conjugated E80.6
  neonatal (transient) — *see* Jaundice, newborn
Hypercalcemia, hypocalciuric, familial E83.52
Hypercalciuria, idiopathic E83.52
Hypercapnia R06.89
  newborn P84
Hypercarotenemia, hypercarotinemia (dietary) E67.1
Hypercementosis K03.4
Hyperchloremia E87.8
Hyperchlorhydria K31.89
  neurotic F45.8
  psychogenic F45.8
Hypercholesterinemia — *see* Hypercholesterolemia
Hypercholesterolemia (essential) (familial) (hereditary)
  (primary) (pure) E78.0
  with hyperglyceridemia, endogenous E78.2

Hypercholesterolemia — *continued*
  dietary counseling and surveillance Z71.3
Hyperchylia gastrica, psychogenic F45.8
Hyperchylomicronemia (familial) (primary) E78.3
  with hyperbetalipoproteinemia E78.3
Hypercoagulable (state) D68.59
  activated protein C resistance D68.51
  antithrombin (III) deficiency D68.59
  factor V Leiden mutation D68.51
  primary NEC D68.59
  protein C deficiency D68.59
  protein S deficiency D68.59
  prothrombin gene mutation D68.52
  secondary D68.69
  specified NEC D68.69
Hypercoagulation (state) D68.59
Hypercorticalism, pituitary-dependent E24.0
Hypercorticosolism — *see* Cushing's, syndrome
Hypercorticosteronism E24.2
  correct substance properly administered — *see* Table
    of Drugs and Chemicals, by drug, adverse effect
  overdose or wrong substance given or taken — *see*
    Table of Drugs and Chemicals, by drug, poison-
    ing
Hypercortisonism E24.2
  correct substance properly administered — *see* Table
    of Drugs and Chemicals, by drug, adverse effect
  overdose or wrong substance given or taken — *see*
    Table of Drugs and Chemicals, by drug, poison-
    ing
Hyperekplexia Q89.8
Hyperelectrolytemia E87.8
Hyperemesis R11.10
  with nausea R11.2
  gravidarum (mild) O21.0
    with
      carbohydrate depletion O21.1
      dehydration O21.1
      electrolyte imbalance O21.1
      metabolic disturbance O21.1
      severe (with metabolic disturbance) O21.1
  projectile R11.12
  psychogenic F45.8
Hyperemia (acute) (passive) R68.89
  anal mucosa K62.89
  bladder N32.89
  cerebral I67.89
  conjunctiva H11.43- ☑
  ear internal, acute — *see* subcategory H83.0 ☑
  enteric K59.8
  eye — *see* Hyperemia, conjunctiva
  eyelid (active) (passive) — *see* Disorder, eyelid, speci-
    fied type NEC
  intestine K59.8
  iris — *see* Disorder, iris, vascular
  kidney N28.89
  labyrinth — *see* subcategory H83.0 ☑
  liver (active) K76.89
  lung (passive) — *see* Edema, lung
  pulmonary (passive) — *see* Edema, lung
  renal N28.89
  retina H35.89
  stomach K31.89
Hyperesthesia (body surface) R20.3
  larynx (reflex) J38.7
    hysterical F44.89
  pharynx (reflex) J39.2
    hysterical F44.89
Hyperestrogenism (drug-induced) (iatrogenic) E28.0
Hyperexplexia Q89.8
Hyperfibrinolysis — *see* Fibrinolysis
Hyperfructosemia E74.19
Hyperfunction
  adrenal cortex, not associated with Cushing's syn-
    drome E27.0
    medulla E27.5
      adrenomedullary E27.5
    virilism E25.9
      congenital E25.0
  ovarian E28.8
  pancreas K86.8
  parathyroid (gland) E21.3
  pituitary (gland) (anterior) E22.9
    specified NEC E22.8
  polyglandular E31.1
  testicular E29.0

Hypergammaglobulinemia D89.2
  polyclonal D89.0
  Waldenström D89.0
Hypergastrinemia E16.4
Hyperglobulinemia R77.1
Hyperglycemia, hyperglycemic (transient) R73.9
  coma — *see* Diabetes, by type, with coma
  postpancreatectomy E89.1
Hyperglyceridemia (endogenous) (essential) (familial)
  (hereditary) (pure) E78.1
  mixed E78.3
Hyperglycinemia (non-ketotic) E72.51
Hypergonadism
  ovarian E28.8
  testicular (primary) (infantile) E29.0
Hyperheparinemia D68.32
Hyperhidrosis, hyperidrosis R61
  focal
    primary L74.519
      axilla L74.510
      face L74.511
      palms L74.512
      soles L74.513
    secondary L74.52
  generalized R61
  localized
    primary L74.519
      axilla L74.510
      face L74.511
      palms L74.512
      soles L74.513
    secondary L74.52
  psychogenic F45.8
  secondary R61
    focal L74.52
Hyperhistidinemia E70.41
Hyperhomocysteinemia E72.11
Hyperhydroxyprolinemia E72.59
Hyperinsulinism (functional) E16.1
  with
    coma (hypoglycemic) E15
    encephalopathy E16.1 [G94]
  ectopic E16.1
  therapeutic misadventure (from administration of in-
    sulin) — *see* subcategory T38.3 ☑
Hyperkalemia E87.5
Hyperkeratosis (*see also* Keratosis) L85.9
  cervix N88.0
  due to yaws (early) (late) (palmar or plantar) A66.3
  follicularis Q82.8
    penetrans (in cutem) L87.0
  palmoplantaris climacterica L85.1
  pinta A67.1
  senile (with pruritus) L57.0
  universalis congenita Q80.8
  vocal cord J38.3
  vulva N90.4
Hyperkinesia, hyperkinetic (disease) (reaction) (syndrome) (childhood) (adolescence) (*see also* Disorder,
  attention-deficit hyperactivity)
  heart I51.89
Hyperleucine-isoleucinemia E71.19
Hyperlipemia, hyperlipidemia E78.5
  combined E78.2
    familial E78.4
  group
    A E78.0
    B E78.1
    C E78.2
    D E78.3
  mixed E78.2
  specified NEC E78.4
Hyperlipidosis E75.6
  hereditary NEC E75.5
Hyperlipoproteinemia E78.5
  Fredrickson's type
    I E78.3
    IIa E78.0
    IIb E78.2
    III E78.2
    IV E78.1
    V E78.3
  low-density-lipoprotein-type (LDL) E78.0
  very-low-density-lipoprotein-type (VLDL) E78.1
Hyperlucent lung, unilateral J43.0
Hyperlysinemia E72.3
Hypermagnesemia E83.41
  neonatal P71.8

Hypermenorrhea N92.0
Hypermethioninemia E72.19
Hypermetropia (congenital) H52.0- ☑
Hypermobility, hypermotility
  cecum — *see* Syndrome, irritable bowel
  coccyx — *see* subcategory M53.2 ☑
  colon — *see* Syndrome, irritable bowel
    psychogenic F45.8
  ileum K58.9
  intestine (*see also* Syndrome, irritable bowel) K58.9
    psychogenic F45.8
  meniscus (knee) — *see* Derangement, knee, meniscus
  scapula — *see* Instability, joint, shoulder
  stomach K31.89
    psychogenic F45.8
  syndrome M35.7
  urethra N36.41
    with intrinsic sphincter deficiency N36.43
Hypernasality R49.21
Hypernatremia E87.0
Hypernephroma C64.- ☑
Hyperopia — *see* Hypermetropia
Hyperorexia nervosa F50.2
Hyperornithinemia E72.4
Hyperosmia R43.1
Hyperosmolality E87.0
Hyperostosis (monomelic) (*see also* Disorder, bone, density and structure, specified NEC)
  ankylosing (spine) M48.10
    cervical region M48.12
    cervicothoracic region M48.13
    lumbar region M48.16
    lumbosacral region M48.17
    multiple sites M48.19
    occipito-atlanto-axial region M48.11
    sacrococcygeal region M48.18
    thoracic region M48.14
    thoracolumbar region M48.15
  cortical (skull) M85.2
    infantile M89.8X- ☑
  frontal, internal of skull M85.2
  interna frontalis M85.2
  skeletal, diffuse idiopathic — *see* Hyperostosis, ankylosing
  skull M85.2
    congenital Q75.8
  vertebral, ankylosing — *see* Hyperostosis, ankylosing
Hyperovarism E28.8
Hyperoxaluria (primary) E72.53
Hyperparathyroidism E21.3
  primary E21.0
  secondary (renal) N25.81
    non-renal E21.1
  specified NEC E21.2
  tertiary E21.2
Hyperpathia R20.8
Hyperperistalsis R19.2
  psychogenic F45.8
Hyperpermeability, capillary I78.8
Hyperphagia R63.2
Hyperphenylalaninemia NEC E70.1
Hyperphoria (alternating) H50.53
Hyperphosphatemia E83.39
Hyperpiesis, hyperpiesia — *see* Hypertension
Hyperpigmentation (*see also* Pigmentation)
  melanin NEC L81.4
  postinflammatory L81.0
Hyperpinealism E34.8
Hyperpituitarism E22.9
Hyperplasia, hyperplastic
  adenoids J35.2
  adrenal (capsule) (cortex) (gland) E27.8
    with
      sexual precocity (male) E25.9
        congenital E25.0
      virilism, adrenal E25.9
        congenital E25.0
      virilization (female) E25.9
        congenital E25.0
    congenital E25.0
    salt-losing E25.0
  adrenomedullary E27.5
  angiolymphoid, eosinophilia (ALHE) D18.01
  appendix (lymphoid) K38.0
  artery, fibromuscular I77.3
  bone (*see also* Hypertrophy, bone)
    marrow D75.89

Hyperplasia, hyperplastic — *continued*
  breast (*see also* Hypertrophy, breast)
    ductal (atypical) N60.9- ☑
  C-cell, thyroid E07.0
  cementation (tooth) (teeth) K03.4
  cervical gland R59.0
  cervix (uteri) (basal cell) (endometrium) (polypoid) (*see also* Dysplasia, cervix)
    congenital Q51.828
  clitoris, congenital Q52.6
  denture K06.2
  endocervicitis N72
  endometrium, endometrial (adenomatous) (benign) (cystic) (glandular) (glandular-cystic) (polypoid) N85.00
    with atypia N85.02
    cervix — *see* Dysplasia, cervix
    complex (without atypia) N85.01
    simple (without atypia) N85.01
  epithelial L85.9
    focal, oral, including tongue K13.29
    nipple N62
    skin L85.9
    tongue K13.29
    vaginal wall N89.3
  erythroid D75.89
  fibromuscular of artery (carotid) (renal) I77.3
  genital
    female NEC N94.89
    male N50.8
  gingiva K06.1
  glandularis cystica uteri (interstitialis) (*see also* Hyperplasia, endometrial) N85.00
  gum K06.1
  hymen, congenital Q52.4
  irritative, edentulous (alveolar) K06.2
  jaw M26.09
    alveolar M26.79
      lower M26.03
        alveolar M26.72
      upper M26.01
        alveolar M26.71
  kidney (congenital) Q63.3
  labia N90.6
    epithelial N90.3
  liver (congenital) Q44.7
    nodular, focal K76.89
  lymph gland or node R59.9
  mandible, mandibular M26.03
    alveolar M26.72
    unilateral condylar M27.8
  maxilla, maxillary M26.01
    alveolar M26.71
  myometrium, myometrial N85.2
  neuroendocrine cell, of infancy J84.841
  nose
    lymphoid J34.89
    polypoid J33.9
  oral mucosa (irritative) K13.6
  organ or site, congenital NEC — *see* Anomaly, by site
  ovary N83.8
  palate, papillary (irritative) K13.6
  pancreatic islet cells E16.9
    alpha E16.8
      with excess
        gastrin E16.4
        glucagon E16.3
    beta E16.1
  parathyroid (gland) E21.0
  pharynx (lymphoid) J39.2
  prostate (adenofibromatous) (nodular) N40.0
    with lower urinary tract symptoms (LUTS) N40.1
    without lower urinary tract symtpoms (LUTS) N40.0
  renal artery I77.89
  reticulo-endothelial (cell) D75.89
  salivary gland (any) K11.1
  Schimmelbusch's — *see* Mastopathy, cystic
  suprarenal capsule (gland) E27.8
  thymus (gland) (persistent) E32.0
  thyroid (gland) — *see* Goiter
  tonsils (faucial) (infective) (lingual) (lymphoid) J35.1
    with adenoids J35.3
  unilateral condylar M27.8
  uterus, uterine N85.2
    endometrium (glandular) (*see also* Hyperplasia, endometrial) N85.00
  vulva N90.6
    epithelial N90.3

Hyperpnea — *see* Hyperventilation
Hyperpotassemia E87.5
Hyperprebetalipoproteinemia (familial) E78.1
Hyperprolactinemia E22.1
Hyperprolinemia (type I) (type II) E72.59
Hyperproteinemia E88.09
Hyperprothrombinemia, causing coagulation factor deficiency D68.4
Hyperpyrexia R50.9
  heat (effects) T67.0 ☑
  malignant, due to anesthetic T88.3 ☑
  rheumatic — *see* Fever, rheumatic
  unknown origin R50.9
Hyper-reflexia R29.2
Hypersalivation K11.7
Hypersecretion
  ACTH (not associated with Cushing's syndrome) E27.0
    pituitary E24.0
  adrenaline E27.5
  adrenomedullary E27.5
  androgen (testicular) E29.0
    ovarian (drug-induced) (iatrogenic) E28.1
  calcitonin E07.0
  catecholamine E27.5
  corticoadrenal E24.9
  cortisol E24.9
  epinephrine E27.5
  estrogen E28.0
  gastric K31.89
    psychogenic F45.8
  gastrin E16.4
  glucagon E16.3
  hormone(s)
    ACTH (not associated with Cushing's syndrome) E27.0
      pituitary E24.0
    antidiuretic E22.2
    growth E22.0
    intestinal NEC E34.1
    ovarian androgen E28.1
    pituitary E22.9
    testicular E29.0
    thyroid stimulating E05.80
      with thyroid storm E05.81
  insulin — *see* Hyperinsulinism
  lacrimal glands — *see* Epiphora
  medulloadrenal E27.5
  milk O92.6
  ovarian androgens E28.1
  salivary gland (any) K11.7
  thyrocalcitonin E07.0
  upper respiratory J39.8
Hypersegmentation, leukocytic, hereditary D72.0
Hypersensitive, hypersensitiveness, hypersensitivity (*see also* Allergy)
  carotid sinus G90.01
  colon — *see* Irritable, colon
  drug T88.7 ☑
  gastrointestinal K52.2
    psychogenic F45.8
  labyrinth — *see* subcategory H83.2 ☑
  pain R20.8
  pneumonitis — *see* Pneumonitis, allergic
  reaction T78.40 ☑
    upper respiratory tract NEC J39.3
Hypersomnia (organic) G47.10
  due to
    alcohol
      abuse F10.182
      dependence F10.282
      use F10.982
    amphetamines
      abuse F15.182
      dependence F15.282
      use F15.982
    caffeine
      abuse F15.182
      dependence F15.282
      use F15.982
    cocaine
      abuse F14.182
      dependence F14.282
      use F14.982
    drug NEC
      abuse F19.182
      dependence F19.282
      use F19.982
    medical condition G47.14

☑ **Additional Character Required** — Refer to the Tabular List for Character Selection   🔻 **Subterms under main terms may continue to next column or page**

Hypersomnia — continued
 due to — continued
  mental disorder F51.13
  opioid
   abuse F11.182
   dependence F11.282
   use F11.982
  psychoactive substance NEC
   abuse F19.182
   dependence F19.282
   use F19.982
  sedative, hypnotic, or anxiolytic
   abuse F13.182
   dependence F13.282
   use F13.982
  stimulant NEC
   abuse F15.182
   dependence F15.282
   use F15.982
 idiopathic G47.11
  with long sleep time G47.11
  without long sleep time G47.12
 menstrual related G47.13
 nonorganic origin F51.11
  specified NEC F51.19
 not due to a substance or known physiological condition F51.11
  specified NEC F51.19
 primary F51.11
 recurrent G47.13
 specified NEC G47.19
Hypersplenia, hypersplenism D73.1
Hyperstimulation, ovaries (associated with induced ovulation) N98.1
Hypersusceptibility — see Allergy
Hypertelorism (ocular) (orbital) Q75.2
Hypertension, hypertensive (accelerated) (benign) (essential) (idiopathic) (malignant) (systemic) I10
 with
  heart involvement (conditions in I51.4 - I51.9 due to hypertension) — see Hypertension, heart
  kidney involvement — see Hypertension, kidney
 benign, intracranial G93.2
 borderline R03.0
 cardiorenal (disease) I13.10
  with heart failure I13.0
   with stage 1 through stage 4 chronic kidney disease I13.0
   with stage 5 or end stage renal disease I13.2
  without heart failure I13.10
   with stage 1 through stage 4 chronic kidney disease I13.10
   with stage 5 or end stage renal disease I13.11
 cardiovascular
  disease (arteriosclerotic) (sclerotic) — see Hypertension, heart
  renal (disease) — see Hypertension, cardiorenal
 chronic venous — see Hypertension, venous (chronic)
 complicating
  childbirth (labor) O10.92
   with
    heart disease O10.12
     with renal disease O10.32
    renal disease O10.22
     with heart disease O10.32
   essential O10.02
   secondary O10.42
  pregnancy O16.- ☑
   with edema (see also Pre-eclampsia) O14.9- ☑
   gestational (pregnancy induced) (transient) (without proteinuria) O13.- ☑
   with proteinuria O14.9- ☑
    mild pre-eclampsia O14.0- ☑
    moderate pre-eclampsia O14.0- ☑
    severe pre-eclampsia O14.1- ☑
     with hemolysis, elevated liver enzymes and low platelet count (HELLP) O14.2- ☑
   pre-existing O10.91- ☑
    with
     heart disease O10.11- ☑
      with renal disease O10.31- ☑
     pre-eclampsia O11.- ☑
     renal disease O10.21- ☑
      with heart disease O10.31- ☑
    essential O10.01- ☑
    secondary O10.41- ☑

Hypertension, hypertensive — continued
 complicating — continued
  puerperium, pre-existing O10.93
   with
    heart disease O10.13
     with renal disease O10.33
    renal disease O10.23
     with heart disease O10.33
   essential O10.03
   pregnancy-induced O13.9
   secondary O10.43
 due to
  endocrine disorders I15.2
  pheochromocytoma I15.2
  renal disorders NEC I15.1
   arterial I15.0
  renovascular disorders I15.0
  specified disease NEC I15.8
 encephalopathy I67.4
 gestational (without significant proteinuria) (pregnancy-induced) (transient) O13.- ☑
  with significant proteinuria — see Pre-eclampsia
 Goldblatt's I70.1
 heart (disease) (conditions in I51.4-I51.9 due to hypertension) I11.9
  with
   heart failure (congestive) I11.0
   kidney disease (chronic) — see Hypertension, cardiorenal
 intracranial (benign) G93.2
 kidney I12.9
  with
   heart disease — see Hypertension, cardiorenal
   stage 1 through stage 4 chronic kidney disease I12.9
   stage 5 chronic kidney disease (CKD) or end stage renal disease (ESRD) I12.0
 lesser circulation I27.0
 newborn P29.2
  pulmonary (persistent) P29.3
 ocular H40.05- ☑
 pancreatic duct — code to underlying condition
  with chronic pancreatitis K86.1
 portal (due to chronic liver disease) (idiopathic) K76.6
  gastropathy K31.89
  in (due to) schistosomiasis (bilharziasis) B65.9 [K77]
 postoperative I97.3
 psychogenic F45.8
 pulmonary (artery) (secondary) NEC I27.2
  with
   cor pulmonale (chronic) I27.2
    acute I26.09
   right heart ventricular strain/failure I27.2
    acute I26.09
  of newborn (persistent) P29.3
  primary (idiopathic) I27.0
 renal — see Hypertension, kidney
 renovascular I15.0
 secondary NEC I15.9
  due to
   endocrine disorders I15.2
   pheochromocytoma I15.2
   renal disorders NEC I15.1
    arterial I15.0
   renovascular disorders I15.0
  specified NEC I15.8
 venous (chronic)
  due to
   deep vein thrombosis — see Syndrome, post-thrombotic
  idiopathic I87.309
   with
    inflammation I87.32- ☑
     with ulcer I87.33- ☑
    specified complication NEC I87.39- ☑
    ulcer I87.31- ☑
     with inflammation I87.33- ☑
    asymptomatic I87.30- ☑
Hypertensive urgency — see Hypertension
Hyperthecosis ovary E28.8
Hyperthermia (of unknown origin) (see also Hyperpyrexia)
 malignant, due to anesthesia T88.3 ☑
 newborn P81.9
  environmental P81.0
Hyperthyroid (recurrent) — see Hyperthyroidism

Hyperthyroidism (latent) (pre-adult) (recurrent) E05.90
 with
  goiter (diffuse) E05.00
   with thyroid storm E05.01
   nodular (multinodular) E05.20
    with thyroid storm E05.21
    uninodular E05.10
     with thyroid storm E05.11
  storm E05.91
 due to ectopic thyroid tissue E05.30
  with thyroid storm E05.31
 neonatal, transitory P72.1
 specified NEC E05.80
  with thyroid storm E05.81
Hypertony, hypertonia, hypertonicity
 bladder N31.8
 congenital P94.1
 stomach K31.89
  psychogenic F45.8
 uterus, uterine (contractions) (complicating delivery) O62.4
Hypertrichosis L68.9
 congenital Q84.2
 eyelid H02.869
  left H02.866
   lower H02.865
   upper H02.864
  right H02.863
   lower H02.862
   upper H02.861
 lanuginosa Q84.2
  acquired L68.1
 localized L68.2
 specified NEC L68.8
Hypertriglyceridemia, essential E78.1
Hypertrophy, hypertrophic
 adenofibromatous, prostate — see Enlargement, enlarged, prostate
 adenoids (infective) J35.2
  with tonsils J35.3
 adrenal cortex E27.8
 alveolar process or ridge — see Anomaly, alveolar
 anal papillae K62.89
 artery I77.89
  congenital NEC Q27.8
   digestive system Q27.8
   lower limb Q27.8
   specified site NEC Q27.8
   upper limb Q27.8
 auricular — see Hypertrophy, cardiac
 Bartholin's gland N75.8
 bile duct (common) (hepatic) K83.8
 bladder (sphincter) (trigone) N32.89
 bone M89.30
  carpus M89.34- ☑
  clavicle M89.31- ☑
  femur M89.35- ☑
  fibula M89.36- ☑
  finger M89.34- ☑
  humerus M89.32- ☑
  ilium M89.359
  ischium M89.359
  metacarpus M89.34- ☑
  metatarsus M89.37- ☑
  multiple sites M89.39
  neck M89.38
  radius M89.33- ☑
  rib M89.38
  scapula M89.31- ☑
  skull M89.38
  tarsus M89.37- ☑
  tibia M89.36- ☑
  toe M89.37- ☑
  ulna M89.33- ☑
  vertebra M89.38
 brain G93.89
 breast N62
  cystic — see Mastopathy, cystic
  newborn P83.4
  pubertal, massive N62
  puerperal, postpartum — see Disorder, breast, specified type NEC
  senile (parenchymatous) N62
 cardiac (chronic) (idiopathic) I51.7
  with rheumatic fever (conditions in I00)
   active I01.8
   inactive or quiescent (with chorea) I09.89
  congenital NEC Q24.8

⬚ Subterms under main terms may continue to next column or page　　　☑ Additional Character Required — Refer to the Tabular List for Character Selection　　　169

Hypersomnia — Hypertrophy, hypertrophic

Hypertrophy, hypertrophic — *continued*
cardiac — *continued*
  fatty — *see* Degeneration, myocardial
  hypertensive — *see* Hypertension, heart
  rheumatic (with chorea) I09.89
    active or acute I01.8
      with chorea I02.0
  valve — *see* Endocarditis
cartilage — *see* Disorder, cartilage, specified type NEC
cecum — *see* Megacolon
cervix (uteri) N88.8
  congenital Q51.828
  elongation N88.4
clitoris (cirrhotic) N90.89
  congenital Q52.6
colon (*see also* Megacolon)
  congenital Q43.2
conjunctiva, lymphoid H11.89
corpora cavernosa N48.89
cystic duct K82.8
duodenum K31.89
endometrium (glandular) (*see also* Hyperplasia, endometrial) N85.00
  cervix N88.8
epididymis N50.8
esophageal hiatus (congenital) Q79.1
  with hernia — *see* Hernia, hiatal
eyelid — *see* Disorder, eyelid, specified type NEC
fat pad E65
  knee (infrapatellar) (popliteal) (prepatellar) (retropatellar) M79.4
foot (congenital) Q74.2
frenulum, frenum (tongue) K14.8
  lip K13.0
gallbladder K82.8
gastric mucosa K29.60
  with bleeding K29.61
gland, glandular R59.9
  generalized R59.1
  localized R59.0
gum (mucous membrane) K06.1
heart (idiopathic) (*see also* Hypertrophy, cardiac)
  valve (*see also* Endocarditis) I38
hemifacial Q67.4
hepatic — *see* Hypertrophy, liver
hiatus (esophageal) Q79.1
hilus gland R59.0
hymen, congenital Q52.4
ileum K63.89
intestine NEC K63.89
jejunum K63.89
kidney (compensatory) N28.81
  congenital Q63.3
labium (majus) (minus) N90.6
ligament — *see* Disorder, ligament
lingual tonsil (infective) J35.1
  with adenoids J35.3
lip K13.0
  congenital Q18.6
liver R16.0
  acute K76.89
  cirrhotic — *see* Cirrhosis, liver
  congenital Q44.7
  fatty — *see* Fatty, liver
lymph, lymphatic gland R59.9
  generalized R59.1
  localized R59.0
  tuberculous — *see* Tuberculosis, lymph gland
mammary gland — *see* Hypertrophy, breast
Meckel's diverticulum (congenital) Q43.0
  malignant — *see* Table of Neoplasms, small intestine, malignant
median bar — *see* Hyperplasia, prostate
meibomian gland — *see* Chalazion
meniscus, knee, congenital Q74.1
metatarsal head — *see* Hypertrophy, bone, metatarsus
metatarsus — *see* Hypertrophy, bone, metatarsus
mucous membrane
  alveolar ridge K06.2
  gum K06.1
  nose (turbinate) J34.3
muscle M62.89
muscular coat, artery I77.89
myocardium (*see also* Hypertrophy, cardiac)
  idiopathic I42.2
myometrium N85.2
nail L60.2
  congenital Q84.5

Hypertrophy, hypertrophic — *continued*
nasal J34.89
  alae J34.89
  bone J34.89
  cartilage J34.89
  mucous membrane (septum) J34.3
  sinus J34.89
  turbinate J34.3
nasopharynx, lymphoid (infectional) (tissue) (wall) J35.2
nipple N62
organ or site, congenital NEC — *see* Anomaly, by site
ovary N83.8
palate (hard) M27.8
  soft K13.79
pancreas, congenital Q45.3
parathyroid (gland) E21.0
parotid gland K11.1
penis N48.89
pharyngeal tonsil J35.2
pharynx J39.2
  lymphoid (infectional) (tissue) (wall) J35.2
pituitary (anterior) (fossa) (gland) E23.6
prepuce (congenital) N47.8
  female N90.89
prostate — *see* Enlargement, enlarged, prostate
  congenital Q55.4
pseudomuscular G71.0
pylorus (adult) (muscle) (sphincter) K31.1
  congenital or infantile Q40.0
rectal, rectum (sphincter) K62.89
rhinitis (turbinate) J31.0
salivary gland (any) K11.1
  congenital Q38.4
scaphoid (tarsal) — *see* Hypertrophy, bone, tarsus
scar L91.0
scrotum N50.8
seminal vesicle N50.8
sigmoid — *see* Megacolon
skin L91.9
  specified NEC L91.8
spermatic cord N50.8
spleen — *see* Splenomegaly
spondylitis — *see* Spondylosis
stomach K31.89
sublingual gland K11.1
submandibular gland K11.1
suprarenal cortex (gland) E27.8
synovial NEC M67.20
  acromioclavicular M67.21- ☑
  ankle M67.27- ☑
  elbow M67.22- ☑
  foot M67.27- ☑
  hand M67.24- ☑
  hip M67.25- ☑
  knee M67.26- ☑
  multiple sites M67.29
  specified site NEC M67.28
  wrist M67.23- ☑
tendon — *see* Disorder, tendon, specified type NEC
testis N44.8
  congenital Q55.29
thymic, thymus (gland) (congenital) E32.0
thyroid (gland) — *see* Goiter
toe (congenital) Q74.2
  acquired (*see also* Deformity, toe, specified NEC)
tongue K14.8
  congenital Q38.2
  papillae (foliate) K14.3
tonsils (faucial) (infective) (lingual) (lymphoid) J35.1
  with adenoids J35.3
tunica vaginalis N50.8
ureter N28.89
urethra N36.8
uterus N85.2
  neck (with elongation) N88.4
  puerperal O90.89
uvula K13.79
vagina N89.8
vas deferens N50.8
vein I87.8
ventricle, ventricular (heart) (*see also* Hypertrophy, cardiac)
  congenital Q24.8
  in tetralogy of Fallot Q21.3
verumontanum N36.8
vocal cord J38.3

Hypertrophy, hypertrophic — *continued*
vulva N90.6
  stasis (nonfilarial) N90.6
Hypertropia H50.2- ☑
Hypertyrosinemia E70.21
Hyperuricemia (asymptomatic) E79.0
Hypervalinemia E71.19
Hyperventilation (tetany) R06.4
  hysterical F45.8
  psychogenic F45.8
  syndrome F45.8
Hypervitaminosis (dietary) NEC E67.8
  A E67.0
    administered as drug (prolonged intake) — *see* Table of Drugs and Chemicals, vitamins, adverse effect
    overdose or wrong substance given or taken — *see* Table of Drugs and Chemicals, vitamins, poisoning
  B6 E67.2
  D E67.3
    administered as drug (prolonged intake) — *see* Table of Drugs and Chemicals, vitamins, adverse effect
    overdose or wrong substance given or taken — *see* Table of Drugs and Chemicals, vitamins, poisoning
  K E67.8
    administered as drug (prolonged intake) — *see* Table of Drugs and Chemicals, vitamins, adverse effect
    overdose or wrong substance given or taken — *see* Table of Drugs and Chemicals, vitamins, poisoning
Hypervolemia E87.70
  specified NEC E87.79
Hypesthesia R20.1
  cornea — *see* Anesthesia, cornea
Hyphema H21.0- ☑
  traumatic S05.1- ☑
Hypoacidity, gastric K31.89
  psychogenic F45.8
Hypoadrenalism, hypoadrenia E27.40
  primary E27.1
  tuberculous A18.7
Hypoadrenocorticism E27.40
  pituitary E23.0
  primary E27.1
Hypoalbuminemia E88.09
Hypoaldosteronism E27.40
Hypoalphalipoproteinemia E78.6
Hypobarism T70.29 ☑
Hypobaropathy T70.29 ☑
Hypobetalipoproteinemia (familial) E78.6
Hypocalcemia E83.51
  dietary E58
  neonatal P71.1
    due to cow's milk P71.0
  phosphate-loading (newborn) P71.1
Hypochloremia E87.8
Hypochlorhydria K31.89
  neurotic F45.8
  psychogenic F45.8
Hypochondria, hypochondriac, hypochondriasis (reaction) F45.21
  sleep F51.03
Hypochondrogenesis Q77.0
Hypochondroplasia Q77.4
Hypochromasia, blood cells D50.8
Hypodontia — *see* Anodontia
Hypoeosinophilia D72.89
Hypoesthesia R20.1
Hypofibrinogenemia D68.8
  acquired D65
  congenital (hereditary) D68.2
Hypofunction
  adrenocortical E27.40
    drug-induced E27.3
    postprocedural E89.6
    primary E27.1
  adrenomedullary, postprocedural E89.6
  cerebral R29.818
  corticoadrenal NEC E27.40
  intestinal K59.8
  labyrinth — *see* subcategory H83.2 ☑
  ovary E28.39
  pituitary (gland) (anterior) E23.0

Index

Hypertrophy, hypertrophic — Hypofunction

Hypofunction — *continued*
  testicular E29.1
    postprocedural (postsurgical) (postirradiation) (iatrogenic) E89.5
Hypogalactia O92.4
Hypogammaglobulinemia (*see also* Agammaglobulinemia) D80.1
  hereditary D80.0
  nonfamilial D80.1
  transient, of infancy D80.7
Hypogenitalism (congenital) — *see* Hypogonadism
Hypoglossia Q38.3
Hypoglycemia (spontaneous) E16.2
  coma E15
    diabetic — *see* Diabetes, coma
  diabetic — *see* Diabetes, hypoglycemia
  dietary counseling and surveillance Z71.3
  drug-induced E16.0
    with coma (nondiabetic) E15
  due to insulin E16.0
    with coma (nondiabetic) E15
    therapeutic misadventure — *see* subcategory T38.3 ☑
  functional, nonhyperinsulinemic E16.1
  iatrogenic E16.0
    with coma (nondiabetic) E15
  in infant of diabetic mother P70.1
    gestational diabetes P70.0
  infantile E16.1
  leucine-induced E71.19
  neonatal (transitory) P70.4
    iatrogenic P70.3
  reactive (not drug-induced) E16.1
  transitory neonatal P70.4
Hypogonadism
  female E28.39
  hypogonadotropic E23.0
  male E29.1
  ovarian (primary) E28.39
  pituitary E23.0
  testicular (primary) E29.1
Hypohidrosis, hypoidrosis L74.4
Hypoinsulinemia, postprocedural E89.1
Hypokalemia E87.6
Hypoleukocytosis — *see* Agranulocytosis
Hypolipoproteinemia (alpha) (beta) E78.6
Hypomagnesemia E83.42
  neonatal P71.2
Hypomania, hypomanic reaction F30.8
Hypomenorrhea — *see* Oligomenorrhea
Hypometabolism R63.8
Hypomotility
  gastrointestinal (tract) K31.89
    psychogenic F45.8
  intestine K59.8
    psychogenic F45.8
  stomach K31.89
    psychogenic F45.8
Hyponasality R49.22
Hyponatremia E87.1
Hypo-osmolality E87.1
Hypo-ovarianism, hypo-ovarism E28.39
Hypoparathyroidism E20.9
  familial E20.8
  idiopathic E20.0
  neonatal, transitory P71.4
  postprocedural E89.2
  specified NEC E20.8
Hypoperfusion (in)
  newborn P96.89
Hypopharyngitis — *see* Laryngopharyngitis
Hypophoria H50.53
Hypophosphatemia, hypophosphatasia (acquired) (congenital) (renal) E83.39
  familial E83.31
Hypophyseal, hypophysis (*see also* condition)
  dwarfism E23.0
  gigantism E22.0
Hypopiesis — *see* Hypotension
Hypopinealism E34.8
Hypopituitarism (juvenile) E23.0
  drug-induced E23.1
  due to
    hypophysectomy E89.3
    radiotherapy E89.3
  iatrogenic NEC E23.1
  postirradiation E89.3

Hypopituitarism — *continued*
  postpartum E23.0
  postprocedural E89.3
Hypoplasia, hypoplastic
  adrenal (gland), congenital Q89.1
  alimentary tract, congenital Q45.8
    upper Q40.8
  anus, anal (canal) Q42.3
    with fistula Q42.2
  aorta, aortic Q25.4
    ascending, in hypoplastic left heart syndrome Q23.4
    valve Q23.1
      in hypoplastic left heart syndrome Q23.4
  areola, congenital Q83.8
  arm (congenital) — *see* Defect, reduction, upper limb
  artery (peripheral) Q27.8
    brain (congenital) Q28.3
    coronary Q24.5
    digestive system Q27.8
    lower limb Q27.8
    pulmonary Q25.79
      functional, unilateral J43.0
    retinal (congenital) Q14.1
    specified site NEC Q27.8
    umbilical Q27.0
    upper limb Q27.8
  auditory canal Q17.8
    causing impairment of hearing Q16.9
  biliary duct or passage Q44.5
  bone NOS Q79.9
    face Q75.8
    marrow D61.9
      megakaryocytic D69.49
    skull — *see* Hypoplasia, skull
  brain Q02
    gyri Q04.3
    part of Q04.3
  breast (areola) N64.82
  bronchus Q32.4
  cardiac Q24.8
  carpus — *see* Defect, reduction, upper limb, specified type NEC
  cartilage hair Q78.5
  cecum Q42.8
  cementum K00.4
  cephalic Q02
  cerebellum Q04.3
  cervix (uteri), congenital Q51.821
  clavicle (congenital) Q74.0
  coccyx Q76.49
  colon Q42.9
    specified NEC Q42.8
  corpus callosum Q04.0
  cricoid cartilage Q31.2
  digestive organ(s) or tract NEC Q45.8
    upper (congenital) Q40.8
  ear (auricle) (lobe) Q17.2
    middle Q16.4
  enamel of teeth (neonatal) (postnatal) (prenatal) K00.4
  endocrine (gland) NEC Q89.2
  endometrium N85.8
  epididymis (congenital) Q55.4
  epiglottis Q31.2
  erythroid, congenital D61.01
  esophagus (congenital) Q39.8
  eustachian tube Q17.8
  eye Q11.2
  eyelid (congenital) Q10.3
  face Q18.8
    bone(s) Q75.8
  femur (congenital) — *see* Defect, reduction, lower limb, specified type NEC
  fibula (congenital) — *see* Defect, reduction, lower limb, specified type NEC
  finger (congenital) — *see* Defect, reduction, upper limb, specified type NEC
  focal dermal Q82.8
  foot — *see* Defect, reduction, lower limb, specified type NEC
  gallbladder Q44.0
  genitalia, genital organ(s)
    female, congenital Q52.8
      external Q52.79
      internal NEC Q52.8
    in adiposogenital dystrophy E23.6
  glottis Q31.2
  hair Q84.2

Hypoplasia, hypoplastic — *continued*
  hand (congenital) — *see* Defect, reduction, upper limb, specified type NEC
  heart Q24.8
  humerus (congenital) — *see* Defect, reduction, upper limb, specified type NEC
  intestine (small) Q41.9
    large Q42.9
      specified NEC Q42.8
  jaw M26.09
    alveolar M26.79
    lower M26.04
      alveolar M26.74
    upper M26.02
      alveolar M26.73
  kidney(s) Q60.5
    bilateral Q60.4
    unilateral Q60.3
  labium (majus) (minus), congenital Q52.79
  larynx Q31.2
  left heart syndrome Q23.4
  leg (congenital) — *see* Defect, reduction, lower limb
  limb Q73.8
    lower (congenital) — *see* Defect, reduction, lower limb
    upper (congenital) — *see* Defect, reduction, upper limb
  liver Q44.7
  lung (lobe) (not associated with short gestation) Q33.6
    associated with immaturity, low birth weight, prematurity, or short gestation P28.0
  mammary (areola), congenital Q83.8
  mandible, mandibular M26.04
    alveolar M26.74
    unilateral condylar M27.8
  maxillary M26.02
    alveolar M26.73
  medullary D61.9
  megakaryocytic D69.49
  metacarpus — *see* Defect, reduction, upper limb, specified type NEC
  metatarsus — *see* Defect, reduction, lower limb, specified type NEC
  muscle Q79.8
  nail(s) Q84.6
  nose, nasal Q30.1
  optic nerve H47.03- ☑
  osseous meatus (ear) Q17.8
  ovary, congenital Q50.39
  pancreas Q45.0
  parathyroid (gland) Q89.2
  parotid gland Q38.4
  patella Q74.1
  pelvis, pelvic girdle Q74.2
  penis (congenital) Q55.62
  peripheral vascular system Q27.8
    digestive system Q27.8
    lower limb Q27.8
    specified site NEC Q27.8
    upper limb Q27.8
  pituitary (gland) (congenital) Q89.2
  pulmonary (not associated with short gestation) Q33.6
    artery, functional J43.0
    associated with short gestation P28.0
  radioulnar — *see* Defect, reduction, upper limb, specified type NEC
  radius — *see* Defect, reduction, upper limb
  rectum Q42.1
    with fistula Q42.0
  respiratory system NEC Q34.8
  rib Q76.6
  right heart syndrome Q22.6
  sacrum Q76.49
  scapula Q74.0
  scrotum Q55.1
  shoulder girdle Q74.0
  skin Q82.8
  skull (bone) Q75.8
    with
      anencephaly Q00.0
      encephalocele — *see* Encephalocele
      hydrocephalus Q03.9
        with spina bifida — *see* Spina bifida, by site, with hydrocephalus
      microcephaly Q02
  spinal (cord) (ventral horn cell) Q06.1
  spine Q76.49
  sternum Q76.7

Hypoplasia, hypoplastic — *continued*
  tarsus — *see* Defect, reduction, lower limb, specified type NEC
  testis Q55.1
  thymic, with immunodeficiency D82.1
  thymus (gland) Q89.2
    with immunodeficiency D82.1
  thyroid (gland) E03.1
    cartilage Q31.2
  tibiofibular (congenital) — *see* Defect, reduction, lower limb, specified type NEC
  toe — *see* Defect, reduction, lower limb, specified type NEC
  tongue Q38.3
  Turner's K00.4
  ulna (congenital) — *see* Defect, reduction, upper limb
  umbilical artery Q27.0
  unilateral condylar M27.8
  ureter Q62.8
  uterus, congenital Q51.811
  vagina Q52.4
  vascular NEC peripheral Q27.8
    brain Q28.3
    digestive system Q27.8
    lower limb Q27.8
    specified site NEC Q27.8
    upper limb Q27.8
  vein(s) (peripheral) Q27.8
    brain Q28.3
    digestive system Q27.8
    great Q26.8
    lower limb Q27.8
    specified site NEC Q27.8
    upper limb Q27.8
  vena cava (inferior) (superior) Q26.8
  vertebra Q76.49
  vulva, congenital Q52.79
  zonule (ciliary) Q12.8
Hypopotassemia E87.6
Hypoproconvertinemia, congenital (hereditary) D68.2
Hypoproteinemia E77.8
Hypoprothrombinemia (congenital) (hereditary) (idiopathic) D68.2
  acquired D68.4
  newborn, transient P61.6
Hypoptyalism K11.7
Hypopyon (eye) (anterior chamber) — *see* Iridocyclitis, acute, hypopyon
Hypopyrexia R68.0
Hyporeflexia R29.2
Hyposecretion
  ACTH E23.0
  antidiuretic hormone E23.2
  ovary E28.39
  salivary gland (any) K11.7
  vasopressin E23.2
Hyposegmentation, leukocytic, hereditary D72.0
Hyposiderinemia D50.9
Hypospadias Q54.9
  balanic Q54.0
  coronal Q54.0
  glandular Q54.0
  penile Q54.1
  penoscrotal Q54.2
  perineal Q54.3
  specified NEC Q54.8
Hypospermatogenesis — *see* Oligospermia
Hyposplenism D73.0
Hypostasis pulmonary, passive — *see* Edema, lung
Hypostatic — *see* condition
Hyposthenuria N28.89
Hypotension (arterial) (constitutional) I95.9
  chronic I95.89
  drug-induced I95.2
  due to (of) hemodialysis I95.3
  iatrogenic I95.89
  idiopathic (permanent) I95.0
  intracranial, following ventricular shunting (ventriculostomy) G97.2
  intra-dialytic I95.3
  maternal, syndrome (following labor and delivery) O26.5- ☑
  neurogenic, orthostatic G90.3
  orthostatic (chronic) I95.1
    due to drugs I95.2
    neurogenic G90.3
  postoperative I95.81
  postural I95.1

Hypotension — *continued*
  specified NEC I95.89
Hypothermia (accidental) T68 ☑
  due to anesthesia, anesthetic T88.51 ☑
  low environmental temperature T68 ☑
  neonatal P80.9
    environmental (mild) NEC P80.8
    mild P80.8
    severe (chronic) (cold injury syndrome) P80.0
    specified NEC P80.8
  not associated with low environmental temperature R68.0
Hypothyroidism (acquired) E03.9
  congenital (without goiter) E03.1
    with goiter (diffuse) E03.0
  due to
    exogenous substance NEC E03.2
    iodine-deficiency, acquired E01.8
      subclinical E02
    irradiation therapy E89.0
    medicament NEC E03.2
    P-aminosalicylic acid (PAS) E03.2
    phenylbutazone E03.2
    resorcinol E03.2
    sulfonamide E03.2
    surgery E89.0
    thiourea group drugs E03.2
  iatrogenic NEC E03.2
  iodine-deficiency (acquired) E01.8
    congenital — *see* Syndrome, iodine- deficiency, congenital
    subclinical E02
  neonatal, transitory P72.2
  postinfectious E03.3
  postirradiation E89.0
  postprocedural E89.0
  postsurgical E89.0
  specified NEC E03.8
  subclinical, iodine-deficiency related E02
Hypotonia, hypotonicity, hypotony
  bladder N31.2
  congenital (benign) P94.2
  eye — *see* Disorder, globe, hypotony
Hypotrichosis — *see* Alopecia
Hypotropia H50.2- ☑
Hypoventilation R06.89
  congenital central alveolar G47.35
  sleep related
    idiopathic nonobstructive alveolar G47.34
    in conditions classified elsewhere G47.36
Hypovitaminosis — *see* Deficiency, vitamin
Hypovolemia E86.1
  surgical shock T81.19 ☑
  traumatic (shock) T79.4 ☑
Hypoxemia R09.02
  newborn P84
  sleep related, in conditions classified elsewhere G47.36
Hypoxia (*see also* Anoxia) R09.02
  cerebral, during a procedure NEC G97.81
    postprocedural NEC G97.82
  intrauterine P84
  myocardial — *see* Insufficiency, coronary
  newborn P84
  sleep-related G47.34
Hypsarrhythmia — *see* Epilepsy, generalized, specified NEC
Hysteralgia, pregnant uterus O26.89- ☑
Hysteria, hysterical (conversion) (dissociative state) F44.9
  anxiety F41.8
  convulsions F44.5
  psychosis, acute F44.9
Hysteroepilepsy F44.5

I

Ichthyoparasitism due to Vandellia cirrhosa B88.8
Ichthyosis (congenital) Q80.9
  acquired L85.0
  fetalis Q80.4
  hystrix Q80.8
  lamellar Q80.2
  lingual K13.29
  palmaris and plantaris Q82.8
  simplex Q80.0
  vera Q80.8
  vulgaris Q80.0

Ichthyosis — *continued*
  X-linked Q80.1
Ichthyotoxism — *see* Poisoning, fish
  bacterial — *see* Intoxication, foodborne
Icteroanemia, hemolytic (acquired) D59.9
  congenital — *see* Spherocytosis
Icterus (*see also* Jaundice)
  conjunctiva R17
  gravis, newborn P55.0
  hematogenous (acquired) D59.9
  hemolytic (acquired) D59.9
    congenital — *see* Spherocytosis
  hemorrhagic (acute) (leptospiral) (spirochetal) A27.0
    newborn P53
  infectious B15.9
    with hepatic coma B15.0
    leptospiral A27.0
    spirochetal A27.0
  neonatorum — *see* Jaundice, newborn
  newborn P59.9
  spirochetal A27.0
Ictus solaris, solis T67.0 ☑
Id reaction (due to bacteria) L30.2
Ideation
  homicidal R45.850
  suicidal R45.851
Identity disorder (child) F64.9
  gender role F64.2
  psychosexual F64.2
Idioglossia F80.0
Idiopathic — *see* condition
Idiot, idiocy (congenital) F73
  amaurotic (Bielschowsky(-Jansky)) (family) (infantile (late)) (Juvenile (late)) (Vogt-Spielmeyer) E75.4
  microcephalic Q02
IgE asthma J45.909
IIAC (idiopathic infantile arterial calcification) Q28.8
Ileitis (chronic) (noninfectious) (*see also* Enteritis) K52.9
  backwash — *see* Pancolitis, ulcerative (chronic)
  infectious A09
  regional (ulcerative) — *see* Enteritis, regional, small intestine
  segmental — *see* Enteritis, regional
  terminal (ulcerative) — *see* Enteritis, regional, small intestine
Ileocolitis (*see also* Enteritis) K52.9
  infectious A09
  regional — *see* Enteritis, regional
Ileostomy
  attention to Z43.2
  malfunctioning K94.13
  status Z93.2
    with complication — *see* Complications, enterostomy
Ileotyphus — *see* Typhoid
Ileum — *see* condition
Ileus (bowel) (colon) (inhibitory) (intestine) K56.7
  adynamic K56.0
  due to gallstone (in intestine) K56.3
  duodenal (chronic) K31.5
  gallstone K56.3
  mechanical NEC K56.69
  meconium P76.0
    in cystic fibrosis E84.11
    meaning meconium plug (without cystic fibrosis) P76.0
  myxedema K59.8
  neurogenic K56.0
    Hirschsprung's disease or megacolon Q43.1
  newborn
    due to meconium P76.0
      in cystic fibrosis E84.11
      meaning meconium plug (without cystic fibrosis) P76.0
    transitory P76.1
  obstructive K56.69
  paralytic K56.0
Iliac — *see* condition
Iliotibial band syndrome M76.3- ☑
Illiteracy Z55.0
Illness (*see also* Disease) R69
  manic-depressive — *see* Disorder, bipolar
Imbalance R26.89
  autonomic G90.8
  constituents of food intake E63.1
  electrolyte E87.8

Imbalance — continued
- electrolyte — continued
  - with
    - abortion — see Abortion by type, complicated by, electrolyte imbalance
    - molar pregnancy O08.8
  - due to hyperemesis gravidarum O21.1
  - following ectopic or molar pregnancy O08.5
  - neonatal, transitory NEC P74.4
    - potassium P74.3
    - sodium P74.2
- endocrine E34.9
- eye muscle NOS H50.9
- hormone E34.9
- hysterical F44.4
- labyrinth — see subcategory H83.2 ☑
- posture R29.3
- protein-energy — see Malnutrition
- sympathetic G90.8

Imbecile, imbecility (I.Q. 35-49) F71
Imbedding, intrauterine device T83.39 ☑
Imbibition, cholesterol (gallbladder) K82.4
Imbrication, teeth,, fully erupted M26.30
Imerslund (-Gräsbeck) **syndrome** D51.1
Immature (see also Immaturity)
- birth (less than 37 completed weeks) — see Preterm, newborn
  - extremely (less than 28 completed weeks) — see Immaturity, extreme
- personality F60.89

Immaturity (less than 37 completed weeks) (see also Preterm, newborn)
- extreme of newborn (less than 28 completed weeks) (less than 196 completed days of gestation) (unspecified weeks of gestation) P07.20
  - gestational age
    - less than 23 completed weeks P07.21
    - 23 completed weeks (23 weeks, 0 days through 23 weeks, 6 days) P07.22
    - 24 completed weeks (24 weeks, 0 days through 24 weeks, 6 days) P07.23
    - 25 completed weeks (25 weeks, 0 days through 25 weeks, 6 days) P07.24
    - 26 completed weeks (26 weeks, 0 days through 26 weeks, 6 days) P07.25
    - 27 completed weeks (27 weeks, 0 days through 27 weeks, 6 days) P07.26
- fetus or infant light-for-dates — see Light-for-dates
- lung, newborn P28.0
- organ or site NEC — see Hypoplasia
- pulmonary, newborn P28.0
- reaction F60.89
- sexual (female) (male), after puberty E30.0

Immersion T75.1 ☑
- foot T69.02- ☑
- hand T69.01- ☑

Immobile, immobility
- complete, due to severe physical disability or frailty R53.2
- intestine K59.8
- syndrome (paraplegic) M62.3

Immune reconstitution (inflammatory) syndrome [IRIS] D89.3
Immunization (see also Vaccination)
- ABO — see Incompatibility, ABO
  - in newborn P55.1
- complication — see Complications, vaccination
- encounter for Z23
- not done (not carried out) Z28.9
  - because (of)
    - acute illness of patient Z28.01
    - allergy to vaccine (or component) Z28.04
    - caregiver refusal Z28.82
    - chronic illness of patient Z28.02
    - contraindication NEC Z28.09
    - group pressure Z28.1
    - guardian refusal Z28.82
    - immune compromised state of patient Z28.03
    - parent refusal Z28.82
    - patient had disease being vaccinated against Z28.81
    - patient refusal Z28.21
    - patient's belief Z28.1
    - religious beliefs of patient Z28.1
    - specified reason NEC Z28.89
      - of patient Z28.29
    - unspecified patient reason Z28.20

Immunization — continued
- Rh factor
  - affecting management of pregnancy NEC O36.09- ☑
    - anti-D antibody O36.01- ☑
  - from transfusion — see Complication(s), transfusion, incompatibility reaction, Rh (factor)
Immunocytoma C83.0- ☑
Immunodeficiency D84.9
- with
  - adenosine-deaminase deficiency D81.3
  - antibody defects D80.9
    - specified type NEC D80.8
  - hyperimmunoglobulinemia D80.6
  - increased immunoglobulin M (IgM) D80.5
  - major defect D82.9
    - specified type NEC D82.8
  - partial albinism D82.8
  - short-limbed stature D82.2
  - thrombocytopenia and eczema D82.0
- antibody with
  - hyperimmunoglobulinemia D80.6
  - near-normal immunoglobulins D80.6
- autosomal recessive, Swiss type D80.0
- combined D81.9
  - biotin-dependent carboxylase D81.819
    - biotinidase D81.810
    - holocarboxylase synthetase D81.818
    - specified type NEC D81.818
  - severe (SCID) D81.9
    - with
      - low or normal B-cell numbers D81.2
      - low T- and B-cell numbers D81.1
      - reticular dysgenesis D81.0
  - specified type NEC D81.89
- common variable D83.9
  - with
    - abnormalities of B-cell numbers and function D83.0
    - autoantibodies to B- or T-cells D83.2
    - immunoregulatory T-cell disorders D83.1
  - specified type NEC D83.8
- following hereditary defective response to Epstein-Barr virus (EBV) D82.3
- selective, immunoglobulin
  - A (IgA) D80.2
  - G (IgG) (subclasses) D80.3
  - M (IgM) D80.4
- severe combined (SCID) D81.9
- specified type NEC D84.8
- X-linked, with increased IgM D80.5
Immunotherapy (encounter for)
- antineoplastic Z51.12
Impaction, impacted
- bowel, colon, rectum (see also Impaction, fecal) K56.49
  - by gallstone K56.3
- calculus — see Calculus
- cerumen (ear) (external) H61.2- ☑
- cuspid — see Impaction, tooth
- dental (same or adjacent tooth) K01.1
- fecal, feces K56.41
- fracture — see Fracture, by site
- gallbladder — see Calculus, gallbladder
- gallstone(s) — see Calculus, gallbladder
  - bile duct (common) (hepatic) — see Calculus, bile duct
  - cystic duct — see Calculus, gallbladder
  - in intestine, with obstruction (any part) K56.3
- intestine (calculous) NEC (see also Impaction, fecal) K56.49
  - gallstone, with ileus K56.3
- intrauterine device (IUD) T83.39 ☑
- molar — see Impaction, tooth
- shoulder, causing obstructed labor O66.0
- tooth, teeth K01.1
- turbinate J34.89
Impaired, impairment (function)
- auditory discrimination — see Abnormal, auditory perception
- cognitive, mild, so stated G31.84
- dual sensory Z73.82
- fasting glucose R73.01
- glucose tolerance (oral) R73.02
- hearing — see Deafness
- heart — see Disease, heart
- kidney N28.9
  - disorder resulting from N25.9
    - specified NEC N25.89

Impaired, impairment — continued
- liver K72.90
  - with coma K72.91
- mastication K08.8
- mild cognitive, so stated G31.84
- mobility
  - ear ossicles — see Ankylosis, ear ossicles
  - requiring care provider Z74.09
- myocardium, myocardial — see Insufficiency, myocardial
- rectal sphincter R19.8
- renal (acute) (chronic) N28.9
  - disorder resulting from N25.9
    - specified NEC N25.89
- vision NEC H54.7
  - both eyes H54.3
Impediment, speech R47.9
- psychogenic (childhood) F98.8
- slurring R47.81
- specified NEC R47.89
Impending
- coronary syndrome I20.0
- delirium tremens F10.239
- myocardial infarction I20.0
Imperception auditory (acquired) (see also Deafness)
- congenital H93.25
Imperfect
- aeration, lung (newborn) NEC — see Atelectasis
- closure (congenital)
  - alimentary tract NEC Q45.8
    - lower Q43.8
    - upper Q40.8
  - atrioventricular ostium Q21.2
  - atrium (secundum) Q21.1
  - branchial cleft or sinus Q18.0
  - choroid Q14.3
  - cricoid cartilage Q31.8
  - cusps, heart valve NEC Q24.8
    - pulmonary Q22.3
  - ductus
    - arteriosus Q25.0
    - Botalli Q25.0
  - ear drum (causing impairment of hearing) Q16.4
  - esophagus with communication to bronchus or trachea Q39.1
  - eyelid Q10.3
  - foramen
    - botalli Q21.1
    - ovale Q21.1
  - genitalia, genital organ(s) or system
    - female Q52.8
      - external Q52.79
      - internal NEC Q52.8
    - male Q55.8
  - glottis Q31.8
  - interatrial ostium or septum Q21.1
  - interauricular ostium or septum Q21.1
  - interventricular ostium or septum Q21.0
  - larynx Q31.8
  - lip — see Cleft, lip
  - nasal septum Q30.3
  - nose Q30.2
  - omphalomesenteric duct Q43.0
  - optic nerve entry Q14.2
  - organ or site not listed — see Anomaly, by site
  - ostium
    - interatrial Q21.1
    - interauricular Q21.1
    - interventricular Q21.0
  - palate — see Cleft, palate
  - preauricular sinus Q18.1
  - retina Q14.1
  - roof of orbit Q75.8
  - sclera Q13.5
  - septum
    - aorticopulmonary Q21.4
    - atrial (secundum) Q21.1
    - between aorta and pulmonary artery Q21.4
    - heart Q21.9
    - interatrial (secundum) Q21.1
    - interauricular (secundum) Q21.1
    - interventricular Q21.0
      - in tetralogy of Fallot Q21.3
    - nasal Q30.3
    - ventricular Q21.0
      - with pulmonary stenosis or atresia, dextraposition of aorta, and hypertrophy of right ventricle Q21.3

Imperfect — *continued*
  closure — *continued*
    septum — *continued*
      ventricular — *continued*
        in tetralogy of Fallot Q21.3
      skull Q75.0
        with
          anencephaly Q00.0
          encephalocele — *see* Encephalocele
          hydrocephalus Q03.9
            with spina bifida — *see* Spina bifida, by
              site, with hydrocephalus
          microcephaly Q02
      spine (with meningocele) — *see* Spina bifida
      trachea Q32.1
      tympanic membrane (causing impairment of
        hearing) Q16.4
      uterus Q51.818
      vitelline duct Q43.0
    erection — *see* Dysfunction, sexual, male, erectile
    fusion — *see* Imperfect, closure
    inflation, lung (newborn) — *see* Atelectasis
    posture R29.3
    rotation, intestine Q43.3
    septum, ventricular Q21.0
Imperfectly descended testis — *see* Cryptorchid
Imperforate (congenital) (*see also* Atresia)
  anus Q42.3
    with fistula Q42.2
  cervix (uteri) Q51.828
  esophagus Q39.0
    with tracheoesophageal fistula Q39.1
  hymen Q52.3
  jejunum Q41.1
  pharynx Q38.8
  rectum Q42.1
    with fistula Q42.0
  urethra Q64.39
  vagina Q52.4
Impervious (congenital) (*see also* Atresia)
  anus Q42.3
    with fistula Q42.2
  bile duct Q44.2
  esophagus Q39.0
    with tracheoesophageal fistula Q39.1
  intestine (small) Q41.9
    large Q42.9
      specified NEC Q42.8
  rectum Q42.1
    with fistula Q42.0
  ureter — *see* Atresia, ureter
  urethra Q64.39
Impetiginization of dermatoses L01.1
Impetigo (any organism) (any site) (circinate) (contagiosa) (simplex) (vulgaris) L01.00
  Bockhart's L01.02
  bullous, bullosa L01.03
  external ear L01.00 [H62.40]
  follicularis L01.02
  furfuracea L30.5
  herpetiformis L40.1
    nonobstetrical L40.1
  neonatorum L01.03
  nonbullous L01.01
  specified type NEC L01.09
  ulcerative L01.09
Impingement (on teeth)
  soft tissue
    anterior M26.81
    posterior M26.82
Implant, endometrial N80.9
Implantation
  anomalous — *see* Anomaly, by site
    ureter Q62.63
  cyst
    external area or site (skin) NEC L72.0
    iris — *see* Cyst, iris, implantation
    vagina N89.8
    vulva N90.7
  dermoid (cyst) — *see* Implantation, cyst
Impotence (sexual) N52.9
  counseling Z70.1
  organic origin (*see also* Dysfunction, sexual, male,
    erectile) N52.9
  psychogenic F52.21
Impression, basilar Q75.8
Imprisonment, anxiety concerning Z65.1
Improper care (child) (newborn) — *see* Maltreatment

Improperly tied umbilical cord (causing hemorrhage)
  P51.8
Impulsiveness (impulsive) R45.87
Inability to swallow — *see* Aphagia
Inaccessible, inaccessibility
  health care NEC Z75.3
    due to
      waiting period Z75.2
        for admission to facility elsewhere Z75.1
    other helping agencies Z75.4
Inactive — *see* condition
Inadequate, inadequacy
  aesthetics of dental restoration K08.56
  biologic, constitutional, functional, or social F60.7
  development
    child R62.50
    genitalia
      after puberty NEC E30.0
      congenital
        female Q52.8
          external Q52.79
          internal Q52.8
        male Q55.8
    lungs Q33.6
      associated with short gestation P28.0
    organ or site not listed — *see* Anomaly, by site
  diet (causing nutritional deficiency) E63.9
  eating habits Z72.4
  environment, household Z59.1
  family support Z63.8
  food (supply) NEC Z59.4
    hunger effects T73.0 ☑
  functional F60.7
  household care, due to
    family member
      handicapped or ill Z74.2
      on vacation Z75.5
      temporarily away from home Z74.2
    technical defects in home Z59.1
    temporary absence from home of person rendering
      care Z74.2
  housing (heating) (space) Z59.1
  income (financial) Z59.6
  intrafamilial communication Z63.8
  material resources Z59.9
  mental — *see* Disability, intellectual
  parental supervision or control of child Z62.0
  personality F60.7
  pulmonary
    function R06.89
      newborn P28.5
    ventilation, newborn P28.5
  sample of cytologic smear
    anus R85.615
    cervix R87.615
    vagina R87.625
  social F60.7
    insurance Z59.7
    skills NEC Z73.4
  supervision of child by parent Z62.0
  teaching affecting education Z55.8
  welfare support Z59.7
Inanition R64
  with edema — *see* Malnutrition, severe
  due to
    deprivation of food T73.0 ☑
    malnutrition — *see* Malnutrition
  fever R50.9
Inappropriate
  change in quantitative human chorionic gonadotropin
    (hCG) in early pregnancy O02.81
  diet or eating habits Z72.4
  level of quantitative human chorionic gonadotropin
    (hCG) for gestational age in early pregnancy
    O02.81
  secretion
    antidiuretic hormone (ADH) (excessive) E22.2
      deficiency E23.2
    pituitary (posterior) E22.2
Inattention at or after birth — *see* Neglect
Incarceration, incarcerated
  enterocele K46.0
    gangrenous K46.1
  epiplocele K46.0
    gangrenous K46.1
  exophthalmos K42.0
    gangrenous K42.1

Incarceration, incarcerated — *continued*
  hernia (*see also* Hernia, by site, with
    obstruction)
    with gangrene — *see* Hernia, by site, with gan-
      grene
  iris, in wound — *see* Injury, eye, laceration, with pro-
    lapse
  lens, in wound — *see* Injury, eye, laceration, with
    prolapse
  omphalocele K42.0
  prison, anxiety concerning Z65.1
  rupture — *see* Hernia, by site
  sarcoepiplocele K46.0
    gangrenous K46.1
  sarcoepiplomphalocele K42.0
    with gangrene K42.1
  uterus N85.8
    gravid O34.51- ☑
      causing obstructed labor O65.5
Incised wound
  external — *see* Laceration
  internal organs — *see* Injury, by site
Incision, incisional
  hernia K43.2
    with
      gangrene (and obstruction) K43.1
      obstruction K43.0
    surgical, complication — *see* Complications, surgical
      procedure
    traumatic
      external — *see* Laceration
      internal organs — *see* Injury, by site
Inclusion
  azurophilic leukocytic D72.0
  blennorrhea (neonatal) (newborn) P39.1
  gallbladder in liver (congenital) Q44.1
Incompatibility
  ABO
    affecting management of pregnancy O36.11- ☑
      anti-A sensitization O36.11- ☑
      anti-B sensitization O36.19- ☑
      specified NEC O36.19- ☑
    infusion or transfusion reaction — *see* Complica-
      tion(s), transfusion, incompatibility reaction,
      ABO
    newborn P55.1
  blood (group) (Duffy) (K(ell)) (Kidd) (Lewis) (M) (S) NEC
    affecting management of pregnancy O36.11- ☑
      anti-A sensitization O36.11- ☑
      anti-B sensitization O36.19- ☑
    infusion or transfusion reaction T80.89 ☑
    newborn P55.8
  divorce or estrangement Z63.5
  Rh (blood group) (factor) Z31.82
    affecting management of pregnancy NEC
      O36.09- ☑
      anti-D antibody O36.01- ☑
    infusion or transfusion reaction — *see* Complica-
      tion(s), transfusion, incompatibility reaction,
      Rh (factor)
    newborn P55.0
  rhesus — *see* Incompatibility, Rh
Incompetency, incompetent, incompetence
  annular
    aortic (valve) — *see* Insufficiency, aortic
    mitral (valve) I34.0
    pulmonary valve (heart) I37.1
  aortic (valve) — *see* Insufficiency, aortic
  cardiac valve — *see* Endocarditis
  cervix, cervical (os) N88.3
    in pregnancy O34.3- ☑
  chronotropic I45.89
    with
      autonomic dysfunction G90.8
      ischemic heart disease I25.89
      left ventricular dysfunction I51.89
      sinus node dysfunction I49.8
  esophagogastric (junction) (sphincter) K22.0
  mitral (valve) — *see* Insufficiency, mitral
  pelvic fundus N81.89
  pubocervical tissue N81.82
  pulmonary valve (heart) I37.1
    congenital Q22.3
  rectovaginal tissue N81.83
  tricuspid (annular) (valve) — *see* Insufficiency, tricuspid
  valvular — *see* Endocarditis
    congenital Q24.8

Incompetency, incompetent, incompetence —
 continued
 vein, venous (saphenous) (varicose) — *see* Varix, leg
Incomplete (*see also* condition)
 bladder, emptying R33.9
 defecation R15.0
 expansion lungs (newborn) NEC — *see* Atelectasis
 rotation, intestine Q43.3
Inconclusive
 diagnostic imaging due to excess body fat of patient
  R93.9
 findings on diagnostic imaging of breast NEC R92.8
 mammogram (due to dense breasts) R92.2
Incontinence R32
 anal sphincter R15.9
 feces R15.9
  nonorganic origin F98.1
 overflow N39.490
 psychogenic F45.8
 rectal R15.9
 reflex N39.498
 stress (female) (male) N39.3
  and urge N39.46
 urethral sphincter R32
 urge N39.41
  and stress (female) (male) N39.46
 urine (urinary) R32
  continuous N39.45
  due to cognitive impairment, or severe physical
   disability or immobility R39.81
  functional R39.81
  mixed (stress and urge) N39.46
  nocturnal N39.44
  nonorganic origin F98.0
  overflow N39.490
  post dribbling N39.43
  reflex N39.498
  specified NEC N39.498
  stress (female) (male) N39.3
   and urge N39.46
  total N39.498
  unaware N39.42
  urge N39.41
   and stress (female) (male) N39.46
Incontinentia pigmenti Q82.3
Incoordinate, incoordination
 esophageal-pharyngeal (newborn) — *see* Dysphagia
 muscular R27.8
 uterus (action) (contractions) (complicating delivery)
  O62.4
Increase, increased
 abnormal, in development R63.8
 androgens (ovarian) E28.1
 anticoagulants (antithrombin) (anti-VIIIa) (anti-IXa)
  (anti-Xa) (anti-XIa) — *see* Circulating anticoagulants
 cold sense R20.8
 estrogen E28.0
 function
  adrenal
   cortex — *see* Cushing's, syndrome
   medulla E27.5
  pituitary (gland) (anterior) (lobe) E22.9
   posterior E22.2
 heat sense R20.8
 intracranial pressure (benign) G93.2
 permeability, capillaries I78.8
 pressure, intracranial G93.2
 secretion
  gastrin E16.4
  glucagon E16.3
  pancreas, endocrine E16.9
   growth hormone-releasing hormone E16.8
   pancreatic polypeptide E16.8
   somatostatin E16.8
   vasoactive-intestinal polypeptide E16.8
 sphericity, lens Q12.4
 splenic activity D73.1
 venous pressure I87.8
  portal K76.6
Increta placenta O43.22- ☑
Incrustation, cornea, foreign body (lead)(zinc) — *see*
 Foreign body, cornea
Incyclophoria H50.54
Incyclotropia — *see* Cyclotropia
Indeterminate sex Q56.4
India rubber skin Q82.8

Indigestion (acid) (bilious) (functional) K30
 catarrhal K31.89
 due to decomposed food NOS A05.9
 nervous F45.8
 psychogenic F45.8
Indirect — *see* condition
Induratio penis plastica N48.6
Induration, indurated
 brain G93.89
 breast (fibrous) N64.51
  puerperal, postpartum O92.29
 broad ligament N83.8
 chancre
  anus A51.1
  congenital A50.07
  extragenital NEC A51.2
 corpora cavernosa (penis) (plastic) N48.6
 liver (chronic) K76.89
 lung (black) (chronic) (fibroid) (*see also* Fibrosis, lung)
  J84.10
  essential brown J84.03
 penile (plastic) N48.6
 phlebitic — *see* Phlebitis
 skin R23.4
Inebriety (without dependence) — *see* Alcohol, intoxication
Inefficiency, kidney N28.9
Inelasticity, skin R23.4
Inequality, leg (length) (acquired) (*see also* Deformity,
 limb, unequal length)
 congenital — *see* Defect, reduction, lower limb
 lower leg — *see* Deformity, limb, unequal length
Inertia
 bladder (neurogenic) N31.2
 stomach K31.89
  psychogenic F45.8
 uterus, uterine during labor O62.2
  during latent phase of labor O62.0
  primary O62.0
  secondary O62.1
 vesical (neurogenic) N31.2
Infancy, infantile, infantilism (*see also* condition)
 celiac K90.0
 genitalia, genitals (after puberty) E30.0
 Herter's (nontropical sprue) K90.0
 intestinal K90.0
 Lorain E23.0
 pancreatic K86.8
 pelvis M95.5
  with disproportion (fetopelvic) O33.1
   causing obstructed labor O65.1
 pituitary E23.0
 renal N25.0
 uterus — *see* Infantile, genitalia
Infant(s) (*see also* Infancy)
 excessive crying R68.11
 irritable child R68.12
 lack of care — *see* Neglect
 liveborn (singleton) Z38.2
  born in hospital Z38.00
   by cesarean Z38.01
  born outside hospital Z38.1
  multiple NEC Z38.8
   born in hospital Z38.68
    by cesarean Z38.69
   born outside hospital Z38.7
  quadruplet Z38.8
   born in hospital Z38.63
    by cesarean Z38.64
   born outside hospital Z38.7
  quintuplet Z38.8
   born in hospital Z38.65
    by cesarean Z38.66
   born outside hospital Z38.7
  triplet Z38.8
   born in hospital Z38.61
    by cesarean Z38.62
   born outside hospital Z38.7
  twin Z38.5
   born in hospital Z38.30
    by cesarean Z38.31
   born outside hospital Z38.4
 of diabetic mother (syndrome of) P70.1
  gestational diabetes P70.0
Infantile (*see also* condition)
 genitalia, genitals E30.0
 os, uterine E30.0
 penis E30.0

Infantile — *continued*
 testis E29.1
 uterus E30.0
Infantilism — *see* Infancy
Infarct, infarction
 adrenal (capsule) (gland) E27.49
 appendices epiploicae K55.0
 bowel K55.0
 brain (stem) — *see* Infarct, cerebral
 breast N64.89
 brewer's (kidney) N28.0
 cardiac — *see* Infarct, myocardium
 cerebellar — *see* Infarct, cerebral
 cerebral (*see also* Occlusion, artery cerebral or precerebral, with infarction) I63.9
  aborted I63.9
  cortical I63.9
  due to
   cerebral venous thrombosis, nonpyogenic I63.6
   embolism
    cerebral arteries I63.4- ☑
    precerebral arteries I63.1- ☑
   occlusion NEC
    cerebral arteries I63.5- ☑
    precerebral arteries I63.2- ☑
   stenosis NEC
    cerebral arteries I63.5- ☑
    precerebral arteries I63.2- ☑
   thrombosis
    cerebral artery I63.3- ☑
    precerebral artery I63.0- ☑
  intraoperative
   during cardiac surgery I97.810
   during other surgery I97.811
  postprocedural
   following cardiac surgery I97.820
   following other surgery I97.821
  specified NEC I63.8
 colon (acute) (agnogenic) (embolic) (hemorrhagic)
  (nonocclusive) (nonthrombotic) (occlusive)
  (segmental) (thrombotic) (with gangrene) K55.0
 coronary artery — *see* Infarct, myocardium
 embolic — *see* Embolism
 fallopian tube N83.8
 gallbladder K82.8
 heart — *see* Infarct, myocardium
 hepatic K76.3
 hypophysis (anterior lobe) E23.6
 impending (myocardium) I20.0
 intestine (acute) (agnogenic) (embolic) (hemorrhagic)
  (nonocclusive) (nonthrombotic) (occlusive)
  (thrombotic) (with gangrene) K55.0
 kidney N28.0
 liver K76.3
 lung (embolic) (thrombotic) — *see* Embolism, pulmonary
 lymph node I89.8
 mesentery, mesenteric (embolic) (thrombotic) (with
  gangrene) K55.0
 muscle (ischemic) M62.20
  ankle M62.27- ☑
  foot M62.27- ☑
  forearm M62.23- ☑
  hand M62.24- ☑
  lower leg M62.26- ☑
  pelvic region M62.25- ☑
  shoulder region M62.21- ☑
  specified site NEC M62.28
  thigh M62.25- ☑
  upper arm M62.22- ☑
 myocardium, myocardial (acute) (with stated duration
  of 4 weeks or less) I21.3
  diagnosed on ECG, but presenting no symptoms
   I25.2
  healed or old I25.2
  intraoperative
   during cardiac surgery I97.790
   during other surgery I97.791
  non-Q wave I21.4
  non-ST elevation (NSTEMI) I21.4
   subsequent I22.2
  nontransmural I21.4
  past (diagnosed on ECG or other investigation, but
   currently presenting no symptoms) I25.2
  postprocedural
   following cardiac surgery I97.190
   following other surgery I97.191
  Q wave (see also, Infarct, myocardium, by site) I21.3

Infarct, infarction — *continued*
  myocardium, myocardial — *continued*
    ST elevation (STEMI) I21.3
      anterior (anteroapical) (anterolateral) (anteroseptal) (Q wave) (wall) I21.09
        subsequent I22.0
      inferior (diaphragmatic) (inferolateral) (inferoposterior) (wall) NEC I21.19
        subsequent I22.1
      inferoposterior transmural (Q wave) I21.11
      involving
        coronary artery of anterior wall NEC I21.09
        coronary artery of inferior wall NEC I21.19
        diagonal coronary artery I21.02
        left anterior descending coronary artery I21.02
        left circumflex coronary artery I21.21
        left main coronary artery I21.01
        oblique marginal coronary artery I21.21
        right coronary artery I21.11
      lateral (apical-lateral) (basal-lateral) (high) I21.29
        subsequent I22.8
      posterior (posterobasal) (posterolateral) (posteroseptal) (true) I21.29
        subsequent I22.8
      septal I21.29
        subsequent I22.8
      specified NEC I21.29
        subsequent I22.8
      subsequent I22.9
    subsequent (recurrent) (reinfarction) I22.9
      anterior (anteroapical) (anterolateral) (anteroseptal) (wall) I22.0
      diaphragmatic (wall) I22.1
      inferior (diaphragmatic) (inferolateral) (inferoposterior) (wall) I22.1
      lateral (apical-lateral) (basal-lateral) (high) I22.8
      non-ST elevation (NSTEMI) I22.2
      posterior (posterobasal) (posterolateral) (posteroseptal) (true) I22.8
      septal I22.8
      specified NEC I22.8
      ST elevation I22.9
        anterior (anteroapical) (anterolateral) (anteroseptal) (wall) I22.0
        inferior (diaphragmatic) (inferolateral) (inferoposterior) (wall) I22.1
        specified NEC I22.8
      subendocardial I22.2
      transmural I22.9
        anterior (anteroapical) (anterolateral) (anteroseptal) (wall) I22.0
        diaphragmatic (wall) I22.1
        inferior (diaphragmatic) (inferolateral) (inferoposterior) (wall) I22.1
        lateral (apical-lateral) (basal-lateral) (high) I22.8
        posterior (posterobasal) (posterolateral) (posteroseptal) (true) I22.8
        specified NEC I22.8
    syphilitic A52.06
    transmural I21.3
      anterior (anteroapical) (anterolateral) (anteroseptal) (Q wave) (wall) NEC I21.09
      inferior (diaphragmatic) (inferolateral) (inferoposterior) (Q wave) (wall) NEC I21.19
      inferoposterior (Q wave) I21.11
      lateral (apical-lateral) (basal-lateral) (high) NEC I21.29
      posterior (posterobasal) (posterolateral) (posteroseptal) (true) NEC I21.29
      septal NEC I21.29
      specified NEC I21.29
  nontransmural I21.4
  omentum K55.0
  ovary N83.8
  pancreas K86.8
  papillary muscle — *see* Infarct, myocardium
  parathyroid gland E21.4
  pituitary (gland) E23.6
  placenta O43.81- ☑
  prostate N42.89
  pulmonary (artery) (vein) (hemorrhagic) — *see* Embolism, pulmonary
  renal (embolic) (thrombotic) N28.0
  retina, retinal (artery) — *see* Occlusion, artery, retina
  spinal (cord) (acute) (embolic) (nonembolic) G95.11

Infarct, infarction — *continued*
  spleen D73.5
    embolic or thrombotic I74.8
  subendocardial (acute) (nontransmural) I21.4
  suprarenal (capsule) (gland) E27.49
  testis N50.1
  thrombotic (*see also* Thrombosis)
    artery, arterial — *see* Embolism
  thyroid (gland) E07.89
  ventricle (heart) — *see* Infarct, myocardium
Infecting — *see* condition
Infection, infected, infective (opportunistic) B99.9
  with
    drug resistant organism — *see* Resistance (to), drug (*see also* specific organism)
    lymphangitis — *see* Lymphangitis
    organ dysfunction (acute) R65.20
      with septic shock R65.21
  abscess (skin) — *code by* site under Abscess
  Absidia — *see* Mucormycosis
  Acanthamoeba — *see* Acanthamebiasis
  Acanthocheilonema (perstans) (streptocerca) B74.4
  accessory sinus (chronic) — *see* Sinusitis
  achorion — *see* Dermatophytosis
  Acremonium falciforme B47.0
  acromioclavicular M00.9
  Actinobacillus (actinomycetem-comitans) A28.8
    mallei A24.0
    muris A25.1
  Actinomadura B47.1
  Actinomyces (israelii) (*see also* Actinomycosis) A42.9
  Actinomycetales — *see* Actinomycosis
  actinomycotic NOS — *see* Actinomycosis
  adenoid (and tonsil) J03.90
    chronic J35.02
  adenovirus NEC
    as cause of disease classified elsewhere B97.0
    unspecified nature or site B34.0
  aerogenes capsulatus A48.0
  aertrycke — *see* Infection, salmonella
  alimentary canal NOS — *see* Enteritis, infectious
  Allescheria boydii B48.2
  Alternaria B48.8
  alveolus, alveolar (process) K04.7
  Ameba, amebic (histolytica) — *see* Amebiasis
  amniotic fluid, sac or cavity O41.10- ☑
    chorioamnionitis O41.12- ☑
    placentitis O41.14- ☑
  amputation stump (surgical) — *see* Complication, amputation stump, infection
  Ancylostoma (duodenalis) B76.0
  Anisakiasis, Anisakis larvae B81.0
  anthrax — *see* Anthrax
  antrum (chronic) — *see* Sinusitis, maxillary
  anus, anal (papillae) (sphincter) K62.89
  arbovirus (arbor virus) A94
    specified type NEC A93.8
  artificial insemination N98.0
  Ascaris lumbricoides — *see* Ascariasis
  Ascomycetes B47.0
  Aspergillus (flavus) (fumigatus) (terreus) — *see* Aspergillosis
  atypical
    acid-fast (bacilli) — *see* Mycobacterium, atypical
    mycobacteria — *see* Mycobacterium, atypical
    virus A81.9
      specified type NEC A81.89
  auditory meatus (external) — *see* Otitis, externa, infective
  auricle (ear) — *see* Otitis, externa, infective
  axillary gland (lymph) L04.2
  Bacillus A49.9
    abortus A23.1
    anthracis — *see* Anthrax
    Ducrey's (any location) A57
    Flexner's A03.1
    Friedländer's NEC A49.8
    gas (gangrene) A48.0
    mallei A24.0
    melitensis A23.0
    paratyphoid, paratyphosus A01.4
      A A01.1
      B A01.2
      C A01.3
    Shiga (-Kruse) A03.0
    suipestifer — *see* Infection, salmonella
    swimming pool A31.1

Infection, infected, infective — *continued*
  Bacillus — *continued*
    typhosa A01.00
    welchii — *see* Gangrene, gas
  bacterial NOS A49.9
    as cause of disease classified elsewhere B96.89
      Bacteroides fragilis [B. fragilis] B96.6
      Clostridium perfringens [C. perfringens] B96.7
      Enterobacter sakazakii B96.89
      Enterococcus B95.2
      Escherichia coli [E. coli] (*see also* Escherichia coli) B96.20
      Helicobacter pylori [H.pylori] B96.81
      Hemophilus influenzae [H. influenzae] B96.3
      Klebsiella pneumoniae [K. pneumoniae] B96.1
      Mycoplasma pneumoniae [M. pneumoniae] B96.0
      Proteus (mirabilis) (morganii) B96.4
      Pseudomonas (aeruginosa) (mallei) (pseudomallei) B96.5
      Staphylococcus B95.8
        aureus (methicillin susceptible) (MSSA) B95.61
        methicillin resistant (MRSA) B95.62
        specified NEC B95.7
      Streptococcus B95.5
        group A B95.0
        group B B95.1
        pneumoniae B95.3
        specified NEC B95.4
      Vibrio vulnificus B96.82
    specified NEC A48.8
  Bacterium
    paratyphosum A01.4
      A A01.1
      B A01.2
      C A01.3
    typhosum A01.00
  Bacteroides NEC A49.8
    fragilis, as cause of disease classified elsewhere B96.6
  Balantidium coli A07.0
  Bartholin's gland N75.8
  Basidiobolus B46.8
  bile duct (common) (hepatic) — *see* Cholangitis
  bladder — *see* Cystitis
  Blastomyces, blastomycotic (*see also* Blastomycosis)
    brasiliensis — *see* Paracoccidioidomycosis
    dermatitidis — *see* Blastomycosis
    European — *see* Cryptococcosis
    Loboi B48.0
    North American B40.9
    South American — *see* Paracoccidioidomycosis
  bleb, postprocedure — *see* Blebitis
  bone — *see* Osteomyelitis
  Bordetella — *see* Whooping cough
  Borrelia bergdorfi A69.20
  brain (*see also* Encephalitis) G04.90
    membranes — *see* Meningitis
    septic G06.0
      meninges — *see* Meningitis, bacterial
  branchial cyst Q18.0
  breast — *see* Mastitis
  bronchus — *see* Bronchitis
  Brucella A23.9
    abortus A23.1
    canis A23.3
    melitensis A23.0
    mixed A23.8
    specified NEC A23.8
    suis A23.2
  Brugia (malayi) B74.1
    timori B74.2
  bursa — *see* Bursitis, infective
  buttocks (skin) L08.9
  Campylobacter, intestinal A04.5
    as cause of disease classified elsewhere B96.81
  Candida (albicans) (tropicalis) — *see* Candidiasis
  candiru B88.8
  Capillaria (intestinal) B81.1
    hepatica B83.8
    philippinensis B81.1
  cartilage — *see* Disorder, cartilage, specified type NEC
  cat liver fluke B66.0
  catheter-related bloodstream (CRBSI) T80.211 ☑
  cellulitis — *code by* site under Cellulitis
  central line-associated T80.219 ☑
    bloodstream (CLABSI) T80.211 ☑

☑ **Additional Character Required** — Refer to the Tabular List for Character Selection   Subterms under main terms may continue to next column or page

Infection, infected, infective — *continued*

central line-associated — *continued*
  specified NEC T80.218 ☑
Cephalosporium falciforme B47.0
cerebrospinal — *see* Meningitis
cervical gland (lymph) L04.0
cervix — *see* Cervicitis
cesarean delivery wound (puerperal) O86.0
cestodes — *see* Infestation, cestodes
chest J22
Chilomastix (intestinal) A07.8
Chlamydia, chlamydial A74.9
  anus A56.3
  genitourinary tract A56.2
    lower A56.00
    specified NEC A56.19
  lymphogranuloma A55
  pharynx A56.4
  psittaci A70
  rectum A56.3
  sexually transmitted NEC A56.8
cholera — *see* Cholera
Cladosporium
  bantianum (brain abscess) B43.1
  carrionii B43.0
  castellanii B36.1
  trichoides (brain abscess) B43.1
  werneckii B36.1
Clonorchis (sinensis) (liver) B66.1
Clostridium NEC
  bifermentans A48.0
  botulinum (food poisoning) A05.1
    infant A48.51
    wound A48.52
  difficile
    as cause of disease classified elsewhere B96.89
    foodborne (disease) A04.7
    gas gangrene A48.0
    necrotizing enterocolitis A04.7
    sepsis A41.4
  gas-forming NEC A48.0
  histolyticum A48.0
  novyi, causing gas gangrene A48.0
  oedematiens A48.0
  perfringens
    as cause of disease classified elsewhere B96.7
    due to food A05.2
    foodborne (disease) A05.2
    gas gangrene A48.0
    sepsis A41.4
  septicum, causing gas gangrene A48.0
  sordellii, causing gas gangrene A48.0
  welchii
    as cause of disease classified elsewhere B96.7
    foodborne (disease) A05.2
    gas gangrene A48.0
    necrotizing enteritis A05.2
    sepsis A41.4
Coccidioides (immitis) — *see* Coccidioidomycosis
colon — *see* Enteritis, infectious
colostomy K94.02
common duct — *see* Cholangitis
congenital P39.9
  Candida (albicans) P37.5
  cytomegalovirus P35.1
  hepatitis, viral P35.3
  herpes simplex P35.2
  infectious or parasitic disease P37.9
    specified NEC P37.8
  listeriosis (disseminated) P37.2
  malaria NEC P37.4
    falciparum P37.3
  Plasmodium falciparum P37.3
  poliomyelitis P35.8
  rubella P35.0
  skin P39.4
  toxoplasmosis (acute) (subacute) (chronic) P37.1
  tuberculosis P37.0
  urinary (tract) P39.3
  vaccinia P35.8
  virus P35.9
    specified type NEC P35.8
Conidiobolus B46.8
coronavirus NEC B34.2
  as cause of disease classified elsewhere B97.29
  severe acute respiratory syndrome (SARS associated) B97.21
corpus luteum — *see* Salpingo-oophoritis

Infection, infected, infective — *continued*

Corynebacterium diphtheriae — *see* Diphtheria
cotia virus B08.8
Coxiella burnetii A78
coxsackie — *see* Coxsackie
Cryptococcus neoformans — *see* Cryptococcosis
Cryptosporidium A07.2
Cunninghamella — *see* Mucormycosis
cyst — *see* Cyst
cystic duct (*see also* Cholecystitis) K81.9
Cysticercus cellulosae — *see* Cysticercosis
cytomegalovirus, cytomegaloviral B25.9
  congenital P35.1
  maternal, maternal care for (suspected) damage to fetus O35.3 ☑
  mononucleosis B27.10
    with
      complication NEC B27.19
      meningitis B27.12
      polyneuropathy B27.11
delta-agent (acute), in hepatitis B carrier B17.0
dental (pulpal origin) K04.7
Deuteromycetes B47.0
Dicrocoelium dendriticum B66.2
Dipetalonema (perstans) (streptocerca) B74.4
diphtherial — *see* Diphtheria
Diphyllobothrium (adult) (latum) (pacificum) B70.0
  larval B70.1
Diplogonoporus (grandis) B71.8
Dipylidium caninum B67.4
Dirofilaria B74.8
Dracunculus medinensis B72
Drechslera (hawaiiensis) B43.8
Ducrey Haemophilus (any location) A57
due to or resulting from
  artificial insemination N98.0
  central venous catheter T80.219 ☑
    bloodstream T80.211 ☑
    exit or insertion site T80.212 ☑
    localized T80.212 ☑
    port or reservoir T80.212 ☑
    specified NEC T80.218 ☑
    tunnel T80.212 ☑
  device, implant or graft (*see also* Complications, by site and type, infection or inflammation) T85.79 ☑
    arterial graft NEC T82.7 ☑
    breast (implant) T85.79 ☑
    catheter NEC T85.79 ☑
      dialysis (renal) T82.7 ☑
        intraperitoneal T85.71 ☑
      infusion NEC T82.7 ☑
        spinal (epidural) (subdural) T85.79 ☑
      urinary (indwelling) T83.51 ☑
    electronic (electrode) (pulse generator) (stimulator)
      bone T84.7 ☑
      cardiac T82.7 ☑
      nervous system (brain) (peripheral nerve) (spinal) T85.79 ☑
      urinary T83.59 ☑
    fixation, internal (orthopedic) NEC — *see* Complication, fixation device, infection
    gastrointestinal (bile duct) (esophagus) T85.79 ☑
    genital NEC T83.6 ☑
    heart NEC T82.7 ☑
      valve (prosthesis) T82.6 ☑
        graft T82.7 ☑
    joint prosthesis — *see* Complication, joint prosthesis, infection
    ocular (corneal graft) (orbital implant) NEC T85.79 ☑
    orthopedic NEC T84.7 ☑
    specified NEC T85.79 ☑
    urinary NEC T83.59 ☑
    vascular NEC T82.7 ☑
    ventricular intracranial shunt T85.79 ☑
  Hickman catheter T80.219 ☑
    bloodstream T80.211 ☑
    localized T80.212 ☑
    specified NEC T80.218 ☑
  immunization or vaccination T88.0 ☑
  infusion, injection or transfusion NEC T80.29 ☑
  injury NEC — *code by* site under Wound, open

Infection, infected, infective — *continued*

due to or resulting from — *continued*
  peripherally inserted central catheter (PICC) T80.219 ☑
    bloodstream T80.211 ☑
    localized T80.212 ☑
    specified NEC T80.218 ☑
  portacath (port-a-cath) T80.219 ☑
    bloodstream T80.211 ☑
    localized T80.212 ☑
    specified NEC T80.218 ☑
  surgery T81.4 ☑
  triple lumen catheter T80.219 ☑
    bloodstream T80.211 ☑
    localized T80.212 ☑
    specified NEC T80.218 ☑
  umbilical venous catheter T80.219 ☑
    bloodstream T80.211 ☑
    localized T80.212 ☑
    specified NEC T80.218 ☑
during labor NEC O75.3
ear (middle) (*see also* Otitis media)
  external — *see* Otitis, externa, infective
  inner — *see* subcategory H83.0 ☑
Eberthella typhosa A01.00
Echinococcus — *see* Echinococcus
echovirus
  as cause of disease classified elsewhere B97.12
  unspecified nature or site B34.1
endocardium I33.0
endocervix — *see* Cervicitis
Entamoeba — *see* Amebiasis
enteric — *see* Enteritis, infectious
Enterobacter sakazakii B96.89
Enterobius vermicularis B80
enterostomy K94.12
enterovirus B34.1
  as cause of disease classified elsewhere B97.10
    coxsackievirus B97.11
    echovirus B97.12
    specified NEC B97.19
Entomophthora B46.8
Epidermophyton — *see* Dermatophytosis
epididymis — *see* Epididymitis
episiotomy (puerperal) O86.0
Erysipelothrix (insidiosa) (rhusiopathiae) — *see* Erysipeloid
erythema infectiosum B08.3
Escherichia (E.) coli NEC A49.8
  as cause of disease classified elsewhere (*see also* Escherichia coli) B96.20
  congenital P39.8
    sepsis P36.4
  generalized A41.51
  intestinal — *see* Enteritis, infectious, due to, Escherichia coli
ethmoidal (chronic) (sinus) — *see* Sinusitis, ethmoidal
eustachian tube (ear) — *see* Salpingitis, eustachian
external auditory canal (meatus) NEC — *see* Otitis, externa, infective
eye (purulent) — *see* Endophthalmitis, purulent
eyelid — *see* Inflammation, eyelid
fallopian tube — *see* Salpingo-oophoritis
Fasciola (gigantica) (hepatica) (indica) B66.3
Fasciolopsis (buski) B66.5
filarial — *see* Infestation, filarial
finger (skin) L08.9
  nail L03.01- ☑
    fungus B35.1
fish tapeworm B70.0
  larval B70.1
flagellate, intestinal A07.9
fluke — *see* Infestation, fluke
focal
  teeth (pulpal origin) K04.7
  tonsils J35.01
Fonsecaea (compactum) (pedrosoi) B43.0
food — *see* Intoxication, foodborne
foot (skin) L08.9
  dermatophytic fungus B35.3
Francisella tularensis — *see* Tularemia
frontal (sinus) (chronic) — *see* Sinusitis, frontal
fungus NOS B49
  beard B35.0
  dermatophytic — *see* Dermatophytosis
  foot B35.3
  groin B35.6

Infection, infected, infective — *continued*
  fungus — *continued*
    hand B35.2
    nail B35.1
    pathogenic to compromised host only B48.8
    perianal (area) B35.6
    scalp B35.0
    skin B36.9
      foot B35.3
      hand B35.2
      toenails B35.1
  Fusarium B48.8
  gallbladder — *see* Cholecystitis
  gas bacillus — *see* Gangrene, gas
  gastrointestinal — *see* Enteritis, infectious
  generalized NEC — *see* Sepsis
  genital organ or tract
    female — *see* Disease, pelvis, inflammatory
    male N49.9
      multiple sites N49.8
      specified NEC N49.8
  Ghon tubercle, primary A15.7
  Giardia lamblia A07.1
  gingiva (chronic) K05.10
    acute K05.00
      nonplaque induced K05.01
      plaque induced K05.00
    nonplaque induced K05.11
    plaque induced K05.10
  glanders A24.0
  glenosporopsis B48.0
  Gnathostoma (spinigerum) B83.1
  Gongylonema B83.8
  gonococcal — *see* Gonococcus
  gram-negative bacilli NOS A49.9
  guinea worm B72
  gum (chronic) K05.10
    acute K05.00
      nonplaque induced K05.01
      plaque induced K05.00
    nonplaque induced K05.11
    plaque induced K05.10
  Haemophilus — *see* Infection, Hemophilus
  heart — *see* Carditis
  Helicobacter pylori A04.8
    as cause of disease classified elsewhere B96.81
  helminths B83.9
    intestinal B82.0
      mixed (types classifiable to more than one of
        the titles B65.0–B81.3 and B81.8) B81.4
      specified type NEC B81.8
    specified type NEC B83.8
  Hemophilus
    aegyptius, systemic A48.4
    ducrey (any location) A57
    generalized A41.3
    influenzae NEC A49.2
      as cause of disease classified elsewhere B96.3
  herpes (simplex) (*see also* Herpes)
    congenital P35.2
    disseminated B00.7
    zoster B02.9
  herpesvirus, herpesviral — *see* Herpes
  Heterophyes (heterophyes) B66.8
  hip (joint) NEC M00.9
    due to internal joint prosthesis
      left T84.52 ☑
      right T84.51 ☑
    skin NEC L08.9
  Histoplasma — *see* Histoplasmosis
    American B39.4
    capsulatum B39.4
  hookworm B76.9
  human
    papilloma virus A63.0
    T-cell lymphotropic virus type-1 (HTLV-1) B33.3
  hydrocele N43.0
  Hymenolepis B71.0
  hypopharynx — *see* Pharyngitis
  inguinal (lymph) glands L04.1
    due to soft chancre A57
  intervertebral disc, pyogenic M46.30
    cervical region M46.32
    cervicothoracic region M46.33
    lumbar region M46.36
    lumbosacral region M46.37
    multiple sites M46.39
    occipito-atlanto-axial region M46.31

Infection, infected, infective — *continued*
  intervertebral disc, pyogenic — *continued*
    sacrococcygeal region M46.38
    thoracic region M46.34
    thoracolumbar region M46.35
  intestine, intestinal — *see* Enteritis, infectious
    specified NEC A08.8
  intra-amniotic affecting newborn NEC P39.2
  Isospora belli or hominis A07.3
  Japanese B encephalitis A83.0
  jaw (bone) (lower) (upper) M27.2
  joint NEC M00.9
    due to internal joint prosthesis T84.50 ☑
  kidney (cortex) (hematogenous) N15.9
    with calculus N20.0
      with hydronephrosis N13.6
    following ectopic gestation O08.83
    pelvis and ureter (cystic) N28.85
    puerperal (postpartum) O86.21
    specified NEC N15.8
  Klebsiella (K.) pneumoniae NEC A49.8
    as cause of disease classified elsewhere B96.1
  knee (joint) NEC M00.9
    due to internal joint prosthesis
      left T84.54 ☑
      right T84.53 ☑
    joint M00.9
    skin L08.9
  Koch's — *see* Tuberculosis
  labia (majora) (minora) (acute) — *see* Vulvitis
  lacrimal
    gland — *see* Dacryoadenitis
    passages (duct) (sac) — *see* Inflammation, lacrimal,
      passages
  lancet fluke B66.2
  larynx NEC J38.7
  leg (skin) NOS L08.9
  Legionella pneumophila A48.1
    nonpneumonic A48.2
  Leishmania (*see also* Leishmaniasis)
    aethiopica B55.1
    braziliensis B55.2
    chagasi B55.0
    donovani B55.0
    infantum B55.0
    major B55.1
    mexicana B55.1
    tropica B55.1
  lentivirus, as cause of disease classified elsewhere
    B97.31
  Leptosphaeria senegalensis B47.0
  Leptospira interrogans A27.9
    autumnalis A27.89
    canicola A27.89
    hebdomadis A27.89
    icterohaemorrhagiae A27.0
    pomona A27.89
    specified type NEC A27.89
  leptospirochetal NEC — *see* Leptospirosis
  Listeria monocytogenes (*see also* Listeriosis)
    congenital P37.2
  Loa loa B74.3
    with conjunctival infestation B74.3
    eyelid B74.3
  Loboa loboi B48.0
  local, skin (staphylococcal) (streptococcal) L08.9
    abscess — *code by* site under Abscess
    cellulitis — *code by* site under Cellulitis
    specified NEC L08.89
    ulcer — *see* Ulcer, skin
  Loefflerella mallei A24.0
  lung (*see also* Pneumonia) J18.9
    atypical Mycobacterium A31.0
    spirochetal A69.8
    tuberculous — *see* Tuberculosis, pulmonary
    virus — *see* Pneumonia, viral
  lymph gland (*see also* Lymphadenitis, acute)
    mesenteric I88.0
  lymphoid tissue, base of tongue or posterior pharynx,
    NEC (chronic) J35.03
  Madurella (grisea) (mycetomii) B47.0
  major
    following ectopic or molar pregnancy O08.0
    puerperal, postpartum, childbirth O85
  Malassezia furfur B36.0
  Malleomyces
    mallei A24.0
    pseudomallei (whitmori) — *see* Melioidosis

Infection, infected, infective — *continued*
  mammary gland N61
  Mansonella (ozzardi) (perstans) (streptocerca) B74.4
  mastoid — *see* Mastoiditis
  maxilla, maxillary M27.2
    sinus (chronic) — *see* Sinusitis, maxillary
  mediastinum J98.5
  Medina (worm) B72
  meibomian cyst or gland — *see* Hordeolum
  meninges — *see* Meningitis, bacterial
  meningococcal (*see also* condition) A39.9
    adrenals A39.1
    brain A39.81
    cerebrospinal A39.0
    conjunctiva A39.89
    endocardium A39.51
    heart A39.50
      endocardium A39.51
      myocardium A39.52
      pericardium A39.53
    joint A39.83
    meninges A39.0
    meningococcemia A39.4
      acute A39.2
      chronic A39.3
    myocardium A39.52
    pericardium A39.53
    retrobulbar neuritis A39.82
    specified site NEC A39.89
  mesenteric lymph nodes or glands NEC I88.0
  Metagonimus B66.8
  metatarsophalangeal M00.9
  methicillin
    resistant Staphylococcus aureus (MRSA) A49.02
    susceptible Staphylococcus aureus (MSSA) A49.01
  Microsporum, microsporic — *see* Dermatophytosis
  mixed flora (bacterial) NEC A49.8
  Monilia — *see* Candidiasis
  Monosporium apiospermum B48.2
  mouth, parasitic B37.0
  Mucor — *see* Mucormycosis
  muscle NEC — *see* Myositis, infective
  mycelium NOS B49
  mycetoma B47.9
    actinomycotic NEC B47.1
    mycotic NEC B47.0
  Mycobacterium, mycobacterial — *see* Mycobacterium
  Mycoplasma NEC A49.3
    pneumoniae, as cause of disease classified else-
      where B96.0
  mycotic NOS B49
    pathogenic to compromised host only B48.8
    skin NOS B36.9
  myocardium NEC I40.0
  nail (chronic)
    with lymphangitis — *see* Lymphangitis, acute,
      digit
    finger L03.01- ☑
      fungus B35.1
    ingrowing L60.0
    toe L03.03- ☑
      fungus B35.1
  nasal sinus (chronic) — *see* Sinusitis
  nasopharynx — *see* Nasopharyngitis
  navel L08.82
  Necator americanus B76.1
  Neisseria — *see* Gonococcus
  Neotestudina rosatii B47.0
  newborn P39.9
    intra-amniotic NEC P39.2
    skin P39.4
    specified type NEC P39.8
  nipple N61
    associated with
      lactation O91.03
      pregnancy O91.01- ☑
      puerperium O91.02
  Nocardia — *see* Nocardiosis
  obstetrical surgical wound (puerperal) O86.0
  Oesophagostomum (apiostomum) B81.8
  Oestrus ovis — *see* Myiasis
  Oidium albicans B37.9
  Onchocerca (volvulus) — *see* Onchocerciasis
  oncovirus, as cause of disease classified elsewhere
    B97.32
  operation wound T81.4 ☑
  Opisthorchis (felineus) (viverrini) B66.0
  orbit, orbital — *see* Inflammation, orbit

  ☑ **Additional Character Required — Refer to the Tabular List for Character Selection**   ▽ Subterms under main terms may continue to next column or page

Infection, infected, infective — *continued*
orthopoxvirus NEC B08.09
ovary — *see* Salpingo-oophoritis
Oxyuris vermicularis B80
pancreas (acute) K85.9
 abscess — *see* Pancreatitis, acute
 specified NEC K85.8
papillomavirus, as cause of disease classified elsewhere
 B97.7
papovavirus NEC B34.4
Paracoccidioides brasiliensis — *see* Paracoccidioidomycosis
Paragonimus (westermani) B66.4
parainfluenza virus B34.8
parameningococcus NOS A39.9
parapoxvirus B08.60
 specified NEC B08.69
parasitic B89
Parastrongylus
 cantonensis B83.2
 costaricensis B81.3
 paratyphoid A01.4
  Type A A01.1
  Type B A01.2
  Type C A01.3
paraurethral ducts N34.2
parotid gland — *see* Sialoadenitis
parvovirus NEC B34.3
 as cause of disease classified elsewhere B97.6
Pasteurella NEC A28.0
 multocida A28.0
 pestis — *see* Plague
 pseudotuberculosis A28.0
 septica (cat bite) (dog bite) A28.0
 tularensis — *see* Tularemia
pelvic, female — *see* Disease, pelvis, inflammatory
Penicillium (marneffei) B48.4
penis (glans) (retention) NEC N48.29
periapical K04.5
peridental, periodontal K05.20
 generalized K05.22
 localized K05.21
perinatal period P39.9
 specified type NEC P39.8
perineal repair (puerperal) O86.0
periorbital — *see* Inflammation, orbit
perirectal K62.89
perirenal — *see* Infection, kidney
peritoneal — *see* Peritonitis
periureteral N28.89
Petriellidium boydii B48.2
pharynx (*see also* Pharyngitis)
 coxsackievirus B08.5
 posterior, lymphoid (chronic) J35.03
Phialophora
 gougerotii (subcutaneous abscess or cyst) B43.2
 jeanselmei (subcutaneous abscess or cyst) B43.2
 verrucosa (skin) B43.0
Piedraia hortae B36.3
pinta A67.9
 intermediate A67.1
 late A67.2
 mixed A67.3
 primary A67.0
pinworm B80
pityrosporum furfur B36.0
pleuro-pneumonia-like organism (PPLO) NEC A49.3
 as cause of disease classified elsewhere B96.0
pneumococcus, pneumococcal NEC A49.1
 as cause of disease classified elsewhere B95.3
 generalized (purulent) A40.3
  with pneumonia J13
Pneumocystis carinii (pneumonia) B59
Pneumocystis jiroveci (pneumonia) B59
port or reservoir T80.212 ☑
postoperative T81.4 ☑
postoperative wound T81.4 ☑
postprocedural T81.4 ☑
postvaccinal T88.0 ☑
prepuce NEC N47.7
 with penile inflammation N47.6
prion — *see* Disease, prion, central nervous system
prostate (capsule) — *see* Prostatitis
Proteus (mirabilis) (morganii) (vulgaris) NEC A49.8
 as cause of disease classified elsewhere B96.4
protozoal NEC B64
 intestinal A07.9
  specified NEC A07.8

Infection, infected, infective — *continued*
protozoal — *continued*
 specified NEC B60.8
Pseudoallescheria boydii B48.2
Pseudomonas NEC A49.8
 as cause of disease classified elsewhere B96.5
 mallei A24.0
 pneumonia J15.1
 pseudomallei — *see* Melioidosis
puerperal O86.4
 genitourinary tract NEC O86.89
 major or generalized O85
 minor O86.4
 specified NEC O86.89
pulmonary — *see* Infection, lung
purulent — *see* Abscess
Pyrenochaeta romeroi B47.0
Q fever A78
rectum (sphincter) K62.89
renal (*see also* Infection, kidney)
 pelvis and ureter (cystic) N28.85
reovirus, as cause of disease classified elsewhere B97.5
respiratory (tract) NEC J98.8
 acute J22
 chronic J98.8
 influenzal (upper) (acute) — *see* Influenza, with,
  respiratory manifestations NEC
 lower (acute) J22
  chronic — *see* Bronchitis, chronic
 rhinovirus J00
 syncytial virus, as cause of disease classified elsewhere B97.4
 upper (acute) NOS J06.9
  chronic J39.8
  streptococcal J06.9
  viral NOS J06.9
resulting from
 presence of internal prosthesis, implant, graft —
  see Complications, by site and type, infection
retortamoniasis A07.8
retroperitoneal NEC K68.9
retrovirus B33.3
 as cause of disease classified elsewhere B97.30
  human
   immunodeficiency, type 2 (HIV 2) B97.35
   T-cell lymphotropic
    type I (HTLV-I) B97.33
    type II (HTLV-II) B97.34
  lentivirus B97.31
  oncovirus B97.32
  specified NEC B97.39
Rhinosporidium (seeberi) B48.1
rhinovirus
 as cause of disease classified elsewhere B97.89
 unspecified nature or site B34.8
Rhizopus — *see* Mucormycosis
rickettsial NOS A79.9
roundworm (large) NEC B82.0
 Ascariasis (*see also* Ascariasis) B77.9
rubella — *see* Rubella
Saccharomyces — *see* Candidiasis
salivary duct or gland (any) — *see* Sialoadenitis
Salmonella (aertrycke) (arizonae) (callinarum)
 (cholerae-suis) (enteritidis) (suipestifer) (typhimurium) A02.9
 with
  (gastro)enteritis A02.0
  sepsis A02.1
  specified manifestation NEC A02.8
 due to food (poisoning) A02.9
 hirschfeldii A01.3
 localized A02.20
  arthritis A02.23
  meningitis A02.21
  osteomyelitis A02.24
  pneumonia A02.22
  pyelonephritis A02.25
  specified NEC A02.29
 paratyphi A01.4
  A A01.1
  B A01.2
  C A01.3
 schottmuelleri A01.2
 typhi, typhosa — *see* Typhoid
Sarcocystis A07.8
scabies B86
Schistosoma — *see* Infestation, Schistosoma
scrotum (acute) NEC N49.2

Infection, infected, infective — *continued*
seminal vesicle — *see* Vesiculitis
septic
 localized, skin — *see* Abscess
sheep liver fluke B66.3
Shigella A03.9
 boydii A03.2
 dysenteriae A03.0
 flexneri A03.1
 group
  A A03.0
  B A03.1
  C A03.2
  D A03.3
 Schmitz (-Stutzer) A03.0
 schmitzii A03.0
 shigae A03.0
 sonnei A03.3
 specified NEC A03.8
shoulder (joint) NEC M00.9
 due to internal joint prosthesis T84.59 ☑
 skin NEC L08.9
sinus (accessory) (chronic) (nasal) (*see also* Sinusitis)
 pilonidal — *see* Sinus, pilonidal
 skin NEC L08.89
Skene's duct or gland — *see* Urethritis
skin (local) (staphylococcal) (streptococcal) L08.9
 abscess — *code by* site under Abscess
 cellulitis — *code by* site under Cellulitis
 due to fungus B36.9
  specified type NEC B36.8
 mycotic B36.9
  specified type NEC B36.8
 newborn P39.4
 ulcer — *see* Ulcer, skin
slow virus A81.9
 specified NEC A81.89
Sparganum (mansoni) (proliferum) (baxteri) B70.1
specific (*see also* Syphilis)
 to perinatal period — *see* Infection, congenital
specified NEC B99.8
spermatic cord NEC N49.1
sphenoidal (sinus) — *see* Sinusitis, sphenoidal
spinal cord NOS (*see also* Myelitis) G04.91
 abscess G06.1
 meninges — *see* Meningitis
 streptococcal G04.89
Spirillum A25.0
spirochetal NOS A69.9
 lung A69.8
 specified NEC A69.8
Spirometra larvae B70.1
spleen D73.89
Sporotrichum, Sporothrix (schenckii) — *see* Sporotrichosis
staphylococcal, unspecified site
 as cause of disease classified elsewhere B95.8
  aureus (methicillin susceptible) (MSSA) B95.61
   methicillin resistant (MRSA) B95.62
  specified NEC B95.7
 aureus (methicillin susceptible) (MSSA) A49.01
  methicillin resistant (MRSA) A49.02
 food poisoning A05.0
 generalized (purulent) A41.2
 pneumonia — *see* Pneumonia, staphylococcal
Stellantchasmus falcatus B66.8
streptobacillus moniliformis A25.1
streptococcal NEC A49.1
 as cause of disease classified elsewhere B95.5
 B genitourinary complicating
  childbirth O98.82
  pregnancy O98.81- ☑
  puerperium O98.83
 congenital
  sepsis P36.10
   group B P36.0
   specified NEC P36.19
 generalized (purulent) A40.9
Streptomyces B47.1
Strongyloides (stercoralis) — *see* Strongyloidiasis
stump (amputation) (surgical) — *see* Complication,
 amputation stump, infection
subcutaneous tissue, local L08.9
suipestifer — *see* Infection, salmonella
swimming pool bacillus A31.1
Taenia — *see* Infestation, Taenia
Taeniarhynchus saginatus B68.1
tapeworm — *see* Infestation, tapeworm

Infection, infected, infective — *continued*
- tendon (sheath) — *see* Tenosynovitis, infective NEC
- Ternidens diminutus B81.8
- testis — *see* Orchitis
- threadworm B80
- throat — *see* Pharyngitis
- thyroglossal duct K14.8
- toe (skin) L08.9
    - cellulitis L03.03- ☑
        - fungus B35.1
    - nail L03.03- ☑
        - fungus B35.1
- tongue NEC K14.0
    - parasitic B37.0
- tonsil (and adenoid) (faucial) (lingual) (pharyngeal) — *see* Tonsillitis
- tooth, teeth K04.7
    - periapical K04.7
    - peridental, periodontal K05.20
        - generalized K05.22
        - localized K05.21
    - pulp K04.0
    - socket M27.3
- TORCH — *see* Infection, congenital
    - without active infection P00.2
- Torula histolytica — *see* Cryptococcosis
- Toxocara (canis) (cati) (felis) B83.0
- Toxoplasma gondii — *see* Toxoplasma
- trachea, chronic J42
- trematode NEC — *see* Infestation, fluke
- trench fever A79.0
- Treponema pallidum — *see* Syphilis
- Trichinella (spiralis) B75
- Trichomonas A59.9
    - cervix A59.09
    - intestine A07.8
    - prostate A59.02
    - specified site NEC A59.8
    - urethra A59.03
    - urogenitalis A59.00
    - vagina A59.01
    - vulva A59.01
- Trichophyton, trichophytic — *see* Dermatophytosis
- Trichosporon (beigelii) cutaneum B36.2
- Trichostrongylus B81.2
- Trichuris (trichiura) B79
- Trombicula (irritans) B88.0
- Trypanosoma
    - brucei
        - gambiense B56.0
        - rhodesiense B56.1
    - cruzi — *see* Chagas' disease
- tubal — *see* Salpingo-oophoritis
- tuberculous NEC — *see* Tuberculosis
- tubo-ovarian — *see* Salpingo-oophoritis
- tunica vaginalis N49.1
- tunnel T80.212 ☑
- tympanic membrane NEC — *see* Myringitis
- typhoid (abortive) (ambulant) (bacillus) — *see* Typhoid
- typhus A75.9
    - flea-borne A75.2
    - mite-borne A75.3
    - recrudescent A75.1
    - tick-borne A77.9
        - African A77.1
        - North Asian A77.2
- umbilicus L08.82
- ureter N28.86
- urethra — *see* Urethritis
- urinary (tract) N39.0
    - bladder — *see* Cystitis
    - complicating
        - pregnancy O23.4- ☑
            - specified type NEC O23.3- ☑
    - kidney — *see* Infection, kidney
    - newborn P39.3
    - puerperal (postpartum) O86.20
    - tuberculous A18.13
    - urethra — *see* Urethritis
- uterus, uterine — *see* Endometritis
- vaccination T88.0 ☑
- vaccinia not from vaccination B08.011
- vagina (acute) — *see* Vaginitis
- varicella B01.9
- varicose veins — *see* Varix
- vas deferens NEC N49.1
- vesical — *see* Cystitis

Infection, infected, infective — *continued*
- Vibrio
    - cholerae A00.0
        - El Tor A00.1
    - parahaemolyticus (food poisoning) A05.3
    - vulnificus
        - as cause of disease classified elsewhere B96.82
        - foodborne intoxication A05.5
- Vincent's (gum) (mouth) (tonsil) A69.1
- virus, viral NOS B34.9
    - adenovirus
        - as cause of disease classified elsewhere B97.0
        - unspecified nature or site B34.0
    - arborvirus, arbovirus arthropod-borne A94
    - as cause of disease classified elsewhere B97.89
        - adenovirus B97.0
        - coronavirus B97.29
            - SARS-associated B97.21
        - coxsackievirus B97.11
        - echovirus B97.12
        - enterovirus B97.10
            - coxsackievirus B97.11
            - echovirus B97.12
            - specified NEC B97.19
        - human
            - immunodeficiency, type 2 (HIV 2) B97.35
            - metapneumovirus B97.81
            - T-cell lymphotropic,
                - type I (HTLV-I) B97.33
                - type II (HTLV-II) B97.34
        - papillomavirus B97.7
        - parvovirus B97.6
        - reovirus B97.5
        - respiratory syncytial B97.4
        - retrovirus B97.30
            - human
                - immunodeficiency, type 2 (HIV 2) B97.35
                - T-cell lymphotropic,
                    - type I (HTLV-I) B97.33
                    - type II (HTLV-II) B97.34
            - lentivirus B97.31
            - oncovirus B97.32
            - specified NEC B97.39
        - specified NEC B97.89
    - central nervous system A89
        - atypical A81.9
            - specified NEC A81.89
        - enterovirus NEC A88.8
            - meningitis A87.0
        - slow virus A81.9
            - specified NEC A81.89
        - specified NEC A88.8
    - chest J98.8
    - cotia B08.8
    - coxsackie (*see also* Infection, coxsackie) B34.1
        - as cause of disease classified elsewhere B97.11
    - ECHO
        - as cause of disease classified elsewhere B97.12
        - unspecified nature or site B34.1
    - encephalitis, tick-borne A84.9
    - enterovirus, as cause of disease classified elsewhere B97.10
        - coxsackievirus B97.11
        - echovirus B97.12
        - specified NEC B97.19
    - exanthem NOS B09
    - human metapneumovirus as cause of disease classified elsewhere B97.81
    - human papilloma as cause of disease classified elsewhere B97.7
    - intestine — *see* Enteritis, viral
    - respiratory syncytial
        - as cause of disease classified elsewhere B97.4
        - bronchopneumonia J12.1
        - common cold syndrome J00
        - nasopharyngitis (acute) J00
    - rhinovirus
        - as cause of disease classified elsewhere B97.89
        - unspecified nature or site B34.8
    - slow A81.9
        - specified NEC A81.89
    - specified type NEC B33.8
        - as cause of disease classified elsewhere B97.89
        - unspecified nature or site B34.8
    - unspecified nature or site B34.9
    - West Nile — *see* Virus, West Nile
- vulva (acute) — *see* Vulvitis
- West Nile — *see* Virus, West Nile

Infection, infected, infective — *continued*
- whipworm B79
- worms B83.9
    - specified type NEC B83.8
- Wuchereria (bancrofti) B74.0
    - malayi B74.1
- yatapoxvirus B08.70
    - specified NEC B08.79
- yeast (*see also* Candidiasis) B37.9
- yellow fever — *see* Fever, yellow
- Yersinia
    - enterocolitica (intestinal) A04.6
    - pestis — *see* Plague
    - pseudotuberculosis A28.2
- Zeis' gland — *see* Hordeolum
- zoonotic bacterial NOS A28.9
- Zopfia senegalensis B47.0

Infective, infectious — *see* condition

Infertility
- female N97.9
    - age-related N97.8
    - associated with
        - anovulation N97.0
        - cervical (mucus) disease or anomaly N88.3
        - congenital anomaly
            - cervix N88.3
            - fallopian tube N97.1
            - uterus N97.2
            - vagina N97.8
        - dysmucorrhea N88.3
        - fallopian tube disease or anomaly N97.1
        - pituitary-hypothalamic origin E23.0
        - specified origin NEC N97.8
        - Stein-Leventhal syndrome E28.2
        - uterine disease or anomaly N97.2
        - vaginal disease or anomaly N97.8
    - due to
        - cervical anomaly N88.3
        - fallopian tube anomaly N97.1
        - ovarian failure E28.39
        - Stein-Leventhal syndrome E28.2
        - uterine anomaly N97.2
        - vaginal anomaly N97.8
    - nonimplantation N97.2
    - origin
        - cervical N88.3
        - tubal (block) (occlusion) (stenosis) N97.1
        - uterine N97.2
        - vaginal N97.8
- male N46.9
    - azoospermia N46.01
        - extratesticular cause N46.029
            - drug therapy N46.021
            - efferent duct obstruction N46.023
            - infection N46.022
            - radiation N46.024
            - specified cause NEC N46.029
            - systemic disease N46.025
    - oligospermia N46.11
        - extratesticular cause N46.129
            - drug therapy N46.121
            - efferent duct obstruction N46.123
            - infection N46.122
            - radiation N46.124
            - specified cause NEC N46.129
            - systemic disease N46.125
    - specified type NEC N46.8

Infestation B88.9
- Acanthocheilonema (perstans) (streptocerca) B74.4
- Acariasis B88.0
    - demodex folliculorum B88.0
    - sarcoptes scabiei B86
    - trombiculae B88.0
- Agamofilaria streptocerca B74.4
- Ancylostoma, ankylostoma (braziliense) (caninum) (ceylanicum) (duodenale) B76.0
    - americanum B76.1
    - new world B76.1
- Anisakis larvae, anisakiasis B81.0
- arthropod NEC B88.2
- Ascaris lumbricoides — *see* Ascariasis
- Balantidium coli A07.0
- beef tapeworm B68.1
- Bothriocephalus (latus) B70.0
    - larval B70.1
- broad tapeworm B70.0
    - larval B70.1
- Brugia (malayi) B74.1

Infestation — continued
- Brugia (malayi) B74.1
  - timori B74.2
- candiru B88.8
- Capillaria
  - hepatica B83.8
  - philippinensis B81.1
- cat liver fluke B66.0
- cestodes B71.9
  - diphyllobothrium — see Infestation, diphyllobothrium
  - dipylidiasis B71.1
  - hymenolepiasis B71.0
  - specified type NEC B71.8
- chigger B88.0
- chigo, chigoe B88.1
- Clonorchis (sinensis) (liver) B66.1
- coccidial A07.3
- crab-lice B85.3
- Cysticercus cellulosae — see Cysticercosis
- Demodex (folliculorum) B88.0
- Dermanyssus gallinae B88.0
- Dermatobia (hominis) — see Myiasis
- Dibothriocephalus (latus) B70.0
  - larval B70.1
- Dicrocoelium dendriticum B66.2
- Diphyllobothrium (adult) (latum) (intestinal) (pacificum) B70.0
  - larval B70.1
- Diplogonoporus (grandis) B71.8
- Dipylidium caninum B67.4
- Distoma hepaticum B66.3
- dog tapeworm B67.4
- Dracunculus medinensis B72
- dragon worm B72
- dwarf tapeworm B71.0
- Echinococcus — see Echinococcus
- Echinostomum ilocanum B66.8
- Entamoeba (histolytica) — see Infection, Ameba
- Enterobius vermicularis B80
- eyelid
  - in (due to)
    - leishmaniasis B55.1
    - loiasis B74.3
    - onchocerciasis B73.09
    - phthriasis B85.3
    - parasitic NOS B89
- eyeworm B74.3
- Fasciola (gigantica) (hepatica) (indica) B66.3
- Fasciolopsis (buski) (intestine) B66.5
- filarial B74.9
  - bancroftian B74.0
  - conjunctiva B74.9
  - due to
    - Acanthocheilonema (perstans) (streptocerca) B74.4
    - Brugia (malayi) B74.1
      - timori B74.2
    - Dracunculus medinensis B72
    - guinea worm B72
    - loa loa B74.3
    - Mansonella (ozzardi) (perstans) (streptocerca) B74.4
    - Onchocerca volvulus B73.00
      - eye B73.00
      - eyelid B73.09
    - Wuchereria (bancrofti) B74.0
  - Malayan B74.1
  - ozzardi B74.4
  - specified type NEC B74.8
- fish tapeworm B70.0
  - larval B70.1
- fluke B66.9
  - blood NOS — see Schistosomiasis
  - cat liver B66.0
  - intestinal B66.5
  - lancet B66.2
  - liver (sheep) B66.3
    - cat B66.0
    - Chinese B66.1
    - due to clonorchiasis B66.1
    - oriental B66.1
  - lung (oriental) B66.4
  - sheep liver B66.3
  - specified type NEC B66.8
- fly larvae — see Myiasis
- Gasterophilus (intestinalis) — see Myiasis
- Gastrodiscoides hominis B66.8

Infestation — continued
- Giardia lamblia A07.1
- Gnathostoma (spinigerum) B83.1
- Gongylonema B83.8
- guinea worm B72
- helminth B83.9
  - angiostrongyliasis B83.2
    - intestinal B81.3
  - gnathostomiasis B83.1
  - hirudiniasis, internal B83.4
  - intestinal B82.0
    - angiostrongyliasis B81.3
    - anisakiasis B81.0
    - ascariasis — see Ascariasis
    - capillariasis B81.1
    - cysticercosis — see Cysticercosis
    - diphyllobothriasis — see Infestation, diphyllobothriasis
    - dracunculiasis B72
    - echinococcus — see Echinococcosis
    - enterobiasis B80
    - filariasis — see Infestation, filarial
    - fluke — see Infestation, fluke
    - hookworm — see Infestation, hookworm
    - mixed (types classifiable to more than one of the titles B65.0-B81.3 and B81.8) B81.4
    - onchocerciasis — see Onchocerciasis
    - schistosomiasis — see Infestation, schistosoma
    - specified
      - cestode NEC — see Infestation, cestode type NEC B81.8
    - strongyloidiasis — see Strongyloidiasis
    - taenia — see Infestation, taenia
    - trichinellosis B75
    - trichostrongyliasis B81.2
    - trichuriasis B79
  - specified type NEC B83.8
  - syngamiasis B83.3
  - visceral larva migrans B83.0
- Heterophyes (heterophyes) B66.8
- hookworm B76.9
  - ancylostomiasis B76.0
  - necatoriasis B76.1
  - specified type NEC B76.8
- Hymenolepis (diminuta) (nana) B71.0
- intestinal NEC B82.9
- leeches (aquatic) (land) — see Hirudiniasis
- Leishmania — see Leishmaniasis
- lice, louse — see Infestation, Pediculus
- Linguatula B88.8
- Liponyssoides sanguineus B88.0
- Loa loa B74.3
  - conjunctival B74.3
  - eyelid B74.3
- louse — see Infestation, Pediculus
- maggots — see Myiasis
- Mansonella (ozzardi) (perstans) (streptocerca) B74.4
- Medina (worm) B72
- Metagonimus (yokogawai) B66.8
- microfilaria streptocerca — see Onchocerciasis
  - eye B73.00
  - eyelid B73.09
- mites B88.9
  - scabic B86
- Monilia (albicans) — see Candidiasis
- mouth B37.0
- Necator americanus B76.1
- nematode NEC (intestinal) B82.0
  - Ancylostoma B76.0
  - conjunctiva NEC B83.9
  - Enterobius vermicularis B80
  - Gnathostoma spinigerum B83.1
  - physaloptera B80
  - specified NEC B81.8
  - trichostrongylus B81.2
  - trichuris (trichuria) B79
- Oesophagostomum (apiostomum) B81.8
- Oestrus ovis (see also Myiasis) B87.9
- Onchocerca (volvulus) — see Onchocerciasis
- Opisthorchis (felineus) (viverrini) B66.0
- orbit, parasitic NOS B89
- Oxyuris vermicularis B80
- Paragonimus (westermani) B66.4
- parasite, parasitic B89
  - eyelid B89
  - intestinal NOS B82.9
  - mouth B37.0
  - skin B88.9

Infestation — continued
- parasite, parasitic — continued
  - tongue B37.0
- Parastrongylus
  - cantonensis B83.2
  - costaricensis B81.3
- Pediculus B85.2
  - body B85.1
  - capitis (humanus) (any site) B85.0
  - corporis (humanus) (any site) B85.1
  - head B85.0
  - mixed (classifiable to more than one of the titles B85.0 - B85.3) B85.4
  - pubis (any site) B85.3
- Pentastoma B88.8
- Phthirus (pubis) (any site) B85.3
  - with any infestation classifiable to B85.0 - B85.2 B85.4
- pinworm B80
- pork tapeworm (adult) B68.0
- protozoal NEC B64
  - intestinal A07.9
    - specified NEC A07.8
  - specified NEC B60.8
- pubic, louse B85.3
- rat tapeworm B71.0
- red bug B88.0
- roundworm (large) NEC B82.0
  - Ascariasis (see also Ascariasis) B77.9
- sandflea B88.1
- Sarcoptes scabiei B86
- scabies B86
- Schistosoma B65.9
  - bovis B65.8
  - cercariae B65.3
  - haematobium B65.0
  - intercalatum B65.8
  - japonicum B65.2
  - mansoni B65.1
  - mattheei B65.8
  - mekongi B65.8
  - specified type NEC B65.8
  - spindale B65.8
- screw worms — see Myiasis
- skin NOS B88.9
- Sparganum (mansoni) (proliferum) (baxteri) B70.1
  - larval B70.1
- specified type NEC B88.8
- Spirometra larvae B70.1
- Stellantchasmus falcatus B66.8
- Strongyloides stercoralis — see Strongyloidiasis
- Taenia B68.9
  - diminuta B71.0
  - echinococcus — see Echinococcus
  - mediocanellata B68.1
  - nana B71.0
  - saginata B68.1
  - solium (intestinal form) B68.0
    - larval form — see Cysticercosis
- Taeniarhynchus saginatus B68.1
- tapeworm B71.9
  - beef B68.1
  - broad B70.0
    - larval B70.1
  - dog B67.4
  - dwarf B71.0
  - fish B70.0
    - larval B70.1
  - pork B68.0
  - rat B71.0
- Ternidens diminutus B81.8
- Tetranychus molestissimus B88.0
- threadworm B80
- tongue B37.0
- Toxocara (canis) (cati) (felis) B83.0
- trematode(s) NEC — see Infestation, fluke
- Trichinella (spiralis) B75
- Trichocephalus B79
- Trichomonas — see Trichomoniasis
- Trichostrongylus B81.2
- Trichuris (trichiura) B79
- Trombicula (irritans) B88.0
- Tunga penetrans B88.1
- Uncinaria americana B76.1
- Vandellia cirrhosa B88.8
- whipworm B79
- worms B83.9
  - intestinal B82.0

Infestation — *continued*
  Wuchereria (bancrofti) B74.0
Infiltrate, infiltration
  amyloid (generalized) (localized) — *see* Amyloidosis
  calcareous NEC R89.7
    localized — *see* Degeneration, by site
  calcium salt R89.7
  cardiac
    fatty — *see* Degeneration, myocardial
    glycogenic E74.02 [I43]
  corneal — *see* Edema, cornea
  eyelid — *see* Inflammation, eyelid
  glycogen, glycogenic — *see* Disease, glycogen storage
  heart, cardiac
    fatty — *see* Degeneration, myocardial
    glycogenic E74.02 [I43]
  inflammatory in vitreous H43.89
  kidney N28.89
  leukemic — *see* Leukemia
  liver K76.89
    fatty — *see* Fatty, liver NEC
    glycogen (*see also* Disease, glycogen storage)
      E74.03 [K77]
  lung R91.8
    eosinophilic J82
  lymphatic (*see also* Leukemia, lymphatic) C91.9- ☑
    gland I88.9
  muscle, fatty M62.89
  myocardium, myocardial
    fatty — *see* Degeneration, myocardial
    glycogenic E74.02 [I43]
  on chest x-ray R91.8
  pulmonary R91.8
    with eosinophilia J82
  skin (lymphocytic) L98.6
  thymus (gland) (fatty) E32.8
  urine R39.0
  vesicant agent
    antineoplastic chemotherapy T80.810 ☑
    other agent NEC T80.818 ☑
  vitreous body H43.89
Infirmity R68.89
  senile R54
Inflammation, inflamed, inflammatory (with exudation)
  abducent (nerve) — *see* Strabismus, paralytic, sixth nerve
  accessory sinus (chronic) — *see* Sinusitis
  adrenal (gland) E27.8
  alveoli, teeth M27.3
    scorbutic E54
  anal canal, anus K62.89
  antrum (chronic) — *see* Sinusitis, maxillary
  appendix — *see* Appendicitis
  arachnoid — *see* Meningitis
  areola N61
    puerperal, postpartum or gestational — *see* Infection, nipple
  areolar tissue NOS L08.9
  artery — *see* Arteritis
  auditory meatus (external) — *see* Otitis, externa
  Bartholin's gland N75.8
  bile duct (common) (hepatic) or passage — *see* Cholangitis
  bladder — *see* Cystitis
  bone — *see* Osteomyelitis
  brain (*see also* Encephalitis)
    membrane — *see* Meningitis
  breast N61
    puerperal, postpartum, gestational — *see* Mastitis, obstetric
  broad ligament — *see* Disease, pelvis, inflammatory
  bronchi — *see* Bronchitis
  catarrhal J00
  cecum — *see* Appendicitis
  cerebral (*see also* Encephalitis)
    membrane — *see* Meningitis
  cerebrospinal
    meningococcal A39.0
  cervix (uteri) — *see* Cervicitis
  chest J98.8
  chorioretinal H30.9- ☑
    cyclitis — *see* Cyclitis
    disseminated H30.10- ☑
      generalized H30.13- ☑
      peripheral H30.12- ☑
      posterior pole H30.11- ☑

Inflammation, inflamed, inflammatory — *continued*
  chorioretinal — *continued*
    epitheliopathy — *see* Epitheliopathy
    focal H30.00- ☑
      juxtapapillary H30.01- ☑
      macular H30.04- ☑
      paramacular — *see* Inflammation, chorioretinal, focal, macular
      peripheral H30.03- ☑
      posterior pole H30.02- ☑
    specified type NEC H30.89- ☑
  choroid — *see* Inflammation, chorioretinal
  chronic, postmastoidectomy cavity — *see* Complications, postmastoidectomy, inflammation
  colon — *see* Enteritis
  connective tissue (diffuse) NEC — *see* Disorder, soft tissue, specified type NEC
  cornea — *see* Keratitis
  corpora cavernosa N48.29
  cranial nerve — *see* Disorder, nerve, cranial
  Douglas' cul-de-sac or pouch (chronic) N73.0
  due to device, implant or graft (*see also* Complications, by site and type, infection or inflammation)
    arterial graft T82.7 ☑
    breast (implant) T85.79 ☑
    catheter T85.79 ☑
      dialysis (renal) T82.7 ☑
        intraperitoneal T85.71 ☑
      infusion T82.7 ☑
        spinal (epidural) (subdural) T85.79 ☑
      urinary (indwelling) T83.51 ☑
    electronic (electrode) (pulse generator) (stimulator)
      bone T84.7 ☑
      cardiac T82.7 ☑
      nervous system (brain) (peripheral nerve) (spinal) T85.79 ☑
      urinary T83.59 ☑
    fixation, internal (orthopedic) NEC — *see* Complication, fixation device, infection
    gastrointestinal (bile duct) (esophagus) T85.79 ☑
    genital NEC T83.6 ☑
    heart NEC T82.7 ☑
      valve (prosthesis) T82.6 ☑
        graft T82.7 ☑
    joint prosthesis — *see* Complication, joint prosthesis, infection
    ocular (corneal graft) (orbital implant) NEC T85.79 ☑
    orthopedic NEC T84.7 ☑
    specified NEC T85.79 ☑
    urinary NEC T83.59 ☑
    vascular NEC T82.7 ☑
    ventricular intracranial shunt T85.79 ☑
  duodenum K29.80
    with bleeding K29.81
  dura mater — *see* Meningitis
  ear (middle) (*see also* Otitis, media)
    external — *see* Otitis, externa
    inner — *see* subcategory H83.0 ☑
  epididymis — *see* Epididymitis
  esophagus K20.9
  ethmoidal (sinus) (chronic) — *see* Sinusitis, ethmoidal
  eustachian tube (catarrhal) — *see* Salpingitis, eustachian
  eyelid H01.9
    abscess — *see* Abscess, eyelid
    blepharitis — *see* Blepharitis
    chalazion — *see* Chalazion
    dermatosis (noninfectious) — *see* Dermatosis, eyelid
    hordeolum — *see* Hordeolum
    specified NEC H01.8
  fallopian tube — *see* Salpingo-oophoritis
  fascia — *see* Myositis
  follicular, pharynx J31.2
  frontal (sinus) (chronic) — *see* Sinusitis, frontal
  gallbladder — *see* Cholecystitis
  gastric — *see* Gastritis
  gastrointestinal — *see* Enteritis
  genital organ (internal) (diffuse)
    female — *see* Disease, pelvis, inflammatory
    male N49.9
      multiple sites N49.8
      specified NEC N49.8
  gland (lymph) — *see* Lymphadenitis

Inflammation, inflamed, inflammatory — *continued*
  glottis — *see* Laryngitis
  granular, pharynx J31.2
  gum K05.10
    nonplaque induced K05.11
    plaque induced K05.10
  heart — *see* Carditis
  hepatic duct — *see* Cholangitis
  ileoanal (internal) pouch K91.850
  ileum (*see also* Enteritis)
    regional or terminal — *see* Enteritis, regional
  intestinal pouch K91.850
  intestine (any part) — *see* Enteritis
  jaw (acute) (bone) (chronic) (lower) (suppurative) (upper) M27.2
  joint NEC — *see* Arthritis
    sacroiliac M46.1
  kidney — *see* Nephritis
  knee (joint) M13.169
    tuberculous A18.02
  labium (majus) (minus) — *see* Vulvitis
  lacrimal
    gland — *see* Dacryoadenitis
    passages (duct) (sac) (*see also* Dacryocystitis)
      canaliculitis — *see* Canaliculitis, lacrimal
  larynx — *see* Laryngitis
  leg NOS L08.9
  lip K13.0
  liver (capsule) (*see also* Hepatitis)
    chronic K73.9
    suppurative K75.0
  lung (acute) (*see also* Pneumonia)
    chronic J98.4
  lymph gland or node — *see* Lymphadenitis
  lymphatic vessel — *see* Lymphangitis
  maxilla, maxillary M27.2
    sinus (chronic) — *see* Sinusitis, maxillary
  membranes of brain or spinal cord — *see* Meningitis
  meninges — *see* Meningitis
  mouth K12.1
  muscle — *see* Myositis
  myocardium — *see* Myocarditis
  nasal sinus (chronic) — *see* Sinusitis
  nasopharynx — *see* Nasopharyngitis
  navel L08.82
  nerve NEC — *see* Neuralgia
  nipple N61
    puerperal, postpartum or gestational — *see* Infection, nipple
  nose — *see* Rhinitis
  oculomotor (nerve) — *see* Strabismus, paralytic, third nerve
  optic nerve — *see* Neuritis, optic
  orbit (chronic) H05.10
    acute H05.00
      abscess — *see* Abscess, orbit
      cellulitis — *see* Cellulitis, orbit
      osteomyelitis — *see* Osteomyelitis, orbit
      periostitis — *see* Periostitis, orbital
      tenonitis — *see* Tenonitis, eye
    granuloma — *see* Granuloma, orbit
    myositis — *see* Myositis, orbital
  ovary — *see* Salpingo-oophoritis
  oviduct — *see* Salpingo-oophoritis
  pancreas (acute) — *see* Pancreatitis
  parametrium N73.0
  parotid region L08.9
  pelvis, female — *see* Disease, pelvis, inflammatory
  penis (corpora cavernosa) N48.29
  perianal K62.89
  pericardium — *see* Pericarditis
  perineum (female) (male) L08.9
  perirectal K62.89
  peritoneum — *see* Peritonitis
  periuterine — *see* Disease, pelvis, inflammatory
  perivesical — *see* Cystitis
  petrous bone (acute) (chronic) — *see* Petrositis
  pharynx (acute) — *see* Pharyngitis
  pia mater — *see* Meningitis
  pleura — *see* Pleurisy
  polyp, colon (*see also* Polyp, colon, inflammatory) K51.40
  prostate (*see also* Prostatitis)
    specified type NEC N41.8
  rectosigmoid — *see* Rectosigmoiditis
  rectum (*see also* Proctitis) K62.89

Inflammation, inflamed, inflammatory — *continued*
  respiratory, upper (*see also* Infection, respiratory, upper) J06.9
    acute, due to radiation J70.0
    chronic, due to external agent — *see* condition, respiratory, chronic, due to
    due to
      chemicals, gases, fumes or vapors (inhalation) J68.2
      radiation J70.1
  retina — *see* Chorioretinitis
  retrocecal — *see* Appendicitis
  retroperitoneal — *see* Peritonitis
  salivary duct or gland (any) (suppurative) — *see* Sialoadenitis
  scorbutic, alveoli, teeth E54
  scrotum N49.2
  seminal vesicle — *see* Vesiculitis
  sigmoid — *see* Enteritis
  sinus — *see* Sinusitis
  Skene's duct or gland — *see* Urethritis
  skin L08.9
  spermatic cord N49.1
  sphenoidal (sinus) — *see* Sinusitis, sphenoidal
  spinal
    cord — *see* Encephalitis
    membrane — *see* Meningitis
    nerve — *see* Disorder, nerve
  spine — *see* Spondylopathy, inflammatory
  spleen (capsule) D73.89
  stomach — *see* Gastritis
  subcutaneous tissue L08.9
  suprarenal (gland) E27.8
  synovial — *see* Tenosynovitis
  tendon (sheath) NEC — *see* Tenosynovitis
  testis — *see* Orchitis
  throat (acute) — *see* Pharyngitis
  thymus (gland) E32.8
  thyroid (gland) — *see* Thyroiditis
  tongue K14.0
  tonsil — *see* Tonsillitis
  trachea — *see* Tracheitis
  trochlear (nerve) — *see* Strabismus, paralytic, fourth nerve
  tubal — *see* Salpingo-oophoritis
  tuberculous NEC — *see* Tuberculosis
  tubo-ovarian — *see* Salpingo-oophoritis
  tunica vaginalis N49.1
  tympanic membrane — *see* Tympanitis
  umbilicus, umbilical L08.82
  uterine ligament — *see* Disease, pelvis, inflammatory
  uterus (catarrhal) — *see* Endometritis
  uveal tract (anterior) NOS (*see also* Iridocyclitis)
    posterior — *see* Chorioretinitis
  vagina — *see* Vaginitis
  vas deferens N49.1
  vein (*see also* Phlebitis)
    intracranial or intraspinal (septic) G08
    thrombotic I80.9
      leg — *see* Phlebitis, leg
      lower extremity — *see* Phlebitis, leg
  vocal cord J38.3
  vulva — *see* Vulvitis
  Wharton's duct (suppurative) — *see* Sialoadenitis
Inflation, lung, imperfect (newborn) — *see* Atelectasis
Influenza (bronchial) (epidemic) (respiratory (upper)) (unidentified influenza virus) J11.1
  with
    digestive manifestations J11.2
    encephalopathy J11.81
    enteritis J11.2
    gastroenteritis J11.2
    gastrointestinal manifestations J11.2
    laryngitis J11.1
    myocarditis J11.82
    otitis media J11.83
    pharyngitis J11.1
    pneumonia J11.00
      specified type J11.08
    respiratory manifestations NEC J11.1
    specified manifestation NEC J11.89
  A/H5N1 (*see also* Influenza, due to, identified novel influenza A virus) J09.X2
  avian (*see also* Influenza, due to, identified novel influenza A virus) J09.X2

Influenza — *continued*
  bird (*see also* Influenza, due to, identified novel influenza A virus) J09.X2
  due to
    avian (*see also* Influenza, due to, identified novel influenza A virus) J09.X2
    identified influenza virus NEC J10.1
      with
        digestive manifestations J10.2
        encephalopathy J10.81
        enteritis J10.2
        gastroenteritis J10.2
        gastrointestinal manifestations J10.2
        laryngitis J10.1
        myocarditis J10.82
        otitis media J10.83
        pharyngitis J10.1
        pneumonia (unspecified type) J10.00
          with same identified influenza virus J10.01
          specified type NEC J10.08
        respiratory manifestations NEC J10.1
        specified manifestation NEC J10.89
    identified novel influenza A virus J09.X2
      with
        digestive manifestations J09.X3
        encephalopathy J09.X9
        enteritis J09.X3
        gastroenteritis J09.X3
        gastrointestinal manifestations J09.X3
        laryngitis J09.X2
        myocarditis J09.X9
        otitis media J09.X9
        pharyngitis J09.X2
        pneumonia J09.X1
        respiratory manifestations NEC J09.X2
        specified manifestation NEC J09.X9
        upper respiratory symptoms J09.X2
  novel (2009) H1N1 influenza (*see also* Influenza, due to, identified influenza virus NEC) J10.1
  novel influenza A/H1N1 (*see also* Influenza, due to, identified influenza virus NEC) J10.1
  of other animal origin, not bird or swine (*see also* Influenza, due to, identified novel influenza A virus) J09.X2
  swine (viruses that normally cause infections in pigs) (*see also* Influenza, due to, identified novel influenza A virus) J09.X2
Influenzal — *see* Influenza
Influenza-like disease — *see* Influenza
Infraction, Freiberg's (metatarsal head) — *see* Osteochondrosis, juvenile, metatarsus
Infraeruption of tooth (teeth) M26.34
Infusion complication, misadventure, or reaction — *see* Complications, infusion
Ingestion
  chemical — *see* Table of Drugs and Chemicals, by substance, poisoning
  drug or medicament
    correct substance properly administered — *see* Table of Drugs and Chemicals, by drug, adverse effect
    overdose or wrong substance given or taken — *see* Table of Drugs and Chemicals, by drug, poisoning
  foreign body — *see* Foreign body, alimentary tract
  tularemia A21.3
Ingrowing
  hair (beard) L73.1
  nail (finger) (toe) L60.0
Inguinal (*see also* condition)
  testicle Q53.9
    bilateral Q53.21
    unilateral Q53.11
Inhalation
  anthrax A22.1
  flame T27.3 ☑
  food or foreign body — *see* Foreign body, by site
  gases, fumes, or vapors NEC T59.9- ☑
    specified agent — *see* Table of Drugs and Chemicals, by substance
  liquid or vomitus — *see* Asphyxia
  meconium (newborn) P24.00
    with
      with respiratory symptoms P24.01
      pneumonia (pneumonitis) P24.01
  mucus — *see* Asphyxia, mucus

Inhalation — *continued*
  oil or gasoline (causing suffocation) — *see* Foreign body, by site
  smoke J70.5
    due to chemicals, gases, fumes and vapors J68.9
  steam — *see* Toxicity, vapors
  stomach contents or secretions — *see* Foreign body, by site
    due to anesthesia (general) (local) or other sedation T88.59
      in labor and delivery O74.0
      in pregnancy O29.01- ☑
      postpartum, puerperal O89.01
Inhibition, orgasm
  female F52.31
  male F52.32
Inhibitor, systemic lupus erythematosus (presence of) D68.62
Iniencephalus, iniencephaly Q00.2
Injection, traumatic jet (air) (industrial) (water) (paint or dye) T70.4 ☑
Injury (*see also* specified injury type) T14.90
  abdomen, abdominal S39.91 ☑
    blood vessel — *see* Injury, blood vessel, abdomen
    cavity — *see* Injury, intra-abdominal
    contusion S30.1 ☑
    internal — *see* Injury, intra-abdominal
    intra-abdominal organ — *see* Injury, intra-abdominal
    nerve — *see* Injury, nerve, abdomen
    open — *see* Wound, open, abdomen
    specified NEC S39.81 ☑
    superficial — *see* Injury, superficial, abdomen
  Achilles tendon S86.00- ☑
    laceration S86.02- ☑
    specified type NEC S86.09- ☑
    strain S86.01- ☑
  acoustic, resulting in deafness — *see* Injury, nerve, acoustic
  adrenal (gland) S37.819 ☑
    contusion S37.812 ☑
    laceration S37.813 ☑
    specified type NEC S37.818 ☑
  alveolar (process) S09.93 ☑
  ankle S99.91- ☑
    contusion — *see* Contusion, ankle
    dislocation — *see* Dislocation, ankle
    fracture — *see* Fracture, ankle
    nerve — *see* Injury, nerve, ankle
    open — *see* Wound, open, ankle
    specified type NEC S99.81- ☑
    sprain — *see* Sprain, ankle
    superficial — *see* Injury, superficial, ankle
  anterior chamber, eye — *see* Injury, eye, specified site NEC
  anus — *see* Injury, abdomen
  aorta (thoracic) S25.00 ☑
    abdominal S35.00 ☑
      laceration (minor) (superficial) S35.01 ☑
        major S35.02 ☑
      specified type NEC S35.09 ☑
    laceration (minor) (superficial) S25.01 ☑
      major S25.02 ☑
    specified type NEC S25.09 ☑
  arm (upper) S49.9- ☑
    blood vessel — *see* Injury, blood vessel, arm
    contusion — *see* Contusion, arm, upper
    fracture — *see* Fracture, humerus
    lower — *see* Injury, forearm
    muscle — *see* Injury, muscle, shoulder
    nerve — *see* Injury, nerve, arm
    open — *see* Wound, open, arm
    specified type NEC S49.8- ☑
    superficial — *see* Injury, superficial, arm
  artery (complicating trauma) (*see also* Injury, blood vessel, by site)
    cerebral or meningeal — *see* Injury, intracranial
  auditory canal (external) (meatus) S09.91 ☑
  auricle, auris, ear S09.91 ☑
  axilla — *see* Injury, shoulder
  back — *see* Injury, back, lower
  bile duct S36.13 ☑
  birth (*see also* Birth, injury) P15.9
  bladder (sphincter) S37.20 ☑
    at delivery O71.5
    contusion S37.22 ☑

Injury — *continued*
  bladder — *continued*
    laceration S37.23 ☑
    obstetrical trauma O71.5
    specified type NEC S37.29 ☑
  blast (air) (hydraulic) (immersion) (underwater) NEC
      T14.8
    acoustic nerve trauma — *see* Injury, nerve, acoustic
    bladder — *see* Injury, bladder
    brain — *see* Concussion
    colon — *see* Injury, intestine, large
    ear (primary) S09.31- ☑
      secondary S09.39- ☑
    generalized T70.8 ☑
    lung — *see* Injury, intrathoracic, lung
    multiple body organs T70.8 ☑
    peritoneum S36.81 ☑
    rectum S36.61 ☑
    retroperitoneum S36.898 ☑
    small intestine S36.419 ☑
      duodenum S36.410 ☑
      specified site NEC S36.418 ☑
    specified
      intra-abdominal organ NEC S36.898 ☑
      pelvic organ NEC S37.899 ☑
  blood vessel NEC T14.8
    abdomen S35.9 ☑
      aorta — *see* Injury, aorta, abdominal
      celiac artery — *see* Injury, blood vessel, celiac
          artery
      iliac vessel — *see* Injury, blood vessel, iliac
      laceration S35.91 ☑
      mesenteric vessel — *see* Injury, mesenteric
      portal vein — *see* Injury, blood vessel, portal
          vein
      renal vessel — *see* Injury, blood vessel, renal
      specified vessel NEC S35.8X- ☑
      splenic vessel — *see* Injury, blood vessel,
          splenic
      vena cava — *see* Injury, vena cava, inferior
    ankle — *see* Injury, blood vessel, foot
    aorta (abdominal) (thoracic) — *see* Injury, aorta
    arm (upper) NEC S45.90- ☑
      forearm — *see* Injury, blood vessel, forearm
      laceration S45.91- ☑
      specified
        site NEC S45.80- ☑
          laceration S45.81- ☑
          specified type NEC S45.89- ☑
        type NEC S45.99- ☑
      superficial vein S45.30- ☑
        laceration S45.31- ☑
        specified type NEC S45.39- ☑
    axillary
      artery S45.00- ☑
        laceration S45.01- ☑
        specified type NEC S45.09- ☑
      vein S45.20- ☑
        laceration S45.21- ☑
        specified type NEC S45.29- ☑
    azygos vein — *see* Injury, blood vessel, thoracic,
        specified site NEC
    brachial
      artery S45.10- ☑
        laceration S45.11- ☑
        specified type NEC S45.19- ☑
      vein S45.20- ☑
        laceration S45.219 ☑
        specified type NEC S45.29- ☑
    carotid artery (common) (external) (internal, ex-
        tracranial) S15.00- ☑
      internal, intracranial S06.8- ☑
      laceration (minor) (superficial) S15.01- ☑
        major S15.02- ☑
      specified type NEC S15.09- ☑
    celiac artery S35.219 ☑
      branch S35.299 ☑
        laceration (minor) (superficial) S35.291 ☑
          major S35.292 ☑
        specified NEC S35.298 ☑
      laceration (minor) (superficial) S35.211 ☑
        major S35.212 ☑
      specified type NEC S35.218 ☑
    cerebral — *see* Injury, intracranial
    deep plantar — *see* Injury, blood vessel, plantar
        artery

Injury — *continued*
  blood vessel — *continued*
    digital (hand) — *see* Injury, blood vessel, finger
    dorsal
      artery (foot) S95.00- ☑
        laceration S95.01- ☑
        specified type NEC S95.09- ☑
      vein (foot) S95.20- ☑
        laceration S95.21- ☑
        specified type NEC S95.29- ☑
    due to accidental laceration during procedure —
        see Laceration, accidental complicating
        surgery
    extremity — *see* Injury, blood vessel, limb
    femoral
      artery (common) (superficial) S75.00- ☑
        laceration (minor) (superficial) S75.01- ☑
          major S75.02- ☑
        specified type NEC S75.09- ☑
      vein (hip level) (thigh level) S75.10- ☑
        laceration (minor) (superficial) S75.11- ☑
          major S75.12- ☑
        specified type NEC S75.19- ☑
    finger S65.50- ☑
      index S65.50- ☑
        laceration S65.51- ☑
        specified type NEC S65.59- ☑
      laceration S65.51- ☑
      little S65.50- ☑
        laceration S65.51- ☑
        specified type NEC S65.59- ☑
      middle S65.50- ☑
        laceration S65.51- ☑
        specified type NEC S65.59- ☑
      specified type NEC S65.59- ☑
      thumb — *see* Injury, blood vessel, thumb
    foot S95.90- ☑
      dorsal
        artery — *see* Injury, blood vessel, dorsal,
            artery
        vein — *see* Injury, blood vessel, dorsal, vein
      laceration S95.91- ☑
      plantar artery — *see* Injury, blood vessel, plan-
          tar artery
      specified
        site NEC S95.80- ☑
          laceration S95.81- ☑
          specified type NEC S95.89- ☑
        specified type NEC S95.99- ☑
    forearm S55.90- ☑
      laceration S55.91- ☑
      radial artery — *see* Injury, blood vessel, radial
          artery
      specified
        site NEC S55.80- ☑
          laceration S55.81- ☑
          specified type NEC S55.89- ☑
        type NEC S55.99- ☑
      ulnar artery — *see* Injury, blood vessel, ulnar
          artery
      vein S55.20- ☑
        laceration S55.21- ☑
        specified type NEC S55.29- ☑
    gastric
      artery — *see* Injury, mesenteric, artery, branch
      vein — *see* Injury, blood vessel, abdomen
    gastroduodenal artery — *see* Injury, mesenteric,
        artery, branch
    greater saphenous vein (lower leg level) S85.30- ☑
      hip (and thigh) level S75.20- ☑
        laceration (minor) (superficial) S75.21- ☑
          major S75.22- ☑
        specified type NEC S75.29- ☑
      laceration S85.31- ☑
      specified type NEC S85.39- ☑
    hand (level) S65.90- ☑
      finger — *see* Injury, blood vessel, finger
      laceration S65.91- ☑
      palmar arch — *see* Injury, blood vessel, palmar
          arch
      radial artery — *see* Injury, blood vessel, radial
          artery, hand
      specified
        site NEC S65.80- ☑
          laceration S65.81- ☑
          specified type NEC S65.89- ☑

Injury — *continued*
  blood vessel — *continued*
    hand — *continued*
      specified — *continued*
        type NEC S65.99- ☑
      thumb — *see* Injury, blood vessel, thumb
      ulnar artery — *see* Injury, blood vessel, ulnar
          artery, hand
    head S09.0 ☑
      intracranial — *see* Injury, intracranial
      multiple S09.0 ☑
    hepatic
      artery — *see* Injury, mesenteric, artery
      vein — *see* Injury, vena cava, inferior
    hip S75.90- ☑
      femoral artery — *see* Injury, blood vessel,
          femoral, artery
      femoral vein — *see* Injury, blood vessel,
          femoral, vein
      greater saphenous vein — *see* Injury, blood
          vessel, greater saphenous, hip level
      laceration S75.91- ☑
      specified
        site NEC S75.80- ☑
          laceration S75.81- ☑
          specified type NEC S75.89- ☑
        type NEC S75.99- ☑
    hypogastric (artery) (vein) — *see* Injury, blood
        vessel, iliac
    iliac S35.5- ☑
      artery S35.51- ☑
      specified vessel NEC S35.5- ☑
      uterine vessel — *see* Injury, blood vessel, uter-
          ine
      vein S35.51- ☑
    innominate — *see* Injury, blood vessel, thoracic,
        innominate
    intercostal (artery) (vein) — *see* Injury, blood vessel,
        thoracic, intercostal
    jugular vein (external) S15.20- ☑
      internal S15.30- ☑
        laceration (minor) (superficial) S15.31- ☑
          major S15.32- ☑
        specified type NEC S15.39- ☑
      laceration (minor) (superficial) S15.21- ☑
        major S15.22- ☑
      specified type NEC S15.29- ☑
    leg (level) (lower) S85.90- ☑
      greater saphenous — *see* Injury, blood vessel,
          greater saphenous
      laceration S85.91- ☑
      lesser saphenous — *see* Injury, blood vessel,
          lesser saphenous
      peroneal artery — *see* Injury, blood vessel,
          peroneal artery
      popliteal
        artery — *see* Injury, blood vessel, popliteal,
            artery
        vein — *see* Injury, blood vessel, popliteal,
            vein
      specified
        site NEC S85.80- ☑
          laceration S85.81- ☑
          specified type NEC S85.89- ☑
        type NEC S85.99- ☑
      thigh — *see* Injury, blood vessel, hip
      tibial artery — *see* Injury, blood vessel, tibial
          artery
    lesser saphenous vein (lower leg level) S85.40- ☑
      laceration S85.41- ☑
      specified type NEC S85.49- ☑
    limb
      lower — *see* Injury, blood vessel, leg
      upper — *see* Injury, blood vessel, arm
    lower back — *see* Injury, blood vessel, abdomen
      specified NEC — *see* Injury, blood vessel, ab-
          domen, specified, site NEC
    mammary (artery) (vein) — *see* Injury, blood vessel,
        thoracic, specified site NEC
    mesenteric (inferior) (superior)
      artery — *see* Injury, mesenteric, artery
      vein — *see* Injury, blood vessel, mesenteric,
          vein
    neck S15.9 ☑
      specified site NEC S15.8 ☑
    ovarian (artery) (vein) — *see* subcategory S35.8 ☑

☑ **Additional Character Required** — **Refer to the Tabular List for Character Selection**   ▽ **Subterms under main terms may continue to next column or page**

Injury — *continued*
  blood vessel — *continued*
    palmar arch (superficial) S65.20- ☑
      deep S65.30- ☑
        laceration S65.31- ☑
        specified type NEC S65.39- ☑
      laceration S65.21- ☑
      specified type NEC S65.29- ☑
    pelvis — *see* Injury, blood vessel, abdomen
      specified NEC — *see* Injury, blood vessel, abdomen, specified, site NEC
    peroneal artery S85.20- ☑
      laceration S85.21- ☑
      specified type NEC S85.29- ☑
    plantar artery (deep) (foot) S95.10- ☑
      laceration S95.11- ☑
      specified type NEC S95.19- ☑
    popliteal
      artery S85.00- ☑
        laceration S85.01- ☑
        specified type NEC S85.09- ☑
      vein S85.50- ☑
        laceration S85.51- ☑
        specified type NEC S85.59- ☑
    portal vein S35.319
      laceration S35.311 ☑
      specified type NEC S35.318 ☑
    precerebral — *see* Injury, blood vessel, neck
    pulmonary (artery) (vein) — *see* Injury, blood vessel, thoracic, pulmonary
    radial artery (forearm level) S55.10- ☑
      hand and wrist (level) S65.10- ☑
        laceration S65.11- ☑
        specified type NEC S65.19- ☑
      laceration S55.11- ☑
      specified type NEC S55.19- ☑
    renal
      artery S35.40- ☑
        laceration S35.41- ☑
        specified NEC S35.49- ☑
      vein S35.40- ☑
        laceration S35.41- ☑
        specified NEC S35.49- ☑
    saphenous vein (greater) (lower leg level) — *see* Injury, blood vessel, greater saphenous
      hip and thigh level — *see* Injury, blood vessel, greater saphenous, hip level
      lesser — *see* Injury, blood vessel, lesser saphenous
    shoulder
      specified NEC — *see* Injury, blood vessel, arm, specified site NEC
      superficial vein — *see* Injury, blood vessel, arm, superficial vein
    specified NEC T14.8
    splenic
      artery — *see* Injury, blood vessel, celiac artery, branch
      vein S35.329 ☑
        laceration S35.321 ☑
        specified NEC S35.328 ☑
    subclavian — *see* Injury, blood vessel, thoracic, innominate
    thigh — *see* Injury, blood vessel, hip
    thoracic S25.90 ☑
      aorta S25.00 ☑
        laceration (minor) (superficial) S25.01 ☑
          major S25.02 ☑
        specified type NEC S25.09 ☑
      azygos vein — *see* Injury, blood vessel, thoracic, specified, site NEC
      innominate
        artery S25.10- ☑
          laceration (minor) (superficial) S25.11- ☑
            major S25.12- ☑
          specified type NEC S25.19- ☑
        vein S25.30- ☑
          laceration (minor) (superficial) S25.31- ☑
            major S25.32- ☑
          specified type NEC S25.39- ☑
      intercostal S25.50- ☑
        laceration S25.51- ☑
        specified type NEC S25.59- ☑
      laceration S25.91 ☑

Injury — *continued*
  blood vessel — *continued*
    thoracic — *continued*
      mammary vessel — *see* Injury, blood vessel, thoracic, specified, site NEC
      pulmonary S25.40- ☑
        laceration (minor) (superficial) S25.41- ☑
          major S25.42- ☑
        specified type NEC S25.49- ☑
      specified
        site NEC S25.80- ☑
          laceration S25.81 ☑
          specified type NEC S25.89 ☑
        type NEC S25.99 ☑
      subclavian — *see* Injury, blood vessel, thoracic, innominate
      vena cava (superior) S25.20 ☑
        laceration (minor) (superficial) S25.21 ☑
          major S25.22 ☑
        specified type NEC S25.29 ☑
    thumb S65.40- ☑
      laceration S65.41- ☑
      specified type NEC S65.49- ☑
    tibial artery S85.10- ☑
      anterior S85.13- ☑
        laceration S85.14- ☑
        specified injury NEC S85.15- ☑
      laceration S85.11- ☑
      posterior S85.16- ☑
        laceration S85.17- ☑
        specified injury NEC S85.18- ☑
      specified injury NEC S85.12- ☑
    ulnar artery (forearm level) S55.00- ☑
      hand and wrist (level) S65.00- ☑
        laceration S65.01- ☑
        specified type NEC S65.09- ☑
      laceration S55.01- ☑
      specified type NEC S55.09- ☑
    upper arm (level) — *see* Injury, blood vessel, arm
    superficial vein — *see* Injury, blood vessel, arm, superficial vein
    uterine S35.5- ☑
      artery S35.53- ☑
      vein S35.53- ☑
    vena cava — *see* Injury, vena cava
    vertebral artery S15.10- ☑
      laceration (minor) (superficial) S15.11- ☑
        major S15.12- ☑
      specified type NEC S15.19- ☑
    wrist (level) — *see* Injury, blood vessel, hand
  brachial plexus S14.3 ☑
    newborn P14.3
  brain (traumatic) S06.9- ☑
    diffuse (axonal) S06.2X- ☑
    focal S06.30- ☑
    traumatic — *see* category S06 ☑
  brainstem S06.38- ☑
  breast NOS S29.9 ☑
  broad ligament — *see* Injury, pelvic organ, specified site NEC
  bronchus, bronchi — *see* Injury, intrathoracic, bronchus
  brow S09.90 ☑
  buttock S39.92 ☑
  canthus, eye S05.90 ☑
  cardiac plexus — *see* Injury, nerve, thorax, sympathetic
  cauda equina S34.3 ☑
  cavernous sinus — *see* Injury, intracranial
  cecum — *see* Injury, colon
  celiac ganglion or plexus — *see* Injury, nerve, lumbosacral, sympathetic
  cerebellum — *see* Injury, intracranial
  cerebral — *see* Injury, intracranial
  cervix (uteri) — *see* Injury, uterus
  cheek (wall) S09.93 ☑
  chest — *see* Injury, thorax
  childbirth (newborn) (*see also* Birth, injury)
    maternal NEC O71.9
  chin S09.93 ☑
  choroid (eye) — *see* Injury, eye, specified site NEC
  clitoris S39.94 ☑
  coccyx (*see also* Injury, back, lower)
    complicating delivery O71.6
  colon — *see* Injury, intestine, large
  common bile duct — *see* Injury, liver
  conjunctiva (superficial) — *see* Injury, eye, conjunctiva

Injury — *continued*
  conus medullaris — *see* Injury, spinal, sacral
  cord
    spermatic (pelvic region) S37.898 ☑
      scrotal region S39.848 ☑
    spinal — *see* Injury, spinal cord, by region
  cornea — *see* Injury, eye, specified site NEC
    abrasion — *see* Injury, eye, cornea, abrasion
  cortex (cerebral) (*see also* Injury, intracranial)
    visual — *see* Injury, nerve, optic
  costal region NEC S29.9 ☑
  costochondral NEC S29.9 ☑
  cranial
    cavity — *see* Injury, intracranial
    nerve — *see* Injury, nerve, cranial
  crushing — *see* Crush
  cutaneous sensory nerve
  cystic duct — *see* Injury, liver
  deep tissue — *see* Contusion, by site
    meaning pressure ulcer — *see* Ulcer, pressure, unstageable, by site
  delivery (newborn) P15.9
    maternal NEC O71.9
  Descemet's membrane — *see* Injury, eyeball, penetrating
  diaphragm — *see* Injury, intrathoracic, diaphragm
  duodenum — *see* Injury, intestine, small, duodenum
  ear (auricle) (external) (canal) S09.91 ☑
    abrasion — *see* Abrasion, ear
    bite — *see* Bite, ear
    blister — *see* Blister, ear
    bruise — *see* Contusion, ear
    contusion — *see* Contusion, ear
    external constriction — *see* Constriction, external, ear
    hematoma — *see* Hematoma, ear
    inner — *see* Injury, ear, middle
    laceration — *see* Laceration, ear
    middle S09.30- ☑
      blast — *see* Injury, blast, ear
      specified NEC S09.39- ☑
    puncture — *see* Puncture, ear
    superficial — *see* Injury, superficial, ear
  eighth cranial nerve (acoustic or auditory) — *see* Injury, nerve, acoustic
  elbow S59.90- ☑
    contusion — *see* Contusion, elbow
    dislocation — *see* Dislocation, elbow
    fracture — *see* Fracture, ulna, upper end
    open — *see* Wound, open, elbow
    specified NEC S59.80- ☑
    sprain — *see* Sprain, elbow
    superficial — *see* Injury, superficial, elbow
  eleventh cranial nerve (accessory) — *see* Injury, nerve, accessory
  epididymis S39.94 ☑
  epigastric region S39.91 ☑
  epiglottis NEC S19.89 ☑
  esophageal plexus — *see* Injury, nerve, thorax, sympathetic
  esophagus (thoracic part) (*see also* Injury, intrathoracic, esophagus)
    cervical NEC S19.85 ☑
  eustachian tube S09.30 ☑
  eye S05.9- ☑
    avulsion S05.7- ☑
    ball — *see* Injury, eyeball
    conjunctiva S05.0- ☑
    cornea
      abrasion S05.0- ☑
      laceration S05.3- ☑
        with prolapse S05.2- ☑
    lacrimal apparatus S05.8X- ☑
    orbit penetration S05.4- ☑
    specified site NEC S05.8X- ☑
  eyeball S05.8X- ☑
    contusion S05.1- ☑
    penetrating S05.6- ☑
      with
        foreign body S05.5- ☑
        prolapse or loss of intraocular tissue S05.2- ☑
        without prolapse or loss of intraocular tissue S05.3- ☑
    specified type NEC S05.8- ☑
  eyebrow S09.93 ☑

⬗ Subterms under main terms may continue to next column or page   ☑ Additional Character Required — Refer to the Tabular List for Character Selection   **185**

Injury — Injury

Injury — *continued*
  eyelid S09.93 ☑
    abrasion — *see* Abrasion, eyelid
    contusion — *see* Contusion, eyelid
    open — *see* Wound, open, eyelid
  face S09.93 ☑
  fallopian tube S37.509 ☑
    bilateral S37.502 ☑
      blast injury S37.512 ☑
      contusion S37.522 ☑
      laceration S37.532 ☑
      specified type NEC S37.592 ☑
    blast injury (primary) S37.519 ☑
      bilateral S37.512 ☑
      secondary — *see* Injury, fallopian tube, specified type NEC
      unilateral S37.511 ☑
    contusion S37.529 ☑
      bilateral S37.522 ☑
      unilateral S37.521 ☑
    laceration S37.539 ☑
      bilateral S37.532 ☑
      unilateral S37.531 ☑
    specified type NEC S37.599 ☑
      bilateral S37.592 ☑
      unilateral S37.591 ☑
    unilateral S37.501 ☑
      blast injury S37.511 ☑
      contusion S37.521 ☑
      laceration S37.531 ☑
      specified type NEC S37.591 ☑
  fascia — *see* Injury, muscle
  fifth cranial nerve (trigeminal) — *see* Injury, nerve, trigeminal
  finger (nail) S69.9- ☑
    blood vessel — *see* Injury, blood vessel, finger
    contusion — *see* Contusion, finger
    dislocation — *see* Dislocation, finger
    fracture — *see* Fracture, finger
    muscle — *see* Injury, muscle, finger
    nerve — *see* Injury, nerve, digital, finger
    open — *see* Wound, open, finger
    specified NEC S69.8- ☑
    sprain — *see* Sprain, finger
    superficial — *see* Injury, superficial, finger
  first cranial nerve (olfactory) — *see* Injury, nerve, olfactory
  flank — *see* Injury, abdomen
  foot S99.92- ☑
    blood vessel — *see* Injury, blood vessel, foot
    contusion — *see* Contusion, foot
    dislocation — *see* Dislocation, foot
    fracture — *see* Fracture, foot
    muscle — *see* Injury, muscle, foot
    open — *see* Wound, open, foot
    specified type NEC S99.82- ☑
    sprain — *see* Sprain, foot
    superficial — *see* Injury, superficial, foot
  forceps NOS P15.9
  forearm S59.91- ☑
    blood vessel — *see* Injury, blood vessel, forearm
    contusion — *see* Contusion, forearm
    fracture — *see* Fracture, forearm
    muscle — *see* Injury, muscle, forearm
    nerve — *see* Injury, nerve, forearm
    open — *see* Wound, open, forearm
    specified NEC S59.81- ☑
    superficial — *see* Injury, superficial, forearm
  forehead S09.90 ☑
  fourth cranial nerve (trochlear) — *see* Injury, nerve, trochlear
  gallbladder S36.129 ☑
    contusion S36.122 ☑
    laceration S36.123 ☑
    specified NEC S36.128 ☑
  ganglion
    celiac, coeliac — *see* Injury, nerve, lumbosacral, sympathetic
    gasserian — *see* Injury, nerve, trigeminal
    stellate — *see* Injury, nerve, thorax, sympathetic
    thoracic sympathetic — *see* Injury, nerve, thorax, sympathetic
  gasserian ganglion — *see* Injury, nerve, trigeminal
  gastric artery — *see* Injury, blood vessel, celiac artery, branch

Injury — *continued*
  gastroduodenal artery — *see* Injury, blood vessel, celiac artery, branch
  gastrointestinal tract — *see* Injury, intra-abdominal
    with open wound into abdominal cavity — *see* Wound, open, with penetration into peritoneal cavity
    colon — *see* Injury, intestine, large
    rectum — *see* Injury, intestine, large, rectum
      with open wound into abdominal cavity S36.61
    small intestine — *see* Injury, intestine, small
    specified site NEC — *see* Injury, intra-abdominal, specified, site NEC
    stomach — *see* Injury, stomach
  genital organ(s)
    external S39.94 ☑
      specified NEC S39.848 ☑
    internal S37.90 ☑
      fallopian tube — *see* Injury, fallopian tube
      ovary — *see* Injury, ovary
      prostate — *see* Injury, prostate
      seminal vesicle — *see* Injury, pelvis, organ, specified site NEC
      uterus — *see* Injury, uterus
      vas deferens — *see* Injury, pelvis, organ, specified site NEC
    obstetrical trauma O71.9
  gland
    lacrimal laceration — *see* Injury, eye, specified site NEC
    salivary S09.90 ☑
    thyroid NEC S19.84 ☑
  globe (eye) S05.90 ☑
    specified NEC S05.8X- ☑
  groin — *see* Injury, abdomen
  gum S09.90 ☑
  hand S69.9- ☑
    blood vessel — *see* Injury, blood vessel, hand
    contusion — *see* Contusion, hand
    fracture — *see* Fracture, hand
    muscle — *see* Injury, muscle, hand
    nerve — *see* Injury, nerve, hand
    open — *see* Wound, open, hand
    specified NEC S69.8- ☑
    sprain — *see* Sprain, hand
    superficial — *see* Injury, superficial, hand
  head S09.90 ☑
    with loss of consciousness S06.9- ☑
    specified NEC S09.8 ☑
  heart S26.90 ☑
    with hemopericardium S26.00 ☑
      contusion S26.01 ☑
      laceration (mild) S26.020 ☑
        major S26.022 ☑
        moderate S26.021 ☑
      specified type NEC S26.09 ☑
    without hemopericardium S26.10 ☑
      contusion S26.11 ☑
      laceration S26.12 ☑
      specified type NEC S26.19 ☑
    contusion S26.91 ☑
    laceration S26.92 ☑
    specified type NEC S26.99 ☑
  heel — *see* Injury, foot
  hepatic
    artery — *see* Injury, blood vessel, celiac artery, branch
    duct — *see* Injury, liver
    vein — *see* Injury, vena cava, inferior
  hip S79.91- ☑
    blood vessel — *see* Injury, blood vessel, hip
    contusion — *see* Contusion, hip
    dislocation — *see* Dislocation, hip
    fracture — *see* Fracture, femur, neck
    muscle — *see* Injury, muscle, hip
    nerve — *see* Injury, nerve, hip
    open — *see* Wound, open, hip
    specified NEC S79.81- ☑
    sprain — *see* Sprain, hip
    superficial — *see* Injury, superficial, hip
  hymen S39.94 ☑
  hypogastric
    blood vessel — *see* Injury, blood vessel, iliac
    plexus — *see* Injury, nerve, lumbosacral, sympathetic

Injury — *continued*
  ileum — *see* Injury, intestine, small
  iliac region S39.91 ☑
  instrumental (during surgery) — *see* Laceration, accidental complicating surgery
    birth injury — *see* Birth, injury
    nonsurgical — *see* Injury, by site
    obstetrical O71.9
      bladder O71.5
      cervix O71.3
      high vaginal O71.4
      perineal NOS O70.9
      urethra O71.5
      uterus O71.5
        with rupture or perforation O71.1
  internal T14.8
    aorta — *see* Injury, aorta
    bladder (sphincter) — *see* Injury, bladder
      with
        ectopic or molar pregnancy O08.6
        following ectopic or molar pregnancy O08.6
        obstetrical trauma O71.5
    bronchus, bronchi — *see* Injury, intrathoracic, bronchus
    cecum — *see* Injury, intestine, large
    cervix (uteri) (*see also* Injury, uterus)
      with ectopic or molar pregnancy O08.6
      following ectopic or molar pregnancy O08.6
      obstetrical trauma O71.3
    chest — *see* Injury, intrathoracic
    gastrointestinal tract — *see* Injury, intra-abdominal
    heart — *see* Injury, heart
    intestine NEC — *see* Injury, intestine
    intrauterine — *see* Injury, uterus
    mesentery — *see* Injury, intra-abdominal, specified, site NEC
    pelvis, pelvic (organ) S37.90 ☑
      following ectopic or molar pregnancy (subsequent episode) O08.6
      obstetrical trauma NEC O71.5
        rupture or perforation O71.1
      specified NEC S39.83 ☑
    rectum — *see* Injury, intestine, large, rectum
    stomach — *see* Injury, stomach
    ureter — *see* Injury, ureter
    urethra (sphincter) following ectopic or molar pregnancy O08.6
    uterus — *see* Injury, uterus
  interscapular area — *see* Injury, thorax
  intestine
    large S36.509 ☑
      ascending (right) S36.500 ☑
        blast injury (primary) S36.510 ☑
          secondary S36.590 ☑
        contusion S36.520 ☑
        laceration S36.530 ☑
        specified type NEC S36.590 ☑
      blast injury (primary) S36.519 ☑
        ascending (right) S36.510 ☑
        descending (left) S36.512 ☑
        rectum S36.61
        sigmoid S36.513 ☑
        specified site NEC S36.518 ☑
        transverse S36.511 ☑
      contusion S36.529 ☑
        ascending (right) S36.520 ☑
        descending (left) S36.522 ☑
        rectum S36.62 ☑
        sigmoid S36.523 ☑
        specified site NEC S36.528 ☑
        transverse S36.521 ☑
      descending (left) S36.502 ☑
        blast injury (primary) S36.512 ☑
          secondary S36.592 ☑
        contusion S36.522 ☑
        laceration S36.532 ☑
        specified type NEC S36.592 ☑
      laceration S36.539 ☑
        ascending (right) S36.530 ☑
        descending (left) S36.532 ☑
        rectum S36.63 ☑
        sigmoid S36.533 ☑
        specified site NEC S36.538 ☑
        transverse S36.531 ☑
      rectum S36.60 ☑
        blast injury (primary) S36.61 ☑

☑ **Additional Character Required — Refer to the Tabular List for Character Selection**
    ▽ **Subterms under main terms may continue to next column or page**

Injury — *continued*
  intestine — *continued*
    large — *continued*
      rectum — *continued*
        blast injury — *continued*
          secondary S36.69 ☑
        contusion S36.62 ☑
        laceration S36.63 ☑
        specified type NEC S36.69 ☑
      sigmoid S36.503 ☑
        blast injury (primary) S36.513 ☑
          secondary S36.593 ☑
        contusion S36.523 ☑
        laceration S36.533 ☑
        specified type NEC S36.593 ☑
      specified
        site NEC S36.508 ☑
          blast injury (primary) S36.518 ☑
            secondary S36.598 ☑
          contusion S36.528 ☑
          laceration S36.538 ☑
          specified type NEC S36.598 ☑
        type NEC S36.599 ☑
          ascending (right) S36.590 ☑
          descending (left) S36.592 ☑
          rectum S36.69 ☑
          sigmoid S36.593 ☑
          specified site NEC S36.598 ☑
          transverse S36.591 ☑
      transverse S36.501 ☑
        blast injury (primary) S36.511 ☑
          secondary S36.591 ☑
        contusion S36.521 ☑
        laceration S36.531 ☑
        specified type NEC S36.591 ☑
    small S36.409 ☑
      blast injury (primary) S36.419 ☑
        duodenum S36.410 ☑
        secondary S36.499 ☑
          duodenum S36.490 ☑
          specified site NEC S36.498 ☑
        specified site NEC S36.418 ☑
      contusion S36.429 ☑
        duodenum S36.420 ☑
        specified site NEC S36.428 ☑
      duodenum S36.400 ☑
        blast injury (primary) S36.410 ☑
          secondary S36.490 ☑
        contusion S36.420 ☑
        laceration S36.430 ☑
        specified NEC S36.490 ☑
      laceration S36.439 ☑
        duodenum S36.430 ☑
        specified site NEC S36.438 ☑
      specified
        site NEC S36.408 ☑
        type NEC S36.499 ☑
          duodenum S36.490 ☑
          specified site NEC S36.498 ☑
  intra-abdominal S36.90 ☑
    adrenal gland — *see* Injury, adrenal gland
    bladder — *see* Injury, bladder
    colon — *see* Injury, intestine, large
    contusion S36.92 ☑
    fallopian tube — *see* Injury, fallopian tube
    gallbladder — *see* Injury, gallbladder
    intestine — *see* Injury, intestine
    kidney — *see* Injury, kidney
    laceration S36.93 ☑
    liver — *see* Injury, liver
    ovary — *see* Injury, ovary
    pancreas — *see* Injury, pancreas
    pelvic NOS S37.90 ☑
    peritoneum — *see* Injury, intra-abdominal, speci-
      fied, site NEC
    prostate — *see* Injury, prostate
    rectum — *see* Injury, intestine, large, rectum
    retroperitoneum — *see* Injury, intra-abdominal,
      specified, site NEC
    seminal vesicle — *see* Injury, pelvis, organ, speci-
      fied site NEC
    small intestine — *see* Injury, intestine, small

Injury — *continued*
  intra-abdominal — *continued*
    specified
      pelvic S37.90 ☑
        specified
          site NEC S37.899 ☑
            specified type NEC S37.898 ☑
          type NEC S37.99 ☑
      site NEC S36.899 ☑
        contusion S36.892 ☑
        laceration S36.893 ☑
        specified type NEC S36.898 ☑
      type NEC S36.99 ☑
    spleen — *see* Injury, spleen
    stomach — *see* Injury, stomach
    ureter — *see* Injury, ureter
    urethra — *see* Injury, urethra
    uterus — *see* Injury, uterus
    vas deferens — *see* Injury, pelvis, organ, specified
      site NEC
  intracranial (traumatic) S06.9- ☑
    cerebellar hemorrhage, traumatic — *see* Injury,
      intracranial, focal
    cerebral edema, traumatic S06.1X- ☑
      diffuse S06.1X- ☑
      focal S06.1X- ☑
    diffuse (axonal) S06.2X- ☑
    epidural hemorrhage (traumatic) S06.4X- ☑
    focal brain injury S06.30- ☑
      contusion — *see* Contusion, cerebral
      laceration — *see* Laceration, cerebral
      intracerebral hemorrhage, traumatic S06.36- ☑
        left side S06.35- ☑
        right side S06.34- ☑
    subarachnoid hemorrhage, traumatic S06.6X- ☑
    subdural hemorrhage, traumatic S06.5X- ☑
  intraocular — *see* Injury, eyeball, penetrating
  intrathoracic S27.9 ☑
    bronchus S27.409 ☑
      bilateral S27.402 ☑
      blast injury (primary) S27.419 ☑
        bilateral S27.412 ☑
        secondary — *see* Injury, intrathoracic,
          bronchus, specified type NEC
        unilateral S27.411 ☑
      contusion S27.429 ☑
        bilateral S27.422 ☑
        unilateral S27.421 ☑
      laceration S27.439 ☑
        bilateral S27.432 ☑
        unilateral S27.431 ☑
      specified type NEC S27.499 ☑
        bilateral S27.492 ☑
        unilateral S27.491 ☑
      unilateral S27.401 ☑
    diaphragm S27.809 ☑
      contusion S27.802 ☑
      laceration S27.803 ☑
      specified type NEC S27.808 ☑
    esophagus (thoracic) S27.819 ☑
      contusion S27.812 ☑
      laceration S27.813 ☑
      specified type NEC S27.818 ☑
    heart — *see* Injury, heart
    hemopneumothorax S27.2 ☑
    hemothorax S27.1 ☑
    lung S27.309 ☑
      aspiration J69.0
      bilateral S27.302 ☑
      blast injury (primary) S27.319 ☑
        bilateral S27.312 ☑
        secondary — *see* Injury, intrathoracic, lung,
          specified type NEC
        unilateral S27.311 ☑
      contusion S27.329 ☑
        bilateral S27.322 ☑
        unilateral S27.321 ☑
      laceration S27.339 ☑
        bilateral S27.332 ☑
        unilateral S27.331 ☑
      specified type NEC S27.399 ☑
        bilateral S27.392 ☑
        unilateral S27.391 ☑
      unilateral S27.301 ☑
    pleura S27.60 ☑
      laceration S27.63 ☑

Injury — *continued*
  intrathoracic — *continued*
    pleura — *continued*
      specified type NEC S27.69 ☑
      pneumothorax S27.0 ☑
      specified organ NEC S27.899 ☑
        contusion S27.892 ☑
        laceration S27.893 ☑
        specified type NEC S27.898 ☑
      thoracic duct — *see* Injury, intrathoracic, specified
        organ NEC
      thymus gland — *see* Injury, intrathoracic, specified
        organ NEC
      trachea, thoracic S27.50 ☑
        blast (primary) S27.51 ☑
        contusion S27.52 ☑
        laceration S27.53 ☑
        specified type NEC S27.59 ☑
  iris — *see* Injury, eye, specified site NEC
    penetrating — *see* Injury, eyeball, penetrating
  jaw S09.93 ☑
  jejunum — *see* Injury, intestine, small
  joint NOS T14.8
    old or residual — *see* Disorder, joint, specified type
      NEC
  kidney S37.00- ☑
    acute (nontraumatic) N17.9
    contusion — *see* Contusion, kidney
    laceration — *see* Laceration, kidney
    specified NEC S37.09- ☑
  knee S89.9- ☑
    contusion — *see* Contusion, knee
    dislocation — *see* Dislocation, knee
    meniscus (lateral) (medial) — *see* Sprain, knee,
      specified site NEC
      old injury or tear — *see* Derangement, knee,
        meniscus, due to old injury
    open — *see* Wound, open, knee
    specified NEC S89.8- ☑
    sprain — *see* Sprain, knee
    superficial — *see* Injury, superficial, knee
  labium (majus) (minus) S39.94 ☑
  labyrinth, ear S09.30- ☑
  lacrimal apparatus, duct, gland, or sac — *see* Injury,
    eye, specified site NEC
  larynx NEC S19.81 ☑
  leg (lower) S89.9- ☑
    blood vessel — *see* Injury, blood vessel, leg
    contusion — *see* Contusion, leg
    fracture — *see* Fracture, leg
    muscle — *see* Injury, muscle, leg
    nerve — *see* Injury, nerve, leg
    open — *see* Wound, open, leg
    specified NEC S89.8- ☑
    superficial — *see* Injury, superficial, leg
  lens, eye — *see* Injury, eye, specified site NEC
    penetrating — *see* Injury, eyeball, penetrating
  limb NEC T14.8
  lip S09.93 ☑
  liver S36.119 ☑
    contusion S36.112 ☑
    laceration S36.113 ☑
      major (stellate) S36.116 ☑
      minor S36.114 ☑
      moderate S36.115 ☑
    specified NEC S36.118 ☑
  lower back S39.92 ☑
    specified NEC S39.82 ☑
  lumbar, lumbosacral (region) S39.92 ☑
    plexus — *see* Injury, lumbosacral plexus
  lumbosacral plexus S34.4 ☑
  lung (*see also* Injury, intrathoracic, lung)
    aspiration J69.0
    transfusion-related (TRALI) J95.84
  lymphatic thoracic duct — *see* Injury, intrathoracic,
    specified organ NEC
  malar region S09.93 ☑
  mastoid region S09.90 ☑
  maxilla S09.93 ☑
  mediastinum — *see* Injury, intrathoracic, specified
    organ NEC
  membrane, brain — *see* Injury, intracranial
  meningeal artery — *see* Injury, intracranial, subdural
    hemorrhage
  meninges (cerebral) — *see* Injury, intracranial

Injury — *continued*
  mesenteric
    artery
      branch S35.299 ☑
        laceration (minor) (superficial) S35.291 ☑
          major S35.292 ☑
        specified NEC S35.298 ☑
      inferior S35.239 ☑
        laceration (minor) (superficial) S35.231 ☑
          major S35.232 ☑
        specified NEC S35.238 ☑
      superior S35.229 ☑
        laceration (minor) (superficial) S35.221 ☑
          major S35.222 ☑
        specified NEC S35.228 ☑
    plexus (inferior) (superior) — *see* Injury, nerve, lumbosacral, sympathetic
    vein
      inferior S35.349 ☑
        laceration S35.341 ☑
        specified NEC S35.348 ☑
      superior S35.339 ☑
        laceration S35.331 ☑
        specified NEC S35.338 ☑
  mesentery — *see* Injury, intra-abdominal, specified site NEC
  mesosalpinx — *see* Injury, pelvic organ, specified site NEC
  middle ear S09.30- ☑
  midthoracic region NOS S29.9 ☑
  mouth S09.93 ☑
  multiple NOS T07
  muscle (and fascia) (and tendon)
    abdomen S39.001 ☑
      laceration S39.021 ☑
      specified type NEC S39.091 ☑
      strain S39.011 ☑
    abductor
      thumb, forearm level — *see* Injury, muscle, thumb, abductor
    adductor
      thigh S76.20- ☑
        laceration S76.22- ☑
        specified type NEC S76.29- ☑
        strain S76.21- ☑
    ankle — *see* Injury, muscle, foot
    anterior muscle group, at leg level (lower) S86.20- ☑
      laceration S86.22- ☑
      specified type NEC S86.29- ☑
      strain S86.21- ☑
    arm (upper) — *see* Injury, muscle, shoulder
    biceps (parts NEC) S46.20- ☑
      laceration S46.22- ☑
      long head S46.10- ☑
        laceration S46.12- ☑
        specified type NEC S46.19- ☑
        strain S46.11- ☑
      specified type NEC S46.29- ☑
      strain S46.21- ☑
    extensor
      finger(s) (other than thumb) — *see* Injury, muscle, finger by site, extensor
      forearm level, specified NEC — *see* Injury, muscle, forearm, extensor
      thumb — *see* Injury, muscle, thumb, extensor
      toe (large) (ankle level) (foot level) — *see* Injury, muscle, toe, extensor
    finger
      extensor (forearm level) S56.40- ☑
        hand level S66.309 ☑
          laceration S66.329 ☑
          specified type NEC S66.399 ☑
          strain S66.319 ☑
        laceration S56.429 ☑
        specified type NEC S56.499 ☑
        strain S56.419 ☑
      flexor (forearm level) S56.10- ☑
        hand level S66.109 ☑
          laceration S66.129 ☑
          specified type NEC S66.199 ☑
          strain S66.119 ☑
        laceration S56.129 ☑
        specified type NEC S56.199 ☑
        strain S56.119 ☑

Injury — *continued*
  muscle — *continued*
    finger — *continued*
      index
        extensor (forearm level)
          hand level S66.308 ☑
            laceration S66.32- ☑
            specified type NEC S66.39- ☑
            strain S66.31- ☑
          specified type NEC S56.492- ☑
        flexor (forearm level)
          hand level S66.108 ☑
            laceration S66.12- ☑
            specified type NEC S66.19- ☑
            strain S66.11- ☑
          specified type NEC S56.19- ☑
          strain S56.11- ☑
        intrinsic S66.50- ☑
          laceration S66.52- ☑
          specified type NEC S66.59- ☑
          strain S66.51- ☑
      intrinsic S66.509 ☑
        laceration S66.529 ☑
        specified type NEC S66.599 ☑
        strain S66.519 ☑
      little
        extensor (forearm level)
          hand level S66.30- ☑
            laceration S66.32- ☑
            specified type NEC S66.39- ☑
            strain S66.31- ☑
          laceration S56.42- ☑
          specified type NEC S56.49- ☑
          strain S56.41- ☑
        flexor (forearm level)
          hand level S66.10- ☑
            laceration S66.12- ☑
            specified type NEC S66.19- ☑
            strain S66.11- ☑
          laceration S56.12- ☑
          specified type NEC S56.19- ☑
          strain S56.11- ☑
        intrinsic S66.50- ☑
          laceration S66.52- ☑
          specified type NEC S66.59- ☑
          strain S66.51- ☑
      middle
        extensor (forearm level)
          hand level S66.30- ☑
            laceration S66.32- ☑
            specified type NEC S66.39- ☑
            strain S66.31- ☑
          laceration S56.42- ☑
          specified type NEC S56.49- ☑
          strain S56.41- ☑
        flexor (forearm level)
          hand level S66.10- ☑
            laceration S66.12- ☑
            specified type NEC S66.19- ☑
            strain S66.11- ☑
          laceration S56.12- ☑
          specified type NEC S56.19- ☑
          strain S56.11- ☑
        intrinsic S66.50- ☑
          laceration S66.52- ☑
          specified type NEC S66.59- ☑
          strain S66.51- ☑
      ring
        extensor (forearm level)
          hand level S66.30- ☑
            laceration S66.32- ☑
            specified type NEC S66.39- ☑
            strain S66.31- ☑
          laceration S56.42- ☑
          specified type NEC S56.49- ☑
          strain S56.41- ☑
        flexor (forearm level)
          hand level S66.10- ☑
            laceration S66.12- ☑
            specified type NEC S66.19- ☑
            strain S66.11- ☑
          laceration S56.12- ☑
          specified type NEC S56.19- ☑
          strain S56.11- ☑
        intrinsic S66.50- ☑
          laceration S66.52- ☑

Injury — *continued*
  muscle — *continued*
    finger — *continued*
      ring — *continued*
        intrinsic — *continued*
          specified type NEC S66.59- ☑
          strain S66.51- ☑
    flexor
      finger(s) (other than thumb) — *see* Injury, muscle, finger
      forearm level, specified NEC — *see* Injury, muscle, forearm, flexor
      thumb — *see* Injury, muscle, thumb, flexor
      toe (long) (ankle level) (foot level) — *see* Injury, muscle, toe, flexor
    foot S96.90- ☑
      intrinsic S96.20- ☑
        laceration S96.22- ☑
        specified type NEC S96.29- ☑
        strain S96.21- ☑
      laceration S96.92- ☑
      long extensor, toe — *see* Injury, muscle, toe, extensor
      long flexor, toe — *see* Injury, muscle, toe, flexor
      specified
        site NEC S96.80- ☑
          laceration S96.82- ☑
          specified type NEC S96.89- ☑
          strain S96.81- ☑
        type S96.99- ☑
      strain S96.91- ☑
    forearm (level) S56.90- ☑
      extensor S56.50- ☑
        laceration S56.52- ☑
        specified type NEC S56.59- ☑
        strain S56.51- ☑
      flexor S56.20- ☑
        laceration S56.22- ☑
        specified type NEC S56.29- ☑
        strain S56.21- ☑
      laceration S56.92- ☑
      specified S56.99- ☑
        site NEC S56.80- ☑
          laceration S56.82- ☑
          strain S56.81- ☑
          type NEC S56.89- ☑
      strain S56.91- ☑
    hand (level) S66.90- ☑
      laceration S66.92- ☑
      specified
        site NEC S66.80- ☑
          laceration S66.82- ☑
          specified type NEC S66.89- ☑
          strain S66.81- ☑
          type NEC S66.99- ☑
      strain S66.91- ☑
    head S09.10- ☑
      laceration S09.12 ☑
      specified type NEC S09.19 ☑
      strain S09.11 ☑
    hip NEC S76.00- ☑
      laceration S76.02- ☑
      specified type NEC S76.09- ☑
      strain S76.01- ☑
    intrinsic
      ankle and foot level — *see* Injury, muscle, foot, intrinsic
      finger (other than thumb) — *see* Injury, muscle, finger by site, intrinsic
      foot (level) — *see* Injury, muscle, foot, intrinsic
      thumb — *see* Injury, muscle, thumb, intrinsic
    leg (level) (lower) S86.90- ☑
      Achilles tendon — *see* Injury, Achilles tendon
      anterior muscle group — *see* Injury, muscle, anterior muscle group
      laceration S86.92- ☑
      peroneal muscle group — *see* Injury, muscle, peroneal muscle group
      posterior muscle group — *see* Injury, muscle, posterior muscle group, leg level
      specified
        site NEC S86.80- ☑
          laceration S86.82- ☑
          specified type NEC S86.89- ☑
          strain S86.81- ☑
          type NEC S86.99- ☑

☑ Additional Character Required — Refer to the Tabular List for Character Selection   ▽ Subterms under main terms may continue to next column or page

Injury — continued
  muscle — continued
    leg — continued
      strain S86.91- ☑
      long
        extensor toe, at ankle and foot level — see Injury, muscle, toe, extensor
        flexor, toe, at ankle and foot level — see Injury, muscle, toe, flexor
        head, biceps — see Injury, muscle, biceps, long head
      lower back S39.002 ☑
        laceration S39.022 ☑
        specified type NEC S39.092 ☑
        strain S39.012 ☑
      neck (level) S16.9 ☑
        laceration S16.2 ☑
        specified type NEC S16.8 ☑
        strain S16.1 ☑
      pelvis S39.003 ☑
        laceration S39.023 ☑
        specified type NEC S39.093 ☑
        strain S39.013 ☑
      peroneal muscle group, at leg level (lower) S86.30- ☑
        laceration S86.32- ☑
        specified type NEC S86.39- ☑
        strain S86.31- ☑
      posterior muscle (group)
        leg level (lower) S86.10- ☑
          laceration S86.12- ☑
          specified type NEC S86.19- ☑
          strain S86.11- ☑
        thigh level S76.30- ☑
          laceration S76.32- ☑
          specified type NEC S76.39- ☑
          strain S76.31- ☑
      quadriceps (thigh) S76.10- ☑
        laceration S76.12- ☑
        specified type NEC S76.19- ☑
        strain S76.11- ☑
      shoulder S46.90- ☑
        laceration S46.92- ☑
        rotator cuff — see Injury, rotator cuff
        specified site NEC S46.80- ☑
          laceration S46.82- ☑
          specified type NEC S46.89- ☑
          strain S46.81- ☑
        specified type NEC S46.99- ☑
        strain S46.91- ☑
      thigh NEC (level) S76.90- ☑
        adductor — see Injury, muscle, adductor, thigh
        laceration S76.92- ☑
        posterior muscle (group) — see Injury, muscle, posterior muscle, thigh level
        quadriceps — see Injury, muscle, quadriceps
        specified
          site NEC S76.80- ☑
            laceration S76.82- ☑
            specified type NEC S76.89- ☑
            strain S76.81- ☑
          type NEC S76.99- ☑
        strain S76.91- ☑
      thorax (level) S29.009 ☑
        back wall S29.002 ☑
        front wall S29.001 ☑
        laceration S29.029 ☑
          back wall S29.022 ☑
          front wall S29.021 ☑
        specified type NEC S29.099 ☑
          back wall S29.092 ☑
          front wall S29.091 ☑
        strain S29.019 ☑
          back wall S29.012 ☑
          front wall S29.011 ☑
      thumb
        abductor (forearm level) S56.30- ☑
          laceration S56.32- ☑
          specified type NEC S56.39- ☑
          strain S56.31- ☑
        extensor (forearm level) S56.30- ☑
          hand level S66.20- ☑
            laceration S66.22- ☑
            specified type NEC S66.29- ☑
            strain S66.21- ☑
          laceration S56.32- ☑

Injury — continued
  muscle — continued
    thumb — continued
      extensor — continued
        specified type NEC S56.39- ☑
        strain S56.31- ☑
      flexor (forearm level) S56.00- ☑
        hand level S66.00- ☑
          laceration S66.02- ☑
          specified type NEC S66.09- ☑
          strain S66.01- ☑
        laceration S56.02- ☑
        specified type NEC S56.09- ☑
        strain S56.01- ☑
        wrist level — see Injury, muscle, thumb, flexor, hand level
      intrinsic S66.40- ☑
        laceration S66.42- ☑
        specified type NEC S66.49- ☑
        strain S66.41- ☑
    toe (see also Injury, muscle, foot)
      extensor, long S96.10- ☑
        laceration S96.12- ☑
        specified type NEC S96.19- ☑
        strain S96.11- ☑
      flexor, long S96.00- ☑
        laceration S96.02- ☑
        specified type NEC S96.09- ☑
        strain S96.01- ☑
    triceps S46.30- ☑
      laceration S46.32- ☑
      specified type NEC S46.39- ☑
      strain S46.31- ☑
    wrist (and hand) level — see Injury, muscle, hand
  musculocutaneous nerve — see Injury, nerve, musculocutaneous
  myocardium — see Injury, heart
  nape — see Injury, neck
  nasal (septum) (sinus) S09.92 ☑
  nasopharynx S09.92 ☑
  neck S19.9 ☑
    specified NEC S19.80 ☑
      specified site NEC S19.89 ☑
  nerve NEC T14.8
    abdomen S34.9 ☑
      peripheral S34.6 ☑
      specified site NEC S34.8 ☑
    abducens S04.4- ☑
      contusion S04.4- ☑
      laceration S04.4- ☑
      specified type NEC S04.4- ☑
    abducent — see Injury, nerve, abducens
    accessory S04.7- ☑
      contusion S04.7- ☑
      laceration S04.7- ☑
      specified type NEC S04.7- ☑
    acoustic S04.6- ☑
      contusion S04.6- ☑
      laceration S04.6- ☑
      specified type NEC S04.6- ☑
    ankle S94.9- ☑
      cutaneous sensory S94.3- ☑
      specified site NEC — see subcategory S94.8 ☑
    anterior crural, femoral — see Injury, nerve, femoral
    arm (upper) S44.9- ☑
      axillary — see Injury, nerve, axillary
      cutaneous — see Injury, nerve, cutaneous, arm
      median — see Injury, nerve, median, upper arm
      musculocutaneous — see Injury, nerve, musculocutaneous
      radial — see Injury, nerve, radial, upper arm
      specified site NEC — see subcategory S44.8 ☑
      ulnar — see Injury, nerve, ulnar, arm
    auditory — see Injury, nerve, acoustic
    axillary S44.3- ☑
    brachial plexus — see Injury, brachial plexus
    cervical sympathetic S14.5 ☑
    cranial S04.9 ☑
      contusion S04.9 ☑
      eighth (acoustic or auditory) — see Injury, nerve, acoustic
      eleventh (accessory) — see Injury, nerve, accessory
      fifth (trigeminal) — see Injury, nerve, trigeminal
      first (olfactory) — see Injury, nerve, olfactory
      fourth (trochlear) — see Injury, nerve, trochlear

Injury — continued
  nerve — continued
    cranial — continued
      laceration S04.9 ☑
      ninth (glossopharyngeal) — see Injury, nerve, glossopharyngeal
      second (optic) — see Injury, nerve, optic
      seventh (facial) — see Injury, nerve, facial
      sixth (abducent) — see Injury, nerve, abducens
      specified
        nerve NEC S04.89- ☑
          contusion S04.89- ☑
          laceration S04.89- ☑
          specified type NEC S04.89- ☑
        type NEC S04.9 ☑
      tenth (pneumogastric or vagus) — see Injury, nerve, vagus
      third (oculomotor) — see Injury, nerve, oculomotor
      twelfth (hypoglossal) — see Injury, nerve, hypoglossal
    cutaneous sensory
      ankle (level) S94.3- ☑
      arm (upper) (level) S44.5- ☑
      foot (level) — see Injury, nerve, cutaneous sensory, ankle
      forearm (level) S54.3- ☑
      hip (level) S74.2- ☑
      leg (lower level) S84.2- ☑
      shoulder (level) — see Injury, nerve, cutaneous sensory, arm
      thigh (level) — see Injury, nerve, cutaneous sensory, hip
    deep peroneal — see Injury, nerve, peroneal, foot
    digital
      finger S64.4- ☑
        index S64.49- ☑
        little S64.49- ☑
        middle S64.49- ☑
        ring S64.49- ☑
      thumb S64.3- ☑
      toe — see Injury, nerve, ankle, specified site NEC
    eighth cranial (acoustic or auditory) — see Injury, nerve, acoustic
    eleventh cranial (accessory) — see Injury, nerve, accessory
    facial S04.5- ☑
      contusion S04.5- ☑
      laceration S04.5- ☑
      newborn P11.3
      specified type NEC S04.5- ☑
    femoral (hip level) (thigh level) S74.1- ☑
    fifth cranial (trigeminal) — see Injury, nerve, trigeminal
    finger (digital) — see Injury, nerve, digital, finger
    first cranial (olfactory) — see Injury, nerve, olfactory
    foot S94.9- ☑
      cutaneous sensory S94.3- ☑
      deep peroneal S94.2- ☑
      lateral plantar S94.0- ☑
      medial plantar S94.1- ☑
      specified site NEC — see subcategory S94.8 ☑
    forearm (level) S54.9- ☑
      cutaneous sensory — see Injury, nerve, cutaneous sensory, forearm
      median — see Injury, nerve, median
      radial — see Injury, nerve, radial
      specified site NEC — see subcategory S54.8 ☑
      ulnar — see Injury, nerve, ulnar
    fourth cranial (trochlear) — see Injury, nerve, trochlear
    glossopharyngeal S04.89- ☑
      specified type NEC S04.89- ☑
    hand S64.9- ☑
      median — see Injury, nerve, median, hand
      radial — see Injury, nerve, radial, hand
      specified NEC — see subcategory S64.8 ☑
      ulnar — see Injury, nerve, ulnar, hand
    hip (level) S74.9- ☑
      cutaneous sensory — see Injury, nerve, cutaneous sensory, hip
      femoral — see Injury, nerve, femoral
      sciatic — see Injury, nerve, sciatic
      specified site NEC — see subcategory S74.8 ☑

Injury — continued
 nerve — continued
  hypoglossal S04.89- ☑
   specified type NEC S04.89- ☑
  lateral plantar S94.0- ☑
  leg (lower) S84.9- ☑
   cutaneous sensory — see Injury, nerve, cutaneous sensory, leg
   peroneal — see Injury, nerve, peroneal
   specified site NEC — see subcategory S84.8 ☑
   tibial — see Injury, nerve, tibial
   upper — see Injury, nerve, thigh
  lower
   back — see Injury, nerve, abdomen, specified site NEC
    peripheral — see Injury, nerve, abdomen, peripheral
   limb — see Injury, nerve, leg
  lumbar plexus — see Injury, nerve, lumbosacral, sympathetic
  lumbar spinal — see Injury, nerve, spinal, lumbar
  lumbosacral
   plexus — see Injury, nerve, lumbosacral, sympathetic
   sympathetic S34.5 ☑
  medial plantar S94.1- ☑
  median (forearm level) S54.1- ☑
   hand (level) S64.1- ☑
   upper arm (level) S44.1- ☑
   wrist (level) — see Injury, nerve, median, hand
  musculocutaneous S44.4- ☑
  musculospiral (upper arm level) — see Injury, nerve, radial, upper arm
  neck S14.9 ☑
   peripheral S14.4 ☑
   specified site NEC S14.8 ☑
   sympathetic S14.5 ☑
  ninth cranial (glossopharyngeal) — see Injury, nerve, glossopharyngeal
  oculomotor S04.1- ☑
   contusion S04.1- ☑
   laceration S04.1- ☑
   specified type NEC S04.1- ☑
  olfactory S04.81- ☑
   specified type NEC S04.81- ☑
  optic S04.01- ☑
   contusion S04.01- ☑
   laceration S04.01- ☑
   specified type NEC S04.01- ☑
  pelvic girdle — see Injury, nerve, hip
  pelvis — see Injury, nerve, abdomen, specified site NEC
   peripheral — see Injury, nerve, abdomen, peripheral
  peripheral NEC T14.8
   abdomen — see Injury, nerve, abdomen, peripheral
   lower back — see Injury, nerve, abdomen, peripheral
   neck — see Injury, nerve, neck, peripheral
   pelvis — see Injury, nerve, abdomen, peripheral
   specified NEC T14.8
  peroneal (lower leg level) S84.1- ☑
   foot S94.2- ☑
  plexus
   brachial — see Injury, brachial plexus
   celiac, coeliac — see Injury, nerve, lumbosacral, sympathetic
   mesenteric, inferior — see Injury, nerve, lumbosacral, sympathetic
   sacral — see Injury, lumbosacral plexus
   spinal
    brachial — see Injury, brachial plexus
    lumbosacral — see Injury, lumbosacral plexus
  pneumogastric — see Injury, nerve, vagus
  radial (forearm level) S54.2- ☑
   hand (level) S64.2- ☑
   upper arm (level) S44.2- ☑
   wrist (level) — see Injury, nerve, radial, hand
  root — see Injury, nerve, spinal, root
  sacral plexus — see Injury, lumbosacral plexus
  sacral spinal — see Injury, nerve, spinal, sacral
  sciatic (hip level) (thigh level) S74.0- ☑
  second cranial (optic) — see Injury, nerve, optic
  seventh cranial (facial) — see Injury, nerve, facial

Injury — continued
 nerve — continued
  shoulder — see Injury, nerve, arm
  sixth cranial (abducent) — see Injury, nerve, abducens
  spinal
   plexus — see Injury, nerve, plexus, spinal
   root
    cervical S14.2 ☑
    dorsal S24.2 ☑
    lumbar S34.21 ☑
    sacral S34.22 ☑
    thoracic — see Injury, nerve, spinal, root, dorsal
  splanchnic — see Injury, nerve, lumbosacral, sympathetic
  sympathetic NEC — see Injury, nerve, lumbosacral, sympathetic
   cervical — see Injury, nerve, cervical sympathetic
  tenth cranial (pneumogastric or vagus) — see Injury, nerve, vagus
  thigh (level) — see Injury, nerve, hip
   cutaneous sensory — see Injury, nerve, cutaneous sensory, hip
   femoral — see Injury, nerve, femoral
   sciatic — see Injury, nerve, sciatic
   specified NEC — see Injury, nerve, hip
  third cranial (oculomotor) — see Injury, nerve, oculomotor
  thorax S24.9 ☑
   peripheral S24.3 ☑
   specified site NEC S24.8 ☑
   sympathetic S24.4 ☑
  thumb, digital — see Injury, nerve, digital, thumb
  tibial (lower leg level) (posterior) S84.0- ☑
  toe — see Injury, nerve, ankle
  trigeminal S04.3- ☑
   contusion S04.3- ☑
   laceration S04.3- ☑
   specified type NEC S04.3- ☑
  trochlear S04.2- ☑
   contusion S04.2- ☑
   laceration S04.2- ☑
   specified type NEC S04.2- ☑
  twelfth cranial (hypoglossal) — see Injury, nerve, hypoglossal
  ulnar (forearm level) S54.0- ☑
   arm (upper) (level) S44.0- ☑
   hand (level) S64.0- ☑
   wrist (level) — see Injury, nerve, ulnar, hand
  vagus S04.89- ☑
   specified type NEC S04.89- ☑
  wrist (level) — see Injury, nerve, hand
 ninth cranial nerve (glossopharyngeal) — see Injury, nerve, glossopharyngeal
 nose (septum) S09.92 ☑
 obstetrical O71.9
  specified NEC O71.89
 occipital (region) (scalp) S09.90 ☑
  lobe — see Injury, intracranial
 optic chiasm S04.02 ☑
 optic radiation S04.03- ☑
 optic tract and pathways S04.03- ☑
 orbit, orbital (region) — see Injury, eye
  penetrating (with foreign body) — see Injury, eye, orbit, penetrating
  specified NEC — see Injury, eye, specified site NEC
 ovary, ovarian S37.409 ☑
  bilateral S37.402 ☑
   contusion S37.422 ☑
   laceration S37.432 ☑
   specified type NEC S37.492 ☑
  blood vessel — see Injury, blood vessel, ovarian
  contusion S37.429 ☑
   bilateral S37.422 ☑
   unilateral S37.421 ☑
  laceration S37.439 ☑
   bilateral S37.432 ☑
   unilateral S37.431 ☑
  specified type NEC S37.499 ☑
   bilateral S37.492 ☑
   unilateral S37.491 ☑
  unilateral S37.401 ☑
   contusion S37.421 ☑
   laceration S37.431 ☑

Injury — continued
 ovary, ovarian — continued
  unilateral — continued
   specified type NEC S37.491 ☑
 palate (hard) (soft) S09.93 ☑
 pancreas S36.209 ☑
  body S36.201 ☑
   contusion S36.221 ☑
   laceration S36.231 ☑
    major S36.261 ☑
    minor S36.241 ☑
    moderate S36.251 ☑
   specified type NEC S36.291 ☑
  contusion S36.229 ☑
  head S36.200 ☑
   contusion S36.220 ☑
   laceration S36.230 ☑
    major S36.260 ☑
    minor S36.240 ☑
    moderate S36.250 ☑
   specified type NEC S36.290 ☑
  laceration S36.239 ☑
   major S36.269 ☑
   minor S36.249 ☑
   moderate S36.259 ☑
  specified type NEC S36.299 ☑
  tail S36.202 ☑
   contusion S36.222 ☑
   laceration S36.232 ☑
    major S36.262 ☑
    minor S36.242 ☑
    moderate S36.252 ☑
   specified type NEC S36.292 ☑
 parietal (region) (scalp) S09.90 ☑
  lobe — see Injury, intracranial
 patellar ligament (tendon) S76.10- ☑
  laceration S76.12- ☑
  specified NEC S76.19- ☑
  strain S76.11- ☑
 pelvis, pelvic (floor) S39.93 ☑
  complicating delivery O70.1
  joint or ligament, complicating delivery O71.6
  organ S37.90 ☑
   with ectopic or molar pregnancy O08.6
   complication of abortion — see Abortion
   contusion S37.92 ☑
   following ectopic or molar pregnancy O08.6
   laceration S37.93 ☑
   obstetrical trauma NEC O71.5
   specified
    site NEC S37.899 ☑
     contusion S37.892 ☑
     laceration S37.893 ☑
     specified type NEC S37.898 ☑
    type NEC S37.99 ☑
  specified NEC S39.83 ☑
 penis S39.94 ☑
 perineum S39.94 ☑
 peritoneum S36.81 ☑
  laceration S36.893 ☑
 periurethral tissue — see Injury, urethra
  complicating delivery O71.82
 phalanges
  foot — see Injury, foot
  hand — see Injury, hand
 pharynx NEC S19.85 ☑
 pleura — see Injury, intrathoracic, pleura
 plexus
  brachial — see Injury, brachial plexus
  cardiac — see Injury, nerve, thorax, sympathetic
  celiac, coeliac — see Injury, nerve, lumbosacral, sympathetic
  esophageal — see Injury, nerve, thorax, sympathetic
  hypogastric — see Injury, nerve, lumbosacral, sympathetic
  lumbar, lumbosacral — see Injury, lumbosacral plexus
  mesenteric — see Injury, nerve, lumbosacral, sympathetic
  pulmonary — see Injury, nerve, thorax, sympathetic
 postcardiac surgery (syndrome) I97.0
 prepuce S39.94 ☑
 prostate S37.829 ☑
  contusion S37.822 ☑

Injury — *continued*
  prostate — *continued*
    laceration S37.823 ☑
    specified type NEC S37.828 ☑
  pubic region S39.94 ☑
  pudendum S39.94 ☑
  pulmonary plexus — *see* Injury, nerve, thorax, sympathetic
  rectovaginal septum NEC S39.83 ☑
  rectum — *see* Injury, intestine, large, rectum
  retina — *see* Injury, eye, specified site NEC
    penetrating — *see* Injury, eyeball, penetrating
  retroperitoneal — *see* Injury, intra-abdominal, specified site NEC
  rotator cuff (muscle(s)) (tendon(s)) S46.00- ☑
    laceration S46.02-
    specified type NEC S46.09- ☑
    strain S46.01- ☑
  round ligament — *see* Injury, pelvic organ, specified site NEC
  sacral plexus — *see* Injury, lumbosacral plexus
  salivary duct or gland S09.93 ☑
  scalp S09.90 ☑
    newborn (birth injury) P12.9
      due to monitoring (electrode) (sampling incision) P12.4
      specified NEC P12.89
        caput succedaneum P12.81
  scapular region — *see* Injury, shoulder
  sclera — *see* Injury, eye, specified site NEC
    penetrating — *see* Injury, eyeball, penetrating
  scrotum S39.94 ☑
  second cranial nerve (optic) — *see* Injury, nerve, optic
  seminal vesicle — *see* Injury, pelvic organ, specified site NEC
  seventh cranial nerve (facial) — *see* Injury, nerve, facial
  shoulder S49.9- ☑
    blood vessel — *see* Injury, blood vessel, arm
    contusion — *see* Contusion, shoulder
    dislocation — *see* Dislocation, shoulder
    fracture — *see* Fracture, shoulder
    muscle — *see* Injury, muscle, shoulder
    nerve — *see* Injury, nerve, shoulder
    open — *see* Wound, open, shoulder
    specified type NEC S49.8- ☑
    sprain — *see* Sprain, shoulder girdle
    superficial — *see* Injury, superficial, shoulder
  sinus
    cavernous — *see* Injury, intracranial
    nasal S09.92 ☑
  sixth cranial nerve (abducent) — *see* Injury, nerve, abducens
  skeleton, birth injury P13.9
    specified part NEC P13.8
  skin NEC T14.8
    surface intact — *see* Injury, superficial
  skull NEC S09.90 ☑
  specified NEC T14.8
  spermatic cord (pelvic region) S37.898 ☑
    scrotal region S39.848 ☑
  spinal (cord)
    cervical (neck) S14.109 ☑
      anterior cord syndrome S14.139 ☑
        C1 level S14.131 ☑
        C2 level S14.132 ☑
        C3 level S14.133 ☑
        C4 level S14.134 ☑
        C5 level S14.135 ☑
        C6 level S14.136 ☑
        C7 level S14.137 ☑
        C8 level S14.138 ☑
      Brown-Séquard syndrome S14.149 ☑
        C1 level S14.141 ☑
        C2 level S14.142 ☑
        C3 level S14.143 ☑
        C4 level S14.144 ☑
        C5 level S14.145 ☑
        C6 level S14.146 ☑
        C7 level S14.147 ☑
        C8 level S14.148 ☑
      C1 level S14.101 ☑
      C2 level S14.102 ☑
      C3 level S14.103 ☑
      C4 level S14.104 ☑
      C5 level S14.105 ☑
      C6 level S14.106 ☑

Injury — *continued*
  spinal — *continued*
    cervical — *continued*
      C7 level S14.107 ☑
      C8 level S14.108 ☑
      central cord syndrome S14.129 ☑
        C1 level S14.121 ☑
        C2 level S14.122 ☑
        C3 level S14.123 ☑
        C4 level S14.124 ☑
        C5 level S14.125 ☑
        C6 level S14.126 ☑
        C7 level S14.127 ☑
        C8 level S14.128 ☑
      complete lesion S14.119 ☑
        C1 level S14.111 ☑
        C2 level S14.112 ☑
        C3 level S14.113 ☑
        C4 level S14.114 ☑
        C5 level S14.115 ☑
        C6 level S14.116 ☑
        C7 level S14.117 ☑
        C8 level S14.118 ☑
      concussion S14.0 ☑
      edema S14.0 ☑
      incomplete lesion specified NEC S14.159 ☑
        C1 level S14.151 ☑
        C2 level S14.152 ☑
        C3 level S14.153 ☑
        C4 level S14.154 ☑
        C5 level S14.155 ☑
        C6 level S14.156 ☑
        C7 level S14.157 ☑
        C8 level S14.158 ☑
      posterior cord syndrome S14.159 ☑
        C1 level S14.151 ☑
        C2 level S14.152 ☑
        C3 level S14.153 ☑
        C4 level S14.154 ☑
        C5 level S14.155 ☑
        C6 level S14.156 ☑
        C7 level S14.157 ☑
        C8 level S14.158 ☑
    dorsal — *see* Injury, spinal, thoracic
    lumbar S34.109 ☑
      complete lesion S34.119 ☑
        L1 level S34.111 ☑
        L2 level S34.112 ☑
        L3 level S34.113 ☑
        L4 level S34.114 ☑
        L5 level S34.115 ☑
      concussion S34.01 ☑
      edema S34.01 ☑
      incomplete lesion S34.129 ☑
        L1 level S34.121 ☑
        L2 level S34.122 ☑
        L3 level S34.123 ☑
        L4 level S34.124 ☑
        L5 level S34.125 ☑
      L1 level S34.101 ☑
      L2 level S34.102 ☑
      L3 level S34.103 ☑
      L4 level S34.104 ☑
      L5 level S34.105 ☑
    nerve root NEC
      cervical — *see* Injury, nerve, spinal, root, cervical
      dorsal — *see* Injury, nerve, spinal, root, dorsal
      lumbar S34.21 ☑
      sacral S34.22 ☑
      thoracic — *see* Injury, nerve, spinal, root, dorsal
    plexus
      brachial — *see* Injury, brachial plexus
      lumbosacral — *see* Injury, lumbosacral plexus
    sacral S34.139 ☑
      complete lesion S34.131 ☑
      incomplete lesion S34.132 ☑
    thoracic S24.109 ☑
      anterior cord syndrome S24.139 ☑
        T1 level S24.131 ☑
        T2-T6 level S24.132 ☑
        T7-T10 level S24.133 ☑
        T11-T12 level S24.134 ☑
      Brown-Séquard syndrome S24.149 ☑
        T1 level S24.141 ☑

Injury — *continued*
  spinal — *continued*
    thoracic — *continued*
      Brown-Séquard syndrome — *continued*
        T2-T6 level S24.142 ☑
        T7-T10 level S24.143 ☑
        T11-T12 level S24.144 ☑
      complete lesion S24.119 ☑
        T1 level S24.111 ☑
        T2-T6 level S24.112 ☑
        T7-T10 level S24.113 ☑
        T11-T12 level S24.114 ☑
      concussion S24.0 ☑
      edema S24.0 ☑
      incomplete lesion specified NEC S24.159 ☑
        T1 level S24.151 ☑
        T2-T6 level S24.152 ☑
        T7-T10 level S24.153 ☑
        T11-T12 level S24.154 ☑
      posterior cord syndrome S24.159 ☑
        T1 level S24.151 ☑
        T2-T6 level S24.152 ☑
        T7-T10 level S24.153 ☑
        T11-T12 level S24.154 ☑
      T1 level S24.101 ☑
      T2-T6 level S24.102 ☑
      T7-T10 level S24.103 ☑
      T11-T12 level S24.104 ☑
  splanchnic nerve — *see* Injury, nerve, lumbosacral, sympathetic
  spleen S36.00 ☑
    contusion S36.029 ☑
      major S36.021 ☑
      minor S36.020 ☑
    laceration S36.039 ☑
      major (massive) (stellate) S36.032 ☑
      moderate S36.031 ☑
      superficial (capsular) (minor) S36.030 ☑
    specified type NEC S36.09 ☑
  splenic artery — *see* Injury, blood vessel, celiac artery, branch
  stellate ganglion — *see* Injury, nerve, thorax, sympathetic
  sternal region S29.9 ☑
  stomach S36.30 ☑
    contusion S36.32 ☑
    laceration S36.33 ☑
    specified type NEC S36.39 ☑
  subconjunctival — *see* Injury, eye, conjunctiva
  subcutaneous NEC T14.8
  submaxillary region S09.93 ☑
  submental region S09.93 ☑
  subungual
    fingers — *see* Injury, hand
    toes — *see* Injury, foot
  superficial NEC T14.8
    abdomen, abdominal (wall) S30.92 ☑
      abrasion S30.811 ☑
      bite S30.871 ☑
        insect S30.861 ☑
      contusion S30.1 ☑
      external constriction S30.841 ☑
      foreign body S30.851 ☑
    abrasion — *see* Abrasion, by site
    adnexa, eye NEC — *see* Injury, eye, specified site NEC
    alveolar process — *see* Injury, superficial, oral cavity
    ankle S90.91- ☑
      abrasion — *see* Abrasion, ankle
      bite — *see* Bite, ankle
      blister — *see* Blister, ankle
      contusion — *see* Contusion, ankle
      external constriction — *see* Constriction, external, ankle
      foreign body — *see* Foreign body, superficial, ankle
    anus S30.98 ☑
    arm (upper) S40.92- ☑
      abrasion — *see* Abrasion, arm
      bite — *see* Bite, superficial, arm
      blister — *see* Blister, arm (upper)
      contusion — *see* Contusion, arm
      external constriction — *see* Constriction, external, arm

Injury — *continued*
  superficial — *continued*
    arm — *continued*
      foreign body — *see* Foreign body, superficial, arm
    auditory canal (external) (meatus) — *see* Injury, superficial, ear
    auricle — *see* Injury, superficial, ear
    axilla — *see* Injury, superficial, arm
    back (*see also* Injury, superficial, thorax, back)
      lower S30.91 ☑
        abrasion S30.810 ☑
        contusion S30.0 ☑
        external constriction S30.840 ☑
        superficial
          bite NEC S30.870 ☑
            insect S30.860 ☑
          foreign body S30.850 ☑
    bite NEC — *see* Bite, superficial NEC, by site
    blister — *see* Blister, by site
    breast S20.10- ☑
      abrasion — *see* Abrasion, breast
      bite — *see* Bite, superficial, breast
      contusion — *see* Contusion, breast
      external constriction — *see* Constriction, external, breast
      foreign body — *see* Foreign body, superficial, breast
    brow — *see* Injury, superficial, head, specified NEC
    buttock S30.91 ☑
    calf — *see* Injury, superficial, leg
    canthus, eye — *see* Injury, superficial, periocular area
    cheek (external) — *see* Injury, superficial, head, specified NEC
      internal — *see* Injury, superficial, oral cavity
    chest wall — *see* Injury, superficial, thorax
    chin — *see* Injury, superficial, head NEC
    clitoris S30.95 ☑
    conjunctiva — *see* Injury, eye, conjunctiva
      with foreign body (in conjunctival sac) — *see* Foreign body, conjunctival sac
    contusion — *see* Contusion, by site
    costal region — *see* Injury, superficial, thorax
    digit(s)
      hand — *see* Injury, superficial, finger
    ear (auricle) (canal) (external) S00.40- ☑
      abrasion — *see* Abrasion, ear
      bite — *see* Bite, superficial, ear
      contusion — *see* Contusion, ear
      external constriction — *see* Constriction, external, ear
      foreign body — *see* Foreign body, superficial, ear
    elbow S50.90- ☑
      abrasion — *see* Abrasion, elbow
      bite — *see* Bite, superficial, elbow
      blister — *see* Blister, elbow
      contusion — *see* Contusion, elbow
      external constriction — *see* Constriction, external, elbow
      foreign body — *see* Foreign body, superficial, elbow
    epididymis S30.94 ☑
    epigastric region S30.92 ☑
    epiglottis — *see* Injury, superficial, throat
    esophagus
      cervical — *see* Injury, superficial, throat
    external constriction — *see* Constriction, external, by site
    extremity NEC T14.8
    eyeball NEC — *see* Injury, eye, specified site NEC
    eyebrow — *see* Injury, superficial, periocular area
    eyelid S00.20- ☑
      abrasion — *see* Abrasion, eyelid
      bite — *see* Bite, superficial, eyelid
      contusion — *see* Contusion, eyelid
      external constriction — *see* Constriction, external, eyelid
      foreign body — *see* Foreign body, superficial, eyelid
    face NEC — *see* Injury, superficial, head, specified NEC
    finger(s) S60.949 ☑
      abrasion — *see* Abrasion, finger
      bite — *see* Bite, superficial, finger

Injury — *continued*
  superficial — *continued*
    finger(s) — *continued*
      blister — *see* Blister, finger
      contusion — *see* Contusion, finger
      external constriction — *see* Constriction, external, finger
      foreign body — *see* Foreign body, superficial, finger
      index S60.94- ☑
      insect bite — *see* Bite, by site, superficial, insect
      little S60.94- ☑
      middle S60.94- ☑
      ring S60.94- ☑
    flank S30.92 ☑
    foot S90.92- ☑
      abrasion — *see* Abrasion, foot
      bite — *see* Bite, foot
      blister — *see* Blister, foot
      contusion — *see* Contusion, foot
      external constriction — *see* Constriction, external, foot
      foreign body — *see* Foreign body, superficial, foot
    forearm S50.91- ☑
      abrasion — *see* Abrasion, forearm
      bite — *see* Bite, forearm, superficial
      blister — *see* Blister, forearm
      contusion — *see* Contusion, forearm
      elbow only — *see* Injury, superficial, elbow
      external constriction — *see* Constriction, external, forearm
      foreign body — *see* Foreign body, superficial, forearm
    forehead — *see* Injury, superficial, head NEC
    foreign body — *see* Foreign body, superficial
    genital organs, external
      female S30.97 ☑
      male S30.96 ☑
    globe (eye) — *see* Injury, eye, specified site NEC
    groin S30.92 ☑
    gum — *see* Injury, superficial, oral cavity
    hand S60.92- ☑
      abrasion — *see* Abrasion, hand
      bite — *see* Bite, superficial, hand
      contusion — *see* Contusion, hand
      external constriction — *see* Constriction, external, hand
      foreign body — *see* Foreign body, superficial, hand
    head S00.90 ☑
      ear — *see* Injury, superficial, ear
      eyelid — *see* Injury, superficial, eyelid
      nose S00.30 ☑
      oral cavity S00.502 ☑
      scalp S00.00 ☑
      specified site NEC S00.80 ☑
    heel — *see* Injury, superficial, foot
    hip S70.91- ☑
      abrasion — *see* Abrasion, hip
      bite — *see* Bite, superficial, hip
      blister — *see* Blister, hip
      contusion — *see* Contusion, hip
      external constriction — *see* Constriction, external, hip
      foreign body — *see* Foreign body, superficial, hip
    iliac region — *see* Injury, superficial, abdomen
    inguinal region — *see* Injury, superficial, abdomen
    insect bite — *see* Bite, by site, superficial, insect
    interscapular region — *see* Injury, superficial, thorax, back
    jaw — *see* Injury, superficial, head, specified NEC
    knee S80.91- ☑
      abrasion — *see* Abrasion, knee
      bite — *see* Bite, superficial, knee
      blister — *see* Blister, knee
      contusion — *see* Contusion, knee
      external constriction — *see* Constriction, external, knee
      foreign body — *see* Foreign body, superficial, knee
    labium (majus) (minus) S30.95 ☑
    lacrimal (apparatus) (gland) (sac) — *see* Injury, eye, specified site NEC
    larynx — *see* Injury, superficial, throat

Injury — *continued*
  superficial — *continued*
    leg (lower) S80.92- ☑
      abrasion — *see* Abrasion, leg
      bite — *see* Bite, superficial, leg
      contusion — *see* Contusion, leg
      external constriction — *see* Constriction, external, leg
      foreign body — *see* Foreign body, superficial, leg
      knee — *see* Injury, superficial, knee
    limb NEC T14.8
    lip S00.501 ☑
    lower back S30.91 ☑
    lumbar region S30.91 ☑
    malar region — *see* Injury, superficial, head, specified NEC
    mammary — *see* Injury, superficial, breast
    mastoid region — *see* Injury, superficial, head, specified NEC
    mouth — *see* Injury, superficial, oral cavity
    muscle NEC T14.8
    nail NEC T14.8
      finger — *see* Injury, superficial, finger
      toe — *see* Injury, superficial, toe
    nasal (septum) — *see* Injury, superficial, nose
    neck S10.90 ☑
      specified site NEC S10.80 ☑
    nose (septum) S00.30 ☑
    occipital region — *see* Injury, superficial, scalp
    oral cavity S00.502 ☑
    orbital region — *see* Injury, superficial, periocular area
    palate — *see* Injury, superficial, oral cavity
    palm — *see* Injury, superficial, hand
    parietal region — *see* Injury, superficial, scalp
    pelvis S30.91 ☑
      girdle — *see* Injury, superficial, hip
    penis S30.93 ☑
    perineum
      female S30.95 ☑
      male S30.91 ☑
    periocular area S00.20- ☑
      abrasion — *see* Abrasion, eyelid
      bite — *see* Bite, superficial, eyelid
      contusion — *see* Contusion, eyelid
      external constriction — *see* Constriction, external, eyelid
      foreign body — *see* Foreign body, superficial, eyelid
    phalanges
      finger — *see* Injury, superficial, finger
      toe — *see* Injury, superficial, toe
    pharynx — *see* Injury, superficial, throat
    pinna — *see* Injury, superficial, ear
    popliteal space — *see* Injury, superficial, knee
    prepuce S30.93 ☑
    pubic region S30.91 ☑
    pudendum
      female S30.97 ☑
      male S30.96 ☑
    sacral region S30.91 ☑
    scalp S00.00 ☑
    scapular region — *see* Injury, superficial, shoulder
    sclera — *see* Injury, eye, specified site NEC
    scrotum S30.94 ☑
    shin — *see* Injury, superficial, leg
    shoulder S40.91- ☑
      abrasion — *see* Abrasion, shoulder
      bite — *see* Bite, superficial, shoulder
      blister — *see* Blister, shoulder
      contusion — *see* Contusion, shoulder
      external constriction — *see* Constriction, external, shoulder
      foreign body — *see* Foreign body, superficial, shoulder
    skin NEC T14.8
    sternal region — *see* Injury, superficial, thorax, front
    subconjunctival — *see* Injury, eye, specified site NEC
    subcutaneous NEC T14.8
    submaxillary region — *see* Injury, superficial, head, specified NEC
    submental region — *see* Injury, superficial, head, specified NEC

☑ **Additional Character Required — Refer to the Tabular List for Character Selection**   ⬇ **Subterms under main terms may continue to next column or page**

Injury — *continued*
  superficial — *continued*
    subungual
      finger(s) — *see* Injury, superficial, finger
      toe(s) — *see* Injury, superficial, toe
    supraclavicular fossa — *see* Injury, superficial, neck
    supraorbital — *see* Injury, superficial, head, specified NEC
    temple — *see* Injury, superficial, head, specified NEC
    temporal region — *see* Injury, superficial, head, specified NEC
    testis S30.94 ☑
    thigh S70.92- ☑
      abrasion — *see* Abrasion, thigh
      bite — *see* Bite, superficial, thigh
      blister — *see* Blister, thigh
      contusion — *see* Contusion, thigh
      external constriction — *see* Constriction, external, thigh
      foreign body — *see* Foreign body, superficial, thigh
    thorax, thoracic (wall) S20.90 ☑
      abrasion — *see* Abrasion, thorax
      back S20.40- ☑
      bite — *see* Bite, thorax, superficial
      blister — *see* Blister, thorax
      contusion — *see* Contusion, thorax
      external constriction — *see* Constriction, external, thorax
      foreign body — *see* Foreign body, superficial, thorax
      front S20.30- ☑
    throat S10.10 ☑
      abrasion S10.11 ☑
      bite S10.17 ☑
        insect S10.16 ☑
      blister S10.12 ☑
      contusion S10.0 ☑
      external constriction S10.14 ☑
      foreign body S10.15 ☑
    thumb S60.93- ☑
      abrasion — *see* Abrasion, thumb
      bite — *see* Bite, superficial, thumb
      blister — *see* Blister, thumb
      contusion — *see* Contusion, thumb
      external constriction — *see* Constriction, external, thumb
      foreign body — *see* Foreign body, superficial, thumb
      insect bite — *see* Bite, by site, superficial, insect
      specified type NEC S60.39 ☑
    toe(s) S90.93- ☑
      abrasion — *see* Abrasion, toe
      bite — *see* Bite, toe
      blister — *see* Blister, toe
      contusion — *see* Contusion, toe
      external constriction — *see* Constriction, external, toe
      foreign body — *see* Foreign body, superficial, toe
      great S90.93- ☑
    tongue — *see* Injury, superficial, oral cavity
    tooth, teeth — *see* Injury, superficial, oral cavity
    trachea S10.10 ☑
    tunica vaginalis S30.94 ☑
    tympanum, tympanic membrane — *see* Injury, superficial, ear
    uvula — *see* Injury, superficial, oral cavity
    vagina S30.95 ☑
    vocal cords — *see* Injury, superficial, throat
    vulva S30.95 ☑
    wrist S60.91- ☑
  supraclavicular region — *see* Injury, neck
  supraorbital S09.93 ☑
  suprarenal gland (multiple) — *see* Injury, adrenal
  surgical complication (external or internal site) — *see* Laceration, accidental complicating surgery
  temple S09.90 ☑
  temporal region S09.90 ☑
  tendon (*see also* Injury, muscle, by site)
    abdomen — *see* Injury, muscle, abdomen
    Achilles — *see* Injury, Achilles tendon
    lower back — *see* Injury, muscle, lower back
    pelvic organs — *see* Injury, muscle, pelvis

Injury — *continued*
  tenth cranial nerve (pneumogastric or vagus) — *see* Injury, nerve, vagus
  testis S39.94 ☑
  thigh S79.92- ☑
    blood vessel — *see* Injury, blood vessel, hip
    contusion — *see* Contusion, thigh
    fracture — *see* Fracture, femur
    muscle — *see* Injury, muscle, thigh
    nerve — *see* Injury, nerve, thigh
    open — *see* Wound, open, thigh
    specified NEC S79.82- ☑
    superficial — *see* Injury, superficial, thigh
  third cranial nerve (oculomotor) — *see* Injury, nerve, oculomotor
  thorax, thoracic S29.9 ☑
    blood vessel — *see* Injury, blood vessel, thorax
    cavity — *see* Injury, intrathoracic
    dislocation — *see* Dislocation, thorax
    external (wall) S29.9 ☑
      contusion — *see* Contusion, thorax
      nerve — *see* Injury, nerve, thorax
      open — *see* Wound, open, thorax
      specified NEC S29.8 ☑
      sprain — *see* Sprain, thorax
      superficial — *see* Injury, superficial, thorax
    fracture — *see* Fracture, thorax
    internal — *see* Injury, intrathoracic
    intrathoracic organ — *see* Injury, intrathoracic
    sympathetic ganglion — *see* Injury, nerve, thorax, sympathetic
  throat (*see also* Injury, neck) S19.9 ☑
  thumb S69.9- ☑
    blood vessel — *see* Injury, blood vessel, thumb
    contusion — *see* Contusion, thumb
    dislocation — *see* Dislocation, thumb
    fracture — *see* Fracture, thumb
    muscle — *see* Injury, muscle, thumb
    nerve — *see* Injury, nerve, digital, thumb
    open — *see* Wound, open, thumb
    specified NEC S69.8- ☑
    sprain — *see* Sprain, thumb
    superficial — *see* Injury, superficial, thumb
  thymus (gland) — *see* Injury, intrathoracic, specified organ NEC
  thyroid (gland) NEC S19.84 ☑
  toe S99.92- ☑
    contusion — *see* Contusion, toe
    dislocation — *see* Dislocation, toe
    fracture — *see* Fracture, toe
    muscle — *see* Injury, muscle, toe
    open — *see* Wound, open, toe
    specified type NEC S99.82- ☑
    sprain — *see* Sprain, toe
    superficial — *see* Injury, superficial, toe
  tongue S09.93 ☑
  tonsil S09.93 ☑
  tooth S09.93 ☑
  trachea (cervical) NEC S19.82 ☑
    thoracic — *see* Injury, intrathoracic, trachea, thoracic
  transfusion-related acute lung (TRALI) J95.84
  tunica vaginalis S39.94 ☑
  twelfth cranial nerve (hypoglossal) — *see* Injury, nerve, hypoglossal
  ureter S37.10 ☑
    contusion S37.12 ☑
    laceration S37.13 ☑
    specified type NEC S37.19 ☑
  urethra (sphincter) S37.30 ☑
    at delivery O71.5
    contusion S37.32 ☑
    laceration S37.33 ☑
    specified type NEC S37.39 ☑
  urinary organ S37.90 ☑
    contusion S37.92 ☑
    laceration S37.93 ☑
    specified
      site NEC S37.899 ☑
        contusion S37.892 ☑
        laceration S37.893 ☑
        specified type NEC S37.898 ☑
      type NEC S37.99 ☑
  uterus, uterine S37.60 ☑
    with ectopic or molar pregnancy O08.6
    blood vessel — *see* Injury, blood vessel, iliac

Injury — *continued*
  uterus, uterine — *continued*
    contusion S37.62 ☑
    laceration S37.63 ☑
      cervix at delivery O71.3
    rupture associated with obstetrics — *see* Rupture, uterus
    specified type NEC S37.69 ☑
  uvula S09.93 ☑
  vagina S39.93 ☑
    abrasion S30.814 ☑
    bite S31.45 ☑
      insect S30.864 ☑
      superficial NEC S30.874 ☑
    contusion S30.23 ☑
    crush S38.03 ☑
    during delivery — *see* Laceration, vagina, during delivery
    external constriction S30.844 ☑
    insect bite S30.864 ☑
    laceration S31.41 ☑
      with foreign body S31.42 ☑
    open wound S31.40 ☑
    puncture S31.43 ☑
      with foreign body S31.44 ☑
    superficial S30.95 ☑
      foreign body S30.854 ☑
  vas deferens — *see* Injury, pelvic organ, specified site NEC
  vascular NEC T14.8
  vein — *see* Injury, blood vessel
  vena cava (superior) S25.20 ☑
    inferior S35.10 ☑
      laceration (minor) (superficial) S35.11 ☑
        major S35.12 ☑
      specified type NEC S35.19 ☑
    laceration (minor) (superficial) S25.21 ☑
      major S25.22 ☑
    specified type NEC S25.29 ☑
  vesical (sphincter) — *see* Injury, bladder
  visual cortex S04.04- ☑
  vitreous (humor) S05.90 ☑
    specified NEC S05.8X- ☑
  vocal cord NEC S19.83 ☑
  vulva S39.94 ☑
    abrasion S30.814 ☑
    bite S31.45 ☑
      insect S30.864 ☑
      superficial NEC S30.874 ☑
    contusion S30.23 ☑
    crush S38.03 ☑
    during delivery — *see* Laceration, perineum, female, during delivery
    external constriction S30.844 ☑
    insect bite S30.864 ☑
    laceration S31.41 ☑
      with foreign body S31.42 ☑
    open wound S31.40 ☑
    puncture S31.43 ☑
      with foreign body S31.44 ☑
    superficial S30.95 ☑
      foreign body S30.854 ☑
  whiplash (cervical spine) S13.4 ☑
  wrist S69.9- ☑
    blood vessel — *see* Injury, blood vessel, hand
    contusion — *see* Contusion, wrist
    dislocation — *see* Dislocation, wrist
    fracture — *see* Fracture, wrist
    muscle — *see* Injury, muscle, hand
    nerve — *see* Injury, nerve, hand
    open — *see* Wound, open, wrist
    specified NEC S69.8- ☑
    sprain — *see* Sprain, wrist
    superficial — *see* Injury, superficial, wrist
Inoculation (*see also* Vaccination)
  complication or reaction — *see* Complications, vaccination
Insanity, insane (*see also* Psychosis)
  adolescent — *see* Schizophrenia
  confusional F28
    acute or subacute F05
  delusional F22
  senile F03 ☑
Insect
  bite — *see* Bite, by site, superficial, insect

Insect — continued
   venomous, poisoning NEC (by) — see Venom, arthropod
Insensitivity
   adrenocorticotropin hormone (ACTH) E27.49
   androgen E34.50
      complete E34.51
      partial E34.52
Insertion
   cord (umbilical) lateral or velamentous O43.12- ☑
   intrauterine contraceptive device (encounter for) —
      see Intrauterine contraceptive device
Insolation (sunstroke) T67.0 ☑
Insomnia (organic) G47.00
   without objective findings F51.02
   adjustment F51.02
   adjustment disorder F51.02
   behavioral, of childhood Z73.819
      combined type Z73.812
      limit setting type Z73.811
      sleep-onset association type Z73.810
   childhood Z73.819
   chronic F51.04
      somatized tension F51.04
   conditioned F51.04
   due to
      alcohol
         abuse F10.182
         dependence F10.282
         use F10.982
      amphetamines
         abuse F15.182
         dependence F15.282
         use F15.982
      anxiety disorder F51.05
      caffeine
         abuse F15.182
         dependence F15.282
         use F15.982
      cocaine
         abuse F14.182
         dependence F14.282
         use F14.982
      depression F51.05
      drug NEC
         abuse F19.182
         dependence F19.282
         use F19.982
      medical condition G47.01
      mental disorder NEC F51.05
      opioid
         abuse F11.182
         dependence F11.282
         use F11.982
      psychoactive substance NEC
         abuse F19.182
         dependence F19.182
         use F19.982
      sedative, hypnotic, or anxiolytic
         abuse F13.182
         dependence F13.282
         use F13.982
      stimulant NEC
         abuse F15.182
         dependence F15.282
         use F15.982
   fatal familial (FFI) A81.83
   idiopathic F51.01
   learned F51.3
   nonorganic origin F51.01
   not due to a substance or known physiological condition F51.01
      specified NEC F51.09
   paradoxical F51.03
   primary F51.01
   psychiatric F51.05
   psychophysiologic F51.04
   related to psychopathology F51.05
   short-term F51.02
   specified NEC G47.09
   stress-related F51.02
   transient F51.02
Inspiration
   food or foreign body — see Foreign body, by site
   mucus — see Asphyxia, mucus
Inspissated bile syndrome (newborn) P59.1
Instability
   emotional (excessive) F60.3

Instability — continued
   joint (post-traumatic) M25.30
      ankle M25.37- ☑
      due to old ligament injury — see Disorder, ligament
      elbow M25.32- ☑
      flail — see Flail, joint
      foot M25.37- ☑
      hand M25.34- ☑
      hip M25.35- ☑
      knee M25.36- ☑
      lumbosacral — see subcategory M53.2 ☑
      prosthesis — see Complications, joint prosthesis, mechanical, displacement, by site
      sacroiliac — see subcategory M53.2 ☑
      secondary to
         old ligament injury — see Disorder, ligament
         removal of joint prosthesis M96.89
      shoulder (region) M25.31- ☑
      spine — see subcategory M53.2 ☑
      wrist M25.33- ☑
   knee (chronic) M23.5- ☑
   lumbosacral — see subcategory M53.2 ☑
   nervous F48.8
   personality (emotional) F60.3
   spine — see Instability, joint, spine
   vasomotor R55
Institutional syndrome (childhood) F94.2
Institutionalization, affecting child Z62.22
   disinhibited attachment F94.2
Insufficiency, insufficient
   accommodation, old age H52.4
   adrenal (gland) E27.40
      primary E27.1
   adrenocortical E27.40
      drug-induced E27.3
      iatrogenic E27.3
      primary E27.1
   anterior (occlusal) guidance M26.54
   anus K62.89
   aortic (valve) I35.1
      with
         mitral (valve) disease I08.0
            with tricuspid (valve) disease I08.3
         stenosis I35.2
         tricuspid (valve) disease I08.2
            with mitral (valve) disease I08.3
      congenital Q23.1
      rheumatic I06.1
         with
            mitral (valve) disease I08.0
               with tricuspid (valve) disease I08.3
            stenosis I06.2
               with mitral (valve) disease I08.0
                  with tricuspid (valve) disease I08.3
            tricuspid (valve) disease I08.2
               with mitral (valve) disease I08.3
      specified cause NEC I35.1
      syphilitic A52.03
   arterial I77.1
      basilar G45.0
      carotid (hemispheric) G45.1
      cerebral I67.81
      coronary (acute or subacute) I24.8
      mesenteric K55.1
      peripheral I73.9
      precerebral (multiple) (bilateral) G45.2
      vertebral G45.0
   arteriovenous I99.8
   biliary K83.8
   cardiac (see also Insufficiency, myocardial)
      due to presence of (cardiac) prosthesis I97.11- ☑
      postprocedural I97.11- ☑
   cardiorenal, hypertensive I13.2
   cardiovascular — see Disease, cardiovascular
   cerebrovascular (acute) I67.81
      with transient focal neurological signs and symptoms G45.8
   circulatory NEC I99.8
      newborn P29.89
   convergence H51.11
   coronary (acute or subacute) I24.8
      chronic or with a stated duration of over 4 weeks I25.89
   corticoadrenal E27.40
      primary E27.1
   dietary E63.9
   divergence H51.8

Insufficiency, insufficient — continued
   food T73.0 ☑
   gastroesophageal K22.8
   gonadal
      ovary E28.39
      testis E29.1
   heart (see also Insufficiency, myocardial)
      newborn P29.0
      valve — see Endocarditis
   hepatic — see Failure, hepatic
   idiopathic autonomic G90.09
   interocclusal distance of fully erupted teeth (ridge) M26.36
   kidney N28.9
      acute N28.9
      chronic N18.9
   lacrimal (secretion) H04.12- ☑
      passages — see Stenosis, lacrimal
   liver — see Failure, hepatic
   lung — see Insufficiency, pulmonary
   mental (congenital) — see Disability, intellectual
   mesenteric K55.1
   mitral (valve) I34.0
      with
         aortic valve disease I08.0
            with tricuspid (valve) disease I08.3
         obstruction or stenosis I05.2
            with aortic valve disease I08.0
         tricuspid (valve) disease I08.1
            with aortic (valve) disease I08.3
      congenital Q23.3
      rheumatic I05.1
         with
            aortic valve disease I08.0
               with tricuspid (valve) disease I08.3
            obstruction or stenosis I05.2
               with aortic valve disease I08.0
                  with tricuspid (valve) disease I08.3
            tricuspid (valve) disease I08.1
               with aortic (valve) disease I08.3
      active or acute I01.1
         with chorea, rheumatic (Sydenham's) I02.0
      specified cause, except rheumatic I34.0
   muscle (see also Disease, muscle)
      heart — see Insufficiency, myocardial
      ocular NEC H50.9
   myocardial, myocardium (with arteriosclerosis) I50.9
      with
         rheumatic fever (conditions in I00) I09.0
            active, acute or subacute I01.2
               with chorea I02.0
            inactive or quiescent (with chorea) I09.0
      congenital Q24.8
      hypertensive — see Hypertension, heart
      newborn P29.0
      rheumatic I09.0
         active, acute, or subacute I01.2
      syphilitic A52.06
   nourishment T73.0 ☑
   pancreatic K86.8
   parathyroid (gland) E20.9
   peripheral vascular (arterial) I73.9
   pituitary E23.0
   placental (mother) O36.51- ☑
   platelets D69.6
   prenatal care affecting management of pregnancy O09.3- ☑
   progressive pluriglandular E31.0
   pulmonary J98.4
      acute, following surgery (nonthoracic) J95.2
         thoracic J95.1
      chronic, following surgery J95.3
      following
         shock J98.4
         trauma J98.4
      newborn P28.5
      valve I37.1
         with stenosis I37.2
         congenital Q22.2
         rheumatic I09.89
            with aortic, mitral or tricuspid (valve) disease I08.8
   pyloric K31.89
   renal (acute) N28.9
      chronic N18.9
   respiratory R06.89
      newborn P28.5
   rotation — see Malrotation

Insufficiency, insufficient — continued
  sleep syndrome F51.12
  social insurance Z59.7
  suprarenal E27.40
    primary E27.1
  tarso-orbital fascia, congenital Q10.3
  testis E29.1
  thyroid (gland) (acquired) E03.9
    congenital E03.1
  tricuspid (valve) (rheumatic) I07.1
    with
      aortic (valve) disease I08.2
        with mitral (valve) disease I08.3
      mitral (valve) disease I08.1
        with aortic (valve) disease I08.3
      obstruction or stenosis I07.2
        with aortic (valve) disease I08.2
          with mitral (valve) disease I08.3
    congenital Q22.8
    nonrheumatic I36.1
      with stenosis I36.2
  urethral sphincter R32
  valve, valvular (heart) — see Endocarditis
    congenital Q24.8
  vascular I99.8
    intestine K55.9
      acute K55.0
    mesenteric K55.1
    peripheral I73.9
    renal — see Hypertension, kidney
  velopharyngeal
    acquired K13.79
    congenital Q38.8
  venous (chronic) (peripheral) I87.2
  ventricular — see Insufficiency, myocardial
  welfare support Z59.7
Insufflation, fallopian Z31.41
Insular — see condition
Insulinoma
  pancreas
    benign D13.7
    malignant C25.4
    uncertain behavior D37.8
  specified site
    benign — see Neoplasm, by site, benign
    malignant — see Neoplasm, by site, malignant
    uncertain behavior — see Neoplasm, by site, uncertain behavior
  unspecified site
    benign D13.7
    malignant C25.4
    uncertain behavior D37.8
Insuloma — see Insulinoma
Interference
  balancing side M26.56
  non-working side M26.56
Intermenstrual — see condition
Intermittent — see condition
Internal — see condition
Interrogation
  cardiac defibrillator (automatic) (implantable) Z45.02
  cardiac pacemaker Z45.018
  cardiac (event) (loop) recorder Z45.09
  infusion pump (implanted) (intrathecal) Z45.1
  neurostimulator Z46.2
Interruption
  bundle of His I44.30
  phase-shift, sleep cycle — see Disorder, sleep, circadian rhythm
  sleep phase-shift, or 24 hour sleep-wake cycle — see Disorder, sleep, circadian rhythm
Interstitial — see condition
Intertrigo L30.4
  labialis K13.0
Intervertebral disc — see condition
Intestine, intestinal — see condition
Intolerance
  carbohydrate K90.4
  disaccharide, hereditary E73.0
  fat NEC K90.4
    pancreatic K90.3
  food K90.4
    dietary counseling and surveillance Z71.3
  fructose E74.10
    hereditary E74.12
  glucose (-galactose) E74.39
  gluten K90.0

Intolerance — continued
  lactose E73.9
    specified NEC E73.8
  lysine E72.3
  milk NEC K90.4
    lactose E73.9
  protein K90.4
  starch NEC K90.4
  sucrose (-isomaltose) E74.31
Intoxicated NEC (without dependence) — see Alcohol, intoxication
Intoxication
  acid E87.2
  alcoholic (acute) (without dependence) — see Alcohol, intoxication
  alimentary canal K52.1
  amphetamine (without dependence) — see Abuse, drug, stimulant, with intoxication
    with dependence — see Dependence, drug, stimulant, with intoxication
  anxiolytic (acute) (without dependence) — see Abuse, drug, sedative, with intoxication
    with dependence — see Dependence, drug, sedative, with intoxication
  caffeine (acute) (without dependence) — see Abuse, drug, stimulant, with intoxication
    with dependence — see Dependence, drug, stimulant, with intoxication
  cannabinoids (acute) (without dependence) — see Abuse, drug, cannabis, with intoxication
    with dependence — see Dependence, drug, cannabis, with intoxication
  chemical — see Table of Drugs and Chemicals
    via placenta or breast milk — see - Absorption, chemical, through placenta
  cocaine (acute) (without dependence) — see Abuse, drug, cocaine, with intoxication
    with dependence — see Dependence, drug, cocaine, with intoxication
  drug
    acute (without dependence) — see Abuse, drug, by type with intoxication
      with dependence — see Dependence, drug, by type with intoxication
    addictive
      via placenta or breast milk — see Absorption, drug, addictive, through placenta
    newborn P93.8
      gray baby syndrome P93.0
    overdose or wrong substance given or taken — see Table of Drugs and Chemicals, by drug, poisoning
  enteric K52.1
  foodborne A05.9
    bacterial A05.9
    classical (Clostridium botulinum) A05.1
    due to
      Bacillus cereus A05.4
      bacterium A05.9
        specified NEC A05.8
      Clostridium
        botulinum A05.1
        perfringens A05.2
        welchii A05.2
      Salmonella A02.9
        with
          (gastro)enteritis A02.0
          localized infection(s) A02.20
            arthritis A02.23
            meningitis A02.21
            osteomyelitis A02.24
            pneumonia A02.22
            pyelonephritis A02.25
            specified NEC A02.29
          sepsis A02.1
          specified manifestation NEC A02.8
      Staphylococcus A05.0
      Vibrio
        parahaemolyticus A05.3
        vulnificus A05.5
    enterotoxin, staphylococcal A05.0
    noxious — see Poisoning, food, noxious
  gastrointestinal K52.1
  hallucinogenic (without dependence) — see Abuse, drug, hallucinogen, with intoxication
    with dependence — see Dependence, drug, hallucinogen, with intoxication

Intoxication — continued
  hypnotic (acute) (without dependence) — see Abuse, drug, sedative, with intoxication
    with dependence — see Dependence, drug, sedative, with intoxication
  inhalant (acute) (without dependence) — see Abuse, drug, inhalant, with intoxication
    with dependence — see Dependence, drug, inhalant, with intoxication
  meaning
    inebriation — see category F10 ☑
    poisoning — see Table of Drugs and Chemicals
  methyl alcohol (acute) (without dependence) — see Alcohol, intoxication
  opioid (acute) (without dependence) — see Abuse, drug, opioid, with intoxication
    with dependence — see Dependence, drug, opioid, with intoxication
  pathologic NEC (without dependence) — see Alcohol, intoxication
  phencyclidine (without dependence) — see Abuse, drug, psychoactive NEC, with intoxication
    with dependence — see Dependence, drug, psychoactive NEC, with intoxication
  potassium (K) E87.5
  psychoactive substance NEC (without dependence) — see Abuse, drug, psychoactive NEC, with intoxication
    with dependence — see Dependence, drug, psychoactive NEC, with intoxication
  sedative (acute) (without dependence) — see Abuse, drug, sedative, with intoxication
    with dependence — see Dependence, drug, sedative, with intoxication
  serum (see also Reaction, serum) T80.69 ☑
  uremic — see Uremia
  volatile solvents (acute) (without dependence) — see Abuse, drug, inhalant, with intoxication
    with dependence — see Dependence, drug, inhalant, with intoxication
  water E87.79
Intracranial — see condition
Intrahepatic gallbladder Q44.1
Intraligamentous — see condition
Intrathoracic (see also condition)
  kidney Q63.2
Intrauterine contraceptive device
  checking Z30.431
  in situ Z97.5
  insertion Z30.430
    immediately following removal Z30.433
  management Z30.431
  reinsertion Z30.433
  removal Z30.432
  replacement Z30.433
  retention in pregnancy O26.3- ☑
Intraventricular — see condition
Intrinsic deformity — see Deformity
Intubation, difficult or failed T88.4 ☑
Intumescence, lens (eye) (cataract) — see Cataract
Intussusception (bowel) (colon) (enteric) (ileocecal) (ileocolic) (intestine) (rectum) K56.1
  appendix K38.8
  congenital Q43.8
  ureter (with obstruction) N13.5
Invagination (bowel, colon, intestine or rectum) K56.1
Inversion
  albumin-globulin (A-G) ratio E88.09
  bladder N32.89
  cecum — see Intussusception
  cervix N88.8
  chromosome in normal individual Q95.1
  circadian rhythm — see Disorder, sleep, circadian rhythm
  nipple N64.59
    congenital Q83.8
    gestational — see Retraction, nipple
    puerperal, postpartum — see Retraction, nipple
  nyctohemeral rhythm — see Disorder, sleep, circadian rhythm
  optic papilla Q14.2
  organ or site, congenital NEC — see Anomaly, by site
  sleep rhythm — see Disorder, sleep, circadian rhythm
  testis (congenital) Q55.29
  uterus (chronic) (postinfectional) (postpartal, old) N85.5
    postpartum O71.2

Inversion — *continued*
   vagina (posthysterectomy) N99.3
   ventricular Q20.5
Investigation (*see also* Examination) Z04.9
   clinical research subject (control) (normal comparison)
      (participant) Z00.6
Involuntary movement, abnormal R25.9
Involution, involutional (*see also* condition)
   breast, cystic — *see* Dysplasia, mammary, specified
      type NEC
   depression (single episode) F32.8
     recurrent episode F33.9
   melancholia (recurrent episode) (single episode) F32.8
   ovary, senile — *see* Atrophy, ovary
   thymus failure E32.8
I.Q.
   under 20 F73
   20-34 F72
   35-49 F71
   50-69 F70
IRDS (type I) P22.0
   type II P22.1
Irideremia Q13.1
Iridis rubeosis — *see* Disorder, iris, vascular
Iridochoroiditis (panuveitis) — *see* Panuveitis
Iridocyclitis H20.9
   acute H20.0- ☑
     hypopyon H20.05- ☑
     primary H20.01- ☑
     recurrent H20.02- ☑
     secondary (noninfectious) H20.04- ☑
       infectious H20.03- ☑
   chronic H20.1- ☑
   due to allergy — *see* Iridocyclitis, acute, secondary
   endogenous — *see* Iridocyclitis, acute, primary
   Fuchs' — *see* Cyclitis, Fuchs' heterochromic
   gonococcal A54.32
   granulomatous — *see* Iridocyclitis, chronic
   herpes, herpetic (simplex) B00.51
     zoster B02.32
   hypopyon — *see* Iridocyclitis, acute, hypopyon
   in (due to)
     ankylosing spondylitis M45.9
     gonococcal infection A54.32
     herpes (simplex) virus B00.51
      zoster B02.32
     infectious disease NOS B99 ☑
     parasitic disease NOS B89 [H22]
     sarcoidosis D86.83
     syphilis A51.43
     tuberculosis A18.54
     zoster B02.32
   lens-induced H20.2- ☑
   nongranulomatous — *see* Iridocyclitis, acute
   recurrent — *see* Iridocyclitis, acute, recurrent
   rheumatic — *see* Iridocyclitis, chronic
   subacute — *see* Iridocyclitis, acute
   sympathetic — *see* Uveitis, sympathetic
   syphilitic (secondary) A51.43
   tuberculous (chronic) A18.54
   Vogt-Koyanagi H20.82- ☑
Iridocyclochoroiditis (panuveitis) — *see* Panuveitis
Iridodialysis H21.53- ☑
Iridodonesis H21.89
Iridoplegia (complete) (partial) (reflex) H57.09
Iridoschisis H21.25- ☑
Iris (*see also* condition)
   bombé — *see* Membrane, pupillary
Iritis (*see also* Iridocyclitis)
   chronic — *see* Iridocyclitis, chronic
   diabetic — *see* E08-E13 with .39
   due to
     herpes simplex B00.51
     leprosy A30.9 [H22]
   gonococcal A54.32
   gouty M10.9
   granulomatous — *see* Iridocyclitis, chronic
   lens induced — *see* Iridocyclitis, lens-induced
   papulosa (syphilitic) A52.71
   rheumatic — *see* Iridocyclitis, chronic
   syphilitic (secondary) A51.43
     congenital (early) A50.01
     late A52.71
   tuberculous A18.54
Iron — *see* condition
Iron-miner's lung J63.4
Irradiated enamel (tooth, teeth) K03.89

Irradiation effects, adverse T66 ☑
Irreducible, irreducibility — *see* condition
Irregular, irregularity
   action, heart I49.9
   alveolar process K08.8
   bleeding N92.6
   breathing R06.89
   contour of cornea (acquired) — *see* Deformity, cornea
     congenital Q13.4
   contour, reconstructed breast N65.0
   dentin (in pulp) K04.3
   eye movements H55.89
     nystagmus — *see* Nystagmus
     saccadic H55.81
   labor O62.2
   menstruation (cause unknown) N92.6
   periods N92.6
   prostate N42.9
   pupil — *see* Abnormality, pupillary
   reconstructed breast N65.0
   respiratory R06.89
   septum (nasal) J34.2
   shape, organ or site, congenital NEC — *see* Distortion
   sleep-wake pattern (rhythm) G47.23
Irritable, irritability R45.4
   bladder N32.89
   bowel (syndrome) K58.9
     with diarrhea K58.0
     psychogenic F45.8
   bronchial — *see* Bronchitis
   cerebral, in newborn P91.3
   colon K58.9
     with diarrhea K58.0
     psychogenic F45.8
   duodenum K59.8
   heart (psychogenic) F45.8
   hip — *see* Derangement, joint, specified type NEC, hip
   ileum K59.8
   infant R68.12
   jejunum K59.8
   rectum K59.8
   stomach K31.89
     psychogenic F45.8
   sympathetic G90.8
   urethra N36.8
Irritation
   anus K62.89
   axillary nerve G54.0
   bladder N32.89
   brachial plexus G54.0
   bronchial — *see* Bronchitis
   cervical plexus G54.2
   cervix — *see* Cervicitis
   choroid, sympathetic — *see* Endophthalmitis
   cranial nerve — *see* Disorder, nerve, cranial
   gastric K31.89
     psychogenic F45.8
   globe, sympathetic — *see* Uveitis, sympathetic
   labyrinth — *see* subcategory H83.2 ☑
   lumbosacral plexus G54.1
   meninges (traumatic) — *see* Injury, intracranial
     nontraumatic — *see* Meningismus
   nerve — *see* Disorder, nerve
   nervous R45.0
   penis N48.89
   perineum NEC L29.3
   peripheral autonomic nervous system G90.8
   peritoneum — *see* Peritonitis
   pharynx J39.2
   plantar nerve — *see* Lesion, nerve, plantar
   spinal (cord) (traumatic) (*see also* Injury, spinal cord,
     by region)
     nerve G58.9
      root NEC — *see* Radiculopathy
     nontraumatic — *see* Myelopathy
   stomach K31.89
     psychogenic F45.8
   sympathetic nerve NEC G90.8
   ulnar nerve — *see* Lesion, nerve, ulnar
   vagina N89.8
Ischemia, ischemic I99.8
   bowel (transient)
     acute K55.0
     chronic K55.1
     due to mesenteric artery insufficiency K55.1
   brain — *see* Ischemia, cerebral
   cardiac (see Disease, heart, ischemic)
   cardiomyopathy I25.5

Ischemia, ischemic — *continued*
   cerebral (chronic) (generalized) I67.82
     arteriosclerotic I67.2
     intermittent G45.9
     newborn P91.0
     recurrent focal G45.8
     transient G45.9
   colon chronic (due to mesenteric artery insufficiency)
     K55.1
   coronary — *see* Disease, heart, ischemic
   demand (coronary) (*see also* Angina) I24.8
   heart (chronic or with a stated duration of over 4
     weeks) I25.9
     acute or with a stated duration of 4 weeks or less
      I24.9
     subacute I24.9
   infarction, muscle — *see* Infarct, muscle
   intestine (large) (small) (transient) K55.9
     acute K55.0
     chronic K55.1
     due to mesenteric artery insufficiency K55.1
   kidney N28.0
   mesenteric, acute K55.0
   muscle, traumatic T79.6 ☑
   myocardium, myocardial (chronic or with a stated
     duration of over 4 weeks) I25.9
     acute, without myocardial infarction I24.0
     silent (asymptomatic) I25.6
     transient of newborn P29.4
   renal N28.0
   retina, retinal — *see* Occlusion, artery, retina
   small bowel
     acute K55.0
     chronic K55.1
     due to mesenteric artery insufficiency K55.1
   spinal cord G95.11
   subendocardial — *see* Insufficiency, coronary
   supply (coronary) (*see also* Angina) I25.9
     due to vasospasm I20.1
Ischial spine — *see* condition
Ischialgia — *see* Sciatica
Ischiopagus Q89.4
Ischium, ischial — *see* condition
Ischuria R34
Iselin's disease or osteochondrosis — *see* Osteochon-
   drosis, juvenile, metatarsus
Islands of
   parotid tissue in
     lymph nodes Q38.6
     neck structures Q38.6
   submaxillary glands in
     fascia Q38.6
     lymph nodes Q38.6
     neck muscles Q38.6
Islet cell tumor, pancreas D13.7
Isoimmunization NEC (*see also* Incompatibility)
   affecting management of pregnancy (ABO) (with hy-
     drops fetalis) O36.11- ☑
     anti-A sensitization O36.11- ☑
     anti-B sensitization O36.19- ☑
     anti-c sensitization O36.09- ☑
     anti-C sensitization O36.09- ☑
     anti-E sensitization O36.09- ☑
     anti-e sensitization O36.09- ☑
     Rh NEC O36.09- ☑
      anti-D antibody O36.01- ☑
     specified NEC O36.19- ☑
   newborn P55.9
     with
      hydrops fetalis P56.0
      kernicterus P57.0
     ABO (blood groups) P55.1
     Rhesus (Rh) factor P55.0
     specified type NEC P55.8
Isolation, isolated
   dwelling Z59.8
   family Z63.79
   social Z60.4
Isoleucinosis E71.19
Isomerism atrial appendages (with asplenia or
   polysplenia) Q20.6
Isosporiasis, isosporosis A07.3
Isovaleric acidemia E71.110
Issue of
   medical certificate Z02.79
     for disability determination Z02.71

196

☑ Additional Character Required — Refer to the Tabular List for Character Selection   ▽ Subterms under main terms may continue to next column or page

Issue of — *continued*
  repeat prescription (appliance) (glasses) (medicinal substance, medicament, medicine) Z76.0
    contraception — *see* Contraception
Itch, itching (*see also* Pruritus)
  baker's L23.6
  barber's B35.0
  bricklayer's L24.5
  cheese B88.0
  clam digger's B65.3
  coolie B76.9
  copra B88.0
  dew B76.9
  dhobi B35.6
  filarial — *see* Infestation, filarial
  grain B88.0
  grocer's B88.0
  ground B76.9
  harvest B88.0
  jock B35.6
  Malabar B35.5
    beard B35.0
    foot B35.3
    scalp B35.0
  meaning scabies B86
  Norwegian B86
  perianal L29.0
  poultrymen's B88.0
  sarcoptic B86
  scabies B86
  scrub B88.0
  straw B88.0
  swimmer's B65.3
  water B76.9
  winter L29.8
Ivemark's syndrome (asplenia with congenital heart disease) Q89.01
Ivory bones Q78.2
Ixodiasis NEC B88.8

J

Jaccoud's syndrome — *see* Arthropathy, postrheumatic, chronic
Jackson's
  membrane Q43.3
  paralysis or syndrome G83.89
  veil Q43.3
Jacquet's dermatitis (diaper dermatitis) L22
Jadassohn-Pellizari's disease or anetoderma L90.2
Jadassohn's
  blue nevus — *see* Nevus
  intraepidermal epithelioma — *see* Neoplasm, skin, benign
Jaffe-Lichtenstein (-Uehlinger) **syndrome** — *see* Dysplasia, fibrous, bone NEC
Jakob-Creutzfeldt disease or syndrome — *see* Creutzfeldt-Jakob disease or syndrome
Jaksch-Luzet disease D64.89
Jamaican
  neuropathy G92
  paraplegic tropical ataxic-spastic syndrome G92
Janet's disease F48.8
Janiceps Q89.4
Jansky-Bielschowsky amaurotic idiocy E75.4
Japanese
  B-type encephalitis A83.0
  river fever A75.3
Jaundice (yellow) R17
  acholuric (familial) (splenomegalic) (*see also* Spherocytosis)
    acquired D59.8
  breast-milk (inhibitor) P59.3
  catarrhal (acute) B15.9
    with hepatic coma B15.0
  cholestatic (benign) R17
  due to or associated with
    delayed conjugation P59.8
      associated with (due to) preterm delivery P59.0
    preterm delivery P59.0
  epidemic (catarrhal) B15.9
    with hepatic coma B15.0
    leptospiral A27.0
    spirochetal A27.0
  familial nonhemolytic (congenital) (Gilbert) E80.4
    Crigler-Najjar E80.5
  febrile (acute) B15.9
    with hepatic coma B15.0

Jaundice — *continued*
  febrile — *continued*
    leptospiral A27.0
    spirochetal A27.0
  hematogenous D59.9
  hemolytic (acquired) D59.9
    congenital — *see* Spherocytosis
  hemorrhagic (acute) (leptospiral) (spirochetal) A27.0
  infectious (acute) (subacute) B15.9
    with hepatic coma B15.0
    leptospiral A27.0
    spirochetal A27.0
  leptospiral (hemorrhagic) A27.0
  malignant (without coma) K72.90
    with coma K72.91
  neonatal — *see* Jaundice, newborn
  newborn P59.9
    due to or associated with
      ABO
        antibodies P55.1
        incompatibility, maternal/fetal P55.1
        isoimmunization P55.1
      absence or deficiency of enzyme system for bilirubin conjugation (congenital) P59.8
      bleeding P58.1
      breast milk inhibitors to conjugation P59.3
        associated with preterm delivery P59.0
      bruising P58.0
      Crigler-Najjar syndrome E80.5
      delayed conjugation P59.8
        associated with preterm delivery P59.0
      drugs or toxins
        given to newborn P58.42
        transmitted from mother P58.41
      excessive hemolysis P58.9
        due to
          bleeding P58.1
          bruising P58.0
          drugs or toxins
            given to newborn P58.42
            transmitted from mother P58.41
          infection P58.2
          polycythemia P58.3
          swallowed maternal blood P58.5
        specified type NEC P58.8
      galactosemia E74.21
      Gilbert syndrome E80.4
      hemolytic disease P55.9
        ABO isoimmunization P55.1
        Rh isoimmunization P55.0
        specified NEC P55.8
      hepatocellular damage P59.20
        specified NEC P59.29
      hereditary hemolytic anemia P58.8
      hypothyroidism, congenital E03.1
      incompatibility, maternal/fetal NOS P55.9
      infection P58.2
      inspissated bile syndrome P59.1
      isoimmunization NOS P55.9
      mucoviscidosis E84.9
      polycythemia P58.3
      preterm delivery P59.0
      Rh
        antibodies P55.0
        incompatibility, maternal/fetal P55.0
        isoimmunization P55.0
      specified cause NEC P59.8
      swallowed maternal blood P58.5
    spherocytosis (congenital) D58.0
  nonhemolytic congenital familial (Gilbert) E80.4
  nuclear, newborn (*see also* Kernicterus of newborn) P57.9
  obstructive (*see also* Obstruction, bile duct) K83.1
  post-immunization — *see* Hepatitis, viral, type, B
  post-transfusion — *see* Hepatitis, viral, type, B
  regurgitation (*see also* Obstruction, bile duct) K83.1
  serum (homologous) (prophylactic) (therapeutic) — *see* Hepatitis, viral, type, B
  spirochetal (hemorrhagic) A27.0
  symptomatic R17
    newborn P59.9
Jaw — *see* condition
Jaw-winking phenomenon or syndrome Q07.8
Jealousy
  alcoholic F10.988
  childhood F93.8
  sibling F93.8
Jejunitis — *see* Enteritis

Jejunostomy status Z93.4
Jejunum, jejunal — *see* condition
Jensen's disease — *see* Inflammation, chorioretinal, focal, juxtapapillary
Jerks, myoclonic G25.3
Jervell-Lange-Nielsen syndrome I45.81
Jeune's disease Q77.2
Jigger disease B88.1
Job's syndrome (chronic granulomatous disease) D71
Joint (*see also* condition)
  mice — *see* Loose, body, joint
    knee M23.4-
Jordan's anomaly or syndrome D72.0
Joseph-Diamond-Blackfan anemia (congenital hypoplastic) D61.01
Jungle yellow fever A95.0
Jüngling's disease — *see* Sarcoidosis
Juvenile — *see* condition

K

Kahler's disease C90.0- ☑
Kakke E51.11
Kala-azar B55.0
Kallmann's syndrome E23.0
Kanner's syndrome (autism) — *see* Psychosis, childhood
Kaposi's
  dermatosis (xeroderma pigmentosum) Q82.1
  lichen ruber L44.0
    acuminatus L44.0
  sarcoma
    colon C46.4
    connective tissue C46.1
    gastrointestinal organ C46.4
    lung C46.5- ☑
    lymph node (multiple) C46.3
    palate (hard) (soft) C46.2
    rectum C46.4
    skin (multiple sites) C46.0
    specified site NEC C46.7
    stomach C46.4
    unspecified site C46.9
  varicelliform eruption B00.0
    vaccinia T88.1 ☑
Kartagener's syndrome or triad (sinusitis, bronchiectasis, situs inversus) Q89.3
Karyotype
  with abnormality except iso (Xq) Q96.2
  45,X Q96.0
  46,X
    iso (Xq) Q96.1
  46,XX Q98.3
    with streak gonads Q50.32
    hermaphrodite (true) Q99.1
    male Q98.3
  46,XY
    with streak gonads Q56.1
    female Q97.3
    hermaphrodite (true) Q99.1
  47,XXX Q97.0
  47,XXY Q98.0
  47,XYY Q98.5
Kaschin-Beck disease — *see* Disease, Kaschin-Beck
Katayama's disease or fever B65.2
Kawasaki's syndrome M30.3
Kayser-Fleischer ring (cornea) (pseudosclerosis) H18.04- ☑
Kaznelson's syndrome (congenital hypoplastic anemia) D61.01
Kearns-Sayre syndrome H49.81- ☑
Kedani fever A75.3
Kelis L91.0
Kelly (-Patterson) **syndrome** (sideropenic dysphagia) D50.1
Keloid, cheloid L91.0
  acne L73.0
  Addison's L94.0
  cornea — *see* Opacity, cornea
  Hawkin's L91.0
  scar L91.0
Keloma L91.0
Kenya fever A77.1
Keratectasia (*see also* Ectasia, cornea)
  congenital Q13.4
Keratinization of alveolar ridge mucosa
  excessive K13.23
  minimal K13.22

Keratinized residual ridge mucosa
- excessive K13.23
- minimal K13.22

Keratitis (nodular) (nonulcerative) (simple) (zonular) H16.9
- with ulceration (central) (marginal) (perforated) (ring) — see Ulcer, cornea
- actinic — see Photokeratitis
- arborescens (herpes simplex) B00.52
- areolar H16.11- ☑
- bullosa H16.8
- deep H16.309
  - specified type NEC H16.399
- dendritic (a) (herpes simplex) B00.52
- disciform (is) (herpes simplex) B00.52
  - varicella B01.81
- filamentary H16.12- ☑
- gonococcal (congenital or prenatal) A54.33
- herpes, herpetic (simplex) B00.52
  - zoster B02.33
- in (due to)
  - acanthamebiasis B60.13
  - adenovirus B30.0
  - exanthema (see also Exanthem) B09
  - herpes (simplex) virus B00.52
  - measles B05.81
  - syphilis A50.31
  - tuberculosis A18.52
  - zoster B02.33
- interstitial (nonsyphilitic) H16.30- ☑
  - diffuse H16.32- ☑
  - herpes, herpetic (simplex) B00.52
    - zoster B02.33
  - sclerosing H16.33- ☑
  - specified type NEC H16.39- ☑
  - syphilitic (congenital) (late) A50.31
  - tuberculous A18.52
- macular H16.11- ☑
- nummular H16.11- ☑
- oyster shuckers' H16.8
- parenchymatous — see Keratitis, interstitial
- petrificans H16.8
- postmeasles B05.81
- punctata
  - leprosa A30.9 [H16.14-] ☑
  - syphilitic (profunda) A50.31
- punctate H16.14- ☑
- purulent H16.8
- rosacea L71.8
- sclerosing H16.33- ☑
- specified type NEC H16.8
- stellate H16.11- ☑
- striate H16.11- ☑
- superficial H16.10- ☑
  - with conjunctivitis — see Keratoconjunctivitis
  - due to light — see Photokeratitis
- suppurative H16.8
- syphilitic (congenital) (prenatal) A50.31
- trachomatous A71.1
  - sequelae B94.0
- tuberculous A18.52
- vesicular H16.8
- xerotic (see also Keratomalacia) H16.8
  - vitamin A deficiency E50.4

Keratoacanthoma L85.8
Keratocele — see Descemetocele
Keratoconjunctivitis H16.20- ☑
- Acanthamoeba B60.13
- adenoviral B30.0
- epidemic B30.0
- exposure H16.21- ☑
- herpes, herpetic (simplex) B00.52
  - zoster B02.33
- in exanthema (see also Exanthem) B09
- infectious B30.0
- lagophthalmic — see Keratoconjunctivitis, specified type NEC
- neurotrophic H16.23- ☑
- phlyctenular H16.25- ☑
- postmeasles B05.81
- shipyard B30.0
- sicca (Sjogren's) M35.0- ☑
  - not Sjogren's H16.22- ☑
- specified type NEC H16.29- ☑
- tuberculous (phlyctenular) A18.52
- vernal H16.26- ☑

Keratoconus H18.60- ☑

Keratoconus H18.60- ☑
- congenital Q13.4
- stable H18.61- ☑
- unstable H18.62- ☑

Keratocyst (dental) (odontogenic) — see Cyst, calcifying odontogenic

Keratoderma, keratodermia (congenital) (palmaris et plantaris) (symmetrical) Q82.8
- acquired L85.1
  - in diseases classified elsewhere L86
- climactericum L85.1
- gonococcal A54.89
- gonorrheal A54.89
- punctata L85.2
- Reiter's — see Reiter's disease

Keratodermatocele — see Descemetocele
Keratoglobus H18.79 ☑
- congenital Q15.8
  - with glaucoma Q15.0

Keratohemia — see Pigmentation, cornea, stromal
Keratoiritis (see also Iridocyclitis)
- syphilitic A50.39
- tuberculous A18.54

Keratoma L57.0
- palmaris and plantaris hereditarium Q82.8
- senile L57.0

Keratomalacia H18.44- ☑
- vitamin A deficiency E50.4

Keratomegaly Q13.4
Keratomycosis B49
- nigrans, nigricans (palmaris) B36.1

Keratopathy H18.9
- band H18.42- ☑
- bullous (aphakic), following cataract surgery H59.01- ☑
- bullous H18.1- ☑

Keratoscleritis, tuberculous A18.52
Keratosis L57.0
- actinic L57.0
- arsenical L85.8
- congenital, specified NEC Q80.8
- female genital NEC N94.89
- follicularis Q82.8
  - acquired L11.0
  - congenita Q82.8
  - et parafollicularis in cutem penetrans L87.0
  - spinulosa (decalvans) Q82.8
  - vitamin A deficiency E50.8
- gonococcal A54.89
- male genital (external) N50.8
- nigricans L83
- obturans, external ear (canal) — see Cholesteatoma, external ear
- palmaris et plantaris (inherited) (symmetrical) Q82.8
  - acquired L85.1
- penile N48.89
- pharynx J39.2
- pilaris, acquired L85.8
- punctata (palmaris et plantaris) L85.2
- scrotal N50.8
- seborrheic L82.1
  - inflamed L82.0
- senile L57.0
- solar L57.0
- tonsillaris J35.8
- vagina N89.4
- vegetans Q82.8
- vitamin A deficiency E50.8
- vocal cord J38.3

Kerato-uveitis — see Iridocyclitis
Kerion (celsi) B35.0
Kernicterus of newborn (not due to isoimmunization) P57.9
- due to isoimmunization (conditions in P55.0-P55.9) P57.0
- specified type NEC P57.8

Kerunoparalysis T75.09 ☑
Keshan disease E59
Ketoacidosis E87.2
- diabetic — see Diabetes, by type, with ketoacidosis

Ketonuria R82.4
Ketosis NEC E88.89
- diabetic — see Diabetes, by type, with with ketoacidosis

Kew Garden fever A79.1
Kidney — see condition

Kienböck's disease (see also Osteochondrosis, juvenile, hand, carpal lunate)
- adult M93.1

Kimmelstiel (-Wilson) **disease** — see Diabetes, Kimmelstiel (-Wilson) disease

Kink, kinking
- artery I77.1
- hair (acquired) L67.8
- ileum or intestine — see Obstruction, intestine
- Lane's — see Obstruction, intestine
- organ or site, congenital NEC — see Anomaly, by site
- ureter (pelvic junction) N13.5
  - with
    - hydronephrosis N13.1
      - with infection N13.6
    - pyelonephritis (chronic) N11.1
  - congenital Q62.39
- vein(s) I87.8
  - caval I87.1
  - peripheral I87.1

Kinnier Wilson's disease (hepatolenticular degeneration) E83.01
Kissing spine M48.20
- cervical region M48.22
- cervicothoracic region M48.23
- lumbar region M48.26
- lumbosacral region M48.27
- occipito-atlanto-axial region M48.21
- thoracic region M48.24
- thoracolumbar region M48.25

Klatskin's tumor C22.1
Klauder's disease A26.8
Klebs' disease (see also Glomerulonephritis) N05- ☑
Klebsiella (K.) **pneumoniae, as cause of disease classified elsewhere** B96.1
Klein (e)-**Levin syndrome** G47.13
Kleptomania F63.2
Klinefelter's syndrome Q98.4
- karyotype 47,XXY Q98.0
- male with more than two X chromosomes Q98.1

Klippel-Feil deficiency, disease, or syndrome (brevicollis) Q76.1
Klippel's disease I67.2
Klippel-Trenaunay (-Weber) **syndrome** Q87.2
Klumpke (-Déjerine) **palsy, paralysis** (birth) (newborn) P14.1
Knee — see condition
Knock knee (acquired) M21.06- ☑
- congenital Q74.1

Knot(s)
- intestinal, syndrome (volvulus) K56.2
- surfer S89.8- ☑
- umbilical cord (true) O69.2 ☑

Knotting (of)
- hair L67.8
- intestine K56.2

Knuckle pad (Garrod's) M72.1
Koch's
- infection — see Tuberculosis
- relapsing fever A68.9

Koch-Weeks' conjunctivitis — see Conjunctivitis, acute, mucopurulent
Köebner's syndrome Q81.8
Köenig's disease (osteochondritis dissecans) — see Osteochondritis, dissecans
Köhler-Pellegrini-Steida disease or syndrome (calcification, knee joint) — see Bursitis, tibial collateral
Köhler's disease
- patellar — see Osteochondrosis, juvenile, patella
- tarsal navicular — see Osteochondrosis, juvenile, tarsus

Koilonychia L60.3
- congenital Q84.6

Kojevnikov's, epilepsy — see Kozhevnikof's epilepsy
Koplik's spots B05.9
Kopp's asthma E32.8
Korsakoff's (Wernicke) **disease, psychosis or syndrome** (alcoholic) F10.96
- with dependence F10.26
- drug-induced
  - due to drug abuse — see Abuse, drug, by type, with amnestic disorder
  - due to drug dependence — see Dependence, drug, by type, with amnestic disorder
- nonalcoholic F04

Korsakov's disease, psychosis or syndrome — see Korsakoff's disease

Keratinized residual ridge mucosa — Korsakov's disease, psychosis or syndrome

Korsakow's disease, psychosis or syndrome — *see* Korsakoff's disease
Kostmann's disease or syndrome (infantile genetic agranulocytosis) — *see* Agranulocytosis
Kozhevnikof's epilepsy G40.109
  intractable G40.119
    with status epilepticus G40.111
    without status epilepticus G40.119
  not intractable G40.109
    with status epilepticus G40.101
    without status epilepticus G40.109
Krabbe's
  disease E75.23
  syndrome, congenital muscle hypoplasia Q79.8
Kraepelin-Morel disease — *see* Schizophrenia
Kraft-Weber-Dimitri disease Q85.8
Kraurosis
  ani K62.89
  penis N48.0
  vagina N89.8
  vulva N90.4
Kreotoxism A05.9
Krukenberg's
  spindle — *see* Pigmentation, cornea, posterior
  tumor C79.6- ☑
Kufs' disease E75.4
Kugelberg-Welander disease G12.1
Kuhnt-Junius degeneration (see also Degeneration, macula) H35.32
Kümmell's disease or spondylitis — *see* Spondylopathy, traumatic
Kupffer cell sarcoma C22.3
Kuru A81.81
Kussmaul's
  disease M30.0
  respiration E87.2
    in diabetic acidosis — *see* Diabetes, by type, with ketoacidosis
Kwashiorkor E40
  marasmic, marasmus type E42
Kyasanur Forest disease A98.2
Kyphoscoliosis, kyphoscoliotic (acquired) (see also Scoliosis) M41.9
  congenital Q67.5
  heart (disease) I27.1
  sequelae of rickets E64.3
  tuberculous A18.01
Kyphosis, kyphotic (acquired) M40.209
  cervical region M40.202
  cervicothoracic region M40.203
  congenital Q76.419
    cervical region Q76.412
    cervicothoracic region Q76.413
    occipito-atlanto-axial region Q76.411
    thoracic region Q76.414
    thoracolumbar region Q76.415
  Morquio-Brailsford type (spinal) (see also subcategory M49.8) E76.219
  postlaminectomy M96.3
  postradiation therapy M96.2
  postural (adolescent) M40.00
    cervicothoracic region M40.03
    thoracic region M40.04
    thoracolumbar region M40.05
  secondary NEC M40.10
    cervical region M40.12
    cervicothoracic region M40.13
    thoracic region M40.14
    thoracolumbar region M40.15
  sequelae of rickets E64.3
  specified type NEC M40.299
    cervical region M40.292
    cervicothoracic region M40.293
    thoracic region M40.294
    thoracolumbar region M40.295
  syphilitic, congenital A50.56
  thoracic region M40.204
  thoracolumbar region M40.205
  tuberculous A18.01
Kyrle disease L87.0

L

Labia, labium — *see* condition
Labile
  blood pressure R09.89
  vasomotor system I73.9

Labioglossal paralysis G12.29
Labium leporinum — *see* Cleft, lip
Labor — *see* Delivery
Labored breathing — *see* Hyperventilation
Labyrinthitis (circumscribed) (destructive) (diffuse) (inner ear) (latent) (purulent) (suppurative) (see also subcategory) H83.0 ☑
  syphilitic A52.79
Laceration
  with abortion — *see* Abortion, by type, complicated by laceration of pelvic organs
  abdomen, abdominal
    wall S31.119 ☑
      with
        foreign body S31.129 ☑
        penetration into peritoneal cavity S31.619 ☑
          with foreign body S31.629 ☑
      epigastric region S31.112 ☑
        with
          foreign body S31.122 ☑
          penetration into peritoneal cavity S31.612 ☑
            with foreign body S31.622 ☑
      left
        lower quadrant S31.114 ☑
          with
            foreign body S31.124 ☑
            penetration into peritoneal cavity S31.614 ☑
              with foreign body S31.624 ☑
        upper quadrant S31.111 ☑
          with
            foreign body S31.121 ☑
            penetration into peritoneal cavity S31.611 ☑
              with foreign body S31.621 ☑
      periumbilic region S31.115 ☑
        with
          foreign body S31.125 ☑
          penetration into peritoneal cavity S31.615 ☑
            with foreign body S31.625 ☑
      right
        lower quadrant S31.113 ☑
          with
            foreign body S31.123 ☑
            penetration into peritoneal cavity S31.613 ☑
              with foreign body S31.623 ☑
        upper quadrant S31.110 ☑
          with
            foreign body S31.120 ☑
            penetration into peritoneal cavity S31.610 ☑
              with foreign body S31.620 ☑
  accidental, complicating surgery — *see* Complications, surgical, accidental puncture or laceration
  Achilles tendon S86.02- ☑
  adrenal gland S37.813 ☑
  alveolar (process) — *see* Laceration, oral cavity
  ankle S91.01- ☑
    with
      foreign body S91.02- ☑
  antecubital space — *see* Laceration, elbow
  anus (sphincter) S31.831 ☑
    with
      ectopic or molar pregnancy O08.6
      foreign body S31.832 ☑
    complicating delivery — *see* Delivery, complicated, by, laceration, anus (sphincter)
    following ectopic or molar pregnancy O08.6
    nontraumatic, nonpuerperal — *see* Fissure, anus
  arm (upper) S41.11- ☑
    with foreign body S41.12- ☑
    lower — *see* Laceration, forearm
  auditory canal (external) (meatus) — *see* Laceration, ear
  auricle, ear — *see* Laceration, ear
  axilla — *see* Laceration, arm
  back (see also Laceration, thorax, back)
    lower S31.010 ☑
      with
        foreign body S31.020 ☑
        with penetration into retroperitoneal space S31.021 ☑

Laceration — *continued*
  back (see also Laceration, thorax, back) — *continued*
    lower — *continued*
      with — *continued*
        penetration into retroperitoneal space S31.011 ☑
  bile duct S36.13 ☑
  bladder S37.23 ☑
    with ectopic or molar pregnancy O08.6
    following ectopic or molar pregnancy O08.6
    obstetrical trauma O71.5
  blood vessel — *see* Injury, blood vessel
  bowel (see also Laceration, intestine)
    with ectopic or molar pregnancy O08.6
    complicating abortion — *see* Abortion, by type, complicated by, specified condition NEC
    following ectopic or molar pregnancy O08.6
    obstetrical trauma O71.5
  brain (any part) (cortex) (diffuse) (membrane) (see also Injury, intracranial, diffuse)
    during birth P10.8
      with hemorrhage P10.1
    focal — *see* Injury, intracranial, focal brain injury
  brainstem S06.38- ☑
  breast S21.01- ☑
    with foreign body S21.02- ☑
  broad ligament S37.893 ☑
    with ectopic or molar pregnancy O08.6
    following ectopic or molar pregnancy O08.6
    laceration syndrome N83.8
    obstetrical trauma O71.6
    syndrome (laceration) N83.8
  buttock S31.801 ☑
    with foreign body S31.802 ☑
    left S31.821 ☑
      with foreign body S31.822 ☑
    right S31.811 ☑
      with foreign body S31.812 ☑
  calf — *see* Laceration, leg
  canaliculus lacrimalis — *see* Laceration, eyelid
  canthus, eye — *see* Laceration, eyelid
  capsule, joint — *see* Sprain
  causing eversion of cervix uteri (old) N86
  central (perineal), complicating delivery O70.9
  cerebellum, traumatic S06.37- ☑
  cerebral S06.33- ☑
    during birth P10.8
      with hemorrhage P10.1
    left side S06.32- ☑
    right side S06.31- ☑
  cervix (uteri)
    with ectopic or molar pregnancy O08.6
    following ectopic or molar pregnancy O08.6
    nonpuerperal, nontraumatic N88.1
    obstetrical trauma (current) O71.3
    old (postpartal) N88.1
    traumatic S37.63 ☑
  cheek (external) S01.41- ☑
    with foreign body S01.42- ☑
    internal — *see* Laceration, oral cavity
  chest wall — *see* Laceration, thorax
  chin — *see* Laceration, head, specified site NEC
  chordae tendinae NEC I51.1
    concurrent with acute myocardial infarction — *see* Infarct, myocardium
    following acute myocardial infarction (current complication) I23.4
  clitoris — *see* Laceration, vulva
  colon — *see* Laceration, intestine, large, colon
  common bile duct S36.13 ☑
  cortex (cerebral) — *see* Injury, intracranial, diffuse
  costal region — *see* Laceration, thorax
  cystic duct S36.13 ☑
  diaphragm S27.803 ☑
  digit(s)
    foot — *see* Laceration, toe
    hand — *see* Laceration, finger
  duodenum S36.430 ☑
  ear (canal) (external) S01.31- ☑
    with foreign body S01.32- ☑
    drum S09.2- ☑
  elbow S51.01- ☑
    with
      foreign body S51.02- ☑
  epididymis — *see* Laceration, testis

Laceration — *continued*
  epigastric region — *see* Laceration, abdomen, wall,
    epigastric region
  esophagus K22.8
    traumatic
      cervical S11.21 ☑
        with foreign body S11.22 ☑
      thoracic S27.813 ☑
  eye (ball) S05.3- ☑
    with prolapse or loss of intraocular tissue S05.2- ☑
    penetrating S05.6- ☑
  eyebrow — *see* Laceration, eyelid
  eyelid S01.11- ☑
    with foreign body S01.12- ☑
  face NEC — *see* Laceration, head, specified site NEC
  fallopian tube S37.539 ☑
    bilateral S37.532 ☑
    unilateral S37.531 ☑
  finger(s) S61.219 ☑
    with
      damage to nail S61.319 ☑
        with
          foreign body S61.329 ☑
      foreign body S61.229 ☑
    index S61.218 ☑
      with
        damage to nail S61.318 ☑
          with
            foreign body S61.328 ☑
        foreign body S61.228 ☑
      left S61.211 ☑
        with
          damage to nail S61.311 ☑
            with
              foreign body S61.321 ☑
          foreign body S61.221 ☑
      right S61.210 ☑
        with
          damage to nail S61.310 ☑
            with
              foreign body S61.320 ☑
          foreign body S61.220 ☑
    little S61.218 ☑
      with
        damage to nail S61.318 ☑
          with
            foreign body S61.328 ☑
        foreign body S61.228 ☑
      left S61.217 ☑
        with
          damage to nail S61.317 ☑
            with
              foreign body S61.327 ☑
          foreign body S61.227 ☑
      right S61.216 ☑
        with
          damage to nail S61.316 ☑
            with
              foreign body S61.326 ☑
          foreign body S61.226 ☑
    middle S61.218 ☑
      with
        damage to nail S61.318 ☑
          with
            foreign body S61.328 ☑
        foreign body S61.228 ☑
      left S61.213 ☑
        with
          damage to nail S61.313 ☑
            with
              foreign body S61.323 ☑
          foreign body S61.223 ☑
      right S61.212 ☑
        with
          damage to nail S61.312 ☑
            with
              foreign body S61.322 ☑
          foreign body S61.222 ☑
    ring S61.218 ☑
      with
        damage to nail S61.318 ☑
          with
            foreign body S61.328 ☑
        foreign body S61.228 ☑

Laceration — *continued*
  finger(s) — *continued*
    ring — *continued*
      left S61.215 ☑
        with
          damage to nail S61.315 ☑
            with
              foreign body S61.325 ☑
          foreign body S61.225 ☑
      right S61.214 ☑
        with
          damage to nail S61.314 ☑
            with
              foreign body S61.324 ☑
          foreign body S61.224 ☑
  flank S31.119 ☑
    with foreign body S31.129 ☑
  foot (except toe(s) alone) S91.319 ☑
    with foreign body S91.329 ☑
    left S91.312 ☑
      with foreign body S91.322 ☑
    right S91.311 ☑
      with foreign body S91.321 ☑
    toe — *see* Laceration, toe
  forearm S51.819 ☑
    with
      foreign body S51.829 ☑
    elbow only — *see* Laceration, elbow
    left S51.812 ☑
      with
        foreign body S51.822 ☑
    right S51.811 ☑
      with
        foreign body S51.821 ☑
  forehead S01.81 ☑
    with foreign body S01.82 ☑
  fourchette O70.0
    with ectopic or molar pregnancy O08.6
    complicating delivery O70.0
    following ectopic or molar pregnancy O08.6
  gallbladder S36.123 ☑
  genital organs, external
    female S31.512 ☑
      with foreign body S31.522 ☑
      vagina — *see* Laceration, vagina
      vulva — *see* Laceration, vulva
    male S31.511 ☑
      with foreign body S31.521 ☑
      penis — *see* Laceration, penis
      scrotum — *see* Laceration, scrotum
      testis — *see* Laceration, testis
  groin — *see* Laceration, abdomen, wall
  gum — *see* Laceration, oral cavity
  hand S61.419 ☑
    with
      foreign body S61.429 ☑
    finger — *see* Laceration, finger
    left S61.412 ☑
      with
        foreign body S61.422 ☑
    right S61.411 ☑
      with
        foreign body S61.421 ☑
    thumb — *see* Laceration, thumb
  head S01.91 ☑
    with foreign body S01.92 ☑
    cheek — *see* Laceration, cheek
    ear — *see* Laceration, ear
    eyelid — *see* Laceration, eyelid
    lip — *see* Laceration, lip
    nose — *see* Laceration, nose
    oral cavity — *see* Laceration, oral cavity
    scalp S01.01 ☑
      with foreign body S01.02 ☑
    specified site NEC S01.81 ☑
      with foreign body S01.82 ☑
    temporomandibular area — *see* Laceration, cheek
  heart — *see* Injury, heart, laceration
  heel — *see* Laceration, foot
  hepatic duct S36.13 ☑
  hip S71.019 ☑
    with foreign body S71.029 ☑
    left S71.012 ☑
      with foreign body S71.022 ☑
    right S71.011 ☑
      with foreign body S71.021 ☑

Laceration — *continued*
  hymen — *see* Laceration, vagina
  hypochondrium — *see* Laceration, abdomen, wall
  hypogastric region — *see* Laceration, abdomen, wall
  ileum S36.438 ☑
  inguinal region — *see* Laceration, abdomen, wall
  instep — *see* Laceration, foot
  internal organ — *see* Injury, by site
  interscapular region — *see* Laceration, thorax, back
  intestine
    large
      colon S36.539 ☑
        ascending S36.530 ☑
        descending S36.532 ☑
        sigmoid S36.533 ☑
        specified site NEC S36.538 ☑
      rectum S36.63 ☑
        transverse S36.531 ☑
    small S36.439 ☑
      duodenum S36.430 ☑
      specified site NEC S36.438 ☑
  intra-abdominal organ S36.93 ☑
    intestine — *see* Laceration, intestine
    liver — *see* Laceration, liver
    pancreas — *see* Laceration, pancreas
    peritoneum S36.81 ☑
    specified site NEC S36.893 ☑
    spleen — *see* Laceration, spleen
    stomach — *see* Laceration, stomach
  intracranial NEC (*see also* Injury, intracranial, diffuse)
    birth injury P10.9
  jaw — *see* Laceration, head, specified site NEC
  jejunum S36.438 ☑
  joint capsule — *see* Sprain, by site
  kidney S37.03- ☑
    major (greater than 3 cm) (massive) (stellate)
      S37.06- ☑
    minor (less than 1 cm) S37.04- ☑
    moderate (1 to 3 cm) S37.05- ☑
    multiple S37.06- ☑
  knee S81.01- ☑
    with foreign body S81.02- ☑
  labium (majus) (minus) — *see* Laceration, vulva
  lacrimal duct — *see* Laceration, eyelid
  large intestine — *see* Laceration, intestine, large
  larynx S11.011 ☑
    with foreign body S11.012 ☑
  leg (lower) S81.819 ☑
    with foreign body S81.829 ☑
    foot — *see* Laceration, foot
    knee — *see* Laceration, knee
    left S81.812 ☑
      with foreign body S81.822 ☑
    right S81.811 ☑
      with foreign body S81.821 ☑
    upper — *see* Laceration, thigh
  ligament — *see* Sprain
  lip S01.511 ☑
    with foreign body S01.521 ☑
  liver S36.113 ☑
    major (stellate) S36.116 ☑
    minor S36.114 ☑
    moderate S36.115 ☑
  loin — *see* Laceration, abdomen, wall
  lower back — *see* Laceration, back, lower
  lumbar region — *see* Laceration, back, lower
  lung S27.339 ☑
    bilateral S27.332 ☑
    unilateral S27.331 ☑
  malar region — *see* Laceration, head, specified site
    NEC
  mammary — *see* Laceration, breast
  mastoid region — *see* Laceration, head, specified site
    NEC
  meninges — *see* Injury, intracranial, diffuse
  meniscus — *see* Tear, meniscus
  mesentery S36.893 ☑
  mesosalpinx S37.893 ☑
  mouth — *see* Laceration, oral cavity
  muscle — *see* Injury, muscle, by site, laceration
  nail
    finger — *see* Laceration, finger, with damage to
      nail
    toe — *see* Laceration, toe, with damage to nail
  nasal (septum) (sinus) — *see* Laceration, nose

☑ **Additional Character Required — Refer to the Tabular List for Character Selection**   ▽ **Subterms under main terms may continue to next column or page**

Laceration — *continued*
- nasopharynx — *see* Laceration, head, specified site NEC
- neck S11.91 ☑
  - with foreign body S11.92 ☑
  - involving
    - cervical esophagus S11.21 ☑
      - with foreign body S11.22 ☑
    - larynx — *see* Laceration, larynx
    - pharynx — *see* Laceration, pharynx
    - thyroid gland — *see* Laceration, thyroid gland
    - trachea — *see* Laceration, trachea
  - specified site NEC S11.81 ☑
    - with foreign body S11.82 ☑
- nerve — *see* Injury, nerve
- nose (septum) (sinus) S01.21 ☑
  - with foreign body S01.22 ☑
- ocular NOS S05.3- ☑
  - adnexa NOS S01.11- ☑
- oral cavity S01.512 ☑
  - with foreign body S01.522 ☑
- orbit (eye) — *see* Wound, open, ocular, orbit
- ovary S37.439 ☑
  - bilateral S37.432 ☑
  - unilateral S37.431 ☑
- palate — *see* Laceration, oral cavity
- palm — *see* Laceration, hand
- pancreas S36.239 ☑
- pelvic S31.010 ☑
  - with
    - foreign body S31.020 ☑
      - penetration into retroperitoneal cavity S31.021 ☑
    - penetration into retroperitoneal cavity S31.011 ☑
  - floor (*see also* Laceration, back, lower)
    - with ectopic or molar pregnancy O08.6
    - complicating delivery O70.1
    - following ectopic or molar pregnancy O08.6
    - old (postpartal) N81.89
  - organ S37.93 ☑
- penis S31.21 ☑
  - with foreign body S31.22 ☑
- perineum
  - female S31.41 ☑
    - with
      - ectopic or molar pregnancy O08.6
      - foreign body S31.42 ☑
    - during delivery O70.9
      - first degree O70.0
      - fourth degree O70.3
      - second degree O70.1
      - third degree O70.2
    - old (postpartal) N81.89
    - postpartal N81.89
    - secondary (postpartal) O90.1
  - male S31.119 ☑
    - with foreign body S31.129 ☑
- periocular area (with or without lacrimal passages) — *see* Laceration, eyelid
- peritoneum S36.893 ☑
- periumbilic region — *see* Laceration, abdomen, wall, periumbilic
- periurethral tissue — *see* Laceration, urethra
- phalanges
  - finger — *see* Laceration, finger
  - toe — *see* Laceration, toe
- pharynx S11.21 ☑
  - with foreign body S11.22 ☑
- pinna — *see* Laceration, ear
- popliteal space — *see* Laceration, knee
- prepuce — *see* Laceration, penis
- prostate S37.823 ☑
- pubic region S31.119 ☑
  - with foreign body S31.129 ☑
- pudendum — *see* Laceration, genital organs, external
- rectovaginal septum — *see* Laceration, vagina
- rectum S36.63 ☑
- retroperitoneum S36.893 ☑
- round ligament S37.893 ☑
- sacral region — *see* Laceration, back, lower
- sacroiliac region — *see* Laceration, back, lower
- salivary gland — *see* Laceration, oral cavity
- scalp S01.01 ☑
  - with foreign body S01.02 ☑
- scapular region — *see* Laceration, shoulder

Laceration — *continued*
- scrotum S31.31 ☑
  - with foreign body S31.32 ☑
- seminal vesicle S37.893 ☑
- shin — *see* Laceration, leg
- shoulder S41.019 ☑
  - with foreign body S41.029 ☑
  - left S41.012 ☑
    - with foreign body S41.022 ☑
  - right S41.011 ☑
    - with foreign body S41.021 ☑
- small intestine — *see* Laceration, intestine, small
- spermatic cord — *see* Laceration, testis
- spinal cord (meninges) (*see also* Injury, spinal cord, by region)
  - due to injury at birth P11.5
  - newborn (birth injury) P11.5
- spleen S36.039 ☑
  - major (massive) (stellate) S36.032 ☑
  - moderate S36.031 ☑
  - superficial (minor) S36.030 ☑
- sternal region — *see* Laceration, thorax, front
- stomach S36.33 ☑
- submaxillary region — *see* Laceration, head, specified site NEC
- submental region — *see* Laceration, head, specified site NEC
- subungual
  - finger(s) — *see* Laceration, finger, with damage to nail
  - toe(s) — *see* Laceration, toe, with damage to nail
- suprarenal gland — *see* Laceration, adrenal gland
- temple, temporal region — *see* Laceration, head, specified site NEC
- temporomandibular area — *see* Laceration, cheek
- tendon — *see* Injury, muscle, by site, laceration
  - Achilles S86.02- ☑
- tentorium cerebelli — *see* Injury, intracranial, diffuse
- testis S31.31 ☑
  - with foreign body S31.32 ☑
- thigh S71.11- ☑
  - with foreign body S71.12- ☑
- thorax, thoracic (wall) S21.91 ☑
  - with foreign body S21.92 ☑
  - back S21.22- ☑
    - with penetration into thoracic cavity S21.42- ☑
  - front S21.12- ☑
    - with penetration into thoracic cavity S21.32- ☑
  - back S21.21- ☑
    - with
      - foreign body S21.22- ☑
        - with penetration into thoracic cavity S21.42- ☑
      - penetration into thoracic cavity S21.41- ☑
  - breast — *see* Laceration, breast
  - front S21.11- ☑
    - with
      - foreign body S21.12- ☑
        - with penetration into thoracic cavity S21.32- ☑
      - penetration into thoracic cavity S21.31- ☑
- thumb S61.019 ☑
  - with
    - damage to nail S61.119 ☑
      - with foreign body S61.129 ☑
    - foreign body S61.029 ☑
  - left S61.012 ☑
    - with
      - damage to nail S61.112 ☑
        - with foreign body S61.122 ☑
      - foreign body S61.022 ☑
  - right S61.011 ☑
    - with
      - damage to nail S61.111 ☑
        - with foreign body S61.121 ☑
      - foreign body S61.021 ☑
- thyroid gland S11.11 ☑
  - with foreign body S11.12 ☑

Laceration — *continued*
- toe(s) S91.119 ☑
  - with
    - damage to nail S91.219 ☑
      - with foreign body S91.229 ☑
    - foreign body S91.129 ☑
  - great S91.113 ☑
    - with
      - damage to nail S91.213 ☑
        - with foreign body S91.223 ☑
      - foreign body S91.123 ☑
    - left S91.112 ☑
      - with
        - damage to nail S91.212 ☑
          - with foreign body S91.222 ☑
        - foreign body S91.122 ☑
    - right S91.111 ☑
      - with
        - damage to nail S91.211 ☑
          - with foreign body S91.221 ☑
        - foreign body S91.121 ☑
  - lesser S91.116 ☑
    - with
      - damage to nail S91.216 ☑
        - with foreign body S91.226 ☑
      - foreign body S91.126 ☑
    - left S91.115 ☑
      - with
        - damage to nail S91.215 ☑
          - with foreign body S91.225 ☑
        - foreign body S91.125 ☑
    - right S91.114 ☑
      - with
        - damage to nail S91.214 ☑
          - with foreign body S91.224 ☑
        - foreign body S91.124 ☑
- tongue — *see* Laceration, oral cavity
- trachea S11.021 ☑
  - with foreign body S11.022 ☑
- tunica vaginalis — *see* Laceration, testis
- tympanum, tympanic membrane — *see* Laceration, ear, drum
- umbilical region S31.115 ☑
  - with foreign body S31.125 ☑
- ureter S37.13 ☑
- urethra S37.33 ☑
  - with or following ectopic or molar pregnancy O08.6
  - obstetrical trauma O71.5
- urinary organ NEC S37.893 ☑
- uterus S37.63 ☑
  - with ectopic or molar pregnancy O08.6
  - following ectopic or molar pregnancy O08.6
  - nonpuerperal, nontraumatic N85.8
  - obstetrical trauma NEC O71.81
  - old (postpartal) N85.8
- uvula — *see* Laceration, oral cavity
- vagina S31.41 ☑
  - with
    - ectopic or molar pregnancy O08.6
    - foreign body S31.42 ☑
  - during delivery O71.4
    - with perineal laceration — *see* Laceration, perineum, female, during delivery
  - following ectopic or molar pregnancy O08.6
  - nonpuerperal, nontraumatic N89.8
  - old (postpartal) N89.8
- vas deferens S37.893 ☑
- vesical — *see* Laceration, bladder
- vocal cords S11.031 ☑
  - with foreign body S11.032 ☑
- vulva S31.41 ☑
  - with
    - ectopic or molar pregnancy O08.6
    - foreign body S31.42 ☑
  - complicating delivery O70.0
  - following ectopic or molar pregnancy O08.6
  - nonpuerperal, nontraumatic N90.89
  - old (postpartal) N90.89

Laceration — *continued*
  wrist S61.519 ☑
    with
      foreign body S61.529 ☑
    left S61.512 ☑
      with
        foreign body S61.522 ☑
    right S61.511 ☑
      with
        foreign body S61.521 ☑
Lack of
  achievement in school Z55.3
  adequate
    food Z59.4
    intermaxillary vertical dimension of fully erupted
      teeth M26.36
    sleep Z72.820
  appetite (see Anorexia) R63.0
  awareness R41.9
  care
    in home Z74.2
    of infant (at or after birth) T76.02 ☑
      confirmed T74.02 ☑
  cognitive functions R41.9
  coordination R27.9
    ataxia R27.0
    specified type NEC R27.8
  development (physiological) R62.50
    failure to thrive (child over 28 days old) R62.51
      adult R62.7
      newborn P92.6
    short stature R62.52
    specified type NEC R62.59
  energy R53.83
  financial resources Z59.6
  food T73.0 ☑
  growth R62.52
  heating Z59.1
  housing (permanent) (temporary) Z59.0
    adequate Z59.1
  learning experiences in childhood Z62.898
  leisure time (affecting life-style) Z73.2
  material resources Z59.9
  memory (see also Amnesia)
    mild, following organic brain damage F06.8
  ovulation N97.0
  parental supervision or control of child Z62.0
  person able to render necessary care Z74.2
  physical exercise Z72.3
  play experience in childhood Z62.898
  posterior occlusal support M26.57
  relaxation (affecting life-style) Z73.2
  sexual
    desire F52.0
    enjoyment F52.1
  shelter Z59.0
  sleep (adequate) Z72.820
  supervision of child by parent Z62.0
  support, posterior occlusal M26.57
  water T73.1 ☑
Lacrimal — *see* condition
Lacrimation, abnormal — *see* Epiphora
Lacrimonasal duct — *see* condition
Lactation, lactating (breast) (puerperal, postpartum)
  associated
    cracked nipple O92.13
    retracted nipple O92.03
  defective O92.4
  disorder NEC O92.79
  excessive O92.6
  failed (complete) O92.3
    partial O92.4
  mastitis NEC — *see* Mastitis, obstetric
  mother (care and/or examination) Z39.1
  nonpuerperal N64.3
Lacticemia, excessive E87.2
Lacunar skull Q75.8
Laennec's cirrhosis K74.69
  alcoholic K70.30
    with ascites K70.31
Lafora's disease — *see* Epilepsy, generalized, idiopathic
Lag, lid (nervous) — *see* Retraction, lid
Lagophthalmos (eyelid) (nervous) H02.209
  cicatricial H02.219
    left H02.216
      lower H02.215
      upper H02.214

Lagophthalmos — *continued*
  cicatricial — *continued*
    right H02.213
      lower H02.212
      upper H02.211
  keratoconjunctivitis — *see* Keratoconjunctivitis
  left H02.206
    lower H02.205
    upper H02.204
  mechanical H02.229
    left H02.226
      lower H02.225
      upper H02.224
    right H02.223
      lower H02.222
      upper H02.221
  paralytic H02.239
    left H02.236
      lower H02.235
      upper H02.234
    right H02.233
      lower H02.232
      upper H02.231
  right H02.203
    lower H02.202
    upper H02.201
Laki-Lorand factor deficiency — *see* Defect, coagulation, specified type NEC
Lalling F80.0
Lambert-Eaton syndrome — *see* Syndrome, Lambert-Eaton
Lambliasis, lambliosis A07.1
Landau-Kleffner syndrome — *see* Epilepsy, specified NEC
Landouzy-Déjérine dystrophy or facioscapulohumeral atrophy G71.0
Landouzy's disease (icterohemorrhagic leptospirosis) A27.0
Landry-Guillain-Barré, syndrome or paralysis G61.0
Landry's disease or paralysis G61.0
Lane's
  band Q43.3
  kink — *see* Obstruction, intestine
  syndrome K90.2
Langdon Down syndrome — *see* Trisomy, 21
Lapsed immunization schedule status Z28.3
Large
  baby (regardless of gestational age) (4000g to 4499g) P08.1
  ear, congenital Q17.1
  physiological cup Q14.2
  stature R68.89
Large-for-dates NEC (infant) (4000g to 4499g) P08.1
  affecting management of pregnancy O36.6- ☑
  exceptionally (4500g or more) P08.0
Larsen-Johansson disease orosteochondrosis — *see* Osteochondrosis, juvenile, patella
Larsen's syndrome (flattened facies and multiple congenital dislocations) Q74.8
Larva migrans
  cutaneous B76.9
    Ancylostoma B76.0
  visceral B83.0
Laryngeal — *see* condition
Laryngismus (stridulus) J38.5
  congenital P28.89
  diphtheritic A36.2
Laryngitis (acute) (edematous) (fibrinous) (infective) (infiltrative) (malignant) (membranous) (phlegmonous) (pneumococcal) (pseudomembranous) (septic) (subglottic) (suppurative) (ulcerative) J04.0
  with
    influenza, flu, or grippe — *see* Influenza, with, laryngitis
    tracheitis (acute) — *see* Laryngotracheitis
  atrophic J37.0
  catarrhal J37.0
  chronic J37.0
    with tracheitis (chronic) J37.1
  diphtheritic A36.2
  due to external agent — *see* Inflammation, respiratory, upper, due to
  H. influenzae J04.0
  Hemophilus influenzae J04.0
  hypertrophic J37.0
  influenzal — *see* Influenza, with, respiratory manifestations NEC
  obstructive J05.0

Laryngitis — *continued*
  sicca J37.0
  spasmodic J05.0
    acute J04.0
  streptococcal J04.0
  stridulous J05.0
  syphilitic (late) A52.73
    congenital A50.59 [J99]
      early A50.03 [J99]
  tuberculous A15.5
  Vincent's A69.1
Laryngocele (congenital) (ventricular) Q31.3
Laryngofissure J38.7
  congenital Q31.8
Laryngomalacia (congenital) Q31.5
Laryngopharyngitis (acute) J06.0
  chronic J37.0
  due to external agent — *see* Inflammation, respiratory, upper, due to
Laryngoplegia J38.00
  bilateral J38.02
  unilateral J38.01
Laryngoptosis J38.7
Laryngospasm J38.5
Laryngostenosis J38.6
Laryngotracheitis (acute) (Infectional) (infective) (viral) J04.2
  atrophic J37.1
  catarrhal J37.1
  chronic J37.1
  diphtheritic A36.2
  due to external agent — *see* Inflammation, respiratory, upper, due to
  Hemophilus influenzae J04.2
  hypertrophic J37.1
  influenzal — *see* Influenza, with, respiratory manifestations NEC
  pachydermic J38.7
  sicca J37.1
  spasmodic J38.5
    acute J05.0
  streptococcal J04.2
  stridulous J38.5
  syphilitic (late) A52.73
    congenital A50.59 [J99]
      early A50.03 [J99]
  tuberculous A15.5
  Vincent's A69.1
Laryngotracheobronchitis — *see* Bronchitis
Larynx, laryngeal — *see* condition
Lassa fever A96.2
Lassitude — *see* Weakness
Late
  talker R62.0
  walker R62.0
Late effect(s) — *see* Sequelae
Latent — *see* condition
Laterocession — *see* Lateroversion
Lateroflexion — *see* Lateroversion
Lateroversion
  cervix — *see* Lateroversion, uterus
  uterus, uterine (cervix) (postinfectional) (postpartal, old) N85.4
    congenital Q51.818
    in pregnancy or childbirth O34.59- ☑
Lathyrism — *see* Poisoning, food, noxious, plant
Launois' syndrome (pituitary gigantism) E22.0
Launois-Bensaude adenolipomatosis E88.89
Laurence-Moon (-Bardet)-**Biedl syndrome** Q87.89
Lax, laxity (see also Relaxation)
  ligament (ous) (see also Disorder, ligament)
    familial M35.7
    knee — *see* Derangement, knee
  skin (acquired) L57.4
    congenital Q82.8
Laxative habit F55.2
Lazy leukocyte syndrome D70.8
Lead miner's lung J63.6
Leak, leakage
  air NEC J93.82
    postprocedural J95.812
  amniotic fluid — *see* Rupture, membranes, premature
  blood (microscopic), fetal, into maternal circulation
    affecting management of pregnancy — *see* Pregnancy, complicated by
  cerebrospinal fluid G96.0
    from spinal (lumbar) puncture G97.0

☑ **Additional Character Required** — Refer to the Tabular List for Character Selection   ▽ Subterms under main terms may continue to next column or page

Leak, leakage — *continued*
  device, implant or graft (*see also* Complications, by
    site and type, mechanical)
    arterial graft NEC — *see* Complication, cardiovas-
      cular device, mechanical, vascular
    breast (implant) T85.43 ☑
    catheter NEC T85.638 ☑
      dialysis (renal) T82.43 ☑
        intraperitoneal T85.631 ☑
      infusion NEC T82.534 ☑
        spinal (epidural) (subdural) T85.630 ☑
      urinary, indwelling T83.038 ☑
        cystostomy T83.030 ☑
    gastrointestinal — *see* Complications, prosthetic
      device, mechanical, gastrointestinal device
    genital NEC T83.498 ☑
      penile prosthesis T83.490 ☑
    heart NEC — *see* Complication, cardiovascular de-
      vice, mechanical
    joint prosthesis — *see* Complications, joint prosthe-
      sis, mechanical, specified NEC, by site
    ocular NEC — *see* Complications, prosthetic device,
      mechanical, ocular device
    orthopedic NEC — *see* Complication, orthopedic,
      device, mechanical
    persistent air J93.82
    specified NEC T85.638 ☑
    urinary NEC (*see also* Complication, genitourinary,
      device, urinary, mechanical)
      graft T83.23 ☑
    vascular NEC — *see* Complication, cardiovascular
      device, mechanical
    ventricular intracranial shunt T85.03 ☑
  urine — *see* Incontinence
Leaky heart — *see* Endocarditis
Learning defect (specific) F81.9
Leather bottle stomach C16.9
Leber's
  congenital amaurosis H35.50
  optic atrophy (hereditary) H47.22
Lederer's anemia D59.1
Leeches (external) — *see* Hirudiniasis
Leg — *see* condition
Legg (-Calvé)-**Perthes disease, syndrome or osteo-**
  chondrosis M91.1- ☑
Legionellosis A48.1
  nonpneumonic A48.2
Legionnaires'
  disease A48.1
    nonpneumonic A48.2
  pneumonia A48.1
Leigh's disease G31.82
Leiner's disease L21.1
Leiofibromyoma — *see* Leiomyoma
Leiomyoblastoma — *see* Neoplasm, connective tissue,
  benign
Leiomyofibroma (*see also* Neoplasm, connective tissue,
  benign)
  uterus (cervix) (corpus) D25.9
Leiomyoma (*see also* Neoplasm, connective tissue, benign)
  bizarre — *see* Neoplasm, connective tissue, benign
  cellular — *see* Neoplasm, connective tissue, benign
  epithelioid — *see* Neoplasm, connective tissue, benign
  uterus (cervix) (corpus) D25.9
    intramural D25.1
    submucous D25.0
    subserosal D25.2
  vascular — *see* Neoplasm, connective tissue, benign
Leiomyoma, leiomyomatosis (intravascular) — *see*
  Neoplasm, connective tissue, uncertain behavior
Leiomyosarcoma (*see also* Neoplasm, connective tissue,
  malignant)
  epithelioid — *see* Neoplasm, connective tissue, malig-
    nant
  myxoid — *see* Neoplasm, connective tissue, malignant
Leishmaniasis B55.9
  American (mucocutaneous) B55.2
    cutaneous B55.1
  Asian Desert B55.1
  Brazilian B55.2
  cutaneous (any type) B55.1
  dermal (*see also* Leishmaniasis, cutaneous)
    post-kala-azar B55.0
  eyelid B55.1
  infantile B55.0
  Mediterranean B55.0

Leishmaniasis — *continued*
  mucocutaneous (American) (New World) B55.2
  naso-oral B55.2
  nasopharyngeal B55.2
  old world B55.1
  tegumentaria diffusa B55.1
  visceral B55.0
Leishmanoid, dermal (*see also* Leishmaniasis, cutaneous)
  post-kala-azar B55.0
Lenegre's disease I44.2
Lengthening, leg — *see* Deformity, limb, unequal length
Lennert's lymphoma — *see* Lymphoma, Lennert's
Lennox-Gastaut syndrome G40.812
  intractable G40.814
    with status epilepticus G40.813
    without status epilepticus G40.814
  not intractable G40.812
    with status epilepticus G40.811
    without status epilepticus G40.812
Lens — *see* condition
Lenticonus (anterior) (posterior) (congenital) Q12.8
Lenticular degeneration, progressive E83.01
Lentiglobus (posterior) (congenital) Q12.8
Lentigo (congenital) L81.4
  maligna (*see also* Melanoma, in situ)
    melanoma — *see* Melanoma
Lentivirus, as cause of disease classified elsewhere
  B97.31
Leontiasis
  ossium M85.2
  syphilitic (late) A52.78
    congenital A50.59
Lepothrix A48.8
Lepra — *see* Leprosy
Leprechaunism E34.8
Leprosy A30.- ☑
  with muscle disorder A30.9 [M63.80]
    ankle A30.9 [M63.87-] ☑
    foot A30.9 [M63.87-] ☑
    forearm A30.9 [M63.83-] ☑
    hand A30.9 [M63.84-] ☑
    lower leg A30.9 [M63.86-] ☑
    multiple sites A30.9 [M63.89]
    pelvic region A30.9 [M63.85-] ☑
    shoulder region A30.9 [M63.81-] ☑
    specified site NEC A30.9 [M63.88]
    thigh A30.9 [M63.85-] ☑
    upper arm A30.9 [M63.82-] ☑
  anesthetic A30.9
  BB A30.3
  BL A30.4
  borderline (infiltrated) (neuritic) A30.3
    lepromatous A30.4
    tuberculoid A30.2
  BT A30.2
  dimorphous (infiltrated) (neuritic) A30.3
  I A30.0
  indeterminate (macular) (neuritic) A30.0
  lepromatous (diffuse) (infiltrated) (macular) (neuritic)
    (nodular) A30.5
  LL A30.5
  macular (early) (neuritic) (simple) A30.9
  maculoanesthetic A30.9
  mixed A30.3
  neural A30.9
  nodular A30.5
  primary neuritic A30.3
  specified type NEC A30.8
  TT A30.1
  tuberculoid (major) (minor) A30.1
Leptocytosis, hereditary D56.9
Leptomeningitis (chronic) (circumscribed) (hemorrhagic)
  (nonsuppurative) — *see* Meningitis
Leptomeningopathy G96.19
Leptospiral — *see* condition
Leptospirochetal — *see* condition
Leptospirosis A27.9
  canicola A27.89
  due to Leptospira interrogans serovar icterohaemor-
    rhagiae A27.0
  icterohemorrhagica A27.0
  pomona A27.89
  Weil's disease A27.0
Leptus dermatitis B88.0
Leriche's syndrome (aortic bifurcation occlusion) I74.09
Leri's pleonosteosis Q78.8

Leri-Weill syndrome Q77.8
Lermoyez' syndrome — *see* Vertigo, peripheral NEC
Lesch-Nyhan syndrome E79.1
Leser-Trélat disease L82.1
  inflamed L82.0
Lesion(s) (nontraumatic)
  abducens nerve — *see* Strabismus, paralytic, sixth
    nerve
  alveolar process K08.9
  angiocentric immunoproliferative D47.Z9 (*following*
    D47.4)
  anorectal K62.9
  aortic (valve) I35.9
  auditory nerve — *see* subcategory H93.3 ☑
  basal ganglion G25.9
  bile duct — *see* Disease, bile duct
  biomechanical M99.9
    specified type NEC M99.89
      abdomen M99.89
      acromioclavicular M99.87
      cervical region M99.81
      cervicothoracic M99.81
      costochondral M99.88
      costovertebral M99.88
      head region M99.80
      hip M99.85
      lower extremity M99.86
      lumbar region M99.83
      lumbosacral M99.83
      occipitocervical M99.80
      pelvic region M99.85
      pubic M99.85
      rib cage M99.88
      sacral region M99.84
      sacrococcygeal M99.84
      sacroiliac M99.84
      specified NEC M99.89
      sternochondral M99.88
      sternoclavicular M99.87
      thoracic region M99.82
      thoracolumbar M99.82
      upper extremity M99.87
  bladder N32.9
  bone — *see* Disorder, bone
  brachial plexus G54.0
  brain G93.9
    congenital Q04.9
    vascular I67.9
      degenerative I67.9
      hypertensive I67.4
  buccal cavity K13.79
  calcified — *see* Calcification
  canthus — *see* Disorder, eyelid
  carate — *see* Pinta, lesions
  cardia K22.9
  cardiac (*see also* Disease, heart) I51.9
    congenital Q24.9
    valvular — *see* Endocarditis
  cauda equina G83.4
  cecum K63.9
  cerebral — *see* Lesion, brain
  cerebrovascular I67.9
    degenerative I67.9
    hypertensive I67.4
  cervical (nerve) root NEC G54.2
  chiasmal — *see* Disorder, optic, chiasm
  chorda tympani G51.8
  coin, lung R91.1
  colon K63.9
  congenital — *see* Anomaly, by site
  conjunctiva H11.9
  conus medullaris — *see* Injury, conus medullaris
  coronary artery — *see* Ischemia, heart
  cranial nerve G52.9
    eighth — *see* Disorder, ear
    eleventh G52.9
    fifth G50.9
    first G52.0
    fourth — *see* Strabismus, paralytic, fourth nerve
    seventh G51.9
    sixth — *see* Strabismus, paralytic, sixth nerve
    tenth G52.2
    twelfth G52.3
  cystic — *see* Cyst
  degenerative — *see* Degeneration
  duodenum K31.9
  edentulous (alveolar) ridge, associated with trauma,
    due to traumatic occlusion K06.2

Lesion(s) — *continued*
en coup de sabre L94.1
eyelid — *see* Disorder, eyelid
gasserian ganglion G50.8
gastric K31.9
gastroduodenal K31.9
gastrointestinal K63.9
gingiva, associated with trauma K06.2
glomerular
    focal and segmental (*see also* N00-N07 with fourth character .1) N05.1
    minimal change (*see also* N00-N07 with fourth character .0) N05.0
heart (organic) — *see* Disease, heart
hyperchromic, due to pinta (carate) A67.1
hyperkeratotic — *see* Hyperkeratosis
hypothalamic E23.7
ileocecal K63.9
ileum K63.9
iliohypogastric nerve G57.8- ☑
inflammatory — *see* Inflammation
intestine K63.9
intracerebral — *see* Lesion, brain
intrachiasmal (optic) — *see* Disorder, optic, chiasm
intracranial, space-occupying R90.0
joint — *see* Disorder, joint
    sacroiliac (old) M53.3
keratotic — *see* Keratosis
kidney — *see* Disease, renal
laryngeal nerve (recurrent) G52.2
lip K13.0
liver K76.9
lumbosacral
    plexus G54.1
    root (nerve) NEC G54.4
lung (coin) R91.1
maxillary sinus J32.0
mitral I05.9
Morel-Lavallée — *see* Hematoma, by site
motor cortex NEC G93.89
mouth K13.79
nerve G58.9
    femoral G57.2- ☑
    median G56.1- ☑
        carpal tunnel syndrome — *see* Syndrome, carpal tunnel
    plantar G57.6- ☑
    popliteal (lateral) G57.3- ☑
        medial G57.4- ☑
    radial G56.3- ☑
    sciatic G57.0- ☑
    spinal — *see* Injury, nerve, spinal
    ulnar G56.2- ☑
nervous system, congenital Q07.9
nonallopathic — *see* Lesion, biomechanical
nose (internal) J34.89
obstructive — *see* Obstruction
obturator nerve G57.8- ☑
oral mucosa K13.70
organ or site NEC — *see* Disease, by site
osteolytic — *see* Osteolysis
peptic K27.9
periodontal, due to traumatic occlusion K05.5
pharynx J39.2
pigment, pigmented (skin) L81.9
pinta — *see* Pinta, lesions
polypoid — *see* Polyp
prechiasmal (optic) — *see* Disorder, optic, chiasm
primary (*see also* Syphilis, primary) A51.0
    carate A67.0
    pinta A67.0
    yaws A66.0
pulmonary J98.4
    valve I37.9
pylorus K31.9
rectosigmoid K63.9
retina, retinal H35.9
sacroiliac (joint) (old) M53.3
salivary gland K11.9
    benign lymphoepithelial K11.8
saphenous nerve G57.8- ☑
sciatic nerve G57.0- ☑
secondary — *see* Syphilis, secondary
shoulder (region) M75.9- ☑
    specified NEC M75.8- ☑
sigmoid K63.9
sinus (accessory) (nasal) J34.89

Lesion(s) — *continued*
skin L98.9
    suppurative L08.0
SLAP S43.43- ☑
spinal cord G95.9
    congenital Q06.9
spleen D73.89
stomach K31.9
superior glenoid labrum S43.43- ☑
syphilitic — *see* Syphilis
tertiary — *see* Syphilis, tertiary
thoracic root (nerve) NEC G54.3
tonsillar fossa J35.9
tooth, teeth K08.9
    white spot
        chewing surface K02.51
        pit and fissure surface K02.51
        smooth surface K02.61
traumatic — *see specific type of injury by site*
tricuspid (valve) I07.9
    nonrheumatic I36.9
trigeminal nerve G50.9
ulcerated or ulcerative — *see* Ulcer, skin
uterus N85.9
vagus nerve G52.2
valvular — *see* Endocarditis
vascular I99.9
    affecting central nervous system I67.9
    following trauma NEC T14.8
    umbilical cord, complicating delivery O69.5 ☑
warty — *see* Verruca
white spot (tooth)
    chewing surface K02.51
    pit and fissure surface K02.51
    smooth surface K02.61
Lethargic — *see* condition
Lethargy R53.83
Letterer-Siwe's disease C96.0
Leukemia, leukemic C95.9- ☑
acute basophilic C94.8- ☑
acute bilineal C95.0- ☑
acute erythroid C94.0- ☑
acute lymphoblastic C91.0- ☑
acute megakaryoblastic C94.2- ☑
acute megakaryocytic C94.2- ☑
acute mixed lineage C95.0- ☑
acute monoblastic (monoblastic/monocytic) C93.0- ☑
acute monocytic (monoblastic/monocytic) C93.0- ☑
acute myeloblastic (minimal differentiation) (with maturation) C92.0- ☑
acute myeloid
    with
        11q23-abnormality C92.6- ☑
        dysplasia of remaining hematopoesis and/or myelodysplastic disease in its history C92.A- ☑ (*following* C92.6)
        multilineage dysplasia C92.A- ☑ (*following* C92.6)
        variation of MLL-gene C92.6- ☑
    M6 (a)(b) C94.0- ☑
    M7 C94.2- ☑
acute myelomonocytic C92.5- ☑
acute promyelocytic C92.4- ☑
adult T-cell (HTLV-1-associated) (acute variant) (chronic variant) (lymphomatoid variant) (smouldering variant) C91.5- ☑
aggressive NK-cell C94.8- ☑
AML (1/ETO) (M0) (M1) (M2) (without a FAB classification) C92.0- ☑
AML M3 C92.4- ☑
AML M4 (Eo with inv(16) or t(16;16)) C92.5- ☑
AML M5 C93.0- ☑
AML M5a C93.0- ☑
AML M5b C93.0- ☑
AML Me with t (15;17) and variants C92.4- ☑
atypical chronic myeloid, BCR/ABL-negative C92.2- ☑
biphenotypic acute C95.0- ☑
blast cell C95.0- ☑
Burkitt-type, mature B-cell C91.A- ☑ (*following* C91.6)
chronic lymphocytic, of B-cell type C91.1- ☑
chronic monocytic C93.1- ☑
chronic myelogenous (Philadelphia chromosome (Ph1) positive) (t(9;22)) (q34;q11) (with crisis of blast cells) C92.1- ☑
chronic myeloid, BCR/ABL-positive C92.1- ☑
    atypical, BCR/ABL-negative C92.2- ☑
chronic myelomonocytic C93.1- ☑

Leukemia, leukemic — *continued*
chronic neutrophilic D47.1
CMML (-1) (-2) (with eosinophilia) C93.1- ☑
granulocytic (*see also* Category C92) C92.9- ☑
hairy cell C91.4- ☑
juvenile myelomonocytic C93.3- ☑
lymphoid C91.9- ☑
    specified NEC C91.Z- ☑ (*following* C91.6)
mast cell C94.3- ☑
mature B-cell, Burkitt-type C91.A- ☑ (*following* C91.6)
monocytic (subacute) C93.9- ☑
    specified NEC C93.Z- ☑ (*following* C93.3)
myelogenous (*see also* Category C92) C92.9- ☑
myeloid C92.9- ☑
    specified NEC C92.Z- ☑ (*following* C92.6)
plasma cell C90.1- ☑
plasmacytic C90.1- ☑
prolymphocytic
    of B-cell type C91.3- ☑
    of T-cell type C91.6- ☑
specified NEC C94.8- ☑
stem cell, of unclear lineage C95.0- ☑
subacute lymphocytic C91.9- ☑
T-cell large granular lymphocytic C91.Z- ☑ (*following* C91.6)
unspecified cell type C95.9- ☑
    acute C95.0- ☑
    chronic C95.1- ☑
Leukemoid reaction (*see also* Reaction, leukemoid) D72.823
Leukoaraiosis (hypertensive) I67.81
Leukoariosis — *see* Leukoaraiosis
Leukocoria — *see* Disorder, globe, degenerated condition, leucocoria
Leukocytopenia D72.819
Leukocytosis D72.829
eosinophilic D72.1
Leukoderma, leukodermia NEC L81.5
syphilitic A51.39
    late A52.79
Leukodystrophy E75.29
Leukoedema, oral epithelium K13.29
Leukoencephalitis G04.81
acute (subacute) hemorrhagic G36.1
    postimmunization or postvaccinal G04.02
postinfectious G04.01
subacute sclerosing A81.1
van Bogaert's (sclerosing) A81.1
Leukoencephalopathy (*see also* Encephalopathy) G93.49
Binswanger's I67.3
heroin vapor G92
metachromatic E75.25
multifocal (progressive) A81.2
postimmunization and postvaccinal G04.02
progressive multifocal A81.2
reversible, posterior G93.6
van Bogaert's (sclerosing) A81.1
vascular, progressive I67.3
Leukoerythroblastosis D75.9
Leukokeratosis (*see also* Leukoplakia)
mouth K13.21
nicotina palati K13.24
oral mucosa K13.21
tongue K13.21
vocal cord J38.3
Leukokraurosis vulva (e) N90.4
Leukoma (cornea) (*see also* Opacity, cornea)
adherent H17.0- ☑
interfering with central vision — *see* Opacity, cornea, central
Leukomalacia, cerebral, newborn P91.2
periventricular P91.2
Leukomelanopathy, hereditary D72.0
Leukonychia (punctata) (striata) L60.8
congenital Q84.4
Leukopathia unguium L60.8
congenital Q84.4
Leukopenia D72.819
basophilic D72.818
chemotherapy (cancer) induced D70.1
congenital D70.0
cyclic D70.0
drug induced NEC D70.2
    due to cytoreductive cancer chemotherapy D70.1
eosinophilic D72.818
familial D70.0

Leukopenia — *continued*
infantile genetic D70.0
malignant D70.9
periodic D70.0
transitory neonatal P61.5
Leukopenic — *see* condition
Leukoplakia
anus K62.89
bladder (postinfectional) N32.89
buccal K13.21
cervix (uteri) N88.0
esophagus K22.8
gingiva K13.21
hairy (oral mucosa) (tongue) K13.3
kidney (pelvis) N28.89
larynx J38.7
lip K13.21
mouth K13.21
oral epithelium, including tongue (mucosa) K13.21
palate K13.21
pelvis (kidney) N28.89
penis (infectional) N48.0
rectum K62.89
syphilitic (late) A52.79
tongue K13.21
ureter (postinfectional) N28.89
urethra (postinfectional) N36.8
uterus N85.8
vagina N89.4
vocal cord J38.3
vulva N90.4
Leukorrhea N89.8
due to Trichomonas (vaginalis) A59.00
trichomonal A59.00
Leukosarcoma C85.9- ☑
Levocardia (isolated) Q24.1
with situs inversus Q89.3
Levotransposition Q20.5
Lev's disease or syndrome (acquired complete heart
     block) I44.2
Levulosuria — *see* Fructosuria
Levulosuria — *see* Fructosuria
Levurid L30.2
Lewy body (ies) (dementia) (disease) G31.83
Leyden-Moebius dystrophy G71.0
Leydig cell
carcinoma
specified site — *see* Neoplasm, malignant, by site
unspecified site
female C56.9
male C62.9- ☑
tumor
benign
specified site — *see* Neoplasm, benign, by site
unspecified site
female D27.- ☑
male D29.2- ☑
malignant
specified site — *see* Neoplasm, malignant, by
     site
unspecified site
female C56.- ☑
male C62.9- ☑
specified site — *see* Neoplasm, uncertain behavior,
     by site
unspecified site
female D39.1- ☑
male D40.1- ☑
Leydig-Sertoli cell tumor
specified site — *see* Neoplasm, benign, by site
unspecified site
female D27.- ☑
male D29.2- ☑
LGSIL (Low grade squamous intraepithelial lesion on cy-
     tologic smear of)
anus R85.612
cervix R87.612
vagina R87.622
Liar, pathologic F60.2
Libido
decreased R68.82
Libman-Sacks disease M32.11
Lice (infestation) B85.2
body (Pediculus corporis) B85.1
crab B85.3
head (Pediculus capitis) B85.0
mixed (classifiable to more than one of the titles B85.0-
     B85.3) B85.4

Lice — *continued*
pubic (Phthirus pubis) B85.3
Lichen L28.0
albus L90.0
penis N48.0
vulva N90.4
amyloidosis E85.4 [L99]
atrophicus L90.0
penis N48.0
vulva N90.4
congenital Q82.8
myxedematosus L98.5
nitidus L44.1
pilaris Q82.8
acquired L85.8
planopilaris L66.1
planus (chronicus) L43.9
annularis L43.8
bullous L43.1
follicular L66.1
hypertrophic L43.0
moniliformis L44.3
of Wilson L43.9
specified NEC L43.8
subacute (active) L43.3
tropicus L43.3
ruber
acuminatus L44.0
moniliformis L44.3
planus L43.9
sclerosus (et atrophicus) L90.0
penis N48.0
vulva N90.4
scrofulosus (primary) (tuberculous) A18.4
simplex (chronicus) (circumscriptus) L28.0
striatus L44.2
urticatus L28.2
Lichenification L28.0
Lichenoides tuberculosis (primary) A18.4
Lichtheim's disease or syndrome — *see* Degeneration,
     combined
Lien migrans D73.89
Ligament — *see* condition
Light
for gestational age — *see* Light for dates
headedness R42
Light-for-dates (infant) P05.00
with weight of
1000-1249 grams P05.04
1250-1499 grams P05.05
1500-1749 grams P05.06
1750-1999 grams P05.07
2000-2499 grams P05.08
499 grams or less P05.01
500-749 grams P05.02
750-999 grams P05.03
affecting management of pregnancy O36.59- ☑
and small-for-dates — *see* Small for dates
Lightning (effects) (stroke) (struck by) T75.00 ☑
burn — *see* Burn
foot E53.8
shock T75.01 ☑
specified effect NEC T75.09 ☑
Lightwood-Albright syndrome N25.89
Lightwood's disease or syndrome (renal tubular acido-
     sis) N25.89
Lignac (-de Toni) (-Fanconi) (-Debré) **disease or syn-**
     drome E72.09
with cystinosis E72.04
Ligneous thyroiditis E06.5
Likoff's syndrome I20.8
Limb — *see* condition
Limbic epilepsy personality syndrome F07.0
Limitation, limited
activities due to disability Z73.6
cardiac reserve — *see* Disease, heart
eye muscle duction, traumatic — *see* Strabismus,
     mechanical
mandibular range of motion M26.52
Lindau (-von Hippel) **disease** Q85.8
Line(s)
Beau's L60.4
Harris' — *see* Arrest, epiphyseal
Hudson's (cornea) — *see* Pigmentation, cornea, ante-
     rior
Stähli's (cornea) — *see* Pigmentation, cornea, anterior
Linea corneae senilis — *see* Change, cornea, senile

Lingua
geographica K14.1
nigra (villosa) K14.3
plicata K14.5
tylosis K13.29
Lingual — *see* condition
Linguatulosis B88.8
Linitis (gastric) **plastica** C16.9
Lip — *see* condition
Lipedema — *see* Edema
Lipemia (*see also* Hyperlipidemia)
retina, retinalis E78.3
Lipidosis E75.6
cerebral (infantile) (juvenile) (late) E75.4
cerebroretinal E75.4
cerebroside E75.22
cholesterol (cerebral) E75.5
glycolipid E75.21
hepatosplenomegalic E78.3
sphingomyelin — *see* Niemann-Pick disease or syn-
     drome
sulfatide E75.29
Lipoadenoma — *see* Neoplasm, benign, by site
Lipoblastoma — *see* Lipoma
Lipoblastomatosis — *see* Lipoma
Lipochondrodystrophy E76.01
Lipochrome histiocytosis (familial) D71
Lipodermatosclerosis — *see* Varix, leg, with, inflamma-
     tion
ulcerated — *see* Varix, leg, with, ulcer, with inflamma-
     tion by site
Lipodystrophia progressiva E88.1
Lipodystrophy (progressive) E88.1
insulin E88.1
intestinal K90.81
mesenteric K65.4
Lipofibroma — *see* Lipoma
Lipofuscinosis, neuronal (with ceroidosis) E75.4
Lipogranuloma, sclerosing L92.8
Lipogranulomatosis E78.89
Lipoid (*see also* condition)
histiocytosis D76.3
essential E75.29
nephrosis N04.9
proteinosis of Urbach E78.89
Lipoidemia — *see* Hyperlipidemia
Lipoidosis — *see* Lipidosis
Lipoma D17.9
fetal D17.9
fat cell D17.9
infiltrating D17.9
intramuscular D17.9
pleomorphic D17.9
site classification
arms (skin) (subcutaneous) D17.2- ☑
connective tissue D17.30
intra-abdominal D17.5
intrathoracic D17.4
peritoneum D17.79
retroperitoneum D17.79
specified site NEC D17.39
spermatic cord D17.6
face (skin) (subcutaneous) D17.0
genitourinary organ NEC D17.72
head (skin) (subcutaneous) D17.0
intra-abdominal D17.5
intrathoracic D17.4
kidney D17.71
legs (skin) (subcutaneous) D17.2- ☑
neck (skin) (subcutaneous) D17.0
peritoneum D17.79
retroperitoneum D17.79
skin D17.30
specified site NEC D17.39
specified site NEC D17.79
spermatic cord D17.6
subcutaneous D17.30
specified site NEC D17.39
trunk (skin) (subcutaneous) D17.1
unspecified D17.9
spindle cell D17.9
Lipomatosis E88.2
dolorosa (Dercum) E88.2
fetal — *see* Lipoma
Launois-Bensaude E88.89
Lipomyoma — *see* Lipoma
Lipomyxoma — *see* Lipoma

Lipomyxosarcoma — see Neoplasm, connective tissue, malignant
Lipoprotein metabolism disorder E78.9
Lipoproteinemia E78.5
  broad-beta E78.2
  floating-beta E78.2
  hyper-pre-beta E78.1
Liposarcoma (see also Neoplasm, connective tissue, malignant)
  dedifferentiated — see Neoplasm, connective tissue, malignant
  differentiated type — see Neoplasm, connective tissue, malignant
  embryonal — see Neoplasm, connective tissue, malignant
  mixed type — see Neoplasm, connective tissue, malignant
  myxoid — see Neoplasm, connective tissue, malignant
  pleomorphic — see Neoplasm, connective tissue, malignant
  round cell — see Neoplasm, connective tissue, malignant
  well differentiated type — see Neoplasm, connective tissue, malignant
Liposynovitis prepatellaris E88.89
Lipping, cervix N86
Lipschütz disease or ulcer N76.6
Lipuria R82.0
  schistosomiasis (bilharziasis) B65.0
Lisping F80.0
Lissauer's paralysis A52.17
Lissencephalia, lissencephaly Q04.3
Listeriosis, listerellosis A32.9
  congenital (disseminated) P37.2
  cutaneous A32.0
  neonatal, newborn (disseminated) P37.2
  oculoglandular A32.81
  specified NEC A32.89
Lithemia E79.0
Lithiasis — see Calculus
Lithosis J62.8
Lithuria R82.99
Litigation, anxiety concerning Z65.3
Little leaguer's elbow — see Epicondylitis, medial
Little's disease G80.9
Littre's
  gland — see condition
  hernia — see Hernia, abdomen
Littritis — see Urethritis
Livedo (annularis) (racemosa) (reticularis) R23.1
Liver — see condition
Living alone (problems with) Z60.2
  with handicapped person Z74.2
Lloyd's syndrome — see Adenomatosis, endocrine
Loa loa, loaiasis, loasis B74.3
Lobar — see condition
Lobomycosis B48.0
Lobo's disease B48.0
Lobotomy syndrome F07.0
Lobstein (-Ekman) **disease or syndrome** Q78.0
Lobster-claw hand Q71.6- ☑
Lobulation (congenital) (see also Anomaly, by site)
  kidney, Q63.1
  liver, abnormal Q44.7
  spleen Q89.09
Lobule, lobular — see condition
Local, localized — see condition
Locked twins causing obstructed labor O66.1
Locked-in state G83.5
Locking
  joint — see Derangement, joint, specified type NEC
    knee — see Derangement, knee
Lockjaw — see Tetanus
Löffler's
  endocarditis I42.3
  eosinophilia J82
  pneumonia J82
  syndrome (eosinophilic pneumonitis) J82
Loiasis (with conjunctival infestation) (eyelid) B74.3
Lone Star fever A77.0
Long
  labor O63.9
    first stage O63.0
    second stage O63.1
  QT syndrome I45.81
Longitudinal stripes or grooves, nails L60.8
  congenital Q84.6

Long-term (current) (prophylactic) **drug therapy** (use of)
  agents affecting estrogen receptors and estrogen levels NEC Z79.818
  anastrozole (Arimidex) Z79.811
  antibiotics Z79.2
    short-term use — omit code
  anticoagulants Z79.01
  anti-inflammatory, non-steroidal (NSAID) Z79.1
  antiplatelet Z79.02
  antithrombotics Z79.02
  aromatase inhibitors Z79.811
  aspirin Z79.82
  birth control pill or patch Z79.3
  bisphosphonates Z79.83
  contraceptive, oral Z79.3
  drug, specified NEC Z79.899
  estrogen receptor downregulators Z79.818
  Evista Z79.810
  exemestane (Aromasin) Z79.811
  Fareston Z79.810
  fulvestrant (Faslodex) Z79.818
  gonadotropin-releasing hormone (GnRH) agonist Z79.818
  goserelin acetate (Zoladex) Z79.818
  hormone replacement (postmenopausal) Z79.890
  insulin Z79.4
  letrozole (Femara) Z79.811
  leuprolide acetate (leuprorelin) (Lupron) Z79.818
  megestrol acetate (Megace) Z79.818
  methadone for pain management Z79.891
  Nolvadex Z79.810
  non-steroidal anti-inflammatories (NSAID) Z79.1
  opiate analgesic Z79.891
  oral contraceptive Z79.3
  raloxifene (Evista) Z79.810
  selective estrogen receptor modulators (SERMs) Z79.810
  steroids
    inhaled Z79.51
    systemic Z79.52
  tamoxifen (Nolvadex) Z79.810
  toremifene (Fareston) Z79.810
Loop
  intestine — see Volvulus
  vascular on papilla (optic) Q14.2
Loose (see also condition)
  body
    joint M24.00
      ankle M24.07- ☑
      elbow M24.02- ☑
      hand M24.04- ☑
      hip M24.05- ☑
      knee M23.4- ☑
      shoulder (region) M24.01- ☑
      specified site NEC M24.08
      toe M24.07- ☑
      vertebra M24.08
      wrist M24.03- ☑
    knee M23.4- ☑
    sheath, tendon — see Disorder, tendon, specified type NEC
  cartilage — see Loose, body, joint
  tooth, teeth K08.8
Loosening
  aseptic
    joint prosthesis — see Complications, joint prosthesis, mechanical, loosening, by site
  epiphysis — see Osteochondropathy
  mechanical
    joint prosthesis — see Complications, joint prosthesis, mechanical, loosening, by site
Looser-Milkman (-Debray) **syndrome** M83.8
Lop ear (deformity) Q17.3
Lorain (-Levi) **short stature syndrome** E23.0
Lordosis M40.50
  acquired — see Lordosis, specified type NEC
  congenital Q76.429
    lumbar region Q76.426
    lumbosacral region Q76.427
    sacral region Q76.428
    sacrococcygeal region Q76.428
    thoracolumbar region Q76.425
  lumbar region M40.56
  lumbosacral region M40.57
  postsurgical M96.4
  postural — see Lordosis, specified type NEC
  rachitic (late effect) (sequelae) E64.3

Lordosis — continued
  sequelae of rickets E64.3
  specified type NEC M40.40
    lumbar region M40.46
    lumbosacral region M40.47
    thoracolumbar region M40.45
  thoracolumbar region M40.55
  tuberculous A18.01
Loss (of)
  appetite (see Anorexia) R63.0
    hysterical F50.8
    nonorganic origin F50.8
    psychogenic F50.8
  blood — see Hemorrhage
  consciousness, transient R55
    traumatic — see Injury, intracranial
  control, sphincter, rectum R15.9
    nonorganic origin F98.1
  elasticity, skin R23.4
  family (member) in childhood Z62.898
  fluid (acute) E86.9
    with
      hypernatremia E87.0
      hyponatremia E87.1
  function of labyrinth — see subcategory H83.2 ☑
  hair, nonscarring — see Alopecia
  hearing (see also Deafness)
    central NOS H90.5
    neural NOS H90.5
    perceptive NOS H90.5
    sensorineural NOS H90.5
    sensory NOS H90.5
  height R29.890
  limb or member, traumatic, current — see Amputation, traumatic
  love relationship in childhood Z62.898
  memory (see also Amnesia)
    mild, following organic brain damage F06.8
  mind — see Psychosis
  occlusal vertical dimension of fully erupted teeth M26.37
  organ or part — see Absence, by site, acquired
  ossicles, ear (partial) H74.32- ☑
  parent in childhood Z63.4
  pregnancy, recurrent N96
    without current pregnancy N96
    care in current pregnancy O26.2- ☑
  recurrent pregnancy — see Loss, pregnancy, recurrent
  self-esteem, in childhood Z62.898
  sense of
    smell — see Disturbance, sensation, smell
    taste — see Disturbance, sensation, taste
    touch R20.8
  sensory R44.9
    dissociative F44.6
  sexual desire F52.0
  sight (acquired) (complete) (congenital) — see Blindness
  substance of
    bone — see Disorder, bone, density and structure, specified NEC
    cartilage — see Disorder, cartilage, specified type NEC
      auricle (ear) — see Disorder, pinna, specified type NEC
    vitreous (humor) H15.89
  tooth, teeth — see Absence, teeth, acquired
  vision, visual H54.7
    both eyes H54.3
    one eye H54.60
      left (normal vision on right) H54.62
      right (normal vision on left) H54.61
    specified as blindness — see Blindness
    subjective
      sudden H53.13- ☑
      transient H53.12- ☑
  vitreous — see Prolapse, vitreous
  voice — see Aphonia
  weight (abnormal) (cause unknown) R63.4
Louis-Bar syndrome (ataxia-telangiectasia) G11.3
Louping ill (encephalitis) A84.8
Louse, lousiness — see Lice
Low
  achiever, school Z55.3
  back syndrome M54.5
  basal metabolic rate R94.8
  birthweight (2499 grams or less) P07.10

☑ **Additional Character Required** — Refer to the Tabular List for Character Selection   ▽ **Subterms under main terms may continue to next column or page**

Low — *continued*
  birthweight — *continued*
    with weight of
      1000-1249 grams P07.14
      1250-1499 grams P07.15
      1500-1749 grams P07.16
      1750-1999 grams P07.17
      2000-2499 grams P07.18
    extreme (999 grams or less) P07.00
      with weight of
        499 grams or less P07.01
        500-749 grams P07.02
        750-999 grams P07.03
    for gestational age — *see* Light for dates
  blood pressure (*see also* Hypotension)
    reading (incidental) (isolated) (nonspecific) R03.1
  cardiac reserve — *see* Disease, heart
  function (*see also* Hypofunction)
    kidney N28.9
  hematocrit D64.9
  hemoglobin D64.9
  income Z59.6
  level of literacy Z55.0
  lying
    kidney N28.89
    organ or site, congenital — *see* Malposition, congenital
  output syndrome (cardiac) — *see* Failure, heart
  platelets (blood) — *see* Thrombocytopenia
  reserve, kidney N28.89
  salt syndrome E87.1
  self esteem R45.81
  set ears Q17.4
  vision H54.2
    one eye (other eye normal) H54.50
      left (normal vision on right) H54.52
      other eye blind — *see* Blindness
      right (normal vision on left) H54.51
Low-density-lipoprotein-type (LDL) **hyperlipoproteinemia** E78.0
Lowe's syndrome E72.03
Lown-Ganong-Levine syndrome I45.6
LSD reaction (acute) (without dependence) F16.90
  with dependence F16.20
L-shaped kidney Q63.8
Ludwig's angina or disease K12.2
Lues (venerea), **luetic** — *see* Syphilis
Luetscher's syndrome (dehydration) E86.0
Lumbago, lumbalgia M54.5
  with sciatica M54.4- ☑
    due to intervertebral disc disorder M51.17
  due to displacement, intervertebral disc M51.27
    with sciatica M51.17
Lumbar — *see* condition
Lumbarization, vertebra, congenital Q76.49
Lumbermen's itch B88.0
Lump — *see* Mass
Lunacy — *see* Psychosis
Lung — *see* condition
Lupoid (miliary) **of Boeck** D86.3
Lupus
  anticoagulant D68.62
    with
      hemorrhagic disorder D68.312
      hypercoagulable state D68.62
      finding without diagnosis R76.0
  discoid (local) L93.0
  erythematosus (discoid) (local) L93.0
    disseminated — *see* Lupus, erythematosus, systemic
    eyelid H01.129
      left H01.126
        lower H01.125
        upper H01.124
      right H01.123
        lower H01.122
        upper H01.121
    profundus L93.2
    specified NEC L93.2
    subacute cutaneous L93.1
    systemic M32.9
      with organ or system involvement M32.10
        endocarditis M32.11
        lung M32.13
        pericarditis M32.12
        renal (glomerular) M32.14
          tubulo-interstitial M32.15
        specified organ or system NEC M32.19

Lupus — *continued*
  erythematosus — *continued*
    systemic — *continued*
      drug-induced M32.0
      inhibitor (presence of) D68.62
        with
          hemorrhagic disorder D68.312
          hypercoagulable state D68.62
          finding without diagnosis R76.0
      specified NEC M32.8
  exedens A18.4
  hydralazine M32.0
    correct substance properly administered — *see* Table of Drugs and Chemicals, by drug, adverse effect
    overdose or wrong substance given or taken — *see* Table of Drugs and Chemicals, by drug, poisoning
  nephritis (chronic) M32.14
  nontuberculous, not disseminated L93.0
  panniculitis L93.2
  pernio (Besnier) D86.3
  systemic — *see* Lupus, erythematosus, systemic
  tuberculous A18.4
    eyelid A18.4
  vulgaris A18.4
    eyelid A18.4
Luteinoma D27.- ☑
Lutembacher's disease or syndrome (atrial septal defect with mitral stenosis) Q21.1
Luteoma D27.- ☑
Lutz (-Splendore-de Almeida) **disease** — *see* Paracoccidioidomycosis
Luxation (*see also* Dislocation)
  eyeball (nontraumatic) — *see* Luxation, globe
    birth injury P15.3
  globe, nontraumatic H44.82- ☑
  lacrimal gland — *see* Dislocation, lacrimal gland
  lens (old) (partial) (spontaneous)
    congenital Q12.1
    syphilitic A50.39
Lycanthropy F22
Lyell's syndrome L51.2
  due to drug L51.2
    correct substance properly administered — *see* Table of Drugs and Chemicals, by drug, adverse effect
    overdose or wrong substance given or taken — *see* Table of Drugs and Chemicals, by drug, poisoning
Lyme disease A69.20
Lymph
  gland or node — *see* condition
  scrotum — *see* Infestation, filarial
Lymphadenitis I88.9
  with ectopic or molar pregnancy O08.0
  acute L04.9
    axilla L04.2
    face L04.0
    head L04.0
    hip L04.3
    limb
      lower L04.3
      upper L04.2
    neck L04.0
    shoulder L04.2
    specified site NEC L04.8
    trunk L04.1
  anthracosis (occupational) J60
  any site, except mesenteric I88.9
    chronic I88.1
    subacute I88.1
  breast
    gestational — *see* Mastitis, obstetric
    puerperal, postpartum (nonpurulent) O91.22
  chancroidal (congenital) A57
  chronic I88.1
    mesenteric I88.0
  due to
    Brugia (malayi) B74.1
      timori B74.2
    chlamydial lymphogranuloma A55
    diphtheria (toxin) A36.89
    lymphogranuloma venereum A55
    Wuchereria bancrofti B74.0
  following ectopic or molar pregnancy O08.0
  gonorrheal A54.89
  infective — *see* Lymphadenitis, acute

Lymphadenitis — *continued*
  mesenteric (acute) (chronic) (nonspecific) (subacute) I88.0
    due to Salmonella typhi A01.09
    tuberculous A18.39
  mycobacterial A31.8
  purulent — *see* Lymphadenitis, acute
  pyogenic — *see* Lymphadenitis, acute
  regional, nonbacterial I88.8
  septic — *see* Lymphadenitis, acute
  subacute, unspecified site I88.1
  suppurative — *see* Lymphadenitis, acute
  syphilitic (early) (secondary) A51.49
    late A52.79
  tuberculous — *see* Tuberculosis, lymph gland
  venereal (chlamydial) A55
Lymphadenoid goiter E06.3
Lymphadenopathy (generalized) R59.1
  angioimmunoblastic, with dysproteinemia (AILD) C86.5
  due to toxoplasmosis (acquired) B58.89
    congenital (acute) (subacute) (chronic) P37.1
  localized R59.0
  syphilitic (early) (secondary) A51.49
Lymphadenosis R59.1
Lymphangiectasis I89.0
  conjunctiva H11.89
  postinfectional I89.0
  scrotum I89.0
Lymphangiectatic elephantiasis, nonfilarial I89.0
Lymphangioendothelioma D18.1
  malignant — *see* Neoplasm, connective tissue, malignant
Lymphangioleiomyomatosis J84.81
Lymphangioma D18.1
  capillary D18.1
  cavernous D18.1
  cystic D18.1
  malignant — *see* Neoplasm, connective tissue, malignant
Lymphangiomyoma D18.1
Lymphangiomyomatosis J84.81
Lymphangiosarcoma — *see* Neoplasm, connective tissue, malignant
Lymphangitis I89.1
  with
    abscess — *code by* site under Abscess
    cellulitis — *code by* site under Cellulitis
    ectopic or molar pregnancy O08.0
  acute L03.91
    abdominal wall L03.321
    ankle — *see* Lymphangitis, acute, lower limb
    arm — *see* Lymphangitis, acute, upper limb
    auricle (ear) — *see* Lymphangitis, acute, ear
    axilla L03.12- ☑
    back (any part) L03.322
    buttock L03.327
    cervical (meaning neck) L03.222
    cheek (external) L03.212
    chest wall L03.323
    digit
      finger — *see* Lymphangitis, acute, finger
      toe — *see* Lymphangitis, acute, toe
    ear (external) H60.1- ☑
    external auditory canal — *see* Lymphangitis, acute, ear
    eyelid — *see* Abscess, eyelid
    face NEC L03.212
    finger (intrathecal) (periosteal) (subcutaneous) (subcuticular) L03.02- ☑
    foot — *see* Lymphangitis, acute, lower limb
    gluteal (region) L03.327
    groin L03.324
    hand — *see* Lymphangitis, acute, upper limb
    head NEC L03.891
      face (any part, except ear, eye and nose) L03.212
    heel — *see* Lymphangitis, acute, lower limb
    hip — *see* Lymphangitis, acute, lower limb
    jaw (region) L03.212
    knee — *see* Lymphangitis, acute, lower limb
    leg — *see* Lymphangitis, acute, lower limb
    lower limb L03.12- ☑
      toe — *see* Lymphangitis, acute, toe
    navel L03.326
    neck (region) L03.222
    orbit, orbital — *see* Cellulitis, orbit

Lymphangitis — *continued*
  acute — *continued*
    pectoral (region) L03.323
    perineal, perineum L03.325
    scalp (any part) L03.891
    shoulder — *see* Lymphangitis, acute, upper limb
    specified site NEC L03.898
    thigh — *see* Lymphangitis, acute, lower limb
    thumb (intrathecal) (periosteal) (subcutaneous) (subcuticular) — *see* Lymphangitis, acute, finger
    toe (intrathecal) (periosteal) (subcutaneous) (subcuticular) L03.04- ☑
    trunk L03.329
      abdominal wall L03.321
      back (any part) L03.322
      buttock L03.327
      chest wall L03.323
      groin L03.324
      perineal, perineum L03.325
      umbilicus L03.326
    umbilicus L03.326
    upper limb L03.12- ☑
      axilla — *see* Lymphangitis, acute, axilla
      finger — *see* Lymphangitis, acute, finger
      thumb — *see* Lymphangitis, acute, finger
      wrist — *see* Lymphangitis, acute, upper limb
  breast
    gestational — *see* Mastitis, obstetric
  chancroidal A57
  chronic (any site) I89.1
  due to
    Brugia (malayi) B74.1
      timori B74.2
    Wuchereria bancrofti B74.0
  following ectopic or molar pregnancy O08.89
  penis
    acute N48.29
    gonococcal (acute) (chronic) A54.09
  puerperal, postpartum, childbirth O86.89
  strumous, tuberculous A18.2
  subacute (any site) I89.1
  tuberculous — *see* Tuberculosis, lymph gland
Lymphatic (vessel) — *see* condition
Lymphatism E32.8
Lymphectasia I89.0
Lymphedema (acquired) (*see also* Elephantiasis)
  congenital Q82.0
  hereditary (chronic) (idiopathic) Q82.0
  postmastectomy I97.2
  praecox I89.0
  secondary I89.0
  surgical NEC I97.89
    postmastectomy (syndrome) I97.2
Lymphoblastic — *see* condition
Lymphoblastoma (diffuse) — *see* Lymphoma, lymphoblastic (diffuse)
  giant follicular — *see* Lymphoma, lymphoblastic (diffuse)
  macrofollicular — *see* Lymphoma, lymphoblastic (diffuse)
Lymphocele I89.8
Lymphocytic
  chorioencephalitis (acute) (serous) A87.2
  choriomeningitis (acute) (serous) A87.2
  meningoencephalitis A87.2
Lymphocytoma, benign cutis L98.8
Lymphocytopenia D72.810
Lymphocytosis (symptomatic) D72.820
  infectious (acute) B33.8
Lymphoepithelioma — *see* Neoplasm, malignant, by site
Lymphogranuloma (malignant) (*see also* Lymphoma, Hodgkin)
  chlamydial A55
  inguinale A55
  venereum (any site) (chlamydial) (with stricture of rectum) A55
Lymphogranulomatosis (malignant) (*see also* Lymphoma, Hodgkin)
  benign (Boeck's sarcoid) (Schaumann's) D86.1
Lymphohistiocytosis, hemophagocytic (familial) D76.1
Lymphoid — *see* condition
Lymphoma (of) (malignant) C85.90
  adult T-cell (HTLV-1-associated) (acute variant) (chronic variant) (lymphomatoid variant) (smouldering variant) C91.5- ☑

Lymphoma — *continued*
  anaplastic large cell
    ALK-negative C84.7- ☑
    ALK-positive C84.6- ☑
    CD30-positive C84.6- ☑
    primary cutaneous C86.6
  angioimmunoblastic T-cell C86.5
  BALT C88.4
  B-cell C85.1- ☑
  blastic NK-cell C86.4
  B-precursor C83.5- ☑
  bronchial-associated lymphoid tissue [BALT-lymphoma] C88.4
  Burkitt (atypical) C83.7- ☑
  Burkitt-like C83.7- ☑
  centrocytic C83.1- ☑
  cutaneous follicle center C82.6- ☑
  cutaneous T-cell C84.A- ☑ (*following* C84.7)
  diffuse follicle center C82.5 ☑
  diffuse large cell C83.3- ☑
    anaplastic C83.3- ☑
    B-cell C83.3- ☑
    CD30-positive C83.3- ☑
    centroblastic C83.3- ☑
    immunoblastic C83.3- ☑
    plasmablastic C83.3- ☑
    subtype not specified C83.3- ☑
    T-cell rich C83.3- ☑
  enteropathy-type (associated) (intestinal) T-cell C86.2
  extranodal marginal zone B-cell lymphoma of mucosa-associated lymphoid tissue [MALT-lymphoma] C88.4
  extranodal NK/T-cell, nasal type C86.0
  follicular C82.9- ☑
    grade
      I C82.0- ☑
      II C82.1- ☑
      III C82.2- ☑
      IIIa C82.3- ☑
      IIIb C82.4- ☑
    specified NEC C82.8- ☑
  hepatosplenic T-cell (alpha-beta) (gamma-delta) C86.1
  histiocytic C85.9- ☑
    true C96.A (*following* C96.6)
  Hodgkin C81.9
    classical C81.7- ☑
      lymphocyte depleted C81.3- ☑
      lymphocyte-rich C81.4- ☑
      mixed cellularity C81.2- ☑
      nodular sclerosis C81.1- ☑
      specified NEC C81.7- ☑
    lymphocyte depleted classical C81.3- ☑
    lymphocyte-rich classical C81.4- ☑
    mixed cellularity classical C81.2- ☑
    nodular
      lymphocyte predominant C81.0- ☑
      sclerosis classical C81.1- ☑
  intravascular large B-cell C83.8- ☑
  Lennert's C84.4- ☑
  lymphoblastic (diffuse) C83.5- ☑
  lymphoblastic B-cell C83.5- ☑
  lymphoblastic T-cell C83.5- ☑
  lymphoepithelioid C84.4- ☑
  lymphoplasmacytic C83.0- ☑
    with IgM-production C88.0
  MALT C88.4
  mantle cell C83.1- ☑
  mature T-cell NEC C84.4- ☑
  mature T/NK-cell C84.9- ☑
    specified NEC C84.Z- ☑ (*following* C84.7)
  mediastinal (thymic) large B-cell C85.2- ☑
  Mediterranean C88.3
  mucosa-associated lymphoid tissue [MALT-lymphoma] C88.4
  NK/T cell C84.9- ☑
  nodal marginal zone C83.0- ☑
  non-follicular (diffuse) C83.9- ☑
    specified NEC C83.8- ☑
  non-Hodgkin (*see also* Lymphoma, by type) C85.9- ☑
    specified NEC C85.8- ☑
  non-leukemic variant of B-CLL C83.0- ☑
  peripheral T-cell, not classified C84.4- ☑
  primary cutaneous
    anaplastic large cell C86.6
    CD30-positive large T-cell C86.6
  primary effusion B-cell C83.8- ☑

Lymphoma — *continued*
  SALT C88.4
  skin-associated lymphoid tissue [SALT-lymphoma] C88.4
  small cell B-cell C83.0- ☑
  splenic marginal zone C83.0- ☑
  subcutaneous panniculitis-like T-cell C86.3
  T-precursor C83.5- ☑
  true histiocytic C96.A (*following* C96.6)
Lymphomatosis — *see* Lymphoma
Lymphopathia venereum, veneris A55
Lymphopenia D72.810
Lymphoplasmacytic leukemia — *see* Leukemia, chronic lymphocytic, B-cell type
Lymphoproliferation, X-linked disease D82.3
Lymphoreticulosis, benign (of inoculation) A28.1
Lymphorrhea I89.8
Lymphosarcoma (diffuse) (*see also* Lymphoma) C85.9- ☑
Lymphostasis I89.8
Lypemania — *see* Melancholia
Lysine and hydroxylysine metabolism disorder E72.3
Lyssa — *see* Rabies

M

Macacus ear Q17.3
Maceration, wet feet, tropical (syndrome) T69.02- ☑
MacLeod's syndrome J43.0
Macrocephalia, macrocephaly Q75.3
Macrocheilia, macrochilia (congenital) Q18.6
Macrocolon (*see also* Megacolon) Q43.1
Macrocornea Q15.8
  with glaucoma Q15.0
Macrocytic — *see* condition
Macrocytosis D75.89
Macrodactylia, macrodactylism (fingers) (thumbs) Q74.0
  toes Q74.2
Macrodontia K00.2
Macrogenia M26.05
Macrogenitosomia (adrenal) (male) (praecox) E25.9
  congenital E25.0
Macroglobulinemia (idiopathic) (primary) C88.0
  monoclonal (essential) D47.2
  Waldenström C88.0
Macroglossia (congenital) Q38.2
  acquired K14.8
Macrognathia, macrognathism (congenital) (mandibular) (maxillary) M26.09
Macrogyria (congenital) Q04.8
Macrohydrocephalus — *see* Hydrocephalus
Macromastia — *see* Hypertrophy, breast
Macrophthalmos Q11.3
  in congenital glaucoma Q15.0
Macropsia H53.15
Macrosigmoid K59.3
  congenital Q43.2
Macrospondylitis , acromegalic E22.0
Macrostomia (congenital) Q18.4
Macrotia (external ear) (congenital) Q17.1
Macula
  cornea, corneal — *see* Opacity, cornea
  degeneration (atrophic) (exudative) (senile) (*see also* Degeneration, macula)
    hereditary — *see* Dystrophy, retina
Maculae ceruleae B85.1
Maculopathy, toxic — *see* Degeneration, macula, toxic
Madarosis (eyelid) H02.729
  left H02.726
    lower H02.725
    upper H02.724
  right H02.723
    lower H02.722
    upper H02.721
Madelung's
  deformity (radius) Q74.0
  disease
    radial deformity Q74.0
    symmetrical lipomas, neck E88.89
Madness — *see* Psychosis
Madura
  foot B47.9
    actinomycotic B47.1
    mycotic B47.0
Maduromycosis B47.0
Maffucci's syndrome Q78.4

☑ **Additional Character Required** — Refer to the Tabular List for Character Selection   ▽ **Subterms under main terms may continue to next column or page**

Magnesium metabolism disorder — *see* Disorder,
  metabolism, magnesium
Main en griffe (acquired) (*see also* Deformity, limb,
  clawhand)
  congenital Q74.0
Maintenance (encounter for)
  antineoplastic chemotherapy Z51.11
  antineoplastic radiation therapy Z51.0
  methadone F11.20
Majocchi's
  disease L81.7
  granuloma B35.8
Major — *see* condition
Mal de los pintos — *see* Pinta
Mal de mer T75.3 ☑
Malabar itch (any site) B35.5
Malabsorption K90.9
  calcium K90.89
  carbohydrate K90.4
  disaccharide E73.9
  fat K90.4
  galactose E74.20
  glucose (-galactose) E74.39
  intestinal K90.9
    specified NEC K90.89
  isomaltose E74.31
  lactose E73.9
  methionine E72.19
  monosaccharide E74.39
  postgastrectomy K91.2
  postsurgical K91.2
  protein K90.4
  starch K90.4
  sucrose E74.39
  syndrome K90.9
    postsurgical K91.2
Malacia, bone (adult) M83.9
  juvenile — *see* Rickets
Malacoplakia
  bladder N32.89
  pelvis (kidney) N28.89
  ureter N28.89
  urethra N36.8
Malacosteon, juvenile — *see* Rickets
Maladaptation — *see* Maladjustment
Maladie de Roger Q21.0
Maladjustment
  conjugal Z63.0
    involving divorce or estrangement Z63.5
  educational Z55.4
  family Z63.9
  marital Z63.0
    involving divorce or estrangement Z63.5
  occupational NEC Z56.89
  simple, adult — *see* Disorder, adjustment
  situational — *see* Disorder, adjustment
  social Z60.9
    due to
      acculturation difficulty Z60.3
      discrimination and persecution (perceived)
        Z60.5
      exclusion and isolation Z60.4
      life-cycle (phase of life) transition Z60.0
      rejection Z60.4
      specified reason NEC Z60.8
Malaise R53.81
Malakoplakia — *see* Malacoplakia
Malaria, malarial (fever) B54
  with
    blackwater fever B50.8
      hemoglobinuric (bilious) B50.8
    hemoglobinuria B50.8
  accidentally induced (therapeutically) — *code by* type
    under Malaria
  algid B50.9
  cerebral B50.0 [G94]
  clinically diagnosed (without parasitological confirma-
    tion) B54
  congenital NEC P37.4
    falciparum P37.3
  congestion, congestive B54
  continued (fever) B50.9
  estivo-autumnal B50.9
  falciparum B50.9
    with complications NEC B50.8
      cerebral B50.0 [G94]
    severe B50.8
  hemorrhagic B54

Malaria, malarial — *continued*
  malariae B52.9
    with
      complications NEC B52.8
      glomerular disorder B52.0
  malignant (tertian) — *see* Malaria, falciparum
  mixed infections — *code to* first listed type in B50-B53
  ovale B53.0
  parasitologically confirmed NEC B53.8
  pernicious, acute — *see* Malaria, falciparum
  Plasmodium (P.)
    falciparum NEC — *see* Malaria, falciparum
    malariae NEC B52.9
      with Plasmodium
        falciparum (and or vivax) — *see* Malaria,
          falciparum
        vivax (*see also* Malaria, vivax)
          and falciparum — *see* Malaria, falci-
            parum
    ovale B53.0
      with Plasmodium malariae (*see also* Malaria,
        malariae)
        and vivax (*see also* Malaria, vivax)
          and falciparum — *see* Malaria, falci-
            parum
    simian B53.1
      with Plasmodium malariae (*see also* Malaria,
        malariae)
        and vivax (*see also* Malaria, vivax)
          and falciparum — *see* Malaria, falci-
            parum
    vivax NEC B51.9
      with Plasmodium falciparum — *see* Malaria,
        falciparum
  quartan — *see* Malaria, malariae
  quotidian — *see* Malaria, falciparum
  recurrent B54
  remittent B54
  specified type NEC (parasitologically confirmed) B53.8
  spleen B54
  subtertian (fever) — *see* Malaria, falciparum
  tertian (benign) (*see also* Malaria, vivax)
    malignant B50.9
  tropical B50.9
  typhoid B54
  vivax B51.9
    with
      complications NEC B51.8
      ruptured spleen B51.0
Malassez's disease (cystic) N50.8
Malassimilation K90.9
Maldescent, testis Q53.9
  bilateral Q53.20
    abdominal Q53.21
    perineal Q53.22
  unilateral Q53.10
    abdominal Q53.11
    perineal Q53.12
Maldevelopment (*see also* Anomaly)
  brain Q07.9
  colon Q43.9
  hip Q74.2
    congenital dislocation Q65.2
      bilateral Q65.1
      unilateral Q65.0- ☑
  mastoid process Q75.8
  middle ear Q16.4
    except ossicles Q16.4
    ossicles Q16.3
  ossicles Q16.3
  spine Q76.49
  toe Q74.2
Male type pelvis Q74.2
  with disproportion (fetopelvic) O33.3 ☑
    causing obstructed labor O65.3
Malformation (congenital) (*see also* Anomaly)
  adrenal gland Q89.1
  affecting multiple systems with skeletal changes NEC
    Q87.5
  alimentary tract Q45.9
    specified type NEC Q45.8
    upper Q40.9
      specified type NEC Q40.8
  aorta Q25.9
    atresia Q25.2
    coarctation (preductal) (postductal) Q25.1
    patent ductus arteriosus Q25.0
    specified type NEC Q25.4

Malformation — *continued*
  aorta — *continued*
    stenosis (supravalvular) Q25.3
  aortic valve Q23.9
    specified NEC Q23.8
  arteriovenous, aneurysmatic (congenital) Q27.30
    brain Q28.2
    cerebral Q28.2
    peripheral Q27.30
      digestive system Q27.33
      lower limb Q27.32
      other specified site Q27.39
      renal vessel Q27.34
      upper limb Q27.31
    precerebral vessels (nonruptured) Q28.0
  auricle
    ear (congenital) Q17.3
      acquired H61.119
        left H61.112
          with right H61.113
        right H61.111
          with left H61.113
  bile duct Q44.5
  bladder Q64.79
    aplasia Q64.5
    diverticulum Q64.6
    exstrophy — *see* Exstrophy, bladder
    neck obstruction Q64.31
  bone Q79.9
    face Q75.9
      specified type NEC Q75.8
    skull Q75.9
      specified type NEC Q75.8
  brain (multiple) Q04.9
    arteriovenous Q28.2
    specified type NEC Q04.8
  branchial cleft Q18.2
  breast Q83.9
    specified type NEC Q83.8
  broad ligament Q50.6
  bronchus Q32.4
  bursa Q79.9
  cardiac
    chambers Q20.9
      specified type NEC Q20.8
    septum Q21.9
      specified type NEC Q21.8
  cerebral Q04.9
    vessels Q28.3
  cervix uteri Q51.9
    specified type NEC Q51.828
  Chiari
    Type I G93.5
    Type II Q07.01
  choroid (congenital) Q14.3
    plexus Q07.8
  circulatory system Q28.9
  cochlea Q16.5
  cornea Q13.4
  coronary vessels Q24.5
  corpus callosum (congenital) Q04.0
  diaphragm Q79.1
  digestive system NEC, specified type NEC Q45.8
  dura Q07.9
    brain Q04.9
    spinal Q06.9
  ear Q17.9
    causing impairment of hearing Q16.9
    external Q17.9
      accessory auricle Q17.0
      causing impairment of hearing Q16.9
        absence of
          auditory canal Q16.1
          auricle Q16.0
      macrotia Q17.1
      microtia Q17.2
      misplacement Q17.4
      misshapen NEC Q17.3
      prominence Q17.5
      specified type NEC Q17.8
    inner Q16.5
    middle Q16.4
      absence of eustachian tube Q16.2
      ossicles (fusion) Q16.3
    ossicles Q16.3
    specified type NEC Q17.8
  epididymis Q55.4

Malformation — *continued*
esophagus Q39.9
  specified type NEC Q39.8
eye Q15.9
  lid Q10.3
  specified NEC Q15.8
fallopian tube Q50.6
genital organ — *see* Anomaly, genitalia
great
  artery Q25.9
    aorta — *see* Malformation, aorta
    pulmonary artery — *see* Malformation, pul-
      monary, artery
    specified type NEC Q25.8
  vein Q26.9
    anomalous
      portal venous connection Q26.5
      pulmonary venous connection Q26.4
        partial Q26.3
        total Q26.2
    persistent left superior vena cava Q26.1
    portal vein-hepatic artery fistula Q26.6
    specified type NEC Q26.8
    vena cava stenosis, congenital Q26.0
gum Q38.6
hair Q84.2
heart Q24.9
  specified type NEC Q24.8
integument Q84.9
  specified type NEC Q84.8
internal ear Q16.5
intestine Q43.9
  specified type NEC Q43.8
iris Q13.2
joint Q74.9
  ankle Q74.2
  lumbosacral Q76.49
  sacroiliac Q74.2
  specified type NEC Q74.8
kidney Q63.9
  accessory Q63.0
  giant Q63.3
  horseshoe Q63.1
  hydronephrosis Q62.0
  malposition Q63.2
  specified type NEC Q63.8
lacrimal apparatus Q10.6
lingual Q38.3
lip Q38.0
liver Q44.7
lung Q33.9
meninges or membrane (congenital) Q07.9
  cerebral Q04.8
  spinal (cord) Q06.9
middle ear Q16.4
  ossicles Q16.3
mitral valve Q23.9
  specified NEC Q23.8
Mondini's (congenital) (malformation, cochlea) Q16.5
mouth (congenital) Q38.6
multiple types NEC Q89.7
musculoskeletal system Q79.9
myocardium Q24.8
nail Q84.6
nervous system (central) Q07.9
nose Q30.9
  specified type NEC Q30.8
optic disc Q14.2
orbit Q10.7
ovary Q50.39
palate Q38.5
parathyroid gland Q89.2
pelvic organs or tissues NEC
  in pregnancy or childbirth O34.8- ☑
    causing obstructed labor O65.5
penis Q55.69
  aplasia Q55.5
  curvature (lateral) Q55.61
  hypoplasia Q55.62
pericardium Q24.8
peripheral vascular system Q27.9
  specified type NEC Q27.8
pharynx Q38.8
precerebral vessels Q28.1
prostate Q55.4
pulmonary
  arteriovenous Q25.72

Malformation — *continued*
pulmonary — *continued*
  artery Q25.9
    atresia Q25.5
    specified type NEC Q25.79
    stenosis Q25.6
  valve Q22.3
renal artery Q27.2
respiratory system Q34.9
retina Q14.1
scrotum — *see* Malformation, testis and scrotum
seminal vesicles Q55.4
sense organs NEC Q07.9
skin Q82.9
  specified NEC Q89.8
spinal
  cord Q06.9
  nerve root Q07.8
spine Q76.49
  kyphosis — *see* Kyphosis, congenital
  lordosis — *see* Lordosis, congenital
spleen Q89.09
stomach Q40.3
  specified type NEC Q40.2
teeth, tooth K00.9
tendon Q79.9
testis and scrotum Q55.20
  aplasia Q55.0
  hypoplasia Q55.1
  polyorchism Q55.21
  retractile testis Q55.22
  scrotal transposition Q55.23
  specified NEC Q55.29
thorax, bony Q76.9
throat Q38.8
thyroid gland Q89.2
tongue (congenital) Q38.3
  hypertrophy Q38.2
  tie Q38.1
trachea Q32.1
tricuspid valve Q22.9
  specified type NEC Q22.8
umbilical cord NEC (complicating delivery) O69.89 ☑
umbilicus Q89.9
ureter Q62.8
  agenesis Q62.4
  duplication Q62.5
  malposition — *see* Malposition, congenital, ureter
  obstructive defect — *see* Defect, obstructive, ureter
  vesico-uretero-renal reflux Q62.7
urethra Q64.79
  aplasia Q64.5
  duplication Q64.74
  posterior valves Q64.2
  prolapse Q64.71
  stricture Q64.32
urinary system Q64.9
uterus Q51.9
  specified type NEC Q51.818
vagina Q52.4
vas deferens Q55.4
  atresia Q55.3
vascular system, peripheral Q27.9
venous — *see* Anomaly, vein(s)
vulva Q52.70
Malfunction (*see also* Dysfunction)
cardiac electronic device T82.119 ☑
  electrode T82.110 ☑
  pulse generator T82.111 ☑
  specified type NEC T82.118 ☑
catheter device NEC T85.618 ☑
  cystostomy T83.010 ☑
  dialysis (renal) (vascular) T82.41 ☑
    intraperitoneal T85.611 ☑
  infusion NEC T82.514 ☑
    spinal (epidural) (subdural) T85.610 ☑
  urinary, indwelling T83.018 ☑
colostomy K94.03
  valve K94.03
cystostomy (stoma) N99.512
  catheter T83.010 ☑
enteric stoma K94.13
enterostomy K94.13
esophagostomy K94.33
gastroenteric K31.89
gastrostomy K94.23
ileostomy K94.13
  valve K94.13

Malfunction — *continued*
jejunostomy K94.13
pacemaker — *see* Malfunction, cardiac electronic device
prosthetic device, internal — *see* Complications,
  prosthetic device, by site, mechanical
tracheostomy J95.03
urinary device NEC — *see* Complication, genitourinary,
  device, urinary, mechanical
valve
  colostomy K94.03
  heart T82.09 ☑
  ileostomy K94.13
vascular graft or shunt NEC — *see* Complication, cardiovascular device, mechanical, vascular
ventricular (communicating shunt) T85.01 ☑
Malherbe's tumor — *see* Neoplasm, skin, benign
Malibu disease L98.8
Malignancy (*see also* Neoplasm, malignant, by site)
unspecified site (primary) C80.1
Malignant — *see* condition
Malingerer, malingering Z76.5
Mallet finger (acquired) — *see* Deformity, finger, mallet
  finger
congenital Q74.0
sequelae of rickets E64.3
Malleus A24.0
Mallory's bodies R89.7
Mallory-Weiss syndrome K22.6
Malnutrition E46
degree
  first E44.1
  mild (protein) E44.1
  moderate (protein) E44.0
  second E44.0
  severe (protein-energy) E43
    intermediate form E42
      with
        kwashiorkor (and marasmus) E42
        marasmus E41
  third E43
following gastrointestinal surgery K91.2
intrauterine
  light-for-dates — *see* Light for dates
  small-for-dates — *see* Small for dates
lack of care, or neglect (child) (infant) T76.02 ☑
  confirmed T74.02 ☑
malignant E40
protein E46
  calorie E46
    mild E44.1
    moderate E44.0
    severe E43
      intermediate form E42
        with
          kwashiorkor (and marasmus) E42
          marasmus E41
  energy E46
    mild E44.1
    moderate E44.0
    severe E43
      intermediate form E42
        with
          kwashiorkor (and marasmus) E42
          marasmus E41
severe (protein-energy) E43
  with
    kwashiorkor (and marasmus) E42
    marasmus E41
Malocclusion (teeth) M26.4
Angle's M26.219
  class I M26.211
  class II M26.212
  class III M26.213
due to
  abnormal swallowing M26.59
  mouth breathing M26.59
  tongue, lip or finger habits M26.59
temporomandibular (joint) M26.69
Malposition
cervix — *see* Malposition, uterus
congenital
  adrenal (gland) Q89.1
  alimentary tract Q45.8
    lower Q43.8
    upper Q40.8
  aorta Q25.4
  appendix Q43.8

☑ Additional Character Required — Refer to the Tabular List for Character Selection   ▽ Subterms under main terms may continue to next column or page

Malposition — *continued*
  congenital — *continued*
    arterial trunk Q20.0
    artery (peripheral) Q27.8
      coronary Q24.5
      digestive system Q27.8
      lower limb Q27.8
      pulmonary Q25.79
      specified site NEC Q27.8
      upper limb Q27.8
    auditory canal Q17.8
      causing impairment of hearing Q16.9
    auricle (ear) Q17.4
      causing impairment of hearing Q16.9
      cervical Q18.2
    biliary duct or passage Q44.5
    bladder (mucosa) — *see* Exstrophy, bladder
    brachial plexus Q07.8
    brain tissue Q04.8
    breast Q83.8
    bronchus Q32.4
    cecum Q43.8
    clavicle Q74.0
    colon Q43.8
    digestive organ or tract NEC Q45.8
      lower Q43.8
      upper Q40.8
    ear (auricle) (external) Q17.4
      ossicles Q16.3
    endocrine (gland) NEC Q89.2
    epiglottis Q31.8
    eustachian tube Q17.8
    eye Q15.8
    facial features Q18.8
    fallopian tube Q50.6
    finger(s) Q68.1
      supernumerary Q69.0
    foot Q66.9
    gallbladder Q44.1
    gastrointestinal tract Q45.8
    genitalia, genital organ(s) or tract
      female Q52.8
        external Q52.79
        internal NEC Q52.8
      male Q55.8
    glottis Q31.8
    hand Q68.1
    heart Q24.8
      dextrocardia Q24.0
        with complete transposition of viscera Q89.3
    hepatic duct Q44.5
    hip (joint) Q65.89
    intestine (large) (small) Q43.8
      with anomalous adhesions, fixation or malrotation Q43.3
    joint NEC Q68.8
    kidney Q63.2
    larynx Q31.8
    limb Q68.8
      lower Q68.8
      upper Q68.8
    liver Q44.7
    lung (lobe) Q33.8
    nail(s) Q84.6
    nerve Q07.8
    nervous system NEC Q07.8
    nose, nasal (septum) Q30.8
    organ or site not listed — *see* Anomaly, by site
    ovary Q50.39
    pancreas Q45.3
    parathyroid (gland) Q89.2
    patella Q74.1
    peripheral vascular system Q27.8
    pituitary (gland) Q89.2
    respiratory organ or system NEC Q34.8
    rib (cage) Q76.6
      supernumerary in cervical region Q76.5
    scapula Q74.0
    shoulder Q74.0
    spinal cord Q06.8
    spleen Q89.09
    sternum NEC Q76.7
    stomach Q40.2
    symphysis pubis Q74.2
    thymus (gland) Q89.2
    thyroid (gland) (tissue) Q89.2
      cartilage Q31.8

Malposition — *continued*
  congenital — *continued*
    toe(s) Q66.9
      supernumerary Q69.2
    tongue Q38.3
    trachea Q32.1
    ureter Q62.60
      deviation Q62.61
      displacement Q62.62
      ectopia Q62.63
      specified type NEC Q62.69
    uterus Q51.818
    vein(s) (peripheral) Q27.8
      great Q26.8
    vena cava (inferior) (superior) Q26.8
  device, implant or graft (*see also* Complications, by site and type, mechanical) T85.628 ☑
    arterial graft NEC — *see* Complication, cardiovascular device, mechanical, vascular
    breast (implant) T85.42 ☑
    catheter NEC T85.628 ☑
      cystostomy T83.020 ☑
      dialysis (renal) T82.42 ☑
        intraperitoneal T85.621 ☑
      infusion NEC T82.524 ☑
        spinal (epidural) (subdural) T85.620 ☑
      urinary, indwelling T83.028 ☑
    electronic (electrode) (pulse generator) (stimulator)
      bone T84.320 ☑
      cardiac T82.129 ☑
        electrode T82.120 ☑
        pulse generator T82.121 ☑
        specified type NEC T82.128 ☑
      nervous system — *see* Complication, prosthetic device, mechanical, electronic nervous system stimulator
      urinary — *see* Complication, genitourinary, device, urinary, mechanical
    fixation, internal (orthopedic) NEC — *see* Complication, fixation device, mechanical
    gastrointestinal — *see* Complications, prosthetic device, mechanical, gastrointestinal device
    genital NEC T83.428 ☑
      intrauterine contraceptive device T83.32 ☑
      penile prosthesis T83.420 ☑
    heart NEC — *see* Complication, cardiovascular device, mechanical
    joint prosthesis — *see* Complication, joint prosthesis, mechanical
    ocular NEC — *see* Complications, prosthetic device, mechanical, ocular device
    orthopedic NEC — *see* Complication, orthopedic, device, mechanical
    specified NEC T85.628 ☑
    urinary NEC (*see also* Complication, genitourinary, device, urinary, mechanical)
      graft T83.22 ☑
    vascular NEC — *see* Complication, cardiovascular device, mechanical
    ventricular intracranial shunt T85.02 ☑
  fetus — *see* Pregnancy, complicated by (management affected by), presentation, fetal
  gallbladder K82.8
  gastrointestinal tract, congenital Q45.8
  heart, congenital NEC Q24.8
  joint prosthesis — *see* Complications, joint prosthesis, mechanical, displacement, by site
  stomach K31.89
    congenital Q40.2
  tooth, teeth, fully erupted M26.30
  uterus (acute) (acquired) (adherent) (asymptomatic) (postinfectional) (postpartal, old) N85.4
    anteflexion or anteversion N85.4
      congenital Q51.818
    flexion N85.4
      lateral — *see* Lateroversion, uterus
    inversion N85.5
    lateral (flexion) (version) — *see* Lateroversion, uterus
      in pregnancy or childbirth — *see* subcategory O34.5 ☑
    retroflexion or retroversion — *see* Retroversion, uterus
Malposture R29.3
Malrotation
  cecum Q43.3
  colon Q43.3

Malrotation — *continued*
  intestine Q43.3
  kidney Q63.2
Malta fever — *see* Brucellosis
Maltreatment
  adult
    abandonment
      confirmed T74.01 ☑
      suspected T76.01 ☑
    confirmed T74.91 ☑
    history of Z91.419
    neglect
      confirmed T74.01 ☑
      suspected T76.01 ☑
    physical abuse
      confirmed T74.11 ☑
      suspected T76.11 ☑
    psychological abuse
      confirmed T74.31 ☑
      history of Z91.411
      suspected T76.31 ☑
    sexual abuse
      confirmed T74.21 ☑
      suspected T76.21 ☑
    suspected T76.91 ☑
  child
    abandonment
      confirmed T74.02 ☑
      suspected T76.02 ☑
    confirmed T74.92 ☑
    history of — *see* History, personal (of), abuse
    neglect
      confirmed T74.02 ☑
      history of — *see* History, personal (of), abuse
      suspected T76.02 ☑
    physical abuse
      confirmed T74.12 ☑
      history of — *see* History, personal (of), abuse
      suspected T76.12 ☑
    psychological abuse
      confirmed T74.32 ☑
      history of — *see* History, personal (of), abuse
      suspected T76.32 ☑
    sexual abuse
      confirmed T74.22 ☑
      history of — *see* History, personal (of), abuse
      suspected T76.22 ☑
    suspected T76.92 ☑
  personal history of Z91.89
Maltworker's lung J67.4
Malunion, fracture — *see* Fracture, by site
Mammillitis N61
  puerperal, postpartum O91.02
Mammitis — *see* Mastitis
Mammogram (examination) Z12.39
  routine Z12.31
Mammoplasia N62
Management (of)
  bone conduction hearing device (implanted) Z45.320
  cardiac pacemaker NEC Z45.018
  cerebrospinal fluid drainage device Z45.41
  cochlear device (implanted) Z45.321
  contraceptive Z30.9
    specified NEC Z30.8
  implanted device Z45.9
    specified NEC Z45.89
  infusion pump Z45.1
  procreative Z31.9
    male factor infertility in female Z31.81
    specified NEC Z31.89
  prosthesis (external) (*see also* Fitting) Z44.9
    implanted Z45.9
      specified NEC Z45.89
  renal dialysis catheter Z49.01
  vascular access device Z45.2
Mangled — *see* specified injury by site
Mania (monopolar) (*see also* Disorder, mood, manic episode)
  with psychotic symptoms F30.2
  without psychotic symptoms F30.10
    mild F30.11
    moderate F30.12
    severe F30.13
  Bell's F30.8
  chronic (recurrent) F31.89
  hysterical F44.89
  puerperal F30.8

Mania — *continued*
  recurrent F31.89
Manic-depressive insanity, psychosis, or syndrome — *see* Disorder, bipolar
Mannosidosis E77.1
Mansonelliasis, mansonellosis B74.4
Manson's
  disease B65.1
  schistosomiasis B65.1
Manual — *see* condition
Maple-bark-stripper's lung (disease) J67.6
Maple-syrup-urine disease E71.0
Marable's syndrome (celiac artery compression) I77.4
Marasmus E41
  due to malnutrition E41
  intestinal E41
  nutritional E41
  senile R54
  tuberculous NEC — *see* Tuberculosis
Marble
  bones Q78.2
  skin R23.8
Marburg virus disease A98.3
March
  fracture — *see* Fracture, traumatic, stress, by site
  hemoglobinuria D59.6
Marchesani (-Weill) **syndrome** Q87.0
Marchiafava (-Bignami) **syndrome or disease** G37.1
Marchiafava-Micheli syndrome D59.5
Marcus Gunn's syndrome Q07.8
Marfan's syndrome — *see* Syndrome, Marfan's
Marie-Bamberger disease — *see* Osteoarthropathy, hypertrophic, specified NEC
Marie-Charcot-Tooth neuropathic muscular atrophy G60.0
Marie's
  cerebellar ataxia (late-onset) G11.2
  disease or syndrome (acromegaly) E22.0
Marie-Strümpell arthritis, disease or spondylitis — *see* Spondylitis, ankylosing
Marion's disease (bladder neck obstruction) N32.0
Marital conflict Z63.0
Mark
  port wine Q82.5
  raspberry Q82.5
  strawberry Q82.5
  stretch L90.6
  tattoo L81.8
Marker heterochromatin — *see* Extra, marker chromosomes
Maroteaux-Lamy syndrome (mild) (severe) E76.29
Marrow (bone)
  arrest D61.9
  poor function D75.89
Marseilles fever A77.1
Marsh fever — *see* Malaria
Marshall's (hidrotic) **ectodermal dysplasia** Q82.4
Marsh's disease (exophthalmic goiter) E05.00
  with storm E05.01
Masculinization (female) **with adrenal hyperplasia** E25.9
  congenital E25.0
Masculinovoblastoma D27.- ☑
Masochism (sexual) F65.51
Mason's lung J62.8
Mass
  abdominal R19.00
    epigastric R19.06
    generalized R19.07
    left lower quadrant R19.04
    left upper quadrant R19.02
    periumbilic R19.05
    right lower quadrant R19.03
    right upper quadrant R19.01
    specified site NEC R19.09
  breast N63
  chest R22.2
  cystic — *see* Cyst
  ear H93.8- ☑
  head R22.0
  intra-abdominal (diffuse) (generalized) — *see* Mass, abdominal
  kidney N28.89
  liver R16.0
  localized (skin) R22.9
    chest R22.2
    head R22.0

Mass — *continued*
  localized — *continued*
    limb
      lower R22.4- ☑
      upper R22.3- ☑
    neck R22.1
    trunk R22.2
  lung R91.8
  malignant — *see* Neoplasm, malignant, by site
  neck R22.1
  pelvic (diffuse) (generalized) — *see* Mass, abdominal
  specified organ NEC — *see* Disease, by site
  splenic R16.1
  substernal thyroid — *see* Goiter
  superficial (localized) R22.9
  umbilical (diffuse) (generalized) R19.09
Massive — *see* condition
Mast cell
  disease, systemic tissue D47.0
  leukemia C94.3- ☑
  sarcoma C96.2
  tumor D47.0
    malignant C96.2
Mastalgia N64.4
Masters-Allen syndrome N83.8
Mastitis (acute) (diffuse) (nonpuerperal) (subacute) N61
  chronic (cystic) — *see* Mastopathy, cystic
  cystic (Schimmelbusch's type) — *see* Mastopathy, cystic
  fibrocystic — *see* Mastopathy, cystic
  infective N61
    newborn P39.0
  interstitial, gestational or puerperal — *see* Mastitis, obstetric
  neonatal (noninfective) P83.4
    infective P39.0
  obstetric (interstitial) (nonpurulent)
    associated with
      lactation O91.23
      pregnancy O91.21- ☑
      puerperium O91.22
    purulent
      associated with
        lactation O91.13
        pregnancy O91.11- ☑
        puerperium O91.12
  periductal — *see* Ectasia, mammary duct
  phlegmonous — *see* Mastopathy, cystic
  plasma cell — *see* Ectasia, mammary duct
Mastocytoma D47.0
  malignant C96.2
Mastocytosis Q82.2
  aggressive systemic C96.2
  indolent systemic D47.0
  malignant C96.2
  systemic, associated with clonal hematopoetic non-mast-cell disease (SM-AHNMD) D47.0
Mastodynia N64.4
Mastoid — *see* condition
Mastoidalgia — *see* subcategory H92.0 ☑
Mastoiditis (coalescent) (hemorrhagic) (suppurative) H70.9- ☑
  acute, subacute H70.00- ☑
    complicated NEC H70.09- ☑
    subperiosteal H70.01- ☑
  chronic (necrotic) (recurrent) H70.1- ☑
  in (due to)
    infectious disease NEC B99 ☑ [H75.0-] ☑
    parasitic disease NEC B89 [H75.0-] ☑
    tuberculosis A18.03
  petrositis — *see* Petrositis
  postauricular fistula — *see* Fistula, postauricular
  specified NEC H70.89- ☑
  tuberculous A18.03
Mastopathy, mastopathia N64.9
  chronica cystica — *see* Mastopathy, cystic
  cystic (chronic) (diffuse) N60.1- ☑
    with epithelial proliferation N60.3- ☑
  diffuse cystic — *see* Mastopathy, cystic
  estrogenic, oestrogenica N64.89
  ovarian origin N64.89
Mastoplasia, mastoplastia N62
Masturbation (excessive) F98.8
Maternal care (for) — *see* Pregnancy (complicated by) (management affected by)
Matheiu's disease (leptospiral jaundice) A27.0

Mauclaire's disease or osteochondrosis — *see* Osteochondrosis, juvenile, hand, metacarpal
Maxcy's disease A75.2
Maxilla, maxillary — *see* condition
May (-Hegglin) **anomaly or syndrome** D72.0
McArdle (-Schmid)(-Pearson) **disease** (glycogen storage) E74.04
McCune-Albright syndrome Q78.1
McQuarrie's syndrome (idiopathic familial hypoglycemia) E16.2
Meadow's syndrome Q86.1
Measles (black) (hemorrhagic) (suppressed) B05.9
  with
    complications NEC B05.89
    encephalitis B05.0
    intestinal complications B05.4
    keratitis (keratoconjunctivitis) B05.81
    meningitis B05.1
    otitis media B05.3
    pneumonia B05.2
  French — *see* Rubella
  German — *see* Rubella
  Liberty — *see* Rubella
Meatitis, urethral — *see* Urethritis
Meatus, meatal — *see* condition
Meat-wrappers' asthma J68.9
Meckel-Gruber syndrome Q61.9
Meckel's diverticulitis, diverticulum (displaced) (hypertrophic) Q43.0
  malignant — *see* Table of Neoplasms, small intestine, malignant
Meconium
  ileus, newborn P76.0
    in cystic fibrosis E84.11
    meaning meconium plug (without cystic fibrosis) P76.0
  obstruction, newborn P76.0
    due to fecaliths P76.0
    in mucoviscidosis E84.11
  peritonitis P78.0
  plug syndrome (newborn) NEC P76.0
Median (*see also* condition)
  arcuate ligament syndrome I77.4
  bar (prostate) (vesical orifice) — *see* Hyperplasia, prostate
  rhomboid glossitis K14.2
Mediastinal shift R93.8
Mediastinitis (acute) (chronic) J98.5
  syphilitic A52.73
  tuberculous A15.8
Mediastinopericarditis (*see also* Pericarditis)
  acute I30.9
  adhesive I31.0
  chronic I31.8
  rheumatic I09.2
Mediastinum, mediastinal — *see* condition
Medicine poisoning — *see* Table of Drugs and Chemicals, by drug, poisoning
Mediterranean
  fever — *see* Brucellosis
    familial E85.0
    tick A77.1
  kala-azar B55.0
  leishmaniasis B55.0
  tick fever A77.1
Medulla — *see* condition
Medullary cystic kidney Q61.5
Medullated fibers
  optic (nerve) Q14.8
  retina Q14.1
Medulloblastoma
  desmoplastic C71.6
  specified site — *see* Neoplasm, malignant, by site
  unspecified site C71.6
Medulloepithelioma (*see also* Neoplasm, malignant, by site)
  teratoid — *see* Neoplasm, malignant, by site
Medullomyoblastoma
  specified site — *see* Neoplasm, malignant, by site
  unspecified site C71.6
Meekeren-Ehlers-Danlos syndrome Q79.6
Megacolon (acquired) (functional) (not Hirschsprung's disease) (in) K59.3
  Chagas' disease B57.32
  congenital, congenitum (aganglionic) Q43.1
  Hirschsprung's (disease) Q43.1

Megacolon — *continued*
    toxic NEC K59.3
        due to Clostridium difficile A04.7
Megaesophagus (functional) K22.0
    congenital Q39.5
    in (due to) Chagas' disease B57.31
Megalencephaly Q04.5
Megalerythema (epidemic) B08.3
Megaloappendix Q43.8
Megalocephalus, megalocephaly NEC Q75.3
Megalocornea Q15.8
    with glaucoma Q15.0
Megalocytic anemia D53.1
Megalodactylia (fingers) (thumbs) (congenital) Q74.0
    toes Q74.2
Megaloduodenum Q43.8
Megaloesophagus (functional) K22.0
    congenital Q39.5
Megalogastria (acquired) K31.89
    congenital Q40.2
Megalophthalmos Q11.3
Megalopsia H53.15
Megalosplenia — *see* Splenomegaly
Megaloureter N28.82
    congenital Q62.2
Megarectum K62.89
Megasigmoid K59.3
    congenital Q43.2
Megaureter N28.82
    congenital Q62.2
Megavitamin-B6 syndrome E67.2
Megrim — *see* Migraine
Meibomian
    cyst, infected — *see* Hordeolum
    gland — *see* condition
    sty, stye — *see* Hordeolum
Meibomitis — *see* Hordeolum
Meige-Milroy disease (chronic hereditary edema) Q82.0
Meige's syndrome Q82.0
Melalgia, nutritional E53.8
Melancholia F32.9
    climacteric (single episode) F32.8
        recurrent episode F33.9
    hypochondriac F45.29
    intermittent (single episode) F32.8
        recurrent episode F33.9
    involutional (single episode) F32.8
        recurrent episode F33.9
    menopausal (single episode) F32.8
        recurrent episode F33.9
    puerperal F32.8
    reactive (emotional stress or trauma) F32.3
    recurrent F33.9
    senile F03 ☑
    stuporous (single episode) F32.8
        recurrent episode F33.9
Melanemia R79.89
Melanoameloblastoma — *see* Neoplasm, bone, benign
Melanoblastoma — *see* Melanoma
Melanocarcinoma — *see* Melanoma
Melanocytoma, eyeball D31.4- ☑
Melanocytosis, neurocutaneous Q82.8
Melanoderma, melanodermia L81.4
Melanodontia, infantile K03.89
Melanodontoclasia K03.89
Melanoepithelioma — *see* Melanoma
Melanoma (malignant) C43.9
    acral lentiginous, malignant — *see* Melanoma, skin, by site
    amelanotic — *see* Melanoma, skin, by site
    balloon cell — *see* Melanoma, skin, by site
    benign — *see* Nevus
    desmoplastic, malignant — *see* Melanoma, skin, by site
    epithelioid cell — *see* Melanoma, skin, by site
        with spindle cell, mixed — *see* Melanoma, skin, by site
    in
        giant pigmented nevus — *see* Melanoma, skin, by site
        Hutchinson's melanotic freckle — *see* Melanoma, skin, by site
        junctional nevus — *see* Melanoma, skin, by site
        precancerous melanosis — *see* Melanoma, skin, by site
    in situ D03.9
        abdominal wall D03.59

Melanoma — *continued*
    in situ — *continued*
        ala nasi D03.39
        ankle D03.7- ☑
        anus, anal (margin) (skin) D03.51
        arm D03.6- ☑
        auditory canal D03.2- ☑
        auricle (ear) D03.2- ☑
        auricular canal (external) D03.2- ☑
        axilla, axillary fold D03.59
        back D03.59
        breast D03.52
        brow D03.39
        buttock D03.59
        canthus (eye) D03.1- ☑
        cheek (external) D03.39
        chest wall D03.59
        chin D03.39
        choroid D03.8
        conjunctiva D03.8
        ear (external) D03.2- ☑
        external meatus (ear) D03.2- ☑
        eye D03.8
        eyebrow D03.39
        eyelid (lower) (upper) D03.1- ☑
        face D03.30
            specified NEC D03.39
        female genital organ (external) NEC D03.8
        finger D03.6- ☑
        flank D03.59
        foot D03.7- ☑
        forearm D03.6- ☑
        forehead D03.39
        foreskin D03.8
        gluteal region D03.59
        groin D03.59
        hand D03.6- ☑
        heel D03.7- ☑
        helix D03.2- ☑
        hip D03.7- ☑
        interscapular region D03.59
        iris D03.8
        jaw D03.39
        knee D03.7- ☑
        labium (majus) (minus) D03.8
        lacrimal gland D03.8
        leg D03.7- ☑
        lip (lower) (upper) D03.0
        lower limb NEC D03.7- ☑
        male genital organ (external) NEC D03.8
        nail D03.9
            finger D03.6- ☑
            toe D03.7- ☑
        neck D03.4
        nose (external) D03.39
        orbit D03.8
        penis D03.8
        perianal skin D03.51
        perineum D03.51
        pinna D03.2- ☑
        popliteal fossa or space D03.7- ☑
        prepuce D03.8
        pudendum D03.8
        retina D03.8
        retrobulbar D03.8
        scalp D03.4
        scrotum D03.8
        shoulder D03.6- ☑
        specified site NEC D03.8
        submammary fold D03.52
        temple D03.39
        thigh D03.7- ☑
        toe D03.7- ☑
        trunk NEC D03.59
        umbilicus D03.59
        upper limb NEC D03.6- ☑
        vulva D03.8
    juvenile — *see* Nevus
    malignant, of soft parts except skin — *see* Neoplasm, connective tissue, malignant
    metastatic
        breast C79.81
        genital organ C79.82
        specified site NEC C79.89
    neurotropic, malignant — *see* Melanoma, skin, by site
    nodular — *see* Melanoma, skin, by site
    regressing, malignant — *see* Melanoma, skin, by site

Melanoma — *continued*
    skin C43.9
        abdominal wall C43.59
        ala nasi C43.31
        ankle C43.7- ☑
        anus, anal (skin) C43.51
        arm C43.6- ☑
        auditory canal (external) C43.2- ☑
        auricle (ear) C43.2- ☑
        auricular canal (external) C43.2- ☑
        axilla, axillary fold C43.59
        back C43.59
        breast (female) (male) C43.52
        brow C43.39
        buttock C43.59
        canthus (eye) C43.1- ☑
        cheek (external) C43.39
        chest wall C43.59
        chin C43.39
        ear (external) C43.2- ☑
        elbow C43.6- ☑
        external meatus (ear) C43.2- ☑
        eyebrow C43.39
        eyelid (lower) (upper) C43.1- ☑
        face C43.30
            specified NEC C43.39
        female genital organ (external) NEC C51.9
        finger C43.6- ☑
        flank C43.59
        foot C43.7- ☑
        forearm C43.6- ☑
        forehead C43.39
        foreskin C60.0
        glabella C43.39
        gluteal region C43.59
        groin C43.59
        hand C43.6- ☑
        heel C43.7- ☑
        helix C43.2- ☑
        hip C43.7- ☑
        interscapular region C43.59
        jaw (external) C43.39
        knee C43.7- ☑
        labium C51.9
            majus C51.0
            minus C51.1
        leg C43.7- ☑
        lip (lower) (upper) C43.0
        lower limb NEC C43.7- ☑
        male genital organ (external) NEC C63.9
        nail
            finger C43.6- ☑
            toe C43.7- ☑
        nasolabial groove C43.39
        nates C43.59
        neck C43.4
        nose (external) C43.31
        overlapping site C43.8
        palpebra C43.1- ☑
        penis C60.9
        perianal skin C43.51
        perineum C43.51
        pinna C43.2- ☑
        popliteal fossa or space C43.7- ☑
        prepuce C60.0
        pudendum C51.9
        scalp C43.4
        scrotum C63.2
        shoulder C43.6- ☑
        skin NEC C43.9
        submammary fold C43.52
        temple C43.39
        thigh C43.7- ☑
        toe C43.7- ☑
        trunk NEC C43.59
        umbilicus C43.59
        upper limb NEC C43.6- ☑
        vulva C51.9
            overlapping sites C51.8
    spindle cell
        with epithelioid, mixed — *see* Melanoma, skin, by site
        type A C69.4- ☑
        type B C69.4- ☑
    superficial spreading — *see* Melanoma, skin, by site
Melanosarcoma (*see also* Melanoma)
    epithelioid cell — *see* Melanoma

Melanosis L81.4
  addisonian E27.1
    tuberculous A18.7
  adrenal E27.1
  colon K63.89
  conjunctiva — *see* Pigmentation, conjunctiva
    congenital Q13.89
  cornea (presenile) (senile) (*see also* Pigmentation, cornea)
    congenital Q13.4
  eye NEC H57.8
    congenital Q15.8
  lenticularis progressiva Q82.1
  liver K76.89
  precancerous (*see also* Melanoma, in situ)
    malignant melanoma in — *see* Melanoma
  Riehl's L81.4
  sclera H15.89
    congenital Q13.89
  suprarenal E27.1
  tar L81.4
  toxic L81.4
Melanuria R82.99
MELAS syndrome E88.41
Melasma L81.1
  adrenal (gland) E27.1
  suprarenal (gland) E27.1
Melena K92.1
  with ulcer — *code by* site under Ulcer, with hemorrhage K27.4
  due to swallowed maternal blood P78.2
  newborn, neonatal P54.1
    due to swallowed maternal blood P78.2
Meleney's
  gangrene (cutaneous) — *see* Ulcer, skin
  ulcer (chronic undermining) — *see* Ulcer, skin
Melioidosis A24.9
  acute A24.1
  chronic A24.2
  fulminating A24.1
  pneumonia A24.1
  pulmonary (chronic) A24.2
    acute A24.1
    subacute A24.2
  sepsis A24.1
  specified NEC A24.3
  subacute A24.2
Melitensis, febris A23.0
Melkersson (-Rosenthal) **syndrome** G51.2
Mellitus, diabetes — *see* Diabetes
Melorheostosis (bone) — *see* Disorder, bone, density and structure, specified NEC
Meloschisis Q18.4
Melotia Q17.4
Membrana
  capsularis lentis posterior Q13.89
  epipapillaris Q14.2
Membranacea placenta O43.19- ☑
Membranaceous uterus N85.8
Membrane(s), membranous (*see also* condition)
  cyclitic — *see* Membrane, pupillary
  folds, congenital — *see* Web
  Jackson's Q43.3
  over face of newborn P28.9
  premature rupture — *see* Rupture, membranes, premature
  pupillary H21.4- ☑
    persistent Q13.89
  retained (with hemorrhage) (complicating delivery) O72.2
    without hemorrhage O73.1
  secondary cataract — *see* Cataract, secondary
  unruptured (causing asphyxia) — *see* Asphyxia, newborn
  vitreous — *see* Opacity, vitreous, membranes and strands
Membranitis — *see* Chorioamnionitis
Memory disturbance, lack or loss (*see also* Amnesia)
  mild, following organic brain damage F06.8
Menadione deficiency E56.1
Menarche
  delayed E30.0
  precocious E30.1
Mendacity, pathologic F60.2
Mendelson's syndrome (due to anesthesia) J95.4
  in labor and delivery O74.0
  in pregnancy O29.01- ☑

Mendelson's syndrome — *continued*
  obstetric O74.0
  postpartum, puerperal O89.01
Ménétrier's disease or syndrome K29.60
  with bleeding K29.61
Ménière's disease, syndrome or vertigo H81.0- ☑
Meninges, meningeal — *see* condition
Meningioma (*see also* Neoplasm, meninges, benign)
  angioblastic — *see* Neoplasm, meninges, benign
  angiomatous — *see* Neoplasm, meninges, benign
  endotheliomatous — *see* Neoplasm, meninges, benign
  fibroblastic — *see* Neoplasm, meninges, benign
  fibrous — *see* Neoplasm, meninges, benign
  hemangioblastic — *see* Neoplasm, meninges, benign
  hemangiopericytic — *see* Neoplasm, meninges, benign
  malignant — *see* Neoplasm, meninges, malignant
  meningiothelial — *see* Neoplasm, meninges, benign
  meningotheliomatous — *see* Neoplasm, meninges, benign
  mixed — *see* Neoplasm, meninges, benign
  multiple — *see* Neoplasm, meninges, uncertain behavior
  papillary — *see* Neoplasm, meninges, uncertain behavior
  psammomatous — *see* Neoplasm, meninges, benign
  syncytial — *see* Neoplasm, meninges, benign
  transitional — *see* Neoplasm, meninges, benign
Meningiomatosis (diffuse) — *see* Neoplasm, meninges, uncertain behavior
Meningism — *see* Meningismus
Meningismus (infectional) (pneumococcal) R29.1
  due to serum or vaccine R29.1
  influenzal — *see* Influenza, with, manifestations NEC
Meningitis (basal) (basic) (brain) (cerebral) (cervical) (congestive) (diffuse) (hemorrhagic) (infantile) (membranous) (metastatic) (nonspecific) (pontine) (progressive) (simple) (spinal) (subacute) (sympathetic) (toxic) G03.9
  abacterial G03.0
  actinomycotic A42.81
  adenoviral A87.1
  arbovirus A87.8
  aseptic (acute) G03.0
  bacterial G00.9
    Escherichia coli (E. coli) G00.8
    Friedländer (bacillus) G00.8
    gram-negative G00.9
    H. influenzae G00.0
    Klebsiella G00.8
    pneumococcal G00.1
    specified organism NEC G00.8
    staphylococcal G00.3
    streptococcal (acute) G00.2
  benign recurrent (Mollaret) G03.2
  candidal B37.5
  caseous (tuberculous) A17.0
  cerebrospinal A39.0
  chronic NEC G03.1
  clear cerebrospinal fluid NEC G03.0
  coxsackievirus A87.0
  cryptococcal B45.1
  diplococcal (gram positive) A39.0
  echovirus A87.0
  enteroviral A87.0
  eosinophilic B83.2
  epidemic NEC A39.0
  Escherichia coli (E. coli) G00.8
  fibrinopurulent G00.9
    specified organism NEC G00.8
  Friedländer (bacillus) G00.8
  gonococcal A54.81
  gram-negative cocci G00.9
  gram-positive cocci G00.9
  H. influenzae G00.0
  Haemophilus (influenzae) G00.0
  in (due to)
    adenovirus A87.1
    African trypanosomiasis B56.9 [G02]
    anthrax A22.8
    bacterial disease NEC A48.8 [G01]
    Chagas' disease (chronic) B57.41
    chickenpox B01.0
    coccidioidomycosis B38.4
    Diplococcus pneumoniae G00.1
    enterovirus A87.0
    herpes (simplex) virus B00.3
      zoster B02.1

Meningitis — *continued*
  in — *continued*
    infectious mononucleosis B27.92
    leptospirosis A27.81
    Listeria monocytogenes A32.11
    Lyme disease A69.21
    measles B05.1
    mumps (virus) B26.1
    neurosyphilis (late) A52.13
    parasitic disease NEC B89 [G02]
    poliovirus A80.9 [G02]
    preventive immunization, inoculation or vaccination G03.8
    rubella B06.02
    Salmonella infection A02.21
    specified cause NEC G03.8
    typhoid fever A01.01
    varicella B01.0
    viral disease NEC A87.8
    whooping cough A37.90
    zoster B02.1
  infectious G00.9
  influenzal (H. influenzae) G00.0
  Klebsiella G00.8
  leptospiral (aseptic) A27.81
  lymphocytic (acute) (benign) (serous) A87.2
  meningococcal A39.0
  Mima polymorpha G00.8
  Mollaret (benign recurrent) G03.2
  monilial B37.5
  mycotic NEC B49 [G02]
  Neisseria A39.0
  nonbacterial G03.0
  nonpyogenic NEC G03.0
  ossificans G96.19
  pneumococcal G00.1
  poliovirus A80.9 [G02]
  postmeasles B05.1
  purulent G00.9
    specified organism NEC G00.8
  pyogenic G00.9
    specified organism NEC G00.8
  Salmonella (arizonae) (Cholerae-Suis) (enteritidis) (typhimurium) A02.21
  septic G00.9
    specified organism NEC G00.8
  serosa circumscripta NEC G03.0
  serous NEC G93.2
  specified organism NEC G00.8
  sporotrichosis B42.81
  staphylococcal G00.3
  sterile G03.0
  streptococcal (acute) G00.2
  suppurative G00.9
    specified organism NEC G00.8
  syphilitic (late) (tertiary) A52.13
    acute A51.41
    congenital A50.41
    secondary A51.41
  Torula histolytica (cryptococcal) B45.1
  traumatic (complication of injury) T79.8 ☑
  tuberculous A17.0
  typhoid A01.01
  viral NEC A87.9
  Yersinia pestis A20.3
Meningocele (spinal) (*see also* Spina bifida)
  with hydrocephalus — *see* Spina bifida, by site, with hydrocephalus
  acquired (traumatic) G96.19
  cerebral — *see* Encephalocele
Meningocerebritis — *see* Meningoencephalitis
Meningococcemia A39.4
  acute A39.2
  chronic A39.3
Meningococcus, meningococcal (*see also* condition) A39.9
  adrenalitis, hemorrhagic A39.1
  carrier (suspected) of Z22.31
  meningitis (cerebrospinal) A39.0
Meningoencephalitis (*see also* Encephalitis) G04.90
  acute NEC (*see also* Encephalitis, viral) A86
  bacterial NEC G04.2
  California A83.5
  diphasic A84.1
  eosinophilic B83.2
  epidemic A39.81
  herpesviral, herpetic B00.4
    due to herpesvirus 6 B10.01

Meningoencephalitis — *continued*
  herpesviral, herpetic — *continued*
    due to herpesvirus 7 B10.09
    specified NEC B10.09
  in (due to)
    blastomycosis NEC B40.81
    diseases classified elsewhere G05.3
    free-living amebae B60.2
    H. influenzae G00.0
    Hemophilus influenzae (H .influenzae) G04.2
    herpes B00.4
      due to herpesvirus 6 B10.01
      due to herpesvirus 7 B10.09
      specified NEC B10.09
    Lyme disease A69.22
    mercury — *see* subcategory T56.1 ☑
    mumps B26.2
    Naegleria (amebae) (organisms) (fowleri) B60.2
    Parastrongylus cantonensis B83.2
    toxoplasmosis (acquired) B58.2
      congenital P37.1
  infectious (acute) (viral) A86
  influenzal (H. influenzae) G04.2
  Listeria monocytogenes A32.12
  lymphocytic (serous) A87.2
  mumps B26.2
  parasitic NEC B89 [G05.3]
  pneumococcal G00.1
  primary amebic B60.2
  specific (syphilitic) A52.14
  specified organism NEC G04.81
  staphylococcal G04.2
  streptococcal G04.2
  syphilitic A52.14
  toxic NEC G92
    due to mercury — *see* subcategory T56.1 ☑
  tuberculous A17.82
  virus NEC A86
Meningoencephalocele (*see also* Encephalocele)
  syphilitic A52.19
    congenital A50.49
Meningoencephalomyelitis (*see also* Meningoen-cephalitis)
  acute NEC (viral) A86
    disseminated G04.00
      postimmunization or postvaccination G04.02
      postinfectious G04.01
  due to
    actinomycosis A42.82
    Torula B45.1
    Toxoplasma or toxoplasmosis (acquired) B58.2
      congenital P37.1
  postimmunization or postvaccination G04.02
Meningoencephalomyelopathy G96.9
Meningoencephalopathy G96.9
Meningomyelitis (*see also* Meningoencephalitis)
  bacterial NEC G04.2
  blastomycotic NEC B40.81
  cryptococcal B45.1
  in diseases classified elsewhere G05.4
  meningococcal A39.81
  syphilitic A52.14
  tuberculous A17.82
Meningomyelocele (*see also* Spina bifida)
  syphilitic A52.19
Meningomyeloneuritis — *see* Meningoencephalitis
Meningoradiculitis — *see* Meningitis
Meningovascular — *see* condition
Menkes' disease or syndrome E83.09
  meaning maple-syrup-urine disease E71.0
Menometrorrhagia N92.1
Menopause, menopausal (asymptomatic) (state) Z78.0
  arthritis (any site) NEC — *see* Arthritis, specified form NEC
  bleeding N92.4
  depression (single episode) F32.8
    agitated (single episode) F32.2
      recurrent episode F33.9
    psychotic (single episode) F32.8
      recurrent episode F33.9
    recurrent episode F33.9
  melancholia (single episode) F32.8
    recurrent episode F33.9
  paranoid state F22
  premature E28.319
    asymptomatic E28.319
      postirradiation E89.40
      postsurgical E89.40

Menopause, menopausal — *continued*
  premature — *continued*
    symptomatic E28.310
      postirradiation E89.41
      postsurgical E89.41
  psychosis NEC F28
  symptomatic N95.1
  toxic polyarthritis NEC — *see* Arthritis, specified form NEC
Menorrhagia (primary) N92.0
  climacteric N92.4
    menopausal N92.4
  menopausal N92.4
  postclimacteric N95.0
  postmenopausal N95.0
  preclimacteric or premenopausal N92.4
  pubertal (menses retained) N92.2
Menostaxis N92.0
Menses, retention N94.89
Menstrual — *see* Menstruation
Menstruation
  absent — *see* Amenorrhea
  anovulatory N97.0
  cycle, irregular N92.6
  delayed N91.0
  disorder N93.9
    psychogenic F45.8
  during pregnancy O20.8
  excessive (with regular cycle) N92.0
    with irregular cycle N92.1
    at puberty N92.2
  frequent N92.0
  infrequent — *see* Oligomenorrhea
  irregular N92.6
    specified NEC N92.5
  latent N92.5
  membranous N92.5
  painful (*see also* Dysmenorrhea) N94.6
    primary N94.4
    psychogenic F45.8
    secondary N94.5
  passage of clots N92.0
  precocious E30.1
  protracted N92.5
  rare — *see* Oligomenorrhea
  retained N94.89
  retrograde N92.5
  scanty — *see* Oligomenorrhea
  suppression N94.89
  vicarious (nasal) N94.89
Mental (*see also* condition)
  deficiency — *see* Disability, intellectual
  deterioration — *see* Psychosis
  disorder — *see* Disorder, mental
  exhaustion F48.8
  insufficiency (congenital) — *see* Disability, intellectual
  observation without need for further medical care Z03.89
  retardation — *see* Disability, intellectual
  subnormality — *see* Disability, intellectuall
  upset — *see* Disorder, mental
Meralgia paresthetica G57.1- ☑
Mercurial — *see* condition
Mercurialism — *see* subcategory T56.1 ☑
Merkel cell tumor — *see* Carcinoma, Merkel cell
Merocele — *see* Hernia, femoral
Meromelia
  lower limb — *see* Defect, reduction, lower limb
    intercalary
      femur — *see* Defect, reduction, lower limb, specified type NEC
      tibiofibular (complete) (incomplete) — *see* Defect, reduction, lower limb
  upper limb — *see* Defect, reduction, upper limb
    intercalary, humeral, radioulnar — *see* Agenesis, arm, with hand present
MERRF syndrome (myoclonic epilepsy associated with ragged-red fiber) E88.42
Merzbacher-Pelizaeus disease E75.29
Mesaortitis — *see* Aortitis
Mesarteritis — *see* Arteritis
Mesencephalitis — *see* Encephalitis
Mesenchymoma (*see also* Neoplasm, connective tissue, uncertain behavior)
  benign — *see* Neoplasm, connective tissue, benign
  malignant — *see* Neoplasm, connective tissue, malignant

Mesenteritis
  retractile K65.4
  sclerosing K65.4
Mesentery, mesenteric — *see* condition
Mesiodens, mesiodentes K00.1
Mesio-occlusion M26.213
Mesocolon — *see* condition
Mesonephroma (malignant) — *see* Neoplasm, malignant, by site
  benign — *see* Neoplasm, benign, by site
Mesophlebitis — *see* Phlebitis
Mesostromal dysgenesia Q13.89
Mesothelioma (malignant) C45.9
  benign
    mesentery D19.1
    mesocolon D19.1
    omentum D19.1
    peritoneum D19.1
    pleura D19.0
    specified site NEC D19.7
    unspecified site D19.9
  biphasic C45.9
    benign
      mesentery D19.1
      mesocolon D19.1
      omentum D19.1
      peritoneum D19.1
      pleura D19.0
      specified site NEC D19.7
      unspecified site D19.9
  cystic D48.4
  epithelioid C45.9
    benign
      mesentery D19.1
      mesocolon D19.1
      omentum D19.1
      peritoneum D19.1
      pleura D19.0
      specified site NEC D19.7
      unspecified site D19.9
  fibrous C45.9
    benign
      mesentery D19.1
      mesocolon D19.1
      omentum D19.1
      peritoneum D19.1
      pleura D19.0
      specified site NEC D19.7
      unspecified site D19.9
  site classification
    liver C45.7
    lung C45.7
    mediastinum C45.7
    mesentery C45.1
    mesocolon C45.1
    omentum C45.1
    pericardium C45.2
    peritoneum C45.1
    pleura C45.0
      parietal C45.0
    retroperitoneum C45.7
    specified site NEC C45.7
    unspecified C45.9
Metabolic syndrome E88.81
Metagonimiasis B66.8
Metagonimus infestation (intestine) B66.8
Metal
  pigmentation L81.8
  polisher's disease J62.8
Metamorphopsia H53.15
Metaplasia
  apocrine (breast) — *see* Dysplasia, mammary, specified type NEC
  cervix (squamous) — *see* Dysplasia, cervix
  endometrium (squamous) (uterus) N85.8
  esophagus
  kidney (pelvis) (squamous) N28.89
  myelogenous D73.1
  myeloid (agnogenic) (megakaryocytic) D73.1
  spleen D73.1
  squamous cell, bladder N32.89
Metastasis, metastatic
  abscess — *see* Abscess
  calcification E83.59
  cancer
    from specified site — *see* Neoplasm, malignant, by site

Metastasis, metastatic — *continued*
   cancer — *continued*
      to specified site — *see* Neoplasm, secondary, by
         site
      deposits (in) — *see* Neoplasm, secondary, by site
      disease (*see also* Neoplasm, secondary, by site) C79.9
      spread (to) — *see* Neoplasm, secondary, by site
Metastrongyliasis B83.8
Metatarsalgia M77.4- ☑
   anterior G57.6- ☑
   Morton's G57.6- ☑
Metatarsus, metatarsal (*see also* condition)
   valgus (abductus), congenital Q66.6
   varus (adductus) (congenital) Q66.2
Methadone use F11.20
Methemoglobinemia D74.9
   acquired (with sulfhemoglobinemia) D74.8
   congenital D74.0
   enzymatic (congenital) D74.0
   Hb M disease D74.0
   hereditary D74.0
   toxic D74.8
Methemoglobinuria — *see* Hemoglobinuria
Methioninemia E72.19
Methylmalonic acidemia E71.120
Metritis (catarrhal) (hemorrhagic) (septic) (suppurative)
      (*see also* Endometritis)
   cervical — *see* Cervicitis
Metropathia hemorrhagica N93.8
Metroperitonitis — *see* Peritonitis, pelvic, female
Metrorrhagia N92.1
   climacteric N92.4
   menopausal N92.4
   postpartum NEC (atonic) (following delivery of placen-
      ta) O72.1
      delayed or secondary O72.2
   preclimacteric or premenopausal N92.4
   psychogenic F45.8
Metrorrhexis — *see* Rupture, uterus
Metrosalpingitis N70.91
Metrostaxis N93.8
Metrovaginitis — *see* Endometritis
Meyer-Schwickerath and Weyers syndrome Q87.0
Meynert's amentia (nonalcoholic) F04
   alcoholic F10.96
      with dependence F10.26
Mibelli's disease (porokeratosis) Q82.8
Mice, joint — *see* Loose, body, joint
   knee M23.4- ☑
Micrencephalon, micrencephaly Q02
Microalbuminuria R80.9
Microaneurysm, retinal (*see also* Disorder, retina, mi-
      croaneurysms)
   diabetic — *see* E08-E13 with .31
Microangiopathy (peripheral) I73.9
   thrombotic M31.1
Microcalcifications, breast R92.0
Microcephalus, microcephalic, microcephaly Q02
   due to toxoplasmosis (congenital) P37.1
Microcheilia Q18.7
Microcolon (congenital) Q43.8
Microcornea (congenital) Q13.4
Microcytic — *see* condition
Microdeletions NEC Q93.88
Microdontia K00.2
Microdrepanocytosis D57.40
   with crisis (vasoocclusive pain) D57.419
      with
         acute chest syndrome D57.411
         splenic sequestration D57.412
Microembolism
   atherothrombotic — *see* Atheroembolism
   retinal — *see* Occlusion, artery, retina
Microencephalon Q02
Microfilaria streptocerca infestation — *see* Onchocer-
      ciasis
Microgastria (congenital) Q40.2
Microgenia M26.06
Microgenitalia, congenital
   female Q52.8
   male Q55.8
Microglioma — *see* Lymphoma, non-Hodgkin, specified
      NEC
Microglossia (congenital) Q38.3
Micrognathia, micrognathism (congenital)
      (mandibular) (maxillary) M26.09
Microgyria (congenital) Q04.3

Microinfarct of heart — *see* Insufficiency, coronary
Microlentia (congenital) Q12.8
Microlithiasis, alveolar, pulmonary J84.02
Micromastia N64.82
Micromyelia (congenital) Q06.8
Micropenis Q55.62
Microphakia (congenital) Q12.8
Microphthalmos, microphthalmia (congenital) Q11.2
   due to toxoplasmosis P37.1
Micropsia H53.15
Microscopic polyangiitis (polyarteritis) M31.7
Microsporidiosis B60.8
   intestinal A07.8
Microsporon furfur infestation B36.0
Microsporosis (*see also* Dermatophytosis)
   nigra B36.1
Microstomia (congenital) Q18.5
Microtia (congenital) (external ear) Q17.2
Microtropia H50.40
Microvillus inclusion disease (MVD) (MVID) Q43.8
Micturition
   disorder NEC R39.19
      psychogenic F45.8
   frequency R35.0
      psychogenic F45.8
   hesitancy R39.11
   incomplete emptying R39.14
   nocturnal R35.1
   painful R30.9
      dysuria R30.0
      psychogenic F45.8
      tenesmus R30.1
   poor stream R39.12
   split stream R39.13
   straining R39.16
   urgency R39.15
Mid plane — *see* condition
Middle
   ear — *see* condition
   lobe (right) syndrome J98.19
Miescher's elastoma L87.2
Mietens' syndrome Q87.2
Migraine (idiopathic) G43.909
   with aura (acute-onset) (prolonged) (typical) (without
         headache) G43.109
      with refractory migraine G43.119
         with status migrainosus G43.111
         without status migrainosus G43.119
      without mention of refractory migraine G43.109
         with status migrainosus G43.101
         without status migrainosus G43.109
      intractable G43.119
         with status migrainosus G43.111
         without status migrainosus G43.119
      not intractable G43.109
         with status migrainosus G43.101
         without status migrainosus G43.109
      persistent G43.509
         with cerebral infarction G43.609
            with refractory migraine G43.619
               with status migrainosus G43.611
               without status migrainosus G43.619
            without refractory migraine G43.609
               with status migrainosus G43.601
               without status migrainosus G43.609
            intractable G43.619
               with status migrainosus G43.611
               without status migrainosus G43.619
            not intractable G43.609
               with status migrainosus G43.601
               without status migrainosus G43.609
         without cerebral infarction G43.509
            with refractory migraine G43.519
               with status migrainosus G43.511
               without status migrainosus G43.519
            without refractory migraine G43.509
               with status migrainosus G43.501
               without status migrainosus G43.509
            intractable G43.519
               with status migrainosus G43.511
               without status migrainosus G43.519
            not intractable G43.509
               with status migrainosus G43.501
               without status migrainosus G43.509
   with refractory migraine G43.919
      with status migrainosus G43.911
      without status migrainosus G43.919

Migraine — *continued*
   without aura G43.009
      with refractory migraine G43.019
         with status migrainosus G43.011
         without status migrainosus G43.019
      without mention of refractory migraine G43.009
         with status migrainosus G43.001
         without status migrainosus G43.009
      chronic G43.709
         with refractory migraine G43.719
            with status migrainosus G43.711
            without status migrainosus G43.719
         without refractory migraine G43.709
            with status migrainosus G43.701
            without status migrainosus G43.709
         intractable
            with status migrainosus G43.711
            without status migrainosus G43.719
         not intractable
            with status migrainosus G43.701
            without status migrainosus G43.709
      intractable
         with status migrainosus G43.011
         without status migrainosus G43.019
      not intractable
         with status migrainosus G43.001
         without status migrainosus G43.009
   without refractory migraine G43.909
      with status migrainosus G43.901
      without status migrainosus G43.919
   abdominal G43.D0 (*following* G43.7)
      with refractory migraine G43.D1 (*following* G43.7)
      without refractory migraine G43.D0 (*following*
         G43.7)
      intractable G43.D1 (*following* G43.7)
      not intractable G43.D0 (*following* G43.7)
   basilar — *see* Migraine, with aura
   classical — *see* Migraine, with aura
   common — *see* Migraine, without aura
   complicated G43.109
   equivalents — *see* Migraine, with aura
   familiar — *see* Migraine, hemiplegic
   hemiplegic G43.409
      with refractory migraine G43.419
         with status migrainosus G43.411
         without status migrainosus G43.419
      without refractory migraine G43.409
         with status migrainosus G43.401
         without status migrainosus G43.409
      intractable G43.419
         with status migrainosus G43.411
         without status migrainosus G43.419
      not intractable G43.409
         with status migrainosus G43.401
         without status migrainosus G43.409
   intractable G43.919
      with status migrainosus G43.911
      without status migrainosus G43.919
   menstrual G43.829
      with refractory migraine G43.839
         with status migrainosus G43.831
         without status migrainosus G43.839
      without refractory migraine G43.829
         with status migrainosus G43.821
         without status migrainosus G43.829
      intractable G43.839
         with status migrainosus G43.831
         without status migrainosus G43.839
      not intractable 4G43.829
         with status migrainosus G43.821
         without status migrainosus G43.829
   menstrually related — *see* Migraine, menstrual
   not intractable G43.909
      with status migrainosus G43.901
      without status migrainosus G43.919
   ophthalmoplegic G43.B0 (*following* G43.7)
      with refractory migraine G43.B1 (*following* G43.7)
      without refractory migraine G43.B0 (*following*
         G43.7)
      intractable G43.B1 (*following* G43.7)
      not intractable G43.B0 (*following* G43.7)
   persistent aura (with, without) cerebral infarction —
      see Migraine, with aura, persistent
   preceded or accompanied by transient focal neurolog-
      ical phenomena — *see* Migraine, with aura
   pre-menstrual — *see* Migraine, menstrual
   pure menstrual — *see* Migraine, menstrual
   retinal — *see* Migraine, with aura

Migraine — *continued*
  specified NEC G43.8Ø9
    intractable G43.819
      with status migrainosus G43.811
      without status migrainosus G43.819
    not intractable G43.8Ø9
      with status migrainosus G43.8Ø1
      without status migrainosus G43.8Ø9
  sporadic — *see* Migraine, hemiplegic
  transformed — *see* Migraine, without aura, chronic
  triggered seizures — *see* Migraine, with aura
Migrant, social Z59.Ø
Migration, anxiety concerning Z6Ø.3
Migratory, migrating (*see also* condition)
  person Z59.Ø
  testis Q55.29
Mikity-Wilson disease or syndrome P27.Ø
Mikulicz' disease or syndrome K11.8
Miliaria L74.3
  alba L74.1
  apocrine L75.2
  crystallina L74.1
  profunda L74.2
  rubra L74.Ø
  tropicalis L74.2
Miliary — *see* condition
Milium L72.Ø
  colloid L57.8
Milk
  crust L21.Ø
  excessive secretion O92.6
  poisoning — *see* Poisoning, food, noxious
  retention O92.79
  sickness — *see* Poisoning, food, noxious
  spots I31.Ø
Milk-alkali disease or syndrome E83.52
Milk-leg (deep vessels) (nonpuerperal) — *see* Embolism, vein, lower extremity
  complicating pregnancy O22.3- ☑
  puerperal, postpartum, childbirth O87.1
Milkman's disease or syndrome M83.8
Milky urine — *see* Chyluria
Millard-Gubler (-Foville) **paralysis or syndrome** G46.3
Millar's asthma J38.5
Miller Fisher syndrome G61.Ø
Mills' disease — *see* Hemiplegia
Millstone maker's pneumoconiosis J62.8
Milroy's disease (chronic hereditary edema) Q82.Ø
Minamata disease T26.1- ☑
Miners' asthma or lung J6Ø
Minkowski-Chauffard syndrome — *see* Spherocytosis
Minor — *see* condition
Minor's disease (hematomyelia) G95.19
Minot's disease (hemorrhagic disease), newborn P53
Minot-von Willebrand-Jurgens disease or syndrome (angiohemophilia) D68.Ø
Minus (and plus) **hand** (intrinsic) — *see* Deformity, limb, specified type NEC, forearm
Miosis (pupil) H57.Ø3
Mirizzi's syndrome (hepatic duct stenosis) K83.1
Mirror writing F81.Ø
Misadventure (of) (prophylactic) (therapeutic) (*see also* Complications) T88.9 ☑
  administration of insulin (by accident) — *see* subcategory T38.3 ☑
  infusion — *see* Complications, infusion
  local applications (of fomentations, plasters, etc.) T88.9 ☑
    burn or scald — *see* Burn
    specified NEC T88.8 ☑
  medical care (early) (late) T88.9 ☑
    adverse effect of drugs or chemicals — *see* Table of Drugs and Chemicals
    burn or scald — *see* Burn
    specified NEC T88.8 ☑
  specified NEC T88.8 ☑
  surgical procedure (early) (late) — *see* Complications, surgical procedure
  transfusion — *see* Complications, transfusion
  vaccination or other immunological procedure — *see* Complications, vaccination
Miscarriage O03.9
Misdirection, aqueous H4Ø.83- ☑
Misperception, sleep state F51.Ø2
Misplaced, misplacement
  ear Q17.4

Misplaced, misplacement — *continued*
  kidney (acquired) N28.89
    congenital Q63.2
  organ or site, congenital NEC — *see* Malposition, congenital
Missed
  abortion O02.1
  delivery O36.4 ☑
Missing — *see* Absence
Misuse of drugs F19.99
Mitchell's disease (erythromelalgia) I73.81
Mite(s) (infestation) B88.9
  diarrhea B88.Ø
  grain (itch) B88.Ø
  hair follicle (itch) B88.Ø
  in sputum B88.Ø
Mitral — *see* condition
Mittelschmerz N94.Ø
Mixed — *see* condition
MNGIE (Mitochondrial Neurogastrointestinal Encephalopathy) **syndrome** E88.49
Mobile, mobility
  cecum Q43.3
  excessive — *see* Hypermobility
  gallbladder, congenital Q44.1
  kidney N28.89
  organ or site, congenital NEC — *see* Malposition, congenital
Mobitz heart block (atrioventricular) I44.1
Moebius, Möbius
  disease (ophthalmoplegic migraine) — *see* Migraine, ophthalmoplegic
  syndrome Q87.Ø
    congenital oculofacial paralysis (with other anomalies) Q87.Ø
    ophthalmoplegic migraine — *see* Migraine, ophthalmoplegic
Moeller's glossitis K14.Ø
Mohr's syndrome (Types I and II) Q87.Ø
Mola destruens D39.2
Molar pregnancy O02.Ø
Molarization of premolars KØØ.2
Molding, head (during birth) — *omit code*
Mole (pigmented) (*see also* Nevus)
  blood O02.Ø
  Breus' O02.Ø
  cancerous — *see* Melanoma
  carneous O02.Ø
  destructive D39.2
  fleshy O02.Ø
  hydatid, hydatidiform (benign) (complicating pregnancy) (delivered) (undelivered) O01.9
    classical O01.Ø
    complete O01.Ø
    incomplete O01.1
    invasive D39.2
    malignant D39.2
    partial O01.1
  intrauterine O02.Ø
  invasive (hydatidiform) D39.2
  malignant
    meaning
      malignant hydatidiform mole D39.2
      melanoma — *see* Melanoma
  nonhydatidiform O02.Ø
  nonpigmented — *see* Nevus
  pregnancy NEC O02.Ø
  skin — *see* Nevus
  tubal O00.1
  vesicular — *see* Mole, hydatidiform
Molimen, molimina (menstrual) N94.3
Molluscum contagiosum (epitheliale) BØ8.1
Mönckeberg's arteriosclerosis, disease, or sclerosis — *see* Arteriosclerosis, extremities
Mondini's malformation (cochlea) Q16.5
Mondor's disease I8Ø.8
Monge's disease T7Ø.29 ☑
Monilethrix (congenital) Q84.1
Moniliasis (*see also* Candidiasis) B37.9
  neonatal P37.5
Monitoring (encounter for)
  therapeutic drug level Z51.81
Monkey malaria B53.1
Monkeypox BØ4
Monoarthritis M13.1Ø
  ankle M13.17- ☑
  elbow M13.12- ☑

Monoarthritis — *continued*
  foot joint M13.17- ☑
  hand joint M13.14- ☑
  hip M13.15- ☑
  knee M13.16- ☑
  shoulder M13.11- ☑
  wrist M13.13- ☑
Monoblastic — *see* condition
Monochromat (ism), monochromatopsia (acquired) (congenital) H53.51
Monocytic — *see* condition
Monocytopenia D72.818
Monocytosis (symptomatic) D72.821
Monomania — *see* Psychosis
Mononeuritis G58.9
  cranial nerve — *see* Disorder, nerve, cranial
  femoral nerve G57.2- ☑
  lateral
    cutaneous nerve of thigh G57.1- ☑
    popliteal nerve G57.3- ☑
  lower limb G57.9- ☑
    specified nerve NEC G57.8- ☑
  medial popliteal nerve G57.4- ☑
  median nerve G56.1- ☑
  multiplex G58.7
  plantar nerve G57.6- ☑
  posterior tibial nerve G57.5- ☑
  radial nerve G56.3- ☑
  sciatic nerve G57.Ø- ☑
  specified NEC G58.8
  tibial nerve G57.4- ☑
  ulnar nerve G56.2- ☑
  upper limb G56.9- ☑
    specified nerve NEC G56.8- ☑
  vestibular — *see* subcategory H93.3 ☑
Mononeuropathy G58.9
  carpal tunnel syndrome — *see* Syndrome, carpal tunnel
  diabetic NEC — *see* EØ8-E13 with .41
  femoral nerve — *see* Lesion, nerve, femoral
  ilioinguinal nerve G57.8- ☑
  in diseases classified elsewhere — *see* category G59
  intercostal G58.Ø
  lower limb G57.9- ☑
    causalgia — *see* Causalgia, lower limb
    femoral nerve — *see* Lesion, nerve, femoral
    meralgia paresthetica G57.1- ☑
    plantar nerve — *see* Lesion, nerve, plantar
    popliteal nerve — *see* Lesion, nerve, popliteal
    sciatic nerve — *see* Lesion, nerve, sciatic
    specified NEC G57.8- ☑
    tarsal tunnel syndrome — *see* Syndrome, tarsal tunnel
  median nerve — *see* Lesion, nerve, median
  multiplex G58.7
  obturator nerve G57.8- ☑
  popliteal nerve — *see* Lesion, nerve, popliteal
  radial nerve — *see* Lesion, nerve, radial
  saphenous nerve G57.8- ☑
  specified NEC G58.8
  tarsal tunnel syndrome — *see* Syndrome, tarsal tunnel
  tuberculous A17.83
  ulnar nerve — *see* Lesion, nerve, ulnar
  upper limb G56.9- ☑
    carpal tunnel syndrome — *see* Syndrome, carpal tunnel
    causalgia — *see* Causalgia
    median nerve — *see* Lesion, nerve, median
    radial nerve — *see* Lesion, nerve, radial
    specified site NEC G56.8- ☑
    ulnar nerve — *see* Lesion, nerve, ulnar
Mononucleosis, infectious B27.9Ø
  with
    complication NEC B27.99
    meningitis B27.92
    polyneuropathy B27.91
  cytomegaloviral B27.1Ø
    with
      complication NEC B27.19
      meningitis B27.12
      polyneuropathy B27.11
  Epstein-Barr (virus) B27.ØØ
    with
      complication NEC B27.Ø9
      meningitis B27.Ø2
      polyneuropathy B27.Ø1

Mononucleosis, infectious — *continued*
  gammaherpesviral B27.00
    with
      complication NEC B27.09
      meningitis B27.02
      polyneuropathy B27.01
    specified NEC B27.80
      with
        complication NEC B27.89
        meningitis B27.82
        polyneuropathy B27.81
Monoplegia G83.3- ☑
  congenital (cerebral) G80.8
    spastic G80.1
  embolic (current episode) I63.4 ☑
  following
    cerebrovascular disease
      cerebral infarction
        lower limb I69.34- ☑
        upper limb I69.33- ☑
      intracerebral hemorrhage
        lower limb I69.14- ☑
        upper limb I69.13- ☑
      lower limb I69.94- ☑
      nontraumatic intracranial hemorrhage NEC
        lower limb I69.24- ☑
        upper limb I69.23- ☑
      specified disease NEC
        lower limb I69.84- ☑
        upper limb I69.83- ☑
      stroke NOS
        lower limb I69.34- ☑
        upper limb I69.33- ☑
      subarachnoid hemorrhage
        lower limb I69.04- ☑
        upper limb I69.03- ☑
      upper limb I69.93- ☑
  hysterical (transient) F44.4
  lower limb G83.1- ☑
  psychogenic (conversion reaction) F44.4
  thrombotic (current episode) I63.3 ☑
  transient R29.818
  upper limb G83.2- ☑
Monorchism, monorchidism Q55.0
Monosomy (*see also* Deletion, chromosome) Q93.9
  specified NEC Q93.89
  whole chromosome
    meiotic nondisjunction Q93.0
    mitotic nondisjunction Q93.1
    mosaicism Q93.1
  X Q96.9
Monster, monstrosity (single) Q89.7
  acephalic Q00.0
  twin Q89.4
Monteggia's fracture (-dislocation) S52.27- ☑
Mooren's ulcer (cornea) — *see* Ulcer, cornea, Mooren's
Moore's syndrome — *see* Epilepsy, specified NEC
Mooser-Neill reaction A75.2
Mooser's bodies A75.2
Morbidity not stated or unknown R69
Morbilli — *see* Measles
Morbus (*see also* Disease)
  angelicus, anglorum E55.0
  Beigel B36.2
  caducus — *see* Epilepsy
  celiacus K90.0
  comitialis — *see* Epilepsy
  cordis (*see also* Disease, heart) I51.9
    valvulorum — *see* Endocarditis
  coxae senilis M16.9
    tuberculous A18.02
  hemorrhagicus neonatorum P53
  maculosus neonatorum P54.5
Morel (-Stewart)(-Morgagni) **syndrome** M85.2
Morel-Kraepelin disease — *see* Schizophrenia
Morel-Moore syndrome M85.2
Morgagni's
  cyst, organ, hydatid, or appendage
    female Q50.5
    male (epididymal) Q55.4
      testicular Q55.29
  syndrome M85.2
Morgagni-Stewart-Morel syndrome M85.2
Morgagni-Stokes-Adams syndrome I45.9
Morgagni-Turner (-Albright) **syndrome** Q96.9
Moria F07.0
Moron (I.Q. 50-69) F70

Morphea L94.0
Morphinism (without remission) F11.20
  with remission F11.21
Morphinomania (without remission) F11.20
  with remission F11.21
Morquio (-Ullrich)(-Brailsford) **disease or syndrome** —
  see Mucopolysaccharidosis
Mortification (dry) (moist) — *see* Gangrene
Morton's metatarsalgia (neuralgia)(neuroma) (syndrome) G57.6- ☑
Morvan's disease or syndrome G60.8
Mosaicism, mosaic (autosomal) (chromosomal)
  45,X/46,XX Q96.3
  45,X/other cell lines NEC with abnormal sex chromosome Q96.4
  sex chromosome
    female Q97.8
    lines with various numbers of X chromosomes Q97.2
    male Q98.7
  XY Q96.3
Moschowitz' disease M31.1
Mother yaw A66.0
Motion sickness (from travel, any vehicle) (from roundabouts or swings) T75.3 ☑
Mottled, mottling, teeth (enamel) (endemic) (nonendemic) K00.3
Mounier-Kuhn syndrome Q32.4
  with bronchiectasis J47.9
    exacerbation (acute) J47.1
    lower respiratory infection J47.0
  acquired J98.09
    with bronchiectasis J47.9
      with
        exacerbation (acute) J47.1
        lower respiratory infection J47.0
Mountain
  sickness T70.29 ☑
    with polycythemia , acquired (acute) D75.1
  tick fever A93.2
Mouse, joint — *see* Loose, body, joint
  knee M23.4- ☑
Mouth — *see* condition
Movable
  coccyx — *see* subcategory M53.2 ☑
  kidney N28.89
    congenital Q63.8
  spleen D73.89
Movements, dystonic R25.8
Moyamoya disease I67.5
MRSA (Methicillin resistant Staphylococcus aureus)
  infection A49.02
    as the cause of diseases classified elsewhere B95.62
  sepsis A41.02
MSSA (Methicillin susceptible Staphylococcus aureus)
  infection A49.01
    as the cause of diseases classified elsewhere B95.61
  sepsis A41.01
Mucha-Habermann disease L41.0
Mucinosis (cutaneous) (focal) (papular) (skin) L98.5
  oral K13.79
Mucocele
  appendix K38.8
  buccal cavity K13.79
  gallbladder K82.1
  lacrimal sac, chronic H04.43- ☑
  nasal sinus J34.1
  nose J34.1
  salivary gland (any) K11.6
  sinus (accessory) (nasal) J34.1
  turbinate (bone) (middle) (nasal) J34.1
  uterus N85.8
Mucolipidosis
  I E77.1
  II, III E77.0
  IV E75.11
Mucopolysaccharidosis E76.3
  beta-gluduronidase deficiency E76.29
  cardiopathy E76.3 [I52]
  Hunter's syndrome E76.1
  Hurler's syndrome E76.01
  Hurler-Scheie syndrome E76.02
  Maroteaux-Lamy syndrome E76.29
  Morquio syndrome E76.219
    A E76.210
    B E76.211
    classic E76.210

Mucopolysaccharidosis — *continued*
  Sanfilippo syndrome E76.22
  Scheie's syndrome E76.03
  specified NEC E76.29
  type
    I
      Hurler's syndrome E76.01
      Hurler-Scheie syndrome E76.02
      Scheie's syndrome E76.03
    II E76.1
    III E76.22
    IV E76.219
    IVA E76.210
    IVB E76.211
    VI E76.29
    VII E76.29
Mucormycosis B46.5
  cutaneous B46.3
  disseminated B46.4
  gastrointestinal B46.2
  generalized B46.4
  pulmonary B46.0
  rhinocerebral B46.1
  skin B46.3
  subcutaneous B46.3
Mucositis (ulcerative) K12.30
  due to drugs NEC K12.32
  gastrointestinal K92.81
  mouth (oral) (oropharyngeal) K12.30
    due to antineoplastic therapy K12.31
    due to drugs NEC K12.32
    due to radiation K12.33
    specified NEC K12.39
    viral K12.39
  nasal J34.81
  oral cavity — *see* Mucositis, mouth
  oral soft tissues — *see* Mucositis, mouth
  vagina and vulva N76.81
Mucositis necroticans agranulocytica — *see* Agranulocytosis
Mucous (*see also* condition)
  patches (syphilitic) A51.39
    congenital A50.07
Mucoviscidosis E84.9
  with meconium obstruction E84.11
Mucus
  asphyxia or suffocation — *see* Asphyxia, mucus
  in stool R19.5
  plug — *see* Asphyxia, mucus
Muguet B37.0
Mulberry molars (congenital syphilis) A50.52
Müllerian mixed tumor
  specified site — *see* Neoplasm, malignant, by site
  unspecified site C54.9
Multicystic kidney (development) Q61.4
Multiparity (grand) Z64.1
  affecting management of pregnancy, labor and delivery (supervision only) O09.4- ☑
  requiring contraceptive management — *see* Contraception
Multipartita placenta O43.19- ☑
Multiple, multiplex (*see also* condition)
  digits (congenital) Q69.9
  endocrine neoplasia — *see* Neoplasia, endocrine, multiple (MEN)
  personality F44.81
Mumps B26.9
  arthritis B26.85
  complication NEC B26.89
  encephalitis B26.2
  hepatitis B26.81
  meningitis (aseptic) B26.1
  meningoencephalitis B26.2
  myocarditis B26.82
  oophoritis B26.89
  orchitis B26.0
  pancreatitis B26.3
  polyneuropathy B26.84
Mumu (*see also* Infestation, filarial) B74.9 [N51]
Münchhausen's syndrome — *see* Disorder, factitious
Münchmeyer's syndrome — *see* Myositis, ossificans, progressiva
Mural — *see* condition
Murmur (cardiac) (heart) (organic) R01.1
  abdominal R19.15
  aortic (valve) — *see* Endocarditis, aortic
  benign R01.0
  diastolic — *see* Endocarditis

☑ **Additional Character Required** — Refer to the Tabular List for Character Selection   ◥ Subterms under main terms may continue to next column or page

Murmur — *continued*
Flint I35.1
functional R01.0
Graham Steell I37.1
innocent R01.0
mitral (valve) — *see* Insufficiency, mitral
nonorganic R01.0
presystolic, mitral — *see* Insufficiency, mitral
pulmonic (valve) I37.8
systolic (valvular) — *see* Endocarditis
tricuspid (valve) I07.9
valvular — *see* Endocarditis
Murri's disease (intermittent hemoglobinuria) D59.6
Muscle, muscular (*see also* condition)
carnitine (palmityltransferase) deficiency E71.314
Musculoneuralgia — *see* Neuralgia
Mushrooming hip — *see* Derangement, joint, specified
NEC, hip
Mushroom-workers' (pickers') **disease or lung** J67.5
Mutation(s)
factor V Leiden D68.51
prothrombin gene D68.52
surfactant, of lung J84.83
Mutism (*see also* Aphasia)
deaf (acquired) (congenital) NEC H91.3
elective (adjustment reaction) (childhood) F94.0
hysterical F44.4
selective (childhood) F94.0
MVD (microvillus inclusion disease) Q43.8
MVID (microvillus inclusion disease) Q43.8
Myalgia M79.1
epidemic (cervical) B33.0
traumatic NEC T14.8
Myasthenia G70.9
congenital G70.2
cordis — *see* Failure, heart
developmental G70.2
gravis G70.00
with exacerbation (acute) G70.01
in crisis G70.01
neonatal, transient P94.0
pseudoparalytica G70.00
with exacerbation (acute) G70.01
in crisis G70.01
stomach, psychogenic F45.8
syndrome
in
diabetes mellitus — *see* E08-E13 with .44
neoplastic disease (*see also* Neoplasm)
D49.9 [G73.3]
pernicious anemia D51.0 [G73.3]
thyrotoxicosis E05.90 [G73.3]
with thyroid storm E05.91 [G73.3]
Myasthenic M62.81
Mycelium infection B49
Mycetismus — *see* Poisoning, food, noxious, mushroom
Mycetoma B47.9
actinomycotic B47.1
bone (mycotic) B47.9 [M90.80]
eumycotic B47.0
foot B47.9
actinomycotic B47.1
mycotic B47.0
madurae NEC B47.9
mycotic B47.0
maduromycotic B47.0
mycotic B47.0
nocardial B47.1
Mycobacteriosis — *see* Mycobacterium
Mycobacterium, mycobacterial (infection) A31.9
anonymous A31.9
atypical A31.9
cutaneous A31.1
pulmonary A31.0
tuberculous — *see* Tuberculosis, pulmonary
specified site NEC A31.8
avium (intracellulare complex) A31.0
balnei A31.1
Battey A31.0
chelonei A31.8
cutaneous A31.1
extrapulmonary systemic A31.8
fortuitum A31.8
intracellulare (Battey bacillus) A31.0
kakaferifu A31.8
kansasii (yellow bacillus) A31.0
kasongo A31.8
leprae (*see also* Leprosy) A30.9

Mycobacterium, mycobacterial — *continued*
luciflavum A31.1
marinum (M. balnei) A31.1
nonspecific — *see* Mycobacterium, atypical
pulmonary (atypical) A31.0
tuberculous — *see* Tuberculosis, pulmonary
scrofulaceum A31.8
simiae A31.8
systemic, extrapulmonary A31.8
szulgai A31.8
terrae A31.8
triviale A31.8
tuberculosis (human, bovine) — *see* Tuberculosis
ulcerans A31.1
xenopi A31.8
Mycoplasma (M.) **pneumoniae, as cause of disease
classified elsewhere** B96.0
Mycosis, mycotic B49
cutaneous NEC B36.9
ear B36.8
fungoides (extranodal) (solid organ) C84.0- ☑
mouth B37.0
nails B35.1
opportunistic B48.8
skin NEC B36.9
specified NEC B48.8
stomatitis B37.0
vagina, vaginitis (candidal) B37.3
Mydriasis (pupil) H57.04
Myelatelia Q06.1
Myelinolysis, pontine, central G37.2
Myelitis (acute) (ascending) (childhood) (chronic) (descending) (diffuse) (disseminated) (idiopathic)
(pressure) (progressive) (spinal cord) (subacute)
(*see also* Encephalitis) G04.91
herpes simplex B00.82
herpes zoster B02.24
in diseases classified elsewhere G05.4
necrotizing, subacute G37.4
optic neuritis in G36.0
postchickenpox B01.12
postherpetic B02.24
postimmunization G04.02
postinfectious NEC G04.89
postvaccinal G04.02
specified NEC G04.89
syphilitic (transverse) A52.14
toxic G92
transverse (in demyelinating diseases of central nervous system) G37.3
tuberculous A17.82
varicella B01.12
Myeloblastic — *see* condition
Myeloblastoma
granular cell (*see also* Neoplasm, connective tissue)
malignant — *see* Neoplasm, connective tissue,
malignant
tongue D10.1
Myelocele — *see* Spina bifida
Myelocystocele — *see* Spina bifida
Myelocytic — *see* condition
Myelodysplasia D46.9
specified NEC D46.Z (*following* D46.4)
spinal cord (congenital) Q06.1
Myelodysplastic syndrome D46.9
with
5q deletion D46.C (*following* D46.2)
isolated del (5q) chromosomal abnormality D46.C
(*following* D46.2)
specified NEC D46.Z (*following* D46.4)
Myeloencephalitis — *see* Encephalitis
Myelofibrosis D75.81
with myeloid metaplasia D47.4
acute C94.4- ☑
idiopathic (chronic) D47.4
primary D47.1
secondary D75.81
in myeloproliferative disease D47.4
Myelogenous — *see* condition
Myeloid — *see* condition
Myelokathexis D70.9
Myeloleukodystrophy E75.29
Myelolipoma — *see* Lipoma
Myeloma (multiple) C90.0- ☑
monostotic C90.3 ☑
plasma cell C90.0- ☑
plasma cell C90.0- ☑

Myeloma — *continued*
solitary (*see also* Plasmacytoma, solitary) C90.3- ☑
Myelomalacia G95.89
Myelomatosis C90.0- ☑
Myelomeningitis — *see* Meningoencephalitis
Myelomeningocele (spinal cord) — *see* Spina bifida
Myelo-osteo-musculodysplasia hereditaria Q79.8
Myelopathic
anemia D64.89
muscle atrophy — *see* Atrophy, muscle, spinal
pain syndrome G89.0
Myelopathy (spinal cord) G95.9
drug-induced G95.89
in (due to)
degeneration or displacement, intervertebral disc
NEC — *see* Disorder, disc, with, myelopathy
infection — *see* Encephalitis
intervertebral disc disorder (*see also* Disorder, disc,
with, myelopathy)
mercury — *see* subcategory T56.1 ☑
neoplastic disease (*see also* Neoplasm)
D49.9 [G99.2]
pernicious anemia D51.0 [G99.2]
spondylosis — *see* Spondylosis, with myelopathy
NEC
necrotic (subacute) (vascular) G95.19
radiation-induced G95.89
spondylogenic NEC — *see* Spondylosis, with
myelopathy NEC
toxic G95.89
transverse, acute G37.3
vascular G95.19
vitamin B12 E53.8 [G32.0]
Myelophthisis D61.82
Myeloradiculitis G04.91
Myeloradiculodysplasia (spinal) Q06.1
Myelosarcoma C92.3- ☑
Myelosclerosis D75.89
with myeloid metaplasia D47.4
disseminated, of nervous system G35
megakaryocytic D47.4
with myeloid metaplasia D47.4
Myelosis
acute C92.0- ☑
aleukemic C92.9- ☑
chronic D47.1
erythremic (acute) C94.0- ☑
megakaryocytic C94.2- ☑
nonleukemic D72.828
subacute C92.9- ☑
Myiasis (cavernous) B87.9
aural B87.4
creeping B87.0
cutaneous B87.0
dermal B87.0
ear (external) (middle) B87.4
eye B87.2
genitourinary B87.81
intestinal B87.82
laryngeal B87.3
nasopharyngeal B87.3
ocular B87.2
orbit B87.2
skin B87.0
specified site NEC B87.89
traumatic B87.1
wound B87.1
Myoadenoma, prostate — *see* Hyperplasia, prostate
Myoblastoma
granular cell (*see also* Neoplasm, connective tissue,
benign)
malignant — *see* Neoplasm, connective tissue,
malignant
tongue D10.1
Myocardial — *see* condition
Myocardiopathy (congestive) (constrictive) (familial)
(hypertrophic nonobstructive) (idiopathic) (infiltrative) (obstructive) (primary) (restrictive) (sporadic)
(*see also* Cardiomyopathy) I42.9
alcoholic I42.6
cobalt-beer I42.6
glycogen storage E74.02 [I43]
hypertrophic obstructive I42.1
in (due to)
beriberi E51.12
cardiac glycogenosis E74.02 [I43]
Friedreich's ataxia G11.1 [I43]

Myocardiopathy — *continued*
  in — *continued*
    myotonia atrophica G71.11 [I43]
    progressive muscular dystrophy G71.0 [I43]
  obscure (African) I42.8
  secondary I42.9
  thyrotoxic E05.90 [I43]
    with storm E05.91 [I43]
  toxic NEC I42.7
Myocarditis (with arteriosclerosis)(chronic)(fibroid) (interstitial) (old) (progressive) (senile) I51.4
  with
    rheumatic fever (conditions in I00) I09.0
      active — *see* Myocarditis, acute, rheumatic
      inactive or quiescent (with chorea) I09.0
  active I40.9
    rheumatic I01.2
      with chorea (acute) (rheumatic) (Sydenham's) I02.0
  acute or subacute (interstitial) I40.9
    due to
      streptococcus (beta-hemolytic) I01.2
    idiopathic I40.1
    rheumatic I01.2
      with chorea (acute) (rheumatic) (Sydenham's) I02.0
    specified NEC I40.8
  aseptic of newborn B33.22
  bacterial (acute) I40.0
  Coxsackie (virus) B33.22
  diphtheritic A36.81
  eosinophilic I40.1
  epidemic of newborn (Coxsackie) B33.22
  Fiedler's (acute) (isolated) I40.1
  giant cell (acute) (subacute) I40.1
  gonococcal A54.83
  granulomatous (idiopathic) (isolated) (nonspecific) I40.1
  hypertensive — *see* Hypertension, heart
  idiopathic (granulomatous) I40.1
  in (due to)
    diphtheria A36.81
    epidemic louse-borne typhus A75.0 [I41]
    Lyme disease A69.29
    sarcoidosis D86.85
    scarlet fever A38.1
    toxoplasmosis (acquired) B58.81
    typhoid A01.02
    typhus NEC A75.9 [I41]
  infective I40.0
  influenzal — *see* Influenza, with, myocarditis
  isolated (acute) I40.1
  meningococcal A39.52
  mumps B26.82
  nonrheumatic, active I40.9
  parenchymatous I40.9
  pneumococcal I40.0
  rheumatic (chronic) (inactive) (with chorea) I09.0
    active or acute I01.2
      with chorea (acute) (rheumatic) (Sydenham's) I02.0
  rheumatoid — *see* Rheumatoid, carditis
  septic I40.0
  staphylococcal I40.0
  suppurative I40.0
  syphilitic (chronic) A52.06
  toxic I40.8
    rheumatic — *see* Myocarditis, acute, rheumatic
  tuberculous A18.84
  typhoid A01.02
  valvular — *see* Endocarditis
  virus, viral I40.0
    of newborn (Coxsackie) B33.22
Myocardium, myocardial — *see* condition
Myocardosis — *see* Cardiomyopathy
Myoclonus, myoclonic, myoclonia (familial) (essential) (multifocal) (simplex) G25.3
  drug-induced G25.3
  epilepsy (*see also* Epilepsy, generalized, specified NEC) G40.4- ☑
    familial (progressive) G25.3
  epileptica G40.409
    with status epilepticus G40.401
  facial G51.3
  familial progressive G25.3
  Friedreich's G25.3
  jerks G25.3
  massive G25.3

Myoclonus, myoclonic, myoclonia — *continued*
  palatal G25.3
  pharyngeal G25.3
Myocytolysis I51.5
Myodiastasis — *see* Diastasis, muscle
Myoendocarditis — *see* Endocarditis
Myoepithelioma — *see* Neoplasm, benign, by site
Myofasciitis (acute) — *see* Myositis
Myofibroma (*see also* Neoplasm, connective tissue, benign)
  uterus (cervix) (corpus) — *see* Leiomyoma
Myofibromatosis D48.1
  infantile Q89.8
Myofibrosis M62.89
  heart — *see* Myocarditis
  scapulohumeral — *see* Lesion, shoulder, specified NEC
Myofibrositis M79.7
  scapulohumeral — *see* Lesion, shoulder, specified NEC
Myoglobulinuria, myoglobinuria (primary) R82.1
Myokymia, facial G51.4
Myolipoma — *see* Lipoma
Myoma (*see also* Neoplasm, connective tissue, benign)
  malignant — *see* Neoplasm, connective tissue, malignant
  prostate D29.1
  uterus (cervix) (corpus) — *see* Leiomyoma
Myomalacia M62.89
Myometritis — *see* Endometritis
Myometrium — *see* condition
Myonecrosis, clostridial A48.0
Myopathy G72.9
  acute
    necrotizing G72.81
      quadriplegic G72.81
  alcoholic G72.1
  benign congenital G71.2
  central core G71.2
  centronuclear G71.2
  congenital (benign) G71.2
  critical illness G72.81
  distal G71.0
  drug-induced G72.0
  endocrine NEC E34.9 [G73.7]
  extraocular muscles H05.82- ☑
  facioscapulohumeral G71.0
  hereditary G71.9
    specified NEC G71.8
  immune NEC G72.49
  in (due to)
    Addison's disease E27.1 [G73.7]
    alcohol G72.1
    amyloidosis E85.0 [G73.7]
    cretinism E00.9 [G73.7]
    Cushing's syndrome E24.9 [G73.7]
    drugs G72.0
    endocrine disease NEC E34.9 [G73.7]
    giant cell arteritis M31.6 [G73.7]
    glycogen storage disease E74.00 [G73.7]
    hyperadrenocorticism E24.9 [G73.7]
    hyperparathyroidism E21.3 [G73.7]
    hypoparathyroidism E20.9 [G73.7]
    hypopituitarism E23.0 [G73.7]
    hypothyroidism E03.9 [G73.7]
    infectious disease NEC B99 ☑ [G73.7]
    lipid storage disease E75.6 [G73.7]
    metabolic disease NEC E88.9 [G73.7]
    myxedema E03.9 [G73.7]
    parasitic disease NEC B89 [G73.7]
    polyarteritis nodosa M30.0 [G73.7]
    rheumatoid arthritis — *see* Rheumatoid, myopathy
    sarcoidosis D86.87
    scleroderma M34.82
    sicca syndrome M35.03
    Sjögren's syndrome M35.03
    systemic lupus erythematosus M32.19
    thyrotoxicosis (hyperthyroidism) E05.90 [G73.7]
      with thyroid storm E05.91 [G73.7]
    toxic agent NEC G72.2
  inflammatory NEC G72.49
  intensive care (ICU) G72.81
  limb-girdle G71.0
  mitochondrial NEC G71.3
  myotubular G71.2
  mytonic, proximal (PROMM) G71.11
  nemaline G71.2
  ocular G71.0
  oculopharyngeal G71.0
  of critical illness G72.81

Myopathy — *continued*
  primary G71.9
    specified NEC G71.8
  progressive NEC G72.89
  proximal myotonic (PROMM) G71.11
  rod G71.2
  scapulohumeral G71.0
  specified NEC G72.89
  toxic G72.2
Myopericarditis (*see also* Pericarditis)
  chronic rheumatic I09.2
Myopia (axial) (congenital) H52.1- ☑
  degenerative (malignant) H44.2- ☑
  malignant H44.2- ☑
  pernicious H44.2- ☑
  progressive high (degenerative) H44.2- ☑
Myosarcoma — *see* Neoplasm, connective tissue, malignant
Myosis (pupil) H57.03
  stromal (endolymphatic) D39.0
Myositis M60.9
  clostridial A48.0
  due to posture — *see* Myositis, specified type NEC
  epidemic B33.0
  fibrosa or fibrous (chronic), Volkmann's T79.6 ☑
  foreign body granuloma — *see* Granuloma, foreign body
  in (due to)
    bilharziasis B65.9 [M63.8-] ☑
    cysticercosis B69.81
    leprosy A30.9 [M63.8-] ☑
    mycosis B49 [M63.8-] ☑
    sarcoidosis D86.87
    schistosomiasis B65.9 [M63.8-] ☑
    syphilis
      late A52.78
      secondary A51.49
    toxoplasmosis (acquired) B58.82
    trichinellosis B75 [M63.8-] ☑
    tuberculosis A18.09
  inclusion body [IBM] G72.41
  infective M60.009
    arm M60.002
      left M60.001
      right M60.000
    leg M60.005
      left M60.004
      right M60.003
    lower limb M60.005
      ankle M60.07- ☑
      foot M60.07- ☑
      lower leg M60.06- ☑
      thigh M60.05- ☑
      toe M60.07- ☑
    multiple sites M60.09
    specified site NEC M60.08
    upper limb M60.002
      finger M60.04- ☑
      forearm M60.03- ☑
      hand M60.04- ☑
      shoulder region M60.01- ☑
      upper arm M60.02- ☑
  interstitial M60.10
    ankle M60.17- ☑
    foot M60.17- ☑
    forearm M60.13- ☑
    hand M60.14- ☑
    lower leg M60.16- ☑
    multiple sites M60.19
    shoulder region M60.11- ☑
    specified site NEC M60.18
    thigh M60.15- ☑
    upper arm M60.12- ☑
  mycotic B49 [M63.8-] ☑
  orbital, chronic H05.12- ☑
  ossificans or ossifying (circumscripta) (*see also* Ossification, muscle, specified NEC)
    in (due to)
      burns M61.30
        ankle M61.37- ☑
        foot M61.37- ☑
        forearm M61.33- ☑
        hand M61.34- ☑
        lower leg M61.36- ☑
        multiple sites M61.39
        pelvic region M61.35- ☑
        shoulder region M61.31- ☑

  ☑ Additional Character Required — Refer to the Tabular List for Character Selection   ▽ Subterms under main terms may continue to next column or page

Myositis — *continued*
  ossificans or ossifying (*see also* Ossification, muscle, specified) — *continued*
    in — *continued*
      burns — *continued*
        specified site NEC M61.38
        thigh M61.35- ☑
        upper arm M61.32- ☑
      quadriplegia or paraplegia M61.20
        ankle M61.27- ☑
        foot M61.27- ☑
        forearm M61.23- ☑
        hand M61.24- ☑
        lower leg M61.26- ☑
        multiple sites M61.29
        pelvic region M61.25- ☑
        shoulder region M61.21- ☑
        specified site NEC M61.28
        thigh M61.25- ☑
        upper arm M61.22- ☑
    progressiva M61.10
      ankle M61.17- ☑
      finger M61.14- ☑
      foot M61.17- ☑
      forearm M61.13- ☑
      hand M61.14- ☑
      lower leg M61.16- ☑
      multiple sites M61.19
      pelvic region M61.15- ☑
      shoulder region M61.11- ☑
      specified site NEC M61.18
      thigh M61.15- ☑
      toe M61.17- ☑
      upper arm M61.12- ☑
    traumatica M61.00
      ankle M61.07- ☑
      foot M61.07- ☑
      forearm M61.03- ☑
      hand M61.04- ☑

Myositis — *continued*
  ossificans or ossifying (*see also* Ossification, muscle, specified) — *continued*
    traumatica — *continued*
      lower leg M61.06- ☑
      multiple sites M61.09
      pelvic region M61.05- ☑
      shoulder region M61.01- ☑
      specified site NEC M61.08
      thigh M61.05- ☑
      upper arm M61.02- ☑
  purulent — *see* Myositis, infective
  specified type NEC M60.80
    ankle M60.87- ☑
    foot M60.87- ☑
    forearm M60.83- ☑
    hand M60.84- ☑
    lower leg M60.86- ☑
    multiple sites M60.89
    pelvic region M60.85- ☑
    shoulder region M60.81- ☑
    specified site NEC M60.88
    thigh M60.85- ☑
    upper arm M60.82- ☑
  suppurative — *see* Myositis, infective
  traumatic (old) — *see* Myositis, specified type NEC
Myospasia impulsiva F95.2
Myotonia (acquisita) (intermittens) M62.89
  atrophica G71.11
  chondrodystrophic G71.13
  congenita (acetazolamide responsive) (dominant) (recessive) G71.12
  drug-induced G71.14
  dystrophica G71.11
  fluctuans G71.19
  levior G71.12
  permanens G71.19
  symptomatic G71.19

Myotonic pupil — *see* Anomaly, pupil, function, tonic pupil
Myriapodiasis B88.2
Myringitis H73.2- ☑
  with otitis media — *see* Otitis, media
  acute H73.00- ☑
    bullous H73.01- ☑
    specified NEC H73.09- ☑
  bullous — *see* Myringitis, acute, bullous
  chronic H73.1- ☑
Mysophobia F40.228
Mytilotoxism — *see* Poisoning, fish
Myxadenitis labialis K13.0
Myxedema (adult) (idiocy) (infantile) (juvenile) (*see also* Hypothyroidism) E03.9
  circumscribed E05.90
    with storm E05.91
  coma E03.5
  congenital E00.1
  cutis L98.5
  localized (pretibial) E05.90
    with storm E05.91
  papular L98.5
Myxochondrosarcoma — *see* Neoplasm, cartilage, malignant
Myxofibroma — *see* Neoplasm, connective tissue, benign
  odontogenic — *see* Cyst, calcifying odontogenic
Myxofibrosarcoma — *see* Neoplasm, connective tissue, malignant
Myxolipoma D17.9
Myxoliposarcoma — *see* Neoplasm, connective tissue, malignant
Myxoma (*see also* Neoplasm, connective tissue, benign)
  nerve sheath — *see* Neoplasm, nerve, benign
  odontogenic — *see* Cyst, calcifying odontogenic
Myxosarcoma — *see* Neoplasm, connective tissue, malignant

▽ **Subterms under main terms may continue to next column or page**   ☑ **Additional Character Required — Refer to the Tabular List for Character Selection**   **221**

Myositis — Myxosarcoma

N

Naegeli's
  disease Q82.8
  leukemia, monocytic C93.1- ☑
Naegleriasis (with meningoencephalitis) B60.2
Naffziger's syndrome G54.0
Naga sore — see Ulcer, skin
Nägele's pelvis M95.5
  with disproportion (fetopelvic) O33.0
    causing obstructed labor O65.0
Nail (see also condition)
  biting F98.8
  patella syndrome Q87.2
Nanism, nanosomia — see Dwarfism
Nanophyetiasis B66.8
Nanukayami A27.89
Napkin rash L22
Narcolepsy G47.419
  with cataplexy G47.411
  in conditions classified elsewhere G47.429
    with cataplexy G47.421
Narcosis R06.89
Narcotism — see Dependence
NARP (Neuropathy, Ataxia and Retinitis pigmentosa)
  syndrome E88.49
Narrow
  anterior chamber angle H40.03- ☑
  pelvis — see Contraction, pelvis
Narrowing (see also Stenosis)
  artery I77.1
    auditory, internal I65.8
    basilar — see Occlusion, artery, basilar
    carotid — see Occlusion, artery, carotid
    cerebellar — see Occlusion, artery, cerebellar
    cerebral — see Occlusion artery, cerebral
    choroidal — see Occlusion, artery, cerebral, specified NEC
    communicating posterior — see Occlusion, artery, cerebral, specified NEC
    coronary (see also Disease, heart, ischemic, atherosclerotic)
      congenital Q24.5
        syphilitic A50.54 [I52]
      due to syphilis NEC A52.06
    hypophyseal — see Occlusion, artery, cerebral, specified NEC
    pontine — see Occlusion, artery, cerebral, specified NEC
    precerebral — see Occlusion, artery, precerebral
    vertebral — see Occlusion, artery, vertebral
  auditory canal (external) — see Stenosis, external ear canal
  eustachian tube — see Obstruction, eustachian tube
  eyelid — see Disorder, eyelid function
  larynx J38.6
  mesenteric artery K55.0
  palate M26.89
  palpebral fissure — see Disorder, eyelid function
  ureter N13.5
    with infection N13.6
  urethra — see Stricture, urethra
Narrowness, abnormal, eyelid Q10.3
Nasal — see condition
Nasolachrymal, nasolacrimal — see condition
Nasopharyngeal (see also condition)
  pituitary gland Q89.2
  torticollis M43.6
Nasopharyngitis (acute) (infective) (streptococcal) (subacute) J00
  chronic (suppurative) (ulcerative) J31.1
Nasopharynx, nasopharyngeal — see condition
Natal tooth, teeth K00.6
Nausea (without vomiting) R11.0
  with vomiting R11.2
  gravidarum — see Hyperemesis, gravidarum
  marina T75.3 ☑
  navalis T75.3 ☑
Navel — see condition
Neapolitan fever — see Brucellosis

Near drowning T75.1 ☑
Nearsightedness — see Myopia
Near-syncope R55
Nebula, cornea — see Opacity, cornea
Necator americanus infestation B76.1
Necatoriasis B76.1
Neck — see condition
Necrobiosis R68.89
  lipoidica NEC L92.1
    with diabetes — see E08-E13 with .620
Necrolysis, toxic epidermal L51.2
  due to drug
    correct substance properly administered — see Table of Drugs and Chemicals, by drug, adverse effect
    overdose or wrong substance given or taken — see Table of Drugs and Chemicals, by drug, poisoning
Necrophilia F65.89
Necrosis, necrotic (ischemic) (see also Gangrene)
  adrenal (capsule) (gland) E27.49
  amputation stump (surgical) (late) T87.50
    arm T87.5- ☑
    leg T87.5- ☑
  antrum J32.0
  aorta (hyaline) (see also Aneurysm, aorta)
    cystic medial — see Dissection, aorta
  artery I77.5
  bladder (aseptic) (sphincter) N32.89
  bone (see also Osteonecrosis) M87.9
    aseptic or avascular — see Osteonecrosis
      idiopathic M87.00
    ethmoid J32.2
    jaw M27.2
    tuberculous — see Tuberculosis, bone
  brain I67.89
  breast (aseptic) (fat) (segmental) N64.1
  bronchus J98.09
  central nervous system NEC I67.89
  cerebellar I67.89
  cerebral I67.89
  colon K55.0
  cornea H18.40
  cortical (acute) (renal) N17.1
  cystic medial (aorta) — see Dissection, aorta
  dental pulp K04.1
  esophagus K22.8
  ethmoid (bone) J32.2
  eyelid — see Disorder, eyelid, degenerative
  fat, fatty (generalized) (see also Disorder, soft tissue, specified type NEC)
    abdominal wall K65.4
    breast (aseptic) (segmental) N64.1
    localized — see Degeneration, by site, fatty
    mesentery K65.4
    omentum K65.4
    pancreas K86.8
    peritoneum K65.4
    skin (subcutaneous), newborn P83.0
    subcutaneous, due to birth injury P15.6
  gallbladder — see Cholecystitis, acute
  heart — see Infarct, myocardium
  hip, aseptic or avascular — see Osteonecrosis, by type, femur
  intestine (acute) (hemorrhagic) (massive) K55.0
  jaw M27.2
  kidney (bilateral) N28.0
    acute N17.9
    cortical (acute) (bilateral) N17.1
      with ectopic or molar pregnancy O08.4
    medullary (bilateral) (in acute renal failure) (papillary) N17.2
    papillary (bilateral) (in acute renal failure) N17.2
    tubular (acute) N17.0
      with ectopic or molar pregnancy O08.4
      complicating
        abortion — see Abortion, by type, complicated by, tubular necrosis
        ectopic or molar pregnancy O08.4
        pregnancy — see Pregnancy, complicated by, diseases of, specified type or system NEC

Necrosis, necrotic — continued
  kidney — continued
    tubular — continued
      following ectopic or molar pregnancy O08.4
      traumatic T79.5 ☑
  larynx J38.7
  liver (with hepatic failure) (cell) — see Failure, hepatic
    hemorrhagic, central K76.2
  lung J85.0
  lymphatic gland — see Lymphadenitis, acute
  mammary gland (fat) (segmental) N64.1
  mastoid (chronic) — see Mastoiditis, chronic
  medullary (acute) (renal) N17.2
  mesentery K55.0
    fat K65.4
  mitral valve — see Insufficiency, mitral
  myocardium, myocardial — see Infarct, myocardium
  nose J34.0
  omentum (with mesenteric infarction) K55.0
    fat K65.4
  orbit, orbital — see Osteomyelitis, orbit
  ossicles, ear — see Abnormal, ear ossicles
  ovary N70.92
  pancreas (aseptic) (duct) (fat) K86.8
    acute (infective) — see Pancreatitis, acute
    infective — see Pancreatitis, acute
  papillary (acute) (renal) N17.2
  perineum N90.89
  peritoneum (with mesenteric infarction) K55.0
    fat K65.4
  pharynx J02.9
    in granulocytopenia — see Neutropenia
    Vincent's A69.1
  phosphorus — see subcategory T54.2 ☑
  pituitary (gland) (postpartum) (Sheehan) E23.0
  pressure — see Ulcer, pressure, by site
  pulmonary J85.0
  pulp (dental) K04.1
  radiation — see Necrosis, by site
  radium — see Necrosis, by site
  renal — see Necrosis, kidney
  sclera H15.89
  scrotum N50.8
  skin or subcutaneous tissue NEC I96
  spine, spinal (column) (see also Osteonecrosis, by type, vertebra)
    cord G95.19
  spleen D73.5
  stomach K31.89
  stomatitis (ulcerative) A69.0
  subcutaneous fat, newborn P83.8
  subendocardial (acute) I21.4
    chronic I25.89
  suprarenal (capsule) (gland) E27.49
  testis N50.8
  thymus (gland) E32.8
  tonsil J35.8
  trachea J39.8
  tuberculous NEC — see Tuberculosis
  tubular (acute) (anoxic) (renal) (toxic) N17.0
    postprocedural N99.0
  vagina N89.8
  vertebra (see also Osteonecrosis, by type, vertebra)
    tuberculous A18.01
  vulva N90.89
  X-ray — see Necrosis, by site
Necrospermia — see Infertility, male
Need (for)
  care provider because (of)
    assistance with personal care Z74.1
    continuous supervision required Z74.3
    impaired mobility Z74.09
    no other household member able to render care Z74.2
    specified reason NEC Z74.8
  immunization — see Vaccination
  vaccination — see Vaccination
Neglect
  adult
    confirmed T74.01 ☑
    history of Z91.412
    suspected T76.01 ☑

☑ **Additional Character Required** — Refer to the Tabular List for Character Selection   ⬮ **Subterms under main terms may continue to next column or page**

Neglect — *continued*
- child (childhood)
  - confirmed T74.02 ☑
  - history of Z62.812
  - suspected T76.02 ☑
- emotional, in childhood Z62.898
- hemispatial R41.4
- left-sided R41.4
- sensory R41.4
- visuospatial R41.4

Neisserian infection NEC — *see* Gonococcus
Nelaton's syndrome G60.8
Nelson's syndrome E24.1
Nematodiasis (intestinal) B82.0
- Ancylostoma B76.0

Neonatal (*see also* Newborn)
- acne L70.4
- bradycardia P29.12
- screening, abnormal findings on P09
- tachycardia P29.11
- tooth, teeth K00.6

Neonatorum — *see* condition
Neoplasia
- endocrine, multiple (MEN) E31.20
  - type I E31.21
  - type IIA E31.22
  - type IIB E31.23
- intraepithelial (histologically confirmed)
  - anal (AIN) (histologically confirmed) K62.82
    - grade I K62.82
    - grade II K62.82
    - severe D01.3
  - cervical glandular (histologically confirmed) D06.9
  - cervix (uteri) (CIN) (histologically confirmed) N87.9
    - glandular D06.9
    - grade I N87.0
    - grade II N87.1
    - grade III (severe dysplasia) (*see also* Carcinoma, cervix uteri, in situ) D06.9
  - prostate (histologically confirmed) (PIN I) (PIN II) N42.3
    - grade I N42.3
    - grade II N42.3
    - severe D07.5
  - vagina (histologically confirmed) (VAIN) N89.3
    - grade I N89.0
    - grade II N89.1
    - grade III (severe dysplasia) D07.2
  - vulva (histologically confirmed) (VIN) N90.3
    - grade I N90.0
    - grade II N90.1
    - grade III (severe dysplasia) D07.1

Neoplasm, neoplastic (*see also* Table of Neoplasms)
- lipomatous, benign — *see* Lipoma

Neovascularization
- ciliary body — *see* Disorder, iris, vascular
- cornea H16.40- ☑
  - deep H16.44- ☑
  - ghost vessels — *see* Ghost, vessels
  - localized H16.43- ☑
  - pannus — *see* Pannus
- iris — *see* Disorder, iris, vascular
- retina H35.05- ☑

Nephralgia N23
Nephritis, nephritic (albuminuric) (azotemic) (congenital) (disseminated) (epithelial) (familial) (focal) (granulomatous) (hemorrhagic) (infantile) (nonsuppurative, excretory) (uremic) N05.9
- with
  - dense deposit disease N05.6
  - diffuse
    - crescentic glomerulonephritis N05.7
    - endocapillary proliferative glomerulonephritis N05.4
    - membranous glomerulonephritis N05.2
    - mesangial proliferative glomerulonephritis N05.3
    - mesangiocapillary glomerulonephritis N05.5
  - edema — *see* Nephrosis
  - focal and segmental glomerular lesions N05.1
  - foot process disease N04.9
  - glomerular lesion
    - diffuse sclerosing N05.8
    - hypocomplementemic — *see* Nephritis, membranoproliferative
    - IgA — *see* Nephropathy, IgA
    - lobular, lobulonodular — *see* Nephritis, membranoproliferative

Nephritis, nephritic — *continued*
- with — *continued*
  - glomerular lesion — *continued*
    - nodular — *see* Nephritis, membranoproliferative
  - lesion of
    - glomerulonephritis, proliferative N05.8
    - renal necrosis N05.9
  - minor glomerular abnormality N05.0
  - specified morphological changes NEC N05.8
- acute N00.9
  - with
    - dense deposit disease N00.6
    - diffuse
      - crescentic glomerulonephritis N00.7
      - endocapillary proliferative glomerulonephritis N00.4
      - membranous glomerulonephritis N00.2
      - mesangial proliferative glomerulonephritis N00.3
      - mesangiocapillary glomerulonephritis N00.5
    - focal and segmental glomerular lesions N00.1
    - minor glomerular abnormality N00.0
    - specified morphological changes NEC N00.8
- amyloid E85.4 [N08]
- antiglomerular basement membrane (anti-GBM) antibody NEC
  - in Goodpasture's syndrome M31.0
- antitubular basement membrane (tubulo-interstitial) NEC N12
  - toxic — *see* Nephropathy, toxic
- arteriolar — *see* Hypertension, kidney
- arteriosclerotic — *see* Hypertension, kidney
- ascending — *see* Nephritis, tubulo-interstitial
- atrophic N03.9
- Balkan (endemic) N15.0
- calculous, calculus — *see* Calculus, kidney
- cardiac — *see* Hypertension, kidney
- cardiovascular — *see* Hypertension, kidney
- chronic N03.9
  - with
    - dense deposit disease N03.6
    - diffuse
      - crescentic glomerulonephritis N03.7
      - endocapillary proliferative glomerulonephritis N03.4
      - membranous glomerulonephritis N03.2
      - mesangial proliferative glomerulonephritis N03.3
      - mesangiocapillary glomerulonephritis N03.5
    - focal and segmental glomerular lesions N03.1
    - minor glomerular abnormality N03.0
    - specified morphological changes NEC N03.8
  - arteriosclerotic — *see* Hypertension, kidney
- cirrhotic N26.9
- complicating pregnancy O26.83- ☑
- croupous N00.9
- degenerative — *see* Nephrosis
- diffuse sclerosing N05.8
- due to
  - diabetes mellitus — *see* E08-E13 with .21
  - subacute bacterial endocarditis I33.0
  - systemic lupus erythematosus (chronic) M32.14
  - typhoid fever A01.09
- gonococcal (acute) (chronic) A54.21
- hypocomplementemic — *see* Nephritis, membranoproliferative
- IgA — *see* Nephropathy, IgA
- immune complex (circulating) NEC N05.8
- infective — *see* Nephritis, tubulo-interstitial
- interstitial — *see* Nephritis, tubulo-interstitial
- lead N14.3
- membranoproliferative (diffuse) (type 1 or 3) (*see also* N00-N07 with fourth character .5) N05.5
  - type 2 (*see also* N00-N07 with fourth character .6) N05.6
- minimal change N05.0
- necrotic, necrotizing NEC (*see also* N00-N07 with fourth character .8) N05.8
- nephrotic — *see* Nephrosis
- nodular — *see* Nephritis, membranoproliferative
- polycystic Q61.3
  - adult type Q61.2
  - autosomal
    - dominant Q61.2
    - recessive NEC Q61.19
  - childhood type NEC Q61.19
  - infantile type NEC Q61.19

Nephritis, nephritic — *continued*
- poststreptococcal N05.9
  - acute N05.9
  - chronic N03.9
  - rapidly progressive N01.9
- proliferative NEC (*see also* N00-N07 with fourth character .8) N05.8
- purulent — *see* Nephritis, tubulo-interstitial
- rapidly progressive N01.9
  - with
    - dense deposit disease N01.6
    - diffuse
      - crescentic glomerulonephritis N01.7
      - endocapillary proliferative glomerulonephritis N01.4
      - membranous glomerulonephritis N01.2
      - mesangial proliferative glomerulonephritis N01.3
      - mesangiocapillary glomerulonephritis N01.5
    - focal and segmental glomerular lesions N01.1
    - minor glomerular abnormality N01.0
    - specified morphological changes NEC N01.8
- salt losing or wasting NEC N28.89
- saturnine N14.3
- sclerosing, diffuse N05.8
- septic — *see* Nephritis, tubulo-interstitial
- specified pathology NEC (*see also* N00-N07 with fourth character .8) N05.8
- subacute N01.9
- suppurative — *see* Nephritis, tubulo-interstitial
- syphilitic (late) A52.75
  - congenital A50.59 [N08]
  - early (secondary) A51.44
- toxic — *see* Nephropathy, toxic
- tubal, tubular — *see* Nephritis, tubulo-interstitial
- tuberculous A18.11
- tubulo-interstitial (in) N12
  - acute (infectious) N10
  - chronic (infectious) N11.9
    - nonobstructive N11.8
      - reflux-associated N11.0
    - obstructive N11.1
    - specified NEC N11.8
  - due to
    - brucellosis A23.9 [N16]
    - cryoglobulinemia D89.1 [N16]
    - glycogen storage disease E74.00 [N16]
    - Sjögren's syndrome M35.04
- vascular — *see* Hypertension, kidney
- war N00.9

Nephroblastoma (epithelial) (mesenchymal) C64- ☑
Nephrocalcinosis E83.59 [N29]
Nephrocystitis, pustular — *see* Nephritis, tubulo-interstitial
Nephrolithiasis (congenital) (pelvis) (recurrent) (*see also* Calculus, kidney)
Nephroma C64- ☑
- mesoblastic D41.0- ☑

Nephronephritis — *see* Nephrosis
Nephronophthisis Q61.5
Nephropathia epidemica A98.5
Nephropathy (*see also* Nephritis) N28.9
- with
  - edema — *see* Nephrosis
  - glomerular lesion — *see* Glomerulonephritis
- amyloid, hereditary E85.0
- analgesic N14.0
  - with medullary necrosis, acute N17.2
- Balkan (endemic) N15.0
- chemical — *see* Nephropathy, toxic
- diabetic — *see* E08-E13 with .21
- drug-induced N14.2
  - specified NEC N14.1
- focal and segmental hyalinosis or sclerosis N02.1
- heavy metal-induced N14.3
- hereditary NEC N07.9
  - with
    - dense deposit disease N07.6
    - diffuse
      - crescentic glomerulonephritis N07.7
      - endocapillary proliferative glomerulonephritis N07.4
      - membranous glomerulonephritis N07.2
      - mesangial proliferative glomerulonephritis N07.3
      - mesangiocapillary glomerulonephritis N07.5
    - focal and segmental glomerular lesions N07.1
    - minor glomerular abnormality N07.0

⬙ **Subterms under main terms may continue to next column or page**   ☑ **Additional Character Required — Refer to the Tabular List for Character Selection**   **223**

Neglect — Nephropathy

Nephropathy — *continued*
  hereditary — *continued*
    with — *continued*
      specified morphological changes NEC N07.8
  hypercalcemic N25.89
  hypertensive — *see* Hypertension, kidney
  hypokalemic (vacuolar) N25.89
  IgA N02.8
    with glomerular lesion N02.9
      focal and segmental hyalinosis or sclerosis
        N02.1
      membranoproliferative (diffuse) N02.5
      membranous (diffuse) N02.2
      mesangial proliferative (diffuse) N02.3
      mesangiocapillary (diffuse) N02.5
      proliferative NEC N02.8
      specified pathology NEC N02.8
  lead N14.3
  membranoproliferative (diffuse) N02.5
  membranous (diffuse) N02.2
  mesangial (IgA/IgG) — *see* Nephropathy, IgA
    proliferative (diffuse) N02.3
  mesangiocapillary (diffuse) N02.5
  obstructive N13.8
  phenacetin N17.2
  phosphate-losing N25.0
  potassium depletion N25.89
  pregnancy-related O26.83- ☑
  proliferative NEC (*see also* N00-N07 with fourth char-
    acter .8) N05.8
  protein-losing N25.89
  saturnine N14.3
  sickle-cell D57.- ☑ [N08]
  toxic NEC N14.4
    due to
      drugs N14.2
        analgesic N14.0
          specified NEC N14.1
        heavy metals N14.3
  vasomotor N17.0
  water-losing N25.89
Nephroptosis N28.83
Nephropyosis — *see* Abscess, kidney
Nephrorrhagia N28.89
Nephrosclerosis (arteriolar)(arteriosclerotic) (chronic)
  (hyaline) (*see also* Hypertension, kidney)
  hyperplastic — *see* Hypertension, kidney
  senile N26.9
Nephrosis, nephrotic (Epstein's) (syndrome) (congenital)
  N04.9
  with
    foot process disease N04.9
    glomerular lesion N04.1
    hypocomplementemic N04.5
  acute N04.9
  anoxic — *see* Nephrosis, tubular
  chemical — *see* Nephrosis, tubular
  cholemic K76.7
  diabetic — *see* E08-E13 with .21
  Finnish type (congenital) Q89.8
  hemoglobin N10
  hemoglobinuric — *see* Nephrosis, tubular
  in
    amyloidosis E85.4 [N08]
    diabetes mellitus — *see* E08-E13 with .21
    epidemic hemorrhagic fever A98.5
    malaria (malariae) B52.0
  ischemic — *see* Nephrosis, tubular
  lipoid N04.9
  lower nephron — *see* Nephrosis, tubular
  malarial (malariae) B52.0
  minimal change N04.0
  myoglobin N10
  necrotizing — *see* Nephrosis, tubular
  osmotic (sucrose) N25.89
  radiation N04.9
  syphilitic (late) A52.75
  toxic — *see* Nephrosis, tubular
  tubular (acute) N17.0
    postprocedural N99.0
    radiation N04.9
Nephrosonephritis, hemorrhagic (endemic) A98.5
Nephrostomy
  attention to Z43.6
  status Z93.6
Nerve (*see also* condition)
  injury — *see* Injury, nerve, by body site
Nerves R45.0

Nervous (*see also* condition) R45.0
  heart F45.8
  stomach F45.8
  tension R45.0
Nervousness R45.0
Nesidioblastoma
  pancreas D13.7
  specified site NEC — *see* Neoplasm, benign, by site
  unspecified site D13.7
Nettleship's syndrome Q82.2
Neumann's disease or syndrome L10.1
Neuralgia, neuralgic (acute) M79.2
  accessory (nerve) G52.8
  acoustic (nerve) — *see* subcategory H93.3 ☑
  auditory (nerve) — *see* subcategory H93.3 ☑
  ciliary G44.009
    intractable G44.001
    not intractable G44.009
  cranial
    nerve (*see also* Disorder, nerve, cranial)
      fifth or trigeminal — *see* Neuralgia, trigeminal
    postherpetic, postzoster B02.29
  ear — *see* subcategory H92.0 ☑
  facialis vera G51.1
  Fothergill's — *see* Neuralgia, trigeminal
  glossopharyngeal (nerve) G52.1
  Horton's G44.009
    intractable G44.091
    not intractable G44.099
  Hunt's B02.21
  hypoglossal (nerve) G52.3
  infraorbital — *see* Neuralgia, trigeminal
  malarial — *see* Malaria
  migrainous G44.009
    intractable G44.001
    not intractable G44.009
  Morton's G57.6- ☑
  nerve, cranial — *see* Disorder, nerve, cranial
  nose G52.0
  occipital M54.81
  olfactory G52.0
  penis N48.9
  perineum R10.2
  postherpetic NEC B02.29
    trigeminal B02.22
  pubic region R10.2
  scrotum R10.2
  Sluder's G44.89
  specified nerve NEC G58.8
  spermatic cord R10.2
  sphenopalatine (ganglion) G90.09
  trifacial — *see* Neuralgia, trigeminal
  trigeminal G50.0
    postherpetic, postzoster B02.22
  vagus (nerve) G52.2
  writer's F48.8
    organic G25.89
Neurapraxia — *see* Injury, nerve
Neurasthenia F48.8
  cardiac F45.8
  gastric F45.8
  heart F45.8
Neurilemmoma (*see also* Neoplasm, nerve, benign)
  acoustic (nerve) D33.3
  malignant (*see also* Neoplasm, nerve, malignant)
    acoustic (nerve) C72.4- ☑
Neurilemmosarcoma — *see* Neoplasm, nerve, malignant
Neurinoma — *see* Neoplasm, nerve, benign
Neurinomatosis — *see* Neoplasm, nerve, uncertain behavior
Neuritis (rheumatoid) M79.2
  abducens (nerve) — *see* Strabismus, paralytic, sixth
    nerve
  accessory (nerve) G52.8
  acoustic (nerve) (*see also* subcategory) H93.3 ☑
    in (due to)
      infectious disease NEC B99 ☑ [H94.0-] ☑
      parasitic disease NEC B89 [H94.0-] ☑
    syphilitic A52.15
  alcoholic G62.1
    with psychosis — *see* Psychosis, alcoholic
  amyloid, any site E85.4 [G63]
  auditory (nerve) — *see* subcategory H93.3 ☑
  brachial — *see* Radiculopathy
    due to displacement, intervertebral disc — *see*
      Disorder, disc, cervical, with neuritis

Neuritis — *continued*
  cranial nerve
    due to Lyme disease A69.22
    eighth or acoustic or auditory — *see* subcategory
      H93.3 ☑
    eleventh or accessory G52.8
    fifth or trigeminal G51.0
    first or olfactory G52.0
    fourth or trochlear — *see* Strabismus, paralytic,
      fourth nerve
    second or optic — *see* Neuritis, optic
    seventh or facial G51.8
      newborn (birth injury) P11.3
    sixth or abducent — *see* Strabismus, paralytic, sixth
      nerve
    tenth or vagus G52.2
    third or oculomotor — *see* Strabismus, paralytic,
      third nerve
    twelfth or hypoglossal G52.3
  Déjérine-Sottas G60.0
  diabetic (mononeuropathy) — *see* E08-E13 with .41
    polyneuropathy — *see* E08-E13 with .42
  due to
    beriberi E51.11
    displacement, prolapse or rupture, intervertebral
      disc — *see* Disorder, disc, with, radiculopathy
    herniation, nucleus pulposus M51.9 [G55]
  endemic E51.11
  facial G51.8
    newborn (birth injury) P11.3
  general — *see* Polyneuropathy
  geniculate ganglion G51.1
    due to herpes (zoster) B02.21
  gouty M10.00 [G63]
  hypoglossal (nerve) G52.3
  ilioinguinal (nerve) G57.9- ☑
  infectious (multiple) NEC G61.0
  interstitial hypertrophic progressive G60.0
  lumbar M54.16
  lumbosacral M54.17
  multiple (*see also* Polyneuropathy)
    endemic E51.11
    infective, acute G61.0
  multiplex endemica E51.11
  nerve root — *see* Radiculopathy
  oculomotor (nerve) — *see* Strabismus, paralytic, third
    nerve
  olfactory nerve G52.0
  optic (nerve) (hereditary) (sympathetic) H46.9
    with demyelination G36.0
    in myelitis G36.0
    nutritional H46.2
    papillitis — *see* Papillitis, optic
    retrobulbar H46.1- ☑
    specified type NEC H46.8
    toxic H46.3
  peripheral (nerve) G62.9
    multiple — *see* Polyneuropathy
    single — *see* Mononeuritis
  pneumogastric (nerve) G52.2
  postherpetic, postzoster B02.29
  progressive hypertrophic interstitial G60.0
  retrobulbar (*see also* Neuritis, optic, retrobulbar)
    in (due to)
      late syphilis A52.15
      meningococcal infection A39.82
    meningococcal A39.82
    syphilitic A52.15
  sciatic (nerve) (*see also* Sciatica)
    due to displacement of intervertebral disc — *see*
      Disorder, disc, with, radiculopathy
  serum (*see also* Reaction, serum) T80.69 ☑
  shoulder-girdle G54.5
  specified nerve NEC G58.8
  spinal (nerve) root — *see* Radiculopathy
  syphilitic A52.15
  thenar (median) G56.1- ☑
  thoracic M54.14
  toxic NEC G62.2
  trochlear (nerve) — *see* Strabismus, paralytic, fourth
    nerve
  vagus (nerve) G52.2
Neuroastrocytoma — *see* Neoplasm, uncertain behavior, by site
Neuroavitaminosis E56.9 [G99.8]
Neuroblastoma
  olfactory C30.0
  specified site — *see* Neoplasm, malignant, by site

Neuroblastoma — *continued*
  unspecified site C74.90
Neurochorioretinitis — *see* Chorioretinitis
Neurocirculatory asthenia F45.8
Neurocysticercosis B69.0
Neurocytoma — *see* Neoplasm, benign, by site
Neurodermatitis (circumscribed) (circumscripta) (local) L28.0
  atopic L20.81
  diffuse (Brocq) L20.81
  disseminated L20.81
Neuroencephalomyelopathy, optic G36.0
Neuroepithelioma (*see also* Neoplasm, malignant, by site)
  olfactory C30.0
Neurofibroma (*see also* Neoplasm, nerve, benign)
  melanotic — *see* Neoplasm, nerve, benign
  multiple — *see* Neurofibromatosis
  plexiform — *see* Neoplasm, nerve, benign
Neurofibromatosis (multiple) (nonmalignant) Q85.00
  acoustic Q85.02
  malignant — *see* Neoplasm, nerve, malignant
  specified NEC Q85.09
  type 1 (von Recklinghausen) Q85.01
  type 2 Q85.02
Neurofibrosarcoma — *see* Neoplasm, nerve, malignant
Neurogenic (*see also* condition)
  bladder (*see also* Dysfunction, bladder, neuromuscular) N31.9
    cauda equina syndrome G83.4
  bowel NEC K59.2
  heart F45.8
Neuroglioma — *see* Neoplasm, uncertain behavior, by site
Neurolabyrinthitis (of Dix and Hallpike) — *see* Neuronitis, vestibular
Neurolathyrism — *see* Poisoning, food, noxious, plant
Neuroleprosy A30.9
Neuroma (*see also* Neoplasm, nerve, benign)
  acoustic (nerve) D33.3
  amputation (stump) (traumatic) (surgical complication) (late) T87.3- ☑
    arm T87.3- ☑
    leg T87.3- ☑
  digital (toe) G57.6- ☑
  interdigital (toe) G58.8
    lower limb G57.8- ☑
    upper limb G56.8- ☑
  intermetatarsal G57.8- ☑
  Morton's G57.6- ☑
  nonneoplastic
    arm G56.9- ☑
    leg G57.9- ☑
    lower extremity G57.9- ☑
    upper extremity G56.9- ☑
  optic (nerve) D33.3
  plantar G57.6- ☑
  plexiform — *see* Neoplasm, nerve, benign
  surgical (nonneoplastic)
    arm G56.9- ☑
    leg G57.9- ☑
    lower extremity G57.9- ☑
    upper extremity G56.9- ☑
Neuromyalgia — *see* Neuralgia
Neuromyasthenia (epidemic) (postinfectious) G93.3
Neuromyelitis G36.9
  ascending G61.0
  optica G36.0
Neuromyopathy G70.9
  paraneoplastic D49.9 [G13.0]
Neuromyotonia (Isaacs) G71.19
Neuronevus — *see* Nevus
Neuronitis G58.9
  ascending (acute) G57.2- ☑
  vestibular H81.2- ☑
Neuroparalytic — *see* condition
Neuropathy, neuropathic G62.9
  acute motor G62.81
  alcoholic G62.1
    with psychosis — *see* Psychosis, alcoholic
  arm G56.9- ☑
  autonomic, peripheral — *see* Neuropathy, peripheral, autonomic
  axillary G56.9- ☑
  bladder N31.9
    atonic (motor) (sensory) N31.2
    autonomous N31.2

Neuropathy, neuropathic — *continued*
  bladder — *continued*
    flaccid N31.2
    nonreflex N31.2
    reflex N31.1
    uninhibited N31.0
  brachial plexus G54.0
  cervical plexus G54.2
  chronic
    progressive segmentally demyelinating G62.89
    relapsing demyelinating G62.89
  Déjérine-Sottas G60.0
  diabetic — *see* E08-E13 with .40
    mononeuropathy — *see* E08-E13 with .41
    polyneuropathy — *see* E08-E13 with .42
  entrapment G58.9
    iliohypogastric nerve G57.8- ☑
    ilioinguinal nerve G57.8- ☑
    lateral cutaneous nerve of thigh G57.1- ☑
    median nerve G56.0- ☑
    obturator nerve G57.8- ☑
    peroneal nerve G57.3- ☑
    posterior tibial nerve G57.5- ☑
    saphenous nerve G57.8- ☑
    ulnar nerve G56.2- ☑
  facial nerve G51.9
  hereditary G60.9
    motor and sensory (types I-IV) G60.0
    sensory G60.8
    specified NEC G60.8
  hypertrophic G60.0
    Charcot-Marie-Tooth G60.0
    Déjérine-Sottas G60.0
    interstitial progressive G60.0
    of infancy G60.0
    Refsum G60.1
  idiopathic G60.9
    progressive G60.3
    specified NEC G60.8
  in association with hereditary ataxia G60.2
  intercostal G58.0
  ischemic — *see* Disorder, nerve
  Jamaica (ginger) G62.2
  leg NEC G57.9- ☑
  lower extremity G57.9- ☑
  lumbar plexus G54.1
  median nerve G56.1- ☑
  motor and sensory (*see also* Polyneuropathy)
    hereditary (types I-IV) G60.0
  multiple (acute) (chronic) — *see* Polyneuropathy
  optic (nerve) (*see also* Neuritis, optic)
    ischemic H47.01- ☑
  paraneoplastic (sensorial) (Denny Brown) D49.9 [G13.0]
  peripheral (nerve) (*see also* Polyneuropathy) G62.9
    autonomic G90.9
      idiopathic G90.09
      in (due to)
        amyloidosis E85.4 [G99.0]
        diabetes mellitus — *see* E08-E13 with .43
        endocrine disease NEC E34.9 [G99.0]
        gout M10.00 [G99.0]
        hyperthyroidism E05.90 [G99.0]
          with thyroid storm E05.91 [G99.0]
        metabolic disease NEC E88.9 [G99.0]
    idiopathic G60.9
      progressive G60.3
    in (due to)
      antitetanus serum G62.0
      arsenic G62.2
      drugs NEC G62.0
      lead G62.2
      organophosphate compounds G62.2
      toxic agent NEC G62.2
  plantar nerves G57.6- ☑
  progressive
    hypertrophic interstitial G60.0
    inflammatory G62.81
  radicular NEC — *see* Radiculopathy
  sacral plexus G54.1
  sciatic G57.0- ☑
  serum G61.1
  toxic NEC G62.2
  trigeminal sensory G50.8
  ulnar nerve G56.2- ☑
  uremic N18.9 [G63]
  vitamin B12 E53.8 [G63]
    with anemia (pernicious) D51.0 [G63]
      due to dietary deficiency D51.3 [G63]

Neurophthisis (*see also* Disorder, nerve)
  peripheral, diabetic — *see* E08-E13 with .42
Neuroretinitis — *see* Chorioretinitis
Neuroretinopathy, hereditary optic H47.22
Neurosarcoma — *see* Neoplasm, nerve, malignant
Neurosclerosis — *see* Disorder, nerve
Neurosis, neurotic F48.9
  anankastic F42
  anxiety (state) F41.1
    panic type F41.0
  asthenic F48.8
  bladder F45.8
  cardiac (reflex) F45.8
  cardiovascular F45.8
  character F60.9
  colon F45.8
  compensation F68.1 ☑
  compulsive, compulsion F42
  conversion F44.9
  craft F48.8
  cutaneous F45.8
  depersonalization F48.1
  depressive (reaction) (type) F34.1
  environmental F48.8
  excoriation L98.1
  fatigue F48.8
  functional — *see* Disorder, somatoform
  gastric F45.8
  gastrointestinal F45.8
  heart F45.8
  hypochondriacal F45.21
  hysterical F44.9
  incoordination F45.8
    larynx F45.8
    vocal cord F45.8
  intestine F45.8
  larynx (sensory) F45.8
    hysterical F44.4
  mixed NEC F48.8
  musculoskeletal F45.8
  obsessional F42
  obsessive-compulsive F42
  occupational F48.8
  ocular NEC F45.8
  organ — *see* Disorder, somatoform
  pharynx F45.8
  phobic F40.9
  posttraumatic (situational) F43.10
    acute F43.11
    chronic F43.12
  psychasthenic (type) F48.8
  railroad F48.8
  rectum F45.8
  respiratory F45.8
  rumination F45.8
  sexual F65.9
  situational F48.8
  social F40.10
    generalized F40.11
  specified type NEC F48.8
  state F48.9
    with depersonalization episode F48.1
  stomach F45.8
  traumatic F43.10
    acute F43.11
    chronic F43.12
  vasomotor F45.8
  visceral F45.8
  war F48.8
Neurospongioblastosis diffusa Q85.1
Neurosyphilis (arrested) (early) (gumma) (late) (latent) (recurrent) (relapse) A52.3
  with ataxia (cerebellar) (locomotor) (spastic) (spinal) A52.19
  aneurysm (cerebral) A52.05
  arachnoid (adhesive) A52.13
  arteritis (any artery) (cerebral) A52.04
  asymptomatic A52.2
  congenital A50.40
  dura (mater) A52.13
  general paresis A52.17
  hemorrhagic A52.05
  juvenile (asymptomatic) (meningeal) A50.40
  leptomeninges (aseptic) A52.13
  meningeal, meninges (adhesive) A52.13
  meningitis A52.13
  meningovascular (diffuse) A52.13
  optic atrophy A52.15

▽ Subterms under main terms may continue to next column or page   ☑ Additional Character Required — Refer to the Tabular List for Character Selection   225

Neuroblastoma — Neurosyphilis

Neurosyphilis — *continued*
  parenchymatous (degenerative) A52.19
  paresis, paretic A52.17
    juvenile A50.45
  remission in (sustained) A52.3
  serological (without symptoms) A52.2
  specified nature or site NEC A52.19
  tabes, tabetic (dorsalis) A52.11
    juvenile A50.45
  taboparesis A52.17
    juvenile A50.45
  thrombosis (cerebral) A52.05
  vascular (cerebral) NEC A52.05
Neurothekeoma — *see* Neoplasm, nerve, benign
Neurotic — *see* Neurosis
Neurotoxemia — *see* Toxemia
Neutroclusion M26.211
Neutropenia, neutropenic (chronic) (genetic) (idiopathic) (immune) (infantile) (malignant) (pernicious) (splenic) D70.9
  congenital (primary) D70.0
  cyclic D70.4
  cytoreductive cancer chemotherapy sequela D70.1
  drug-induced D70.2
    due to cytoreductive cancer chemotherapy D70.1
  due to infection D70.3
  fever D70.9
  neonatal, transitory (isoimmune) (maternal transfer) P61.5
  periodic D70.4
  secondary (cyclic) (periodic) (splenic) D70.4
    drug-induced D70.2
      due to cytoreductive cancer chemotherapy D70.1
  toxic D70.8
Neutrophilia, hereditary giant D72.0
Nevocarcinoma — *see* Melanoma
Nevus D22.9
  achromic — *see* Neoplasm, skin, benign
  amelanotic — *see* Neoplasm, skin, benign
  angiomatous D18.00
    intra-abdominal D18.03
    intracranial D18.02
    skin D18.01
    specified site NEC D18.09
  araneus I78.1
  balloon cell — *see* Neoplasm, skin, benign
  bathing trunk D48.5
  blue — *see* Neoplasm, skin, benign
    cellular — *see* Neoplasm, skin, benign
    giant — *see* Neoplasm, skin, benign
    Jadassohn's — *see* Neoplasm, skin, benign
    malignant — *see* Melanoma
  capillary D18.00
    intra-abdominal D18.03
    intracranial D18.02
    skin D18.01
    specified site NEC D18.09
  cavernous D18.00
    intra-abdominal D18.03
    intracranial D18.02
    skin D18.01
    specified site NEC D18.09
  cellular — *see* Neoplasm, skin, benign
    blue — *see* Neoplasm, skin, benign
  choroid D31.3- ☑
  comedonicus Q82.5
  conjunctiva D31.0- ☑
  dermal — *see* Neoplasm, skin, benign
    with epidermal nevus — *see* Neoplasm, skin, benign
  dysplastic — *see* Neoplasm, skin, benign
  eye D31.9- ☑
  flammeus Q82.5
  hemangiomatous D18.00
    intra-abdominal D18.03
    intracranial D18.02
    skin D18.01
    specified site NEC D18.09
  iris D31.4- ☑
  lacrimal gland D31.5- ☑
  lymphatic D18.1
  magnocellular
    specified site — *see* Neoplasm, benign, by site
    unspecified site D31.40
  malignant — *see* Melanoma
  meaning hemangioma D18.00
    intra-abdominal D18.03

Nevus — *continued*
  meaning hemangioma — *continued*
    intracranial D18.02
    skin D18.01
    specified site NEC D18.09
  mouth (mucosa) D10.30
    specified site NEC D10.39
    white sponge Q38.6
  multiplex Q85.1
  non-neoplastic I78.1
  oral mucosa D10.30
    specified site NEC D10.39
    white sponge Q38.6
  orbit D31.6- ☑
  pigmented
    giant (*see also* Neoplasm, skin, uncertain behavior) D48.5
      malignant melanoma in — *see* Melanoma
  portwine Q82.5
  retina D31.2- ☑
  retrobulbar D31.6- ☑
  sanguineous Q82.5
  senile I78.1
  skin D22.9
    abdominal wall D22.5
    ala nasi D22.39
    ankle D22.7- ☑
    anus, anal D22.5
    arm D22.6- ☑
    auditory canal (external) D22.2- ☑
    auricle (ear) D22.2- ☑
    auricular canal (external) D22.2- ☑
    axilla, axillary fold D22.5
    back D22.5
    breast D22.5
    brow D22.39
    buttock D22.5
    canthus (eye) D22.1- ☑
    cheek (external) D22.39
    chest wall D22.5
    chin D22.39
    ear (external) D22.2- ☑
    external meatus (ear) D22.2- ☑
    eyebrow D22.39
    eyelid (lower) (upper) D22.1- ☑
    face D22.30
      specified NEC D22.39
    female genital organ (external) NEC D28.0
    finger D22.6- ☑
    flank D22.5
    foot D22.7- ☑
    forearm D22.6- ☑
    forehead D22.39
    foreskin D29.0
    genital organ (external) NEC
      female D28.0
      male D29.9
    gluteal region D22.5
    groin D22.5
    hand D22.6- ☑
    heel D22.7- ☑
    helix D22.2- ☑
    hip D22.7- ☑
    interscapular region D22.5
    jaw D22.39
    knee D22.7- ☑
    labium (majus) (minus) D28.0
    leg D22.7- ☑
    lip (lower) (upper) D22.0
    lower limb D22.7- ☑
    male genital organ (external) D29.9
    nail D22.9
      finger D22.6- ☑
      toe D22.7- ☑
    nasolabial groove D22.39
    nates D22.5
    neck D22.4
    nose (external) D22.39
    palpebra D22.1- ☑
    penis D29.0
    perianal skin D22.5
    perineum D22.5
    pinna D22.2- ☑
    popliteal fossa or space D22.7- ☑
    prepuce D29.0
    pudendum D28.0
    scalp D22.4

Nevus — *continued*
  skin — *continued*
    scrotum D29.4
    shoulder D22.6- ☑
    submammary fold D22.5
    temple D22.39
    thigh D22.7- ☑
    toe D22.7- ☑
    trunk NEC D22.5
    umbilicus D22.5
    upper limb D22.6- ☑
    vulva D28.0
  specified site NEC — *see* Neoplasm, by site, benign
  spider I78.1
  stellar I78.1
  strawberry Q82.5
  Sutton's — *see* Neoplasm, skin, benign
  unius lateris Q82.5
  Unna's Q82.5
  vascular Q82.5
  verrucous Q82.5
Newborn (infant) (liveborn) (singleton) Z38.2
  abstinence syndrome P96.1
  acne L70.4
  affected by (suspected to be)
    abnormalities of membranes P02.9
      specified NEC P02.8
    abruptio placenta P02.1
    amino-acid metabolic disorder, transitory P74.8
    amniocentesis (while in utero) P00.6
    amnionitis P02.7
    apparent life threatening event (ALTE) R68.13
    bleeding (into)
      cerebral cortex P52.22
      germinal matrix P52.0
      ventricles P52.1
    breech delivery P03.0
    cardiac arrest P29.81
    cardiomyopathy I42.8
      congenital I42.4
    cerebral ischemia P91.0
    Cesarean delivery P03.4
    chemotherapy agents P04.1
    chorioamnionitis P02.7
    cocaine (crack) P04.41
    complications of labor and delivery P03.9
      specified NEC P03.89
    compression of umbilical cord NEC P02.5
    contracted pelvis P03.1
    delivery P03.9
      Cesarean P03.4
      forceps P03.2
      vacuum extractor P03.3
    entanglement (knot) in umbilical cord P02.5
    environmental chemicals P04.6
    fetal (intrauterine)
      growth retardation P05.9
      malnutrition not light or small for gestational age P05.2
    forceps delivery P03.2
    heart rate abnormalities
      bradycardia P29.12
      intrauterine P03.819
        before onset of labor P03.810
        during labor P03.811
      tachycardia P29.11
    hemorrhage (antepartum) P02.1
      cerebellar (nontraumatic) P52.6
      intracerebral (nontraumatic) P52.4
      intracranial (nontraumatic) P52.9
        specified NEC P52.8
      intraventricular (nontraumatic) P52.3
        grade 1 P52.0
        grade 2 P52.1
        grade 3 P52.21
        grade 4 P52.22
      posterior fossa (nontraumatic) P52.6
      subarachnoid (nontraumatic) P52.5
      subependymal P52.0
        with intracerebral extension P52.22
        with intraventricular extension P52.1
          with enlargment of ventricles P52.21
        without intraventricular extension P52.0
    hypoxic ischemic encephalopathy [HIE] P91.60
      mild P91.61
      moderate P91.62
      severe P91.63
    induction of labor P03.89

☑ **Additional Character Required** — Refer to the Tabular List for Character Selection   ▽ **Subterms under main terms may continue to next column or page**

Newborn — *continued*
  affected by — *continued*
    intestinal perforation P78.0
    intrauterine (fetal) blood loss P50.9
      due to (from)
        cut end of co-twin cord P50.5
        hemorrhage into
          co-twin P50.3
            maternal circulation P50.4
          placenta P50.2
        ruptured cord blood P50.1
        vasa previa P50.0
      specified NEC P50.8
    intrauterine (fetal) hemorrhage P50.9
    intrauterine (in utero) procedure P96.5
    malpresentation (malposition) NEC P03.1
    maternal (complication of) (use of)
      alcohol P04.3
      analgesia (maternal) P04.0
      anesthesia (maternal) P04.0
      blood loss P02.1
      circulatory disease P00.3
      condition P00.9
        specified NEC P00.89
      delivery P03.9
        Cesarean P03.4
        forceps P03.2
        vacuum extractor P03.3
      diabetes mellitus (pre-existing) P70.1
      disorder P00.9
        specified NEC P00.89
      drugs (addictive) (illegal) NEC P04.49
      ectopic pregnancy P01.4
      gestational diabetes P70.0
      hemorrhage P02.1
      hypertensive disorder P00.0
      incompetent cervix P01.0
      infectious disease P00.2
      injury P00.5
      labor and delivery P03.9
      malpresentation before labor P01.7
      maternal death P01.6
      medical procedure P00.7
      medication P04.1
      multiple pregnancy P01.5
      nutritional disorder P00.4
      oligohydramnios P01.2
      parasitic disease P00.2
      periodontal disease P00.81
      placenta previa P02.0
      polyhydramnios P01.3
      precipitate delivery P03.5
      pregnancy P01.9
        specified P01.8
      premature rupture of membranes P01.1
      renal disease P00.1
      respiratory disease P00.3
      surgical procedure P00.6
      urinary tract disease P00.1
      uterine contraction (abnormal) P03.6
    meconium peritonitis P78.0
    medication (legal) (maternal use) (prescribed) P04.1
    membrane abnormalities P02.9
      specified NEC P02.8
    membranitis P02.7
    methamphetamine(s) P04.49
    mixed metabolic and respiratory acidosis P84
    neonatal abstinence syndrome P96.1
    noxious substances transmitted via placenta or
      breast milk P04.9
      specified NEC P04.8
    nutritional supplements P04.5
    placenta previa P02.0
    placental
      abnormality (functional) (morphological)
        P02.20
        specified NEC P02.29
      dysfunction P02.29
      infarction P02.29
      insufficiency P02.29
      separation NEC P02.1
      transfusion syndromes P02.3
    placentitis P02.7
    precipitate delivery P03.5
    prolapsed cord P02.4
    respiratory arrest P28.81
    slow intrauterine growth P05.9
    tobacco P04.2

Newborn — *continued*
  affected by — *continued*
    twin to twin transplacental transfusion P02.3
    umbilical cord (tightly) around neck P02.5
    umbilical cord condition P02.60
      short cord P02.69
      specified NEC P02.69
    uterine contractions (abnormal) P03.6
    vasa previa P02.69
      from intrauterine blood loss P50.0
  apnea P28.3
    obstructive P28.4
    primary P28.3
    specified P28.4
  born in hospital Z38.00
    by cesarean Z38.01
  born outside hospital Z38.1
  breast buds P96.89
  breast engorgement P83.4
  check-up — *see* Newborn, examination
  convulsion P90
  dehydration P74.1
  examination
    8 to 28 days old Z00.111
    under 8 days old Z00.110
  fever P81.9
    environmentally-induced P81.0
  hyperbilirubinemia P59.9
    of prematurity P59.0
  hypernatremia P74.2
  hyponatremia P74.2
  infection P39.9
    candidal P37.5
    specified NEC P39.8
    urinary tract P39.3
  jaundice P59.8
    due to
      breast milk inhibitor P59.3
      hepatocellular damage P59.20
        specified NEC P59.29
      preterm delivery P59.0
    of prematurity P59.0
    specified NEC P59.8
  late metabolic acidosis P74.0
  mastitis P39.0
    infective P39.0
    noninfective P83.4
  multiple born NEC Z38.8
    born in hospital Z38.68
      by cesarean Z38.69
    born outside hospital Z38.7
  omphalitis P38.9
    with mild hemorrhage P38.1
    without hemorrhage P38.9
  post-term P08.21
  prolonged gestation (over 42 completed weeks)
    P08.22
  quadruplet Z38.8
    born in hospital Z38.63
      by cesarean Z38.64
    born outside hospital Z38.7
  quintuplet Z38.8
    born in hospital Z38.65
      by cesarean Z38.66
    born outside hospital Z38.7
  seizure P90
  sepsis (congenital) P36.9
    due to
      anaerobes NEC P36.5
      Escherichia coli P36.4
      Staphylococcus P36.30
        aureus P36.2
        specified NEC P36.39
      Streptococcus P36.10
        group B P36.0
        specified NEC P36.19
      specified NEC P36.8
  triplet Z38.8
    born in hospital Z38.61
      by cesarean Z38.62
    born outside hospital Z38.7
  twin Z38.5
    born in hospital Z38.30
      by cesarean Z38.31
    born outside hospital Z38.4
  vomiting P92.09
    bilious P92.01
  weight check Z00.111

Newcastle conjunctivitis or disease B30.8
Nezelof's syndrome (pure alymphocytosis) D81.4
Niacin (amide) **deficiency** E52
Nicolas (-Durand)-**Favre disease** A55
Nicotine — *see* Tobacco
Nicotinic acid deficiency E52
Niemann-Pick disease or syndrome E75.249
  specified NEC E75.248
  type
    A E75.240
    B E75.241
    C E75.242
    D E75.243
Night
  blindness — *see* Blindness, night
  sweats R61
  terrors (child) F51.4
Nightmares (REM sleep type) F51.5
Nipple — *see* condition
Nisbet's chancre A57
Nishimoto (-Takeuchi) **disease** I67.5
Nitritoid crisis or reaction — *see* Crisis, nitritoid
Nitrosohemoglobinemia D74.8
Njovera A65
Nocardiosis, nocardiasis A43.9
  cutaneous A43.1
  lung A43.0
  pneumonia A43.0
  pulmonary A43.0
  specified site NEC A43.8
Nocturia R35.1
  psychogenic F45.8
Nocturnal — *see* condition
Nodal rhythm I49.8
Node(s) (*see also* Nodule)
  Bouchard's (with arthropathy) M15.2
  Haygarth's M15.8
  Heberden's (with arthropathy) M15.1
  larynx J38.7
  lymph — *see* condition
  milker's B08.03
  Osler's I33.0
  Schmorl's — *see* Schmorl's disease
  singer's J38.2
  teacher's J38.2
  tuberculous — *see* Tuberculosis, lymph gland
  vocal cord J38.2
Nodule(s), **nodular**
  actinomycotic — *see* Actinomycosis
  breast NEC N63
  colloid (cystic), thyroid E04.1
  cutaneous — *see* Swelling, localized
  endometrial (stromal) D26.1
  Haygarth's M15.8
  inflammatory — *see* Inflammation
  juxta-articular
    syphilitic A52.77
    yaws A66.7
  larynx J38.7
  lung, solitary (subsegmental branch of the bronchial
    tree) R91.1
    multiple R91.8
  milker's B08.03
  prostate N40.2
    with lower urinary tract symptoms (LUTS) N40.3
    without lower urinary tract symtpoms (LUTS) N40.2
  pulmonary, solitary (subsegmental branch of the
    bronchial tree) R91.1
  retrocardiac R09.89
  rheumatoid M06.30
    ankle M06.37- ☑
    elbow M06.32- ☑
    foot joint M06.37- ☑
    hand joint M06.34- ☑
    hip M06.35- ☑
    knee M06.36- ☑
    multiple site M06.39
    shoulder M06.31- ☑
    vertebra M06.38
    wrist M06.33- ☑
  scrotum (inflammatory) N49.2
  singer's J38.2
  solitary, lung (subsegmental branch of the bronchial
    tree) R91.1
    multiple R91.8
  subcutaneous — *see* Swelling, localized
  teacher's J38.2

Nodule(s), **nodular** — *continued*
thyroid (cold) (gland) (nontoxic) E04.1
with thyrotoxicosis E05.20
with thyroid storm E05.21
toxic or with hyperthyroidism E05.20
with thyroid storm E05.21
vocal cord J38.2
Noma (gangrenous) (hospital) (infective) A69.0
auricle I96
mouth A69.0
pudendi N76.89
vulvae N76.89
Nomad, nomadism Z59.0
Nonautoimmune hemolytic anemia D59.4
drug-induced D59.2
Nonclosure (*see also* Imperfect, closure)
ductus arteriosus (Botallo's) Q25.0
foramen
botalli Q21.1
ovale Q21.1
Noncompliance Z91.19
with
dialysis Z91.15
dietary regimen Z91.11
medical treatment Z91.19
medication regimen NEC Z91.14
underdosing (*see also* Table of Drugs and
Chemicals, categories T36-T50, with final
character 6) Z91.14
intentional NEC Z91.128
due to financial hardship of patient
Z91.120
unintentional NEC Z91.138
due to patient's age related debility
Z91.130
renal dialysis Z91.15
Nondescent (congenital) (*see also* Malposition, congenital)
cecum Q43.3
colon Q43.3
testicle Q53.9
bilateral Q53.20
abdominal Q53.21
perineal Q53.22
unilateral Q53.10
abdominal Q53.11
perineal Q53.12
Nondevelopment
brain Q02
part of Q04.3
heart Q24.8
organ or site, congenital NEC — *see* Hypoplasia
Nonengagement
head NEC O32.4 ☑
in labor, causing obstructed labor O64.8 ☑
Nonexanthematous tick fever A93.2
Nonexpansion, lung (newborn) P28.0
Nonfunctioning
cystic duct (*see also* Disease, gallbladder) K82.8
gallbladder (*see also* Disease, gallbladder) K82.8
kidney N28.9
labyrinth — *see* subcategory H83.2 ☑
Non-Hodgkin lymphoma NEC — *see* Lymphoma, non-Hodgkin
Nonimplantation, ovum N97.2
Noninsufflation, fallopian tube N97.1
Non-ketotic hyperglycinemia E72.51
Nonne-Milroy syndrome Q82.0
Nonovulation N97.0
Nonpatent fallopian tube N97.1
Nonpneumatization, lung NEC P28.0
Nonrotation — *see* Malrotation
Nonsecretion, urine — *see* Anuria
Nonunion
fracture — *see* Fracture, by site
organ or site, congenital NEC — *see* Imperfect, closure
symphysis pubis, congenital Q74.2
Nonvisualization, gallbladder R93.2
Nonvital, nonvitalized tooth K04.99
Non-working side interference M26.56
Noonan's syndrome Q87.1
Normocytic anemia (infectional) due to blood loss
(chronic) D50.0
acute D62
Norrie's disease (congenital) Q15.8
North American blastomycosis B40.9
Norwegian itch B86

Nose, nasal — *see* condition
Nosebleed R04.0
Nose-picking F98.8
Nosomania F45.21
Nosophobia F45.22
Nostalgia F43.20
Notch of iris Q13.2
Notching nose, congenital (tip) Q30.2
Nothnagel's
syndrome — *see* Strabismus, paralytic, third nerve
vasomotor acroparesthesia I73.89
Novy's relapsing fever A68.9
louse-borne A68.0
tick-borne A68.1
Noxious
foodstuffs, poisoning by — *see* Poisoning, food, noxious, plant
substances transmitted through placenta or breast
milk P04.9
Nucleus pulposus — *see* condition
Numbness R20.0
Nuns' knee — *see* Bursitis, prepatellar
Nursemaid's elbow S53.03- ☑
Nutcracker esophagus K22.4
Nutmeg liver K76.1
Nutrient element deficiency E61.9
specified NEC E61.8
Nutrition deficient or insufficient (*see also* Malnutrition) E46
due to
insufficient food T73.0 ☑
lack of
care (child) T76.02 ☑
adult T76.01 ☑
food T73.0 ☑
Nutritional stunting E45
Nyctalopia (night blindness) — *see* Blindness, night
Nycturia R35.1
psychogenic F45.8
Nymphomania F52.8
Nystagmus H55.00
benign paroxysmal — *see* Vertigo, benign paroxysmal
central positional H81.4- ☑
congenital H55.01
dissociated H55.04
latent H55.02
miners' H55.09
positional
benign paroxysmal H81.4- ☑
central H81.4- ☑
specified form NEC H55.09
visual deprivation H55.03

O

Obermeyer's relapsing fever (European) A68.0
Obesity E66.9
with alveolar hyperventilation E66.2
adrenal E27.8
complicating
childbirth O99.214
pregnancy O99.21- ☑
puerperium O99.215
constitutional E66.8
dietary counseling and surveillance Z71.3
drug-induced E66.1
due to
drug E66.1
excess calories E66.09
morbid E66.01
severe E66.01
endocrine E66.8
endogenous E66.8
familial E66.8
glandular E66.8
hypothyroid — *see* Hypothyroidism
morbid E66.01
with alveolar hypoventilation E66.2
due to excess calories E66.01
nutritional E66.09
pituitary E23.6
severe E66.01
specified type NEC E66.8
Oblique — *see* condition
Obliteration
appendix (lumen) K38.8
artery I77.1

Obliteration — *continued*
bile duct (noncalculous) K83.1
common duct (noncalculous) K83.1
cystic duct — *see* Obstruction, gallbladder
disease, arteriolar I77.1
endometrium N85.8
eye, anterior chamber — *see* Disorder, globe, hypotony
fallopian tube N97.1
lymphatic vessel I89.0
due to mastectomy I97.2
organ or site, congenital NEC — *see* Atresia, by site
ureter N13.5
with infection N13.6
urethra — *see* Stricture, urethra
vein I87.8
vestibule (oral) K08.8
Observation (following) (for) (without need for further
medical care) Z04.9
accident NEC Z04.3
at work Z04.2
transport Z04.1
adverse effect of drug Z03.6
alleged rape or sexual assault (victim), ruled out
adult Z04.41
child Z04.42
criminal assault Z04.8
development state
adolescent Z00.3
period of rapid growth in childhood Z00.2
puberty Z00.3
disease, specified NEC Z03.89
following work accident Z04.2
growth and development state — *see* Observation,
development state
injuries (accidental) NEC (*see also* Observation, accident)
newborn (for suspected condition, ruled out) — *see* -
Newborn, affected by (suspected to be), maternal (complication of) (use of)
postpartum
immediately after delivery Z39.0
routine follow-up Z39.2
pregnancy (normal) (without complication) Z34.9- ☑
high risk O09.9- ☑
suicide attempt, alleged NEC Z03.89
self-poisoning Z03.6
suspected, ruled out (*see also* Suspected condition,
ruled out)
abuse, physical
adult Z04.71
child Z04.72
accident at work Z04.2
adult battering victim Z04.71
child battering victim Z04.72
condition NEC Z03.89
newborn — *see* Newborn, affected by (suspected to be), maternal (complication of) (use of)
drug poisoning or adverse effect Z03.6
exposure (to)
anthrax Z03.810
biological agent NEC Z03.818
inflicted injury NEC Z04.8
suicide attempt, alleged Z03.89
self-poisoning Z03.6
toxic effects from ingested substance (drug) (poison) Z03.6
toxic effects from ingested substance (drug) (poison)
Z03.6
Obsession, obsessional state F42
Obsessive-compulsive neurosis or reaction F42
Obstetric embolism, septic — *see* Embolism, obstetric,
septic
Obstetrical trauma (complicating delivery) O71.9
with or following ectopic or molar pregnancy O08.6
specified type NEC O71.89
Obstipation — *see* Constipation
Obstruction, obstructed, obstructive
airway J98.8
with
allergic alveolitis J67.9
asthma J45.909
with
exacerbation (acute) J45.901
status asthmaticus J45.902
bronchiectasis J47.9

☑ **Additional Character Required** — Refer to the Tabular List for Character Selection   ▽ **Subterms under main terms may continue to next column or page**

Obstruction, obstructed, obstructive — *continued*
airway — *continued*
  with
    bronchiectasis — *continued*
      with — *continued*
        exacerbation (acute) J47.1
        lower respiratory infection J47.0
    bronchitis (chronic) J44.9
    emphysema J43.9
    chronic J44.9
      with
        allergic alveolitis — *see* Pneumonitis, hypersensitivity
        bronchiectasis J47.9
          with
            exacerbation (acute) J47.1
            lower respiratory infection J47.0
  due to
    foreign body — *see* Foreign body, by site, causing asphyxia
    inhalation of fumes or vapors J68.9
    laryngospasm J38.5
ampulla of Vater K83.1
aortic (heart) (valve) — *see* Stenosis, aortic
aortoiliac I74.09
aqueduct of Sylvius G91.1
  congenital Q03.0
    with spina bifida — *see* Spina bifida, by site, with hydrocephalus
Arnold-Chiari — *see* Arnold-Chiari disease
artery (*see also* Embolism, artery) I74.9
  basilar (complete) (partial) — *see* Occlusion, artery, basilar
  carotid (complete) (partial) — *see* Occlusion, artery, carotid
  cerebellar — *see* Occlusion, artery, cerebellar
  cerebral (anterior) (middle) (posterior) — *see* Occlusion, artery, cerebral
  precerebral — *see* Occlusion, artery, precerebral
  renal N28.0
  retinal NEC — *see* Occlusion, artery, retina
  vertebral (complete) (partial) — *see* Occlusion, artery, vertebral
band (intestinal) K56.69
bile duct or passage (common) (hepatic) (noncalculous) K83.1
  with calculus K80.51
  congenital (causing jaundice) Q44.3
biliary (duct) (tract) K83.1
  gallbladder K82.0
bladder-neck (acquired) N32.0
  congenital Q64.31
  due to hyperplasia (hypertrophy) of prostate — *see* Hyperplasia, prostate
bowel — *see* Obstruction, intestine
bronchus J98.09
canal, ear — *see* Stenosis, external ear canal
cardia K22.2
caval veins (inferior) (superior) I87.1
cecum — *see* Obstruction, intestine
circulatory I99.8
colon — *see* Obstruction, intestine
common duct (noncalculous) K83.1
coronary (artery) — *see* Occlusion, coronary
cystic duct (*see also* Obstruction, gallbladder)
  with calculus K80.21
device, implant or graft (*see also* Complications, by site and type, mechanical) T85.698 ☑
  arterial graft NEC — *see* Complication, cardiovascular device, mechanical, vascular
  catheter NEC T85.628 ☑
    cystostomy T83.090 ☑
    dialysis (renal) T82.49 ☑
      intraperitoneal T85.691 ☑
    infusion NEC T82.594 ☑
      spinal (epidural) (subdural) T85.690 ☑
    urinary, indwelling T83.098 ☑
  due to infection T85.79 ☑
  gastrointestinal — *see* Complications, prosthetic device, mechanical, gastrointestinal device
  genital NEC T83.498 ☑
    intrauterine contraceptive device T83.39 ☑
    penile prosthesis T83.490 ☑
  heart NEC — *see* Complication, cardiovascular device, mechanical
  joint prosthesis — *see* Complications, joint prosthesis, mechanical, specified NEC, by site

Obstruction, obstructed, obstructive — *continued*
device, implant or graft (*see also* Complications, by site and type, mechanical) — *continued*
  orthopedic NEC — *see* Complication, orthopedic, device, mechanical
  specified NEC T85.628 ☑
  urinary NEC (*see also* Complication, genitourinary, device, urinary, mechanical)
    graft T83.29 ☑
  vascular NEC — *see* Complication, cardiovascular device, mechanical
  ventricular intracranial shunt T85.09 ☑
due to foreign body accidentally left in operative wound T81.529 ☑
duodenum K31.5
ejaculatory duct N50.8
esophagus K22.2
eustachian tube (complete) (partial) H68.10- ☑
  cartilagenous (extrinsic) H68.13- ☑
    intrinsic H68.12- ☑
  osseous H68.11- ☑
fallopian tube (bilateral) N97.1
fecal K56.41
  with hernia — *see* Hernia, by site, with obstruction
foramen of Monro (congenital) Q03.8
  with spina bifida — *see* Spina bifida, by site, with hydrocephalus
foreign body — *see* Foreign body
gallbladder K82.0
  with calculus, stones K80.21
  congenital Q44.1
gastric outlet K31.1
gastrointestinal — *see* Obstruction, intestine
hepatic K76.89
  duct (noncalculous) K83.1
ileum — *see* Obstruction, intestine
iliofemoral (artery) I74.5
intestine K56.60
  with
    adhesions (intestinal) (peritoneal) K56.5
  adynamic K56.0
  by gallstone K56.3
  congenital (small) Q41.9
    large Q42.9
      specified part NEC Q42.8
  neurogenic K56.0
    Hirschsprung's disease or megacolon Q43.1
  newborn P76.9
    due to
      fecaliths P76.8
      inspissated milk P76.2
      meconium (plug) P76.0
        in mucoviscidosis E84.11
    specified NEC P76.8
  postoperative K91.3
  reflex K56.0
  specified NEC K56.69
  volvulus K56.2
intracardiac ball valve prosthesis T82.09 ☑
jejunum — *see* Obstruction, intestine
joint prosthesis — *see* Complications, joint prosthesis, mechanical, specified NEC, by site
kidney (calices) N28.89
labor — *see* Delivery
lacrimal (passages) (duct)
  by
    dacryolith — *see* Dacryolith
    stenosis — *see* Stenosis, lacrimal
  congenital Q10.5
  neonatal H04.53- ☑
lacrimonasal duct — *see* Obstruction, lacrimal
lacteal, with steatorrhea K90.2
laryngitis — *see* Laryngitis
larynx NEC J38.6
  congenital Q31.8
lung J98.4
  disease, chronic J44.9
lymphatic I89.0
meconium (plug)
  newborn P76.0
    due to fecaliths P76.0
    in mucoviscidosis E84.11
mitral — *see* Stenosis, mitral
nasal J34.89
nasolacrimal duct (*see also* Obstruction, lacrimal)
  congenital Q10.5
nasopharynx J39.2
nose J34.89

Obstruction, obstructed, obstructive — *continued*
organ or site, congenital NEC — *see* Atresia, by site
pancreatic duct K86.8
parotid duct or gland K11.8
pelviureteral junction N13.5
  congenital Q62.39
pharynx J39.2
portal (circulation) (vein) I81
prostate (*see also* Hyperplasia, prostate)
  valve (urinary) N32.0
pulmonary valve (heart) I37.0
pyelonephritis (chronic) N11.1
pylorus
  adult K31.1
  congenital or infantile Q40.0
rectosigmoid — *see* Obstruction, intestine
rectum K62.4
renal N28.89
  outflow N13.8
  pelvis, congenital Q62.39
respiratory J98.8
  chronic J44.9
retinal (vessels) H34.9
salivary duct (any) K11.8
  with calculus K11.5
sigmoid — *see* Obstruction, intestine
sinus (accessory) (nasal) J34.89
Stensen's duct K11.8
stomach NEC K31.89
  acute K31.0
  congenital Q40.2
  due to pylorospasm K31.3
submandibular duct K11.8
submaxillary gland K11.8
  with calculus K11.5
thoracic duct I89.0
thrombotic — *see* Thrombosis
trachea J39.8
tracheostomy airway J95.03
tricuspid (valve) — *see* Stenosis, tricuspid
upper respiratory, congenital Q34.8
ureter (functional) (pelvic junction) NEC N13.5
  with
    hydronephrosis N13.1
      with infection N13.6
    pyelonephritis (chronic) N11.1
  congenital Q62.39
  due to calculus — *see* Calculus, ureter
urethra NEC N36.8
  congenital Q64.39
urinary (moderate) N13.9
  due to hyperplasia (hypertrophy) of prostate — *see* Hyperplasia, prostate
  organ or tract (lower) N13.9
  prostatic valve N32.0
  specified NEC N13.8
uropathy N13.9
uterus N85.8
vagina N89.5
valvular — *see* Endocarditis
vein, venous I87.1
  caval (inferior) (superior) I87.1
  thrombotic — *see* Thrombosis
vena cava (inferior) (superior) I87.1
vesical NEC N32.0
vesicourethral orifice N32.0
  congenital Q64.31
vessel NEC I99.8
Obturator — *see* condition
Occlusal wear, teeth K03.0
Occlusio pupillae — *see* Membrane, pupillary
Occlusion, occluded
anus K62.4
  congenital Q42.3
    with fistula Q42.2
aortoiliac (chronic) I74.09
aqueduct of Sylvius G91.1
  congenital Q03.0
    with spina bifida — *see* Spina bifida, by site, with hydrocephalus
artery (*see also* Embolism, artery) I74.9
  auditory, internal I65.8
  basilar I65.1
    with
      infarction I63.22
        due to
          embolism I63.12
          thrombosis I63.02

Occlusion, occluded — *continued*
artery (*see also* Embolism, artery) — *continued*
brain or cerebral I66.9
with infarction (due to) I63.5 ☑
embolism I63.4 ☑
thrombosis I63.3 ☑
carotid I65.2- ☑
with
infarction I63.23- ☑
due to
embolism I63.13- ☑
thrombosis I63.03- ☑
cerebellar (anterior inferior) (posterior inferior) (superior) I66.3
with infarction I63.54- ☑
due to
embolism I63.44- ☑
thrombosis I63.34- ☑
cerebral I66.9
with infarction I63.50
due to
embolism I63.40
specified NEC I63.49
thrombosis I63.30
specified NEC I63.39
anterior I66.1- ☑
with infarction I63.52- ☑
due to
embolism I63.42- ☑
thrombosis I63.32- ☑
middle I66.0- ☑
with infarction I63.51- ☑
due to
embolism I63.41- ☑
thrombosis I63.31- ☑
posterior I66.2- ☑
with infarction I63.53- ☑
due to
embolism I63.43- ☑
thrombosis I63.33- ☑
specified NEC I66.8
with infarction I63.59
due to
embolism I63.4 ☑
thrombosis I63.3 ☑
choroidal (anterior) — *see* Occlusion, artery, precerebral, specified NEC
communicating posterior — *see* Occlusion, artery, cerebral, specified NEC
complete
coronary I25.82
extremities I70.92
coronary (acute) (thrombotic) (without myocardial infarction) I24.0
with myocardial infarction — *see* Infarction, myocardium
chronic total I25.82
complete I25.82
healed or old I25.2
total (chronic) I25.82
hypophyseal — *see* Occlusion, artery, precerebral, specified NEC
iliac I74.5
lower extremities due to stenosis or stricture I77.1
mesenteric (embolic) (thrombotic) K55.0
perforating — *see* Occlusion, artery, cerebral, specified NEC
peripheral I77.9
thrombotic or embolic I74.4
pontine — *see* Occlusion, artery, cerebral, specified NEC
precerebral I65.9
with infarction I63.20
due to
embolism I63.10
specified NEC I63.19
thrombosis I63.00
specified NEC I63.09
specified NEC I63.29
basilar — *see* Occlusion, artery, basilar
carotid — *see* Occlusion, artery, carotid
puerperal O88.23
specified NEC I65.8
with infarction I63.29
due to
embolism I63.19
thrombosis I63.00

artery (*see also* Embolism, artery) — *continued*
precerebral — *continued*
vertebral — *see* Occlusion, artery, vertebral
renal N28.0
retinal
branch H34.23- ☑
central H34.1- ☑
partial H34.21- ☑
transient H34.0- ☑
spinal — *see* Occlusion, artery, precerebral, vertebral
total (chronic)
coronary I25.82
extremities I70.92
vertebral I65.0- ☑
with
infarction I63.21- ☑
due to
embolism I63.11- ☑
thrombosis I63.01- ☑
basilar artery — *see* Occlusion, artery, basilar
bile duct (common) (hepatic) (noncalculous) K83.1
bowel — *see* Obstruction, intestine
carotid (artery) (common) (internal) — *see* Occlusion, artery, carotid
centric (of teeth) M26.59
maximum intercuspation discrepancy M26.55
cerebellar (artery) — *see* Occlusion, artery, cerebellar
cerebral (artery) — *see* Occlusion, artery, cerebral
cerebrovascular (*see also* Occlusion, artery, cerebral)
with infarction I63.5 ☑
cervical canal — *see* Stricture, cervix
cervix (uteri) — *see* Stricture, cervix
choanal Q30.0
choroidal (artery) — *see* Occlusion, artery, precerebral, specified NEC
colon — *see* Obstruction, intestine
communicating posterior artery — *see* Occlusion, artery, precerebral, specified NEC
coronary (artery) (vein) (thrombotic) (*see also* Infarct, myocardium)
chronic total I25.82
healed or old I25.2
not resulting in infarction I24.0
total (chronic) I25.82
cystic duct — *see* Obstruction, gallbladder
embolic — *see* Embolism
fallopian tube N97.1
congenital Q50.6
gallbladder (*see also* Obstruction, gallbladder)
congenital (causing jaundice) Q44.1
gingiva, traumatic K06.2
hymen N89.6
congenital Q52.3
hypophyseal (artery) — *see* Occlusion, artery, precerebral, specified NEC
iliac artery I74.5
intestine — *see* Obstruction, intestine
lacrimal passages — *see* Obstruction, lacrimal
lung J98.4
lymph or lymphatic channel I89.0
mammary duct N64.89
mesenteric artery (embolic) (thrombotic) K55.0
nose J34.89
congenital Q30.0
organ or site, congenital NEC — *see* Atresia, by site
oviduct N97.1
congenital Q50.6
peripheral arteries
due to stricture or stenosis I77.1
upper extremity I74.2
pontine (artery) — *see* Occlusion, artery, precerebral, specified NEC
posterior lingual, of mandibular teeth M26.29
precerebral artery — *see* Occlusion, artery, precerebral
punctum lacrimale — *see* Obstruction, lacrimal
pupil — *see* Membrane, pupillary
pylorus, adult (*see also* Stricture, pylorus) K31.1
renal artery N28.0
retina, retinal
artery — *see* Occlusion, artery, retinal
vein (central) H34.81- ☑
engorgement H34.82- ☑
tributary H34.83- ☑
vessels H34.9

Occlusion, occluded — *continued*
spinal artery — *see* Occlusion, artery, precerebral, vertebral
teeth (mandibular) (posterior lingual) M26.29
thoracic duct I89.0
thrombotic — *see* Thrombosis, artery
traumatic
edentulous (alveolar) ridge K06.2
gingiva K06.2
periodontal K05.5
tubal N97.1
ureter (complete) (partial) N13.5
congenital Q62.10
ureteropelvic junction N13.5
congenital Q62.11
ureterovesical orifice N13.5
congenital Q62.12
urethra — *see* Stricture, urethra
uterus N85.8
vagina N89.5
vascular NEC I99.8
vein — *see* Thrombosis
retinal — *see* Occlusion, retinal, vein
vena cava (inferior) (superior) — *see* Embolism, vena cava
ventricle (brain) NEC G91.1
vertebral (artery) — *see* Occlusion, artery, vertebral
vessel (blood) I99.8
vulva N90.5
Occult
blood in feces (stools) R19.5
Occupational
problems NEC Z56.89
Ochlophobia — *see* Agoraphobia
Ochronosis (endogenous) E70.29
Ocular muscle — *see* condition
Oculogyric crisis or disturbance H51.8
psychogenic F45.8
Oculomotor syndrome H51.9
Oculopathy
syphilitic NEC A52.71
congenital
early A50.01
late A50.30
early (secondary) A51.43
late A52.71
Oddi's sphincter spasm K83.4
Odontalgia K08.8
Odontoameloblastoma — *see* Cyst, calcifying odontogenic
Odontoclasia K03.89
Odontodysplasia, regional K00.4
Odontogenesis imperfecta K00.5
Odontoma (ameloblastic) (complex) (compound) (fibroameloblastic) — *see* Cyst, calcifying odontogenic
Odontomyelitis (closed) (open) K04.0
Odontorrhagia K08.8
Odontosarcoma, ameloblastic C41.1
upper jaw (bone) C41.0
Oestriasis — *see* Myiasis
Oguchi's disease H53.63
Ohara's disease — *see* Tularemia
Oidiomycosis — *see* Candidiasis
Oidium albicans infection — *see* Candidiasis
Old age (without mention of debility) R54
dementia F03 ☑
Old (previous) **myocardial infarction** I25.2
Olfactory — *see* condition
Oligemia — *see* Anemia
Oligoastrocytoma
specified site — *see* Neoplasm, malignant, by site
unspecified site C71.9
Oligocythemia D64.9
Oligodendroblastoma
specified site — *see* Neoplasm, malignant
unspecified site C71.9
Oligodendroglioma
anaplastic type
specified site — *see* Neoplasm, malignant, by site
unspecified site C71.9
specified site — *see* Neoplasm, malignant, by site
unspecified site C71.9
Oligodontia — *see* Anodontia
Oligoencephalon Q02
Oligohidrosis L74.4
Oligohydramnios O41.0- ☑
Oligohydrosis L74.4

☑ Additional Character Required — Refer to the Tabular List for Character Selection
Subterms under main terms may continue to next column or page

Oligomenorrhea N91.5
  primary N91.3
  secondary N91.4
Oligophrenia (*see also* Disability, intellectual)
  phenylpyruvic E70.0
Oligospermia N46.11
  due to
    drug therapy N46.121
    efferent duct obstruction N46.123
    infection N46.122
    radiation N46.124
    specified cause NEC N46.129
    systemic disease N46.125
Oligotrichia — *see* Alopecia
Oliguria R34
  postprocedural N99.0
  with, complicating or following ectopic or molar
    pregnancy O08.4
Ollier's disease Q78.4
Omenotocele — *see* Hernia, abdomen, specified site
  NEC
Omentitis — *see* Peritonitis
Omentum, omental — *see* condition
Omphalitis (congenital) (newborn) P38.9
  with mild hemorrhage P38.1
  without hemorrhage P38.9
  not of newborn L08.82
  tetanus A33
Omphalocele Q79.2
Omphalomesenteric duct, persistent Q43.0
Omphalorrhagia, newborn P51.9
Omsk hemorrhagic fever A98.1
Onanism (excessive) F98.8
Onchocerciasis, onchocercosis B73.1
  with
    eye disease B73.00
      endophthalmitis B73.01
      eyelid B73.09
      glaucoma B73.02
      specified NEC B73.09
    eyelid B73.09
    eye NEC B73.00
Oncocytoma — *see* Neoplasm, benign, by site
Oncovirus, as cause of disease classified elsewhere
  B97.32
Ondine's curse — *see* Apnea, sleep
Oneirophrenia F23
Onychauxis L60.2
  congenital Q84.5
Onychia (*see also* Cellulitis, digit)
  with lymphangitis — *see* Lymphangitis, acute, digit
  candidal B37.2
  dermatophytic B35.1
Onychitis (*see also* Cellulitis, digit)
  with lymphangitis — *see* Lymphangitis, acute, digit
Onychocryptosis L60.0
Onychodystrophy L60.3
  congenital Q84.6
Onychogryphosis, onychogryposis L60.2
Onycholysis L60.1
Onychomadesis L60.8
Onychomalacia L60.3
Onychomycosis (finger) (toe) B35.1
Onycho-osteodysplasia Q79.8
Onychophagia F98.8
Onychophosis L60.8
Onychoptosis L60.8
Onychorrhexis L60.3
  congenital Q84.6
Onychoschizia L60.3
Onyxis (finger) (toe) L60.0
Onyxitis (*see also* Cellulitis, digit)
  with lymphangitis — *see* Lymphangitis, acute, digit
Oophoritis (cystic) (infectional) (interstitial) N70.92
  with salpingitis N70.93
  acute N70.02
    with salpingitis N70.03
  chronic N70.12
    with salpingitis N70.13
  complicating abortion — *see* Abortion, by type, com-
    plicated by, oophoritis
Oophorocele N83.4
Opacity, opacities
  cornea H17.- ☑
    central H17.1- ☑
    congenital Q13.3
    degenerative — *see* Degeneration, cornea

Opacity, opacities — *continued*
  cornea — *continued*
    hereditary — *see* Dystrophy, cornea
    inflammatory — *see* Keratitis
    minor H17.81- ☑
    peripheral H17.82- ☑
    sequelae of trachoma (healed) B94.0
    specified NEC H17.89
  enamel (teeth) (fluoride) (nonfluoride) K00.3
  lens — *see* Cataract
  snowball — *see* Deposit, crystalline
  vitreous (humor) NEC H43.39- ☑
    congenital Q14.0
    membranes and strands H43.31- ☑
Opalescent dentin (hereditary) K00.5
Open, opening
  abnormal, organ or site, congenital — *see* Imperfect,
    closure
  angle with
    borderline
      findings
        high risk H40.02- ☑
        low risk H40.01- ☑
      intraocular pressure H40.00- ☑
    cupping of discs H40.01- ☑
    glaucoma (primary) — *see* Glaucoma, open angle
  bite
    anterior M26.220
    posterior M26.221
  false — *see* Imperfect, closure
  margin on tooth restoration K08.51
  restoration margins of tooth K08.51
  wound — *see* Wound, open
Operational fatigue F48.8
Operative — *see* condition
Operculitis — *see* Periodontitis
Operculum — *see* Break, retina
Ophiasis L63.2
Ophthalmia (*see also* Conjunctivitis) H10.9
  actinic rays — *see* Photokeratitis
  allergic (acute) — *see* Conjunctivitis, acute, atopic
  blennorrhagic (gonococcal) (neonatorum) A54.31
  diphtheritic A36.86
  Egyptian A71.1
  electrica — *see* Photokeratitis
  gonococcal (neonatorum) A54.31
  metastatic — *see* Endophthalmitis, purulent
  migraine — *see* Migraine, ophthalmoplegic
  neonatorum, newborn P39.1
    gonococcal A54.31
  nodosa H16.24- ☑
  purulent — *see* Conjunctivitis, acute, mucopurulent
  spring — *see* Conjunctivitis, acute, atopic
  sympathetic — *see* Uveitis, sympathetic
Ophthalmitis — *see* Ophthalmia
Ophthalmocele (congenital) Q15.8
Ophthalmoneuromyelitis G36.0
Ophthalmoplegia (*see also* Strabismus, paralytic)
  anterior internuclear — *see* Ophthalmoplegia, inter-
    nuclear
  ataxia-areflexia G61.0
  diabetic — *see* E08-E13 with .39
  exophthalmic E05.00
    with thyroid storm E05.01
  external H49.88- ☑
    progressive H49.4- ☑
      with pigmentary retinopathy — *see* Kearns-
        Sayre syndrome
    total H49.3- ☑
  internal (complete) (total) H52.51- ☑
  internuclear H51.2- ☑
  migraine — *see* Migraine, ophthalmoplegic
  Parinaud's H49.88- ☑
  progressive external — *see* Ophthalmoplegia, external,
    progressive
  supranuclear, progressive G23.1
  total (external) — *see* Ophthalmoplegia, external, total
Opioid(s)
  abuse — *see* Abuse, drug, opioids
  dependence — *see* Dependence, drug, opioids
Opisthognathism M26.09
Opisthorchiasis (felineus) (viverrini) B66.0
Opitz' disease D73.2
Opiumism — *see* Dependence, drug, opioid
Oppenheim's disease G70.2
Oppenheim-Urbach disease (necrobiosis lipoidica dia-
  beticorum) — *see* E08-E13 with .620

Optic nerve — *see* condition
Orbit — *see* condition
Orchioblastoma C62.9- ☑
Orchitis (gangrenous) (nonspecific) (septic) (suppurative)
  N45.2
  blennorrhagic (gonococcal) (acute) (chronic) A54.23
  chlamydial A56.19
  filarial (*see also* Infestation, filarial) B74.9 [N51]
  gonococcal (acute) (chronic) A54.23
  mumps B26.0
  syphilitic A52.76
  tuberculous A18.15
Orf (virus disease) B08.02
Organic (*see also* condition)
  brain syndrome F09
  heart — *see* Disease, heart
  mental disorder F09
  psychosis F09
Orgasm
  anejaculatory N53.13
Oriental
  bilharziasis B65.2
  schistosomiasis B65.2
Orifice — *see* condition
Origin of both great vessels from right ventricle
  Q20.1
Ormond's disease (with ureteral obstruction) N13.5
  with infection N13.6
Ornithine metabolism disorder E72.4
Ornithinemia (Type I) (Type II) E72.4
Ornithosis A70
Orotaciduria, oroticaciduria (congenital) (hereditary)
  (pyrimidine deficiency) E79.8
  anemia D53.0
Orthodontics
  adjustment Z46.4
  fitting Z46.4
Orthopnea R06.01
Orthopoxvirus B08.09
  specified NEC B08.09
Os, uterus — *see* condition
Osgood-Schlatter disease or osteochondrosis — *see*
  Osteochondrosis, juvenile, tibia
Osler (-Weber)-**Rendu disease** I78.0
Osler's nodes I33.0
Osmidrosis L75.0
Osseous — *see* condition
Ossification
  artery — *see* Arteriosclerosis
  auricle (ear) — *see* Disorder, pinna, specified type NEC
  bronchial J98.09
  cardiac — *see* Degeneration, myocardial
  cartilage (senile) — *see* Disorder, cartilage, specified
    type NEC
  coronary (artery) — *see* Disease, heart, ischemic,
    atherosclerotic
  diaphragm J98.6
  ear, middle — *see* Otosclerosis
  falx cerebri G96.19
  fontanel, premature Q75.0
  heart (*see also* Degeneration, myocardial)
    valve — *see* Endocarditis
  larynx J38.7
  ligament — *see* Disorder, tendon, specified type NEC
    posterior longitudinal — *see* Spondylopathy,
      specified NEC
  meninges (cerebral) (spinal) G96.19
  multiple, eccentric centers — *see* Disorder, bone, de-
    velopment or growth
  muscle (*see also* Calcification, muscle)
    due to burns — *see* Myositis, ossificans, in, burns
    paralytic — *see* Myositis, ossificans, in, quadriplegia
    progressive — *see* Myositis, ossificans, progressiva
    specified NEC M61.50
      ankle M61.57- ☑
      foot M61.57- ☑
      forearm M61.53- ☑
      hand M61.54- ☑
      lower leg M61.56- ☑
      multiple sites M61.59
      pelvic region M61.55- ☑
      shoulder region M61.51- ☑
      specified site NEC M61.58
      thigh M61.55- ☑
      upper arm M61.52- ☑
    traumatic — *see* Myositis, ossificans, traumatica

Ossification — *continued*
  myocardium, myocardial — *see* Degeneration, myocardial
  penis N48.89
  periarticular — *see* Disorder, joint, specified type NEC
  pinna — *see* Disorder, pinna, specified type NEC
  rider's bone — *see* Ossification, muscle, specified NEC
  sclera H15.89
  subperiosteal, post-traumatic M89.8X- ☑
  tendon — *see* Disorder, tendon, specified type NEC
  trachea J39.8
  tympanic membrane — *see* Disorder, tympanic membrane, specified NEC
  vitreous (humor) — *see* Deposit, crystalline
Osteitis (*see also* Osteomyelitis)
  alveolar M27.3
  condensans M85.30
    ankle M85.37- ☑
    foot M85.37- ☑
    forearm M85.33- ☑
    hand M85.34- ☑
    lower leg M85.36- ☑
    multiple site M85.39
    neck M85.38
    rib M85.38
    shoulder M85.31- ☑
    skull M85.38
    specified site NEC M85.38
    thigh M85.35- ☑
    toe M85.37- ☑
    upper arm M85.32- ☑
    vertebra M85.38
  deformans M88.9
    in (due to)
      malignant neoplasm of bone C41.9 [M90.60]
      neoplastic disease (*see also* Neoplasm) D49.9 [M90.60]
        carpus D49.9 [M90.64-] ☑
        clavicle D49.9 [M90.61-] ☑
        femur D49.9 [M90.65-] ☑
        fibula D49.9 [M90.66-] ☑
        finger D49.9 [M90.64-] ☑
        humerus D49.9 [M90.62-] ☑
        ilium D49.9 [M90.65-] ☑
        ischium D49.9 [M90.65-] ☑
        metacarpus D49.9 [M90.64-] ☑
        metatarsus D49.9 [M90.67-] ☑
        multiple sites D49.9 [M90.69]
        neck D49.9 [M90.68]
        radius D49.9 [M90.63-] ☑
        rib D49.9 [M90.68]
        scapula D49.9 [M90.61-] ☑
        skull D49.9 [M90.68]
        tarsus D49.9 [M90.67-] ☑
        tibia D49.9 [M90.66-] ☑
        toe D49.9 [M90.67-] ☑
        ulna D49.9 [M90.63-] ☑
        vertebra D49.9 [M90.68]
    skull M88.0
    specified NEC — *see* Paget's disease, bone, by site
    vertebra M88.1
  due to yaws A66.6
  fibrosa NEC — *see* Cyst, bone, by site
    circumscripta — *see* Dysplasia, fibrous, bone NEC
    cystica (generalisata) E21.0
    disseminata Q78.1
    osteoplastica E21.0
  fragilitans Q78.0
  Garr's (sclerosing) — *see* Osteomyelitis, specified type NEC
  jaw (acute) (chronic) (lower) (suppurative) (upper) M27.2
  parathyroid E21.0
  petrous bone (acute) (chronic) — *see* Petrositis
  sclerotic, nonsuppurative — *see* Osteomyelitis, specified type NEC
  tuberculosa A18.09
    cystica D86.89
    multiplex cystoides D86.89
Osteoarthritis M19.90
  ankle M19.07- ☑
  elbow M19.02- ☑
  foot joint M19.07- ☑
  generalized M15.9
    erosive M15.4
    primary M15.0
    specified NEC M15.8

Osteoarthritis — *continued*
  hand joint M19.04- ☑
    first carpometacarpal joint M18.9
  hip M16.1- ☑
    bilateral M16.0
    due to hip dysplasia (unilateral) M16.3- ☑
      bilateral M16.2
  interphalangeal
    distal (Heberden) M15.1
    proximal (Bouchard) M15.2
  knee M17.9
    bilateral M17.0
  post-traumatic NEC M19.92
    ankle M19.17- ☑
    elbow M19.12- ☑
    foot joint M19.17- ☑
    hand joint M19.14- ☑
      first carpometacarpal joint M18.3- ☑
        bilateral M18.2
    hip M16.5- ☑
      bilateral M16.4
    knee M17.3- ☑
      bilateral M17.2
    shoulder M19.11- ☑
    wrist M19.13- ☑
  primary M19.91
    ankle M19.07- ☑
    elbow M19.02- ☑
    foot joint M19.07- ☑
    hand joint M19.04- ☑
      first carpometacarpal joint M18.1- ☑
        bilateral M18.0
    hip M16.1- ☑
      bilateral M16.0
    knee M17.1- ☑
      bilateral M17.0
    shoulder M19.01- ☑
    spine — *see* Spondylosis
    wrist M19.03- ☑
  secondary M19.93
    ankle M19.27- ☑
    elbow M19.22- ☑
    foot joint M19.27- ☑
    hand joint M19.24- ☑
      first carpometacarpal joint M18.5- ☑
        bilateral M18.4
    hip M16.7
      bilateral M16.6
    knee M17.5
      bilateral M17.4
    multiple M15.3
    shoulder M19.21- ☑
    spine — *see* Spondylosis
    wrist M19.23- ☑
  shoulder M19.01- ☑
  spine — *see* Spondylosis
  wrist M19.03- ☑
Osteoarthropathy (hypertrophic) M19.90
  ankle — *see* Osteoarthritis, primary, ankle
  elbow — *see* Osteoarthritis, primary, elbow
  foot joint — *see* Osteoarthritis, primary, foot
  hand joint — *see* Osteoarthritis, primary, hand joint
  knee joint — *see* Osteoarthritis, primary, knee
  multiple site — *see* Osteoarthritis, primary, multiple joint
  pulmonary (*see also* Osteoarthropathy, specified type NEC)
    hypertrophic — *see* Osteoarthropathy, hypertrophic, specified type NEC
  secondary — *see* Osteoarthropathy, specified type NEC
  secondary hypertrophic — *see* Osteoarthropathy, specified type NEC
  shoulder — *see* Osteoarthritis, primary, shoulder
  specified joint NEC — *see* Osteoarthritis, primary, specified joint NEC
  specified type NEC M89.40
    carpus M89.44- ☑
    clavicle M89.41- ☑
    femur M89.45- ☑
    fibula M89.46- ☑
    finger M89.44- ☑
    humerus M89.42- ☑
    ilium M89.459
    ischium M89.459
    metacarpus M89.44- ☑

Osteoarthropathy — *continued*
  specified type — *continued*
    metatarsus M89.47- ☑
    multiple sites M89.49
    neck M89.48
    radius M89.43- ☑
    rib M89.48
    scapula M89.41- ☑
    skull M89.48
    tarsus M89.47- ☑
    tibia M89.46- ☑
    toe M89.47- ☑
    ulna M89.43- ☑
    vertebra M89.48
  spine — *see* Spondylosis
  wrist — *see* Osteoarthritis, primary, wrist
Osteoarthrosis (degenerative) (hypertrophic) (joint) (*see also* Osteoarthritis)
  deformans alkaptonurica E70.29 [M36.0]
  erosive M15.4
  generalized M15.9
    primary M15.0
  polyarticular M15.9
  spine — *see* Spondylosis
Osteoblastoma — *see* Neoplasm, bone, benign
  aggressive — *see* Neoplasm, bone, uncertain behavior
Osteochondritis (*see also* Osteochondropathy, by site)
  Brailsford's — *see* Osteochondrosis, juvenile, radius
  dissecans M93.20
    ankle M93.27- ☑
    elbow M93.22- ☑
    foot M93.27- ☑
    hand M93.24- ☑
    hip M93.25- ☑
    knee M93.26- ☑
    multiple sites M93.29
    shoulder joint M93.21- ☑
    specified site NEC M93.28
    wrist M93.23- ☑
  juvenile M92.9
    patellar — *see* Osteochondrosis, juvenile, patella
  syphilitic (congenital) (early) A50.02 [M90.80]
    ankle A50.02 [M90.87-] ☑
    elbow A50.02 [M90.82-] ☑
    foot A50.02 [M90.87-] ☑
    forearm A50.02 [M90.83-] ☑
    hand A50.02 [M90.84-] ☑
    hip A50.02 [M90.85-] ☑
    knee A50.02 [M90.86-] ☑
    multiple sites A50.02 [M90.89]
    shoulder joint A50.02 [M90.81-] ☑
    specified site NEC A50.02 [M90.88]
Osteochondroarthrosis deformans endemica — *see* Disease, Kaschin-Beck
Osteochondrodysplasia Q78.9
  with defects of growth of tubular bones and spine Q77.9
    specified NEC Q77.8
  specified NEC Q78.8
Osteochondrodystrophy E78.9
Osteochondrolysis — *see* Osteochondritis, dissecans
Osteochondroma — *see* Neoplasm, bone, benign
Osteochondromatosis D48.0
  syndrome Q78.4
Osteochondromyxosarcoma — *see* Neoplasm, bone, malignant
Osteochondropathy M93.90
  ankle M93.97- ☑
  elbow M93.92- ☑
  foot M93.97- ☑
  hand M93.94- ☑
  hip M93.95- ☑
  Kienböck's disease of adults M93.1
  knee M93.96- ☑
  multiple joints M93.99
  osteochondritis dissecans — *see* Osteochondritis, dissecans
  osteochondrosis — *see* Osteochondrosis
  shoulder region M93.91- ☑
  slipped upper femoral epiphysis — *see* Slipped, epiphysis, upper femoral
  specified joint NEC M93.98
  specified type NEC M93.80
    ankle M93.87- ☑
    elbow M93.82- ☑
    foot M93.87- ☑

Osteochondropathy — *continued*
  specified type — *continued*
    hand M93.84- ☑
    hip M93.85- ☑
    knee M93.86- ☑
    multiple joints M93.89
    shoulder region M93.81- ☑
    specified joint NEC M93.88
    wrist M93.83- ☑
  syphilitic, congenital
    early A50.02 [M90.80]
    late A50.56 [M90.80]
  wrist M93.93- ☑
Osteochondrosarcoma — *see* Neoplasm, bone, malignant
Osteochondrosis (*see also* Osteochondropathy, by site)
  acetabulum (juvenile) M91.0
  adult — *see* Osteochondropathy, specified type NEC, by site
  astragalus (juvenile) — *see* Osteochondrosis, juvenile, tarsus
  Blount's — *see* Osteochondrosis, juvenile, tibia
  Buchanan's M91.0
  Burns' — *see* Osteochondrosis, juvenile, ulna
  calcaneus (juvenile) — *see* Osteochondrosis, juvenile, tarsus
  capitular epiphysis (femur) (juvenile) — *see* Legg-Calvé-Perthes disease
  carpal (juvenile) (lunate) (scaphoid) — *see* Osteochondrosis, juvenile, hand, carpal lunate
    adult M93.1
  coxae juvenilis — *see* Legg-Calvé-Perthes disease
  deformans juvenilis, coxae — *see* Legg-Calvé-Perthes disease
  Diaz's — *see* Osteochondrosis, juvenile, tarsus
  dissecans (knee) (shoulder) — *see* Osteochondritis, dissecans
  femoral capital epiphysis (juvenile) — *see* Legg-Calvé-Perthes disease
  femur (head), juvenile — *see* Legg-Calvé-Perthes disease
  fibula (juvenile) — *see* Osteochondrosis, juvenile, fibula
  foot NEC (juvenile) M92.8
  Freiberg's — *see* Osteochondrosis, juvenile, metatarsus
  Haas' (juvenile) — *see* Osteochondrosis, juvenile, humerus
  Haglund's — *see* Osteochondrosis, juvenile, tarsus
  hip (juvenile) — *see* Legg-Calvé-Perthes disease
  humerus (capitulum) (head) (juvenile) — *see* Osteochondrosis, juvenile, humerus
  ilium, iliac crest (juvenile) M91.0
  ischiopubic synchondrosis M91.0
  Iselin's — *see* Osteochondrosis, juvenile, metatarsus
  juvenile, juvenilis M92.9
    after congenital dislocation of hip reduction — *see* Osteochondrosis, juvenile, hip, specified NEC
    arm — *see* Osteochondrosis, juvenile, upper limb NEC
    capitular epiphysis (femur) — *see* Legg-Calvé-Perthes disease
    clavicle, sternal epiphysis — *see* Osteochondrosis, juvenile, upper limb NEC
    coxae — *see* Legg-Calvé-Perthes disease
    deformans M92.9
    fibula M92.5- ☑
    foot NEC M92.8
    hand M92.20- ☑
      carpal lunate M92.21- ☑
      metacarpal head M92.22- ☑
      specified site NEC M92.29- ☑
    head of femur — *see* Legg-Calvé-Perthes disease
    hip and pelvis M91.9- ☑
      coxa plana — *see* Coxa, plana
      femoral head — *see* Legg-Calvé-Perthes disease
      pelvis M91.0
      pseudocoxalgia — *see* Pseudocoxalgia
      specified NEC M91.8- ☑
    humerus M92.0- ☑
    limb
      lower NEC M92.8
      upper NEC — *see* Osteochondrosis, juvenile, upper limb NEC
    medial cuneiform bone — *see* Osteochondrosis, juvenile, tarsus
    metatarsus M92.7- ☑
    patella M92.4- ☑

Osteochondrosis — *continued*
  juvenile, juvenilis — *continued*
    radius M92.1- ☑
    specified site NEC M92.8
    spine M42.00
      cervical region M42.02
      cervicothoracic region M42.03
      lumbar region M42.06
      lumbosacral region M42.07
      multiple sites M42.09
      occipito-atlanto-axial region M42.01
      sacrococcygeal region M42.08
      thoracic region M42.04
      thoracolumbar region M42.05
    tarsus M92.6- ☑
    tibia M92.5- ☑
    ulna M92.1- ☑
    upper limb NEC M92.3- ☑
    vertebra (body) (epiphyseal plates) (Calvé's) (Scheuermann's) — *see* Osteochondrosis, juvenile, spine
  Kienböck's — *see* Osteochondrosis, juvenile, hand, carpal lunate
    adult M93.1
  Köhler's
    patellar — *see* Osteochondrosis, juvenile, patella
    tarsal navicular — *see* Osteochondrosis, juvenile, tarsus
  Legg-Perthes (-Calvé)(-Waldenström) — *see* Legg-Calvé-Perthes disease
  limb
    lower NEC (juvenile) M92.8
    upper NEC (juvenile) — *see* Osteochondrosis, juvenile, upper limb NEC
  lunate bone (carpal) (juvenile) (*see also* Osteochondrosis, juvenile, hand, carpal lunate)
    adult M93.1
  Mauclaire's — *see* Osteochondrosis, juvenile, hand, metacarpal
  metacarpal (head) (juvenile) — *see* Osteochondrosis, juvenile, hand, metacarpal
  metatarsus (fifth) (head) (juvenile) (second) — *see* Osteochondrosis, juvenile, metatarsus
  navicular (juvenile) — *see* Osteochondrosis, juvenile, tarsus
  os
    calcis (juvenile) — *see* Osteochondrosis, juvenile, tarsus
    tibiale externum (juvenile) — *see* Osteochondrosis, juvenile, tarsus
  Osgood-Schlatter — *see* Osteochondrosis, juvenile, tibia
  Panner's — *see* Osteochondrosis, juvenile, humerus
  patellar center (juvenile) (primary) (secondary) — *see* Osteochondrosis, juvenile, patella
  pelvis (juvenile) M91.0
  Pierson's M91.0
  radius (head) (juvenile) — *see* Osteochondrosis, juvenile, radius
  Scheuermann's — *see* Osteochondrosis, juvenile, spine
  Sever's — *see* Osteochondrosis, juvenile, tarsus
  Sinding-Larsen — *see* Osteochondrosis, juvenile, patella
  spine M42.9
    adult M42.10
      cervical region M42.12
      cervicothoracic region M42.13
      lumbar region M42.16
      lumbosacral region M42.17
      multiple sites M42.19
      occipito-atlanto-axial region M42.11
      sacrococcygeal region M42.18
      thoracic region M42.14
      thoracolumbar region M42.15
    juvenile — *see* Osteochondrosis, juvenile, spine
  symphysis pubis (juvenile) M91.0
  syphilitic (congenital) A50.02
  talus (juvenile) — *see* Osteochondrosis, juvenile, tarsus
  tarsus (navicular) (juvenile) — *see* Osteochondrosis, juvenile, tarsus
  tibia (proximal) (tubercle) (juvenile) — *see* Osteochondrosis, juvenile, tibia
  tuberculous — *see* Tuberculosis, bone
  ulna (lower) (juvenile) — *see* Osteochondrosis, juvenile, ulna
  van Neck's M91.0
  vertebral — *see* Osteochondrosis, spine

Osteoclastoma D48.0
  malignant — *see* Neoplasm, bone, malignant
Osteodynia — *see* Disorder, bone, specified type NEC
Osteodystrophy Q78.9
  azotemic N25.0
  congenital Q78.9
  parathyroid, secondary E21.1
  renal N25.0
Osteofibroma — *see* Neoplasm, bone, benign
Osteofibrosarcoma — *see* Neoplasm, bone, malignant
Osteogenesis imperfecta Q78.0
Osteogenic — *see* condition
Osteolysis M89.50
  carpus M89.54- ☑
  clavicle M89.51- ☑
  femur M89.55- ☑
  fibula M89.56- ☑
  finger M89.54- ☑
  humerus M89.52- ☑
  ilium M89.559
  ischium M89.559
  joint prosthesis (periprosthetic) — *see* Complications, joint prosthesis, mechanical, periprosthetic, osteolysis, by site
  metacarpus M89.54- ☑
  metatarsus M89.57- ☑
  multiple sites M89.59
  neck M89.58
  periprosthetic — *see* Complications, joint prosthesis, mechanical, periprosthetic, osteolysis, by site
  radius M89.53- ☑
  rib M89.58
  scapula M89.51- ☑
  skull M89.58
  tarsus M89.57- ☑
  tibia M89.56- ☑
  toe M89.57- ☑
  ulna M89.53- ☑
  vertebra M89.58
Osteoma (*see also* Neoplasm, bone, benign)
  osteoid (*see also* Neoplasm, bone, benign)
    giant — *see* Neoplasm, bone, benign
Osteomalacia M83.9
  adult M83.9
    drug-induced NEC M83.5
    due to
      malabsorption (postsurgical) M83.2
      malnutrition M83.3
    specified NEC M83.8
  aluminium-induced M83.4
  infantile — *see* Rickets
  juvenile — *see* Rickets
  oncogenic E83.89
  pelvis M83.8
  puerperal M83.0
  senile M83.1
  vitamin-D-resistant in adults E83.31 [M90.8-] ☑
    carpus E83.31 [M90.84-] ☑
    clavicle E83.31 [M90.81-] ☑
    femur E83.31 [M90.85-] ☑
    fibula E83.31 [M90.86-] ☑
    finger E83.31 [M90.84-] ☑
    humerus E83.31 [M90.82-] ☑
    ilium E83.31 [M90.859]
    ischium E83.31 [M90.859]
    metacarpus E83.31 [M90.84-] ☑
    metatarsus E83.31 [M90.87-] ☑
    multiple sites E83.31 [M90.89]
    neck E83.31 [M90.88]
    radius E83.31 [M90.83-] ☑
    rib E83.31 [M90.88]
    scapula E83.31 [M90.819]
    skull E83.31 [M90.88]
    tarsus E83.31 [M90.879]
    tibia E83.31 [M90.869]
    toe E83.31 [M90.879]
    ulna E83.31 [M90.839]
    vertebra E83.31 [M90.88]
Osteomyelitis (general) (infective) (localized) (neonatal) (purulent) (septic) (staphylococcal) (streptococcal) (suppurative) (with periostitis) M86.9
  acute M86.10
    carpus M86.14- ☑
    clavicle M86.11- ☑
    femur M86.15- ☑
    fibula M86.16- ☑
    finger M86.14- ☑

Osteomyelitis — *continued*
  acute — *continued*
    hematogenous M86.00
      carpus M86.04- ☑
      clavicle M86.01- ☑
      femur M86.05- ☑
      fibula M86.06- ☑
      finger M86.04- ☑
      humerus M86.02- ☑
      ilium M86.059
      ischium M86.059
      mandible M27.2
      metacarpus M86.04- ☑
      metatarsus M86.07- ☑
      multiple sites M86.09
      neck M86.08
      orbit H05.02- ☑
      petrous bone — *see* Petrositis
      radius M86.03- ☑
      rib M86.08
      scapula M86.01- ☑
      skull M86.08
      tarsus M86.07- ☑
      tibia M86.06- ☑
      toe M86.07- ☑
      ulna M86.03- ☑
      vertebra — *see* Osteomyelitis, vertebra
    humerus M86.12- ☑
    ilium M86.159
    ischium M86.159
    mandible M27.2
    metacarpus M86.14- ☑
    metatarsus M86.17- ☑
    multiple sites M86.19
    neck M86.18
    orbit H05.02- ☑
    petrous bone — *see* Petrositis
    radius M86.13- ☑
    rib M86.18
    scapula M86.11- ☑
    skull M86.18
    tarsus M86.17- ☑
    tibia M86.16- ☑
    toe M86.17- ☑
    ulna M86.13- ☑
    vertebra — *see* Osteomyelitis, vertebra
  chronic (or old) M86.60
    with draining sinus M86.40
      carpus M86.44- ☑
      clavicle M86.41- ☑
      femur M86.45- ☑
      fibula M86.46- ☑
      finger M86.44- ☑
      humerus M86.42- ☑
      ilium M86.459
      ischium M86.459
      mandible M27.2
      metacarpus M86.44- ☑
      metatarsus M86.47- ☑
      multiple sites M86.49
      neck M86.48
      orbit H05.02- ☑
      petrous bone — *see* Petrositis
      radius M86.43- ☑
      rib M86.48
      scapula M86.41- ☑
      skull M86.48
      tarsus M86.47- ☑
      tibia M86.46- ☑
      toe M86.47- ☑
      ulna M86.43- ☑
      vertebra — *see* Osteomyelitis, vertebra
    carpus M86.64- ☑
    clavicle M86.61- ☑
    femur M86.65- ☑
    fibula M86.66- ☑
    finger M86.64- ☑
    hematogenous NEC M86.50
      carpus M86.54- ☑
      clavicle M86.51- ☑
      femur M86.55- ☑
      fibula M86.56- ☑
      finger M86.54- ☑
      humerus M86.52- ☑
      ilium M86.559
      ischium M86.559

Osteomyelitis — *continued*
  chronic — *continued*
    hematogenous — *continued*
      mandible M27.2
      metacarpus M86.54- ☑
      metatarsus M86.57- ☑
      multifocal M86.30
        carpus M86.34- ☑
        clavicle M86.31- ☑
        femur M86.35- ☑
        fibula M86.36- ☑
        finger M86.34- ☑
        humerus M86.32- ☑
        ilium M86.359
        ischium M86.359
        metacarpus M86.34- ☑
        metatarsus M86.37- ☑
        multiple sites M86.39
        neck M86.38
        radius M86.33- ☑
        rib M86.38
        scapula M86.31- ☑
        skull M86.38
        tarsus M86.37- ☑
        tibia M86.36- ☑
        toe M86.37- ☑
        ulna M86.33- ☑
        vertebra — *see* Osteomyelitis, vertebra
      multiple sites M86.59
      neck M86.58
      orbit H05.02- ☑
      petrous bone — *see* Petrositis
      radius M86.53- ☑
      rib M86.58
      scapula M86.51- ☑
      skull M86.58
      tarsus M86.57- ☑
      tibia M86.56- ☑
      toe M86.57- ☑
      ulna M86.53- ☑
      vertebra — *see* Osteomyelitis, vertebra
    humerus M86.62- ☑
    ilium M86.659
    ischium M86.659
    mandible M27.2
    metacarpus M86.64- ☑
    metatarsus M86.67- ☑
    multifocal — *see* Osteomyelitis, chronic, hematogenous, multifocal
    multiple sites M86.69
    neck M86.68
    orbit H05.02- ☑
    petrous bone — *see* Petrositis
    radius M86.63- ☑
    rib M86.68
    scapula M86.61- ☑
    skull M86.68
    tarsus M86.67- ☑
    tibia M86.66- ☑
    toe M86.67- ☑
    ulna M86.63- ☑
    vertebra — *see* Osteomyelitis, vertebra
  echinococcal B67.2
  Garr's — *see* Osteomyelitis, specified type NEC
  jaw (acute) (chronic) (lower) (neonatal) (suppurative) (upper) M27.2
  nonsuppurating — *see* Osteomyelitis, specified type NEC
  orbit H05.02- ☑
  petrous bone — *see* Petrositis
  Salmonella (arizonae) (cholerae-suis) (enteritidis) (typhimurium) A02.24
  sclerosing, nonsuppurative — *see* Osteomyelitis, specified type NEC
  specified type NEC (*see also* subcategory) M86.8X- ☑
    mandible M27.2
    orbit H05.02- ☑
    petrous bone — *see* Petrositis
    vertebra — *see* Osteomyelitis, vertebra
  subacute M86.20
    carpus M86.24- ☑
    clavicle M86.21- ☑
    femur M86.25- ☑
    fibula M86.26- ☑
    finger M86.24- ☑
    humerus M86.22- ☑

Osteomyelitis — *continued*
  subacute — *continued*
    mandible M27.2
    metacarpus M86.24- ☑
    metatarsus M86.27- ☑
    multiple sites M86.29
    neck M86.28
    orbit H05.02- ☑
    petrous bone — *see* Petrositis
    radius M86.23- ☑
    rib M86.28
    scapula M86.21- ☑
    skull M86.28
    tarsus M86.27- ☑
    tibia M86.26- ☑
    toe M86.27- ☑
    ulna M86.23- ☑
    vertebra — *see* Osteomyelitis, vertebra
  syphilitic A52.77
    congenital (early) A50.02 [M90.80]
  tuberculous — *see* Tuberculosis, bone
  typhoid A01.05
  vertebra M46.20
    cervical region M46.22
    cervicothoracic region M46.23
    lumbar region M46.26
    lumbosacral region M46.27
    occipito-atlanto-axial region M46.21
    sacrococcygeal region M46.28
    thoracic region M46.24
    thoracolumbar region M46.25
Osteomyelofibrosis D75.89
Osteomyelosclerosis D75.89
Osteonecrosis M87.9
  due to
    drugs — *see* Osteonecrosis, secondary, due to, drugs
    trauma — *see* Osteonecrosis, secondary, due to, trauma
  idiopathic aseptic M87.00
    ankle M87.07- ☑
    carpus M87.03- ☑
    clavicle M87.01- ☑
    femur M87.05- ☑
    fibula M87.06- ☑
    finger M87.04- ☑
    humerus M87.02- ☑
    ilium M87.050
    ischium M87.050
    metacarpus M87.04- ☑
    metatarsus M87.07- ☑
    multiple sites M87.09
    neck M87.08
    pelvis M87.050
    radius M87.03- ☑
    rib M87.08
    scapula M87.01- ☑
    skull M87.08
    tarsus M87.07- ☑
    tibia M87.06- ☑
    toe M87.07- ☑
    ulna M87.03- ☑
    vertebra M87.08
  secondary NEC M87.30
    carpus M87.33- ☑
    clavicle M87.31- ☑
    due to
      drugs M87.10
        carpus M87.13- ☑
        clavicle M87.11- ☑
        femur M87.15- ☑
        fibula M87.16- ☑
        finger M87.14- ☑
        humerus M87.12- ☑
        ilium M87.159
        ischium M87.159
        jaw M87.180
        metacarpus M87.14- ☑
        metatarsus M87.17- ☑
        multiple sites M87.19
        neck M87.18 ☑
        radius M87.13- ☑
        rib M87.18 ☑
        scapula M87.11- ☑
        skull M87.18 ☑
        tarsus M87.17- ☑
        tibia M87.16- ☑

☑ Additional Character Required — Refer to the Tabular List for Character Selection   ▽ Subterms under main terms may continue to next column or page

Osteonecrosis — continued
  secondary — continued
    due to — continued
      drugs — continued
        toe M87.17- ☑
        ulna M87.13- ☑
        vertebra M87.18 ☑
      hemoglobinopathy NEC D58.2 [M90.50]
        carpus D58.2 [M90.54-] ☑
        clavicle D58.2 [M90.51-] ☑
        femur D58.2 [M90.55-] ☑
        fibula D58.2 [M90.56-] ☑
        finger D58.2 [M90.54-] ☑
        humerus D58.2 [M90.52-] ☑
        ilium D58.2 [M90.55-] ☑
        ischium D58.2 [M90.55-] ☑
        metacarpus D58.2 [M90.54-] ☑
        metatarsus D58.2 [M90.57-] ☑
        multiple sites D58.2 [M90.58]
        neck D58.2 [M90.58]
        radius D58.2 [M90.53-] ☑
        rib D58.2 [M90.58]
        scapula D58.2 [M90.51-] ☑
        skull D58.2 [M90.58]
        tarsus D58.2 [M90.57-] ☑
        tibia D58.2 [M90.56-] ☑
        toe D58.2 [M90.57-] ☑
        ulna D58.2 [M90.53-] ☑
        vertebra D58.2 [M90.58]
      trauma (previous) M87.20
        carpus M87.23- ☑
        clavicle M87.21- ☑
        femur M87.25- ☑
        fibula M87.26- ☑
        finger M87.24- ☑
        humerus M87.22- ☑
        ilium M87.25- ☑
        ischium M87.25- ☑
        metacarpus M87.24- ☑
        metatarsus M87.27- ☑
        multiple sites M87.29
        neck M87.28
        radius M87.23- ☑
        rib M87.28
        scapula M87.21- ☑
        skull M87.28
        tarsus M87.27- ☑
        tibia M87.26- ☑
        toe M87.27- ☑
        ulna M87.23- ☑
        vertebra M87.28
  femur M87.35- ☑
  fibula M87.36- ☑
  finger M87.34- ☑
  humerus M87.32- ☑
  ilium M87.350
  in
    caisson disease T70.3 ☑ [M90.50]
      carpus T70.3 ☑ [M90.54-] ☑
      clavicle T70.3 ☑ [M90.51-] ☑
      femur T70.3 ☑ [M90.55-] ☑
      fibula T70.3 ☑ [M90.56-] ☑
      finger T70.3 ☑ [M90.54-] ☑
      humerus T70.3 ☑ [M90.52-] ☑
      ilium T70.3 ☑ [M90.55-] ☑
      ischium T70.3 ☑ [M90.55-] ☑
      metacarpus T70.3 ☑ [M90.54-] ☑
      metatarsus T70.3 ☑ [M90.57-] ☑
      multiple sites T70.3 ☑ [M90.59]
      neck T70.3 ☑ [M90.58]
      radius T70.3 ☑ [M90.53-] ☑
      rib T70.3 ☑ [M90.58]
      scapula T70.3 ☑ [M90.51-] ☑
      skull T70.3 ☑ [M90.58]
      tarsus T70.3 ☑ [M90.57-] ☑
      tibia T70.3 ☑ [M90.56-] ☑
      toe T70.3 ☑ [M90.57-] ☑
      ulna T70.3 ☑ [M90.53-] ☑
      vertebra T70.3 ☑ [M90.58]
  ischium M87.350
  metacarpus M87.34- ☑
  metatarsus M87.37- ☑
  multiple site M87.39
  neck M87.38
  radius M87.33- ☑
  rib M87.38

Osteonecrosis — continued
  secondary — continued
    scapula M87.319
    skull M87.38
    tarsus M87.379
    tibia M87.366
    toe M87.379
    ulna M87.33- ☑
    vertebra M87.38
  specified type NEC M87.80
    carpus M87.83- ☑
    clavicle M87.81- ☑
    femur M87.85- ☑
    fibula M87.86- ☑
    finger M87.84- ☑
    humerus M87.82- ☑
    ilium M87.85- ☑
    ischium M87.85- ☑
    metacarpus M87.84- ☑
    metatarsus M87.87- ☑
    multiple sites M87.89
    neck M87.88
    radius M87.83- ☑
    rib M87.88
    scapula M87.81- ☑
    skull M87.88
    tarsus M87.87- ☑
    tibia M87.86- ☑
    toe M87.87- ☑
    ulna M87.83- ☑
    vertebra M87.88

Osteo-onycho-arthro-dysplasia Q79.8
Osteo-onychodysplasia, hereditary Q79.8
Osteopathia condensans disseminata Q78.8
Osteopathy (see also Osteomyelitis, Osteonecrosis, Osteoporosis)
  after poliomyelitis M89.60
    carpus M89.64- ☑
    clavicle M89.61- ☑
    femur M89.65- ☑
    fibula M89.66- ☑
    finger M89.64- ☑
    humerus M89.62- ☑
    ilium M89.659
    ischium M89.659
    metacarpus M89.64- ☑
    metatarsus M89.67- ☑
    multiple sites M89.69
    neck M89.68
    radius M89.63- ☑
    rib M89.68
    scapula M89.61- ☑
    skull M89.68
    tarsus M89.67- ☑
    tibia M89.66- ☑
    toe M89.67- ☑
    ulna M89.63- ☑
    vertebra M89.68
  in (due to)
    renal osteodystrophy N25.0
    specified diseases classified elsewhere — see subcategory M90.8 ☑
Osteopenia M85.8- ☑
  borderline M85.8- ☑
Osteoperiostitis — see Osteomyelitis, specified type NEC
Osteopetrosis (familial) Q78.2
Osteophyte M25.70
  ankle M25.77- ☑
  elbow M25.72- ☑
  foot joint M25.77- ☑
  hand joint M25.74- ☑
  hip M25.75- ☑
  knee M25.76- ☑
  shoulder M25.71- ☑
  spine M25.78
  vertebrae M25.78
  wrist M25.73- ☑
Osteopoikilosis Q78.8
Osteoporosis (female) (male) M81.0
  with current pathological fracture M80.00 ☑
  age-related M81.0
    with current pathologic fracture M80.00 ☑
      carpus M80.04- ☑
      clavicle M80.01- ☑
      fibula M80.06- ☑

Osteoporosis — continued
  age-related — continued
    with current pathologic fracture — continued
      finger M80.04- ☑
      humerus M80.02- ☑
      ilium M80.05- ☑
      ischium M80.05- ☑
      metacarpus M80.04- ☑
      metatarsus M80.07- ☑
      pelvis M80.05- ☑
      radius M80.03- ☑
      scapula M80.01- ☑
      tarsus M80.07- ☑
      tibia M80.06- ☑
      toe M80.07- ☑
      ulna M80.03- ☑
      vertebra M80.08 ☑
  disuse M81.8
    with current pathological fracture M80.80 ☑
      carpus M80.84- ☑
      clavicle M80.81- ☑
      fibula M80.86- ☑
      finger M80.84- ☑
      humerus M80.82- ☑
      ilium M80.85- ☑
      ischium M80.85- ☑
      metacarpus M80.84- ☑
      metatarsus M80.87- ☑
      pelvis M80.85- ☑
      radius M80.83- ☑
      scapula M80.81- ☑
      tarsus M80.87- ☑
      tibia M80.86- ☑
      toe M80.87- ☑
      ulna M80.83- ☑
      vertebra M80.88 ☑
  drug-induced — see Osteoporosis, specified type NEC
  idiopathic — see Osteoporosis, specified type NEC
  involutional — see Osteoporosis, age-related
  Lequesne M81.6
  localized M81.6
  postmenopausal M81.0
    with pathological fracture M80.00 ☑
      carpus M80.04- ☑
      clavicle M80.01- ☑
      fibula M80.06- ☑
      finger M80.04- ☑
      humerus M80.02- ☑
      ilium M80.05- ☑
      ischium M80.05- ☑
      metacarpus M80.04- ☑
      metatarsus M80.07- ☑
      pelvis M80.05- ☑
      radius M80.03- ☑
      scapula M80.01- ☑
      tarsus M80.07- ☑
      tibia M80.06- ☑
      toe M80.07- ☑
      ulna M80.03- ☑
      vertebra M80.08 ☑
  postoophorectomy — see Osteoporosis, specified type NEC
  postsurgical malabsorption — see Osteoporosis, specified type NEC
  post-traumatic — see Osteoporosis, specified type NEC
  senile — see Osteoporosis, age-related
  specified type NEC M81.8
    with pathological fracture M80.80 ☑
      carpus M80.84- ☑
      clavicle M80.81- ☑
      fibula M80.86- ☑
      finger M80.84- ☑
      humerus M80.82- ☑
      ilium M80.85- ☑
      ischium M80.85- ☑
      metacarpus M80.84- ☑
      metatarsus M80.87- ☑
      pelvis M80.85- ☑
      radius M80.83- ☑
      scapula M80.81- ☑
      tarsus M80.87- ☑
      tibia M80.86- ☑
      toe M80.87- ☑
      ulna M80.83- ☑
      vertebra M80.88 ☑

Index

Osteonecrosis — Osteoporosis

Osteopsathyrosis (idiopathica) Q78.0
Osteoradionecrosis, jaw (acute) (chronic) (lower) (suppurative) (upper) M27.2
Osteosarcoma (any form) — *see* Neoplasm, bone, malignant
Osteosclerosis Q78.2
  acquired M85.8- ☑
  congenita Q77.4
  fragilitas (generalisata) Q78.2
  myelofibrosis D75.81
Osteosclerotic anemia D64.89
Osteosis
  cutis L94.2
  renal fibrocystic N25.0
Österreicher-Turner syndrome Q87.2
Ostium
  atrioventriculare commune Q21.2
  primum (arteriosum) (defect) (persistent) Q21.2
  secundum (arteriosum) (defect) (patent) (persistent) Q21.1
Ostrum-Furst syndrome Q75.8
Otalgia H92.0 ☑
Otitis (acute) H66.90
  with effusion (*see also* Otitis, media, nonsuppurative)
    purulent — *see* Otitis, media, suppurative
  adhesive — *see* subcategory H74.1 ☑
  chronic (*see also* Otitis, media, chronic)
    with effusion (*see also* Otitis, media, nonsuppurative, chronic)
  externa H60.9- ☑
    abscess — *see* Abscess, ear, external
    acute (noninfective) H60.50- ☑
      actinic H60.51- ☑
      chemical H60.52- ☑
      contact H60.53- ☑
      eczematoid H60.54- ☑
      infective — *see* Otitis, externa, infective
      reactive H60.55- ☑
      specified NEC H60.59- ☑
    cellulitis — *see* Cellulitis, ear
    chronic H60.6- ☑
    diffuse — *see* Otitis, externa, infective, diffuse
    hemorrhagic — *see* Otitis, externa, infective, hemorrhagic
    in (due to)
      aspergillosis B44.89
      candidiasis B37.84
      erysipelas A46 [H62.40]
      herpes (simplex) virus infection B00.1
        zoster B02.8
      impetigo L01.00 [H62.40]
      infectious disease NEC B99 ☑ [H62.4-] ☑
      mycosis NEC B36.9 [H62.40]
      parasitic disease NEC B89 [H62.40]
      viral disease NEC B34.9 [H62.40]
      zoster B02.8
    infective NEC H60.39- ☑
      abscess — *see* Abscess, ear, external
      cellulitis — *see* Cellulitis, ear
      diffuse H60.31- ☑
      hemorrhagic H60.32- ☑
      swimmer's ear — *see* Swimmer's, ear
    malignant H60.2- ☑
    mycotic B36.9 [H62.40]
    necrotizing — *see* Otitis, externa, malignant
    Pseudomonas aeruginosa — *see* Otitis, externa, malignant
    reactive — *see* Otitis, externa, acute, reactive
    specified NEC — *see* subcategory H60.8 ☑
    tropical B36.8
  insidiosa — *see* Otosclerosis
  interna H83.0 ☑
  media (hemorrhagic) (staphylococcal) (streptococcal) H66.9-
    with effusion (nonpurulent) — *see* Otitis, media, nonsuppurative
    acute, subacute H66.90
      allergic — *see* Otitis, media, nonsuppurative, acute, allergic
      exudative — *see* Otitis, media, nonsuppurative, acute
      mucoid — *see* Otitis, media, nonsuppurative, acute
      necrotizing (*see also* Otitis, media, suppurative, acute)
        in
          measles B05.3

Otitis — *continued*
  media — *continued*
    acute, subacute — *continued*
      necrotizing (*see also* Otitis, media, suppurative, acute) — *continued*
        in — *continued*
          scarlet fever A38.0
      nonsuppurative NEC — *see* Otitis, media, nonsuppurative, acute
      purulent — *see* Otitis, media, suppurative, acute
      sanguinous — *see* Otitis, media, nonsuppurative, acute
      secretory — *see* Otitis, media, nonsuppurative, acute, serous
      seromucinous — *see* Otitis, media, nonsuppurative, acute
      serous — *see* Otitis, media, nonsuppurative, acute, serous
      suppurative — *see* Otitis, media, suppurative, acute
    allergic — *see* Otitis, media, nonsuppurative
    catarrhal — *see* Otitis, media, nonsuppurative
    chronic H66.90
      with effusion (nonpurulent) — *see* Otitis, media, nonsuppurative, chronic
      allergic — *see* Otitis, media, nonsuppurative, chronic, allergic
      benign suppurative — *see* Otitis, media, suppurative, chronic, tubotympanic
      catarrhal — *see* Otitis, media, nonsuppurative, chronic, serous
      exudative — *see* Otitis, media, nonsuppurative, chronic
      mucinous — *see* Otitis, media, nonsuppurative, chronic, mucoid
      mucoid — *see* Otitis, media, nonsuppurative, chronic, mucoid
      nonsuppurative NEC — *see* Otitis, media, nonsuppurative, chronic
      purulent — *see* Otitis, media, suppurative, chronic
      secretory — *see* Otitis, media, nonsuppurative, chronic, mucoid
      seromucinous — *see* Otitis, media, nonsuppurative, chronic
      serous — *see* Otitis, media, nonsuppurative, chronic, serous
      suppurative — *see* Otitis, media, suppurative, chronic
      transudative — *see* Otitis, media, nonsuppurative, chronic, mucoid
    exudative — *see* Otitis, media, nonsuppurative
    in (due to) (with)
      influenza — *see* Influenza, with, otitis media
      measles B05.3
      scarlet fever A38.0
      tuberculosis A18.6
      viral disease NEC B34.- ☑ [H67.-] ☑
    mucoid — *see* Otitis, media, nonsuppurative
    nonsuppurative H65.9- ☑
      acute or subacute NEC H65.19- ☑
        allergic H65.11- ☑
          recurrent H65.11- ☑
        recurrent H65.19- ☑
        secretory — *see* Otitis, media, nonsuppurative, serous
        serous H65.0- ☑
          recurrent H65.0- ☑
      chronic H65.49- ☑
        allergic H65.41- ☑
        mucoid H65.3- ☑
        serous H65.2- ☑
    postmeasles B05.3
    purulent — *see* Otitis, media, suppurative
    secretory — *see* Otitis, media, nonsuppurative
    seromucinous — *see* Otitis, media, nonsuppurative
    serous — *see* Otitis, media, nonsuppurative
    suppurative H66.4- ☑
      acute H66.00- ☑
        with rupture of ear drum H66.01- ☑
        recurrent H66.00- ☑
          with rupture of ear drum H66.01- ☑
      chronic (*see also* subcategory) H66.3
        atticoantral H66.2- ☑
        benign — *see* Otitis, media, suppurative, chronic, tubotympanic

Otitis — *continued*
  media — *continued*
    suppurative — *continued*
      chronic (*see also* subcategory) — *continued*
        tubotympanic H66.1- ☑
      transudative — *see* Otitis, media, nonsuppurative
      tuberculous A18.6
Otocephaly Q18.2
Otolith syndrome — *see* subcategory H81.8 ☑
Otomycosis (diffuse) **NEC** B36.9 [H62.40]
  in
    aspergillosis B44.89
    candidiasis B37.84
    moniliasis B37.84
Otoporosis — *see* Otosclerosis
Otorrhagia (nontraumatic) H92.2- ☑
  traumatic — *code by* Type of injury
Otorrhea H92.1- ☑
  cerebrospinal G96.0
Otosclerosis (general) H80.9- ☑
  cochlear (endosteal) H80.2- ☑
  involving
    otic capsule — *see* Otosclerosis, cochlear
    oval window
      nonobliterative H80.0- ☑
      obliterative H80.1- ☑
    round window — *see* Otosclerosis, cochlear
  nonobliterative — *see* Otosclerosis, involving, oval window, nonobliterative
  obliterative — *see* Otosclerosis, involving, oval window, obliterative
  specified NEC H80.8- ☑
Otospongiosis — *see* Otosclerosis
Otto's disease or pelvis M24.7
Outcome of delivery Z37.9
  multiple births Z37.9
    all liveborn Z37.50
      quadruplets Z37.52
      quintuplets Z37.53
      sextuplets Z37.54
      specified number NEC Z37.59
      triplets Z37.51
    all stillborn Z37.7
    some liveborn Z37.60
      quadruplets Z37.62
      quintuplets Z37.63
      sextuplets Z37.64
      specified number NEC Z37.69
      triplets Z37.61
  single NEC Z37.9
    liveborn Z37.0
    stillborn Z37.1
  twins NEC Z37.9
    both liveborn Z37.2
    both stillborn Z37.4
    one liveborn, one stillborn Z37.3
Outlet — *see* condition
Ovalocytosis (congenital) (hereditary) — *see* Elliptocytosis
Ovarian — *see* Condition
Ovariocele N83.4
Ovaritis (cystic) — *see* Oophoritis
Ovary, ovarian (*see also* condition)
  resistant syndrome E28.39
  vein syndrome N13.8
Overactive (*see also* Hyperfunction)
  adrenal cortex NEC E27.0
  bladder N32.81
  hypothalamus E23.3
  thyroid — *see* Hyperthyroidism
Overactivity R46.3
  child — *see* Disorder, attention-deficit hyperactivity
Overbite (deep) (excessive) (horizontal) (vertical) M26.29
Overbreathing — *see* Hyperventilation
Overconscientious personality F60.5
Overdevelopment — *see* Hypertrophy
Overdistension — *see* Distension
Overdose, overdosage (drug) — *see* Table of Drugs and Chemicals, by drug, poisoning
Overeating R63.2
  nonorganic origin F50.8
  psychogenic F50.8
Overexertion (effects) (exhaustion) T73.3 ☑
Overexposure (effects) T73.9 ☑
  exhaustion T73.2 ☑
Overfeeding — *see* Overeating
  newborn P92.4

Overfill, endodontic M27.52
Overgrowth, bone — *see* Hypertrophy, bone
Overhanging of dental restorative material (unrepairable) K08.52
Overheated (places) (effects) — *see* Heat
Overjet (excessive horizontal) M26.23
Overlaid, overlying (suffocation) — *see* Asphyxia, traumatic, due to mechanical threat
Overlap, excessive horizontal (teeth) M26.23
Overlapping toe (acquired) (*see also* Deformity, toe, specified NEC)
   congenital (fifth toe) Q66.89
Overload
   circulatory, due to transfusion (blood) (blood components) (TACO) E87.71
   fluid E87.70
      due to transfusion (blood) (blood components) E87.71
      specified NEC E87.79
   iron, due to repeated red blood cell transfusions E83.111
   potassium (K) E87.5
   sodium (Na) E87.0
Overnutrition — *see* Hyperalimentation
Overproduction (*see also* Hypersecretion)
   ACTH E27.0
   catecholamine E27.5
   growth hormone E22.0
Overprotection, child by parent Z62.1
Overriding
   aorta Q25.4
   finger (acquired) — *see* Deformity, finger
      congenital Q68.1
   toe (acquired) (*see also* Deformity, toe, specified NEC)
      congenital Q66.89
Overstrained R53.83
   heart — *see* Hypertrophy, cardiac
Overuse, muscle NEC M70.8- ☑
Overweight E66.3
Overworked R53.83
Oviduct — *see* condition
Ovotestis Q56.0
Ovulation (cycle)
   failure or lack of N97.0
   pain N94.0
Ovum — *see* condition
Owren's disease or syndrome (parahemophilia) D68.2
Ox heart — *see* Hypertrophy, cardiac
Oxalosis E72.53
Oxaluria E72.53
Oxycephaly, oxycephalic Q75.0
   syphilitic, congenital A50.02
Oxyuriasis B80
Oxyuris vermicularis (infestation) B80
Ozena J31.0

P

Pachyderma, pachydermia L85.9
   larynx (verrucosa) J38.7
Pachydermatocele (congenital) Q82.8
Pachydermoperiostosis (*see also* Osteoarthropathy, hypertrophic, specified type NEC)
   clubbed nail M89.40 [L62]
Pachygyria Q04.3
Pachymeningitis (adhesive) (basal) (brain) (cervical) (chronic)(circumscribed) (external) (fibrous) (hemorrhagic) (hypertrophic) (internal) (purulent) (spinal) (suppurative) — *see* Meningitis
Pachyonychia (congenital) Q84.5
Pacinian tumor — *see* Neoplasm, skin, benign
Pad, knuckle or Garrod's M72.1
Paget's disease
   with infiltrating duct carcinoma — *see* Neoplasm, breast, malignant
   bone M88.9
      carpus M88.84- ☑
      clavicle M88.81- ☑
      femur M88.85- ☑
      fibula M88.86- ☑
      finger M88.84- ☑
      humerus M88.82- ☑
      ilium M88.85- ☑
      in neoplastic disease — *see* Osteitis, deformans, in neoplastic disease
      ischium M88.85- ☑
      metacarpus M88.84- ☑

Paget's disease — *continued*
   bone — *continued*
      metatarsus M88.87- ☑
      multiple sites M88.89
      neck M88.88
      radius M88.83- ☑
      rib M88.88
      scapula M88.81- ☑
      skull M88.0
      tarsus M88.87- ☑
      tibia M88.86- ☑
      toe M88.87- ☑
      ulna M88.83- ☑
      vertebra M88.88
   breast (female) C50.01- ☑
      male C50.02- ☑
   extramammary (*see also* Neoplasm, skin, malignant)
      anus C21.0
         margin C44.590
         skin C44.590
   intraductal carcinoma — *see* Neoplasm, breast, malignant
   malignant — *see* Neoplasm, skin, malignant
      breast (female) C50.01- ☑
         male C50.02- ☑
      unspecified site (female) C50.01- ☑
         male C50.02- ☑
   mammary — *see* Paget's disease, breast
   nipple — *see* Paget's disease, breast
   osteitis deformans — *see* Paget's disease, bone
Paget-Schroetter syndrome I82.890
Pain(s) (*see also* Painful) R52
   abdominal R10.9
      colic R10.83
      generalized R10.84
         with acute abdomen R10.0
      lower R10.30
         left quadrant R10.32
         pelvic or perineal R10.2
         periumbilical R10.33
         right quadrant R10.31
      rebound — *see* Tenderness, abdominal, rebound
      severe with abdominal rigidity R10.0
      tenderness — *see* Tenderness, abdominal
      upper R10.10
         epigastric R10.13
         left quadrant R10.12
         right quadrant R10.11
   acute R52
      due to trauma G89.11
      neoplasm related G89.3
      postprocedural NEC G89.18
      post-thoracotomy G89.12
      specified by site — *code to* Pain, by site
   adnexa (uteri) R10.2
   anginoid — *see* Pain, precordial
   anus K62.89
   arm — *see* Pain, limb, upper
   axillary (axilla) M79.62- ☑
   back (postural) M54.9
   bladder R39.89
      associated with micturition — *see* Micturition, painful
   bone — *see* Disorder, bone, specified type NEC
   breast N64.4
   broad ligament R10.2
   cancer associated (acute) (chronic) G89.3
   cecum — *see* Pain, abdominal
   cervicobrachial M53.1
   chest (central) R07.9
      anterior wall R07.89
      atypical R07.89
      ischemic I20.9
      musculoskeletal R07.89
      non-cardiac R07.89
      on breathing R07.1
      pleurodynia R07.81
      precordial R07.2
      wall (anterior) R07.89
   chronic G89.29
      associated with significant psychosocial dysfunction G89.4
      due to trauma G89.21
      neoplasm related G89.3
      postoperative NEC G89.28
      postprocedural NEC G89.28
      post-thoracotomy G89.22

Pain(s) — *continued*
   chronic — *continued*
      specified NEC G89.29
   coccyx M53.3
   colon — *see* Pain, abdominal
   coronary — *see* Angina
   costochondral R07.1
   diaphragm R07.1
   due to cancer G89.3
   due to device, implant or graft (*see also* Complications, by site and type, specified NEC) T85.84 ☑
      arterial graft NEC T82.848 ☑
      breast (implant) T85.84 ☑
      catheter NEC T85.84 ☑
         dialysis (renal) T82.848 ☑
            intraperitoneal T85.84 ☑
         infusion NEC T82.848 ☑
            spinal (epidural) (subdural) T85.84 ☑
         urinary (indwelling) T83.84 ☑
      electronic (electrode) (pulse generator) (stimulator)
         bone T84.84 ☑
         cardiac T82.847 ☑
         nervous system (brain) (peripheral nerve) (spinal) T85.84 ☑
         urinary T83.84 ☑
      fixation, internal (orthopedic) NEC T84.84 ☑
      gastrointestinal (bile duct) (esophagus) T85.84 ☑
      genital NEC T83.84 ☑
      heart NEC T82.847 ☑
      infusion NEC T85.84 ☑
      joint prosthesis T84.84 ☑
      ocular (corneal graft) (orbital implant) NEC T85.84 ☑
      orthopedic NEC T84.84 ☑
      specified NEC T85.84 ☑
      urinary NEC T83.84 ☑
      vascular NEC T82.848 ☑
      ventricular intracranial shunt T85.84 ☑
   due to malignancy (primary) (secondary) G89.3
   ear — *see* subcategory H92.0 ☑
   epigastric, epigastrium R10.13
   eye — *see* Pain, ocular
   face, facial R51
      atypical G50.1
   female genital organs NEC N94.89
   finger — *see* Pain, limb, upper
   flank — *see* Pain, abdominal
   foot — *see* Pain, limb, lower
   gallbladder K82.9
   gas (intestinal) R14.1
   gastric — *see* Pain, abdominal
   generalized NOS R52
   genital organ
      female N94.89
      male N50.8
   groin — *see* Pain, abdominal, lower
   hand — *see* Pain, limb, upper
   head — *see* Headache
   heart — *see* Pain, precordial
   infra-orbital — *see* Neuralgia, trigeminal
   intercostal R07.82
   intermenstrual N94.0
   jaw R68.84
   joint M25.50
      ankle M25.57- ☑
      elbow M25.52- ☑
      finger M79.64- ☑
      foot M79.67- ☑
      hand M79.64- ☑
      hip M25.55- ☑
      knee M25.56- ☑
      shoulder M25.51- ☑
      toe M79.67- ☑
      wrist M25.53- ☑
   kidney N23
   laryngeal R07.0
   leg — *see* Pain, limb, lower
   limb M79.609
      lower M79.60- ☑
         foot M79.67- ☑
         lower leg M79.66- ☑
         thigh M79.65- ☑
         toe M79.67- ☑
      upper M79.60- ☑
         axilla M79.62- ☑
         finger M79.64- ☑

Pain(s) — *continued*
  limb — *continued*
    upper — *continued*
      forearm M79.63- ☑
      hand M79.64- ☑
      upper arm M79.62- ☑
  loin M54.5
  low back M54.5
  lumbar region M54.5
  mandibular R68.84
  mastoid — *see* subcategory H92.0 ☑
  maxilla R68.84
  menstrual (*see also* Dysmenorrhea) N94.6
  metacarpophalangeal (joint) — *see* Pain, joint, hand
  metatarsophalangeal (joint) — *see* Pain, joint, foot
  mouth K13.79
  muscle — *see* Myalgia
  musculoskeletal (*see also* Pain, by site) M79.1
  myofascial M79.1
  nasal J34.89
  nasopharynx J39.2
  neck NEC M54.2
  nerve NEC — *see* Neuralgia
  neuromuscular — *see* Neuralgia
  nose J34.89
  ocular H57.1- ☑
  ophthalmic — *see* Pain, ocular
  orbital region — *see* Pain, ocular
  ovary N94.89
  over heart — *see* Pain, precordial
  ovulation N94.0
  pelvic (female) R10.2
  penis N48.89
  pericardial — *see* Pain, precordial
  perineal, perineum R10.2
  pharynx J39.2
  pleura, pleural, pleuritic R07.81
  postoperative NOS G89.18
  postprocedural NOS G89.18
  post-thoracotomy G89.12
  precordial (region) R07.2
  premenstrual N94.3
  psychogenic (persistent) (any site) F45.41
  radicular (spinal) — *see* Radiculopathy
  rectum K62.89
  respiration R07.1
  retrosternal R07.2
  rheumatoid, muscular — *see* Myalgia
  rib R07.81
  root (spinal) — *see* Radiculopathy
  round ligament (stretch) R10.2
  sacroiliac M53.3
  sciatic — *see* Sciatica
  scrotum N50.8
  seminal vesicle N50.8
  shoulder M25.51- ☑
  spermatic cord N50.8
  spinal root — *see* Radiculopathy
  spine M54.9
    cervical M54.2
    low back M54.5
      with sciatica M54.4- ☑
    thoracic M54.6
  stomach — *see* Pain, abdominal
  substernal R07.2
  temporomandibular (joint) M26.62
  testis N50.8
  thoracic spine M54.6
    with radicular and visceral pain M54.14
  throat R07.0
  tibia — *see* Pain, limb, lower
  toe — *see* Pain, limb, lower
  tongue K14.6
  tooth K08.8
  trigeminal — *see* Neuralgia, trigeminal
  tumor associated G89.3
  ureter N23
  urinary (organ) (system) N23
  uterus NEC N94.89
  vagina R10.2
  vertebrogenic (syndrome) M54.89
  vesical R39.89
    associated with micturition — *see* Micturition, painful
  vulva R10.2
Painful (*see also* Pain)
  coitus
    female N94.1

Painful — *continued*
  coitus — *continued*
    male N53.12
    psychogenic F52.6
  ejaculation (semen) N53.12
    psychogenic F52.6
  erection — *see* Priapism
  feet syndrome E53.8
  joint replacement (hip) (knee) T84.84 ☑
  menstruation — *see* Dysmenorrhea
    psychogenic F45.8
  micturition — *see* Micturition, painful
  respiration R07.1
  scar NEC L90.5
  wire sutures T81.89 ☑
Painter's colic — *see* subcategory T56.0 ☑
Palate — *see* condition
Palatoplegia K13.79
Palatoschisis — *see* Cleft, palate
Palilalia R48.8
Palliative care Z51.5
Pallor R23.1
  optic disc, temporal — *see* Atrophy, optic
Palmar (*see also* condition)
  fascia — *see* condition
Palpable
  cecum K63.89
  kidney N28.89
  ovary N83.8
  prostate N42.9
  spleen — *see* Splenomegaly
Palpitations (heart) R00.2
  psychogenic F45.8
Palsy (*see also* Paralysis) G83.9
  atrophic diffuse (progressive) G12.22
  Bell's (*see also* Palsy, facial)
    newborn P11.3
  brachial plexus NEC G54.0
    newborn (birth injury) P14.3
  brain — *see* Palsy, cerebral
  bulbar (progressive) (chronic) G12.22
    of childhood (Fazio-Londe) G12.1
    pseudo NEC G12.29
    supranuclear (progressive) G23.1
  cerebral (congenital) G80.9
    ataxic G80.4
    athetoid G80.3
    choreathetoid G80.3
    diplegic G80.8
      spastic G80.1
    dyskinetic G80.3
      athetoid G80.3
      choreathetoid G80.3
      distonic G80.3
    dystonic G80.3
    hemiplegic G80.8
      spastic G80.2
    mixed G80.8
    monoplegic G80.8
      spastic G80.1
    paraplegic G80.8
      spastic G80.1
    quadriplegic G80.8
      spastic G80.0
    spastic G80.1
      diplegic G80.1
      hemiplegic G80.2
      monoplegic G80.1
      quadriplegic G80.0
      specified NEC G80.1
      tetraplegic G80.0
    specified NEC G80.8
    syphilitic A52.12
      congenital A50.49
    tetraplegic G80.8
      spastic G80.0
  cranial nerve (*see also* Disorder, nerve, cranial)
    multiple G52.7
      in
        infectious disease B99 ☑ [G53]
        neoplastic disease (*see also* Neoplasm)
          D49.9 [G53]
        parasitic disease B89 [G53]
        sarcoidosis D86.82
  creeping G12.22
  diver's T70.3 ☑
  Erb's P14.0

Palsy — *continued*
  facial G51.0
    newborn (birth injury) P11.3
  glossopharyngeal G52.1
  Klumpke (-Déjérine) P14.1
  lead — *see* subcategory T56.0 ☑
  median nerve (tardy) G56.1- ☑
  nerve G58.9
    specified NEC G58.8
  peroneal nerve (acute) (tardy) G57.3- ☑
  progressive supranuclear G23.1
  pseudobulbar NEC G12.29
  radial nerve (acute) G56.3- ☑
  seventh nerve (*see also* Palsy, facial)
    newborn P11.3
  shaking — *see* Parkinsonism
  spastic (cerebral) (spinal) G80.1
  ulnar nerve (tardy) G56.2- ☑
  wasting G12.29
Paludism — *see* Malaria
Panangiitis M30.0
Panaris, panaritium (*see also* Cellulitis, digit)
  with lymphangitis — *see* Lymphangitis, acute, digit
Panarteritis nodosa M30.0
  brain or cerebral I67.7
Pancake heart R93.1
  with cor pulmonale (chronic) I27.81
Pancarditis (acute) (chronic) I51.89
  rheumatic I09.89
    active or acute I01.8
Pancoast's syndrome or tumor C34.1- ☑
Pancolitis, ulcerative (chronic) K51.00
  with
    abscess K51.014
    complication K51.019
    fistula K51.013
    obstruction K51.012
    rectal bleeding K51.011
    specified complication NEC K51.018
Pancreas, pancreatic — *see* condition
Pancreatitis (annular) (apoplectic) (calcareous) (edematous) (hemorrhagic) (malignant) (recurrent) (subacute) (suppurative) K85.9
  acute K85.9
    alcohol induced K85.2
    biliary K85.1
    drug induced K85.3
    gallstone K85.1
    idiopathic K85.0
    specified NEC K85.8
  chronic (infectious) K86.1
    alcohol-induced K86.0
    recurrent K86.1
    relapsing K86.1
  cystic (chronic) K86.1
  cytomegaloviral B25.2
  fibrous (chronic) K86.1
  gallstone K85.1
  gangrenous K85.8
  interstitial (chronic) K86.1
    acute K85.8
  mumps B26.3
  recurrent (chronic) K86.1
  relapsing, chronic K86.1
  syphilitic A52.74
Pancreatoblastoma — *see* Neoplasm, pancreas, malignant
Pancreolithiasis K86.8
Pancytolysis D75.89
Pancytopenia (acquired) D61.818
  with
    malformations D61.09
    myelodysplastic syndrome — *see* Syndrome, myelodysplastic
  antineoplastic chemotherapy induced D61.810
  congenital D61.09
  drug-induced NEC D61.811
Panencephalitis, subacute, sclerosing A81.1
Panhematopenia D61.9
  congenital D61.09
  constitutional D61.09
  splenic, primary D73.1
Panhemocytopenia D61.9
  congenital D61.09
  constitutional D61.09
Panhypogonadism E29.1
Panhypopituitarism E23.0
  prepubertal E23.0

☑ **Additional Character Required** — **Refer to the Tabular List for Character Selection**   ⚏ **Subterms under main terms may continue to next column or page**

Panic (attack) (state) F41.0
　reaction to exceptional stress (transient) F43.0
Panmyelopathy, familial, constitutional D61.09
Panmyelophthisis D61.82
　congenital D61.09
Panmyelosis (acute) (with myelofibrosis) C94.4- ☑
Panner's disease — see Osteochondrosis, juvenile, humerus
Panneuritis endemica E51.11
Panniculitis (nodular) (nonsuppurative) M79.3
　back M54.00
　　cervical region M54.02
　　cervicothoracic region M54.03
　　lumbar region M54.06
　　lumbosacral region M54.07
　　multiple sites M54.09
　　occipito-atlanto-axial region M54.01
　　sacrococcygeal region M54.08
　　thoracic region M54.04
　　thoracolumbar region M54.05
　lupus L93.2
　mesenteric K65.4
　neck M54.02
　　cervicothoracic region M54.03
　　occipito-atlanto-axial region M54.01
　relapsing M35.6
Panniculus adiposus (abdominal) E65
Pannus (allergic) (cornea) (degenerativus) (keratic) H16.42- ☑
　abdominal (symptomatic) E65
　trachomatosus, trachomatous (active) A71.1
Panophthalmitis H44.01- ☑
Pansinusitis (chronic) (hyperplastic) (nonpurulent) (purulent) J32.4
　acute J01.40
　　recurrent J01.41
　tuberculous A15.8
Panuveitis (sympathetic) H44.11- ☑
Panvalvular disease I08.9
　specified NEC I08.8
Papanicolaou smear, cervix Z12.4
　as part of routine gynecological examination Z01.419
　　with abnormal findings Z01.411
　for suspected neoplasm Z12.4
　nonspecific abnormal finding R87.619
　routine Z01.419
　　with abnormal findings Z01.411
Papilledema (choked disc) H47.10
　associated with
　　decreased ocular pressure H47.12
　　increased intracranial pressure H47.11
　　retinal disorder H47.13
　Foster-Kennedy syndrome H47.14- ☑
Papillitis H46.00
　anus K62.89
　chronic lingual K14.4
　necrotizing, kidney N17.2
　optic H46.0- ☑
　rectum K62.89
　renal, necrotizing N17.2
　tongue K14.0
Papilloma (see also Neoplasm, benign, by site)
　acuminatum (female) (male) (anogenital) A63.0
　benign pinta (primary) A67.0
　bladder (urinary) (transitional cell) D41.4
　choroid plexus (lateral ventricle) (third ventricle) D33.0
　　anaplastic C71.5
　　fourth ventricle D33.1
　　malignant C71.5
　renal pelvis (transitional cell) D41.1- ☑
　　benign D30.1- ☑
　Schneiderian
　　specified site — see Neoplasm, benign, by site
　　unspecified site D14.0
　serous surface
　　borderline malignancy
　　　specified site — see Neoplasm, uncertain behavior, by site
　　　unspecified site D39.10
　　specified site — see Neoplasm, benign, by site
　　unspecified site D27.9
　transitional (cell)
　　bladder (urinary) D41.4
　　inverted type — see Neoplasm, uncertain behavior, by site
　　renal pelvis D41.1- ☑
　　ureter D41.2- ☑

Papilloma — continued
　ureter (transitional cell) D41.2- ☑
　　benign D30.2- ☑
　urothelial — see Neoplasm, uncertain behavior, by site
　villous — see Neoplasm, uncertain behavior, by site
　　adenocarcinoma in — see Neoplasm, malignant, by site
　　in situ — see Neoplasm, in situ
　yaws, plantar or palmar A66.1
Papillomata, multiple, of yaws A66.1
Papillomatosis (see also Neoplasm, benign, by site)
　confluent and reticulated L83
　cystic, breast — see Mastopathy, cystic
　ductal, breast — see Mastopathy, cystic
　intraductal (diffuse) — see Neoplasm, benign, by site
　subareolar duct D24- ☑
Papillomavirus, as cause of disease classified elsewhere B97.7
Papillon-Léage and Psaume syndrome Q87.0
Papule(s) R23.8
　carate (primary) A67.0
　fibrous, of nose D22.39
　Gottron's L94.4
　pinta (primary) A67.0
Papulosis
　lymphomatoid C86.6
　malignant I77.89
Papyraceous fetus O31.0- ☑
Para-albuminemia E88.09
Paracephalus Q89.7
Parachute mitral valve Q23.2
Paracoccidioidomycosis B41.9
　disseminated B41.7
　generalized B41.7
　mucocutaneous-lymphangitic B41.8
　pulmonary B41.0
　specified NEC B41.8
　visceral B41.8
Paradentosis K05.4
Paraffinoma T88.8 ☑
Paraganglioma D44.7
　adrenal D35.0- ☑
　　malignant C74.1- ☑
　aortic body D44.7
　　malignant C75.5
　carotid body D44.6
　　malignant C75.4
　chromaffin (see also Neoplasm, benign, by site)
　　malignant — see Neoplasm, malignant, by site
　extra-adrenal D44.7
　　malignant C75.5
　　　specified site — see Neoplasm, malignant, by site
　　　unspecified site C75.5
　　specified site — see Neoplasm, uncertain behavior, by site
　　unspecified site D44.7
　gangliocytic D13.2
　　specified site — see Neoplasm, benign, by site
　　unspecified site D13.2
　glomus jugulare D44.7
　　malignant C75.5
　jugular D44.7
　malignant C75.5
　　specified site — see Neoplasm, malignant, by site
　　unspecified site C75.5
　nonchromaffin D44.7
　　malignant C75.5
　　　specified site — see Neoplasm, malignant, by site
　　　unspecified site C75.5
　　specified site — see Neoplasm, uncertain behavior, by site
　　unspecified site D44.7
　parasympathetic D44.7
　　specified site — see Neoplasm, uncertain behavior, by site
　　unspecified site D44.7
　specified site — see Neoplasm, uncertain behavior, malignant
　sympathetic D44.7
　　specified site — see Neoplasm, uncertain behavior, by site
　　unspecified site D44.7
　unspecified site D44.7

Parageusia R43.2
　psychogenic F45.8
Paragonimiasis B66.4
Paragranuloma, Hodgkin — see Lymphoma, Hodgkin, classical, specified NEC
Parahemophilia (see also Defect, coagulation) D68.2
Parakeratosis R23.4
　variegata L41.0
Paralysis, paralytic (complete) (incomplete) G83.9
　with
　　syphilis A52.17
　abducens, abducent (nerve) — see Strabismus, paralytic, sixth nerve
　abductor, lower extremity G57.9- ☑
　accessory nerve G52.8
　accommodation (see also Paresis, of accommodation)
　　hysterical F44.89
　acoustic nerve (except Deafness) H93.3 ☑
　agitans (see also Parkinsonism) G20
　　arteriosclerotic G21.4
　alternating (oculomotor) G83.89
　amyotrophic G12.21
　ankle G57.9- ☑
　anus (sphincter) K62.89
　arm — see Monoplegia, upper limb
　ascending (spinal), acute G61.0
　association G12.29
　asthenic bulbar G70.00
　　with exacerbation (acute) G70.01
　　in crisis G70.01
　ataxic (hereditary) G11.9
　　general (syphilitic) A52.17
　atrophic G58.9
　　infantile, acute — see Poliomyelitis, paralytic
　　progressive G12.22
　　spinal (acute) — see Poliomyelitis, paralytic
　axillary G54.0
　Babinski-Nageotte's G83.89
　Bell's G51.0
　　newborn P11.3
　Benedikt's G46.3
　birth injury P14.9
　　spinal cord P11.5
　bladder (neurogenic) (sphincter) N31.2
　bowel, colon or intestine K56.0
　brachial plexus G54.0
　　birth injury P14.3
　　newborn (birth injury) P14.3
　brain G83.9
　　diplegia G83.0
　　triplegia G83.89
　bronchial J98.09
　Brown-Séquard G83.81
　bulbar (chronic) (progressive) G12.22
　　infantile — see Poliomyelitis, paralytic
　　poliomyelitic — see Poliomyelitis, paralytic
　　pseudo G12.29
　bulbospinal G70.00
　　with exacerbation (acute) G70.01
　　in crisis G70.01
　cardiac (see also Failure, heart) I50.9
　cerebrocerebellar, diplegic G80.1
　cervical
　　plexus G54.2
　　sympathetic G90.09
　Céstan-Chenais G46.3
　Charcot-Marie-Tooth type G60.0
　Clark's G80.9
　colon K56.0
　compressed air T70.3 ☑
　compression
　　arm G56.9- ☑
　　leg G57.9- ☑
　　lower extremity G57.9- ☑
　　upper extremity G56.9- ☑
　congenital (cerebral) — see Palsy, cerebral
　conjugate movement (gaze) (of eye) H51.0
　　cortical (nuclear) (supranuclear) H51.0
　cordis — see Failure, heart
　cranial or cerebral nerve G52.9
　creeping G12.22
　crossed leg G83.89
　crutch — see Injury, brachial plexus
　deglutition R13.0
　　hysterical F44.4
　dementia A52.17
　descending (spinal) NEC G12.29

Paralysis, paralytic — *continued*
- diaphragm (flaccid) J98.6
  - due to accidental dissection of phrenic nerve during procedure — *see* Puncture, accidental complicating surgery
- digestive organs NEC K59.8
- diplegic — *see* Diplegia
- divergence (nuclear) H51.8
- diver's T70.3 ☑
- Duchenne's
  - birth injury P14.0
  - due to or associated with
    - motor neuron disease G12.22
    - muscular dystrophy G71.0
  - due to intracranial or spinal birth injury — *see* Palsy, cerebral
- embolic (current episode) I63.4 ☑
- Erb (-Duchenne) (birth) (newborn) P14.0
- Erb's syphilitic spastic spinal A52.17
- esophagus K22.8
- eye muscle (extrinsic) H49.9
  - intrinsic (*see also* Paresis, of accommodation)
- facial (nerve) G51.0
  - birth injury P11.3
  - congenital P11.3
  - following operation NEC — *see* Puncture, accidental complicating surgery
  - newborn (birth injury) P11.3
- familial (recurrent) (periodic) G72.3
  - spastic G11.4
- fauces J39.2
- finger G56.9- ☑
- gait R26.1
- gastric nerve (nondiabetic) G52.2
- gaze, conjugate H51.0
- general (progressive) (syphilitic) A52.17
  - juvenile A50.45
- glottis J38.00
  - bilateral J38.02
  - unilateral J38.01
- gluteal G54.1
- Gubler (-Millard) G46.3
- hand — *see* Monoplegia, upper limb
- heart — *see* Arrest, cardiac
- hemiplegic — *see* Hemiplegia
- hyperkalemic periodic (familial) G72.3
- hypoglossal (nerve) G52.3
- hypokalemic periodic G72.3
- hysterical F44.4
- ileus K56.0
- infantile (*see also* Poliomyelitis, paralytic) A80.30
  - bulbar — *see* Poliomyelitis, paralytic
  - cerebral — *see* Palsy, cerebral
  - spastic — *see* Palsy, cerebral, spastic
- infective — *see* Poliomyelitis, paralytic
- inferior nuclear G83.9
- internuclear — *see* Ophthalmoplegia, internuclear
- intestine K56.0
- iris H57.09
  - due to diphtheria (toxin) A36.89
- ischemic, Volkmann's (complicating trauma) T79.6 ☑
- Jackson's G83.89
- jake — *see* Poisoning, food, noxious, plant
- Jamaica ginger (jake) G62.2
- juvenile general A50.45
- Klumpke (-Déjérine) (birth) (newborn) P14.1
- labioglossal (laryngeal) (pharyngeal) G12.29
- Landry's G61.0
- laryngeal nerve (recurrent) (superior) (unilateral) J38.00
  - bilateral J38.02
  - unilateral J38.01
- larynx J38.00
  - bilateral J38.02
  - due to diphtheria (toxin) A36.2
  - unilateral J38.01
- lateral G12.21
- lead T56.0 ☑
- left side — *see* Hemiplegia
- leg G83.1- ☑
  - both — *see* Paraplegia
  - crossed G83.89
  - hysterical F44.4
  - psychogenic F44.4
  - transient or transitory R29.818
    - traumatic NEC — *see* Injury, nerve, leg
- levator palpebrae superioris — *see* Blepharoptosis, paralytic
- limb — *see* Monoplegia

Paralysis, paralytic — *continued*
- lip K13.0
- Lissauer's A52.17
- lower limb — *see* Monoplegia, lower limb
  - both — *see* Paraplegia
- lung J98.4
- median nerve G56.1- ☑
- medullary (tegmental) G83.89
- mesencephalic NEC G83.89
  - tegmental G83.89
- middle alternating G83.89
- Millard-Gubler-Foville G46.3
- monoplegic — *see* Monoplegia
- motor G83.9
- muscle, muscular NEC G72.89
  - due to nerve lesion G58.9
  - eye (extrinsic) H49.9
    - intrinsic — *see* Paresis, of accommodation
    - oblique — *see* Strabismus, paralytic, fourth nerve
  - iris sphincter H21.9
  - ischemic (Volkmann's) (complicating trauma) T79.6 ☑
  - progressive G12.21
  - pseudohypertrophic G71.0
- musculocutaneous nerve G56.9- ☑
- musculospiral G56.9- ☑
- nerve (*see also* Disorder, nerve)
  - abducent — *see* Strabismus, paralytic, sixth nerve
  - accessory G52.8
  - auditory (except Deafness) H93.3 ☑
  - birth injury P14.9
  - cranial or cerebral G52.9
  - facial G51.0
    - birth injury P11.3
    - congenital P11.3
    - newborn (birth injury) P11.3
  - fourth or trochlear — *see* Strabismus, paralytic, fourth nerve
  - newborn (birth injury) P14.9
  - oculomotor — *see* Strabismus, paralytic, third nerve
  - phrenic (birth injury) P14.2
  - radial G56.3- ☑
  - seventh or facial G51.0
    - newborn (birth injury) P11.3
  - sixth or abducent — *see* Strabismus, paralytic, sixth nerve
  - syphilitic A52.15
  - third or oculomotor — *see* Strabismus, paralytic, third nerve
  - trigeminal G50.9
  - trochlear — *see* Strabismus, paralytic, fourth nerve
  - ulnar G56.2- ☑
- normokalemic periodic G72.3
- ocular H49.9
  - alternating G83.89
- oculofacial, congenital (Moebius) Q87.0
- oculomotor (external bilateral) (nerve) — *see* Strabismus, paralytic, third nerve
- palate (soft) K13.79
- paratrigeminal G50.9
- periodic (familial) (hyperkalemic) (hypokalemic) (myotonic) (normokalemic) (potassium sensitive) (secondary) G72.3
- peripheral autonomic nervous system — *see* Neuropathy, peripheral, autonomic
- peroneal (nerve) G57.3- ☑
- pharynx J39.2
- phrenic nerve G56.8- ☑
- plantar nerve(s) G57.6- ☑
- pneumogastric nerve G52.2
- poliomyelitis (current) — *see* Poliomyelitis, paralytic
- popliteal nerve G57.3- ☑
- postepileptic transitory G83.84
- progressive (atrophic) (bulbar) (spinal) G12.22
  - general A52.17
  - infantile acute — *see* Poliomyelitis, paralytic
  - supranuclear G23.1
- pseudobulbar G12.29
- pseudohypertrophic (muscle) G71.0
- psychogenic F44.4
- quadriceps G57.9- ☑
- quadriplegic — *see* Tetraplegia
- radial nerve G56.3- ☑
- rectus muscle (eye) H49.9
- recurrent isolated sleep G47.53

Paralysis, paralytic — *continued*
- respiratory (muscle) (system) (tract) R06.81
  - center NEC G93.89
  - congenital P28.89
  - newborn P28.89
- right side — *see* Hemiplegia
- saturnine T56.0 ☑
- sciatic nerve G57.0- ☑
- senile G83.9
- shaking — *see* Parkinsonism
- shoulder G56.9- ☑
- sleep, recurrent isolated G47.53
- spastic G83.9
  - cerebral — *see* Palsy, cerebral, spastic
  - congenital (cerebral) — *see* Palsy, cerebral, spastic
  - familial G11.4
  - hereditary G11.4
  - quadriplegic G80.0
  - syphilitic (spinal) A52.17
- sphincter, bladder — *see* Paralysis, bladder
- spinal (cord) G83.9
  - accessory nerve G52.8
  - acute — *see* Poliomyelitis, paralytic
  - ascending acute G61.0
  - atrophic (acute) (*see also* Poliomyelitis, paralytic) spastic, syphilitic A52.17
  - congenital NEC — *see* Palsy, cerebral
  - hereditary G95.89
  - infantile — *see* Poliomyelitis, paralytic
  - progressive G12.21
  - sequelae NEC G83.89
- sternomastoid G52.8
- stomach K31.84
  - diabetic — *see* Diabetes, by type, with gastroparesis
  - nerve G52.2
    - diabetic — *see* Diabetes, by type, with gastroparesis
- stroke — *see* Infarct, brain
- subcapsularis G56.8- ☑
- supranuclear (progressive) G23.1
- sympathetic G90.8
  - cervical G90.09
  - nervous system — *see* Neuropathy, peripheral, autonomic
- syndrome G83.9
  - specified NEC G83.89
- syphilitic spastic spinal (Erb's) A52.17
- thigh G57.9- ☑
- throat J39.2
  - diphtheritic A36.0
  - muscle J39.2
- thrombotic (current episode) I63.3 ☑
- thumb G56.9- ☑
- tick — *see* Toxicity, venom, arthropod, specified NEC
- Todd's (postepileptic transitory paralysis) G83.84
- toe G57.6- ☑
- tongue K14.8
- transient R29.5
  - arm or leg NEC R29.818
  - traumatic NEC — *see* Injury, nerve
- trapezius G52.8
- traumatic, transient NEC — *see* Injury, nerve
- trembling — *see* Parkinsonism
- triceps brachii G56.9- ☑
- trigeminal nerve G50.9
- trochlear (nerve) — *see* Strabismus, paralytic, fourth nerve
- ulnar nerve G56.2- ☑
- upper limb — *see* Monoplegia, upper limb
- uremic N18.9 [G99.8]
- uveoparotitic D86.89
- uvula K13.79
  - postdiphtheritic A36.0
- vagus nerve G52.2
- vasomotor NEC G90.8
- velum palati K13.79
- vesical — *see* Paralysis, bladder
- vestibular nerve (except Vertigo) H93.3 ☑
- vocal cords J38.00
  - bilateral J38.02
  - unilateral J38.01
- Volkmann's (complicating trauma) T79.6 ☑
- wasting G12.29
- Weber's G46.3
- wrist G56.9- ☑

Paramedial urethrovesical orifice Q64.79

☑ **Additional Character Required** — **Refer to the Tabular List for Character Selection**   ▽ **Subterms under main terms may continue to next column or page**

Paramenia N92.6
Parametritis (*see also* Disease, pelvis, inflammatory) N73.2
  acute N73.0
  complicating abortion — *see* Abortion, by type, complicated by, parametritis
Parametrium, parametric — *see* condition
Paramnesia — *see* Amnesia
Paramolar K00.1
Paramyloidosis E85.8
Paramyoclonus multiplex G25.3
Paramyotonia (congenita) G71.19
Parangi — *see* Yaws
Paranoia (querulans) F22
  senile F03 ☑
Paranoid
  dementia (senile) F03 ☑
    praecox — *see* Schizophrenia
  personality F60.0
  psychosis (climacteric) (involutional) (menopausal) F22
    psychogenic (acute) F23
    senile F03 ☑
  reaction (acute) F23
    chronic F22
  schizophrenia F20.0
  state (climacteric) (involutional) (menopausal) (simple) F22
    senile F03 ☑
  tendencies F60.0
  traits F60.0
  trends F60.0
  type, psychopathic personality F60.0
Paraparesis — *see* Paraplegia
Paraphasia R47.02
Paraphilia F65.9
Paraphimosis (congenital) N47.2
  chancroidal A57
Paraphrenia, paraphrenic (late) F22
  schizophrenia F20.0
Paraplegia (lower) G82.20
  ataxic — *see* Degeneration, combined, spinal cord
  complete G82.21
  congenital (cerebral) G80.8
    spastic G80.1
  familial spastic G11.4
  functional (hysterical) F44.4
  hereditary, spastic G11.4
  hysterical F44.4
  incomplete G82.22
  Pott's A18.01
  psychogenic F44.4
  spastic
    Erb's spinal, syphilitic A52.17
    hereditary G11.4
    tropical G04.1
  syphilitic (spastic) A52.17
  tropical spastic G04.1
Parapoxvirus B08.60
  specified NEC B08.69
Paraproteinemia D89.2
  benign (familial) D89.2
  monoclonal D47.2
  secondary to malignant disease D47.2
Parapsoriasis L41.9
  en plaques L41.4
  guttata L41.1
  large plaque L41.4
  retiform, retiformis L41.5
  small plaque L41.3
  specified NEC L41.8
  varioliformis (acuta) L41.0
Parasitic (*see also* condition)
  disease NEC B89
  stomatitis B37.0
  sycosis (beard) (scalp) B35.0
  twin Q89.4
Parasitism B89
  intestinal B82.9
  skin B88.9
  specified — *see* Infestation
Parasitophobia F40.218
Parasomnia G47.50
  due to
    alcohol
      abuse F10.182
      dependence F10.282

Parasomnia — *continued*
  due to — *continued*
    alcohol — *continued*
      use F10.982
    amphetamines
      abuse F15.182
      dependence F15.282
      use F15.982
    caffeine
      abuse F15.182
      dependence F15.282
      use F15.982
    cocaine
      abuse F14.182
      dependence F14.282
      use F14.982
    drug NEC
      abuse F19.182
      dependence F19.282
      use F19.982
    opioid
      abuse F11.182
      dependence F11.282
      use F11.982
    psychoactive substance NEC
      abuse F19.182
      dependence F19.282
      use F19.982
    sedative, hypnotic, or anxiolytic
      abuse F13.182
      dependence F13.282
      use F13.982
    stimulant NEC
      abuse F15.182
      dependence F15.282
      use F15.982
  in conditions classified elsewhere G47.54
  nonorganic origin F51.8
  organic G47.50
  specified NEC G47.59
Paraspadias Q54.9
Paraspasmus facialis G51.8
Parasuicide (attempt)
  history of (personal) Z91.5
    in family Z81.8
Parathyroid gland — *see* condition
Parathyroid tetany E20.9
Paratrachoma A74.0
Paratyphilitis — *see* Appendicitis
Paratyphoid (fever) — *see* Fever, paratyphoid
Paratyphus — *see* Fever, paratyphoid
Paraurethral duct Q64.79
  nonorganic origin F51.5
Paraurethritis (*see also* Urethritis)
  gonococcal (acute) (chronic) (with abscess) A54.1
Paravaccinia NEC B08.04
Paravaginitis — *see* Vaginitis
Parencephalitis (*see also* Encephalitis)
  sequelae G09
Parent-child conflict — *see* Conflict, parent-child
  estrangement NEC Z62.890
Paresis (*see also* Paralysis)
  accommodation — *see* Paresis, of accommodation
  Bernhardt's G57.1- ☑
  bladder (sphincter) (*see also* Paralysis, bladder)
    tabetic A52.17
  bowel, colon or intestine K56.0
  extrinsic muscle, eye H49.9
  general (progressive) (syphilitic) A52.17
    juvenile A50.45
  heart — *see* Failure, heart
  insane (syphilitic) A52.17
  juvenile (general) A50.45
  of accommodation H52.52- ☑
  peripheral progressive (idiopathic) G60.3
  pseudohypertrophic G71.0
  senile G83.9
  syphilitic (general) A52.17
    congenital A50.45
  vesical NEC N31.2
Paresthesia (*see also* Disturbance, sensation)
  Bernhardt G57.1- ☑
Paretic — *see* condition
Parinaud's
  conjunctivitis H10.89
  oculoglandular syndrome H10.89
  ophthalmoplegia H49.88- ☑

Parkinsonism (idiopathic) (primary) G20
  with neurogenic orthostatic hypotension (symptomatic) G90.3
  arteriosclerotic G21.4
  dementia G31.83 [F02.80]
    with behavioral disturbance G31.83 [F02.81]
  due to
    drugs NEC G21.19
      neuroleptic G21.11
  neuroleptic induced G21.11
  postencephalitic G21.3
  secondary G21.9
    due to
      arteriosclerosis G21.4
      drugs NEC G21.19
        neuroleptic G21.11
      encephalitis G21.3
      external agents NEC G21.2
      syphilis A52.19
    specified NEC G21.8
  syphilitic A52.19
  treatment-induced NEC G21.19
  vascular G21.4
Parkinson's disease, syndrome or tremor — *see* Parkinsonism
Parodontitis — *see* Periodontitis
Parodontosis K05.4
Paronychia (*see also* Cellulitis, digit)
  with lymphangitis — *see* Lymphangitis, acute, digit
  candidal (chronic) B37.2
  tuberculous (primary) A18.4
Parorexia (psychogenic) F50.8
Parosmia R43.1
  psychogenic F45.8
Parotid gland — *see* condition
Parotitis, parotiditis (allergic)(nonspecific toxic) (purulent) (septic) (suppurative) (*see also* Sialoadenitis)
  epidemic — *see* Mumps
  infectious — *see* Mumps
  postoperative K91.89
  surgical K91.89
Parrot fever A70
Parrot's disease (early congenital syphilitic pseudoparalysis) A50.02
Parry-Romberg syndrome G51.8
Parry's disease or syndrome E05.00
  with thyroid storm E05.01
Pars planitis — *see* Cyclitis
Parsonage (-Aldren)-**Turner syndrome** G54.5
Parson's disease (exophthalmic goiter) E05.00
  with thyroid storm E05.01
Particolored infant Q82.8
Parturition — *see* Delivery
Parulis K04.7
  with sinus K04.6
Parvovirus, as cause of disease classified elsewhere B97.6
Pasini and Pierini's atrophoderma L90.3
Passage
  false, urethra N36.5
  meconium (newborn) during delivery P03.82
  of sounds or bougies — *see* Attention to, artificial, opening
Passive — *see* condition
  smoking Z77.22
Pasteurella septica A28.0
Pasteurellosis — *see* Infection, Pasteurella
PAT (paroxysmal atrial tachycardia) I47.1
Patau's syndrome — *see* Trisomy, 13
Patches
  mucous (syphilitic) A51.39
    congenital A50.07
  smokers' (mouth) K13.24
Patellar — *see* condition
Patent (*see also* Imperfect, closure)
  canal of Nuck Q52.4
  cervix N88.3
  ductus arteriosus or Botallo's Q25.0
  foramen
    botalli Q21.1
    ovale Q21.1
  interauricular septum Q21.1
  interventricular septum Q21.0
  omphalomesenteric duct Q43.0
  os (uteri) — *see* Patent, cervix
  ostium secundum Q21.1
  urachus Q64.4

Patent — *continued*
vitelline duct Q43.0
Paterson (-Brown)(-Kelly) **syndrome or web** D50.1
Pathologic, pathological (*see also* condition)
asphyxia R09.01
fire-setting F63.1
gambling F63.0
ovum O02.0
resorption, tooth K03.3
stealing F63.2
Pathology (of) — *see* Disease
periradicular, associated with previous endodontic
treatment NEC M27.59
Pattern, sleep-wake, irregular G47.23
Patulous (*see also* Imperfect, closure (congenital))
alimentary tract Q45.8
lower Q43.8
upper Q40.8
eustachian tube H69.0- ☑
Pause, sinoatrial I49.5
Paxton's disease B36.2
Pearl(s)
enamel K00.2
Epstein's K09.8
Pearl-worker's disease — *see* Osteomyelitis, specified
type NEC
Pectenosis K62.4
Pectoral — *see* condition
Pectus
carinatum (congenital) Q67.7
acquired M95.4
rachitic sequelae (late effect) E64.3
excavatum (congenital) Q67.6
acquired M95.4
rachitic sequelae (late effect) E64.3
recurvatum (congenital) Q67.6
Pedatrophia E41
Pederosis F65.4
Pediculosis (infestation) B85.2
capitis (head-louse) (any site) B85.0
corporis (body-louse) (any site) B85.1
eyelid B85.0
mixed (classifiable to more than one of the titles B85.0-
B85.3) B85.4
pubis (pubic louse) (any site) B85.3
vestimenti B85.1
vulvae B85.3
Pediculus (infestation) — *see* Pediculosis
Pedophilia F65.4
Peg-shaped teeth K00.2
Pelade — *see* Alopecia, areata
Pelger-Huët anomaly or syndrome D72.0
Peliosis (rheumatica) D69.0
hepatis K76.4
with toxic liver disease K71.8
Pelizaeus-Merzbacher disease E75.29
Pellagra (alcoholic) (with polyneuropathy) E52
**Pellagra-cerebellar-ataxia-renal aminoaciduria
syndrome** E72.02
Pellegrini (-Stieda) **disease or syndrome** — *see* Bursitis,
tibial collateral
Pellizzi's syndrome E34.8
Pel's crisis A52.11
Pelvic (*see also* condition)
examination (periodic) (routine) Z01.419
with abnormal findings Z01.411
kidney, congenital Q63.2
Pelviolithiasis — *see* Calculus, kidney
Pelviperitonitis (*see also* Peritonitis, pelvic)
gonococcal A54.24
puerperal O85
Pelvis — *see* condition or type
Pemphigoid L12.9
benign, mucous membrane L12.1
bullous L12.0
cicatricial L12.1
juvenile L12.2
ocular L12.1
specified NEC L12.8
Pemphigus L10.9
benign familial (chronic) Q82.8
Brazilian L10.3
circinatus L13.0
conjunctiva L12.1
drug-induced L10.5
erythematosus L10.4
foliaceous L10.2

Pemphigus — *continued*
gangrenous — *see* Gangrene
neonatorum L01.03
ocular L12.1
paraneoplastic L10.81
specified NEC L10.89
syphilitic (congenital) A50.06
vegetans L10.1
vulgaris L10.0
wildfire L10.3
Pendred's syndrome E07.1
Pendulous
abdomen, in pregnancy — *see* Pregnancy, complicated by, abnormal, pelvic organs or tissues NEC
breast N64.89
Penetrating wound (*see also* Puncture)
with internal injury — *see* Injury, by site
eyeball — *see* Puncture, eyeball
orbit (with or without foreign body) — *see* Puncture,
orbit
uterus by instrument with or following ectopic or
molar pregnancy O08.6
Penicillosis B48.4
Penis — *see* condition
Penitis N48.29
Pentalogy of Fallot Q21.8
Pentasomy X syndrome Q97.1
Pentosuria (essential) E74.8
Percreta placenta - O43.23 ☑
Peregrinating patient — *see* Disorder, factitious
Perforation, perforated (nontraumatic) (of)
accidental during procedure (blood vessel) (nerve)
(organ) — *see* Complication, accidental puncture or laceration
antrum — *see* Sinusitis, maxillary
appendix K35.2
atrial septum, multiple Q21.1
attic, ear — *see* Perforation, tympanum, attic
bile duct (common) (hepatic) K83.2
cystic K82.2
bladder (urinary)
with or following ectopic or molar pregnancy O08.6
obstetrical trauma O71.5
traumatic S37.29 ☑
at delivery O71.5
bowel K63.1
with or following ectopic or molar pregnancy O08.6
newborn P78.0
obstetrical trauma O71.5
traumatic — *see* Laceration, intestine
broad ligament N83.8
with or following ectopic or molar pregnancy O08.6
obstetrical trauma O71.6
by
device, implant or graft (*see also* Complications,
by site and type, mechanical) T85.628 ☑
arterial graft NEC — *see* Complication, cardiovascular device, mechanical, vascular
breast (implant) T85.49 ☑
catheter NEC T85.698 ☑
cystostomy T83.090 ☑
dialysis (renal) T82.49 ☑
intraperitoneal T85.691 ☑
infusion NEC T82.594 ☑
spinal (epidural) (subdural) T85.690 ☑
electronic (electrode) (pulse generator) (stimulator)
bone T84.390 ☑
cardiac T82.199 ☑
electrode T82.190 ☑
pulse generator T82.191 ☑
specified type NEC T82.198 ☑
nervous system — *see* Complication, prosthetic device, mechanical, electronic
nervous system stimulator
urinary — *see* Complication, genitourinary,
device, urinary, mechanical
fixation, internal (orthopedic) NEC — *see*
Complication, fixation device, mechanical
gastrointestinal — *see* Complications, prosthetic device, mechanical, gastrointestinal
device
genital NEC T83.498 ☑
intrauterine contraceptive device T83.39 ☑
penile prosthesis T83.490 ☑
heart NEC — *see* Complication, cardiovascular
device, mechanical

Perforation, perforated — *continued*
by — *continued*
device, implant or graft (*see also* Complications, by
site and type, mechanical) — *continued*
joint prosthesis — *see* Complications, joint
prosthesis, mechanical, specified NEC, by
site
ocular NEC — *see* Complications, prosthetic
device, mechanical, ocular device
orthopedic NEC — *see* Complication, orthopedic, device, mechanical
specified NEC T85.628 ☑
urinary, indwelling T83.098 ☑
urinary NEC (*see also* Complication, genitourinary, device, urinary, mechanical)
graft T83.29 ☑
vascular NEC — *see* Complication, cardiovascular device, mechanical
ventricular intracranial shunt T85.09 ☑
foreign body left accidentally in operative wound
T81.539 ☑
instrument (any) during a procedure, accidental
— *see* Puncture, accidental complicating
surgery
cecum K35.2
cervix (uteri) N88.8
with or following ectopic or molar pregnancy O08.6
obstetrical trauma O71.3
colon K63.1
newborn P78.0
obstetrical trauma O71.5
traumatic — *see* Laceration, intestine, large
common duct (bile) K83.2
cornea (due to ulceration) — *see* Ulcer, cornea, perforated
cystic duct K82.2
diverticulum (intestine) K57.80
with bleeding K57.81
large intestine K57.20
with
bleeding K57.21
small intestine K57.40
with bleeding K57.41
small intestine K57.00
with
bleeding K57.01
large intestine K57.40
with bleeding K57.41
ear drum — *see* Perforation, tympanum
esophagus K22.3
ethmoidal sinus — *see* Sinusitis, ethmoidal
frontal sinus — *see* Sinusitis, frontal
gallbladder K82.2
heart valve — *see* Endocarditis
ileum K63.1
newborn P78.0
obstetrical trauma O71.5
traumatic — *see* Laceration, intestine, small
instrumental, surgical (accidental) (blood vessel)
(nerve) (organ) — *see* Puncture, accidental
complicating surgery
intestine NEC K63.1
with ectopic or molar pregnancy O08.6
newborn P78.0
obstetrical trauma O71.5
traumatic — *see* Laceration, intestine
ulcerative NEC K63.1
newborn P78.0
jejunum, jejunal K63.1
obstetrical trauma O71.5
traumatic — *see* Laceration, intestine, small
ulcer — *see* Ulcer, gastrojejunal, with perforation
joint prosthesis — *see* Complications, joint prosthesis,
mechanical, specified NEC, by site
mastoid (antrum) (cell) — *see* Disorder, mastoid,
specified NEC
maxillary sinus — *see* Sinusitis, maxillary
membrana tympani — *see* Perforation, tympanum
nasal
septum J34.89
congenital Q30.3
syphilitic A52.73
sinus J34.89
congenital Q30.8
due to sinusitis — *see* Sinusitis
palate (*see also* Cleft, palate) Q35.9
syphilitic A52.79

☑ **Additional Character Required — Refer to the Tabular List for Character Selection**   ▽ **Subterms under main terms may continue to next column or page**

Perforation, perforated — *continued*
  palatine vault (*see also* Cleft, palate, hard) Q35.1
    syphilitic A52.79
      congenital A50.59
  pars flaccida (ear drum) — *see* Perforation, tympanum, attic
  pelvic
    floor S31.030 ☑
      with
        ectopic or molar pregnancy O08.6
        penetration into retroperitoneal space S31.031
        retained foreign body S31.040 ☑
          with penetration into retroperitoneal space S31.041 ☑
      following ectopic or molar pregnancy O08.6
      obstetrical trauma O70.1
    organ S37.99 ☑
      adrenal gland S37.818 ☑
      bladder — *see* Perforation, bladder
      fallopian tube S37.599 ☑
        bilateral S37.592 ☑
        unilateral S37.591 ☑
      kidney S37.09- ☑
      obstetrical trauma O71.5
      ovary S37.499 ☑
        bilateral S37.492 ☑
        unilateral S37.491 ☑
      prostate S37.828 ☑
      specified organ NEC S37.898 ☑
      ureter — *see* Perforation, ureter
      urethra — *see* Perforation, urethra
      uterus — *see* Perforation, uterus
  perineum — *see* Laceration, perineum
  pharynx J39.2
  rectum K63.1
    newborn P78.0
    obstetrical trauma O71.5
    traumatic S36.63
  root canal space due to endodontic treatment M27.51
  sigmoid K63.1
    newborn P78.0
    obstetrical trauma O71.5
    traumatic S36.533 ☑
  sinus (accessory) (chronic) (nasal) J34.89
  sphenoidal sinus — *see* Sinusitis, sphenoidal
  surgical (accidental) (by instrument) (blood vessel) (nerve) (organ) — *see* Puncture, accidental complicating surgery
  traumatic
    external — *see* Puncture
    eye — *see* Puncture, eyeball
    internal organ — *see* Injury, by site
  tympanum, tympanic (membrane) (persistent post-traumatic) (postinflammatory) H72.9- ☑
    attic H72.1- ☑
      multiple — *see* Perforation, tympanum, multiple
      total — *see* Perforation, tympanum, total
    central H72.0- ☑
      multiple — *see* Perforation, tympanum, multiple
      total — *see* Perforation, tympanum, total
    marginal NEC — *see* subcategory H72.2 ☑
    multiple H72.81- ☑
    pars flaccida — *see* Perforation, tympanum, attic
    total H72.82- ☑
    traumatic, current episode S09.2- ☑
  typhoid, gastrointestinal — *see* Typhoid
  ulcer — *see* Ulcer, by site, with perforation
  ureter N28.89
    traumatic S37.19 ☑
  urethra N36.8
    with ectopic or molar pregnancy O08.6
    following ectopic or molar pregnancy O08.6
    obstetrical trauma O71.5
    traumatic S37.39 ☑
      at delivery O71.5
  uterus
    with ectopic or molar pregnancy O08.6
    by intrauterine contraceptive device T83.39
    following ectopic or molar pregnancy O08.6
    obstetrical trauma O71.1
    traumatic S37.69 ☑
      obstetric O71.1
  uvula K13.79
    syphilitic A52.79

Perforation, perforated — *continued*
  vagina O71.4
    obstetrical trauma O71.4
    other trauma — *see* Puncture, vagina
Periadenitis mucosa necrotica recurrens K12.0
Periappendicitis (acute) — *see* Appendicitis
Periarteritis nodosa (disseminated) (infectious) (necrotizing) M30.0
Periarthritis (joint) (*see also* Enthesopathy)
  Duplay's M75.0- ☑
  gonococcal A54.42
  humeroscapularis — *see* Capsulitis, adhesive
  scapulohumeral — *see* Capsulitis, adhesive
  shoulder — *see* Capsulitis, adhesive
  wrist M77.2- ☑
Periarthrosis (angioneural) — *see* Enthesopathy
Pericapsulitis, adhesive (shoulder) — *see* Capsulitis, adhesive
Pericarditis (with decompensation) (with effusion) I31.9
  with rheumatic fever (conditions in I00)
    active — *see* Pericarditis, rheumatic
    inactive or quiescent I09.2
  acute (hemorrhagic) (nonrheumatic) (Sicca) I30.9
    with chorea (acute) (rheumatic) (Sydenham's) I02.0
    benign I30.8
    nonspecific I30.0
    rheumatic I01.0
      with chorea (acute) (Sydenham's) I02.0
  adhesive or adherent (chronic) (external) (internal) I31.0
    acute — *see* Pericarditis, acute
    rheumatic I09.2
  bacterial (acute) (subacute) (with serous or seropurulent effusion) I30.1
  calcareous I31.1
  cholesterol (chronic) I31.8
    acute I30.9
  chronic (nonrheumatic) I31.9
    rheumatic I09.2
  constrictive (chronic) I31.1
  coxsackie B33.23
  fibrinocaseous (tuberculous) A18.84
  fibrinopurulent I30.1
  fibrinous I30.8
  fibrous I31.0
  gonococcal A54.83
  idiopathic I30.0
  in systemic lupus erythematosus M32.12
  infective I30.1
  meningococcal A39.53
  neoplastic (chronic) I31.8
    acute I30.9
  obliterans, obliterating I31.0
  plastic I31.0
  pneumococcal I30.1
  postinfarction I24.1
  purulent I30.1
  rheumatic (active) (acute) (with effusion) (with pneumonia) I01.0
    with chorea (acute) (rheumatic) (Sydenham's) I02.0
    chronic or inactive (with chorea) I09.2
  rheumatoid — *see* Rheumatoid, carditis
  septic I30.1
  serofibrinous I30.8
  staphylococcal I30.1
  streptococcal I30.1
  suppurative I30.1
  syphilitic A52.06
  tuberculous A18.84
  uremic N18.9 [I32]
  viral I30.1
Pericardium, pericardial — *see* condition
Pericellulitis — *see* Cellulitis
Pericementitis (chronic) (suppurative) (*see also* Periodontitis)
  acute K05.20
    generalized K05.22
    localized K05.21
Perichondritis
  auricle — *see* Perichondritis, ear
  bronchus J98.09
  ear (external) H61.00- ☑
    acute H61.01- ☑
    chronic H61.02- ☑
  external auditory canal — *see* Perichondritis, ear
  larynx J38.7
    syphilitic A52.73
    typhoid A01.09

Perichondritis — *continued*
  nose J34.89
  pinna — *see* Perichondritis, ear
  trachea J39.8
Periclasia K05.4
Pericoronitis — *see* Periodontitis
Pericystitis N30.90
  with hematuria N30.91
Peridiverticulitis (intestine) K57.92
  cecum — *see* Diverticulitis, intestine, large
  colon — *see* Diverticulitis, intestine, large
  duodenum — *see* Diverticulitis, intestine, small
  intestine — *see* Diverticulitis, intestine
  jejunum — *see* Diverticulitis, intestine, small
  rectosigmoid — *see* Diverticulitis, intestine, large
  rectum — *see* Diverticulitis, intestine, large
  sigmoid — *see* Diverticulitis, intestine, large
Periendocarditis — *see* Endocarditis
Periepididymitis N45.1
Perifolliculitis L01.02
  abscedens, caput, scalp L66.3
  capitis, abscedens (et suffodiens) L66.3
  superficial pustular L01.02
Perihepatitis K65.8
Perilabyrinthitis (acute) — *see* subcategory H83.0 ☑
Perimeningitis — *see* Meningitis
Perimetritis — *see* Endometritis
Perimetrosalpingitis — *see* Salpingo-oophoritis
Perineocele N81.81
Perinephric, perinephritic — *see* condition
Perinephritis (*see also* Infection, kidney)
  purulent — *see* Abscess, kidney
Perineum, perineal — *see* condition
Perineuritis NEC — *see* Neuralgia
Periodic — *see* condition
Periodontitis (chronic) (complex) (compound) (local) (simplex) K05.30
  acute K05.20
    generalized K05.22
    localized K05.21
  apical K04.5
    acute (pulpal origin) K04.4
  generalized K05.32
  localized K05.31
Periodontoclasia K05.4
Periodontosis (juvenile) K05.4
Periods (*see also* Menstruation)
  heavy N92.0
  irregular N92.6
  shortened intervals (irregular) N92.1
Perionychia (*see also* Cellulitis, digit)
  with lymphangitis — *see* Lymphangitis, acute, digit
Perioophoritis — *see* Salpingo-oophoritis
Periorchitis N45.2
Periosteum, periosteal — *see* condition
Periostitis (albuminosa) (circumscribed) (diffuse) (infective) (monomelic) (*see also* Osteomyelitis)
  alveolar M27.3
  alveolodental M27.3
  dental M27.3
  gonorrheal A54.43
  jaw (lower) (upper) M27.2
  orbit H05.03- ☑
  syphilitic A52.77
    congenital (early) A50.02 [M90.80]
    secondary A51.46
  tuberculous — *see* Tuberculosis, bone
  yaws (hypertrophic) (early) (late) A66.6 [M90.80]
Periostosis (hyperplastic) (*see also* Disorder, bone, specified type NEC)
  with osteomyelitis — *see* Osteomyelitis, specified type NEC
Peripartum
  cardiomyopathy O90.3
Periphlebitis — *see* Phlebitis
Periproctitis K62.89
Periprostatitis — *see* Prostatitis
Perirectal — *see* condition
Perirenal — *see* condition
Perisalpingitis — *see* Salpingo-oophoritis
Perisplenitis (infectional) D73.89
Peristalsis, visible or reversed R19.2
Peritendinitis — *see* Enthesopathy
Peritoneum, peritoneal — *see* condition
Peritonitis (adhesive) (bacterial) (fibrinous) (hemorrhagic) (idiopathic) (localized) (perforative) (primary) (with adhesions) (with effusion) K65.9

Peritonitis — *continued*
  with or following
    abscess K65.1
    appendicitis K35.2
      with perforation or rupture K35.2
      generalized K35.2
      localized K35.3
    diverticular disease (intestine) K57.80
      with bleeding K57.81
    ectopic or molar pregnancy O08.0
    large intestine K57.20
      with
        bleeding K57.21
        small intestine K57.40
          with bleeding K57.41
      small intestine K57.00
        with
          bleeding K57.01
          large intestine K57.40
            with bleeding K57.41
  acute (generalized) K65.0
  aseptic T81.61 ☑
  bile, biliary K65.3
  chemical T81.61 ☑
  chlamydial A74.81
  chronic proliferative K65.8
  complicating abortion — *see* Abortion, by type, complicated by, pelvic peritonitis
  congenital P78.1
  diaphragmatic K65.0
  diffuse K65.0
  diphtheritic A36.89
  disseminated K65.0
  due to
    bile K65.3
    foreign
      body or object accidentally left during a procedure (instrument) (sponge) (swab) T81.599 ☑
      substance accidentally left during a procedure (chemical) (powder) (talc) T81.61 ☑
    talc T81.61 ☑
    urine K65.8
  eosinophilic K65.8
    acute K65.0
  fibrocaseous (tuberculous) A18.31
  fibropurulent K65.0
  following ectopic or molar pregnancy O08.0
  general (ized) K65.0
  gonococcal A54.85
  meconium (newborn) P78.0
  neonatal P78.1
    meconium P78.0
  pancreatic K65.0
  paroxysmal, familial E85.0
    benign E85.0
  pelvic
    female N73.5
      acute N73.3
      chronic N73.4
        with adhesions N73.6
    male K65.0
  periodic, familial E85.0
  proliferative, chronic K65.8
  puerperal, postpartum, childbirth O85
  purulent K65.0
  septic K65.0
  specified NEC K65.8
  spontaneous bacterial K65.2
  subdiaphragmatic K65.0
  subphrenic K65.0
  suppurative K65.0
  syphilitic A52.74
    congenital (early) A50.08 [K67]
  talc T81.61 ☑
  tuberculous A18.31
  urine K65.8
Peritonsillar — *see* condition
Peritonsillitis J36
Perityphlitis K37
Periureteritis N28.89
Periurethral — *see* condition
Periurethritis (gangrenous) — *see* Urethritis
Periuterine — *see* condition
Perivaginitis — *see* Vaginitis
Perivasculitis, retinal H35.06- ☑
Perivasitis (chronic) N49.1
Perivesiculitis (seminal) — *see* Vesiculitis

Perlèche NEC K13.0
  due to
    candidiasis B37.83
    moniliasis B37.83
    riboflavin deficiency E53.0
    vitamin B2 (riboflavin) deficiency E53.0
Pernicious — *see* condition
Pernio, perniosis T69.1 ☑
Perpetrator (of abuse) — *see* Index to External Causes of Injury, Perpetrator
Persecution
  delusion F22
  social Z60.5
Perseveration (tonic) R48.8
Persistence, persistent (congenital)
  anal membrane Q42.3
    with fistula Q42.2
  arteria stapedia Q16.3
  atrioventricular canal Q21.2
  branchial cleft Q18.0
  bulbus cordis in left ventricle Q21.8
  canal of Cloquet Q14.0
  capsule (opaque) Q12.8
  cilioretinal artery or vein Q14.8
  cloaca Q43.7
  communication — *see* Fistula, congenital
  convolutions
    aortic arch Q25.4
    fallopian tube Q50.6
    oviduct Q50.6
    uterine tube Q50.6
  double aortic arch Q25.4
  ductus arteriosus (Botalli) Q25.0
  fetal
    circulation P29.3
    form of cervix (uteri) Q51.828
    hemoglobin, hereditary (HPFH) D56.4
  foramen
    Botalli Q21.1
    ovale Q21.1
  Gartner's duct Q52.4
  hemoglobin, fetal (hereditary) (HPFH) D56.4
  hyaloid
    artery (generally incomplete) Q14.0
    system Q14.8
  hymen, in pregnancy or childbirth — *see* Pregnancy, complicated by, abnormal, vulva
  lanugo Q84.2
  left
    posterior cardinal vein Q26.8
    root with right arch of aorta Q25.4
    superior vena cava Q26.1
  Meckel's diverticulum Q43.0
    malignant — *see* Table of Neoplasms, small intestine, malignant
  mucosal disease (middle ear) — *see* Otitis, media, suppurative, chronic, tubotympanic
  nail(s), anomalous Q84.6
  omphalomesenteric duct Q43.0
  organ or site not listed — *see* Anomaly, by site
  ostium
    atrioventriculare commune Q21.2
    primum Q21.2
    secundum Q21.1
  ovarian rests in fallopian tube Q50.6
  pancreatic tissue in intestinal tract Q43.8
  primary (deciduous)
    teeth K00.6
    vitreous hyperplasia Q14.0
  pupillary membrane Q13.89
  rhesus (Rh) titer — *see* Complication(s), transfusion, incompatibility reaction, Rh (factor)
  right aortic arch Q25.4
  sinus
    urogenitalis
      female Q52.8
      male Q55.8
    venosus with imperfect incorporation in right auricle Q26.8
  thymus (gland) (hyperplasia) E32.0
  thyroglossal duct Q89.2
  thyrolingual duct Q89.2
  truncus arteriosus or communis Q20.0
  tunica vasculosa lentis Q12.2
  umbilical sinus Q64.4
  urachus Q64.4
  vitelline duct Q43.0

Person (with)
  admitted for clinical research, as a control subject (normal comparison) (participant) Z00.6
  awaiting admission to adequate facility elsewhere Z75.1
  concern (normal) about sick person in family Z63.6
  consulting on behalf of another Z71.0
  feigning illness Z76.5
  living (in)
    without
      adequate housing (heating) (space) Z59.1
      housing (permanent) (temporary) Z59.0
      person able to render necessary care Z74.2
      shelter Z59.0
    alone Z60.2
    boarding school Z59.3
    residential institution Z59.3
  on waiting list Z75.1
  sick or handicapped in family Z63.6
Personality (disorder) F60.9
  accentuation of traits (type A pattern) Z73.1
  affective F34.0
  aggressive F60.3
  amoral F60.2
  anacastic, anankastic F60.5
  antisocial F60.2
  anxious F60.6
  asocial F60.2
  asthenic F60.7
  avoidant F60.6
  borderline F60.3
  change due to organic condition (enduring) F07.0
  compulsive F60.5
  cycloid F34.0
  cyclothymic F34.0
  dependent F60.7
  depressive F34.1
  dissocial F60.2
  dual F44.81
  eccentric F60.89
  emotionally unstable F60.3
  expansive paranoid F60.0
  explosive F60.3
  fanatic F60.0
  haltlose type F60.89
  histrionic F60.4
  hyperthymic F34.0
  hypothymic F34.1
  hysterical F60.4
  immature F60.89
  inadequate F60.7
  labile (emotional) F60.3
  mixed (nonspecific) F60.81
  morally defective F60.2
  multiple F44.81
  narcissistic F60.81
  obsessional F60.5
  obsessive (-compulsive) F60.5
  organic F07.0
  overconscientious F60.5
  paranoid F60.0
  passive (-dependent) F60.7
  passive-aggressive F60.89
  pathologic F60.9
  pattern defect or disturbance F60.9
  pseudopsychopathic (organic) F07.0
  pseudoretarded (organic) F07.0
  psychoinfantile F60.4
  psychoneurotic NEC F60.89
  psychopathic F60.2
  querulant F60.0
  sadistic F60.89
  schizoid F60.1
  self-defeating F60.7
  sensitive paranoid F60.0
  sociopathic (amoral) (antisocial) (asocial) (dissocial) F60.2
  specified NEC F60.89
  type A Z73.1
  unstable (emotional) F60.3
Perthes' disease — *see* Legg-Calvé-Perthes disease
Pertussis (*see also* Whooping cough) A37.90
Perversion, perverted
  appetite F50.8
    psychogenic F50.8
  function
    pituitary gland E23.2
      posterior lobe E22.2

Perversion, perverted — *continued*
sense of smell and taste R43.8
psychogenic F45.8
sexual — *see* Deviation, sexual
Pervious, congenital (*see also* Imperfect, closure)
ductus arteriosus Q25.0
Pes (congenital) (*see also* Talipes)
acquired (*see also* Deformity, limb, foot, specified NEC)
planus — *see* Deformity, limb, flat foot
adductus Q66.89
cavus Q66.7
deformity NEC, acquired — *see* Deformity, limb, foot, specified NEC
planus (acquired) (any degree) (*see also* Deformity, limb, flat foot)
rachitic sequelae (late effect) E64.3
valgus Q66.6
Pest, pestis — *see* Plague
Petechia, petechiae R23.3
newborn P54.5
Petechial typhus A75.9
Peter's anomaly Q13.4
Petit mal seizure — *see* Epilepsy, generalized, specified NEC
Petit's hernia — *see* Hernia, abdomen, specified site NEC
Petrellidosis B48.2
Petrositis H70.20- ☑
acute H70.21- ☑
chronic H70.22- ☑
Peutz-Jeghers disease or syndrome Q85.8
Peyronie's disease N48.6
Pfeiffer's disease — *see* Mononucleosis, infectious
Phagedena (dry) (moist) (sloughing) (*see also* Gangrene)
geometric L88
penis N48.29
tropical — *see* Ulcer, skin
vulva N76.6
Phagedenic — *see* condition
Phakoma H35.89
Phakomatosis (*see also* specific eponymous syndromes) Q85.9
Bourneville's Q85.1
specified NEC Q85.8
Phantom limb syndrome (without pain) G54.7
with pain G54.6
Pharyngeal pouch syndrome D82.1
Pharyngitis (acute) (catarrhal) (gangrenous) (infective) (malignant) (membranous) (phlegmonous) (pseudomembranous) (simple) (subacute) (suppurative) (ulcerative) (viral) J02.9
with influenza, flu, or grippe — *see* Influenza, with, pharyngitis
aphthous B08.5
atrophic J31.2
chlamydial A56.4
chronic (atrophic) (granular) (hypertrophic) J31.2
coxsackievirus B08.5
diphtheritic A36.0
enteroviral vesicular B08.5
follicular (chronic) J31.2
fusospirochetal A69.1
gonococcal A54.5
granular (chronic) J31.2
herpesviral B00.2
hypertrophic J31.2
infectional, chronic J31.2
influenzal — *see* Influenza, with, respiratory manifestations NEC
lymphonodular, acute (enteroviral) B08.8
pneumococcal J02.8
purulent J02.9
putrid J02.9
septic J02.0
sicca J31.2
specified organism NEC J02.8
staphylococcal J02.8
streptococcal J02.0
syphilitic, congenital (early) A50.03
tuberculous A15.8
vesicular, enteroviral B08.5
viral NEC J02.8
Pharyngoconjunctivitis, viral B30.2
Pharyngolaryngitis (acute) J06.0
chronic J37.0
Pharyngoplegia J39.2
Pharyngotonsillitis, herpesviral B00.2

Pharyngotracheitis, chronic J42
Pharynx, pharyngeal — *see* condition
Phenomenon
Arthus' — *see* Arthus' phenomenon
jaw-winking Q07.8
lupus erythematosus (LE) cell M32.9
Raynaud's (secondary) I73.00
with gangrene I73.01
vasomotor R55
vasospastic I73.9
vasovagal R55
Wenckebach's I44.1
Phenylketonuria E70.1
classical E70.0
maternal E70.1
Pheochromoblastoma
specified site — *see* Neoplasm, malignant, by site
unspecified site C74.10
Pheochromocytoma
malignant
specified site — *see* Neoplasm, malignant, by site
unspecified site C74.10
specified site — *see* Neoplasm, benign, by site
unspecified site D35.00
Pheohyphomycosis — *see* Chromomycosis
Pheomycosis — *see* Chromomycosis
Phimosis (congenital) (due to infection) N47.1
chancroidal A57
Phlebectasia (*see also* Varix)
congenital Q27.4
Phlebitis (infective) (pyemic) (septic) (suppurative) I80.9
antepartum — *see* Thrombophlebitis, antepartum
blue — *see* Phlebitis, leg, deep
breast, superficial I80.8
cavernous (venous) sinus — *see* Phlebitis, intracranial (venous) sinus
cerebral (venous) sinus — *see* Phlebitis, intracranial (venous) sinus
chest wall, superficial I80.8
cranial (venous) sinus — *see* Phlebitis, intracranial (venous) sinus
deep (vessels) — *see* Phlebitis, leg, deep
due to implanted device — *see* Complications, by site and type, specified NEC
during or resulting from a procedure T81.72 ☑
femoral vein (superficial) I80.1- ☑
femoropopliteal vein I80.0- ☑
gestational — *see* Phlebopathy, gestational
hepatic veins I80.8
iliofemoral — *see* Phlebitis, femoral vein
intracranial (venous) sinus (any) G08
nonpyogenic I67.6
intraspinal venous sinuses and veins G08
nonpyogenic G95.19
lateral (venous) sinus — *see* Phlebitis, intracranial (venous) sinus
leg I80.3
antepartum — *see* Thrombophlebitis, antepartum
deep (vessels) NEC I80.20- ☑
iliac I80.21- ☑
popliteal vein I80.22- ☑
specified vessel NEC I80.29- ☑
tibial vein I80.23- ☑
femoral vein (superficial) I80.1- ☑
superficial (vessels) I80.0- ☑
longitudinal sinus — *see* Phlebitis, intracranial (venous) sinus
lower limb — *see* Phlebitis, leg
migrans, migrating (superficial) I82.1
pelvic
with ectopic or molar pregnancy O08.0
following ectopic or molar pregnancy O08.0
puerperal, postpartum O87.1
popliteal vein — *see* Phlebitis, leg, deep, popliteal
portal (vein) K75.1
postoperative T81.72 ☑
pregnancy — *see* Thrombophlebitis, antepartum
puerperal, postpartum, childbirth O87.0
deep O87.1
pelvic O87.1
superficial O87.0
retina — *see* Vasculitis, retina
saphenous (accessory) (great) (long) (small) — *see* Phlebitis, leg, superficial
sinus (meninges) — *see* Phlebitis, intracranial (venous) sinus
specified site NEC I80.8

Phlebitis — *continued*
syphilitic A52.09
tibial vein — *see* Phlebitis, leg, deep, tibial
ulcerative I80.9
leg — *see* Phlebitis, leg
umbilicus I80.8
uterus (septic) — *see* Endometritis
varicose (leg) (lower limb) — *see* Varix, leg, with, inflammation
Phlebofibrosis I87.8
Phleboliths I87.8
Phlebopathy,
gestational O22.9- ☑
puerperal O87.9
Phlebosclerosis I87.8
Phlebothrombosis (*see also* Thrombosis)
antepartum — *see* Thrombophlebitis, antepartum
pregnancy — *see* Thrombophlebitis, antepartum
puerperal — *see* Thrombophlebitis, puerperal
Phlebotomus fever A93.1
Phlegmasia
alba dolens O87.1
nonpuerperal — *see* Phlebitis, femoral vein
cerulea dolens — *see* Phlebitis, leg, deep
Phlegmon — *see* Abscess
Phlegmonous — *see* condition
Phlyctenulosis (allergic) (keratoconjunctivitis) (nontuberculous) (*see also* Keratoconjunctivitis)
cornea — *see* Keratoconjunctivitis
tuberculous A18.52
Phobia, phobic F40.9
animal F40.218
spiders F40.210
examination F40.298
reaction F40.9
simple F40.298
social F40.10
generalized F40.11
specific (isolated) F40.298
animal F40.218
spiders F40.210
blood F40.230
injection F40.231
injury F40.233
men F40.290
natural environment F40.228
thunderstorms F40.220
situational F40.248
bridges F40.242
closed in spaces F40.240
flying F40.243
heights F40.241
specified focus NEC F40.298
transfusion F40.231
women F40.291
specified NEC F40.8
medical care NEC F40.232
state F40.9
Phocas' disease — *see* Mastopathy, cystic
Phocomelia Q73.1
lower limb — *see* Agenesis, leg, with foot present
upper limb — *see* Agenesis, arm, with hand present
Phoria H50.50
Phosphate-losing tubular disorder N25.0
Phosphatemia E83.39
Phosphaturia E83.39
Photodermatitis (sun) L56.8
chronic L57.8
due to drug L56.8
light other than sun L59.8
Photokeratitis H16.13- ☑
Photophobia H53.14- ☑
Photophthalmia — *see* Photokeratitis
Photopsia H53.19
Photoretinitis — *see* Retinopathy, solar
Photosensitivity, photosensitization (sun) skin L56.8
light other than sun L59.8
Phrenitis — *see* Encephalitis
Phrynoderma (vitamin A deficiency) E50.8
Phthiriasis (pubis) B85.3
with any infestation classifiable to B85.0-B85.2 B85.4
Phthirus infestation — *see* Phthiriasis
Phthisis (*see also* Tuberculosis)
bulbi (infectional) — *see* Disorder, globe, degenerated condition, atrophy
eyeball (due to infection) — *see* Disorder, globe, degenerated condition, atrophy

Phycomycosis — *see* Zygomycosis
Physalopteriasis B81.8
Physical restraint status Z78.1
Phytobezoar T18.9 ☑
  intestine T18.3 ☑
  stomach T18.2 ☑
Pian — *see* Yaws
Pianoma A66.1
Pica F50.8
  in adults F50.8
  infant or child F98.3
Picking, nose F98.8
Pick-Niemann disease — *see* Niemann-Pick disease or
  syndrome
Pick's
  cerebral atrophy G31.01 [F02.80]
   with behavioral disturbance G31.01 [F02.81]
  disease or syndrome (brain) G31.01 [F02.80]
   with behavioral disturbance G31.01 [F02.81]
Pickwickian syndrome E66.2
Piebaldism E70.39
Piedra (beard) (scalp) B36.8
  black B36.3
  white B36.2
Pierre Robin deformity or syndrome Q87.0
Pierson's disease or osteochondrosis M91.0
Pig-bel A05.2
Pigeon
  breast or chest (acquired) M95.4
   congenital Q67.7
   rachitic sequelae (late effect) E64.3
  breeder's disease or lung J67.2
  fancier's disease or lung J67.2
  toe — *see* Deformity, toe, specified NEC
Pigmentation (abnormal) (anomaly) L81.9
  conjunctiva H11.13- ☑
  cornea (anterior) H18.01- ☑
   posterior H18.05- ☑
   stromal H18.06- ☑
  diminished melanin formation NEC L81.6
  iron L81.8
  lids, congenital Q82.8
  limbus corneae — *see* Pigmentation, cornea
  metals L81.8
  optic papilla, congenital Q14.2
  retina, congenital (grouped) (nevoid) Q14.1
  scrotum, congenital Q82.8
  tattoo L81.8
Piles (*see also* Hemorrhoids) K64.9
Pili
  annulati or torti (congenital) Q84.1
  incarnati L73.1
Pill roller hand (intrinsic) — *see* Parkinsonism
Pilomatrixoma — *see* Neoplasm, skin, benign
  malignant — *see* Neoplasm, skin, malignant
Pilonidal — *see* condition
Pimple R23.8
Pinched nerve — *see* Neuropathy, entrapment
Pindborg tumor — *see* Cyst, calcifying odontogenic
Pineal body or gland — *see* condition
Pinealoblastoma C75.3
Pinealoma D44.5
  malignant C75.3
Pineoblastoma C75.3
Pineocytoma D44.5
Pinguecula H11.15- ☑
Pingueculitis H10.81- ☑
Pinhole meatus (*see also* Stricture, urethra) N35.9
Pink
  disease — *see* subcategory T56.1 ☑
  eye — *see* Conjunctivitis, acute, mucopurulent
Pinkus' disease (lichen nitidus) L44.1
Pinpoint
  meatus — *see* Stricture, urethra
  os (uteri) — *see* Stricture, cervix
Pins and needles R20.2
Pinta A67.9
  cardiovascular lesions A67.2
  chancre (primary) A67.0
  erythematous plaques A67.1
  hyperchromic lesions A67.1
  hyperkeratosis A67.1
  lesions A67.9
   cardiovascular A67.2
   hyperchromic A67.1
   intermediate A67.1
   late A67.2

Pinta — *continued*
  lesions — *continued*
   mixed A67.3
   primary A67.0
   skin (achromic) (cicatricial) (dyschromic) A67.2
    hyperchromic A67.1
    mixed (achromic and hyperchromic) A67.3
  papule (primary) A67.0
  skin lesions (achromic) (cicatricial) (dyschromic) A67.2
   hyperchromic A67.1
   mixed (achromic and hyperchromic) A67.3
  vitiligo A67.2
Pintids A67.1
Pinworm (disease) (infection) (infestation) B80
Piroplasmosis B60.0
Pistol wound — *see* Gunshot wound
Pitchers' elbow — *see* Derangement, joint, specified
  type NEC, elbow
Pithecoid pelvis Q74.2
  with disproportion (fetopelvic) O33.0
   causing obstructed labor O65.0
Pithiatism F48.8
Pitted — *see* Pitting
Pitting (*see also* Edema) R60.9
  lip R60.0
  nail L60.8
  teeth K00.4
Pituitary gland — *see* condition
Pituitary-snuff-taker's disease J67.8
Pityriasis (capitis) L21.0
  alba L30.5
  circinata (et maculata) L42
  furfuracea L21.0
  Hebra's L26
  lichenoides L41.0
   chronica L41.1
   et varioliformis (acuta) L41.0
  maculata (et circinata) L30.5
  nigra B36.1
  pilaris, Hebra's L44.0
  rosea L42
  rotunda L44.8
  rubra (Hebra) pilaris L44.0
  simplex L30.5
  specified type NEC L30.5
  streptogenes L30.5
  versicolor (scrotal) B36.0
Placenta, placental — *see* Pregnancy, complicated by
  (care of) (management affected by), specified condition
Placentitis O41.14- ☑
Plagiocephaly Q67.3
Plague A20.9
  abortive A20.8
  ambulatory A20.8
  asymptomatic A20.8
  bubonic A20.0
  cellulocutaneous A20.1
  cutaneobubonic A20.1
  lymphatic gland A20.0
  meningitis A20.3
  pharyngeal A20.8
  pneumonic (primary) (secondary) A20.2
  pulmonary, pulmonic A20.2
  septicemic A20.7
  tonsillar A20.8
   septicemic A20.7
Planning, family
  contraception Z30.9
  procreation Z31.69
Plaque(s)
  artery, arterial — *see* Arteriosclerosis
  calcareous — *see* Calcification
  coronary, lipid rich I25.83
  epicardial I31.8
  erythematous, of pinta A67.1
  Hollenhorst's — *see* Occlusion, artery, retina
  lipid rich, coronary I25.83
  pleural (without asbestos) J92.9
   with asbestos J92.0
  tongue K13.29
Plasmacytoma C90.3- ☑
  extramedullary C90.2- ☑
  medullary C90.0- ☑
  solitary C90.3- ☑
Plasmacytopenia D72.818
Plasmacytosis D72.822
Plaster ulcer — *see* Ulcer, pressure, by site

Plateau iris syndrome (post-iridectomy) (postprocedu-
  ral) (without glaucoma) H21.82
  with glaucoma H40.22- ☑
Platybasia Q75.8
Platyonychia (congenital) Q84.6
  acquired L60.8
Platypelloid pelvis M95.5
  with disproportion (fetopelvic) O33.0
   causing obstructed labor O65.0
  congenital Q74.2
Platyspondylisis Q76.49
Plaut (-Vincent) **disease** (*see also* Vincent's) A69.1
Plethora R23.2
  newborn P61.1
Pleura, pleural — *see* condition
Pleuralgia R07.81
Pleurisy (acute) (adhesive) (chronic) (costal) (diaphragmatic) (double) (dry) (fibrinous) (fibrous) (interlobar)
  (latent) (plastic) (primary) (residual) (sicca) (sterile)
  (subacute) (unresolved) R09.1
  with
   adherent pleura J86.0
   effusion J90
    chylous, chyliform J94.0
    tuberculous (non primary) A15.6
     primary (progressive) A15.7
   tuberculosis — *see* Pleurisy, tuberculous (non pri-
    mary)
  encysted — *see* Pleurisy, with effusion
  exudative — *see* Pleurisy, with effusion
  fibrinopurulent, fibropurulent — *see* Pyothorax
  hemorrhagic — *see* Hemothorax
  pneumococcal J90
  purulent — *see* Pyothorax
  septic — *see* Pyothorax
  serofibrinous — *see* Pleurisy, with effusion
  seropurulent — *see* Pyothorax
  serous — *see* Pleurisy, with effusion
  staphylococcal J86.9
  streptococcal J90
  suppurative — *see* Pyothorax
  traumatic (post) (current) — *see* Injury, intrathoracic,
   pleura
  tuberculous (with effusion) (non primary) A15.6
   primary (progressive) A15.7
Pleuritis sicca — *see* Pleurisy
Pleurobronchopneumonia — *see* Pneumonia, broncho-
Pleurodynia R07.81
  epidemic B33.0
  viral B33.0
Pleuropericarditis (*see also* Pericarditis)
  acute I30.9
Pleuropneumonia (acute) (bilateral) (double) (septic)
  (*see also* Pneumonia) J18.8
  chronic — *see* Fibrosis, lung
Pleuro-pneumonia-like-organism (PPLO), as cause of
  disease classified elsewhere B96.0
Pleurorrhea — *see* Pleurisy, with effusion
Plexitis, brachial G54.0
Plica
  polonica B85.0
  syndrome, knee M67.5- ☑
  tonsil J35.8
Plicated tongue K14.5
Plug
  bronchus NEC J98.09
  meconium (newborn) NEC syndrome P76.0
  mucus — *see* Asphyxia, mucus
Plumbism — *see* subcategory T56.0 ☑
Plummer's disease E05.20
  with thyroid storm E05.21
Plummer-Vinson syndrome D50.1
Pluricarential syndrome of infancy E40
Plus (and minus) **hand** (intrinsic) — *see* Deformity, limb,
  specified type NEC, forearm
Pneumathemia — *see* Air, embolism
Pneumatic hammer (drill) syndrome T75.21 ☑
Pneumatocele (lung) J98.4
  intracranial G93.89
  tension J44.9
Pneumatosis
  cystoides intestinalis K63.89
  intestinalis K63.89
  peritonei K66.8
Pneumaturia R39.89
Pneumoblastoma — *see* Neoplasm, lung, malignant
Pneumocephalus G93.89

☑ **Additional Character Required — Refer to the Tabular List for Character Selection** ▽ **Subterms under main terms may continue to next column or page**

Pneumococcemia A40.3
Pneumococcus, pneumococcal — *see* condition
Pneumoconiosis (due to) (inhalation of) J64
   with tuberculosis (any type in A15) J65
   aluminum J63.0
   asbestos J61
   bagasse, bagassosis J67.1
   bauxite J63.1
   beryllium J63.2
   coal miners' (simple) J60
   coalworkers' (simple) J60
   collier's J60
   cotton dust J66.0
   diatomite (diatomaceous earth) J62.8
   dust
     inorganic NEC J63.6
     lime J62.8
     marble J62.8
     organic NEC J66.8
   fumes or vapors (from silo) J68.9
   graphite J63.3
   grinder's J62.8
   kaolin J62.8
   mica J62.8
   millstone maker's J62.8
   mineral fibers NEC J61
   miner's J60
   moldy hay J67.0
   potter's J62.8
   rheumatoid — *see* Rheumatoid, lung
   sandblaster's J62.8
   silica, silicate NEC J62.8
     with carbon J60
   stonemason's J62.8
   talc (dust) J62.0
Pneumocystis carinii pneumonia B59
Pneumocystis jiroveci (pneumonia) B59
Pneumocystosis (with pneumonia) B59
Pneumohemopericardium I31.2
Pneumohemothorax J94.2
   traumatic S27.2 ☑
Pneumohydropericardium — *see* Pericarditis
Pneumohydrothorax — *see* Hydrothorax
Pneumomediastinum J98.2
   congenital or perinatal P25.2
Pneumomycosis B49 [J99]
Pneumonia (acute) (double) (migratory) (purulent)
   (septic) (unresolved) J18.9
   with
     influenza — *see* Influenza, with, pneumonia
     lung abscess J85.1
       due to specified organism — *see* Pneumonia,
         in (due to)
   adenoviral J12.0
   adynamic J18.2
   alba A50.04
   allergic (eosinophilic) J82
   alveolar — *see* Pneumonia, lobar
   anaerobes J15.8
   anthrax A22.1
   apex, apical — *see* Pneumonia, lobar
   Ascaris B77.81
   aspiration J69.0
     due to
       aspiration of microorganisms
         bacterial J15.9
         viral J12.9
       food (regurgitated) J69.0
       gastric secretions J69.0
       milk (regurgitated) J69.0
       oils, essences J69.1
       solids, liquids NEC J69.8
       vomitus J69.0
     newborn P24.81
       amniotic fluid (clear) P24.11
       blood P24.21
       food (regurgitated) P24.31
       liquor (amnii) P24.11
       meconium P24.01
       milk P24.31
       mucus P24.11
       specified NEC P24.81
       stomach contents P24.31
     postprocedural J95.4
   atypical NEC J18.9
   bacillus J15.9
     specified NEC J15.8

Pneumonia — *continued*
   bacterial J15.9
     specified NEC J15.8
   Bacteroides (fragilis) (oralis) (melaninogenicus) J15.8
   basal, basic, basilar — *see* Pneumonia, by type
   bronchiolitis obliterans organized (BOOP) J84.89
   broncho-, bronchial (confluent) (croupous) (diffuse)
     (disseminated) (hemorrhagic) (involving lobes)
     (lobar) (terminal) J18.0
     allergic (eosinophilic) J82
     aspiration — *see* Pneumonia, aspiration
     bacterial J15.9
       specified NEC J15.8
     chronic — *see* Fibrosis, lung
     diplococcal J13
     Eaton's agent J15.7
     Escherichia coli (E. coli) J15.5
     Friedländer's bacillus J15.0
     Hemophilus influenzae J14
     hypostatic J18.2
     inhalation (*see also* Pneumonia, aspiration)
       due to fumes or vapors (chemical) J68.0
       of oils or essences J69.1
     Klebsiella (pneumoniae) J15.0
     lipid, lipoid J69.1
       endogenous J84.89
     Mycoplasma (pneumoniae) J15.7
     pleuro-pneumonia-like-organisms (PPLO) J15.7
     pneumococcal J13
     Proteus J15.6
     Pseudomonas J15.1
     Serratia marcescens J15.6
     specified organism NEC J16.8
     staphylococcal — *see* Pneumonia, staphylococcal
     streptococcal NEC J15.4
       group B J15.3
       pneumoniae J13
     viral, virus — *see* Pneumonia, viral
   Butyrivibrio (fibriosolvens) J15.8
   Candida B37.1
   caseous — *see* Tuberculosis, pulmonary
   catarrhal — *see* Pneumonia, broncho
   chlamydial J16.0
     congenital P23.1
   cholesterol J84.89
   cirrhotic (chronic) — *see* Fibrosis, lung
   Clostridium (haemolyticum) (novyi) J15.8
   confluent — *see* Pneumonia, broncho
   congenital (infective) P23.9
     due to
       bacterium NEC P23.6
       Chlamydia P23.1
       Escherichia coli P23.4
       Haemophilus influenzae P23.6
       infective organism NEC P23.8
       Klebsiella pneumoniae P23.6
       Mycoplasma P23.6
       Pseudomonas P23.5
       Staphylococcus P23.2
       Streptococcus (except group B) P23.6
         group B P23.3
       viral agent P23.0
     specified NEC P23.8
   croupous — *see* Pneumonia, lobar
   cryptogenic organizing J84.116
   cytomegalic inclusion B25.0
   cytomegaloviral B25.0
   deglutition — *see* Pneumonia, aspiration
   desquamative interstitial J84.117
   diffuse — *see* Pneumonia, broncho
   diplococcal, diplococcus (broncho-) (lobar) J13
   disseminated (focal) — *see* Pneumonia, broncho
   Eaton's agent J15.7
   embolic, embolism — *see* Embolism, pulmonary
   Enterobacter J15.6
   eosinophilic J82
   Escherichia coli (E. coli) J15.5
   Eubacterium J15.8
   fibrinous — *see* Pneumonia, lobar
   fibroid, fibrous (chronic) — *see* Fibrosis, lung
   Friedländer's bacillus J15.0
   Fusobacterium (nucleatum) J15.8
   gangrenous J85.0
   giant cell (measles) B05.2
   gonococcal A54.84
   gram-negative bacteria NEC J15.6
     anaerobic J15.8
   Hemophilus influenzae (broncho) (lobar) J14

Pneumonia — *continued*
   human metapneumovirus J12.3
   hypostatic (broncho) (lobar) J18.2
   in (due to)
     actinomycosis A42.0
     adenovirus J12.0
     anthrax A22.1
     ascariasis B77.81
     aspergillosis B44.9
     Bacillus anthracis A22.1
     Bacterium anitratum J15.6
     candidiasis B37.1
     chickenpox B01.2
     Chlamydia J16.0
       neonatal P23.1
     coccidioidomycosis B38.2
       acute B38.0
       chronic B38.1
     cytomegalovirus disease B25.0
     Diplococcus (pneumoniae) J13
     Eaton's agent J15.7
     Enterobacter J15.6
     Escherichia coli (E. coli) J15.5
     Friedländer's bacillus J15.0
     fumes and vapors (chemical) (inhalation) J68.0
     gonorrhea A54.84
     Hemophilus influenzae (H. influenzae) J14
     Herellea J15.6
     histoplasmosis B39.2
       acute B39.0
       chronic B39.1
     human metapneumovirus J12.3
     Klebsiella (pneumoniae) J15.0
     measles B05.2
     Mycoplasma (pneumoniae) J15.7
     nocardiosis, nocardiasis A43.0
     ornithosis A70
     parainfluenza virus J12.2
     pleuro-pneumonia-like-organism (PPLO) J15.7
     pneumococcal J13
     pneumocystosis (Pneumocystis carinii) (Pneumo-
       cystis jiroveci) B59
     Proteus J15.6
     Pseudomonas NEC J15.1
       pseudomallei A24.1
     psittacosis A70
     Q fever A78
     respiratory syncytial virus J12.1
     rheumatic fever I00 [J17]
     rubella B06.81
     Salmonella (infection) A02.22
       typhi A01.03
     schistosomiasis B65.9 [J17]
     Serratia marcescens J15.6
     specified
       bacterium NEC J15.8
       organism NEC J16.8
     spirochetal NEC A69.8
     Staphylococcus J15.20
       aureus (methicillin susceptible) (MSSA) J15.211
         methicillin resistant (MRSA) J15.212
       specified NEC J15.29
     Streptococcus J15.4
       group B J15.3
       pneumoniae J13
       specified NEC J15.4
     toxoplasmosis B58.3
     tularemia A21.2
     typhoid (fever) A01.03
     varicella B01.2
     virus — *see* Pneumonia, viral
     whooping cough A37.91
       due to
         Bordetella parapertussis A37.11
         Bordetella pertussis A37.01
         specified NEC A37.81
     Yersinia pestis A20.2
   inhalation of food or vomit — *see* Pneumonia, aspira-
     tion
   interstitial J84.9
     chronic J84.111
     desquamative J84.117
     due to
       collagen vascular disease J84.17
       known underlying cause J84.17
     idiopathic NOS J84.111
     in disease classified elsewhere J84.17

Pneumonia — *continued*
 interstitial — *continued*
  lymphocytic (due to collagen vascular disease) (in diseases classified elsewhere) J84.17
  lymphoid J84.2
  non-specific J84.89
   due to
    collagen vascular disease J84.17
    known underlying cause J84.17
   idiopathic J84.113
   in diseases classified elsewhere J84.17
  plasma cell B59
  pseudomonas J15.1
  usual J84.112
   due to collagen vascular disease J84.17
   idiopathic J84.112
   in diseases classified elsewhere J84.17
 Klebsiella (pneumoniae) J15.0
 lipid, lipoid (exogenous) J69.1
  endogenous J84.89
 lobar (disseminated) (double) (interstitial) J18.1
  bacterial J15.9
   specified NEC J15.8
  chronic — *see* Fibrosis, lung
  Escherichia coli (E. coli) J15.5
  Friedländer's bacillus J15.0
  Hemophilus influenzae J14
  hypostatic J18.2
  Klebsiella (pneumoniae) J15.0
  pneumococcal J13
  Proteus J15.6
  Pseudomonas J15.1
  specified organism NEC J16.8
  staphylococcal — *see* Pneumonia, staphylococcal
  streptococcal NEC J15.4
  Streptococcus pneumoniae J13
  viral, virus — *see* Pneumonia, viral
 lobular — *see* Pneumonia, broncho
 Löffler's J82
 lymphoid interstitial J84.2
 massive — *see* Pneumonia, lobar
 meconium P24.01
 MSSA (methicillin susceptible Staphylococcus aureus) J15.211
 multilobar — *see* Pneumonia, by type
 Mycoplasma (pneumoniae) J15.7
 necrotic J85.0
 neonatal P23.9
  aspiration — *see* Aspiration, by substance, with pneumonia
 nitrogen dioxide J68.9
 organizing J84.89
  due to
   collagen vascular disease J84.17
   known underlying cause J84.17
   in diseases classified elsewhere J84.17
 orthostatic J18.2
 parainfluenza virus J12.2
 parenchymatous — *see* Fibrosis, lung
 passive J18.2
 patchy — *see* Pneumonia, broncho
 Peptococcus J15.8
 Peptostreptococcus J15.8
 plasma cell (of infants) B59
 pleurolobar — *see* Pneumonia, lobar
 pleuro-pneumonia-like organism (PPLO) J15.7
 pneumococcal (broncho) (lobar) J13
 Pneumocystis (carinii) (jiroveci) B59
 postinfectional NEC B99 ☑ [J17]
 postmeasles B05.2
 Proteus J15.6
 Pseudomonas J15.1
 psittacosis A70
 radiation J70.0
 respiratory syncytial virus J12.1
 resulting from a procedure J95.89
 rheumatic I00 [J17]
 Salmonella (arizonae) (cholerae-suis) (enteritidis) (typhimurium) A02.22
  typhi A01.03
  typhoid fever A01.03
 SARS-associated coronavirus J12.81
 segmented, segmental — *see* Pneumonia, broncho-
 Serratia marcescens J15.6
 specified NEC J18.8
  bacterium NEC J15.8
  organism NEC J16.8
  virus NEC J12.89

Pneumonia — *continued*
 spirochetal NEC A69.8
 staphylococcal (broncho) (lobar) J15.20
  aureus (methicillin susceptible) (MSSA) J15.211
   methicillin resistant (MRSA) J15.212
  specified NEC J15.29
 static, stasis J18.2
 streptococcal NEC (broncho) (lobar) J15.4
  group
   A J15.4
   B J15.3
   specified NEC J15.4
 Streptococcus pneumoniae J13
 syphilitic, congenital (early) A50.04
 traumatic (complication) (early) (secondary) T79.8 ☑
 tuberculous (any) — *see* Tuberculosis, pulmonary
 tularemic A21.2
 varicella B01.2
 Veillonella J15.8
 ventilator associated J95.851
 viral, virus (broncho) (interstitial) (lobar) J12.9
  adenoviral J12.0
  congenital P23.0
  human metapneumovirus J12.3
  parainfluenza J12.2
  respiratory syncytial J12.1
  SARS-associated coronavirus J12.81
  specified NEC J12.89
 white (congenital) A50.04
Pneumonic — *see* condition
Pneumonitis (acute) (primary) (*see also* Pneumonia)
 air-conditioner J67.7
 allergic (due to) J67.9
  organic dust NEC J67.8
  red cedar dust J67.8
  sequoiosis J67.8
  wood dust J67.8
 aspiration J69.0
  due to
   anesthesia J95.4
    during
     labor and delivery O74.0
     pregnancy O29.01- ☑
     puerperium O89.01
   fumes or gases J68.0
  obstetric O74.0
 chemical (due to gases, fumes or vapors) (inhalation) J68.0
  due to anesthesia J95.4
 cholesterol J84.89
 chronic — *see* Fibrosis, lung
 congenital rubella P35.0
 crack (cocaine) J68.0
 due to
  beryllium J68.0
  cadmium J68.0
  crack (cocaine) J68.0
  detergent J69.8
  fluorocarbon-polymer J68.0
  food, vomit (aspiration) J69.0
  fumes or vapors J68.0
  gases, fumes or vapors (inhalation) J68.0
  inhalation
   blood J69.8
   essences J69.1
   food (regurgitated), milk, vomit J69.0
   oils, essences J69.1
   saliva J69.0
   solids, liquids NEC J69.8
  manganese J68.0
  nitrogen dioxide J68.0
  oils, essences J69.1
  solids, liquids NEC J69.8
  toxoplasmosis (acquired) B58.3
   congenital P37.1
  vanadium J68.0
  ventilator J95.851
 eosinophilic J82
 hypersensitivity J67.9
  air conditioner lung J67.7
  bagassosis J67.1
  bird fancier's lung J67.2
  farmer's lung J67.0
  maltworker's lung J67.4
  maple bark-stripper's lung J67.6
  mushroom worker's lung J67.5
  specified organic dust NEC J67.8
  suberosis J67.3

Pneumonitis — *continued*
 interstitial (chronic) J84.89
  acute J84.114
  lymphoid J84.2
  non-specific J84.89
   idiopathic J84.113
 lymphoid, interstitial J84.2
 meconium P24.01
 postanesthetic J95.4
  correct substance properly administered — *see* Table of Drugs and Chemicals, by drug, adverse effect
  in labor and delivery O74.0
  in pregnancy O29.01- ☑
  obstetric O74.0
  overdose or wrong substance given or taken (by accident) — *see* Table of Drugs and Chemicals, by drug, poisoning
  postpartum, puerperal O89.01
 postoperative J95.4
  obstetric O74.0
 radiation J70.0
 rubella, congenital P35.0
 ventilation (air-conditioning) J67.7
 ventilator associated J95.851
 wood-dust J67.8
Pneumonoconiosis — *see* Pneumoconiosis
Pneumoparotid K11.8
Pneumopathy NEC J98.4
 alveolar J84.09
 due to organic dust NEC J66.8
 parietoalveolar J84.09
Pneumopericarditis (*see also* Pericarditis)
 acute I30.9
Pneumopericardium (*see also* Pericarditis)
 congenital P25.3
 newborn P25.3
 traumatic (post) — *see* Injury, heart
Pneumophagia (psychogenic) F45.8
Pneumopleurisy, pneumopleuritis (*see also* Pneumonia) J18.8
Pneumopyopericardium I30.1
Pneumopyothorax — *see* Pyopneumothorax
 with fistula J86.0
Pneumorrhagia (*see also* Hemorrhage, lung)
 tuberculous — *see* Tuberculosis, pulmonary
Pneumothorax NOS J93.9
 acute J93.83
 chronic J93.81
 congenital P25.1
 perinatal period P25.1
 postprocedural J95.811
 specified NEC J93.83
 spontaneous NOS J93.83
  newborn P25.1
  primary J93.11
  secondary J93.12
  tension J93.0
 tense valvular, infectional J93.0
 tension (spontaneous) J93.0
 traumatic S27.0 ☑
  with hemothorax S27.2 ☑
 tuberculous — *see* Tuberculosis, pulmonary
Podagra (*see also* Gout) M10.9
Podencephalus Q01.9
Poikilocytosis R71.8
Poikiloderma L81.6
 Civatte's L57.3
 congenital Q82.8
 vasculare atrophicans L94.5
Poikilodermatomyositis M33.10
 with
  myopathy M33.12
  respiratory involvement M33.11
  specified organ involvement NEC M33.19
Pointed ear (congenital) Q17.3
Poison ivy, oak, sumac or other plant dermatitis (allergic) (contact) L23.7
Poisoning (acute) (*see also* Table of Drugs and Chemicals)
 algae and toxins T65.82- ☑
 Bacillus B (aertrycke) (cholerae (suis)) (paratyphosus) (suipestifer) A02.9
  botulinus A05.1
 bacterial toxins A05.9
 berries, noxious — *see* Poisoning, food, noxious, berries
 botulism A05.1
 ciguatera fish T61.0- ☑

Poisoning — *continued*
- Clostridium botulinum A05.1
- death-cap (Amanita phalloides) (Amanita verna) — *see* Poisoning, food, noxious, mushrooms
- drug — *see* Table of Drugs and Chemicals, by drug, poisoning
- epidemic, fish (noxious) — *see* Poisoning, seafood
  - bacterial A05.9
- fava bean D55.0
- fish (noxious) T61.9- ☑
  - bacterial — *see* Intoxication, foodborne, by agent
  - ciguatera fish — *see* Poisoning, ciguatera fish
  - scombroid fish — *see* Poisoning, scombroid fish
  - specified type NEC T61.77- ☑
- food (acute) (diseased) (infected) (noxious) NEC T62.9- ☑
  - bacterial — *see* Intoxication, foodborne, by agent
  - due to
    - Bacillus (aertrycke) (choleraesuis) (paratyphosus) (suipestifer) A02.9
      - botulinus A05.1
    - Clostridium (perfringens) (Welchii) A05.2
    - salmonella (aertrycke) (callinarum) (choleraesuis) (enteritidis) (paratyphi) (suipestifer) A02.9
      - with
        - gastroenteritis A02.0
        - sepsis A02.1
    - staphylococcus A05.0
    - Vibrio
      - parahaemolyticus A05.3
      - vulnificus A05.5
  - noxious or naturally toxic T62.9- ☑
    - berries — *see* subcategory T62.1 ☑
    - fish — *see* Poisoning, seafood
    - mushrooms — *see* subcategory T62.0X ☑
    - plants NEC — *see* subcategory T62.2X ☑
    - seafood — *see* Poisoning, seafood
    - specified NEC — *see* subcategory T62.8X ☑
- ichthyotoxism — *see* Poisoning, seafood
- kreotoxism, food A05.9
- latex T65.81- ☑
- lead T56.0- ☑
- mushroom — *see* Poisoning, food, noxious, mushroom
- mussels (*see also* Poisoning, shellfish)
  - bacterial — *see* Intoxication, foodborne, by agent
- nicotine (tobacco) T65.2- ☑
- noxious foodstuffs — *see* Poisoning, food, noxious
- plants, noxious — *see* Poisoning, food, noxious, plants NEC
- ptomaine — *see* Poisoning, food
- radiation J70.0
- Salmonella (arizonae) (cholerae-suis) (enteritidis) (typhimurium) A02.9
- scombroid fish T61.1- ☑
- seafood (noxious) T61.9- ☑
  - bacterial — *see* Intoxication, foodborne, by agent
  - fish — *see* Poisoning, fish
  - shellfish — *see* Poisoning, shellfish
  - specified NEC — *see* subcategory T61.8X ☑
- shellfish (amnesic) (azaspiracid) (diarrheic) (neurotoxic) (noxious) (paralytic) T61.78- ☑
  - bacterial — *see* Intoxication, foodborne, by agent
  - ciguatera mollusk — *see* Poisoning, ciguatera fish
- specified substance NEC T65.891 ☑
- Staphylococcus, food A05.0
- tobacco (nicotine) T65.2- ☑
- water E87.79

Poker spine — *see* Spondylitis, ankylosing
Poland syndrome Q79.8
Polioencephalitis (acute) (bulbar) A80.9
- inferior G12.22
- influenzal — *see* Influenza, with, encephalopathy
- superior hemorrhagic (acute) (Wernicke's) E51.2
- Wernicke's E51.2

Polioencephalomyelitis (acute) (anterior) A80.9
- with beriberi E51.2

Polioencephalopathy, superior hemorrhagic E51.2
- with
  - beriberi E51.11
  - pellagra E52

Poliomeningoencephalitis — *see* Meningoencephalitis
Poliomyelitis (acute) (anterior) (epidemic) A80.9
- with paralysis (bulbar) — *see* Poliomyelitis, paralytic
- abortive A80.4
- ascending (progressive) — *see* Poliomyelitis, paralytic
- bulbar (paralytic) — *see* Poliomyelitis, paralytic

Poliomyelitis — *continued*
- congenital P35.8
- nonepidemic A80.9
- nonparalytic A80.4
- paralytic A80.30
  - specified NEC A80.39
  - vaccine-associated A80.0
  - wild virus
    - imported A80.1
    - indigenous A80.2
- spinal, acute A80.9

Poliosis (eyebrow) (eyelashes) L67.1
- circumscripta, acquired L67.1

Pollakiuria R35.0
- psychogenic F45.8

Pollinosis J30.1
Pollitzer's disease L73.2
Polyadenitis (*see also* Lymphadenitis)
- malignant A20.0

Polyalgia M79.89
Polyangiitis M30.0
- microscopic M31.7
- overlap syndrome M30.8

Polyarteritis
- microscopic M31.7
- nodosa M30.0
  - with lung involvement M30.1
  - juvenile M30.2
  - related condition NEC M30.8

Polyarthralgia — *see* Pain, joint
Polyarthritis, polyarthropathy (*see also* Arthritis) M13.0
- due to or associated with other specified conditions — *see* Arthritis
- epidemic (Australian) (with exanthema) B33.1
- infective — *see* Arthritis, pyogenic or pyemic
- inflammatory M06.4
- juvenile (chronic) (seronegative) M08.3
- migratory — *see* Fever, rheumatic
- rheumatic, acute — *see* Fever, rheumatic

Polyarthrosis M15.9
- post-traumatic M15.3
- primary M15.0
- specified NEC M15.8

Polycarential syndrome of infancy E40
Polychondritis (atrophic) (chronic) (*see also* Disorder, cartilage, specified type NEC)
- relapsing M94.1

Polycoria Q13.2
Polycystic (disease)
- degeneration, kidney Q61.3
  - autosomal dominant (adult type) Q61.2
  - autosomal recessive (infantile type) NEC Q61.19
- kidney Q61.3
  - autosomal
    - dominant Q61.2
    - recessive NEC Q61.19
  - autosomal dominant (adult type) Q61.2
  - autosomal recessive (childhood type) NEC Q61.19
  - infantile type NEC Q61.19
- liver Q44.6
- lung J98.4
  - congenital Q33.0
- ovary, ovaries E28.2
- spleen Q89.09

Polycythemia (secondary) D75.1
- acquired D75.1
- benign (familial) D75.0
- due to
  - donor twin P61.1
  - erythropoietin D75.1
  - fall in plasma volume D75.1
  - high altitude D75.1
  - maternal-fetal transfusion P61.1
  - stress D75.1
- emotional D75.1
- erythropoietin D75.1
- familial (benign) D75.0
- Gaisböck's (hypertonica) D75.1
- high altitude D75.1
- hypertonica D75.1
- hypoxemic D75.1
- neonatorum P61.1
- nephrogenous D75.1
- relative D75.1
- secondary D75.1
- spurious D75.1
- stress D75.1
- vera D45

Polycytosis cryptogenica D75.1
Polydactylism, polydactyly Q69.9
- toes Q69.2

Polydipsia R63.1
Polydystrophy, pseudo-Hurler E77.0
Polyembryoma — *see* Neoplasm, malignant, by site
Polyglandular
- deficiency E31.0
- dyscrasia E31.9
- dysfunction E31.9
- syndrome E31.8

Polyhydramnios O40.- ☑
Polymastia Q83.1
Polymenorrhea N92.0
Polymyalgia M35.3
- arteritica, giant cell M31.5
- rheumatica M35.3
  - with giant cell arteritis M31.5

Polymyositis (acute) (chronic) (hemorrhagic) M33.20
- with
  - myopathy M33.22
  - respiratory involvement M33.21
  - skin involvement — *see* Dermatopolymyositis
  - specified organ involvement NEC M33.29
- ossificans (generalisata) (progressiva) — *see* Myositis, ossificans, progressiva

Polyneuritis, polyneuritic (*see also* Polyneuropathy)
- acute (post-)infective G61.0
- alcoholic G62.1
- cranialis G52.7
- demyelinating, chronic inflammatory (CIDP) G61.81
- diabetic — *see* Diabetes, polyneuropathy
- diphtheritic A36.83
- due to lack of vitamin NEC E56.9 [G63]
- endemic E51.11
- erythredema — *see* subcategory T56.1 ☑
- febrile, acute G61.0
- hereditary ataxic G60.1
- idiopathic, acute G61.0
- infective (acute) G61.0
- inflammatory, chronic demyelinating (CIDP) G61.81
- nutritional E63.9 [G63]
- postinfective (acute) G61.0
- specified NEC G62.89

Polyneuropathy (peripheral) G62.9
- alcoholic G62.1
- amyloid (Portuguese) E85.1 [G63]
- arsenical G62.2
- critical illness G62.81
- demyelinating, chronic inflammatory (CIDP) G61.81
- diabetic — *see* Diabetes, polyneuropathy
- drug-induced G62.0
- hereditary G60.9
  - specified NEC G60.8
- idiopathic G60.9
  - progressive G60.3
- in (due to)
  - alcohol G62.1
    - sequelae G65.2
  - amyloidosis, familial (Portuguese) E85.1 [G63]
  - antitetanus serum G61.1
  - arsenic G62.2
    - sequelae G65.2
  - avitaminosis NEC E56.9 [G63]
  - beriberi E51.11
  - collagen vascular disease NEC M35.9 [G63]
  - deficiency (of)
    - B (-complex) vitamins E53.9 [G63]
    - vitamin B6 E53.1 [G63]
  - diabetes — *see* Diabetes, polyneuropathy
  - diphtheria A36.83
  - drug or medicament G62.0
    - correct substance properly administered — *see* Table of Drugs and Chemicals, by drug, adverse effect
    - overdose or wrong substance given or taken — *see* Table of Drugs and Chemicals, by drug, poisoning
  - endocrine disease NEC E34.9 [G63]
  - herpes zoster B02.23
  - hypoglycemia E16.2 [G63]
  - infectious
    - disease NEC B99 ☑ [G63]
    - mononucleosis B27.91
  - lack of vitamin NEC E56.9 [G63]
  - lead G62.2
    - sequelae G65.2
  - leprosy A30.9 [G63]

▽ Subterms under main terms may continue to next column or page   ☑ Additional Character Required — Refer to the Tabular List for Character Selection   **249**

Poisoning — Polyneuropathy

Polyneuropathy — continued
  in — continued
    Lyme disease A69.22
    metabolic disease NEC E88.9 [G63]
    microscopic polyangiitis M31.7 [G63]
    mumps B26.84
    neoplastic disease (see also Neoplasm) D49.9 [G63]
    nutritional deficiency NEC E63.9 [G63]
    organophosphate compounds G62.2
      sequelae G65.2
    parasitic disease NEC B89 [G63]
    pellagra E52 [G63]
    polyarteritis nodosa M30.0
    porphyria E80.20 [G63]
    radiation G62.82
    rheumatoid arthritis — see Rheumatoid, polyneu-
      ropathy
    sarcoidosis D86.89
    serum G61.1
    syphilis (late) A52.15
      congenital A50.43
    systemic
      connective tissue disorder M35.9 [G63]
      lupus erythematosus M32.19
    toxic agent NEC G62.2
      sequelae G65.2
    triorthocresyl phosphate G62.2
      sequelae G65.2
    tuberculosis A17.89
    uremia N18.9 [G63]
    vitamin B12 deficiency E53.8 [G63]
      with anemia (pernicious) D51.0 [G63]
        due to dietary deficiency D51.3 [G63]
    zoster B02.23
  inflammatory G61.9
    chronic demyelinating (CIDP) G61.81
    sequelae G65.1
    specified NEC G61.89
  lead G62.2
    sequelae G65.2
  nutritional NEC E63.9 [G63]
  postherpetic (zoster) B02.23
  progressive G60.3
  radiation-induced G62.82
  sensory (hereditary) (idiopathic) G60.8
  specified NEC G62.89
  syphilitic (late) A52.15
    congenital A50.43
Polyopia H53.8
Polyorchism, polyorchidism Q55.21
Polyosteoarthritis (see also Osteoarthritis, generalized)
    M15.9
  post-traumatic M15.3
  specified NEC M15.8
Polyostotic fibrous dysplasia Q78.1
Polyotia Q17.0
Polyp, polypus
  accessory sinus J33.8
  adenocarcinoma in — see Neoplasm, malignant, by
    site
  adenocarcinoma in situ in — see Neoplasm, in situ, by
    site
  adenoid tissue J33.0
  adenomatous (see also Neoplasm, benign, by site)
    adenocarcinoma in — see Neoplasm, malignant,
      by site
    adenocarcinoma in situ in — see Neoplasm, in situ,
      by site
    carcinoma in — see Neoplasm, malignant, by site
    carcinoma in situ in — see Neoplasm, in situ, by
      site
    multiple — see Neoplasm, benign
      adenocarcinoma in — see Neoplasm, malig-
        nant, by site
      adenocarcinoma in situ in — see Neoplasm, in
        situ, by site
  antrum J33.8
  anus, anal (canal) K62.0
  Bartholin's gland N84.3
  bladder D41.4
  carcinoma in — see Neoplasm, malignant, by site
  carcinoma in situ in — see Neoplasm, in situ, by site
  cecum D12.0
  cervix (uteri) N84.1
    in pregnancy or childbirth — see Pregnancy,
      complicated by, abnormal, cervix
    mucous N84.1
    nonneoplastic N84.1

Polyp, polypus — continued
  choanal J33.0
  cholesterol K82.4
  clitoris N84.3
  colon K63.5
    adenomatous D12.6
    ascending D12.2
    cecum D12.0
    descending D12.4
    inflammatory K51.40
      with
        abscess K51.414
        complication K51.419
          specified NEC K51.418
        fistula K51.413
        intestinal obstruction K51.412
        rectal bleeding K51.411
    sigmoid D12.5
    transverse D12.3
  corpus uteri N84.0
  dental K04.0
  duodenum K31.7
  ear (middle) H74.4- ☑
  endometrium N84.0
  ethmoidal (sinus) J33.8
  fallopian tube N84.8
  female genital tract N84.9
    specified NEC N84.8
  frontal (sinus) J33.8
  gallbladder K82.4
  gingiva, gum K06.8
  labia, labium (majus) (minus) N84.3
  larynx (mucous) J38.1
    adenomatous D14.1
  malignant — see Neoplasm, malignant, by site
  maxillary (sinus) J33.8
  middle ear — see Polyp, ear (middle)
  myometrium N84.0
  nares
    anterior J33.9
    posterior J33.9
  nasal (mucous) J33.9
    cavity J33.0
    septum J33.0
  nasopharyngeal J33.0
  nose (mucous) J33.9
  oviduct N84.8
  pharynx J39.2
  placenta O90.89
  prostate — see Enlargement, enlarged, prostate
  pudenda, pudendum N84.3
  pulpal (dental) K04.0
  rectum (nonadenomatous) K62.1
    adenomatous — see Polyp, adenomatous
  septum (nasal) J33.0
  sinus (accessory) (ethmoidal) (frontal) (maxillary)
    (sphenoidal) J33.8
  sphenoidal (sinus) J33.8
  stomach K31.7
    adenomatous D13.1
  tube, fallopian N84.8
  turbinate, mucous membrane J33.8
  umbilical, newborn P83.6
  ureter N28.89
  urethra N36.2
  uterus (body) (corpus) (mucous) N84.0
    cervix N84.1
    in pregnancy or childbirth — see Pregnancy,
      complicated by, tumor, uterus
  vagina N84.2
  vocal cord (mucous) J38.1
  vulva N84.3
Polyphagia R63.2
Polyploidy Q92.7
Polypoid — see condition
Polyposis (see also Polyp)
  coli (adenomatous) D12.6
    adenocarcinoma in C18.9
    adenocarcinoma in situ in — see Neoplasm, in situ,
      by site
    carcinoma in C18.9
  colon (adenomatous) D12.6
  familial D12.6
    adenocarcinoma in situ in — see Neoplasm, in situ,
      by site
  intestinal (adenomatous) D12.6
  malignant lymphomatous C83.1- ☑

Polyposis — continued
  multiple, adenomatous (see also Neoplasm, benign)
    D36.9
Polyradiculitis — see Polyneuropathy
Polyradiculoneuropathy (acute) (postinfective) (seg-
    mentally demyelinating) G61.0
Polyserositis
  due to pericarditis I31.1
  pericardial I31.1
  periodic, familial E85.0
  tuberculous A19.9
    acute A19.1
    chronic A19.8
Polysplenia syndrome Q89.09
Polysyndactyly (see also Syndactylism, syndactyly) Q70.4
Polytrichia L68.3
Polyunguia Q84.6
Polyuria R35.8
  nocturnal R35.1
  psychogenic F45.8
Pompe's disease (glycogen storage) E74.02
Pompholyx L30.1
Poncet's disease (tuberculous rheumatism) A18.09
Pond fracture — see Fracture, skull
Ponos B55.0
Pons, pontine — see condition
Poor
  aesthetic of existing restoration of tooth K08.56
  contractions, labor O62.2
  gingival margin to tooth restoration K08.51
  personal hygiene R46.0
  prenatal care, affecting management of pregnancy
    — see Pregnancy, complicated by, insufficient,
    prenatal care
  sucking reflex (newborn) R29.2
  urinary stream R39.12
  vision NEC H54.7
Poradenitis, nostras inguinalis or venerea A55
Porencephaly (congenital) (developmental) (true) Q04.6
  acquired G93.0
  nondevelopmental G93.0
  traumatic (post) F07.89
Porocephaliasis B88.8
Porokeratosis Q82.8
Poroma, eccrine — see Neoplasm, skin, benign
Porphyria (South African) E80.20
  acquired E80.20
  acute intermittent (hepatic) (Swedish) E80.21
  cutanea tarda (hereditary) (symptomatic) E80.1
  due to drugs E80.20
    correct substance properly administered — see
      Table of Drugs and Chemicals, by drug, ad-
      verse effect
    overdose or wrong substance given or taken —
      see Table of Drugs and Chemicals, by drug,
      poisoning
  erythropoietic (congenital) (hereditary) E80.0
  hepatocutaneous type E80.1
  secondary E80.20
  toxic NEC E80.20
  variegata E80.20
Porphyrinuria — see Porphyria
Porphyruria — see Porphyria
Port wine nevus, mark, or stain Q82.5
Portal — see condition
Posadas-Wernicke disease B38.9
Positive
  culture (nonspecific)
    blood R78.81
    bronchial washings R84.5
    cerebrospinal fluid R83.5
    cervix uteri R87.5
    nasal secretions R84.5
    nipple discharge R89.5
    nose R84.5
      staphylococcus (Methicillin susceptible) Z22.321
        Methicillin resistant Z22.322
    peritoneal fluid R85.5
    pleural fluid R84.5
    prostatic secretions R86.5
    saliva R85.5
    seminal fluid R86.5
    sputum R84.5
    synovial fluid R89.5
    throat scrapings R84.5
    urine R82.7
    vagina R87.5
    vulva R87.5

☑ **Additional Character Required** — Refer to the Tabular List for Character Selection   ▽ Subterms under main terms may continue to next column or page

Positive — *continued*
  culture — *continued*
    wound secretions R89.5
    PPD (skin test) R76.11
    serology for syphilis A53.0
      with signs or symptoms — *code as* Syphilis, by site and stage
      false R76.8
    skin test, tuberculin (without active tuberculosis) R76.11
    test, human immunodeficiency virus (HIV) R75
    VDRL A53.0
      with signs or symptoms — *code by* site and stage under Syphilis A53.9
    Wassermann reaction A53.0
Postcardiotomy syndrome I97.0
Postcaval ureter Q62.62
Postcholecystectomy syndrome K91.5
Postclimacteric bleeding N95.0
Postcommissurotomy syndrome I97.0
Postconcussional syndrome F07.81
Postcontusional syndrome F07.81
Postcricoid region — *see* condition
Post-dates (40-42 weeks) (pregnancy) (mother) O48.0
  more than 42 weeks gestation O48.1
Postencephalitic syndrome F07.89
Posterior — *see* condition
Posterolateral sclerosis (spinal cord) — *see* Degeneration, combined
Postexanthematous — *see* condition
Postfebrile — *see* condition
Postgastrectomy dumping syndrome K91.1
Posthemiplegic chorea — *see* Monoplegia
Posthemorrhagic anemia (chronic) D50.0
  acute D62
  newborn P61.3
Postherpetic neuralgia (zoster) B02.29
  trigeminal B02.22
Posthitis N47.7
Postimmunization complication or reaction — *see* Complications, vaccination
Postinfectious — *see* condition
Postlaminectomy syndrome NEC M96.1
Postleukotomy syndrome F07.0
Postmastectomy lymphedema (syndrome) I97.2
Postmaturity, postmature (over 42 weeks)
  maternal (over 42 weeks gestation) O48.1
  newborn P08.22
Postmeasles complication NEC (*see also* condition) B05.89
Postmenopausal
  endometrium (atrophic) N95.8
    suppurative (*see also* Endometritis) N71.9
  osteoporosis — *see* Osteoporosis, postmenopausal
Postnasal drip R09.82
  due to
    allergic rhinitis — *see* Rhinitis, allergic
    common cold J00
    gastroesophageal reflux — *see* Reflux, gastroesophageal
    nasopharyngitis — *see* Nasopharyngitis
    other known condition — *code to* condition
    sinusitis — *see* Sinusitis
Postnatal — *see* condition
Postoperative (postprocedural) — *see* Complication, postoperative
  pneumothorax, therapeutic Z98.3
  state NEC Z98.89
Postpancreatectomy hyperglycemia E89.1
Postpartum — *see* Puerperal
Postphlebitic syndrome — *see* Syndrome, postthrombotic
Postpolio (myelitic) **syndrome** G14
Postpoliomyelitic (*see also* condition)
  osteopathy — *see* Osteopathy, after poliomyelitis
Postprocedural (*see also* Postoperative)
  hypoinsulinemia E89.1
Postschizophrenic depression F32.8
Postsurgery status (*see also* Status (post))
  pneumothorax, therapeutic Z98.3
Post-term (40-42 weeks) (pregnancy) (mother) O48.0
  infant P08.21
  more than 42 weeks gestation (mother) O48.1
Post-traumatic brain syndrome, nonpsychotic F07.81
Post-typhoid abscess A01.09
Postures, hysterical F44.2

Postvaccinal reaction or complication — *see* Complications, vaccination
Postvalvulotomy syndrome I97.0
Potain's
  disease (pulmonary edema) — *see* Edema, lung
  syndrome (gastrectasis with dyspepsia) K31.0
Potter's
  asthma J62.8
  facies Q60.6
  lung J62.8
  syndrome (with renal agenesis) Q60.6
Pott's
  curvature (spinal) A18.01
  disease or paraplegia A18.01
  spinal curvature A18.01
  tumor, puffy — *see* Osteomyelitis, specified type NEC
Pouch
  bronchus Q32.4
  Douglas' — *see* condition
  esophagus, esophageal, congenital Q39.6
    acquired K22.5
  gastric K31.4
  Hartmann's K82.8
  pharynx, pharyngeal (congenital) Q38.7
Pouchitis K91.850
Poultrymen's itch B88.0
Poverty NEC Z59.6
  extreme Z59.5
Poxvirus NEC B08.8
Prader-Willi syndrome Q87.1
Preauricular appendage or tag Q17.0
Prebetalipoproteinemia (acquired) (essential) (familial) (hereditary) (primary) (secondary) E78.1
  with chylomicronemia E78.3
Precipitate labor or delivery O62.3
Preclimacteric bleeding (menorrhagia) N92.4
Precocious
  adrenarche E30.1
  menarche E30.1
  menstruation E30.1
  pubarche E30.1
  puberty E30.1
    central E22.8
  sexual development NEC E30.1
  thelarche E30.8
Precocity, sexual (constitutional) (cryptogenic) (female) (idiopathic) (male) E30.1
  with adrenal hyperplasia E25.9
    congenital E25.0
Precordial pain R07.2
Predeciduous teeth K00.2
Prediabetes, prediabetic R73.09
  complicating
    pregnancy — *see* Pregnancy, complicated by, diseases of, specified type or system NEC
    puerperium O99.89
Predislocation status of hip at birth Q65.6
Pre-eclampsia O14.9- ☑
  with pre-existing hypertension — *see* Hypertension, complicating pregnancy, pre-existing, with, preeclampsia
  mild O14.0- ☑
  moderate O14.0- ☑
  severe O14.1- ☑
    with hemolysis, elevated liver enzymes and low platelet count (HELLP) O14.2- ☑
Pre-eruptive color change, teeth, tooth K00.8
Pre-excitation atrioventricular conduction I45.6
Preglaucoma H40.00- ☑
Pregnancy (single) (uterine) (*see also* Delivery and Puerperal)

> *Note: The Tabular must be reviewed for assignment of appropriate seventh character for multiple gestation codes in Chapter 15*

> *Note: The Tabular must be reviewed for assignment of the appropriate character indicating the trimester of the pregnancy*

  abdominal (ectopic) O00.0
    with viable fetus O36.7- ☑
  ampullar O00.1
  biochemical O02.81
  broad ligament O00.8
  cervical O00.8
  chemical O02.81

Pregnancy — *continued*
  complicated by (care of) (management affected by)
    abnormal, abnormality
      cervix O34.4- ☑
        causing obstructed labor O65.5
      cord (umbilical) O69.9 ☑
      findings on antenatal screening of mother O28.9
        biochemical O28.1
        chromosomal O28.5
        cytological O28.2
        genetic O28.5
        hematological O28.0
        radiological O28.4
        specified NEC O28.8
        ultrasonic O28.3
      glucose (tolerance) NEC O99.810
      pelvic organs O34.9- ☑
        specified NEC O34.8- ☑
          causing obstructed labor O65.5
      pelvis (bony) (major) NEC O33.0
      perineum O34.7- ☑
      position
        placenta O44.1- ☑
          without hemorrhage O44.0- ☑
        uterus O34.59- ☑
      uterus O34.59- ☑
        causing obstructed labor O65.5
        congenital O34.0- ☑
      vagina O34.6- ☑
        causing obstructed labor O65.5
      vulva O34.7- ☑
        causing obstructed labor O65.5
    abruptio placentae — *see* Abruptio placentae
    abscess or cellulitis
      bladder O23.1- ☑
      breast O91.11- ☑
      genital organ or tract O23.9- ☑
    abuse
      physical O9A.31 ☑ (*following* O99)
      psychological O9A.51 ☑ (*following* O99)
      sexual O9A.41 ☑ (*following* O99)
    adverse effect anesthesia O29.9- ☑
      aspiration pneumonitis O29.01- ☑
      cardiac arrest O29.11- ☑
      cardiac complication NEC O29.19- ☑
      cardiac failure O29.12- ☑
      central nervous system complication NEC O29.29- ☑
      cerebral anoxia O29.21- ☑
      failed or difficult intubation O29.6- ☑
      inhalation of stomach contents or secretions NOS O29.01- ☑
      local, toxic reaction O29.3X ☑
      Mendelson's syndrome O29.01- ☑
      pressure collapse of lung O29.02- ☑
      pulmonary complications NEC O29.09- ☑
      specified NEC O29.8X- ☑
      spinal and epidural type NEC O29.5X ☑
        induced headache O29.4- ☑
    albuminuria O12.1- ☑
    alcohol use O99.31- ☑
    amnionitis O41.12- ☑
    anaphylactoid syndrome of pregnancy O88.01- ☑
    anemia (conditions in D50-D64) (pre-existing) O99.01- ☑
      complicating the puerperium O99.03
    antepartum hemorrhage O46.9- ☑
      with coagulation defect — *see* Hemorrhage, antepartum, with coagulation defect
      specified NEC O46.8X- ☑
    appendicitis O99.61- ☑
    atrophy (yellow) (acute) liver (subacute) O26.61- ☑
    bariatric surgery status O99.84- ☑
    bicornis or bicornuate uterus O34.59- ☑
    biliary tract problems O26.61- ☑
    breech presentation O32.1 ☑
    cardiovascular diseases (conditions in I00-I09, I20-I52, I70-I99) O99.41- ☑
    cerebrovascular disorders (conditions in I60-I69) O99.41- ☑
    cervical shortening O26.87- ☑
    cervicitis O23.51- ☑
    chloasma (gravidarum) O26.89- ☑
    cholecystitis O99.61- ☑
    cholestasis (intrahepatic) O26.61- ☑

Pregnancy — *continued*
  complicated by — *continued*
    chorioamnionitis O41.12- ☑
    circulatory system disorder (conditions in I00-I09, I20-I99, O99.41-)
    compound presentation O32.6 ☑
    conjoined twins O30.02- ☑
    connective system disorders (conditions in M00-M99) O99.89
    contracted pelvis (general) O33.1
      inlet O33.2
      outlet O33.3 ☑
    convulsions (eclamptic) (uremic) (*see also* Eclampsia) O15.9
    cracked nipple O92.11- ☑
    cystitis O23.1- ☑
    cystocele O34.8- ☑
    death of fetus (near term) O36.4 ☑
      early pregnancy O02.1
      of one fetus or more in multiple gestation O31.2- ☑
    deciduitis O41.14- ☑
    decreased fetal movement O36.81- ☑
    dental problems O99.61- ☑
    diabetes (mellitus) O24.91- ☑
      gestational (pregnancy induced) — *see* Diabetes, gestational
      pre-existing O24.31- ☑
        specified NEC O24.81- ☑
        type 1 O24.01- ☑
        type 2 O24.11- ☑
    digestive system disorders (conditions in K00-K93) O99.61- ☑
    diseases of — *see* Pregnancy, complicated by, specified body system disease
      biliary tract O26.61- ☑
      blood NEC (conditions in D65-D77) O99.11- ☑
      liver O26.61- ☑
      specified NEC O99.89
    disorders of — *see* Pregnancy, complicated by, specified body system disorder
      amniotic fluid and membranes O41.9- ☑
        specified NEC O41.8X- ☑
      biliary tract O26.61- ☑
      ear and mastoid process (conditions in H60-H95) O99.89
      eye and adnexa (conditions in H00-H59) O99.89
      liver O26.61- ☑
      skin (conditions in L00-L99) O99.71- ☑
      specified NEC O99.89
    displacement, uterus NEC O34.59- ☑
      causing obstructed labor O65.5
    disproportion (due to) O33.9
      fetal deformities NEC O33.7
      generally contracted pelvis O33.1
      hydrocephalic fetus O33.6 ☑
      inlet contraction of pelvis O33.2
      mixed maternal and fetal origin O33.4 ☑
      specified NEC O33.8
    double uterus O34.59- ☑
      causing obstructed labor O65.5
    drug use (conditions in F11-F19) O99.32- ☑
    eclampsia, eclamptic (coma) (convulsions) (delirium) (nephritis) (uremia) (*see also* Eclampsia) O15.- ☑
    ectopic pregnancy — *see* Pregnancy, ectopic
    edema O12.0- ☑
      with
        gestational hypertension, mild (*see also* Preeclampsia) O14.0- ☑
        proteinuria O12.2- ☑
    effusion, amniotic fluid — *see* Pregnancy, complicated by, premature rupture of membranes
    elderly
      multigravida O09.52- ☑
      primigravida O09.51- ☑
    embolism (*see also* Embolism, obstetric, pregnancy) O88.- ☑
    endocrine diseases NEC O99.28- ☑
    endometritis O86.12
    excessive weight gain O26.0- ☑
    exhaustion O26.81- ☑
      during labor and delivery O75.81
    face presentation O32.3 ☑
    failed induction of labor O61.9
      instrumental O61.1
      mechanical O61.1

Pregnancy — *continued*
  complicated by — *continued*
    failed induction of labor — *continued*
      medical O61.0
      specified NEC O61.8
      surgical O61.1
    failed or difficult intubation for anesthesia O29.6- ☑
    false labor (pains) O47.9
      at or after 37 completed weeks of pregnancy O47.1
      before 37 completed weeks of pregnancy O47.0- ☑
    fatigue O26.81- ☑
      during labor and delivery O75.81
    fatty metamorphosis of liver O26.61- ☑
    female genital mutilation O34.8- ☑ [N90.81-] ☑
    fetal (maternal care for)
      abnormality or damage O35.9
        acid-base balance O68
        specified type NEC O35.8 ☑
      acidemia O68
      acidosis O68
      alkalosis O68
      anemia and thrombocytopenia O36.82- ☑
      anencephaly O35.0
      chromosomal abnormality (conditions in Q90-Q99) O35.1 ☑
      conjoined twins O30.02- ☑
      damage from
        amniocentesis O35.7 ☑
        biopsy procedures O35.7 ☑
        drug addiction O35.5 ☑
        hematological investigation O35.7 ☑
        intrauterine contraceptive device O35.7 ☑
        maternal
          alcohol addiction O35.4 ☑
          cytomegalovirus infection O35.3 ☑
          disease NEC O35.8 ☑
          drug addiction O35.5 ☑
          listeriosis O35.8 ☑
          rubella O35.3 ☑
          toxoplasmosis O35.8 ☑
          viral infection O35.3 ☑
        medical procedure NEC O35.7 ☑
        radiation O35.6 ☑
      death (near term) O36.4 ☑
        early pregnancy O02.1
      decreased movement O36.81- ☑
      disproportion due to deformity (fetal) O33.7
      excessive growth (large for dates) O36.6- ☑
      growth retardation O36.59- ☑
        light for dates O36.59- ☑
        small for dates O36.59- ☑
      heart rate irregularity (bradycardia) (decelerations) (tachycardia) O76
      hereditary disease O35.2 ☑
      hydrocephalus O35.0
      intrauterine death O36.4 ☑
      poor growth O36.59- ☑
        light for dates O36.59- ☑
        small for dates O36.59- ☑
      problem O36.9- ☑
        specified NEC O36.89- ☑
      reduction (elective) O31.3- ☑
      selective termination O31.3- ☑
      spina bifida O35.0
      thrombocytopenia O36.82- ☑
    fibroid (tumor) (uterus) O34.1- ☑
    fissure of nipple O92.11- ☑
    gallstones O99.61- ☑
    gastric banding status O99.84- ☑
    gastric bypass status O99.84- ☑
    genital herpes (asymptomatic) (history of) (inactive) O98.51- ☑
    genital tract infection O23.9- ☑
    glomerular diseases (conditions in N00-N07) O26.83- ☑
      with hypertension, pre-existing — *see* Hypertension, complicating, pregnancy, pre-existing, with, renal disease
    gonorrhea O98.21- ☑
    grand multiparity O09.4 ☑
    habitual aborter — *see* Pregnancy, complicated by, recurrent pregnancy loss

Pregnancy — *continued*
  complicated by — *continued*
    HELLP syndrome (hemolysis, elevated liver enzymes and low platelet count) O14.2- ☑
    hemorrhage
      antepartum — *see* Hemorrhage, antepartum
      before 20 completed weeks gestation O20.9
        specified NEC O20.8
        due to premature separation, placenta (*see also* Abruptio placentae) O45.9- ☑
      early O20.9
        specified NEC O20.8
      threatened abortion O20.0
    hemorrhoids O22.4- ☑
    hepatitis (viral) O98.41- ☑
    herniation of uterus O34.59- ☑
    high
      head at term O32.4 ☑
      risk — *see* Supervision (of) (for), high-risk
    history of in utero procedure during previous pregnancy O09.82- ☑
    HIV O98.71- ☑
    human immunodeficiency virus (HIV) disease O98.71- ☑
    hydatidiform mole (*see also* Mole, hydatidiform) O01.9
    hydramnios O40.- ☑
    hydrocephalic fetus (disproportion) O33.6 ☑
    hydrops
      amnii O40.- ☑
      fetalis O36.2- ☑
        associated with isoimmunization (*see also* Pregnancy, complicated by, isoimmunization) O36.11- ☑
    hydrorrhea O42.90
    hyperemesis (gravidarum) (mild) (*see also* Hyperemesis, gravidarum) O21.0
    hypertension — *see* Hypertension, complicating pregnancy
    hypertensive
      heart and renal disease, pre-existing — *see* Hypertension, complicating, pregnancy, pre-existing, with, heart disease, with renal disease
      heart disease, pre-existing — *see* Hypertension, complicating, pregnancy, pre-existing, with, heart disease
      renal disease, pre-existing — *see* Hypertension, complicating, pregnancy, pre-existing, with, renal disease
    hypotension O26.5- ☑
    immune disorders NEC (conditions in D80-D89) O99.11- ☑
    incarceration, uterus O34.51- ☑
    incompetent cervix O34.3- ☑
    inconclusive fetal viability O36.80 ☑
    infection(s) O98.91- ☑
      amniotic fluid or sac O41.10- ☑
      bladder O23.1- ☑
      carrier state NEC O99.830
        streptococcus B O99.820
      genital organ or tract O23.9- ☑
        specified NEC O23.59- ☑
      genitourinary tract O23.9- ☑
      gonorrhea O98.21- ☑
      hepatitis (viral) O98.41- ☑
      HIV O98.71- ☑
      human immunodeficiency virus (HIV) O98.71- ☑
      kidney O23.0- ☑
      nipple O91.01- ☑
      parasitic disease O98.91- ☑
        specified NEC O98.81- ☑
      protozoal disease O98.61- ☑
      sexually transmitted NEC O98.31- ☑
      specified type NEC O98.81- ☑
      syphilis O98.11- ☑
      tuberculosis O98.01- ☑
      urethra O23.2- ☑
      urinary (tract) O23.4- ☑
        specified NEC O23.3- ☑
      viral disease O98.51- ☑
    injury or poisoning (conditions in S00-T88) O9A.21- ☑ (*following* O99)
    due to abuse
      physical O9A.31- ☑ (*following* O99)

Pregnancy — *continued*
  complicated by — *continued*
    injury or poisoning — *continued*
      due to abuse — *continued*
        psychological O9A.51- ☑ (*following* O99)
        sexual O9A.41- ☑ (*following* O99)
    insufficient
      prenatal care O09.3- ☑
      weight gain O26.1- ☑
    insulin resistance O26.89 ☑
    intrauterine fetal death (near term) O36.4 ☑
      early pregnancy O02.1
      multiple gestation (one fetus or more)
        O31.2- ☑
    isoimmunization O36.11- ☑
      anti-A sensitization O36.11- ☑
      anti-B sensitization O36.19- ☑
      Rh O36.09- ☑
        anti-D antibody O36.01- ☑
      specified NEC O36.19- ☑
    laceration of uterus NEC O71.81
    malformation
      placenta, placental (vessel) O43.10- ☑
        specified NEC O43.19- ☑
      uterus (congenital) O34.0- ☑
    malnutrition (conditions in E40-E46) O25.1- ☑
    maternal hypotension syndrome O26.5- ☑
    mental disorders (conditions in F01-F09, F20-F99)
      O99.34-
      alcohol use O99.31- ☑
      drug use O99.32- ☑
      smoking O99.33- ☑
    mentum presentation O32.3
    metabolic disorders O99.28- ☑
    missed
      abortion O02.1
      delivery O36.4 ☑
    multiple gestations O30.9- ☑
      conjoined twins O30.02- ☑
      quadruplet — *see* Pregnancy, quadruplet
      specified complication NEC O31.8X- ☑
      specified number of multiples NEC — *see*
        Pregnancy, multiple (gestation), specified
        NEC
      triplet — *see* Pregnancy, triplet
      twin — *see* Pregnancy, twin
    musculoskeletal condition (conditions is M00-M99)
      O99.89
    necrosis, liver (conditions in K72) O26.61- ☑
    neoplasm
      benign
        cervix O34.4- ☑
        corpus uteri O34.1- ☑
        uterus O34.1- ☑
      malignant O9A.11- ☑ (*following* O99)
    nephropathy NEC O26.83- ☑
    nervous system condition (conditions in G00-G99)
      O99.35-
    nutritional diseases NEC O99.28- ☑
    obesity (pre-existing) O99.21- ☑
    obesity surgery status O99.84- ☑
    oblique lie or presentation O32.2 ☑
    older mother — *see* Pregnancy, complicated by,
      elderly
    oligohydramnios O41.0- ☑
      with premature rupture of membranes (*see also*
        Pregnancy, complicated by, premature
        rupture of membranes) O42.- ☑
    onset (spontaneous) of labor after 37 completed
      weeks of gestation but before 39 completed
      weeks gestation, with delivery by (planned)
      cesarean section O75.82
    oophoritis O23.52- ☑
    overdose, drug (*see also* Table of Drugs and
      Chemicals, by drug, poisoning) O9A.21- ☑
      (*following* O99)
    oversize fetus O33.5 ☑
    papyraceous fetus O31.0- ☑
    pelvic inflammatory disease O99.89
    periodontal disease O99.61- ☑
    peripheral neuritis O26.82- ☑
    peritoneal (pelvic) adhesions O99.89
    phlebitis O22.9- ☑
    phlebopathy O22.9- ☑
    phlebothrombosis (superficial) O22.2- ☑
      deep O22.3- ☑

Pregnancy — *continued*
  complicated by — *continued*
    placenta accreta O43.21- ☑
    placenta increta O43.22- ☑
    placenta percreta O43.23- ☑
    placenta previa O44.1- ☑
      without hemorrhage O44.0- ☑
    placental disorder O43.9- ☑
      specified NEC O43.89- ☑
    placental dysfunction O43.89- ☑
    placental infarction O43.81- ☑
    placental insufficiency O36.51- ☑
    placental transfusion syndromes
      fetomaternal O43.01- ☑
      fetus to fetus O43.02- ☑
      maternofetal O43.01- ☑
    placentitis O41.14- ☑
    pneumonia O99.51- ☑
    poisoning (*see also* Table of Drugs and Chemicals)
      O9A.21 ☑ (*following* O99)
    polyhydramnios O40- ☑
    polymorphic eruption of pregnancy O26.86
    poor obstetric history NEC O09.29- ☑
    postmaturity (post-term) (40 to 42 weeks) O48.0
      more than 42 completed weeks gestation
        (prolonged) O48.1
    pre-eclampsia O14.9- ☑
      mild O14.0- ☑
      moderate O14.0- ☑
      severe O14.1- ☑
        with hemolysis, elevated liver enzymes and
          low platelet count (HELLP) O14.2- ☑
    premature labor — *see* Pregnancy, complicated
      by, preterm labor
    premature rupture of membranes O42.90
      with onset of labor
        after 24 hours O42.10
          after 37 weeks gestation O42.12
          pre-term (before 37 completed weeks
            of gestation) O42.11- ☑
        within 24 hours O42.00
          after 37 weeks gestation O42.02
          pre-term (before 37 completed weeks
            of gestation) O42.01- ☑
      after 37 weeks gestation O42.92
      full-term O42.92
      pre-term (before 37 completed weeks of gesta-
        tion) O42.91- ☑
    premature separation of placenta (*see also* Abrup-
      tio placentae) O45.9- ☑
    presentation, fetal — *see* Delivery, complicated
      by, malposition
    preterm delivery O60.10 ☑
    preterm labor
      with delivery O60.10 ☑
        preterm O60.10 ☑
        term O60.20 ☑
      without delivery O60.00
        second trimester O60.02
        third trimester O60.03
      second trimester
        with preterm delivery
          second trimester O60.12 ☑
          third trimester O60.13 ☑
        with term delivery O60.22 ☑
        without delivery O60.02
      third trimester
        with term delivery O60.23 ☑
        with third trimester preterm delivery
          O60.14 ☑
        without delivery O60.03
    previous history of — *see* Pregnancy, supervision
      of, high-risk
    prolapse, uterus O34.52- ☑
    proteinuria (gestational) O12.1- ☑
      with edema O12.2- ☑
    pruritic urticarial papules and plaques of pregnancy
      (PUPPP) O26.86
    pruritus (neurogenic) O26.89- ☑
    psychosis or psychoneurosis (puerperal) F53
    ptyalism O26.89- ☑
    PUPPP (pruritic urticarial papules and plaques of
      pregnancy) O26.86
    pyelitis O23.0- ☑
    recurrent pregnancy loss O26.2- ☑

Pregnancy — *continued*
  complicated by — *continued*
    renal disease or failure NEC O26.83- ☑
      with secondary hypertension, pre-existing —
        see Hypertension, complicating, pregnan-
        cy, pre-existing, secondary
      hypertensive, pre-existing — *see* Hypertension,
        complicating, pregnancy, pre-existing,
        with, renal disease
    respiratory condition (conditions in J00-J99)
      O99.51- ☑
    retained, retention
      dead ovum O02.0
      intrauterine contraceptive device O26.3- ☑
    retroversion, uterus O34.53- ☑
    Rh immunization, incompatibility or sensitization
      NEC O36.09- ☑
      anti-D antibody O36.01- ☑
    rupture
      amnion (premature) (*see also* Pregnancy, com-
        plicated by, premature rupture of mem-
        branes) O42- ☑
      membranes (premature) (*see also* Pregnancy,
        complicated by, premature rupture of
        membranes) O42- ☑
      uterus (during labor) O71.1
        before onset of labor O71.0- ☑
    salivation (excessive) O26.89- ☑
    salpingitis O23.52- ☑
    salpingo-oophoritis O23.52- ☑
    sepsis (conditions in A40, A41) O98.81- ☑
    size date discrepancy (uterine) O26.84- ☑
    skin condition (conditions in L00-L99) O99.71- ☑
    smoking (tobacco) O99.33- ☑
    social problem O09.7- ☑
    specified condition NEC O26.89- ☑
    spotting O26.85- ☑
    streptococcus B carrier state O99.820
    subluxation of symphysis (pubis) O26.71- ☑
    syphilis (conditions in A50-A53) O98.11- ☑
    threatened
      abortion O20.0
      labor O47.9
        at or after 37 completed weeks of gestation
          O47.1
        before 37 completed weeks of gestation
          O47.0- ☑
    thrombophlebitis (superficial) O22.2- ☑
    thrombosis O22.9- ☑
      cerebral venous O22.5- ☑
      cerebrovenous sinus O22.5- ☑
      deep O22.3- ☑
    torsion of uterus O34.59- ☑
    toxemia O14.9- ☑
    transverse lie or presentation O32.2 ☑
    tuberculosis (conditions in A15-A19) O98.01- ☑
    tumor (benign)
      cervix O34.4- ☑
      malignant O9A.11- ☑ (*following* O99)
      uterus O34.1- ☑
    unstable lie O32.0 ☑
    upper respiratory infection O99.51- ☑
    urethritis O23.2- ☑
    uterine size date discrepancy O26.84- ☑
    vaginitis or vulvitis O23.59- ☑
    varicose veins (lower extremities) O22.0- ☑
      genitals O22.1- ☑
      legs O22.0- ☑
      perineal O22.1- ☑
      vaginal or vulval O22.1- ☑
    venereal disease NEC (conditions in A63.8)
      O98.31- ☑
    venous disorders O22.9- ☑
      specified NEC O22.8X- ☑
    very young mother — *see* Pregnancy, complicated
      by, young mother
    viral diseases (conditions in A80-B09, B25-B34)
      O98.51- ☑
    vomiting O21.9
      due to diseases classified elsewhere O21.8
      hyperemesis gravidarum (mild) (*see also* Hyper-
        emesis, gravidarum) O21.0
      late (occurring after 20 weeks of gestation)
        O21.2
    young mother
      multigravida O09.62- ☑

Pregnancy — *continued*
  complicated by — *continued*
    young mother — *continued*
      primigravida O09.61- ☑
  complicated NOS O26.9- ☑
  concealed O09.3- ☑
  continuing following
    elective fetal reduction of one or more fetus
      O31.3- ☑
    intrauterine death of one or more fetus O31.2- ☑
    spontaneous abortion of one or more fetus
      O31.1- ☑
  cornual O00.8
  ectopic (ruptured) O00.9
    abdominal O00.0
      with viable fetus O36.7- ☑
    cervical O00.8
    complicated (by) O08.9
      afibrinogenemia O08.1
      cardiac arrest O08.81
      chemical damage of pelvic organ(s) O08.6
      circulatory collapse O08.3
      defibrination syndrome O08.1
      electrolyte imbalance O08.5
      embolism (amniotic fluid) (blood clot) (pul-
        monary) (septic) O08.2
      endometritis O08.0
      genital tract and pelvic infection O08.0
      hemorrhage (delayed) (excessive) O08.1
      infection
        genital tract or pelvic O08.0
        kidney O08.83
        urinary tract O08.3
      intravascular coagulation O08.1
      laceration of pelvic organ(s) O08.6
      metabolic disorder O08.5
      oliguria O08.4
      oophoritis O08.0
      parametritis O08.0
      pelvic peritonitis O08.0
      perforation of pelvic organ(s) O08.6
      renal failure or shutdown O08.4
      salpingitis or salpingo-oophoritis O08.0
      sepsis O08.82
      shock O08.83
        septic O08.82
      specified condition NEC O08.89
      tubular necrosis (renal) O08.4
      uremia O08.4
      urinary infection O08.83
      venous complication NEC O08.7
        embolism O08.2
    cornual O00.8
    intraligamentous O00.8
    mural O00.8
    ovarian O00.2
    specified site NEC O00.8
    tubal (ruptured) O00.1
  examination (normal) Z34.9- ☑
    first Z34.0- ☑
    high-risk — *see* Pregnancy, supervision of, high-
      risk
    specified Z34.8- ☑
  extrauterine — *see* Pregnancy, ectopic
  fallopian O00.1
  false F45.8
  hidden O09.3- ☑
  high-risk — *see* Pregnancy, supervision of, high-risk
  incidental finding Z33.1
  interstitial O00.8
  intraligamentous O00.8
  intramural O00.8
  intraperitoneal O00.0
  isthmian O00.1
  mesometric (mural) O00.8
  molar NEC O02.0
    complicated (by) O08.9
      afibrinogenemia O08.1
      cardiac arrest O08.81
      chemical damage of pelvic organ(s) O08.6
      circulatory collapse O08.3
      defibrination syndrome O08.1
      electrolyte imbalance O08.5
      embolism (amniotic fluid) (blood clot) (pul-
        monary) (septic) O08.2
      endometritis O08.0
      genital tract and pelvic infection O08.0
      hemorrhage (delayed) (excessive) O08.1

Pregnancy — *continued*
  molar — *continued*
    complicated — *continued*
      infection
        genital tract or pelvic O08.0
        kidney O08.83
        urinary tract O08.83
      intravascular coagulation O08.1
      laceration of pelvic organ(s) O08.6
      metabolic disorder O08.5
      oliguria O08.4
      oophoritis O08.0
      parametritis O08.0
      pelvic peritonitis O08.0
      perforation of pelvic organ(s) O08.6
      renal failure or shutdown O08.4
      salpingitis or salpingo-oophoritis O08.0
      sepsis O08.82
      shock O08.3
        septic O08.82
      specified condition NEC O08.89
      tubular necrosis (renal) O08.4
      uremia O08.4
      urinary infection O08.83
      venous complication NEC O08.7
        embolism O08.2
    hydatiform (*see also* Mole, hydatidiform) O01.9
  multiple (gestation) O30.9- ☑
    greater than quadruplets — *see* Pregnancy, multi-
      ple (gestation), specified NEC
    specified NEC O30.80- ☑
      with
        two or more monoamniotic fetuses
          O30.82- ☑
        two or more monochorionic fetuses
          O30.81- ☑
      two or more monoamniotic fetuses O30.82- ☑
      two or more monochorionic fetuses O30.81- ☑
      unable to determine number of placenta and
        number of amniotic sacs O30.89- ☑
      unspecified number of placenta and unspeci-
        fied number of amniotic sacs O30.80- ☑
  mural O00.8
  normal (supervision of) Z34.9- ☑
    first Z34.0- ☑
    high-risk — *see* Pregnancy, supervision of, high-
      risk
    specified Z34.8- ☑
  ovarian O00.2
  postmature (40 to 42 weeks) O48.0
    more than 42 weeks gestation O48.1
  post-term (40 to 42 weeks) O48.0
  prenatal care only Z34.9- ☑
    first Z34.0- ☑
    high-risk — *see* Pregnancy, supervision of, high-
      risk
    specified Z34.8- ☑
  prolonged (more than 42 weeks gestation) O48.1
  quadruplet O30.20- ☑
    with
      two or more monoamniotic fetuses O30.22- ☑
      two or more monochorionic fetuses O30.21- ☑
    two or more monoamniotic fetuses O30.22- ☑
    two or more monochorionic fetuses O30.21- ☑
    unable to determine number of placenta and
      number of amniotic sacs O30.29- ☑
    unspecified number of placenta and unspecified
      number of amniotic sacs O30.20- ☑
  quintuplet — *see* Pregnancy, multiple (gestation),
    specified NEC
  sextuplet — *see* Pregnancy, multiple (gestation),
    specified NEC
  supervision of
    concealed pregnancy O09.3- ☑
    elderly mother
      multigravida O09.52- ☑
      primigravida O09.51- ☑
    hidden pregnancy O09.3- ☑
    high-risk O09.9- ☑
      due to (history of)
        ectopic pregnancy O09.1- ☑
        elderly — *see* Pregnancy, supervision, elder-
          ly mother
        grand multiparity O09.4 ☑
        in utero procedure during previous pregnan-
          cy O09.82- ☑
        in vitro fertilization O09.81- ☑

Pregnancy — *continued*
  supervision of — *continued*
    high-risk — *continued*
      due to — *continued*
        infertility O09.0- ☑
        insufficient prenatal care O09.3- ☑
        molar pregnancy O09.1- ☑
        multiple previous pregnancies O09.4- ☑
        older mother — *see* Pregnancy, supervision
          of, elderly mother
        poor reproductive or obstetric history NEC
          O09.29- ☑
        pre-term labor O09.21- ☑
        previous
          neonatal death O09.29- ☑
        social problems O09.7- ☑
        specified NEC O09.89- ☑
        very young mother — *see* Pregnancy, super-
          vision, young mother
      resulting from in vitro fertilization O09.81- ☑
    normal Z34.9- ☑
      first Z34.0- ☑
      specified NEC Z34.8- ☑
    young mother
      multigravida O09.62- ☑
      primigravida O09.61- ☑
  triplet O30.10- ☑
    with
      two or more monoamniotic fetuses O30.12- ☑
      two or more monochrorionic fetuses O30.11- ☑
    two or more monoamniotic fetuses O30.12- ☑
    two or more monochrorionic fetuses O30.11- ☑
    unable to determine number of placenta and
      number of amniotic sacs O30.19- ☑
    unspecified number of placenta and unspecified
      number of amniotic sacs O30.10- ☑
  tubal (with abortion) (with rupture) O00.1
  twin O30.00- ☑
    conjoined O30.02- ☑
    dichorionic/diamniotic (two placenta, two amniotic
      sacs) O30.04- ☑
    monochorionic/diamniotic (one placenta, two
      amniotic sacs) O30.03- ☑
    monochorionic/monoamniotic (one placenta, one
      amniotic sac) O30.01- ☑
    unable to determine number of placenta and
      number of amniotic sacs O30.09- ☑
    unspecified number of placenta and unspecified
      number of amniotic sacs O30.00- ☑
  unwanted Z64.0
  weeks of gestation
    8 weeks Z3A.08 (*following* Z36)
    9 weeks Z3A.09 (*following* Z36)
    10 weeks Z3A.10 (*following* Z36)
    11 weeks Z3A.11 (*following* Z36)
    12 weeks Z3A.12 (*following* Z36)
    13 weeks Z3A.13 (*following* Z36)
    14 weeks Z3A.14 (*following* Z36)
    15 weeks Z3A.15 (*following* Z36)
    16 weeks Z3A.16 (*following* Z36)
    17 weeks Z3A.17 (*following* Z36)
    18 weeks Z3A.18 (*following* Z36)
    19 weeks Z3A.19 (*following* Z36)
    20 weeks Z3A.20 (*following* Z36)
    21 weeks Z3A.21 (*following* Z36)
    22 weeks Z3A.22 (*following* Z36)
    23 weeks Z3A.23 (*following* Z36)
    24 weeks Z3A.24 (*following* Z36)
    25 weeks Z3A.25 (*following* Z36)
    26 weeks Z3A.26 (*following* Z36)
    27 weeks Z3A.27 (*following* Z36)
    28 weeks Z3A.28 (*following* Z36)
    29 weeks Z3A.29 (*following* Z36)
    30 weeks Z3A.30 (*following* Z36)
    31 weeks Z3A.31 (*following* Z36)
    32 weeks Z3A.32 (*following* Z36)
    33 weeks Z3A.33 (*following* Z36)
    34 weeks Z3A.34 (*following* Z36)
    35 weeks Z3A.35 (*following* Z36)
    36 weeks Z3A.36 (*following* Z36)
    37 weeks Z3A.37 (*following* Z36)
    38 weeks Z3A.38 (*following* Z36)
    39 weeks Z3A.39 (*following* Z36)
    40 weeks Z3A.40 (*following* Z36)
    41 weeks Z3A.41 (*following* Z36)
    42 weeks Z3A.42 (*following* Z36)

☑ **Additional Character Required — Refer to the Tabular List for Character Selection**   ⬇ **Subterms under main terms may continue to next column or page**

Pregnancy — *continued*
  weeks of gestation — *continued*
    greater than 42 weeks Z3A.49 (*following* Z36)
    less than 8 weeks Z3A.01 (*following* Z36)
    not specified Z3A.00 (*following* Z36)
Preiser's disease — *see* Osteonecrosis, secondary, due to, trauma, metacarpus
Pre-kwashiorkor — *see* Malnutrition, severe
Preleukemia (syndrome) D46.9
Preluxation, hip, congenital Q65.6
Premature (*see also* condition)
  adrenarche E27.0
  aging E34.8
  beats I49.40
    atrial I49.1
    auricular I49.1
    supraventricular I49.1
  birth NEC — *see* Preterm, newborn
  closure, foramen ovale Q21.8
  contraction
    atrial I49.1
    atrioventricular I49.2
    auricular I49.1
    auriculoventricular I49.49
    heart (extrasystole) I49.49
    junctional I49.2
    ventricular I49.3
  delivery (*see also* Pregnancy, complicated by, preterm labor) O60.10 ☑
  ejaculation F52.4
  infant NEC — *see* Preterm, newborn
    light-for-dates — *see* Light for dates
  labor — *see* Pregnancy, complicated by, preterm labor
  lungs P28.0
  menopause E28.319
    asymptomatic E28.319
    symptomatic E28.310
  newborn
    less than 37 completed weeks — *see* Preterm, newborn
    extreme (less than 28 completed weeks) — *see* Immaturity, extreme
  puberty E30.1
  rupture membranes or amnion — *see* Pregnancy, complicated by, premature rupture of membranes
  senility E34.8
  thelarche E30.8
  ventricular systole I49.3
Prematurity NEC (less than 37 completed weeks) — *see* Preterm, newborn
  extreme (less than 28 completed weeks) — *see* Immaturity, extreme
Premenstrual
  dysphoric disorder (PMDD) N94.3
  tension (syndrome) N94.3
Premolarization, cuspids K00.2
Prenatal
  care, normal pregnancy — *see* Pregnancy, normal
  screening of mother Z36
  teeth K00.6
Preparatory care for subsequent treatment NEC
  for dialysis Z49.01
    peritoneal Z49.02
Prepartum — *see* condition
Preponderance, left or right ventricular I51.7
Prepuce — *see* condition
PRES (posterior reversible encephalopathy syndrome) I67.83
Presbycardia R54
Presbycusis, presbyacusia H91.1- ☑
Presbyesophagus K22.8
Presbyophrenia F03 ☑
Presbyopia H52.4
Prescription of contraceptives (initial) Z30.019
  emergency (postcoital) Z30.012
  implantable subdermal Z30.019
  injectable Z30.013
  intrauterine contraceptive device Z30.014
  pills Z30.011
  postcoital (emergency) Z30.012
  repeat Z30.40
    implantable subdermal Z30.49
    injectable Z30.42
    pills Z30.41
    specified type NEC Z30.49
  specified type NEC Z30.018

Presence (of)
  ankle-joint implant (functional) (prosthesis) Z96.66- ☑
  aortocoronary (bypass) graft Z95.1
  arterial-venous shunt (dialysis) Z99.2
  artificial
    eye (globe) Z97.0
    heart (fully implantable) (mechanical) Z95.812
      valve Z95.2
    larynx Z96.3
    lens (intraocular) Z96.1
    limb (complete) (partial) Z97.1- ☑
      arm Z97.1- ☑
        bilateral Z97.15
      leg Z97.1- ☑
        bilateral Z97.16
  audiological implant (functional) Z96.29
  bladder implant (functional) Z96.0
  bone
    conduction hearing device Z96.29
    implant (functional) NEC Z96.7
    joint (prosthesis) — *see* Presence, joint implant
  cardiac
    defibrillator (functional) (with synchronous cardiac pacemaker) Z95.810
    implant or graft Z95.9
      specified type NEC Z95.818
    pacemaker Z95.0
  cerebrospinal fluid drainage device Z98.2
  cochlear implant (functional) Z96.21
  contact lens (es) Z97.3
  coronary artery graft or prosthesis Z95.5
  CSF shunt Z98.2
  dental prosthesis device Z97.2
  dentures Z97.2
  device (external) NEC Z97.8
    cardiac NEC Z95.818
    heart assist Z95.811
    implanted (functional) Z96.9
      specified NEC Z96.89
    prosthetic Z97.8
  ear implant Z96.20
    cochlear implant Z96.21
    myringotomy tube Z96.22
    specified type NEC Z96.29
  elbow-joint implant (functional) (prosthesis) Z96.62- ☑
  endocrine implant (functional) NEC Z96.49
  eustachian tube stent or device (functional) Z96.29
  external hearing-aid or device Z97.4
  finger-joint implant (functional) (prosthetic) Z96.69- ☑
  functional implant Z96.9
    specified NEC Z96.89
  graft
    cardiac NEC Z95.818
    vascular NEC Z95.828
  hearing-aid or device (external) Z97.4
    implant (bone) (cochlear) (functional) Z96.21
  heart assist device Z95.811
  heart valve implant (functional) Z95.2
    prosthetic Z95.2
    specified type NEC Z95.4
    xenogenic Z95.3
  hip-joint implant (functional) (prosthesis) Z96.64- ☑
  implanted device (artificial) (functional) (prosthetic) Z96.9
    automatic cardiac defibrillator (with synchronous cardiac pacemaker) Z95.810
    cardiac pacemaker Z95.0
    cochlear Z96.21
    dental Z96.5
    heart Z95.812
    heart valve Z95.2
      prosthetic Z95.2
      specified NEC Z95.4
      xenogenic Z95.3
    insulin pump Z96.41
    intraocular lens Z96.1
    joint Z96.60
      ankle Z96.66- ☑
      elbow Z96.62- ☑
      finger Z96.69- ☑
      hip Z96.64- ☑
      knee Z96.65- ☑
      shoulder Z96.61- ☑
      specified NEC Z96.698
      wrist Z96.63- ☑
    larynx Z96.3
    myringotomy tube Z96.22

Presence — *continued*
  implanted device — *continued*
    otological Z96.20
      cochlear Z96.21
      eustachian stent Z96.29
      myringotomy Z96.22
      specified NEC Z96.29
      stapes Z96.29
    skin Z96.81
    skull plate Z96.7
    specified NEC Z96.89
    urogenital Z96.0
  insulin pump (functional) Z96.41
  intestinal bypass or anastomosis Z98.0
  intraocular lens (functional) Z96.1
  intrauterine contraceptive device (IUD) Z97.5
  intravascular implant (functional) (prosthetic) NEC Z95.9
    coronary artery Z95.5
    defibrillator (with synchronous cardiac pacemaker) Z95.810
    peripheral vessel (with angioplasty) Z95.820
  joint implant (prosthetic) (any) Z96.60
    ankle — *see* Presence, ankle joint implant
    elbow — *see* Presence, elbow joint implant
    finger — *see* Presence, finger joint implant
    hip — *see* Presence, hip joint implant
    knee — *see* Presence, knee joint implant
    shoulder — *see* Presence, shoulder joint implant
    specified joint NEC Z96.698
    wrist — *see* Presence, wrist joint implant
  knee-joint implant (functional) (prosthesis) Z96.65- ☑
  laryngeal implant (functional) Z96.3
  mandibular implant (dental) Z96.5
  myringotomy tube(s) Z96.22
  orthopedic-joint implant (prosthetic) (any) — *see* Presence, joint implant
  otological implant (functional) Z96.29
  shoulder-joint implant (functional) (prosthesis) Z96.61- ☑
  skull-plate implant Z96.7
  spectacles Z97.3
  stapes implant (functional) Z96.29
  systemic lupus erythematosus [SLE] inhibitor D68.62
  tendon implant (functional) (graft) Z96.7
  tooth root(s) implant Z96.5
  ureteral stent Z96.0
  urethral stent Z96.0
  urogenital implant (functional) Z96.0
  vascular implant or device Z95.9
    access port device Z95.828
    specified type NEC Z95.828
  wrist-joint implant (functional) (prosthesis) Z96.63- ☑
Presenile (*see also* condition)
  dementia F03 ☑
  premature aging E34.8
Presentation, fetal — *see* Delivery, complicated by, malposition
Prespondylolisthesis (congenital) Q76.2
Pressure
  area, skin — *see* Ulcer, pressure, by site
  brachial plexus G54.0
  brain G93.5
    injury at birth NEC P11.1
  cerebral — *see* Pressure, brain
  chest R07.89
  cone, tentorial G93.5
  hyposystolic (*see also* Hypotension)
    incidental reading, without diagnosis of hypotension R03.1
  increased
    intracranial (benign) G93.2
      injury at birth P11.0
    intraocular H40.05- ☑
  lumbosacral plexus G54.1
  mediastinum J98.5
  necrosis (chronic) — *see* Ulcer, pressure, by site
  parental, inappropriate (excessive) Z62.6
  sore (chronic) — *see* Ulcer, pressure, by site
  spinal cord G95.20
  ulcer (chronic) — *see* Ulcer, pressure, by site
  venous, increased I87.8
Pre-syncope R55
Preterm
  delivery (*see also* Pregnancy, complicated by, preterm labor) O60.10 ☑
  labor — *see* Pregnancy, complicated by, preterm labor

Preterm — *continued*
 newborn (infant) P07.30
  gestational age
   28 completed weeks (28 weeks, 0 days through 28 weeks, 6 days) P07.31
   29 completed weeks (29 weeks, 0 days through 29 weeks, 6 days) P07.32
   30 completed weeks (30 weeks, 0 days through 30 weeks, 6 days) P07.33
   31 completed weeks (31 weeks, 0 days through 31 weeks, 6 days) P07.34
   32 completed weeks (32 weeks, 0 days through 32 weeks, 6 days) P07.35
   33 completed weeks (33 weeks, 0 days through 33 weeks, 6 days) P07.36
   34 completed weeks (34 weeks, 0 days through 34 weeks, 6 days) P07.37
   35 completed weeks (35 weeks, 0 days through 35 weeks, 6 days) P07.38
   36 completed weeks (36 weeks, 0 days through 36 weeks, 6 days) P07.39
Previa
 placenta (low) (marginal) (partial) (total) (with hemorrhage) O44.1- ☑
  without hemorrhage O44.0- ☑
 vasa O69.4 ☑
Priapism N48.30
 due to
  disease classified elsewhere N48.32
  drug N48.33
  specified cause NEC N48.39
  trauma N48.31
Prickling sensation (skin) R20.2
Prickly heat L74.0
Primary — *see* condition
Primigravida
 elderly, affecting management of pregnancy, labor and delivery (supervision only) — *see* Pregnancy, complicated by, elderly, primigravida
 older, affecting management of pregnancy, labor and delivery (supervision only) — *see* Pregnancy, complicated by, elderly, primigravida
 very young, affecting management of pregnancy, labor and delivery (supervision only) — *see* Pregnancy, complicated by, young mother, primigravida
Primipara
 elderly, affecting management of pregnancy, labor and delivery (supervision only) — *see* Pregnancy, complicated by, elderly, primigravida
 older, affecting management of pregnancy, labor and delivery (supervision only) — *see* Pregnancy, complicated by, elderly, primigravida
 very young, affecting management of pregnancy, labor and delivery (supervision only) — *see* Pregnancy, complicated by, young mother, primigravida
Primus varus (bilateral) Q66.2
PRIND (Prolonged reversible ischemic neurologic deficit) I63.9
Pringle's disease (tuberous sclerosis) Q85.1
Prinzmetal angina I20.1
Prizefighter ear — *see* Cauliflower ear
Problem (with) (related to)
 academic Z55.8
 acculturation Z60.3
 adjustment (to)
  change of job Z56.1
  life-cycle transition Z60.0
  pension Z60.0
  retirement Z60.0
 adopted child Z62.821
 alcoholism in family Z63.72
 atypical parenting situation Z62.9
 bankruptcy Z59.8
 behavioral (adult) F69
  drug seeking Z72.89
 birth of sibling affecting child Z62.898
 care (of)
  provider dependency Z74.9
   specified NEC Z74.8
  sick or handicapped person in family or household Z63.6
 child
  abuse (affecting the child) — *see* Maltreatment, child
  custody or support proceedings Z65.3
  in care of non-parental family member Z62.21
  in foster care Z62.21
  in welfare custody Z62.21

Problem — *continued*
 child — *continued*
  living in orphanage or group home Z62.22
 child-rearing Z62.9
  specified NEC Z62.898
 communication (developmental) F80.9
 conflict or discord (with)
  boss Z56.4
  classmates Z55.4
  counselor Z64.4
  employer Z56.4
  family Z63.9
   specified NEC Z63.8
  probation officer Z64.4
  social worker Z64.4
  teachers Z55.4
  workmates Z56.4
 conviction in legal proceedings Z65.0
  with imprisonment Z65.1
 counselor Z64.4
 creditors Z59.8
 digestive K92.9
 drug addict in family Z63.72
 ear — *see* Disorder, ear
 economic Z59.9
  affecting care Z59.9
  specified NEC Z59.8
 education Z55.9
  specified NEC Z55.8
 employment Z56.9
  change of job Z56.1
  discord Z56.4
  environment Z56.5
  sexual harassment Z56.81
  specified NEC Z56.89
  stressful schedule Z56.3
  stress NEC Z56.6
  threat of job loss Z56.2
  unemployment Z56.0
 enuresis, child F98.0
 eye H57.9
 failed examinations (school) Z55.2
 falling Z91.81
 family (*see also* Disruption, family) Z63.9
  specified NEC Z63.8
 feeding (elderly) (infant) R63.3
  newborn P92.9
   breast P92.5
   overfeeding P92.4
   slow P92.2
   specified NEC P92.8
   underfeeding P92.3
  nonorganic F50.8
 finance Z59.9
  specified NEC Z59.8
 foreclosure on loan Z59.8
 foster child Z62.822
 frightening experience(s) in childhood Z62.898
 genital NEC
  female N94.9
  male N50.9
 health care Z75.9
  specified NEC Z75.8
 hearing — *see* Deafness
 homelessness Z59.0
 housing Z59.9
  inadequate Z59.1
  isolated Z59.8
  specified NEC Z59.8
 identity (of childhood) F93.8
 illegitimate pregnancy (unwanted) Z64.0
 illiteracy Z55.0
 impaired mobility Z74.09
 imprisonment or incarceration Z65.1
 inadequate teaching affecting education Z55.8
 inappropriate (excessive) parental pressure Z62.6
 influencing health status NEC Z78.9
 in-law Z63.1
 institutionalization, affecting child Z62.22
 intrafamilial communication Z63.8
 jealousy, child F93.8
 landlord Z59.2
 language (developmental) F80.9
 learning (developmental) F81.9
 legal Z65.3
  conviction without imprisonment Z65.0
  imprisonment Z65.1
  release from prison Z65.2

Problem — *continued*
 life-management Z73.9
  specified NEC Z73.89
 life-style Z72.9
  gambling Z72.6
  high-risk sexual behavior (heterosexual) Z72.51
   bisexual Z72.53
   homosexual Z72.52
  inappropriate eating habits Z72.4
  self-damaging behavior NEC Z72.89
  specified NEC Z72.89
  tobacco use Z72.0
 literacy Z55.9
  low level Z55.0
  specified NEC Z55.8
 living alone Z60.2
 lodgers Z59.2
 loss of love relationship in childhood Z62.898
 marital Z63.0
  involving
   divorce Z63.5
   estrangement Z63.5
   gender identity F66
 mastication K08.8
 medical
  care, within family Z63.6
  facilities Z75.9
   specified NEC Z75.8
 mental F48.9
 multiparity Z64.1
 negative life events in childhood Z62.9
  altered pattern of family relationships Z62.898
  frightening experience Z62.898
  loss of
   love relationship Z62.898
   self-esteem Z62.898
  physical abuse (alleged) — *see* Maltreatment, child
  removal from home Z62.29
  specified event NEC Z62.898
 neighbor Z59.2
 neurological NEC R29.818
 new step-parent affecting child Z62.898
 none (feared complaint unfounded) Z71.1
 occupational NEC Z56.89
 parent-child — *see* Conflict, parent-child
 personal hygiene Z91.89
 personality F69
 phase-of-life transition, adjustment Z60.0
 presence of sick or disabled person in family or household Z63.79
  needing care Z63.6
 primary support group (family) Z63.9
  specified NEC Z63.8
 probation officer Z64.4
 psychiatric F99
 psychosexual (development) F66
 psychosocial Z65.9
  specified NEC Z65.8
 relationship Z63.9
  childhood F93.8
 release from prison Z65.2
 removal from home affecting child Z62.29
 seeking and accepting known hazardous and harmful
  behavioral or psychological interventions Z65.8
  chemical, nutritional or physical interventions Z65.8
 sexual function (nonorganic) F52.9
 sight H54.7
 sleep disorder, child F51.9
 smell — *see* Disturbance, sensation, smell
 social
  environment Z60.9
   specified NEC Z60.8
  exclusion and rejection Z60.4
  worker Z64.4
 speech R47.9
  developmental F80.9
  specified NEC R47.89
 swallowing — *see* Dysphagia
 taste — *see* Disturbance, sensation, taste
 tic, child F95.0
 underachievement in school Z55.3
 unemployment Z56.0
  threatened Z56.2
 unwanted pregnancy Z64.0
 upbringing Z62.9
  specified NEC Z62.898
 urinary N39.9
 voice production R47.89

Problem — *continued*
  work schedule (stressful) Z56.3
Procedure (surgical)
  for purpose other than remedying health state Z41.9
    specified NEC Z41.8
  not done Z53.9
    because of
      administrative reasons Z53.8
      contraindication Z53.09
        smoking Z53.01
      patient's decision Z53.20
        for reasons of belief or group pressure Z53.1
        left against medical advice (AMA) Z53.21
        specified reason NEC Z53.29
      specified reason NEC Z53.8
Procidentia (uteri) N81.3
Proctalgia K62.89
  fugax K59.4
  spasmodic K59.4
Proctitis K62.89
  amebic (acute) A06.0
  chlamydial A56.3
  gonococcal A54.6
  granulomatous — *see* Enteritis, regional, large intestine
  herpetic A60.1
  radiation K62.7
  tuberculous A18.32
  ulcerative (chronic) K51.20
    with
      complication K51.219
        abscess K51.214
        fistula K51.213
        obstruction K51.212
        rectal bleeding K51.211
        specified NEC K51.218
Proctocele
  female (without uterine prolapse) N81.6
    with uterine prolapse N81.2
      complete N81.3
  male K62.3
Proctocolitis, mucosal — *see* Rectosigmoiditis, ulcerative
Proctoptosis K62.3
Proctorrhagia K62.5
Proctosigmoiditis K63.89
  ulcerative (chronic) — *see* Rectosigmoiditis, ulcerative
Proctospasm K59.4
  psychogenic F45.8
Profichet's disease — *see* Disorder, soft tissue, specified type NEC
Progeria E34.8
Prognathism (mandibular) (maxillary) M26.19
Progonoma (melanotic) — *see* Neoplasm, benign, by site
Progressive — *see* condition
Prolactinoma
  specified site — *see* Neoplasm, benign, by site
  unspecified site D35.2
Prolapse, prolapsed
  anus, anal (canal) (sphincter) K62.2
  arm or hand O32.2 ☑
    causing obstructed labor O64.4 ☑
  bladder (mucosa) (sphincter) (acquired)
    congenital Q79.4
    female — *see* Cystocele
    male N32.89
  breast implant (prosthetic) T85.49 ☑
  cecostomy K94.09
  cecum K63.4
  cervix, cervical (hypertrophied) N81.2
    anterior lip, obstructing labor O65.5
    congenital Q51.828
    postpartal, old N81.2
    stump N81.85
  ciliary body (traumatic) — *see* Laceration, eye(ball), with prolapse or loss of interocular tissue
  colon (pedunculated) K63.4
  colostomy K94.09
  disc (intervertebral) — *see* Displacement, intervertebral disc
  eye implant (orbital) T85.398 ☑
    lens (ocular) — *see* Complications, intraocular lens
  fallopian tube N83.4
  gastric (mucosa) K31.89
  genital, female N81.9
    specified NEC N81.89
  globe, nontraumatic — *see* Luxation, globe

Prolapse, prolapsed — *continued*
  ileostomy bud K94.19
  intervertebral disc — *see* Displacement, intervertebral disc
  intestine (small) K63.4
  iris (traumatic) — *see* Laceration, eye(ball), with prolapse or loss of interocular tissue
    nontraumatic H21.89
  kidney N28.83
    congenital Q63.2
  laryngeal muscles or ventricle J38.7
  liver K76.89
  meatus urinarius N36.8
  mitral (valve) I34.1
  ocular lens implant — *see* Complications, intraocular lens
  organ or site, congenital NEC — *see* Malposition, congenital
  ovary N83.4
  pelvic floor, female N81.89
  perineum, female N81.89
  rectum (mucosa) (sphincter) K62.3
    due to trichuris trichuria B79
  spleen D73.89
  stomach K31.89
  umbilical cord
    complicating delivery O69.0 ☑
  urachus, congenital Q64.4
  ureter N28.89
    with obstruction N13.5
      with infection N13.6
  ureterovesical orifice N28.89
  urethra (acquired) (infected) (mucosa) N36.8
    congenital Q64.71
  urinary meatus N36.8
    congenital Q64.72
  uterovaginal N81.4
    complete N81.3
    incomplete N81.2
  uterus (with prolapse of vagina) N81.4
    complete N81.3
    congenital Q51.818
    first degree N81.2
    in pregnancy or childbirth — *see* Pregnancy, complicated by, abnormal, uterus
    incomplete N81.2
    postpartal (old) N81.4
    second degree N81.2
    third degree N81.3
  uveal (traumatic) — *see* Laceration, eye(ball), with prolapse or loss of interocular tissue
  vagina (anterior) (wall) — *see* Cystocele
    with prolapse of uterus N81.4
      complete N81.3
      incomplete N81.2
    posterior wall N81.6
    posthysterectomy N99.3
  vitreous (humor) H43.0- ☑
    in wound — *see* Laceration, eye(ball), with prolapse or loss of interocular tissue
  womb — *see* Prolapse, uterus
Prolapsus, female N81.9
  specified NEC N81.89
Proliferation(s)
  primary cutaneous CD30-positive large T-cell C86.6
Proliferative — *see* condition
Prolonged, prolongation (of)
  bleeding (time) (idiopathic) R79.1
  coagulation (time) R79.1
  gestation (over 42 completed weeks)
    mother O48.1
    newborn P08.22
  interval I44.0
  labor O63.9
    first stage O63.0
    second stage O63.1
  partial thromboplastin time (PTT) R79.1
  pregnancy (more than 42 weeks gestation) O48.1
  prothrombin time R79.1
  QT interval I45.81
  uterine contractions in labor O62.4
Prominence, prominent
  auricle (congenital) (ear) Q17.5
  ischial spine or sacral promontory
    with disproportion (fetopelvic) O33.0
      causing obstructed labor O65.0
  nose (congenital) acquired M95.0
Promiscuity — *see* High, risk, sexual behavior

Pronation
  ankle — *see* Deformity, limb, foot, specified NEC
  foot (*see also* Deformity, limb, foot, specified NEC)
    congenital Q74.2
Prophylactic
  administration of
    antibiotics, long-term Z79.2
      short-term use — *omit code*
    drug (*see also* Long-term (current) drug therapy (use of)) Z79.899
  medication Z79.899
  organ removal (for neoplasia management) Z40.00
    breast Z40.01
    ovary Z40.02
    specified site NEC Z40.09
  surgery Z40.9
    for risk factors related to malignant neoplasm — *see* Prophylactic, organ removal
    specified NEC Z40.8
  vaccination Z23
Propionic acidemia E71.121
Proptosis (ocular) (*see also* Exophthalmos)
  thyroid — *see* Hyperthyroidism, with goiter
Prosecution, anxiety concerning Z65.3
Prosopagnosia R48.3
Prostadynia N42.81
Prostate, prostatic — *see* condition
Prostatism — *see* Hyperplasia, prostate
Prostatitis (congestive) (suppurative) (with cystitis) N41.9
  acute N41.0
  cavitary N41.8
  chronic N41.1
  diverticular N41.8
  due to Trichomonas (vaginalis) A59.02
  fibrous N41.1
  gonococcal (acute) (chronic) A54.22
  granulomatous N41.4
  hypertrophic N41.1
  subacute N41.1
  trichomonal A59.02
  tuberculous A18.14
Prostatocystitis N41.3
Prostatorrhea N42.89
Prostatosis N42.82
Prostration R53.83
  heat (*see also* Heat, exhaustion)
    anhydrotic T67.3 ☑
    due to
      salt (and water) depletion T67.4 ☑
      water depletion T67.3 ☑
  nervous F48.8
  senile R54
Protanomaly (anomalous trichromat) H53.54
Protanopia (complete) (incomplete) H53.54
Protection (against) (from) — *see* Prophylactic
Protein
  deficiency NEC — *see* Malnutrition
  malnutrition — *see* Malnutrition
  sickness (*see also* Reaction, serum) T80.69 ☑
Proteinemia R77.9
Proteinosis
  alveolar (pulmonary) J84.01
  lipid or lipoid (of Urbach) E78.89
Proteinuria R80.9
  Bence Jones R80.3
  complicating pregnancy — *see* Proteinuria, gestational
  gestational O12.1- ☑
    with edema O12.2- ☑
  idiopathic R80.0
  isolated R80.0
    with glomerular lesion N06.9
      dense deposit disease N06.6
      diffuse
        crescentic glomerulonephritis N06.7
        endocapillary proliferative glomerulonephritis N06.4
        mesangiocapillary glomerulonephritis N06.5
      focal and segmental hyalinosis or sclerosis N06.1
      membranous (diffuse) N06.2
      mesangial proliferative (diffuse) N06.3
      minimal change N06.0
      specified pathology NEC N06.8
  orthostatic R80.2
    with glomerular lesion — *see* Proteinuria, isolated, with glomerular lesion

Proteinuria — *continued*
  persistent R80.1
    with glomerular lesion — *see* Proteinuria, isolated,
      with glomerular lesion
  postural R80.2
    with glomerular lesion — *see* Proteinuria, isolated,
      with glomerular lesion
  pre-eclamptic — *see* Pre-eclampsia
  specified type NEC R80.8
Proteolysis, pathologic D65
Proteus (mirabilis) (morganii), **as cause of disease classified elsewhere** B96.4
Prothrombin gene mutation D68.52
Protoporphyria, erythropoietic E80.0
Protozoal (*see also* condition)
  disease B64
    specified NEC B60.8
Protrusion, protrusio
  acetabuli M24.7
  acetabulum (into pelvis) M24.7
  device, implant or graft (*see also* Complications, by
    site and type, mechanical) T85.698 ☑
    arterial graft NEC — *see* Complication, cardiovas-
      cular device, mechanical, vascular
    breast (implant) T85.49
    catheter NEC T85.698 ☑
      cystostomy T83.090 ☑
      dialysis (renal) T82.49 ☑
        intraperitoneal T85.691 ☑
      infusion NEC T82.594 ☑
        spinal (epidural) (subdural) T85.690 ☑
      urinary, indwelling T83.098 ☑
    electronic (electrode) (pulse generator) (stimulator)
      bone T84.390 ☑
      nervous system — *see* Complication, prosthetic
        device, mechanical, electronic nervous
        system stimulator
    fixation, internal (orthopedic) NEC — *see* Compli-
      cation, fixation device, mechanical
    gastrointestinal — *see* Complications, prosthetic
      device, mechanical, gastrointestinal device
    genital NEC T83.498 ☑
      intrauterine contraceptive device T83.39 ☑
      penile prosthesis T83.490 ☑
    heart NEC — *see* Complication, cardiovascular de-
      vice, mechanical
    joint prosthesis — *see* Complications, joint prosthe-
      sis, mechanical, specified NEC, by site
    ocular NEC — *see* Complications, prosthetic device,
      mechanical, ocular device
    orthopedic NEC — *see* Complication, orthopedic,
      device, mechanical
    specified NEC T85.628 ☑
    urinary NEC (*see also* Complication, genitourinary,
      device, urinary, mechanical)
      graft T83.29 ☑
    vascular NEC — *see* Complication, cardiovascular
      device, mechanical
    ventricular intracranial shunt T85.09 ☑
  intervertebral disc — *see* Displacement, intervertebral
    disc
  joint prosthesis — *see* Complications, joint prosthesis,
    mechanical, specified NEC, by site
  nucleus pulposus — *see* Displacement, intervertebral
    disc
Prune belly (syndrome) Q79.4
Prurigo (ferox) (gravis) (Hebrae) (Hebra's) (mitis) (simplex)
  L28.2
  Besnier's L20.0
  estivalis L56.4
  nodularis L28.1
  psychogenic F45.8
Pruritus, pruritic (essential) L29.9
  ani, anus L29.0
    psychogenic F45.8
  anogenital L29.3
    psychogenic F45.8
  due to onchocerca volvulus B73.1
  gravidarum — *see* Pregnancy, complicated by, speci-
    fied pregnancy-related condition NEC
  hiemalis L29.8
  neurogenic (any site) F45.8
  perianal L29.0
  psychogenic (any site) F45.8
  scroti, scrotum L29.1
    psychogenic F45.8
  senile, senilis L29.8

Pruritus, pruritic — *continued*
  specified NEC L29.8
    psychogenic F45.8
  Trichomonas A59.9
  vulva, vulvae L29.2
    psychogenic F45.8
Pseudarthrosis, pseudoarthrosis (bone) — *see*
  Nonunion, fracture
  clavicle, congenital Q74.0
  joint, following fusion or arthrodesis M96.0
Pseudoaneurysm — *see* Aneurysm
Pseudoangina (pectoris) — *see* Angina
Pseudoangioma I81
Pseudoarteriosus Q28.8
Pseudoarthrosis — *see* Pseudarthrosis
Pseudobulbar affect (PBA) F48.8
Pseudochromhidrosis L67.8
Pseudocirrhosis, liver, pericardial I31.1
Pseudocowpox B08.03
Pseudocoxalgia M91.3- ☑
Pseudocroup J38.5
Pseudo-Cushing's syndrome, alcohol-induced E24.4
Pseudocyesis F45.8
Pseudocyst
  lung J98.4
  pancreas K86.3
  retina — *see* Cyst, retina
Pseudoelephantiasis neuroarthritica Q82.0
Pseudoexfoliation, capsule (lens) — *see* Cataract,
  specified NEC
Pseudofolliculitis barbae L73.1
Pseudoglioma H44.89
Pseudohemophilia (Bernuth's) (hereditary) (type B)
  D68.0
  Type A D69.8
  vascular D69.8
Pseudohermaphroditism Q56.3
  adrenal E25.8
  female Q56.2
    with adrenocortical disorder E25.8
    without adrenocortical disorder Q56.2
      adrenal, congenital E25.0
  male Q56.1
    with
      5-alpha-reductase deficiency E29.1
      adrenocortical disorder E25.8
      androgen resistance E34.51
      cleft scrotum Q56.1
      feminizing testis E34.51
    without gonadal disorder Q56.1
      adrenal E25.8
Pseudo-Hurler's polydystrophy E77.0
Pseudohydrocephalus G93.2
Pseudohypertrophic muscular dystrophy (Erb's) G71.0
Pseudohypertrophy, muscle G71.0
Pseudohypoparathyroidism E20.1
Pseudoinsomnia F51.03
Pseudoleukemia, infantile D64.89
Pseudomembranous — *see* condition
Pseudomeningocele (cerebral) (infective) (post-traumat-
  ic) G96.19
  postprocedural (spinal) G97.82
Pseudomenses (newborn) P54.6
Pseudomenstruation (newborn) P54.6
Pseudomonas
  aeruginosa, as cause of disease classified elsewhere
    B96.5
  mallei infection A24.0
    as cause of disease classified elsewhere B96.5
  pseudomallei, as cause of disease classified elsewhere
    B96.5
Pseudomyotonia G71.19
Pseudomyxoma peritonei C78.6
Pseudoneuritis, optic (nerve) (disc) (papilla), **congeni-
  tal** Q14.2
Pseudo-obstruction intestine (acute) (chronic) (idio-
  pathic) (intermittent secondary) (primary) K59.8
Pseudopapilledema H47.33- ☑
  congenital Q14.2
Pseudoparalysis
  arm or leg R29.818
  atonic, congenital P94.2
Pseudopelade L66.0
Pseudophakia Z96.1
Pseudopolyarthritis, rhizomelic M35.3
Pseudopolycythemia D75.1
Pseudopseudohypoparathyroidism E20.1

Pseudopterygium H11.81- ☑
Pseudoptosis (eyelid) — *see* Blepharochalasis
Pseudopuberty, precocious
  female heterosexual E25.8
  male isosexual E25.8
Pseudorickets (renal) N25.0
Pseudorubella B08.20
Pseudosclerema, newborn P83.8
Pseudosclerosis (brain)
  Jakob's — *see* Creutzfeldt-Jakob disease or syndrome
    of Westphal (Strümpell) E83.01
  spastic — *see* Creutzfeldt-Jakob disease or syndrome
Pseudotetanus — *see* Convulsions
Pseudotetany R29.0
  hysterical F44.5
Pseudotruncus arteriosus Q25.4
Pseudotuberculosis A28.2
  enterocolitis A04.8
  pasteurella (infection) A28.0
Pseudotumor
  cerebri G93.2
  orbital H05.11 ☑
Pseudoxanthoma elasticum Q82.8
Psilosis (sprue) (tropical) K90.1
  nontropical K90.0
Psittacosis A70
Psoitis M60.88
Psoriasis L40.9
  arthropathic L40.50
    arthritis mutilans L40.52
    distal interphalangeal L40.51
    juvenile L40.54
    other specified L40.59
    spondylitis L40.53
  buccal K13.29
  flexural L40.8
  guttate L40.4
  mouth K13.29
  nummular L40.0
  plaque L40.0
  psychogenic F54
  pustular (generalized) L40.1
    palmaris et plantaris L40.3
  specified NEC L40.8
  vulgaris L40.0
Psychasthenia F48.8
Psychiatric disorder or problem F99
Psychogenic (*see also* condition)
  factors associated with physical conditions F54
**Psychological and behavioral factors affecting
  medical condition** F59
Psychoneurosis, psychoneurotic (*see also* Neurosis)
  anxiety (state) F41.1
  depersonalization F48.1
  hypochondriacal F45.21
  hysteria F44.9
  neurasthenic F48.8
  personality NEC F60.89
Psychopathy, psychopathic
  affectionless F94.2
  autistic F84.5
  constitution, post-traumatic F07.81
  personality — *see* Disorder, personality
  sexual — *see* Deviation, sexual
  state F60.2
Psychosexual identity disorder of childhood F64.2
Psychosis, psychotic F29
  acute (transient) F23
    hysterical F44.9
  affective — *see* Disorder, mood
  alcoholic F10.959
    with
      abuse F10.159
      anxiety disorder F10.980
        with
          abuse F10.180
          dependence F10.280
      delirium tremens F10.231
      delusions F10.950
        with
          abuse F10.150
          dependence F10.250
      dementia F10.97
        with dependence F10.27
      dependence F10.259

Psychosis, psychotic — *continued*
alcoholic — *continued*
  with — *continued*
    hallucinosis F10.951
      with
        abuse F10.151
        dependence F10.251
    mood disorder F10.94
      with
        abuse F10.14
        dependence F10.24
    paranoia F10.950
      with
        abuse F10.150
        dependence F10.250
    persisting amnesia F10.96
      with dependence F10.26
  amnestic confabulatory F10.96
    with dependence F10.26
  delirium tremens F10.231
  Korsakoff's, Korsakov's, Korsakow's F10.26
  paranoid type F10.950
    with
      abuse F10.150
      dependence F10.250
anergastic — *see* Psychosis, organic
arteriosclerotic (simple type) (uncomplicated) F01.50
  with behavioral disturbance F01.51
childhood F84.0
  atypical F84.8
climacteric — *see* Psychosis, involutional
confusional F29
  acute or subacute F05
  reactive F23
cycloid F23
depressive — *see* Disorder, depressive
disintegrative (childhood) F84.3
drug-induced — *see* F11-F19 with .X59
  paranoid and hallucinatory states — *see* F11-F19
    with .X50 or .X51
due to or associated with
  addiction, drug — *see* F11-F19 with .X59
  dependence
    alcohol F10.259
    drug — *see* F11-F19 with .X59
  epilepsy F06.8
  Huntington's chorea F06.8
  ischemia, cerebrovascular (generalized) F06.8
  multiple sclerosis F06.8
  physical disease F06.8
  presenile dementia F03 ☑
  senile dementia F03 ☑
  vascular disease (arteriosclerotic) (cerebral) F01.50
    with behavioral disturbance F01.51
epileptic F06.8
episode F23
  due to or associated with physical condition F06.8
exhaustive F43.0
hallucinatory, chronic F28
hypomanic F30.8
hysterical (acute) F44.9
induced F24
infantile F84.0
  atypical F84.8
infective (acute) (subacute) F05
involutional F28
  depressive — *see* Disorder, depressive
  melancholic — *see* Disorder, depressive
  paranoid (state) F22
Korsakoff's, Korsakov's, Korsakow's (nonalcoholic) F04
  alcoholic F10.96
    in dependence F10.26
  induced by other psychoactive substance — *see*
    categories F11-F19 with .X5X
mania, manic (single episode) F30.2
  recurrent type F31.89
manic-depressive — *see* Disorder, mood
menopausal — *see* Psychosis, involutional
mixed schizophrenic and affective F25.8
multi-infarct (cerebrovascular) F01.50
  with behavioral disturbance F01.51
nonorganic F29
  specified NEC F28
organic F09
  due to or associated with
    arteriosclerosis (cerebral) — *see* Psychosis, ar-
      teriosclerotic

Psychosis, psychotic — *continued*
organic — *continued*
  due to or associated with — *continued*
    cerebrovascular disease, arteriosclerotic — *see*
      Psychosis, arteriosclerotic
    childbirth — *see* Psychosis, puerperal
    Creutzfeldt-Jakob disease or syndrome — *see*
      Creutzfeldt-Jakob disease or syndrome
    dependence, alcohol F10.259
    disease
      alcoholic liver F10.259
      brain, arteriosclerotic — *see* Psychosis, arte-
        riosclerotic
      cerebrovascular F01.50
        with behavioral disturbance F01.51
      Creutzfeldt-Jakob — *see* Creutzfeldt-Jakob
        disease or syndrome
      endocrine or metabolic F06.8
        acute or subacute F05
      liver, alcoholic F10.259
    epilepsy transient (acute) F05
    infection
      brain (intracranial) F06.8
        acute or subacute F05
    intoxication
      alcoholic (acute) F10.259
      drug F11-F19 with .X59
    ischemia, cerebrovascular (generalized) — *see*
      Psychosis, arteriosclerotic
    puerperium — *see* Psychosis, puerperal
    trauma, brain (birth) (from electric current)
      (surgical) F06.8
      acute or subacute F05
  infective F06.8
    acute or subacute F05
  post-traumatic F06.8
    acute or subacute F05
paranoiac F22
paranoid (climacteric) (involutional) (menopausal) F22
  psychogenic (acute) F23
  schizophrenic F20.0
  senile F03 ☑
postpartum F53
presbyophrenic (type) F03 ☑
presenile F03 ☑
psychogenic (paranoid) F23
  depressive F32.3
puerperal F53
  specified type — *see* Psychosis, by type
reactive (brief) (transient) (emotional stress) (psychological trauma) F23
  depressive F32.3
    recurrent F33.3
  excitative type F30.8
schizoaffective F25.9
  depressive type F25.1
  manic type F25.0
schizophrenia, schizophrenic — *see* Schizophrenia
schizophrenia-like, in epilepsy F06.2
schizophreniform F20.81
  affective type F25.9
  brief F23
  confusional type F23
  depressive type F25.1
  manic type F25.0
  mixed type F25.0
senile NEC F03 ☑
  depressed or paranoid type F03 ☑
  simple deterioration F03 ☑
  specified type — *code to* condition
shared F24
situational (reactive) F23
symbiotic (childhood) F84.3
symptomatic F09
Psychosomatic — *see* Disorder, psychosomatic
Psychosyndrome, organic F07.9
Psychotic episode due to or associated with physical
  condition F06.8
Pterygium (eye) H11.00- ☑
  amyloid H11.01- ☑
  central H11.02- ☑
  colli Q18.3
  double H11.03- ☑
  peripheral
    progressive H11.05- ☑
    stationary H11.04- ☑
  recurrent H11.06- ☑

Ptilosis (eyelid) — *see* Madarosis
Ptomaine (poisoning) — *see* Poisoning, food
Ptosis (*see also* Blepharoptosis)
  adiposa (false) — *see* Blepharoptosis
  breast N64.81
  cecum K63.4
  colon K63.4
  congenital (eyelid) Q10.0
    specified site NEC — *see* Anomaly, by site
  eyelid — *see* Blepharoptosis
    congenital Q10.0
  gastric K31.89
  intestine K63.4
  kidney N28.83
  liver K76.89
  renal N28.83
  splanchnic K63.4
  spleen D73.89
  stomach K31.89
  viscera K63.4
PTP D69.51
Ptyalism (periodic) K11.7
  hysterical F45.8
  pregnancy — *see* Pregnancy, complicated by, specified
    pregnancy-related condition NEC
  psychogenic F45.8
Ptyalolithiasis K11.5
Pubarche, precocious E30.1
Pubertas praecox E30.1
Puberty (development state) Z00.3
  bleeding (excessive) N92.2
  delayed E30.0
  precocious (constitutional) (cryptogenic) (idiopathic)
    E30.1
    central E22.8
    due to
      ovarian hyperfunction E28.1
        estrogen E28.0
      testicular hyperfunction E29.0
  premature E30.1
    due to
      adrenal cortical hyperfunction E25.8
      pineal tumor E34.8
      pituitary (anterior) hyperfunction E22.8
Puckering, macula — *see* Degeneration, macula, puckering
Pudenda, pudendum — *see* condition
Puente's disease (simple glandular cheilitis) K13.0
Puerperal, puerperium (complicated by, complications)
  abnormal glucose (tolerance test) O99.815
  abscess
    areola O91.02
      associated with lactation O91.03
    Bartholin's gland O86.19
    breast O91.12
      associated with lactation O91.13
    cervix (uteri) O86.11
    genital organ NEC O86.19
    kidney O86.21
    mammary O91.12
      associated with lactation O91.13
    nipple O91.02
      associated with lactation O91.03
    peritoneum O85
    subareolar O91.12
      associated with lactation O91.13
    urinary tract — *see* Puerperal, infection, urinary
    uterus O86.12
    vagina (wall) O86.13
    vaginorectal O86.13
    vulvovaginal gland O86.13
  adnexitis O86.19
  afibrinogenemia, or other coagulation defect O72.3
  albuminuria (acute) (subacute) — *see* Proteinuria,
    gestational
  alcohol use O99.315
  anemia O90.81
    pre-existing (pre-pregnancy) O99.03
  anesthetic death O89.8
  apoplexy O99.43
  bariatric surgery status O99.845
  blood disorder NEC O99.13
  blood dyscrasia O72.3
  cardiomyopathy O90.3
  cerebrovascular disorder (conditions in I60-I69) O99.43
  cervicitis O86.11
  circulatory system disorder O99.43
  coagulopathy (any) O72.3

Puerperal, puerperium — *continued*
- complications O90.9
  - specified NEC O90.89
- convulsions — *see* Eclampsia
- cystitis O86.22
- cystopyelitis O86.29
- delirium NEC F05
- diabetes O24.93
  - gestational — *see* Puerperal, gestational diabetes
  - pre-existing O24.33
    - specified NEC O24.83
    - type 1 O24.03
    - type 2 O24.13
- digestive system disorder O99.63
- disease O90.9
  - breast NEC O92.29
  - cerebrovascular (acute) O99.43
  - nonobstetric NEC O99.89
  - tubo-ovarian O86.19
  - Valsuani's O99.03
- disorder O90.9
  - biliary tract O26.63
  - lactation O92.70
  - liver O26.63
  - nonobstetric NEC O99.89
- disruption
  - cesarean wound O90.0
  - episiotomy wound O90.1
  - perineal laceration wound O90.1
- drug use O99.325
- eclampsia (with pre-existing hypertension) O15.2
- embolism (pulmonary) (blood clot) — *see* Embolism, obstetric, puerperal
- endocrine, nutritional or metabolic disease NEC O99.285
- endophlebitis — *see* Puerperal, phlebitis
- endotrachelitis O86.11
- failure
  - lactation (complete) O92.3
    - partial O92.4
  - renal, acute O90.4
- fever (of unknown origin) O86.4
  - septic O85
- fissure, nipple O92.12
  - associated with lactation O92.13
- fistula
  - breast (due to mastitis) O91.12
    - associated with lactation O91.13
  - nipple O91.02
    - associated with lactation O91.03
- galactophoritis O91.22
  - associated with lactation O91.23
- galactorrhea O92.6
- gastric banding status O99.845
- gastric bypass status O99.845
- gastrointestinal disease NEC O99.63
- gestational diabetes O24.439
  - diet controlled O24.430
  - insulin (and diet) controlled O24.434
- gonorrhea O98.23
- hematoma, subdural O99.43
- hemiplegia, cerebral O99.355
  - due to cerebrovascular disorder O99.43
- hemorrhage O72.1
  - brain O99.43
  - bulbar O99.43
  - cerebellar O99.43
  - cerebral O99.43
  - cortical O99.43
  - delayed or secondary O72.2
  - extradural O99.43
  - internal capsule O99.43
  - intracranial O99.43
  - intrapontine O99.43
  - meningeal O99.43
  - pontine O99.43
  - retained placenta O72.0
  - subarachnoid O99.43
  - subcortical O99.43
  - subdural O99.43
  - third stage O72.0
  - uterine, delayed O72.2
  - ventricular O99.43
- hemorrhoids O87.2
- hepatorenal syndrome O90.4
- hypertension — *see* Hypertension, complicating, puerperium
- hypertrophy, breast O92.29

Puerperal, puerperium — *continued*
- induration breast (fibrous) O92.29
- infection O86.4
  - cervix O86.11
  - generalized O85
  - genital tract NEC O86.19
    - obstetric surgical wound O86.0
  - kidney (bacillus coli) O86.21
  - maternal O98.93
    - carrier state NEC O99.835
    - gonorrhea O98.23
    - human immunodeficiency virus (HIV) O98.73
    - protozoal O98.63
    - sexually transmitted NEC O98.33
    - specified NEC O98.83
    - streptococcus B carrier state O99.825
    - syphilis O98.13
    - tuberculosis O98.03
    - viral hepatitis O98.43
    - viral NEC O98.53
  - nipple O91.02
    - associated with lactation O91.03
  - peritoneum O85
  - renal O86.21
  - specified NEC O86.89
  - urinary (asymptomatic) (tract) NEC O86.20
    - bladder O86.22
    - kidney O86.21
    - specified site NEC O86.29
    - urethra O86.22
  - vagina O86.13
  - vein — *see* Puerperal, phlebitis
- ischemia, cerebral O99.43
- lymphangitis O86.89
  - breast O91.22
    - associated with lactation O91.23
- malignancy O9A.13 (*following* O99)
- malnutrition O25.3
- mammillitis O91.02
  - associated with lactation O91.03
- mammitis O91.22
  - associated with lactation O91.23
- mania F30.8
- mastitis O91.22
  - associated with lactation O91.23
  - purulent O91.12
    - associated with lactation O91.13
- melancholia — *see* Disorder, depressive
- mental disorder NEC O99.345
- metroperitonitis O85
- metrorrhagia — *see* Hemorrhage, postpartum
- metrosalpingitis O86.19
- metrovaginitis O86.13
- milk leg O87.1
- monoplegia, cerebral O99.43
- mood disturbance O90.6
- necrosis, liver (acute) (subacute) (conditions in subcategory K72.0) O26.63
  - with renal failure O90.4
- nervous system disorder O99.355
- obesity (pre-existing prior to pregnancy) O99.215
- obesity surgery status O99.845
- occlusion, precerebral artery O99.43
- paralysis
  - bladder (sphincter) O90.89
  - cerebral O99.43
- paralytic stroke O99.43
- parametritis O85
- paravaginitis O86.13
- pelviperitonitis O85
- perimetritis O86.12
- perimetrosalpingitis O86.19
- perinephritis O86.21
- periphlebitis — *see* Puerperal phlebitis
- peritoneal infection O85
- peritonitis (pelvic) O85
- perivaginitis O86.13
- phlebitis O87.0
  - deep O87.1
  - pelvic O87.1
  - superficial O87.0
- phlebothrombosis, deep O87.1
- phlegmasia alba dolens O87.1
- placental polyp O90.89
- pneumonia, embolic — *see* Embolism, obstetric, puerperal
- pre-eclampsia — *see* Pre-eclampsia
- psychosis F53

Puerperal, puerperium — *continued*
- pyelitis O86.21
- pyelocystitis O86.29
- pyelonephritis O86.21
- pyelonephrosis O86.21
- pyemia O85
- pyocystitis O86.29
- pyohemia O85
- pyometra O86.12
- pyonephritis O86.21
- pyosalpingitis O86.19
- pyrexia (of unknown origin) O86.4
- renal
  - disease NEC O90.89
  - failure O90.4
- respiratory disease NEC O99.53
- retention
  - decidua — *see* Retention, decidua
  - placenta O72.0
  - secundines — *see* Retention, secundines
- retrated nipple O92.02
- salpingo-ovaritis O86.19
- salpingoperitonitis O85
- secondary perineal tear O90.1
- sepsis (pelvic) O85
- sepsis O85
- septic thrombophlebitis O86.81
- skin disorder NEC O99.73
- specified condition NEC O99.89
- stroke O99.43
- subinvolution (uterus) O90.89
- subluxation of symphysis (pubis) O26.73
- suppuration — *see* Puerperal, abscess
- tetanus A34
- thelitis O91.02
  - associated with lactation O91.03
- thrombocytopenia O72.3
- thrombophlebitis (superficial) O87.0
  - deep O87.1
  - pelvic O87.1
  - septic O86.81
- thrombosis (venous) — *see* Thrombosis, puerperal
- thyroiditis O90.5
- toxemia (eclamptic) (pre-eclamptic) (with convulsions) O15.2
- trauma, non-obstetric O9A.23 (*following* O99)
  - caused by abuse (physical) (suspected) O9A.33 (*following* O99)
    - confirmed O9A.33 (*following* O99)
    - psychological (suspected) O9A.53 (*following* O99)
      - confirmed O9A.53 (*following* O99)
    - sexual (suspected) O9A.43 (*following* O99)
      - confirmed O9A.43 (*following* O99)
- uremia (due to renal failure) O90.4
- urethritis O86.22
- vaginitis O86.13
- varicose veins (legs) O87.4
  - vulva or perineum O87.8
- venous O87.9
- vulvitis O86.19
- vulvovaginitis O86.13
- white leg O87.1

Puerperium — *see* Puerperal

Pulmolithiasis J98.4

Pulmonary — *see* condition

Pulpitis (acute) (anachoretic) (chronic) (hyperplastic) (irreversible) (putrescent) (reversible) (suppurative) (ulcerative) K04.0

Pulpless tooth K04.99

Pulse
- alternating R00.8
- bigeminal R00.8
- fast R00.0
- feeble, rapid due to shock following injury T79.4 ☑
- rapid R00.0
- weak R09.89

Pulsus alternans or trigeminus R00.8

Punch drunk F07.81

Punctum lacrimale occlusion — *see* Obstruction, lacrimal

Puncture
- abdomen, abdominal
  - wall S31.139 ☑
    - with
      - foreign body S31.149 ☑

Puncture — *continued*
  abdomen, abdominal — *continued*
    wall — *continued*
      with — *continued*
        penetration into peritoneal cavity
          S31.639 ☑
          with foreign body S31.649 ☑
        epigastric region S31.132 ☑
          with
            foreign body S31.142 ☑
            penetration into peritoneal cavity
              S31.632 ☑
              with foreign body S31.642 ☑
        left
          lower quadrant S31.134 ☑
            with
              foreign body S31.144 ☑
              penetration into peritoneal cavity
                S31.634 ☑
                with foreign body S31.644 ☑
          upper quadrant S31.131 ☑
            with
              foreign body S31.141 ☑
              penetration into peritoneal cavity
                S31.631 ☑
                with foreign body S31.641 ☑
        periumbilic region S31.135 ☑
          with
            foreign body S31.145 ☑
            penetration into peritoneal cavity
              S31.635 ☑
              with foreign body S31.645 ☑
        right
          lower quadrant S31.133 ☑
            with
              foreign body S31.143 ☑
              penetration into peritoneal cavity
                S31.633 ☑
                with foreign body S31.643 ☑
          upper quadrant S31.130 ☑
            with
              foreign body S31.140 ☑
              penetration into peritoneal cavity
                S31.630 ☑
                with foreign body S31.640 ☑
  accidental, complicating surgery — *see* Complication,
    accidental puncture or laceration
  alveolar (process) — *see* Puncture, oral cavity
  ankle S91.039 ☑
    with
      foreign body S91.049 ☑
    left S91.032 ☑
      with
        foreign body S91.042 ☑
    right S91.031 ☑
      with
        foreign body S91.041 ☑
  anus S31.833 ☑
    with foreign body S31.834 ☑
  arm (upper) S41.139 ☑
    with foreign body S41.149 ☑
    left S41.132 ☑
      with foreign body S41.142 ☑
    lower — *see* Puncture, forearm
    right S41.131 ☑
      with foreign body S41.141 ☑
  auditory canal (external) (meatus) — *see* Puncture,
    ear
  auricle, ear — *see* Puncture, ear
  axilla — *see* Puncture, arm
  back (*see also* Puncture, thorax, back)
    lower S31.030 ☑
      with
        foreign body S31.040 ☑
          with penetration into retroperitoneal
            space S31.041 ☑
        penetration into retroperitoneal space
          S31.031 ☑
  bladder (traumatic) S37.29 ☑
    nontraumatic N32.89
  breast S21.039 ☑
    with foreign body S21.049 ☑
    left S21.032 ☑
      with foreign body S21.042 ☑
    right S21.031 ☑
      with foreign body S21.041 ☑

Puncture — *continued*
  buttock S31.803 ☑
    with foreign body S31.804 ☑
    left S31.823 ☑
      with foreign body S31.824 ☑
    right S31.813 ☑
      with foreign body S31.814 ☑
  by
    device, implant or graft — *see* Complications, by
      site and type, mechanical
    foreign body left accidentally in operative wound
      T81.539 ☑
    instrument (any) during a procedure, accidental
      — *see* Puncture, accidental complicating
      surgery
  calf — *see* Puncture, leg
  canaliculus lacrimalis — *see* Puncture, eyelid
  canthus, eye — *see* Puncture, eyelid
  cervical esophagus S11.23 ☑
    with foreign body S11.24 ☑
  cheek (external) S01.439 ☑
    with foreign body S01.449 ☑
    internal — *see* Puncture, oral cavity
    left S01.432 ☑
      with foreign body S01.442 ☑
    right S01.431 ☑
      with foreign body S01.441 ☑
  chest wall — *see* Puncture, thorax
  chin — *see* Puncture, head, specified site NEC
  clitoris — *see* Puncture, vulva
  costal region — *see* Puncture, thorax
  digit(s)
    foot — *see* Puncture, toe
    hand — *see* Puncture, finger
  ear (canal) (external) S01.339 ☑
    with foreign body S01.349 ☑
    drum S09.2- ☑
    left S01.332 ☑
      with foreign body S01.342 ☑
    right S01.331 ☑
      with foreign body S01.341 ☑
  elbow S51.039 ☑
    with
      foreign body S51.049 ☑
    left S51.032 ☑
      with
        foreign body S51.042 ☑
    right S51.031 ☑
      with
        foreign body S51.041 ☑
  epididymis — *see* Puncture, testis
  epigastric region — *see* Puncture, abdomen, wall,
    epigastric
  epiglottis S11.83 ☑
    with foreign body S11.84 ☑
  esophagus
    cervical S11.23 ☑
      with foreign body S11.24 ☑
    thoracic S27.818 ☑
  eyeball S05.6- ☑
    with foreign body S05.5- ☑
  eyebrow — *see* Puncture, eyelid
  eyelid S01.13- ☑
    with foreign body S01.14- ☑
    left S01.132 ☑
      with foreign body S01.142 ☑
    right S01.131 ☑
      with foreign body S01.141 ☑
  face NEC — *see* Puncture, head, specified site NEC
  finger(s) S61.239 ☑
    with
      damage to nail S61.339 ☑
        with
          foreign body S61.349 ☑
      foreign body S61.249 ☑
    index S61.238 ☑
      with
        damage to nail S61.338 ☑
          with
            foreign body S61.348 ☑
        foreign body S61.248 ☑
      left S61.231 ☑
        with
          damage to nail S61.331 ☑
            with
              foreign body S61.341 ☑

Puncture — *continued*
  finger(s) — *continued*
    index — *continued*
      left — *continued*
        with — *continued*
          foreign body S61.241 ☑
      right S61.230 ☑
        with
          damage to nail S61.330 ☑
            with
              foreign body S61.340 ☑
            foreign body S61.240 ☑
    little S61.238 ☑
      with
        damage to nail S61.338 ☑
          with
            foreign body S61.348 ☑
        foreign body S61.248 ☑
      left S61.237 ☑
        with
          damage to nail S61.337 ☑
            with
              foreign body S61.347 ☑
            foreign body S61.247 ☑
      right S61.236 ☑
        with
          damage to nail S61.336 ☑
            with
              foreign body S61.346 ☑
            foreign body S61.246 ☑
    middle S61.238 ☑
      with
        damage to nail S61.338 ☑
          with
            foreign body S61.348 ☑
        foreign body S61.248 ☑
      left S61.233 ☑
        with
          damage to nail S61.333 ☑
            with
              foreign body S61.343 ☑
            foreign body S61.243 ☑
      right S61.232 ☑
        with
          damage to nail S61.332 ☑
            with
              foreign body S61.342 ☑
            foreign body S61.242 ☑
    ring S61.238 ☑
      with
        damage to nail S61.338 ☑
          with
            foreign body S61.348 ☑
        foreign body S61.248 ☑
      left S61.235 ☑
        with
          damage to nail S61.335 ☑
            with
              foreign body S61.345 ☑
            foreign body S61.245 ☑
      right S61.234 ☑
        with
          damage to nail S61.334 ☑
            with
              foreign body S61.344 ☑
            foreign body S61.244 ☑
  flank S31.139 ☑
    with foreign body S31.149 ☑
  foot (except toe(s) alone) S91.339 ☑
    with foreign body S91.349 ☑
    left S91.332 ☑
      with foreign body S91.342 ☑
    right S91.331 ☑
      with foreign body S91.341 ☑
    toe — *see* Puncture, toe
  forearm S51.839 ☑
    with
      foreign body S51.849 ☑
    elbow only — *see* Puncture, elbow
    left S51.832 ☑
      with
        foreign body S51.842 ☑
    right S51.831 ☑
      with
        foreign body S51.841 ☑
  forehead — *see* Puncture, head, specified site NEC

Puncture — *continued*
  genital organs, external
    female S31.532 ☑
      with foreign body S31.542 ☑
      vagina — *see* Puncture, vagina
      vulva — *see* Puncture, vulva
    male S31.531 ☑
      with foreign body S31.541 ☑
      penis — *see* Puncture, penis
      scrotum — *see* Puncture, scrotum
      testis — *see* Puncture, testis
  groin — *see* Puncture, abdomen, wall
  gum — *see* Puncture, oral cavity
  hand S61.439 ☑
    with
      foreign body S61.449 ☑
    finger — *see* Puncture, finger
    left S61.432 ☑
      with
        foreign body S61.442 ☑
    right S61.431 ☑
      with
        foreign body S61.441 ☑
    thumb — *see* Puncture, thumb
  head S01.93 ☑
    with foreign body S01.94 ☑
    cheek — *see* Puncture, cheek
    ear — *see* Puncture, ear
    eyelid — *see* Puncture, eyelid
    lip — *see* Puncture, oral cavity
    nose — *see* Puncture, nose
    oral cavity — *see* Puncture, oral cavity
    scalp S01.03 ☑
      with foreign body S01.04 ☑
    specified site NEC S01.83 ☑
      with foreign body S01.84 ☑
    temporomandibular area — *see* Puncture, cheek
  heart S26.99 ☑
    with hemopericardium S26.09 ☑
    without hemopericardium S26.19 ☑
  heel — *see* Puncture, foot
  hip S71.039 ☑
    with foreign body S71.049 ☑
    left S71.032 ☑
      with foreign body S71.042 ☑
    right S71.031 ☑
      with foreign body S71.041 ☑
  hymen — *see* Puncture, vagina
  hypochondrium — *see* Puncture, abdomen, wall
  hypogastric region — *see* Puncture, abdomen, wall
  inguinal region — *see* Puncture, abdomen, wall
  instep — *see* Puncture, foot
  internal organs — *see* Injury, by site
  interscapular region — *see* Puncture, thorax, back
  intestine
    large
      colon S36.599 ☑
        ascending S36.590 ☑
        descending S36.592 ☑
        sigmoid S36.593 ☑
        specified site NEC S36.598 ☑
        transverse S36.591 ☑
      rectum S36.69 ☑
    small S36.499 ☑
      duodenum S36.490 ☑
      specified site NEC S36.498 ☑
  intra-abdominal organ S36.99 ☑
    gallbladder S36.128 ☑
    intestine — *see* Puncture, intestine
    liver S36.118 ☑
    pancreas — *see* Puncture, pancreas
    peritoneum S36.81 ☑
    specified site NEC S36.898 ☑
    spleen S36.09 ☑
    stomach S36.39 ☑
  jaw — *see* Puncture, head, specified site NEC
  knee S81.039 ☑
    with foreign body S81.049 ☑
    left S81.032 ☑
      with foreign body S81.042 ☑
    right S81.031 ☑
      with foreign body S81.041 ☑
  labium (majus) (minus) — *see* Puncture, vulva
  lacrimal duct — *see* Puncture, eyelid
  larynx S11.013 ☑
    with foreign body S11.014 ☑

Puncture — *continued*
  leg (lower) S81.839 ☑
    with foreign body S81.849 ☑
    foot — *see* Puncture, foot
    knee — *see* Puncture, knee
    left S81.832 ☑
      with foreign body S81.842 ☑
    right S81.831 ☑
      with foreign body S81.841 ☑
    upper — *see* Puncture, thigh
  lip S01.531 ☑
    with foreign body S01.541 ☑
  loin — *see* Puncture, abdomen, wall
  lower back — *see* Puncture, back, lower
  lumbar region — *see* Puncture, back, lower
  malar region — *see* Puncture, head, specified site NEC
  mammary — *see* Puncture, breast
  mastoid region — *see* Puncture, head, specified site NEC
  mouth — *see* Puncture, oral cavity
  nail
    finger — *see* Puncture, finger, with damage to nail
    toe — *see* Puncture, toe, with damage to nail
  nasal (septum) (sinus) — *see* Puncture, nose
  nasopharynx — *see* Puncture, head, specified site NEC
  neck S11.93 ☑
    with foreign body S11.94 ☑
    involving
      cervical esophagus — *see* Puncture, cervical esophagus
      larynx — *see* Puncture, larynx
      pharynx — *see* Puncture, pharynx
      thyroid gland — *see* Puncture, thyroid gland
      trachea — *see* Puncture, trachea
    specified site NEC S11.83 ☑
      with foreign body S11.84 ☑
  nose (septum) (sinus) S01.23 ☑
    with foreign body S01.24 ☑
  ocular — *see* Puncture, eyeball
  oral cavity S01.532 ☑
    with foreign body S01.542 ☑
  orbit S05.4- ☑
  palate — *see* Puncture, oral cavity
  palm — *see* Puncture, hand
  pancreas S36.299 ☑
    body S36.291 ☑
    head S36.290 ☑
    tail S36.292 ☑
  pelvis — *see* Puncture, back, lower
  penis S31.23 ☑
    with foreign body S31.24 ☑
  perineum
    female S31.43 ☑
      with foreign body S31.44 ☑
    male S31.139 ☑
      with foreign body S31.149 ☑
  periocular area (with or without lacrimal passages) — *see* Puncture, eyelid
  phalanges
    finger — *see* Puncture, finger
    toe — *see* Puncture, toe
  pharynx S11.23 ☑
    with foreign body S11.24 ☑
  pinna — *see* Puncture, ear
  popliteal space — *see* Puncture, knee
  prepuce — *see* Puncture, penis
  pubic region S31.139 ☑
    with foreign body S31.149 ☑
  pudendum — *see* Puncture, genital organs, external
  rectovaginal septum — *see* Puncture, vagina
  sacral region — *see* Puncture, back, lower
  sacroiliac region — *see* Puncture, back, lower
  salivary gland — *see* Puncture, oral cavity
  scalp S01.03 ☑
    with foreign body S01.04 ☑
  scapular region — *see* Puncture, shoulder
  scrotum S31.33 ☑
    with foreign body S31.34 ☑
  shin — *see* Puncture, leg
  shoulder S41.039 ☑
    with foreign body S41.049 ☑
    left S41.032 ☑
      with foreign body S41.042 ☑
    right S41.031 ☑
      with foreign body S41.041 ☑
  spermatic cord — *see* Puncture, testis

Puncture — *continued*
  sternal region — *see* Puncture, thorax, front
  submaxillary region — *see* Puncture, head, specified site NEC
  submental region — *see* Puncture, head, specified site NEC
  subungual
    finger(s) — *see* Puncture, finger, with damage to nail
    toe — *see* Puncture, toe, with damage to nail
  supraclavicular fossa — *see* Puncture, neck, specified site NEC
  temple, temporal region — *see* Puncture, head, specified site NEC
  temporomandibular area — *see* Puncture, cheek
  testis S31.33 ☑
    with foreign body S31.34 ☑
  thigh S71.139 ☑
    with foreign body S71.149 ☑
    left S71.132 ☑
      with foreign body S71.142 ☑
    right S71.131 ☑
      with foreign body S71.141 ☑
  thorax, thoracic (wall) S21.93 ☑
    with foreign body S21.94 ☑
    back S21.23- ☑
      with
        foreign body S21.24- ☑
          with penetration S21.44 ☑
        penetration S21.43 ☑
    breast — *see* Puncture, breast
    front S21.13- ☑
      with
        foreign body S21.14- ☑
          with penetration S21.34 ☑
        penetration S21.33 ☑
  throat — *see* Puncture, neck
  thumb S61.039 ☑
    with
      damage to nail S61.139 ☑
        with
          foreign body S61.149 ☑
      foreign body S61.049 ☑
    left S61.032 ☑
      with
        damage to nail S61.132 ☑
          with
            foreign body S61.142 ☑
        foreign body S61.042 ☑
    right S61.031 ☑
      with
        damage to nail S61.131 ☑
          with
            foreign body S61.141 ☑
        foreign body S61.041 ☑
  thyroid gland S11.13 ☑
    with foreign body S11.14 ☑
  toe(s) S91.139 ☑
    with
      damage to nail S91.239 ☑
        with
          foreign body S91.249 ☑
      foreign body S91.149 ☑
    great S91.133 ☑
      with
        damage to nail S91.233 ☑
          with
            foreign body S91.243 ☑
        foreign body S91.143 ☑
      left S91.132 ☑
        with
          damage to nail S91.232 ☑
            with
              foreign body S91.242 ☑
          foreign body S91.142 ☑
      right S91.131 ☑
        with
          damage to nail S91.231 ☑
            with
              foreign body S91.241 ☑
          foreign body S91.141 ☑
    lesser S91.136 ☑
      with
        damage to nail S91.236 ☑
          with
            foreign body S91.246 ☑

☑ **Additional Character Required** — Refer to the Tabular List for Character Selection   ▼ Subterms under main terms may continue to next column or page

Puncture — *continued*
  toe(s) — *continued*
    lesser — *continued*
      with — *continued*
        foreign body S91.146 ☑
      left S91.135 ☑
        with
          damage to nail S91.235 ☑
            with
              foreign body S91.245 ☑
          foreign body S91.145 ☑
      right S91.134 ☑
        with
          damage to nail S91.234 ☑
            with
              foreign body S91.244 ☑
          foreign body S91.144 ☑
  tongue — *see* Puncture, oral cavity
  trachea S11.023 ☑
    with foreign body S11.024 ☑
  tunica vaginalis — *see* Puncture, testis
  tympanum, tympanic membrane S09.2- ☑
  umbilical region S31.135 ☑
    with foreign body S31.145 ☑
  uvula — *see* Puncture, oral cavity
  vagina S31.43 ☑
    with foreign body S31.44 ☑
  vocal cords S11.033 ☑
    with foreign body S11.034 ☑
  vulva S31.43 ☑
    with foreign body S31.44 ☑
  wrist S61.539 ☑
    with
      foreign body S61.549 ☑
    left S61.532 ☑
      with
        foreign body S61.542 ☑
    right S61.531 ☑
      with
        foreign body S61.541 ☑
PUO (pyrexia of unknown origin) R50.9
Pupillary membrane (persistent) Q13.89
Pupillotonia — *see* Anomaly, pupil, function, tonic pupil
Purpura D69.2
  abdominal D69.0
  allergic D69.0
  anaphylactoid D69.0
  annularis telangiectodes L81.7
  arthritic D69.0
  autoerythrocyte sensitization D69.2
  autoimmune D69.0
  bacterial D69.0
  Bateman's (senile) D69.2
  capillary fragility (hereditary) (idiopathic) D69.8
  cryoglobulinemic D89.1
  Devil's pinches D69.2
  fibrinolytic — *see* Fibrinolysis
  fulminans, fulminous D65
  gangrenous D65
  hemorrhagic, hemorrhagica D69.3
    not due to thrombocytopenia D69.0
  Henoch (-Schönlein) (allergic) D69.0
  hypergammaglobulinemic (benign) (Waldenström)
    D89.0
  idiopathic (thrombocytopenic) D69.3
    nonthrombocytopenic D69.0
  immune thrombocytopenic D69.3
  infectious D69.0
  malignant D69.0
  neonatorum P54.5
  nervosa D69.0
  newborn P54.5
  nonthrombocytopenic D69.2
    hemorrhagic D69.0
    idiopathic D69.0
  nonthrombopenic D69.2
  peliosis rheumatica D69.0
  posttransfusion (post-transfusion) (from (fresh) whole
    blood or blood products) D69.51
  primary D69.49
  red cell membrane sensitivity D69.2
  rheumatica D69.0
  Schönlein (-Henoch) (allergic) D69.0
  scorbutic E54 [D77]
  senile D69.2
  simplex D69.2
  symptomatica D69.0

Purpura — *continued*
  telangiectasia annularis L81.7
  thrombocytopenic D69.49
    congenital D69.42
    hemorrhagic D69.3
    hereditary D69.42
    idiopathic D69.3
    immune D69.3
    neonatal, transitory P61.0
    thrombotic M31.1
  thrombohemolytic — *see* Fibrinolysis
  thrombolytic — *see* Fibrinolysis
  thrombopenic D69.49
  thrombotic, thrombocytopenic M31.1
  toxic D69.0
  vascular D69.0
  visceral symptoms D69.0
Purpuric spots R23.3
Purulent — *see* condition
Pus
  in
    stool R19.5
    urine N39.0
  tube (rupture) — *see* Salpingo-oophoritis
Pustular rash L08.0
Pustule (nonmalignant) L08.9
  malignant A22.0
Pustulosis palmaris et plantaris L40.3
Putnam (-Dana) disease or syndrome — *see* Degeneration, combined
Putrescent pulp (dental) K04.1
Pyarthritis, pyarthrosis — *see* Arthritis, pyogenic or pyemic
  tuberculous — *see* Tuberculosis, joint
Pyelectasis — *see* Hydronephrosis
Pyelitis (congenital) (uremic) (*see also* Pyelonephritis)
  with
    calculus — *see* category N20 ☑
      with hydronephrosis N13.2
    contracted kidney N11.9
  acute N10
  chronic N11.9
    with calculus — *see* category N20 ☑
      with hydronephrosis N13.2
  cystica N28.84
  puerperal (postpartum) O86.21
  tuberculous A18.11
Pyelocystitis — *see* Pyelonephritis
Pyelonephritis (*see also* Nephritis, tubulo-interstitial)
  with
    calculus — *see* category N20 ☑
      with hydronephrosis N13.2
    contracted kidney N11.9
  acute N10
  calculous — *see* category N20 ☑
    with hydronephrosis N13.2
  chronic N11.9
    with calculus — *see* category N20 ☑
      with hydronephrosis N13.2
    associated with ureteral obstruction or stricture
      N11.1
    nonobstructive N11.8
      with reflux (vesicoureteral) N11.0
    obstructive N11.1
    specified NEC N11.8
  in (due to)
    brucellosis A23.9 [N16]
    cryoglobulinemia (mixed) D89.1 [N16]
    cystinosis E72.04
    diphtheria A36.84
    glycogen storage disease E74.09 [N16]
    leukemia NEC C95.9- ☑ [N16]
    lymphoma NEC C85.90 [N16]
    multiple myeloma C90.0- ☑ [N16]
    obstruction N11.1
    Salmonella infection A02.25
    sarcoidosis D86.84
    sepsis A41.9 [N16]
    Sjögren's disease M35.04
    toxoplasmosis B58.83
    transplant rejection T86.91 [N16]
    Wilson's disease E83.01 [N16]
  nonobstructive N12
    with reflux (vesicoureteral) N11.0
    chronic N11.8
  syphilitic A52.75
Pyelonephrosis (obstructive) N11.1
  chronic N11.9

Pyelophlebitis I80.8
Pyeloureteritis cystica N28.85
Pyemia, pyemic (fever) (infection) (purulent) (*see also* Sepsis)
  joint — *see* Arthritis, pyogenic or pyemic
  liver K75.1
  pneumococcal A40.3
  portal K75.1
  postvaccinal T88.0 ☑
  puerperal, postpartum, childbirth O85
  specified organism NEC A41.89
  tuberculous — *see* Tuberculosis, miliary
Pygopagus Q89.4
Pyknoepilepsy (idiopathic) — *see* Pyknolepsy
Pyknolepsy G40.A09 (following G40.3)
  intractable G40.A19 (following G40.3)
    with status epilepticus G40.A11 (following G40.3)
    without status epilepticus G40.A19 (following
      G40.3)
  not intractable G40.A09 (following G40.3)
    with status epilepticus G40.A01 (following G40.3)
    without status epilepticus G40.A09 (following
      G40.3)
Pylephlebitis K75.1
Pyle's syndrome Q78.5
Pylethrombophlebitis K75.1
Pylethrombosis K75.1
Pyloritis K29.90
  with bleeding K29.91
Pylorospasm (reflex) **NEC** K31.3
  congenital or infantile Q40.0
  neurotic F45.8
  newborn Q40.0
  psychogenic F45.8
Pylorus, pyloric — *see* condition
Pyoarthrosis — *see* Arthritis, pyogenic or pyemic
Pyocele
  mastoid — *see* Mastoiditis, acute
  sinus (accessory) — *see* Sinusitis
  turbinate (bone) J32.9
  urethra (*see also* Urethritis) N34.0
Pyocolpos — *see* Vaginitis
Pyocystitis N30.80
  with hematuria N30.81
Pyoderma, pyodermia L08.0
  gangrenosum L88
  newborn P39.4
  phagedenic L88
  vegetans L08.81
Pyodermatitis L08.0
  vegetans L08.81
Pyogenic — *see* condition
Pyohydronephrosis N13.6
Pyometra, pyometrium, pyometritis — *see* Endometritis
Pyomyositis (tropical) — *see* Myositis, infective
Pyonephritis N12
Pyonephrosis N13.6
  tuberculous A18.11
Pyo-oophoritis — *see* Salpingo-oophoritis
Pyo-ovarium — *see* Salpingo-oophoritis
Pyopericarditis, pyopericardium I30.1
Pyophlebitis — *see* Phlebitis
Pyopneumopericardium I30.1
Pyopneumothorax (infective) J86.9
  with fistula J86.0
  tuberculous NEC A15.6
Pyosalpinx, pyosalpingitis (*see also* Salpingo-oophoritis)
Pyothorax J86.9
  with fistula J86.0
  tuberculous NEC A15.6
Pyoureter N28.89
  tuberculous A18.11
Pyramidopallidonigral syndrome G20
Pyrexia (of unknown origin) R50.9
  atmospheric T67.0 ☑
  during labor NEC O75.2
  heat T67.0 ☑
  newborn P81.9
    environmentally-induced P81.0
  persistent R50.9
  puerperal O86.4
Pyroglobulinemia NEC E88.09
Pyromania F63.1
Pyrosis R12
Pyuria (bacterial) N39.0

Q

Q fever A78
  with pneumonia A78
Quadricuspid aortic valve Q23.8
Quadrilateral fever A78
Quadriparesis — *see* Quadriplegia
  meaning muscle weakness M62.81
Quadriplegia G82.50
  complete
    C1-C4 level G82.51
    C5-C7 level G82.53
  congenital (cerebral) (spinal) G80.8
    spastic G80.0
  embolic (current episode) I63.4 ☑
  functional R53.2
  incomplete
    C1-C4 level G82.52
    C5-C7 level G82.54
  thrombotic (current episode) I63.3 ☑
  traumatic — *code to* injury with seventh character S
    current episode — *see* Injury, spinal (cord), cervical
Quadruplet, pregnancy — *see* Pregnancy, quadruplet
Quarrelsomeness F60.3
Queensland fever A77.3
Quervain's disease M65.4
  thyroid E06.1
Queyrat's erythroplasia D07.4
  penis D07.4
  specified site — *see* Neoplasm, skin, in situ
  unspecified site D07.4
Quincke's disease or edema T78.3 ☑
  hereditary D84.1
Quinsy (gangrenous) J36
Quintan fever A79.0
Quintuplet, pregnancy — *see* Pregnancy, quintuplet

R

Rabbit fever — *see* Tularemia
Rabies A82.9
  contact Z20.3
  exposure to Z20.3
  inoculation reaction — *see* Complications, vaccination
  sylvatic A82.0
  urban A82.1
Rachischisis — *see* Spina bifida
Rachitic (*see also* condition)
  deformities of spine (late effect) (sequelae) E64.3
  pelvis (late effect) (sequelae) E64.3
    with disproportion (fetopelvic) O33.0
      causing obstructed labor O65.0
Rachitis, rachitism (acute) (tarda) (*see also* Rickets)
  renalis N25.0
  sequelae E64.3
Radial nerve — *see* condition
Radiation
  burn — *see* Burn
  effects NOS T66 ☑
  sickness NOS T66 ☑
  therapy, encounter for Z51.0
Radiculitis (pressure) (vertebrogenic) — *see* Radiculopathy
Radiculomyelitis (*see also* Encephalitis)
  toxic, due to
    Clostridium tetani A35
    Corynebacterium diphtheriae A36.82
Radiculopathy M54.10
  cervical region M54.12
  cervicothoracic region M54.13
  due to
    disc disorder
      C3 M50.11
      C4 M50.11
      C5 M50.12
      C6 M50.12
      C7 M50.12
      C8 M50.13
    displacement of intervertebral disc — *see* Disorder, disc, with, radiculopathy
  leg M54.1- ☑
  lumbar region M54.16
  lumbosacral region M54.17
  occipito-atlanto-axial region M54.11
  postherpetic B02.29
  sacrococcygeal region M54.18

Radiculopathy — *continued*
  syphilitic A52.11
  thoracic region (with visceral pain) M54.14
  thoracolumbar region M54.15
Radiodermal burns (acute, chronic, or occupational) — *see* Burn
Radiodermatitis L58.9
  acute L58.0
  chronic L58.1
Radiotherapy session Z51.0
Rage, meaning rabies — *see* Rabies
Ragpicker's disease A22.1
Ragsorter's disease A22.1
Raillietiniasis B71.8
Railroad neurosis F48.8
Railway spine F48.8
Raised (*see also* Elevated)
  antibody titer R76.0
Rake teeth, tooth M26.39
Rales R09.89
Ramifying renal pelvis Q63.8
Ramsay-Hunt disease or syndrome (*see also* Hunt's disease) B02.21
  meaning dyssynergia cerebellaris myoclonica G11.1
Ranula K11.6
  congenital Q38.4
Rape
  adult
    confirmed T74.21 ☑
    suspected T76.21 ☑
  alleged, observation or examination, ruled out
    adult Z04.41
    child Z04.42
  child
    confirmed T74.22 ☑
    suspected T76.22 ☑
Rapid
  feeble pulse, due to shock, following injury T79.4 ☑
  heart (beat) R00.0
    psychogenic F45.8
  second stage (delivery) O62.3
  time-zone change syndrome — *see* Disorder, sleep, circadian rhythm, psychogenic
Rarefaction, bone — *see* Disorder, bone, density and structure, specified NEC
Rash (toxic) R21
  canker A38.9
  diaper L22
  drug (internal use) L27.0
    contact (*see also* Dermatitis, due to, drugs, external) L25.1
  following immunization T88.1 ☑
  food — *see* Dermatitis, due to, food
  heat L74.0
  napkin (psoriasiform) L22
  nettle — *see* Urticaria
  pustular L08.0
  rose R21
    epidemic B06.9
  scarlet A38.9
  serum (*see also* Reaction, serum) T80.69 ☑
  wandering tongue K14.1
Rasmussen aneurysm — *see* Tuberculosis, pulmonary
Rasmussen encephalitis G04.81
Rat-bite fever A25.9
  due to Streptobacillus moniliformis A25.1
  spirochetal (morsus muris) A25.0
Rathke's pouch tumor D44.3
Raymond (-Céstan) **syndrome** I65.8
Raynaud's disease, phenomenon or syndrome (secondary) I73.00
  with gangrene (symmetric) I73.01
RDS (newborn) (type I) P22.0
  type II P22.1
Reaction (*see also* Disorder)
  adaptation — *see* Disorder, adjustment
  adjustment (anxiety) (conduct disorder) (depressiveness) (distress) — *see* Disorder, adjustment
    with
      mutism, elective (child) (adolescent) F94.0
  adverse
    food (any) (ingested) NEC T78.1 ☑
      anaphylactic — *see* Shock, anaphylactic, due to food
  affective — *see* Disorder, mood
  allergic — *see* Allergy
  anaphylactic — *see* Shock, anaphylactic

Reaction — *continued*
  anaphylactoid — *see* Shock, anaphylactic
  anesthesia — *see* Anesthesia, complication
  antitoxin (prophylactic) (therapeutic) — *see* Complications, vaccination
  anxiety F41.1
  Arthus — *see* Arthus' phenomenon
  asthenic F48.8
  combat and operational stress F43.0
  compulsive F42
  conversion F44.9
  crisis, acute F43.0
  deoxyribonuclease (DNA) (DNase) hypersensitivity D69.2
  depressive (single episode) F32.9
    affective (single episode) F31.4
      recurrent episode F33.9
    neurotic F34.1
    psychoneurotic F34.1
    psychotic F32.3
    recurrent — *see* Disorder, depressive, recurrent
  dissociative F44.9
  drug NEC T88.7 ☑
    addictive — *see* Dependence, drug
      transmitted via placenta or breast milk — *see* Absorption, drug, addictive, through placenta
    allergic — *see* Allergy, drug
    lichenoid L43.2
    newborn P93.8
      gray baby syndrome P93.0
    overdose or poisoning (by accident) — *see* Table of Drugs and Chemicals, by drug, poisoning
    photoallergic L56.1
    phototoxic L56.0
    withdrawal — *see* Dependence, by drug, with, withdrawal
      infant of dependent mother P96.1
      newborn P96.1
    wrong substance given or taken (by accident) — *see* Table of Drugs and Chemicals, by drug, poisoning
  fear F40.9
    child (abnormal) F93.8
  febrile nonhemolytic transfusion (FNHTR) R50.84
  fluid loss, cerebrospinal G97.1
  foreign
    body NEC — *see* Granuloma, foreign body
      in operative wound (inadvertently left) — *see* Foreign body, accidentally left during a procedure
    substance accidentally left during a procedure (chemical) (powder) (talc) T81.60 ☑
      aseptic peritonitis T81.61 ☑
      body or object (instrument) (sponge) (swab) — *see* Foreign body, accidentally left during a procedure
      specified reaction NEC T81.69 ☑
  grief — *see* Disorder, adjustment
  Herxheimer's R68.89
  hyperkinetic — *see* Hyperkinesia
  hypochondriacal F45.20
  hypoglycemic, due to insulin E16.0
    with coma (diabetic) — *see* Diabetes, coma nondiabetic E15
    therapeutic misadventure — *see* subcategory T38.3 ☑
  hypomanic F30.8
  hysterical F44.9
  immunization — *see* Complications, vaccination
  incompatibility
    ABO blood group (infusion) (transfusion) — *see* Complication(s), transfusion, incompatibility reaction, ABO
      delayed serologic T80.39 ☑
    minor blood group (Duffy) (E) (K(ell)) (Kidd) (Lewis) (M) (N) (P) (S) T80.89 ☑
    Rh (factor) (infusion) (transfusion) — *see* Complication(s), transfusion, incompatibility reaction, Rh (factor)
  inflammatory — *see* Infection
  infusion — *see* Complications, infusion
  inoculation (immune serum) — *see* Complications, vaccination
  insulin T38.3- ☑
  involutional psychotic — *see* Disorder, depressive

Reaction — *continued*
  leukemoid D72.823
    basophilic D72.823
    lymphocytic D72.823
    monocytic D72.823
    myelocytic D72.823
    neutrophilic D72.823
  LSD (acute)
    due to drug abuse — *see* Abuse, drug, hallucinogen
    due to drug dependence — *see* Dependence, drug, hallucinogen
  lumbar puncture G97.1
  manic-depressive — *see* Disorder, bipolar
  neurasthenic F48.8
  neurogenic — *see* Neurosis
  neurotic F48.9
  neurotic-depressive F34.1
  nitritoid — *see* Crisis, nitritoid
  nonspecific
    to
      cell mediated immunity measurement of gamma interferon antigen response without active tuberculosis R76.12
      QuantiFERON-TB test (QFT) without active tuberculosis R76.12
      tuberculin test (*see also* Reaction, tuberculin skin test) R76.11
  obsessive-compulsive F42
  organic, acute or subacute — *see* Delirium
  paranoid (acute) F23
    chronic F22
    senile F03 ☑
  passive dependency F60.7
  phobic F40.9
  post-traumatic stress, uncomplicated Z73.3
  psychogenic F99
  psychoneurotic (*see also* Neurosis)
    compulsive F42
    depersonalization F48.1
    depressive F34.1
    hypochondriacal F45.20
    neurasthenic F48.8
    obsessive F42
  psychophysiologic — *see* Disorder, somatoform
  psychosomatic — *see* Disorder, somatoform
  psychotic — *see* Psychosis
  scarlet fever toxin — *see* Complications, vaccination
  schizophrenic F23
    acute (brief) (undifferentiated) F23
    latent F21
    undifferentiated (acute) (brief) F23
  serological for syphilis — *see* Serology for syphilis
  serum T80.69 ☑
    anaphylactic (immediate) (*see also* Shock, anaphylactic) T80.59 ☑
    specified reaction NEC
      due to
        administration of blood and blood products T80.61 ☑
        immunization T80.62 ☑
        serum specified NEC T80.69 ☑
        vaccination T80.62 ☑
  situational — *see* Disorder, adjustment
  somatization — *see* Disorder, somatoform
  spinal puncture G97.1
  stress (severe) F43.9
    acute (agitation) ("daze") (disorientation) (disturbance of consciousness) (flight reaction) (fugue) F43.0
    specified NEC F43.8
  surgical procedure — *see* Complications, surgical procedure
  tetanus antitoxin — *see* Complications, vaccination
  toxic, to local anesthesia T81.89 ☑
    in labor and delivery O74.4
    in pregnancy O29.3X- ☑
    postpartum, puerperal O89.3
  toxin-antitoxin — *see* Complications, vaccination
  transfusion (blood) (bone marrow) (lymphocytes) (allergic) — *see* Complications, transfusion
  tuberculin skin test, abnormal R76.11
  vaccination (any) — *see* Complications, vaccination
  withdrawing, child or adolescent F93.8
Reactive airway disease — *see* Asthma
Reactive depression — *see* Reaction, depressive

Rearrangement
  chromosomal
    balanced (in) Q95.9
      abnormal individual (autosomal) Q95.2
        non-sex (autosomal) chromosomes Q95.2
        sex/non-sex chromosomes Q95.3
      specified NEC Q95.8
Recalcitrant patient — *see* Noncompliance
Recanalization, thrombus — *see* Thrombosis
Recession, receding
  chamber angle (eye) H21.55- ☑
  chin M26.09
  gingival (generalized) (localized) (postinfective) (postoperative) K06.0
Recklinghausen disease Q85.01
  bones E21.0
Reclus' disease (cystic) — *see* Mastopathy, cystic
Recrudescent typhus (fever) A75.1
Recruitment, auditory H93.21- ☑
Rectalgia K62.89
Rectitis K62.89
Rectocele
  female (without uterine prolapse) N81.6
    with uterine prolapse N81.4
      incomplete N81.2
  in pregnancy — *see* Pregnancy, complicated by, abnormal, pelvic organs or tissues NEC
  male K62.3
Rectosigmoid junction — *see* condition
Rectosigmoiditis K63.89
  ulcerative (chronic) K51.30
    with
      complication K51.319
        abscess K51.314
        fistula K51.313
        obstruction K51.312
        rectal bleeding K51.311
        specified NEC K51.318
Rectourethral — *see* condition
Rectovaginal — *see* condition
Rectovesical — *see* condition
Rectum, rectal — *see* condition
Recurrent — *see* condition
  pregnancy loss — *see* Loss (of), pregnancy, recurrent
Red bugs B88.0
Red tide (*see also* Table of Drugs and Chemicals) T65.82- ☑
Red-cedar lung or pneumonitis J67.8
Reduced
  mobility Z74.09
  ventilatory or vital capacity R94.2
Redundant, redundancy
  anus (congenital) Q43.8
  clitoris N90.89
  colon (congenital) Q43.8
  foreskin (congenital) N47.8
  intestine (congenital) Q43.8
  labia N90.6
  organ or site, congenital NEC — *see* Accessory
  panniculus (abdominal) E65
  prepuce (congenital) N47.8
  pylorus K31.89
  rectum (congenital) Q43.8
  scrotum N50.8
  sigmoid (congenital) Q43.8
  skin (of face) L57.4
    eyelids — *see* Blepharochalasis
  stomach K31.89
Reduplication — *see* Duplication
Reflex R29.2
  hyperactive gag J39.2
  pupillary, abnormal — *see* Anomaly, pupil, function
  vasoconstriction I73.9
  vasovagal R55
Reflux K21.9
  acid K21.9
  esophageal K21.9
    with esophagitis K21.0
    newborn P78.83
  gastroesophageal K21.9
    with esophagitis K21.0
  mitral — *see* Insufficiency, mitral
  ureteral — *see* Reflux, vesicoureteral

Reflux — *continued*
  vesicoureteral (with scarring) N13.70
    with
      nephropathy N13.729
        with hydroureter N13.739
          bilateral N13.732
          unilateral N13.731
        without hydroureter N13.729
          bilateral N13.722
          unilateral N13.721
        bilateral N13.722
        unilateral N13.721
      pyelonephritis (chronic) N11.0
    without nephropathy N13.71
    congenital Q62.7
Reforming, artificial openings — *see* Attention to, artificial, opening
Refractive error — *see* Disorder, refraction
Refsum's disease or syndrome G60.1
Refusal of
  food, psychogenic F50.8
  treatment (because of) Z53.20
    left against medical advice (AMA) Z53.21
    patient's decision NEC Z53.29
    reasons of belief or group pressure Z53.1
Regional — *see* condition
Regurgitation R11.10
  aortic (valve) — *see* Insufficiency, aortic
  food (*see also* Vomiting)
    with reswallowing — *see* Rumination
    newborn P92.1
  gastric contents — *see* Vomiting
  heart — *see* Endocarditis
  mitral (valve) — *see* Insufficiency, mitral
    congenital Q23.3
  myocardial — *see* Endocarditis
  pulmonary (valve) (heart) I37.1
    congenital Q22.2
    syphilitic A52.03
  tricuspid — *see* Insufficiency, tricuspid
  valve, valvular — *see* Endocarditis
    congenital Q24.8
  vesicoureteral — *see* Reflux, vesicoureteral
Reichmann's disease or syndrome K31.89
Reifenstein syndrome E34.52
Reinsertion, contraceptive device Z30.433
Reiter's disease, syndrome, or urethritis M02.30
  ankle M02.37- ☑
  elbow M02.32- ☑
  foot joint M02.37- ☑
  hand joint M02.34- ☑
  hip M02.35- ☑
  knee M02.36- ☑
  multiple site M02.39
  shoulder M02.31- ☑
  vertebra M02.38
  wrist M02.33- ☑
Rejection
  food, psychogenic F50.8
  transplant T86.91
    bone T86.830
      marrow T86.01
    cornea T86.840
    heart T86.21
      with lung(s) T86.31
    intestine T86.850
    kidney T86.11
    liver T86.41
    lung(s) T86.810
      with heart T86.31
    organ (immune or nonimmune cause) T86.91
    pancreas T86.890
    skin (allograft) (autograft) T86.820
    specified NEC T86.890
    stem cell (peripheral blood) (umbilical cord) T86.5
Relapsing fever A68.9
  Carter's (Asiatic) A68.1
  Dutton's (West African) A68.1
  Koch's A68.9
  louse-borne (epidemic) A68.0
  Novy's (American) A68.1
  Obermeyers's (European) A68.0
  Spirillum A68.9
  tick-borne (endemic) A68.1
Relationship
  occlusal
    open anterior M26.220

Relationship — *continued*
  occlusal — *continued*
    open posterior M26.221
Relaxation
  anus (sphincter) K62.89
    psychogenic F45.8
  arch (foot) (*see also* Deformity, limb, flat foot)
  back ligaments — *see* Instability, joint, spine
  bladder (sphincter) N31.2
  cardioesophageal K21.9
  cervix — *see* Incompetency, cervix
  diaphragm J98.6
  joint (capsule) (ligament) (paralytic) — *see* Flail, joint
    congenital NEC Q74.8
  lumbosacral (joint) — *see* subcategory M53.2 ☑
  pelvic floor N81.89
  perineum N81.89
  posture R29.3
  rectum (sphincter) K62.89
  sacroiliac (joint) — *see* subcategory M53.2 ☑
  scrotum N50.8
  urethra (sphincter) N36.44
  vesical N31.2
Release from prison, anxiety concerning Z65.2
Remains
  canal of Cloquet Q14.0
  capsule (opaque) Q14.8
Remittent fever (malarial) B54
Remnant
  canal of Cloquet Q14.0
  capsule (opaque) Q14.8
  cervix, cervical stump (acquired) (postoperative) N88.8
  cystic duct, postcholecystectomy K91.5
  fingernail L60.8
    congenital Q84.6
  meniscus, knee — *see* Derangement, knee, meniscus,
    specified NEC
  thyroglossal duct Q89.2
  tonsil J35.8
    infected (chronic) J35.01
  urachus Q64.4
Removal (from) (of)
  artificial
    arm Z44.00- ☑
      complete Z44.01- ☑
      partial Z44.02- ☑
    eye Z44.2- ☑
    leg Z44.10- ☑
      complete Z44.11- ☑
      partial Z44.12- ☑
  breast implant Z45.81 ☑
  cardiac pulse generator (battery) (end-of-life) Z45.010
  catheter (urinary) (indwelling) Z46.6
    from artificial opening — *see* Attention to, artificial,
      opening
    non-vascular Z46.82
    vascular NEC Z45.2
  device Z46.9
    contraceptive Z30.432
    implanted NEC Z45.89
    specified NEC Z46.89
  drains Z48.03
  dressing (nonsurgical) Z48.00
    surgical Z48.01
  external
    fixation device — *code to* fracture with seventh
      character D
    prosthesis, prosthetic device Z44.9
      breast Z44.3- ☑
      specified NEC Z44.8
  home in childhood (to foster home or institution)
    Z62.29
  ileostomy Z43.2
  insulin pump Z46.81
  myringotomy device (stent) (tube) Z45.82
  nervous system device NEC Z46.2
    brain neuropacemaker Z46.2
    visual substitution device Z46.2
      implanted Z45.31
  non-vascular catheter Z46.82
  organ, prophylactic (for neoplasia management) —
    see Prophylactic, organ removal
  orthodontic device Z46.4
  staples Z48.02
  stent
    ureteral Z46.6
  suture Z48.02
  urinary device Z46.6

Removal — *continued*
  vascular access device or catheter Z45.2
Ren
  arcuatus Q63.1
  mobile, mobilis N28.89
    congenital Q63.8
  unguliformis Q63.1
Renal — *see* condition
Rendu-Osler-Weber disease or syndrome I78.0
Reninoma D41.0- ☑
Renon-Delille syndrome E23.3
Reovirus, as cause of disease classified elsewhere
    B97.5
Repeated falls NEC R29.6
Replaced chromosome by dicentric ring Q93.2
Replacement by artificial or mechanical device or
    prosthesis of
  bladder Z96.0
  blood vessel NEC Z95.820
  bone NEC Z96.7
  cochlea Z96.21
  coronary artery Z95.5
  eustachian tube Z96.29
  eye globe Z97.0
  heart Z95.812
    valve Z95.2
      prosthetic Z95.2
      specified NEC Z95.4
      xenogenic Z95.3
  intestine Z96.89
  joint Z96.60
    hip — *see* Presence, hip joint implant
    knee — *see* Presence, knee joint implant
    specified site NEC Z96.698
  larynx Z96.3
  lens Z96.1
  limb(s) — *see* Presence, artificial, limb
  mandible NEC (for tooth root implant(s)) Z96.5
  organ NEC Z96.89
  peripheral vessel NEC Z95.828
  stapes Z96.29
  teeth Z97.2
  tendon Z96.7
  tissue NEC Z96.89
  tooth root(s) Z96.5
  vessel NEC Z95.828
    coronary (artery) Z95.5
Request for expert evidence Z04.8
Reserve, decreased or low
  cardiac — *see* Disease, heart
  kidney N28.89
Residual (*see also* condition)
  ovary syndrome N99.83
  state, schizophrenic F20.5
  urine R39.19
Resistance, resistant (to)
  activated protein C D68.51
  complicating pregnancy O26.89 ☑
  insulin E88.81
  organism(s)
    to
      drug
        aminoglycosides Z16.29
        amoxicillin Z16.11
        ampicillin Z16.11
        antibiotic(s) Z16.20
          multiple Z16.24
          specified NEC Z16.29
        antifungal Z16.32
        antimicrobial (single) Z16.30
          multiple Z16.35
          specified NEC Z16.39
        antimycbacterial (single) Z16.341
          multiple Z16.342
        antiparasitic Z16.31
        antiviral Z16.33
        beta lactam antibiotics Z16.10
          specified NEC Z16.19
        cephalosporins Z16.19
        extended beta lactamase (ESBL) Z16.12
        fluoroquinolones Z16.23
        macrolides Z16.29
        methicillin — *see* MRSA
        multiple drugs (MDRO)
          antibiotics Z16.24
        penicillins Z16.11
        quinine (and related compounds) Z16.31
        quinolones Z16.23

Resistance, resistant — *continued*
  organism(s) — *continued*
    to — *continued*
      drug — *continued*
        sulfonamides Z16.29
        tetracyclines Z16.29
        tuberculostatics (single) Z16.341
          multiple Z16.342
        vancomycin Z16.21
          related antibiotics Z16.22
  thyroid hormone E07.89
Resorption
  dental (roots) K03.3
    alveoli M26.79
  teeth (external) (internal) (pathological) (roots) K03.3
Respiration
  Cheyne-Stokes R06.3
  decreased due to shock, following injury T79.4 ☑
  disorder of, psychogenic F45.8
  insufficient, or poor R06.89
    newborn P28.5
  painful R07.1
  sighing, psychogenic F45.8
Respiratory (*see also* condition)
  distress syndrome (newborn) (type I) P22.0
    type II P22.1
  syncytial virus, as cause of disease classified elsewhere
    B97.4
Respite care Z75.5
Response (drug)
  photoallergic L56.1
  phototoxic L56.0
Restless legs (syndrome) G25.81
Restlessness R45.1
Restoration (of)
  dental
    aesthetically inadequate or displeasing K08.56
    defective K08.50
      specified NEC K08.59
    failure of marginal integrity K08.51
    failure of periodontal anatomical intergrity K08.54
  organ continuity from previous sterilization (tubuplas-
    ty) (vasoplasty) Z31.0
    aftercare Z31.42
  tooth (existing)
    contours biologically incompatible with oral health
      K08.54
      open margins K08.51
      overhanging K08.52
      poor aesthetic K08.56
      poor gingival margins K08.51
    unsatisfactory, of tooth K08.50
      specified NEC K08.59
Restorative material (dental)
  allergy to K08.55
  fractured K08.539
    with loss of material K08.531
    without loss of material K08.530
  unrepairable overhanging of K08.52
Restriction of housing space Z59.1
Rests, ovarian, in fallopian tube Q50.6
Restzustand (schizophrenic) F20.5
Retained (*see also* Retention)
  cholelithiasis following cholecystectomy K91.86
  foreign body fragments (type of) Z18.9
    acrylics Z18.2
    animal quill(s) or spines Z18.31
    cement Z18.83
    concrete Z18.83
    crystalline Z18.83
    depleted isotope Z18.09
    depleted uranium Z18.01
    diethylhexylphthalates Z18.2
    glass Z18.81
    isocyanate Z18.2
    magnetic metal Z18.11
    metal Z18.10
    nonmagnectic metal Z18.12
    nontherapeutic radioactive Z18.09
    organic NEC Z18.39
    plastic Z18.2
    quill(s) (animal) Z18.31
    radioactive (nontherapeutic) NEC Z18.09
    specified NEC Z18.89
    spine(s) (animal) Z18.31
    stone Z18.83
    tooth (teeth) Z18.32
    wood Z18.33

☑ **Additional Character Required** — **Refer to the Tabular List for Character Selection** ⬇ **Subterms under main terms may continue to next column or page**

Retained — continued
- fragments (type of) Z18.9
  - acrylics Z18.2
  - animal quill(s) or spines Z18.31
  - cement Z18.83
  - concrete Z18.83
  - crystalline Z18.83
  - depleted isotope Z18.09
  - depleted uranium Z18.01
  - diethylhexylphthalates Z18.2
  - glass Z18.81
  - isocyanate Z18.2
  - magnetic metal Z18.11
  - metal Z18.10
  - nonmagnectic metal Z18.12
  - nontherapeutic radioactive Z18.09
  - organic NEC Z18.39
  - plastic Z18.2
  - quill(s) (animal) Z18.31
  - radioactive (nontherapeutic) NEC Z18.09
  - specified NEC Z18.89
  - spine(s) (animal) Z18.31
  - stone Z18.83
  - tooth (teeth) Z18.32
  - wood Z18.33
- gallstones, following cholecystectomy K91.86

Retardation
- development, developmental, specific — see Disorder, developmental
- endochondral bone growth — see Disorder, bone, development or growth
- growth R62.50
  - due to malnutrition E45
- mental — see Disability, intellectual
- motor function, specific F82
- physical (child) R62.52
  - due to malnutrition E45
- reading (specific) F81.0
- spelling (specific) (without reading disorder) F81.81

Retching — see Vomiting

Retention (see also Retained)
- bladder — see Retention, urine
- carbon dioxide E87.2
- cholelithiasis following cholecystectomy K91.86
- cyst — see Cyst
- dead
  - fetus (at or near term) (mother) O36.4 ☑
    - early fetal death O02.1
  - ovum O02.0
- decidua (fragments) (following delivery) (with hemorrhage) O72.2
  - without hemorrhage O73.1
- deciduous tooth K00.6
- dental root K08.3
- fecal — see Constipation
- fetus
  - dead O36.4 ☑
    - early O02.1
- fluid R60.9
- foreign body (see also Foreign body, retained)
  - current trauma — code as Foreign body, by site or type
- gallstones, following cholecystectomy K91.86
- gastric K31.89
- intrauterine contraceptive device, in pregnancy — see Pregnancy, complicated by, retention, intrauterine device
- membranes (complicating delivery) (with hemorrhage) O72.2
  - with abortion — see Abortion, by type
  - without hemorrhage O73.1
- meniscus — see Derangement, meniscus
- menses N94.89
- milk (puerperal, postpartum) O92.79
- nitrogen, extrarenal R39.2
- ovary syndrome N99.83
- placenta (total) (with hemorrhage) O72.0
  - without hemorrhage O73.0
  - portions or fragments (with hemorrhage) O72.2
    - without hemorrhage O73.1
- products of conception
  - early pregnancy (dead fetus) O02.1
  - following
    - delivery (with hemorrhage) O72.2
      - without hemorrhage O73.1
- secundines (following delivery) (with hemorrhage) O72.0
  - without hemorrhage O73.0

Retention — continued
- secundines — continued
  - complicating puerperium (delayed hemorrhage) O72.2
  - partial O72.2
    - without hemorrhage O73.1
- smegma, clitoris N90.89
- urine R33.9
  - drug-induced R33.0
  - due to hyperplasia (hypertrophy) of prostate — see Hyperplasia, prostate
  - organic R33.8
    - drug-induced R33.0
  - psychogenic F45.8
  - specified NEC R33.8
- water (in tissues) — see Edema

Reticulation, dust — see Pneumoconiosis

Reticulocytosis R70.1

Reticuloendotheliosis
- acute infantile C96.0
- leukemic C91.4- ☑
- malignant C96.9
- nonlipid C96.0

Reticulohistiocytoma (giant-cell) D76.3

Reticuloid, actinic L57.1

Reticulosis (skin)
- acute of infancy C96.0
- hemophagocytic, familial D76.1
- histiocytic medullary C96.9
- lipomelanotic I89.8
- malignant (midline) C86.0
- nonlipid C96.0
- polymorphic C83.8- ☑
- Sézary — see Sézary disease

Retina, retinal (see also condition)
- dark area D49.81

Retinitis (see also Inflammation, chorioretinal)
- albuminurica N18.9 [H32]
- diabetic — see Diabetes, retinitis
- disciformis — see Degeneration, macula
- focal — see Inflammation, chorioretinal, focal
- gravidarum — see Pregnancy, complicated by, specified pregnancy-related condition NEC
- juxtapapillaris — see Inflammation, chorioretinal, focal, juxtapapillary
- luetic — see Retinitis, syphilitic
- pigmentosa H35.52
- proliferans — see Disorder, globe, degenerative, specified type NEC
- proliferating — see Disorder, globe, degenerative, specified type NEC
- renal N18.9 [H32]
- syphilitic (early) (secondary) A51.43
  - central, recurrent A52.71
  - congenital (early) A50.01 [H32]
  - late A52.71
- tuberculous A18.53

Retinoblastoma C69.2- ☑
- differentiated C69.2- ☑
- undifferentiated C69.2- ☑

Retinochoroiditis (see also Inflammation, chorioretinal)
- disseminated — see Inflammation, chorioretinal, disseminated
  - syphilitic A52.71
- focal — see Inflammation, chorioretinal
- juxtapapillaris — see Inflammation, chorioretinal, focal, juxtapapillary

Retinopathy (background) H35.00
- arteriosclerotic I70.8 [H35.0-] ☑
- atherosclerotic I70.8 [H35.0-] ☑
- central serous — see Chorioretinopathy, central serous
- Coats H35.02- ☑
- diabetic — see Diabetes, retinopathy
- exudative H35.02- ☑
- hypertensive H35.03- ☑
- in (due to)
  - diabetes — see Diabetes, retinopathy
  - sickle-cell disorders D57.- ☑ [H36]
- of prematurity H35.10- ☑
  - stage 0 H35.11- ☑
  - stage 1 H35.12- ☑
  - stage 2 H35.13- ☑
  - stage 3 H35.14- ☑
  - stage 4 H35.15- ☑
  - stage 5 H35.16- ☑
- pigmentary, congenital — see Dystrophy, retina

Retinopathy — continued
- proliferative NEC H35.2- ☑
  - diabetic — see Diabetes, retinopathy, proliferative
  - sickle-cell D57.- ☑ [H36]
- solar H31.02- ☑

Retinoschisis H33.10- ☑
- congenital Q14.1
- specified type NEC H33.19- ☑

Retortamoniasis A07.8

Retractile testis Q55.22

Retraction
- cervix — see Retroversion, uterus
- drum (membrane) — see Disorder, tympanic membrane, specified NEC
- finger — see Deformity, finger
- lid H02.539
  - left H02.536
    - lower H02.535
    - upper H02.534
  - right H02.533
    - lower H02.532
    - upper H02.531
- lung J98.4
- mediastinum J98.5
- nipple N64.53
  - associated with
    - lactation O92.03
    - pregnancy O92.01- ☑
    - puerperium O92.02
  - congenital Q83.8
- palmar fascia M72.0
- pleura — see Pleurisy
- ring, uterus (Bandl's) (pathological) O62.4
- sternum (congenital) Q76.7
  - acquired M95.4
- uterus — see Retroversion, uterus
- valve (heart) — see Endocarditis

Retrobulbar — see condition

Retrocecal — see condition

Retrocession — see Retroversion

Retrodisplacement — see Retroversion

Retroflection, retroflexion — see Retroversion

Retrognathia, retrognathism (mandibular) (maxillary) M26.19

Retrograde menstruation N92.5

Retroperineal — see condition

Retroperitoneal — see condition

Retroperitonitis K68.9

Retropharyngeal — see condition

Retroplacental — see condition

Retroposition — see Retroversion

Retroprosthetic membrane T85.398 ☑

Retrosternal thyroid (congenital) Q89.2

Retroversion, retroverted
- cervix — see Retroversion, uterus
- female NEC — see Retroversion, uterus
- iris H21.89
- testis (congenital) Q55.29
- uterus (acquired) (acute) (any degree) (asymptomatic) (cervix) (postinfectional) (postpartal, old) N85.4
  - congenital Q51.818
  - in pregnancy O34.53- ☑

Retrovirus, as cause of disease classified elsewhere B97.30
- human
  - immunodeficiency, type 2 (HIV 2) B97.35
  - T-cell lymphotropic
    - type I (HTLV-I) B97.33
    - type II (HTLV-II) B97.34
- lentivirus B97.31
- oncovirus B97.32
- specified NEC B97.39

Retrusion, premaxilla (developmental) M26.09

Rett's disease or syndrome F84.2

Reverse peristalsis R19.2

Reye's syndrome G93.7

Rh (factor)
- hemolytic disease (newborn) P55.0
- incompatibility, immunization or sensitization
  - affecting management of pregnancy NEC O36.09- ☑
    - anti-D antibody O36.01- ☑
  - newborn P55.0
  - transfusion reaction — see Complication(s), transfusion, incompatibility reaction, Rh (factor)
- negative mother affecting newborn P55.0

Index

Retained — Rh

Rh — *continued*
  titer elevated — *see* Complication(s), transfusion, incompatibility reaction, Rh (factor)
  transfusion reaction — *see* Complication(s), transfusion, incompatibility reaction, Rh (factor)
Rhabdomyolysis (idiopathic) NEC M62.82
  traumatic T79.6 ☑
Rhabdomyoma (*see also* Neoplasm, connective tissue, benign)
  adult — *see* Neoplasm, connective tissue, benign
  fetal — *see* Neoplasm, connective tissue, benign
  glycogenic — *see* Neoplasm, connective tissue, benign
Rhabdomyosarcoma (any type) — *see* Neoplasm, connective tissue, malignant
Rhabdosarcoma — *see* Rhabdomyosarcoma
Rhesus (factor) **incompatibility** — *see* Rh, incompatibility
Rheumatic (acute) (subacute) (chronic)
  adherent pericardium I09.2
  coronary arteritis I01.9
  degeneration, myocardium I09.0
  fever (acute) — *see* Fever, rheumatic
  heart — *see* Disease, heart, rheumatic
  myocardial degeneration — *see* Degeneration, myocardium
  myocarditis (chronic) (inactive) (with chorea) I09.0
    with chorea (acute) (rheumatic) (Sydenham's) I02.0
    active or acute I01.2
  pancarditis, acute I01.8
    with chorea (acute (rheumatic) Sydenham's) I02.0
  pericarditis (active) (acute) (with effusion) (with pneumonia) I01.0
    with chorea (acute) (rheumatic) (Sydenham's) I02.0
  chronic or inactive I09.2
  pneumonia I00 [J17]
  torticollis M43.6
  typhoid fever A01.09
Rheumatism (articular) (neuralgic) (nonarticular) M79.0
  gout — *see* Arthritis, rheumatoid
  intercostal, meaning Tietze's disease M94.0
  palindromic (any site) M12.30
    ankle M12.37- ☑
    elbow M12.32- ☑
    foot joint M12.37- ☑
    hand joint M12.34- ☑
    hip M12.35- ☑
    knee M12.36- ☑
    multiple site M12.39
    shoulder M12.31- ☑
    specified joint NEC M12.38
    vertebrae M12.38
    wrist M12.33- ☑
  sciatic M54.4- ☑
Rheumatoid (*see also* condition)
  arthritis (*see also* Arthritis, rheumatoid)
    with involvement of organs NEC M05.60
      ankle M05.67- ☑
      elbow M05.62- ☑
      foot joint M05.67- ☑
      hand joint M05.64- ☑
      hip M05.65- ☑
      knee M05.66- ☑
      multiple site M05.69
      shoulder M05.61- ☑
      vertebra — *see* Spondylitis, ankylosing
      wrist M05.63- ☑
    seronegative — *see* Arthritis, rheumatoid, seronegative
    seropositive — *see* Arthritis, rheumatoid, seropositive
  carditis M05.30
    ankle M05.37- ☑
    elbow M05.32- ☑
    foot joint M05.37- ☑
    hand joint M05.34- ☑
    hip M05.35- ☑
    knee M05.36- ☑
    multiple site M05.39
    shoulder M05.31- ☑
    vertebra — *see* Spondylitis, ankylosing
    wrist M05.33- ☑
  endocarditis — *see* Rheumatoid, carditis
  lung (disease) M05.10
    ankle M05.17- ☑
    elbow M05.12- ☑
    foot joint M05.17- ☑
    hand joint M05.14- ☑

Rheumatoid — *continued*
  lung — *continued*
    hip M05.15- ☑
    knee M05.16- ☑
    multiple site M05.19
    shoulder M05.11- ☑
    vertebra — *see* Spondylitis, ankylosing
    wrist M05.13- ☑
  myocarditis — *see* Rheumatoid, carditis
  myopathy M05.40
    ankle M05.47- ☑
    elbow M05.42- ☑
    foot joint M05.47- ☑
    hand joint M05.44- ☑
    hip M05.45- ☑
    knee M05.46- ☑
    multiple site M05.49
    shoulder M05.41- ☑
    vertebra — *see* Spondylitis, ankylosing
    wrist M05.43- ☑
  pericarditis — *see* Rheumatoid, carditis
  polyarthritis — *see* Arthritis, rheumatoid
  polyneuropathy M05.50
    ankle M05.57- ☑
    elbow M05.52- ☑
    foot joint M05.57- ☑
    hand joint M05.54- ☑
    hip M05.55- ☑
    knee M05.56- ☑
    multiple site M05.59
    shoulder M05.51- ☑
    vertebra — *see* Spondylitis, ankylosing
    wrist M05.53- ☑
  vasculitis M05.20
    ankle M05.27- ☑
    elbow M05.22- ☑
    foot joint M05.27- ☑
    hand joint M05.24- ☑
    hip M05.25- ☑
    knee M05.26- ☑
    multiple site M05.29
    shoulder M05.21- ☑
    vertebra — *see* Spondylitis, ankylosing
    wrist M05.23- ☑
Rhinitis (atrophic) (catarrhal) (chronic) (croupous) (fibrinous) (granulomatous) (hyperplastic) (hypertrophic) (membranous) (obstructive) (purulent) (suppurative) (ulcerative) J31.0
  with
    sore throat — *see* Nasopharyngitis
  acute J00
  allergic J30.9
    with asthma J45.909
      with
        exacerbation (acute) J45.901
        status asthmaticus J45.902
    due to
      food J30.5
      pollen J30.1
    nonseasonal J30.89
    perennial J30.89
    seasonal NEC J30.2
    specified NEC J30.89
  infective J00
  pneumococcal J00
  syphilitic A52.73
    congenital A50.05 [J99]
  tuberculous A15.8
  vasomotor J30.0
Rhinoantritis (chronic) — *see* Sinusitis, maxillary
Rhinodacryolith — *see* Dacryolith
Rhinolith (nasal sinus) J34.89
Rhinomegaly J34.89
Rhinopharyngitis (acute) (subacute) (*see also* Nasopharyngitis)
  chronic J31.1
  destructive ulcerating A66.5
  mutilans A66.5
Rhinophyma L71.1
Rhinorrhea J34.89
  cerebrospinal (fluid) G96.0
  paroxysmal — *see* Rhinitis, allergic
  spasmodic — *see* Rhinitis, allergic
Rhinosalpingitis — *see* Salpingitis, eustachian
Rhinoscleroma A48.8
Rhinosporidiosis B48.1
Rhinovirus infection NEC B34.8

Rhizomelic chondrodysplasia punctata E71.540
Rhythm
  atrioventricular nodal I49.8
  disorder I49.9
    coronary sinus I49.8
    ectopic I49.8
    nodal I49.8
  escape I49.9
  heart, abnormal I49.9
  idioventricular I44.2
  nodal I49.8
  sleep, inversion G47.2- ☑
    nonorganic origin — *see* Disorder, sleep, circadian rhythm, psychogenic
Rhytidosis facialis L98.8
Rib (*see also* condition)
  cervical Q76.5
Riboflavin deficiency E53.0
Rice bodies (*see also* Loose, body, joint)
  knee M23.4- ☑
Richter syndrome — *see* Leukemia, chronic lymphocytic, B-cell type
Richter's hernia — *see* Hernia, abdomen, with obstruction
Ricinism — *see* Poisoning, food, noxious, plant
Rickets (active) (acute) (adolescent) (chest wall) (congenital) (current) (infantile) (intestinal) E55.0
  adult — *see* Osteomalacia
  celiac K90.0
  hypophosphatemic with nephrotic-glycosuric dwarfism E72.09
  inactive E64.3
  kidney N25.0
  renal N25.0
  sequelae, any E64.3
  vitamin-D-resistant E83.31 [M90.80]
Rickettsial disease A79.9
  specified type NEC A79.89
Rickettsialpox (Rickettsia akari) A79.1
Rickettsiosis A79.9
  due to
    Ehrlichia sennetsu A79.81
    Rickettsia akari (rickettsialpox) A79.1
  specified type NEC A79.89
  tick-borne A77.9
  vesicular A79.1
Rider's bone — *see* Ossification, muscle, specified NEC
Ridge, alveolus (*see also* condition)
  flabby K06.8
Ridged ear, congenital Q17.3
Riedel's
  lobe, liver Q44.7
  struma, thyroiditis or disease E06.5
Rieger's anomaly or syndrome Q13.81
Riehl's melanosis L81.4
Rietti-Greppi-Micheli anemia D56.9
Rieux's hernia — *see* Hernia, abdomen, specified site NEC
Riga (-Fede) **disease** K14.0
Riggs' disease — *see* Periodontitis
Right middle lobe syndrome J98.11
Rigid, rigidity (*see also* condition)
  abdominal R19.30
    with severe abdominal pain R10.0
    epigastric R19.36
    generalized R19.37
    left lower quadrant R19.34
    left upper quadrant R19.32
    periumbilic R19.35
    right lower quadrant R19.33
    right upper quadrant R19.31
  articular, multiple, congenital Q68.8
  cervix (uteri) in pregnancy — *see* Pregnancy, complicated by, abnormal, cervix
  hymen (acquired) (congenital) N89.6
  nuchal R29.1
  pelvic floor in pregnancy — *see* Pregnancy, complicated by, abnormal, pelvic organs or tissues NEC
  perineum or vulva in pregnancy — *see* Pregnancy, complicated by, abnormal, vulva
  spine — *see* Dorsopathy, specified NEC
  vagina in pregnancy — *see* Pregnancy, complicated by, abnormal, vagina
Rigors R68.89
  with fever R50.9
Riley-Day syndrome G90.1
RIND (reversible ischemic neurologic deficit) I63.9

☑ **Additional Character Required — Refer to the Tabular List for Character Selection**   ▽ Subterms under main terms may continue to next column or page

Ring(s)
aorta (vascular) Q25.4
Bandl's O62.4
contraction, complicating delivery O62.4
esophageal, lower (muscular) K22.2
Fleischer's (cornea) H18.04- ☑
hymenal, tight (acquired) (congenital) N89.6
Kayser-Fleischer (cornea) H18.04- ☑
retraction, uterus, pathological O62.4
Schatzki's (esophagus) (lower) K22.2
   congenital Q39.3
Soemmerring's — see Cataract, secondary
vascular (congenital) Q25.8
   aorta Q25.4

Ringed hair (congenital) Q84.1

Ringworm B35.9
beard B35.0
black dot B35.0
body B35.4
Burmese B35.5
corporeal B35.4
foot B35.3
groin B35.6
hand B35.2
honeycomb B35.0
nails B35.1
perianal (area) B35.6
scalp B35.0
specified NEC B35.8
Tokelau B35.5

Rise, venous pressure I87.8

Risk, suicidal
meaning personal history of attempted suicide Z91.5
meaning suicidal ideation — see Ideation, suicidal

Ritter's disease L00

Rivalry, sibling Z62.891

Rivalta's disease A42.2

River blindness B73.01

Robert's pelvis Q74.2
with disproportion (fetopelvic) O33.0
   causing obstructed labor O65.0

Robin (-Pierre) **syndrome** Q87.0

Robinow-Silvermann-Smith syndrome Q87.1

Robinson's (hidrotic) **ectodermal dysplasia or syndrome** Q82.4

Robles' disease B73.01

Rocky Mountain (spotted) **fever** A77.0

Roetheln — see Rubella

Roger's disease Q21.0

Rokitansky-Aschoff sinuses (gallbladder) K82.8

Rolando's fracture (displaced) S62.22- ☑
nondisplaced S62.22- ☑

Romano-Ward (prolonged QT interval) **syndrome** I45.81

Romberg's disease or syndrome G51.8

Roof, mouth — see condition

Rosacea L71.9
acne L71.9
keratitis L71.8
specified NEC L71.8

Rosary, rachitic E55.0

Rose
cold J30.1
fever J30.1
rash R21
   epidemic B06.9

Rosenbach's erysipeloid A26.0

Rosenthal's disease or syndrome D68.1

Roseola B09
infantum B08.20
   due to human herpesvirus 6 B08.21
   due to human herpesvirus 7 B08.22

Ross River disease or fever B33.1

Rossbach's disease K31.89
psychogenic F45.8

Rostan's asthma (cardiac) — see Failure, ventricular, left

Rotation
anomalous, incomplete or insufficient, intestine Q43.3
cecum (congenital) Q43.3
colon (congenital) Q43.3
spine, incomplete or insufficient — see Dorsopathy,
   deforming, specified NEC
tooth, teeth, fully erupted M26.35
vertebra, incomplete or insufficient — see Dorsopathy,
   deforming, specified NEC

Rotes Quérol disease or syndrome — see Hyperostosis,
   ankylosing

Roth (-Bernhardt) **disease or syndrome** — see Meralgia
   paraesthetica

Rothmund (-Thomson) **syndrome** Q82.8

Rotor's disease or syndrome E80.6

Round
back (with wedging of vertebrae) — see Kyphosis
   sequelae (late effect) of rickets E64.3
worms (large) (infestation) NEC B82.0
   Ascariasis (see also Ascariasis) B77.9

Roussy-Lévy syndrome G60.0

Rubella (German measles) B06.9
complication NEC B06.09
   neurological B06.00
congenital P35.0
contact Z20.4
exposure to Z20.4
maternal
   care for (suspected) damage to fetus O35.3 ☑
   manifest rubella in infant P35.0
   suspected damage to fetus affecting management
      of pregnancy O35.3 ☑
specified complications NEC B06.89

Rubeola (meaning measles) — see Measles
meaning rubella — see Rubella

Rubeosis, iris — see Disorder, iris, vascular

Rubinstein-Taybi syndrome Q87.2

Rudimentary (congenital) (see also Agenesis)
arm — see Defect, reduction, upper limb
bone Q79.9
cervix uteri Q51.828
eye Q11.2
lobule of ear Q17.3
patella Q74.1
respiratory organs in thoracopagus Q89.4
tracheal bronchus Q32.4
uterus Q51.818
   in male Q56.1
vagina Q52.0

Ruled out condition — see Observation, suspected

Rumination R11.10
with nausea R11.2
disorder of infancy F98.21
neurotic F42
newborn P92.1
obsessional F42
psychogenic F42

Runeberg's disease D51.0

Runny nose R09.89

Rupia (syphilitic) A51.39
congenital A50.06
tertiary A52.79

Rupture, ruptured
abscess (spontaneous) — code by site under Abscess
aneurysm — see Aneurysm
anus (sphincter) — see Laceration, anus
aorta, aortic I71.8
   abdominal I71.3
   arch I71.1
   ascending I71.1
   descending I71.8
      abdominal I71.3
      thoracic I71.1
   syphilitic A52.01
   thoracoabdominal I71.5
   thorax, thoracic I71.1
   transverse I71.1
   traumatic — see Injury, aorta, laceration, major
   valve or cusp (see also Endocarditis, aortic) I35.8
appendix (with peritonitis) K35.2
arteriovenous fistula, brain I60.8
artery I77.2
   brain — see Hemorrhage, intracranial, intracerebral
   coronary — see Infarct, myocardium
   heart — see Infarct, myocardium
   pulmonary I28.8
   traumatic (complication) — see Injury, blood vessel
bile duct (common) (hepatic) K83.2
   cystic K82.2
bladder (sphincter) (nontraumatic) (spontaneous)
   N32.89
   following ectopic or molar pregnancy O08.6
   obstetrical trauma O71.5
   traumatic S37.29 ☑
blood vessel (see also Hemorrhage)
   brain — see Hemorrhage, intracranial, intracerebral
   heart — see Infarct, myocardium

Rupture, ruptured — continued
blood vessel (see also Hemorrhage) — continued
   traumatic (complication) — see Injury, blood ves-
      sel, laceration, major, by site
bone — see Fracture
bowel (nontraumatic) K63.1
brain
   aneurysm (congenital) (see also Hemorrhage, in-
      tracranial, subarachnoid)
      syphilitic A52.05
   hemorrhagic — see Hemorrhage, intracranial, in-
      tracerebral
capillaries I78.8
cardiac (auricle) (ventricle) (wall) I23.3
   with hemopericardium I23.0
   infectional I40.9
   traumatic — see Injury, heart
cartilage (articular) (current) (see also Sprain)
   knee S83.3- ☑
   semilunar — see Tear, meniscus
cecum (with peritonitis) K65.0
   with peritoneal abscess K35.3
   traumatic S36.598 ☑
celiac artery, traumatic — see Injury, blood vessel,
   celiac artery, laceration, major
cerebral aneurysm (congenital) (see Hemorrhage, intracranial, subarachnoid)
cervix (uteri)
   with ectopic or molar pregnancy O08.6
   following ectopic or molar pregnancy O08.6
   obstetrical trauma O71.3
   traumatic S37.69 ☑
chordae tendineae NEC I51.1
   concurrent with acute myocardial infarction — see
      Infarct, myocardium
   following acute myocardial infarction (current
      complication) I23.4
choroid (direct) (indirect) (traumatic) H31.32- ☑
circle of Willis I60.6
colon (nontraumatic) K63.1
   traumatic — see Injury, intestine, large
cornea (traumatic) — see Injury, eye, laceration
coronary (artery) (thrombotic) — see Infarct, myocardium
corpus luteum (infected) (ovary) N83.1
cyst — see Cyst
cystic duct K82.2
Descemet's membrane — see Change, corneal membrane, Descemet's, rupture
   traumatic — see Injury, eye, laceration
diaphragm, traumatic — see Injury, intrathoracic, diaphragm
disc — see Rupture, intervertebral disc
diverticulum (intestine) K57.80
   with bleeding K57.81
   bladder N32.3
   large intestine K57.20
      with
         bleeding K57.21
         small intestine K57.40
            with bleeding K57.41
   small intestine K57.00
      with
         bleeding K57.01
         large intestine K57.40
            with bleeding K57.41
duodenal stump K31.89
ear drum (nontraumatic) (see also Perforation, tympanum)
   traumatic S09.2- ☑
   due to blast injury — see Injury, blast, ear
esophagus K22.3
eye (without prolapse or loss of intraocular tissue) —
   see Injury, eye, laceration
fallopian tube NEC (nonobstetric) (nontraumatic) N83.8
   due to pregnancy O00.1
fontanel P13.1
gallbladder K82.2
   traumatic S36.128 ☑
gastric (see also Rupture, stomach)
   vessel K92.2
globe (eye) (traumatic) — see Injury, eye, laceration
graafian follicle (hematoma) N83.0
heart — see Rupture, cardiac
hymen (nontraumatic) (nonintentional) N89.8
internal organ, traumatic — see Injury, by site

Rupture, ruptured — *continued*
  intervertebral disc — *see* Displacement, intervertebral
    disc
    traumatic — *see* Rupture, traumatic, intervertebral
      disc
  intestine NEC (nontraumatic) K63.1
    traumatic — *see* Injury, intestine
  iris (*see also* Abnormality, pupillary)
    traumatic — *see* Injury, eye, laceration
  joint capsule, traumatic — *see* Sprain
  kidney (traumatic) S37.06- ☑
    birth injury P15.8
    nontraumatic N28.89
  lacrimal duct (traumatic) — *see* Injury, eye, specified
    site NEC
  lens (cataract) (traumatic) — *see* Cataract, traumatic
  ligament, traumatic — *see* Rupture, traumatic, liga-
    ment, by site
  liver S36.116 ☑
    birth injury P15.0
  lymphatic vessel I89.8
  marginal sinus (placental) (with hemorrhage) — *see*
    Hemorrhage, antepartum, specified cause NEC
  membrana tympani (nontraumatic) — *see* Perforation,
    tympanum
  membranes (spontaneous)
    artificial
      delayed delivery following O75.5
    delayed delivery following — *see* Pregnancy,
      complicated by, premature rupture of
      membranes
  meningeal artery I60.8
  meniscus (knee) (*see also* Tear, meniscus)
    old — *see* Derangement, meniscus
    site other than knee — *code as* Sprain
  mesenteric artery, traumatic — *see* Injury, mesenteric,
    artery, laceration, major
  mesentery (nontraumatic) K66.8
    traumatic — *see* Injury, intra-abdominal, specified,
      site NEC
  mitral (valve) I34.8
  muscle (traumatic) (*see also* Strain)
    diastasis — *see* Diastasis, muscle
    nontraumatic M62.10
      ankle M62.17- ☑
      foot M62.17- ☑
      forearm M62.13- ☑
      hand M62.14- ☑
      lower leg M62.16- ☑
      pelvic region M62.15- ☑
      shoulder region M62.11- ☑
      specified site NEC M62.18
      thigh M62.15- ☑
      upper arm M62.12- ☑
    traumatic — *see* Strain, by site
  musculotendinous junction NEC, nontraumatic — *see*
    Rupture, tendon, spontaneous
  mycotic aneurysm causing cerebral hemorrhage —
    see Hemorrhage, intracranial, subarachnoid
  myocardium, myocardial — *see* Rupture, cardiac
    traumatic — *see* Injury, heart
  nontraumatic, meaning hernia — *see* Hernia
  obstructed — *see* Hernia, by site, obstructed
  operation wound — *see* Disruption, wound, operation
  ovary, ovarian N83.8
    corpus luteum cyst N83.1
    follicle (graafian) N83.0
  oviduct (nonobstetric) (nontraumatic) N83.8
    due to pregnancy O00.1
  pancreas (nontraumatic) K86.8
    traumatic S36.299 ☑
  papillary muscle NEC I51.2
    following acute myocardial infarction (current
      complication) I23.5
  pelvic
    floor, complicating delivery O70.1
    organ NEC, obstetrical trauma O71.5
  perineum (nonobstetric) (nontraumatic) N90.89
    complicating delivery — *see* Delivery, complicated,
      by, laceration, anus (sphincter)
  postoperative wound — *see* Disruption, wound, oper-
    ation
  prostate (traumatic) S37.828 ☑
  pulmonary
    artery I28.8
    valve (heart) I37.8
    vein I28.8

Rupture, ruptured — *continued*
  pulmonary — *continued*
    vessel I28.8
  pus tube — *see* Salpingitis
  pyosalpinx — *see* Salpingitis
  rectum (nontraumatic) K63.1
    traumatic S36.69 ☑
  retina, retinal (traumatic) (without detachment) (*see*
    also Break, retina)
    with detachment — *see* Detachment, retina, with
      retinal, break
  rotator cuff (nontraumatic) M75.10- ☑
    complete M75.12- ☑
    incomplete M75.11- ☑
  sclera — *see* Injury, eye, laceration
  sigmoid (nontraumatic) K63.1
    traumatic S36.593 ☑
  spinal cord (*see also* Injury, spinal cord, by region)
    due to injury at birth P11.5
    newborn (birth injury) P11.5
  spleen (traumatic) S36.09 ☑
    birth injury P15.1
    congenital (birth injury) P15.1
    due to P. vivax malaria B51.0
    nontraumatic D73.5
    spontaneous D73.5
  splenic vein R58
    traumatic — *see* Injury, blood vessel, splenic vein
  stomach (nontraumatic) (spontaneous) K31.89
    traumatic S36.39 ☑
  supraspinatus (complete) (incomplete) (nontraumatic)
    — *see* Tear, rotator cuff
  symphysis pubis
    obstetric O71.6
    traumatic S33.4 ☑
  synovium (cyst) M66.10
    ankle M66.17- ☑
    elbow M66.12- ☑
    finger M66.14- ☑
    foot M66.17- ☑
    forearm M66.13- ☑
    hand M66.14- ☑
    pelvic region M66.15- ☑
    shoulder region M66.11- ☑
    specified site NEC M66.18
    thigh M66.15- ☑
    toe M66.17- ☑
    upper arm M66.12- ☑
    wrist M66.13- ☑
  tendon (traumatic) — *see* Strain
    nontraumatic (spontaneous) M66.9
      ankle M66.87- ☑
      extensor M66.20
        ankle M66.27- ☑
        foot M66.27- ☑
        forearm M66.23- ☑
        hand M66.24- ☑
        lower leg M66.26- ☑
        multiple sites M66.29
        pelvic region M66.25- ☑
        shoulder region M66.21- ☑
        specified site NEC M66.28
        thigh M66.25- ☑
        upper arm M66.22- ☑
      flexor M66.30
        ankle M66.37- ☑
        foot M66.37- ☑
        forearm M66.33- ☑
        hand M66.34- ☑
        lower leg M66.36- ☑
        multiple sites M66.39
        pelvic region M66.35- ☑
        shoulder region M66.31- ☑
        specified site NEC M66.38
        thigh M66.35- ☑
        upper arm M66.32- ☑
      foot M66.87- ☑
      forearm M66.83- ☑
      hand M66.84- ☑
      lower leg M66.86- ☑
      multiple sites M66.89
      pelvic region M66.85- ☑
      shoulder region M66.81- ☑
      specified
        site NEC M66.88
        tendon M66.80

Rupture, ruptured — *continued*
  tendon — *see* Strain — *continued*
    nontraumatic — *continued*
      thigh M66.85- ☑
      upper arm M66.82- ☑
  thoracic duct I89.8
  tonsil J35.8
  traumatic
    aorta — *see* Injury, aorta, laceration, major
    diaphragm — *see* Injury, intrathoracic, diaphragm
    external site — *see* Wound, open, by site
    eye — *see* Injury, eye, laceration
    internal organ — *see* Injury, by site
    intervertebral disc
      cervical S13.0 ☑
      lumbar S33.0 ☑
      thoracic S23.0 ☑
    kidney S37.06- ☑
    ligament (*see also* Sprain)
      ankle — *see* Sprain, ankle
      carpus — *see* Rupture, traumatic, ligament,
        wrist
      collateral (hand) — *see* Rupture, traumatic,
        ligament, finger, collateral
      finger (metacarpophalangeal) (interphalangeal)
        S63.40- ☑
        collateral S63.41- ☑
          index S63.41- ☑
          little S63.41- ☑
          middle S63.41- ☑
          ring S63.41- ☑
        index S63.40- ☑
        little S63.40- ☑
        middle S63.40- ☑
        palmar S63.42- ☑
          index S63.42- ☑
          little S63.42- ☑
          middle S63.42- ☑
          ring S63.42- ☑
        ring S63.40- ☑
        specified site NEC S63.499 ☑
          index S63.49- ☑
          little S63.49- ☑
          middle S63.49- ☑
          ring S63.49- ☑
        volar plate S63.43- ☑
          index S63.43- ☑
          little S63.43- ☑
          middle S63.43- ☑
          ring S63.43- ☑
      foot — *see* Sprain, foot
      radial collateral S53.2- ☑
      radiocarpal — *see* Rupture, traumatic, ligament,
        wrist, radiocarpal
      ulnar collateral S53.3- ☑
      ulnocarpal — *see* Rupture, traumatic, ligament,
        wrist, ulnocarpal
      wrist S63.30- ☑
        collateral S63.31- ☑
        radiocarpal S63.32- ☑
        specified site NEC S63.39- ☑
        ulnocarpal (palmar) S63.33- ☑
    liver S36.116 ☑
    membrana tympani — *see* Rupture, ear drum,
      traumatic
    muscle or tendon — *see* Strain
    myocardium — *see* Injury, heart
    pancreas S36.299 ☑
    rectum S36.69 ☑
    sigmoid S36.593 ☑
    spleen S36.09 ☑
    stomach S36.39 ☑
    symphysis pubis S33.4 ☑
    tympanum, tympanic (membrane) — *see* Rupture,
      ear drum, traumatic
    ureter S37.19 ☑
    uterus S37.69 ☑
    vagina — *see* Injury, vagina
    vena cava — *see* Injury, vena cava, laceration, ma-
      jor
  tricuspid (heart) (valve) I07.8
  tube, tubal (nonobstetric) (nontraumatic) N83.8
    abscess — *see* Salpingitis
    due to pregnancy O00.1

☑ **Additional Character Required** — **Refer to the Tabular List for Character Selection**
▼ **Subterms under main terms may continue to next column or page**

Rupture, ruptured — continued

  tympanum, tympanic (membrane) (nontraumatic)
    (see also Perforation, tympanic membrane)
    H72.9- ☑

    traumatic — see Rupture, ear drum, traumatic

  umbilical cord, complicating delivery O69.89 ☑

  ureter (traumatic) S37.19 ☑

    nontraumatic N28.89

  urethra (nontraumatic) N36.8

    with ectopic or molar pregnancy O08.6

    following ectopic or molar pregnancy O08.6

    obstetrical trauma O71.5

    traumatic S37.39 ☑

  uterosacral ligament (nonobstetric) (nontraumatic)
    N83.8

  uterus (traumatic) S37.69 ☑

    before labor O71.0- ☑

    during or after labor O71.1

    nonpuerperal, nontraumatic N85.8

    pregnant (during labor) O71.1

      before labor O71.0- ☑

  vagina — see Injury, vagina

  valve, valvular (heart) — see Endocarditis

  varicose vein — see Varix

  varix — see Varix

  vena cava R58

    traumatic — see Injury, vena cava, laceration, major

  vesical (urinary) N32.89

  vessel (blood) R58

    pulmonary I28.8

    traumatic — see Injury, blood vessel

  viscus R19.8

  vulva complicating delivery O70.0

Russell-Silver syndrome Q87.1

Russian spring-summer type encephalitis A84.0

Rust's disease (tuberculous cervical spondylitis) A18.01

Ruvalcaba-Myhre-Smith syndrome E71.440

Rytand-Lipsitch syndrome I44.2

S

Saber, sabre shin or tibia (syphilitic) A50.56 [M90.8-] ☑

Sac lacrimal — see condition

Saccharomyces infection B37.9

Saccharopinuria E72.3

Saccular — see condition

Sacculation

  aorta (nonsyphilitic) — see Aneurysm, aorta

  bladder N32.3

  intralaryngeal (congenital) (ventricular) Q31.3

  larynx (congenital) (ventricular) Q31.3

  organ or site, congenital — see Distortion

  pregnant uterus — see Pregnancy, complicated by,
    abnormal, uterus

  ureter N28.89

  urethra N36.1

  vesical N32.3

Sachs' amaurotic familial idiocy or disease E75.02

Sachs-Tay disease E75.02

Sacks-Libman disease M32.11

Sacralgia M53.3

Sacralization Q76.49

Sacrodynia M53.3

Sacroiliac joint — see condition

Sacroiliitis NEC M46.1

Sacrum — see condition

Saddle

  back — see Lordosis

  embolus

    abdominal aorta I74.01

    pulmonary artery I26.92

      with acute cor pulmonale I26.02

  injury — code to condition

  nose M95.0

    due to syphilis A50.57

Sadism (sexual) F65.52

Sadness, postpartal O90.6

Sadomasochism F65.50

Saemisch's ulcer (cornea) — see Ulcer, cornea, central

Sahib disease B55.0

Sailors' skin L57.8

Saint

  Anthony's fire — see Erysipelas

  triad — see Hernia, diaphragm

  Vitus' dance — see Chorea, Sydenham's

Salaam

  attack(s) — see Epilepsy, spasms

Salaam — continued

  tic R25.8

Salicylism

  abuse F55.8

  overdose or wrong substance given — see Table of
    Drugs and Chemicals, by drug, poisoning

Salivary duct or gland — see condition

Salivation, excessive K11.7

Salmonella — see Infection, Salmonella

Salmonellosis A02.0

Salpingitis (catarrhal) (fallopian tube) (nodular) (pseud-
  ofollicular) (purulent) (septic) N70.91

  with oophoritis N70.93

  acute N70.01

    with oophoritis N70.03

  chlamydial A56.11

  chronic N70.11

    with oophoritis N70.13

  complicating abortion — see Abortion, by type, com-
    plicated by, salpingitis

  ear — see Salpingitis, eustachian

  eustachian (tube) H68.00- ☑

    acute H68.01- ☑

    chronic H68.02- ☑

  follicularis N70.11

    with oophoritis N70.13

  gonococcal (acute) (chronic) A54.24

  interstitial, chronic N70.11

    with oophoritis N70.13

  isthmica nodosa N70.11

    with oophoritis N70.13

  specific (gonococcal) (acute) (chronic) A54.24

  tuberculous (acute) (chronic) A18.17

  venereal (gonococcal) (acute) (chronic) A54.24

Salpingocele N83.4

Salpingo-oophoritis (catarrhal) (purulent) (ruptured)
  (septic) (suppurative) N70.93

  acute N70.03

    with ectopic or molar pregnancy O08.0

    following ectopic or molar pregnancy O08.0

    gonococcal A54.24

  chronic N70.13

  following ectopic or molar pregnancy O08.0

  gonococcal (acute) (chronic) A54.24

  puerperal O86.19

  specific (gonococcal) (acute) (chronic) A54.24

  subacute N70.03

  tuberculous (acute) (chronic) A18.17

  venereal (gonococcal) (acute) (chronic) A54.24

Salpingo-ovaritis — see Salpingo-oophoritis

Salpingoperitonitis — see Salpingo-oophoritis

Salzmann's nodular dystrophy — see Degeneration,
  cornea, nodular

Sampson's cyst or tumor N80.1

San Joaquin (Valley) **fever** B38.0

Sandblaster's asthma, lung or pneumoconiosis J62.8

Sander's disease (paranoia) F22

Sandfly fever A93.1

Sandhoff's disease E75.01

Sanfilippo (Type B) (Type C) (Type D) **syndrome** E76.22

Sanger-Brown ataxia G11.2

Sao Paulo fever or typhus A77.0

Saponification, mesenteric K65.8

Sarcocele (benign)

  syphilitic A52.76

    congenital A50.59

Sarcocystosis A07.8

Sarcoepiplocele — see Hernia

Sarcoepiplomphalocele Q79.2

Sarcoid (see also Sarcoidosis)

  arthropathy D86.86

  Boeck's D86.9

  Darier-Roussy D86.3

  iridocyclitis D86.83

  meningitis D86.81

  myocarditis D86.85

  myositis D86.87

  pyelonephritis D86.84

  Spiegler-Fendt L08.89

Sarcoidosis D86.9

  with

    cranial nerve palsies D86.82

    hepatic granuloma D86.89

    polyarthritis D86.86

    tubulo-interstitial nephropathy D86.84

  combined sites NEC D86.89

Sarcoidosis — continued

  lung D86.0

    and lymph nodes D86.2

  lymph nodes D86.1

    and lung D86.2

  meninges D86.81

  skin D86.3

  specified type NEC D86.89

Sarcoma (of) (see also Neoplasm, connective tissue, malignant)

  alveolar soft part — see Neoplasm, connective tissue,
    malignant

  ameloblastic C41.1

    upper jaw (bone) C41.0

  botryoid — see Neoplasm, connective tissue, malig-
    nant

  botryoides — see Neoplasm, connective tissue, malig-
    nant

  cerebellar C71.6

    circumscribed (arachnoidal) C71.6

  circumscribed (arachnoidal) cerebellar C71.6

  clear cell (see also Neoplasm, connective tissue, malig-
    nant)

    kidney C64.- ☑

  dendritic cells (accessory cells) C96.4

  embryonal — see Neoplasm, connective tissue, malig-
    nant

  endometrial (stromal) C54.1

    isthmus C54.0

  epithelioid (cell) — see Neoplasm, connective tissue,
    malignant

  Ewing's — see Neoplasm, bone, malignant

  follicular dendritic cell C96.4

  germinoblastic (diffuse) — see Lymphoma, diffuse
    large cell

    follicular — see Lymphoma, follicular, specified
      NEC

  giant cell (except of bone) (see also Neoplasm, connec-
    tive tissue, malignant)

    bone — see Neoplasm, bone, malignant

  glomoid — see Neoplasm, connective tissue, malig-
    nant

  granulocytic C92.3- ☑

  hemangioendothelial — see Neoplasm, connective
    tissue, malignant

  hemorrhagic, multiple — see Sarcoma, Kaposi's

  histiocytic C96.A (following C96.6)

  Hodgkin — see Lymphoma, Hodgkin

  immunoblastic (diffuse) — see Lymphoma, diffuse
    large cell

  interdigitating dendritic cell C96.4

  Kaposi's

    colon C46.4

    connective tissue C46.1

    gastrointestinal organ C46.4

    lung C46.5- ☑

    lymph node(s) C46.3

    palate (hard) (soft) C46.2

    rectum C46.4

    skin C46.0

    specified site NEC C46.7

    stomach C46.4

    unspecified site C46.9

  Kupffer cell C22.3

  Langerhans cell C96.4

  leptomeningeal — see Neoplasm, meninges, malig-
    nant

  liver NEC C22.4

  lymphangioendothelial — see Neoplasm, connective
    tissue, malignant

  lymphoblastic — see Lymphoma, lymphoblastic (dif-
    fuse)

  lymphocytic — see Lymphoma, small cell B-cell

  mast cell C96.2

  melanotic — see Melanoma

  meningeal — see Neoplasm, meninges, malignant

  meningothelial — see Neoplasm, meninges, malignant

  mesenchymal (see also Neoplasm, connective tissue,
    malignant)

    mixed — see Neoplasm, connective tissue, malig-
      nant

  mesothelial — see Mesothelioma

  monstrocellular

    specified site — see Neoplasm, malignant, by site

    unspecified site C71.9

  myeloid C92.3- ☑

  neurogenic — see Neoplasm, nerve, malignant

▽ Subterms under main terms may continue to next column or page   ☑ Additional Character Required — Refer to the Tabular List for Character Selection   271

Rupture, ruptured — Sarcoma

Sarcoma — *continued*
odontogenic C41.1
upper jaw (bone) C41.0
osteoblastic — *see* Neoplasm, bone, malignant
osteogenic (*see also* Neoplasm, bone, malignant)
juxtacortical — *see* Neoplasm, bone, malignant
periosteal — *see* Neoplasm, bone, malignant
periosteal (*see also* Neoplasm, bone, malignant)
osteogenic — *see* Neoplasm, bone, malignant
pleomorphic cell — *see* Neoplasm, connective tissue, malignant
reticulum cell (diffuse) — *see* Lymphoma, diffuse large cell
nodular — *see* Lymphoma, follicular
pleomorphic cell type — *see* Lymphoma, diffuse large cell
rhabdoid — *see* Neoplasm, malignant, by site
round cell — *see* Neoplasm, connective tissue, malignant
small cell — *see* Neoplasm, connective tissue, malignant
soft tissue — *see* Neoplasm, connective tissue, malignant
spindle cell — *see* Neoplasm, connective tissue, malignant
stromal (endometrial) C54.1
isthmus C54.0
synovial (*see also* Neoplasm, connective tissue, malignant)
biphasic — *see* Neoplasm, connective tissue, malignant
epithelioid cell — *see* Neoplasm, connective tissue, malignant
spindle cell — *see* Neoplasm, connective tissue, malignant
Sarcomatosis
meningeal — *see* Neoplasm, meninges, malignant
specified site NEC — *see* Neoplasm, connective tissue, malignant
unspecified site C80.1
Sarcosinemia E72.59
Sarcosporidiosis (intestinal) A07.8
Satiety, early R68.81
Saturnine — *see* condition
Saturnism
overdose or wrong substance given or taken — *see* Table of Drugs and Chemicals, by drug, poisoning
Satyriasis F52.8
Sauriasis — *see* Ichthyosis
SBE (subacute bacterial endocarditis) I33.0
Scabies (any site) B86
Scabs R23.4
Scaglietti-Dagnini syndrome E22.0
Scald — *see* Burn
Scalenus anticus (anterior) **syndrome** G54.0
Scales R23.4
Scaling, skin R23.4
Scalp — *see* condition
Scapegoating affecting child Z62.3
Scaphocephaly Q75.0
Scapulalgia M89.8X1
Scapulohumeral myopathy G71.0
Scar, scarring (*see also* Cicatrix) L90.5
adherent L90.5
atrophic L90.5
cervix
in pregnancy or childbirth — *see* Pregnancy, complicated by, abnormal cervix
cheloid L91.0
chorioretinal H31.00- ☑
posterior pole macula H31.01- ☑
postsurgical H59.81- ☑
solar retinopathy H31.02- ☑
specified type NEC H31.09- ☑
choroid — *see* Scar, chorioretinal
conjunctiva H11.24- ☑
cornea H17.9
xerophthalmic (*see also* Opacity, cornea)
vitamin A deficiency E50.6
duodenum, obstructive K31.5
hypertrophic L91.0
keloid L91.0
labia N90.89
lung (base) J98.4
macula — *see* Scar, chorioretinal, posterior pole
muscle M62.89

Scar, scarring — *continued*
myocardium, myocardial I25.2
painful L90.5
posterior pole (eye) — *see* Scar, chorioretinal, posterior pole
retina — *see* Scar, chorioretinal
trachea J39.8
uterus N85.8
in pregnancy O34.29
vagina N89.8
postoperative N99.2
vulva N90.89
Scarabiasis B88.2
Scarlatina (anginosa) (maligna) (ulcerosa) A38.9
myocarditis (acute) A38.1
old — *see* Myocarditis
otitis media A38.0
Scarlet fever (albuminuria) (angina) A38.9
Schamberg's disease (progressive pigmentary dermatosis) L81.7
Schatzki's ring (acquired) (esophagus) (lower) K22.2
congenital Q39.3
Schaufenster krankheit I20.8
Schaumann's
benign lymphogranulomatosis D86.1
disease or syndrome — *see* Sarcoidosis
Scheie's syndrome E76.03
Schenck's disease B42.1
Scheuermann's disease or osteochondrosis — *see* Osteochondrosis, juvenile, spine
Schilder (-Flatau) **disease** G37.0
Schilling-type monocytic leukemia C93.0- ☑
Schimmelbusch's disease, cystic mastitis, or hyperplasia — *see* Mastopathy, cystic
Schistosoma infestation — *see* Infestation, Schistosoma
Schistosomiasis B65.9
with muscle disorder B65.9 [M63.80]
ankle B65.9 [M63.87-] ☑
foot B65.9 [M63.87-] ☑
forearm B65.9 [M63.83-] ☑
hand B65.9 [M63.84-] ☑
lower leg B65.9 [M63.86-] ☑
multiple sites B65.9 [M63.89]
pelvic region B65.9 [M63.85-] ☑
shoulder region B65.9 [M63.81-] ☑
specified site NEC B65.9 [M63.88]
thigh B65.9 [M63.85-] ☑
upper arm B65.9 [M63.82-] ☑
Asiatic B65.2
bladder B65.0
chestermani B65.8
colon B65.1
cutaneous B65.3
due to
S. haematobium B65.0
S. japonicum B65.2
S. mansoni B65.1
S. mattheii B65.8
Eastern B65.2
genitourinary tract B65.0
intestinal B65.1
lung NEC B65.9 [J99]
pneumonia B65.9 [J17]
Manson's (intestinal) B65.1
oriental B65.2
pulmonary NEC B65.9 [J99]
pneumonia B65.9
Schistosoma
haematobium B65.0
japonicum B65.2
mansoni B65.1
specified type NEC B65.8
urinary B65.0
vesical B65.0
Schizencephaly Q04.6
Schizoaffective psychosis F25.9
Schizodontia K00.2
Schizoid personality F60.1
Schizophrenia, schizophrenic F20.9
acute (brief) (undifferentiated) F23
atypical (form) F20.3
borderline F21
catalepsy F20.2
catatonic (type) (excited) (withdrawn) F20.2
cenesthopathic, cenesthesiopathic F20.89
childhood type F84.5
chronic undifferentiated F20.5

Schizophrenia, schizophrenic — *continued*
cyclic F25.0
disorganized (type) F20.1
flexibilitas cerea F20.2
hebephrenic (type) F20.1
incipient F21
latent F21
negative type F20.5
paranoid (type) F20.0
paraphrenic F20.0
post-psychotic depression F32.8
prepsychotic F21
prodromal F21
pseudoneurotic F21
pseudopsychopathic F21
reaction F23
residual (state) (type) F20.5
restzustand F20.5
schizoaffective (type) — *see* Psychosis, schizoaffective
simple (type) F20.89
simplex F20.89
specified type NEC F20.89
stupor F20.2
syndrome of childhood F84.5
undifferentiated (type) F20.3
chronic F20.5
Schizothymia (persistent) F60.1
Schlatter-Osgood disease or osteochondrosis — *see* Osteochondrosis, juvenile, tibia
Schlatter's tibia — *see* Osteochondrosis, juvenile, tibia
Schmidt's syndrome (polyglandular, autoimmune) E31.0
Schmincke's carcinoma or tumor — *see* Neoplasm, nasopharynx, malignant
Schmitz (-Stutzer) **dysentery** A03.0
Schmorl's disease or nodes
lumbar region M51.46
lumbosacral region M51.47
sacrococcygeal region M53.3
thoracic region M51.44
thoracolumbar region M51.45
Schneiderian
papilloma — *see* Neoplasm, nasopharynx, benign
specified site — *see* Neoplasm, benign, by site
unspecified site D14.0
specified site — *see* Neoplasm, malignant, by site
unspecified site C30.0
Scholte's syndrome (malignant carcinoid) E34.0
Scholz (-Bielchowsky-Henneberg) **disease or syndrome** E75.25
Schönlein (-Henoch) disease or purpura (primary) (rheumatic) D69.0
Schottmuller's disease A01.4
Schroeder's syndrome (endocrine hypertensive) E27.0
Schüller-Christian disease or syndrome C96.5
Schultze's type acroparesthesia, simple I73.89
Schultz's disease or syndrome — *see* Agranulocytosis
Schwalbe-Ziehen-Oppenheim disease G24.1
Schwannoma (*see also* Neoplasm, nerve, benign)
malignant (*see also* Neoplasm, nerve, malignant)
with rhabdomyoblastic differentiation — *see* Neoplasm, nerve, malignant
melanocytic — *see* Neoplasm, nerve, benign
pigmented — *see* Neoplasm, nerve, benign
Schwannomatosis Q85.03
Schwartz (-Jampel) **syndrome** G71.13
Schwartz-Bartter syndrome E22.2
Schweniger-Buzzi anetoderma L90.1
Sciatic — *see* condition
Sciatica (infective)
with lumbago M54.4- ☑
due to intervertebral disc disorder — *see* Disorder, disc, with, radiculopathy
due to displacement of intervertebral disc (with lumbago) — *see* Disorder, disc, with, radiculopathy
wallet M54.3- ☑
Scimitar syndrome Q26.8
Sclera — *see* condition
Sclerectasia H15.84- ☑
Scleredema
adultorum — *see* Sclerosis, systemic
Buschke's — *see* Sclerosis, systemic
newborn P83.0
Sclerema (adiposum) (edematosum) (neonatorum) (newborn) P83.0
adultorum — *see* Sclerosis, systemic
Scleriasis — *see* Scleroderma

Scleritis H15.00- ☑
  with corneal involvement H15.04- ☑
  anterior H15.01- ☑
  brawny H15.02- ☑
  in (due to) zoster B02.34
  posterior H15.03- ☑
  specified type NEC H15.09- ☑
  syphilitic A52.71
  tuberculous (nodular) A18.51
Sclerochoroiditis H31.8
Scleroconjunctivitis — *see* Scleritis
Sclerocystic ovary syndrome E28.2
Sclerodactyly, sclerodactylia L94.3
Scleroderma, sclerodermia (acrosclerotic) (diffuse)
  (generalized) (progressive) (pulmonary) (*see also*
  Sclerosis, systemic) M34.9
  circumscribed L94.0
  linear L94.1
  localized L94.0
  newborn P83.8
  systemic M34.9
Sclerokeratitis H16.8
  tuberculous A18.52
Scleroma nasi A48.8
Scleromalacia (perforans) H15.05- ☑
Scleromyxedema L98.5
Sclérose en plaques G35
Sclerosis, sclerotic
  adrenal (gland) E27.8
  Alzheimer's — *see* Disease, Alzheimer's
  amyotrophic (lateral) G12.21
  aorta, aortic I70.0
    valve — *see* Endocarditis, aortic
  artery, arterial, arteriolar, arteriovascular — *see* Arteriosclerosis
  ascending multiple G35
  brain (generalized) (lobular) G37.9
    artery, arterial I67.2
    diffuse G37.0
    disseminated G35
    insular G35
    Krabbe's E75.23
    miliary G35
    multiple G35
    presenile (Alzheimer's) — *see* Disease, Alzheimer's,
      early onset
    senile (arteriosclerotic) I67.2
    stem, multiple G35
    tuberous Q85.1
  bulbar, multiple G35
  bundle of His I44.39
  cardiac — *see* Disease, heart, ischemic, atherosclerotic
  cardiorenal — *see* Hypertension, cardiorenal
  cardiovascular (*see also* Disease, cardiovascular)
    renal — *see* Hypertension, cardiorenal
  cerebellar — *see* Sclerosis, brain
  cerebral — *see* Sclerosis, brain
  cerebrospinal (disseminated) (multiple) G35
  cerebrovascular I67.2
  choroid — *see* Degeneration, choroid
  combined (spinal cord) (*see also* Degeneration, combined)
    multiple G35
  concentric (Balo) G37.5
  cornea — *see* Opacity, cornea
  coronary (artery) I25.10
    with angina pectoris — *see* Arteriosclerosis, coronary (artery),
  corpus cavernosum
    female N90.89
    male N48.6
  diffuse (brain) (spinal cord) G37.0
  disseminated G35
  dorsal G35
  dorsolateral (spinal cord) — *see* Degeneration, combined
  endometrium N85.5
  extrapyramidal G25.9
  eye, nuclear (senile) — *see* Cataract, senile, nuclear
  focal and segmental (glomerular) (*see also* N00-N07
    with fourth character .1) N05.1
  Friedreich's (spinal cord) G11.1
  funicular (spermatic cord) N50.8
  general (vascular) — *see* Arteriosclerosis
  gland (lymphatic) I89.8
  hepatic K74.1
    alcoholic K70.2

Sclerosis, sclerotic — *continued*
  hereditary
    cerebellar G11.9
    spinal (Friedreich's ataxia) G11.1
  hippocampal G93.81
  insular G35
  kidney — *see* Sclerosis, renal
  larynx J38.7
  lateral (amyotrophic) (descending) (primary) (spinal)
    G12.21
  lens, senile nuclear — *see* Cataract, senile, nuclear
  liver K74.1
    with fibrosis K74.2
      alcoholic K70.2
    alcoholic K70.2
    cardiac K76.1
  lung — *see* Fibrosis, lung
  mastoid — *see* Mastoiditis, chronic
  mesial temporal G93.81
  mitral I05.8
  Mönckeberg's (medial) — *see* Arteriosclerosis, extremities
  multiple (brain stem) (cerebral) (generalized) (spinal
    cord) G35
  myocardium, myocardial — *see* Disease, heart, ischemic, atherosclerotic
  nuclear (senile), eye — *see* Cataract, senile, nuclear
  ovary N83.8
  pancreas K86.8
  penis N48.6
  peripheral arteries — *see* Arteriosclerosis, extremities
  plaques G35
  pluriglandular E31.8
  polyglandular E31.8
  posterolateral (spinal cord) — *see* Degeneration,
    combined
  presenile (Alzheimer's) — *see* Disease, Alzheimer's,
    early onset
  primary, lateral G12.29
  progressive, systemic M34.0
  pulmonary — *see* Fibrosis, lung
    artery I27.0
    valve (heart) — *see* Endocarditis, pulmonary
  renal N26.9
    with
      cystine storage disease E72.09
      hypertensive heart disease (conditions in I11)
        — *see* Hypertension, cardiorenal
      arteriolar (hyaline) (hyperplastic) — *see* Hypertension, kidney
  retina (senile) (vascular) H35.00
  senile (vascular) — *see* Arteriosclerosis
  spinal (cord) (progressive) G95.89
    ascending G61.0
    combined (*see also* Degeneration, combined)
      multiple G35
      syphilitic A52.11
    disseminated G35
    dorsolateral — *see* Degeneration, combined
    hereditary (Friedreich's) (mixed form) G11.1
    lateral (amyotrophic) G12.21
    multiple G35
    posterior (syphilitic) A52.11
  stomach K31.89
  subendocardial, congenital I42.4
  systemic M34.9
    with
      lung involvement M34.81
      myopathy M34.82
      polyneuropathy M34.83
    drug-induced M34.2
    due to chemicals NEC M34.2
    progressive M34.0
    specified NEC M34.89
  temporal (mesial) G93.81
  tricuspid (heart) (valve) I07.8
  tuberous (brain) Q85.1
  tympanic membrane — *see* Disorder, tympanic
    membrane, specified NEC
  valve, valvular (heart) — *see* Endocarditis
  vascular — *see* Arteriosclerosis
  vein I87.8
Scoliosis (acquired) (postural) M41.9
  adolescent (idiopathic) — *see* Scoliosis, idiopathic,
    juvenile
  congenital Q67.5
    due to bony malformation Q76.3
    failure of segmentation (hemivertebra) Q76.3

Scoliosis — *continued*
  congenital — *continued*
    hemivertebra fusion Q76.3
    postural Q67.5
  idiopathic M41.20
    adolescent M41.129
      cervical region M41.122
      cervicothoracic region M41.123
      lumbar region M41.126
      lumbosacral region M41.127
      thoracic region M41.124
      thoracolumbar region M41.125
    cervical region M41.22
    cervicothoracic region M41.23
    infantile M41.00
      cervical region M41.02
      cervicothoracic region M41.03
      lumbar region M41.06
      lumbosacral region M41.07
      sacrococcygeal region M41.08
      thoracic region M41.04
      thoracolumbar region M41.05
    juvenile M41.119
      cervical region M41.112
      cervicothoracic region M41.113
      lumbar region M41.116
      lumbosacral region M41.117
      thoracic region M41.114
      thoracolumbar region M41.115
    lumbar region M41.26
    lumbosacral region M41.27
    thoracic region M41.24
    thoracolumbar region M41.25
  neuromuscular M41.40
    cervical region M41.42
    cervicothoracic region M41.43
    lumbar region M41.46
    lumbosacral region M41.47
    occipito-atlanto-axial region M41.41
    thoracic region M41.44
    thoracolumbar region M41.45
  paralytic — *see* Scoliosis, neuromuscular
  postradiation therapy M96.5
  rachitic (late effect or sequelae) E64.3 [M49.80]
    cervical region E64.3 [M49.82]
    cervicothoracic region E64.3 [M49.83]
    lumbar region E64.3 [M49.86]
    lumbosacral region E64.3 [M49.87]
    multiple sites E64.3 [M49.89]
    occipito-atlanto-axial region E64.3 [M49.81]
    sacrococcygeal region E64.3 [M49.88]
    thoracic region E64.3 [M49.84]
    thoracolumbar region E64.3 [M49.85]
  sciatic M54.4- ☑
  secondary (to) NEC M41.50
    cerebral palsy, Friedreich's ataxia, poliomyelitis,
      neuromuscular disorders — *see* Scoliosis,
      neuromuscular
    cervical region M41.52
    cervicothoracic region M41.53
    lumbar region M41.56
    lumbosacral region M41.57
    thoracic region M41.54
    thoracolumbar region M41.55
  specified form NEC M41.80
    cervical region M41.82
    cervicothoracic region M41.83
    lumbar region M41.86
    lumbosacral region M41.87
    thoracic region M41.84
    thoracolumbar region M41.85
  thoracogenic M41.30
    thoracic region M41.34
    thoracolumbar region M41.35
  tuberculous A18.01
Scoliotic pelvis
  with disproportion (fetopelvic) O33.0
    causing obstructed labor O65.0
Scorbutus, scorbutic (*see also* Scurvy)
  anemia D53.2
Scotoma (arcuate) (Bjerrum) (central) (ring) (*see also*
  Defect, visual field, localized, scotoma)
  scintillating H53.19
Scratch — *see* Abrasion
Scratchy throat R09.89
Screening (for) Z13.9
  alcoholism Z13.89
  anemia Z13.0

Screening — *continued*
anomaly, congenital Z13.89
antenatal, of mother Z36
arterial hypertension Z13.6
arthropod-borne viral disease NEC Z11.59
bacteriuria, asymptomatic Z13.89
behavioral disorder Z13.89
brain injury, traumatic Z13.850
bronchitis, chronic Z13.83
brucellosis Z11.2
cardiovascular disorder Z13.6
cataract Z13.5
chlamydial diseases Z11.8
cholera Z11.0
chromosomal abnormalities (nonprocreative) NEC
    Z13.79
colonoscopy Z12.11
congenital
    dislocation of hip Z13.89
    eye disorder Z13.5
    malformation or deformation Z13.89
contamination NEC Z13.88
cystic fibrosis Z13.228
dengue fever Z11.59
dental disorder Z13.84
depression Z13.89
developmental handicap Z13.4
    in early childhood Z13.4
diabetes mellitus Z13.1
diphtheria Z11.2
disability, intellectual Z13.4
disease or disorder Z13.9
    bacterial NEC Z11.2
        intestinal infectious Z11.0
        respiratory tuberculosis Z11.1
    blood or blood-forming organ Z13.0
    cardiovascular Z13.6
    Chagas' Z11.6
    chlamydial Z11.8
    dental Z13.89
    developmental Z13.4
    digestive tract NEC Z13.818
        lower GI Z13.811
        upper GI Z13.810
    ear Z13.5
    endocrine Z13.29
    eye Z13.5
    genitourinary Z13.89
    heart Z13.6
    human immunodeficiency virus (HIV) infection
        Z11.4
    immunity Z13.0
    infection
        intestinal Z11.0
            specified NEC Z11.6
    infectious Z11.9
    mental Z13.89
    metabolic Z13.228
    neurological Z13.89
    nutritional Z13.21
        metabolic Z13.228
            lipoid disorders Z13.220
    protozoal Z11.6
        intestinal Z11.0
    respiratory Z13.83
    rheumatic Z13.828
    rickettsial Z11.8
    sexually-transmitted NEC Z11.3
        human immunodeficiency virus (HIV) Z11.4
    sickle-cell (trait) Z13.0
    skin Z13.89
    specified NEC Z13.89
    spirochetal Z11.8
    thyroid Z13.29
    vascular Z13.6
    venereal Z11.3
    viral NEC Z11.59
        human immunodeficiency virus (HIV) Z11.4
        intestinal Z11.0
elevated titer Z13.89
emphysema Z13.83
encephalitis, viral (mosquito- or tick-borne) Z11.59
exposure to contaminants (toxic) Z13.88
fever
    dengue Z11.59
    hemorrhagic Z11.59
    yellow Z11.59
filariasis Z11.6

Screening — *continued*
galactosemia Z13.228
gastrointestinal condition Z13.818
genetic (nonprocreative) - for procreative manage-
      ment — *see* Testing, genetic, for procreative
      management
    disease carrier status (nonprocreative) Z13.71
    specified NEC (nonprocreative) Z13.79
genitourinary condition Z13.89
glaucoma Z13.5
gonorrhea Z11.3
gout Z13.89
helminthiasis (intestinal) Z11.6
hematopoietic malignancy Z12.89
hemoglobinopathies NEC Z13.0
hemorrhagic fever Z11.59
Hodgkin disease Z12.89
human immunodeficiency virus (HIV) Z11.4
human papillomavirus Z11.51
hypertension Z13.6
immunity disorders Z13.0
infection
    mycotic Z11.8
    parasitic Z11.8
ingestion of radioactive substance Z13.88
intellectual disability Z13.4
intestinal
    helminthiasis Z11.6
    infectious disease Z11.0
leishmaniasis Z11.6
leprosy Z11.2
leptospirosis Z11.8
leukemia Z12.89
lymphoma Z12.89
malaria Z11.6
malnutrition Z13.29
    metabolic Z13.228
    nutritional Z13.21
measles Z11.59
mental disorder Z13.89
metabolic errors, inborn Z13.228
multiphasic Z13.89
musculoskeletal disorder Z13.828
    osteoporosis Z13.820
mycoses Z11.8
myocardial infarction (acute) Z13.6
neoplasm (malignant) (of) Z12.9
    bladder Z12.6
    blood Z12.89
    breast Z12.39
        routine mammogram Z12.31
    cervix Z12.4
    colon Z12.11
    genitourinary organs NEC Z12.79
        bladder Z12.6
        cervix Z12.4
        ovary Z12.73
        prostate Z12.5
        testis Z12.71
        vagina Z12.72
    hematopoietic system Z12.89
    intestinal tract Z12.10
        colon Z12.11
        rectum Z12.12
        small intestine Z12.13
    lung Z12.2
    lymph (glands) Z12.89
    nervous system Z12.82
    oral cavity Z12.81
    prostate Z12.5
    rectum Z12.12
    respiratory organs Z12.2
    skin Z12.83
    small intestine Z12.13
    specified site NEC Z12.89
    stomach Z12.0
nephropathy Z13.89
nervous system disorders NEC Z13.858
neurological condition Z13.89
osteoporosis Z13.820
parasitic infestation Z11.9
    specified NEC Z11.8
phenylketonuria Z13.228
plague Z11.2
poisoning (chemical) (heavy metal) Z13.88
poliomyelitis Z11.59
postnatal, chromosomal abnormalities Z13.89
prenatal, of mother Z36

Screening — *continued*
protozoal disease Z11.6
    intestinal Z11.0
pulmonary tuberculosis Z11.1
radiation exposure Z13.88
respiratory condition Z13.83
respiratory tuberculosis Z11.1
rheumatoid arthritis Z13.828
rubella Z11.59
schistosomiasis Z11.6
sexually-transmitted disease NEC Z11.3
    human immunodeficiency virus (HIV) Z11.4
sickle-cell disease or trait Z13.0
skin condition Z13.89
sleeping sickness Z11.6
special Z13.9
    specified NEC Z13.89
syphilis Z11.3
tetanus Z11.2
trachoma Z11.8
traumatic brain injury Z13.850
trypanosomiasis Z11.6
tuberculosis, respiratory Z11.1
venereal disease Z11.3
viral encephalitis (mosquito- or tick-borne) Z11.59
whooping cough Z11.2
worms, intestinal Z11.6
yaws Z11.8
yellow fever Z11.59
Scrofula, scrofulosis (tuberculosis of cervical lymph
    glands) A18.2
Scrofulide (primary) (tuberculous) A18.4
Scrofuloderma, scrofulodermia (any site) (primary)
    A18.4
Scrofulosus lichen (primary) (tuberculous) A18.4
Scrofulous — *see* condition
Scrotal tongue K14.5
Scrotum — *see* condition
Scurvy, scorbutic E54
    anemia D53.2
    gum E54
    infantile E54
    rickets E55.0 [M90.80]
Sealpox B08.62
Seasickness T75.3 ☑
Seatworm (infection) (infestation) B80
Sebaceous (*see also* condition)
    cyst — *see* Cyst, sebaceous
Seborrhea, seborrheic L21.9
    capillitii R23.8
    capitis L21.0
    dermatitis L21.9
        infantile L21.1
    eczema L21.9
        infantile L21.1
    sicca L21.0
Seckel's syndrome Q87.1
Seclusion, pupil — *see* Membrane, pupillary
Second hand tobacco smoke exposure (acute)
    (chronic) Z77.22
    in the perinatal period P96.81
Secondary
    dentin (in pulp) K04.3
    neoplasm, secondaries — *see* Table of Neoplasms,
        secondary
Secretion
    antidiuretic hormone, inappropriate E22.2
    catecholamine, by pheochromocytoma E27.5
    hormone
        antidiuretic, inappropriate (syndrome) E22.2
        by
            carcinoid tumor E34.0
            pheochromocytoma E27.5
        ectopic NEC E34.2
    urinary
        excessive R35.8
        suppression R34
Section
    nerve, traumatic — *see* Injury, nerve
Segmentation, incomplete (congenital) (*see also* Fu-
    sion)
    bone NEC Q78.8
    lumbosacral (joint) (vertebra) Q76.49
Seitelberger's syndrome (infantile neuraxonal dystro-
    phy) G31.89
Seizure(s) (*see also* Convulsions) R56.9
    akinetic — *see* Epilepsy, generalized, specified NEC
    atonic — *see* Epilepsy, generalized, specified NEC

☑ **Additional Character Required — Refer to the Tabular List for Character Selection**   ▼ Subterms under main terms may continue to next column or page

Seizure(s) — *continued*
  autonomic (hysterical) F44.5
  convulsive — *see* Convulsions
  cortical (focal) (motor) — *see* Epilepsy, localization-
     related, symptomatic, with simple partial
     seizures
  disorder (*see also* Epilepsy) G40.909
  due to stroke — *see* Sequelae (of), disease, cerebrovas-
     cular, by type, specified NEC
  epileptic — *see* Epilepsy
  febrile (simple) R56.00
    with status epilepticus G40.901
    complex (atypical) (complicated) R56.01
      with status epilepticus G40.901
  grand mal G40.409
    intractable G40.419
      with status epilepticus G40.411
      without status epilepticus G40.419
    not intractable G40.409
      with status epilepticus G40.401
      without status epilepticus G40.409
  heart — *see* Disease, heart
  hysterical F44.5
  intractable G40.919
    with status epilepticus G40.911
  Jacksonian (focal) (motor type) (sensory type) — *see*
     Epilepsy, localization-related, symptomatic, with
     simple partial seizures
  newborn P90
  nonspecific epileptic
    atonic — *see* Epilepsy, generalized, specified NEC
    clonic — *see* Epilepsy, generalized, specified NEC
    myoclonic — *see* Epilepsy, generalized, specified
      NEC
    tonic — *see* Epilepsy, generalized, specified NEC
    tonic-clonic — *see* Epilepsy, generalized, specified
      NEC
  partial, developing into secondarily generalized
    seizures
    complex — *see* Epilepsy, localization-related,
     symptomatic, with complex partial seizures
    simple — *see* Epilepsy, localization-related, symp-
     tomatic, with simple partial seizures
  petit mal G40.409
    intractable G40.419
      with status epilepticus G40.411
      without status epilepticus G40.419
    not intractable G40.409
      with status epilepticus G40.401
      without status epilepticus G40.409
  post traumatic R56.1
  recurrent G40.909
  specified NEC G40.89
  uncinate — *see* Epilepsy, localization-related, symp-
    tomatic, with complex partial seizures
Selenium deficiency, dietary E59
Self-damaging behavior (life-style) Z72.89
Self-harm (attempted)
  history (personal) Z91.5
    in family Z81.8
Self-mutilation (attempted)
  history (personal) Z91.5
    in family Z81.8
Self-poisoning
  history (personal) Z91.5
    in family Z81.8
  observation following (alleged) attempt Z03.6
Semicoma R40.1
Seminal vesiculitis N49.0
Seminoma C62.9- ☑
  specified site — *see* Neoplasm, malignant, by site
Senear-Usher disease or syndrome L10.4
Senectus R54
Senescence (without mention of psychosis) R54
Senile, senility (*see also* condition) R41.81
  with
    acute confusional state F05
    mental changes NOS F03 ☑
    psychosis NEC — *see* Psychosis, senile
  asthenia R54
  cervix (atrophic) N88.8
  debility R54
  endometrium (atrophic) N85.8
  fallopian tube (atrophic) — *see* Atrophy, fallopian tube
  heart (failure) R54
  ovary (atrophic) — *see* Atrophy, ovary
  premature E34.8

Senile, senility — *continued*
  vagina, vaginitis (atrophic) N95.2
  wart L82.1
Sensation
  burning (skin) R20.8
    tongue K14.6
  loss of R20.8
  prickling (skin) R20.2
  tingling (skin) R20.2
Sense loss
  smell — *see* Disturbance, sensation, smell
  taste — *see* Disturbance, sensation, taste
  touch R20.8
Sensibility disturbance (cortical) (deep) (vibratory)
  R20.9
Sensitive, sensitivity (*see also* Allergy)
  carotid sinus G90.01
  child (excessive) F93.8
  cold, autoimmune D59.1
  dentin K03.89
  latex Z91.040
  methemoglobin D74.8
  tuberculin, without clinical or radiological symptoms
    R76.11
  visual
    glare H53.71
    impaired contrast H53.72
Sensitiver Beziehungswahn F22
Sensitization, auto-erythrocytic D69.2
Separation
  anxiety, abnormal (of childhood) F93.0
  apophysis, traumatic — *code as* Fracture, by site
  choroid — *see* Detachment, choroid
  epiphysis, epiphyseal
    nontraumatic (*see also* Osteochondropathy, speci-
     fied type NEC)
      upper femoral — *see* Slipped, epiphysis, upper
      femoral
    traumatic — *code as* Fracture, by site
  fracture — *see* Fracture
  infundibulum cardiac from right ventricle by a partition
    Q24.3
  joint (traumatic) (current) — *code by* site under Dislo-
    cation
  pubic bone, obstetrical trauma O71.6
  retina, retinal — *see* Detachment, retina
  symphysis pubis, obstetrical trauma O71.6
  tracheal ring, incomplete, congenital Q32.1
Sepsis (generalized) (unspecified organism) A41.9
  with
    organ dysfunction (acute) (multiple) R65.20
      with septic shock R65.21
  actinomycotic A42.7
  adrenal hemorrhage syndrome (meningococcal) A39.1
  anaerobic A41.4
  Bacillus anthracis A22.7
  Brucella (*see also* Brucellosis) A23.9
  candidal B37.7
  cryptogenic A41.9
  due to device, implant or graft T85.79 ☑
    arterial graft NEC T82.7 ☑
    breast (implant) T85.79 ☑
    catheter NEC T85.79 ☑
      dialysis (renal) T82.7 ☑
        intraperitoneal T85.71 ☑
      infusion NEC T82.7 ☑
        spinal (epidural) (subdural) T85.79 ☑
      urinary (indwelling) T83.51 ☑
    ectopic or molar pregnancy O08.82
    electronic (electrode) (pulse generator) (stimulator)
      bone T84.7 ☑
      cardiac T82.7 ☑
      nervous system (brain) (peripheral nerve)
        (spinal) T85.79 ☑
      urinary T83.59 ☑
    fixation, internal (orthopedic) — *see* Complication,
      fixation device, infection
    gastrointestinal (bile duct) (esophagus) T85.79 ☑
    genital T83.6 ☑
    heart NEC T82.7 ☑
      valve (prosthesis) T82.6 ☑
        graft T82.7 ☑
    joint prosthesis — *see* Complication, joint prosthe-
      sis, infection
    ocular (corneal graft) (orbital implant) T85.79 ☑
    orthopedic NEC T84.7 ☑

Sepsis — *continued*
  due to device, implant or graft — *continued*
    orthopedic — *continued*
      fixation device, internal — *see* Complication,
        fixation device, infection
      specified NEC T85.79 ☑
      vascular T82.7 ☑
      ventricular intracranial shunt T85.79 ☑
  during labor O75.3
  Enterococcus A41.81
  Erysipelothrix (rhusiopathiae) (erysipeloid) A26.7
  Escherichia coli (E. coli) A41.5 ☑
  extraintestinal yersiniosis A28.2
  following
    abortion (subsequent episode) O08.0
      current episode — *see* Abortion
    ectopic or molar pregnancy O08.82
    immunization T88.0 ☑
    infusion, therapeutic injection or transfusion NEC
      T80.29 ☑
  gangrenous A41.9
  gonococcal A54.86
  Gram-negative (organism) A41.5 ☑
    anaerobic A41.4
  Haemophilus influenzae A41.3
  herpesviral B00.7
  intra-abdominal K65.1
  intraocular — *see* Endophthalmitis, purulent
  Listeria monocytogenes A32.7
  localized — *code to* specific localized infection
    in operation wound T81.4 ☑
    skin — *see* Abscess
  malleus A24.0
  melioidosis A24.1
  meningeal — *see* Meningitis
  meningococcal A39.4
    acute A39.2
    chronic A39.3
  MSSA (Methicillin susceptible Staphylococcus aureus)
    A41.01
  newborn P36.9
    due to
      anaerobes NEC P36.5
      Escherichia coli P36.4
      Staphylococcus P36.30
        aureus P36.2
        specified NEC P36.39
      Streptococcus P36.10
        group B P36.0
        specified NEC P36.19
    specified NEC P36.8
  Pasteurella multocida A28.0
  pelvic, puerperal, postpartum, childbirth O85
  pneumococcal A40.3
  postprocedural T81.4 ☑
  puerperal, postpartum, childbirth (pelvic) O85
  Salmonella (arizonae) (cholerae-suis) (enteritidis) (ty-
    phimurium) A02.1
  severe R65.20
    with septic shock R65.21
  Shigella (*see also* Dysentery, bacillary) A03.9
  skin, localized — *see* Abscess
  specified organism NEC A41.89
  Staphylococcus, staphylococcal A41.2
    aureus (methicillin susceptible) (MSSA) A41.01
      methicillin resistant (MRSA) A41.02
    coagulase-negative A41.1
    specified NEC A41.1
  Streptococcus, streptococcal A40.9
    agalactiae A40.1
    group
      A A40.0
      B A40.1
      D A41.81
    neonatal P36.10
      group B P36.0
      specified NEC P36.19
    pneumoniae A40.3
    pyogenes A40.0
    specified NEC A40.8
  tracheostomy stoma J95.02
  tularemic A21.7
  umbilical, umbilical cord (newborn) — *see* Sepsis,
    newborn
  Yersinia pestis A20.7
Septate — *see* Septum

Septic — *see* condition
arm — *see* Cellulitis, upper limb
with lymphangitis — *see* Lymphangitis, acute, upper limb
embolus — *see* Embolism
finger — *see* Cellulitis, digit
with lymphangitis — *see* Lymphangitis, acute, digit
foot — *see* Cellulitis, lower limb
with lymphangitis — *see* Lymphangitis, acute, lower limb
gallbladder (acute) K81.0
hand — *see* Cellulitis, upper limb
with lymphangitis — *see* Lymphangitis, acute, upper limb
joint — *see* Arthritis, pyogenic or pyemic
leg — *see* Cellulitis, lower limb
with lymphangitis — *see* Lymphangitis, acute, lower limb
nail (*see also* Cellulitis, digit)
with lymphangitis — *see* Lymphangitis, acute, digit
sore (*see also* Abscess)
throat J02.0
streptococcal J02.0
spleen (acute) D73.89
teeth, tooth (pulpal origin) K04.4
throat — *see* Pharyngitis
thrombus — *see* Thrombosis
toe — *see* Cellulitis, digit
with lymphangitis — *see* Lymphangitis, acute, digit
tonsils, chronic J35.01
with adenoiditis J35.03
uterus — *see* Endometritis
Septicemia A41.9
meaning sepsis — *see* Sepsis
Septum, septate (congenital) (*see also* Anomaly, by site)
anal Q42.3
with fistula Q42.2
aqueduct of Sylvius Q03.0
with spina bifida — *see* Spina bifida, by site, with hydrocephalus
uterus (complete) (partial) Q51.2
vagina Q52.10
in pregnancy — *see* Pregnancy, complicated by, abnormal vagina
causing obstructed labor O65.5
longitudinal (with or without obstruction) Q52.12
transverse Q52.11
Sequelae (of) (*see also* condition)
abscess, intracranial or intraspinal (conditions in G06) G09
amputation — *code to* injury with seventh character S
burn and corrosion — *code to* injury with seventh character S
calcium deficiency E64.8
cerebrovascular disease — *see* Sequelae, disease, cerebrovascular
childbirth O94
contusion — *code to* injury with seventh character S
corrosion — *see* Sequelae, burn and corrosion
crushing injury — *code to* injury with seventh character S
disease
cerebrovascular I69.90
alteration of sensation I69.998
aphasia I69.920
apraxia I69.990
ataxia I69.993
cognitive deficits I69.91
disturbance of vision I69.998
dysarthria I69.922
dysphagia I69.991
dysphasia I69.921
facial droop I69.992
facial weakness I69.992
fluency disorder I69.923
hemiplegia I69.95- ☑
hemorrhage
intracerebral — *see* Sequelae, hemorrhage, intracerebral
intracranial, nontraumatic NEC — *see* Sequelae, hemorrhage, intracranial, nontraumatic

Sequelae — *continued*
disease — *continued*
cerebrovascular — *continued*
hemorrhage — *continued*
subarachnoid — *see* Sequelae, hemorrhage, subarachnoid
language deficit I69.928
monoplegia
lower limb I69.84- ☑
upper limb I69.93- ☑
paralytic syndrome I69.96- ☑
specified effect NEC I69.998
specified type NEC I69.80
alteration of sensation I69.898
aphasia I69.820
apraxia I69.890
ataxia I69.893
cognitive deficits I69.81
disturbance of vision I69.898
dysarthria I69.822
dysphagia I69.891
dysphasia I69.821
facial droop I69.892
facial weakness I69.892
fluency disorder I69.823
hemiplegia I69.85- ☑
language deficit I69.828
monoplegia
lower limb I69.84- ☑
upper limb I69.83- ☑
paralytic syndrome I69.86- ☑
specified effect NEC I69.898
speech deficit I69.928
speech deficit I69.828
stroke NOS — *see* Sequelae, stroke NOS
dislocation — *code to* injury with seventh character S
encephalitis or encephalomyelitis (conditions in G04) G09
in infectious disease NEC B94.8
viral B94.1
external cause — *code to* injury with seventh character S
foreign body entering natural orifice — *code to* injury with seventh character S
fracture — *code to* injury with seventh character S
frostbite — *code to* injury with seventh character S
Hansen's disease B92
hemorrhage
intracerebral I69.10
alteration of sensation I69.198
aphasia I69.120
apraxia I69.190
ataxia I69.193
cognitive deficits I69.11
disturbance of vision I69.198
dysarthria I69.122
dysphagia I69.191
dysphasia I69.121
facial droop I69.192
facial weakness I69.192
fluency disorder I69.123
hemiplegia I69.15- ☑
language deficit NEC I69.128
monoplegia
lower limb I69.14- ☑
upper limb I69.13- ☑
paralytic syndrome I69.16- ☑
specified effect NEC I69.198
speech deficit NEC I69.128
intracranial, nontraumatic NEC I69.20
alteration of sensation I69.298
aphasia I69.220
apraxia I69.290
ataxia I69.293
cognitive deficits I69.21
disturbance of vision I69.298
dysarthria I69.222
dysphagia I69.291
dysphasia I69.221
facial droop I69.292
facial weakness I69.292
fluency disorder I69.223
hemiplegia I69.25- ☑
language deficit NEC I69.228
monoplegia
lower limb I69.24- ☑
upper limb I69.23- ☑
paralytic syndrome I69.26- ☑

Sequelae — *continued*
hemorrhage — *continued*
intracranial, nontraumatic — *continued*
specified effect NEC I69.298
speech deficit NEC I69.228
subarachnoid I69.00
alteration of sensation I69.098
aphasia I69.020
apraxia I69.090
ataxia I69.093
cognitive deficits I69.01
disturbance of vision I69.098
dysarthria I69.022
dysphagia I69.091
dysphasia I69.021
facial droop I69.092
facial weakness I69.092
fluency disorder I69.023
hemiplegia I69.05- ☑
language deficit NEC I69.028
monoplegia
lower limb I69.04- ☑
upper limb I69.03- ☑
paralytic syndrome I69.06- ☑
specified effect NEC I69.098
speech deficit NEC I69.028
hepatitis, viral B94.2
hyperalimentation E68
infarction
cerebral I69.30
alteration of sensation I69.398
aphasia I69.320
apraxia I69.390
ataxia I69.393
cognitive deficits I69.31
disturbance of vision I69.398
dysarthria I69.322
dysphagia I69.391
dysphasia I69.321
facial droop I69.392
facial weakness I69.392
fluency disorder I69.323
hemiplegia I69.35- ☑
language deficit NEC I69.328
monoplegia
lower limb I69.34- ☑
upper limb I69.33- ☑
paralytic syndrome I69.36- ☑
specified effect NEC I69.398
speech deficit NEC I69.328
infection, pyogenic, intracranial or intraspinal G09
infectious disease B94.9
specified NEC B94.8
injury — *code to* injury with seventh character S
leprosy B92
meningitis
bacterial (conditions in G00) G09
other or unspecified cause (conditions in G03) G09
muscle (and tendon) injury — *code to* injury with seventh character S
myelitis — *see* Sequelae, encephalitis
niacin deficiency E64.8
nutritional deficiency E64.9
specified NEC E64.8
obstetrical condition O94
parasitic disease B94.9
phlebitis or thrombophlebitis of intracranial or intraspinal venous sinuses and veins (conditions in G08) G09
poisoning — *code to* poisoning with seventh character S
nonmedicinal substance — *see* Sequelae, toxic effect, nonmedicinal substance
poliomyelitis (acute) B91
pregnancy O94
protein-energy malnutrition E64.0
puerperium O94
rickets E64.3
selenium deficiency E64.8
sprain and strain — *code to* injury with seventh character S
stroke NOS I69.30
alteration in sensation I69.398
aphasia I69.320
apraxia I69.390
ataxia I69.393
cognitive deficits I69.31
disturbance of vision I69.398

Sequelae — *continued*
  stroke — *continued*
    dysarthria I69.322
    dysphagia I69.391
    dysphasia I69.321
    facial droop I69.392
    facial weakness I69.392
    hemiplegia I69.35- ☑
    language deficit NEC I69.328
    monoplegia
      lower limb I69.34- ☑
      upper limb I69.33- ☑
    paralytic syndrome I69.36- ☑
    specified effect NEC I69.398
    speech deficit NEC I69.328
  tendon and muscle injury — *code to* injury with seventh character S
  thiamine deficiency E64.8
  trachoma B94.0
  tuberculosis B90.9
    bones and joints B90.2
    central nervous system B90.0
    genitourinary B90.1
    pulmonary (respiratory) B90.9
    specified organs NEC B90.8
  viral
    encephalitis B94.1
    hepatitis B94.2
  vitamin deficiency NEC E64.8
    A E64.1
    B E64.8
    C E64.2
  wound, open — *code to* injury with seventh character S

Sequestration (*see also* Sequestrum)
  lung, congenital Q33.2

Sequestrum
  bone — *see* Osteomyelitis, chronic
  dental M27.2
  jaw bone M27.2
  orbit — *see* Osteomyelitis, orbit
  sinus (accessory) (nasal) — *see* Sinusitis

Sequoiosis lung or pneumonitis J67.8

Serology for syphilis
  doubtful
    with signs or symptoms — *code by* site and stage under Syphilis
    follow-up of latent syphilis — *see* Syphilis, latent
  negative, with signs or symptoms — *code by* site and stage under Syphilis
  positive A53.0
    with signs or symptoms — *code by* site and stage under Syphilis
    reactivated A53.0

Seroma (*see also* Hematoma)
  traumatic, secondary and recurrent T79.2 ☑

Seropurulent — *see* condition

Serositis, multiple K65.8
  pericardial I31.1
  peritoneal K65.8

Serous — *see* condition

Sertoli cell
  adenoma
    specified site — *see* Neoplasm, benign, by site
    unspecified site
      female D27.9
      male D29.20
  carcinoma
    specified site — *see* Neoplasm, malignant, by site
    unspecified site (male) C62.9- ☑
      female C56.9
  tumor
    with lipid storage
      specified site — *see* Neoplasm, benign, by site
      unspecified site
        female D27.9
        male D29.20
    specified site — *see* Neoplasm, benign, by site
    unspecified site
      female D27.9
      male D29.20

Sertoli-Leydig cell tumor — *see* Neoplasm, benign, by site
  specified site — *see* Neoplasm, benign, by site
  unspecified site
    female D27.9
    male D29.20

Serum
  allergy, allergic reaction (*see also* Reaction, serum) T80.69 ☑
    shock (*see also* Shock, anaphylactic) T80.59 ☑
  arthritis (*see also* Reaction, serum) T80.69 ☑
  complication or reaction NEC (*see also* Reaction, serum) T80.69 ☑
  disease NEC (*see also* Reaction, serum) T80.69 ☑
  hepatitis (*see also* Hepatitis, viral, type B)
    carrier (suspected) of Z22.51
  intoxication (*see also* Reaction, serum) T80.69 ☑
  neuritis (*see also* Reaction, serum) T80.69 ☑
  neuropathy G61.1
  poisoning NEC (*see also* Reaction, serum) T80.69 ☑
  rash NEC (*see also* Reaction, serum) T80.69 ☑
  reaction NEC (*see also* Reaction, serum) T80.69 ☑
  sickness NEC (*see also* Reaction, serum) T80.69 ☑
  urticaria (*see also* Reaction, serum) T80.69 ☑

Sesamoiditis M25.8- ☑

Severe sepsis R65.20
  with septic shock R65.21

Sever's disease or osteochondrosis — *see* Osteochondrosis, juvenile, tarsus

Sex
  chromosome mosaics Q97.8
    lines with various numbers of X chromosomes Q97.2
  education Z70.8
  reassignment surgery status Z87.890

Sextuplet pregnancy — *see* Pregnancy, sextuplet

Sexual
  function, disorder of (psychogenic) F52.9
  immaturity (female) (male) E30.0
  impotence (psychogenic) organic origin NEC — *see* Dysfunction, sexual, male
  precocity (constitutional) (cryptogenic)(female) (idiopathic) (male) E30.1

Sexuality, pathologic — *see* Deviation, sexual

Sézary disease C84.1- ☑

Shadow, lung R91.8

Shaking palsy or paralysis — *see* Parkinsonism

Shallowness, acetabulum — *see* Derangement, joint, specified type NEC, hip

Shaver's disease J63.1

Sheath (tendon) — *see* condition

Sheathing, retinal vessels H35.01- ☑

Shedding
  nail L60.8
  premature, primary (deciduous) teeth K00.6

Sheehan's disease or syndrome E23.0

Shelf, rectal K62.89

Shell teeth K00.5

Shellshock (current) F43.0
  lasting state — *see* Disorder, post-traumatic stress

Shield kidney Q63.1

Shift
  auditory threshold (temporary) H93.24- ☑
  mediastinal R93.8

Shifting sleep-work schedule (affecting sleep) G47.26

Shiga (-Kruse) **dysentery** A03.0

Shiga's bacillus A03.0

Shigella (dysentery) — *see* Dysentery, bacillary

Shigellosis A03.9
  Group A A03.0
  Group B A03.1
  Group C A03.2
  Group D A03.3

Shin splints S86.89- ☑

Shingles — *see* Herpes, zoster

Shipyard disease or eye B30.0

Shirodkar suture, in pregnancy — *see* Pregnancy, complicated by, incompetent cervix

Shock R57.9
  with ectopic or molar pregnancy O08.3
  adrenal (cortical) (Addisonian) E27.2
  adverse food reaction (anaphylactic) — *see* Shock, anaphylactic, due to food
  allergic — *see* Shock, anaphylactic
  anaphylactic T78.2 ☑
    chemical — *see* Table of Drugs and Chemicals
    due to drug or medicinal substance
      correct substance properly administered T88.6 ☑
      overdose or wrong substance given or taken (by accident) — *see* Table of Drugs and Chemicals, by drug, poisoning

Shock — *continued*
  anaphylactic — *continued*
    due to food (nonpoisonous) T78.00 ☑
      additives T78.06 ☑
      dairy products T78.07 ☑
      eggs T78.08 ☑
      fish T78.03 ☑
        shellfish T78.02 ☑
      fruit T78.04 ☑
      milk T78.07 ☑
      nuts T78.05 ☑
        peanuts T78.01 ☑
      peanuts T78.01 ☑
      seeds T78.05 ☑
      specified type NEC T78.09 ☑
      vegetable T78.04 ☑
    following sting(s) — *see* Venom
    immunization T80.52 ☑
    serum T80.59 ☑
      blood and blood products T80.51 ☑
      immunization T80.52 ☑
      specified NEC T80.59 ☑
      vaccination T80.52 ☑
  anaphylactoid — *see* Shock, anaphylactic
  anesthetic
    correct substance properly administered T88.2 ☑
    overdose or wrong substance given or taken — *see* Table of Drugs and Chemicals, by drug, poisoning
      specified anesthetic — *see* Table of Drugs and Chemicals, by drug, poisoning
  cardiogenic R57.0
  chemical substance — *see* Table of Drugs and Chemicals
  complicating ectopic or molar pregnancy O08.3
  culture — *see* Disorder, adjustment
  drug
    due to correct substance properly administered T88.6 ☑
    overdose or wrong substance given or taken (by accident) — *see* Table of Drugs and Chemicals, by drug, poisoning
  during or after labor and delivery O75.1
  electric T75.4 ☑
    (taser) T75.4 ☑
  endotoxic R65.21
    postprocedural (during or resulting from a procedure, not elsewhere classified) T81.12 ☑
  following
    ectopic or molar pregnancy O08.3
    injury (immediate) (delayed) T79.4 ☑
    labor and delivery O75.1
  food (anaphylactic) — *see* Shock, anaphylactic, due to food
  from electroshock gun (taser) T75.4 ☑
  gram-negative R65.21
    postprocedural (during or resulting from a procedure, not elsewhere classified) T81.12 ☑
  hematologic R57.8
  hemorrhagic
    surgery (intraoperative) (postoperative) T81.19 ☑
    trauma T79.4 ☑
  hypovolemic R57.1
    surgical T81.19 ☑
    traumatic T79.4 ☑
  insulin E15
    therapeutic misadventure — *see* subcategory T38.3 ☑
  kidney N17.0
    traumatic (following crushing) T79.5 ☑
  lightning T75.01 ☑
  lung J80
  obstetric O75.1
    with ectopic or molar pregnancy O08.3
    following ectopic or molar pregnancy O08.3
  pleural (surgical) T81.19 ☑
    due to trauma T79.4 ☑
  postprocedural (postoperative) T81.10 ☑
    with ectopic or molar pregnancy O08.3
    cardiogenic T81.11 ☑
    endotoxic T81.12 ☑
    following ectopic or molar pregnancy O08.3
    gram-negative T81.12 ☑
    hypovolemic T81.19 ☑
    septic T81.12 ☑
    specified type NEC T81.19 ☑

Shock — *continued*
  psychic F43.0
  septic (due to severe sepsis) R65.21
  specified NEC R57.8
  surgical T81.10 ☑
  taser gun (taser) T75.4 ☑
  therapeutic misadventure NEC T81.10 ☑
  thyroxin
    overdose or wrong substance given or taken —
        see Table of Drugs and Chemicals, by drug,
        poisoning
  toxic, syndrome A48.3
  transfusion — *see* Complications, transfusion
  traumatic (immediate) (delayed) T79.4 ☑
Shoemaker's chest M95.4
Short, shortening, shortness
  arm (acquired) (*see also* Deformity, limb, unequal
        length)
    congenital Q71.01 ☑
    forearm — *see* Deformity, limb, unequal length
  bowel syndrome K91.2
  breath R06.02
  cervical (complicating pregnancy) O26.87- ☑
    non-gravid uterus N88.3
  common bile duct, congenital Q44.5
  cord (umbilical), complicating delivery O69.3 ☑
  cystic duct, congenital Q44.5
  esophagus (congenital) Q39.8
  femur (acquired) — *see* Deformity, limb, unequal
        length, femur
    congenital — *see* Defect, reduction, lower limb,
        longitudinal, femur
  frenum, frenulum, linguae (congenital) Q38.1
  hip (acquired) (*see also* Deformity, limb, unequal
        length)
    congenital Q65.89
  leg (acquired) (*see also* Deformity, limb, unequal
        length)
    congenital Q72.81- ☑
    lower leg (*see also* Deformity, limb, unequal length)
  limbed stature, with immunodeficiency D82.2
  lower limb (acquired) (*see also* Deformity, limb, un-
        equal length)
    congenital Q72.81- ☑
  organ or site, congenital NEC — *see* Distortion
  palate, congenital Q38.5
  radius (acquired) (*see also* Deformity, limb, unequal
        length)
    congenital — *see* Defect, reduction, upper limb,
        longitudinal, radius
  rib syndrome Q77.2
  stature (child) (hereditary) (idiopathic) NEC R62.52
    constitutional E34.3
    due to endocrine disorder E34.3
    Laron-type E34.3
  tendon (*see also* Contraction, tendon)
    with contracture of joint — *see* Contraction, joint
    Achilles (acquired) M67.0- ☑
      congenital Q66.89
    congenital Q79.8
  thigh (acquired) (*see also* Deformity, limb, unequal
        length, femur)
    congenital — *see* Defect, reduction, lower limb,
        longitudinal, femur
  tibialis anterior (tendon) — *see* Contraction, tendon
  umbilical cord
    complicating delivery O69.3 ☑
  upper limb, congenital — *see* Defect, reduction, upper
        limb, specified type NEC
  urethra N36.8
  uvula, congenital Q38.5
  vagina (congenital) Q52.4
Shortsightedness — *see* Myopia
Shoshin (acute fulminating beriberi) E51.11
Shoulder — *see* condition
Shovel-shaped incisors K00.2
Shower, thromboembolic — *see* Embolism
Shunt
  arterial-venous (dialysis) Z99.2
  arteriovenous, pulmonary (acquired) I28.0
    congenital Q25.72
  cerebral ventricle (communicating) in situ Z98.2
  surgical, prosthetic, with complications — *see* Compli-
        cations, cardiovascular, device or implant
Shutdown, renal N28.9
Shy-Drager syndrome G90.3

Sialadenitis, sialadenosis (any gland) (chronic) (period-
    ic) (suppurative) — *see* Sialoadenitis
Sialectasia K11.8
Sialidosis E77.1
Sialitis, silitis (any gland) (chronic) (suppurative) — *see*
    Sialoadenitis
Sialoadenitis (any gland) (periodic) (suppurative) K11.20
  acute K11.21
    recurrent K11.22
  chronic K11.23
Sialoadenopathy K11.9
Sialoangitis — *see* Sialoadenitis
Sialodochitis (fibrinosa) — *see* Sialoadenitis
Sialodocholithiasis K11.5
Sialolithiasis K11.5
Sialometaplasia, necrotizing K11.8
Sialorrhea (*see also* Ptyalism)
  periodic — *see* Sialoadenitis
Sialosis K11.7
Siamese twin Q89.4
Sibling rivalry Z62.891
Sicard's syndrome G52.7
Sicca syndrome M35.00
  with
    keratoconjunctivitis M35.01
    lung involvement M35.02
    myopathy M35.03
    renal tubulo-interstitial disorders M35.04
  specified organ involvement NEC M35.09
Sick R69
  or handicapped person in family Z63.79
    needing care at home Z63.6
  sinus (syndrome) I49.5
Sick-euthyroid syndrome E07.81
Sickle-cell
  anemia — *see* Disease, sickle-cell
  trait D57.3
Sicklemia (*see also* Disease, sickle-cell)
  trait D57.3
Sickness
  air (travel) T75.3 ☑
  airplane T75.3 ☑
  alpine T70.29 ☑
  altitude T70.20 ☑
  Andes T70.29 ☑
  aviator's T70.29 ☑
  balloon T70.29 ☑
  car T75.3 ☑
  compressed air T70.3 ☑
  decompression T70.3 ☑
  green D50.8
  milk — *see* Poisoning, food, noxious
  motion T75.3 ☑
  mountain T70.29 ☑
    acute D75.1
  protein (*see also* Reaction, serum) T80.69 ☑
  radiation T66 ☑
  roundabout (motion) T75.3 ☑
  sea T75.3 ☑
  serum NEC (*see also* Reaction, serum) T80.69 ☑
  sleeping (African) B56.9
    by Trypanosoma B56.9
      brucei
        gambiense B56.0
        rhodesiense B56.1
    East African B56.1
    Gambian B56.0
    Rhodesian B56.1
    West African B56.0
  swing (motion) T75.3 ☑
  train (railway) (travel) T75.3 ☑
  travel (any vehicle) T75.3 ☑
Sideropenia — *see* Anemia, iron deficiency
Siderosilicosis J62.8
Siderosis (lung) J63.4
  eye (globe) — *see* Disorder, globe, degenerative,
        siderosis
Siemens' syndrome (ectodermal dysplasia) Q82.8
Sighing R06.89
  psychogenic F45.8
Sigmoid (*see also* condition)
  flexure — *see* condition
  kidney Q63.1
Sigmoiditis (*see also* Enteritis) K52.9
  infectious A09
  noninfectious K52.9
Silfversköld's syndrome Q78.9

Silicosiderosis J62.8
Silicosis, silicotic (simple) (complicated) J62.8
  with tuberculosis J65
Silicotuberculosis J65
Silo-fillers' disease J68.8
  bronchitis J68.0
  pneumonitis J68.0
  pulmonary edema J68.1
Silver's syndrome Q87.1
Simian malaria B53.1
Simmonds' cachexia or disease E23.0
Simons' disease or syndrome (progressive lipodystro-
    phy) E88.1
Simple, simplex — *see* condition
Simulation, conscious (of illness) Z76.5
Simultanagnosia (asimultagnosia) R48.3
Sin Nombre virus disease (Hantavirus) (cardio)-pul-
    monary syndrome) B33.4
Sinding-Larsen disease or osteochondrosis — *see*
    Osteochondrosis, juvenile, patella
Singapore hemorrhagic fever A91
Singer's node or nodule J38.2
Single
  atrium Q21.2
  coronary artery Q24.5
  umbilical artery Q27.0
  ventricle Q20.4
Singultus R06.6
  epidemicus B33.0
Sinus (*see also* Fistula)
  abdominal K63.89
  arrest I45.5
  arrhythmia I49.8
  bradycardia R00.1
  branchial cleft (internal) (external) Q18.0
  coccygeal — *see* Sinus, pilonidal
  dental K04.6
  dermal (congenital) Q06.8
    with abscess Q06.8
    coccygeal, pilonidal — *see* Sinus, coccygeal
  infected, skin NEC L08.89
  marginal, ruptured or bleeding — *see* Hemorrhage,
        antepartum, specified cause NEC
  medial, face and neck Q18.8
  pause I45.5
  pericranii Q01.9
  pilonidal (infected) (rectum) L05.92
    with abscess L05.02
  preauricular Q18.1
  rectovaginal N82.3
  Rokitansky-Aschoff (gallbladder) K82.8
  sacrococcygeal (dermoid) (infected) — *see* Sinus, pi-
        lonidal
  tachycardia R00.0
    paroxysmal I47.1
  tarsi syndrome M25.57- ☑
  testis N50.8
  tract (postinfective) — *see* Fistula
  urachus Q64.4
Sinusitis (accessory) (chronic) (hyperplastic) (nasal)
    (nonpurulent) (purulent) J32.9
  acute J01.90
    ethmoidal J01.20
      recurrent J01.21
    frontal J01.10
      recurrent J01.11
    involving more than one sinus, other than pansi-
        nusitis J01.80
      recurrent J01.81
    maxillary J01.00
      recurrent J01.01
    pansinusitis J01.40
      recurrent J01.41
    recurrent J01.91
    specified NEC J01.80
      recurrent J01.81
    sphenoidal J01.30
      recurrent J01.31
  allergic — *see* Rhinitis, allergic
  due to high altitude T70.1 ☑
  ethmoidal J32.2
    acute J01.20
      recurrent J01.21
  frontal J32.1
    acute J01.10
      recurrent J01.11
  influenzal — *see* Influenza, with, respiratory manifes-
        tations NEC

☑ **Additional Character Required** — **Refer to the Tabular List for Character Selection**   ⚐ **Subterms under main terms may continue to next column or page**

Sinusitis — *continued*
    involving more than one sinus but not pansinusitis
        J32.8
        acute J01.80
            recurrent J01.81
        maxillary J32.0
            acute J01.00
                recurrent J01.01
        sphenoidal J32.3
            acute J01.30
                recurrent J01.31
        tuberculous, any sinus A15.8
Sinusitis-bronchiectasis-situs inversus (syndrome) (triad) Q89.3
Sipple's syndrome E31.22
Sirenomelia (syndrome) Q87.2
Siriasis T67.0 ☑
Sirkari's disease B55.0
Siti A65
Situation, psychiatric F99
Situational
    disturbance (transient) — *see* Disorder, adjustment
        acute F43.0
    maladjustment — *see* Disorder, adjustment
    reaction — *see* Disorder, adjustment
        acute F43.0
Situs inversus or transversus (abdominalis) (thoracis) Q89.3
Sixth disease B08.20
    due to human herpesvirus 6 B08.21
    due to human herpesvirus 7 B08.22
Sjögren-Larsson syndrome Q87.1
Sjögren's syndrome or disease — *see* Sicca syndrome
Skeletal — *see* condition
Skene's gland — *see* condition
Skenitis — *see* Urethritis
Skerljevo A65
Skevas-Zerfus disease — *see* Toxicity, venom, marine animal, sea anemone
Skin (*see also* condition)
    clammy R23.1
    donor — *see* Donor, skin
    hidebound M35.9
Slate-dressers' or slate-miners' lung J62.8
Sleep
    apnea — *see* Apnea, sleep
    deprivation Z72.820
    disorder or disturbance G47.9
        child F51.9
        nonorganic origin F51.9
        specified NEC G47.8
    disturbance G47.9
        nonorganic origin F51.9
    drunkenness F51.9
    rhythm inversion G47.2- ☑
    terrors F51.4
    walking F51.3
        hysterical F44.89
Sleep hygiene
    abuse Z72.821
    inadequate Z72.821
    poor Z72.821
Sleeping sickness — *see* Sickness, sleeping
Sleeplessness — *see* Insomnia
    menopausal N95.1
Sleep-wake schedule disorder G47.20
Slim disease (in HIV infection) B20
Slipped, slipping
    epiphysis (traumatic) (*see also* Osteochondropathy, specified type NEC)
        capital femoral (traumatic)
            acute (on chronic) S79.01- ☑
        current traumatic — *code as* Fracture, by site
        upper femoral (nontraumatic) M93.00- ☑
            acute M93.01- ☑
                on chronic M93.03- ☑
            chronic M93.02- ☑
    intervertebral disc — *see* Displacement, intervertebral disc
    ligature, umbilical P51.8
    patella — *see* Disorder, patella, derangement NEC
    rib M89.8X8
    sacroiliac joint — *see* subcategory M53.2 ☑
    tendon — *see* Disorder, tendon
    ulnar nerve, nontraumatic — *see* Lesion, nerve, ulnar
    vertebra NEC — *see* Spondylolisthesis
Slocumb's syndrome E27.0

Sloughing (multiple) (phagedena) (skin) (*see also* Gangrene)
    abscess — *see* Abscess
    appendix K38.8
    fascia — *see* Disorder, soft tissue, specified type NEC
    scrotum N50.8
    tendon — *see* Disorder, tendon
    transplanted organ — *see* Rejection, transplant
    ulcer — *see* Ulcer, skin
Slow
    feeding, newborn P92.2
    flow syndrome, coronary I20.8
    heart (beat) R00.1
Slowing, urinary stream R39.19
Sluder's neuralgia (syndrome) G44.89
Slurred, slurring speech R47.81
Small (ness)
    for gestational age — *see* Small for dates
    introitus, vagina N89.6
    kidney (unknown cause) N27.9
        bilateral N27.1
        unilateral N27.0
    ovary (congenital) Q50.39
    pelvis
        with disproportion (fetopelvic) O33.1
            causing obstructed labor O65.1
    uterus N85.8
    white kidney N03.9
Small-and-light-for-dates — *see* Small for dates
Small-for-dates (infant) P05.10
    with weight of
        1000-1249 grams P05.14
        1250-1499 grams P05.15
        1500-1749 grams P05.16
        1750-1999 grams P05.17
        2000-2499 grams P05.18
        499 grams or less P05.11
        500-749 grams P05.12
        750-999 grams P05.13
Smallpox B03
Smearing, fecal R15.1
Smith-Lemli-Opitz syndrome E78.72
Smith's fracture S52.54- ☑
Smoker — *see* Dependence, drug, nicotine
Smoker's
    bronchitis J41.0
    cough J41.0
    palate K13.24
    throat J31.2
    tongue K13.24
Smoking
    passive Z77.22
Smothering spells R06.81
Snaggle teeth, tooth M26.39
Snapping
    finger — *see* Trigger finger
    hip — *see* Derangement, joint, specified type NEC, hip
        involving the iliotiblial band M76.3- ☑
    knee — *see* Derangement, knee
        involving the iliotiblial band M76.3- ☑
Sneddon-Wilkinson disease or syndrome (sub-corneal pustular dermatosis) L13.1
Sneezing (intractable) R06.7
Sniffing
    cocaine
        abuse — *see* Abuse, drug, cocaine
        dependence — *see* Dependence, drug, cocaine
    gasoline
        abuse — *see* Abuse, drug, inhalant
        dependence — *see* Dependence, drug, inhalant
    glue (airplane)
        abuse — *see* Abuse, drug, inhalant
        drug dependence — *see* Dependence, drug, inhalant
Sniffles
    newborn P28.89
Snoring R06.83
Snow blindness — *see* Photokeratitis
Snuffles (non-syphilitic) R06.5
    newborn P28.89
    syphilitic (infant) A50.05 [J99]
Social
    exclusion Z60.4
        due to discrimination or persecution (perceived) Z60.5
    migrant Z59.0
        acculturation difficulty Z60.3

Social — *continued*
    rejection Z60.4
        due to discrimination or persecution Z60.5
    role conflict NEC Z73.5
    skills inadequacy NEC Z73.4
    transplantation Z60.3
Sodoku A25.0
Soemmerring's ring — *see* Cataract, secondary
Soft (*see also* condition)
    nails L60.3
Softening
    bone — *see* Osteomalacia
    brain (necrotic) (progressive) G93.89
        congenital Q04.8
        embolic I63.4 ☑
        hemorrhagic — *see* Hemorrhage, intracranial, intracerebral
        occlusive I63.5 ☑
        thrombotic I63.3 ☑
    cartilage M94.2-
        patella M22.4- ☑
    cerebellar — *see* Softening, brain
    cerebral — *see* Softening, brain
    cerebrospinal — *see* Softening, brain
    myocardial, heart — *see* Degeneration, myocardial
    spinal cord G95.89
    stomach K31.89
Soldier's
    heart F45.8
    patches I31.0
Solitary
    cyst, kidney N28.1
    kidney, congenital Q60.0
Solvent abuse — *see* Abuse, drug, inhalant
    dependence — *see* Dependence, drug, inhalant
Somatization reaction, somatic reaction — *see* Disorder, somatoform
Somnambulism F51.3
    hysterical F44.89
Somnolence R40.0
    nonorganic origin F51.11
Sonne dysentery A03.3
Soor B37.0
Sore
    bed — *see* Ulcer, pressure, by site
    chiclero B55.1
    Delhi B55.1
    desert — *see* Ulcer, skin
    eye H57.1- ☑
    Lahore B55.1
    mouth K13.79
        canker K12.0
    muscle M79.1
    Naga — *see* Ulcer, skin
    of skin — *see* Ulcer, skin
    oriental B55.1
    pressure — *see* Ulcer, pressure, by site
    skin L98.9
    soft A57
    throat (acute) (*see also* Pharyngitis)
        with influenza, flu, or grippe — *see* Influenza, with, respiratory manifestations NEC
        chronic J31.2
        coxsackie (virus) B08.5
        diphtheritic A36.0
        herpesviral B00.2
        influenzal — *see* Influenza, with, respiratory manifestations NEC
        septic J02.0
        streptococcal (ulcerative) J02.0
        viral NEC J02.8
            coxsackie B08.5
    tropical — *see* Ulcer, skin
    veldt — *see* Ulcer, skin
Soto's syndrome (cerebral gigantism) Q87.3
South African cardiomyopathy syndrome I42.8
Southeast Asian hemorrhagic fever A91
Spacing
    abnormal, tooth, teeth, fully erupted M26.30
    excessive, tooth, fully erupted M26.32
Spade-like hand (congenital) Q68.1
Spading nail L60.8
    congenital Q84.6
Spanish collar N47.1
Sparganosis B70.1
Spasm(s), **spastic, spasticity** (*see also* condition) R25.2
    accommodation — *see* Spasm, of accommodation

Spasm(s), spastic, spasticity — *continued*
  ampulla of Vater K83.4
  anus, ani (sphincter) (reflex) K59.4
    psychogenic F45.8
  artery I73.9
    cerebral G45.9
  Bell's G51.3
  bladder (sphincter, external or internal) N32.89
    psychogenic F45.8
  bronchus, bronchiole J98.01
  cardia K22.0
  cardiac I20.1
  carpopedal — *see* Tetany
  cerebral (arteries) (vascular) G45.9
  cervix, complicating delivery O62.4
  ciliary body (of accommodation) — *see* Spasm, of accommodation
  colon K58.9
    with diarrhea K58.0
    psychogenic F45.8
  common duct K83.8
  compulsive — *see* Tic
  conjugate H51.8
  coronary (artery) I20.1
  diaphragm (reflex) R06.6
    epidemic B33.0
    psychogenic F45.8
  duodenum K59.8
  epidemic diaphragmatic (transient) B33.0
  esophagus (diffuse) K22.4
    psychogenic F45.8
  facial G51.3
  fallopian tube N83.8
  gastrointestinal (tract) K31.89
    psychogenic F45.8
  glottis J38.5
    hysterical F44.4
    psychogenic F45.8
      conversion reaction F44.4
    reflex through recurrent laryngeal nerve J38.5
  habit — *see* Tic
  heart I20.1
  hemifacial (clonic) G51.3
  hourglass — *see* Contraction, hourglass
  hysterical F44.4
  infantile — *see* Epilepsy, spasms
  inferior oblique, eye H51.8
  intestinal (*see also* Syndrome, irritable bowel) K58.9
    psychogenic F45.8
  larynx, laryngeal J38.5
    hysterical F44.4
    psychogenic F45.8
      conversion reaction F44.4
  levator palpebrae superioris — *see* Disorder, eyelid function
  muscle NEC M62.838
    back M62.830
  nerve, trigeminal G51.0
  nervous F45.8
  nodding F98.4
  occupational F48.8
  oculogyric H51.8
    psychogenic F45.8
  of accommodation H52.53- ☑
  ophthalmic artery — *see* Occlusion, artery, retina
  perineal, female N94.89
  peroneo-extensor (*see also* Deformity, limb, flat foot)
  pharynx (reflex) J39.2
    hysterical F45.8
    psychogenic F45.8
  psychogenic F45.8
  pylorus NEC K31.3
    adult hypertrophic K31.89
    congenital or infantile Q40.0
    psychogenic F45.8
  rectum (sphincter) K59.4
    psychogenic F45.8
  retinal (artery) — *see* Occlusion, artery, retina
  sigmoid (*see also* Syndrome, irritable bowel) K58.9
    psychogenic F45.8
  sphincter of Oddi K83.4
  stomach K31.89
    neurotic F45.8
  throat J39.2
    hysterical F45.8
    psychogenic F45.8
  tic F95.9
    chronic F95.1

Spasm(s), spastic, spasticity — *continued*
  tic — *continued*
    transient of childhood F95.0
  tongue K14.8
  torsion (progressive) G24.1
  trigeminal nerve — *see* Neuralgia, trigeminal
  ureter N13.5
  urethra (sphincter) N35.9
  uterus N85.8
    complicating labor O62.4
  vagina N94.2
    psychogenic F52.5
  vascular I73.9
  vasomotor I73.9
  vein NEC I87.8
  viscera — *see* Pain, abdominal
Spasmodic — *see* condition
Spasmophilia — *see* Tetany
Spasmus nutans F98.4
Spastic, spasticity (*see also* Spasm)
  child (cerebral) (congenital) (paralysis) G80.1
Speaker's throat R49.8
Specific, specified — *see* condition
Speech
  defect, disorder, disturbance, impediment R47.9
    psychogenic, in childhood and adolescence F98.8
    slurring R47.81
    specified NEC R47.89
Spencer's disease A08.19
Spens' syndrome (syncope with heart block) I45.9
Sperm counts (fertility testing) Z31.41
  postvasectomy Z30.8
  reversal Z31.42
Spermatic cord — *see* condition
Spermatocele N43.40
  congenital Q55.4
  multiple N43.42
  single N43.41
Spermatocystitis N49.0
Spermatocytoma C62.9- ☑
  specified site — *see* Neoplasm, malignant, by site
Spermatorrhea N50.8
Sphacelus — *see* Gangrene
Sphenoidal — *see* condition
Sphenoiditis (chronic) — *see* Sinusitis, sphenoidal
Sphenopalatine ganglion neuralgia G90.09
Sphericity, increased, lens (congenital) Q12.4
Spherocytosis (congenital) (familial) (hereditary) D58.0
  hemoglobin disease D58.0
  sickle-cell (disease) D57.8- ☑
Spherophakia Q12.4
Sphincter — *see* condition
Sphincteritis, sphincter of Oddi — *see* Cholangitis
Sphingolipidosis E75.3
  specified NEC E75.29
Sphingomyelinosis E75.3
Spicule tooth K00.2
Spider
  bite — *see* Toxicity, venom, spider
  fingers — *see* Syndrome, Marfan's
  nevus I78.1
  toes — *see* Syndrome, Marfan's
  vascular I78.1
Spiegler-Fendt
  benign lymphocytoma L98.8
  sarcoid L08.89
Spielmeyer-Vogt disease E75.4
Spina bifida (aperta) Q05.9
  with hydrocephalus NEC Q05.4
  cervical Q05.5
    with hydrocephalus Q05.0
  dorsal Q05.6
    with hydrocephalus Q05.1
  lumbar Q05.7
    with hydrocephalus Q05.2
  lumbosacral Q05.7
    with hydrocephalus Q05.2
  occulta Q76.0
  sacral Q05.8
    with hydrocephalus Q05.3
  thoracic Q05.6
    with hydrocephalus Q05.1
  thoracolumbar Q05.6
    with hydrocephalus Q05.1
Spindle, Krukenberg's — *see* Pigmentation, cornea, posterior
Spine, spinal — *see* condition

Spiradenoma (eccrine) — *see* Neoplasm, skin, benign
Spirillosis A25.0
Spirillum
  minus A25.0
  obermeieri infection A68.0
Spirochetal — *see* condition
Spirochetosis A69.9
  arthritic, arthritica A69.9
  bronchopulmonary A69.8
  icterohemorrhagic A27.0
  lung A69.8
Spirometrosis B70.1
Spitting blood — *see* Hemoptysis
Splanchnoptosis K63.4
Spleen, splenic — *see* condition
Splenectasis — *see* Splenomegaly
Splenitis (interstitial) (malignant) (nonspecific) D73.89
  malarial (*see also* Malaria) B54 [D77]
  tuberculous A18.85
Splenocele D73.89
Splenomegaly, splenomegalia (Bengal) (cryptogenic) (idiopathic) (tropical) R16.1
  with hepatomegaly R16.2
  cirrhotic D73.2
  congenital Q89.09
  congestive, chronic D73.2
  Egyptian B65.1
  Gaucher's E75.22
  malarial (*see also* Malaria) B54 [D77]
  neutropenic D73.81
  Niemann-Pick — *see* Niemann-Pick disease or syndrome
  siderotic D73.2
  syphilitic A52.79
    congenital (early) A50.08 [D77]
Splenopathy D73.9
Splenoptosis D73.89
Splenosis D73.89
Splinter — *see* Foreign body, superficial, by site
Split, splitting
  foot Q72.7- ☑
  heart sounds R01.2
  lip, congenital — *see* Cleft, lip
  nails L60.3
  urinary stream R39.13
Spondylarthrosis — *see* Spondylosis
Spondylitis (chronic) (*see also* Spondylopathy, inflammatory)
  ankylopoietica — *see* Spondylitis, ankylosing
  ankylosing (chronic) M45.9
    with lung involvement M45.9 [J99]
    cervical region M45.2
    cervicothoracic region M45.3
    juvenile M08.1
    lumbar region M45.6
    lumbosacral region M45.7
    multiple sites M45.0
    occipito-atlanto-axial region M45.1
    sacrococcygeal region M45.8
    thoracic region M45.4
    thoracolumbar region M45.5
  atrophic (ligamentous) — *see* Spondylitis, ankylosing
  deformans (chronic) — *see* Spondylosis
  gonococcal A54.41
  gouty M10.08
  in (due to)
    brucellosis A23.9 [M49.80]
      cervical region A23.9 [M49.82]
      cervicothoracic region A23.9 [M49.83]
      lumbar region A23.9 [M49.86]
      lumbosacral region A23.9 [M49.87]
      multiple sites A23.9 [M49.89]
      occipito-atlanto-axial region A23.9 [M49.81]
      sacrococcygeal region A23.9 [M49.88]
      thoracic region A23.9 [M49.84]
      thoracolumbar region A23.9 [M49.85]
    enterobacteria (*see also* subcategory M49.8) A04.9
    tuberculosis A18.01
  infectious NEC — *see* Spondylopathy, infective
  juvenile ankylosing (chronic) M08.1
  Kümmell's — *see* Spondylopathy, traumatic
  Marie-Strümpell — *see* Spondylitis, ankylosing
  muscularis — *see* Spondylopathy, specified NEC
  psoriatic L40.53
  rheumatoid — *see* Spondylitis, ankylosing
  rhizomelica — *see* Spondylitis, ankylosing
  sacroiliac NEC M46.1

☑ **Additional Character Required** — **Refer to the Tabular List for Character Selection**   ▽ Subterms under main terms may continue to next column or page

Spondylitis — continued
  senescent, senile — see Spondylosis
  traumatic (chronic) or post-traumatic — see Spondylopathy, traumatic
  tuberculous A18.01
  typhosa A01.05
Spondylolisthesis (acquired) (degenerative) M43.10
  with disproportion (fetopelvic) O33.0
    causing obstructed labor O65.0
  cervical region M43.12
  cervicothoracic region M43.13
  congenital Q76.2
  lumbar region M43.16
  lumbosacral region M43.17
  multiple sites M43.19
  occipito-atlanto-axial region M43.11
  sacrococcygeal region M43.18
  thoracic region M43.14
  thoracolumbar region M43.15
  traumatic (old) M43.10
    acute
      fifth cervical (displaced) S12.430 ☑
        nondisplaced S12.431 ☑
        specified type NEC (displaced) S12.450 ☑
          nondisplaced S12.451 ☑
        type III S12.44 ☑
      fourth cervical (displaced) S12.330 ☑
        nondisplaced S12.331 ☑
        specified type NEC (displaced) S12.350 ☑
          nondisplaced S12.351 ☑
        type III S12.34 ☑
      second cervical (displaced) S12.130 ☑
        nondisplaced S12.131 ☑
        specified type NEC (displaced) S12.150 ☑
          nondisplaced S12.151 ☑
        type III S12.14 ☑
      seventh cervical (displaced) S12.630 ☑
        nondisplaced S12.631 ☑
        specified type NEC (displaced) S12.650 ☑
          nondisplaced S12.651 ☑
        type III S12.64 ☑
      sixth cervical (displaced) S12.530 ☑
        nondisplaced S12.531 ☑
        specified type NEC (displaced) S12.550 ☑
          nondisplaced S12.551 ☑
        type III S12.54 ☑
      third cervical (displaced) S12.230 ☑
        nondisplaced S12.231 ☑
        specified type NEC (displaced) S12.250 ☑
          nondisplaced S12.251 ☑
        type III S12.24 ☑
Spondylolysis (acquired) M43.00
  cervical region M43.02
  cervicothoracic region M43.03
  congenital Q76.2
  lumbar region M43.06
  lumbosacral region M43.07
    with disproportion (fetopelvic) O33.0
      causing obstructed labor O65.8
  multiple sites M43.09
  occipito-atlanto-axial region M43.01
  sacrococcygeal region M43.08
  thoracic region M43.04
  thoracolumbar region M43.05
Spondylopathy M48.9
  infective NEC M46.50
    cervical region M46.52
    cervicothoracic region M46.53
    lumbar region M46.56
    lumbosacral region M46.57
    multiple sites M46.59
    occipito-atlanto-axial region M46.51
    sacrococcygeal region M46.58
    thoracic region M46.54
    thoracolumbar region M46.55
  inflammatory M46.90
    cervical region M46.92
    cervicothoracic region M46.93
    lumbar region M46.96
    lumbosacral region M46.97
    multiple sites M46.99
    occipito-atlanto-axial region M46.91
    sacrococcygeal region M46.98
    specified type NEC M46.80
      cervical region M46.82
      cervicothoracic region M46.83
      lumbar region M46.86

Spondylopathy — continued
  inflammatory — continued
    specified type — continued
      lumbosacral region M46.87
      multiple sites M46.89
      occipito-atlanto-axial region M46.81
      sacrococcygeal region M46.88
      thoracic region M46.84
      thoracolumbar region M46.85
    thoracic region M46.94
    thoracolumbar region M46.95
  neuropathic, in
    syringomyelia and syringobulbia G95.0
    tabes dorsalis A52.11
  specified NEC — see subcategory M48.8 ☑
  traumatic M48.30
    cervical region M48.32
    cervicothoracic region M48.33
    lumbar region M48.36
    lumbosacral region M48.37
    occipito-atlanto-axial region M48.31
    sacrococcygeal region M48.38
    thoracic region M48.34
    thoracolumbar region M48.35
Spondylosis M47.9
  with
    disproportion (fetopelvic) O33.0
      causing obstructed labor O65.0
    myelopathy NEC M47.10
      cervical region M47.12
      cervicothoracic region M47.13
      lumbar region M47.16
      occipito-atlanto-axial region M47.11
      thoracic region M47.14
      thoracolumbar region M47.15
    radiculopathy M47.20
      cervical region M47.22
      cervicothoracic region M47.23
      lumbar region M47.26
      lumbosacral region M47.27
      occipito-atlanto-axial region M47.21
      sacrococcygeal region M47.28
      thoracic region M47.24
      thoracolumbar region M47.25
  without myelopathy or radiculopathy M47.819
    cervical region M47.812
    cervicothoracic region M47.813
    lumbar region M47.816
    lumbosacral region M47.817
    occipito-atlanto-axial region M47.811
    sacrococcygeal region M47.818
    thoracic region M47.814
    thoracolumbar region M47.815
  specified NEC M47.899
    cervical region M47.892
    cervicothoracic region M47.893
    lumbar region M47.896
    lumbosacral region M47.897
    occipito-atlanto-axial region M47.891
    sacrococcygeal region M47.898
    thoracic region M47.894
    thoracolumbar region M47.895
  traumatic — see Spondylopathy, traumatic
Sponge
  inadvertently left in operation wound — see Foreign body, accidentally left during a procedure
  kidney (medullary) Q61.5
Sponge-diver's disease — see Toxicity, venom, marine animal, sea anemone
Spongioblastoma (any type) — see Neoplasm, malignant, by site
  specified site — see Neoplasm, malignant, by site
  unspecified site C71.9
Spongioneuroblastoma — see Neoplasm, malignant, by site
Spontaneous (see also condition)
  fracture (cause unknown) — see Fracture, pathological
Spoon nail L60.3
  congenital Q84.6
Sporadic — see condition
Sporothrix schenckii infection — see Sporotrichosis
Sporotrichosis B42.9
  arthritis B42.82
  disseminated B42.7
  generalized B42.7
  lymphocutaneous (fixed) (progressive) B42.1
  pulmonary B42.0
  specified NEC B42.89

Spots, spotting (in) (of)
  Bitot's (see also Pigmentation, conjunctiva)
    in the young child E50.1
    vitamin A deficiency E50.1
  café, au lait L81.3
  Cayenne pepper I78.1
  cotton wool, retina — see Occlusion, artery, retina
  de Morgan's (senile angiomas) I78.1
  Fuchs' black (myopic) H44.2- ☑
  intermenstrual (regular) N92.0
    irregular N92.1
  Koplik's B05.9
  liver L81.4
  pregnancy O26.85- ☑
  purpuric R23.3
  ruby I78.1
Spotted fever — see Fever, spotted N92.3
Sprain (joint) (ligament)
  acromioclavicular joint or ligament S43.5- ☑
  ankle S93.40- ☑
    calcaneofibular ligament S93.41- ☑
    deltoid ligament S93.42- ☑
    internal collateral ligament — see Sprain, ankle, specified ligament NEC
    specified ligament NEC S93.49- ☑
    talofibular ligament — see Sprain, ankle, specified ligament NEC
    tibiofibular ligament S93.43- ☑
  anterior longitudinal, cervical S13.4 ☑
  atlas, atlanto-axial, atlanto-occipital S13.4 ☑
  breast bone — see Sprain, sternum
  calcaneofibular — see Sprain, ankle
  carpal — see Sprain, wrist
  carpometacarpal — see Sprain, hand, specified site NEC
  cartilage
    costal S23.41 ☑
    semilunar (knee) — see Sprain, knee, specified site NEC
      with current tear — see Tear, meniscus
    thyroid region S13.5 ☑
    xiphoid — see Sprain, sternum
  cervical, cervicodorsal, cervicothoracic S13.4 ☑
  chondrosternal S23.421 ☑
  coracoclavicular S43.8- ☑
  coracohumeral S43.41- ☑
  coronary, knee — see Sprain, knee, specified site NEC
  costal cartilage S23.41 ☑
  cricoarytenoid articulation or ligament S13.5 ☑
  cricothyroid articulation S13.5 ☑
  cruciate, knee — see Sprain, knee, cruciate
  deltoid, ankle — see Sprain, ankle
  dorsal (spine) S23.3 ☑
  elbow S53.40- ☑
    radial collateral ligament S53.43- ☑
    radiohumeral S53.41- ☑
    rupture
      radial collateral ligament — see Rupture, traumatic, ligament, radial collateral
      ulnar collateral ligament — see Rupture, traumatic, ligament, ulnar collateral
    specified type NEC S53.49- ☑
    ulnar collateral ligament S53.44- ☑
    ulnohumeral S53.42- ☑
  femur, head — see Sprain, hip
  fibular collateral, knee — see Sprain, knee, collateral
  fibulocalcaneal — see Sprain, ankle
  finger(s) S63.61- ☑
    index S63.61- ☑
    interphalangeal (joint) S63.63- ☑
      index S63.63- ☑
      little S63.63- ☑
      middle S63.63- ☑
      ring S63.63- ☑
    little S63.61- ☑
    metacarpophalangeal (joint) S63.65- ☑
    middle S63.61- ☑
    ring S63.61- ☑
    specified site NEC S63.69- ☑
      index S63.69- ☑
      little S63.69- ☑
      middle S63.69- ☑
      ring S63.69- ☑
  foot S93.60- ☑
    specified ligament NEC S93.69- ☑
    tarsal ligament S93.61- ☑

▽ Subterms under main terms may continue to next column or page   ☑ Additional Character Required — Refer to the Tabular List for Character Selection   281

Spondylitis — Sprain

Sprain — continued
foot — continued
tarsometatarsal ligament S93.62- ☑
toe — see Sprain, toe
hand S63.9- ☑
finger — see Sprain, finger
specified site NEC — see subcategory S63.8 ☑
thumb — see Sprain, thumb
head S03.9 ☑
hip S73.10- ☑
iliofemoral ligament S73.11- ☑
ischiocapsular (ligament) S73.12- ☑
specified NEC S73.19- ☑
iliofemoral — see Sprain, hip
innominate
acetabulum — see Sprain, hip
sacral junction S33.6 ☑
internal
collateral, ankle — see Sprain, ankle
semilunar cartilage — see Sprain, knee, specified
site NEC
interphalangeal
finger — see Sprain, finger, interphalangeal (joint)
toe — see Sprain, toe, interphalangeal joint
ischiocapsular — see Sprain, hip
ischiofemoral — see Sprain, hip
jaw (articular disc) (cartilage) (meniscus) S03.4 ☑
old M26.69
knee S83.9- ☑
collateral ligament S83.40- ☑
lateral (fibular) S83.42- ☑
medial (tibial) S83.41- ☑
cruciate ligament S83.50- ☑
anterior S83.51- ☑
posterior S83.52- ☑
lateral (fibular) collateral ligament S83.42- ☑
medial (tibial) collateral ligament S83.41- ☑
patellar ligament S76.11- ☑
specified site NEC S83.8X- ☑
superior tibiofibular joint (ligament) S83.6- ☑
lateral collateral, knee — see Sprain, knee, collateral
lumbar (spine) S33.5 ☑
lumbosacral S33.9 ☑
mandible (articular disc) S03.4 ☑
old M26.69
medial collateral, knee — see Sprain, knee, collateral
meniscus
jaw S03.4 ☑
old M26.69
knee — see Sprain, knee, specified site NEC
with current tear — see Tear, meniscus
old — see Derangement, knee, meniscus,
due to old tear
mandible S03.4 ☑
old M26.69
metacarpal (distal) (proximal) — see Sprain, hand,
specified site NEC
metacarpophalangeal — see Sprain, finger, metacarpophalangeal (joint)
metatarsophalangeal — see Sprain, toe, metatarsophalangeal joint
midcarpal — see Sprain, hand, specified site NEC
midtarsal — see Sprain, foot, specified site NEC
neck S13.9 ☑
anterior longitudinal cervical ligament S13.4 ☑
atlanto-axial joint S13.4 ☑
atlanto-occipital joint S13.4 ☑
cervical spine S13.4 ☑
cricoarytenoid ligament S13.5 ☑
cricothyroid ligament S13.5 ☑
specified site NEC S13.8 ☑
thyroid region (cartilage) S13.5 ☑
nose S03.8 ☑
orbicular, hip — see Sprain, hip
patella — see Sprain, knee, specified site NEC
patellar ligament S76.11- ☑
pelvis NEC S33.8 ☑
phalanx
finger — see Sprain, finger
toe — see Sprain, toe
pubofemoral — see Sprain, hip
radiocarpal — see Sprain, wrist
radiohumeral — see Sprain, elbow
radius, collateral — see Rupture, traumatic, ligament,
radial collateral
rib (cage) S23.41 ☑

Sprain — continued
rotator cuff (capsule) S43.42- ☑
sacroiliac (region)
chronic or old — see subcategory M53.2 ☑
joint S33.6 ☑
scaphoid (hand) — see Sprain, hand, specified site
NEC
scapula (r) — see Sprain, shoulder girdle, specified site
NEC
semilunar cartilage (knee) — see Sprain, knee, specified site NEC
with current tear — see Tear, meniscus
old — see Derangement, knee, meniscus, due
to old tear
shoulder joint S43.40- ☑
acromioclavicular joint (ligament) — see Sprain,
acromioclavicular joint
blade — see Sprain, shoulder, girdle, specified site
NEC
coracoclavicular joint (ligament) — see Sprain,
coracoclavicular joint
coracohumeral ligament — see Sprain, coracohumeral joint
girdle S43.9- ☑
specified site NEC S43.8- ☑
rotator cuff — see Sprain, rotator cuff
specified site NEC S43.49- ☑
sternoclavicular joint (ligament) — see Sprain,
sternoclavicular joint
spine
cervical S13.4 ☑
lumbar S33.5 ☑
thoracic S23.3 ☑
sternoclavicular joint S43.6- ☑
sternum S23.429 ☑
chondrosternal joint S23.421 ☑
specified site NEC S23.428 ☑
sternoclavicular (joint) (ligament) S23.420 ☑
symphysis
jaw S03.4 ☑
old M26.69
mandibular S03.4 ☑
old M26.69
talofibular — see Sprain, ankle
tarsal — see Sprain, foot, specified site NEC
tarsometatarsal — see Sprain, foot, specified site NEC
temporomandibular S03.4 ☑
old M26.69
thorax S23.9 ☑
ribs S23.41 ☑
specified site NEC S23.8 ☑
spine S23.3 ☑
sternum — see Sprain, sternum
thumb S63.60- ☑
interphalangeal (joint) S63.62- ☑
metacarpophalangeal (joint) S63.64- ☑
specified site NEC S63.68- ☑
thyroid cartilage or region S13.5 ☑
tibia (proximal end) — see Sprain, knee, specified site
NEC
tibial collateral, knee — see Sprain, knee, collateral
tibiofibular
distal — see Sprain, ankle
superior — see Sprain, knee, specified site NEC
toe(s) S93.50- ☑
great S93.50- ☑
interphalangeal joint S93.51- ☑
great S93.51- ☑
lesser S93.51- ☑
lesser S93.50- ☑
metatarsophalangeal joint S93.52- ☑
great S93.52- ☑
lesser S93.52- ☑
ulna, collateral — see Rupture, traumatic, ligament,
ulnar collateral
ulnohumeral — see Sprain, elbow
wrist S63.50- ☑
carpal S63.51- ☑
radiocarpal S63.52- ☑
specified site NEC S63.59- ☑
xiphoid cartilage — see Sprain, sternum
Sprengel's deformity (congenital) Q74.0
Sprue (tropical) K90.1
celiac K90.0
idiopathic K90.0
meaning thrush B37.0

Sprue — continued
nontropical K90.0
Spur, bone (see also Enthesopathy)
calcaneal M77.3- ☑
iliac crest M76.2- ☑
nose (septum) J34.89
Spurway's syndrome Q78.0
Sputum
abnormal (amount) (color) (odor) (purulent) R09.3
blood-stained R04.2
excessive (cause unknown) R09.3
Squamous (see also condition)
epithelium in
cervical canal (congenital) Q51.828
uterine mucosa (congenital) Q51.818
Squashed nose M95.0
congenital Q67.4
Squeeze, diver's T70.3 ☑
Squint (see also Strabismus)
accommodative — see Strabismus, convergent concomitant
St. Hubert's disease A82.9
Stab (see also Laceration)
internal organs — see Injury, by site
Stafne's cyst or cavity M27.0
Staggering gait R26.0
hysterical F44.4
Staghorn calculus — see Calculus, kidney
Stähli's line (cornea) (pigment) — see Pigmentation,
cornea, anterior
Stain, staining
meconium (newborn) P96.83
port wine Q82.5
tooth, teeth (hard tissues) (extrinsic) K03.6
due to
accretions K03.6
deposits (betel) (black) (green) (materia alba)
(orange) (soft) (tobacco) K03.6
metals (copper) (silver) K03.7
nicotine K03.6
pulpal bleeding K03.7
tobacco K03.6
intrinsic K00.8
Stammering (see also Disorder, fluency) F80.81
Standstill
auricular I45.5
cardiac — see Arrest, cardiac
sinoatrial I45.5
ventricular — see Arrest, cardiac
Stannosis J63.5
Stanton's disease — see Melioidosis
Staphylitis (acute) (catarrhal) (chronic) (gangrenous)
(membranous) (suppurative) (ulcerative) K12.2
Staphylococcal scalded skin syndrome L00
Staphylococcemia A41.2
Staphylococcus, staphylococcal (see also condition)
as cause of disease classified elsewhere B95.8
aureus (methicillin susceptible) (MSSA) B95.61
methicillin resistant (MRSA) B95.62
specified NEC, as cause of disease classified elsewhere
B95.7
Staphyloma (sclera)
cornea H18.72- ☑
equatorial H15.81- ☑
localized (anterior) H15.82- ☑
posticum H15.83- ☑
ring H15.85- ☑
Stargardt's disease — see Dystrophy, retina
Starvation (inanition) (due to lack of food) T73.0 ☑
edema — see Malnutrition, severe
Stasis
bile (noncalculous) K83.1
bronchus J98.09
with infection — see Bronchitis
cardiac — see Failure, heart, congestive
cecum K59.8
colon K59.8
dermatitis — see Varix, leg, with, inflammation
duodenal K31.5
eczema — see Varix, leg, with, inflammation
edema — see Hypertension, venous (chronic), idiopathic
foot T69.0- ☑
ileocecal coil K59.8
ileum K59.8
intestinal K59.8
jejunum K59.8

282
☑ **Additional Character Required — Refer to the Tabular List for Character Selection**
☑ **Subterms under main terms may continue to next column or page**

Stasis — *continued*
kidney N19
liver (cirrhotic) K76.1
lymphatic I89.8
pneumonia J18.2
pulmonary — *see* Edema, lung
rectal K59.8
renal N19
  tubular N17.0
ulcer — *see* Varix, leg, with, ulcer
  without varicose veins I87.2
urine — *see* Retention, urine
venous I87.8
State (of)
affective and paranoid, mixed, organic psychotic F06.8
agitated R45.1
  acute reaction to stress F43.0
anxiety (neurotic) F41.1
apprehension F41.1
burn-out Z73.0
climacteric, female Z78.0
  symptomatic N95.1
compulsive F42
  mixed with obsessional thoughts F42
confusional (psychogenic) F44.89
  acute (*see also* Delirium)
    with
      arteriosclerotic dementia F01.50
        with behavioral disturbance F01.51
      senility or dementia F05
    alcoholic F10.231
    epileptic F05
    reactive (from emotional stress, psychological
      trauma) F44.89
    subacute — *see* Delirium
convulsive — *see* Convulsions
crisis F43.0
depressive F32.9
  neurotic F34.1
dissociative F44.9
emotional shock (stress) R45.7
hypercoagulation — *see* Hypercoagulable
locked-in G83.5
menopausal Z78.0
  symptomatic N95.1
neurotic F48.9
  with depersonalization F48.1
obsessional F42
oneiroid (schizophrenia-like) F23
organic
  hallucinatory (nonalcoholic) F06.0
  paranoid (-hallucinatory) F06.2
panic F41.0
paranoid F22
  climacteric F22
  involutional F22
  menopausal F22
  organic F06.2
  senile F03 ☑
  simple F22
persistent vegetative R40.3
phobic F40.9
postleukotomy F07.0
pregnant, incidental Z33.1
psychogenic, twilight F44.89
psychopathic (constitutional) F60.2
psychotic, organic (*see also* Psychosis, organic)
  mixed paranoid and affective F06.8
  senile or presenile F03 ☑
  transient NEC F06.8
    with
      depression F06.31
      hallucinations F06.0
residual schizophrenic F20.5
restlessness R45.1
stress (emotional) R45.7
tension (mental) F48.9
  specified NEC F48.8
transient organic psychotic NEC F06.8
  depressive type F06.31
  hallucinatory type F06.30
twilight
  epileptic F05
  psychogenic F44.89
vegetative, persistent R40.3
vital exhaustion Z73.0
withdrawal, — *see* Withdrawal, state

Status (post) (*see also* Presence (of))
absence, epileptic — *see* Epilepsy, by type, with status
  epilepticus
administration of tPA (rtPA) in a different facility
  within the last 24 hours prior to admission to
  current facility Z92.82
adrenalectomy (unilateral) (bilateral) E89.6
anastomosis Z98.0
anginosus I20.9
angioplasty (peripheral) Z98.62
  with implant Z95.820
  coronary artery Z98.61
    with implant Z95.5
aortocoronary bypass Z95.1
arthrodesis Z98.1
artificial opening (of) Z93.9
  gastrointestinal tract Z93.4
  specified NEC Z93.8
  urinary tract Z93.6
  vagina Z93.8
asthmaticus — *see* Asthma, by type, with status asthmaticus
awaiting organ transplant Z76.82
bariatric surgery Z98.84
bed confinement Z74.01
bleb, filtering (vitreous), after glaucoma surgery Z98.83
breast implant Z98.82
  removal Z98.86
cataract extraction Z98.4- ☑
cholecystectomy Z90.49
clitorectomy N90.811
  with excision of labia minora N90.812
colectomy (complete) (partial) Z90.49
colonization — *see* Carrier (suspected) of
colostomy Z93.3
convulsivus idiopathicus — *see* Epilepsy, by type, with
  status epilepticus
coronary artery angioplasty — *see* Status, angioplasty,
  coronary artery
cystectomy (urinary bladder) Z90.6
cystostomy Z93.50
  appendico-vesicostomy Z93.52
  cutaneous Z93.51
  specified NEC Z93.59
delinquent immunization Z28.3
dental Z98.818
  crown Z98.811
  fillings Z98.811
  restoration Z98.811
  sealant Z98.810
  specified NEC Z98.818
deployment (current) (military) Z56.82
dialysis (hemodialysis) (peritoneal) Z99.2
do not resuscitate (DNR) Z66
donor — *see* Donor
embedded fragments — *see* Retained, foreign body
  fragments (type of)
embedded splinter — *see* Retained, foreign body
  fragments (type of)
enterostomy Z93.4
epileptic, epilepticus (*see also* Epilepsy, by type, with
  status epilepticus) G40.901
estrogen receptor
  negative Z17.1
  positive Z17.0
female genital cutting — *see* Female genital mutilation
  status
female genital mutilation — *see* Female genital mutilation status
filtering (vitreous) bleb after glaucoma surgery Z98.83
gastrectomy (complete) (partial) Z90.3
gastric banding Z98.84
gastric bypass for obesity Z98.84
gastrostomy Z93.1
human immunodeficiency virus (HIV) infection,
  asymptomatic Z21
hysterectomy (complete) (total) Z90.710
  partial (with remaining cervial stump) Z90.711
ileostomy Z93.2
implant
  breast Z98.82
infibulation N90.813
intestinal bypass Z98.0
jejunostomy Z93.4
lapsed immunization schedule Z28.3
laryngectomy Z90.02
lymphaticus E32.8
marmoratus G80.3

Status — *continued*
mastectomy (unilateral) (bilateral) Z90.1- ☑
military deployment status (current) Z56.82
  in theater or in support of military war, peacekeep-
    ing and humanitarian operations Z56.82
nephrectomy (unilateral) (bilateral) Z90.5
nephrostomy Z93.6
obesity surgery Z98.84
oophorectomy
  bilateral Z90.722
  unilateral Z90.721
organ replacement
  by artificial or mechanical device or prosthesis of
    artery Z95.828
    bladder Z96.0
    blood vessel Z95.828
    breast Z97.8
    eye globe Z97.0
    heart Z95.812
      valve Z95.2
    intestine Z97.8
    joint Z96.60
      hip — *see* Presence, hip joint implant
      knee — *see* Presence, knee joint implant
      specified site NEC Z96.698
    kidney Z97.8
    larynx Z96.3
    lens Z96.1
    limbs — *see* Presence, artificial, limb
    liver Z97.8
    lung Z97.8
    pancreas Z97.8
  by organ transplant (heterologous)(homologous)
    — *see* Transplant
pacemaker
  brain Z96.89
  cardiac Z95.0
  specified NEC Z96.89
pancreatectomy Z90.410
  complete Z90.410
  partial Z90.411
  total Z90.410
physical restraint Z78.1
pneumonectomy (complete) (partial) Z90.2
pneumothorax, therapeutic Z98.3
postcommotio cerebri F07.81
postoperative (postprocedural) NEC Z98.89
  breast implant Z98.82
  dental Z98.818
    crown Z98.811
    fillings Z98.811
    restoration Z98.811
    sealant Z98.810
    specified NEC Z98.818
  pneumothorax, therapeutic Z98.3
postpartum (routine follow-up) Z39.2
  care immediately after delivery Z39.0
postsurgical (postprocedural) NEC Z98.89
  pneumothorax, therapeutic Z98.3
pregnancy, incidental Z33.1
prosthesis coronary angioplasty Z95.5
pseudophakia Z96.1
renal dialysis (hemodialysis) (peritoneal) Z99.2
retained foreign body — *see* Retained, foreign body
  fragments (type of)
reversed jejunal transposition (for bypass) Z98.0
salpingo-oophorectomy
  bilateral Z90.722
  unilateral Z90.721
sex reassignment surgery status Z87.890
shunt
  arteriovenous (for dialysis) Z99.2
  cerebrospinal fluid Z98.2
  ventricular (communicating) (for drainage) Z98.2
splenectomy Z90.81
thymicolymphaticus E32.8
thymicus E32.8
thymolymphaticus E32.8
thyroidectomy (hypothyroidism) E89.0
tooth (teeth) extraction (*see also* Absence, teeth, acquired) K08.409
tPA (rtPA) administration in a different facility within
  the last 24 hours prior to admission to current
  facility Z92.82
tracheostomy Z93.0
transplant — *see* Transplant
  organ removed Z98.85
tubal ligation Z98.51

Status — *continued*
  underimmunization Z28.3
  ureterostomy Z93.6
  urethrostomy Z93.6
  vagina, artificial Z93.8
  vasectomy Z98.52
  wheelchair confinement Z99.3
Stealing
  child problem F91.8
  in company with others Z72.810
  pathological (compulsive) F63.2
Steam burn — *see* Burn
Steatocystoma multiplex L72.2
Steatohepatitis (nonalcoholic) (NASH) K75.81
Steatoma L72.3
  eyelid (cystic) — *see* Dermatosis, eyelid
  infected — *see* Hordeolum
Steatorrhea (chronic) K90.4
  with lacteal obstruction K90.2
  idiopathic (adult) (infantile) K90.0
  pancreatic K90.3
  primary K90.0
  tropical K90.1
Steatosis E88.89
  heart — *see* Degeneration, myocardial
  kidney N28.89
  liver NEC K76.0
Steele-Richardson-Olszewski disease or syndrome G23.1
Steinbrocker's syndrome G90.8
Steinert's disease G71.11
Stein-Leventhal syndrome E28.2
Stein's syndrome E28.2
STEMI (*see also* Infarct, myocardium, ST elevation) I21.3
Stenocardia I20.8
Stenocephaly Q75.8
Stenosis, stenotic (cicatricial) (*see also* Stricture)
  ampulla of Vater K83.1
  anus, anal (canal) (sphincter) K62.4
    and rectum K62.4
    congenital Q42.3
      with fistula Q42.2
  aorta (ascending) (supraventricular) (congenital) Q25.3
    arteriosclerotic I70.0
    calcified I70.0
  aortic (valve) I35.0
    with insufficiency I35.2
    congenital Q23.0
    rheumatic I06.0
      with
        incompetency, insufficiency or regurgitation I06.2
          with mitral (valve) disease I08.0
            with tricuspid (valve) disease I08.3
          mitral (valve) disease I08.0
            with tricuspid (valve) disease I08.3
          tricuspid (valve) disease I08.2
            with mitral (valve) disease I08.3
    specified cause NEC I35.0
    syphilitic A52.03
  aqueduct of Sylvius (congenital) Q03.0
    with spina bifida — *see* Spina bifida, by site, with hydrocephalus
    acquired G91.1
  artery NEC (*see also* Arteriosclerosis) I77.1
    celiac I77.4
    cerebral — *see* Occlusion, artery, cerebral
    extremities — *see* Arteriosclerosis, extremities
    precerebral — *see* Occlusion, artery, precerebral
    pulmonary (congenital) Q25.6
      acquired I28.8
    renal I70.1
  bile duct (common) (hepatic) K83.1
    congenital Q44.3
  bladder-neck (acquired) N32.0
    congenital Q64.31
  brain G93.89
  bronchus J98.09
    congenital Q32.3
    syphilitic A52.72
  cardia (stomach) K22.2
    congenital Q39.3
  cardiovascular — *see* Disease, cardiovascular
  caudal M48.08
  cervix, cervical (canal) N88.2
    congenital Q51.828
    in pregnancy or childbirth — *see* Pregnancy, complicated by, abnormal cervix

Stenosis, stenotic — *continued*
  colon (*see also* Obstruction, intestine)
    congenital Q42.9
      specified NEC Q42.8
  colostomy K94.03
  common (bile) duct K83.1
    congenital Q44.3
  coronary (artery) — *see* Disease, heart, ischemic, atherosclerotic
  cystic duct — *see* Obstruction, gallbladder
  due to presence of device, implant or graft (*see also* Complications, by site and type, specified NEC) T85.85 ☑
    arterial graft NEC T82.858 ☑
    breast (implant) T85.85 ☑
    catheter T85.85 ☑
      dialysis (renal) T82.858 ☑
        intraperitoneal T85.85 ☑
      infusion NEC T82.858 ☑
        spinal (epidural) (subdural) T85.85 ☑
      urinary (indwelling) T83.85 ☑
    fixation, internal (orthopedic) NEC T84.85 ☑
    gastrointestinal (bile duct) (esophagus) T85.85 ☑
    genital NEC T83.85 ☑
    heart NEC T82.857 ☑
    joint prosthesis T84.85 ☑
    ocular (corneal graft) (orbital implant) NEC T85.85 ☑
    orthopedic NEC T84.85 ☑
    specified NEC T85.85 ☑
    urinary NEC T83.85 ☑
    vascular NEC T82.858 ☑
    ventricular intracranial shunt T85.85 ☑
  duodenum K31.5
    congenital Q41.0
  ejaculatory duct NEC N50.8
  endocervical os — *see* Stenosis, cervix
  enterostomy K94.13
  esophagus K22.2
    congenital Q39.3
    syphilitic A52.79
      congenital A50.59 [K23]
  eustachian tube — *see* Obstruction, eustachian tube
  external ear canal (acquired) H61.30- ☑
    congenital Q16.1
    due to
      inflammation H61.32- ☑
      trauma H61.31- ☑
    postprocedural H95.81- ☑
    specified cause NEC H61.39- ☑
  gallbladder — *see* Obstruction, gallbladder
  glottis J38.6
  heart valve (congenital) Q24.8
    aortic Q23.0
    mitral Q23.2
    pulmonary Q22.1
    tricuspid Q22.4
  hepatic duct K83.1
  hymen N89.6
  hypertrophic subaortic (idiopathic) I42.1
  ileum K56.69
    congenital Q41.2
  infundibulum cardia Q24.3
  intervertebral foramina (*see also* Lesion, biomechanical, specified NEC)
    connective tissue M99.79
      abdomen M99.79
      cervical region M99.71
      cervicothoracic M99.71
      head region M99.70
      lumbar region M99.73
      lumbosacral M99.73
      occipitocervical M99.70
      sacral region M99.74
      sacrococcygeal M99.74
      sacroiliac M99.74
      specified NEC M99.79
      thoracic region M99.72
      thoracolumbar M99.72
    disc M99.79
      abdomen M99.79
      cervical region M99.71
      cervicothoracic M99.71
      head region M99.70
      lower extremity M99.76
      lumbar region M99.73
      lumbosacral M99.73

Stenosis, stenotic — *continued*
  intervertebral foramina (*see also* Lesion, biomechanical, specified) — *continued*
    disc — *continued*
      occipitocervical M99.70
      pelvic M99.75
      rib cage M99.78
      sacral region M99.74
      sacrococcygeal M99.74
      sacroiliac M99.74
      specified NEC M99.79
      thoracic region M99.72
      thoracolumbar M99.72
      upper extremity M99.77
    osseous M99.69
      abdomen M99.69
      cervical region M99.61
      cervicothoracic M99.61
      head region M99.60
      lower extremity M99.66
      lumbar region M99.63
      lumbosacral M99.63
      occipitocervical M99.60
      pelvic M99.65
      rib cage M99.68
      sacral region M99.64
      sacrococcygeal M99.64
      sacroiliac M99.64
      specified NEC M99.69
      thoracic region M99.62
      thoracolumbar M99.62
      upper extremity M99.67
    subluxation — *see* Stenosis, intervertebral foramina, osseous
  intestine (*see also* Obstruction, intestine)
    congenital (small) Q41.9
      large Q42.9
        specified NEC Q42.8
      specified NEC Q41.8
  jejunum K56.69
    congenital Q41.1
  lacrimal (passage)
    canaliculi H04.54- ☑
    congenital Q10.5
    duct H04.55- ☑
    punctum H04.56- ☑
    sac H04.57- ☑
  lacrimonasal duct — *see* Stenosis, lacrimal, duct
    congenital Q10.5
  larynx J38.6
    congenital NEC Q31.8
      subglottic Q31.1
    syphilitic A52.73
      congenital A50.59 [J99]
  mitral (chronic) (inactive) (valve) I05.0
    with
      aortic valve disease I08.0
      incompetency, insufficiency or regurgitation I05.2
    active or acute I01.1
      with rheumatic or Sydenham's chorea I02.0
    congenital Q23.2
    specified cause, except rheumatic I34.2
    syphilitic A52.03
  myocardium, myocardial (*see also* Degeneration, myocardial)
    hypertrophic subaortic (idiopathic) I42.1
  nares (anterior) (posterior) J34.89
    congenital Q30.0
  nasal duct (*see also* Stenosis, lacrimal, duct)
    congenital Q10.5
  nasolacrimal duct (*see also* Stenosis, lacrimal, duct)
    congenital Q10.5
  neural canal (*see also* Lesion, biomechanical, specified NEC)
    connective tissue M99.49
      abdomen M99.49
      cervical region M99.41
      cervicothoracic M99.41
      head region M99.40
      lower extremity M99.46
      lumbar region M99.43
      lumbosacral M99.43
      occipitocervical M99.40
      pelvic M99.45
      rib cage M99.48
      sacral region M99.44
      sacrococcygeal M99.44

☑ **Additional Character Required — Refer to the Tabular List for Character Selection** ▽ Subterms under main terms may continue to next column or page

Stenosis, stenotic — *continued*
　neural canal (*see also* Lesion, biomechanical, specified)
　　— *continued*
　　connective tissue — *continued*
　　　sacroiliac M99.44
　　　specified NEC M99.49
　　　thoracic region M99.42
　　　thoracolumbar M99.42
　　　upper extremity M99.47
　　intervertebral disc M99.59
　　　abdomen M99.59
　　　cervical region M99.51
　　　cervicothoracic M99.51
　　　head region M99.50
　　　lower extremity M99.56
　　　lumbar region M99.53
　　　lumbosacral M99.53
　　　occipitocervical M99.50
　　　pelvic M99.55
　　　rib cage M99.58
　　　sacral region M99.54
　　　sacrococcygeal M99.54
　　　sacroiliac M99.54
　　　specified NEC M99.59
　　　thoracic region M99.52
　　　thoracolumbar M99.52
　　　upper extremity M99.57
　　osseous M99.39
　　　abdomen M99.39
　　　cervical region M99.31
　　　cervicothoracic M99.31
　　　head region M99.30
　　　lower extremity M99.36
　　　lumbar region M99.33
　　　lumbosacral M99.33
　　　occipitocervical M99.30
　　　pelvic M99.35
　　　rib cage M99.38
　　　sacral region M99.34
　　　sacrococcygeal M99.34
　　　sacroiliac M99.34
　　　specified NEC M99.39
　　　thoracic region M99.32
　　　thoracolumbar M99.32
　　　upper extremity M99.37
　　subluxation M99.29
　　　cervical region M99.21
　　　cervicothoracic M99.21
　　　head region M99.20
　　　lower extremity M99.26
　　　lumbar region M99.23
　　　lumbosacral M99.23
　　　occipitocervical M99.20
　　　pelvic M99.25
　　　rib cage M99.28
　　　sacral region M99.24
　　　sacrococcygeal M99.24
　　　sacroiliac M99.24
　　　specified NEC M99.29
　　　thoracic region M99.22
　　　thoracolumbar M99.22
　　　upper extremity M99.27
　organ or site, congenital NEC — *see* Atresia, by site
　papilla of Vater K83.1
　pulmonary (artery) (congenital) Q25.6
　　with ventricular septal defect, transposition of
　　　aorta, and hypertrophy of right ventricle
　　　Q21.3
　　acquired I28.8
　　in tetralogy of Fallot Q21.3
　　infundibular Q24.3
　　subvalvular Q24.3
　　supravalvular Q25.6
　　valve I37.0
　　　with insufficiency I37.2
　　　congenital Q22.1
　　　rheumatic I09.89
　　　　with aortic, mitral or tricuspid (valve) disease
　　　　　I08.8
　　vein, acquired I28.8
　　vessel NEC I28.8
　pulmonic (congenital) Q22.1
　　infundibular Q24.3
　　subvalvular Q24.3
　pylorus (hypertrophic) (acquired) K31.1
　　adult K31.1
　　congenital Q40.0
　　infantile Q40.0

Stenosis, stenotic — *continued*
　rectum (sphincter) — *see* Stricture, rectum
　renal artery I70.1
　　congenital Q27.1
　salivary duct (any) K11.8
　sphincter of Oddi K83.1
　spinal M48.00
　　cervical region M48.02
　　cervicothoracic region M48.03
　　lumbar region M48.06
　　lumbosacral region M48.07
　　occipito-atlanto-axial region M48.01
　　sacrococcygeal region M48.08
　　thoracic region M48.04
　　thoracolumbar region M48.05
　stomach, hourglass K31.2
　subaortic (congenital) Q24.4
　　hypertrophic (idiopathic) I42.1
　subglottic J38.6
　　congenital Q31.1
　　postprocedural J95.5
　trachea J39.8
　　congenital Q32.1
　　syphilitic A52.73
　　tuberculous NEC A15.5
　tracheostomy J95.03
　tricuspid (valve) I07.0
　　with
　　　aortic (valve) disease I08.2
　　　incompetency, insufficiency or regurgitation
　　　　I07.2
　　　　with aortic (valve) disease I08.2
　　　　　with mitral (valve) disease I08.3
　　　mitral (valve) disease I08.1
　　　　with aortic (valve) disease I08.3
　　congenital Q22.4
　　nonrheumatic I36.0
　　　with insufficiency I36.2
　tubal N97.1
　ureter — *see* Atresia, ureter
　ureteropelvic junction, congenital Q62.11
　ureterovesical orifice, congenital Q62.12
　urethra (valve) (*see also* Stricture, urethra)
　　congenital Q64.32
　urinary meatus, congenital Q64.33
　vagina N89.5
　　congenital Q52.4
　　in pregnancy — *see* Pregnancy, complicated by,
　　　abnormal vagina
　　　causing obstructed labor O65.5
　valve (cardiac) (heart) (*see also* Endocarditis) I38
　　congenital Q24.8
　　　aortic Q23.0
　　　mitral Q23.2
　　　pulmonary Q22.1
　　　tricuspid Q22.4
　vena cava (inferior) (superior) I87.1
　　congenital Q26.0
　vesicourethral orifice Q64.31
　vulva N90.5

Stent jail T82.897 ☑
Stercolith (impaction) K56.41
　appendix K38.1
Stercoraceous, stercoral ulcer K63.3
　anus or rectum K62.6
Stereotypies NEC F98.4
Sterility — *see* Infertility
Sterilization — *see* Encounter (for), sterilization
Sternalgia — *see* Angina
Sternopagus Q89.4
Sternum bifidum Q76.7
Steroid
　effects (adverse) (adrenocortical) (iatrogenic)
　　cushingoid E24.2
　　　correct substance properly administered — *see*
　　　　Table of Drugs and Chemicals, by drug,
　　　　adverse effect
　　　overdose or wrong substance given or taken
　　　　— *see* Table of Drugs and Chemicals, by
　　　　drug, poisoning
　　diabetes — *see* subcategory E09 ☑
　　　correct substance properly administered — *see*
　　　　Table of Drugs and Chemicals, by drug,
　　　　adverse effect
　　　overdose or wrong substance given or taken
　　　　— *see* Table of Drugs and Chemicals, by
　　　　drug, poisoning
　　fever R50.2

Steroid — *continued*
　effects — *continued*
　　insufficiency E27.3
　　　correct substance properly administered — *see*
　　　　Table of Drugs and Chemicals, by drug,
　　　　adverse effect
　　　overdose or wrong substance given or taken
　　　　— *see* Table of Drugs and Chemicals, by
　　　　drug, poisoning
　　responder H40.04- ☑
Stevens-Johnson disease or syndrome L51.1
　toxic epidermal necrolysis overlap L51.3
Stewart-Morel syndrome M85.2
Sticker's disease B08.3
Sticky eye — *see* Conjunctivitis, acute, mucopurulent
Stieda's disease — *see* Bursitis, tibial collateral
Stiff neck — *see* Torticollis
Stiff-man syndrome G25.82
Stiffness, joint NEC M25.60
　ankle M25.67- ☑
　ankylosis — *see* Ankylosis, joint
　contracture — *see* Contraction, joint
　elbow M25.62- ☑
　foot M25.67- ☑
　hand M25.64- ☑
　hip M25.65- ☑
　knee M25.66- ☑
　shoulder M25.61- ☑
　wrist M25.63- ☑
Stigmata congenital syphilis A50.59
Stillbirth P95
Still-Felty syndrome — *see* Felty's syndrome
Still's disease or syndrome (juvenile) M08.20
　adult-onset M06.1
　ankle M08.27- ☑
　elbow M08.22- ☑
　foot joint M08.27- ☑
　hand joint M08.24- ☑
　hip M08.25- ☑
　knee M08.26- ☑
　multiple site M08.29
　shoulder M08.21- ☑
　vertebra M08.28
　wrist M08.23- ☑
Stimulation, ovary E28.1
Sting (venomous) (with allergic or anaphylactic shock)
　　— *see* Table of Drugs and Chemicals, by animal or
　　substance, poisoning
Stippled epiphyses Q78.8
Stitch
　abscess T81.4 ☑
　burst (in operation wound) — *see* Disruption, wound,
　　operation
Stokes' disease E05.00
　with thyroid storm E05.01
Stokes-Adams disease or syndrome I45.9
Stokvis (-Talma) **disease** D74.8
Stoma malfunction
　colostomy K94.03
　enterostomy K94.13
　gastrostomy K94.23
　ileostomy K94.13
　tracheostomy J95.03
Stomach — *see* condition
Stomatitis (denture) (ulcerative) K12.1
　angular K13.0
　　due to dietary or vitamin deficiency E53.0
　aphthous K12.0
　bovine B08.61
　candidal B37.0
　catarrhal K12.1
　diphtheritic A36.89
　due to
　　dietary deficiency E53.0
　　thrush B37.0
　　vitamin deficiency
　　　B group NEC E53.9
　　　B2 (riboflavin) E53.0
　epidemic B08.8
　epizootic B08.8
　follicular K12.1
　gangrenous A69.0
　Geotrichum B48.3
　herpesviral, herpetic B00.2
　herpetiformis K12.0
　malignant K12.1
　membranous acute K12.1

▽ **Subterms under main terms may continue to next column or page**　　☑ **Additional Character Required** — Refer to the Tabular List for Character Selection　　**285**

Stenosis, stenotic — Stomatitis

Stomatitis — *continued*
  monilial B37.Ø
  mycotic B37.Ø
  necrotizing ulcerative A69.Ø
  parasitic B37.Ø
  septic K12.1
  spirochetal A69.1
  suppurative (acute) K12.2
  ulceromembranous A69.1
  vesicular K12.1
    with exanthem (enteroviral) BØ8.4
    virus disease A93.8
  Vincent's A69.1
Stomatocytosis D58.8
Stomatomycosis B37.Ø
Stomatorrhagia K13.79
Stone(s) (*see also* Calculus)
  bladder (diverticulum) N21.Ø
  cystine E72.Ø9
  heart syndrome I5Ø.1
  kidney N2Ø.Ø
  prostate N42.Ø
  pulpal (dental) KØ4.2
  renal N2Ø.Ø
  salivary gland or duct (any) K11.5
  urethra (impacted) N21.1
  urinary (duct) (impacted) (passage) N2Ø.9
    bladder (diverticulum) N21.Ø
    lower tract N21.9
    specified NEC N21.8
  xanthine E79.8 [N22]
Stonecutter's lung J62.8
Stonemason's asthma, disease, lung or pneumoco-niosis J62.8
Stoppage
  heart — *see* Arrest, cardiac
  urine — *see* Retention, urine
Storm, thyroid — *see* Thyrotoxicosis
Strabismus (congenital) (nonparalytic) H5Ø.9
  concomitant H5Ø.4Ø
    convergent — *see* Strabismus, convergent concomitant
    divergent — *see* Strabismus, divergent concomitant
  convergent concomitant H5Ø.ØØ
    accommodative component H5Ø.43
    alternating H5Ø.Ø5
      with
        A pattern H5Ø.Ø6
        specified nonconcomitances NEC H5Ø.Ø8
        V pattern H5Ø.Ø7
    monocular H5Ø.Ø1- ☑
      with
        A pattern H5Ø.Ø2- ☑
        specified nonconcomitances NEC H5Ø.Ø4- ☑
        V pattern H5Ø.Ø3- ☑
      intermittent H5Ø.31- ☑
        alternating H5Ø.32
  cyclotropia H5Ø.1- ☑
  divergent concomitant H5Ø.1Ø
    alternating H5Ø.15
      with
        A pattern H5Ø.16
        specified noncomitances NEC H5Ø.18
        V pattern H5Ø.17
    monocular H5Ø.11- ☑
      with
        A pattern H5Ø.12- ☑
        specified noncomitances NEC H5Ø.14- ☑
        V pattern H5Ø.13- ☑
      intermittent H5Ø.33 ☑
        alternating H5Ø.34
  Duane's syndrome H5Ø.81- ☑
  due to adhesions, scars H5Ø.69
  heterophoria H5Ø.5Ø
    alternating H5Ø.55
    cyclophoria H5Ø.54
    esophoria H5Ø.51
    exophoria H5Ø.52
    vertical H5Ø.53
  heterotropia H5Ø.4Ø
    intermittent H5Ø.3Ø
  hypertropia H5Ø.2- ☑
  hypotropia — *see* Hypertropia
  latent H5Ø.5Ø
  mechanical H5Ø.6Ø
    Brown's sheath syndrome H5Ø.61- ☑

Strabismus — *continued*
  mechanical — *continued*
    specified type NEC H5Ø.69
  monofixation syndrome H5Ø.42
  paralytic H49.9
    abducens nerve H49.2- ☑
    fourth nerve H49.1- ☑
    Kearns-Sayre syndrome H49.81- ☑
    ophthalmoplegia (external)
      progressive H49.4- ☑
        with pigmentary retinopathy H49.81- ☑
      total H49.3- ☑
    sixth nerve H49.2- ☑
    specified type NEC H49.88- ☑
    third nerve H49.Ø- ☑
    trochlear nerve H49.1- ☑
  specified type NEC H5Ø.89
  vertical H5Ø.2- ☑
Strain
  back S39.Ø12 ☑
  cervical S16.1 ☑
  eye NEC — *see* Disturbance, vision, subjective
  heart — *see* Disease, heart
  low back S39.Ø12 ☑
  mental NOS Z73.3
    work-related Z56.6
  muscle (tendon) — *see* Injury, muscle, by site, strain
  neck S16.1 ☑
  physical NOS Z73.3
    work-related Z56.6
  postural (*see also* Disorder, soft tissue, due to use)
  psychological NEC Z73.3
  tendon — *see* Injury, muscle, by site, strain
Straining, on urination R39.16
Strand, vitreous — *see* Opacity, vitreous, membranes and strands
Strangulation, strangulated (*see also* Asphyxia, traumatic)
  appendix K38.8
  bladder-neck N32.Ø
  bowel or colon K56.2
  food or foreign body — *see* Foreign body, by site
  hemorrhoids — *see* Hemorrhoids, with complication
  hernia (*see also* Hernia, by site, with obstruction)
    with gangrene — *see* Hernia, by site, with gangrene
  intestine (large) (small) K56.2
    with hernia (*see also* Hernia, by site, with obstruction)
      with gangrene — *see* Hernia, by site, with gangrene
  mesentery K56.2
  mucus — *see* Asphyxia, mucus
  omentum K56.2
  organ or site, congenital NEC — *see* Atresia, by site
  ovary — *see* Torsion, ovary
  penis N48.89
    foreign body T19.4 ☑
  rupture — *see* Hernia, by site, with obstruction
  stomach due to hernia (*see also* Hernia, by site, with obstruction)
    with gangrene — *see* Hernia, by site, with gangrene
  vesicourethral orifice N32.Ø
Strangury R3Ø.Ø
Straw itch B88.Ø
Strawberry
  gallbladder K82.4
  mark Q82.5
  tongue (red) (white) K14.3
Streak(s)
  macula, angioid H35.33
  ovarian Q5Ø.32
Strephosymbolia F81.Ø
  secondary to organic lesion R48.8
Streptobacillary fever A25.1
Streptobacillosis A25.1
Streptobacillus moniliformis A25.1
Streptococcus, streptococcal (*see also* condition)
  as cause of disease classified elsewhere B95.5
  group
    A, as cause of disease classified elsewhere B95.Ø
    B, as cause of disease classified elsewhere B95.1
    D, as cause of disease classified elsewhere B95.2
  pneumoniae, as cause of disease classified elsewhere B95.3

Streptococcus, streptococcal — *continued*
  specified NEC, as cause of disease classified elsewhere B95.4
Streptomycosis B47.1
Streptotrichosis A48.8
Stress F43.9
  family — *see* Disruption, family
  fetal P84
    complicating pregnancy O77.9
      due to drug administration O77.1
  mental NEC Z73.3
    work-related Z56.6
  physical NEC Z73.3
    work-related Z56.6
  polycythemia D75.1
  reaction (*see also* Reaction, stress) F43.9
  work schedule Z56.3
Stretching, nerve — *see* Injury, nerve
Striae albicantes, atrophicae or distensae (cutis) L9Ø.6
Stricture (*see also* Stenosis)
  ampulla of Vater K83.1
  anus (sphincter) K62.4
    congenital Q42.3
      with fistula Q42.2
    infantile Q42.3
      with fistula Q42.2
  aorta (ascending) (congenital) Q25.3
    arteriosclerotic I7Ø.Ø
    calcified I7Ø.Ø
    supravalvular, congenital Q25.3
  aortic (valve) — *see* Stenosis, aortic
  aqueduct of Sylvius (congenital) QØ3.Ø
    with spina bifida — *see* Spina bifida, by site, with hydrocephalus
    acquired G91.1
  artery I77.1
    basilar — *see* Occlusion, artery, basilar
    carotid — *see* Occlusion, artery, carotid
    celiac I77.4
    congenital (peripheral) Q27.8
      cerebral Q28.3
      coronary Q24.5
      digestive system Q27.8
      lower limb Q27.8
      retinal Q14.1
      specified site NEC Q27.8
      umbilical Q27.Ø
      upper limb Q27.8
    coronary — *see* Disease, heart, ischemic, atherosclerotic
      congenital Q24.5
    precerebral — *see* Occlusion, artery, precerebral
    pulmonary (congenital) Q25.6
      acquired I28.8
    renal I7Ø.1
    vertebral — *see* Occlusion, artery, vertebral
  auditory canal (external) (congenital)
    acquired — *see* Stenosis, external ear canal
  bile duct (common) (hepatic) K83.1
    congenital Q44.3
    postoperative K91.89
  bladder N32.89
    neck N32.Ø
  bowel — *see* Obstruction, intestine
  brain G93.89
  bronchus J98.Ø9
    congenital Q32.3
    syphilitic A52.72
  cardia (stomach) K22.2
    congenital Q39.3
  cardiac (*see also* Disease, heart)
    orifice (stomach) K22.2
  cecum — *see* Obstruction, intestine
  cervix, cervical (canal) N88.2
    congenital Q51.828
    in pregnancy — *see* Pregnancy, complicated by, abnormal cervix
      causing obstructed labor O65.5
  colon (*see also* Obstruction, intestine)
    congenital Q42.9
      specified NEC Q42.8
  colostomy K94.Ø3
  common (bile) duct K83.1
  coronary (artery) — *see* Disease, heart, ischemic, atherosclerotic
  cystic duct — *see* Obstruction, gallbladder
  digestive organs NEC, congenital Q45.8

Stricture — *continued*
- duodenum K31.5
  - congenital Q41.0
- ear canal (external) (congenital) Q16.1
  - acquired — *see* Stricture, auditory canal, acquired
- ejaculatory duct N50.8
- enterostomy K94.13
- esophagus K22.2
  - congenital Q39.3
  - syphilitic A52.79
    - congenital A50.59 [K23]
- eustachian tube (*see also* Obstruction, eustachian tube)
  - congenital Q17.8
- fallopian tube N97.1
  - gonococcal A54.24
  - tuberculous A18.17
- gallbladder — *see* Obstruction, gallbladder
- glottis J38.6
- heart (*see also* Disease, heart)
  - valve (*see also* Endocarditis) I38
    - aortic Q23.0
    - mitral Q23.4
    - pulmonary Q22.1
    - tricuspid Q22.4
- hepatic duct K83.1
- hourglass, of stomach K31.2
- hymen N89.6
- hypopharynx J39.2
- ileum K56.69
  - congenital Q41.2
- intestine (*see also* Obstruction, intestine)
  - congenital (small) Q41.9
    - large Q42.9
      - specified NEC Q42.8
    - specified NEC Q41.8
  - ischemic K55.1
- jejunum K56.69
  - congenital Q41.1
- lacrimal passages (*see also* Stenosis, lacrimal)
  - congenital Q10.5
- larynx J38.6
  - congenital NEC Q31.8
    - subglottic Q31.1
  - syphilitic A52.73
    - congenital A50.59 [J99]
- meatus
  - ear (congenital) Q16.1
    - acquired — *see* Stricture, auditory canal, acquired
  - osseous (ear) (congenital) Q16.1
    - acquired — *see* Stricture, auditory canal, acquired
  - urinarius (*see also* Stricture, urethra)
    - congenital Q64.33
- mitral (valve) — *see* Stenosis, mitral
- myocardium, myocardial I51.5
  - hypertrophic subaortic (idiopathic) I42.1
- nares (anterior) (posterior) J34.89
  - congenital Q30.0
- nasal duct (*see also* Stenosis, lacrimal, duct)
  - congenital Q10.5
- nasolacrimal duct (*see also* Stenosis, lacrimal, duct)
  - congenital Q10.5
- nasopharynx J39.2
  - syphilitic A52.73
- nose J34.89
  - congenital Q30.0
- nostril (anterior) (posterior) J34.89
  - congenital Q30.0
  - syphilitic A52.73
    - congenital A50.59 [J99]
- organ or site, congenital NEC — *see* Atresia, by site
- os uteri — *see* Stricture, cervix
- osseous meatus (ear) (congenital) Q16.1
  - acquired — *see* Stricture, auditory canal, acquired
- oviduct — *see* Stricture, fallopian tube
- pelviureteric junction (congenital) Q62.11
- penis, by foreign body T19.4 ☑
- pharynx J39.2
- prostate N42.89
- pulmonary, pulmonic
  - artery (congenital) Q25.6
    - acquired I28.8
    - noncongenital I28.8
  - infundibulum (congenital) Q24.3
    - valve I37.0
      - congenital Q22.1
  - vein, acquired I28.8

Stricture — *continued*
- pulmonary, pulmonic — *continued*
  - vessel NEC I28.8
- punctum lacrimale (*see also* Stenosis, lacrimal, punctum)
  - congenital Q10.5
- pylorus (hypertrophic) K31.1
  - adult K31.1
  - congenital Q40.0
  - infantile Q40.0
- rectosigmoid K56.69
- rectum (sphincter) K62.4
  - congenital Q42.1
    - with fistula Q42.0
  - due to
    - chlamydial lymphogranuloma A55
    - irradiation K91.89
    - lymphogranuloma venereum A55
  - gonococcal A54.6
  - inflammatory (chlamydial) A55
  - syphilitic A52.74
  - tuberculous A18.32
- renal artery I70.1
  - congenital Q27.1
- salivary duct or gland (any) K11.8
- sigmoid (flexure) — *see* Obstruction, intestine
- spermatic cord N50.8
- stoma (following) (of)
  - colostomy K94.03
  - enterostomy K94.13
  - gastrostomy K94.23
  - ileostomy K94.13
  - tracheostomy J95.03
- stomach K31.89
  - congenital Q40.2
  - hourglass K31.2
- subaortic Q24.4
  - hypertrophic (acquired) (idiopathic) I42.1
- subglottic J38.6
- syphilitic NEC A52.79
- trachea J39.8
  - congenital Q32.1
  - syphilitic A52.73
  - tuberculous NEC A15.5
- tracheostomy J95.03
- tricuspid (valve) — *see* Stenosis, tricuspid
- tunica vaginalis N50.8
- ureter (postoperative) N13.5
  - with
    - hydronephrosis N13.1
      - with infection N13.6
    - pyelonephritis (chronic) N11.1
  - congenital — *see* Atresia, ureter
  - tuberculous A18.11
- ureteropelvic junction (congenital) Q62.11
- ureterovesical orifice N13.5
  - with infection N13.6
- urethra (organic) (spasmodic) N35.9
  - associated with schistosomiasis B65.0 [N37]
  - congenital Q64.39
    - valvular (posterior) Q64.2
  - due to
    - infection — *see* Stricture, urethra, postinfective
    - trauma — *see* Stricture, urethra, post-traumatic
  - gonococcal, gonorrheal A54.01
  - infective NEC — *see* Stricture, urethra, postinfective
  - late effect (sequelae) of injury — *see* Stricture, urethra, post-traumatic
  - postcatheterization — *see* Stricture, urethra, postprocedural
  - postinfective NEC
    - female N35.12
    - male N35.119
      - anterior urethra N35.114
      - bulbous urethra N35.112
      - meatal N35.111
      - membranous urethra N35.113
  - postobstetric N35.021
  - postoperative — *see* Stricture, urethra, postprocedural
  - postprocedural
    - female N99.12
    - male N99.114
      - anterior urethra N99.113
      - bulbous urethra N99.111
      - meatal N99.110
      - membranous urethra N99.112

Stricture — *continued*
- urethra — *continued*
  - post-traumatic
    - female N35.028
      - due to childbirth N35.021
    - male N35.014
      - anterior urethra N35.013
      - bulbous urethra N35.011
      - meatal N35.010
      - membranous urethra N35.012
    - sequela (late effect) of
      - childbirth N35.021
      - injury — *see* Stricture, urethra, post-traumatic
  - specified cause NEC N35.8
  - syphilitic A52.76
  - traumatic — *see* Stricture, urethra, post-traumatic
  - valvular (posterior), congenital Q64.2
- urinary meatus — *see* Stricture, urethra
- uterus, uterine (synechiae) N85.6
  - os (external) (internal) — *see* Stricture, cervix
- vagina (outlet) — *see* Stenosis, vagina
- valve (cardiac) (heart) (*see also* Endocarditis)
  - congenital
    - aortic Q23.0
    - mitral Q23.2
    - pulmonary Q22.1
    - tricuspid Q22.4
- vas deferens N50.8
  - congenital Q55.4
- vein I87.1
- vena cava (inferior) (superior) NEC I87.1
  - congenital Q26.0
- vesicourethral orifice N32.0
  - congenital Q64.31
- vulva (acquired) N90.5
Stridor R06.1
- congenital (larynx) P28.89
Stridulous — *see* condition
Stroke (apoplectic) (brain) (embolic) (ischemic) (paralytic) (thrombotic) I63.9
- epileptic — *see* Epilepsy
- heat T67.0 ☑
- in evolution I63.9
- intraoperative
  - during cardiac surgery I97.810
  - during other surgery I97.811
- lightning — *see* Lightning
- meaning
  - cerebral hemorrhage — *code to* Hemorrhage, intracranial
  - cerebral infarction — *code to* Infarction, cerebral
- postprocedural
  - following cardiac surgery I97.820
  - following other surgery I97.821
- unspecified (NOS) I63.9
Stromatosis, endometrial D39.0
Strongyloidiasis, strongyloidosis B78.9
- cutaneous B78.1
- disseminated B78.7
- intestinal B78.0
Strophulus pruriginosus L28.2
Struck by lightning — *see* Lightning
Struma (*see also* Goiter)
- Hashimoto E06.3
- lymphomatosa E06.3
- nodosa (simplex) E04.9
  - endemic E01.2
    - multinodular E01.1
  - multinodular E04.2
    - iodine-deficiency related E01.1
  - toxic or with hyperthyroidism E05.20
    - with thyroid storm E05.21
    - multinodular E05.20
      - with thyroid storm E05.21
    - uninodular E05.10
      - with thyroid storm E05.11
  - toxicosa E05.20
    - with thyroid storm E05.21
    - multinodular E05.20
      - with thyroid storm E05.21
    - uninodular E05.10
      - with thyroid storm E05.11
  - uninodular E04.1
- ovarii D27.- ☑
- Riedel's E06.5
Strumipriva cachexia E03.4
Strümpell-Marie spine — *see* Spondylitis, ankylosing
Strümpell-Westphal pseudosclerosis E83.01

Stuart deficiency disease (factor X) D68.2
Stuart-Prower factor deficiency (factor X) D68.2
Student's elbow — *see* Bursitis, elbow, olecranon
Stump — *see* Amputation
Stunting, nutritional E45
Stupor (catatonic) R40.1
   depressive F32.8
   dissociative F44.2
   manic F30.2
   manic-depressive F31.89
   psychogenic (anergic) F44.2
   reaction to exceptional stress (transient) F43.0
Sturge (-Weber) (-Dimitri) (-Kalischer) **disease or syn-**
     drome Q85.8
Stuttering F80.81
   adult onset F98.5
   childhood onset F80.81
   following cerebrovascular disease — *see* Disorder,
     fluency, following cerebrovascular disease
   in conditions classified elsewhere R47.82
Sty, stye (external) (internal) (meibomian) (zeisian) —
   see Hordeolum
Subacidity, gastric K31.89
   psychogenic F45.8
Subacute — *see* condition
Subarachnoid — *see* condition
Subcortical — *see* condition
Subcostal syndrome, nerve compression — *see*
   Mononeuropathy, upper limb, specified site NEC
Subcutaneous, subcuticular — *see* condition
Subdural — *see* condition
Subendocardium — *see* condition
Subependymoma
   specified site — *see* Neoplasm, uncertain behavior,
     by site
   unspecified site D43.2
Suberosis J67.3
Subglossitis — *see* Glossitis
Subhemophilia D66
Subinvolution
   breast (postlactational) (postpuerperal) N64.89
   puerperal O90.89
   uterus (chronic) (nonpuerperal) N85.3
     puerperal O90.89
Sublingual — *see* condition
Sublinguitis — *see* Sialoadenitis
Subluxatable hip Q65.6
Subluxation (*see also* Dislocation)
   acromioclavicular S43.11- ☑
   ankle S93.0- ☑
   atlantoaxial, recurrent M43.4
     with myelopathy M43.3
   carpometacarpal (joint) NEC S63.05- ☑
     thumb S63.04- ☑
   complex, vertebral — *see* Complex, subluxation
   congenital (*see also* Malposition, congenital)
     hip — *see* Dislocation, hip, congenital, partial
     joint (excluding hip)
       lower limb Q68.8
       shoulder Q68.8
       upper limb Q68.8
   elbow (traumatic) S53.10- ☑
     anterior S53.11- ☑
     lateral S53.14- ☑
     medial S53.13- ☑
     posterior S53.12- ☑
     specified type NEC S53.19- ☑
   finger S63.20- ☑
     index S63.20- ☑
     interphalangeal S63.22- ☑
       distal S63.24- ☑
         index S63.24- ☑
         little S63.24- ☑
         middle S63.24- ☑
         ring S63.24- ☑
       index S63.22- ☑
       little S63.22- ☑
       middle S63.22- ☑
       proximal S63.23- ☑
         index S63.23- ☑
         little S63.23- ☑
         middle S63.23- ☑
         ring S63.23- ☑
       ring S63.22- ☑
     little S63.20- ☑

Subluxation — *continued*
   finger — *continued*
     metacarpophalangeal S63.21- ☑
       index S63.21- ☑
       little S63.21- ☑
       middle S63.21- ☑
       ring S63.21- ☑
     middle S63.20- ☑
     ring S63.20- ☑
   foot S93.30- ☑
     specified site NEC S93.33- ☑
     tarsal joint S93.31- ☑
     tarsometatarsal joint S93.32- ☑
     toe — *see* Subluxation, toe
   hip S73.00- ☑
     anterior S73.03- ☑
     obturator S73.02- ☑
     central S73.04- ☑
     posterior S73.01- ☑
   interphalangeal (joint)
     finger S63.22- ☑
       distal joint S63.24- ☑
         index S63.24- ☑
         little S63.24- ☑
         middle S63.24- ☑
         ring S63.24- ☑
       index S63.22- ☑
       little S63.22- ☑
       middle S63.22- ☑
       proximal joint S63.23- ☑
         index S63.23- ☑
         little S63.23- ☑
         middle S63.23- ☑
         ring S63.23- ☑
       ring S63.22- ☑
     thumb S63.12- ☑
       distal joint S63.14- ☑
       proximal joint S63.13- ☑
     toe S93.13- ☑
       great S93.13- ☑
       lesser S93.13- ☑
   joint prosthesis — *see* Complications, joint prosthesis,
     mechanical, displacement, by site
   knee S83.10- ☑
     cap — *see* Subluxation, patella
     patella — *see* Subluxation, patella
     proximal tibia
       anteriorly S83.11- ☑
       laterally S83.14- ☑
       medially S83.13- ☑
       posteriorly S83.12- ☑
     specified type NEC S83.19- ☑
   lens — *see* Dislocation, lens, partial
   ligament, traumatic — *see* Sprain, by site
   metacarpal (bone)
     proximal end S63.06- ☑
   metacarpophalangeal (joint)
     finger S63.21- ☑
       index S63.21- ☑
       little S63.21- ☑
       middle S63.21- ☑
       ring S63.21- ☑
     thumb S63.11- ☑
   metatarsophalangeal joint S93.14- ☑
     great toe S93.14- ☑
     lesser toe S93.14- ☑
   midcarpal (joint) S63.03- ☑
   patella S83.00- ☑
     lateral S83.01- ☑
     recurrent (nontraumatic) — *see* Dislocation,
       patella, recurrent, incomplete
     specified type NEC S83.09- ☑
   pathological — *see* Dislocation, pathological
   radial head S53.00- ☑
     anterior S53.01- ☑
     nursemaid's elbow S53.03- ☑
     posterior S53.02- ☑
     specified type NEC S53.09- ☑
   radiocarpal (joint) S63.02- ☑
   radioulnar (joint)
     distal S63.01- ☑
     proximal — *see* Subluxation, elbow
   shoulder
     congenital Q68.8
     girdle S43.30- ☑
       scapula S43.31- ☑

Subluxation — *continued*
   shoulder — *continued*
     girdle — *continued*
       specified site NEC S43.39- ☑
     traumatic S43.00- ☑
       anterior S43.01- ☑
       inferior S43.03- ☑
       posterior S43.02- ☑
       specified type NEC S43.08- ☑
   sternoclavicular (joint) S43.20- ☑
     anterior S43.21- ☑
     posterior S43.22- ☑
   symphysis (pubis)
   thumb S63.103 ☑
     interphalangeal joint — *see* Subluxation, interpha-
       langeal (joint), thumb
     metacarpophalangeal joint — *see* Subluxation,
       metacarpophalangeal (joint), thumb
   toe(s) S93.10- ☑
     great S93.10- ☑
       interphalangeal joint S93.13- ☑
       metatarsophalangeal joint S93.14- ☑
     interphalangeal joint S93.13- ☑
     lesser S93.10- ☑
       interphalangeal joint S93.13- ☑
       metatarsophalangeal joint S93.14- ☑
     metatarsophalangeal joint S93.149 ☑
   ulna
     distal end S63.07- ☑
     proximal end — *see* Subluxation, elbow
   ulnohumeral joint — *see* Subluxation, elbow
   vertebral
     recurrent NEC — *see* subcategory M43.5 ☑
     traumatic
       cervical S13.100 ☑
         atlantoaxial joint S13.120 ☑
         atlantooccipital joint S13.110 ☑
         atloidooccipital joint S13.110 ☑
         joint between
           C0 and C1 S13.110 ☑
           C1 and C2 S13.120 ☑
           C2 and C3 S13.130 ☑
           C3 and C4 S13.140 ☑
           C4 and C5 S13.150 ☑
           C5 and C6 S13.160 ☑
           C6 and C7 S13.170 ☑
           C7 and T1 S13.180 ☑
         occipitoatloid joint S13.110 ☑
       lumbar S33.100 ☑
         joint between
           L1 and L2 S33.110 ☑
           L2 and L3 S33.120 ☑
           L3 and L4 S33.130 ☑
           L4 and L5 S33.140 ☑
       thoracic S23.100 ☑
         joint between
           T1 and T2 S23.110 ☑
           T2 and T3 S23.120 ☑
           T3 and T4 S23.122 ☑
           T4 and T5 S23.130 ☑
           T5 and T6 S23.132 ☑
           T6 and T7 S23.140 ☑
           T7 and T8 S23.142 ☑
           T8 and T9 S23.150 ☑
           T9 and T10 S23.152 ☑
           T10 and T11 S23.160 ☑
           T11 and T12 S23.162 ☑
           T12 and L1 S23.170 ☑
   wrist (carpal bone) S63.00- ☑
     carpometacarpal joint — *see* Subluxation, car-
       pometacarpal (joint)
     distal radioulnar joint — *see* Subluxation, radioul-
       nar (joint), distal
     metacarpal bone, proximal — *see* Subluxation,
       metacarpal (bone), proximal end
     midcarpal — *see* Subluxation, midcarpal (joint)
     radiocarpal joint — *see* Subluxation, radiocarpal
       (joint)
     recurrent — *see* Dislocation, recurrent, wrist
     specified site NEC S63.09- ☑
     ulna — *see* Subluxation, ulna, distal end
Submaxillary — *see* condition
Submersion (fatal) (nonfatal) T75.1 ☑
Submucous — *see* condition
Subnormal, subnormality
   accommodation (old age) H52.4

Index

Stuart deficiency disease — Subnormal, subnormality

Subnormal, subnormality — *continued*
    mental — *see* Disability, intellectual
    temperature (accidental) T68 ☑
Subphrenic — *see* condition
Subscapular nerve — *see* condition
Subseptus uterus Q51.2
Subsiding appendicitis K36
Substernal thyroid E04.9
    congenital Q89.2
Substitution disorder F44.9
Subtentorial — *see* condition
Subthyroidism (acquired) (*see also* Hypothyroidism)
    congenital E03.1
Succenturiate placenta O43.19- ☑
Sucking thumb, child (excessive) F98.8
Sudamen, sudamina L74.1
Sudanese kala-azar B55.0
Sudden
    hearing loss — *see* Deafness, sudden
    heart failure — *see* Failure, heart
Sudeck's atrophy, disease, or syndrome — *see* Algo-
    neurodystrophy
Suffocation — *see* Asphyxia, traumatic
Sugar
    blood
        high (transient) R73.9
        low (transient) E16.2
    in urine R81
Suicide, suicidal (attempted) T14.91
    by poisoning — *see* Table of Drugs and Chemicals
    history of (personal) Z91.5
        in family Z81.8
    ideation — *see* Ideation, suicidal
    risk
        meaning personal history of attempted suicide
            Z91.5
        meaning suicidal ideation — *see* Ideation, suicidal
    tendencies
        meaning personal history of attempted suicide
            Z91.5
        meaning suicidal ideation — *see* Ideation, suicidal
    trauma — *see* nature of injury by site
Suipestifer infection — *see* Infection, salmonella
Sulfhemoglobinemia, sulphemoglobinemia (ac-
    quired) (with methemoglobinemia) D74.8
Sumatran mite fever A75.3
Summer — *see* condition
Sunburn L55.9
    first degree L55.0
    second degree L55.1
    third degree L55.2
SUNCT (short lasting unilateral neuralgiform headache
    with conjunctival injection and tearing) G44.059
    intractable G44.051
    not intractable G44.059
Sunken acetabulum — *see* Derangement, joint, speci-
    fied type NEC, hip
Sunstroke T67.0 ☑
Superfecundation — *see* Pregnancy, multiple
Superfetation — *see* Pregnancy, multiple
Superinvolution (uterus) N85.8
Supernumerary (congenital)
    aortic cusps Q23.8
    auditory ossicles Q16.3
    bone Q79.8
    breast Q83.1
    carpal bones Q74.0
    cusps, heart valve NEC Q24.8
        aortic Q23.8
        mitral Q23.2
        pulmonary Q22.3
    digit(s) Q69.9
    ear (lobule) Q17.0
    fallopian tube Q50.6
    finger Q69.0
    hymen Q52.4
    kidney Q63.0
    lacrimonasal duct Q10.6
    lobule (ear) Q17.0
    mitral cusps Q23.2
    muscle Q79.8
    nipple(s) Q83.3
    organ or site not listed — *see* Accessory
    ossicles, auditory Q16.3
    ovary Q50.31
    oviduct Q50.6
    pulmonary, pulmonic cusps Q22.3

Supernumerary — *continued*
    rib Q76.6
        cervical or first (syndrome) Q76.5
    roots (of teeth) K00.2
    spleen Q89.09
    tarsal bones Q74.2
    teeth K00.1
    testis Q55.29
    thumb Q69.1
    toe Q69.2
    uterus Q51.2
    vagina Q52.1 ☑
    vertebra Q76.49
Supervision (of)
    contraceptive — *see* Prescription, contraceptives
    dietary (for) Z71.3
        allergy (food) Z71.3
        colitis Z71.3
        diabetes mellitus Z71.3
        food allergy or intolerance Z71.3
        gastritis Z71.3
        hypercholesterolemia Z71.3
        hypoglycemia Z71.3
        intolerance (food) Z71.3
        obesity Z71.3
        specified NEC Z71.3
    healthy infant or child Z76.2
        foundling Z76.1
    high-risk pregnancy — *see* Pregnancy, complicated
        by, high, risk
    lactation Z39.1
    pregnancy — *see* Pregnancy, supervision of
Supplemental teeth K00.1
Suppression
    binocular vision H53.34
    lactation O92.5
    menstruation N94.89
    ovarian secretion E28.39
    renal N28.9
    urine, urinary secretion R34
Suppuration, suppurative (*see also* condition)
    accessory sinus (chronic) — *see* Sinusitis
    adrenal gland
    antrum (chronic) — *see* Sinusitis, maxillary
    bladder — *see* Cystitis
    brain G06.0
        sequelae G09
    breast N61
        puerperal, postpartum or gestational — *see* Masti-
            tis, obstetric, purulent
    dental periosteum M27.3
    ear (middle) (*see also* Otitis, media)
        external NEC — *see* Otitis, externa, infective
        internal — *see* subcategory H83.0 ☑
    ethmoidal (chronic) (sinus) — *see* Sinusitis, ethmoidal
    fallopian tube — *see* Salpingo-oophoritis
    frontal (chronic) (sinus) — *see* Sinusitis, frontal
    gallbladder (acute) K81.0
    gum K05.20
        generalized K05.22
        localized K05.21
    intracranial G06.0
    joint — *see* Arthritis, pyogenic or pyemic
    labyrinthine — *see* subcategory H83.0 ☑
    lung — *see* Abscess, lung
    mammary gland N61
        puerperal, postpartum O91.12
            associated with lactation O91.13
    maxilla, maxillary M27.2
        sinus (chronic) — *see* Sinusitis, maxillary
    muscle — *see* Myositis, infective
    nasal sinus (chronic) — *see* Sinusitis
    pancreas, acute K85.8
    parotid gland — *see* Sialoadenitis
    pelvis, pelvic
        female — *see* Disease, pelvis, inflammatory
        male K65.0
    pericranial — *see* Osteomyelitis
    salivary duct or gland (any) — *see* Sialoadenitis
    sinus (accessory) (chronic) (nasal) — *see* Sinusitis
    sphenoidal sinus (chronic) — *see* Sinusitis, sphenoidal
    thymus (gland) E32.1
    thyroid (gland) E06.0
    tonsil — *see* Tonsillitis
    uterus — *see* Endometritis
Supraeruption of tooth (teeth) M26.34

Supraglottitis J04.30
    with obstruction J04.31
Suprarenal (gland) — *see* condition
Suprascapular nerve — *see* condition
Suprasellar — *see* condition
Surfer's knots or nodules S89.8- ☑
Surgical
    emphysema T81.82 ☑
    procedures, complication or misadventure — *see*
        Complications, surgical procedures
    shock T81.10 ☑
Surveillance (of) (for) (*see also* Observation)
    alcohol abuse Z71.41
    contraceptive — *see* Prescription, contraceptives
    dietary Z71.3
    drug abuse Z71.51
Susceptibility to disease, genetic Z15.89
    malignant neoplasm Z15.09
        breast Z15.01
        endometrium Z15.04
        ovary Z15.02
        prostate Z15.03
        specified NEC Z15.09
    multiple endocrine neoplasia Z15.81
Suspected condition, ruled out (*see also* Observation,
    suspected)
    amniotic cavity and membrane Z03.71
    cervical shortening Z03.75
    fetal anomaly Z03.73
    fetal growth Z03.74
    maternal and fetal conditions NEC Z03.79
    oligohydramnios Z03.71
    placental problem Z03.72
    polyhydramnios Z03.71
Suspended uterus
    in pregnancy or childbirth — *see* Pregnancy, compli-
        cated by, abnormal uterus
Sutton's nevus D22.9
Suture
    burst (in operation wound) T81.31 ☑
        external operation wound T81.31 ☑
        internal operation wound T81.32 ☑
    inadvertently left in operation wound — *see* Foreign
        body, accidentally left during a procedure
    removal Z48.02
Swab inadvertently left in operation wound — *see*
    Foreign body, accidentally left during a procedure
Swallowed, swallowing
    difficulty — *see* Dysphagia
    foreign body — *see* Foreign body, alimentary tract
Swan-neck deformity (finger) — *see* Deformity, finger,
    swan-neck
Swearing, compulsive F42
    in Gilles de la Tourette's syndrome F95.2
Sweat, sweats
    fetid L75.0
    night R61
Sweating, excessive R61
Sweeley-Klionsky disease E75.21
Sweet's disease or dermatosis L98.2
Swelling (of) R60.9
    abdomen, abdominal (not referable to any particular
        organ) — *see* Mass, abdominal
    ankle — *see* Effusion, joint, ankle
    arm M79.89
        forearm M79.89
    breast N63
    Calabar B74.3
    cervical gland R59.0
    chest, localized R22.2
    ear H93.8- ☑
    extremity (lower) (upper) — *see* Disorder, soft tissue,
        specified type NEC
    finger M79.89
    foot M79.89
    glands R59.9
        generalized R59.1
        localized R59.0
    hand M79.89
    head (localized) R22.0
    inflammatory — *see* Inflammation
    intra-abdominal — *see* Mass, abdominal
    joint — *see* Effusion, joint
    leg M79.89
        lower M79.89
    limb — *see* Disorder, soft tissue, specified type NEC

▽ Subterms under main terms may continue to next column or page   ☑ Additional Character Required — Refer to the Tabular List for Character Selection   **289**

Subnormal, subnormality — Swelling

Swelling — continued
  localized (skin) R22.9
    chest R22.2
    head R22.0
    limb
      lower — see Mass, localized, limb, lower
      upper — see Mass, localized, limb, upper
    neck R22.1
    trunk R22.2
  neck (localized) R22.1
  pelvic — see Mass, abdominal
  scrotum N50.8
  splenic — see Splenomegaly
  testis N50.8
  toe M79.89
  umbilical R19.09
  wandering, due to Gnathostoma (spinigerum) B83.1
  white — see Tuberculosis, arthritis
Swift (-Feer) disease
  overdose or wrong substance given or taken — see Table of Drugs and Chemicals, by drug, poisoning
Swimmer's
  cramp T75.1 ☑
  ear H60.33- ☑
  itch B65.3
Swimming in the head R42
Swollen — see Swelling
Swyer syndrome Q99.1
Sycosis L73.8
  barbae (not parasitic) L73.8
  contagiosa (mycotic) B35.0
  lupoides L73.8
  mycotic B35.0
  parasitic B35.0
  vulgaris L73.8
Sydenham's chorea — see Chorea, Sydenham's
Sylvatic yellow fever A95.0
Sylvest's disease B33.0
Symblepharon H11.23- ☑
  congenital Q10.3
Symond's syndrome G93.2
Sympathetic — see condition
Sympatheticotonia G90.8
Sympathicoblastoma
  specified site — see Neoplasm, malignant, by site
  unspecified site C74.90
Sympathogonioma — see Sympathicoblastoma
Symphalangy (fingers) (toes) Q70.9
Symptoms NEC R68.89
  breast NEC N64.59
  development NEC R63.8
  factitious, self-induced — see Disorder, factitious
  genital organs, female R10.2
  involving
    abdomen NEC R19.8
    appearance NEC R46.89
    awareness R41.9
      altered mental status R41.82
      amnesia — see Amnesia
      borderline intellectual functioning R41.83
      coma — see Coma
      disorientation R41.0
      neurologic neglect syndrome R41.4
      senile cognitive decline R41.81
      specified symptom NEC R41.89
    behavior NEC R46.89
    cardiovascular system NEC R09.89
    chest NEC R09.89
    circulatory system NEC R09.89
    cognitive functions R41.9
      altered mental status R41.82
      amnesia — see Amnesia
      borderline intellectual functioning R41.83
      coma — see Coma
      disorientation R41.0
      neurologic neglect syndrome R41.4
      senile cognitive decline R41.81
      specified symptom NEC R41.89
    development NEC R62.50
    digestive system NEC R19.8
    emotional state NEC R45.89
      emotional lability R45.86
    food and fluid intake R63.8
    general perceptions and sensations R44.9
      specified NEC R44.8
    musculoskeletal system R29.91

Symptoms — continued
  involving — continued
    musculoskeletal system R29.91
      specified NEC R29.898
    nervous system R29.90
      specified NEC R29.818
    pelvis NEC R19.8
    respiratory system NEC R09.89
    skin and integument R23.9
    urinary system R39.9
  menopausal N95.1
  metabolism NEC R63.8
  neurotic F48.8
  of infancy R68.19
  pelvis NEC, female R10.2
  skin and integument NEC R23.9
  subcutaneous tissue NEC R23.9
Sympus Q74.2
Syncephalus Q89.4
Synchondrosis
  abnormal (congenital) Q78.8
  ischiopubic M91.0
Synchysis (scintillans) (senile) (vitreous body) H43.89
Syncope (near) (pre-) R55
  anginosa I20.8
  bradycardia R00.1
  cardiac R55
  carotid sinus G90.01
  due to spinal (lumbar) puncture G97.1
  heart R55
  heat T67.1 ☑
  laryngeal R05
  psychogenic F48.8
  tussive R05
  vasoconstriction R55
  vasodepressor R55
  vasomotor R55
  vasovagal R55
Syndactylism, syndactyly Q70.9
  complex (with synostosis)
    fingers Q70.0- ☑
    toes Q70.2- ☑
  simple (without synostosis)
    fingers Q70.1- ☑
    toes Q70.3- ☑
Syndrome (see also Disease)
  48,XXXX Q97.1
  49,XXXXX Q97.1
  5q minus NOS D46.C (following D46.2)
  abdominal
    acute R10.0
    muscle deficiency Q79.4
  abnormal innervation H02.519
    left H02.516
      lower H02.515
      upper H02.514
    right H02.513
      lower H02.512
      upper H02.511
  abstinence, neonatal P96.1
  acid pulmonary aspiration, obstetric O74.0
  acquired immunodeficiency — see Human, immunodeficiency virus (HIV) disease
  acute abdominal R10.0
  acute respiratory distress (adult) (child) J80
  Adair-Dighton Q78.0
  Adams-Stokes (-Morgagni) I45.9
  adiposogenital E23.6
  adrenal
    hemorrhage (meningococcal) A39.1
    meningococcic A39.1
  adrenocortical — see Cushing's, syndrome
  adrenogenital E25.9
    congenital, associated with enzyme deficiency E25.0
  afferent loop NEC K91.89
  Alagille's Q44.7
  alcohol withdrawal (without convulsions) — see Dependence, alcohol, with, withdrawal
  Alder's D72.0
  Aldrich (-Wiskott) D82.0
  alien hand R41.4
  Alport Q87.81
  alveolar hypoventilation E66.2
  alveolocapillary block J84.10
  amnesic, amnestic (confabulatory) (due to) — see Disorder, amnesic
  amyostatic (Wilson's disease) E83.01

Syndrome — continued
  androgen insensitivity E34.50
    complete E34.51
    partial E34.52
  androgen resistance (see also Syndrome, androgen insensitivity) E34.50
  Angelman Q93.5
  anginal — see Angina
  ankyloglossia superior Q38.1
  anterior
    chest wall R07.89
    cord G83.82
    spinal artery G95.19
      compression M47.019
        cervical region M47.012
        cervicothoracic region M47.013
        lumbar region M47.016
        occipito-atlanto-axial region M47.011
        thoracic region M47.014
        thoracolumbar region M47.015
    tibial M76.81- ☑
  antibody deficiency D80.9
    agammaglobulinemic D80.1
      hereditary D80.0
    congenital D80.0
    hypogammaglobulinemic D80.1
      hereditary D80.0
  anticardiolipin (-antibody) D68.61
  antiphospholipid (-antibody) D68.61
  aortic
    arch M31.4
    bifurcation I74.09
  aortomesenteric duodenum occlusion K31.5
  apical ballooning (transient left ventricular) I51.81
  arcuate ligament I77.4
  argentaffin, argintaffinoma E34.0
  Arnold-Chiari — see Arnold-Chiari disease
  Arrillaga-Ayerza I27.0
  Asherman's N85.6
  aspiration, of newborn — see Aspiration, by substance, with pneumonia
    meconium P24.01
  ataxia-telangiectasia G11.3
  auriculotemporal G50.8
  autoerythrocyte sensitization (Gardner-Diamond) D69.2
  autoimmune lymphoproliferative [ALPS] D89.82
  autoimmune polyglandular E31.0
  autosomal — see Abnormal, autosomes
  Avellis' G46.8
  Ayerza (-Arrillaga) I27.0
  Babinski-Nageotte G83.89
  Bakwin-Krida Q79.8
  bare lymphocyte D81.6
  Barré-Guillain G61.0
  Barré-Liéou M53.0
  Barrett's — see Barrett's, esophagus
  Barsony-Polgar K22.4
  Bársony-Teschendorf K22.4
  Barth E78.71
  Bartter's E26.81
  basal cell nevus Q87.89
  Basedow's E05.00
    with thyroid storm E05.01
  basilar artery G45.0
  Batten-Steinert G71.11
  battered
    baby or child — see Maltreatment, child, physical abuse
    spouse — see Maltreatment, adult, physical abuse
  Beals Q87.40
  Beau's I51.5
  Beck's I65.8
  Benedikt's G46.3
  Béquez César (-Steinbrinck-Chédiak-Higashi) E70.330
  Bernhardt-Roth — see Meralgia paresthetica
  Bernheim's I50.9
  big spleen D73.1
  bilateral polycystic ovarian E28.2
  Bing-Horton's — see Horton's headache
  Birt-Hogg-Dube syndrome Q87.89
  Björck (-Thorsen) E34.0
  black
    lung J60
    widow spider bite — see Toxicity, venom, spider, black widow
  Blackfan-Diamond D61.01

Syndrome — *continued*
- blind loop K90.2
  - congenital Q43.8
  - postsurgical K91.2
- blue sclera Q78.0
- blue toe I75.02- ☑
- Boder-Sedgewick G11.3
- Boerhaave's K22.3
- Borjeson Forssman Lehmann Q89.8
- Bouillaud's I01.9
- Bourneville (-Pringle) Q85.1
- Bouveret (-Hoffman) I47.9
- brachial plexus G54.0
- bradycardia-tachycardia I49.5
- brain (nonpsychotic) F09
  - with psychosis, psychotic reaction F09
  - acute or subacute — *see* Delirium
  - congenital — *see* Disability, intellectual
  - organic F09
    - post-traumatic (nonpsychotic) F07.81
      - psychotic F09
  - personality change F07.0
  - postcontusional F07.81
  - post-traumatic, nonpsychotic F07.81
  - psycho-organic F09
  - psychotic F06.8
- brain stem stroke G46.3
- Brandt's (acrodermatitis enteropathica) E83.2
- broad ligament laceration N83.8
- Brock's J98.11
- bronze baby P83.8
- Brown-Sequard G83.81
- bubbly lung P27.0
- Buchem's M85.2
- Budd-Chiari I82.0
- bulbar (progressive) G12.22
- Bürger-Grütz E78.3
- Burke's K86.8
- Burnett's (milk-alkali) E83.52
- burning feet E53.9
- Bywaters' T79.5 ☑
- Call-Fleming I67.841
- carbohydrate-deficient glycoprotein (CDGS) E77.8
- carcinogenic thrombophlebitis I82.1
- carcinoid E34.0
- cardiac asthma I50.1
- cardiacos negros I27.0
- cardiofaciocutaneous Q87.89
- cardiopulmonary-obesity E66.2
- cardiorenal — *see* Hypertension, cardiorenal
- cardiorespiratory distress (idiopathic), newborn P22.0
- cardiovascular renal — *see* Hypertension, cardiorenal
- carotid
  - artery (hemispheric) (internal) G45.1
  - body G90.01
  - sinus G90.01
- carpal tunnel G56.0- ☑
- Cassidy (-Scholte) E34.0
- cat cry Q93.4
- cat eye Q92.8
- cauda equina G83.4
- causalgia — *see* Causalgia
- celiac K90.0
  - artery compression I77.4
  - axis I77.4
- central pain G89.0
- cerebellar
  - hereditary G11.9
  - stroke G46.4
- cerebellomedullary malformation — *see* Spina bifida
- cerebral
  - artery
    - anterior G46.1
    - middle G46.0
    - posterior G46.2
  - gigantism E22.0
- cervical (root) M53.1
  - disc — *see* Disorder, disc, cervical, with neuritis
  - fusion Q76.1
  - posterior, sympathicus M53.0
  - rib Q76.5
  - sympathetic paralysis G90.2
- cervicobrachial (diffuse) M53.1
- cervicocranial M53.0
- cervicodorsal outlet G54.2
- cervicothoracic outlet G54.0
- Céstan (-Raymond) I65.8

Syndrome — *continued*
- Charcot's (angina cruris) (intermittent claudication) I73.9
- Charcot-Weiss-Baker G90.09
- CHARGE Q89.8
- Chédiak-Higashi (-Steinbrinck) E70.330
- chest wall R07.1
- Chiari's (hepatic vein thrombosis) I82.0
- Chilaiditi's Q43.3
- child maltreatment — *see* Maltreatment, child
- chondrocostal junction M94.0
- chondroectodermal dysplasia Q77.6
- chromosome 4 short arm deletion Q93.3
- chromosome 5 short arm deletion Q93.4
- chronic
  - pain G89.4
    - personality F68.8
- Clarke-Hadfield K86.8
- Clerambault's automatism G93.89
- Clouston's (hidrotic ectodermal dysplasia) Q82.4
- clumsiness, clumsy child F82
- cluster headache G44.009
  - intractable G44.001
  - not intractable G44.009
- Coffin-Lowry Q89.8
- cold injury (newborn) P80.0
- combined immunity deficiency D81.9
- compartment (deep) (posterior) (traumatic) T79.A0 ☑ (*following* T79.7)
  - abdomen T79.A3 ☑ (*following* T79.7)
  - lower extremity (hip, buttock, thigh, leg, foot, toes) T79.A2 ☑ (*following* T79.7)
  - nontraumatic
    - abdomen M79.A3 (*following* M79.7)
    - lower extremity (hip, buttock, thigh, leg, foot, toes) M79.A2- ☑ (*following* M79.7)
    - specified site NEC M79.A9 (*following* M79.7)
    - upper extremity (shoulder, arm, forearm, wrist, hand, fingers) M79.A1- ☑ (*following* M79.7)
  - postprocedural — *see* Syndrome, compartment, nontraumatic
  - specified site NEC T79.A9 ☑ (*following* T79.7)
  - upper extremity (shoulder, arm, forearm, wrist, hand, fingers) T79.A1 ☑ (*following* T79.7)
- complex regional pain — *see* Syndrome, pain, complex regional
- compression T79.5 ☑
  - anterior spinal — *see* Syndrome, anterior, spinal artery, compression
  - cauda equina G83.4
  - celiac artery I77.4
  - vertebral artery M47.029
    - cervical region M47.022
    - occipito-atlanto-axial region M47.021
- concussion F07.81
- congenital
  - affecting multiple systems NEC Q87.89
  - central alveolar hypoventilation G47.35
  - facial diplegia Q87.0
  - muscular hypertrophy-cerebral Q87.89
  - oculo-auriculovertebral Q87.0
  - oculofacial diplegia (Moebius) Q87.0
  - rubella (manifest) P35.0
- congestion-fibrosis (pelvic), female N94.89
- congestive dysmenorrhea N94.6
- connective tissue M35.9
  - overlap NEC M35.1
- Conn's E26.01
- conus medullaris G95.81
- cord
  - anterior G83.82
  - posterior G83.83
- coronary
  - acute NEC I24.9
  - insufficiency or intermediate I20.0
  - slow flow I20.8
- Costen's (complex) M26.69
- costochondral junction M94.0
- costoclavicular G54.0
- costovertebral E22.0
- Cowden Q85.8
- craniovertebral M53.0
- Creutzfeldt-Jakob — *see* Creutzfeldt-Jakob disease or syndrome
- crib death R99
- cricopharyngeal — *see* Dysphagia
- cri-du-chat Q93.4

Syndrome — *continued*
- croup J05.0
- CRPS I — *see* Syndrome, pain, complex regional I
- crush T79.5 ☑
- cryptophthalmos Q87.0
- cubital tunnel — *see* Lesion, nerve, ulnar
- Curschmann (-Batten) (-Steinert) G71.11
- Cushing's E24.9
  - alcohol-induced E24.4
  - drug-induced E24.2
  - due to
    - alcohol
    - drugs E24.2
    - ectopic ACTH E24.3
    - overproduction of pituitary ACTH E24.0
  - overdose or wrong substance given or taken — *see* Table of Drugs and Chemicals, by drug, poisoning
  - pituitary-dependent E24.0
  - specified type NEC E24.8
- cystic duct stump K91.5
- Dana-Putnam D51.0
- Danbolt (-Cross) (acrodermatitis enteropathica) E83.2
- Dandy-Walker Q03.1
  - with spina bifida Q07.01
- Danlos' Q79.8
- De Quervain E34.51
- de Toni-Fanconi (-Debré) E72.09
  - with cystinosis E72.04
- defibrination (*see also* Fibrinolysis)
  - with
    - antepartum hemorrhage — *see* Hemorrhage, antepartum, with coagulation defect
    - intrapartum hemorrhage — *see* Hemorrhage, complicating, delivery
  - newborn P60
  - postpartum O72.3
- Degos' I77.89
- Déjérine-Roussy G89.0
- delayed sleep phase G47.21
- demyelinating G37.9
- dependence — *see* F10-F19 with fourth character .2
- depersonalization (-derealization) F48.1
- di George's D82.1
- diabetes mellitus in newborn infant P70.2
- diabetes mellitus-hypertension-nephrosis — *see* Diabetes, nephrosis
- diabetes-nephrosis — *see* Diabetes, nephrosis
- diabetic amyotrophy — *see* Diabetes, amyotrophy
- Diamond-Blackfan D61.01
- Diamond-Gardener D69.2
- DIC (diffuse or disseminated intravascular coagulopathy) D65
- Dighton's Q78.0
- disequilibrium E87.8
- Döhle body-panmyelopathic D72.0
- dorsolateral medullary G46.4
- double athetosis G80.3
- Down (*see also* Down syndrome) Q90.9
- Dresbach's (elliptocytosis) D58.1
- Dressler's (postmyocardial infarction) I24.1
  - postcardiotomy I97.0
- drug withdrawal, infant of dependent mother P96.1
- dry eye H04.12- ☑
- due to abnormality
  - chromosomal Q99.9
    - sex
      - female phenotype Q97.9
      - male phenotype Q98.9
    - specified NEC Q99.8
- dumping (postgastrectomy) K91.1
  - nonsurgical K31.89
- Dupré's (meningism) R29.1
- dysmetabolic X E88.81
- dyspraxia, developmental F82
- Eagle-Barrett Q79.4
- Eaton-Lambert — *see* Syndrome, Lambert-Eaton
- Ebstein's Q22.5
- ectopic ACTH E24.3
- eczema-thrombocytopenia D82.0
- Eddowes' Q78.8
- effort (psychogenic) F45.8
- Ehlers-Danlos Q79.6
- Eisenmenger's I27.89
- Ekman's Q78.0
- electric feet E53.8
- Ellis-van Creveld Q77.6
- empty nest Z60.0

Syndrome — *continued*
  endocrine-hypertensive E27.0
  entrapment — *see* Neuropathy, entrapment
  eosinophilia-myalgia M35.8
  epileptic (*see also* Epilepsy, by type)
    absence G40.A09 (*following* G40.3)
      intractable G40.A19 (*following* G40.3)
        with status epilepticus G40.A11 (*following* G40.3)
        without status epilepticus G40.A19 (*following* G40.3)
      not intractable G40.A09 (*following* G40.3)
        with status epilepticus G40.A01 (*following* G40.3)
        without status epilepticus G40.A09 (*following* G40.3)
  Erdheim-Chester (ECD) E88.89
  Erdheim's E22.0
  erythrocyte fragmentation D59.4
  Evans D69.41
  exhaustion F48.8
  extrapyramidal G25.9
    specified NEC G25.89
  eye retraction — *see* Strabismus
  eyelid-malar-mandible Q87.0
  Faber's D50.9
  facial pain, paroxysmal G50.0
  Fallot's Q21.3
  familial eczema-thrombocytopenia (Wiskott-Aldrich) D82.0
  Fanconi (-de Toni) (-Debré) E72.09
    with cystinosis E72.04
  Fanconi's (anemia) (congenital pancytopenia) D61.09
  fatigue
    chronic R53.82
    psychogenic F48.8
  faulty bowel habit K59.3
  Feil-Klippel (brevicollis) Q76.1
  Felty's — *see* Felty's syndrome
  fertile eunuch E23.0
  fetal
    alcohol (dysmorphic) Q86.0
    hydantoin Q86.1
  Fiedler's I40.1
  first arch Q87.0
  fish odor E72.8
  Fisher's G61.0
  Fitzhugh-Curtis
    due to
      Chlamydia trachomatis A74.81
      Neisseria gonorrhorea (gonococcal peritonitis) A54.85
  Fitz's K85.8
  Flajani (-Basedow) E05.00
    with thyroid storm E05.01
  flatback — *see* Flatback syndrome
  floppy
    baby P94.2
    iris (intraoeprative) (IFIS) H21.81
    mitral valve I34.1
  flush E34.0
  Foix-Alajouanine G95.19
  Fong's Q79.8
  foramen magnum G93.5
  Foster-Kennedy H47.14- ☑
  Foville's (peduncular) G46.3
  fragile X Q99.2
  Franceschetti Q75.4
  Frey's
    auriculotemporal G50.8
    hyperhidrosis L74.52
  Friderichsen-Waterhouse A39.1
  Froin's G95.89
  frontal lobe F07.0
  Fukuhara E88.49
  functional
    bowel K59.9
    prepubertal castrate E29.1
  Gaisböck's D75.1
  ganglion (basal ganglia brain) G25.9
    geniculi G51.1
  Gardner-Diamond D69.2
  gastroesophageal
    junction K22.0
    laceration-hemorrhage K22.6
  gastrojejunal loop obstruction K91.89
  Gee-Herter-Heubner K90.0

Syndrome — *continued*
  Gelineau's G47.419
    with cataplexy G47.411
  genito-anorectal A55
  Gerstmann-Sträussler-Scheinker (GSS) A81.82
  Gianotti-Crosti L44.4
  giant platelet (Bernard-Soulier) D69.1
  Gilles de la Tourette's F95.2
  goiter-deafness E07.1
  Goldberg Q89.8
  Goldberg-Maxwell E34.51
  Good's D83.8
  Gopalan' (burning feet) E53.8
  Gorlin's Q87.89
  Gougerot-Blum L81.7
  Gouley's I31.1
  Gower's R55
  gray or grey (newborn) P93.0
    platelet D69.1
  Gubler-Millard G46.3
  Guillain-Barré (-Strohl) G61.0
  gustatory sweating G50.8
  Hadfield-Clarke K86.8
  hair tourniquet — *see* Constriction, external, by site
  Hamman's J98.19
  hand-foot L27.1
  hand-shoulder G90.8
  hantavirus (cardio)-pulmonary (HPS) (HCPS) B33.4
  happy puppet Q93.5
  Harada's H30.81- ☑
  Hayem-Faber D50.9
  headache NEC G44.89
    complicated NEC G44.59
  Heberden's I20.8
  Hedinger's E34.0
  Hegglin's D72.0
  HELLP (hemolysis, elevated liver enzymes and low platelet count) O14.2- ☑
  hemolytic-uremic D59.3
  hemophagocytic, infection-associated D76.2
  Henoch-Schönlein D69.0
  hepatic flexure K59.8
  hepatopulmonary K76.81
  hepatorenal K76.7
    following delivery O90.4
    postoperative or postprocedural K91.83
    postpartum, puerperal O90.4
  hepatourologic K76.7
  Herter (-Gee) (nontropical sprue) K90.0
  Heubner-Herter K90.0
  Heyd's K76.7
  Hilger's G90.09
  histamine-like (fish poisoning) — *see* Poisoning, fish
  histiocytic D76.3
  histiocytosis NEC D76.3
  HIV infection, acute B20
  Hoffmann-Werdnig G12.0
  Hollander-Simons E88.1
  Hoppe-Goldflam G70.00
    with exacerbation (acute) G70.01
    in crisis G70.01
  Horner's G90.2
  hungry bone E83.81
  hunterian glossitis D51.0
  Hutchinson's triad A50.53
  hyperabduction G54.0
  hyperammonemia-hyperornithinemia-homocitrullinemia E72.4
  hypereosinophilic (idiopathic) D72.1
  hyperimmunoglobulin E (IgE) D82.4
  hyperkalemic E87.5
  hyperkinetic — *see* Hyperkinesia
  hypermobility M35.7
  hypernatremia E87.0
  hyperosmolarity E87.0
  hyperperfusion G97.82
  hypersplenic D73.1
  hypertransfusion, newborn P61.1
  hyperventilation F45.8
  hyperviscosity (of serum)
    polycythemic D75.1
    sclerothymic D58.8
  hypoglycemic (familial) (neonatal) E16.2
  hypokalemic E87.6
  hyponatremic E87.1
  hypopituitarism E23.0
  hypoplastic left-heart Q23.4
  hypopotassemia E87.6

Syndrome — *continued*
  hyposmolality E87.1
  hypotension, maternal O26.5- ☑
  hypothenar hammer I73.89
  ICF (intravascular coagulation-fibrinolysis) D65
  idiopathic
    cardiorespiratory distress, newborn P22.0
    nephrotic (infantile) N04.9
  iliotibial band M76.3- ☑
  immobility, immobilization (paraplegic) M62.3
  immune reconstitution D89.3
  immune reconstitution inflammatory [IRIS] D89.3
  immunity deficiency, combined D81.9
  immunodeficiency
    acquired — *see* Human, immunodeficiency virus (HIV) disease
    combined D81.9
  impending coronary I20.0
  impingement, shoulder M75.4- ☑
  inappropriate secretion of antidiuretic hormone E22.2
  infant
    gestational diabetes P70.0
    of diabetic mother P70.1
  infantilism (pituitary) E23.0
  inferior vena cava I87.1
  inspissated bile (newborn) P59.1
  institutional (childhood) F94.2
  insufficient sleep F51.12
  intermediate coronary (artery) I20.0
  interspinous ligament — *see* Spondylopathy, specified NEC
  intestinal
    carcinoid E34.0
    knot K56.2
  intravascular coagulation-fibrinolysis (ICF) D65
  iodine-deficiency, congenital E00.9
    type
      mixed E00.2
      myxedematous E00.1
      neurological E00.0
  IRDS (idiopathic respiratory distress, newborn) P22.0
  irritable
    bowel K58.9
      with diarrhea K58.0
      psychogenic F45.8
    heart (psychogenic) F45.8
    weakness F48.8
  ischemic bowel (transient) K55.9
    chronic K55.1
    due to mesenteric artery insufficiency K55.1
  IVC (intravascular coagulopathy) D65
  Ivemark's Q89.01
  Jaccoud's — *see* Arthropathy, postrheumatic, chronic
  Jackson's G83.89
  Jakob-Creutzfeldt — *see* Creutzfeldt-Jakob disease or syndrome
  jaw-winking Q07.8
  Jervell-Lange-Nielsen I45.81
  jet lag G47.25
  Job's D71
  Joseph-Diamond-Blackfan D61.01
  jugular foramen G52.7
  Kabuki Q89.8
  Kanner's (autism) F84.0
  Kartagener's Q89.3
  Kelly's D50.1
  Kimmelsteil-Wilson — *see* Diabetes, specified type, with Kimmelsteil-Wilson disease
  Klein (e)-Levine G47.13
  Klippel-Feil (brevicollis) Q76.1
  Köhler-Pellegrini-Steida — *see* Bursitis, tibial collateral
  König's K59.8
  Korsakoff (-Wernicke) (nonalcoholic) F04
    alcoholic F10.26
  Kostmann's D70.0
  Krabbe's congenital muscle hypoplasia Q79.8
  labyrinthine — *see* subcategory H83.2 ☑
  lacunar NEC G46.7
  Lambert-Eaton G70.80
    in
      neoplastic disease G73.1
      specified disease NEC G70.81
  Landau-Kleffner — *see* Epilepsy, specified NEC
  Larsen's Q74.8
  lateral
    cutaneous nerve of thigh G57.1- ☑
    medullary G46.4
  Launois' E22.0

Syndrome — *continued*
- lazy
  - leukocyte D70.8
  - posture M62.3
- Lemiere I80.8
- Lennox-Gastaut G40.812
  - intractable G40.814
    - with status epilepticus G40.813
    - without status epilepticus G40.814
  - not intractable G40.812
    - with status epilepticus G40.811
    - without status epilepticus G40.812
- lenticular, progressive E83.01
- Leopold-Levi's E05.90
- Lev's I44.2
- Lichtheim's D51.0
- Li-Fraumeni Z15.01
- Lightwood's N25.89
- Lignac (de Toni) (-Fanconi) (-Debré) E72.09
  - with cystinosis E72.04
- Likoff's I20.8
- limbic epilepsy personality F07.0
- liver-kidney K76.7
- lobotomy F07.0
- Loffler's J82
- long arm 18 or 21 deletion Q93.89
- long QT I45.81
- Louis-Barré G11.3
- low
  - atmospheric pressure T70.29 ☑
  - back M54.5
  - output (cardiac) I50.9
- lower radicular, newborn (birth injury) P14.8
- Luetscher's (dehydration) E86.0
- Lupus anticoagulant D68.62
- Lutembacher's Q21.1
- macrophage activation D76.1
  - due to infection D76.2
- magnesium-deficiency R29.0
- Mal de Debarquement R42
- malabsorption K90.9
  - postsurgical K91.2
- malformation, congenital, due to
  - alcohol Q86.0
  - exogenous cause NEC Q86.8
  - hydantoin Q86.1
  - warfarin Q86.2
- malignant
  - carcinoid E34.0
  - neuroleptic G21.0
- Mallory-Weiss K22.6
- mandibulofacial dysostosis Q75.4
- manic-depressive — *see* Disorder, bipolar, affective
- maple-syrup-urine E71.0
- Marable's I77.4
- Marfan's Q87.40
  - with
    - cardiovascular manifestations Q87.418
      - aortic dilation Q87.410
    - ocular manifestations Q87.42
    - skeletal manifestations Q87.43
- Marie's (acromegaly) E22.0
- maternal hypotension — *see* Syndrome, hypotension, maternal
- May (-Hegglin) D72.0
- McArdle (-Schmidt) (-Pearson) E74.04
- McQuarrie's E16.2
- meconium plug (newborn) P76.0
- median arcuate ligament I77.4
- Meekeren-Ehlers-Danlos Q79.6
- megavitamin-B6 E67.2
- Meige G24.4
- MELAS E88.41
- Mendelson's O74.0
- MERRF (myoclonic epilepsy associated with ragged-red fibers) E88.42
- mesenteric
  - artery (superior) K55.1
  - vascular insufficiency K55.1
- metabolic E88.81
- metastatic carcinoid E34.0
- micrognathia-glossoptosis Q87.0
- midbrain NEC G93.89
- middle lobe (lung) J98.19
- middle radicular G54.0
- migraine (*see also* Migraine) G43.909
- Mikulicz' K11.8
- milk-alkali E83.52

Syndrome — *continued*
- Millard-Gubler G46.3
- Miller-Dieker Q93.88
- Miller-Fisher G61.0
- Minkowski-Chauffard D58.0
- Mirizzi's K83.1
- MNGIE (Mitochondrial Neurogastrointestinal Encephalopathy) E88.49
- Möbius, ophthalmoplegic migraine — *see* Migraine, ophthalmoplegic
- monofixation H50.42
- Morel-Moore M85.2
- Morel-Morgagni M85.2
- Morgagni (-Morel) (-Stewart) M85.2
- Morgagni-Adams-Stokes I45.9
- Mounier-Kuhn Q32.4
  - with bronchiectasis J47.9
    - with
      - exacerbation (acute) J47.1
      - lower respiratory infection J47.0
  - acquired J98.09
    - with bronchiectasis J47.9
      - with
        - exacerbation (acute) J47.1
        - lower respiratory infection J47.0
- mucocutaneous lymph node (acute febrile) (MCLS) M30.3
- multiple endocrine neoplasia (MEN) — *see* Neoplasia, endocrine, multiple (MEN)
- multiple operations — *see* Disorder, factitious
- myasthenic G70.9
  - in
    - diabetes mellitus — *see* Diabetes, amyotrophy
    - endocrine disease NEC E34.9 [G73.3]
    - neoplastic disease (*see also* Neoplasm) D49.9 [G73.3]
    - thyrotoxicosis (hyperthyroidism) E05.90 [G73.3]
      - with thyroid storm E05.91 [G73.3]
- myelodysplastic D46.9
  - with
    - 5q deletion D46.C (*following* D46.2)
    - isolated del (5q) chromosomal abnormality D46.C (*following* D46.2)
    - lesions, low grade D46.20
    - specified NEC D46.Z (*following* D46.4)
- myelopathic pain G89.0
- myeloproliferative (chronic) D47.1
- myofascial pain M79.1
- Naffziger's G54.0
- nail patella Q87.2
- NARP (Neuropathy, Ataxia and Retinitis pigmentosa) E88.49
- neonatal abstinence P96.1
- nephritic (*see also* Nephritis)
  - with edema — *see* Nephrosis
  - acute N00.9
  - chronic N03.9
  - rapidly progressive N01.9
- nephrotic (congenital) (*see also* Nephrosis) N04.9
  - with
    - dense deposit disease N04.6
    - diffuse
      - crescentic glomerulonephritis N04.7
      - endocapillary proliferative glomerulonephritis N04.4
      - membranous glomerulonephritis N04.2
      - mesangial proliferative glomerulonephritis N04.3
      - mesangiocapillary glomerulonephritis N04.5
    - focal and segmental glomerular lesions N04.1
    - minor glomerular abnormality N04.0
    - specified morphological changes NEC N04.8
  - diabetic — *see* Diabetes, nephrosis
- neurologic neglect R41.4
- Nezelof's D81.4
- Nonne-Milroy-Meige Q82.0
- Nothnagel's vasomotor acroparesthesia I73.89
- oculomotor H51.9
- ophthalmoplegia-cerebellar ataxia — *see* Strabismus, paralytic, third nerve
- oral-facial-digital Q87.0
- organic
  - affective F06.30
  - amnesic (not alcohol- or drug-induced) F04
  - brain F09
  - depressive F06.31
  - hallucinosis F06.0
  - personality F07.0

Syndrome — *continued*
- Ormond's N13.5
- oro-facial-digital Q87.0
- os trigonum Q68.8
- Osler-Weber-Rendu I78.0
- osteoporosis-osteomalacia M83.8
- Osterreicher-Turner Q79.8
- otolith — *see* subcategory H81.8 ☑
- oto-palatal-digital Q87.0
- outlet (thoracic) G54.0
- ovary
  - polycystic E28.2
  - resistant E28.39
  - sclerocystic E28.2
- Owren's D68.2
- Paget-Schroetter I82.890
- pain (*see also* Pain)
  - complex regional I G90.50
    - lower limb G90.52- ☑
    - specified site NEC G90.59
    - upper limb G90.51- ☑
  - complex regional II — *see* Causalgia
- painful
  - bruising D69.2
  - feet E53.8
  - prostate N42.81
- paralysis agitans — *see* Parkinsonism
- paralytic G83.9
  - specified NEC G83.89
- Parinaud's H51.0
- parkinsonian — *see* Parkinsonism
- Parkinson's — *see* Parkinsonism
- paroxysmal facial pain G50.0
- Parry's E05.00
  - with thyroid storm E05.01
- Parsonage (-Aldren)-Turner G54.5
- patella clunk M25.86- ☑
- Paterson (-Brown) (-Kelly) D50.1
- pectoral girdle I77.89
- pectoralis minor I77.89
- Pelger-Huet D72.0
- pellagra-cerebellar ataxia-renal aminoaciduria E72.02
- pellagroid E52
- Pellegrini-Stieda — *see* Bursitis, tibial collateral
- pelvic congestion-fibrosis, female N94.89
- penta X Q97.1
- peptic ulcer — *see* Ulcer, peptic
- perabduction I77.89
- periodic headache, in adults and children — *see* Headache, periodic syndromes in adults and children
- periurethral fibrosis N13.5
- phantom limb (without pain) G54.7
  - with pain G54.6
- pharyngeal pouch D82.1
- Pick's (heart) (liver) I31.1
- Pickwickian E66.2
- PIE (pulmonary infiltration with eosinophilia) J82
- pigmentary pallidal degeneration (progressive) G23.0
- pineal E34.8
- pituitary E22.0
- placental transfusion — *see* Pregnancy, complicated by, placental transfusion syndromes
- plantar fascia M72.2
- plateau iris (post-iridectomy) (postprocedural) H21.82
- Plummer-Vinson D50.1
- pluricarential of infancy E40
- plurideficiency E40
- pluriglandular (compensatory) E31.8
  - autoimmune E31.0
- pneumatic hammer T75.21 ☑
- polyangiitis overlap M30.8
- polycarential of infancy E40
- polyglandular E31.8
  - autoimmune E31.0
- polysplenia Q89.09
- pontine NEC G93.89
- popliteal
  - artery entrapment I77.89
  - web Q87.89
- post chemoembolization — *code to* associated conditions
- postcardiac injury
  - postcardiotomy I97.0
  - postmyocardial infarction I24.1
- postcardiotomy I97.0
- postcholecystectomy K91.5
- postcommissurotomy I97.0

Syndrome — *continued*
  postconcussional F07.81
  postcontusional F07.81
  postencephalitic F07.89
  posterior
    cervical sympathetic M53.0
    cord G83.83
    fossa compression G93.5
    reversible encephalopathy (PRES) I67.83
  postgastrectomy (dumping) K91.1
  postgastric surgery K91.1
  postinfarction I24.1
  postlaminectomy NEC M96.1
  postleukotomy F07.0
  postmastectomy lymphedema I97.2
  postmyocardial infarction I24.1
  postoperative NEC T81.9 ☑
    blind loop K90.2
  postpartum panhypopituitary (Sheehan) E23.0
  postpolio (myelitic) G14
  postthrombotic I87.009
    with
      inflammation I87.02- ☑
        with ulcer I87.03- ☑
      specified complication NEC I87.09- ☑
      ulcer I87.01- ☑
        with inflammation I87.03- ☑
    asymptomatic I87.00- ☑
  postvagotomy K91.1
  postvalvulotomy I97.0
  postviral NEC G93.3
    fatigue G93.3
  Potain's K31.0
  potassium intoxication E87.5
  precerebral artery (multiple) (bilateral) G45.2
  preinfarction I20.0
  preleukemic D46.9
  premature senility E34.8
  premenstrual dysphoric N94.3
  premenstrual tension N94.3
  Prinzmetal-Massumi R07.1
  prune belly Q79.4
  pseudo -Turner's Q87.1
  pseudocarpal tunnel (sublimis) — *see* Syndrome,
    carpal tunnel
  pseudoparalytica G70.00
    with exacerbation (acute) G70.01
    in crisis G70.01
  psycho-organic (nonpsychotic severity) F07.9
    acute or subacute F05
    depressive type F06.31
    hallucinatory type F06.0
    nonpsychotic severity F07.0
    specified NEC F07.89
  pulmonary
    arteriosclerosis I27.0
    dysmaturity (Wilson-Mikity) P27.0
    hypoperfusion (idiopathic) P22.0
    renal (hemorrhagic) (Goodpasture's) M31.0
  pure
    motor lacunar G46.5
    sensory lacunar G46.6
  Putnam-Dana D51.0
  pyramidopallidonigral G20
  pyriformis — *see* Lesion, nerve, sciatic
  QT interval prolongation I45.81
  radicular NEC — *see* Radiculopathy
    upper limbs, newborn (birth injury) P14.3
  rapid time-zone change G47.25
  Rasmussen G04.81
  Raymond (-Céstan) I65.8
  Raynaud's I73.00
    with gangrene I73.01
  RDS (respiratory distress syndrome, newborn) P22.0
  reactive airways dysfunction J68.3
  Refsum's G60.1
  Reifenstein E34.52
  renal glomerulohyalinosis-diabetic — *see* Diabetes,
    nephrosis
  Rendu-Osler-Weber I78.0
  residual ovary N99.83
  resistant ovary E28.39
  respiratory
    distress
      acute J80
        adult J80
        child J80

Syndrome — *continued*
  respiratory — *continued*
    distress — *continued*
      newborn (idiopathic) (type I) P22.0
        type II P22.1
  restless legs G25.81
  retinoblastoma (familial) C69.2 ☑
  retroperitoneal fibrosis N13.5
  retroviral seroconversion (acute) Z21
  Reye's G93.7
  Richter — *see* Leukemia, chronic lymphocytic, B-cell
    type
  Ridley's I50.1
  right
    heart, hypoplastic Q22.6
    ventricular obstruction — *see* Failure, heart, con-
      gestive
  Romano-Ward (prolonged QT interval) I45.81
  rotator cuff, shoulder (*see also* Tear, rotator cuff)
    M75.10- ☑
  Rotes Quérol — *see* Hyperostosis, ankylosing
  Roth — *see* Meralgia paresthetica
  rubella (congenital) P35.0
  Ruvalcaba-Myhre-Smith E71.440
  Rytand-Lipsitch I44.2
  salt
    depletion E87.1
      due to heat NEC T67.8 ☑
        causing heat exhaustion or prostration
          T67.4 ☑
    low E87.1
  salt-losing N28.89
  Scaglietti-Dagnini E22.0
  scalenus anticus (anterior) G54.0
  scapulocostal — *see* Mononeuropathy, upper limb,
    specified site NEC
  scapuloperoneal G71.0
  schizophrenic, of childhood NEC F84.5
  Schnitzler D47.2
  Scholte's E34.0
  Schroeder's E27.0
  Schüller-Christian C96.5
  Schwachman's — *see* Syndrome, Shwachman's
  Schwartz (-Jampel) G71.13
  Schwartz-Bartter E22.2
  scimitar Q26.8
  sclerocystic ovary E28.2
  Seitelberger's G31.89
  septicemic adrenal hemorrhage A39.1
  seroconversion, retroviral (acute) Z21
  serous meningitis G93.2
  severe acute respiratory (SARS) J12.81
  shaken infant T74.4 ☑
  shock (traumatic) T79.4 ☑
    kidney N17.0
      following crush injury T79.5 ☑
    toxic A48.3
  shock-lung J80
  Shone's — *code to* specific anomalies
  short
    bowel K91.2
    rib Q77.2
  shoulder-hand — *see* Algoneurodystrophy
  Shwachman's D70.4
  sicca — *see* Sicca syndrome
  sick
    cell E87.1
    sinus I49.5
  sick-euthyroid E07.81
  sideropenic D50.1
  Siemens' ectodermal dysplasia Q82.4
  Silfversköld's Q78.9
  Simons' E88.1
  sinus tarsi M25.57- ☑
  sinusitis-bronchiectasis-situs inversus Q89.3
  Sipple's E31.22
  sirenomelia Q87.2
  Slocumb's E27.0
  slow flow, coronary I20.8
  Sluder's G44.89
  Smith-Magenis Q93.88
  Sneddon-Wilkinson L13.1
  Sotos' E22.0
  South African cardiomyopathy I42.8
  spasmodic
    upward movement, eyes H51.8
    winking F95.8
  Spen's I45.9

Syndrome — *continued*
  splenic
    agenesis Q89.01
    flexure K59.8
    neutropenia D73.81
  Spurway's Q78.0
  staphylococcal scalded skin L00
  Stein-Leventhal E28.2
  Stein's E28.2
  Stevens-Johnson syndrome L51.1
    toxic epidermal necrolysis overlap L51.3
  Stewart-Morel M85.2
  Stickler Q89.8
  stiff baby Q89.8
  stiff man G25.82
  Still-Felty — *see* Felty's syndrome
  Stokes (-Adams) I45.9
  stone heart I50.1
  straight back, congenital Q76.49
  subclavian steal G45.8
  subcoracoid-pectoralis minor G54.0
  subcostal nerve compression I77.89
  subphrenic interposition Q43.3
  superior
    cerebellar artery I63.8
    mesenteric artery K55.1
    semi-circular canal dehiscence H83.8X- ☑
    vena cava I87.1
  supine hypotensive (maternal) — *see* Syndrome, hy-
    potension, maternal
  suprarenal cortical E27.0
  supraspinatus (*see also* Tear, rotator cuff) M75.10- ☑
  Susac G93.49
  swallowed blood P78.2
  sweat retention L74.0
  Swyer Q99.1
  Symond's G93.2
  sympathetic
    cervical paralysis G90.2
    pelvic, female N94.89
  systemic inflammatory response (SIRS), of non-infec-
    tious origin (without organ dysfunction) R65.10
    with acute organ dysfunction R65.11
  tachycardia-bradycardia I49.5
  takotsubo I51.81
  TAR (thrombocytopenia with absent radius) Q87.2
  tarsal tunnel G57.5- ☑
  teething K00.7
  tegmental G93.89
  telangiectasic-pigmentation-cataract Q82.8
  temporal pyramidal apex — *see* Otitis, media, suppu-
    rative, acute
  temporomandibular joint-pain-dysfunction M26.62
  Terry's H44.2- ☑
  testicular feminization (*see also* Syndrome, androgen
    insensitivity) E34.51
  thalamic pain (hyperesthetic) G89.0
  thoracic outlet (compression) G54.0
  Thorson-Björck E34.0
  thrombocytopenia with absent radius (TAR) Q87.2
  thyroid-adrenocortical insufficiency E31.0
  tibial
    anterior M76.81- ☑
    posterior M76.82- ☑
  Tietze's M94.0
  time-zone (rapid) G47.25
  Toni-Fanconi E72.09
    with cystinosis E72.04
  Touraine's Q79.8
  tourniquet — *see* Constriction, external, by site
  toxic shock A48.3
  transient left ventricular apical ballooning I51.81
  traumatic vasospastic T75.22 ☑
  Treacher Collins Q75.4
  triple X, female Q97.0
  trisomy Q92.9
    13 Q91.7
      meiotic nondisjunction Q91.4
      mitotic nondisjunction Q91.5
      mosaicism Q91.5
      translocation Q91.6
    18 Q91.3
      meiotic nondisjunction Q91.0
      mitotic nondisjunction Q91.1
      mosaicism Q91.1
      translocation Q91.2
    20 (q)(p) Q92.8

☑ **Additional Character Required — Refer to the Tabular List for Character Selection**   🔻 **Subterms under main terms may continue to next column or page**

Syndrome — *continued*
  trisomy — *continued*
    21 Q90.9
      meiotic nondisjunction Q90.0
      mitotic nondisjunction Q90.1
      mosaicism Q90.1
      translocation Q90.2
    22 Q92.8
  tropical wet feet T69.0- ☑
  Trousseau's I82.1
  tumor lysis (following antineoplastic chemotherapy) (spontaneous) NEC E88.3
  Twiddler's (due to)
    automatic implantable defibrillator T82.198 ☑
    cardiac pacemaker T82.198 ☑
  Unverricht (-Lundborg) — *see* Epilepsy, generalized, idiopathic
  upward gaze H51.8
  uremia, chronic (*see also* Disease, kidney, chronic) N18.9
  urethral N34.3
  urethro-oculo-articular — *see* Reiter's disease
  urohepatic K76.7
  vago-hypoglossal G52.7
  van Buchem's M85.2
  van der Hoeve's Q78.0
  vascular NEC in cerebrovascular disease G46.8
  vasoconstriction, reversible cerebrovascular I67.841
  vasomotor I73.9
  vasospastic (traumatic) T75.22 ☑
  vasovagal R55
  VATER Q87.2
  velo-cardio-facial Q93.81
  vena cava (inferior) (superior) (obstruction) I87.1
  vertebral
    artery G45.0
      compression — *see* Syndrome, anterior, spinal artery, compression
    steal G45.0
  vertebro-basilar artery G45.0
  vertebrogenic (pain) M54.89
  vertiginous — *see* Disorder, vestibular function
  Vinson-Plummer D50.1
  virus B34.9
  visceral larva migrans B83.0
  visual disorientation H53.8
  vitamin B6 deficiency E53.1
  vitreal corneal H59.01- ☑
  vitreous (touch) H59.01- ☑
  Vogt-Koyanagi H20.82- ☑
  Volkmann's T79.6 ☑
  von Schroetter's I82.890
  von Willebrand (-Jürgen) D68.0
  Waldenström-Kjellberg D50.1
  Wallenberg's G46.3
  water retention E87.79
  Waterhouse (-Friderichsen) A39.1
  Weber-Gubler G46.3
  Weber-Leyden G46.3
  Weber's G46.3
  Wegener's M31.30
    with
      kidney involvement M31.31
      lung involvement M31.30
        with kidney involvement M31.31
  Weingarten's (tropical eosinophilia) J82
  Weiss-Baker G90.09
  Werdnig-Hoffman G12.0
  Wermer's E31.21
  Werner's E34.8
  Wernicke-Korsakoff (nonalcoholic) F04
    alcoholic F10.26
  Westphal-Strümpell E83.01
  West's — *see* Epilepsy, spasms
  wet
    feet (maceration) (tropical) T69.0- ☑
    lung, newborn P22.1
  whiplash S13.4 ☑
  whistling face Q87.0
  Wilkie's K55.1
  Wilkinson-Sneddon L13.1
  Willebrand (-Jürgens) D68.0
  Wilson's (hepatolenticular degeneration) E83.01
  Wiskott-Aldrich D82.0
  withdrawal — *see* Withdrawal, state
    drug
      infant of dependent mother P96.1
      therapeutic use, newborn P96.2

Syndrome — *continued*
  Woakes' (ethmoiditis) J33.1
  Wright's (hyperabduction) I77.89
  X I20.9
  XXXX Q97.1
  XXXXX Q97.1
  XXXXY Q98.1
  XXY Q98.0
  yellow nail L60.5
  Zahorsky's B08.5
  Zellweger syndrome E71.510
  Zellweger-like syndrome E71.541
Synechia (anterior) (iris) (posterior) (pupil) (*see also* Adhesions, iris)
  intra-uterine (traumatic) N85.6
Synesthesia R20.8
Syngamiasis, syngamosis B83.3
Synodontia K00.2
Synorchidism, synorchism Q55.1
Synostosis (congenital) Q78.8
  astragalo-scaphoid Q74.2
  radioulnar Q74.0
Synovial sarcoma — *see* Neoplasm, connective tissue, malignant
Synovioma (malignant) (*see also* Neoplasm, connective tissue, malignant)
  benign — *see* Neoplasm, connective tissue, benign
Synoviosarcoma — *see* Neoplasm, connective tissue, malignant
Synovitis (*see also* Tenosynovitis)
  crepitant
    hand M70.0- ☑
    wrist M70.03- ☑
  gonococcal A54.49
  gouty — *see* Gout, idiopathic
  in (due to)
    crystals M65.8- ☑
    gonorrhea A54.49
    syphilis (late) A52.78
    use, overuse, pressure — *see* Disorder, soft tissue, due to use
  infective NEC — *see* Tenosynovitis, infective NEC
  specified NEC — *see* Tenosynovitis, specified type NEC
  syphilitic A52.78
    congenital (early) A50.02
  toxic — *see* Synovitis, transient
  transient M67.3- ☑
    ankle M67.37- ☑
    elbow M67.32- ☑
    foot joint M67.37- ☑
    hand joint M67.34- ☑
    hip M67.35- ☑
    knee M67.36- ☑
    multiple site M67.39
    pelvic region M67.35- ☑
    shoulder M67.31- ☑
    specified joint NEC M67.38
    wrist M67.33- ☑
  traumatic, current — *see* Sprain
  tuberculous — *see* Tuberculosis, synovitis
  villonodular (pigmented) M12.2- ☑
    ankle M12.27- ☑
    elbow M12.22- ☑
    foot joint M12.27- ☑
    hand joint M12.24- ☑
    hip M12.25- ☑
    knee M12.26- ☑
    multiple site M12.29
    pelvic region M12.25- ☑
    shoulder M12.21- ☑
    specified joint NEC M12.28
    vertebrae M12.28
    wrist M12.23- ☑
Syphilid A51.39
  congenital A50.06
  newborn A50.06
  tubercular (late) A52.79
Syphilis, syphilitic (acquired) A53.9
  abdomen (late) A52.79
  acoustic nerve A52.15
  adenopathy (secondary) A51.49
  adrenal (gland) (with cortical hypofunction) A52.79
  age under 2 years NOS (*see also* Syphilis, congenital, early)
    acquired A51.9
  alopecia (secondary) A51.32
  anemia (late) A52.79 [D63.8]

Syphilis, syphilitic — *continued*
  aneurysm (aorta) (ruptured) A52.01
    central nervous system A52.05
    congenital A50.54 [I79.0]
  anus (late) A52.74
    primary A51.1
    secondary A51.39
  aorta (arch) (abdominal) (thoracic) A52.02
    aneurysm A52.01
  aortic (insufficiency) (regurgitation) (stenosis) A52.03
    aneurysm A52.01
  arachnoid (adhesive) (cerebral) (spinal) A52.13
  asymptomatic — *see* Syphilis, latent
  ataxia (locomotor) A52.11
  atrophoderma maculatum A51.39
  auricular fibrillation A52.06
  bladder (late) A52.76
  bone A52.77
    secondary A51.46
  brain A52.17
  breast (late) A52.79
  bronchus (late) A52.72
  bubo (primary) A51.0
  bulbar palsy A52.19
  bursa (late) A52.78
  cardiac decompensation A52.06
  cardiovascular A52.00
  central nervous system (late) (recurrent) (relapse) (tertiary) A52.3
    with
      ataxia A52.11
      general paralysis A52.17
        juvenile A50.45
      paresis (general) A52.17
        juvenile A50.45
      tabes (dorsalis) A52.11
        juvenile A50.45
      taboparesis A52.17
        juvenile A50.45
    aneurysm A52.05
    congenital A50.40
      juvenile A50.40
    remission in (sustained) A52.3
    serology doubtful, negative, or positive A52.3
    specified nature or site NEC A52.19
    vascular A52.05
  cerebral A52.17
    meningovascular A52.13
    nerves (multiple palsies) A52.15
    sclerosis A52.17
    thrombosis A52.05
  cerebrospinal (tabetic type) A52.12
  cerebrovascular A52.05
  cervix (late) A52.76
  chancre (multiple) A51.0
    extragenital A51.2
    Rollet's A51.0
  Charcot's joint A52.16
  chorioretinitis A51.43
    congenital A50.01
    late A52.71
    prenatal A50.01
  choroiditis — *see* Syphilitic chorioretinitis
  choroidoretinitis — *see* Syphilitic chorioretinitis
  ciliary body (secondary) A51.43
    late A52.71
  colon (late) A52.74
  combined spinal sclerosis A52.11
  condyloma (latum) A51.31
  congenital A50.9
    with
      paresis (general) A50.45
      tabes (dorsalis) A50.45
      taboparesis A50.45
    early, or less than 2 years after birth NEC A50.2
      with manifestations — *see* Syphilis, congenital, early, symptomatic
      latent (without manifestations) A50.1
        negative spinal fluid test A50.1
        serology positive A50.1
      symptomatic A50.09
        cutaneous A50.06
        mucocutaneous A50.07
        oculopathy A50.01
        osteochondropathy A50.02
        pharyngitis A50.03
        pneumonia A50.04
        rhinitis A50.05

Syphilis, syphilitic — *continued*
  congenital — *continued*
    early, or less than 2 years after birth — *continued*
      symptomatic — *continued*
        visceral A50.08
    chorioretinitis, choroiditis A50.01 [H32]
    interstitial keratitis A50.31
    juvenile neurosyphilis A50.45
    late, or 2 years or more after birth NEC A50.7
      chorioretinitis, choroiditis A50.32
      interstitial keratitis A50.31
      juvenile neurosyphilis A50.45
      latent (without manifestations) A50.6
        negative spinal fluid test A50.6
        serology positive A50.6
      symptomatic or with manifestations NEC
          A50.59
        arthropathy A50.55
        cardiovascular A50.54
        Clutton's joints A50.51
        Hutchinson's teeth A50.52
        Hutchinson's triad A50.53
        osteochondropathy A50.56
        saddle nose A50.57
  conjugal A53.9
    tabes A52.11
  conjunctiva (late) A52.71
  contact Z20.2
  cord bladder A52.19
  cornea, late A52.71
  coronary (artery) (sclerosis) A52.06
  coryza, congenital A50.05
  cranial nerve A52.15
    multiple palsies A52.15
  cutaneous — *see* Syphilis, skin
  dacryocystitis (late) A52.71
  degeneration, spinal cord A52.12
  dementia paralytica A52.17
    juvenilis A50.45
  destruction of bone A52.77
  dilatation, aorta A52.01
  due to blood transfusion A53.9
  dura mater A52.13
  ear A52.79
    inner A52.79
      nerve (eighth) A52.15
      neurorecurrence A52.15
  early A51.9
    cardiovascular A52.00
    central nervous system A52.3
    latent (without manifestations) (less than 2 years
        after infection) A51.5
      negative spinal fluid test A51.5
      serological relapse after treatment A51.5
      serology positive A51.5
    relapse (treated, untreated) A51.9
    skin A51.39
    symptomatic A51.9
      extragenital chancre A51.2
      primary, except extragenital chancre A51.0
      secondary (*see also* Syphilis, secondary) A51.39
        relapse (treated, untreated) A51.49
      ulcer A51.39
  eighth nerve (neuritis) A52.15
  endemic A65
  endocarditis A52.03
    aortic A52.03
    pulmonary A52.03
  epididymis (late) A52.76
  epiglottis (late) A52.73
  epiphysitis (congenital) (early) A50.02
  episcleritis (late) A52.71
  esophagus A52.79
  eustachian tube A52.73
  exposure to Z20.2
  eye A52.71
  eyelid (late) (with gumma) A52.71
  fallopian tube (late) A52.76
  fracture A52.77
  gallbladder (late) A52.74
  gastric (polyposis) (late) A52.74
  general A53.9
    paralysis A52.17
      juvenile A50.45
  genital (primary) A51.0
  glaucoma A52.71

Syphilis, syphilitic — *continued*
  gumma NEC A52.79
    cardiovascular system A52.00
    central nervous system A52.3
    congenital A50.59
  heart (block) (decompensation) (disease) (failure)
      A52.06 [I52]
    valve NEC A52.03
  hemianesthesia A52.19
  hemianopsia A52.71
  hemiparesis A52.17
  hemiplegia A52.17
  hepatic artery A52.09
  hepatis A52.74
  hepatomegaly, congenital A50.08
  hereditaria tarda — *see* Syphilis, congenital, late
  hereditary — *see* Syphilis, congenital
  Hutchinson's teeth A50.52
  hyalitis A52.71
  inactive — *see* Syphilis, latent
  infantum — *see* Syphilis, congenital
  inherited — *see* Syphilis, congenital
  internal ear A52.79
  intestine (late) A52.74
  iris, iritis (secondary) A51.43
    late A52.71
  joint (late) A52.77
  keratitis (congenital) (interstitial) (late) A50.31
  kidney (late) A52.75
  lacrimal passages (late) A52.71
  larynx (late) A52.73
  late A52.9
    cardiovascular A52.00
    central nervous system A52.3
    kidney A52.75
    latent or 2 years or more after infection (without
        manifestations) A52.8
      negative spinal fluid test A52.8
      serology positive A52.8
    paresis A52.17
    specified site NEC A52.79
    symptomatic or with manifestations A52.79
    tabes A52.11
  latent A53.0
    with signs or symptoms — *code by* site and stage
        under Syphilis
    early, or less than 2 years after infection A51.5
    central nervous system A52.2
    date of infection unspecified A53.0
    follow-up of latent syphilis A53.0
      date of infection unspecified A53.0
      late, or 2 years or more after infection A52.8
    late, or 2 years or more after infection A52.8
    positive serology (only finding) A53.0
      early, or less than 2 years after infection A51.5
      date of infection unspecified A53.0
      late, or 2 years or more after infection A52.8
  lens (late) A52.71
  leukoderma A51.39
    late A52.79
  lienitis A52.79
  lip A51.39
    chancre (primary) A51.2
    late A52.79
  Lissauer's paralysis A52.17
  liver A52.74
  locomotor ataxia A52.11
  lung A52.72
  lymph gland (early) (secondary) A51.49
    late A52.79
  lymphadenitis (secondary) A51.49
  macular atrophy of skin A51.39
    striated A52.79
  mediastinum (late) A52.73
  meninges (adhesive) (brain) (spinal cord) A52.13
  meningitis A52.13
    acute (secondary) A51.41
    congenital A50.41
  meningoencephalitis A52.14
  meningovascular A52.13
    congenital A50.41
  mesarteritis A52.09
    brain A52.04
  middle ear A52.77
  mitral stenosis A52.03
  monoplegia A52.17
  mouth (secondary) A51.39
    late A52.79

Syphilis, syphilitic — *continued*
  mucocutaneous (secondary) A51.39
    late A52.79
  mucous
    membrane (secondary) A51.39
      late A52.79
    patches A51.39
      congenital A50.07
  mulberry molars A50.52
  muscle A52.78
  myocardium A52.06
  nasal sinus (late) A52.73
  neonatorum — *see* Syphilis, congenital
  nephrotic syndrome (secondary) A51.44
  nerve palsy (any cranial nerve) A52.15
    multiple A52.15
  nervous system, central A52.3
  neuritis A52.15
    acoustic A52.15
  neurorecidive of retina A52.19
  neuroretinitis A52.19
  newborn — *see* Syphilis, congenital
  nodular superficial (late) A52.79
  nonvenereal A65
  nose (late) A52.73
    saddle back deformity A50.57
  occlusive arterial disease A52.09
  oculopathy A52.71
  ophthalmic (late) A52.71
  optic nerve (atrophy) (neuritis) (papilla) A52.15
  orbit (late) A52.71
  organic A53.9
  osseous (late) A52.77
  osteochondritis (congenital) (early) A50.02 [M90.80]
  osteoporosis A52.77
  ovary (late) A52.76
  oviduct (late) A52.76
  palate (late) A52.79
  pancreas (late) A52.74
  paralysis A52.17
    general A52.17
      juvenile A50.45
  paresis (general) A52.17
    juvenile A50.45
  paresthesia A52.19
  Parkinson's disease or syndrome A52.19
  paroxysmal tachycardia A52.06
  pemphigus (congenital) A50.06
  penis (chancre) A51.0
    late A52.76
  pericardium A52.06
  perichondritis, larynx (late) A52.73
  periosteum (late) A52.77
    congenital (early) A50.02 [M90.80]
    early (secondary) A51.46
  peripheral nerve A52.79
  petrous bone (late) A52.77
  pharynx (late) A52.73
    secondary A51.39
  pituitary (gland) A52.79
  pleura (late) A52.73
  pneumonia, white A50.04
  pontine lesion A52.17
  portal vein A52.09
  primary A51.0
    anal A51.1
    and secondary — *see* Syphilis, secondary
    central nervous system A52.3
    extragenital chancre NEC A51.2
    fingers A51.2
    genital A51.0
    lip A51.2
    specified site NEC A51.2
    tonsils A51.2
  prostate (late) A52.76
  ptosis (eyelid) A52.71
  pulmonary (late) A52.72
    artery A52.09
  pyelonephritis (late) A52.75
  recently acquired, symptomatic A51.9
  rectum (late) A52.74
  respiratory tract (late) A52.73
  retina, late A52.71
  retrobulbar neuritis A52.15
  salpingitis A52.76
  sclera (late) A52.71
  sclerosis
    cerebral A52.17

Syphilis, syphilitic — *continued*
  sclerosis — *continued*
    coronary A52.06
    multiple A52.11
  scotoma (central) A52.71
  scrotum (late) A52.76
  secondary (and primary) A51.49
    adenopathy A51.49
    anus A51.39
    bone A51.46
    chorioretinitis, choroiditis A51.43
    hepatitis A51.45
    liver A51.45
    lymphadenitis A51.49
    meningitis (acute) A51.41
    mouth A51.39
    mucous membranes A51.39
    periosteum, periostitis A51.46
    pharynx A51.39
    relapse (treated, untreated) A51.49
    skin A51.39
    specified form NEC A51.49
    tonsil A51.39
    ulcer A51.39
    viscera NEC A51.49
    vulva A51.39
  seminal vesicle (late) A52.76
  seronegative with signs or symptoms — *code by* site
        and stage under Syphilis
  seropositive
    with signs or symptoms — *code by* site and stage
        under Syphilis
    follow-up of latent syphilis — *see* Syphilis, latent
    only finding — *see* Syphilis, latent
  seventh nerve (paralysis) A52.15
  sinus, sinusitis (late) A52.73
  skeletal system A52.77
  skin (with ulceration) (early) (secondary) A51.39
    late or tertiary A52.79
  small intestine A52.74
  spastic spinal paralysis A52.17
  spermatic cord (late) A52.76
  spinal (cord) A52.12

Syphilis, syphilitic — *continued*
  spleen A52.79
  splenomegaly A52.79
  spondylitis A52.77
  staphyloma A52.71
  stigmata (congenital) A50.59
  stomach A52.74
  synovium A52.78
  tabes dorsalis (late) A52.11
    juvenile A50.45
  tabetic type A52.11
    juvenile A50.45
  taboparesis A52.17
    juvenile A50.45
  tachycardia A52.06
  tendon (late) A52.78
  tertiary A52.9
    with symptoms NEC A52.79
    cardiovascular A52.00
    central nervous system A52.3
    multiple NEC A52.79
    specified site NEC A52.79
  testis A52.76
  thorax A52.73
  throat A52.73
  thymus (gland) (late) A52.79
  thyroid (late) A52.79
  tongue (late) A52.79
  tonsil (lingual) (late) A52.73
    primary A51.2
    secondary A51.39
  trachea (late) A52.73
  tunica vaginalis (late) A52.76
  ulcer (any site) (early) (secondary) A51.39
    late A52.79
    perforating A52.79
      foot A52.11
  urethra (late) A52.76
  urogenital (late) A52.76
  uterus (late) A52.76
  uveal tract (secondary) A51.43
    late A52.71

Syphilis, syphilitic — *continued*
  uveitis (secondary) A51.43
    late A52.71
  uvula (late) (perforated) A52.79
  vagina A51.0
    late A52.76
  valvulitis NEC A52.03
  vascular A52.00
    brain (cerebral) A52.05
  ventriculi A52.74
  vesicae urinariae (late) A52.76
  viscera (abdominal) (late) A52.74
    secondary A51.49
  vitreous (opacities) (late) A52.71
    hemorrhage A52.71
  vulva A51.0
    late A52.76
    secondary A51.39
Syphiloma A52.79
  cardiovascular system A52.00
  central nervous system A52.3
  circulatory system A52.00
  congenital A50.59
Syphilophobia F45.29
Syringadenoma (*see also* Neoplasm, skin, benign)
  papillary — *see* Neoplasm, skin, benign
Syringobulbia G95.0
Syringocystadenoma — *see* Neoplasm, skin, benign
  papillary — *see* Neoplasm, skin, benign
Syringoma (*see also* Neoplasm, skin, benign)
  chondroid — *see* Neoplasm, skin, benign
Syringomyelia G95.0
Syringomyelitis — *see* Encephalitis
Syringomyelocele — *see* Spina bifida
Syringopontia G95.0
System, systemic (*see also* condition)
  disease, combined — *see* Degeneration, combined
  inflammatory response syndrome (SIRS) of non-infec-
        tious origin (without organ dysfunction) R65.10
    with acute organ dysfunction R65.11
  lupus erythematosus M32.9
    inhibitor present D68.62

T

Tabacism, tabacosis, tabagism (see also Poisoning, tobacco)
  meaning dependence (without remission) F17.200
    with
      disorder F17.299
        remission F17.211
        specified disorder NEC F17.298
        withdrawal F17.203
Tabardillo A75.9
  flea-borne A75.2
  louse-borne A75.0
Tabes, tabetic A52.10
  with
    central nervous system syphilis A52.10
    Charcot's joint A52.16
    cord bladder A52.19
    crisis, viscera (any) A52.19
    paralysis, general A52.17
    paresis (general) A52.17
    perforating ulcer (foot) A52.19
  arthropathy (Charcot) A52.16
  bladder A52.19
  bone A52.11
  cerebrospinal A52.12
  congenital A50.45
  conjugal A52.10
  dorsalis A52.11
    juvenile A50.49
  juvenile A50.49
  latent A52.19
  mesenterica A18.39
  paralysis, insane, general A52.17
  spasmodic A52.17
  syphilis (cerebrospinal) A52.12
Taboparalysis A52.17
Taboparesis (remission) A52.17
  juvenile A50.45
TAC (trigeminal autonomic cephalgia) **NEC** G44.099
  intractable G44.091
  not intractable G44.099
Tache noir S60.22- ☑
Tachyalimentation K91.2
Tachyarrhythmia, tachyrhythmia — see Tachycardia
Tachycardia R00.0
  atrial (paroxysmal) I47.1
  auricular I47.1
  AV nodal re-entry (re-entrant) I47.1
  junctional (paroxysmal) I47.1
  newborn P29.11
  nodal (paroxysmal) I47.1
  non-paroxysmal AV nodal I45.89
  paroxysmal (sustained) (nonsustained) I47.9
    with sinus bradycardia I49.5
    atrial (PAT) I47.1
    atrioventricular (AV) (re-entrant) I47.1
      psychogenic F54
    junctional I47.1
      ectopic I47.1
    nodal I47.1
    psychogenic (atrial) (supraventricular) (ventricular) F54
    supraventricular (sustained) I47.1
      psychogenic F54
    ventricular I47.2
      psychogenic F54
  psychogenic F45.8
  sick sinus I49.5
  sinoauricular NOS R00.0
    paroxysmal I47.1
  sinus [sinusal] NOS R00.0
    paroxysmal I47.1
  supraventricular I47.1
  ventricular (paroxysmal) (sustained) I47.2
    psychogenic F54
Tachygastria K31.89
Tachypnea R06.82
  hysterical F45.8
  newborn (idiopathic) (transitory) P22.1
  psychogenic F45.8
  transitory, of newborn P22.1

TACO (transfusion associated circulatory overload) E87.71
Taenia (infection) (infestation) B68.9
  diminuta B71.0
  echinococcal infestation B67.90
  mediocanellata B68.1
  nana B71.0
  saginata B68.1
  solium (intestinal form) B68.0
    larval form — see Cysticercosis
Taeniasis (intestine) — see Taenia
Tag (hypertrophied skin) (infected) L91.8
  adenoid J35.8
  anus K64.4
  hemorrhoidal K64.4
  hymen N89.8
  perineal N90.89
  preauricular Q17.0
  sentinel K64.4
  skin L91.8
    accessory (congenital) Q82.8
    anus K64.4
    congenital Q82.8
    preauricular Q17.0
  tonsil J35.8
  urethra, urethral N36.8
  vulva N90.89
Tahyna fever B33.8
Takahara's disease E80.3
Takayasu's disease or syndrome M31.4
Talcosis (pulmonary) J62.0
Talipes (congenital) Q66.89
  acquired, planus — see Deformity, limb, flat foot
  asymmetric Q66.89
  calcaneovalgus Q66.4
  calcaneovarus Q66.1
  calcaneus Q66.89
  cavus Q66.7
  equinovalgus Q66.6
  equinovarus Q66.0
  equinus Q66.89
  percavus Q66.7
  planovalgus Q66.6
  planus (acquired) (any degree) (see also Deformity, limb, flat foot)
    congenital Q66.5- ☑
    due to rickets (sequelae) E64.3
  valgus Q66.6
  varus Q66.3
Tall stature, constitutional E34.4
Talma's disease M62.89
Talon noir S90.3- ☑
  hand S60.22- ☑
  heel S90.3- ☑
  toe S90.1- ☑
Tamponade, heart I31.4
Tanapox (virus disease) B08.71
Tangier disease E78.6
Tantrum, child problem F91.8
Tapeworm (infection) (infestation) — see Infestation, tapeworm
Tapia's syndrome G52.7
TAR (thrombocytopenia with absent radius) **syndrome** Q87.2
Tarral-Besnier disease L44.0
Tarsal tunnel syndrome — see Syndrome, tarsal tunnel
Tarsalgia — see Pain, limb, lower
Tarsitis (eyelid) H01.8
  syphilitic A52.71
  tuberculous A18.4
Tartar (teeth) (dental calculus) K03.6
Tattoo (mark) L81.8
Tauri's disease E74.09
Taurodontism K00.2
Taussig-Bing syndrome Q20.1
Taybi's syndrome Q87.2
Tay-Sachs amaurotic familial idiocy or disease E75.02
TBI (traumatic brain injury) — see category S06 ☑
Teacher's node or nodule J38.2
Tear, torn (traumatic) (see also Laceration)
  with abortion — see Abortion
  annular fibrosis M51.35
  anus, anal (sphincter) S31.831 ☑

Tear, torn — continued
  anus, anal — continued
    complicating delivery
      with third degree perineal laceration O70.2
        with mucosa O70.3
      without third degree perineal laceration O70.4
    nontraumatic (healed) (old) K62.81
  articular cartilage, old — see Derangement, joint, articular cartilage, by site
  bladder
    with ectopic or molar pregnancy O08.6
    following ectopic or molar pregnancy O08.6
    obstetrical O71.5
    traumatic — see Injury, bladder
  bowel
    with ectopic or molar pregnancy O08.6
    following ectopic or molar pregnancy O08.6
    obstetrical trauma O71.5
  broad ligament
    with ectopic or molar pregnancy O08.6
    following ectopic or molar pregnancy O08.6
    obstetrical trauma O71.6
  bucket handle (knee) (meniscus) — see Tear, meniscus
  capsule, joint — see Sprain
  cartilage (see also Sprain)
    articular, old — see Derangement, joint, articular cartilage, by site
  cervix
    with ectopic or molar pregnancy O08.6
    following ectopic or molar pregnancy O08.6
    obstetrical trauma (current) O71.3
    old N88.1
    traumatic — see Injury, uterus
  dural G97.41
    nontraumatic G96.11
  internal organ — see Injury, by site
  knee cartilage
    articular (current) S83.3- ☑
    old — see Derangement, knee, meniscus, due to old tear
  ligament — see Sprain
  meniscus (knee) (current injury) S83.209 ☑
    bucket-handle S83.20- ☑
    lateral
      bucket-handle S83.25- ☑
      complex S83.27- ☑
      peripheral S83.26- ☑
      specified type NEC S83.28- ☑
    medial
      bucket-handle S83.21- ☑
      complex S83.23- ☑
      peripheral S83.22- ☑
      specified type NEC S83.24- ☑
    old — see Derangement, knee, meniscus, due to old tear
    site other than knee — code as Sprain
    specified type NEC S83.20- ☑
  muscle — see Strain
  pelvic
    floor, complicating delivery O70.1
    organ NEC, obstetrical trauma O71.5
      with ectopic or molar pregnancy O08.6
      following ectopic or molar pregnancy O08.6
  perineal, secondary O90.1
  periurethral tissue, obstetrical trauma O71.82
    with ectopic or molar pregnancy O08.6
    following ectopic or molar pregnancy O08.6
  rectovaginal septum — see Laceration, vagina
  retina, retinal (without detachment) (horseshoe) (see also Break, retina, horseshoe)
    with detachment — see Detachment, retina, with retinal, break
  rotator cuff (nontraumatic) M75.10- ☑
    complete M75.12- ☑
    incomplete M75.11- ☑
    traumatic S46.01- ☑
      capsule S43.42- ☑
  semilunar cartilage, knee — see Tear, meniscus
  supraspinatus (complete) (incomplete) (nontraumatic) (see also Tear, rotator cuff) M75.10- ☑
  tendon — see Strain
  tentorial, at birth P10.4

Tear, torn — *continued*
  umbilical cord
    complicating delivery O69.89 ☑
  urethra
    with ectopic or molar pregnancy O08.6
    following ectopic or molar pregnancy O08.6
    obstetrical trauma O71.5
  uterus — *see* Injury, uterus
  vagina — *see* Laceration, vagina
  vessel, from catheter — *see* Puncture, accidental complicating surgery
  vulva, complicating delivery O70.0
Tear-stone — *see* Dacryolith
Teeth (*see also* condition)
  grinding
    psychogenic F45.8
    sleep related G47.63
Teething (syndrome) K00.7
Telangiectasia, telangiectasis (verrucous) I78.1
  ataxic (cerebellar) (Louis-Bar) G11.3
  familial I78.0
  hemorrhagic, hereditary (congenital) (senile) I78.0
  hereditary, hemorrhagic (congenital) (senile) I78.0
  juxtafoveal H35.07- ☑
  macular H35.07- ☑
  parafoveal H35.07- ☑
  retinal (idiopathic) (juxtafoveal) (macular) (parafoveal) H35.07- ☑
  spider I78.1
Telephone scatologia F65.89
Telescoped bowel or intestine K56.1
  congenital Q43.8
Temperature
  body, high (of unknown origin) R50.9
  cold, trauma from T69.9 ☑
    newborn P80.0
    specified effect NEC T69.8 ☑
Temple — *see* condition
Temporal — *see* condition
Temporomandibular joint pain-dysfunction syndrome M26.62
Temporosphenoidal — *see* condition
Tendency
  bleeding — *see* Defect, coagulation
  suicide
    meaning personal history of attempted suicide Z91.5
    meaning suicidal ideation — *see* Ideation, suicidal
  to fall R29.6
Tenderness, abdominal R10.819
  epigastric R10.816
  generalized R10.817
  left lower quadrant R10.814
  left upper quadrant R10.812
  periumbilic R10.815
  rebound R10.829
    epigastric R10.826
    generalized R10.827
    left lower quadrant R10.824
    left upper quadrant R10.822
    periumbilic R10.825
    right lower quadrant R10.823
    right upper quadrant R10.821
  right lower quadrant R10.813
  right upper quadrant R10.811
Tendinitis, tendonitis (*see also* Enthesopathy)
  Achilles M76.6- ☑
  adhesive — *see* Tenosynovitis, specified type NEC
    shoulder — *see* Capsulitis, adhesive
  bicipital M75.2- ☑
  calcific M65.2- ☑
    ankle M65.27- ☑
    foot M65.27- ☑
    forearm M65.23- ☑
    hand M65.24- ☑
    lower leg M65.26- ☑
    multiple sites M65.29
    pelvic region M65.25- ☑
    shoulder M75.3- ☑
    specified site NEC M65.28
    thigh M65.25- ☑
    upper arm M65.22- ☑
  due to use, overuse, pressure (*see also* Disorder, soft tissue, due to use)
    specified NEC — *see* Disorder, soft tissue, due to use, specified NEC
  gluteal M76.0- ☑

Tendinitis, tendonitis — *continued*
  patellar M76.5- ☑
  peroneal M76.7- ☑
  psoas M76.1- ☑
  tibial (posterior) M76.82- ☑
    anterior M76.81- ☑
  trochanteric — *see* Bursitis, hip, trochanteric
Tendon — *see* condition
Tendosynovitis — *see* Tenosynovitis
Tenesmus (rectal) R19.8
  vesical R30.1
Tennis elbow — *see* Epicondylitis, lateral
Tenonitis (*see also* Tenosynovitis)
  eye (capsule) H05.04- ☑
Tenontosynovitis — *see* Tenosynovitis
Tenontothecitis — *see* Tenosynovitis
Tenophyte — *see* Disorder, synovium, specified type NEC
Tenosynovitis (*see also* Synovitis) M65.9
  adhesive — *see* Tenosynovitis, specified type NEC
    shoulder — *see* Capsulitis, adhesive
  bicipital (calcifying) — *see* Tendinitis, bicipital
  gonococcal A54.49
  in (due to)
    crystals M65.8- ☑
    gonorrhea A54.49
    syphilis (late) A52.78
    use, overuse, pressure (*see also* Disorder, soft tissue, due to use)
      specified NEC — *see* Disorder, soft tissue, due to use, specified NEC
  infective NEC M65.1- ☑
    ankle M65.17- ☑
    foot M65.17- ☑
    forearm M65.13- ☑
    hand M65.14- ☑
    lower leg M65.16- ☑
    multiple sites M65.19
    pelvic region M65.15- ☑
    shoulder region M65.11- ☑
    specified site NEC M65.18
    thigh M65.15- ☑
    upper arm M65.12- ☑
  radial styloid M65.4
  shoulder region M65.81- ☑
    adhesive — *see* Capsulitis, adhesive
  specified type NEC M65.88
    ankle M65.87- ☑
    foot M65.87- ☑
    forearm M65.83- ☑
    hand M65.84- ☑
    lower leg M65.86- ☑
    multiple sites M65.89
    pelvic region M65.85- ☑
    shoulder region M65.81- ☑
    specified site NEC M65.88
    thigh M65.85- ☑
    upper arm M65.82- ☑
  tuberculous — *see* Tuberculosis, tenosynovitis
Tenovaginitis — *see* Tenosynovitis
Tension
  arterial, high (*see also* Hypertension)
    without diagnosis of hypertension R03.0
  headache G44.209
    intractable G44.201
    not intractable G44.209
  nervous R45.0
  pneumothorax J93.0
  premenstrual N94.3
  state (mental) F48.9
Tentorium — *see* condition
Teratencephalus Q89.8
Teratism Q89.7
Teratoblastoma (malignant) — *see* Neoplasm, malignant, by site
Teratocarcinoma (*see also* Neoplasm, malignant, by site)
  liver C22.7
Teratoma (solid) (*see also* Neoplasm, uncertain behavior, by site)
  with embryonal carcinoma, mixed — *see* Neoplasm, malignant, by site
  with malignant transformation — *see* Neoplasm, malignant, by site
  adult (cystic) — *see* Neoplasm, benign, by site
  benign — *see* Neoplasm, benign, by site

Teratoma — *continued*
  combined with choriocarcinoma — *see* Neoplasm, malignant, by site
  cystic (adult) — *see* Neoplasm, benign, by site
  differentiated — *see* Neoplasm, benign, by site
  embryonal (*see also* Neoplasm, malignant, by site)
    liver C22.7
  immature — *see* Neoplasm, malignant, by site
  liver C22.7
    adult, benign, cystic, differentiated type or mature D13.4
  malignant (*see also* Neoplasm, malignant, by site)
    anaplastic — *see* Neoplasm, malignant, by site
    intermediate — *see* Neoplasm, malignant, by site
      specified site — *see* Neoplasm, malignant, by site
      unspecified site C62.90
    undifferentiated — *see* Neoplasm, malignant, by site
  mature — *see* Neoplasm, uncertain behavior, by site
    malignant — *see* Neoplasm, by site, malignant, by site
  ovary D27.- ☑
    embryonal, immature or malignant C56- ☑
  solid — *see* Neoplasm, uncertain behavior, by site
  testis C62.9- ☑
    adult, benign, cystic, differentiated type or mature D29.2- ☑
    scrotal C62.1- ☑
    undescended C62.0- ☑
Termination
  anomalous (*see also* Malposition, congenital)
    right pulmonary vein Q26.3
  pregnancy, elective Z33.2
Ternidens diminutus infestation B81.8
Ternidensiasis B81.8
Terror(s) night (child) F51.4
Terrorism, victim of Z65.4
Terry's syndrome H44.2- ☑
Tertiary — *see* condition
Test, tests, testing (for)
  adequacy (for dialysis)
    hemodialysis Z49.31
    peritoneal Z49.32
  blood pressure Z01.30
    abnormal reading — *see* Blood, pressure
  blood typing Z01.83
    Rh typing Z01.83
  blood-alcohol Z04.8
    positive — *see* Findings, abnormal, in blood
  blood-drug Z04.8
    positive — *see* Findings, abnormal, in blood
  cardiac pulse generator (battery) Z45.010
  fertility Z31.41
  genetic
    disease carrier status for procreative management
      female Z31.430
      male Z31.440
    male partner of patient with recurrent pregnancy loss Z31.441
    procreative management NEC
      female Z31.438
      male Z31.448
  hearing Z01.10
    with abnormal findings NEC Z01.118
  HIV (human immunodeficiency virus)
    nonconclusive (in infants) R75
    positive Z21
    seropositive Z21
  immunity status Z01.84
  intelligence NEC Z01.89
  laboratory (as part of a general medical examination) Z00.00
    with abnormal finding Z00.01
    for medicolegal reason NEC Z04.8
  male partner of patient with recurrent pregnancy loss Z31.441
  Mantoux (for tuberculosis) Z11.1
    abnormal result R76.11
  pregnancy, positive first pregnancy — *see* Pregnancy, normal, first
  procreative Z31.49
    fertility Z31.41
  skin, diagnostic
    allergy Z01.82
      special screening examination — *see* Screening, by name of disease

Test, tests, testing — *continued*
  skin, diagnostic — *continued*
    Mantoux Z11.1
    tuberculin Z11.1
  specified NEC Z01.89
  tuberculin Z11.1
    abnormal result R76.11
  vision Z01.00
    with abnormal findings Z01.01
  Wassermann Z11.3
    positive — *see* Serology for syphilis, positive
Testicle, testicular, testis (*see also* condition)
  feminization syndrome (*see also* Syndrome, androgen
      insensitivity) E34.51
  migrans Q55.29
Tetanus, tetanic (cephalic) (convulsions) A35
  with
    abortion A34
    ectopic or molar pregnancy O08.0
  following ectopic or molar pregnancy O08.0
  inoculation reaction (due to serum) — *see* Complica-
      tions, vaccination
  neonatorum A33
  obstetrical A34
  puerperal, postpartum, childbirth A34
Tetany (due to) R29.0
  alkalosis E87.3
  associated with rickets E55.0
  convulsions R29.0
    hysterical F44.5
  functional (hysterical) F44.5
  hyperkinetic R29.0
    hysterical F44.5
  hyperpnea R06.4
    hysterical F44.5
    psychogenic F45.8
  hyperventilation (*see also* Hyperventilation) R06.4
    hysterical F44.5
  neonatal (without calcium or magnesium deficiency)
      P71.3
  parathyroid (gland) E20.9
  parathyroprival E89.2
  post- (para)thyroidectomy E89.2
  postoperative E89.2
  pseudotetany R29.0
  psychogenic (conversion reaction) F44.5
Tetralogy of Fallot Q21.3
Tetraplegia (chronic) (*see also* Quadriplegia) G82.50
Thailand hemorrhagic fever A91
Thalassanemia — *see* Thalassemia
Thalassemia (anemia) (disease) D56.9
  with other hemoglobinopathy D56.8
  alpha (major) (severe) (triple gene defect) D56.0
    minor D56.3
    silent carrier D56.3
    trait D56.3
  beta (severe) D56.1
    homozygous D56.1
    major D56.1
    minor D56.3
    trait D56.3
  delta-beta (homozygous) D56.2
    minor D56.3
    trait D56.3
  dominant D56.8
  hemoglobin
    C D56.8
    E-beta D56.5
  intermedia D56.1
  major D56.1
  minor D56.3
  mixed D56.8
  sickle-cell — *see* Disease, sickle-cell, thalassemia
  specified type NEC D56.8
  trait D56.3
  variants D56.8
Thanatophoric dwarfism or short stature Q77.1
Thaysen-Gee disease (nontropical sprue) K90.0
Thaysen's disease K90.0
Thecoma D27- ☑
  luteinized D27- ☑
  malignant C56- ☑
Thelarche, premature E30.8
Thelaziasis B83.8
Thelitis N61
  puerperal, postpartum or gestational — *see* Infection,
      nipple
Therapeutic — *see* condition

Therapy
  drug, long-term (current) (prophylactic)
    agents affecting estrogen receptors and estrogen
        levels NEC Z79.818
    anastrozole (Arimidex) Z79.811
    antibiotics Z79.2
      short-term use — *omit code*
    anticoagulants Z79.01
    anti-inflammatory Z79.1
    antiplatelet Z79.02
    antithrombotics Z79.02
    aromatase inhibitors Z79.811
    aspirin Z79.82
    birth control pill or patch Z79.3
    bisphosphonates Z79.83
    contraceptive, oral Z79.3
    drug, specified NEC Z79.899
    estrogen receptor downregulators Z79.818
    Evista Z79.810
    exemestane (Aromasin) Z79.811
    Fareston Z79.810
    fulvestrant (Faslodex) Z79.818
    gonadotropin-releasing hormone (GnRH) agonist
        Z79.818
    goserelin acetate (Zoladex) Z79.818
    hormone replacement (postmenopausal) Z79.890
    insulin Z79.4
    letrozole (Femara) Z79.811
    leuprolide acetate (leuprorelin) (Lupron) Z79.818
    megestrol acetate (Megace) Z79.818
    methadone
      for pain management Z79.891
      maintenance therapy F11.20
    Nolvadex Z79.810
    opiate analgesic Z79.891
    oral contraceptive Z79.3
    raloxifene (Evista) Z79.810
    selective estrogen receptor modulators (SERMs)
        Z79.810
    short term — *omit code*
    steroids
      inhaled Z79.51
      systemic Z79.52
    tamoxifen (Nolvadex) Z79.810
    toremifene (Fareston) Z79.810
Thermic — *see* condition
Thermography (abnormal) (*see also* Abnormal, diagnos-
    tic imaging) R93.8
  breast R92.8
Thermoplegia T67.0 ☑
Thesaurismosis, glycogen — *see* Disease, glycogen
    storage
Thiamin deficiency E51.9
  specified NEC E51.8
Thiaminic deficiency with beriberi E51.11
Thibierge-Weissenbach syndrome — *see* Sclerosis,
    systemic
Thickening
  bone — *see* Hypertrophy, bone
  breast N64.59
  endometrium R93.8
  epidermal L85.9
    specified NEC L85.8
  hymen N89.6
  larynx J38.7
  nail L60.2
    congenital Q84.5
  periosteal — *see* Hypertrophy, bone
  pleura J92.9
    with asbestos J92.0
  skin R23.4
  subepiglottic J38.7
  tongue K14.8
  valve, heart — *see* Endocarditis
Thigh — *see* condition
Thinning vertebra — *see* Spondylopathy, specified NEC
Thirst, excessive R63.1
  due to deprivation of water T73.1 ☑
Thomsen disease G71.12
Thoracic (*see also* condition)
  kidney Q63.2
  outlet syndrome G54.0
Thoracogastroschisis (congenital) Q79.8
Thoracopagus Q89.4
Thorax — *see* condition
Thorn's syndrome N28.89
Thorson-Björck syndrome E34.0
Threadworm (infection) (infestation) B80

Threatened
  abortion O20.0
    with subsequent abortion O03.9
  job loss, anxiety concerning Z56.2
  labor (without delivery) O47.9
    after 37 completed weeks of gestation O47.1
    before 37 completed weeks of gestation O47.0- ☑
  loss of job, anxiety concerning Z56.2
  miscarriage O20.0
  unemployment, anxiety concerning Z56.2
Three-day fever A93.1
Threshers' lung J67.0
Thrix annulata (congenital) Q84.1
Throat — *see* condition
Thrombasthenia (Glanzmann) (hemorrhagic) (heredi-
    tary) D69.1
Thromboangiitis I73.1
  obliterans (general) I73.1
    cerebral I67.89
    vessels
      brain I67.89
      spinal cord I67.89
Thromboarteritis — *see* Arteritis
Thromboasthenia (Glanzmann) (hemorrhagic) (heredi-
    tary) D69.1
Thrombocytasthenia (Glanzmann) D69.1
Thrombocythemia (essential) (hemorrhagic) (idiopathic)
    (primary) D47.3
Thrombocytopathy (dystrophic) (granulopenic) D69.1
Thrombocytopenia, thrombocytopenic D69.6
  with absent radius (TAR) Q87.2
  congenital D69.42
  dilutional D69.59
  due to
    (massive) blood transfusion D69.59
    drugs D69.59
    extracorporeal circulation of blood D69.59
    platelet alloimmunization D69.59
  essential D69.3
  heparin induced (HIT) D75.82
  hereditary D69.42
  idiopathic D69.3
  neonatal, transitory P61.0
    due to
      exchange transfusion P61.0
      idiopathic maternal thrombocytopenia P61.0
      isoimmunization P61.0
  primary NEC D69.49
    idiopathic D69.3
  puerperal, postpartum O72.3
  secondary D69.59
  transient neonatal P61.0
Thrombocytosis, essential D47.3
  primary D47.3
Thromboembolism — *see* Embolism
Thrombopathy (Bernard-Soulier) D69.1
  constitutional D68.0
  Willebrand-Jurgens D68.0
Thrombopenia — *see* Thrombocytopenia
Thrombophilia D68.59
  primary NEC D68.59
  secondary NEC D68.69
  specified NEC D68.69
Thrombophlebitis I80.9
  antepartum O22.2- ☑
    deep O22.3- ☑
    superficial O22.2- ☑
  cavernous (venous) sinus G08
    complicating pregnancy O22.5- ☑
    nonpyogenic I67.6
  cerebral (sinus) (vein) G08
    nonpyogenic I67.6
    sequelae G09
  due to implanted device — *see* Complications, by site
      and type, specified NEC
  during or resulting from a procedure NEC T81.72 ☑
  femoral vein (superficial) I80.1- ☑
  femoropopliteal vein I80.0- ☑
  hepatic (vein) I80.8
  idiopathic, recurrent I82.1
  iliofemoral I80.1- ☑
  intracranial venous sinus (any) G08
    nonpyogenic I67.6
    sequelae G09
  intraspinal venous sinuses and veins G08
    nonpyogenic G95.19
  lateral (venous) sinus G08
    nonpyogenic I67.6

Thrombophlebitis — *continued*
leg I80.299
superficial I80.0- ☑
longitudinal (venous) sinus G08
nonpyogenic I67.6
lower extremity I80.299
migrans, migrating I82.1
pelvic
with ectopic or molar pregnancy O08.0
following ectopic or molar pregnancy O08.0
puerperal O87.1
popliteal vein — *see* Phlebitis, leg, deep, popliteal
portal (vein) K75.1
postoperative T81.72 ☑
pregnancy — *see* Thrombophlebitis, antepartum
puerperal, postpartum, childbirth O87.0
deep O87.1
pelvic O87.1
septic O86.81
superficial O87.0
saphenous (greater) (lesser) I80.0- ☑
sinus (intracranial) G08
nonpyogenic I67.6
specified site NEC I80.8
tibial vein I80.23- ☑

Thrombosis, thrombotic (bland) (multiple) (progressive)
(silent) (vessel) I82.90
anal K64.5
antepartum — *see* Thrombophlebitis, antepartum
aorta, aortic I74.10
abdominal I74.09
saddle I74.01
bifurcation I74.09
saddle I74.01
specified site NEC I74.19
terminal I74.09
thoracic I74.11
valve — *see* Endocarditis, aortic
apoplexy I63.3 ☑
artery, arteries (postinfectional) I74.9
auditory, internal — *see* Occlusion, artery, precerebral, specified NEC
basilar — *see* Occlusion, artery, basilar
carotid (common) (internal) — *see* Occlusion, artery, carotid
cerebellar (anterior inferior) (posterior inferior) (superior) — *see* Occlusion, artery, cerebellar
cerebral — *see* Occlusion, artery, cerebral
choroidal (anterior) — *see* Occlusion, artery, cerebral, specified NEC
communicating, posterior — *see* Occlusion, artery, cerebral, specified NEC
coronary (see also Infarct, myocardium)
not resulting in infarction I24.0
hepatic I74.8
hypophyseal — *see* Occlusion, artery, cerebral, specified NEC
iliac I74.5
limb I74.4
lower I74.3
upper I74.2
meningeal, anterior or posterior — *see* Occlusion, artery, cerebral, specified NEC
mesenteric (with gangrene) K55.0
ophthalmic — *see* Occlusion, artery, retina
pontine — *see* Occlusion, artery, cerebral, specified NEC
precerebral — *see* Occlusion, artery, precerebral
pulmonary (iatrogenic) — *see* Embolism, pulmonary
renal N28.0
retinal — *see* Occlusion, artery, retina
spinal, anterior or posterior G95.11
traumatic NEC T14.8
vertebral — *see* Occlusion, artery, vertebral
atrium, auricular (see also Infarct, myocardium)
following acute myocardial infarction (current complication) I23.6
not resulting in infarction I24.0
basilar (artery) — *see* Occlusion, artery, basilar
brain (artery) (stem) (see also Occlusion, artery, cerebral)
due to syphilis A52.05
puerperal O99.43
sinus — *see* Thrombosis, intracranial venous sinus
capillary I78.8

Thrombosis, thrombotic — *continued*
cardiac (see also Infarct, myocardium)
not resulting in infarction I24.0
valve — *see* Endocarditis
carotid (artery) (common) (internal) — *see* Occlusion, artery, carotid
cavernous (venous) sinus — *see* Thrombosis, intracranial venous sinus
cerebellar artery (anterior inferior) (posterior inferior) (superior) I66.3
cerebral (artery) — *see* Occlusion, artery, cerebral
cerebrovenous sinus (see also Thrombosis, intracranial venous sinus)
puerperium O87.3
chronic I82.91
coronary (artery) (vein) (see also Infarct, myocardium)
not resulting in infarction I24.0
corpus cavernosum N48.89
cortical I66.9
deep — *see* Embolism, vein, lower extremity
due to device, implant or graft (see also Complications, by site and type, specified NEC) T85.86 ☑
arterial graft NEC T82.868 ☑
breast (implant) T85.86 ☑
catheter NEC T85.86 ☑
dialysis (renal) T82.868 ☑
intraperitoneal T85.86 ☑
infusion NEC T82.868 ☑
spinal (epidural) (subdural) T85.86 ☑
urinary (indwelling) T83.86 ☑
electronic (electrode) (pulse generator) (stimulator)
bone T84.86 ☑
cardiac T82.867 ☑
nervous system (brain) (peripheral nerve) (spinal) T85.86 ☑
urinary T83.86 ☑
fixation, internal (orthopedic) NEC T84.86 ☑
gastrointestinal (bile duct) (esophagus) T85.86 ☑
genital NEC T83.86 ☑
heart T82.867 ☑
joint prosthesis T84.86 ☑
ocular (corneal graft) (orbital implant) NEC T85.86 ☑
orthopedic NEC T84.86 ☑
specified NEC T85.86 ☑
urinary NEC T83.86 ☑
vascular NEC T82.868 ☑
ventricular intracranial shunt T85.86 ☑
during the puerperium — *see* Thrombosis, puerperal
endocardial (see also Infarct, myocardium)
not resulting in infarction I24.0
eye — *see* Occlusion, retina
genital organ
female NEC N94.89
pregnancy — *see* Thrombophlebitis, antepartum
male N50.1
gestational — *see* Phlebopathy, gestational
heart (chamber) (see also Infarct, myocardium)
not resulting in infarction I24.0
hepatic (vein) I82.0
artery I74.8
history (of) Z86.718
intestine (with gangrene) K55.0
intracardiac NEC (apical) (atrial) (auricular) (ventricular) (old) I51.3
intracranial (arterial) I66.9
venous sinus (any) G08
nonpyogenic origin I67.6
puerperium O87.3
intramural (see also Infarct, myocardium)
not resulting in infarction I24.0
intraspinal venous sinuses and veins G08
nonpyogenic G95.19
kidney (artery) N28.0
lateral (venous) sinus — *see* Thrombosis, intracranial venous sinus
leg — *see* Thrombosis, vein, lower extremity
arterial I74.3
liver (venous) I82.0
artery I74.8
portal vein I81
longitudinal (venous) sinus — *see* Thrombosis, intracranial venous sinus
lower limb — *see* Thrombosis, vein, lower extremity
lung (iatrogenic) (postoperative) — *see* Embolism, pulmonary

Thrombosis, thrombotic — *continued*
meninges (brain) (arterial) I66.8
mesenteric (artery) (with gangrene) K55.0
vein (inferior) (superior) I81
mitral I34.8
mural (see also Infarct, myocardium)
due to syphilis A52.06
not resulting in infarction I24.0
omentum (with gangrene) K55.0
ophthalmic — *see* Occlusion, retina
pampiniform plexus (male) N50.1
parietal (see also Infarct, myocardium)
not resulting in infarction I24.0
penis, superficial vein N48.81
perianal venous K64.5
peripheral arteries I74.4
upper I74.2
personal history (of) Z86.718
portal I81
due to syphilis A52.09
precerebral artery — *see* Occlusion, artery, precerebral
puerperal, postpartum O87.0
brain (artery) O99.43
venous (sinus) O87.3
cardiac O99.43
cerebral (artery) O99.43
venous (sinus) O87.3
superficial O87.0
pulmonary (artery) (iatrogenic) (postoperative) (vein) — *see* Embolism, pulmonary
renal (artery) N28.0
vein I82.3
resulting from presence of device, implant or graft — *see* Complications, by site and type, specified NEC
retina, retinal — *see* Occlusion, retina
scrotum N50.1
seminal vesicle N50.1
sigmoid (venous) sinus — *see* Thrombosis, intracranial venous sinus
sinus, intracranial (any) — *see* Thrombosis, intracranial venous sinus
specified site NEC I82.890
chronic I82.891
spermatic cord N50.1
spinal cord (arterial) G95.11
due to syphilis A52.09
pyogenic origin G06.1
spleen, splenic D73.5
artery I74.8
testis N50.1
traumatic NEC T14.8
tricuspid I07.8
tumor — *see* Neoplasm, unspecified behavior, by site
tunica vaginalis N50.1
umbilical cord (vessels), complicating delivery O69.5 ☑
vas deferens N50.1
vein (acute) I82.90
antecubital I82.61- ☑
chronic I82.71- ☑
axillary I82.A1- ☑ (following I82.7)
chronic I82.A2- ☑ (following I82.7)
basilic I82.61- ☑
chronic I82.71- ☑
brachial I82.62- ☑
chronic I82.72- ☑
brachiocephalic (innominate) I82.290
chronic I82.291
cephalic I82.61- ☑
chronic I82.71- ☑
cerebral, nonpyogenic I67.6
chronic I82.91
deep (DVT) I82.40- ☑
calf I82.4Z- ☑
chronic I82.5Z- ☑
lower leg I82.4Z- ☑
chronic I82.5Z- ☑
thigh I82.4Y- ☑
chronic I82.5Y- ☑
upper leg I82.4Y ☑
chronic I82.5y--
femoral I82.41- ☑
chronic I82.51- ☑
iliac (iliofemoral) I82.42- ☑
chronic I82.52- ☑
innominate I82.290
chronic I82.291

Thrombosis, thrombotic *continued*
  vein — *continued*
    internal jugular I82.C1- ☑ (*following* I82.7)
      chronic I82.C2- ☑ (*following* I82.7)
    lower extremity
      deep I82.40- ☑
        chronic I82.50- ☑
        specified NEC I82.49- ☑
          chronic NEC I82.59- ☑
      distal
        deep I82.4Z- ☑
      proximal
        deep I82.4Y- ☑
          chronic I82.5Y- ☑
      superficial I82.81- ☑
    perianal K64.5
    popliteal I82.43- ☑
      chronic I82.53- ☑
    radial I02.62- ☑
      chronic I82.72- ☑
    renal I82.3
    saphenous (greater) (lesser) I82.81- ☑
    specified NEC I82.890
      chronic NEC I82.891
    subclavian I82.B1- ☑ (*following* I82.7)
      chronic I82.B2- ☑ (*following* I82.7)
    thoracic NEC I82.290
      chronic I82.291
    tibial I82.44- ☑
      chronic I82.54- ☑
    ulnar I82.62- ☑
      chronic I82.72- ☑
    upper extremity I82.60- ☑
      chronic I82.70- ☑
      deep I82.62- ☑
        chronic I82.72- ☑
      superficial I82.61- ☑
        chronic I82.71- ☑
  vena cava
    inferior I82.220
      chronic I82.221
    superior I82.210
      chronic I82.211
  venous, perianal K64.5
  ventricle (*see also* Infarct, myocardium)
    following acute myocardial infarction (current complication) I23.6
    not resulting in infarction I24.0
Thrombus — *see* Thrombosis
Thrush (*see also* Candidiasis)
  newborn P37.5
  oral B37.0
  vaginal B37.3
Thumb (*see also* condition)
  sucking (child problem) F98.8
Thymitis E32.8
Thymoma (benign) D15.0
  malignant C37
Thymus, thymic (gland) — *see* condition
Thyrocele — *see* Goiter
Thyroglossal (*see also* condition)
  cyst Q89.2
  duct, persistent Q89.2
Thyroid (gland) (body) (*see also* condition)
  hormone resistance E07.89
  lingual Q89.2
  nodule (cystic) (nontoxic) (single) E04.1
Thyroiditis E06.9
  acute (nonsuppurative) (pyogenic) (suppurative) E06.0
  autoimmune E06.3
  chronic (nonspecific) (sclerosing) E06.5
    with thyrotoxicosis, transient E06.2
    fibrous E06.5
    lymphadenoid E06.3
    lymphocytic E06.3
    lymphoid E06.3
  de Quervain's E06.1
  drug-induced E06.4
  fibrous (chronic) E06.5
  giant-cell (follicular) E06.1
  granulomatous (de Quervain) (subacute) E06.1
  Hashimoto's (struma lymphomatosa) E06.3
  iatrogenic E06.4
  ligneous E06.5
  lymphocytic (chronic) E06.3
  lymphoid E06.3
  lymphomatous E06.3

Thyroiditis — *continued*
  nonsuppurative E06.1
  postpartum, puerperal O90.5
  pseudotuberculous E06.1
  pyogenic E06.0
  radiation E06.4
  Riedel's E06.5
  subacute (granulomatous) E06.1
  suppurative E06.0
  tuberculous A18.81
  viral E06.1
  woody E06.5
Thyrolingual duct, persistent Q89.2
Thyromegaly E01.0
Thyrotoxic
  crisis — *see* Thyrotoxicosis
  heart disease or failure (*see also* Thyrotoxicosis) E05.90 [I43]
    with thyroid storm E05.91 [I43]
  storm — *see* Thyrotoxicosis
Thyrotoxicosis (recurrent) E05.90
  with
    goiter (diffuse) E05.00
      with thyroid storm E05.01
      adenomatous uninodular E05.10
        with thyroid storm E05.11
      multinodular E05.20
        with thyroid storm E05.21
      nodular E05.20
        with thyroid storm E05.21
      uninodular E05.10
        with thyroid storm E05.11
    infiltrative
      dermopathy E05.00
        with thyroid storm E05.01
      ophthalmopathy E05.00
        with thyroid storm E05.01
    single thyroid nodule E05.10
      with thyroid storm E05.11
    thyroid storm E05.91
  due to
    ectopic thyroid nodule or tissue E05.30
      with thyroid storm E05.31
    ingestion of (excessive) thyroid material E05.40
      with thyroid storm E05.41
    overproduction of thyroid-stimulating hormone E05.80
      with thyroid storm E05.81
    specified cause NEC E05.80
      with thyroid storm E05.81
  factitia E05.40
    with thyroid storm E05.41
  heart E05.90 [I43]
    with thyroid storm E05.91 [I43]
    failure E05.90 [I43]
  neonatal (transient) P72.1
  transient with chronic thyroiditis E06.2
Tibia vara — *see* Osteochondrosis, juvenile, tibia
Tic (disorder) F95.9
  breathing F95.8
  child problem F95.0
  compulsive F95.1
  de la Tourette F95.2
  degenerative (generalized) (localized) G25.69
    facial G25.69
  disorder
    chronic
      motor F95.1
      vocal F95.1
    combined vocal and multiple motor F95.2
    transient F95.0
  douloureux G50.0
    atypical G50.1
    postherpetic, postzoster B02.22
  drug-induced G25.61
  eyelid F95.8
  habit F95.9
    chronic F95.1
    transient of childhood F95.0
  lid, transient of childhood F95.0
  motor-verbal F95.2
  occupational F48.8
  orbicularis F95.8
    transient of childhood F95.0
  organic origin G25.69
  postchoreic G25.69
  psychogenic, compulsive F95.1
  salaam R25.8

Tic — *continued*
  spasm (motor or vocal) F95.9
    chronic F95.1
    transient of childhood F95.0
  specified NEC F95.8
Tick-borne — *see* condition
Tietze's disease or syndrome M94.0
Tight, tightness
  anus K62.89
  chest R07.89
  fascia (lata) M62.89
  foreskin (congenital) N47.1
  hymen, hymenal ring N89.6
  introitus (acquired) (congenital) N89.6
  rectal sphincter K62.89
  tendon — *see* Short, tendon
  urethral sphincter N35.9
Tilting vertebra — *see* Dorsopathy, deforming, specified NEC
Timidity, child F93.8
Tinea (intersecta) (tarsi) B35.9
  amiantacea L44.8
  asbestina B35.0
  barbae B35.0
  beard B35.0
  black dot B35.0
  blanca B36.2
  capitis B35.0
  corporis B35.4
  cruris B35.6
  flava B36.0
  foot B35.3
  furfuracea B36.0
  imbricata (Tokelau) B35.5
  kerion B35.0
  manuum B35.2
  microsporic — *see* Dermatophytosis
  nigra B36.1
  nodosa — *see* Piedra
  pedis B35.3
  scalp B35.0
  specified site NEC B35.8
  sycosis B35.0
  tonsurans B35.0
  trichophytic — *see* Dermatophytosis
  unguium B35.1
  versicolor B36.0
Tingling sensation (skin) R20.2
Tin-miner's lung J63.5
Tinnitus (audible) (aurium) (subjective) — *see* subcategory H93.1 ☑
Tipped tooth (teeth) M26.33
Tipping
  pelvis M95.5
    with disproportion (fetopelvic) O33.0
      causing obstructed labor O65.0
  tooth (teeth), fully erupted M26.33
Tiredness R53.83
Tissue — *see* condition
Tobacco (nicotine)
  dependence — *see* Dependence, drug, nicotine
  harmful use Z72.0
  heart — *see* Tobacco, toxic effect
  maternal use, affecting newborn P04.2
  toxic effect — *see* Table of Drugs and Chemicals, by substance, poisoning
    chewing tobacco — *see* Table of Drugs and Chemicals, by substance, poisoning
    cigarettes — *see* Table of Drugs and Chemicals, by substance, poisoning
  use Z72.0
    complicating
      childbirth O99.334
      pregnancy O99.33- ☑
      puerperium O99.335
    counseling and surveillance Z71.6
  withdrawal state — *see* Dependence, drug, nicotine
Tocopherol deficiency E56.0
Todd's
  cirrhosis K74.3
  paralysis (postepileptic) (transitory) G83.84
Toe — *see* condition
Toilet, artificial opening — *see* Attention to, artificial, opening
Tokelau (ringworm) B35.5
Tollwut — *see* Rabies
Tommaselli's disease R31.9

Tommaselli's disease — continued
   correct substance properly administered — see Table
         of Drugs and Chemicals, by drug, adverse effect
   overdose or wrong substance given or taken — see
         Table of Drugs and Chemicals, by drug, poison-
         ing
Tongue (see also condition)
   tie Q38.1
Tonic pupil — see Anomaly, pupil, function, tonic pupil
Toni-Fanconi syndrome (cystinosis) E72.09
   with cystinosis E72.04
Tonsil — see condition
Tonsillitis (acute) (catarrhal) (croupous) (follicular)
         (gangrenous) (infective) (lacunar) (lingual) (malig-
         nant) (membranous) (parenchymatous) (phleg-
         monous) (pseudomembranous) (purulent) (septic)
         (subacute) (suppurative) (toxic) (ulcerative) (vesicu-
         lar) (viral) J03.90
   chronic J35.01
      with adenoiditis J35.03
   diphtheritic A36.0
   hypertrophic J35.01
      with adenoiditis J35.03
   recurrent J03.91
   specified organism NEC J03.80
      recurrent J03.81
   staphylococcal J03.80
      recurrent J03.81
   streptococcal J03.00
      recurrent J03.01
   tuberculous A15.8
   Vincent's A69.1
Tooth, teeth — see condition
Toothache K08.8
Topagnosis R20.8
Tophi — see Gout, chronic
TORCH infection — see Infection, congenital
   without active infection P00.2
Torn — see Tear
Tornwaldt's cyst or disease J39.2
Torsion
   accessory tube — see Torsion, fallopian tube
   adnexa (female) — see Torsion, fallopian tube
   aorta, acquired I77.1
   appendix epididymis N44.04
   appendix testis N44.03
   bile duct (common) (hepatic) K83.8
      congenital Q44.5
   bowel, colon or intestine K56.2
   cervix — see Malposition, uterus
   cystic duct K82.8
   dystonia — see Dystonia, torsion
   epididymis (appendix) N44.04
   fallopian tube N83.52
      with ovary N83.53
   gallbladder K82.8
      congenital Q44.1
   hydatid of Morgagni
      female N83.52
      male N44.03
   kidney (pedicle) (leading to infarction) N28.0
   Meckel's diverticulum (congenital) Q43.0
      malignant — see Table of Neoplasms, small intes-
            tine, malignant
   mesentery K56.2
   omentum K56.2
   organ or site, congenital NEC — see Anomaly, by site
   ovary (pedicle) N83.51
      with fallopian tube N83.53
      congenital Q50.2
   oviduct — see Torsion, fallopian tube
   penis (acquired) N48.82
      congenital Q55.63
   spasm — see Dystonia, torsion
   spermatic cord N44.02
      extravaginal N44.01
      intravaginal N44.02
   spleen D73.5
   testis, testicle N44.00
      appendix N44.03
   tibia — see Deformity, limb, specified type NEC, lower
         leg
   uterus — see Malposition, uterus
Torticollis (intermittent) (spastic) M43.6
   congenital (sternomastoid) Q68.0
   due to birth injury P15.8
   hysterical F44.4
   ocular R29.891

Torticollis — continued
   psychogenic F45.8
      conversion reaction F44.4
   rheumatic M43.6
   rheumatoid M06.88
   spasmodic G24.3
   traumatic, current S13.4 ☑
Tortipelvis G24.1
Tortuous
   artery I77.1
   organ or site, congenital NEC — see Distortion
   retinal vessel, congenital Q14.1
   ureter N13.8
   urethra N36.8
   vein — see Varix
Torture, victim of Z65.4
Torula, torular (histolytica) (infection) — see Cryptococ-
      cosis
Torulosis — see Cryptococcosis
Torus (mandibularis) (palatinus) M27.0
   fracture — see Fracture, by site, torus
Touraine's syndrome Q79.8
Tourette's syndrome F95.2
Tourniquet syndrome — see Constriction, external, by
      site
Tower skull Q75.0
   with exophthalmos Q87.0
Toxemia R68.89
   bacterial — see Sepsis
   burn — see Burn
   eclamptic (with pre-existing hypertension) — see
         Eclampsia
   erysipelatous — see Erysipelas
   fatigue R68.89
   food — see Poisoning, food
   gastrointestinal K52.1
   intestinal K52.1
   kidney — see Uremia
   malarial — see Malaria
   myocardial — see Myocarditis, toxic
   of pregnancy — see Pre-eclampsia
   pre-eclamptic — see Pre-eclampsia
   small intestine K52.1
   staphylococcal, due to food A05.0
   stasis R68.89
   uremic — see Uremia
   urinary — see Uremia
Toxemica cerebropathia psychica (nonalcoholic) F04
   alcoholic — see Alcohol, amnestic disorder
Toxic (poisoning) (see also condition) T65.91 ☑
   effect — see Table of Drugs and Chemicals, by sub-
         stance, poisoning
   shock syndrome A48.3
   thyroid (gland) — see Thyrotoxicosis
Toxicemia — see Toxemia
Toxicity — see Table of Drugs and Chemicals, by sub-
      stance, poisoning
   fava bean D55.0
   food, noxious — see Poisoning, food
   from drug or nonmedicinal substance — see Table of
         Drugs and Chemicals, by drug
Toxicosis (see also Toxemia)
   capillary, hemorrhagic D69.0
Toxinfection, gastrointestinal K52.1
Toxocariasis B83.0
Toxoplasma, toxoplasmosis (acquired) B58.9
   with
      hepatitis B58.1
      meningoencephalitis B58.2
      ocular involvement B58.00
      other organ involvement B58.89
      pneumonia, pneumonitis B58.3
   congenital (acute) (subacute) (chronic) P37.1
   maternal, manifest toxoplasmosis in infant (acute)
         (subacute) (chronic) P37.1
tPA (rtPA) **administration in a different facility within
      the last 24 hours prior to admission to current
      facility** Z92.82
Trabeculation, bladder N32.89
Trachea — see condition
Tracheitis (catarrhal) (infantile) (membranous) (plastic)
      (septal) (suppurative) (viral) J04.10
   with
      bronchitis (15 years of age and above) J40
         acute or subacute — see Bronchitis, acute
         chronic J42
         tuberculous NEC A15.5

Tracheitis — continued
   with — continued
      bronchitis — continued
         under 15 years of age J20.9
      laryngitis (acute) J04.2
         chronic J37.1
         tuberculous NEC A15.5
   acute J04.10
      with obstruction J04.11
   chronic J42
      with
         bronchitis (chronic) J42
         laryngitis (chronic) J37.1
   diphtheritic (membranous) A36.89
   due to external agent — see Inflammation, respiratory,
         upper, due to
   syphilitic A52.73
   tuberculous A15.5
Trachelitis (nonvenereal) — see Cervicitis
Tracheobronchial — see condition
Tracheobronchitis (15 years of age and above) (see also
      Bronchitis)
   due to
      Bordetella bronchiseptica A37.80
         with pneumonia A37.81
      Francisella tularensis A21.8
Tracheobronchomegaly Q32.4
   with bronchiectasis J47.9
      with
         exacerbation (acute) J47.1
         lower respiratory infection J47.0
   acquired J98.09
      with bronchiectasis J47.9
         with
            exacerbation (acute) J47.1
            lower respiratory infection J47.0
Tracheobronchopneumonitis — see Pneumonia,
      broncho-
Tracheocele (external) (internal) J39.8
   congenital Q32.1
Tracheomalacia J39.8
   congenital Q32.0
Tracheopharyngitis (acute) J06.9
   chronic J42
   due to external agent — see Inflammation, respiratory,
         upper, due to
Tracheostenosis J39.8
Tracheostomy
   complication — see Complication, tracheostomy
   status Z93.0
      attention to Z43.0
      malfunctioning J95.03
Trachoma, trachomatous A71.9
   active (stage) A71.1
   contraction of conjunctiva A71.1
   dubium A71.0
   healed or sequelae B94.0
   initial (stage) A71.0
   pannus A71.1
   Türck's J37.0
Traction, vitreomacular H43.82- ☑
Train sickness T75.3 ☑
Trait(s)
   Hb-S D57.3
   hemoglobin
      abnormal NEC D58.2
         with thalassemia D56.3
      C — see Disease, hemoglobin C
      S (Hb-S) D57.3
   Lepore D56.3
   personality, accentuated Z73.1
   sickle-cell D57.3
      with elliptocytosis or spherocytosis D57.3
   type A personality Z73.1
Tramp Z59.0
Trance R41.89
   hysterical F44.89
Transaminasemia R74.0
Transection
   abdomen (partial) S38.3 ☑
   aorta (incomplete) (see also Injury, aorta)
      complete — see Injury, aorta, laceration, major
   carotid artery (incomplete) (see also Injury, blood
         vessel, carotid, laceration)
      complete — see Injury, blood vessel, carotid, lacer-
            ation, major
   celiac artery (incomplete) S35.211 ☑

Transection — *continued*
  celiac artery — *continued*
    branch (incomplete) S35.291 ☑
      complete S35.292 ☑
    complete S35.212 ☑
  innominate
    artery (incomplete) (*see also* Injury, blood vessel, thoracic, innominate, artery, laceration)
      complete — *see* Injury, blood vessel, thoracic, innominate, artery, laceration, major
    vein (incomplete) (*see also* Injury, blood vessel, thoracic, innominate, vein, laceration)
      complete — *see* Injury, blood vessel, thoracic, innominate, vein, laceration, major
  jugular vein (external) (incomplete) (*see also* Injury, blood vessel, jugular vein, laceration)
    complete — *see* Injury, blood vessel, jugular vein, laceration, major
    internal (incomplete) (*see also* Injury, blood vessel, jugular vein, internal, laceration)
      complete — *see* Injury, blood vessel, jugular vein, internal, laceration, major
  mesenteric artery (incomplete) (*see also* Injury, mesenteric, artery, laceration)
    complete — *see* Injury, mesenteric artery, laceration, major
  pulmonary vessel (incomplete) (*see also* Injury, blood vessel, thoracic, pulmonary, laceration)
    complete — *see* Injury, blood vessel, thoracic, pulmonary, laceration, major
  subclavian — *see* Transection, innominate
  vena cava (incomplete) (*see also* Injury, vena cava)
    complete — *see* Injury, vena cava, laceration, major
  vertebral artery (incomplete) (*see also* Injury, blood vessel, vertebral, laceration)
    complete — *see* Injury, blood vessel, vertebral, laceration, major
Transfusion
  associated (red blood cell) hemochromatosis E83.111
  blood
    ABO incompatible — *see* Complication(s), transfusion, incompatibility reaction, ABO
    minor blood group (Duffy) (E) (K(ell)) (Kidd) (Lewis) (M) (N) (P) (S) T80.89 ☑
    reaction or complication — *see* Complications, transfusion
  fetomaternal (mother) — *see* Pregnancy, complicated by, placenta, transfusion syndrome
  maternofetal (mother) — *see* Pregnancy, complicated by, placenta, transfusion syndrome
  placental (syndrome) (mother) — *see* Pregnancy, complicated by, placenta, transfusion syndrome
  reaction (adverse) — *see* Complications, transfusion
  related acute lung injury (TRALI) J95.84
  twin-to-twin — *see* Pregnancy, complicated by, placenta, transfusion syndrome, fetus to fetus
Transient (meaning homeless) (*see also* condition) Z59.0
Translocation
  balanced autosomal Q95.9
    in normal individual Q95.0
  chromosomes NEC Q99.8
    balanced and insertion in normal individual Q95.0
  Down syndrome Q90.2
  trisomy
    13 Q91.6
    18 Q91.2
    21 Q90.2
Translucency, iris — *see* Degeneration, iris
Transmission of chemical substances through the placenta — *see* Absorption, chemical, through placenta
Transparency, lung, unilateral J43.0
Transplant (ed) (status) Z94.9
  awaiting organ Z76.82
  bone Z94.6
    marrow Z94.81
  candidate Z76.82
  complication — *see* Complication, transplant
  cornea Z94.7
  heart Z94.1
    and lung(s) Z94.3
    valve Z95.2
      prosthetic Z95.2
      specified NEC Z95.4
      xenogenic Z95.3
  intestine Z94.82
  kidney Z94.0

Transplant — *continued*
  liver Z94.4
  lung(s) Z94.2
    and heart Z94.3
  organ (failure) (infection) (rejection) Z94.9
    removal status Z98.85
  pancreas Z94.83
  skin Z94.5
  social Z60.3
  specified organ or tissue NEC Z94.89
  stem cells Z94.84
  tissue Z94.9
Transplants, ovarian, endometrial N80.1
Transposed — *see* Transposition
Transposition (congenital) (*see also* Malposition, congenital)
  abdominal viscera Q89.3
  aorta (dextra) Q20.3
  appendix Q43.8
  colon Q43.8
  corrected Q20.5
  great vessels (complete) (partial) Q20.3
  heart Q24.0
    with complete transposition of viscera Q89.3
  intestine (large) (small) Q43.8
  reversed jejunal (for bypass) (status) Z98.0
  scrotum Q55.23
  stomach Q40.2
    with general transposition of viscera Q89.3
  tooth, teeth, fully erupted M26.30
  vessels, great (complete) (partial) Q20.3
  viscera (abdominal) (thoracic) Q89.3
Transsexualism F64.1
Transverse (*see also* condition)
  arrest (deep), in labor O64.0 ☑
  lie (mother) O32.2 ☑
    causing obstructed labor O64.8 ☑
Transvestism, transvestitism (dual-role) F64.1
  fetishistic F65.1
Trapped placenta (with hemorrhage) O72.0
  without hemorrhage O73.0
Trauma, traumatism (*see also* Injury)
  acoustic — *see* subcategory H83.3 ☑
  birth — *see* Birth, injury
  complicating ectopic or molar pregnancy O08.6
  during delivery O71.9
  following ectopic or molar pregnancy O08.6
  obstetric O71.9
    specified NEC O71.89
Traumatic (*see also* condition)
  brain injury — *see* category S06 ☑
Treacher Collins syndrome Q75.4
Treitz's hernia — *see* Hernia, abdomen, specified site NEC
Trematode infestation — *see* Infestation, fluke
Trematodiasis — *see* Infestation, fluke
Trembling paralysis — *see* Parkinsonism
Tremor(s) R25.1
  drug induced G25.1
  essential (benign) G25.0
  familial G25.0
  hereditary G25.0
  hysterical F44.4
  intention G25.2
  medication induced postural G25.1
  mercurial — *see* subcategory T56.1 ☑
  Parkinson's — *see* Parkinsonism
  psychogenic (conversion reaction) F44.4
  senilis R54
  specified type NEC G25.2
Trench
  fever A79.0
  foot — *see* Immersion, foot
  mouth A69.1
Treponema pallidum infection — *see* Syphilis
Treponematosis
  due to
    T. pallidum — *see* Syphilis
    T. pertenue — *see* Yaws
Triad
  Hutchinson's (congenital syphilis) A50.53
  Kartagener's Q89.3
  Saint's — *see* Hernia, diaphragm
Trichiasis (eyelid) H02.059
  with entropion — *see* Entropion
  left H02.056
    lower H02.055

Trichiasis *continued*
  left — *continued*
    upper H02.054
  right H02.053
    lower H02.052
    upper H02.051
Trichinella spiralis (infection) (infestation) B75
Trichinellosis, trichiniasis, trichinelliasis, trichinosis B75
  with muscle disorder B75 [M63.80]
    ankle B75 [M63.87-] ☑
    foot B75 [M63.87-] ☑
    forearm B75 [M63.83-] ☑
    hand B75 [M63.84-] ☑
    lower leg B75 [M63.86-] ☑
    multiple sites B75 [M63.89]
    pelvic region B75 [M63.85-] ☑
    shoulder region B75 [M63.81-] ☑
    specified site NEC B75 [M63.88]
    thigh B75 [M63.85-] ☑
    upper arm B75 [M63.82-] ☑
Trichobezoar T18.9 ☑
  intestine T18.3 ☑
  stomach T18.2 ☑
Trichocephaliasis, trichocephalosis B79
Trichocephalus infestation B79
Trichoclasis L67.8
Trichoepithelioma (*see also* Neoplasm, skin, benign)
  malignant — *see* Neoplasm, skin, malignant
Trichofolliculoma — *see* Neoplasm, skin, benign
Tricholemmoma — *see* Neoplasm, skin, benign
Trichomoniasis A59.9
  bladder A59.03
  cervix A59.09
  intestinal A07.8
  prostate A59.02
  seminal vesicles A59.09
  specified site NEC A59.8
  urethra A59.03
  urogenitalis A59.00
  vagina A59.01
  vulva A59.01
Trichomycosis
  axillaris A48.8
  nodosa, nodularis B36.8
Trichonodosis L67.8
Trichophytid, trichophyton infection — *see* Dermatophytosis
Trichophytobezoar T18.9 ☑
  intestine T18.3 ☑
  stomach T18.2 ☑
Trichophytosis — *see* Dermatophytosis
Trichoptilosis L67.8
Trichorrhexis (nodosa) (invaginata) L67.0
Trichosis axillaris A48.8
Trichosporosis nodosa B36.2
Trichostasis spinulosa (congenital) Q84.1
Trichostrongyliasis, trichostrongylosis (small intestine) B81.2
Trichostrongylus infection B81.2
Trichotillomania F63.3
Trichromat, trichromatopsia, anomalous (congenital) H53.55
Trichuriasis B79
Trichuris trichiura (infection) (infestation) (any site) B79
Tricuspid (valve) — *see* condition
Trifid (*see also* Accessory)
  kidney (pelvis) Q63.8
  tongue Q38.3
Trigeminal neuralgia — *see* Neuralgia, trigeminal
Trigeminy R00.8
Trigger finger (acquired) M65.30
  congenital Q74.0
  index finger M65.32- ☑
  little finger M65.35- ☑
  middle finger M65.33- ☑
  ring finger M65.34- ☑
  thumb M65.31- ☑
Trigonitis (bladder) (chronic) (pseudomembranous) N30.30
  with hematuria N30.31
Trigonocephaly Q75.0
Trilocular heart — *see* Cor triloculare
Trimethylaminuria E72.52
Tripartite placenta O43.19- ☑
Triphalangeal thumb Q74.0

Triple (*see also* Accessory)
  kidneys Q63.0
  uteri Q51.818
  X, female Q97.0
Triplegia G83.89
  congenital G80.8
Triplet (newborn) (*see also* Newborn, triplet)
  complicating pregnancy — *see* Pregnancy, triplet
Triplication — *see* Accessory
Triploidy Q92.7
Trismus R25.2
  neonatorum A33
  newborn A33
Trisomy (syndrome) Q92.9
  13 (partial) Q91.7
    meiotic nondisjunction Q91.4
    mitotic nondisjunction Q91.5
    mosaicism Q91.5
    translocation Q91.6
  18 (partial) Q91.3
    meiotic nondisjunction Q91.0
    mitotic nondisjunction Q91.1
    mosaicism Q91.1
    translocation Q91.2
  20 Q92.8
  21 (partial) Q90.9
    meiotic nondisjunction Q90.0
    mitotic nondisjunction Q90.1
    mosaicism Q90.1
    translocation Q90.2
  22 Q92.8
  autosomes Q92.9
  chromosome specified NEC Q92.8
    partial Q92.2
      due to unbalanced translocation Q92.5
    specified NEC Q92.8
    whole (nonsex chromosome)
      meiotic nondisjunction Q92.0
      mitotic nondisjunction Q92.1
      mosaicism Q92.1
  due to
    dicentrics — *see* Extra, marker chromosomes
    extra rings — *see* Extra, marker chromosomes
    isochromosomes — *see* Extra, marker chromo-
      somes
  specified NEC Q92.8
  whole chromosome Q92.9
    meiotic nondisjunction Q92.0
    mitotic nondisjunction Q92.1
    mosaicism Q92.1
    partial Q92.9
    specified NEC Q92.8
Tritanomaly, tritanopia H53.55
Trombiculosis, trombiculiasis, trombidiosis B88.0
Trophedema (congenital) (hereditary) Q82.0
Trophoblastic disease (*see also* Mole, hydatidiform)
  O01.9
Tropholymphedema Q82.0
Trophoneurosis NEC G96.8
  disseminated M34.9
Tropical — *see* condition
Trouble (*see also* Disease)
  heart — *see* Disease, heart
  kidney — *see* Disease, renal
  nervous R45.0
  sinus — *see* Sinusitis
Trousseau's syndrome (thrombophlebitis migrans) I82.1
Truancy, childhood
  from school Z72.810
Truncus
  arteriosus (persistent) Q20.0
  communis Q20.0
Trunk — *see* condition
Trypanosomiasis
  African B56.9
    by Trypanosoma brucei
      gambiense B56.0
      rhodesiense B56.1
  American — *see* Chagas' disease
  Brazilian — *see* Chagas' disease
  by Trypanosoma
    brucei gambiense B56.0
    brucei rhodesiense B56.1
    cruzi — *see* Chagas' disease
  gambiensis, Gambian B56.0
  rhodesiensis, Rhodesian B56.1
  South American — *see* Chagas' disease
  where

Trypanosomiasis — *continued*
  where — *continued*
    African trypanosomiasis is prevalent B56.9
    Chagas' disease is prevalent B57.2
T-shaped incisors K00.2
Tsutsugamushi (disease) (fever) A75.3
Tube, tubal, tubular — *see* condition
Tubercle (*see also* Tuberculosis)
  brain, solitary A17.81
  Darwin's Q17.8
  Ghon, primary infection A15.7
Tuberculid, tuberculide (indurating, subcutaneous)
  (lichenoid) (miliary) (papulonecrotic) (primary) (skin)
  A18.4
Tuberculoma (*see also* Tuberculosis)
  brain A17.81
  meninges (cerebral) (spinal) A17.1
  spinal cord A17.81
Tuberculosis, tubercular, tuberculous (calcification)
  (calcified) (caseous) (chromogenic acid-fast bacilli)
  (degeneration) (fibrocaseous) (fistula) (interstitial)
  (isolated circumscribed lesions) (necrosis)
  (parenchymatous) (ulcerative) A15.9
  with pneumoconiosis (any condition in J60-J64) J65
  abdomen (lymph gland) A18.39
  abscess (respiratory) A15.9
    bone A18.03
      hip A18.02
      knee A18.02
      sacrum A18.01
      specified site NEC A18.03
      spinal A18.01
      vertebra A18.01
    brain A17.81
    breast A18.89
    Cowper's gland A18.15
    dura (mater) (cerebral) (spinal) A17.81
    epidural (cerebral) (spinal) A17.81
    female pelvis A18.17
    frontal sinus A15.8
    genital organs NEC A18.10
    genitourinary A18.10
    gland (lymphatic) — *see* Tuberculosis, lymph gland
    hip A18.02
    intestine A18.32
    ischiorectal A18.32
    joint NEC A18.02
      hip A18.02
      knee A18.02
      specified NEC A18.02
      vertebral A18.01
    kidney A18.11
    knee A18.02
    latent R76.11
    lumbar (spine) A18.01
    lung — *see* Tuberculosis, pulmonary
    meninges (cerebral) (spinal) A17.0
    muscle A18.09
    perianal (fistula) A18.32
    perinephritic A18.11
    perirectal A18.32
    rectum A18.32
    retropharyngeal A15.8
    sacrum A18.01
    scrofulous A18.2
    scrotum A18.15
    skin (primary) A18.4
    spinal cord A17.81
    spine or vertebra (column) A18.01
    subdiaphragmatic A18.31
    testis A18.15
    urinary A18.13
    uterus A18.17
  accessory sinus — *see* Tuberculosis, sinus
  Addison's disease A18.7
  adenitis — *see* Tuberculosis, lymph gland
  adenoids A15.8
  adenopathy — *see* Tuberculosis, lymph gland
  adherent pericardium A18.84
  adnexa (uteri) A18.17
  adrenal (capsule) (gland) A18.7
  alimentary canal A18.32
  anemia A18.89
  ankle (joint) (bone) A18.02
  anus A18.32
  apex, apical — *see* Tuberculosis, pulmonary
  appendicitis, appendix A18.32
  arachnoid A17.0

Tuberculosis, tubercular, tuberculous — *continued*
  artery, arteritis A18.89
    cerebral A18.89
  arthritis (chronic) (synovial) A18.02
    spine or vertebra (column) A18.01
  articular — *see* Tuberculosis, joint
  ascites A18.31
  asthma — *see* Tuberculosis, pulmonary
  axilla, axillary (gland) A18.2
  bladder A18.12
  bone A18.03
    hip A18.02
    knee A18.02
    limb NEC A18.03
    sacrum A18.01
    spine or vertebral column A18.01
  bowel (miliary) A18.32
  brain A17.81
  breast A18.89
  broad ligament A18.17
  bronchi, bronchial, bronchus A15.5
    ectasia, ectasis (bronchiectasis) — *see* Tuberculosis,
      pulmonary
    fistula A15.5
      primary (progressive) A15.7
    gland or node A15.4
      primary (progressive) A15.7
    lymph gland or node A15.4
      primary (progressive) A15.7
  bronchiectasis — *see* Tuberculosis, pulmonary
  bronchitis A15.5
  bronchopleural A15.6
  bronchopneumonia, bronchopneumonic — *see* Tuber-
    culosis, pulmonary
  bronchorrhagia A15.5
  bronchotracheal A15.5
  bronze disease A18.7
  buccal cavity A18.83
  bulbourethral gland A18.15
  bursa A18.09
  cachexia A15.9
  cardiomyopathy A18.84
  caries — *see* Tuberculosis, bone
  cartilage A18.02
    intervertebral A18.01
  catarrhal — *see* Tuberculosis, respiratory
  cecum A18.32
  cellulitis (primary) A18.4
  cerebellum A17.81
  cerebral, cerebrum A17.81
  cerebrospinal A17.81
    meninges A17.0
  cervical (lymph gland or node) A18.2
  cervicitis, cervix (uteri) A18.16
  chest — *see* Tuberculosis, respiratory
  chorioretinitis A18.53
  choroid, choroiditis A18.53
  ciliary body A18.54
  colitis A18.32
  collier's J65
  colliquativa (primary) A18.4
  colon A18.32
  complex, primary A15.7
  congenital P37.0
  conjunctiva A18.59
  connective tissue (systemic) A18.89
  contact Z20.1
  cornea (ulcer) A18.52
  Cowper's gland A18.15
  coxae A18.02
  coxalgia A18.02
  cul-de-sac of Douglas A18.17
  curvature, spine A18.01
  cutis (colliquativa) (primary) A18.4
  cyst, ovary A18.18
  cystitis A18.12
  dactylitis A18.03
  diarrhea A18.32
  diffuse — *see* Tuberculosis, miliary
  digestive tract A18.32
  disseminated — *see* Tuberculosis, miliary
  duodenum A18.32
  dura (mater) (cerebral) (spinal) A17.0
    abscess (cerebral) (spinal) A17.81
  dysentery A18.32
  ear (inner) (middle) A18.6
    bone A18.03
    external (primary) A18.4

ear — *continued*
skin (primary) A18.4
elbow A18.02
emphysema — *see* Tuberculosis, pulmonary
empyema A15.6
encephalitis A17.82
endarteritis A18.89
endocarditis A18.84
aortic A18.84
mitral A18.84
pulmonary A18.84
tricuspid A18.84
endocrine glands NEC A18.82
endometrium A18.17
enteric, enterica, enteritis A18.32
enterocolitis A18.32
epididymis, epididymitis A18.15
epidural abscess (cerebral) (spinal) A17.81
epiglottis A15.5
episcleritis A18.51
erythema (induratum) (nodosum) (primary) A18.4
esophagus A18.83
eustachian tube A18.6
exposure (to) Z20.1
exudative — *see* Tuberculosis, pulmonary
eye A18.50
eyelid (primary) (lupus) A18.4
fallopian tube (acute) (chronic) A18.17
fascia A18.09
fauces A15.8
female pelvic inflammatory disease A18.17
finger A18.03
first infection A15.7
gallbladder A18.83
ganglion A18.09
gastritis A18.83
gastrocolic fistula A18.32
gastroenteritis A18.32
gastrointestinal tract A18.32
general, generalized — *see* Tuberculosis, miliary
genital organs A18.10
genitourinary A18.10
genu A18.02
glandula suprarenalis A18.7
glandular, general A18.2
glottis A15.5
grinder's J65
gum A18.83
hand A18.03
heart A18.84
hematogenous — *see* Tuberculosis, miliary
hemoptysis — *see* Tuberculosis, pulmonary
hemorrhage NEC — *see* Tuberculosis, pulmonary
hemothorax A15.6
hepatitis A18.83
hilar lymph nodes A15.4
primary (progressive) A15.7
hip (joint) (disease) (bone) A18.02
hydropneumothorax A15.6
hydrothorax A15.6
hypoadrenalism A18.7
hypopharynx A15.8
ileocecal (hyperplastic) A18.32
ileocolitis A18.32
ileum A18.32
iliac spine (superior) A18.03
immunological findings only A15.7
indurativa (primary) A18.4
infantile A15.7
infection A15.9
without clinical manifestations A15.7
infraclavicular gland A18.2
inguinal gland A18.2
inguinalis A18.2
intestine (any part) A18.32
iridocyclitis A18.54
iris, iritis A18.54
ischiorectal A18.32
jaw A18.03
jejunum A18.32
joint A18.02
vertebral A18.01
keratitis (interstitial) A18.52
keratoconjunctivitis A18.52
kidney A18.11
knee (joint) A18.02
kyphosis, kyphoscoliosis A18.01

laryngitis A15.5
larynx A15.5
latent R76.11
leptomeninges, leptomeningitis (cerebral) (spinal) A17.0
lichenoides (primary) A18.4
linguae A18.83
lip A18.83
liver A18.83
lordosis A18.01
lung — *see* Tuberculosis, pulmonary
lupus vulgaris A18.4
lymph gland or node (peripheral) A18.2
abdomen A18.39
bronchial A15.4
primary (progressive) A15.7
cervical A18.2
hilar A15.4
primary (progressive) A15.7
intrathoracic A15.4
primary (progressive) A15.7
mediastinal A15.4
primary (progressive) A15.7
mesenteric A18.39
retroperitoneal A18.39
tracheobronchial A15.4
primary (progressive) A15.7
lymphadenitis — *see* Tuberculosis, lymph gland
lymphangitis — *see* Tuberculosis, lymph gland
lymphatic (gland) (vessel) — *see* Tuberculosis, lymph gland
mammary gland A18.89
marasmus A15.9
mastoiditis A18.03
mediastinal lymph gland or node A15.4
primary (progressive) A15.7
mediastinitis A15.8
primary (progressive) A15.7
mediastinum A15.8
primary (progressive) A15.7
medulla A17.81
melanosis, Addisonian A18.7
meninges, meningitis (basilar) (cerebral) (cerebrospinal) (spinal) A17.0
meningoencephalitis A17.82
mesentery, mesenteric (gland or node) A18.39
miliary A19.9
acute A19.2
multiple sites A19.1
single specified site A19.0
chronic A19.8
specified NEC A19.8
millstone makers' J65
miner's J65
molder's J65
mouth A18.83
multiple A19.9
acute A19.1
chronic A19.8
muscle A18.09
myelitis A17.82
myocardium, myocarditis A18.84
nasal (passage) (sinus) A15.8
nasopharynx A15.8
neck gland A18.2
nephritis A18.11
nerve (mononeuropathy) A17.83
nervous system A17.9
nose (septum) A15.8
ocular A18.50
omentum A18.31
oophoritis (acute) (chronic) A18.17
optic (nerve trunk) (papilla) A18.59
orbit A18.59
orchitis A18.15
organ, specified NEC A18.89
osseous — *see* Tuberculosis, bone
osteitis — *see* Tuberculosis, bone
osteomyelitis — *see* Tuberculosis, bone
otitis media A18.6
ovary, ovaritis (acute) (chronic) A18.17
oviduct (acute) (chronic) A18.17
pachymeningitis A17.0
palate (soft) A18.83
pancreas A18.83
papulonecrotic (a) (primary) A18.4
parathyroid glands A18.82

paronychia (primary) A18.4
parotid gland or region A18.83
pelvis (bony) A18.03
penis A18.15
peribronchitis A15.5
pericardium, pericarditis A18.84
perichondritis, larynx A15.5
periostitis — *see* Tuberculosis, bone
perirectal fistula A18.32
peritoneum NEC A18.31
peritonitis A18.31
pharynx, pharyngitis A15.8
phlyctenulosis (keratoconjunctivitis) A18.52
phthisis NEC — *see* Tuberculosis, pulmonary
pituitary gland A18.82
pleura, pleural, pleurisy, pleuritis (fibrinous) (obliterative) (purulent) (simple plastic) (with effusion) A15.6
primary (progressive) A15.7
pneumonia, pneumonic — *see* Tuberculosis, pulmonary
pneumothorax (spontaneous) (tense valvular) — *see* Tuberculosis, pulmonary
polyneuropathy A17.89
polyserositis A19.9
acute A19.1
chronic A19.8
potter's J65
prepuce A18.15
primary (complex) A15.7
proctitis A18.32
prostate, prostatitis A18.14
pulmonalis — *see* Tuberculosis, pulmonary
pulmonary (cavitated) (fibrotic) (infiltrative) (nodular) A15.0
childhood type or first infection A15.7
primary (complex) A15.7
pyelitis A18.11
pyelonephritis A18.11
pyemia — *see* Tuberculosis, miliary
pyonephrosis A18.11
pyopneumothorax A15.6
pyothorax A15.6
rectum (fistula) (with abscess) A18.32
reinfection stage — *see* Tuberculosis, pulmonary
renal A18.11
renis A18.11
respiratory A15.9
primary A15.7
specified site NEC A15.8
retina, retinitis A18.53
retroperitoneal (lymph gland or node) A18.39
rheumatism NEC A18.09
rhinitis A15.8
sacroiliac (joint) A18.01
sacrum A18.01
salivary gland A18.83
salpingitis (acute) (chronic) A18.17
sandblaster's J65
sclera A18.51
scoliosis A18.01
scrofulous A18.2
scrotum A18.15
seminal tract or vesicle A18.15
senile A15.9
septic — *see* Tuberculosis, miliary
shoulder (joint) A18.02
blade A18.03
sigmoid A18.32
sinus (any nasal) A15.8
bone A18.03
epididymis A18.15
skeletal NEC A18.03
skin (any site) (primary) A18.4
small intestine A18.32
soft palate A18.83
spermatic cord A18.15
spine, spinal (column) A18.01
cord A17.81
medulla A17.81
membrane A17.0
meninges A17.0
spleen, splenitis A18.85
spondylitis A18.01
sternoclavicular joint A18.02
stomach A18.83
stonemason's J65

☑ **Additional Character Required** — **Refer to the Tabular List for Character Selection**
▼ Subterms under main terms may continue to next column or page

Tuberculosis, tubercular, tuberculous — *continued*
  subcutaneous tissue (cellular) (primary) A18.4
  subcutis (primary) A18.4
  subdeltoid bursa A18.83
  submaxillary (region) A18.83
  supraclavicular gland A18.2
  suprarenal (capsule) (gland) A18.7
  swelling, joint (*see also* category M01) (*see also* Tuberculosis, joint) A18.02
  symphysis pubis A18.02
  synovitis A18.09
    articular A18.02
    spine or vertebra A18.01
  systemic — *see* Tuberculosis, miliary
  tarsitis A18.4
  tendon (sheath) — *see* Tuberculosis, tenosynovitis
  tenosynovitis A18.09
    spine or vertebra A18.01
  testis A18.15
  throat A15.8
  thymus gland A18.82
  thyroid gland A18.81
  tongue A18.83
  tonsil, tonsillitis A15.8
  trachea, tracheal A15.5
    lymph gland or node A15.4
      primary (progressive) A15.7
  tracheobronchial A15.5
    lymph gland or node A15.4
      primary (progressive) A15.7
  tubal (acute) (chronic) A18.17
  tunica vaginalis A18.15
  ulcer (skin) (primary) A18.4
    bowel or intestine A18.32
    specified NEC — *see* Tuberculosis, by site
  unspecified site A15.9
  ureter A18.11
  urethra, urethral (gland) A18.13
  urinary organ or tract A18.13
  uterus A18.17
  uveal tract A18.54
  uvula A18.83
  vagina A18.18
  vas deferens A18.15
  verruca, verrucosa (cutis) (primary) A18.4
  vertebra (column) A18.01
  vesiculitis A18.15
  vulva A18.18
  wrist (joint) A18.02
Tuberculum
  Carabelli — *see* Excludes Note at K00.2
  occlusal — *see* Excludes Note at K00.2
  paramolare K00.2
Tuberosity, enitre maxillary M26.07
Tuberous sclerosis (brain) Q85.1
Tubo-ovarian — *see* condition
Tuboplasty, after previous sterilization Z31.0
  aftercare Z31.42
Tubotympanitis, catarrhal (chronic) — *see* Otitis, media, nonsuppurative, chronic, serous
Tularemia A21.9
  with
    conjunctivitis A21.1
    pneumonia A21.2
  abdominal A21.3
  bronchopneumonic A21.2
  conjunctivitis A21.1
  cryptogenic A21.3
  enteric A21.3
  gastrointestinal A21.3
  generalized A21.7
  ingestion A21.3
  intestinal A21.3
  oculoglandular A21.1
  ophthalmic A21.1
  pneumonia (any), pneumonic A21.2
  pulmonary A21.2
  sepsis A21.7
  specified NEC A21.8
  typhoidal A21.7
  ulceroglandular A21.0
Tularensis conjunctivitis A21.1
Tumefaction (*see also* Swelling)
  liver — *see* Hypertrophy, liver
Tumor (*see also* Neoplasm, unspecified behavior, by site)
  acinar cell — *see* Neoplasm, uncertain behavior, by site

Tumor — *continued*
  acinic cell — *see* Neoplasm, uncertain behavior, by site
  adenocarcinoid — *see* Neoplasm, malignant, by site
  adenomatoid (*see also* Neoplasm, benign, by site)
    odontogenic — *see* Cyst, calcifying odontogenic
  adnexal (skin) — *see* Neoplasm, skin, benign, by site
  adrenal
    cortical (benign) D35.0- ☑
      malignant C74.0- ☑
    rest — *see* Neoplasm, benign, by site
  alpha-cell
    malignant
      pancreas C25.4
      specified site NEC — *see* Neoplasm, malignant, by site
      unspecified site C25.4
    pancreas D13.7
    specified site NEC — *see* Neoplasm, benign, by site
    unspecified site D13.7
  aneurysmal — *see* Aneurysm
  aortic body D44.7
    malignant C75.5
  Askin's — *see* Neoplasm, connective tissue, malignant
  basal cell (*see also* Neoplasm, skin, uncertain behavior) D48.5
  Bednar — *see* Neoplasm, skin, malignant
  benign (unclassified) — *see* Neoplasm, benign, by site
  beta-cell
    malignant
      pancreas C25.4
      specified site NEC — *see* Neoplasm, malignant, by site
      unspecified site C25.4
    pancreas D13.7
    specified site NEC — *see* Neoplasm, benign, by site
    unspecified site D13.7
  Brenner D27.9
    borderline malignancy D39.1- ☑
    malignant C56- ☑
    proliferating D39.1- ☑
  bronchial alveolar, intravascular D38.1
  Brooke's — *see* Neoplasm, skin, benign
  brown fat — *see* Lipoma
  Burkitt — *see* Lymphoma, Burkitt
  calcifying epithelial odontogenic — *see* Cyst, calcifying odontogenic
  carcinoid
    benign D3A.00 (*following* D36)
      appendix D3A.020 (*following* D36)
      ascending colon D3A.022 (*following* D36)
      bronchus (lung) D3A.090 (*following* D36)
      cecum D3A.021 (*following* D36)
      colon D3A.029 (*following* D36)
      descending colon D3A.024 (*following* D36)
      duodenum D3A.010 (*following* D36)
      foregut NOS D3A.094 (*following* D36)
      hindgut NOS D3A.096 (*following* D36)
      ileum D3A.012 (*following* D36)
      jejunum D3A.011 (*following* D36)
      kidney D3A.093 (*following* D36)
      large intestine D3A.029 (*following* D36)
      lung (bronchus) D3A.090 (*following* D36)
      midgut NOS D3A.095 (*following* D36)
      rectum D3A.026 (*following* D36)
      sigmoid colon D3A.025 (*following* D36)
      small intestine D3A.019 (*following* D36)
      specified NEC D3A.098 (*following* D36)
      stomach D3A.092 (*following* D36)
      thymus D3A.091 (*following* D36)
      transverse colon D3A.023 (*following* D36)
    malignant C7A.00 (*following* C75)
      appendix C7A.020 (*following* C75)
      ascending colon C7A.022 (*following* C75)
      bronchus (lung) C7A.090 (*following* C75)
      cecum C7A.021 (*following* C75)
      colon C7A.029 (*following* C75)
      descending colon C7A.024 (*following* C75)
      duodenum C7A.010 (*following* C75)
      foregut NOS C7A.094 (*following* C75)
      hindgut NOS C7A.096 (*following* C75)
      ileum C7A.012 (*following* C75)
      jejunum C7A.011 (*following* C75)
      kidney C7A.093 (*following* C75)
      large intestine C7A.029 (*following* C75)
      lung (bronchus) C7A.090 (*following* C75)
      midgut NOS C7A.095 (*following* C75)
      rectum C7A.026 (*following* C75)

Tumor — *continued*
  carcinoid — *continued*
    malignant — *continued*
      sigmoid colon C7A.025 (*following* C75)
      small intestine C7A.019 (*following* C75)
      specified NEC C7A.098 (*following* C75)
      stomach C7A.092 (*following* C75)
      thymus C7A.091 (*following* C75)
      transverse colon C7A.023 (*following* C75)
    mesentery metastasis C7B.04 (*following* C75)
    secondary C7B.00 (*following* C75)
      bone C7B.03 (*following* C75)
      distant lymph nodes C7B.01 (*following* C75)
      liver C7B.02 (*following* C75)
      peritoneum C7B.04 (*following* C75)
      specified NEC C7B.09 (*following* C75)
  carotid body D44.6
    malignant C75.4
  cells (*see also* Neoplasm, unspecified behavior, by site)
    benign — *see* Neoplasm, benign, by site
    malignant — *see* Neoplasm, malignant, by site
    uncertain whether benign or malignant — *see* Neoplasm, uncertain behavior, by site
  cervix, in pregnancy or childbirth — *see* Pregnancy, complicated by, tumor, cervix
  chondromatous giant cell — *see* Neoplasm, bone, benign
  chromaffin (*see also* Neoplasm, benign, by site)
    malignant — *see* Neoplasm, malignant, by site
  Cock's peculiar L72.3
  Codman's — *see* Neoplasm, bone, benign
  dentigerous, mixed — *see* Cyst, calcifying odontogenic
  dermoid — *see* Neoplasm, benign, by site
    with malignant transformation C56- ☑
  desmoid (extra-abdominal) (*see also* Neoplasm, connective tissue, uncertain behavior)
    abdominal — *see* Neoplasm, connective tissue, uncertain behavior
  embolus — *see* Neoplasm, secondary, by site
  embryonal (mixed) (*see also* Neoplasm, uncertain behavior, by site)
    liver C22.7
  endodermal sinus
    specified site — *see* Neoplasm, malignant, by site
    unspecified site
      female C56.- ☑
      male C62.90
  epithelial
    benign — *see* Neoplasm, benign, by site
    malignant — *see* Neoplasm, malignant, by site
  Ewing's — *see* Neoplasm, bone, malignant, by site
  fatty — *see* Lipoma
  fibroid — *see* Leiomyoma
  G cell
    malignant
      pancreas C25.4
      specified site NEC — *see* Neoplasm, malignant, by site
      unspecified site C25.4
    specified site — *see* Neoplasm, uncertain behavior, by site
    unspecified site D37.8
  germ cell (*see also* Neoplasm, malignant, by site)
    mixed — *see* Neoplasm, malignant, by site
  ghost cell, odontogenic — *see* Cyst, calcifying odontogenic
  giant cell (*see also* Neoplasm, uncertain behavior, by site)
    bone D48.0
      malignant — *see* Neoplasm, bone, malignant
    chondromatous — *see* Neoplasm, bone, benign
    malignant — *see* Neoplasm, malignant, by site
    soft parts — *see* Neoplasm, connective tissue, uncertain behavior
      malignant — *see* Neoplasm, connective tissue, malignant
  glomus D18.00
    intra-abdominal D18.03
    intracranial D18.02
    jugulare D44.7
      malignant C75.5
    skin D18.01
    specified site NEC D18.09
  gonadal stromal — *see* Neoplasm, uncertain behavior, by site

Tumor — *continued*
  granular cell (*see also* Neoplasm, connective tissue, benign)
    malignant — *see* Neoplasm, connective tissue, malignant
  granulosa cell D39.1- ☑
    juvenile D39.1- ☑
    malignant C56- ☑
  granulosa cell-theca cell D39.1- ☑
    malignant C56- ☑
  Grawitz's C64- ☑
  hemorrhoidal — *see* Hemorrhoids
  hilar cell D27- ☑
  hilus cell D27- ☑
  Hurthle cell (benign) D34
    malignant C73
  hydatid — *see* Echinococcus
  hypernephroid (*see also* Neoplasm, uncertain behavior, by site)
  interstitial cell (*see also* Neoplasm, uncertain behavior, by site)
    benign — *see* Neoplasm, benign, by site
    malignant — *see* Neoplasm, malignant, by site
  intravascular bronchial alveolar D38.1
  islet cell — *see* Neoplasm, benign, by site
    malignant — *see* Neoplasm, malignant, by site
      pancreas C25.4
      specified site NEC — *see* Neoplasm, malignant, by site
      unspecified site C25.4
    pancreas D13.7
    specified site NEC — *see* Neoplasm, benign, by site
    unspecified site D13.7
  juxtaglomerular D41.0- ☑
  Klatskin's C22.1
  Krukenberg's C79.6- ☑
  Leydig cell — *see* Neoplasm, uncertain behavior, by site
    benign — *see* Neoplasm, benign, by site
      specified site — *see* Neoplasm, benign, by site
      unspecified site
        female D27.9
        male D29.20
    malignant — *see* Neoplasm, malignant, by site
      specified site — *see* Neoplasm, malignant, by site
      unspecified site
        female C56.9
        male C62.90
    specified site — *see* Neoplasm, uncertain behavior, by site
    unspecified site
      female D39.10
      male D40.10
  lipid cell, ovary D27- ☑
  lipoid cell, ovary D27- ☑
  malignant (*see also* Neoplasm, malignant, by site) C80.1
    fusiform cell (type) C80.1
    giant cell (type) C80.1
    localized, plasma cell — *see* Plasmacytoma, solitary
    mixed NEC C80.1
    small cell (type) C80.1
    spindle cell (type) C80.1
    unclassified C80.1
  mast cell D47.0
    malignant C96.2
  melanotic, neuroectodermal — *see* Neoplasm, benign, by site
  Merkel cell — *see* Carcinoma, Merkel cell
  mesenchymal
    malignant — *see* Neoplasm, connective tissue, malignant
    mixed — *see* Neoplasm, connective tissue, uncertain behavior
  mesodermal, mixed (*see also* Neoplasm, malignant, by site)
    liver C22.4
  mesonephric (*see also* Neoplasm, uncertain behavior, by site)
    malignant — *see* Neoplasm, malignant, by site
  metastatic
    from specified site — *see* Neoplasm, malignant, by site
    of specified site — *see* Neoplasm, malignant, by site

Tumor — *continued*
  metastatic — *continued*
    to specified site — *see* Neoplasm, secondary, by site
  mixed NEC (*see also* Neoplasm, benign, by site)
    malignant — *see* Neoplasm, malignant, by site
  mucinous of low malignant potential
    specified site — *see* Neoplasm, malignant, by site
    unspecified site C56.9
  mucocarcinoid
    specified site — *see* Neoplasm, malignant, by site
    unspecified site C18.1
  mucoepidermoid — *see* Neoplasm, uncertain behavior, by site
  Müllerian, mixed
    specified site — *see* Neoplasm, malignant, by site
    unspecified site C54.9
  myoepithelial — *see* Neoplasm, benign, by site
  neuroectodermal (peripheral) — *see* Neoplasm, malignant, by site
    primitive
      specified site — *see* Neoplasm, malignant, by site
      unspecified site C71.9
  neuroendocrine D3A.8 (*following* D36)
    malignant poorly differentiated C7A.1 (*following* C75)
    secondary NEC C7B.8 (*following* C75)
    specified NEC C7A.8 (*following* C75)
  neurogenic olfactory C30.0
  nonencapsulated sclerosing C73
  odontogenic (adenomatoid) (benign) (calcifying epithelial) (keratocystic) (squamous) — *see* Cyst, calcifying odontogenic
    malignant C41.1
      upper jaw (bone) C41.0
  ovarian stromal D39.1- ☑
  ovary, in pregnancy — *see* Pregnancy, complicated by
  pacinian — *see* Neoplasm, skin, benign
  Pancoast's — *see* Pancoast's syndrome
  papillary (*see also* Papilloma)
    cystic D37.9
    mucinous of low malignant potential C56- ☑
      specified site — *see* Neoplasm, malignant, by site
      unspecified site C56.9
    serous of low malignant potential
      specified site — *see* Neoplasm, malignant, by site
      unspecified site C56.9
  pelvic, in pregnancy or childbirth — *see* Pregnancy, complicated by
  phantom F45.8
  phyllodes D48.6- ☑
    benign D24- ☑
    malignant — *see* Neoplasm, breast, malignant
  Pindborg — *see* Cyst, calcifying odontogenic
  placental site trophoblastic D39.2
  plasma cell (malignant) (localized) — *see* Plasmacytoma, solitary
  polyvesicular vitelline
    specified site — *see* Neoplasm, malignant, by site
    unspecified site
      female C56.9
      male C62.90
  Pott's puffy — *see* Osteomyelitis, specified NEC
  Rathke's pouch D44.3
  retinal anlage — *see* Neoplasm, benign, by site
  salivary gland type, mixed — *see* Neoplasm, salivary gland, benign
    malignant — *see* Neoplasm, salivary gland, malignant
  Sampson's N80.1
  Schmincke's — *see* Neoplasm, nasopharynx, malignant
  sclerosing stromal D27- ☑
  sebaceous — *see* Cyst, sebaceous
  secondary — *see* Neoplasm, secondary, by site
    carcinoid C7B.00 (*following* C75)
      bone C7B.03 (*following* C75)
      distant lymph nodes C7B.01 (*following* C75)
      liver C7B.02 (*following* C75)
      peritoneum C7B.04 (*following* C75)
      specified NEC C7B.09 (*following* C75)
    neuroendocrine NEC C7B.8 (*following* C75)
  serous of low malignant potential
    specified site — *see* Neoplasm, malignant, by site

Tumor — *continued*
  serous of low malignant potential — *continued*
    unspecified site C56.9
  Sertoli cell — *see* Neoplasm, benign, by site
    with lipid storage
      specified site — *see* Neoplasm, benign, by site
      unspecified site
        female D27.9
        male D29.20
    specified site — *see* Neoplasm, benign, by site
    unspecified site
      female D27.9
      male D29.20
  Sertoli-Leydig cell — *see* Neoplasm, benign, by site
    specified site — *see* Neoplasm, benign, by site
    unspecified site
      female D27.9
      male D29.20
  sex cord (-stromal) — *see* Neoplasm, uncertain behavior, by site
    with annular tubules D39.1- ☑
  skin appendage — *see* Neoplasm, skin, benign
  smooth muscle — *see* Neoplasm, connective tissue, uncertain behavior
  soft tissue
    benign — *see* Neoplasm, connective tissue, benign
    malignant — *see* Neoplasm, connective tissue, malignant
  sternomastoid (congenital) Q68.0
  stromal
    endometrial D39.0
    gastric D48.1
      benign D21.4
      malignant C16.9
      uncertain behavior D48.1
    gastrointestinal
      benign D21.4
      malignant C49.4
      uncertain behavior D48.1
    intestine
      benign D21.4
      malignant C49.4
      uncertain behavior D48.1
    ovarian D39.1- ☑
    stomach
      benign D21.4
      malignant C16.9
      uncertain behavior D48.1
  sweat gland (*see also* Neoplasm, skin, uncertain behavior)
    benign — *see* Neoplasm, skin, benign
    malignant — *see* Neoplasm, skin, malignant
  syphilitic, brain A52.17
  testicular D40.10
  testicular stromal D40.1- ☑
  theca cell D27.- ☑
  theca cell-granulosa cell D39.1- ☑
  Triton, malignant — *see* Neoplasm, nerve, malignant
  trophoblastic, placental site D39.2
  turban D23.4
  uterus (body), in pregnancy or childbirth — *see* Pregnancy, complicated by, tumor, uterus
  vagina, in pregnancy or childbirth — *see* Pregnancy, complicated by
  varicose — *see* Varix
  von Recklinghausen's — *see* Neurofibromatosis
  vulva or perineum, in pregnancy or childbirth — *see* Pregnancy, complicated by
    causing obstructed labor O65.5
  Warthin's — *see* Neoplasm, salivary gland, benign
  Wilms' C64- ☑
  yolk sac — *see* Neoplasm, malignant, by site
    specified site — *see* Neoplasm, malignant, by site
    unspecified site
      female C56.9
      male C62.90
Tumor lysis syndrome (following antineoplastic chemotherapy) (spontaneous) NEC E88.3
Tumorlet — *see* Neoplasm, uncertain behavior, by site
Tungiasis B88.1
Tunica vasculosa lentis Q12.2
Turban tumor D23.4
Türck's trachoma J37.0
Turner-Kieser syndrome Q79.8
Turner-like syndrome Q87.1
Turner's
  hypoplasia (tooth) K00.4

☑ **Additional Character Required — Refer to the Tabular List for Character Selection**   ▽ **Subterms under main terms may continue to next column or page**

Turner's — *continued*
  syndrome Q96.9
    specified NEC Q96.8
  tooth K00.4
Turner-Ullrich syndrome Q96.9
Tussis convulsiva — *see* Whooping cough
Twiddler's syndrome (due to)
  automatic implantable defibrillatorT82.198
  cardiac pacemaker T82.198 ☑
Twilight state
  epileptic F05
  psychogenic F44.89
Twin (newborn) (*see also* Newborn, twin)
  conjoined Q89.4
  pregnancy — *see* Pregnancy, twin, conjoined
Twinning, teeth K00.2
Twist, twisted
  bowel, colon or intestine K56.2
  hair (congenital) Q84.1
  mesentery K56.2
  omentum K56.2
  organ or site, congenital NEC — *see* Anomaly, by site
  ovarian pedicle — *see* Torsion, ovary
Twitching R25.3
Tylosis (acquired) L84
  buccalis K13.29
  linguae K13.29
  palmaris et plantaris (congenital) (inherited) Q82.8
    acquired L85.1
Tympanism R14.0
Tympanites (abdominal) (intestinal) R14.0
Tympanitis — *see* Myringitis
Tympanosclerosis H74.0 ☑
Tympanum — *see* condition
Tympany
  abdomen R14.0
  chest R09.89
Type A behavior pattern Z73.1
Typhlitis — *see* Appendicitis
Typhoenteritis — *see* Typhoid
Typhoid (abortive) (ambulant) (any site) (clinical) (fever) (hemorrhagic) (infection) (intermittent) (malignant) (rheumatic) (Widal negative) A01.00
  with pneumonia A01.03
  abdominal A01.09
  arthritis A01.04
  carrier (suspected) of Z22.0
  cholecystitis (current) A01.09
  endocarditis A01.02
  heart involvement A01.02
  inoculation reaction — *see* Complications, vaccination
  meningitis A01.01
  mesenteric lymph nodes A01.09
  myocarditis A01.02
  osteomyelitis A01.05
  perichondritis, larynx A01.09
  pneumonia A01.03
  specified NEC A01.09
  spine A01.05
  ulcer (perforating) A01.09
Typhomalaria (fever) — *see* Malaria
Typhomania A01.00
Typhoperitonitis A01.09
Typhus (fever) A75.9
  abdominal, abdominalis — *see* Typhoid
  African tick A77.1
  amarillic A95.9
  brain A75.9 [G94]
  cerebral A75.9 [G94]
  classical A75.0
  due to Rickettsia
    prowazekii A75.0
      recrudescent A75.1
    tsutsugamushi A75.3
    typhi A75.2
  endemic (flea-borne) A75.2
  epidemic (louse-borne) A75.0
  exanthematicus SAI A75.0
    brilii SAI A75.1
    mexicanus SAI A75.2
    typhus murinus SAI A75.2
  exanthematic NEC A75.0
  flea-borne A75.2
  India tick A77.1
  Kenya (tick) A77.1
  louse-borne A75.0
  Mexican A75.2
  mite-borne A75.3

Typhus — *continued*
  murine A75.2
  North Asian tick-borne A77.2
  petechial A75.9
  Queensland tick A77.3
  rat A75.2
  recrudescent A75.1
  recurrens — *see* Fever, relapsing
  Sao Paulo A77.0
  scrub (China) (India) (Malaysia) (New Guinea) A75.3
  shop (of Malaysia) A75.2
  Siberian tick A77.2
  tick-borne A77.9
  tropical (mite-borne) A75.3
Tyrosinemia E70.21
  newborn, transitory P74.5
Tyrosinosis E70.21
Tyrosinuria E70.29

U

Uhl's anomaly or disease Q24.8
Ulcer, ulcerated, ulcerating, ulceration, ulcerative
  alveolar process M27.3
  amebic (intestine) A06.1
    skin A06.7
  anastomotic — *see* Ulcer, gastrojejunal
  anorectal K62.6
  antral — *see* Ulcer, stomach
  anus (sphincter) (solitary) K62.6
  aorta — *see* Aneurysm
  aphthous (oral) (recurrent) K12.0
    genital organ(s)
      female N76.6
      male N50.8
  artery I77.2
  atrophic — *see* Ulcer, skin
    decubitus — *see* Ulcer, pressure, by site
  back L98.429
    with
      bone necrosis L98.424
      exposed fat layer L98.422
      muscle necrosis L98.423
      skin breakdown only L98.421
  Barrett's (esophagus) K22.10
    with bleeding K22.11
  bile duct (common) (hepatic) K83.8
  bladder (solitary) (sphincter) NEC N32.89
    bilharzial B65.9 [N33]
    in schistosomiasis (bilharzial) B65.9 [N33]
    submucosal — *see* Cystitis, interstitial
    tuberculous A18.12
  bleeding K27.4
  bone — *see* Osteomyelitis, specified type NEC
  bowel — *see* Ulcer, intestine
  breast N61
  bronchus J98.09
  buccal (cavity) (traumatic) K12.1
  Buruli A31.1
  buttock L98.419
    with
      bone necrosis L98.414
      exposed fat layer L98.412
      muscle necrosis L98.413
      skin breakdown only L98.411
  cancerous — *see* Neoplasm, malignant, by site
  cardia K22.10
    with bleeding K22.11
  cardioesophageal (peptic) K22.10
    with bleeding K22.11
  cecum — *see* Ulcer, intestine
  cervix (uteri) (decubitus) (trophic) N86
    with cervicitis N72
  chancroidal A57
  chiclero B55.1
  chronic (cause unknown) — *see* Ulcer, skin
  Cochin-China B55.1
  colon — *see* Ulcer, intestine
  conjunctiva H10.89
  cornea H16.00- ☑
    with hypopyon H16.03- ☑
    central H16.01- ☑
    dendritic (herpes simplex) B00.52
    marginal H16.04- ☑
    Mooren's H16.05- ☑
    mycotic H16.06- ☑
    perforated H16.07- ☑

Ulcer, ulcerated, ulcerating, ulceration, ulcerative — *continued*
  cornea — *continued*
    ring H16.02- ☑
    tuberculous (phlyctenular) A18.52
  corpus cavernosum (chronic) N48.5
  crural — *see* Ulcer, lower limb
  Curling's — *see* Ulcer, peptic, acute
  Cushing's — *see* Ulcer, peptic, acute
  cystic duct K82.8
  cystitis (interstitial) — *see* Cystitis, interstitial
  decubitus — *see* Ulcer, pressure, by site
  dendritic, cornea (herpes simplex) B00.52
  diabetes, diabetic — *see* Diabetes, ulcer
  Dieulafoy's K25.0
  due to
    infection NEC — *see* Ulcer, skin
    radiation NEC L59.8
    trophic disturbance (any region) — *see* Ulcer, skin
    X-ray L58.1
  duodenum, duodenal (eroded) (peptic) K26.9
    with
      hemorrhage K26.4
        and perforation K26.6
      perforation K26.5
    acute K26.3
      with
        hemorrhage K26.0
          and perforation K26.2
        perforation K26.1
    chronic K26.7
      with
        hemorrhage K26.4
          and perforation K26.6
        perforation K26.5
  dysenteric A09
  elusive — *see* Cystitis, interstitial
  endocarditis (acute) (chronic) (subacute) I28.8
  epiglottis J38.7
  esophagus (peptic) K22.10
    with bleeding K22.11
    due to
      aspirin K22.10
        with bleeding K22.11
      gastrointestinal reflux disease K21.0
      ingestion of chemical or medicament K22.10
        with bleeding K22.11
      fungal K22.10
        with bleeding K22.11
      infective K22.10
        with bleeding K22.11
      varicose — *see* Varix, esophagus
  eyelid (region) H01.8
  fauces J39.2
  Fenwick (-Hunner) (solitary) — *see* Cystitis, interstitial
  fistulous — *see* Ulcer, skin
  foot (indolent) (trophic) — *see* Ulcer, lower limb
  frambesial, initial A66.0
  frenum (tongue) K14.0
  gallbladder or duct K82.8
  gangrenous — *see* Gangrene
  gastric — *see* Ulcer, stomach
  gastrocolic — *see* Ulcer, gastrojejunal
  gastroduodenal — *see* Ulcer, peptic
  gastroesophageal — *see* Ulcer, stomach
  gastrointestinal — *see* Ulcer, gastrojejunal
  gastrojejunal (peptic) K28.9
    with
      hemorrhage K28.4
        and perforation K28.6
      perforation K28.5
    acute K28.3
      with
        hemorrhage K28.0
          and perforation K28.2
        perforation K28.1
    chronic K28.7
      with
        hemorrhage K28.4
          and perforation K28.6
        perforation K28.5
  gastrojejunocolic — *see* Ulcer, gastrojejunal
  gingiva K06.8
  gingivitis K05.10
    nonplaque induced K05.11
    plaque induced K05.10
  glottis J38.7
  granuloma of pudenda A58

Ulcer, ulcerated, ulcerating, ulceration, ulcerative
  — continued
  gum K06.8
  gumma, due to yaws A66.4
  heel — see Ulcer, lower limb
  hemorrhoid (see also Hemorrhoids, by degree) K64.8
  Hunner's — see Cystitis, interstitial
  hypopharynx J39.2
  hypopyon (chronic) (subacute) — see Ulcer, cornea, with hypopyon
  hypostaticum — see Ulcer, varicose
  ileum — see Ulcer, intestine
  intestine, intestinal K63.3
    with perforation K63.1
    amebic A06.1
    duodenal — see Ulcer, duodenum
    granulocytopenic (with hemorrhage) — see Neutropenia
    marginal — see Ulcer, gastrojejunal
    perforating K63.1
      newborn P78.0
    primary, small intestine K63.3
    rectum K62.6
    stercoraceous, stercoral K63.3
    tuberculous A18.32
    typhoid (fever) — see Typhoid
    varicose I86.8
  jejunum, jejunal — see Ulcer, gastrojejunal
  keratitis — see Ulcer, cornea
  knee — see Ulcer, lower limb
  labium (majus) (minus) N76.6
  laryngitis — see Laryngitis
  larynx (aphthous) (contact) J38.7
    diphtheritic A36.2
  leg — see Ulcer, lower limb
  lip K13.0
  Lipschütz's N76.6
  lower limb (atrophic) (chronic) (neurogenic) (perforating) (pyogenic) (trophic) (tropical) L97.909
    with
      bone necrosis L97.904
      exposed fat layer L97.902
      muscle necrosis L97.903
      skin breakdown only L97.901
    ankle L97.309
      with
        bone necrosis L97.304
        exposed fat layer L97.302
        muscle necrosis L97.303
        skin breakdown only L97.301
      left L97.329
        with
          bone necrosis L97.324
          exposed fat layer L97.322
          muscle necrosis L97.323
          skin breakdown only L97.321
      right L97.319
        with
          bone necrosis L97.314
          exposed fat layer L97.312
          muscle necrosis L97.313
          skin breakdown only L97.311
    calf L97.209
      with
        bone necrosis L97.204
        exposed fat layer L97.202
        muscle necrosis L97.203
        skin breakdown only L97.201
      left L97.229
        with
          bone necrosis L97.224
          exposed fat layer L97.222
          muscle necrosis L97.223
          skin breakdown only L97.221
      right L97.219
        with
          bone necrosis L97.214
          exposed fat layer L97.212
          muscle necrosis L97.213
          skin breakdown only L97.211
    decubitus — see Ulcer, pressure, by site
    foot specified NEC L97.509
      with
        bone necrosis L97.504
        exposed fat layer L97.502
        muscle necrosis L97.503
        skin breakdown only L97.501
      left L97.529

Ulcer, ulcerated, ulcerating, ulceration, ulcerative
  — continued
  lower limb — continued
    foot specified — continued
      left — continued
        with
          bone necrosis L97.524
          exposed fat layer L97.522
          muscle necrosis L97.523
          skin breakdown only L97.521
      right L97.519
        with
          bone necrosis L97.514
          exposed fat layer L97.512
          muscle necrosis L97.513
          skin breakdown only L97.511
    heel L97.409
      with
        bone necrosis L97.404
        exposed fat layer L97.402
        muscle necrosis L97.403
        skin breakdown only L97.401
      left L97.429
        with
          bone necrosis L97.424
          exposed fat layer L97.422
          muscle necrosis L97.423
          skin breakdown only L97.421
      right L97.419
        with
          bone necrosis L97.414
          exposed fat layer L97.412
          muscle necrosis L97.413
          skin breakdown only L97.411
    left L97.929
      with
        bone necrosis L97.924
        exposed fat layer L97.922
        muscle necrosis L97.923
        skin breakdown only L97.921
    leprous A30.1
    lower leg NOS L97.909
      with
        bone necrosis L97.904
        exposed fat layer L97.902
        muscle necrosis L97.903
        skin breakdown only L97.901
      left L97.929
        with
          bone necrosis L97.924
          exposed fat layer L97.922
          muscle necrosis L97.923
          skin breakdown only L97.921
      right L97.919
        with
          bone necrosis L97.914
          exposed fat layer L97.912
          muscle necrosis L97.913
          skin breakdown only L97.911
    specified site NEC L97.809
      with
        bone necrosis L97.804
        exposed fat layer L97.802
        muscle necrosis L97.803
        skin breakdown only L97.801
      left L97.829
        with
          bone necrosis L97.824
          exposed fat layer L97.822
          muscle necrosis L97.823
          skin breakdown only L97.821
      right L97.819
        with
          bone necrosis L97.814
          exposed fat layer L97.812
          muscle necrosis L97.813
          skin breakdown only L97.811
    midfoot L97.409
      with
        bone necrosis L97.404
        exposed fat layer L97.402
        muscle necrosis L97.403
        skin breakdown only L97.401
      left L97.429
        with
          bone necrosis L97.424
          exposed fat layer L97.422
          muscle necrosis L97.423

Ulcer, ulcerated, ulcerating, ulceration, ulcerative
  — continued
  lower limb — continued
    midfoot — continued
      left — continued
        with — continued
          skin breakdown only L97.421
      right L97.419
        with
          bone necrosis L97.414
          exposed fat layer L97.412
          muscle necrosis L97.413
          skin breakdown only L97.411
    right L97.919
      with
        bone necrosis L97.914
        exposed fat layer L97.912
        muscle necrosis L97.913
        skin breakdown only L97.911
    syphilitic A52.19
    thigh L97.109
      with
        bone necrosis L97.104
        exposed fat layer L97.102
        muscle necrosis L97.103
        skin breakdown only L97.101
      left L97.129
        with
          bone necrosis L97.124
          exposed fat layer L97.122
          muscle necrosis L97.123
          skin breakdown only L97.121
      right L97.119
        with
          bone necrosis L97.114
          exposed fat layer L97.112
          muscle necrosis L97.113
          skin breakdown only L97.111
    toe L97.509
      with
        bone necrosis L97.504
        exposed fat layer L97.502
        muscle necrosis L97.503
        skin breakdown only L97.501
      left L97.529
        with
          bone necrosis L97.524
          exposed fat layer L97.522
          muscle necrosis L97.523
          skin breakdown only L97.521
      right L97.519
        with
          bone necrosis L97.514
          exposed fat layer L97.512
          muscle necrosis L97.513
          skin breakdown only L97.511
    varicose — see Varix, leg, with, ulcer
  luetic — see Ulcer, syphilitic
  lung J98.4
    tuberculous — see Tuberculosis, pulmonary
  malignant — see Neoplasm, malignant, by site
  marginal NEC — see Ulcer, gastrojejunal
  meatus (urinarius) N34.2
  Meckel's diverticulum Q43.0
    malignant — see Table of Neoplasms, small intestine, malignant
  Meleney's (chronic undermining) — see Ulcer, skin
  Mooren's (cornea) — see Ulcer, cornea, Mooren's
  mycobacterial (skin) A31.1
  nasopharynx J39.2
  neck, uterus N86
  neurogenic NEC — see Ulcer, skin
  nose, nasal (passage) (infective) (septum) J34.0
    skin — see Ulcer, skin
    spirochetal A69.8
    varicose (bleeding) I86.8
  oral mucosa (traumatic) K12.1
  palate (soft) K12.1
  penis (chronic) N48.5
  peptic (site unspecified) K27.9
    with
      hemorrhage K27.4
        and perforation K27.6
      perforation K27.5
    acute K27.3
      with
        hemorrhage K27.0
          and perforation K27.2

☑ **Additional Character Required** — Refer to the Tabular List for Character Selection   ⬇ **Subterms under main terms may continue to next column or page**

Ulcer, ulcerated, ulcerating, ulceration, ulcerative
— *continued*
peptic — *continued*
  acute — *continued*
    with — *continued*
      perforation K27.1
  chronic K27.7
    with
      hemorrhage K27.4
        and perforation K27.6
      perforation K27.5
  esophagus K22.10
    with bleeding K22.11
  newborn P78.82
perforating K27.5
  skin — *see* Ulcer, skin
peritonsillar J35.8
phagedenic (tropical) — *see* Ulcer, skin
pharynx J39.2
phlebitis — *see* Phlebitis
plaster — *see* Ulcer, pressure, by site
popliteal space — *see* Ulcer, lower limb
postpyloric — *see* Ulcer, duodenum
prepuce N47.7
prepyloric — *see* Ulcer, stomach
pressure (pressure area) L89.9- ☑
  ankle L89.5- ☑
  back L89.1- ☑
  buttock L89.3- ☑
  coccyx L89.15- ☑
  contiguous site of back, buttock, hip L89.4- ☑
  elbow L89.0- ☑
  face L89.81- ☑
  head L89.81- ☑
  heel L89.6- ☑
  hip L89.2- ☑
  sacral region (tailbone) L89.15- ☑
  specified site NEC L89.89- ☑
  stage 1 (healing) (pre-ulcer skin changes limited
    to persistent focal edema)
    ankle L89.5- ☑
    back L89.1- ☑
    buttock L89.3- ☑
    coccyx L89.15- ☑
    contiguous site of back, buttock, hip L89.4- ☑
    elbow L89.0- ☑
    face L89.81- ☑
    head L89.81- ☑
    heel L89.6- ☑
    hip L89.2- ☑
    sacral region (tailbone) L89.15- ☑
    specified site NEC L89.89- ☑
  stage 2 (healing) (abrasion, blister, partial thickness
    skin loss involving epidermis and/or dermis)
    ankle L89.5- ☑
    back L89.1- ☑
    buttock L89.3- ☑
    coccyx L89.15- ☑
    contiguous site of back, buttock, hip L89.4- ☑
    elbow L89.0- ☑
    face L89.81- ☑
    head L89.81- ☑
    heel L89.6- ☑
    hip L89.2- ☑
    sacral region (tailbone) L89.15- ☑
    specified site NEC L89.89- ☑
  stage 3 (healing) (full thickness skin loss involving
    damage or necrosis of subcutaneous tissue)
    ankle L89.5- ☑
    back L89.1- ☑
    buttock L89.3- ☑
    coccyx L89.15- ☑
    contiguous site of back, buttock, hip L89.4- ☑
    elbow L89.0- ☑
    face L89.81- ☑
    head L89.81- ☑
    heel L89.6- ☑
    hip L89.2- ☑
    sacral region (tailbone) L89.15- ☑
    specified site NEC L89.89- ☑
  stage 4 (healing) (necrosis of soft tissues through
    to underlying muscle, tendon, or bone)
    ankle L89.5- ☑
    back L89.1- ☑
    buttock L89.3- ☑
    coccyx L89.15- ☑

Ulcer, ulcerated, ulcerating, ulceration, ulcerative
— *continued*
pressure — *continued*
  stage 4 — *continued*
    contiguous site of back, buttock, hip L89.4- ☑
    elbow L89.0- ☑
    face L89.81- ☑
    head L89.81- ☑
    heel L89.6- ☑
    hip L89.2- ☑
    sacral region (tailbone) L89.15- ☑
    specified site NEC L89.89- ☑
  unspecified stage
    ankle L89.5- ☑
    back L89.1- ☑
    buttock L89.3- ☑
    coccyx L89.15- ☑
    contiguous site of back, buttock, hip L89.4- ☑
    elbow L89.0- ☑
    face L89.81- ☑
    head L89.81- ☑
    heel L89.6- ☑
    hip L89.2- ☑
    sacral region (tailbone) L89.15- ☑
    specified site NEC L89.89- ☑
  unstageable
    ankle L89.5- ☑
    back L89.1- ☑
    buttock L89.3- ☑
    coccyx L89.15- ☑
    contiguous site of back, buttock, hip L89.4- ☑
    elbow L89.0- ☑
    face L89.81- ☑
    head L89.81- ☑
    heel L89.6- ☑
    hip L89.2- ☑
    sacral region (tailbone) L89.15- ☑
    specified site NEC L89.89- ☑
  primary of intestine K63.3
    with perforation K63.1
prostate N41.9
pyloric — *see* Ulcer, stomach
rectosigmoid K63.3
  with perforation K63.1
rectum (sphincter) (solitary) K62.6
  stercoraceous, stercoral K62.6
retina — *see* Inflammation, chorioretinal
rodent (*see also* Neoplasm, skin, malignant)
sclera — *see* Scleritis
scrofulous (tuberculous) A18.2
scrotum N50.8
  tuberculous A18.15
  varicose I86.1
seminal vesicle N50.8
sigmoid — *see* Ulcer, intestine
skin (atrophic) (chronic) (neurogenic) (non-healing)
  (perforating) (pyogenic) (trophic) (tropical)
  L98.499
  with gangrene — *see* Gangrene
  amebic A06.7
  back — *see* Ulcer, back
  buttock — *see* Ulcer, buttock
  decubitus — *see* Ulcer, pressure
  lower limb — *see* Ulcer, lower limb
  mycobacterial A31.1
  specified site NEC L98.499
    with
      bone necrosis L98.494
      exposed fat layer L98.492
      muscle necrosis L98.493
      skin breakdown only L98.491
  tuberculous (primary) A18.4
  varicose — *see* Ulcer, varicose
sloughing — *see* Ulcer, skin
solitary, anus or rectum (sphincter) K62.6
sore throat J02.9
  streptococcal J02.0
spermatic cord N50.8
spine (tuberculous) A18.01
stasis (venous) — *see* Varix, leg, with, ulcer
  without varicose veins I87.2
stercoraceous, stercoral K63.3
  with perforation K63.1
  anus or rectum K62.6
stoma, stomal — *see* Ulcer, gastrojejunal
stomach (eroded) (peptic) (round) K25.9
  with

Ulcer, ulcerated, ulcerating, ulceration, ulcerative
— *continued*
stomach — *continued*
  with — *continued*
    hemorrhage K25.4
      and perforation K25.6
    perforation K25.5
  acute K25.3
    with
      hemorrhage K25.0
        and perforation K25.2
      perforation K25.1
  chronic K25.7
    with
      hemorrhage K25.4
        and perforation K25.6
      perforation K25.5
stomal — *see* Ulcer, gastrojejunal
stomatitis K12.1
stress — *see* Ulcer, peptic
strumous (tuberculous) A18.2
submucosal, bladder — *see* Cystitis, interstitial
syphilitic (any site) (early) (secondary) A51.39
  late A52.79
    perforating A52.79
      foot A52.11
testis N50.8
thigh — *see* Ulcer, lower limb
throat J39.2
  diphtheritic A36.0
toe — *see* Ulcer, lower limb
tongue (traumatic) K14.0
tonsil J35.8
  diphtheritic A36.0
trachea J39.8
trophic — *see* Ulcer, skin
tropical — *see* Ulcer, skin
tuberculous — *see* Tuberculosis, ulcer
tunica vaginalis N50.8
turbinate J34.89
typhoid (perforating) — *see* Typhoid
unspecified site — *see* Ulcer, skin
urethra (meatus) — *see* Urethritis
uterus N85.8
  cervix N86
    with cervicitis N72
  neck N86
    with cervicitis N72
vagina N76.5
  in Behçet's disease M35.2 [N77.0]
  pessary N89.8
valve, heart I33.0
varicose (lower limb, any part) (*see also* Varix, leg, with,
  ulcer)
  broad ligament I86.2
  esophagus — *see* Varix, esophagus
  inflamed or infected — *see* Varix, leg, with ulcer,
    with inflammation
  nasal septum I86.8
  perineum I86.3
  scrotum I86.1
  specified site NEC I86.8
  sublingual I86.0
  vulva I86.3
vas deferens N50.8
vulva (acute) (infectional) N76.6
  in (due to)
    Behçet's disease M35.2 [N77.0]
    herpesviral (herpes simplex) infection A60.04
    tuberculosis A18.18
vulvobuccal, recurring N76.6
X-ray L58.1
yaws A66.4
Ulcerosa scarlatina A38.8
Ulcus (*see also* Ulcer)
cutis tuberculosum A18.4
duodeni — *see* Ulcer, duodenum
durum (syphilitic) A51.0
  extragenital A51.2
gastrojejunale — *see* Ulcer, gastrojejunal
hypostaticum — *see* Ulcer, varicose
molle (cutis) (skin) A57
serpens corneae — *see* Ulcer, cornea, central
ventriculi — *see* Ulcer, stomach
Ulegyria Q04.8
Ulerythema
ophryogenes, congenital Q84.2
sycosiforme L73.8

Ullrich (-Bonnevie)(-Turner) **syndrome** Q87.1
Ullrich-Feichtiger syndrome Q87.0
Ulnar — *see* condition
Ulorrhagia, ulorrhea K06.8
Umbilicus, umbilical — *see* condition
Unacceptable
    contours of tooth K08.54
    morphology of tooth K08.54
Unavailability (of)
    bed at medical facility Z75.1
    health service-related agencies Z75.4
    medical facilities (at) Z75.3
        due to
            investigation by social service agency Z75.2
            lack of services at home Z75.0
            remoteness from facility Z75.3
                waiting list Z75.1
        home Z75.0
        outpatient clinic Z75.3
    schooling Z55.1
    social service agencies Z75.4
Uncinaria americana infestation B76.1
Uncinariasis B76.9
Uncongenial work Z56.5
Unconscious (ness) — *see* Coma
Under observation — *see* Observation
Underachievement in school Z55.3
Underdevelopment (*see also* Undeveloped)
    nose Q30.1
    sexual E30.0
Underdosing (*see also* Table of Drugs and Chemicals,
        categories T36-T50, with final character 6) Z91.14
    intentional NEC Z91.128
        due to financial hardship of patient Z91.120
    unintentional NEC Z91.138
        due to patient's age related debility Z91.130
Underfeeding, newborn P92.3
Underfill, endodontic M27.53
Underimmunization status Z28.3
Undernourishment — *see* Malnutrition
Undernutrition — *see* Malnutrition
Underweight R63.6
    for gestational age — *see* Light for dates
Underwood's disease P83.0
Undescended (*see also* Malposition, congenital)
    cecum Q43.3
    colon Q43.3
    testicle — *see* Cryptorchid
Undeveloped, undevelopment (*see also* Hypoplasia)
    brain (congenital) Q02
    cerebral (congenital) Q02
    heart Q24.8
    lung Q33.6
    testis E29.1
    uterus E30.0
Undiagnosed (disease) R69
Undulant fever — *see* Brucellosis
Unemployment, anxiety concerning Z56.0
    threatened Z56.2
Unequal length (acquired) (limb) (*see also* Deformity,
        limb, unequal length)
    leg (*see also* Deformity, limb, unequal length)
        congenital Q72.9- ☑
Unextracted dental root K08.3
Unguis incarnatus L60.0
Unhappiness R45.2
Unhealthy lifestyle Z72.9
Unicornate uterus Q51.4
Unilateral (*see also* condition)
    development, breast N64.89
    organ or site, congenital NEC — *see* Agenesis, by site
Unilocular heart Q20.8
Union, abnormal (*see also* Fusion)
    larynx and trachea Q34.8
Universal mesentery Q43.3
**Unrepairable overhanging of dental restorative
        materials** K08.52
Unsatisfactory
    restoration of tooth K08.50
        specified NEC K08.59
    sample of cytologic smear
        anus R85.615
        cervix R87.615
        vagina R87.625
    surroundings Z59.1
        work Z56.5
Unsoundness of mind — *see* Psychosis

Unstable
    back NEC — *see* Instability, joint, spine
    hip (congenital) Q65.6
        acquired — *see* Derangement, joint, specified type
            NEC, hip
    joint — *see* Instability, joint
        secondary to removal of joint prosthesis M96.89
    lie (mother) O32.0 ☑
    lumbosacral joint (congenital)
        acquired — *see* subcategory M53.2 ☑
    sacroiliac — *see* subcategory M53.2 ☑
    spine NEC — *see* Instability, joint, spine
Unsteadiness on feet R26.81
Untruthfulness, child problem F91.8
Unverricht (-Lundborg) **disease or epilepsy** — *see*
        Epilepsy, generalized, idiopathic
Unwanted pregnancy Z64.0
Upbringing, institutional Z62.22
    away from parents NEC Z62.29
    in care of non-parental family member Z62.21
    in foster care Z62.21
    in orphanage or group home Z62.22
    in welfare custody Z62.21
Upper respiratory — *see* condition
Upset
    gastric K30
    gastrointestinal K30
        psychogenic F45.8
    intestinal (large) (small) K59.9
        psychogenic F45.8
    menstruation N93.9
    mental F48.9
    stomach K30
        psychogenic F45.8
Urachus (*see also* condition)
    patent or persistent Q64.4
Urbach-Oppenheim disease (necrobiosis lipoidica dia-
        beticorum) — *see* E08-E13 with .620
Urbach's lipoid proteinosis E78.89
Urbach-Wiethe disease E78.89
Urban yellow fever A95.1
Urea
    blood, high — *see* Uremia
    cycle metabolism disorder — *see* Disorder, urea cycle
        metabolism
Uremia, uremic N19
    with
        ectopic or molar pregnancy O08.4
        polyneuropathy N18.9 [G63]
    chronic (*see also* Disease, kidney, chronic) N18.9
        due to hypertension — *see* Hypertensive, kidney
    complicating
        ectopic or molar pregnancy O08.4
    congenital P96.0
    extrarenal R39.2
    following ectopic or molar pregnancy O08.4
    newborn P96.0
    prerenal R39.2
Ureter, ureteral — *see* condition
Ureteralgia N23
Ureterectasis — *see* Hydroureter
Ureteritis N28.89
    cystica N28.86
    due to calculus N20.1
        with calculus, kidney N20.2
            with hydronephrosis N13.2
    gonococcal (acute) (chronic) A54.21
    nonspecific N28.89
Ureterocele N28.89
    congenital (orthotopic) Q62.31
        ectopic Q62.32
Ureterolith, ureterolithiasis — *see* Calculus, ureter
Ureterostomy
    attention to Z43.6
    status Z93.6
Urethra, urethral — *see* condition
Urethralgia R39.89
Urethritis (anterior) (posterior) N34.2
    calculous N21.1
    candidal B37.41
    chlamydial A56.01
    diplococcal (gonococcal) A54.01
        with abscess (accessory gland) (periurethral) A54.1
    gonococcal A54.01
        with abscess (accessory gland) (periurethral) A54.1
    nongonococcal N34.1
        Reiter's — *see* Reiter's disease

Urethritis — *continued*
    nonspecific N34.1
    nonvenereal N34.1
    postmenopausal N34.2
    puerperal O86.22
    Reiter's — *see* Reiter's disease
    specified NEC N34.2
    trichomonal or due to Trichomonas (vaginalis) A59.03
Urethrocele N81.0
    with
        cystocele — *see* Cystocele
        prolapse of uterus — *see* Prolapse, uterus
Urethrolithiasis (with colic or infection) N21.1
Urethrorectal — *see* condition
Urethrorrhagia N36.8
Urethrorrhea R36.9
Urethrostomy
    attention to Z43.6
    status Z93.6
Urethrotrigonitis — *see* Trigonitis
Urethrovaginal — *see* condition
Urgency
    fecal R15.2
    hypertensive — *see* Hypertension
    urinary N39.41
Urhidrosis, uridrosis L74.8
Uric acid in blood (increased) E79.0
Uricacidemia (asymptomatic) E79.0
Uricemia (asymptomatic) E79.0
Uricosuria R82.99
Urinary — *see* condition
Urination
    frequent R35.0
    painful R30.9
Urine
    blood in — *see* Hematuria
    discharge, excessive R35.8
    enuresis, nonorganic origin F98.0
    extravasation R39.0
    frequency R35.0
    incontinence R32
        nonorganic origin F98.0
    intermittent stream R39.19
    pus in N39.0
    retention or stasis R33.9
        organic R33.8
            drug-induced R33.0
        psychogenic F45.8
    secretion
        deficient R34
        excessive R35.8
        frequency R35.0
    stream
        intermittent R39.19
        slowing R39.19
        splitting R39.13
        weak R39.12
Urinemia — *see* Uremia
Urinoma, urethra N36.8
Uroarthritis, infectious (Reiter's) — *see* Reiter's disease
Urodialysis R34
Urolithiasis — *see* Calculus, urinary
Uronephrosis — *see* Hydronephrosis
Uropathy N39.9
    obstructive N13.9
        specified NEC N13.8
    reflux N13.9
        specified NEC N13.8
    vesicoureteral reflux-associated — *see* Reflux, vesi-
        coureteral
Urosepsis — *code to* condition
Urticaria L50.9
    with angioneurotic edema T78.3 ☑
        hereditary D84.1
    allergic L50.0
    cholinergic L50.5
    chronic L50.8
    cold, familial L50.2
    contact L50.6
    dermatographic L50.3
    due to
        cold or heat L50.2
        drugs L50.0
        food L50.0
        inhalants L50.0
        plants L50.6
        serum (*see also* Reaction, serum) T80.69 ☑

☑ **Additional Character Required** — Refer to the Tabular List for Character Selection   ▽ **Subterms under main terms may continue to next column or page**

Urticaria — *continued*
  factitial L50.3
  giant T78.3 ☑
    hereditary D84.1
  gigantea T78.3 ☑
  idiopathic L50.1
  larynx T78.3 ☑
    hereditary D84.1
  neonatorum P83.8
  nonallergic L50.1
  papulosa (Hebra) L28.2
  pigmentosa Q82.2
  recurrent periodic L50.8
  serum (*see also* Reaction, serum) T80.69 ☑
  solar L56.3
  specified type NEC L50.8
  thermal (cold) (heat) L50.2
  vibratory L50.4
  xanthelasmoidea Q82.2
Use (of)
  alcohol F10.99
    with sleep disorder F10.982
    harmful — *see* Abuse, alcohol
  amphetamines — *see* Use, stimulant NEC
  caffeine — *see* Use, stimulant NEC
  cannabis F12.90
    with
      anxiety disorder F12.980
      intoxication F12.929
        with
          delirium F12.921
          perceptual disturbance F12.922
        uncomplicated F12.920
      other specified disorder F12.988
      psychosis F12.959
        delusions F12.950
        hallucinations F12.951
      unspecified disorder F12.99
  cocaine F14.90
    with
      anxiety disorder F14.980
      intoxication F14.929
        with
          delirium F14.921
          perceptual disturbance F14.922
        uncomplicated F14.920
      other specified disorder F14.988
      psychosis F14.959
        delusions F14.950
        hallucinations F14.951
      sexual dysfunction F14.981
      sleep disorder F14.982
      unspecified disorder F14.99
    harmful — *see* Abuse, drug, cocaine
  drug(s) NEC F19.90
    with sleep disorder F19.982
    harmful — *see* Abuse, drug, by type
  hallucinogen NEC F16.90
    with
      anxiety disorder F16.980
      intoxication F16.929
        with
          delirium F16.921
        uncomplicated F16.920
      mood disorder F16.94
      other specified disorder F16.988
      perception disorder (flashbacks) F16.983
      psychosis F16.959
        delusions F16.950
        hallucinations F16.951
      unspecified disorder F16.99
    harmful — *see* Abuse, drug, hallucinogen NEC
  inhalants F18.90
    with
      anxiety disorder F18.980
      intoxication F18.929
        with delirium F18.921
        uncomplicated F18.920
      mood disorder F18.94
      other specified disorder F18.988
      persisting dementia F18.97
      psychosis F18.959
        delusions F18.950
        hallucinations F18.951
      unspecified disorder F18.99
    harmful — *see* Abuse, drug, inhalant
  methadone F11.20

Use — *continued*
  nonprescribed drugs F19.90
    harmful — *see* Abuse, non-psychoactive substance
  opioid F11.90
    with
      disorder F11.99
        mood F11.94
        sleep F11.982
        specified type NEC F11.988
      intoxication F11.929
        with
          delirium F11.921
          perceptual disturbance F11.922
        uncomplicated F11.920
      withdrawal F11.93
    harmful — *see* Abuse, drug, opioid
  patent medicines F19.90
    harmful — *see* Abuse, non-psychoactive substance
  psychoactive drug NEC F19.90
    with
      anxiety disorder F19.980
      intoxication F19.929
        with
          delirium F19.921
          perceptual disturbance F19.922
        uncomplicated F19.920
      mood disorder F19.94
      other specified disorder F19.988
      persisting
        amnestic disorder F19.96
        dementia F19.97
      psychosis F19.959
        delusions F19.950
        hallucinations F19.951
      sexual dysfunction F19.981
      sleep disorder F19.982
      unspecified disorder F19.99
      withdrawal F19.939
        with
          delirium F19.931
          perceptual disturbance F19.932
        uncomplicated F19.930
    harmful — *see* Abuse, drug NEC, psychoactive NEC
  sedative, hypnotic, or anxiolytic F13.90
    with
      anxiety disorder F13.980
      intoxication F13.929
        with
          delirium F13.921
        uncomplicated F13.920
      other specified disorder F13.988
      persisting
        amnestic disorder F13.96
        dementia F13.97
      psychosis F13.959
        delusions F13.950
        hallucinations F13.951
      sexual dysfunction F13.981
      sleep disorder F13.982
      unspecified disorder F13.99
    harmful — *see* Abuse, drug, sedative, hypnotic, or anxiolytic
  stimulant NEC F15.90
    with
      anxiety disorder F15.980
      intoxication F15.929
        with
          delirium F15.921
          perceptual disturbance F15.922
        uncomplicated F15.920
      mood disorder F15.94
      other specified disorder F15.988
      psychosis F15.959
        delusions F15.950
        hallucinations F15.951
      sexual dysfunction F15.981
      sleep disorder F15.982
      unspecified disorder F15.99
      withdrawal F15.93
    harmful — *see* Abuse, drug, stimulant NEC
  tobacco Z72.0
    with dependence — *see* Dependence, drug, nicotine
  volatile solvents (*see also* Use, inhalant) F18.90
    harmful — *see* Abuse, drug, inhalant
Usher-Senear disease or syndrome L10.4
Uta B55.1
Uteromegaly N85.2

Uterovaginal — *see* condition
Uterovesical — *see* condition
Uveal — *see* condition
Uveitis (anterior) (*see also* Iridocyclitis)
  acute — *see* Iridocyclitis, acute
  chronic — *see* Iridocyclitis, chronic
  due to toxoplasmosis (acquired) B58.09
    congenital P37.1
  granulomatous — *see* Iridocyclitis, chronic
  heterochromic — *see* Cyclitis, Fuchs' heterochromic
  lens-induced — *see* Iridocyclitis, lens-induced
  posterior — *see* Chorioretinitis
  sympathetic H44.13- ☑
  syphilitic (secondary) A51.43
    congenital (early) A50.01
    late A52.71
  tuberculous A18.54
Uveoencephalitis — *see* Inflammation, chorioretinal
Uveokeratitis — *see* Iridocyclitis
Uveoparotitis D86.89
Uvula — *see* condition
Uvulitis (acute) (catarrhal) (chronic) (membranous) (suppurative) (ulcerative) K12.2

V

Vaccination (prophylactic)
  complication or reaction — *see* Complications, vaccination
  delayed Z28.9
  encounter for Z23
  not done — *see* Immunization, not done, because (of)
Vaccinia (generalized) (localized) T88.1 ☑
  without vaccination B08.011
  congenital P35.8
Vacuum, in sinus (accessory) (nasal) J34.89
Vagabond, vagabondage Z59.0
Vagabond's disease B85.1
Vagina, vaginal — *see* condition
Vaginalitis (tunica) (testis) N49.1
Vaginismus (reflex) N94.2
  functional F52.5
  nonorganic F52.5
  psychogenic F52.5
  secondary N94.2
Vaginitis (acute) (circumscribed) (diffuse) (emphysematous) (nonvenereal) (ulcerative) N76.0
  with ectopic or molar pregnancy O08.0
  ambic A06.82
  atrophic, postmenopausal N95.2
  bacterial N76.0
  blennorrhagic (gonococcal) A54.02
  candidal B37.3
  chlamydial A56.02
  chronic N76.1
  due to Trichomonas (vaginalis) A59.01
  following ectopic or molar pregnancy O08.0
  gonococcal A54.02
    with abscess (accessory gland) (periurethral) A54.1
  granuloma A58
  in (due to)
    candidiasis B37.3
    herpesviral (herpes simplex) infection A60.04
    pinworm infection B80 [N77.1]
  monilial B37.3
  mycotic (candidal) B37.3
  postmenopausal atrophic N95.2
  puerperal (postpartum) O86.13
  senile (atrophic) N95.2
  subacute or chronic N76.1
  syphilitic (early) A51.0
    late A52.76
  trichomonal A59.01
  tuberculous A18.18
Vaginosis — *see* Vaginitis
Vagotonia G52.2
Vagrancy Z59.0
VAIN — *see* Neoplasia, intraepithelial, vagina
Vallecula — *see* condition
Valley fever B38.0
Valsuani's disease — *see* Anemia, obstetric
Valve, valvular (formation) (*see also* condition)
  cerebral ventricle (communicating) in situ Z98.2
  cervix, internal os Q51.828
  congenital NEC — *see* Atresia, by site
  ureter (pelvic junction) (vesical orifice) Q62.39
  urethra (congenital) (posterior) Q64.2

Valvulitis (chronic) — *see* Endocarditis
Valvulopathy — *see* Endocarditis
Van Bogaert's leukoencephalopathy (sclerosing) (subacute) A81.1
Van Bogaert-Scherer-Epstein disease or syndrome E75.5
Van Buchem's syndrome M85.2
Van Creveld-von Gierke disease E74.01
Van der Hoeve (-de Kleyn) **syndrome** Q78.0
Van der Woude's syndrome Q38.0
Van Neck's disease or osteochondrosis M91.0
Vanishing lung J44.9
Vapor asphyxia or suffocation T59.9 ☑
   specified agent — *see* Table of Drugs and Chemicals
Variance, lethal ball, prosthetic heart valve T82.09 ☑
Variants, thalassemic D56.8
Variations in hair color L67.1
Varicella B01.9
   with
      complications NEC B01.89
      encephalitis B01.11
      encephalomyelitis B01.11
      meningitis B01.0
      myelitis B01.12
      pneumonia B01.2
   congenital P35.8
Varices — *see* Varix
Varicocele (scrotum) (thrombosed) I86.1
   ovary I86.2
   perineum I86.3
   spermatic cord (ulcerated) I86.1
Varicose
   aneurysm (ruptured) I77.0
   dermatitis — *see* Varix, leg, with, inflammation
   eczema — *see* Varix, leg, with, inflammation
   phlebitis — *see* Varix, with, inflammation
   tumor — *see* Varix
   ulcer (lower limb, any part) (*see also* Varix, leg, with, ulcer)
      anus (*see also* Hemorrhoids) K64.8
      esophagus — *see* Varix, esophagus
      inflamed or infected — *see* Varix, leg, with ulcer, with inflammation
      nasal septum I86.8
      perineum I86.3
      scrotum I86.1
      specified site NEC I86.8
   vein — *see* Varix
   vessel — *see* Varix, leg
Varicosis, varicosities, varicosity — *see* Varix
Variola (major) (minor) B03
Varioloid B03
Varix (lower limb) (ruptured) I83.90
   with
      edema I83.899
      inflammation I83.10
         with ulcer (venous) I83.209
      pain I83.819
      specified complication NEC I83.899
      stasis dermatitis I83.10
         with ulcer (venous) I83.209
      swelling I83.899
      ulcer I83.009
         with inflammation I83.209
   aneurysmal I77.0
   asymptomatic I83.9- ☑
   bladder I86.2
   broad ligament I86.2
   complicating
      childbirth (lower extremity) O87.4
         anus or rectum O87.2
         genital (vagina, vulva or perineum) O87.8
      pregnancy (lower extremity) O22.0- ☑
         anus or rectum O22.4- ☑
         genital (vagina, vulva or perineum) O22.1- ☑
      puerperium (lower extremity) O87.4
         anus or rectum O87.2
         genital (vagina, vulva, perineum) O87.8
   congenital (any site) Q27.8
   esophagus (idiopathic) (primary) (ulcerated) I85.00
      bleeding I85.01
      congenital Q27.8
      in (due to)
         alcoholic liver disease I85.10
            bleeding I85.11
         cirrhosis of liver I85.10
            bleeding I85.11

Varix — *continued*
   esophagus — *continued*
      in — *continued*
         portal hypertension I85.10
            bleeding I85.11
         schistosomiasis I85.10
            bleeding I85.11
         toxic liver disease I85.10
            bleeding I85.11
      secondary I85.10
         bleeding I85.11
   gastric I86.4
   inflamed or infected I83.10
      ulcerated I83.209
   labia (majora) I86.3
   leg (asymptomatic) I83.90
      with
         edema I83.899
         inflammation I83.10
            with ulcer — *see* Varix, leg, with, ulcer, with inflammation by site
         pain I83.819
         specified complication NEC I83.899
         swelling I83.899
         ulcer I83.009
            with inflammation I83.209
            ankle I83.003
               with inflammation I83.203
            calf I83.002
               with inflammation I83.202
            foot NEC I83.005
               with inflammation I83.205
            heel I83.004
               with inflammation I83.204
            lower leg NEC I83.008
               with inflammation I83.208
            midfoot I83.004
               with inflammation I83.204
            thigh I83.001
               with inflammation I83.201
      bilateral (asymptomatic) I83.93
        with
           edema I83.893
           pain I83.813
           specified complication NEC I83.893
           swelling I83.893
           ulcer I83.009
             with inflammation I83.209
      left (asymptomatic) I83.92
        with
           edema I83.892
           inflammation I83.12
             with ulcer — *see* Varix, leg, with, ulcer, with inflammation by site
           pain I83.812
           specified complication NEC I83.892
           swelling I83.892
           ulcer I83.029
             with inflammation I83.229
             ankle I83.023
               with inflammation I83.223
             calf I83.022
               with inflammation I83.222
             foot NEC I83.025
               with inflammation I83.225
             heel I83.024
               with inflammation I83.224
             lower leg NEC I83.028
               with inflammation I83.228
             midfoot I83.024
               with inflammation I83.224
             thigh I83.021
               with inflammation I83.221
      right (asymptomatic) I83.91
        with
           edema I83.891
           inflammation I83.11
             with ulcer — *see* Varix, leg, with, ulcer, with inflammation by site
           pain I83.811
           specified complication NEC I83.891
           swelling I83.891
           ulcer I83.019
             with inflammation I83.219
             ankle I83.013
               with inflammation I83.213
             calf I83.012
               with inflammation I83.212

Varix — *continued*
   leg — *continued*
      right — *continued*
         with — *continued*
           ulcer — *continued*
             foot NEC I83.015
               with inflammation I83.215
             heel I83.014
               with inflammation I83.214
             lower leg NEC I83.018
               with inflammation I83.218
             midfoot I83.014
               with inflammation I83.214
             thigh I83.011
               with inflammation I83.211
   nasal septum I86.8
   orbit I86.8
      congenital Q27.8
   ovary I86.2
   papillary I78.1
   pelvis I86.2
   perineum I86.3
   pharynx I86.8
   placenta O43.89- ☑
   renal papilla I86.8
   retina H35.09
   scrotum (ulcerated) I86.1
   sigmoid colon I86.8
   specified site NEC I86.8
   spinal (cord) (vessels) I86.8
   spleen, splenic (vein) (with phlebolith) I86.8
   stomach I86.4
   sublingual I86.0
   ulcerated I83.009
      inflamed or infected I83.209
   uterine ligament I86.2
   vagina I86.8
   vocal cord I86.8
   vulva I86.3
Vas deferens — *see* condition
Vas deferentitis N49.1
Vasa previa O69.4 ☑
   hemorrhage from, affecting newborn P50.0
Vascular (*see also* condition)
   loop on optic papilla Q14.2
   spasm I73.9
   spider I78.1
Vascularization, cornea — *see* Neovascularization, cornea
Vasculitis I77.6
   allergic D69.0
   cryoglobulinemic D89.1
   disseminated I77.6
   hypocomplementemic M31.8
   kidney I77.89
   livedoid L95.0
   nodular L95.8
   retina H35.06- ☑
   rheumatic — *see* Fever, rheumatic
   rheumatoid — *see* Rheumatoid, vasculitis
   skin (limited to) L95.9
      specified NEC L95.8
Vasculopathy, necrotizing M31.9
   cardiac allograft T86.290
   specified NEC M31.8
Vasitis (nodosa) N49.1
   tuberculous A18.15
Vasodilation I73.9
Vasomotor — *see* condition
Vasoplasty, after previous sterilization Z31.0
   aftercare Z31.42
Vasospasm (vasoconstriction) I73.9
   cerebral (cerebrovascular) (artery) I67.848
      reversible I67.841
   coronary I20.1
   nerve
      arm — *see* Mononeuropathy, upper limb
      brachial plexus G54.0
      cervical plexus G54.2
      leg — *see* Mononeuropathy, lower limb
      peripheral NOS I73.9
   retina (artery) — *see* Occlusion, artery, retina
Vasospastic — *see* condition
Vasovagal attack (paroxysmal) R55
   psychogenic F45.8
VATER syndrome Q87.2
Vater's ampulla — *see* condition

☑ Additional Character Required — Refer to the Tabular List for Character Selection   ▽ Subterms under main terms may continue to next column or page

Vegetation, vegetative
  adenoid (nasal fossa) J35.8
  endocarditis (acute) (any valve) (subacute) I33.0
  heart (mycotic) (valve) I33.0
Veil
  Jackson's Q43.3
Vein, venous — *see* condition
Veldt sore — *see* Ulcer, skin
Velpeau's hernia — *see* Hernia, femoral
Venereal
  bubo A55
  disease A64
  granuloma inguinale A58
  lymphogranuloma (Durand-Nicolas-Favre) A55
Venofibrosis I87.8
Venom, venomous — *see* Table of Drugs and Chemicals, by animal or substance, poisoning
Venous — *see* condition
Ventilator lung, newborn P27.8
Ventral — *see* condition
Ventricle, ventricular (*see also* condition)
  escape I49.3
  inversion Q20.5
Ventriculitis (cerebral) (*see also* Encephalitis) G04.90
Ventriculostomy status Z98.2
Vernet's syndrome G52.7
Verneuil's disease (syphilitic bursitis) A52.78
Verruca (due to HPV) (filiformis) (simplex) (viral) (vulgaris) B07.9
  acuminata A63.0
  necrogenica (primary) (tuberculosa) A18.4
  plana B07.8
  plantaris B07.0
  seborrheica L82.1
    inflamed L82.0
  senile (seborrheic) L82.1
    inflamed L82.0
  tuberculosa (primary) A18.4
  venereal A63.0
Verrucosities — *see* Verruca
Verruga peruana, peruviana A44.1
Version
  with extraction
  cervix — *see* Malposition, uterus
  uterus (postinfectional) (postpartal, old) — *see* Malposition, uterus
Vertebra, vertebral — *see* condition
Vertical talus (congenital) Q66.80
  left foot Q66.82
  right foot Q66.81
Vertigo R42
  auditory — *see* Vertigo, aural
  aural H81.31- ☑
  benign paroxysmal (positional) H81.1- ☑
  central (origin) H81.4- ☑
  cerebral H81.4- ☑
  Dix and Hallpike (epidemic) — *see* Neuronitis, vestibular
  due to infrasound T75.23 ☑
  epidemic A88.1
    Dix and Hallpike — *see* Neuronitis, vestibular
    Pedersen's — *see* Neuronitis, vestibular
    vestibular neuronitis — *see* Neuronitis, vestibular
  hysterical F44.89
  infrasound T75.23 ☑
  labyrinthine — *see* subcategory H81.0 ☑
  laryngeal R05
  malignant positional H81.4- ☑
  Ménière's — *see* subcategory H81.0 ☑
  menopausal N95.1
  otogenic — *see* Vertigo, aural
  paroxysmal positional, benign — *see* Vertigo, benign paroxysmal
  Pedersen's (epidemic) — *see* Neuronitis, vestibular
  peripheral NEC H81.39- ☑
  positional
    benign paroxysmal — *see* Vertigo, benign paroxysmal
    malignant H81.4- ☑
Very-low-density-lipoprotein-type (VLDL) **hyperlipoproteinemia** E78.1
Vesania — *see* Psychosis
Vesical — *see* condition
Vesicle
  cutaneous R23.8
  seminal — *see* condition
  skin R23.8

Vesicocolic — *see* condition
Vesicoperineal — *see* condition
Vesicorectal — *see* condition
Vesicourethrorectal — *see* condition
Vesicovaginal — *see* condition
Vesicular — *see* condition
Vesiculitis (seminal) N49.0
  amebic A06.82
  gonorrheal (acute) (chronic) A54.23
  trichomonal A59.09
  tuberculous A18.15
Vestibulitis (ear) (*see also* subcategory) H83.0 ☑
  nose (external) J34.89
  vulvar N94.810
Vestibulopathy , acute peripheral (recurrent) — *see* Neuronitis, vestibular
Vestige, vestigial (*see also* Persistence)
  branchial Q18.0
  structures in vitreous Q14.0
Vibration
  adverse effects T75.20 ☑
    pneumatic hammer syndrome T75.21 ☑
    specified effect NEC T75.29 ☑
    vasospastic syndrome T75.22 ☑
    vertigo from infrasound T75.23 ☑
  exposure (occupational) Z57.7
  vertigo T75.23 ☑
Vibriosis A28.9
Victim (of)
  crime Z65.4
  disaster Z65.5
  terrorism Z65.4
  torture Z65.4
  war Z65.5
Vidal's disease L28.0
Villaret's syndrome G52.7
Villous — *see* condition
VIN — *see* Neoplasia, intraepithelial, vulva
Vincent's infection (angina) (gingivitis) A69.1
  stomatitis NEC A69.1
Vinson-Plummer syndrome D50.1
Violence, physical R45.6
Viosterol deficiency — *see* Deficiency, calciferol
Vipoma — *see* Neoplasm, malignant, by site
Viremia B34.9
Virilism (adrenal) E25.9
  congenital E25.0
Virilization (female) (suprarenal) E25.9
  congenital E25.0
  isosexual E28.2
Virulent bubo A57
Virus, viral (*see also* condition)
  as cause of disease classified elsewhere B97.89
  cytomegalovirus B25.9
  human immunodeficiency (HIV) — *see* Human, immunodeficiency virus (HIV) disease
  infection — *see* Infection, virus
  specified NEC B34.8
  swine influenza (viruses that normally cause infections in pigs) (*see also* Influenza, due to, identified novel influenza A virus) J09.X2
  West Nile (fever) A92.30
    with
      complications NEC A92.39
      cranial nerve disorders A92.32
      encephalitis A92.31
      encephalomyelitis A92.31
      neurologic manifestation NEC A92.32
      optic neuritis A92.32
      polyradiculitis A92.32
Viscera, visceral — *see* condition
Visceroptosis K63.4
Visible peristalsis R19.2
Vision, visual
  binocular, suppression H53.34
  blurred, blurring H53.8
    hysterical F44.6
  defect, defective NEC H54.7
  disorientation (syndrome) H53.8
  disturbance H53.9
    hysterical F44.6
  double H53.2
  examination Z01.00
    with abnormal findings Z01.01
  field, limitation (defect) — *see* Defect, visual field
  hallucinations R44.1
  halos H53.19

Vision, visual — *continued*
  loss — *see* Loss, vision
    sudden — *see* Disturbance, vision, subjective, loss, sudden
  low (both eyes) — *see* Low, vision
  perception, simultaneous without fusion H53.33
Vitality, lack or want of R53.83
  newborn P96.89
Vitamin deficiency — *see* Deficiency, vitamin
Vitelline duct, persistent Q43.0
Vitiligo L80
  eyelid H02.739
    left H02.736
      lower H02.735
      upper H02.734
    right H02.733
      lower H02.732
      upper H02.731
  pinta A67.2
  vulva N90.89
Vitreal corneal syndrome H59.01- ☑
Vitreoretinopathy, proliferative (*see also* Retinopathy, proliferative)
  with retinal detachment — *see* Detachment, retina, traction
Vitreous (*see also* condition)
  touch syndrome — *see* Complication, postprocedural, following cataract surgery
Vocal cord — *see* condition
Vogt-Koyanagi syndrome H20.82- ☑
Vogt's disease or syndrome G80.3
Vogt-Spielmeyer amaurotic idiocy or disease E75.4
Voice
  change R49.9
    specified NEC R49.8
  loss — *see* Aphonia
Volhynian fever A79.0
Volkmann's ischemic contracture or paralysis (complicating trauma) T79.6 ☑
Volvulus (bowel) (colon) (duodenum) (intestine) K56.2
  with perforation K56.2
  congenital Q43.8
  fallopian tube — *see* Torsion, fallopian tube
  oviduct — *see* Torsion, fallopian tube
  stomach (due to absence of gastrocolic ligament) K31.89
Vomiting R11.10
  with nausea R11.2
  without nausea R11.11
  asphyxia — *see* Foreign body, by site, causing asphyxia, gastric contents
  bilious (cause unknown) R11.14
    following gastro-intestinal surgery K91.0
    in newborn P92.01
  blood — *see* Hematemesis
  causing asphyxia, choking, or suffocation — *see* Foreign body, by site
  cyclical G43.A0 (*following* G43.7)
    with refractory migraine G43.A1 (*following* G43.7)
    without refractory migraine G43.A0 (*following* G43.7)
    intractable G43.A1 (*following* G43.7)
    not intractable G43.A0 (*following* G43.7)
    psychogenic F50.8
  fecal mater R11.13
  following gastrointestinal surgery K91.0
    psychogenic F50.8
  functional K31.89
  hysterical F50.8
  nervous F50.8
  neurotic F50.8
  newborn NEC P92.09
    bilious P92.01
  periodic R11.10
    psychogenic F50.8
  projectile R11.12
  psychogenic F50.8
  uremic — *see* Uremia
Vomito negro — *see* Fever, yellow
Von Bezold's abscess — *see* Mastoiditis, acute
Von Economo-Cruchet disease A85.8
Von Eulenburg's disease G71.19
Von Gierke's disease E74.01
Von Hippel (-Lindau) **disease or syndrome** Q85.8
Von Jaksch's anemia or disease D64.89

Index

Vegetation, vegetative — Von Jaksch's anemia or disease

Von Recklinghausen
  disease (neurofibromatosis) Q85.01
    bones E21.0
Von Schroetter's syndrome I82.890
Von Willebrand (-Jurgens)(-Minot) **disease or syndrome** D68.0
Von Zumbusch's disease L40.1
Voyeurism F65.3
Vrolik's disease Q78.0
Vulva — *see* condition
Vulvismus N94.2
Vulvitis (acute) (allergic) (atrophic) (hypertrophic) (intertriginous) (senile) N76.2
  with ectopic or molar pregnancy O08.0
  adhesive, congenital Q52.79
  blennorrhagic (gonococcal) A54.02
  candidal B37.3
  chlamydial A56.02
  due to Haemophilus ducreyi A57
  following ectopic or molar pregnancy O08.0
  gonococcal A54.02
    with abscess (accessory gland) (periurethral) A54.1
  herpesviral A60.04
  leukoplakic N90.4
  monilial B37.3
  puerperal (postpartum) O86.19
  subacute or chronic N76.3
  syphilitic (early) A51.0
    late A52.76
  trichomonal A59.01
  tuberculous A18.18
Vulvodynia N94.819
  specified NEC N94.818
Vulvorectal — *see* condition
Vulvovaginitis (acute) — *see* Vaginitis

W

Waiting list, person on Z75.1
  for organ transplant Z76.82
  undergoing social agency investigation Z75.2
Waldenström
  hypergammaglobulinemia D89.0
  syndrome or macroglobulinemia C88.0
Waldenström-Kjellberg syndrome D50.1
Walking
  difficulty R26.2
    psychogenic F44.4
  sleep F51.3
    hysterical F44.89
Wall, abdominal — *see* condition
Wallenberg's disease or syndrome G46.3
Wallgren's disease I87.8
Wandering
  gallbladder, congenital Q44.1
  in diseases classified elsewhere Z91.83
  kidney, congenital Q63.8
  organ or site, congenital NEC — *see* Malposition, congenital, by site
  pacemaker (heart) I49.8
  spleen D73.89
War neurosis F48.8
Wart (due to HPV) (filiform) (infectious) (viral) B07.9
  anogenital region (venereal) A63.0
  common B07.8
  external genital organs (venereal) A63.0
  flat B07.8
  Hassal-Henle's (of cornea) H18.49
  Peruvian A44.1
  plantar B07.0
  prosector (tuberculous) A18.4
  seborrheic L82.1
    inflamed L82.0
  senile (seborrheic) L82.1
    inflamed L82.0
  tuberculous A18.4
  venereal A63.0
Warthin's tumor — *see* Neoplasm, salivary gland, benign
Wassilieff's disease A27.0
Wasting
  disease R64
    due to malnutrition E41
  extreme (due to malnutrition) E41
  muscle NEC — *see* Atrophy, muscle
Water
  clefts (senile cataract) — *see* Cataract, senile, incipient
  deprivation of T73.1 ☑

Water — *continued*
  intoxication E87.79
  itch B76.9
  lack of T73.1 ☑
  loading E87.70
  on
    brain — *see* Hydrocephalus
    chest J94.8
  poisoning E87.79
Waterbrash R12
Waterhouse (-Friderichsen) **syndrome or disease** (meningococcal) A39.1
Water-losing nephritis N25.89
Watermelon stomach K31.819
  with hemorrhage K31.811
  without hemorrhage K31.819
Watsoniasis B66.8
Wax in ear — *see* Impaction, cerumen
Weak, weakening, weakness (generalized) R53.1
  arches (acquired) (*see also* Deformity, limb, flat foot)
  bladder (sphincter) R32
  facial R29.810
    following
      cerebrovascular disease I69.992
        cerebral infarction I69.392
        intracerebral hemorrhage I69.192
        nontraumatic intracranial hemorrhage NEC I69.292
        specified disease NEC I69.892
        stroke I69.392
        subarachnoid hemorrhage I69.092
  foot (double) — *see* Weak, arches
  heart, cardiac — *see* Failure, heart
  mind F70
  muscle M62.81
  myocardium — *see* Failure, heart
  newborn P96.89
  pelvic fundus N81.89
  pubocervical tissue N81.82
  rectovaginal tissue N81.83
  senile R54
  urinary stream R39.12
  valvular — *see* Endocarditis
Wear, worn (with normal or routine use)
  articular bearing surface of internal joint prosthesis — *see* Complications, joint prosthesis, mechanical, wear of articular bearing surfaces, by site
  device, implant or graft — *see* Complications, by site, mechanical complication
  tooth, teeth (approximal) (hard tissues) (interproximal) (occlusal) K03.0
Weather, weathered
  effects of
    cold T69.9 ☑
      specified effect NEC T69.8 ☑
    hot — *see* Heat
    skin L57.8
Weaver's syndrome Q87.3
Web, webbed (congenital)
  duodenal Q43.8
  esophagus Q39.4
  fingers Q70.1- ☑
  larynx (glottic) (subglottic) Q31.0
  neck (pterygium colli) Q18.3
  Paterson-Kelly D50.1
  popliteal syndrome Q87.89
  toes Q70.3- ☑
Weber-Christian disease M35.6
Weber-Cockayne syndrome (epidermolysis bullosa) Q81.8
Weber-Gubler syndrome G46.3
Weber-Leyden syndrome G46.3
Weber-Osler syndrome I78.0
Weber's paralysis or syndrome G46.3
Wedge-shaped or wedging vertebra — *see* Collapse, vertebra NEC
Wegener's granulomatosis or syndrome M31.30
  with
    kidney involvement M31.31
    lung involvement M31.30
      with kidney involvement M31.31
Wegner's disease A50.02
Weight
  1000-2499 grams at birth (low) — *see* Low, birthweight
  999 grams or less at birth (extremely low) — *see* Low, birthweight, extreme

Weight — *continued*
  gain (abnormal) (excessive) R63.5
    in pregnancy — *see* Pregnancy, complicated by, excessive weight gain
    low — *see* Pregnancy, complicated by, insufficient, weight gain
  loss (abnormal) (cause unknown) R63.4
Weightlessness (effect of) T75.82 ☑
Weil (I)-**Marchesani syndrome** Q87.1
Weil's disease A27.0
Weingarten's syndrome J82
Weir Mitchell's disease I73.81
Weiss-Baker syndrome G90.09
Wells' disease L98.3
Wen — *see* Cyst, sebaceous
Wenckebach's block or phenomenon I44.1
Werdnig-Hoffmann syndrome (muscular atrophy) G12.0
Werlhof's disease D69.3
Wermer's disease or syndrome E31.21
Werner-His disease A79.0
Werner's disease or syndrome E34.8
Wernicke-Korsakoff's syndrome or psychosis (alcoholic) F10.96
  with dependence F10.26
  drug-induced
    due to drug abuse — *see* Abuse, drug, by type, with amnestic disorder
    due to drug dependence — *see* Dependence, drug, by type, with amnestic disorder
  nonalcoholic F04
Wernicke-Posadas disease B38.9
Wernicke's
  developmental aphasia F80.2
  disease or syndrome E51.2
  encephalopathy E51.2
  polioencephalitis, superior E51.2
West African fever B50.8
Westphal-Strümpell syndrome E83.01
West's syndrome — *see* Epilepsy, spasms
Wet
  feet, tropical (maceration) (syndrome) — *see* Immersion, foot
  lung (syndrome), newborn P22.1
Wharton's duct — *see* condition
Wheal — *see* Urticaria
Wheezing R06.2
Whiplash injury S13.4 ☑
Whipple's disease (*see also* subcategory M14.8-) K90.81
Whipworm (disease) (infection) (infestation) B79
Whistling face Q87.0
White (*see also* condition)
  kidney, small N03.9
  leg, puerperal, postpartum, childbirth O87.1
  mouth B37.0
  patches of mouth K13.29
  spot lesions, teeth
    chewing surface K02.51
    pit and fissure surface K02.51
    smooth surface K02.61
Whitehead L70.0
Whitlow (*see also* Cellulitis, digit)
  with lymphangitis — *see* Lymphangitis, acute, digit
  herpesviral B00.89
Whitmore's disease or fever — *see* Melioidosis
Whooping cough A37.90
  with pneumonia A37.91
    due to Bordetella
      bronchiseptica A37.81
      parapertussis A37.11
      pertussis A37.01
    specified organism NEC A37.81
  due to
    Bordetella
      bronchiseptica A37.80
        with pneumonia A37.81
      parapertussis A37.10
        with pneumonia A37.11
      pertussis A37.00
        with pneumonia A37.01
      specified NEC A37.80
        with pneumonia A37.81
Wichman's asthma J38.5
Wide cranial sutures, newborn P96.3
Widening aorta — *see* Ectasia, aorta
  with aneurysm — *see* Aneurysm, aorta
Wilkie's disease or syndrome K55.1

☑ **Additional Character Required** — Refer to the Tabular List for Character Selection   ▽ **Subterms under main terms may continue to next column or page**

Wilkinson-Sneddon disease or syndrome L13.1
Willebrand (-Jürgens) **thrombopathy** D68.0
Willige-Hunt disease or syndrome G23.1
Wilms' tumor C64- ☑
Wilson-Mikity syndrome P27.0
Wilson's
  disease or syndrome E83.01
  hepatolenticular degeneration E83.01
  lichen ruber L43.9
Window (see also Imperfect, closure)
  aorticopulmonary Q21.4
Winter — see condition
Wiskott-Aldrich syndrome D82.0
Withdrawal state (see also Dependence, drug by type, with withdrawal)
  newborn
    correct therapeutic substance properly administered P96.2
    infant of dependent mother P96.1
    therapeutic substance, neonatal P96.2
Witts' anemia D50.8
Witzelsucht F07.0
Woakes' ethmoiditis or syndrome J33.1
Wolff-Hirschorn syndrome Q93.3
Wolff-Parkinson-White syndrome I45.6
Wolhynian fever A79.0
Wolman's disease E75.5
Wood lung or pneumonitis J67.8
Woolly, wooly hair (congenital) (nevus) Q84.1
Woolsorter's disease A22.1
Word
  blindness (congenital) (developmental) F81.0
  deafness (congenital) (developmental) H93.25
Worm(s) (infection) (infestation) (see also Infestation, helminth)
  guinea B72
  in intestine NEC B82.0
Worm-eaten soles A66.3
Worn out — see Exhaustion
  cardiac
    defibrillator (with synchronous cardiace pacemaker) Z45.02
    pacemaker
      battery Z45.010
      lead Z45.018
  device, implant or graft — see Complications, by site, mechanical
Worried well Z71.1
Worries R45.82
Wound, open
  abdomen, abdominal
    wall S31.109 ☑
      with penetration into peritoneal cavity S31.609 ☑
      bite — see Bite, abdomen, wall
      epigastric region S31.102 ☑
        with penetration into peritoneal cavity S31.602 ☑
        bite — see Bite, abdomen, wall, epigastric region
        laceration — see Laceration, abdomen, wall, epigastric region
        puncture — see Puncture, abdomen, wall, epigastric region
      laceration — see Laceration, abdomen, wall
      left
        lower quadrant S31.104 ☑
          with penetration into peritoneal cavity S31.604 ☑
          bite — see Bite, abdomen, wall, left, lower quadrant
          laceration — see Laceration, abdomen, wall, left, lower quadrant
          puncture — see Puncture, abdomen, wall, left, lower quadrant
        upper quadrant S31.101 ☑
          with penetration into peritoneal cavity S31.601 ☑
          bite — see Bite, abdomen, wall, left, upper quadrant
          laceration — see Laceration, abdomen, wall, left, upper quadrant
          puncture — see Puncture, abdomen, wall, left, upper quadrant
      periumbilic region S31.105 ☑
        with penetration into peritoneal cavity S31.605 ☑

Wound, open — continued
  abdomen, abdominal — continued
    wall — continued
      periumbilic region — continued
        bite — see Bite, abdomen, wall, periumbilic region
        laceration — see Laceration, abdomen, wall, periumbilic region
        puncture — see Puncture, abdomen, wall, periumbilic region
      puncture — see Puncture, abdomen, wall
      right
        lower quadrant S31.103 ☑
          with penetration into peritoneal cavity S31.603 ☑
          bite — see Bite, abdomen, wall, right, lower quadrant
          laceration — see Laceration, abdomen, wall, right, lower quadrant
          puncture — see Puncture, abdomen, wall, right, lower quadrant
        upper quadrant S31.100 ☑
          with penetration into peritoneal cavity S31.600 ☑
          bite — see Bite, abdomen, wall, right, upper quadrant
          laceration — see Laceration, abdomen, wall, right, upper quadrant
          puncture — see Puncture, abdomen, wall, right, upper quadrant
  alveolar (process) — see Wound, open, oral cavity
  ankle S91.00- ☑
    bite — see Bite, ankle
    laceration — see Laceration, ankle
    puncture — see Puncture, ankle
  antecubital space — see Wound, open, elbow
  anterior chamber, eye — see Wound, open, ocular
  anus S31.839 ☑
    bite S31.835 ☑
    laceration — see Laceration, anus
    puncture — see Puncture, anus
  arm (upper) S41.10- ☑
    with amputation — see Amputation, traumatic, arm
    bite — see Bite, arm
    forearm — see Wound, open, forearm
    laceration — see Laceration, arm
    puncture — see Puncture, arm
  auditory canal (external) (meatus) — see Wound, open, ear
  auricle, ear — see Wound, open, ear
  axilla — see Wound, open, arm
  back (see also Wound, open, thorax, back)
    lower S31.000 ☑
      with penetration into retroperitoneal space S31.001 ☑
      bite — see Bite, back, lower
      laceration — see Laceration, back, lower
      puncture — see Puncture, back, lower
  bite — see Bite
  blood vessel — see Injury, blood vessel
  breast S21.00- ☑
    with amputation — see Amputation, traumatic, breast
    bite — see Bite, breast
    laceration — see Laceration, breast
    puncture — see Puncture, breast
  buttock S31.809 ☑
    bite — see Bite, buttock
    laceration — see Laceration, buttock
    left S31.829 ☑
    puncture — see Puncture, buttock
    right S31.819 ☑
  calf — see Wound, open, leg
  canaliculus lacrimalis — see Wound, open, eyelid
  canthus, eye — see Wound, open, eyelid
  cervical esophagus S11.20 ☑
    bite S11.25 ☑
    laceration — see Laceration, esophagus, traumatic, cervical
    puncture — see Puncture, cervical esophagus
  cheek (external) S01.40- ☑
    bite — see Bite, cheek
    internal — see Wound, open, oral cavity
    laceration — see Laceration, cheek
    puncture — see Puncture, cheek

Wound, open — continued
  chest wall — see Wound, open, thorax
  chin — see Wound, open, head, specified site NEC
  choroid — see Wound, open, ocular
  ciliary body (eye) — see Wound, open, ocular
  clitoris S31.40 ☑
    with amputation — see Amputation, traumatic, clitoris
    bite S31.45 ☑
    laceration — see Laceration, vulva
    puncture — see Puncture, vulva
  conjunctiva — see Wound, open, ocular
  cornea — see Wound, open, ocular
  costal region — see Wound, open, thorax
  Descemet's membrane — see Wound, open, ocular
  digit(s)
    foot — see Wound, open, toe
    hand — see Wound, open, finger
  ear (canal) (external) S01.30- ☑
    with amputation — see Amputation, traumatic, ear
    bite — see Bite, ear
    drum S09.2- ☑
    laceration — see Laceration, ear
    puncture — see Puncture, ear
  elbow S51.00- ☑
    bite — see Bite, elbow
    laceration — see Laceration, elbow
    puncture — see Puncture, elbow
  epididymis — see Wound, open, testis
  epigastric region S31.102 ☑
    with penetration into peritoneal cavity S31.602 ☑
    bite — see Bite, abdomen, wall, epigastric region
    laceration — see Laceration, abdomen, wall, epigastric region
    puncture — see Puncture, abdomen, wall, epigastric region
  epiglottis — see Wound, open, neck, specified site NEC
  esophagus (thoracic) S27.819 ☑
    cervical — see Wound, open, cervical esophagus
    laceration S27.813 ☑
    specified type NEC S27.818 ☑
  eye — see Wound, open, ocular
  eyeball — see Wound, open, ocular
  eyebrow — see Wound, open, eyelid
  eyelid S01.10- ☑
    bite — see Bite, eyelid
    laceration — see Laceration, eyelid
    puncture — see Puncture, eyelid
  face NEC — see Wound, open, head, specified site NEC
  finger(s) S61.209 ☑
    with
      amputation — see Amputation, traumatic, finger
      damage to nail S61.309 ☑
    bite — see Bite, finger
    index S61.208 ☑
      with
        damage to nail S61.308 ☑
      left S61.201 ☑
        with
          damage to nail S61.301 ☑
      right S61.200 ☑
        with
          damage to nail S61.300 ☑
    laceration — see Laceration, finger
    little S61.208 ☑
      with
        damage to nail S61.308 ☑
      left S61.207 ☑
        with damage to nail S61.307 ☑
      right S61.206 ☑
        with damage to nail S61.306 ☑
    middle S61.208 ☑
      with
        damage to nail S61.308 ☑
      left S61.203 ☑
        with damage to nail S61.303 ☑
      right S61.202 ☑
        with damage to nail S61.302 ☑
    puncture — see Puncture, finger
    ring S61.208 ☑
      with
        damage to nail S61.308 ☑

Wound, open — *continued*
   finger(s) — *continued*
      ring — *continued*
         left S61.205 ☑
            with damage to nail S61.305 ☑
         right S61.204 ☑
            with damage to nail S61.304 ☑
   flank — *see* Wound, open, abdomen, wall
   foot (except toe(s) alone) S91.30- ☑
      with amputation — *see* Amputation, traumatic, foot
      bite — *see* Bite, foot
      laceration — *see* Laceration, foot
      puncture — *see* Puncture, foot
      toe — *see* Wound, open, toe
   forearm S51.80- ☑
      with
         amputation — *see* Amputation, traumatic, forearm
      bite — *see* Bite, forearm
      elbow only — *see* Wound, open, elbow
      laceration — *see* Laceration, forearm
      puncture — *see* Puncture, forearm
   forehead — *see* Wound, open, head, specified site NEC
   genital organs, external
      with amputation — *see* Amputation, traumatic, genital organs
      bite — *see* Bite, genital organ
      female S31.502 ☑
         vagina S31.40 ☑
         vulva S31.40 ☑
      laceration — *see* Laceration, genital organ
      male S31.501 ☑
         penis S31.20 ☑
         scrotum S31.30 ☑
         testes S31.30 ☑
      puncture — *see* Puncture, genital organ
   globe (eye) — *see* Wound, open, ocular
   groin — *see* Wound, open, abdomen, wall
   gum — *see* Wound, open, oral cavity
   hand S61.40- ☑
      with
         amputation — *see* Amputation, traumatic, hand
      bite — *see* Bite, hand
      finger(s) — *see* Wound, open, finger
      laceration — *see* Laceration, hand
      puncture — *see* Puncture, hand
      thumb — *see* Wound, open, thumb
   head S01.90 ☑
      bite — *see* Bite, head
      cheek — *see* Wound, open, cheek
      ear — *see* Wound, open, ear
      eyelid — *see* Wound, open, eyelid
      laceration — *see* Laceration, head
      lip — *see* Wound, open, lip
      nose S01.20 ☑
      oral cavity — *see* Wound, open, oral cavity
      puncture — *see* Puncture, head
      scalp — *see* Wound, open, scalp
      specified site NEC S01.80 ☑
      temporomandibular area — *see* Wound, open, cheek
   heel — *see* Wound, open, foot
   hip S71.00- ☑
      with amputation — *see* Amputation, traumatic, hip
      bite — *see* Bite, hip
      laceration — *see* Laceration, hip
      puncture — *see* Puncture, hip
   hymen S31.40 ☑
      bite — *see* Bite, vulva
      laceration — *see* Laceration, vagina
      puncture — *see* Puncture, vagina
   hypochondrium S31.109 ☑
      bite — *see* Bite, hypochondrium
      laceration — *see* Laceration, hypochondrium
      puncture — *see* Puncture, hypochondrium
   hypogastric region S31.109 ☑
      bite — *see* Bite, hypogastric region
      laceration — *see* Laceration, hypogastric region
      puncture — *see* Puncture, hypogastric region
   iliac (region) — *see* Wound, open, inguinal region
   inguinal region S31.109 ☑
      bite — *see* Bite, abdomen, wall, lower quadrant
      laceration — *see* Laceration, inguinal region

Wound, open — *continued*
   inguinal region — *continued*
      puncture — *see* Puncture, inguinal region
   instep — *see* Wound, open, foot
   interscapular region — *see* Wound, open, thorax, back
   intraocular — *see* Wound, open, ocular
   iris — *see* Wound, open, ocular
   jaw — *see* Wound, open, head, specified site NEC
   knee S81.00- ☑
      bite — *see* Bite, knee
      laceration — *see* Laceration, knee
      puncture — *see* Puncture, knee
   labium (majus) (minus) — *see* Wound, open, vulva
   laceration — *see* Laceration, by site
   lacrimal duct — *see* Wound, open, eyelid
   larynx S11.019 ☑
      bite — *see* Bite, larynx
      laceration — *see* Laceration, larynx
      puncture — *see* Puncture, larynx
   left
      lower quadrant S31.104 ☑
         with penetration into peritoneal cavity S31.604 ☑
         bite — *see* Bite, abdomen, wall, left, lower quadrant
         laceration — *see* Laceration, abdomen, wall, left, lower quadrant
         puncture — *see* Puncture, abdomen, wall, left, lower quadrant
      upper quadrant S31.101 ☑
         with penetration into peritoneal cavity S31.601 ☑
         bite — *see* Bite, abdomen, wall, left, upper quadrant
         laceration — *see* Laceration, abdomen, wall, left, upper quadrant
         puncture — *see* Puncture, abdomen, wall, left, upper quadrant
   leg (lower) S81.80- ☑
      with amputation — *see* Amputation, traumatic, leg
      ankle — *see* Wound, open, ankle
      bite — *see* Bite, leg
      foot — *see* Wound, open, foot
      knee — *see* Wound, open, knee
      laceration — *see* Laceration, leg
      puncture — *see* Puncture, leg
      toe — *see* Wound, open, toe
      upper — *see* Wound, open, thigh
   lip S01.501 ☑
      bite — *see* Bite, lip
      laceration — *see* Laceration, lip
      puncture — *see* Puncture, lip
   loin S31.109 ☑
      bite — *see* Bite, abdomen, wall
      laceration — *see* Laceration, loin
      puncture — *see* Puncture, loin
   lower back — *see* Wound, open, back, lower
   lumbar region — *see* Wound, open, back, lower
   malar region — *see* Wound, open, head, specified site NEC
   mammary — *see* Wound, open, breast
   mastoid region — *see* Wound, open, head, specified site NEC
   mouth — *see* Wound, open, oral cavity
   nail
      finger — *see* Wound, open, finger, with damage to nail
      toe — *see* Wound, open, toe, with damage to nail
   nape (neck) — *see* Wound, open, neck
   nasal (septum) (sinus) — *see* Wound, open, nose
   nasopharynx — *see* Wound, open, head, specified site NEC
   neck S11.90 ☑
      bite — *see* Bite, neck
      involving
         cervical esophagus S11.20 ☑
         larynx — *see* Wound, open, larynx
         pharynx S11.20 ☑
         thyroid S11.10 ☑
         trachea (cervical) S11.029 ☑
            bite — *see* Bite, trachea
            laceration S11.021 ☑
               with foreign body S11.022 ☑
            puncture S11.023 ☑
               with foreign body S11.024 ☑

Wound, open — *continued*
   neck — *continued*
      laceration — *see* Laceration, neck
      puncture — *see* Puncture, neck
      specified site NEC S11.80 ☑
         specified type NEC S11.89 ☑
   nose (septum) (sinus) S01.20 ☑
      with amputation — *see* Amputation, traumatic, nose
      bite — *see* Bite, nose
      laceration — *see* Laceration, nose
      puncture — *see* Puncture, nose
   ocular S05.90 ☑
      avulsion (traumatic enucleation) S05.7- ☑
      eyeball S05.6- ☑
         with foreign body S05.5- ☑
      eyelid — *see* Wound, open, eyelid
      laceration and rupture S05.3- ☑
         with prolapse or loss of intraocular tissue S05.2- ☑
      orbit (penetrating) (with or without foreign body) S05.4- ☑
      periocular area — *see* Wound, open, eyelid
      specified NEC S05.8X- ☑
   oral cavity S01.502 ☑
      bite S01.552 ☑
      laceration — *see* Laceration, oral cavity
      puncture — *see* Puncture, oral cavity
   orbit — *see* Wound, open, ocular, orbit
   palate — *see* Wound, open, oral cavity
   palm — *see* Wound, open, hand
   pelvis, pelvic (*see also* Wound, open, back, lower)
      girdle — *see* Wound, open, hip
   penetrating — *see* Puncture, by site
   penis S31.20 ☑
      with amputation — *see* Amputation, traumatic, penis
      bite S31.25 ☑
      laceration — *see* Laceration, penis
      puncture — *see* Puncture, penis
   perineum
      bite — *see* Bite, perineum
      female S31.502 ☑
      laceration — *see* Laceration, perineum
      male S31.501 ☑
      puncture — *see* Puncture, perineum
   periocular area (with or without lacrimal passages) — *see* Wound, open, eyelid
   periumbilic region S31.105 ☑
      with penetration into peritoneal cavity S31.605 ☑
      bite — *see* Bite, abdomen, wall, periumbilic region
      laceration — *see* Laceration, abdomen, wall, periumbilic region
      puncture — *see* Puncture, abdomen, wall, periumbilic region
   phalanges
      finger — *see* Wound, open, finger
      toe — *see* Wound, open, toe
   pharynx S11.20 ☑
   pinna — *see* Wound, open, ear
   popliteal space — *see* Wound, open, knee
   prepuce — *see* Wound, open, penis
   pubic region — *see* Wound, open, back, lower
   pudendum — *see* Wound, open, genital organs, external
   puncture wound — *see* Puncture
   rectovaginal septum — *see* Wound, open, vagina
   right
      lower quadrant S31.103 ☑
         with penetration into peritoneal cavity S31.603 ☑
         bite — *see* Bite, abdomen, wall, right, lower quadrant
         laceration — *see* Laceration, abdomen, wall, right, lower quadrant
         puncture — *see* Puncture, abdomen, wall, right, lower quadrant
      upper quadrant S31.100 ☑
         with penetration into peritoneal cavity S31.600 ☑
         bite — *see* Bite, abdomen, wall, right, upper quadrant
         laceration — *see* Laceration, abdomen, wall, right, upper quadrant
         puncture — *see* Puncture, abdomen, wall, right, upper quadrant

Wound, open — *continued*
  sacral region — *see* Wound, open, back, lower
  sacroiliac region — *see* Wound, open, back, lower
  salivary gland — *see* Wound, open, oral cavity
  scalp S01.00 ☑
    bite S01.05 ☑
    laceration — *see* Laceration, scalp
    puncture — *see* Puncture, scalp
  scalpel, newborn (birth injury) P15.8
  scapular region — *see* Wound, open, shoulder
  sclera — *see* Wound, open, ocular
  scrotum S31.30 ☑
    with amputation — *see* Amputation, traumatic, scrotum
    bite S31.35 ☑
    laceration — *see* Laceration, scrotum
    puncture — *see* Puncture, scrotum
  shin — *see* Wound, open, leg
  shoulder S41.00- ☑
    with amputation — *see* Amputation, traumatic, arm
    bite — *see* Bite, shoulder
    laceration — *see* Laceration, shoulder
    puncture — *see* Puncture, shoulder
  skin NOS T14.8
  spermatic cord — *see* Wound, open, testis
  sternal region — *see* Wound, open, thorax, front wall
  submaxillary region — *see* Wound, open, head, specified site NEC
  submental region — *see* Wound, open, head, specified site NEC
  subungual
    finger(s) — *see* Wound, open, finger
    toe(s) — *see* Wound, open, toe
  supraclavicular region — *see* Wound, open, neck, specified site NEC
  temple, temporal region — *see* Wound, open, head, specified site NEC
  temporomandibular area — *see* Wound, open, cheek
  testis S31.30 ☑
    with amputation — *see* Amputation, traumatic, testes
    bite S31.35 ☑
    laceration — *see* Laceration, testis
    puncture — *see* Puncture, testis
  thigh S71.10- ☑
    with amputation — *see* Amputation, traumatic, hip
    bite — *see* Bite, thigh
    laceration — *see* Laceration, thigh
    puncture — *see* Puncture, thigh
  thorax, thoracic (wall) S21.90 ☑
    back S21.20- ☑
      with penetration S21.40 ☑
    bite — *see* Bite, thorax
    breast — *see* Wound, open, breast
    front S21.10- ☑
      with penetration S21.30 ☑
    laceration — *see* Laceration, thorax
    puncture — *see* Puncture, thorax
  throat — *see* Wound, open, neck
  thumb S61.009 ☑
    with
      amputation — *see* Amputation, traumatic, thumb
      damage to nail S61.109 ☑
    bite — *see* Bite, thumb
    laceration — *see* Laceration, thumb
    left S61.002 ☑
      with
        damage to nail S61.102 ☑
    puncture — *see* Puncture, thumb
    right S61.001 ☑
      with
        damage to nail S61.101 ☑
  thyroid (gland) — *see* Wound, open, neck, thyroid
  toe(s) S91.109 ☑
    with
      amputation — *see* Amputation, traumatic, toe
      damage to nail S91.209 ☑
    bite — *see* Bite, toe
    great S91.103 ☑
      with
        damage to nail S91.203 ☑

Wound, open — *continued*
  toe(s) — *continued*
    great — *continued*
      left S91.102 ☑
        with
          damage to nail S91.202 ☑
      right S91.101 ☑
        with
          damage to nail S91.201 ☑
      laceration — *see* Laceration, toe
    lesser S91.106 ☑
      with
        damage to nail S91.206 ☑
      left S91.105 ☑
        with
          damage to nail S91.205 ☑
      right S91.104 ☑
        with
          damage to nail S91.204 ☑
    puncture — *see* Puncture, toe
  tongue — *see* Wound, open, oral cavity
  trachea (cervical region) — *see* Wound, open, neck, trachea
  tunica vaginalis — *see* Wound, open, testis
  tympanum, tympanic membrane S09.2- ☑
    laceration — *see* Laceration, ear, drum
    puncture — *see* Puncture, tympanum
  umbilical region — *see* Wound, open, abdomen, wall, periumbilic region
  uvula — *see* Wound, open, oral cavity
  vagina S31.40 ☑
    bite S31.45 ☑
    laceration — *see* Laceration, vagina
    puncture — *see* Puncture, vagina
  vitreous (humor) — *see* Wound, open, ocular
  vocal cord S11.039 ☑
    bite — *see* Bite, vocal cord
    laceration S11.031 ☑
      with foreign body S11.032 ☑
    puncture S11.033 ☑
      with foreign body S11.034 ☑
  vulva S31.40 ☑
    with amputation — *see* Amputation, traumatic, vulva
    bite S31.45 ☑
    laceration — *see* Laceration, vulva
    puncture — *see* Puncture, vulva
  wrist S61.50- ☑
    bite — *see* Bite, wrist
    laceration — *see* Laceration, wrist
    puncture — *see* Puncture, wrist
Wound, superficial — *see* Injury (*see also* specified injury type)
Wright's syndrome G54.0
Wrist — *see* condition
Wrong drug (by accident) (given in error) — *see* Table of Drugs and Chemicals, by drug, poisoning
Wry neck — *see* Torticollis
Wuchereria (bancrofti) **infestation** B74.0
Wuchereriasis B74.0
Wuchernde Struma Langhans C73

X

Xanthelasma (eyelid) (palpebrarum) H02.60
  left H02.66
    lower H02.65
    upper H02.64
  right H02.63
    lower H02.62
    upper H02.61
Xanthelasmatosis (essential) E78.2
Xanthinuria, hereditary E79.8
Xanthoastrocytoma
  specified site — *see* Neoplasm, malignant, by site
  unspecified site C71.9
Xanthofibroma — *see* Neoplasm, connective tissue, benign
Xanthogranuloma D76.3
Xanthoma(s), xanthomatosis (primary) (familial) (hereditary) E75.5
  with
    hyperlipoproteinemia
      Type I E78.3
      Type III E78.2
      Type IV E78.1

Xanthoma(s), xanthomatosis — *continued*
  with — *continued*
    hyperlipoproteinemia — *continued*
      Type V E78.3
  bone (generalisata) C96.5
  cerebrotendinous E75.5
  cutaneotendinous E75.5
  disseminatum (skin) E78.2
  eruptive E78.2
  hypercholesterinemic E78.0
  hypercholesterolemic E78.0
  hyperlipidemic E78.5
  joint E75.5
  multiple (skin) E78.2
  tendon (sheath) E75.5
  tuberosum E78.2
  tuberous E78.2
  tubo-eruptive E78.2
  verrucous, oral mucosa K13.4
Xanthosis R23.8
Xenophobia F40.10
Xeroderma (*see also* Ichthyosis)
  acquired L85.0
  eyelid H01.149
    left H01.146
      lower H01.145
      upper H01.144
    right H01.143
      lower H01.142
      upper H01.141
  pigmentosum Q82.1
  vitamin A deficiency E50.8
Xerophthalmia (vitamin A deficiency) E50.7
  unrelated to vitamin A deficiency — *see* Keratoconjunctivitis
Xerosis
  conjunctiva H11.14- ☑
    with Bitot's spots (*see also* Pigmentation, conjunctiva)
      vitamin A deficiency E50.1
    vitamin A deficiency E50.0
  cornea H18.89- ☑
    with ulceration — *see* Ulcer, cornea
      vitamin A deficiency E50.3
    vitamin A deficiency E50.2
  cutis L85.3
  skin L85.3
Xerostomia K11.7
Xiphopagus Q89.4
XO syndrome Q96.9
X-ray (of)
  abnormal findings — *see* Abnormal, diagnostic imaging
  breast (mammogram) (routine) Z12.31
  chest
    routine (as part of a general medical examination) Z00.00
      with abnormal findings Z00.01
  routine (as part of a general medical examination) Z00.00
    with abnormal findings Z00.01
XXXXY syndrome Q98.1
XXY syndrome Q98.0

Y

Yaba pox (virus disease) B08.72
Yatapoxvirus B08.70
  specified NEC B08.79
Yawning R06.89
  psychogenic F45.8
Yaws A66.9
  cutaneous, less than five years after infection A66.2
  bone lesions A66.6
  butter A66.1
  chancre A66.0
  early (cutaneous) (macular) (maculopapular) (micropapular) (papular) A66.2
    frambeside A66.2
    skin lesions NEC A66.2
  eyelid A66.2
  ganglion A66.6
  gangosis, gangosa A66.5
  gumma, gummata A66.4
    bone A66.6
  gummatous
    frambeside A66.4
    osteitis A66.6

Index

Yaws — Zymotic

Yaws — *continued*
  gummatous — *continued*
    periostitis A66.6
  hydrarthrosis (*see also* subcategory M14.8-) A66.6
  hyperkeratosis (early) (late) A66.3
  initial lesions A66.0
  joint lesions (*see also* subcategory M14.8-) A66.6
  juxta-articular nodules A66.7
  late nodular (ulcerated) A66.4
  latent (without clinical manifestations) (with positive serology) A66.8
  mother A66.0
  mucosal A66.7
  multiple papillomata A66.1
  nodular, late (ulcerated) A66.4
  osteitis A66.6
  papilloma, plantar or palmar A66.1
  periostitis (hypertrophic) A66.6

Yaws — *continued*
  specified NEC A66.7
  ulcers A66.4
  wet crab A66.1
Yeast infection (*see also* Candidiasis) B37.9
Yellow
  atrophy (liver) — *see* Failure, hepatic
  fever — *see* Fever, yellow
  jack — *see* Fever, yellow
  jaundice — *see* Jaundice
  nail syndrome L60.5
Yersiniosis (*see also* Infection, Yersinia)
  extraintestinal A28.2
  intestinal A04.6

Z

Zahorsky's syndrome (herpangina) B08.5

Zellweger's syndrome Q87.89
Zenker's diverticulum (esophagus) K22.5
Ziehen-Oppenheim disease G24.1
Zieve's syndrome K70.0
Zinc
  deficiency, dietary E60
  metabolism disorder E83.2
Zollinger-Ellison syndrome E16.4
Zona — *see* Herpes, zoster
Zoophobia F40.218
Zoster (herpes) — *see* Herpes, zoster
Zygomycosis B46.9
  specified NEC B46.8
Zymotic — *see* condition

☑ **Additional Character Required — Refer to the Tabular List for Character Selection**   ▽ **Subterms under main terms may continue to next column or page**

ICD-10-CM Neoplasm Table

	Malignant Primary	Malignant Secondary	Ca in situ	Benign	Uncertain	Unspecified Behavior

Note: The list below gives the code number for neoplasms by anatomical site. For each site there are six possible code numbers according to whether the neoplasm in question is malignant, benign, in situ, of uncertain behavior, or of unspecified nature. The description of the neoplasm will often indicate which of the six columns is appropriate; e.g., malignant melanoma of skin, benign fibroadenoma of breast, carcinoma in situ of cervix uteri. Where such descriptors are not present, the remainder of the Index should be consulted where guidance is given to the appropriate column for each morphological (histological) variety listed; e.g., Mesonephroma – see Neoplasm, malignant; Embryoma (see also Neoplasm, uncertain behavior); Disease, Bowen's – see Neoplasm, skin, in situ. However, the guidance in the Index can be overridden if one of the descriptors mentioned above is present; e.g., malignant adenoma of colon is coded to C18.9 and not to D12.6 as the adjective "malignant" overrides the Index entry "Adenoma (see also Neoplasm, benign)." Codes listed with a dash -, following the code have a required 5th character for laterality. The tabular list must be reviewed for the complete code.

	Malignant Primary	Malignant Secondary	Ca in situ	Benign	Uncertain	Unspecified Behavior
Neoplasm, neoplastic	C80.1	C79.9	D09.9	D36.9	D48.9	D49.9
abdomen,						
abdominal	C76.2	C79.8-✓	D09.8	D36.7	D48.7	D49.89
cavity	C76.2	C79.8-✓	D09.8	D36.7	D48.7	D49.89
organ	C76.2	C79.8-✓	D09.8	D36.7	D48.7	D49.89
viscera	C76.2	C79.8-✓	D09.8	D36.7	D48.7	D49.89
wall — see also Neoplasm, abdomen, wall,						
skin	C44.509	C79.2	D04.5	D23.5	D48.5	D49.2
connective tissue	C49.4	C79.8-✓	—	D21.4	D48.1	D49.2
skin	C44.509	—	—	—	—	—
basal cell carcinoma	C44.519	—	—	—	—	—
specified type NEC	C44.599	—	—	—	—	—
squamous cell carcinoma	C44.529	—	—	—	—	—
abdominopelvic	C76.8	C79.8-✓	—	D36.7	D48.7	D49.89
accessory sinus — see Neoplasm, sinus						
acoustic nerve	C72.4-✓	C79.49	—	D33.3	D43.3	D49.7
adenoid (pharynx) (tissue)	C11.1	C79.89	D00.08	D10.6	D37.05	D49.0
adipose tissue — see also Neoplasm, connective tissue	C49.4	C79.89	—	D21.9	D48.1	D49.2
adnexa (uterine)	C57.4	C79.89	D07.39	D28.7	D39.8	D49.5
adrenal	C74.9-✓	C79.7-✓	D09.3	D35.0-✓	D44.1-✓	D49.7
capsule	C74.9-✓	C79.7-✓	D09.3	D35.0-✓	D44.1-✓	D49.7
cortex	C74.0-✓	C79.7-✓	D09.3	D35.0-✓	D44.1-✓	D49.7
gland	C74.9-✓	C79.7-✓	D09.3	D35.0-✓	D44.1-✓	D49.7
medulla	C74.1-✓	C79.7-✓	D09.3	D35.0-✓	D44.1-✓	D49.7
ala nasi (external) — see also Neoplasm, skin, nose	C44.301	C79.2	D04.39	D23.39	D48.5	D49.2
alimentary canal or tract NEC	C26.9	C78.80	D01.9	D13.9	D37.9	D49.0
alveolar	C03.9	C79.89	D00.03	D10.39	D37.09	D49.0
mucosa	C03.9	C79.89	D00.03	D10.39	D37.09	D49.0
lower	C03.1	C79.89	D00.03	D10.39	D37.09	D49.0
upper	C03.0	C79.89	D00.03	D10.39	D37.09	D49.0
ridge or process	C41.1	C79.51	—	D16.5	D48.0	D49.2
carcinoma	C03.9	C79.8-✓	—	—	—	—
lower	C03.1	C79.8-✓	—	—	—	—
upper	C03.0	C79.8-✓	—	—	—	—
lower	C41.1	C79.51	—	D16.5	D48.0	D49.2
mucosa	C03.9	C79.89	D00.03	D10.39	D37.09	D49.0
lower	C03.1	C79.89	D00.03	D10.39	D37.09	D49.0
upper	C03.0	C79.89	D00.03	D10.39	D37.09	D49.0
upper	C41.0	C79.51	—	D16.4	D48.0	D49.2
sulcus	C06.1	C79.89	D00.02	D10.39	D37.09	D49.0
alveolus	C03.9	C79.89	D00.03	D10.39	D37.09	D49.0
lower	C03.1	C79.89	D00.03	D10.39	D37.09	D49.0
upper	C03.0	C79.89	D00.03	D10.39	D37.09	D49.0
ampulla of Vater	C24.1	C78.89	D01.5	D13.5	D37.6	D49.0
ankle NEC	C76.5-✓	C79.89	D04.7-✓	D36.7	D48.7	D49.89

Neoplasm, neoplastic — continued	Malignant Primary	Malignant Secondary	Ca in situ	Benign	Uncertain	Unspecified Behavior
anorectum, anorectal (junction)	C21.8	C78.5	D01.3	D12.9	D37.8	D49.0
antecubital fossa or space	C76.4-✓	C79.89	D04.6-✓	D36.7	D48.7	D49.89
antrum (Highmore) (maxillary)	C31.0	C78.39	D02.3	D14.0	D38.5	D49.1
pyloric	C16.3	C78.89	D00.2	D13.1	D37.1	D49.0
tympanicum	C30.1	C78.39	D02.3	D14.0	D38.5	D49.1
anus, anal	C21.0	C78.5	D01.3	D12.9	D37.8	D49.0
canal	C21.1	C78.5	D01.3	D12.9	D37.8	D49.0
cloacogenic zone	C21.2	C78.5	D01.3	D12.9	D37.8	D49.0
margin — see also Neoplasm, anus, skin	C44.500	C79.2	D04.5	D23.5	D48.5	D49.2
overlapping lesion with rectosigmoid junction or rectum	C21.8	—	—	—	—	—
skin	C44.500	C79.2	D04.5	D23.5	D48.5	D49.2
basal cell carcinoma	C44.510	—	—	—	—	—
specified type NEC	C44.590	—	—	—	—	—
squamous cell carcinoma	C44.520	—	—	—	—	—
sphincter	C21.1	C78.5	D01.3	D12.9	D37.8	D49.0
aorta (thoracic)	C49.3	C79.89	—	D21.3	D48.1	D49.2
abdominal	C49.4	C79.89	—	D21.4	D48.1	D49.2
aortic body	C75.5	C79.89	—	D35.6	D44.7	D49.7
aponeurosis	C49.9	C79.89	—	D21.9	D48.1	D49.2
palmar	C49.1-✓	C79.89	—	D21.1-✓	D48.1	D49.2
plantar	C49.2-✓	C79.89	—	D21.2-✓	D48.1	D49.2
appendix	C18.1	C78.5	D01.0	D12.1	D37.3	D49.0
arachnoid	C70.9	C79.49	—	D32.9	D42.9	D49.7
cerebral	C70.0	C79.32	—	D32.0	D42.0	D49.7
spinal	C70.1	C79.49	—	D32.1	D42.1	D49.7
areola	C50.0-✓	C79.81	D05-✓	D24-✓	D48.6-✓	D49.3
arm NEC	C76.4-✓	C79.89	D04.6-✓	D36.7	D48.7	D49.89
artery — see Neoplasm, connective tissue						
aryepiglottic fold	C13.1	C79.89	D00.08	D10.7	D37.05	D49.0
hypopharyngeal aspect	C13.1	C79.89	D00.08	D10.7	D37.05	D49.0
laryngeal aspect	C32.1	C78.39	D02.0	D14.1	D38.0	D49.1
marginal zone	C13.1	C79.89	D00.08	D10.7	D37.05	D49.0
arytenoid (cartilage)	C32.3	C78.39	D02.0	D14.1	D38.0	D49.1
fold — see Neoplasm, aryepiglottic						
associated with transplanted organ	C80.2	—	—	—	—	—
atlas	C41.2	C79.51	—	D16.6	D48.0	D49.2
atrium, cardiac	C38.0	C79.89	—	D15.1	D48.7	D49.89
auditory						
canal (external) (skin) A81	C44.20-✓	C79.2	D04.2-✓	D23.2-✓	D48.5	D49.2
internal	C30.1	C78.39	D02.3	D14.0	D38.5	D49.1
nerve	C72.4-✓	C79.49	—	D33.3	D43.3	D49.7
tube	C30.1	C78.39	D02.3	D14.0	D38.5	D49.1
opening	C11.2	C79.89	D00.08	D10.6	D37.05	D49.0
auricle, ear — see also Neoplasm, skin, ear	C44.20-✓	C79.2	D04.2-✓	D23.2-✓	D48.5	D49.2
auricular canal (external) — see also Neoplasm, skin, ear	C44.20-✓	C79.2	D04.2-✓	D23.2-✓	D48.5	D49.2
internal	C30.1	C78.39	D02.3	D14.0	D38.5	D49.2
autonomic nerve or nervous system NEC (see Neoplasm, nerve, peripheral)						
axilla, axillary	C76.1	C79.89	D09.8	D36.7	D48.7	D49.89
fold — see also Neoplasm, skin, trunk	C44.509	C79.2	D04.5	D23.5	D48.5	D49.2
back NEC	C76.8	C79.89	D04.5	D36.7	D48.7	D49.89

Neoplasm, neoplastic — continued

	Malignant Primary	Malignant Secondary	Ca in situ	Benign	Uncertain	Unspecified Behavior
Bartholin's gland	C51.0	C79.82	D07.1	D28.0	D39.8	D49.5
basal ganglia	C71.0	C79.31	—	D33.0	D43.0	D49.6
basis pedunculi	C71.7	C79.31	—	D33.1	D43.1	D49.6
bile or biliary (tract)	C24.9	C78.89	D01.5	D13.5	D37.6	D49.0
canaliculi (biliferi) (intrahepatic)	C22.1	C78.7	D01.5	D13.4	D37.6	D49.0
canals, interlobular	C22.1	C78.89	D01.5	D13.4	D37.6	D49.0
duct or passage (common) (cystic) (extrahepatic)	C24.0	C78.89	D01.5	D13.5	D37.6	D49.0
interlobular	C22.1	C78.89	D01.5	D13.4	D37.6	D49.0
intrahepatic	C22.1	C78.7	D01.5	D13.4	D37.6	D49.0
and extrahepatic	C24.8	C78.89	D01.5	D13.5	D37.6	D49.0
bladder (urinary)	C67.9	C79.11	D09.0	D30.3	D41.4	D49.4
dome	C67.1	C79.11	D09.0	D30.3	D41.4	D49.4
neck	C67.5	C79.11	D09.0	D30.3	D41.4	D49.4
orifice	C67.9	C79.11	D09.0	D30.3	D41.4	D49.4
ureteric	C67.6	C79.11	D09.0	D30.3	D41.4	D49.4
urethral	C67.5	C79.11	D09.0	D30.3	D41.4	D49.4
overlapping lesion	C67.8	—	—	—	—	—
sphincter	C67.8	C79.11	D09.0	D30.3	D41.4	D49.4
trigone	C67.0	C79.11	D09.0	D30.3	D41.4	D49.4
urachus	C67.7	C79.11	D09.0	D30.3	D41.4	D49.4
wall	C67.9	C79.11	D09.0	D30.3	D41.4	D49.4
anterior	C67.3	C79.11	D09.0	D30.3	D41.4	D49.4
lateral	C67.2	C79.11	D09.0	D30.3	D41.4	D49.4
posterior	C67.4	C79.11	D09.0	D30.3	D41.4	D49.4
blood vessel — see Neoplasm, connective tissue						
bone (periosteum)	C41.9	C79.51	—	D16.9	D48.0	D49.2
acetabulum	C41.4	C79.51	—	D16.8	D48.0	D49.2
ankle	C40.3-☑	C79.51	—	D16.3-☑	—	—
arm NEC	C40.0-☑	C79.51	—	D16.0-☑	—	—
astragalus	C40.3-☑	C79.51	—	D16.3-☑	—	—
atlas	C41.2	C79.51	—	D16.6	D48.0	D49.2
axis	C41.2	C79.51	—	D16.6	D48.0	D49.2
back NEC	C41.2	C79.51	—	D16.6	D48.0	D49.2
calcaneus	C40.3-☑	C79.51	—	D16.3-☑	—	—
calvarium	C41.0	C79.51	—	D16.4	D48.0	D49.2
carpus (any)	C40.1-☑	C79.51	—	D16.1-☑	—	—
cartilage NEC	C41.9	C79.51	—	D16.9	D48.0	D49.2
clavicle	C41.3	C79.51	—	D16.7	D48.0	D49.2
clivus	C41.0	C79.51	—	D16.4	D48.0	D49.2
coccygeal vertebra	C41.4	C79.51	—	D16.8	D48.0	D49.2
coccyx	C41.4	C79.51	—	D16.8	D48.0	D49.2
costal cartilage	C41.3	C79.51	—	D16.7	D48.0	D49.2
costovertebral joint	C41.3	C79.51	—	D16.7	D48.0	D49.2
cranial	C41.0	C79.51	—	D16.4	D48.0	D49.2
cuboid	C40.3-☑	C79.51	—	D16.3-☑	—	—
cuneiform	C41.9	C79.51	—	D16.9	D48.0	D49.2
elbow	C40.0-☑	C79.51	—	D16.0-☑	—	—
ethmoid (labyrinth)	C41.0	C79.51	—	D16.4	D48.0	D49.2
face	C41.0	C79.51	—	D16.4	D48.0	D49.2
femur (any part)	C40.2-☑	C79.51	—	D16.2-☑	—	—
fibula (any part)	C40.2-☑	C79.51	—	D16.2-☑	—	—
finger (any)	C40.1-☑	C79.51	—	D16.1-☑	—	—
foot	C40.3-☑	C79.51	—	D16.3-☑	—	—
forearm	C40.0-☑	C79.51	—	D16.0-☑	—	—
frontal	C41.0	C79.51	—	D16.4	D48.0	D49.2
hand	C40.1-☑	C79.51	—	D16.1-☑	—	—
heel	C40.3-☑	C79.51	—	D16.3-☑	—	—
hip	C41.4	C79.51	—	D16.8	D48.0	D49.2
humerus (any part)	C40.0-☑	C79.51	—	D16.0-☑	—	—
hyoid	C41.0	C79.51	—	D16.4	D48.0	D49.2
ilium	C41.4	C79.51	—	D16.8	D48.0	D49.2
innominate	C41.4	C79.51	—	D16.8	D48.0	D49.2
intervertebral cartilage or disc	C41.2	C79.51	—	D16.6	D48.0	D49.2
ischium	C41.4	C79.51	—	D16.8	D48.0	D49.2
jaw (lower)	C41.1	C79.51	—	D16.5	D48.0	D49.2
knee	C40.2-☑	C79.51	—	D16.2-☑	—	—
leg NEC	C40.2-☑	C79.51	—	D16.2-☑	—	—
limb NEC	C40.9-☑	C79.51	—	D16.9	—	—

Neoplasm, neoplastic — continued

	Malignant Primary	Malignant Secondary	Ca in situ	Benign	Uncertain	Unspecified Behavior
bone — continued						
limb — continued						
lower (long bones)	C40.2-☑	C79.51	—	D16.2-☑	—	—
short bones	C40.3-☑	C79.51	—	D16.3-☑	—	—
upper (long bones)	C40.0-☑	C79.51	—	D16.0-☑	—	—
short bones	C40.1-☑	C79.51	—	D16.1-☑	—	—
malar	C41.0	C79.51	—	D16.4	D48.0	D49.2
mandible	C41.1	C79.51	—	D16.5	D48.0	D49.2
marrow NEC (any bone)	C96.9	C79.52	—	—	D47.9	D49.89
mastoid	C41.0	C79.51	—	D16.4	D48.0	D49.2
maxilla, maxillary (superior)	C41.0	C79.51	—	D16.4	D48.0	D49.2
inferior	C41.1	C79.51	—	D16.5	D48.0	D49.2
metacarpus (any)	C40.1-☑	C79.51	—	D16.1-☑	—	—
metatarsus (any)	C40.3-☑	C79.51	—	D16.3-☑	—	—
navicular						
ankle	C40.3-☑	C79.51	—	—	—	—
hand	C40.1-☑	C79.51	—	—	—	—
nose, nasal	C41.0	C79.51	—	D16.4	D48.0	D49.2
occipital	C41.0	C79.51	—	D16.4	D48.0	D49.2
orbit	C41.0	C79.51	—	D16.4	D48.0	D49.2
overlapping sites	C40.8-☑	—	—	—	—	—
parietal	C41.0	C79.51	—	D16.4	D48.0	D49.2
patella	C40.2-☑	C79.51	—	—	—	—
pelvic	C41.4	C79.51	—	D16.8	D48.0	D49.2
phalanges						
foot	C40.3-☑	C79.51	—	—	—	—
hand	C40.1-☑	C79.51	—	—	—	—
pubic	C41.4	C79.51	—	D16.8	D48.0	D49.2
radius (any part)	C40.0-☑	C79.51	—	D16.0-☑	—	—
rib	C41.3	C79.51	—	D16.7	D48.0	D49.2
sacral vertebra	C41.4	C79.51	—	D16.8	D48.0	D49.2
sacrum	C41.4	C79.51	—	D16.8	D48.0	D49.2
scaphoid						
of ankle	C40.3-☑	C79.51	—	—	—	—
of hand	C40.1-☑	C79.51	—	—	—	—
scapula (any part)	C40.0-☑	C79.51	--	D16.0-☑	—	—
sella turcica	C41.0	C79.51	—	D16.4	D48.0	D49.2
shoulder	C40.0-☑	C79.51	—	D16.0-☑	—	—
skull	C41.0	C79.51	—	D16.4	D48.0	D49.2
sphenoid	C41.0	C79.51	—	D16.4	D48.0	D49.2
spine, spinal (column)	C41.2	C79.51	—	D16.6	D48.0	D49.2
coccyx	C41.4	C79.51	—	D16.8	D48.0	D49.2
sacrum	C41.4	C79.51	—	D16.8	D48.0	D49.2
sternum	C41.3	C79.51	—	D16.7	D48.0	D49.2
tarsus (any)	C40.3-☑	C79.51	—	—	—	—
temporal	C41.0	C79.51	—	D16.4	D48.0	D49.2
thumb	C40.1-☑	C79.51	—	—	—	—
tibia (any part)	C40.2-☑	C79.51	—	—	—	—
toe (any)	C40.3-☑	C79.51	—	—	—	—
trapezium	C40.1-☑	C79.51	—	—	—	—
trapezoid	C40.1-☑	C79.51	—	—	—	—
turbinate	C41.0	C79.51	—	D16.4	D48.0	D49.2
ulna (any part)	C40.0-☑	C79.51	—	D16.0-☑	—	—
unciform	C40.1-☑	C79.51	—	—	—	—
vertebra (column)	C41.2	C79.51	—	D16.6	D48.0	D49.2
coccyx	C41.4	C79.51	—	D16.8	D48.0	D49.2
sacrum	C41.4	C79.51	—	D16.8	D48.0	D49.2
vomer	C41.0	C79.51	—	D16.4	D48.0	D49.2
wrist	C40.1-☑	C79.51	—	—	—	—
xiphoid process	C41.3	C79.51	—	D16.7	D48.0	D49.2
zygomatic	C41.0	C79.51	—	D16.4	D48.0	D49.2
book-leaf (mouth) — ventral surface of tongue and floor of mouth	C06.89	C79.89	D00.00	D10.39	D37.09	D49.0
bowel — see Neoplasm, intestine						
brachial plexus	C47.1-☑	C79.89	—	D36.12	D48.2	D49.2
brain NEC	C71.9	C79.31	—	D33.2	D43.2	D49.6
basal ganglia	C71.0	C79.31	—	D33.0	D43.0	D49.6
cerebellopontine angle	C71.6	C79.31	—	D33.1	D43.1	D49.6
cerebellum NOS	C71.6	C79.31	—	D33.1	D43.1	D49.6
cerebrum	C71.0	C79.31	—	D33.0	D43.0	D49.6

☑ **Additional Character Required — Refer to the Tabular List for Character Selection**   ▽ **Subterms under main terms may continue to next column or page**

Neoplasm Table

	Malignant Primary	Malignant Secondary	Ca in situ	Benign	Uncertain	Unspecified Behavior
Neoplasm, neoplastic — *continued*						
brain — *continued*						
choroid plexus	C71.7	C79.31	—	D33.1	D43.1	D49.6
corpus callosum	C71.8	C79.31	—	D33.2	D43.2	D49.6
corpus striatum	C71.0	C79.31	—	D33.0	D43.0	D49.6
cortex (cerebral)	C71.0	C79.31	—	D33.0	D43.0	D49.6
frontal lobe	C71.1	C79.31	—	D33.0	D43.0	D49.6
globus pallidus	C71.0	C79.31	—	D33.0	D43.0	D49.6
hippocampus	C71.2	C79.31	—	D33.0	D43.0	D49.6
hypothalamus	C71.0	C79.31	—	D33.0	D43.0	D49.6
internal capsule	C71.0	C79.31	—	D33.0	D43.0	D49.6
medulla oblongata	C71.7	C79.31	—	D33.1	D43.1	D49.6
meninges	C70.0	C79.32	—	D32.0	D42.0	D49.7
midbrain	C71.7	C79.31	—	D33.1	D43.1	D49.6
occipital lobe	C71.4	C79.31	—	D33.0	D43.0	D49.6
overlapping lesion	C71.8	C79.31	—	—	—	—
parietal lobe	C71.3	C79.31	—	D33.0	D43.0	D49.6
peduncle	C71.7	C79.31	—	D33.1	D43.1	D49.6
pons	C71.7	C79.31	—	D33.1	D43.1	D49.6
stem	C71.7	C79.31	—	D33.1	D43.1	D49.6
tapetum	C71.8	C79.31	—	D33.2	D43.2	D49.6
temporal lobe	C71.2	C79.31	—	D33.0	D43.0	D49.6
thalamus	C71.0	C79.31	—	D33.0	D43.0	D49.6
uncus	C71.2	C79.31	—	D33.0	D43.0	D49.6
ventricle (floor)	C71.5	C79.31	—	D33.0	D43.0	D49.6
fourth	C71.7	C79.31	—	D33.1	D43.1	D49.6
branchial (cleft) (cyst) (vestiges)	C10.4	C79.89	D00.08	D10.5	D37.05	D49.0
breast (connective tissue) (glandular tissue) (soft parts)	C50.9-☑	C79.81	D05.-☑	D24.-☑	D48.6-☑	D49.3
areola	C50.0-☑	C79.81	D05.-☑	D24.-☑	D48.6-☑	D49.3
axillary tail	C50.6-☑	C79.81	D05.-☑	D24.-☑	D48.6-☑	D49.3
central portion	C50.1-☑	C79.81	D05.-☑	D24.-☑	D48.6-☑	D49.3
inner	C50.8-☑	C79.81	D05.-☑	D24.-☑	D48.6-☑	D49.3
lower	C50.8-☑	C79.81	D05.-☑	D24.-☑	D48.6-☑	D49.3
lower-inner quadrant	C50.3-☑	C79.81	D05.-☑	D24.-☑	D48.6-☑	D49.3
lower-outer quadrant	C50.5-☑	C79.81	D05.-☑	D24.-☑	D48.6-☑	D49.3
mastectomy site (skin) — *see also* Neoplasm, breast, skin	C44.501	C79.2	—	—	—	—
specified as breast tissue	C50.8-☑	C79.81	—	—	—	—
midline	C50.8-☑	C79.81	D05.-☑	D24.-☑	D48.6-☑	D49.3
nipple	C50.0-☑	C79.81	D05.-☑	D24.-☑	D48.6-☑	D49.3
outer	C50.8-☑	C79.81	D05.-☑	D24.-☑	D48.6-☑	D49.3
overlapping lesion	C50.8-☑	—	—	—	—	—
skin	C44.501	C79.2	D04.5	D23.5	D48.5	D49.2
basal cell carcinoma	C44.511	—	—	—	—	—
specified type NEC	C44.591	—	—	—	—	—
squamous cell carcinoma	C44.521	—	—	—	—	—
tail (axillary)	C50.6-☑	C79.81	D05.-☑	D24.-☑	D48.6-☑	D49.3
upper	C50.8-☑	C79.81	D05.-☑	D24.-☑	D48.6-☑	D49.3
upper-inner quadrant	C50.2-☑	C79.81	D05.-☑	D24.-☑	D48.6-☑	D49.3
upper-outer quadrant	C50.4-☑	C79.81	D05.-☑	D24.-☑	D48.6-☑	D49.3
broad ligament	C57.1-☑	C79.82	D07.39	D28.2	D39.8	D49.5
bronchiogenic, bronchogenic (lung)	C34.9-☑	C78.0-☑	D02.2-☑	D14.3-☑	D38.1	D49.1
bronchiole	C34.9-☑	C78.0-☑	D02.2-☑	D14.3-☑	D38.1	D49.1
bronchus	C34.9-☑	C78.0-☑	D02.2-☑	D14.3-☑	D38.1	D49.1
carina	C34.0-☑	C78.0-☑	D02.2-☑	D14.3-☑	D38.1	D49.1
lower lobe of lung	C34.3-☑	C78.0-☑	D02.2-☑	D14.3-☑	D38.1	D49.1
main	C34.0-☑	C78.0-☑	D02.2-☑	D14.3-☑	D38.1	D49.1
middle lobe of lung	C34.2	C78.0-☑	D02.21	D14.31	D38.1	D49.1
overlapping lesion	C34.8-☑	—	—	—	—	—
upper lobe of lung	C34.1-☑	C78.0-☑	D02.2-☑	D14.3-☑	D38.1	D49.1
brow	C44.309	C79.2	D04.39	D23.39	D48.5	D49.2
basal cell carcinoma	C44.319	—	—	—	—	—
specified type NEC	C44.399	—	—	—	—	—

	Malignant Primary	Malignant Secondary	Ca in situ	Benign	Uncertain	Unspecified Behavior
Neoplasm, neoplastic — *continued*						
brow — *continued*						
squamous cell carcinoma	C44.329	—	—	—	—	—
buccal (cavity)	C06.9	C79.89	D00.00	D10.39	D37.09	D49.0
commissure	C06.0	C79.89	D00.02	D10.39	D37.09	D49.0
groove (lower) (upper)	C06.1	C79.89	D00.02	D10.39	D37.09	D49.0
mucosa	C06.0	C79.89	D00.02	D10.39	D37.09	D49.0
sulcus (lower) (upper)	C06.1	C79.89	D00.02	D10.39	D37.09	D49.0
bulbourethral gland	C68.0	C79.19	D09.19	D30.4	D41.3	D49.5
bursa — *see* Neoplasm, connective tissue						
buttock NEC	C76.3	C79.89	D04.5	D36.7	D48.7	D49.89
calf	C76.5-☑	C79.89	D04.7-☑	D36.7	D48.7	D49.89
calvarium	C41.0	C79.51	—	D16.4	D48.0	D49.2
calyx, renal	C65.-☑	C79.0-☑	D09.19	D30.1-☑	D41.1-☑	D49.5
canal						
anal	C21.1	C78.5	D01.3	D12.9	D37.8	D49.0
auditory (external) — *see also* Neoplasm, skin, ear	C44.20-☑	C79.2	D04.2-☑	D23.2-☑	D48.5	D49.2
auricular (external) — *see also* Neoplasm, skin, ear	C44.20-☑	C79.2	D04.2-☑	D23.2-☑	D48.5	D49.2
canaliculi, biliary (biliferi) (intrahepatic)	C22.1	C78.7	D01.5	D13.4	D37.6	D49.0
canthus (eye) (inner) (outer)	C44.10-☑	C79.2	D04.1-☑	D23.1-☑	D48.5	D49.2
basal cell carcinoma	C44.11-☑	—	—	—	—	—
specified type NEC	C44.19-☑	—	—	—	—	—
squamous cell carcinoma	C44.12-☑	—	—	—	—	—
capillary — *see* Neoplasm, connective tissue						
caput coli	C18.0	C78.5	D01.0	D12.0	D37.4	D49.0
carcinoid — *see* Tumor, carcinoid						
cardia (gastric)	C16.0	C78.89	D00.2	D13.1	D37.1	D49.0
cardiac orifice (stomach)	C16.0	C78.89	D00.2	D13.1	D37.1	D49.0
cardio-esophageal junction	C16.0	C78.89	D00.2	D13.1	D37.1	D49.0
cardio-esophagus	C16.0	C78.89	D00.2	D13.1	D37.1	D49.0
carina (bronchus)	C34.0-☑	C78.0-☑	D02.2-☑	D14.3-☑	D38.1	D49.1
carotid (artery)	C49.0	C79.89	—	D21.0	D48.1	D49.2
body	C75.4	C79.89	—	D35.5	D44.6	D49.7
carpus (any bone)	C40.1-☑	C79.51	—	D16.1-☑	—	—
cartilage (articular) (joint) NEC — *see also* Neoplasm, bone	C41.9	C79.51	—	D16.9	D48.0	D49.2
arytenoid	C32.3	C78.39	D02.0	D14.1	D38.0	D49.1
auricular	C49.0	C79.89	—	D21.0	D48.1	D49.2
bronchi	C34.0-☑	C78.39	—	D14.3-☑	D38.1	D49.1
costal	C41.3	C79.51	—	D16.7	D48.0	D49.2
cricoid	C32.3	C78.39	D02.0	D14.1	D38.0	D49.1
cuneiform	C32.3	C78.39	D02.0	D14.1	D38.0	D49.1
ear (external)	C49.0	C79.89	—	D21.0	D48.1	D49.2
ensiform	C41.3	C79.51	—	D16.7	D48.0	D49.2
epiglottis	C32.1	C78.39	D02.0	D14.1	D38.0	D49.1
anterior surface	C10.1	C79.89	D00.08	D10.5	D37.05	D49.0
eyelid	C49.0	C79.89	—	D21.0	D48.1	D49.2
intervertebral	C41.2	C79.51	—	D16.6	D48.0	D49.2
larynx, laryngeal	C32.3	C78.39	D02.0	D14.1	D38.0	D49.1
nose, nasal	C30.0	C78.39	D02.3	D14.0	D38.5	D49.1
pinna	C49.0	C79.89	—	D21.0	D48.1	D49.2
rib	C41.3	C79.51	—	D16.7	D48.0	D49.2
semilunar (knee)	C40.2-☑	C79.51	—	D16.2-☑	D48.0	D49.2
thyroid	C32.3	C78.39	D02.0	D14.1	D38.0	D49.1
trachea	C33	C78.39	D02.1	D14.2	D38.1	D49.1
cauda equina	C72.1	C79.49	—	D33.4	D43.4	D49.7
cavity						
buccal	C06.9	C79.89	D00.00	D10.30	D37.09	D49.0
nasal	C30.0	C78.39	D02.3	D14.0	D38.5	D49.1
oral	C06.9	C79.89	D00.00	D10.30	D37.09	D49.0
peritoneal	C48.2	C78.6	—	D20.1	D48.4	D49.0
tympanic	C30.1	C78.39	D02.3	D14.0	D38.5	D49.1
cecum	C18.0	C78.5	D01.0	D12.0	D37.4	D49.0

Neoplasm Table

Neoplasm, central nervous system — Neoplasm, connective tissue NEC

Neoplasm, neoplastic — *continued*	Malignant Primary	Malignant Secondary	Ca in situ	Benign	Uncertain	Unspecified Behavior
central nervous system	C72.9	C79.40	—	—	—	—
cerebellopontine (angle)	C71.6	C79.31	—	D33.1	D43.1	D49.6
cerebellum, cerebellar	C71.6	C79.31	—	D33.1	D43.1	D49.6
cerebrum, cerebral (cortex) (hemisphere) (white matter)	C71.0	C79.31	—	D33.0	D43.0	D49.6
meninges	C70.0	C79.32	—	D32.0	D42.0	D49.7
peduncle	C71.7	C79.31	—	D33.1	D43.1	D49.6
ventricle	C71.5	C79.31	—	D33.0	D43.0	D49.6
fourth	C71.7	C79.31	—	D33.1	D43.1	D49.6
cervical region	C76.0	C79.89	D09.8	D36.7	D48.7	D49.89
cervix (cervical) (uteri) (uterus)	C53.9	C79.82	D06.9	D26.0	D39.0	D49.5
canal	C53.0	C79.82	D06.0	D26.0	D39.0	D49.5
endocervix (canal) (gland)	C53.0	C79.82	D06.0	D26.0	D39.0	D49.5
exocervix	C53.1	C79.82	D06.1	D26.0	D39.0	D49.5
external os	C53.1	C79.82	D06.1	D26.0	D39.0	D49.5
internal os	C53.0	C79.82	D06.0	D26.0	D39.0	D49.5
nabothian gland	C53.0	C79.82	D06.0	D26.0	D39.0	D49.5
overlapping lesion	C53.8	—	—	—	—	—
squamocolumnar junction	C53.8	C79.82	D06.7	D26.0	D39.0	D49.5
stump	C53.8	C79.82	D06.7	D26.0	D39.0	D49.5
cheek	C76.0	C79.89	D09.8	D36.7	D48.7	D49.89
external	C44.309	C79.2	D04.39	D23.39	D48.5	D49.2
basal cell carcinoma	C44.319	—	—	—	—	—
specified type NEC	C44.399	—	—	—	—	—
squamous cell carcinoma	C44.329	—	—	—	—	—
inner aspect	C06.0	C79.89	D00.02	D10.39	D37.09	D49.0
internal	C06.0	C79.89	D00.02	D10.39	D37.09	D49.0
mucosa	C06.0	C79.89	D00.02	D10.39	D37.09	D49.0
chest (wall) NEC	C76.1	C79.89	D09.8	D36.7	D48.7	D49.89
chiasma opticum	C72.3-✓	C79.49	—	D33.3	D43.3	D49.7
chin	C44.309	C79.2	D04.39	D23.39	D48.5	D49.2
basal cell carcinoma	C44.319	—	—	—	—	—
specified type NEC	C44.399	—	—	—	—	—
squamous cell carcinoma	C44.329	—	—	—	—	—
choana	C11.3	C79.89	D00.08	D10.6	D37.05	D49.0
cholangiole	C22.1	C78.89	D01.5	D13.4	D37.6	D49.0
choledochal duct	C24.0	C78.89	D01.5	D13.5	D37.6	D49.0
choroid	C69.3-✓	C79.49	D09.2-✓	D31.3-✓	D48.7	D49.81
plexus	C71.5	C79.31	—	D33.0	D43.0	D49.6
ciliary body	C69.4-✓	C79.49	D09.2-✓	D31.4-✓	D48.7	D49.89
clavicle	C41.3	C79.51	—	D16.7	D48.0	D49.2
clitoris	C51.2	C79.82	D07.1	D28.0	D39.8	D49.5
clivus	C41.0	C79.51	—	D16.4	D48.0	D49.2
cloacogenic zone	C21.2	C78.5	D01.3	D12.9	D37.8	D49.0
coccygeal						
body or glomus	C49.5	C79.89	—	D21.5	D48.1	D49.2
vertebra	C41.4	C79.51	—	D16.8	D48.0	D49.2
coccyx	C41.4	C79.51	—	D16.8	D48.0	D49.2
colon — *see also* Neoplasm, intestine, large	C18.9	C78.5	—	—	—	—
with rectum	C19	C78.5	D01.1	D12.7	D37.5	D49.0
columnella — *see also* Neoplasm, skin, face	C44.390	C79.2	D04.39	D23.39	D48.5	D49.2
column, spinal — *see* Neoplasm, spine						
commissure						
labial, lip	C00.6	C79.89	D00.01	D10.39	D37.01	D49.0
laryngeal	C32.0	C78.39	D02.0	D14.1	D38.0	D49.1
common (bile) duct	C24.0	C78.89	D01.5	D13.5	D37.6	D49.0
concha — *see also* Neoplasm, skin, ear	C44.20-✓	C79.2	D04.2-✓	D23.2-✓	D48.5	D49.2
nose	C30.0	C78.39	D02.3	D14.0	D38.5	D49.1
conjunctiva	C69.0-✓	C79.49	D09.2-✓	D31.0-✓	D48.7	D49.89

Neoplasm, neoplastic — *continued*	Malignant Primary	Malignant Secondary	Ca in situ	Benign	Uncertain	Unspecified Behavior
connective tissue NEC	C49.9	C79.89	—	D21.9	D48.1	D49.2

Note: For neoplasms of connective tissue (blood vessel, bursa, fascia, ligament, muscle, peripheral nerves, sympathetic and parasympathetic nerves and ganglia, synovia, tendon, etc.) or of morphological types that indicate connective tissue, code according to the list under "Neoplasm, connective tissue". For sites that do not appear in this list, code to neoplasm of that site; e.g., fibrosarcoma, pancreas (C25.9)

Note: Morphological types that indicate connective tissue appear in their proper place in the alphabetic index with the instruction "see Neoplasm, connective tissue ...."

	Malignant Primary	Malignant Secondary	Ca in situ	Benign	Uncertain	Unspecified Behavior
abdomen	C49.4	C79.89	—	D21.4	D48.1	D49.2
abdominal wall	C49.4	C79.89	—	D21.4	D48.1	D49.2
ankle	C49.2-✓	C79.89	—	D21.2-✓	D48.1	D49.2
antecubital fossa or space	C49.1-✓	C79.89	—	D21.1-✓	D48.1	D49.2
arm	C49.1-✓	C79.89	—	D21.1-✓	D48.1	D49.2
auricle (ear)	C49.0	C79.89	—	D21.0	D48.1	D49.2
axilla	C49.3	C79.89	—	D21.3	D48.1	D49.2
back	C49.6	C79.89	—	D21.6	D48.1	D49.2
breast — *see* Neoplasm, breast						
buttock	C49.5	C79.89	—	D21.5	D48.1	D49.2
calf	C49.2-✓	C79.89	—	D21.2-✓	D48.1	D49.2
cervical region	C49.0	C79.89	—	D21.0	D48.1	D49.2
cheek	C49.0	C79.89	—	D21.0	D48.1	D49.2
chest (wall)	C49.3	C79.89	—	D21.3	D48.1	D49.2
chin	C49.0	C79.89	—	D21.0	D48.1	D49.2
diaphragm	C49.3	C79.89	—	D21.3	D48.1	D49.2
ear (external)	C49.0	C79.89	—	D21.0	D48.1	D49.2
elbow	C49.1-✓	C79.89	—	D21.1-✓	D48.1	D49.2
extrarectal	C49.5	C79.89	—	D21.5	D48.1	D49.2
extremity	C49.9	C79.89	—	D21.9	D48.1	D49.2
lower	C49.2-✓	C79.89	—	D21.2-✓	D48.1	D49.2
upper	C49.1-✓	C79.89	—	D21.1-✓	D48.1	D49.2
eyelid	C49.0	C79.89	—	D21.0	D48.1	D49.2
face	C49.0	C79.89	—	D21.0	D48.1	D49.2
finger	C49.1-✓	C79.89	—	D21.1-✓	D48.1	D49.2
flank	C49.6	C79.89	—	D21.6	D48.1	D49.2
foot	C49.2-✓	C79.89	—	D21.2-✓	D48.1	D49.2
forearm	C49.1-✓	C79.89	—	D21.1-✓	D48.1	D49.2
forehead	C49.0	C79.89	—	D21.0	D48.1	D49.2
gastric	C49.4	C79.89	—	D21.4	D48.1	D49.2
gastrointestinal	C49.4	C79.89	—	D21.4	D48.1	D49.2
gluteal region	C49.5	C79.89	—	D21.5	D48.1	D49.2
great vessels NEC	C49.3	C79.89	—	D21.3	D48.1	D49.2
groin	C49.5	C79.89	—	D21.5	D48.1	D49.2
hand	C49.1-✓	C79.89	—	D21.1-✓	D48.1	D49.2
head	C49.0	C79.89	—	D21.0	D48.1	D49.2
heel	C49.2-✓	C79.89	—	D21.2-✓	D48.1	D49.2
hip	C49.2-✓	C79.89	—	D21.2-✓	D48.1	D49.2
hypochondrium	C49.4	C79.89	—	D21.4	D48.1	D49.2
iliopsoas muscle	C49.5	C79.89	—	D21.5	D48.1	D49.2
infraclavicular region	C49.3	C79.89	—	D21.3	D48.1	D49.2
inguinal (canal) (region)	C49.5	C79.89	—	D21.5	D48.1	D49.2
intestinal	C49.4	C79.89	—	D21.4	D48.1	D49.2
intrathoracic	C49.3	C79.89	—	D21.3	D48.1	D49.2
ischiorectal fossa	C49.5	C79.89	—	D21.5	D48.1	D49.2
jaw	C03.9	C79.89	D00.03	D10.39	D48.1	D49.0
knee	C49.2-✓	C79.89	—	D21.2-✓	D48.1	D49.2
leg	C49.2-✓	C79.89	—	D21.2-✓	D48.1	D49.2
limb NEC	C49.9	C79.89	—	D21.9	D48.1	D49.2
lower	C49.2-✓	C79.89	—	D21.2-✓	D48.1	D49.2
upper	C49.1-✓	C79.89	—	D21.1-✓	D48.1	D49.2
nates	C49.5	C79.89	—	D21.5	D48.1	D49.2
neck	C49.0	C79.89	—	D21.0	D48.1	D49.2
orbit	C69.6-✓	C79.49	D09.2-✓	D31.6-✓	D48.1	D49.89
overlapping lesion	C49.8	—	—	—	—	—
pararectal	C49.5	C79.89	—	D21.5	D48.1	D49.2
para-urethral	C49.5	C79.89	—	D21.5	D48.1	D49.2
paravaginal	C49.5	C79.89	—	D21.5	D48.1	D49.2
pelvis (floor)	C49.5	C79.89	—	D21.5	D48.1	D49.2
pelvo-abdominal	C49.8	C79.89	—	D21.6	D48.1	D49.2
perineum	C49.5	C79.89	—	D21.5	D48.1	D49.2
perirectal (tissue)	C49.5	C79.89	—	D21.5	D48.1	D49.2

Neoplasm, neoplastic —	Malignant Primary	Malignant Secondary	Ca in situ	Benign	Uncertain	Unspecified Behavior
continued						
connective tissue —						
continued						
periurethral						
(tissue)	C49.5	C79.89	—	D21.5	D48.1	D49.2
popliteal fossa or						
space	C49.2-☑	C79.89	—	D21.2-☑	D48.1	D49.2
presacral	C49.5	C79.89	—	D21.5	D48.1	D49.2
psoas muscle	C49.4	C79.89	—	D21.4	D48.1	D49.2
pterygoid fossa	C49.0	C79.89	—	D21.0	D48.1	D49.2
rectovaginal septum or						
wall	C49.5	C79.89	—	D21.5	D48.1	D49.2
rectovesical	C49.5	C79.89	—	D21.5	D48.1	D49.2
retroperitoneum	C48.0	C78.6	—	D20.0	D48.3	D49.0
sacrococcygeal						
region	C49.5	C79.89	—	D21.5	D48.1	D49.2
scalp	C49.0	C79.89	—	D21.0	D48.1	D49.2
scapular region	C49.3	C79.89	—	D21.3	D48.1	D49.2
shoulder	C49.1-☑	C79.89	—	D21.1-☑	D48.1	D49.2
skin (dermis) NEC — *see*						
also Neoplasm, skin,						
by site	C44.90	C79.2	D04.9	D23.9	D48.5	D49.2
stomach	C49.4	C79.89	—	D21.4	D48.1	D49.2
submental	C49.0	C79.89	—	D21.0	D48.1	D49.2
supraclavicular						
region	C49.0	C79.89	—	D21.0	D48.1	D49.2
temple	C49.0	C79.89	—	D21.0	D48.1	D49.2
temporal region	C49.0	C79.89	—	D21.0	D48.1	D49.2
thigh	C49.2-☑	C79.89	—	D21.2-☑	D48.1	D49.2
thoracic (duct)						
(wall)	C49.3	C79.89	—	D21.3	D48.1	D49.2
thorax	C49.3	C79.89	—	D21.3	D48.1	D49.2
thumb	C49.1-☑	C79.89	—	D21.1-☑	D48.1	D49.2
toe	C49.2-☑	C79.89	—	D21.2-☑	D48.1	D49.2
trunk	C49.6	C79.89	—	D21.6	D48.1	D49.2
umbilicus	C49.4	C79.89	—	D21.4	D48.1	D49.2
vesicorectal	C49.5	C79.89	—	D21.5	D48.1	D49.2
wrist	C49.1-☑	C79.89	—	D21.1-☑	D48.1	D49.2
conus medullaris	C72.0	C79.49	—	D33.4	D43.4	D49.7
cord (true) (vocal)	C32.0	C78.39	D02.0	D14.1	D38.0	D49.1
false	C32.1	C78.39	D02.0	D14.1	D38.0	D49.1
spermatic	C63.1-☑	C79.82	D07.69	D29.8	D40.8	D49.5
spinal (cervical)						
(lumbar)						
(thoracic)	C72.0	C79.49	—	D33.4	D43.4	D49.7
cornea (limbus)	C69.1-☑	C79.49	D09.2-☑	D31.1-☑	D48.7	D49.89
corpus						
albicans	C56.-☑	C79.6-☑	D07.39	D27.-☑	D39.1-☑	D49.5
callosum, brain	C71.0	C79.31	—	D33.2	D43.2	D49.6
cavernosum	C60.2	C79.82	D07.4	D29.0	D40.8	D49.5
gastric	C16.2	C78.89	D00.2	D13.1	D37.1	D49.0
overlapping sites	C54.8	—	—	—	—	—
penis	C60.2	C79.82	D07.4	D29.0	D40.8	D49.5
striatum,						
cerebrum	C71.0	C79.31	—	D33.0	D43.0	D49.6
uteri	C54.9	C79.82	D07.0	D26.1	D39.0	D49.5
isthmus	C54.0	C79.82	D07.0	D26.1	D39.0	D49.5
cortex						
adrenal	C74.0-☑	C79.7-☑	D09.3	D35.0-☑	D44.1-☑	D49.7
cerebral	C71.0	C79.31	—	D33.0	D43.0	D49.6
costal cartilage	C41.3	C79.51	—	D16.7	D48.0	D49.2
costovertebral joint	C41.3	C79.51	—	D16.7	D48.0	D49.2
Cowper's gland	C68.0	C79.19	D09.19	D30.4	D41.3	D49.5
cranial (fossa, any)	C71.9	C79.31	—	D33.2	D43.2	D49.6
meninges	C70.0	C79.32	—	D32.0	D42.0	D49.7
nerve	C72.50	C79.49	—	D33.3	D43.3	D49.7
specified NEC	C72.59	C79.49	—	D33.3	D43.3	D49.7
craniobuccal pouch	C75.2	C79.89	D09.3	D35.2	D44.3	D49.7
craniopharyngeal (duct)						
(pouch)	C75.2	C79.89	D09.3	D35.3	D44.4	D49.7
cricoid	C13.0	C79.89	D00.08	D10.7	D37.05	D49.0
cartilage	C32.3	C78.39	D02.0	D14.1	D38.0	D49.1
cricopharynx	C13.0	C79.89	D00.08	D10.7	D37.05	D49.0
crypt of Morgagni	C21.8	C78.5	D01.3	D12.9	D37.8	D49.0
crystalline lens	C69.4-☑	C79.49	D09.2-☑	D31.4-☑	D48.7	D49.89
cul-de-sac						
(Douglas')	C48.1	C78.6	—	D20.1	D48.4	D49.0
cuneiform cartilage	C32.3	C78.39	D02.0	D14.1	D38.0	D49.1
cutaneous — *see*						
Neoplasm, skin						
cutis — *see* Neoplasm,						
skin						

Neoplasm, neoplastic —	Malignant Primary	Malignant Secondary	Ca in situ	Benign	Uncertain	Unspecified Behavior
continued						
cystic (bile) duct						
(common)	C24.0	C78.89	D01.5	D13.5	D37.6	D49.0
dermis — *see* Neoplasm,						
skin						
diaphragm	C49.3	C79.89	—	D21.3	D48.1	D49.2
digestive organs, system,						
tube, or tract						
NEC	C26.9	C78.89	D01.9	D13.9	D37.9	D49.0
disc, intervertebral	C41.2	C79.51	—	D16.6	D48.0	D49.2
disease, generalized	C80.0	—	—	—	—	—
disseminated	C80.0	—	—	—	—	—
Douglas' cul-de-sac or						
pouch	C48.1	C78.6	—	D20.1	D48.4	D49.0
duodenojejunal						
junction	C17.8	C78.4	D01.49	D13.39	D37.2	D49.0
duodenum	C17.0	C78.4	D01.49	D13.2	D37.2	D49.0
dura (cranial)						
(mater)	C70.9	C79.49	—	D32.9	D42.9	D49.7
cerebral	C70.0	C79.32	—	D32.0	D42.0	D49.7
spinal	C70.1	C79.49	—	D32.1	D42.1	D49.7
ear (external) — *see also*						
Neoplasm, skin,						
ear	C44.20-☑	C79.2	D04.2-☑	D23.2-☑	D48.5	D49.2
auricle or auris — *see*						
also Neoplasm, skin,						
ear	C44.20-☑	C79.2	D04.2-☑	D23.2-☑	D48.5	D49.2
canal, external — *see*						
also Neoplasm, skin,						
ear	C44.20-☑	C79.2	D04.2-☑	D23.2-☑	D48.5	D49.2
cartilage	C49.0	C79.89	—	D21.0	D48.1	D49.2
external meatus — *see*						
also Neoplasm, skin,						
ear	C44.20-☑	C79.2	D04.2-☑	D23.2-☑	D48.5	D49.2
inner	C30.1	C78.39	D02.3	D14.0	D38.5	D49.1
lobule — *see also*						
Neoplasm, skin,						
ear	C44.20-☑	C79.2	D04.2-☑	D23.2-☑	D48.5	D49.2
middle	C30.1	C78.39	D02.3	D14.0	D38.5	D49.1
overlapping lesion with						
accessory						
sinuses	C31.8	—	—	—	—	—
skin	C44.20-☑	C79.2	D04.2-☑	D23.2-☑	D48.5	D49.2
basal cell						
carcinoma	C44.21-☑	—	—	—	—	—
specified type						
NEC	C44.29-☑	—	—	—	—	—
squamous cell						
carcinoma	C44.22-☑	—	—	—	—	—
earlobe	C44.20-☑	C79.2	D04.2-☑	D23.2-☑	D48.5	D49.2
basal cell						
carcinoma	C44.21-☑	—	—	—	—	—
specified type NEC	C44.29-☑	—	—	—	—	—
squamous cell						
carcinoma	C44.22-☑	—	—	—	—	—
ejaculatory duct	C63.7	C79.82	D07.69	D29.8	D40.8	D49.5
elbow NEC	C76.4-☑	C79.89	D04.6-☑	D36.7	D48.7	D49.89
endocardium	C38.0	C79.89	—	D15.1	D48.7	D49.89
endocervix (canal)						
(gland)	C53.0	C79.82	D06.0	D26.0	D39.0	D49.5
endocrine gland						
NEC	C75.9	C79.89	D09.3	D35.9	D44.9	D49.7
pluriglandular	C75.8	C79.89	D09.3	D35.7	D44.9	D49.7
endometrium (gland)						
(stroma)	C54.1	C79.82	D07.0	D26.1	D39.0	D49.5
ensiform cartilage	C41.3	C79.51	—	D16.7	D48.0	D49.2
enteric — *see* Neoplasm,						
intestine						
ependyma (brain)	C71.5	C79.31	—	D33.0	D43.0	D49.6
fourth ventricle	C71.7	C79.31	—	D33.1	D43.1	D49.6
epicardium	C38.0	C79.89	—	D15.1	D48.7	D49.89
epidermis — *see* Neoplasm,						
epididymis	C63.0-☑	C79.82	D07.69	D29.3-☑	D40.8	D49.5
epidural	C72.9	C79.49	—	D33.9	D43.9	D49.7
epiglottis	C32.1	C78.39	D02.0	D14.1	D38.0	D49.1
anterior aspect or						
surface	C10.1	C79.89	D00.08	D10.5	D37.05	D49.0
cartilage	C32.3	C78.39	D02.0	D14.1	D38.0	D49.1
free border						
(margin)	C10.1	C79.89	D00.08	D10.5	D37.05	D49.0
junctional region	C10.8	C79.89	D00.08	D10.5	D37.05	D49.0
posterior (laryngeal)						
surface	C32.1	C78.39	D02.0	D14.1	D38.0	D49.1

Neoplasm, neoplastic — continued

epiglottis — continued	Malignant Primary	Malignant Secondary	Ca in situ	Benign	Uncertain	Unspecified Behavior
suprahyoid portion	C32.1	C78.39	D02.0	D14.1	D38.0	D49.1
esophagogastric junction	C16.0	C78.89	D00.2	D13.1	D37.1	D49.0
esophagus	C15.9	C78.89	D00.1	D13.0	D37.8	D49.0
abdominal	C15.5	C78.89	D00.1	D13.0	D37.8	D49.0
cervical	C15.3	C78.89	D00.1	D13.0	D37.8	D49.0
distal (third)	C15.5	C78.89	D00.1	D13.0	D37.8	D49.0
lower (third)	C15.5	C78.89	D00.1	D13.0	D37.8	D49.0
middle (third)	C15.4	C78.89	D00.1	D13.0	D37.8	D49.0
overlapping lesion	C15.8	—	—	—	—	—
proximal (third)	C15.3	C78.89	D00.1	D13.0	D37.8	D49.0
thoracic	C15.4	C78.89	D00.1	D13.0	D37.8	D49.0
upper (third)	C15.3	C78.89	D00.1	D13.0	D37.8	D49.0
ethmoid (sinus)	C31.1	C78.39	D02.3	D14.0	D38.5	D49.1
bone or labyrinth	C41.0	C79.51	—	D16.4	D48.0	D49.2
eustachian tube	C30.1	C78.39	D02.3	D14.0	D38.5	D49.1
exocervix	C53.1	C79.82	D06.1	D26.0	D39.0	D49.5
external						
meatus (ear) — see also Neoplasm, skin, ear	C44.20-☑	C79.2	D04.2-☑	D23.2-☑	D48.5	D49.2
os, cervix uteri	C53.1	C79.82	D06.1	D26.0	D39.0	D49.5
extradural	C72.9	C79.49	—	D33.9	D43.9	D49.7
extrahepatic (bile) duct	C24.0	C78.89	D01.5	D13.5	D37.6	D49.0
overlapping lesion with gallbladder	C24.8	—	—	—	—	—
extraocular muscle	C69.6-☑	C79.49	D09.2-☑	D31.6-☑	D48.7	D49.89
extrarectal	C76.3	C79.89	D09.8	D36.7	D48.7	D49.89
extremity	C76.8	C79.89	D04.8	D36.7	D48.7	D49.89
lower	C76.5-☑	C79.89	D04.7-☑	D36.7	D48.7	D49.89
upper	C76.4-☑	C79.89	D04.6-☑	D36.7	D48.7	D49.89
eyeball	C69.9-☑	C79.49	D09.2-☑	D31.9-☑	D48.7	D49.89
eyebrow	C44.309	C79.2	D04.39	D23.39	D48.5	D49.2
basal cell carcinoma	C44.319	—	—	—	—	—
specified type NEC	C44.399	—	—	—	—	—
squamous cell carcinoma	C44.329	—	—	—	—	—
eyelid (lower) (skin) (upper)	C44.10-☑	—	—	—	—	—
basal cell carcinoma	C44.11-☑	—	—	—	—	—
cartilage	C49.0	C79.89	—	D21.0	D48.1	D49.2
specified type NEC	C44.19-☑	—	—	—	—	—
squamous cell carcinoma	C44.12-☑	—	—	—	—	—
eye NEC	C69.9-☑	C79.49	D09.2-☑	D31.9-☑	D48.7	D49.89
overlapping sites	C69.8-☑	—	—	—	—	—
face NEC	C76.0	C79.89	D04.39	D36.7	D48.7	D49.89
fallopian tube (accessory)	C57.0-☑	C79.82	D07.39	D28.2	D39.8	D49.5
falx (cerebella) (cerebri)	C70.0	C79.32	—	D32.0	D42.0	D49.7
fascia — see also Neoplasm, connective tissue						
palmar	C49.1-☑	C79.89	—	D21.1-☑	D48.1	D49.2
plantar	C49.2-☑	C79.89	—	D21.2-☑	D48.1	D49.2
fatty tissue — see Neoplasm, connective tissue						
fauces, faucial NEC	C10.9	C79.89	D00.08	D10.5	D37.05	D49.0
pillars	C09.1	C79.89	D00.08	D10.5	D37.05	D49.0
tonsil	C09.9	C79.89	D00.08	D10.5	D37.05	D49.0
femur (any part)	C40.2-☑	—	—	D16.2-☑	—	—
fetal membrane	C58	C79.82	D07.0	D26.7	D39.2	D49.5
fibrous tissue — see Neoplasm, connective tissue						
fibula (any part)	C40.2-☑	C79.51	—	D16.2-☑	—	—
filum terminale	C72.0	C79.49	—	D33.4	D43.4	D49.7
finger NEC	C76.4-☑	C79.89	D04.6-☑	D36.7	D48.7	D49.89
flank NEC	C76.8	C79.89	D04.5	D36.7	D48.7	D49.89
follicle, nabothian	C53.0	C79.82	D06.0	D26.0	D39.0	D49.5
foot NEC	C76.5-☑	C79.89	D04.7-☑	D36.7	D48.7	D49.89
forearm NEC	C76.4-☑	C79.89	D04.6-☑	D36.7	D48.7	D49.89
forehead (skin)	C44.309	C79.2	D04.39	D23.39	D48.5	D49.2

Neoplasm, neoplastic — continued

forehead — continued	Malignant Primary	Malignant Secondary	Ca in situ	Benign	Uncertain	Unspecified Behavior
basal cell carcinoma	C44.319	—	—	—	—	—
specified type NEC	C44.399	—	—	—	—	—
squamous cell carcinoma	C44.329	—	—	—	—	—
foreskin	C60.0	C79.82	D07.4	D29.0	D40.8	D49.5
fornix						
pharyngeal	C11.3	C79.89	D00.08	D10.6	D37.05	D49.0
vagina	C52	C79.82	D07.2	D28.1	D39.8	D49.5
fossa (of)						
anterior (cranial)	C71.9	C79.31	—	D33.2	D43.2	D49.6
cranial	C71.9	C79.31	—	D33.2	D43.2	D49.6
ischiorectal	C76.3	C79.89	D09.8	D36.7	D48.7	D49.89
middle (cranial)	C71.9	C79.31	—	D33.2	D43.2	D49.6
piriform	C12	C79.89	D00.08	D10.7	D37.05	D49.0
pituitary	C75.1	C79.89	D09.3	D35.2	D44.3	D49.7
posterior (cranial)	C71.9	C79.31	—	D33.2	D43.2	D49.6
pterygoid	C49.0	C79.89	—	D21.0	D48.1	D49.2
pyriform	C12	C79.89	D00.08	D10.7	D37.05	D49.0
Rosenmuller	C11.2	C79.89	D00.08	D10.6	D37.05	D49.0
tonsillar	C09.0	C79.89	D00.08	D10.5	D37.05	D49.0
fourchette	C51.9	C79.82	D07.1	D28.0	D39.8	D49.5
frenulum						
labii — see Neoplasm, lip, internal						
linguae	C02.2	C79.89	D00.07	D10.1	D37.02	D49.0
frontal						
bone	C41.0	C79.51	—	D16.4	D48.0	D49.2
lobe, brain	C71.1	C79.31	—	D33.0	D43.0	D49.6
pole	C71.1	C79.31	—	D33.0	D43.0	D49.6
sinus	C31.2	C78.39	D02.3	D14.0	D38.5	D49.1
fundus						
stomach	C16.1	C78.89	D00.2	D13.1	D37.1	D49.0
uterus	C54.3	C79.82	D07.0	D26.1	D39.0	D49.5
gallbladder	C23	C78.89	D01.5	D13.5	D37.6	D49.0
overlapping lesion with extrahepatic bile ducts	C24.8	—	—	—	—	—
gall duct (extrahepatic)	C24.0	C78.89	D01.5	D13.5	D37.6	D49.0
intrahepatic	C22.1	C78.7	D01.5	D13.4	D37.6	D49.0
ganglia — see also Neoplasm, nerve, peripheral	C47.9	C79.89	—	D36.10	D48.2	D49.2
basal	C71.0	C79.31	—	D33.0	D43.0	D49.6
cranial nerve	C72.50	C79.49	—	D33.3	D43.3	D49.7
Gartner's duct	C52	C79.82	D07.2	D28.1	D39.8	D49.5
gastric — see Neoplasm, stomach						
gastrocolic	C26.9	C78.89	D01.9	D13.9	D37.9	D49.0
gastroesophageal junction	C16.0	C78.89	D00.2	D13.1	D37.1	D49.0
gastrointestinal (tract) NEC	C26.9	C78.89	D01.9	D13.9	D37.9	D49.0
generalized	C80.0	—	—	—	—	—
genital organ or tract						
female NEC	C57.9	C79.82	D07.30	D28.9	D39.9	D49.5
overlapping lesion	C57.8	—	—	—	—	—
specified site NEC	C57.7	C79.82	D07.39	D28.7	D39.8	D49.5
male NEC	C63.9	C79.82	D07.60	D29.9	D40.9	D49.5
overlapping lesion	C63.8	—	—	—	—	—
specified site NEC	C63.7	C79.82	D07.69	D29.8	D40.8	D49.5
genitourinary tract						
female	C57.9	C79.82	D07.30	D28.9	D39.9	D49.5
male	C63.9	C79.82	D07.60	D29.9	D40.9	D49.5
gingiva (alveolar) (marginal)	C03.9	C79.89	D00.03	D10.39	D37.09	D49.0
lower	C03.1	C79.89	D00.03	D10.39	D37.09	D49.0
mandibular	C03.1	C79.89	D00.03	D10.39	D37.09	D49.0
maxillary	C03.0	C79.89	D00.03	D10.39	D37.09	D49.0
upper	C03.0	C79.89	D00.03	D10.39	D37.09	D49.0
gland, glandular (lymphatic) (system) — see also Neoplasm, lymph gland						
endocrine NEC	C75.9	C79.89	D09.3	D35.9	D44.9	D49.7

☑ Additional Character Required — Refer to the Tabular List for Character Selection   ▽ Subterms under main terms may continue to next column or page

	Malignant Primary	Malignant Secondary	Ca in situ	Benign	Uncertain	Unspecified Behavior
Neoplasm, neoplastic — *continued*						
gland, glandular — *see also* Neoplasm, lymph gland — *continued*						
salivary — *see* Neoplasm, salivary gland						
glans penis	C60.1	C79.82	D07.4	D29.0	D40.8	D49.5
globus pallidus	C71.0	C79.31	—	D33.0	D43.0	D49.6
glomus						
coccygeal	C49.5	C79.89	—	D21.5	D48.1	D49.2
jugularis	C75.5	C79.89	—	D35.6	D44.7	D49.7
glosso-epiglottic fold(s)	C10.1	C79.89	D00.08	D10.5	D37.05	D49.0
glossopalatine fold	C09.1	C79.89	D00.08	D10.5	D37.05	D49.0
glossopharyngeal sulcus	C09.0	C79.89	D00.08	D10.5	D37.05	D49.0
glottis	C32.0	C78.39	D02.0	D14.1	D38.0	D49.1
gluteal region	C76.3	C79.89	D04.5	D36.7	D48.7	D49.89
great vessels NEC	C49.3	C79.89	—	D21.3	D48.1	D49.2
groin NEC	C76.3	C79.89	D04.5	D36.7	D48.7	D49.89
gum	C03.9	C79.89	D00.03	D10.39	D37.09	D49.0
lower	C03.1	C79.89	D00.03	D10.39	D37.09	D49.0
upper	C03.0	C79.89	D00.03	D10.39	D37.09	D49.0
hand NEC	C76.4-☑	C79.89	D04.6-☑	D36.7	D48.7	D49.89
head NEC	C76.0	C79.89	D04.4	D36.7	D48.7	D49.89
heart	C38.0	C79.89	—	D15.1	D48.7	D49.89
heel NEC	C76.5-☑	C79.89	D04.7-☑	D36.7	D48.7	D49.89
helix — *see also* Neoplasm, skin, ear	C44.20-☑	C79.2	D04.2-☑	D23.2-☑	D48.5	D49.2
hematopoietic, hemopoietic tissue NEC	C96.9	—	—	—	—	—
specified NEC	C96.Z	—	—	—	—	—
hemisphere, cerebral	C71.0	C79.31	—	D33.0	D43.0	D49.6
hemorrhoidal zone	C21.1	C78.5	D01.3	D12.9	D37.8	D49.0
hepatic — *see also* Index to disease, by histology	C22.9	C78.7	D01.5	D13.4	D37.6	D49.0
duct (bile)	C24.0	C78.89	D01.5	D13.5	D37.6	D49.0
flexure (colon)	C18.3	C78.5	D01.0	D12.3	D37.4	D49.0
primary	C22.8	C78.7	D01.5	D13.4	D37.6	D49.0
hepatobiliary	C24.9	C78.89	D01.5	D13.5	D37.6	D49.0
hepatoblastoma	C22.2	C78.7	D01.5	D13.4	D37.6	D49.0
hepatoma	C22.0	C78.7	D01.5	D13.4	D37.6	D49.0
hilus of lung	C34.0-☑	C78.0-☑	D02.2-☑	D14.3-☑	D38.1	D49.1
hippocampus, brain	C71.2	C79.31	—	D33.0	D43.0	D49.6
hip NEC	C76.5-☑	C79.89	D04.7-☑	D36.7	D48.7	D49.89
humerus (any part)	C40.0-☑	C79.51	—	D16.0-☑	—	D49.2
hymen	C52	C79.82	D07.2	D28.1	D39.8	D49.5
hypopharynx, hypopharyngeal NEC	C13.9	C79.89	D00.08	D10.7	D37.05	D49.0
overlapping lesion	C13.8	—	—	—	—	—
postcricoid region	C13.0	C79.89	D00.08	D10.7	D37.05	D49.0
posterior wall	C13.2	C79.89	D00.08	D10.7	D37.05	D49.0
pyriform fossa (sinus)	C12	C79.89	D00.08	D10.7	D37.05	D49.0
hypophysis	C75.1	C79.89	D09.3	D35.2	D44.3	D49.7
hypothalamus	C71.0	C79.31	—	D33.0	D43.0	D49.6
ileocecum, ileocecal (coil) (junction) (valve)	C18.0	C78.5	D01.0	D12.0	D37.4	D49.0
ileum	C17.2	C78.4	D01.49	D13.39	D37.2	D49.0
ilium	C41.4	C79.51	—	D16.8	D48.0	D49.2
immunoproliferative NEC	C88.9	—	—	—	—	—
infraclavicular (region)	C76.1	C79.89	D04.5	D36.7	D48.7	D49.89
inguinal (region)	C76.3	C79.89	D04.5	D36.7	D48.7	D49.89
insula	C71.0	C79.31	—	D33.0	D43.0	D49.6
insular tissue (pancreas)	C25.4	C78.89	D01.7	D13.7	D37.8	D49.0
brain	C71.0	C79.31	—	D33.0	D43.0	D49.6
interarytenoid fold	C13.1	C78.39	D00.08	D10.7	D37.05	D49.0
hypopharyngeal aspect	C13.1	C79.89	D00.08	D10.7	D37.05	D49.0
laryngeal aspect	C32.1	C78.39	D02.0	D14.1	D38.0	D49.1
marginal zone	C13.1	C79.89	D00.08	D10.7	D37.05	D49.0
interdental papillae	C03.9	C79.89	D00.03	D10.39	D37.09	D49.0

	Malignant Primary	Malignant Secondary	Ca in situ	Benign	Uncertain	Unspecified Behavior
Neoplasm, neoplastic — *continued*						
interdental papillae — *continued*						
lower	C03.1	C79.89	D00.03	D10.39	D37.09	D49.0
upper	C03.0	C79.89	D00.03	D10.39	D37.09	D49.0
internal						
capsule	C71.0	C79.31	—	D33.0	D43.0	D49.6
os (cervix)	C53.0	C79.82	D06.0	D26.0	D39.0	D49.5
intervertebral cartilage or disc	C41.2	C79.51	—	D16.6	D48.0	D49.2
intestine, intestinal	C26.0	C78.80	D01.40	D13.9	D37.8	D49.0
large	C18.9	C78.5	D01.0	D12.6	D37.4	D49.0
appendix	C18.1	C78.5	D01.0	D12.1	D37.3	D49.0
caput coli	C18.0	C78.5	D01.0	D12.0	D37.4	D49.0
cecum	C18.0	C78.5	D01.0	D12.0	D37.4	D49.0
colon	C18.9	C78.5	D01.0	D12.6	D37.4	D49.0
and rectum	C19	C78.5	D01.1	D12.7	D37.5	D49.0
ascending	C18.2	C78.5	D01.0	D12.2	D37.4	D49.0
caput	C18.0	C78.5	D01.0	D12.0	D37.4	D49.0
descending	C18.6	C78.5	D01.0	D12.4	D37.4	D49.0
distal	C18.6	C78.5	D01.0	D12.4	D37.4	D49.0
left	C18.6	C78.5	D01.0	D12.4	D37.4	D49.0
overlapping lesion	C18.8	—	—	—	—	—
pelvic	C18.7	C78.5	D01.0	D12.5	D37.4	D49.0
right	C18.2	C78.5	D01.0	D12.2	D37.4	D49.0
sigmoid (flexure)	C18.7	C78.5	D01.0	D12.5	D37.4	D49.0
transverse	C18.4	C78.5	D01.0	D12.3	D37.4	D49.0
hepatic flexure	C18.3	C78.5	D01.0	D12.3	D37.4	D49.0
ileocecum, ileocecal (coil) (valve)	C18.0	C78.5	D01.0	D12.0	D37.4	D49.0
overlapping lesion	C18.8	—	—	—	—	—
sigmoid flexure (lower) (upper)	C18.7	C78.5	D01.0	D12.5	D37.4	D49.0
splenic flexure	C18.5	C78.5	D01.0	D12.3	D37.4	D49.0
small	C17.9	C78.4	D01.40	D13.30	D37.2	D49.0
duodenum	C17.0	C78.4	D01.49	D13.2	D37.2	D49.0
ileum	C17.2	C78.4	D01.49	D13.39	D37.2	D49.0
jejunum	C17.1	C78.4	D01.49	D13.39	D37.2	D49.0
overlapping lesion	C17.8	—	—	—	—	—
tract NEC	C26.0	C78.89	D01.40	D13.9	D37.8	D49.0
intra-abdominal	C76.2	C79.89	D09.8	D36.7	D48.7	D49.89
intracranial NEC	C71.9	C79.31	—	D33.2	D43.2	D49.6
intrahepatic (bile) duct	C22.1	C78.7	D01.5	D13.4	D37.6	D49.0
intraocular	C69.9-☑	C79.49	D09.2-☑	D31.9-☑	D48.7	D49.89
intraorbital	C69.6-☑	C79.49	D09.2-☑	D31.6-☑	D48.7	D49.89
intrasellar	C75.1	C79.89	D09.3	D35.2	D44.3	D49.7
intrathoracic (cavity) (organs)	C76.1	C79.89	D09.8	D15.9	D48.7	D49.89
specified NEC	C76.1	C79.89	D09.8	D15.7	—	—
iris	C69.4-☑	C79.49	D09.2-☑	D31.4-☑	D48.7	D49.89
ischiorectal (fossa)	C76.3	C79.89	D09.8	D36.7	D48.7	D49.89
ischium	C41.4	C79.51	—	D16.8	D48.0	D49.2
island of Reil	C71.0	C79.31	—	D33.0	D43.0	D49.6
islands or islets of Langerhans	C25.4	C78.89	D01.7	D13.7	D37.8	D49.0
isthmus uteri	C54.0	C79.82	D07.0	D26.1	D39.0	D49.5
jaw	C76.0	C79.89	D09.8	D36.7	D48.7	D49.89
bone	C41.1	C79.51	—	D16.5	D48.0	D49.2
lower	C41.1	C79.51	—	D16.5	—	—
upper	C41.0	C79.51	—	D16.4	—	—
carcinoma (any type) (lower) (upper)	C76.0	C79.89	—	—	—	—
skin — *see also* Neoplasm, skin, face	C44.309	C79.2	D04.39	D23.39	D48.5	D49.2
soft tissues	C03.9	C79.89	D00.03	D10.39	D37.09	D49.0
lower	C03.1	C79.89	D00.03	D10.39	D37.09	D49.0
upper	C03.0	C79.89	D00.03	D10.39	D37.09	D49.0
jejunum	C17.1	C78.4	D01.49	D13.39	D37.2	D49.0
joint NEC — *see also* Neoplasm, bone	C41.9	C79.51	—	D16.9	D48.0	D49.2
acromioclavicular	C40.0-☑	C79.51	—	D16.0-☑	—	—

Neoplasm Table

Neoplasm, joint NEC — Neoplasm, lung

Neoplasm, neoplastic —	Malignant Primary	Malignant Secondary	Ca in situ	Benign	Uncertain	Unspecified Behavior
continued						
joint — *see also*						
Neoplasm, bone —						
continued						
bursa or synovial						
membrane — *see*						
Neoplasm,						
connective tissue						
costovertebral	C41.3	C79.51	—	D16.7	D48.0	D49.2
sternocostal	C41.3	C79.51	—	D16.7	D48.0	D49.2
temporomandibular	C41.1	C79.51	—	D16.5	D48.0	D49.2
junction						
anorectal	C21.8	C78.5	D01.3	D12.9	D37.8	D49.0
cardioesophageal	C16.0	C78.89	D00.2	D13.1	D37.1	D49.0
esophagogastric	C16.0	C78.89	D00.2	D13.1	D37.1	D49.0
gastroesophageal	C16.0	C78.89	D00.2	D13.1	D37.1	D49.0
hard and soft						
palate	C05.9	C79.89	D00.00	D10.39	D37.09	D49.0
ileocecal	C18.0	C78.5	D01.0	D12.0	D37.4	D49.0
pelvirectal	C19	C78.5	D01.1	D12.7	D37.5	D49.0
pelviureteric	C65.-☑	C79.0-☑	D09.19	D30.1-☑	D41.1-☑	D49.5
rectosigmoid	C19	C78.5	D01.1	D12.7	D37.5	D49.0
squamocolumnar, of						
cervix	C53.8	C79.82	D06.7	D26.0	D39.0	D49.5
Kaposi's sarcoma — *see*						
Kaposi's, sarcoma						
kidney						
(parenchymal)	C64.-☑	C79.0-☑	D09.19	D30.0-☑	D41.0-☑	D49.5
calyx	C65.-☑	C79.0-☑	D09.19	D30.1-☑	D41.1-☑	D49.5
hilus	C65.-☑	C79.0-☑	D09.19	D30.1-☑	D41.1-☑	D49.5
pelvis	C65.-☑	C79.0-☑	D09.19	D30.1-☑	D41.1-☑	D49.5
knee NEC	C76.5-☑	C79.89	D04.7-☑	D36.7	D48.7	D49.89
labia (skin)	C51.9	C79.82	D07.1	D28.0	D39.8	D49.5
majora	C51.0	C79.82	D07.1	D28.0	D39.8	D49.5
minora	C51.1	C79.82	D07.1	D28.0	D39.8	D49.5
labial — *see also*						
Neoplasm, lip	C00.9	C79.89	D00.01	D10.0	D37.01	D49.0
sulcus (lower)						
(upper)	C06.1	C79.89	D00.02	D10.39	D37.09	D49.0
labium (skin)	C51.9	C79.82	D07.1	D28.0	D39.8	D49.5
majus	C51.0	C79.82	D07.1	D28.0	D39.8	D49.5
minus	C51.1	C79.82	D07.1	D28.0	D39.8	D49.5
lacrimal						
canaliculi	C69.5-☑	C79.49	D09.2-☑	D31.5-☑	D48.7	D49.89
duct (nasal)	C69.5-☑	C79.49	D09.2-☑	D31.5-☑	D48.7	D49.89
gland	C69.5-☑	C79.49	D09.2-☑	D31.5-☑	D48.7	D49.89
punctum	C69.5-☑	C79.49	D09.2-☑	D31.5-☑	D48.7	D49.89
sac	C69.5-☑	C79.49	D09.2-☑	D31.5-☑	D48.7	D49.89
Langerhans, islands or						
islets	C25.4	C78.89	D01.7	D13.7	D37.8	D49.0
laryngopharynx	C13.9	C79.89	D00.08	D10.7	D37.05	D49.0
larynx, laryngeal						
NEC	C32.9	C78.39	D02.0	D14.1	D38.0	D49.1
aryepiglottic fold	C32.1	C78.39	D02.0	D14.1	D38.0	D49.1
cartilage (arytenoid)						
(cricoid)						
(cuneiform)						
(thyroid)	C32.3	C78.39	D02.0	D14.1	D38.0	D49.1
commissure (anterior)						
(posterior)	C32.0	C78.39	D02.0	D14.1	D38.0	D49.1
extrinsic NEC	C32.1	C78.39	D02.0	D14.1	D38.0	D49.1
meaning						
hypopharynx	C13.9	C79.89	D00.08	D10.7	D37.05	D49.0
interarytenoid fold	C32.1	C78.39	D02.0	D14.1	D38.0	D49.1
intrinsic	C32.0	C78.39	D02.0	D14.1	D38.0	D49.1
overlapping lesion	C32.8	—	—	—	—	—
ventricular band	C32.1	C78.39	D02.0	D14.1	D38.0	D49.1
leg NEC	C76.5-☑	C79.89	D04.7-☑	D36.7	D48.7	D49.89
lens, crystalline	C69.4-☑	C79.49	D09.2-☑	D31.4-☑	D48.7	D49.89
lid (lower) (upper)	C44.10-☑	C79.2	D04.1-☑	D23.1-☑	D48.5	D49.2
basal cell						
carcinoma	C44.11-☑	—	—	—	—	—
specified type NEC	C44.19-☑	—	—	—	—	—
squamous cell						
carcinoma	C44.12-☑	—	—	—	—	—
ligament — *see also*						
Neoplasm, connective						
tissue						

Neoplasm, neoplastic —	Malignant Primary	Malignant Secondary	Ca in situ	Benign	Uncertain	Unspecified Behavior
continued						
ligament — *see also*						
Neoplasm, connective						
tissue — *continued*						
broad	C57.1-☑	C79.82	D07.39	D28.2	D39.8	D49.5
Mackenrodt's	C57.7	C79.82	D07.39	D28.7	D39.8	D49.5
non-uterine — *see*						
Neoplasm,						
connective tissue						
round	C57.2-☑	C79.82	—	D28.2	D39.8	D49.5
sacro-uterine	C57.3	C79.82	—	D28.2	D39.8	D49.5
uterine	C57.3	C79.82	—	D28.2	D39.8	D49.5
utero-ovarian	C57.7	C79.82	D07.39	D28.2	D39.8	D49.5
uterosacral	C57.3	C79.82	—	D28.2	D39.8	D49.5
limb	C76.8	C79.89	D04.8	D36.7	D48.7	D49.89
lower	C76.5-☑	C79.89	D04.7-☑	D36.7	D48.7	D49.89
upper	C76.4-☑	C79.89	D04.6-☑	D36.7	D48.7	D49.89
limbus of cornea	C69.1-☑	C79.49	D09.2-☑	D31.1-☑	D48.7	D49.89
lingual NEC — *see also*						
Neoplasm,						
tongue	C02.9	C79.89	D00.07	D10.1	D37.02	D49.0
lingula, lung	C34.1-☑	C78.0-☑	D02.2-☑	D14.3-☑	D38.1	D49.1
lip	C00.9	C79.89	D00.01	D10.0	D37.01	D49.0
buccal aspect — *see*						
Neoplasm, lip,						
internal						
commissure	C00.6	C79.89	D00.01	D10.0	D37.01	D49.0
external	C00.2	C79.89	D00.01	D10.0	D37.01	D49.0
lower	C00.1	C79.89	D00.01	D10.0	D37.01	D49.0
upper	C00.0	C79.89	D00.01	D10.0	D37.01	D49.0
frenulum — *see*						
Neoplasm, lip,						
internal						
inner aspect — *see*						
Neoplasm, lip,						
internal						
internal	C00.5	C79.89	D00.01	D10.0	D37.01	D49.0
lower	C00.4	C79.89	D00.01	D10.0	D37.01	D49.0
upper	C00.3	C79.89	D00.01	D10.0	D37.01	D49.0
lipstick area	C00.2	C79.89	D00.01	D10.0	D37.01	D49.0
lower	C00.1	C79.89	D00.01	D10.0	D37.01	D49.0
upper	C00.0	C79.89	D00.01	D10.0	D37.01	D49.0
lower	C00.1	C79.89	D00.01	D10.0	D37.01	D49.0
internal	C00.4	C79.89	D00.01	D10.0	D37.01	D49.0
mucosa — *see*						
Neoplasm, lip,						
internal						
oral aspect — *see*						
Neoplasm, lip,						
internal						
overlapping lesion	C00.8	—	—	—	—	—
with oral cavity or						
pharynx	C14.8	—	—	—	—	—
skin (commissure)						
(lower)						
(upper)	C44.00	C79.2	D04.0	D23.0	D48.5	D49.2
basal cell						
carcinoma	C44.01	—	—	—	—	—
specified type						
NEC	C44.09	—	—	—	—	—
squamous cell						
carcinoma	C44.02	—	—	—	—	—
upper	C00.0	C79.89	D00.01	D10.0	D37.01	D49.0
internal	C00.3	C79.89	D00.01	D10.0	D37.01	D49.0
vermilion border	C00.2	C79.89	D00.01	D10.0	D37.01	D49.0
lower	C00.1	C79.89	D00.01	D10.0	D37.01	D49.0
upper	C00.0	C79.89	D00.01	D10.0	D37.01	D49.0
lipomatous — *see*						
Lipoma, by site						
liver — *see also* Index to						
disease, by						
histology	C22.9	C78.7	D01.5	D13.4	D37.6	D49.0
primary	C22.8	C78.7	D01.5	D13.4	D37.6	D49.0
lumbosacral plexus	C47.5	C79.89	—	D36.16	D48.2	D49.2
lung	C34.9-☑	C78.0-☑	D02.2-☑	D14.3-☑	D38.1	D49.1
azygos lobe	C34.1-☑	C78.0-☑	D02.2-☑	D14.3-☑	D38.1	D49.1
carina	C34.0-☑	C78.0-☑	D02.2-☑	D14.3-☑	D38.1	D49.1
hilus	C34.0-☑	C78.0-☑	D02.2-☑	D14.3-☑	D38.1	D49.1
lingula	C34.1-☑	C78.0-☑	D02.2-☑	D14.3-☑	D38.1	D49.1
lobe NEC	C34.9-☑	C78.0-☑	D02.2-☑	D14.3-☑	D38.1	D49.1
lower lobe	C34.3-☑	C78.0-☑	D02.2-☑	D14.3-☑	D38.1	D49.1

☑ **Additional Character Required — Refer to the Tabular List for Character Selection**   ▽ Subterms under main terms may continue to next column or page

Neoplasm, neoplastic — continued	Malignant Primary	Malignant Secondary	Ca in situ	Benign	Uncertain	Unspecified Behavior
lung — *continued*						
main bronchus	C34.0-☑	C78.0-☑	D02.2-☑	D14.3-☑	D38.1	D49.1
mesothelioma — *see* Mesothelioma						
middle lobe	C34.2	C78.0-☑	D02.21	D14.31	D38.1	D49.1
overlapping lesion	C34.8-☑	—	—	—	—	—
upper lobe	C34.1-☑	C78.0-☑	D02.2-☑	D14.3-☑	D38.1	D49.1
lymph, lymphatic channel						
NEC	C49.9	C79.89	—	D21.9	D48.1	D49.2
gland (secondary)	—	C77.9	—	D36.0	D48.7	D49.89
abdominal	—	C77.2	—	D36.0	D48.7	D49.89
aortic	—	C77.2	—	D36.0	D48.7	D49.89
arm	—	C77.3	—	D36.0	D48.7	D49.89
auricular (anterior) (posterior)	—	C77.0	—	D36.0	D48.7	D49.89
axilla, axillary	—	C77.3	—	D36.0	D48.7	D49.89
brachial	—	C77.3	—	D36.0	D48.7	D49.89
bronchial	—	C77.1	—	D36.0	D48.7	D49.89
bronchopulmonary	—	C77.1	—	D36.0	D48.7	D49.89
celiac	—	C77.2	—	D36.0	D48.7	D49.89
cervical	—	C77.0	—	D36.0	D48.7	D49.89
cervicofacial	—	C77.0	—	D36.0	D48.7	D49.89
Cloquet	—	C77.4	—	D36.0	D48.7	D49.89
colic	—	C77.2	—	D36.0	D48.7	D49.89
common duct	—	C77.2	—	D36.0	D48.7	D49.89
cubital	—	C77.3	—	D36.0	D48.7	D49.89
diaphragmatic	—	C77.1	—	D36.0	D48.7	D49.89
epigastric, inferior	—	C77.1	—	D36.0	D48.7	D49.89
epitrochlear	—	C77.3	—	D36.0	D48.7	D49.89
esophageal	—	C77.1	—	D36.0	D48.7	D49.89
face	—	C77.0	—	D36.0	D48.7	D49.89
femoral	—	C77.4	—	D36.0	D48.7	D49.89
gastric	—	C77.2	—	D36.0	D48.7	D49.89
groin	—	C77.4	—	D36.0	D48.7	D49.89
head	—	C77.0	—	D36.0	D48.7	D49.89
hepatic	—	C77.2	—	D36.0	D48.7	D49.89
hilar (pulmonary)	—	C77.1	—	D36.0	D48.7	D49.89
splenic	—	C77.2	—	D36.0	D48.7	D49.89
hypogastric	—	C77.5	—	D36.0	D48.7	D49.89
ileocolic	—	C77.2	—	D36.0	D48.7	D49.89
iliac	—	C77.5	—	D36.0	D48.7	D49.89
infraclavicular	—	C77.3	—	D36.0	D48.7	D49.89
inguina, inguinal	—	C77.4	—	D36.0	D48.7	D49.89
innominate	—	C77.1	—	D36.0	D48.7	D49.89
intercostal	—	C77.1	—	D36.0	D48.7	D49.89
intestinal	—	C77.2	—	D36.0	D48.7	D49.89
intrabdominal	—	C77.2	—	D36.0	D48.7	D49.89
intrapelvic	—	C77.5	—	D36.0	D48.7	D49.89
intrathoracic	—	C77.1	—	D36.0	D48.7	D49.89
jugular	—	C77.0	—	D36.0	D48.7	D49.89
leg	—	C77.4	—	D36.0	D48.7	D49.89
limb						
lower	—	C77.4	—	D36.0	D48.7	D49.89
upper	—	C77.3	—	D36.0	D48.7	D49.89
lower limb	—	C77.4	—	D36.0	D48.7	D49.89
lumbar	—	C77.2	—	D36.0	D48.7	D49.89
mandibular	—	C77.0	—	D36.0	D48.7	D49.89
mediastinal	—	C77.1	—	D36.0	D48.7	D49.89
mesenteric (inferior) (superior)	—	C77.2	—	D36.0	D48.7	D49.89
midcolic	—	C77.2	—	D36.0	D48.7	D49.89
multiple sites in categories C77.0 - C77.5	—	C77.8	—	D36.0	D48.7	D49.89
neck	—	C77.0	—	D36.0	D48.7	D49.89
obturator	—	C77.5	—	D36.0	D48.7	D49.89
occipital	—	C77.0	—	D36.0	D48.7	D49.89
pancreatic	—	C77.2	—	D36.0	D48.7	D49.89
para-aortic	—	C77.2	—	D36.0	D48.7	D49.89
paracervical	—	C77.5	—	D36.0	D48.7	D49.89
parametrial	—	C77.5	—	D36.0	D48.7	D49.89
parasternal	—	C77.1	—	D36.0	D48.7	D49.89
parotid	—	C77.0	—	D36.0	D48.7	D49.89
pectoral	—	C77.3	—	D36.0	D48.7	D49.89
pelvic	—	C77.5	—	D36.0	D48.7	D49.89
peri-aortic	—	C77.2	—	D36.0	D48.7	D49.89
peripancreatic	—	C77.2	—	D36.0	D48.7	D49.89
popliteal	—	C77.4	—	D36.0	D48.7	D49.89
porta hepatis	—	C77.2	—	D36.0	D48.7	D49.89

Neoplasm, neoplastic — continued	Malignant Primary	Malignant Secondary	Ca in situ	Benign	Uncertain	Unspecified Behavior
lymph, lymphatic channel — *continued*						
gland — *continued*						
portal	—	C77.2	—	D36.0	D48.7	D49.89
preauricular	—	C77.0	—	D36.0	D48.7	D49.89
prelaryngeal	—	C77.0	—	D36.0	D48.7	D49.89
presymphysial	—	C77.5	—	D36.0	D48.7	D49.89
pretracheal	—	C77.0	—	D36.0	D48.7	D49.89
primary (any site)						
NEC	C96.9	—	—	—	—	—
pulmonary (hiler)	—	C77.1	—	D36.0	D48.7	D49.89
pyloric	—	C77.2	—	D36.0	D48.7	D49.89
retroperitoneal	—	C77.2	—	D36.0	D48.7	D49.89
retropharyngeal	—	C77.0	—	D36.0	D48.7	D49.89
Rosenmuller's	—	C77.4	—	D36.0	D48.7	D49.89
sacral	—	C77.5	—	D36.0	D48.7	D49.89
scalene	—	C77.0	—	D36.0	D48.7	D49.89
site NEC	—	C77.9	—	D36.0	D48.7	D49.89
splenic (hilar)	—	C77.2	—	D36.0	D48.7	D49.89
subclavicular	—	C77.3	—	D36.0	D48.7	D49.89
subinguinal	—	C77.4	—	D36.0	D48.7	D49.89
sublingual	—	C77.0	—	D36.0	D48.7	D49.89
submandibular	—	C77.0	—	D36.0	D48.7	D49.89
submaxillary	—	C77.0	—	D36.0	D48.7	D49.89
submental	—	C77.0	—	D36.0	D48.7	D49.89
subscapular	—	C77.3	—	D36.0	D48.7	D49.89
supraclavicular	—	C77.0	—	D36.0	D48.7	D49.89
thoracic	—	C77.1	—	D36.0	D48.7	D49.89
tibial	—	C77.4	—	D36.0	D48.7	D49.89
tracheal	—	C77.1	—	D36.0	D48.7	D49.89
tracheobronchial	—	C77.1	—	D36.0	D48.7	D49.89
upper limb	—	C77.3	—	D36.0	D48.7	D49.89
Virchow's	—	C77.0	—	D36.0	D48.7	D49.89
node — *see also* Neoplasm, lymph gland						
primary NEC	C96.9	—	—	—	—	—
vessel — *see also* Neoplasm, connective tissue	C49.9	C79.89	—	D21.9	D48.1	D49.2
Mackenrodt's ligament	C57.7	C79.82	D07.39	D28.7	D39.8	D49.5
malar	C41.0	C79.51	—	D16.4	D48.0	D49.2
region — *see* Neoplasm, cheek						
mammary gland — *see* Neoplasm, breast						
mandible	C41.1	C79.51	—	D16.5	D48.0	D49.2
alveolar						
mucosa (carcinoma)	C03.1	C79.89	D00.03	D10.39	D37.09	D49.0
ridge or process	C41.1	C79.51	—	D16.5	D48.0	D49.2
marrow (bone) NEC	C96.9	C79.52	—	—	D47.9	D49.89
mastectomy site (skin) — *see also* Neoplasm, breast, skin	C44.501	C79.2	—	—	—	—
specified as breast tissue	C50.8-☑	C79.81	—	—	—	—
mastoid (air cells) (antrum) (cavity)	C30.1	C78.39	D02.3	D14.0	D38.5	D49.1
bone or process	C41.0	C79.51	—	D16.4	D48.0	D49.2
maxilla, maxillary (superior)	C41.0	C79.51	—	D16.4	D48.0	D49.2
alveolar						
mucosa	C03.0	C79.89	D00.03	D10.39	D37.09	D49.0
ridge or process (carcinoma)	C41.0	C79.51	—	D16.4	D48.0	D49.2
antrum	C31.0	C78.39	D02.3	D14.0	D38.5	D49.1
carcinoma	C03.0	C79.51	—	—	—	—
inferior — *see* Neoplasm, mandible						
sinus	C31.0	C78.39	D02.3	D14.0	D38.5	D49.1
meatus external (ear) — *see also* Neoplasm, skin, ear	C44.20-☑	C79.2	D04.2-☑	D23.2-☑	D48.5	D49.2
Meckel diverticulum, malignant	C17.3	C78.4	D01.49	D13.39	D37.2	D49.0

▽ Subterms under main terms may continue to next column or page   ☑ Additional Character Required — Refer to the Tabular List for Character Selection

Neoplasm Table

Neoplasm, mediastinum, mediastinal — Neoplasm, nerve

	Malignant Primary	Malignant Secondary	Ca in situ	Benign	Uncertain	Unspecified Behavior
Neoplasm, neoplastic — *continued*						
mediastinum, mediastinal	C38.3	C78.1	—	D15.2	D38.3	D49.89
anterior	C38.1	C78.1	—	D15.2	D38.3	D49.89
posterior	C38.2	C78.1	—	D15.2	D38.3	D49.89
medulla						
adrenal	C74.1-☑	C79.7-☑	D09.3	D35.0-☑	D44.1-☑	D49.7
oblongata	C71.7	C79.31		D33.1	D43.1	D49.6
meibomian gland	C44.10-☑	C79.2	D04.1-☑	D23.1-☑	D48.5	D49.2
basal cell carcinoma	C44.11-☑	—	—	—	—	—
specified type NEC	C44.19-☑	—	—	—	—	—
squamous cell carcinoma	C44.12-☑	—	—	—	—	—
melanoma — *see* Melanoma						
meninges	C70.9	C79.49	—	D32.9	D42.9	D49.7
brain	C70.0	C79.32	—	D32.0	D42.0	D49.7
cerebral	C70.0	C79.32	—	D32.0	D42.0	D49.7
crainial	C70.0	C79.32	—	D32.0	D42.0	D49.7
intracranial	C70.0	C79.32	—	D32.0	D42.0	D49.7
spinal (cord)	C70.1	C79.49	—	D32.1	D42.1	D49.7
meniscus, knee joint (lateral) (medial)	C40.2-☑	C79.51		D16.2-☑	D48.0	D49.2
Merkel cell — *see* Carcinoma, Merkel cell						
mesentery, mesenteric	C48.1	C78.6	—	D20.1	D48.4	D49.0
mesoappendix	C48.1	C78.6	—	D20.1	D48.4	D49.0
mesocolon	C48.1	C78.6	—	D20.1	D48.4	D49.0
mesopharynx — *see* Neoplasm, oropharynx						
mesosalpinx	C57.1-☑	C79.82	D07.39	D28.2	D39.8	D49.5
mesothelial tissue — *see* Mesothelioma						
mesothelioma — *see* Mesothelioma						
mesovarium	C57.1-☑	C79.82	D07.39	D28.2	D39.8	D49.5
metacarpus (any bone)	C40.1-☑	C79.51		D16.1-☑	—	—
metastatic NEC — *see also* Neoplasm, by site, secondary	—	C79.9	—	—	—	—
metatarsus (any bone)	C40.3-☑	C79.51		D16.3-☑	—	—
midbrain	C71.7	C79.31		D33.1	D43.1	D49.6
milk duct — *see* Neoplasm, breast						
mons						
pubis	C51.9	C79.82	D07.1	D28.0	D39.8	D49.5
veneris	C51.9	C79.82	D07.1	D28.0	D39.8	D49.5
motor tract	C72.9	C79.49	—	D33.9	D43.9	D49.7
brain	C71.9	C79.31		D33.2	D43.2	D49.6
cauda equina	C72.1	C79.49	—	D33.4	D43.4	D49.7
spinal	C72.0	C79.49	—	D33.4	D43.4	D49.7
mouth	C06.9	C79.89	D00.00	D10.30	D37.09	D49.0
book-leaf	C06.89	C79.89	—	—	—	—
floor	C04.9	C79.89	D00.06	D10.2	D37.09	D49.0
anterior portion	C04.0	C79.89	D00.06	D10.2	D37.09	D49.0
lateral portion	C04.1	C79.89	D00.06	D10.2	D37.09	D49.0
overlapping lesion	C04.8	—	—	—	—	—
overlapping NEC	C06.80	—	—	—	—	—
roof	C05.9	C79.89	D00.00	D10.39	D37.09	D49.0
specified part NEC	C06.89	C79.89	D00.00	D10.39	D37.09	D49.0
vestibule	C06.1	C79.89	D00.00	D10.39	D37.09	D49.0
mucosa						
alveolar (ridge or process)	C03.9	C79.89	D00.03	D10.39	D37.09	D49.0
lower	C03.1	C79.89	D00.03	D10.39	D37.09	D49.0
upper	C03.0	C79.89	D00.03	D10.39	D37.09	D49.0
buccal	C06.0	C79.89	D00.02	D10.39	D37.09	D49.0
cheek	C06.0	C79.89	D00.02	D10.39	D37.09	D49.0
lip — *see* Neoplasm, lip, internal						
nasal	C30.0	C78.39	D02.3	D14.0	D38.5	D49.1
oral	C06.0	C79.89	D00.02	D10.39	D37.09	D49.0
Mullerian duct						
female	C57.7	C79.82	D07.39	D28.7	D39.8	D49.5
male	C63.7	C79.82	D07.69	D29.8	D40.8	D49.5

	Malignant Primary	Malignant Secondary	Ca in situ	Benign	Uncertain	Unspecified Behavior
Neoplasm, neoplastic — *continued*						
muscle — *see also* Neoplasm, connective tissue						
extraocular	C69.6-☑	C79.49	D09.2-☑	D31.6-☑	D48.7	D49.89
myocardium	C38.0	C79.89	—	D15.1	D48.7	D49.89
myometrium	C54.2	C79.82	D07.0	D26.1	D39.0	D49.5
myopericardium	C38.0	C79.89	—	D15.1	D48.7	D49.89
nabothian gland (follicle)	C53.0	C79.82	D06.0	D26.0	D39.0	D49.5
nail — *see also* Neoplasm, skin, limb	C44.90	C79.2	D04.9	D23.9	D48.5	D49.2
finger — *see also* Neoplasm, skin, limb, upper	C44.60-☑	C79.2	D04.6-☑	D23.6-☑	D48.5	D49.2
toe — *see also* Neoplasm, skin, limb, lower	C44.70-☑	C79.2	D04.7-☑	D23.7-☑	D48.5	D49.2
nares, naris (anterior) (posterior)	C30.0	C78.39	D02.3	D14.0	D38.5	D49.1
nasal — *see* Neoplasm, nose						
nasolabial groove — *see also* Neoplasm, skin, face	C44.309	C79.2	D04.39	D23.39	D48.5	D49.2
nasolacrimal duct	C69.5-☑	C79.49	D09.2-☑	D31.5-☑	D48.7	D49.89
nasopharynx, nasopharyngeal	C11.9	C79.89	D00.08	D10.6	D37.05	D49.0
floor	C11.3	C79.89	D00.08	D10.6	D37.05	D49.0
overlapping lesion	C11.8	—	—	—	—	—
roof	C11.0	C79.89	D00.08	D10.6	D37.05	D49.0
wall	C11.9	C79.89	D00.08	D10.6	D37.05	D49.0
anterior	C11.3	C79.89	D00.08	D10.6	D37.05	D49.0
lateral	C11.2	C79.89	D00.08	D10.6	D37.05	D49.0
posterior	C11.1	C79.89	D00.08	D10.6	D37.05	D49.0
superior	C11.0	C79.89	D00.08	D10.6	D37.05	D49.0
nates — *see also* Neoplasm, skin, trunk	C44.509	C79.2	D04.5	D23.5	D48.5	D49.2
neck NEC	C76.0	C79.89	D09.8	D36.7	D48.7	D49.89
skin	C44.40	—	—	—	—	—
basal cell carcinoma	C44.41	—	—	—	—	—
specified type NEC	C44.49	—	—	—	—	—
squamous cell carcinoma	C44.42	—	—	—	—	—
nerve (ganglion)	C47.9	C79.89	—	D36.10	D48.2	D49.2
abducens	C72.59	C79.49	—	D33.3	D43.3	D49.7
accessory (spinal)	C72.59	C79.49	—	D33.3	D43.3	D49.7
acoustic	C72.4-☑	C79.49	—	D33.3	D43.3	D49.7
auditory	C72.4-☑	C79.49	—	D33.3	D43.3	D49.7
autonomic NEC — *see also* Neoplasm, nerve, peripheral	C47.9	C79.89		D36.10	D48.2	D49.2
brachial	C47.1-☑	C79.89		D36.12	D48.2	D49.2
cranial	C72.50	C79.49	—	D33.3	D43.3	D49.7
specified NEC	C72.59	C79.49	—	D33.3	D43.3	D49.7
facial	C72.59	C79.49	—	D33.3	D43.3	D49.7
femoral	C47.2-☑	C79.89		D36.13	D48.2	D49.2
ganglion NEC — *see also* Neoplasm, nerve, peripheral	C47.9	C79.89		D36.10	D48.2	D49.2
glossopharyngeal	C72.59	C79.49	—	D33.3	D43.3	D49.7
hypoglossal	C72.59	C79.49	—	D33.3	D43.3	D49.7
intercostal	C47.3	C79.89	—	D36.14	D48.2	D49.2
lumbar	C47.6	C79.89	—	D36.17	D48.2	D49.2
median	C47.1-☑	C79.89		D36.12	D48.2	D49.2
obturator	C47.2-☑	C79.89		D36.13	D48.2	D49.2
oculomotor	C72.59	C79.49	—	D33.3	D43.3	D49.7
olfactory	C47.2-☑	C79.49	—	D33.3	D43.3	D49.7
optic	C72.3-☑	C79.49	—	D33.3	D43.3	D49.7
parasympathetic NEC	C47.9	C79.89	—	D36.10	D48.2	D49.2
peripheral NEC	C47.9	C79.89	—	D36.10	D48.2	D49.2
abdomen	C47.4	C79.89	—	D36.15	D48.2	D49.2
abdominal wall	C47.4	C79.89	—	D36.15	D48.2	D49.2
ankle	C47.2-☑	C79.89	—	D36.13	D48.2	D49.2

☑ **Additional Character Required** — Refer to the Tabular List for Character Selection ▽ Subterms under main terms may continue to next column or page

	Malignant Primary	Malignant Secondary	Ca in situ	Benign	Uncertain	Unspecified Behavior
Neoplasm, neoplastic —						
continued						
nerve — *continued*						
peripheral — *continued*						
antecubital fossa or						
space	C47.1-☑	C79.89	—	D36.12	D48.2	D49.2
arm	C47.1-☑	C79.89	—	D36.12	D48.2	D49.2
auricle (ear)	C47.0	C79.89	—	D36.11	D48.2	D49.2
axilla	C47.3	C79.89	—	D36.12	D48.2	D49.2
back	C47.6	C79.89	—	D36.17	D48.2	D49.2
buttock	C47.5	C79.89	—	D36.16	D48.2	D49.2
calf	C47.2-☑	C79.89	—	D36.13	D48.2	D49.2
cervical region	C47.0	C79.89	—	D36.11	D48.2	D49.2
cheek	C47.0	C79.89	—	D36.11	D48.2	D49.2
chest (wall)	C47.3	C79.89	—	D36.14	D48.2	D49.2
chin	C47.0	C79.89	—	D36.11	D48.2	D49.2
ear (external)	C47.0	C79.89	—	D36.11	D48.2	D49.2
elbow	C47.1-☑	C79.89	—	D36.12	D48.2	D49.2
extrarectal	C47.5	C79.89	—	D36.16	D48.2	D49.2
extremity	C47.9	C79.89	—	D36.10	D48.2	D49.2
lower	C47.2-☑	C79.89	—	D36.13	D48.2	D49.2
upper	C47.1-☑	C79.89	—	D36.12	D48.2	D49.2
eyelid	C47.0	C79.89	—	D36.11	D48.2	D49.2
face	C47.0	C79.89	—	D36.11	D48.2	D49.2
finger	C47.1-☑	C79.89	—	D36.12	D48.2	D49.2
flank	C47.6	C79.89	—	D36.17	D48.2	D49.2
foot	C47.2-☑	C79.89	—	D36.13	D48.2	D49.2
forearm	C47.1-☑	C79.89	—	D36.12	D48.2	D49.2
forehead	C47.0	C79.89	—	D36.11	D48.2	D49.2
gluteal region	C47.5	C79.89	—	D36.16	D48.2	D49.2
groin	C47.5	C79.89	—	D36.16	D48.2	D49.2
hand	C47.1-☑	C79.89	—	D36.12	D48.2	D49.2
head	C47.0	C79.89	—	D36.11	D48.2	D49.2
heel	C47.2-☑	C79.89	—	D36.13	D48.2	D49.2
hip	C47.2-☑	C79.89	—	D36.13	D48.2	D49.2
infraclavicular						
region	C47.3	C79.89	—	D36.14	D48.2	D49.2
inguinal (canal)						
(region)	C47.5	C79.89	—	D36.16	D48.2	D49.2
intrathoracic	C47.3	C79.89	—	D36.14	D48.2	D49.2
ischiorectal						
fossa	C47.5	C79.89	—	D36.16	D48.2	D49.2
knee	C47.2-☑	C79.89	—	D36.13	D48.2	D49.2
leg	C47.2-☑	C79.89	—	D36.13	D48.2	D49.2
limb NEC	C47.9	C79.89	—	D36.10	D48.2	D49.2
lower	C47.2-☑	C79.89	—	D36.13	D48.2	D49.2
upper	C47.1-☑	C79.89	—	D36.12	D48.2	D49.2
nates	C47.5	C79.89	—	D36.16	D48.2	D49.2
neck	C47.0	C79.89	—	D36.11	D48.2	D49.2
orbit	C69.6-☑	C79.49	—	D31.6-☑	D48.7	D49.2
pararectal	C47.5	C79.89	—	D36.16	D48.2	D49.2
paraurethral	C47.5	C79.89	—	D36.16	D48.2	D49.2
paravaginal	C47.5	C79.89	—	D36.16	D48.2	D49.2
pelvis (floor)	C47.5	C79.89	—	D36.16	D48.2	D49.2
pelvoabdominal	C47.8	C79.89	—	D36.17	D48.2	D49.2
perineum	C47.5	C79.89	—	D36.16	D48.2	D49.2
perirectal						
(tissue)	C47.5	C79.89	—	D36.16	D48.2	D49.2
periurethral						
(tissue)	C47.5	C79.89	—	D36.16	D48.2	D49.2
popliteal fossa or						
space	C47.2-☑	C79.89	—	D36.13	D48.2	D49.2
presacral	C47.5	C79.89	—	D36.16	D48.2	D49.2
pterygoid fossa	C47.0	C79.89	—	D36.11	D48.2	D49.2
rectovaginal septum						
or wall	C47.5	C79.89	—	D36.16	D48.2	D49.2
rectovesical	C47.5	C79.89	—	D36.16	D48.2	D49.2
sacrococcygeal						
region	C47.5	C79.89	—	D36.16	D48.2	D49.2
scalp	C47.0	C79.89	—	D36.11	D48.2	D49.2
scapular region	C47.3	C79.89	—	D36.14	D48.2	D49.2
shoulder	C47.1-☑	C79.89	—	D36.12	D48.2	D49.2
submental	C47.0	C79.89	—	D36.11	D48.2	D49.2
supraclavicular						
region	C47.0	C79.89	—	D36.11	D48.2	D49.2
temple	C47.0	C79.89	—	D36.11	D48.2	D49.2
temporal region	C47.0	C79.89	—	D36.11	D48.2	D49.2
thigh	C47.2-☑	C79.89	—	D36.13	D48.2	D49.2
thoracic (duct)						
(wall)	C47.3	C79.89	—	D36.14	D48.2	D49.2
thorax	C47.3	C79.89	—	D36.14	D48.2	D49.2
thumb	C47.1-☑	C79.89	—	D36.12	D48.2	D49.2

	Malignant Primary	Malignant Secondary	Ca in situ	Benign	Uncertain	Unspecified Behavior
Neoplasm, neoplastic —						
continued						
nerve — *continued*						
peripheral — *continued*						
toe	C47.2-☑	C79.89	—	D36.13	D48.2	D49.2
trunk	C47.6	C79.89	—	D36.17	D48.2	D49.2
umbilicus	C47.4	C79.89	—	D36.15	D48.2	D49.2
vesicorectal	C47.5	C79.89	—	D36.16	D48.2	D49.2
wrist	C47.1-☑	C79.89	—	D36.12	D48.2	D49.2
radial	C47.1-☑	C79.89	—	D36.12	D48.2	D49.2
sacral	C47.5	C79.89	—	D36.16	D48.2	D49.2
sciatic	C47.2-☑	C79.89	—	D36.13	D48.2	D49.2
spinal NEC	C47.9	C79.89	—	D36.10	D48.2	D49.2
accessory	C72.59	C79.49	—	D33.3	D43.3	D49.7
sympathetic NEC — *see*						
also Neoplasm,						
nerve,						
peripheral	C47.9	C79.89	—	D36.10	D48.2	D49.2
trigeminal	C72.59	C79.49	—	D33.3	D43.3	D49.7
trochlear	C72.59	C79.49	—	D33.3	D43.3	D49.7
ulnar	C47.1-☑	C79.89	—	D36.12	D48.2	D49.2
vagus	C72.59	C79.49	—	D33.3	D43.3	D49.7
nervous system						
(central)	C72.9	C79.40	—	D33.9	D43.9	D49.7
autonomic — *see*						
Neoplasm, nerve,						
peripheral						
parasympathetic — *see*						
Neoplasm, nerve,						
peripheral						
specified site NEC		C79.49	—	D33.7	D43.8	—
sympathetic — *see*						
Neoplasm, nerve,						
peripheral						
nevus — *see* Nevus						
nipple	C50.0-☑	C79.81	D05.-☑	D24.-☑	—	—
nose, nasal	C76.0	C79.89	D09.8	D36.7	D48.7	D49.89
ala (external) (nasi) —						
see also Neoplasm,						
nose, skin	C44.301	C79.2	D04.39	D23.39	D48.5	D49.2
bone	C41.0	C79.51	—	D16.4	D48.0	D49.2
cartilage	C30.0	C78.39	D02.3	D14.0	D38.5	D49.1
cavity	C30.0	C78.39	D02.3	D14.0	D38.5	D49.1
choana	C11.3	C79.89	D00.08	D10.6	D37.05	D49.0
external (skin) — *see*						
also Neoplasm,						
nose, skin	C44.301	C79.2	D04.39	D23.39	D48.5	D49.2
fossa	C30.0	C78.39	D02.3	D14.0	D38.5	D49.1
internal	C30.0	C78.39	D02.3	D14.0	D38.5	D49.1
mucosa	C30.0	C78.39	D02.3	D14.0	D38.5	D49.1
septum	C30.0	C78.39	D02.3	D14.0	D38.5	D49.1
posterior margin	C11.3	C79.89	D00.08	D10.6	D37.05	D49.0
sinus — *see* Neoplasm,						
sinus						
skin	C44.301	C79.2	D04.39	D23.39	D48.5	D49.2
basal cell						
carcinoma	C44.311	—	—	—	—	—
specified type						
NEC	C44.391	—	—	—	—	—
squamous cell						
carcinoma	C44.321	—	—	—	—	—
turbinate						
(mucosa)	C30.0	C78.39	D02.3	D14.0	D38.5	D49.1
bone	C41.0	C79.51	—	D16.4	D48.0	D49.2
vestibule	C30.0	C78.39	D02.3	D14.0	D38.5	D49.1
nostril	C30.0	C78.39	D02.3	D14.0	D38.5	D49.1
nucleus pulposus	C41.2	C79.51	—	D16.6	D48.0	D49.2
occipital						
bone	C41.0	C79.51	—	D16.4	D48.0	D49.2
lobe or pole, brain	C71.4	C79.31	—	D33.0	D43.0	D49.6
odontogenic — *see*						
Neoplasm, jaw bone						
olfactory nerve or						
bulb	C72.2-☑	C79.49	—	D33.3	D43.3	D49.7
olive (brain)	C71.7	C79.31	—	D33.1	D43.1	D49.6
omentum	C48.1	C78.6	—	D20.1	D48.4	D49.0
operculum (brain)	C71.0	C79.31	—	D33.0	D43.0	D49.6
optic nerve, chiasm, or						
tract	C72.3-☑	C79.49	—	D33.3	D43.3	D49.7
oral (cavity)	C06.9	C79.89	D00.00	D10.30	D37.09	D49.0
ill-defined	C14.8	C79.89	D00.00	D10.30	D37.09	D49.0
mucosa	C06.0	C79.89	D00.02	D10.39	D37.09	D49.0

Neoplasm Table

Neoplasm, nerve — Neoplasm, oral

	Malignant Primary	Malignant Secondary	Ca in situ	Benign	Uncertain	Unspecified Behavior
Neoplasm, neoplastic —						
continued						
orbit	C69.6-✓	C79.49	D09.2-✓	D31.6-✓	D48.7	D49.89
autonomic nerve	C69.6-✓	C79.49	—	D31.6-✓	D48.7	D49.2
bone	C41.0	C79.51	—	D16.4	D48.0	D49.2
eye	C69.6-✓	C79.49	D09.2-✓	D31.6-✓	D48.7	D49.89
peripheral nerves	C69.6-✓	C79.49	—	D31.6-✓	D48.7	D49.2
soft parts	C69.6-✓	C79.49	D09.2-✓	D31.6-✓	D48.7	D49.89
organ of						
Zuckerkandl	C75.5	C79.89	—	D35.6	D44.7	D49.7
oropharynx	C10.9	C79.89	D00.08	D10.5	D37.05	D49.0
branchial cleft						
(vestige)	C10.4	C79.89	D00.08	D10.5	D37.05	D49.0
junctional region	C10.8	C79.89	D00.08	D10.5	D37.05	D49.0
lateral wall	C10.2	C79.89	D00.08	D10.5	D37.05	D49.0
overlapping lesion	C10.8	—	—	—	—	—
pillars or fauces	C09.1	C79.89	D00.08	D10.5	D37.05	D49.0
posterior wall	C10.3	C79.89	D00.08	D10.5	D37.05	D49.0
vallecula	C10.0	C79.89	D00.08	D10.5	D37.05	D49.0
os						
external	C53.1	C79.82	D06.1	D26.0	D39.0	D49.5
internal	C53.0	C79.82	D06.0	D26.0	D39.0	D49.5
ovary	C56.-✓	C79.6-✓	D07.39	D27.-✓	D39.1-✓	D49.5
oviduct	C57.0-✓	C79.82	D07.39	D28.2	D39.8	D49.5
palate	C05.9	C79.89	D00.00	D10.39	D37.09	D49.0
hard	C05.0	C79.89	D00.05	D10.39	D37.09	D49.0
junction of hard and						
soft palate	C05.9	C79.89	D00.00	D10.39	D37.09	D49.0
overlapping						
lesions	C05.8	—	—	—	—	—
soft	C05.1	C79.89	D00.04	D10.39	D37.09	D49.0
nasopharyngeal						
surface	C11.3	C79.89	D00.08	D10.6	D37.05	D49.0
posterior surface	C11.3	C79.89	D00.08	D10.6	D37.05	D49.0
superior surface	C11.3	C79.89	D00.08	D10.6	D37.05	D49.0
palatoglossal arch	C09.1	C79.89	D00.00	D10.5	D37.09	D49.0
palatopharyngeal						
arch	C09.1	C79.89	D00.00	D10.5	D37.09	D49.0
pallium	C71.0	C79.31	—	D33.0	D43.0	D49.6
palpebra	C44.10-✓	C79.2	D04.1-✓	D23.1-✓	D48.5	D49.2
basal cell						
carcinoma	C44.11-✓	—	—	—	—	—
specified type NEC	C44.19-✓	—	—	—	—	—
squamous cell						
carcinoma	C44.12-✓	—	—	—	—	—
pancreas	C25.9	C78.89	D01.7	D13.6	D37.8	D49.0
body	C25.1	C78.89	D01.7	D13.6	D37.8	D49.0
duct (of Santorini) (of						
Wirsung)	C25.3	C78.89	D01.7	D13.6	D37.8	D49.0
ectopic tissue	C25.7	C78.89	—	D13.6	D37.8	D49.0
head	C25.0	C78.89	D01.7	D13.6	D37.8	D49.0
islet cells	C25.4	C78.89	D01.7	D13.7	D37.8	D49.0
neck	C25.7	C78.89	D01.7	D13.6	D37.8	D49.0
overlapping lesion	C25.8	—	—	—	—	—
tail	C25.2	C78.89	D01.7	D13.6	D37.8	D49.0
para-aortic body	C75.5	C79.89	—	D35.6	D44.7	D49.7
paraganglion NEC	C75.5	C79.89	—	D35.6	D44.7	D49.7
parametrium	C57.3	C79.82	—	D28.2	D39.8	D49.5
paranephric	C48.0	C78.6	—	D20.0	D48.3	D49.0
pararectal	C76.3	C79.89	—	D36.7	D48.7	D49.89
parasagittal (region)	C76.0	C79.89	D09.8	D36.7	D48.7	D49.89
parasellar	C72.9	C79.49	—	D33.9	D43.8	D49.7
parathyroid (gland)	C75.0	C79.89	D09.3	D35.1	D44.2	D49.7
paraurethral	C76.3	C79.89	—	D36.7	D48.7	D49.89
gland	C68.1	C79.19	D09.19	D30.8	D41.8	D49.5
paravaginal	C76.3	C79.89	—	D36.7	D48.7	D49.89
parenchyma, kidney	C64.-✓	C79.0-✓	D09.19	D30.0-✓	D41.0-✓	D49.5
parietal						
bone	C41.0	C79.51	—	D16.4	D48.0	D49.2
lobe, brain	C71.3	C79.31	—	D33.0	D43.0	D49.6
parootid (duct)	C57.1-✓	C79.82	D07.39	D28.2	D39.8	D49.5
parotid (duct)						
(gland)	C07	C79.89	D00.00	D11.0	D37.030	D49.0
parovarium	C57.1-✓	C79.82	D07.39	D28.2	D39.8	D49.5
patella	C40.20	C79.51	—	—	—	—
peduncle, cerebral	C71.7	C79.31	—	D33.1	D43.1	D49.6
pelvirectal junction	C19	C78.5	D01.1	D12.7	D37.5	D49.0
pelvis, pelvic	C76.3	C79.89	D09.8	D36.7	D48.7	D49.89
bone	C41.4	C79.51	—	D16.8	D48.0	D49.2
floor	C76.3	C79.89	D09.8	D36.7	D48.7	D49.89
renal	C65.-✓	C79.0-✓	D09.19	D30.1-✓	D41.1-✓	D49.5
viscera	C76.3	C79.89	D09.8	D36.7	D48.7	D49.89

	Malignant Primary	Malignant Secondary	Ca in situ	Benign	Uncertain	Unspecified Behavior
Neoplasm, neoplastic —						
continued						
pelvis, pelvic — *continued*						
wall	C76.3	C79.89	D09.8	D36.7	D48.7	D49.89
pelvo-abdominal	C76.8	C79.89	D09.8	D36.7	D48.7	D49.89
penis	C60.9	C79.82	D07.4	D29.0	D40.8	D49.5
body	C60.2	C79.82	D07.4	D29.0	D40.8	D49.5
corpus						
(cavernosum)	C60.2	C79.82	D07.4	D29.0	D40.8	D49.5
glans	C60.1	C79.82	D07.4	D29.0	D40.8	D49.5
overlapping sites	C60.8	—	—	—	—	—
skin NEC	C60.9	C79.82	D07.4	D29.0	D40.8	D49.5
periadrenal (tissue)	C48.0	C78.6	—	D20.0	D48.3	D49.0
perianal (skin) — *see also*						
Neoplasm, anus,						
skin	C44.500	C79.2	D04.5	D23.5	D48.5	D49.2
pericardium	C38.0	C79.89	—	D15.1	D48.7	D49.89
perinephric	C48.0	C78.6	—	D20.0	D48.3	D49.0
perineum	C76.3	C79.89	D09.8	D36.7	D48.7	D49.89
periodontal tissue						
NEC	C03.9	C79.89	D00.03	D10.39	D37.09	D49.0
periosteum — *see*						
Neoplasm, bone						
peripancreatic	C48.0	C78.6	—	D20.0	D48.3	D49.0
peripheral nerve						
NEC	C47.9	C79.89	—	D36.10	D48.2	D49.2
perirectal (tissue)	C76.3	C79.89	—	D36.7	D48.7	D49.89
perirenal (tissue)	C48.0	C78.6	—	D20.0	D48.3	D49.0
peritoneum, peritoneal						
(cavity)	C48.2	C78.6	—	D20.1	D48.4	D49.0
benign mesothelial						
tissue — *see*						
Mesothelioma,						
benign						
overlapping lesion						
with digestive						
organs	C26.9	—	—	—	—	—
parietal	C48.1	C78.6	—	D20.1	D48.4	D49.0
pelvic	C48.1	C78.6	—	D20.1	D48.4	D49.0
specified part NEC	C48.1	C78.6	—	D20.1	D48.4	D49.0
peritonsillar (tissue)	C76.0	C79.89	D09.8	D36.7	D48.7	D49.89
periurethral tissue	C76.3	C79.89	—	D36.7	D48.7	D49.89
phalanges						
foot	C40.3-✓	C79.51	—	D16.3-✓	—	—
hand	C40.1-✓	C79.51	—	D16.1-✓	—	—
pharynx, pharyngeal	C14.0	C79.89	D00.08	D10.9	D37.05	D49.0
bursa	C11.1	C79.89	D00.08	D10.6	D37.05	D49.0
fornix	C11.3	C79.89	D00.08	D10.6	D37.05	D49.0
recess	C11.2	C79.89	D00.08	D10.6	D37.05	D49.0
region	C14.0	C79.89	D00.08	D10.9	D37.05	D49.0
tonsil	C11.1	C79.89	D00.08	D10.6	D37.05	D49.0
wall (lateral)						
(posterior)	C14.0	C79.89	D00.08	D10.9	D37.05	D49.0
pia mater	C70.9	C79.40	—	D32.9	D42.9	D49.7
cerebral	C70.0	C79.32	—	D32.0	D42.0	D49.7
cranial	C70.0	C79.32	—	D32.0	D42.0	D49.7
spinal	C70.1	C79.49	—	D32.1	D42.1	D49.7
pillars of fauces	C09.1	C79.89	D00.08	D10.5	D37.05	D49.0
pineal (body)						
(gland)	C75.3	C79.89	D09.3	D35.4	D44.5	D49.7
pinna (ear) NEC — *see*						
also Neoplasm, skin,						
ear	C44.20-✓	C79.2	D04.2-✓	D23.2-✓	D48.5	D49.2
piriform fossa or						
sinus	C12	C79.89	D00.08	D10.7	D37.05	D49.0
pituitary (body) (fossa)						
(gland) (lobe)	C75.1	C79.89	D09.3	D35.2	D44.3	D49.7
placenta	C58	C79.82	D07.0	D26.7	D39.2	D49.5
pleura, pleural						
(cavity)	C38.4	C78.2	—	D19.0	D38.2	D49.1
overlapping lesion with						
heart or						
mediastinum	C38.8	—	—	—	—	—
parietal	C38.4	C78.2	—	D19.0	D38.2	D49.1
visceral	C38.4	C78.2	—	D19.0	D38.2	D49.1
plexus						
brachial	C47.1-✓	C79.89	—	D36.12	D48.2	D49.2
cervical	C47.0	C79.89	—	D36.11	D48.2	D49.2
choroid	C71.5	C79.31	—	D33.0	D43.0	D49.6
lumbosacral	C47.5	C79.89	—	D36.16	D48.2	D49.2
sacral	C47.5	C79.89	—	D36.16	D48.2	D49.2
pluriendocrine	C75.8	C79.89	D09.3	D35.7	D44.9	D49.7

✓ **Additional Character Required** — Refer to the Tabular List for Character Selection   ▽ Subterms under main terms may continue to next column or page

Neoplasm Table

Neoplasm, neoplastic — *continued*

	Malignant Primary	Malignant Secondary	Ca in situ	Benign	Uncertain	Unspecified Behavior
pole						
frontal	C71.1	C79.31	—	D33.0	D43.0	D49.6
occipital	C71.4	C79.31	—	D33.0	D43.0	D49.6
pons (varolii)	C71.7	C79.31	—	D33.1	D43.1	D49.6
popliteal fossa or space	C76.5-☑	C79.89	D04.7-☑	D36.7	D48.7	D49.89
postcricoid (region)	C13.0	C79.89	D00.08	D10.7	D37.05	D49.0
posterior fossa (cranial)	C71.9	C79.31	—	D33.2	D43.2	D49.6
postnasal space	C11.9	C79.89	D00.08	D10.6	D37.05	D49.0
prepuce	C60.0	C79.82	D07.4	D29.0	D40.8	D49.5
prepylorus	C16.4	C78.89	D00.2	D13.1	D37.1	D49.0
presacral (region)	C76.3	C79.89	—	D36.7	D48.7	D49.89
prostate (gland)	C61	C79.82	D07.5	D29.1	D40.0	D49.5
utricle	C68.0	C79.19	D09.19	D30.4	D41.3	D49.5
pterygoid fossa	C49.0	C79.89	—	D21.0	D48.1	D49.2
pubic bone	C41.4	C79.51	—	D16.8	D48.0	D49.2
pudenda, pudendum (female)	C51.9	C79.82	D07.1	D28.0	D39.8	D49.5
pulmonary — *see also* Neoplasm, lung	C34.9-☑	C78.0-☑	D02.2-☑	D14.3-☑	D38.1	D49.1
putamen	C71.0	C79.31	—	D33.0	D43.0	D49.6
pyloric						
antrum	C16.3	C78.89	D00.2	D13.1	D37.1	D49.0
canal	C16.4	C78.89	D00.2	D13.1	D37.1	D49.0
pylorus	C16.4	C78.89	D00.2	D13.1	D37.1	D49.0
pyramid (brain)	C71.7	C79.31	—	D33.1	D43.1	D49.6
pyriform fossa or sinus	C12	C79.89	D00.08	D10.7	D37.05	D49.0
radius (any part)	C40.0-☑	C79.51	—	D16.0-☑	—	—
Rathke's pouch	C75.1	C79.89	D09.3	D35.2	D44.3	D49.7
rectosigmoid (junction)	C19	C78.5	D01.1	D12.7	D37.5	D49.0
overlapping lesion with anus or rectum	C21.8	—	—	—	—	—
rectouterine pouch	C48.1	C78.6	—	D20.1	D48.4	D49.0
rectovaginal septum or wall	C76.3	C79.89	D09.8	D36.7	D48.7	D49.89
rectovesical septum	C76.3	C79.89	D09.8	D36.7	D48.7	D49.89
rectum (ampulla)	C20	C78.5	D01.2	D12.8	D37.5	D49.0
and colon	C19	C78.5	D01.1	D12.7	D37.5	D49.0
overlapping lesion with anus or rectosigmoid junction	C21.8	—	—	—	—	—
renal	C64.-☑	C79.0-☑	D09.19	D30.0-☑	D41.0-☑	D49.5
calyx	C65.-☑	C79.0-☑	D09.19	D30.1-☑	D41.1-☑	D49.5
hilus	C65.-☑	C79.0-☑	D09.19	D30.1-☑	D41.1-☑	D49.5
parenchyma	C64.-☑	C79.0-☑	D09.19	D30.0-☑	D41.0-☑	D49.5
pelvis	C65.-☑	C79.0-☑	D09.19	D30.1-☑	D41.1-☑	D49.5
respiratory						
organs or system NEC	C39.9	C78.30	D02.4	D14.4	D38.6	D49.1
tract NEC	C39.9	C78.30	D02.4	D14.4	D38.5	D49.1
upper	C39.0	C78.30	D02.4	D14.4	D38.5	D49.1
retina	C69.2-☑	C79.49	D09.2-☑	D31.2-☑	D48.7	D49.81
retrobulbar	C69.6-☑	C79.49	—	D31.6-☑	D48.7	D49.89
retrocecal	C48.0	C78.6	—	D20.0	D48.3	D49.0
retromolar (area) (triangle) (trigone)	C06.2	C79.89	D00.00	D10.39	D37.09	D49.0
retro-orbital	C76.0	C79.89	D09.8	D36.7	D48.7	D49.89
retroperitoneal (space) (tissue)	C48.0	C78.6	—	D20.0	D48.3	D49.0
retroperitoneum	C48.0	C78.6	—	D20.0	D48.3	D49.0
retropharyngeal	C14.0	C79.89	D00.08	D10.9	D37.05	D49.0
retrovesical (septum)	C76.3	C79.89	D09.8	D36.7	D48.7	D49.89
rhinencephalon	C71.0	C79.31	—	D33.0	D43.0	D49.6
rib	C41.3	C79.51	—	D16.7	D48.0	D49.2
Rosenmuller's fossa	C11.2	C79.89	D00.08	D10.6	D37.05	D49.0
round ligament	C57.2-☑	C79.82	—	D28.2	D39.8	D49.5
sacrococcyx, sacrococcygeal region	C41.4	C79.51	—	D16.8	D48.0	D49.2
	C76.3	C79.89	D09.8	D36.7	D48.7	D49.89
sacrouterine ligament	C57.3	C79.82	—	D28.2	D39.8	D49.5
sacrum, sacral (vertebra)	C41.4	C79.51	—	D16.8	D48.0	D49.2

Neoplasm, neoplastic — *continued*

	Malignant Primary	Malignant Secondary	Ca in situ	Benign	Uncertain	Unspecified Behavior
salivary gland or duct (major)	C08.9	C79.89	D00.00	D11.9	D37.039	D49.0
minor NEC	C06.9	C79.89	D00.00	D10.39	D37.04	D49.0
overlapping lesion	C08.9	—	—	—	—	—
parotid	C07	C79.89	D00.00	D11.0	D37.030	D49.0
pluriglandular	C08.9	C79.89	D00.00	D11.9	D37.039	D49.0
sublingual	C08.1	C79.89	D00.00	D11.7	D37.031	D49.0
submandibular	C08.0	C79.89	D00.00	D11.7	D37.032	D49.0
submaxillary	C08.0	C79.89	D00.00	D11.7	D37.032	D49.0
salpinx (uterine)	C57.0-☑	C79.82	D07.39	D28.2	D39.8	D49.5
Santorini's duct	C25.3	C78.89	D01.7	D13.6	D37.8	D49.0
scalp	C44.40	C79.2	D04.4	D23.4	D48.5	D49.2
basal cell carcinoma	C44.41	—	—	—	—	—
specified type NEC	C44.49	—	—	—	—	—
squamous cell carcinoma	C44.42	—	—	—	—	—
scapula (any part)	C40.0-☑	C79.51	—	D16.0-☑	—	—
scapular region	C76.1	C79.89	D09.8	D36.7	D48.7	D49.89
scar NEC — *see also* Neoplasm, skin, by site	C44.90	C79.2	D04.9	D23.9	D48.5	D49.2
sciatic nerve	C47.2-☑	C79.89	—	D36.13	D48.2	D49.2
sclera	C69.4-☑	C79.49	D09.2-☑	D31.4-☑	D48.7	D49.89
scrotum (skin)	C63.2	C79.82	D07.61	D29.4	D40.8	D49.5
sebaceous gland — *see* Neoplasm, skin						
sella turcica	C75.1	C79.89	D09.3	D35.2	D44.3	D49.7
bone	C41.0	C79.51	—	D16.4	D48.0	D49.2
semilunar cartilage (knee)	C40.2-☑	C79.51	—	D16.2-☑	D48.0	D49.2
seminal vesicle	C63.7	C79.82	D07.69	D29.8	D40.8	D49.5
septum						
nasal	C30.0	C78.39	D02.3	D14.0	D38.5	D49.1
posterior margin	C11.3	C79.89	D00.08	D10.6	D37.05	D49.0
rectovaginal	C76.3	C79.89	D09.8	D36.7	D48.7	D49.89
rectovesical	C76.3	C79.89	D09.8	D36.7	D48.7	D49.89
urethrovaginal	C57.9	C79.82	D07.30	D28.9	D39.9	D49.5
vesicovaginal	C57.9	C79.82	D07.30	D28.9	D39.9	D49.5
shoulder NEC	C76.4-☑	C79.89	D04.6-☑	D36.7	D48.7	D49.89
sigmoid flexure (lower) (upper)	C18.7	C78.5	D01.0	D12.5	D37.4	D49.0
sinus (accessory)	C31.9	C78.39	D02.3	D14.0	D38.5	D49.1
bone (any)	C41.0	C79.51	—	D16.4	D48.0	D49.2
ethmoidal	C31.1	C78.39	D02.3	D14.0	D38.5	D49.1
frontal	C31.2	C78.39	D02.3	D14.0	D38.5	D49.1
maxillary	C31.0	C78.39	D02.3	D14.0	D38.5	D49.1
nasal, paranasal NEC	C31.9	C78.39	D02.3	D14.0	D38.5	D49.1
overlapping lesion	C31.8	—	—	—	—	—
pyriform	C12	C79.89	D00.08	D10.7	D37.05	D49.0
sphenoid	C31.3	C78.39	D02.3	D14.0	D38.5	D49.1
skeleton, skeletal NEC	C41.9	C79.51	—	D16.9	D48.0	D49.2
Skene's gland	C68.1	C79.19	D09.19	D30.8	D41.8	D49.5
skin NOS	C44.90	C79.2	D04.9	D23.9	D48.5	D49.2
abdominal wall	C44.509	C79.2	D04.5	D23.5	D48.5	D49.2
basal cell carcinoma	C44.519	—	—	—	—	—
specified type NEC	C44.599	—	—	—	—	—
squamous cell carcinoma	C44.529	—	—	—	—	—
ala nasi — *see also* Neoplasm, nose, skin	C44.301	C79.2	D04.39	D23.39	D48.5	D49.2
ankle — *see also* Neoplasm, skin, limb, lower	C44.70-☑	C79.2	D04.7-☑	D23.7-☑	D48.5	D49.2
antecubital space — *see also* Neoplasm, skin, limb, upper	C44.60-☑	C79.2	D04.6-☑	D23.6-☑	D48.5	D49.2
anus	C44.500	C79.2	D04.5	D23.5	D48.5	D49.2
basal cell carcinoma	C44.510	—	—	—	—	—
specified type NEC	C44.590	—	—	—	—	—
squamous cell carcinoma	C44.520	—	—	—	—	—

Neoplasm, pole — Neoplasm, skin NOS

Neoplasm, neoplastic — continued

	Malignant Primary	Malignant Secondary	Ca in situ	Benign	Uncertain	Unspecified Behavior
skin — continued						
arm — see also Neoplasm, skin, limb, upper	C44.60-☑	C79.2	D04.6-☑	D23.6-☑	D48.5	D49.2
auditory canal (external) — see also Neoplasm, skin, ear	C44.20-☑	C79.2	D04.2-☑	D23.2-☑	D48.5	D49.2
auricle (ear) — see also Neoplasm, skin, ear	C44.20-☑	C79.2	D04.2-☑	D23.2-☑	D48.5	D49.2
auricular canal (external) — see also Neoplasm, skin, ear	C44.20-☑	C79.2	D04.2-☑	D23.2-☑	D48.5	D49.2
axilla, axillary fold — see also Neoplasm, skin, trunk	C44.509	C79.2	D04.5	D23.5	D48.5	D49.2
back — see also Neoplasm, skin, trunk	C44.509	C79.2	D04.5	D23.5	D48.5	D49.2
basal cell carcinoma	C44.91	—	—	—	—	—
breast	C44.501	C79.2	D04.5	D23.5	D48.5	D49.2
basal cell carcinoma	C44.511	—	—	—	—	—
specified type NEC	C44.591	—	—	—	—	—
squamous cell carcinoma	C44.521	—	—	—	—	—
brow — see also Neoplasm, skin, face	C44.309	C79.2	D04.39	D23.39	D48.5	D49.2
buttock — see also Neoplasm, skin, trunk	C44.509	C79.2	D04.5	D23.5	D48.5	D49.2
calf — see also Neoplasm, skin, limb, lower	C44.70-☑	C79.2	D04.7-☑	D23.7-☑	D48.5	D49.2
canthus (eye) (inner) (outer)	C44.10-☑	C79.2	D04.1-☑	D23.1-☑	D48.5	D49.2
basal cell carcinoma	C44.11-☑	—	—	—	—	—
specified type NEC	C44.19-☑	—	—	—	—	—
squamous cell carcinoma	C44.12-☑	—	—	—	—	—
cervical region — see also Neoplasm, skin, neck	C44.40	C79.2	D04.4	D23.4	D48.5	D49.2
cheek (external) — see also Neoplasm, skin, face	C44.309	C79.2	D04.39	D23.39	D48.5	D49.2
chest (wall) — see also Neoplasm, skin, trunk	C44.509	C79.2	D04.5	D23.5	D48.5	D49.2
chin — see also Neoplasm, skin, face	C44.309	C79.2	D04.39	D23.39	D48.5	D49.2
clavicular area — see also Neoplasm, skin, trunk	C44.509	C79.2	D04.5	D23.5	D48.5	D49.2
clitoris	C51.2	C79.82	D07.1	D28.0	D39.8	D49.5
columnella — see also Neoplasm, skin, face	C44.309	C79.2	D04.39	D23.39	D48.5	D49.2
concha — see also Neoplasm, skin, ear	C44.20-☑	C79.2	D04.2-☑	D23.2-☑	D48.5	D49.2
ear (external)	C44.20-☑	C79.2	D04.2-☑	D23.2-☑	D48.5	D49.2
basal cell carcinoma	C44.21-☑	—	—	—	—	—
specified type NEC	C44.29-☑	—	—	—	—	—
squamous cell carcinoma	C44.22-☑	—	—	—	—	—
elbow — see also Neoplasm, skin, limb, upper	C44.60-☑	C79.2	D04.6-☑	D23.6-☑	D48.5	D49.2

Neoplasm, neoplastic — continued

	Malignant Primary	Malignant Secondary	Ca in situ	Benign	Uncertain	Unspecified Behavior
skin — continued						
eyebrow — see also Neoplasm, skin, face	C44.309	C79.2	D04.39	D23.39	D48.5	D49.2
eyelid	C44.10-☑	C79.2	D04.1-☑	D23.1-☑	D48.5	D49.2
basal cell carcinoma	C44.11-☑	—	—	—	—	—
specified type NEC	C44.19-☑	—	—	—	—	—
squamous cell carcinoma	C44.12-☑	—	—	—	—	—
face NOS	C44.300	C79.2	D04.30	D23.30	D48.5	D49.2
basal cell carcinoma	C44.310	—	—	—	—	—
specified type NEC	C44.390	—	—	—	—	—
squamous cell carcinoma	C44.320	—	—	—	—	—
female genital organs (external)	C51.9	C79.82	D07.1	D28.0	D39.8	D49.5
clitoris	C51.2	C79.82	D07.1	D28.0	D39.8	D49.5
labium NEC	C51.9	C79.82	D07.1	D28.0	D39.8	D49.5
majus	C51.0	C79.82	D07.1	D28.0	D39.8	D49.5
minus	C51.1	C79.82	D07.1	D28.0	D39.8	D49.5
pudendum	C51.9	C79.82	D07.1	D28.0	D39.8	D49.5
vulva	C51.9	C79.82	D07.1	D28.0	D39.8	D49.5
finger — see also Neoplasm, skin, limb, upper	C44.60-☑	C79.2	D04.6-☑	D23.6-☑	D48.5	D49.2
flank — see also Neoplasm, skin, trunk	C44.509	C79.2	D04.5	D23.5	D48.5	D49.2
foot — see also Neoplasm, skin, limb, lower	C44.70-☑	C79.2	D04.7-☑	D23.7-☑	D48.5	D49.2
forearm — see also Neoplasm, skin, limb, upper	C44.60-☑	C79.2	D04.6-☑	D23.6-☑	D48.5	D49.2
forehead — see also Neoplasm, skin, face	C44.309	C79.2	D04.39	D23.39	D48.5	D49.2
glabella — see also Neoplasm, skin, face	C44.309	C79.2	D04.39	D23.39	D48.5	D49.2
gluteal region — see also Neoplasm, skin, trunk	C44.509	C79.2	D04.5	D23.5	D48.5	D49.2
groin — see also Neoplasm, skin, trunk	C44.509	C79.2	D04.5	D23.5	D48.5	D49.2
hand — see also Neoplasm, skin, limb, upper	C44.60-☑	C79.2	D04.6-☑	D23.6-☑	D48.5	D49.2
head NEC — see also Neoplasm, skin, scalp	C44.40	C79.2	D04.4	D23.4	D48.5	D49.2
heel — see also Neoplasm, skin, limb, lower	C44.70-☑	C79.2	D04.7-☑	D23.7-☑	D48.5	D49.2
helix — see also Neoplasm, skin, ear	C44.20-☑	C79.2	D04.2-☑	D23.2-☑	D48.5	D49.2
hip — see also Neoplasm, skin, limb, lower	C44.70-☑	C79.2	D04.7-☑	D23.7-☑	D48.5	D49.2
infraclavicular region — see also Neoplasm, skin, trunk	C44.509	C79.2	D04.5	D23.5	D48.5	D49.2
inguinal region — see also Neoplasm, skin, trunk	C44.509	C79.2	D04.5	D23.5	D48.5	D49.2
jaw — see also Neoplasm, skin, face	C44.309	C79.2	D04.39	D23.39	D48.5	D49.2
Kaposi's sarcoma — see Kaposi's, sarcoma, skin						
knee — see also Neoplasm, skin, limb, lower	C44.70-☑	C79.2	D04.7-☑	D23.7-☑	D48.5	D49.2

☑ Additional Character Required — Refer to the Tabular List for Character Selection   ▽ Subterms under main terms may continue to next column or page

Neoplasm, neoplastic — continued	Malignant Primary	Malignant Secondary	Ca in situ	Benign	Uncertain	Unspecified Behavior
skin — continued						
labia						
majora	C51.0	C79.82	D07.1	D28.0	D39.8	D49.5
minora	C51.1	C79.82	D07.1	D28.0	D39.8	D49.5
leg — see also Neoplasm, skin, limb, lower	C44.70-☑	C79.2	D04.7-☑	D23.7-☑	D48.5	D49.2
lid (lower) (upper)	C44.10-☑	C79.2	D04.1-☑	D23.1-☑	D48.5	D49.2
basal cell carcinoma	C44.11-☑	—	—	—	—	—
specified type NEC	C44.19-☑	—	—	—	—	—
squamous cell carcinoma	C44.12-☑	—	—	—	—	—
limb NEC	C44.90	C79.2	D04.9	D23.9	D48.5	D49.2
basal cell carcinoma	C44.91					
lower	C44.70-☑	C79.2	D04.7-☑	D23.7-☑	D48.5	D49.2
basal cell carcinoma	C44.71-☑					
specified type NEC	C44.79-☑					
squamous cell carcinoma	C44.72-☑					
upper	C44.60-☑	C79.2	D04.6-☑	D23.6-☑	D48.5	D49.2
basal cell carcinoma	C44.61-☑					
specified type NEC	C44.69-☑					
squamous cell carcinoma	C44.62-☑					
lip (lower) (upper)	C44.00	C79.2	D04.0	D23.0	D48.5	D49.2
basal cell carcinoma	C44.01					
specified type NEC	C44.09					
squamous cell carcinoma	C44.02					
male genital organs	C63.9	C79.82	D07.60	D29.9	D40.8	D49.5
penis	C60.9	C79.82	D07.4	D29.0	D40.8	D49.5
prepuce	C60.0	C79.82	D07.4	D29.0	D40.8	D49.5
scrotum	C63.2	C79.82	D07.61	D29.4	D40.8	D49.5
mastectomy site (skin) — see also Neoplasm, skin, breast	C44.501	C79.2	—	—	—	—
specified as breast tissue	C50.8-☑	C79.81	—	—	—	—
meatus, acoustic (external) — see also Neoplasm, skin, ear	C44.20-☑	C79.2	D04.2-☑	D23.2-☑	D48.5	D49.2
melanotic — see Melanoma						
Merkel cell — see Carcinoma, Merkel cell						
nates — see also Neoplasm, skin, trunk	C44.509	C79.2	D04.5	D23.5	D48.5	D49.2
neck	C44.40	C79.2	D04.4	D23.4	D48.5	D49.2
basal cell carcinoma	C44.41	—				
specified type NEC	C44.49					
squamous cell carcinoma	C44.42					
nevus — see Nevus, skin						
nose (external) — see also Neoplasm, nose, skin	C44.301	C79.2	D04.39	D23.39	D48.5	D49.2
overlapping lesion	C44.80	—	—	—	—	—
basal cell carcinoma	C44.81					
specified type NEC	C44.89					
squamous cell carcinoma	C44.82	—	—	—	—	—

Neoplasm, neoplastic — continued	Malignant Primary	Malignant Secondary	Ca in situ	Benign	Uncertain	Unspecified Behavior
skin — continued						
palm — see also Neoplasm, skin, limb, upper	C44.60-☑	C79.2	D04.6-☑	D23.6-☑	D48.5	D49.2
palpebra	C44.10-☑	C79.2	D04.1-☑	D23.1-☑	D48.5	D49.2
basal cell carcinoma	C44.11-☑	—	—	—	—	—
specified type NEC	C44.19-☑	—	—	—	—	—
squamous cell carcinoma	C44.12-☑	—	—	—	—	—
penis NEC	C60.9	C79.82	D07.4	D29.0	D40.8	D49.5
perianal — see also Neoplasm, skin, anus	C44.500	C79.2	D04.5	D23.5	D48.5	D49.2
perineum — see also Neoplasm, skin, anus	C44.500	C79.2	D04.5	D23.5	D48.5	D49.2
pinna — see also Neoplasm, skin, ear	C44.20-☑	C79.2	D04.2-☑	D23.2-☑	D48.5	D49.2
plantar — see also Neoplasm, skin, limb, lower	C44.70-☑	C79.2	D04.7-☑	D23.7-☑	D48.5	D49.2
popliteal fossa or space — see also Neoplasm, skin, limb, lower	C44.70-☑	C79.2	D04.7-☑	D23.7-☑	D48.5	D49.2
prepuce	C60.0	C79.82	D07.4	D29.0	D40.8	D49.5
pubes — see also Neoplasm, skin, trunk	C44.509	C79.2	D04.5	D23.5	D48.5	D49.2
sacrococcygeal region — see also Neoplasm, skin, trunk	C44.509	C79.2	D04.5	D23.5	D48.5	D49.2
scalp	C44.40	C79.2	D04.4	D23.4	D48.5	D49.2
basal cell carcinoma	C44.41	—	—	—	—	—
specified type NEC	C44.49					
squamous cell carcinoma	C44.42					
scapular region — see also Neoplasm, skin, trunk	C44.509	C79.2	D04.5	D23.5	D48.5	D49.2
scrotum	C63.2	C79.82	D07.61	D29.4	D40.8	D49.5
shoulder — see also Neoplasm, skin, limb, upper	C44.60-☑	C79.2	D04.6-☑	D23.6-☑	D48.5	D49.2
sole (foot) — see also Neoplasm, skin, limb, lower	C44.70-☑	C79.2	D04.7-☑	D23.7-☑	D48.5	D49.2
specified sites NEC	C44.80	C79.2	D04.8	D23.9	D48.5	D49.2
basal cell carcinoma	C44.81	—	—	—	—	—
specified type NEC	C44.89	—	—	—	—	—
squamous cell carcinoma	C44.82	—	—	—	—	—
specified type NEC	C44.99	—	—	—	—	—
squamous cell carcinoma	C44.92	—	—	—	—	—
submammary fold — see also Neoplasm, skin, trunk	C44.509	C79.2	D04.5	D23.5	D48.5	D49.2
supraclavicular region — see also Neoplasm, skin, neck	C44.40	C79.2	D04.4	D23.4	D48.5	D49.2
temple — see also Neoplasm, skin, face	C44.309	C79.2	D04.39	D23.39	D48.5	D49.2
thigh — see also Neoplasm, skin, limb, lower	C44.70-☑	C79.2	D04.7-☑	D23.7-☑	D48.5	D49.2
thoracic wall — see also Neoplasm, skin, trunk	C44.509	C79.2	D04.5	D23.5	D48.5	D49.2

Neoplasm, neoplastic — continued

skin — continued	Malignant Primary	Malignant Secondary	Ca in situ	Benign	Uncertain	Unspecified Behavior
thumb — see also Neoplasm, skin, limb, upper	C44.60-✓	C79.2	D04.6-✓	D23.6-✓	D48.5	D49.2
toe — see also Neoplasm, skin, limb, lower	C44.70-✓	C79.2	D04.7-✓	D23.7-✓	D48.5	D49.2
tragus — see also Neoplasm, skin, ear	C44.20-✓	C79.2	D04.2-✓	D23.2-✓	D48.5	D49.2
trunk	C44.509	C79.2	D04.5	D23.5	D48.5	D49.2
basal cell carcinoma	C44.519	—	—	—	—	—
specified type NEC	C44.599	—	—	—	—	—
squamous cell carcinoma	C44.529	—	—	—	—	—
umbilicus — see also Neoplasm, skin, trunk	C44.509	C79.2	D04.5	D23.5	D48.5	D49.2
vulva	C51.9	C79.82	D07.1	D28.0	D39.8	D49.5
overlapping lesion	C51.8	—	—	—	—	—
wrist — see also Neoplasm, skin, limb, upper	C44.60-✓	C79.2	D04.6-✓	D23.6-✓	D48.5	D49.2
skull	C41.0	C79.51	—	D16.4	D48.0	D49.2
soft parts or tissues — see Neoplasm, connective tissue						
specified site NEC	C76.8	C79.89	D09.8	D36.7	D48.7	D49.89
spermatic cord	C63.1-✓	C79.82	D07.69	D29.8	D40.8	D49.5
sphenoid	C31.3	C78.39	D02.3	D14.0	D38.5	D49.1
bone	C41.0	C79.51	—	D16.4	D48.0	D49.2
sinus	C31.3	C78.39	D02.3	D14.0	D38.5	D49.1
sphincter						
anal	C21.1	C78.5	D01.3	D12.9	D37.8	D49.0
of Oddi	C24.0	C78.89	D01.5	D13.5	D37.6	D49.0
spine, spinal (column)	C41.2	C79.51	—	D16.6	D48.0	D49.2
bulb	C71.7	C79.31	—	D33.1	D43.1	D49.6
coccyx	C41.4	C79.51	—	D16.8	D48.0	D49.2
cord (cervical) (lumbar) (sacral) (thoracic)	C72.0	C79.49	—	D33.4	D43.4	D49.7
dura mater	C70.1	C79.49	—	D32.1	D42.1	D49.7
lumbosacral	C41.2	C79.51	—	D16.6	D48.0	D49.2
marrow NEC	C96.9	C79.52	—	—	D47.9	D49.89
membrane	C70.1	C79.49	—	D32.1	D42.1	D49.7
meninges	C70.1	C79.49	—	D32.1	D42.1	D49.7
nerve (root)	C47.9	C79.89	—	D36.10	D48.2	D49.2
pia mater	C70.1	C79.49	—	D32.1	D42.1	D49.7
root	C47.9	C79.89	—	D36.10	D48.2	D49.2
sacrum	C41.4	C79.51	—	D16.8	D48.0	D49.2
spleen, splenic NEC	C26.1	C78.89	D01.7	D13.9	D37.8	D49.0
flexure (colon)	C18.5	C78.5	D01.0	D12.3	D37.4	D49.0
stem, brain	C71.7	C79.31	—	D33.1	D43.1	D49.6
Stensen's duct	C07	C79.89	D00.00	D11.0	D37.030	D49.0
sternum	C41.3	C79.51	—	D16.7	D48.0	D49.2
stomach	C16.9	C78.89	D00.2	D13.1	D37.1	D49.0
antrum (pyloric)	C16.3	C78.89	D00.2	D13.1	D37.1	D49.0
body	C16.2	C78.89	D00.2	D13.1	D37.1	D49.0
cardia	C16.0	C78.89	D00.2	D13.1	D37.1	D49.0
cardiac orifice	C16.0	C78.89	D00.2	D13.1	D37.1	D49.0
corpus	C16.2	C78.89	D00.2	D13.1	D37.1	D49.0
fundus	C16.1	C78.89	D00.2	D13.1	D37.1	D49.0
greater curvature NEC	C16.6	C78.89	D00.2	D13.1	D37.1	D49.0
lesser curvature NEC	C16.5	C78.89	D00.2	D13.1	D37.1	D49.0
overlapping lesion	C16.8	—	—	—	—	—
prepylorus	C16.4	C78.89	D00.2	D13.1	D37.1	D49.0
pylorus	C16.4	C78.89	D00.2	D13.1	D37.1	D49.0
wall NEC	C16.9	C78.89	D00.2	D13.1	D37.1	D49.0
anterior NEC	C16.8	C78.89	D00.2	D13.1	D37.1	D49.0
posterior NEC	C16.8	C78.89	D00.2	D13.1	D37.1	D49.0
stroma, endometrial	C54.1	C79.82	D07.0	D26.1	D39.0	D49.5
stump, cervical	C53.8	C79.82	D06.7	D26.0	D39.0	D49.5

Neoplasm, neoplastic — continued

	Malignant Primary	Malignant Secondary	Ca in situ	Benign	Uncertain	Unspecified Behavior
subcutaneous (nodule) (tissue) NEC — see Neoplasm, connective tissue						
subdural	C70.9	C79.32	—	D32.9	D42.9	D49.7
subglottis, subglottic	C32.2	C78.39	D02.0	D14.1	D38.0	D49.1
sublingual	C04.9	C79.89	D00.06	D10.2	D37.09	D49.0
gland or duct	C08.1	C79.89	D00.00	D11.7	D37.031	D49.0
submandibular gland	C08.0	C79.89	D00.00	D11.7	D37.032	D49.0
submaxillary gland or duct	C08.0	C79.89	D00.00	D11.7	D37.032	D49.0
submental	C76.0	C79.89	D09.8	D36.7	D48.7	D49.89
subpleural	C34.9-✓	C78.0-✓	D02.2-✓	D14.3-✓	D38.1	D49.1
substernal	C38.1	C78.1	—	D15.2	D38.3	D49.89
sudoriferous, sudoriparous gland, site unspecified	C44.90	C79.2	D04.9	D23.9	D48.5	D49.2
specified site — see Neoplasm, skin						
supraclavicular region	C76.0	C79.89	D09.8	D36.7	D48.7	D49.89
supraglottis	C32.1	C78.39	D02.0	D14.1	D38.0	D49.1
suprarenal	C74.9-✓	C79.7-✓	D09.3	D35.0-✓	D44.1-✓	D49.7
capsule	C74.9-✓	C79.7-✓	D09.3	D35.0-✓	D44.1-✓	D49.7
cortex	C74.0-✓	C79.7-✓	D09.3	D35.0-✓	D44.1-✓	D49.7
gland	C74.9-✓	C79.7-✓	D09.3	D35.0-✓	D44.1-✓	D49.7
medulla	C74.1-✓	C79.7-✓	D09.3	D35.0-✓	D44.1-✓	D49.7
suprasellar (region)	C71.9	C79.31	—	D33.2	D43.2	D49.6
supratentorial (brain) NEC	C71.0	C79.31	—	D33.0	D43.0	D49.6
sweat gland (apocrine) (eccrine), site unspecified	C44.90	C79.2	D04.9	D23.9	D48.5	D49.2
specified site — see Neoplasm, skin						
sympathetic nerve or nervous system NEC	C47.9	C79.89	—	D36.10	D48.2	D49.2
symphysis pubis	C41.4	C79.51	—	D16.8	D48.0	D49.2
synovial membrane — see Neoplasm, connective tissue						
tapetum, brain	C71.8	C79.31	—	D33.2	D43.2	D49.6
tarsus (any bone)	C40.3-✓	C79.51	—	D16.3-✓	—	—
temple (skin) — see also Neoplasm, skin, face	C44.309	C79.2	D04.39	D23.39	D48.5	D49.2
temporal						
bone	C41.0	C79.51	—	D16.4	D48.0	D49.2
lobe or pole	C71.2	C79.31	—	D33.0	D43.0	D49.6
region	C76.0	C79.89	D09.8	D36.7	D48.7	D49.89
skin — see also Neoplasm, skin, face	C44.309	C79.2	D04.39	D23.39	D48.5	D49.2
tendon (sheath) — see Neoplasm, connective tissue						
tentorium (cerebelli)	C70.0	C79.32	—	D32.0	D42.0	D49.7
testis, testes	C62.9-✓	C79.82	D07.69	D29.2-✓	D40.1-✓	D49.5
descended	C62.1-✓	C79.82	D07.69	D29.2-✓	D40.1-✓	D49.5
ectopic	C62.0-✓	C79.82	D07.69	D29.2-✓	D40.1-✓	D49.5
retained	C62.0-✓	C79.82	D07.69	D29.2-✓	D40.1-✓	D49.5
scrotal	C62.1-✓	C79.82	D07.69	D29.2-✓	D40.1-✓	D49.5
undescended	C62.0-✓	C79.82	D07.69	D29.2-✓	D40.1-✓	D49.5
unspecified whether descended or undescended	C62.9-✓	C79.82	D07.69	D29.2-✓	D40.1-✓	D49.5
thalamus	C71.0	C79.31	—	D33.0	D43.0	D49.6
thigh NEC	C76.5-✓	C79.89	D04.7-✓	D36.7	D48.7	D49.89
thorax, thoracic (cavity) (organs NEC)	C76.1	C79.89	D09.8	D36.7	D48.7	D49.89
duct	C49.3	C79.89	—	D21.3	D48.1	D49.2
wall NEC	C76.1	C79.89	D09.8	D36.7	D48.7	D49.89
throat	C14.0	C79.89	D00.08	D10.9	D37.05	D49.0
thumb NEC	C76.4-✓	C79.89	D04.6-✓	D36.7	D48.7	D49.89
thymus (gland)	C37	C79.89	D09.3	D15.0	D38.4	D49.89
thyroglossal duct	C73	C79.89	D09.3	D34	D44.0	D49.7

✓ **Additional Character Required — Refer to the Tabular List for Character Selection**   ▽ **Subterms under main terms may continue to next column or page**

Neoplasm, neoplastic — continued

	Malignant Primary	Malignant Secondary	Ca in situ	Benign	Uncertain	Unspecified Behavior
thyroid (gland)	C73	C79.89	D09.3	D34	D44.0	D49.7
cartilage	C32.3	C78.39	D02.0	D14.1	D38.0	D49.1
tibia (any part)	C40.2-☑	C79.51	—	D16.2-☑	D48.0	D49.2
toe NEC	C76.5-☑	C79.89	D04.7-☑	D36.7	D48.7	D49.89
tongue	C02.9	C79.89	D00.07	D10.1	D37.02	D49.0
anterior (two-thirds) NEC	C02.3	C79.89	D00.07	D10.1	D37.02	D49.0
dorsal surface	C02.0	C79.89	D00.07	D10.1	D37.02	D49.0
ventral surface	C02.2	C79.89	D00.07	D10.1	D37.02	D49.0
base (dorsal surface)	C01	C79.89	D00.07	D10.1	D37.02	D49.0
border (lateral)	C02.1	C79.89	D00.07	D10.1	D37.02	D49.0
dorsal surface NEC	C02.0	C79.89	D00.07	D10.1	D37.02	D49.0
fixed part NEC	C01	C79.89	D00.07	D10.1	D37.02	D49.0
foramen cecum	C02.0	C79.89	D00.07	D10.1	D37.02	D49.0
frenulum linguae	C02.2	C79.89	D00.07	D10.1	D37.02	D49.0
junctional zone	C02.8	C79.89	D00.07	D10.1	D37.02	D49.0
margin (lateral)	C02.1	C79.89	D00.07	D10.1	D37.02	D49.0
midline NEC	C02.0	C79.89	D00.07	D10.1	D37.02	D49.0
mobile part NEC	C02.3	C79.89	D00.07	D10.1	D37.02	D49.0
overlapping lesion	C02.8	—	—	—	—	—
posterior (third)	C01	C79.89	D00.07	D10.1	D37.02	D49.0
root	C01	C79.89	D00.07	D10.1	D37.02	D49.0
surface (dorsal)	C02.0	C79.89	D00.07	D10.1	D37.02	D49.0
base	C01	C79.89	D00.07	D10.1	D37.02	D49.0
ventral	C02.2	C79.89	D00.07	D10.1	D37.02	D49.0
tip	C02.1	C79.89	D00.07	D10.1	D37.02	D49.0
tonsil	C02.4	C79.89	D00.07	D10.1	D37.02	D49.0
tonsil	C09.9	C79.89	D00.08	D10.4	D37.05	D49.0
fauces, faucial	C09.9	C79.89	D00.08	D10.4	D37.05	D49.0
lingual	C02.4	C79.89	D00.07	D10.1	D37.02	D49.0
overlapping sites	C09.8	—	—	—	—	—
palatine	C09.9	C79.89	D00.08	D10.4	D37.05	D49.0
pharyngeal	C11.1	C79.89	D00.08	D10.6	D37.05	D49.0
pillar (anterior) (posterior)	C09.1	C79.89	D00.08	D10.5	D37.05	D49.0
tonsillar fossa	C09.0	C79.89	D00.08	D10.5	D37.05	D49.0
tooth socket NEC	C03.9	C79.89	D00.03	D10.39	D37.09	D49.0
trachea (cartilage) (mucosa)	C33	C78.39	D02.1	D14.2	D38.1	D49.1
overlapping lesion with bronchus or lung	C34.8-☑	—	—	—	—	—
tracheobronchial	C34.8-☑	C78.39	D02.1	D14.2	D38.1	D49.1
overlapping lesion with lung	C34.8-☑	—	—	—	—	—
tragus — see also Neoplasm, skin, ear	C44.20-☑	C79.2	D04.2-☑	D23.2-☑	D48.5	D49.2
trunk NEC	C76.8	C79.89	D04.5	D36.7	D48.7	D49.89
tubo-ovarian	C57.8	C79.82	D07.39	D28.7	D39.8	D49.5
tunica vaginalis	C63.7	C79.82	D07.69	D29.8	D40.8	D49.5
turbinate (bone)	C41.0	C79.51	—	D16.4	D48.0	D49.2
nasal	C30.0	C78.39	D02.3	D14.0	D38.5	D49.1
tympanic cavity	C30.1	C78.39	D02.3	D14.0	D38.5	D49.1
ulna (any part)	C40.0-☑	C79.51	—	D16.0-☑	D48.0	D49.2
umbilicus, umbilical — see also Neoplasm, skin, trunk	C44.509	C79.2	D04.5	D23.5	D48.5	D49.2
uncus, brain	C71.2	C79.31	—	D33.0	D43.0	D49.6
unknown site or unspecified	C80.1	C79.9	D09.9	D36.9	D48.9	D49.9
urachus	C67.7	C79.11	D09.0	D30.3	D41.4	D49.4
ureter-bladder (junction)	C67.6	C79.11	D09.0	D30.3	D41.4	D49.4
ureter, ureteral	C66.-☑	C79.19	D09.19	D30.2-☑	D41.2-☑	D49.5
orifice (bladder)	C67.6	C79.11	D09.0	D30.3	D41.4	D49.4
urethra, urethral (gland)	C68.0	C79.19	D09.19	D30.4	D41.3	D49.5
orifice, internal	C67.5	C79.11	D09.0	D30.3	D41.4	D49.4
urethrovaginal (septum)	C57.9	C79.82	D07.30	D28.9	D39.8	D49.5
urinary organ or system	C68.9	C79.10	D09.10	D30.9	D41.9	D49.5
bladder — see Neoplasm, bladder						
overlapping lesion	C68.8	—	—	—	—	—
specified sites NEC	C68.8	C79.19	D09.19	D30.8	D41.8	D49.5
utero-ovarian	C57.8	C79.82	D07.39	D28.7	D39.8	D49.5
ligament	C57.1-☑	C79.82	D07.39	D28.2	D39.8	D49.5
uterosacral ligament	C57.3	C79.82	—	D28.2	D39.8	D49.5
uterus, uteri, uterine	C55	C79.82	D07.0	D26.9	D39.0	D49.5
adnexa NEC	C57.4	C79.82	D07.39	D28.7	D39.8	D49.5
body	C54.9	C79.82	D07.0	D26.1	D39.0	D49.5
cervix	C53.9	C79.82	D06.9	D26.0	D39.0	D49.5
cornu	C54.9	C79.82	D07.0	D26.1	D39.0	D49.5
corpus	C54.9	C79.82	D07.0	D26.1	D39.0	D49.5
endocervix (canal) (gland)	C53.0	C79.82	D06.0	D26.0	D39.0	D49.5
endometrium	C54.1	C79.82	D07.0	D26.1	D39.0	D49.5
exocervix	C53.1	C79.82	D06.1	D26.0	D39.0	D49.5
external os	C53.1	C79.82	D06.1	D26.0	D39.0	D49.5
fundus	C54.3	C79.82	D07.0	D26.1	D39.0	D49.5
internal os	C53.0	C79.82	D06.0	D26.0	D39.0	D49.5
isthmus	C54.0	C79.82	D07.0	D26.1	D39.0	D49.5
ligament	C57.3	C79.82	—	D28.2	D39.2	D49.5
broad	C57.1-☑	C79.82	D07.39	D28.2	D39.8	D49.5
round	C57.2-☑	C79.82	—	D28.2	D39.8	D49.5
lower segment	C54.0	C79.82	D07.0	D26.1	D39.0	D49.5
myometrium	C54.2	C79.82	D07.0	D26.1	D39.0	D49.5
overlapping sites	C54.8	—	—	—	—	—
squamocolumnar junction	C53.8	C79.82	D06.7	D26.0	D39.0	D49.5
tube	C57.0-☑	C79.82	D07.39	D28.2	D39.8	D49.5
utricle, prostatic	C68.0	C79.19	D09.19	D30.4	D41.3	D49.5
uveal tract	C69.4-☑	C79.49	D09.2-☑	D31.4-☑	D48.7	D49.89
uvula	C05.2	C79.89	D00.04	D10.39	D37.09	D49.0
vagina, vaginal (fornix) (vault) (wall)	C52	C79.82	D07.2	D28.1	D39.8	D49.5
vaginovesical	C57.9	C79.82	D07.30	D28.9	D39.9	D49.5
septum	C57.9	C79.82	D07.30	D28.9	D39.9	D49.5
vallecula (epiglottis)	C10.0	C79.89	D00.08	D10.5	D37.05	D49.0
vascular — see Neoplasm, connective tissue						
vas deferens	C63.1-☑	C79.82	D07.69	D29.8	D40.8	D49.5
Vater's ampulla	C24.1	C78.89	D01.5	D13.5	D37.6	D49.0
vein, venous — see Neoplasm, connective tissue						
vena cava (abdominal) (inferior)	C49.4	C79.89	—	D21.4	D48.1	D49.2
superior	C49.3	C79.89	—	D21.3	D48.1	D49.2
ventricle (cerebral) (floor) (lateral) (third)	C71.5	C79.31	—	D33.0	D43.0	D49.6
cardiac (left) (right)	C38.0	C79.89	—	D15.1	D48.7	D49.89
fourth	C71.7	C79.31	—	D33.1	D43.1	D49.6
ventricular band of larynx	C32.1	C78.39	D02.0	D14.1	D38.0	D49.1
ventriculus — see Neoplasm, stomach						
vermillion border — see Neoplasm, lip						
vermis, cerebellum	C71.6	C79.31	—	D33.1	D43.1	D49.6
vertebra (column)	C41.2	C79.51	—	D16.6	D48.0	D49.2
coccyx	C41.4	C79.51	—	D16.8	D48.0	D49.2
marrow NEC	C96.9	C79.52	—	—	D47.9	D49.89
sacrum	C41.4	C79.51	—	D16.8	D48.0	D49.2
vesical — see Neoplasm, bladder						
vesicle, seminal	C63.7	C79.82	D07.69	D29.8	D40.8	D49.5
vesicocervical tissue	C57.9	C79.82	D07.30	D28.9	D39.9	D49.5
vesicorectal	C76.3	C79.82	D09.8	D36.7	D48.7	D49.89
vesicovaginal	C57.9	C79.82	D07.30	D28.9	D39.9	D49.5
septum	C57.9	C79.82	D07.30	D28.9	D39.8	D49.5
vessel (blood) — see Neoplasm, connective tissue						
vestibular gland, greater	C51.0	C79.82	D07.1	D28.0	D39.8	D49.5
vestibule						
mouth	C06.1	C79.89	D00.00	D10.39	D37.09	D49.0
nose	C30.0	C78.39	D02.3	D14.0	D38.5	D49.1
Virchow's gland	C77.0	C77.0	—	D36.0	D48.7	D49.89
viscera NEC	C76.8	C79.89	D09.8	D36.7	D48.7	D49.89
vocal cords (true)	C32.0	C78.39	D02.0	D14.1	D38.0	D49.1
false	C32.1	C78.39	D02.0	D14.1	D38.0	D49.1
vomer	C41.0	C79.51	—	D16.4	D48.0	D49.2
vulva	C51.9	C79.82	D07.1	D28.0	D39.8	D49.5
vulvovaginal gland	C51.0	C79.82	D07.1	D28.0	D39.8	D49.5
Waldeyer's ring	C14.2	C79.89	D00.08	D10.9	D37.05	D49.0
Wharton's duct	C08.0	C79.89	D00.00	D11.7	D37.032	D49.0

▽ **Subterms under main terms may continue to next column or page**   ☑ **Additional Character Required — Refer to the Tabular List for Character Selection**

	Malignant Primary	Malignant Secondary	Ca in situ	Benign	Uncertain	Unspecified Behavior
Neoplasm, neoplastic — *continued*						
white matter (central) (cerebral)	C71.0	C79.31	—	D33.0	D43.0	D49.6
windpipe	C33	C78.39	D02.1	D14.2	D38.1	D49.1
Wirsung's duct	C25.3	C78.89	D01.7	D13.6	D37.8	D49.0
wolffian (body) (duct)						
female	C57.7	C79.82	D07.39	D28.7	D39.8	D49.5
male	C63.7	C79.82	D07.69	D29.8	D40.8	D49.5
womb — *see* Neoplasm, uterus						
wrist NEC	C76.4-☑	C79.89	D04.6-☑	D36.7	D48.7	D49.89
xiphoid process	C41.3	C79.51	—	D16.7	D48.0	D49.2
Zuckerkandl organ	C75.5	C79.89	—	D35.6	D44.7	D49.7

☑ **Additional Character Required — Refer to the Tabular List for Character Selection** ▽ **Subterms under main terms may continue to next column or page**

ICD-10-CM Table of Drugs and Chemicals

Substance	Poisoning, Accidental (unintentional)	Poisoning, Intentional Self-harm	Poisoning, Assault	Poisoning, Undetermined	Adverse Effect	Under-dosing
14-Hydroxydihydromorphinone	T40.2X1	T40.2X2	T40.2X3	T40.2X4	T40.2X5	T40.2X6
1-Propanol	T51.3X1	T51.3X2	T51.3X3	T51.3X4	—	—
2,3,7,8-Tetrachlorodibenzo-p-dioxin	T53.7X1	T53.7X2	T53.7X3	T53.7X4	—	—
2,4,5-T (trichlorophenoxyacetic acid)	T60.1X1	T60.1X2	T60.1X3	T60.1X4	—	—
2,4,5-Trichlorophenoxyacetic acid	T60.3X1	T60.3X2	T60.3X3	T60.3X4	—	—
2,4-D (dichlorophenoxyacetic acid)	T60.3X1	T60.3X2	T60.3X3	T60.3X4	—	—
2,4-Toluene diisocyanate	T65.0X1	T65.0X2	T65.0X3	T65.0X4	—	—
2-Deoxy-5-fluorouridine	T45.1X1	T45.1X2	T45.1X3	T45.1X4	T45.1X5	T45.1X6
2-Ethoxyethanol	T52.3X1	T52.3X2	T52.3X3	T52.3X4	—	—
2-Methoxyethanol	T52.3X1	T52.3X2	T52.3X3	T52.3X4	—	—
2-Propanol	T51.2X1	T51.2X2	T51.2X3	T51.2X4	—	—
4-Aminobutyric acid	T43.8X1	T43.8X2	T43.8X3	T43.8X4	T43.8X5	T43.8X6
4-Aminophenol derivatives	T39.1X1	T39.1X2	T39.1X3	T39.1X4	T39.1X5	T39.1X6
5-Deoxy-5-fluorouridine	T45.1X1	T45.1X2	T45.1X3	T45.1X4	T45.1X5	T45.1X6
5-Methoxypsoralen (5-MOP)	T50.991	T50.992	T50.993	T50.994	T50.995	T50.996
8-Aminoquinoline drugs	T37.2X1	T37.2X2	T37.2X3	T37.2X4	T37.2X5	T37.2X6
8-Methoxypsoralen (8-MOP)	T50.991	T50.992	T50.993	T50.994	T50.995	T50.996
ABOB	T37.5X1	T37.5X2	T37.5X3	T37.5X4	T37.5X5	T37.5X6
Abrine	T62.2X1	T62.2X2	T62.2X3	T62.2X4	—	—
Abrus (seed)	T62.2X1	T62.2X2	T62.2X3	T62.2X4	—	—
Absinthe	T51.0X1	T51.0X2	T51.0X3	T51.0X4	—	—
beverage	T51.0X1	T51.0X2	T51.0X3	T51.0X4	—	—
Acaricide	T60.8X1	T60.8X2	T60.8X3	T60.8X4	—	—
Acebutolol	T44.7X1	T44.7X2	T44.7X3	T44.7X4	T44.7X5	T44.7X6
Acecarbromal	T42.6X1	T42.6X2	T42.6X3	T42.6X4	T42.6X5	T42.6X6
Aceclidine	T44.1X1	T44.1X2	T44.1X3	T44.1X4	T44.1X5	T44.1X6
Acedapsone	T37.0X1	T37.0X2	T37.0X3	T37.0X4	T37.0X5	T37.0X6
Acefylline piperazine	T48.6X1	T48.6X2	T48.6X3	T48.6X4	T48.6X5	T48.6X6
Acemorphan	T40.2X1	T40.2X2	T40.2X3	T40.2X4	T40.2X5	T40.2X6
Acenocoumarin	T45.511	T45.512	T45.513	T45.514	T45.515	T45.516
Acenocoumarol	T45.511	T45.512	T45.513	T45.514	T45.515	T45.516
Acepifylline	T48.6X1	T48.6X2	T48.6X3	T48.6X4	T48.6X5	T48.6X6
Acepromazine	T43.3X1	T43.3X2	T43.3X3	T43.3X4	T43.3X5	T43.3X6
Acesulfamethoxypyridazine	T37.0X1	T37.0X2	T37.0X3	T37.0X4	T37.0X5	T37.0X6
Acetal	T52.8X1	T52.8X2	T52.8X3	T52.8X4	—	—
Acetaldehyde (vapor)	T52.8X1	T52.8X2	T52.8X3	T52.8X4	—	—
liquid	T65.891	T65.892	T65.893	T65.894	—	—
Acetaminophen	T39.1X1	T39.1X2	T39.1X3	T39.1X4	T39.1X5	T39.1X6
Acetaminosalol	T39.1X1	T39.1X2	T39.1X3	T39.1X4	T39.1X5	T39.1X6
Acetanilide	T39.1X1	T39.1X2	T39.1X3	T39.1X4	T39.1X5	T39.1X6
Acetarsol	T37.3X1	T37.3X2	T37.3X3	T37.3X4	T37.3X5	T37.3X6
Acetazolamide	T50.2X1	T50.2X2	T50.2X3	T50.2X4	T50.2X5	T50.2X6
Acetiamine	T45.2X1	T45.2X2	T45.2X3	T45.2X4	T45.2X5	T45.2X6
Acetic						
acid	T54.2X1	T54.2X2	T54.2X3	T54.2X4	—	—
with sodium acetate (ointment)	T49.3X1	T49.3X2	T49.3X3	T49.3X4	T49.3X5	T49.3X6
ester (solvent)(vapor)	T52.8X1	T52.8X2	T52.8X3	T52.8X4	—	—
irrigating solution	T50.3X1	T50.3X2	T50.3X3	T50.3X4	T50.3X5	T50.3X6
medicinal (lotion)	T49.2X1	T49.2X2	T49.2X3	T49.2X4	T49.2X5	T49.2X6
anhydride	T65.891	T65.892	T65.893	T65.894	—	—
ether (vapor)	T52.8X1	T52.8X2	T52.8X3	T52.8X4	—	—
Acetohexamide	T38.3X1	T38.3X2	T38.3X3	T38.3X4	T38.3X5	T38.3X6
Acetohydroxamic acid	T50.991	T50.992	T50.993	T50.994	T50.995	T50.996
Acetomenaphthone	T45.7X1	T45.7X2	T45.7X3	T45.7X4	T45.7X5	T45.7X6
Acetomorphine	T40.1X1	T40.1X2	T40.1X3	T40.1X4	—	—
Acetone (oils)	T52.4X1	T52.4X2	T52.4X3	T52.4X4	—	—
chlorinated	T52.4X1	T52.4X2	T52.4X3	T52.4X4	—	—
vapor	T52.4X1	T52.4X2	T52.4X3	T52.4X4	—	—
Acetonitrile	T52.8X1	T52.8X2	T52.8X3	T52.8X4	—	—
Acetophenazine	T43.3X1	T43.3X2	T43.3X3	T43.3X4	T43.3X5	T43.3X6
Acetophenetedin	T39.1X1	T39.1X2	T39.1X3	T39.1X4	T39.1X5	T39.1X6
Acetophenone	T52.4X1	T52.4X2	T52.4X3	T52.4X4	—	—
Acetorphine	T40.2X1	T40.2X2	T40.2X3	T40.2X4	—	—
Acetosulfone (sodium)	T37.1X1	T37.1X2	T37.1X3	T37.1X4	T37.1X5	T37.1X6
Acetrizoate (sodium)	T50.8X1	T50.8X2	T50.8X3	T50.8X4	T50.8X5	T50.8X6
Acetrizoic acid	T50.8X1	T50.8X2	T50.8X3	T50.8X4	T50.8X5	T50.8X6
Acetyl						
bromide	T53.6X1	T53.6X2	T53.6X3	T53.6X4	—	—
chloride	T53.6X1	T53.6X2	T53.6X3	T53.6X4	—	—
Acetylcarbromal	T42.6X1	T42.6X2	T42.6X3	T42.6X4	T42.6X5	T42.6X6
Acetylcholine						
chloride	T44.1X1	T44.1X2	T44.1X3	T44.1X4	T44.1X5	T44.1X6
derivative	T44.1X1	T44.1X2	T44.1X3	T44.1X4	T44.1X5	T44.1X6
Acetylcysteine	T48.4X1	T48.4X2	T48.4X3	T48.4X4	T48.4X5	T48.4X6
Acetyldigitoxin	T46.0X1	T46.0X2	T46.0X3	T46.0X4	T46.0X5	T46.0X6
Acetyldigoxin	T46.0X1	T46.0X2	T46.0X3	T46.0X4	T46.0X5	T46.0X6
Acetyldihydrocodeine	T40.2X1	T40.2X2	T40.2X3	T40.2X4	—	—
Acetyldihydrocodeinone	T40.2X1	T40.2X2	T40.2X3	T40.2X4	—	—
Acetylene (gas)	T59.891	T59.892	T59.893	T59.894	—	—
dichloride	T53.6X1	T53.6X2	T53.6X3	T53.6X4	—	—
incomplete combustion of	T58.11	T58.12	T58.13	T58.14	—	—
industrial	T59.891	T59.892	T59.893	T59.894	—	—
tetrachloride	T53.6X1	T53.6X2	T53.6X3	T53.6X4	—	—
vapor	T53.6X1	T53.6X2	T53.6X3	T53.6X4	—	—
Acetylpheneturide	T42.6X1	T42.6X2	T42.6X3	T42.6X4	T42.6X5	T42.6X6
Acetylphenylhydrazine	T39.8X1	T39.8X2	T39.8X3	T39.8X4	T39.8X5	T39.8X6
Acetylsalicylic acid (salts)	T39.011	T39.012	T39.013	T39.014	T39.015	T39.016
enteric coated	T39.011	T39.012	T39.013	T39.014	T39.015	T39.016
Acetylsulfamethoxypyridazine	T37.0X1	T37.0X2	T37.0X3	T37.0X4	T37.0X5	T37.0X6
Achromycin	T36.4X1	T36.4X2	T36.4X3	T36.4X4	T36.4X5	T36.4X6
ophthalmic preparation	T49.5X1	T49.5X2	T49.5X3	T49.5X4	T49.5X5	T49.5X6
topical NEC	T49.0X1	T49.0X2	T49.0X3	T49.0X4	T49.0X5	T49.0X6
Aciclovir	T37.5X1	T37.5X2	T37.5X3	T37.5X4	T37.5X5	T37.5X6
Acidifying agent NEC	T50.901	T50.902	T50.903	T50.904	T50.905	T50.906
Acid (corrosive) NEC	T54.2X1	T54.2X2	T54.2X3	T54.2X4	—	—
Acipimox	T46.6X1	T46.6X2	T46.6X3	T46.6X4	T46.6X5	T46.6X6
Acitretin	T50.991	T50.992	T50.993	T50.994	T50.995	T50.996
Aclarubicin	T45.1X1	T45.1X2	T45.1X3	T45.1X4	T45.1X5	T45.1X6
Aclatonium napadisilate	T48.1X1	T48.1X2	T48.1X3	T48.1X4	T48.1X5	T48.1X6
Aconite (wild)	T46.991	T46.992	T46.993	T46.994	T46.995	T46.996
Aconitine	T46.991	T46.992	T46.993	T46.994	T46.995	T46.996
Aconitum ferox	T46.991	T46.992	T46.993	T46.994	T46.995	T46.996
Acridine	T65.6X1	T65.6X2	T65.6X3	T65.6X4	—	—
vapor	T59.891	T59.892	T59.893	T59.894	—	—
Acriflavine	T37.91	T37.92	T37.93	T37.94	T37.95	T37.96
Acriflavinium chloride	T49.0X1	T49.0X2	T49.0X3	T49.0X4	T49.0X5	T49.0X6
Acrinol	T49.0X1	T49.0X2	T49.0X3	T49.0X4	T49.0X5	T49.0X6
Acrisorcin	T49.0X1	T49.0X2	T49.0X3	T49.0X4	T49.0X5	T49.0X6
Acrivastine	T45.0X1	T45.0X2	T45.0X3	T45.0X4	T45.0X5	T45.0X6
Acrolein (gas)	T59.891	T59.892	T59.893	T59.894	—	—
liquid	T54.1X1	T54.1X2	T54.1X3	T54.1X4	—	—
Acrylamide	T65.891	T65.892	T65.893	T65.894	—	—
Acrylic resin	T49.3X1	T49.3X2	T49.3X3	T49.3X4	T49.3X5	T49.3X6
Acrylonitrile	T65.891	T65.892	T65.893	T65.894	—	—
Actaea spicata	T62.2X1	T62.2X2	T62.2X3	T62.2X4	—	—
berry	T62.1X1	T62.1X2	T62.1X3	T62.1X4	—	—
Acterol	T37.3X1	T37.3X2	T37.3X3	T37.3X4	T37.3X5	T37.3X6
ACTH	T38.811	T38.812	T38.813	T38.814	T38.815	T38.816
Actinomycin C	T45.1X1	T45.1X2	T45.1X3	T45.1X4	T45.1X5	T45.1X6
Actinomycin D	T45.1X1	T45.1X2	T45.1X3	T45.1X4	T45.1X5	T45.1X6
Activated charcoal — see also Charcoal, medicinal	T47.6X1	T47.6X2	T47.6X3	T47.6X4	T47.6X5	T47.6X6
Acyclovir	T37.5X1	T37.5X2	T37.5X3	T37.5X4	T37.5X5	T37.5X6
Adenine	T45.2X1	T45.2X2	T45.2X3	T45.2X4	T45.2X5	T45.2X6
arabinoside	T37.5X1	T37.5X2	T37.5X3	T37.5X4	T37.5X5	T37.5X6
Adenosine (phosphate)	T46.2X1	T46.2X2	T46.2X3	T46.2X4	T46.2X5	T46.2X6
ADH	T38.891	T38.892	T38.893	T38.894	T38.895	T38.896
Adhesive NEC	T65.891	T65.892	T65.893	T65.894	—	—
Adicillin	T36.0X1	T36.0X2	T36.0X3	T36.0X4	T36.0X5	T36.0X6
Adiphenine	T44.3X1	T44.3X2	T44.3X3	T44.3X4	T44.3X5	T44.3X6
Adipiodone	T50.8X1	T50.8X2	T50.8X3	T50.8X4	T50.8X5	T50.8X6
Adjunct, pharmaceutical	T50.901	T50.902	T50.903	T50.904	T50.905	T50.906
Adrenal (extract, cortex or medulla) (glucocorticoids) (hormones) (mineralocorticoids)	T38.0X1	T38.0X2	T38.0X3	T38.0X4	T38.0X5	T38.0X6
ENT agent	T49.6X1	T49.6X2	T49.6X3	T49.6X4	T49.6X5	T49.6X6
ophthalmic preparation	T49.5X1	T49.5X2	T49.5X3	T49.5X4	T49.5X5	T49.5X6
topical NEC	T49.0X1	T49.0X2	T49.0X3	T49.0X4	T49.0X5	T49.0X6
Adrenalin — see Adrenaline						
Adrenaline	T44.5X1	T44.5X2	T44.5X3	T44.5X4	T44.5X5	T44.5X6
Adrenergic NEC	T44.901	T44.902	T44.903	T44.904	T44.905	T44.906
blocking agent NEC	T44.8X1	T44.8X2	T44.8X3	T44.8X4	T44.8X5	T44.8X6
beta, heart	T44.7X1	T44.7X2	T44.7X3	T44.7X4	T44.7X5	T44.7X6
specified NEC	T44.991	T44.992	T44.993	T44.994	T44.995	T44.996
Adrenochrome						
derivative	T46.991	T46.992	T46.993	T46.994	T46.995	T46.996

Substance	Poisoning, Accidental (unintentional)	Poisoning, Intentional Self-harm	Poisoning, Assault	Poisoning, Undetermined	Adverse Effect	Underdosing
Adrenochrome — continued						
(mono) semicarbazone	T46.991	T46.992	T46.993	T46.994	T46.995	T46.996
Adrenocorticotrophic hormone	T38.811	T38.812	T38.813	T38.814	T38.815	T38.816
Adrenocorticotrophin	T38.811	T38.812	T38.813	T38.814	T38.815	T38.816
Adriamycin	T45.1X1	T45.1X2	T45.1X3	T45.1X4	T45.1X5	T45.1X6
Aerosol spray NEC	T65.91	T65.92	T65.93	T65.94		
Aerosporin	T36.8X1	T36.8X2	T36.8X3	T36.8X4	T36.8X5	T36.8X6
ENT agent	T49.6X1	T49.6X2	T49.6X3	T49.6X4	T49.6X5	T49.6X6
ophthalmic preparation	T49.5X1	T49.5X2	T49.5X3	T49.5X4	T49.5X5	T49.5X6
topical NEC	T49.0X1	T49.0X2	T49.0X3	T49.0X4	T49.0X5	T49.0X6
Aethusa cynapium	T62.2X1	T62.2X2	T62.2X3	T62.2X4		
Afghanistan black	T40.7X1	T40.7X2	T40.7X3	T40.7X4	T40.7X5	T40.7X6
Aflatoxin	T64.01	T64.02	T64.03	T64.04		
Afloqualone	T42.8X1	T42.8X2	T42.8X3	T42.8X4	T42.8X5	T42.8X6
African boxwood	T62.2X1	T62.2X2	T62.2X3	T62.2X4		
Agar	T47.4X1	T47.4X2	T47.4X3	T47.4X4	T47.4X5	T47.4X6
Agonist						
predominantly						
alpha-adrenoreceptor	T44.4X1	T44.4X2	T44.4X3	T44.4X4	T44.4X5	T44.4X6
beta-adrenoreceptor	T44.5X1	T44.5X2	T44.5X3	T44.5X4	T44.5X5	T44.5X6
Agricultural agent NEC	T65.91	T65.92	T65.93	T65.94	—	—
Agrypnal	T42.3X1	T42.3X2	T42.3X3	T42.3X4	T42.3X5	T42.3X6
AHLG	T50.Z11	T50.Z12	T50.Z13	T50.Z14	T50.Z15	T50.Z16
Air contaminant(s), source/type NOS	T65.91	T65.92	T65.93	T65.94	—	—
Ajmaline	T46.2X1	T46.2X2	T46.2X3	T46.2X4	T46.2X5	T46.2X6
Akee	T62.1X1	T62.1X2	T62.1X3	T62.1X4	—	—
Akrinol	T49.0X1	T49.0X2	T49.0X3	T49.0X4	T49.0X5	T49.0X6
Akritoin	T37.8X1	T37.8X2	T37.8X3	T37.8X4	T37.8X5	T37.8X6
Alacepril	T46.4X1	T46.4X2	T46.4X3	T46.4X4	T46.4X5	T46.4X6
Alantolactone	T37.4X1	T37.4X2	T37.4X3	T37.4X4	T37.4X5	T37.4X6
Albamycin	T36.8X1	T36.8X2	T36.8X3	T36.8X4	T36.8X5	T36.8X6
Albendazole	T37.4X1	T37.4X2	T37.4X3	T37.4X4	T37.4X5	T37.4X6
Albumin						
bovine	T45.8X1	T45.8X2	T45.8X3	T45.8X4	T45.8X5	T45.8X6
human serum	T45.8X1	T45.8X2	T45.8X3	T45.8X4	T45.8X5	T45.8X6
salt-poor	T45.8X1	T45.8X2	T45.8X3	T45.8X4	T45.8X5	T45.8X6
normal human serum	T45.8X1	T45.8X2	T45.8X3	T45.8X4	T45.8X5	T45.8X6
Albuterol	T48.6X1	T48.6X2	T48.6X3	T48.6X4	T48.6X5	T48.6X6
Albutoin	T42.0X1	T42.0X2	T42.0X3	T42.0X4	T42.0X5	T42.0X6
Alclometasone	T49.0X1	T49.0X2	T49.0X3	T49.0X4	T49.0X5	T49.0X6
Alcohol	T51.91	T51.92	T51.93	T51.94	—	—
absolute	T51.0X1	T51.0X2	T51.0X3	T51.0X4		
beverage	T51.0X1	T51.0X2	T51.0X3	T51.0X4		
allyl	T51.8X1	T51.8X2	T51.8X3	T51.8X4		
amyl	T51.3X1	T51.3X2	T51.3X3	T51.3X4		
antifreeze	T51.1X1	T51.1X2	T51.1X3	T51.1X4		
beverage	T51.0X1	T51.0X2	T51.0X3	T51.0X4		
butyl	T51.3X1	T51.3X2	T51.3X3	T51.3X4		
dehydrated	T51.0X1	T51.0X2	T51.0X3	T51.0X4		
beverage	T51.0X1	T51.0X2	T51.0X3	T51.0X4		
denatured	T51.0X1	T51.0X2	T51.0X3	T51.0X4	—	—
deterrent NEC	T50.6X1	T50.6X2	T50.6X3	T50.6X4	T50.6X5	T50.6X6
diagnostic (gastric function)	T50.8X1	T50.8X2	T50.8X3	T50.8X4	T50.8X5	T50.8X6
ethyl	T51.0X1	T51.0X2	T51.0X3	T51.0X4	—	—
beverage	T51.0X1	T51.0X2	T51.0X3	T51.0X4	—	—
grain	T51.0X1	T51.0X2	T51.0X3	T51.0X4	—	—
beverage	T51.0X1	T51.0X2	T51.0X3	T51.0X4	—	—
industrial	T51.0X1	T51.0X2	T51.0X3	T51.0X4	—	—
isopropyl	T51.2X1	T51.2X2	T51.2X3	T51.2X4		
methyl	T51.1X1	T51.1X2	T51.1X3	T51.1X4		
preparation for consumption	T51.0X1	T51.0X2	T51.0X3	T51.0X4	—	—
propyl	T51.3X1	T51.3X2	T51.3X3	T51.3X4	—	—
secondary	T51.2X1	T51.2X2	T51.2X3	T51.2X4	—	—
radiator	T51.1X1	T51.1X2	T51.1X3	T51.1X4	—	—
rubbing	T51.2X1	T51.2X2	T51.2X3	T51.2X4	—	—
specified type NEC	T51.8X1	T51.8X2	T51.8X3	T51.8X4	—	—
surgical	T51.0X1	T51.0X2	T51.0X3	T51.0X4	—	—
vapor (from any type of Alcohol)	T59.891	T59.892	T59.893	T59.894		
wood	T51.1X1	T51.1X2	T51.1X3	T51.1X4	—	—
Alcuronium (chloride)	T48.1X1	T48.1X2	T48.1X3	T48.1X4	T48.1X5	T48.1X6
Aldactone	T50.0X1	T50.0X2	T50.0X3	T50.0X4	T50.0X5	T50.0X6
Aldesulfone sodium	T37.1X1	T37.1X2	T37.1X3	T37.1X4	T37.1X5	T37.1X6
Aldicarb	T60.0X1	T60.0X2	T60.0X3	T60.0X4		
Aldomet	T46.5X1	T46.5X2	T46.5X3	T46.5X4	T46.5X5	T46.5X6
Aldosterone	T50.0X1	T50.0X2	T50.0X3	T50.0X4	T50.0X5	T50.0X6
Aldrin (dust)	T60.1X1	T60.1X2	T60.1X3	T60.1X4	—	—
Aleve — see Naproxen						
Alexitol sodium	T47.1X1	T47.1X2		T47.1X4	T47.1X5	T47.1X6
Alfacalcidol	T45.2X1	T45.2X2	T45.2X3	T45.2X4	T45.2X5	T45.2X6
Alfadolone	T41.1X1	T41.1X2	T41.1X3	T41.1X4	T41.1X5	T41.1X6
Alfaxalone	T41.1X1	T41.1X2	T41.1X3	T41.1X4	T41.1X5	T41.1X6
Alfentanil	T40.4X1	T40.4X2	T40.4X3	T40.4X4	T40.4X5	T40.4X6
Alfuzosin (hydrochloride)	T44.8X1	T44.8X2	T44.8X3	T44.8X4	T44.8X5	T44.8X6
Algae (harmful) (toxin)	T65.821	T65.822	T65.823	T65.824	—	—
Algeldrate	T47.1X1	T47.1X2	T47.1X3	T47.1X4	T47.1X5	T47.1X6
Algin	T47.8X1	T47.8X2	T47.8X3	T47.8X4	T47.8X5	T47.8X6
Alglucerase	T45.3X1	T45.3X2	T45.3X3	T45.3X4	T45.3X5	T45.3X6
Alidase	T45.3X1	T45.3X2	T45.3X3	T45.3X4	T45.3X5	T45.3X6
Alimemazine	T43.3X1	T43.3X2	T43.3X3	T43.3X4	T43.3X5	T43.3X6
Aliphatic thiocyanates	T65.0X1	T65.0X2	T65.0X3	T65.0X4	—	—
Alizapride	T45.0X1	T45.0X2	T45.0X3	T45.0X4	T45.0X5	T45.0X6
Alkali (caustic)	T54.3X1	T54.3X2	T54.3X3	T54.3X1		
Alkaline antiseptic solution (aromatic)	T49.6X1	T49.6X2	T49.6X3	T49.6X4	T49.6X5	T49.6X6
Alkalinizing agents (medicinal)	T50.901	T50.902	T50.903	T50.904	T50.905	T50.906
Alkalizing agent NEC	T50.901	T50.902	T50.903	T50.904	T50.905	T50.906
Alka-seltzer	T39.011	T39.012	T39.013	T39.014	T39.015	T39.016
Alkavervir	T46.5X1	T46.5X2	T46.5X3	T46.5X4	T46.5X5	T46.5X6
Alkonium (bromide)	T49.0X1	T49.0X2	T49.0X3	T49.0X4	T49.0X5	T49.0X6
Alkylating drug NEC	T45.1X1	T45.1X2	T45.1X3	T45.1X4	T45.1X5	T45.1X6
antimyeloproliferative	T45.1X1	T45.1X2	T45.1X3	T45.1X4	T45.1X5	T45.1X6
lymphatic	T45.1X1	T45.1X2	T45.1X3	T45.1X4	T45.1X5	T45.1X6
Alkylisocyanate	T65.0X1	T65.0X2	T65.0X3	T65.0X4	—	—
Allantoin	T49.4X1	T49.4X2	T49.4X3	T49.4X4	T49.4X5	T49.4X6
Allegron	T43.011	T43.012	T43.013	T43.014	T43.015	T43.016
Allethrin	T49.0X1	T49.0X2	T49.0X3	T49.0X4	T49.0X5	T49.0X6
Allobarbital	T42.3X1	T42.3X2	T42.3X3	T42.3X4	T42.3X5	T42.3X6
Allopurinol	T50.4X1	T50.4X2	T50.4X3	T50.4X4	T50.4X5	T50.4X6
Allyl						
alcohol	T51.8X1	T51.8X2	T51.8X3	T51.8X4	—	—
disulfide	T46.6X1	T46.6X2	T46.6X3	T46.6X4	T46.6X5	T46.6X6
Allylestrenol	T38.5X1	T38.5X2	T38.5X3	T38.5X4	T38.5X5	T38.5X6
Allylisopropylacetylurea	T42.6X1	T42.6X2	T42.6X3	T42.6X4	T42.6X5	T42.6X6
Allylisopropylmalonylurea	T42.3X1	T42.3X2	T42.3X3	T42.3X4	T42.3X5	T42.3X6
Allylthiourea	T49.3X1	T49.3X2	T49.3X3	T49.3X4	T49.3X5	T49.3X6
Allyltribromide	T42.6X1	T42.6X2	T42.6X3	T42.6X4	T42.6X5	T42.6X6
Allypropymal	T42.3X1	T42.3X2	T42.3X3	T42.3X4	T42.3X5	T42.3X6
Almagate	T47.1X1	T47.1X2	T47.1X3	T47.1X4	T47.1X5	T47.1X6
Almasilate	T47.1X1	T47.1X2	T47.1X3	T47.1X4	T47.1X5	T47.1X6
Almitrine	T50.7X1	T50.7X2	T50.7X3	T50.7X4	T50.7X5	T50.7X6
Aloes	T47.2X1	T47.2X2	T47.2X3	T47.2X4	T47.2X5	T47.2X6
Aloglutamol	T47.1X1	T47.1X2	T47.1X3	T47.1X4	T47.1X5	T47.1X6
Aloin	T47.2X1	T47.2X2	T47.2X3	T47.2X4	T47.2X5	T47.2X6
Aloxidone	T42.2X1	T42.2X2	T42.2X3	T42.2X4	T42.2X5	T42.2X6
Alpha						
acetyldigoxin	T46.0X1	T46.0X2	T46.0X3	T46.0X4	T46.0X5	T46.0X6
adrenergic blocking drug	T44.6X1	T44.6X2	T44.6X3	T44.6X4	T44.6X5	T44.6X6
amylase	T45.3X1	T45.3X2	T45.3X3	T45.3X4	T45.3X5	T45.3X6
tocoferol (acetate)	T45.2X1	T45.2X2	T45.2X3	T45.2X4	T45.2X5	T45.2X6
tocopherol	T45.2X1	T45.2X2	T45.2X3	T45.2X4	T45.2X5	T45.2X6
Alphadolone	T41.1X1	T41.1X2	T41.1X3	T41.1X4	T41.1X5	T41.1X6
Alphaprodine	T40.4X1	T40.4X2	T40.4X3	T40.4X4	T40.4X5	T40.4X6
Alphaxalone	T41.1X1	T41.1X2	T41.1X3	T41.1X4	T41.1X5	T41.1X6
Alprazolam	T42.4X1	T42.4X2	T42.4X3	T42.4X4	T42.4X5	T42.4X6
Alprenolol	T44.7X1	T44.7X2	T44.7X3	T44.7X4	T44.7X5	T44.7X6
Alprostadil	T46.7X1	T46.7X2	T46.7X3	T46.7X4	T46.7X5	T46.7X6
Alsactide	T38.811	T38.812	T38.813	T38.814	T38.815	T38.816
Alseroxylon	T46.5X1	T46.5X2	T46.5X3	T46.5X4	T46.5X5	T46.5X6
Alteplase	T45.611	T45.612	T45.613	T45.614	T45.615	T45.616
Altizide	T50.2X1	T50.2X2	T50.2X3	T50.2X4	T50.2X5	T50.2X6
Altretamine	T45.1X1	T45.1X2	T45.1X3	T45.1X4	T45.1X5	T45.1X6
Alum (medicinal)	T49.4X1	T49.4X2	T49.4X3	T49.4X4	T49.4X5	T49.4X6
nonmedicinal (ammonium) (potassium)	T56.891	T56.892	T56.893	T56.894	—	—
Aluminium, aluminum						
acetate	T49.2X1	T49.2X2	T49.2X3	T49.2X4	T49.2X5	T49.2X6
solution	T49.0X1	T49.0X2	T49.0X3	T49.0X4	T49.0X5	T49.0X6
aspirin	T39.011	T39.012	T39.013	T39.014	T39.015	T39.016
bis (acetylsalicylate)	T39.011	T39.012	T39.013	T39.014	T39.015	T39.016
carbonate (gel, basic)	T47.1X1	T47.1X2	T47.1X3	T47.1X4	T47.1X5	T47.1X6
chlorhydroxide-complex	T47.1X1	T47.1X2	T47.1X3	T47.1X4	T47.1X5	T47.1X6
chloride	T49.2X1	T49.2X2	T49.2X3	T49.2X4	T49.2X5	T49.2X6
clofibrate	T46.6X1	T46.6X2	T46.6X3	T46.6X4	T46.6X5	T46.6X6
diacetate	T49.2X1	T49.2X2	T49.2X3	T49.2X4	T49.2X5	T49.2X6
glycinate	T47.1X1	T47.1X2	T47.1X3	T47.1X4	T47.1X5	T47.1X6
hydroxide (gel)	T47.1X1	T47.1X2	T47.1X3	T47.1X4	T47.1X5	T47.1X6
hydroxide-magnesium carb. gel	T47.1X1	T47.1X2	T47.1X3	T47.1X4	T47.1X5	T47.1X6
magnesium silicate	T47.1X1	T47.1X2	T47.1X3	T47.1X4	T47.1X5	T47.1X6
nicotinate	T46.7X1	T46.7X2	T46.7X3	T46.7X4	T46.7X5	T46.7X6

Additional Character May Be Required — Refer to the Tabular List for Character Selection ▽ Subterms under main terms may continue to next column or page

Substance	Poisoning, Accidental (unintentional)	Poisoning, Intentional Self-harm	Poisoning, Assault	Poisoning, Undetermined	Adverse Effect	Under-dosing
Aluminium, aluminum — *continued*						
ointment (surgical) (topical)	T49.3X1	T49.3X2	T49.3X3	T49.3X4	T49.3X5	T49.3X6
phosphate	T47.1X1	T47.1X2	T47.1X3	T47.1X4	T47.1X5	T47.1X6
salicylate	T39.Ø91	T39.Ø92	T39.Ø93	T39.Ø94	T39.Ø95	T39.Ø96
silicate	T47.1X1	T47.1X2	T47.1X3	T47.1X4	T47.1X5	T47.1X6
sodium silicate	T47.1X1	T47.1X2	T47.1X3	T47.1X4	T47.1X5	T47.1X6
subacetate	T49.2X1	T49.2X2	T49.2X3	T49.2X4	T49.2X5	T49.2X6
sulfate	T49.ØX1	T49.ØX2	T49.ØX3	T49.ØX4	T49.ØX5	T49.ØX6
tannate	T47.6X1	T47.6X2	T47.6X3	T47.6X4	T47.6X5	T47.6X6
topical NEC	T49.3X1	T49.3X2	T49.3X3	T49.3X4	T49.3X5	T49.3X6
Alurate	T42.3X1	T42.3X2	T42.3X3	T42.3X4	T42.3X5	T42.3X6
Alverine	T44.3X1	T44.3X2	T44.3X3	T44.3X4	T44.3X5	T44.3X6
Alvodine	T4Ø.2X1	T4Ø.2X2	T4Ø.2X3	T4Ø.2X4	T4Ø.2X5	T4Ø.2X6
Amanita phalloides	T62.ØX1	T62.ØX2	T62.ØX3	T62.ØX4	—	—
Amanitine	T62.ØX1	T62.ØX2	T62.ØX3	T62.ØX4	—	—
Amantadine	T42.8X1	T42.8X2	T42.8X3	T42.8X4	T42.8X5	T42.8X6
Ambazone	T49.6X1	T49.6X2	T49.6X3	T49.6X4	T49.6X5	T49.6X6
Ambenonium (chloride)	T44.ØX1	T44.ØX2	T44.ØX3	T44.ØX4	T44.ØX5	T44.ØX6
Ambroxol	T48.4X1	T48.4X2	T48.4X3	T48.4X4	T48.4X5	T48.4X6
Ambuphylline	T48.6X1	T48.6X2	T48.6X3	T48.6X4	T48.6X5	T48.6X6
Ambutonium bromide	T44.3X1	T44.3X2	T44.3X3	T44.3X4	T44.3X5	T44.3X6
Amcinonide	T49.ØX1	T49.ØX2	T49.ØX3	T49.ØX4	T49.ØX5	T49.ØX6
Amdinocilline	T36.ØX1	T36.ØX2	T36.ØX3	T36.ØX4	T36.ØX5	T36.ØX6
Ametazole	T5Ø.8X1	T5Ø.8X2	T5Ø.8X3	T5Ø.8X4	T5Ø.8X5	T5Ø.8X6
Amethocaine	T41.3X1	T41.3X2	T41.3X3	T41.3X4	T41.3X5	T41.3X6
regional	T41.3X1	T41.3X2	T41.3X3	T41.3X4	T41.3X5	T41.3X6
spinal	T41.3X1	T41.3X2	T41.3X3	T41.3X4	T41.3X5	T41.3X6
Amethopterin	T45.1X1	T45.1X2	T45.1X3	T45.1X4	T45.1X5	T45.1X6
Amezinium metilsulfate	T44.991	T44.992	T44.993	T44.994	T44.995	T44.996
Amfebutamone	T43.291	T43.292	T43.293	T43.294	T43.295	T43.296
Amfepramone	T5Ø.5X1	T5Ø.5X2	T5Ø.5X3	T5Ø.5X4	T5Ø.5X5	T5Ø.5X6
Amfetamine	T43.621	T43.622	T43.623	T43.624	T43.625	T43.626
Amfetaminil	T43.621	T43.622	T43.623	T43.624	T43.625	T43.626
Amfomycin	T36.8X1	T36.8X2	T36.8X3	T36.8X4	T36.8X5	T36.8X6
Amidefrine mesilate	T48.5X1	T48.5X2	T48.5X3	T48.5X4	T48.5X5	T48.5X6
Amidone	T4Ø.3X1	T4Ø.3X2	T4Ø.3X3	T4Ø.3X4	T4Ø.3X5	T4Ø.3X6
Amidopyrine	T39.2X1	T39.2X2	T39.2X3	T39.2X4	T39.2X5	T39.2X6
Amidotrizoate	T5Ø.8X1	T5Ø.8X2	T5Ø.8X3	T5Ø.8X4	T5Ø.8X5	T5Ø.8X6
Amiflamine	T43.1X1	T43.1X2	T43.1X3	T43.1X4	T43.1X5	T43.1X6
Amikacin	T36.5X1	T36.5X2	T36.5X3	T36.5X4	T36.5X5	T36.5X6
Amikhelline	T46.3X1	T46.3X2	T46.3X3	T46.3X4	T46.3X5	T46.3X6
Amiloride	T5Ø.2X1	T5Ø.2X2	T5Ø.2X3	T5Ø.2X4	T5Ø.2X5	T5Ø.2X6
Aminacrine	T49.ØX1	T49.ØX2	T49.ØX3	T49.ØX4	T49.ØX5	T49.ØX6
Amineptine	T43.Ø11	T43.Ø12	T43.Ø13	T43.Ø14	T43.Ø15	T43.Ø16
Aminitrozole	T37.3X1	T37.3X2	T37.3X3	T37.3X4	T37.3X5	T37.3X6
Aminoacetic acid (derivatives)	T5Ø.3X1	T5Ø.3X2	T5Ø.3X3	T5Ø.3X4	T5Ø.3X5	T5Ø.3X6
Amino acids	T5Ø.3X1	T5Ø.3X2	T5Ø.3X3	T5Ø.3X4	T5Ø.3X5	T5Ø.3X6
Aminoacridine	T49.ØX1	T49.ØX2	T49.ØX3	T49.ØX4	T49.ØX5	T49.ØX6
Aminobenzoic acid (-p)	T49.3X1	T49.3X2	T49.3X3	T49.3X4	T49.3X5	T49.3X6
Aminocaproic acid	T45.621	T45.622	T45.623	T45.624	T45.625	T45.626
Aminoethylisothiourium	T45.8X1	T45.8X2	T45.8X3	T45.8X4	T45.8X5	T45.8X6
Aminofenazone	T39.2X1	T39.2X2	T39.2X3	T39.2X4	T39.2X5	T39.2X6
Aminoglutethimide	T45.1X1	T45.1X2	T45.1X3	T45.1X4	T45.1X5	T45.1X6
Aminohippuric acid	T5Ø.8X1	T5Ø.8X2	T5Ø.8X3	T5Ø.8X4	T5Ø.8X5	T5Ø.8X6
Aminomethylbenzoic acid	T45.691	T45.692	T45.693	T45.694	T45.695	T45.696
Aminometradine	T5Ø.2X1	T5Ø.2X2	T5Ø.2X3	T5Ø.2X4	T5Ø.2X5	T5Ø.2X6
Aminopentamide	T44.3X1	T44.3X2	T44.3X3	T44.3X4	T44.3X5	T44.3X6
Aminophenazone	T39.2X1	T39.2X2	T39.2X3	T39.2X4	T39.2X5	T39.2X6
Aminophenol	T54.ØX1	T54.ØX2	T54.ØX3	T54.ØX4	—	—
Aminophenylpyridone	T43.591	T43.592	T43.593	T43.594	T43.595	T43.596
Aminophylline	T48.6X1	T48.6X2	T48.6X3	T48.6X4	T48.6X5	T48.6X6
Aminopterin sodium	T45.1X1	T45.1X2	T45.1X3	T45.1X4	T45.1X5	T45.1X6
Aminopyrine	T39.2X1	T39.2X2	T39.2X3	T39.2X4	T39.2X5	T39.2X6
Aminorex	T5Ø.5X1	T5Ø.5X2	T5Ø.5X3	T5Ø.5X4	T5Ø.5X5	T5Ø.5X6
Aminosalicylic acid	T37.1X1	T37.1X2	T37.1X3	T37.1X4	T37.1X5	T37.1X6
Aminosalylum	T37.1X1	T37.1X2	T37.1X3	T37.1X4	T37.1X5	T37.1X6
Amiodarone	T46.2X1	T46.2X2	T46.2X3	T46.2X4	T46.2X5	T46.2X6
Amiphenazole	T5Ø.7X1	T5Ø.7X2	T5Ø.7X3	T5Ø.7X4	T5Ø.7X5	T5Ø.7X6
Amiquinsin	T46.5X1	T46.5X2	T46.5X3	T46.5X4	T46.5X5	T46.5X6
Amisometradine	T5Ø.2X1	T5Ø.2X2	T5Ø.2X3	T5Ø.2X4	T5Ø.2X5	T5Ø.2X6
Amisulpride	T43.591	T43.592	T43.593	T43.594	T43.595	T43.596
Amitriptyline	T43.Ø11	T43.Ø12	T43.Ø13	T43.Ø14	T43.Ø15	T43.Ø16
Amitriptylinoxide	T43.Ø11	T43.Ø12	T43.Ø13	T43.Ø14	T43.Ø15	T43.Ø16
Amlexanox	T48.6X1	T48.6X2	T48.6X3	T48.6X4	T48.6X5	T48.6X6
Ammonia (fumes) (gas) (vapor)	T59.891	T59.892	T59.893	T59.894	—	—
aromatic spirit	T48.991	T48.992	T48.993	T48.994	T48.995	T48.996
liquid (household)	T54.3X1	T54.3X2	T54.3X3	T54.3X4	—	—
Ammoniated mercury	T49.ØX1	T49.ØX2	T49.ØX3	T49.ØX4	T49.ØX5	T49.ØX6
Ammonium						
acid tartrate	T49.5X1	T49.5X2	T49.5X3	T49.5X4	T49.5X5	T49.5X6
Ammonium — *continued*						
bromide	T42.6X1	T42.6X2	T42.6X3	T42.6X4	T42.6X5	T42.6X6
carbonate	T54.3X1	T54.3X2	T54.3X3	T54.3X4	—	—
chloride	T5Ø.991	T5Ø.992	T5Ø.993	T5Ø.994	T5Ø.995	T5Ø.996
expectorant	T48.4X1	T48.4X2	T48.4X3	T48.4X4	T48.4X5	T48.4X6
compounds (household) NEC	T54.3X1	T54.3X2	T54.3X3	T54.3X4	—	—
fumes (any usage)	T59.891	T59.892	T59.893	T59.894	—	—
industrial	T54.3X1	T54.3X2	T54.3X3	T54.3X4	—	—
ichthyosulronate	T49.4X1	T49.4X2	T49.4X3	T49.4X4	T49.4X5	T49.4X6
mandelate	T37.91	T37.92	T37.93	T37.94	T37.95	T37.96
sulfamate	T6Ø.3X1	T6Ø.3X2	T6Ø.3X3	T6Ø.3X4	—	—
sulfonate resin	T47.8X1	T47.8X2	T47.8X3	T47.8X4	T47.8X5	T47.8X6
Amobarbital (sodium)	T42.3X1	T42.3X2	T42.3X3	T42.3X4	T42.3X5	T42.3X6
Amodiaquine	T37.2X1	T37.2X2	T37.2X3	T37.2X4	T37.2X5	T37.2X6
Amopyroquin (e)	T37.2X1	T37.2X2	T37.2X3	T37.2X4	T37.2X5	T37.2X6
Amoxapine	T43.Ø11	T43.Ø12	T43.Ø13	T43.Ø14	T43.Ø15	T43.Ø16
Amoxicillin	T36.ØX1	T36.ØX2	T36.ØX3	T36.ØX4	T36.ØX5	T36.ØX6
Amperozide	T43.591	T43.592	T43.593	T43.594	T43.595	T43.596
Amphenidone	T43.591	T43.592	T43.593	T43.594	T43.595	T43.596
Amphetamine NEC	T43.621	T43.622	T43.623	T43.624	T43.625	T43.626
Amphomycin	T36.8X1	T36.8X2	T36.8X3	T36.8X4	T36.8X5	T36.8X6
Amphotalide	T37.4X1	T37.4X2	T37.4X3	T37.4X4	T37.4X5	T37.4X6
Amphotericin B	T36.7X1	T36.7X2	T36.7X3	T36.7X4	T36.7X5	T36.7X6
topical	T49.ØX1	T49.ØX2	T49.ØX3	T49.ØX4	T49.ØX5	T49.ØX6
Ampicillin	T36.ØX1	T36.ØX2	T36.ØX3	T36.ØX4	T36.ØX5	T36.ØX6
Amprotropine	T44.3X1	T44.3X2	T44.3X3	T44.3X4	T44.3X5	T44.3X6
Amsacrine	T45.1X1	T45.1X2	T45.1X3	T45.1X4	T45.1X5	T45.1X6
Amygdaline	T62.2X1	T62.2X2	T62.2X3	T62.2X4	—	—
Amyl						
acetate	T52.8X1	T52.8X2	T52.8X3	T52.8X4	—	—
vapor	T59.891	T59.892	T59.893	T59.894	—	—
alcohol	T51.3X1	T51.3X2	T51.3X3	T51.3X4	—	—
chloride	T53.6X1	T53.6X2	T53.6X3	T53.6X4	—	—
formate	T52.8X1	T52.8X2	T52.8X3	T52.8X4	—	—
nitrite	T46.3X1	T46.3X2	T46.3X3	T46.3X4	T46.3X5	T46.3X6
propionate	T65.891	T65.892	T65.893	T65.894	—	—
Amylase	T47.5X1	T47.5X2	T47.5X3	T47.5X4	T47.5X5	T47.5X6
Amyleine, regional	T41.3X1	T41.3X2	T41.3X3	T41.3X4	T41.3X5	T41.3X6
Amylene						
dichloride	T53.6X1	T53.6X2	T53.6X3	T53.6X4	—	—
hydrate	T51.3X1	T51.3X2	T51.3X3	T51.3X4	—	—
Amylmetacresol	T49.6X1	T49.6X2	T49.6X3	T49.6X4	T49.6X5	T49.6X6
Amylobarbitone	T42.3X1	T42.3X2	T42.3X3	T42.3X4	T42.3X5	T42.3X6
Amylocaine, regional	T41.3X1	T41.3X2	T41.3X3	T41.3X4	T41.3X5	T41.3X6
infiltration (subcutaneous)	T41.3X1	T41.3X2	T41.3X3	T41.3X4	T41.3X5	T41.3X6
nerve block (peripheral) (plexus)	T41.3X1	T41.3X2	T41.3X3	T41.3X4	T41.3X5	T41.3X6
spinal	T41.3X1	T41.3X2	T41.3X3	T41.3X4	T41.3X5	T41.3X6
topical (surface)	T41.3X1	T41.3X2	T41.3X3	T41.3X4	T41.3X5	T41.3X6
Amylopectin	T47.6X1	T47.6X2	T47.6X3	T47.6X4	T47.6X5	T47.6X6
Amytal (sodium)	T42.3X1	T42.3X2	T42.3X3	T42.3X4	T42.3X5	T42.3X6
Anabolic steroid	T38.7X1	T38.7X2	T38.7X3	T38.7X4	T38.7X5	T38.7X6
Analeptic NEC	T5Ø.7X1	T5Ø.7X2	T5Ø.7X3	T5Ø.7X4	T5Ø.7X5	T5Ø.7X6
Analgesic	T39.91	T39.92	T39.93	T39.94	T39.95	T39.96
anti-inflammatory NEC	T39.91	T39.92	T39.93	T39.94	T39.95	T39.96
propionic acid derivative	T39.311	T39.312	T39.313	T39.314	T39.315	T39.316
antirheumatic NEC	T39.4X1	T39.4X2	T39.4X3	T39.4X4	T39.4X5	T39.4X6
aromatic NEC	T39.1X1	T39.1X2	T39.1X3	T39.1X4	T39.1X5	T39.1X6
narcotic NEC	T4Ø.6Ø1	T4Ø.6Ø2	T4Ø.6Ø3	T4Ø.6Ø4	T4Ø.6Ø5	T4Ø.6Ø6
combination	T4Ø.6Ø1	T4Ø.6Ø2	T4Ø.6Ø3	T4Ø.6Ø4	T4Ø.6Ø5	T4Ø.6Ø6
obstetric	T4Ø.6Ø1	T4Ø.6Ø2	T4Ø.6Ø3	T4Ø.6Ø4	T4Ø.6Ø5	T4Ø.6Ø6
non-narcotic NEC	T39.91	T39.92	T39.93	T39.94	T39.95	T39.96
combination	T39.91	T39.92	T39.93	T39.94	T39.95	T39.96
pyrazole	T39.2X1	T39.2X2	T39.2X3	T39.2X4	T39.2X5	T39.2X6
specified NEC	T39.8X1	T39.8X2	T39.8X3	T39.8X4	T39.8X5	T39.8X6
Analgin	T39.2X1	T39.2X2	T39.2X3	T39.2X4	T39.2X5	T39.2X6
Anamirta cocculus	T62.1X1	T62.1X2	T62.1X3	T62.1X4	—	—
Ancillin	T36.ØX1	T36.ØX2	T36.ØX3	T36.ØX4	T36.ØX5	T36.ØX6
Ancrod	T45.691	T45.692	T45.693	T45.694	T45.695	T45.696
Androgen	T38.7X1	T38.7X2	T38.7X3	T38.7X4	T38.7X5	T38.7X6
Androgen-estrogen mixture	T38.7X1	T38.7X2	T38.7X3	T38.7X4	T38.7X5	T38.7X6
Androstalone	T38.7X1	T38.7X2	T38.7X3	T38.7X4	T38.7X5	T38.7X6
Androstanolone	T38.7X1	T38.7X2	T38.7X3	T38.7X4	T38.7X5	T38.7X6
Androsterone	T38.7X1	T38.7X2	T38.7X3	T38.7X4	T38.7X5	T38.7X6
Anemone pulsatilla	T62.2X1	T62.2X2	T62.2X3	T62.2X4	—	—
Anesthesia						
caudal	T41.3X1	T41.3X2	T41.3X3	T41.3X4	T41.3X5	T41.3X6
endotracheal	T41.ØX1	T41.ØX2	T41.ØX3	T41.ØX4	T41.ØX5	T41.ØX6
epidural	T41.3X1	T41.3X2	T41.3X3	T41.3X4	T41.3X5	T41.3X6
inhalation	T41.ØX1	T41.ØX2	T41.ØX3	T41.ØX4	T41.ØX5	T41.ØX6
local	T41.3X1	T41.3X2	T41.3X3	T41.3X4	T41.3X5	T41.3X6

Anesthesia ICD-10-CM 2016

Table of Drugs and Chemicals

Substance	Poisoning, Accidental (unintentional)	Poisoning, Intentional Self-harm	Poisoning, Assault	Poisoning, Undetermined	Adverse Effect	Under-dosing
Anesthesia — *continued*						
mucosal	T41.3X1	T41.3X2	T41.3X3	T41.3X4	T41.3X5	T41.3X6
muscle relaxation	T48.1X1	T48.1X2	T48.1X3	T48.1X4	T48.1X5	T48.1X6
nerve blocking	T41.3X1	T41.3X2	T41.3X3	T41.3X4	T41.3X5	T41.3X6
plexus blocking	T41.3X1	T41.3X2	T41.3X3	T41.3X4	T41.3X5	T41.3X6
potentiated	T41.2Ø1	T41.2Ø2	T41.2Ø3	T41.2Ø4	T41.2Ø5	T41.2Ø6
rectal	T41.2Ø1	T41.2Ø2	T41.2Ø3	T41.2Ø4	T41.2Ø5	T41.2Ø6
general	T41.2Ø1	T41.2Ø2	T41.2Ø3	T41.2Ø4	T41.2Ø5	T41.2Ø6
local	T41.3X1	T41.3X2	T41.3X3	T41.3X4	T41.3X5	T41.3X6
regional	T41.3X1	T41.3X2	T41.3X3	T41.3X4	T41.3X5	T41.3X6
surface	T41.3X1	T41.3X2	T41.3X3	T41.3X4	T41.3X5	T41.3X6
Anesthetic NEC — *see also* Anesthesia	T41.41	T41.42	T41.43	T41.44	T41.45	T41.46
with muscle relaxant	T41.2Ø1	T41.2Ø2	T41.2Ø3	T41.2Ø4	T41.2Ø5	T41.2Ø6
general	T41.2Ø1	T41.2Ø2	T41.2Ø3	T41.2Ø4	T41.2Ø5	T41.2Ø6
local	T41.3X1	T41.3X2	T41.3X3	T41.3X4	T41.3X5	T41.3X6
gaseous NEC	T41.ØX1	T41.ØX2	T41.ØX3	T41.ØX4	T41.ØX5	T41.ØX6
general NEC	T41.2Ø1	T41.2Ø2	T41.2Ø3	T41.2Ø4	T41.2Ø5	T41.2Ø6
halogenated hydrocarbon derivatives NEC	T41.ØX1	T41.ØX2	T41.ØX3	T41.ØX4	T41.ØX5	T41.ØX6
infiltration NEC	T41.3X1	T41.3X2	T41.3X3	T41.3X4	T41.3X5	T41.3X6
intravenous NEC	T41.1X1	T41.1X2	T41.1X3	T41.1X4	T41.1X5	T41.1X6
local NEC	T41.3X1	T41.3X2	T41.3X3	T41.3X4	T41.3X5	T41.3X6
rectal	T41.2Ø1	T41.2Ø2	T41.2Ø3	T41.2Ø4	T41.2Ø5	T41.2Ø6
general	T41.2Ø1	T41.2Ø2	T41.2Ø3	T41.2Ø4	T41.2Ø5	T41.2Ø6
local	T41.3X1	T41.3X2	T41.3X3	T41.3X4	T41.3X5	T41.3X6
regional NEC	T41.3X1	T41.3X2	T41.3X3	T41.3X4	T41.3X5	T41.3X6
spinal NEC	T41.3X1	T41.3X2	T41.3X3	T41.3X4	T41.3X5	T41.3X6
thiobarbiturate	T41.1X1	T41.1X2	T41.1X3	T41.1X4	T41.1X5	T41.1X6
topical	T41.3X1	T41.3X2	T41.3X3	T41.3X4	T41.3X5	T41.3X6
Aneurine	T45.2X1	T45.2X2	T45.2X3	T45.2X4	T45.2X5	T45.2X6
Angio-Conray	T5Ø.8X1	T5Ø.8X2	T5Ø.8X3	T5Ø.8X4	T5Ø.8X5	T5Ø.8X6
Angiotensin	T44.5X1	T44.5X2	T44.5X3	T44.5X4	T44.5X5	T44.5X6
Angiotensinamide	T44.991	T44.992	T44.993	T44.994	T44.995	T44.996
Anhydrohydroxy-progesterone	T38.5X1	T38.5X2	T38.5X3	T38.5X4	T38.5X5	T38.5X6
Anhydron	T5Ø.2X1	T5Ø.2X2	T5Ø.2X3	T5Ø.2X4	T5Ø.2X5	T5Ø.2X6
Anileridine	T4Ø.4X1	T4Ø.4X2	T4Ø.4X3	T4Ø.4X4	T4Ø.4X5	T4Ø.4X6
Aniline (dye) (liquid)	T65.3X1	T65.3X2	T65.3X3	T65.3X4	—	—
analgesic	T39.1X1	T39.1X2	T39.1X3	T39.1X4	T39.1X5	T39.1X6
derivatives, therapeutic NEC	T39.1X1	T39.1X2	T39.1X3	T39.1X4	T39.1X5	T39.1X6
vapor	T65.3X1	T65.3X2	T65.3X3	T65.3X4	—	—
Aniscoropine	T44.3X1	T44.3X2	T44.3X3	T44.3X4	T44.3X5	T44.3X6
Anise oil	T47.5X1	T47.5X2	T47.5X3	T47.5X4	T47.5X5	T47.5X6
Anisidine	T65.3X1	T65.3X2	T65.3X3	T65.3X4	—	—
Anisindione	T45.511	T45.512	T45.513	T45.514	T45.515	T45.516
Anisotropine methyl-bromide	T44.3X1	T44.3X2	T44.3X3	T44.3X4	T44.3X5	T44.3X6
Anistreplase	T45.611	T45.612	T45.613	T45.614	T45.615	T45.616
Anorexiant (central)	T5Ø.5X1	T5Ø.5X2	T5Ø.5X3	T5Ø.5X4	T5Ø.5X5	T5Ø.5X6
Anorexic agents	T5Ø.5X1	T5Ø.5X2	T5Ø.5X3	T5Ø.5X4	T5Ø.5X5	T5Ø.5X6
Ansamycin	T36.6X1	T36.6X2	T36.6X3	T36.6X4	T36.6X5	T36.6X6
Ant (bite) (sting)	T63.421	T63.422	T63.423	T63.424	—	—
Antabuse	T5Ø.6X1	T5Ø.6X2	T5Ø.6X3	T5Ø.6X4	T5Ø.6X5	T5Ø.6X6
Antacid NEC	T47.1X1	T47.1X2	T47.1X3	T47.1X4	T47.1X5	T47.1X6
Antagonist						
Aldosterone	T5Ø.ØX1	T5Ø.ØX2	T5Ø.ØX3	T5Ø.ØX4	T5Ø.ØX5	T5Ø.ØX6
alpha-adrenoreceptor	T44.6X1	T44.6X2	T44.6X3	T44.6X4	T44.6X5	T44.6X6
anticoagulant	T45.7X1	T45.7X2	T45.7X3	T45.7X4	T45.7X5	T45.7X6
beta-adrenoreceptor	T44.7X1	T44.7X2	T44.7X3	T44.7X4	T44.7X5	T44.7X6
extrapyramidal NEC	T44.3X1	T44.3X2	T44.3X3	T44.3X4	T44.3X5	T44.3X6
folic acid	T45.1X1	T45.1X2	T45.1X3	T45.1X4	T45.1X5	T45.1X6
H2 receptor	T47.ØX1	T47.ØX2	T47.ØX3	T47.ØX4	T47.ØX5	T47.ØX6
heavy metal	T45.8X1	T45.8X2	T45.8X3	T45.8X4	T45.8X5	T45.8X6
narcotic analgesic	T5Ø.7X1	T5Ø.7X2	T5Ø.7X3	T5Ø.7X4	T5Ø.7X5	T5Ø.7X6
opiate	T5Ø.7X1	T5Ø.7X2	T5Ø.7X3	T5Ø.7X4	T5Ø.7X5	T5Ø.7X6
pyrimidine	T45.1X1	T45.1X2	T45.1X3	T45.1X4	T45.1X5	T45.1X6
serotonin	T46.5X1	T46.5X2	T46.5X3	T46.5X4	T46.5X5	T46.5X6
Antazolin (e)	T45.ØX1	T45.ØX2	T45.ØX3	T45.ØX4	T45.ØX5	T45.ØX6
Anterior pituitary hormone NEC	T38.811	T38.812	T38.813	T38.814	T38.815	T38.816
Anthelmintic NEC	T37.4X1	T37.4X2	T37.4X3	T37.4X4	T37.4X5	T37.4X6
Anthiolimine	T37.4X1	T37.4X2	T37.4X3	T37.4X4	T37.4X5	T37.4X6
Anthralin	T49.4X1	T49.4X2	T49.4X3	T49.4X4	T49.4X5	T49.4X6
Anthramycin	T45.1X1	T45.1X2	T45.1X3	T45.1X4	T45.1X5	T45.1X6
Antiadrenergic NEC	T44.8X1	T44.8X2	T44.8X3	T44.8X4	T44.8X5	T44.8X6
Antiallergic NEC	T45.ØX1	T45.ØX2	T45.ØX3	T45.ØX4	T45.ØX5	T45.ØX6
Antiandrogen NEC	T38.6X1	T38.6X2	T38.6X3	T38.6X4	T38.6X5	T38.6X6
Anti-anemic (drug) (preparation)	T45.8X1	T45.8X2	T45.8X3	T45.8X4	T45.8X5	T45.8X6
Antianxiety drug NEC	T43.5Ø1	T43.5Ø2	T43.5Ø3	T43.5Ø4	T43.5Ø5	T43.5Ø6
Antiaris toxicaria	T65.891	T65.892	T65.893	T65.894	—	—
Antiarteriosclerotic drug	T46.6X1	T46.6X2	T46.6X3	T46.6X4	T46.6X5	T46.6X6

Substance	Poisoning, Accidental (unintentional)	Poisoning, Intentional Self-harm	Poisoning, Assault	Poisoning, Undetermined	Adverse Effect	Under-dosing
Antiasthmatic drug NEC	T48.6X1	T48.6X2	T48.6X3	T48.6X4	T48.6X5	T48.6X6
Antibiotic NEC	T36.91	T36.92	T36.93	T36.94	T36.95	T36.96
aminoglycoside	T36.5X1	T36.5X2	T36.5X3	T36.5X4	T36.5X5	T36.5X6
anticancer	T45.1X1	T45.1X2	T45.1X3	T45.1X4	T45.1X5	T45.1X6
antifungal	T36.7X1	T36.7X2	T36.7X3	T36.7X4	T36.7X5	T36.7X6
antimycobacterial	T36.5X1	T36.5X2	T36.5X3	T36.5X4	T36.5X5	T36.5X6
antineoplastic	T45.1X1	T45.1X2	T45.1X3	T45.1X4	T45.1X5	T45.1X6
b-lactam NEC	T36.1X1	T36.1X2	T36.1X3	T36.1X4	T36.1X5	T36.1X6
cephalosporin (group)	T36.1X1	T36.1X2	T36.1X3	T36.1X4	T36.1X5	T36.1X6
chloramphenicol (group)	T36.2X1	T36.2X2	T36.2X3	T36.2X4	T36.2X5	T36.2X6
ENT	T49.6X1	T49.6X2	T49.6X3	T49.6X4	T49.6X5	T49.6X6
eye	T49.5X1	T49.5X2	T49.5X3	T49.5X4	T49.5X5	T49.5X6
fungicidal (local)	T49.ØX1	T49.ØX2	T49.ØX3	T49.ØX4	T49.ØX5	T49.ØX6
intestinal	T36.8X1	T36.8X2	T36.8X3	T36.8X4	T36.8X5	T36.8X6
local	T49.ØX1	T49.ØX2	T49.ØX3	T49.ØX4	T49.ØX5	T49.ØX6
macrolides	T36.3X1	T36.3X2	T36.3X3	T36.3X4	T36.3X5	T36.3X6
polypeptide	T36.8X1	T36.8X2	T36.8X3	T36.8X4	T36.8X5	T36.8X6
specified NEC	T36.8X1	T36.8X2	T36.8X3	T36.8X4	T36.8X5	T36.8X6
tetracycline (group)	T36.4X1	T36.4X2	T36.4X3	T36.4X4	T36.4X5	T36.4X6
throat	T49.6X1	T49.6X2	T49.6X3	T49.6X4	T49.6X5	T49.6X6
Anticancer agents NEC	T45.1X1	T45.1X2	T45.1X3	T45.1X4	T45.1X5	T45.1X6
Anticholesterolemic drug NEC	T46.6X1	T46.6X2	T46.6X3	T46.6X4	T46.6X5	T46.6X6
Anticholinergic NEC	T44.3X1	T44.3X2	T44.3X3	T44.3X4	T44.3X5	T44.3X6
Anticholinesterase	T44.ØX1	T44.ØX2	T44.ØX3	T44.ØX4	T44.ØX5	T44.ØX6
organophosphorus	T44.ØX1	T44.ØX2	T44.ØX3	T44.ØX4	T44.ØX5	T44.ØX6
insecticide	T6Ø.ØX1	T6Ø.ØX2	T6Ø.ØX3	T6Ø.ØX4	—	—
nerve gas	T59.891	T59.892	T59.893	T59.894	—	—
reversible	T44.ØX1	T44.ØX2	T44.ØX3	T44.ØX4	T44.ØX5	T44.ØX6
ophthalmological	T49.5X1	T49.5X2	T49.5X3	T49.5X4	T49.5X5	T49.5X6
Anticoagulant NEC	T45.511	T45.512	T45.513	T45.514	T45.515	T45.516
Antagonist	T45.7X1	T45.7X2	T45.7X3	T45.7X4	T45.7X5	T45.7X6
Anti-common-cold drug NEC	T48.5X1	T48.5X2	T48.5X3	T48.5X4	T48.5X5	T48.5X6
Anticonvulsant	T42.71	T42.72	T42.73	T42.74	T42.75	T42.76
barbiturate	T42.3X1	T42.3X2	T42.3X3	T42.3X4	T42.3X5	T42.3X6
combination (with barbiturate)	T42.3X1	T42.3X2	T42.3X3	T42.3X4	T42.3X5	T42.3X6
hydantoin	T42.ØX1	T42.ØX2	T42.ØX3	T42.ØX4	T42.ØX5	T42.ØX6
hypnotic NEC	T42.6X1	T42.6X2	T42.6X3	T42.6X4	T42.6X5	T42.6X6
oxazolidinedione	T42.2X1	T42.2X2	T42.2X3	T42.2X4	T42.2X5	T42.2X6
pyrimidinedione	T42.6X1	T42.6X2	T42.6X3	T42.6X4	T42.6X5	T42.6X6
specified NEC	T42.6X1	T42.6X2	T42.6X3	T42.6X4	T42.6X5	T42.6X6
succinimide	T42.2X1	T42.2X2	T42.2X3	T42.2X4	T42.2X5	T42.2X6
Antidepressant	T43.2Ø1	T43.2Ø2	T43.2Ø3	T43.2Ø4	T43.2Ø5	T43.2Ø6
monoamine oxidase inhibitor	T43.1X1	T43.1X2	T43.1X3	T43.1X4	T43.1X5	T43.1X6
selective serotonin norepinephrine reuptake inhibitor	T43.211	T43.212	T43.213	T43.214	T43.215	T43.216
selective serotonin reuptake inhibitor	T43.221	T43.222	T43.223	T43.224	T43.225	T43.226
specified NEC	T43.291	T43.292	T43.293	T43.294	T43.295	T43.296
tetracyclic	T43.Ø21	T43.Ø22	T43.Ø23	T43.Ø24	T43.Ø25	T43.Ø26
triazolopyridine	T43.211	T43.212	T43.213	T43.214	T43.215	T43.216
tricyclic	T43.Ø11	T43.Ø12	T43.Ø13	T43.Ø14	T43.Ø15	T43.Ø16
Antidiabetic NEC	T38.3X1	T38.3X2	T38.3X3	T38.3X4	T38.3X5	T38.3X6
biguanide	T38.3X1	T38.3X2	T38.3X3	T38.3X4	T38.3X5	T38.3X6
and sulfonyl combined	T38.3X1	T38.3X2	T38.3X3	T38.3X4	T38.3X5	T38.3X6
combined	T38.3X1	T38.3X2	T38.3X3	T38.3X4	T38.3X5	T38.3X6
sulfonylurea	T38.3X1	T38.3X2	T38.3X3	T38.3X4	T38.3X5	T38.3X6
Antidiarrheal drug NEC	T47.6X1	T47.6X2	T47.6X3	T47.6X4	T47.6X5	T47.6X6
absorbent	T47.6X1	T47.6X2	T47.6X3	T47.6X4	T47.6X5	T47.6X6
Anti-D immunoglobulin (human)	T5Ø.Z11	T5Ø.Z12	T5Ø.Z13	T5Ø.Z14	T5Ø.Z15	T5Ø.Z16
Antidiphtheria serum	T5Ø.Z11	T5Ø.Z12	T5Ø.Z13	T5Ø.Z14	T5Ø.Z15	T5Ø.Z16
Antidiuretic hormone	T38.891	T38.892	T38.893	T38.894	T38.895	T38.896
Antidote NEC	T5Ø.6X1	T5Ø.6X2	T5Ø.6X3	T5Ø.6X4	T5Ø.6X5	T5Ø.6X6
heavy metal	T45.8X1	T45.8X2	T45.8X3	T45.8X4	T45.8X5	T45.8X6
Antidysrhythmic NEC	T46.2X1	T46.2X2	T46.2X3	T46.2X4	T46.2X5	T46.2X6
Antiemetic drug	T45.ØX1	T45.ØX2	T45.ØX3	T45.ØX4	T45.ØX5	T45.ØX6
Antiepilepsy agent	T42.71	T42.72	T42.73	T42.74	T42.75	T42.76
combination	T42.5X1	T42.5X2	T42.5X3	T42.5X4	T42.5X5	T42.5X6
mixed	T42.5X1	T42.5X2	T42.5X3	T42.5X4	T42.5X5	T42.5X6
specified, NEC	T42.6X1	T42.6X2	T42.6X3	T42.6X4	T42.6X5	T42.6X6
Antiestrogen NEC	T38.6X1	T38.6X2	T38.6X3	T38.6X4	T38.6X5	T38.6X6
Antifertility pill	T38.4X1	T38.4X2	T38.4X3	T38.4X4	T38.4X5	T38.4X6
Antifibrinolytic drug	T45.621	T45.622	T45.623	T45.624	T45.625	T45.626
Antifilarial drug	T37.4X1	T37.4X2	T37.4X3	T37.4X4	T37.4X5	T37.4X6
Antiflatulent	T47.5X1	T47.5X2	T47.5X3	T47.5X4	T47.5X5	T47.5X6
Antifreeze	T65.91	T65.92	T65.93	T65.94	—	—
alcohol	T51.1X1	T51.1X2	T51.1X3	T51.1X4	—	—
ethylene glycol	T51.8X1	T51.8X2	T51.8X3	T51.8X4	—	—

Substance	Poisoning, Accidental (unintentional)	Poisoning, Intentional Self-harm	Poisoning, Assault	Poisoning, Undetermined	Adverse Effect	Under-dosing
Antifungal						
antibiotic (systemic)	T36.7X1	T36.7X2	T36.7X3	T36.7X4	T36.7X5	T36.7X6
anti-infective NEC	T37.91	T37.92	T37.93	T37.94	T37.95	T37.96
disinfectant, local	T49.ØX1	T49.ØX2	T49.ØX3	T49.ØX4	T49.ØX5	T49.ØX6
nonmedicinal (spray)	T6Ø.3X1	T6Ø.3X2	T6Ø.3X3	T6Ø.3X4	—	—
topical	T49.ØX1	T49.ØX2	T49.ØX3	T49.ØX4	T49.ØX5	T49.ØX6
Anti-gastric-secretion drug NEC	T47.1X1	T47.1X2	T47.1X3	T47.1X4	T47.1X5	T47.1X6
Antigonadotrophin NEC	T38.6X1	T38.6X2	T38.6X3	T38.6X4	T38.6X5	T38.6X6
Antihallucinogen	T43.5Ø1	T43.5Ø2	T43.5Ø3	T43.5Ø4	T43.5Ø5	T43.5Ø6
Antihelmintics	T37.4X1	T37.4X2	T37.4X3	T37.4X4	T37.4X5	T37.4X6
Antihemophilic						
factor	T45.8X1	T45.8X2	T45.8X3	T45.8X4	T45.8X5	T45.8X6
fraction	T45.8X1	T45.8X2	T45.8X3	T45.8X4	T45.8X5	T45.8X6
globulin concentrate	T45.7X1	T45.7X2	T45.7X3	T45.7X4	T45.7X5	T45.7X6
human plasma	T45.8X1	T45.8X2	T45.8X3	T45.8X4	T45.8X5	T45.8X6
plasma, dried	T45.7X1	T45.7X2	T45.7X3	T45.7X4	T45.7X5	T45.7X6
Antihemorrhoidal preparation	T49.2X1	T49.2X2	T49.2X3	T49.2X4	T49.2X5	T49.2X6
Antiheparin drug	T45.7X1	T45.7X2	T45.7X3	T45.7X4	T45.7X5	T45.7X6
Antihistamine	T45.ØX1	T45.ØX2	T45.ØX3	T45.ØX4	T45.ØX5	T45.ØX6
Antihookworm drug	T37.4X1	T37.4X2	T37.4X3	T37.4X4	T37.4X5	T37.4X6
Anti-human lymphocytic globulin	T5Ø.Z11	T5Ø.Z12	T5Ø.Z13	T5Ø.Z14	T5Ø.Z15	T5Ø.Z16
Antihyperlipidemic drug	T46.6X1	T46.6X2	T46.6X3	T46.6X4	T46.6X5	T46.6X6
Antihypertensive drug NEC	T46.5X1	T46.5X2	T46.5X3	T46.5X4	T46.5X5	T46.5X6
Anti-infective NEC	T37.91	T37.92	T37.93	T37.94	T37.95	T37.96
anthelmintic	T37.4X1	T37.4X2	T37.4X3	T37.4X4	T37.4X5	T37.4X6
antibiotics	T36.91	T36.92	T36.93	T36.94	T36.95	T36.96
specified NEC	T36.8X1	T36.8X2	T36.8X3	T36.8X4	T36.8X5	T36.8X6
antimalarial	T37.2X1	T37.2X2	T37.2X3	T37.2X4	T37.2X5	T37.2X6
antimycobacterial NEC	T37.1X1	T37.1X2	T37.1X3	T37.1X4	T37.1X5	T37.1X6
antibiotics	T36.5X1	T36.5X2	T36.5X3	T36.5X4	T36.5X5	T36.5X6
antiprotozoal NEC	T37.3X1	T37.3X2	T37.3X3	T37.3X4	T37.3X5	T37.3X6
blood	T37.2X1	T37.2X2	T37.2X3	T37.2X4	T37.2X5	T37.2X6
antiviral	T37.5X1	T37.5X2	T37.5X3	T37.5X4	T37.5X5	T37.5X6
arsenical	T37.8X1	T37.8X2	T37.8X3	T37.8X4	T37.8X5	T37.8X6
bismuth, local	T49.ØX1	T49.ØX2	T49.ØX3	T49.ØX4	T49.ØX5	T49.ØX6
ENT	T49.6X1	T49.6X2	T49.6X3	T49.6X4	T49.6X5	T49.6X6
eye NEC	T49.5X1	T49.5X2	T49.5X3	T49.5X4	T49.5X5	T49.5X6
heavy metals NEC	T37.8X1	T37.8X2	T37.8X3	T37.8X4	T37.8X5	T37.8X6
local NEC	T49.ØX1	T49.ØX2	T49.ØX3	T49.ØX4	T49.ØX5	T49.ØX6
specified NEC	T49.ØX1	T49.ØX2	T49.ØX3	T49.ØX4	T49.ØX5	T49.ØX6
mixed	T37.91	T37.92	T37.93	T37.94	T37.95	T37.96
ophthalmic preparation	T49.5X1	T49.5X2	T49.5X3	T49.5X4	T49.5X5	T49.5X6
topical NEC	T49.ØX1	T49.ØX2	T49.ØX3	T49.ØX4	T49.ØX5	T49.ØX6
Anti-inflammatory drug NEC	T39.391	T39.392	T39.393	T39.394	T39.395	T39.396
local	T49.ØX1	T49.ØX2	T49.ØX3	T49.ØX4	T49.ØX5	T49.ØX6
nonsteroidal NEC	T39.391	T39.392	T39.393	T39.394	T39.395	T39.396
propionic acid derivative	T39.311	T39.312	T39.313	T39.314	T39.315	T39.316
specified NEC	T39.391	T39.392	T39.393	T39.394	T39.395	T39.396
Antikaluretic	T5Ø.3X1	T5Ø.3X2	T5Ø.3X3	T5Ø.3X4	T5Ø.3X5	T5Ø.3X6
Antiknock (tetraethyl lead)	T56.ØX1	T56.ØX2	T56.ØX3	T56.ØX4	—	—
Antilipemic drug NEC	T46.6X1	T46.6X2	T46.6X3	T46.6X4	T46.6X5	T46.6X6
Antimalarial	T37.2X1	T37.2X2	T37.2X3	T37.2X4	T37.2X5	T37.2X6
prophylactic NEC	T37.2X1	T37.2X2	T37.2X3	T37.2X4	T37.2X5	T37.2X6
pyrimidine derivative	T37.2X1	T37.2X2	T37.2X3	T37.2X4	T37.2X5	T37.2X6
Antimetabolite	T45.1X1	T45.1X2	T45.1X3	T45.1X4	T45.1X5	T45.1X6
Antimitotic agent	T45.1X1	T45.1X2	T45.1X3	T45.1X4	T45.1X5	T45.1X6
Antimony (compounds) (vapor) **NEC**	T56.891	T56.892	T56.893	T56.894	—	—
anti-infectives	T37.8X1	T37.8X2	T37.8X3	T37.8X4	T37.8X5	T37.8X6
dimercaptosuccinate	T37.3X1	T37.3X2	T37.3X3	T37.3X4	T37.3X5	T37.3X6
hydride	T56.891	T56.892	T56.893	T56.894	—	—
pesticide (vapor)	T6Ø.8X1	T6Ø.8X2	T6Ø.8X3	T6Ø.8X4	—	—
potassium (sodium) tartrate	T37.8X1	T37.8X2	T37.8X3	T37.8X4	T37.8X5	T37.8X6
sodium dimercaptosuccinate	T37.3X1	T37.3X2	T37.3X3	T37.3X4	T37.3X5	T37.3X6
tartrated	T37.8X1	T37.8X2	T37.8X3	T37.8X4	T37.8X5	T37.8X6
Antimuscarinic NEC	T44.3X1	T44.3X2	T44.3X3	T44.3X4	T44.3X5	T44.3X6
Antimycobacterial drug NEC	T37.1X1	T37.1X2	T37.1X3	T37.1X4	T37.1X5	T37.1X6
antibiotics	T36.5X1	T36.5X2	T36.5X3	T36.5X4	T36.5X5	T36.5X6
combination	T37.1X1	T37.1X2	T37.1X3	T37.1X4	T37.1X5	T37.1X6
Antinausea drug	T45.ØX1	T45.ØX2	T45.ØX3	T45.ØX4	T45.ØX5	T45.ØX6
Antinematode drug	T37.4X1	T37.4X2	T37.4X3	T37.4X4	T37.4X5	T37.4X6
Antineoplastic NEC	T45.1X1	T45.1X2	T45.1X3	T45.1X4	T45.1X5	T45.1X6
alkaloidal	T45.1X1	T45.1X2	T45.1X3	T45.1X4	T45.1X5	T45.1X6
antibiotics	T45.1X1	T45.1X2	T45.1X3	T45.1X4	T45.1X5	T45.1X6
combination	T45.1X1	T45.1X2	T45.1X3	T45.1X4	T45.1X5	T45.1X6
estrogen	T38.5X1	T38.5X2	T38.5X3	T38.5X4	T38.5X5	T38.5X6

Substance	Poisoning, Accidental (unintentional)	Poisoning, Intentional Self-harm	Poisoning, Assault	Poisoning, Undetermined	Adverse Effect	Under-dosing
Antineoplastic — *continued*						
steroid	T38.7X1	T38.7X2	T38.7X3	T38.7X4	T38.7X5	T38.7X6
Antiparasitic drug (systemic)	T37.91	T37.92	T37.93	T37.94	T37.95	T37.96
local	T49.ØX1	T49.ØX2	T49.ØX3	T49.ØX4	T49.ØX5	T49.ØX6
specified NEC	T37.8X1	T37.8X2	T37.8X3	T37.8X4	T37.8X5	T37.8X6
Antiparkinsonism drug NEC	T42.8X1	T42.8X2	T42.8X3	T42.8X4	T42.8X5	T42.8X6
Antiperspirant NEC	T49.2X1	T49.2X2	T49.2X3	T49.2X4	T49.2X5	T49.2X6
Antiphlogistic NEC	T39.4X1	T39.4X2	T39.4X3	T39.4X4	T39.4X5	T39.4X6
Antiplatyhelmintic drug	T37.4X1	T37.4X2	T37.4X3	T37.4X4	T37.4X5	T37.4X6
Antiprotozoal drug NEC	T37.3X1	T37.3X2	T37.3X3	T37.3X4	T37.3X5	T37.3X6
blood	T37.2X1	T37.2X2	T37.2X3	T37.2X4	T37.2X5	T37.2X6
local	T49.ØX1	T49.ØX2	T49.ØX3	T49.ØX4	T49.ØX5	T49.ØX6
Antipruritic drug NEC	T49.1X1	T49.1X2	T49.1X3	T49.1X4	T49.1X5	T49.1X6
Antipsychotic drug	T43.5Ø1	T43.5Ø2	T43.5Ø3	T43.5Ø4	T43.5Ø5	T43.5Ø6
specified NEC	T43.591	T43.592	T43.593	T43.594	T43.595	T43.596
Antipyretic	T39.91	T39.92	T39.93	T39.94	T39.95	T39.96
specified NEC	T39.8X1	T39.8X2	T39.8X3	T39.8X4	T39.8X5	T39.8X6
Antipyrine	T39.2X1	T39.2X2	T39.2X3	T39.2X4	T39.2X5	T39.2X6
Antirabies hyperimmune serum	T5Ø.Z11	T5Ø.Z12	T5Ø.Z13	T5Ø.Z14	T5Ø.Z15	T5Ø.Z16
Antirheumatic NEC	T39.4X1	T39.4X2	T39.4X3	T39.4X4	T39.4X5	T39.4X6
Antirigidity drug NEC	T42.8X1	T42.8X2	T42.8X3	T42.8X4	T42.8X5	T42.8X6
Antischistosomal drug	T37.4X1	T37.4X2	T37.4X3	T37.4X4	T37.4X5	T37.4X6
Antiscorpion sera	T5Ø.Z11	T5Ø.Z12	T5Ø.Z13	T5Ø.Z14	T5Ø.Z15	T5Ø.Z16
Antiseborrheics	T49.4X1	T49.4X2	T49.4X3	T49.4X4	T49.4X5	T49.4X6
Antiseptics (external) (medicinal)	T49.ØX1	T49.ØX2	T49.ØX3	T49.ØX4	T49.ØX5	T49.ØX6
Antistine	T45.ØX1	T45.ØX2	T45.ØX3	T45.ØX4	T45.ØX5	T45.ØX6
Antitapeworm drug	T37.4X1	T37.4X2	T37.4X3	T37.4X4	T37.4X5	T37.4X6
Antitetanus immunoglobulin	T5Ø.Z11	T5Ø.Z12	T5Ø.Z13	T5Ø.Z14	T5Ø.Z15	T5Ø.Z16
Antithyroid drug NEC	T38.2X1	T38.2X2	T38.2X3	T38.2X4	T38.2X5	T38.2X6
Antitoxin	T5Ø.Z11	T5Ø.Z12	T5Ø.Z13	T5Ø.Z14	T5Ø.Z15	T5Ø.Z16
diphtheria	T5Ø.Z11	T5Ø.Z12	T5Ø.Z13	T5Ø.Z14	T5Ø.Z15	T5Ø.Z16
gas gangrene	T5Ø.Z11	T5Ø.Z12	T5Ø.Z13	T5Ø.Z14	T5Ø.Z15	T5Ø.Z16
tetanus	T5Ø.Z11	T5Ø.Z12	T5Ø.Z13	T5Ø.Z14	T5Ø.Z15	T5Ø.Z16
Antitrichomonal drug	T37.3X1	T37.3X2	T37.3X3	T37.3X4	T37.3X5	T37.3X6
Antituberculars	T37.1X1	T37.1X2	T37.1X3	T37.1X4	T37.1X5	T37.1X6
antibiotics	T36.5X1	T36.5X2	T36.5X3	T36.5X4	T36.5X5	T36.5X6
Antitussive NEC	T48.3X1	T48.3X2	T48.3X3	T48.3X4	T48.3X5	T48.3X6
codeine mixture	T4Ø.2X1	T4Ø.2X2	T4Ø.2X3	T4Ø.2X4	T4Ø.2X5	T4Ø.2X6
opiate	T4Ø.2X1	T4Ø.2X2	T4Ø.2X3	T4Ø.2X4	T4Ø.2X5	T4Ø.2X6
Antivaricose drug	T46.8X1	T46.8X2	T46.8X3	T46.8X4	T46.8X5	T46.8X6
Antivenin, antivenom (sera)	T5Ø.Z11	T5Ø.Z12	T5Ø.Z13	T5Ø.Z14	T5Ø.Z15	T5Ø.Z16
crotaline	T5Ø.Z11	T5Ø.Z12	T5Ø.Z13	T5Ø.Z14	T5Ø.Z15	T5Ø.Z16
spider bite	T5Ø.Z11	T5Ø.Z12	T5Ø.Z13	T5Ø.Z14	T5Ø.Z15	T5Ø.Z16
Antivertigo drug	T45.ØX1	T45.ØX2	T45.ØX3	T45.ØX4	T45.ØX5	T45.ØX6
Antiviral drug NEC	T37.5X1	T37.5X2	T37.5X3	T37.5X4	T37.5X5	T37.5X6
eye	T49.5X1	T49.5X2	T49.5X3	T49.5X4	T49.5X5	T49.5X6
Antiwhipworm drug	T37.4X1	T37.4X2	T37.4X3	T37.4X4	T37.4X5	T37.4X6
Ant poison — *see* Insecticide						
Antrol — *see also* by specific chemical substance	T6Ø.91	T6Ø.92	T6Ø.93	T6Ø.94	—	—
fungicide	T6Ø.91	T6Ø.92	T6Ø.93	T6Ø.94	—	—
ANTU (alpha naphthylthiourea)	T6Ø.4X1	T6Ø.4X2	T6Ø.4X3	T6Ø.4X4	—	—
Apalcillin	T36.ØX1	T36.ØX2	T36.ØX3	T36.ØX4	T36.ØX5	T36.ØX6
APC	T48.5X1	T48.5X2	T48.5X3	T48.5X4	T48.5X5	T48.5X6
Aplonidine	T44.4X1	T44.4X2	T44.4X3	T44.4X4	T44.4X5	T44.4X6
Apomorphine	T47.7X1	T47.7X2	T47.7X3	T47.7X4	T47.7X5	T47.7X6
Appetite depressants, central	T5Ø.5X1	T5Ø.5X2	T5Ø.5X3	T5Ø.5X4	T5Ø.5X5	T5Ø.5X6
Apraclonidine (hydrochloride)	T44.4X1	T44.4X2	T44.4X3	T44.4X4	T44.4X5	T44.4X6
Apresoline	T46.5X1	T46.5X2	T46.5X3	T46.5X4	T46.5X5	T46.5X6
Aprindine	T46.2X1	T46.2X2	T46.2X3	T46.2X4	T46.2X5	T46.2X6
Aprobarbital	T42.3X1	T42.3X2	T42.3X3	T42.3X4	T42.3X5	T42.3X6
Apronalide	T42.6X1	T42.6X2	T42.6X3	T42.6X4	T42.6X5	T42.6X6
Aprotinin	T45.621	T45.622	T45.623	T45.624	T45.625	T45.626
Aptocaine	T41.3X1	T41.3X2	T41.3X3	T41.3X4	T41.3X5	T41.3X6
Aqua fortis	T54.2X1	T54.2X2	T54.2X3	T54.2X4	—	—
Ara-A	T37.5X1	T37.5X2	T37.5X3	T37.5X4	T37.5X5	T37.5X6
Ara-C	T45.1X1	T45.1X2	T45.1X3	T45.1X4	T45.1X5	T45.1X6
Arachis oil	T49.3X1	T49.3X2	T49.3X3	T49.3X4	T49.3X5	T49.3X6
cathartic	T47.4X1	T47.4X2	T47.4X3	T47.4X4	T47.4X5	T47.4X6
Aralen	T37.2X1	T37.2X2	T37.2X3	T37.2X4	T37.2X5	T37.2X6
Arecoline	T44.1X1	T44.1X2	T44.1X3	T44.1X4	T44.1X5	T44.1X6
Arginine	T5Ø.991	T5Ø.992	T5Ø.993	T5Ø.994	T5Ø.995	T5Ø.996
glutamate	T5Ø.991	T5Ø.992	T5Ø.993	T5Ø.994	T5Ø.995	T5Ø.996
Argyrol	T49.ØX1	T49.ØX2	T49.ØX3	T49.ØX4	T49.ØX5	T49.ØX6
ENT agent	T49.6X1	T49.6X2	T49.6X3	T49.6X4	T49.6X5	T49.6X6

Substance	Poisoning, Accidental (unintentional)	Poisoning, Intentional Self-harm	Poisoning, Assault	Poisoning, Undetermined	Adverse Effect	Under-dosing
Argyrol — *continued*						
ophthalmic preparation	T49.5X1	T49.5X2	T49.5X3	T49.5X4	T49.5X5	T49.5X6
Aristocort	T38.ØX1	T38.ØX2	T38.ØX3	T38.ØX4	T38.ØX5	T38.ØX6
ENT agent	T49.6X1	T49.6X2	T49.6X3	T49.6X4	T49.6X5	T49.6X6
ophthalmic preparation	T49.5X1	T49.5X2	T49.5X3	T49.5X4	T49.5X5	T49.5X6
topical NEC	T49.ØX1	T49.ØX2	T49.ØX3	T49.ØX4	T49.ØX5	T49.ØX6
Aromatics, corrosive	T54.1X1	T54.1X2	T54.1X3	T54.1X4	—	—
disinfectants	T54.1X1	T54.1X2	T54.1X3	T54.1X4	—	—
Arsenate of lead	T57.ØX1	T57.ØX2	T57.ØX3	T57.ØX4	—	—
herbicide	T57.ØX1	T57.ØX2	T57.ØX3	T57.ØX4	—	—
Arsenic, arsenicals (compounds) (dust) (vapor) **NEC**	T57.ØX1	T57.ØX2	T57.ØX3	T57.ØX4	—	—
anti-infectives	T37.8X1	T37.8X2	T37.8X3	T37.8X4	T37.8X5	T37.8X6
pesticide (dust) (fumes)	T57.ØX1	T57.ØX2	T57.ØX3	T57.ØX4	—	—
Arsine (gas)	T57.ØX1	T57.ØX2	T57.ØX3	T57.ØX4	—	—
Arsphenamine (silver)	T37.8X1	T37.8X2	T37.8X3	T37.8X4	T37.8X5	T37.8X6
Arsthinol	T37.3X1	T37.3X2	T37.3X3	T37.3X4	T37.3X5	T37.3X6
Artane	T44.3X1	T44.3X2	T44.3X3	T44.3X4	T44.3X5	T44.3X6
Arthropod (venomous) **NEC**	T63.481	T63.482	T63.483	T63.484	—	—
Articaine	T41.3X1	T41.3X2	T41.3X3	T41.3X4	T41.3X5	T41.3X6
Asbestos	T57.8X1	T57.8X2	T57.8X3	T57.8X4	—	—
Ascaridole	T37.4X1	T37.4X2	T37.4X3	T37.4X4	T37.4X5	T37.4X6
Ascorbic acid	T45.2X1	T45.2X2	T45.2X3	T45.2X4	T45.2X5	T45.2X6
Asiaticoside	T49.ØX1	T49.ØX2	T49.ØX3	T49.ØX4	T49.ØX5	T49.ØX6
Asparaginase	T45.1X1	T45.1X2	T45.1X3	T45.1X4	T45.1X5	T45.1X6
Aspidium (oleoresin)	T37.4X1	T37.4X2	T37.4X3	T37.4X4	T37.4X5	T37.4X6
Aspirin (aluminum) (soluble)	T39.Ø11	T39.Ø12	T39.Ø13	T39.Ø14	T39.Ø15	T39.Ø16
Aspoxicillin	T36.ØX1	T36.ØX2	T36.ØX3	T36.ØX4	T36.ØX5	T36.ØX6
Astemizole	T45.ØX1	T45.ØX2	T45.ØX3	T45.ØX4	T45.ØX5	T45.ØX6
Astringent (local)	T49.2X1	T49.2X2	T49.2X3	T49.2X4	T49.2X5	T49.2X6
specified NEC	T49.2X1	T49.2X2	T49.2X3	T49.2X4	T49.2X5	T49.2X6
Astromicin	T36.5X1	T36.5X2	T36.5X3	T36.5X4	T36.5X5	T36.5X6
Ataractic drug NEC	T43.5Ø1	T43.5Ø2	T43.5Ø3	T43.5Ø4	T43.5Ø5	T43.5Ø6
Atenolol	T44.7X1	T44.7X2	T44.7X3	T44.7X4	T44.7X5	T44.7X6
Atonia drug, intestinal	T47.4X1	T47.4X2	T47.4X3	T47.4X4	T47.4X5	T47.4X6
Atophan	T5Ø.4X1	T5Ø.4X2	T5Ø.4X3	T5Ø.4X4	T5Ø.4X5	T5Ø.4X6
Atracurium besilate	T48.1X1	T48.1X2	T48.1X3	T48.1X4	T48.1X5	T48.1X6
Atropine	T44.3X1	T44.3X2	T44.3X3	T44.3X4	T44.3X5	T44.3X6
derivative	T44.3X1	T44.3X2	T44.3X3	T44.3X4	T44.3X5	T44.3X6
methonitrate	T44.3X1	T44.3X2	T44.3X3	T44.3X4	T44.3X5	T44.3X6
Attapulgite	T47.6X1	T47.6X2	T47.6X3	T47.6X4	T47.6X5	T47.6X6
Auramine	T65.891	T65.892	T65.893	T65.894	—	—
dye	T65.6X1	T65.6X2	T65.6X3	T65.6X4	—	—
fungicide	T6Ø.3X1	T6Ø.3X2	T6Ø.3X3	T6Ø.3X4	—	—
Auranofin	T39.4X1	T39.4X2	T39.4X3	T39.4X4	T39.4X5	T39.4X6
Aurantiin	T46.991	T46.992	T46.993	T46.994	T46.995	T46.996
Aureomycin	T36.4X1	T36.4X2	T36.4X3	T36.4X4	T36.4X5	T36.4X6
ophthalmic preparation	T49.5X1	T49.5X2	T49.5X3	T49.5X4	T49.5X5	T49.5X6
topical NEC	T49.ØX1	T49.ØX2	T49.ØX3	T49.ØX4	T49.ØX5	T49.ØX6
Aurothioglucose	T39.4X1	T39.4X2	T39.4X3	T39.4X4	T39.4X5	T39.4X6
Aurothioglycanide	T39.4X1	T39.4X2	T39.4X3	T39.4X4	T39.4X5	T39.4X6
Aurothiomalate sodium	T39.4X1	T39.4X2	T39.4X3	T39.4X4	T39.4X5	T39.4X6
Aurotioprol	T39.4X1	T39.4X2	T39.4X3	T39.4X4	T39.4X5	T39.4X6
Automobile fuel	T52.ØX1	T52.ØX2	T52.ØX3	T52.ØX4	—	—
Autonomic nervous system agent NEC	T44.9Ø1	T44.9Ø2	T44.9Ø3	T44.9Ø4	T44.9Ø5	T44.9Ø6
Avlosulfon	T37.1X1	T37.1X2	T37.1X3	T37.1X4	T37.1X5	T37.1X6
Avomine	T42.6X1	T42.6X2	T42.6X3	T42.6X4	T42.6X5	T42.6X6
Axerophthol	T45.2X1	T45.2X2	T45.2X3	T45.2X4	T45.2X5	T45.2X6
Azacitidine	T45.1X1	T45.1X2	T45.1X3	T45.1X4	T45.1X5	T45.1X6
Azacyclonol	T43.591	T43.592	T43.593	T43.594	T43.595	T43.596
Azadirachta	T6Ø.2X1	T6Ø.2X2	T6Ø.2X3	T6Ø.2X4	—	—
Azanidazole	T37.3X1	T37.3X2	T37.3X3	T37.3X4	T37.3X5	T37.3X6
Azapetine	T46.7X1	T46.7X2	T46.7X3	T46.7X4	T46.7X5	T46.7X6
Azapropazone	T39.2X1	T39.2X2	T39.2X3	T39.2X4	T39.2X5	T39.2X6
Azaribine	T45.1X1	T45.1X2	T45.1X3	T45.1X4	T45.1X5	T45.1X6
Azaserine	T45.1X1	T45.1X2	T45.1X3	T45.1X4	T45.1X5	T45.1X6
Azatadine	T45.ØX1	T45.ØX2	T45.ØX3	T45.ØX4	T45.ØX5	T45.ØX6
Azatepa	T45.1X1	T45.1X2	T45.1X3	T45.1X4	T45.1X5	T45.1X6
Azathioprine	T45.1X1	T45.1X2	T45.1X3	T45.1X4	T45.1X5	T45.1X6
Azelaic acid	T49.ØX1	T49.ØX2	T49.ØX3	T49.ØX4	T49.ØX5	T49.ØX6
Azelastine	T45.ØX1	T45.ØX2	T45.ØX3	T45.ØX4	T45.ØX5	T45.ØX6
Azidocillin	T36.ØX1	T36.ØX2	T36.ØX3	T36.ØX4	T36.ØX5	T36.ØX6
Azidothymidine	T37.5X1	T37.5X2	T37.5X3	T37.5X4	T37.5X5	T37.5X6
Azinphos (ethyl) (methyl)	T6Ø.ØX1	T6Ø.ØX2	T6Ø.ØX3	T6Ø.ØX4	—	—
Aziridine (chelating)	T54.1X1	T54.1X2	T54.1X3	T54.1X4	—	—
Azithromycin	T36.3X1	T36.3X2	T36.3X3	T36.3X4	T36.3X5	T36.3X6
Azlocillin	T36.ØX1	T36.ØX2	T36.ØX3	T36.ØX4	T36.ØX5	T36.ØX6
Azobenzene smoke	T65.3X1	T65.3X2	T65.3X3	T65.3X4	—	—
acaricide	T6Ø.8X1	T6Ø.8X2	T6Ø.8X3	T6Ø.8X4	—	—
Azosulfamide	T37.ØX1	T37.ØX2	T37.ØX3	T37.ØX4	T37.ØX5	T37.ØX6
AZT	T37.5X1	T37.5X2	T37.5X3	T37.5X4	T37.5X5	T37.5X6
Aztreonam	T36.1X1	T36.1X2	T36.1X3	T36.1X4	T36.1X5	T36.1X6

Substance	Poisoning, Accidental (unintentional)	Poisoning, Intentional Self-harm	Poisoning, Assault	Poisoning, Undetermined	Adverse Effect	Under-dosing
Azulfidine	T37.ØX1	T37.ØX2	T37.ØX3	T37.ØX4	T37.ØX5	T37.ØX6
Azuresin	T5Ø.8X1	T5Ø.8X2	T5Ø.8X3	T5Ø.8X4	T5Ø.8X5	T5Ø.8X6
b-acetyldigoxin	T46.ØX1	T46.ØX2	T46.ØX3	T46.ØX4	T46.ØX5	T46.ØX6
P-Acetamidophenol	T39.1X1	T39.1X2	T39.1X3	T39.1X4	T39.1X5	T39.1X6
Bacampicillin	T36.ØX1	T36.ØX2	T36.ØX3	T36.ØX4	T36.ØX5	T36.ØX6
Bacillus						
lactobacillus	T47.8X1	T47.8X2	T47.8X3	T47.8X4	T47.8X5	T47.8X6
subtilis	T47.6X1	T47.6X2	T47.6X3	T47.6X4	T47.6X5	T47.6X6
Bacimycin	T49.ØX1	T49.ØX2	T49.ØX3	T49.ØX4	T49.ØX5	T49.ØX6
ophthalmic preparation	T49.5X1	T49.5X2	T49.5X3	T49.5X4	T49.5X5	T49.5X6
Bacitracin zinc	T49.ØX1	T49.ØX2	T49.ØX3	T49.ØX4	T49.ØX5	T49.ØX6
with neomycin	T49.ØX1	T49.ØX2	T49.ØX3	T49.ØX4	T49.ØX5	T49.ØX6
ENT agent	T49.6X1	T49.6X2	T49.6X3	T49.6X4	T49.6X5	T49.6X6
ophthalmic preparation	T49.5X1	T49.5X2	T49.5X3	T49.5X4	T49.5X5	T49.5X6
topical NEC	T49.ØX1	T49.ØX2	T49.ØX3	T49.ØX4	T49.ØX5	T49.ØX6
Baclofen	T42.8X1	T42.8X2	T42.8X3	T42.8X4	T42.8X5	T42.8X6
Baking soda	T5Ø.991	T5Ø.992	T5Ø.993	T5Ø.994	T5Ø.995	T5Ø.996
BAL	T45.8X1	T45.8X2	T45.8X3	T45.8X4	T45.8X5	T45.8X6
Bambuterol	T48.6X1	T48.6X2	T48.6X3	T48.6X4	T48.6X5	T48.6X6
Bamethan (sulfate)	T46.7X1	T46.7X2	T46.7X3	T46.7X4	T46.7X5	T46.7X6
Bamifylline	T48.6X1	T48.6X2	T48.6X3	T48.6X4	T48.6X5	T48.6X6
Bamipine	T45.ØX1	T45.ØX2	T45.ØX3	T45.ØX4	T45.ØX5	T45.ØX6
Baneberry — *see* Actaea spicata						
Banewort — *see* Belladonna						
Barbenyl	T42.3X1	T42.3X2	T42.3X3	T42.3X4	T42.3X5	T42.3X6
Barbexaclone	T42.6X1	T42.6X2	T42.6X3	T42.6X4	T42.6X5	T42.6X6
Barbital	T42.3X1	T42.3X2	T42.3X3	T42.3X4	T42.3X5	T42.3X6
sodium	T42.3X1	T42.3X2	T42.3X3	T42.3X4	T42.3X5	T42.3X6
Barbitone	T42.3X1	T42.3X2	T42.3X3	T42.3X4	T42.3X5	T42.3X6
Barbiturate NEC	T42.3X1	T42.3X2	T42.3X3	T42.3X4	T42.3X5	T42.3X6
with tranquilizer	T42.3X1	T42.3X2	T42.3X3	T42.3X4	T42.3X5	T42.3X6
anesthetic (intravenous)	T41.1X1	T41.1X2	T41.1X3	T41.1X4	T41.1X5	T41.1X6
Barium (carbonate) (chloride) (sulfite)	T57.8X1	T57.8X2	T57.8X3	T57.8X4	—	—
diagnostic agent	T5Ø.8X1	T5Ø.8X2	T5Ø.8X3	T5Ø.8X4	T5Ø.8X5	T5Ø.8X6
pesticide	T6Ø.4X1	T6Ø.4X2	T6Ø.4X3	T6Ø.4X4	—	—
rodenticide	T6Ø.4X1	T6Ø.4X2	T6Ø.4X3	T6Ø.4X4	—	—
sulfate (medicinal)	T5Ø.8X1	T5Ø.8X2	T5Ø.8X3	T5Ø.8X4	T5Ø.8X5	T5Ø.8X6
Barrier cream	T49.3X1	T49.3X2	T49.3X3	T49.3X4	T49.3X5	T49.3X6
Basic fuchsin	T49.ØX1	T49.ØX2	T49.ØX3	T49.ØX4	T49.ØX5	T49.ØX6
Battery acid or fluid	T54.2X1	T54.2X2	T54.2X3	T54.2X4	—	—
Bay rum	T51.8X1	T51.8X2	T51.8X3	T51.8X4	—	—
b-benzalbutyramide	T46.6X1	T46.6X2	T46.6X3	T46.6X4	T46.6X5	T46.6X6
BCG (vaccine)	T5Ø.A91	T5Ø.A92	T5Ø.A93	T5Ø.A94	T5Ø.A95	T5Ø.A96
BCNU	T45.1X1	T45.1X2	T45.1X3	T45.1X4	T45.1X5	T45.1X6
Bearsfoot	T62.2X1	T62.2X2	T62.2X3	T62.2X4	—	—
Beclamide	T42.6X1	T42.6X2	T42.6X3	T42.6X4	T42.6X5	T42.6X6
Beclomethasone	T44.5X1	T44.5X2	T44.5X3	T44.5X4	T44.5X5	T44.5X6
Bee (sting) (venom)	T63.441	T63.442	T63.443	T63.444	—	—
Befunolol	T49.5X1	T49.5X2	T49.5X3	T49.5X4	T49.5X5	T49.5X6
Bekanamycin	T36.5X1	T36.5X2	T36.5X3	T36.5X4	T36.5X5	T36.5X6
Belladonna — *see also* Nightshade						
alkaloids	T44.3X1	T44.3X2	T44.3X3	T44.3X4	T44.3X5	T44.3X6
extract	T44.3X1	T44.3X2	T44.3X3	T44.3X4	T44.3X5	T44.3X6
herb	T44.3X1	T44.3X2	T44.3X3	T44.3X4	T44.3X5	T44.3X6
Bemegride	T5Ø.7X1	T5Ø.7X2	T5Ø.7X3	T5Ø.7X4	T5Ø.7X5	T5Ø.7X6
Benactyzine	T44.3X1	T44.3X2	T44.3X3	T44.3X4	T44.3X5	T44.3X6
Benadryl	T45.ØX1	T45.ØX2	T45.ØX3	T45.ØX4	T45.ØX5	T45.ØX6
Benaprizine	T44.3X1	T44.3X2	T44.3X3	T44.3X4	T44.3X5	T44.3X6
Benazepril	T46.4X1	T46.4X2	T46.4X3	T46.4X4	T46.4X5	T46.4X6
Bencyclane	T46.7X1	T46.7X2	T46.7X3	T46.7X4	T46.7X5	T46.7X6
Bendazol	T46.3X1	T46.3X2	T46.3X3	T46.3X4	T46.3X5	T46.3X6
Bendrofluazide	T5Ø.2X1	T5Ø.2X2	T5Ø.2X3	T5Ø.2X4	T5Ø.2X5	T5Ø.2X6
Bendroflumethiazide	T5Ø.2X1	T5Ø.2X2	T5Ø.2X3	T5Ø.2X4	T5Ø.2X5	T5Ø.2X6
Benemid	T5Ø.4X1	T5Ø.4X2	T5Ø.4X3	T5Ø.4X4	T5Ø.4X5	T5Ø.4X6
Benethamine penicillin	T36.ØX1	T36.ØX2	T36.ØX3	T36.ØX4	T36.ØX5	T36.ØX6
Benexate	T47.1X1	T47.1X2	T47.1X3	T47.1X4	T47.1X5	T47.1X6
Benfluorex	T46.6X1	T46.6X2	T46.6X3	T46.6X4	T46.6X5	T46.6X6
Benfotiamine	T45.2X1	T45.2X2	T45.2X3	T45.2X4	T45.2X5	T45.2X6
Benisone	T49.ØX1	T49.ØX2	T49.ØX3	T49.ØX4	T49.ØX5	T49.ØX6
Benomyl	T6Ø.ØX1	T6Ø.ØX2	T6Ø.ØX3	T6Ø.ØX4	—	—
Benoquin	T49.8X1	T49.8X2	T49.8X3	T49.8X4	T49.8X5	T49.8X6
Benoxinate	T41.3X1	T41.3X2	T41.3X3	T41.3X4	T41.3X5	T41.3X6
Benperidol	T43.4X1	T43.4X2	T43.4X3	T43.4X4	T43.4X5	T43.4X6
Benproperine	T48.3X1	T48.3X2	T48.3X3	T48.3X4	T48.3X5	T48.3X6
Benserazide	T42.8X1	T42.8X2	T42.8X3	T42.8X4	T42.8X5	T42.8X6
Bentazepam	T42.4X1	T42.4X2	T42.4X3	T42.4X4	T42.4X5	T42.4X6
Bentiromide	T5Ø.8X1	T5Ø.8X2	T5Ø.8X3	T5Ø.8X4	T5Ø.8X5	T5Ø.8X6
Bentonite	T49.3X1	T49.3X2	T49.3X3	T49.3X4	T49.3X5	T49.3X6
Benzalbutyramide	T46.6X1	T46.6X2	T46.6X3	T46.6X4	T46.6X5	T46.6X6
Benzalkonium (chloride)	T49.ØX1	T49.ØX2	T49.ØX3	T49.ØX4	T49.ØX5	T49.ØX6
ophthalmic preparation	T49.5X1	T49.5X2	T49.5X3	T49.5X4	T49.5X5	T49.5X6

Substance	Poisoning, Accidental (unintentional)	Poisoning, Intentional Self-harm	Poisoning, Assault	Poisoning, Undetermined	Adverse Effect	Under-dosing
Benzamidosalicylate	T37.1X1	T37.1X2	T37.1X3	T37.1X4	T37.1X5	T37.1X6
(calcium)						
Benzamine	T41.3X1	T41.3X2	T41.3X3	T41.3X4	T41.3X5	T41.3X6
lactate	T49.1X1	T49.1X2	T49.1X3	T49.1X4	T49.1X5	T49.1X6
Benzamphetamine	T5Ø.5X1	T5Ø.5X2	T5Ø.5X3	T5Ø.5X4	T5Ø.5X5	T5Ø.5X6
Benzapril hydrochloride	T46.5X1	T46.5X2	T46.5X3	T46.5X4	T46.5X5	T46.5X6
Benzathine benzylpenicillin	T36.ØX1	T36.ØX2	T36.ØX3	T36.ØX4	T36.ØX5	T36.ØX6
Benzathine penicillin	T36.ØX1	T36.ØX2	T36.ØX3	T36.ØX4	T36.ØX5	T36.ØX6
Benzatropine	T42.8X1	T42.8X2	T42.8X3	T42.8X4	T42.8X5	T42.8X6
Benzbromarone	T5Ø.4X1	T5Ø.4X2	T5Ø.4X3	T5Ø.4X4	T5Ø.4X5	T5Ø.4X6
Benzcarbimine	T45.1X1	T45.1X2	T45.1X3	T45.1X4	T45.1X5	T45.1X6
Benzedrex	T44.991	T44.992	T44.993	T44.994	T44.995	T44.996
Benzedrine (amphetamine)	T43.621	T43.622	T43.623	T43.624	T43.625	T43.626
Benzenamine	T65.3X1	T65.3X2	T65.3X3	T65.3X4	—	—
Benzene	T52.1X1	T52.1X2	T52.1X3	T52.1X4	—	—
homologues (acetyl) (dimethyl) (methyl) (solvent)	T52.2X1	T52.2X2	T52.2X3	T52.2X4	—	—
Benzethonium (chloride)	T49.ØX1	T49.ØX2	T49.ØX3	T49.ØX4	T49.ØX5	T49.ØX6
Benzfetamine	T5Ø.5X1	T5Ø.5X2	T5Ø.5X3	T5Ø.5X4	T5Ø.5X5	T5Ø.5X6
Benzhexol	T44.3X1	T44.3X2	T44.3X3	T44.3X4	T44.3X5	T44.3X6
Benzhydramine (chloride)	T45.ØX1	T45.ØX2	T45.ØX3	T45.ØX4	T45.ØX5	T45.ØX6
Benzidine	T65.891	T65.892	T65.893	T65.894	—	—
Benzilonium bromide	T44.3X1	T44.3X2	T44.3X3	T44.3X4	T44.3X5	T44.3X6
Benzimidazole	T6Ø.3X1	T6Ø.3X2	T6Ø.3X3	T6Ø.3X4	—	—
Benzin (e) — *see* Ligroin						
Benziodarone	T46.3X1	T46.3X2	T46.3X3	T46.3X4	T46.3X5	T46.3X6
Benznidazole	T37.3X1	T37.3X2	T37.3X3	T37.3X4	T37.3X5	T37.3X6
Benzocaine	T41.3X1	T41.3X2	T41.3X3	T41.3X4	T41.3X5	T41.3X6
Benzodiapin	T42.4X1	T42.4X2	T42.4X3	T42.4X4	T42.4X5	T42.4X6
Benzodiazepine NEC	T42.4X1	T42.4X2	T42.4X3	T42.4X4	T42.4X5	T42.4X6
Benzoic acid	T49.ØX1	T49.ØX2	T49.ØX3	T49.ØX4	T49.ØX5	T49.ØX6
with salicylic acid	T49.ØX1	T49.ØX2	T49.ØX3	T49.ØX4	T49.ØX5	T49.ØX6
Benzoin (tincture)	T48.5X1	T48.5X2	T48.5X3	T48.5X4	T48.5X5	T48.5X6
Benzol (benzene)	T52.1X1	T52.1X2	T52.1X3	T52.1X4	—	—
vapor	T52.ØX1	T52.ØX2	T52.ØX3	T52.ØX4	—	—
Benzomorphan	T4Ø.2X1	T4Ø.2X2	T4Ø.2X3	T4Ø.2X4	T4Ø.2X5	T4Ø.2X6
Benzonatate	T48.3X1	T48.3X2	T48.3X3	T48.3X4	T48.3X5	T48.3X6
Benzophenones	T49.3X1	T49.3X2	T49.3X3	T49.3X4	T49.3X5	T49.3X6
Benzopyrone	T46.991	T46.992	T46.993	T46.994	T46.995	T46.996
Benzothiadiazides	T5Ø.2X1	T5Ø.2X2	T5Ø.2X3	T5Ø.2X4	T5Ø.2X5	T5Ø.2X6
Benzoxonium chloride	T49.ØX1	T49.ØX2	T49.ØX3	T49.ØX4	T49.ØX5	T49.ØX6
Benzoylpas calcium	T37.1X1	T37.1X2	T37.1X3	T37.1X4	T37.1X5	T37.1X6
Benzoyl peroxide	T49.ØX1	T49.ØX2	T49.ØX3	T49.ØX4	T49.ØX5	T49.ØX6
Benzperidin	T43.591	T43.592	T43.593	T43.594	T43.595	T43.596
Benzperidol	T43.591	T43.592	T43.593	T43.594	T43.595	T43.596
Benzphetamine	T5Ø.5X1	T5Ø.5X2	T5Ø.5X3	T5Ø.5X4	T5Ø.5X5	T5Ø.5X6
Benzpyrinium bromide	T44.1X1	T44.1X2	T44.1X3	T44.1X4	T44.1X5	T44.1X6
Benzquinamide	T45.ØX1	T45.ØX2	T45.ØX3	T45.ØX4	T45.ØX5	T45.ØX6
Benzthiazide	T5Ø.2X1	T5Ø.2X2	T5Ø.2X3	T5Ø.2X4	T5Ø.2X5	T5Ø.2X6
Benztropine						
anticholinergic	T44.3X1	T44.3X2	T44.3X3	T44.3X4	T44.3X5	T44.3X6
antiparkinson	T42.8X1	T42.8X2	T42.8X3	T42.8X4	T42.8X5	T42.8X6
Benzydamine	T49.ØX1	T49.ØX2	T49.ØX3	T49.ØX4	T49.ØX5	T49.ØX6
Benzyl						
acetate	T52.8X1	T52.8X2	T52.8X3	T52.8X4	—	—
alcohol	T49.ØX1	T49.ØX2	T49.ØX3	T49.ØX4	T49.ØX5	T49.ØX6
benzoate	T49.ØX1	T49.ØX2	T49.ØX3	T49.ØX4	T49.ØX5	T49.ØX6
Benzoic acid	T49.ØX1	T49.ØX2	T49.ØX3	T49.ØX4	T49.ØX5	T49.ØX6
morphine	T4Ø.2X1	T4Ø.2X2	T4Ø.2X3	T4Ø.2X4	—	—
nicotinate	T46.6X1	T46.6X2	T46.6X3	T46.6X4	T46.6X5	T46.6X6
penicillin	T36.ØX1	T36.ØX2	T36.ØX3	T36.ØX4	T36.ØX5	T36.ØX6
Benzylhydrochlorthiazide	T5Ø.2X1	T5Ø.2X2	T5Ø.2X3	T5Ø.2X4	T5Ø.2X5	T5Ø.2X6
Benzylpenicillin	T36.ØX1	T36.ØX2	T36.ØX3	T36.ØX4	T36.ØX5	T36.ØX6
Benzylthiouracil	T38.2X1	T38.2X2	T38.2X3	T38.2X4	T38.2X5	T38.2X6
Bephenium hydroxynaphthoate	T37.4X1	T37.4X2	T37.4X3	T37.4X4	T37.4X5	T37.4X6
Bepridil	T46.1X1	T46.1X2	T46.1X3	T46.1X4	T46.1X5	T46.1X6
Bergamot oil	T65.891	T65.892	T65.893	T65.894	—	—
Bergapten	T5Ø.991	T5Ø.992	T5Ø.993	T5Ø.994	T5Ø.995	T5Ø.996
Berries, poisonous	T62.1X1	T62.1X2	T62.1X3	T62.1X4	—	—
Beryllium (compounds)	T56.7X1	T56.7X2	T56.7X3	T56.7X4	—	—
beta adrenergic blocking agent, heart	T44.7X1	T44.7X2	T44.7X3	T44.7X4	T44.7X5	T44.7X6
Betacarotene	T45.2X1	T45.2X2	T45.2X3	T45.2X4	T45.2X5	T45.2X6
Beta-Chlor	T42.6X1	T42.6X2	T42.6X3	T42.6X4	T42.6X5	T42.6X6
Betahistine	T46.7X1	T46.7X2	T46.7X3	T46.7X4	T46.7X5	T46.7X6
Betaine	T47.5X1	T47.5X2	T47.5X3	T47.5X4	T47.5X5	T47.5X6
Betamethasone	T49.ØX1	T49.ØX2	T49.ØX3	T49.ØX4	T49.ØX5	T49.ØX6
topical	T49.ØX1	T49.ØX2	T49.ØX3	T49.ØX4	T49.ØX5	T49.ØX6
Betamicin	T36.8X1	T36.8X2	T36.8X3	T36.8X4	T36.8X5	T36.8X6
Betanidine	T46.5X1	T46.5X2	T46.5X3	T46.5X4	T46.5X5	T46.5X6
Betaxolol	T44.7X1	T44.7X2	T44.7X3	T44.7X4	T44.7X5	T44.7X6

Substance	Poisoning, Accidental (unintentional)	Poisoning, Intentional Self-harm	Poisoning, Assault	Poisoning, Undetermined	Adverse Effect	Under-dosing
Betazole	T5Ø.8X1	T5Ø.8X2	T5Ø.8X3	T5Ø.8X4	T5Ø.8X5	T5Ø.8X6
Bethanechol	T44.1X1	T44.1X2	T44.1X3	T44.1X4	T44.1X5	T44.1X6
chloride	T44.1X1	T44.1X2	T44.1X3	T44.1X4	T44.1X5	T44.1X6
Bethanidine	T46.5X1	T46.5X2	T46.5X3	T46.5X4	T46.5X5	T46.5X6
Betoxycaine	T41.3X1	T41.3X2	T41.3X3	T41.3X4	T41.3X5	T41.3X6
Betula oil	T49.3X1	T49.3X2	T49.3X3	T49.3X4	T49.3X5	T49.3X6
Bevantolol	T44.7X1	T44.7X2	T44.7X3	T44.7X4	T44.7X5	T44.7X6
Bevonium metilsulfate	T44.3X1	T44.3X2	T44.3X3	T44.3X4	T44.3X5	T44.3X6
Bezafibrate	T46.6X1	T46.6X2	T46.6X3	T46.6X4	T46.6X5	T46.6X6
Bezitramide	T4Ø.4X1	T4Ø.4X2	T4Ø.4X3	T4Ø.4X4	T4Ø.4X5	T4Ø.4X6
BHA	T5Ø.991	T5Ø.992	T5Ø.993	T5Ø.994	T5Ø.995	T5Ø.996
Bhang	T4Ø.7X1	T4Ø.7X2	T4Ø.7X3	T4Ø.7X4	T4Ø.7X5	T4Ø.7X6
BHC (medicinal)	T49.ØX1	T49.ØX2	T49.ØX3	T49.ØX4	T49.ØX5	T49.ØX6
nonmedicinal (vapor)	T53.6X1	T53.6X2	T53.6X3	T53.6X4	—	—
Bialamicol	T37.3X1	T37.3X2	T37.3X3	T37.3X4	T37.3X5	T37.3X6
Bibenzonium bromide	T48.3X1	T48.3X2	T48.3X3	T48.3X4	T48.3X5	T48.3X6
Bibrocathol	T49.5X1	T49.5X2	T49.5X3	T49.5X4	T49.5X5	T49.5X6
Bichloride of mercury — *see* Mercury, chloride						
Bichromates (calcium) (potassium)(sodium) (crystals)	T57.8X1	T57.8X2	T57.8X3	T57.8X4	—	—
fumes	T56.2X1	T56.2X2	T56.2X3	T56.2X4	—	—
Biclotymol	T49.6X1	T49.6X2	T49.6X3	T49.6X4	T49.6X5	T49.6X6
Bicucculine	T5Ø.7X1	T5Ø.7X2	T5Ø.7X3	T5Ø.7X4	T5Ø.7X5	T5Ø.7X6
Bifemelane	T43.291	T43.292	T43.293	T43.294	T43.295	T43.296
Biguanide derivatives, oral	T38.3X1	T38.3X2	T38.3X3	T38.3X4	T38.3X5	T38.3X6
Bile salts	T47.5X1	T47.5X2	T47.5X3	T47.5X4	T47.5X5	T47.5X6
Biligrafin	T5Ø.8X1	T5Ø.8X2	T5Ø.8X3	T5Ø.8X4	T5Ø.8X5	T5Ø.8X6
Bilopaque	T5Ø.8X1	T5Ø.8X2	T5Ø.8X3	T5Ø.8X4	T5Ø.8X5	T5Ø.8X6
Binifibrate	T46.6X1	T46.6X2	T46.6X3	T46.6X4	T46.6X5	T46.6X6
Binitrobenzol	T65.3X1	T65.3X2	T65.3X3	T65.3X4	—	—
Bioflavonoid(s)	T46.991	T46.992	T46.993	T46.994	T46.995	T46.996
Biological substance NEC	T5Ø.9Ø1	T5Ø.9Ø2	T5Ø.9Ø3	T5Ø.9Ø4	T5Ø.9Ø5	T5Ø.9Ø6
Biotin	T45.2X1	T45.2X2	T45.2X3	T45.2X4	T45.2X5	T45.2X6
Biperiden	T44.3X1	T44.3X2	T44.3X3	T44.3X4	T44.3X5	T44.3X6
Bisacodyl	T47.2X1	T47.2X2	T47.2X3	T47.2X4	T47.2X5	T47.2X6
Bisbentiamine	T45.2X1	T45.2X2	T45.2X3	T45.2X4	T45.2X5	T45.2X6
Bisbutiamine	T45.2X1	T45.2X2	T45.2X3	T45.2X4	T45.2X5	T45.2X6
Bisdequalinium (salts) (diacetate)	T49.6X1	T49.6X2	T49.6X3	T49.6X4	T49.6X5	T49.6X6
Bishydroxycoumarin	T45.511	T45.512	T45.513	T45.514	T45.515	T45.516
Bismarsen	T37.8X1	T37.8X2	T37.8X3	T37.8X4	T37.8X5	T37.8X6
Bismuth salts	T47.6X1	T47.6X2	T47.6X3	T47.6X4	T47.6X5	T47.6X6
aluminate	T47.1X1	T47.1X2	T47.1X3	T47.1X4	T47.1X5	T47.1X6
anti-infectives	T37.8X1	T37.8X2	T37.8X3	T37.8X4	T37.8X5	T37.8X6
formic iodide	T49.ØX1	T49.ØX2	T49.ØX3	T49.ØX4	T49.ØX5	T49.ØX6
glycolylarsenate	T49.ØX1	T49.ØX2	T49.ØX3	T49.ØX4	T49.ØX5	T49.ØX6
nonmedicinal (compounds) NEC	T65.91	T65.92	T65.93	T65.94	—	—
subcarbonate	T47.6X1	T47.6X2	T47.6X3	T47.6X4	T47.6X5	T47.6X6
subsalicylate	T37.8X1	T37.8X2	T37.8X3	T37.8X4	T37.8X5	T37.8X6
sulfarsphenamine	T37.8X1	T37.8X2	T37.8X3	T37.8X4	T37.8X5	T37.8X6
Bisoprolol	T44.7X1	T44.7X2	T44.7X3	T44.7X4	T44.7X5	T44.7X6
Bisoxatin	T47.2X1	T47.2X2	T47.2X3	T47.2X4	T47.2X5	T47.2X6
Bisulepin (hydrochloride)	T45.ØX1	T45.ØX2	T45.ØX3	T45.ØX4	T45.ØX5	T45.ØX6
Bithionol	T37.8X1	T37.8X2	T37.8X3	T37.8X4	T37.8X5	T37.8X6
anthelminthic	T37.4X1	T37.4X2	T37.4X3	T37.4X4	T37.4X5	T37.4X6
Bitolterol	T48.6X1	T48.6X2	T48.6X3	T48.6X4	T48.6X5	T48.6X6
Bitoscanate	T37.4X1	T37.4X2	T37.4X3	T37.4X4	T37.4X5	T37.4X6
Bitter almond oil	T62.8X1	T62.8X2	T62.8X3	T62.8X4	—	—
Bittersweet	T62.2X1	T62.2X2	T62.2X3	T62.2X4	—	—
Black						
flag	T6Ø.91	T6Ø.92	T6Ø.93	T6Ø.94	—	—
henbane	T62.2X1	T62.2X2	T62.2X3	T62.2X4	—	—
leaf (40)	T6Ø.91	T6Ø.92	T6Ø.93	T6Ø.94	—	—
widow spider (bite)	T63.311	T63.312	T63.313	T63.314	—	—
antivenin	T5Ø.Z11	T5Ø.Z12	T5Ø.Z13	T5Ø.Z14	T5Ø.Z15	T5Ø.Z16
Blast furnace gas (carbon monoxide from)	T58.8X1	T58.8X2	T58.8X3	T58.8X4	—	—
Bleach	T54.91	T54.92	T54.93	T54.94	—	—
Bleaching agent (medicinal)	T49.4X1	T49.4X2	T49.4X3	T49.4X4	T49.4X5	T49.4X6
Bleomycin	T45.1X1	T45.1X2	T45.1X3	T45.1X4	T45.1X5	T45.1X6
Blockain	T41.3X1	T41.3X2	T41.3X3	T41.3X4	T41.3X5	T41.3X6
infiltration (subcutaneous)	T41.3X1	T41.3X2	T41.3X3	T41.3X4	T41.3X5	T41.3X6
nerve block (peripheral) (plexus)	T41.3X1	T41.3X2	T41.3X3	T41.3X4	T41.3X5	T41.3X6
topical (surface)	T41.3X1	T41.3X2	T41.3X3	T41.3X4	T41.3X5	T41.3X6
Blockers, calcium channel	T46.1X1	T46.1X2	T46.1X3	T46.1X4	T46.1X5	T46.1X6
Blood (derivatives) (natural) (plasma) (whole)	T45.8X1	T45.8X2	T45.8X3	T45.8X4	T45.8X5	T45.8X6
dried	T45.8X1	T45.8X2	T45.8X3	T45.8X4	T45.8X5	T45.8X6
drug affecting NEC	T45.91	T45.92	T45.93	T45.94	T45.95	T45.96

Subterms under main terms may continue to next column or page
Additional Character May Be Required — Refer to the Tabular List for Character Selection
345

Blood ICD-10-CM 2016

Table of Drugs and Chemicals

Substance	Poisoning, Accidental (unintentional)	Poisoning, Intentional Self-harm	Poisoning, Assault	Poisoning, Undetermined	Adverse Effect	Under-dosing
Blood — *continued*						
expander NEC	T45.8X1	T45.8X2	T45.8X3	T45.8X4	T45.8X5	T45.8X6
fraction NEC	T45.8X1	T45.8X2	T45.8X3	T45.8X4	T45.8X5	T45.8X6
substitute (macromolecular)	T45.8X1	T45.8X2	T45.8X3	T45.8X4	T45.8X5	T45.8X6
Blue velvet	T4Ø.2X1	T4Ø.2X2	T4Ø.2X3	T4Ø.2X4	—	—
Bone meal	T62.8X1	T62.8X2	T62.8X3	T62.8X4	—	—
Bonine	T45.ØX1	T45.ØX2	T45.ØX3	T45.ØX4	T45.ØX5	T45.ØX6
Bopindolol	T44.7X1	T44.7X2	T44.7X3	T44.7X4	T44.7X5	T44.7X6
Boracic acid	T49.ØX1	T49.ØX2	T49.ØX3	T49.ØX4	T49.ØX5	T49.ØX6
ENT agent	T49.6X1	T49.6X2	T49.6X3	T49.6X4	T49.6X5	T49.6X6
ophthalmic preparation	T49.5X1	T49.5X2	T49.5X3	T49.5X4	T49.5X5	T49.5X6
Borane complex	T57.8X1	T57.8X2	T57.8X3	T57.8X4	—	—
Borate(s)	T57.8X1	T57.8X2	T57.8X3	T57.8X4	—	—
buffer	T5Ø.991	T5Ø.992	T5Ø.993	T5Ø.994	T5Ø.995	T5Ø.996
cleanser	T54.91	T54.92	T54.93	T54.94	—	—
sodium	T57.8X1	T57.8X2	T57.8X3	T57.8X4	—	—
Borax (cleanser)	T54.91	T54.92	T54.93	T54.94	—	—
Bordeaux mixture	T6Ø.3X1	T6Ø.3X2	T6Ø.3X3	T6Ø.3X4	—	—
Boric acid	T49.ØX1	T49.ØX2	T49.ØX3	T49.ØX4	T49.ØX5	T49.ØX6
ENT agent	T49.6X1	T49.6X2	T49.6X3	T49.6X4	T49.6X5	T49.6X6
ophthalmic preparation	T49.5X1	T49.5X2	T49.5X3	T49.5X4	T49.5X5	T49.5X6
Bornaprine	T44.3X1	T44.3X2	T44.3X3	T44.3X4	T44.3X5	T44.3X6
Boron	T57.8X1	T57.8X2	T57.8X3	T57.8X4	—	—
hydride NEC	T57.8X1	T57.8X2	T57.8X3	T57.8X4	—	—
fumes or gas	T57.8X1	T57.8X2	T57.8X3	T57.8X4	—	—
trifluoride	T59.891	T59.892	T59.893	T59.894	—	—
Botox	T48.291	T48.292	T48.293	T48.294	T48.295	T48.296
Botulinus anti-toxin (type A, B)	T5Ø.Z11	T5Ø.Z12	T5Ø.Z13	T5Ø.Z14	T5Ø.Z15	T5Ø.Z16
Brake fluid vapor	T59.891	T59.892	T59.893	T59.894	—	—
Brallobarbital	T42.3X1	T42.3X2	T42.3X3	T42.3X4	T42.3X5	T42.3X6
Bran (wheat)	T47.4X1	T47.4X2	T47.4X3	T47.4X4	T47.4X5	T47.4X6
Brass (fumes)	T56.891	T56.892	T56.893	T56.894	—	—
Brasso	T52.ØX1	T52.ØX2	T52.ØX3	T52.ØX4	—	—
Bretylium tosilate	T46.2X1	T46.2X2	T46.2X3	T46.2X4	T46.2X5	T46.2X6
Brevital (sodium)	T41.1X1	T41.1X2	T41.1X3	T41.1X4	T41.1X5	T41.1X6
Brinase	T45.3X1	T45.3X2	T45.3X3	T45.3X4	T45.3X5	T45.3X6
British antilewisite	T45.8X1	T45.8X2	T45.8X3	T45.8X4	T45.8X5	T45.8X6
Brodifacoum	T6Ø.4X1	T6Ø.4X2	T6Ø.4X3	T6Ø.4X4	—	—
Bromal (hydrate)	T42.6X1	T42.6X2	T42.6X3	T42.6X4	T42.6X5	T42.6X6
Bromazepam	T42.4X1	T42.4X2	T42.4X3	T42.4X4	T42.4X5	T42.4X6
Bromazine	T45.ØX1	T45.ØX2	T45.ØX3	T45.ØX4	T45.ØX5	T45.ØX6
Brombenzylcyanide	T59.3X1	T59.3X2	T59.3X3	T59.3X4	—	—
Bromelains	T45.3X1	T45.3X2	T45.3X3	T45.3X4	T45.3X5	T45.3X6
Bromethalin	T6Ø.4X1	T6Ø.4X2	T6Ø.4X3	T6Ø.4X4	—	—
Bromhexine	T48.4X1	T48.4X2	T48.4X3	T48.4X4	T48.4X5	T48.4X6
Bromide salts	T42.6X1	T42.6X2	T42.6X3	T42.6X4	T42.6X5	T42.6X6
Bromindione	T45.511	T45.512	T45.513	T45.514	T45.515	T45.516
Bromine						
compounds (medicinal)	T42.6X1	T42.6X2	T42.6X3	T42.6X4	T42.6X5	T42.6X6
sedative	T42.6X1	T42.6X2	T42.6X3	T42.6X4	T42.6X5	T42.6X6
vapor	T59.891	T59.892	T59.893	T59.894	—	—
Bromisoval	T42.6X1	T42.6X2	T42.6X3	T42.6X4	T42.6X5	T42.6X6
Bromisovalum	T42.6X1	T42.6X2	T42.6X3	T42.6X4	T42.6X5	T42.6X6
Bromobenzylcyanide	T59.3X1	T59.3X2	T59.3X3	T59.3X4	—	—
Bromochlorosalicylani-lide	T49.ØX1	T49.ØX2	T49.ØX3	T49.ØX4	T49.ØX5	T49.ØX6
Bromocriptine	T42.8X1	T42.8X2	T42.8X3	T42.8X4	T42.8X5	T42.8X6
Bromodiphenhydramine	T45.ØX1	T45.ØX2	T45.ØX3	T45.ØX4	T45.ØX5	T45.ØX6
Bromoform	T42.6X1	T42.6X2	T42.6X3	T42.6X4	T42.6X5	T42.6X6
Bromophenol blue reagent	T5Ø.991	T5Ø.992	T5Ø.993	T5Ø.994	T5Ø.995	T5Ø.996
Bromopride	T47.8X1	T47.8X2	T47.8X3	T47.8X4	T47.8X5	T47.8X6
Bromosalicylchloranitide	T49.ØX1	T49.ØX2	T49.ØX3	T49.ØX4	T49.ØX5	T49.ØX6
Bromosalicylhydroxamic acid	T37.1X1	T37.1X2	T37.1X3	T37.1X4	T37.1X5	T37.1X6
Bromo-seltzer	T39.1X1	T39.1X2	T39.1X3	T39.1X4	T39.1X5	T39.1X6
Bromoxynil	T6Ø.3X1	T6Ø.3X2	T6Ø.3X3	T6Ø.3X4	—	—
Bromperidol	T43.4X1	T43.4X2	T43.4X3	T43.4X4	T43.4X5	T43.4X6
Brompheniramine	T45.ØX1	T45.ØX2	T45.ØX3	T45.ØX4	T45.ØX5	T45.ØX6
Bromsulfophthalein	T5Ø.8X1	T5Ø.8X2	T5Ø.8X3	T5Ø.8X4	T5Ø.8X5	T5Ø.8X6
Bromural	T42.6X1	T42.6X2	T42.6X3	T42.6X4	T42.6X5	T42.6X6
Bromvaletone	T42.6X1	T42.6X2	T42.6X3	T42.6X4	T42.6X5	T42.6X6
Bronchodilator NEC	T48.6X1	T48.6X2	T48.6X3	T48.6X4	T48.6X5	T48.6X6
Brotizolam	T42.4X1	T42.4X2	T42.4X3	T42.4X4	T42.4X5	T42.4X6
Brovincamine	T46.7X1	T46.7X2	T46.7X3	T46.7X4	T46.7X5	T46.7X6
Brown recluse spider (bite) (venom)	T63.331	T63.332	T63.333	T63.334	—	—
Brown spider (bite) (venom)	T63.391	T63.392	T63.393	T63.394	—	—
Broxaterol	T48.6X1	T48.6X2	T48.6X3	T48.6X4	T48.6X5	T48.6X6
Broxuridine	T45.1X1	T45.1X2	T45.1X3	T45.1X4	T45.1X5	T45.1X6
Broxyquinoline	T37.8X1	T37.8X2	T37.8X3	T37.8X4	T37.8X5	T37.8X6
Bruceine	T48.291	T48.292	T48.293	T48.294	T48.295	T48.296
Brucia	T62.2X1	T62.2X2	T62.2X3	T62.2X4	—	—

Substance	Poisoning, Accidental (unintentional)	Poisoning, Intentional Self-harm	Poisoning, Assault	Poisoning, Undetermined	Adverse Effect	Under-dosing
Brucine	T65.1X1	T65.1X2	T65.1X3	T65.1X4	—	—
Brunswick green — *see* Copper						
Bruten — *see* Ibuprofen						
Bryonia	T47.2X1	T47.2X2	T47.2X3	T47.2X4	T47.2X5	T47.2X6
Buclizine	T45.ØX1	T45.ØX2	T45.ØX3	T45.ØX4	T45.ØX5	T45.ØX6
Buclosamide	T49.ØX1	T49.ØX2	T49.ØX3	T49.ØX4	T49.ØX5	T49.ØX6
Budesonide	T44.5X1	T44.5X2	T44.5X3	T44.5X4	T44.5X5	T44.5X6
Budralazine	T46.5X1	T46.5X2	T46.5X3	T46.5X4	T46.5X5	T46.5X6
Bufferin	T39.Ø11	T39.Ø12	T39.Ø13	T39.Ø14	T39.Ø15	T39.Ø16
Buflomedil	T46.7X1	T46.7X2	T46.7X3	T46.7X4	T46.7X5	T46.7X6
Buformin	T38.3X1	T38.3X2	T38.3X3	T38.3X4	T38.3X5	T38.3X6
Bufotenine	T4Ø.991	T4Ø.992	T4Ø.993	T4Ø.994	—	—
Bufrolin	T48.6X1	T48.6X2	T48.6X3	T48.6X4	T48.6X5	T48.6X6
Bufylline	T48.6X1	T48.6X2	T48.6X3	T48.6X4	T48.6X5	T48.6X6
Bulk filler	T5Ø.5X1	T5Ø.5X2	T5Ø.5X3	T5Ø.5X4	T5Ø.5X5	T5Ø.5X6
cathartic	T47.4X1	T47.4X2	T47.4X3	T47.4X4	T47.4X5	T47.4X6
Bumetanide	T5Ø.1X1	T5Ø.1X2	T5Ø.1X3	T5Ø.1X4	T5Ø.1X5	T5Ø.1X6
Bunaftine	T46.2X1	T46.2X2	T46.2X3	T46.2X4	T46.2X5	T46.2X6
Bunamiodyl	T5Ø.8X1	T5Ø.8X2	T5Ø.8X3	T5Ø.8X4	T5Ø.8X5	T5Ø.8X6
Bunazosin	T44.6X1	T44.6X2	T44.6X3	T44.6X4	T44.6X5	T44.6X6
Bunitrolol	T44.7X1	T44.7X2	T44.7X3	T44.7X4	T44.7X5	T44.7X6
Buphenine	T46.7X1	T46.7X2	T46.7X3	T46.7X4	T46.7X5	T46.7X6
Bupivacaine	T41.3X1	T41.3X2	T41.3X3	T41.3X4	T41.3X5	T41.3X6
infiltration (subcutaneous)	T41.3X1	T41.3X2	T41.3X3	T41.3X4	T41.3X5	T41.3X6
nerve block (peripheral) (plexus)	T41.3X1	T41.3X2	T41.3X3	T41.3X4	T41.3X5	T41.3X6
spinal	T41.3X1	T41.3X2	T41.3X3	T41.3X4	T41.3X5	T41.3X6
Bupranolol	T44.7X1	T44.7X2	T44.7X3	T44.7X4	T44.7X5	T44.7X6
Buprenorphine	T4Ø.4X1	T4Ø.4X2	T4Ø.4X3	T4Ø.4X4	T4Ø.4X5	T4Ø.4X6
Bupropion	T43.291	T43.292	T43.293	T43.294	T43.295	T43.296
Burimamide	T47.1X1	T47.1X2	T47.1X3	T47.1X4	T47.1X5	T47.1X6
Buserelin	T38.891	T38.892	T38.893	T38.894	T38.895	T38.896
Buspirone	T43.591	T43.592	T43.593	T43.594	T43.595	T43.596
Busulfan, busulphan	T45.1X1	T45.1X2	T45.1X3	T45.1X4	T45.1X5	T45.1X6
Butabarbital (sodium)	T42.3X1	T42.3X2	T42.3X3	T42.3X4	T42.3X5	T42.3X6
Butabarbitone	T42.3X1	T42.3X2	T42.3X3	T42.3X4	T42.3X5	T42.3X6
Butabarpal	T42.3X1	T42.3X2	T42.3X3	T42.3X4	T42.3X5	T42.3X6
Butacaine	T41.3X1	T41.3X2	T41.3X3	T41.3X4	T41.3X5	T41.3X6
Butalamine	T46.7X1	T46.7X2	T46.7X3	T46.7X4	T46.7X5	T46.7X6
Butalbital	T42.3X1	T42.3X2	T42.3X3	T42.3X4	T42.3X5	T42.3X6
Butallylonal	T42.3X1	T42.3X2	T42.3X3	T42.3X4	T42.3X5	T42.3X6
Butamben	T41.3X1	T41.3X2	T41.3X3	T41.3X4	T41.3X5	T41.3X6
Butamirate	T48.3X1	T48.3X2	T48.3X3	T48.3X4	T48.3X5	T48.3X6
Butane (distributed in mobile container)	T59.891	T59.892	T59.893	T59.894	—	—
distributed through pipes	T59.891	T59.892	T59.893	T59.894	—	—
incomplete combustion	T58.11	T58.12	T58.13	T58.14	—	—
Butanilicaine	T41.3X1	T41.3X2	T41.3X3	T41.3X4	T41.3X5	T41.3X6
Butanol	T51.3X1	T51.3X2	T51.3X3	T51.3X4	—	—
Butanone, 2-butanone	T52.4X1	T52.4X2	T52.4X3	T52.4X4	—	—
Butantrone	T49.4X1	T49.4X2	T49.4X3	T49.4X4	T49.4X5	T49.4X6
Butaperazine	T43.3X1	T43.3X2	T43.3X3	T43.3X4	T43.3X5	T43.3X6
Butazolidin	T39.2X1	T39.2X2	T39.2X3	T39.2X4	T39.2X5	T39.2X6
Butetamate	T48.6X1	T48.6X2	T48.6X3	T48.6X4	T48.6X5	T48.6X6
Butethal	T42.3X1	T42.3X2	T42.3X3	T42.3X4	T42.3X5	T42.3X6
Butethamate	T44.3X1	T44.3X2	T44.3X3	T44.3X4	T44.3X5	T44.3X6
Buthalitone (sodium)	T41.1X1	T41.1X2	T41.1X3	T41.1X4	T41.1X5	T41.1X6
Butisol (sodium)	T42.3X1	T42.3X2	T42.3X3	T42.3X4	T42.3X5	T42.3X6
Butizide	T5Ø.2X1	T5Ø.2X2	T5Ø.2X3	T5Ø.2X4	T5Ø.2X5	T5Ø.2X6
Butobarbital	T42.3X1	T42.3X2	T42.3X3	T42.3X4	T42.3X5	T42.3X6
sodium	T42.3X1	T42.3X2	T42.3X3	T42.3X4	T42.3X5	T42.3X6
Butobarbitone	T42.3X1	T42.3X2	T42.3X3	T42.3X4	T42.3X5	T42.3X6
Butoconazole (nitrate)	T49.ØX1	T49.ØX2	T49.ØX3	T49.ØX4	T49.ØX5	T49.ØX6
Butorphanol	T4Ø.4X1	T4Ø.4X2	T4Ø.4X3	T4Ø.4X4	T4Ø.4X5	T4Ø.4X6
Butriptyline	T43.Ø11	T43.Ø12	T43.Ø13	T43.Ø14	T43.Ø15	T43.Ø16
Butropium bromide	T44.3X1	T44.3X2	T44.3X3	T44.3X4	T44.3X5	T44.3X6
Buttercups	T62.2X1	T62.2X2	T62.2X3	T62.2X4	—	—
Butter of antimony — *see* Antimony						
Butyl						
acetate (secondary)	T52.8X1	T52.8X2	T52.8X3	T52.8X4	—	—
alcohol	T51.3X1	T51.3X2	T51.3X3	T51.3X4	—	—
aminobenzoate	T41.3X1	T41.3X2	T41.3X3	T41.3X4	T41.3X5	T41.3X6
butyrate	T52.8X1	T52.8X2	T52.8X3	T52.8X4	—	—
carbinol	T51.3X1	T51.3X2	T51.3X3	T51.3X4	—	—
carbitol	T52.3X1	T52.3X2	T52.3X3	T52.3X4	—	—
cellosolve	T52.3X1	T52.3X2	T52.3X3	T52.3X4	—	—
chloral (hydrate)	T42.6X1	T42.6X2	T42.6X3	T42.6X4	T42.6X5	T42.6X6
formate	T52.8X1	T52.8X2	T52.8X3	T52.8X4	—	—
lactate	T52.8X1	T52.8X2	T52.8X3	T52.8X4	—	—
propionate	T52.8X1	T52.8X2	T52.8X3	T52.8X4	—	—
scopolamine bromide	T44.3X1	T44.3X2	T44.3X3	T44.3X4	T44.3X5	T44.3X6
thiobarbital sodium	T41.1X1	T41.1X2	T41.1X3	T41.1X4	T41.1X5	T41.1X6

Blood — Butyl

346 Additional Character May Be Required — Refer to the Tabular List for Character Selection Subterms under main terms may continue to next column or page

Substance	Poisoning, Accidental (unintentional)	Poisoning, Intentional Self-harm	Poisoning, Assault	Poisoning, Undetermined	Adverse Effect	Under-dosing
Butylated hydroxyanisole	T50.991	T50.992	T50.993	T50.994	T50.995	T50.996
Butylchloral hydrate	T42.6X1	T42.6X2	T42.6X3	T42.6X4	T42.6X5	T42.6X6
Butyltoluene	T52.2X1	T52.2X2	T52.2X3	T52.2X4	—	—
Butyn	T41.3X1	T41.3X2	T41.3X3	T41.3X4	T41.3X5	T41.3X6
Butyrophenone (-based tranquilizers)	T43.4X1	T43.4X2	T43.4X3	T43.4X4	T43.4X5	T43.4X6
Cabergoline	T42.8X1	T42.8X2	T42.8X3	T42.8X4	T42.8X5	T42.8X6
Cacodyl, cacodylic acid	T57.0X1	T57.0X2	T57.0X3	T57.0X4	—	—
Cactinomycin	T45.1X1	T45.1X2	T45.1X3	T45.1X4	T45.1X5	T45.1X6
Cade oil	T49.4X1	T49.4X2	T49.4X3	T49.4X4	T49.4X5	T49.4X6
Cadexomer iodine	T49.0X1	T49.0X2	T49.0X3	T49.0X4	T49.0X5	T49.0X6
Cadmium (chloride) (fumes) (oxide)	T56.3X1	T56.3X2	T56.3X3	T56.3X4	—	—
sulfide (medicinal) NEC	T49.4X1	T49.4X2	T49.4X3	T49.4X4	T49.4X5	T49.4X6
Cadralazine	T46.5X1	T46.5X2	T46.5X3	T46.5X4	T46.5X5	T46.5X6
Caffeine	T43.611	T43.612	T43.613	T43.614	T43.615	T43.616
Calabar bean	T62.2X1	T62.2X2	T62.2X3	T62.2X4	—	—
Caladium seguinum	T62.2X1	T62.2X2	T62.2X3	T62.2X4	—	—
Calamine (lotion)	T49.3X1	T49.3X2	T49.3X3	T49.3X4	T49.3X5	T49.3X6
Calcifediol	T45.2X1	T45.2X2	T45.2X3	T45.2X4	T45.2X5	T45.2X6
Calciferol	T45.2X1	T45.2X2	T45.2X3	T45.2X4	T45.2X5	T45.2X6
Calcitonin	T50.991	T50.992	T50.993	T50.994	T50.995	T50.996
Calcitriol	T45.2X1	T45.2X2	T45.2X3	T45.2X4	T45.2X5	T45.2X6
Calcium	T50.3X1	T50.3X2	T50.3X3	T50.3X4	T50.3X5	T50.3X6
actylsalicylate	T39.011	T39.012	T39.013	T39.014	T39.015	T39.016
benzamidosalicylate	T37.1X1	T37.1X2	T37.1X3	T37.1X4	T37.1X5	T37.1X6
bromide	T42.6X1	T42.6X2	T42.6X3	T42.6X4	T42.6X5	T42.6X6
bromolactobionate	T42.6X1	T42.6X2	T42.6X3	T42.6X4	T42.6X5	T42.6X6
carbaspirin	T39.011	T39.012	T39.013	T39.014	T39.015	T39.016
carbimide	T50.6X1	T50.6X2	T50.6X3	T50.6X4	T50.6X5	T50.6X6
carbonate	T47.1X1	T47.1X2	T47.1X3	T47.1X4	T47.1X5	T47.1X6
chloride	T50.991	T50.992	T50.993	T50.994	T50.995	T50.996
anhydrous	T50.991	T50.992	T50.993	T50.994	T50.995	T50.996
cyanide	T57.8X1	T57.8X2	T57.8X3	T57.8X4	—	—
dioctyl sulfosuccinate	T47.4X1	T47.4X2	T47.4X3	T47.4X4	T47.4X5	T47.4X6
disodium edathamil	T45.8X1	T45.8X2	T45.8X3	T45.8X4	T45.8X5	T45.8X6
disodium edetate	T45.8X1	T45.8X2	T45.8X3	T45.8X4	T45.8X5	T45.8X6
dobesilate	T46.991	T46.992	T46.993	T46.994	T46.995	T46.996
EDTA	T45.8X1	T45.8X2	T45.8X3	T45.8X4	T45.8X5	T45.8X6
ferrous citrate	T45.4X1	T45.4X2	T45.4X3	T45.4X4	T45.4X5	T45.4X6
folinate	T45.8X1	T45.8X2	T45.8X3	T45.8X4	T45.8X5	T45.8X6
glubionate	T50.3X1	T50.3X2	T50.3X3	T50.3X4	T50.3X5	T50.3X6
gluconate	T50.3X1	T50.3X2	T50.3X3	T50.3X4	T50.3X5	T50.3X6
gluconogalactogluconate	T50.3X1	T50.3X2	T50.3X3	T50.3X4	T50.3X5	T50.3X6
hydrate, hydroxide	T54.3X1	T54.3X2	T54.3X3	T54.3X4	—	—
hypochlorite	T54.3X1	T54.3X2	T54.3X3	T54.3X4	—	—
iodide	T48.4X1	T48.4X2	T48.4X3	T48.4X4	T48.4X5	T48.4X6
ipodate	T50.8X1	T50.8X2	T50.8X3	T50.8X4	T50.8X5	T50.8X6
lactate	T50.3X1	T50.3X2	T50.3X3	T50.3X4	T50.3X5	T50.3X6
leucovorin	T45.8X1	T45.8X2	T45.8X3	T45.8X4	T45.8X5	T45.8X6
mandelate	T37.91	T37.92	T37.93	T37.94	T37.95	T37.96
oxide	T54.3X1	T54.3X2	T54.3X3	T54.3X4	—	—
pantothenate	T45.2X1	T45.2X2	T45.2X3	T45.2X4	T45.2X5	T45.2X6
phosphate	T50.3X1	T50.3X2	T50.3X3	T50.3X4	T50.3X5	T50.3X6
salicylate	T39.091	T39.092	T39.093	T39.094	T39.095	T39.096
salts	T50.3X1	T50.3X2	T50.3X3	T50.3X4	T50.3X5	T50.3X6
Calculus-dissolving drug	T50.991	T50.992	T50.993	T50.994	T50.995	T50.996
Calomel	T49.0X1	T49.0X2	T49.0X3	T49.0X4	T49.0X5	T49.0X6
Caloric agent	T50.3X1	T50.3X2	T50.3X3	T50.3X4	T50.3X5	T50.3X6
Calusterone	T38.7X1	T38.7X2	T38.7X3	T38.7X4	T38.7X5	T38.7X6
Camazepam	T42.4X1	T42.4X2	T42.4X3	T42.4X4	T42.4X5	T42.4X6
Camomile	T49.0X1	T49.0X2	T49.0X3	T49.0X4	T49.0X5	T49.0X6
Camoquin	T37.2X1	T37.2X2	T37.2X3	T37.2X4	T37.2X5	T37.2X6
Camphor						
insecticide	T60.2X1	T60.2X2	T60.2X3	T60.2X4	—	—
medicinal	T49.8X1	T49.8X2	T49.8X3	T49.8X4	T49.8X5	T49.8X6
Camylofin	T44.3X1	T44.3X2	T44.3X3	T44.3X4	T44.3X5	T44.3X6
Cancer chemotherapy drug regimen	T45.1X1	T45.1X2	T45.1X3	T45.1X4	T45.1X5	T45.1X6
Candeptin	T49.0X1	T49.0X2	T49.0X3	T49.0X4	T49.0X5	T49.0X6
Candicidin	T49.0X1	T49.0X2	T49.0X3	T49.0X4	T49.0X5	T49.0X6
Cannabinol	T40.7X1	T40.7X2	T40.7X3	T40.7X4	T40.7X5	T40.7X6
Cannabis (derivatives)	T40.7X1	T40.7X2	T40.7X3	T40.7X4	T40.7X5	T40.7X6
Canned heat	T51.1X1	T51.1X2	T51.1X3	T51.1X4	—	—
Canrenoic acid	T50.0X1	T50.0X2	T50.0X3	T50.0X4	T50.0X5	T50.0X6
Canrenone	T50.0X1	T50.0X2	T50.0X3	T50.0X4	T50.0X5	T50.0X6
Cantharides, cantharidin, cantharis	T49.8X1	T49.8X2	T49.8X3	T49.8X4	T49.8X5	T49.8X6
Canthaxanthin	T50.991	T50.992	T50.993	T50.994	T50.995	T50.996
Capillary-active drug NEC	T46.901	T46.902	T46.903	T46.904	T46.905	T46.906
Capreomycin	T36.8X1	T36.8X2	T36.8X3	T36.8X4	T36.8X5	T36.8X6
Capsicum	T49.4X1	T49.4X2	T49.4X3	T49.4X4	T49.4X5	T49.4X6
Captafol	T60.3X1	T60.3X2	T60.3X3	T60.3X4	—	—
Captan	T60.3X1	T60.3X2	T60.3X3	T60.3X4	—	—
Captodiame, captodiamine	T43.591	T43.592	T43.593	T43.594	T43.595	T43.596
Captopril	T46.4X1	T46.4X2	T46.4X3	T46.4X4	T46.4X5	T46.4X6
Caramiphen	T44.3X1	T44.3X2	T44.3X3	T44.3X4	T44.3X5	T44.3X6
Carazolol	T44.7X1	T44.7X2	T44.7X3	T44.7X4	T44.7X5	T44.7X6
Carbachol	T44.1X1	T44.1X2	T44.1X3	T44.1X4	T44.1X5	T44.1X6
Carbacrylamine (resin)	T50.3X1	T50.3X2	T50.3X3	T50.3X4	T50.3X5	T50.3X6
Carbamate (insecticide)	T60.0X1	T60.0X2	T60.0X3	T60.0X4	—	—
Carbamate (sedative)	T42.6X1	T42.6X2	T42.6X3	T42.6X4	T42.6X5	T42.6X6
herbicide	T60.0X1	T60.0X2	T60.0X3	T60.0X4	—	—
insecticide	T60.0X1	T60.0X2	T60.0X3	T60.0X4	—	—
Carbamazepine	T42.1X1	T42.1X2	T42.1X3	T42.1X4	T42.1X5	T42.1X6
Carbamide	T47.3X1	T47.3X2	T47.3X3	T47.3X4	T47.3X5	T47.3X6
peroxide	T49.0X1	T49.0X2	T49.0X3	T49.0X4	T49.0X5	T49.0X6
topical	T49.8X1	T49.8X2	T49.8X3	T49.8X4	T49.8X5	T49.8X6
Carbamylcholine chloride	T44.1X1	T44.1X2	T44.1X3	T44.1X4	T44.1X5	T44.1X6
Carbaril	T60.0X1	T60.0X2	T60.0X3	T60.0X4	—	—
Carbarsone	T37.3X1	T37.3X2	T37.3X3	T37.3X4	T37.3X5	T37.3X6
Carbaryl	T60.0X1	T60.0X2	T60.0X3	T60.0X4	—	—
Carbaspirin	T39.011	T39.012	T39.013	T39.014	T39.015	T39.016
Carbazochrome (salicylate) (sodium sulfonate)	T49.4X1	T49.4X2	T49.4X3	T49.4X4	T49.4X5	T49.4X6
Carbenicillin	T36.0X1	T36.0X2	T36.0X3	T36.0X4	T36.0X5	T36.0X6
Carbenoxolone	T47.1X1	T47.1X2	T47.1X3	T47.1X4	T47.1X5	T47.1X6
Carbetapentane	T48.3X1	T48.3X2	T48.3X3	T48.3X4	T48.3X5	T48.3X6
Carbethyl salicylate	T39.091	T39.092	T39.093	T39.094	T39.095	T39.096
Carbidopa (with levodopa)	T42.8X1	T42.8X2	T42.8X3	T42.8X4	T42.8X5	T42.8X6
Carbimazole	T38.2X1	T38.2X2	T38.2X3	T38.2X4	T38.2X5	T38.2X6
Carbinol	T51.1X1	T51.1X2	T51.1X3	T51.1X4	—	—
Carbinoxamine	T45.0X1	T45.0X2	T45.0X3	T45.0X4	T45.0X5	T45.0X6
Carbiphene	T39.8X1	T39.8X2	T39.8X3	T39.8X4	T39.8X5	T39.8X6
Carbitol	T52.3X1	T52.3X2	T52.3X3	T52.3X4	—	—
Carbocaine	T41.3X1	T41.3X2	T41.3X3	T41.3X4	T41.3X5	T41.3X6
infiltration (subcutaneous)	T41.3X1	T41.3X2	T41.3X3	T41.3X4	T41.3X5	T41.3X6
nerve block (peripheral) (plexus)	T41.3X1	T41.3X2	T41.3X3	T41.3X4	T41.3X5	T41.3X6
topical (surface)	T41.3X1	T41.3X2	T41.3X3	T41.3X4	T41.3X5	T41.3X6
Carbocisteine	T48.4X1	T48.4X2	T48.4X3	T48.4X4	T48.4X5	T48.4X6
Carbocromen	T46.3X1	T46.3X2	T46.3X3	T46.3X4	T46.3X5	T46.3X6
Carbol fuchsin	T49.0X1	T49.0X2	T49.0X3	T49.0X4	T49.0X5	T49.0X6
Carbolic acid — see also Phenol	T54.0X1	T54.0X2	T54.0X3	T54.0X4	—	—
Carbolonium (bromide)	T48.1X1	T48.1X2	T48.1X3	T48.1X4	T48.1X5	T48.1X6
Carbo medicinalis	T47.6X1	T47.6X2	T47.6X3	T47.6X4	T47.6X5	T47.6X6
Carbomycin	T36.8X1	T36.8X2	T36.8X3	T36.8X4	T36.8X5	T36.8X6
Carbon						
bisulfide (liquid)	T65.4X1	T65.4X2	T65.4X3	T65.4X4	—	—
vapor	T65.4X1	T65.4X2	T65.4X3	T65.4X4	—	—
dioxide (gas)	T59.7X1	T59.7X2	T59.7X3	T59.7X4	—	—
medicinal	T41.5X1	T41.5X2	T41.5X3	T41.5X4	T41.5X5	T41.5X6
nonmedicinal	T59.7X1	T59.7X2	T59.7X3	T59.7X4	—	—
snow	T49.4X1	T49.4X2	T49.4X3	T49.4X4	T49.4X5	T49.4X6
disulfide (liquid)	T65.4X1	T65.4X2	T65.4X3	T65.4X4	—	—
vapor	T65.4X1	T65.4X2	T65.4X3	T65.4X4	—	—
monoxide (from incomplete combustion)	T58.91	T58.92	T58.93	T58.94	—	—
blast furnace gas	T58.8X1	T58.8X2	T58.8X3	T58.8X4	—	—
butane (distributed in mobile container)	T58.11	T58.12	T58.13	T58.14	—	—
distributed through pipes	T58.11	T58.12	T58.13	T58.14	—	—
charcoal fumes	T58.2X1	T58.2X2	T58.2X3	T58.2X4	—	—
coal	T58.2X1	T58.2X2	T58.2X3	T58.2X4	—	—
coke (in domestic stoves, fireplaces)	T58.2X1	T58.2X2	T58.2X3	T58.2X4	—	—
exhaust gas (motor) not in transit	T58.01	T58.02	T58.03	T58.04	—	—
combustion engine, any not in watercraft	T58.01	T58.02	T58.03	T58.04	—	—
farm tractor, not in transit	T58.01	T58.02	T58.03	T58.04	—	—
gas engine	T58.01	T58.02	T58.03	T58.04	—	—
motor pump	T58.01	T58.02	T58.03	T58.04	—	—
motor vehicle, not in transit	T58.01	T58.02	T58.03	T58.04	—	—
fuel (in domestic use)	T58.2X1	T58.2X2	T58.2X3	T58.2X4	—	—
gas (piped)	T58.11	T58.12	T58.13	T58.14	—	—
in mobile container	T58.11	T58.12	T58.13	T58.14	—	—
piped (natural)	T58.11	T58.12	T58.13	T58.14	—	—
utility	T58.11	T58.12	T58.13	T58.14	—	—
in mobile container	T58.11	T58.12	T58.13	T58.14	—	—
gas (piped)	T58.11	T58.12	T58.13	T58.14	—	—
illuminating gas	T58.11	T58.12	T58.13	T58.14	—	—

Subterms under main terms may continue to next column or page

Additional Character May Be Required — Refer to the Tabular List for Character Selection

Substance	Poisoning, Accidental (unintentional)	Poisoning, Intentional Self-harm	Poisoning, Assault	Poisoning, Undetermined	Adverse Effect	Under-dosing
Carbon — *continued*						
monoxide — *continued*						
industrial fuels or gases, any	T58.8X1	T58.8X2	T58.8X3	T58.8X4	—	—
kerosene (in domestic stoves, fireplaces)	T58.2X1	T58.2X2	T58.2X3	T58.2X4	—	—
kiln gas or vapor	T58.8X1	T58.8X2	T58.8X3	T58.8X4	—	—
motor exhaust gas, not in transit	T58.Ø1	T58.Ø2	T58.Ø3	T58.Ø4	—	—
piped gas (manufactured) (natural)	T58.11	T58.12	T58.13	T58.14	—	—
producer gas	T58.8X1	T58.8X2	T58.8X3	T58.8X4	—	—
propane (distributed in mobile container)	T58.11	T58.12	T58.13	T58.14	—	—
distributed through pipes	T58.11	T58.12	T58.13	T58.14	—	—
solid (in domestic stoves, fireplaces)	T58.2X1	T58.2X2	T58.2X3	T58.2X4	—	—
specified source NEC	T58.8X1	T58.8X2	T58.8X3	T58.8X4	—	—
stove gas	T58.11	T58.12	T58.13	T58.14	—	—
piped	T58.11	T58.12	T58.13	T58.14	—	—
utility gas	T58.11	T58.12	T58.13	T58.14	—	—
piped	T58.11	T58.12	T58.13	T58.14	—	—
water gas	T58.11	T58.12	T58.13	T58.14	—	—
wood (in domestic stoves, fireplaces)	T58.2X1	T58.2X2	T58.2X3	T58.2X4	—	—
tetrachloride (vapor) NEC	T53.ØX1	T53.ØX2	T53.ØX3	T53.ØX4	—	—
liquid (cleansing agent) NEC	T53.ØX1	T53.ØX2	T53.ØX3	T53.ØX4	—	—
solvent	T53.ØX1	T53.ØX2	T53.ØX3	T53.ØX4	—	—
Carbonic acid gas	T59.7X1	T59.7X2	T59.7X3	T59.7X4	—	—
anhydrase inhibitor NEC	T5Ø.2X1	T5Ø.2X2	T5Ø.2X3	T5Ø.2X4	T5Ø.2X5	T5Ø.2X6
Carbophenothion	T6Ø.ØX1	T6Ø.ØX2	T6Ø.ØX3	T6Ø.ØX4	—	—
Carboplatin	T45.1X1	T45.1X2	T45.1X3	T45.1X4	T45.1X5	T45.1X6
Carboprost	T48.ØX1	T48.ØX2	T48.ØX3	T48.ØX4	T48.ØX5	T48.ØX6
Carboquone	T45.1X1	T45.1X2	T45.1X3	T45.1X4	T45.1X5	T45.1X6
Carbowax	T49.3X1	T49.3X2	T49.3X3	T49.3X4	T49.3X5	T49.3X6
Carboxymethylcellulose	T47.4X1	T47.4X2	T47.4X3	T47.4X4	T47.4X5	T47.4X6
Carbrital	T42.3X1	T42.3X2	T42.3X3	T42.3X4	T42.3X5	T42.3X6
Carbromal	T42.6X1	T42.6X2	T42.6X3	T42.6X4	T42.6X5	T42.6X6
Carbutamide	T38.3X1	T38.3X2	T38.3X3	T38.3X4	T38.3X5	T38.3X6
Carbuterol	T48.6X1	T48.6X2	T48.6X3	T48.6X4	T48.6X5	T48.6X6
Cardiac						
depressants	T46.2X1	T46.2X2	T46.2X3	T46.2X4	T46.2X5	T46.2X6
rhythm regulator	T46.2X1	T46.2X2	T46.2X3	T46.2X4	T46.2X5	T46.2X6
specified NEC	T46.2X1	T46.2X2	T46.2X3	T46.2X4	T46.2X5	T46.2X6
Cardiografin	T5Ø.8X1	T5Ø.8X2	T5Ø.8X3	T5Ø.8X4	T5Ø.8X5	T5Ø.8X6
Cardiogreen	T5Ø.8X1	T5Ø.8X2	T5Ø.8X3	T5Ø.8X4	T5Ø.8X5	T5Ø.8X6
Cardiotonic (glycoside) **NEC**	T46.ØX1	T46.ØX2	T46.ØX3	T46.ØX4	T46.ØX5	T46.ØX6
Cardiovascular drug NEC	T46.9Ø1	T46.9Ø2	T46.9Ø3	T46.9Ø4	T46.9Ø5	T46.9Ø6
Cardrase	T5Ø.2X1	T5Ø.2X2	T5Ø.2X3	T5Ø.2X4	T5Ø.2X5	T5Ø.2X6
Carfecillin	T36.ØX1	T36.ØX2	T36.ØX3	T36.ØX4	T36.ØX5	T36.ØX6
Carfenazine	T43.3X1	T43.3X2	T43.3X3	T43.3X4	T43.3X5	T43.3X6
Carfusin	T49.ØX1	T49.ØX2	T49.ØX3	T49.ØX4	T49.ØX5	T49.ØX6
Carindacillin	T36.ØX1	T36.ØX2	T36.ØX3	T36.ØX4	T36.ØX5	T36.ØX6
Carisoprodol	T42.8X1	T42.8X2	T42.8X3	T42.8X4	T42.8X5	T42.8X6
Carmellose	T47.4X1	T47.4X2	T47.4X3	T47.4X4	T47.4X5	T47.4X6
Carminative	T47.5X1	T47.5X2	T47.5X3	T47.5X4	T47.5X5	T47.5X6
Carmofur	T45.1X1	T45.1X2	T45.1X3	T45.1X4	T45.1X5	T45.1X6
Carmustine	T45.1X1	T45.1X2	T45.1X3	T45.1X4	T45.1X5	T45.1X6
Carotene	T45.2X1	T45.2X2	T45.2X3	T45.2X4	T45.2X5	T45.2X6
Carphenazine	T43.3X1	T43.3X2	T43.3X3	T43.3X4	T43.3X5	T43.3X6
Carpipramine	T42.4X1	T42.4X2	T42.4X3	T42.4X4	T42.4X5	T42.4X6
Carprofen	T39.311	T39.312	T39.313	T39.314	T39.315	T39.316
Carpronium chloride	T44.3X1	T44.3X2	T44.3X3	T44.3X4	T44.3X5	T44.3X6
Carrageenan	T47.8X1	T47.8X2	T47.8X3	T47.8X4	T47.8X5	T47.8X6
Carteolol	T44.7X1	T44.7X2	T44.7X3	T44.7X4	T44.7X5	T44.7X6
Carter's Little Pills	T47.2X1	T47.2X2	T47.2X3	T47.2X4	T47.2X5	T47.2X6
Cascara (sagrada)	T47.2X1	T47.2X2	T47.2X3	T47.2X4	T47.2X5	T47.2X6
Cassava	T62.2X1	T62.2X2	T62.2X3	T62.2X4	—	—
Castellani's paint	T49.ØX1	T49.ØX2	T49.ØX3	T49.ØX4	T49.ØX5	T49.ØX6
Castor						
bean	T62.2X1	T62.2X2	T62.2X3	T62.2X4	—	—
oil	T47.2X1	T47.2X2	T47.2X3	T47.2X4	T47.2X5	T47.2X6
Catalase	T45.3X1	T45.3X2	T45.3X3	T45.3X4	T45.3X5	T45.3X6
Caterpillar (sting)	T63.431	T63.432	T63.433	T63.434	—	—
Catha (edulis) (tea)	T43.691	T43.692	T43.693	T43.694	—	—
Cathartic NEC	T47.4X1	T47.4X2	T47.4X3	T47.4X4	T47.4X5	T47.4X6
anthacene derivative	T47.2X1	T47.2X2	T47.2X3	T47.2X4	T47.2X5	T47.2X6
bulk	T47.4X1	T47.4X2	T47.4X3	T47.4X4	T47.4X5	T47.4X6
contact	T47.2X1	T47.2X2	T47.2X3	T47.2X4	T47.2X5	T47.2X6
emollient NEC	T47.4X1	T47.4X2	T47.4X3	T47.4X4	T47.4X5	T47.4X6
irritant NEC	T47.2X1	T47.2X2	T47.2X3	T47.2X4	T47.2X5	T47.2X6

Substance	Poisoning, Accidental (unintentional)	Poisoning, Intentional Self-harm	Poisoning, Assault	Poisoning, Undetermined	Adverse Effect	Under-dosing
Cathartic — *continued*						
mucilage	T47.4X1	T47.4X2	T47.4X3	T47.4X4	T47.4X5	T47.4X6
saline	T47.3X1	T47.3X2	T47.3X3	T47.3X4	T47.3X5	T47.3X6
vegetable	T47.2X1	T47.2X2	T47.2X3	T47.2X4	T47.2X5	T47.2X6
Cathine	T5Ø.5X1	T5Ø.5X2	T5Ø.5X3	T5Ø.5X4	T5Ø.5X5	T5Ø.5X6
Cathomycin	T36.8X1	T36.8X2	T36.8X3	T36.8X4	T36.8X5	T36.8X6
Cation exchange resin	T5Ø.3X1	T5Ø.3X2	T5Ø.3X3	T5Ø.3X4	T5Ø.3X5	T5Ø.3X6
Caustic(s) **NEC**	T54.91	T54.92	T54.93	T54.94	—	—
alkali	T54.3X1	T54.3X2	T54.3X3	T54.3X4	—	—
hydroxide	T54.3X1	T54.3X2	T54.3X3	T54.3X4	—	—
potash	T54.3X1	T54.3X2	T54.3X3	T54.3X4	—	—
soda	T54.3X1	T54.3X2	T54.3X3	T54.3X4	—	—
specified NEC	T54.91	T54.92	T54.93	T54.94	—	—
Ceepryn	T49.ØX1	T49.ØX2	T49.ØX3	T49.ØX4	T49.ØX5	T49.ØX6
ENT agent	T49.6X1	T49.6X2	T49.6X3	T49.6X4	T49.6X5	T49.6X6
lozenges	T49.6X1	T49.6X2	T49.6X3	T49.6X4	T49.6X5	T49.6X6
Cefacetrile	T36.1X1	T36.1X2	T36.1X3	T36.1X4	T36.1X5	T36.1X6
Cefaclor	T36.1X1	T36.1X2	T36.1X3	T36.1X4	T36.1X5	T36.1X6
Cefadroxil	T36.1X1	T36.1X2	T36.1X3	T36.1X4	T36.1X5	T36.1X6
Cefalexin	T36.1X1	T36.1X2	T36.1X3	T36.1X4	T36.1X5	T36.1X6
Cefaloglycin	T36.1X1	T36.1X2	T36.1X3	T36.1X4	T36.1X5	T36.1X6
Cefaloridine	T36.1X1	T36.1X2	T36.1X3	T36.1X4	T36.1X5	T36.1X6
Cefalosporins	T36.1X1	T36.1X2	T36.1X3	T36.1X4	T36.1X5	T36.1X6
Cefalotin	T36.1X1	T36.1X2	T36.1X3	T36.1X4	T36.1X5	T36.1X6
Cefamandole	T36.1X1	T36.1X2	T36.1X3	T36.1X4	T36.1X5	T36.1X6
Cefamycin antibiotic	T36.1X1	T36.1X2	T36.1X3	T36.1X4	T36.1X5	T36.1X6
Cefapirin	T36.1X1	T36.1X2	T36.1X3	T36.1X4	T36.1X5	T36.1X6
Cefatrizine	T36.1X1	T36.1X2	T36.1X3	T36.1X4	T36.1X5	T36.1X6
Cefazedone	T36.1X1	T36.1X2	T36.1X3	T36.1X4	T36.1X5	T36.1X6
Cefazolin	T36.1X1	T36.1X2	T36.1X3	T36.1X4	T36.1X5	T36.1X6
Cefbuperazone	T36.1X1	T36.1X2	T36.1X3	T36.1X4	T36.1X5	T36.1X6
Cefetamet	T36.1X1	T36.1X2	T36.1X3	T36.1X4	T36.1X5	T36.1X6
Cefixime	T36.1X1	T36.1X2	T36.1X3	T36.1X4	T36.1X5	T36.1X6
Cefmenoxime	T36.1X1	T36.1X2	T36.1X3	T36.1X4	T36.1X5	T36.1X6
Cefmetazole	T36.1X1	T36.1X2	T36.1X3	T36.1X4	T36.1X5	T36.1X6
Cefminox	T36.1X1	T36.1X2	T36.1X3	T36.1X4	T36.1X5	T36.1X6
Cefonicid	T36.1X1	T36.1X2	T36.1X3	T36.1X4	T36.1X5	T36.1X6
Cefoperazone	T36.1X1	T36.1X2	T36.1X3	T36.1X4	T36.1X5	T36.1X6
Ceforanide	T36.1X1	T36.1X2	T36.1X3	T36.1X4	T36.1X5	T36.1X6
Cefotaxime	T36.1X1	T36.1X2	T36.1X3	T36.1X4	T36.1X5	T36.1X6
Cefotetan	T36.1X1	T36.1X2	T36.1X3	T36.1X4	T36.1X5	T36.1X6
Cefotiam	T36.1X1	T36.1X2	T36.1X3	T36.1X4	T36.1X5	T36.1X6
Cefoxitin	T36.1X1	T36.1X2	T36.1X3	T36.1X4	T36.1X5	T36.1X6
Cefpimizole	T36.1X1	T36.1X2	T36.1X3	T36.1X4	T36.1X5	T36.1X6
Cefpiramide	T36.1X1	T36.1X2	T36.1X3	T36.1X4	T36.1X5	T36.1X6
Cefradine	T36.1X1	T36.1X2	T36.1X3	T36.1X4	T36.1X5	T36.1X6
Cefroxadine	T36.1X1	T36.1X2	T36.1X3	T36.1X4	T36.1X5	T36.1X6
Cefsulodin	T36.1X1	T36.1X2	T36.1X3	T36.1X4	T36.1X5	T36.1X6
Ceftazidime	T36.1X1	T36.1X2	T36.1X3	T36.1X4	T36.1X5	T36.1X6
Cefteram	T36.1X1	T36.1X2	T36.1X3	T36.1X4	T36.1X5	T36.1X6
Ceftezole	T36.1X1	T36.1X2	T36.1X3	T36.1X4	T36.1X5	T36.1X6
Ceftizoxime	T36.1X1	T36.1X2	T36.1X3	T36.1X4	T36.1X5	T36.1X6
Ceftriaxone	T36.1X1	T36.1X2	T36.1X3	T36.1X4	T36.1X5	T36.1X6
Cefuroxime	T36.1X1	T36.1X2	T36.1X3	T36.1X4	T36.1X5	T36.1X6
Cefuzonam	T36.1X1	T36.1X2	T36.1X3	T36.1X4	T36.1X5	T36.1X6
Celestone	T38.ØX1	T38.ØX2	T38.ØX3	T38.ØX4	T38.ØX5	T38.ØX6
topical	T49.ØX1	T49.ØX2	T49.ØX3	T49.ØX4	T49.ØX5	T49.ØX6
Celiprolol	T44.7X1	T44.7X2	T44.7X3	T44.7X4	T44.7X5	T44.7X6
Cellosolve	T52.91	T52.92	T52.93	T52.94	—	—
Cell stimulants and proliferants	T49.8X1	T49.8X2	T49.8X3	T49.8X4	T49.8X5	T49.8X6
Cellulose						
cathartic	T47.4X1	T47.4X2	T47.4X3	T47.4X4	T47.4X5	T47.4X6
hydroxyethyl	T47.4X1	T47.4X2	T47.4X3	T47.4X4	T47.4X5	T47.4X6
nitrates (topical)	T49.3X1	T49.3X2	T49.3X3	T49.3X4	T49.3X5	T49.3X6
oxidized	T49.4X1	T49.4X2	T49.4X3	T49.4X4	T49.4X5	T49.4X6
Centipede (bite)	T63.411	T63.412	T63.413	T63.414	—	—
Central nervous system						
depressants	T42.71	T42.72	T42.73	T42.74	T42.75	T42.76
anesthetic (general) NEC	T41.2Ø1	T41.2Ø2	T41.2Ø3	T41.2Ø4	T41.2Ø5	T41.2Ø6
gases NEC	T41.ØX1	T41.ØX2	T41.ØX3	T41.ØX4	T41.ØX5	T41.ØX6
intravenous	T41.1X1	T41.1X2	T41.1X3	T41.1X4	T41.1X5	T41.1X6
barbiturates	T42.3X1	T42.3X2	T42.3X3	T42.3X4	T42.3X5	T42.3X6
benzodiazepines	T42.4X1	T42.4X2	T42.4X3	T42.4X4	T42.4X5	T42.4X6
bromides	T42.6X1	T42.6X2	T42.6X3	T42.6X4	T42.6X5	T42.6X6
cannabis sativa	T4Ø.7X1	T4Ø.7X2	T4Ø.7X3	T4Ø.7X4	T4Ø.7X5	T4Ø.7X6
chloral hydrate	T42.6X1	T42.6X2	T42.6X3	T42.6X4	T42.6X5	T42.6X6
ethanol	T51.ØX1	T51.ØX2	T51.ØX3	T51.ØX4	—	—
hallucinogenics	T4Ø.9Ø1	T4Ø.9Ø2	T4Ø.9Ø3	T4Ø.9Ø4	T4Ø.9Ø5	T4Ø.9Ø6
hypnotics	T42.71	T42.72	T42.73	T42.74	T42.75	T42.76
specified NEC	T42.6X1	T42.6X2	T42.6X3	T42.6X4	T42.6X5	T42.6X6
muscle relaxants	T42.8X1	T42.8X2	T42.8X3	T42.8X4	T42.8X5	T42.8X6
paraldehyde	T42.6X1	T42.6X2	T42.6X3	T42.6X4	T42.6X5	T42.6X6

Substance	Poisoning, Accidental (unintentional)	Poisoning, Intentional Self-harm	Poisoning, Assault	Poisoning, Undetermined	Adverse Effect	Under-dosing
Central nervous system — *continued*						
depressants — *continued*						
sedatives; sedative-hypnotics	T42.71	T42.72	T42.73	T42.74	T42.75	T42.76
mixed NEC	T42.6X1	T42.6X2	T42.6X3	T42.6X4	T42.6X5	T42.6X6
specified NEC	T42.6X1	T42.6X2	T42.6X3	T42.6X4	T42.6X5	T42.6X6
muscle-tone depressants	T42.8X1	T42.8X2	T42.8X3	T42.8X4	T42.8X5	T42.8X6
stimulants	T43.6Ø1	T43.6Ø2	T43.6Ø3	T43.6Ø4	T43.6Ø5	T43.6Ø6
amphetamines	T43.621	T43.622	T43.623	T43.624	T43.625	T43.626
analeptics	T5Ø.7X1	T5Ø.7X2	T5Ø.7X3	T5Ø.7X4	T5Ø.7X5	T5Ø.7X6
antidepressants	T43.2Ø1	T43.2Ø2	T43.2Ø3	T43.2Ø4	T43.2Ø5	T43.2Ø6
opiate antagonists	T5Ø.7X1	T5Ø.7X2	T5Ø.7X3	T5Ø.7X4	T5Ø.7X5	T5Ø.7X6
specified NEC	T43.691	T43.692	T43.693	T43.694	T43.695	T43.696
Cephalexin	T36.1X1	T36.1X2	T36.1X3	T36.1X4	T36.1X5	T36.1X6
Cephaloglycin	T36.1X1	T36.1X2	T36.1X3	T36.1X4	T36.1X5	T36.1X6
Cephaloridine	T36.1X1	T36.1X2	T36.1X3	T36.1X4	T36.1X5	T36.1X6
Cephalosporins	T36.1X1	T36.1X2	T36.1X3	T36.1X4	T36.1X5	T36.1X6
N (adicillin)	T36.ØX1	T36.ØX2	T36.ØX3	T36.ØX4	T36.ØX5	T36.ØX6
Cephalothin	T36.1X1	T36.1X2	T36.1X3	T36.1X4	T36.1X5	T36.1X6
Cephalotin	T36.1X1	T36.1X2	T36.1X3	T36.1X4	T36.1X5	T36.1X6
Cephradine	T36.1X1	T36.1X2	T36.1X3	T36.1X4	T36.1X5	T36.1X6
Cerbera (odallam)	T62.2X1	T62.2X2	T62.2X3	T62.2X4	—	—
Cerberin	T46.ØX1	T46.ØX2	T46.ØX3	T46.ØX4	T46.ØX5	T46.ØX6
Cerebral stimulants	T43.6Ø1	T43.6Ø2	T43.6Ø3	T43.6Ø4	T43.6Ø5	T43.6Ø6
psychotherapeutic	T43.6Ø1	T43.6Ø2	T43.6Ø3	T43.6Ø4	T43.6Ø5	T43.6Ø6
specified NEC	T43.691	T43.692	T43.693	T43.694	T43.695	T43.696
Cerium oxalate	T45.ØX1	T45.ØX2	T45.ØX3	T45.ØX4	T45.ØX5	T45.ØX6
Cerous oxalate	T45.ØX1	T45.ØX2	T45.ØX3	T45.ØX4	T45.ØX5	T45.ØX6
Ceruletide	T5Ø.8X1	T5Ø.8X2	T5Ø.8X3	T5Ø.8X4	T5Ø.8X5	T5Ø.8X6
Cetalkonium (chloride)	T49.ØX1	T49.ØX2	T49.ØX3	T49.ØX4	T49.ØX5	T49.ØX6
Cethexonium chloride	T49.ØX1	T49.ØX2	T49.ØX3	T49.ØX4	T49.ØX5	T49.ØX6
Cetiedil	T46.7X1	T46.7X2	T46.7X3	T46.7X4	T46.7X5	T46.7X6
Cetirizine	T45.ØX1	T45.ØX2	T45.ØX3	T45.ØX4	T45.ØX5	T45.ØX6
Cetomacrogol	T5Ø.991	T5Ø.992	T5Ø.993	T5Ø.994	T5Ø.995	T5Ø.996
Cetotiamine	T45.2X1	T45.2X2	T45.2X3	T45.2X4	T45.2X5	T45.2X6
Cetoxime	T45.ØX1	T45.ØX2	T45.ØX3	T45.ØX4	T45.ØX5	T45.ØX6
Cetraxate	T47.1X1	T47.1X2	T47.1X3	T47.1X4	T47.1X5	T47.1X6
Cetrimide	T49.ØX1	T49.ØX2	T49.ØX3	T49.ØX4	T49.ØX5	T49.ØX6
Cetrimonium (bromide)	T49.ØX1	T49.ØX2	T49.ØX3	T49.ØX4	T49.ØX5	T49.ØX6
Cetylpyridinium chloride	T49.ØX1	T49.ØX2	T49.ØX3	T49.ØX4	T49.ØX5	T49.ØX6
ENT agent	T49.6X1	T49.6X2	T49.6X3	T49.6X4	T49.6X5	T49.6X6
lozenges	T49.6X1	T49.6X2	T49.6X3	T49.6X4	T49.6X5	T49.6X6
Cevadilla — *see* Sabadilla						
Cevitamic acid	T45.2X1	T45.2X2	T45.2X3	T45.2X4	T45.2X5	T45.2X6
Chalk, precipitated	T47.1X1	T47.1X2	T47.1X3	T47.1X4	T47.1X5	T47.1X6
Chamomile	T49.ØX1	T49.ØX2	T49.ØX3	T49.ØX4	T49.ØX5	T49.ØX6
Ch'an su	T46.ØX1	T46.ØX2	T46.ØX3	T46.ØX4	T46.ØX5	T46.ØX6
Charcoal	T47.6X1	T47.6X2	T47.6X3	T47.6X4	T47.6X5	T47.6X6
activated — *see also* Charcoal, medicinal	T47.6X1	T47.6X2	T47.6X3	T47.6X4	T47.6X5	T47.6X6
fumes (Carbon monoxide)	T58.2X1	T58.2X2	T58.2X3	T58.2X4	—	—
industrial	T58.8X1	T58.8X2	T58.8X3	T58.8X4	—	—
medicinal (activated)	T47.6X1	T47.6X2	T47.6X3	T47.6X4	T47.6X5	T47.6X6
antidiarrheal	T47.6X1	T47.6X2	T47.6X3	T47.6X4	T47.6X5	T47.6X6
poison control	T47.8X1	T47.8X2	T47.8X3	T47.8X4	T47.8X5	T47.8X6
specified use other than for diarrhea	T47.8X1	T47.8X2	T47.8X3	T47.8X4	T47.8X5	T47.8X6
topical	T49.8X1	T49.8X2	T49.8X3	T49.8X4	T49.8X5	T49.8X6
Chaulmosulfone	T37.1X1	T37.1X2	T37.1X3	T37.1X4	T37.1X5	T37.1X6
Chelating agent NEC	T5Ø.6X1	T5Ø.6X2	T5Ø.6X3	T5Ø.6X4	T5Ø.6X5	T5Ø.6X6
Chelidonium majus	T62.2X1	T62.2X2	T62.2X3	T62.2X4	—	—
Chemical substance NEC	T65.91	T65.92	T65.93	T65.94	—	—
Chenodeoxycholic acid	T47.5X1	T47.5X2	T47.5X3	T47.5X4	T47.5X5	T47.5X6
Chenodiol	T47.5X1	T47.5X2	T47.5X3	T47.5X4	T47.5X5	T47.5X6
Chenopodium	T37.4X1	T37.4X2	T37.4X3	T37.4X4	T37.4X5	T37.4X6
Cherry laurel	T62.2X1	T62.2X2	T62.2X3	T62.2X4	—	—
Chinidin (e)	T46.2X1	T46.2X2	T46.2X3	T46.2X4	T46.2X5	T46.2X6
Chiniofon	T37.8X1	T37.8X2	T37.8X3	T37.8X4	T37.8X5	T37.8X6
Chlophedianol	T48.3X1	T48.3X2	T48.3X3	T48.3X4	T48.3X5	T48.3X6
Chloral	T42.6X1	T42.6X2	T42.6X3	T42.6X4	T42.6X5	T42.6X6
derivative	T42.6X1	T42.6X2	T42.6X3	T42.6X4	T42.6X5	T42.6X6
hydrate	T42.6X1	T42.6X2	T42.6X3	T42.6X4	T42.6X5	T42.6X6
Chloralamide	T42.6X1	T42.6X2	T42.6X3	T42.6X4	T42.6X5	T42.6X6
Chloralodol	T42.6X1	T42.6X2	T42.6X3	T42.6X4	T42.6X5	T42.6X6
Chloralose	T6Ø.4X1	T6Ø.4X2	T6Ø.4X3	T6Ø.4X4	—	—
Chlorambucil	T45.1X1	T45.1X2	T45.1X3	T45.1X4	T45.1X5	T45.1X6
Chloramine	T57.8X1	T57.8X2	T57.8X3	T57.8X4	—	—
T	T49.ØX1	T49.ØX2	T49.ØX3	T49.ØX4	T49.ØX5	T49.ØX6
topical	T49.ØX1	T49.ØX2	T49.ØX3	T49.ØX4	T49.ØX5	T49.ØX6
Chloramphenicol	T36.2X1	T36.2X2	T36.2X3	T36.2X4	T36.2X5	T36.2X6
ENT agent	T49.6X1	T49.6X2	T49.6X3	T49.6X4	T49.6X5	T49.6X6
ophthalmic preparation	T49.5X1	T49.5X2	T49.5X3	T49.5X4	T49.5X5	T49.5X6

Substance	Poisoning, Accidental (unintentional)	Poisoning, Intentional Self-harm	Poisoning, Assault	Poisoning, Undetermined	Adverse Effect	Under-dosing
Chloramphenicol — *continued*						
topical NEC	T49.ØX1	T49.ØX2	T49.ØX3	T49.ØX4	T49.ØX5	T49.ØX6
Chlorate (potassium) (sodium) **NEC**	T6Ø.3X1	T6Ø.3X2	T6Ø.3X3	T6Ø.3X4	—	—
herbicide	T6Ø.3X1	T6Ø.3X2	T6Ø.3X3	T6Ø.3X4	—	—
Chlorazanil	T5Ø.2X1	T5Ø.2X2	T5Ø.2X3	T5Ø.2X4	T5Ø.2X5	T5Ø.2X6
Chlorbenzene, chlorbenzol	T53.7X1	T53.7X2	T53.7X3	T53.7X4	—	—
Chlorbenzoxamine	T44.3X1	T44.3X2	T44.3X3	T44.3X4	T44.3X5	T44.3X6
Chlorbutol	T42.6X1	T42.6X2	T42.6X3	T42.6X4	T42.6X5	T42.6X6
Chlorcyclizine	T45.ØX1	T45.ØX2	T45.ØX3	T45.ØX4	T45.ØX5	T45.ØX6
Chlordan (e) (dust)	T6Ø.1X1	T6Ø.1X2	T6Ø.1X3	T6Ø.1X4	—	—
Chlordantoin	T49.ØX1	T49.ØX2	T49.ØX3	T49.ØX4	T49.ØX5	T49.ØX6
Chlordiazepoxide	T42.4X1	T42.4X2	T42.4X3	T42.4X4	T42.4X5	T42.4X6
Chlordiethyl benzamide	T49.3X1	T49.3X2	T49.3X3	T49.3X4	T49.3X5	T49.3X6
Chloresium	T49.8X1	T49.8X2	T49.8X3	T49.8X4	T49.8X5	T49.8X6
Chlorethiazol	T42.6X1	T42.6X2	T42.6X3	T42.6X4	T42.6X5	T42.6X6
Chlorethyl — *see* Ethyl chloride						
Chloretone	T42.6X1	T42.6X2	T42.6X3	T42.6X4	T42.6X5	T42.6X6
Chlorex	T53.6X1	T53.6X2	T53.6X3	T53.6X4	—	—
insecticide	T6Ø.1X1	T6Ø.1X2	T6Ø.1X3	T6Ø.1X4	—	—
Chlorfenvinphos	T6Ø.ØX1	T6Ø.ØX2	T6Ø.ØX3	T6Ø.ØX4	—	—
Chlorhexadol	T42.6X1	T42.6X2	T42.6X3	T42.6X4	T42.6X5	T42.6X6
Chlorhexamide	T45.1X1	T45.1X2	T45.1X3	T45.1X4	T45.1X5	T45.1X6
Chlorhexidine	T49.ØX1	T49.ØX2	T49.ØX3	T49.ØX4	T49.ØX5	T49.ØX6
Chlorhydroxyquinolin	T49.ØX1	T49.ØX2	T49.ØX3	T49.ØX4	T49.ØX5	T49.ØX6
Chloride of lime (bleach)	T54.3X1	T54.3X2	T54.3X3	T54.3X4	—	—
Chlorimipramine	T43.Ø11	T43.Ø12	T43.Ø13	T43.Ø14	T43.Ø15	T43.Ø16
Chlorinated						
camphene	T53.6X1	T53.6X2	T53.6X3	T53.6X4	—	—
diphenyl	T53.7X1	T53.7X2	T53.7X3	T53.7X4	—	—
hydrocarbons NEC	T53.91	T53.92	T53.93	T53.94	—	—
solvents	T53.91	T53.92	T53.93	T53.94	—	—
lime (bleach)	T54.3X1	T54.3X2	T54.3X3	T54.3X4	—	—
and boric acid solution	T49.ØX1	T49.ØX2	T49.ØX3	T49.ØX4	T49.ØX5	T49.ØX6
naphthalene (insecticide)	T6Ø.1X1	T6Ø.1X2	T6Ø.1X3	T6Ø.1X4	—	—
industrial (non-pesticide)	T53.7X1	T53.7X2	T53.7X3	T53.7X4	—	—
pesticide NEC	T6Ø.8X1	T6Ø.8X2	T6Ø.8X3	T6Ø.8X4	—	—
soda — *see also* sodium hypochlorite						
solution	T49.ØX1	T49.ØX2	T49.ØX3	T49.ØX4	T49.ØX5	T49.ØX6
Chlorine (fumes) (gas)	T59.4X1	T59.4X2	T59.4X3	T59.4X4	—	—
bleach	T54.3X1	T54.3X2	T54.3X3	T54.3X4	—	—
compound gas NEC	T59.4X1	T59.4X2	T59.4X3	T59.4X4	—	—
disinfectant	T59.4X1	T59.4X2	T59.4X3	T59.4X4	—	—
releasing agents NEC	T59.4X1	T59.4X2	T59.4X3	T59.4X4	—	—
Chlorisondamine chloride	T46.991	T46.992	T46.993	T46.994	T46.995	T46.996
Chlormadinone	T38.5X1	T38.5X2	T38.5X3	T38.5X4	T38.5X5	T38.5X6
Chlormephos	T6Ø.ØX1	T6Ø.ØX2	T6Ø.ØX3	T6Ø.ØX4	—	—
Chlormerodrin	T5Ø.2X1	T5Ø.2X2	T5Ø.2X3	T5Ø.2X4	T5Ø.2X5	T5Ø.2X6
Chlormethiazole	T42.6X1	T42.6X2	T42.6X3	T42.6X4	T42.6X5	T42.6X6
Chlormethine	T45.1X1	T45.1X2	T45.1X3	T45.1X4	T45.1X5	T45.1X6
Chlormethylenecycline	T36.4X1	T36.4X2	T36.4X3	T36.4X4	T36.4X5	T36.4X6
Chlormezanone	T42.6X1	T42.6X2	T42.6X3	T42.6X4	T42.6X5	T42.6X6
Chloroacetic acid	T6Ø.3X1	T6Ø.3X2	T6Ø.3X3	T6Ø.3X4	—	—
Chloroacetone	T59.3X1	T59.3X2	T59.3X3	T59.3X4	—	—
Chloroacetophenone	T59.3X1	T59.3X2	T59.3X3	T59.3X4	—	—
Chloroaniline	T53.7X1	T53.7X2	T53.7X3	T53.7X4	—	—
Chlorobenzene, chlorobenzol	T53.7X1	T53.7X2	T53.7X3	T53.7X4	—	—
Chlorobromomethane (fire extinguisher)	T53.6X1	T53.6X2	T53.6X3	T53.6X4	—	—
Chlorobutanol	T49.ØX1	T49.ØX2	T49.ØX3	T49.ØX4	T49.ØX5	T49.ØX6
Chlorocresol	T49.ØX1	T49.ØX2	T49.ØX3	T49.ØX4	T49.ØX5	T49.ØX6
Chlorodehydromethyltestosterone	T38.7X1	T38.7X2	T38.7X3	T38.7X4	T38.7X5	T38.7X6
Chlorodinitrobenzene	T53.7X1	T53.7X2	T53.7X3	T53.7X4	—	—
dust or vapor	T53.7X1	T53.7X2	T53.7X3	T53.7X4	—	—
Chlorodiphenyl	T53.7X1	T53.7X2	T53.7X3	T53.7X4	—	—
Chloroethane — *see* Ethyl chloride						
Chloroethylene	T53.6X1	T53.6X2	T53.6X3	T53.6X4	—	—
Chlorofluorocarbons	T53.5X1	T53.5X2	T53.5X3	T53.5X4	—	—
Chloroform (fumes) (vapor)	T53.1X1	T53.1X2	T53.1X3	T53.1X4	—	—
anesthetic	T41.ØX1	T41.ØX2	T41.ØX3	T41.ØX4	T41.ØX5	T41.ØX6
solvent	T53.1X1	T53.1X2	T53.1X3	T53.1X4	—	—
water, concentrated	T41.ØX1	T41.ØX2	T41.ØX3	T41.ØX4	T41.ØX5	T41.ØX6
Chloroguanide	T37.2X1	T37.2X2	T37.2X3	T37.2X4	T37.2X5	T37.2X6
Chloromycetin	T36.2X1	T36.2X2	T36.2X3	T36.2X4	T36.2X5	T36.2X6
ENT agent	T49.6X1	T49.6X2	T49.6X3	T49.6X4	T49.6X5	T49.6X6
ophthalmic preparation	T49.5X1	T49.5X2	T49.5X3	T49.5X4	T49.5X5	T49.5X6
otic solution	T49.6X1	T49.6X2	T49.6X3	T49.6X4	T49.6X5	T49.6X6
topical NEC	T49.ØX1	T49.ØX2	T49.ØX3	T49.ØX4	T49.ØX5	T49.ØX6
Chloronitrobenzene	T53.7X1	T53.7X2	T53.7X3	T53.7X4	—	—
dust or vapor	T53.7X1	T53.7X2	T53.7X3	T53.7X4	—	—

Substance	Poisoning, Accidental (unintentional)	Poisoning, Intentional Self-harm	Poisoning, Assault	Poisoning, Undetermined	Adverse Effect	Under-dosing
Chlorophacinone	T6Ø.4X1	T6Ø.4X2	T6Ø.4X3	T6Ø.4X4	—	—
Chlorophenol	T53.7X1	T53.7X2	T53.7X3	T53.7X4	—	—
Chlorophenothane	T6Ø.1X1	T6Ø.1X2	T6Ø.1X3	T6Ø.1X4	—	—
Chlorophyll	T5Ø.991	T5Ø.992	T5Ø.993	T5Ø.994	T5Ø.995	T5Ø.996
Chloropicrin (fumes)	T53.6X1	T53.6X2	T53.6X3	T53.6X4	—	—
fumigant	T6Ø.8X1	T6Ø.8X2	T6Ø.8X3	T6Ø.8X4	—	—
fungicide	T6Ø.3X1	T6Ø.3X2	T6Ø.3X3	T6Ø.3X4	—	—
pesticide	T6Ø.8X1	T6Ø.8X2	T6Ø.8X3	T6Ø.8X4	—	—
Chloroprocaine	T41.3X1	T41.3X2	T41.3X3	T41.3X4	T41.3X5	T41.3X6
infiltration (subcutaneous)	T41.3X1	T41.3X2	T41.3X3	T41.3X4	T41.3X5	T41.3X6
nerve block (peripheral) (plexus)	T41.3X1	T41.3X2	T41.3X3	T41.3X4	T41.3X5	T41.3X6
spinal	T41.3X1	T41.3X2	T41.3X3	T41.3X4	T41.3X5	T41.3X6
Chloroptic	T49.5X1	T49.5X2	T49.5X3	T49.5X4	T49.5X5	T49.5X6
Chloropurine	T45.1X1	T45.1X2	T45.1X3	T45.1X4	T45.1X5	T45.1X6
Chloropyramine	T45.ØX1	T45.ØX2	T45.ØX3	T45.ØX4	T45.ØX5	T45.ØX6
Chloropyrifos	T6Ø.ØX1	T6Ø.ØX2	T6Ø.ØX3	T6Ø.ØX4	—	—
Chloropyrilene	T45.ØX1	T45.ØX2	T45.ØX3	T45.ØX4	T45.ØX5	T45.ØX6
Chloroquine	T37.2X1	T37.2X2	T37.2X3	T37.2X4	T37.2X5	T37.2X6
Chlorothalonil	T6Ø.3X1	T6Ø.3X2	T6Ø.3X3	T6Ø.3X4	—	—
Chlorothen	T45.ØX1	T45.ØX2	T45.ØX3	T45.ØX4	T45.ØX5	T45.ØX6
Chlorothiazide	T5Ø.2X1	T5Ø.2X2	T5Ø.2X3	T5Ø.2X4	T5Ø.2X5	T5Ø.2X6
Chlorothymol	T49.4X1	T49.4X2	T49.4X3	T49.4X4	T49.4X5	T49.4X6
Chlorotrianisene	T38.5X1	T38.5X2	T38.5X3	T38.5X4	T38.5X5	T38.5X6
Chlorovinyldichloroarsine, not in war	T57.ØX1	T57.ØX2	T57.ØX3	T57.ØX4	—	—
Chloroxine	T49.4X1	T49.4X2	T49.4X3	T49.4X4	T49.4X5	T49.4X6
Chloroxylenol	T49.ØX1	T49.ØX2	T49.ØX3	T49.ØX4	T49.ØX5	T49.ØX6
Chlorphenamine	T45.ØX1	T45.ØX2	T45.ØX3	T45.ØX4	T45.ØX5	T45.ØX6
Chlorphenesin	T42.8X1	T42.8X2	T42.8X3	T42.8X4	T42.8X5	T42.8X6
topical (antifungal)	T49.ØX1	T49.ØX2	T49.ØX3	T49.ØX4	T49.ØX5	T49.ØX6
Chlorpheniramine	T45.ØX1	T45.ØX2	T45.ØX3	T45.ØX4	T45.ØX5	T45.ØX6
Chlorphenoxamine	T45.ØX1	T45.ØX2	T45.ØX3	T45.ØX4	T45.ØX5	T45.ØX6
Chlorphentermine	T5Ø.5X1	T5Ø.5X2	T5Ø.5X3	T5Ø.5X4	T5Ø.5X5	T5Ø.5X6
Chlorprocaine — *see* Chloroprocaine						
Chlorproguanil	T37.2X1	T37.2X2	T37.2X3	T37.2X4	T37.2X5	T37.2X6
Chlorpromazine	T43.3X1	T43.3X2	T43.3X3	T43.3X4	T43.3X5	T43.3X6
Chlorpropamide	T38.3X1	T38.3X2	T38.3X3	T38.3X4	T38.3X5	T38.3X6
Chlorprothixene	T43.4X1	T43.4X2	T43.4X3	T43.4X4	T43.4X5	T43.4X6
Chlorquinaldol	T49.ØX1	T49.ØX2	T49.ØX3	T49.ØX4	T49.ØX5	T49.ØX6
Chlorquinol	T49.ØX1	T49.ØX2	T49.ØX3	T49.ØX4	T49.ØX5	T49.ØX6
Chlortalidone	T5Ø.2X1	T5Ø.2X2	T5Ø.2X3	T5Ø.2X4	T5Ø.2X5	T5Ø.2X6
Chlortetracycline	T36.4X1	T36.4X2	T36.4X3	T36.4X4	T36.4X5	T36.4X6
Chlorthalidone	T5Ø.2X1	T5Ø.2X2	T5Ø.2X3	T5Ø.2X4	T5Ø.2X5	T5Ø.2X6
Chlorthion	T6Ø.ØX1	T6Ø.ØX2	T6Ø.ØX3	T6Ø.ØX4	—	—
Chlorthiophos	T6Ø.ØX1	T6Ø.ØX2	T6Ø.ØX3	T6Ø.ØX4	—	—
Chlortrianisene	T38.5X1	T38.5X2	T38.5X3	T38.5X4	T38.5X5	T38.5X6
Chlor-Trimeton	T45.ØX1	T45.ØX2	T45.ØX3	T45.ØX4	T45.ØX5	T45.ØX6
Chlorzoxazone	T42.8X1	T42.8X2	T42.8X3	T42.8X4	T42.8X5	T42.8X6
Choke damp	T59.7X1	T59.7X2	T59.7X3	T59.7X4	—	—
Cholagogues	T47.5X1	T47.5X2	T47.5X3	T47.5X4	T47.5X5	T47.5X6
Cholebrine	T5Ø.8X1	T5Ø.8X2	T5Ø.8X3	T5Ø.8X4	T5Ø.8X5	T5Ø.8X6
Cholecalciferol	T45.2X1	T45.2X2	T45.2X3	T45.2X4	T45.2X5	T45.2X6
Cholecystokinin	T5Ø.8X1	T5Ø.8X2	T5Ø.8X3	T5Ø.8X4	T5Ø.8X5	T5Ø.8X6
Cholera vaccine	T5Ø.A91	T5Ø.A92	T5Ø.A93	T5Ø.A94	T5Ø.A95	T5Ø.A96
Choleretic	T47.5X1	T47.5X2	T47.5X3	T47.5X4	T47.5X5	T47.5X6
Cholesterol-lowering agents	T46.6X1	T46.6X2	T46.6X3	T46.6X4	T46.6X5	T46.6X6
Cholestyramine (resin)	T46.6X1	T46.6X2	T46.6X3	T46.6X4	T46.6X5	T46.6X6
Cholic acid	T47.5X1	T47.5X2	T47.5X3	T47.5X4	T47.5X5	T47.5X6
Choline	T48.6X1	T48.6X2	T48.6X3	T48.6X4	T48.6X5	T48.6X6
chloride	T5Ø.991	T5Ø.992	T5Ø.993	T5Ø.994	T5Ø.995	T5Ø.996
dihydrogen citrate	T5Ø.991	T5Ø.992	T5Ø.993	T5Ø.994	T5Ø.995	T5Ø.996
salicylate	T39.Ø91	T39.Ø92	T39.Ø93	T39.Ø94	T39.Ø95	T39.Ø96
theophyllinate	T48.6X1	T48.6X2	T48.6X3	T48.6X4	T48.6X5	T48.6X6
Cholinergic (drug) NEC	T44.1X1	T44.1X2	T44.1X3	T44.1X4	T44.1X5	T44.1X6
muscle tone enhancer	T44.1X1	T44.1X2	T44.1X3	T44.1X4	T44.1X5	T44.1X6
organophosphorus	T44.ØX1	T44.ØX2	T44.ØX3	T44.ØX4	T44.ØX5	T44.ØX6
insecticide	T6Ø.ØX1	T6Ø.ØX2	T6Ø.ØX3	T6Ø.ØX4	—	—
nerve gas	T59.891	T59.892	T59.893	T59.894	—	—
trimethyl ammonium propanediol	T44.1X1	T44.1X2	T44.1X3	T44.1X4	T44.1X5	T44.1X6
Cholinesterase reactivator	T5Ø.6X1	T5Ø.6X2	T5Ø.6X3	T5Ø.6X4	T5Ø.6X5	T5Ø.6X6
Cholografin	T5Ø.8X1	T5Ø.8X2	T5Ø.8X3	T5Ø.8X4	T5Ø.8X5	T5Ø.8X6
Chorionic gonadotropin	T38.891	T38.892	T38.893	T38.894	T38.895	T38.896
Chromate	T56.2X1	T56.2X2	T56.2X3	T56.2X4	—	—
dust or mist	T56.2X1	T56.2X2	T56.2X3	T56.2X4	—	—
lead — *see also* lead	T56.ØX1	T56.ØX2	T56.ØX3	T56.ØX4	—	—
paint	T56.ØX1	T56.ØX2	T56.ØX3	T56.ØX4	—	—
Chromic						
acid	T56.2X1	T56.2X2	T56.2X3	T56.2X4	—	—
dust or mist	T56.2X1	T56.2X2	T56.2X3	T56.2X4	—	—

Substance	Poisoning, Accidental (unintentional)	Poisoning, Intentional Self-harm	Poisoning, Assault	Poisoning, Undetermined	Adverse Effect	Under-dosing
Chromic — *continued*						
phosphate 32P	T45.1X1	T45.1X2	T45.1X3	T45.1X4	T45.1X5	T45.1X6
Chromium	T56.2X1	T56.2X2	T56.2X3	T56.2X4	—	—
compounds — *see* Chromate						
sesquioxide	T5Ø.8X1	T5Ø.8X2	T5Ø.8X3	T5Ø.8X4	T5Ø.8X5	T5Ø.8X6
Chromomycin A3	T45.1X1	T45.1X2	T45.1X3	T45.1X4	T45.1X5	T45.1X6
Chromonar	T46.3X1	T46.3X2	T46.3X3	T46.3X4	T46.3X5	T46.3X6
Chromyl chloride	T56.2X1	T56.2X2	T56.2X3	T56.2X4	—	—
Chrysarobin	T49.4X1	T49.4X2	T49.4X3	T49.4X4	T49.4X5	T49.4X6
Chrysazin	T47.2X1	T47.2X2	T47.2X3	T47.2X4	T47.2X5	T47.2X6
Chymar	T45.3X1	T45.3X2	T45.3X3	T45.3X4	T45.3X5	T45.3X6
ophthalmic preparation	T49.5X1	T49.5X2	T49.5X3	T49.5X4	T49.5X5	T49.5X6
Chymopapain	T45.3X1	T45.3X2	T45.3X3	T45.3X4	T45.3X5	T45.3X6
Chymotrypsin	T45.3X1	T45.3X2	T45.3X3	T45.3X4	T45.3X5	T45.3X6
ophthalmic preparation	T49.5X1	T49.5X2	T49.5X3	T49.5X4	T49.5X5	T49.5X6
Cianidanol	T5Ø.991	T5Ø.992	T5Ø.993	T5Ø.994	T5Ø.995	T5Ø.996
Cianopramine	T43.Ø11	T43.Ø12	T43.Ø13	T43.Ø14	T43.Ø15	T43.Ø16
Cibenzoline	T46.2X1	T46.2X2	T46.2X3	T46.2X4	T46.2X5	T46.2X6
Ciclacillin	T36.ØX1	T36.ØX2	T36.ØX3	T36.ØX4	T36.ØX5	T36.ØX6
Ciclobarbital — *see* Hexobarbital						
Ciclonicate	T46.7X1	T46.7X2	T46.7X3	T46.7X4	T46.7X5	T46.7X6
Ciclopirox (olamine)	T49.ØX1	T49.ØX2	T49.ØX3	T49.ØX4	T49.ØX5	T49.ØX6
Ciclosporin	T45.1X1	T45.1X2	T45.1X3	T45.1X4	T45.1X5	T45.1X6
Cicuta maculata or virosa	T62.2X1	T62.2X2	T62.2X3	T62.2X4	—	—
Cicutoxin	T62.2X1	T62.2X2	T62.2X3	T62.2X4	—	—
Cigarette lighter fluid	T52.ØX1	T52.ØX2	T52.ØX3	T52.ØX4	—	—
Cigarettes (tobacco)	T65.221	T65.222	T65.223	T65.224	—	—
Ciguatoxin	T61.Ø1	T61.Ø2	T61.Ø3	T61.Ø4	—	—
Cilazapril	T46.4X1	T46.4X2	T46.4X3	T46.4X4	T46.4X5	T46.4X6
Cimetidine	T47.ØX1	T47.ØX2	T47.ØX3	T47.ØX4	T47.ØX5	T47.ØX6
Cimetropium bromide	T44.3X1	T44.3X2	T44.3X3	T44.3X4	T44.3X5	T44.3X6
Cinchocaine	T41.3X1	T41.3X2	T41.3X3	T41.3X4	T41.3X5	T41.3X6
topical (surface)	T41.3X1	T41.3X2	T41.3X3	T41.3X4	T41.3X5	T41.3X6
Cinchona	T37.2X1	T37.2X2	T37.2X3	T37.2X4	T37.2X5	T37.2X6
Cinchonine alkaloids	T37.2X1	T37.2X2	T37.2X3	T37.2X4	T37.2X5	T37.2X6
Cinchophen	T5Ø.4X1	T5Ø.4X2	T5Ø.4X3	T5Ø.4X4	T5Ø.4X5	T5Ø.4X6
Cinepazide	T46.7X1	T46.7X2	T46.7X3	T46.7X4	T46.7X5	T46.7X6
Cinnamedrine	T48.5X1	T48.5X2	T48.5X3	T48.5X4	T48.5X5	T48.5X6
Cinnarizine	T45.ØX1	T45.ØX2	T45.ØX3	T45.ØX4	T45.ØX5	T45.ØX6
Cinoxacin	T37.8X1	T37.8X2	T37.8X3	T37.8X4	T37.8X5	T37.8X6
Ciprofibrate	T46.6X1	T46.6X2	T46.6X3	T46.6X4	T46.6X5	T46.6X6
Ciprofloxacin	T36.8X1	T36.8X2	T36.8X3	T36.8X4	T36.8X5	T36.8X6
Cisapride	T47.8X1	T47.8X2	T47.8X3	T47.8X4	T47.8X5	T47.8X6
Cisplatin	T45.1X1	T45.1X2	T45.1X3	T45.1X4	T45.1X5	T45.1X6
Citalopram	T43.221	T43.222	T43.223	T43.224	T43.225	T43.226
Citanest	T41.3X1	T41.3X2	T41.3X3	T41.3X4	T41.3X5	T41.3X6
infiltration (subcutaneous)	T41.3X1	T41.3X2	T41.3X3	T41.3X4	T41.3X5	T41.3X6
nerve block (peripheral) (plexus)	T41.3X1	T41.3X2	T41.3X3	T41.3X4	T41.3X5	T41.3X6
Citric acid	T47.5X1	T47.5X2	T47.5X3	T47.5X4	T47.5X5	T47.5X6
Citrovorum (factor)	T45.8X1	T45.8X2	T45.8X3	T45.8X4	T45.8X5	T45.8X6
Claviceps purpurea	T62.2X1	T62.2X2	T62.2X3	T62.2X4	—	—
Clavulanic acid	T36.1X1	T36.1X2	T36.1X3	T36.1X4	T36.1X5	T36.1X6
Cleaner, cleansing agent, type not specified	T65.891	T65.892	T65.893	T65.894	—	—
of paint or varnish	T52.91	T52.92	T52.93	T52.94	—	—
specified type NEC	T65.891	T65.892	T65.893	T65.894	—	—
Clebopride	T47.8X1	T47.8X2	T47.8X3	T47.8X4	T47.8X5	T47.8X6
Clefamide	T37.3X1	T37.3X2	T37.3X3	T37.3X4	T37.3X5	T37.3X6
Clemastine	T45.ØX1	T45.ØX2	T45.ØX3	T45.ØX4	T45.ØX5	T45.ØX6
Clematis vitalba	T62.2X1	T62.2X2	T62.2X3	T62.2X4	—	—
Clemizole	T45.ØX1	T45.ØX2	T45.ØX3	T45.ØX4	T45.ØX5	T45.ØX6
penicillin	T36.ØX1	T36.ØX2	T36.ØX3	T36.ØX4	T36.ØX5	T36.ØX6
Clenbuterol	T48.6X1	T48.6X2	T48.6X3	T48.6X4	T48.6X5	T48.6X6
Clidinium bromide	T44.3X1	T44.3X2	T44.3X3	T44.3X4	T44.3X5	T44.3X6
Clindamycin	T36.8X1	T36.8X2	T36.8X3	T36.8X4	T36.8X5	T36.8X6
Clinofibrate	T46.6X1	T46.6X2	T46.6X3	T46.6X4	T46.6X5	T46.6X6
Clioquinol	T37.8X1	T37.8X2	T37.8X3	T37.8X4	T37.8X5	T37.8X6
Cliradon	T4Ø.2X1	T4Ø.2X2	T4Ø.2X3	T4Ø.2X4	—	—
Clobazam	T42.4X1	T42.4X2	T42.4X3	T42.4X4	T42.4X5	T42.4X6
Clobenzorex	T5Ø.5X1	T5Ø.5X2	T5Ø.5X3	T5Ø.5X4	T5Ø.5X5	T5Ø.5X6
Clobetasol	T49.ØX1	T49.ØX2	T49.ØX3	T49.ØX4	T49.ØX5	T49.ØX6
Clobetasone	T49.ØX1	T49.ØX2	T49.ØX3	T49.ØX4	T49.ØX5	T49.ØX6
Clobutinol	T48.3X1	T48.3X2	T48.3X3	T48.3X4	T48.3X5	T48.3X6
Clocortolone	T38.ØX1	T38.ØX2	T38.ØX3	T38.ØX4	T38.ØX5	T38.ØX6
Clodantoin	T49.ØX1	T49.ØX2	T49.ØX3	T49.ØX4	T49.ØX5	T49.ØX6
Clodronic acid	T5Ø.991	T5Ø.992	T5Ø.993	T5Ø.994	T5Ø.995	T5Ø.996
Clofazimine	T37.1X1	T37.1X2	T37.1X3	T37.1X4	T37.1X5	T37.1X6
Clofedanol	T48.3X1	T48.3X2	T48.3X3	T48.3X4	T48.3X5	T48.3X6
Clofenamide	T5Ø.2X1	T5Ø.2X2	T5Ø.2X3	T5Ø.2X4	T5Ø.2X5	T5Ø.2X6
Clofenotane	T49.ØX1	T49.ØX2	T49.ØX3	T49.ØX4	T49.ØX5	T49.ØX6
Clofezone	T39.2X1	T39.2X2	T39.2X3	T39.2X4	T39.2X5	T39.2X6
Clofibrate	T46.6X1	T46.6X2	T46.6X3	T46.6X4	T46.6X5	T46.6X6

Substance	Poisoning, Accidental (unintentional)	Poisoning, Intentional Self-harm	Poisoning, Assault	Poisoning, Undetermined	Adverse Effect	Under-dosing
Clofibride	T46.6X1	T46.6X2	T46.6X3	T46.6X4	T46.6X5	T46.6X6
Cloforex	T50.5X1	T50.5X2	T50.5X3	T50.5X4	T50.5X5	T50.5X6
Clomethiazole	T42.6X1	T42.6X2	T42.6X3	T42.6X4	T42.6X5	T42.6X6
Clometocillin	T36.0X1	T36.0X2	T36.0X3	T36.0X4	T36.0X5	T36.0X6
Clomifene	T38.5X1	T38.5X2	T38.5X3	T38.5X4	T38.5X5	T38.5X6
Clomiphene	T38.5X1	T38.5X2	T38.5X3	T38.5X4	T38.5X5	T38.5X6
Clomipramine	T43.011	T43.012	T43.013	T43.014	T43.015	T43.016
Clomocycline	T36.4X1	T36.4X2	T36.4X3	T36.4X4	T36.4X5	T36.4X6
Clonazepam	T42.4X1	T42.4X2	T42.4X3	T42.4X4	T42.4X5	T42.4X6
Clonidine	T46.5X1	T46.5X2	T46.5X3	T46.5X4	T46.5X5	T46.5X6
Clonixin	T39.8X1	T39.8X2	T39.8X3	T39.8X4	T39.8X5	T39.8X6
Clopamide	T50.2X1	T50.2X2	T50.2X3	T50.2X4	T50.2X5	T50.2X6
Clopenthixol	T43.4X1	T43.4X2	T43.4X3	T43.4X4	T43.4X5	T43.4X6
Cloperastine	T48.3X1	T48.3X2	T48.3X3	T48.3X4	T48.3X5	T48.3X6
Clophedianol	T48.3X1	T48.3X2	T48.3X3	T48.3X4	T48.3X5	T48.3X6
Cloponone	T36.2X1	T36.2X2	T36.2X3	T36.2X4	T36.2X5	T36.2X6
Cloprednol	T38.0X1	T38.0X2	T38.0X3	T38.0X4	T38.0X5	T38.0X6
Cloral betaine	T42.6X1	T42.6X2	T42.6X3	T42.6X4	T42.6X5	T42.6X6
Cloramfenicol	T36.2X1	T36.2X2	T36.2X3	T36.2X4	T36.2X5	T36.2X6
Clorazepate (dipotassium)	T42.4X1	T42.4X2	T42.4X3	T42.4X4	T42.4X5	T42.4X6
Clorexolone	T50.2X1	T50.2X2	T50.2X3	T50.2X4	T50.2X5	T50.2X6
Clorfenamine	T45.0X1	T45.0X2	T45.0X3	T45.0X4	T45.0X5	T45.0X6
Clorgiline	T43.1X1	T43.1X2	T43.1X3	T43.1X4	T43.1X5	T43.1X6
Clorotepine	T44.3X1	T44.3X2	T44.3X3	T44.3X4	T44.3X5	T44.3X6
Clorox (bleach)	T54.91	T54.92	T54.93	T54.94	—	—
Clorprenaline	T48.6X1	T48.6X2	T48.6X3	T48.6X4	T48.6X5	T48.6X6
Clortermine	T50.5X1	T50.5X2	T50.5X3	T50.5X4	T50.5X5	T50.5X6
Clotiapine	T43.591	T43.592	T43.593	T43.594	T43.595	T43.596
Clotiazepam	T42.4X1	T42.4X2	T42.4X3	T42.4X4	T42.4X5	T42.4X6
Clotibric acid	T46.6X1	T46.6X2	T46.6X3	T46.6X4	T46.6X5	T46.6X6
Clotrimazole	T49.0X1	T49.0X2	T49.0X3	T49.0X4	T49.0X5	T49.0X6
Cloxacillin	T36.0X1	T36.0X2	T36.0X3	T36.0X4	T36.0X5	T36.0X6
Cloxazolam	T42.4X1	T42.4X2	T42.4X3	T42.4X4	T42.4X5	T42.4X6
Cloxiquine	T49.0X1	T49.0X2	T49.0X3	T49.0X4	T49.0X5	T49.0X6
Clozapine	T42.4X1	T42.4X2	T42.4X3	T42.4X4	T42.4X5	T42.4X6
Coagulant NEC	T45.7X1	T45.7X2	T45.7X3	T45.7X4	T45.7X5	T45.7X6
Coal (carbon monoxide from) — see also Carbon, monoxide, coal	T58.2X1	T58.2X2	T58.2X3	T58.2X4	—	—
oil — see Kerosene						
tar	T49.1X1	T49.1X2	T49.1X3	T49.1X4	T49.1X5	T49.1X6
fumes	T59.891	T59.892	T59.893	T59.894	—	—
medicinal (ointment)	T49.4X1	T49.4X2	T49.4X3	T49.4X4	T49.4X5	T49.4X6
analgesics NEC	T39.2X1	T39.2X2	T39.2X3	T39.2X4	T39.2X5	T39.2X6
naphtha (solvent)	T52.0X1	T52.0X2	T52.0X3	T52.0X4	—	—
Cobalamine	T45.2X1	T45.2X2	T45.2X3	T45.2X4	T45.2X5	T45.2X6
Cobalt (nonmedicinal) (fumes) (industrial)	T56.891	T56.892	T56.893	T56.894	—	—
medicinal (trace) (chloride)	T45.8X1	T45.8X2	T45.8X3	T45.8X4	T45.8X5	T45.8X6
Cobra (venom)	T63.041	T63.042	T63.043	T63.044	—	—
Coca (leaf)	T40.5X1	T40.5X2	T40.5X3	T40.5X4	T40.5X5	T40.5X6
Cocaine	T40.5X1	T40.5X2	T40.5X3	T40.5X4	T40.5X5	T40.5X6
topical anesthetic	T41.3X1	T41.3X2	T41.3X3	T41.3X4	T41.3X5	T41.3X6
Cocarboxylase	T45.3X1	T45.3X2	T45.3X3	T45.3X4	T45.3X5	T45.3X6
Coccidioidin	T50.8X1	T50.8X2	T50.8X3	T50.8X4	T50.8X5	T50.8X6
Cocculus indicus	T62.1X1	T62.1X2	T62.1X3	T62.1X4	—	—
Cochineal	T65.6X1	T65.6X2	T65.6X3	T65.6X4	—	—
medicinal products	T50.991	T50.992	T50.993	T50.994	T50.995	T50.996
Codeine	T40.2X1	T40.2X2	T40.2X3	T40.2X4	T40.2X5	T40.2X6
Cod-liver oil	T45.2X1	T45.2X2	T45.2X3	T45.2X4	T45.2X5	T45.2X6
Coenzyme A	T50.991	T50.992	T50.993	T50.994	T50.995	T50.996
Coffee	T62.8X1	T62.8X2	T62.8X3	T62.8X4	—	—
Cogalactoisomerase	T50.991	T50.992	T50.993	T50.994	T50.995	T50.996
Cogentin	T44.3X1	T44.3X2	T44.3X3	T44.3X4	T44.3X5	T44.3X6
Coke fumes or gas (carbon monoxide)	T58.2X1	T58.2X2	T58.2X3	T58.2X4	—	—
industrial use	T58.8X1	T58.8X2	T58.8X3	T58.8X4	—	—
Colace	T47.4X1	T47.4X2	T47.4X3	T47.4X4	T47.4X5	T47.4X6
Colaspase	T45.1X1	T45.1X2	T45.1X3	T45.1X4	T45.1X5	T45.1X6
Colchicine	T50.4X1	T50.4X2	T50.4X3	T50.4X4	T50.4X5	T50.4X6
Colchicum	T62.2X1	T62.2X2	T62.2X3	T62.2X4	—	—
Cold cream	T49.3X1	T49.3X2	T49.3X3	T49.3X4	T49.3X5	T49.3X6
Colecalciferol	T45.2X1	T45.2X2	T45.2X3	T45.2X4	T45.2X5	T45.2X6
Colestipol	T46.6X1	T46.6X2	T46.6X3	T46.6X4	T46.6X5	T46.6X6
Colestyramine	T46.6X1	T46.6X2	T46.6X3	T46.6X4	T46.6X5	T46.6X6
Colimycin	T36.8X1	T36.8X2	T36.8X3	T36.8X4	T36.8X5	T36.8X6
Colistimethate	T36.8X1	T36.8X2	T36.8X3	T36.8X4	T36.8X5	T36.8X6
Colistin	T36.8X1	T36.8X2	T36.8X3	T36.8X4	T36.8X5	T36.8X6
sulfate (eye preparation)	T49.5X1	T49.5X2	T49.5X3	T49.5X4	T49.5X5	T49.5X6
Collagen	T50.991	T50.992	T50.993	T50.994	T50.995	T50.996
Collagenase	T49.4X1	T49.4X2	T49.4X3	T49.4X4	T49.4X5	T49.4X6
Collodion	T49.3X1	T49.3X2	T49.3X3	T49.3X4	T49.3X5	T49.3X6
Colocynth	T47.2X1	T47.2X2	T47.2X3	T47.2X4	T47.2X5	T47.2X6

Substance	Poisoning, Accidental (unintentional)	Poisoning, Intentional Self-harm	Poisoning, Assault	Poisoning, Undetermined	Adverse Effect	Under-dosing
Colophony adhesive	T49.3X1	T49.3X2	T49.3X3	T49.3X4	T49.3X5	T49.3X6
Colorant — see also Dye						
Colorant	T50.991	T50.992	T50.993	T50.994	T50.995	T50.996
Coloring matter — see Dye(s)						
Combustion gas (after combustion) — see Carbon, monoxide						
prior to combustion	T59.891	T59.892	T59.893	T59.894	—	—
Compazine	T43.3X1	T43.3X2	T43.3X3	T43.3X4	T43.3X5	T43.3X6
Compound						
1080 (sodium fluoroacetate)	T60.4X1	T60.4X2	T60.4X3	T60.4X4	—	—
269 (endrin)	T60.1X1	T60.1X2	T60.1X3	T60.1X4	—	—
3422 (parathion)	T60.0X1	T60.0X2	T60.0X3	T60.0X4	—	—
3911 (phorate)	T60.0X1	T60.0X2	T60.0X3	T60.0X4	—	—
3956 (toxaphene)	T60.1X1	T60.1X2	T60.1X3	T60.1X4	—	—
4049 (malathion)	T60.0X1	T60.0X2	T60.0X3	T60.0X4	—	—
4069 (malathion)	T60.0X1	T60.0X2	T60.0X3	T60.0X4	—	—
4124 (dicapthon)	T60.0X1	T60.0X2	T60.0X3	T60.0X4	—	—
42 (warfarin)	T60.4X1	T60.4X2	T60.4X3	T60.4X4	—	—
497 (dieldrin)	T60.1X1	T60.1X2	T60.1X3	T60.1X4	—	—
E (cortisone)	T38.0X1	T38.0X2	T38.0X3	T38.0X4	T38.0X5	T38.0X6
F (hydrocortisone)	T38.0X1	T38.0X2	T38.0X3	T38.0X4	T38.0X5	T38.0X6
Congener, anabolic	T38.7X1	T38.7X2	T38.7X3	T38.7X4	T38.7X5	T38.7X6
Congo red	T50.8X1	T50.8X2	T50.8X3	T50.8X4	T50.8X5	T50.8X6
Coniine, conine	T62.2X1	T62.2X2	T62.2X3	T62.2X4	—	—
Conium (maculatum)	T62.2X1	T62.2X2	T62.2X3	T62.2X4	—	—
Conjugated estrogenic substances	T38.5X1	T38.5X2	T38.5X3	T38.5X4	T38.5X5	T38.5X6
Contac	T48.5X1	T48.5X2	T48.5X3	T48.5X4	T48.5X5	T48.5X6
Contact lens solution	T49.5X1	T49.5X2	T49.5X3	T49.5X4	T49.5X5	T49.5X6
Contraceptive (oral)	T38.4X1	T38.4X2	T38.4X3	T38.4X4	T38.4X5	T38.4X6
vaginal	T49.8X1	T49.8X2	T49.8X3	T49.8X4	T49.8X5	T49.8X6
Contrast medium, radiography	T50.8X1	T50.8X2	T50.8X3	T50.8X4	T50.8X5	T50.8X6
Convallaria glycosides	T46.0X1	T46.0X2	T46.0X3	T46.0X4	T46.0X5	T46.0X6
Convallaria majalis	T62.2X1	T62.2X2	T62.2X3	T62.2X4	—	—
berry	T62.1X1	T62.1X2	T62.1X3	T62.1X4	—	—
Copperhead snake (bite) (venom)	T63.061	T63.062	T63.063	T63.064	—	—
Copper (dust) (fumes) (nonmedicinal) NEC	T56.4X1	T56.4X2	T56.4X3	T56.4X4	—	—
arsenate, arsenite	T57.0X1	T57.0X2	T57.0X3	T57.0X4	—	—
insecticide	T60.2X1	T60.2X2	T60.2X3	T60.2X4	—	—
emetic	T47.7X1	T47.7X2	T47.7X3	T47.7X4	T47.7X5	T47.7X6
fungicide	T60.3X1	T60.3X2	T60.3X3	T60.3X4	—	—
gluconate	T49.0X1	T49.0X2	T49.0X3	T49.0X4	T49.0X5	T49.0X6
insecticide	T60.2X1	T60.2X2	T60.2X3	T60.2X4	—	—
medicinal (trace)	T45.8X1	T45.8X2	T45.8X3	T45.8X4	T45.8X5	T45.8X6
oleate	T49.0X1	T49.0X2	T49.0X3	T49.0X4	T49.0X5	T49.0X6
sulfate	T56.4X1	T56.4X2	T56.4X3	T56.4X4	—	—
cupric	T56.4X1	T56.4X2	T56.4X3	T56.4X4	—	—
fungicide	T60.3X1	T60.3X2	T60.3X3	T60.3X4	—	—
medicinal						
ear	T49.6X1	T49.6X2	T49.6X3	T49.6X4	T49.6X5	T49.6X6
emetic	T47.7X1	T47.7X2	T47.7X3	T47.7X4	T47.7X5	T47.7X6
eye	T49.5X1	T49.5X2	T49.5X3	T49.5X4	T49.5X5	T49.5X6
cuprous	T56.4X1	T56.4X2	T56.4X3	T56.4X4	—	—
fungicide	T60.3X1	T60.3X2	T60.3X3	T60.3X4	—	—
medicinal						
ear	T49.6X1	T49.6X2	T49.6X3	T49.6X4	T49.6X5	T49.6X6
emetic	T47.7X1	T47.7X2	T47.7X3	T47.7X4	T47.7X5	T47.7X6
eye	T49.5X1	T49.5X2	T49.5X3	T49.5X4	T49.5X5	T49.5X6
Coral (sting)	T63.691	T63.692	T63.693	T63.694	—	—
snake (bite) (venom)	T63.021	T63.022	T63.023	T63.024	—	—
Corbadrine	T49.6X1	T49.6X2	T49.6X3	T49.6X4	T49.6X5	T49.6X6
Cordite	T65.891	T65.892	T65.893	T65.894	—	—
vapor	T59.891	T59.892	T59.893	T59.894	—	—
Cordran	T49.0X1	T49.0X2	T49.0X3	T49.0X4	T49.0X5	T49.0X6
Corn cures	T49.4X1	T49.4X2	T49.4X3	T49.4X4	T49.4X5	T49.4X6
Cornhusker's lotion	T49.3X1	T49.3X2	T49.3X3	T49.3X4	T49.3X5	T49.3X6
Corn starch	T49.3X1	T49.3X2	T49.3X3	T49.3X4	T49.3X5	T49.3X6
Coronary vasodilator NEC	T46.3X1	T46.3X2	T46.3X3	T46.3X4	T46.3X5	T46.3X6
Corrosive NEC	T54.91	T54.92	T54.93	T54.94	—	—
acid NEC	T54.2X1	T54.2X2	T54.2X3	T54.2X4	—	—
aromatics	T54.1X1	T54.1X2	T54.1X3	T54.1X4	—	—
disinfectant	T54.1X1	T54.1X2	T54.1X3	T54.1X4	—	—
fumes NEC	T54.91	T54.92	T54.93	T54.94	—	—
specified NEC	T54.91	T54.92	T54.93	T54.94	—	—
sublimate	T56.1X1	T56.1X2	T56.1X3	T56.1X4	—	—
Cortate	T38.0X1	T38.0X2	T38.0X3	T38.0X4	T38.0X5	T38.0X6
Cort-Dome	T38.0X1	T38.0X2	T38.0X3	T38.0X4	T38.0X5	T38.0X6
ENT agent	T49.6X1	T49.6X2	T49.6X3	T49.6X4	T49.6X5	T49.6X6
ophthalmic preparation	T49.5X1	T49.5X2	T49.5X3	T49.5X4	T49.5X5	T49.5X6

Cort-Dome ICD-10-CM 2016

Table of Drugs and Chemicals

Cort-Dome — Dantron

Substance	Poisoning, Accidental (unintentional)	Poisoning, Intentional Self-harm	Poisoning, Assault	Poisoning, Undetermined	Adverse Effect	Under-dosing
Cort-Dome — *continued*						
topical NEC	T49.ØX1	T49.ØX2	T49.ØX3	T49.ØX4	T49.ØX5	T49.ØX6
Cortef	T38.ØX1	T38.ØX2	T38.ØX3	T38.ØX4	T38.ØX5	T38.ØX6
ENT agent	T49.6X1	T49.6X2	T49.6X3	T49.6X4	T49.6X5	T49.6X6
ophthalmic preparation	T49.5X1	T49.5X2	T49.5X3	T49.5X4	T49.5X5	T49.5X6
topical NEC	T49.ØX1	T49.ØX2	T49.ØX3	T49.ØX4	T49.ØX5	T49.ØX6
Corticosteroid	T38.ØX1	T38.ØX2	T38.ØX3	T38.ØX4	T38.ØX5	T38.ØX6
ENT agent	T49.6X1	T49.6X2	T49.6X3	T49.6X4	T49.6X5	T49.6X6
mineral	T5Ø.ØX1	T5Ø.ØX2	T5Ø.ØX3	T5Ø.ØX4	T5Ø.ØX5	T5Ø.ØX6
ophthalmic	T49.5X1	T49.5X2	T49.5X3	T49.5X4	T49.5X5	T49.5X6
topical NEC	T49.ØX1	T49.ØX2	T49.ØX3	T49.ØX4	T49.ØX5	T49.ØX6
Corticotropin	T38.811	T38.812	T38.813	T38.814	T38.815	T38.816
Cortisol	T49.ØX1	T49.ØX2	T49.ØX3	T49.ØX4	T49.ØX5	T49.ØX6
ENT agent	T49.6X1	T49.6X2	T49.6X3	T49.6X4	T49.6X5	T49.6X6
ophthalmic preparation	T49.5X1	T49.5X2	T49.5X3	T49.5X4	T49.5X5	T49.5X6
topical NEC	T49.ØX1	T49.ØX2	T49.ØX3	T49.ØX4	T49.ØX5	T49.ØX6
Cortisone (acetate)	T38.ØX1	T38.ØX2	T38.ØX3	T38.ØX4	T38.ØX5	T38.ØX6
ENT agent	T49.6X1	T49.6X2	T49.6X3	T49.6X4	T49.6X5	T49.6X6
ophthalmic preparation	T49.5X1	T49.5X2	T49.5X3	T49.5X4	T49.5X5	T49.5X6
topical NEC	T49.ØX1	T49.ØX2	T49.ØX3	T49.ØX4	T49.ØX5	T49.ØX6
Cortivazol	T38.ØX1	T38.ØX2	T38.ØX3	T38.ØX4	T38.ØX5	T38.ØX6
Cortogen	T38.ØX1	T38.ØX2	T38.ØX3	T38.ØX4	T38.ØX5	T38.ØX6
ENT agent	T49.6X1	T49.6X2	T49.6X3	T49.6X4	T49.6X5	T49.6X6
ophthalmic preparation	T49.5X1	T49.5X2	T49.5X3	T49.5X4	T49.5X5	T49.5X6
Cortone	T38.ØX1	T38.ØX2	T38.ØX3	T38.ØX4	T38.ØX5	T38.ØX6
ENT agent	T49.6X1	T49.6X2	T49.6X3	T49.6X4	T49.6X5	T49.6X6
ophthalmic preparation	T49.5X1	T49.5X2	T49.5X3	T49.5X4	T49.5X5	T49.5X6
Cortril	T38.ØX1	T38.ØX2	T38.ØX3	T38.ØX4	T38.ØX5	T38.ØX6
ENT agent	T49.6X1	T49.6X2	T49.6X3	T49.6X4	T49.6X5	T49.6X6
ophthalmic preparation	T49.5X1	T49.5X2	T49.5X3	T49.5X4	T49.5X5	T49.5X6
topical NEC	T49.ØX1	T49.ØX2	T49.ØX3	T49.ØX4	T49.ØX5	T49.ØX6
Corynebacterium parvum	T45.1X1	T45.1X2	T45.1X3	T45.1X4	T45.1X5	T45.1X6
Cosmetic preparation	T49.8X1	T49.8X2	T49.8X3	T49.8X4	T49.8X5	T49.8X6
Cosmetics	T49.8X1	T49.8X2	T49.8X3	T49.8X4	T49.8X5	T49.8X6
Cosyntropin	T38.811	T38.812	T38.813	T38.814	T38.815	T38.816
Cotarnine	T45.7X1	T45.7X2	T45.7X3	T45.7X4	T45.7X5	T45.7X6
Co-trimoxazole	T36.8X1	T36.8X2	T36.8X3	T36.8X4	T36.8X5	T36.8X6
Cottonseed oil	T49.3X1	T49.3X2	T49.3X3	T49.3X4	T49.3X5	T49.3X6
Cough mixture (syrup)	T48.4X1	T48.4X2	T48.4X3	T48.4X4	T48.4X5	T48.4X6
containing opiates	T4Ø.2X1	T4Ø.2X2	T4Ø.2X3	T4Ø.2X4	T4Ø.2X5	T4Ø.2X6
expectorants	T48.4X1	T48.4X2	T48.4X3	T48.4X4	T48.4X5	T48.4X6
Coumadin	T45.511	T45.512	T45.513	T45.514	T45.515	T45.516
rodenticide	T6Ø.4X1	T6Ø.4X2	T6Ø.4X3	T6Ø.4X4	—	—
Coumaphos	T6Ø.ØX1	T6Ø.ØX2	T6Ø.ØX3	T6Ø.ØX4	—	—
Coumarin	T45.511	T45.512	T45.513	T45.514	T45.515	T45.516
Coumetarol	T45.511	T45.512	T45.513	T45.514	T45.515	T45.516
Cowbane	T62.2X1	T62.2X2	T62.2X3	T62.2X4	—	—
Cozyme	T45.2X1	T45.2X2	T45.2X3	T45.2X4	T45.2X5	T45.2X6
Crack	T4Ø.5X1	T4Ø.5X2	T4Ø.5X3	T4Ø.5X4	—	—
Crataegus extract	T46.ØX1	T46.ØX2	T46.ØX3	T46.ØX4	T46.ØX5	T46.ØX6
Creolin	T54.1X1	T54.1X2	T54.1X3	T54.1X4	—	—
disinfectant	T54.1X1	T54.1X2	T54.1X3	T54.1X4	—	—
Creosol (compound)	T49.ØX1	T49.ØX2	T49.ØX3	T49.ØX4	T49.ØX5	T49.ØX6
Creosote (coal tar) (beechwood)	T49.ØX1	T49.ØX2	T49.ØX3	T49.ØX4	T49.ØX5	T49.ØX6
medicinal (expectorant)	T48.4X1	T48.4X2	T48.4X3	T48.4X4	T48.4X5	T48.4X6
syrup	T48.4X1	T48.4X2	T48.4X3	T48.4X4	T48.4X5	T48.4X6
Cresol(s)	T49.ØX1	T49.ØX2	T49.ØX3	T49.ØX4	T49.ØX5	T49.ØX6
and soap solution	T49.ØX1	T49.ØX2	T49.ØX3	T49.ØX4	T49.ØX5	T49.ØX6
Cresyl acetate	T49.ØX1	T49.ØX2	T49.ØX3	T49.ØX4	T49.ØX5	T49.ØX6
Cresylic acid	T49.ØX1	T49.ØX2	T49.ØX3	T49.ØX4	T49.ØX5	T49.ØX6
Crimidine	T6Ø.4X1	T6Ø.4X2	T6Ø.4X3	T6Ø.4X4	—	—
Croconazole	T37.8X1	T37.8X2	T37.8X3	T37.8X4	T37.8X5	T37.8X6
Cromoglicic acid	T48.6X1	T48.6X2	T48.6X3	T48.6X4	T48.6X5	T48.6X6
Cromolyn	T48.6X1	T48.6X2	T48.6X3	T48.6X4	T48.6X5	T48.6X6
Cromonar	T46.3X1	T46.3X2	T46.3X3	T46.3X4	T46.3X5	T46.3X6
Cropropamide	T39.8X1	T39.8X2	T39.8X3	T39.8X4	T39.8X5	T39.8X6
with crotethamide	T5Ø.7X1	T5Ø.7X2	T5Ø.7X3	T5Ø.7X4	T5Ø.7X5	T5Ø.7X6
Crotamiton	T49.ØX1	T49.ØX2	T49.ØX3	T49.ØX4	T49.ØX5	T49.ØX6
Crotethamide	T39.8X1	T39.8X2	T39.8X3	T39.8X4	T39.8X5	T39.8X6
with cropropamide	T5Ø.7X1	T5Ø.7X2	T5Ø.7X3	T5Ø.7X4	T5Ø.7X5	T5Ø.7X6
Croton (oil)	T47.2X1	T47.2X2	T47.2X3	T47.2X4	T47.2X5	T47.2X6
chloral	T42.6X1	T42.6X2	T42.6X3	T42.6X4	T42.6X5	T42.6X6
Crude oil	T52.ØX1	T52.ØX2	T52.ØX3	T52.ØX4	—	—
Cryogenine	T39.8X1	T39.8X2	T39.8X3	T39.8X4	T39.8X5	T39.8X6
Cryolite (vapor)	T6Ø.1X1	T6Ø.1X2	T6Ø.1X3	T6Ø.1X4	—	—
insecticide	T6Ø.1X1	T6Ø.1X2	T6Ø.1X3	T6Ø.1X4	—	—
Cryptenamine (tannates)	T46.5X1	T46.5X2	T46.5X3	T46.5X4	T46.5X5	T46.5X6
Crystal violet	T49.ØX1	T49.ØX2	T49.ØX3	T49.ØX4	T49.ØX5	T49.ØX6
Cuckoopint	T62.2X1	T62.2X2	T62.2X3	T62.2X4	—	—
Cumetharol	T45.511	T45.512	T45.513	T45.514	T45.515	T45.516
Cupric						
acetate	T6Ø.3X1	T6Ø.3X2	T6Ø.3X3	T6Ø.3X4	—	—

Substance	Poisoning, Accidental (unintentional)	Poisoning, Intentional Self-harm	Poisoning, Assault	Poisoning, Undetermined	Adverse Effect	Under-dosing
Cupric — *continued*						
acetoarsenite	T57.ØX1	T57.ØX2	T57.ØX3	T57.ØX4	—	—
arsenate	T57.ØX1	T57.ØX2	T57.ØX3	T57.ØX4	—	—
gluconate	T49.ØX1	T49.ØX2	T49.ØX3	T49.ØX4	T49.ØX5	T49.ØX6
oleate	T49.ØX1	T49.ØX2	T49.ØX3	T49.ØX4	T49.ØX5	T49.ØX6
sulfate	T56.4X1	T56.4X2	T56.4X3	T56.4X4	—	—
Cuprous sulfate — *see also* Copper sulfate	T56.4X1	T56.4X2	T56.4X3	T56.4X4	—	—
Curare, curarine	T48.1X1	T48.1X2	T48.1X3	T48.1X4	T48.1X5	T48.1X6
Cyamemazine	T43.3X1	T43.3X2	T43.3X3	T43.3X4	T43.3X5	T43.3X6
Cyamopsis tetragonoloba	T46.6X1	T46.6X2	T46.6X3	T46.6X4	T46.6X5	T46.6X6
Cyanacetyl hydrazide	T37.1X1	T37.1X2	T37.1X3	T37.1X4	T37.1X5	T37.1X6
Cyanic acid (gas)	T59.891	T59.892	T59.893	T59.894	—	—
Cyanide(s) (compounds) (potassium) (sodium) **NEC**	T65.ØX1	T65.ØX2	T65.ØX3	T65.ØX4	—	—
dust or gas (inhalation) NEC	T57.3X1	T57.3X2	T57.3X3	T57.3X4	—	—
fumigant	T65.ØX1	T65.ØX2	T65.ØX3	T65.ØX4	—	—
hydrogen	T57.3X1	T57.3X2	T57.3X3	T57.3X4	—	—
mercuric — *see* Mercury						
pesticide (dust) (fumes)	T65.ØX1	T65.ØX2	T65.ØX3	T65.ØX4	—	—
Cyanoacrylate adhesive	T49.3X1	T49.3X2	T49.3X3	T49.3X4	T49.3X5	T49.3X6
Cyanocobalamin	T45.8X1	T45.8X2	T45.8X3	T45.8X4	T45.8X5	T45.8X6
Cyanogen (chloride) (gas) **NEC**	T59.891	T59.892	T59.893	T59.894	—	—
Cyclacillin	T36.ØX1	T36.ØX2	T36.ØX3	T36.ØX4	T36.ØX5	T36.ØX6
Cyclaine	T41.3X1	T41.3X2	T41.3X3	T41.3X4	T41.3X5	T41.3X6
Cyclamate	T5Ø.991	T5Ø.992	T5Ø.993	T5Ø.994	T5Ø.995	T5Ø.996
Cyclamen europaeum	T62.2X1	T62.2X2	T62.2X3	T62.2X4	—	—
Cyclandelate	T46.7X1	T46.7X2	T46.7X3	T46.7X4	T46.7X5	T46.7X6
Cyclazocine	T5Ø.7X1	T5Ø.7X2	T5Ø.7X3	T5Ø.7X4	T5Ø.7X5	T5Ø.7X6
Cyclizine	T45.ØX1	T45.ØX2	T45.ØX3	T45.ØX4	T45.ØX5	T45.ØX6
Cyclobarbital	T42.3X1	T42.3X2	T42.3X3	T42.3X4	T42.3X5	T42.3X6
Cyclobarbitone	T42.3X1	T42.3X2	T42.3X3	T42.3X4	T42.3X5	T42.3X6
Cyclobenzaprine	T48.1X1	T48.1X2	T48.1X3	T48.1X4	T48.1X5	T48.1X6
Cyclodrine	T44.3X1	T44.3X2	T44.3X3	T44.3X4	T44.3X5	T44.3X6
Cycloguanil embonate	T37.2X1	T37.2X2	T37.2X3	T37.2X4	T37.2X5	T37.2X6
Cyclohexane	T52.8X1	T52.8X2	T52.8X3	T52.8X4	—	—
Cyclohexanol	T51.8X1	T51.8X2	T51.8X3	T51.8X4	—	—
Cyclohexanone	T52.4X1	T52.4X2	T52.4X3	T52.4X4	—	—
Cycloheximide	T6Ø.3X1	T6Ø.3X2	T6Ø.3X3	T6Ø.3X4	—	—
Cyclohexyl acetate	T52.8X1	T52.8X2	T52.8X3	T52.8X4	—	—
Cycloleucin	T45.1X1	T45.1X2	T45.1X3	T45.1X4	T45.1X5	T45.1X6
Cyclomethycaine	T41.3X1	T41.3X2	T41.3X3	T41.3X4	T41.3X5	T41.3X6
Cyclopentamine	T44.4X1	T44.4X2	T44.4X3	T44.4X4	T44.4X5	T44.4X6
Cyclopenthiazide	T5Ø.2X1	T5Ø.2X2	T5Ø.2X3	T5Ø.2X4	T5Ø.2X5	T5Ø.2X6
Cyclopentolate	T44.3X1	T44.3X2	T44.3X3	T44.3X4	T44.3X5	T44.3X6
Cyclophosphamide	T45.1X1	T45.1X2	T45.1X3	T45.1X4	T45.1X5	T45.1X6
Cycloplegic drug	T49.5X1	T49.5X2	T49.5X3	T49.5X4	T49.5X5	T49.5X6
Cyclopropane	T41.291	T41.292	T41.293	T41.294	T41.295	T41.296
Cyclopyrabital	T39.8X1	T39.8X2	T39.8X3	T39.8X4	T39.8X5	T39.8X6
Cycloserine	T37.1X1	T37.1X2	T37.1X3	T37.1X4	T37.1X5	T37.1X6
Cyclosporin	T45.1X1	T45.1X2	T45.1X3	T45.1X4	T45.1X5	T45.1X6
Cyclothiazide	T5Ø.2X1	T5Ø.2X2	T5Ø.2X3	T5Ø.2X4	T5Ø.2X5	T5Ø.2X6
Cycrimine	T44.3X1	T44.3X2	T44.3X3	T44.3X4	T44.3X5	T44.3X6
Cyhalothrin	T6Ø.1X1	T6Ø.1X2	T6Ø.1X3	T6Ø.1X4	—	—
Cymarin	T46.ØX1	T46.ØX2	T46.ØX3	T46.ØX4	T46.ØX5	T46.ØX6
Cypermethrin	T6Ø.1X1	T6Ø.1X2	T6Ø.1X3	T6Ø.1X4	—	—
Cyphenothrin	T6Ø.2X1	T6Ø.2X2	T6Ø.2X3	T6Ø.2X4	—	—
Cyproheptadine	T45.ØX1	T45.ØX2	T45.ØX3	T45.ØX4	T45.ØX5	T45.ØX6
Cyproterone	T38.6X1	T38.6X2	T38.6X3	T38.6X4	T38.6X5	T38.6X6
Cysteamine	T5Ø.6X1	T5Ø.6X2	T5Ø.6X3	T5Ø.6X4	T5Ø.6X5	T5Ø.6X6
Cytarabine	T45.1X1	T45.1X2	T45.1X3	T45.1X4	T45.1X5	T45.1X6
Cytisus						
laburnum	T62.2X1	T62.2X2	T62.2X3	T62.2X4	—	—
scoparius	T62.2X1	T62.2X2	T62.2X3	T62.2X4	—	—
Cytochrome C	T47.5X1	T47.5X2	T47.5X3	T47.5X4	T47.5X5	T47.5X6
Cytomel	T38.1X1	T38.1X2	T38.1X3	T38.1X4	T38.1X5	T38.1X6
Cytosine arabinoside	T45.1X1	T45.1X2	T45.1X3	T45.1X4	T45.1X5	T45.1X6
Cytoxan	T45.1X1	T45.1X2	T45.1X3	T45.1X4	T45.1X5	T45.1X6
Cytozyme	T45.7X1	T45.7X2	T45.7X3	T45.7X4	T45.7X5	T45.7X6
S-Carboxymethylcysteine	T48.4X1	T48.4X2	T48.4X3	T48.4X4	T48.4X5	T48.4X6
Dacarbazine	T45.1X1	T45.1X2	T45.1X3	T45.1X4	T45.1X5	T45.1X6
Dactinomycin	T45.1X1	T45.1X2	T45.1X3	T45.1X4	T45.1X5	T45.1X6
DADPS	T37.1X1	T37.1X2	T37.1X3	T37.1X4	T37.1X5	T37.1X6
Dakin's solution	T49.ØX1	T49.ØX2	T49.ØX3	T49.ØX4	T49.ØX5	T49.ØX6
Dalapon (sodium)	T6Ø.3X1	T6Ø.3X2	T6Ø.3X3	T6Ø.3X4	—	—
Dalmane	T42.4X1	T42.4X2	T42.4X3	T42.4X4	T42.4X5	T42.4X6
Danazol	T38.6X1	T38.6X2	T38.6X3	T38.6X4	T38.6X5	T38.6X6
Danilone	T45.511	T45.512	T45.513	T45.514	T45.515	T45.516
Danthron	T47.2X1	T47.2X2	T47.2X3	T47.2X4	T47.2X5	T47.2X6
Dantrolene	T42.8X1	T42.8X2	T42.8X3	T42.8X4	T42.8X5	T42.8X6
Dantron	T47.2X1	T47.2X2	T47.2X3	T47.2X4	T47.2X5	T47.2X6

Substance	Poisoning, Accidental (unintentional)	Poisoning, Intentional Self-harm	Poisoning, Assault	Poisoning, Undetermined	Adverse Effect	Under-dosing
Daphne (gnidium) (mezereum)	T62.2X1	T62.2X2	T62.2X3	T62.2X4	—	—
berry	T62.1X1	T62.1X2	T62.1X3	T62.1X4	—	—
Dapsone	T37.1X1	T37.1X2	T37.1X3	T37.1X4	T37.1X5	T37.1X6
Daraprim	T37.2X1	T37.2X2	T37.2X3	T37.2X4	T37.2X5	T37.2X6
Darnel	T62.2X1	T62.2X2	T62.2X3	T62.2X4	—	—
Darvon	T39.8X1	T39.8X2	T39.8X3	T39.8X4	T39.8X5	T39.8X6
Daunomycin	T45.1X1	T45.1X2	T45.1X3	T45.1X4	T45.1X5	T45.1X6
Daunorubicin	T45.1X1	T45.1X2	T45.1X3	T45.1X4	T45.1X5	T45.1X6
DBI	T38.3X1	T38.3X2	T38.3X3	T38.3X4	T38.3X5	T38.3X6
D-Con	T60.91	T60.92	T60.93	T60.94	—	—
insecticide	T60.2X1	T60.2X2	T60.2X3	T60.2X4	—	—
rodenticide	T60.4X1	T60.4X2	T60.4X3	T60.4X4	—	—
DDAVP	T38.891	T38.892	T38.893	T38.894	T38.895	T38.896
DDE (bis(chlorophenyl)-dichloroethylene)	T60.2X1	T60.2X2	T60.2X3	T60.2X4	—	—
DDS	T37.1X1	T37.1X2	T37.1X3	T37.1X4	T37.1X5	T37.1X6
DDT (dust)	T60.1X1	T60.1X2	T60.1X3	T60.1X4	—	—
Deadly nightshade — see also Belladonna	T62.2X1	T62.2X2	T62.2X3	T62.2X4	—	—
berry	T62.1X1	T62.1X2	T62.1X3	T62.1X4	—	—
Deamino-D-arginine vasopressin	T38.891	T38.892	T38.893	T38.894	T38.895	T38.896
Deanol (aceglumate)	T50.991	T50.992	T50.993	T50.994	T50.995	T50.996
Debrisoquine	T46.5X1	T46.5X2	T46.5X3	T46.5X4	T46.5X5	T46.5X6
Decaborane	T57.8X1	T57.8X2	T57.8X3	T57.8X4	—	—
fumes	T59.891	T59.892	T59.893	T59.894	—	—
Decadron	T38.0X1	T38.0X2	T38.0X3	T38.0X4	T38.0X5	T38.0X6
ENT agent	T49.6X1	T49.6X2	T49.6X3	T49.6X4	T49.6X5	T49.6X6
ophthalmic preparation	T49.5X1	T49.5X2	T49.5X3	T49.5X4	T49.5X5	T49.5X6
topical NEC	T49.0X1	T49.0X2	T49.0X3	T49.0X4	T49.0X5	T49.0X6
Decahydronaphthalene	T52.8X1	T52.8X2	T52.8X3	T52.8X4	—	—
Decalin	T52.8X1	T52.8X2	T52.8X3	T52.8X4	—	—
Decamethonium (bromide)	T48.1X1	T48.1X2	T48.1X3	T48.1X4	T48.1X5	T48.1X6
Decholin	T47.5X1	T47.5X2	T47.5X3	T47.5X4	T47.5X5	T47.5X6
Declomycin	T36.4X1	T36.4X2	T36.4X3	T36.4X4	T36.4X5	T36.4X6
Decongestant, nasal (mucosa)	T48.5X1	T48.5X2	T48.5X3	T48.5X4	T48.5X5	T48.5X6
combination	T48.5X1	T48.5X2	T48.5X3	T48.5X4	T48.5X5	T48.5X6
Deet	T60.8X1	T60.8X2	T60.8X3	T60.8X4	—	—
Deferoxamine	T45.8X1	T45.8X2	T45.8X3	T45.8X4	T45.8X5	T45.8X6
Deflazacort	T38.0X1	T38.0X2	T38.0X3	T38.0X4	T38.0X5	T38.0X6
Deglycyrrhizinized extract of licorice	T48.4X1	T48.4X2	T48.4X3	T48.4X4	T48.4X5	T48.4X6
Dehydrocholic acid	T47.5X1	T47.5X2	T47.5X3	T47.5X4	T47.5X5	T47.5X6
Dehydroemetine	T37.3X1	T37.3X2	T37.3X3	T37.3X4	T37.3X5	T37.3X6
Dekalin	T52.8X1	T52.8X2	T52.8X3	T52.8X4	—	—
Delalutin	T38.5X1	T38.5X2	T38.5X3	T38.5X4	T38.5X5	T38.5X6
Delorazepam	T42.4X1	T42.4X2	T42.4X3	T42.4X4	T42.4X5	T42.4X6
Delphinium	T62.2X1	T62.2X2	T62.2X3	T62.2X4	—	—
Deltamethrin	T60.1X1	T60.1X2	T60.1X3	T60.1X4	—	—
Deltasone	T38.0X1	T38.0X2	T38.0X3	T38.0X4	T38.0X5	T38.0X6
Delta	T38.0X1	T38.0X2	T38.0X3	T38.0X4	T38.0X5	T38.0X6
Delvinal	T42.3X1	T42.3X2	T42.3X3	T42.3X4	T42.3X5	T42.3X6
Demecarium (bromide)	T49.5X1	T49.5X2	T49.5X3	T49.5X4	T49.5X5	T49.5X6
Demeclocycline	T36.4X1	T36.4X2	T36.4X3	T36.4X4	T36.4X5	T36.4X6
Demecolcine	T45.1X1	T45.1X2	T45.1X3	T45.1X4	T45.1X5	T45.1X6
Demegestone	T38.5X1	T38.5X2	T38.5X3	T38.5X4	T38.5X5	T38.5X6
Demelanizing agents	T49.8X1	T49.8X2	T49.8X3	T49.8X4	T49.8X5	T49.8X6
Demephion -O and -S	T60.0X1	T60.0X2	T60.0X3	T60.0X4	—	—
Demerol	T40.2X1	T40.2X2	T40.2X3	T40.2X4	T40.2X5	T40.2X6
Demethylchlortetracycline	T36.4X1	T36.4X2	T36.4X3	T36.4X4	T36.4X5	T36.4X6
Demethyltetracycline	T36.4X1	T36.4X2	T36.4X3	T36.4X4	T36.4X5	T36.4X6
Demeton -O and -S	T60.0X1	T60.0X2	T60.0X3	T60.0X4	—	—
Demulcent (external)	T49.3X1	T49.3X2	T49.3X3	T49.3X4	T49.3X5	T49.3X6
specified NEC	T49.3X1	T49.3X2	T49.3X3	T49.3X4	T49.3X5	T49.3X6
Demulen	T38.4X1	T38.4X2	T38.4X3	T38.4X4	T38.4X5	T38.4X6
Denatured alcohol	T51.0X1	T51.0X2	T51.0X3	T51.0X4	—	—
Dendrid	T49.5X1	T49.5X2	T49.5X3	T49.5X4	T49.5X5	T49.5X6
Dental drug, topical application NEC	T49.7X1	T49.7X2	T49.7X3	T49.7X4	T49.7X5	T49.7X6
Dentifrice	T49.7X1	T49.7X2	T49.7X3	T49.7X4	T49.7X5	T49.7X6
Deodorant spray (feminine hygiene)	T49.8X1	T49.8X2	T49.8X3	T49.8X4	T49.8X5	T49.8X6
Deoxycortone	T50.0X1	T50.0X2	T50.0X3	T50.0X4	T50.0X5	T50.0X6
Deoxyribonuclease (pancreatic)	T45.3X1	T45.3X2	T45.3X3	T45.3X4	T45.3X5	T45.3X6
Depilatory	T49.4X1	T49.4X2	T49.4X3	T49.4X4	T49.4X5	T49.4X6
Deprenalin	T42.8X1	T42.8X2	T42.8X3	T42.8X4	T42.8X5	T42.8X6
Deprenyl	T42.8X1	T42.8X2	T42.8X3	T42.8X4	T42.8X5	T42.8X6
Depressant						
appetite (central)	T50.5X1	T50.5X2	T50.5X3	T50.5X4	T50.5X5	T50.5X6
cardiac	T46.2X1	T46.2X2	T46.2X3	T46.2X4	T46.2X5	T46.2X6

Substance	Poisoning, Accidental (unintentional)	Poisoning, Intentional Self-harm	Poisoning, Assault	Poisoning, Undetermined	Adverse Effect	Under-dosing
Depressant — continued						
central nervous system (anesthetic) — see also Central nervous system, depressants	T42.71	T42.72	T42.73	T42.74	T42.75	T42.76
general anesthetic	T41.201	T41.202	T41.203	T41.204	T41.205	T41.206
muscle tone	T42.8X1	T42.8X2	T42.8X3	T42.8X4	T42.8X5	T42.8X6
muscle tone, central	T42.8X1	T42.8X2	T42.8X3	T42.8X4	T42.8X5	T42.8X6
psychotherapeutic	T43.501	T43.502	T43.503	T43.504	T43.505	T43.506
Depressant, appetite	T50.5X1	T50.5X2	T50.5X3	T50.5X4	T50.5X5	T50.5X6
Deptropine	T45.0X1	T45.0X2	T45.0X3	T45.0X4	T45.0X5	T45.0X6
Dequalinium (chloride)	T49.0X1	T49.0X2	T49.0X3	T49.0X4	T49.0X5	T49.0X6
Derris root	T60.2X1	T60.2X2	T60.2X3	T60.2X4	—	—
Deserpidine	T46.5X1	T46.5X2	T46.5X3	T46.5X4	T46.5X5	T46.5X6
Desferrioxamine	T45.8X1	T45.8X2	T45.8X3	T45.8X4	T45.8X5	T45.8X6
Desipramine	T43.011	T43.012	T43.013	T43.014	T43.015	T43.016
Deslanoside	T46.0X1	T46.0X2	T46.0X3	T46.0X4	T46.0X5	T46.0X6
Desloughing agent	T49.4X1	T49.4X2	T49.4X3	T49.4X4	T49.4X5	T49.4X6
Desmethylimipramine	T43.011	T43.012	T43.013	T43.014	T43.015	T43.016
Desmopressin	T38.891	T38.892	T38.893	T38.894	T38.895	T38.896
Desocodeine	T40.2X1	T40.2X2	T40.2X3	T40.2X4	T40.2X5	T40.2X6
Desogestrel	T38.5X1	T38.5X2	T38.5X3	T38.5X4	T38.5X5	T38.5X6
Desomorphine	T40.2X1	T40.2X2	T40.2X3	T40.2X4	—	—
Desonide	T49.0X1	T49.0X2	T49.0X3	T49.0X4	T49.0X5	T49.0X6
Desoximetasone	T49.0X1	T49.0X2	T49.0X3	T49.0X4	T49.0X5	T49.0X6
Desoxycorticosteroid	T50.0X1	T50.0X2	T50.0X3	T50.0X4	T50.0X5	T50.0X6
Desoxycortone	T50.0X1	T50.0X2	T50.0X3	T50.0X4	T50.0X5	T50.0X6
Desoxyephedrine	T43.621	T43.622	T43.623	T43.624	T43.625	T43.626
Detaxtran	T46.6X1	T46.6X2	T46.6X3	T46.6X4	T46.6X5	T46.6X6
Detergent	T49.2X1	T49.2X2	T49.2X3	T49.2X4	T49.2X5	T49.2X6
external medication	T49.2X1	T49.2X2	T49.2X3	T49.2X4	T49.2X5	T49.2X6
local	T49.2X1	T49.2X2	T49.2X3	T49.2X4	T49.2X5	T49.2X6
medicinal	T49.2X1	T49.2X2	T49.2X3	T49.2X4	T49.2X5	T49.2X6
nonmedicinal	T55.1X1	T55.1X2	T55.1X3	T55.1X4	—	—
specified NEC	T55.1X1	T55.1X2	T55.1X3	T55.1X4	—	—
Deterrent, alcohol	T50.6X1	T50.6X2	T50.6X3	T50.6X4	T50.6X5	T50.6X6
Detoxifying agent	T50.6X1	T50.6X2	T50.6X3	T50.6X4	T50.6X5	T50.6X6
Detrothyronine	T38.1X1	T38.1X2	T38.1X3	T38.1X4	T38.1X5	T38.1X6
Dettol (external medication)	T49.0X1	T49.0X2	T49.0X3	T49.0X4	T49.0X5	T49.0X6
Dexamethasone	T38.0X1	T38.0X2	T38.0X3	T38.0X4	T38.0X5	T38.0X6
ENT agent	T49.6X1	T49.6X2	T49.6X3	T49.6X4	T49.6X5	T49.6X6
ophthalmic preparation	T49.5X1	T49.5X2	T49.5X3	T49.5X4	T49.5X5	T49.5X6
topical NEC	T49.0X1	T49.0X2	T49.0X3	T49.0X4	T49.0X5	T49.0X6
Dexamfetamine	T43.621	T43.622	T43.623	T43.624	T43.625	T43.626
Dexamphetamine	T43.621	T43.622	T43.623	T43.624	T43.625	T43.626
Dexbrompheniramine	T45.0X1	T45.0X2	T45.0X3	T45.0X4	T45.0X5	T45.0X6
Dexchlorpheniramine	T45.0X1	T45.0X2	T45.0X3	T45.0X4	T45.0X5	T45.0X6
Dexedrine	T43.621	T43.622	T43.623	T43.624	T43.625	T43.626
Dexetimide	T44.3X1	T44.3X2	T44.3X3	T44.3X4	T44.3X5	T44.3X6
Dexfenfluramine	T50.5X1	T50.5X2	T50.5X3	T50.5X4	T50.5X5	T50.5X6
Dexpanthenol	T45.2X1	T45.2X2	T45.2X3	T45.2X4	T45.2X5	T45.2X6
Dextran (40) (70) (150)	T45.8X1	T45.8X2	T45.8X3	T45.8X4	T45.8X5	T45.8X6
Dextriferron	T45.4X1	T45.4X2	T45.4X3	T45.4X4	T45.4X5	T45.4X6
Dextroamphetamine	T43.621	T43.622	T43.623	T43.624	T43.625	T43.626
Dextro calcium pantothenate	T45.2X1	T45.2X2	T45.2X3	T45.2X4	T45.2X5	T45.2X6
Dextromethorphan	T48.3X1	T48.3X2	T48.3X3	T48.3X4	T48.3X5	T48.3X6
Dextromoramide	T40.4X1	T40.4X2	T40.4X3	T40.4X4	—	—
topical	T49.8X1	T49.8X2	T49.8X3	T49.8X4	T49.8X5	T49.8X6
Dextro pantothenyl alcohol	T45.2X1	T45.2X2	T45.2X3	T45.2X4	T45.2X5	T45.2X6
Dextropropoxyphene	T40.4X1	T40.4X2	T40.4X3	T40.4X4	T40.4X5	T40.4X6
Dextrorphan	T40.2X1	T40.2X2	T40.2X3	T40.2X4	T40.2X5	T40.2X6
Dextrose	T50.3X1	T50.3X2	T50.3X3	T50.3X4	T50.3X5	T50.3X6
concentrated solution, intravenous	T46.8X1	T46.8X2	T46.8X3	T46.8X4	T46.8X5	T46.8X6
Dextrothyroxin	T38.1X1	T38.1X2	T38.1X3	T38.1X4	T38.1X5	T38.1X6
Dextrothyroxine sodium	T38.1X1	T38.1X2	T38.1X3	T38.1X4	T38.1X5	T38.1X6
DFP	T44.0X1	T44.0X2	T44.0X3	T44.0X4	T44.0X5	T44.0X6
DHE	T37.3X1	T37.3X2	T37.3X3	T37.3X4	T37.3X5	T37.3X6
45	T46.5X1	T46.5X2	T46.5X3	T46.5X4	T46.5X5	T46.5X6
Diabinese	T38.3X1	T38.3X2	T38.3X3	T38.3X4	T38.3X5	T38.3X6
Diacetone alcohol	T52.4X1	T52.4X2	T52.4X3	T52.4X4	—	—
Diacetyl monoxime	T50.991	T50.992	T50.993	T50.994	—	—
Diacetylmorphine	T40.1X1	T40.1X2	T40.1X3	T40.1X4	—	—
Diachylon plaster	T49.4X1	T49.4X2	T49.4X3	T49.4X4	T49.4X5	T49.4X6
Diaethylstilboestrolum	T38.5X1	T38.5X2	T38.5X3	T38.5X4	T38.5X5	T38.5X6
Diagnostic agent NEC	T50.8X1	T50.8X2	T50.8X3	T50.8X4	T50.8X5	T50.8X6
Dial (soap)	T49.2X1	T49.2X2	T49.2X3	T49.2X4	T49.2X5	T49.2X6
sedative	T42.3X1	T42.3X2	T42.3X3	T42.3X4	T42.3X5	T42.3X6
Dialkyl carbonate	T52.91	T52.92	T52.93	T52.94	—	—
Diallylbarbituric acid	T42.3X1	T42.3X2	T42.3X3	T42.3X4	T42.3X5	T42.3X6
Diallymal	T42.3X1	T42.3X2	T42.3X3	T42.3X4	T42.3X5	T42.3X6

Substance	Poisoning, Accidental (unintentional)	Poisoning, Intentional Self-harm	Poisoning, Assault	Poisoning, Undetermined	Adverse Effect	Under-dosing
Dialysis solution (intraperitoneal)	T5Ø.3X1	T5Ø.3X2	T5Ø.3X3	T5Ø.3X4	T5Ø.3X5	T5Ø.3X6
Diaminodiphenylsulfone	T37.1X1	T37.1X2	T37.1X3	T37.1X4	T37.1X5	T37.1X6
Diamorphine	T4Ø.1X1	T4Ø.1X2	T4Ø.1X3	T4Ø.1X4	—	—
Diamox	T5Ø.2X1	T5Ø.2X2	T5Ø.2X3	T5Ø.2X4	T5Ø.2X5	T5Ø.2X6
Diamthazole	T49.ØX1	T49.ØX2	T49.ØX3	T49.ØX4	T49.ØX5	T49.ØX6
Dianthone	T47.2X1	T47.2X2	T47.2X3	T47.2X4	T47.2X5	T47.2X6
Diaphenylsulfone	T37.ØX1	T37.ØX2	T37.ØX3	T37.ØX4	T37.ØX5	T37.ØX6
Diasone (sodium)	T37.1X1	T37.1X2	T37.1X3	T37.1X4	T37.1X5	T37.1X6
Diastase	T47.5X1	T47.5X2	T47.5X3	T47.5X4	T47.5X5	T47.5X6
Diatrizoate	T5Ø.8X1	T5Ø.8X2	T5Ø.8X3	T5Ø.8X4	T5Ø.8X5	T5Ø.8X6
Diazepam	T42.4X1	T42.4X2	T42.4X3	T42.4X4	T42.4X5	T42.4X6
Diazinon	T6Ø.ØX1	T6Ø.ØX2	T6Ø.ØX3	T6Ø.ØX4	—	—
Diazomethane (gas)	T59.891	T59.892	T59.893	T59.894	—	—
Diazoxide	T46.5X1	T46.5X2	T46.5X3	T46.5X4	T46.5X5	T46.5X6
Dibekacin	T36.5X1	T36.5X2	T36.5X3	T36.5X4	T36.5X5	T36.5X6
Dibenamine	T44.6X1	T44.6X2	T44.6X3	T44.6X4	T44.6X5	T44.6X6
Dibenzepin	T43.Ø11	T43.Ø12	T43.Ø13	T43.Ø14	T43.Ø15	T43.Ø16
Dibenzheptropine	T45.ØX1	T45.ØX2	T45.ØX3	T45.ØX4	T45.ØX5	T45.ØX6
Dibenzyline	T44.6X1	T44.6X2	T44.6X3	T44.6X4	T44.6X5	T44.6X6
Diborane (gas)	T59.891	T59.892	T59.893	T59.894	—	—
Dibromochloropropane	T6Ø.8X1	T6Ø.8X2	T6Ø.8X3	T6Ø.8X4	—	—
Dibromodulcitol	T45.1X1	T45.1X2	T45.1X3	T45.1X4	T45.1X5	T45.1X6
Dibromoethane	T53.6X1	T53.6X2	T53.6X3	T53.6X4	—	—
Dibromomannitol	T45.1X1	T45.1X2	T45.1X3	T45.1X4	T45.1X5	T45.1X6
Dibromopropamidine isethionate	T49.ØX1	T49.ØX2	T49.ØX3	T49.ØX4	T49.ØX5	T49.ØX6
Dibrompropamidine	T49.ØX1	T49.ØX2	T49.ØX3	T49.ØX4	T49.ØX5	T49.ØX6
Dibucaine	T41.3X1	T41.3X2	T41.3X3	T41.3X4	T41.3X5	T41.3X6
topical (surface)	T41.3X1	T41.3X2	T41.3X3	T41.3X4	T41.3X5	T41.3X6
Dibunate sodium	T48.3X1	T48.3X2	T48.3X3	T48.3X4	T48.3X5	T48.3X6
Dibutoline sulfate	T44.3X1	T44.3X2	T44.3X3	T44.3X4	T44.3X5	T44.3X6
Dicamba	T6Ø.3X1	T6Ø.3X2	T6Ø.3X3	T6Ø.3X4	—	—
Dicapthon	T6Ø.ØX1	T6Ø.ØX2	T6Ø.ØX3	T6Ø.ØX4	—	—
Dichlobenil	T6Ø.3X1	T6Ø.3X2	T6Ø.3X3	T6Ø.3X4	—	—
Dichlone	T6Ø.3X1	T6Ø.3X2	T6Ø.3X3	T6Ø.3X4	—	—
Dichloralphenozone	T42.6X1	T42.6X2	T42.6X3	T42.6X4	T42.6X5	T42.6X6
Dichlorbenzidine	T65.3X1	T65.3X2	T65.3X3	T65.3X4	—	—
Dichlorhydrin	T52.8X1	T52.8X2	T52.8X3	T52.8X4	—	—
Dichlorhydroxyquinoline	T37.8X1	T37.8X2	T37.8X3	T37.8X4	T37.8X5	T37.8X6
Dichlorobenzene	T53.7X1	T53.7X2	T53.7X3	T53.7X4	—	—
Dichlorobenzyl alcohol	T49.6X1	T49.6X2	T49.6X3	T49.6X4	T49.6X5	T49.6X6
Dichlorodifluoromethane	T53.5X1	T53.5X2	T53.5X3	T53.5X4	—	—
Dichloroethane	T52.8X1	T52.8X2	T52.8X3	T52.8X4	—	—
Dichloroethylene	T53.6X1	T53.6X2	T53.6X3	T53.6X4	—	—
Dichloroethyl sulfide, not in war	T59.891	T59.892	T59.893	T59.894	—	—
Dichloroformoxine, not in war	T59.891	T59.892	T59.893	T59.894	—	—
Dichlorohydrin, alpha-dichlorohydrin	T52.8X1	T52.8X2	T52.8X3	T52.8X4	—	—
Dichloromethane (solvent)	T53.4X1	T53.4X2	T53.4X3	T53.4X4	—	—
vapor	T53.4X1	T53.4X2	T53.4X3	T53.4X4	—	—
Dichloronaphthoquinone	T6Ø.3X1	T6Ø.3X2	T6Ø.3X3	T6Ø.3X4	—	—
Dichlorophen	T37.4X1	T37.4X2	T37.4X3	T37.4X4	T37.4X5	T37.4X6
Dichloropropene	T6Ø.3X1	T6Ø.3X2	T6Ø.3X3	T6Ø.3X4	—	—
Dichloropropionic acid	T6Ø.3X1	T6Ø.3X2	T6Ø.3X3	T6Ø.3X4	—	—
Dichlorphenamide	T5Ø.2X1	T5Ø.2X2	T5Ø.2X3	T5Ø.2X4	T5Ø.2X5	T5Ø.2X6
Dichlorvos	T6Ø.ØX1	T6Ø.ØX2	T6Ø.ØX3	T6Ø.ØX4	—	—
Diclofenac	T39.391	T39.392	T39.393	T39.394	T39.395	T39.396
Diclofenamide	T5Ø.2X1	T5Ø.2X2	T5Ø.2X3	T5Ø.2X4	T5Ø.2X5	T5Ø.2X6
Diclofensine	T43.291	T43.292	T43.293	T43.294	T43.295	T43.296
Diclonixine	T39.8X1	T39.8X2	T39.8X3	T39.8X4	T39.8X5	T39.8X6
Dicloxacillin	T36.ØX1	T36.ØX2	T36.ØX3	T36.ØX4	T36.ØX5	T36.ØX6
Dicophane	T49.ØX1	T49.ØX2	T49.ØX3	T49.ØX4	T49.ØX5	T49.ØX6
Dicoumarol, dicoumarin, dicumarol	T45.511	T45.512	T45.513	T45.514	T45.515	T45.516
Dicrotophos	T6Ø.ØX1	T6Ø.ØX2	T6Ø.ØX3	T6Ø.ØX4	—	—
Dicyanogen (gas)	T65.ØX1	T65.ØX2	T65.ØX3	T65.ØX4	—	—
Dicyclomine	T44.3X1	T44.3X2	T44.3X3	T44.3X4	T44.3X5	T44.3X6
Dicycloverine	T44.3X1	T44.3X2	T44.3X3	T44.3X4	T44.3X5	T44.3X6
Dideoxycytidine	T37.5X1	T37.5X2	T37.5X3	T37.5X4	T37.5X5	T37.5X6
Dideoxyinosine	T37.5X1	T37.5X2	T37.5X3	T37.5X4	T37.5X5	T37.5X6
Dieldrin (vapor)	T6Ø.1X1	T6Ø.1X2	T6Ø.1X3	T6Ø.1X4	—	—
Diemal	T42.3X1	T42.3X2	T42.3X3	T42.3X4	T42.3X5	T42.3X6
Dienestrol	T38.5X1	T38.5X2	T38.5X3	T38.5X4	T38.5X5	T38.5X6
Dienoestrol	T38.5X1	T38.5X2	T38.5X3	T38.5X4	T38.5X5	T38.5X6
Dietetic drug NEC	T5Ø.9Ø1	T5Ø.9Ø2	T5Ø.9Ø3	T5Ø.9Ø4	T5Ø.9Ø5	T5Ø.9Ø6
Diethazine	T42.8X1	T42.8X2	T42.8X3	T42.8X4	T42.8X5	T42.8X6
Diethyl						
barbituric acid	T42.3X1	T42.3X2	T42.3X3	T42.3X4	T42.3X5	T42.3X6
carbamazine	T37.4X1	T37.4X2	T37.4X3	T37.4X4	T37.4X5	T37.4X6
carbinol	T51.3X1	T51.3X2	T51.3X3	T51.3X4	—	—

Substance	Poisoning, Accidental (unintentional)	Poisoning, Intentional Self-harm	Poisoning, Assault	Poisoning, Undetermined	Adverse Effect	Under-dosing
Diethyl — *continued*						
carbonate	T52.8X1	T52.8X2	T52.8X3	T52.8X4	—	—
ether (vapor) — *see also* ether	T41.ØX1	T41.ØX2	T41.ØX3	T41.ØX4	T41.ØX5	T41.ØX6
oxide	T52.8X1	T52.8X2	T52.8X3	T52.8X4	—	—
propion	T5Ø.5X1	T5Ø.5X2	T5Ø.5X3	T5Ø.5X4	T5Ø.5X5	T5Ø.5X6
stilbestrol	T38.5X1	T38.5X2	T38.5X3	T38.5X4	T38.5X5	T38.5X6
toluamide (nonmedicinal)	T6Ø.8X1	T6Ø.8X2	T6Ø.8X3	T6Ø.8X4	—	—
medicinal	T49.3X1	T49.3X2	T49.3X3	T49.3X4	T49.3X5	T49.3X6
Diethylcarbamazine	T37.4X1	T37.4X2	T37.4X3	T37.4X4	T37.4X5	T37.4X6
Diethylene						
dioxide	T52.8X1	T52.8X2	T52.8X3	T52.8X4	—	—
glycol (monoacetate) (monobutyl ether) (monoethyl ether)	T52.3X1	T52.3X2	T52.3X3	T52.3X4	—	—
Diethylhexylphthalate	T65.891	T65.892	T65.893	T65.894	—	—
Diethylpropion	T5Ø.5X1	T5Ø.5X2	T5Ø.5X3	T5Ø.5X4	T5Ø.5X5	T5Ø.5X6
Diethylstilbestrol	T38.5X1	T38.5X2	T38.5X3	T38.5X4	T38.5X5	T38.5X6
Diethylstilboestrol	T38.5X1	T38.5X2	T38.5X3	T38.5X4	T38.5X5	T38.5X6
Diethylsulfone-diethylmethane	T42.6X1	T42.6X2	T42.6X3	T42.6X4	T42.6X5	T42.6X6
Diethyltoluamide	T49.ØX1	T49.ØX2	T49.ØX3	T49.ØX4	T49.ØX5	T49.ØX6
Diethyltryptamine (DET)	T4Ø.991	T4Ø.992	T4Ø.993	T4Ø.994	—	—
Difebarbamate	T42.3X1	T42.3X2	T42.3X3	T42.3X4	T42.3X5	T42.3X6
Difencloxazine	T4Ø.2X1	T4Ø.2X2	T4Ø.2X3	T4Ø.2X4	T4Ø.2X5	T4Ø.2X6
Difenidol	T45.ØX1	T45.ØX2	T45.ØX3	T45.ØX4	T45.ØX5	T45.ØX6
Difenoxin	T47.6X1	T47.6X2	T47.6X3	T47.6X4	T47.6X5	T47.6X6
Difetarsone	T37.3X1	T37.3X2	T37.3X3	T37.3X4	T37.3X5	T37.3X6
Diffusin	T45.3X1	T45.3X2	T45.3X3	T45.3X4	T45.3X5	T45.3X6
Diflorasone	T49.ØX1	T49.ØX2	T49.ØX3	T49.ØX4	T49.ØX5	T49.ØX6
Diflos	T44.ØX1	T44.ØX2	T44.ØX3	T44.ØX4	T44.ØX5	T44.ØX6
Diflubenzuron	T6Ø.1X1	T6Ø.1X2	T6Ø.1X3	T6Ø.1X4	—	—
Diflucortolone	T49.ØX1	T49.ØX2	T49.ØX3	T49.ØX4	T49.ØX5	T49.ØX6
Diflunisal	T39.Ø91	T39.Ø92	T39.Ø93	T39.Ø94	T39.Ø95	T39.Ø96
Difluoromethyldopa	T42.8X1	T42.8X2	T42.8X3	T42.8X4	T42.8X5	T42.8X6
Difluorophate	T44.ØX1	T44.ØX2	T44.ØX3	T44.ØX4	T44.ØX5	T44.ØX6
Digestant NEC	T47.5X1	T47.5X2	T47.5X3	T47.5X4	T47.5X5	T47.5X6
Digitalin (e)	T46.ØX1	T46.ØX2	T46.ØX3	T46.ØX4	T46.ØX5	T46.ØX6
Digitalis (leaf)(glycoside)	T46.ØX1	T46.ØX2	T46.ØX3	T46.ØX4	T46.ØX5	T46.ØX6
lanata	T46.ØX1	T46.ØX2	T46.ØX3	T46.ØX4	T46.ØX5	T46.ØX6
purpurea	T46.ØX1	T46.ØX2	T46.ØX3	T46.ØX4	T46.ØX5	T46.ØX6
Digitoxin	T46.ØX1	T46.ØX2	T46.ØX3	T46.ØX4	T46.ØX5	T46.ØX6
Digitoxose	T46.ØX1	T46.ØX2	T46.ØX3	T46.ØX4	T46.ØX5	T46.ØX6
Digoxin	T46.ØX1	T46.ØX2	T46.ØX3	T46.ØX4	T46.ØX5	T46.ØX6
Digoxine	T46.ØX1	T46.ØX2	T46.ØX3	T46.ØX4	T46.ØX5	T46.ØX6
Dihydralazine	T46.5X1	T46.5X2	T46.5X3	T46.5X4	T46.5X5	T46.5X6
Dihydrazine	T46.5X1	T46.5X2	T46.5X3	T46.5X4	T46.5X5	T46.5X6
Dihydrocodeine	T4Ø.2X1	T4Ø.2X2	T4Ø.2X3	T4Ø.2X4	T4Ø.2X5	T4Ø.2X6
Dihydrocodeinone	T4Ø.2X1	T4Ø.2X2	T4Ø.2X3	T4Ø.2X4	T4Ø.2X5	T4Ø.2X6
Dihydroergocornine	T46.7X1	T46.7X2	T46.7X3	T46.7X4	T46.7X5	T46.7X6
Dihydroergocristine (mesilate)	T46.7X1	T46.7X2	T46.7X3	T46.7X4	T46.7X5	T46.7X6
Dihydroergokryptine	T46.7X1	T46.7X2	T46.7X3	T46.7X4	T46.7X5	T46.7X6
Dihydroergotamine	T46.5X1	T46.5X2	T46.5X3	T46.5X4	T46.5X5	T46.5X6
Dihydroergotoxine	T46.7X1	T46.7X2	T46.7X3	T46.7X4	T46.7X5	T46.7X6
mesilate	T46.7X1	T46.7X2	T46.7X3	T46.7X4	T46.7X5	T46.7X6
Dihydrohydroxycodeinone	T4Ø.2X1	T4Ø.2X2	T4Ø.2X3	T4Ø.2X4	T4Ø.2X5	T4Ø.2X6
Dihydrohydroxymorphinone	T4Ø.2X1	T4Ø.2X2	T4Ø.2X3	T4Ø.2X4	T4Ø.2X5	T4Ø.2X6
Dihydroisocodeine	T4Ø.2X1	T4Ø.2X2	T4Ø.2X3	T4Ø.2X4	T4Ø.2X5	T4Ø.2X6
Dihydromorphine	T4Ø.2X1	T4Ø.2X2	T4Ø.2X3	T4Ø.2X4	—	—
Dihydromorphinone	T4Ø.2X1	T4Ø.2X2	T4Ø.2X3	T4Ø.2X4	T4Ø.2X5	T4Ø.2X6
Dihydrostreptomycin	T36.5X1	T36.5X2	T36.5X3	T36.5X4	T36.5X5	T36.5X6
Dihydrotachysterol	T45.2X1	T45.2X2	T45.2X3	T45.2X4	T45.2X5	T45.2X6
Dihydroxyaluminum aminoacetate	T47.1X1	T47.1X2	T47.1X3	T47.1X4	T47.1X5	T47.1X6
Dihydroxyaluminum sodium carbonate	T47.1X1	T47.1X2	T47.1X3	T47.1X4	T47.1X5	T47.1X6
Dihydroxyanthraquinone	T47.2X1	T47.2X2	T47.2X3	T47.2X4	T47.2X5	T47.2X6
Dihydroxycodeinone	T4Ø.2X1	T4Ø.2X2	T4Ø.2X3	T4Ø.2X4	T4Ø.2X5	T4Ø.2X6
Dihydroxypropyl theophylline	T5Ø.2X1	T5Ø.2X2	T5Ø.2X3	T5Ø.2X4	T5Ø.2X5	T5Ø.2X6
Diiodohydroxyquin	T37.8X1	T37.8X2	T37.8X3	T37.8X4	T37.8X5	T37.8X6
topical	T49.ØX1	T49.ØX2	T49.ØX3	T49.ØX4	T49.ØX5	T49.ØX6
Diiodohydroxyquinoline	T37.8X1	T37.8X2	T37.8X3	T37.8X4	T37.8X5	T37.8X6
Diiodotyrosine	T38.2X1	T38.2X2	T38.2X3	T38.2X4	T38.2X5	T38.2X6
Diisopromine	T44.3X1	T44.3X2	T44.3X3	T44.3X4	T44.3X5	T44.3X6
Diisopropylamine	T46.3X1	T46.3X2	T46.3X3	T46.3X4	T46.3X5	T46.3X6
Diisopropylfluorophosphonate	T44.ØX1	T44.ØX2	T44.ØX3	T44.ØX4	T44.ØX5	T44.ØX6
Dilantin	T42.ØX1	T42.ØX2	T42.ØX3	T42.ØX4	T42.ØX5	T42.ØX6
Dilaudid	T4Ø.2X1	T4Ø.2X2	T4Ø.2X3	T4Ø.2X4	T4Ø.2X5	T4Ø.2X6
Dilazep	T46.3X1	T46.3X2	T46.3X3	T46.3X4	T46.3X5	T46.3X6
Dill	T47.5X1	T47.5X2	T47.5X3	T47.5X4	T47.5X5	T47.5X6
Diloxanide	T37.3X1	T37.3X2	T37.3X3	T37.3X4	T37.3X5	T37.3X6
Diltiazem	T46.1X1	T46.1X2	T46.1X3	T46.1X4	T46.1X5	T46.1X6

Substance	Poisoning, Accidental (unintentional)	Poisoning, Intentional Self-harm	Poisoning, Assault	Poisoning, Undetermined	Adverse Effect	Under-dosing
Dimazole	T49.0X1	T49.0X2	T49.0X3	T49.0X4	T49.0X5	T49.0X6
Dimefline	T50.7X1	T50.7X2	T50.7X3	T50.7X4	T50.7X5	T50.7X6
Dimefox	T60.0X1	T60.0X2	T60.0X3	T60.0X4	—	—
Dimemorfan	T48.3X1	T48.3X2	T48.3X3	T48.3X4	T48.3X5	T48.3X6
Dimenhydrinate	T45.0X1	T45.0X2	T45.0X3	T45.0X4	T45.0X5	T45.0X6
Dimercaprol (British anti-lewisite)	T45.8X1	T45.8X2	T45.8X3	T45.8X4	T45.8X5	T45.8X6
Dimercaptopropanol	T45.8X1	T45.8X2	T45.8X3	T45.8X4	T45.8X5	T45.8X6
Dimestrol	T38.5X1	T38.5X2	T38.5X3	T38.5X4	T38.5X5	T38.5X6
Dimetane	T45.0X1	T45.0X2	T45.0X3	T45.0X4	T45.0X5	T45.0X6
Dimethicone	T47.1X1	T47.1X2	T47.1X3	T47.1X4	T47.1X5	T47.1X6
Dimethindene	T45.0X1	T45.0X2	T45.0X3	T45.0X4	T45.0X5	T45.0X6
Dimethisoquin	T49.1X1	T49.1X2	T49.1X3	T49.1X4	T49.1X5	T49.1X6
Dimethisterone	T38.5X1	T38.5X2	T38.5X3	T38.5X4	T38.5X5	T38.5X6
Dimethoate	T60.0X1	T60.0X2	T60.0X3	T60.0X4	—	—
Dimethocaine	T41.3X1	T41.3X2	T41.3X3	T41.3X4	T41.3X5	T41.3X6
Dimethoxanate	T48.3X1	T48.3X2	T48.3X3	T48.3X4	T48.3X5	T48.3X6
Dimethyl						
arsine, arsinic acid	T57.0X1	T57.0X2	T57.0X3	T57.0X4	—	—
carbinol	T51.2X1	T51.2X2	T51.2X3	T51.2X4	—	—
carbonate	T52.8X1	T52.8X2	T52.8X3	T52.8X4	—	—
diguanide	T38.3X1	T38.3X2	T38.3X3	T38.3X4	T38.3X5	T38.3X6
ketone	T52.4X1	T52.4X2	T52.4X3	T52.4X4	—	—
vapor	T52.4X1	T52.4X2	T52.4X3	T52.4X4	—	—
meperidine	T40.2X1	T40.2X2	T40.2X3	T40.2X4	T40.2X5	T40.2X6
parathion	T60.0X1	T60.0X2	T60.0X3	T60.0X4	—	—
phthlate	T49.3X1	T49.3X2	T49.3X3	T49.3X4	T49.3X5	T49.3X6
polysiloxane	T47.8X1	T47.8X2	T47.8X3	T47.8X4	T47.8X5	T47.8X6
sulfate (fumes)	T59.891	T59.892	T59.893	T59.894	—	—
liquid	T65.891	T65.892	T65.893	T65.894	—	—
sulfoxide (nonmedicinal)	T52.8X1	T52.8X2	T52.8X3	T52.8X4	—	—
medicinal	T49.4X1	T49.4X2	T49.4X3	T49.4X4	T49.4X5	T49.4X6
tryptamine	T40.991	T40.992	T40.993	T40.994	—	—
tubocurarine	T48.1X1	T48.1X2	T48.1X3	T48.1X4	T48.1X5	T48.1X6
Dimethylamine sulfate	T49.4X1	T49.4X2	T49.4X3	T49.4X4	T49.4X5	T49.4X6
Dimethylformamide	T52.8X1	T52.8X2	T52.8X3	T52.8X4	—	—
Dimethyltubocurarinium chloride	T48.1X1	T48.1X2	T48.1X3	T48.1X4	T48.1X5	T48.1X6
Dimeticone	T47.1X1	T47.1X2	T47.1X3	T47.1X4	T47.1X5	T47.1X6
Dimetilan	T60.0X1	T60.0X2	T60.0X3	T60.0X4	—	—
Dimetindene	T45.0X1	T45.0X2	T45.0X3	T45.0X4	T45.0X5	T45.0X6
Dimetotiazine	T43.3X1	T43.3X2	T43.3X3	T43.3X4	T43.3X5	T43.3X6
Dimorpholamine	T50.7X1	T50.7X2	T50.7X3	T50.7X4	T50.7X5	T50.7X6
Dimoxyline	T46.3X1	T46.3X2	T46.3X3	T46.3X4	T46.3X5	T46.3X6
Dinitrobenzene	T65.3X1	T65.3X2	T65.3X3	T65.3X4	—	—
vapor	T59.891	T59.892	T59.893	T59.894	—	—
Dinitrobenzol	T65.3X1	T65.3X2	T65.3X3	T65.3X4	—	—
vapor	T59.891	T59.892	T59.893	T59.894	—	—
Dinitrobutylphenol	T65.3X1	T65.3X2	T65.3X3	T65.3X4	—	—
Dinitro (-ortho-)cresol (pesticide) (spray)	T65.3X1	T65.3X2	T65.3X3	T65.3X4	—	—
Dinitrocyclohexylphenol	T65.3X1	T65.3X2	T65.3X3	T65.3X4	—	—
Dinitrophenol	T65.3X1	T65.3X2	T65.3X3	T65.3X4	—	—
Dinoprost	T48.0X1	T48.0X2	T48.0X3	T48.0X4	T48.0X5	T48.0X6
Dinoprostone	T48.0X1	T48.0X2	T48.0X3	T48.0X4	T48.0X5	T48.0X6
Dinoseb	T60.3X1	T60.3X2	T60.3X3	T60.3X4	—	—
Dioctyl sulfosuccinate (calcium) (sodium)	T47.4X1	T47.4X2	T47.4X3	T47.4X4	T47.4X5	T47.4X6
Diodone	T50.8X1	T50.8X2	T50.8X3	T50.8X4	T50.8X5	T50.8X6
Diodoquin	T37.8X1	T37.8X2	T37.8X3	T37.8X4	T37.8X5	T37.8X6
Dionin	T40.2X1	T40.2X2	T40.2X3	T40.2X4	T40.2X5	T40.2X6
Diosmin	T46.991	T46.992	T46.993	T46.994	T46.995	T46.996
Dioxane	T52.8X1	T52.8X2	T52.8X3	T52.8X4	—	—
Dioxathion	T60.0X1	T60.0X2	T60.0X3	T60.0X4	—	—
Dioxin	T53.7X1	T53.7X2	T53.7X3	T53.7X4	—	—
Dioxopromethazine	T43.3X1	T43.3X2	T43.3X3	T43.3X4	T43.3X5	T43.3X6
Dioxyline	T46.3X1	T46.3X2	T46.3X3	T46.3X4	T46.3X5	T46.3X6
Dipentene	T52.8X1	T52.8X2	T52.8X3	T52.8X4	—	—
Diperodon	T41.3X1	T41.3X2	T41.3X3	T41.3X4	T41.3X5	T41.3X6
Diphacinone	T60.4X1	T60.4X2	T60.4X3	T60.4X4	—	—
Diphemanil	T44.3X1	T44.3X2	T44.3X3	T44.3X4	T44.3X5	T44.3X6
metilsulfate	T44.3X1	T44.3X2	T44.3X3	T44.3X4	T44.3X5	T44.3X6
Diphenadione	T45.511	T45.512	T45.513	T45.514	T45.515	T45.516
rodenticide	T60.4X1	T60.4X2	T60.4X3	T60.4X4	—	—
Diphenhydramine	T45.0X1	T45.0X2	T45.0X3	T45.0X4	T45.0X5	T45.0X6
Diphenidol	T45.0X1	T45.0X2	T45.0X3	T45.0X4	T45.0X5	T45.0X6
Diphenoxylate	T47.6X1	T47.6X2	T47.6X3	T47.6X4	T47.6X5	T47.6X6
Diphenylamine	T65.3X1	T65.3X2	T65.3X3	T65.3X4	—	—
Diphenylbutazone	T39.2X1	T39.2X2	T39.2X3	T39.2X4	T39.2X5	T39.2X6
Diphenylchloroarsine, not in war	T57.0X1	T57.0X2	T57.0X3	T57.0X4	—	—
Diphenylhydantoin	T42.0X1	T42.0X2	T42.0X3	T42.0X4	T42.0X5	T42.0X6
Diphenylmethane dye	T52.1X1	T52.1X2	T52.1X3	T52.1X4	—	—
Diphenylpyraline	T45.0X1	T45.0X2	T45.0X3	T45.0X4	T45.0X5	T45.0X6
Diphtheria						
antitoxin	T50.Z11	T50.Z12	T50.Z13	T50.Z14	T50.Z15	T50.Z16
toxoid	T50.A91	T50.A92	T50.A93	T50.A94	T50.A95	T50.A96
with tetanus toxoid	T50.A21	T50.A22	T50.A23	T50.A24	T50.A25	T50.A26
with pertussis component	T50.A11	T50.A12	T50.A13	T50.A14	T50.A15	T50.A16
vaccine	T50.A91	T50.A92	T50.A93	T50.A94	T50.A95	T50.A96
combination						
without pertussis	T50.A21	T50.A22	T50.A23	T50.A24	T50.A25	T50.A26
including pertussis	T50.A11	T50.A12	T50.A13	T50.A14	T50.A15	T50.A16
Diphylline	T50.2X1	T50.2X2	T50.2X3	T50.2X4	T50.2X5	T50.2X6
Dipipanone	T40.4X1	T40.4X2	T40.4X3	T40.4X4	—	—
Dipivefrine	T49.5X1	T49.5X2	T49.5X3	T49.5X4	T49.5X5	T49.5X6
Diplovax	T50.B91	T50.B92	T50.B93	T50.B94	T50.B95	T50.B96
Diprophylline	T50.2X1	T50.2X2	T50.2X3	T50.2X4	T50.2X5	T50.2X6
Dipropyline	T48.291	T48.292	T48.293	T48.294	T48.295	T48.296
Dipyridamole	T46.3X1	T46.3X2	T46.3X3	T46.3X4	T46.3X5	T46.3X6
Dipyrone	T39.2X1	T39.2X2	T39.2X3	T39.2X4	T39.2X5	T39.2X6
Diquat (dibromide)	T60.3X1	T60.3X2	T60.3X3	T60.3X4	—	—
Disinfectant	T65.891	T65.892	T65.893	T65.894	—	—
alkaline	T54.3X1	T54.3X2	T54.3X3	T54.3X4	—	—
aromatic	T54.1X1	T54.1X2	T54.1X3	T54.1X4	—	—
intestinal	T37.8X1	T37.8X2	T37.8X3	T37.8X4	T37.8X5	T37.8X6
Disipal	T42.8X1	T42.8X2	T42.8X3	T42.8X4	T42.8X5	T42.8X6
Disodium edetate	T50.6X1	T50.6X2	T50.6X3	T50.6X4	T50.6X5	T50.6X6
Disoprofol	T41.291	T41.292	T41.293	T41.294	T41.295	T41.296
Disopyramide	T46.2X1	T46.2X2	T46.2X3	T46.2X4	T46.2X5	T46.2X6
Distigmine (bromide)	T44.0X1	T44.0X2	T44.0X3	T44.0X4	T44.0X5	T44.0X6
Disulfamide	T50.2X1	T50.2X2	T50.2X3	T50.2X4	T50.2X5	T50.2X6
Disulfanilamide	T37.0X1	T37.0X2	T37.0X3	T37.0X4	T37.0X5	T37.0X6
Disulfiram	T50.6X1	T50.6X2	T50.6X3	T50.6X4	T50.6X5	T50.6X6
Disulfoton	T60.0X1	T60.0X2	T60.0X3	T60.0X4	—	—
Dithiazanine iodide	T37.4X1	T37.4X2	T37.4X3	T37.4X4	T37.4X5	T37.4X6
Dithiocarbamate	T60.0X1	T60.0X2	T60.0X3	T60.0X4	—	—
Dithranol	T49.4X1	T49.4X2	T49.4X3	T49.4X4	T49.4X5	T49.4X6
Diucardin	T50.2X1	T50.2X2	T50.2X3	T50.2X4	T50.2X5	T50.2X6
Diupres	T50.2X1	T50.2X2	T50.2X3	T50.2X4	T50.2X5	T50.2X6
Diuretic NEC	T50.2X1	T50.2X2	T50.2X3	T50.2X4	T50.2X5	T50.2X6
benzothiadiazine	T50.2X1	T50.2X2	T50.2X3	T50.2X4	T50.2X5	T50.2X6
carbonic acid anhydrase inhibitors	T50.2X1	T50.2X2	T50.2X3	T50.2X4	T50.2X5	T50.2X6
furfuryl NEC	T50.2X1	T50.2X2	T50.2X3	T50.2X4	T50.2X5	T50.2X6
loop (high-ceiling)	T50.1X1	T50.1X2	T50.1X3	T50.1X4	T50.1X5	T50.1X6
mercurial NEC	T50.2X1	T50.2X2	T50.2X3	T50.2X4	T50.2X5	T50.2X6
osmotic	T50.2X1	T50.2X2	T50.2X3	T50.2X4	T50.2X5	T50.2X6
purine NEC	T50.2X1	T50.2X2	T50.2X3	T50.2X4	T50.2X5	T50.2X6
saluretic NEC	T50.2X1	T50.2X2	T50.2X3	T50.2X4	T50.2X5	T50.2X6
sulfonamide	T50.2X1	T50.2X2	T50.2X3	T50.2X4	T50.2X5	T50.2X6
thiazide NEC	T50.2X1	T50.2X2	T50.2X3	T50.2X4	T50.2X5	T50.2X6
xanthine	T50.2X1	T50.2X2	T50.2X3	T50.2X4	T50.2X5	T50.2X6
Diurgin	T50.2X1	T50.2X2	T50.2X3	T50.2X4	T50.2X5	T50.2X6
Diuril	T50.2X1	T50.2X2	T50.2X3	T50.2X4	T50.2X5	T50.2X6
Diuron	T60.3X1	T60.3X2	T60.3X3	T60.3X4	—	—
Divalproex	T42.6X1	T42.6X2	T42.6X3	T42.6X4	T42.6X5	T42.6X6
Divinyl ether	T41.0X1	T41.0X2	T41.0X3	T41.0X4	T41.0X5	T41.0X6
Dixanthogen	T49.0X1	T49.0X2	T49.0X3	T49.0X4	T49.0X5	T49.0X6
Dixyrazine	T43.3X1	T43.3X2	T43.3X3	T43.3X4	T43.3X5	T43.3X6
D-lysergic acid diethylamide	T40.8X1	T40.8X2	T40.8X3	T40.8X4	—	—
DMCT	T36.4X1	T36.4X2	T36.4X3	T36.4X4	T36.4X5	T36.4X6
DMSO — *see* Dimethyl sulfoxide						
DNBP	T60.3X1	T60.3X2	T60.3X3	T60.3X4	—	—
DNOC	T65.3X1	T65.3X2	T65.3X3	T65.3X4	—	—
Dobutamine	T44.5X1	T44.5X2	T44.5X3	T44.5X4	T44.5X5	T44.5X6
DOCA	T38.0X1	T38.0X2	T38.0X3	T38.0X4	T38.0X5	T38.0X6
Docusate sodium	T47.4X1	T47.4X2	T47.4X3	T47.4X4	T47.4X5	T47.4X6
Dodicin	T49.0X1	T49.0X2	T49.0X3	T49.0X4	T49.0X5	T49.0X6
Dofamium chloride	T49.0X1	T49.0X2	T49.0X3	T49.0X4	T49.0X5	T49.0X6
Dolophine	T40.3X1	T40.3X2	T40.3X3	T40.3X4	T40.3X5	T40.3X6
Doloxene	T39.8X1	T39.8X2	T39.8X3	T39.8X4	T39.8X5	T39.8X6
Domestic gas (after combustion) — *see* Gas, utility						
prior to combustion	T59.891	T59.892	T59.893	T59.894	—	—
Domiodol	T48.4X1	T48.4X2	T48.4X3	T48.4X4	T48.4X5	T48.4X6
Domiphen (bromide)	T49.0X1	T49.0X2	T49.0X3	T49.0X4	T49.0X5	T49.0X6
Domperidone	T45.0X1	T45.0X2	T45.0X3	T45.0X4	T45.0X5	T45.0X6
Dopa	T42.8X1	T42.8X2	T42.8X3	T42.8X4	T42.8X5	T42.8X6
Dopamine	T44.991	T44.992	T44.993	T44.994	T44.995	T44.996
Doriden	T42.6X1	T42.6X2	T42.6X3	T42.6X4	T42.6X5	T42.6X6
Dormiral	T42.3X1	T42.3X2	T42.3X3	T42.3X4	T42.3X5	T42.3X6
Dormison	T42.6X1	T42.6X2	T42.6X3	T42.6X4	T42.6X5	T42.6X6
Dornase	T48.4X1	T48.4X2	T48.4X3	T48.4X4	T48.4X5	T48.4X6

▽ Subterms under main terms may continue to next column or page   Additional Character May Be Required — Refer to the Tabular List for Character Selection

Table of Drugs and Chemicals

Substance	Poisoning, Accidental (unintentional)	Poisoning, Intentional Self-harm	Poisoning, Assault	Poisoning, Undetermined	Adverse Effect	Under-dosing
Dorsacaine	T41.3X1	T41.3X2	T41.3X3	T41.3X4	T41.3X5	T41.3X6
Dosulepin	T43.Ø11	T43.Ø12	T43.Ø13	T43.Ø14	T43.Ø15	T43.Ø16
Dothiepin	T43.Ø11	T43.Ø12	T43.Ø13	T43.Ø14	T43.Ø15	T43.Ø16
Doxantrazole	T48.6X1	T48.6X2	T48.6X3	T48.6X4	T48.6X5	T48.6X6
Doxapram	T5Ø.7X1	T5Ø.7X2	T5Ø.7X3	T5Ø.7X4	T5Ø.7X5	T5Ø.7X6
Doxazosin	T44.6X1	T44.6X2	T44.6X3	T44.6X4	T44.6X5	T44.6X6
Doxepin	T43.Ø11	T43.Ø12	T43.Ø13	T43.Ø14	T43.Ø15	T43.Ø16
Doxifluridine	T45.1X1	T45.1X2	T45.1X3	T45.1X4	T45.1X5	T45.1X6
Doxorubicin	T45.1X1	T45.1X2	T45.1X3	T45.1X4	T45.1X5	T45.1X6
Doxycycline	T36.4X1	T36.4X2	T36.4X3	T36.4X4	T36.4X5	T36.4X6
Doxylamine	T45.ØX1	T45.ØX2	T45.ØX3	T45.ØX4	T45.ØX5	T45.ØX6
Dramamine	T45.ØX1	T45.ØX2	T45.ØX3	T45.ØX4	T45.ØX5	T45.ØX6
Drano (drain cleaner)	T54.3X1	T54.3X2	T54.3X3	T54.3X4	—	—
Dressing, live pulp	T49.7X1	T49.7X2	T49.7X3	T49.7X4	T49.7X5	T49.7X6
Drocode	T4Ø.2X1	T4Ø.2X2	T4Ø.2X3	T4Ø.2X4	T4Ø.2X5	T4Ø.2X6
Dromoran	T4Ø.2X1	T4Ø.2X2	T4Ø.2X3	T4Ø.2X4	T4Ø.2X5	T4Ø.2X6
Dromostanolone	T38.7X1	T38.7X2	T38.7X3	T38.7X4	T38.7X5	T38.7X6
Dronabinol	T4Ø.7X1	T4Ø.7X2	T4Ø.7X3	T4Ø.7X4	T4Ø.7X5	T4Ø.7X6
Droperidol	T43.591	T43.592	T43.593	T43.594	T43.595	T43.596
Dropropizine	T48.3X1	T48.3X2	T48.3X3	T48.3X4	T48.3X5	T48.3X6
Drostanolone	T38.7X1	T38.7X2	T38.7X3	T38.7X4	T38.7X5	T38.7X6
Drotaverine	T44.3X1	T44.3X2	T44.3X3	T44.3X4	T44.3X5	T44.3X6
Drotrecogin alfa	T45.511	T45.512	T45.513	T45.514	T45.515	T45.516
Drug NEC	T5Ø.9Ø1	T5Ø.9Ø2	T5Ø.9Ø3	T5Ø.9Ø4	T5Ø.9Ø5	T5Ø.9Ø6
specified NEC	T5Ø.991	T5Ø.992	T5Ø.993	T5Ø.994	T5Ø.995	T5Ø.996
DTIC	T45.1X1	T45.1X2	T45.1X3	T45.1X4	T45.1X5	T45.1X6
Duboisine	T44.3X1	T44.3X2	T44.3X3	T44.3X4	T44.3X5	T44.3X6
Dulcolax	T47.2X1	T47.2X2	T47.2X3	T47.2X4	T47.2X5	T47.2X6
Duponol (C) (EP)	T49.2X1	T49.2X2	T49.2X3	T49.2X4	T49.2X5	T49.2X6
Durabolin	T38.7X1	T38.7X2	T38.7X3	T38.7X4	T38.7X5	T38.7X6
Dyclone	T41.3X1	T41.3X2	T41.3X3	T41.3X4	T41.3X5	T41.3X6
Dyclonine	T41.3X1	T41.3X2	T41.3X3	T41.3X4	T41.3X5	T41.3X6
Dydrogesterone	T38.5X1	T38.5X2	T38.5X3	T38.5X4	T38.5X5	T38.5X6
Dye NEC	T65.6X1	T65.6X2	T65.6X3	T65.6X4	—	—
antiseptic	T49.ØX1	T49.ØX2	T49.ØX3	T49.ØX4	T49.ØX5	T49.ØX6
diagnostic agents	T5Ø.8X1	T5Ø.8X2	T5Ø.8X3	T5Ø.8X4	T5Ø.8X5	T5Ø.8X6
pharmaceutical NEC	T5Ø.9Ø1	T5Ø.9Ø2	T5Ø.9Ø3	T5Ø.9Ø4	T5Ø.9Ø5	T5Ø.9Ø6
Dyflos	T44.ØX1	T44.ØX2	T44.ØX3	T44.ØX4	T44.ØX5	T44.ØX6
Dymelor	T38.3X1	T38.3X2	T38.3X3	T38.3X4	T38.3X5	T38.3X6
Dynamite	T65.3X1	T65.3X2	T65.3X3	T65.3X4	—	—
fumes	T59.891	T59.892	T59.893	T59.894	—	—
Dyphylline	T44.3X1	T44.3X2	T44.3X3	T44.3X4	T44.3X5	T44.3X6
b-eucaine	T49.1X1	T49.1X2	T49.1X3	T49.1X4	T49.1X5	T49.1X6
Ear drug NEC	T49.6X1	T49.6X2	T49.6X3	T49.6X4	T49.6X5	T49.6X6
Ear preparations	T49.6X1	T49.6X2	T49.6X3	T49.6X4	T49.6X5	T49.6X6
Echothiophate, echothiopate, ecothiopate	T49.5X1	T49.5X2	T49.5X3	T49.5X4	T49.5X5	T49.5X6
Econazole	T49.ØX1	T49.ØX2	T49.ØX3	T49.ØX4	T49.ØX5	T49.ØX6
Ecothiopate iodide	T49.5X1	T49.5X2	T49.5X3	T49.5X4	T49.5X5	T49.5X6
Ecstasy	T43.621	T43.622	T43.623	T43.624	T43.625	T43.626
Ectylurea	T42.6X1	T42.6X2	T42.6X3	T42.6X4	T42.6X5	T42.6X6
Edathamil disodium	T45.8X1	T45.8X2	T45.8X3	T45.8X4	T45.8X5	T45.8X6
Edecrin	T5Ø.1X1	T5Ø.1X2	T5Ø.1X3	T5Ø.1X4	T5Ø.1X5	T5Ø.1X6
Edetate, disodium (calcium)	T45.8X1	T45.8X2	T45.8X3	T45.8X4	T45.8X5	T45.8X6
Edoxudine	T49.5X1	T49.5X2	T49.5X3	T49.5X4	T49.5X5	T49.5X6
Edrophonium	T44.ØX1	T44.ØX2	T44.ØX3	T44.ØX4	T44.ØX5	T44.ØX6
chloride	T44.ØX1	T44.ØX2	T44.ØX3	T44.ØX4	T44.ØX5	T44.ØX6
EDTA	T5Ø.6X1	T5Ø.6X2	T5Ø.6X3	T5Ø.6X4	T5Ø.6X5	T5Ø.6X6
Eflornithine	T37.2X1	T37.2X2	T37.2X3	T37.2X4	T37.2X5	T37.2X6
Efloxate	T46.3X1	T46.3X2	T46.3X3	T46.3X4	T46.3X5	T46.3X6
Elase	T49.8X1	T49.8X2	T49.8X3	T49.8X4	T49.8X5	T49.8X6
Elastase	T47.5X1	T47.5X2	T47.5X3	T47.5X4	T47.5X5	T47.5X6
Elaterium	T47.2X1	T47.2X2	T47.2X3	T47.2X4	T47.2X5	T47.2X6
Elcatonin	T5Ø.991	T5Ø.992	T5Ø.993	T5Ø.994	T5Ø.995	T5Ø.996
Elder	T62.2X1	T62.2X2	T62.2X3	T62.2X4	—	—
berry, (unripe)	T62.1X1	T62.1X2	T62.1X3	T62.1X4	—	—
Electrolyte balance drug	T5Ø.3X1	T5Ø.3X2	T5Ø.3X3	T5Ø.3X4	T5Ø.3X5	T5Ø.3X6
Electrolytes NEC	T5Ø.3X1	T5Ø.3X2	T5Ø.3X3	T5Ø.3X4	T5Ø.3X5	T5Ø.3X6
Electrolytic agent NEC	T5Ø.3X1	T5Ø.3X2	T5Ø.3X3	T5Ø.3X4	T5Ø.3X5	T5Ø.3X6
Elemental diet	T5Ø.9Ø1	T5Ø.9Ø2	T5Ø.9Ø3	T5Ø.9Ø4	T5Ø.9Ø5	T5Ø.9Ø6
Elliptinium acetate	T45.1X1	T45.1X2	T45.1X3	T45.1X4	T45.1X5	T45.1X6
Embramine	T45.ØX1	T45.ØX2	T45.ØX3	T45.ØX4	T45.ØX5	T45.ØX6
Emepronium (salts)	T44.3X1	T44.3X2	T44.3X3	T44.3X4	T44.3X5	T44.3X6
bromide	T44.3X1	T44.3X2	T44.3X3	T44.3X4	T44.3X5	T44.3X6
Emetic NEC	T47.7X1	T47.7X2	T47.7X3	T47.7X4	T47.7X5	T47.7X6
Emetine	T37.3X1	T37.3X2	T37.3X3	T37.3X4	T37.3X5	T37.3X6
Emollient NEC	T49.3X1	T49.3X2	T49.3X3	T49.3X4	T49.3X5	T49.3X6
Emorfazone	T39.8X1	T39.8X2	T39.8X3	T39.8X4	T39.8X5	T39.8X6
Emylcamate	T43.591	T43.592	T43.593	T43.594	T43.595	T43.596
Enalapril	T46.4X1	T46.4X2	T46.4X3	T46.4X4	T46.4X5	T46.4X6
Enalaprilat	T46.4X1	T46.4X2	T46.4X3	T46.4X4	T46.4X5	T46.4X6
Encainide	T46.2X1	T46.2X2	T46.2X3	T46.2X4	T46.2X5	T46.2X6
Endocaine	T41.3X1	T41.3X2	T41.3X3	T41.3X4	T41.3X5	T41.3X6
Endosulfan	T6Ø.2X1	T6Ø.2X2	T6Ø.2X3	T6Ø.2X4	—	—
Endothall	T6Ø.3X1	T6Ø.3X2	T6Ø.3X3	T6Ø.3X4	—	—
Endralazine	T46.5X1	T46.5X2	T46.5X3	T46.5X4	T46.5X5	T46.5X6
Endrin	T6Ø.1X1	T6Ø.1X2	T6Ø.1X3	T6Ø.1X4	—	—
Enflurane	T41.ØX1	T41.ØX2	T41.ØX3	T41.ØX4	T41.ØX5	T41.ØX6
Enhexymal	T42.3X1	T42.3X2	T42.3X3	T42.3X4	T42.3X5	T42.3X6
Enocitabine	T45.1X1	T45.1X2	T45.1X3	T45.1X4	T45.1X5	T45.1X6
Enovid	T38.4X1	T38.4X2	T38.4X3	T38.4X4	T38.4X5	T38.4X6
Enoxacin	T36.8X1	T36.8X2	T36.8X3	T36.8X4	T36.8X5	T36.8X6
Enoxaparin (sodium)	T45.511	T45.512	T45.513	T45.514	T45.515	T45.516
Enpiprazole	T43.591	T43.592	T43.593	T43.594	T43.595	T43.596
Enprofylline	T48.6X1	T48.6X2	T48.6X3	T48.6X4	T48.6X5	T48.6X6
Enprostil	T47.1X1	T47.1X2	T47.1X3	T47.1X4	T47.1X5	T47.1X6
Enterogastrone	T38.891	T38.892	T38.893	T38.894	T38.895	T38.896
ENT preparations (anti-infectives)	T49.6X1	T49.6X2	T49.6X3	T49.6X4	T49.6X5	T49.6X6
Enviomycin	T36.8X1	T36.8X2	T36.8X3	T36.8X4	T36.8X5	T36.8X6
Enzodase	T45.3X1	T45.3X2	T45.3X3	T45.3X4	T45.3X5	T45.3X6
Enzyme NEC	T45.3X1	T45.3X2	T45.3X3	T45.3X4	T45.3X5	T45.3X6
depolymerizing	T49.8X1	T49.8X2	T49.8X3	T49.8X4	T49.8X5	T49.8X6
fibrolytic	T45.3X1	T45.3X2	T45.3X3	T45.3X4	T45.3X5	T45.3X6
gastric	T47.5X1	T47.5X2	T47.5X3	T47.5X4	T47.5X5	T47.5X6
intestinal	T47.5X1	T47.5X2	T47.5X3	T47.5X4	T47.5X5	T47.5X6
local action	T49.4X1	T49.4X2	T49.4X3	T49.4X4	T49.4X5	T49.4X6
proteolytic	T49.4X1	T49.4X2	T49.4X3	T49.4X4	T49.4X5	T49.4X6
thrombolytic	T45.3X1	T45.3X2	T45.3X3	T45.3X4	T45.3X5	T45.3X6
EPAB	T41.3X1	T41.3X2	T41.3X3	T41.3X4	T41.3X5	T41.3X6
Epanutin	T42.ØX1	T42.ØX2	T42.ØX3	T42.ØX4	T42.ØX5	T42.ØX6
Ephedra	T44.991	T44.992	T44.993	T44.994	T44.995	T44.996
Ephedrine	T44.991	T44.992	T44.993	T44.994	T44.995	T44.996
Epichlorhydrin, epichlorohydrin	T52.8X1	T52.8X2	T52.8X3	T52.8X4	—	—
Epicillin	T36.ØX1	T36.ØX2	T36.ØX3	T36.ØX4	T36.ØX5	T36.ØX6
Epiestriol	T38.5X1	T38.5X2	T38.5X3	T38.5X4	T38.5X5	T38.5X6
Epilim — *see* Sodium valproate						
Epimestrol	T38.5X1	T38.5X2	T38.5X3	T38.5X4	T38.5X5	T38.5X6
Epinephrine	T44.5X1	T44.5X2	T44.5X3	T44.5X4	T44.5X5	T44.5X6
Epirubicin	T45.1X1	T45.1X2	T45.1X3	T45.1X4	T45.1X5	T45.1X6
Epitiostanol	T38.7X1	T38.7X2	T38.7X3	T38.7X4	T38.7X5	T38.7X6
Epitizide	T5Ø.2X1	T5Ø.2X2	T5Ø.2X3	T5Ø.2X4	T5Ø.2X5	T5Ø.2X6
EPN	T6Ø.ØX1	T6Ø.ØX2	T6Ø.ØX3	T6Ø.ØX4	—	—
EPO	T45.8X1	T45.8X2	T45.8X3	T45.8X4	T45.8X5	T45.8X6
Epoetin alpha	T45.8X1	T45.8X2	T45.8X3	T45.8X4	T45.8X5	T45.8X6
Epomediol	T5Ø.991	T5Ø.992	T5Ø.993	T5Ø.994	T5Ø.995	T5Ø.996
Epoprostenol	T45.521	T45.522	T45.523	T45.524	T45.525	T45.526
Epoxy resin	T65.891	T65.892	T65.893	T65.894	—	—
Eprazinone	T48.4X1	T48.4X2	T48.4X3	T48.4X4	T48.4X5	T48.4X6
Epsilon aminocaproic acid	T45.621	T45.622	T45.623	T45.624	T45.625	T45.626
Epsom salt	T47.3X1	T47.3X2	T47.3X3	T47.3X4	T47.3X5	T47.3X6
Eptazocine	T4Ø.4X1	T4Ø.4X2	T4Ø.4X3	T4Ø.4X4	T4Ø.4X5	T4Ø.4X6
Equanil	T43.591	T43.592	T43.593	T43.594	T43.595	T43.596
Equisetum	T62.2X1	T62.2X2	T62.2X3	T62.2X4	—	—
diuretic	T5Ø.2X1	T5Ø.2X2	T5Ø.2X3	T5Ø.2X4	T5Ø.2X5	T5Ø.2X6
Ergobasine	T48.ØX1	T48.ØX2	T48.ØX3	T48.ØX4	T48.ØX5	T48.ØX6
Ergocalciferol	T45.2X1	T45.2X2	T45.2X3	T45.2X4	T45.2X5	T45.2X6
Ergoloid mesylates	T46.7X1	T46.7X2	T46.7X3	T46.7X4	T46.7X5	T46.7X6
Ergometrine	T48.ØX1	T48.ØX2	T48.ØX3	T48.ØX4	T48.ØX5	T48.ØX6
Ergonovine	T48.ØX1	T48.ØX2	T48.ØX3	T48.ØX4	T48.ØX5	T48.ØX6
Ergotamine	T46.5X1	T46.5X2	T46.5X3	T46.5X4	T46.5X5	T46.5X6
Ergotocine	T48.ØX1	T48.ØX2	T48.ØX3	T48.ØX4	T48.ØX5	T48.ØX6
Ergotrate	T48.ØX1	T48.ØX2	T48.ØX3	T48.ØX4	T48.ØX5	T48.ØX6
Ergot NEC	T64.81	T64.82	T64.83	T64.84	—	—
derivative	T48.ØX1	T48.ØX2	T48.ØX3	T48.ØX4	T48.ØX5	T48.ØX6
medicinal (alkaloids)	T48.ØX1	T48.ØX2	T48.ØX3	T48.ØX4	T48.ØX5	T48.ØX6
prepared	T48.ØX1	T48.ØX2	T48.ØX3	T48.ØX4	T48.ØX5	T48.ØX6
Eritrityl tetranitrate	T46.3X1	T46.3X2	T46.3X3	T46.3X4	T46.3X5	T46.3X6
Erythrityl tetranitrate	T46.3X1	T46.3X2	T46.3X3	T46.3X4	T46.3X5	T46.3X6
Erythrol tetranitrate	T46.3X1	T46.3X2	T46.3X3	T46.3X4	T46.3X5	T46.3X6
Erythromycin (salts)	T36.3X1	T36.3X2	T36.3X3	T36.3X4	T36.3X5	T36.3X6
ophthalmic preparation	T49.5X1	T49.5X2	T49.5X3	T49.5X4	T49.5X5	T49.5X6
topical NEC	T49.ØX1	T49.ØX2	T49.ØX3	T49.ØX4	T49.ØX5	T49.ØX6
Erythropoietin	T45.8X1	T45.8X2	T45.8X3	T45.8X4	T45.8X5	T45.8X6
human	T45.8X1	T45.8X2	T45.8X3	T45.8X4	T45.8X5	T45.8X6
Escin	T46.991	T46.992	T46.993	T46.994	T46.995	T46.996
Esculin	T45.2X1	T45.2X2	T45.2X3	T45.2X4	T45.2X5	T45.2X6
Esculoside	T45.2X1	T45.2X2	T45.2X3	T45.2X4	T45.2X5	T45.2X6
ESDT (ether-soluble tar distillate)	T49.1X1	T49.1X2	T49.1X3	T49.1X4	T49.1X5	T49.1X6
Eserine	T49.5X1	T49.5X2	T49.5X3	T49.5X4	T49.5X5	T49.5X6
Esflurbiprofen	T39.311	T39.312	T39.313	T39.314	T39.315	T39.316
Eskabarb	T42.3X1	T42.3X2	T42.3X3	T42.3X4	T42.3X5	T42.3X6
Eskalith	T43.8X1	T43.8X2	T43.8X3	T43.8X4	T43.8X5	T43.8X6
Esmolol	T44.7X1	T44.7X2	T44.7X3	T44.7X4	T44.7X5	T44.7X6

Dorsacaine — Esmolol

356 Additional Character May Be Required — Refer to the Tabular List for Character Selection Subterms under main terms may continue to next column or page

Substance	Poisoning, Accidental (unintentional)	Poisoning, Intentional Self-harm	Poisoning, Assault	Poisoning, Undetermined	Adverse Effect	Under-dosing
Estanozolol	T38.7X1	T38.7X2	T38.7X3	T38.7X4	T38.7X5	T38.7X6
Estazolam	T42.4X1	T42.4X2	T42.4X3	T42.4X4	T42.4X5	T42.4X6
Estradiol	T38.5X1	T38.5X2	T38.5X3	T38.5X4	T38.5X5	T38.5X6
with testosterone	T38.7X1	T38.7X2	T38.7X3	T38.7X4	T38.7X5	T38.7X6
benzoate	T38.5X1	T38.5X2	T38.5X3	T38.5X4	T38.5X5	T38.5X6
Estramustine	T45.1X1	T45.1X2	T45.1X3	T45.1X4	T45.1X5	T45.1X6
Estriol	T38.5X1	T38.5X2	T38.5X3	T38.5X4	T38.5X5	T38.5X6
Estrogen	T38.5X1	T38.5X2	T38.5X3	T38.5X4	T38.5X5	T38.5X6
with progesterone	T38.5X1	T38.5X2	T38.5X3	T38.5X4	T38.5X5	T38.5X6
conjugated	T38.5X1	T38.5X2	T38.5X3	T38.5X4	T38.5X5	T38.5X6
Estrone	T38.5X1	T38.5X2	T38.5X3	T38.5X4	T38.5X5	T38.5X6
Estropipate	T38.5X1	T38.5X2	T38.5X3	T38.5X4	T38.5X5	T38.5X6
Etacrynate sodium	T5Ø.1X1	T5Ø.1X2	T5Ø.1X3	T5Ø.1X4	T5Ø.1X5	T5Ø.1X6
Etacrynic acid	T5Ø.1X1	T5Ø.1X2	T5Ø.1X3	T5Ø.1X4	T5Ø.1X5	T5Ø.1X6
Etafedrine	T48.6X1	T48.6X2	T48.6X3	T48.6X4	T48.6X5	T48.6X6
Etafenone	T46.3X1	T46.3X2	T46.3X3	T46.3X4	T46.3X5	T46.3X6
Etambutol	T37.1X1	T37.1X2	T37.1X3	T37.1X4	T37.1X5	T37.1X6
Etamiphyllin	T48.6X1	T48.6X2	T48.6X3	T48.6X4	T48.6X5	T48.6X6
Etamivan	T5Ø.7X1	T5Ø.7X2	T5Ø.7X3	T5Ø.7X4	T5Ø.7X5	T5Ø.7X6
Etamsylate	T45.7X1	T45.7X2	T45.7X3	T45.7X4	T45.7X5	T45.7X6
Etebenecid	T5Ø.4X1	T5Ø.4X2	T5Ø.4X3	T5Ø.4X4	T5Ø.4X5	T5Ø.4X6
Ethacridine	T49.ØX1	T49.ØX2	T49.ØX3	T49.ØX4	T49.ØX5	T49.ØX6
Ethacrynic acid	T5Ø.1X1	T5Ø.1X2	T5Ø.1X3	T5Ø.1X4	T5Ø.1X5	T5Ø.1X6
Ethadione	T42.2X1	T42.2X2	T42.2X3	T42.2X4	T42.2X5	T42.2X6
Ethambutol	T37.1X1	T37.1X2	T37.1X3	T37.1X4	T37.1X5	T37.1X6
Ethamide	T5Ø.2X1	T5Ø.2X2	T5Ø.2X3	T5Ø.2X4	T5Ø.2X5	T5Ø.2X6
Ethamivan	T5Ø.7X1	T5Ø.7X2	T5Ø.7X3	T5Ø.7X4	T5Ø.7X5	T5Ø.7X6
Ethamsylate	T45.7X1	T45.7X2	T45.7X3	T45.7X4	T45.7X5	T45.7X6
Ethanol	T51.ØX1	T51.ØX2	T51.ØX3	T51.ØX4	—	—
beverage	T51.ØX1	T51.ØX2	T51.ØX3	T51.ØX4	—	—
Ethanolamine oleate	T46.8X1	T46.8X2	T46.8X3	T46.8X4	T46.8X5	T46.8X6
Ethaverine	T44.3X1	T44.3X2	T44.3X3	T44.3X4	T44.3X5	T44.3X6
Ethchlorvynol	T42.6X1	T42.6X2	T42.6X3	T42.6X4	T42.6X5	T42.6X6
Ethebenecid	T5Ø.4X1	T5Ø.4X2	T5Ø.4X3	T5Ø.4X4	T5Ø.4X5	T5Ø.4X6
Ether (vapor)	T41.ØX1	T41.ØX2	T41.ØX3	T41.ØX4	T41.ØX5	T41.ØX6
anesthetic	T41.ØX1	T41.ØX2	T41.ØX3	T41.ØX4	T41.ØX5	T41.ØX6
divinyl	T41.ØX1	T41.ØX2	T41.ØX3	T41.ØX4	T41.ØX5	T41.ØX6
ethyl (medicinal)	T41.ØX1	T41.ØX2	T41.ØX3	T41.ØX4	T41.ØX5	T41.ØX6
nonmedicinal	T52.8X1	T52.8X2	T52.8X3	T52.8X4	—	—
petroleum — *see* Ligroin						
solvent	T52.8X1	T52.8X2	T52.8X3	T52.8X4	—	—
Ethiazide	T5Ø.2X1	T5Ø.2X2	T5Ø.2X3	T5Ø.2X4	T5Ø.2X5	T5Ø.2X6
Ethidium chloride (vapor)	T59.891	T59.892	T59.893	T59.894	—	—
Ethinamate	T42.6X1	T42.6X2	T42.6X3	T42.6X4	T42.6X5	T42.6X6
Ethinylestradiol, ethinyloestradiol	T38.5X1	T38.5X2	T38.5X3	T38.5X4	T38.5X5	T38.5X6
with						
levonorgestrel	T38.4X1	T38.4X2	T38.4X3	T38.4X4	T38.4X5	T38.4X6
norethisterone	T38.4X1	T38.4X2	T38.4X3	T38.4X4	T38.4X5	T38.4X6
Ethiodized oil (131 I)	T5Ø.8X1	T5Ø.8X2	T5Ø.8X3	T5Ø.8X4	T5Ø.8X5	T5Ø.8X6
Ethion	T6Ø.ØX1	T6Ø.ØX2	T6Ø.ØX3	T6Ø.ØX4	—	—
Ethionamide	T37.1X1	T37.1X2	T37.1X3	T37.1X4	T37.1X5	T37.1X6
Ethioniamide	T37.1X1	T37.1X2	T37.1X3	T37.1X4	T37.1X5	T37.1X6
Ethisterone	T38.5X1	T38.5X2	T38.5X3	T38.5X4	T38.5X5	T38.5X6
Ethobral	T42.3X1	T42.3X2	T42.3X3	T42.3X4	T42.3X5	T42.3X6
Ethocaine (infiltration) (topical)	T41.3X1	T41.3X2	T41.3X3	T41.3X4	T41.3X5	T41.3X6
nerve block (peripheral) (plexus)	T41.3X1	T41.3X2	T41.3X3	T41.3X4	T41.3X5	T41.3X6
spinal	T41.3X1	T41.3X2	T41.3X3	T41.3X4	T41.3X5	T41.3X6
Ethoheptazine	T4Ø.4X1	T4Ø.4X2	T4Ø.4X3	T4Ø.4X4	T4Ø.4X5	T4Ø.4X6
Ethopropazine	T44.3X1	T44.3X2	T44.3X3	T44.3X4	T44.3X5	T44.3X6
Ethosuximide	T42.2X1	T42.2X2	T42.2X3	T42.2X4	T42.2X5	T42.2X6
Ethotoin	T42.ØX1	T42.ØX2	T42.ØX3	T42.ØX4	T42.ØX5	T42.ØX6
Ethoxazene	T37.91	T37.92	T37.93	T37.94	T37.95	T37.96
Ethoxazorutoside	T46.991	T46.992	T46.993	T46.994	T46.995	T46.996
Ethoxzolamide	T5Ø.2X1	T5Ø.2X2	T5Ø.2X3	T5Ø.2X4	T5Ø.2X5	T5Ø.2X6
Ethyl						
acetate	T52.8X1	T52.8X2	T52.8X3	T52.8X4	—	—
alcohol	T51.ØX1	T51.ØX2	T51.ØX3	T51.ØX4	—	—
beverage	T51.ØX1	T51.ØX2	T51.ØX3	T51.ØX4	—	—
aldehyde (vapor)	T59.891	T59.892	T59.893	T59.894	—	—
liquid	T52.8X1	T52.8X2	T52.8X3	T52.8X4	—	—
aminobenzoate	T41.3X1	T41.3X2	T41.3X3	T41.3X4	T41.3X5	T41.3X6
aminophenothiazine	T43.3X1	T43.3X2	T43.3X3	T43.3X4	T43.3X5	T43.3X6
benzoate	T52.8X1	T52.8X2	T52.8X3	T52.8X4	—	—
biscoumacetate	T45.511	T45.512	T45.513	T45.514	T45.515	T45.516
bromide (anesthetic)	T41.ØX1	T41.ØX2	T41.ØX3	T41.ØX4	T41.ØX5	T41.ØX6
carbamate	T45.1X1	T45.1X2	T45.1X3	T45.1X4	T45.1X5	T45.1X6
carbinol	T51.3X1	T51.3X2	T51.3X3	T51.3X4	—	—
carbonate	T52.8X1	T52.8X2	T52.8X3	T52.8X4	—	—
chaulmoograte	T37.1X1	T37.1X2	T37.1X3	T37.1X4	T37.1X5	T37.1X6
chloride (anesthetic)	T41.ØX1	T41.ØX2	T41.ØX3	T41.ØX4	T41.ØX5	T41.ØX6
Ethyl — *continued*						
chloride — *continued*						
anesthetic (local)	T41.3X1	T41.3X2	T41.3X3	T41.3X4	T41.3X5	T41.3X6
inhaled	T41.ØX1	T41.ØX2	T41.ØX3	T41.ØX4	T41.ØX5	T41.ØX6
local	T49.4X1	T49.4X2	T49.4X3	T49.4X4	T49.4X5	T49.4X6
solvent	T53.6X1	T53.6X2	T53.6X3	T53.6X4	—	—
dibunate	T48.3X1	T48.3X2	T48.3X3	T48.3X4	T48.3X5	T48.3X6
dichloroarsine (vapor)	T57.ØX1	T57.ØX2	T57.ØX3	T57.ØX4	—	—
estranol	T38.7X1	T38.7X2	T38.7X3	T38.7X4	T38.7X5	T38.7X6
ether — *see also* ether	T52.8X1	T52.8X2	T52.8X3	T52.8X4	—	—
formate NEC (solvent)	T52.ØX1	T52.ØX2	T52.ØX3	T52.ØX4	—	—
fumarate	T49.4X1	T49.4X2	T49.4X3	T49.4X4	T49.4X5	T49.4X6
hydroxyisobutyrate NEC (solvent)	T52.8X1	T52.8X2	T52.8X3	T52.8X4	—	—
iodoacetate	T59.3X1	T59.3X2	T59.3X3	T59.3X4	—	—
lactate NEC (solvent)	T52.8X1	T52.8X2	T52.8X3	T52.8X4	—	—
loflazepate	T42.4X1	T42.4X2	T42.4X3	T42.4X4	T42.4X5	T42.4X6
mercuric chloride	T56.1X1	T56.1X2	T56.1X3	T56.1X4	—	—
methylcarbinol	T51.8X1	T51.8X2	T51.8X3	T51.8X4	—	—
morphine	T4Ø.2X1	T4Ø.2X2	T4Ø.2X3	T4Ø.2X4	T4Ø.2X5	T4Ø.2X6
noradrenaline	T48.6X1	T48.6X2	T48.6X3	T48.6X4	T48.6X5	T48.6X6
oxybutyrate NEC (solvent)	T52.8X1	T52.8X2	T52.8X3	T52.8X4	—	—
Ethylene (gas)	T59.891	T59.892	T59.893	T59.894	—	—
anesthetic (general)	T41.ØX1	T41.ØX2	T41.ØX3	T41.ØX4	T41.ØX5	T41.ØX6
chlorohydrin	T52.8X1	T52.8X2	T52.8X3	T52.8X4	—	—
vapor	T53.6X1	T53.6X2	T53.6X3	T53.6X4	—	—
dichloride	T52.8X1	T52.8X2	T52.8X3	T52.8X4	—	—
vapor	T53.6X1	T53.6X2	T53.6X3	T53.6X4	—	—
dinitrate	T52.3X1	T52.3X2	T52.3X3	T52.3X4	—	—
glycol(s)	T52.8X1	T52.8X2	T52.8X3	T52.8X4	—	—
dinitrate	T52.3X1	T52.3X2	T52.3X3	T52.3X4	—	—
monobutyl ether	T52.3X1	T52.3X2	T52.3X3	T52.3X4	—	—
imine	T54.1X1	T54.1X2	T54.1X3	T54.1X4	—	—
oxide (fumigant) (nonmedicinal)	T59.891	T59.892	T59.893	T59.894	—	—
medicinal	T49.ØX1	T49.ØX2	T49.ØX3	T49.ØX4	T49.ØX5	T49.ØX6
Ethylenediaminetetra-acetic acid	T5Ø.6X1	T5Ø.6X2	T5Ø.6X3	T5Ø.6X4	T5Ø.6X5	T5Ø.6X6
Ethylenediamine theophylline	T48.6X1	T48.6X2	T48.6X3	T48.6X4	T48.6X5	T48.6X6
Ethylenedinitrilotetra-acetate	T5Ø.6X1	T5Ø.6X2	T5Ø.6X3	T5Ø.6X4	T5Ø.6X5	T5Ø.6X6
Ethylestrenol	T38.7X1	T38.7X2	T38.7X3	T38.7X4	T38.7X5	T38.7X6
Ethylhydroxycellulose	T47.4X1	T47.4X2	T47.4X3	T47.4X4	T47.4X5	T47.4X6
Ethylidene						
chloride NEC	T53.6X1	T53.6X2	T53.6X3	T53.6X4	—	—
diacetate	T6Ø.3X1	T6Ø.3X2	T6Ø.3X3	T6Ø.3X4	—	—
dicoumarin	T45.511	T45.512	T45.513	T45.514	T45.515	T45.516
dicoumarol	T45.511	T45.512	T45.513	T45.514	T45.515	T45.516
diethyl ether	T52.ØX1	T52.ØX2	T52.ØX3	T52.ØX4	—	—
Ethylmorphine	T4Ø.2X1	T4Ø.2X2	T4Ø.2X3	T4Ø.2X4	T4Ø.2X5	T4Ø.2X6
Ethylnorepinephrine	T48.6X1	T48.6X2	T48.6X3	T48.6X4	T48.6X5	T48.6X6
Ethylparachlorophen-oxyisobutyrate	T46.6X1	T46.6X2	T46.6X3	T46.6X4	T46.6X5	T46.6X6
Ethynodiol	T38.4X1	T38.4X2	T38.4X3	T38.4X4	T38.4X5	T38.4X6
with mestranol diacetate	T38.4X1	T38.4X2	T38.4X3	T38.4X4	T38.4X5	T38.4X6
Etidocaine	T41.3X1	T41.3X2	T41.3X3	T41.3X4	T41.3X5	T41.3X6
infiltration (subcutaneous)	T41.3X1	T41.3X2	T41.3X3	T41.3X4	T41.3X5	T41.3X6
nerve (peripheral) (plexus)	T41.3X1	T41.3X2	T41.3X3	T41.3X4	T41.3X5	T41.3X6
Etidronate	T5Ø.991	T5Ø.992	T5Ø.993	T5Ø.994	T5Ø.995	T5Ø.996
Etidronic acid (disodium salt)	T5Ø.991	T5Ø.992	T5Ø.993	T5Ø.994	T5Ø.995	T5Ø.996
Etifoxine	T42.6X1	T42.6X2	T42.6X3	T42.6X4	T42.6X5	T42.6X6
Etilefrine	T44.4X1	T44.4X2	T44.4X3	T44.4X4	T44.4X5	T44.4X6
Etilfen	T42.3X1	T42.3X2	T42.3X3	T42.3X4	T42.3X5	T42.3X6
Etinodiol	T38.4X1	T38.4X2	T38.4X3	T38.4X4	T38.4X5	T38.4X6
Etiroxate	T46.6X1	T46.6X2	T46.6X3	T46.6X4	T46.6X5	T46.6X6
Etizolam	T42.4X1	T42.4X2	T42.4X3	T42.4X4	T42.4X5	T42.4X6
Etodolac	T39.391	T39.392	T39.393	T39.394	T39.395	T39.396
Etofamide	T37.3X1	T37.3X2	T37.3X3	T37.3X4	T37.3X5	T37.3X6
Etofibrate	T46.6X1	T46.6X2	T46.6X3	T46.6X4	T46.6X5	T46.6X6
Etofylline	T46.7X1	T46.7X2	T46.7X3	T46.7X4	T46.7X5	T46.7X6
clofibrate	T46.6X1	T46.6X2	T46.6X3	T46.6X4	T46.6X5	T46.6X6
Etoglucid	T45.1X1	T45.1X2	T45.1X3	T45.1X4	T45.1X5	T45.1X6
Etomidate	T41.1X1	T41.1X2	T41.1X3	T41.1X4	T41.1X5	T41.1X6
Etomide	T39.8X1	T39.8X2	T39.8X3	T39.8X4	T39.8X5	T39.8X6
Etomidoline	T44.3X1	T44.3X2	T44.3X3	T44.3X4	T44.3X5	T44.3X6
Etoposide	T45.1X1	T45.1X2	T45.1X3	T45.1X4	T45.1X5	T45.1X6
Etorphine	T4Ø.2X1	T4Ø.2X2	T4Ø.2X3	T4Ø.2X4	T4Ø.2X5	T4Ø.2X6
Etoval	T42.3X1	T42.3X2	T42.3X3	T42.3X4	T42.3X5	T42.3X6
Etozolin	T5Ø.1X1	T5Ø.1X2	T5Ø.1X3	T5Ø.1X4	T5Ø.1X5	T5Ø.1X6
Etretinate	T5Ø.991	T5Ø.992	T5Ø.993	T5Ø.994	T5Ø.995	T5Ø.996
Etryptamine	T43.691	T43.692	T43.693	T43.694	T43.695	T43.696
Etybenzatropine	T44.3X1	T44.3X2	T44.3X3	T44.3X4	T44.3X5	T44.3X6

Subterms under main terms may continue to next column or page

Additional Character May Be Required — Refer to the Tabular List for Character Selection

357

Substance	Poisoning, Accidental (unintentional)	Poisoning, Intentional Self-harm	Poisoning, Assault	Poisoning, Undetermined	Adverse Effect	Under-dosing
Etynodiol	T38.4X1	T38.4X2	T38.4X3	T38.4X4	T38.4X5	T38.4X6
Eucaine	T41.3X1	T41.3X2	T41.3X3	T41.3X4	T41.3X5	T41.3X6
Eucalyptus oil	T49.7X1	T49.7X2	T49.7X3	T49.7X4	T49.7X5	T49.7X6
Eucatropine	T49.5X1	T49.5X2	T49.5X3	T49.5X4	T49.5X5	T49.5X6
Eucodal	T4Ø.2X1	T4Ø.2X2	T4Ø.2X3	T4Ø.2X4	T4Ø.2X5	T4Ø.2X6
Euneryl	T42.3X1	T42.3X2	T42.3X3	T42.3X4	T42.3X5	T42.3X6
Euphthalmine	T44.3X1	T44.3X2	T44.3X3	T44.3X4	T44.3X5	T44.3X6
Eurax	T49.ØX1	T49.ØX2	T49.ØX3	T49.ØX4	T49.ØX5	T49.ØX6
Euresol	T49.4X1	T49.4X2	T49.4X3	T49.4X4	T49.4X5	T49.4X6
Euthroid	T38.1X1	T38.1X2	T38.1X3	T38.1X4	T38.1X5	T38.1X6
Evans blue	T5Ø.8X1	T5Ø.8X2	T5Ø.8X3	T5Ø.8X4	T5Ø.8X5	T5Ø.8X6
Evipal	T42.3X1	T42.3X2	T42.3X3	T42.3X4	T42.3X5	T42.3X6
sodium	T41.1X1	T41.1X2	T41.1X3	T41.1X4	T41.1X5	T41.1X6
Evipan	T42.3X1	T42.3X2	T42.3X3	T42.3X4	T42.3X5	T42.3X6
sodium	T41.1X1	T41.1X2	T41.1X3	T41.1X4	T41.1X5	T41.1X6
Exalamide	T49.ØX1	T49.ØX2	T49.ØX3	T49.ØX4	T49.ØX5	T49.ØX6
Exalgin	T39.1X1	T39.1X2	T39.1X3	T39.1X4	T39.1X5	T39.1X6
Excipients, pharmaceutical	T5Ø.9Ø1	T5Ø.9Ø2	T5Ø.9Ø3	T5Ø.9Ø4	T5Ø.9Ø5	T5Ø.9Ø6
Exhaust gas (engine) (motor vehicle)	T58.Ø1	T58.Ø2	T58.Ø3	T58.Ø4	—	—
Ex-Lax (phenolphthalein)	T47.2X1	T47.2X2	T47.2X3	T47.2X4	T47.2X5	T47.2X6
Expectorant NEC	T48.4X1	T48.4X2	T48.4X3	T48.4X4	T48.4X5	T48.4X6
Extended insulin zinc suspension	T38.3X1	T38.3X2	T38.3X3	T38.3X4	T38.3X5	T38.3X6
External medications (skin) (mucous membrane)	T49.91	T49.92	T49.93	T49.94	T49.95	T49.96
dental agent	T49.7X1	T49.7X2	T49.7X3	T49.7X4	T49.7X5	T49.7X6
ENT agent	T49.6X1	T49.6X2	T49.6X3	T49.6X4	T49.6X5	T49.6X6
ophthalmic preparation	T49.5X1	T49.5X2	T49.5X3	T49.5X4	T49.5X5	T49.5X6
specified NEC	T49.8X1	T49.8X2	T49.8X3	T49.8X4	T49.8X5	T49.8X6
Extrapyramidal antagonist NEC	T44.3X1	T44.3X2	T44.3X3	T44.3X4	T44.3X5	T44.3X6
Eye agents (anti-infective)	T49.5X1	T49.5X2	T49.5X3	T49.5X4	T49.5X5	T49.5X6
Eye drug NEC	T49.5X1	T49.5X2	T49.5X3	T49.5X4	T49.5X5	T49.5X6
FAC (fluorouracil + doxorubicin + cyclophosphamide)	T45.1X1	T45.1X2	T45.1X3	T45.1X4	T45.1X5	T45.1X6
Factor						
I (fibrinogen)	T45.8X1	T45.8X2	T45.8X3	T45.8X4	T45.8X5	T45.8X6
III (thromboplastin)	T45.8X1	T45.8X2	T45.8X3	T45.8X4	T45.8X5	T45.8X6
IX complex	T45.7X1	T45.7X2	T45.7X3	T45.7X4	T45.7X5	T45.7X6
human	T45.8X1	T45.8X2	T45.8X3	T45.8X4	T45.8X5	T45.8X6
VIII (antihemophilic Factor) (concentrate)	T45.8X1	T45.8X2	T45.8X3	T45.8X4	T45.8X5	T45.8X6
Famotidine	T47.ØX1	T47.ØX2	T47.ØX3	T47.ØX4	T47.ØX5	T47.ØX6
Fat suspension, intravenous	T5Ø.991	T5Ø.992	T5Ø.993	T5Ø.994	T5Ø.995	T5Ø.996
Fazadinium bromide	T48.1X1	T48.1X2	T48.1X3	T48.1X4	T48.1X5	T48.1X6
Febarbamate	T42.3X1	T42.3X2	T42.3X3	T42.3X4	T42.3X5	T42.3X6
Fecal softener	T47.4X1	T47.4X2	T47.4X3	T47.4X4	T47.4X5	T47.4X6
Fedrilate	T48.3X1	T48.3X2	T48.3X3	T48.3X4	T48.3X5	T48.3X6
Felodipine	T46.1X1	T46.1X2	T46.1X3	T46.1X4	T46.1X5	T46.1X6
Felypressin	T38.891	T38.892	T38.893	T38.894	T38.895	T38.896
Femoxetine	T43.221	T43.222	T43.223	T43.224	T43.225	T43.226
Fenalcomine	T46.3X1	T46.3X2	T46.3X3	T46.3X4	T46.3X5	T46.3X6
Fenamisal	T37.1X1	T37.1X2	T37.1X3	T37.1X4	T37.1X5	T37.1X6
Fenazone	T39.2X1	T39.2X2	T39.2X3	T39.2X4	T39.2X5	T39.2X6
Fenbendazole	T37.4X1	T37.4X2	T37.4X3	T37.4X4	T37.4X5	T37.4X6
Fenbutrazate	T5Ø.5X1	T5Ø.5X2	T5Ø.5X3	T5Ø.5X4	T5Ø.5X5	T5Ø.5X6
Fencamfamine	T43.691	T43.692	T43.693	T43.694	T43.695	T43.696
Fendiline	T46.1X1	T46.1X2	T46.1X3	T46.1X4	T46.1X5	T46.1X6
Fenetylline	T43.691	T43.692	T43.693	T43.694	T43.695	T43.696
Fenflumizole	T39.391	T39.392	T39.393	T39.394	T39.395	T39.396
Fenfluramine	T5Ø.5X1	T5Ø.5X2	T5Ø.5X3	T5Ø.5X4	T5Ø.5X5	T5Ø.5X6
Fenobarbital	T42.3X1	T42.3X2	T42.3X3	T42.3X4	T42.3X5	T42.3X6
Fenofibrate	T46.6X1	T46.6X2	T46.6X3	T46.6X4	T46.6X5	T46.6X6
Fenoprofen	T39.311	T39.312	T39.313	T39.314	T39.315	T39.316
Fenoterol	T48.6X1	T48.6X2	T48.6X3	T48.6X4	T48.6X5	T48.6X6
Fenoverine	T44.3X1	T44.3X2	T44.3X3	T44.3X4	T44.3X5	T44.3X6
Fenoxazoline	T48.5X1	T48.5X2	T48.5X3	T48.5X4	T48.5X5	T48.5X6
Fenproporex	T5Ø.5X1	T5Ø.5X2	T5Ø.5X3	T5Ø.5X4	T5Ø.5X5	T5Ø.5X6
Fenquizone	T5Ø.2X1	T5Ø.2X2	T5Ø.2X3	T5Ø.2X4	T5Ø.2X5	T5Ø.2X6
Fentanyl	T4Ø.4X1	T4Ø.4X2	T4Ø.4X3	T4Ø.4X4	T4Ø.4X5	T4Ø.4X6
Fentazin	T43.3X1	T43.3X2	T43.3X3	T43.3X4	T43.3X5	T43.3X6
Fenthion	T6Ø.ØX1	T6Ø.ØX2	T6Ø.ØX3	T6Ø.ØX4	—	—
Fenticlor	T49.ØX1	T49.ØX2	T49.ØX3	T49.ØX4	T49.ØX5	T49.ØX6
Fenylbutazone	T39.2X1	T39.2X2	T39.2X3	T39.2X4	T39.2X5	T39.2X6
Feprazone	T39.2X1	T39.2X2	T39.2X3	T39.2X4	T39.2X5	T39.2X6
Fer de lance (bite) (venom)	T63.Ø61	T63.Ø62	T63.Ø63	T63.Ø64	—	—
Ferric — *see also* Iron						
chloride	T45.4X1	T45.4X2	T45.4X3	T45.4X4	T45.4X5	T45.4X6
citrate	T45.4X1	T45.4X2	T45.4X3	T45.4X4	T45.4X5	T45.4X6
hydroxide						
colloidal	T45.4X1	T45.4X2	T45.4X3	T45.4X4	T45.4X5	T45.4X6

Substance	Poisoning, Accidental (unintentional)	Poisoning, Intentional Self-harm	Poisoning, Assault	Poisoning, Undetermined	Adverse Effect	Under-dosing
Ferric — *see also* Iron — *continued*						
hydroxide — *continued*						
polymaltose	T45.4X1	T45.4X2	T45.4X3	T45.4X4	T45.4X5	T45.4X6
pyrophosphate	T45.4X1	T45.4X2	T45.4X3	T45.4X4	T45.4X5	T45.4X6
Ferritin	T45.4X1	T45.4X2	T45.4X3	T45.4X4	T45.4X5	T45.4X6
Ferrocholinate	T45.4X1	T45.4X2	T45.4X3	T45.4X4	T45.4X5	T45.4X6
Ferrodextrane	T45.4X1	T45.4X2	T45.4X3	T45.4X4	T45.4X5	T45.4X6
Ferropolimaler	T45.4X1	T45.4X2	T45.4X3	T45.4X4	T45.4X5	T45.4X6
Ferrous — *see also* Iron						
phosphate	T45.4X1	T45.4X2	T45.4X3	T45.4X4	T45.4X5	T45.4X6
salt	T45.4X1	T45.4X2	T45.4X3	T45.4X4	T45.4X5	T45.4X6
with folic acid	T45.4X1	T45.4X2	T45.4X3	T45.4X4	T45.4X5	T45.4X6
Ferrous fumerate, gluconate, lactate, salt NEC, sulfate (medicinal)	T45.4X1	T45.4X2	T45.4X3	T45.4X4	T45.4X5	T45.4X6
Ferrovanadium (fumes)	T59.891	T59.892	T59.893	T59.894	—	—
Ferrum — *see* Iron						
Fertilizers NEC	T65.891	T65.892	T65.893	T65.894	—	—
with herbicide mixture	T6Ø.3X1	T6Ø.3X2	T6Ø.3X3	T6Ø.3X4	—	—
Fetoxilate	T47.6X1	T47.6X2	T47.6X3	T47.6X4	T47.6X5	T47.6X6
Fiber, dietary	T47.4X1	T47.4X2	T47.4X3	T47.4X4	T47.4X5	T47.4X6
Fiberglass	T65.831	T65.832	T65.833	T65.834	—	—
Fibrinogen (human)	T45.8X1	T45.8X2	T45.8X3	T45.8X4	T45.8X5	T45.8X6
Fibrinolysin (human)	T45.691	T45.692	T45.693	T45.694	T45.695	T45.696
Fibrinolysis						
affecting drug	T45.6Ø1	T45.6Ø2	T45.6Ø3	T45.6Ø4	T45.6Ø5	T45.6Ø6
inhibitor NEC	T45.621	T45.622	T45.623	T45.624	T45.625	T45.626
Fibrinolytic drug	T45.611	T45.612	T45.613	T45.614	T45.615	T45.616
Filix mas	T37.4X1	T37.4X2	T37.4X3	T37.4X4	T37.4X5	T37.4X6
Filtering cream	T49.3X1	T49.3X2	T49.3X3	T49.3X4	T49.3X5	T49.3X6
Fiorinal	T39.Ø11	T39.Ø12	T39.Ø13	T39.Ø14	T39.Ø15	T39.Ø16
Firedamp	T59.891	T59.892	T59.893	T59.894	—	—
Fish, noxious, nonbacterial	T61.91	T61.92	T61.93	T61.94	—	—
ciguatera	T61.Ø1	T61.Ø2	T61.Ø3	T61.Ø4	—	—
scombroid	T61.11	T61.12	T61.13	T61.14	—	—
shell	T61.781	T61.782	T61.783	T61.784	—	—
specified NEC	T61.771	T61.772	T61.773	T61.774	—	—
Flagyl	T37.3X1	T37.3X2	T37.3X3	T37.3X4	T37.3X5	T37.3X6
Flavine adenine dinucleotide	T45.2X1	T45.2X2	T45.2X3	T45.2X4	T45.2X5	T45.2X6
Flavodic acid	T46.991	T46.992	T46.993	T46.994	T46.995	T46.996
Flavoxate	T44.3X1	T44.3X2	T44.3X3	T44.3X4	T44.3X5	T44.3X6
Flaxedil	T48.1X1	T48.1X2	T48.1X3	T48.1X4	T48.1X5	T48.1X6
Flaxseed (medicinal)	T49.3X1	T49.3X2	T49.3X3	T49.3X4	T49.3X5	T49.3X6
Flecainide	T46.2X1	T46.2X2	T46.2X3	T46.2X4	T46.2X5	T46.2X6
Fleroxacin	T36.8X1	T36.8X2	T36.8X3	T36.8X4	T36.8X5	T36.8X6
Floctafenine	T39.8X1	T39.8X2	T39.8X3	T39.8X4	T39.8X5	T39.8X6
Flomax	T44.6X1	T44.6X2	T44.6X3	T44.6X4	T44.6X5	T44.6X6
Flomoxef	T36.1X1	T36.1X2	T36.1X3	T36.1X4	T36.1X5	T36.1X6
Flopropione	T44.3X1	T44.3X2	T44.3X3	T44.3X4	T44.3X5	T44.3X6
Florantyrone	T47.5X1	T47.5X2	T47.5X3	T47.5X4	T47.5X5	T47.5X6
Floraquin	T37.8X1	T37.8X2	T37.8X3	T37.8X4	T37.8X5	T37.8X6
Florinef	T38.ØX1	T38.ØX2	T38.ØX3	T38.ØX4	T38.ØX5	T38.ØX6
ENT agent	T49.6X1	T49.6X2	T49.6X3	T49.6X4	T49.6X5	T49.6X6
ophthalmic preparation	T49.5X1	T49.5X2	T49.5X3	T49.5X4	T49.5X5	T49.5X6
topical NEC	T49.ØX1	T49.ØX2	T49.ØX3	T49.ØX4	T49.ØX5	T49.ØX6
Flowers of sulfur	T49.4X1	T49.4X2	T49.4X3	T49.4X4	T49.4X5	T49.4X6
Floxuridine	T45.1X1	T45.1X2	T45.1X3	T45.1X4	T45.1X5	T45.1X6
Fluanisone	T43.4X1	T43.4X2	T43.4X3	T43.4X4	T43.4X5	T43.4X6
Flubendazole	T37.4X1	T37.4X2	T37.4X3	T37.4X4	T37.4X5	T37.4X6
Fluclorolone acetonide	T49.ØX1	T49.ØX2	T49.ØX3	T49.ØX4	T49.ØX5	T49.ØX6
Flucloxacillin	T36.ØX1	T36.ØX2	T36.ØX3	T36.ØX4	T36.ØX5	T36.ØX6
Fluconazole	T37.8X1	T37.8X2	T37.8X3	T37.8X4	T37.8X5	T37.8X6
Flucytosine	T37.8X1	T37.8X2	T37.8X3	T37.8X4	T37.8X5	T37.8X6
Fludeoxyglucose (18F)	T5Ø.8X1	T5Ø.8X2	T5Ø.8X3	T5Ø.8X4	T5Ø.8X5	T5Ø.8X6
Fludiazepam	T42.4X1	T42.4X2	T42.4X3	T42.4X4	T42.4X5	T42.4X6
Fludrocortisone	T5Ø.ØX1	T5Ø.ØX2	T5Ø.ØX3	T5Ø.ØX4	T5Ø.ØX5	T5Ø.ØX6
ENT agent	T49.6X1	T49.6X2	T49.6X3	T49.6X4	T49.6X5	T49.6X6
ophthalmic preparation	T49.5X1	T49.5X2	T49.5X3	T49.5X4	T49.5X5	T49.5X6
topical NEC	T49.ØX1	T49.ØX2	T49.ØX3	T49.ØX4	T49.ØX5	T49.ØX6
Fludroxycortide	T49.ØX1	T49.ØX2	T49.ØX3	T49.ØX4	T49.ØX5	T49.ØX6
Flufenamic acid	T39.391	T39.392	T39.393	T39.394	T39.395	T39.396
Fluindione	T45.511	T45.512	T45.513	T45.514	T45.515	T45.516
Flumequine	T37.8X1	T37.8X2	T37.8X3	T37.8X4	T37.8X5	T37.8X6
Flumethasone	T49.ØX1	T49.ØX2	T49.ØX3	T49.ØX4	T49.ØX5	T49.ØX6
Flumethiazide	T5Ø.2X1	T5Ø.2X2	T5Ø.2X3	T5Ø.2X4	T5Ø.2X5	T5Ø.2X6
Flumidin	T37.5X1	T37.5X2	T37.5X3	T37.5X4	T37.5X5	T37.5X6
Flunarizine	T46.7X1	T46.7X2	T46.7X3	T46.7X4	T46.7X5	T46.7X6
Flunidazole	T37.8X1	T37.8X2	T37.8X3	T37.8X4	T37.8X5	T37.8X6
Flunisolide	T48.6X1	T48.6X2	T48.6X3	T48.6X4	T48.6X5	T48.6X6
Flunitrazepam	T42.4X1	T42.4X2	T42.4X3	T42.4X4	T42.4X5	T42.4X6
Fluocinolone (acetonide)	T49.ØX1	T49.ØX2	T49.ØX3	T49.ØX4	T49.ØX5	T49.ØX6
Fluocinonide	T49.ØX1	T49.ØX2	T49.ØX3	T49.ØX4	T49.ØX5	T49.ØX6

Substance	Poisoning, Accidental (unintentional)	Poisoning, Intentional Self-harm	Poisoning, Assault	Poisoning, Undetermined	Adverse Effect	Under-dosing
Fluocortin (butyl)	T49.0X1	T49.0X2	T49.0X3	T49.0X4	T49.0X5	T49.0X6
Fluocortolone	T49.0X1	T49.0X2	T49.0X3	T49.0X4	T49.0X5	T49.0X6
Fluohydrocortisone	T38.0X1	T38.0X2	T38.0X3	T38.0X4	T38.0X5	T38.0X6
ENT agent	T49.6X1	T49.6X2	T49.6X3	T49.6X4	T49.6X5	T49.6X6
ophthalmic preparation	T49.5X1	T49.5X2	T49.5X3	T49.5X4	T49.5X5	T49.5X6
topical NEC	T49.0X1	T49.0X2	T49.0X3	T49.0X4	T49.0X5	T49.0X6
Fluonid	T49.0X1	T49.0X2	T49.0X3	T49.0X4	T49.0X5	T49.0X6
Fluopromazine	T43.3X1	T43.3X2	T43.3X3	T43.3X4	T43.3X5	T43.3X6
Fluoracetate	T60.8X1	T60.8X2	T60.8X3	T60.8X4	—	—
Fluorescein	T50.8X1	T50.8X2	T50.8X3	T50.8X4	T50.8X5	T50.8X6
Fluorhydrocortisone	T50.0X1	T50.0X2	T50.0X3	T50.0X4	T50.0X5	T50.0X6
Fluoride (nonmedicinal) (pesticide) (sodium) NEC	T60.8X1	T60.8X2	T60.8X3	T60.8X4	—	—
hydrogen — see Hydrofluoric acid						
medicinal NEC	T50.991	T50.992	T50.993	T50.994	T50.995	T50.996
dental use	T49.7X1	T49.7X2	T49.7X3	T49.7X4	T49.7X5	T49.7X6
not pesticide NEC	T54.91	T54.92	T54.93	T54.94	—	—
stannous	T49.7X1	T49.7X2	T49.7X3	T49.7X4	T49.7X5	T49.7X6
Fluorinated corticosteroids	T38.0X1	T38.0X2	T38.0X3	T38.0X4	T38.0X5	T38.0X6
Fluorine (gas)	T59.5X1	T59.5X2	T59.5X3	T59.5X4	—	—
salt — see Fluoride(s)						
Fluoristan	T49.7X1	T49.7X2	T49.7X3	T49.7X4	T49.7X5	T49.7X6
Fluormetholone	T49.0X1	T49.0X2	T49.0X3	T49.0X4	T49.0X5	T49.0X6
Fluoroacetate	T60.8X1	T60.8X2	T60.8X3	T60.8X4	—	—
Fluorocarbon monomer	T53.6X1	T53.6X2	T53.6X3	T53.6X4	—	—
Fluorocytosine	T37.8X1	T37.8X2	T37.8X3	T37.8X4	T37.8X5	T37.8X6
Fluorodeoxyuridine	T45.1X1	T45.1X2	T45.1X3	T45.1X4	T45.1X5	T45.1X6
Fluorometholone	T49.0X1	T49.0X2	T49.0X3	T49.0X4	T49.0X5	T49.0X6
ophthalmic preparation	T49.5X1	T49.5X2	T49.5X3	T49.5X4	T49.5X5	T49.5X6
Fluorophosphate insecticide	T60.0X1	T60.0X2	T60.0X3	T60.0X4	—	—
Fluorosol	T46.3X1	T46.3X2	T46.3X3	T46.3X4	T46.3X5	T46.3X6
Fluorouracil	T45.1X1	T45.1X2	T45.1X3	T45.1X4	T45.1X5	T45.1X6
Fluorphenylalanine	T49.5X1	T49.5X2	T49.5X3	T49.5X4	T49.5X5	T49.5X6
Fluothane	T41.0X1	T41.0X2	T41.0X3	T41.0X4	T41.0X5	T41.0X6
Fluoxetine	T43.221	T43.222	T43.223	T43.224	T43.225	T43.226
Fluoxymesterone	T38.7X1	T38.7X2	T38.7X3	T38.7X4	T38.7X5	T38.7X6
Flupenthixol	T43.4X1	T43.4X2	T43.4X3	T43.4X4	T43.4X5	T43.4X6
Flupentixol	T43.4X1	T43.4X2	T43.4X3	T43.4X4	T43.4X5	T43.4X6
Fluphenazine	T43.3X1	T43.3X2	T43.3X3	T43.3X4	T43.3X5	T43.3X6
Fluprednidene	T49.0X1	T49.0X2	T49.0X3	T49.0X4	T49.0X5	T49.0X6
Fluprednisolone	T38.0X1	T38.0X2	T38.0X3	T38.0X4	T38.0X5	T38.0X6
Fluradoline	T39.8X1	T39.8X2	T39.8X3	T39.8X4	T39.8X5	T39.8X6
Flurandrenolide	T49.0X1	T49.0X2	T49.0X3	T49.0X4	T49.0X5	T49.0X6
Flurandrenolone	T49.0X1	T49.0X2	T49.0X3	T49.0X4	T49.0X5	T49.0X6
Flurazepam	T42.4X1	T42.4X2	T42.4X3	T42.4X4	T42.4X5	T42.4X6
Flurbiprofen	T39.311	T39.312	T39.313	T39.314	T39.315	T39.316
Flurobate	T49.0X1	T49.0X2	T49.0X3	T49.0X4	T49.0X5	T49.0X6
Fluroxene	T41.0X1	T41.0X2	T41.0X3	T41.0X4	T41.0X5	T41.0X6
Fluspirilene	T43.591	T43.592	T43.593	T43.594	T43.595	T43.596
Flutamide	T38.6X1	T38.6X2	T38.6X3	T38.6X4	T38.6X5	T38.6X6
Flutazolam	T42.4X1	T42.4X2	T42.4X3	T42.4X4	T42.4X5	T42.4X6
Fluticasone propionate	T49.1X1	T49.1X2	T49.1X3	T49.1X4	T49.1X5	T49.1X6
Flutoprazepam	T42.4X1	T42.4X2	T42.4X3	T42.4X4	T42.4X5	T42.4X6
Flutropium bromide	T48.6X1	T48.6X2	T48.6X3	T48.6X4	T48.6X5	T48.6X6
Fluvoxamine	T43.221	T43.222	T43.223	T43.224	T43.225	T43.226
Folacin	T45.8X1	T45.8X2	T45.8X3	T45.8X4	T45.8X5	T45.8X6
Folic acid	T45.8X1	T45.8X2	T45.8X3	T45.8X4	T45.8X5	T45.8X6
with ferrous salt	T45.2X1	T45.2X2	T45.2X3	T45.2X4	T45.2X5	T45.2X6
antagonist	T45.1X1	T45.1X2	T45.1X3	T45.1X4	T45.1X5	T45.1X6
Folinic acid	T45.8X1	T45.8X2	T45.8X3	T45.8X4	T45.8X5	T45.8X6
Folium stramoniae	T48.6X1	T48.6X2	T48.6X3	T48.6X4	T48.6X5	T48.6X6
Follicle-stimulating hormone, human	T38.811	T38.812	T38.813	T38.814	T38.815	T38.816
Folpet	T60.3X1	T60.3X2	T60.3X3	T60.3X4	—	—
Fominoben	T48.3X1	T48.3X2	T48.3X3	T48.3X4	T48.3X5	T48.3X6
Food, foodstuffs, noxious, nonbacterial, NEC	T62.91	T62.92	T62.93	T62.94	—	—
berries	T62.1X1	T62.1X2	T62.1X3	T62.1X4	—	—
fish — see also Fish	T61.91	T61.92	T61.93	T61.94	—	—
mushrooms	T62.0X1	T62.0X2	T62.0X3	T62.0X4	—	—
plants	T62.2X1	T62.2X2	T62.2X3	T62.2X4	—	—
seafood	T61.91	T61.92	T61.93	T61.94	—	—
specified NEC	T61.8X1	T61.8X2	T61.8X3	T61.8X4	—	—
seeds	T62.2X1	T62.2X2	T62.2X3	T62.2X4	—	—
shellfish	T61.781	T61.782	T61.783	T61.784	—	—
specified NEC	T62.8X1	T62.8X2	T62.8X3	T62.8X4	—	—
Fool's parsley	T62.2X1	T62.2X2	T62.2X3	T62.2X4	—	—
Formaldehyde (solution), gas or vapor	T59.2X1	T59.2X2	T59.2X3	T59.2X4	—	—
fungicide	T60.3X1	T60.3X2	T60.3X3	T60.3X4	—	—

Substance	Poisoning, Accidental (unintentional)	Poisoning, Intentional Self-harm	Poisoning, Assault	Poisoning, Undetermined	Adverse Effect	Under-dosing
Formalin	T59.2X1	T59.2X2	T59.2X3	T59.2X4	—	—
fungicide	T60.3X1	T60.3X2	T60.3X3	T60.3X4	—	—
vapor	T59.2X1	T59.2X2	T59.2X3	T59.2X4	—	—
Formic acid	T54.2X1	T54.2X2	T54.2X3	T54.2X4	—	—
vapor	T59.891	T59.892	T59.893	T59.894	—	—
Foscarnet sodium	T37.5X1	T37.5X2	T37.5X3	T37.5X4	T37.5X5	T37.5X6
Fosfestrol	T38.5X1	T38.5X2	T38.5X3	T38.5X4	T38.5X5	T38.5X6
Fosfomycin	T36.8X1	T36.8X2	T36.8X3	T36.8X4	T36.8X5	T36.8X6
Fosfonet sodium	T37.5X1	T37.5X2	T37.5X3	T37.5X4	T37.5X5	T37.5X6
Fosinopril	T46.4X1	T46.4X2	T46.4X3	T46.4X4	T46.4X5	T46.4X6
sodium	T46.4X1	T46.4X2	T46.4X3	T46.4X4	T46.4X5	T46.4X6
Fowler's solution	T57.0X1	T57.0X2	T57.0X3	T57.0X4	—	—
Foxglove	T62.2X1	T62.2X2	T62.2X3	T62.2X4	—	—
Framycetin	T36.5X1	T36.5X2	T36.5X3	T36.5X4	T36.5X5	T36.5X6
Frangula	T47.2X1	T47.2X2	T47.2X3	T47.2X4	T47.2X5	T47.2X6
extract	T47.2X1	T47.2X2	T47.2X3	T47.2X4	T47.2X5	T47.2X6
Frei antigen	T50.8X1	T50.8X2	T50.8X3	T50.8X4	T50.8X5	T50.8X6
Freon	T53.5X1	T53.5X2	T53.5X3	T53.5X4	—	—
Fructose	T50.3X1	T50.3X2	T50.3X3	T50.3X4	T50.3X5	T50.3X6
Frusemide	T50.1X1	T50.1X2	T50.1X3	T50.1X4	T50.1X5	T50.1X6
FSH	T38.811	T38.812	T38.813	T38.814	T38.815	T38.816
Ftorafur	T45.1X1	T45.1X2	T45.1X3	T45.1X4	T45.1X5	T45.1X6
Fuel						
automobile	T52.0X1	T52.0X2	T52.0X3	T52.0X4	—	—
exhaust gas, not in transit	T58.01	T58.02	T58.03	T58.04	—	—
vapor NEC	T52.0X1	T52.0X2	T52.0X3	T52.0X4	—	—
gas (domestic use) — see also Carbon, monoxide, fuel, utility	T59.891	T59.892	T59.893	T59.894	—	—
utility	T59.891	T59.892	T59.893	T59.894	—	—
incomplete combustion of — see Carbon, monoxide, fuel, utility						
in mobile container	T59.891	T59.892	T59.893	T59.894	—	—
piped (natural)	T59.891	T59.892	T59.893	T59.894	—	—
industrial, incomplete combustion	T58.8X1	T58.8X2	T58.8X3	T58.8X4	—	—
Fugillin	T36.8X1	T36.8X2	T36.8X3	T36.8X4	T36.8X5	T36.8X6
Fulminate of mercury	T56.1X1	T56.1X2	T56.1X3	T56.1X4	—	—
Fulvicin	T36.7X1	T36.7X2	T36.7X3	T36.7X4	T36.7X5	T36.7X6
Fumadil	T36.8X1	T36.8X2	T36.8X3	T36.8X4	T36.8X5	T36.8X6
Fumagillin	T36.8X1	T36.8X2	T36.8X3	T36.8X4	T36.8X5	T36.8X6
Fumaric acid	T49.4X1	T49.4X2	T49.4X3	T49.4X4	T49.4X5	T49.4X6
Fumes (from)	T59.91	T59.92	T59.93	T59.94	—	—
carbon monoxide — see Carbon, monoxide						
charcoal (domestic use) — see Charcoal, fumes						
chloroform — see Chloroform						
coke (in domestic stoves, fireplaces) — see Coke fumes						
corrosive NEC	T54.91	T54.92	T54.93	T54.94	—	—
ether — see ether						
freons	T53.5X1	T53.5X2	T53.5X3	T53.5X4	—	—
hydrocarbons	T59.891	T59.892	T59.893	T59.894	—	—
petroleum (liquefied)	T59.891	T59.892	T59.893	T59.894	—	—
distributed through pipes (pure or mixed with air)	T59.891	T59.892	T59.893	T59.894	—	—
lead — see lead						
metal — see Metals, or the specified metal						
nitrogen dioxide	T59.0X1	T59.0X2	T59.0X3	T59.0X4	—	—
pesticides — see Pesticides						
petroleum (liquefied)	T59.891	T59.892	T59.893	T59.894	—	—
distributed through pipes (pure or mixed with air)	T59.891	T59.892	T59.893	T59.894	—	—
polyester	T59.891	T59.892	T59.893	T59.894	—	—
specified source NEC — see also substance specified	T59.891	T59.892	T59.893	T59.894	—	—
sulfur dioxide	T59.1X1	T59.1X2	T59.1X3	T59.1X4	—	—
Fumigant NEC	T60.91	T60.92	T60.93	T60.94	—	—
Fungicide NEC (nonmedicinal)	T60.3X1	T60.3X2	T60.3X3	T60.3X4	—	—
Fungi, noxious, used as food	T62.0X1	T62.0X2	T62.0X3	T62.0X4	—	—
Fungizone	T36.7X1	T36.7X2	T36.7X3	T36.7X4	T36.7X5	T36.7X6
topical	T49.0X1	T49.0X2	T49.0X3	T49.0X4	T49.0X5	T49.0X6
Furacin	T49.0X1	T49.0X2	T49.0X3	T49.0X4	T49.0X5	T49.0X6
Furadantin	T37.91	T37.92	T37.93	T37.94	T37.95	T37.96
Furazolidone	T37.8X1	T37.8X2	T37.8X3	T37.8X4	T37.8X5	T37.8X6

Substance	Poisoning, Accidental (unintentional)	Poisoning, Intentional Self-harm	Poisoning, Assault	Poisoning, Undetermined	Adverse Effect	Under-dosing
Furazolium chloride	T49.0X1	T49.0X2	T49.0X3	T49.0X4	T49.0X5	T49.0X6
Furfural	T52.8X1	T52.8X2	T52.8X3	T52.8X4	—	—
Furnace (coal burning) (domestic), gas from	T58.2X1	T58.2X2	T58.2X3	T58.2X4	—	—
industrial	T58.8X1	T58.8X2	T58.8X3	T58.8X4	—	—
Furniture polish	T65.891	T65.892	T65.893	T65.894	—	—
Furosemide	T50.1X1	T50.1X2	T50.1X3	T50.1X4	T50.1X5	T50.1X6
Furoxone	T37.91	T37.92	T37.93	T37.94	T37.95	T37.96
Fursultiamine	T45.2X1	T45.2X2	T45.2X3	T45.2X4	T45.2X5	T45.2X6
Fusafungine	T36.8X1	T36.8X2	T36.8X3	T36.8X4	T36.8X5	T36.8X6
Fusel oil (any) (amyl) (butyl) (propyl), vapor	T51.3X1	T51.3X2	T51.3X3	T51.3X4	—	—
Fusidate (ethanolamine) (sodium)	T36.8X1	T36.8X2	T36.8X3	T36.8X4	T36.8X5	T36.8X6
Fusidic acid	T36.8X1	T36.8X2	T36.8X3	T36.8X4	T36.8X5	T36.8X6
Fytic acid, nonasodium	T50.6X1	T50.6X2	T50.6X3	T50.6X4	T50.6X5	T50.6X6
b-Galactosidase	T47.5X1	T47.5X2	T47.5X3	T47.5X4	T47.5X5	T47.5X6
GABA	T43.8X1	T43.8X2	T43.8X3	T43.8X4	T43.8X5	T43.8X6
Gadopentetic acid	T50.8X1	T50.8X2	T50.8X3	T50.8X4	T50.8X5	T50.8X6
Galactose	T50.3X1	T50.3X2	T50.3X3	T50.3X4	T50.3X5	T50.3X6
Galantamine	T44.0X1	T44.0X2	T44.0X3	T44.0X4	T44.0X5	T44.0X6
Gallamine (triethiodide)	T48.1X1	T48.1X2	T48.1X3	T48.1X4	T48.1X5	T48.1X6
Gallium citrate	T50.991	T50.992	T50.993	T50.994	T50.995	T50.996
Gallopamil	T46.1X1	T46.1X2	T46.1X3	T46.1X4	T46.1X5	T46.1X6
Gamboge	T47.2X1	T47.2X2	T47.2X3	T47.2X4	T47.2X5	T47.2X6
Gamimune	T50.Z11	T50.Z12	T50.Z13	T50.Z14	T50.Z15	T50.Z16
Gamma-aminobutyric acid	T43.8X1	T43.8X2	T43.8X3	T43.8X4	T43.8X5	T43.8X6
Gamma-benzene hexachloride (medicinal)	T49.0X1	T49.0X2	T49.0X3	T49.0X4	T49.0X5	T49.0X6
nonmedicinal, vapor	T53.6X1	T53.6X2	T53.6X3	T53.6X4	—	—
Gamma-BHC (medicinal) — see also Gamma-benzene hexachloride	T49.0X1	T49.0X2	T49.0X3	T49.0X4	T49.0X5	T49.0X6
Gamma globulin	T50.Z11	T50.Z12	T50.Z13	T50.Z14	T50.Z15	T50.Z16
Gamulin	T50.Z11	T50.Z12	T50.Z13	T50.Z14	T50.Z15	T50.Z16
Ganciclovir (sodium)	T37.5X1	T37.5X2	T37.5X3	T37.5X4	T37.5X5	T37.5X6
Ganglionic blocking drug NEC	T44.2X1	T44.2X2	T44.2X3	T44.2X4	T44.2X5	T44.2X6
specified NEC	T44.2X1	T44.2X2	T44.2X3	T44.2X4	T44.2X5	T44.2X6
Ganja	T40.7X1	T40.7X2	T40.7X3	T40.7X4	T40.7X5	T40.7X6
Garamycin	T36.5X1	T36.5X2	T36.5X3	T36.5X4	T36.5X5	T36.5X6
ophthalmic preparation	T49.5X1	T49.5X2	T49.5X3	T49.5X4	T49.5X5	T49.5X6
topical NEC	T49.0X1	T49.0X2	T49.0X3	T49.0X4	T49.0X5	T49.0X6
Gardenal	T42.3X1	T42.3X2	T42.3X3	T42.3X4	T42.3X5	T42.3X6
Gardepanyl	T42.3X1	T42.3X2	T42.3X3	T42.3X4	T42.3X5	T42.3X6
Gas	T59.91	T59.92	T59.93	T59.94	—	—
acetylene	T59.891	T59.892	T59.893	T59.894	—	—
incomplete combustion of	T58.11	T58.12	T58.13	T58.14	—	—
air contaminants, source or type not specified	T59.91	T59.92	T59.93	T59.94	—	—
anesthetic	T41.0X1	T41.0X2	T41.0X3	T41.0X4	T41.0X5	T41.0X6
blast furnace	T58.8X1	T58.8X2	T58.8X3	T58.8X4	—	—
butane — see butane						
carbon monoxide — see Carbon, monoxide						
chlorine	T59.4X1	T59.4X2	T59.4X3	T59.4X4	—	—
coal	T58.2X1	T58.2X2	T58.2X3	T58.2X4	—	—
cyanide	T57.3X1	T57.3X2	T57.3X3	T57.3X4	—	—
dicyanogen	T65.0X1	T65.0X2	T65.0X3	T65.0X4	—	—
domestic — see Domestic gas						
exhaust	T58.01	T58.02	T58.03	T58.04	—	—
from utility (for cooking, heating, or lighting) (after combustion) — see Carbon, monoxide, fuel, utility						
prior to combustion	T59.891	T59.892	T59.893	T59.894	—	—
from wood- or coal-burning stove or fireplace	T58.2X1	T58.2X2	T58.2X3	T58.2X4	—	—
fuel (domestic use) (after combustion) — see also Carbon, monoxide, fuel						
industrial use	T58.8X1	T58.8X2	T58.8X3	T58.8X4	—	—
prior to combustion	T59.891	T59.892	T59.893	T59.894	—	—
utility	T59.891	T59.892	T59.893	T59.894	—	—
incomplete combustion of — see Carbon, monoxide, fuel, utility						
in mobile container	T59.891	T59.892	T59.893	T59.894	—	—
piped (natural)	T59.891	T59.892	T59.893	T59.894	—	—
garage	T58.01	T58.02	T58.03	T58.04	—	—

Substance	Poisoning, Accidental (unintentional)	Poisoning, Intentional Self-harm	Poisoning, Assault	Poisoning, Undetermined	Adverse Effect	Under-dosing
Gas — continued						
hydrocarbon NEC	T59.891	T59.892	T59.893	T59.894	—	—
incomplete combustion of — see Carbon, monoxide, fuel, utility						
liquefied — see butane						
piped	T59.891	T59.892	T59.893	T59.894	—	—
hydrocyanic acid	T65.0X1	T65.0X2	T65.0X3	T65.0X4	—	—
illuminating (after combustion)	T58.11	T58.12	T58.13	T58.14	—	—
prior to combustion	T59.891	T59.892	T59.893	T59.894	—	—
incomplete combustion, any — see Carbon, monoxide						
kiln	T58.8X1	T58.8X2	T58.8X3	T58.8X4	—	—
lacrimogenic	T59.3X1	T59.3X2	T59.3X3	T59.3X4	—	—
liquefied petroleum — see butane						
marsh	T59.891	T59.892	T59.893	T59.894	—	—
motor exhaust, not in transit	T58.01	T58.02	T58.03	T58.04	—	—
mustard, not in war	T59.891	T59.892	T59.893	T59.894	—	—
natural	T59.891	T59.892	T59.893	T59.894	—	—
nerve, not in war	T59.91	T59.92	T59.93	T59.94	—	—
oil	T52.0X1	T52.0X2	T52.0X3	T52.0X4	—	—
petroleum (liquefied) (distributed in mobile containers)	T59.891	T59.892	T59.893	T59.894	—	—
piped (pure or mixed with air)	T59.891	T59.892	T59.893	T59.894	—	—
piped (manufactured) (natural) NEC	T59.891	T59.892	T59.893	T59.894	—	—
producer	T58.8X1	T58.8X2	T58.8X3	T58.8X4	—	—
propane — see propane						
refrigerant (chlorofluoro-carbon)	T53.5X1	T53.5X2	T53.5X3	T53.5X4	—	—
not chlorofluoro-carbon	T59.891	T59.892	T59.893	T59.894	—	—
sewer	T59.91	T59.92	T59.93	T59.94	—	—
specified source NEC	T59.91	T59.92	T59.93	T59.94	—	—
stove (after combustion)	T58.11	T58.12	T58.13	T58.14	—	—
prior to combustion	T59.891	T59.892	T59.893	T59.894	—	—
tear	T59.3X1	T59.3X2	T59.3X3	T59.3X4	—	—
therapeutic	T41.5X1	T41.5X2	T41.5X3	T41.5X4	T41.5X5	T41.5X6
utility (for cooking, heating, or lighting) (piped) NEC	T59.891	T59.892	T59.893	T59.894	—	—
incomplete combustion of — see Carbon, monoxide, fuel, utilty						
in mobile container	T59.891	T59.892	T59.893	T59.894	—	—
piped (natural)	T59.891	T59.892	T59.893	T59.894	—	—
water	T58.11	T58.12	T58.13	T58.14	—	—
incomplete combustion of — see Carbon, monoxide, fuel, utility						
Gaseous substance — see Gas						
Gasoline	T52.0X1	T52.0X2	T52.0X3	T52.0X4	—	—
vapor	T52.0X1	T52.0X2	T52.0X3	T52.0X4	—	—
Gastric enzymes	T47.5X1	T47.5X2	T47.5X3	T47.5X4	T47.5X5	T47.5X6
Gastrografin	T50.8X1	T50.8X2	T50.8X3	T50.8X4	T50.8X5	T50.8X6
Gastrointestinal drug	T47.91	T47.92	T47.93	T47.94	T47.95	T47.96
biological	T47.8X1	T47.8X2	T47.8X3	T47.8X4	T47.8X5	T47.8X6
specified NEC	T47.8X1	T47.8X2	T47.8X3	T47.8X4	T47.8X5	T47.8X6
Gaultheria procumbens	T62.2X1	T62.2X2	T62.2X3	T62.2X4	—	—
Gefarnate	T44.3X1	T44.3X2	T44.3X3	T44.3X4	T44.3X5	T44.3X6
Gelatin (intravenous)	T45.8X1	T45.8X2	T45.8X3	T45.8X4	T45.8X5	T45.8X6
absorbable (sponge)	T45.7X1	T45.7X2	T45.7X3	T45.7X4	T45.7X5	T45.7X6
Gelfilm	T49.8X1	T49.8X2	T49.8X3	T49.8X4	T49.8X5	T49.8X6
Gelfoam	T45.7X1	T45.7X2	T45.7X3	T45.7X4	T45.7X5	T45.7X6
Gelsemine	T50.991	T50.992	T50.993	T50.994	T50.995	T50.996
Gelsemium (sempervirens)	T62.2X1	T62.2X2	T62.2X3	T62.2X4	—	—
Gemeprost	T48.0X1	T48.0X2	T48.0X3	T48.0X4	T48.0X5	T48.0X6
Gemfibrozil	T46.6X1	T46.6X2	T46.6X3	T46.6X4	T46.6X5	T46.6X6
Gemonil	T42.3X1	T42.3X2	T42.3X3	T42.3X4	T42.3X5	T42.3X6
Gentamicin	T36.5X1	T36.5X2	T36.5X3	T36.5X4	T36.5X5	T36.5X6
ophthalmic preparation	T49.5X1	T49.5X2	T49.5X3	T49.5X4	T49.5X5	T49.5X6
topical NEC	T49.0X1	T49.0X2	T49.0X3	T49.0X4	T49.0X5	T49.0X6
Gentian	T47.5X1	T47.5X2	T47.5X3	T47.5X4	T47.5X5	T47.5X6
violet	T49.0X1	T49.0X2	T49.0X3	T49.0X4	T49.0X5	T49.0X6
Gepefrine	T44.4X1	T44.4X2	T44.4X3	T44.4X4	T44.4X5	T44.4X6
Gestonorone caproate	T38.5X1	T38.5X2	T38.5X3	T38.5X4	T38.5X5	T38.5X6
Gexane	T49.0X1	T49.0X2	T49.0X3	T49.0X4	T49.0X5	T49.0X6
Gila monster (venom)	T63.111	T63.112	T63.113	T63.114	—	—
Ginger	T47.5X1	T47.5X2	T47.5X3	T47.5X4	T47.5X5	T47.5X6
Jamaica — see Jamaica, ginger						

Substance	Poisoning, Accidental (unintentional)	Poisoning, Intentional Self-harm	Poisoning, Assault	Poisoning, Undetermined	Adverse Effect	Under-dosing
Gitalin	T46.ØX1	T46.ØX2	T46.ØX3	T46.ØX4	T46.ØX5	T46.ØX6
amorphous	T46.ØX1	T46.ØX2	T46.ØX3	T46.ØX4	T46.ØX5	T46.ØX6
Gitaloxin	T46.ØX1	T46.ØX2	T46.ØX3	T46.ØX4	T46.ØX5	T46.ØX6
Gitoxin	T46.ØX1	T46.ØX2	T46.ØX3	T46.ØX4	T46.ØX5	T46.ØX6
Glafenine	T39.8X1	T39.8X2	T39.8X3	T39.8X4	T39.8X5	T39.8X6
Glandular extract (medicinal) **NEC**	T5Ø.Z91	T5Ø.Z92	T5Ø.Z93	T5Ø.Z94	T5Ø.Z95	T5Ø.Z96
Glaucarubin	T37.3X1	T37.3X2	T37.3X3	T37.3X4	T37.3X5	T37.3X6
Glibenclamide	T38.3X1	T38.3X2	T38.3X3	T38.3X4	T38.3X5	T38.3X6
Glibornuride	T38.3X1	T38.3X2	T38.3X3	T38.3X4	T38.3X5	T38.3X6
Gliclazide	T38.3X1	T38.3X2	T38.3X3	T38.3X4	T38.3X5	T38.3X6
Glimidine	T38.3X1	T38.3X2	T38.3X3	T38.3X4	T38.3X5	T38.3X6
Glipizide	T38.3X1	T38.3X2	T38.3X3	T38.3X4	T38.3X5	T38.3X6
Gliquidone	T38.3X1	T38.3X2	T38.3X3	T38.3X4	T38.3X5	T38.3X6
Glisolamide	T38.3X1	T38.3X2	T38.3X3	T38.3X4	T38.3X5	T38.3X6
Glisoxepide	T38.3X1	T38.3X2	T38.3X3	T38.3X4	T38.3X5	T38.3X6
Globin zinc insulin	T38.3X1	T38.3X2	T38.3X3	T38.3X4	T38.3X5	T38.3X6
Globulin						
antilymphocytic	T5Ø.Z11	T5Ø.Z12	T5Ø.Z13	T5Ø.Z14	T5Ø.Z15	T5Ø.Z16
antirhesus	T5Ø.Z11	T5Ø.Z12	T5Ø.Z13	T5Ø.Z14	T5Ø.Z15	T5Ø.Z16
antivenin	T5Ø.Z11	T5Ø.Z12	T5Ø.Z13	T5Ø.Z14	T5Ø.Z15	T5Ø.Z16
antiviral	T5Ø.Z11	T5Ø.Z12	T5Ø.Z13	T5Ø.Z14	T5Ø.Z15	T5Ø.Z16
Glucagon	T38.3X1	T38.3X2	T38.3X3	T38.3X4	T38.3X5	T38.3X6
Glucocorticoids	T38.ØX1	T38.ØX2	T38.ØX3	T38.ØX4	T38.ØX5	T38.ØX6
Glucocorticosteroid	T38.ØX1	T38.ØX2	T38.ØX3	T38.ØX4	T38.ØX5	T38.ØX6
Gluconic acid	T5Ø.991	T5Ø.992	T5Ø.993	T5Ø.994	T5Ø.995	T5Ø.996
Glucosamine sulfate	T39.4X1	T39.4X2	T39.4X3	T39.4X4	T39.4X5	T39.4X6
Glucose	T5Ø.3X1	T5Ø.3X2	T5Ø.3X3	T5Ø.3X4	T5Ø.3X5	T5Ø.3X6
with sodium chloride	T5Ø.3X1	T5Ø.3X2	T5Ø.3X3	T5Ø.3X4	T5Ø.3X5	T5Ø.3X6
Glucosulfone sodium	T37.1X1	T37.1X2	T37.1X3	T37.1X4	T37.1X5	T37.1X6
Glucurolactone	T47.8X1	T47.8X2	T47.8X3	T47.8X4	T47.8X5	T47.8X6
Glue NEC	T52.8X1	T52.8X2	T52.8X3	T52.8X4	—	—
Glutamic acid	T47.5X1	T47.5X2	T47.5X3	T47.5X4	T47.5X5	T47.5X6
Glutaral (medicinal)	T49.ØX1	T49.ØX2	T49.ØX3	T49.ØX4	T49.ØX5	T49.ØX6
nonmedicinal	T65.891	T65.892	T65.893	T65.894	—	—
Glutaraldehyde (nonmedicinal)	T65.891	T65.892	T65.893	T65.894	—	—
medicinal	T49.ØX1	T49.ØX2	T49.ØX3	T49.ØX4	T49.ØX5	T49.ØX6
Glutathione	T5Ø.6X1	T5Ø.6X2	T5Ø.6X3	T5Ø.6X4	T5Ø.6X5	T5Ø.6X6
Glutethimide	T42.6X1	T42.6X2	T42.6X3	T42.6X4	T42.6X5	T42.6X6
Glyburide	T38.3X1	T38.3X2	T38.3X3	T38.3X4	T38.3X5	T38.3X6
Glycerin	T47.4X1	T47.4X2	T47.4X3	T47.4X4	T47.4X5	T47.4X6
Glycerol	T47.4X1	T47.4X2	T47.4X3	T47.4X4	T47.4X5	T47.4X6
borax	T49.6X1	T49.6X2	T49.6X3	T49.6X4	T49.6X5	T49.6X6
intravenous	T5Ø.3X1	T5Ø.3X2	T5Ø.3X3	T5Ø.3X4	T5Ø.3X5	T5Ø.3X6
iodinated	T48.4X1	T48.4X2	T48.4X3	T48.4X4	T48.4X5	T48.4X6
Glycerophosphate	T5Ø.991	T5Ø.992	T5Ø.993	T5Ø.994	T5Ø.995	T5Ø.996
Glyceryl						
gualacolate	T48.4X1	T48.4X2	T48.4X3	T48.4X4	T48.4X5	T48.4X6
nitrate	T46.3X1	T46.3X2	T46.3X3	T46.3X4	T46.3X5	T46.3X6
triacetate (topical)	T49.ØX1	T49.ØX2	T49.ØX3	T49.ØX4	T49.ØX5	T49.ØX6
trinitrate	T46.3X1	T46.3X2	T46.3X3	T46.3X4	T46.3X5	T46.3X6
Glycine	T5Ø.3X1	T5Ø.3X2	T5Ø.3X3	T5Ø.3X4	T5Ø.3X5	T5Ø.3X6
Glyclopyramide	T38.3X1	T38.3X2	T38.3X3	T38.3X4	T38.3X5	T38.3X6
Glycobiarsol	T37.3X1	T37.3X2	T37.3X3	T37.3X4	T37.3X5	T37.3X6
Glycols (ether)	T52.3X1	T52.3X2	T52.3X3	T52.3X4	—	—
Glyconiazide	T37.1X1	T37.1X2	T37.1X3	T37.1X4	T37.1X5	T37.1X6
Glycopyrrolate	T44.3X1	T44.3X2	T44.3X3	T44.3X4	T44.3X5	T44.3X6
Glycopyrronium	T44.3X1	T44.3X2	T44.3X3	T44.3X4	T44.3X5	T44.3X6
bromide	T44.3X1	T44.3X2	T44.3X3	T44.3X4	T44.3X5	T44.3X6
Glycoside, cardiac (stimulant)	T46.ØX1	T46.ØX2	T46.ØX3	T46.ØX4	T46.ØX5	T46.ØX6
Glycyclamide	T38.3X1	T38.3X2	T38.3X3	T38.3X4	T38.3X5	T38.3X6
Glycyrrhiza extract	T48.4X1	T48.4X2	T48.4X3	T48.4X4	T48.4X5	T48.4X6
Glycyrrhizic acid	T48.4X1	T48.4X2	T48.4X3	T48.4X4	T48.4X5	T48.4X6
Glycyrrhizinate potassium	T48.4X1	T48.4X2	T48.4X3	T48.4X4	T48.4X5	T48.4X6
Glymidine sodium	T38.3X1	T38.3X2	T38.3X3	T38.3X4	T38.3X5	T38.3X6
Glyphosate	T6Ø.3X1	T6Ø.3X2	T6Ø.3X3	T6Ø.3X4	—	—
Glyphylline	T48.6X1	T48.6X2	T48.6X3	T48.6X4	T48.6X5	T48.6X6
Gold						
colloidal (I98Au)	T45.1X1	T45.1X2	T45.1X3	T45.1X4	T45.1X5	T45.1X6
salts	T39.4X1	T39.4X2	T39.4X3	T39.4X4	T39.4X5	T39.4X6
Golden sulfide of antimony	T56.891	T56.892	T56.893	T56.894	—	—
Goldylocks	T62.2X1	T62.2X2	T62.2X3	T62.2X4	—	—
Gonadal tissue extract	T38.9Ø1	T38.9Ø2	T38.9Ø3	T38.9Ø4	T38.9Ø5	T38.9Ø6
female	T38.5X1	T38.5X2	T38.5X3	T38.5X4	T38.5X5	T38.5X6
male	T38.7X1	T38.7X2	T38.7X3	T38.7X4	T38.7X5	T38.7X6
Gonadorelin	T38.891	T38.892	T38.893	T38.894	T38.895	T38.896
Gonadotropin	T38.891	T38.892	T38.893	T38.894	T38.895	T38.896
chorionic	T38.891	T38.892	T38.893	T38.894	T38.895	T38.896
pituitary	T38.811	T38.812	T38.813	T38.814	T38.815	T38.816
Goserelin	T45.1X1	T45.1X2	T45.1X3	T45.1X4	T45.1X5	T45.1X6
Grain alcohol	T51.ØX1	T51.ØX2	T51.ØX3	T51.ØX4	—	—
Gramicidin	T49.ØX1	T49.ØX2	T49.ØX3	T49.ØX4	T49.ØX5	T49.ØX6
Granisetron	T45.ØX1	T45.ØX2	T45.ØX3	T45.ØX4	T45.ØX5	T45.ØX6
Gratiola officinalis	T62.2X1	T62.2X2	T62.2X3	T62.2X4	—	—
Grease	T65.891	T65.892	T65.893	T65.894	—	—
Green hellebore	T62.2X1	T62.2X2	T62.2X3	T62.2X4	—	—
Green soap	T49.2X1	T49.2X2	T49.2X3	T49.2X4	T49.2X5	T49.2X6
Grifulvin	T36.7X1	T36.7X2	T36.7X3	T36.7X4	T36.7X5	T36.7X6
Griseofulvin	T36.7X1	T36.7X2	T36.7X3	T36.7X4	T36.7X5	T36.7X6
Growth hormone	T38.811	T38.812	T38.813	T38.814	T38.815	T38.816
Guaiacol derivatives	T48.4X1	T48.4X2	T48.4X3	T48.4X4	T48.4X5	T48.4X6
Guaiac reagent	T5Ø.991	T5Ø.992	T5Ø.993	T5Ø.994	T5Ø.995	T5Ø.996
Guaifenesin	T48.4X1	T48.4X2	T48.4X3	T48.4X4	T48.4X5	T48.4X6
Guaimesal	T48.4X1	T48.4X2	T48.4X3	T48.4X4	T48.4X5	T48.4X6
Guaiphenesin	T48.4X1	T48.4X2	T48.4X3	T48.4X4	T48.4X5	T48.4X6
Guamecycline	T36.4X1	T36.4X2	T36.4X3	T36.4X4	T36.4X5	T36.4X6
Guanabenz	T46.5X1	T46.5X2	T46.5X3	T46.5X4	T46.5X5	T46.5X6
Guanacline	T46.5X1	T46.5X2	T46.5X3	T46.5X4	T46.5X5	T46.5X6
Guanadrel	T46.5X1	T46.5X2	T46.5X3	T46.5X4	T46.5X5	T46.5X6
Guanatol	T37.2X1	T37.2X2	T37.2X3	T37.2X4	T37.2X5	T37.2X6
Guanethidine	T46.5X1	T46.5X2	T46.5X3	T46.5X4	T46.5X5	T46.5X6
Guanfacine	T46.5X1	T46.5X2	T46.5X3	T46.5X4	T46.5X5	T46.5X6
Guano	T65.891	T65.892	T65.893	T65.894	—	—
Guanochlor	T46.5X1	T46.5X2	T46.5X3	T46.5X4	T46.5X5	T46.5X6
Guanoclor	T46.5X1	T46.5X2	T46.5X3	T46.5X4	T46.5X5	T46.5X6
Guanoctine	T46.5X1	T46.5X2	T46.5X3	T46.5X4	T46.5X5	T46.5X6
Guanoxabenz	T46.5X1	T46.5X2	T46.5X3	T46.5X4	T46.5X5	T46.5X6
Guanoxan	T46.5X1	T46.5X2	T46.5X3	T46.5X4	T46.5X5	T46.5X6
Guar gum (medicinal)	T46.6X1	T46.6X2	T46.6X3	T46.6X4	T46.6X5	T46.6X6
Hachimycin	T36.7X1	T36.7X2	T36.7X3	T36.7X4	T36.7X5	T36.7X6
Hair						
dye	T49.4X1	T49.4X2	T49.4X3	T49.4X4	T49.4X5	T49.4X6
preparation NEC	T49.4X1	T49.4X2	T49.4X3	T49.4X4	T49.4X5	T49.4X6
Halazepam	T42.4X1	T42.4X2	T42.4X3	T42.4X4	T42.4X5	T42.4X6
Halcinolone	T49.ØX1	T49.ØX2	T49.ØX3	T49.ØX4	T49.ØX5	T49.ØX6
Halcinonide	T49.ØX1	T49.ØX2	T49.ØX3	T49.ØX4	T49.ØX5	T49.ØX6
Halethazole	T49.ØX1	T49.ØX2	T49.ØX3	T49.ØX4	T49.ØX5	T49.ØX6
Hallucinogen NEC	T4Ø.9Ø1	T4Ø.9Ø2	T4Ø.9Ø3	T4Ø.9Ø4	T4Ø.9Ø5	T4Ø.9Ø6
Halofantrine	T37.2X1	T37.2X2	T37.2X3	T37.2X4	T37.2X5	T37.2X6
Halofenate	T46.6X1	T46.6X2	T46.6X3	T46.6X4	T46.6X5	T46.6X6
Halometasone	T49.ØX1	T49.ØX2	T49.ØX3	T49.ØX4	T49.ØX5	T49.ØX6
Haloperidol	T43.4X1	T43.4X2	T43.4X3	T43.4X4	T43.4X5	T43.4X6
Haloprogin	T49.ØX1	T49.ØX2	T49.ØX3	T49.ØX4	T49.ØX5	T49.ØX6
Halotex	T49.ØX1	T49.ØX2	T49.ØX3	T49.ØX4	T49.ØX5	T49.ØX6
Halothane	T41.ØX1	T41.ØX2	T41.ØX3	T41.ØX4	T41.ØX5	T41.ØX6
Haloxazolam	T42.4X1	T42.4X2	T42.4X3	T42.4X4	T42.4X5	T42.4X6
Halquinols	T49.ØX1	T49.ØX2	T49.ØX3	T49.ØX4	T49.ØX5	T49.ØX6
Hamamelis	T49.2X1	T49.2X2	T49.2X3	T49.2X4	T49.2X5	T49.2X6
Haptendextran	T45.8X1	T45.8X2	T45.8X3	T45.8X4	T45.8X5	T45.8X6
Harmonyl	T46.5X1	T46.5X2	T46.5X3	T46.5X4	T46.5X5	T46.5X6
Hartmann's solution	T5Ø.3X1	T5Ø.3X2	T5Ø.3X3	T5Ø.3X4	T5Ø.3X5	T5Ø.3X6
Hashish	T4Ø.7X1	T4Ø.7X2	T4Ø.7X3	T4Ø.7X4	T4Ø.7X5	T4Ø.7X6
Hawaiian Woodrose seeds	T4Ø.991	T4Ø.992	T4Ø.993	T4Ø.994	—	—
HCB	T6Ø.3X1	T6Ø.3X2	T6Ø.3X3	T6Ø.3X4	—	—
HCH	T53.6X1	T53.6X2	T53.6X3	T53.6X4	—	—
medicinal	T49.ØX1	T49.ØX2	T49.ØX3	T49.ØX4	T49.ØX5	T49.ØX6
HCN	T57.3X1	T57.3X2	T57.3X3	T57.3X4	—	—
Headache cures, drugs, powders NEC	T5Ø.9Ø1	T5Ø.9Ø2	T5Ø.9Ø3	T5Ø.9Ø4	T5Ø.9Ø5	T5Ø.9Ø6
Heavenly Blue (morning glory)	T4Ø.991	T4Ø.992	T4Ø.993	T4Ø.994	—	—
Heavy metal antidote	T45.8X1	T45.8X2	T45.8X3	T45.8X4	T45.8X5	T45.8X6
Hedaquinium	T49.ØX1	T49.ØX2	T49.ØX3	T49.ØX4	T49.ØX5	T49.ØX6
Hedge hyssop	T62.2X1	T62.2X2	T62.2X3	T62.2X4	—	—
Heet	T49.8X1	T49.8X2	T49.8X3	T49.8X4	T49.8X5	T49.8X6
Helenin	T37.4X1	T37.4X2	T37.4X3	T37.4X4	T37.4X5	T37.4X6
Helium (nonmedicinal) **NEC**	T59.891	T59.892	T59.893	T59.894	—	—
medicinal	T48.991	T48.992	T48.993	T48.994	T48.995	T48.996
Hellebore (black) (green) (white)	T62.2X1	T62.2X2	T62.2X3	T62.2X4	—	—
Hematin	T45.8X1	T45.8X2	T45.8X3	T45.8X4	T45.8X5	T45.8X6
Hematinic preparation	T45.8X1	T45.8X2	T45.8X3	T45.8X4	T45.8X5	T45.8X6
Hematological agent	T45.91	T45.92	T45.93	T45.94	T45.95	T45.96
specified NEC	T45.8X1	T45.8X2	T45.8X3	T45.8X4	T45.8X5	T45.8X6
Hemlock	T62.2X1	T62.2X2	T62.2X3	T62.2X4	—	—
Hemostatic	T45.621	T45.622	T45.623	T45.624	T45.625	T45.626
drug, systemic	T45.621	T45.622	T45.623	T45.624	T45.625	T45.626
Hemostyptic	T49.4X1	T49.4X2	T49.4X3	T49.4X4	T49.4X5	T49.4X6
Henbane	T62.2X1	T62.2X2	T62.2X3	T62.2X4	—	—
Heparin (sodium)	T45.511	T45.512	T45.513	T45.514	T45.515	T45.516
action reverser	T45.7X1	T45.7X2	T45.7X3	T45.7X4	T45.7X5	T45.7X6
Heparin-fraction	T45.511	T45.512	T45.513	T45.514	T45.515	T45.516
Heparinoid (systemic)	T45.511	T45.512	T45.513	T45.514	T45.515	T45.516

Subterms under main terms may continue to next column or page

Additional Character May Be Required — Refer to the Tabular List for Character Selection

361

Table of Drugs and Chemicals

Gitalin — Heparinoid

Substance	Poisoning, Accidental (unintentional)	Poisoning, Intentional Self-harm	Poisoning, Assault	Poisoning, Undetermined	Adverse Effect	Under-dosing
Hepatic secretion stimulant	T47.8X1	T47.8X2	T47.8X3	T47.8X4	T47.8X5	T47.8X6
Hepatitis B						
immune globulin	T5Ø.Z11	T5Ø.Z12	T5Ø.Z13	T5Ø.Z14	T5Ø.Z15	T5Ø.Z16
vaccine	T5Ø.B91	T5Ø.B92	T5Ø.B93	T5Ø.B94	T5Ø.B95	T5Ø.B96
Hepronicate	T46.7X1	T46.7X2	T46.7X3	T46.7X4	T46.7X5	T46.7X6
Heptabarb	T42.3X1	T42.3X2	T42.3X3	T42.3X4	T42.3X5	T42.3X6
Heptabarbital	T42.3X1	T42.3X2	T42.3X3	T42.3X4	T42.3X5	T42.3X6
Heptabarbitone	T42.3X1	T42.3X2	T42.3X3	T42.3X4	T42.3X5	T42.3X6
Heptachlor	T6Ø.1X1	T6Ø.1X2	T6Ø.1X3	T6Ø.1X4	—	—
Heptalgin	T4Ø.2X1	T4Ø.2X2	T4Ø.2X3	T4Ø.2X4	T4Ø.2X5	T4Ø.2X6
Heptaminol	T46.3X1	T46.3X2	T46.3X3	T46.3X4	T46.3X5	T46.3X6
Herbicide NEC	T6Ø.3X1	T6Ø.3X2	T6Ø.3X3	T6Ø.3X4	—	—
Heroin	T4Ø.1X1	T4Ø.1X2	T4Ø.1X3	T4Ø.1X4	—	—
Herplex	T49.5X1	T49.5X2	T49.5X3	T49.5X4	T49.5X5	T49.5X6
HES	T45.8X1	T45.8X2	T45.8X3	T45.8X4	T45.8X5	T45.8X6
Hesperidin	T46.991	T46.992	T46.993	T46.994	T46.995	T46.996
Hetacillin	T36.ØX1	T36.ØX2	T36.ØX3	T36.ØX4	T36.ØX5	T36.ØX6
Hetastarch	T45.8X1	T45.8X2	T45.8X3	T45.8X4	T45.8X5	T45.8X6
HETP	T6Ø.ØX1	T6Ø.ØX2	T6Ø.ØX3	T6Ø.ØX4	—	—
Hexachlorobenzene (vapor)	T6Ø.3X1	T6Ø.3X2	T6Ø.3X3	T6Ø.3X4	—	—
Hexachlorocyclohexane	T53.6X1	T53.6X2	T53.6X3	T53.6X4	—	—
Hexachlorophene	T49.ØX1	T49.ØX2	T49.ØX3	T49.ØX4	T49.ØX5	T49.ØX6
Hexadiline	T46.3X1	T46.3X2	T46.3X3	T46.3X4	T46.3X5	T46.3X6
Hexadimethrine (bromide)	T45.7X1	T45.7X2	T45.7X3	T45.7X4	T45.7X5	T45.7X6
Hexadylamine	T46.3X1	T46.3X2	T46.3X3	T46.3X4	T46.3X5	T46.3X6
Hexaethyl tetraphosphate	T6Ø.ØX1	T6Ø.ØX2	T6Ø.ØX3	T6Ø.ØX4	—	—
Hexafluorenium bromide	T48.1X1	T48.1X2	T48.1X3	T48.1X4	T48.1X5	T48.1X6
Hexafluronium (bromide)	T48.1X1	T48.1X2	T48.1X3	T48.1X4	T48.1X5	T48.1X6
Hexa-germ	T49.2X1	T49.2X2	T49.2X3	T49.2X4	T49.2X5	T49.2X6
Hexahydrobenzol	T52.8X1	T52.8X2	T52.8X3	T52.8X4	—	—
Hexahydrocresol(s)	T51.8X1	T51.8X2	T51.8X3	T51.8X4	—	—
arsenide	T57.ØX1	T57.ØX2	T57.ØX3	T57.ØX4	—	—
arseniurated	T57.ØX1	T57.ØX2	T57.ØX3	T57.ØX4	—	—
cyanide	T57.3X1	T57.3X2	T57.3X3	T57.3X4	—	—
gas	T59.891	T59.892	T59.893	T59.894	—	—
Fluoride (liquid)	T57.8X1	T57.8X2	T57.8X3	T57.8X4	—	—
vapor	T59.891	T59.892	T59.893	T59.894	—	—
phophorated	T6Ø.ØX1	T6Ø.ØX2	T6Ø.ØX3	T6Ø.ØX4	—	—
sulfate	T57.8X1	T57.8X2	T57.8X3	T57.8X4	—	—
sulfide (gas)	T59.6X1	T59.6X2	T59.6X3	T59.6X4	—	—
arseniurated	T57.ØX1	T57.ØX2	T57.ØX3	T57.ØX4	—	—
sulfurated	T57.8X1	T57.8X2	T57.8X3	T57.8X4	—	—
Hexahydrophenol	T51.8X1	T51.8X2	T51.8X3	T51.8X4	—	—
Hexalen	T51.8X1	T51.8X2	T51.8X3	T51.8X4	—	—
Hexamethonium bromide	T44.2X1	T44.2X2	T44.2X3	T44.2X4	T44.2X5	T44.2X6
Hexamethylene	T52.8X1	T52.8X2	T52.8X3	T52.8X4	—	—
Hexamethylmelamine	T45.1X1	T45.1X2	T45.1X3	T45.1X4	T45.1X5	T45.1X6
Hexamidine	T49.ØX1	T49.ØX2	T49.ØX3	T49.ØX4	T49.ØX5	T49.ØX6
Hexamine (mandelate)	T37.8X1	T37.8X2	T37.8X3	T37.8X4	T37.8X5	T37.8X6
Hexanone, 2-hexanone	T52.4X1	T52.4X2	T52.4X3	T52.4X4	—	—
Hexanuorenium	T48.1X1	T48.1X2	T48.1X3	T48.1X4	T48.1X5	T48.1X6
Hexapropymate	T42.6X1	T42.6X2	T42.6X3	T42.6X4	T42.6X5	T42.6X6
Hexasonium iodide	T44.3X1	T44.3X2	T44.3X3	T44.3X4	T44.3X5	T44.3X6
Hexcarbacholine bromide	T48.1X1	T48.1X2	T48.1X3	T48.1X4	T48.1X5	T48.1X6
Hexemal	T42.3X1	T42.3X2	T42.3X3	T42.3X4	T42.3X5	T42.3X6
Hexestrol	T38.5X1	T38.5X2	T38.5X3	T38.5X4	T38.5X5	T38.5X6
Hexethal (sodium)	T42.3X1	T42.3X2	T42.3X3	T42.3X4	T42.3X5	T42.3X6
Hexetidine	T37.8X1	T37.8X2	T37.8X3	T37.8X4	T37.8X5	T37.8X6
Hexobarbital	T42.3X1	T42.3X2	T42.3X3	T42.3X4	T42.3X5	T42.3X6
rectal	T41.291	T41.292	T41.293	T41.294	T41.295	T41.296
sodium	T41.1X1	T41.1X2	T41.1X3	T41.1X4	T41.1X5	T41.1X6
Hexobendine	T46.3X1	T46.3X2	T46.3X3	T46.3X4	T46.3X5	T46.3X6
Hexocyclium	T44.3X1	T44.3X2	T44.3X3	T44.3X4	T44.3X5	T44.3X6
metilsulfate	T44.3X1	T44.3X2	T44.3X3	T44.3X4	T44.3X5	T44.3X6
Hexoestrol	T38.5X1	T38.5X2	T38.5X3	T38.5X4	T38.5X5	T38.5X6
Hexone	T52.4X1	T52.4X2	T52.4X3	T52.4X4	—	—
Hexoprenaline	T48.6X1	T48.6X2	T48.6X3	T48.6X4	T48.6X5	T48.6X6
Hexylcaine	T41.3X1	T41.3X2	T41.3X3	T41.3X4	T41.3X5	T41.3X6
Hexylresorcinol	T52.2X1	T52.2X2	T52.2X3	T52.2X4	—	—
HGH (human growth hormone)	T38.811	T38.812	T38.813	T38.814	T38.815	T38.816
Hinkle's pills	T47.2X1	T47.2X2	T47.2X3	T47.2X4	T47.2X5	T47.2X6
Histalog	T5Ø.8X1	T5Ø.8X2	T5Ø.8X3	T5Ø.8X4	T5Ø.8X5	T5Ø.8X6
Histamine (phosphate)	T5Ø.8X1	T5Ø.8X2	T5Ø.8X3	T5Ø.8X4	T5Ø.8X5	T5Ø.8X6
Histoplasmin	T5Ø.8X1	T5Ø.8X2	T5Ø.8X3	T5Ø.8X4	T5Ø.8X5	T5Ø.8X6
Holly berries	T62.2X1	T62.2X2	T62.2X3	T62.2X4	—	—
Homatropine	T44.3X1	T44.3X2	T44.3X3	T44.3X4	T44.3X5	T44.3X6
methylbromide	T44.3X1	T44.3X2	T44.3X3	T44.3X4	T44.3X5	T44.3X6
Homochlorcyclizine	T45.ØX1	T45.ØX2	T45.ØX3	T45.ØX4	T45.ØX5	T45.ØX6
Homosalate	T49.3X1	T49.3X2	T49.3X3	T49.3X4	T49.3X5	T49.3X6
Homo-tet	T5Ø.Z11	T5Ø.Z12	T5Ø.Z13	T5Ø.Z14	T5Ø.Z15	T5Ø.Z16

Substance	Poisoning, Accidental (unintentional)	Poisoning, Intentional Self-harm	Poisoning, Assault	Poisoning, Undetermined	Adverse Effect	Under-dosing
Hormone	T38.8Ø1	T38.8Ø2	T38.8Ø3	T38.8Ø4	T38.8Ø5	T38.8Ø6
adrenal cortical steroids	T38.ØX1	T38.ØX2	T38.ØX3	T38.ØX4	T38.ØX5	T38.ØX6
androgenic	T38.7X1	T38.7X2	T38.7X3	T38.7X4	T38.7X5	T38.7X6
anterior pituitary NEC	T38.811	T38.812	T38.813	T38.814	T38.815	T38.816
antidiabetic agents	T38.3X1	T38.3X2	T38.3X3	T38.3X4	T38.3X5	T38.3X6
antidiuretic	T38.891	T38.892	T38.893	T38.894	T38.895	T38.896
cancer therapy	T45.1X1	T45.1X2	T45.1X3	T45.1X4	T45.1X5	T45.1X6
follicle stimulating	T38.811	T38.812	T38.813	T38.814	T38.815	T38.816
gonadotropic	T38.891	T38.892	T38.893	T38.894	T38.895	T38.896
pituitary	T38.811	T38.812	T38.813	T38.814	T38.815	T38.816
growth	T38.811	T38.812	T38.813	T38.814	T38.815	T38.816
luteinizing	T38.811	T38.812	T38.813	T38.814	T38.815	T38.816
ovarian	T38.5X1	T38.5X2	T38.5X3	T38.5X4	T38.5X5	T38.5X6
oxytocic	T48.ØX1	T48.ØX2	T48.ØX3	T48.ØX4	T48.ØX5	T48.ØX6
parathyroid (derivatives)	T5Ø.991	T5Ø.992	T5Ø.993	T5Ø.994	T5Ø.995	T5Ø.996
pituitary (posterior) NEC	T38.891	T38.892	T38.893	T38.894	T38.895	T38.896
anterior	T38.811	T38.812	T38.813	T38.814	T38.815	T38.816
specified, NEC	T38.891	T38.892	T38.893	T38.894	T38.895	T38.896
thyroid	T38.1X1	T38.1X2	T38.1X3	T38.1X4	T38.1X5	T38.1X6
Hornet (sting)	T63.451	T63.452	T63.453	T63.454	—	—
Horse anti-human lymphocytic serum	T5Ø.Z11	T5Ø.Z12	T5Ø.Z13	T5Ø.Z14	T5Ø.Z15	T5Ø.Z16
Horticulture agent NEC	T65.91	T65.92	T65.93	T65.94	—	—
with pesticide	T6Ø.91	T6Ø.92	T6Ø.93	T6Ø.94	—	—
Human						
albumin	T45.8X1	T45.8X2	T45.8X3	T45.8X4	T45.8X5	T45.8X6
growth hormone (HGH)	T38.811	T38.812	T38.813	T38.814	T38.815	T38.816
immune serum	T5Ø.Z11	T5Ø.Z12	T5Ø.Z13	T5Ø.Z14	T5Ø.Z15	T5Ø.Z16
Hyaluronidase	T45.3X1	T45.3X2	T45.3X3	T45.3X4	T45.3X5	T45.3X6
Hyazyme	T45.3X1	T45.3X2	T45.3X3	T45.3X4	T45.3X5	T45.3X6
Hycodan	T4Ø.2X1	T4Ø.2X2	T4Ø.2X3	T4Ø.2X4	T4Ø.2X5	T4Ø.2X6
Hydantoin derivative NEC	T42.ØX1	T42.ØX2	T42.ØX3	T42.ØX4	T42.ØX5	T42.ØX6
Hydeltra	T38.ØX1	T38.ØX2	T38.ØX3	T38.ØX4	T38.ØX5	T38.ØX6
Hydergine	T44.6X1	T44.6X2	T44.6X3	T44.6X4	T44.6X5	T44.6X6
Hydrabamine penicillin	T36.ØX1	T36.ØX2	T36.ØX3	T36.ØX4	T36.ØX5	T36.ØX6
Hydralazine	T46.5X1	T46.5X2	T46.5X3	T46.5X4	T46.5X5	T46.5X6
Hydrargaphen	T49.ØX1	T49.ØX2	T49.ØX3	T49.ØX4	T49.ØX5	T49.ØX6
Hydrargyri aminochloridum	T49.ØX1	T49.ØX2	T49.ØX3	T49.ØX4	T49.ØX5	T49.ØX6
Hydrastine	T48.291	T48.292	T48.293	T48.294	T48.295	T48.296
Hydrazine	T54.1X1	T54.1X2	T54.1X3	T54.1X4	—	—
monoamine oxidase inhibitors	T43.1X1	T43.1X2	T43.1X3	T43.1X4	T43.1X5	T43.1X6
Hydrazoic acid, azides	T54.2X1	T54.2X2	T54.2X3	T54.2X4	—	—
Hydriodic acid	T48.4X1	T48.4X2	T48.4X3	T48.4X4	T48.4X5	T48.4X6
Hydrocarbon gas	T59.891	T59.892	T59.893	T59.894	—	—
incomplete combustion of — *see* Carbon, monoxide, fuel, utility						
liquefied (mobile container)	T59.891	T59.892	T59.893	T59.894	—	—
piped (natural)	T59.891	T59.892	T59.893	T59.894	—	—
Hydrochloric acid (liquid)	T54.2X1	T54.2X2	T54.2X3	T54.2X4	—	—
medicinal (digestant)	T47.5X1	T47.5X2	T47.5X3	T47.5X4	T47.5X5	T47.5X6
vapor	T59.891	T59.892	T59.893	T59.894	—	—
Hydrochlorothiazide	T5Ø.2X1	T5Ø.2X2	T5Ø.2X3	T5Ø.2X4	T5Ø.2X5	T5Ø.2X6
Hydrocodone	T4Ø.2X1	T4Ø.2X2	T4Ø.2X3	T4Ø.2X4	T4Ø.2X5	T4Ø.2X6
Hydrocortisone (derivatives)	T49.ØX1	T49.ØX2	T49.ØX3	T49.ØX4	T49.ØX5	T49.ØX6
aceponate	T49.ØX1	T49.ØX2	T49.ØX3	T49.ØX4	T49.ØX5	T49.ØX6
ENT agent	T49.6X1	T49.6X2	T49.6X3	T49.6X4	T49.6X5	T49.6X6
ophthalmic preparation	T49.5X1	T49.5X2	T49.5X3	T49.5X4	T49.5X5	T49.5X6
topical NEC	T49.ØX1	T49.ØX2	T49.ØX3	T49.ØX4	T49.ØX5	T49.ØX6
Hydrocortone	T38.ØX1	T38.ØX2	T38.ØX3	T38.ØX4	T38.ØX5	T38.ØX6
ENT agent	T49.6X1	T49.6X2	T49.6X3	T49.6X4	T49.6X5	T49.6X6
ophthalmic preparation	T49.5X1	T49.5X2	T49.5X3	T49.5X4	T49.5X5	T49.5X6
topical NEC	T49.ØX1	T49.ØX2	T49.ØX3	T49.ØX4	T49.ØX5	T49.ØX6
Hydrocyanic acid (liquid)	T57.3X1	T57.3X2	T57.3X3	T57.3X4	—	—
gas	T65.ØX1	T65.ØX2	T65.ØX3	T65.ØX4	—	—
Hydroflumethiazide	T5Ø.2X1	T5Ø.2X2	T5Ø.2X3	T5Ø.2X4	T5Ø.2X5	T5Ø.2X6
Hydrofluoric acid (liquid)	T54.2X1	T54.2X2	T54.2X3	T54.2X4	—	—
vapor	T59.891	T59.892	T59.893	T59.894	—	—
Hydrogen	T59.891	T59.892	T59.893	T59.894	—	—
arsenide	T57.ØX1	T57.ØX2	T57.ØX3	T57.ØX4	—	—
arseniureted	T57.ØX1	T57.ØX2	T57.ØX3	T57.ØX4	—	—
chloride	T57.8X1	T57.8X2	T57.8X3	T57.8X4	—	—
cyanide (salts)	T57.3X1	T57.3X2	T57.3X3	T57.3X4	—	—
gas	T57.3X1	T57.3X2	T57.3X3	T57.3X4	—	—
Fluoride	T59.5X1	T59.5X2	T59.5X3	T59.5X4	—	—
vapor	T59.5X1	T59.5X2	T59.5X3	T59.5X4	—	—
peroxide	T49.ØX1	T49.ØX2	T49.ØX3	T49.ØX4	T49.ØX5	T49.ØX6
phosphureted	T57.1X1	T57.1X2	T57.1X3	T57.1X4	—	—
sulfide	T59.6X1	T59.6X2	T59.6X3	T59.6X4	—	—
arseniureted	T57.ØX1	T57.ØX2	T57.ØX3	T57.ØX4	—	—
sulfureted	T59.6X1	T59.6X2	T59.6X3	T59.6X4	—	—

Substance	Poisoning, Accidental (unintentional)	Poisoning, Intentional Self-harm	Poisoning, Assault	Poisoning, Undetermined	Adverse Effect	Under-dosing
Hydromethylpyridine	T46.7X1	T46.7X2	T46.7X3	T46.7X4	T46.7X5	T46.7X6
Hydromorphinol	T40.2X1	T40.2X2	T40.2X3	T40.2X4	—	—
Hydromorphinone	T40.2X1	T40.2X2	T40.2X3	T40.2X4	T40.2X5	T40.2X6
Hydromorphone	T40.2X1	T40.2X2	T40.2X3	T40.2X4	T40.2X5	T40.2X6
Hydromox	T50.2X1	T50.2X2	T50.2X3	T50.2X4	T50.2X5	T50.2X6
Hydrophilic lotion	T49.3X1	T49.3X2	T49.3X3	T49.3X4	T49.3X5	T49.3X6
Hydroquinidine	T46.2X1	T46.2X2	T46.2X3	T46.2X4	T46.2X5	T46.2X6
Hydroquinone	T52.2X1	T52.2X2	T52.2X3	T52.2X4	—	—
vapor	T59.891	T59.892	T59.893	T59.894	—	—
Hydrosulfuric acid (gas)	T59.6X1	T59.6X2	T59.6X3	T59.6X4	—	—
Hydrotalcite	T47.1X1	T47.1X2	T47.1X3	T47.1X4	T47.1X5	T47.1X6
Hydrous wool fat	T49.3X1	T49.3X2	T49.3X3	T49.3X4	T49.3X5	T49.3X6
Hydroxide, caustic	T54.3X1	T54.3X2	T54.3X3	T54.3X4	—	—
Hydroxocobalamin	T45.8X1	T45.8X2	T45.8X3	T45.8X4	T45.8X5	T45.8X6
Hydroxyamphetamine	T49.5X1	T49.5X2	T49.5X3	T49.5X4	T49.5X5	T49.5X6
Hydroxycarbamide	T45.1X1	T45.1X2	T45.1X3	T45.1X4	T45.1X5	T45.1X6
Hydroxychloroquine	T37.8X1	T37.8X2	T37.8X3	T37.8X4	T37.8X5	T37.8X6
Hydroxydihydrocodeinone	T40.2X1	T40.2X2	T40.2X3	T40.2X4	T40.2X5	T40.2X6
Hydroxyestrone	T38.5X1	T38.5X2	T38.5X3	T38.5X4	T38.5X5	T38.5X6
Hydroxyethyl starch	T45.8X1	T45.8X2	T45.8X3	T45.8X4	T45.8X5	T45.8X6
Hydroxymethylpentanone	T52.4X1	T52.4X2	T52.4X3	T52.4X4	—	—
Hydroxyphenamate	T43.591	T43.592	T43.593	T43.594	T43.595	T43.596
Hydroxyphenylbutazone	T39.2X1	T39.2X2	T39.2X3	T39.2X4	T39.2X5	T39.2X6
Hydroxyprogesterone	T38.5X1	T38.5X2	T38.5X3	T38.5X4	T38.5X5	T38.5X6
caproate	T38.5X1	T38.5X2	T38.5X3	T38.5X4	T38.5X5	T38.5X6
Hydroxyquinoline (derivatives) NEC	T37.8X1	T37.8X2	T37.8X3	T37.8X4	T37.8X5	T37.8X6
Hydroxystilbamidine	T37.3X1	T37.3X2	T37.3X3	T37.3X4	T37.3X5	T37.3X6
Hydroxytoluene (nonmedicinal)	T54.0X1	T54.0X2	T54.0X3	T54.0X4	—	—
medicinal	T49.0X1	T49.0X2	T49.0X3	T49.0X4	T49.0X5	T49.0X6
Hydroxyurea	T45.1X1	T45.1X2	T45.1X3	T45.1X4	T45.1X5	T45.1X6
Hydroxyzine	T43.591	T43.592	T43.593	T43.594	T43.595	T43.596
Hyoscine	T44.3X1	T44.3X2	T44.3X3	T44.3X4	T44.3X5	T44.3X6
Hyoscyamine	T44.3X1	T44.3X2	T44.3X3	T44.3X4	T44.3X5	T44.3X6
Hyoscyamus	T44.3X1	T44.3X2	T44.3X3	T44.3X4	T44.3X5	T44.3X6
dry extract	T44.3X1	T44.3X2	T44.3X3	T44.3X4	T44.3X5	T44.3X6
Hypaque	T50.8X1	T50.8X2	T50.8X3	T50.8X4	T50.8X5	T50.8X6
Hypertussis	T50.Z11	T50.Z12	T50.Z13	T50.Z14	T50.Z15	T50.Z16
Hypnotic	T42.71	T42.72	T42.73	T42.74	T42.75	T42.76
anticonvulsant	T42.71	T42.72	T42.73	T42.74	T42.75	T42.76
specified NEC	T42.6X1	T42.6X2	T42.6X3	T42.6X4	T42.6X5	T42.6X6
Hypochlorite	T49.0X1	T49.0X2	T49.0X3	T49.0X4	T49.0X5	T49.0X6
Hypophysis, posterior	T38.891	T38.892	T38.893	T38.894	T38.895	T38.896
Hypotensive NEC	T46.5X1	T46.5X2	T46.5X3	T46.5X4	T46.5X5	T46.5X6
Hypromellose	T49.5X1	T49.5X2	T49.5X3	T49.5X4	T49.5X5	T49.5X6
Ibacitabine	T37.5X1	T37.5X2	T37.5X3	T37.5X4	T37.5X5	T37.5X6
Ibopamine	T44.991	T44.992	T44.993	T44.994	T44.995	T44.996
Ibufenac	T39.311	T39.312	T39.313	T39.314	T39.315	T39.316
Ibuprofen	T39.311	T39.312	T39.313	T39.314	T39.315	T39.316
Ibuproxam	T39.311	T39.312	T39.313	T39.314	T39.315	T39.316
Ibuterol	T48.6X1	T48.6X2	T48.6X3	T48.6X4	T48.6X5	T48.6X6
Ichthammol	T49.0X1	T49.0X2	T49.0X3	T49.0X4	T49.0X5	T49.0X6
Ichthyol	T49.4X1	T49.4X2	T49.4X3	T49.4X4	T49.4X5	T49.4X6
Idarubicin	T45.1X1	T45.1X2	T45.1X3	T45.1X4	T45.1X5	T45.1X6
Idrocilamide	T42.8X1	T42.8X2	T42.8X3	T42.8X4	T42.8X5	T42.8X6
Ifenprodil	T46.7X1	T46.7X2	T46.7X3	T46.7X4	T46.7X5	T46.7X6
Ifosfamide	T45.1X1	T45.1X2	T45.1X3	T45.1X4	T45.1X5	T45.1X6
Iletin	T38.3X1	T38.3X2	T38.3X3	T38.3X4	T38.3X5	T38.3X6
Ilex	T62.2X1	T62.2X2	T62.2X3	T62.2X4	—	—
Illuminating gas (after combustion)	T58.11	T58.12	T58.13	T58.14	—	—
prior to combustion	T59.891	T59.892	T59.893	T59.894	—	—
Ilopan	T45.2X1	T45.2X2	T45.2X3	T45.2X4	T45.2X5	T45.2X6
Iloprost	T46.7X1	T46.7X2	T46.7X3	T46.7X4	T46.7X5	T46.7X6
Ilotycin	T36.3X1	T36.3X2	T36.3X3	T36.3X4	T36.3X5	T36.3X6
ophthalmic preparation	T49.5X1	T49.5X2	T49.5X3	T49.5X4	T49.5X5	T49.5X6
topical NEC	T49.0X1	T49.0X2	T49.0X3	T49.0X4	T49.0X5	T49.0X6
Imidazole-4-carboxamide	T45.1X1	T45.1X2	T45.1X3	T45.1X4	T45.1X5	T45.1X6
Iminostilbene	T42.1X1	T42.1X2	T42.1X3	T42.1X4	T42.1X5	T42.1X6
Imipenem	T36.0X1	T36.0X2	T36.0X3	T36.0X4	T36.0X5	T36.0X6
Imipramine	T43.011	T43.012	T43.013	T43.014	T43.015	T43.016
Immu-G	T50.Z11	T50.Z12	T50.Z13	T50.Z14	T50.Z15	T50.Z16
Immuglobin	T50.Z11	T50.Z12	T50.Z13	T50.Z14	T50.Z15	T50.Z16
Immune						
globulin	T50.Z11	T50.Z12	T50.Z13	T50.Z14	T50.Z15	T50.Z16
serum globulin	T50.Z11	T50.Z12	T50.Z13	T50.Z14	T50.Z15	T50.Z16
Immunoglobin human (intravenous) (normal)	T50.Z11	T50.Z12	T50.Z13	T50.Z14	T50.Z15	T50.Z16
unmodified	T50.Z11	T50.Z12	T50.Z13	T50.Z14	T50.Z15	T50.Z16
Immunosuppressive drug	T45.1X1	T45.1X2	T45.1X3	T45.1X4	T45.1X5	T45.1X6
Immu-tetanus	T50.Z11	T50.Z12	T50.Z13	T50.Z14	T50.Z15	T50.Z16
Indalpine	T43.221	T43.222	T43.223	T43.224	T43.225	T43.226
Indanazoline	T48.5X1	T48.5X2	T48.5X3	T48.5X4	T48.5X5	T48.5X6
Indandione (derivatives)	T45.511	T45.512	T45.513	T45.514	T45.515	T45.516
Indapamide	T46.5X1	T46.5X2	T46.5X3	T46.5X4	T46.5X5	T46.5X6
Indendione (derivatives)	T45.511	T45.512	T45.513	T45.514	T45.515	T45.516
Indenolol	T44.7X1	T44.7X2	T44.7X3	T44.7X4	T44.7X5	T44.7X6
Inderal	T44.7X1	T44.7X2	T44.7X3	T44.7X4	T44.7X5	T44.7X6
Indian						
hemp	T40.7X1	T40.7X2	T40.7X3	T40.7X4	T40.7X5	T40.7X6
tobacco	T62.2X1	T62.2X2	T62.2X3	T62.2X4	—	—
Indigo carmine	T50.8X1	T50.8X2	T50.8X3	T50.8X4	T50.8X5	T50.8X6
Indobufen	T45.521	T45.522	T45.523	T45.524	T45.525	T45.526
Indocin	T39.2X1	T39.2X2	T39.2X3	T39.2X4	T39.2X5	T39.2X6
Indocyanine green	T50.8X1	T50.8X2	T50.8X3	T50.8X4	T50.8X5	T50.8X6
Indometacin	T39.391	T39.392	T39.393	T39.394	T39.395	T39.396
Indomethacin	T39.391	T39.392	T39.393	T39.394	T39.395	T39.396
farnesil	T39.4X1	T39.4X2	T39.4X3	T39.4X4	T39.4X5	T39.4X6
Indoramin	T44.6X1	T44.6X2	T44.6X3	T44.6X4	T44.6X5	T44.6X6
Industrial						
alcohol	T51.0X1	T51.0X2	T51.0X3	T51.0X4	—	—
fumes	T59.891	T59.892	T59.893	T59.894	—	—
solvents (fumes) (vapors)	T52.91	T52.92	T52.93	T52.94	—	—
Influenza vaccine	T50.B91	T50.B92	T50.B93	T50.B94	T50.B95	T50.B96
Ingested substance NEC	T65.91	T65.92	T65.93	T65.94	—	—
INH	T37.1X1	T37.1X2	T37.1X3	T37.1X4	T37.1X5	T37.1X6
Inhalation, gas (noxious) — see Gas						
Inhibitor						
angiotensin-converting enzyme	T46.4X1	T46.4X2	T46.4X3	T46.4X4	T46.4X5	T46.4X6
carbonic anhydrase	T50.2X1	T50.2X2	T50.2X3	T50.2X4	T50.2X5	T50.2X6
fibrinolysis	T45.621	T45.622	T45.623	T45.624	T45.625	T45.626
monoamine oxidase NEC	T43.1X1	T43.1X2	T43.1X3	T43.1X4	T43.1X5	T43.1X6
hydrazine	T43.1X1	T43.1X2	T43.1X3	T43.1X4	T43.1X5	T43.1X6
postsynaptic	T43.8X1	T43.8X2	T43.8X3	T43.8X4	T43.8X5	T43.8X6
prothrombin synthesis	T45.511	T45.512	T45.513	T45.514	T45.515	T45.516
Ink	T65.891	T65.892	T65.893	T65.894	—	—
Inorganic substance NEC	T57.91	T57.92	T57.93	T57.94	—	—
Inosine pranobex	T37.5X1	T37.5X2	T37.5X3	T37.5X4	T37.5X5	T37.5X6
Inositol	T50.991	T50.992	T50.993	T50.994	T50.995	T50.996
nicotinate	T46.7X1	T46.7X2	T46.7X3	T46.7X4	T46.7X5	T46.7X6
Inproquone	T45.1X1	T45.1X2	T45.1X3	T45.1X4	T45.1X5	T45.1X6
Insecticide NEC	T60.91	T60.92	T60.93	T60.94	—	—
carbamate	T60.0X1	T60.0X2	T60.0X3	T60.0X4	—	—
chlorinated	T60.1X1	T60.1X2	T60.1X3	T60.1X4	—	—
mixed	T60.91	T60.92	T60.93	T60.94	—	—
organochlorine	T60.1X1	T60.1X2	T60.1X3	T60.1X4	—	—
organophosphorus	T60.0X1	T60.0X2	T60.0X3	T60.0X4	—	—
Insect (sting), venomous	T63.481	T63.482	T63.483	T63.484		
ant	T63.421	T63.422	T63.423	T63.424		
bee	T63.441	T63.442	T63.443	T63.444		
caterpillar	T63.431	T63.432	T63.433	T63.434		
hornet	T63.451	T63.452	T63.453	T63.454		
wasp	T63.461	T63.462	T63.463	T63.464		
Insular tissue extract	T38.3X1	T38.3X2	T38.3X3	T38.3X4	T38.3X5	T38.3X6
Insulin (amorphous) (globin) (isophane) (Lente) (NPH) (Semilente) (Ultralente)	T38.3X1	T38.3X2	T38.3X3	T38.3X4	T38.3X5	T38.3X6
defalan	T38.3X1	T38.3X2	T38.3X3	T38.3X4	T38.3X5	T38.3X6
human	T38.3X1	T38.3X2	T38.3X3	T38.3X4	T38.3X5	T38.3X6
injection, soluble	T38.3X1	T38.3X2	T38.3X3	T38.3X4	T38.3X5	T38.3X6
biphasic	T38.3X1	T38.3X2	T38.3X3	T38.3X4	T38.3X5	T38.3X6
intermediate acting	T38.3X1	T38.3X2	T38.3X3	T38.3X4	T38.3X5	T38.3X6
protamine zinc	T38.3X1	T38.3X2	T38.3X3	T38.3X4	T38.3X5	T38.3X6
slow acting	T38.3X1	T38.3X2	T38.3X3	T38.3X4	T38.3X5	T38.3X6
zinc						
protamine injection	T38.3X1	T38.3X2	T38.3X3	T38.3X4	T38.3X5	T38.3X6
suspension (amorphous) (crystalline)	T38.3X1	T38.3X2	T38.3X3	T38.3X4	T38.3X5	T38.3X6
Interferon (alpha) (beta) (gamma)	T37.5X1	T37.5X2	T37.5X3	T37.5X4	T37.5X5	T37.5X6
Intestinal motility control drug	T47.6X1	T47.6X2	T47.6X3	T47.6X4	T47.6X5	T47.6X6
biological	T47.8X1	T47.8X2	T47.8X3	T47.8X4	T47.8X5	T47.8X6
Intranarcon	T41.1X1	T41.1X2	T41.1X3	T41.1X4	T41.1X5	T41.1X6
Intravenous						
amino acids	T50.991	T50.992	T50.993	T50.994	T50.995	T50.996
fat suspension	T50.991	T50.992	T50.993	T50.994	T50.995	T50.996
Inulin	T50.8X1	T50.8X2	T50.8X3	T50.8X4	T50.8X5	T50.8X6
Invert sugar	T50.3X1	T50.3X2	T50.3X3	T50.3X4	T50.3X5	T50.3X6
Inza — see Naproxen						
Iobenzamic acid	T50.8X1	T50.8X2	T50.8X3	T50.8X4	T50.8X5	T50.8X6
Iocarmic acid	T50.8X1	T50.8X2	T50.8X3	T50.8X4	T50.8X5	T50.8X6
Iocetamic acid	T50.8X1	T50.8X2	T50.8X3	T50.8X4	T50.8X5	T50.8X6

Table of Drugs and Chemicals

Hydromethylpyridine — Iocetamic acid

Substance	Poisoning, Accidental (unintentional)	Poisoning, Intentional Self-harm	Poisoning, Assault	Poisoning, Undetermined	Adverse Effect	Under-dosing
Iodamide	T5Ø.8X1	T5Ø.8X2	T5Ø.8X3	T5Ø.8X4	T5Ø.8X5	T5Ø.8X6
Iodide NEC — *see also* Iodine	T49.ØX1	T49.ØX2	T49.ØX3	T49.ØX4	T49.ØX5	T49.ØX6
mercury (ointment)	T49.ØX1	T49.ØX2	T49.ØX3	T49.ØX4	T49.ØX5	T49.ØX6
methylate	T49.ØX1	T49.ØX2	T49.ØX3	T49.ØX4	T49.ØX5	T49.ØX6
potassium (expectorant) NEC	T48.4X1	T48.4X2	T48.4X3	T48.4X4	T48.4X5	T48.4X6
Iodinated						
contrast medium	T5Ø.8X1	T5Ø.8X2	T5Ø.8X3	T5Ø.8X4	T5Ø.8X5	T5Ø.8X6
glycerol	T48.4X1	T48.4X2	T48.4X3	T48.4X4	T48.4X5	T48.4X6
human serum albumin (131I)	T5Ø.8X1	T5Ø.8X2	T5Ø.8X3	T5Ø.8X4	T5Ø.8X5	T5Ø.8X6
Iodine (antiseptic, external) (tincture) **NEC**	T49.ØX1	T49.ØX2	T49.ØX3	T49.ØX4	T49.ØX5	T49.ØX6
125 — *see also* Radiation sickness, and Exposure to radioactivce isotopes	T5Ø.8X1	T5Ø.8X2	T5Ø.8X3	T5Ø.8X4	T5Ø.8X5	T5Ø.8X6
therapeutic	T5Ø.991	T5Ø.992	T5Ø.993	T5Ø.994	T5Ø.995	T5Ø.996
131 — *see also* Radiation sickness, and Exposure to radioactivce isotopes	T5Ø.8X1	T5Ø.8X2	T5Ø.8X3	T5Ø.8X4	T5Ø.8X5	T5Ø.8X6
therapeutic	T38.2X1	T38.2X2	T38.2X3	T38.2X4	T38.2X5	T38.2X6
diagnostic	T5Ø.8X1	T5Ø.8X2	T5Ø.8X3	T5Ø.8X4	T5Ø.8X5	T5Ø.8X6
for thyroid conditions (antithyroid)	T38.2X1	T38.2X2	T38.2X3	T38.2X4	T38.2X5	T38.2X6
solution	T49.ØX1	T49.ØX2	T49.ØX3	T49.ØX4	T49.ØX5	T49.ØX6
vapor	T59.891	T59.892	T59.893	T59.894	—	—
Iodipamide	T5Ø.8X1	T5Ø.8X2	T5Ø.8X3	T5Ø.8X4	T5Ø.8X5	T5Ø.8X6
Iodized (poppy seed) oil	T5Ø.8X1	T5Ø.8X2	T5Ø.8X3	T5Ø.8X4	T5Ø.8X5	T5Ø.8X6
Iodobismitol	T37.8X1	T37.8X2	T37.8X3	T37.8X4	T37.8X5	T37.8X6
Iodochlorhydroxyquin	T37.8X1	T37.8X2	T37.8X3	T37.8X4	T37.8X5	T37.8X6
topical	T49.ØX1	T49.ØX2	T49.ØX3	T49.ØX4	T49.ØX5	T49.ØX6
Iodochlorhydroxyquinoline	T37.8X1	T37.8X2	T37.8X3	T37.8X4	T37.8X5	T37.8X6
Iodocholesterol (131I)	T5Ø.8X1	T5Ø.8X2	T5Ø.8X3	T5Ø.8X4	T5Ø.8X5	T5Ø.8X6
Iodoform	T49.ØX1	T49.ØX2	T49.ØX3	T49.ØX4	T49.ØX5	T49.ØX6
Iodohippuric acid	T5Ø.8X1	T5Ø.8X2	T5Ø.8X3	T5Ø.8X4	T5Ø.8X5	T5Ø.8X6
Iodopanoic acid	T5Ø.8X1	T5Ø.8X2	T5Ø.8X3	T5Ø.8X4	T5Ø.8X5	T5Ø.8X6
Iodophthalein (sodium)	T5Ø.8X1	T5Ø.8X2	T5Ø.8X3	T5Ø.8X4	T5Ø.8X5	T5Ø.8X6
Iodopyracet	T5Ø.8X1	T5Ø.8X2	T5Ø.8X3	T5Ø.8X4	T5Ø.8X5	T5Ø.8X6
Iodoquinol	T37.8X1	T37.8X2	T37.8X3	T37.8X4	T37.8X5	T37.8X6
Iodoxamic acid	T5Ø.8X1	T5Ø.8X2	T5Ø.8X3	T5Ø.8X4	T5Ø.8X5	T5Ø.8X6
Iofendylate	T5Ø.8X1	T5Ø.8X2	T5Ø.8X3	T5Ø.8X4	T5Ø.8X5	T5Ø.8X6
Ioglycamic acid	T5Ø.8X1	T5Ø.8X2	T5Ø.8X3	T5Ø.8X4	T5Ø.8X5	T5Ø.8X6
Iohexol	T5Ø.8X1	T5Ø.8X2	T5Ø.8X3	T5Ø.8X4	T5Ø.8X5	T5Ø.8X6
Ion exchange resin						
anion	T47.8X1	T47.8X2	T47.8X3	T47.8X4	T47.8X5	T47.8X6
cation	T5Ø.3X1	T5Ø.3X2	T5Ø.3X3	T5Ø.3X4	T5Ø.3X5	T5Ø.3X6
cholestyramine	T46.6X1	T46.6X2	T46.6X3	T46.6X4	T46.6X5	T46.6X6
intestinal	T47.8X1	T47.8X2	T47.8X3	T47.8X4	T47.8X5	T47.8X6
Iopamidol	T5Ø.8X1	T5Ø.8X2	T5Ø.8X3	T5Ø.8X4	T5Ø.8X5	T5Ø.8X6
Iopanoic acid	T5Ø.8X1	T5Ø.8X2	T5Ø.8X3	T5Ø.8X4	T5Ø.8X5	T5Ø.8X6
Iophenoic acid	T5Ø.8X1	T5Ø.8X2	T5Ø.8X3	T5Ø.8X4	T5Ø.8X5	T5Ø.8X6
Iopodate, sodium	T5Ø.8X1	T5Ø.8X2	T5Ø.8X3	T5Ø.8X4	T5Ø.8X5	T5Ø.8X6
Iopodic acid	T5Ø.8X1	T5Ø.8X2	T5Ø.8X3	T5Ø.8X4	T5Ø.8X5	T5Ø.8X6
Iopromide	T5Ø.8X1	T5Ø.8X2	T5Ø.8X3	T5Ø.8X4	T5Ø.8X5	T5Ø.8X6
Iopydol	T5Ø.8X1	T5Ø.8X2	T5Ø.8X3	T5Ø.8X4	T5Ø.8X5	T5Ø.8X6
Iotalamic acid	T5Ø.8X1	T5Ø.8X2	T5Ø.8X3	T5Ø.8X4	T5Ø.8X5	T5Ø.8X6
Iothalamate	T5Ø.8X1	T5Ø.8X2	T5Ø.8X3	T5Ø.8X4	T5Ø.8X5	T5Ø.8X6
Iothiouracil	T38.2X1	T38.2X2	T38.2X3	T38.2X4	T38.2X5	T38.2X6
Iotrol	T5Ø.8X1	T5Ø.8X2	T5Ø.8X3	T5Ø.8X4	T5Ø.8X5	T5Ø.8X6
Iotrolan	T5Ø.8X1	T5Ø.8X2	T5Ø.8X3	T5Ø.8X4	T5Ø.8X5	T5Ø.8X6
Iotroxate	T5Ø.8X1	T5Ø.8X2	T5Ø.8X3	T5Ø.8X4	T5Ø.8X5	T5Ø.8X6
Iotroxic acid	T5Ø.8X1	T5Ø.8X2	T5Ø.8X3	T5Ø.8X4	T5Ø.8X5	T5Ø.8X6
Ioversol	T5Ø.8X1	T5Ø.8X2	T5Ø.8X3	T5Ø.8X4	T5Ø.8X5	T5Ø.8X6
Ioxaglate	T5Ø.8X1	T5Ø.8X2	T5Ø.8X3	T5Ø.8X4	T5Ø.8X5	T5Ø.8X6
Ioxaglic acid	T5Ø.8X1	T5Ø.8X2	T5Ø.8X3	T5Ø.8X4	T5Ø.8X5	T5Ø.8X6
Ioxitalamic acid	T5Ø.8X1	T5Ø.8X2	T5Ø.8X3	T5Ø.8X4	T5Ø.8X5	T5Ø.8X6
Ipecac	T47.7X1	T47.7X2	T47.7X3	T47.7X4	T47.7X5	T47.7X6
Ipecacuanha	T48.4X1	T48.4X2	T48.4X3	T48.4X4	T48.4X5	T48.4X6
Ipodate, calcium	T5Ø.8X1	T5Ø.8X2	T5Ø.8X3	T5Ø.8X4	T5Ø.8X5	T5Ø.8X6
Ipral	T42.3X1	T42.3X2	T42.3X3	T42.3X4	T42.3X5	T42.3X6
Ipratropium (bromide)	T48.6X1	T48.6X2	T48.6X3	T48.6X4	T48.6X5	T48.6X6
Ipriflavone	T46.3X1	T46.3X2	T46.3X3	T46.3X4	T46.3X5	T46.3X6
Iprindole	T43.Ø11	T43.Ø12	T43.Ø13	T43.Ø14	T43.Ø15	T43.Ø16
Iproclozide	T43.1X1	T43.1X2	T43.1X3	T43.1X4	T43.1X5	T43.1X6
Iprofenin	T5Ø.8X1	T5Ø.8X2	T5Ø.8X3	T5Ø.8X4	T5Ø.8X5	T5Ø.8X6
Iproheptine	T49.2X1	T49.2X2	T49.2X3	T49.2X4	T49.2X5	T49.2X6
Iproniazid	T43.1X1	T43.1X2	T43.1X3	T43.1X4	T43.1X5	T43.1X6
Iproplatin	T45.1X1	T45.1X2	T45.1X3	T45.1X4	T45.1X5	T45.1X6
Iproveratril	T46.1X1	T46.1X2	T46.1X3	T46.1X4	T46.1X5	T46.1X6
Iron (compounds) (medicinal) **NEC**	T45.4X1	T45.4X2	T45.4X3	T45.4X4	T45.4X5	T45.4X6
ammonium	T45.4X1	T45.4X2	T45.4X3	T45.4X4	T45.4X5	T45.4X6
dextran injection	T45.4X1	T45.4X2	T45.4X3	T45.4X4	T45.4X5	T45.4X6

Substance	Poisoning, Accidental (unintentional)	Poisoning, Intentional Self-harm	Poisoning, Assault	Poisoning, Undetermined	Adverse Effect	Under-dosing
Iron (compounds) (medicinal) **NEC** — *continued*						
nonmedicinal	T56.891	T56.892	T56.893	T56.894	—	—
salts	T45.4X1	T45.4X2	T45.4X3	T45.4X4	T45.4X5	T45.4X6
sorbitex	T45.4X1	T45.4X2	T45.4X3	T45.4X4	T45.4X5	T45.4X6
sorbitol citric acid complex	T45.4X1	T45.4X2	T45.4X3	T45.4X4	T45.4X5	T45.4X6
Irrigating fluid (vaginal)	T49.8X1	T49.8X2	T49.8X3	T49.8X4	T49.8X5	T49.8X6
eye	T49.5X1	T49.5X2	T49.5X3	T49.5X4	T49.5X5	T49.5X6
Isepamicin	T36.5X1	T36.5X2	T36.5X3	T36.5X4	T36.5X5	T36.5X6
Isoaminile (citrate)	T48.3X1	T48.3X2	T48.3X3	T48.3X4	T48.3X5	T48.3X6
Isoamyl nitrite	T46.3X1	T46.3X2	T46.3X3	T46.3X4	T46.3X5	T46.3X6
Isobenzan	T6Ø.1X1	T6Ø.1X2	T6Ø.1X3	T6Ø.1X4	—	—
Isobutyl acetate	T52.8X1	T52.8X2	T52.8X3	T52.8X4	—	—
Isocarboxazid	T43.1X1	T43.1X2	T43.1X3	T43.1X4	T43.1X5	T43.1X6
Isoconazole	T49.ØX1	T49.ØX2	T49.ØX3	T49.ØX4	T49.ØX5	T49.ØX6
Isocyanate	T65.ØX1	T65.ØX2	T65.ØX3	T65.ØX4	—	—
Isoephedrine	T44.991	T44.992	T44.993	T44.994	T44.995	T44.996
Isoetarine	T48.6X1	T48.6X2	T48.6X3	T48.6X4	T48.6X5	T48.6X6
Isoethadione	T42.2X1	T42.2X2	T42.2X3	T42.2X4	T42.2X5	T42.2X6
Isoetharine	T44.5X1	T44.5X2	T44.5X3	T44.5X4	T44.5X5	T44.5X6
Isoflurane	T41.ØX1	T41.ØX2	T41.ØX3	T41.ØX4	T41.ØX5	T41.ØX6
Isoflurophate	T44.ØX1	T44.ØX2	T44.ØX3	T44.ØX4	T44.ØX5	T44.ØX6
Isomaltose, ferric complex	T45.4X1	T45.4X2	T45.4X3	T45.4X4	T45.4X5	T45.4X6
Isometheptene	T44.3X1	T44.3X2	T44.3X3	T44.3X4	T44.3X5	T44.3X6
Isoniazid	T37.1X1	T37.1X2	T37.1X3	T37.1X4	T37.1X5	T37.1X6
with						
rifampicin	T36.6X1	T36.6X2	T36.6X3	T36.6X4	T36.6X5	T36.6X6
thioacetazone	T37.1X1	T37.1X2	T37.1X3	T37.1X4	T37.1X5	T37.1X6
Isonicotinic acid hydrazide	T37.1X1	T37.1X2	T37.1X3	T37.1X4	T37.1X5	T37.1X6
Isonipecaine	T4Ø.4X1	T4Ø.4X2	T4Ø.4X3	T4Ø.4X4	T4Ø.4X5	T4Ø.4X6
Isopentaquine	T37.2X1	T37.2X2	T37.2X3	T37.2X4	T37.2X5	T37.2X6
Isophane insulin	T38.3X1	T38.3X2	T38.3X3	T38.3X4	T38.3X5	T38.3X6
Isophorone	T65.891	T65.892	T65.893	T65.894	—	—
Isophosphamide	T45.1X1	T45.1X2	T45.1X3	T45.1X4	T45.1X5	T45.1X6
Isopregnenone	T38.5X1	T38.5X2	T38.5X3	T38.5X4	T38.5X5	T38.5X6
Isoprenaline	T48.6X1	T48.6X2	T48.6X3	T48.6X4	T48.6X5	T48.6X6
Isopromethazine	T43.3X1	T43.3X2	T43.3X3	T43.3X4	T43.3X5	T43.3X6
Isopropamide	T44.3X1	T44.3X2	T44.3X3	T44.3X4	T44.3X5	T44.3X6
iodide	T44.3X1	T44.3X2	T44.3X3	T44.3X4	T44.3X5	T44.3X6
Isopropanol	T51.2X1	T51.2X2	T51.2X3	T51.2X4	—	—
Isopropyl						
acetate	T52.8X1	T52.8X2	T52.8X3	T52.8X4	—	—
alcohol	T51.2X1	T51.2X2	T51.2X3	T51.2X4	—	—
medicinal	T49.4X1	T49.4X2	T49.4X3	T49.4X4	T49.4X5	T49.4X6
ether	T52.8X1	T52.8X2	T52.8X3	T52.8X4	—	—
Isopropylaminophenazone	T39.2X1	T39.2X2	T39.2X3	T39.2X4	T39.2X5	T39.2X6
Isoproterenol	T48.6X1	T48.6X2	T48.6X3	T48.6X4	T48.6X5	T48.6X6
Isosorbide dinitrate	T46.3X1	T46.3X2	T46.3X3	T46.3X4	T46.3X5	T46.3X6
Isothipendyl	T45.ØX1	T45.ØX2	T45.ØX3	T45.ØX4	T45.ØX5	T45.ØX6
Isotretinoin	T5Ø.991	T5Ø.992	T5Ø.993	T5Ø.994	T5Ø.995	T5Ø.996
Isoxazolyl penicillin	T36.ØX1	T36.ØX2	T36.ØX3	T36.ØX4	T36.ØX5	T36.ØX6
Isoxicam	T39.391	T39.392	T39.393	T39.394	T39.395	T39.396
Isoxsuprine	T46.7X1	T46.7X2	T46.7X3	T46.7X4	T46.7X5	T46.7X6
Ispagula	T47.4X1	T47.4X2	T47.4X3	T47.4X4	T47.4X5	T47.4X6
husk	T47.4X1	T47.4X2	T47.4X3	T47.4X4	T47.4X5	T47.4X6
Isradipine	T46.1X1	T46.1X2	T46.1X3	T46.1X4	T46.1X5	T46.1X6
I-thyroxine sodium	T38.1X1	T38.1X2	T38.1X3	T38.1X4	T38.1X5	T38.1X6
Itraconazole	T37.8X1	T37.8X2	T37.8X3	T37.8X4	T37.8X5	T37.8X6
Itramin tosilate	T46.3X1	T46.3X2	T46.3X3	T46.3X4	T46.3X5	T46.3X6
Ivermectin	T37.4X1	T37.4X2	T37.4X3	T37.4X4	T37.4X5	T37.4X6
Izoniazid	T37.1X1	T37.1X2	T37.1X3	T37.1X4	T37.1X5	T37.1X6
with thioacetazone	T37.1X1	T37.1X2	T37.1X3	T37.1X4	T37.1X5	T37.1X6
Jalap	T47.2X1	T47.2X2	T47.2X3	T47.2X4	T47.2X5	T47.2X6
Jamaica						
dogwood (bark)	T39.8X1	T39.8X2	T39.8X3	T39.8X4	T39.8X5	T39.8X6
ginger	T65.891	T65.892	T65.893	T65.894	—	—
root	T62.2X1	T62.2X2	T62.2X3	T62.2X4	—	—
Jatropha	T62.2X1	T62.2X2	T62.2X3	T62.2X4	—	—
curcas	T62.2X1	T62.2X2	T62.2X3	T62.2X4	—	—
Jectofer	T45.4X1	T45.4X2	T45.4X3	T45.4X4	T45.4X5	T45.4X6
Jellyfish (sting)	T63.621	T63.622	T63.623	T63.624	—	—
Jequirity (bean)	T62.2X1	T62.2X2	T62.2X3	T62.2X4	—	—
Jimson weed (stramonium)	T62.2X1	T62.2X2	T62.2X3	T62.2X4	—	—
seeds	T62.2X1	T62.2X2	T62.2X3	T62.2X4	—	—
Josamycin	T36.3X1	T36.3X2	T36.3X3	T36.3X4	T36.3X5	T36.3X6
Juniper tar	T49.1X1	T49.1X2	T49.1X3	T49.1X4	T49.1X5	T49.1X6
Kallidinogenase	T46.7X1	T46.7X2	T46.7X3	T46.7X4	T46.7X5	T46.7X6
Kallikrein	T46.7X1	T46.7X2	T46.7X3	T46.7X4	T46.7X5	T46.7X6
Kanamycin	T36.5X1	T36.5X2	T36.5X3	T36.5X4	T36.5X5	T36.5X6
Kantrex	T36.5X1	T36.5X2	T36.5X3	T36.5X4	T36.5X5	T36.5X6
Kaolin	T47.6X1	T47.6X2	T47.6X3	T47.6X4	T47.6X5	T47.6X6
light	T47.6X1	T47.6X2	T47.6X3	T47.6X4	T47.6X5	T47.6X6
Karaya (gum)	T47.4X1	T47.4X2	T47.4X3	T47.4X4	T47.4X5	T47.4X6

Substance	Poisoning, Accidental (unintentional)	Poisoning, Intentional Self-harm	Poisoning, Assault	Poisoning, Undetermined	Adverse Effect	Under-dosing
Kebuzone	T39.2X1	T39.2X2	T39.2X3	T39.2X4	T39.2X5	T39.2X6
Kelevan	T60.1X1	T60.1X2	T60.1X3	T60.1X4	—	—
Kemithal	T41.1X1	T41.1X2	T41.1X3	T41.1X4	T41.1X5	T41.1X6
Kenacort	T38.0X1	T38.0X2	T38.0X3	T38.0X4	T38.0X5	T38.0X6
Keratolytic drug NEC	T49.4X1	T49.4X2	T49.4X3	T49.4X4	T49.4X5	T49.4X6
anthracene	T49.4X1	T49.4X2	T49.4X3	T49.4X4	T49.4X5	T49.4X6
Keratoplastic NEC	T49.4X1	T49.4X2	T49.4X3	T49.4X4	T49.4X5	T49.4X6
Kerosene, kerosine (fuel) (solvent) NEC	T52.0X1	T52.0X2	T52.0X3	T52.0X4	—	—
insecticide	T52.0X1	T52.0X2	T52.0X3	T52.0X4	—	—
vapor	T52.0X1	T52.0X2	T52.0X3	T52.0X4	—	—
Ketamine	T41.291	T41.292	T41.293	T41.294	T41.295	T41.296
Ketazolam	T42.4X1	T42.4X2	T42.4X3	T42.4X4	T42.4X5	T42.4X6
Ketazon	T39.2X1	T39.2X2	T39.2X3	T39.2X4	T39.2X5	T39.2X6
Ketobemidone	T40.4X1	T40.4X2	T40.4X3	T40.4X4	—	—
Ketoconazole	T49.0X1	T49.0X2	T49.0X3	T49.0X4	T49.0X5	T49.0X6
Ketols	T52.4X1	T52.4X2	T52.4X3	T52.4X4	—	—
Ketone oils	T52.4X1	T52.4X2	T52.4X3	T52.4X4	—	—
Ketoprofen	T39.311	T39.312	T39.313	T39.314	T39.315	T39.316
Ketorolac	T39.8X1	T39.8X2	T39.8X3	T39.8X4	T39.8X5	T39.8X6
Ketotifen	T45.0X1	T45.0X2	T45.0X3	T45.0X4	T45.0X5	T45.0X6
Khat	T43.691	T43.692	T43.693	T43.694	—	—
Khellin	T46.3X1	T46.3X2	T46.3X3	T46.3X4	T46.3X5	T46.3X6
Khelloside	T46.3X1	T46.3X2	T46.3X3	T46.3X4	T46.3X5	T46.3X6
Kiln gas or vapor (carbon monoxide)	T58.8X1	T58.8X2	T58.8X3	T58.8X4	—	—
Kitasamycin	T36.3X1	T36.3X2	T36.3X3	T36.3X4	T36.3X5	T36.3X6
Konsyl	T47.4X1	T47.4X2	T47.4X3	T47.4X4	T47.4X5	T47.4X6
Kosam seed	T62.2X1	T62.2X2	T62.2X3	T62.2X4	—	—
Krait (venom)	T63.091	T63.092	T63.093	T63.094	—	—
Kwell (insecticide)	T60.1X1	T60.1X2	T60.1X3	T60.1X4	—	—
anti-infective (topical)	T49.0X1	T49.0X2	T49.0X3	T49.0X4	T49.0X5	T49.0X6
Labetalol	T44.8X1	T44.8X2	T44.8X3	T44.8X4	T44.8X5	T44.8X6
Laburnum (seeds)	T62.2X1	T62.2X2	T62.2X3	T62.2X4	—	—
leaves	T62.2X1	T62.2X2	T62.2X3	T62.2X4	—	—
Lachesine	T49.5X1	T49.5X2	T49.5X3	T49.5X4	T49.5X5	T49.5X6
Lacidipine	T46.5X1	T46.5X2	T46.5X3	T46.5X4	T46.5X5	T46.5X6
Lacquer	T65.6X1	T65.6X2	T65.6X3	T65.6X4	—	—
Lacrimogenic gas	T59.3X1	T59.3X2	T59.3X3	T59.3X4	—	—
Lactated potassic saline	T50.3X1	T50.3X2	T50.3X3	T50.3X4	T50.3X5	T50.3X6
Lactic acid	T49.8X1	T49.8X2	T49.8X3	T49.8X4	T49.8X5	T49.8X6
Lactobacillus						
acidophilus	T47.6X1	T47.6X2	T47.6X3	T47.6X4	T47.6X5	T47.6X6
compound	T47.6X1	T47.6X2	T47.6X3	T47.6X4	T47.6X5	T47.6X6
bifidus, lyophilized	T47.6X1	T47.6X2	T47.6X3	T47.6X4	T47.6X5	T47.6X6
bulgaricus	T47.6X1	T47.6X2	T47.6X3	T47.6X4	T47.6X5	T47.6X6
sporogenes	T47.6X1	T47.6X2	T47.6X3	T47.6X4	T47.6X5	T47.6X6
Lactoflavin	T45.2X1	T45.2X2	T45.2X3	T45.2X4	T45.2X5	T45.2X6
Lactose (as excipient)	T50.901	T50.902	T50.903	T50.904	T50.905	T50.906
Lactuca (virosa) (extract)	T42.6X1	T42.6X2	T42.6X3	T42.6X4	T42.6X5	T42.6X6
Lactucarium	T42.6X1	T42.6X2	T42.6X3	T42.6X4	T42.6X5	T42.6X6
Lactulose	T47.3X1	T47.3X2	T47.3X3	T47.3X4	T47.3X5	T47.3X6
Laevo — see Levo-						
Lanatosides	T46.0X1	T46.0X2	T46.0X3	T46.0X4	T46.0X5	T46.0X6
Lanolin	T49.3X1	T49.3X2	T49.3X3	T49.3X4	T49.3X5	T49.3X6
Largactil	T43.3X1	T43.3X2	T43.3X3	T43.3X4	T43.3X5	T43.3X6
Larkspur	T62.2X1	T62.2X2	T62.2X3	T62.2X4	—	—
Laroxyl	T43.011	T43.012	T43.013	T43.014	T43.015	T43.016
Lasix	T50.1X1	T50.1X2	T50.1X3	T50.1X4	T50.1X5	T50.1X6
Lassar's paste	T49.4X1	T49.4X2	T49.4X3	T49.4X4	T49.4X5	T49.4X6
Latamoxef	T36.1X1	T36.1X2	T36.1X3	T36.1X4	T36.1X5	T36.1X6
Latex	T65.811	T65.812	T65.813	T65.814	—	—
Lathyrus (seed)	T62.2X1	T62.2X2	T62.2X3	T62.2X4	—	—
Laudanum	T40.0X1	T40.0X2	T40.0X3	T40.0X4	T40.0X5	T40.0X6
Laudexium	T48.1X1	T48.1X2	T48.1X3	T48.1X4	T48.1X5	T48.1X6
Laughing gas	T41.0X1	T41.0X2	T41.0X3	T41.0X4	T41.0X5	T41.0X6
Laurel, black or cherry	T62.2X1	T62.2X2	T62.2X3	T62.2X4	—	—
Laurolinium	T49.0X1	T49.0X2	T49.0X3	T49.0X4	T49.0X5	T49.0X6
Lauryl sulfoacetate	T49.2X1	T49.2X2	T49.2X3	T49.2X4	T49.2X5	T49.2X6
Laxative NEC	T47.4X1	T47.4X2	T47.4X3	T47.4X4	T47.4X5	T47.4X6
osmotic	T47.3X1	T47.3X2	T47.3X3	T47.3X4	T47.3X5	T47.3X6
saline	T47.3X1	T47.3X2	T47.3X3	T47.3X4	T47.3X5	T47.3X6
stimulant	T47.2X1	T47.2X2	T47.2X3	T47.2X4	T47.2X5	T47.2X6
L-dopa	T42.8X1	T42.8X2	T42.8X3	T42.8X4	T42.8X5	T42.8X6
Lead (dust) (fumes) (vapor) NEC	T56.0X1	T56.0X2	T56.0X3	T56.0X4	—	—
acetate	T49.2X1	T49.2X2	T49.2X3	T49.2X4	T49.2X5	T49.2X6
alkyl (fuel additive)	T56.0X1	T56.0X2	T56.0X3	T56.0X4	—	—
anti-infectives	T37.8X1	T37.8X2	T37.8X3	T37.8X4	T37.8X5	T37.8X6
antiknock compound (tetraethyl)	T56.0X1	T56.0X2	T56.0X3	T56.0X4	—	—

Substance	Poisoning, Accidental (unintentional)	Poisoning, Intentional Self-harm	Poisoning, Assault	Poisoning, Undetermined	Adverse Effect	Under-dosing
Lead (dust) (fumes) (vapor) NEC — continued						
arsenate, arsenite (dust)(herbicide) (insecticide) (vapor)	T57.0X1	T57.0X2	T57.0X3	T57.0X4	—	—
carbonate	T56.0X1	T56.0X2	T56.0X3	T56.0X4	—	—
paint	T56.0X1	T56.0X2	T56.0X3	T56.0X4	—	—
chromate	T56.0X1	T56.0X2	T56.0X3	T56.0X4	—	—
paint	T56.0X1	T56.0X2	T56.0X3	T56.0X4	—	—
dioxide	T56.0X1	T56.0X2	T56.0X3	T56.0X4	—	—
inorganic	T56.0X1	T56.0X2	T56.0X3	T56.0X4	—	—
iodide	T56.0X1	T56.0X2	T56.0X3	T56.0X4	—	—
pigment (paint)	T56.0X1	T56.0X2	T56.0X3	T56.0X4	—	—
monoxide (dust)	T56.0X1	T56.0X2	T56.0X3	T56.0X4	—	—
paint	T56.0X1	T56.0X2	T56.0X3	T56.0X4	—	—
organic	T56.0X1	T56.0X2	T56.0X3	T56.0X4	—	—
oxide	T56.0X1	T56.0X2	T56.0X3	T56.0X4	—	—
paint	T56.0X1	T56.0X2	T56.0X3	T56.0X4	—	—
paint	T56.0X1	T56.0X2	T56.0X3	T56.0X4	—	—
salts	T56.0X1	T56.0X2	T56.0X3	T56.0X4	—	—
specified compound NEC	T56.0X1	T56.0X2	T56.0X3	T56.0X4	—	—
tetra-ethyl	T56.0X1	T56.0X2	T56.0X3	T56.0X4	—	—
Lebanese red	T40.7X1	T40.7X2	T40.7X3	T40.7X4	T40.7X5	T40.7X6
Lefetamine	T39.8X1	T39.8X2	T39.8X3	T39.8X4	T39.8X5	T39.8X6
Lenperone	T43.4X1	T43.4X2	T43.4X3	T43.4X4	T43.4X5	T43.4X6
Lente lietin (insulin)	T38.3X1	T38.3X2	T38.3X3	T38.3X4	T38.3X5	T38.3X6
Leptazol	T50.7X1	T50.7X2	T50.7X3	T50.7X4	T50.7X5	T50.7X6
Leptophos	T60.0X1	T60.0X2	T60.0X3	T60.0X4	—	—
Leritine	T40.2X1	T40.2X2	T40.2X3	T40.2X4	T40.2X5	T40.2X6
Letosteine	T48.4X1	T48.4X2	T48.4X3	T48.4X4	T48.4X5	T48.4X6
Letter	T38.1X1	T38.1X2	T38.1X3	T38.1X4	T38.1X5	T38.1X6
Lettuce opium	T42.6X1	T42.6X2	T42.6X3	T42.6X4	T42.6X5	T42.6X6
Leucinocaine	T41.3X1	T41.3X2	T41.3X3	T41.3X4	T41.3X5	T41.3X6
Leucocianidol	T46.991	T46.992	T46.993	T46.994	T46.995	T46.996
Leucovorin (factor)	T45.8X1	T45.8X2	T45.8X3	T45.8X4	T45.8X5	T45.8X6
Leukeran	T45.1X1	T45.1X2	T45.1X3	T45.1X4	T45.1X5	T45.1X6
Leuprolide	T38.891	T38.892	T38.893	T38.894	T38.895	T38.896
Levalbuterol	T48.6X1	T48.6X2	T48.6X3	T48.6X4	T48.6X5	T48.6X6
Levallorphan	T50.7X1	T50.7X2	T50.7X3	T50.7X4	T50.7X5	T50.7X6
Levamisole	T37.4X1	T37.4X2	T37.4X3	T37.4X4	T37.4X5	T37.4X6
Levanil	T42.6X1	T42.6X2	T42.6X3	T42.6X4	T42.6X5	T42.6X6
Levarterenol	T44.4X1	T44.4X2	T44.4X3	T44.4X4	T44.4X5	T44.4X6
Levdropropizine	T48.3X1	T48.3X2	T48.3X3	T48.3X4	T48.3X5	T48.3X6
Levobunolol	T49.5X1	T49.5X2	T49.5X3	T49.5X4	T49.5X5	T49.5X6
Levocabastine (hydrochloride)	T45.0X1	T45.0X2	T45.0X3	T45.0X4	T45.0X5	T45.0X6
Levocarnitine	T50.991	T50.992	T50.993	T50.994	T50.995	T50.996
Levodopa	T42.8X1	T42.8X2	T42.8X3	T42.8X4	T42.8X5	T42.8X6
with carbidopa	T42.8X1	T42.8X2	T42.8X3	T42.8X4	T42.8X5	T42.8X6
Levo-dromoran	T40.2X1	T40.2X2	T40.2X3	T40.2X4	T40.2X5	T40.2X6
Levoglutamide	T50.991	T50.992	T50.993	T50.994	T50.995	T50.996
Levoid	T38.1X1	T38.1X2	T38.1X3	T38.1X4	T38.1X5	T38.1X6
Levo-isomethadone	T40.3X1	T40.3X2	T40.3X3	T40.3X4	T40.3X5	T40.3X6
Levomepromazine	T43.3X1	T43.3X2	T43.3X3	T43.3X4	T43.3X5	T43.3X6
Levonordefrin	T49.6X1	T49.6X2	T49.6X3	T49.6X4	T49.6X5	T49.6X6
Levonorgestrel	T38.4X1	T38.4X2	T38.4X3	T38.4X4	T38.4X5	T38.4X6
with ethinylestradiol	T38.5X1	T38.5X2	T38.5X3	T38.5X4	T38.5X5	T38.5X6
Levopromazine	T43.3X1	T43.3X2	T43.3X3	T43.3X4	T43.3X5	T43.3X6
Levoprome	T42.6X1	T42.6X2	T42.6X3	T42.6X4	T42.6X5	T42.6X6
Levopropoxyphene	T40.4X1	T40.4X2	T40.4X3	T40.4X4	T40.4X5	T40.4X6
Levopropylhexedrine	T50.5X1	T50.5X2	T50.5X3	T50.5X4	T50.5X5	T50.5X6
Levoproxyphylline	T48.6X1	T48.6X2	T48.6X3	T48.6X4	T48.6X5	T48.6X6
Levorphanol	T40.4X1	T40.4X2	T40.4X3	T40.4X4	T40.4X5	T40.4X6
Levothyroxine	T38.1X1	T38.1X2	T38.1X3	T38.1X4	T38.1X5	T38.1X6
sodium	T38.1X1	T38.1X2	T38.1X3	T38.1X4	T38.1X5	T38.1X6
Levsin	T44.3X1	T44.3X2	T44.3X3	T44.3X4	T44.3X5	T44.3X6
Levulose	T50.3X1	T50.3X2	T50.3X3	T50.3X4	T50.3X5	T50.3X6
Lewisite (gas), not in war	T57.0X1	T57.0X2	T57.0X3	T57.0X4	—	—
Librium	T42.4X1	T42.4X2	T42.4X3	T42.4X4	T42.4X5	T42.4X6
Lidex	T49.0X1	T49.0X2	T49.0X3	T49.0X4	T49.0X5	T49.0X6
Lidocaine	T41.3X1	T41.3X2	T41.3X3	T41.3X4	T41.3X5	T41.3X6
regional	T41.3X1	T41.3X2	T41.3X3	T41.3X4	T41.3X5	T41.3X6
spinal	T41.3X1	T41.3X2	T41.3X3	T41.3X4	T41.3X5	T41.3X6
Lidofenin	T50.8X1	T50.8X2	T50.8X3	T50.8X4	T50.8X5	T50.8X6
Lidoflazine	T46.1X1	T46.1X2	T46.1X3	T46.1X4	T46.1X5	T46.1X6
Lighter fluid	T52.0X1	T52.0X2	T52.0X3	T52.0X4	—	—
Lignin hemicellulose	T47.6X1	T47.6X2	T47.6X3	T47.6X4	T47.6X5	T47.6X6
Lignocaine	T41.3X1	T41.3X2	T41.3X3	T41.3X4	T41.3X5	T41.3X6
regional	T41.3X1	T41.3X2	T41.3X3	T41.3X4	T41.3X5	T41.3X6
spinal	T41.3X1	T41.3X2	T41.3X3	T41.3X4	T41.3X5	T41.3X6
Ligroin (e) (solvent)	T52.0X1	T52.0X2	T52.0X3	T52.0X4	—	—
vapor	T59.891	T59.892	T59.893	T59.894	—	—
Ligustrum vulgare	T62.2X1	T62.2X2	T62.2X3	T62.2X4	—	—

Substance	Poisoning, Accidental (unintentional)	Poisoning, Intentional Self-harm	Poisoning, Assault	Poisoning, Undetermined	Adverse Effect	Under-dosing
Lily of the valley	T62.2X1	T62.2X2	T62.2X3	T62.2X4	—	—
Lime (chloride)	T54.3X1	T54.3X2	T54.3X3	T54.3X4	—	—
Limonene	T52.8X1	T52.8X2	T52.8X3	T52.8X4	—	—
Lincomycin	T36.8X1	T36.8X2	T36.8X3	T36.8X4	T36.8X5	T36.8X6
Lindane (insecticide) (nonmedicinal) (vapor)	T53.6X1	T53.6X2	T53.6X3	T53.6X4	—	—
medicinal	T49.ØX1	T49.ØX2	T49.ØX3	T49.ØX4	T49.ØX5	T49.ØX6
Liniments NEC	T49.91	T49.92	T49.93	T49.94	T49.95	T49.96
Linoleic acid	T46.6X1	T46.6X2	T46.6X3	T46.6X4	T46.6X5	T46.6X6
Linolenic acid	T46.6X1	T46.6X2	T46.6X3	T46.6X4	T46.6X5	T46.6X6
Linseed	T47.4X1	T47.4X2	T47.4X3	T47.4X4	T47.4X5	T47.4X6
Liothyronine	T38.1X1	T38.1X2	T38.1X3	T38.1X4	T38.1X5	T38.1X6
Liotrix	T38.1X1	T38.1X2	T38.1X3	T38.1X4	T38.1X5	T38.1X6
Lipancreatin	T47.5X1	T47.5X2	T47.5X3	T47.5X4	T47.5X5	T47.5X6
Lipo-alprostadil	T46.7X1	T46.7X2	T46.7X3	T46.7X4	T46.7X5	T46.7X6
Lipo-Lutin	T38.5X1	T38.5X2	T38.5X3	T38.5X4	T38.5X5	T38.5X6
Lipotropic drug NEC	T5Ø.9Ø1	T5Ø.9Ø2	T5Ø.9Ø3	T5Ø.9Ø4	T5Ø.9Ø5	T5Ø.9Ø6
Liquefied petroleum gases	T59.891	T59.892	T59.893	T59.894	—	—
piped (pure or mixed with air)	T59.891	T59.892	T59.893	T59.894	—	—
Liquid						
paraffin	T47.4X1	T47.4X2	T47.4X3	T47.4X4	T47.4X5	T47.4X6
petrolatum	T47.4X1	T47.4X2	T47.4X3	T47.4X4	T47.4X5	T47.4X6
topical	T49.3X1	T49.3X2	T49.3X3	T49.3X4	T49.3X5	T49.3X6
specified NEC	T65.891	T65.892	T65.893	T65.894	—	—
substance	T65.91	T65.92	T65.93	T65.94	—	—
Liquor creosolis compositus	T65.891	T65.892	T65.893	T65.894	—	—
Liquorice	T48.4X1	T48.4X2	T48.4X3	T48.4X4	T48.4X5	T48.4X6
extract	T47.8X1	T47.8X2	T47.8X3	T47.8X4	T47.8X5	T47.8X6
Lisinopril	T46.4X1	T46.4X2	T46.4X3	T46.4X4	T46.4X5	T46.4X6
Lisuride	T42.8X1	T42.8X2	T42.8X3	T42.8X4	T42.8X5	T42.8X6
Lithane	T43.8X1	T43.8X2	T43.8X3	T43.8X4	T43.8X5	T43.8X6
Lithium	T56.891	T56.892	T56.893	T56.894	—	—
gluconate	T43.591	T43.592	T43.593	T43.594	T43.595	T43.596
salts (carbonate)	T43.591	T43.592	T43.593	T43.594	T43.595	T43.596
Lithonate	T43.8X1	T43.8X2	T43.8X3	T43.8X4	T43.8X5	T43.8X6
Liver						
extract	T45.8X1	T45.8X2	T45.8X3	T45.8X4	T45.8X5	T45.8X6
for parenteral use	T45.8X1	T45.8X2	T45.8X3	T45.8X4	T45.8X5	T45.8X6
fraction 1	T45.8X1	T45.8X2	T45.8X3	T45.8X4	T45.8X5	T45.8X6
hydrolysate	T45.8X1	T45.8X2	T45.8X3	T45.8X4	T45.8X5	T45.8X6
Lizard (bite) (venom)	T63.121	T63.122	T63.123	T63.124	—	—
LMD	T45.8X1	T45.8X2	T45.8X3	T45.8X4	T45.8X5	T45.8X6
Lobelia	T62.2X1	T62.2X2	T62.2X3	T62.2X4	—	—
Lobeline	T5Ø.7X1	T5Ø.7X2	T5Ø.7X3	T5Ø.7X4	T5Ø.7X5	T5Ø.7X6
Local action drug NEC	T49.8X1	T49.8X2	T49.8X3	T49.8X4	T49.8X5	T49.8X6
Locorten	T49.ØX1	T49.ØX2	T49.ØX3	T49.ØX4	T49.ØX5	T49.ØX6
Lofepramine	T43.Ø11	T43.Ø12	T43.Ø13	T43.Ø14	T43.Ø15	T43.Ø16
Lolium temulentum	T62.2X1	T62.2X2	T62.2X3	T62.2X4	—	—
Lomotil	T47.6X1	T47.6X2	T47.6X3	T47.6X4	T47.6X5	T47.6X6
Lomustine	T45.1X1	T45.1X2	T45.1X3	T45.1X4	T45.1X5	T45.1X6
Lonidamine	T45.1X1	T45.1X2	T45.1X3	T45.1X4	T45.1X5	T45.1X6
Loperamide	T47.6X1	T47.6X2	T47.6X3	T47.6X4	T47.6X5	T47.6X6
Loprazolam	T42.4X1	T42.4X2	T42.4X3	T42.4X4	T42.4X5	T42.4X6
Lorajmine	T46.2X1	T46.2X2	T46.2X3	T46.2X4	T46.2X5	T46.2X6
Loratidine	T45.ØX1	T45.ØX2	T45.ØX3	T45.ØX4	T45.ØX5	T45.ØX6
Lorazepam	T42.4X1	T42.4X2	T42.4X3	T42.4X4	T42.4X5	T42.4X6
Lorcainide	T46.2X1	T46.2X2	T46.2X3	T46.2X4	T46.2X5	T46.2X6
Lormetazepam	T42.4X1	T42.4X2	T42.4X3	T42.4X4	T42.4X5	T42.4X6
Lotions NEC	T49.91	T49.92	T49.93	T49.94	T49.95	T49.96
Lotusate	T42.3X1	T42.3X2	T42.3X3	T42.3X4	T42.3X5	T42.3X6
Lovastatin	T46.6X1	T46.6X2	T46.6X3	T46.6X4	T46.6X5	T46.6X6
Lowila	T49.2X1	T49.2X2	T49.2X3	T49.2X4	T49.2X5	T49.2X6
Loxapine	T43.591	T43.592	T43.593	T43.594	T43.595	T43.596
Lozenges (throat)	T49.6X1	T49.6X2	T49.6X3	T49.6X4	T49.6X5	T49.6X6
LSD	T4Ø.8X1	T4Ø.8X2	T4Ø.8X3	T4Ø.8X4	—	—
L-Tryptophan — *see* amino acid						
Lubricant, eye	T49.5X1	T49.5X2	T49.5X3	T49.5X4	T49.5X5	T49.5X6
Lubricating oil NEC	T52.ØX1	T52.ØX2	T52.ØX3	T52.ØX4	—	—
Lucanthone	T37.4X1	T37.4X2	T37.4X3	T37.4X4	T37.4X5	T37.4X6
Luminal	T42.3X1	T42.3X2	T42.3X3	T42.3X4	T42.3X5	T42.3X6
Lung irritant (gas) **NEC**	T59.91	T59.92	T59.93	T59.94	—	—
Luteinizing hormone	T38.811	T38.812	T38.813	T38.814	T38.815	T38.816
Lutocylol	T38.5X1	T38.5X2	T38.5X3	T38.5X4	T38.5X5	T38.5X6
Lutromone	T38.5X1	T38.5X2	T38.5X3	T38.5X4	T38.5X5	T38.5X6
Lututrin	T48.291	T48.292	T48.293	T48.294	T48.295	T48.296
Lye (concentrated)	T54.3X1	T54.3X2	T54.3X3	T54.3X4	—	—
Lygranum (skin test)	T5Ø.8X1	T5Ø.8X2	T5Ø.8X3	T5Ø.8X4	T5Ø.8X5	T5Ø.8X6
Lymecycline	T36.4X1	T36.4X2	T36.4X3	T36.4X4	T36.4X5	T36.4X6
Lymphogranuloma venereum antigen	T5Ø.8X1	T5Ø.8X2	T5Ø.8X3	T5Ø.8X4	T5Ø.8X5	T5Ø.8X6
Lynestrenol	T38.4X1	T38.4X2	T38.4X3	T38.4X4	T38.4X5	T38.4X6

Substance	Poisoning, Accidental (unintentional)	Poisoning, Intentional Self-harm	Poisoning, Assault	Poisoning, Undetermined	Adverse Effect	Under-dosing
Lyovac Sodium Edecrin	T5Ø.1X1	T5Ø.1X2	T5Ø.1X3	T5Ø.1X4	T5Ø.1X5	T5Ø.1X6
Lypressin	T38.891	T38.892	T38.893	T38.894	T38.895	T38.896
Lysergic acid diethylamide	T4Ø.8X1	T4Ø.8X2	T4Ø.8X3	T4Ø.8X4	—	—
Lysergide	T4Ø.8X1	T4Ø.8X2	T4Ø.8X3	T4Ø.8X4	—	—
Lysine vasopressin	T38.891	T38.892	T38.893	T38.894	T38.895	T38.896
Lysol	T54.1X1	T54.1X2	T54.1X3	T54.1X4	—	—
Lysozyme	T49.ØX1	T49.ØX2	T49.ØX3	T49.ØX4	T49.ØX5	T49.ØX6
Lytta (vitatta)	T49.8X1	T49.8X2	T49.8X3	T49.8X4	T49.8X5	T49.8X6
Mace	T59.3X1	T59.3X2	T59.3X3	T59.3X4	—	—
Macrogol	T5Ø.991	T5Ø.992	T5Ø.993	T5Ø.994	T5Ø.995	T5Ø.996
Macrolide						
anabolic drug	T38.7X1	T38.7X2	T38.7X3	T38.7X4	T38.7X5	T38.7X6
antibiotic	T36.3X1	T36.3X2	T36.3X3	T36.3X4	T36.3X5	T36.3X6
Mafenide	T49.ØX1	T49.ØX2	T49.ØX3	T49.ØX4	T49.ØX5	T49.ØX6
Magaldrate	T47.1X1	T47.1X2	T47.1X3	T47.1X4	T47.1X5	T47.1X6
Magic mushroom	T4Ø.991	T4Ø.992	T4Ø.993	T4Ø.994	—	—
Magnamycin	T36.8X1	T36.8X2	T36.8X3	T36.8X4	T36.8X5	T36.8X6
Magnesia magma	T47.1X1	T47.1X2	T47.1X3	T47.1X4	T47.1X5	T47.1X6
Magnesium NEC	T56.891	T56.892	T56.893	T56.894	—	—
carbonate	T47.1X1	T47.1X2	T47.1X3	T47.1X4	T47.1X5	T47.1X6
citrate	T47.4X1	T47.4X2	T47.4X3	T47.4X4	T47.4X5	T47.4X6
hydroxide	T47.1X1	T47.1X2	T47.1X3	T47.1X4	T47.1X5	T47.1X6
oxide	T47.1X1	T47.1X2	T47.1X3	T47.1X4	T47.1X5	T47.1X6
peroxide	T49.ØX1	T49.ØX2	T49.ØX3	T49.ØX4	T49.ØX5	T49.ØX6
salicylate	T39.Ø91	T39.Ø92	T39.Ø93	T39.Ø94	T39.Ø95	T39.Ø96
silicofluoride	T5Ø.3X1	T5Ø.3X2	T5Ø.3X3	T5Ø.3X4	T5Ø.3X5	T5Ø.3X6
sulfate	T47.4X1	T47.4X2	T47.4X3	T47.4X4	T47.4X5	T47.4X6
thiosulfate	T45.ØX1	T45.ØX2	T45.ØX3	T45.ØX4	T45.ØX5	T45.ØX6
trisilicate	T47.1X1	T47.1X2	T47.1X3	T47.1X4	T47.1X5	T47.1X6
Malathion (medicinal)	T49.ØX1	T49.ØX2	T49.ØX3	T49.ØX4	T49.ØX5	T49.ØX6
insecticide	T6Ø.ØX1	T6Ø.ØX2	T6Ø.ØX3	T6Ø.ØX4	—	—
Male fern extract	T37.4X1	T37.4X2	T37.4X3	T37.4X4	T37.4X5	T37.4X6
M-AMSA	T45.1X1	T45.1X2	T45.1X3	T45.1X4	T45.1X5	T45.1X6
Mandelic acid	T37.8X1	T37.8X2	T37.8X3	T37.8X4	T37.8X5	T37.8X6
Manganese (dioxide) (salts)	T57.2X1	T57.2X2	T57.2X3	T57.2X4	—	—
medicinal	T5Ø.991	T5Ø.992	T5Ø.993	T5Ø.994	T5Ø.995	T5Ø.996
Mannitol	T47.3X1	T47.3X2	T47.3X3	T47.3X4	T47.3X5	T47.3X6
hexanitrate	T46.3X1	T46.3X2	T46.3X3	T46.3X4	T46.3X5	T46.3X6
Mannomustine	T45.1X1	T45.1X2	T45.1X3	T45.1X4	T45.1X5	T45.1X6
MAO inhibitors	T43.1X1	T43.1X2	T43.1X3	T43.1X4	T43.1X5	T43.1X6
Mapharsen	T37.8X1	T37.8X2	T37.8X3	T37.8X4	T37.8X5	T37.8X6
Maphenide	T49.ØX1	T49.ØX2	T49.ØX3	T49.ØX4	T49.ØX5	T49.ØX6
Maprotiline	T43.Ø21	T43.Ø22	T43.Ø23	T43.Ø24	T43.Ø25	T43.Ø26
Marcaine	T41.3X1	T41.3X2	T41.3X3	T41.3X4	T41.3X5	T41.3X6
infiltration (subcutaneous)	T41.3X1	T41.3X2	T41.3X3	T41.3X4	T41.3X5	T41.3X6
nerve block (peripheral) (plexus)	T41.3X1	T41.3X2	T41.3X3	T41.3X4	T41.3X5	T41.3X6
Marezine	T45.ØX1	T45.ØX2	T45.ØX3	T45.ØX4	T45.ØX5	T45.ØX6
Marihuana	T4Ø.7X1	T4Ø.7X2	T4Ø.7X3	T4Ø.7X4	T4Ø.7X5	T4Ø.7X6
Marijuana	T4Ø.7X1	T4Ø.7X2	T4Ø.7X3	T4Ø.7X4	T4Ø.7X5	T4Ø.7X6
Marine (sting)	T63.691	T63.692	T63.693	T63.694	—	—
animals (sting)	T63.691	T63.692	T63.693	T63.694	—	—
plants (sting)	T63.711	T63.712	T63.713	T63.714	—	—
Marplan	T43.1X1	T43.1X2	T43.1X3	T43.1X4	T43.1X5	T43.1X6
Marsh gas	T59.891	T59.892	T59.893	T59.894	—	—
Marsilid	T43.1X1	T43.1X2	T43.1X3	T43.1X4	T43.1X5	T43.1X6
Matulane	T45.1X1	T45.1X2	T45.1X3	T45.1X4	T45.1X5	T45.1X6
Mazindol	T5Ø.5X1	T5Ø.5X2	T5Ø.5X3	T5Ø.5X4	T5Ø.5X5	T5Ø.5X6
MCPA	T6Ø.3X1	T6Ø.3X2	T6Ø.3X3	T6Ø.3X4	—	—
MDMA	T43.621	T43.622	T43.623	T43.624	T43.625	T43.626
Meadow saffron	T62.2X1	T62.2X2	T62.2X3	T62.2X4	—	—
Measles virus vaccine (attenuated)	T5Ø.B91	T5Ø.B92	T5Ø.B93	T5Ø.B94	T5Ø.B95	T5Ø.B96
Meat, noxious	T62.8X1	T62.8X2	T62.8X3	T62.8X4	—	—
Meballymal	T42.3X1	T42.3X2	T42.3X3	T42.3X4	T42.3X5	T42.3X6
Mebanazine	T43.1X1	T43.1X2	T43.1X3	T43.1X4	T43.1X5	T43.1X6
Mebaral	T42.3X1	T42.3X2	T42.3X3	T42.3X4	T42.3X5	T42.3X6
Mebendazole	T37.4X1	T37.4X2	T37.4X3	T37.4X4	T37.4X5	T37.4X6
Mebeverine	T44.3X1	T44.3X2	T44.3X3	T44.3X4	T44.3X5	T44.3X6
Mebhydrolin	T45.ØX1	T45.ØX2	T45.ØX3	T45.ØX4	T45.ØX5	T45.ØX6
Mebumal	T42.3X1	T42.3X2	T42.3X3	T42.3X4	T42.3X5	T42.3X6
Mebutamate	T43.591	T43.592	T43.593	T43.594	T43.595	T43.596
Mecamylamine	T44.2X1	T44.2X2	T44.2X3	T44.2X4	T44.2X5	T44.2X6
Mechlorethamine	T45.1X1	T45.1X2	T45.1X3	T45.1X4	T45.1X5	T45.1X6
Mecillinam	T36.ØX1	T36.ØX2	T36.ØX3	T36.ØX4	T36.ØX5	T36.ØX6
Meclizine (hydrochloride)	T45.ØX1	T45.ØX2	T45.ØX3	T45.ØX4	T45.ØX5	T45.ØX6
Meclocycline	T36.4X1	T36.4X2	T36.4X3	T36.4X4	T36.4X5	T36.4X6
Meclofenamate	T39.391	T39.392	T39.393	T39.394	T39.395	T39.396
Meclofenamic acid	T39.391	T39.392	T39.393	T39.394	T39.395	T39.396
Meclofenoxate	T43.691	T43.692	T43.693	T43.694	T43.695	T43.696
Meclozine	T45.ØX1	T45.ØX2	T45.ØX3	T45.ØX4	T45.ØX5	T45.ØX6
Mecobalamin	T45.8X1	T45.8X2	T45.8X3	T45.8X4	T45.8X5	T45.8X6
Mecoprop	T6Ø.3X1	T6Ø.3X2	T6Ø.3X3	T6Ø.3X4	—	—

Lily of the valley — Mecoprop

366 Additional Character May Be Required — Refer to the Tabular List for Character Selection
Subterms under main terms may continue to next column or page

Substance	Poisoning, Accidental (unintentional)	Poisoning, Intentional Self-harm	Poisoning, Assault	Poisoning, Undetermined	Adverse Effect	Under-dosing
Mecrilate	T49.3X1	T49.3X2	T49.3X3	T49.3X4	T49.3X5	T49.3X6
Mecysteine	T48.4X1	T48.4X2	T48.4X3	T48.4X4	T48.4X5	T48.4X6
Medazepam	T42.4X1	T42.4X2	T42.4X3	T42.4X4	T42.4X5	T42.4X6
Medicament NEC	T50.901	T50.902	T50.903	T50.904	T50.905	T50.906
Medinal	T42.3X1	T42.3X2	T42.3X3	T42.3X4	T42.3X5	T42.3X6
Medomin	T42.3X1	T42.3X2	T42.3X3	T42.3X4	T42.3X5	T42.3X6
Medrogestone	T38.5X1	T38.5X2	T38.5X3	T38.5X4	T38.5X5	T38.5X6
Medroxalol	T44.8X1	T44.8X2	T44.8X3	T44.8X4	T44.8X5	T44.8X6
Medroxyprogesterone acetate (depot)	T38.5X1	T38.5X2	T38.5X3	T38.5X4	T38.5X5	T38.5X6
Medrysone	T49.0X1	T49.0X2	T49.0X3	T49.0X4	T49.0X5	T49.0X6
Mefenamic acid	T39.391	T39.392	T39.393	T39.394	T39.395	T39.396
Mefenorex	T50.5X1	T50.5X2	T50.5X3	T50.5X4	T50.5X5	T50.5X6
Mefloquine	T37.2X1	T37.2X2	T37.2X3	T37.2X4	T37.2X5	T37.2X6
Mefruside	T50.2X1	T50.2X2	T50.2X3	T50.2X4	T50.2X5	T50.2X6
Megahallucinogen	T40.901	T40.902	T40.903	T40.904	T40.905	T40.906
Megestrol	T38.5X1	T38.5X2	T38.5X3	T38.5X4	T38.5X5	T38.5X6
Meglumine						
antimoniate	T37.8X1	T37.8X2	T37.8X3	T37.8X4	T37.8X5	T37.8X6
diatrizoate	T50.8X1	T50.8X2	T50.8X3	T50.8X4	T50.8X5	T50.8X6
iodipamide	T50.8X1	T50.8X2	T50.8X3	T50.8X4	T50.8X5	T50.8X6
iotroxate	T50.8X1	T50.8X2	T50.8X3	T50.8X4	T50.8X5	T50.8X6
MEK (methyl ethyl ketone)	T52.4X1	T52.4X2	T52.4X3	T52.4X4	—	—
Meladinin	T49.3X1	T49.3X2	T49.3X3	T49.3X4	T49.3X5	T49.3X6
Meladrazine	T44.3X1	T44.3X2	T44.3X3	T44.3X4	T44.3X5	T44.3X6
Melaleuca alternifolia oil	T49.0X1	T49.0X2	T49.0X3	T49.0X4	T49.0X5	T49.0X6
Melanizing agents	T49.3X1	T49.3X2	T49.3X3	T49.3X4	T49.3X5	T49.3X6
Melanocyte-stimulating hormone	T38.891	T38.892	T38.893	T38.894	T38.895	T38.896
Melarsonyl potassium	T37.3X1	T37.3X2	T37.3X3	T37.3X4	T37.3X5	T37.3X6
Melarsoprol	T37.3X1	T37.3X2	T37.3X3	T37.3X4	T37.3X5	T37.3X6
Melia azedarach	T62.2X1	T62.2X2	T62.2X3	T62.2X4	—	—
Melitracen	T43.011	T43.012	T43.013	T43.014	T43.015	T43.016
Mellaril	T43.3X1	T43.3X2	T43.3X3	T43.3X4	T43.3X5	T43.3X6
Meloxine	T49.3X1	T49.3X2	T49.3X3	T49.3X4	T49.3X5	T49.3X6
Melperone	T43.4X1	T43.4X2	T43.4X3	T43.4X4	T43.4X5	T43.4X6
Melphalan	T45.1X1	T45.1X2	T45.1X3	T45.1X4	T45.1X5	T45.1X6
Memantine	T43.8X1	T43.8X2	T43.8X3	T43.8X4	T43.8X5	T43.8X6
Menadiol	T45.7X1	T45.7X2	T45.7X3	T45.7X4	T45.7X5	T45.7X6
sodium sulfate	T45.7X1	T45.7X2	T45.7X3	T45.7X4	T45.7X5	T45.7X6
Menadione	T45.7X1	T45.7X2	T45.7X3	T45.7X4	T45.7X5	T45.7X6
sodium bisulfite	T45.7X1	T45.7X2	T45.7X3	T45.7X4	T45.7X5	T45.7X6
Menaphthone	T45.7X1	T45.7X2	T45.7X3	T45.7X4	T45.7X5	T45.7X6
Menaquinone	T45.7X1	T45.7X2	T45.7X3	T45.7X4	T45.7X5	T45.7X6
Menatetrenone	T45.7X1	T45.7X2	T45.7X3	T45.7X4	T45.7X5	T45.7X6
Meningococcal vaccine	T50.A91	T50.A92	T50.A93	T50.A94	T50.A95	T50.A96
Menningovax (-AC) (-C)	T50.A91	T50.A92	T50.A93	T50.A94	T50.A95	T50.A96
Menotropins	T38.811	T38.812	T38.813	T38.814	T38.815	T38.816
Menthol	T48.5X1	T48.5X2	T48.5X3	T48.5X4	T48.5X5	T48.5X6
Mepacrine	T37.2X1	T37.2X2	T37.2X3	T37.2X4	T37.2X5	T37.2X6
Meparfynol	T42.6X1	T42.6X2	T42.6X3	T42.6X4	T42.6X5	T42.6X6
Mepartricin	T36.7X1	T36.7X2	T36.7X3	T36.7X4	T36.7X5	T36.7X6
Mepazine	T43.3X1	T43.3X2	T43.3X3	T43.3X4	T43.3X5	T43.3X6
Mepenzolate	T44.3X1	T44.3X2	T44.3X3	T44.3X4	T44.3X5	T44.3X6
bromide	T44.3X1	T44.3X2	T44.3X3	T44.3X4	T44.3X5	T44.3X6
Meperidine	T40.4X1	T40.4X2	T40.4X3	T40.4X4	T40.4X5	T40.4X6
Mephebarbital	T42.3X1	T42.3X2	T42.3X3	T42.3X4	T42.3X5	T42.3X6
Mephenamin (e)	T42.8X1	T42.8X2	T42.8X3	T42.8X4	T42.8X5	T42.8X6
Mephenesin	T42.8X1	T42.8X2	T42.8X3	T42.8X4	T42.8X5	T42.8X6
Mephenhydramine	T45.0X1	T45.0X2	T45.0X3	T45.0X4	T45.0X5	T45.0X6
Mephenoxalone	T42.8X1	T42.8X2	T42.8X3	T42.8X4	T42.8X5	T42.8X6
Mephentermine	T44.991	T44.992	T44.993	T44.994	T44.995	T44.996
Mephenytoin	T42.0X1	T42.0X2	T42.0X3	T42.0X4	T42.0X5	T42.0X6
with phenobarbital	T42.3X1	T42.3X2	T42.3X3	T42.3X4	T42.3X5	T42.3X6
Mephobarbital	T42.3X1	T42.3X2	T42.3X3	T42.3X4	T42.3X5	T42.3X6
Mephosfolan	T60.0X1	T60.0X2	T60.0X3	T60.0X4	—	—
Mepindolol	T44.7X1	T44.7X2	T44.7X3	T44.7X4	T44.7X5	T44.7X6
Mepiperphenidol	T44.3X1	T44.3X2	T44.3X3	T44.3X4	T44.3X5	T44.3X6
Mepitiostane	T38.7X1	T38.7X2	T38.7X3	T38.7X4	T38.7X5	T38.7X6
Mepivacaine	T41.3X1	T41.3X2	T41.3X3	T41.3X4	T41.3X5	T41.3X6
epidural	T41.3X1	T41.3X2	T41.3X3	T41.3X4	T41.3X5	T41.3X6
Meprednisone	T38.0X1	T38.0X2	T38.0X3	T38.0X4	T38.0X5	T38.0X6
Meprobam	T43.591	T43.592	T43.593	T43.594	T43.595	T43.596
Meprobamate	T43.591	T43.592	T43.593	T43.594	T43.595	T43.596
Meproscillarin	T46.0X1	T46.0X2	T46.0X3	T46.0X4	T46.0X5	T46.0X6
Meprylcaine	T41.3X1	T41.3X2	T41.3X3	T41.3X4	T41.3X5	T41.3X6
Meptazinol	T39.8X1	T39.8X2	T39.8X3	T39.8X4	T39.8X5	T39.8X6
Mepyramine	T45.0X1	T45.0X2	T45.0X3	T45.0X4	T45.0X5	T45.0X6
Mequitazine	T43.3X1	T43.3X2	T43.3X3	T43.3X4	T43.3X5	T43.3X6
Meralluride	T50.2X1	T50.2X2	T50.2X3	T50.2X4	T50.2X5	T50.2X6
Merbaphen	T50.2X1	T50.2X2	T50.2X3	T50.2X4	T50.2X5	T50.2X6
Merbromin	T49.0X1	T49.0X2	T49.0X3	T49.0X4	T49.0X5	T49.0X6

Substance	Poisoning, Accidental (unintentional)	Poisoning, Intentional Self-harm	Poisoning, Assault	Poisoning, Undetermined	Adverse Effect	Under-dosing
Mercaptobenzothiazole salts	T49.0X1	T49.0X2	T49.0X3	T49.0X4	T49.0X5	T49.0X6
Mercaptomerin	T50.2X1	T50.2X2	T50.2X3	T50.2X4	T50.2X5	T50.2X6
Mercaptopurine	T45.1X1	T45.1X2	T45.1X3	T45.1X4	T45.1X5	T45.1X6
Mercumatilin	T50.2X1	T50.2X2	T50.2X3	T50.2X4	T50.2X5	T50.2X6
Mercuramide	T50.2X1	T50.2X2	T50.2X3	T50.2X4	T50.2X5	T50.2X6
Mercurochrome	T49.0X1	T49.0X2	T49.0X3	T49.0X4	T49.0X5	T49.0X6
Mercurophylline	T50.2X1	T50.2X2	T50.2X3	T50.2X4	T50.2X5	T50.2X6
Mercury, mercurial, mercuric, mercurous (compounds) (cyanide) (fumes) (nonmedicinal) (vapor) **NEC**	T56.1X1	T56.1X2	T56.1X3	T56.1X4	—	—
ammoniated	T49.0X1	T49.0X2	T49.0X3	T49.0X4	T49.0X5	T49.0X6
anti-infective						
local	T49.0X1	T49.0X2	T49.0X3	T49.0X4	T49.0X5	T49.0X6
systemic	T37.8X1	T37.8X2	T37.8X3	T37.8X4	T37.8X5	T37.8X6
topical	T49.0X1	T49.0X2	T49.0X3	T49.0X4	T49.0X5	T49.0X6
chloride (ammoniated)	T49.0X1	T49.0X2	T49.0X3	T49.0X4	T49.0X5	T49.0X6
fungicide	T56.1X1	T56.1X2	T56.1X3	T56.1X4	—	—
diuretic NEC	T50.2X1	T50.2X2	T50.2X3	T50.2X4	T50.2X5	T50.2X6
fungicide	T56.1X1	T56.1X2	T56.1X3	T56.1X4	—	—
organic (fungicide)	T56.1X1	T56.1X2	T56.1X3	T56.1X4	—	—
oxide, yellow	T49.0X1	T49.0X2	T49.0X3	T49.0X4	T49.0X5	T49.0X6
Mersalyl	T50.2X1	T50.2X2	T50.2X3	T50.2X4	T50.2X5	T50.2X6
Merthiolate	T49.0X1	T49.0X2	T49.0X3	T49.0X4	T49.0X5	T49.0X6
ophthalmic preparation	T49.5X1	T49.5X2	T49.5X3	T49.5X4	T49.5X5	T49.5X6
Meruvax	T50.B91	T50.B92	T50.B93	T50.B94	T50.B95	T50.B96
Mesalazine	T47.8X1	T47.8X2	T47.8X3	T47.8X4	T47.8X5	T47.8X6
Mescal buttons	T40.991	T40.992	T40.993	T40.994	—	—
Mescaline	T40.991	T40.992	T40.993	T40.994	—	—
Mesna	T48.4X1	T48.4X2	T48.4X3	T48.4X4	T48.4X5	T48.4X6
Mesoglycan	T46.6X1	T46.6X2	T46.6X3	T46.6X4	T46.6X5	T46.6X6
Mesoridazine	T43.3X1	T43.3X2	T43.3X3	T43.3X4	T43.3X5	T43.3X6
Mestanolone	T38.7X1	T38.7X2	T38.7X3	T38.7X4	T38.7X5	T38.7X6
Mesterolone	T38.7X1	T38.7X2	T38.7X3	T38.7X4	T38.7X5	T38.7X6
Mestranol	T38.5X1	T38.5X2	T38.5X3	T38.5X4	T38.5X5	T38.5X6
Mesulergine	T42.8X1	T42.8X2	T42.8X3	T42.8X4	T42.8X5	T42.8X6
Mesulfen	T49.0X1	T49.0X2	T49.0X3	T49.0X4	T49.0X5	T49.0X6
Mesuximide	T42.2X1	T42.2X2	T42.2X3	T42.2X4	T42.2X5	T42.2X6
Metabutethamine	T41.3X1	T41.3X2	T41.3X3	T41.3X4	T41.3X5	T41.3X6
Metactesylacetate	T49.0X1	T49.0X2	T49.0X3	T49.0X4	T49.0X5	T49.0X6
Metacycline	T36.4X1	T36.4X2	T36.4X3	T36.4X4	T36.4X5	T36.4X6
Metaldehyde (snail killer) **NEC**	T60.8X1	T60.8X2	T60.8X3	T60.8X4	—	—
Metals (heavy) (nonmedicinal)	T56.91	T56.92	T56.93	T56.94	—	—
dust, fumes, or vapor NEC	T56.91	T56.92	T56.93	T56.94	—	—
light NEC	T56.91	T56.92	T56.93	T56.94	—	—
dust, fumes, or vapor NEC	T56.91	T56.92	T56.93	T56.94	—	—
specified NEC	T56.891	T56.892	T56.893	T56.894	—	—
thallium	T56.811	T56.812	T56.813	T56.814	—	—
Metamfetamine	T43.621	T43.622	T43.623	T43.624	T43.625	T43.626
Metamizole sodium	T39.2X1	T39.2X2	T39.2X3	T39.2X4	T39.2X5	T39.2X6
Metampicillin	T36.0X1	T36.0X2	T36.0X3	T36.0X4	T36.0X5	T36.0X6
Metamucil	T47.4X1	T47.4X2	T47.4X3	T47.4X4	T47.4X5	T47.4X6
Metandienone	T38.7X1	T38.7X2	T38.7X3	T38.7X4	T38.7X5	T38.7X6
Metandrostenolone	T38.7X1	T38.7X2	T38.7X3	T38.7X4	T38.7X5	T38.7X6
Metaphen	T49.0X1	T49.0X2	T49.0X3	T49.0X4	T49.0X5	T49.0X6
Metaphos	T60.0X1	T60.0X2	T60.0X3	T60.0X4	—	—
Metapramine	T43.011	T43.012	T43.013	T43.014	T43.015	T43.016
Metaproterenol	T48.291	T48.292	T48.293	T48.294	T48.295	T48.296
Metaraminol	T44.4X1	T44.4X2	T44.4X3	T44.4X4	T44.4X5	T44.4X6
Metaxalone	T42.8X1	T42.8X2	T42.8X3	T42.8X4	T42.8X5	T42.8X6
Metenolone	T38.7X1	T38.7X2	T38.7X3	T38.7X4	T38.7X5	T38.7X6
Metergoline	T42.8X1	T42.8X2	T42.8X3	T42.8X4	T42.8X5	T42.8X6
Metescufylline	T46.991	T46.992	T46.993	T46.994	T46.995	T46.996
Metetoin	T42.0X1	T42.0X2	T42.0X3	T42.0X4	T42.0X5	T42.0X6
Metformin	T38.3X1	T38.3X2	T38.3X3	T38.3X4	T38.3X5	T38.3X6
Methacholine	T44.1X1	T44.1X2	T44.1X3	T44.1X4	T44.1X5	T44.1X6
Methacycline	T36.4X1	T36.4X2	T36.4X3	T36.4X4	T36.4X5	T36.4X6
Methadone	T40.3X1	T40.3X2	T40.3X3	T40.3X4	T40.3X5	T40.3X6
Methallenestril	T38.5X1	T38.5X2	T38.5X3	T38.5X4	T38.5X5	T38.5X6
Methallenoestril	T38.5X1	T38.5X2	T38.5X3	T38.5X4	T38.5X5	T38.5X6
Methamphetamine	T43.621	T43.622	T43.623	T43.624	T43.625	T43.626
Methampyrone	T39.2X1	T39.2X2	T39.2X3	T39.2X4	T39.2X5	T39.2X6
Methandienone	T38.7X1	T38.7X2	T38.7X3	T38.7X4	T38.7X5	T38.7X6
Methandriol	T38.7X1	T38.7X2	T38.7X3	T38.7X4	T38.7X5	T38.7X6
Methandrostenolone	T38.7X1	T38.7X2	T38.7X3	T38.7X4	T38.7X5	T38.7X6
Methane	T59.891	T59.892	T59.893	T59.894	—	—
Methanethiol	T59.891	T59.892	T59.893	T59.894	—	—
Methaniazide	T37.1X1	T37.1X2	T37.1X3	T37.1X4	T37.1X5	T37.1X6
Methanol (vapor)	T51.1X1	T51.1X2	T51.1X3	T51.1X4	—	—

Methantheline ICD-10-CM 2016

Table of Drugs and Chemicals

Substance	Poisoning, Accidental (unintentional)	Poisoning, Intentional Self-harm	Poisoning, Assault	Poisoning, Undetermined	Adverse Effect	Under-dosing
Methantheline	T44.3X1	T44.3X2	T44.3X3	T44.3X4	T44.3X5	T44.3X6
Methanthelinium bromide	T44.3X1	T44.3X2	T44.3X3	T44.3X4	T44.3X5	T44.3X6
Methaphenilene	T45.ØX1	T45.ØX2	T45.ØX3	T45.ØX4	T45.ØX5	T45.ØX6
Methapyrilene	T45.ØX1	T45.ØX2	T45.ØX3	T45.ØX4	T45.ØX5	T45.ØX6
Methaqualone (compound)	T42.6X1	T42.6X2	T42.6X3	T42.6X4	T42.6X5	T42.6X6
Metharbital	T42.3X1	T42.3X2	T42.3X3	T42.3X4	T42.3X5	T42.3X6
Methazolamide	T5Ø.2X1	T5Ø.2X2	T5Ø.2X3	T5Ø.2X4	T5Ø.2X5	T5Ø.2X6
Methdilazine	T43.3X1	T43.3X2	T43.3X3	T43.3X4	T43.3X5	T43.3X6
Methedrine	T43.621	T43.622	T43.623	T43.624	T43.625	T43.626
Methenamine (mandelate)	T37.8X1	T37.8X2	T37.8X3	T37.8X4	T37.8X5	T37.8X6
Methenolone	T38.7X1	T38.7X2	T38.7X3	T38.7X4	T38.7X5	T38.7X6
Methergine	T48.ØX1	T48.ØX2	T48.ØX3	T48.ØX4	T48.ØX5	T48.ØX6
Methetoin	T42.ØX1	T42.ØX2	T42.ØX3	T42.ØX4	T42.ØX5	T42.ØX6
Methiacil	T38.2X1	T38.2X2	T38.2X3	T38.2X4	T38.2X5	T38.2X6
Methicillin	T36.ØX1	T36.ØX2	T36.ØX3	T36.ØX4	T36.ØX5	T36.ØX6
Methimazole	T38.2X1	T38.2X2	T38.2X3	T38.2X4	T38.2X5	T38.2X6
Methiodal sodium	T5Ø.8X1	T5Ø.8X2	T5Ø.8X3	T5Ø.8X4	T5Ø.8X5	T5Ø.8X6
Methionine	T5Ø.991	T5Ø.992	T5Ø.993	T5Ø.994	T5Ø.995	T5Ø.996
Methisazone	T37.5X1	T37.5X2	T37.5X3	T37.5X4	T37.5X5	T37.5X6
Methisoprinol	T37.5X1	T37.5X2	T37.5X3	T37.5X4	T37.5X5	T37.5X6
Methitural	T42.3X1	T42.3X2	T42.3X3	T42.3X4	T42.3X5	T42.3X6
Methixene	T44.3X1	T44.3X2	T44.3X3	T44.3X4	T44.3X5	T44.3X6
Methobarbital, methobarbitone	T42.3X1	T42.3X2	T42.3X3	T42.3X4	T42.3X5	T42.3X6
Methocarbamol	T42.8X1	T42.8X2	T42.8X3	T42.8X4	T42.8X5	T42.8X6
skeletal muscle relaxant	T48.1X1	T48.1X2	T48.1X3	T48.1X4	T48.1X5	T48.1X6
Methohexital	T41.1X1	T41.1X2	T41.1X3	T41.1X4	T41.1X5	T41.1X6
Methohexitone	T41.1X1	T41.1X2	T41.1X3	T41.1X4	T41.1X5	T41.1X6
Methoin	T42.ØX1	T42.ØX2	T42.ØX3	T42.ØX4	T42.ØX5	T42.ØX6
Methopholine	T39.8X1	T39.8X2	T39.8X3	T39.8X4	T39.8X5	T39.8X6
Methopromazine	T43.3X1	T43.3X2	T43.3X3	T43.3X4	T43.3X5	T43.3X6
Methorate	T48.3X1	T48.3X2	T48.3X3	T48.3X4	T48.3X5	T48.3X6
Methoserpidine	T46.5X1	T46.5X2	T46.5X3	T46.5X4	T46.5X5	T46.5X6
Methotrexate	T45.1X1	T45.1X2	T45.1X3	T45.1X4	T45.1X5	T45.1X6
Methotrimeprazine	T43.3X1	T43.3X2	T43.3X3	T43.3X4	T43.3X5	T43.3X6
Methoxa-Dome	T49.3X1	T49.3X2	T49.3X3	T49.3X4	T49.3X5	T49.3X6
Methoxamine	T44.4X1	T44.4X2	T44.4X3	T44.4X4	T44.4X5	T44.4X6
Methoxsalen	T5Ø.991	T5Ø.992	T5Ø.993	T5Ø.994	T5Ø.995	T5Ø.996
Methoxyaniline	T65.3X1	T65.3X2	T65.3X3	T65.3X4	—	—
Methoxybenzyl penicillin	T36.ØX1	T36.ØX2	T36.ØX3	T36.ØX4	T36.ØX5	T36.ØX6
Methoxychlor	T53.7X1	T53.7X2	T53.7X3	T53.7X4	—	—
Methoxy-DDT	T53.7X1	T53.7X2	T53.7X3	T53.7X4	—	—
Methoxyflurane	T41.ØX1	T41.ØX2	T41.ØX3	T41.ØX4	T41.ØX5	T41.ØX6
Methoxyphenamine	T48.6X1	T48.6X2	T48.6X3	T48.6X4	T48.6X5	T48.6X6
Methoxypromazine	T43.3X1	T43.3X2	T43.3X3	T43.3X4	T43.3X5	T43.3X6
Methscopolamine bromide	T44.3X1	T44.3X2	T44.3X3	T44.3X4	T44.3X5	T44.3X6
Methsuximide	T42.2X1	T42.2X2	T42.2X3	T42.2X4	T42.2X5	T42.2X6
Methyclothiazide	T5Ø.2X1	T5Ø.2X2	T5Ø.2X3	T5Ø.2X4	T5Ø.2X5	T5Ø.2X6
Methyl						
acetate	T52.4X1	T52.4X2	T52.4X3	T52.4X4	—	—
acetone	T52.4X1	T52.4X2	T52.4X3	T52.4X4	—	—
acrylate	T65.891	T65.892	T65.893	T65.894	—	—
alcohol	T51.1X1	T51.1X2	T51.1X3	T51.1X4	—	—
aminophenol	T65.3X1	T65.3X2	T65.3X3	T65.3X4	—	—
amphetamine	T43.621	T43.622	T43.623	T43.624	T43.625	T43.626
androstanolone	T38.7X1	T38.7X2	T38.7X3	T38.7X4	T38.7X5	T38.7X6
atropine	T44.3X1	T44.3X2	T44.3X3	T44.3X4	T44.3X5	T44.3X6
benzene	T52.2X1	T52.2X2	T52.2X3	T52.2X4	—	—
benzoate	T52.8X1	T52.8X2	T52.8X3	T52.8X4	—	—
benzol	T52.2X1	T52.2X2	T52.2X3	T52.2X4	—	—
bromide (gas)	T59.891	T59.892	T59.893	T59.894	—	—
fumigant	T6Ø.8X1	T6Ø.8X2	T6Ø.8X3	T6Ø.8X4	—	—
butanol	T51.3X1	T51.3X2	T51.3X3	T51.3X4	—	—
carbinol	T51.1X1	T51.1X2	T51.1X3	T51.1X4	—	—
carbonate	T52.8X1	T52.8X2	T52.8X3	T52.8X4	—	—
CCNU	T45.1X1	T45.1X2	T45.1X3	T45.1X4	T45.1X5	T45.1X6
cellosolve	T52.91	T52.92	T52.93	T52.94	—	—
cellulose	T47.4X1	T47.4X2	T47.4X3	T47.4X4	T47.4X5	T47.4X6
chloride (gas)	T59.891	T59.892	T59.893	T59.894	—	—
chloroformate	T59.3X1	T59.3X2	T59.3X3	T59.3X4	—	—
cyclohexane	T52.8X1	T52.8X2	T52.8X3	T52.8X4	—	—
cyclohexanol	T51.8X1	T51.8X2	T51.8X3	T51.8X4	—	—
cyclohexanone	T52.8X1	T52.8X2	T52.8X3	T52.8X4	—	—
cyclohexyl acetate	T52.8X1	T52.8X2	T52.8X3	T52.8X4	—	—
demeton	T6Ø.ØX1	T6Ø.ØX2	T6Ø.ØX3	T6Ø.ØX4	—	—
dihydromorphinone	T4Ø.2X1	T4Ø.2X2	T4Ø.2X3	T4Ø.2X4	T4Ø.2X5	T4Ø.2X6
ergometrine	T48.ØX1	T48.ØX2	T48.ØX3	T48.ØX4	T48.ØX5	T48.ØX6
ergonovine	T48.ØX1	T48.ØX2	T48.ØX3	T48.ØX4	T48.ØX5	T48.ØX6
ethyl ketone	T52.4X1	T52.4X2	T52.4X3	T52.4X4	—	—
glucamine antimonate	T37.8X1	T37.8X2	T37.8X3	T37.8X4	T37.8X5	T37.8X6
hydrazine	T65.891	T65.892	T65.893	T65.894	—	—
iodide	T65.891	T65.892	T65.893	T65.894	—	—
isobutyl ketone	T52.4X1	T52.4X2	T52.4X3	T52.4X4	—	—

Substance	Poisoning, Accidental (unintentional)	Poisoning, Intentional Self-harm	Poisoning, Assault	Poisoning, Undetermined	Adverse Effect	Under-dosing
Methyl — *continued*						
isothiocyanate	T6Ø.3X1	T6Ø.3X2	T6Ø.3X3	T6Ø.3X4	—	—
mercaptan	T59.891	T59.892	T59.893	T59.894	—	—
morphine NEC	T4Ø.2X1	T4Ø.2X2	T4Ø.2X3	T4Ø.2X4	T4Ø.2X5	T4Ø.2X6
nicotinate	T49.4X1	T49.4X2	T49.4X3	T49.4X4	T49.4X5	T49.4X6
paraben	T49.ØX1	T49.ØX2	T49.ØX3	T49.ØX4	T49.ØX5	T49.ØX6
parafynol	T42.6X1	T42.6X2	T42.6X3	T42.6X4	T42.6X5	T42.6X6
parathion	T6Ø.ØX1	T6Ø.ØX2	T6Ø.ØX3	T6Ø.ØX4	—	—
peridol	T43.4X1	T43.4X2	T43.4X3	T43.4X4	T43.4X5	T43.4X6
phenidate	T43.631	T43.632	T43.633	T43.634	T43.635	T43.636
prednisolone	T38.ØX1	T38.ØX2	T38.ØX3	T38.ØX4	T38.ØX5	T38.ØX6
ENT agent	T49.6X1	T49.6X2	T49.6X3	T49.6X4	T49.6X5	T49.6X6
ophthalmic preparation	T49.5X1	T49.5X2	T49.5X3	T49.5X4	T49.5X5	T49.5X6
topical NEC	T49.ØX1	T49.ØX2	T49.ØX3	T49.ØX4	T49.ØX5	T49.ØX6
propylcarbinol	T51.3X1	T51.3X2	T51.3X3	T51.3X4	—	—
rosaniline NEC	T49.ØX1	T49.ØX2	T49.ØX3	T49.ØX4	T49.ØX5	T49.ØX6
salicylate	T49.2X1	T49.2X2	T49.2X3	T49.2X4	T49.2X5	T49.2X6
sulfate (fumes)	T59.891	T59.892	T59.893	T59.894	—	—
liquid	T52.8X1	T52.8X2	T52.8X3	T52.8X4	—	—
sulfonal	T42.6X1	T42.6X2	T42.6X3	T42.6X4	T42.6X5	T42.6X6
testosterone	T38.7X1	T38.7X2	T38.7X3	T38.7X4	T38.7X5	T38.7X6
thiouracil	T38.2X1	T38.2X2	T38.2X3	T38.2X4	T38.2X5	T38.2X6
Methylamphetamine	T43.621	T43.622	T43.623	T43.624	T43.625	T43.626
Methylated spirit	T51.1X1	T51.1X2	T51.1X3	T51.1X4	—	—
Methylatropine nitrate	T44.3X1	T44.3X2	T44.3X3	T44.3X4	T44.3X5	T44.3X6
Methylbenactyzium bromide	T44.3X1	T44.3X2	T44.3X3	T44.3X4	T44.3X5	T44.3X6
Methylbenzethonium chloride	T49.ØX1	T49.ØX2	T49.ØX3	T49.ØX4	T49.ØX5	T49.ØX6
Methylcellulose	T47.4X1	T47.4X2	T47.4X3	T47.4X4	T47.4X5	T47.4X6
laxative	T47.4X1	T47.4X2	T47.4X3	T47.4X4	T47.4X5	T47.4X6
Methylchlorophenoxyacetic acid	T6Ø.3X1	T6Ø.3X2	T6Ø.3X3	T6Ø.3X4	—	—
Methyldopa	T46.5X1	T46.5X2	T46.5X3	T46.5X4	T46.5X5	T46.5X6
Methyldopate	T46.5X1	T46.5X2	T46.5X3	T46.5X4	T46.5X5	T46.5X6
Methylene						
blue	T5Ø.6X1	T5Ø.6X2	T5Ø.6X3	T5Ø.6X4	T5Ø.6X5	T5Ø.6X6
chloride or dichloride (solvent) NEC	T53.4X1	T53.4X2	T53.4X3	T53.4X4	—	—
Methylenedioxyamphetamine	T43.621	T43.622	T43.623	T43.624	T43.625	T43.626
Methylenedioxymethamphetamine	T43.621	T43.622	T43.623	T43.624	T43.625	T43.626
Methylergometrine	T48.ØX1	T48.ØX2	T48.ØX3	T48.ØX4	T48.ØX5	T48.ØX6
Methylergonovine	T48.ØX1	T48.ØX2	T48.ØX3	T48.ØX4	T48.ØX5	T48.ØX6
Methylestrenolone	T38.5X1	T38.5X2	T38.5X3	T38.5X4	T38.5X5	T38.5X6
Methylethyl cellulose	T5Ø.991	T5Ø.992	T5Ø.993	T5Ø.994	T5Ø.995	T5Ø.996
Methylhexabital	T42.3X1	T42.3X2	T42.3X3	T42.3X4	T42.3X5	T42.3X6
Methylmorphine	T4Ø.2X1	T4Ø.2X2	T4Ø.2X3	T4Ø.2X4	T4Ø.2X5	T4Ø.2X6
Methylparaben (ophthalmic)	T49.5X1	T49.5X2	T49.5X3	T49.5X4	T49.5X5	T49.5X6
Methylparafynol	T42.6X1	T42.6X2	T42.6X3	T42.6X4	T42.6X5	T42.6X6
Methylpentynol, methylpenthynol	T42.6X1	T42.6X2	T42.6X3	T42.6X4	T42.6X5	T42.6X6
Methylphenidate	T43.631	T43.632	T43.633	T43.634	T43.635	T43.636
Methylphenobarbital	T42.3X1	T42.3X2	T42.3X3	T42.3X4	T42.3X5	T42.3X6
Methylpolysiloxane	T47.1X1	T47.1X2	T47.1X3	T47.1X4	T47.1X5	T47.1X6
Methylprednisolone — *see* Methyl, prednisolone						
Methylrosaniline	T49.ØX1	T49.ØX2	T49.ØX3	T49.ØX4	T49.ØX5	T49.ØX6
Methylrosanilinium chloride	T49.ØX1	T49.ØX2	T49.ØX3	T49.ØX4	T49.ØX5	T49.ØX6
Methyltestosterone	T38.7X1	T38.7X2	T38.7X3	T38.7X4	T38.7X5	T38.7X6
Methylthionine chloride	T5Ø.6X1	T5Ø.6X2	T5Ø.6X3	T5Ø.6X4	T5Ø.6X5	T5Ø.6X6
Methylthioninium chloride	T5Ø.6X1	T5Ø.6X2	T5Ø.6X3	T5Ø.6X4	T5Ø.6X5	T5Ø.6X6
Methylthiouracil	T38.2X1	T38.2X2	T38.2X3	T38.2X4	T38.2X5	T38.2X6
Methyprylon	T42.6X1	T42.6X2	T42.6X3	T42.6X4	T42.6X5	T42.6X6
Methysergide	T46.5X1	T46.5X2	T46.5X3	T46.5X4	T46.5X5	T46.5X6
Metiamide	T47.1X1	T47.1X2	T47.1X3	T47.1X4	T47.1X5	T47.1X6
Meticillin	T36.ØX1	T36.ØX2	T36.ØX3	T36.ØX4	T36.ØX5	T36.ØX6
Meticrane	T5Ø.2X1	T5Ø.2X2	T5Ø.2X3	T5Ø.2X4	T5Ø.2X5	T5Ø.2X6
Metildigoxin	T46.ØX1	T46.ØX2	T46.ØX3	T46.ØX4	T46.ØX5	T46.ØX6
Metipranolol	T49.5X1	T49.5X2	T49.5X3	T49.5X4	T49.5X5	T49.5X6
Metirosine	T46.5X1	T46.5X2	T46.5X3	T46.5X4	T46.5X5	T46.5X6
Metisazone	T37.5X1	T37.5X2	T37.5X3	T37.5X4	T37.5X5	T37.5X6
Metixene	T44.3X1	T44.3X2	T44.3X3	T44.3X4	T44.3X5	T44.3X6
Metizoline	T48.5X1	T48.5X2	T48.5X3	T48.5X4	T48.5X5	T48.5X6
Metoclopramide	T45.ØX1	T45.ØX2	T45.ØX3	T45.ØX4	T45.ØX5	T45.ØX6
Metofenazate	T43.3X1	T43.3X2	T43.3X3	T43.3X4	T43.3X5	T43.3X6
Metofoline	T39.8X1	T39.8X2	T39.8X3	T39.8X4	T39.8X5	T39.8X6
Metolazone	T5Ø.2X1	T5Ø.2X2	T5Ø.2X3	T5Ø.2X4	T5Ø.2X5	T5Ø.2X6
Metopon	T4Ø.2X1	T4Ø.2X2	T4Ø.2X3	T4Ø.2X4	T4Ø.2X5	T4Ø.2X6
Metoprine	T45.1X1	T45.1X2	T45.1X3	T45.1X4	T45.1X5	T45.1X6
Metoprolol	T44.7X1	T44.7X2	T44.7X3	T44.7X4	T44.7X5	T44.7X6
Metrifonate	T6Ø.ØX1	T6Ø.ØX2	T6Ø.ØX3	T6Ø.ØX4	—	—

Table of Drugs and Chemicals

Substance	Poisoning, Accidental (unintentional)	Poisoning, Intentional Self-harm	Poisoning, Assault	Poisoning, Undetermined	Adverse Effect	Under-dosing
Metrizamide	T50.8X1	T50.8X2	T50.8X3	T50.8X4	T50.8X5	T50.8X6
Metrizoic acid	T50.8X1	T50.8X2	T50.8X3	T50.8X4	T50.8X5	T50.8X6
Metronidazole	T37.8X1	T37.8X2	T37.8X3	T37.8X4	T37.8X5	T37.8X6
Metycaine	T41.3X1	T41.3X2	T41.3X3	T41.3X4	T41.3X5	T41.3X6
infiltration (subcutaneous)	T41.3X1	T41.3X2	T41.3X3	T41.3X4	T41.3X5	T41.3X6
nerve block (peripheral) (plexus)	T41.3X1	T41.3X2	T41.3X3	T41.3X4	T41.3X5	T41.3X6
topical (surface)	T41.3X1	T41.3X2	T41.3X3	T41.3X4	T41.3X5	T41.3X6
Metyrapone	T50.8X1	T50.8X2	T50.8X3	T50.8X4	T50.8X5	T50.8X6
Mevinphos	T60.0X1	T60.0X2	T60.0X3	T60.0X4	—	—
Mexazolam	T42.4X1	T42.4X2	T42.4X3	T42.4X4	T42.4X5	T42.4X6
Mexenone	T49.3X1	T49.3X2	T49.3X3	T49.3X4	T49.3X5	T49.3X6
Mexiletine	T46.2X1	T46.2X2	T46.2X3	T46.2X4	T46.2X5	T46.2X6
Mezereon	T62.2X1	T62.2X2	T62.2X3	T62.2X4	—	—
berries	T62.1X1	T62.1X2	T62.1X3	T62.1X4	—	—
Mezlocillin	T36.0X1	T36.0X2	T36.0X3	T36.0X4	T36.0X5	T36.0X6
Mianserin	T43.021	T43.022	T43.023	T43.024	T43.025	T43.026
Micatin	T49.0X1	T49.0X2	T49.0X3	T49.0X4	T49.0X5	T49.0X6
Miconazole	T49.0X1	T49.0X2	T49.0X3	T49.0X4	T49.0X5	T49.0X6
Micronomicin	T36.5X1	T36.5X2	T36.5X3	T36.5X4	T36.5X5	T36.5X6
Midazolam	T42.4X1	T42.4X2	T42.4X3	T42.4X4	T42.4X5	T42.4X6
Midecamycin	T36.3X1	T36.3X2	T36.3X3	T36.3X4	T36.3X5	T36.3X6
Mifepristone	T38.6X1	T38.6X2	T38.6X3	T38.6X4	T38.6X5	T38.6X6
Milk of magnesia	T47.1X1	T47.1X2	T47.1X3	T47.1X4	T47.1X5	T47.1X6
Millipede (tropical) (venomous)	T63.411	T63.412	T63.413	T63.414	—	—
Miltown	T43.591	T43.592	T43.593	T43.594	T43.595	T43.596
Milverine	T44.3X1	T44.3X2	T44.3X3	T44.3X4	T44.3X5	T44.3X6
Minaprine	T43.291	T43.292	T43.293	T43.294	T43.295	T43.296
Minaxolone	T41.291	T41.292	T41.293	T41.294	T41.295	T41.296
Mineral						
acids	T54.2X1	T54.2X2	T54.2X3	T54.2X4	—	—
oil (laxative)(medicinal)	T47.4X1	T47.4X2	T47.4X3	T47.4X4	T47.4X5	T47.4X6
emulsion	T47.2X1	T47.2X2	T47.2X3	T47.2X4	T47.2X5	T47.2X6
nonmedicinal	T52.0X1	T52.0X2	T52.0X3	T52.0X4	—	—
topical	T49.3X1	T49.3X2	T49.3X3	T49.3X4	T49.3X5	T49.3X6
salt NEC	T50.3X1	T50.3X2	T50.3X3	T50.3X4	T50.3X5	T50.3X6
spirits	T52.0X1	T52.0X2	T52.0X3	T52.0X4	—	—
Mineralocorticosteroid	T50.0X1	T50.0X2	T50.0X3	T50.0X4	T50.0X5	T50.0X6
Minocycline	T36.4X1	T36.4X2	T36.4X3	T36.4X4	T36.4X5	T36.4X6
Minoxidil	T46.7X1	T46.7X2	T46.7X3	T46.7X4	T46.7X5	T46.7X6
Miokamycin	T36.3X1	T36.3X2	T36.3X3	T36.3X4	T36.3X5	T36.3X6
Miotic drug	T49.5X1	T49.5X2	T49.5X3	T49.5X4	T49.5X5	T49.5X6
Mipafox	T60.0X1	T60.0X2	T60.0X3	T60.0X4	—	—
Mirex	T60.1X1	T60.1X2	T60.1X3	T60.1X4	—	—
Mirtazapine	T43.021	T43.022	T43.023	T43.024	T43.025	T43.026
Misonidazole	T37.3X1	T37.3X2	T37.3X3	T37.3X4	T37.3X5	T37.3X6
Misoprostol	T47.1X1	T47.1X2	T47.1X3	T47.1X4	T47.1X5	T47.1X6
Mithramycin	T45.1X1	T45.1X2	T45.1X3	T45.1X4	T45.1X5	T45.1X6
Mitobronitol	T45.1X1	T45.1X2	T45.1X3	T45.1X4	T45.1X5	T45.1X6
Mitoguazone	T45.1X1	T45.1X2	T45.1X3	T45.1X4	T45.1X5	T45.1X6
Mitolactol	T45.1X1	T45.1X2	T45.1X3	T45.1X4	T45.1X5	T45.1X6
Mitomycin	T45.1X1	T45.1X2	T45.1X3	T45.1X4	T45.1X5	T45.1X6
Mitopodozide	T45.1X1	T45.1X2	T45.1X3	T45.1X4	T45.1X5	T45.1X6
Mitotane	T45.1X1	T45.1X2	T45.1X3	T45.1X4	T45.1X5	T45.1X6
Mitoxantrone	T45.1X1	T45.1X2	T45.1X3	T45.1X4	T45.1X5	T45.1X6
Mivacurium chloride	T48.1X1	T48.1X2	T48.1X3	T48.1X4	T48.1X5	T48.1X6
Miyari bacteria	T47.6X1	T47.6X2	T47.6X3	T47.6X4	T47.6X5	T47.6X6
Moclobemide	T43.1X1	T43.1X2	T43.1X3	T43.1X4	T43.1X5	T43.1X6
Moderil	T46.5X1	T46.5X2	T46.5X3	T46.5X4	T46.5X5	T46.5X6
Mofebutazone	T39.2X1	T39.2X2	T39.2X3	T39.2X4	T39.2X5	T39.2X6
Mogadon — see Nitrazepam						
Molindone	T43.591	T43.592	T43.593	T43.594	T43.595	T43.596
Molsidomine	T46.3X1	T46.3X2	T46.3X3	T46.3X4	T46.3X5	T46.3X6
Mometasone	T49.0X1	T49.0X2	T49.0X3	T49.0X4	T49.0X5	T49.0X6
Monistat	T49.0X1	T49.0X2	T49.0X3	T49.0X4	T49.0X5	T49.0X6
Monkshood	T62.2X1	T62.2X2	T62.2X3	T62.2X4	—	—
Monoamine oxidase inhibitor NEC	T43.1X1	T43.1X2	T43.1X3	T43.1X4	T43.1X5	T43.1X6
hydrazine	T43.1X1	T43.1X2	T43.1X3	T43.1X4	T43.1X5	T43.1X6
Monobenzone	T49.4X1	T49.4X2	T49.4X3	T49.4X4	T49.4X5	T49.4X6
Monochloroacetic acid	T60.3X1	T60.3X2	T60.3X3	T60.3X4	—	—
Monochlorobenzene	T53.7X1	T53.7X2	T53.7X3	T53.7X4	—	—
Monoethanolamine	T46.8X1	T46.8X2	T46.8X3	T46.8X4	T46.8X5	T46.8X6
oleate	T46.8X1	T46.8X2	T46.8X3	T46.8X4	T46.8X5	T46.8X6
Monooctanoin	T50.991	T50.992	T50.993	T50.994	T50.995	T50.996
Monophenylbutazone	T39.2X1	T39.2X2	T39.2X3	T39.2X4	T39.2X5	T39.2X6
Monosodium glutamate	T65.891	T65.892	T65.893	T65.894	—	—
Monosulfiram	T49.0X1	T49.0X2	T49.0X3	T49.0X4	T49.0X5	T49.0X6
Monoxide, carbon — see Carbon, monoxide						
Monoxidine hydrochloride	T46.1X1	T46.1X2	T46.1X3	T46.1X4	T46.1X5	T46.1X6
Monuron	T60.3X1	T60.3X2	T60.3X3	T60.3X4	—	—

Substance	Poisoning, Accidental (unintentional)	Poisoning, Intentional Self-harm	Poisoning, Assault	Poisoning, Undetermined	Adverse Effect	Under-dosing
Moperone	T43.4X1	T43.4X2	T43.4X3	T43.4X4	T43.4X5	T43.4X6
Mopidamol	T45.1X1	T45.1X2	T45.1X3	T45.1X4	T45.1X5	T45.1X6
MOPP (mechloreth-amine + vincristine + prednisone + procarba-zine)	T45.1X1	T45.1X2	T45.1X3	T45.1X4	T45.1X5	T45.1X6
Morfin	T40.2X1	T40.2X2	T40.2X3	T40.2X4	T40.2X5	T40.2X6
Morinamide	T37.1X1	T37.1X2	T37.1X3	T37.1X4	T37.1X5	T37.1X6
Morning glory seeds	T40.991	T40.992	T40.993	T40.994		
Moroxydine	T37.5X1	T37.5X2	T37.5X3	T37.5X4	T37.5X5	T37.5X6
Morphazinamide	T37.1X1	T37.1X2	T37.1X3	T37.1X4	T37.1X5	T37.1X6
Morphine	T40.2X1	T40.2X2	T40.2X3	T40.2X4	T40.2X5	T40.2X6
antagonist	T50.7X1	T50.7X2	T50.7X3	T50.7X4	T50.7X5	T50.7X6
Morpholinylethylmorphine	T40.2X1	T40.2X2	T40.2X3	T40.2X4		
Morsuximide	T42.2X1	T42.2X2	T42.2X3	T42.2X4	T42.2X5	T42.2X6
Mosapramine	T43.591	T43.592	T43.593	T43.594	T43.595	T43.596
Moth balls — see also Pesticides	T60.2X1	T60.2X2	T60.2X3	T60.2X4		
naphthalene	T60.2X1	T60.2X2	T60.2X3	T60.2X4	—	—
paradichlorobenzene	T60.1X1	T60.1X2	T60.1X3	T60.1X4	—	—
Motor exhaust gas	T58.01	T58.02	T58.03	T58.04		
Mouthwash (antiseptic) (zinc chloride)	T49.6X1	T49.6X2	T49.6X3	T49.6X4	T49.6X5	T49.6X6
Moxastine	T45.0X1	T45.0X2	T45.0X3	T45.0X4	T45.0X5	T45.0X6
Moxaverine	T44.3X1	T44.3X2	T44.3X3	T44.3X4	T44.3X5	T44.3X6
Moxisylyte	T46.7X1	T46.7X2	T46.7X3	T46.7X4	T46.7X5	T46.7X6
Mucilage, plant	T47.4X1	T47.4X2	T47.4X3	T47.4X4	T47.4X5	T47.4X6
Mucolytic drug	T48.4X1	T48.4X2	T48.4X3	T48.4X4	T48.4X5	T48.4X6
Mucomyst	T48.4X1	T48.4X2	T48.4X3	T48.4X4	T48.4X5	T48.4X6
Mucous membrane agents (external)	T49.91	T49.92	T49.93	T49.94	T49.95	T49.96
specified NEC	T49.8X1	T49.8X2	T49.8X3	T49.8X4	T49.8X5	T49.8X6
Mumps						
immune globulin (human)	T50.Z11	T50.Z12	T50.Z13	T50.Z14	T50.Z15	T50.Z16
skin test antigen	T50.8X1	T50.8X2	T50.8X3	T50.8X4	T50.8X5	T50.8X6
vaccine	T50.B91	T50.B92	T50.B93	T50.B94	T50.B95	T50.B96
Mumpsvax	T50.B91	T50.B92	T50.B93	T50.B94	T50.B95	T50.B96
Mupirocin	T49.0X1	T49.0X2	T49.0X3	T49.0X4	T49.0X5	T49.0X6
Muriatic acid — see Hydrochloric acid						
Muromonab-CD3	T45.1X1	T45.1X2	T45.1X3	T45.1X4	T45.1X5	T45.1X6
Muscle-action drug NEC	T48.201	T48.202	T48.203	T48.204	T48.205	T48.206
Muscle affecting agents NEC	T48.201	T48.202	T48.203	T48.204	T48.205	T48.206
oxytocic	T48.0X1	T48.0X2	T48.0X3	T48.0X4	T48.0X5	T48.0X6
relaxants	T48.201	T48.202	T48.203	T48.204	T48.205	T48.206
central nervous system	T42.8X1	T42.8X2	T42.8X3	T42.8X4	T42.8X5	T42.8X6
skeletal	T48.1X1	T48.1X2	T48.1X3	T48.1X4	T48.1X5	T48.1X6
smooth	T44.3X1	T44.3X2	T44.3X3	T44.3X4	T44.3X5	T44.3X6
Muscle relaxant — see Relaxant, muscle						
Muscle-tone depressant, central NEC	T42.8X1	T42.8X2	T42.8X3	T42.8X4	T42.8X5	T42.8X6
specified NEC	T42.8X1	T42.8X2	T42.8X3	T42.8X4	T42.8X5	T42.8X6
Mushroom, noxious	T62.0X1	T62.0X2	T62.0X3	T62.0X4	—	—
Mussel, noxious	T61.781	T61.782	T61.783	T61.784	—	—
Mustard (emetic)	T47.7X1	T47.7X2	T47.7X3	T47.7X4	T47.7X5	T47.7X6
black	T47.7X1	T47.7X2	T47.7X3	T47.7X4	T47.7X5	T47.7X6
gas, not in war	T59.91	T59.92	T59.93	T59.94		
nitrogen	T45.1X1	T45.1X2	T45.1X3	T45.1X4	T45.1X5	T45.1X6
Mustine	T45.1X1	T45.1X2	T45.1X3	T45.1X4	T45.1X5	T45.1X6
M-vac	T45.1X1	T45.1X2	T45.1X3	T45.1X4	T45.1X5	T45.1X6
Mycifradin	T36.5X1	T36.5X2	T36.5X3	T36.5X4	T36.5X5	T36.5X6
topical	T49.0X1	T49.0X2	T49.0X3	T49.0X4	T49.0X5	T49.0X6
Mycitracin	T36.8X1	T36.8X2	T36.8X3	T36.8X4	T36.8X5	T36.8X6
ophthalmic preparation	T49.5X1	T49.5X2	T49.5X3	T49.5X4	T49.5X5	T49.5X6
Mycostatin	T36.7X1	T36.7X2	T36.7X3	T36.7X4	T36.7X5	T36.7X6
topical	T49.0X1	T49.0X2	T49.0X3	T49.0X4	T49.0X5	T49.0X6
Mycotoxins	T64.81	T64.82	T64.83	T64.84	—	—
aflatoxin	T64.01	T64.02	T64.03	T64.04	—	—
specified NEC	T64.81	T64.82	T64.83	T64.84	—	—
Mydriacyl	T44.3X1	T44.3X2	T44.3X3	T44.3X4	T44.3X5	T44.3X6
Mydriatic drug	T49.5X1	T49.5X2	T49.5X3	T49.5X4	T49.5X5	T49.5X6
Myelobromal	T45.1X1	T45.1X2	T45.1X3	T45.1X4	T45.1X5	T45.1X6
Myleran	T45.1X1	T45.1X2	T45.1X3	T45.1X4	T45.1X5	T45.1X6
Myochrysin (e)	T39.2X1	T39.2X2	T39.2X3	T39.2X4	T39.2X5	T39.2X6
Myoneural blocking agents	T48.1X1	T48.1X2	T48.1X3	T48.1X4	T48.1X5	T48.1X6
Myralact	T49.0X1	T49.0X2	T49.0X3	T49.0X4	T49.0X5	T49.0X6
Myristica fragrans	T62.2X1	T62.2X2	T62.2X3	T62.2X4	—	—
Myristicin	T65.891	T65.892	T65.893	T65.894	—	—
Mysoline	T42.3X1	T42.3X2	T42.3X3	T42.3X4	T42.3X5	T42.3X6
Nabilone	T40.7X1	T40.7X2	T40.7X3	T40.7X4	T40.7X5	T40.7X6
Nabumetone	T39.391	T39.392	T39.393	T39.394	T39.395	T39.396
Nadolol	T44.7X1	T44.7X2	T44.7X3	T44.7X4	T44.7X5	T44.7X6

Metrizamide — Nadolol

Substance	Poisoning, Accidental (unintentional)	Poisoning, Intentional Self-harm	Poisoning, Assault	Poisoning, Undetermined	Adverse Effect	Under-dosing
Nafcillin	T36.ØX1	T36.ØX2	T36.ØX3	T36.ØX4	T36.ØX5	T36.ØX6
Nafoxidine	T38.6X1	T38.6X2	T38.6X3	T38.6X4	T38.6X5	T38.6X6
Naftazone	T46.991	T46.992	T46.993	T46.994	T46.995	T46.996
Naftidrofuryl (oxalate)	T46.7X1	T46.7X2	T46.7X3	T46.7X4	T46.7X5	T46.7X6
Naftifine	T49.ØX1	T49.ØX2	T49.ØX3	T49.ØX4	T49.ØX5	T49.ØX6
Nail polish remover	T52.91	T52.92	T52.93	T52.94	—	—
Nalbuphine	T4Ø.4X1	T4Ø.4X2	T4Ø.4X3	T4Ø.4X4	T4Ø.4X5	T4Ø.4X6
Naled	T6Ø.ØX1	T6Ø.ØX2	T6Ø.ØX3	T6Ø.ØX4	—	—
Nalidixic acid	T37.8X1	T37.8X2	T37.8X3	T37.8X4	T37.8X5	T37.8X6
Nalorphine	T5Ø.7X1	T5Ø.7X2	T5Ø.7X3	T5Ø.7X4	T5Ø.7X5	T5Ø.7X6
Naloxone	T5Ø.7X1	T5Ø.7X2	T5Ø.7X3	T5Ø.7X4	T5Ø.7X5	T5Ø.7X6
Naltrexone	T5Ø.7X1	T5Ø.7X2	T5Ø.7X3	T5Ø.7X4	T5Ø.7X5	T5Ø.7X6
Namenda	T43.8X1	T43.8X2	T43.8X3	T43.8X4	T43.8X5	T43.8X6
Nandrolone	T38.7X1	T38.7X2	T38.7X3	T38.7X4	T38.7X5	T38.7X6
Naphazoline	T48.5X1	T48.5X2	T48.5X3	T48.5X4	T48.5X5	T48.5X6
Naphtha (painters') (petroleum)	T52.ØX1	T52.ØX2	T52.ØX3	T52.ØX4	—	—
solvent	T52.ØX1	T52.ØX2	T52.ØX3	T52.ØX4	—	—
vapor	T52.ØX1	T52.ØX2	T52.ØX3	T52.ØX4	—	—
Naphthalene (non-chlorinated)	T6Ø.2X1	T6Ø.2X2	T6Ø.2X3	T6Ø.2X4	—	—
chlorinated	T6Ø.1X1	T6Ø.1X2	T6Ø.1X3	T6Ø.1X4	—	—
vapor	T6Ø.1X1	T6Ø.1X2	T6Ø.1X3	T6Ø.1X4	—	—
insecticide or moth repellent	T6Ø.2X1	T6Ø.2X2	T6Ø.2X3	T6Ø.2X4	—	—
chlorinated	T6Ø.1X1	T6Ø.1X2	T6Ø.1X3	T6Ø.1X4	—	—
vapor	T6Ø.2X1	T6Ø.2X2	T6Ø.2X3	T6Ø.2X4	—	—
chlorinated	T6Ø.1X1	T6Ø.1X2	T6Ø.1X3	T6Ø.1X4	—	—
Naphthol	T65.891	T65.892	T65.893	T65.894	—	—
Naphthylamine	T65.891	T65.892	T65.893	T65.894	—	—
Naphthylthiourea (ANTU)	T6Ø.4X1	T6Ø.4X2	T6Ø.4X3	T6Ø.4X4	—	—
Naprosyn — *see* Naproxen						
Naproxen	T39.311	T39.312	T39.313	T39.314	T39.315	T39.316
Narcotic (drug)	T4Ø.6Ø1	T4Ø.6Ø2	T4Ø.6Ø3	T4Ø.6Ø4	T4Ø.6Ø5	T4Ø.6Ø6
analgesic NEC	T4Ø.6Ø1	T4Ø.6Ø2	T4Ø.6Ø3	T4Ø.6Ø4	T4Ø.6Ø5	T4Ø.6Ø6
antagonist	T5Ø.7X1	T5Ø.7X2	T5Ø.7X3	T5Ø.7X4	T5Ø.7X5	T5Ø.7X6
specified NEC	T4Ø.691	T4Ø.692	T4Ø.693	T4Ø.694	T4Ø.695	T4Ø.696
synthetic	T4Ø.4X1	T4Ø.4X2	T4Ø.4X3	T4Ø.4X4	T4Ø.4X5	T4Ø.4X6
Narcotine	T48.3X1	T48.3X2	T48.3X3	T48.3X4	T48.3X5	T48.3X6
Nardil	T43.1X1	T43.1X2	T43.1X3	T43.1X4	T43.1X5	T43.1X6
Nasal drug NEC	T49.6X1	T49.6X2	T49.6X3	T49.6X4	T49.6X5	T49.6X6
Natamycin	T49.ØX1	T49.ØX2	T49.ØX3	T49.ØX4	T49.ØX5	T49.ØX6
Natrium cyanide — *see* Cyanide(s)						
Natural						
blood (product)	T45.8X1	T45.8X2	T45.8X3	T45.8X4	T45.8X5	T45.8X6
gas (piped)	T59.891	T59.892	T59.893	T59.894	—	—
incomplete combustion	T58.11	T58.12	T58.13	T58.14	—	—
Nealbarbital	T42.3X1	T42.3X2	T42.3X3	T42.3X4	T42.3X5	T42.3X6
Nectadon	T48.3X1	T48.3X2	T48.3X3	T48.3X4	T48.3X5	T48.3X6
Nedocromil	T48.6X1	T48.6X2	T48.6X3	T48.6X4	T48.6X5	T48.6X6
Nefopam	T39.8X1	T39.8X2	T39.8X3	T39.8X4	T39.8X5	T39.8X6
Nematocyst (sting)	T63.691	T63.692	T63.693	T63.694	—	—
Nembutal	T42.3X1	T42.3X2	T42.3X3	T42.3X4	T42.3X5	T42.3X6
Nemonapride	T43.591	T43.592	T43.593	T43.594	T43.595	T43.596
Neoarsphenamine	T37.8X1	T37.8X2	T37.8X3	T37.8X4	T37.8X5	T37.8X6
Neocinchophen	T5Ø.4X1	T5Ø.4X2	T5Ø.4X3	T5Ø.4X4	T5Ø.4X5	T5Ø.4X6
Neomycin (derivatives)	T36.5X1	T36.5X2	T36.5X3	T36.5X4	T36.5X5	T36.5X6
with						
bacitracin	T49.ØX1	T49.ØX2	T49.ØX3	T49.ØX4	T49.ØX5	T49.ØX6
neostigmine	T44.ØX1	T44.ØX2	T44.ØX3	T44.ØX4	T44.ØX5	T44.ØX6
ENT agent	T49.6X1	T49.6X2	T49.6X3	T49.6X4	T49.6X5	T49.6X6
ophthalmic preparation	T49.5X1	T49.5X2	T49.5X3	T49.5X4	T49.5X5	T49.5X6
topical NEC	T49.ØX1	T49.ØX2	T49.ØX3	T49.ØX4	T49.ØX5	T49.ØX6
Neonal	T42.3X1	T42.3X2	T42.3X3	T42.3X4	T42.3X5	T42.3X6
Neoprontosil	T37.ØX1	T37.ØX2	T37.ØX3	T37.ØX4	T37.ØX5	T37.ØX6
Neosalvarsan	T37.8X1	T37.8X2	T37.8X3	T37.8X4	T37.8X5	T37.8X6
Neosilversalvarsan	T37.8X1	T37.8X2	T37.8X3	T37.8X4	T37.8X5	T37.8X6
Neosporin	T36.8X1	T36.8X2	T36.8X3	T36.8X4	T36.8X5	T36.8X6
ENT agent	T49.6X1	T49.6X2	T49.6X3	T49.6X4	T49.6X5	T49.6X6
opthalmic preparation	T49.5X1	T49.5X2	T49.5X3	T49.5X4	T49.5X5	T49.5X6
topical NEC	T49.ØX1	T49.ØX2	T49.ØX3	T49.ØX4	T49.ØX5	T49.ØX6
Neostigmine bromide	T44.ØX1	T44.ØX2	T44.ØX3	T44.ØX4	T44.ØX5	T44.ØX6
Neraval	T42.3X1	T42.3X2	T42.3X3	T42.3X4	T42.3X5	T42.3X6
Neravan	T42.3X1	T42.3X2	T42.3X3	T42.3X4	T42.3X5	T42.3X6
Nerium oleander	T62.2X1	T62.2X2	T62.2X3	T62.2X4	—	—
Nerve gas, not in war	T59.91	T59.92	T59.93	T59.94	—	—
Nesacaine	T41.3X1	T41.3X2	T41.3X3	T41.3X4	T41.3X5	T41.3X6
infiltration (subcutaneous)	T41.3X1	T41.3X2	T41.3X3	T41.3X4	T41.3X5	T41.3X6
nerve block (peripheral) (plexus)	T41.3X1	T41.3X2	T41.3X3	T41.3X4	T41.3X5	T41.3X6
Netilmicin	T36.5X1	T36.5X2	T36.5X3	T36.5X4	T36.5X5	T36.5X6
Neurobarb	T42.3X1	T42.3X2	T42.3X3	T42.3X4	T42.3X5	T42.3X6

Substance	Poisoning, Accidental (unintentional)	Poisoning, Intentional Self-harm	Poisoning, Assault	Poisoning, Undetermined	Adverse Effect	Under-dosing
Neuroleptic drug NEC	T43.5Ø1	T43.5Ø2	T43.5Ø3	T43.5Ø4	T43.5Ø5	T43.5Ø6
Neuromuscular blocking drug	T48.1X1	T48.1X2	T48.1X3	T48.1X4	T48.1X5	T48.1X6
Neutral insulin injection	T38.3X1	T38.3X2	T38.3X3	T38.3X4	T38.3X5	T38.3X6
Neutral spirits	T51.ØX1	T51.ØX2	T51.ØX3	T51.ØX4	—	—
beverage	T51.ØX1	T51.ØX2	T51.ØX3	T51.ØX4	—	—
Niacin	T46.7X1	T46.7X2	T46.7X3	T46.7X4	T46.7X5	T46.7X6
Niacinamide	T45.2X1	T45.2X2	T45.2X3	T45.2X4	T45.2X5	T45.2X6
Nialamide	T43.1X1	T43.1X2	T43.1X3	T43.1X4	T43.1X5	T43.1X6
Niaprazine	T42.6X1	T42.6X2	T42.6X3	T42.6X4	T42.6X5	T42.6X6
Nicametate	T46.7X1	T46.7X2	T46.7X3	T46.7X4	T46.7X5	T46.7X6
Nicardipine	T46.1X1	T46.1X2	T46.1X3	T46.1X4	T46.1X5	T46.1X6
Nicergoline	T46.7X1	T46.7X2	T46.7X3	T46.7X4	T46.7X5	T46.7X6
Nickel (carbonyl) (tetra-carbonyl) (fumes) (vapor)	T56.891	T56.892	T56.893	T56.894	—	—
Nickelocene	T56.891	T56.892	T56.893	T56.894	—	—
Niclosamide	T37.4X1	T37.4X2	T37.4X3	T37.4X4	T37.4X5	T37.4X6
Nicofuranose	T46.7X1	T46.7X2	T46.7X3	T46.7X4	T46.7X5	T46.7X6
Nicomorphine	T4Ø.2X1	T4Ø.2X2	T4Ø.2X3	T4Ø.2X4	—	—
Nicorandil	T46.3X1	T46.3X2	T46.3X3	T46.3X4	T46.3X5	T46.3X6
Nicotiana (plant)	T62.2X1	T62.2X2	T62.2X3	T62.2X4	—	—
Nicotinamide	T45.2X1	T45.2X2	T45.2X3	T45.2X4	T45.2X5	T45.2X6
Nicotine (insecticide) (spray) (sulfate) **NEC**	T6Ø.2X1	T6Ø.2X2	T6Ø.2X3	T6Ø.2X4	—	—
from tobacco	T65.291	T65.292	T65.293	T65.294	—	—
cigarettes	T65.221	T65.222	T65.223	T65.224	—	—
not insecticide	T65.291	T65.292	T65.293	T65.294	—	—
Nicotinic acid	T46.7X1	T46.7X2	T46.7X3	T46.7X4	T46.7X5	T46.7X6
Nicotinyl alcohol	T46.7X1	T46.7X2	T46.7X3	T46.7X4	T46.7X5	T46.7X6
Nicoumalone	T45.511	T45.512	T45.513	T45.514	T45.515	T45.516
Nifedipine	T46.1X1	T46.1X2	T46.1X3	T46.1X4	T46.1X5	T46.1X6
Nifenazone	T39.2X1	T39.2X2	T39.2X3	T39.2X4	T39.2X5	T39.2X6
Nifuraldezone	T37.91	T37.92	T37.93	T37.94	T37.95	T37.96
Nifuratel	T37.8X1	T37.8X2	T37.8X3	T37.8X4	T37.8X5	T37.8X6
Nifurtimox	T37.3X1	T37.3X2	T37.3X3	T37.3X4	T37.3X5	T37.3X6
Nifurtoinol	T37.8X1	T37.8X2	T37.8X3	T37.8X4	T37.8X5	T37.8X6
Nightshade, deadly (solanum) — *see also* Belladonna	T62.2X1	T62.2X2	T62.2X3	T62.2X4	—	—
berry	T62.1X1	T62.1X2	T62.1X3	T62.1X4	—	—
Nikethamide	T5Ø.7X1	T5Ø.7X2	T5Ø.7X3	T5Ø.7X4	T5Ø.7X5	T5Ø.7X6
Nilstat	T36.7X1	T36.7X2	T36.7X3	T36.7X4	T36.7X5	T36.7X6
topical	T49.ØX1	T49.ØX2	T49.ØX3	T49.ØX4	T49.ØX5	T49.ØX6
Nilutamide	T38.6X1	T38.6X2	T38.6X3	T38.6X4	T38.6X5	T38.6X6
Nimesulide	T39.391	T39.392	T39.393	T39.394	T39.395	T39.396
Nimetazepam	T42.4X1	T42.4X2	T42.4X3	T42.4X4	T42.4X5	T42.4X6
Nimodipine	T46.1X1	T46.1X2	T46.1X3	T46.1X4	T46.1X5	T46.1X6
Nimorazole	T37.3X1	T37.3X2	T37.3X3	T37.3X4	T37.3X5	T37.3X6
Nimustine	T45.1X1	T45.1X2	T45.1X3	T45.1X4	T45.1X5	T45.1X6
Niridazole	T37.4X1	T37.4X2	T37.4X3	T37.4X4	T37.4X5	T37.4X6
Nisentil	T4Ø.2X1	T4Ø.2X2	T4Ø.2X3	T4Ø.2X4	T4Ø.2X5	T4Ø.2X6
Nisoldipine	T46.1X1	T46.1X2	T46.1X3	T46.1X4	T46.1X5	T46.1X6
Nitramine	T65.3X1	T65.3X2	T65.3X3	T65.3X4	—	—
Nitrate, organic	T46.3X1	T46.3X2	T46.3X3	T46.3X4	T46.3X5	T46.3X6
Nitrazepam	T42.4X1	T42.4X2	T42.4X3	T42.4X4	T42.4X5	T42.4X6
Nitrefazole	T5Ø.6X1	T5Ø.6X2	T5Ø.6X3	T5Ø.6X4	T5Ø.6X5	T5Ø.6X6
Nitrendipine	T46.1X1	T46.1X2	T46.1X3	T46.1X4	T46.1X5	T46.1X6
Nitric						
acid (liquid)	T54.2X1	T54.2X2	T54.2X3	T54.2X4	—	—
vapor	T59.891	T59.892	T59.893	T59.894	—	—
oxide (gas)	T59.ØX1	T59.ØX2	T59.ØX3	T59.ØX4	—	—
Nitrimidazine	T37.3X1	T37.3X2	T37.3X3	T37.3X4	T37.3X5	T37.3X6
Nitrite, amyl (medicinal) (vapor)	T46.3X1	T46.3X2	T46.3X3	T46.3X4	T46.3X5	T46.3X6
Nitroaniline	T65.3X1	T65.3X2	T65.3X3	T65.3X4	—	—
vapor	T59.891	T59.892	T59.893	T59.894	—	—
Nitrobenzene, nitrobenzol	T65.3X1	T65.3X2	T65.3X3	T65.3X4	—	—
vapor	T65.3X1	T65.3X2	T65.3X3	T65.3X4	—	—
Nitrocellulose	T65.891	T65.892	T65.893	T65.894	—	—
lacquer	T65.891	T65.892	T65.893	T65.894	—	—
Nitrodiphenyl	T65.3X1	T65.3X2	T65.3X3	T65.3X4	—	—
Nitrofural	T49.ØX1	T49.ØX2	T49.ØX3	T49.ØX4	T49.ØX5	T49.ØX6
Nitrofurantoin	T37.8X1	T37.8X2	T37.8X3	T37.8X4	T37.8X5	T37.8X6
Nitrofurazone	T49.ØX1	T49.ØX2	T49.ØX3	T49.ØX4	T49.ØX5	T49.ØX6
Nitrogen	T59.ØX1	T59.ØX2	T59.ØX3	T59.ØX4	—	—
mustard	T45.1X1	T45.1X2	T45.1X3	T45.1X4	T45.1X5	T45.1X6
Nitroglycerin, nitroglycerol (medicinal)	T46.3X1	T46.3X2	T46.3X3	T46.3X4	T46.3X5	T46.3X6
nonmedicinal	T65.5X1	T65.5X2	T65.5X3	T65.5X4	—	—
fumes	T65.5X1	T65.5X2	T65.5X3	T65.5X4	—	—
Nitroglycol	T52.3X1	T52.3X2	T52.3X3	T52.3X4	—	—
Nitrohydrochloric acid	T54.2X1	T54.2X2	T54.2X3	T54.2X4	—	—
Nitromersol	T49.ØX1	T49.ØX2	T49.ØX3	T49.ØX4	T49.ØX5	T49.ØX6
Nitronaphthalene	T65.891	T65.892	T65.893	T65.894	—	—

Substance	Poisoning, Accidental (unintentional)	Poisoning, Intentional Self-harm	Poisoning, Assault	Poisoning, Undetermined	Adverse Effect	Under-dosing
Nitrophenol	T54.ØX1	T54.ØX2	T54.ØX3	T54.ØX4	—	—
Nitropropane	T52.8X1	T52.8X2	T52.8X3	T52.8X4	—	—
Nitroprusside	T46.5X1	T46.5X2	T46.5X3	T46.5X4	T46.5X5	T46.5X6
Nitrosodimethylamine	T65.3X1	T65.3X2	T65.3X3	T65.3X4	—	—
Nitrothiazol	T37.4X1	T37.4X2	T37.4X3	T37.4X4	T37.4X5	T37.4X6
Nitrotoluene, nitrotoluol	T65.3X1	T65.3X2	T65.3X3	T65.3X4	—	—
vapor	T65.3X1	T65.3X2	T65.3X3	T65.3X4	—	—
Nitrous						
acid (liquid)	T54.2X1	T54.2X2	T54.2X3	T54.2X4	—	—
fumes	T59.891	T59.892	T59.893	T59.894	—	—
ether spirit	T46.3X1	T46.3X2	T46.3X3	T46.3X4	T46.3X5	T46.3X6
oxide	T41.ØX1	T41.ØX2	T41.ØX3	T41.ØX4	T41.ØX5	T41.ØX6
Nitroxoline	T37.8X1	T37.8X2	T37.8X3	T37.8X4	T37.8X5	T37.8X6
Nitrozone	T49.ØX1	T49.ØX2	T49.ØX3	T49.ØX4	T49.ØX5	T49.ØX6
Nizatidine	T47.ØX1	T47.ØX2	T47.ØX3	T47.ØX4	T47.ØX5	T47.ØX6
Nizofenone	T43.8X1	T43.8X2	T43.8X3	T43.8X4	T43.8X5	T43.8X6
Noctec	T42.6X1	T42.6X2	T42.6X3	T42.6X4	T42.6X5	T42.6X6
Noludar	T42.6X1	T42.6X2	T42.6X3	T42.6X4	T42.6X5	T42.6X6
Nomegestrol	T38.5X1	T38.5X2	T38.5X3	T38.5X4	T38.5X5	T38.5X6
Nomifensine	T43.291	T43.292	T43.293	T43.294	T43.295	T43.296
Nonoxinol	T49.8X1	T49.8X2	T49.8X3	T49.8X4	T49.8X5	T49.8X6
Nonylphenoxy (polyethoxyethanol)	T49.8X1	T49.8X2	T49.8X3	T49.8X4	T49.8X5	T49.8X6
Noptil	T42.3X1	T42.3X2	T42.3X3	T42.3X4	T42.3X5	T42.3X6
Noradrenaline	T44.4X1	T44.4X2	T44.4X3	T44.4X4	T44.4X5	T44.4X6
Noramidopyrine	T39.2X1	T39.2X2	T39.2X3	T39.2X4	T39.2X5	T39.2X6
methanesulfonate sodium	T39.2X1	T39.2X2	T39.2X3	T39.2X4	T39.2X5	T39.2X6
Norbormide	T6Ø.4X1	T6Ø.4X2	T6Ø.4X3	T6Ø.4X4	—	—
Nordazepam	T42.4X1	T42.4X2	T42.4X3	T42.4X4	T42.4X5	T42.4X6
Norepinephrine	T44.4X1	T44.4X2	T44.4X3	T44.4X4	T44.4X5	T44.4X6
Norethandrolone	T38.7X1	T38.7X2	T38.7X3	T38.7X4	T38.7X5	T38.7X6
Norethindrone	T38.4X1	T38.4X2	T38.4X3	T38.4X4	T38.4X5	T38.4X6
Norethisterone (acetate) (enantate)	T38.4X1	T38.4X2	T38.4X3	T38.4X4	T38.4X5	T38.4X6
with ethinylestradiol	T38.5X1	T38.5X2	T38.5X3	T38.5X4	T38.5X5	T38.5X6
Noretynodrel	T38.5X1	T38.5X2	T38.5X3	T38.5X4	T38.5X5	T38.5X6
Norfenefrine	T44.4X1	T44.4X2	T44.4X3	T44.4X4	T44.4X5	T44.4X6
Norfloxacin	T36.8X1	T36.8X2	T36.8X3	T36.8X4	T36.8X5	T36.8X6
Norgestrel	T38.4X1	T38.4X2	T38.4X3	T38.4X4	T38.4X5	T38.4X6
Norgestrienone	T38.4X1	T38.4X2	T38.4X3	T38.4X4	T38.4X5	T38.4X6
Norlestrin	T38.4X1	T38.4X2	T38.4X3	T38.4X4	T38.4X5	T38.4X6
Norlutin	T38.4X1	T38.4X2	T38.4X3	T38.4X4	T38.4X5	T38.4X6
Normal serum albumin (human), salt-poor	T45.8X1	T45.8X2	T45.8X3	T45.8X4	T45.8X5	T45.8X6
Normethandrone	T38.5X1	T38.5X2	T38.5X3	T38.5X4	T38.5X5	T38.5X6
Normison — *see* Benzodiazepines						
Normorphine	T4Ø.2X1	T4Ø.2X2	T4Ø.2X3	T4Ø.2X4	—	—
Norpseudoephedrine	T5Ø.5X1	T5Ø.5X2	T5Ø.5X3	T5Ø.5X4	T5Ø.5X5	T5Ø.5X6
Nortestosterone (furanpropionate)	T38.7X1	T38.7X2	T38.7X3	T38.7X4	T38.7X5	T38.7X6
Nortriptyline	T43.Ø11	T43.Ø12	T43.Ø13	T43.Ø14	T43.Ø15	T43.Ø16
Noscapine	T48.3X1	T48.3X2	T48.3X3	T48.3X4	T48.3X5	T48.3X6
Nose preparations	T49.6X1	T49.6X2	T49.6X3	T49.6X4	T49.6X5	T49.6X6
Novobiocin	T36.5X1	T36.5X2	T36.5X3	T36.5X4	T36.5X5	T36.5X6
Novocain (infiltration) (topical)	T41.3X1	T41.3X2	T41.3X3	T41.3X4	T41.3X5	T41.3X6
nerve block (peripheral) (plexus)	T41.3X1	T41.3X2	T41.3X3	T41.3X4	T41.3X5	T41.3X6
spinal	T41.3X1	T41.3X2	T41.3X3	T41.3X4	T41.3X5	T41.3X6
Noxious foodstuff	T62.91	T62.92	T62.93	T62.94	—	—
specified NEC	T62.8X1	T62.8X2	T62.8X3	T62.8X4	—	—
Noxiptiline	T43.Ø11	T43.Ø12	T43.Ø13	T43.Ø14	T43.Ø15	T43.Ø16
Noxytiolin	T49.ØX1	T49.ØX2	T49.ØX3	T49.ØX4	T49.ØX5	T49.ØX6
NPH Iletin (insulin)	T38.3X1	T38.3X2	T38.3X3	T38.3X4	T38.3X5	T38.3X6
Numorphan	T4Ø.2X1	T4Ø.2X2	T4Ø.2X3	T4Ø.2X4	T4Ø.2X5	T4Ø.2X6
Nunol	T42.3X1	T42.3X2	T42.3X3	T42.3X4	T42.3X5	T42.3X6
Nupercaine (spinal anesthetic)	T41.3X1	T41.3X2	T41.3X3	T41.3X4	T41.3X5	T41.3X6
topical (surface)	T41.3X1	T41.3X2	T41.3X3	T41.3X4	T41.3X5	T41.3X6
Nutmeg oil (liniment)	T49.3X1	T49.3X2	T49.3X3	T49.3X4	T49.3X5	T49.3X6
Nutritional supplement	T5Ø.9Ø1	T5Ø.9Ø2	T5Ø.9Ø3	T5Ø.9Ø4	T5Ø.9Ø5	T5Ø.9Ø6
Nux vomica	T65.1X1	T65.1X2	T65.1X3	T65.1X4	—	—
Nydrazid	T37.1X1	T37.1X2	T37.1X3	T37.1X4	T37.1X5	T37.1X6
Nylidrin	T46.7X1	T46.7X2	T46.7X3	T46.7X4	T46.7X5	T46.7X6
Nystatin	T36.7X1	T36.7X2	T36.7X3	T36.7X4	T36.7X5	T36.7X6
topical	T49.ØX1	T49.ØX2	T49.ØX3	T49.ØX4	T49.ØX5	T49.ØX6
Nytol	T45.ØX1	T45.ØX2	T45.ØX3	T45.ØX4	T45.ØX5	T45.ØX6
Obidoxime chloride	T5Ø.6X1	T5Ø.6X2	T5Ø.6X3	T5Ø.6X4	T5Ø.6X5	T5Ø.6X6
Octafonium (chloride)	T49.3X1	T49.3X2	T49.3X3	T49.3X4	T49.3X5	T49.3X6
Octamethyl pyrophosphoramide	T6Ø.ØX1	T6Ø.ØX2	T6Ø.ØX3	T6Ø.ØX4	—	—
Octanoin	T5Ø.991	T5Ø.992	T5Ø.993	T5Ø.994	T5Ø.995	T5Ø.996

Substance	Poisoning, Accidental (unintentional)	Poisoning, Intentional Self-harm	Poisoning, Assault	Poisoning, Undetermined	Adverse Effect	Under-dosing
Octatropine methylbromide	T44.3X1	T44.3X2	T44.3X3	T44.3X4	T44.3X5	T44.3X6
Octotiamine	T45.2X1	T45.2X2	T45.2X3	T45.2X4	T45.2X5	T45.2X6
Octoxinol (9)	T49.8X1	T49.8X2	T49.8X3	T49.8X4	T49.8X5	T49.8X6
Octreotide	T38.991	T38.992	T38.993	T38.994	T38.995	T38.996
Octyl nitrite	T46.3X1	T46.3X2	T46.3X3	T46.3X4	T46.3X5	T46.3X6
Oestradiol	T38.5X1	T38.5X2	T38.5X3	T38.5X4	T38.5X5	T38.5X6
Oestriol	T38.5X1	T38.5X2	T38.5X3	T38.5X4	T38.5X5	T38.5X6
Oestrogen	T38.5X1	T38.5X2	T38.5X3	T38.5X4	T38.5X5	T38.5X6
Oestrone	T38.5X1	T38.5X2	T38.5X3	T38.5X4	T38.5X5	T38.5X6
Ofloxacin	T36.8X1	T36.8X2	T36.8X3	T36.8X4	T36.8X5	T36.8X6
Oil (of)	T65.891	T65.892	T65.893	T65.894	—	—
bitter almond	T62.8X1	T62.8X2	T62.8X3	T62.8X4	—	—
cloves	T49.7X1	T49.7X2	T49.7X3	T49.7X4	T49.7X5	T49.7X6
colors	T65.6X1	T65.6X2	T65.6X3	T65.6X4	—	—
fumes	T59.891	T59.892	T59.893	T59.894	—	—
lubricating	T52.ØX1	T52.ØX2	T52.ØX3	T52.ØX4	—	—
Niobe	T52.8X1	T52.8X2	T52.8X3	T52.8X4	—	—
vitriol (liquid)	T54.2X1	T54.2X2	T54.2X3	T54.2X4	—	—
fumes	T54.2X1	T54.2X2	T54.2X3	T54.2X4	—	—
wintergreen (bitter) NEC	T49.3X1	T49.3X2	T49.3X3	T49.3X4	T49.3X5	T49.3X6
Oily preparation (for skin)	T49.3X1	T49.3X2	T49.3X3	T49.3X4	T49.3X5	T49.3X6
Ointment NEC	T49.3X1	T49.3X2	T49.3X3	T49.3X4	T49.3X5	T49.3X6
Olanzapine	T43.591	T43.592	T43.593	T43.594	T43.595	T43.596
Oleander	T62.2X1	T62.2X2	T62.2X3	T62.2X4	—	—
Oleandomycin	T36.3X1	T36.3X2	T36.3X3	T36.3X4	T36.3X5	T36.3X6
Oleandrin	T46.ØX1	T46.ØX2	T46.ØX3	T46.ØX4	T46.ØX5	T46.ØX6
Oleic acid	T46.6X1	T46.6X2	T46.6X3	T46.6X4	T46.6X5	T46.6X6
Oleovitamin A	T45.2X1	T45.2X2	T45.2X3	T45.2X4	T45.2X5	T45.2X6
Oleum ricini	T47.2X1	T47.2X2	T47.2X3	T47.2X4	T47.2X5	T47.2X6
Olive oil (medicinal) **NEC**	T47.4X1	T47.4X2	T47.4X3	T47.4X4	T47.4X5	T47.4X6
Olivomycin	T45.1X1	T45.1X2	T45.1X3	T45.1X4	T45.1X5	T45.1X6
Olsalazine	T47.8X1	T47.8X2	T47.8X3	T47.8X4	T47.8X5	T47.8X6
Omeprazole	T47.1X1	T47.1X2	T47.1X3	T47.1X4	T47.1X5	T47.1X6
OMPA	T6Ø.ØX1	T6Ø.ØX2	T6Ø.ØX3	T6Ø.ØX4	—	—
Oncovin	T45.1X1	T45.1X2	T45.1X3	T45.1X4	T45.1X5	T45.1X6
Ondansetron	T45.ØX1	T45.ØX2	T45.ØX3	T45.ØX4	T45.ØX5	T45.ØX6
Ophthaine	T41.3X1	T41.3X2	T41.3X3	T41.3X4	T41.3X5	T41.3X6
Ophthetic	T41.3X1	T41.3X2	T41.3X3	T41.3X4	T41.3X5	T41.3X6
Opiate NEC	T4Ø.6Ø1	T4Ø.6Ø2	T4Ø.6Ø3	T4Ø.6Ø4	T4Ø.6Ø5	T4Ø.6Ø6
antagonists	T5Ø.7X1	T5Ø.7X2	T5Ø.7X3	T5Ø.7X4	T5Ø.7X5	T5Ø.7X6
Opioid NEC	T4Ø.2X1	T4Ø.2X2	T4Ø.2X3	T4Ø.2X4	T4Ø.2X5	T4Ø.2X6
Opipramol	T43.Ø11	T43.Ø12	T43.Ø13	T43.Ø14	T43.Ø15	T43.Ø16
Opium alkaloids (total)	T4Ø.ØX1	T4Ø.ØX2	T4Ø.ØX3	T4Ø.ØX4	T4Ø.ØX5	T4Ø.ØX6
standardized powdered	T4Ø.ØX1	T4Ø.ØX2	T4Ø.ØX3	T4Ø.ØX4	T4Ø.ØX5	T4Ø.ØX6
tincture (camphorated)	T4Ø.ØX1	T4Ø.ØX2	T4Ø.ØX3	T4Ø.ØX4	T4Ø.ØX5	T4Ø.ØX6
Oracon	T38.4X1	T38.4X2	T38.4X3	T38.4X4	T38.4X5	T38.4X6
Oragrafin	T5Ø.8X1	T5Ø.8X2	T5Ø.8X3	T5Ø.8X4	T5Ø.8X5	T5Ø.8X6
Oral contraceptives	T38.4X1	T38.4X2	T38.4X3	T38.4X4	T38.4X5	T38.4X6
Oral rehydration salts	T5Ø.3X1	T5Ø.3X2	T5Ø.3X3	T5Ø.3X4	T5Ø.3X5	T5Ø.3X6
Orazamide	T5Ø.991	T5Ø.992	T5Ø.993	T5Ø.994	T5Ø.995	T5Ø.996
Orciprenaline	T48.291	T48.292	T48.293	T48.294	T48.295	T48.296
Organidin	T48.4X1	T48.4X2	T48.4X3	T48.4X4	T48.4X5	T48.4X6
Organonitrate NEC	T46.3X1	T46.3X2	T46.3X3	T46.3X4	T46.3X5	T46.3X6
Organophosphates	T6Ø.ØX1	T6Ø.ØX2	T6Ø.ØX3	T6Ø.ØX4	—	—
Orimune	T5Ø.B91	T5Ø.B92	T5Ø.B93	T5Ø.B94	T5Ø.B95	T5Ø.B96
Orinase	T38.3X1	T38.3X2	T38.3X3	T38.3X4	T38.3X5	T38.3X6
Ormeloxifene	T38.6X1	T38.6X2	T38.6X3	T38.6X4	T38.6X5	T38.6X6
Ornidazole	T37.3X1	T37.3X2	T37.3X3	T37.3X4	T37.3X5	T37.3X6
Ornithine aspartate	T5Ø.991	T5Ø.992	T5Ø.993	T5Ø.994	T5Ø.995	T5Ø.996
Ornoprostil	T47.1X1	T47.1X2	T47.1X3	T47.1X4	T47.1X5	T47.1X6
Orphenadrine (hydrochloride)	T42.8X1	T42.8X2	T42.8X3	T42.8X4	T42.8X5	T42.8X6
Ortal (sodium)	T42.3X1	T42.3X2	T42.3X3	T42.3X4	T42.3X5	T42.3X6
Orthoboric acid	T49.ØX1	T49.ØX2	T49.ØX3	T49.ØX4	T49.ØX5	T49.ØX6
ENT agent	T49.6X1	T49.6X2	T49.6X3	T49.6X4	T49.6X5	T49.6X6
ophthalmic preparation	T49.5X1	T49.5X2	T49.5X3	T49.5X4	T49.5X5	T49.5X6
Orthocaine	T41.3X1	T41.3X2	T41.3X3	T41.3X4	T41.3X5	T41.3X6
Orthodichlorobenzene	T53.7X1	T53.7X2	T53.7X3	T53.7X4	—	—
Ortho-Novum	T38.4X1	T38.4X2	T38.4X3	T38.4X4	T38.4X5	T38.4X6
Orthotolidine (reagent)	T54.2X1	T54.2X2	T54.2X3	T54.2X4	—	—
Osmic acid (liquid)	T54.2X1	T54.2X2	T54.2X3	T54.2X4	—	—
fumes	T54.2X1	T54.2X2	T54.2X3	T54.2X4	—	—
Osmotic diuretics	T5Ø.2X1	T5Ø.2X2	T5Ø.2X3	T5Ø.2X4	T5Ø.2X5	T5Ø.2X6
Otilonium bromide	T44.3X1	T44.3X2	T44.3X3	T44.3X4	T44.3X5	T44.3X6
Otorhinolaryngological drug NEC	T49.6X1	T49.6X2	T49.6X3	T49.6X4	T49.6X5	T49.6X6
Ouabain (e)	T46.ØX1	T46.ØX2	T46.ØX3	T46.ØX4	T46.ØX5	T46.ØX6
Ovarian						
hormone	T38.5X1	T38.5X2	T38.5X3	T38.5X4	T38.5X5	T38.5X6
stimulant	T38.5X1	T38.5X2	T38.5X3	T38.5X4	T38.5X5	T38.5X6
Ovral	T38.4X1	T38.4X2	T38.4X3	T38.4X4	T38.4X5	T38.4X6
Ovulen	T38.4X1	T38.4X2	T38.4X3	T38.4X4	T38.4X5	T38.4X6

Subterms under main terms may continue to next column or page Additional Character May Be Required — Refer to the Tabular List for Character Selection 371

Substance	Poisoning, Accidental (unintentional)	Poisoning, Intentional Self-harm	Poisoning, Assault	Poisoning, Undetermined	Adverse Effect	Under-dosing
Oxacillin	T36.ØX1	T36.ØX2	T36.ØX3	T36.ØX4	T36.ØX5	T36.ØX6
Oxalic acid	T54.2X1	T54.2X2	T54.2X3	T54.2X4	—	—
ammonium salt	T5Ø.991	T5Ø.992	T5Ø.993	T5Ø.994	T5Ø.995	T5Ø.996
Oxamniquine	T37.4X1	T37.4X2	T37.4X3	T37.4X4	T37.4X5	T37.4X6
Oxanamide	T43.591	T43.592	T43.593	T43.594	T43.595	T43.596
Oxandrolone	T38.7X1	T38.7X2	T38.7X3	T38.7X4	T38.7X5	T38.7X6
Oxantel	T37.4X1	T37.4X2	T37.4X3	T37.4X4	T37.4X5	T37.4X6
Oxapium iodide	T44.3X1	T44.3X2	T44.3X3	T44.3X4	T44.3X5	T44.3X6
Oxaprotiline	T43.Ø21	T43.Ø22	T43.Ø23	T43.Ø24	T43.Ø25	T43.Ø26
Oxaprozin	T39.311	T39.312	T39.313	T39.314	T39.315	T39.316
Oxatomide	T45.ØX1	T45.ØX2	T45.ØX3	T45.ØX4	T45.ØX5	T45.ØX6
Oxazepam	T42.4X1	T42.4X2	T42.4X3	T42.4X4	T42.4X5	T42.4X6
Oxazimedrine	T5Ø.5X1	T5Ø.5X2	T5Ø.5X3	T5Ø.5X4	T5Ø.5X5	T5Ø.5X6
Oxazolam	T42.4X1	T42.4X2	T42.4X3	T42.4X4	T42.4X5	T42.4X6
Oxazolidine derivatives	T42.2X1	T42.2X2	T42.2X3	T42.2X4	T42.2X5	T42.2X6
Oxazolidinedione (derivative)	T42.2X1	T42.2X2	T42.2X3	T42.2X4	T42.2X5	T42.2X6
Ox bile extract	T47.5X1	T47.5X2	T47.5X3	T47.5X4	T47.5X5	T47.5X6
Oxcarbazepine	T42.1X1	T42.1X2	T42.1X3	T42.1X4	T42.1X5	T42.1X6
Oxedrine	T44.4X1	T44.4X2	T44.4X3	T44.4X4	T44.4X5	T44.4X6
Oxeladin (citrate)	T48.3X1	T48.3X2	T48.3X3	T48.3X4	T48.3X5	T48.3X6
Oxendolone	T38.5X1	T38.5X2	T38.5X3	T38.5X4	T38.5X5	T38.5X6
Oxetacaine	T41.3X1	T41.3X2	T41.3X3	T41.3X4	T41.3X5	T41.3X6
Oxethazine	T41.3X1	T41.3X2	T41.3X3	T41.3X4	T41.3X5	T41.3X6
Oxetorone	T39.8X1	T39.8X2	T39.8X3	T39.8X4	T39.8X5	T39.8X6
Oxiconazole	T49.ØX1	T49.ØX2	T49.ØX3	T49.ØX4	T49.ØX5	T49.ØX6
Oxidizing agent NEC	T54.91	T54.92	T54.93	T54.94	—	—
Oxipurinol	T5Ø.4X1	T5Ø.4X2	T5Ø.4X3	T5Ø.4X4	T5Ø.4X5	T5Ø.4X6
Oxitriptan	T43.291	T43.292	T43.293	T43.294	T43.295	T43.296
Oxitropium bromide	T48.6X1	T48.6X2	T48.6X3	T48.6X4	T48.6X5	T48.6X6
Oxodipine	T46.1X1	T46.1X2	T46.1X3	T46.1X4	T46.1X5	T46.1X6
Oxolamine	T48.3X1	T48.3X2	T48.3X3	T48.3X4	T48.3X5	T48.3X6
Oxolinic acid	T37.8X1	T37.8X2	T37.8X3	T37.8X4	T37.8X5	T37.8X6
Oxomemazine	T43.3X1	T43.3X2	T43.3X3	T43.3X4	T43.3X5	T43.3X6
Oxophenarsine	T37.3X1	T37.3X2	T37.3X3	T37.3X4	T37.3X5	T37.3X6
Oxprenolol	T44.7X1	T44.7X2	T44.7X3	T44.7X4	T44.7X5	T44.7X6
Oxsoralen	T49.3X1	T49.3X2	T49.3X3	T49.3X4	T49.3X5	T49.3X6
Oxtriphylline	T48.6X1	T48.6X2	T48.6X3	T48.6X4	T48.6X5	T48.6X6
Oxybate sodium	T41.291	T41.292	T41.293	T41.294	T41.295	T41.296
Oxybuprocaine	T41.3X1	T41.3X2	T41.3X3	T41.3X4	T41.3X5	T41.3X6
Oxybutynin	T44.3X1	T44.3X2	T44.3X3	T44.3X4	T44.3X5	T44.3X6
Oxychlorosene	T49.ØX1	T49.ØX2	T49.ØX3	T49.ØX4	T49.ØX5	T49.ØX6
Oxycodone	T4Ø.2X1	T4Ø.2X2	T4Ø.2X3	T4Ø.2X4	T4Ø.2X5	T4Ø.2X6
Oxyfedrine	T46.3X1	T46.3X2	T46.3X3	T46.3X4	T46.3X5	T46.3X6
Oxygen	T41.5X1	T41.5X2	T41.5X3	T41.5X4	T41.5X5	T41.5X6
Oxylone	T49.ØX1	T49.ØX2	T49.ØX3	T49.ØX4	T49.ØX5	T49.ØX6
ophthalmic preparation	T49.5X1	T49.5X2	T49.5X3	T49.5X4	T49.5X5	T49.5X6
Oxymesterone	T38.7X1	T38.7X2	T38.7X3	T38.7X4	T38.7X5	T38.7X6
Oxymetazoline	T48.5X1	T48.5X2	T48.5X3	T48.5X4	T48.5X5	T48.5X6
Oxymetholone	T38.7X1	T38.7X2	T38.7X3	T38.7X4	T38.7X5	T38.7X6
Oxymorphone	T4Ø.2X1	T4Ø.2X2	T4Ø.2X3	T4Ø.2X4	T4Ø.2X5	T4Ø.2X6
Oxypertine	T43.591	T43.592	T43.593	T43.594	T43.595	T43.596
Oxyphenbutazone	T39.2X1	T39.2X2	T39.2X3	T39.2X4	T39.2X5	T39.2X6
Oxyphencyclimine	T44.3X1	T44.3X2	T44.3X3	T44.3X4	T44.3X5	T44.3X6
Oxyphenisatine	T47.2X1	T47.2X2	T47.2X3	T47.2X4	T47.2X5	T47.2X6
Oxyphenonium bromide	T44.3X1	T44.3X2	T44.3X3	T44.3X4	T44.3X5	T44.3X6
Oxypolygelatin	T45.8X1	T45.8X2	T45.8X3	T45.8X4	T45.8X5	T45.8X6
Oxyquinoline (derivatives)	T37.8X1	T37.8X2	T37.8X3	T37.8X4	T37.8X5	T37.8X6
Oxytetracycline	T36.4X1	T36.4X2	T36.4X3	T36.4X4	T36.4X5	T36.4X6
Oxytocic drug NEC	T48.ØX1	T48.ØX2	T48.ØX3	T48.ØX4	T48.ØX5	T48.ØX6
Oxytocin (synthetic)	T48.ØX1	T48.ØX2	T48.ØX3	T48.ØX4	T48.ØX5	T48.ØX6
Ozone	T59.891	T59.892	T59.893	T59.894	—	—
PABA	T49.3X1	T49.3X2	T49.3X3	T49.3X4	T49.3X5	T49.3X6
Packed red cells	T45.8X1	T45.8X2	T45.8X3	T45.8X4	T45.8X5	T45.8X6
Padimate	T49.3X1	T49.3X2	T49.3X3	T49.3X4	T49.3X5	T49.3X6
Paint NEC	T65.6X1	T65.6X2	T65.6X3	T65.6X4	—	—
cleaner	T52.91	T52.92	T52.93	T52.94	—	—
fumes NEC	T59.891	T59.892	T59.893	T59.894	—	—
lead (fumes)	T56.ØX1	T56.ØX2	T56.ØX3	T56.ØX4	—	—
solvent NEC	T52.8X1	T52.8X2	T52.8X3	T52.8X4	—	—
stripper	T52.8X1	T52.8X2	T52.8X3	T52.8X4	—	—
Palfium	T4Ø.2X1	T4Ø.2X2	T4Ø.2X3	T4Ø.2X4	—	—
Palm kernel oil	T5Ø.991	T5Ø.992	T5Ø.993	T5Ø.994	T5Ø.995	T5Ø.996
Paludrine	T37.2X1	T37.2X2	T37.2X3	T37.2X4	T37.2X5	T37.2X6
PAM (pralidoxime)	T5Ø.6X1	T5Ø.6X2	T5Ø.6X3	T5Ø.6X4	T5Ø.6X5	T5Ø.6X6
Pamaquine (naphthoute)	T37.2X1	T37.2X2	T37.2X3	T37.2X4	T37.2X5	T37.2X6
Panadol	T39.1X1	T39.1X2	T39.1X3	T39.1X4	T39.1X5	T39.1X6
Pancreatic						
digestive secretion stimulant	T47.8X1	T47.8X2	T47.8X3	T47.8X4	T47.8X5	T47.8X6
dornase	T45.3X1	T45.3X2	T45.3X3	T45.3X4	T45.3X5	T45.3X6
Pancreatin	T47.5X1	T47.5X2	T47.5X3	T47.5X4	T47.5X5	T47.5X6
Pancrelipase	T47.5X1	T47.5X2	T47.5X3	T47.5X4	T47.5X5	T47.5X6
Pancuronium (bromide)	T48.1X1	T48.1X2	T48.1X3	T48.1X4	T48.1X5	T48.1X6
Pangamic acid	T45.2X1	T45.2X2	T45.2X3	T45.2X4	T45.2X5	T45.2X6
Panthenol	T45.2X1	T45.2X2	T45.2X3	T45.2X4	T45.2X5	T45.2X6
topical	T49.8X1	T49.8X2	T49.8X3	T49.8X4	T49.8X5	T49.8X6
Pantopon	T4Ø.ØX1	T4Ø.ØX2	T4Ø.ØX3	T4Ø.ØX4	T4Ø.ØX5	T4Ø.ØX6
Pantothenic acid	T45.2X1	T45.2X2	T45.2X3	T45.2X4	T45.2X5	T45.2X6
Panwarfin	T45.511	T45.512	T45.513	T45.514	T45.515	T45.516
Papain	T47.5X1	T47.5X2	T47.5X3	T47.5X4	T47.5X5	T47.5X6
digestant	T47.5X1	T47.5X2	T47.5X3	T47.5X4	T47.5X5	T47.5X6
Papaveretum	T4Ø.ØX1	T4Ø.ØX2	T4Ø.ØX3	T4Ø.ØX4	T4Ø.ØX5	T4Ø.ØX6
Papaverine	T44.3X1	T44.3X2	T44.3X3	T44.3X4	T44.3X5	T44.3X6
Para-acetamidophenol	T39.1X1	T39.1X2	T39.1X3	T39.1X4	T39.1X5	T39.1X6
Para-aminobenzoic acid	T49.3X1	T49.3X2	T49.3X3	T49.3X4	T49.3X5	T49.3X6
Para aminophenol derivatives	T39.1X1	T39.1X2	T39.1X3	T39.1X4	T39.1X5	T39.1X6
Para-aminosalicylic acid	T37.1X1	T37.1X2	T37.1X3	T37.1X4	T37.1X5	T37.1X6
Paracetaldehyde	T42.6X1	T42.6X2	T42.6X3	T42.6X4	T42.6X5	T42.6X6
Paracetamol	T39.1X1	T39.1X2	T39.1X3	T39.1X4	T39.1X5	T39.1X6
Parachlorophenol (camphorated)	T49.ØX1	T49.ØX2	T49.ØX3	T49.ØX4	T49.ØX5	T49.ØX6
Paracodin	T4Ø.2X1	T4Ø.2X2	T4Ø.2X3	T4Ø.2X4	T4Ø.2X5	T4Ø.2X6
Paradione	T42.2X1	T42.2X2	T42.2X3	T42.2X4	T42.2X5	T42.2X6
Paraffin(s) (wax)	T52.ØX1	T52.ØX2	T52.ØX3	T52.ØX4	—	—
liquid (medicinal)	T47.4X1	T47.4X2	T47.4X3	T47.4X4	T47.4X5	T47.4X6
nonmedicinal	T52.ØX1	T52.ØX2	T52.ØX3	T52.ØX4	—	—
Paraformaldehyde	T6Ø.3X1	T6Ø.3X2	T6Ø.3X3	T6Ø.3X4	—	—
Paraldehyde	T42.6X1	T42.6X2	T42.6X3	T42.6X4	T42.6X5	T42.6X6
Paramethadione	T42.2X1	T42.2X2	T42.2X3	T42.2X4	T42.2X5	T42.2X6
Paramethasone	T38.ØX1	T38.ØX2	T38.ØX3	T38.ØX4	T38.ØX5	T38.ØX6
acetate	T49.ØX1	T49.ØX2	T49.ØX3	T49.ØX4	T49.ØX5	T49.ØX6
Paraoxon	T6Ø.ØX1	T6Ø.ØX2	T6Ø.ØX3	T6Ø.ØX4	—	—
Paraquat	T6Ø.3X1	T6Ø.3X2	T6Ø.3X3	T6Ø.3X4	—	—
Parasympatholytic NEC	T44.3X1	T44.3X2	T44.3X3	T44.3X4	T44.3X5	T44.3X6
Parasympathomimetic drug NEC	T44.1X1	T44.1X2	T44.1X3	T44.1X4	T44.1X5	T44.1X6
Parathion	T6Ø.ØX1	T6Ø.ØX2	T6Ø.ØX3	T6Ø.ØX4	—	—
Parathormone	T5Ø.991	T5Ø.992	T5Ø.993	T5Ø.994	T5Ø.995	T5Ø.996
Parathyroid extract	T5Ø.991	T5Ø.992	T5Ø.993	T5Ø.994	T5Ø.995	T5Ø.996
Paratyphoid vaccine	T5Ø.A91	T5Ø.A92	T5Ø.A93	T5Ø.A94	T5Ø.A95	T5Ø.A96
Paredrine	T44.4X1	T44.4X2	T44.4X3	T44.4X4	T44.4X5	T44.4X6
Paregoric	T4Ø.ØX1	T4Ø.ØX2	T4Ø.ØX3	T4Ø.ØX4	T4Ø.ØX5	T4Ø.ØX6
Pargyline	T46.5X1	T46.5X2	T46.5X3	T46.5X4	T46.5X5	T46.5X6
Paris green	T57.ØX1	T57.ØX2	T57.ØX3	T57.ØX4	—	—
insecticide	T57.ØX1	T57.ØX2	T57.ØX3	T57.ØX4	—	—
Parnate	T43.1X1	T43.1X2	T43.1X3	T43.1X4	T43.1X5	T43.1X6
Paromomycin	T36.5X1	T36.5X2	T36.5X3	T36.5X4	T36.5X5	T36.5X6
Paroxypropione	T45.1X1	T45.1X2	T45.1X3	T45.1X4	T45.1X5	T45.1X6
Parzone	T4Ø.2X1	T4Ø.2X2	T4Ø.2X3	T4Ø.2X4	T4Ø.2X5	T4Ø.2X6
PAS	T37.1X1	T37.1X2	T37.1X3	T37.1X4	T37.1X5	T37.1X6
Pasiniazid	T37.1X1	T37.1X2	T37.1X3	T37.1X4	T37.1X5	T37.1X6
PBB (polybrominated biphenyls)	T65.891	T65.892	T65.893	T65.894	—	—
PCB	T65.891	T65.892	T65.893	T65.894	—	—
PCP						
meaning pentachlorophenol	T6Ø.1X1	T6Ø.1X2	T6Ø.1X3	T6Ø.1X4	—	—
fungicide	T6Ø.3X1	T6Ø.3X2	T6Ø.3X3	T6Ø.3X4	—	—
herbicide	T6Ø.3X1	T6Ø.3X2	T6Ø.3X3	T6Ø.3X4	—	—
insecticide	T6Ø.1X1	T6Ø.1X2	T6Ø.1X3	T6Ø.1X4	—	—
meaning phencyclidine	T4Ø.991	T4Ø.992	T4Ø.993	T4Ø.994	—	—
Peach kernel oil (emulsion)	T47.4X1	T47.4X2	T47.4X3	T47.4X4	T47.4X5	T47.4X6
Peanut oil (emulsion) **NEC**	T47.4X1	T47.4X2	T47.4X3	T47.4X4	T47.4X5	T47.4X6
topical	T49.3X1	T49.3X2	T49.3X3	T49.3X4	T49.3X5	T49.3X6
Pearly Gates (morning glory seeds)	T4Ø.991	T4Ø.992	T4Ø.993	T4Ø.994	—	—
Pecazine	T43.3X1	T43.3X2	T43.3X3	T43.3X4	T43.3X5	T43.3X6
Pectin	T47.6X1	T47.6X2	T47.6X3	T47.6X4	T47.6X5	T47.6X6
Pefloxacin	T37.8X1	T37.8X2	T37.8X3	T37.8X4	T37.8X5	T37.8X6
Pegademase, bovine	T5Ø.Z91	T5Ø.Z92	T5Ø.Z93	T5Ø.Z94	T5Ø.Z95	T5Ø.Z96
Pelletierine tannate	T37.4X1	T37.4X2	T37.4X3	T37.4X4	T37.4X5	T37.4X6
Pemirolast (potassium)	T48.6X1	T48.6X2	T48.6X3	T48.6X4	T48.6X5	T48.6X6
Pemoline	T5Ø.7X1	T5Ø.7X2	T5Ø.7X3	T5Ø.7X4	T5Ø.7X5	T5Ø.7X6
Pempidine	T44.2X1	T44.2X2	T44.2X3	T44.2X4	T44.2X5	T44.2X6
Penamecillin	T36.ØX1	T36.ØX2	T36.ØX3	T36.ØX4	T36.ØX5	T36.ØX6
Penbutolol	T44.7X1	T44.7X2	T44.7X3	T44.7X4	T44.7X5	T44.7X6
Penethamate	T36.ØX1	T36.ØX2	T36.ØX3	T36.ØX4	T36.ØX5	T36.ØX6
Penfluridol	T43.591	T43.592	T43.593	T43.594	T43.595	T43.596
Penflutizide	T5Ø.2X1	T5Ø.2X2	T5Ø.2X3	T5Ø.2X4	T5Ø.2X5	T5Ø.2X6
Pengitoxin	T46.ØX1	T46.ØX2	T46.ØX3	T46.ØX4	T46.ØX5	T46.ØX6
Penicillamine	T5Ø.6X1	T5Ø.6X2	T5Ø.6X3	T5Ø.6X4	T5Ø.6X5	T5Ø.6X6
Penicillin (any)	T36.ØX1	T36.ØX2	T36.ØX3	T36.ØX4	T36.ØX5	T36.ØX6
Penicillinase	T45.3X1	T45.3X2	T45.3X3	T45.3X4	T45.3X5	T45.3X6
Penicilloyl polylysine	T5Ø.8X1	T5Ø.8X2	T5Ø.8X3	T5Ø.8X4	T5Ø.8X5	T5Ø.8X6

Substance	Poisoning, Accidental (unintentional)	Poisoning, Intentional Self-harm	Poisoning, Assault	Poisoning, Undetermined	Adverse Effect	Under-dosing
Penimepicycline	T36.4X1	T36.4X2	T36.4X3	T36.4X4	T36.4X5	T36.4X6
Pentachloroethane	T53.6X1	T53.6X2	T53.6X3	T53.6X4	—	—
Pentachloronaphthalene	T53.7X1	T53.7X2	T53.7X3	T53.7X4	—	—
Pentachlorophenol	T60.1X1	T60.1X2	T60.1X3	T60.1X4	—	—
(pesticide)						
fungicide	T60.3X1	T60.3X2	T60.3X3	T60.3X4	—	—
herbicide	T60.3X1	T60.3X2	T60.3X3	T60.3X4	—	—
insecticide	T60.1X1	T60.1X2	T60.1X3	T60.1X4	—	—
Pentaerythritol	T46.3X1	T46.3X2	T46.3X3	T46.3X4	T46.3X5	T46.3X6
chloral	T42.6X1	T42.6X2	T42.6X3	T42.6X4	T42.6X5	T42.6X6
tetranitrate NEC	T46.3X1	T46.3X2	T46.3X3	T46.3X4	T46.3X5	T46.3X6
Pentaerythrityl tetranitrate	T46.3X1	T46.3X2	T46.3X3	T46.3X4	T46.3X5	T46.3X6
Pentagastrin	T50.8X1	T50.8X2	T50.8X3	T50.8X4	T50.8X5	T50.8X6
Pentalin	T53.6X1	T53.6X2	T53.6X3	T53.6X4	—	—
Pentamethonium bromide	T44.2X1	T44.2X2	T44.2X3	T44.2X4	T44.2X5	T44.2X6
Pentamidine	T37.3X1	T37.3X2	T37.3X3	T37.3X4	T37.3X5	T37.3X6
Pentanol	T51.3X1	T51.3X2	T51.3X3	T51.3X4	—	—
Pentapyrrolinium (bitartrate)	T44.2X1	T44.2X2	T44.2X3	T44.2X4	T44.2X5	T44.2X6
Pentaquine	T37.2X1	T37.2X2	T37.2X3	T37.2X4	T37.2X5	T37.2X6
Pentazocine	T40.4X1	T40.4X2	T40.4X3	T40.4X4	T40.4X5	T40.4X6
Pentetrazole	T50.7X1	T50.7X2	T50.7X3	T50.7X4	T50.7X5	T50.7X6
Penthienate bromide	T44.3X1	T44.3X2	T44.3X3	T44.3X4	T44.3X5	T44.3X6
Pentifylline	T46.7X1	T46.7X2	T46.7X3	T46.7X4	T46.7X5	T46.7X6
Pentobarbital	T42.3X1	T42.3X2	T42.3X3	T42.3X4	T42.3X5	T42.3X6
sodium	T42.3X1	T42.3X2	T42.3X3	T42.3X4	T42.3X5	T42.3X6
Pentobarbitone	T42.3X1	T42.3X2	T42.3X3	T42.3X4	T42.3X5	T42.3X6
Pentolonium tartrate	T44.2X1	T44.2X2	T44.2X3	T44.2X4	T44.2X5	T44.2X6
Pentosan polysulfate (sodium)	T39.8X1	T39.8X2	T39.8X3	T39.8X4	T39.8X5	T39.8X6
Pentostatin	T45.1X1	T45.1X2	T45.1X3	T45.1X4	T45.1X5	T45.1X6
Pentothal	T41.1X1	T41.1X2	T41.1X3	T41.1X4	T41.1X5	T41.1X6
Pentoxifylline	T46.7X1	T46.7X2	T46.7X3	T46.7X4	T46.7X5	T46.7X6
Pentoxyverine	T48.3X1	T48.3X2	T48.3X3	T48.3X4	T48.3X5	T48.3X6
Pentrinat	T46.3X1	T46.3X2	T46.3X3	T46.3X4	T46.3X5	T46.3X6
Pentylenetetrazole	T50.7X1	T50.7X2	T50.7X3	T50.7X4	T50.7X5	T50.7X6
Pentylsalicylamide	T37.1X1	T37.1X2	T37.1X3	T37.1X4	T37.1X5	T37.1X6
Pentymal	T42.3X1	T42.3X2	T42.3X3	T42.3X4	T42.3X5	T42.3X6
Peplomycin	T45.1X1	T45.1X2	T45.1X3	T45.1X4	T45.1X5	T45.1X6
Peppermint (oil)	T47.5X1	T47.5X2	T47.5X3	T47.5X4	T47.5X5	T47.5X6
Pepsin	T47.5X1	T47.5X2	T47.5X3	T47.5X4	T47.5X5	T47.5X6
digestant	T47.5X1	T47.5X2	T47.5X3	T47.5X4	T47.5X5	T47.5X6
Pepstatin	T47.1X1	T47.1X2	T47.1X3	T47.1X4	T47.1X5	T47.1X6
Peptavlon	T50.8X1	T50.8X2	T50.8X3	T50.8X4	T50.8X5	T50.8X6
Perazine	T43.3X1	T43.3X2	T43.3X3	T43.3X4	T43.3X5	T43.3X6
Percaine (spinal)	T41.3X1	T41.3X2	T41.3X3	T41.3X4	T41.3X5	T41.3X6
topical (surface)	T41.3X1	T41.3X2	T41.3X3	T41.3X4	T41.3X5	T41.3X6
Perchloroethylene	T53.3X1	T53.3X2	T53.3X3	T53.3X4	—	—
medicinal	T37.4X1	T37.4X2	T37.4X3	T37.4X4	T37.4X5	T37.4X6
vapor	T53.3X1	T53.3X2	T53.3X3	T53.3X4	—	—
Percodan	T40.2X1	T40.2X2	T40.2X3	T40.2X4	T40.2X5	T40.2X6
Percogesic — see also acetaminophen	T45.0X1	T45.0X2	T45.0X3	T45.0X4	T45.0X5	T45.0X6
Percorten	T38.0X1	T38.0X2	T38.0X3	T38.0X4	T38.0X5	T38.0X6
Pergolide	T42.8X1	T42.8X2	T42.8X3	T42.8X4	T42.8X5	T42.8X6
Pergonal	T38.811	T38.812	T38.813	T38.814	T38.815	T38.816
Perhexilene	T46.3X1	T46.3X2	T46.3X3	T46.3X4	T46.3X5	T46.3X6
Perhexiline (maleate)	T46.3X1	T46.3X2	T46.3X3	T46.3X4	T46.3X5	T46.3X6
Periactin	T45.0X1	T45.0X2	T45.0X3	T45.0X4	T45.0X5	T45.0X6
Periciazine	T43.3X1	T43.3X2	T43.3X3	T43.3X4	T43.3X5	T43.3X6
Periclor	T42.6X1	T42.6X2	T42.6X3	T42.6X4	T42.6X5	T42.6X6
Perindopril	T46.4X1	T46.4X2	T46.4X3	T46.4X4	T46.4X5	T46.4X6
Perisoxal	T39.8X1	T39.8X2	T39.8X3	T39.8X4	T39.8X5	T39.8X6
Peritoneal dialysis solution	T50.3X1	T50.3X2	T50.3X3	T50.3X4	T50.3X5	T50.3X6
Peritrate	T46.3X1	T46.3X2	T46.3X3	T46.3X4	T46.3X5	T46.3X6
Perlapine	T42.4X1	T42.4X2	T42.4X3	T42.4X4	T42.4X5	T42.4X6
Permanganate	T65.891	T65.892	T65.893	T65.894	—	—
Permethrin	T60.1X1	T60.1X2	T60.1X3	T60.1X4	—	—
Pernocton	T42.3X1	T42.3X2	T42.3X3	T42.3X4	T42.3X5	T42.3X6
Pernoston	T42.3X1	T42.3X2	T42.3X3	T42.3X4	T42.3X5	T42.3X6
Peronine	T40.2X1	T40.2X2	T40.2X3	T40.2X4	—	—
Perphenazine	T43.3X1	T43.3X2	T43.3X3	T43.3X4	T43.3X5	T43.3X6
Pertofrane	T43.011	T43.012	T43.013	T43.014	T43.015	T43.016
Pertussis						
immune serum (human)	T50.Z11	T50.Z12	T50.Z13	T50.Z14	T50.Z15	T50.Z16
vaccine (with diphtheria toxoid) (with tetanus toxoid)	T50.A11	T50.A12	T50.A13	T50.A14	T50.A15	T50.A16
Peruvian balsam	T49.0X1	T49.0X2	T49.0X3	T49.0X4	T49.0X5	T49.0X6
Peruvoside	T46.0X1	T46.0X2	T46.0X3	T46.0X4	T46.0X5	T46.0X6
Pesticide (dust) (fumes) (vapor) NEC	T60.91	T60.92	T60.93	T60.94	—	—
arsenic	T57.0X1	T57.0X2	T57.0X3	T57.0X4	—	—

Substance	Poisoning, Accidental (unintentional)	Poisoning, Intentional Self-harm	Poisoning, Assault	Poisoning, Undetermined	Adverse Effect	Under-dosing
Pesticide (dust) (fumes) (vapor) NEC — continued						
chlorinated	T60.1X1	T60.1X2	T60.1X3	T60.1X4	—	—
cyanide	T65.0X1	T65.0X2	T65.0X3	T65.0X4	—	—
kerosene	T52.0X1	T52.0X2	T52.0X3	T52.0X4	—	—
mixture (of compounds)	T60.91	T60.92	T60.93	T60.94	—	—
naphthalene	T60.2X1	T60.2X2	T60.2X3	T60.2X4	—	—
organochlorine (compounds)	T60.1X1	T60.1X2	T60.1X3	T60.1X4	—	—
petroleum (distillate) (products) NEC	T60.8X1	T60.8X2	T60.8X3	T60.8X4	—	—
specified ingredient NEC	T60.8X1	T60.8X2	T60.8X3	T60.8X4	—	—
strychnine	T65.1X1	T65.1X2	T65.1X3	T65.1X4	—	—
thallium	T60.4X1	T60.4X2	T60.4X3	T60.4X4	—	—
Pethidine	T40.4X1	T40.4X2	T40.4X3	T40.4X4	T40.4X5	T40.4X6
Petrichloral	T42.6X1	T42.6X2	T42.6X3	T42.6X4	T42.6X5	T42.6X6
Petrol	T52.0X1	T52.0X2	T52.0X3	T52.0X4	—	—
vapor	T52.0X1	T52.0X2	T52.0X3	T52.0X4	—	—
Petrolatum	T49.3X1	T49.3X2	T49.3X3	T49.3X4	T49.3X5	T49.3X6
hydrophilic	T49.3X1	T49.3X2	T49.3X3	T49.3X4	T49.3X5	T49.3X6
liquid	T47.4X1	T47.4X2	T47.4X3	T47.4X4	T47.4X5	T47.4X6
topical	T49.3X1	T49.3X2	T49.3X3	T49.3X4	T49.3X5	T49.3X6
nonmedicinal	T52.0X1	T52.0X2	T52.0X3	T52.0X4	—	—
red veterinary	T49.3X1	T49.3X2	T49.3X3	T49.3X4	T49.3X5	T49.3X6
white	T49.3X1	T49.3X2	T49.3X3	T49.3X4	T49.3X5	T49.3X6
Petroleum (products) NEC	T52.0X1	T52.0X2	T52.0X3	T52.0X4	—	—
benzine(s) — see Ligroin						
ether — see Ligroin						
jelly — see Petrolatum						
naphtha — see Ligroin						
pesticide	T60.8X1	T60.8X2	T60.8X3	T60.8X4	—	—
solids	T52.0X1	T52.0X2	T52.0X3	T52.0X4	—	—
solvents	T52.0X1	T52.0X2	T52.0X3	T52.0X4	—	—
vapor	T52.0X1	T52.0X2	T52.0X3	T52.0X4	—	—
Peyote	T40.991	T40.992	T40.993	T40.994	—	—
Phanodorm, phanodorn	T42.3X1	T42.3X2	T42.3X3	T42.3X4	T42.3X5	T42.3X6
Phanquinone	T37.3X1	T37.3X2	T37.3X3	T37.3X4	T37.3X5	T37.3X6
Phanquone	T37.3X1	T37.3X2	T37.3X3	T37.3X4	T37.3X5	T37.3X6
Pharmaceutical						
adjunct NEC	T50.901	T50.902	T50.903	T50.904	T50.905	T50.906
excipient NEC	T50.901	T50.902	T50.903	T50.904	T50.905	T50.906
sweetener	T50.901	T50.902	T50.903	T50.904	T50.905	T50.906
viscous agent	T50.901	T50.902	T50.903	T50.904	T50.905	T50.906
Phemitone	T42.3X1	T42.3X2	T42.3X3	T42.3X4	T42.3X5	T42.3X6
Phenacaine	T41.3X1	T41.3X2	T41.3X3	T41.3X4	T41.3X5	T41.3X6
Phenacemide	T42.6X1	T42.6X2	T42.6X3	T42.6X4	T42.6X5	T42.6X6
Phenacetin	T39.1X1	T39.1X2	T39.1X3	T39.1X4	T39.1X5	T39.1X6
Phenadoxone	T40.2X1	T40.2X2	T40.2X3	T40.2X4	—	—
Phenaglycodol	T43.591	T43.592	T43.593	T43.594	T43.595	T43.596
Phenantoin	T42.0X1	T42.0X2	T42.0X3	T42.0X4	T42.0X5	T42.0X6
Phenaphthazine reagent	T50.991	T50.992	T50.993	T50.994	T50.995	T50.996
Phenazocine	T40.4X1	T40.4X2	T40.4X3	T40.4X4	T40.4X5	T40.4X6
Phenazone	T39.2X1	T39.2X2	T39.2X3	T39.2X4	T39.2X5	T39.2X6
Phenazopyridine	T39.8X1	T39.8X2	T39.8X3	T39.8X4	T39.8X5	T39.8X6
Phenbenicillin	T36.0X1	T36.0X2	T36.0X3	T36.0X4	T36.0X5	T36.0X6
Phenbutrazate	T50.5X1	T50.5X2	T50.5X3	T50.5X4	T50.5X5	T50.5X6
Phencyclidine	T40.991	T40.992	T40.993	T40.994	T40.995	T40.996
Phendimetrazine	T50.5X1	T50.5X2	T50.5X3	T50.5X4	T50.5X5	T50.5X6
Phenelzine	T43.1X1	T43.1X2	T43.1X3	T43.1X4	T43.1X5	T43.1X6
Phenemal	T42.3X1	T42.3X2	T42.3X3	T42.3X4	T42.3X5	T42.3X6
Phenergan	T42.6X1	T42.6X2	T42.6X3	T42.6X4	T42.6X5	T42.6X6
Pheneticillin	T36.0X1	T36.0X2	T36.0X3	T36.0X4	T36.0X5	T36.0X6
Pheneturide	T42.6X1	T42.6X2	T42.6X3	T42.6X4	T42.6X5	T42.6X6
Phenformin	T38.3X1	T38.3X2	T38.3X3	T38.3X4	T38.3X5	T38.3X6
Phenglutarimide	T44.3X1	T44.3X2	T44.3X3	T44.3X4	T44.3X5	T44.3X6
Phenicarbazide	T39.8X1	T39.8X2	T39.8X3	T39.8X4	T39.8X5	T39.8X6
Phenindamine	T45.0X1	T45.0X2	T45.0X3	T45.0X4	T45.0X5	T45.0X6
Phenindione	T45.511	T45.512	T45.513	T45.514	T45.515	T45.516
Pheniprazine	T43.1X1	T43.1X2	T43.1X3	T43.1X4	T43.1X5	T43.1X6
Pheniramine	T45.0X1	T45.0X2	T45.0X3	T45.0X4	T45.0X5	T45.0X6
Phenisatin	T47.2X1	T47.2X2	T47.2X3	T47.2X4	T47.2X5	T47.2X6
Phenmetrazine	T50.5X1	T50.5X2	T50.5X3	T50.5X4	T50.5X5	T50.5X6
Phenobal	T42.3X1	T42.3X2	T42.3X3	T42.3X4	T42.3X5	T42.3X6
Phenobarbital	T42.3X1	T42.3X2	T42.3X3	T42.3X4	T42.3X5	T42.3X6
with						
mephenytoin	T42.3X1	T42.3X2	T42.3X3	T42.3X4	T42.3X5	T42.3X6
phenytoin	T42.3X1	T42.3X2	T42.3X3	T42.3X4	T42.3X5	T42.3X6
sodium	T42.3X1	T42.3X2	T42.3X3	T42.3X4	T42.3X5	T42.3X6
Phenobarbitone	T42.3X1	T42.3X2	T42.3X3	T42.3X4	T42.3X5	T42.3X6
Phenobutiodil	T50.8X1	T50.8X2	T50.8X3	T50.8X4	T50.8X5	T50.8X6
Phenoctide	T49.0X1	T49.0X2	T49.0X3	T49.0X4	T49.0X5	T49.0X6
Phenol	T49.0X1	T49.0X2	T49.0X3	T49.0X4	T49.0X5	T49.0X6
disinfectant	T54.0X1	T54.0X2	T54.0X3	T54.0X4	—	—

Phenol ICD-10-CM 2016

Table of Drugs and Chemicals

Substance	Poisoning, Accidental (unintentional)	Poisoning, Intentional Self-harm	Poisoning, Assault	Poisoning, Undetermined	Adverse Effect	Under-dosing
Phenol — *continued*						
in oil injection	T46.8X1	T46.8X2	T46.8X3	T46.8X4	T46.8X5	T46.8X6
medicinal	T49.1X1	T49.1X2	T49.1X3	T49.1X4	T49.1X5	T49.1X6
nonmedicinal NEC	T54.0X1	T54.0X2	T54.0X3	T54.0X4	—	—
pesticide	T60.8X1	T60.8X2	T60.8X3	T60.8X4	—	—
red	T50.8X1	T50.8X2	T50.8X3	T50.8X4	T50.8X5	T50.8X6
Phenolic preparation	T49.1X1	T49.1X2	T49.1X3	T49.1X4	T49.1X5	T49.1X6
Phenolphthalein	T47.2X1	T47.2X2	T47.2X3	T47.2X4	T47.2X5	T47.2X6
Phenolsulfonphthalein	T50.8X1	T50.8X2	T50.8X3	T50.8X4	T50.8X5	T50.8X6
Phenomorphan	T40.2X1	T40.2X2	T40.2X3	T40.2X4	—	—
Phenonyl	T42.3X1	T42.3X2	T42.3X3	T42.3X4	T42.3X5	T42.3X6
Phenoperidine	T40.4X1	T40.4X2	T40.4X3	T40.4X4	—	—
Phenopyrazone	T46.991	T46.992	T46.993	T46.994	T46.995	T46.996
Phenoquin	T50.4X1	T50.4X2	T50.4X3	T50.4X4	T50.4X5	T50.4X6
Phenothiazine (psychotropic) **NEC**	T43.3X1	T43.3X2	T43.3X3	T43.3X4	T43.3X5	T43.3X6
insecticide	T60.2X1	T60.2X2	T60.2X3	T60.2X4	—	—
Phenothrin	T49.0X1	T49.0X2	T49.0X3	T49.0X4	T49.0X5	T49.0X6
Phenoxybenzamine	T46.7X1	T46.7X2	T46.7X3	T46.7X4	T46.7X5	T46.7X6
Phenoxyethanol	T49.0X1	T49.0X2	T49.0X3	T49.0X4	T49.0X5	T49.0X6
Phenoxymethyl penicillin	T36.0X1	T36.0X2	T36.0X3	T36.0X4	T36.0X5	T36.0X6
Phenprobamate	T42.8X1	T42.8X2	T42.8X3	T42.8X4	T42.8X5	T42.8X6
Phenprocoumon	T45.511	T45.512	T45.513	T45.514	T45.515	T45.516
Phensuximide	T42.2X1	T42.2X2	T42.2X3	T42.2X4	T42.2X5	T42.2X6
Phentermine	T50.5X1	T50.5X2	T50.5X3	T50.5X4	T50.5X5	T50.5X6
Phenthicillin	T36.0X1	T36.0X2	T36.0X3	T36.0X4	T36.0X5	T36.0X6
Phentolamine	T46.7X1	T46.7X2	T46.7X3	T46.7X4	T46.7X5	T46.7X6
Phenyl						
butazone	T39.2X1	T39.2X2	T39.2X3	T39.2X4	T39.2X5	T39.2X6
enediamine	T65.3X1	T65.3X2	T65.3X3	T65.3X4	—	—
hydrazine	T65.3X1	T65.3X2	T65.3X3	T65.3X4	—	—
antineoplastic	T45.1X1	T45.1X2	T45.1X3	T45.1X4	T45.1X5	T45.1X6
mercuric compounds — *see* Mercury						
salicylate	T49.3X1	T49.3X2	T49.3X3	T49.3X4	T49.3X5	T49.3X6
Phenylalanine mustard	T45.1X1	T45.1X2	T45.1X3	T45.1X4	T45.1X5	T45.1X6
Phenylbutazone	T39.2X1	T39.2X2	T39.2X3	T39.2X4	T39.2X5	T39.2X6
Phenylenediamine	T65.3X1	T65.3X2	T65.3X3	T65.3X4	—	—
Phenylephrine	T44.4X1	T44.4X2	T44.4X3	T44.4X4	T44.4X5	T44.4X6
Phenylethylbiguanide	T38.3X1	T38.3X2	T38.3X3	T38.3X4	T38.3X5	T38.3X6
Phenylmercuric						
acetate	T49.0X1	T49.0X2	T49.0X3	T49.0X4	T49.0X5	T49.0X6
borate	T49.0X1	T49.0X2	T49.0X3	T49.0X4	T49.0X5	T49.0X6
nitrate	T49.0X1	T49.0X2	T49.0X3	T49.0X4	T49.0X5	T49.0X6
Phenylmethylbarbitone	T42.3X1	T42.3X2	T42.3X3	T42.3X4	T42.3X5	T42.3X6
Phenylpropanol	T47.5X1	T47.5X2	T47.5X3	T47.5X4	T47.5X5	T47.5X6
Phenylpropanolamine	T44.991	T44.992	T44.993	T44.994	T44.995	T44.996
Phenylsulfthion	T60.0X1	T60.0X2	T60.0X3	T60.0X4	—	—
Phenyltoloxamine	T45.0X1	T45.0X2	T45.0X3	T45.0X4	T45.0X5	T45.0X6
Phenyramidol, phenyramidon	T39.8X1	T39.8X2	T39.8X3	T39.8X4	T39.8X5	T39.8X6
Phenytoin	T42.0X1	T42.0X2	T42.0X3	T42.0X4	T42.0X5	T42.0X6
with Phenobarbital	T42.3X1	T42.3X2	T42.3X3	T42.3X4	T42.3X5	T42.3X6
pHisoHex	T49.2X1	T49.2X2	T49.2X3	T49.2X4	T49.2X5	T49.2X6
Pholcodine	T48.3X1	T48.3X2	T48.3X3	T48.3X4	T48.3X5	T48.3X6
Pholedrine	T46.991	T46.992	T46.993	T46.994	T46.995	T46.996
Phorate	T60.0X1	T60.0X2	T60.0X3	T60.0X4	—	—
Phosdrin	T60.0X1	T60.0X2	T60.0X3	T60.0X4	—	—
Phosfolan	T60.0X1	T60.0X2	T60.0X3	T60.0X4	—	—
Phosgene (gas)	T59.891	T59.892	T59.893	T59.894	—	—
Phosphamidon	T60.0X1	T60.0X2	T60.0X3	T60.0X4	—	—
Phosphate	T65.891	T65.892	T65.893	T65.894	—	—
laxative	T47.4X1	T47.4X2	T47.4X3	T47.4X4	T47.4X5	T47.4X6
organic	T60.0X1	T60.0X2	T60.0X3	T60.0X4	—	—
solvent	T52.91	T52.92	T52.93	T52.94	—	—
tricresyl	T65.891	T65.892	T65.893	T65.894	—	—
Phosphine	T57.1X1	T57.1X2	T57.1X3	T57.1X4	—	—
fumigant	T57.1X1	T57.1X2	T57.1X3	T57.1X4	—	—
Phospholine	T49.5X1	T49.5X2	T49.5X3	T49.5X4	T49.5X5	T49.5X6
Phosphoric acid	T54.2X1	T54.2X2	T54.2X3	T54.2X4	—	—
Phosphorus (compound) **NEC**	T57.1X1	T57.1X2	T57.1X3	T57.1X4	—	—
pesticide	T60.0X1	T60.0X2	T60.0X3	T60.0X4	—	—
Phthalates	T65.891	T65.892	T65.893	T65.894	—	—
Phthalic anhydride	T65.891	T65.892	T65.893	T65.894	—	—
Phthalimidoglutarimide	T42.6X1	T42.6X2	T42.6X3	T42.6X4	T42.6X5	T42.6X6
Phthalylsulfathiazole	T37.0X1	T37.0X2	T37.0X3	T37.0X4	T37.0X5	T37.0X6
Phylloquinone	T45.7X1	T45.7X2	T45.7X3	T45.7X4	T45.7X5	T45.7X6
Physeptone	T40.3X1	T40.3X2	T40.3X3	T40.3X4	T40.3X5	T40.3X6
Physostigma venenosum	T62.2X1	T62.2X2	T62.2X3	T62.2X4	—	—
Physostigmine	T49.5X1	T49.5X2	T49.5X3	T49.5X4	T49.5X5	T49.5X6
Phytolacca decandra	T62.2X1	T62.2X2	T62.2X3	T62.2X4	—	—
berries	T62.1X1	T62.1X2	T62.1X3	T62.1X4	—	—

Substance	Poisoning, Accidental (unintentional)	Poisoning, Intentional Self-harm	Poisoning, Assault	Poisoning, Undetermined	Adverse Effect	Under-dosing
Phytomenadione	T45.7X1	T45.7X2	T45.7X3	T45.7X4	T45.7X5	T45.7X6
Phytonadione	T45.7X1	T45.7X2	T45.7X3	T45.7X4	T45.7X5	T45.7X6
Picoperine	T48.3X1	T48.3X2	T48.3X3	T48.3X4	T48.3X5	T48.3X6
Picosulfate (sodium)	T47.2X1	T47.2X2	T47.2X3	T47.2X4	T47.2X5	T47.2X6
Picric (acid)	T54.2X1	T54.2X2	T54.2X3	T54.2X4	—	—
Picrotoxin	T50.7X1	T50.7X2	T50.7X3	T50.7X4	T50.7X5	T50.7X6
Piketoprofen	T49.0X1	T49.0X2	T49.0X3	T49.0X4	T49.0X5	T49.0X6
Pilocarpine	T44.1X1	T44.1X2	T44.1X3	T44.1X4	T44.1X5	T44.1X6
Pilocarpus (jaborandi) extract	T44.1X1	T44.1X2	T44.1X3	T44.1X4	T44.1X5	T44.1X6
Pilsicainide (hydrochloride)	T46.2X1	T46.2X2	T46.2X3	T46.2X4	T46.2X5	T46.2X6
Pimaricin	T36.7X1	T36.7X2	T36.7X3	T36.7X4	T36.7X5	T36.7X6
Pimeclone	T50.7X1	T50.7X2	T50.7X3	T50.7X4	T50.7X5	T50.7X6
Pimelic ketone	T52.8X1	T52.8X2	T52.8X3	T52.8X4	—	—
Pimethixene	T45.0X1	T45.0X2	T45.0X3	T45.0X4	T45.0X5	T45.0X6
Piminodine	T40.2X1	T40.2X2	T40.2X3	T40.2X4	T40.2X5	T40.2X6
Pimozide	T43.591	T43.592	T43.593	T43.594	T43.595	T43.596
Pinacidil	T46.5X1	T46.5X2	T46.5X3	T46.5X4	T46.5X5	T46.5X6
Pinaverium bromide	T44.3X1	T44.3X2	T44.3X3	T44.3X4	T44.3X5	T44.3X6
Pinazepam	T42.4X1	T42.4X2	T42.4X3	T42.4X4	T42.4X5	T42.4X6
Pindolol	T44.7X1	T44.7X2	T44.7X3	T44.7X4	T44.7X5	T44.7X6
Pindone	T60.4X1	T60.4X2	T60.4X3	T60.4X4	—	—
Pine oil (disinfectant)	T65.891	T65.892	T65.893	T65.894	—	—
Pinkroot	T37.4X1	T37.4X2	T37.4X3	T37.4X4	T37.4X5	T37.4X6
Pipadone	T40.2X1	T40.2X2	T40.2X3	T40.2X4	—	—
Pipamazine	T45.0X1	T45.0X2	T45.0X3	T45.0X4	T45.0X5	T45.0X6
Pipamperone	T43.4X1	T43.4X2	T43.4X3	T43.4X4	T43.4X5	T43.4X6
Pipazetate	T48.3X1	T48.3X2	T48.3X3	T48.3X4	T48.3X5	T48.3X6
Pipemidic acid	T37.8X1	T37.8X2	T37.8X3	T37.8X4	T37.8X5	T37.8X6
Pipenzolate bromide	T44.3X1	T44.3X2	T44.3X3	T44.3X4	T44.3X5	T44.3X6
Piperacetazine	T43.3X1	T43.3X2	T43.3X3	T43.3X4	T43.3X5	T43.3X6
Piperacillin	T36.0X1	T36.0X2	T36.0X3	T36.0X4	T36.0X5	T36.0X6
Piperazine	T37.4X1	T37.4X2	T37.4X3	T37.4X4	T37.4X5	T37.4X6
estrone sulfate	T38.5X1	T38.5X2	T38.5X3	T38.5X4	T38.5X5	T38.5X6
Piper cubeba	T62.2X1	T62.2X2	T62.2X3	T62.2X4	—	—
Piperidione	T48.3X1	T48.3X2	T48.3X3	T48.3X4	T48.3X5	T48.3X6
Piperidolate	T44.3X1	T44.3X2	T44.3X3	T44.3X4	T44.3X5	T44.3X6
Piperocaine	T41.3X1	T41.3X2	T41.3X3	T41.3X4	T41.3X5	T41.3X6
infiltration (subcutaneous)	T41.3X1	T41.3X2	T41.3X3	T41.3X4	T41.3X5	T41.3X6
nerve block (peripheral) (plexus)	T41.3X1	T41.3X2	T41.3X3	T41.3X4	T41.3X5	T41.3X6
topical (surface)	T41.3X1	T41.3X2	T41.3X3	T41.3X4	T41.3X5	T41.3X6
Piperonyl butoxide	T60.8X1	T60.8X2	T60.8X3	T60.8X4	—	—
Pipethanate	T44.3X1	T44.3X2	T44.3X3	T44.3X4	T44.3X5	T44.3X6
Pipobroman	T45.1X1	T45.1X2	T45.1X3	T45.1X4	T45.1X5	T45.1X6
Pipotiazine	T43.3X1	T43.3X2	T43.3X3	T43.3X4	T43.3X5	T43.3X6
Pipoxizine	T45.0X1	T45.0X2	T45.0X3	T45.0X4	T45.0X5	T45.0X6
Pipradrol	T43.691	T43.692	T43.693	T43.694	T43.695	T43.696
Piprinhydrinate	T45.0X1	T45.0X2	T45.0X3	T45.0X4	T45.0X5	T45.0X6
Pirarubicin	T45.1X1	T45.1X2	T45.1X3	T45.1X4	T45.1X5	T45.1X6
Pirazinamide	T37.1X1	T37.1X2	T37.1X3	T37.1X4	T37.1X5	T37.1X6
Pirbuterol	T48.6X1	T48.6X2	T48.6X3	T48.6X4	T48.6X5	T48.6X6
Pirenzepine	T47.1X1	T47.1X2	T47.1X3	T47.1X4	T47.1X5	T47.1X6
Piretanide	T50.1X1	T50.1X2	T50.1X3	T50.1X4	T50.1X5	T50.1X6
Piribedil	T42.8X1	T42.8X2	T42.8X3	T42.8X4	T42.8X5	T42.8X6
Piridoxilate	T46.3X1	T46.3X2	T46.3X3	T46.3X4	T46.3X5	T46.3X6
Piritramide	T40.4X1	T40.4X2	T40.4X3	T40.4X4	—	—
Piromidic acid	T37.8X1	T37.8X2	T37.8X3	T37.8X4	T37.8X5	T37.8X6
Piroxicam	T39.391	T39.392	T39.393	T39.394	T39.395	T39.396
beta-cyclodextrin complex	T39.8X1	T39.8X2	T39.8X3	T39.8X4	T39.8X5	T39.8X6
Pirozadil	T46.6X1	T46.6X2	T46.6X3	T46.6X4	T46.6X5	T46.6X6
Piscidia (bark) (erythrina)	T39.8X1	T39.8X2	T39.8X3	T39.8X4	T39.8X5	T39.8X6
Pitch	T65.891	T65.892	T65.893	T65.894	—	—
Pitkin's solution	T41.3X1	T41.3X2	T41.3X3	T41.3X4	T41.3X5	T41.3X6
Pitocin	T48.0X1	T48.0X2	T48.0X3	T48.0X4	T48.0X5	T48.0X6
Pitressin (tannate)	T38.891	T38.892	T38.893	T38.894	T38.895	T38.896
Pituitary extracts (posterior)	T38.891	T38.892	T38.893	T38.894	T38.895	T38.896
anterior	T38.811	T38.812	T38.813	T38.814	T38.815	T38.816
Pituitrin	T38.891	T38.892	T38.893	T38.894	T38.895	T38.896
Pivampicillin	T36.0X1	T36.0X2	T36.0X3	T36.0X4	T36.0X5	T36.0X6
Pivmecillinam	T36.0X1	T36.0X2	T36.0X3	T36.0X4	T36.0X5	T36.0X6
Placental hormone	T38.891	T38.892	T38.893	T38.894	T38.895	T38.896
Placidyl	T42.6X1	T42.6X2	T42.6X3	T42.6X4	T42.6X5	T42.6X6
Plague vaccine	T50.A91	T50.A92	T50.A93	T50.A94	T50.A95	T50.A96
Plant						
food or fertilizer NEC	T65.891	T65.892	T65.893	T65.894	—	—
containing herbicide	T60.3X1	T60.3X2	T60.3X3	T60.3X4	—	—
noxious, used as food	T62.2X1	T62.2X2	T62.2X3	T62.2X4	—	—
berries	T62.1X1	T62.1X2	T62.1X3	T62.1X4	—	—
seeds	T62.2X1	T62.2X2	T62.2X3	T62.2X4	—	—
specified type NEC	T62.2X1	T62.2X2	T62.2X3	T62.2X4	—	—
Plasma	T45.8X1	T45.8X2	T45.8X3	T45.8X4	T45.8X5	T45.8X6
expander NEC	T45.8X1	T45.8X2	T45.8X3	T45.8X4	T45.8X5	T45.8X6

Substance	Poisoning, Accidental (unintentional)	Poisoning, Intentional Self-harm	Poisoning, Assault	Poisoning, Undetermined	Adverse Effect	Under-dosing
Plasma — *continued*						
protein fraction (human)	T45.8X1	T45.8X2	T45.8X3	T45.8X4	T45.8X5	T45.8X6
Plasmanate	T45.8X1	T45.8X2	T45.8X3	T45.8X4	T45.8X5	T45.8X6
Plasminogen (tissue) activator	T45.611	T45.612	T45.613	T45.614	T45.615	T45.616
Plaster dressing	T49.3X1	T49.3X2	T49.3X3	T49.3X4	T49.3X5	T49.3X6
Plastic dressing	T49.3X1	T49.3X2	T49.3X3	T49.3X4	T49.3X5	T49.3X6
Plegicil	T43.3X1	T43.3X2	T43.3X3	T43.3X4	T43.3X5	T43.3X6
Plicamycin	T45.1X1	T45.1X2	T45.1X3	T45.1X4	T45.1X5	T45.1X6
Podophyllotoxin	T49.8X1	T49.8X2	T49.8X3	T49.8X4	T49.8X5	T49.8X6
Podophyllum (resin)	T49.4X1	T49.4X2	T49.4X3	T49.4X4	T49.4X5	T49.4X6
Poisonous berries	T62.1X1	T62.1X2	T62.1X3	T62.1X4	—	—
Poison NEC	T65.91	T65.92	T65.93	T65.94	—	—
Pokeweed (any part)	T62.2X1	T62.2X2	T62.2X3	T62.2X4	—	—
Poldine metilsulfate	T44.3X1	T44.3X2	T44.3X3	T44.3X4	T44.3X5	T44.3X6
Polidexide (sulfate)	T46.6X1	T46.6X2	T46.6X3	T46.6X4	T46.6X5	T46.6X6
Polidocanol	T46.8X1	T46.8X2	T46.8X3	T46.8X4	T46.8X5	T46.8X6
Poliomyelitis vaccine	T50.B91	T50.B92	T50.B93	T50.B94	T50.B95	T50.B96
Polish (car) (floor) (furniture) (metal) (porcelain) (silver)	T65.891	T65.892	T65.893	T65.894	—	—
abrasive	T65.891	T65.892	T65.893	T65.894	—	—
porcelain	T65.891	T65.892	T65.893	T65.894	—	—
Poloxalkol	T47.4X1	T47.4X2	T47.4X3	T47.4X4	T47.4X5	T47.4X6
Poloxamer	T47.4X1	T47.4X2	T47.4X3	T47.4X4	T47.4X5	T47.4X6
Polyaminostyrene resins	T50.3X1	T50.3X2	T50.3X3	T50.3X4	T50.3X5	T50.3X6
Polycarbophil	T47.4X1	T47.4X2	T47.4X3	T47.4X4	T47.4X5	T47.4X6
Polychlorinated biphenyl	T65.891	T65.892	T65.893	T65.894	—	—
Polycycline	T36.4X1	T36.4X2	T36.4X3	T36.4X4	T36.4X5	T36.4X6
Polyester fumes	T59.891	T59.892	T59.893	T59.894	—	—
Polyester resin hardener	T52.91	T52.92	T52.93	T52.94	—	—
fumes	T59.891	T59.892	T59.893	T59.894	—	—
Polyestradiol phosphate	T38.5X1	T38.5X2	T38.5X3	T38.5X4	T38.5X5	T38.5X6
Polyethanolamine alkyl sulfate	T49.2X1	T49.2X2	T49.2X3	T49.2X4	T49.2X5	T49.2X6
Polyethylene adhesive	T49.3X1	T49.3X2	T49.3X3	T49.3X4	T49.3X5	T49.3X6
Polyferose	T45.4X1	T45.4X2	T45.4X3	T45.4X4	T45.4X5	T45.4X6
Polygeline	T45.8X1	T45.8X2	T45.8X3	T45.8X4	T45.8X5	T45.8X6
Polymyxin	T36.8X1	T36.8X2	T36.8X3	T36.8X4	T36.8X5	T36.8X6
B	T36.8X1	T36.8X2	T36.8X3	T36.8X4	T36.8X5	T36.8X6
ENT agent	T49.6X1	T49.6X2	T49.6X3	T49.6X4	T49.6X5	T49.6X6
ophthalmic preparation	T49.5X1	T49.5X2	T49.5X3	T49.5X4	T49.5X5	T49.5X6
topical NEC	T49.0X1	T49.0X2	T49.0X3	T49.0X4	T49.0X5	T49.0X6
E sulfate (eye preparation)	T49.5X1	T49.5X2	T49.5X3	T49.5X4	T49.5X5	T49.5X6
Polynoxylin	T49.0X1	T49.0X2	T49.0X3	T49.0X4	T49.0X5	T49.0X6
Polyoestradiol phosphate	T38.5X1	T38.5X2	T38.5X3	T38.5X4	T38.5X5	T38.5X6
Polyoxymethyleneurea	T49.0X1	T49.0X2	T49.0X3	T49.0X4	T49.0X5	T49.0X6
Polysilane	T47.8X1	T47.8X2	T47.8X3	T47.8X4	T47.8X5	T47.8X6
Polytetrafluoroethylene (inhaled)	T59.891	T59.892	T59.893	T59.894	—	—
Polythiazide	T50.2X1	T50.2X2	T50.2X3	T50.2X4	T50.2X5	T50.2X6
Polyvidone	T45.8X1	T45.8X2	T45.8X3	T45.8X4	T45.8X5	T45.8X6
Polyvinylpyrrolidone	T45.8X1	T45.8X2	T45.8X3	T45.8X4	T45.8X5	T45.8X6
Pontocaine (hydrochloride) (infiltration) (topical)	T41.3X1	T41.3X2	T41.3X3	T41.3X4	T41.3X5	T41.3X6
nerve block (peripheral) (plexus)	T41.3X1	T41.3X2	T41.3X3	T41.3X4	T41.3X5	T41.3X6
spinal	T41.3X1	T41.3X2	T41.3X3	T41.3X4	T41.3X5	T41.3X6
Porfiromycin	T45.1X1	T45.1X2	T45.1X3	T45.1X4	T45.1X5	T45.1X6
Posterior pituitary hormone NEC	T38.891	T38.892	T38.893	T38.894	T38.895	T38.896
Pot	T40.7X1	T40.7X2	T40.7X3	T40.7X4	T40.7X5	T40.7X6
Potash (caustic)	T54.3X1	T54.3X2	T54.3X3	T54.3X4	—	—
Potassic saline injection (lactated)	T50.3X1	T50.3X2	T50.3X3	T50.3X4	T50.3X5	T50.3X6
Potassium-removing resin	T50.3X1	T50.3X2	T50.3X3	T50.3X4	T50.3X5	T50.3X6
Potassium-retaining drug	T50.3X1	T50.3X2	T50.3X3	T50.3X4	T50.3X5	T50.3X6
Potassium (salts) **NEC**	T50.3X1	T50.3X2	T50.3X3	T50.3X4	T50.3X5	T50.3X6
aminobenzoate	T45.8X1	T45.8X2	T45.8X3	T45.8X4	T45.8X5	T45.8X6
aminosalicylate	T37.1X1	T37.1X2	T37.1X3	T37.1X4	T37.1X5	T37.1X6
antimony 'tartrate'	T37.8X1	T37.8X2	T37.8X3	T37.8X4	T37.8X5	T37.8X6
arsenite (solution)	T57.0X1	T57.0X2	T57.0X3	T57.0X4	—	—
bichromate	T56.2X1	T56.2X2	T56.2X3	T56.2X4	—	—
bisulfate	T47.3X1	T47.3X2	T47.3X3	T47.3X4	T47.3X5	T47.3X6
bromide	T42.6X1	T42.6X2	T42.6X3	T42.6X4	T42.6X5	T42.6X6
canrenoate	T50.0X1	T50.0X2	T50.0X3	T50.0X4	T50.0X5	T50.0X6
carbonate	T54.3X1	T54.3X2	T54.3X3	T54.3X4	—	—
chlorate NEC	T65.891	T65.892	T65.893	T65.894	—	—
chloride	T50.3X1	T50.3X2	T50.3X3	T50.3X4	T50.3X5	T50.3X6
citrate	T50.991	T50.992	T50.993	T50.994	T50.995	T50.996
cyanide	T65.0X1	T65.0X2	T65.0X3	T65.0X4	—	—
ferric hexacyanoferrate (medicinal)	T50.6X1	T50.6X2	T50.6X3	T50.6X4	T50.6X5	T50.6X6
nonmedicinal	T65.891	T65.892	T65.893	T65.894	—	—

Substance	Poisoning, Accidental (unintentional)	Poisoning, Intentional Self-harm	Poisoning, Assault	Poisoning, Undetermined	Adverse Effect	Under-dosing
Potassium (salts) **NEC** — *continued*						
Fluoride	T57.8X1	T57.8X2	T57.8X3	T57.8X4	—	—
glucaldrate	T47.1X1	T47.1X2	T47.1X3	T47.1X4	T47.1X5	T47.1X6
hydroxide	T54.3X1	T54.3X2	T54.3X3	T54.3X4	—	—
iodate	T49.0X1	T49.0X2	T49.0X3	T49.0X4	T49.0X5	T49.0X6
iodide	T48.4X1	T48.4X2	T48.4X3	T48.4X4	T48.4X5	T48.4X6
nitrate	T57.8X1	T57.8X2	T57.8X3	T57.8X4	—	—
oxalate	T65.891	T65.892	T65.893	T65.894	—	—
perchlorate (nonmedicinal) NEC	T65.891	T65.892	T65.893	T65.894	—	—
antithyroid	T38.2X1	T38.2X2	T38.2X3	T38.2X4	T38.2X5	T38.2X6
medicinal	T38.2X1	T38.2X2	T38.2X3	T38.2X4	T38.2X5	T38.2X6
Permanganate (nonmedicinal)	T65.891	T65.892	T65.893	T65.894	—	—
medicinal	T49.0X1	T49.0X2	T49.0X3	T49.0X4	T49.0X5	T49.0X6
sulfate	T47.2X1	T47.2X2	T47.2X3	T47.2X4	T47.2X5	T47.2X6
Povidone	T45.8X1	T45.8X2	T45.8X3	T45.8X4	T45.8X5	T45.8X6
iodine	T49.0X1	T49.0X2	T49.0X3	T49.0X4	T49.0X5	T49.0X6
Practolol	T44.7X1	T44.7X2	T44.7X3	T44.7X4	T44.7X5	T44.7X6
Prajmalium bitartrate	T46.2X1	T46.2X2	T46.2X3	T46.2X4	T46.2X5	T46.2X6
Pralidoxime (iodide)	T50.6X1	T50.6X2	T50.6X3	T50.6X4	T50.6X5	T50.6X6
chloride	T50.6X1	T50.6X2	T50.6X3	T50.6X4	T50.6X5	T50.6X6
Pramiverine	T44.3X1	T44.3X2	T44.3X3	T44.3X4	T44.3X5	T44.3X6
Pramocaine	T49.1X1	T49.1X2	T49.1X3	T49.1X4	T49.1X5	T49.1X6
Pramoxine	T49.1X1	T49.1X2	T49.1X3	T49.1X4	T49.1X5	T49.1X6
Prasterone	T38.7X1	T38.7X2	T38.7X3	T38.7X4	T38.7X5	T38.7X6
Pravastatin	T46.6X1	T46.6X2	T46.6X3	T46.6X4	T46.6X5	T46.6X6
Prazepam	T42.4X1	T42.4X2	T42.4X3	T42.4X4	T42.4X5	T42.4X6
Praziquantel	T37.4X1	T37.4X2	T37.4X3	T37.4X4	T37.4X5	T37.4X6
Prazitone	T43.291	T43.292	T43.293	T43.294	T43.295	T43.296
Prazosin	T44.6X1	T44.6X2	T44.6X3	T44.6X4	T44.6X5	T44.6X6
Prednicarbate	T49.0X1	T49.0X2	T49.0X3	T49.0X4	T49.0X5	T49.0X6
Prednimustine	T45.1X1	T45.1X2	T45.1X3	T45.1X4	T45.1X5	T45.1X6
Prednisolone	T38.0X1	T38.0X2	T38.0X3	T38.0X4	T38.0X5	T38.0X6
ENT agent	T49.6X1	T49.6X2	T49.6X3	T49.6X4	T49.6X5	T49.6X6
ophthalmic preparation	T49.5X1	T49.5X2	T49.5X3	T49.5X4	T49.5X5	T49.5X6
steaglate	T49.0X1	T49.0X2	T49.0X3	T49.0X4	T49.0X5	T49.0X6
topical NEC	T49.0X1	T49.0X2	T49.0X3	T49.0X4	T49.0X5	T49.0X6
Prednisone	T38.0X1	T38.0X2	T38.0X3	T38.0X4	T38.0X5	T38.0X6
Prednylidene	T38.0X1	T38.0X2	T38.0X3	T38.0X4	T38.0X5	T38.0X6
Pregnandiol	T38.5X1	T38.5X2	T38.5X3	T38.5X4	T38.5X5	T38.5X6
Pregneninolone	T38.5X1	T38.5X2	T38.5X3	T38.5X4	T38.5X5	T38.5X6
Preludin	T43.691	T43.692	T43.693	T43.694	T43.695	T43.696
Premarin	T38.5X1	T38.5X2	T38.5X3	T38.5X4	T38.5X5	T38.5X6
Premedication anesthetic	T41.201	T41.202	T41.203	T41.204	T41.205	T41.206
Prenalterol	T44.5X1	T44.5X2	T44.5X3	T44.5X4	T44.5X5	T44.5X6
Prenoxdiazine	T48.3X1	T48.3X2	T48.3X3	T48.3X4	T48.3X5	T48.3X6
Prenylamine	T46.3X1	T46.3X2	T46.3X3	T46.3X4	T46.3X5	T46.3X6
Preparation H	T49.8X1	T49.8X2	T49.8X3	T49.8X4	T49.8X5	T49.8X6
Preparation, local	T49.4X1	T49.4X2	T49.4X3	T49.4X4	T49.4X5	T49.4X6
Preservative (nonmedicinal)	T65.891	T65.892	T65.893	T65.894	—	—
medicinal	T50.901	T50.902	T50.903	T50.904	T50.905	T50.906
wood	T60.91	T60.92	T60.93	T60.94	—	—
Prethcamide	T50.7X1	T50.7X2	T50.7X3	T50.7X4	T50.7X5	T50.7X6
Pride of China	T62.2X1	T62.2X2	T62.2X3	T62.2X4	—	—
Pridinol	T44.3X1	T44.3X2	T44.3X3	T44.3X4	T44.3X5	T44.3X6
Prifinium bromide	T44.3X1	T44.3X2	T44.3X3	T44.3X4	T44.3X5	T44.3X6
Prilocaine	T41.3X1	T41.3X2	T41.3X3	T41.3X4	T41.3X5	T41.3X6
infiltration (subcutaneous)	T41.3X1	T41.3X2	T41.3X3	T41.3X4	T41.3X5	T41.3X6
nerve block (peripheral) (plexus)	T41.3X1	T41.3X2	T41.3X3	T41.3X4	T41.3X5	T41.3X6
regional	T41.3X1	T41.3X2	T41.3X3	T41.3X4	T41.3X5	T41.3X6
Primaquine	T37.2X1	T37.2X2	T37.2X3	T37.2X4	T37.2X5	T37.2X6
Primidone	T42.6X1	T42.6X2	T42.6X3	T42.6X4	T42.6X5	T42.6X6
Primula (veris)	T62.2X1	T62.2X2	T62.2X3	T62.2X4	—	—
Prinadol	T40.2X1	T40.2X2	T40.2X3	T40.2X4	T40.2X5	T40.2X6
Priscol, Priscoline	T44.6X1	T44.6X2	T44.6X3	T44.6X4	T44.6X5	T44.6X6
Pristinamycin	T36.3X1	T36.3X2	T36.3X3	T36.3X4	T36.3X5	T36.3X6
Privet	T62.2X1	T62.2X2	T62.2X3	T62.2X4	—	—
berries	T62.1X1	T62.1X2	T62.1X3	T62.1X4	—	—
Privine	T44.4X1	T44.4X2	T44.4X3	T44.4X4	T44.4X5	T44.4X6
Pro-Banthine	T44.3X1	T44.3X2	T44.3X3	T44.3X4	T44.3X5	T44.3X6
Probarbital	T42.3X1	T42.3X2	T42.3X3	T42.3X4	T42.3X5	T42.3X6
Probenecid	T50.4X1	T50.4X2	T50.4X3	T50.4X4	T50.4X5	T50.4X6
Probucol	T46.6X1	T46.6X2	T46.6X3	T46.6X4	T46.6X5	T46.6X6
Procainamide	T46.2X1	T46.2X2	T46.2X3	T46.2X4	T46.2X5	T46.2X6
Procaine	T41.3X1	T41.3X2	T41.3X3	T41.3X4	T41.3X5	T41.3X6
benzylpenicillin	T36.0X1	T36.0X2	T36.0X3	T36.0X4	T36.0X5	T36.0X6
nerve block (periphreal) (plexus)	T41.3X1	T41.3X2	T41.3X3	T41.3X4	T41.3X5	T41.3X6
penicillin G	T36.0X1	T36.0X2	T36.0X3	T36.0X4	T36.0X5	T36.0X6
regional	T41.3X1	T41.3X2	T41.3X3	T41.3X4	T41.3X5	T41.3X6

Subterms under main terms may continue to next column or page Additional Character May Be Required — Refer to the Tabular List for Character Selection 375

Substance	Poisoning, Accidental (unintentional)	Poisoning, Intentional Self-harm	Poisoning, Assault	Poisoning, Undetermined	Adverse Effect	Underdosing
Procaine — *continued*						
spinal	T41.3X1	T41.3X2	T41.3X3	T41.3X4	T41.3X5	T41.3X6
Procalmidol	T43.591	T43.592	T43.593	T43.594	T43.595	T43.596
Procarbazine	T45.1X1	T45.1X2	T45.1X3	T45.1X4	T45.1X5	T45.1X6
Procaterol	T44.5X1	T44.5X2	T44.5X3	T44.5X4	T44.5X5	T44.5X6
Prochlorperazine	T43.3X1	T43.3X2	T43.3X3	T43.3X4	T43.3X5	T43.3X6
Procyclidine	T44.3X1	T44.3X2	T44.3X3	T44.3X4	T44.3X5	T44.3X6
Producer gas	T58.8X1	T58.8X2	T58.8X3	T58.8X4	—	—
Profadol	T40.4X1	T40.4X2	T40.4X3	T40.4X4	T40.4X5	T40.4X6
Profenamine	T44.3X1	T44.3X2	T44.3X3	T44.3X4	T44.3X5	T44.3X6
Profenil	T44.3X1	T44.3X2	T44.3X3	T44.3X4	T44.3X5	T44.3X6
Proflavine	T49.0X1	T49.0X2	T49.0X3	T49.0X4	T49.0X5	T49.0X6
Progabide	T42.6X1	T42.6X2	T42.6X3	T42.6X4	T42.6X5	T42.6X6
Progesterone	T38.5X1	T38.5X2	T38.5X3	T38.5X4	T38.5X5	T38.5X6
Progestin	T38.5X1	T38.5X2	T38.5X3	T38.5X4	T38.5X5	T38.5X6
oral contraceptive	T38.4X1	T38.4X2	T38.4X3	T38.4X4	T38.4X5	T38.4X6
Progestogen NEC	T38.5X1	T38.5X2	T38.5X3	T38.5X4	T38.5X5	T38.5X6
Progestone	T38.5X1	T38.5X2	T38.5X3	T38.5X4	T38.5X5	T38.5X6
Proglumide	T47.1X1	T47.1X2	T47.1X3	T47.1X4	T47.1X5	T47.1X6
Proguanil	T37.2X1	T37.2X2	T37.2X3	T37.2X4	T37.2X5	T37.2X6
Prolactin	T38.811	T38.812	T38.813	T38.814	T38.815	T38.816
Prolintane	T43.691	T43.692	T43.693	T43.694	T43.695	T43.696
Proloid	T38.1X1	T38.1X2	T38.1X3	T38.1X4	T38.1X5	T38.1X6
Proluton	T38.5X1	T38.5X2	T38.5X3	T38.5X4	T38.5X5	T38.5X6
Promacetin	T37.1X1	T37.1X2	T37.1X3	T37.1X4	T37.1X5	T37.1X6
Promazine	T43.3X1	T43.3X2	T43.3X3	T43.3X4	T43.3X5	T43.3X6
Promedol	T40.2X1	T40.2X2	T40.2X3	T40.2X4	—	—
Promegestone	T38.5X1	T38.5X2	T38.5X3	T38.5X4	T38.5X5	T38.5X6
Promethazine (teoclate)	T43.3X1	T43.3X2	T43.3X3	T43.3X4	T43.3X5	T43.3X6
Promin	T37.1X1	T37.1X2	T37.1X3	T37.1X4	T37.1X5	T37.1X6
Pronase	T45.3X1	T45.3X2	T45.3X3	T45.3X4	T45.3X5	T45.3X6
Pronestyl (hydrochloride)	T46.2X1	T46.2X2	T46.2X3	T46.2X4	T46.2X5	T46.2X6
Pronetalol	T44.7X1	T44.7X2	T44.7X3	T44.7X4	T44.7X5	T44.7X6
Prontosil	T37.0X1	T37.0X2	T37.0X3	T37.0X4	T37.0X5	T37.0X6
Propachlor	T60.3X1	T60.3X2	T60.3X3	T60.3X4	—	—
Propafenone	T46.2X1	T46.2X2	T46.2X3	T46.2X4	T46.2X5	T46.2X6
Propallylonal	T42.3X1	T42.3X2	T42.3X3	T42.3X4	T42.3X5	T42.3X6
Propamidine	T49.0X1	T49.0X2	T49.0X3	T49.0X4	T49.0X5	T49.0X6
Propane (distributed in mobile container)	T59.891	T59.892	T59.893	T59.894		
distributed through pipes	T59.891	T59.892	T59.893	T59.894	—	—
incomplete combustion	T58.11	T58.12	T58.13	T58.14	—	—
Propanidid	T41.291	T41.292	T41.293	T41.294	T41.295	T41.296
Propanil	T60.3X1	T60.3X2	T60.3X3	T60.3X4	—	—
Propantheline	T44.3X1	T44.3X2	T44.3X3	T44.3X4	T44.3X5	T44.3X6
bromide	T44.3X1	T44.3X2	T44.3X3	T44.3X4	T44.3X5	T44.3X6
Proparacaine	T41.3X1	T41.3X2	T41.3X3	T41.3X4	T41.3X5	T41.3X6
Propatylnitrate	T46.3X1	T46.3X2	T46.3X3	T46.3X4	T46.3X5	T46.3X6
Propicillin	T36.0X1	T36.0X2	T36.0X3	T36.0X4	T36.0X5	T36.0X6
Propiolactone	T49.0X1	T49.0X2	T49.0X3	T49.0X4	T49.0X5	T49.0X6
Propiomazine	T45.0X1	T45.0X2	T45.0X3	T45.0X4	T45.0X5	T45.0X6
Propionaidehyde (medicinal)	T42.6X1	T42.6X2	T42.6X3	T42.6X4	T42.6X5	T42.6X6
Propionate (calcium) (sodium)	T49.0X1	T49.0X2	T49.0X3	T49.0X4	T49.0X5	T49.0X6
Propion gel	T49.0X1	T49.0X2	T49.0X3	T49.0X4	T49.0X5	T49.0X6
Propitocaine	T41.3X1	T41.3X2	T41.3X3	T41.3X4	T41.3X5	T41.3X6
infiltration (subcutaneous)	T41.3X1	T41.3X2	T41.3X3	T41.3X4	T41.3X5	T41.3X6
nerve block (peripheral) (plexus)	T41.3X1	T41.3X2	T41.3X3	T41.3X4	T41.3X5	T41.3X6
Propofol	T41.291	T41.292	T41.293	T41.294	T41.295	T41.296
Propoxur	T60.0X1	T60.0X2	T60.0X3	T60.0X4	—	—
Propoxycaine	T41.3X1	T41.3X2	T41.3X3	T41.3X4	T41.3X5	T41.3X6
infiltration (subcutaneous)	T41.3X1	T41.3X2	T41.3X3	T41.3X4	T41.3X5	T41.3X6
nerve block (peripheral) (plexus)	T41.3X1	T41.3X2	T41.3X3	T41.3X4	T41.3X5	T41.3X6
topical (surface)	T41.3X1	T41.3X2	T41.3X3	T41.3X4	T41.3X5	T41.3X6
Propoxyphene	T40.4X1	T40.4X2	T40.4X3	T40.4X4	T40.4X5	T40.4X6
Propranolol	T44.7X1	T44.7X2	T44.7X3	T44.7X4	T44.7X5	T44.7X6
Propyl						
alcohol	T51.3X1	T51.3X2	T51.3X3	T51.3X4	—	—
carbinol	T51.3X1	T51.3X2	T51.3X3	T51.3X4	—	—
hexadrine	T44.4X1	T44.4X2	T44.4X3	T44.4X4	T44.4X5	T44.4X6
iodone	T50.8X1	T50.8X2	T50.8X3	T50.8X4	T50.8X5	T50.8X6
thiouracil	T38.2X1	T38.2X2	T38.2X3	T38.2X4	T38.2X5	T38.2X6
Propylaminophenothiazine	T43.3X1	T43.3X2	T43.3X3	T43.3X4	T43.3X5	T43.3X6
Propylene	T59.891	T59.892	T59.893	T59.894		
Propylhexedrine	T48.5X1	T48.5X2	T48.5X3	T48.5X4	T48.5X5	T48.5X6
Propyliodone	T50.8X1	T50.8X2	T50.8X3	T50.8X4	T50.8X5	T50.8X6
Propylparaben (ophthalmic)	T49.5X1	T49.5X2	T49.5X3	T49.5X4	T49.5X5	T49.5X6
Propylthiouracil	T38.2X1	T38.2X2	T38.2X3	T38.2X4	T38.2X5	T38.2X6
Propyphenazone	T39.2X1	T39.2X2	T39.2X3	T39.2X4	T39.2X5	T39.2X6
Proquazone	T39.391	T39.392	T39.393	T39.394	T39.395	T39.396

Substance	Poisoning, Accidental (unintentional)	Poisoning, Intentional Self-harm	Poisoning, Assault	Poisoning, Undetermined	Adverse Effect	Underdosing
Proscillaridin	T46.0X1	T46.0X2	T46.0X3	T46.0X4	T46.0X5	T46.0X6
Prostacyclin	T45.521	T45.522	T45.523	T45.524	T45.525	T45.526
Prostaglandin (I2)	T45.521	T45.522	T45.523	T45.524	T45.525	T45.526
E1	T46.7X1	T46.7X2	T46.7X3	T46.7X4	T46.7X5	T46.7X6
E2	T48.0X1	T48.0X2	T48.0X3	T48.0X4	T48.0X5	T48.0X6
F2 alpha	T48.0X1	T48.0X2	T48.0X3	T48.0X4	T48.0X5	T48.0X6
Prostigmin	T44.0X1	T44.0X2	T44.0X3	T44.0X4	T44.0X5	T44.0X6
Prosultiamine	T45.2X1	T45.2X2	T45.2X3	T45.2X4	T45.2X5	T45.2X6
Protamine sulfate	T45.7X1	T45.7X2	T45.7X3	T45.7X4	T45.7X5	T45.7X6
zinc insulin	T38.3X1	T38.3X2	T38.3X3	T38.3X4	T38.3X5	T38.3X6
Protease	T47.5X1	T47.5X2	T47.5X3	T47.5X4	T47.5X5	T47.5X6
Protectant, skin NEC	T49.3X1	T49.3X2	T49.3X3	T49.3X4	T49.3X5	T49.3X6
Protein hydrolysate	T50.991	T50.992	T50.993	T50.994	T50.995	T50.996
Prothiaden — *see* Dothiepin hydrochloride						
Prothionamide	T37.1X1	T37.1X2	T37.1X3	T37.1X4	T37.1X5	T37.1X6
Prothipendyl	T43.591	T43.592	T43.593	T43.594	T43.595	T43.596
Prothoate	T60.0X1	T60.0X2	T60.0X3	T60.0X4	—	—
Prothrombin						
activator	T45.7X1	T45.7X2	T45.7X3	T45.7X4	T45.7X5	T45.7X6
synthesis inhibitor	T45.511	T45.512	T45.513	T45.514	T45.515	T45.516
Protionamide	T37.1X1	T37.1X2	T37.1X3	T37.1X4	T37.1X5	T37.1X6
Protirelin	T38.891	T38.892	T38.893	T38.894	T38.895	T38.896
Protokylol	T48.6X1	T48.6X2	T48.6X3	T48.6X4	T48.6X5	T48.6X6
Protopam	T50.6X1	T50.6X2	T50.6X3	T50.6X4	T50.6X5	T50.6X6
Protoveratrine(s) (A) (B)	T46.5X1	T46.5X2	T46.5X3	T46.5X4	T46.5X5	T46.5X6
Protriptyline	T43.011	T43.012	T43.013	T43.014	T43.015	T43.016
Provera	T38.5X1	T38.5X2	T38.5X3	T38.5X4	T38.5X5	T38.5X6
Provitamin A	T45.2X1	T45.2X2	T45.2X3	T45.2X4	T45.2X5	T45.2X6
Proxibarbal	T42.3X1	T42.3X2	T42.3X3	T42.3X4	T42.3X5	T42.3X6
Proxymetacaine	T41.3X1	T41.3X2	T41.3X3	T41.3X4	T41.3X5	T41.3X6
Proxyphylline	T48.6X1	T48.6X2	T48.6X3	T48.6X4	T48.6X5	T48.6X6
Prozac — *see* Fluoxetine hydrochloride						
Prunus						
laurocerasus	T62.2X1	T62.2X2	T62.2X3	T62.2X4	—	—
virginiana	T62.2X1	T62.2X2	T62.2X3	T62.2X4	—	—
Prussian blue						
commercial	T65.891	T65.892	T65.893	T65.894	—	—
therapeutic	T50.6X1	T50.6X2	T50.6X3	T50.6X4	T50.6X5	T50.6X6
Prussic acid	T65.0X1	T65.0X2	T65.0X3	T65.0X4	—	—
vapor	T57.3X1	T57.3X2	T57.3X3	T57.3X4	—	—
Pseudoephedrine	T44.991	T44.992	T44.993	T44.994	T44.995	T44.996
Psilocin	T40.991	T40.992	T40.993	T40.994	—	—
Psilocybin	T40.991	T40.992	T40.993	T40.994	—	—
Psilocybine	T40.991	T40.992	T40.993	T40.994	—	—
Psoralene (nonmedicinal)	T65.891	T65.892	T65.893	T65.894	—	—
Psoralens (medicinal)	T50.991	T50.992	T50.993	T50.994	T50.995	T50.996
PSP (phenolsulfonphthalein)	T50.8X1	T50.8X2	T50.8X3	T50.8X4	T50.8X5	T50.8X6
Psychodysleptic drug NEC	T40.901	T40.902	T40.903	T40.904	T40.905	T40.906
Psychostimulant	T43.601	T43.602	T43.603	T43.604	T43.605	T43.606
amphetamine	T43.621	T43.622	T43.623	T43.624	T43.625	T43.626
caffeine	T43.611	T43.612	T43.613	T43.614	T43.615	T43.616
methylphenidate	T43.631	T43.632	T43.633	T43.634	T43.635	T43.636
specified NEC	T43.691	T43.692	T43.693	T43.694	T43.695	T43.696
Psychotherapeutic drug NEC	T43.91	T43.92	T43.93	T43.94	T43.95	T43.96
antidepressants — *see also* Antidepressant	T43.201	T43.202	T43.203	T43.204	T43.205	T43.206
specified NEC	T43.8X1	T43.8X2	T43.8X3	T43.8X4	T43.8X5	T43.8X6
tranquilizers NEC	T43.501	T43.502	T43.503	T43.504	T43.505	T43.506
Psychotomimetic agents	T40.901	T40.902	T40.903	T40.904	T40.905	T40.906
Psychotropic drug NEC	T43.91	T43.92	T43.93	T43.94	T43.95	T43.96
specified NEC	T43.8X1	T43.8X2	T43.8X3	T43.8X4	T43.8X5	T43.8X6
Psyllium hydrophilic mucilloid	T47.4X1	T47.4X2	T47.4X3	T47.4X4	T47.4X5	T47.4X6
Pteroylglutamic acid	T45.8X1	T45.8X2	T45.8X3	T45.8X4	T45.8X5	T45.8X6
Pteroyltriglutamate	T45.1X1	T45.1X2	T45.1X3	T45.1X4	T45.1X5	T45.1X6
PTFE — *see* Polytetrafluoroethylene						
Pulp						
devitalizing paste	T49.7X1	T49.7X2	T49.7X3	T49.7X4	T49.7X5	T49.7X6
dressing	T49.7X1	T49.7X2	T49.7X3	T49.7X4	T49.7X5	T49.7X6
Pulsatilla	T62.2X1	T62.2X2	T62.2X3	T62.2X4	—	—
Pumpkin seed extract	T37.4X1	T37.4X2	T37.4X3	T37.4X4	T37.4X5	T37.4X6
Purex (bleach)	T54.91	T54.92	T54.93	T54.94	—	—
Purgative NEC — *see also* Cathartic	T47.4X1	T47.4X2	T47.4X3	T47.4X4	T47.4X5	T47.4X6
Purine analogue (antineoplastic)	T45.1X1	T45.1X2	T45.1X3	T45.1X4	T45.1X5	T45.1X6
Purine diuretics	T50.2X1	T50.2X2	T50.2X3	T50.2X4	T50.2X5	T50.2X6
Purinethol	T45.1X1	T45.1X2	T45.1X3	T45.1X4	T45.1X5	T45.1X6
PVP	T45.8X1	T45.8X2	T45.8X3	T45.8X4	T45.8X5	T45.8X6

Substance	Poisoning, Accidental (unintentional)	Poisoning, Intentional Self-harm	Poisoning, Assault	Poisoning, Undetermined	Adverse Effect	Under-dosing
Pyrabital	T39.8X1	T39.8X2	T39.8X3	T39.8X4	T39.8X5	T39.8X6
Pyramidon	T39.2X1	T39.2X2	T39.2X3	T39.2X4	T39.2X5	T39.2X6
Pyrantel	T37.4X1	T37.4X2	T37.4X3	T37.4X4	T37.4X5	T37.4X6
Pyrathiazine	T45.ØX1	T45.ØX2	T45.ØX3	T45.ØX4	T45.ØX5	T45.ØX6
Pyrazinamide	T37.1X1	T37.1X2	T37.1X3	T37.1X4	T37.1X5	T37.1X6
Pyrazinoic acid (amide)	T37.1X1	T37.1X2	T37.1X3	T37.1X4	T37.1X5	T37.1X6
Pyrazole (derivatives)	T39.2X1	T39.2X2	T39.2X3	T39.2X4	T39.2X5	T39.2X6
Pyrazolone analgesic NEC	T39.2X1	T39.2X2	T39.2X3	T39.2X4	T39.2X5	T39.2X6
Pyrethrin, pyrethrum (nonmedicinal)	T6Ø.2X1	T6Ø.2X2	T6Ø.2X3	T6Ø.2X4	—	—
Pyrethrum extract	T49.ØX1	T49.ØX2	T49.ØX3	T49.ØX4	T49.ØX5	T49.ØX6
Pyribenzamine	T45.ØX1	T45.ØX2	T45.ØX3	T45.ØX4	T45.ØX5	T45.ØX6
Pyridine	T52.8X1	T52.8X2	T52.8X3	T52.8X4	—	—
aldoxime methiodide	T5Ø.6X1	T5Ø.6X2	T5Ø.6X3	T5Ø.6X4	T5Ø.6X5	T5Ø.6X6
aldoxime methyl chloride	T5Ø.6X1	T5Ø.6X2	T5Ø.6X3	T5Ø.6X4	T5Ø.6X5	T5Ø.6X6
vapor	T59.891	T59.892	T59.893	T59.894	—	—
Pyridium	T39.8X1	T39.8X2	T39.8X3	T39.8X4	T39.8X5	T39.8X6
Pyridostigmine bromide	T44.ØX1	T44.ØX2	T44.ØX3	T44.ØX4	T44.ØX5	T44.ØX6
Pyridoxal phosphate	T45.2X1	T45.2X2	T45.2X3	T45.2X4	T45.2X5	T45.2X6
Pyridoxine	T45.2X1	T45.2X2	T45.2X3	T45.2X4	T45.2X5	T45.2X6
Pyrilamine	T45.ØX1	T45.ØX2	T45.ØX3	T45.ØX4	T45.ØX5	T45.ØX6
Pyrimethamine	T37.2X1	T37.2X2	T37.2X3	T37.2X4	T37.2X5	T37.2X6
with sulfadoxine	T37.2X1	T37.2X2	T37.2X3	T37.2X4	T37.2X5	T37.2X6
Pyrimidine antagonist	T45.1X1	T45.1X2	T45.1X3	T45.1X4	T45.1X5	T45.1X6
Pyriminil	T6Ø.4X1	T6Ø.4X2	T6Ø.4X3	T6Ø.4X4	—	—
Pyrithione zinc	T49.4X1	T49.4X2	T49.4X3	T49.4X4	T49.4X5	T49.4X6
Pyrithyldione	T42.6X1	T42.6X2	T42.6X3	T42.6X4	T42.6X5	T42.6X6
Pyrogallic acid	T49.ØX1	T49.ØX2	T49.ØX3	T49.ØX4	T49.ØX5	T49.ØX6
Pyrogallol	T49.ØX1	T49.ØX2	T49.ØX3	T49.ØX4	T49.ØX5	T49.ØX6
Pyroxylin	T49.3X1	T49.3X2	T49.3X3	T49.3X4	T49.3X5	T49.3X6
Pyrrobutamine	T45.ØX1	T45.ØX2	T45.ØX3	T45.ØX4	T45.ØX5	T45.ØX6
Pyrrolizidine alkaloids	T62.8X1	T62.8X2	T62.8X3	T62.8X4	—	—
Pyrvinium chloride	T37.4X1	T37.4X2	T37.4X3	T37.4X4	T37.4X5	T37.4X6
PZI	T38.3X1	T38.3X2	T38.3X3	T38.3X4	T38.3X5	T38.3X6
Quaalude	T42.6X1	T42.6X2	T42.6X3	T42.6X4	T42.6X5	T42.6X6
Quarternary ammonium						
anti-infective	T49.ØX1	T49.ØX2	T49.ØX3	T49.ØX4	T49.ØX5	T49.ØX6
ganglion blocking	T44.2X1	T44.2X2	T44.2X3	T44.2X4	T44.2X5	T44.2X6
parasympatholytic	T44.3X1	T44.3X2	T44.3X3	T44.3X4	T44.3X5	T44.3X6
Quazepam	T42.4X1	T42.4X2	T42.4X3	T42.4X4	T42.4X5	T42.4X6
Quicklime	T54.3X1	T54.3X2	T54.3X3	T54.3X4	—	—
Quillaja extract	T48.4X1	T48.4X2	T48.4X3	T48.4X4	T48.4X5	T48.4X6
Quinacrine	T37.2X1	T37.2X2	T37.2X3	T37.2X4	T37.2X5	T37.2X6
Quinaglute	T46.2X1	T46.2X2	T46.2X3	T46.2X4	T46.2X5	T46.2X6
Quinalbarbital	T42.3X1	T42.3X2	T42.3X3	T42.3X4	T42.3X5	T42.3X6
Quinalbarbitone sodium	T42.3X1	T42.3X2	T42.3X3	T42.3X4	T42.3X5	T42.3X6
Quinalphos	T6Ø.ØX1	T6Ø.ØX2	T6Ø.ØX3	T6Ø.ØX4	—	—
Quinapril	T46.4X1	T46.4X2	T46.4X3	T46.4X4	T46.4X5	T46.4X6
Quinestradiol	T38.5X1	T38.5X2	T38.5X3	T38.5X4	T38.5X5	T38.5X6
Quinestradol	T38.5X1	T38.5X2	T38.5X3	T38.5X4	T38.5X5	T38.5X6
Quinestrol	T38.5X1	T38.5X2	T38.5X3	T38.5X4	T38.5X5	T38.5X6
Quinethazone	T5Ø.2X1	T5Ø.2X2	T5Ø.2X3	T5Ø.2X4	T5Ø.2X5	T5Ø.2X6
Quingestanol	T38.4X1	T38.4X2	T38.4X3	T38.4X4	T38.4X5	T38.4X6
Quinidine	T46.2X1	T46.2X2	T46.2X3	T46.2X4	T46.2X5	T46.2X6
Quinine	T37.2X1	T37.2X2	T37.2X3	T37.2X4	T37.2X5	T37.2X6
Quiniobine	T37.8X1	T37.8X2	T37.8X3	T37.8X4	T37.8X5	T37.8X6
Quinisocaine	T49.1X1	T49.1X2	T49.1X3	T49.1X4	T49.1X5	T49.1X6
Quinocide	T37.2X1	T37.2X2	T37.2X3	T37.2X4	T37.2X5	T37.2X6
Quinoline (derivatives) **NEC**	T37.8X1	T37.8X2	T37.8X3	T37.8X4	T37.8X5	T37.8X6
Quinupramine	T43.Ø11	T43.Ø12	T43.Ø13	T43.Ø14	T43.Ø15	T43.Ø16
Quotane	T41.3X1	T41.3X2	T41.3X3	T41.3X4	T41.3X5	T41.3X6
Rabies						
immune globulin (human)	T5Ø.Z11	T5Ø.Z12	T5Ø.Z13	T5Ø.Z14	T5Ø.Z15	T5Ø.Z16
vaccine	T5Ø.B91	T5Ø.B92	T5Ø.B93	T5Ø.B94	T5Ø.B95	T5Ø.B96
Racemoramide	T4Ø.2X1	T4Ø.2X2	T4Ø.2X3	T4Ø.2X4	—	—
Racemorphan	T4Ø.2X1	T4Ø.2X2	T4Ø.2X3	T4Ø.2X4	T4Ø.2X5	T4Ø.2X6
Racepinefrin	T44.5X1	T44.5X2	T44.5X3	T44.5X4	T44.5X5	T44.5X6
Raclopride	T43.591	T43.592	T43.593	T43.594	T43.595	T43.596
Radiator alcohol	T51.1X1	T51.1X2	T51.1X3	T51.1X4	—	—
Radioactive drug NEC	T5Ø.8X1	T5Ø.8X2	T5Ø.8X3	T5Ø.8X4	T5Ø.8X5	T5Ø.8X6
Radio-opaque (drugs) (materials)	T5Ø.8X1	T5Ø.8X2	T5Ø.8X3	T5Ø.8X4	T5Ø.8X5	T5Ø.8X6
Ramifenazone	T39.2X1	T39.2X2	T39.2X3	T39.2X4	T39.2X5	T39.2X6
Ramipril	T46.4X1	T46.4X2	T46.4X3	T46.4X4	T46.4X5	T46.4X6
Ranitidine	T47.ØX1	T47.ØX2	T47.ØX3	T47.ØX4	T47.ØX5	T47.ØX6
Ranunculus	T62.2X1	T62.2X2	T62.2X3	T62.2X4	—	—
Rat poison NEC	T6Ø.4X1	T6Ø.4X2	T6Ø.4X3	T6Ø.4X4	—	—
Rattlesnake (venom)	T63.Ø11	T63.Ø12	T63.Ø13	T63.Ø14	—	—
Raubasine	T46.7X1	T46.7X2	T46.7X3	T46.7X4	T46.7X5	T46.7X6
Raudixin	T46.5X1	T46.5X2	T46.5X3	T46.5X4	T46.5X5	T46.5X6
Rautensin	T46.5X1	T46.5X2	T46.5X3	T46.5X4	T46.5X5	T46.5X6
Rautina	T46.5X1	T46.5X2	T46.5X3	T46.5X4	T46.5X5	T46.5X6
Rautotal	T46.5X1	T46.5X2	T46.5X3	T46.5X4	T46.5X5	T46.5X6

Substance	Poisoning, Accidental (unintentional)	Poisoning, Intentional Self-harm	Poisoning, Assault	Poisoning, Undetermined	Adverse Effect	Under-dosing
Rauwiloid	T46.5X1	T46.5X2	T46.5X3	T46.5X4	T46.5X5	T46.5X6
Rauwoldin	T46.5X1	T46.5X2	T46.5X3	T46.5X4	T46.5X5	T46.5X6
Rauwolfia (alkaloids)	T46.5X1	T46.5X2	T46.5X3	T46.5X4	T46.5X5	T46.5X6
Razoxane	T45.1X1	T45.1X2	T45.1X3	T45.1X4	T45.1X5	T45.1X6
Realgar	T57.ØX1	T57.ØX2	T57.ØX3	T57.ØX4	—	—
Recombinant (R) — *see* specific protein						
Red blood cells, packed	T45.8X1	T45.8X2	T45.8X3	T45.8X4	T45.8X5	T45.8X6
Red squill (scilliroside)	T6Ø.4X1	T6Ø.4X2	T6Ø.4X3	T6Ø.4X4	—	—
Reducing agent, industrial NEC	T65.891	T65.892	T65.893	T65.894	—	—
Refrigerant gas (chlorofluorocarbon)	T53.5X1	T53.5X2	T53.5X3	T53.5X4	—	—
not chlorofluorocarbon	T59.891	T59.892	T59.893	T59.894	—	—
Regroton	T5Ø.2X1	T5Ø.2X2	T5Ø.2X3	T5Ø.2X4	T5Ø.2X5	T5Ø.2X6
Rehydration salts (oral)	T5Ø.3X1	T5Ø.3X2	T5Ø.3X3	T5Ø.3X4	T5Ø.3X5	T5Ø.3X6
Rela	T42.8X1	T42.8X2	T42.8X3	T42.8X4	T42.8X5	T42.8X6
Relaxant, muscle						
anesthetic	T48.1X1	T48.1X2	T48.1X3	T48.1X4	T48.1X5	T48.1X6
central nervous system	T42.8X1	T42.8X2	T42.8X3	T42.8X4	T42.8X5	T42.8X6
skeletal NEC	T48.1X1	T48.1X2	T48.1X3	T48.1X4	T48.1X5	T48.1X6
smooth NEC	T44.3X1	T44.3X2	T44.3X3	T44.3X4	T44.3X5	T44.3X6
Remoxipride	T43.591	T43.592	T43.593	T43.594	T43.595	T43.596
Renese	T5Ø.2X1	T5Ø.2X2	T5Ø.2X3	T5Ø.2X4	T5Ø.2X5	T5Ø.2X6
Renografin	T5Ø.8X1	T5Ø.8X2	T5Ø.8X3	T5Ø.8X4	T5Ø.8X5	T5Ø.8X6
Replacement solution	T5Ø.3X1	T5Ø.3X2	T5Ø.3X3	T5Ø.3X4	T5Ø.3X5	T5Ø.3X6
Reproterol	T48.6X1	T48.6X2	T48.6X3	T48.6X4	T48.6X5	T48.6X6
Rescinnamine	T46.5X1	T46.5X2	T46.5X3	T46.5X4	T46.5X5	T46.5X6
Reserpin (e)	T46.5X1	T46.5X2	T46.5X3	T46.5X4	T46.5X5	T46.5X6
Resorcin, resorcinol (nonmedicinal)	T65.891	T65.892	T65.893	T65.894	—	—
medicinal	T49.4X1	T49.4X2	T49.4X3	T49.4X4	T49.4X5	T49.4X6
Respaire	T48.4X1	T48.4X2	T48.4X3	T48.4X4	T48.4X5	T48.4X6
Respiratory drug NEC	T48.9Ø1	T48.9Ø2	T48.9Ø3	T48.9Ø4	T48.9Ø5	T48.9Ø6
antiasthmatic NEC	T48.6X1	T48.6X2	T48.6X3	T48.6X4	T48.6X5	T48.6X6
anti-common-cold NEC	T48.5X1	T48.5X2	T48.5X3	T48.5X4	T48.5X5	T48.5X6
expectorant NEC	T48.4X1	T48.4X2	T48.4X3	T48.4X4	T48.4X5	T48.4X6
stimulant	T48.9Ø1	T48.9Ø2	T48.9Ø3	T48.9Ø4	T48.9Ø5	T48.9Ø6
Retinoic acid	T49.ØX1	T49.ØX2	T49.ØX3	T49.ØX4	T49.ØX5	T49.ØX6
Retinol	T45.2X1	T45.2X2	T45.2X3	T45.2X4	T45.2X5	T45.2X6
Rh (D) **immune globulin** (human)	T5Ø.Z11	T5Ø.Z12	T5Ø.Z13	T5Ø.Z14	T5Ø.Z15	T5Ø.Z16
Rhodine	T39.Ø11	T39.Ø12	T39.Ø13	T39.Ø14	T39.Ø15	T39.Ø16
RhoGAM	T5Ø.Z11	T5Ø.Z12	T5Ø.Z13	T5Ø.Z14	T5Ø.Z15	T5Ø.Z16
Rhubarb						
dry extract	T47.2X1	T47.2X2	T47.2X3	T47.2X4	T47.2X5	T47.2X6
tincture, compound	T47.2X1	T47.2X2	T47.2X3	T47.2X4	T47.2X5	T47.2X6
Ribavirin	T37.5X1	T37.5X2	T37.5X3	T37.5X4	T37.5X5	T37.5X6
Riboflavin	T45.2X1	T45.2X2	T45.2X3	T45.2X4	T45.2X5	T45.2X6
Ribostamycin	T36.5X1	T36.5X2	T36.5X3	T36.5X4	T36.5X5	T36.5X6
Ricin	T62.2X1	T62.2X2	T62.2X3	T62.2X4	—	—
Ricinus communis	T62.2X1	T62.2X2	T62.2X3	T62.2X4	—	—
Rickettsial vaccine NEC	T5Ø.A91	T5Ø.A92	T5Ø.A93	T5Ø.A94	T5Ø.A95	T5Ø.A96
Rifabutin	T36.6X1	T36.6X2	T36.6X3	T36.6X4	T36.6X5	T36.6X6
Rifamide	T36.6X1	T36.6X2	T36.6X3	T36.6X4	T36.6X5	T36.6X6
Rifampicin	T36.6X1	T36.6X2	T36.6X3	T36.6X4	T36.6X5	T36.6X6
with isoniazid	T37.1X1	T37.1X2	T37.1X3	T37.1X4	T37.1X5	T37.1X6
Rifampin	T36.6X1	T36.6X2	T36.6X3	T36.6X4	T36.6X5	T36.6X6
Rifamycin	T36.6X1	T36.6X2	T36.6X3	T36.6X4	T36.6X5	T36.6X6
Rifaximin	T36.6X1	T36.6X2	T36.6X3	T36.6X4	T36.6X5	T36.6X6
Rimantadine	T37.5X1	T37.5X2	T37.5X3	T37.5X4	T37.5X5	T37.5X6
Rimazolium metilsulfate	T39.8X1	T39.8X2	T39.8X3	T39.8X4	T39.8X5	T39.8X6
Rimifon	T37.1X1	T37.1X2	T37.1X3	T37.1X4	T37.1X5	T37.1X6
Rimiterol	T48.6X1	T48.6X2	T48.6X3	T48.6X4	T48.6X5	T48.6X6
Ringer (lactate) **solution**	T5Ø.3X1	T5Ø.3X2	T5Ø.3X3	T5Ø.3X4	T5Ø.3X5	T5Ø.3X6
Ristocetin	T36.8X1	T36.8X2	T36.8X3	T36.8X4	T36.8X5	T36.8X6
Ritalin	T43.631	T43.632	T43.633	T43.634	T43.635	T43.636
Ritodrine	T44.5X1	T44.5X2	T44.5X3	T44.5X4	T44.5X5	T44.5X6
Roach killer — *see* Insecticide						
Rociverine	T44.3X1	T44.3X2	T44.3X3	T44.3X4	T44.3X5	T44.3X6
Rocky Mountain spotted fever vaccine	T5Ø.A91	T5Ø.A92	T5Ø.A93	T5Ø.A94	T5Ø.A95	T5Ø.A96
Rodenticide NEC	T6Ø.4X1	T6Ø.4X2	T6Ø.4X3	T6Ø.4X4	—	—
Rohypnol	T42.4X1	T42.4X2	T42.4X3	T42.4X4	T42.4X5	T42.4X6
Rokitamycin	T36.3X1	T36.3X2	T36.3X3	T36.3X4	T36.3X5	T36.3X6
Rolaids	T47.1X1	T47.1X2	T47.1X3	T47.1X4	T47.1X5	T47.1X6
Rolitetracycline	T36.4X1	T36.4X2	T36.4X3	T36.4X4	T36.4X5	T36.4X6
Romilar	T48.3X1	T48.3X2	T48.3X3	T48.3X4	T48.3X5	T48.3X6
Ronifibrate	T46.6X1	T46.6X2	T46.6X3	T46.6X4	T46.6X5	T46.6X6
Rosaprostol	T47.1X1	T47.1X2	T47.1X3	T47.1X4	T47.1X5	T47.1X6
Rose bengal sodium (131I)	T5Ø.8X1	T5Ø.8X2	T5Ø.8X3	T5Ø.8X4	T5Ø.8X5	T5Ø.8X6
Rose water ointment	T49.3X1	T49.3X2	T49.3X3	T49.3X4	T49.3X5	T49.3X6
Rosoxacin	T37.8X1	T37.8X2	T37.8X3	T37.8X4	T37.8X5	T37.8X6

Table of Drugs and Chemicals

Substance	Poisoning, Accidental (unintentional)	Poisoning, Intentional Self-harm	Poisoning, Assault	Poisoning, Undetermined	Adverse Effect	Under-dosing
Rotenone	T6Ø.2X1	T6Ø.2X2	T6Ø.2X3	T6Ø.2X4	—	—
Rotoxamine	T45.ØX1	T45.ØX2	T45.ØX3	T45.ØX4	T45.ØX5	T45.ØX6
Rough-on-rats	T6Ø.4X1	T6Ø.4X2	T6Ø.4X3	T6Ø.4X4	—	—
Roxatidine	T47.ØX1	T47.ØX2	T47.ØX3	T47.ØX4	T47.ØX5	T47.ØX6
Roxithromycin	T36.3X1	T36.3X2	T36.3X3	T36.3X4	T36.3X5	T36.3X6
Rt-PA	T45.611	T45.612	T45.613	T45.614	T45.615	T45.616
Rubbing alcohol	T51.2X1	T51.2X2	T51.2X3	T51.2X4	—	—
Rubefacient	T49.4X1	T49.4X2	T49.4X3	T49.4X4	T49.4X5	T49.4X6
Rubella vaccine	T5Ø.B91	T5Ø.B92	T5Ø.B93	T5Ø.B94	T5Ø.B95	T5Ø.B96
Rubeola vaccine	T5Ø.B91	T5Ø.B92	T5Ø.B93	T5Ø.B94	T5Ø.B95	T5Ø.B96
Rubidium chloride Rb82	T5Ø.8X1	T5Ø.8X2	T5Ø.8X3	T5Ø.8X4	T5Ø.8X5	T5Ø.8X6
Rubidomycin	T45.1X1	T45.1X2	T45.1X3	T45.1X4	T45.1X5	T45.1X6
Rue	T62.2X1	T62.2X2	T62.2X3	T62.2X4	—	—
Rufocromomycin	T45.1X1	T45.1X2	T45.1X3	T45.1X4	T45.1X5	T45.1X6
Russel's viper venin	T45.7X1	T45.7X2	T45.7X3	T45.7X4	T45.7X5	T45.7X6
Ruta (graveolens)	T62.2X1	T62.2X2	T62.2X3	T62.2X4	—	—
Rutinum	T46.991	T46.992	T46.993	T46.994	T46.995	T46.996
Rutoside	T46.991	T46.992	T46.993	T46.994	T46.995	T46.996
b-sitosterol(s)	T46.6X1	T46.6X2	T46.6X3	T46.6X4	T46.6X5	T46.6X6
Sabadilla (plant)	T62.2X1	T62.2X2	T62.2X3	T62.2X4	—	—
pesticide	T6Ø.2X1	T6Ø.2X2	T6Ø.2X3	T6Ø.2X4	—	—
Saccharated iron oxide	T45.8X1	T45.8X2	T45.8X3	T45.8X4	T45.8X5	T45.8X6
Saccharin	T5Ø.9Ø1	T5Ø.9Ø2	T5Ø.9Ø3	T5Ø.9Ø4	T5Ø.9Ø5	T5Ø.9Ø6
Saccharomyces boulardii	T47.6X1	T47.6X2	T47.6X3	T47.6X4	T47.6X5	T47.6X6
Safflower oil	T46.6X1	T46.6X2	T46.6X3	T46.6X4	T46.6X5	T46.6X6
Safrazine	T43.1X1	T43.1X2	T43.1X3	T43.1X4	T43.1X5	T43.1X6
Salazosulfapyridine	T37.ØX1	T37.ØX2	T37.ØX3	T37.ØX4	T37.ØX5	T37.ØX6
Salbutamol	T48.6X1	T48.6X2	T48.6X3	T48.6X4	T48.6X5	T48.6X6
Salicylamide	T39.Ø91	T39.Ø92	T39.Ø93	T39.Ø94	T39.Ø95	T39.Ø96
Salicylate NEC	T39.Ø91	T39.Ø92	T39.Ø93	T39.Ø94	T39.Ø95	T39.Ø96
methyl	T49.3X1	T49.3X2	T49.3X3	T49.3X4	T49.3X5	T49.3X6
theobromine calcium	T5Ø.2X1	T5Ø.2X2	T5Ø.2X3	T5Ø.2X4	T5Ø.2X5	T5Ø.2X6
Salicylazosulfapyridine	T37.ØX1	T37.ØX2	T37.ØX3	T37.ØX4	T37.ØX5	T37.ØX6
Salicylhydroxamic acid	T49.ØX1	T49.ØX2	T49.ØX3	T49.ØX4	T49.ØX5	T49.ØX6
Salicylic acid	T49.4X1	T49.4X2	T49.4X3	T49.4X4	T49.4X5	T49.4X6
with benzoic acid	T49.4X1	T49.4X2	T49.4X3	T49.4X4	T49.4X5	T49.4X6
congeners	T39.Ø91	T39.Ø92	T39.Ø93	T39.Ø94	T39.Ø95	T39.Ø96
derivative	T39.Ø91	T39.Ø92	T39.Ø93	T39.Ø94	T39.Ø95	T39.Ø96
salts	T39.Ø91	T39.Ø92	T39.Ø93	T39.Ø94	T39.Ø95	T39.Ø96
Salinazid	T37.1X1	T37.1X2	T37.1X3	T37.1X4	T37.1X5	T37.1X6
Salmeterol	T48.6X1	T48.6X2	T48.6X3	T48.6X4	T48.6X5	T48.6X6
Salol	T49.3X1	T49.3X2	T49.3X3	T49.3X4	T49.3X5	T49.3X6
Salsalate	T39.Ø91	T39.Ø92	T39.Ø93	T39.Ø94	T39.Ø95	T39.Ø96
Salt-replacing drug	T5Ø.9Ø1	T5Ø.9Ø2	T5Ø.9Ø3	T5Ø.9Ø4	T5Ø.9Ø5	T5Ø.9Ø6
Salt-retaining mineralocorticoid	T5Ø.ØX1	T5Ø.ØX2	T5Ø.ØX3	T5Ø.ØX4	T5Ø.ØX5	T5Ø.ØX6
Salt substitute	T5Ø.9Ø1	T5Ø.9Ø2	T5Ø.9Ø3	T5Ø.9Ø4	T5Ø.9Ø5	T5Ø.9Ø6
Saluretic NEC	T5Ø.2X1	T5Ø.2X2	T5Ø.2X3	T5Ø.2X4	T5Ø.2X5	T5Ø.2X6
Saluron	T5Ø.2X1	T5Ø.2X2	T5Ø.2X3	T5Ø.2X4	T5Ø.2X5	T5Ø.2X6
Salvarsan 606 (neosilver) (silver)	T37.8X1	T37.8X2	T37.8X3	T37.8X4	T37.8X5	T37.8X6
Sambucus canadensis	T62.2X1	T62.2X2	T62.2X3	T62.2X4	—	—
berry	T62.1X1	T62.1X2	T62.1X3	T62.1X4	—	—
Sandril	T46.5X1	T46.5X2	T46.5X3	T46.5X4	T46.5X5	T46.5X6
Sanguinaria canadensis	T62.2X1	T62.2X2	T62.2X3	T62.2X4	—	—
Saniflush (cleaner)	T54.2X1	T54.2X2	T54.2X3	T54.2X4	—	—
Santonin	T37.4X1	T37.4X2	T37.4X3	T37.4X4	T37.4X5	T37.4X6
Santyl	T49.8X1	T49.8X2	T49.8X3	T49.8X4	T49.8X5	T49.8X6
Saralasin	T46.5X1	T46.5X2	T46.5X3	T46.5X4	T46.5X5	T46.5X6
Sarcolysin	T45.1X1	T45.1X2	T45.1X3	T45.1X4	T45.1X5	T45.1X6
Sarkomycin	T45.1X1	T45.1X2	T45.1X3	T45.1X4	T45.1X5	T45.1X6
Saroten	T43.Ø11	T43.Ø12	T43.Ø13	T43.Ø14	T43.Ø15	T43.Ø16
Saturnine — *see* Lead						
Savin (oil)	T49.4X1	T49.4X2	T49.4X3	T49.4X4	T49.4X5	T49.4X6
Scammony	T47.2X1	T47.2X2	T47.2X3	T47.2X4	T47.2X5	T47.2X6
Scarlet red	T49.8X1	T49.8X2	T49.8X3	T49.8X4	T49.8X5	T49.8X6
Scheele's green	T57.ØX1	T57.ØX2	T57.ØX3	T57.ØX4	—	—
insecticide	T57.ØX1	T57.ØX2	T57.ØX3	T57.ØX4	—	—
Schizontozide (blood) (tissue)	T37.2X1	T37.2X2	T37.2X3	T37.2X4	T37.2X5	T37.2X6
Schradan	T6Ø.ØX1	T6Ø.ØX2	T6Ø.ØX3	T6Ø.ØX4	—	—
Schweinfurth green	T57.ØX1	T57.ØX2	T57.ØX3	T57.ØX4	—	—
insecticide	T57.ØX1	T57.ØX2	T57.ØX3	T57.ØX4	—	—
Scilla, rat poison	T6Ø.4X1	T6Ø.4X2	T6Ø.4X3	T6Ø.4X4	—	—
Scillaren	T6Ø.4X1	T6Ø.4X2	T6Ø.4X3	T6Ø.4X4	—	—
Sclerosing agent	T46.8X1	T46.8X2	T46.8X3	T46.8X4	T46.8X5	T46.8X6
Scombrotoxin	T61.11	T61.12	T61.13	T61.14	—	—
Scopolamine	T44.3X1	T44.3X2	T44.3X3	T44.3X4	T44.3X5	T44.3X6
Scopolia extract	T44.3X1	T44.3X2	T44.3X3	T44.3X4	T44.3X5	T44.3X6
Scouring powder	T65.891	T65.892	T65.893	T65.894	—	—
Sea						
anemone (sting)	T63.631	T63.632	T63.633	T63.634	—	—
cucumber (sting)	T63.691	T63.692	T63.693	T63.694	—	—
Sea — *continued*						
snake (bite) (venom)	T63.Ø91	T63.Ø92	T63.Ø93	T63.Ø94	—	—
urchin spine (puncture)	T63.691	T63.692	T63.693	T63.694	—	—
Seafood	T61.91	T61.92	T61.93	T61.94	—	—
specified NEC	T61.8X1	T61.8X2	T61.8X3	T61.8X4	—	—
Secbutabarbital	T42.3X1	T42.3X2	T42.3X3	T42.3X4	T42.3X5	T42.3X6
Secbutabarbitone	T42.3X1	T42.3X2	T42.3X3	T42.3X4	T42.3X5	T42.3X6
Secnidazole	T37.3X1	T37.3X2	T37.3X3	T37.3X4	T37.3X5	T37.3X6
Secobarbital	T42.3X1	T42.3X2	T42.3X3	T42.3X4	T42.3X5	T42.3X6
Seconal	T42.3X1	T42.3X2	T42.3X3	T42.3X4	T42.3X5	T42.3X6
Secretin	T5Ø.8X1	T5Ø.8X2	T5Ø.8X3	T5Ø.8X4	T5Ø.8X5	T5Ø.8X6
Sedative NEC	T42.71	T42.72	T42.73	T42.74	T42.75	T42.76
mixed NEC	T42.6X1	T42.6X2	T42.6X3	T42.6X4	T42.6X5	T42.6X6
Sedormid	T42.6X1	T42.6X2	T42.6X3	T42.6X4	T42.6X5	T42.6X6
Seed disinfectant or dressing	T6Ø.8X1	T6Ø.8X2	T6Ø.8X3	T6Ø.8X4	—	—
Seeds (poisonous)	T62.2X1	T62.2X2	T62.2X3	T62.2X4	—	—
Selegiline	T42.8X1	T42.8X2	T42.8X3	T42.8X4	T42.8X5	T42.8X6
Selenium NEC	T56.891	T56.892	T56.893	T56.894	—	—
disulfide or sulfide	T49.4X1	T49.4X2	T49.4X3	T49.4X4	T49.4X5	T49.4X6
fumes	T59.891	T59.892	T59.893	T59.894	—	—
sulfide	T49.4X1	T49.4X2	T49.4X3	T49.4X4	T49.4X5	T49.4X6
Selenomethionine (75Se)	T5Ø.8X1	T5Ø.8X2	T5Ø.8X3	T5Ø.8X4	T5Ø.8X5	T5Ø.8X6
Selsun	T49.4X1	T49.4X2	T49.4X3	T49.4X4	T49.4X5	T49.4X6
Semustine	T45.1X1	T45.1X2	T45.1X3	T45.1X4	T45.1X5	T45.1X6
Senega syrup	T48.4X1	T48.4X2	T48.4X3	T48.4X4	T48.4X5	T48.4X6
Senna	T47.2X1	T47.2X2	T47.2X3	T47.2X4	T47.2X5	T47.2X6
Sennoside A+B	T47.2X1	T47.2X2	T47.2X3	T47.2X4	T47.2X5	T47.2X6
Septisol	T49.2X1	T49.2X2	T49.2X3	T49.2X4	T49.2X5	T49.2X6
Seractide	T38.811	T38.812	T38.813	T38.814	T38.815	T38.816
Serax	T42.4X1	T42.4X2	T42.4X3	T42.4X4	T42.4X5	T42.4X6
Serenesil	T42.6X1	T42.6X2	T42.6X3	T42.6X4	T42.6X5	T42.6X6
Serenium (hydrochloride)	T37.91	T37.92	T37.93	T37.94	T37.95	T37.96
Serepax — *see* Oxazepam						
Sermorelin	T38.891	T38.892	T38.893	T38.894	T38.895	T38.896
Sernyl	T41.1X1	T41.1X2	T41.1X3	T41.1X4	T41.1X5	T41.1X6
Serotonin	T5Ø.991	T5Ø.992	T5Ø.993	T5Ø.994	T5Ø.995	T5Ø.996
Serpasil	T46.5X1	T46.5X2	T46.5X3	T46.5X4	T46.5X5	T46.5X6
Serrapeptase	T45.3X1	T45.3X2	T45.3X3	T45.3X4	T45.3X5	T45.3X6
Serum						
antibotulinus	T5Ø.Z11	T5Ø.Z12	T5Ø.Z13	T5Ø.Z14	T5Ø.Z15	T5Ø.Z16
anticytotoxic	T5Ø.Z11	T5Ø.Z12	T5Ø.Z13	T5Ø.Z14	T5Ø.Z15	T5Ø.Z16
antidiphtheria	T5Ø.Z11	T5Ø.Z12	T5Ø.Z13	T5Ø.Z14	T5Ø.Z15	T5Ø.Z16
antimeningococcus	T5Ø.Z11	T5Ø.Z12	T5Ø.Z13	T5Ø.Z14	T5Ø.Z15	T5Ø.Z16
anti-Rh	T5Ø.Z11	T5Ø.Z12	T5Ø.Z13	T5Ø.Z14	T5Ø.Z15	T5Ø.Z16
anti-snake-bite	T5Ø.Z11	T5Ø.Z12	T5Ø.Z13	T5Ø.Z14	T5Ø.Z15	T5Ø.Z16
antitetanic	T5Ø.Z11	T5Ø.Z12	T5Ø.Z13	T5Ø.Z14	T5Ø.Z15	T5Ø.Z16
antitoxic	T5Ø.Z11	T5Ø.Z12	T5Ø.Z13	T5Ø.Z14	T5Ø.Z15	T5Ø.Z16
complement (inhibitor)	T45.8X1	T45.8X2	T45.8X3	T45.8X4	T45.8X5	T45.8X6
convalescent	T5Ø.Z11	T5Ø.Z12	T5Ø.Z13	T5Ø.Z14	T5Ø.Z15	T5Ø.Z16
hemolytic complement	T45.8X1	T45.8X2	T45.8X3	T45.8X4	T45.8X5	T45.8X6
immune (human)	T5Ø.Z11	T5Ø.Z12	T5Ø.Z13	T5Ø.Z14	T5Ø.Z15	T5Ø.Z16
protective NEC	T5Ø.Z11	T5Ø.Z12	T5Ø.Z13	T5Ø.Z14	T5Ø.Z15	T5Ø.Z16
Setastine	T45.ØX1	T45.ØX2	T45.ØX3	T45.ØX4	T45.ØX5	T45.ØX6
Setoperone	T43.591	T43.592	T43.593	T43.594	T43.595	T43.596
Sewer gas	T59.91	T59.92	T59.93	T59.94	—	—
Shampoo	T55.ØX1	T55.ØX2	T55.ØX3	T55.ØX4	—	—
Shellfish, noxious, nonbacterial	T61.781	T61.782	T61.783	T61.784	—	—
Sildenafil	T46.7X1	T46.7X2	T46.7X3	T46.7X4	T46.7X5	T46.7X6
Silibinin	T5Ø.991	T5Ø.992	T5Ø.993	T5Ø.994	T5Ø.995	T5Ø.996
Silicone NEC	T65.891	T65.892	T65.893	T65.894	—	—
medicinal	T49.3X1	T49.3X2	T49.3X3	T49.3X4	T49.3X5	T49.3X6
Silvadene	T49.ØX1	T49.ØX2	T49.ØX3	T49.ØX4	T49.ØX5	T49.ØX6
Silver	T49.ØX1	T49.ØX2	T49.ØX3	T49.ØX4	T49.ØX5	T49.ØX6
anti-infectives	T49.ØX1	T49.ØX2	T49.ØX3	T49.ØX4	T49.ØX5	T49.ØX6
arsphenamine	T37.8X1	T37.8X2	T37.8X3	T37.8X4	T37.8X5	T37.8X6
colloidal	T49.ØX1	T49.ØX2	T49.ØX3	T49.ØX4	T49.ØX5	T49.ØX6
nitrate	T49.ØX1	T49.ØX2	T49.ØX3	T49.ØX4	T49.ØX5	T49.ØX6
ophthalmic preparation	T49.5X1	T49.5X2	T49.5X3	T49.5X4	T49.5X5	T49.5X6
toughened (keratolytic)	T49.4X1	T49.4X2	T49.4X3	T49.4X4	T49.4X5	T49.4X6
nonmedicinal (dust)	T56.891	T56.892	T56.893	T56.894	—	—
protein	T49.5X1	T49.5X2	T49.5X3	T49.5X4	T49.5X5	T49.5X6
salvarsan	T37.8X1	T37.8X2	T37.8X3	T37.8X4	T37.8X5	T37.8X6
sulfadiazine	T49.4X1	T49.4X2	T49.4X3	T49.4X4	T49.4X5	T49.4X6
Silymarin	T5Ø.991	T5Ø.992	T5Ø.993	T5Ø.994	T5Ø.995	T5Ø.996
Simaldrate	T47.1X1	T47.1X2	T47.1X3	T47.1X4	T47.1X5	T47.1X6
Simazine	T6Ø.3X1	T6Ø.3X2	T6Ø.3X3	T6Ø.3X4	—	—
Simethicone	T47.1X1	T47.1X2	T47.1X3	T47.1X4	T47.1X5	T47.1X6
Simfibrate	T46.6X1	T46.6X2	T46.6X3	T46.6X4	T46.6X5	T46.6X6
Simvastatin	T46.6X1	T46.6X2	T46.6X3	T46.6X4	T46.6X5	T46.6X6
Sincalide	T5Ø.8X1	T5Ø.8X2	T5Ø.8X3	T5Ø.8X4	T5Ø.8X5	T5Ø.8X6
Sinequan	T43.Ø11	T43.Ø12	T43.Ø13	T43.Ø14	T43.Ø15	T43.Ø16

Rotenone — Sinequan

378 Additional Character May Be Required — Refer to the Tabular List for Character Selection ▽ Subterms under main terms may continue to next column or page

Substance	Poisoning, Accidental (unintentional)	Poisoning, Intentional Self-harm	Poisoning, Assault	Poisoning, Undetermined	Adverse Effect	Under-dosing
Singoserp	T46.5X1	T46.5X2	T46.5X3	T46.5X4	T46.5X5	T46.5X6
Sintrom	T45.511	T45.512	T45.513	T45.514	T45.515	T45.516
Sisomicin	T36.5X1	T36.5X2	T36.5X3	T36.5X4	T36.5X5	T36.5X6
Sitosterols	T46.6X1	T46.6X2	T46.6X3	T46.6X4	T46.6X5	T46.6X6
Skeletal muscle relaxants	T48.1X1	T48.1X2	T48.1X3	T48.1X4	T48.1X5	T48.1X6
Skin						
agents (external)	T49.91	T49.92	T49.93	T49.94	T49.95	T49.96
specified NEC	T49.8X1	T49.8X2	T49.8X3	T49.8X4	T49.8X5	T49.8X6
test antigen	T50.8X1	T50.8X2	T50.8X3	T50.8X4	T50.8X5	T50.8X6
Sleep-eze	T45.0X1	T45.0X2	T45.0X3	T45.0X4	T45.0X5	T45.0X6
Sleeping draught, pill	T42.71	T42.72	T42.73	T42.74	T42.75	T42.76
Smallpox vaccine	T50.B11	T50.B12	T50.B13	T50.B14	T50.B15	T50.B16
Smelter fumes NEC	T56.91	T56.92	T56.93	T56.94	—	—
Smog	T59.1X1	T59.1X2	T59.1X3	T59.1X4	—	—
Smoke NEC	T59.811	T59.812	T59.813	T59.814	—	—
Smooth muscle relaxant	T44.3X1	T44.3X2	T44.3X3	T44.3X4	T44.3X5	T44.3X6
Snail killer NEC	T60.8X1	T60.8X2	T60.8X3	T60.8X4	—	—
Snake venom or bite	T63.001	T63.002	T63.003	T63.004	—	—
hemocoagulase	T45.7X1	T45.7X2	T45.7X3	T45.7X4	T45.7X5	T45.7X6
Snuff	T65.211	T65.212	T65.213	T65.214	—	—
Soap (powder) (product)	T55.0X1	T55.0X2	T55.0X3	T55.0X4	—	—
enema	T47.4X1	T47.4X2	T47.4X3	T47.4X4	T47.4X5	T47.4X6
medicinal, soft	T49.2X1	T49.2X2	T49.2X3	T49.2X4	T49.2X5	T49.2X6
superfatted	T49.2X1	T49.2X2	T49.2X3	T49.2X4	T49.2X5	T49.2X6
Sobrerol	T48.4X1	T48.4X2	T48.4X3	T48.4X4	T48.4X5	T48.4X6
Soda (caustic)	T54.3X1	T54.3X2	T54.3X3	T54.3X4	—	—
bicarb	T47.1X1	T47.1X2	T47.1X3	T47.1X4	T47.1X5	T47.1X6
chlorinated — *see* Sodium, hypochlorite						
Sodium						
acetosulfone	T37.1X1	T37.1X2	T37.1X3	T37.1X4	T37.1X5	T37.1X6
acetrizoate	T50.8X1	T50.8X2	T50.8X3	T50.8X4	T50.8X5	T50.8X6
acid phosphate	T50.3X1	T50.3X2	T50.3X3	T50.3X4	T50.3X5	T50.3X6
alginate	T47.8X1	T47.8X2	T47.8X3	T47.8X4	T47.8X5	T47.8X6
amidotrizoate	T50.8X1	T50.8X2	T50.8X3	T50.8X4	T50.8X5	T50.8X6
aminopterin	T45.1X1	T45.1X2	T45.1X3	T45.1X4	T45.1X5	T45.1X6
amylosulfate	T47.8X1	T47.8X2	T47.8X3	T47.8X4	T47.8X5	T47.8X6
amytal	T42.3X1	T42.3X2	T42.3X3	T42.3X4	T42.3X5	T42.3X6
antimony gluconate	T37.3X1	T37.3X2	T37.3X3	T37.3X4	T37.3X5	T37.3X6
arsenate	T57.0X1	T57.0X2	T57.0X3	T57.0X4	—	—
aurothiomalate	T39.4X1	T39.4X2	T39.4X3	T39.4X4	T39.4X5	T39.4X6
aurothiosulfate	T39.4X1	T39.4X2	T39.4X3	T39.4X4	T39.4X5	T39.4X6
barbiturate	T42.3X1	T42.3X2	T42.3X3	T42.3X4	T42.3X5	T42.3X6
basic phosphate	T47.4X1	T47.4X2	T47.4X3	T47.4X4	T47.4X5	T47.4X6
bicarbonate	T47.1X1	T47.1X2	T47.1X3	T47.1X4	T47.1X5	T47.1X6
bichromate	T57.8X1	T57.8X2	T57.8X3	T57.8X4	—	—
biphosphate	T50.3X1	T50.3X2	T50.3X3	T50.3X4	T50.3X5	T50.3X6
bisulfate	T65.891	T65.892	T65.893	T65.894	—	—
borate						
cleanser	T57.8X1	T57.8X2	T57.8X3	T57.8X4	—	—
eye	T49.5X1	T49.5X2	T49.5X3	T49.5X4	T49.5X5	T49.5X6
therapeutic	T49.8X1	T49.8X2	T49.8X3	T49.8X4	T49.8X5	T49.8X6
bromide	T42.6X1	T42.6X2	T42.6X3	T42.6X4	T42.6X5	T42.6X6
cacodylate (nonmedicinal) NEC	T50.8X1	T50.8X2	T50.8X3	T50.8X4	T50.8X5	T50.8X6
anti-infective	T37.8X1	T37.8X2	T37.8X3	T37.8X4	T37.8X5	T37.8X6
herbicide	T60.3X1	T60.3X2	T60.3X3	T60.3X4	—	—
calcium edetate	T45.8X1	T45.8X2	T45.8X3	T45.8X4	T45.8X5	T45.8X6
carbonate NEC	T54.3X1	T54.3X2	T54.3X3	T54.3X4	—	—
chlorate NEC	T65.891	T65.892	T65.893	T65.894	—	—
herbicide	T54.91	T54.92	T54.93	T54.94	—	—
chloride	T50.3X1	T50.3X2	T50.3X3	T50.3X4	T50.3X5	T50.3X6
with glucose	T50.3X1	T50.3X2	T50.3X3	T50.3X4	T50.3X5	T50.3X6
chromate	T65.891	T65.892	T65.893	T65.894	—	—
citrate	T50.991	T50.992	T50.993	T50.994	T50.995	T50.996
cromoglicate	T48.6X1	T48.6X2	T48.6X3	T48.6X4	T48.6X5	T48.6X6
cyanide	T65.0X1	T65.0X2	T65.0X3	T65.0X4	—	—
cyclamate	T50.3X1	T50.3X2	T50.3X3	T50.3X4	T50.3X5	T50.3X6
dehydrocholate	T45.8X1	T45.8X2	T45.8X3	T45.8X4	T45.8X5	T45.8X6
diatrizoate	T50.8X1	T50.8X2	T50.8X3	T50.8X4	T50.8X5	T50.8X6
dibunate	T48.4X1	T48.4X2	T48.4X3	T48.4X4	T48.4X5	T48.4X6
dioctyl sulfosuccinate	T47.4X1	T47.4X2	T47.4X3	T47.4X4	T47.4X5	T47.4X6
dipantoyl ferrate	T45.8X1	T45.8X2	T45.8X3	T45.8X4	T45.8X5	T45.8X6
edetate	T45.8X1	T45.8X2	T45.8X3	T45.8X4	T45.8X5	T45.8X6
ethacrynate	T50.1X1	T50.1X2	T50.1X3	T50.1X4	T50.1X5	T50.1X6
feredetate	T45.8X1	T45.8X2	T45.8X3	T45.8X4	T45.8X5	T45.8X6
Fluoride — *see* Fluoride						
fluoroacetate (dust) (pesticide)	T60.4X1	T60.4X2	T60.4X3	T60.4X4	—	—
free salt	T50.3X1	T50.3X2	T50.3X3	T50.3X4	T50.3X5	T50.3X6
fusidate	T36.8X1	T36.8X2	T36.8X3	T36.8X4	T36.8X5	T36.8X6
glucaldrate	T47.1X1	T47.1X2	T47.1X3	T47.1X4	T47.1X5	T47.1X6
glucosulfone	T37.1X1	T37.1X2	T37.1X3	T37.1X4	T37.1X5	T37.1X6

Substance	Poisoning, Accidental (unintentional)	Poisoning, Intentional Self-harm	Poisoning, Assault	Poisoning, Undetermined	Adverse Effect	Under-dosing
Sodium — *continued*						
glutamate	T45.8X1	T45.8X2	T45.8X3	T45.8X4	T45.8X5	T45.8X6
hydrogen carbonate	T50.3X1	T50.3X2	T50.3X3	T50.3X4	T50.3X5	T50.3X6
hydroxide	T54.3X1	T54.3X2	T54.3X3	T54.3X4	—	—
hypochlorite (bleach) NEC	T54.3X1	T54.3X2	T54.3X3	T54.3X4	—	—
disinfectant	T54.3X1	T54.3X2	T54.3X3	T54.3X4	—	—
medicinal (anti-infective) (external)	T49.0X1	T49.0X2	T49.0X3	T49.0X4	T49.0X5	T49.0X6
vapor	T54.3X1	T54.3X2	T54.3X3	T54.3X4	—	—
hyposulfite	T49.0X1	T49.0X2	T49.0X3	T49.0X4	T49.0X5	T49.0X6
indigotin disulfonate	T50.8X1	T50.8X2	T50.8X3	T50.8X4	T50.8X5	T50.8X6
iodide	T50.991	T50.992	T50.993	T50.994	T50.995	T50.996
I-131	T50.8X1	T50.8X2	T50.8X3	T50.8X4	T50.8X5	T50.8X6
therapeutic	T38.2X1	T38.2X2	T38.2X3	T38.2X4	T38.2X5	T38.2X6
iodohippurate (131I)	T50.8X1	T50.8X2	T50.8X3	T50.8X4	T50.8X5	T50.8X6
iopodate	T50.8X1	T50.8X2	T50.8X3	T50.8X4	T50.8X5	T50.8X6
iothalamate	T50.8X1	T50.8X2	T50.8X3	T50.8X4	T50.8X5	T50.8X6
iron edetate	T45.4X1	T45.4X2	T45.4X3	T45.4X4	T45.4X5	T45.4X6
lactate (compound solution)	T45.8X1	T45.8X2	T45.8X3	T45.8X4	T45.8X5	T45.8X6
lauryl (sulfate)	T49.2X1	T49.2X2	T49.2X3	T49.2X4	T49.2X5	T49.2X6
L-triiodothyronine	T38.1X1	T38.1X2	T38.1X3	T38.1X4	T38.1X5	T38.1X6
magnesium citrate	T50.991	T50.992	T50.993	T50.994	T50.995	T50.996
mersalate	T50.2X1	T50.2X2	T50.2X3	T50.2X4	T50.2X5	T50.2X6
metasilicate	T65.891	T65.892	T65.893	T65.894	—	—
metrizoate	T50.8X1	T50.8X2	T50.8X3	T50.8X4	T50.8X5	T50.8X6
monofluoroacetate (pesticide)	T60.1X1	T60.1X2	T60.1X3	T60.1X4	—	—
morrhuate	T46.8X1	T46.8X2	T46.8X3	T46.8X4	T46.8X5	T46.8X6
nafcillin	T36.0X1	T36.0X2	T36.0X3	T36.0X4	T36.0X5	T36.0X6
nitrate (oxidizing agent)	T65.891	T65.892	T65.893	T65.894	—	—
nitrite	T50.6X1	T50.6X2	T50.6X3	T50.6X4	T50.6X5	T50.6X6
nitroferricyanide	T46.5X1	T46.5X2	T46.5X3	T46.5X4	T46.5X5	T46.5X6
nitroprusside	T46.5X1	T46.5X2	T46.5X3	T46.5X4	T46.5X5	T46.5X6
oxalate	T65.891	T65.892	T65.893	T65.894	—	—
oxide/peroxide	T65.891	T65.892	T65.893	T65.894	—	—
oxybate	T41.291	T41.292	T41.293	T41.294	T41.295	T41.296
para-aminohippurate	T50.8X1	T50.8X2	T50.8X3	T50.8X4	T50.8X5	T50.8X6
perborate (nonmedicinal) NEC	T65.891	T65.892	T65.893	T65.894	—	—
medicinal	T49.0X1	T49.0X2	T49.0X3	T49.0X4	T49.0X5	T49.0X6
soap	T55.0X1	T55.0X2	T55.0X3	T55.0X4	—	—
percarbonate — *see* Sodium, perborate						
pertechnetate Tc99m	T50.8X1	T50.8X2	T50.8X3	T50.8X4	T50.8X5	T50.8X6
phosphate						
cellulose	T45.8X1	T45.8X2	T45.8X3	T45.8X4	T45.8X5	T45.8X6
dibasic	T47.2X1	T47.2X2	T47.2X3	T47.2X4	T47.2X5	T47.2X6
monobasic	T47.2X1	T47.2X2	T47.2X3	T47.2X4	T47.2X5	T47.2X6
phytate	T50.6X1	T50.6X2	T50.6X3	T50.6X4	T50.6X5	T50.6X6
picosulfate	T47.2X1	T47.2X2	T47.2X3	T47.2X4	T47.2X5	T47.2X6
polyhydroxyaluminium monocarbonate	T47.1X1	T47.1X2	T47.1X3	T47.1X4	T47.1X5	T47.1X6
polystyrene sulfonate	T50.3X1	T50.3X2	T50.3X3	T50.3X4	T50.3X5	T50.3X6
propionate	T49.0X1	T49.0X2	T49.0X3	T49.0X4	T49.0X5	T49.0X6
propyl hydroxybenzoate	T50.991	T50.992	T50.993	T50.994	T50.995	T50.996
psylliate	T46.8X1	T46.8X2	T46.8X3	T46.8X4	T46.8X5	T46.8X6
removing resins	T50.3X1	T50.3X2	T50.3X3	T50.3X4	T50.3X5	T50.3X6
salicylate	T39.091	T39.092	T39.093	T39.094	T39.095	T39.096
salt NEC	T50.3X1	T50.3X2	T50.3X3	T50.3X4	T50.3X5	T50.3X6
selenate	T60.2X1	T60.2X2	T60.2X3	T60.2X4	—	—
stibogluconate	T37.3X1	T37.3X2	T37.3X3	T37.3X4	T37.3X5	T37.3X6
sulfate	T47.4X1	T47.4X2	T47.4X3	T47.4X4	T47.4X5	T47.4X6
sulfoxone	T37.1X1	T37.1X2	T37.1X3	T37.1X4	T37.1X5	T37.1X6
tetradecyl sulfate	T46.8X1	T46.8X2	T46.8X3	T46.8X4	T46.8X5	T46.8X6
thiopental	T41.1X1	T41.1X2	T41.1X3	T41.1X4	T41.1X5	T41.1X6
thiosalicylate	T39.091	T39.092	T39.093	T39.094	T39.095	T39.096
thiosulfate	T50.6X1	T50.6X2	T50.6X3	T50.6X4	T50.6X5	T50.6X6
tolbutamide	T38.3X1	T38.3X2	T38.3X3	T38.3X4	T38.3X5	T38.3X6
(L)-triiodothyronine	T38.1X1	T38.1X2	T38.1X3	T38.1X4	T38.1X5	T38.1X6
tyropanoate	T50.8X1	T50.8X2	T50.8X3	T50.8X4	T50.8X5	T50.8X6
valproate	T42.6X1	T42.6X2	T42.6X3	T42.6X4	T42.6X5	T42.6X6
versenate	T50.6X1	T50.6X2	T50.6X3	T50.6X4	T50.6X5	T50.6X6
Sodium-free salt	T50.901	T50.902	T50.903	T50.904	T50.905	T50.906
Sodium-removing resin	T50.3X1	T50.3X2	T50.3X3	T50.3X4	T50.3X5	T50.3X6
Soft soap	T55.0X1	T55.0X2	T55.0X3	T55.0X4	—	—
Solanine	T62.2X1	T62.2X2	T62.2X3	T62.2X4	—	—
berries	T62.1X1	T62.1X2	T62.1X3	T62.1X4	—	—
Solanum dulcamara	T62.2X1	T62.2X2	T62.2X3	T62.2X4	—	—
berries	T62.1X1	T62.1X2	T62.1X3	T62.1X4	—	—
Solapsone	T37.1X1	T37.1X2	T37.1X3	T37.1X4	T37.1X5	T37.1X6
Solar lotion	T49.3X1	T49.3X2	T49.3X3	T49.3X4	T49.3X5	T49.3X6
Solasulfone	T37.1X1	T37.1X2	T37.1X3	T37.1X4	T37.1X5	T37.1X6

Substance	Poisoning, Accidental (unintentional)	Poisoning, Intentional Self-harm	Poisoning, Assault	Poisoning, Undetermined	Adverse Effect	Under-dosing
Soldering fluid	T65.891	T65.892	T65.893	T65.894	—	—
Solid substance	T65.91	T65.92	T65.93	T65.94	—	—
specified NEC	T65.891	T65.892	T65.893	T65.894	—	—
Solvent, industrial NEC	T52.91	T52.92	T52.93	T52.94	—	—
naphtha	T52.ØX1	T52.ØX2	T52.ØX3	T52.ØX4	—	—
petroleum	T52.ØX1	T52.ØX2	T52.ØX3	T52.ØX4	—	—
specified NEC	T52.8X1	T52.8X2	T52.8X3	T52.8X4	—	—
Soma	T42.8X1	T42.8X2	T42.8X3	T42.8X4	T42.8X5	T42.8X6
Somatorelin	T38.891	T38.892	T38.893	T38.894	T38.895	T38.896
Somatostatin	T38.991	T38.992	T38.993	T38.994	T38.995	T38.996
Somatotropin	T38.811	T38.812	T38.813	T38.814	T38.815	T38.816
Somatrem	T38.811	T38.812	T38.813	T38.814	T38.815	T38.816
Somatropin	T38.811	T38.812	T38.813	T38.814	T38.815	T38.816
Sominex	T45.ØX1	T45.ØX2	T45.ØX3	T45.ØX4	T45.ØX5	T45.ØX6
Somnos	T42.6X1	T42.6X2	T42.6X3	T42.6X4	T42.6X5	T42.6X6
Somonal	T42.3X1	T42.3X2	T42.3X3	T42.3X4	T42.3X5	T42.3X6
Soneryl	T42.3X1	T42.3X2	T42.3X3	T42.3X4	T42.3X5	T42.3X6
Soothing syrup	T5Ø.9Ø1	T5Ø.9Ø2	T5Ø.9Ø3	T5Ø.9Ø4	T5Ø.9Ø5	T5Ø.9Ø6
Sopor	T42.6X1	T42.6X2	T42.6X3	T42.6X4	T42.6X5	T42.6X6
Soporific	T42.71	T42.72	T42.73	T42.74	T42.75	T42.76
Soporific drug	T42.71	T42.72	T42.73	T42.74	T42.75	T42.76
specified type NEC	T42.6X1	T42.6X2	T42.6X3	T42.6X4	T42.6X5	T42.6X6
Sorbide nitrate	T46.3X1	T46.3X2	T46.3X3	T46.3X4	T46.3X5	T46.3X6
Sorbitol	T47.4X1	T47.4X2	T47.4X3	T47.4X4	T47.4X5	T47.4X6
Sotalol	T44.7X1	T44.7X2	T44.7X3	T44.7X4	T44.7X5	T44.7X6
Sotradecol	T46.8X1	T46.8X2	T46.8X3	T46.8X4	T46.8X5	T46.8X6
Soysterol	T46.6X1	T46.6X2	T46.6X3	T46.6X4	T46.6X5	T46.6X6
Spacoline	T44.3X1	T44.3X2	T44.3X3	T44.3X4	T44.3X5	T44.3X6
Spanish fly	T49.8X1	T49.8X2	T49.8X3	T49.8X4	T49.8X5	T49.8X6
Sparine	T43.3X1	T43.3X2	T43.3X3	T43.3X4	T43.3X5	T43.3X6
Sparteine	T48.ØX1	T48.ØX2	T48.ØX3	T48.ØX4	T48.ØX5	T48.ØX6
Spasmolytic						
anticholinergics	T44.3X1	T44.3X2	T44.3X3	T44.3X4	T44.3X5	T44.3X6
autonomic	T44.3X1	T44.3X2	T44.3X3	T44.3X4	T44.3X5	T44.3X6
bronchial NEC	T48.6X1	T48.6X2	T48.6X3	T48.6X4	T48.6X5	T48.6X6
quaternary ammonium	T44.3X1	T44.3X2	T44.3X3	T44.3X4	T44.3X5	T44.3X6
skeletal muscle NEC	T48.1X1	T48.1X2	T48.1X3	T48.1X4	T48.1X5	T48.1X6
Spectinomycin	T36.5X1	T36.5X2	T36.5X3	T36.5X4	T36.5X5	T36.5X6
Speed	T43.621	T43.622	T43.623	T43.624	T43.625	T43.626
Spermicide	T49.8X1	T49.8X2	T49.8X3	T49.8X4	T49.8X5	T49.8X6
Spider (bite) (venom)	T63.391	T63.392	T63.393	T63.394	—	—
antivenin	T5Ø.Z11	T5Ø.Z12	T5Ø.Z13	T5Ø.Z14	T5Ø.Z15	T5Ø.Z16
Spigelia (root)	T37.4X1	T37.4X2	T37.4X3	T37.4X4	T37.4X5	T37.4X6
Spindle inactivator	T5Ø.4X1	T5Ø.4X2	T5Ø.4X3	T5Ø.4X4	T5Ø.4X5	T5Ø.4X6
Spiperone	T43.4X1	T43.4X2	T43.4X3	T43.4X4	T43.4X5	T43.4X6
Spiramycin	T36.3X1	T36.3X2	T36.3X3	T36.3X4	T36.3X5	T36.3X6
Spirapril	T46.4X1	T46.4X2	T46.4X3	T46.4X4	T46.4X5	T46.4X6
Spirilene	T43.591	T43.592	T43.593	T43.594	T43.595	T43.596
Spirit(s) (neutral) **NEC**	T51.ØX1	T51.ØX2	T51.ØX3	T51.ØX4	—	—
beverage	T51.ØX1	T51.ØX2	T51.ØX3	T51.ØX4	—	—
industrial	T51.ØX1	T51.ØX2	T51.ØX3	T51.ØX4	—	—
mineral	T52.ØX1	T52.ØX2	T52.ØX3	T52.ØX4	—	—
of salt — *see* Hydrochloric acid						
surgical	T51.ØX1	T51.ØX2	T51.ØX3	T51.ØX4	—	—
Spironolactone	T5Ø.ØX1	T5Ø.ØX2	T5Ø.ØX3	T5Ø.ØX4	T5Ø.ØX5	T5Ø.ØX6
Spiroperidol	T43.4X1	T43.4X2	T43.4X3	T43.4X4	T43.4X5	T43.4X6
Sponge, absorbable (gelatin)	T45.7X1	T45.7X2	T45.7X3	T45.7X4	T45.7X5	T45.7X6
Sporostacin	T49.ØX1	T49.ØX2	T49.ØX3	T49.ØX4	T49.ØX5	T49.ØX6
Spray (aerosol)	T65.91	T65.92	T65.93	T65.94	—	—
cosmetic	T65.891	T65.892	T65.893	T65.894	—	—
medicinal NEC	T5Ø.9Ø1	T5Ø.9Ø2	T5Ø.9Ø3	T5Ø.9Ø4	T5Ø.9Ø5	T5Ø.9Ø6
pesticides — *see* Pesticides						
specified content — *see* specific substance						
Spurge flax	T62.2X1	T62.2X2	T62.2X3	T62.2X4	—	—
Spurges	T62.2X1	T62.2X2	T62.2X3	T62.2X4	—	—
Sputum viscosity-lowering drug	T48.4X1	T48.4X2	T48.4X3	T48.4X4	T48.4X5	T48.4X6
Squill	T46.ØX1	T46.ØX2	T46.ØX3	T46.ØX4	T46.ØX5	T46.ØX6
rat poison	T6Ø.4X1	T6Ø.4X2	T6Ø.4X3	T6Ø.4X4	—	—
Squirting cucumber (cathartic)	T47.2X1	T47.2X2	T47.2X3	T47.2X4	T47.2X5	T47.2X6
Stains	T65.6X1	T65.6X2	T65.6X3	T65.6X4	—	—
Stannous fluoride	T49.7X1	T49.7X2	T49.7X3	T49.7X4	T49.7X5	T49.7X6
Stanolone	T38.7X1	T38.7X2	T38.7X3	T38.7X4	T38.7X5	T38.7X6
Stanozolol	T38.7X1	T38.7X2	T38.7X3	T38.7X4	T38.7X5	T38.7X6
Staphisagria or stavesacre (pediculicide)	T49.ØX1	T49.ØX2	T49.ØX3	T49.ØX4	T49.ØX5	T49.ØX6
Starch	T5Ø.9Ø1	T5Ø.9Ø2	T5Ø.9Ø3	T5Ø.9Ø4	T5Ø.9Ø5	T5Ø.9Ø6
Stelazine	T43.3X1	T43.3X2	T43.3X3	T43.3X4	T43.3X5	T43.3X6
Stemetil	T43.3X1	T43.3X2	T43.3X3	T43.3X4	T43.3X5	T43.3X6
Stepronin	T48.4X1	T48.4X2	T48.4X3	T48.4X4	T48.4X5	T48.4X6

Substance	Poisoning, Accidental (unintentional)	Poisoning, Intentional Self-harm	Poisoning, Assault	Poisoning, Undetermined	Adverse Effect	Under-dosing
Sterculia	T47.4X1	T47.4X2	T47.4X3	T47.4X4	T47.4X5	T47.4X6
Sternutator gas	T59.891	T59.892	T59.893	T59.894	—	—
Steroid	T38.ØX1	T38.ØX2	T38.ØX3	T38.ØX4	T38.ØX5	T38.ØX6
anabolic	T38.7X1	T38.7X2	T38.7X3	T38.7X4	T38.7X5	T38.7X6
androgenic	T38.7X1	T38.7X2	T38.7X3	T38.7X4	T38.7X5	T38.7X6
antineoplastic, hormone	T38.7X1	T38.7X2	T38.7X3	T38.7X4	T38.7X5	T38.7X6
estrogen	T38.5X1	T38.5X2	T38.5X3	T38.5X4	T38.5X5	T38.5X6
ENT agent	T49.6X1	T49.6X2	T49.6X3	T49.6X4	T49.6X5	T49.6X6
ophthalmic preparation	T49.5X1	T49.5X2	T49.5X3	T49.5X4	T49.5X5	T49.5X6
topical NEC	T49.ØX1	T49.ØX2	T49.ØX3	T49.ØX4	T49.ØX5	T49.ØX6
Stibine	T56.891	T56.892	T56.893	T56.894	—	—
Stibogluconate	T37.3X1	T37.3X2	T37.3X3	T37.3X4	T37.3X5	T37.3X6
Stibophen	T37.4X1	T37.4X2	T37.4X3	T37.4X4	T37.4X5	T37.4X6
Stilbamidine (isetionate)	T37.3X1	T37.3X2	T37.3X3	T37.3X4	T37.3X5	T37.3X6
Stilbestrol	T38.5X1	T38.5X2	T38.5X3	T38.5X4	T38.5X5	T38.5X6
Stilboestrol	T38.5X1	T38.5X2	T38.5X3	T38.5X4	T38.5X5	T38.5X6
Stimulant						
central nervous system — *see also* Psychostimulant	T43.6Ø1	T43.6Ø2	T43.6Ø3	T43.6Ø4	T43.6Ø5	T43.6Ø6
analeptics	T5Ø.7X1	T5Ø.7X2	T5Ø.7X3	T5Ø.7X4	T5Ø.7X5	T5Ø.7X6
opiate antagonist	T5Ø.7X1	T5Ø.7X2	T5Ø.7X3	T5Ø.7X4	T5Ø.7X5	T5Ø.7X6
psychotherapeutic NEC — *see also* Psychotherapeutic drug	T43.6Ø1	T43.6Ø2	T43.6Ø3	T43.6Ø4	T43.6Ø5	T43.6Ø6
specified NEC	T43.691	T43.692	T43.693	T43.694	T43.695	T43.696
respiratory	T48.9Ø1	T48.9Ø2	T48.9Ø3	T48.9Ø4	T48.9Ø5	T48.9Ø6
Stone-dissolving drug	T5Ø.9Ø1	T5Ø.9Ø2	T5Ø.9Ø3	T5Ø.9Ø4	T5Ø.9Ø5	T5Ø.9Ø6
Storage battery (cells) (acid)	T54.2X1	T54.2X2	T54.2X3	T54.2X4	—	—
Stovaine	T41.3X1	T41.3X2	T41.3X3	T41.3X4	T41.3X5	T41.3X6
infiltration (subcutaneous)	T41.3X1	T41.3X2	T41.3X3	T41.3X4	T41.3X5	T41.3X6
nerve block (peripheral) (plexus)	T41.3X1	T41.3X2	T41.3X3	T41.3X4	T41.3X5	T41.3X6
spinal	T41.3X1	T41.3X2	T41.3X3	T41.3X4	T41.3X5	T41.3X6
topical (surface)	T41.3X1	T41.3X2	T41.3X3	T41.3X4	T41.3X5	T41.3X6
Stovarsal	T37.8X1	T37.8X2	T37.8X3	T37.8X4	T37.8X5	T37.8X6
Stove gas — *see* Gas, stove						
Stoxil	T49.5X1	T49.5X2	T49.5X3	T49.5X4	T49.5X5	T49.5X6
Stramonium	T48.6X1	T48.6X2	T48.6X3	T48.6X4	T48.6X5	T48.6X6
natural state	T62.2X1	T62.2X2	T62.2X3	T62.2X4	—	—
Streptodornase	T45.3X1	T45.3X2	T45.3X3	T45.3X4	T45.3X5	T45.3X6
Streptoduocin	T36.5X1	T36.5X2	T36.5X3	T36.5X4	T36.5X5	T36.5X6
Streptokinase	T45.611	T45.612	T45.613	T45.614	T45.615	T45.616
Streptomycin (derivative)	T36.5X1	T36.5X2	T36.5X3	T36.5X4	T36.5X5	T36.5X6
Streptonivicin	T36.5X1	T36.5X2	T36.5X3	T36.5X4	T36.5X5	T36.5X6
Streptovarycin	T36.5X1	T36.5X2	T36.5X3	T36.5X4	T36.5X5	T36.5X6
Streptozocin	T45.1X1	T45.1X2	T45.1X3	T45.1X4	T45.1X5	T45.1X6
Streptozotocin	T45.1X1	T45.1X2	T45.1X3	T45.1X4	T45.1X5	T45.1X6
Stripper (paint) (solvent)	T52.8X1	T52.8X2	T52.8X3	T52.8X4	—	—
Strobane	T6Ø.1X1	T6Ø.1X2	T6Ø.1X3	T6Ø.1X4	—	—
Strofantina	T46.ØX1	T46.ØX2	T46.ØX3	T46.ØX4	T46.ØX5	T46.ØX6
Strophanthin (g) (k)	T46.ØX1	T46.ØX2	T46.ØX3	T46.ØX4	T46.ØX5	T46.ØX6
Strophanthus	T46.ØX1	T46.ØX2	T46.ØX3	T46.ØX4	T46.ØX5	T46.ØX6
Strophantin	T46.ØX1	T46.ØX2	T46.ØX3	T46.ØX4	T46.ØX5	T46.ØX6
Strophantin-g	T46.ØX1	T46.ØX2	T46.ØX3	T46.ØX4	T46.ØX5	T46.ØX6
Strychnine (nonmedicinal) (pesticide) (salts)	T65.1X1	T65.1X2	T65.1X3	T65.1X4	—	—
medicinal	T48.291	T48.292	T48.293	T48.294	T48.295	T48.296
Strychnos (ignatii) — *see* Strychnine						
Styramate	T42.8X1	T42.8X2	T42.8X3	T42.8X4	T42.8X5	T42.8X6
Styrene	T65.891	T65.892	T65.893	T65.894	—	—
Succinimide, antiepileptic or anticonvulsant	T42.2X1	T42.2X2	T42.2X3	T42.2X4	T42.2X5	T42.2X6
mercuric — *see* Mercury						
Succinylcholine	T48.1X1	T48.1X2	T48.1X3	T48.1X4	T48.1X5	T48.1X6
Succinylsulfathiazole	T37.ØX1	T37.ØX2	T37.ØX3	T37.ØX4	T37.ØX5	T37.ØX6
Sucralfate	T47.1X1	T47.1X2	T47.1X3	T47.1X4	T47.1X5	T47.1X6
Sucrose	T5Ø.3X1	T5Ø.3X2	T5Ø.3X3	T5Ø.3X4	T5Ø.3X5	T5Ø.3X6
Sufentanil	T4Ø.4X1	T4Ø.4X2	T4Ø.4X3	T4Ø.4X4	T4Ø.4X5	T4Ø.4X6
Sulbactam	T36.ØX1	T36.ØX2	T36.ØX3	T36.ØX4	T36.ØX5	T36.ØX6
Sulbenicillin	T36.ØX1	T36.ØX2	T36.ØX3	T36.ØX4	T36.ØX5	T36.ØX6
Sulbentine	T49.ØX1	T49.ØX2	T49.ØX3	T49.ØX4	T49.ØX5	T49.ØX6
Sulfacetamide	T49.ØX1	T49.ØX2	T49.ØX3	T49.ØX4	T49.ØX5	T49.ØX6
ophthalmic preparation	T49.5X1	T49.5X2	T49.5X3	T49.5X4	T49.5X5	T49.5X6
Sulfachlorpyridazine	T37.ØX1	T37.ØX2	T37.ØX3	T37.ØX4	T37.ØX5	T37.ØX6
Sulfacitine	T37.ØX1	T37.ØX2	T37.ØX3	T37.ØX4	T37.ØX5	T37.ØX6
Sulfadiasulfone sodium	T37.ØX1	T37.ØX2	T37.ØX3	T37.ØX4	T37.ØX5	T37.ØX6
Sulfadiazine	T37.ØX1	T37.ØX2	T37.ØX3	T37.ØX4	T37.ØX5	T37.ØX6
silver (topical)	T49.ØX1	T49.ØX2	T49.ØX3	T49.ØX4	T49.ØX5	T49.ØX6
Sulfadimethoxine	T37.ØX1	T37.ØX2	T37.ØX3	T37.ØX4	T37.ØX5	T37.ØX6
Sulfadimidine	T37.ØX1	T37.ØX2	T37.ØX3	T37.ØX4	T37.ØX5	T37.ØX6
Sulfadoxine	T37.ØX1	T37.ØX2	T37.ØX3	T37.ØX4	T37.ØX5	T37.ØX6
with pyrimethamine	T37.2X1	T37.2X2	T37.2X3	T37.2X4	T37.2X5	T37.2X6

380 **Additional Character May Be Required — Refer to the Tabular List for Character Selection** **Subterms under main terms may continue to next column or page**

Substance	Poisoning, Accidental (unintentional)	Poisoning, Intentional Self-harm	Poisoning, Assault	Poisoning, Undetermined	Adverse Effect	Under-dosing
Sulfaethidole	T37.ØX1	T37.ØX2	T37.ØX3	T37.ØX4	T37.ØX5	T37.ØX6
Sulfafurazole	T37.ØX1	T37.ØX2	T37.ØX3	T37.ØX4	T37.ØX5	T37.ØX6
Sulfaguanidine	T37.ØX1	T37.ØX2	T37.ØX3	T37.ØX4	T37.ØX5	T37.ØX6
Sulfalene	T37.ØX1	T37.ØX2	T37.ØX3	T37.ØX4	T37.ØX5	T37.ØX6
Sulfaloxate	T37.ØX1	T37.ØX2	T37.ØX3	T37.ØX4	T37.ØX5	T37.ØX6
Sulfaloxic acid	T37.ØX1	T37.ØX2	T37.ØX3	T37.ØX4	T37.ØX5	T37.ØX6
Sulfamazone	T39.2X1	T39.2X2	T39.2X3	T39.2X4	T39.2X5	T39.2X6
Sulfamerazine	T37.ØX1	T37.ØX2	T37.ØX3	T37.ØX4	T37.ØX5	T37.ØX6
Sulfameter	T37.ØX1	T37.ØX2	T37.ØX3	T37.ØX4	T37.ØX5	T37.ØX6
Sulfamethazine	T37.ØX1	T37.ØX2	T37.ØX3	T37.ØX4	T37.ØX5	T37.ØX6
Sulfamethizole	T37.ØX1	T37.ØX2	T37.ØX3	T37.ØX4	T37.ØX5	T37.ØX6
Sulfamethoxazole	T37.ØX1	T37.ØX2	T37.ØX3	T37.ØX4	T37.ØX5	T37.ØX6
with trimethoprim	T36.8X1	T36.8X2	T36.8X3	T36.8X4	T36.8X5	T36.8X6
Sulfamethoxydiazine	T37.ØX1	T37.ØX2	T37.ØX3	T37.ØX4	T37.ØX5	T37.ØX6
Sulfamethoxypyridazine	T37.ØX1	T37.ØX2	T37.ØX3	T37.ØX4	T37.ØX5	T37.ØX6
Sulfamethylthiazole	T37.ØX1	T37.ØX2	T37.ØX3	T37.ØX4	T37.ØX5	T37.ØX6
Sulfametoxydiazine	T37.ØX1	T37.ØX2	T37.ØX3	T37.ØX4	T37.ØX5	T37.ØX6
Sulfamidopyrine	T39.2X1	T39.2X2	T39.2X3	T39.2X4	T39.2X5	T39.2X6
Sulfamonomethoxine	T37.ØX1	T37.ØX2	T37.ØX3	T37.ØX4	T37.ØX5	T37.ØX6
Sulfamoxole	T37.ØX1	T37.ØX2	T37.ØX3	T37.ØX4	T37.ØX5	T37.ØX6
Sulfamylon	T49.ØX1	T49.ØX2	T49.ØX3	T49.ØX4	T49.ØX5	T49.ØX6
Sulfan blue (diagnostic dye)	T5Ø.8X1	T5Ø.8X2	T5Ø.8X3	T5Ø.8X4	T5Ø.8X5	T5Ø.8X6
Sulfanilamide	T37.ØX1	T37.ØX2	T37.ØX3	T37.ØX4	T37.ØX5	T37.ØX6
Sulfanilylguanidine	T37.ØX1	T37.ØX2	T37.ØX3	T37.ØX4	T37.ØX5	T37.ØX6
Sulfaperin	T37.ØX1	T37.ØX2	T37.ØX3	T37.ØX4	T37.ØX5	T37.ØX6
Sulfaphenazole	T37.ØX1	T37.ØX2	T37.ØX3	T37.ØX4	T37.ØX5	T37.ØX6
Sulfaphenylthiazole	T37.ØX1	T37.ØX2	T37.ØX3	T37.ØX4	T37.ØX5	T37.ØX6
Sulfaproxyline	T37.ØX1	T37.ØX2	T37.ØX3	T37.ØX4	T37.ØX5	T37.ØX6
Sulfapyridine	T37.ØX1	T37.ØX2	T37.ØX3	T37.ØX4	T37.ØX5	T37.ØX6
Sulfapyrimidine	T37.ØX1	T37.ØX2	T37.ØX3	T37.ØX4	T37.ØX5	T37.ØX6
Sulfarsphenamine	T37.8X1	T37.8X2	T37.8X3	T37.8X4	T37.8X5	T37.8X6
Sulfasalazine	T37.ØX1	T37.ØX2	T37.ØX3	T37.ØX4	T37.ØX5	T37.ØX6
Sulfasuxidine	T37.ØX1	T37.ØX2	T37.ØX3	T37.ØX4	T37.ØX5	T37.ØX6
Sulfasymazine	T37.ØX1	T37.ØX2	T37.ØX3	T37.ØX4	T37.ØX5	T37.ØX6
Sulfated amylopectin	T47.8X1	T47.8X2	T47.8X3	T47.8X4	T47.8X5	T47.8X6
Sulfathiazole	T37.ØX1	T37.ØX2	T37.ØX3	T37.ØX4	T37.ØX5	T37.ØX6
Sulfatostearate	T49.2X1	T49.2X2	T49.2X3	T49.2X4	T49.2X5	T49.2X6
Sulfinpyrazone	T5Ø.4X1	T5Ø.4X2	T5Ø.4X3	T5Ø.4X4	T5Ø.4X5	T5Ø.4X6
Sulfiram	T49.ØX1	T49.ØX2	T49.ØX3	T49.ØX4	T49.ØX5	T49.ØX6
Sulfisomidine	T37.ØX1	T37.ØX2	T37.ØX3	T37.ØX4	T37.ØX5	T37.ØX6
Sulfisoxazole	T37.ØX1	T37.ØX2	T37.ØX3	T37.ØX4	T37.ØX5	T37.ØX6
ophthalmic preparation	T49.5X1	T49.5X2	T49.5X3	T49.5X4	T49.5X5	T49.5X6
Sulfobromophthalein (sodium)	T5Ø.8X1	T5Ø.8X2	T5Ø.8X3	T5Ø.8X4	T5Ø.8X5	T5Ø.8X6
Sulfobromphthalein	T5Ø.8X1	T5Ø.8X2	T5Ø.8X3	T5Ø.8X4	T5Ø.8X5	T5Ø.8X6
Sulfogaiacol	T48.4X1	T48.4X2	T48.4X3	T48.4X4	T48.4X5	T48.4X6
Sulfomyxin	T36.8X1	T36.8X2	T36.8X3	T36.8X4	T36.8X5	T36.8X6
Sulfonal	T42.6X1	T42.6X2	T42.6X3	T42.6X4	T42.6X5	T42.6X6
Sulfonamide NEC	T37.ØX1	T37.ØX2	T37.ØX3	T37.ØX4	T37.ØX5	T37.ØX6
eye	T49.5X1	T49.5X2	T49.5X3	T49.5X4	T49.5X5	T49.5X6
Sulfonazide	T37.1X1	T37.1X2	T37.1X3	T37.1X4	T37.1X5	T37.1X6
Sulfones	T37.1X1	T37.1X2	T37.1X3	T37.1X4	T37.1X5	T37.1X6
Sulfonethylmethane	T42.6X1	T42.6X2	T42.6X3	T42.6X4	T42.6X5	T42.6X6
Sulfonmethane	T42.6X1	T42.6X2	T42.6X3	T42.6X4	T42.6X5	T42.6X6
Sulfonphthal, sulfonphthol	T5Ø.8X1	T5Ø.8X2	T5Ø.8X3	T5Ø.8X4	T5Ø.8X5	T5Ø.8X6
Sulfonylurea derivatives, oral	T38.3X1	T38.3X2	T38.3X3	T38.3X4	T38.3X5	T38.3X6
Sulforidazine	T43.3X1	T43.3X2	T43.3X3	T43.3X4	T43.3X5	T43.3X6
Sulfoxone	T37.1X1	T37.1X2	T37.1X3	T37.1X4	T37.1X5	T37.1X6
Sulfuric acid	T54.2X1	T54.2X2	T54.2X3	T54.2X4	—	—
Sulfur, sulfurated, sulfuric, sulfurous, sulfuryl (compounds NEC) (medicinal)	T49.4X1	T49.4X2	T49.4X3	T49.4X4	T49.4X5	T49.4X6
acid	T54.2X1	T54.2X2	T54.2X3	T54.2X4	—	—
dioxide (gas)	T59.1X1	T59.1X2	T59.1X3	T59.1X4	—	—
ether — *see* Ether(s)						
hydrogen	T59.6X1	T59.6X2	T59.6X3	T59.6X4	—	—
medicinal (keratolytic) (ointment) NEC	T49.4X1	T49.4X2	T49.4X3	T49.4X4	T49.4X5	T49.4X6
ointment	T49.ØX1	T49.ØX2	T49.ØX3	T49.ØX4	T49.ØX5	T49.ØX6
pesticide (vapor)	T6Ø.91	T6Ø.92	T6Ø.93	T6Ø.94	—	—
vapor NEC	T59.891	T59.892	T59.893	T59.894	—	—
Sulglicotide	T47.1X1	T47.1X2	T47.1X3	T47.1X4	T47.1X5	T47.1X6
Sulindac	T39.391	T39.392	T39.393	T39.394	T39.395	T39.396
Sulisatin	T47.2X1	T47.2X2	T47.2X3	T47.2X4	T47.2X5	T47.2X6
Sulisobenzone	T49.3X1	T49.3X2	T49.3X3	T49.3X4	T49.3X5	T49.3X6
Sulkowitch's reagent	T5Ø.8X1	T5Ø.8X2	T5Ø.8X3	T5Ø.8X4	T5Ø.8X5	T5Ø.8X6
Sulmetozine	T44.3X1	T44.3X2	T44.3X3	T44.3X4	T44.3X5	T44.3X6
Suloctidil	T46.7X1	T46.7X2	T46.7X3	T46.7X4	T46.7X5	T46.7X6
Sulph- — *see also* Sulf-						
Sulphadiazine	T37.ØX1	T37.ØX2	T37.ØX3	T37.ØX4	T37.ØX5	T37.ØX6
Sulphadimethoxine	T37.ØX1	T37.ØX2	T37.ØX3	T37.ØX4	T37.ØX5	T37.ØX6
Sulphadimidine	T37.ØX1	T37.ØX2	T37.ØX3	T37.ØX4	T37.ØX5	T37.ØX6
Sulphadione	T37.1X1	T37.1X2	T37.1X3	T37.1X4	T37.1X5	T37.1X6
Sulphafurazole	T37.ØX1	T37.ØX2	T37.ØX3	T37.ØX4	T37.ØX5	T37.ØX6
Sulphamethizole	T37.ØX1	T37.ØX2	T37.ØX3	T37.ØX4	T37.ØX5	T37.ØX6
Sulphamethoxazole	T37.ØX1	T37.ØX2	T37.ØX3	T37.ØX4	T37.ØX5	T37.ØX6
Sulphan blue	T5Ø.8X1	T5Ø.8X2	T5Ø.8X3	T5Ø.8X4	T5Ø.8X5	T5Ø.8X6
Sulphaphenazole	T37.ØX1	T37.ØX2	T37.ØX3	T37.ØX4	T37.ØX5	T37.ØX6
Sulphapyridine	T37.ØX1	T37.ØX2	T37.ØX3	T37.ØX4	T37.ØX5	T37.ØX6
Sulphasalazine	T37.ØX1	T37.ØX2	T37.ØX3	T37.ØX4	T37.ØX5	T37.ØX6
Sulphinpyrazone	T5Ø.4X1	T5Ø.4X2	T5Ø.4X3	T5Ø.4X4	T5Ø.4X5	T5Ø.4X6
Sulpiride	T43.591	T43.592	T43.593	T43.594	T43.595	T43.596
Sulprostone	T48.ØX1	T48.ØX2	T48.ØX3	T48.ØX4	T48.ØX5	T48.ØX6
Sulpyrine	T39.2X1	T39.2X2	T39.2X3	T39.2X4	T39.2X5	T39.2X6
Sultamicillin	T36.ØX1	T36.ØX2	T36.ØX3	T36.ØX4	T36.ØX5	T36.ØX6
Sulthiame	T42.6X1	T42.6X2	T42.6X3	T42.6X4	T42.6X5	T42.6X6
Sultiame	T42.6X1	T42.6X2	T42.6X3	T42.6X4	T42.6X5	T42.6X6
Sultopride	T43.591	T43.592	T43.593	T43.594	T43.595	T43.596
Sumatriptan	T39.8X1	T39.8X2	T39.8X3	T39.8X4	T39.8X5	T39.8X6
Sunflower seed oil	T46.6X1	T46.6X2	T46.6X3	T46.6X4	T46.6X5	T46.6X6
Superinone	T48.4X1	T48.4X2	T48.4X3	T48.4X4	T48.4X5	T48.4X6
Suprofen	T39.311	T39.312	T39.313	T39.314	T39.315	T39.316
Suramin (sodium)	T37.4X1	T37.4X2	T37.4X3	T37.4X4	T37.4X5	T37.4X6
Surfacaine	T41.3X1	T41.3X2	T41.3X3	T41.3X4	T41.3X5	T41.3X6
Surital	T41.1X1	T41.1X2	T41.1X3	T41.1X4	T41.1X5	T41.1X6
Sutilains	T45.3X1	T45.3X2	T45.3X3	T45.3X4	T45.3X5	T45.3X6
Suxamethonium (chloride)	T48.1X1	T48.1X2	T48.1X3	T48.1X4	T48.1X5	T48.1X6
Suxethonium (chloride)	T48.1X1	T48.1X2	T48.1X3	T48.1X4	T48.1X5	T48.1X6
Suxibuzone	T39.2X1	T39.2X2	T39.2X3	T39.2X4	T39.2X5	T39.2X6
Sweetener	T5Ø.9Ø1	T5Ø.9Ø2	T5Ø.9Ø3	T5Ø.9Ø4	T5Ø.9Ø5	T5Ø.9Ø6
Sweet niter spirit	T46.3X1	T46.3X2	T46.3X3	T46.3X4	T46.3X5	T46.3X6
Sweet oil (birch)	T49.3X1	T49.3X2	T49.3X3	T49.3X4	T49.3X5	T49.3X6
Sym-dichloroethyl ether	T53.6X1	T53.6X2	T53.6X3	T53.6X4	—	—
Sympatholytic NEC	T44.8X1	T44.8X2	T44.8X3	T44.8X4	T44.8X5	T44.8X6
haloalkylamine	T44.8X1	T44.8X2	T44.8X3	T44.8X4	T44.8X5	T44.8X6
Sympathomimetic NEC	T44.9Ø1	T44.9Ø2	T44.9Ø3	T44.9Ø4	T44.9Ø5	T44.9Ø6
anti-common-cold	T48.5X1	T48.5X2	T48.5X3	T48.5X4	T48.5X5	T48.5X6
bronchodilator	T48.6X1	T48.6X2	T48.6X3	T48.6X4	T48.6X5	T48.6X6
specified NEC	T44.991	T44.992	T44.993	T44.994	T44.995	T44.996
Synagis	T5Ø.B91	T5Ø.B92	T5Ø.B93	T5Ø.B94	T5Ø.B95	T5Ø.B96
Synalar	T49.ØX1	T49.ØX2	T49.ØX3	T49.ØX4	T49.ØX5	T49.ØX6
Synthroid	T38.1X1	T38.1X2	T38.1X3	T38.1X4	T38.1X5	T38.1X6
Syntocinon	T48.ØX1	T48.ØX2	T48.ØX3	T48.ØX4	T48.ØX5	T48.ØX6
Syrosingopine	T46.5X1	T46.5X2	T46.5X3	T46.5X4	T46.5X5	T46.5X6
Systemic drug	T45.91	T45.92	T45.93	T45.94	T45.95	T45.96
specified NEC	T45.8X1	T45.8X2	T45.8X3	T45.8X4	T45.8X5	T45.8X6
Tablets — *see also* specified substance	T5Ø.9Ø1	T5Ø.9Ø2	T5Ø.9Ø3	T5Ø.9Ø4	T5Ø.9Ø5	T5Ø.9Ø6
Tace	T38.5X1	T38.5X2	T38.5X3	T38.5X4	T38.5X5	T38.5X6
Tacrine	T44.ØX1	T44.ØX2	T44.ØX3	T44.ØX4	T44.ØX5	T44.ØX6
Tadalafil	T46.7X1	T46.7X2	T46.7X3	T46.7X4	T46.7X5	T46.7X6
Talampicillin	T36.ØX1	T36.ØX2	T36.ØX3	T36.ØX4	T36.ØX5	T36.ØX6
Talbutal	T42.3X1	T42.3X2	T42.3X3	T42.3X4	T42.3X5	T42.3X6
Talc powder	T49.3X1	T49.3X2	T49.3X3	T49.3X4	T49.3X5	T49.3X6
Talcum	T49.3X1	T49.3X2	T49.3X3	T49.3X4	T49.3X5	T49.3X6
Taleranol	T38.6X1	T38.6X2	T38.6X3	T38.6X4	T38.6X5	T38.6X6
Tamoxifen	T38.6X1	T38.6X2	T38.6X3	T38.6X4	T38.6X5	T38.6X6
Tamsulosin	T44.6X1	T44.6X2	T44.6X3	T44.6X4	T44.6X5	T44.6X6
Tandearil, tanderil	T39.2X1	T39.2X2	T39.2X3	T39.2X4	T39.2X5	T39.2X6
Tannic acid	T49.2X1	T49.2X2	T49.2X3	T49.2X4	T49.2X5	T49.2X6
medicinal (astringent)	T49.2X1	T49.2X2	T49.2X3	T49.2X4	T49.2X5	T49.2X6
Tannin — *see* Tannic acid						
Tansy	T62.2X1	T62.2X2	T62.2X3	T62.2X4	—	—
TAO	T36.3X1	T36.3X2	T36.3X3	T36.3X4	T36.3X5	T36.3X6
Tapazole	T38.2X1	T38.2X2	T38.2X3	T38.2X4	T38.2X5	T38.2X6
Taractan	T43.591	T43.592	T43.593	T43.594	T43.595	T43.596
Tarantula (venomous)	T63.321	T63.322	T63.323	T63.324	—	—
Tartar emetic	T37.8X1	T37.8X2	T37.8X3	T37.8X4	T37.8X5	T37.8X6
Tartaric acid	T65.891	T65.892	T65.893	T65.894	—	—
Tartrated antimony (anti-infective)	T37.8X1	T37.8X2	T37.8X3	T37.8X4	T37.8X5	T37.8X6
Tartrate, laxative	T47.4X1	T47.4X2	T47.4X3	T47.4X4	T47.4X5	T47.4X6
Tar NEC	T52.ØX1	T52.ØX2	T52.ØX3	T52.ØX4	—	—
camphor	T6Ø.1X1	T6Ø.1X2	T6Ø.1X3	T6Ø.1X4	—	—
distillate	T49.1X1	T49.1X2	T49.1X3	T49.1X4	T49.1X5	T49.1X6
fumes	T59.891	T59.892	T59.893	T59.894	—	—
medicinal	T49.1X1	T49.1X2	T49.1X3	T49.1X4	T49.1X5	T49.1X6
ointment	T49.1X1	T49.1X2	T49.1X3	T49.1X4	T49.1X5	T49.1X6
Tauromustine	T45.1X1	T45.1X2	T45.1X3	T45.1X4	T45.1X5	T45.1X6
TCA — *see* Trichloroacetic acid						
TCDD	T53.7X1	T53.7X2	T53.7X3	T53.7X4	—	—
TDI (vapor)	T65.ØX1	T65.ØX2	T65.ØX3	T65.ØX4	—	—
Tear						
gas	T59.3X1	T59.3X2	T59.3X3	T59.3X4	—	—

Substance	Poisoning, Accidental (unintentional)	Poisoning, Intentional Self-harm	Poisoning, Assault	Poisoning, Undetermined	Adverse Effect	Under-dosing
Tear — *continued*						
solution	T49.5X1	T49.5X2	T49.5X3	T49.5X4	T49.5X5	T49.5X6
Teclothiazide	T5Ø.2X1	T5Ø.2X2	T5Ø.2X3	T5Ø.2X4	T5Ø.2X5	T5Ø.2X6
Teclozan	T37.3X1	T37.3X2	T37.3X3	T37.3X4	T37.3X5	T37.3X6
Tegafur	T45.1X1	T45.1X2	T45.1X3	T45.1X4	T45.1X5	T45.1X6
Tegretol	T42.1X1	T42.1X2	T42.1X3	T42.1X4	T42.1X5	T42.1X6
Teicoplanin	T36.8X1	T36.8X2	T36.8X3	T36.8X4	T36.8X5	T36.8X6
Telepaque	T5Ø.8X1	T5Ø.8X2	T5Ø.8X3	T5Ø.8X4	T5Ø.8X5	T5Ø.8X6
Tellurium	T56.891	T56.892	T56.893	T56.894	—	—
fumes	T56.891	T56.892	T56.893	T56.894	—	—
TEM	T45.1X1	T45.1X2	T45.1X3	T45.1X4	T45.1X5	T45.1X6
Temazepam	T42.4X1	T42.4X2	T42.4X3	T42.4X4	T42.4X5	T42.4X6
Temocillin	T36.ØX1	T36.ØX2	T36.ØX3	T36.ØX4	T36.ØX5	T36.ØX6
Tenamfetamine	T43.621	T43.622	T43.623	T43.624	T43.625	T43.626
Teniposide	T45.1X1	T45.1X2	T45.1X3	T45.1X4	T45.1X5	T45.1X6
Tenitramine	T46.3X1	T46.3X2	T46.3X3	T46.3X4	T46.3X5	T46.3X6
Tenoglicin	T48.4X1	T48.4X2	T48.4X3	T48.4X4	T48.4X5	T48.4X6
Tenonitrozole	T37.3X1	T37.3X2	T37.3X3	T37.3X4	T37.3X5	T37.3X6
Tenoxicam	T39.391	T39.392	T39.393	T39.394	T39.395	T39.396
TEPA	T45.1X1	T45.1X2	T45.1X3	T45.1X4	T45.1X5	T45.1X6
TEPP	T6Ø.ØX1	T6Ø.ØX2	T6Ø.ØX3	T6Ø.ØX4	—	—
Teprotide	T46.5X1	T46.5X2	T46.5X3	T46.5X4	T46.5X5	T46.5X6
Terazosin	T44.6X1	T44.6X2	T44.6X3	T44.6X4	T44.6X5	T44.6X6
Terbufos	T6Ø.ØX1	T6Ø.ØX2	T6Ø.ØX3	T6Ø.ØX4	—	—
Terbutaline	T48.6X1	T48.6X2	T48.6X3	T48.6X4	T48.6X5	T48.6X6
Terconazole	T49.ØX1	T49.ØX2	T49.ØX3	T49.ØX4	T49.ØX5	T49.ØX6
Terfenadine	T45.ØX1	T45.ØX2	T45.ØX3	T45.ØX4	T45.ØX5	T45.ØX6
Teriparatide (acetate)	T5Ø.991	T5Ø.992	T5Ø.993	T5Ø.994	T5Ø.995	T5Ø.996
Terizidone	T37.1X1	T37.1X2	T37.1X3	T37.1X4	T37.1X5	T37.1X6
Terlipressin	T38.891	T38.892	T38.893	T38.894	T38.895	T38.896
Terodiline	T46.3X1	T46.3X2	T46.3X3	T46.3X4	T46.3X5	T46.3X6
Teroxalene	T37.4X1	T37.4X2	T37.4X3	T37.4X4	T37.4X5	T37.4X6
Terpin (cis) **hydrate**	T48.4X1	T48.4X2	T48.4X3	T48.4X4	T48.4X5	T48.4X6
Terramycin	T36.4X1	T36.4X2	T36.4X3	T36.4X4	T36.4X5	T36.4X6
Tertatolol	T44.7X1	T44.7X2	T44.7X3	T44.7X4	T44.7X5	T44.7X6
Tessalon	T48.3X1	T48.3X2	T48.3X3	T48.3X4	T48.3X5	T48.3X6
Testolactone	T38.7X1	T38.7X2	T38.7X3	T38.7X4	T38.7X5	T38.7X6
Testosterone	T38.7X1	T38.7X2	T38.7X3	T38.7X4	T38.7X5	T38.7X6
Tetanus toxoid or vaccine	T5Ø.A91	T5Ø.A92	T5Ø.A93	T5Ø.A94	T5Ø.A95	T5Ø.A96
antitoxin	T5Ø.Z11	T5Ø.Z12	T5Ø.Z13	T5Ø.Z14	T5Ø.Z15	T5Ø.Z16
immune globulin (human)	T5Ø.Z11	T5Ø.Z12	T5Ø.Z13	T5Ø.Z14	T5Ø.Z15	T5Ø.Z16
toxoid	T5Ø.A91	T5Ø.A92	T5Ø.A93	T5Ø.A94	T5Ø.A95	T5Ø.A96
with diphtheria toxoid	T5Ø.A21	T5Ø.A22	T5Ø.A23	T5Ø.A24	T5Ø.A25	T5Ø.A26
with pertussis	T5Ø.A11	T5Ø.A12	T5Ø.A13	T5Ø.A14	T5Ø.A15	T5Ø.A16
Tetrabenazine	T43.591	T43.592	T43.593	T43.594	T43.595	T43.596
Tetracaine	T41.3X1	T41.3X2	T41.3X3	T41.3X4	T41.3X5	T41.3X6
nerve block (peripheral) (plexus)	T41.3X1	T41.3X2	T41.3X3	T41.3X4	T41.3X5	T41.3X6
regional	T41.3X1	T41.3X2	T41.3X3	T41.3X4	T41.3X5	T41.3X6
spinal	T41.3X1	T41.3X2	T41.3X3	T41.3X4	T41.3X5	T41.3X6
Tetrachlorethylene — *see* Tetrachloroethylene						
Tetrachlormethiazide	T5Ø.2X1	T5Ø.2X2	T5Ø.2X3	T5Ø.2X4	T5Ø.2X5	T5Ø.2X6
Tetrachloroethane	T53.6X1	T53.6X2	T53.6X3	T53.6X4	—	—
vapor	T53.6X1	T53.6X2	T53.6X3	T53.6X4	—	—
paint or varnish	T53.6X1	T53.6X2	T53.6X3	T53.6X4	—	—
Tetrachloroethylene (liquid)	T53.3X1	T53.3X2	T53.3X3	T53.3X4	—	—
medicinal	T37.4X1	T37.4X2	T37.4X3	T37.4X4	T37.4X5	T37.4X6
vapor	T53.3X1	T53.3X2	T53.3X3	T53.3X4	—	—
Tetrachloromethane — *see* Carbon tetrachloride						
Tetracosactide	T38.811	T38.812	T38.813	T38.814	T38.815	T38.816
Tetracosactrin	T38.811	T38.812	T38.813	T38.814	T38.815	T38.816
Tetracycline	T36.4X1	T36.4X2	T36.4X3	T36.4X4	T36.4X5	T36.4X6
ophthalmic preparation	T49.5X1	T49.5X2	T49.5X3	T49.5X4	T49.5X5	T49.5X6
topical NEC	T49.ØX1	T49.ØX2	T49.ØX3	T49.ØX4	T49.ØX5	T49.ØX6
Tetradifon	T6Ø.8X1	T6Ø.8X2	T6Ø.8X3	T6Ø.8X4	—	—
Tetradotoxin	T61.771	T61.772	T61.773	T61.774	—	—
Tetraethyl						
lead	T56.ØX1	T56.ØX2	T56.ØX3	T56.ØX4	—	—
pyrophosphate	T6Ø.ØX1	T6Ø.ØX2	T6Ø.ØX3	T6Ø.ØX4	—	—
Tetraethylammonium chloride	T44.2X1	T44.2X2	T44.2X3	T44.2X4	T44.2X5	T44.2X6
Tetraethylthiuram disulfide	T5Ø.6X1	T5Ø.6X2	T5Ø.6X3	T5Ø.6X4	T5Ø.6X5	T5Ø.6X6
Tetrahydroaminoacridine	T44.ØX1	T44.ØX2	T44.ØX3	T44.ØX4	T44.ØX5	T44.ØX6
Tetrahydrocannabinol	T4Ø.7X1	T4Ø.7X2	T4Ø.7X3	T4Ø.7X4	T4Ø.7X5	T4Ø.7X6
Tetrahydrofuran	T52.8X1	T52.8X2	T52.8X3	T52.8X4	—	—
Tetrahydronaphthalene	T52.8X1	T52.8X2	T52.8X3	T52.8X4	—	—
Tetrahydrozoline	T49.5X1	T49.5X2	T49.5X3	T49.5X4	T49.5X5	T49.5X6
Tetralin	T52.8X1	T52.8X2	T52.8X3	T52.8X4	—	—
Tetramethrin	T6Ø.2X1	T6Ø.2X2	T6Ø.2X3	T6Ø.2X4	—	—
Tetramethylthiuram (disulfide) NEC	T6Ø.3X1	T6Ø.3X2	T6Ø.3X3	T6Ø.3X4	—	—
medicinal	T49.ØX1	T49.ØX2	T49.ØX3	T49.ØX4	T49.ØX5	T49.ØX6
Tetramisole	T37.4X1	T37.4X2	T37.4X3	T37.4X4	T37.4X5	T37.4X6
Tetranicotinoyl fructose	T46.7X1	T46.7X2	T46.7X3	T46.7X4	T46.7X5	T46.7X6
Tetrazepam	T42.4X1	T42.4X2	T42.4X3	T42.4X4	T42.4X5	T42.4X6
Tetronal	T42.6X1	T42.6X2	T42.6X3	T42.6X4	T42.6X5	T42.6X6
Tetryl	T65.3X1	T65.3X2	T65.3X3	T65.3X4	—	—
Tetrylammonium chloride	T44.2X1	T44.2X2	T44.2X3	T44.2X4	T44.2X5	T44.2X6
Tetryzoline	T49.5X1	T49.5X2	T49.5X3	T49.5X4	T49.5X5	T49.5X6
Thalidomide	T45.1X1	T45.1X2	T45.1X3	T45.1X4	T45.1X5	T45.1X6
Thallium (compounds) (dust) NEC	T56.811	T56.812	T56.813	T56.814	—	—
pesticide	T6Ø.4X1	T6Ø.4X2	T6Ø.4X3	T6Ø.4X4	—	—
THC	T4Ø.7X1	T4Ø.7X2	T4Ø.7X3	T4Ø.7X4	T4Ø.7X5	T4Ø.7X6
Thebacon	T48.3X1	T48.3X2	T48.3X3	T48.3X4	T48.3X5	T48.3X6
Thebaine	T4Ø.2X1	T4Ø.2X2	T4Ø.2X3	T4Ø.2X4	T4Ø.2X5	T4Ø.2X6
Thenoic acid	T49.6X1	T49.6X2	T49.6X3	T49.6X4	T49.6X5	T49.6X6
Thenyldiamine	T45.ØX1	T45.ØX2	T45.ØX3	T45.ØX4	T45.ØX5	T45.ØX6
Theobromine (calcium salicylate)	T48.6X1	T48.6X2	T48.6X3	T48.6X4	T48.6X5	T48.6X6
sodium salicylate	T48.6X1	T48.6X2	T48.6X3	T48.6X4	T48.6X5	T48.6X6
Theophyllamine	T48.6X1	T48.6X2	T48.6X3	T48.6X4	T48.6X5	T48.6X6
Theophylline	T48.6X1	T48.6X2	T48.6X3	T48.6X4	T48.6X5	T48.6X6
aminobenzoic acid	T48.6X1	T48.6X2	T48.6X3	T48.6X4	T48.6X5	T48.6X6
ethylenediamine	T48.6X1	T48.6X2	T48.6X3	T48.6X4	T48.6X5	T48.6X6
piperazine p-amino-benzoate	T48.6X1	T48.6X2	T48.6X3	T48.6X4	T48.6X5	T48.6X6
Thiabendazole	T37.4X1	T37.4X2	T37.4X3	T37.4X4	T37.4X5	T37.4X6
Thialbarbital	T41.1X1	T41.1X2	T41.1X3	T41.1X4	T41.1X5	T41.1X6
Thiamazole	T38.2X1	T38.2X2	T38.2X3	T38.2X4	T38.2X5	T38.2X6
Thiambutosine	T37.1X1	T37.1X2	T37.1X3	T37.1X4	T37.1X5	T37.1X6
Thiamine	T45.2X1	T45.2X2	T45.2X3	T45.2X4	T45.2X5	T45.2X6
Thiamphenicol	T36.2X1	T36.2X2	T36.2X3	T36.2X4	T36.2X5	T36.2X6
Thiamylal	T41.1X1	T41.1X2	T41.1X3	T41.1X4	T41.1X5	T41.1X6
sodium	T41.1X1	T41.1X2	T41.1X3	T41.1X4	T41.1X5	T41.1X6
Thiazesim	T43.291	T43.292	T43.293	T43.294	T43.295	T43.296
Thiazides (diuretics)	T5Ø.2X1	T5Ø.2X2	T5Ø.2X3	T5Ø.2X4	T5Ø.2X5	T5Ø.2X6
Thiazinamium metilsulfate	T43.3X1	T43.3X2	T43.3X3	T43.3X4	T43.3X5	T43.3X6
Thiethylperazine	T43.3X1	T43.3X2	T43.3X3	T43.3X4	T43.3X5	T43.3X6
Thimerosal	T49.ØX1	T49.ØX2	T49.ØX3	T49.ØX4	T49.ØX5	T49.ØX6
ophthalmic preparation	T49.5X1	T49.5X2	T49.5X3	T49.5X4	T49.5X5	T49.5X6
Thioacetazone	T37.1X1	T37.1X2	T37.1X3	T37.1X4	T37.1X5	T37.1X6
with isoniazid	T37.1X1	T37.1X2	T37.1X3	T37.1X4	T37.1X5	T37.1X6
Thiobarbital sodium	T41.1X1	T41.1X2	T41.1X3	T41.1X4	T41.1X5	T41.1X6
Thiobarbiturate anesthetic	T41.1X1	T41.1X2	T41.1X3	T41.1X4	T41.1X5	T41.1X6
Thiobismol	T37.8X1	T37.8X2	T37.8X3	T37.8X4	T37.8X5	T37.8X6
Thiobutabarbital sodium	T41.1X1	T41.1X2	T41.1X3	T41.1X4	T41.1X5	T41.1X6
Thiocarbamate (insecticide)	T6Ø.ØX1	T6Ø.ØX2	T6Ø.ØX3	T6Ø.ØX4	—	—
Thiocarbamide	T38.2X1	T38.2X2	T38.2X3	T38.2X4	T38.2X5	T38.2X6
Thiocarbarsone	T37.8X1	T37.8X2	T37.8X3	T37.8X4	T37.8X5	T37.8X6
Thiocarlide	T37.1X1	T37.1X2	T37.1X3	T37.1X4	T37.1X5	T37.1X6
Thioctamide	T5Ø.991	T5Ø.992	T5Ø.993	T5Ø.994	T5Ø.995	T5Ø.996
Thioctic acid	T5Ø.991	T5Ø.992	T5Ø.993	T5Ø.994	T5Ø.995	T5Ø.996
Thiofos	T6Ø.ØX1	T6Ø.ØX2	T6Ø.ØX3	T6Ø.ØX4	—	—
Thioglycolate	T49.4X1	T49.4X2	T49.4X3	T49.4X4	T49.4X5	T49.4X6
Thioglycolic acid	T65.891	T65.892	T65.893	T65.894	—	—
Thioguanine	T45.1X1	T45.1X2	T45.1X3	T45.1X4	T45.1X5	T45.1X6
Thiomercaptomerin	T5Ø.2X1	T5Ø.2X2	T5Ø.2X3	T5Ø.2X4	T5Ø.2X5	T5Ø.2X6
Thiomerin	T5Ø.2X1	T5Ø.2X2	T5Ø.2X3	T5Ø.2X4	T5Ø.2X5	T5Ø.2X6
Thiomersal	T49.ØX1	T49.ØX2	T49.ØX3	T49.ØX4	T49.ØX5	T49.ØX6
Thionazin	T6Ø.ØX1	T6Ø.ØX2	T6Ø.ØX3	T6Ø.ØX4	—	—
Thiopental (sodium)	T41.1X1	T41.1X2	T41.1X3	T41.1X4	T41.1X5	T41.1X6
Thiopentone (sodium)	T41.1X1	T41.1X2	T41.1X3	T41.1X4	T41.1X5	T41.1X6
Thiopropazate	T43.3X1	T43.3X2	T43.3X3	T43.3X4	T43.3X5	T43.3X6
Thioproperazine	T43.3X1	T43.3X2	T43.3X3	T43.3X4	T43.3X5	T43.3X6
Thioridazine	T43.3X1	T43.3X2	T43.3X3	T43.3X4	T43.3X5	T43.3X6
Thiosinamine	T49.3X1	T49.3X2	T49.3X3	T49.3X4	T49.3X5	T49.3X6
Thiotepa	T45.1X1	T45.1X2	T45.1X3	T45.1X4	T45.1X5	T45.1X6
Thiothixene	T43.4X1	T43.4X2	T43.4X3	T43.4X4	T43.4X5	T43.4X6
Thiouracil (benzyl) (methyl) (propyl)	T38.2X1	T38.2X2	T38.2X3	T38.2X4	T38.2X5	T38.2X6
Thiourea	T38.2X1	T38.2X2	T38.2X3	T38.2X4	T38.2X5	T38.2X6
Thiphenamil	T44.3X1	T44.3X2	T44.3X3	T44.3X4	T44.3X5	T44.3X6
Thiram	T6Ø.3X1	T6Ø.3X2	T6Ø.3X3	T6Ø.3X4	—	—
medicinal	T49.2X1	T49.2X2	T49.2X3	T49.2X4	T49.2X5	T49.2X6
Thonzylamine (systemic)	T45.ØX1	T45.ØX2	T45.ØX3	T45.ØX4	T45.ØX5	T45.ØX6
mucosal decongestant	T48.5X1	T48.5X2	T48.5X3	T48.5X4	T48.5X5	T48.5X6
Thorazine	T43.3X1	T43.3X2	T43.3X3	T43.3X4	T43.3X5	T43.3X6
Thorium dioxide suspension	T5Ø.8X1	T5Ø.8X2	T5Ø.8X3	T5Ø.8X4	T5Ø.8X5	T5Ø.8X6
Thornapple	T62.2X1	T62.2X2	T62.2X3	T62.2X4	—	—
Throat drug NEC	T49.6X1	T49.6X2	T49.6X3	T49.6X4	T49.6X5	T49.6X6

Substance	Poisoning, Accidental (unintentional)	Poisoning, Intentional Self-harm	Poisoning, Assault	Poisoning, Undetermined	Adverse Effect	Under-dosing
Thrombin	T45.7X1	T45.7X2	T45.7X3	T45.7X4	T45.7X5	T45.7X6
Thrombolysin	T45.611	T45.612	T45.613	T45.614	T45.615	T45.616
Thromboplastin	T45.7X1	T45.7X2	T45.7X3	T45.7X4	T45.7X5	T45.7X6
Thurfyl nicotinate	T46.7X1	T46.7X2	T46.7X3	T46.7X4	T46.7X5	T46.7X6
Thymol	T49.ØX1	T49.ØX2	T49.ØX3	T49.ØX4	T49.ØX5	T49.ØX6
Thymopentin	T37.5X1	T37.5X2	T37.5X3	T37.5X4	T37.5X5	T37.5X6
Thymoxamine	T46.7X1	T46.7X2	T46.7X3	T46.7X4	T46.7X5	T46.7X6
Thymus extract	T38.891	T38.892	T38.893	T38.894	T38.895	T38.896
Thyreotrophic hormone	T38.811	T38.812	T38.813	T38.814	T38.815	T38.816
Thyroglobulin	T38.1X1	T38.1X2	T38.1X3	T38.1X4	T38.1X5	T38.1X6
Thyroid (hormone)	T38.1X1	T38.1X2	T38.1X3	T38.1X4	T38.1X5	T38.1X6
Thyrolar	T38.1X1	T38.1X2	T38.1X3	T38.1X4	T38.1X5	T38.1X6
Thyrotrophin	T38.811	T38.812	T38.813	T38.814	T38.815	T38.816
Thyrotropic hormone	T38.811	T38.812	T38.813	T38.814	T38.815	T38.816
Thyroxine	T38.1X1	T38.1X2	T38.1X3	T38.1X4	T38.1X5	T38.1X6
Tiabendazole	T37.4X1	T37.4X2	T37.4X3	T37.4X4	T37.4X5	T37.4X6
Tiamizide	T5Ø.2X1	T5Ø.2X2	T5Ø.2X3	T5Ø.2X4	T5Ø.2X5	T5Ø.2X6
Tianeptine	T43.291	T43.292	T43.293	T43.294	T43.295	T43.296
Tiapamil	T46.1X1	T46.1X2	T46.1X3	T46.1X4	T46.1X5	T46.1X6
Tiapride	T43.591	T43.592	T43.593	T43.594	T43.595	T43.596
Tiaprofenic acid	T39.311	T39.312	T39.313	T39.314	T39.315	T39.316
Tiaramide	T39.8X1	T39.8X2	T39.8X3	T39.8X4	T39.8X5	T39.8X6
Ticarcillin	T36.ØX1	T36.ØX2	T36.ØX3	T36.ØX4	T36.ØX5	T36.ØX6
Ticlatone	T49.ØX1	T49.ØX2	T49.ØX3	T49.ØX4	T49.ØX5	T49.ØX6
Ticlopidine	T45.521	T45.522	T45.523	T45.524	T45.525	T45.526
Ticrynafen	T5Ø.1X1	T5Ø.1X2	T5Ø.1X3	T5Ø.1X4	T5Ø.1X5	T5Ø.1X6
Tidiacic	T5Ø.991	T5Ø.992	T5Ø.993	T5Ø.994	T5Ø.995	T5Ø.996
Tiemonium	T44.3X1	T44.3X2	T44.3X3	T44.3X4	T44.3X5	T44.3X6
iodide	T44.3X1	T44.3X2	T44.3X3	T44.3X4	T44.3X5	T44.3X6
Tienilic acid	T5Ø.1X1	T5Ø.1X2	T5Ø.1X3	T5Ø.1X4	T5Ø.1X5	T5Ø.1X6
Tifenamil	T44.3X1	T44.3X2	T44.3X3	T44.3X4	T44.3X5	T44.3X6
Tigan	T45.ØX1	T45.ØX2	T45.ØX3	T45.ØX4	T45.ØX5	T45.ØX6
Tigloidine	T44.3X1	T44.3X2	T44.3X3	T44.3X4	T44.3X5	T44.3X6
Tilactase	T47.5X1	T47.5X2	T47.5X3	T47.5X4	T47.5X5	T47.5X6
Tiletamine	T41.291	T41.292	T41.293	T41.294	T41.295	T41.296
Tilidine	T4Ø.4X1	T4Ø.4X2	T4Ø.4X3	T4Ø.4X4	—	—
Timepidium bromide	T44.3X1	T44.3X2	T44.3X3	T44.3X4	T44.3X5	T44.3X6
Timiperone	T43.4X1	T43.4X2	T43.4X3	T43.4X4	T43.4X5	T43.4X6
Timolol	T44.7X1	T44.7X2	T44.7X3	T44.7X4	T44.7X5	T44.7X6
Tincture, iodine — *see* Iodine						
Tindal	T43.3X1	T43.3X2	T43.3X3	T43.3X4	T43.3X5	T43.3X6
Tinidazole	T37.3X1	T37.3X2	T37.3X3	T37.3X4	T37.3X5	T37.3X6
Tinoridine	T39.8X1	T39.8X2	T39.8X3	T39.8X4	T39.8X5	T39.8X6
Tin (chloride) (dust) (oxide) **NEC**	T56.6X1	T56.6X2	T56.6X3	T56.6X4	—	—
anti-infectives	T37.8X1	T37.8X2	T37.8X3	T37.8X4	T37.8X5	T37.8X6
Tiocarlide	T37.1X1	T37.1X2	T37.1X3	T37.1X4	T37.1X5	T37.1X6
Tioclomarol	T45.511	T45.512	T45.513	T45.514	T45.515	T45.516
Tioconazole	T49.ØX1	T49.ØX2	T49.ØX3	T49.ØX4	T49.ØX5	T49.ØX6
Tioguanine	T45.1X1	T45.1X2	T45.1X3	T45.1X4	T45.1X5	T45.1X6
Tiopronin	T5Ø.991	T5Ø.992	T5Ø.993	T5Ø.994	T5Ø.995	T5Ø.996
Tiotixene	T43.4X1	T43.4X2	T43.4X3	T43.4X4	T43.4X5	T43.4X6
Tioxolone	T49.4X1	T49.4X2	T49.4X3	T49.4X4	T49.4X5	T49.4X6
Tipepidine	T48.3X1	T48.3X2	T48.3X3	T48.3X4	T48.3X5	T48.3X6
Tiquizium bromide	T44.3X1	T44.3X2	T44.3X3	T44.3X4	T44.3X5	T44.3X6
Tiratricol	T38.1X1	T38.1X2	T38.1X3	T38.1X4	T38.1X5	T38.1X6
Tisopurine	T5Ø.4X1	T5Ø.4X2	T5Ø.4X3	T5Ø.4X4	T5Ø.4X5	T5Ø.4X6
Titanium (compounds) (vapor)	T56.891	T56.892	T56.893	T56.894	—	—
dioxide	T49.3X1	T49.3X2	T49.3X3	T49.3X4	T49.3X5	T49.3X6
ointment	T49.3X1	T49.3X2	T49.3X3	T49.3X4	T49.3X5	T49.3X6
oxide	T49.3X1	T49.3X2	T49.3X3	T49.3X4	T49.3X5	T49.3X6
tetrachloride	T56.891	T56.892	T56.893	T56.894	—	—
Titanocene	T56.891	T56.892	T56.893	T56.894	—	—
Titroid	T38.1X1	T38.1X2	T38.1X3	T38.1X4	T38.1X5	T38.1X6
Tizanidine	T42.8X1	T42.8X2	T42.8X3	T42.8X4	T42.8X5	T42.8X6
TMTD	T6Ø.3X1	T6Ø.3X2	T6Ø.3X3	T6Ø.3X4	—	—
TNT (fumes)	T65.3X1	T65.3X2	T65.3X3	T65.3X4	—	—
Toadstool	T62.ØX1	T62.ØX2	T62.ØX3	T62.ØX4	—	—
Tobacco NEC	T65.291	T65.292	T65.293	T65.294	—	—
cigarettes	T65.221	T65.222	T65.223	T65.224	—	—
Indian	T62.2X1	T62.2X2	T62.2X3	T62.2X4	—	—
smoke, second-hand	T65.221	T65.222	T65.223	T65.224	—	—
Tobramycin	T36.5X1	T36.5X2	T36.5X3	T36.5X4	T36.5X5	T36.5X6
Tocainide	T46.2X1	T46.2X2	T46.2X3	T46.2X4	T46.2X5	T46.2X6
Tocoferol	T45.2X1	T45.2X2	T45.2X3	T45.2X4	T45.2X5	T45.2X6
Tocopherol	T45.2X1	T45.2X2	T45.2X3	T45.2X4	T45.2X5	T45.2X6
acetate	T45.2X1	T45.2X2	T45.2X3	T45.2X4	T45.2X5	T45.2X6
Tocosamine	T48.ØX1	T48.ØX2	T48.ØX3	T48.ØX4	T48.ØX5	T48.ØX6
Todralazine	T46.5X1	T46.5X2	T46.5X3	T46.5X4	T46.5X5	T46.5X6
Tofisopam	T42.4X1	T42.4X2	T42.4X3	T42.4X4	T42.4X5	T42.4X6
Tofranil	T43.Ø11	T43.Ø12	T43.Ø13	T43.Ø14	T43.Ø15	T43.Ø16
Toilet deodorizer	T65.891	T65.892	T65.893	T65.894	—	—

Substance	Poisoning, Accidental (unintentional)	Poisoning, Intentional Self-harm	Poisoning, Assault	Poisoning, Undetermined	Adverse Effect	Under-dosing
Tolamolol	T44.7X1	T44.7X2	T44.7X3	T44.7X4	T44.7X5	T44.7X6
Tolazamide	T38.3X1	T38.3X2	T38.3X3	T38.3X4	T38.3X5	T38.3X6
Tolazoline	T46.7X1	T46.7X2	T46.7X3	T46.7X4	T46.7X5	T46.7X6
Tolbutamide (sodium)	T38.3X1	T38.3X2	T38.3X3	T38.3X4	T38.3X5	T38.3X6
Tolciclate	T49.ØX1	T49.ØX2	T49.ØX3	T49.ØX4	T49.ØX5	T49.ØX6
Tolmetin	T39.391	T39.392	T39.393	T39.394	T39.395	T39.396
Tolnaftate	T49.ØX1	T49.ØX2	T49.ØX3	T49.ØX4	T49.ØX5	T49.ØX6
Tolonidine	T46.5X1	T46.5X2	T46.5X3	T46.5X4	T46.5X5	T46.5X6
Toloxatone	T42.6X1	T42.6X2	T42.6X3	T42.6X4	T42.6X5	T42.6X6
Tolperisone	T44.3X1	T44.3X2	T44.3X3	T44.3X4	T44.3X5	T44.3X6
Tolserol	T42.8X1	T42.8X2	T42.8X3	T42.8X4	T42.8X5	T42.8X6
Toluene (liquid)	T52.2X1	T52.2X2	T52.2X3	T52.2X4	—	—
diisocyanate	T65.ØX1	T65.ØX2	T65.ØX3	T65.ØX4	—	—
Toluidine	T65.891	T65.892	T65.893	T65.894	—	—
vapor	T59.891	T59.892	T59.893	T59.894	—	—
Toluol (liquid)	T52.2X1	T52.2X2	T52.2X3	T52.2X4	—	—
vapor	T52.2X1	T52.2X2	T52.2X3	T52.2X4	—	—
Toluylenediamine	T65.3X1	T65.3X2	T65.3X3	T65.3X4	—	—
Tolylene-2,4-diisocyanate	T65.ØX1	T65.ØX2	T65.ØX3	T65.ØX4	—	—
Tonic NEC	T5Ø.9Ø1	T5Ø.9Ø2	T5Ø.9Ø3	T5Ø.9Ø4	T5Ø.9Ø5	T5Ø.9Ø6
Topical action drug NEC	T49.91	T49.92	T49.93	T49.94	T49.95	T49.96
ear, nose or throat	T49.6X1	T49.6X2	T49.6X3	T49.6X4	T49.6X5	T49.6X6
eye	T49.5X1	T49.5X2	T49.5X3	T49.5X4	T49.5X5	T49.5X6
skin	T49.91	T49.92	T49.93	T49.94	T49.95	T49.96
specified NEC	T49.8X1	T49.8X2	T49.8X3	T49.8X4	T49.8X5	T49.8X6
Toquizine	T44.3X1	T44.3X2	T44.3X3	T44.3X4	T44.3X5	T44.3X6
Toremifene	T38.6X1	T38.6X2	T38.6X3	T38.6X4	T38.6X5	T38.6X6
Tosylchloramide sodium	T49.8X1	T49.8X2	T49.8X3	T49.8X4	T49.8X5	T49.8X6
Toxaphene (dust) (spray)	T6Ø.1X1	T6Ø.1X2	T6Ø.1X3	T6Ø.1X4	—	—
Toxin, diphtheria (Schick Test)	T5Ø.8X1	T5Ø.8X2	T5Ø.8X3	T5Ø.8X4	T5Ø.8X5	T5Ø.8X6
Toxoid						
combined	T5Ø.A21	T5Ø.A22	T5Ø.A23	T5Ø.A24	T5Ø.A25	T5Ø.A26
diphtheria	T5Ø.A91	T5Ø.A92	T5Ø.A93	T5Ø.A94	T5Ø.A95	T5Ø.A96
tetanus	T5Ø.A91	T5Ø.A92	T5Ø.A93	T5Ø.A94	T5Ø.A95	T5Ø.A96
Trace element NEC	T45.8X1	T45.8X2	T45.8X3	T45.8X4	T45.8X5	T45.8X6
Tractor fuel NEC	T52.ØX1	T52.ØX2	T52.ØX3	T52.ØX4	—	—
Tragacanth	T5Ø.991	T5Ø.992	T5Ø.993	T5Ø.994	T5Ø.995	T5Ø.996
Tramadol	T4Ø.4X1	T4Ø.4X2	T4Ø.4X3	T4Ø.4X4	T4Ø.4X5	T4Ø.4X6
Tramazoline	T48.5X1	T48.5X2	T48.5X3	T48.5X4	T48.5X5	T48.5X6
Tranexamic acid	T45.621	T45.622	T45.623	T45.624	T45.625	T45.626
Tranilast	T45.ØX1	T45.ØX2	T45.ØX3	T45.ØX4	T45.ØX5	T45.ØX6
Tranquilizer NEC	T43.5Ø1	T43.5Ø2	T43.5Ø3	T43.5Ø4	T43.5Ø5	T43.5Ø6
with hypnotic or sedative	T42.6X1	T42.6X2	T42.6X3	T42.6X4	T42.6X5	T42.6X6
benzodiazepine NEC	T42.4X1	T42.4X2	T42.4X3	T42.4X4	T42.4X5	T42.4X6
butyrophenone NEC	T43.4X1	T43.4X2	T43.4X3	T43.4X4	T43.4X5	T43.4X6
carbamate	T43.591	T43.592	T43.593	T43.594	T43.595	T43.596
dimethylamine	T43.3X1	T43.3X2	T43.3X3	T43.3X4	T43.3X5	T43.3X6
ethylamine	T43.3X1	T43.3X2	T43.3X3	T43.3X4	T43.3X5	T43.3X6
hydroxyzine	T43.591	T43.592	T43.593	T43.594	T43.595	T43.596
major NEC	T43.5Ø1	T43.5Ø2	T43.5Ø3	T43.5Ø4	T43.5Ø5	T43.5Ø6
penothiazine NEC	T43.3X1	T43.3X2	T43.3X3	T43.3X4	T43.3X5	T43.3X6
phenothiazine-based	T43.3X1	T43.3X2	T43.3X3	T43.3X4	T43.3X5	T43.3X6
piperazine NEC	T43.3X1	T43.3X2	T43.3X3	T43.3X4	T43.3X5	T43.3X6
piperidine	T43.3X1	T43.3X2	T43.3X3	T43.3X4	T43.3X5	T43.3X6
propylamine	T43.3X1	T43.3X2	T43.3X3	T43.3X4	T43.3X5	T43.3X6
specified NEC	T43.591	T43.592	T43.593	T43.594	T43.595	T43.596
thioxanthene NEC	T43.591	T43.592	T43.593	T43.594	T43.595	T43.596
Tranxene	T42.4X1	T42.4X2	T42.4X3	T42.4X4	T42.4X5	T42.4X6
Tranylcypromine	T43.1X1	T43.1X2	T43.1X3	T43.1X4	T43.1X5	T43.1X6
Trapidil	T46.3X1	T46.3X2	T46.3X3	T46.3X4	T46.3X5	T46.3X6
Trasentine	T44.3X1	T44.3X2	T44.3X3	T44.3X4	T44.3X5	T44.3X6
Travert	T5Ø.3X1	T5Ø.3X2	T5Ø.3X3	T5Ø.3X4	T5Ø.3X5	T5Ø.3X6
Trazodone	T43.211	T43.212	T43.213	T43.214	T43.215	T43.216
Trecator	T37.1X1	T37.1X2	T37.1X3	T37.1X4	T37.1X5	T37.1X6
Treosulfan	T45.1X1	T45.1X2	T45.1X3	T45.1X4	T45.1X5	T45.1X6
Tretamine	T45.1X1	T45.1X2	T45.1X3	T45.1X4	T45.1X5	T45.1X6
Tretinoin	T49.ØX1	T49.ØX2	T49.ØX3	T49.ØX4	T49.ØX5	T49.ØX6
Tretoquinol	T48.6X1	T48.6X2	T48.6X3	T48.6X4	T48.6X5	T48.6X6
Triacetin	T49.ØX1	T49.ØX2	T49.ØX3	T49.ØX4	T49.ØX5	T49.ØX6
Triacetoxyanthracene	T49.4X1	T49.4X2	T49.4X3	T49.4X4	T49.4X5	T49.4X6
Triacetyloleandomycin	T36.3X1	T36.3X2	T36.3X3	T36.3X4	T36.3X5	T36.3X6
Triamcinolone	T49.ØX1	T49.ØX2	T49.ØX3	T49.ØX4	T49.ØX5	T49.ØX6
ENT agent	T49.6X1	T49.6X2	T49.6X3	T49.6X4	T49.6X5	T49.6X6
hexacetonide	T49.ØX1	T49.ØX2	T49.ØX3	T49.ØX4	T49.ØX5	T49.ØX6
ophthalmic preparation	T49.5X1	T49.5X2	T49.5X3	T49.5X4	T49.5X5	T49.5X6
topical NEC	T49.ØX1	T49.ØX2	T49.ØX3	T49.ØX4	T49.ØX5	T49.ØX6
Triampyzine	T44.3X1	T44.3X2	T44.3X3	T44.3X4	T44.3X5	T44.3X6
Triamterene	T5Ø.2X1	T5Ø.2X2	T5Ø.2X3	T5Ø.2X4	T5Ø.2X5	T5Ø.2X6
Triazine (herbicide)	T6Ø.3X1	T6Ø.3X2	T6Ø.3X3	T6Ø.3X4	—	—
Triaziquone	T45.1X1	T45.1X2	T45.1X3	T45.1X4	T45.1X5	T45.1X6
Triazolam	T42.4X1	T42.4X2	T42.4X3	T42.4X4	T42.4X5	T42.4X6
Triazole (herbicide)	T6Ø.3X1	T6Ø.3X2	T6Ø.3X3	T6Ø.3X4	—	—

Substance	Poisoning, Accidental (unintentional)	Poisoning, Intentional Self-harm	Poisoning, Assault	Poisoning, Undetermined	Adverse Effect	Under-dosing
Tribenoside	T46.991	T46.992	T46.993	T46.994	T46.995	T46.996
Tribromacetaldehyde	T42.6X1	T42.6X2	T42.6X3	T42.6X4	T42.6X5	T42.6X6
Tribromoethanol, rectal	T41.291	T41.292	T41.293	T41.294	T41.295	T41.296
Tribromomethane	T42.6X1	T42.6X2	T42.6X3	T42.6X4	T42.6X5	T42.6X6
Trichlorethane	T53.2X1	T53.2X2	T53.2X3	T53.2X4	—	—
Trichlorethylene	T53.2X1	T53.2X2	T53.2X3	T53.2X4	—	—
Trichlorfon	T6Ø.ØX1	T6Ø.ØX2	T6Ø.ØX3	T6Ø.ØX4	—	—
Trichlormethiazide	T5Ø.2X1	T5Ø.2X2	T5Ø.2X3	T5Ø.2X4	T5Ø.2X5	T5Ø.2X6
Trichlormethine	T45.1X1	T45.1X2	T45.1X3	T45.1X4	T45.1X5	T45.1X6
Trichloroacetic acid, Trichloracetic acid	T54.2X1	T54.2X2	T54.2X3	T54.2X4	—	—
medicinal	T49.4X1	T49.4X2	T49.4X3	T49.4X4	T49.4X5	T49.4X6
Trichloroethane	T53.2X1	T53.2X2	T53.2X3	T53.2X4	—	—
Trichloroethanol	T42.6X1	T42.6X2	T42.6X3	T42.6X4	T42.6X5	T42.6X6
Trichloroethylene (liquid) (vapor)	T53.2X1	T53.2X2	T53.2X3	T53.2X4	—	—
anesthetic (gas)	T41.ØX1	T41.ØX2	T41.ØX3	T41.ØX4	T41.ØX5	T41.ØX6
vapor NEC	T53.2X1	T53.2X2	T53.2X3	T53.2X4	—	—
Trichloroethyl phosphate	T42.6X1	T42.6X2	T42.6X3	T42.6X4	T42.6X5	T42.6X6
Trichlorofluoromethane NEC	T53.5X1	T53.5X2	T53.5X3	T53.5X4	—	—
Trichloronate	T6Ø.ØX1	T6Ø.ØX2	T6Ø.ØX3	T6Ø.ØX4	—	—
Trichloropropane	T53.6X1	T53.6X2	T53.6X3	T53.6X4	—	—
Trichlorotriethylamine	T45.1X1	T45.1X2	T45.1X3	T45.1X4	T45.1X5	T45.1X6
Trichomonacides NEC	T37.3X1	T37.3X2	T37.3X3	T37.3X4	T37.3X5	T37.3X6
Trichomycin	T36.7X1	T36.7X2	T36.7X3	T36.7X4	T36.7X5	T36.7X6
Triclobisonium chloride	T49.ØX1	T49.ØX2	T49.ØX3	T49.ØX4	T49.ØX5	T49.ØX6
Triclocarban	T49.ØX1	T49.ØX2	T49.ØX3	T49.ØX4	T49.ØX5	T49.ØX6
Triclofos	T42.6X1	T42.6X2	T42.6X3	T42.6X4	T42.6X5	T42.6X6
Triclosan	T49.ØX1	T49.ØX2	T49.ØX3	T49.ØX4	T49.ØX5	T49.ØX6
Tricresyl phosphate	T65.891	T65.892	T65.893	T65.894	—	—
solvent	T52.91	T52.92	T52.93	T52.94	—	—
Tricyclamol chloride	T44.3X1	T44.3X2	T44.3X3	T44.3X4	T44.3X5	T44.3X6
Tridesilon	T49.ØX1	T49.ØX2	T49.ØX3	T49.ØX4	T49.ØX5	T49.ØX6
Tridihexethyl iodide	T44.3X1	T44.3X2	T44.3X3	T44.3X4	T44.3X5	T44.3X6
Tridione	T42.2X1	T42.2X2	T42.2X3	T42.2X4	T42.2X5	T42.2X6
Trientine	T45.8X1	T45.8X2	T45.8X3	T45.8X4	T45.8X5	T45.8X6
Triethanolamine NEC	T54.3X1	T54.3X2	T54.3X3	T54.3X4	—	—
detergent	T54.3X1	T54.3X2	T54.3X3	T54.3X4	—	—
trinitrate (biphosphate)	T46.3X1	T46.3X2	T46.3X3	T46.3X4	T46.3X5	T46.3X6
Triethanomelamine	T45.1X1	T45.1X2	T45.1X3	T45.1X4	T45.1X5	T45.1X6
Triethylenemelamine	T45.1X1	T45.1X2	T45.1X3	T45.1X4	T45.1X5	T45.1X6
Triethylenephosphoramide	T45.1X1	T45.1X2	T45.1X3	T45.1X4	T45.1X5	T45.1X6
Triethylenethiophosphoramide	T45.1X1	T45.1X2	T45.1X3	T45.1X4	T45.1X5	T45.1X6
Trifluoperazine	T43.3X1	T43.3X2	T43.3X3	T43.3X4	T43.3X5	T43.3X6
Trifluoroethyl vinyl ether	T41.ØX1	T41.ØX2	T41.ØX3	T41.ØX4	T41.ØX5	T41.ØX6
Trifluperidol	T43.4X1	T43.4X2	T43.4X3	T43.4X4	T43.4X5	T43.4X6
Triflupromazine	T43.3X1	T43.3X2	T43.3X3	T43.3X4	T43.3X5	T43.3X6
Trifluridine	T37.5X1	T37.5X2	T37.5X3	T37.5X4	T37.5X5	T37.5X6
Triflusal	T45.521	T45.522	T45.523	T45.524	T45.525	T45.526
Trihexyphenidyl	T44.3X1	T44.3X2	T44.3X3	T44.3X4	T44.3X5	T44.3X6
Triiodothyronine	T38.1X1	T38.1X2	T38.1X3	T38.1X4	T38.1X5	T38.1X6
Trilene	T41.ØX1	T41.ØX2	T41.ØX3	T41.ØX4	T41.ØX5	T41.ØX6
Trilostane	T38.991	T38.992	T38.993	T38.994	T38.995	T38.996
Trimebutine	T44.3X1	T44.3X2	T44.3X3	T44.3X4	T44.3X5	T44.3X6
Trimecaine	T41.3X1	T41.3X2	T41.3X3	T41.3X4	T41.3X5	T41.3X6
Trimeprazine (tartrate)	T44.3X1	T44.3X2	T44.3X3	T44.3X4	T44.3X5	T44.3X6
Trimetaphan camsilate	T44.2X1	T44.2X2	T44.2X3	T44.2X4	T44.2X5	T44.2X6
Trimetazidine	T46.7X1	T46.7X2	T46.7X3	T46.7X4	T46.7X5	T46.7X6
Trimethadione	T42.2X1	T42.2X2	T42.2X3	T42.2X4	T42.2X5	T42.2X6
Trimethaphan	T44.2X1	T44.2X2	T44.2X3	T44.2X4	T44.2X5	T44.2X6
Trimethidinium	T44.2X1	T44.2X2	T44.2X3	T44.2X4	T44.2X5	T44.2X6
Trimethobenzamide	T45.ØX1	T45.ØX2	T45.ØX3	T45.ØX4	T45.ØX5	T45.ØX6
Trimethoprim	T37.8X1	T37.8X2	T37.8X3	T37.8X4	T37.8X5	T37.8X6
with sulfamethoxazole	T36.8X1	T36.8X2	T36.8X3	T36.8X4	T36.8X5	T36.8X6
Trimethylcarbinol	T51.3X1	T51.3X2	T51.3X3	T51.3X4	—	—
Trimethylpsoralen	T49.3X1	T49.3X2	T49.3X3	T49.3X4	T49.3X5	T49.3X6
Trimeton	T45.ØX1	T45.ØX2	T45.ØX3	T45.ØX4	T45.ØX5	T45.ØX6
Trimetrexate	T45.1X1	T45.1X2	T45.1X3	T45.1X4	T45.1X5	T45.1X6
Trimipramine	T43.Ø11	T43.Ø12	T43.Ø13	T43.Ø14	T43.Ø15	T43.Ø16
Trimustine	T45.1X1	T45.1X2	T45.1X3	T45.1X4	T45.1X5	T45.1X6
Trinitrine	T46.3X1	T46.3X2	T46.3X3	T46.3X4	T46.3X5	T46.3X6
Trinitrobenzol	T65.3X1	T65.3X2	T65.3X3	T65.3X4	—	—
Trinitrophenol	T65.3X1	T65.3X2	T65.3X3	T65.3X4	—	—
Trinitrotoluene (fumes)	T65.3X1	T65.3X2	T65.3X3	T65.3X4	—	—
Trional	T42.6X1	T42.6X2	T42.6X3	T42.6X4	T42.6X5	T42.6X6
Triorthocresyl phosphate	T65.891	T65.892	T65.893	T65.894	—	—
Trioxide of arsenic	T57.ØX1	T57.ØX2	T57.ØX3	T57.ØX4	—	—
Trioxysalen	T49.4X1	T49.4X2	T49.4X3	T49.4X4	T49.4X5	T49.4X6
Tripamide	T5Ø.2X1	T5Ø.2X2	T5Ø.2X3	T5Ø.2X4	T5Ø.2X5	T5Ø.2X6
Triparanol	T46.6X1	T46.6X2	T46.6X3	T46.6X4	T46.6X5	T46.6X6
Tripelennamine	T45.ØX1	T45.ØX2	T45.ØX3	T45.ØX4	T45.ØX5	T45.ØX6
Triperiden	T44.3X1	T44.3X2	T44.3X3	T44.3X4	T44.3X5	T44.3X6

Substance	Poisoning, Accidental (unintentional)	Poisoning, Intentional Self-harm	Poisoning, Assault	Poisoning, Undetermined	Adverse Effect	Under-dosing
Triperidol	T43.4X1	T43.4X2	T43.4X3	T43.4X4	T43.4X5	T43.4X6
Triphenylphosphate	T65.891	T65.892	T65.893	T65.894	—	—
Triple						
bromides	T42.6X1	T42.6X2	T42.6X3	T42.6X4	T42.6X5	T42.6X6
carbonate	T47.1X1	T47.1X2	T47.1X3	T47.1X4	T47.1X5	T47.1X6
vaccine						
DPT	T5Ø.A11	T5Ø.A12	T5Ø.A13	T5Ø.A14	T5Ø.A15	T5Ø.A16
including pertussis	T5Ø.A11	T5Ø.A12	T5Ø.A13	T5Ø.A14	T5Ø.A15	T5Ø.A16
MMR	T5Ø.B91	T5Ø.B92	T5Ø.B93	T5Ø.B94	T5Ø.B95	T5Ø.B96
Triprolidine	T45.ØX1	T45.ØX2	T45.ØX3	T45.ØX4	T45.ØX5	T45.ØX6
Trisodium hydrogen edetate	T5Ø.6X1	T5Ø.6X2	T5Ø.6X3	T5Ø.6X4	T5Ø.6X5	T5Ø.6X6
Trisoralen	T49.3X1	T49.3X2	T49.3X3	T49.3X4	T49.3X5	T49.3X6
Trisulfapyrimidines	T37.ØX1	T37.ØX2	T37.ØX3	T37.ØX4	T37.ØX5	T37.ØX6
Trithiozine	T44.3X1	T44.3X2	T44.3X3	T44.3X4	T44.3X5	T44.3X6
Tritiozine	T44.3X1	T44.3X2	T44.3X3	T44.3X4	T44.3X5	T44.3X6
Tritoqualine	T45.ØX1	T45.ØX2	T45.ØX3	T45.ØX4	T45.ØX5	T45.ØX6
Trofosfamide	T45.1X1	T45.1X2	T45.1X3	T45.1X4	T45.1X5	T45.1X6
Troleandomycin	T36.3X1	T36.3X2	T36.3X3	T36.3X4	T36.3X5	T36.3X6
Trolnitrate (phosphate)	T46.3X1	T46.3X2	T46.3X3	T46.3X4	T46.3X5	T46.3X6
Tromantadine	T37.5X1	T37.5X2	T37.5X3	T37.5X4	T37.5X5	T37.5X6
Trometamol	T5Ø.2X1	T5Ø.2X2	T5Ø.2X3	T5Ø.2X4	T5Ø.2X5	T5Ø.2X6
Tromethamine	T5Ø.2X1	T5Ø.2X2	T5Ø.2X3	T5Ø.2X4	T5Ø.2X5	T5Ø.2X6
Tronothane	T41.3X1	T41.3X2	T41.3X3	T41.3X4	T41.3X5	T41.3X6
Tropacine	T44.3X1	T44.3X2	T44.3X3	T44.3X4	T44.3X5	T44.3X6
Tropatepine	T44.3X1	T44.3X2	T44.3X3	T44.3X4	T44.3X5	T44.3X6
Tropicamide	T44.3X1	T44.3X2	T44.3X3	T44.3X4	T44.3X5	T44.3X6
Trospium chloride	T44.3X1	T44.3X2	T44.3X3	T44.3X4	T44.3X5	T44.3X6
Troxerutin	T46.991	T46.992	T46.993	T46.994	T46.995	T46.996
Troxidone	T42.2X1	T42.2X2	T42.2X3	T42.2X4	T42.2X5	T42.2X6
Tryparsamide	T37.3X1	T37.3X2	T37.3X3	T37.3X4	T37.3X5	T37.3X6
Trypsin	T45.3X1	T45.3X2	T45.3X3	T45.3X4	T45.3X5	T45.3X6
Tryptizol	T43.Ø11	T43.Ø12	T43.Ø13	T43.Ø14	T43.Ø15	T43.Ø16
TSH	T38.811	T38.812	T38.813	T38.814	T38.815	T38.816
Tuaminoheptane	T48.5X1	T48.5X2	T48.5X3	T48.5X4	T48.5X5	T48.5X6
Tuberculin, purified protein derivative (PPD)	T5Ø.8X1	T5Ø.8X2	T5Ø.8X3	T5Ø.8X4	T5Ø.8X5	T5Ø.8X6
Tubocurare	T48.1X1	T48.1X2	T48.1X3	T48.1X4	T48.1X5	T48.1X6
Tubocurarine (chloride)	T48.1X1	T48.1X2	T48.1X3	T48.1X4	T48.1X5	T48.1X6
Tulobuterol	T48.6X1	T48.6X2	T48.6X3	T48.6X4	T48.6X5	T48.6X6
Turpentine (spirits of)	T52.8X1	T52.8X2	T52.8X3	T52.8X4	—	—
vapor	T52.8X1	T52.8X2	T52.8X3	T52.8X4	—	—
Tybamate	T43.591	T43.592	T43.593	T43.594	T43.595	T43.596
Tyloxapol	T48.4X1	T48.4X2	T48.4X3	T48.4X4	T48.4X5	T48.4X6
Tymazoline	T48.5X1	T48.5X2	T48.5X3	T48.5X4	T48.5X5	T48.5X6
Typhoid-paratyphoid vaccine	T5Ø.A91	T5Ø.A92	T5Ø.A93	T5Ø.A94	T5Ø.A95	T5Ø.A96
Typhus vaccine	T5Ø.A91	T5Ø.A92	T5Ø.A93	T5Ø.A94	T5Ø.A95	T5Ø.A96
Tyropanoate	T5Ø.8X1	T5Ø.8X2	T5Ø.8X3	T5Ø.8X4	T5Ø.8X5	T5Ø.8X6
Tyrothricin	T49.6X1	T49.6X2	T49.6X3	T49.6X4	T49.6X5	T49.6X6
ENT agent	T49.6X1	T49.6X2	T49.6X3	T49.6X4	T49.6X5	T49.6X6
ophthalmic preparation	T49.5X1	T49.5X2	T49.5X3	T49.5X4	T49.5X5	T49.5X6
Ufenamate	T39.391	T39.392	T39.393	T39.394	T39.395	T39.396
Ultraviolet light protectant	T49.3X1	T49.3X2	T49.3X3	T49.3X4	T49.3X5	T49.3X6
Undecenoic acid	T49.ØX1	T49.ØX2	T49.ØX3	T49.ØX4	T49.ØX5	T49.ØX6
Undecoylium	T49.ØX1	T49.ØX2	T49.ØX3	T49.ØX4	T49.ØX5	T49.ØX6
Undecylenic acid (derivatives)	T49.ØX1	T49.ØX2	T49.ØX3	T49.ØX4	T49.ØX5	T49.ØX6
Unna's boot	T49.3X1	T49.3X2	T49.3X3	T49.3X4	T49.3X5	T49.3X6
Unsaturated fatty acid	T46.6X1	T46.6X2	T46.6X3	T46.6X4	T46.6X5	T46.6X6
Uracil mustard	T45.1X1	T45.1X2	T45.1X3	T45.1X4	T45.1X5	T45.1X6
Uramustine	T45.1X1	T45.1X2	T45.1X3	T45.1X4	T45.1X5	T45.1X6
Urapidil	T46.5X1	T46.5X2	T46.5X3	T46.5X4	T46.5X5	T46.5X6
Urari	T48.1X1	T48.1X2	T48.1X3	T48.1X4	T48.1X5	T48.1X6
Urate oxidase	T5Ø.4X1	T5Ø.4X2	T5Ø.4X3	T5Ø.4X4	T5Ø.4X5	T5Ø.4X6
Urea	T47.3X1	T47.3X2	T47.3X3	T47.3X4	T47.3X5	T47.3X6
peroxide	T49.ØX1	T49.ØX2	T49.ØX3	T49.ØX4	T49.ØX5	T49.ØX6
stibamine	T37.4X1	T37.4X2	T37.4X3	T37.4X4	T37.4X5	T37.4X6
topical	T49.8X1	T49.8X2	T49.8X3	T49.8X4	T49.8X5	T49.8X6
Urethane	T45.1X1	T45.1X2	T45.1X3	T45.1X4	T45.1X5	T45.1X6
Urginea (maritima) (scilla) — *see* Squill						
Uric acid metabolism drug NEC	T5Ø.4X1	T5Ø.4X2	T5Ø.4X3	T5Ø.4X4	T5Ø.4X5	T5Ø.4X6
Uricosuric agent	T5Ø.4X1	T5Ø.4X2	T5Ø.4X3	T5Ø.4X4	T5Ø.4X5	T5Ø.4X6
Urinary anti-infective	T37.8X1	T37.8X2	T37.8X3	T37.8X4	T37.8X5	T37.8X6
Urofollitropin	T38.811	T38.812	T38.813	T38.814	T38.815	T38.816
Urokinase	T45.611	T45.612	T45.613	T45.614	T45.615	T45.616
Urokon	T5Ø.8X1	T5Ø.8X2	T5Ø.8X3	T5Ø.8X4	T5Ø.8X5	T5Ø.8X6
Ursodeoxycholic acid	T5Ø.991	T5Ø.992	T5Ø.993	T5Ø.994	T5Ø.995	T5Ø.996
Ursodiol	T5Ø.991	T5Ø.992	T5Ø.993	T5Ø.994	T5Ø.995	T5Ø.996
Urtica	T62.2X1	T62.2X2	T62.2X3	T62.2X4	—	—
Utility gas — *see* Gas, utility						

Substance	Poisoning, Accidental (unintentional)	Poisoning, Intentional Self-harm	Poisoning, Assault	Poisoning, Undetermined	Adverse Effect	Under-dosing
Vaccine NEC	T50.Z91	T50.Z92	T50.Z93	T50.Z94	T50.Z95	T50.Z96
antineoplastic	T50.Z91	T50.Z92	T50.Z93	T50.Z94	T50.Z95	T50.Z96
bacterial NEC	T50.A91	T50.A92	T50.A93	T50.A94	T50.A95	T50.A96
with						
other bacterial	T50.A21	T50.A22	T50.A23	T50.A24	T50.A25	T50.A26
component						
pertussis component	T50.A11	T50.A12	T50.A13	T50.A14	T50.A15	T50.A16
viral-rickettsial	T50.A21	T50.A22	T50.A23	T50.A24	T50.A25	T50.A26
component						
mixed NEC	T50.A21	T50.A22	T50.A23	T50.A24	T50.A25	T50.A26
BCG	T50.A91	T50.A92	T50.A93	T50.A94	T50.A95	T50.A96
cholera	T50.A91	T50.A92	T50.A93	T50.A94	T50.A95	T50.A96
diphtheria	T50.A91	T50.A92	T50.A93	T50.A94	T50.A95	T50.A96
with tetanus	T50.A21	T50.A22	T50.A23	T50.A24	T50.A25	T50.A26
and pertussis	T50.A11	T50.A12	T50.A13	T50.A14	T50.A15	T50.A16
influenza	T50.B91	T50.B92	T50.B93	T50.B94	T50.B95	T50.B96
measles	T50.B91	T50.B92	T50.B93	T50.B94	T50.B95	T50.B96
with mumps and rubella	T50.B91	T50.B92	T50.B93	T50.B94	T50.B95	T50.B96
meningococcal	T50.A91	T50.A92	T50.A93	T50.A94	T50.A95	T50.A96
mumps	T50.B91	T50.B92	T50.B93	T50.B94	T50.B95	T50.B96
paratyphoid	T50.A91	T50.A92	T50.A93	T50.A94	T50.A95	T50.A96
pertussis	T50.A11	T50.A12	T50.A13	T50.A14	T50.A15	T50.A16
with diphtheria	T50.A11	T50.A12	T50.A13	T50.A14	T50.A15	T50.A16
and tetanus	T50.A11	T50.A12	T50.A13	T50.A14	T50.A15	T50.A16
with other component	T50.A11	T50.A12	T50.A13	T50.A14	T50.A15	T50.A16
plague	T50.A91	T50.A92	T50.A93	T50.A94	T50.A95	T50.A96
poliomyelitis	T50.B91	T50.B92	T50.B93	T50.B94	T50.B95	T50.B96
poliovirus	T50.B91	T50.B92	T50.B93	T50.B94	T50.B95	T50.B96
rabies	T50.B91	T50.B92	T50.B93	T50.B94	T50.B95	T50.B96
respiratory syncytial virus	T50.B91	T50.B92	T50.B93	T50.B94	T50.B95	T50.B96
rickettsial NEC	T50.A91	T50.A92	T50.A93	T50.A94	T50.A95	T50.A96
with						
bacterial component	T50.A21	T50.A22	T50.A23	T50.A24	T50.A25	T50.A26
Rocky Mountain spotted	T50.A91	T50.A92	T50.A93	T50.A94	T50.A95	T50.A96
fever						
rubella	T50.B91	T50.B92	T50.B93	T50.B94	T50.B95	T50.B96
sabin oral	T50.B91	T50.B92	T50.B93	T50.B94	T50.B95	T50.B96
smallpox	T50.B11	T50.B12	T50.B13	T50.B14	T50.B15	T50.B16
TAB	T50.A91	T50.A92	T50.A93	T50.A94	T50.A95	T50.A96
tetanus	T50.A91	T50.A92	T50.A93	T50.A94	T50.A95	T50.A96
typhoid	T50.A91	T50.A92	T50.A93	T50.A94	T50.A95	T50.A96
typhus	T50.A91	T50.A92	T50.A93	T50.A94	T50.A95	T50.A96
viral NEC	T50.B91	T50.B92	T50.B93	T50.B94	T50.B95	T50.B96
yellow fever	T50.B91	T50.B92	T50.B93	T50.B94	T50.B95	T50.B96
Vaccinia immune globulin	T50.Z11	T50.Z12	T50.Z13	T50.Z14	T50.Z15	T50.Z16
Vaginal contraceptives	T49.8X1	T49.8X2	T49.8X3	T49.8X4	T49.8X5	T49.8X6
Valerian						
root	T42.6X1	T42.6X2	T42.6X3	T42.6X4	T42.6X5	T42.6X6
tincture	T42.6X1	T42.6X2	T42.6X3	T42.6X4	T42.6X5	T42.6X6
Valethamate bromide	T44.3X1	T44.3X2	T44.3X3	T44.3X4	T44.3X5	T44.3X6
Valisone	T49.0X1	T49.0X2	T49.0X3	T49.0X4	T49.0X5	T49.0X6
Valium	T42.4X1	T42.4X2	T42.4X3	T42.4X4	T42.4X5	T42.4X6
Valmid	T42.6X1	T42.6X2	T42.6X3	T42.6X4	T42.6X5	T42.6X6
Valnoctamide	T42.6X1	T42.6X2	T42.6X3	T42.6X4	T42.6X5	T42.6X6
Valproate (sodium)	T42.6X1	T42.6X2	T42.6X3	T42.6X4	T42.6X5	T42.6X6
Valproic acid	T42.6X1	T42.6X2	T42.6X3	T42.6X4	T42.6X5	T42.6X6
Valpromide	T42.6X1	T42.6X2	T42.6X3	T42.6X4	T42.6X5	T42.6X6
Vanadium	T56.891	T56.892	T56.893	T56.894	—	—
Vancomycin	T36.8X1	T36.8X2	T36.8X3	T36.8X4	T36.8X5	T36.8X6
Vapor — *see also* Gas	T59.91	T59.92	T59.93	T59.94	—	—
kiln (carbon monoxide)	T58.8X1	T58.8X2	T58.8X3	T58.8X4	—	—
lead — *see* lead						
specified source NEC	T59.891	T59.892	T59.893	T59.894	—	—
Vardenafil	T46.7X1	T46.7X2	T46.7X3	T46.7X4	T46.7X5	T46.7X6
Varicose reduction drug	T46.8X1	T46.8X2	T46.8X3	T46.8X4	T46.8X5	T46.8X6
Varnish	T65.4X1	T65.4X2	T65.4X3	T65.4X4	—	—
cleaner	T52.91	T52.92	T52.93	T52.94	—	—
Vaseline	T49.3X1	T49.3X2	T49.3X3	T49.3X4	T49.3X5	T49.3X6
Vasodilan	T46.7X1	T46.7X2	T46.7X3	T46.7X4	T46.7X5	T46.7X6
Vasodilator						
coronary NEC	T46.3X1	T46.3X2	T46.3X3	T46.3X4	T46.3X5	T46.3X6
peripheral NEC	T46.7X1	T46.7X2	T46.7X3	T46.7X4	T46.7X5	T46.7X6
Vasopressin	T38.891	T38.892	T38.893	T38.894	T38.895	T38.896
Vasopressor drugs	T38.891	T38.892	T38.893	T38.894	T38.895	T38.896
Vecuronium bromide	T48.1X1	T48.1X2	T48.1X3	T48.1X4	T48.1X5	T48.1X6
Vegetable extract,	T49.2X1	T49.2X2	T49.2X3	T49.2X4	T49.2X5	T49.2X6
astringent						
Venlafaxine	T43.211	T43.212	T43.213	T43.214	T43.215	T43.216
Venom, venomous (bite)	T63.91	T63.92	T63.93	T63.94	—	—
(sting)						
amphibian NEC	T63.831	T63.832	T63.833	T63.834	—	—
animal NEC	T63.891	T63.892	T63.893	T63.894	—	—
ant	T63.421	T63.422	T63.423	T63.424	—	—

Substance	Poisoning, Accidental (unintentional)	Poisoning, Intentional Self-harm	Poisoning, Assault	Poisoning, Undetermined	Adverse Effect	Under-dosing
Venom, venomous — *continued*						
arthropod NEC	T63.481	T63.482	T63.483	T63.484	—	—
bee	T63.441	T63.442	T63.443	T63.444	—	—
centipede	T63.411	T63.412	T63.413	T63.414	—	—
fish	T63.591	T63.592	T63.593	T63.594	—	—
frog	T63.811	T63.812	T63.813	T63.814	—	—
hornet	T63.451	T63.452	T63.453	T63.454	—	—
insect NEC	T63.481	T63.482	T63.483	T63.484	—	—
lizard	T63.121	T63.122	T63.123	T63.124	—	—
marine						
animals	T63.691	T63.692	T63.693	T63.694	—	—
bluebottle	T63.611	T63.612	T63.613	T63.614	—	—
jellyfish NEC	T63.621	T63.622	T63.623	T63.624	—	—
Portugese Man-o-war	T63.611	T63.612	T63.613	T63.614	—	—
sea anemone	T63.631	T63.632	T63.633	T63.634	—	—
specified NEC	T63.691	T63.692	T63.693	T63.694	—	—
fish	T63.591	T63.592	T63.593	T63.594	—	—
plants	T63.711	T63.712	T63.713	T63.714	—	—
sting ray	T63.511	T63.512	T63.513	T63.514	—	—
millipede (tropical)	T63.411	T63.412	T63.413	T63.414	—	—
plant NEC	T63.791	T63.792	T63.793	T63.794	—	—
marine	T63.711	T63.712	T63.713	T63.714	—	—
reptile	T63.191	T63.192	T63.193	T63.194	—	—
gila monster	T63.111	T63.112	T63.113	T63.114	—	—
lizard NEC	T63.121	T63.122	T63.123	T63.124	—	—
scorpion	T63.2X1	T63.2X2	T63.2X3	T63.2X4	—	—
snake	T63.001	T63.002	T63.003	T63.004	—	—
African NEC	T63.081	T63.082	T63.083	T63.084	—	—
American (North) (South) NEC	T63.061	T63.062	T63.063	T63.064	—	—
Asian	T63.081	T63.082	T63.083	T63.084	—	—
Australian	T63.071	T63.072	T63.073	T63.074	—	—
cobra	T63.041	T63.042	T63.043	T63.044	—	—
coral snake	T63.021	T63.022	T63.023	T63.024	—	—
rattlesnake	T63.011	T63.012	T63.013	T63.014	—	—
specified NEC	T63.091	T63.092	T63.093	T63.094	—	—
taipan	T63.031	T63.032	T63.033	T63.034	—	—
specified NEC	T63.891	T63.892	T63.893	T63.894	—	—
spider	T63.301	T63.302	T63.303	T63.304	—	—
black widow	T63.311	T63.312	T63.313	T63.314	—	—
brown recluse	T63.331	T63.332	T63.333	T63.334	—	—
specified NEC	T63.391	T63.392	T63.393	T63.394	—	—
tarantula	T63.321	T63.322	T63.323	T63.324	—	—
sting ray	T63.511	T63.512	T63.513	T63.514	—	—
toad	T63.821	T63.822	T63.823	T63.824	—	—
wasp	T63.461	T63.462	T63.463	T63.464	—	—
Venous sclerosing drug NEC	T46.8X1	T46.8X2	T46.8X3	T46.8X4	T46.8X5	T46.8X6
Ventolin — *see* Albuterol						
Veramon	T42.3X1	T42.3X2	T42.3X3	T42.3X4	T42.3X5	T42.3X6
Verapamil	T46.1X1	T46.1X2	T46.1X3	T46.1X4	T46.1X5	T46.1X6
Veratrine	T46.5X1	T46.5X2	T46.5X3	T46.5X4	T46.5X5	T46.5X6
Veratrum						
album	T62.2X1	T62.2X2	T62.2X3	T62.2X4	—	—
alkaloids	T46.5X1	T46.5X2	T46.5X3	T46.5X4	T46.5X5	T46.5X6
viride	T62.2X1	T62.2X2	T62.2X3	T62.2X4	—	—
Verdigris	T60.3X1	T60.3X2	T60.3X3	T60.3X4	—	—
Veronal	T42.3X1	T42.3X2	T42.3X3	T42.3X4	T42.3X5	T42.3X6
Veroxil	T37.4X1	T37.4X2	T37.4X3	T37.4X4	T37.4X5	T37.4X6
Versenate	T50.6X1	T50.6X2	T50.6X3	T50.6X4	T50.6X5	T50.6X6
Versidyne	T39.8X1	T39.8X2	T39.8X3	T39.8X4	T39.8X5	T39.8X6
Vetrabutine	T48.0X1	T48.0X2	T48.0X3	T48.0X4	T48.0X5	T48.0X6
Vidarabine	T37.5X1	T37.5X2	T37.5X3	T37.5X4	T37.5X5	T37.5X6
Vienna						
green	T57.0X1	T57.0X2	T57.0X3	T57.0X4	—	—
insecticide	T60.2X1	T60.2X2	T60.2X3	T60.2X4	—	—
red	T57.0X1	T57.0X2	T57.0X3	T57.0X4	—	—
pharmaceutical dye	T50.991	T50.992	T50.993	T50.994	T50.995	T50.996
Vigabatrin	T42.6X1	T42.6X2	T42.6X3	T42.6X4	T42.6X5	T42.6X6
Viloxazine	T43.291	T43.292	T43.293	T43.294	T43.295	T43.296
Viminol	T39.8X1	T39.8X2	T39.8X3	T39.8X4	T39.8X5	T39.8X6
Vinbarbital, vinbarbitone	T42.3X1	T42.3X2	T42.3X3	T42.3X4	T42.3X5	T42.3X6
Vinblastine	T45.1X1	T45.1X2	T45.1X3	T45.1X4	T45.1X5	T45.1X6
Vinburnine	T46.7X1	T46.7X2	T46.7X3	T46.7X4	T46.7X5	T46.7X6
Vincamine	T45.1X1	T45.1X2	T45.1X3	T45.1X4	T45.1X5	T45.1X6
Vincristine	T45.1X1	T45.1X2	T45.1X3	T45.1X4	T45.1X5	T45.1X6
Vindesine	T45.1X1	T45.1X2	T45.1X3	T45.1X4	T45.1X5	T45.1X6
Vinesthene, vinethene	T41.0X1	T41.0X2	T41.0X3	T41.0X4	T41.0X5	T41.0X6
Vinorelbine tartrate	T45.1X1	T45.1X2	T45.1X3	T45.1X4	T45.1X5	T45.1X6
Vinpocetine	T46.7X1	T46.7X2	T46.7X3	T46.7X4	T46.7X5	T46.7X6
Vinyl						
acetate	T65.891	T65.892	T65.893	T65.894	—	—
bital	T42.3X1	T42.3X2	T42.3X3	T42.3X4	T42.3X5	T42.3X6

Substance	Poisoning, Accidental (unintentional)	Poisoning, Intentional Self-harm	Poisoning, Assault	Poisoning, Undetermined	Adverse Effect	Under-dosing
Vinyl — *continued*						
bromide	T65.891	T65.892	T65.893	T65.894	—	—
chloride	T59.891	T59.892	T59.893	T59.894	—	—
ether	T41.0X1	T41.0X2	T41.0X3	T41.0X4	T41.0X5	T41.0X6
Vinylbital	T42.3X1	T42.3X2	T42.3X3	T42.3X4	T42.3X5	T42.3X6
Vinylidene chloride	T65.891	T65.892	T65.893	T65.894	—	—
Vioform	T37.8X1	T37.8X2	T37.8X3	T37.8X4	T37.8X5	T37.8X6
topical	T49.0X1	T49.0X2	T49.0X3	T49.0X4	T49.0X5	T49.0X6
Viomycin	T36.8X1	T36.8X2	T36.8X3	T36.8X4	T36.8X5	T36.8X6
Viosterol	T45.2X1	T45.2X2	T45.2X3	T45.2X4	T45.2X5	T45.2X6
Viper (venom)	T63.091	T63.092	T63.093	T63.094	—	—
Viprynium	T37.4X1	T37.4X2	T37.4X3	T37.4X4	T37.4X5	T37.4X6
Viquidil	T46.7X1	T46.7X2	T46.7X3	T46.7X4	T46.7X5	T46.7X6
Viral vaccine NEC	T50.B91	T50.B92	T50.B93	T50.B94	T50.B95	T50.B96
Virginiamycin	T36.8X1	T36.8X2	T36.8X3	T36.8X4	T36.8X5	T36.8X6
Virugon	T37.5X1	T37.5X2	T37.5X3	T37.5X4	T37.5X5	T37.5X6
Viscous agent	T50.901	T50.902	T50.903	T50.904	T50.905	T50.906
Visine	T49.5X1	T49.5X2	T49.5X3	T49.5X4	T49.5X5	T49.5X6
Visnadine	T46.3X1	T46.3X2	T46.3X3	T46.3X4	T46.3X5	T46.3X6
Vitamin NEC	T45.2X1	T45.2X2	T45.2X3	T45.2X4	T45.2X5	T45.2X6
A	T45.2X1	T45.2X2	T45.2X3	T45.2X4	T45.2X5	T45.2X6
B1	T45.2X1	T45.2X2	T45.2X3	T45.2X4	T45.2X5	T45.2X6
B2	T45.2X1	T45.2X2	T45.2X3	T45.2X4	T45.2X5	T45.2X6
B6	T45.2X1	T45.2X2	T45.2X3	T45.2X4	T45.2X5	T45.2X6
B12	T45.2X1	T45.2X2	T45.2X3	T45.2X4	T45.2X5	T45.2X6
B15	T45.2X1	T45.2X2	T45.2X3	T45.2X4	T45.2X5	T45.2X6
B NEC	T45.2X1	T45.2X2	T45.2X3	T45.2X4	T45.2X5	T45.2X6
nicotinic acid	T46.7X1	T46.7X2	T46.7X3	T46.7X4	T46.7X5	T46.7X6
C	T45.2X1	T45.2X2	T45.2X3	T45.2X4	T45.2X5	T45.2X6
D	T45.2X1	T45.2X2	T45.2X3	T45.2X4	T45.2X5	T45.2X6
D2	T45.2X1	T45.2X2	T45.2X3	T45.2X4	T45.2X5	T45.2X6
D3	T45.2X1	T45.2X2	T45.2X3	T45.2X4	T45.2X5	T45.2X6
E	T45.2X1	T45.2X2	T45.2X3	T45.2X4	T45.2X5	T45.2X6
E acetate	T45.2X1	T45.2X2	T45.2X3	T45.2X4	T45.2X5	T45.2X6
hematopoietic	T45.8X1	T45.8X2	T45.8X3	T45.8X4	T45.8X5	T45.8X6
K1	T45.7X1	T45.7X2	T45.7X3	T45.7X4	T45.7X5	T45.7X6
K2	T45.7X1	T45.7X2	T45.7X3	T45.7X4	T45.7X5	T45.7X6
K NEC	T45.7X1	T45.7X2	T45.7X3	T45.7X4	T45.7X5	T45.7X6
PP	T45.2X1	T45.2X2	T45.2X3	T45.2X4	T45.2X5	T45.2X6
ulceroprotectant	T47.1X1	T47.1X2	T47.1X3	T47.1X4	T47.1X5	T47.1X6
Vleminckx's solution	T49.4X1	T49.4X2	T49.4X3	T49.4X4	T49.4X5	T49.4X6
Voltaren — *see* Diclofenac sodium						
Warfarin	T45.511	T45.512	T45.513	T45.514	T45.515	T45.516
rodenticide	T60.4X1	T60.4X2	T60.4X3	T60.4X4	—	—
sodium	T60.4X1	T60.4X2	T60.4X3	T60.4X4	—	—
Wasp (sting)	T63.461	T63.462	T63.463	T63.464	—	—
Water						
balance drug	T50.3X1	T50.3X2	T50.3X3	T50.3X4	T50.3X5	T50.3X6
distilled	T50.3X1	T50.3X2	T50.3X3	T50.3X4	T50.3X5	T50.3X6
gas — *see* Gas, water						
incomplete combustion of — *see* Carbon, monoxide, fuel, utility						
hemlock	T62.2X1	T62.2X2	T62.2X3	T62.2X4	—	—
moccasin (venom)	T63.061	T63.062	T63.063	T63.064	—	—
purified	T50.3X1	T50.3X2	T50.3X3	T50.3X4	T50.3X5	T50.3X6
Wax (paraffin) (petroleum)	T52.0X1	T52.0X2	T52.0X3	T52.0X4	—	—
automobile	T65.891	T65.892	T65.893	T65.894	—	—
floor	T52.0X1	T52.0X2	T52.0X3	T52.0X4	—	—
Weed killers NEC	T60.3X1	T60.3X2	T60.3X3	T60.3X4	—	—
Welldorm	T42.6X1	T42.6X2	T42.6X3	T42.6X4	T42.6X5	T42.6X6
White						
arsenic	T57.0X1	T57.0X2	T57.0X3	T57.0X4	—	—
hellebore	T62.2X1	T62.2X2	T62.2X3	T62.2X4	—	—
lotion (keratolytic)	T49.4X1	T49.4X2	T49.4X3	T49.4X4	T49.4X5	T49.4X6
spirit	T52.0X1	T52.0X2	T52.0X3	T52.0X4	—	—
Whitewash	T65.891	T65.892	T65.893	T65.894	—	—
Whole blood (human)	T45.8X1	T45.8X2	T45.8X3	T45.8X4	T45.8X5	T45.8X6
Wild						
black cherry	T62.2X1	T62.2X2	T62.2X3	T62.2X4	—	—
poisonous plants NEC	T62.2X1	T62.2X2	T62.2X3	T62.2X4	—	—
Window cleaning fluid	T65.891	T65.892	T65.893	T65.894	—	—
Wintergreen (oil)	T49.3X1	T49.3X2	T49.3X3	T49.3X4	T49.3X5	T49.3X6
Wisterine	T62.2X1	T62.2X2	T62.2X3	T62.2X4	—	—
Witch hazel	T49.2X1	T49.2X2	T49.2X3	T49.2X4	T49.2X5	T49.2X6
Wood alcohol or spirit	T51.1X1	T51.1X2	T51.1X3	T51.1X4	—	—
Wool fat (hydrous)	T49.3X1	T49.3X2	T49.3X3	T49.3X4	T49.3X5	T49.3X6
Woorali	T48.1X1	T48.1X2	T48.1X3	T48.1X4	T48.1X5	T48.1X6
Wormseed, American	T37.4X1	T37.4X2	T37.4X3	T37.4X4	T37.4X5	T37.4X6
Xamoterol	T44.5X1	T44.5X2	T44.5X3	T44.5X4	T44.5X5	T44.5X6
Xanthine diuretics	T50.2X1	T50.2X2	T50.2X3	T50.2X4	T50.2X5	T50.2X6
Xanthinol nicotinate	T46.7X1	T46.7X2	T46.7X3	T46.7X4	T46.7X5	T46.7X6

Substance	Poisoning, Accidental (unintentional)	Poisoning, Intentional Self-harm	Poisoning, Assault	Poisoning, Undetermined	Adverse Effect	Under-dosing
Xanthotoxin	T49.3X1	T49.3X2	T49.3X3	T49.3X4	T49.3X5	T49.3X6
Xantinol nicotinate	T46.7X1	T46.7X2	T46.7X3	T46.7X4	T46.7X5	T46.7X6
Xantocillin	T36.0X1	T36.0X2	T36.0X3	T36.0X4	T36.0X5	T36.0X6
Xenon (127Xe) (133Xe)	T50.8X1	T50.8X2	T50.8X3	T50.8X4	T50.8X5	T50.8X6
Xenysalate	T49.4X1	T49.4X2	T49.4X3	T49.4X4	T49.4X5	T49.4X6
Xibornol	T37.8X1	T37.8X2	T37.8X3	T37.8X4	T37.8X5	T37.8X6
Xigris	T45.511	T45.512	T45.513	T45.514	T45.515	T45.516
Xipamide	T50.2X1	T50.2X2	T50.2X3	T50.2X4	T50.2X5	T50.2X6
Xylene (vapor)	T52.2X1	T52.2X2	T52.2X3	T52.2X4	—	—
Xylocaine (infiltration) (topical)	T41.3X1	T41.3X2	T41.3X3	T41.3X4	T41.3X5	T41.3X6
nerve block (peripheral) (plexus)	T41.3X1	T41.3X2	T41.3X3	T41.3X4	T41.3X5	T41.3X6
spinal	T41.3X1	T41.3X2	T41.3X3	T41.3X4	T41.3X5	T41.3X6
Xylol (vapor)	T52.2X1	T52.2X2	T52.2X3	T52.2X4	—	—
Xylometazoline	T48.5X1	T48.5X2	T48.5X3	T48.5X4	T48.5X5	T48.5X6
Yeast	T45.2X1	T45.2X2	T45.2X3	T45.2X4	T45.2X5	T45.2X6
dried	T45.2X1	T45.2X2	T45.2X3	T45.2X4	T45.2X5	T45.2X6
Yellow						
fever vaccine	T50.B91	T50.B92	T50.B93	T50.B94	T50.B95	T50.B96
jasmine	T62.2X1	T62.2X2	T62.2X3	T62.2X4	—	—
phenolphthalein	T47.2X1	T47.2X2	T47.2X3	T47.2X4	T47.2X5	T47.2X6
Yew	T62.2X1	T62.2X2	T62.2X3	T62.2X4	—	—
Yohimbic acid	T40.991	T40.992	T40.993	T40.994	T40.995	T40.996
Zactane	T39.8X1	T39.8X2	T39.8X3	T39.8X4	T39.8X5	T39.8X6
Zalcitabine	T37.5X1	T37.5X2	T37.5X3	T37.5X4	T37.5X5	T37.5X6
Zaroxolyn	T50.2X1	T50.2X2	T50.2X3	T50.2X4	T50.2X5	T50.2X6
Zephiran (topical)	T49.0X1	T49.0X2	T49.0X3	T49.0X4	T49.0X5	T49.0X6
ophthalmic preparation	T49.5X1	T49.5X2	T49.5X3	T49.5X4	T49.5X5	T49.5X6
Zeranol	T38.7X1	T38.7X2	T38.7X3	T38.7X4	T38.7X5	T38.7X6
Zerone	T51.1X1	T51.1X2	T51.1X3	T51.1X4	—	—
Zidovudine	T37.5X1	T37.5X2	T37.5X3	T37.5X4	T37.5X5	T37.5X6
Zimeldine	T43.221	T43.222	T43.223	T43.224	T43.225	T43.226
Zinc (compounds) (fumes) (vapor)	T56.5X1	T56.5X2	T56.5X3	T56.5X4	—	—
NEC						
anti-infectives	T49.0X1	T49.0X2	T49.0X3	T49.0X4	T49.0X5	T49.0X6
antivaricose	T46.8X1	T46.8X2	T46.8X3	T46.8X4	T46.8X5	T46.8X6
bacitracin	T49.0X1	T49.0X2	T49.0X3	T49.0X4	T49.0X5	T49.0X6
chloride (mouthwash)	T49.6X1	T49.6X2	T49.6X3	T49.6X4	T49.6X5	T49.6X6
chromate	T56.5X1	T56.5X2	T56.5X3	T56.5X4	—	—
gelatin	T49.3X1	T49.3X2	T49.3X3	T49.3X4	T49.3X5	T49.3X6
oxide	T49.3X1	T49.3X2	T49.3X3	T49.3X4	T49.3X5	T49.3X6
plaster	T49.3X1	T49.3X2	T49.3X3	T49.3X4	T49.3X5	T49.3X6
peroxide	T49.0X1	T49.0X2	T49.0X3	T49.0X4	T49.0X5	T49.0X6
pesticides	T56.5X1	T56.5X2	T56.5X3	T56.5X4	—	—
phosphide	T60.4X1	T60.4X2	T60.4X3	T60.4X4	—	—
pyrithionate	T49.4X1	T49.4X2	T49.4X3	T49.4X4	T49.4X5	T49.4X6
stearate	T49.3X1	T49.3X2	T49.3X3	T49.3X4	T49.3X5	T49.3X6
sulfate	T49.5X1	T49.5X2	T49.5X3	T49.5X4	T49.5X5	T49.5X6
ENT agent	T49.6X1	T49.6X2	T49.6X3	T49.6X4	T49.6X5	T49.6X6
ophthalmic solution	T49.5X1	T49.5X2	T49.5X3	T49.5X4	T49.5X5	T49.5X6
topical NEC	T49.0X1	T49.0X2	T49.0X3	T49.0X4	T49.0X5	T49.0X6
undecylenate	T49.0X1	T49.0X2	T49.0X3	T49.0X4	T49.0X5	T49.0X6
Zineb	T60.0X1	T60.0X2	T60.0X3	T60.0X4	—	—
Zinostatin	T45.1X1	T45.1X2	T45.1X3	T45.1X4	T45.1X5	T45.1X6
Zipeprol	T48.3X1	T48.3X2	T48.3X3	T48.3X4	T48.3X5	T48.3X6
Zofenopril	T46.4X1	T46.4X2	T46.4X3	T46.4X4	T46.4X5	T46.4X6
Zolpidem	T42.6X1	T42.6X2	T42.6X3	T42.6X4	T42.6X5	T42.6X6
Zomepirac	T39.391	T39.392	T39.393	T39.394	T39.395	T39.396
Zopiclone	T42.6X1	T42.6X2	T42.6X3	T42.6X4	T42.6X5	T42.6X6
Zorubicin	T45.1X1	T45.1X2	T45.1X3	T45.1X4	T45.1X5	T45.1X6
Zotepine	T43.591	T43.592	T43.593	T43.594	T43.595	T43.596
Zovant	T45.511	T45.512	T45.513	T45.514	T45.515	T45.516
Zoxazolamine	T42.8X1	T42.8X2	T42.8X3	T42.8X4	T42.8X5	T42.8X6
Zuclopenthixol	T43.4X1	T43.4X2	T43.4X3	T43.4X4	T43.4X5	T43.4X6
Zygadenus (venenosus)	T62.2X1	T62.2X2	T62.2X3	T62.2X4	—	—
Zyprexa	T43.591	T43.592	T43.593	T43.594	T43.595	T43.596

ICD-10-CM Index to External Causes

A

Abandonment (causing exposure to weather conditions) (with intent to injure or kill) NEC X58 ☑
Abuse (adult) (child) (mental) (physical) (sexual) X58 ☑
Accident (to) X58 ☑
  aircraft (in transit) (powered) (see also Accident, transport, aircraft)
    due to, caused by cataclysm — see Forces of nature, by type
  animal-drawn vehicle — see Accident, transport, animal-drawn vehicle occupant
  animal-rider — see Accident, transport, animal-rider
  automobile — see Accident, transport, car occupant
  bare foot water skier V94.4 ☑
  boat, boating (see also Accident, watercraft)
    striking swimmer
      powered V94.11 ☑
      unpowered V94.12 ☑
  bus — see Accident, transport, bus occupant
  cable car, not on rails V98.0 ☑
    on rails — see Accident, transport, streetcar occupant
  car — see Accident, transport, car occupant
  caused by, due to
    animal NEC W64 ☑
    chain hoist W24.0 ☑
    cold (excessive) — see Exposure, cold
    corrosive liquid, substance — see Table of Drugs and Chemicals
    cutting or piercing instrument — see Contact, with, by type of instrument
    drive belt W24.0 ☑
    electric
      current — see Exposure, electric current
      motor (see also Contact, with, by type of machine) W31.3 ☑
      current (of) W86.8 ☑
    environmental factor NEC X58 ☑
    explosive material — see Explosion
    fire, flames — see Exposure, fire
    firearm missile — see Discharge, firearm by type
    heat (excessive) — see Heat
    hot — see Contact, with, hot
    ignition — see Ignition
    lifting device W24.0 ☑
    lightning — see subcategory T75.0 ☑
      causing fire — see Exposure, fire
    machine, machinery — see Contact, with, by type of machine
    natural factor NEC X58 ☑
    pulley (block) W24.0 ☑
    radiation — see Radiation
    steam X13.1 ☑
      inhalation X13.0 ☑
      pipe X16 ☑
    thunderbolt — see subcategory T75.0 ☑
      causing fire — see Exposure, fire
    transmission device W24.1 ☑
  coach — see Accident, transport, bus occupant
  coal car — see Accident, transport, industrial vehicle occupant
  diving (see also Fall, into, water)
    with
      drowning or submersion — see Drowning
  forklift — see Accident, transport, industrial vehicle occupant
  heavy transport vehicle NOS — see Accident, transport, truck occupant
  ice yacht V98.2 ☑
  in
    medical, surgical procedure
      as, or due to misadventure — see Misadventure
      causing an abnormal reaction or later complication without mention of misadventure (see also Complication of or following, by type of procedure) Y84.9
  land yacht V98.1 ☑
  late effect of — see W00-X58 with 7th character S

Accident — continued
  logging car — see Accident, transport, industrial vehicle occupant
  machine, machinery (see also Contact, with, by type of machine)
    on board watercraft V93.69 ☑
      explosion — see Explosion, in, watercraft
      fire — see Burn, on board watercraft
      powered craft V93.63 ☑
        ferry boat V93.61 ☑
        fishing boat V93.62 ☑
        jetskis V93.63 ☑
        liner V93.61 ☑
        merchant ship V93.60 ☑
        passenger ship V93.61 ☑
        sailboat V93.64 ☑
  mine tram — see Accident, transport, industrial vehicle occupant
  mobility scooter (motorized) — see Accident, transport, pedestrian, conveyance, specified type NEC
  motor scooter — see Accident, transport, motorcyclist
  motor vehicle NOS (traffic) (see also Accident, transport) V89.2 ☑
    nontraffic V89.0 ☑
    three-wheeled NOS — see Accident, transport, three-wheeled motor vehicle occupant
  motorcycle NOS — see Accident, transport, motorcyclist
  nonmotor vehicle NOS (nontraffic) (see also Accident, transport) V89.1 ☑
    traffic NOS V89.3 ☑
  nontraffic (victim's mode of transport NOS) V88.9 ☑
    collision (between) V88.7 ☑
      bus and truck V88.5 ☑
      car and:
        bus V88.3 ☑
        pickup V88.2 ☑
        three-wheeled motor vehicle V88.0 ☑
        train V88.6 ☑
        truck V88.4 ☑
        two-wheeled motor vehicle V88.0 ☑
        van V88.2 ☑
      specified vehicle NEC and:
        three-wheeled motor vehicle V88.1 ☑
        two-wheeled motor vehicle V88.1 ☑
    known mode of transport — see Accident, transport, by type of vehicle
    noncollision V88.8 ☑
  on board watercraft V93.89 ☑
    powered craft V93.83 ☑
      ferry boat V93.81 ☑
      fishing boat V93.82 ☑
      jetskis V93.83 ☑
      liner V93.81 ☑
      merchant ship V93.80 ☑
      passenger ship V93.81 ☑
    unpowered craft V93.88 ☑
      canoe V93.85 ☑
      inflatable V93.86 ☑
      in tow
        recreational V94.31 ☑
        specified NEC V94.32 ☑
      kayak V93.85 ☑
      sailboat V93.84 ☑
      surf-board V93.88 ☑
      water skis V93.87 ☑
      windsurfer V93.88 ☑
  parachutist V97.29 ☑
    entangled in object V97.21 ☑
    injured on landing V97.22 ☑
  pedal cycle — see Accident, transport, pedal cyclist
  pedestrian (on foot)
    with
      another pedestrian W51 ☑
        with fall W03 ☑
          due to ice or snow W00.0 ☑
      on pedestrian conveyance NEC V00.09 ☑
      roller skater (in-line) V00.01 ☑
      skate boarder V00.02 ☑
    transport vehicle — see Accident, transport

Accident — continued
  pedestrian — continued
    on pedestrian conveyance — see Accident, transport, pedestrian, conveyance
  pick-up truck or van — see Accident, transport, pickup truck occupant
  quarry truck — see Accident, transport, industrial vehicle occupant
  railway vehicle (any) (in motion) — see Accident, transport, railway vehicle occupant
    due to cataclysm — see Forces of nature, by type
  scooter (non-motorized) — see Accident, transport, pedestrian, conveyance, scooter
  sequelae of — see categories W00-X58 with 7th character S
  skateboard — see Accident, transport, pedestrian, conveyance, skateboard
  ski(ing) — see Accident, transport, pedestrian, conveyance
    lift V98.3 ☑
  specified cause NEC X58 ☑
  streetcar — see Accident, transport, streetcar occupant
  traffic (victim's mode of transport NOS) V87.9 ☑
    collision (between) V87.7 ☑
      bus and truck V87.5 ☑
      car and:
        bus V87.3 ☑
        pickup V87.2 ☑
        three-wheeled motor vehicle V87.0 ☑
        train V87.6 ☑
        truck V87.4 ☑
        two-wheeled motor vehicle V87.0 ☑
        van V87.2 ☑
      specified vehicle NEC and:
        three-wheeled motor vehicle V87.1 ☑
        two-wheeled motor vehicle V87.1 ☑
    known mode of transport — see Accident, transport, by type of vehicle
    noncollision V87.8 ☑
  transport (involving injury to) V99 ☑
    18 wheeler — see Accident, transport, truck occupant
    agricultural vehicle occupant (nontraffic) V84.9 ☑
      driver V84.5 ☑
      hanger-on V84.7 ☑
      passenger V84.6 ☑
      traffic V84.3 ☑
        driver V84.0 ☑
        hanger-on V84.2 ☑
        passenger V84.1 ☑
      while boarding or alighting V84.4 ☑
    aircraft NEC V97.89 ☑
      military NEC V97.818 ☑
        with civilian aircraft V97.810 ☑
        civilian injured by V97.811 ☑
      occupant injured (in)
        nonpowered craft accident V96.9 ☑
          balloon V96.00 ☑
            collision V96.03 ☑
            crash V96.01 ☑
            explosion V96.05 ☑
            fire V96.04 ☑
            forced landing V96.02 ☑
            specified type NEC V96.09 ☑
          glider V96.20 ☑
            collision V96.23 ☑
            crash V96.21 ☑
            explosion V96.25 ☑
            fire V96.24 ☑
            forced landing V96.22 ☑
            specified type NEC V96.29 ☑
          hang glider V96.10 ☑
            collision V96.13 ☑
            crash V96.11 ☑
            explosion V96.15 ☑
            fire V96.14 ☑
            forced landing V96.12 ☑
            specified type NEC V96.19 ☑
          specified craft NEC V96.8 ☑
        powered craft accident V95.9 ☑
          fixed wing NEC

Accident — *continued*
transport — *continued*
aircraft — *continued*
occupant injured — *continued*
powered craft accident — *continued*
fixed wing — *continued*
commercial V95.30 ☑
collision V95.33 ☑
crash V95.31 ☑
explosion V95.35 ☑
fire V95.34 ☑
forced landing V95.32 ☑
specified type NEC V95.39 ☑
private V95.20 ☑
collision V95.23 ☑
crash V95.21 ☑
explosion V95.25 ☑
fire V95.24 ☑
forced landing V95.22 ☑
specified type NEC V95.29 ☑
glider V95.10 ☑
collision V95.13 ☑
crash V95.11 ☑
explosion V95.15 ☑
fire V95.14 ☑
forced landing V95.12 ☑
specified type NEC V95.19 ☑
helicopter V95.00 ☑
collision V95.03 ☑
crash V95.01 ☑
explosion V95.05 ☑
fire V95.04 ☑
forced landing V95.02 ☑
specified type NEC V95.09 ☑
spacecraft V95.40 ☑
collision V95.43 ☑
crash V95.41 ☑
explosion V95.45 ☑
fire V95.44 ☑
forced landing V95.42 ☑
specified type NEC V95.49 ☑
specified craft NEC V95.8 ☑
ultralight V95.10 ☑
collision V95.13 ☑
crash V95.11 ☑
explosion V95.15 ☑
fire V95.14 ☑
forced landing V95.12 ☑
specified type NEC V95.19 ☑
specified accident NEC V97.0 ☑
while boarding or alighting V97.1 ☑
person (injured by)
falling from, in or on aircraft V97.0 ☑
machinery on aircraft V97.89 ☑
on ground with aircraft involvement
V97.39 ☑
rotating propeller V97.32 ☑
struck by object falling from aircraft
V97.31 ☑
sucked into aircraft jet V97.33 ☑
while boarding or alighting aircraft V97.1 ☑
airport (battery-powered) passenger vehicle —
see Accident, transport, industrial vehicle
occupant
all-terrain vehicle occupant (nontraffic) V86.99 ☑
driver V86.59 ☑
dune buggy — see Accident, transport, dune
buggy occupant
hanger-on V86.79 ☑
passenger V86.69 ☑
snowmobile — see Accident, transport, snowmobile occupant
traffic V86.39 ☑
driver V86.09 ☑
hanger-on V86.29 ☑
passenger V86.19 ☑
while boarding or alighting V86.49 ☑
ambulance occupant (traffic) V86.31 ☑
driver V86.01 ☑
hanger-on V86.21 ☑
nontraffic V86.91 ☑
driver V86.51 ☑
hanger-on V86.71 ☑
passenger V86.61 ☑
passenger V86.11 ☑
while boarding or alighting V86.41 ☑

Accident — *continued*
transport — *continued*
animal-drawn vehicle occupant (in) V80.929 ☑
collision (with)
animal V80.12 ☑
being ridden V80.711 ☑
animal-drawn vehicle V80.721 ☑
bus V80.42 ☑
car V80.42 ☑
fixed or stationary object V80.82 ☑
military vehicle V80.920 ☑
nonmotor vehicle V80.791 ☑
pedal cycle V80.22 ☑
pedestrian V80.12 ☑
pickup V80.42 ☑
railway train or vehicle V80.62 ☑
specified motor vehicle NEC V80.52 ☑
streetcar V80.731 ☑
truck V80.42 ☑
two- or three-wheeled motor vehicle
V80.32 ☑
van V80.42 ☑
noncollision V80.02 ☑
specified circumstance NEC V80.928 ☑
animal-rider V80.919 ☑
collision (with)
animal V80.11 ☑
being ridden V80.710 ☑
animal-drawn vehicle V80.720 ☑
bus V80.41 ☑
car V80.41 ☑
fixed or stationary object V80.81 ☑
military vehicle V80.910 ☑
nonmotor vehicle V80.790 ☑
pedal cycle V80.21 ☑
pedestrian V80.11 ☑
pickup V80.41 ☑
railway train or vehicle V80.61 ☑
specified motor vehicle NEC V80.51 ☑
streetcar V80.730 ☑
truck V80.41 ☑
two- or three-wheeled motor vehicle
V80.31 ☑
van V80.41 ☑
noncollision V80.018 ☑
specified as horse rider V80.010 ☑
specified circumstance NEC V80.918 ☑
armored car — see Accident, transport, truck occupant
battery-powered truck (baggage) (mail) — see
Accident, transport, industrial vehicle occupant
bus occupant V79.9 ☑
collision (with)
animal (traffic) V70.9 ☑
being ridden (traffic) V76.9 ☑
nontraffic V76.3 ☑
while boarding or alighting V76.4 ☑
nontraffic V70.3 ☑
while boarding or alighting V70.4 ☑
animal-drawn vehicle (traffic) V76.9 ☑
nontraffic V76.3 ☑
while boarding or alighting V76.4 ☑
bus (traffic) V74.9 ☑
nontraffic V74.3 ☑
while boarding or alighting V74.4 ☑
car (traffic) V73.9 ☑
nontraffic V73.3 ☑
while boarding or alighting V73.4 ☑
motor vehicle NOS (traffic) V79.60 ☑
nontraffic V79.20 ☑
specified type NEC (traffic) V79.69 ☑
nontraffic V79.29 ☑
pedal cycle (traffic) V71.9 ☑
nontraffic V71.3 ☑
while boarding or alighting V71.4 ☑
pickup truck (traffic) V73.9 ☑
nontraffic V73.3 ☑
while boarding or alighting V73.4 ☑
railway vehicle (traffic) V75.9 ☑
nontraffic V75.3 ☑
while boarding or alighting V75.4 ☑
specified vehicle NEC (traffic) V76.9 ☑
nontraffic V76.3 ☑
while boarding or alighting V76.4 ☑
stationary object (traffic) V77.9 ☑

Accident — *continued*
transport — *continued*
bus occupant — *continued*
collision — *continued*
stationary object — *continued*
nontraffic V77.3 ☑
while boarding or alighting V77.4 ☑
streetcar (traffic) V76.9 ☑
nontraffic V76.3 ☑
while boarding or alighting V76.4 ☑
three wheeled motor vehicle (traffic)
V72.9 ☑
nontraffic V72.3 ☑
while boarding or alighting V72.4 ☑
truck (traffic) V74.9 ☑
nontraffic V74.3 ☑
while boarding or alighting V74.4 ☑
two wheeled motor vehicle (traffic) V72.9 ☑
nontraffic V72.3 ☑
while boarding or alighting V72.4 ☑
van (traffic) V73.9 ☑
nontraffic V73.3 ☑
while boarding or alighting V73.4 ☑
driver
collision (with)
animal (traffic) V70.5 ☑
being ridden (traffic) V76.5 ☑
nontraffic V76.0 ☑
nontraffic V70.0 ☑
animal-drawn vehicle (traffic) V76.5 ☑
nontraffic V76.0 ☑
bus (traffic) V74.5 ☑
nontraffic V74.0 ☑
car (traffic) V73.5 ☑
nontraffic V73.0 ☑
motor vehicle NOS (traffic) V79.40 ☑
nontraffic V79.00 ☑
specified type NEC (traffic) V79.49 ☑
nontraffic V79.09 ☑
pedal cycle (traffic) V71.5 ☑
nontraffic V71.0 ☑
pickup truck (traffic) V73.5 ☑
nontraffic V73.0 ☑
railway vehicle (traffic) V75.5 ☑
nontraffic V75.0 ☑
specified vehicle NEC (traffic) V76.5 ☑
nontraffic V76.0 ☑
stationary object (traffic) V77.5 ☑
nontraffic V77.0 ☑
streetcar (traffic) V76.5 ☑
nontraffic V76.0 ☑
three wheeled motor vehicle (traffic)
V72.5 ☑
nontraffic V72.0 ☑
truck (traffic) V74.5 ☑
nontraffic V74.0 ☑
two wheeled motor vehicle (traffic)
V72.5 ☑
nontraffic V72.0 ☑
van (traffic) V73.5 ☑
nontraffic V73.0 ☑
noncollision accident (traffic) V78.5 ☑
nontraffic V78.0 ☑
hanger-on
collision (with)
animal (traffic) V70.7 ☑
being ridden (traffic) V76.7 ☑
nontraffic V76.2 ☑
nontraffic V70.2 ☑
animal-drawn vehicle (traffic) V76.7 ☑
nontraffic V76.2 ☑
bus (traffic) V74.7 ☑
nontraffic V74.2 ☑
car (traffic) V73.7 ☑
nontraffic V73.2 ☑
pedal cycle (traffic) V71.7 ☑
nontraffic V71.2 ☑
pickup truck (traffic) V73.7 ☑
nontraffic V73.2 ☑
railway vehicle (traffic) V75.7 ☑
nontraffic V75.2 ☑
specified vehicle NEC (traffic) V76.7 ☑
nontraffic V76.2 ☑
stationary object (traffic) V77.7 ☑
nontraffic V77.2 ☑
streetcar (traffic) V76.7 ☑

☑ Additional Character Required — Refer to the Tabular List for Character Selection ▽ Subterms under main terms may continue to next column or page

Accident — *continued*
  transport — *continued*
    bus occupant — *continued*
      hanger-on — *continued*
        collision — *continued*
          streetcar — *continued*
            nontraffic V76.2 ☑
          three wheeled motor vehicle (traffic) V72.7 ☑
            nontraffic V72.2 ☑
          truck (traffic) V74.7 ☑
            nontraffic V74.2 ☑
          two wheeled motor vehicle (traffic) V72.7 ☑
            nontraffic V72.2 ☑
          van (traffic) V73.7 ☑
            nontraffic V73.2 ☑
        noncollision accident (traffic) V78.7 ☑
          nontraffic V78.2 ☑
      noncollision accident (traffic) V78.9 ☑
        nontraffic V78.3 ☑
        while boarding or alighting V78.4 ☑
      nontraffic V79.3 ☑
      passenger
        collision (with)
          animal (traffic) V70.6 ☑
            being ridden (traffic) V76.6 ☑
              nontraffic V76.1 ☑
            nontraffic V70.1 ☑
          animal-drawn vehicle (traffic) V76.6 ☑
            nontraffic V76.1 ☑
          bus (traffic) V74.6 ☑
            nontraffic V74.1 ☑
          car (traffic) V73.6 ☑
            nontraffic V73.1 ☑
          motor vehicle NOS (traffic) V79.50 ☑
            nontraffic V79.10 ☑
            specified type NEC (traffic) V79.59 ☑
              nontraffic V79.19 ☑
          pedal cycle (traffic) V71.6 ☑
            nontraffic V71.1 ☑
          pickup truck (traffic) V73.6 ☑
            nontraffic V73.1 ☑
          railway vehicle (traffic) V75.6 ☑
            nontraffic V75.1 ☑
          specified vehicle NEC (traffic) V76.6 ☑
            nontraffic V76.1 ☑
          stationary object (traffic) V77.6 ☑
            nontraffic V77.1 ☑
          streetcar (traffic) V76.6 ☑
            nontraffic V76.1 ☑
          three wheeled motor vehicle (traffic) V72.6 ☑
            nontraffic V72.1 ☑
          truck (traffic) V74.6 ☑
            nontraffic V74.1 ☑
          two wheeled motor vehicle (traffic) V72.6 ☑
            nontraffic V72.1 ☑
          van (traffic) V73.6 ☑
            nontraffic V73.1 ☑
        noncollision accident (traffic) V78.6 ☑
          nontraffic V78.1 ☑
      specified type NEC V79.88 ☑
        military vehicle V79.81 ☑
    cable car, not on rails V98.0 ☑
      on rails — *see* Accident, transport, streetcar occupant
    car occupant V49.9 ☑
      ambulance occupant — *see* Accident, transport, ambulance occupant
      collision (with)
        animal (traffic) V40.9 ☑
          being ridden (traffic) V46.9 ☑
            nontraffic V46.3 ☑
              while boarding or alighting V46.4 ☑
          nontraffic V40.3 ☑
          while boarding or alighting V40.4 ☑
        animal-drawn vehicle (traffic) V46.9 ☑
          nontraffic V46.3 ☑
          while boarding or alighting V46.4 ☑
        bus (traffic) V44.9 ☑
          nontraffic V44.3 ☑
          while boarding or alighting V44.4 ☑
        car (traffic) V43.92 ☑
          nontraffic V43.32 ☑

Accident — *continued*
  transport — *continued*
    car occupant — *continued*
      collision — *continued*
        car — *continued*
          while boarding or alighting V43.42 ☑
        motor vehicle NOS (traffic) V49.60 ☑
          nontraffic V49.20 ☑
          specified type NEC (traffic) V49.69 ☑
            nontraffic V49.29 ☑
        pedal cycle (traffic) V41.9 ☑
          nontraffic V41.3 ☑
          while boarding or alighting V41.4 ☑
        pickup truck (traffic) V43.93 ☑
          nontraffic V43.33 ☑
          while boarding or alighting V43.43 ☑
        railway vehicle (traffic) V45.9 ☑
          nontraffic V45.3 ☑
          while boarding or alighting V45.4 ☑
        specified vehicle NEC (traffic) V46.9 ☑
          nontraffic V46.3 ☑
          while boarding or alighting V46.4 ☑
        sport utility vehicle (traffic) V43.91 ☑
          nontraffic V43.31 ☑
          while boarding or alighting V43.41 ☑
        stationary object (traffic) V47.92 ☑
          nontraffic V47.32 ☑
          while boarding or alighting V47.4 ☑
        streetcar (traffic) V46.9 ☑
          nontraffic V46.3 ☑
          while boarding or alighting V46.4 ☑
        three wheeled motor vehicle (traffic) V42.9 ☑
          nontraffic V42.3 ☑
          while boarding or alighting V42.4 ☑
        truck (traffic) V44.9 ☑
          nontraffic V44.3 ☑
          while boarding or alighting V44.4 ☑
        two wheeled motor vehicle (traffic) V42.9 ☑
          nontraffic V42.3 ☑
          while boarding or alighting V42.4 ☑
        van (traffic) V43.94 ☑
          nontraffic V43.34 ☑
          while boarding or alighting V43.44 ☑
    driver
      collision (with)
        animal (traffic) V40.5 ☑
          being ridden (traffic) V46.5 ☑
            nontraffic V46.0 ☑
          nontraffic V40.0 ☑
        animal-drawn vehicle (traffic) V46.5 ☑
          nontraffic V46.0 ☑
        bus (traffic) V44.5 ☑
          nontraffic V44.0 ☑
        car (traffic) V43.52 ☑
          nontraffic V43.02 ☑
        motor vehicle NOS (traffic) V49.40 ☑
          nontraffic V49.00 ☑
          specified type NEC (traffic) V49.49 ☑
            nontraffic V49.09 ☑
        pedal cycle (traffic) V41.5 ☑
          nontraffic V41.0 ☑
        pickup truck (traffic) V43.53 ☑
          nontraffic V43.03 ☑
        railway vehicle (traffic) V45.5 ☑
          nontraffic V45.0 ☑
        specified vehicle NEC (traffic) V46.5 ☑
          nontraffic V46.0 ☑
        sport utility vehicle (traffic) V43.51 ☑
          nontraffic V43.01 ☑
        stationary object (traffic) V47.52 ☑
          nontraffic V47.02 ☑
        streetcar (traffic) V46.5 ☑
          nontraffic V46.0 ☑
        three wheeled motor vehicle (traffic) V42.5 ☑
          nontraffic V42.0 ☑
        truck (traffic) V44.5 ☑
          nontraffic V44.0 ☑
        two wheeled motor vehicle (traffic) V42.5 ☑
          nontraffic V42.0 ☑
        van (traffic) V43.54 ☑
          nontraffic V43.04 ☑
      noncollision accident (traffic) V48.5 ☑
        nontraffic V48.0 ☑

Accident — *continued*
  transport — *continued*
    car occupant — *continued*
      hanger-on
        collision (with)
          animal (traffic) V40.7 ☑
            being ridden (traffic) V46.7 ☑
              nontraffic V46.2 ☑
            nontraffic V40.2 ☑
          animal-drawn vehicle (traffic) V46.7 ☑
            nontraffic V46.2 ☑
          bus (traffic) V44.7 ☑
            nontraffic V44.2 ☑
          car (traffic) V43.72 ☑
            nontraffic V43.22 ☑
          pedal cycle (traffic) V41.7 ☑
            nontraffic V41.2 ☑
          pickup truck (traffic) V43.73 ☑
            nontraffic V43.23 ☑
          railway vehicle (traffic) V45.7 ☑
            nontraffic V45.2 ☑
          specified vehicle NEC (traffic) V46.7 ☑
            nontraffic V46.2 ☑
          sport utility vehicle (traffic) V43.71 ☑
            nontraffic V43.21 ☑
          stationary object (traffic) V47.7 ☑
            nontraffic V47.2 ☑
          streetcar (traffic) V46.7 ☑
            nontraffic V46.2 ☑
          three wheeled motor vehicle (traffic) V42.7 ☑
            nontraffic V42.2 ☑
          truck (traffic) V44.7 ☑
            nontraffic V44.2 ☑
          two wheeled motor vehicle (traffic) V42.7 ☑
            nontraffic V42.2 ☑
          van (traffic) V43.74 ☑
            nontraffic V43.24 ☑
        noncollision accident (traffic) V48.7 ☑
          nontraffic V48.2 ☑
      noncollision accident (traffic) V48.9 ☑
        nontraffic V48.3 ☑
        while boarding or alighting V48.4 ☑
      nontraffic V49.3 ☑
      passenger
        collision (with)
          animal (traffic) V40.6 ☑
            being ridden (traffic) V46.6 ☑
              nontraffic V46.1 ☑
            nontraffic V40.1 ☑
          animal-drawn vehicle (traffic) V46.6 ☑
            nontraffic V46.1 ☑
          bus (traffic) V44.6 ☑
            nontraffic V44.1 ☑
          car (traffic) V43.62 ☑
            nontraffic V43.12 ☑
          motor vehicle NOS (traffic) V49.50 ☑
            nontraffic V49.10 ☑
            specified type NEC (traffic) V49.59 ☑
              nontraffic V49.19 ☑
          pedal cycle (traffic) V41.6 ☑
            nontraffic V41.1 ☑
          pickup truck (traffic) V43.63 ☑
            nontraffic V43.13 ☑
          railway vehicle (traffic) V45.6 ☑
            nontraffic V45.1 ☑
          specified vehicle NEC (traffic) V46.6 ☑
            nontraffic V46.1 ☑
          sport utility vehicle (traffic) V43.61 ☑
            nontraffic V43.11 ☑
          stationary object (traffic) V47.62 ☑
            nontraffic V47.12 ☑
          streetcar (traffic) V46.6 ☑
            nontraffic V46.1 ☑
          three wheeled motor vehicle (traffic) V42.6 ☑
            nontraffic V42.1 ☑
          truck (traffic) V44.6 ☑
            nontraffic V44.1 ☑
          two wheeled motor vehicle (traffic) V42.6 ☑
            nontraffic V42.1 ☑
          van (traffic) V43.64 ☑
            nontraffic V43.14 ☑
        noncollision accident (traffic) V48.6 ☑

▽ **Subterms under main terms may continue to next column or page**   ☑ **Additional Character Required — Refer to the Tabular List for Character Selection**   **389**

Accident — Accident

Accident — *continued*
  transport — *continued*
    car occupant — *continued*
      passenger — *continued*
        noncollision accident — *continued*
          nontraffic V48.1 ☑
        specified type NEC V49.88 ☑
          military vehicle V49.81 ☑
    coal car — *see* Accident, transport, industrial vehicle occupant
    construction vehicle occupant (nontraffic) V85.9 ☑
      driver V85.5 ☑
      hanger-on V85.7 ☑
      passenger V85.6 ☑
      traffic V85.3 ☑
        driver V85.0 ☑
        hanger-on V85.2 ☑
        passenger V85.1 ☑
      while boarding or alighting V85.4 ☑
    dirt bike rider — *see* Accident, transport, all-terrain vehicle occupant
    due to cataclysm — *see* Forces of nature, by type
    dune buggy occupant (nontraffic) V86.93 ☑
      driver V86.53 ☑
      hanger-on V86.73 ☑
      passenger V86.63 ☑
      traffic V86.33 ☑
        driver V86.03 ☑
        hanger-on V86.23 ☑
        passenger V86.13 ☑
      while boarding or alighting V86.43 ☑
    forklift — *see* Accident, transport, industrial vehicle occupant
    go cart — *see* Accident, transport, all-terrain vehicle occupant
    golf cart — *see* Accident, transport, all-terrain vehicle occupant
    heavy transport vehicle occupant — *see* Accident, transport, truck occupant
    ice yacht V98.2 ☑
    industrial vehicle occupant (nontraffic) V83.9 ☑
      driver V83.5 ☑
      hanger-on V83.7 ☑
      passenger V83.6 ☑
      traffic V83.3 ☑
        driver V83.0 ☑
        hanger-on V83.2 ☑
        passenger V83.1 ☑
      while boarding or alighting V83.4 ☑
    interurban electric car — *see* Accident, transport, streetcar
    land yacht V98.1 ☑
    logging car — *see* Accident, transport, industrial vehicle occupant
    military vehicle occupant (traffic) V86.34 ☑
      driver V86.04 ☑
      hanger-on V86.24 ☑
      nontraffic V86.94 ☑
        driver V86.54 ☑
        hanger-on V86.74 ☑
        passenger V86.64 ☑
      passenger V86.14 ☑
      while boarding or alighting V86.44 ☑
    mine tram — *see* Accident, transport, industrial vehicle occupant
    motor vehicle NEC occupant (traffic) V86.39 ☑
      driver V86.09 ☑
      hanger-on V86.29 ☑
      nontraffic V86.99 ☑
        driver V86.59 ☑
        hanger-on V86.79 ☑
        passenger V86.69 ☑
      passenger V86.19 ☑
      while boarding or alighting V86.49 ☑
    motorcoach — *see* Accident, transport, bus occupant
    motorcyclist V29.9 ☑
      collision (with)
        animal (traffic) V20.9 ☑
          being ridden (traffic) V26.9 ☑
            nontraffic V26.2 ☑
            while boarding or alighting V26.3 ☑
          nontraffic V20.2 ☑
          while boarding or alighting V20.3 ☑
        animal-drawn vehicle (traffic) V26.9 ☑
          nontraffic V26.2 ☑

Accident — *continued*
  transport — *continued*
    motorcyclist — *continued*
      collision — *continued*
        animal-drawn vehicle — *continued*
          while boarding or alighting V26.3 ☑
        bus (traffic) V24.9 ☑
          nontraffic V24.2 ☑
          while boarding or alighting V24.3 ☑
        car (traffic) V23.9 ☑
          nontraffic V23.2 ☑
          while boarding or alighting V23.3 ☑
        motor vehicle NOS (traffic) V29.60 ☑
          nontraffic V29.20 ☑
          specified type NEC (traffic) V29.69 ☑
            nontraffic V29.29 ☑
        pedal cycle (traffic) V21.9 ☑
          nontraffic V21.2 ☑
          while boarding or alighting V21.3 ☑
        pickup truck (traffic) V23.9 ☑
          nontraffic V23.2 ☑
          while boarding or alighting V23.3 ☑
        railway vehicle (traffic) V25.9 ☑
          nontraffic V25.2 ☑
          while boarding or alighting V25.3 ☑
        specified vehicle NEC (traffic) V26.9 ☑
          nontraffic V26.2 ☑
          while boarding or alighting V26.3 ☑
        stationary object (traffic) V27.9 ☑
          nontraffic V27.2 ☑
          while boarding or alighting V27.3 ☑
        streetcar (traffic) V26.9 ☑
          nontraffic V26.2 ☑
          while boarding or alighting V26.3 ☑
        three wheeled motor vehicle (traffic) V22.9 ☑
          nontraffic V22.2 ☑
          while boarding or alighting V22.3 ☑
        truck (traffic) V24.9 ☑
          nontraffic V24.2 ☑
          while boarding or alighting V24.3 ☑
        two wheeled motor vehicle (traffic) V22.9 ☑
          nontraffic V22.2 ☑
          while boarding or alighting V22.3 ☑
        van (traffic) V23.9 ☑
          nontraffic V23.2 ☑
          while boarding or alighting V23.3 ☑
      driver
        collision (with)
          animal (traffic) V20.4 ☑
            being ridden (traffic) V26.4 ☑
              nontraffic V26.0 ☑
            nontraffic V20.0 ☑
          animal-drawn vehicle (traffic) V26.4 ☑
            nontraffic V26.0 ☑
          bus (traffic) V24.4 ☑
            nontraffic V24.0 ☑
          car (traffic) V23.4 ☑
            nontraffic V23.0 ☑
          motor vehicle NOS (traffic) V29.40 ☑
            nontraffic V29.00 ☑
            specified type NEC (traffic) V29.49 ☑
              nontraffic V29.09 ☑
          pedal cycle (traffic) V21.4 ☑
            nontraffic V21.0 ☑
          pickup truck (traffic) V23.4 ☑
            nontraffic V23.0 ☑
          railway vehicle (traffic) V25.4 ☑
            nontraffic V25.0 ☑
          specified vehicle NEC (traffic) V26.4 ☑
            nontraffic V26.0 ☑
          stationary object (traffic) V27.4 ☑
            nontraffic V27.0 ☑
          streetcar (traffic) V26.4 ☑
            nontraffic V26.0 ☑
          three wheeled motor vehicle (traffic) V22.4 ☑
            nontraffic V22.0 ☑
          truck (traffic) V24.4 ☑
            nontraffic V24.0 ☑
          two wheeled motor vehicle (traffic) V22.4 ☑
            nontraffic V22.0 ☑
          van (traffic) V23.4 ☑
            nontraffic V23.0 ☑
        noncollision accident (traffic) V28.4 ☑

Accident — *continued*
  transport — *continued*
    motorcyclist — *continued*
      driver — *continued*
        noncollision accident — *continued*
          nontraffic V28.0 ☑
      noncollision accident (traffic) V28.9 ☑
        nontraffic V28.2 ☑
        while boarding or alighting V28.3 ☑
      nontraffic V29.3 ☑
      passenger
        collision (with)
          animal (traffic) V20.5 ☑
            being ridden (traffic) V26.5 ☑
              nontraffic V26.1 ☑
            nontraffic V20.1 ☑
          animal-drawn vehicle (traffic) V26.5 ☑
            nontraffic V26.1 ☑
          bus (traffic) V24.5 ☑
            nontraffic V24.1 ☑
          car (traffic) V23.5 ☑
            nontraffic V23.1 ☑
          motor vehicle NOS (traffic) V29.50 ☑
            nontraffic V29.10 ☑
            specified type NEC (traffic) V29.59 ☑
              nontraffic V29.19 ☑
          pedal cycle (traffic) V21.5 ☑
            nontraffic V21.1 ☑
          pickup truck (traffic) V23.5 ☑
            nontraffic V23.1 ☑
          railway vehicle (traffic) V25.5 ☑
            nontraffic V25.1 ☑
          specified vehicle NEC (traffic) V26.5 ☑
            nontraffic V26.1 ☑
          stationary object (traffic) V27.5 ☑
            nontraffic V27.1 ☑
          streetcar (traffic) V26.5 ☑
            nontraffic V26.1 ☑
          three wheeled motor vehicle (traffic) V22.5 ☑
            nontraffic V22.1 ☑
          truck (traffic) V24.5 ☑
            nontraffic V24.1 ☑
          two wheeled motor vehicle (traffic) V22.5 ☑
            nontraffic V22.1 ☑
          van (traffic) V23.5 ☑
            nontraffic V23.1 ☑
        noncollision accident (traffic) V28.5 ☑
          nontraffic V28.1 ☑
      specified type NEC V29.88 ☑
      military vehicle V29.81 ☑
    occupant (of)
      aircraft (powered) V95.9 ☑
        fixed wing
          commercial — *see* Accident, transport, aircraft, occupant, powered, fixed wing, commercial
          private — *see* Accident, transport, aircraft, occupant, powered, fixed wing, private
        nonpowered V96.9 ☑
        specified NEC V95.8 ☑
      airport battery-powered vehicle — *see* Accident, transport, industrial vehicle occupant
      all-terrain vehicle (ATV) — *see* Accident, transport, all-terrain vehicle occupant
      animal-drawn vehicle — *see* Accident, transport, animal-drawn vehicle occupant
      automobile — *see* Accident, transport, car occupant
      balloon V96.00 ☑
      battery-powered vehicle — *see* Accident, transport, industrial vehicle occupant
      bicycle — *see* Accident, transport, pedal cyclist
        motorized — *see* Accident, transport, motorcycle rider
      boat NEC — *see* Accident, watercraft
      bulldozer — *see* Accident, transport, construction vehicle occupant
      bus — *see* Accident, transport, bus occupant
      cable car (on rails) (*see also* Accident, transport, streetcar occupant)
        not on rails V98.0 ☑
      car (*see also* Accident, transport, car occupant)

Accident — *continued*
  transport — *continued*
    occupant — *continued*
      car (*see also* Accident, transport, car occupant) — *continued*
        cable (on rails) (*see also* Accident, transport, streetcar occupant)
          not on rails V98.0 ☑
      coach — *see* Accident, transport, bus occupant
      coal-car — *see* Accident, transport, industrial vehicle occupant
      digger — *see* Accident, transport, construction vehicle occupant
      dump truck — *see* Accident, transport, construction vehicle occupant
      earth-leveler — *see* Accident, transport, construction vehicle occupant
      farm machinery (self-propelled) — *see* Accident, transport, agricultural vehicle occupant
      forklift — *see* Accident, transport, industrial vehicle occupant
      glider (unpowered) V96.20 ☑
        hang V96.10 ☑
        powered (microlight) (ultralight) — *see* Accident, transport, aircraft, occupant, powered, glider
      glider (unpowered) NEC V96.20 ☑
      hang-glider V96.10 ☑
      harvester — *see* Accident, transport, agricultural vehicle occupant
      heavy (transport) vehicle — *see* Accident, transport, truck occupant
      helicopter — *see* Accident, transport, aircraft, occupant, helicopter
      ice-yacht V98.2 ☑
      kite (carrying person) V96.8 ☑
      land-yacht V98.1 ☑
      logging car — *see* Accident, transport, industrial vehicle occupant
      mechanical shovel — *see* Accident, transport, construction vehicle occupant
      microlight — *see* Accident, transport, aircraft, occupant, powered, glider
      minibus — *see* Accident, transport, car occupant
      minivan — *see* Accident, transport, car occupant
      moped — *see* Accident, transport, motorcycle
      motor scooter — *see* Accident, transport, motorcycle
      motorcycle (with sidecar) — *see* Accident, transport, motorcycle
      pedal cycle (*see also* Accident, transport, pedal cyclist)
      pick-up (truck) — *see* Accident, transport, pickup truck occupant
      railway (train) (vehicle) (subterranean) (elevated) — *see* Accident, transport, railway vehicle occupant
      rickshaw — *see* Accident, transport, pedal cycle
        motorized — *see* Accident, transport, three-wheeled motor vehicle
        pedal driven — *see* Accident, transport, pedal cyclist
      road-roller — *see* Accident, transport, construction vehicle occupant
      ship NOS V94.9 ☑
      ski-lift (chair) (gondola) V98.3 ☑
      snowmobile — *see* Accident, transport, snowmobile occupant
      spacecraft, spaceship — *see* Accident, transport, aircraft, occupant, spacecraft
      sport utility vehicle — *see* Accident, transport, car occupant
      streetcar (interurban) (operating on public street or highway) — *see* Accident, transport, streetcar occupant
      SUV — *see* Accident, transport, car occupant
      téléférique V98.0 ☑
      three-wheeled vehicle (motorized) (*see also* Accident, transport, three-wheeled motor vehicle occupant)
        nonmotorized — *see* Accident, transport, pedal cycle
      tractor (farm) (and trailer) — *see* Accident, transport, agricultural vehicle occupant

Accident — *continued*
  transport — *continued*
    occupant — *continued*
      train — *see* Accident, transport, railway vehicle occupant
      tram — *see* Accident, transport, streetcar occupant
        in mine or quarry — *see* Accident, transport, industrial vehicle occupant
      tricycle — *see* Accident, transport, pedal cycle
        motorized — *see* Accident, transport, three-wheeled motor vehicle
      trolley — *see* Accident, transport, streetcar occupant
        in mine or quarry — *see* Accident, transport, industrial vehicle occupant
      tub, in mine or quarry — *see* Accident, transport, industrial vehicle occupant
      ultralight — *see* Accident, transport, aircraft, occupant, powered, glider
      van — *see* Accident, transport, van occupant
      vehicle NEC V89.9 ☑
        heavy transport — *see* Accident, transport, truck occupant
        motor (traffic) NEC V89.2 ☑
        nontraffic NEC V89.0 ☑
      watercraft NOS V94.9 ☑
        causing drowning B — *see* Drowning, resulting from accident to boat
    parachutist V97.29 ☑
      after accident to aircraft — *see* Accident, transport, aircraft
      entangled in object V97.21 ☑
      injured on landing V97.22 ☑
    pedal cyclist V19.9 ☑
      collision (with)
        animal (traffic) V10.9 ☑
          being ridden (traffic) V16.9 ☑
            nontraffic V16.2 ☑
            while boarding or alighting V16.3 ☑
          nontraffic V10.2 ☑
          while boarding or alighting V10.3 ☑
        animal-drawn vehicle (traffic) V16.9 ☑
          nontraffic V16.2 ☑
          while boarding or alighting V16.3 ☑
        bus (traffic) V14.9 ☑
          nontraffic V14.2 ☑
          while boarding or alighting V14.3 ☑
        car (traffic) V13.9 ☑
          nontraffic V13.2 ☑
          while boarding or alighting V13.3 ☑
        motor vehicle NOS (traffic) V19.60 ☑
          nontraffic V19.20 ☑
          specified type NEC (traffic) V19.69 ☑
            nontraffic V19.29 ☑
        pedal cycle (traffic) V11.9 ☑
          nontraffic V11.2 ☑
          while boarding or alighting V11.3 ☑
        pickup truck (traffic) V13.9 ☑
          nontraffic V13.2 ☑
          while boarding or alighting V13.3 ☑
        railway vehicle (traffic) V15.9 ☑
          nontraffic V15.2 ☑
          while boarding or alighting V15.3 ☑
        specified vehicle NEC (traffic) V16.9 ☑
          nontraffic V16.2 ☑
          while boarding or alighting V16.3 ☑
        stationary object (traffic) V17.9 ☑
          nontraffic V17.2 ☑
          while boarding or alighting V17.3 ☑
        streetcar (traffic) V16.9 ☑
          nontraffic V16.2 ☑
          while boarding or alighting V16.3 ☑
        three wheeled motor vehicle (traffic) V12.9 ☑
          nontraffic V12.2 ☑
          while boarding or alighting V12.3 ☑
        truck (traffic) V14.9 ☑
          nontraffic V14.2 ☑
          while boarding or alighting V14.3 ☑
        two wheeled motor vehicle (traffic) V12.9 ☑
          nontraffic V12.2 ☑
          while boarding or alighting V12.3 ☑
        van (traffic) V13.9 ☑
          nontraffic V13.2 ☑
          while boarding or alighting V13.3 ☑

Accident — *continued*
  transport — *continued*
    pedal cyclist — *continued*
      driver
        collision (with)
          animal (traffic) V10.4 ☑
            being ridden (traffic) V16.4 ☑
              nontraffic V16.0 ☑
            nontraffic V10.0 ☑
          animal-drawn vehicle (traffic) V16.4 ☑
            nontraffic V16.0 ☑
          bus (traffic) V14.4 ☑
            nontraffic V14.0 ☑
          car (traffic) V13.4 ☑
            nontraffic V13.0 ☑
          motor vehicle NOS (traffic) V19.40 ☑
            nontraffic V19.00 ☑
            specified type NEC (traffic) V19.49 ☑
              nontraffic V19.09 ☑
          pedal cycle (traffic) V11.4 ☑
            nontraffic V11.0 ☑
          pickup truck (traffic) V13.4 ☑
            nontraffic V13.0 ☑
          railway vehicle (traffic) V15.4 ☑
            nontraffic V15.0 ☑
          specified vehicle NEC (traffic) V16.4 ☑
            nontraffic V16.0 ☑
          stationary object (traffic) V17.4 ☑
            nontraffic V17.0 ☑
          streetcar (traffic) V16.4 ☑
            nontraffic V16.0 ☑
          three wheeled motor vehicle (traffic) V12.4 ☑
            nontraffic V12.0 ☑
          truck (traffic) V14.4 ☑
            nontraffic V14.0 ☑
          two wheeled motor vehicle (traffic) V12.4 ☑
            nontraffic V12.0 ☑
          van (traffic) V13.4 ☑
            nontraffic V13.0 ☑
        noncollision accident (traffic) V18.4 ☑
          nontraffic V18.0 ☑
      noncollision accident (traffic) V18.9 ☑
        nontraffic V18.2 ☑
        while boarding or alighting V18.3 ☑
      nontraffic V19.3 ☑
      passenger
        collision (with)
          animal (traffic) V10.5 ☑
            being ridden (traffic) V16.5 ☑
              nontraffic V16.1 ☑
            nontraffic V10.1 ☑
          animal-drawn vehicle (traffic) V16.5 ☑
            nontraffic V16.1 ☑
          bus (traffic) V14.5 ☑
            nontraffic V14.1 ☑
          car (traffic) V13.5 ☑
            nontraffic V13.1 ☑
          motor vehicle NOS (traffic) V19.50 ☑
            nontraffic V19.10 ☑
            specified type NEC (traffic) V19.59 ☑
              nontraffic V19.19 ☑
          pedal cycle (traffic) V11.5 ☑
            nontraffic V11.1 ☑
          pickup truck (traffic) V13.5 ☑
            nontraffic V13.1 ☑
          railway vehicle (traffic) V15.5 ☑
            nontraffic V15.1 ☑
          specified vehicle NEC (traffic) V16.5 ☑
            nontraffic V16.1 ☑
          stationary object (traffic) V17.5 ☑
            nontraffic V17.1 ☑
          streetcar (traffic) V16.5 ☑
            nontraffic V16.1 ☑
          three wheeled motor vehicle (traffic) V12.5 ☑
            nontraffic V12.1 ☑
          truck (traffic) V14.5 ☑
            nontraffic V14.1 ☑
          two wheeled motor vehicle (traffic) V12.5 ☑
            nontraffic V12.1 ☑
          van (traffic) V13.5 ☑
            nontraffic V13.1 ☑
        noncollision accident (traffic) V18.5 ☑

Accident — *continued*
  transport — *continued*
    pedal cyclist — *continued*
      passenger — *continued*
        noncollision accident — *continued*
          nontraffic V18.1 ☑
      specified type NEC V19.88 ☑
      military vehicle V19.81 ☑
    pedestrian
      conveyance (occupant) V09.9 ☑
        babystroller V00.828 ☑
          collision (with) V09.9 ☑
            animal being ridden or animal drawn
              vehicle V06.99 ☑
              nontraffic V06.09 ☑
              traffic V06.19 ☑
            bus or heavy transport V04.99 ☑
              nontraffic V04.09 ☑
              traffic V04.19 ☑
            car V03.99 ☑
              nontraffic V03.09 ☑
              traffic V03.19 ☑
            pedal cycle V01.99 ☑
              nontraffic V01.09 ☑
              traffic V01.19 ☑
            pick-up truck or van V03.99 ☑
              nontraffic V03.09 ☑
              traffic V03.19 ☑
            railway (train) (vehicle) V05.99 ☑
              nontraffic V05.09 ☑
              traffic V05.19 ☑
            stationary object V00.822 ☑
            streetcar V06.99 ☑
              nontraffic V06.09 ☑
              traffic V06.19 ☑
            two- or three-wheeled motor vehicle
              V02.99 ☑
              nontraffic V02.09 ☑
              traffic V02.19 ☑
            vehicle V09.9 ☑
              animal-drawn V06.99 ☑
                nontraffic V06.09 ☑
                traffic V06.19 ☑
              motor
                nontraffic V09.00 ☑
                traffic V09.20 ☑
          fall V00.821 ☑
          nontraffic V09.1 ☑
            involving motor vehicle NEC
              V09.00 ☑
          traffic V09.3 ☑
            involving motor vehicle NEC
              V09.20 ☑
        flat-bottomed NEC V00.388 ☑
          collision (with) V09.9 ☑
            animal being ridden or animal drawn
              vehicle V06.99 ☑
              nontraffic V06.09 ☑
              traffic V06.19 ☑
            bus or heavy transport V04.99 ☑
              nontraffic V04.09 ☑
              traffic V04.19 ☑
            car V03.99 ☑
              nontraffic V03.09 ☑
              traffic V03.19 ☑
            pedal cycle V01.99 ☑
              nontraffic V01.09 ☑
              traffic V01.19 ☑
            pick-up truck or van V03.99 ☑
              nontraffic V03.09 ☑
              traffic V03.19 ☑
            railway (train) (vehicle) V05.99 ☑
              nontraffic V05.09 ☑
              traffic V05.19 ☑
            stationary object V00.382 ☑
            streetcar V06.99 ☑
              nontraffic V06.09 ☑
              traffic V06.19 ☑
            two- or three-wheeled motor vehicle
              V02.99 ☑
              nontraffic V02.09 ☑
              traffic V02.19 ☑
            vehicle V09.9 ☑
              animal-drawn V06.99 ☑
                nontraffic V06.09 ☑
                traffic V06.19 ☑

Accident — *continued*
  transport — *continued*
    pedestrian — *continued*
      conveyance — *continued*
        flat-bottomed — *continued*
          collision — *continued*
            vehicle — *continued*
              motor
                nontraffic V09.00 ☑
                traffic V09.20 ☑
          fall V00.381 ☑
          nontraffic V09.1 ☑
            involving motor vehicle NEC
              V09.00 ☑
          snow
            board — *see* Accident, transport, pedestrian, conveyance, snow board
            ski   *see* Accident, transport, pedestrian, conveyance, skis (snow)
          traffic V09.3 ☑
            involving motor vehicle NEC
              V09.20 ☑
        gliding type NEC V00.288 ☑
          collision (with) V09.9 ☑
            animal being ridden or animal drawn
              vehicle V06.99 ☑
              nontraffic V06.09 ☑
              traffic V06.19 ☑
            bus or heavy transport V04.99 ☑
              nontraffic V04.09 ☑
              traffic V04.19 ☑
            car V03.99 ☑
              nontraffic V03.09 ☑
              traffic V03.19 ☑
            pedal cycle V01.99 ☑
              nontraffic V01.09 ☑
              traffic V01.19 ☑
            pick-up truck or van V03.99 ☑
              nontraffic V03.09 ☑
              traffic V03.19 ☑
            railway (train) (vehicle) V05.99 ☑
              nontraffic V05.09 ☑
              traffic V05.19 ☑
            stationary object V00.282 ☑
            streetcar V06.99 ☑
              nontraffic V06.09 ☑
              traffic V02.19 ☑
            two- or three-wheeled motor vehicle
              V02.99 ☑
              nontraffic V02.09 ☑
              traffic V02.19 ☑
            vehicle V09.9 ☑
              animal-drawn V06.99 ☑
                nontraffic V06.09 ☑
                traffic V06.19 ☑
              motor
                nontraffic V09.00 ☑
                traffic V09.20 ☑
          fall V00.281 ☑
          heelies — *see* Accident, transport, pedestrian, conveyance, heelies
          ice skate — *see* Accident, transport, pedestrian, conveyance, ice skate
          nontraffic V09.1 ☑
            involving motor vehicle NEC
              V09.00 ☑
          sled — *see* Accident, transport, pedestrian, conveyance, sled
          traffic V09.3 ☑
            involving motor vehicle NEC
              V09.20 ☑
          wheelies — *see* Accident, transport, pedestrian, conveyance, heelies
        heelies V00.158 ☑
          colliding with stationary object
            V00.152 ☑
          fall V00.151 ☑
        ice skates V00.218 ☑
          collision (with) V09.9 ☑
            animal being ridden or animal drawn
              vehicle V06.99 ☑
              nontraffic V06.09 ☑
              traffic V06.19 ☑

Accident — *continued*
  transport — *continued*
    pedestrian — *continued*
      conveyance — *continued*
        ice skates — *continued*
          collision — *continued*
            bus or heavy transport V04.99 ☑
              nontraffic V04.09 ☑
              traffic V04.19 ☑
            car V03.99 ☑
              nontraffic V03.09 ☑
              traffic V03.19 ☑
            pedal cycle V01.99 ☑
              nontraffic V01.09 ☑
              traffic V01.19 ☑
            pick-up truck or van V03.99 ☑
              nontraffic V03.09 ☑
              traffic V03.19 ☑
            railway (train) (vehicle) V05.99 ☑
              nontraffic V05.09 ☑
              traffic V05.19 ☑
            stationary object V00.212 ☑
            streetcar V06.99 ☑
              nontraffic V06.09 ☑
              traffic V06.19 ☑
            two- or three-wheeled motor vehicle
              V02.99 ☑
              nontraffic V02.09 ☑
              traffic V02.19 ☑
            vehicle V09.9 ☑
              animal-drawn V06.99 ☑
                nontraffic V06.09 ☑
                traffic V06.19 ☑
              motor
                nontraffic V09.00 ☑
                traffic V09.20 ☑
          fall V00.211 ☑
          nontraffic V09.1 ☑
            involving motor vehicle NEC
              V09.00 ☑
          traffic V09.3 ☑
            involving motor vehicle NEC
              V09.20 ☑
        motorized mobility scooter V00.838 ☑
          collision with stationary object
            V00.832 ☑
          fall from V00.831 ☑
          nontraffic V09.1 ☑
            involving motor vehicle V09.00 ☑
              military V09.01 ☑
              specified type NEC V09.09 ☑
        roller skates (non in-line) V00.128 ☑
          collision (with) V09.9 ☑
            animal being ridden or animal drawn
              vehicle V06.91 ☑
              nontraffic V06.01 ☑
              traffic V06.11 ☑
            bus or heavy transport V04.91 ☑
              nontraffic V04.01 ☑
              traffic V04.11 ☑
            car V03.91 ☑
              nontraffic V03.01 ☑
              traffic V03.11 ☑
            pedal cycle V01.91 ☑
              nontraffic V01.01 ☑
              traffic V01.11 ☑
            pick-up truck or van V03.91 ☑
              nontraffic V03.01 ☑
              traffic V03.11 ☑
            railway (train) (vehicle) V05.91 ☑
              nontraffic V05.01 ☑
              traffic V05.11 ☑
            stationary object V00.122 ☑
            streetcar V06.91 ☑
              nontraffic V06.01 ☑
              traffic V06.11 ☑
            two- or three-wheeled motor vehicle
              V02.91 ☑
              nontraffic V02.01 ☑
              traffic V02.11 ☑
            vehicle V09.9 ☑
              animal-drawn V06.91 ☑
                nontraffic V06.01 ☑
                traffic V06.11 ☑
              motor
                nontraffic V09.00 ☑

   ☑ **Additional Character Required** — Refer to the Tabular List for Character Selection   ▽ **Subterms under main terms may continue to next column or page**

Accident — *continued*
  transport — *continued*
    pedestrian — *continued*
      conveyance — *continued*
        roller skates — *continued*
          collision — *continued*
            vehicle — *continued*
              motor — *continued*
                traffic V09.20 ☑
          fall V09.121 ☑
          in-line V00.118 ☑
            collision — *see also* Accident, transport, pedestrian, conveyance occupant, roller skates, collision
              with stationary object V00.112 ☑
            fall V00.111 ☑
          nontraffic V09.1 ☑
            involving motor vehicle NEC V09.00 ☑
          traffic V09.3 ☑
            involving motor vehicle NEC V09.20 ☑
        rolling shoes V00.158 ☑
          colliding with stationary object V00.152 ☑
          fall V00.151 ☑
        rolling type NEC V00.188 ☑
          collision (with) V09.9 ☑
            animal being ridden or animal drawn vehicle V06.99 ☑
              nontraffic V06.09 ☑
              traffic V06.19 ☑
            bus or heavy transport V04.99 ☑
              nontraffic V04.09 ☑
              traffic V04.19 ☑
            car V03.99 ☑
              nontraffic V03.09 ☑
              traffic V03.19 ☑
            pedal cycle V01.99 ☑
              nontraffic V01.09 ☑
              traffic V01.19 ☑
            pick-up truck or van V03.99 ☑
              nontraffic V03.09 ☑
              traffic V03.19 ☑
            railway (train) (vehicle) V05.99 ☑
              nontraffic V05.09 ☑
              traffic V05.19 ☑
            stationary object V00.182 ☑
            streetcar V06.99 ☑
              nontraffic V06.09 ☑
              traffic V06.19 ☑
            two- or three-wheeled motor vehicle V02.99 ☑
              nontraffic V02.09 ☑
              traffic V02.19 ☑
            vehicle V09.9 ☑
              animal-drawn V06.99 ☑
                nontraffic V06.09 ☑
                traffic V06.19 ☑
              motor
                nontraffic V09.00 ☑
                traffic V09.20 ☑
          fall V00.181 ☑
          in-line roller skate — *see* Accident, transport, pedestrian, conveyance, roller skate, in-line
          nontraffic V09.1 ☑
            involving motor vehicle NEC V09.00 ☑
          roller skate — *see* Accident, transport, pedestrian, conveyance, roller skate
          scooter (non-motorized) — *see* Accident, transport, pedestrian, conveyance, scooter
          skateboard — *see* Accident, transport, pedestrian, conveyance, skateboard
          traffic V09.3 ☑
            involving motor vehicle NEC V09.20 ☑
        scooter (non-motorized) V00.148 ☑
          collision (with) V09.9 ☑
            animal being ridden or animal drawn vehicle V06.99 ☑

Accident — *continued*
  transport — *continued*
    pedestrian — *continued*
      conveyance — *continued*
        scooter — *continued*
          collision — *continued*
            animal being ridden or animal drawn vehicle — *continued*
              nontraffic V06.09 ☑
              traffic V06.19 ☑
            bus or heavy transport V04.99 ☑
              nontraffic V04.09 ☑
              traffic V04.19 ☑
            car V03.99 ☑
              nontraffic V03.09 ☑
              traffic V03.19 ☑
            pedal cycle V01.99 ☑
              nontraffic V01.09 ☑
              traffic V01.19 ☑
            pick-up truck or van V03.99 ☑
              nontraffic V03.09 ☑
              traffic V03.19 ☑
            railway (train) (vehicle) V05.99 ☑
              nontraffic V05.09 ☑
              traffic V05.19 ☑
            stationary object V00.142 ☑
            streetcar V06.99 ☑
              nontraffic V06.09 ☑
              traffic V06.19 ☑
            two- or three-wheeled motor vehicle V02.99 ☑
              nontraffic V02.09 ☑
              traffic V02.19 ☑
            vehicle V09.9 ☑
              animal-drawn V06.99 ☑
                nontraffic V06.09 ☑
                traffic V06.19 ☑
              motor
                nontraffic V09.00 ☑
                traffic V09.20 ☑
          fall V00.141 ☑
          nontraffic V09.1 ☑
            involving motor vehicle NEC V09.00 ☑
          traffic V09.3 ☑
            involving motor vehicle NEC V09.20 ☑
        skate board V00.138 ☑
          collision (with) V09.9 ☑
            animal being ridden or animal drawn vehicle V06.92 ☑
              nontraffic V06.02 ☑
              traffic V06.12 ☑
            bus or heavy transport V04.92 ☑
              nontraffic V04.02 ☑
              traffic V04.12 ☑
            car V03.92 ☑
              nontraffic V03.02 ☑
              traffic V03.12 ☑
            pedal cycle V01.92 ☑
              nontraffic V01.02 ☑
              traffic V01.12 ☑
            pick-up truck or van V03.92 ☑
              nontraffic V03.02 ☑
              traffic V03.12 ☑
            railway (train) (vehicle) V05.92 ☑
              nontraffic V05.02 ☑
              traffic V05.12 ☑
            stationary object V00.132 ☑
            streetcar V06.92 ☑
              nontraffic V06.02 ☑
              traffic V06.12 ☑
            two- or three-wheeled motor vehicle V02.92 ☑
              nontraffic V02.02 ☑
              traffic V02.12 ☑
            vehicle V09.9 ☑
              animal-drawn V06.92 ☑
                nontraffic V06.02 ☑
                traffic V06.12 ☑
              motor
                nontraffic V09.00 ☑
                traffic V09.20 ☑
          fall V00.131 ☑
          nontraffic V09.1 ☑

Accident — *continued*
  transport — *continued*
    pedestrian — *continued*
      conveyance — *continued*
        skate board — *continued*
          nontraffic — *continued*
            involving motor vehicle NEC V09.00 ☑
          traffic V09.3 ☑
            involving motor vehicle NEC V09.20 ☑
        skis (snow) V00.328 ☑
          collision (with) V09.9 ☑
            animal being ridden or animal drawn vehicle V06.99 ☑
              nontraffic V06.09 ☑
              traffic V06.19 ☑
            bus or heavy transport V04.99 ☑
              nontraffic V04.09 ☑
              traffic V04.19 ☑
            car V03.99 ☑
              nontraffic V03.09 ☑
              traffic V03.19 ☑
            pedal cycle V01.99 ☑
              nontraffic V01.09 ☑
              traffic V01.19 ☑
            pick-up truck or van V03.99 ☑
              nontraffic V03.09 ☑
              traffic V03.19 ☑
            railway (train) (vehicle) V05.99 ☑
              nontraffic V05.09 ☑
              traffic V05.19 ☑
            stationary object V00.322 ☑
            streetcar V06.99 ☑
              nontraffic V06.09 ☑
              traffic V06.19 ☑
            two- or three-wheeled motor vehicle V02.99 ☑
              nontraffic V02.09 ☑
              traffic V02.19 ☑
            vehicle V09.9 ☑
              animal-drawn V06.99 ☑
                nontraffic V06.09 ☑
                traffic V06.19 ☑
              motor
                nontraffic V09.00 ☑
                traffic V09.20 ☑
          fall V00.321 ☑
          nontraffic V09.1 ☑
            involving motor vehicle NEC V09.00 ☑
          traffic V09.3 ☑
            involving motor vehicle NEC V09.20 ☑
        sled V00.228 ☑
          collision (with) V09.9 ☑
            animal being ridden or animal drawn vehicle V06.99 ☑
              nontraffic V06.09 ☑
              traffic V06.19 ☑
            bus or heavy transport V04.99 ☑
              nontraffic V04.09 ☑
              traffic V04.19 ☑
            car V03.99 ☑
              nontraffic V03.09 ☑
              traffic V03.19 ☑
            pedal cycle V01.99 ☑
              nontraffic V01.09 ☑
              traffic V01.19 ☑
            pick-up truck or van V03.99 ☑
              nontraffic V03.09 ☑
              traffic V03.19 ☑
            railway (train) (vehicle) V05.99 ☑
              nontraffic V05.09 ☑
              traffic V05.19 ☑
            stationary object V00.222 ☑
            streetcar V06.99 ☑
              nontraffic V06.09 ☑
              traffic V06.19 ☑
            two- or three-wheeled motor vehicle V02.99 ☑
              nontraffic V02.09 ☑
              traffic V02.19 ☑
            vehicle V09.9 ☑
              animal-drawn V06.99 ☑
                nontraffic V06.09 ☑

Accident — *continued*
  transport — *continued*
    pedestrian — *continued*
      conveyance — *continued*
        sled — *continued*
          collision — *continued*
            vehicle — *continued*
              animal-drawn — *continued*
                traffic V06.19 ☑
              motor
                nontraffic V09.00 ☑
                traffic V09.20 ☑
          fall V00.221 ☑
          nontraffic V09.1 ☑
            involving motor vehicle NEC
              V09.00 ☑
          traffic V09.3 ☑
            involving motor vehicle NEC
              V09.20 ☑
        snow board V00.318 ☑
          collision (with) V09.9 ☑
            animal being ridden or animal drawn
              vehicle V06.99 ☑
              nontraffic V06.09 ☑
              traffic V06.19 ☑
            bus or heavy transport V04.99 ☑
              nontraffic V04.09 ☑
              traffic V04.19 ☑
            car V03.99 ☑
              nontraffic V03.09 ☑
              traffic V03.19 ☑
            pedal cycle V01.99 ☑
              nontraffic V01.09 ☑
              traffic V01.19 ☑
            pick-up truck or van V03.99 ☑
              nontraffic V03.09 ☑
              traffic V03.19 ☑
            railway (train) (vehicle) V05.99 ☑
              nontraffic V05.09 ☑
              traffic V05.19 ☑
            stationary object V00.312 ☑
            streetcar V06.99 ☑
              nontraffic V06.09 ☑
              traffic V06.19 ☑
            two- or three-wheeled motor vehicle
              V02.99 ☑
              nontraffic V02.09 ☑
              traffic V02.19 ☑
            vehicle V09.9 ☑
              animal-drawn V06.99 ☑
                nontraffic V06.09 ☑
                traffic V06.19 ☑
              motor
                nontraffic V09.00 ☑
                traffic V09.20 ☑
         fall V00.311 ☑
        nontraffic V09.1 ☑
          involving motor vehicle NEC
            V09.00 ☑
        traffic V09.3 ☑
          involving motor vehicle NEC
            V09.20 ☑
      specified type NEC V00.898 ☑
        collision (with) V09.9 ☑
          animal being ridden or animal drawn
            vehicle V06.99 ☑
              nontraffic V06.09 ☑
              traffic V06.19 ☑
          bus or heavy transport V04.99 ☑
            nontraffic V04.09 ☑
            traffic V04.19 ☑
          car V03.99 ☑
            nontraffic V03.09 ☑
            traffic V03.19 ☑
          pedal cycle V01.99 ☑
            nontraffic V01.09 ☑
            traffic V01.19 ☑
          pick-up truck or van V03.99 ☑
            nontraffic V03.09 ☑
            traffic V03.19 ☑
          railway (train) (vehicle) V05.99 ☑
            nontraffic V05.09 ☑
            traffic V05.19 ☑
          stationary object V00.892 ☑
          streetcar V06.99 ☑
            nontraffic V06.09 ☑

Accident — *continued*
  transport — *continued*
    pedestrian — *continued*
      conveyance — *continued*
        specified type — *continued*
          collision — *continued*
            streetcar — *continued*
              traffic V06.19 ☑
            two- or three-wheeled motor vehicle
              V02.99 ☑
              nontraffic V02.09 ☑
              traffic V02.19 ☑
            vehicle V09.9 ☑
              animal-drawn V06.99 ☑
                nontraffic V06.09 ☑
                traffic V06.19 ☑
              motor
                nontraffic V09.00 ☑
                traffic V09.20 ☑
           fall V00.891 ☑
          nontraffic V09.1 ☑
            involving motor vehicle NEC
              V09.00 ☑
          traffic V09.3 ☑
            involving motor vehicle NEC
              V09.20 ☑
        traffic V09.3 ☑
          involving motor vehicle V09.20 ☑
            military V09.21 ☑
            specified type NEC V09.29 ☑
        wheelchair (powered) V00.818 ☑
          collision (with) V09.9 ☑
            animal being ridden or animal drawn
              vehicle V06.99 ☑
              nontraffic V06.09 ☑
              traffic V06.19 ☑
            bus or heavy transport V04.99 ☑
              nontraffic V04.09 ☑
              traffic V04.19 ☑
            car V03.99 ☑
              nontraffic V03.09 ☑
              traffic V03.19 ☑
            pedal cycle V01.99 ☑
              nontraffic V01.09 ☑
              traffic V01.19 ☑
            pick-up truck or van V03.99 ☑
              nontraffic V03.09 ☑
              traffic V03.19 ☑
            railway (train) (vehicle) V05.99 ☑
              nontraffic V05.09 ☑
              traffic V05.19 ☑
            stationary object V00.812 ☑
            streetcar V06.99 ☑
              nontraffic V06.09 ☑
              traffic V06.19 ☑
            two- or three-wheeled motor vehicle
              V02.99 ☑
              nontraffic V02.09 ☑
              traffic V02.19 ☑
            vehicle V09.9 ☑
              animal-drawn V06.99 ☑
                nontraffic V06.09 ☑
                traffic V06.19 ☑
              motor
                nontraffic V09.00 ☑
                traffic V09.20 ☑
          fall V00.811 ☑
        nontraffic V09.1 ☑
          involving motor vehicle NEC
            V09.00 ☑
        traffic V09.3 ☑
          involving motor vehicle NEC
            V09.20 ☑
      wheeled shoe V00.158 ☑
        colliding with stationary object
          V00.152 ☑
        fall V00.151 ☑
    on foot (*see also* Accident, pedestrian)
      collision (with)
        animal being ridden or animal drawn
          vehicle V06.90 ☑
           nontraffic V06.00 ☑
           traffic V06.10 ☑
        bus or heavy transport V04.90 ☑
          nontraffic V04.00 ☑
          traffic V04.10 ☑

Accident   *continued*
  transport — *continued*
    pedestrian — *continued*
      on foot (*see also* Accident, pedestrian) — *continued*
        collision — *continued*
          car V03.90 ☑
            nontraffic V03.00 ☑
            traffic V03.10 ☑
          pedal cycle V01.90 ☑
            nontraffic V01.00 ☑
            traffic V01.10 ☑
          pick-up truck or van V03.90 ☑
            nontraffic V03.00 ☑
            traffic V03.10 ☑
          railway (train) (vehicle) V05.90 ☑
            nontraffic V05.00 ☑
            traffic V05.10 ☑
          streetcar V06.90 ☑
            nontraffic V06.00 ☑
            traffic V06.10 ☑
          two- or three-wheeled motor vehicle
            V02.90 ☑
            nontraffic V02.00 ☑
            traffic V02.10 ☑
          vehicle V09.9 ☑
            animal-drawn V06.90 ☑
              nontraffic V06.00 ☑
              traffic V06.10 ☑
            motor
        nontraffic V09.1 ☑
          involving motor vehicle V09.00 ☑
            military V09.01 ☑
            specified type NEC V09.09 ☑
        traffic V09.3 ☑
          involving motor vehicle V09.20 ☑
            military V09.21 ☑
            specified type NEC V09.29 ☑
    person NEC (unknown way or transportation)
      V99 ☑
    collision (between)
      bus (with)
        heavy transport vehicle (traffic) V87.5 ☑
          nontraffic V88.5 ☑
      car (with)
        bus (traffic) V87.3 ☑
          nontraffic V88.3 ☑
        heavy transport vehicle (traffic) V87.4 ☑
          nontraffic V88.4 ☑
        nontraffic V88.5 ☑
        pick-up truck or van (traffic) V87.2 ☑
          nontraffic V88.2 ☑
        train or railway vehicle (traffic) V87.6 ☑
          nontraffic V88.6 ☑
        two- or three-wheeled motor vehicle
          (traffic) V87.0 ☑
          nontraffic V88.0 ☑
        motor vehicle (traffic) NEC V87.7 ☑
          nontraffic V88.7 ☑
        two-or three-wheeled vehicle (with) (traffic)
          motor vehicle NEC V87.1 ☑
          nontraffic V88.1 ☑
      nonmotor vehicle (collision) (noncollision)
        (traffic) V87.9 ☑
        nontraffic V88.9 ☑
    pickup truck occupant V59.9 ☑
      collision (with)
        animal (traffic) V50.9 ☑
          being ridden (traffic) V56.9 ☑
           nontraffic V56.3 ☑
           while boarding or alighting V56.4 ☑
          nontraffic V50.3 ☑
          while boarding or alighting V50.4 ☑
        animal-drawn vehicle (traffic) V56.9 ☑
          nontraffic V56.3 ☑
          while boarding or alighting V56.4 ☑
        bus (traffic) V54.9 ☑
          nontraffic V54.3 ☑
          while boarding or alighting V54.4 ☑
        car (traffic) V53.9 ☑
          nontraffic V53.3 ☑
          while boarding or alighting V53.4 ☑
        motor vehicle NOS (traffic) V59.60 ☑
          nontraffic V59.20 ☑
          specified type NEC (traffic) V59.69 ☑
           nontraffic V59.29 ☑

☑ **Additional Character Required — Refer to the Tabular List for Character Selection**   ▽ **Subterms under main terms may continue to next column or page**

Accident — *continued*
  transport — *continued*
    pickup truck occupant — *continued*
      collision — *continued*
        pedal cycle (traffic) V51.9 ☑
          nontraffic V51.3 ☑
          while boarding or alighting V51.4 ☑
        pickup truck (traffic) V53.9 ☑
          nontraffic V53.3 ☑
          while boarding or alighting V53.4 ☑
        railway vehicle (traffic) V55.9 ☑
          nontraffic V55.3 ☑
          while boarding or alighting V55.4 ☑
        specified vehicle NEC (traffic) V56.9 ☑
          nontraffic V56.3 ☑
          while boarding or alighting V56.4 ☑
        stationary object (traffic) V57.9 ☑
          nontraffic V57.3 ☑
          while boarding or alighting V57.4 ☑
        streetcar (traffic) V56.9 ☑
          nontraffic V56.3 ☑
          while boarding or alighting V56.4 ☑
        three wheeled motor vehicle (traffic)
          V52.9 ☑
          nontraffic V52.3 ☑
          while boarding or alighting V52.4 ☑
        truck (traffic) V54.9 ☑
          nontraffic V54.3 ☑
          while boarding or alighting V54.4 ☑
        two wheeled motor vehicle (traffic) V52.9 ☑
          nontraffic V52.3 ☑
          while boarding or alighting V52.4 ☑
        van (traffic) V53.9 ☑
          nontraffic V53.3 ☑
          while boarding or alighting V53.4 ☑
      driver
        collision (with)
          animal (traffic) V50.5 ☑
            being ridden (traffic) V56.5 ☑
              nontraffic V56.0 ☑
            nontraffic V50.0 ☑
          animal-drawn vehicle (traffic) V56.5 ☑
            nontraffic V56.0 ☑
          bus (traffic) V54.5 ☑
            nontraffic V54.0 ☑
          car (traffic) V53.5 ☑
            nontraffic V53.0 ☑
          motor vehicle NOS (traffic) V59.40 ☑
            nontraffic V59.00 ☑
            specified type NEC (traffic) V59.49 ☑
              nontraffic V59.09 ☑
          pedal cycle (traffic) V51.5 ☑
            nontraffic V51.0 ☑
          pickup truck (traffic) V53.5 ☑
            nontraffic V53.0 ☑
          railway vehicle (traffic) V55.5 ☑
            nontraffic V55.0 ☑
          specified vehicle NEC (traffic) V56.5 ☑
            nontraffic V56.0 ☑
          stationary object (traffic) V57.5 ☑
            nontraffic V57.0 ☑
          streetcar (traffic) V56.5 ☑
            nontraffic V56.0 ☑
          three wheeled motor vehicle (traffic)
            V52.5 ☑
            nontraffic V52.0 ☑
          truck (traffic) V54.5 ☑
            nontraffic V54.0 ☑
          two wheeled motor vehicle (traffic)
            V52.5 ☑
            nontraffic V52.0 ☑
          van (traffic) V53.5 ☑
            nontraffic V53.0 ☑
        noncollision accident (traffic) V58.5 ☑
          nontraffic V58.0 ☑
      hanger-on
        collision (with)
          animal (traffic) V50.7 ☑
            being ridden (traffic) V56.7 ☑
              nontraffic V56.2 ☑
            nontraffic V50.2 ☑
          animal-drawn vehicle (traffic) V56.7 ☑
            nontraffic V56.2 ☑
          bus (traffic) V54.7 ☑
            nontraffic V54.2 ☑
          car (traffic) V53.7 ☑

Accident — *continued*
  transport — *continued*
    pickup truck occupant — *continued*
      hanger-on — *continued*
        collision — *continued*
          car — *continued*
            nontraffic V53.2 ☑
          pedal cycle (traffic) V51.7 ☑
            nontraffic V51.2 ☑
          pickup truck (traffic) V53.7 ☑
            nontraffic V53.2 ☑
          railway vehicle (traffic) V55.7 ☑
            nontraffic V55.2 ☑
          specified vehicle NEC (traffic) V56.7 ☑
            nontraffic V56.2 ☑
          stationary object (traffic) V57.7 ☑
            nontraffic V57.2 ☑
          streetcar (traffic) V56.7 ☑
            nontraffic V56.2 ☑
          three wheeled motor vehicle (traffic)
            V52.7 ☑
            nontraffic V52.2 ☑
          truck (traffic) V54.7 ☑
            nontraffic V54.2 ☑
          two wheeled motor vehicle (traffic)
            V52.7 ☑
            nontraffic V52.2 ☑
          van (traffic) V53.7 ☑
            nontraffic V53.2 ☑
        noncollision accident (traffic) V58.7 ☑
          nontraffic V58.2 ☑
      noncollision accident (traffic) V58.9 ☑
        nontraffic V58.3 ☑
        while boarding or alighting V58.4 ☑
      nontraffic V59.3 ☑
      passenger
        collision (with)
          animal (traffic) V50.6 ☑
            being ridden (traffic) V56.6 ☑
              nontraffic V56.1 ☑
            nontraffic V50.1 ☑
          animal-drawn vehicle (traffic) V56.6 ☑
            nontraffic V56.1 ☑
          bus (traffic) V54.6 ☑
            nontraffic V54.1 ☑
          car (traffic) V53.6 ☑
            nontraffic V53.1 ☑
          motor vehicle NOS (traffic) V59.50 ☑
            nontraffic V59.10 ☑
            specified type NEC (traffic) V59.59 ☑
              nontraffic V59.19 ☑
          pedal cycle (traffic) V51.6 ☑
            nontraffic V51.1 ☑
          pickup truck (traffic) V53.6 ☑
            nontraffic V53.1 ☑
          railway vehicle (traffic) V55.6 ☑
            nontraffic V55.1 ☑
          specified vehicle NEC (traffic) V56.6 ☑
            nontraffic V56.1 ☑
          stationary object (traffic) V57.6 ☑
            nontraffic V57.1 ☑
          streetcar (traffic) V56.6 ☑
            nontraffic V56.1 ☑
          three wheeled motor vehicle (traffic)
            V52.6 ☑
            nontraffic V52.1 ☑
          truck (traffic) V54.6 ☑
            nontraffic V54.1 ☑
          two wheeled motor vehicle (traffic)
            V52.6 ☑
            nontraffic V52.1 ☑
          van (traffic) V53.6 ☑
            nontraffic V53.1 ☑
        noncollision accident (traffic) V58.6 ☑
          nontraffic V58.1 ☑
      specified type NEC V59.88 ☑
      military vehicle V59.81 ☑
    quarry truck — *see* Accident, transport, industrial
      vehicle occupant
    race car — *see* Accident, transport, motor vehicle
      NEC occupant
    railway vehicle occupant V81.9 ☑
      collision (with) V81.3 ☑
        motor vehicle (non-military) (traffic)
          V81.1 ☑
          military V81.83 ☑

Accident — *continued*
  transport — *continued*
    railway vehicle occupant — *continued*
      collision — *continued*
        motor vehicle — *continued*
          nontraffic V81.0 ☑
        rolling stock V81.2 ☑
        specified object NEC V81.3 ☑
      during derailment V81.7 ☑
        with antecedent collision B — *see* Accident,
          transport, railway vehicle occupant,
          collision
      explosion V81.81 ☑
      fall (in railway vehicle) V81.5 ☑
        during derailment V81.7 ☑
          with antecedent collision B — *see* Acci-
            dent, transport, railway vehicle
            occupant, collision
        from railway vehicle V81.6 ☑
          during derailment V81.7 ☑
            with antecedent collision B — *see*
              Accident, transport, railway
              vehicle occupant, collision
        while boarding or alighting V81.4 ☑
      fire V81.81 ☑
      object falling onto train V81.82 ☑
      specified type NEC V81.89 ☑
      while boarding or alighting V81.4 ☑
    ski lift V98.3 ☑
    snowmobile occupant (nontraffic) V86.92 ☑
      driver V86.52 ☑
      hanger-on V86.72 ☑
      passenger V86.62 ☑
      traffic V86.32 ☑
        driver V86.02 ☑
        hanger-on V86.22 ☑
        passenger V86.12 ☑
      while boarding or alighting V86.42 ☑
    specified NEC V98.8 ☑
    sport utility vehicle occupant (*see also* Accident,
      transport, car occupant)
      collision (with)
        stationary object (traffic) V47.91 ☑
          nontraffic V47.31 ☑
      driver
        collision (with)
          stationary object (traffic) V47.51 ☑
            nontraffic V47.01 ☑
      passenger
        collision (with)
          stationary object (traffic) V47.61 ☑
            nontraffic V47.11 ☑
    streetcar occupant V82.9 ☑
      collision (with) V82.3 ☑
        motor vehicle (traffic) V82.1 ☑
          nontraffic V82.0 ☑
        rolling stock V82.2 ☑
      during derailment V82.7 ☑
        with antecedent collision B — *see* Accident,
          transport, streetcar occupant, collision
      fall (in streetcar) V82.5 ☑
        during derailment V82.7 ☑
          with antecedent collision B — *see* Acci-
            dent, transport, streetcar occu-
            pant, collision
        from streetcar V82.6 ☑
          during derailment V82.7 ☑
            with antecedent collision B — *see*
              Accident, transport, streetcar
              occupant, collision
        while boarding or alighting V82.4 ☑
      while boarding or alighting V82.4 ☑
      specified type NEC V82.8 ☑
      while boarding or alighting V82.4 ☑
    three-wheeled motor vehicle occupant V39.9 ☑
      collision (with)
        animal (traffic) V30.9 ☑
          being ridden (traffic) V36.9 ☑
            nontraffic V36.3 ☑
            while boarding or alighting V36.4 ☑
          nontraffic V30.3 ☑
          while boarding or alighting V30.4 ☑
        animal-drawn vehicle (traffic) V36.9 ☑
          nontraffic V36.3 ☑
          while boarding or alighting V36.4 ☑
        bus (traffic) V34.9 ☑

Accident — *continued*
  transport — *continued*
    three-wheeled motor vehicle occupant — *continued*
      collision — *continued*
        bus — *continued*
          nontraffic V34.3 ☑
          while boarding or alighting V34.4 ☑
        car (traffic) V33.9 ☑
          nontraffic V33.3 ☑
          while boarding or alighting V33.4 ☑
        motor vehicle NOS (traffic) V39.60 ☑
          nontraffic V39.20 ☑
          specified type NEC (traffic) V39.69 ☑
            nontraffic V39.29 ☑
        pedal cycle (traffic) V31.9 ☑
          nontraffic V31.3 ☑
          while boarding or alighting V31.4 ☑
        pickup truck (traffic) V33.9 ☑
          nontraffic V33.3 ☑
          while boarding or alighting V33.4 ☑
        railway vehicle (traffic) V35.9 ☑
          nontraffic V35.3 ☑
          while boarding or alighting V35.4 ☑
        specified vehicle NEC (traffic) V36.9 ☑
          nontraffic V36.3 ☑
          while boarding or alighting V36.4 ☑
        stationary object (traffic) V37.9 ☑
          nontraffic V37.3 ☑
          while boarding or alighting V37.4 ☑
        streetcar (traffic) V36.9 ☑
          nontraffic V36.3 ☑
          while boarding or alighting V36.4 ☑
        three wheeled motor vehicle (traffic) V32.9 ☑
          nontraffic V32.3 ☑
          while boarding or alighting V32.4 ☑
        truck (traffic) V34.9 ☑
          nontraffic V34.3 ☑
          while boarding or alighting V34.4 ☑
        two wheeled motor vehicle (traffic) V32.9 ☑
          nontraffic V32.3 ☑
          while boarding or alighting V32.4 ☑
        van (traffic) V33.9 ☑
          nontraffic V33.3 ☑
          while boarding or alighting V33.4 ☑
      driver
        collision (with)
          animal (traffic) V30.5 ☑
            being ridden (traffic) V36.5 ☑
              nontraffic V36.0 ☑
            nontraffic V30.0 ☑
          animal-drawn vehicle (traffic) V36.5 ☑
            nontraffic V36.0 ☑
          bus (traffic) V34.5 ☑
            nontraffic V34.0 ☑
          car (traffic) V33.5 ☑
            nontraffic V33.0 ☑
          motor vehicle NOS (traffic) V39.40 ☑
            nontraffic V39.00 ☑
            specified type NEC (traffic) V39.49 ☑
              nontraffic V39.09 ☑
          pedal cycle (traffic) V31.5 ☑
            nontraffic V31.0 ☑
          pickup truck (traffic) V33.5 ☑
            nontraffic V33.0 ☑
          railway vehicle (traffic) V35.5 ☑
            nontraffic V35.0 ☑
          specified vehicle NEC (traffic) V36.5 ☑
            nontraffic V36.0 ☑
          stationary object (traffic) V37.5 ☑
            nontraffic V37.0 ☑
          streetcar (traffic) V36.5 ☑
            nontraffic V36.0 ☑
          three wheeled motor vehicle (traffic) V32.5 ☑
            nontraffic V32.0 ☑
          truck (traffic) V34.5 ☑
            nontraffic V34.0 ☑
          two wheeled motor vehicle (traffic) V32.5 ☑
            nontraffic V32.0 ☑
          van (traffic) V33.5 ☑
            nontraffic V33.0 ☑
        noncollision accident (traffic) V38.5 ☑
          nontraffic V38.0 ☑

Accident — *continued*
  transport — *continued*
    three-wheeled motor vehicle occupant — *continued*
      hanger-on
        collision (with)
          animal (traffic) V30.7 ☑
            being ridden (traffic) V36.7 ☑
              nontraffic V36.2 ☑
            nontraffic V30.2 ☑
          animal-drawn vehicle (traffic) V36.7 ☑
            nontraffic V36.2 ☑
          bus (traffic) V34.7 ☑
            nontraffic V34.2 ☑
          car (traffic) V33.7 ☑
            nontraffic V33.2 ☑
          pedal cycle (traffic) V31.7 ☑
            nontraffic V31.2 ☑
          pickup truck (traffic) V33.7 ☑
            nontraffic V33.2 ☑
          railway vehicle (traffic) V35.7 ☑
            nontraffic V35.2 ☑
          specified vehicle NEC (traffic) V36.7 ☑
            nontraffic V36.2 ☑
          stationary object (traffic) V37.7 ☑
            nontraffic V37.2 ☑
          streetcar (traffic) V36.7 ☑
            nontraffic V36.2 ☑
          three wheeled motor vehicle (traffic) V32.7 ☑
            nontraffic V32.2 ☑
          truck (traffic) V34.7 ☑
            nontraffic V34.2 ☑
          two wheeled motor vehicle (traffic) V32.7 ☑
            nontraffic V32.2 ☑
          van (traffic) V33.7 ☑
            nontraffic V33.2 ☑
        noncollision accident (traffic) V38.7 ☑
          nontraffic V38.2 ☑
      noncollision accident (traffic) V38.9 ☑
        nontraffic V38.3 ☑
        while boarding or alighting V38.4 ☑
      nontraffic V39.3 ☑
      passenger
        collision (with)
          animal (traffic) V30.6 ☑
            being ridden (traffic) V36.6 ☑
              nontraffic V36.1 ☑
            nontraffic V30.1 ☑
          animal-drawn vehicle (traffic) V36.6 ☑
            nontraffic V36.1 ☑
          bus (traffic) V34.6 ☑
            nontraffic V34.1 ☑
          car (traffic) V33.6 ☑
            nontraffic V33.1 ☑
          motor vehicle NOS (traffic) V39.50 ☑
            nontraffic V39.10 ☑
            specified type NEC (traffic) V39.59 ☑
              nontraffic V39.19 ☑
          pedal cycle (traffic) V31.6 ☑
            nontraffic V31.1 ☑
          pickup truck (traffic) V33.6 ☑
            nontraffic V33.1 ☑
          railway vehicle (traffic) V35.6 ☑
            nontraffic V35.1 ☑
          specified vehicle NEC (traffic) V36.6 ☑
            nontraffic V36.1 ☑
          stationary object (traffic) V37.6 ☑
            nontraffic V37.1 ☑
          streetcar (traffic) V36.6 ☑
            nontraffic V36.1 ☑
          three wheeled motor vehicle (traffic) V32.6 ☑
            nontraffic V32.1 ☑
          truck (traffic) V34.6 ☑
            nontraffic V34.1 ☑
          two wheeled motor vehicle (traffic) V32.6 ☑
            nontraffic V32.1 ☑
          van (traffic) V33.6 ☑
            nontraffic V33.1 ☑
        noncollision accident (traffic) V38.6 ☑
          nontraffic V38.1 ☑
      specified type NEC V39.89 ☑
        military vehicle V39.81 ☑

Accident — *continued*
  transport — *continued*
    tractor (farm) (and trailer) — *see* Accident, transport, agricultural vehicle occupant
    tram — *see* Accident, transport, streetcar
      in mine or quarry — *see* Accident, transport, industrial vehicle occupant
    trolley — *see* Accident, transport, streetcar
      in mine or quarry — *see* Accident, transport, industrial vehicle occupant
    truck (heavy) occupant V69.9 ☑
      collision (with)
        animal (traffic) V60.9 ☑
          being ridden (traffic) V66.9 ☑
            nontraffic V66.3 ☑
            while boarding or alighting V66.4 ☑
          nontraffic V60.3 ☑
          while boarding or alighting V60.4 ☑
        animal-drawn vehicle (traffic) V66.9 ☑
          nontraffic V66.3 ☑
          while boarding or alighting V66.4 ☑
        bus (traffic) V64.9 ☑
          nontraffic V64.3 ☑
          while boarding or alighting V64.4 ☑
        car (traffic) V63.9 ☑
          nontraffic V63.3 ☑
          while boarding or alighting V63.4 ☑
        motor vehicle NOS (traffic) V69.60 ☑
          nontraffic V69.20 ☑
          specified type NEC (traffic) V69.69 ☑
            nontraffic V69.29 ☑
        pedal cycle (traffic) V61.9 ☑
          nontraffic V61.3 ☑
          while boarding or alighting V61.4 ☑
        pickup truck (traffic) V63.9 ☑
          nontraffic V63.3 ☑
          while boarding or alighting V63.4 ☑
        railway vehicle (traffic) V65.9 ☑
          nontraffic V65.3 ☑
          while boarding or alighting V65.4 ☑
        specified vehicle NEC (traffic) V66.9 ☑
          nontraffic V66.3 ☑
          while boarding or alighting V66.4 ☑
        stationary object (traffic) V67.9 ☑
          nontraffic V67.3 ☑
          while boarding or alighting V67.4 ☑
        streetcar (traffic) V66.9 ☑
          nontraffic V66.3 ☑
          while boarding or alighting V66.4 ☑
        three wheeled motor vehicle (traffic) V62.9 ☑
          nontraffic V62.3 ☑
          while boarding or alighting V62.4 ☑
        truck (traffic) V64.9 ☑
          nontraffic V64.3 ☑
          while boarding or alighting V64.4 ☑
        two wheeled motor vehicle (traffic) V62.9 ☑
          nontraffic V62.3 ☑
          while boarding or alighting V62.4 ☑
        van (traffic) V63.9 ☑
          nontraffic V63.3 ☑
          while boarding or alighting V63.4 ☑
      driver
        collision (with)
          animal (traffic) V60.5 ☑
            being ridden (traffic) V66.5 ☑
              nontraffic V66.0 ☑
            nontraffic V60.0 ☑
          animal-drawn vehicle (traffic) V66.5 ☑
            nontraffic V66.0 ☑
          bus (traffic) V64.5 ☑
            nontraffic V64.0 ☑
          car (traffic) V63.5 ☑
            nontraffic V63.0 ☑
          motor vehicle NOS (traffic) V69.40 ☑
            nontraffic V69.00 ☑
            specified type NEC (traffic) V69.49 ☑
              nontraffic V69.09 ☑
          pedal cycle (traffic) V61.5 ☑
            nontraffic V61.0 ☑
          pickup truck (traffic) V63.5 ☑
            nontraffic V63.0 ☑
          railway vehicle (traffic) V65.5 ☑
            nontraffic V65.0 ☑
          specified vehicle NEC (traffic) V66.5 ☑
            nontraffic V66.0 ☑

Accident — *continued*
  transport — *continued*
    truck occupant — *continued*
      driver — *continued*
        collision — *continued*
          stationary object (traffic) V67.5 ☑
            nontraffic V67.0 ☑
          streetcar (traffic) V66.5 ☑
            nontraffic V66.0 ☑
          three wheeled motor vehicle (traffic) V62.5 ☑
            nontraffic V62.0 ☑
          truck (traffic) V64.5 ☑
            nontraffic V64.0 ☑
          two wheeled motor vehicle (traffic) V62.5 ☑
            nontraffic V62.0 ☑
          van (traffic) V63.5 ☑
            nontraffic V63.0 ☑
        noncollision accident (traffic) V68.5 ☑
          nontraffic V68.0 ☑
      dump — *see* Accident, transport, construction vehicle occupant
      hanger-on
        collision (with)
          animal (traffic) V60.7 ☑
            being ridden (traffic) V66.7 ☑
              nontraffic V66.2 ☑
            nontraffic V60.2 ☑
          animal-drawn vehicle (traffic) V66.7 ☑
            nontraffic V66.2 ☑
          bus (traffic) V64.7 ☑
            nontraffic V64.2 ☑
          car (traffic) V63.7 ☑
            nontraffic V63.2 ☑
          pedal cycle (traffic) V61.7 ☑
            nontraffic V61.2 ☑
          pickup truck (traffic) V63.7 ☑
            nontraffic V63.2 ☑
          railway vehicle (traffic) V65.7 ☑
            nontraffic V65.2 ☑
          specified vehicle NEC (traffic) V66.7 ☑
            nontraffic V66.2 ☑
          stationary object (traffic) V67.7 ☑
            nontraffic V67.2 ☑
          streetcar (traffic) V66.7 ☑
            nontraffic V66.2 ☑
          three wheeled motor vehicle (traffic) V62.7 ☑
            nontraffic V62.2 ☑
          truck (traffic) V64.7 ☑
            nontraffic V64.2 ☑
          two wheeled motor vehicle (traffic) V62.7 ☑
            nontraffic V62.2 ☑
          van (traffic) V63.7 ☑
            nontraffic V63.2 ☑
        noncollision accident (traffic) V68.7 ☑
          nontraffic V68.2 ☑
      noncollision accident (traffic) V68.9 ☑
        nontraffic V68.3 ☑
        while boarding or alighting V68.4 ☑
      nontraffic V69.3 ☑
      passenger
        collision (with)
          animal (traffic) V60.6 ☑
            being ridden (traffic) V66.6 ☑
              nontraffic V66.1- ☑
            nontraffic V60.1 ☑
          animal-drawn vehicle (traffic) V66.6 ☑
            nontraffic V66.1 ☑
          bus (traffic) V64.6 ☑
            nontraffic V64.1 ☑
          car (traffic) V63.6 ☑
            nontraffic V63.1 ☑
          motor vehicle NOS (traffic) V69.50 ☑
            nontraffic V69.10 ☑
            specified type NEC (traffic) V69.59 ☑
              nontraffic V69.19 ☑
          pedal cycle (traffic) V61.6 ☑
            nontraffic V61.1 ☑
          pickup truck (traffic) V63.6 ☑
            nontraffic V63.1 ☑
          railway vehicle (traffic) V65.6 ☑
            nontraffic V65.1 ☑
          specified vehicle NEC (traffic) V66.6 ☑

Accident — *continued*
  transport — *continued*
    truck occupant — *continued*
      passenger — *continued*
        collision — *continued*
          specified vehicle — *continued*
            nontraffic V66.1 ☑
          stationary object (traffic) V67.6 ☑
            nontraffic V67.1 ☑
          streetcar (traffic) V66.6 ☑
            nontraffic V66.1 ☑
          three wheeled motor vehicle (traffic) V62.6 ☑
            nontraffic V62.1 ☑
          truck (traffic) V64.6 ☑
            nontraffic V64.1 ☑
          two wheeled motor vehicle (traffic) V62.6 ☑
            nontraffic V62.1 ☑
          van (traffic) V63.6 ☑
            nontraffic V63.1 ☑
        noncollision accident (traffic) V68.6 ☑
          nontraffic V68.1 ☑
      pickup — *see* Accident, transport, pickup truck occupant
      specified type NEC V69.88 ☑
        military vehicle V69.81 ☑
    van occupant V59.9 ☑
      collision (with)
        animal (traffic) V50.9 ☑
          being ridden (traffic) V56.9 ☑
            nontraffic V56.3 ☑
            while boarding or alighting V56.4 ☑
          nontraffic V50.3 ☑
          while boarding or alighting V50.4 ☑
        animal-drawn vehicle (traffic) V56.9 ☑
          nontraffic V56.3 ☑
          while boarding or alighting V56.4 ☑
        bus (traffic) V54.9 ☑
          nontraffic V54.3 ☑
          while boarding or alighting V54.4 ☑
        car (traffic) V53.9 ☑
          nontraffic V53.3 ☑
          while boarding or alighting V53.4 ☑
        motor vehicle NOS (traffic) V59.60 ☑
          nontraffic V59.20 ☑
          specified type NEC (traffic) V59.69 ☑
            nontraffic V59.29 ☑
        pedal cycle (traffic) V51.9 ☑
          nontraffic V51.3 ☑
          while boarding or alighting V51.4 ☑
        pickup truck (traffic) V53.9 ☑
          nontraffic V53.3 ☑
          while boarding or alighting V53.4 ☑
        railway vehicle (traffic) V55.9 ☑
          nontraffic V55.3 ☑
          while boarding or alighting V55.4 ☑
        specified vehicle NEC (traffic) V56.9 ☑
          nontraffic V56.3 ☑
          while boarding or alighting V56.4 ☑
        stationary object (traffic) V57.9 ☑
          nontraffic V57.3 ☑
          while boarding or alighting V57.4 ☑
        streetcar (traffic) V56.9 ☑
          nontraffic V56.3 ☑
          while boarding or alighting V56.4 ☑
        three wheeled motor vehicle (traffic) V52.9 ☑
          nontraffic V52.3 ☑
          while boarding or alighting V52.4 ☑
        truck (traffic) V54.9 ☑
          nontraffic V54.3 ☑
          while boarding or alighting V54.4 ☑
        two wheeled motor vehicle (traffic) V52.9 ☑
          nontraffic V52.3 ☑
          while boarding or alighting V52.4 ☑
        van (traffic) V53.9 ☑
          nontraffic V53.3 ☑
          while boarding or alighting V53.4 ☑
      driver
        collision (with)
          animal (traffic) V50.5 ☑
            being ridden (traffic) V56.5 ☑
              nontraffic V56.0 ☑
            nontraffic V50.0 ☑
          animal-drawn vehicle (traffic) V56.5 ☑

Accident — *continued*
  transport — *continued*
    van occupant — *continued*
      driver — *continued*
        collision — *continued*
          animal-drawn vehicle — *continued*
            nontraffic V56.0 ☑
          bus (traffic) V54.5 ☑
            nontraffic V54.0 ☑
          car (traffic) V53.5 ☑
            nontraffic V53.0 ☑
          motor vehicle NOS (traffic) V59.40 ☑
            nontraffic V59.00 ☑
            specified type NEC (traffic) V59.49 ☑
              nontraffic V59.09 ☑
          pedal cycle (traffic) V51.5 ☑
            nontraffic V51.0 ☑
          pickup truck (traffic) V53.5 ☑
            nontraffic V53.0 ☑
          railway vehicle (traffic) V55.5 ☑
            nontraffic V55.0 ☑
          specified vehicle NEC (traffic) V56.5 ☑
            nontraffic V56.0 ☑
          stationary object (traffic) V57.5 ☑
            nontraffic V57.0 ☑
          streetcar (traffic) V56.5 ☑
            nontraffic V56.0 ☑
          three wheeled motor vehicle (traffic) V52.5 ☑
            nontraffic V52.0 ☑
          truck (traffic) V54.5 ☑
            nontraffic V54.0 ☑
          two wheeled motor vehicle (traffic) V52.5 ☑
            nontraffic V52.0 ☑
          van (traffic) V53.5 ☑
            nontraffic V53.0 ☑
        noncollision accident (traffic) V58.5 ☑
          nontraffic V58.0 ☑
      hanger-on
        collision (with)
          animal (traffic) V50.7 ☑
            being ridden (traffic) V56.7 ☑
              nontraffic V56.2 ☑
            nontraffic V50.2 ☑
          animal-drawn vehicle (traffic) V56.7 ☑
            nontraffic V56.2 ☑
          bus (traffic) V54.7 ☑
            nontraffic V54.2 ☑
          car (traffic) V53.7 ☑
            nontraffic V53.2 ☑
          pedal cycle (traffic) V51.7 ☑
            nontraffic V51.2 ☑
          pickup truck (traffic) V53.7 ☑
            nontraffic V53.2 ☑
          railway vehicle (traffic) V55.7 ☑
            nontraffic V55.2 ☑
          specified vehicle NEC (traffic) V56.7 ☑
            nontraffic V56.2 ☑
          stationary object (traffic) V57.7 ☑
            nontraffic V57.2 ☑
          streetcar (traffic) V56.7 ☑
            nontraffic V56.2 ☑
          three wheeled motor vehicle (traffic) V52.7 ☑
            nontraffic V52.2 ☑
          truck (traffic) V54.7 ☑
            nontraffic V54.2 ☑
          two wheeled motor vehicle (traffic) V52.7 ☑
            nontraffic V52.2 ☑
          van (traffic) V53.7 ☑
            nontraffic V53.2 ☑
        noncollision accident (traffic) V58.7 ☑
          nontraffic V58.2 ☑
      noncollision accident (traffic) V58.9 ☑
        nontraffic V58.3 ☑
        while boarding or alighting V58.4 ☑
      nontraffic V59.3 ☑
      passenger
        collision (with)
          animal (traffic) V50.6 ☑
            being ridden (traffic) V56.6 ☑
              nontraffic V56.1 ☑
            nontraffic V50.1 ☑
          animal-drawn vehicle (traffic) V56.6 ☑

⬙ **Subterms under main terms may continue to next column or page**   ☑ **Additional Character Required — Refer to the Tabular List for Character Selection**   **397**

Accident — Accident

Accident — *continued*
  transport — *continued*
    van occupant — *continued*
      passenger — *continued*
        collision — *continued*
          animal-drawn vehicle — *continued*
            nontraffic V56.1 ☑
          bus (traffic) V54.6 ☑
            nontraffic V54.1 ☑
          car (traffic) V53.6 ☑
            nontraffic V53.1 ☑
          motor vehicle NOS (traffic) V59.50 ☑
            nontraffic V59.10 ☑
            specified type NEC (traffic) V59.59 ☑
              nontraffic V59.19 ☑
          pedal cycle (traffic) V51.6 ☑
            nontraffic V51.1 ☑
          pickup truck (traffic) V53.6 ☑
            nontraffic V53.1 ☑
          railway vehicle (traffic) V55.6 ☑
            nontraffic V55.1 ☑
          specified vehicle NEC (traffic) V56.6 ☑
            nontraffic V56.1 ☑
          stationary object (traffic) V57.6 ☑
            nontraffic V57.1 ☑
          streetcar (traffic) V56.6 ☑
            nontraffic V56.1 ☑
          three wheeled motor vehicle (traffic) V52.6 ☑
            nontraffic V52.1 ☑
          truck (traffic) V54.6 ☑
            nontraffic V54.1 ☑
          two wheeled motor vehicle (traffic) V52.6 ☑
            nontraffic V52.1 ☑
          van (traffic) V53.6 ☑
            nontraffic V53.1 ☑
        noncollision accident (traffic) V58.6 ☑
          nontraffic V58.1 ☑
      specified type NEC V59.88 ☑
      military vehicle V59.81 ☑
  watercraft occupant — *see* Accident, watercraft
  vehicle NEC V89.9 ☑
    animal-drawn NEC — *see* Accident, transport, animal-drawn vehicle occupant
    special
      agricultural — *see* Accident, transport, agricultural vehicle occupant
      construction — *see* Accident, transport, construction vehicle occupant
      industrial — *see* Accident, transport, industrial vehicle occupant
      three-wheeled NEC (motorized) — *see* Accident, transport, three-wheeled motor vehicle occupant
  watercraft V94.9 ☑
    causing
      drowning B — *see* Drowning, due to, accident to, watercraft
      injury NEC V91.89 ☑
        crushed between craft and object V91.19 ☑
          powered craft V91.13 ☑
            ferry boat V91.11 ☑
            fishing boat V91.12 ☑
            jetskis V91.13 ☑
            liner V91.11 ☑
            merchant ship V91.10 ☑
            passenger ship V91.11 ☑
          unpowered craft V91.18 ☑
            canoe V91.15 ☑
            inflatable V91.16 ☑
            kayak V91.15 ☑
            sailboat V91.14 ☑
            surf-board V91.18 ☑
            windsurfer V91.18 ☑
        fall on board V91.29 ☑
          powered craft V91.23 ☑
            ferry boat V91.21 ☑
            fishing boat V91.22 ☑
            jetskis V91.23 ☑
            liner V91.21 ☑
            merchant ship V91.20 ☑
            passenger ship V91.21 ☑
          unpowered craft
            canoe V91.25 ☑
            inflatable V91.26 ☑

Accident — *continued*
  watercraft — *continued*
    causing — *continued*
      injury — *continued*
        fall on board — *continued*
          unpowered craft — *continued*
            kayak V91.25 ☑
            sailboat V91.24 ☑
        fire on board causing burn V91.09 ☑
          powered craft V91.03 ☑
            ferry boat V91.01 ☑
            fishing boat V91.02 ☑
            jetskis V91.03 ☑
            liner V91.01 ☑
            merchant ship V91.00 ☑
            passenger ship V91.01 ☑
          unpowered craft V91.08 ☑
            canoe V91.05 ☑
            inflatable V91.06 ☑
            kayak V91.05 ☑
            sailboat V91.04 ☑
            surf-board V91.08 ☑
            water skis V91.07 ☑
            windsurfer V91.08 ☑
        hit by falling object V91.39 ☑
          powered craft V91.33 ☑
            ferry boat V91.31 ☑
            fishing boat V91.32 ☑
            jetskis V91.33 ☑
            liner V91.31 ☑
            merchant ship V91.30 ☑
            passenger ship V91.31 ☑
          unpowered craft V91.38 ☑
            canoe V91.35 ☑
            inflatable V91.36 ☑
            kayak V91.35 ☑
            sailboat V91.34 ☑
            surf-board V91.38 ☑
            water skis V91.37 ☑
            windsurfer V91.38 ☑
        specified type NEC V91.89 ☑
          powered craft V91.83 ☑
            ferry boat V91.81 ☑
            fishing boat V91.82 ☑
            jetskis V91.83 ☑
            liner V91.81 ☑
            merchant ship V91.80 ☑
            passenger ship V91.81 ☑
          unpowered craft V91.88 ☑
            canoe V91.85 ☑
            inflatable V91.86 ☑
            kayak V91.85 ☑
            sailboat V91.84 ☑
            surf-board V91.88 ☑
            water skis V91.87 ☑
            windsurfer V91.88 ☑
      due to, caused by cataclysm — *see* Forces of nature, by type
      military NEC V94.818 ☑
        with civilian watercraft V94.810 ☑
        civilian in water injured by V94.811 ☑
      nonpowered, struck by
        nonpowered vessel V94.22 ☑
        powered vessel V94.21 ☑
      specified type NEC V94.89 ☑
      striking swimmer
        powered V94.11 ☑
        unpowered V94.12 ☑

Acid throwing (assault) Y08.89 ☑
Activity (involving) (of victim at time of event) Y93.9
  aerobic and step exercise (class) Y93.A3 (*following* Y93.7)
  alpine skiing Y93.23
  animal care NEC Y93.K9 (*following* Y93.7)
  arts and handcrafts NEC Y93.D9 (*following* Y93.7)
  athletics played as a team or group NEC Y93.69
  athletics played individually NEC Y93.59
  athletics NEC Y93.79
  baking Y93.G3 (*following* Y93.7)
  ballet Y93.41
  barbells Y93.B3 (*following* Y93.7)
  BASE (Building, Antenna, Span, Earth) jumping Y93.33
  baseball Y93.64
  basketball Y93.67
  bathing (personal) Y93.E1 (*following* Y93.7)
  beach volleyball Y93.68

Activity — *continued*
  bike riding Y93.55
  boogie boarding Y93.18
  bowling Y93.54
  boxing Y93.71
  brass instrument playing Y93.J4 (*following* Y93.7)
  building construction Y93.H3 (*following* Y93.7)
  bungee jumping Y93.34
  calisthenics Y93.A2 (*following* Y93.7)
  canoeing (in calm and turbulent water) Y93.16
  capture the flag Y93.6A
  cardiorespiratory exercise NEC Y93.A9 (*following* Y93.7)
  caregiving (providing) NEC Y93.F9 (*following* Y93.7)
    bathing Y93.F1 (*following* Y93.7)
    lifting Y93.F2 (*following* Y93.7)
  cellular
    communication device Y93.C2 (*following* Y93.7)
    telephone Y93.C2 (*following* Y93.7)
  challenge course Y93.A5 (*following* Y93.7)
  cheerleading Y93.45
  circuit training Y93.A4 (*following* Y93.7)
  cleaning
    floor Y93.E5 (*following* Y93.7)
  climbing NEC Y93.39
    mountain Y93.31
    rock Y93.31
    wall Y93.31
  clothing care and maintenance NEC Y93.E9 (*following* Y93.7)
  combatives Y93.75
  computer
    keyboarding Y93.C1 (*following* Y93.7)
    technology NEC Y93.C9 (*following* Y93.7)
  confidence course Y93.A5 (*following* Y93.7)
  construction (building) Y93.H3 (*following* Y93.7)
  cooking and baking Y93.G3 (*following* Y93.7)
  cool down exercises Y93.A2 (*following* Y93.7)
  cricket Y93.69
  crocheting Y93.D1 (*following* Y93.7)
  cross country skiing Y93.24
  dancing (all types) Y93.41
  digging
    dirt Y93.H1 (*following* Y93.7)
  dirt digging Y93.H1 (*following* Y93.7)
  dishwashing Y93.G1 (*following* Y93.7)
  diving (platform) (springboard) Y93.12
    underwater Y93.15
  dodge ball Y93.6A
  downhill skiing Y93.23
  drum playing Y93.J2 (*following* Y93.7)
  dumbbells Y93.B3 (*following* Y93.7)
  electronic
    devices NEC Y93.C9 (*following* Y93.7)
      hand held interactive Y93.C2 (*following* Y93.7)
    game playing (using) (with)
      interactive device Y93.C2 (*following* Y93.7)
      keyboard or other stationary device Y93.C1 (*following* Y93.7)
  elliptical machine Y93.A1 (*following* Y93.7)
  exercise(s)
    machines ((primarily) for)
      cardiorespiratory conditioning Y93.A1 (*following* Y93.7)
      muscle strengthening Y93.B1 (*following* Y93.7)
    muscle strengthening (non-machine) NEC Y93.B9 (*following* Y93.7)
  external motion NEC Y93.I9 (*following* Y93.7)
    rollercoaster Y93.I1 (*following* Y93.7)
  field hockey Y93.65
  figure skating (pairs) (singles) Y93.21
  flag football Y93.62
  floor mopping and cleaning Y93.E5 (*following* Y93.7)
  food preparation and clean up Y93.G1 (*following* Y93.7)
  football (American) NOS Y93.61
    flag Y93.62
    tackle Y93.61
    touch Y93.62
  four square Y93.6A
  free weights Y93.B3 (*following* Y93.7)
  frisbee (ultimate) Y93.74
  furniture
    building Y93.D3 (*following* Y93.7)
    finishing Y93.D3 (*following* Y93.7)
    repair Y93.D3 (*following* Y93.7)
  game playing (electronic)
    using interactive device Y93.C2 (*following* Y93.7)
    using keyboard or other stationary device Y93.C1 (*following* Y93.7)

Activity — *continued*
- gardening Y93.H2 (*following* Y93.7)
- golf Y93.53
- grass drills Y93.A6 (*following* Y93.7)
- grilling and smoking food Y93.G2 (*following* Y93.7)
- grooming and shearing an animal Y93.K3 (*following* Y93.7)
- guerilla drills Y93.A6 (*following* Y93.7)
- gymnastics (rhythmic) Y93.43
- hand held interactive electronic device Y93.C2 (*following* Y93.7)
- handball Y93.73
- handcrafts NEC Y93.D9 (*following* Y93.7)
- hang gliding Y93.35
- hiking (on level or elevated terrain) Y93.01
- hockey (ice) Y93.22
    - field Y93.65
- horseback riding Y93.52
- household (interior) maintenance NEC Y93.E9 (*following* Y93.7)
- ice NEC Y93.29
    - dancing Y93.21
    - hockey Y93.22
    - skating Y93.21
- inline roller skating Y93.51
- ironing Y93.E4 (*following* Y93.7)
- judo Y93.75
- jumping jacks Y93.A2 (*following* Y93.7)
- jumping rope Y93.56
- jumping (off) NEC Y93.39
    - BASE (Building, Antenna, Span, Earth) Y93.33
    - bungee Y93.34
    - jacks Y93.A2 (*following* Y93.7)
    - rope Y93.56
- karate Y93.75
- kayaking (in calm and turbulent water) Y93.16
- keyboarding (computer) Y93.C1 (*following* Y93.7)
- kickball Y93.6A
- knitting Y93.D1 (*following* Y93.7)
- lacrosse Y93.65
- land maintenance NEC Y93.H9 (*following* Y93.7)
- landscaping Y93.H2 (*following* Y93.7)
- laundry Y93.E2 (*following* Y93.7)
- machines (exercise)
    - primarily for cardiorespiratory conditioning Y93.A1 (*following* Y93.7)
    - primarily for muscle strengthening Y93.B1 (*following* Y93.7)
- maintenance
    - exterior building NEC Y93.H9 (*following* Y93.7)
    - household (interior) NEC Y93.E9 (*following* Y93.7)
    - land Y93.H9 (*following* Y93.7)
    - property Y93.H9 (*following* Y93.7)
- marching (on level or elevated terrain) Y93.01
- martial arts Y93.75
- microwave oven Y93.G3 (*following* Y93.7)
- milking an animal Y93.K2 (*following* Y93.7)
- mopping (floor) Y93.E5 (*following* Y93.7)
- mountain climbing Y93.31
- muscle strengthening
    - exercises (non-machine) NEC Y93.B9 (*following* Y93.7)
    - machines Y93.B1 (*following* Y93.7)
- musical keyboard (electronic) playing Y93.J1 (*following* Y93.7)
- nordic skiing Y93.24
- obstacle course Y93.A5 (*following* Y93.7)
- oven (microwave) Y93.G3 (*following* Y93.7)
- packing up and unpacking in moving to a new residence Y93.E6 (*following* Y93.7)
- parasailing Y93.19
- percussion instrument playing NEC Y93.J2 (*following* Y93.7)
- personal
    - bathing and showering Y93.E1 (*following* Y93.7)
    - hygiene NEC Y93.E8 (*following* Y93.7)
    - showering Y93.E1 (*following* Y93.7)
- physical games generally associated with school recess, summer camp and children Y93.6A
- physical training NEC Y93.A9 (*following* Y93.7)
- piano playing Y93.J1 (*following* Y93.7)
- pilates Y93.B4 (*following* Y93.7)
- platform diving Y93.12
- playing musical instrument
    - brass instrument Y93.J4 (*following* Y93.7)
    - drum Y93.J2 (*following* Y93.7)
    - musical keyboard (electronic) Y93.J1 (*following* Y93.7)

Activity — *continued*
- playing musical instrument — *continued*
    - percussion instrument NEC Y93.J2 (*following* Y93.7)
    - piano Y93.J1 (*following* Y93.7)
    - string instrument Y93.J3 (*following* Y93.7)
    - winds instrument Y93.J4 (*following* Y93.7)
- property maintenance
    - exterior NEC Y93.H9 (*following* Y93.7)
    - interior NEC Y93.E9 (*following* Y93.7)
- pruning (garden and lawn) Y93.H2 (*following* Y93.7)
- pull-ups Y93.B2 (*following* Y93.7)
- push-ups Y93.B2 (*following* Y93.7)
- racquetball Y93.73
- rafting (in calm and turbulent water) Y93.16
- raking (leaves) Y93.H1 (*following* Y93.7)
- rappelling Y93.32
- refereeing a sports activity Y93.81
- residential relocation Y93.E6 (*following* Y93.7)
- rhythmic gymnastics Y93.43
- rhythmic movement NEC Y93.49
- riding
    - horseback Y93.52
    - rollercoaster Y93.I1 (*following* Y93.7)
- rock climbing Y93.31
- roller skating (inline) Y93.51
- rollercoaster riding Y93.I1 (*following* Y93.7)
- rough housing and horseplay Y93.83
- rowing (in calm and turbulent water) Y93.16
- rugby Y93.63
- running Y93.02
- SCUBA diving Y93.15
- sewing Y93.D2 (*following* Y93.7)
- shoveling Y93.H1 (*following* Y93.7)
    - dirt Y93.H1 (*following* Y93.7)
    - snow Y93.H1 (*following* Y93.7)
- showering (personal) Y93.E1 (*following* Y93.7)
- sit-ups Y93.B2 (*following* Y93.7)
- skateboarding Y93.51
- skating (ice) Y93.21
    - roller Y93.51
- skiing (alpine) (downhill) Y93.23
    - cross country Y93.24
    - nordic Y93.24
    - water Y93.17
- sledding (snow) Y93.23
- sleeping (sleep) Y93.84
- smoking and grilling food Y93.G2 (*following* Y93.7)
- snorkeling Y93.15
- snow NEC Y93.29
    - boarding Y93.23
    - shoveling Y93.H1 (*following* Y93.7)
    - sledding Y93.23
    - tubing Y93.23
- soccer Y93.66
- softball Y93.64
- specified NEC Y93.89
- spectator at an event Y93.82
- sports NEC Y93.79
    - sports played as a team or group NEC Y93.69
    - sports played individually NEC Y93.59
- springboard diving Y93.12
- squash Y93.73
- stationary bike Y93.A1 (*following* Y93.7)
- step (stepping) exercise (class) Y93.A3 (*following* Y93.7)
- stepper machine Y93.A1 (*following* Y93.7)
- stove Y93.G3 (*following* Y93.7)
- string instrument playing Y93.J3 (*following* Y93.7)
- surfing Y93.18
    - wind Y93.18
- swimming Y93.11
- tackle football Y93.61
- tap dancing Y93.41
- tennis Y93.73
- tobogganing Y93.23
- touch football Y93.62
- track and field events (non-running) Y93.57
    - running Y93.02
- trampoline Y93.44
- treadmill Y93.A1 (*following* Y93.7)
- trimming shrubs Y93.H2 (*following* Y93.7)
- tubing (in calm and turbulent water) Y93.16
    - snow Y93.23
- ultimate frisbee Y93.74
- underwater diving Y93.15
- unpacking in moving to a new residence Y93.E6 (*following* Y93.7)
- use of stove, oven and microwave oven Y93.G3 (*following* Y93.7)

Activity — *continued*
- vacuuming Y93.E3 (*following* Y93.7)
- volleyball (beach) (court) Y93.68
- wake boarding Y93.17
- walking (on level or elevated terrain) Y93.01
    - an animal Y93.K1 (*following* Y93.7)
- walking an animal Y93.K1 (*following* Y93.7)
- wall climbing Y93.31
- warm up and cool down exercises Y93.A2 (*following* Y93.7)
- water NEC Y93.19
    - aerobics Y93.14
    - craft NEC Y93.19
    - exercise Y93.14
    - polo Y93.13
    - skiing Y93.17
    - sliding Y93.18
    - survival training and testing Y93.19
- weeding (garden and lawn) Y93.H2 (*following* Y93.7)
- wind instrument playing Y93.J4 (*following* Y93.7)
- windsurfing Y93.18
- wrestling Y93.72
- yoga Y93.42

Adverse effect of drugs — *see* Table of Drugs and Chemicals

Aerosinusitis — *see* Air, pressure

After-effect, late — *see* Sequelae

Air
- blast in war operations — *see* War operations, air blast
- pressure
    - change, rapid
        - during
            - ascent W94.29 ☑
                - while (in) (surfacing from)
                    - aircraft W94.23 ☑
                    - deep water diving W94.21 ☑
                    - underground W94.22 ☑
            - descent W94.39 ☑
                - in
                    - aircraft W94.31 ☑
                    - water W94.32 ☑
        - high, prolonged W94.0 ☑
        - low, prolonged W94.12 ☑
            - due to residence or long visit at high altitude W94.11 ☑

Alpine sickness W94.11 ☑

Altitude sickness W94.11 ☑

Anaphylactic shock, anaphylaxis — *see* Table of Drugs and Chemicals

Andes disease W94.11 ☑

Arachnidism, arachnoidism X58 ☑

Arson (with intent to injure or kill) X97 ☑

Asphyxia, asphyxiation
- by
    - food (bone) (seed) — *see* categories T17 and T18 ☑
    - gas (*see also* Table of Drugs and Chemicals)
        - legal
            - execution — *see* Legal, intervention, gas
            - intervention — *see* Legal, intervention, gas
- from
    - fire (*see also* Exposure, fire)
        - in war operations — *see* War operations, fire
    - ignition — *see* Ignition
    - vomitus T17.81 ☑
- in war operations — *see* War operations, restriction of airway

Aspiration
- food (any type) (into respiratory tract) (with asphyxia, obstruction respiratory tract, suffocation) — *see* categories T17 and T18 ☑
- foreign body — *see* Foreign body, aspiration
- vomitus (with asphyxia, obstruction respiratory tract, suffocation) T17.81 ☑

Assassination (attempt) — *see* Assault

Assault (homicidal) (by) (in) Y09
- arson X97 ☑
- bite (of human being) Y04.1 ☑
- bodily force Y04.8 ☑
    - bite Y04.1 ☑
    - bumping into Y04.2 ☑
    - sexual — *see* subcategories T74.0, T76.0 ☑
    - unarmed fight Y04.0 ☑
- bomb X96.9 ☑
    - antipersonnel X96.0 ☑
    - fertilizer X96.3 ☑
    - gasoline X96.1 ☑

▽ **Subterms under main terms may continue to next column or page**   ☑ **Additional Character Required — Refer to the Tabular List for Character Selection**   **399**

Activity — Assault

Assault — *continued*
  bomb — *continued*
    letter X96.2 ☑
    petrol X96.1 ☑
    pipe X96.3 ☑
    specified NEC X96.8 ☑
  brawl (hand) (fists) (foot) (unarmed) Y04.0 ☑
  burning, burns (by fire) NEC X97 ☑
    acid Y08.89 ☑
    caustic, corrosive substance Y08.89 ☑
    chemical from swallowing caustic, corrosive substance — *see* Table of Drugs and Chemicals
    cigarette(s) X97 ☑
    hot object X98.9 ☑
      fluid NEC X98.2 ☑
      household appliance X98.3 ☑
      specified NEC X98.8 ☑
      steam X98.0 ☑
      tap water X98.1 ☑
      vapors X98.0 ☑
    scalding — *see* Assault, burning
    steam X98.0 ☑
    vitriol Y08.89 ☑
  caustic, corrosive substance (gas) Y08.89 ☑
  crashing of
    aircraft Y08.81 ☑
    motor vehicle Y03.8 ☑
      pushed in front of Y02.0 ☑
      run over Y03.0 ☑
      specified NEC Y03.8 ☑
  cutting or piercing instrument X99.9 ☑
    dagger X99.2 ☑
    glass X99.0 ☑
    knife X99.1 ☑
    specified NEC X99.8 ☑
    sword X99.2 ☑
  dagger X99.2 ☑
  drowning (in) X92.9 ☑
    bathtub X92.0 ☑
    natural water X92.3 ☑
    specified NEC X92.8 ☑
    swimming pool X92.1 ☑
      following fall X92.2 ☑
  dynamite X96.8 ☑
  explosive(s) (material) X96.9 ☑
  fight (hand) (fists) (foot) (unarmed) Y04.0 ☑
    with weapon — *see* Assault, by type of weapon
  fire X97 ☑
  firearm X95.9 ☑
    airgun X95.01 ☑
    handgun X93 ☑
    hunting rifle X94.1 ☑
    larger X94.9 ☑
      specified NEC X94.8 ☑
    machine gun X94.2 ☑
    shotgun X94.0 ☑
    specified NEC X95.8 ☑
  from high place Y01 ☑
  gunshot (wound) NEC — *see* Assault, firearm, by type
  incendiary device X97 ☑
  injury Y09
    to child due to criminal abortion attempt NEC Y08.89 ☑
  knife X99.1 ☑
  late effect of — *see* categories X92-Y08 with 7th character S
  placing before moving object NEC Y02.8 ☑
    motor vehicle Y02.0 ☑
  poisoning — *see* categories T36-T65 with 7th character S
  puncture, any part of body — *see* Assault, cutting or piercing instrument
  pushing
    before moving object NEC Y02.8 ☑
      motor vehicle Y02.0 ☑
      subway train Y02.1 ☑
      train Y02.1 ☑
    from high place Y01 ☑
  rape T74.2- ☑
  scalding — *see* Assault, burning
  sequelae of — *see* categories X92-Y08 with 7th character S
  sexual (by bodily force) T74.2- ☑
  shooting — *see* Assault, firearm
  specified means NEC Y08.89 ☑

Assault — *continued*
  stab, any part of body — *see* Assault, cutting or piercing instrument
  steam X98.0 ☑
  striking against
    other person Y04.2 ☑
    sports equipment Y08.09 ☑
      baseball bat Y08.02 ☑
      hockey stick Y08.01 ☑
  struck by
    sports equipment Y08.09 ☑
      baseball bat Y08.02 ☑
      hockey stick Y08.01 ☑
  submersion — *see* Assault, drowning
  violence Y09
  weapon Y09
    blunt Y00 ☑
    cutting or piercing — *see* Assault, cutting or piercing instrument
    firearm — *see* Assault, firearm
  wound Y09
    cutting — *see* Assault, cutting or piercing instrument
    gunshot — *see* Assault, firearm
    knife X99.1 ☑
    piercing — *see* Assault, cutting or piercing instrument
    puncture — *see* Assault, cutting or piercing instrument
    stab — *see* Assault, cutting or piercing instrument
Attack by mammals NEC W55.89 ☑
Avalanche — *see* Landslide
Aviator's disease — *see* Air, pressure

B

Barotitis, barodontalgia, barosinusitis, barotrauma (otitic) (sinus) — *see* Air, pressure
Battered (baby) (child) (person) (syndrome) X58 ☑
Bayonet wound W26.1 ☑
  in
    legal intervention — *see* Legal, intervention, sharp object, bayonet
    war operations — *see* War operations, combat
  stated as undetermined whether accidental or intentional Y28.8 ☑
  suicide (attempt) X78.2 ☑
Bean in nose — *see* categories T17 and T18 ☑
Bed set on fire NEC — *see* Exposure, fire, uncontrolled, building, bed
Beheading (by guillotine)
  homicide X99.9 ☑
  legal execution — *see* Legal, intervention
Bending, injury in — *see* Overexertion
Bends — *see* Air, pressure, change
Bite, bitten by
  alligator W58.01 ☑
  arthropod (nonvenomous) NEC W57 ☑
  bull W55.21 ☑
  cat W55.01 ☑
  cow W55.21 ☑
  crocodile W58.11 ☑
  dog W54.0 ☑
  goat W55.31 ☑
  hoof stock NEC W55.31 ☑
  horse W55.11 ☑
  human being (accidentally) W50.3 ☑
    with intent to injure or kill Y04.1 ☑
    as, or caused by, a crowd or human stampede (with fall) W52 ☑
    assault Y04.1 ☑
    homicide (attempt) Y04.1 ☑
    in
      fight Y04.1 ☑
  insect (nonvenomous) W57 ☑
  lizard (nonvenomous) W59.01 ☑
  mammal NEC W55.81 ☑
  mammal NEC W55.81 ☑
    marine W56.31 ☑
  marine animal (nonvenomous) W56.81 ☑
  millipede W57 ☑
  moray eel W56.51 ☑
  mouse W53.01 ☑
  person(s) (accidentally) W50.3 ☑
    with intent to injure or kill Y04.1 ☑

Bite, bitten by — *continued*
  person(s) — *continued*
    as, or caused by, a crowd or human stampede (with fall) W52 ☑
      assault Y04.1 ☑
      homicide (attempt) Y04.1 ☑
      in
        fight Y04.1 ☑
  pig W55.41 ☑
  raccoon W55.51 ☑
  rat W53.11 ☑
  reptile W59.81 ☑
    lizard W59.01 ☑
    snake W59.11 ☑
    turtle W59.21 ☑
      terrestrial W59.81 ☑
  rodent W53.81 ☑
    mouse W53.01 ☑
    rat W53.11 ☑
    specified NEC W53.81 ☑
    squirrel W53.21 ☑
  shark W56.41 ☑
  sheep W55.31 ☑
  snake (nonvenomous) W59.11 ☑
  spider (nonvenomous) W57 ☑
  squirrel W53.21 ☑
Blast (air) in war operations — *see* War operations, blast
Blizzard X37.2 ☑
Blood alcohol level Y90.9
  less than 20mg/100ml Y90.0
  20-39mg/100ml Y90.1
  40-59mg/100ml Y90.2
  60-79mg/100ml Y90.3
  80-99mg/100ml Y90.4
  100-119mg/100ml Y90.5
  120-199mg/100ml Y90.6
  200-239mg/100ml Y90.7
  presence in blood, level not specified Y90.9
Blow X58 ☑
  by law-enforcing agent, police (on duty) — *see* Legal, intervention, manhandling
    blunt object — *see* Legal, intervention, blunt object
Blowing up — *see* Explosion
Brawl (hand) (fists) (foot) Y04.0 ☑
Breakage (accidental) (part of)
  ladder (causing fall) W11 ☑
  scaffolding (causing fall) W12 ☑
Broken
  glass, contact with — *see* Contact, with, glass
  power line (causing electric shock) W85 ☑
Bumping against, into (accidentally)
  object NEC W22.8 ☑
    with fall — *see* Fall, due to, bumping against, object
    caused by crowd or human stampede (with fall) W52 ☑
    sports equipment W21.9 ☑
  person(s) W51 ☑
    with fall W03 ☑
      due to ice or snow W00.0 ☑
    assault Y04.2 ☑
    caused by, a crowd or human stampede (with fall) W52 ☑
    homicide (attempt) Y04.2 ☑
  sports equipment W21.9 ☑
Burn, burned, burning (accidental) (by) (from) (on)
  acid NEC — *see* Table of Drugs and Chemicals
  bed linen — *see* Exposure, fire, uncontrolled, in building, bed
  blowtorch X08.8 ☑
    with ignition of clothing NEC X06.2 ☑
      nightwear X05 ☑
  bonfire, campfire (controlled) (*see also* Exposure, fire, controlled, not in building)
    uncontrolled — *see* Exposure, fire, uncontrolled, not in building
  candle X08.8 ☑
    with ignition of clothing NEC X06.2 ☑
      nightwear X05 ☑
  caustic liquid, substance (external) (internal) NEC — *see* Table of Drugs and Chemicals
  chemical (external) (internal) (*see also* Table of Drugs and Chemicals)
    in war operations — *see* War operations. fire
  cigar(s) or cigarette(s) X08.8 ☑

☑ **Additional Character Required** — Refer to the Tabular List for Character Selection   ▽ **Subterms under main terms may continue to next column or page**

Burn, burned, burning — *continued*
  cigar(s) or cigarette(s) — *continued*
    with ignition of clothing NEC X06.2 ☑
      nightwear X05 ☑
  clothes, clothing NEC (from controlled fire) X06.2 ☑
    with conflagration — *see* Exposure, fire, uncontrolled, building
      not in building or structure — *see* Exposure, fire, uncontrolled, not in building
  cooker (hot) X15.8 ☑
    stated as undetermined whether accidental or intentional Y27.3 ☑
    suicide (attempt) X77.3 ☑
  electric blanket X16 ☑
  engine (hot) X17 ☑
  fire, flames — *see* Exposure, fire
  flare, Very pistol — *see* Discharge, firearm NEC
  heat
    from appliance (electrical) (household) X15.8 ☑
      cooker X15.8 ☑
      hotplate X15.2 ☑
      kettle X15.8 ☑
      light bulb X15.8 ☑
      saucepan X15.3 ☑
      skillet X15.3 ☑
      stated as undetermined whether accidental or intentional Y27.3 ☑
      stove X15.0 ☑
      suicide (attempt) X77.3 ☑
      toaster X15.1 ☑
    in local application or packing during medical or surgical procedure Y63.5
  heating
    appliance, radiator or pipe X16 ☑
  homicide (attempt) — *see* Assault, burning
  hot
    air X14.1 ☑
    cooker X15.8 ☑
    drink X10.0 ☑
    engine X17 ☑
    fat X10.2 ☑
    fluid NEC X12 ☑
    food X10.1 ☑
    gases X14.1 ☑
    heating appliance X16 ☑
    household appliance NEC X15.8 ☑
    kettle X15.8 ☑
    liquid NEC X12 ☑
    machinery X17 ☑
    metal (molten) (liquid) NEC X18 ☑
    object (not producing fire or flames) NEC X19 ☑
    oil (cooking) X10.2 ☑
    pipe(s) X16 ☑
    radiator X16 ☑
    saucepan (glass) (metal) X15.3 ☑
    stove (kitchen) X15.0 ☑
    substance NEC X19 ☑
      caustic or corrosive NEC — *see* Table of Drugs and Chemicals
    toaster X15.1 ☑
    tool X17 ☑
    vapor X13.1 ☑
    water (tap) — *see* Contact, with, hot, tap water
  hotplate X15.2 ☑
    suicide (attempt) X77.3 ☑
  ignition — *see* Ignition
  in war operations — *see* War operations, fire
  inflicted by other person X97 ☑
    by hot objects, hot vapor, and steam — *see* Assault, burning, hot object
  internal, from swallowed caustic, corrosive liquid, substance — *see* Table of Drugs and Chemicals
  iron (hot) X15.8 ☑
    stated as undetermined whether accidental or intentional Y27.3 ☑
    suicide (attempt) X77.3 ☑
  kettle (hot) X15.8 ☑
    stated as undetermined whether accidental or intentional Y27.3 ☑
    suicide (attempt) X77.3 ☑
  lamp (flame) X08.8 ☑
    with ignition of clothing NEC X06.2 ☑
      nightwear X05 ☑
  lighter (cigar) (cigarette) X08.8 ☑
    with ignition of clothing NEC X06.2 ☑
      nightwear X05 ☑

Burn, burned, burning — *continued*
  lightning — *see* subcategory T75.0 ☑
    causing fire — *see* Exposure, fire
  liquid (boiling) (hot) NEC X12 ☑
    stated as undetermined whether accidental or intentional Y27.2 ☑
    suicide (attempt) X77.2 ☑
  local application of externally applied substance in medical or surgical care Y63.5
  machinery (hot) X17 ☑
  matches X08.8 ☑
    with ignition of clothing NEC X06.2 ☑
      nightwear X05 ☑
  mattress — *see* Exposure, fire, uncontrolled, building, bed
  medicament, externally applied Y63.5
  metal (hot) (liquid) (molten) NEC X18 ☑
  nightwear (nightclothes, nightdress, gown, pajamas, robe) X05 ☑
  object (hot) NEC X19 ☑
  on board watercraft
    due to
      accident to watercraft V91.09 ☑
        powered craft V91.03 ☑
          ferry boat V91.01 ☑
          fishing boat V91.02 ☑
          jetskis V91.03 ☑
          liner V91.01 ☑
          merchant ship V91.00 ☑
          passenger ship V91.01 ☑
        unpowered craft V91.08 ☑
          canoe V91.05 ☑
          inflatable V91.06 ☑
          kayak V91.05 ☑
          sailboat V91.04 ☑
          surf-board V91.08 ☑
          water skis V91.07 ☑
          windsurfer V91.08 ☑
      fire on board V93.09 ☑
        ferry boat V93.01 ☑
        fishing boat V93.02 ☑
        jetskis V93.03 ☑
        liner V93.01 ☑
        merchant ship V93.00 ☑
        passenger ship V93.01 ☑
        powered craft NEC V93.03 ☑
        sailboat V93.04 ☑
      specified heat source NEC on board V93.19 ☑
        ferry boat V93.11 ☑
        fishing boat V93.12 ☑
        jetskis V93.13 ☑
        liner V93.11 ☑
        merchant ship V93.10 ☑
        passenger ship V93.11 ☑
        powered craft NEC V93.13 ☑
        sailboat V93.14 ☑
  pipe (hot) X16 ☑
  smoking X08.8 ☑
    with ignition of clothing NEC X06.2 ☑
      nightwear X05 ☑
  powder — *see* Powder burn
  radiator (hot) X16 ☑
  saucepan (hot) (glass) (metal) X15.3 ☑
    stated as undetermined whether accidental or intentional Y27.3 ☑
    suicide (attempt) X77.3 ☑
  self-inflicted X76 ☑
    stated as undetermined whether accidental or intentional Y26 ☑
  stated as undetermined whether accidental or intentional Y27.0 ☑
  steam X13.1 ☑
    pipe X16 ☑
    stated as undetermined whether accidental or intentional Y27.8 ☑
    stated as undetermined whether accidental or intentional Y27.0 ☑
    suicide (attempt) X77.0 ☑
  stove (hot) (kitchen) X15.0 ☑
    stated as undetermined whether accidental or intentional Y27.3 ☑
    suicide (attempt) X77.3 ☑
  substance (hot) NEC X19 ☑
    boiling X12 ☑
      stated as undetermined whether accidental or intentional Y27.2 ☑

Burn, burned, burning — *continued*
  substance — *continued*
    boiling — *continued*
      suicide (attempt) X77.2 ☑
    molten (metal) X18 ☑
    suicide (attempt) NEC X76 ☑
      hot
        household appliance X77.3 ☑
        object X77.9 ☑
    therapeutic misadventure
      heat in local application or packing during medical or surgical procedure Y63.5
      overdose of radiation Y63.2
  toaster (hot) X15.1 ☑
    stated as undetermined whether accidental or intentional Y27.3 ☑
    suicide (attempt) X77.3 ☑
  tool (hot) X17 ☑
  torch, welding X08.8 ☑
    with ignition of clothing NEC X06.2 ☑
      nightwear X05 ☑
  trash fire (controlled) — *see* Exposure, fire, controlled, not in building
    uncontrolled — *see* Exposure, fire, uncontrolled, not in building
  vapor (hot) X13.1 ☑
    stated as undetermined whether accidental or intentional Y27.0 ☑
    suicide (attempt) X77.0 ☑
  Very pistol — *see* Discharge, firearm NEC
Butted by animal W55.82 ☑
  bull W55.22 ☑
  cow W55.22 ☑
  goat W55.32 ☑
  horse W55.12 ☑
  pig W55.42 ☑
  sheep W55.32 ☑

C

Caisson disease — *see* Air, pressure, change
Campfire (exposure to) (controlled) (*see also* Exposure, fire, controlled, not in building)
  uncontrolled — *see* Exposure, fire, uncontrolled, not in building
Capital punishment (any means) — *see* Legal, intervention
Car sickness T75.3 ☑
Casualty (not due to war) NEC X58 ☑
  war — *see* War operations
Cat
  bite W55.01 ☑
  scratch W55.03 ☑
Cataclysm, cataclysmic (any injury) NEC — *see* Forces of nature
Catching fire — *see* Exposure, fire
Caught
  between
    folding object W23.0 ☑
    objects (moving) (stationary and moving) W23.0 ☑
      and machinery — *see* Contact, with, by type of machine
      stationary W23.1 ☑
    sliding door and door frame W23.0 ☑
  by, in
    machinery (moving parts of) — *see* Contact, with, by type of machine
    washing-machine wringer W23.0 ☑
  under packing crate (due to losing grip) W23.1 ☑
Cave-in caused by cataclysmic earth surface movement or eruption — *see* Landslide
Change(s) in air pressure — *see* Air, pressure, change
Choked, choking (on) (any object except food or vomitus)
  food (bone) (seed) — *see* categories T17 and T18 ☑
  vomitus T17.81- ☑
Civil insurrection — *see* War operations
Cloudburst (any injury) X37.8 ☑
Cold, exposure to (accidental) (excessive) (extreme) (natural) (place) NEC — *see* Exposure, cold
Collapse
  building W20.1 ☑
    burning (uncontrolled fire) X00.2 ☑
  dam or man-made structure (causing earth movement) X36.0 ☑
  machinery — *see* Contact, with, by type of machine

Collapse — *continued*
structure W20.1 ☑
burning (uncontrolled fire) X00.2 ☑
Collision (accidental) NEC (*see also* Accident, transport)
V89.9 ☑
pedestrian W51 ☑
with fall W03 ☑
due to ice or snow W00.0 ☑
involving pedestrian conveyance — *see* Accident, transport, pedestrian, conveyance
and
crowd or human stampede (with fall) W52 ☑
object W22.8 ☑
with fall — *see* Fall, due to, bumping against, object
person(s) — *see* Collision, pedestrian
transport vehicle NEC V89.9 ☑
and
avalanche, fallen or not moving — *see* Accident, transport
falling or moving — *see* Landslide
landslide, fallen or not moving — *see* Accident, transport
falling or moving — *see* Landslide
due to cataclysm — *see* Forces of nature, by type
intentional, purposeful suicide (attempt) — *see* Suicide, collision
Combustion, spontaneous — *see* Ignition
Complication (delayed) **of or following** (medical or surgical procedure) Y84.9
with misadventure — *see* Misadventure
amputation of limb(s) Y83.5
anastomosis (arteriovenous) (blood vessel) (gastrojejunal) (tendon) (natural or artificial material) Y83.2
aspiration (of fluid) Y84.4
tissue Y84.8
biopsy Y84.8
blood
sampling Y84.7
transfusion
procedure Y84.8
bypass Y83.2
catheterization (urinary) Y84.6
cardiac Y84.0
colostomy Y83.3
cystostomy Y83.3
dialysis (kidney) Y84.1
drug — *see* Table of Drugs and Chemicals
due to misadventure — *see* Misadventure
duodenostomy Y83.3
electroshock therapy Y84.3
external stoma, creation of Y83.3
formation of external stoma Y83.3
gastrostomy Y83.3
graft Y83.2
hypothermia (medically-induced) Y84.8
implant, implantation (of)
artificial
internal device (cardiac pacemaker) (electrodes in brain) (heart valve prosthesis) (orthopedic) Y83.1
material or tissue (for anastomosis or bypass) Y83.2
with creation of external stoma Y83.3
natural tissues (for anastomosis or bypass) Y83.2
with creation of external stoma Y83.3
infusion
procedure Y84.8
injection — *see* Table of Drugs and Chemicals
procedure Y84.8
insertion of gastric or duodenal sound Y84.5
insulin-shock therapy Y84.3
paracentesis (abdominal) (thoracic) (aspirative) Y84.4
procedures other than surgical operation — *see* Complication of or following, by type of procedure
radiological procedure or therapy Y84.2
removal of organ (partial) (total) NEC Y83.6
sampling
blood Y84.7
fluid NEC Y84.4
tissue Y84.8
shock therapy Y84.3
surgical operation NEC (*see also* Complication of or following, by type of operation) Y83.9
reconstructive NEC Y83.4
with

Complication (delayed) **of or following** — *continued*
surgical operation (*see also* Complication of or following, by type of operation) — *continued*
reconstructive — *continued*
with — *continued*
anastomosis, bypass or graft Y83.2
formation of external stoma Y83.3
specified NEC Y83.8
transfusion (*see also* Table of Drugs and Chemicals)
procedure Y84.8
transplant, transplantation (heart) (kidney) (liver) (whole organ, any) Y83.0
partial organ Y83.4
ureterostomy Y83.3
vaccination (*see also* Table of Drugs and Chemicals)
procedure Y84.8
Compression
divers' squeeze — *see* Air, pressure, change
trachea by
food (lodged in esophagus) — *see* categories T17 and T18 ☑
vomitus (lodged in esophagus) T17.81- ☑
Conflagration — *see* Exposure, fire, uncontrolled
Constriction (external)
hair W49.01 ☑
jewelry W49.04 ☑
ring W49.04 ☑
rubber band W49.03 ☑
specified item NEC W49.09 ☑
string W49.02 ☑
thread W49.02 ☑
Contact (accidental)
with
abrasive wheel (metalworking) W31.1 ☑
alligator W58.09 ☑
bite W58.01 ☑
crushing W58.03 ☑
strike W58.02 ☑
amphibian W62.9 ☑
frog W62.0 ☑
toad W62.1 ☑
animal (nonvenomous) NEC W64 ☑
marine W56.89 ☑
bite W56.81 ☑
dolphin — *see* Contact, with, dolphin
fish NEC — *see* Contact, with, fish
mammal — *see* Contact, with, mammal, marine
orca — *see* Contact, with, orca
sea lion — *see* Contact, with, sea lion
shark — *see* Contact, with, shark
strike W56.82 ☑
animate mechanical force NEC W64 ☑
arrow W21.89 ☑
not thrown, projected or falling W45.8 ☑
arthropods (nonvenomous) W57 ☑
axe W27.0 ☑
band-saw (industrial) W31.2 ☑
bayonet — *see* Bayonet wound
bee(s) X58 ☑
bench-saw (industrial) W31.2 ☑
bird W61.99 ☑
bite W61.91 ☑
chicken — *see* Contact, with, chicken
duck — *see* Contact, with, duck
goose — *see* Contact, with, goose
macaw — *see* Contact, with, macaw
parrot — *see* Contact, with, parrot
psittacine — *see* Contact, with, psittacine
strike W61.92 ☑
turkey — *see* Contact, with, turkey
blender W29.0 ☑
boiling water X12 ☑
stated as undetermined whether accidental or intentional Y27.2 ☑
suicide (attempt) X77.2 ☑
bore, earth-drilling or mining (land) (seabed) W31.0 ☑
buffalo — *see* Contact, with, hoof stock NEC
bull W55.29 ☑
bite W55.21 ☑
gored W55.22 ☑
strike W55.22 ☑
bumper cars W31.81 ☑
camel — *see* Contact, with, hoof stock NEC

Contact — *continued*
with — *continued*
can
lid W45.2 ☑
opener W27.4 ☑
powered W29.0 ☑
cat W55.09 ☑
bite W55.01 ☑
scratch W55.03 ☑
caterpillar (venomous) X58 ☑
centipede (venomous) X58 ☑
chain
hoist W24.0 ☑
agricultural operations W30.89 ☑
saw W29.3 ☑
chicken W61.39 ☑
peck W61.33 ☑
strike W61.32 ☑
chisel W27.0 ☑
circular saw W31.2 ☑
cobra X58 ☑
combine (harvester) W30.0 ☑
conveyer belt W24.1 ☑
cooker (hot) X15.8 ☑
stated as undetermined whether accidental or intentional Y27.3 ☑
suicide (attempt) X77.3 ☑
coral X58 ☑
cotton gin W31.82 ☑
cow W55.29 ☑
bite W55.21 ☑
strike W55.22 ☑
crane W24.0 ☑
agricultural operations W30.89 ☑
crocodile W58.19 ☑
bite W58.11 ☑
crushing W58.13 ☑
strike W58.12 ☑
dagger W26.1 ☑
stated as undetermined whether accidental or intentional Y28.2 ☑
suicide (attempt) X78.2 ☑
dairy equipment W31.82 ☑
dart W21.89 ☑
not thrown, projected or falling W45.8 ☑
deer — *see* Contact, with, hoof stock NEC
derrick W24.0 ☑
agricultural operations W30.89 ☑
hay W30.2 ☑
dog W54.8 ☑
bite W54.0 ☑
strike W54.1 ☑
dolphin W56.09 ☑
bite W56.01 ☑
strike W56.02 ☑
donkey — *see* Contact, with, hoof stock NEC
drill (powered) W29.8 ☑
earth (land) (seabed) W31.0 ☑
nonpowered W27.8 ☑
drive belt W24.0 ☑
agricultural operations W30.89 ☑
dry ice — *see* Exposure, cold, man-made
dryer (clothes) (powered) (spin) W29.2 ☑
duck W61.69 ☑
bite W61.61 ☑
strike W61.62 ☑
earth (-)
drilling machine (industrial) W31.0 ☑
scraping machine in stationary use W31.83 ☑
edge of stiff paper W45.1 ☑
electric
beater W29.0 ☑
blanket X16 ☑
fan W29.2 ☑
commercial W31.82 ☑
knife W29.1 ☑
mixer W29.0 ☑
elevator (building) W24.0 ☑
agricultural operations W30.89 ☑
grain W30.3 ☑
engine(s), hot NEC X17 ☑
excavating machine W31.0 ☑
farm machine W30.9 ☑
feces — *see* Contact, with, by type of animal
fer de lance X58 ☑

402
☑ **Additional Character Required** — Refer to the Tabular List for Character Selection
⬛ **Subterms under main terms may continue to next column or page**

Contact — *continued*
  with — *continued*
    fish W56.59 ☑
      bite W56.51 ☑
      shark — *see* Contact, with, shark
      strike W56.52 ☑
    flying horses W31.81 ☑
    forging (metalworking) machine W31.1 ☑
    fork W27.4 ☑
    forklift (truck) W24.0 ☑
      agricultural operations W30.89 ☑
    frog W62.0 ☑
    garden
      cultivator (powered) W29.3 ☑
        riding W30.89 ☑
      fork W27.1 ☑
    gas turbine W31.3 ☑
    Gila monster X58 ☑
    giraffe — *see* Contact, with, hoof stock NEC
    glass (sharp) (broken) W25 ☑
      with subsequent fall W18.02 ☑
      assault X99.0 ☑
      due to fall — *see* Fall, by type
      stated as undetermined whether accidental or
        intentional Y28.0 ☑
      suicide (attempt) X78.0 ☑
    goat W55.39 ☑
      bite W55.31 ☑
      strike W55.32 ☑
    goose W61.59 ☑
      bite W61.51 ☑
      strike W61.52 ☑
    hand
      saw W27.0 ☑
      tool (not powered) NEC W27.8 ☑
        powered W29.8 ☑
    harvester W30.0 ☑
    hay-derrick W30.2 ☑
    heating
      appliance (hot) X16 ☑
      pad (electric) X16 ☑
    heat NEC X19 ☑
      from appliance (electrical) (household) — *see*
        Contact, with, hot, household appliance
      heating appliance X16 ☑
    hedge-trimmer (powered) W29.3 ☑
    hoe W27.1 ☑
    hoist (chain) (shaft) NEC W24.0 ☑
      agricultural W30.89 ☑
    hoof stock NEC W55.39 ☑
      bite W55.31 ☑
      strike W55.32 ☑
    hornet(s) X58 ☑
    horse W55.19 ☑
      bite W55.11 ☑
      strike W55.12 ☑
    hot
      air X14.1 ☑
        inhalation X14.0 ☑
      cooker X15.8 ☑
      drinks X10.0 ☑
      engine X17 ☑
      fats X10.2 ☑
      fluids NEC X12 ☑
        assault X98.2 ☑
        suicide (attempt) X77.2 ☑
        undetermined whether accidental or inten-
          tional Y27.2 ☑
      food X10.1 ☑
      gases X14.1 ☑
        inhalation X14.0 ☑
      heating appliance X16 ☑
      household appliance X15.8 ☑
        assault X98.3 ☑
        cooker X15.8 ☑
        hotplate X15.2 ☑
        kettle X15.8 ☑
        light bulb X15.8 ☑
        object NEC X19 ☑
          assault X98.8 ☑
          stated as undetermined whether acciden-
            tal or intentional Y27.9 ☑
          suicide (attempt) X77.8 ☑
        saucepan X15.3 ☑
        skillet X15.3 ☑

Contact — *continued*
  with — *continued*
    hot — *continued*
      household appliance — *continued*
        stated as undetermined whether accidental
          or intentional Y27.3 ☑
        stove X15.0 ☑
        suicide (attempt) X77.3 ☑
        toaster X15.1 ☑
      kettle X15.8 ☑
      light bulb X15.8 ☑
      liquid NEC (*see also* Burn) X12 ☑
        drinks X10.0 ☑
        stated as undetermined whether accidental
          or intentional Y27.2 ☑
        suicide (attempt) X77.2 ☑
        tap water X11.8 ☑
          stated as undetermined whether acciden-
            tal or intentional Y27.1 ☑
          suicide (attempt) X77.1 ☑
      machinery X17 ☑
      metal (molten) (liquid) NEC X18 ☑
      object (not producing fire or flames) NEC X19 ☑
      oil (cooking) X16 ☑
      pipe X16 ☑
      plate X15.2 ☑
      radiator X16 ☑
      saucepan (glass) (metal) X15.3 ☑
      skillet X15.3 ☑
      stove (kitchen) X15.0 ☑
      substance NEC X19 ☑
      tap-water X11.8 ☑
        assault X98.1 ☑
        heated on stove X12 ☑
          stated as undetermined whether whether
            tal or intentional Y27.2 ☑
          suicide (attempt) X77.2 ☑
        in bathtub X11.0 ☑
        running X11.1 ☑
        stated as undetermined whether accidental
          or intentional Y27.1 ☑
        suicide (attempt) X77.1 ☑
      toaster X15.1 ☑
      tool X17 ☑
      vapors X13.1 ☑
        inhalation X13.0 ☑
      water (tap) X11.8 ☑
        boiling X12 ☑
          stated as undetermined whether acciden-
            tal or intentional Y27.2 ☑
          suicide (attempt) X77.2 ☑
        heated on stove X12 ☑
          stated as undetermined whether acciden-
            tal or intentional Y27.2 ☑
          suicide (attempt) X77.2 ☑
        in bathtub X11.0 ☑
        running X11.1 ☑
        stated as undetermined whether accidental
          or intentional Y27.1 ☑
        suicide (attempt) X77.1 ☑
    hotplate X15.2 ☑
    ice-pick W27.4 ☑
    insect (nonvenomous) NEC W57 ☑
    kettle (hot) X15.8 ☑
    knife W26.0 ☑
      assault X99.1 ☑
      electric W29.1 ☑
      stated as undetermined whether accidental or
        intentional Y28.1 ☑
      suicide (attempt) X78.1 ☑
    lathe (metalworking) W31.1 ☑
      turnings W45.8 ☑
      woodworking W31.2 ☑
    lawnmower (powered) (ridden) W28 ☑
      causing electrocution W86.8 ☑
        suicide (attempt) X83.1 ☑
      unpowered W27.1 ☑
    lift, lifting (devices) W24.0 ☑
      agricultural operations W30.89 ☑
      shaft W24.0 ☑
    liquefied gas — *see* Exposure, cold, man-made
    liquid air, hydrogen, nitrogen — *see* Exposure, cold,
      man-made
    lizard (nonvenomous) W59.09 ☑
      bite W59.01 ☑
      strike W59.02 ☑

Contact — *continued*
  with — *continued*
    llama — *see* Contact, with, hoof stock NEC
    macaw W61.19 ☑
      bite W61.11 ☑
      strike W61.12 ☑
    machine, machinery W31.9 ☑
      abrasive wheel W31.1 ☑
      agricultural including animal-powered
        W30.9 ☑
        combine harvester W30.0 ☑
        grain storage elevator W30.3 ☑
        hay derrick W30.2 ☑
        power take-off device W30.1 ☑
        reaper W30.0 ☑
        specified NEC W30.89 ☑
        thresher W30.0 ☑
        transport vehicle, stationary W30.81 ☑
      band saw W31.2 ☑
      bench saw W31.2 ☑
      circular saw W31.2 ☑
      commercial NEC W31.82 ☑
      drilling, metal (industrial) W31.1 ☑
      earth-drilling W31.0 ☑
      earthmoving or scraping W31.89 ☑
      excavating W31.89 ☑
      forging machine W31.1 ☑
      gas turbine W31.3 ☑
      hot X17 ☑
      internal combustion engine W31.3 ☑
      land drill W31.0 ☑
      lathe W31.1 ☑
      lifting (devices) W24.0 ☑
      metal drill W31.1 ☑
      metalworking (industrial) W31.1 ☑
      milling, metal W31.1 ☑
      mining W31.0 ☑
      molding W31.2 ☑
      overhead plane W31.2 ☑
      power press, metal W31.1 ☑
      prime mover W31.3 ☑
      printing W31.89 ☑
      radial saw W31.2 ☑
      recreational W31.81 ☑
      roller-coaster W31.81 ☑
      rolling mill, metal W31.1 ☑
      sander W31.2 ☑
      seabed drill W31.0 ☑
      shaft
        hoist W31.0 ☑
        lift W31.0 ☑
      specified NEC W31.89 ☑
      spinning W31.89 ☑
      steam engine W31.3 ☑
      transmission W24.1 ☑
      undercutter W31.0 ☑
      water driven turbine W31.3 ☑
      weaving W31.89 ☑
      woodworking or forming (industrial) W31.2 ☑
    mammal (feces) (urine) W55.89 ☑
      bull — *see* Contact, with, bull
      cat — *see* Contact, with, cat
      cow — *see* Contact, with, cow
      goat — *see* Contact, with, goat
      hoof stock — *see* Contact, with, hoof stock
      horse — *see* Contact, with, horse
      marine W56.39 ☑
        dolphin — *see* Contact, with, dolphin
        orca — *see* Contact, with, orca
        sea lion — *see* Contact, with, sea lion
        specified NEC W56.39 ☑
          bite W56.31 ☑
          strike W56.32 ☑
      pig — *see* Contact, with, pig
      raccoon — *see* Contact, with, raccoon
      rodent — *see* Contact, with, rodent
      sheep — *see* Contact, with, sheep
      specified NEC W55.89 ☑
        bite W55.81 ☑
        strike W55.82 ☑
    marine
      animal W56.89 ☑
        bite W56.81 ☑
        dolphin — *see* Contact, with, dolphin
        fish NEC — *see* Contact, with, fish

▽ **Subterms under main terms may continue to next column or page**   ☑ **Additional Character Required — Refer to the Tabular List for Character Selection**   **403**

Contact — Contact

Contact — *continued*
  with — *continued*
    marine — *continued*
      animal — *continued*
        mammal — *see* Contact, with, mammal, marine
        orca — *see* Contact, with, orca
        sea lion — *see* Contact, with, sea lion
        shark — *see* Contact, with, shark
        strike W56.82 ☑
    meat
      grinder (domestic) W29.0 ☑
        industrial W31.82 ☑
        nonpowered W27.4 ☑
      slicer (domestic) W29.0 ☑
        industrial W31.82 ☑
    merry go round W31.81 ☑
    metal, hot (liquid) (molten) NEC X18 ☑
    millipede W57 ☑
    nail W45.0 ☑
      gun W29.4 ☑
    needle (sewing) W27.3 ☑
      hypodermic W46.0 ☑
        contaminated W46.1 ☑
    object (blunt) NEC
      hot NEC X19 ☑
      legal intervention — *see* Legal, intervention, blunt object
      sharp NEC W45.8 ☑
        inflicted by other person NEC W45.8 ☑
          stated as
            intentional homicide (attempt) — *see* Assault, cutting or piercing instrument
        legal intervention — *see* Legal, intervention, sharp object
        self-inflicted X78.9 ☑
    orca W56.29 ☑
      bite W56.21 ☑
      strike W56.22 ☑
    overhead plane W31.2 ☑
    paper (as sharp object) W45.1 ☑
    paper-cutter W27.5 ☑
    parrot W61.09 ☑
      bite W61.01 ☑
      strike W61.02 ☑
    pig W55.49 ☑
      bite W55.41 ☑
      strike W55.42 ☑
    pipe, hot X16 ☑
    pitchfork W27.1 ☑
    plane (metal) (wood) W27.0 ☑
      overhead W31.2 ☑
    plant thorns, spines, sharp leaves or other mechanisms W60 ☑
    powered
      garden cultivator W29.3 ☑
      household appliance, implement, or machine W29.8 ☑
      saw (industrial) W31.2 ☑
        hand W29.8 ☑
    printing machine W31.89 ☑
    psittacine bird W61.29 ☑
      bite W61.21 ☑
      macaw — *see* Contact, with, macaw
      parrot — *see* Contact, with, parrot
      strike W61.22 ☑
    pulley (block) (transmission) W24.0 ☑
      agricultural operations W30.89 ☑
    raccoon W55.59 ☑
      bite W55.51 ☑
      strike W55.52 ☑
    radial-saw (industrial) W31.2 ☑
    radiator (hot) X16 ☑
    rake W27.1 ☑
    rattlesnake X58 ☑
    reaper W30.0 ☑
    reptile W59.89 ☑
      lizard — *see* Contact, with, lizard
      snake — *see* Contact, with, snake
      specified NEC W59.89 ☑
        bite W59.81 ☑
        crushing W59.83 ☑
        strike W59.82 ☑
      turtle — *see* Contact, with, turtle
    rivet gun (powered) W29.4 ☑

Contact — *continued*
  with — *continued*
    road scraper — *see* Accident, transport, construction vehicle
    rodent (feces) (urine) W53.89 ☑
      bite W53.81 ☑
      mouse W53.09 ☑
        bite W53.01 ☑
      rat W53.19 ☑
        bite W53.11 ☑
      specified NEC W53.89 ☑
        bite W53.81 ☑
      squirrel W53.29 ☑
        bite W53.21 ☑
    roller coaster W31.81 ☑
    rope NEC W24.0 ☑
      agricultural operations W30.89 ☑
    saliva — *see* Contact, with, by type of animal
    sander W29.8 ☑
      industrial W31.2 ☑
    saucepan (hot) (glass) (metal) X15.3 ☑
    saw W27.0 ☑
      band (industrial) W31.2 ☑
      bench (industrial) W31.2 ☑
      chain W29.3 ☑
      hand W27.0 ☑
    sawing machine, metal W31.1 ☑
    scissors W27.2 ☑
    scorpion X58 ☑
    screwdriver W27.0 ☑
      powered W29.8 ☑
    sea
      anemone, cucumber or urchin (spine) X58 ☑
      lion W56.19 ☑
        bite W56.11 ☑
        strike W56.12 ☑
    serpent — *see* Contact, with, snake, by type
    sewing-machine (electric) (powered) W29.2 ☑
      not powered W27.8 ☑
    shaft (hoist) (lift) (transmission) NEC W24.0 ☑
      agricultural W30.89 ☑
    shark W56.49 ☑
      bite W56.41 ☑
      strike W56.42 ☑
    shears (hand) W27.2 ☑
      powered (industrial) W31.1 ☑
        domestic W29.2 ☑
    sheep W55.39 ☑
      bite W55.31 ☑
      strike W55.32 ☑
    shovel W27.8 ☑
      steam — *see* Accident, transport, construction vehicle
    snake (nonvenomous) W59.19 ☑
      bite W59.11 ☑
      crushing W59.13 ☑
      strike W59.12 ☑
    spade W27.1 ☑
    spider (venomous) X58 ☑
    spin-drier W29.2 ☑
    spinning machine W31.89 ☑
    splinter W45.8 ☑
    sports equipment W21.9 ☑
    staple gun (powered) W29.8 ☑
    steam X13.1 ☑
      engine W31.3 ☑
      inhalation X13.0 ☑
      pipe X16 ☑
      shovel W31.89 ☑
    stove (hot) (kitchen) X15.0 ☑
    substance, hot NEC X19 ☑
      molten (metal) X18 ☑
    sword W26.1 ☑
      assault X99.2 ☑
      stated as undetermined whether accidental or intentional Y28.2 ☑
      suicide (attempt) X78.2 ☑
    tarantula X58 ☑
    thresher W30.0 ☑
    tin can lid W45.2 ☑
    toad W62.1 ☑
    toaster (hot) X15.1 ☑
    tool W27.8 ☑
      hand (not powered) W27.8 ☑
        auger W27.0 ☑

Contact *continued*
  with — *continued*
    tool — *continued*
      hand — *continued*
        axe W27.0 ☑
        can opener W27.4 ☑
        chisel W27.0 ☑
        fork W27.4 ☑
        garden W27.1 ☑
        handsaw W27.0 ☑
        hoe W27.1 ☑
        ice-pick W27.4 ☑
        kitchen utensil W27.4 ☑
        manual
          lawn mower W27.1 ☑
          sewing machine W27.8 ☑
        meat grinder W27.4 ☑
        needle (sewing) W27.3 ☑
          hypodermic W46.0 ☑
            contaminated W46.1 ☑
        paper cutter W27.5 ☑
        pitchfork W27.1 ☑
        rake W27.1 ☑
        scissors W27.2 ☑
        screwdriver W27.0 ☑
        specified NEC W27.8 ☑
        workbench W27.0 ☑
      hot X17 ☑
      powered W29.8 ☑
        blender W29.0 ☑
          commercial W31.82 ☑
        can opener W29.0 ☑
          commercial W31.82 ☑
        chainsaw W29.3 ☑
        clothes dryer W29.2 ☑
          commercial W31.82 ☑
        dishwasher W29.2 ☑
          commercial W31.82 ☑
        edger W29.3 ☑
        electric fan W29.2 ☑
          commercial W31.82 ☑
        electric knife W29.1 ☑
        food processor W29.0 ☑
          commercial W31.82 ☑
        garbage disposal W29.0 ☑
          commercial W31.82 ☑
        garden tool W29.3 ☑
        hedge trimmer W29.3 ☑
        ice maker W29.0 ☑
          commercial W31.82 ☑
        kitchen appliance W29.0 ☑
          commercial W31.82 ☑
        lawn mower W28 ☑
        meat grinder W29.0 ☑
          commercial W31.82 ☑
        mixer W29.0 ☑
          commercial W31.82 ☑
        rototiller W29.3 ☑
        sewing machine W29.2 ☑
          commercial W31.82 ☑
        washing machine W29.2 ☑
          commercial W31.82 ☑
    transmission device (belt, cable, chain, gear, pinion, shaft) W24.1 ☑
      agricultural operations W30.89 ☑
    turbine (gas) (water-driven) W31.3 ☑
    turkey W61.49 ☑
      peck W61.43 ☑
      strike W61.42 ☑
    turtle (nonvenomous) W59.29 ☑
      bite W59.21 ☑
      strike W59.22 ☑
      terrestrial W59.89 ☑
        bite W59.81 ☑
        crushing W59.83 ☑
        strike W59.82 ☑
    under-cutter W31.0 ☑
    urine — *see* Contact, with, by type of animal
    vehicle
      agricultural use (transport) — *see* Accident, transport, agricultural vehicle
        not on public highway W30.81 ☑
      industrial use (transport) — *see* Accident, transport, industrial vehicle
        not on public highway W31.83 ☑

Contact — *continued*
  with — *continued*
    vehicle — *continued*
      off-road use (transport) — *see* Accident, transport, all-terrain or off-road vehicle
        not on public highway W31.83 ☑
      special construction use (transport) — *see* Accident, transport, construction vehicle
        not on public highway W31.83 ☑
    venomous
      animal X58 ☑
      arthropods X58 ☑
      lizard X58 ☑
      marine animal NEC X58 ☑
      marine plant NEC X58 ☑
      millipedes (tropical) X58 ☑
      plant(s) X58 ☑
      snake X58 ☑
      spider X58 ☑
      viper X58 ☑
    washing-machine (powered) W29.2 ☑
    wasp X58 ☑
    weaving-machine W31.89 ☑
    winch W24.0 ☑
      agricultural operations W30.89 ☑
    wire NEC W24.0 ☑
      agricultural operations W30.89 ☑
    wood slivers W45.8 ☑
    yellow jacket X58 ☑
    zebra — *see* Contact, with, hoof stock NEC
Coup de soleil X32 ☑
Crash
  aircraft (in transit) (powered) V95.9 ☑
    balloon V96.01 ☑
    fixed wing NEC (private) V95.21 ☑
      commercial V95.31 ☑
    glider V96.21 ☑
      hang V96.11 ☑
      powered V95.11 ☑
    helicopter V95.01 ☑
    in war operations — *see* War operations, destruction of aircraft
    microlight V95.11 ☑
    nonpowered V96.9 ☑
      specified NEC V96.8 ☑
    powered NEC V95.8 ☑
    stated as
      homicide (attempt) Y08.81 ☑
      suicide (attempt) X83.0 ☑
    ultralight V95.11 ☑
  spacecraft V95.41 ☑
  transport vehicle NEC (*see also* Accident, transport) V89.9 ☑
    homicide (attempt) Y03.8 ☑
    motor NEC (traffic) V89.2 ☑
      homicide (attempt) Y03.8 ☑
      suicide (attempt) — *see* Suicide, collision
Cruelty (mental) (physical) (sexual) X58 ☑
Crushed (accidentally) X58 ☑
  between objects (moving) (stationary and moving) W23.0 ☑
    stationary W23.1 ☑
  by
    alligator W58.03 ☑
    avalanche NEC — *see* Landslide
    cave-in W20.0 ☑
      caused by cataclysmic earth surface movement — *see* Landslide
    crocodile W58.13 ☑
    crowd or human stampede W52 ☑
    falling
      aircraft V97.39 ☑
        in war operations — *see* War operations, destruction of aircraft
      earth, material W20.0 ☑
        caused by cataclysmic earth surface movement — *see* Landslide
      object NEC W20.8 ☑
    landslide NEC — *see* Landslide
    lizard (nonvenomous) W59.09 ☑
    machinery — *see* Contact, with, by type of machine
    reptile NEC W59.89 ☑
    snake (nonvenomous) W59.13 ☑
  in
    machinery — *see* Contact, with, by type of machine

Cut, cutting (any part of body) (accidental) (*see also* Contact, with, by object or machine)
  during medical or surgical treatment as misadventure — *see* Index to Diseases and Injuries, Complications
  homicide (attempt) — *see* Assault, cutting or piercing instrument
  inflicted by other person — *see* Assault, cutting or piercing instrument
  legal
    execution — *see* Legal, intervention
    intervention — *see* Legal, intervention, sharp object
  machine NEC (*see also* Contact, with, by type of machine) W31.9 ☑
  self-inflicted — *see* Suicide, cutting or piercing instrument
  suicide (attempt) — *see* Suicide, cutting or piercing instrument
Cyclone (any injury) X37.1 ☑

D

Decapitation (accidental circumstances) NEC X58 ☑
  homicide X99.9 ☑
  legal execution — *see* Legal, intervention
Dehydration from lack of water X58 ☑
Deprivation X58 ☑
Derailment (accidental)
  railway (rolling stock) (train) (vehicle) (without antecedent collision) V81.7 ☑
    with antecedent collision — *see* Accident, transport, railway vehicle occupant
  streetcar (without antecedent collision) V82.7 ☑
    with antecedent collision — *see* Accident, transport, streetcar occupant
Descent
  parachute (voluntary) (without accident to aircraft) V97.29 ☑
    due to accident to aircraft — *see* Accident, transport, aircraft
Desertion X58 ☑
Destitution X58 ☑
Disability, late effect or sequela of injury — *see* Sequelae
Discharge (accidental)
  airgun W34.010 ☑
    assault X95.01 ☑
    homicide (attempt) X95.01 ☑
    stated as undetermined whether accidental or intentional Y24.0 ☑
    suicide (attempt) X74.01 ☑
  BB gun — *see* Discharge, airgun
  firearm (accidental) W34.00 ☑
    assault X95.9 ☑
    handgun (pistol) (revolver) W32.0 ☑
      assault X93 ☑
      homicide (attempt) X93 ☑
      legal intervention — *see* Legal, intervention, firearm, handgun
      stated as undetermined whether accidental or intentional Y22 ☑
      suicide (attempt) X72 ☑
    homicide (attempt) X95.9 ☑
    hunting rifle W33.02 ☑
      assault X94.1 ☑
      homicide (attempt) X94.1 ☑
      legal intervention
        injuring
          bystander Y35.032 ☑
          law enforcement personnel Y35.031 ☑
          suspect Y35.033 ☑
      stated as undetermined whether accidental or intentional Y23.1 ☑
      suicide (attempt) X73.1 ☑
    larger W33.00 ☑
      assault X94.9 ☑
      homicide (attempt) X94.9 ☑
      hunting rifle — *see* Discharge, firearm, hunting rifle
      legal intervention — *see* Legal, intervention, firearm by type of firearm
      machine gun — *see* Discharge, firearm, machine gun
      shotgun — *see* Discharge, firearm, shotgun
      specified NEC W33.09 ☑

Discharge — *continued*
  firearm — *continued*
    larger — *continued*
      specified — *continued*
        assault X94.8 ☑
        homicide (attempt) X94.8 ☑
        legal intervention
          injuring
            bystander Y35.092 ☑
            law enforcement personnel Y35.091 ☑
            suspect Y35.093 ☑
        stated as undetermined whether accidental or intentional Y23.8 ☑
        suicide (attempt) X73.8 ☑
      stated as undetermined whether accidental or intentional Y23.9 ☑
      suicide (attempt) X73.9 ☑
    legal intervention
      injuring
        bystander Y35.002 ☑
        law enforcement personnel Y35.001 ☑
        suspect Y35.03 ☑
      using rubber bullet
        injuring
          bystander Y35.042 ☑
          law enforcement personnel Y35.041 ☑
          suspect Y35.043 ☑
    machine gun W33.03 ☑
      assault X94.2 ☑
      homicide (attempt) X94.2 ☑
      legal intervention — *see* Legal, intervention, firearm, machine gun
      stated as undetermined whether accidental or intentional Y23.3 ☑
      suicide (attempt) X73.2 ☑
    pellet gun — *see* Discharge, airgun
    shotgun W33.01 ☑
      assault X94.0 ☑
      homicide (attempt) X94.0 ☑
      legal intervention — *see* Legal, intervention, firearm, specified NEC
      stated as undetermined whether accidental or intentional Y23.0 ☑
      suicide (attempt) X73.0 ☑
    specified NEC W34.09 ☑
      assault X95.8 ☑
      homicide (attempt) X95.8 ☑
      legal intervention — *see* Legal, intervention, firearm, specified NEC
      stated as undetermined whether accidental or intentional Y24.8 ☑
      suicide (attempt) X74.8 ☑
    stated as undetermined whether accidental or intentional Y24.9 ☑
    suicide (attempt) X74.9 ☑
    Very pistol W34.09 ☑
      assault X95.8 ☑
      homicide (attempt) X95.8 ☑
      stated as undetermined whether accidental or intentional Y24.8 ☑
      suicide (attempt) X74.8 ☑
  firework(s) W39 ☑
    stated as undetermined whether accidental or intentional Y25 ☑
  gas-operated gun NEC W34.018 ☑
    airgun — *see* Discharge, airgun
    assault X95.09 ☑
    homicide (attempt) X95.09 ☑
    paintball gun — *see* Discharge, paintball gun
    stated as undetermined whether accidental or intentional Y24.8 ☑
    suicide (attempt) X74.09 ☑
  gun NEC (*see also* Discharge, firearm NEC)
    air — *see* Discharge, airgun
    BB — *see* Discharge, airgun
    for single hand use — *see* Discharge, firearm, handgun
    hand — *see* Discharge, firearm, handgun
    machine — *see* Discharge, firearm, machine gun
    other specified — *see* Discharge, firearm NEC
    paintball — *see* Discharge, paintball gun
    pellet — *see* Discharge, airgun
  handgun — *see* Discharge, firearm, handgun
  machine gun — *see* Discharge, firearm, machine gun

Discharge — *continued*
  paintball gun W34.011 ☑
    assault X95.02 ☑
    homicide (attempt) X95.02 ☑
    stated as undetermined whether accidental or intentional Y24.8 ☑
    suicide (attempt) X74.02 ☑
  pistol — *see* Discharge, firearm, handgun
    flare — *see* Discharge, firearm, Very pistol
    pellet — *see* Discharge, airgun
    Very — *see* Discharge, firearm, Very pistol
  revolver — *see* Discharge, firearm, handgun
  rifle (hunting) — *see* Discharge, firearm, hunting rifle
  shotgun — *see* Discharge, firearm, shotgun
  spring-operated gun NEC W34.018 ☑
    assault X95.09 ☑
    homicide (attempt) X95.09 ☑
    stated as undetermined whether accidental or intentional Y24.8 ☑
    suicide (attempt) X74.09 ☑

Disease
  Andes W94.11 ☑
  aviator's — *see* Air, pressure
  range W94.11 ☑

Diver's disease, palsy, paralysis, squeeze — *see* Air, pressure

Diving (into water) — *see* Accident, diving

Dog bite W54.0 ☑

Dragged by transport vehicle NEC (*see also* Accident, transport) V09.9 ☑

Drinking poison (accidental) — *see* Table of Drugs and Chemicals

Dropped (accidentally) **while being carried or supported by other person** W04 ☑

Drowning (accidental) W74 ☑
  assault X92.9 ☑
  due to
    accident (to)
      machinery — *see* Contact, with, by type of machine
      watercraft V90.89 ☑
        burning V90.29 ☑
          powered V90.23 ☑
            fishing boat V90.22 ☑
            jetskis V90.23 ☑
            merchant ship V90.20 ☑
            passenger ship V90.21 ☑
          unpowered V90.28 ☑
            canoe V90.25 ☑
            inflatable V90.26 ☑
            kayak V90.25 ☑
            sailboat V90.24 ☑
            water skis V90.27 ☑
        crushed V90.39 ☑
          powered V90.33 ☑
            fishing boat V90.32 ☑
            jetskis V90.33 ☑
            merchant ship V90.30 ☑
            passenger ship V90.31 ☑
          unpowered V90.38 ☑
            canoe V90.35 ☑
            inflatable V90.36 ☑
            kayak V90.35 ☑
            sailboat V90.34 ☑
            water skis V90.37 ☑
        overturning V90.09 ☑
          powered V90.03 ☑
            fishing boat V90.02 ☑
            jetskis V90.03 ☑
            merchant ship V90.00 ☑
            passenger ship V90.01 ☑
          unpowered V90.08 ☑
            canoe V90.05 ☑
            inflatable V90.06 ☑
            kayak V90.05 ☑
            sailboat V90.04 ☑
        sinking V90.19 ☑
          powered V90.13 ☑
            fishing boat V90.12 ☑
            jetskis V90.13 ☑
            merchant ship V90.10 ☑
            passenger ship V90.11 ☑
          unpowered V90.18 ☑
            canoe V90.15 ☑
            inflatable V90.16 ☑
            kayak V90.15 ☑

Drowning — *continued*
  due to — *continued*
    accident — *continued*
      watercraft — *continued*
        sinking — *continued*
          unpowered — *continued*
            sailboat V90.14 ☑
        specified type NEC V90.89 ☑
          powered V90.83 ☑
            fishing boat V90.82 ☑
            jetskis V90.83 ☑
            merchant ship V90.80 ☑
            passenger ship V90.81 ☑
          unpowered V90.88 ☑
            canoe V90.85 ☑
            inflatable V90.86 ☑
            kayak V90.85 ☑
            sailboat V90.84 ☑
            water skis V90.87 ☑
    avalanche — *see* Landslide
    cataclysmic
      earth surface movement NEC — *see* Forces of nature, earth movement
      storm — *see* Forces of nature, cataclysmic storm
    cloudburst X37.8 ☑
    cyclone X37.1 ☑
    fall overboard (from) V92.09 ☑
      powered craft V92.03 ☑
        ferry boat V92.01 ☑
        fishing boat V92.02 ☑
        jetskis V92.03 ☑
        liner V92.01 ☑
        merchant ship V92.00 ☑
        passenger ship V92.01 ☑
    resulting from
      accident to watercraft — *see* Drowning, due to, accident to, watercraft
      being washed overboard (from) V92.29 ☑
        powered craft V92.23 ☑
          ferry boat V92.21 ☑
          fishing boat V92.22 ☑
          jetskis V92.23 ☑
          liner V92.21 ☑
          merchant ship V92.20 ☑
          passenger ship V92.21 ☑
        unpowered craft V92.28 ☑
          canoe V92.25 ☑
          inflatable V92.26 ☑
          kayak V92.25 ☑
          sailboat V92.24 ☑
          surf-board V92.28 ☑
          water skis V92.27 ☑
          windsurfer V92.28 ☑
      motion of watercraft V92.19 ☑
        powered craft V92.13 ☑
          ferry boat V92.11 ☑
          fishing boat V92.12 ☑
          jetskis V92.13 ☑
          liner V92.11 ☑
          merchant ship V92.10 ☑
          passenger ship V92.11 ☑
        unpowered craft
          canoe V92.15 ☑
          inflatable V92.16 ☑
          kayak V92.15 ☑
          sailboat V92.14 ☑
      unpowered craft V92.08 ☑
        canoe V92.05 ☑
        inflatable V92.06 ☑
        kayak V92.05 ☑
        sailboat V92.04 ☑
        surf-board V92.08 ☑
        water skis V92.07 ☑
        windsurfer V92.08 ☑
    hurricane X37.0 ☑
    jumping into water from watercraft (involved in accident) (*see also* Drowning, due to, accident to, watercraft)
      without accident to or on watercraft W16.711 ☑
    tidal wave NEC — *see* Forces of nature, tidal wave
    torrential rain X37.8 ☑

Drowning — *continued*
  following
    fall
      into
        bathtub W16.211 ☑
        bucket W16.221 ☑
        fountain — *see* Drowning, following, fall, into, water, specified NEC
        quarry — *see* Drowning, following, fall, into, water, specified NEC
        reservoir — *see* Drowning, following, fall, into, water, specified NEC
        swimming-pool W16.011 ☑
          stated as undetermined whether accidental or intentional Y21.3 ☑
          striking
            bottom W16.021 ☑
            wall W16.031 ☑
          suicide (attempt) X71.2 ☑
        water NOS W16.41 ☑
          natural (lake) (open sea) (river) (stream) (pond) W16.111 ☑
            striking
              bottom W16.121 ☑
              side W16.131 ☑
          specified NEC W16.311 ☑
            striking
              bottom W16.321 ☑
              wall W16.331 ☑
      overboard NEC — *see* Drowning, due to, fall overboard
    jump or dive
      from boat W16.711 ☑
        striking bottom W16.721 ☑
      into
        fountain — *see* Drowning, following, jump or dive, into, water, specified NEC
        quarry — *see* Drowning, following, jump or dive, into, water, specified NEC
        reservoir — *see* Drowning, following, jump or dive, into, water, specified NEC
        swimming-pool W16.511 ☑
          striking
            bottom W16.521 ☑
            wall W16.531 ☑
          suicide (attempt) X71.2 ☑
        water NOS W16.91 ☑
          natural (lake) (open sea) (river) (stream) (pond) W16.611 ☑
          specified NEC W16.811 ☑
            bottom W16.821 ☑
            striking
              bottom W16.821 ☑
              wall W16.831 ☑
          striking
            bottom W16.821 ☑
            wall W16.831 ☑
          striking bottom W16.621 ☑
  homicide (attempt) X92.9 ☑
  in
    bathtub (accidental) W65 ☑
      assault X92.0 ☑
      following fall W16.211 ☑
        stated as undetermined whether accidental or intentional Y21.1 ☑
      stated as undetermined whether accidental or intentional Y21.0 ☑
      suicide (attempt) X71.0 ☑
    lake — *see* Drowning, in, natural water
    natural water (lake) (open sea) (river) (stream) (pond) W69 ☑
      assault X92.3 ☑
      following
        dive or jump W16.611 ☑
          striking bottom W16.621 ☑
        fall W16.111 ☑
          striking
            bottom W16.121 ☑
            side W16.131 ☑
      stated as undetermined whether accidental or intentional Y21.4 ☑
      suicide (attempt) X71.3 ☑
    quarry — *see* Drowning, in, specified place NEC
    quenching tank — *see* Drowning, in, specified place NEC
    reservoir — *see* Drowning, in, specified place NEC

Drowning — *continued*
in — *continued*
river — *see* Drowning, in, natural water
sea — *see* Drowning, in, natural water
specified place NEC W73 ☑
assault X92.8 ☑
following
dive or jump W16.811 ☑
striking
bottom W16.821 ☑
wall W16.831 ☑
fall W16.311 ☑
striking
bottom W16.321 ☑
wall W16.331 ☑
stated as undetermined whether accidental or intentional Y21.8 ☑
suicide (attempt) X71.8 ☑
stream — *see* Drowning, in, natural water
swimming-pool W67 ☑
assault X92.1 ☑
following fall X92.2 ☑
following
dive or jump W16.511 ☑
striking
bottom W16.521 ☑
wall W16.531 ☑
fall W16.011 ☑
striking
bottom W16.021 ☑
wall W16.031 ☑
stated as undetermined whether accidental or intentional Y21.2 ☑
following fall Y21.3 ☑
suicide (attempt) X71.1 ☑
following fall X71.2 ☑
war operations — *see* War operations, restriction of airway
resulting from accident to watercraft — *see* Drowning, due to, accident, watercraft
self-inflicted X71.9 ☑
stated as undetermined whether accidental or intentional Y21.9 ☑
suicide (attempt) X71.9 ☑

E

Earth falling (on) W20.0 ☑
caused by cataclysmic earth surface movement or eruption — *see* Landslide
Earth (surface) movement NEC — *see* Forces of nature, earth movement
Earthquake (any injury) X34 ☑
Effect(s) (adverse) **of**
air pressure (any) — *see* Air, pressure
cold, excessive (exposure to) — *see* Exposure, cold
heat (excessive) — *see* Heat
hot place (weather) B — *see* Heat
insolation X30 ☑
late — *see* Sequelae
motion — *see* Motion
nuclear explosion or weapon in war operations — *see* War operations, nuclear weapon
radiation — *see* Radiation
travel — *see* Travel
Electric shock (accidental) (by) (in) — *see* Exposure, electric current
Electrocution (accidental) — *see* Exposure, electric current
Endotracheal tube wrongly placed during anesthetic procedure
Entanglement
in
bed linen, causing suffocation T71 ☑
wheel of pedal cycle V19.88 ☑
Entry of foreign body or material — *see* Foreign body
Environmental pollution related condition — *see* category Z57 ☑
Execution, legal (any method) — *see* Legal, intervention
Exhaustion
cold — *see* Exposure, cold
due to excessive exertion — *see* Overexertion
heat — *see* Heat
Explosion (accidental) (of) (with secondary fire) W40.9 ☑
acetylene W40.1 ☑
aerosol can W36.1 ☑

Explosion — *continued*
air tank (compressed) (in machinery) W36.2 ☑
aircraft (in transit) (powered) NEC V95.9 ☑
balloon V96.05 ☑
fixed wing NEC (private) V95.25 ☑
commercial V95.35 ☑
glider V96.25 ☑
hang V96.15 ☑
powered V95.15 ☑
helicopter V95.05 ☑
in war operations — *see* War operations, destruction of aircraft
microlight V95.15 ☑
nonpowered V96.9 ☑
specified NEC V96.8 ☑
powered NEC V95.8 ☑
stated as
homicide (attempt) Y03.8 ☑
suicide (attempt) X83.0 ☑
ultralight V95.15 ☑
anesthetic gas in operating room W40.1 ☑
antipersonnel bomb W40.8 ☑
assault X96.0 ☑
homicide (attempt) X96.0 ☑
suicide (attempt) X75 ☑
assault X96.9 ☑
bicycle tire W37.0 ☑
blasting (cap) (materials) W40.0 ☑
boiler (machinery), not on transport vehicle W35 ☑
on watercraft — *see* Explosion, in, watercraft
butane W40.1 ☑
caused by other person X96.9 ☑
coal gas W40.1 ☑
detonator W40.0 ☑
dump (munitions) W40.8 ☑
dynamite W40.0 ☑
in
assault X96.8 ☑
homicide (attempt) X96.8 ☑
legal intervention
injuring
bystander Y35.112 ☑
law enforcement personnel Y35.111 ☑
suspect Y35.113 ☑
suicide (attempt) X75 ☑
explosive (material) W40.9 ☑
gas W40.1 ☑
in blasting operation W40.0 ☑
specified NEC W40.8 ☑
in
assault X96.8 ☑
homicide (attempt) X96.8 ☑
legal intervention
injuring
bystander Y35.192 ☑
law enforcement personnel Y35.191 ☑
suspect Y35.193 ☑
suicide (attempt) X75 ☑
factory (munitions) W40.8 ☑
fertilizer bomb W40.8 ☑
assault X96.3 ☑
homicide (attempt) X96.3 ☑
suicide (attempt) X75 ☑
firearm (parts) NEC W34.19 ☑
airgun W34.110 ☑
BB gun W34.110 ☑
gas, air or spring-operated gun NEC W34.118 ☑
hangun W32.1 ☑
hunting rifle W33.12 ☑
larger firearm W33.10 ☑
specified NEC W33.19 ☑
machine gun W33.13 ☑
paintball gun W34.111 ☑
pellet gun W34.110 ☑
shotgun W33.11 ☑
Very pistol [flare] W34.19 ☑
fire-damp W40.1 ☑
fireworks W39 ☑
gas (coal) (explosive) W40.1 ☑
cylinder W36.9 ☑
aerosol can W36.1 ☑
air tank W36.2 ☑
pressurized W36.3 ☑
specified NEC W36.8 ☑

Explosion — *continued*
gasoline (fumes) (tank) not in moving motor vehicle W40.1 ☑
bomb W40.8 ☑
assault X96.1 ☑
homicide (attempt) X96.1 ☑
suicide (attempt) X75 ☑
in motor vehicle — *see* Accident, transport, by type of vehicle
grain store W40.8 ☑
grenade W40.8 ☑
in
assault X96.8 ☑
homicide (attempt) X96.8 ☑
legal intervention
injuring
bystander Y35.192 ☑
law enforcement personnel Y35.191 ☑
suspect Y35.193 ☑
suicide (attempt) X75 ☑
handgun (parts) — *see* Explosion, firearm, hangun (parts)
homicide (attempt) X96.9 ☑
antipersonnel bomb — *see* Explosion, antipersonnel bomb
fertilizer bomb — *see* Explosion, fertilizer bomb
gasoline bomb — *see* Explosion, gasoline bomb
letter bomb — *see* Explosion, letter bomb
pipe bomb — *see* Explosion, pipe bomb
specified NEC X96.8 ☑
hose, pressurized W37.8 ☑
hot water heater, tank (in machinery) W35 ☑
on watercraft — *see* Explosion, in, watercraft
in, on
dump W40.8 ☑
factory W40.8 ☑
mine (of explosive gases) NEC W40.1 ☑
watercraft V93.59 ☑
powered craft V93.53 ☑
ferry boat V93.51 ☑
fishing boat V93.52 ☑
jetskis V93.53 ☑
liner V93.51 ☑
merchant ship V93.50 ☑
passenger ship V93.51 ☑
sailboat V93.54 ☑
letter bomb W40.8 ☑
assault X96.2 ☑
homicide (attempt) X96.2 ☑
suicide (attempt) X75 ☑
machinery (*see also* Contact, with, by type of machine)
on board watercraft — *see* Explosion, in, watercraft
pressure vessel — *see* Explosion, by type of vessel
methane W40.1 ☑
mine W40.1 ☑
missile NEC W40.8 ☑
mortar bomb W40.8 ☑
in
assault X96.8 ☑
homicide (attempt) X96.8 ☑
legal intervention
injuring
bystander Y35.192 ☑
law enforcement personnel Y35.191 ☑
suspect Y35.193 ☑
suicide (attempt) X75 ☑
munitions (dump) (factory) W40.8 ☑
pipe, pressurized W37.8 ☑
bomb W40.8 ☑
assault X96.4 ☑
homicide (attempt) X96.4 ☑
suicide (attempt) X75 ☑
pressure, pressurized
cooker W38 ☑
gas tank (in machinery) W36.3 ☑
hose W37.8 ☑
pipe W37.8 ☑
specified device NEC W38 ☑
tire W37.8 ☑
bicycle W37.0 ☑
vessel (in machinery) W38 ☑
propane W40.1 ☑
self-inflicted X75 ☑
shell (artillery) NEC W40.8 ☑
during war operations — *see* War operations, explosion

Explosion — *continued*
　shell — *continued*
　　in
　　　legal intervention
　　　　injuring
　　　　　bystander Y35.122 ☑
　　　　　law enforcement personnel Y35.121 ☑
　　　　　suspect Y35.123 ☑
　　　　war — *see* War operations, explosion
　spacecraft V95.45 ☑
　stated as undetermined whether accidental or intentional Y25
　steam or water lines (in machinery) W37.8 ☑
　stove W40.9 ☑
　suicide (attempt) X75 ☑
　tire, pressurized W37.8 ☑
　　bicycle W37.0 ☑
　undetermined whether accidental or intentional Y25 ☑
　vehicle tire NEC W37.8 ☑
　　bicycle W37.0 ☑
　war operations — *see* War operations, explosion
Exposure (to) X58 ☑
　air pressure change — *see* Air, pressure
　cold (accidental) (excessive) (extreme) (natural) (place) X31 ☑
　　assault Y08.89 ☑
　　due to
　　　man-made conditions W93.8 ☑
　　　　dry ice (contact) W93.01 ☑
　　　　　inhalation W93.02 ☑
　　　　liquid air (contact) (hydrogen) (nitrogen) W93.11 ☑
　　　　　inhalation W93.12 ☑
　　　　refrigeration unit (deep freeze) W93.2 ☑
　　　　suicide (attempt) X83.2 ☑
　　　　weather (conditions) X31 ☑
　　homicide (attempt) Y08.89 ☑
　　self-inflicted X83.2 ☑
　due to abandonment or neglect X58 ☑
　electric current W86.8 ☑
　　appliance (faulty) W86.8 ☑
　　　domestic W86.0 ☑
　　caused by other person Y08.89 ☑
　　conductor (faulty) W86.1 ☑
　　control apparatus (faulty) W86.1 ☑
　　electric power generating plant, distribution station W86.1 ☑
　　electroshock gun — *see* Exposure, electric current, taser
　　high-voltage cable W85 ☑
　　homicide (attempt) Y08.89 ☑
　　legal execution — *see* Legal, intervention, specified means NEC
　　lightning — *see* subcategory T75.0 ☑
　　live rail W86.8 ☑
　　misadventure in medical or surgical procedure in electroshock therapy Y63.4
　　motor (electric) (faulty) W86.8 ☑
　　　domestic W86.0 ☑
　　self-inflicted X83.1 ☑
　　specified NEC W86.8 ☑
　　　domestic W86.0 ☑
　　stun gun — *see* Exposure, electric current, taser
　　suicide (attempt) X83.1 ☑
　　taser W86.8 ☑
　　　assault Y08.89 ☑
　　　legal intervention — *see* category Y35 ☑
　　　self-harm (intentional) X83.8 ☑
　　　undetermined intent Y33 ☑
　　third rail W86.8 ☑
　　transformer (faulty) W86.1 ☑
　　transmission lines W85 ☑
　environmental tobacco smoke X58 ☑
　excessive
　　cold — *see* Exposure, cold
　　heat (natural) NEC X30 ☑
　　　man-made W92 ☑
　factor(s) NOS X58 ☑
　　environmental NEC X58 ☑
　　　man-made NEC W99 ☑
　　　natural NEC — *see* Forces of nature
　　specified NEC X58 ☑
　fire, flames (accidental) X08.8 ☑
　　assault X97 ☑

Exposure — *continued*
　fire, flames — *continued*
　　campfire — *see* Exposure, fire, controlled, not in building
　　controlled (in)
　　　with ignition (of) clothing (*see also* Ignition, clothes) X06.2 ☑
　　　　nightwear X05 ☑
　　　bonfire — *see* Exposure, fire, controlled, not in building
　　　brazier (in building or structure) (*see also* Exposure, fire, controlled, building)
　　　　not in building or structure — *see* Exposure, fire, controlled, not in building
　　　building or structure X02.0 ☑
　　　　with
　　　　　fall from building X02.3 ☑
　　　　　from building X02.5 ☑
　　　　　injury due to building collapse X02.2 ☑
　　　　　smoke inhalation X02.1 ☑
　　　　hit by object from building X02.4 ☑
　　　　specified mode of injury NEC X02.8 ☑
　　　fireplace, furnace or stove — *see* Exposure, fire, controlled, building
　　　not in building or structure X03.0 ☑
　　　　with
　　　　　fall X03.3 ☑
　　　　　smoke inhalation X03.1 ☑
　　　　hit by object X03.4 ☑
　　　　specified mode of injury NEC X03.8 ☑
　　　trash — *see* Exposure, fire, controlled, not in building
　　fireplace — *see* Exposure, fire, controlled, building
　　fittings or furniture (in building or structure) (uncontrolled) — *see* Exposure, fire, uncontrolled, building
　　forest (uncontrolled) — *see* Exposure, fire, uncontrolled, not in building
　　grass (uncontrolled) — *see* Exposure, fire, uncontrolled, not in building
　　hay (uncontrolled) — *see* Exposure, fire, uncontrolled, not in building
　　homicide (attempt) X97 ☑
　　ignition of highly flammable material X04 ☑
　　in, of, on, starting in
　　　machinery — *see* Contact, with, by type of machine
　　　motor vehicle (in motion) (*see also* Accident, transport, occupant by type of vehicle) V87.8 ☑
　　　　with collision — *see* Collision
　　　railway rolling stock, train, vehicle V81.81 ☑
　　　　with collision — *see* Accident, transport, railway vehicle occupant
　　　street car (in motion) V82.8 ☑
　　　　with collision — *see* Accident, transport, streetcar occupant
　　　transport vehicle NEC (*see also* Accident, transport)
　　　　with collision — *see* Collision
　　　war operations (*see also* War operations, fire)
　　　　from nuclear explosion — *see* War operations, nuclear weapons
　　　watercraft (in transit) (not in transit) V91.09 ☑
　　　　localized — *see* Burn, on board watercraft, due to, fire on board
　　　　powered craft V91.03 ☑
　　　　　ferry boat V91.01 ☑
　　　　　fishing boat V91.02 ☑
　　　　　jet skis V91.03 ☑
　　　　　liner V91.01 ☑
　　　　　merchant ship V91.00 ☑
　　　　　passenger ship V91.01 ☑
　　　　unpowered craft V91.08 ☑
　　　　　canoe V91.05 ☑
　　　　　inflatable V91.06 ☑
　　　　　kayak V91.05 ☑
　　　　　sailboat V91.04 ☑
　　　　　surf-board V91.08 ☑
　　　　　waterskis V91.07 ☑
　　　　　windsurfer V91.08 ☑
　　lumber (uncontrolled) — *see* Exposure, fire, uncontrolled, not in building
　　mine (uncontrolled) — *see* Exposure, fire, uncontrolled, not in building

Exposure — *continued*
　fire, flames — *continued*
　　prairie (uncontrolled) — *see* Exposure, fire, uncontrolled, not in building
　　resulting from
　　　explosion — *see* Explosion
　　　lightning X08.8 ☑
　　self-inflicted X76 ☑
　　specified NEC X08.8 ☑
　　started by other person X97 ☑
　　stated as undetermined whether accidental or intentional X26 ☑
　　stove — *see* Exposure, fire, controlled, building
　　suicide (attempt) X76 ☑
　　tunnel (uncontrolled) — *see* Exposure, fire, uncontrolled, not in building
　　uncontrolled
　　　in building or structure X00.0 ☑
　　　　with
　　　　　fall from building X00.3 ☑
　　　　　injury due to building collapse X00.2 ☑
　　　　　jump from building X00.5 ☑
　　　　　smoke inhalation X00.1 ☑
　　　　bed X08.00 ☑
　　　　　due to
　　　　　　cigarette X08.01 ☑
　　　　　　specified material NEC X08.09 ☑
　　　　furniture NEC X08.20 ☑
　　　　　due to
　　　　　　cigarette X08.21 ☑
　　　　　　specified material NEC X08.29 ☑
　　　　hit by object from building X00.4 ☑
　　　　sofa X08.10 ☑
　　　　　due to
　　　　　　cigarette X08.11 ☑
　　　　　　specified material NEC X08.19 ☑
　　　　specified mode of injury NEC X00.8 ☑
　　　not in building or structure (any) X01.0 ☑
　　　　with
　　　　　fall X01.3 ☑
　　　　　smoke inhalation X01.1 ☑
　　　　hit by object X01.4 ☑
　　　　specified mode of injury NEC X01.8 ☑
　　undetermined whether accidental or intentional Y26 ☑
　forces of nature NEC — *see* Forces of nature
　G-forces (abnormal) W49.9 ☑
　gravitational forces (abnormal) W49.9 ☑
　heat (natural) NEC — *see* Heat
　high-pressure jet (hydraulic) (pneumatic) W49.9 ☑
　hydraulic jet W49.9 ☑
　inanimate mechanical force W49.9 ☑
　jet, high-pressure (hydraulic) (pneumatic) W49.9 ☑
　lightning — *see* subcategory T75.0 ☑
　　causing fire — *see* Exposure, fire
　mechanical forces NEC W49.9 ☑
　　animate NEC W64 ☑
　　inanimate NEC W49.9 ☑
　noise W42.9 ☑
　　supersonic W42.0 ☑
　noxious substance — *see* Table of Drugs and Chemicals
　pneumatic jet W49.9 ☑
　prolonged in deep-freeze unit or refrigerator W93.2 ☑
　radiation — *see* Radiation
　smoke (*see also* Exposure, fire)
　　tobacco, second hand Z77.22
　specified factors NEC X58 ☑
　sunlight X32 ☑
　　man-made (sun lamp) W89.8 ☑
　　　tanning bed W89.1 ☑
　supersonic waves W42.0 ☑
　transmission line(s), electric W85 ☑
　vibration W49.9 ☑
　waves
　　infrasound W49.9 ☑
　　sound W42.9 ☑
　　supersonic W42.0 ☑
　weather NEC — *see* Forces of nature
External cause status Y99.9
　child assisting in compensated work for family Y99.8
　civilian activity done for financial or other compensation Y99.0
　civilian activity done for income or pay Y99.0
　family member assisting in compensated work for other family member Y99.8

☑ **Additional Character Required — Refer to the Tabular List for Character Selection**　　☒ **Subterms under main terms may continue to next column or page**

External cause status — *continued*
 hobby not done for income Y99.8
 leisure activity Y99.8
 military activity Y99.1
 off-duty activity of military personnel Y99.8
 recreation or sport not for income or while a student
  Y99.8
 specified NEC Y99.8
 student activity Y99.8
 volunteer activity Y99.2

F

Factors, supplemental
 alcohol
  blood level
   less than 20mg/100ml Y90.0
   20-39mg/100ml Y90.1
   40-59mg/100ml Y90.2
   60-79mg/100ml Y90.3
   80-99mg/100ml Y90.4
   100-119mg/100ml Y90.5
   120-199mg/100ml Y90.6
   200-239mg/100ml Y90.7
   240mg/100ml or more Y90.8
   presence in blood, level not specified Y90.9
   presence in blood, but level not specified Y90.9
 environmental-pollution-related condition- see Z57 ☑
 nosocomial condition Y95
 work-related condition Y99.0

Failure
 in suture or ligature during surgical procedure Y65.2
 mechanical, of instrument or apparatus (any) (during
  any medical or surgical procedure) Y65.8
 sterile precautions (during medical and surgical care)
  — *see* Misadventure, failure, sterile precautions,
  by type of procedure
 to
  introduce tube or instrument Y65.4
   endotracheal tube during anesthesia Y65.3
  make curve (transport vehicle) NEC — *see* Accident,
   transport
  remove tube or instrument Y65.4

Fall, falling (accidental) W19 ☑
 building W20.1 ☑
  burning (uncontrolled fire) X00.3 ☑
 down
  embankment W17.81 ☑
  escalator W10.0 ☑
  hill W17.81 ☑
  ladder W11 ☑
  ramp W10.2 ☑
  stairs, steps W10.9 ☑
 due to
  bumping against
   object W18.00 ☑
    sharp glass W18.02 ☑
    specified NEC W18.09 ☑
    sports equipment W18.01 ☑
   person W03 ☑
    due to ice or snow W00.0 ☑
    on pedestrian conveyance — *see* Accident,
     transport, pedestrian, conveyance
  collision with another person W03 ☑
   due to ice or snow W00.0 ☑
   involving pedestrian conveyance — *see* Acci-
    dent, transport, pedestrian, conveyance
  grocery cart tipping over W17.82 ☑
  ice or snow W00.9 ☑
   from one level to another W00.2 ☑
    on stairs or steps W00.1 ☑
   involving pedestrian conveyance — *see* Acci-
    dent, transport, pedestrian, conveyance
   on same level W00.0 ☑
  slipping (on moving sidewalk) W01.0 ☑
   with subsequent striking against object
    W01.10 ☑
    furniture W01.190 ☑
    sharp object W01.119 ☑
     glass W01.110 ☑
     power tool or machine W01.111 ☑
     specified NEC W01.118 ☑
    specified NEC W01.198 ☑
  striking against
   object W18.00 ☑
    sharp glass W18.02 ☑
    specified NEC W18.09 ☑

Fall, falling — *continued*
 due to — *continued*
  striking against — *continued*
   object — *continued*
    sports equipment W18.01 ☑
   person W03 ☑
    due to ice or snow W00.0 ☑
    on pedestrian conveyance — *see* Accident,
     transport, pedestrian, conveyance
 earth (with asphyxia or suffocation (by pressure)) —
  see Earth, falling
 from, off, out of
  aircraft NEC (with accident to aircraft NEC) V97.0 ☑
   while boarding or alighting V97.1 ☑
  balcony W13.0 ☑
  bed W06 ☑
  boat, ship, watercraft NEC (with drowning or submersion) — *see* Drowning, due to, fall overboard
   with hitting bottom or object V94.0 ☑
  bridge W13.1 ☑
  building W13.9 ☑
   burning (uncontrolled fire) X00.3 ☑
  cavity W17.2 ☑
  chair W07 ☑
  cherry picker W17.89 ☑
  cliff W15 ☑
  dock W17.4 ☑
  embankment W17.81 ☑
  escalator W10.0 ☑
  flagpole W13.8 ☑
  furniture NEC W08 ☑
  grocery cart W17.82 ☑
  haystack W17.89 ☑
  high place NEC W17.89 ☑
   stated as undetermined whether accidental or
    intentional Y30 ☑
  hole W17.2 ☑
  incline W10.2 ☑
  ladder W11 ☑
  lifting device W17.89 ☑
  machine, machinery (*see also* Contact, with, by
   type of machine)
   not in operation W17.89 ☑
  manhole W17.1 ☑
  mobile elevated work platform [MEWP] W17.89 ☑
  motorized mobility scooter W05.2 ☑
  one level to another NEC W17.89 ☑
   intentional, purposeful, suicide (attempt)
    X80 ☑
   stated as undetermined whether accidental or
    intentional Y30 ☑
  pit W17.2 ☑
  playground equipment W09.8 ☑
   jungle gym W09.2 ☑
   slide W09.0 ☑
   swing W09.1 ☑
  quarry W17.89 ☑
  railing W13.9 ☑
  ramp W10.2 ☑
  roof W13.2 ☑
  scaffolding W12 ☑
  scooter (nonmotorized) W05.1 ☑
   motorized mobility W05.2 ☑
  sky lift W17.89 ☑
  stairs, steps W10.9 ☑
   curb W10.1 ☑
   due to ice or snow W00.1 ☑
   escalator W10.0 ☑
   incline W10.2 ☑
   ramp W10.2 ☑
   sidewalk curb W10.1 ☑
   specified NEC W10.8 ☑
  stepladder W11 ☑
  storm drain W17.1 ☑
  streetcar NEC V82.6 ☑
   with antecedent collision — *see* Accident,
    transport, streetcar occupant
   while boarding or alighting V82.4 ☑
  structure NEC W13.8 ☑
   burning (uncontrolled fire) X00.3 ☑
  table W08 ☑
  toilet W18.11 ☑
   with subsequent striking against object
    W18.12 ☑

Fall, falling — *continued*
 from, off, out of — *continued*
  train NEC V81.6 ☑
   during derailment (without antecedent colli-
    sion) V81.7 ☑
    with antecedent collision — *see* Accident,
     transport, railway vehicle occupant
   while boarding or alighting V81.4 ☑
  transport vehicle after collision — *see* Accident,
   transport, by type of vehicle, collision
  tree W14 ☑
  vehicle (in motion) NEC (*see also* Accident, transport) V89.9 ☑
   motor NEC (*see also* Accident, transport, occu-
    pant, by type of vehicle) V87.8 ☑
   stationary W17.89 ☑
    while boarding or alighting B — *see* Acci-
     dent, transport, by type of vehicle,
     while boarding or alighting
  viaduct W13.8 ☑
  wall W13.8 ☑
  watercraft (*see also* Drowning, due to, fall overboard)
   with hitting bottom or object V94.0 ☑
  well W17.0 ☑
  wheelchair, non-moving W05.0 ☑
   powered — *see* Accident, transport, pedestrian,
    conveyance occupant, specified type NEC
  window W13.4 ☑
 in, on
  aircraft NEC V97.0 ☑
   with accident to aircraft V97.0 ☑
   while boarding or alighting V97.1 ☑
  bathtub (empty) W18.2 ☑
   filled W16.212 ☑
    causing drowning W16.211 ☑
  escalator W10.0 ☑
  incline W10.2 ☑
  ladder W11 ☑
  machine, machinery — *see* Contact, with, by type
   of machine
  object, edged, pointed or sharp (with cut) — *see*
   Fall, by type
  playground equipment W09.8 ☑
   jungle gym W09.2 ☑
   slide W09.0 ☑
   swing W09.1 ☑
  ramp W10.2 ☑
  scaffolding W12 ☑
  shower W18.2 ☑
   causing drowning W16.211 ☑
  staircase, stairs, steps W10.9 ☑
   curb W10.1 ☑
   due to ice or snow W00.1 ☑
   escalator W10.0 ☑
   incline W10.2 ☑
   specified NEC W10.8 ☑
  streetcar (without antecedent collision) V82.5 ☑
   with antecedent collision — *see* Accident,
    transport, streetcar occupant
   while boarding or alighting V82.4 ☑
  train (without antecedent collision) V81.5 ☑
   with antecedent collision — *see* Accident,
    transport, railway vehicle occupant
   during derailment (without antecedent colli-
    sion) V81.7 ☑
    with antecedent collision — *see* Accident,
     transport, railway vehicle occupant
   while boarding or alighting V81.4 ☑
  transport vehicle after collision — *see* Accident,
   transport, by type of vehicle, collision
  watercraft V93.39 ☑
   due to
    accident to craft V91.29 ☑
     powered craft V91.23 ☑
      ferry boat V91.21 ☑
      fishing boat V91.22 ☑
      jetskis V91.23 ☑
      liner V91.21 ☑
      merchant ship V91.20 ☑
      passenger ship V91.21 ☑
     unpowered craft
      canoe V91.25 ☑
      inflatable V91.26 ☑
      kayak V91.25 ☑
      sailboat V91.24 ☑

Fall, falling — *continued*
  in, on — *continued*
    watercraft — *continued*
      powered craft V93.33 ☑
        ferry boat V93.31 ☑
        fishing boat V93.32 ☑
        jetskis V93.33 ☑
        liner V93.31 ☑
        merchant ship V93.30 ☑
        passenger ship V93.31 ☑
      unpowered craft V93.38 ☑
        canoe V93.35 ☑
        inflatable V93.36 ☑
        kayak V93.35 ☑
        sailboat V93.34 ☑
        surf-board V93.38 ☑
        windsurfer V93.38 ☑
  into
    cavity W17.2 ☑
    dock W17.4 ☑
    fire — *see* Exposure, fire, by type
    haystack W17.89 ☑
    hole W17.2 ☑
    lake — *see* Fall, into, water
    lake — *see* Fall, into, water
    manhole W17.1 ☑
    moving part of machinery — *see* Contact, with, by
        type of machine
    ocean — *see* Fall, into, water
    opening in surface NEC W17.89 ☑
    pit W17.2 ☑
    pond — *see* Fall, into, water
    quarry W17.89 ☑
    river — *see* Fall, into, water
    shaft W17.89 ☑
    storm drain W17.1 ☑
    stream — *see* Fall, into, water
    swimming pool (*see also* Fall, into, water, in,
        swimming pool)
      empty W17.3 ☑
    tank W17.89 ☑
    water W16.42 ☑
      causing drowning W16.41 ☑
      from watercraft — *see* Drowning, due to, fall
          overboard
      hitting diving board W21.4 ☑
      in
        bathtub W16.212 ☑
          causing drowning W16.211 ☑
        bucket W16.222 ☑
          causing drowning W16.221 ☑
        natural body of water W16.112 ☑
          causing drowning W16.111 ☑
          striking
            bottom W16.122 ☑
              causing drowning W16.121 ☑
            side W16.132 ☑
              causing drowning W16.131 ☑
        specified water NEC W16.312 ☑
          causing drowning W16.311 ☑
          striking
            bottom W16.322 ☑
              causing drowning W16.321 ☑
            wall W16.332 ☑
              causing drowning W16.331 ☑
        swimming pool W16.012 ☑
          causing drowning W16.011 ☑
          striking
            bottom W16.022 ☑
              causing drowning W16.031 ☑
            wall W16.032 ☑
              causing drowning W16.021 ☑
        utility bucket W16.222 ☑
          causing drowning W16.221 ☑
    well W17.0 ☑
  involving
    bed W06 ☑
    chair W07 ☑
    furniture NEC W08 ☑
    glass — *see* Fall, by type
    playground equipment W09.8 ☑
      jungle gym W09.2 ☑
      slide W09.0 ☑
      swing W09.1 ☑
    roller blades — *see* Accident, transport, pedestrian,
        conveyance

Fall, falling — *continued*
  involving — *continued*
    skateboard(s) — *see* Accident, transport, pedestrian, conveyance
    skates (ice) (in line) (roller) — *see* Accident, transport, pedestrian, conveyance
    skis — *see* Accident, transport, pedestrian, conveyance
    table W08 ☑
    wheelchair, non-moving W05.0 ☑
      powered — *see* Accident, transport, pedestrian, conveyance, specified type NEC
  object — *see* Struck by, object, falling
  off
    toilet W18.11 ☑
      with subsequent striking against object W18.12 ☑
    on same level W18.30 ☑
      due to
        specified NEC W18.39 ☑
        stepping on an object W18.31 ☑
  out of
    bed W06 ☑
    building NEC W13.8 ☑
    chair W07 ☑
    furniture NEC W08 ☑
    wheelchair, non-moving W05.0 ☑
      powered — *see* Accident, transport, pedestrian, conveyance, specified type NEC
    window W13.4 ☑
  over
    animal W01.0 ☑
    cliff W15 ☑
    embankment W17.81 ☑
    small object W01.0 ☑
  rock W20.8 ☑
  same level W18.30 ☑
    from
      being crushed, pushed, or stepped on by a
          crowd or human stampede W52 ☑
      collision, pushing, shoving, by or with other
          person W03 ☑
      slipping, stumbling, tripping W01.0 ☑
    involving ice or snow W00.0 ☑
      involving skates (ice) (roller), skateboard, skis
          — *see* Accident, transport, pedestrian,
          conveyance
  snowslide (avalanche) — *see* Landslide
  stone W20.8 ☑
  structure W20.1 ☑
    burning (uncontrolled fire) X00.3 ☑
  through
    bridge W13.1 ☑
    floor W13.3 ☑
    roof W13.2 ☑
    wall W13.8 ☑
    window W13.4 ☑
  timber W20.8 ☑
  tree (caused by lightning) W20.8 ☑
  while being carried or supported by other person(s)
      W04 ☑
Fallen on by
  animal (not being ridden) NEC W55.89 ☑
Felo-de-se — *see* Suicide
Fight (hand) (fists) (foot) — *see* Assault, fight
Fire (accidental) — *see* Exposure, fire
Firearm discharge — *see* Discharge, firearm
**Fireball effects from nuclear explosion in war oper-
    ations** — *see* War operations, nuclear weapons
Fireworks (explosion) W39 ☑
Flash burns from explosion — *see* Explosion
Flood (any injury) (caused by) X38 ☑
  collapse of man-made structure causing earth move-
      ment X36.0 ☑
  tidal wave — *see* Forces of nature, tidal wave
Food (any type) **in**
  air passages (with asphyxia, obstruction, or suffoca-
      tion) — *see* categories T17 and T18 ☑
  alimentary tract causing asphyxia (due to compression
      of trachea) — *see* categories T17 and T18 ☑
Forces of nature X39.8 ☑
  avalanche X36.1 ☑
    causing transport accident — *see* Accident, trans-
        port, by type of vehicle
  blizzard X37.2 ☑

Forces of nature — *continued*
  cataclysmic storm X37.9 ☑
    with flood X38 ☑
    blizzard X37.2 ☑
    cloudburst X37.8 ☑
    cyclone X37.1 ☑
    dust storm X37.3 ☑
    hurricane X37.0 ☑
    specified storm NEC X37.8 ☑
    storm surge X37.0 ☑
    tornado X37.1 ☑
    twister X37.1 ☑
    typhoon X37.0 ☑
  cloudburst X37.8 ☑
  cold (natural) X31 ☑
  cyclone X37.1 ☑
  dam collapse causing earth movement X36.0 ☑
  dust storm X37.3 ☑
  earth movement X36.1 ☑
    caused by dam or structure collapse X36.0 ☑
    earthquake X34
  earthquake X34
  flood (caused by) X38 ☑
    dam collapse X36.0 ☑
    tidal wave B — *see* Forces of nature, tidal wave
  heat (natural) X30 ☑
  hurricane X37.0 ☑
  landslide X36.1 ☑
    causing transport accident — *see* Accident, trans-
        port, by type of vehicle
  lightning — *see* subcategory T75.0 ☑
    causing fire — *see* Exposure, fire
  mudslide X36.1 ☑
    causing transport accident — *see* Accident, trans-
        port, by type of vehicle
  radiation (natural) X39.08 ☑
    radon X39.01 ☑
  radon X39.01 ☑
  specified force NEC X39.8 ☑
  storm surge X37.0 ☑
  structure collapse causing earth movement X36.0 ☑
  sunlight X32 ☑
  tidal wave X37.41 ☑
    due to
      earthquake X37.41 ☑
      landslide X37.43 ☑
      storm X37.42 ☑
      volcanic eruption X37.41 ☑
  tornado X37.1 ☑
  tsunami X37.41 ☑
  twister X37.1 ☑
  typhoon X37.0 ☑
  volcanic eruption X35 ☑
Foreign body
  aspiration — *see* Index to Diseases and Injuries, For-
      eign body, respiratory tract
  entering through skin W45.8 ☑
    can lid W45.2 ☑
    nail W45.0 ☑
    paper W45.1 ☑
    specified NEC W45.8 ☑
    splinter W45.8 ☑
Forest fire (exposure to) — *see* Exposure, fire, uncon-
    trolled, not in building
Found injured X58 ☑
  from exposure (to) — *see* Exposure
  on
    highway, road(way), street V89.9 ☑
    railway right of way V81.9 ☑
Fracture (circumstances unknown or unspecified) X58 ☑
  due to specified cause NEC X58 ☑
Freezing — *see* Exposure, cold
Frostbite X31 ☑
  due to man-made conditions — *see* Exposure, cold,
      man-made
Frozen — *see* Exposure, cold

G

Gored by bull W55.22 ☑
Gunshot wound W34.00 ☑

H

Hailstones, injured by X39.8 ☑

Hanged herself or himself — *see* Hanging, self-inflicted
Hanging (accidental) (*see also* category) T71 ☑
  legal execution — *see* Legal, intervention, specified
    means NEC
Heat (effects of) (excessive) X30 ☑
  due to
    man-made conditions W92 ☑
      on board watercraft V93.29 ☑
        fishing boat V93.22 ☑
        merchant ship V93.20 ☑
        passenger ship V93.21 ☑
        sailboat V93.24 ☑
        specified powered craft NEC V93.23 ☑
    weather (conditions) X30 ☑
  from
    electric heating apparatus causing burning X16 ☑
    nuclear explosion in war operations — *see* War
      operations, nuclear weapons
  inappropriate in local application or packing in medical
    or surgical procedure Y63.5
Hemorrhage
  delayed following medical or surgical treatment
    without mention of misadventure — *see* Index
    to Diseases and Injuries, Complication(s)
  during medical or surgical treatment as misadventure
    — *see* Index to Diseases and Injuries, Complica-
    tion(s)
High
  altitude (effects) — *see* Air, pressure, low
  level of radioactivity, effects — *see* Radiation
  pressure (effects) — *see* Air, pressure, high
  temperature, effects — *see* Heat
Hit, hitting (accidental) by — *see* Struck by
Hitting against — *see* Striking against
Homicide (attempt) (justifiable) — *see* Assault
Hot
  place, effects (*see also* Heat)
  weather, effects X30 ☑
House fire (uncontrolled) — *see* Exposure, fire, uncon-
  trolled, building
Humidity, causing problem X39.8 ☑
Hunger X58 ☑
Hurricane (any injury) X37.0 ☑
Hypobarism, hypobaropathy — *see* Air, pressure, low

I

Ictus
  caloris (*see also* Heat)
  solaris X30 ☑
Ignition (accidental) (*see also* Exposure, fire) X08.8 ☑
  anesthetic gas in operating room W40.1 ☑
  apparel X06.2 ☑
    from highly flammable material X04 ☑
    nightwear X05 ☑
  bed linen (sheets) (spreads) (pillows) (mattress) — *see*
    Exposure, fire, uncontrolled, building, bed
  benzine X04 ☑
  clothes, clothing NEC (from controlled fire) X06.2 ☑
    from
      highly flammable material X04 ☑
  ether X04 ☑
    in operating room W40.1 ☑
  explosive material — *see* Explosion
  gasoline X04 ☑
  jewelry (plastic) (any) X06.0 ☑
  kerosene X04 ☑
  material
    explosive — *see* Explosion
    highly flammable with secondary explosion X04 ☑
  nightwear X05 ☑
  paraffin X04 ☑
  petrol X04 ☑
Immersion (accidental) (*see also* Drowning)
  hand or foot due to cold (excessive) X31 ☑
Implantation of quills of porcupine W55.89 ☑
Inanition (from) (hunger) X58 ☑
  thirst X58 ☑
Inappropriate operation performed
  correct operation on wrong side or body part (wrong
    side) (wrong site) Y65.53
  operation intended for another patient done on wrong
    patient Y65.52
  wrong operation performed on correct patient Y65.51
Inattention after, at birth (homicidal intent) (infantici-
  dal intent) X58 ☑

Incident, adverse
  device
    anesthesiology Y70.8
      accessory Y70.2
      diagnostic Y70.0
      miscellaneous Y70.8
      monitoring Y70.0
      prosthetic Y70.2
      rehabilitative Y70.1
      surgical Y70.3
      therapeutic Y70.1
    cardiovascular Y71.8
      accessory Y71.2
      diagnostic Y71.0
      miscellaneous Y71.8
      monitoring Y71.0
      prosthetic Y71.2
      rehabilitative Y71.1
      surgical Y71.3
      therapeutic Y71.1
    gastroenterology Y73.8
      accessory Y73.2
      diagnostic Y73.0
      miscellaneous Y73.8
      monitoring Y73.0
      prosthetic Y73.2
      rehabilitative Y73.1
      surgical Y73.3
      therapeutic Y73.1
    general
      hospital Y74.8
        accessory Y74.2
        diagnostic Y74.0
        miscellaneous Y74.8
        monitoring Y74.0
        prosthetic Y74.2
        rehabilitative Y74.1
        surgical Y74.3
        therapeutic Y74.1
      surgical Y81.8
        accessory Y81.2
        diagnostic Y81.0
        miscellaneous Y81.8
        monitoring Y81.0
        prosthetic Y81.2
        rehabilitative Y81.1
        surgical Y81.3
        therapeutic Y81.1
    gynecological Y76.8
      accessory Y76.2
      diagnostic Y76.0
      miscellaneous Y76.8
      monitoring Y76.0
      prosthetic Y76.2
      rehabilitative Y76.1
      surgical Y76.3
      therapeutic Y76.1
    medical Y82.9
      specified type NEC Y82.8
    neurological Y75.8
      accessory Y75.2
      diagnostic Y75.0
      miscellaneous Y75.8
      monitoring Y75.0
      prosthetic Y75.2
      rehabilitative Y75.1
      surgical Y75.3
      therapeutic Y75.1
    obstetrical Y76.8
      accessory Y76.2
      diagnostic Y76.0
      miscellaneous Y76.8
      monitoring Y76.0
      prosthetic Y76.2
      rehabilitative Y76.1
      surgical Y76.3
      therapeutic Y76.1
    ophthalmic Y77.8
      accessory Y77.2
      diagnostic Y77.0
      miscellaneous Y77.8
      monitoring Y77.0
      prosthetic Y77.2
      rehabilitative Y77.1
      surgical Y77.3
      therapeutic Y77.1
    orthopedic Y79.8
      accessory Y79.2

Incident, adverse — *continued*
  device — *continued*
    orthopedic — *continued*
      diagnostic Y79.0
      miscellaneous Y79.8
      monitoring Y79.0
      prosthetic Y79.2
      rehabilitative Y79.1
      surgical Y79.3
      therapeutic Y79.1
    otorhinolaryngological Y72.8
      accessory Y72.2
      diagnostic Y72.0
      miscellaneous Y72.8
      monitoring Y72.0
      prosthetic Y72.2
      rehabilitative Y72.1
      surgical Y72.3
      therapeutic Y72.1
    personal use Y74.8
      accessory Y74.2
      diagnostic Y74.0
      miscellaneous Y74.8
      monitoring Y74.0
      prosthetic Y74.2
      rehabilitative Y74.1
      surgical Y74.3
      therapeutic Y74.1
    physical medicine Y80.8
      accessory Y80.2
      diagnostic Y80.0
      miscellaneous Y80.8
      monitoring Y80.0
      prosthetic Y80.2
      rehabilitative Y80.1
      surgical Y80.3
      therapeutic Y80.1
    plastic surgical Y81.8
      accessory Y81.2
      diagnostic Y81.0
      miscellaneous Y81.8
      monitoring Y81.0
      prosthetic Y81.2
      rehabilitative Y81.1
      surgical Y81.3
      therapeutic Y81.1
    radiological Y78.8
      accessory Y78.2
      diagnostic Y78.0
      miscellaneous Y78.8
      monitoring Y78.0
      prosthetic Y78.2
      rehabilitative Y78.1
      surgical Y78.3
      therapeutic Y78.1
    urology Y73.8
      accessory Y73.2
      diagnostic Y73.0
      miscellaneous Y73.8
      monitoring Y73.0
      prosthetic Y73.2
      rehabilitative Y73.1
      surgical Y73.3
      therapeutic Y73.1
Incineration (accidental) — *see* Exposure, fire
Infanticide — *see* Assault
Infrasound waves (causing injury) W49.9 ☑
Ingestion
  foreign body (causing injury) (with obstruction) — *see*
    Foreign body, alimentary canal
  poisonous
    plant(s) X58 ☑
    substance NEC — *see* Table of Drugs and Chemicals
Inhalation
  excessively cold substance, man-made — *see* Expo-
    sure, cold, man-made
  food (any type) (into respiratory tract) (with asphyxia,
    obstruction respiratory tract, suffocation) — *see*
    categories T17 and T18
  foreign body — *see* Foreign body, aspiration
  gastric contents (with asphyxia, obstruction respiratory
    passage, suffocation) T17.81- ☑
  hot air or gases X14.0 ☑
  liquid air, hydrogen, nitrogen W93.12 ☑
    suicide (attempt) X83.2 ☑
  steam X13.0 ☑
    assault X98.0 ☑

Inhalation — *continued*
  steam — *continued*
    stated as undetermined whether accidental or intentional Y27.0 ☑
    suicide (attempt) X77.0 ☑
  toxic gas — *see* Table of Drugs and Chemicals
  vomitus (with asphyxia, obstruction respiratory passage, suffocation) T17.81- ☑
Injury, injured (accidental(ly)) NOS X58 ☑
  by, caused by, from
    assault — *see* Assault
    law-enforcing agent, police, in course of legal intervention — *see* Legal intervention
    suicide (attempt) X83.8 ☑
  due to, in
    civil insurrection — *see* War operations
    fight (*see also* Assault, fight) Y04.0 ☑
    war operations — *see* War operations
  homicide (*see also* Assault) Y09
  inflicted (by)
    in course of arrest (attempted), suppression of disturbance, maintenance of order, by law-enforcing agents — *see* Legal intervention
    other person
      stated as
        accidental X58 ☑
        intentional, homicide (attempt) — *see* Assault
        undetermined whether accidental or intentional Y33 ☑
    purposely (inflicted) by other person(s) — *see* Assault
  self-inflicted X83.8 ☑
    stated as accidental X58 ☑
  specified cause NEC X58 ☑
  undetermined whether accidental or intentional Y33 ☑
Insolation, effects X30 ☑
Insufficient nourishment X58 ☑
Interruption of respiration (by)
  food (lodged in esophagus) — *see* categories T17 and T18 ☑
  vomitus (lodged in esophagus) T17.81- ☑
Intervention, legal — *see* Legal intervention
Intoxication
  drug — *see* Table of Drugs and Chemicals
  poison — *see* Table of Drugs and Chemicals

J

Jammed (accidentally)
  between objects (moving) (stationary and moving) W23.0 ☑
    stationary W23.1 ☑
Jumped, jumping
  before moving object NEC X81.8 ☑
    motor vehicle X81.0 ☑
    subway train X81.1 ☑
    train X81.1 ☑
    undetermined whether accidental or intentional Y31 ☑
  from
    boat (into water) voluntarily, without accident (to or on boat) W16.712 ☑
      with
        accident to or on boat — *see* Accident, watercraft
        drowning or submersion W16.711 ☑
          suicide (attempt) X71.3 ☑
        striking bottom W16.722 ☑
          causing drowning W16.721 ☑
    building (*see also* Jumped, from, high place) W13.9 ☑
      burning (uncontrolled fire) X00.5 ☑
    high place NEC W17.89 ☑
      suicide (attempt) X80 ☑
      undetermined whether accidental or intentional Y30 ☑
    structure (*see also* Jumped, from, high place) W13.9 ☑
      burning (uncontrolled fire) X00.5 ☑
  into water W16.92 ☑
    causing drowning W16.91 ☑
    from, off watercraft — *see* Jumped, from, boat
    in
      natural body W16.612 ☑
        causing drowning W16.611 ☑

Jumped, jumping — *continued*
  into water — *continued*
    in — *continued*
      natural body — *continued*
        striking bottom W16.622 ☑
          causing drowning W16.621 ☑
      specified place NEC W16.812 ☑
        causing drowning W16.811 ☑
        striking
          bottom W16.822 ☑
            causing drowning W16.821 ☑
          wall W16.832 ☑
            causing drowning W16.831 ☑
      swimming pool W16.512 ☑
        causing drowning W16.511 ☑
        striking
          bottom W16.522 ☑
            causing drowning W16.521 ☑
          wall W16.532 ☑
            causing drowning W16.531 ☑
    suicide (attempt) X71.3 ☑

K

Kicked by
  animal NEC W55.82 ☑
  person(s) (accidentally) W50.1 ☑
    with intent to injure or kill Y04.0 ☑
    as, or caused by, a crowd or human stampede (with fall) W52 ☑
    assault Y04.0 ☑
    homicide (attempt) Y04.0 ☑
    in
      fight Y04.0 ☑
      legal intervention
        injuring
          bystander Y35.812 ☑
          law enforcement personnel Y35.811 ☑
          suspect Y35.813 ☑
Kicking against
  object W22.8 ☑
    sports equipment W21.9 ☑
  stationary wW22.09
    sports equipment W21.89 ☑
  person — *see* Striking against, person
  sports equipment W21.9 ☑
Killed, killing (accidentally) NOS (*see also* Injury) X58 ☑
  in
    action — *see* War operations
    brawl, fight (hand) (fists) (foot) Y04.0 ☑
      by weapon (*see also* Assault)
        cutting, piercing — *see* Assault, cutting or piercing instrument
        firearm — *see* Discharge, firearm, by type, homicide
  self
    stated as
      accident NOS X58 ☑
      suicide — *see* Suicide
      undetermined whether accidental or intentional Y33 ☑
Knocked down (accidentally) (by) NOS X58 ☑
  animal (not being ridden) NEC (*see also* Struck by, by type of animal)
  crowd or human stampede W52 ☑
  person W51 ☑
    in brawl, fight Y04.0 ☑
  transport vehicle NEC (*see also* Accident, transport) V09.9 ☑

L

Laceration NEC — *see* Injury
Lack of
  care (helpless person) (infant) (newborn) X58 ☑
  food except as result of abandonment or neglect X58 ☑
    due to abandonment or neglect X58 ☑
  water except as result of transport accident X58 ☑
    due to transport accident B — *see* Accident, transport, by type
    helpless person, infant, newborn X58 ☑
Landslide (falling on transport vehicle) X36.1 ☑
  caused by collapse of man-made structure X36.0 ☑
Late effect — *see* Sequelae

Legal
  execution (any method) — *see* Legal, intervention
  intervention (by)
    baton — *see* Legal, intervention, blunt object, baton
    bayonet — *see* Legal, intervention, sharp object, bayonet
    blow — *see* Legal, intervention, manhandling
    blunt object
      baton
        injuring
          bystander Y35.312 ☑
          law enforcement personnel Y35.311 ☑
          suspect Y35.313 ☑
      injuring
        bystander Y35.302 ☑
        law enforcement personnel Y35.301 ☑
        suspect Y35.303 ☑
      specified NEC
        injuring
          bystander Y35.392 ☑
          law enforcement personnel Y35.391 ☑
          suspect Y35.393 ☑
      stave
        injuring
          bystander Y35.392 ☑
          law enforcement personnel Y35.391 ☑
          suspect Y35.393 ☑
    bomb — *see* Legal, intervention, explosive
    cutting or piercing instrument — *see* Legal, intervention, sharp object
    dynamite — *see* Legal, intervention, explosive, dynamite
    explosive(s)
      dynamite
        injuring
          bystander Y35.112 ☑
          law enforcement personnel Y35.111 ☑
          suspect Y35.113 ☑
      grenade
        injuring
          bystander Y35.192 ☑
          law enforcement personnel Y35.191 ☑
          suspect Y35.193 ☑
      injuring
        bystander Y35.102 ☑
        law enforcement personnel Y35.101 ☑
        suspect Y35.103 ☑
      mortar bomb
        injuring
          bystander Y35.192 ☑
          law enforcement personnel Y35.191 ☑
          suspect Y35.193 ☑
      shell
        injuring
          bystander Y35.122 ☑
          law enforcement personnel Y35.121 ☑
          suspect Y35.123 ☑
      specified NEC
        injuring
          bystander Y35.192 ☑
          law enforcement personnel Y35.191 ☑
          suspect Y35.193 ☑
    firearm(s) (discharge)
      handgun
        injuring
          bystander Y35.022 ☑
          law enforcement personnel Y35.021 ☑
          suspect Y35.023 ☑
      injuring
        bystander Y35.002 ☑
        law enforcement personnel Y35.001 ☑
        suspect Y35.003 ☑
      machine gun
        injuring
          bystander Y35.012 ☑
          law enforcement personnel Y35.011 ☑
          suspect Y35.013 ☑
      rifle pellet
        injuring
          bystander Y35.032 ☑
          law enforcement personnel Y35.031 ☑
          suspect Y35.033 ☑
      rubber bullet
        injuring
          bystander Y35.042 ☑
          law enforcement personnel Y35.041 ☑

Legal — *continued*
　intervention — *continued*
　　firearm(s) — *continued*
　　　rubber bullet — *continued*
　　　　injuring — *continued*
　　　　　suspect Y35.043 ☑
　　　shotgun — *see* Legal, intervention, firearm, specified NEC
　　　specified NEC
　　　　injuring
　　　　　bystander Y35.092 ☑
　　　　　law enforcement personnel Y35.091 ☑
　　　　　suspect Y35.093 ☑
　　gas (asphyxiation) (poisoning)
　　　injuring
　　　　bystander Y35.202 ☑
　　　　law enforcement personnel Y35.201 ☑
　　　　suspect Y35.203 ☑
　　　specified NEC
　　　　injuring
　　　　　bystander Y35.292 ☑
　　　　　law enforcement personnel Y35.291 ☑
　　　　　suspect Y35.293 ☑
　　　tear gas
　　　　injuring
　　　　　bystander Y35.212 ☑
　　　　　law enforcement personnel Y35.211 ☑
　　　　　suspect Y35.213 ☑
　　grenade — *see* Legal, intervention, explosive, grenade
　　injuring
　　　bystander Y35.92 ☑
　　　law enforcement personnel Y35.91 ☑
　　　suspect Y35.93 ☑
　　late effect (of) — *see* with 7th character S Y35 ☑
　　manhandling
　　　injuring
　　　　bystander Y35.812 ☑
　　　　law enforcement personnel Y35.811 ☑
　　　　suspect Y35.813 ☑
　　sequelae (of) — *see* with 7th character S Y35 ☑
　　sharp objects
　　　bayonet
　　　　injuring
　　　　　bystander Y35.412 ☑
　　　　　law enforcement personnel Y35.411 ☑
　　　　　suspect Y35.413 ☑
　　　injuring
　　　　bystander Y35.402 ☑
　　　　law enforcement personnel Y35.401 ☑
　　　　suspect Y35.403 ☑
　　　specified NEC
　　　　injuring
　　　　　bystander Y35.492 ☑
　　　　　law enforcement personnel Y35.491 ☑
　　　　　suspect Y35.493 ☑
　　specified means NEC
　　　injuring
　　　　bystander Y35.892 ☑
　　　　law enforcement personnel Y35.891 ☑
　　　　suspect Y35.893 ☑
　　stabbing — *see* Legal, intervention, sharp object
　　stave — *see* Legal, intervention, blunt object, stave
　　tear gas — *see* Legal, intervention, gas, tear gas
　　truncheon — *see* Legal, intervention, blunt object, stave
Lightning (shock) (stroke) (struck by) — *see* subcategory T75.0 ☑
　causing fire — *see* Exposure, fire
Loss of control (transport vehicle) NEC — *see* Accident, transport
Lost at sea NOS — *see* Drowning, due to, fall overboard
Low
　pressure (effects) — *see* Air, pressure, low
　temperature (effects) — *see* Exposure, cold
Lying before train, vehicle or other moving object X81.8
　subway train X81.1 ☑
　train X81.1 ☑
　undetermined whether accidental or intentional Y31 ☑
Lynching — *see* Assault

M

Malfunction (mechanism or component) (of)
　firearm W34.10 ☑
　　airgun W34.110 ☑
　　BB gun W34.110 ☑
　　gas, air or spring-operated gun NEC W34.118 ☑
　　handgun W32.1 ☑
　　hunting rifle W33.12 ☑
　　larger firearm W33.10 ☑
　　　specified NEC W33.19 ☑
　　machine gun W33.13 ☑
　　paintball gun W34.111 ☑
　　pellet gun W34.110 ☑
　　shotgun W33.11 ☑
　　specified NEC W34.19 ☑
　　Very pistol [flare] W34.19 ☑
　　handgun — *see* Malfunction, firearm, handgun
Maltreatment — *see* Perpetrator
Mangled (accidentally) NOS X58 ☑
Manhandling (in brawl, fight) Y04.0 ☑
　legal intervention — *see* Legal, intervention, manhandling
Manslaughter (nonaccidental) — *see* Assault
Mauled by animal NEC W55.89 ☑
Medical procedure, complication of (delayed or as an abnormal reaction without mention of misadventure) — *see* Complication of or following, by specified type of procedure
　due to or as a result of misadventure — *see* Misadventure
Melting (due to fire) (*see also* Exposure, fire)
　apparel NEC X06.3 ☑
　clothes, clothing NEC X06.3 ☑
　　nightwear X05 ☑
　fittings or furniture (burning building) (uncontrolled fire) X00.8 ☑
　nightwear X05 ☑
　plastic jewelry X06.1 ☑
Mental cruelty X58 ☑
Military operations (injuries to military and civilians occuring during peacetime on military property and during routine military exercises and operations) (by) (from) (involving) Y37.90- ☑
　air blast Y37.20- ☑
　aircraft
　　destruction — *see* Military operations, destruction of aircraft
　　airway restriction — *see* Military operations, restriction of airways
　asphyxiation — *see* Military operations, restriction of airways
　biological weapons Y37.6X- ☑
　blast Y37.20- ☑
　blast fragments Y37.20- ☑
　blast wave Y37.20- ☑
　blast wind Y37.20- ☑
　bomb Y37.20- ☑
　　dirty Y37.50- ☑
　　gasoline Y37.31- ☑
　　incendiary Y37.31- ☑
　　petrol Y37.31- ☑
　bullet Y37.43- ☑
　　incendiary Y37.32- ☑
　　rubber Y37.41- ☑
　chemical weapons Y37.7X- ☑
　combat
　　hand to hand (unarmed) combat Y37.44- ☑
　　using blunt or piercing object Y37.45- ☑
　conflagration — *see* Military operations, fire
　conventional warfare NEC Y37.49- ☑
　depth-charge Y37.01- ☑
　destruction of aircraft Y37.10- ☑
　　due to
　　　air to air missile Y37.11- ☑
　　　collision with other aircraft Y37.12- ☑
　　　detonation (accidental) of onboard munitions and explosives Y37.14- ☑
　　　enemy fire or explosives Y37.11- ☑
　　　explosive placed on aircraft Y37.11- ☑
　　　onboard fire Y37.13- ☑
　　　rocket propelled grenade [RPG] Y37.11- ☑
　　　small arms fire Y37.11- ☑
　　　surface to air missile Y37.11- ☑
　　specified NEC Y37.19- ☑

Military operations — *continued*
　detonation (accidental) of
　　onboard marine weapons Y37.05- ☑
　　own munitions or munitions launch device Y37.24- ☑
　dirty bomb Y37.50- ☑
　explosion (of) Y37.20- ☑
　　aerial bomb Y37.21- ☑
　　bomb NOS (*see also* Military operations, bomb(s)) Y37.20- ☑
　　fragments Y37.20- ☑
　　grenade Y37.29- ☑
　　guided missile Y37.22- ☑
　　improvised explosive device [IED] (person-borne) (roadside) (vehicle-borne) Y37.23- ☑
　　land mine Y37.29- ☑
　　marine mine (at sea) (in harbor) Y37.02- ☑
　　marine weapon Y37.00- ☑
　　　specified NEC Y37.09- ☑
　　own munitions or munitions launch device (accidental) Y37.24- ☑
　　sea-based artillery shell Y37.03- ☑
　　specified NEC Y37.29- ☑
　　torpedo Y37.04- ☑
　fire Y37.30- ☑
　　specified NEC Y37.39- ☑
　firearms
　　discharge Y37.43- ☑
　　pellets Y37.42- ☑
　flamethrower Y37.33- ☑
　fragments (from) (of)
　　improvised explosive device [IED] (person-borne) (roadside) (vehicle-borne) Y37.26- ☑
　　munitions Y37.25- ☑
　　specified NEC Y37.29- ☑
　　weapons Y37.27- ☑
　friendly fire Y37.92- ☑
　hand to hand (unarmed) combat Y37.44- ☑
　hot substances — *see* Military operations, fire
　incendiary bullet Y37.32- ☑
　nuclear weapon (effects of) Y37.50- ☑
　　acute radiation exposure Y37.54- ☑
　　blast pressure Y37.51- ☑
　　direct blast Y37.51- ☑
　　direct heat Y37.53- ☑
　　fallout exposure Y37.54- ☑
　　fireball Y37.53- ☑
　　indirect blast (struck or crushed by blast debris) (being thrown by blast) Y37.52- ☑
　　ionizing radiation (immediate exposure) Y37.54- ☑
　　nuclear radiation Y37.54- ☑
　　radiation
　　　ionizing (immediate exposure) Y37.54- ☑
　　　nuclear Y37.54- ☑
　　　thermal Y37.53- ☑
　　secondary effects Y37.54- ☑
　　specified NEC Y37.59- ☑
　　thermal radiation Y37.53- ☑
　restriction of air (airway)
　　intentional Y37.46- ☑
　　unintentional Y37.47- ☑
　rubber bullets Y37.41- ☑
　shrapnel NOS Y37.29- ☑
　suffocation — *see* Military operations, restriction of airways
　unconventional warfare NEC Y37.7X- ☑
　underwater blast NOS Y37.00- ☑
　warfare
　　conventional NEC Y37.49- ☑
　　unconventional NEC Y37.7X- ☑
　weapon of mass destruction [WMD] Y37.91- ☑
　weapons
　　biological weapons Y37.6X- ☑
　　chemical Y37.7X- ☑
　　nuclear (effects of) Y37.50- ☑
　　　acute radiation exposure Y37.54- ☑
　　　blast pressure Y37.51- ☑
　　　direct blast Y37.51- ☑
　　　direct heat Y37.53- ☑
　　　fallout exposure Y37.54- ☑
　　　fireball Y37.53- ☑
　　　indirect blast (struck or crushed by blast debris) (being thrown by blast) Y37.52- ☑
　　　radiation
　　　　ionizing (immediate exposure) Y37.54- ☑
　　　　nuclear Y37.54- ☑
　　　　thermal Y37.53- ☑

Military operations — continued
  weapons — continued
    nuclear — continued
      secondary effects Y37.54- ☑
      specified NEC Y37.59- ☑
    of mass destruction [WMD] Y37.91- ☑
Misadventure(s) to patient(s) during surgical or medical care Y69
  contaminated medical or biological substance (blood, drug, fluid) Y64.9
    administered (by) NEC Y64.9
      immunization Y64.1
      infusion Y64.0
      injection Y64.1
      specified means NEC Y64.8
      transfusion Y64.0
      vaccination Y64.1
  excessive amount of blood or other fluid during transfusion or infusion Y63.0
  failure
    in dosage Y63.9
      electroshock therapy Y63.4
      inappropriate temperature (too hot or too cold) in local application and packing Y63.5
      infusion
        excessive amount of fluid Y63.0
        incorrect dilution of fluid Y63.1
      insulin-shock therapy Y63.4
      nonadministration of necessary drug or biological substance Y63.6
      overdose — see Table of Drugs and Chemicals
      radiation, in therapy Y63.2
      radiation
        overdose Y63.2
      specified procedure NEC Y63.8
      transfusion
        excessive amount of blood Y63.0
    mechanical, of instrument or apparatus (any) (during any procedure) Y65.8
    sterile precautions (during procedure) Y62.9
      aspiration of fluid or tissue (by puncture or catheterization, except heart) Y62.6
      biopsy (except needle aspiration) Y62.8
        needle (aspirating) Y62.6
      blood sampling Y62.6
      catheterization Y62.6
        heart Y62.5
      dialysis (kidney) Y62.2
      endoscopic examination Y62.4
      enema Y62.8
      immunization Y62.3
      infusion Y62.1
      injection Y62.3
      needle biopsy Y62.6
      paracentesis (abdominal) (thoracic) Y62.6
      perfusion Y62.2
      puncture (lumbar) Y62.6
      removal of catheter or packing Y62.8
      specified procedure NEC Y62.8
      surgical operation Y62.0
      transfusion Y62.1
      vaccination Y62.3
    suture or ligature during surgical procedure Y65.2
    to introduce or to remove tube or instrument B — see Failure, to
  hemorrhage — see Index to Diseases and Injuries, Complication(s)
  inadvertent exposure of patient to radiation Y63.3
  inappropriate
    operation performed — see Inappropriate operation performed
    temperature (too hot or too cold) in local application or packing Y63.5
  infusion (see also Misadventure, by type, infusion) Y69
    excessive amount of fluid Y63.0
    incorrect dilution of fluid Y63.1
    wrong fluid Y65.1
  mismatched blood in transfusion Y65.0
  nonadministration of necessary drug or biological substance
    overdose — see Table of Drugs and Chemicals
    radiation (in therapy) Y63.2
  perforation — see Index to Diseases and Injuries, Complication(s)
  performance of inappropriate operation — see Inappropriate operation performed
  puncture — see Index to Diseases and Injuries, Complication(s)

Misadventure(s) to patient(s) during surgical or medical care — continued
  specified type NEC Y65.8
    failure
      suture or ligature during surgical operation Y65.2
      to introduce or to remove tube or instrument B — see Failure, to
    infusion of wrong fluid Y65.1
    performance of inappropriate operation — see Inappropriate operation performed
    transfusion of mismatched blood Y65.0
    wrong
      fluid in infusion Y65.1
      placement of endotracheal tube during anesthetic procedure Y65.3
  transfusion — see Misadventure, by type, transfusion
    excessive amount of blood Y63.0
    mismatched blood Y65.0
  wrong
    drug given in error — see Table of Drugs and Chemicals
    fluid in infusion Y65.1
    placement of endotracheal tube during anesthetic procedure Y65.3
Mismatched blood in transfusion Y65.0
Motion sickness T75.3 ☑
Mountain sickness W94.11 ☑
Mudslide (of cataclysmic nature) — see Landslide
Murder (attempt) — see Assault

N

Nail, contact with W45.0 ☑
  gun W29.4 ☑
Neglect (criminal) (homicidal intent) X58 ☑
Noise (causing injury) (pollution) W42.9 ☑
  supersonic W42.0 ☑
Nonadministration (of)
  drug or biological substance (necessary) Y63.6
  surgical and medical care Y66
Nosocomial condition Y95

O

Object
  falling
    from, in, on, hitting
      machinery — see Contact, with, by type of machine
    set in motion by
      accidental explosion or rupture of pressure vessel W38 ☑
      firearm — see Discharge, firearm, by type
      machine(ry) — see Contact, with, by type of machine
Overdose (drug) — see Table of Drugs and Chemicals
  radiation Y63.2
Overexertion — see category Y93 ☑
Overexposure (accidental) (to)
  cold (see also Exposure, cold) X31 ☑
    due to man-made conditions — see Exposure, cold, man-made
  heat (see also Heat) X30 ☑
  radiation — see Radiation
  radioactivity W88.0 ☑
  sun (sunburn) X32 ☑
  weather NEC — see Forces of nature
  wind NEC — see Forces of nature
Overheated — see Heat
Overturning (accidental)
  machinery — see Contact, with, by type of machine
  transport vehicle NEC (see also Accident, transport) V89.9 ☑
  watercraft (causing drowning, submersion) (see also Drowning, due to, accident to, watercraft, overturning)
    causing injury except drowning or submersion B — see Accident, watercraft, causing, injury NEC

P

Parachute descent (voluntary) (without accident to aircraft) V97.29 ☑
Pecked by bird W61.99 ☑

Perforation during medical or surgical treatment as misadventure — see Index to Diseases and Injuries, Complication(s)

Perpetrator, perpetration, of assault, maltreatment and neglect (by) Y07.9
  boyfriend Y07.03
  brother Y07.410
    stepbrother Y07.435
  coach Y07.53
  cousin
    female Y07.491
    male Y07.490
  daycare provider Y07.519
    at-home
      adult care Y07.512
      childcare Y07.510
    care center
      adult care Y07.513
      childcare Y07.511
  family member NEC Y07.499
  father Y07.11
    adoptive Y07.13
    foster Y07.420
    stepfather Y07.430
  foster father Y07.420
  foster mother Y07.421
  girl friend Y07.04
  healthcare provider Y07.529
    mental health Y07.521
    specified NEC Y07.528
  husband Y07.01
  instructor Y07.53
  mother Y07.12
    adoptive Y07.14
    foster Y07.421
    stepmother Y07.433
  nonfamily member Y07.50
    specified NEC Y07.59
  nurse Y07.528
  occupational therapist Y07.528
  partner of parent
    female Y07.434
    male Y07.432
  physical therapist Y07.528
  sister Y07.411
  speech therapist Y07.528
  stepbrother Y07.435
  stepfather Y07.430
  stepmother Y07.433
  stepsister Y07.436
  teacher Y07.53
  wife Y07.02

Piercing — see Contact, with, by type of object or machine

Pinched
  between objects (moving) (stationary and moving) W23.0 ☑
  stationary W23.1 ☑

Pinned under machine(ry) — see Contact, with, by type of machine

Place of occurrence Y92.9
  abandoned house Y92.89
  airplane Y92.813
  airport Y92.520
  ambulatory health services establishment NEC Y92.538
  ambulatory surgery center Y92.530
  amusement park Y92.831
  apartment (co-op) — see Place of occurrence, residence, apartment
  assembly hall Y92.29
  bank Y92.510
  barn Y92.71
  baseball field Y92.320
  basketball court Y92.310
  beach Y92.832
  boarding house — see Place of occurrence, residence, boarding house
  boat Y92.814
  bowling alley Y92.39
  bridge Y92.89
  building under construction Y92.61
  bus Y92.811
    station Y92.521
  cafe Y92.511

Place of occurrence — *continued*
  campsite Y92.833
  campus — *see* Place of occurrence, school
  canal Y92.89
  car Y92.810
  casino Y92.59
  children's home — *see* Place of occurrence, residence,
      institutional, orphanage
  church Y92.22
  cinema Y92.26
  clubhouse Y92.29
  coal pit Y92.64
  college (community) Y92.214
  condominium — *see* Place of occurrence, residence,
      apartment
  construction area — *see* Place of occurrence, industrial
      and construction area
  convalescent home — *see* Place of occurrence, resi-
      dence, institutional, nursing home
  court-house Y92.240
  cricket ground Y92.328
  cultural building Y92.258
    art gallery Y92.250
    museum Y92.251
    music hall Y92.252
    opera house Y92.253
    specified NEC Y92.258
    theater Y92.254
  dancehall Y92.252
  day nursery Y92.210
  dentist office Y92.531
  derelict house Y92.89
  desert Y92.820
  dockyard Y92.62
  dock NOS Y92.89
  doctor's office Y92.531
  dormitory — *see* Place of occurrence, residence, insti-
      tutional, school dormitory
  dry dock Y92.62
  factory (building) (premises) Y92.63
  farm (land under cultivation) (outbuildings) Y92.79
    barn Y92.71
    chicken coop Y92.72
    field Y92.73
    hen house Y92.72
    house — *see* Place of occurrence, residence, house
    orchard Y92.74
    specified NEC Y92.79
  football field Y92.321
  forest Y92.821
  freeway Y92.411
  gallery Y92.250
  garage (commercial) Y92.59
    boarding house Y92.044
    military base Y92.135
    mobile home Y92.025
    nursing home Y92.124
    orphanage Y92.114
    private house Y92.015
    reform school Y92.155
  gas station Y92.524
  gasworks Y92.69
  golf course Y92.39
  gravel pit Y92.64
  grocery Y92.512
  gymnasium Y92.39
  handball court Y92.318
  harbor Y92.89
  harness racing course Y92.39
  healthcare provider office Y92.531
  highway (interstate) Y92.411
  hill Y92.828
  hockey rink Y92.330
  home — *see* Place of occurrence, residence
  hospice — *see* Place of occurrence, residence, institu-
      tional, nursing home
  hospital Y92.239
    cafeteria Y92.233
    corridor Y92.232
    operating room Y92.234
    patient
      bathroom Y92.231
      room Y92.230
    specified NEC Y92.238
  hotel Y92.59
  house (*see also* Place of occurrence, residence)
    abandoned Y92.89
    under construction Y92.61

Place of occurrence — *continued*
  industrial and construction area (yard) Y92.69
    building under construction Y92.61
    dock Y92.62
    dry dock Y92.62
    factory Y92.63
    gasworks Y92.69
    mine Y92.64
    oil rig Y92.65
    pit Y92.64
    power station Y92.69
    shipyard Y92.62
    specified NEC Y92.69
    tunnel under construction Y92.69
    workshop Y92.69
  kindergarten Y92.211
  lacrosse field Y92.328
  lake Y92.828
  library Y92.241
  mall Y92.59
  market Y92.512
  marsh Y92.828
  military
    base — *see* Place of occurrence, residence, institu-
        tional, military base
    training ground Y92.84
  mine Y92.64
  mosque Y92.22
  motel Y92.59
  motorway (interstate) Y92.411
  mountain Y92.828
  movie-house Y92.26
  museum Y92.251
  music-hall Y92.252
  not applicable Y92.9
  nuclear power station Y92.69
  nursing home — *see* Place of occurrence, residence,
      institutional, nursing home
  office building Y92.59
  offshore installation Y92.65
  oil rig Y92.65
  old people's home — *see* Place of occurrence, resi-
      dence, institutional, specified NEC
  opera-house Y92.253
  orphanage — *see* Place of occurrence, residence, insti-
      tutional, orphanage
  outpatient surgery center Y92.530
  park (public) Y92.830
    amusement Y92.831
  parking garage Y92.89
    lot Y92.481
  pavement Y92.480
  physician office Y92.531
  polo field Y92.328
  pond Y92.828
  post office Y92.242
  power station Y92.69
  prairie Y92.828
  prison — *see* Place of occurrence, residence, institu-
      tional, prison
  public
    administration building Y92.248
      city hall Y92.243
      courthouse Y92.240
      library Y92.241
      post office Y92.242
      specified NEC Y92.248
    building NEC Y92.29
    hall Y92.29
    place NOS Y92.89
  race course Y92.39
  radio station Y92.59
  railway line (bridge) Y92.85
  ranch (outbuildings) — *see* Place of occurrence, farm
  recreation area Y92.838
    amusement park Y92.831
    beach Y92.832
    campsite Y92.833
    park (public) Y92.830
    seashore Y92.832
    specified NEC Y92.838
  reform school - — *see* Place of occurrence, residence,
      institutional, reform school
  religious institution Y92.22
  residence (non-institutional) (private) Y92.009
    apartment Y92.039
      bathroom Y92.031
      bedroom Y92.032

Place of occurrence — *continued*
  residence — *continued*
    apartment — *continued*
      kitchen Y92.030
      specified NEC Y92.038
    bathroom Y92.002
    bedroom Y92.003
    boarding house Y92.049
      bathroom Y92.041
      bedroom Y92.042
      driveway Y92.043
      garage Y92.044
      garden Y92.046
      kitchen Y92.040
      specified NEC Y92.048
      swimming pool Y92.045
      yard Y92.046
    dining room Y92.001
    garden Y92.007
    home Y92.009
    house, single family Y92.019
      bathroom Y92.012
      bedroom Y92.013
      dining room Y92.011
      driveway Y92.014
      garage Y92.015
      garden Y92.017
      kitchen Y92.010
      specified NEC Y92.018
      swimming pool Y92.016
      yard Y92.017
    institutional Y92.10
      children's home — *see* Place of occurrence,
        residence, institutional, orphanage
      hospice — *see* Place of occurrence, residence,
        institutional, nursing home
      military base Y92.139
        barracks Y92.133
        garage Y92.135
        garden Y92.137
        kitchen Y92.130
        mess hall Y92.131
        specified NEC Y92.138
        swimming pool Y92.136
        yard Y92.137
      nursing home Y92.129
        bathroom Y92.121
        bedroom Y92.122
        driveway Y92.123
        garage Y92.124
        garden Y92.126
        kitchen Y92.120
        specified NEC Y92.128
        swimming pool Y92.125
        yard Y92.126
      orphanage Y92.119
        bathroom Y92.111
        bedroom Y92.112
        driveway Y92.113
        garage Y92.114
        garden Y92.116
        kitchen Y92.110
        specified NEC Y92.118
        swimming pool Y92.115
        yard Y92.116
      prison Y92.149
        bathroom Y92.142
        cell Y92.143
        courtyard Y92.147
        dining room Y92.141
        kitchen Y92.140
        specified NEC Y92.148
        swimming pool Y92.146
      reform school Y92.159
        bathroom Y92.152
        bedroom Y92.153
        dining room Y92.151
        driveway Y92.154
        garage Y92.155
        garden Y92.157
        kitchen Y92.150
        specified NEC Y92.158
        swimming pool Y92.156
        yard Y92.157
      school dormitory Y92.169
        bathroom Y92.162
        bedroom Y92.163
        dining room Y92.161

Place of occurrence — *continued*
  residence — *continued*
    institutional — *continued*
      school dormitory — *continued*
        kitchen Y92.160
        specified NEC Y92.168
      specified NEC Y92.199
        bathroom Y92.192
        bedroom Y92.193
        dining room Y92.191
        driveway Y92.194
        garage Y92.195
        garden Y92.197
        kitchen Y92.190
        specified NEC Y92.198
        swimming pool Y92.196
        yard Y92.197
    kitchen Y92.000
    mobile home Y92.029
      bathroom Y92.022
      bedroom Y92.023
      dining room Y92.021
      driveway Y92.024
      garage Y92.025
      garden Y92.027
      kitchen Y92.020
      specified NEC Y92.028
      swimming pool Y92.026
      yard Y92.027
    specified place in residence NEC Y92.009
    specified residence type NEC Y92.099
      bathroom Y92.091
      bedroom Y92.092
      driveway Y92.093
      garage Y92.094
      garden Y92.096
      kitchen Y92.090
      specified NEC Y92.098
      swimming pool Y92.095
      yard Y92.096
  restaurant Y92.511
  riding school Y92.39
  river Y92.828
  road Y92.488
  rodeo ring Y92.39
  rugby field Y92.328
  same day surgery center Y92.530
  sand pit Y92.64
  school (private) (public) (state) Y92.219
    college Y92.214
    daycare center Y92.210
    elementary school Y92.211
    high school Y92.213
    kindergarten Y92.211
    middle school Y92.212
    specified NEC Y92.218
    trace school Y92.215
    university Y92.214
    vocational school Y92.215
  sea (shore) Y92.832
  senior citizen center Y92.29
  service area
    airport Y92.520
    bus station Y92.521
    gas station Y92.524
    highway rest stop Y92.523
    railway station Y92.522
  shipyard Y92.62
  shop (commercial) Y92.513
  sidewalk Y92.480
  silo Y92.79
  skating rink (roller) Y92.331
    ice Y92.330
  slaughter house Y92.86
  soccer field Y92.322
  specified place NEC Y92.89
  sports area Y92.39
    athletic
      court Y92.318
        basketball Y92.310
        specified NEC Y92.318
        squash Y92.311
        tennis Y92.312
      field Y92.328
        baseball Y92.320
        cricket ground Y92.328
        football Y92.321
        hockey Y92.328

Place of occurrence — *continued*
  sports area — *continued*
    athletic — *continued*
      field — *continued*
        soccer Y92.322
        specified NEC Y92.328
    golf course Y92.39
    gymnasium Y92.39
    riding school Y92.39
    skating rink (roller) Y92.331
      ice Y92.330
    stadium Y92.39
    swimming pool Y92.34
  squash court Y92.311
  stadium Y92.39
  steeplechasing course Y92.39
  store Y92.512
  stream Y92.828
  street and highway Y92.410
    bike path Y92.482
    freeway Y92.411
    highway ramp Y92.415
    interstate highway Y92.411
    local residential or business street Y92.414
    motorway Y92.411
    parking lot Y92.481
    parkway Y92.412
    sidewalk Y92.480
    specified NEC Y92.488
    state road Y92.413
  subway car Y92.816
  supermarket Y92.512
  swamp Y92.828
  swimming pool (public) Y92.34
    private (at) Y92.095
      boarding house Y92.045
      military base Y92.136
      mobile home Y92.026
      nursing home Y92.125
      orphanage Y92.115
      prison Y92.146
      reform school Y92.156
      single family residence Y92.016
  synagogue Y92.22
  television station Y92.59
  tennis court Y92.312
  theater Y92.254
  trade area Y92.59
    bank Y92.510
    cafe Y92.511
    casino Y92.59
    garage Y92.59
    hotel Y92.59
    market Y92.512
    office building Y92.59
    radio station Y92.59
    restaurant Y92.511
    shop Y92.513
    shopping mall Y92.59
    store Y92.512
    supermarket Y92.512
    television station Y92.59
    warehouse Y92.59
  trailer park, residential — *see* Place of occurrence, residence, mobile home
  trailer site NOS Y92.89
  train Y92.815
    station Y92.522
  truck Y92.812
  tunnel under construction Y92.69
  university Y92.214
  urgent (health) care center Y92.532
  vehicle (transport) Y92.818
    airplane Y92.813
    boat Y92.814
    bus Y92.811
    car Y92.810
    specified NEC Y92.818
    subway car Y92.816
    train Y92.815
    truck Y92.812
  warehouse Y92.59
  water reservoir Y92.89
  wilderness area Y92.828
    desert Y92.820
    forest Y92.821
    marsh Y92.828
    mountain Y92.828

Place of occurrence — *continued*
  wilderness area — *continued*
    prairie Y92.828
    specified NEC Y92.828
    swamp Y92.828
  workshop Y92.69
  yard, private Y92.096
    boarding house Y92.046
    mobile home Y92.027
    single family house Y92.017
  youth center Y92.29
  zoo (zoological garden) Y92.834
Plumbism — *see* Table of Drugs and Chemicals, lead
Poisoning (accidental) (by) (*see also* Table of Drugs and Chemicals)
  by plant, thorns, spines, sharp leaves or other mechanisms NEC X58 ☑
  carbon monoxide
    generated by
      motor vehicle — *see* Accident, transport
      watercraft (in transit) (not in transit) V93.89 ☑
        ferry boat V93.81 ☑
        fishing boat V93.82 ☑
        jet skis V93.83 ☑
        liner V93.81 ☑
        merchant ship V93.80 ☑
        passenger ship V93.81 ☑
        powered craft NEC V93.83 ☑
  caused by injection of poisons into skin by plant thorns, spines, sharp leaves X58 ☑
    marine or sea plants (venomous) X58 ☑
  execution — *see* Legal, intervention, gas
  intervention
    by gas — *see* Legal, intervention, gas
    other specified means — *see* Legal, intervention, specified means NEC
  exhaust gas
    generated by
      motor vehicle — *see* Accident, transport
      watercraft (in transit) (not in transit) V93.89 ☑
        ferry boat V93.81 ☑
        fishing boat V93.82 ☑
        jet skis V93.83 ☑
        liner V93.81 ☑
        merchant ship V93.80 ☑
        passenger ship V93.81 ☑
        powered craft NEC V93.83 ☑
  fumes or smoke due to
    explosion (*see also* Explosion) W40.9 ☑
    fire — *see* Exposure, fire
    ignition — *see* Ignition
  gas
    in legal intervention — *see* Legal, intervention, gas
    legal execution — *see* Legal, intervention, gas
  in war operations — *see* War operations
  legal
Powder burn (by) (from)
  airgun W34.110 ☑
  BB gun W34.110 ☑
  firearm NEC W34.19 ☑
  gas, air or spring-operated gun NEC W34.118 ☑
  handgun W32.1 ☑
  hunting rifle W33.12 ☑
  larger firearm W33.10 ☑
    specified NEC W33.19 ☑
  machine gun W33.13 ☑
  paintball gun W34.111 ☑
  pellet gun W34.110 ☑
  shotgun W33.11 ☑
  Very pistol [flare] W34.19 ☑
Premature cessation (of) **surgical and medical care** Y66
Privation (food) (water) X58 ☑
Procedure (operation)
  correct, on wrong side or body part (wrong side) (wrong site) Y65.53
  intended for another patient done on wrong patient Y65.52
  performed on patient not scheduled for surgery Y65.52
  performed on wrong patient Y65.52
  wrong, performed on correct patient Y65.51
Prolonged
  sitting in transport vehicle — *see* Travel, by type of vehicle
  stay in
    high altitude as cause of anoxia, barodontalgia, barotitis or hypoxia W94.11 ☑

Prolonged — *continued*
  stay in — *continued*
    weightless environment X52 ☑
Pulling, excessive — *see* Overexertion
Puncture, puncturing (*see also* Contact, with, by type of object or machine)
  by
    plant thorns, spines, sharp leaves or other mechanisms NEC W60 ☑
  during medical or surgical treatment as misadventure — *see* Index to Diseases and Injuries, Complication(s)
Pushed, pushing (accidental) (injury in) (overexertion) (*see also* Overexertion)
  by other person(s) (accidental) W51 ☑
    with fall W03 ☑
      due to ice or snow W00.0 ☑
    as, or caused by, a crowd or human stampede (with fall) W52 ☑
    before moving object NEC Y02.8 ☑
      motor vehicle Y02.0 ☑
      subway train Y02.1 ☑
      train Y02.1 ☑
    from
      high place NEC
        in accidental circumstances W17.89 ☑
        stated as
          intentional, homicide (attempt) Y01 ☑
          undetermined whether accidental or intentional Y30 ☑
      transport vehicle NEC (*see also* Accident, transport) V89.9 ☑
        stated as
          intentional, homicide (attempt) Y08.89 ☑

R

Radiation (exposure to)
  arc lamps W89.0 ☑
  atomic power plant (malfunction) NEC W88.1 ☑
  complication of or abnormal reaction to medical radiotherapy Y84.2
  electromagnetic, ionizing W88.0 ☑
  gamma rays W88.1 ☑
  in
    war operations (from or following nuclear explosion) — *see* War operations
  inadvertent exposure of patient (receiving test or therapy) Y63.3
  infrared (heaters and lamps) W90.1 ☑
    excessive heat from W92 ☑
  ionized, ionizing (particles, artificially accelerated)
    radioisotopes W88.1 ☑
    specified NEC W88.8 ☑
    x-rays W88.0 ☑
  isotopes, radioactive — *see* Radiation, radioactive isotopes
  laser(s) W90.2 ☑
    in war operations — *see* War operations
    misadventure in medical care Y63.2
  light sources (man-made visible and ultraviolet) W89.9 ☑
    natural X32 ☑
    specified NEC W89.8 ☑
    tanning bed W89.1 ☑
    welding light W89.0 ☑
  man-made visible light W89.9 ☑
    specified NEC W89.8 ☑
    tanning bed W89.1 ☑
    welding light W89.0 ☑
  microwave W90.8 ☑
  misadventure in medical or surgical procedure Y63.2
  natural NEC X39.08 ☑
    radon X39.01 ☑
  overdose (in medical or surgical procedure) Y63.2
  radar W90.0 ☑
  radioactive isotopes (any) W88.1 ☑
    atomic power plant malfunction W88.1 ☑
    misadventure in medical or surgical treatment Y63.2
  radiofrequency W90.0 ☑
  radium NEC W88.1 ☑
  sun X32 ☑
  ultraviolet (light) (man-made) W89.9 ☑
    natural X32 ☑

Radiation — *continued*
  ultraviolet — *continued*
    specified NEC W89.8 ☑
    tanning bed W89.1 ☑
    welding light W89.0 ☑
  welding arc, torch, or light W89.0 ☑
    excessive heat from W92 ☑
  x-rays (hard) (soft) W88.0 ☑
Range disease W94.11 ☑
Rape (attempted) T74.2- ☑
Rat bite W53.11 ☑
Reaction, abnormal to medical procedure (*see also* Complication of or following, by type of procedure) Y84.9
  with misadventure — *see* Misadventure
  biologicals — *see* Table of Drugs and Chemicals
  drugs — *see* Table of Drugs and Chemicals
  vaccine — *see* Table of Drugs and Chemicals
Recoil
  airgun W34.110 ☑
  BB gun W34.110 ☑
  firearm NEC W34.19 ☑
  gas, air or spring-operated gun NEC W34.118 ☑
  handgun W32.1 ☑
  hunting rifle W33.12 ☑
  larger firearm W33.10 ☑
    specified NEC W33.19 ☑
  machine gun W33.13 ☑
  paintball gun W34.111 ☑
  pellet W34.110 ☑
  shotgun W33.11 ☑
  Very pistol [flare] W34.19 ☑
Reduction in
  atmospheric pressure — *see* Air, pressure, change
Rock falling on or hitting (accidentally) (person) W20.8 ☑
  in cave-in W20.0 ☑
Run over (accidentally) (by)
  animal (not being ridden) NEC W55.89 ☑
  machinery — *see* Contact, with, by specified type of machine
  transport vehicle NEC (*see also* Accident, transport) V09.9 ☑
    intentional homicide (attempt) Y03.0 ☑
    motor NEC V09.20 ☑
      intentional homicide (attempt) Y03.0 ☑
Running
  before moving object X81.8 ☑
    motor vehicle X81.0 ☑
Running off, away
  animal (being ridden) (*see also* Accident, transport) V80.918 ☑
    not being ridden W55.89 ☑
  animal-drawn vehicle NEC (*see also* Accident, transport) V80.928 ☑
  highway, road(way), street
    transport vehicle NEC (*see also* Accident, transport) V89.9 ☑
Rupture pressurized devices — *see* Explosion, by type of device

S

Saturnism — *see* Table of Drugs and Chemicals, lead
Scald, scalding (accidental) (by) (from) (in) X19 ☑
  air (hot) X14.1 ☑
  gases (hot) X14.1 ☑
  homicide (attempt) — *see* Assault, burning, hot object
  inflicted by other person
    stated as intentional, homicide (attempt) — *see* Assault, burning, hot object
  liquid (boiling) (hot) NEC X12 ☑
    stated as undetermined whether accidental or intentional Y27.2 ☑
    suicide (attempt) X77.2 ☑
  local application of externally applied substance in medical or surgical care Y63.5
  metal (molten) (liquid) (hot) NEC X18 ☑
  self-inflicted X77.9 ☑
    stated as undetermined whether accidental or intentional Y27.8 ☑
  steam X13.1 ☑
    assault X98.0 ☑
    stated as undetermined whether accidental or intentional Y27.0 ☑
    suicide (attempt) X77.0 ☑

Scald, scalding — *continued*
  suicide (attempt) X77.9 ☑
  vapor (hot) X13.1 ☑
    assault X98.0 ☑
    stated as undetermined whether accidental or intentional Y27.0 ☑
    suicide (attempt) X77.0 ☑
Scratched by
  cat W55.03 ☑
  person(s) (accidentally) W50.4 ☑
    with intent to injure or kill Y04.0 ☑
    as, or caused by, a crowd or human stampede (with fall) W52 ☑
    assault Y04.0 ☑
    homicide (attempt) Y04.0 ☑
    in
      fight Y04.0 ☑
      legal intervention
        injuring
          bystander Y35.892 ☑
          law enforcement personnel Y35.891 ☑
          suspect Y35.893 ☑
Seasickness T75.3 ☑
Self-harm NEC (*see also* External cause by type, undetermined whether accidental or intentional)
  intentional — *see* Suicide
  poisoning NEC — *see* Table of Drugs and Chemicals, poisoning, accidental
Self-inflicted (injury) **NEC** (*see also* External cause by type, undetermined whether accidental or intentional)
  intentional — *see* Suicide
  poisoning NEC — *see* Table of Drugs and Chemicals, poisoning, accidental
Sequelae (of)
  accident NEC — *see* W00-X58 with 7th character S
  assault (homicidal) (any means) — *see* X92-Y08 with 7th character S
  homicide, attempt (any means) — *see* X92-Y08 with 7th character S
  injury undetermined whether accidentally or purposely inflicted — *see* Y21-Y33 with 7th character S
  intentional self-harm (classifiable to X71-X83) — *see* X71-X83 with 7th character S
  legal intervention — *see* with 7th character S Y35 ☑
  motor vehicle accident — *see* V00-V99 with 7th character S
  suicide, attempt (any means) — *see* X71-X83 with 7th character S
  transport accident — *see* V00-V99 with 7th character S
  war operations — *see* War operations
Shock
  electric — *see* Exposure, electric current
  from electric appliance (any) (faulty) W86.8 ☑
    domestic W86.0 ☑
    suicide (attempt) X83.1 ☑
Shooting, shot (accidental(ly)) (*see also* Discharge, firearm, by type)
  herself or himself — *see* Discharge, firearm by type, self-inflicted
  homicide (attempt) — *see* Discharge, firearm by type, homicide
  in war operations — *see* War operations
  inflicted by other person — *see* Discharge, firearm by type, homicide
    accidental — *see* Discharge, firearm, by type of firearm
  legal
    execution — *see* Legal, intervention, firearm
    intervention — *see* Legal, intervention, firearm
  self-inflicted — *see* Discharge, firearm by type, suicide
    accidental — *see* Discharge, firearm, by type of firearm
  suicide (attempt) — *see* Discharge, firearm by type, suicide
Shoving (accidentally) **by other person** — *see* Pushed, by other person
Sickness
  alpine W94.11 ☑
  motion — *see* Motion
  mountain W94.11 ☑

Sinking (accidental)
  watercraft (causing drowning, submersion) (*see also*
    Drowning, due to, accident to, watercraft, sinking)
    causing injury except drowning or submersion B
      — *see* Accident, watercraft, causing, injury
      NEC
Siriasis X32 ☑
Slashed wrists — *see* Cut, self-inflicted
Slipping (accidental) (on same level) (with fall) W01.0 ☑
  without fall W18.40 ☑
    due to
      specified NEC W18.49 ☑
      stepping from one level to another W18.43 ☑
      stepping into hole or opening W18.42 ☑
      stepping on object W18.41 ☑
  on
    ice W00.0 ☑
      with skates — *see* Accident, transport, pedestri-
      an, conveyance
    mud W01.0 ☑
    oil W01.0 ☑
    snow W00.0 ☑
      with skis — *see* Accident, transport, pedestrian,
      conveyance
    surface (slippery) (wet) NEC W01.0 ☑
Sliver, wood, contact with W45.8 ☑
Smoldering (due to fire) — *see* Exposure, fire
Sodomy (attempted) **by force** T74.2 ☑
Sound waves (causing injury) W42.9 ☑
  supersonic W42.0 ☑
Splinter, contact with W45.8 ☑
Stab, stabbing B — *see* Cut
Starvation X58 ☑
Status of external cause Y99.9
  child assisting in compensated work for family Y99.8
  civilian activity done for financial or other compensa-
    tion Y99.0
  civilian activity done for income or pay Y99.0
  family member assisting in compensated work for
    other family member Y99.8
  hobby not done for income Y99.8
  leisure activity Y99.8
  military activity Y99.1
  off-duty activity of military personnel Y99.8
  recreation or sport not for income or while a student
    Y99.8
  specified NEC Y99.8
  student activity Y99.8
  volunteer activity Y99.2
Stepped on
  by
    animal (not being ridden) NEC W55.89 ☑
    crowd or human stampede W52 ☑
    person W50.0 ☑
Stepping on
  object W22.8 ☑
    with fall W18.31 ☑
    sports equipment W21.9 ☑
    stationary W22.09 ☑
      sports equipment W21.89 ☑
  person W51 ☑
    by crowd or human stampede W52 ☑
  sports equipment W21.9 ☑
Sting
  arthropod, nonvenomous W57 ☑
  insect, nonvenomous W57 ☑
Storm (cataclysmic) B — *see* Forces of nature, cataclysmic
  storm
Straining, excessive — *see* Overexertion
Strangling — *see* Strangulation
Strangulation (accidental) T71 ☑
Strenuous movements — *see* category Y93
Striking against
  airbag (automobile) W22.10 ☑
    driver side W22.11 ☑
    front passenger side W22.12 ☑
    specified NEC W22.19 ☑
  bottom when
    diving or jumping into water (in) W16.822 ☑
      causing drowning W16.821 ☑
      from boat W16.722 ☑
        causing drowning W16.721 ☑
      natural body W16.622 ☑
        causing drowning W16.621 ☑
      swimming pool W16.522 ☑
        causing drowning W16.521 ☑

Striking against — *continued*
  bottom when — *continued*
    falling into water (in) W16.322 ☑
      causing drowning W16.321 ☑
      fountain — *see* Striking against, bottom when,
        falling into water, specified NEC
      natural body W16.122 ☑
        causing drowning W16.121 ☑
      reservoir — *see* Striking against, bottom when,
        falling into water, specified NEC
      specified NEC W16.322 ☑
        causing drowning W16.321 ☑
      swimming pool W16.022 ☑
        causing drowning W16.021 ☑
  diving board (swimming-pool) W21.4 ☑
  object W22.8 ☑
    with
      drowning or submersion — *see* Drowning
      fall — *see* Fall, due to, bumping against, object
    caused by crowd or human stampede (with fall)
      W52 ☑
    furniture W22.03 ☑
    lamppost W22.02 ☑
    sports equipment W21.9 ☑
    stationary W22.09 ☑
      sports equipment W21.89 ☑
    wall W22.01 ☑
  person(s) W51 ☑
    with fall W03 ☑
      due to ice or snow W00.0 ☑
    as, or caused by, a crowd or human stampede (with
      fall) W52 ☑
    assault Y04.2 ☑
    homicide (attempt) Y04.2 ☑
  sports equipment W21.9 ☑
  wall (when) W22.01 ☑
    diving or jumping into water (in) W16.832 ☑
      causing drowning W16.831 ☑
      swimming pool W16.532 ☑
        causing drowning W16.531 ☑
    falling into water (in) W16.332 ☑
      causing drowning W16.331 ☑
      fountain — *see* Striking against, wall when,
        falling into water, specified NEC
      natural body W16.132 ☑
        causing drowning W16.131 ☑
      reservoir — *see* Striking against, wall when,
        falling into water, specified NEC
      specified NEC W16.332 ☑
        causing drowning W16.331 ☑
      swimming pool W16.032 ☑
        causing drowning W16.031 ☑
    swimming pool (when) W22.042 ☑
      causing drowning W22.041 ☑
      diving or jumping into water W16.532 ☑
        causing drowning W16.531 ☑
      falling into water W16.032 ☑
        causing drowning W16.031 ☑
Struck (accidentally) **by**
  airbag (automobile) W22.10 ☑
    driver side W22.11 ☑
    front passenger side W22.12 ☑
    specified NEC W22.19 ☑
  alligator W58.02 ☑
  animal (not being ridden) NEC W55.89 ☑
  avalanche — *see* Landslide
  ball (hit) (thrown) W21.00 ☑
    assault Y08.09 ☑
    baseball W21.03 ☑
    basketball W21.05 ☑
    football W21.01 ☑
    golf ball W21.04 ☑
    soccer W21.02 ☑
    softball W21.07 ☑
    specified NEC W21.09 ☑
    volleyball W21.06 ☑
  bat or racquet
    baseball bat W21.11 ☑
      assault Y08.02 ☑
    golf club W21.13 ☑
      assault Y08.09 ☑
    specified NEC W21.19 ☑
      assault Y08.09 ☑
    tennis racquet W21.12 ☑
      assault Y08.09 ☑

Struck (accidentally) **by** — *continued*
  bullet (*see also* Discharge, firearm by type)
    in war operations — *see* War operations
  crocodile W58.12 ☑
  dog W54.1 ☑
  flare, Very pistol — *see* Discharge, firearm
    NEC
  hailstones X39.8 ☑
  hockey (ice)
    field
      puck W21.221 ☑
      stick W21.211 ☑
    puck W21.220 ☑
    stick W21.210 ☑
    assault Y08.01 ☑
  landslide — *see* Landslide
  law-enforcement agent (on duty) — *see* Legal, inter-
    vention, manhandling
    with blunt object — *see* Legal, intervention, blunt
      object
  lightning T75.0 ☑
    causing fire — *see* Exposure, fire
  machine — *see* Contact, with, by type of machine
  mammal NEC W55.89 ☑
    marine W56.32 ☑
  marine animal W56.82 ☑
  missile
    firearm — *see* Discharge, firearm by type
    in war operations — *see* War operations, missile
  object W22.8 ☑
    blunt W22.8 ☑
      assault Y00 ☑
      suicide (attempt) X79 ☑
      undetermined whether accidental or intention-
        al Y29 ☑
    falling W20.8 ☑
      from, in, on
        building W20.1 ☑
          burning (uncontrolled fire) X00.4 ☑
        cataclysmic
          earth surface movement NEC — *see*
            Landslide
          storm — *see* Forces of nature, cata-
            clysmic storm
        cave-in W20.0 ☑
        earthquake X34 ☑
        machine (in operation) — *see* Contact, with,
          by type of machine
        structure W20.1 ☑
          burning X00.4 ☑
        transport vehicle (in motion) — *see* Acci-
          dent, transport, by type of vehicle
        watercraft V93.49 ☑
          due to
            accident to craft V91.39 ☑
              powered craft V91.33 ☑
                ferry boat V91.31 ☑
                fishing boat V91.32 ☑
                jetskis V91.33 ☑
                liner V91.31 ☑
                merchant ship V91.30 ☑
                passenger ship V91.31 ☑
             unpowered craft V91.38 ☑
                canoe V91.35 ☑
                inflatable V91.36 ☑
                kayak V91.35 ☑
                sailboat V91.34 ☑
                surf-board V91.38 ☑
                windsurfer V91.38 ☑
            powered craft V93.43 ☑
              ferry boat V93.41 ☑
              fishing boat V93.42 ☑
              jetskis V93.43 ☑
              liner V93.41 ☑
              merchant ship V93.40 ☑
              passenger ship V93.41 ☑
            unpowered craft V93.48 ☑
              sailboat V93.44 ☑
              surf-board V93.48 ☑
              windsurfer V93.48 ☑
    moving NEC W20.8 ☑
    projected W20.8 ☑
      assault Y00 ☑
      in sports W21.9 ☑
        assault Y08.09 ☑
        ball W21.00 ☑

☑ Additional Character Required — Refer to the Tabular List for Character Selection   ▽ Subterms under main terms may continue to next column or page

Struck (accidentally) **by** — continued
 object — continued
  projected — continued
   in sports — continued
    ball — continued
     baseball W21.03 ☑
     basketball W21.05 ☑
     football W21.01 ☑
     golf ball W21.04 ☑
     soccer W21.02 ☑
     softball W21.07 ☑
     specified NEC W21.09 ☑
     volleyball W21.06 ☑
    bat or racquet
     baseball bat W21.11 ☑
      assault Y08.02 ☑
     golf club W21.13 ☑
      assault Y08.09 ☑
     specified NEC W21.19 ☑
      assault Y08.09 ☑
     tennis racquet W21.12 ☑
      assault Y08.09 ☑
    hockey (ice)
     field
      puck W21.221 ☑
      stick W21.211 ☑
     puck W21.220 ☑
     stick W21.210 ☑
      assault Y08.01 ☑
    specified NEC W21.89 ☑
  set in motion by explosion — see Explosion
  thrown W20.8 ☑
   assault Y00 ☑
   in sports W21.9 ☑
    assault Y08.09 ☑
    ball W21.00 ☑
     baseball W21.03 ☑
     basketball W21.05 ☑
     football W21.01 ☑
     golf ball W21.04 ☑
     soccer W21.02 ☑
     soft ball W21.07 ☑
     specified NEC W21.09 ☑
     volleyball W21.06 ☑
    bat or racquet
     baseball bat W21.11 ☑
      assault Y08.02 ☑
     golf club W21.13 ☑
      assault Y08.09 ☑
     specified NEC W21.19 ☑
      assault Y08.09 ☑
     tennis racquet W21.12 ☑
      assault Y08.09 ☑
    hockey (ice)
     field
      puck W21.221 ☑
      stick W21.211 ☑
     puck W21.220 ☑
     stick W21.210 ☑
      assault Y08.01 ☑
    specified NEC W21.89 ☑
 other person(s) W50.0 ☑
  with
   blunt object W22.8 ☑
    intentional, homicide (attempt) Y00 ☑
    sports equipment W21.9 ☑
    undetermined whether accidental or intentional Y29 ☑
   fall W03 ☑
    due to ice or snow W00.0 ☑
  as, or caused by, a crowd or human stampede (with fall) W52 ☑
  assault Y04.2 ☑
  homicide (attempt) Y04.2 ☑
  in legal intervention
   injuring
    bystander Y35.812 ☑
    law enforcement personnel Y35.811 ☑
    suspect Y35.813 ☑
  sports equipment W21.9 ☑
  police (on duty) — see Legal, intervention, manhandling
   with blunt object — see Legal, intervention, blunt object
 sports equipment W21.9 ☑
  assault Y08.09 ☑

Struck (accidentally) **by** — continued
 sports equipment — continued
  ball W21.00 ☑
   baseball W21.03 ☑
   basketball W21.05 ☑
   football W21.01 ☑
   golf ball W21.04 ☑
   soccer W21.02 ☑
   soft ball W21.07 ☑
   specified NEC W21.09 ☑
   volleyball W21.06 ☑
  bat or racquet
   baseball bat W21.11 ☑
    assault Y08.02 ☑
   golf club W21.13 ☑
    assault Y08.09 ☑
   specified NEC W21.19 ☑
   tennis racquet W21.12 ☑
    assault Y08.09 ☑
  cleats (shoe) W21.31 ☑
  foot wear NEC W21.39 ☑
  football helmet W21.81 ☑
  hockey (ice)
   field
    puck W21.221 ☑
    stick W21.211 ☑
   puck W21.220 ☑
   stick W21.210 ☑
    assault Y08.01 ☑
  skate blades W21.32 ☑
  specified NEC W21.89 ☑
   assault Y08.09 ☑
 thunderbolt — see subcategory T75.0 ☑
  causing fire — see Exposure, fire
 transport vehicle NEC (see also Accident, transport) V09.9 ☑
  intentional, homicide (attempt) Y03.0 ☑
  motor NEC (see also Accident, transport) V09.20 ☑
   homicide Y03.0 ☑
 vehicle (transport) NEC — see Accident, transport, by type of vehicle
  stationary (falling from jack, hydraulic lift, ramp) W20.8 ☑

Stumbling
 without fall W18.40 ☑
  due to
   specified NEC W18.49 ☑
   stepping from one level to another W18.43 ☑
   stepping into hole or opening W18.42 ☑
   stepping on object W18.41 ☑
  over
   animal NEC W01.0 ☑
    with fall W18.09 ☑
   carpet, rug or (small) object W22.8 ☑
    with fall W18.09 ☑
   person W51 ☑
    with fall W03 ☑
     due to ice or snow W00.0 ☑
Submersion (accidental) — see Drowning
Suffocation (accidental) (by external means) (by pressure) (mechanical) (see also category) T71 ☑
 due to, by
  avalanche — see Landslide
  explosion — see Explosion
  fire — see Exposure, fire
  food, any type (aspiration) (ingestion) (inhalation) — see categories T17 and T18 ☑
  ignition — see Ignition
  landslide — see Landslide
  machine(ry) — see Contact, with, by type of machine
  vomitus (aspiration) (inhalation) T17.81- ☑
 in
  burning building X00.8 ☑
Suicide, suicidal (attempted) (by) X83.8 ☑
 blunt object X79 ☑
 burning, burns X76 ☑
  hot object X77.9 ☑
   fluid NEC X77.2 ☑
   household appliance X77.3 ☑
   specified NEC X77.8 ☑
   steam X77.0 ☑
   tap water X77.1 ☑
   vapors X77.0 ☑
 caustic substance — see Table of Drugs and Chemicals
 cold, extreme X83.2 ☑

Suicide, suicidal — continued
 collision of motor vehicle with
  motor vehicle X82.0 ☑
  specified NEC X82.8 ☑
  train X82.1 ☑
  tree X82.2 ☑
 crashing of aircraft X83.0 ☑
 cut (any part of body) X78.9 ☑
 cutting or piercing instrument X78.9 ☑
  dagger X78.2 ☑
  glass X78.0 ☑
  knife X78.1 ☑
  specified NEC X78.8 ☑
  sword X78.2 ☑
 drowning (in) X71.9 ☑
  bathtub X71.0 ☑
  natural water X71.3 ☑
  specified NEC X71.8 ☑
  swimming pool X71.1 ☑
   following fall X71.2 ☑
 electrocution X83.1 ☑
 explosive(s) (material) X75 ☑
 fire, flames X76
 firearm X74.9 ☑
  airgun X74.01 ☑
  handgun X72
  hunting rifle X73.1 ☑
  larger X73.9 ☑
   specified NEC X73.8 ☑
  machine gun X73.2 ☑
  shotgun X73.0 ☑
  specified NEC X74.8 ☑
 hanging X83.8 ☑
 hot object — see Suicide, burning, hot object
 jumping
  before moving object X81.8 ☑
   motor vehicle X81.0 ☑
   subway train X81.1 ☑
   train X81.1 ☑
  from high place X80 ☑
 late effect of attempt — see X71-X83 with 7th character S
 lying before moving object, train, vehicle X81.8 ☑
 poisoning — see Table of Drugs and Chemicals
 puncture (any part of body) — see Suicide, cutting or piercing instrument
 scald — see Suicide, burning, hot object
 sequelae of attempt — see X71-X83 with 7th character S
 sharp object (any) — see Suicide, cutting or piercing instrument
 shooting — see Suicide, firearm
 specified means NEC X83.8 ☑
 stab (any part of body) — see Suicide, cutting or piercing instrument
 steam, hot vapors X77.0 ☑
 strangulation X83.8 ☑
 submersion — see Suicide, drowning
 suffocation X83.8 ☑
 wound NEC X83.8 ☑
Sunstroke X32 ☑
Supersonic waves (causing injury) W42.0 ☑
Surgical procedure, complication of (delayed or as an abnormal reaction without mention of misadventure) (see also Complication of or following, by type of procedure)
 due to or as a result of misadventure — see Misadventure
Swallowed, swallowing
 foreign body — see Foreign body, alimentary canal
 poison — see Table of Drugs and Chemicals
 substance
  caustic or corrosive — see Table of Drugs and Chemicals
  poisonous — see Table of Drugs and Chemicals

T

Tackle in sport W03 ☑
Terrorism (involving) Y38.80 ☑
 biological weapons Y38.6X- ☑
 chemical weapons Y38.7X- ☑
 conflagration Y38.3X- ☑
 explosion Y38.2X- ☑
  destruction of aircraft Y38.1X- ☑
  marine weapons Y38.0X- ☑

Terrorism — *continued*
  fire Y38.3X- ☑
  firearms Y38.4X- ☑
  hot substances Y38.5X- ☑
  nuclear weapons Y38.5X- ☑
  specified method NEC Y38.89- ☑
Thirst X58 ☑
Threat to breathing
  aspiration — *see* Aspiration
  due to cave-in, falling earth or substance NEC T71 ☑
Thrown (accidentally)
  against part (any) of or object in transport vehicle (in motion) NEC (*see also* Accident, transport)
  from
    high place, homicide (attempt) Y01 ☑
    machinery — *see* Contact, with, by type of machine
    transport vehicle NEC (*see also* Accident, transport) V89.9 ☑
  off — *see* Thrown, from
Thunderbolt — *see* subcategory T75.0 ☑
  causing fire — *see* Exposure, fire
Tidal wave (any injury) NEC — *see* Forces of nature, tidal wave
Took
  overdose (drug) — *see* Table of Drugs and Chemicals
  poison — *see* Table of Drugs and Chemicals
Tornado (any injury) X37.1 ☑
Torrential rain (any injury) X37.8 ☑
Torture X58 ☑
Trampled by animal NEC W55.89 ☑
Trapped (accidentally)
  between objects (moving) (stationary and moving) — *see* Caught
  by part (any) of
    motorcycle V29.88 ☑
    pedal cycle V19.88 ☑
    transport vehicle NEC (*see also* Accident, transport) V89.9 ☑
Travel (effects) (sickness) T75.3 ☑
Tree falling on or hitting (accidentally) (person) W20.8 ☑
Tripping
  without fall W18.40 ☑
    due to
      specified NEC W18.49 ☑
      stepping from one level to another W18.43 ☑
      stepping into hole or opening W18.42 ☑
      stepping on object W18.41 ☑
    over
      animal W01.0 ☑
        with fall W01.0 ☑
      carpet, rug or (small) object W22.8 ☑
        with fall W18.09 ☑
      person W51 ☑
        with fall W03 ☑
          due to ice or snow W00.0 ☑
Twisted by person(s) (accidentally) W50.2 ☑
  with intent to injure or kill Y04.0 ☑
  as, or caused by, a crowd or human stampede (with fall) W52 ☑
  assault Y04.0 ☑
  homicide (attempt) Y04.0 ☑
  in
    fight Y04.0 ☑
    legal intervention — *see* Legal, intervention, manhandling
Twisting, excessive — *see* Overexertion

U

Underdosing of necessary drugs, medicaments or biological substances Y63.6
Undetermined intent (contact) (exposure)
  automobile collision Y32 ☑
  blunt object Y29 ☑
  drowning (submersion) (in) Y21.9 ☑
    bathtub Y21.0 ☑
      after fall Y21.1 ☑
    natural water (lake) (ocean) (pond) (river) (stream) Y21.4 ☑
    specified place NEC Y21.8 ☑
    swimming pool Y21.2 ☑
      after fall Y21.3 ☑
  explosive material Y25 ☑
  fall, jump or push from high place Y30 ☑
  falling, lying or running before moving object Y31 ☑

Undetermined intent — *continued*
  fire Y26 ☑
  firearm discharge Y24.9 ☑
    airgun (BB) (pellet) Y24.0 ☑
    handgun (pistol) (revolver) Y22 ☑
    hunting rifle Y23.1 ☑
    larger Y23.9 ☑
      hunting rifle Y23.1 ☑
      machine gun Y23.3 ☑
      military Y23.2 ☑
      shotgun Y23.0 ☑
      specified type NEC Y23.8 ☑
    machine gun Y23.3 ☑
    military Y23.2 ☑
    shotgun Y23.0 ☑
    specified type NEC Y24.8 ☑
    Very pistol Y24.8 ☑
  hot object Y27.9 ☑
    fluid NEC Y27.2 ☑
    household appliance Y27.3 ☑
    specified object NEC Y27.8 ☑
    steam Y27.0 ☑
    tap water Y27.1 ☑
    vapor Y27.0 ☑
  jump, fall or push from high place Y30 ☑
  lying, falling or running before moving object Y31 ☑
  motor vehicle crash Y32 ☑
  push, fall or jump from high place Y30 ☑
  running, falling or lying before moving object Y31 ☑
  sharp object Y28.9 ☑
    dagger Y28.2 ☑
    glass Y28.0 ☑
    knife Y28.1 ☑
    specified object NEC Y28.8 ☑
    sword Y28.2 ☑
  smoke Y26 ☑
  specified event NEC Y33 ☑

V

Vibration (causing injury) W49.9 ☑
Victim (of)
  avalanche — *see* Landslide
  earth movements NEC — *see* Forces of nature, earth movement
  earthquake X34 ☑
  flood — *see* Flood
  landslide — *see* Landslide
  lightning — *see* subcategory T75.0 ☑
    causing fire — *see* Exposure, fire
  storm (cataclysmic) NEC — *see* Forces of nature, cataclysmic storm
  volcanic eruption X35 ☑
Volcanic eruption (any injury) X35 ☑
Vomitus, gastric contents in air passages (with asphyxia, obstruction or suffocation) T17.81- ☑

W

Walked into stationary object (any) W22.09 ☑
  furniture W22.03 ☑
  lamppost W22.02 ☑
  wall W22.01 ☑
War operations (injuries to military personnel and civilians during war, civil insurrection and peacekeeping missions) (by) (from) (involving) Y36.90 ☑
  after cessation of hostilities Y36.89- ☑
    explosion (of)
      bomb placed during war operations Y36.82- ☑
      mine placed during war operations Y36.81- ☑
      specified NEC Y36.88- ☑
  air blast Y36.20- ☑
  aircraft
    destruction — *see* War operations, destruction of aircraft
    airway restriction — *see* War operations, restriction of airways
  asphyxiation — *see* War operations, restriction of airways
  biological weapons Y36.6X- ☑
  blast Y36.20- ☑
  blast fragments Y36.20- ☑
  blast wave Y36.20- ☑
  blast wind Y36.20- ☑

War operations — *continued*
  bomb Y36.20- ☑
    dirty Y36.50- ☑
    gasoline Y36.31- ☑
    incendiary Y36.31- ☑
    petrol Y36.31- ☑
  bullet Y36.43- ☑
    incendiary Y36.32- ☑
    rubber Y36.41- ☑
  chemical weapons Y36.7X- ☑
  combat
    hand to hand (unarmed) combat Y36.44- ☑
    using blunt or piercing object Y36.45- ☑
  conflagration — *see* War operations, fire
  conventional warfare NEC Y36.49- ☑
  depth-charge Y36.01- ☑
  destruction of aircraft Y36.10- ☑
    due to
      air to air missile Y36.11- ☑
      collision with other aircraft Y36.12- ☑
      detonation (accidental) of onboard munitions and explosives Y36.14- ☑
      enemy fire or explosives Y36.11- ☑
      explosive placed on aircraft Y36.11- ☑
      onboard fire Y36.13- ☑
      rocket propelled grenade [RPG] Y36.11- ☑
      small arms fire Y36.11- ☑
      surface to air missile Y36.11- ☑
    specified NEC Y36.19- ☑
  detonation (accidental) of
    onboard marine weapons Y36.05- ☑
    own munitions or munitions launch device Y36.24- ☑
  dirty bomb Y36.50- ☑
  explosion (of) Y36.20- ☑
    aerial bomb Y36.21- ☑
    after cessation of hostilities
      bomb placed during war operations Y36.82- ☑
      mine placed during war operations Y36.81- ☑
    bomb NOS (*see also* War operations, bomb(s)) Y36.20- ☑
    fragments Y36.20- ☑
    grenade Y36.29- ☑
    guided missile Y36.22- ☑
    improvised explosive device [IED] (person-borne) (roadside) (vehicle-borne) Y36.23- ☑
    land mine Y36.29- ☑
    marine mine (at sea) (in harbor) Y36.02- ☑
    marine weapon Y36.00- ☑
      specified NEC Y36.09- ☑
    own munitions or munitions launch device (accidental) Y36.24- ☑
    sea-based artillery shell Y36.03- ☑
    specified NEC Y36.29- ☑
    torpedo Y36.04- ☑
  fire Y36.30- ☑
    specified NEC Y36.39- ☑
  firearms
    discharge Y36.43- ☑
    pellets Y36.42- ☑
  flamethrower Y36.33- ☑
  fragments (from) (of)
    improvised explosive device [IED] (person-borne) (roadside) (vehicle-borne) Y36.26- ☑
    munitions Y36.25- ☑
    specified NEC Y36.29- ☑
    weapons Y36.27- ☑
  friendly fire Y36.92 ☑
  hand to hand (unarmed) combat Y36.44- ☑
  hot substances — *see* War operations, fire
  incendiary bullet Y36.32- ☑
  nuclear weapon (effects of) Y36.50- ☑
    acute radiation exposure Y36.54- ☑
    blast pressure Y36.51- ☑
    direct blast Y36.51- ☑
    direct heat Y36.53- ☑
    fallout exposure Y36.54- ☑
    fireball Y36.53- ☑
    indirect blast (struck or crushed by blast debris) (being thrown by blast) Y36.52- ☑
    ionizing radiation (immediate exposure) Y36.54- ☑
    nuclear radiation Y36.54- ☑
    radiation
      ionizing (immediate exposure) Y36.54- ☑
      nuclear Y36.54- ☑
      thermal Y36.53- ☑

☑ **Additional Character Required** — **Refer to the Tabular List for Character Selection**
▽ **Subterms under main terms may continue to next column or page**

War operations — *continued*
   nuclear weapon — *continued*
      secondary effects Y36.54- ☑
      specified NEC Y36.59- ☑
      thermal radiation Y36.53- ☑
   restriction of air (airway)
      intentional Y36.46- ☑
      unintentional Y36.47- ☑
   rubber bullets Y36.41- ☑
   shrapnel NOS Y36.29- ☑
   suffocation — *see* War operations, restriction of air-
      ways
   unconventional warfare NEC Y37.7X- ☑
   underwater blast NOS Y36.00- ☑
   warfare
      conventional NEC Y36.49- ☑
      unconventional NEC Y37.7X- ☑
   weapon of mass destruction [WMD] Y36.91 ☑
   weapons
      biological weapons Y36.6X- ☑

War operations — *continued*
   weapons — *continued*
      chemical Y36.7X- ☑
      nuclear (effects of) Y36.50- ☑
         acute radiation exposure Y36.54- ☑
         blast pressure Y36.51- ☑
         direct blast Y36.51- ☑
         direct heat Y36.53- ☑
         fallout exposure Y36.54- ☑
         fireball Y36.53- ☑
         indirect blast (struck or crushed by blast debris)
            (being thrown by blast) Y36.52- ☑
         radiation
            ionizing (immediate exposure) Y36.54- ☑
            nuclear Y36.54- ☑
            thermal Y36.53- ☑
         secondary effects Y36.54- ☑
         specified NEC Y36.59- ☑
   of mass destruction [WMD] Y36.91 ☑

Washed
   away by flood — *see* Flood
   off road by storm (transport vehicle) — *see* Forces of
      nature, cataclysmic storm
Weather exposure NEC — *see* Forces of nature
Weightlessness (causing injury) (effects of) (in spacecraft,
   real or simulated) X52 ☑
Work related condition Y99.0
Wound (accidental) NEC (*see also* Injury) X58 ☑
   battle (*see also* War operations) Y36.90 ☑
   gunshot — *see* Discharge, firearm by type
Wreck transport vehicle NEC (*see also* Accident, transport) V89.9 ☑
Wrong
   device implanted into correct surgical site Y65.51
   fluid in infusion Y65.1
   patient, procedure performed on Y65.52
   procedure (operation) on correct patient Y65.51

External Causes Index

War operations — Wrong

ICD-10-CM Tabular List of Diseases and Injuries

Chapter 1. Certain Infectious and Parasitic Diseases (A00–B99)

Chapter Specific Guidelines with Coding Examples

The chapter specific guidelines from the ICD-10-CM Official Guidelines for Coding and Reporting have been provided below. Along with these guidelines are coding examples, contained in the shaded boxes, that have been developed to help illustrate the coding and/or sequencing guidance found in these guidelines.

a. Human immunodeficiency virus (HIV) infections

1) Code only confirmed cases

Code only confirmed cases of HIV infection/illness. This is an exception to the hospital inpatient guideline Section II, H.

In this context, "confirmation" does not require documentation of positive serology or culture for HIV; the provider's diagnostic statement that the patient is HIV positive, or has an HIV-related illness is sufficient.

> Patient admitted with anemia with possible HIV infection
>
> **D64.9**   **Anemia, unspecified**
>
> *Explanation:* Only the anemia is coded in this scenario because it has not been confirmed that an HIV infection is present. This is an exception to the guideline Section II, H for hospital inpatient coding.

2) Selection and sequencing of HIV codes

(a) Patient admitted for HIV-related condition

If a patient is admitted for an HIV-related condition, the principal diagnosis should be B20, Human immunodeficiency virus [HIV] disease followed by additional diagnosis codes for all reported HIV-related conditions.

> HIV with PCP
>
> **B20**   **Human immunodeficiency virus [HIV] disease**
>
> **B59**   **Pneumocystosis**
>
> *Explanation:* Pneumonia due to *Pneumocystis carinii* is an HIV related condition, so the HIV diagnosis code is reported first, followed by the code for the pneumonia.

(b) Patient with HIV disease admitted for unrelated condition

If a patient with HIV disease is admitted for an unrelated condition (such as a traumatic injury), the code for the unrelated condition (e.g., the nature of injury code) should be the principal diagnosis. Other diagnoses would be B20 followed by additional diagnosis codes for all reported HIV-related conditions.

> Unstable angina, native coronary artery atherosclerosis, HIV
>
> **I25.110**   **Atherosclerotic heart disease of native coronary artery with unstable angina pectoris**
>
> **B20**   **Human immunodeficiency virus [HIV] disease**
>
> *Explanation:* The arteriosclerotic coronary artery disease and the unstable angina are not related to HIV, so those conditions are reported first using a combination code, and HIV is reported secondarily.

(c) Whether the patient is newly diagnosed

Whether the patient is newly diagnosed or has had previous admissions/encounters for HIV conditions is irrelevant to the sequencing decision.

> Newly diagnosed multiple cutaneous Kaposi's sarcoma lesions in previously diagnosed HIV disease
>
> **B20**   **Human immunodeficiency virus [HIV] disease**
>
> **C46.0**   **Kaposi's sarcoma of skin**
>
> *Explanation:* Even though the HIV was diagnosed on a previous encounter, it is still sequenced first when coded with an HIV related condition. Kaposi's sarcoma is an HIV-related condition.

(d) Asymptomatic human immunodeficiency virus

Z21, Asymptomatic human immunodeficiency virus [HIV] infection status, is to be applied when the patient without any documentation of symptoms is listed as being "HIV positive," "known HIV," "HIV test positive," or similar terminology. Do not use this code if the term "AIDS" is used or if the patient is treated for any HIV-related illness or is described as having any condition(s) resulting from his/her HIV positive status; use B20 in these cases.

> Patient admitted with acute appendicitis. Status positive HIV test on Atripla, with no prior symptoms
>
> **K35.80**   **Unspecified acute appendicitis**
>
> **Z21**   **Asymptomatic human immunodeficiency virus [HIV] infection status**
>
> *Explanation:* Code Z21 is sequenced second since documentation indicates that the patient has had a positive HIV test but has been asymptomatic. Being on medication for HIV is not an indication that code B20 is used instead of Z21. Unless there has been documentation that the patient has had current or prior symptoms or HIV-related complications, code B20 is not used. The appendicitis is not an AIDS-related complication and is sequenced first.

(e) Patients with inconclusive HIV serology

Patients with inconclusive HIV serology, but no definitive diagnosis or manifestations of the illness, may be assigned code R75, Inconclusive laboratory evidence of human immunodeficiency virus [HIV].

(f) Previously diagnosed HIV-related illness

Patients with any known prior diagnosis of an HIV-related illness should be coded to B20. Once a patient has developed an HIV-related illness, the patient should always be assigned code B20 on every subsequent admission/encounter. Patients previously diagnosed with any HIV illness (B20) should never be assigned to R75 or Z21, Asymptomatic human immunodeficiency virus [HIV] infection status

(g) HIV infection in pregnancy, childbirth and the puerperium

During pregnancy, childbirth or the puerperium, a patient admitted (or presenting for a health care encounter) because of an HIV-related illness should receive a principal diagnosis code of O98.7-, Human immunodeficiency [HIV] disease complicating pregnancy, childbirth and the puerperium, followed by B20 and the code(s) for the HIV-related illness(es). Codes from Chapter 15 always take sequencing priority.

Patients with asymptomatic HIV infection status admitted (or presenting for a health care encounter) during pregnancy, childbirth, or the puerperium should receive codes of O98.7- and Z21.

(h) Encounters for testing for HIV

If a patient is being seen to determine his/her HIV status, use code Z11.4, Encounter for screening for human immunodeficiency virus [HIV]. Use additional codes for any associated high risk behavior.

If a patient with signs or symptoms is being seen for HIV testing, code the signs and symptoms. An additional counseling code Z71.7, Human immunodeficiency virus [HIV] counseling, may be used if counseling is provided during the encounter for the test.

When a patient returns to be informed of his/her HIV test results and the test result is negative, use code Z71.7, Human immunodeficiency virus [HIV] counseling.

If the results are positive, see previous guidelines and assign codes as appropriate.

b. Infectious agents as the cause of diseases classified to other chapters

Certain infections are classified in chapters other than Chapter 1 and no organism is identified as part of the infection code. In these instances, it is necessary to use an additional code from Chapter 1 to identify the organism. A code from category B95, Streptococcus, Staphylococcus, and Enterococcus as the cause of diseases classified to other chapters, B96, Other bacterial agents as the cause of diseases classified to other chapters, or B97, Viral agents as the cause of diseases classified to other chapters, is to be used as an additional code to identify the organism. An instructional note will be found at the infection code advising that an additional organism code is required.

E. coli UTI

N39.Ø   **Urinary tract infection, site not specified**

B96.2Ø   **Unspecified Escherichia coli [E.coli] as the cause of diseases classified elsewhere**

Explanation: An instructional note under the code for the urinary tract infection indicates to code also the specific organism.

c. Infections resistant to antibiotics

Many bacterial infections are resistant to current antibiotics. It is necessary to identify all infections documented as antibiotic resistant. Assign a code from category Z16, Resistance to antimicrobial drugs, following the infection code only if the infection code does not identify drug resistance.

Antimycobacterial-resistant primary pulmonary tuberculosis

A15.Ø   **Tuberculosis of lung**

Z16.341   **Resistance to single antimycobacterial drug**

Explanation: Code Z16.341 is assigned as a secondary code to represent the antimycobacterial resistance. This code includes resistance to antimycobacterial drug "NOS"; if multiple drug resistance is not specified, classification defaults to the single drug resistance code.

d. Sepsis, severe sepsis, and septic shock

1) Coding of Sepsis and Severe Sepsis

(a) Sepsis

For a diagnosis of sepsis, assign the appropriate code for the underlying systemic infection. If the type of infection or causal organism is not further specified, assign code A41.9, Sepsis, unspecified organism.

A code from subcategory R65.2, Severe sepsis, should not be assigned unless severe sepsis or an associated acute organ dysfunction is documented.

Gram-negative sepsis

A41.5Ø   **Gram-negative sepsis, unspecified**

Staphylococcal sepsis

A41.2   **Sepsis due to unspecified staphylococcus**

Explanation: In both examples above the organism causing the sepsis is identified, therefore A41.9 Sepsis, unspecified organism, would not be appropriate as this code would not capture the highest degree of specificity found in the documentation. Do not use the additional code for severe sepsis unless documented as severe sepsis with acute organ dysfunction.

(i) Negative or inconclusive blood cultures and sepsis

Negative or inconclusive blood cultures do not preclude a diagnosis of sepsis in patients with clinical evidence of the condition; however, the provider should be queried.

(ii) Urosepsis

The term urosepsis is a nonspecific term. It is not to be considered synonymous with sepsis. It has no default code in the Alphabetic Index. Should a provider use this term, he/she must be queried for clarification.

(iii)Sepsis with organ dysfunction

If a patient has sepsis and associated acute organ dysfunction or multiple organ dysfunction (MOD), follow the instructions for coding severe sepsis.

(iv)Acute organ dysfunction that is not clearly associated with the sepsis

If a patient has sepsis and an acute organ dysfunction, but the medical record documentation indicates that the acute organ dysfunction is related to a medical condition other than the sepsis, do not assign a code from subcategory R65.2, Severe sepsis. An acute organ dysfunction must be associated with the sepsis in order to assign the severe sepsis code. If the documentation is not clear as to whether an acute organ dysfunction is related to the sepsis or another medical condition, query the provider.

Sepsis and acute respiratory failure due to COPD exacerbation

A41.9   **Sepsis, unspecified organism**

J44.1   **Chronic obstructive pulmonary disease with (acute) exacerbation**

J96.ØØ   **Acute respiratory failure, unspecified whether with hypoxia or hypercapnia**

Explanation: Although acute organ dysfunction is present in the form of acute respiratory failure, severe sepsis (R65.2) is not coded in this example, as the acute respiratory failure is attributed to the COPD exacerbation rather than the sepsis. Sequencing of these codes would be determined by the circumstances of the admission.

(b) Severe sepsis

The coding of severe sepsis requires a minimum of 2 codes: first a code for the underlying systemic infection, followed by a code from subcategory R65.2, Severe sepsis. If the causal organism is not documented, assign code A41.9, Sepsis, unspecified organism, for the infection. Additional code(s) for the associated acute organ dysfunction are also required.

Due to the complex nature of severe sepsis, some cases may require querying the provider prior to assignment of the codes.

2) Septic shock

(a) Septic shock generally refers to circulatory failure associated with severe sepsis, and therefore, it represents a type of acute organ dysfunction.

For cases of septic shock, the code for the systemic infection should be sequenced first, followed by code R65.21, Severe sepsis with septic shock or code T81.12, Postprocedural septic shock. Any additional codes for the other acute organ dysfunctions should also be assigned. As noted in the sequencing instructions in the Tabular List, the code for septic shock cannot be assigned as a principal diagnosis.

Sepsis with septic shock

A41.9   **Sepsis, unspecified organism**

R65.21   **Severe sepsis with septic shock**

Explanation: Documentation of septic shock automatically implies severe sepsis as it is a form of acute organ dysfunction. Septic shock is not coded as the principal diagnosis; it is always preceded by the code for the systemic infection.

3) Sequencing of severe sepsis

If severe sepsis is present on admission, and meets the definition of principal diagnosis, the underlying systemic infection should be assigned as principal diagnosis followed by the appropriate code from subcategory R65.2 as required by the sequencing rules in the Tabular List. A code from subcategory R65.2 can never be assigned as a principal diagnosis.

When severe sepsis develops during an encounter (it was not present on admission), the underlying systemic infection and the appropriate code from subcategory R65.2 should be assigned as secondary diagnoses.

Severe sepsis may be present on admission, but the diagnosis may not be confirmed until sometime after admission. If the documentation is not clear whether severe sepsis was present on admission, the provider should be queried.

4) Sepsis and severe sepsis with a localized infection

If the reason for admission is both sepsis or severe sepsis and a localized infection, such as pneumonia or cellulitis, a code(s) for the underlying systemic infection should be assigned first and the code for the localized infection should be assigned as a secondary diagnosis. If the patient has severe sepsis, a code from subcategory R65.2 should also be assigned as a secondary diagnosis. If the patient is admitted with a localized infection, such as pneumonia, and sepsis/severe sepsis doesn't develop until after admission, the localized infection should be assigned first, followed by the appropriate sepsis/severe sepsis codes.

Patient presents with acute renal failure due to severe sepsis from *Pseudomonas pneumonia*

A41.9	**Sepsis, unspecified organism**
J15.1	**Pneumonia due to Pseudomonas**
R65.20	**Severe sepsis without septic shock**
N17.9	**Acute kidney failure, unspecified**

Explanation: If all conditions are present on admission, the systemic infection (sepsis) is sequenced first followed by the codes for the localized infection (pneumonia), severe sepsis and any organ dysfunction. If only the pneumonia was present on admission with the sepsis and resulting renal failure developing later in the admission, then the pneumonia would be sequenced first.

5) **Sepsis due to a postprocedural infection**

   (a) **Documentation of causal relationship**

   As with all postprocedural complications, code assignment is based on the provider's documentation of the relationship between the infection and the procedure.

   (b) **Sepsis due to a postprocedural infection**

   For such cases, the postprocedural infection code, such as T80.2, Infections following infusion, transfusion, and therapeutic injection, T81.4, Infection following a procedure, T88.0, Infection following immunization, or O86.0, Infection of obstetric surgical wound, should be coded first, followed by the code for the specific infection. If the patient has severe sepsis, the appropriate code from subcategory R65.2 should also be assigned with the additional code(s) for any acute organ dysfunction.

   (c) **Postprocedural infection and postprocedural septic shock**

   In cases where a postprocedural infection has occurred and has resulted in severe sepsis the code for the precipitating complication such as code T81.4, Infection following a procedure, or O86.0, Infection of obstetrical surgical wound should be coded first followed by code R65.20, Severe sepsis without septic shock. A code for the systemic infection should also be assigned.

   If a postprocedural infection has resulted in postprocedural septic shock, the code for the precipitating complication such as code T81.4, Infection following a procedure, or O86.0, Infection of obstetrical surgical wound should be coded first followed by code T81.12-, Postprocedural septic shock. A code for the systemic infection should also be assigned.

6) **Sepsis and severe sepsis associated with a noninfectious process (condition)**

   In some cases a noninfectious process (condition), such as trauma, may lead to an infection which can result in sepsis or severe sepsis. If sepsis or severe sepsis is documented as associated with a noninfectious condition, such as a burn or serious injury, and this condition meets the definition for principal diagnosis, the code for the noninfectious condition should be sequenced first, followed by the code for the resulting infection. If severe sepsis is present, a code from subcategory R65.2 should also be assigned with any associated organ dysfunction(s) codes. It is not necessary to assign a code from subcategory R65.1, Systemic inflammatory response syndrome (SIRS) of non-infectious origin, for these cases.

   If the infection meets the definition of principal diagnosis, it should be sequenced before the non-infectious condition. When both the associated non-infectious condition and the infection meet the definition of principal diagnosis, either may be assigned as principal diagnosis.

   Only one code from category R65, Symptoms and signs specifically associated with systemic inflammation and infection, should be assigned. Therefore, when a non-infectious condition leads to an infection resulting in severe sepsis, assign the appropriate code from subcategory R65.2, Severe sepsis. Do not additionally assign a code from subcategory R65.1, Systemic inflammatory response syndrome (SIRS) of non-infectious origin.

   See Section I.C.18. SIRS due to non-infectious process

Patient admitted with multiple third-degree burns of upper arm develops severe MSSA sepsis with septic shock, three days into admission

T22.391A	**Burn of third degree of multiple sites of right shoulder and upper arm limb, except wrist and hand, initial encounter**
A41.01	**Sepsis due to methicillin susceptible Staphylococcus aureus**
R65.21	**Severe sepsis with septic shock**

Explanation: Severe sepsis is coded rather than SIRS from R65 because it is documented as a severe systemic infectious response with septic shock to a noninfectious condition. The code for the systemic infection is not used as the principal diagnosis because it was not present on admission. The patient was admitted for the burn injury.

7) **Sepsis and septic shock complicating abortion, pregnancy, childbirth, and the puerperium**

   See Section I.C.15. Sepsis and septic shock complicating abortion, pregnancy, childbirth and the puerperium

8) **Newborn sepsis**

   See Section I.C.16. f. Bacterial sepsis of Newborn

e. **Methicillin resistant *Staphylococcus aureus* (MRSA) conditions**

   1) **Selection and sequencing of MRSA codes**

      (a) **Combination codes for MRSA infection**

      When a patient is diagnosed with an infection that is due to methicillin resistant *Staphylococcus aureus* (MRSA), and that infection has a combination code that includes the causal organism (e.g., sepsis, pneumonia) assign the appropriate combination code for the condition (e.g., code A41.02, Sepsis due to Methicillin resistant Staphylococcus aureus or code J15.212, Pneumonia due to Methicillin resistant Staphylococcus aureus). Do not assign code B95.62, Methicillin resistant Staphylococcus aureus infection as the cause of diseases classified elsewhere, as an additional code, because the combination code includes the type of infection and the MRSA organism. Do not assign a code from subcategory Z16.11, Resistance to penicillins, as an additional diagnosis.

      See Section C.1. for instructions on coding and sequencing of sepsis and severe sepsis.

      (b) **Other codes for MRSA infection**

      When there is documentation of a current infection (e.g., wound infection, stitch abscess, urinary tract infection) due to MRSA, and that infection does not have a combination code that includes the causal organism, assign the appropriate code to identify the condition along with code B95.62, Methicillin resistant Staphylococcus aureus infection as the cause of diseases classified elsewhere for the MRSA infection. Do not assign a code from subcategory Z16.11, Resistance to penicillins.

      (c) **Methicillin susceptible Staphylococcus aureus (MSSA) and MRSA colonization**

      The condition or state of being colonized or carrying MSSA or MRSA is called colonization or carriage, while an individual person is described as being colonized or being a carrier. Colonization means that MSSA or MSRA is present on or in the body without necessarily causing illness. A positive MRSA colonization test might be documented by the provider as "MRSA screen positive" or "MRSA nasal swab positive".

      Assign code Z22.322, Carrier or suspected carrier of Methicillin resistant Staphylococcus aureus, for patients documented as having MRSA colonization. Assign code Z22.321, Carrier or suspected carrier of Methicillin susceptible Staphylococcus aureus, for patient documented as having MSSA colonization. Colonization is not necessarily indicative of a disease process or as the cause of a specific condition the patient may have unless documented as such by the provider.

      (d) **MRSA colonization and infection**

      If a patient is documented as having both MRSA colonization and infection during a hospital admission, code Z22.322, Carrier or suspected carrier of Methicillin resistant Staphylococcus aureus, and a code for the MRSA infection may both be assigned.

Chapter 1. Certain Infectious and Parasitic Diseases (A00-B99)

INCLUDES diseases generally recognized as communicable or transmissible

Use additional code to identify resistance to antimicrobial drugs (Z16.-)

EXCLUDES 1 certain localized infections—see body system-related chapters

EXCLUDES 2 carrier or suspected carrier of infectious disease (Z22.-)

infectious and parasitic diseases specific to the perinatal period (P35-P39)

infectious and parasitic diseases complicating pregnancy, childbirth and the puerperium (O98.-)

influenza and other acute respiratory infections (J00-J22)

This chapter contains the following blocks:

A00-A09	Intestinal infectious diseases
A15-A19	Tuberculosis
A20-A28	Certain zoonotic bacterial diseases
A30-A49	Other bacterial diseases
A50-A64	Infections with a predominantly sexual mode of transmission
A65-A69	Other spirochetal diseases
A70-A74	Other diseases caused by chlamydiae
A75-A79	Rickettsioses
A80-A89	Viral infections of the central nervous system
A90-A99	Arthropod-borne viral fevers and viral hemorrhagic fevers
B00-B09	Viral infections characterized by skin and mucous membrane lesions
B10	Other human herpesviruses
B15-B19	Viral hepatitis
B20	Human immunodeficiency virus [HIV] disease
B25-B34	Other viral diseases
B35-B49	Mycoses
B50-B64	Protozoal diseases
B65-B83	Helminthiases
B85-B89	Pediculosis, acariasis and other infestations
B90-B94	Sequelae of infectious and parasitic diseases
B95-B97	Bacterial and viral infectious agents
B99	Other infectious diseases

Intestinal Infectious Diseases (A00-A09)

✓4ᵗʰ **A00　Cholera**

A00.0　Cholera due to Vibrio cholerae 01, biovar cholerae
Classical cholera

A00.1　Cholera due to Vibrio cholerae 01, biovar eltor
Cholera eltor

A00.9　Cholera, unspecified

✓4ᵗʰ **A01　Typhoid and paratyphoid fevers**

✓5ᵗʰ **A01.0　Typhoid fever**
Infection due to Salmonella typhi

　　A01.00　Typhoid fever, unspecified

　　A01.01　Typhoid meningitis

　　A01.02　Typhoid fever with heart involvement
　　　Typhoid endocarditis
　　　Typhoid myocarditis

　　A01.03　Typhoid pneumonia

　　A01.04　Typhoid arthritis

　　A01.05　Typhoid osteomyelitis

　　A01.09　Typhoid fever with other complications

A01.1　Paratyphoid fever A

A01.2　Paratyphoid fever B

A01.3　Paratyphoid fever C

A01.4　Paratyphoid fever, unspecified
Infection due to Salmonella paratyphi NOS

✓4ᵗʰ **A02　Other salmonella infections**

INCLUDES infection or foodborne intoxication due to any Salmonella species other than S. typhi and S. paratyphi

A02.0　Salmonella enteritis
Salmonellosis

A02.1　Salmonella sepsis

✓5ᵗʰ **A02.2　Localized salmonella infections**

　　A02.20　Localized salmonella infection, unspecified

　　A02.21　Salmonella meningitis

　　A02.22　Salmonella pneumonia

　　A02.23　Salmonella arthritis

　　A02.24　Salmonella osteomyelitis

　　A02.25　Salmonella pyelonephritis
　　　Salmonella tubulo-interstitial nephropathy

　　A02.29　Salmonella with other localized infection

A02.8　Other specified salmonella infections

A02.9　Salmonella infection, unspecified

✓4ᵗʰ **A03　Shigellosis**

A03.0　Shigellosis due to Shigella dysenteriae
Group A shigellosis [Shiga-Kruse dysentery]

A03.1　Shigellosis due to Shigella flexneri
Group B shigellosis

A03.2　Shigellosis due to Shigella boydii
Group C shigellosis

A03.3　Shigellosis due to Shigella sonnei
Group D shigellosis

A03.8　Other shigellosis

A03.9　Shigellosis, unspecified
Bacillary dysentery NOS

✓4ᵗʰ **A04　Other bacterial intestinal infections**

EXCLUDES 1 bacterial foodborne intoxications, NEC (A05.-)
tuberculous enteritis (A18.32)

A04.0　Enteropathogenic Escherichia coli infection

A04.1　Enterotoxigenic Escherichia coli infection

A04.2　Enteroinvasive Escherichia coli infection

A04.3　Enterohemorrhagic Escherichia coli infection

A04.4　Other intestinal Escherichia coli infections
Escherichia coli enteritis NOS

A04.5　Campylobacter enteritis

A04.6　Enteritis due to Yersinia enterocolitica
EXCLUDES 1 extraintestinal yersiniosis (A28.2)

A04.7　Enterocolitis due to Clostridium difficile
Foodborne intoxication by Clostridium difficile
Pseudomembraneous colitis

A04.8　Other specified bacterial intestinal infections

A04.9　Bacterial intestinal infection, unspecified
Bacterial enteritis NOS

✓4ᵗʰ **A05　Other bacterial foodborne intoxications, not elsewhere classified**

EXCLUDES 1 Clostridium difficile foodborne intoxication and infection (A04.7)
Escherichia coli infection (A04.0-A04.4)
listeriosis (A32.-)
salmonella foodborne intoxication and infection (A02.-)
toxic effect of noxious foodstuffs (T61-T62)

A05.0　Foodborne staphylococcal intoxication

A05.1　Botulism food poisoning
Botulism NOS
Classical foodborne intoxication due to Clostridium botulinum
EXCLUDES 1 infant botulism (A48.51)
wound botulism (A48.52)

A05.2　Foodborne Clostridium perfringens [Clostridium welchii] intoxication
Enteritis necroticans
Pig-bel

A05.3　Foodborne Vibrio parahaemolyticus intoxication

A05.4　Foodborne Bacillus cereus intoxication

A05.5　Foodborne Vibrio vulnificus intoxication

A05.8　Other specified bacterial foodborne intoxications

A05.9　Bacterial foodborne intoxication, unspecified

✓4ᵗʰ **A06　Amebiasis**

INCLUDES infection due to Entamoeba histolytica
EXCLUDES 1 other protozoal intestinal diseases (A07.-)
EXCLUDES 2 acanthamebiasis (B60.1-)
Naegleriasis (B60.2)

A06.0　Acute amebic dysentery
Acute amebiasis
Intestinal amebiasis NOS

A06.1　Chronic intestinal amebiasis

A06.2　Amebic nondysenteric colitis

A06.3　Ameboma of intestine
Ameboma NOS

A06.4　Amebic liver abscess
Hepatic amebiasis

A06.5　Amebic lung abscess
Amebic abscess of lung (and liver)

A06.6　Amebic brain abscess
Amebic abscess of brain (and liver) (and lung)

A06.7　Cutaneous amebiasis

✓5ᵗʰ **A06.8　Amebic infection of other sites**

　　A06.81　Amebic cystitis

EXCLUDES 1 Not coded here	**EXCLUDES 2** Not included here	**N** Newborn Age: 0	**P** Pediatric Age: 0-17	**M** Maternity Age: 12-55	**A** Adult Age: 15-124

A06.82 Other amebic genitourinary infections
Amebic balanitis
Amebic vesiculitis
Amebic vulvovaginitis

A06.89 Other amebic infections
Amebic appendicitis
Amebic splenic abscess

A06.9 Amebiasis, unspecified

✓4ᵗʰ **A07 Other protozoal intestinal diseases**

A07.0 Balantidiasis
Balantidial dysentery

A07.1 Giardiasis [lambliasis]

A07.2 Cryptosporidiosis

A07.3 Isosporiasis
Infection due to Isospora belli and Isospora hominis
Intestinal coccidiosis
Isosporosis

A07.4 Cyclosporiasis

A07.8 Other specified protozoal intestinal diseases
Intestinal microsporidiosis
Intestinal trichomoniasis
Sarcocystosis
Sarcosporidiosis

A07.9 Protozoal intestinal disease, unspecified
Flagellate diarrhea   Protozoal diarrhea
Protozoal colitis   Protozoal dysentery

✓4ᵗʰ **A08 Viral and other specified intestinal infections**
EXCLUDES 1   influenza with involvement of gastrointestinal tract (J09.X3, J10.2, J11.2)

A08.0 Rotaviral enteritis

✓5ᵗʰ **A08.1 Acute gastroenteropathy due to Norwalk agent and other small round viruses**

    A08.11 Acute gastroenteropathy due to Norwalk agent
Acute gastroenteropathy due to Norovirus
Acute gastroenteropathy due to Norwalk-like agent

    A08.19 Acute gastroenteropathy due to other small round viruses
Acute gastroenteropathy due to small round virus [SRV] NOS

A08.2 Adenoviral enteritis

✓5ᵗʰ **A08.3 Other viral enteritis**

    A08.31 Calicivirus enteritis

    A08.32 Astrovirus enteritis

    A08.39 Other viral enteritis
Coxsackie virus enteritis
Echovirus enteritis
Enterovirus enteritis NEC
Torovirus enteritis

A08.4 Viral intestinal infection, unspecified
Viral enteritis NOS
Viral gastroenteritis NOS
Viral gastroenteropathy NOS

A08.8 Other specified intestinal infections

A09 Infectious gastroenteritis and colitis, unspecified
Infectious colitis NOS
Infectious enteritis NOS
Infectious gastroenteritis NOS
EXCLUDES 1   colitis NOS (K52.9)
    diarrhea NOS (R19.7)
    enteritis NOS (K52.9)
    gastroenteritis NOS (K52.9)
    noninfective gastroenteritis and colitis, unspecified (K52.9)

Tuberculosis (A15-A19)

INCLUDES   infections due to Mycobacterium tuberculosis and Mycobacterium bovis
EXCLUDES 1   congenital tuberculosis (P37.0)
    nonspecific reaction to test for tuberculosis without active tuberculosis (R76.1-)
    pneumoconiosis associated with tuberculosis, any type in A15 (J65)
    positive PPD (R76.11)
    positive tuberculin skin test without active tuberculosis (R76.11)
    sequelae of tuberculosis (B90.-)
    silicotuberculosis (J65)

✓4ᵗʰ **A15 Respiratory tuberculosis**

A15.0 Tuberculosis of lung
Tuberculous bronchiectasis
Tuberculous fibrosis of lung
Tuberculous pneumonia
Tuberculous pneumothorax

A15.4 Tuberculosis of intrathoracic lymph nodes
Tuberculosis of hilar lymph nodes
Tuberculosis of mediastinal lymph nodes
Tuberculosis of tracheobronchial lymph nodes
EXCLUDES 1   tuberculosis specified as primary (A15.7)

A15.5 Tuberculosis of larynx, trachea and bronchus
Tuberculosis of bronchus
Tuberculosis of glottis
Tuberculosis of larynx
Tuberculosis of trachea

A15.6 Tuberculous pleurisy
Tuberculosis of pleura Tuberculous empyema
EXCLUDES 1   primary respiratory tuberculosis (A15.7)

A15.7 Primary respiratory tuberculosis

A15.8 Other respiratory tuberculosis
Mediastinal tuberculosis
Nasopharyngeal tuberculosis
Tuberculosis of nose
Tuberculosis of sinus [any nasal]

A15.9 Respiratory tuberculosis unspecified

✓4ᵗʰ **A17 Tuberculosis of nervous system**

A17.0 Tuberculous meningitis
Tuberculosis of meninges (cerebral) (spinal)
Tuberculous leptomeningitis
EXCLUDES 1   tuberculous meningoencephalitis (A17.82)

A17.1 Meningeal tuberculoma
Tuberculoma of meninges (cerebral) (spinal)
EXCLUDES 2   tuberculoma of brain and spinal cord (A17.81)

✓5ᵗʰ **A17.8 Other tuberculosis of nervous system**

    A17.81 Tuberculoma of brain and spinal cord
Tuberculous abscess of brain and spinal cord

    A17.82 Tuberculous meningoencephalitis
Tuberculous myelitis

    A17.83 Tuberculous neuritis
Tuberculous mononeuropathy

    A17.89 Other tuberculosis of nervous system
Tuberculous polyneuropathy

A17.9 Tuberculosis of nervous system, unspecified

✓4ᵗʰ **A18 Tuberculosis of other organs**

✓5ᵗʰ **A18.0 Tuberculosis of bones and joints**

    A18.01 Tuberculosis of spine
Pott's disease or curvature of spine
Tuberculous arthritis
Tuberculous osteomyelitis of spine
Tuberculous spondylitis

    A18.02 Tuberculous arthritis of other joints
Tuberculosis of hip (joint)
Tuberculosis of knee (joint)

    A18.03 Tuberculosis of other bones
Tuberculous mastoiditis
Tuberculous osteomyelitis

    A18.09 Other musculoskeletal tuberculosis
Tuberculous myositis
Tuberculous synovitis
Tuberculous tenosynovitis

✓5ᵗʰ **A18.1 Tuberculosis of genitourinary system**

    A18.10 Tuberculosis of genitourinary system, unspecified

    A18.11 Tuberculosis of kidney and ureter

    A18.12 Tuberculosis of bladder

✓ Additional Character Required   ✓x7ᵗʰ Placeholder Alert   Unspecified Dx   Other Specified Dx   Manifestation   ►◄ Revised Text   ● New Code   ▲ Revised Code Title

A18.13 Tuberculosis of other urinary organs
　Tuberculous urethritis

A18.14 Tuberculosis of prostate　　　　　A♂

A18.15 Tuberculosis of other male genital organs　♂

A18.16 Tuberculosis of cervix　　　　　　♀

A18.17 Tuberculous female pelvic inflammatory disease
　Tuberculous endometritis
　Tuberculous oophoritis and salpingitis　♀

A18.18 Tuberculosis of other female genital organs　♀
　Tuberculous ulceration of vulva

A18.2 Tuberculous peripheral lymphadenopathy
　Tuberculous adenitis
　EXCLUDES 2　tuberculosis of bronchial and mediastinal lymph nodes (A15.4)
　　tuberculosis of mesenteric and retroperitoneal lymph nodes (A18.39)
　　tuberculous tracheobronchial adenopathy (A15.4)

✓5th **A18.3 Tuberculosis of** intestines, peritoneum and mesenteric glands

　A18.31 Tuberculous peritonitis
　　Tuberculous ascites

　A18.32 Tuberculous enteritis
　　Tuberculosis of anus and rectum
　　Tuberculosis of intestine (large) (small)

　A18.39 Retroperitoneal tuberculosis
　　Tuberculosis of mesenteric glands
　　Tuberculosis of retroperitoneal (lymph glands)

A18.4 Tuberculosis of skin and subcutaneous tissue
　Erythema induratum, tuberculous
　Lupus excedens
　Lupus vulgaris NOS
　Lupus vulgaris of eyelid
　Scrofuloderma
　Tuberculosis of external ear
　EXCLUDES 2　lupus erythematosus (L93.-)
　　lupus NOS (M32.9)
　　systemic (M32.-)

✓5th **A18.5 Tuberculosis of** eye
　EXCLUDES 2　lupus vulgaris of eyelid (A18.4)

　A18.50 Tuberculosis of eye, unspecified

　A18.51 Tuberculous episcleritis

　A18.52 Tuberculous keratitis
　　Tuberculous interstitial keratitis
　　Tuberculous keratoconjunctivitis (interstitial) (phlyctenular)

　A18.53 Tuberculous chorioretinitis

　A18.54 Tuberculous iridocyclitis

　A18.59 Other tuberculosis of eye
　　Tuberculous conjunctivitis

A18.6 Tuberculosis of (inner) (middle) ear
　Tuberculous otitis media
　EXCLUDES 2　tuberculosis of external ear (A18.4)
　　tuberculous mastoiditis (A18.03)

A18.7 Tuberculosis of adrenal glands
　Tuberculous Addison's disease

✓5th **A18.8 Tuberculosis of** other specified organs

　A18.81 Tuberculosis of thyroid gland

　A18.82 Tuberculosis of other endocrine glands
　　Tuberculosis of pituitary gland
　　Tuberculosis of thymus gland

　A18.83 Tuberculosis of digestive tract organs, **not elsewhere classified**
　　EXCLUDES 1　tuberculosis of intestine (A18.32)

　A18.84 Tuberculosis of heart
　　Tuberculous cardiomyopathy
　　Tuberculous endocarditis
　　Tuberculous myocarditis
　　Tuberculous pericarditis

　A18.85 Tuberculosis of spleen

　A18.89 Tuberculosis of other sites
　　Tuberculosis of muscle
　　Tuberculous cerebral arteritis

✓4th **A19 Miliary tuberculosis**
　INCLUDES　disseminated tuberculosis
　　generalized tuberculosis
　　tuberculous polyserositis

A19.0 Acute miliary tuberculosis of a single specified site

A19.1 Acute miliary tuberculosis of multiple sites

A19.2 Acute miliary tuberculosis, unspecified

A19.8 Other miliary tuberculosis

A19.9 Miliary tuberculosis, unspecified

Certain zoonotic bacterial diseases (A20-A28)

✓4th **A20 Plague**
　INCLUDES　infection due to Yersinia pestis

　A20.0 Bubonic plague

　A20.1 Cellulocutaneous plague

　A20.2 Pneumonic plague

　A20.3 Plague meningitis

　A20.7 Septicemic plague

　A20.8 Other forms of plague
　　Abortive plague
　　Asymptomatic plague
　　Pestis minor

　A20.9 Plague, unspecified

✓4th **A21 Tularemia**
　INCLUDES　deer-fly fever
　　infection due to Francisella tularensis
　　rabbit fever

　A21.0 Ulceroglandular tularemia

　A21.1 Oculoglandular tularemia
　　Ophthalmic tularemia

　A21.2 Pulmonary tularemia

　A21.3 Gastrointestinal tularemia
　　Abdominal tularemia

　A21.7 Generalized tularemia

　A21.8 Other forms of tularemia

　A21.9 Tularemia, unspecified

✓4th **A22 Anthrax**
　INCLUDES　infection due to Bacillus anthracis

　A22.0 Cutaneous anthrax
　　Malignant carbuncle
　　Malignant pustule

　A22.1 Pulmonary anthrax
　　Inhalation anthrax
　　Ragpicker's disease
　　Woolsorter's disease

　A22.2 Gastrointestinal anthrax

　A22.7 Anthrax sepsis

　A22.8 Other forms of anthrax
　　Anthrax meningitis

　A22.9 Anthrax, unspecified

✓4th **A23 Brucellosis**
　Malta fever
　Mediterranean fever
　Undulant fever

　A23.0 Brucellosis due to Brucella melitensis

　A23.1 Brucellosis due to Brucella abortus

　A23.2 Brucellosis due to Brucella suis

　A23.3 Brucellosis due to Brucella canis

　A23.8 Other brucellosis

　A23.9 Brucellosis, unspecified

✓4th **A24 Glanders and melioidosis**

　A24.0 Glanders
　　Infection due to Pseudomonas mallei
　　Malleus

　A24.1 Acute and fulminating melioidosis
　　Melioidosis pneumonia
　　Melioidosis sepsis

　A24.2 Subacute and chronic melioidosis

　A24.3 Other melioidosis

　A24.9 Melioidosis, unspecified
　　Infection due to Pseudomonas pseudomallei NOS
　　Whitmore's disease

✓4th **A25 Rat-bite fevers**

　A25.0 Spirillosis
　　Sodoku

　A25.1 Streptobacillosis
　　Epidemic arthritic erythema
　　Haverhill fever
　　Streptobacillary rat-bite fever

　A25.9 Rat-bite fever, unspecified

EXCLUDES 1 Not coded here　　EXCLUDES 2 Not included here　　N Newborn Age: 0　　P Pediatric Age: 0-17　　M Maternity Age: 12-55　　A Adult Age: 15-124

428
ICD-10-CM 2016

✓4ᵗʰ **A26 Erysipeloid**

A26.0 Cutaneous erysipeloid
Erythema migrans

A26.7 Erysipelothrix sepsis

A26.8 Other forms of erysipeloid

A26.9 Erysipeloid, unspecified

✓4ᵗʰ **A27 Leptospirosis**

A27.0 Leptospirosis icterohemorrhagica
Leptospiral or spirochetal jaundice (hemorrhagic)
Weil's disease

✓5ᵗʰ **A27.8 Other forms of leptospirosis**

A27.81 Aseptic meningitis in leptospirosis

A27.89 Other forms of leptospirosis

A27.9 Leptospirosis, unspecified

✓4ᵗʰ **A28 Other zoonotic bacterial diseases, not elsewhere classified**

A28.0 Pasteurellosis

A28.1 Cat-scratch disease
Cat-scratch fever

A28.2 Extraintestinal yersiniosis
EXCLUDES 1   enteritis due to Yersinia enterocolitica (A04.6)
plague (A20.-)

A28.8 Other specified zoonotic bacterial diseases, not elsewhere classified

A28.9 Zoonotic bacterial disease, unspecified

Other bacterial diseases (A30-A49)

✓4ᵗʰ **A30 Leprosy [Hansen's disease]**
INCLUDES   infection due to Mycobacterium leprae
EXCLUDES 1   sequelae of leprosy (B92)

A30.0 Indeterminate leprosy
I leprosy

A30.1 Tuberculoid leprosy
TT leprosy

A30.2 Borderline tuberculoid leprosy
BT leprosy

A30.3 Borderline leprosy
BB leprosy

A30.4 Borderline lepromatous leprosy
BL leprosy

A30.5 Lepromatous leprosy
LL leprosy

A30.8 Other forms of leprosy

A30.9 Leprosy, unspecified

✓4ᵗʰ **A31 Infection due to other mycobacteria**
EXCLUDES 2   leprosy (A30.-)
tuberculosis (A15-A19)

A31.0 Pulmonary mycobacterial infection
Infection due to Mycobacterium avium
Infection due to Mycobacterium intracellulare [Battey bacillus]
Infection due to Mycobacterium kansasii

A31.1 Cutaneous mycobacterial infection
Buruli ulcer
Infection due to Mycobacterium marinum
Infection due to Mycobacterium ulcerans

A31.2 Disseminated mycobacterium avium-intracellulare complex (DMAC)
MAC sepsis

A31.8 Other mycobacterial infections

A31.9 Mycobacterial infection, unspecified
Atypical mycobacterial infection NOS
Mycobacteriosis NOS

✓4ᵗʰ **A32 Listeriosis**
INCLUDES   listerial foodborne infection
EXCLUDES 1   neonatal (disseminated) listeriosis (P37.2)

A32.0 Cutaneous listeriosis

✓5ᵗʰ **A32.1 Listerial meningitis and meningoencephalitis**

A32.11 Listerial meningitis

A32.12 Listerial meningoencephalitis

A32.7 Listerial sepsis

✓5ᵗʰ **A32.8 Other forms of listeriosis**

A32.81 Oculoglandular listeriosis

A32.82 Listerial endocarditis

A32.89 Other forms of listeriosis
Listerial cerebral arteritis

A32.9 Listeriosis, unspecified

A33 Tetanus neonatorum   N

A34 Obstetrical tetanus   M♀

A35 Other tetanus
Tetanus NOS
EXCLUDES 1   obstetrical tetanus (A34)
tetanus neonatorum (A33)

✓4ᵗʰ **A36 Diphtheria**

A36.0 Pharyngeal diphtheria
Diphtheritic membranous angina
Tonsillar diphtheria

A36.1 Nasopharyngeal diphtheria

A36.2 Laryngeal diphtheria
Diphtheritic laryngotracheitis

A36.3 Cutaneous diphtheria
EXCLUDES 2   erythrasma (L08.1)

✓5ᵗʰ **A36.8 Other diphtheria**

A36.81 Diphtheritic cardiomyopathy
Diphtheritic myocarditis

A36.82 Diphtheritic radiculomyelitis

A36.83 Diphtheritic polyneuritis

A36.84 Diphtheritic tubulo-interstitial nephropathy

A36.85 Diphtheritic cystitis

A36.86 Diphtheritic conjunctivitis

A36.89 Other diphtheritic complications
Diphtheritic peritonitis

A36.9 Diphtheria, unspecified

✓4ᵗʰ **A37 Whooping cough**

✓5ᵗʰ **A37.0 Whooping cough due to Bordetella pertussis**

A37.00 Whooping cough due to Bordetella pertussis without pneumonia

A37.01 Whooping cough due to Bordetella pertussis with pneumonia

✓5ᵗʰ **A37.1 Whooping cough due to Bordetella parapertussis**

A37.10 Whooping cough due to Bordetella parapertussis without pneumonia

A37.11 Whooping cough due to Bordetella parapertussis with pneumonia

✓5ᵗʰ **A37.8 Whooping cough due to other Bordetella species**

A37.80 Whooping cough due to other Bordetella species without pneumonia

A37.81 Whooping cough due to other Bordetella species with pneumonia

✓5ᵗʰ **A37.9 Whooping cough, unspecified species**

A37.90 Whooping cough, unspecified species without pneumonia

A37.91 Whooping cough, unspecified species with pneumonia

✓4ᵗʰ **A38 Scarlet fever**
INCLUDES   scarlatina
EXCLUDES 2   streptococcal sore throat (J02.0)

A38.0 Scarlet fever with otitis media

A38.1 Scarlet fever with myocarditis

A38.8 Scarlet fever with other complications

A38.9 Scarlet fever, uncomplicated
Scarlet fever, NOS

✓4ᵗʰ **A39 Meningococcal infection**

A39.0 Meningococcal meningitis

A39.1 Waterhouse-Friderichsen syndrome
Meningococcal hemorrhagic adrenalitis
Meningococcic adrenal syndrome

A39.2 Acute meningococcemia

A39.3 Chronic meningococcemia

A39.4 Meningococcemia, unspecified

✓5ᵗʰ **A39.5 Meningococcal heart disease**

A39.50 Meningococcal carditis, unspecified

A39.51 Meningococcal endocarditis

A39.52 Meningococcal myocarditis

A39.53 Meningococcal pericarditis

✓5ᵗʰ **A39.8 Other meningococcal infections**

A39.81 Meningococcal encephalitis

✓ Additional Character Required   ✓x7ᵗʰ Placeholder Alert   Unspecified Dx   Other Specified Dx   Manifestation   ►◄ Revised Text   ● New Code   ▲ Revised Code Title

A39.82   **Meningococcal** retrobulbar neuritis

A39.83   **Meningococcal** arthritis

A39.84   **Postmeningococcal** arthritis

A39.89   **Other meningococcal infections**
        Meningococcal conjunctivitis

A39.9   **Meningococcal infection, unspecified**
        Meningococcal disease NOS

✓4ᵗʰ **A40**   **Streptococcal sepsis**
    Code first: postprocedural streptococcal sepsis (T81.4)
          streptococcal sepsis during labor (O75.3)
          streptococcal sepsis following abortion or ectopic or molar
             pregnancy (O03-O07, O08.0)
          streptococcal sepsis following immunization (T88.0)
          streptococcal sepsis following infusion, transfusion or
             therapeutic injection (T80.2-)

     EXCLUDES 1   *neonatal (P36.0-P36.1)*
               puerperal sepsis (O85)
               sepsis due to Streptococcus, group D (A41.81)

A40.0   **Sepsis due to Streptococcus,** group A

A40.1   **Sepsis due to streptococcus,** group B

A40.3   **Sepsis due to Streptococcus** pneumoniae
        Pneumococcal sepsis

A40.8   **Other streptococcal sepsis**

A40.9   **Streptococcal sepsis, unspecified**

✓4ᵗʰ **A41**   **Other sepsis**
    Code first: postprocedural sepsis (T81.4)
          sepsis during labor (O75.3)
          sepsis following abortion, ectopic or molar pregnancy
             (O03-O07, O08.0)
          sepsis following immunization (T88.0)
          sepsis following infusion, transfusion or therapeutic injection
             (T80.2-)

     EXCLUDES 1   *bacteremia NOS (R78.81)*
               neonatal (P36.-)
               puerperal sepsis (O85)
               sepsis NOS (A41.9)
               streptococcal sepsis (A40.-)

     EXCLUDES 2   *sepsis (due to) (in) actinomycotic (A42.7)*
               sepsis (due to) (in) anthrax (A22.7)
               sepsis (due to) (in) candidal (B37.7)
               sepsis (due to) (in) Erysipelothrix (A26.7)
               sepsis (due to) (in) extraintestinal yersiniosis (A28.2)
               sepsis (due to) (in) gonococcal (A54.86)
               sepsis (due to) (in) herpesviral (B00.7)
               sepsis (due to) (in) listerial (A32.7)
               sepsis (due to) (in) melioidosis (A24.1)
               sepsis (due to) (in) meningococcal (A39.2-A39.4)
               sepsis (due to) (in) plague (A20.7)
               sepsis (due to) (in) tularemia (A21.7)
               toxic shock syndrome (A48.3)

     AHA: 2014, 2Q, 13

✓5ᵗʰ **A41.0**   **Sepsis due to Staphylococcus aureus**

       A41.01   **Sepsis due to methicillin susceptible Staphylococcus
aureus**
             MSSA sepsis
             Staphylococcus aureus sepsis NOS

       A41.02   **Sepsis due to methicillin resistant Staphylococcus
aureus**

A41.1   **Sepsis due to other specified staphylococcus**
        Coagulase negative staphylococcus sepsis

A41.2   **Sepsis due to unspecified staphylococcus**

A41.3   **Sepsis due to Hemophilus influenzae**

A41.4   **Sepsis due to anaerobes**
     EXCLUDES 1   *gas gangrene (A48.0)*

✓5ᵗʰ **A41.5**   **Sepsis due to other Gram-negative organisms**

       A41.50   **Gram-negative sepsis, unspecified**
             Gram-negative sepsis NOS

       A41.51   **Sepsis due to Escherichia coli [E. coli]**

       A41.52   **Sepsis due to Pseudomonas**
             Pseudomonas aeroginosa

       A41.53   **Sepsis due to Serratia**

       A41.59   **Other Gram-negative sepsis**

✓5ᵗʰ **A41.8**   **Other specified sepsis**

       A41.81   **Sepsis due to Enterococcus**

       A41.89   **Other specified sepsis**

A41.9   **Sepsis, unspecified organism**
        Septicemia NOS

✓4ᵗʰ **A42**   **Actinomycosis**
     EXCLUDES 1   *actinomycetoma (B47.1)*

A42.0   **Pulmonary actinomycosis**

A42.1   **Abdominal actinomycosis**

A42.2   **Cervicofacial actinomycosis**

A42.7   **Actinomycotic sepsis**

✓5ᵗʰ **A42.8**   **Other forms of actinomycosis**

       A42.81   **Actinomycotic meningitis**

       A42.82   **Actinomycotic encephalitis**

       A42.89   **Other forms of actinomycosis**

A42.9   **Actinomycosis, unspecified**

✓4ᵗʰ **A43**   **Nocardiosis**

A43.0   **Pulmonary nocardiosis**

A43.1   **Cutaneous nocardiosis**

A43.8   **Other forms of nocardiosis**

A43.9   **Nocardiosis, unspecified**

✓4ᵗʰ **A44**   **Bartonellosis**

A44.0   **Systemic bartonellosis**
        Oroya fever

A44.1   **Cutaneous and mucocutaneous bartonellosis**
        Verruga peruana

A44.8   **Other forms of bartonellosis**

A44.9   **Bartonellosis, unspecified**

A46   **Erysipelas**
     EXCLUDES 1   *postpartum or puerperal erysipelas (O86.89)*

✓4ᵗʰ **A48**   **Other bacterial diseases, not elsewhere classified**
     EXCLUDES 1   *actinomycetoma (B47.1)*

A48.0   **Gas gangrene**
        Clostridial cellulitis
        Clostridial myonecrosis

A48.1   **Legionnaires' disease**

A48.2   **Nonpneumonic Legionnaires' disease [Pontiac fever]**

A48.3   **Toxic shock syndrome**
        Use additional code to identify the organism (B95, B96)
     EXCLUDES 1   *endotoxic shock NOS (R57.8)*
               sepsis NOS (A41.9)

A48.4   **Brazilian purpuric fever**
        Systemic Hemophilus aegyptius infection

✓5ᵗʰ **A48.5**   **Other specified botulism**
        Non-foodborne intoxication due to toxins of Clostridium
             botulinum [C. botulinum]
     EXCLUDES 1   *food poisoning due to toxins of Clostridium botulinum
               (A05.1)*

       A48.51   **Infant botulism**   P

       A48.52   **Wound botulism**
             Non-foodborne botulism NOS
             Use additional code for associated wound

A48.8   **Other specified bacterial diseases**

✓4ᵗʰ **A49**   **Bacterial infection of unspecified site**
     EXCLUDES 1   *bacterial agents as the cause of diseases classified elsewhere
               (B95-B96)*
               chlamydial infection NOS (A74.9)
               meningococcal infection NOS (A39.9)
               rickettsial infection NOS (A79.9)
               spirochetal infection NOS (A69.9)

✓5ᵗʰ **A49.0**   **Staphylococcal infection, unspecified site**

       A49.01   **Methicillin susceptible Staphylococcus aureus
infection, unspecified site**
             Methicillin susceptible Staphylococcus aureus (MSSA)
               infection
             Staphylococcus aureus infection NOS

       A49.02   **Methicillin resistant Staphylococcus aureus
infection, unspecified site**
             Methicillin resistant Staphylococcus aureus (MRSA)
               infection

A49.1   **Streptococcal infection, unspecified site**

A49.2   **Hemophilus influenzae infection, unspecified site**

A49.3   **Mycoplasma infection, unspecified site**

A49.8   **Other bacterial infections of unspecified site**

A49.9   **Bacterial infection, unspecified**
     EXCLUDES 1   *bacteremia NOS (R78.81)*

EXCLUDES 1 Not coded here   *EXCLUDES 2* Not included here   N Newborn Age: 0   P Pediatric Age: 0-17   M Maternity Age: 12-55   A Adult Age: 15-124

430   ICD-10-CM 2016

Infections with a predominantly sexual mode of transmission (A50-A64)

> **EXCLUDES 1**　human immunodeficiency virus [HIV] disease (B20)
> nonspecific and nongonococcal urethritis (N34.1)
> Reiter's disease (M02.3-)

✓4th **A50　Congenital syphilis**

　✓5th **A50.0　Early congenital syphilis, symptomatic**
　　　Any congenital syphilitic condition specified as early or manifest less than two years after birth.

　　A50.01　Early congenital syphilitic oculopathy

　　A50.02　Early congenital syphilitic osteochondropathy

　　A50.03　Early congenital syphilitic pharyngitis
　　　Early congenital syphilitic laryngitis

　　A50.04　Early congenital syphilitic pneumonia

　　A50.05　Early congenital syphilitic rhinitis

　　A50.06　Early cutaneous congenital syphilis

　　A50.07　Early mucocutaneous congenital syphilis

　　A50.08　Early visceral congenital syphilis

　　A50.09　Other early congenital syphilis, symptomatic

　A50.1　Early congenital syphilis, latent
　　　Congenital syphilis without clinical manifestations, with positive serological reaction and negative spinal fluid test, less than two years after birth.

　A50.2　Early congenital syphilis, unspecified
　　　Congenital syphilis NOS less than two years after birth.

　✓5th **A50.3　Late congenital syphilitic oculopathy**
　　　EXCLUDES 1　Hutchinson's triad (A50.53)

　　A50.30　Late congenital syphilitic oculopathy, unspecified

　　A50.31　Late congenital syphilitic interstitial keratitis

　　A50.32　Late congenital syphilitic chorioretinitis

　　A50.39　Other late congenital syphilitic oculopathy

　✓5th **A50.4　Late congenital neurosyphilis [juvenile neurosyphilis]**
　　　Use additional code to identify any associated mental disorder
　　　EXCLUDES 1　Hutchinson's triad (A50.53)

　　A50.40　Late congenital neurosyphilis, unspecified
　　　Juvenile neurosyphilis NOS

　　A50.41　Late congenital syphilitic meningitis

　　A50.42　Late congenital syphilitic encephalitis

　　A50.43　Late congenital syphilitic polyneuropathy

　　A50.44　Late congenital syphilitic optic nerve atrophy

　　A50.45　Juvenile general paresis
　　　Dementia paralytica juvenilis
　　　Juvenile tabetoparetic neurosyphilis

　　A50.49　Other late congenital neurosyphilis
　　　Juvenile tabes dorsalis

　✓5th **A50.5　Other late congenital syphilis, symptomatic**
　　　Any congenital syphilitic condition specified as late or manifest two years or more after birth.

　　A50.51　Clutton's joints

　　A50.52　Hutchinson's teeth

　　A50.53　Hutchinson's triad

　　A50.54　Late congenital cardiovascular syphilis

　　A50.55　Late congenital syphilitic arthropathy

　　A50.56　Late congenital syphilitic osteochondropathy

　　A50.57　Syphilitic saddle nose

　　A50.59　Other late congenital syphilis, symptomatic

　A50.6　Late congenital syphilis, latent
　　　Congenital syphilis without clinical manifestations, with positive serological reaction and negative spinal fluid test, two years or more after birth.

　A50.7　Late congenital syphilis, unspecified
　　　Congenital syphilis NOS two years or more after birth.

　A50.9　Congenital syphilis, unspecified

✓4th **A51　Early syphilis**

　A51.0　Primary genital syphilis
　　　Syphilitic chancre NOS

　A51.1　Primary anal syphilis

　A51.2　Primary syphilis of other sites

　✓5th **A51.3　Secondary syphilis of skin and mucous membranes**

　　A51.31　Condyloma latum

　　A51.32　Syphilitic alopecia

　　A51.39　Other secondary syphilis of skin
　　　Syphilitic leukoderma
　　　Syphilitic mucous patch
　　　EXCLUDES 1　late syphilitic leukoderma (A52.79)

　✓5th **A51.4　Other secondary syphilis**

　　A51.41　Secondary syphilitic meningitis

　　A51.42　Secondary syphilitic female pelvic disease　♀

　　A51.43　Secondary syphilitic oculopathy
　　　Secondary syphilitic chorioretinitis
　　　Secondary syphilitic iridocyclitis, iritis
　　　Secondary syphilitic uveitis

　　A51.44　Secondary syphilitic nephritis

　　A51.45　Secondary syphilitic hepatitis

　　A51.46　Secondary syphilitic osteopathy

　　A51.49　Other secondary syphilitic conditions
　　　Secondary syphilitic lymphadenopathy
　　　Secondary syphilitic myositis

　A51.5　Early syphilis, latent
　　　Syphilis (acquired) without clinical manifestations, with positive serological reaction and negative spinal fluid test, less than two years after infection.

　A51.9　Early syphilis, unspecified

✓4th **A52　Late syphilis**

　✓5th **A52.0　Cardiovascular and cerebrovascular syphilis**

　　A52.00　Cardiovascular syphilis, unspecified

　　A52.01　Syphilitic aneurysm of aorta

　　A52.02　Syphilitic aortitis

　　A52.03　Syphilitic endocarditis
　　　Syphilitic aortic valve incompetence or stenosis
　　　Syphilitic mitral valve stenosis
　　　Syphilitic pulmonary valve regurgitation

　　A52.04　Syphilitic cerebral arteritis

　　A52.05　Other cerebrovascular syphilis
　　　Syphilitic cerebral aneurysm (ruptured) (non-ruptured)
　　　Syphilitic cerebral thrombosis

　　A52.06　Other syphilitic heart involvement
　　　Syphilitic coronary artery disease
　　　Syphilitic myocarditis
　　　Syphilitic pericarditis

　　A52.09　Other cardiovascular syphilis

　✓5th **A52.1　Symptomatic neurosyphilis**

　　A52.10　Symptomatic neurosyphilis, unspecified

　　A52.11　Tabes dorsalis
　　　Locomotor ataxia (progressive)
　　　Tabetic neurosyphilis

　　A52.12　Other cerebrospinal syphilis

　　A52.13　Late syphilitic meningitis

　　A52.14　Late syphilitic encephalitis

　　A52.15　Late syphilitic neuropathy
　　　Late syphilitic acoustic neuritis
　　　Late syphilitic optic (nerve) atrophy
　　　Late syphilitic polyneuropathy
　　　Late syphilitic retrobulbar neuritis

　　A52.16　Charcôt's arthropathy (tabetic)

　　A52.17　General paresis
　　　Dementia paralytica

　　A52.19　Other symptomatic neurosyphilis
　　　Syphilitic parkinsonism

　A52.2　Asymptomatic neurosyphilis

　A52.3　Neurosyphilis, unspecified
　　　Gumma (syphilitic)
　　　Syphilis (late)
　　　Syphiloma

　✓5th **A52.7　Other symptomatic late syphilis**

　　A52.71　Late syphilitic oculopathy
　　　Late syphilitic chorioretinitis
　　　Late syphilitic episcleritis

　　A52.72　Syphilis of lung and bronchus

　　A52.73　Symptomatic late syphilis of other respiratory organs

　　A52.74　Syphilis of liver and other viscera
　　　Late syphilitic peritonitis

　　A52.75　Syphilis of kidney and ureter
　　　Syphilitic glomerular disease

✓ Additional Character Required　　✓x7th Placeholder Alert　　Unspecified Dx　　Other Specified Dx　　Manifestation　　▶◀ Revised Text　　● New Code　　▲ Revised Code Title

A52.76 **Other genitourinary symptomatic late syphilis**
Late syphilitic female pelvic inflammatory disease

A52.77 **Syphilis of bone and joint**

A52.78 **Syphilis of other musculoskeletal tissue**
Late syphilitic bursitis
Syphilis [stage unspecified] of bursa
Syphilis [stage unspecified] of muscle
Syphilis [stage unspecified] of synovium
Syphilis [stage unspecified] of tendon

A52.79 **Other symptomatic late syphilis**
Late syphilitic leukoderma
Syphilis of adrenal gland
Syphilis of pituitary gland
Syphilis of thyroid gland
Syphilitic splenomegaly
EXCLUDES 1   syphilitic leukoderma (secondary) (A51.39)

A52.8 **Late syphilis, latent**
Syphilis (acquired) without clinical manifestations, with positive serological reaction and negative spinal fluid test, two years or more after infection

A52.9 **Late syphilis, unspecified**

✓4th **A53 Other and unspecified syphilis**

A53.0 **Latent syphilis, unspecified as early or late**
Latent syphilis NOS
Positive serological reaction for syphilis

A53.9 **Syphilis, unspecified**
Infection due to Treponema pallidum NOS
Syphilis (acquired) NOS
EXCLUDES 1   syphilis NOS under two years of age (A50.2)

✓4th **A54 Gonococcal infection**

✓5th A54.0 **Gonococcal infection of lower genitourinary tract without periurethral or accessory gland abscess**
EXCLUDES 1   gonococcal infection with genitourinary gland abscess (A54.1)
gonococcal infection with periurethral abscess (A54.1)

A54.00 **Gonococcal infection of lower genitourinary tract, unspecified**

A54.01 **Gonococcal cystitis and urethritis, unspecified**

A54.02 **Gonococcal vulvovaginitis, unspecified** ♀

A54.03 **Gonococcal cervicitis, unspecified** ♀

A54.09 **Other gonococcal infection of lower genitourinary tract**

A54.1 **Gonococcal infection of lower genitourinary tract with periurethral and accessory gland abscess**
Gonococcal Bartholin's gland abscess

✓5th A54.2 **Gonococcal pelviperitonitis and other gonococcal genitourinary infection**

A54.21 **Gonococcal infection of kidney and ureter**

A54.22 **Gonococcal prostatitis** ♂

A54.23 **Gonococcal infection of other male genital organs** ♂
Gonococcal epididymitis
Gonococcal orchitis

A54.24 **Gonococcal female pelvic inflammatory disease** ♀
Gonococcal pelviperitonitis
EXCLUDES 1   gonococcal peritonitis (A54.85)

A54.29 **Other gonococcal genitourinary infections**

✓5th A54.3 **Gonococcal infection of eye**

A54.30 **Gonococcal infection of eye, unspecified**

A54.31 **Gonococcal conjunctivitis**
Ophthalmia neonatorum due to gonococcus

A54.32 **Gonococcal iridocyclitis**

A54.33 **Gonococcal keratitis**

A54.39 **Other gonococcal eye infection**
Gonococcal endophthalmia

✓5th A54.4 **Gonococcal infection of musculoskeletal system**

A54.40 **Gonococcal infection of musculoskeletal system, unspecified**

A54.41 **Gonococcal spondylopathy**

A54.42 **Gonococcal arthritis**
EXCLUDES 2   gonococcal infection of spine (A54.41)

A54.43 **Gonococcal osteomyelitis**
EXCLUDES 2   gonococcal infection of spine (A54.41)

A54.49 **Gonococcal infection of other musculoskeletal tissue**
Gonococcal bursitis
Gonococcal myositis
Gonococcal synovitis
Gonococcal tenosynovitis

A54.5 **Gonococcal pharyngitis**

A54.6 **Gonococcal infection of anus and rectum**

✓5th A54.8 **Other gonococcal infections**

A54.81 **Gonococcal meningitis**

A54.82 **Gonococcal brain abscess**

A54.83 **Gonococcal heart infection**
Gonococcal endocarditis
Gonococcal myocarditis
Gonococcal pericarditis

A54.84 **Gonococcal pneumonia**

A54.85 **Gonococcal peritonitis**
EXCLUDES 1   gonococcal pelviperitonitis (A54.24)

A54.86 **Gonococcal sepsis**

A54.89 **Other gonococcal infections**
Gonococcal keratoderma
Gonococcal lymphadenitis

A54.9 **Gonococcal infection, unspecified**

A55 **Chlamydial lymphogranuloma (venereum)**
Climatic or tropical bubo
Durand-Nicolas-Favre disease
Esthiomene
Lymphogranuloma inguinale

✓4th **A56 Other sexually transmitted chlamydial diseases**
INCLUDES   sexually transmitted diseases due to Chlamydia trachomatis
EXCLUDES 1   neonatal chlamydial conjunctivitis (P39.1)
neonatal chlamydial pneumonia (P23.1)
EXCLUDES 2   chlamydial lymphogranuloma (A55)
conditions classified to A74-

✓5th A56.0 **Chlamydial infection of lower genitourinary tract**

A56.00 **Chlamydial infection of lower genitourinary tract, unspecified**

A56.01 **Chlamydial cystitis and urethritis**

A56.02 **Chlamydial vulvovaginitis** ♀

A56.09 **Other chlamydial infection of lower genitourinary tract**
Chlamydial cervicitis

✓5th A56.1 **Chlamydial infection of pelviperitoneum and other genitourinary organs**

A56.11 **Chlamydial female pelvic inflammatory disease** ♀

A56.19 **Other chlamydial genitourinary infection**
Chlamydial epididymitis
Chlamydial orchitis

A56.2 **Chlamydial infection of genitourinary tract, unspecified**

A56.3 **Chlamydial infection of anus and rectum**

A56.4 **Chlamydial infection of pharynx**

A56.8 **Sexually transmitted chlamydial infection of other sites**

A57 **Chancroid**
Ulcus molle

A58 **Granuloma inguinale**
Donovanosis

✓4th **A59 Trichomoniasis**
EXCLUDES 2   intestinal trichomoniasis (A07.8)

✓5th A59.0 **Urogenital trichomoniasis**

A59.00 **Urogenital trichomoniasis, unspecified**
Fluor (vaginalis) due to Trichomonas
Leukorrhea (vaginalis) due to Trichomonas

A59.01 **Trichomonal vulvovaginitis** ♀

A59.02 **Trichomonal prostatitis** ♂

A59.03 **Trichomonal cystitis and urethritis**

A59.09 **Other urogenital trichomoniasis**
Trichomonas cervicitis

A59.8 **Trichomoniasis of other sites**

A59.9 **Trichomoniasis, unspecified**

✓4th **A60 Anogenital herpesviral [herpes simplex] infections**

✓5th A60.0 **Herpesviral infection of genitalia and urogenital tract**

A60.00 **Herpesviral infection of urogenital system, unspecified**

A60.01 **Herpesviral infection of penis** ♂

A60.02 **Herpesviral infection of other male genital organs** ♂

A60.03 **Herpesviral cervicitis** ♀

EXCLUDES 1 Not coded here   *EXCLUDES 2* Not included here   N Newborn Age: 0   P Pediatric Age: 0-17   M Maternity Age: 12-55   A Adult Age: 15-124

A60.04   **Herpesviral vulvovaginitis** ♀
- Herpesviral [herpes simplex] ulceration
- Herpesviral [herpes simplex] vaginitis
- Herpesviral [herpes simplex] vulvitis

A60.09   **Herpesviral infection of other urogenital tract**

A60.1   **Herpesviral infection of perianal skin and rectum**

A60.9   **Anogenital herpesviral infection, unspecified**

✓4ᵗʰ **A63**   **Other predominantly sexually transmitted diseases, not elsewhere classified**
> EXCLUDES 2   *molluscum contagiosum (B08.1)*
> *papilloma of cervix (D26.0)*

A63.0   **Anogenital (venereal) warts**
- Anogenital warts due to (human) papillomavirus [HPV]
- Condyloma acuminatum

A63.8   **Other specified predominantly sexually transmitted diseases**

A64   **Unspecified sexually transmitted disease**

Other spirochetal diseases (A65-A69)

> EXCLUDES 2   *leptospirosis (A27.-)*
> *syphilis (A50-A53)*

A65   **Nonvenereal syphilis**
- Bejel   Njovera
- Endemic syphilis

✓4ᵗʰ **A66**   **Yaws**
> INCLUDES   bouba
> frambesia (tropica)
> pian

A66.0   **Initial lesions of yaws**
- Chancre of yaws
- Frambesia, initial or primary
- Initial frambesial ulcer
- Mother yaw

A66.1   **Multiple papillomata and wet crab yaws**
- Frambesioma
- Pianoma
- Plantar or palmar papilloma of yaws

A66.2   **Other early skin lesions of yaws**
- Cutaneous yaws, less than five years after infection
- Early yaws (cutaneous) (macular) (maculopapular) (micropapular) (papular)
- Frambeside of early yaws

A66.3   **Hyperkeratosis of yaws**
- Ghoul hand
- Hyperkeratosis, palmar or plantar (early) (late) due to yaws
- Worm-eaten soles

A66.4   **Gummata and ulcers of yaws**
- Gummatous frambeside
- Nodular late yaws (ulcerated)

A66.5   **Gangosa**
- Rhinopharyngitis mutilans

A66.6   **Bone and joint lesions of yaws**
- Yaws ganglion   Yaws hydrarthrosis
- Yaws goundou   Yaws osteitis
- Yaws gumma, bone   Yaws periostitis (hypertrophic)
- Yaws gummatous osteitis or periostitis

A66.7   **Other manifestations of yaws**
- Juxta-articular nodules of yaws
- Mucosal yaws

A66.8   **Latent yaws**
- Yaws without clinical manifestations, with positive serology

A66.9   **Yaws, unspecified**

✓4ᵗʰ **A67**   **Pinta [carate]**

A67.0   **Primary lesions of pinta**
- Chancre (primary) of pinta
- Papule (primary) of pinta

A67.1   **Intermediate lesions of pinta**
- Erythematous plaques of pinta
- Hyperchromic lesions of pinta
- Hyperkeratosis of pinta
- Pintids

A67.2   **Late lesions of pinta**
- Achromic skin lesions of pinta
- Cicatricial skin lesions of pinta
- Dyschromic skin lesions of pinta

A67.3   **Mixed lesions of pinta**
- Achromic with hyperchromic skin lesions of pinta [carate]

A67.9   **Pinta, unspecified**

✓4ᵗʰ **A68**   **Relapsing fevers**
> INCLUDES   recurrent fever
> EXCLUDES 2   *Lyme disease (A69.2-)*

A68.0   **Louse-borne relapsing fever**
- Relapsing fever due to Borrelia recurrentis

A68.1   **Tick-borne relapsing fever**
- Relapsing fever due to any Borrelia species other than Borrelia recurrentis

A68.9   **Relapsing fever, unspecified**

✓4ᵗʰ **A69**   **Other spirochetal infections**

A69.0   **Necrotizing ulcerative stomatitis**
- Cancrum oris
- Fusospirochetal gangrene
- Noma
- Stomatitis gangrenosa

A69.1   **Other Vincent's infections**
- Fusospirochetal pharyngitis
- Necrotizing ulcerative (acute) gingivitis
- Necrotizing ulcerative (acute) gingivostomatitis
- Spirochetal stomatitis
- Trench mouth
- Vincent's angina
- Vincent's gingivitis

✓5ᵗʰ **A69.2**   **Lyme disease**
- Erythema chronicum migrans due to Borrelia burgdorferi

     A69.20   **Lyme disease, unspecified**

     A69.21   **Meningitis due to Lyme disease**

     A69.22   **Other neurologic disorders in Lyme disease**
- Cranial neuritis
- Meningoencephalitis
- Polyneuropathy

     A69.23   **Arthritis due to Lyme disease**

     A69.29   **Other conditions associated with Lyme disease**
- Myopericarditis due to Lyme disease

A69.8   **Other specified spirochetal infections**

A69.9   **Spirochetal infection, unspecified**

Other diseases caused by chlamydiae (A70-A74)

> EXCLUDES 1   *sexually transmitted chlamydial diseases (A55-A56)*

A70   **Chlamydia psittaci infections**
- Ornithosis
- Parrot fever
- Psittacosis

✓4ᵗʰ **A71**   **Trachoma**
> EXCLUDES 1   *sequelae of trachoma (B94.0)*

A71.0   **Initial stage of trachoma**
- Trachoma dubium

A71.1   **Active stage of trachoma**
- Granular conjunctivitis (trachomatous)
- Trachomatous follicular conjunctivitis
- Trachomatous pannus

A71.9   **Trachoma, unspecified**

✓4ᵗʰ **A74**   **Other diseases caused by chlamydiae**
> EXCLUDES 1   *neonatal chlamydial conjunctivitis (P39.1)*
> *neonatal chlamydial pneumonia (P23.1)*
> *Reiter's disease (M02.3-)*
> *sexually transmitted chlamydial diseases (A55-A56)*
> EXCLUDES 2   *chlamydial pneumonia (J16.0)*

A74.0   **Chlamydial conjunctivitis**
- Paratrachoma

✓5ᵗʰ **A74.8**   **Other chlamydial diseases**

     A74.81   **Chlamydial peritonitis**

     A74.89   **Other chlamydial diseases**

A74.9   **Chlamydial infection, unspecified**
- Chlamydiosis NOS

Rickettsioses (A75-A79)

✓4ᵗʰ **A75**   **Typhus fever**
> EXCLUDES 1   *rickettsiosis due to Ehrlichia sennetsu (A79.81)*

A75.0   **Epidemic louse-borne typhus fever due to Rickettsia prowazekii**
- Classical typhus (fever)
- Epidemic (louse-borne) typhus

A75.1   **Recrudescent typhus [Brill's disease]**
- Brill-Zinsser disease

✓ Additional Character Required   ✓x7ᵗʰ Placeholder Alert   Unspecified Dx   Other Specified Dx   Manifestation   ▶◀ Revised Text   ● New Code   ▲ Revised Code Title

ICD-10-CM 2016   **433**

A75.2   Typhus fever due to Rickettsia typhi
    Murine (flea-borne) typhus

A75.3   Typhus fever due to Rickettsia tsutsugamushi
    Scrub (mite-borne) typhus
    Tsutsugamushi fever

A75.9   Typhus fever, unspecified
    Typhus (fever) NOS

✓4th A77   Spotted fever [tick-borne rickettsioses]

A77.0   Spotted fever due to Rickettsia rickettsii
    Rocky Mountain spotted fever
    Sao Paulo fever

A77.1   Spotted fever due to Rickettsia conorii
    African tick typhus
    Boutonneuse fever
    India tick typhus
    Kenya tick typhus
    Marseilles fever
    Mediterranean tick fever

A77.2   Spotted fever due to Rickettsia siberica
    North Asian tick fever
    Siberian tick typhus

A77.3   Spotted fever due to Rickettsia australis
    Queensland tick typhus

✓5th **A77.4   Ehrlichiosis**
    EXCLUDES 1   *Rickettsiosis due to Ehrlichia sennetsu (A79.81)*

    A77.40   Ehrlichiosis, unspecified

    A77.41   Ehrlichiosis chafeensis [E. chafeensis]

    A77.49   Other ehrlichiosis

A77.8   Other spotted fevers

A77.9   Spotted fever, unspecified
    Tick-borne typhus NOS

A78   Q fever
    Infection due to Coxiella burnetii
    Nine Mile fever
    Quadrilateral fever

✓4th A79   Other rickettsioses

A79.0   Trench fever
    Quintan fever
    Wolhynian fever

A79.1   Rickettsialpox due to Rickettsia akari
    Kew Garden fever
    Vesicular rickettsiosis

✓5th **A79.8   Other specified rickettsioses**

    A79.81   Rickettsiosis due to Ehrlichia sennetsu

    A79.89   Other specified rickettsioses

A79.9   Rickettsiosis, unspecified
    Rickettsial infection NOS

Viral and prion infections of the central nervous system (A80-A89)

    EXCLUDES 1   *postpolio syndrome (G14)*
            sequelae of poliomyelitis (B91)
            sequelae of viral encephalitis (B94.1)

✓4th A80   Acute poliomyelitis

A80.0   Acute paralytic poliomyelitis, vaccine-associated

A80.1   Acute paralytic poliomyelitis, wild virus, imported

A80.2   Acute paralytic poliomyelitis, wild virus, indigenous

✓5th **A80.3   Acute paralytic poliomyelitis, other and unspecified**

    A80.30   Acute paralytic poliomyelitis, unspecified

    A80.39   Other acute paralytic poliomyelitis

A80.4   Acute nonparalytic poliomyelitis

A80.9   Acute poliomyelitis, unspecified

✓4th A81   Atypical virus infections of central nervous system
    INCLUDES   diseases of the central nervous system caused by prions
    Use additional code to identify:
    dementia with behavioral disturbance (F02.81)
    dementia without behavioral disturbance (F02.80)

✓5th **A81.0   Creutzfeldt-Jakob disease**

    A81.00   Creutzfeldt-Jakob disease, unspecified
       Jakob-Creutzfeldt disease, unspecified

    A81.01   Variant Creutzfeldt-Jakob disease
       vCJD

    A81.09   Other Creutzfeldt-Jakob disease
       CJD
       Familial Creutzfeldt-Jakob disease
       Iatrogenic Creutzfeldt-Jakob disease
       Sporadic Creutzfeldt-Jakob disease
       Subacute spongiform encephalopathy (with dementia)

A81.1   Subacute sclerosing panencephalitis
    Dawson's inclusion body encephalitis
    Van Bogaert's sclerosing leukoencephalopathy

A81.2   Progressive multifocal leukoencephalopathy
    Multifocal leukoencephalopathy NOS

✓5th **A81.8   Other atypical virus infections of central nervous system**

    A81.81   Kuru

    A81.82   Gerstmann-Sträussler-Scheinker syndrome
       GSS syndrome

    A81.83   Fatal familial insomnia
       FFI

    A81.89   Other atypical virus infections of central nervous system

A81.9   Atypical virus infection of central nervous system, unspecified
    Prion diseases of the central nervous system NOS

✓4th A82   Rabies

A82.0   Sylvatic rabies

A82.1   Urban rabies

A82.9   Rabies, unspecified

✓4th A83   Mosquito-borne viral encephalitis
    INCLUDES   mosquito-borne viral meningoencephalitis
    EXCLUDES 2   *Venezuelan equine encephalitis (A92.2)*
            West Nile fever (A92.3-)
            West Nile virus (A92.3-)

A83.0   Japanese encephalitis

A83.1   Western equine encephalitis

A83.2   Eastern equine encephalitis

A83.3   St Louis encephalitis

A83.4   Australian encephalitis
    Kunjin virus disease

A83.5   California encephalitis
    California meningoencephalitis
    La Crosse encephalitis

A83.6   Rocio virus disease

A83.8   Other mosquito-borne viral encephalitis

A83.9   Mosquito-borne viral encephalitis, unspecified

✓4th A84   Tick-borne viral encephalitis
    INCLUDES   tick-borne viral meningoencephalitis

A84.0   Far Eastern tick-borne encephalitis [Russian spring-summer encephalitis]

A84.1   Central European tick-borne encephalitis

A84.8   Other tick-borne viral encephalitis
    Louping ill
    Powassan virus disease

A84.9   Tick-borne viral encephalitis, unspecified

✓4th A85   Other viral encephalitis, not elsewhere classified
    INCLUDES   specified viral encephalomyelitis NEC
            specified viral meningoencephalitis NEC
    EXCLUDES 1   *benign myalgic encephalomyelitis (G93.3)*
            encephalitis due to cytomegalovirus (B25.8)
            encephalitis due to herpesvirus NEC (B10.0-)
            encephalitis due to herpesvirus [herpes simplex] (B00.4)
            encephalitis due to measles virus (B05.0)
            encephalitis due to mumps virus (B26.2)
            encephalitis due to poliomyelitis virus (A80.-)
            encephalitis due to zoster (B02.0)
            lymphocytic choriomeningitis (A87.2)

A85.0   Enteroviral encephalitis
    Enteroviral encephalomyelitis

A85.1   Adenoviral encephalitis
    Adenoviral meningoencephalitis

A85.2   Arthropod-borne viral encephalitis, unspecified
    EXCLUDES 1   *West nile virus with encephalitis (A92.31)*

A85.8   Other specified viral encephalitis
    Encephalitis lethargica
    Von Economo-Cruchet disease

EXCLUDES 1   Not coded here   EXCLUDES 2   Not included here   N Newborn Age: 0   P Pediatric Age: 0-17   M Maternity Age: 12-55   A Adult Age: 15-124

434   ICD-10-CM 2016

A86   Unspecified viral encephalitis
     Viral encephalomyelitis NOS
     Viral meningoencephalitis NOS

✓4ᵗʰ **A87   Viral meningitis**
     EXCLUDES 1   *meningitis due to herpesvirus [herpes simplex] (B00.3)*
           meningitis due to measles virus (B05.1)
           meningitis due to mumps virus (B26.1)
           meningitis due to poliomyelitis virus (A80.-)
           meningitis due to zoster (B02.1)

     A87.0   Enteroviral meningitis
          Coxsackievirus meningitis
          Echovirus meningitis

     A87.1   Adenoviral meningitis

     A87.2   Lymphocytic choriomeningitis
          Lymphocytic meningoencephalitis

     A87.8   Other viral meningitis
     A87.9   Viral meningitis, unspecified

✓4ᵗʰ **A88   Other viral infections of central nervous system, not elsewhere classified**
     EXCLUDES 1   *viral encephalitis NOS (A86)*
           viral meningitis NOS (A87.9)

     A88.0   Enteroviral exanthematous fever [Boston exanthem]
     A88.1   Epidemic vertigo
     A88.8   Other specified viral infections of central nervous system

A89   Unspecified viral infection of central nervous system

Arthropod-borne viral fevers and viral hemorrhagic fevers (A90-A99)

A90   Dengue fever [classical dengue]
     EXCLUDES 1   *dengue hemorrhagic fever (A91)*

A91   Dengue hemorrhagic fever

✓4ᵗʰ **A92   Other mosquito-borne viral fevers**
     EXCLUDES 1   *Ross River disease (B33.1)*

     A92.0   Chikungunya virus disease
          Chikungunya (hemorrhagic) fever

     A92.1   O'nyong-nyong fever

     A92.2   Venezuelan equine fever
          Venezuelan equine encephalitis
          Venezuelan equine encephalomyelitis virus disease

     ✓5ᵗʰ **A92.3   West Nile virus infection**
          West Nile fever

         A92.30   West Nile virus infection, unspecified
              West Nile fever NOS
              West Nile fever without complications
              West Nile virus NOS

         A92.31   West Nile virus infection with encephalitis
              West Nile encephalitis
              West Nile encephalomyelitis

         A92.32   West Nile virus infection with other neurologic manifestation
              Use additional code to specify the neurologic manifestation

         A92.39   West Nile virus infection with other complications
              Use additional code to specify the other conditions

     A92.4   Rift Valley fever
     A92.8   Other specified mosquito-borne viral fevers
     A92.9   Mosquito-borne viral fever, unspecified

✓4ᵗʰ **A93   Other arthropod-borne viral fevers, not elsewhere classified**

     A93.0   Oropouche virus disease
          Oropouche fever

     A93.1   Sandfly fever
          Pappataci fever
          Phlebotomus fever

     A93.2   Colorado tick fever

     A93.8   Other specified arthropod-borne viral fevers
          Piry virus disease
          Vesicular stomatitis virus disease [Indiana fever]

A94   Unspecified arthropod-borne viral fever
     Arboviral fever NOS
     Arbovirus infection NOS

✓4ᵗʰ **A95   Yellow fever**
     A95.0   Sylvatic yellow fever
          Jungle yellow fever
     A95.1   Urban yellow fever

     A95.9   Yellow fever, unspecified

✓4ᵗʰ **A96   Arenaviral hemorrhagic fever**
     A96.0   Junin hemorrhagic fever
          Argentinian hemorrhagic fever

     A96.1   Machupo hemorrhagic fever
          Bolivian hemorrhagic fever

     A96.2   Lassa fever
     A96.8   Other arenaviral hemorrhagic fevers
     A96.9   Arenaviral hemorrhagic fever, unspecified

✓4ᵗʰ **A98   Other viral hemorrhagic fevers, not elsewhere classified**
     EXCLUDES 1   *chikungunya hemorrhagic fever (A92.0)*
           dengue hemorrhagic fever (A91)

     A98.0   Crimean-Congo hemorrhagic fever
          Central Asian hemorrhagic fever

     A98.1   Omsk hemorrhagic fever
     A98.2   Kyasanur Forest disease
     A98.3   Marburg virus disease
     A98.4   Ebola virus disease
     A98.5   Hemorrhagic fever with renal syndrome
          Epidemic hemorrhagic fever
          Korean hemorrhagic fever
          Russian hemorrhagic fever
          Hantaan virus disease
          Hantavirus disease with renal manifestations
          Nephropathia epidemica
          Songo fever
          EXCLUDES 1   *hantavirus (cardio)-pulmonary syndrome (B33.4)*

     A98.8   Other specified viral hemorrhagic fevers

A99   Unspecified viral hemorrhagic fever

Viral infections characterized by skin and mucous membrane lesions (B00-B09)

✓4ᵗʰ **B00   Herpesviral [herpes simplex] infections**
     EXCLUDES 1   *congenital herpesviral infections (P35.2)*
     EXCLUDES 2   *anogenital herpesviral infection (A60.-)*
           gammaherpesviral mononucleosis (B27.0-)
           herpangina (B08.5)

     B00.0   Eczema herpeticum
          Kaposi's varicelliform eruption

     B00.1   Herpesviral vesicular dermatitis
          Herpes simplex facialis
          Herpes simplex labialis
          Herpes simplex otitis externa
          Vesicular dermatitis of ear
          Vesicular dermatitis of lip

     B00.2   Herpesviral gingivostomatitis and pharyngotonsillitis
          Herpesviral pharyngitis

     B00.3   Herpesviral meningitis

     B00.4   Herpesviral encephalitis
          Herpesviral meningoencephalitis
          Simian B disease
          EXCLUDES 1   *herpesviral encephalitis due to herpesvirus 6 and 7 (B10.01, B10.09)*
           non-simplex herpesviral encephalitis (B10.0-)

     ✓5ᵗʰ **B00.5   Herpesviral ocular disease**

         B00.50   Herpesviral ocular disease, unspecified

         B00.51   Herpesviral iridocyclitis
              Herpesviral iritis
              Herpesviral uveitis, anterior

         B00.52   Herpesviral keratitis
              Herpesviral keratoconjunctivitis

         B00.53   Herpesviral conjunctivitis

         B00.59   Other herpesviral disease of eye
              Herpesviral dermatitis of eyelid

     B00.7   Disseminated herpesviral disease
          Herpesviral sepsis

     ✓5ᵗʰ **B00.8   Other forms of herpesviral infections**

         B00.81   Herpesviral hepatitis
         B00.82   Herpes simplex myelitis
         B00.89   Other herpesviral infection
              Herpesviral whitlow

     B00.9   Herpesviral infection, unspecified
          Herpes simplex infection NOS

✓ Additional Character Required   ✓×7ᵗʰ Placeholder Alert   Unspecified Dx   Other Specified Dx   Manifestation   ▶◀ Revised Text   ● New Code   ▲ Revised Code Title

✓4ᵗʰ B01 Varicella [chickenpox]
- **B01.0 Varicella** meningitis
- **✓5ᵗʰ B01.1 Varicella** encephalitis, myelitis and encephalomyelitis
  - Postchickenpox encephalitis, myelitis and encephalomyelitis
  - **B01.11 Varicella** encephalitis and encephalomyelitis
    - Postchickenpox encephalitis and encephalomyelitis
  - **B01.12 Varicella** myelitis
    - Postchickenpox myelitis
- **B01.2 Varicella** pneumonia
- **✓5ᵗʰ B01.8 Varicella with** other complications
  - **B01.81 Varicella** keratitis
  - **B01.89 Other varicella complications**
- **B01.9 Varicella** without complication
  - Varicella NOS

✓4ᵗʰ B02 Zoster [herpes zoster]
> INCLUDES   shingles
>   zona
- **B02.0 Zoster** encephalitis
  - Zoster meningoencephalitis
- **B02.1 Zoster** meningitis
- **✓5ᵗʰ B02.2 Zoster with** other nervous system **involvement**
  - **B02.21 Postherpetic** geniculate ganglionitis
  - **B02.22 Postherpetic** trigeminal neuralgia
  - **B02.23 Postherpetic** polyneuropathy
  - **B02.24 Postherpetic** myelitis
    - Herpes zoster myelitis
  - **B02.29 Other postherpetic nervous system involvement**
    - Postherpetic radiculopathy
- **✓5ᵗʰ B02.3 Zoster** ocular disease
  - **B02.30 Zoster ocular disease, unspecified**
  - **B02.31 Zoster** conjunctivitis
  - **B02.32 Zoster** iridocyclitis
  - **B02.33 Zoster** keratitis
    - Herpes zoster keratoconjunctivitis
  - **B02.34 Zoster** scleritis
  - **B02.39 Other herpes zoster eye disease**
    - Zoster blepharitis
- **B02.7 Disseminated zoster**
- **B02.8 Zoster with** other complications
  - Herpes zoster otitis externa
- **B02.9 Zoster without complications**
  - Zoster NOS

B03 Smallpox
> NOTE
> In 1980 the 33rd World Health Assembly declared that smallpox had been eradicated.
> The classification is maintained for surveillance purposes.

B04 Monkeypox

✓4ᵗʰ B05 Measles
> INCLUDES   morbilli
> EXCLUDES 1   subacute sclerosing panencephalitis (A81.1)
- **B05.0 Measles complicated by** encephalitis
  - Postmeasles encephalitis
- **B05.1 Measles complicated by** meningitis
  - Postmeasles meningitis
- **B05.2 Measles complicated by** pneumonia
  - Postmeasles pneumonia
- **B05.3 Measles complicated by** otitis media
  - Postmeasles otitis media
- **B05.4 Measles with** intestinal **complications**
- **✓5ᵗʰ B05.8 Measles with** other complications
  - **B05.81 Measles** keratitis and keratoconjunctivitis
  - **B05.89 Other measles complications**
- **B05.9 Measles** without complication
  - Measles NOS

✓4ᵗʰ B06 Rubella [German measles]
> EXCLUDES 1   congenital rubella (P35.0)
- **✓5ᵗʰ B06.0 Rubella with** neurological complications
  - **B06.00 Rubella with neurological complication, unspecified**
  - **B06.01 Rubella** encephalitis
    - Rubella meningoencephalitis
  - **B06.02 Rubella** meningitis
  - **B06.09 Other neurological complications of rubella**

✓5ᵗʰ B06.8 Rubella with other complications
- **B06.81 Rubella** pneumonia
- **B06.82 Rubella** arthritis
- **B06.89 Other rubella complications**
B06.9 Rubella without complication
- Rubella NOS

✓4ᵗʰ B07 Viral warts
> INCLUDES   verruca simplex
>   verruca vulgaris
>   viral warts due to human papillomavirus
> EXCLUDES 2   anogenital (venereal) warts (A63.0)
>   papilloma of bladder (D41.4)
>   papilloma of cervix (D26.0)
>   papilloma larynx (D14.1)
- **B07.0 Plantar wart**
  - Verruca plantaris
- **B07.8 Other viral warts**
  - Common wart
  - Flat wart
  - Verruca plana
- **B07.9 Viral wart, unspecified**

✓4ᵗʰ B08 Other viral infections characterized by skin and mucous membrane lesions, not elsewhere classified
> EXCLUDES 1   vesicular stomatitis virus disease (A93.8)
- **✓5ᵗʰ B08.0 Other orthopoxvirus infections**
  > EXCLUDES 2   monkeypox (B04)
  - **✓6ᵗʰ B08.01 Cowpox and vaccinia not from vaccine**
    - **B08.010 Cowpox**
    - **B08.011 Vaccinia not from vaccine**
      > EXCLUDES 1   vaccinia (from vaccination) (generalized) (T88.1)
  - **B08.02 Orf virus disease**
    - Contagious pustular dermatitis
    - Ecthyma contagiosum
  - **B08.03 Pseudocowpox [milker's node]**
  - **B08.04 Paravaccinia, unspecified**
  - **B08.09 Other orthopoxvirus infections**
    - Orthopoxvirus infection NOS
- **B08.1 Molluscum contagiosum**
- **✓5ᵗʰ B08.2 Exanthema subitum [sixth disease]**
  - Roseola infantum
  - **B08.20 Exanthema subitum [sixth disease], unspecified** Ⓟ
    - Roseola infantum, unspecified
  - **B08.21 Exanthema subitum [sixth disease] due to human herpesvirus 6** Ⓟ
    - Roseola infantum due to human herpesvirus 6
  - **B08.22 Exanthema subitum [sixth disease] due to human herpesvirus 7** Ⓟ
    - Roseola infantum due to human herpesvirus 7
- **B08.3 Erythema infectiosum [fifth disease]**
- **B08.4 Enteroviral vesicular stomatitis with exanthem**
  - Hand, foot and mouth disease
- **B08.5 Enteroviral vesicular pharyngitis**
  - Herpangina
- **✓5ᵗʰ B08.6 Parapoxvirus infections**
  - **B08.60 Parapoxvirus infection, unspecified**
  - **B08.61 Bovine stomatitis**
  - **B08.62 Sealpox**
  - **B08.69 Other parapoxvirus infections**
- **✓5ᵗʰ B08.7 Yatapoxvirus infections**
  - **B08.70 Yatapoxvirus infection, unspecified**
  - **B08.71 Tanapox virus disease**
  - **B08.72 Yaba pox virus disease**
    - Yaba monkey tumor disease
  - **B08.79 Other yatapoxvirus infections**
- **B08.8 Other specified viral infections characterized by skin and mucous membrane lesions**
  - Enteroviral lymphonodular pharyngitis
  - Foot-and-mouth disease
  - Poxvirus NEC

B09 Unspecified viral infection characterized by skin and mucous membrane lesions
- Viral enanthema NOS
- Viral exanthema NOS

| EXCLUDES 1 Not coded here | EXCLUDES 2 Not included here | Ⓝ Newborn Age: 0 | Ⓟ Pediatric Age: 0-17 | Ⓜ Maternity Age: 12-55 | Ⓐ Adult Age: 15-124 |

Other human herpesviruses (B10)

☑4ᵗʰ B10 Other human herpesviruses

  EXCLUDES 2   cytomegalovirus (B25.9)
               Epstein-Barr virus (B27.0-)
               herpes NOS (B00.9)
               herpes simplex (B00.-)
               herpes zoster (B02.-)
               human herpesvirus NOS (B00.-)
               human herpesvirus 1 and 2 (B00.-)
               human herpesvirus 3 (B01.-, B02.-)
               human herpesvirus 4 (B27.0-)
               human herpesvirus (B25.-)
               varicella (B01.-)
               zoster (B02.-)

  ☑5ᵗʰ B10.0 Other human herpesvirus encephalitis

    EXCLUDES 2   herpes encephalitis NOS (B00.4)
                 herpes simplex encephalitis (B00.4)
                 human herpesvirus encephalitis (B00.4)
                 simian B herpes virus encephalitis (B00.4)

    B10.01 Human herpesvirus 6 encephalitis

    B10.09 Other human herpesvirus encephalitis
          Human herpesvirus 7 encephalitis

  ☑5ᵗʰ B10.8 Other human herpesvirus infection

    B10.81 Human herpesvirus 6 infection

    B10.82 Human herpesvirus 7 infection

    B10.89 Other human herpesvirus infection
          Human herpesvirus 8 infection
          Kaposi's sarcoma-associated herpesvirus infection

Viral hepatitis (B15-B19)

  EXCLUDES 1   sequelae of viral hepatitis (B94.2)
  EXCLUDES 2   cytomegaloviral hepatitis (B25.1)
               herpesviral [herpes simplex] hepatitis (B00.81)

☑4ᵗʰ B15 Acute hepatitis A

  B15.0 Hepatitis A with hepatic coma

  B15.9 Hepatitis A without hepatic coma
     Hepatitis A (acute)(viral) NOS

☑4ᵗʰ B16 Acute hepatitis B

  B16.0 Acute hepatitis B with delta-agent with hepatic coma

  B16.1 Acute hepatitis B with delta-agent without hepatic coma

  B16.2 Acute hepatitis B without delta-agent with hepatic coma

  B16.9 Acute hepatitis B without delta-agent and without hepatic coma
     Hepatitis B (acute) (viral) NOS

☑4ᵗʰ B17 Other acute viral hepatitis

  B17.0 Acute delta-(super) infection of hepatitis B carrier

  ☑5ᵗʰ B17.1 Acute hepatitis C

    B17.10 Acute hepatitis C without hepatic coma
          Acute hepatitis C NOS

    B17.11 Acute hepatitis C with hepatic coma

  B17.2 Acute hepatitis E

  B17.8 Other specified acute viral hepatitis
     Hepatitis non-A non-B (acute) (viral) NEC

  B17.9 Acute viral hepatitis, unspecified
     Acute viral hepatitis NOS

☑4ᵗʰ B18 Chronic viral hepatitis

  B18.0 Chronic viral hepatitis B with delta-agent

  B18.1 Chronic viral hepatitis B without delta-agent
     Chronic (viral) hepatitis B

  B18.2 Chronic viral hepatitis C

  B18.8 Other chronic viral hepatitis

  B18.9 Chronic viral hepatitis, unspecified

☑4ᵗʰ B19 Unspecified viral hepatitis

  B19.0 Unspecified viral hepatitis with hepatic coma

  ☑5ᵗʰ B19.1 Unspecified viral hepatitis B

    B19.10 Unspecified viral hepatitis B without hepatic coma
          Unspecified viral hepatitis B NOS

    B19.11 Unspecified viral hepatitis B with hepatic coma

  ☑5ᵗʰ B19.2 Unspecified viral hepatitis C

    B19.20 Unspecified viral hepatitis C without hepatic coma
          Viral hepatitis C NOS

    B19.21 Unspecified viral hepatitis C with hepatic coma

  B19.9 Unspecified viral hepatitis without hepatic coma
     Viral hepatitis NOS

Human immunodeficiency virus [HIV] disease (B20)

B20 Human immunodeficiency virus [HIV] disease

  INCLUDES   acquired immune deficiency syndrome [AIDS]
              AIDS-related complex [ARC]
              HIV infection, symptomatic

  Code first human immunodeficiency virus [HIV] disease complicating pregnancy, childbirth and the puerperium, if applicable (O98.7-)

  Use additional code(s) to identify all manifestations of HIV infection

  EXCLUDES 1   asymptomatic human immunodeficiency virus [HIV] infection status (Z21)
               exposure to HIV virus (Z20.6)
               inconclusive serologic evidence of HIV (R75)

Other viral diseases (B25-B34)

☑4ᵗʰ B25 Cytomegaloviral disease

  EXCLUDES 1   congenital cytomegalovirus infection (P35.1)
               cytomegaloviral mononucleosis (B27.1-)

  B25.0 Cytomegaloviral pneumonitis

  B25.1 Cytomegaloviral hepatitis

  B25.2 Cytomegaloviral pancreatitis

  B25.8 Other cytomegaloviral diseases
     Cytomegaloviral encephalitis

  B25.9 Cytomegaloviral disease, unspecified

☑4ᵗʰ B26 Mumps

  INCLUDES   epidemic parotitis
              infectious parotitis

  B26.0 Mumps orchitis   ♂

  B26.1 Mumps meningitis

  B26.2 Mumps encephalitis

  B26.3 Mumps pancreatitis

  ☑5ᵗʰ B26.8 Mumps with other complications

    B26.81 Mumps hepatitis

    B26.82 Mumps myocarditis

    B26.83 Mumps nephritis

    B26.84 Mumps polyneuropathy

    B26.85 Mumps arthritis

    B26.89 Other mumps complications

  B26.9 Mumps without complication
     Mumps NOS
     Mumps parotitis NOS

☑4ᵗʰ B27 Infectious mononucleosis

  INCLUDES   glandular fever
              monocytic angina
              Pfeiffer's disease

  ☑5ᵗʰ B27.0 Gammaherpesviral mononucleosis
     Mononucleosis due to Epstein-Barr virus

    B27.00 Gammaherpesviral mononucleosis without complication

    B27.01 Gammaherpesviral mononucleosis with polyneuropathy

    B27.02 Gammaherpesviral mononucleosis with meningitis

    B27.09 Gammaherpesviral mononucleosis with other complications
          Hepatomegaly in gammaherpesviral mononucleosis

  ☑5ᵗʰ B27.1 Cytomegaloviral mononucleosis

    B27.10 Cytomegaloviral mononucleosis without complications

    B27.11 Cytomegaloviral mononucleosis with polyneuropathy

    B27.12 Cytomegaloviral mononucleosis with meningitis

    B27.19 Cytomegaloviral mononucleosis with other complication
          Hepatomegaly in cytomegaloviral mononucleosis

  ☑5ᵗʰ B27.8 Other infectious mononucleosis

    B27.80 Other infectious mononucleosis without complication

    B27.81 Other infectious mononucleosis with polyneuropathy

    B27.82 Other infectious mononucleosis with meningitis

    B27.89 Other infectious mononucleosis with other complication
          Hepatomegaly in other infectious mononucleosis

☑ Additional Character Required   ☑x7ᵗʰ Placeholder Alert   Unspecified Dx   Other Specified Dx   Manifestation   ▶◀ Revised Text   ● New Code   ▲ Revised Code Title

✓5th **B27.9** Infectious mononucleosis, unspecified

    B27.90 **Infectious mononucleosis, unspecified** without complication

    B27.91 **Infectious mononucleosis, unspecified** with polyneuropathy

    B27.92 **Infectious mononucleosis, unspecified** with meningitis

    B27.99 **Infectious mononucleosis, unspecified with other complication**
        Hepatomegaly in unspecified infectious mononucleosis

✓4th **B30** **Viral conjunctivitis**
    EXCLUDES 1 *herpesviral [herpes simplex] ocular disease (B00.5)*
        ocular zoster (B02.3)

    B30.0 **Keratoconjunctivitis** due to **adenovirus**
        Epidemic keratoconjunctivitis
        Shipyard eye

    B30.1 **Conjunctivitis** due to **adenovirus**
        Acute adenoviral follicular conjunctivitis
        Swimming-pool conjunctivitis

    B30.2 **Viral pharyngoconjunctivitis**

    B30.3 **Acute epidemic hemorrhagic conjunctivitis (enteroviral)**
        Conjunctivitis due to coxsackievirus 24
        Conjunctivitis due to enterovirus 70
        Hemorrhagic conjunctivitis (acute)(epidemic)

    B30.8 **Other viral conjunctivitis**
        Newcastle conjunctivitis

    B30.9 **Viral conjunctivitis, unspecified**

✓4th **B33** **Other viral diseases, not elsewhere classified**

    B33.0 **Epidemic myalgia**
        Bornholm disease

    B33.1 **Ross River disease**
        Epidemic polyarthritis and exanthema
        Ross River fever

    ✓5th **B33.2** **Viral carditis**
        Coxsackie (virus) carditis

        B33.20 **Viral carditis, unspecified**

        B33.21 **Viral endocarditis**

        B33.22 **Viral myocarditis**

        B33.23 **Viral pericarditis**

        B33.24 **Viral cardiomyopathy**

    B33.3 **Retrovirus infections, not elsewhere classified**
        Retrovirus infection NOS

    B33.4 **Hantavirus (cardio)-pulmonary syndrome [HPS] [HCPS]**
        Hantavirus disease with pulmonary manifestations
        Sin nombre virus disease
        Use additional code to identify any associated acute kidney failure (N17.9)
        EXCLUDES 1 *hantavirus disease with renal manifestations (A98.5)*
            hemorrhagic fever with renal manifestations (A98.5)

    B33.8 **Other specified viral diseases**
        EXCLUDES 1 *anogenital human papillomavirus infection (A63.0)*
            viral warts due to human papillomavirus infection (B07)

✓4th **B34** **Viral infection of unspecified site**
    EXCLUDES 1 *anogenital human papillomavirus infection (A63.0)*
        cytomegaloviral disease NOS (B25.9)
        herpesvirus [herpes simplex] infection NOS (B00.9)
        retrovirus infection NOS (B33.3)
        viral agents as the cause of diseases classified elsewhere (B97.-)
        viral warts due to human papillomavirus infection (B07)

    B34.0 **Adenovirus infection, unspecified**

    B34.1 **Enterovirus infection, unspecified**
        Coxsackievirus infection NOS
        Echovirus infection NOS

    B34.2 **Coronavirus infection, unspecified**
        EXCLUDES 1 *pneumonia due to SARS-associated coronavirus (J12.81)*

    B34.3 **Parvovirus infection, unspecified**

    B34.4 **Papovavirus infection, unspecified**

    B34.8 **Other viral infections of unspecified site**

    B34.9 **Viral infection, unspecified**
        Viremia NOS

Mycoses (B35-B49)

EXCLUDES 2 *hypersensitivity pneumonitis due to organic dust (J67.-)*
    mycosis fungoides (C84.0-)

✓4th **B35** **Dermatophytosis**
    INCLUDES favus
        infections due to species of Epidermophyton, Micro-sporum and Trichophyton
        tinea, any type except those in B36-

    B35.0 **Tinea barbae and tinea capitis**
        Beard ringworm
        Kerion
        Scalp ringworm
        Sycosis, mycotic

    B35.1 **Tinea unguium**
        Dermatophytic onychia
        Dermatophytosis of nail
        Onychomycosis
        Ringworm of nails

    B35.2 **Tinea manuum**
        Dermatophytosis of hand
        Hand ringworm

    B35.3 **Tinea pedis**
        Athlete's foot
        Dermatophytosis of foot
        Foot ringworm

    B35.4 **Tinea corporis**
        Ringworm of the body

    B35.5 **Tinea imbricata**
        Tokelau

    B35.6 **Tinea cruris**
        Dhobi itch
        Groin ringworm
        Jock itch

    B35.8 **Other dermatophytoses**
        Disseminated dermatophytosis
        Granulomatous dermatophytosis

    B35.9 **Dermatophytosis, unspecified**
        Ringworm NOS

✓4th **B36** **Other superficial mycoses**

    B36.0 **Pityriasis versicolor**
        Tinea flava
        Tinea versicolor

    B36.1 **Tinea nigra**
        Keratomycosis nigricans palmaris
        Microsporosis nigra
        Pityriasis nigra

    B36.2 **White piedra**
        Tinea blanca

    B36.3 **Black piedra**

    B36.8 **Other specified superficial mycoses**

    B36.9 **Superficial mycosis, unspecified**

✓4th **B37** **Candidiasis**
    INCLUDES candidosis
        moniliasis
    EXCLUDES 1 *neonatal candidiasis (P37.5)*

    B37.0 **Candidal stomatitis**
        Oral thrush

    B37.1 **Pulmonary candidiasis**
        Candidal bronchitis
        Candidal pneumonia

    B37.2 **Candidiasis of skin and nail**
        Candidal onychia
        Candidal paronychia
        EXCLUDES 2 *diaper dermatitis (L22)*

    B37.3 **Candidiasis of vulva and vagina** ♀
        Candidal vulvovaginitis
        Monilial vulvovaginitis
        Vaginal thrush

    ✓5th **B37.4** **Candidiasis of other urogenital sites**

        B37.41 **Candidal cystitis and urethritis**

        B37.42 **Candidal balanitis**

        B37.49 **Other urogenital candidiasis**
            Candidal pyelonephritis

    B37.5 **Candidal meningitis**

    B37.6 **Candidal endocarditis**

EXCLUDES 1 Not coded here   **EXCLUDES 2** Not included here   N Newborn Age: 0   P Pediatric Age: 0-17   M Maternity Age: 12-55   A Adult Age: 15-124

438   ICD-10-CM 2016

B37.7   **Candidal** sepsis
  Disseminated candidiasis
  Systemic candidiasis
  AHA: 2014, 4Q, 46

✓5ᵗʰ **B37.8**   **Candidiasis of** other sites

     B37.81   **Candidal** esophagitis

     B37.82   **Candidal** enteritis
  Candidal proctitis

     B37.83   **Candidal** cheilitis

     B37.84   **Candidal** otitis externa

     B37.89   **Other sites of candidiasis**
  Candidal osteomyelitis

B37.9   **Candidiasis, unspecified**
  Thrush NOS

✓4ᵗʰ **B38**   **Coccidioidomycosis**

     B38.0   Acute pulmonary **coccidioidomycosis**

     B38.1   Chronic pulmonary **coccidioidomycosis**

     B38.2   **Pulmonary coccidioidomycosis, unspecified**

     B38.3   Cutaneous **coccidioidomycosis**

     B38.4   **Coccidioidomycosis** meningitis

     B38.7   Disseminated **coccidioidomycosis**
  Generalized coccidioidomycosis

✓5ᵗʰ **B38.8**   Other forms of **coccidioidomycosis**

     B38.81   Prostatic **coccidioidomycosis**   ♂

     B38.89   **Other forms of coccidioidomycosis**

     B38.9   **Coccidioidomycosis, unspecified**

✓4ᵗʰ **B39**   **Histoplasmosis**
  Code first associated AIDS (B20)
  Use additional code for any associated manifestations, such as:
    endocarditis (I39)
    meningitis (G02)
    pericarditis (I32)
    retinititis (H32)

     B39.0   Acute pulmonary **histoplasmosis capsulati**

     B39.1   Chronic pulmonary **histoplasmosis capsulati**

     B39.2   **Pulmonary histoplasmosis capsulati,** unspecified

     B39.3   Disseminated **histoplasmosis capsulati**
  Generalized histoplasmosis capsulati

     B39.4   **Histoplasmosis** capsulati, unspecified
  American histoplasmosis

     B39.5   **Histoplasmosis** duboisii
  African histoplasmosis

     B39.9   **Histoplasmosis, unspecified**

✓4ᵗʰ **B40**   **Blastomycosis**
  EXCLUDES 1   *Brazilian blastomycosis (B41.-)*
    keloidal blastomycosis (B48.0)

     B40.0   Acute pulmonary **blastomycosis**

     B40.1   Chronic pulmonary **blastomycosis**

     B40.2   **Pulmonary blastomycosis, unspecified**

     B40.3   Cutaneous **blastomycosis**

     B40.7   Disseminated **blastomycosis**
  Generalized blastomycosis

✓5ᵗʰ **B40.8**   Other forms of **blastomycosis**

     B40.81   **Blastomycotic** meningoencephalitis
  Meningomyelitis due to blastomycosis

     B40.89   **Other forms of blastomycosis**

     B40.9   **Blastomycosis, unspecified**

✓4ᵗʰ **B41**   **Paracoccidioidomycosis**
  INCLUDES   Brazilian blastomycosis
    Lutz' disease

     B41.0   Pulmonary **paracoccidioidomycosis**

     B41.7   Disseminated **paracoccidioidomycosis**
  Generalized paracoccidioidomycosis

     B41.8   **Other forms of paracoccidioidomycosis**

     B41.9   **Paracoccidioidomycosis, unspecified**

✓4ᵗʰ **B42**   **Sporotrichosis**

     B42.0   Pulmonary **sporotrichosis**

     B42.1   Lymphocutaneous **sporotrichosis**

     B42.7   Disseminated **sporotrichosis**
  Generalized sporotrichosis

✓5ᵗʰ **B42.8**   Other forms of sporotrichosis

     B42.81   Cerebral **sporotrichosis**
  Meningitis due to sporotrichosis

     B42.82   **Sporotrichosis** arthritis

     B42.89   **Other forms of sporotrichosis**

     B42.9   **Sporotrichosis, unspecified**

✓4ᵗʰ **B43**   **Chromomycosis and pheomycotic abscess**

     B43.0   Cutaneous **chromomycosis**
  Dermatitis verrucosa

     B43.1   Pheomycotic **brain abscess**
  Cerebral chromomycosis

     B43.2   Subcutaneous **pheomycotic** abscess and cyst

     B43.8   **Other forms of chromomycosis**

     B43.9   **Chromomycosis, unspecified**

✓4ᵗʰ **B44**   **Aspergillosis**
  INCLUDES   aspergilloma

     B44.0   Invasive pulmonary **aspergillosis**

     B44.1   **Other pulmonary aspergillosis**

     B44.2   Tonsillar **aspergillosis**

     B44.7   Disseminated **aspergillosis**
  Generalized aspergillosis

✓5ᵗʰ **B44.8**   Other forms of aspergillosis

     B44.81   Allergic bronchopulmonary **aspergillosis**

     B44.89   **Other forms of aspergillosis**

     B44.9   **Aspergillosis, unspecified**

✓4ᵗʰ **B45**   **Cryptococcosis**

     B45.0   Pulmonary **cryptococcosis**

     B45.1   Cerebral **cryptococcosis**
  Cryptococcal meningitis
  Cryptococcosis meningocerebralis

     B45.2   Cutaneous **cryptococcosis**

     B45.3   Osseous **cryptococcosis**

     B45.7   Disseminated **cryptococcosis**
  Generalized cryptococcosis

     B45.8   **Other forms of cryptococcosis**

     B45.9   **Cryptococcosis, unspecified**

✓4ᵗʰ **B46**   **Zygomycosis**

     B46.0   Pulmonary **mucormycosis**

     B46.1   Rhinocerebral **mucormycosis**

     B46.2   Gastrointestinal **mucormycosis**

     B46.3   Cutaneous **mucormycosis**
  Subcutaneous mucormycosis

     B46.4   Disseminated **mucormycosis**
  Generalized mucormycosis

     B46.5   **Mucormycosis, unspecified**

     B46.8   **Other zygomycoses**
  Entomophthoromycosis

     B46.9   **Zygomycosis, unspecified**
  Phycomycosis NOS

✓4ᵗʰ **B47**   **Mycetoma**

     B47.0   Eumycetoma
  Madura foot, mycotic
  Maduromycosis

     B47.1   Actinomycetoma

     B47.9   **Mycetoma, unspecified**
  Madura foot NOS

✓4ᵗʰ **B48**   **Other mycoses, not elsewhere classified**

     B48.0   Lobomycosis
  Keloidal blastomycosis
  Lobo's disease

     B48.1   Rhinosporidiosis

     B48.2   Allescheriasis
  Infection due to Pseudallescheria boydii
  EXCLUDES 1   *eumycetoma (B47.0)*

     B48.3   Geotrichosis
  Geotrichum stomatitis

     B48.4   Penicillosis

✓ Additional Character Required   ✓7ᵗʰ Placeholder Alert   Unspecified Dx   Other Specified Dx   Manifestation   ▶◀ Revised Text   ● New Code   ▲ Revised Code Title

B48.8 **Other specified mycoses**
     Adiaspiromycosis
     Infection of tissue and organs by Alternaria
     Infection of tissue and organs by Drechslera
     Infection of tissue and organs by Fusarium
     Infection of tissue and organs by saprophytic fungi NEC
     AHA: 2014, 4Q, 46; 2014, 2Q, 13

B49 **Unspecified mycosis**
     Fungemia NOS

Protozoal diseases (B50-B64)

EXCLUDES 1   amebiasis (A06.-)
           other protozoal intestinal diseases (A07.-)

✓4ᵗʰ **B50** **Plasmodium falciparum malaria**
     INCLUDES   mixed infections of Plasmodium falciparum with any other
             Plasmodium species

     B50.0 **Plasmodium falciparum malaria with cerebral complications**
           Cerebral malaria NOS

     B50.8 **Other severe and complicated Plasmodium falciparum malaria**
           Severe or complicated Plasmodium falciparum malaria NOS

     B50.9 **Plasmodium falciparum malaria, unspecified**

✓4ᵗʰ **B51** **Plasmodium vivax malaria**
     INCLUDES   mixed infections of Plasmodium vivax with other
             Plasmodium species, except Plasmodium falciparum
     EXCLUDES 1   plasmodium vivax with Plasmodium falciparum (B50.-)

     B51.0 **Plasmodium vivax malaria with rupture of spleen**

     B51.8 **Plasmodium vivax malaria with other complications**

     B51.9 **Plasmodium vivax malaria without complication**
           Plasmodium vivax malaria NOS

✓4ᵗʰ **B52** **Plasmodium malariae malaria**
     INCLUDES   mixed infections of Plasmodium malariae with other
             Plasmodium species, except Plasmodium falciparum
             and Plasmodium vivax
     EXCLUDES 1   Plasmodium falciparum (B50.-)
                Plasmodium vivax (B51.-)

     B52.0 **Plasmodium malariae malaria with nephropathy**

     B52.8 **Plasmodium malariae malaria with other complications**

     B52.9 **Plasmodium malariae malaria without complication**
           Plasmodium malariae malaria NOS

✓4ᵗʰ **B53** **Other specified malaria**
     B53.0 **Plasmodium ovale malaria**
         EXCLUDES 1   Plasmodium ovale with Plasmodium falciparum (B50.-)
                Plasmodium ovale with Plasmodium malariae (B52.-)
                Plasmodium ovale with Plasmodium vivax (B51.-)

     B53.1 **Malaria due to simian plasmodia**
         EXCLUDES 1   Malaria due to simian plasmodia with Plasmodium
                falciparum (B50.-)
                Malaria due to simian plasmodia with Plasmodium
                malariae (B52.-)
                Malaria due to simian plasmodia with Plasmodium
                ovale (B53.0)
                Malaria due to simian plasmodia with Plasmodium
                vivax (B51.-)

     B53.8 **Other malaria, not elsewhere classified**

B54 **Unspecified malaria**

✓4ᵗʰ **B55** **Leishmaniasis**
     B55.0 **Visceral leishmaniasis**
           Kala-azar
           Post-kala-azar dermal leishmaniasis

     B55.1 **Cutaneous leishmaniasis**

     B55.2 **Mucocutaneous leishmaniasis**

     B55.9 **Leishmaniasis, unspecified**

✓4ᵗʰ **B56** **African trypanosomiasis**
     B56.0 **Gambiense trypanosomiasis**
           Infection due to Trypanosoma brucei gambiense
           West African sleeping sickness

     B56.1 **Rhodesiense trypanosomiasis**
           East African sleeping sickness
           Infection due to Trypanosoma brucei rhodesiense

     B56.9 **African trypanosomiasis, unspecified**
           Sleeping sickness NOS

✓4ᵗʰ **B57** **Chagas' disease**
     INCLUDES   American trypanosomiasis
             infection due to Trypanosoma cruzi

     B57.0 **Acute Chagas' disease with heart involvement**
           Acute Chagas' disease with myocarditis

     B57.1 **Acute Chagas' disease without heart involvement**
           Acute Chagas' disease NOS

     B57.2 **Chagas' disease (chronic) with heart involvement**
           American trypanosomiasis NOS
           Chagas' disease (chronic) NOS
           Chagas' disease (chronic) with myocarditis
           Trypanosomiasis NOS

✓5ᵗʰ   **B57.3** **Chagas' disease (chronic) with digestive system involvement**
         B57.30 **Chagas' disease with digestive system involvement, unspecified**
         B57.31 **Megaesophagus in Chagas' disease**
         B57.32 **Megacolon in Chagas' disease**
         B57.39 **Other digestive system involvement in Chagas' disease**

✓5ᵗʰ   **B57.4** **Chagas' disease (chronic) with nervous system involvement**
         B57.40 **Chagas' disease with nervous system involvement, unspecified**
         B57.41 **Meningitis in Chagas' disease**
         B57.42 **Meningoencephalitis in Chagas' disease**
         B57.49 **Other nervous system involvement in Chagas' disease**

     B57.5 **Chagas' disease (chronic) with other organ involvement**

✓4ᵗʰ **B58** **Toxoplasmosis**
     INCLUDES   infection due to Toxoplasma gondii
     EXCLUDES 1   congenital toxoplasmosis (P37.1)

✓5ᵗʰ   **B58.0** **Toxoplasma oculopathy**
         B58.00 **Toxoplasma oculopathy, unspecified**
         B58.01 **Toxoplasma chorioretinitis**
         B58.09 **Other toxoplasma oculopathy**
             Toxoplasma uveitis

     B58.1 **Toxoplasma hepatitis**

     B58.2 **Toxoplasma meningoencephalitis**

     B58.3 **Pulmonary toxoplasmosis**

✓5ᵗʰ   **B58.8** **Toxoplasmosis with other organ involvement**
         B58.81 **Toxoplasma myocarditis**
         B58.82 **Toxoplasma myositis**
         B58.83 **Toxoplasma tubulo-interstitial nephropathy**
             Toxoplasma pyelonephritis
         B58.89 **Toxoplasmosis with other organ involvement**

     B58.9 **Toxoplasmosis, unspecified**

B59 **Pneumocystosis**
     Pneumonia due to Pneumocystis carinii
     Pneumonia due to Pneumocystis jiroveci

✓4ᵗʰ **B60** **Other protozoal diseases, not elsewhere classified**
     EXCLUDES 1   cryptosporidiosis (A07.2)
                intestinal microsporidiosis (A07.8)
                isosporiasis (A07.3)

     B60.0 **Babesiosis**
           Piroplasmosis

✓5ᵗʰ   **B60.1** **Acanthamebiasis**
         B60.10 **Acanthamebiasis, unspecified**
         B60.11 **Meningoencephalitis due to Acanthamoeba (culbertsoni)**
         B60.12 **Conjunctivitis due to Acanthamoeba**
         B60.13 **Keratoconjunctivitis due to Acanthamoeba**
         B60.19 **Other acanthamebic disease**

     B60.2 **Naegleriasis**
           Primary amebic meningoencephalitis

     B60.8 **Other specified protozoal diseases**
           Microsporidiosis

B64 **Unspecified protozoal disease**

EXCLUDES 1 Not coded here   EXCLUDES 2 Not included here   Ⓝ Newborn Age: 0   Ⓟ Pediatric Age: 0-17   Ⓜ Maternity Age: 12-55   Ⓐ Adult Age: 15-124

440   ICD-10-CM 2016

Helminthiases (B65-B83)

✓4ᵗʰ B65   Schistosomiasis [bilharziasis]
    INCLUDES   snail fever

    B65.0   Schistosomiasis due to Schistosoma haematobium [urinary schistosomiasis]

    B65.1   Schistosomiasis due to Schistosoma mansoni [intestinal schistosomiasis]

    B65.2   Schistosomiasis due to Schistosoma japonicum
        Asiatic schistosomiasis

    B65.3   Cercarial dermatitis
        Swimmer's itch

    B65.8   Other schistosomiasis
        Infection due to Schistosoma intercalatum
        Infection due to Schistosoma mattheei
        Infection due to Schistosoma mekongi

    B65.9   Schistosomiasis, unspecified

✓4ᵗʰ B66   Other fluke infections

    B66.0   Opisthorchiasis
        Infection due to cat liver fluke
        Infection due to Opisthorchis (felineus)(viverrini)

    B66.1   Clonorchiasis
        Chinese liver fluke disease
        Infection due to Clonorchis sinensis
        Oriental liver fluke disease

    B66.2   Dicroceliasis
        Infection due to Dicrocoelium dendriticum
        Lancet fluke infection

    B66.3   Fascioliasis
        Infection due to Fasciola gigantica
        Infection due to Fasciola hepatica
        Infection due to Fasciola indica
        Sheep liver fluke disease

    B66.4   Paragonimiasis
        Infection due to Paragonimus species
        Lung fluke disease
        Pulmonary distomiasis

    B66.5   Fasciolopsiasis
        Infection due to Fasciolopsis buski
        Intestinal distomiasis

    B66.8   Other specified fluke infections
        Echinostomiasis
        Heterophyiasis
        Metagonimiasis
        Nanophyetiasis
        Watsoniasis

    B66.9   Fluke infection, unspecified

✓4ᵗʰ B67   Echinococcosis
    INCLUDES   hydatidosis

    B67.0   Echinococcus granulosus infection of liver

    B67.1   Echinococcus granulosus infection of lung

    B67.2   Echinococcus granulosus infection of bone

  ✓5ᵗʰ **B67.3   Echinococcus granulosus infection, other and multiple sites**

      B67.31   Echinococcus granulosus infection, thyroid gland

      B67.32   Echinococcus granulosus infection, multiple sites

      B67.39   Echinococcus granulosus infection, other sites

    B67.4   Echinococcus granulosus infection, unspecified
        Dog tapeworm (infection)

    B67.5   Echinococcus multilocularis infection of liver

  ✓5ᵗʰ **B67.6   Echinococcus multilocularis infection, other and multiple sites**

      B67.61   Echinococcus multilocularis infection, multiple sites

      B67.69   Echinococcus multilocularis infection, other sites

    B67.7   Echinococcus multilocularis infection, unspecified

    B67.8   Echinococcosis, unspecified, of liver

  ✓5ᵗʰ **B67.9   Echinococcosis, other and unspecified**

      B67.90   Echinococcosis, unspecified
          Echinococcosis NOS

      B67.99   Other echinococcosis

✓4ᵗʰ B68   Taeniasis
    EXCLUDES 1   cysticercosis (B69.-)

    B68.0   Taenia solium taeniasis
        Pork tapeworm (infection)

    B68.1   Taenia saginata taeniasis
        Beef tapeworm (infection)
        Infection due to adult tapeworm Taenia saginata

    B68.9   Taeniasis, unspecified

✓4ᵗʰ B69   Cysticercosis
    INCLUDES   cysticerciasis infection due to larval form of Taenia solium

    B69.0   Cysticercosis of central nervous system

    B69.1   Cysticercosis of eye

  ✓5ᵗʰ **B69.8   Cysticercosis of other sites**

      B69.81   Myositis in cysticercosis

      B69.89   Cysticercosis of other sites

    B69.9   Cysticercosis, unspecified

✓4ᵗʰ B70   Diphyllobothriasis and sparganosis

    B70.0   Diphyllobothriasis
        Diphyllobothrium (adult) (latum) (pacificum) infection
        Fish tapeworm (infection)
        EXCLUDES 2   larval diphyllobothriasis (B70.1)

    B70.1   Sparganosis
        Infection due to Sparganum (mansoni) (proliferum)
        Infection due to Spirometra larva
        Larval diphyllobothriasis
        Spirometrosis

✓4ᵗʰ B71   Other cestode infections

    B71.0   Hymenolepiasis
        Dwarf tapeworm infection
        Rat tapeworm (infection)

    B71.1   Dipylidiasis

    B71.8   Other specified cestode infections
        Coenurosis

    B71.9   Cestode infection, unspecified
        Tapeworm (infection) NOS

B72   Dracunculiasis
    INCLUDES   guinea worm infection
              infection due to Dracunculus medinensis

✓4ᵗʰ B73   Onchocerciasis
    INCLUDES   onchocerca volvulus infection
              onchocercosis
              river blindness

  ✓5ᵗʰ **B73.0   Onchocerciasis with eye disease**

      B73.00   Onchocerciasis with eye involvement, unspecified

      B73.01   Onchocerciasis with endophthalmitis

      B73.02   Onchocerciasis with glaucoma

      B73.09   Onchocerciasis with other eye involvement
          Infestation of eyelid due to onchocerciasis

    B73.1   Onchocerciasis without eye disease

✓4ᵗʰ B74   Filariasis
    EXCLUDES 2   onchocerciasis (B73)
              tropical (pulmonary) eosinophilia NOS (J82)

    B74.0   Filariasis due to Wuchereria bancrofti
        Bancroftian elephantiasis
        Bancroftian filariasis

    B74.1   Filariasis due to Brugia malayi

    B74.2   Filariasis due to Brugia timori

    B74.3   Loiasis
        Calabar swelling
        Eyeworm disease of Africa
        Loa loa infection

    B74.4   Mansonelliasis
        Infection due to Mansonella ozzardi
        Infection due to Mansonella perstans
        Infection due to Mansonella streptocerca

    B74.8   Other filariases
        Dirofilariasis

    B74.9   Filariasis, unspecified

B75   Trichinellosis
    INCLUDES   infection due to Trichinella species
              trichiniasis

✓4ᵗʰ B76   Hookworm diseases
    INCLUDES   uncinariasis

    B76.0   Ancylostomiasis
        Infection due to Ancylostoma species

    B76.1   Necatoriasis
        Infection due to Necator americanus

    B76.8   Other hookworm diseases

    B76.9   Hookworm disease, unspecified
        Cutaneous larva migrans NOS

✓ Additional Character Required   ✓ᵀ Placeholder Alert   Unspecified Dx   Other Specified Dx   Manifestation   ▶◀ Revised Text   ● New Code   ▲ Revised Code Title

✓4th **B77 Ascariasis**

INCLUDES ascaridiasis
roundworm infection

B77.0 Ascariasis with intestinal complications

✓5th **B77.8 Ascariasis with other complications**

B77.81 Ascariasis pneumonia

B77.89 Ascariasis with other complications

B77.9 Ascariasis, unspecified

✓4th **B78 Strongyloidiasis**

EXCLUDES 1 trichostrongyliasis (B81.2)

B78.0 Intestinal strongyloidiasis

B78.1 Cutaneous strongyloidiasis

B78.7 Disseminated strongyloidiasis

B78.9 Strongyloidiasis, unspecified

B79 Trichuriasis

INCLUDES trichocephaliasis
whipworm (disease)(infection)

B80 Enterobiasis

INCLUDES oxyuriasis
pinworm infection
threadworm infection

✓4th **B81 Other intestinal helminthiases, not elsewhere classified**

EXCLUDES 1 angiostrongyliasis due to Parastrongylus cantonensis (B83.2)

B81.0 Anisakiasis

Infection due to Anisakis larva

B81.1 Intestinal capillariasis

Capillariasis NOS
Infection due to Capillaria philippinensis

EXCLUDES 2 hepatic capillariasis (B83.8)

B81.2 Trichostrongyliasis

B81.3 Intestinal angiostrongyliasis

Angiostrongyliasis due to Parastrongylus costaricensis

B81.4 Mixed intestinal helminthiases

Infection due to intestinal helminths classified to more than one of the categories B65.0-B81.3 and B81.8
Mixed helminthiasis NOS

B81.8 Other specified intestinal helminthiases

Infection due to Oesophagostomum species [esophagostomiasis]
Infection due to Ternidens diminutus [ternidensiasis]

✓4th **B82 Unspecified intestinal parasitism**

B82.0 Intestinal helminthiasis, unspecified

B82.9 Intestinal parasitism, unspecified

✓4th **B83 Other helminthiases**

EXCLUDES 1 capillariasis NOS (B81.1)

EXCLUDES 2 intestinal capillariasis (B81.1)

B83.0 Visceral larva migrans

Toxocariasis

B83.1 Gnathostomiasis

Wandering swelling

B83.2 Angiostrongyliasis due to Parastrongylus cantonensis

Eosinophilic meningoencephalitis due to Parastrongylus cantonensis

EXCLUDES 2 intestinal angiostrongyliasis (B81.3)

B83.3 Syngamiasis

Syngamosis

B83.4 Internal hirudiniasis

EXCLUDES 2 external hirudiniasis (B88.3)

B83.8 Other specified helminthiases

Acanthocephaliasis
Gongylonemiasis
Hepatic capillariasis
Metastrongyliasis
Thelaziasis

B83.9 Helminthiasis, unspecified

Worms NOS

EXCLUDES 1 intestinal helminthiasis NOS (B82.0)

Pediculosis, acariasis and other infestations (B85-B89)

✓4th **B85 Pediculosis and phthiriasis**

B85.0 Pediculosis due to Pediculus humanus capitis

Head-louse infestation

B85.1 Pediculosis due to Pediculus humanus corporis

Body-louse infestation

B85.2 Pediculosis, unspecified

B85.3 Phthiriasis

Infestation by crab-louse
Infestation by Phthirus pubis

B85.4 Mixed pediculosis and phthiriasis

Infestation classifiable to more than one of the categories B85.0-B85.3

B86 Scabies

Sarcoptic itch

✓4th **B87 Myiasis**

INCLUDES infestation by larva of flies

B87.0 Cutaneous myiasis

Creeping myiasis

B87.1 Wound myiasis

Traumatic myiasis

B87.2 Ocular myiasis

B87.3 Nasopharyngeal myiasis

Laryngeal myiasis

B87.4 Aural myiasis

✓5th **B87.8 Myiasis of other sites**

B87.81 Genitourinary myiasis

B87.82 Intestinal myiasis

B87.89 Myiasis of other sites

B87.9 Myiasis, unspecified

✓4th **B88 Other infestations**

B88.0 Other acariasis

Acarine dermatitis
Dermatitis due to Demodex species
Dermatitis due to Dermanyssus gallinae
Dermatitis due to Liponyssoides sanguineus
Trombiculosis

EXCLUDES 2 scabies (B86)

B88.1 Tungiasis [sandflea infestation]

B88.2 Other arthropod infestations

Scarabiasis

B88.3 External hirudiniasis

Leech infestation NOS

EXCLUDES 2 internal hirudiniasis (B83.4)

B88.8 Other specified infestations

Ichthyoparasitism due to Vandellia cirrhosa
Linguatulosis
Porocephaliasis

B88.9 Infestation, unspecified

Infestation (skin) NOS
Infestation by mites NOS
Skin parasites NOS

B89 Unspecified parasitic disease

Sequelae of infectious and parasitic diseases (B90-B94)

NOTE Categories B90-B94 are to be used to indicate conditions in categories A00-B89 as the cause of sequelae, which are themselves classified elsewhere. The "sequelae" include conditions specified as such; they also include residuals of diseases classifiable to the above categories if there is evidence that the disease itself is no longer present. Codes from these categories are not to be used for chronic infections. Code chronic current infections to active infectious disease as appropriate.

Code first condition resulting from (sequela) the infectious or parasitic disease

✓4th **B90 Sequelae of tuberculosis**

B90.0 Sequelae of central nervous system tuberculosis

B90.1 Sequelae of genitourinary tuberculosis

B90.2 Sequelae of tuberculosis of bones and joints

B90.8 Sequelae of tuberculosis of other organs

EXCLUDES 2 sequelae of respiratory tuberculosis (B90.9)

B90.9 Sequelae of respiratory and unspecified tuberculosis

Sequelae of tuberculosis NOS

B91 Sequelae of poliomyelitis

EXCLUDES 1 postpolio syndrome (G14)

B92 Sequelae of leprosy

✓4th **B94 Sequelae of other and unspecified infectious and parasitic diseases**

B94.0 Sequelae of trachoma

B94.1 Sequelae of viral encephalitis

B94.2 Sequelae of viral hepatitis

B94.8   **Sequelae of other specified infectious and parasitic diseases**

B94.9   **Sequelae of unspecified infectious and parasitic disease**

Bacterial and viral infectious agents (B95-B97)

NOTE   These categories are provided for use as supplementary or additional codes to identify the infectious agent(s) in diseases classified elsewhere.

☑4ᵗʰ **B95   Streptococcus, Staphylococcus, and Enterococcus as the cause of diseases classified elsewhere**

B95.0   **Streptococcus, group A, as the cause of diseases classified elsewhere**

B95.1   **Streptococcus, group B, as the cause of diseases classified elsewhere**

B95.2   **Enterococcus as the cause of diseases classified elsewhere**

B95.3   **Streptococcus pneumoniae as the cause of diseases classified elsewhere**

B95.4   **Other streptococcus as the cause of diseases classified elsewhere**

B95.5   **Unspecified streptococcus as the cause of diseases classified elsewhere**

☑5ᵗʰ B95.6   **Staphylococcus aureus as the cause of diseases classified elsewhere**

B95.61   **Methicillin susceptible Staphylococcus aureus infection as the cause of diseases classified elsewhere**
Methicillin susceptible Staphylococcus aureus (MSSA) infection as the cause of diseases classified elsewhere
Staphylococcus aureus infection NOS as the cause of diseases classified elsewhere

B95.62   **Methicillin resistant Staphylococcus aureus infection as the cause of diseases classified elsewhere**
Methicillin resistant Staphylococcus aureus (MRSA) infection as the cause of diseases classified elsewhere

B95.7   **Other staphylococcus as the cause of diseases classified elsewhere**

B95.8   **Unspecified staphylococcus as the cause of diseases classified elsewhere**

☑4ᵗʰ **B96   Other bacterial agents as the cause of diseases classified elsewhere**

B96.0   **Mycoplasma pneumoniae [M. pneumoniae] as the cause of diseases classified elsewhere**
Pleuro-pneumonia-like-organism [PPLO]

B96.1   **Klebsiella pneumoniae [K. pneumoniae] as the cause of diseases classified elsewhere**

☑5ᵗʰ B96.2   **Escherichia coli [E. coli] as the cause of diseases classified elsewhere**

B96.20   **Unspecified Escherichia coli [E. coli] as the cause of diseases classified elsewhere**
Escherichia coli [E. coli] NOS

B96.21   **Shiga toxin-producing Escherichia coli [E. coli] (STEC) O157 as the cause of diseases classified elsewhere**
E. coli O157:H- (nonmotile) with confirmation of Shiga toxin
E. coli O157 with confirmation of Shiga toxin when H antigen is unknown, or is not H7
O157:H7 Escherichia coli [E.coli] with or without confirmation of Shiga toxin-production
Shiga toxin-producing Escherichia coli [E.coli] O157:H7 with or without confirmation of Shiga toxin-production
STEC O157:H7 with or without confirmation of Shiga toxin-production

B96.22   **Other specified Shiga toxin-producing Escherichia coli [E. coli] (STEC) as the cause of diseases classified elsewhere**
Non-O157 Shiga toxin-producing Escherichia coli [E.coli]
Non-O157 Shiga toxin-producing Escherichia coli [E.coli] with known O group

B96.23   **Unspecified Shiga toxin-producing Escherichia coli [E. coli] (STEC) as the cause of diseases classified elsewhere**
Shiga toxin-producing Escherichia coli [E. coli] with unspecified O group
STEC NOS

B96.29   **Other Escherichia coli [E. coli] as the cause of diseases classified elsewhere**
Non-Shiga toxin-producing E. coli

B96.3   **Hemophilus influenzae [H. influenzae] as the cause of diseases classified elsewhere**

B96.4   **Proteus (mirabilis) (morganii) as the cause of diseases classified elsewhere**

B96.5   **Pseudomonas (aeruginosa) (mallei) (pseudomallei) as the cause of diseases classified elsewhere**
AHA: 2015, 1Q, 18

B96.6   **Bacteroides fragilis [B. fragilis] as the cause of diseases classified elsewhere**

B96.7   **Clostridium perfringens [C. perfringens] as the cause of diseases classified elsewhere**

☑5ᵗʰ B96.8   **Other specified bacterial agents as the cause of diseases classified elsewhere**

B96.81   **Helicobacter pylori [H. pylori] as the cause of diseases classified elsewhere**

B96.82   **Vibrio vulnificus as the cause of diseases classified elsewhere**

B96.89   **Other specified bacterial agents as the cause of diseases classified elsewhere**

☑4ᵗʰ **B97   Viral agents as the cause of diseases classified elsewhere**

B97.0   **Adenovirus as the cause of diseases classified elsewhere**

☑5ᵗʰ B97.1   **Enterovirus as the cause of diseases classified elsewhere**

B97.10   **Unspecified enterovirus as the cause of diseases classified elsewhere**

B97.11   **Coxsackievirus as the cause of diseases classified elsewhere**

B97.12   **Echovirus as the cause of diseases classified elsewhere**

B97.19   **Other enterovirus as the cause of diseases classified elsewhere**

☑5ᵗʰ B97.2   **Coronavirus as the cause of diseases classified elsewhere**

B97.21   **SARS-associated coronavirus as the cause of diseases classified elsewhere**
EXCLUDES 1   *pneumonia due to SARS-associated coronavirus (J12.81)*

B97.29   **Other coronavirus as the cause of diseases classified elsewhere**

☑5ᵗʰ B97.3   **Retrovirus as the cause of diseases classified elsewhere**
EXCLUDES 1   *human immunodeficiency virus [HIV} disease (B20)*

B97.30   **Unspecified retrovirus as the cause of diseases classified elsewhere**

B97.31   **Lentivirus as the cause of diseases classified elsewhere**

B97.32   **Oncovirus as the cause of diseases classified elsewhere**

B97.33   **Human T-cell lymphotrophic virus, type I [HTLV-I] as the cause of diseases classified elsewhere**

B97.34   **Human T-cell lymphotrophic virus, type II [HTLV-II] as the cause of diseases classified elsewhere**

B97.35   **Human immunodeficiency virus, type 2 [HIV 2] as the cause of diseases classified elsewhere**

B97.39   **Other retrovirus as the cause of diseases classified elsewhere**

B97.4   **Respiratory syncytial virus as the cause of diseases classified elsewhere**

B97.5   **Reovirus as the cause of diseases classified elsewhere**

B97.6   **Parvovirus as the cause of diseases classified elsewhere**

B97.7   **Papillomavirus as the cause of diseases classified elsewhere**

☑5ᵗʰ B97.8   **Other viral agents as the cause of diseases classified elsewhere**

B97.81   **Human metapneumovirus as the cause of diseases classified elsewhere**

B97.89   **Other viral agents as the cause of diseases classified elsewhere**

Other infectious diseases (B99)

☑4ᵗʰ **B99   Other and unspecified infectious diseases**

B99.8   **Other infectious disease**

B99.9   **Unspecified infectious disease**

Chapter 2. Neoplasms (C00–D49)

Chapter Specific Guidelines with Coding Examples

The chapter specific guidelines from the ICD-10-CM Official Guidelines for Coding and Reporting have been provided below. Along with these guidelines are coding examples, contained in the shaded boxes, that have been developed to help illustrate the coding and/or sequencing guidance found in these guidelines.

General guidelines

Chapter 2 of the ICD-10-CM contains the codes for most benign and all malignant neoplasms. Certain benign neoplasms, such as prostatic adenomas, may be found in the specific body system chapters. To properly code a neoplasm it is necessary to determine from the record if the neoplasm is benign, in-situ, malignant, or of uncertain histologic behavior. If malignant, any secondary (metastatic) sites should also be determined.

Primary malignant neoplasms overlapping site boundaries

A primary malignant neoplasm that overlaps two or more contiguous (next to each other) sites should be classified to the subcategory/code .8 ('overlapping lesion'), unless the combination is specifically indexed elsewhere. For multiple neoplasms of the same site that are not contiguous such as tumors in different quadrants of the same breast, codes for each site should be assigned.

A 73-year-old white female with a large rapidly growing malignant tumor in the left breast extending from the upper outer quadrant into the axillary tail

C50.812   **Malignant neoplasm of overlapping sites of left female breast**

Explanation: Because this is a single large tumor that overlaps two contiguous sites, a single code for overlapping sites is assigned.

A 52-year old white female with two distinct lesions of the right breast, one (0.5 cm) in the upper outer quadrant and a second (1.5 cm) in the lower outer quadrant; path report indicates both lesions are malignant

C50.411   **Malignant neoplasm of upper-outer quadrant of breast, female**

C50.511   **Malignant neoplasm of lower-outer quadrant of breast, female**

Explanation: This patient has two distinct malignant lesions of right breast in adjacent quadrants. Because the lesions are not contiguous, two codes are reported.

Malignant neoplasm of ectopic tissue

Malignant neoplasms of ectopic tissue are to be coded to the site of origin mentioned, e.g., ectopic pancreatic malignant neoplasms involving the stomach are coded to pancreas, unspecified (C25.9).

The neoplasm table in the Alphabetic Index should be referenced first. However, if the histological term is documented, that term should be referenced first, rather than going immediately to the Neoplasm Table, in order to determine which column in the Neoplasm Table is appropriate. For example, if the documentation indicates "adenoma," refer to the term in the Alphabetic Index to review the entries under this term and the instructional note to "see also neoplasm, by site, benign." The table provides the proper code based on the type of neoplasm and the site. It is important to select the proper column in the table that corresponds to the type of neoplasm. The Tabular List should then be referenced to verify that the correct code has been selected from the table and that a more specific site code does not exist.

See Section I.C.21. Factors influencing health status and contact with health services, Status, for information regarding Z15.0, codes for genetic susceptibility to cancer.

a. Treatment directed at the malignancy

If the treatment is directed at the malignancy, designate the malignancy as the principal diagnosis.

The only exception to this guideline is if a patient admission/encounter is solely for the administration of chemotherapy, immunotherapy or radiation therapy, assign the appropriate Z51.-- code as the first-listed or principal diagnosis, and the diagnosis or problem for which the service is being performed as a secondary diagnosis.

b. Treatment of secondary site

When a patient is admitted because of a primary neoplasm with metastasis and treatment is directed toward the secondary site only, the secondary neoplasm is designated as the principal diagnosis even though the primary malignancy is still present.

Patient with primary prostate cancer with metastasis to lungs admitted for wedge resection of mass in right lung

C78.01   **Secondary malignant neoplasm of right lung**

C61   **Malignant neoplasm of prostate**

Explanation: Since the admission is for treatment of the lung metastasis, the secondary lung metastasis is sequenced before the primary prostate cancer.

c. Coding and sequencing of complications

Coding and sequencing of complications associated with the malignancies or with the therapy thereof are subject to the following guidelines:

1) Anemia associated with malignancy

When admission/encounter is for management of an anemia associated with the malignancy, and the treatment is only for anemia, the appropriate code for the malignancy is sequenced as the principal or first-listed diagnosis followed by the appropriate code for the anemia (such as code D63.0, Anemia in neoplastic disease).

Patient is admitted for treatment of anemia in advanced colon cancer

C18.9   **Malignant neoplasm of colon, unspecified**

D63.0   **Anemia in neoplastic disease**

Explanation: Even though the admission was solely to treat the anemia, this guideline indicates that the code for the malignancy is sequenced first.

2) Anemia associated with chemotherapy, immunotherapy and radiation therapy

When the admission/encounter is for management of an anemia associated with an adverse effect of the administration of chemotherapy or immunotherapy and the only treatment is for the anemia, the anemia code is sequenced first followed by the appropriate codes for the neoplasm and the adverse effect (T45.1X5, Adverse effect of antineoplastic and immunosuppressive drugs).

A 56-year-old Hispanic male with grade II follicular lymphoma involving multiple lymph node sites referred for blood transfusion to treat anemia due to chemotherapy

D64.81   **Anemia due to antineoplastic chemotherapy**

C82.18   **Follicular lymphoma grade II, lymph nodes of multiple sites**

T45.1X5A   **Adverse effect of antineoplastic and immunosuppressive drugs, initial encounter**

Explanation: The code for the anemia is sequenced first followed by the code for the malignant neoplasm and lastly the code for the adverse effect.

When the admission/encounter is for management of an anemia associated with an adverse effect of radiotherapy, the anemia code should be sequenced first, followed by the appropriate neoplasm code and code Y84.2, Radiological procedure and radiotherapy as the cause of abnormal reaction of the patient, or of later complication, without mention of misadventure at the time of the procedure.

A 55-year-old male with a large malignant rectal tumor has been receiving external radiation therapy to shrink the tumor prior to planned surgery. He is admitted today for a blood transfusion to treat anemia related to radiation therapy.

D64.89   **Other specified anemia**

C20   **Malignant neoplasm of rectum**

Y84.2   **Radiological procedure and radiotherapy as the cause of abnormal reaction of the patient, or of later complication, without mention of misadventure at the time of the procedure**

Explanation: The code for the anemia is sequenced first, followed by the code for the malignancy, and lastly the code for the abnormal reaction due to radiotherapy.

3) **Management of dehydration due to the malignancy**

When the admission/encounter is for management of dehydration due to the malignancy and only the dehydration is being treated (intravenous rehydration), the dehydration is sequenced first, followed by the code(s) for the malignancy.

4) **Treatment of a complication resulting from a surgical procedure**

When the admission/encounter is for treatment of a complication resulting from a surgical procedure, designate the complication as the principal or first-listed diagnosis if treatment is directed at resolving the complication.

d. **Primary malignancy previously excised**

When a primary malignancy has been previously excised or eradicated from its site and there is no further treatment directed to that site and there is no evidence of any existing primary malignancy, a code from category Z85, Personal history of malignant neoplasm, should be used to indicate the former site of the malignancy. Any mention of extension, invasion, or metastasis to another site is coded as a secondary malignant neoplasm to that site. The secondary site may be the principal or first-listed with the Z85 code used as a secondary code.

History of breast cancer, left radical mastectomy 18 months ago with no current treatment; bronchoscopy with lung biopsy shows metastatic disease in the right lung

C78.01   **Secondary malignant neoplasm of right lung**

Z85.3   **Personal history of malignant neoplasm of breast**

Explanation: The patient has undergone a diagnostic procedure that revealed metastatic breast cancer in the right lung. The code for the secondary (metastatic) site is sequenced first followed by a personal history code to identify the former site of the primary malignancy.

e. **Admissions/Encounters involving chemotherapy, immunotherapy and radiation therapy**

1) **Episode of care involves surgical removal of neoplasm**

When an episode of care involves the surgical removal of a neoplasm, primary or secondary site, followed by adjunct chemotherapy or radiation treatment during the same episode of care, the code for the neoplasm should be assigned as principal or first-listed diagnosis.

2) **Patient admission/encounter solely for administration of chemotherapy, immunotherapy and radiation therapy**

If a patient admission/encounter is solely for the administration of chemotherapy, immunotherapy or radiation therapy assign code Z51.0, Encounter for antineoplastic radiation therapy, or Z51.11, Encounter for antineoplastic chemotherapy, or Z51.12, Encounter for antineoplastic immunotherapy as the first-listed or principal diagnosis. If a patient receives more than one of these therapies during the same admission more than one of these codes may be assigned, in any sequence.

The malignancy for which the therapy is being administered should be assigned as a secondary diagnosis.

Patient is admitted for second round of rituximab and fludarabine for his chronic B cell lymphocytic leukemia

Z51.11   **Encounter for antineoplastic chemotherapy**

Z51.12   **Encounter for antineoplastic immunotherapy**

C91.10   **Chronic lymphocytic leukemia of B-cell type not having achieved remission**

Explanation: Rituximab is an antineoplastic immunotherapy while fludarabine is an antineoplastic chemotherapy. The two treatments are often used together. The admission was solely for the purpose of administering this treatment and either can be sequenced first, before the neoplastic condition.

3) **Patient admitted for radiation therapy, chemotherapy or immunotherapy and develops complications**

When a patient is admitted for the purpose of radiotherapy, immunotherapy or chemotherapy and develops complications such as uncontrolled nausea and vomiting or dehydration, the principal or first-listed diagnosis is Z51.0, Encounter for antineoplastic radiation therapy, or Z51.11, Encounter for antineoplastic chemotherapy, or Z51.12, Encounter for antineoplastic immunotherapy followed by any codes for the complications.

f. **Admission/encounter to determine extent of malignancy**

When the reason for admission/encounter is to determine the extent of the malignancy, or for a procedure such as paracentesis or thoracentesis, the primary malignancy or appropriate metastatic site is designated as the principal or first-listed diagnosis, even though chemotherapy or radiotherapy is administered.

Patient with left lung cancer with malignant pleural effusion admitted for paracentesis and initiation/administration of chemotherapy

C34.92   **Malignant neoplasm of unspecified part of left bronchus or lung**

J91.0   **Malignant pleural effusion**

Z51.11   **Encounter for antineoplastic chemotherapy**

Explanation: The lung cancer is sequenced before the chemotherapy in this instance because the paracentesis for the malignant effusion is also being performed. An instructional note under the malignant effusion instructs that the lung cancer be sequenced first.

g. **Symptoms, signs, and abnormal findings listed in Chapter 18 associated with neoplasms**

Symptoms, signs, and ill-defined conditions listed in Chapter 18 characteristic of, or associated with, an existing primary or secondary site malignancy cannot be used to replace the malignancy as principal or first-listed diagnosis, regardless of the number of admissions or encounters for treatment and care of the neoplasm.

See Section I.C.21. Factors influencing health status and contact with health services, Encounter for prophylactic organ removal.

h. **Admission/encounter for pain control/management**

See Section I.C.6. for information on coding admission/encounter for pain control/management.

i. **Malignancy in two or more noncontiguous sites**

A patient may have more than one malignant tumor in the same organ. These tumors may represent different primaries or metastatic disease, depending on the site. Should the documentation be unclear, the provider should be queried as to the status of each tumor so that the correct codes can be assigned.

j. **Disseminated malignant neoplasm, unspecified**

Code C80.0, Disseminated malignant neoplasm, unspecified, is for use only in those cases where the patient has advanced metastatic disease and no known primary or secondary sites are specified. It should not be used in place of assigning codes for the primary site and all known secondary sites.

Patient who has had no medical care for many years is seen today and diagnosed with carcinomatosis

C80.0   **Disseminated malignant neoplasm, unspecified**

Explanation: Carcinomatosis NOS is an "includes" note under this code. Should seldom be used but is available for use in cases such as this.

k. Malignant neoplasm without specification of site

Code C80.1, Malignant (primary) neoplasm, unspecified, equates to Cancer, unspecified. This code should only be used when no determination can be made as to the primary site of a malignancy. This code should rarely be used in the inpatient setting.

> Evaluation of painful hip leads to diagnosis of a metastatic bone lesion from an unknown primary neoplasm source
>
> **C79.51**　　**Secondary malignant neoplasm of bone**
>
> **C80.1**　　**Malignant (primary) neoplasm, unspecified**
>
> *Explanation*: If only the secondary site is known, use code C80.1 for the unknown primary site.

l. Sequencing of neoplasm codes

1) Encounter for treatment of primary malignancy

If the reason for the encounter is for treatment of a primary malignancy, assign the malignancy as the principal/first-listed diagnosis. The primary site is to be sequenced first, followed by any metastatic sites.

2) Encounter for treatment of secondary malignancy

When an encounter is for a primary malignancy with metastasis and treatment is directed toward the metastatic (secondary) site(s) only, the metastatic site(s) is designated as the principal/first-listed diagnosis. The primary malignancy is coded as an additional code.

> Patient has primary colon cancer with metastasis to rib and is evaluated for possible excision of portion of rib bone
>
> **C79.51**　　**Secondary malignant neoplasm of bone**
>
> **C18.9**　　**Malignant neoplasm of colon, unspecified**
>
> *Explanation*: The treatment for this encounter is focused on the metastasis to the rib bone rather than the primary colon cancer, thus indicating that the bone metastasis is sequenced as the first-listed code.

3) Malignant neoplasm in a pregnant patient

When a pregnant woman has a malignant neoplasm, a code from subcategory O9A.1-, Malignant neoplasm complicating pregnancy, childbirth, and the puerperium, should be sequenced first, followed by the appropriate code from Chapter 2 to indicate the type of neoplasm.

> A 30-year-old pregnant female in second trimester evaluated for thyroid malignancy
>
> **O9A.112**　　**Malignant neoplasm complicating pregnancy, second trimester**
>
> **C73**　　**Malignant neoplasm of thyroid gland**
>
> *Explanation*: Codes from chapter 15 describing complications of pregnancy are sequenced as first-listed codes, further specified by codes from other chapters such as neoplastic, unless the pregnancy is documented as incidental to the condition. See also guideline 1.C.15.a.1.

4) Encounter for complication associated with a neoplasm

When an encounter is for management of a complication associated with a neoplasm, such as dehydration, and the treatment is only for the complication, the complication is coded first, followed by the appropriate code(s) for the neoplasm.

The exception to this guideline is anemia. When the admission/encounter is for management of an anemia associated with the malignancy, and the treatment is only for anemia, the appropriate code for the malignancy is sequenced as the principal or first-listed diagnosis followed by code D63.0, Anemia in neoplastic disease.

> Patient with pancreatic cancer is seen for initiation of TPN for cancer-related moderate protein-calorie malnutrition
>
> **E44.0**　　**Moderate protein-calorie malnutrition**
>
> **C25.9**　　**Malignant neoplasm of pancreas, unspecified**
>
> *Explanation*: The encounter is to initiate treatment for malnutrition, a common complication of many types of neoplasms, and is sequenced first.

5) Complication from surgical procedure for treatment of a neoplasm

When an encounter is for treatment of a complication resulting from a surgical procedure performed for the treatment of the neoplasm, designate the complication as the principal/first-listed diagnosis. See guideline regarding the coding of a current malignancy versus personal history to determine if the code for the neoplasm should also be assigned.

6) Pathologic fracture due to a neoplasm

When an encounter is for a pathological fracture due to a neoplasm, and the focus of treatment is the fracture, a code from subcategory M84.5, Pathological fracture in neoplastic disease, should be sequenced first, followed by the code for the neoplasm.

If the focus of treatment is the neoplasm with an associated pathological fracture, the neoplasm code should be sequenced first, followed by a code from M84.5 for the pathological fracture.

m. Current malignancy versus personal history of malignancy

When a primary malignancy has been excised but further treatment, such as an additional surgery for the malignancy, radiation therapy or chemotherapy is directed to that site, the primary malignancy code should be used until treatment is completed.

When a primary malignancy has been previously excised or eradicated from its site, there is no further treatment (of the malignancy) directed to that site, and there is no evidence of any existing primary malignancy, a code from category Z85, Personal history of malignant neoplasm, should be used to indicate the former site of the malignancy.

See Section I.C.21. Factors influencing health status and contact with health services, History (of)

> Female patient with ongoing chemotherapy after right mastectomy for breast cancer
>
> **C50.911**　　**Malignant neoplasm of unspecified site of right female breast**
>
> *Explanation*: Even though the breast has been removed, the breast cancer is still being treated with chemotherapy and therefore is still coded as a current condition rather than personal history.

n. Leukemia, multiple myeloma, and malignant plasma cell neoplasms in remission versus personal history

The categories for leukemia, and category C90, Multiple myeloma and malignant plasma cell neoplasms, have codes indicating whether or not the leukemia has achieved remission. There are also codes Z85.6, Personal history of leukemia, and Z85.79, Personal history of other malignant neoplasms of lymphoid, hematopoietic and related tissues. If the documentation is unclear as to whether the leukemia has achieved remission, the provider should be queried.

See Section I.C.21. Factors influencing health status and contact with health services, History (of)

o. Aftercare following surgery for neoplasm

See Section I.C.21. Factors influencing health status and contact with health services, Aftercare

p. Follow-up care for completed treatment of a malignancy

See Section I.C.21. Factors influencing health status and contact with health services, Follow-up

q. Prophylactic organ removal for prevention of malignancy

See Section I.C. 21, Factors influencing health status and contact with health services, Prophylactic organ removal

r. Malignant neoplasm associated with transplanted organ

A malignant neoplasm of a transplanted organ should be coded as a transplant complication. Assign first the appropriate code from category T86.-, Complications of transplanted organs and tissue, followed by code C80.2, Malignant neoplasm associated with transplanted organ. Use an additional code for the specific malignancy.

Chapter 2. Neoplasms (C00-D49)

NOTE

Functional activity

All neoplasms are classified in this chapter, whether they are functionally active or not. An additional code from Chapter 4 may be used, to identify functional activity associated with any neoplasm.

Morphology [Histology]

Chapter 2 classifies neoplasms primarily by site (topography), with broad groupings for behavior, malignant, in situ, benign, etc. The Table of Neoplasms should be used to identify the correct topography code. In a few cases, such as for malignant melanoma and certain neuroendocrine tumors, the morphology (histologic type) is included in the category and codes.

Primary malignant neoplasms overlapping site boundaries

A primary malignant neoplasm that overlaps two or more contiguous (next to each other) sites should be classified to the subcategory/code .8 ("overlapping lesion"), unless the combination is specifically indexed elsewhere. For multiple neoplasms of the same site that are not contiguous, such as tumors in different quadrants of the same breast, codes for each site should be assigned.

Malignant neoplasm of ectopic tissue

Malignant neoplasms of ectopic tissue are to be coded to the site mentioned, e.g., ectopic pancreatic malignant neoplasms are coded to pancreas, unspecified (C25.9).

This chapter contains the following blocks:

C00-C14	Malignant neoplasms of lip, oral cavity and pharynx
C15-C26	Malignant neoplasms of digestive organs
C30-C39	Malignant neoplasms of respiratory and intrathoracic organs
C40-C41	Malignant neoplasms of bone and articular cartilage
C43-C44	Melanoma and other malignant neoplasms of skin
C45-C49	Malignant neoplasms of mesothelial and soft tissue
C50	Malignant neoplasms of breast
C51-C58	Malignant neoplasms of female genital organs
C60-C63	Malignant neoplasms of male genital organs
C64-C68	Malignant neoplasms of urinary tract
C69-C72	Malignant neoplasms of eye, brain and other parts of central nervous system
C73-C75	Malignant neoplasms of thyroid and other endocrine glands
C7A	Malignant neuroendocrine tumors
C7B	Secondary neuroendocrine tumors
C76-C80	Malignant neoplasms of ill-defined, other secondary and unspecified sites
C81-C96	Malignant neoplasms of lymphoid, hematopoietic and related tissue
D00-D09	In situ neoplasms
D10-D36	Benign neoplasms, except benign neuroendocrine tumors
D3A	Benign neuroendocrine tumors
D37-D48	Neoplasms of uncertain behavior, polycythemia vera and myelodysplastic syndromes
D49	Neoplasms of unspecified behavior

MALIGNANT NEOPLASMS (C00-C96)

Malignant neoplasms, stated or presumed to be primary (of specified sites), and certain specified histologies, except neuroendocrine, and of lymphoid, hematopoietic and related tissue (C00-C75)

Malignant neoplasms of lip, oral cavity and pharynx (C00-C14)

✓4ᵗʰ C00 Malignant neoplasm of lip

Use additional code to identify:
    alcohol abuse and dependence (F10.-)
    history of tobacco use (Z87.891)
    tobacco dependence (F17.-)
    tobacco use (Z72.0)
    EXCLUDES 1 *malignant melanoma of lip (C43.0)*
             Merkel cell carcinoma of lip (C4A.0)
             other and unspecified malignant neoplasm of skin of lip (C44.0-)

C00.0 Malignant neoplasm of external upper lip
    Malignant neoplasm of lipstick area of upper lip
    Malignant neoplasm of upper lip NOS
    Malignant neoplasm of vermilion border of upper lip

C00.1 Malignant neoplasm of external lower lip
    Malignant neoplasm of lower lip NOS
    Malignant neoplasm of lipstick area of lower lip
    Malignant neoplasm of vermilion border of lower lip

C00.2 Malignant neoplasm of external lip, unspecified
    Malignant neoplasm of vermilion border of lip NOS

C00.3 Malignant neoplasm of upper lip, inner aspect
    Malignant neoplasm of buccal aspect of upper lip
    Malignant neoplasm of frenulum of upper lip
    Malignant neoplasm of mucosa of upper lip
    Malignant neoplasm of oral aspect of upper lip

C00.4 Malignant neoplasm of lower lip, inner aspect
    Malignant neoplasm of buccal aspect of lower lip
    Malignant neoplasm of frenulum of lower lip
    Malignant neoplasm of mucosa of lower lip
    Malignant neoplasm of oral aspect of lower lip

C00.5 Malignant neoplasm of lip, unspecified, inner aspect
    Malignant neoplasm of buccal aspect of lip, unspecified
    Malignant neoplasm of frenulum of lip, unspecified
    Malignant neoplasm of mucosa of lip, unspecified
    Malignant neoplasm of oral aspect of lip, unspecified

C00.6 Malignant neoplasm of commissure of lip, unspecified

C00.8 Malignant neoplasm of overlapping sites of lip

C00.9 Malignant neoplasm of lip, unspecified

C01 Malignant neoplasm of base of tongue
    Malignant neoplasm of dorsal surface of base of tongue
    Malignant neoplasm of fixed part of tongue NOS
    Malignant neoplasm of posterior third of tongue
    Use additional code to identify:
        alcohol abuse and dependence (F10.-)
        history of tobacco use (Z87.891)
        tobacco dependence (F17.-)
        tobacco use (Z72.0)

✓4ᵗʰ C02 Malignant neoplasm of other and unspecified parts of tongue
    Use additional code to identify:
        alcohol abuse and dependence (F10.-)
        history of tobacco use (Z87.891)
        tobacco dependence (F17.-)
        tobacco use (Z72.0)

C02.0 Malignant neoplasm of dorsal surface of tongue
    Malignant neoplasm of anterior two-thirds of tongue, dorsal surface
    EXCLUDES 2 *malignant neoplasm of dorsal surface of base of tongue (C01)*

C02.1 Malignant neoplasm of border of tongue
    Malignant neoplasm of tip of tongue

C02.2 Malignant neoplasm of ventral surface of tongue
    Malignant neoplasm of anterior two-thirds of tongue, ventral surface
    Malignant neoplasm of frenulum linguae

C02.3 Malignant neoplasm of anterior two-thirds of tongue, part unspecified
    Malignant neoplasm of middle third of tongue NOS
    Malignant neoplasm of mobile part of tongue NOS

C02.4 Malignant neoplasm of lingual tonsil
    EXCLUDES 2 *malignant neoplasm of tonsil NOS (C09.9)*

C02.8 Malignant neoplasm of overlapping sites of tongue
    Malignant neoplasm of two or more contiguous sites of tongue

C02.9 Malignant neoplasm of tongue, unspecified

✓4ᵗʰ C03 Malignant neoplasm of gum
    INCLUDES   malignant neoplasm of alveolar (ridge) mucosa
               malignant neoplasm of gingiva
    Use additional code to identify:
        alcohol abuse and dependence (F10.-)
        history of tobacco use (Z87.891)
        tobacco dependence (F17.-)
        tobacco use (Z72.0)
    EXCLUDES 2 *malignant odontogenic neoplasms (C41.0-C41.1)*

C03.0 Malignant neoplasm of upper gum

C03.1 Malignant neoplasm of lower gum

C03.9 Malignant neoplasm of gum, unspecified

✓4ᵗʰ C04 Malignant neoplasm of floor of mouth
    Use additional code to identify:
        alcohol abuse and dependence (F10.-)
        history of tobacco use (Z87.891)
        tobacco dependence (F17.-)
        tobacco use (Z72.0)

C04.0 Malignant neoplasm of anterior floor of mouth
    Malignant neoplasm of anterior to the premolar-canine junction

C04.1 Malignant neoplasm of lateral floor of mouth

C04.8 Malignant neoplasm of overlapping sites of floor of mouth

C04.9 Malignant neoplasm of floor of mouth, unspecified

☑ Additional Character Required   *v7* Placeholder Alert   Unspecified Dx   Other Specified Dx   Manifestation   ▶◀ Revised Text   ● New Code   ▲ Revised Code Title

ICD-10-CM 2016   447

C00–C04.9

Chapter 2. Neoplasms

C05-C12

✓4ᵗʰ **C05　Malignant neoplasm of** palate
　　Use additional code to identify:
　　　alcohol abuse and dependence (F10.-)
　　　history of tobacco use (Z87.891)
　　　tobacco dependence (F17.-)
　　　tobacco use (Z72.0)
　　EXCLUDES 1　Kaposi's sarcoma of palate (C46.2)

　C05.0　Malignant neoplasm of hard **palate**

　C05.1　Malignant neoplasm of soft **palate**
　　　EXCLUDES 2　malignant neoplasm of nasopharyngeal surface of soft palate (C11.3)

　C05.2　Malignant neoplasm of uvula

　C05.8　Malignant neoplasm of overlapping sites **of palate**

　C05.9　Malignant neoplasm of palate, unspecified
　　　Malignant neoplasm of roof of mouth

✓4ᵗʰ **C06　Malignant neoplasm of** other and unspecified parts of mouth
　　Use additional code to identify:
　　　alcohol abuse and dependence (F10.-)
　　　history of tobacco use (Z87.891)
　　　tobacco dependence (F17.-)
　　　tobacco use (Z72.0)

　C06.0　Malignant neoplasm of cheek mucosa
　　　Malignant neoplasm of buccal mucosa NOS
　　　Malignant neoplasm of internal cheek

　C06.1　Malignant neoplasm of vestibule **of mouth**
　　　Malignant neoplasm of buccal sulcus (upper) (lower)
　　　Malignant neoplasm of labial sulcus (upper) (lower)

　C06.2　Malignant neoplasm of retromolar area

✓5ᵗʰ **C06.8　Malignant neoplasm of** overlapping sites of other and unspecified **parts of mouth**

　　C06.80　Malignant neoplasm of overlapping sites of unspecified parts of mouth

　　C06.89　Malignant neoplasm of overlapping sites of other parts of mouth
　　　　"book leaf" neoplasm [ventral surface of tongue and floor of mouth]

　C06.9　Malignant neoplasm of mouth, unspecified
　　　Malignant neoplasm of minor salivary gland, unspecified site
　　　Malignant neoplasm of oral cavity NOS

C07　Malignant neoplasm of parotid gland
　　Use additional code to identify:
　　　alcohol abuse and dependence (F10.-)
　　　exposure to environmental tobacco smoke (Z77.22)
　　　exposure to tobacco smoke in the perinatal period (P96.81)
　　　history of tobacco use (Z87.891)
　　　occupational exposure to environmental tobacco smoke (Z57.31)
　　　tobacco dependence (F17.-)
　　　tobacco use (Z72.0)

✓4ᵗʰ **C08　Malignant neoplasm of** other and unspecified major salivary glands
　　INCLUDES　malignant neoplasm of salivary ducts
　　Use additional code to identify:
　　　alcohol abuse and dependence (F10.-)
　　　exposure to environmental tobacco smoke (Z77.22)
　　　exposure to tobacco smoke in the perinatal period (P96.81)
　　　history of tobacco use (Z87.891)
　　　occupational exposure to environmental tobacco smoke (Z57.31)
　　　tobacco dependence (F17.-)
　　　tobacco use (Z72.0)
　　EXCLUDES 1　malignant neoplasms of specified minor salivary glands which are classified according to their anatomical location
　　EXCLUDES 2　malignant neoplasms of minor salivary glands NOS (C06.9)
　　　　malignant neoplasm of parotid gland (C07)

　C08.0　Malignant neoplasm of submandibular **gland**
　　　Malignant neoplasm of submaxillary gland

　C08.1　Malignant neoplasm of sublingual **gland**

　C08.9　Malignant neoplasm of major salivary gland**, unspecified**
　　　Malignant neoplasm of salivary gland (major) NOS

✓4ᵗʰ **C09　Malignant neoplasm of** tonsil
　　Use additional code to identify:
　　　alcohol abuse and dependence (F10.-)
　　　exposure to environmental tobacco smoke (Z77.22)
　　　exposure to tobacco smoke in the perinatal period (P96.81)
　　　history of tobacco use (Z87.891)
　　　occupational exposure to environmental tobacco smoke (Z57.31)
　　　tobacco dependence (F17.-)
　　　tobacco use (Z72.0)
　　EXCLUDES 2　malignant neoplasm of lingual tonsil (C02.4)
　　　　malignant neoplasm of pharyngeal tonsil (C11.1)

　C09.0　Malignant neoplasm of tonsillar fossa

　C09.1　Malignant neoplasm of tonsillar pillar **(anterior) (posterior)**

　C09.8　Malignant neoplasm of overlapping sites **of tonsil**

　C09.9　Malignant neoplasm of tonsil, unspecified
　　　Malignant neoplasm of tonsil NOS
　　　Malignant neoplasm of faucial tonsils
　　　Malignant neoplasm of palatine tonsils

✓4ᵗʰ **C10　Malignant neoplasm of** oropharynx
　　Use additional code to identify:
　　　alcohol abuse and dependence (F10.-)
　　　exposure to environmental tobacco smoke (Z77.22)
　　　exposure to tobacco smoke in the perinatal period (P96.81)
　　　history of tobacco use (Z87.891)
　　　occupational exposure to environmental tobacco smoke (Z57.31)
　　　tobacco dependence (F17.-)
　　　tobacco use (Z72.0)
　　EXCLUDES 2　malignant neoplasm of tonsil (C09.-)

　C10.0　Malignant neoplasm of vallecula

　C10.1　Malignant neoplasm of anterior surface of epiglottis
　　　Malignant neoplasm of epiglottis, free border [margin]
　　　Malignant neoplasm of glossoepiglottic fold(s)
　　　EXCLUDES 2　malignant neoplasm of epiglottis (suprahyoid portion) NOS (C32.1)

　C10.2　Malignant neoplasm of lateral wall **of oropharynx**

　C10.3　Malignant neoplasm of posterior wall **of oropharynx**

　C10.4　Malignant neoplasm of branchial cleft
　　　Malignant neoplasm of branchial cyst [site of neoplasm]

　C10.8　Malignant neoplasm of overlapping sites **of oropharynx**
　　　Malignant neoplasm of junctional region of oropharynx

　C10.9　Malignant neoplasm of oropharynx, unspecified

✓4ᵗʰ **C11　Malignant neoplasm of** nasopharynx
　　Use additional code to identify:
　　　exposure to environmental tobacco smoke (Z77.22)
　　　exposure to tobacco smoke in the perinatal period (P96.81)
　　　history of tobacco use (Z87.891)
　　　occupational exposure to environmental tobacco smoke (Z57.31)
　　　tobacco dependence (F17.-)
　　　tobacco use (Z72.0)

　C11.0　Malignant neoplasm of superior wall **of nasopharynx**
　　　Malignant neoplasm of roof of nasopharynx

　C11.1　Malignant neoplasm of posterior wall **of nasopharynx**
　　　Malignant neoplasm of adenoid
　　　Malignant neoplasm of pharyngeal tonsil

　C11.2　Malignant neoplasm of lateral wall **of nasopharynx**
　　　Malignant neoplasm of fossa of Rosenmüller
　　　Malignant neoplasm of opening of auditory tube
　　　Malignant neoplasm of pharyngeal recess

　C11.3　Malignant neoplasm of anterior wall **of nasopharynx**
　　　Malignant neoplasm of floor of nasopharynx
　　　Malignant neoplasm of nasopharyngeal (anterior) (posterior) surface of soft palate
　　　Malignant neoplasm of posterior margin of nasal choana
　　　Malignant neoplasm of posterior margin of nasal septum

　C11.8　Malignant neoplasm of overlapping sites **of nasopharynx**

　C11.9　Malignant neoplasm of nasopharynx, unspecified
　　　Malignant neoplasm of nasopharyngeal wall NOS

C12　Malignant neoplasm of pyriform sinus
　　　Malignant neoplasm of pyriform fossa
　　Use additional code to identify:
　　　exposure to environmental tobacco smoke (Z77.22)
　　　exposure to tobacco smoke in the perinatal period (P96.81)
　　　history of tobacco use (Z87.891)
　　　occupational exposure to environmental tobacco smoke (Z57.31)
　　　tobacco dependence (F17.-)
　　　tobacco use (Z72.0)

EXCLUDES 1 Not coded here　　　**EXCLUDES 2** Not included here　　　Ⓝ Newborn Age: 0　　　Ⓟ Pediatric Age: 0-17　　　Ⓜ Maternity Age: 12-55　　　Ⓐ Adult Age: 15-124

448　　　　　　　　　　　　　　　　　　　　　　　　　　　　　　　　　　　　　　　ICD-10-CM 2016

☑4ᵗʰ **C13 Malignant neoplasm of hypopharynx**
Use additional code to identify:
exposure to environmental tobacco smoke (Z77.22)
exposure to tobacco smoke in the perinatal period (P96.81)
history of tobacco use (Z87.891)
occupational exposure to environmental tobacco smoke (Z57.31)
tobacco dependence (F17.-)
tobacco use (Z72.0)
EXCLUDES 2   *malignant neoplasm of pyriform sinus (C12)*

C13.0 Malignant neoplasm of postcricoid region

C13.1 Malignant neoplasm of aryepiglottic fold, hypopharyngeal aspect
Malignant neoplasm of aryepiglottic fold, marginal zone
Malignant neoplasm of aryepiglottic fold NOS
Malignant neoplasm of interarytenoid fold, marginal zone
Malignant neoplasm of interarytenoid fold NOS
EXCLUDES 2   *malignant neoplasm of aryepiglottic fold or interarytenoid fold, laryngeal aspect (C32.1)*

C13.2 Malignant neoplasm of posterior wall of hypopharynx

C13.8 Malignant neoplasm of overlapping sites of hypopharynx

C13.9 Malignant neoplasm of hypopharynx, unspecified
Malignant neoplasm of hypopharyngeal wall NOS

☑4ᵗʰ **C14 Malignant neoplasm of other and ill-defined sites in the lip, oral cavity and pharynx**
Use additional code to identify:
alcohol abuse and dependence (F10.-)
exposure to environmental tobacco smoke (Z77.22)
exposure to tobacco smoke in the perinatal period (P96.81)
history of tobacco use (Z87.891)
occupational exposure to environmental tobacco smoke (Z57.31)
tobacco dependence (F17.-)
tobacco use (Z72.0)
EXCLUDES 1   *malignant neoplasm of oral cavity NOS (C06.9)*

C14.0 Malignant neoplasm of pharynx, unspecified

C14.2 Malignant neoplasm of Waldeyer's ring

C14.8 Malignant neoplasm of overlapping sites of lip, oral cavity and pharynx
Primary malignant neoplasm of two or more contiguous sites of lip, oral cavity and pharynx
EXCLUDES 1   *"book leaf" neoplasm [ventral surface of tongue and floor of mouth] (C06.89)*

Malignant neoplasms of digestive organs (C15-C26)
EXCLUDES 1   *Kaposi's sarcoma of gastrointestinal sites (C46.4)*

☑4ᵗʰ **C15 Malignant neoplasm of esophagus**
Use additional code to identify:
alcohol abuse and dependence (F10.-)

C15.3 Malignant neoplasm of upper third of esophagus

C15.4 Malignant neoplasm of middle third of esophagus

C15.5 Malignant neoplasm of lower third of esophagus
EXCLUDES 1   *malignant neoplasm of cardio-esophageal junction (C16.0)*

C15.8 Malignant neoplasm of overlapping sites of esophagus

C15.9 Malignant neoplasm of esophagus, unspecified

☑4ᵗʰ **C16 Malignant neoplasm of stomach**
Use additional code to identify:
alcohol abuse and dependence (F10.-)
EXCLUDES 2   *malignant carcinoid tumor of the stomach (C7A.092)*

C16.0 Malignant neoplasm of cardia
Malignant neoplasm of cardiac orifice
Malignant neoplasm of cardio-esophageal junction
Malignant neoplasm of esophagus and stomach
Malignant neoplasm of gastro-esophageal junction

C16.1 Malignant neoplasm of fundus of stomach

C16.2 Malignant neoplasm of body of stomach

C16.3 Malignant neoplasm of pyloric antrum
Malignant neoplasm of gastric antrum

C16.4 Malignant neoplasm of pylorus
Malignant neoplasm of prepylorus
Malignant neoplasm of pyloric canal

C16.5 Malignant neoplasm of lesser curvature of stomach, unspecified
Malignant neoplasm of lesser curvature of stomach, not classifiable to C16.1-C16.4

C16.6 Malignant neoplasm of greater curvature of stomach, unspecified
Malignant neoplasm of greater curvature of stomach, not classifiable to C16.0-C16.4

C16.8 Malignant neoplasm of overlapping sites of stomach

C16.9 Malignant neoplasm of stomach, unspecified
Gastric cancer NOS

☑4ᵗʰ **C17 Malignant neoplasm of small intestine**
EXCLUDES 1   *malignant carcinoid tumors of the small intestine (C7A.01)*

C17.0 Malignant neoplasm of duodenum

C17.1 Malignant neoplasm of jejunum

C17.2 Malignant neoplasm of ileum
EXCLUDES 1   *malignant neoplasm of ileocecal valve (C18.0)*

C17.3 Meckel's diverticulum, malignant
EXCLUDES 1   *Meckel's diverticulum, congenital (Q43.0)*

C17.8 Malignant neoplasm of overlapping sites of small intestine

C17.9 Malignant neoplasm of small intestine, unspecified

☑4ᵗʰ **C18 Malignant neoplasm of colon**
EXCLUDES 1   *malignant carcinoid tumors of the colon (C7A.02-)*

C18.0 Malignant neoplasm of cecum
Malignant neoplasm of ileocecal valve

C18.1 Malignant neoplasm of appendix

C18.2 Malignant neoplasm of ascending colon

C18.3 Malignant neoplasm of hepatic flexure

C18.4 Malignant neoplasm of transverse colon

C18.5 Malignant neoplasm of splenic flexure

C18.6 Malignant neoplasm of descending colon

C18.7 Malignant neoplasm of sigmoid colon
Malignant neoplasm of sigmoid (flexure)
EXCLUDES 1   *malignant neoplasm of rectosigmoid junction (C19)*

C18.8 Malignant neoplasm of overlapping sites of colon

C18.9 Malignant neoplasm of colon, unspecified
Malignant neoplasm of large intestine NOS

C19 Malignant neoplasm of rectosigmoid junction
Malignant neoplasm of colon with rectum
Malignant neoplasm of rectosigmoid (colon)
EXCLUDES 1   *malignant carcinoid tumors of the colon (C7A.02-)*

C20 Malignant neoplasm of rectum
Malignant neoplasm of rectal ampulla
EXCLUDES 1   *malignant carcinoid tumor of the rectum (C7A.026)*

☑4ᵗʰ **C21 Malignant neoplasm of anus and anal canal**
EXCLUDES 2   *malignant carcinoid tumors of the colon (C7A.02-)*
malignant melanoma of anal margin (C43.51)
malignant melanoma of anal skin (C43.51)
malignant melanoma of perianal skin (C43.51)
other and unspecified malignant neoplasm of anal margin (C44.500, C44.510, C44.520, C44.590)
other and unspecified malignant neoplasm of anal skin (C44.500, C44.510, C44.520, C44.590)
other and unspecified malignant neoplasm of perianal skin (C44.500, C44.510, C44.520, C44.590)

C21.0 Malignant neoplasm of anus, unspecified

C21.1 Malignant neoplasm of anal canal
Malignant neoplasm of anal sphincter

C21.2 Malignant neoplasm of cloacogenic zone

C21.8 Malignant neoplasm of overlapping sites of rectum, anus and anal canal
Malignant neoplasm of anorectal junction
Malignant neoplasm of anorectum
Primary malignant neoplasm of two or more contiguous sites of rectum, anus and anal canal

☑4ᵗʰ **C22 Malignant neoplasm of liver and intrahepatic bile ducts**
Use additional code to identify:
alcohol abuse and dependence (F10.-)
hepatitis B (B16.-, B18.0-B18.1)
hepatitis C (B17.1-, B18.2)
EXCLUDES 1   *malignant neoplasm of biliary tract NOS (C24.9)*
secondary malignant neoplasm of liver and intrahepatic bile duct (C78.7)

C22.0 Liver cell carcinoma
Hepatocellular carcinoma
Hepatoma

C22.1 Intrahepatic bile duct carcinoma
Cholangiocarcinoma
EXCLUDES 1   *malignant neoplasm of hepatic duct (C24.0)*

C22.2 Hepatoblastoma

C22.3 Angiosarcoma of liver
Kupffer cell sarcoma

C22.4 Other sarcomas of liver

☑ Additional Character Required   ☑x7ᵗʰ Placeholder Alert   Unspecified Dx   Other Specified Dx   Manifestation   ►◄ Revised Text   ● New Code   ▲ Revised Code Title

Chapter 2. Neoplasms

C22.7-C34.Ø1

C22.7 Other specified carcinomas of liver

C22.8 Malignant neoplasm of liver, primary, unspecified as to type

C22.9 Malignant neoplasm of liver, not specified as primary or secondary

C23 Malignant neoplasm of gallbladder

✓4ᵗʰ **C24** Malignant neoplasm of other and unspecified parts of biliary tract
> EXCLUDES 1   malignant neoplasm of intrahepatic bile duct (C22.1)

C24.Ø Malignant neoplasm of extrahepatic bile duct
Malignant neoplasm of biliary duct or passage NOS
Malignant neoplasm of common bile duct
Malignant neoplasm of cystic duct
Malignant neoplasm of hepatic duct

C24.1 Malignant neoplasm of ampulla of Vater

C24.8 Malignant neoplasm of overlapping sites of biliary tract
Malignant neoplasm involving both intrahepatic and extrahepatic bile ducts
Primary malignant neoplasm of two or more contiguous sites of biliary tract

C24.9 Malignant neoplasm of biliary tract, unspecified

✓4ᵗʰ **C25** Malignant neoplasm of pancreas
Use additional code to identify:
   alcohol abuse and dependence (F1Ø.-)

C25.Ø Malignant neoplasm of head of pancreas

C25.1 Malignant neoplasm of body of pancreas

C25.2 Malignant neoplasm of tail of pancreas

C25.3 Malignant neoplasm of pancreatic duct

C25.4 Malignant neoplasm of endocrine pancreas
Malignant neoplasm of islets of Langerhans
Use additional code to identify any functional activity

C25.7 Malignant neoplasm of other parts of pancreas
Malignant neoplasm of neck of pancreas

C25.8 Malignant neoplasm of overlapping sites of pancreas

C25.9 Malignant neoplasm of pancreas, unspecified

✓4ᵗʰ **C26** Malignant neoplasm of other and ill-defined digestive organs
> EXCLUDES 1   malignant neoplasm of peritoneum and retroperitoneum (C48.-)

C26.Ø Malignant neoplasm of intestinal tract, part unspecified
Malignant neoplasm of intestine NOS

C26.1 Malignant neoplasm of spleen
> EXCLUDES 1   Hodgkin lymphoma (C81.-)
> non-Hodgkin lymphoma (C82-C85)

C26.9 Malignant neoplasm of ill-defined sites within the digestive system
Malignant neoplasm of alimentary canal or tract NOS
Malignant neoplasm of gastrointestinal tract NOS
> EXCLUDES 1   malignant neoplasm of abdominal NOS (C76.2)
> malignant neoplasm of intra-abdominal NOS (C76.2)

Malignant neoplasms of respiratory and intrathoracic organs (C3Ø-C39)

> INCLUDES   malignant neoplasm of middle ear
> EXCLUDES 1   mesothelioma (C45.-)

✓4ᵗʰ **C3Ø** Malignant neoplasm of nasal cavity and middle ear

C3Ø.Ø Malignant neoplasm of nasal cavity
Malignant neoplasm of cartilage of nose
Malignant neoplasm of nasal concha
Malignant neoplasm of internal nose
Malignant neoplasm of septum of nose
Malignant neoplasm of vestibule of nose
> EXCLUDES 1   malignant melanoma of skin of nose (C43.31)
> malignant neoplasm of nasal bone (C41.Ø)
> malignant neoplasm of nose NOS (C76.Ø)
> malignant neoplasm of olfactory bulb (C72.2-)
> malignant neoplasm of posterior margin of nasal septum and choana (C11.3)
> malignant neoplasm of turbinates (C41.Ø)
> other and unspecified malignant neoplasm of skin of nose (C44.3Ø1, C44.311, C44.321, C44.391)

C3Ø.1 Malignant neoplasm of middle ear
Malignant neoplasm of antrum tympanicum
Malignant neoplasm of auditory tube
Malignant neoplasm of eustachian tube
Malignant neoplasm of inner ear
Malignant neoplasm of mastoid air cells
Malignant neoplasm of tympanic cavity
> EXCLUDES 1   malignant melanoma of skin of (external) ear (C43.2-)
> malignant neoplasm of auricular canal (external) (C43.2-,C44.2-)
> malignant neoplasm of bone of ear (meatus) (C41.Ø)
> malignant neoplasm of cartilage of ear (C49.Ø)
> other and unspecified malignant neoplasm of skin of (external) ear (C44.2-)

✓4ᵗʰ **C31** Malignant neoplasm of accessory sinuses

C31.Ø Malignant neoplasm of maxillary sinus
Malignant neoplasm of antrum (Highmore) (maxillary)

C31.1 Malignant neoplasm of ethmoidal sinus

C31.2 Malignant neoplasm of frontal sinus

C31.3 Malignant neoplasm of sphenoid sinus

C31.8 Malignant neoplasm of overlapping sites of accessory sinuses

C31.9 Malignant neoplasm of accessory sinus, unspecified

✓4ᵗʰ **C32** Malignant neoplasm of larynx
Use additional code to identify:
   alcohol abuse and dependence (F1Ø.-)
   exposure to environmental tobacco smoke (Z77.22)
   exposure to tobacco smoke in the perinatal period (P96.81)
   history of tobacco use (Z87.891)
   occupational exposure to environmental tobacco smoke (Z57.31)
   tobacco dependence (F17.-)
   tobacco use (Z72.Ø)

C32.Ø Malignant neoplasm of glottis
Malignant neoplasm of intrinsic larynx
Malignant neoplasm of laryngeal commissure (anterior)(posterior)
Malignant neoplasm of vocal cord (true) NOS

C32.1 Malignant neoplasm of supraglottis
Malignant neoplasm of aryepiglottic fold or interarytenoid fold, laryngeal aspect
Malignant neoplasm of epiglottis (suprahyoid portion) NOS
Malignant neoplasm of extrinsic larynx
Malignant neoplasm of false vocal cord
Malignant neoplasm of posterior (laryngeal) surface of epiglottis
Malignant neoplasm of ventricular bands
> EXCLUDES 2   malignant neoplasm of anterior surface of epiglottis (C1Ø.1)
> malignant neoplasm of aryepiglottic fold or interarytenoid fold, hypopharyngeal aspect (C13.1)
> malignant neoplasm of aryepiglottic fold or interarytenoid fold, marginal zone (C13.1)
> malignant neoplasm of aryepiglottic fold or interarytenoid fold NOS (C13.1)

C32.2 Malignant neoplasm of subglottis

C32.3 Malignant neoplasm of laryngeal cartilage

C32.8 Malignant neoplasm of overlapping sites of larynx

C32.9 Malignant neoplasm of larynx, unspecified

C33 Malignant neoplasm of trachea
Use additional code to identify:
   exposure to environmental tobacco smoke (Z77.22)
   exposure to tobacco smoke in the perinatal period (P96.81)
   history of tobacco use (Z87.891)
   occupational exposure to environmental tobacco smoke (Z57.31)
   tobacco dependence (F17.-)
   tobacco use (Z72.Ø)

✓4ᵗʰ **C34** Malignant neoplasm of bronchus and lung
Use additional code to identify:
   exposure to environmental tobacco smoke (Z77.22)
   exposure to tobacco smoke in the perinatal period (P96.81)
   history of tobacco use (Z87.891)
   occupational exposure to environmental tobacco smoke (Z57.31)
   tobacco dependence (F17.-)
   tobacco use (Z72.Ø)
> EXCLUDES 1   Kaposi's sarcoma of lung (C46.5-)
> malignant carcinoid tumor of the bronchus and lung (C7A.Ø9Ø)

✓5ᵗʰ **C34.Ø** Malignant neoplasm of main bronchus
Malignant neoplasm of carina
Malignant neoplasm of hilus (of lung)

C34.ØØ Malignant neoplasm of unspecified main bronchus

C34.Ø1 Malignant neoplasm of right main bronchus

EXCLUDES 1 Not coded here   EXCLUDES 2 Not included here   N Newborn Age: 0   P Pediatric Age: 0-17   M Maternity Age: 12-55   A Adult Age: 15-124

450   ICD-10-CM 2016

     C34.02   Malignant neoplasm of left main bronchus

✓5ᵗʰ C34.1   Malignant neoplasm of upper lobe, bronchus or lung

     C34.10   Malignant neoplasm of upper lobe, unspecified bronchus or lung

     C34.11   Malignant neoplasm of upper lobe, right bronchus or lung

     C34.12   Malignant neoplasm of upper lobe, left bronchus or lung

   C34.2   Malignant neoplasm of middle lobe, bronchus or lung

✓5ᵗʰ C34.3   Malignant neoplasm of lower lobe, bronchus or lung

     C34.30   Malignant neoplasm of lower lobe, unspecified bronchus or lung

     C34.31   Malignant neoplasm of lower lobe, right bronchus or lung

     C34.32   Malignant neoplasm of lower lobe, left bronchus or lung

✓5ᵗʰ C34.8   Malignant neoplasm of overlapping sites of bronchus and lung

     C34.80   Malignant neoplasm of overlapping sites of unspecified bronchus and lung

     C34.81   Malignant neoplasm of overlapping sites of right bronchus and lung

     C34.82   Malignant neoplasm of overlapping sites of left bronchus and lung

✓5ᵗʰ C34.9   Malignant neoplasm of unspecified part of bronchus or lung

     C34.90   Malignant neoplasm of unspecified part of unspecified bronchus or lung

       Lung cancer NOS

     C34.91   Malignant neoplasm of unspecified part of right bronchus or lung

     C34.92   Malignant neoplasm of unspecified part of left bronchus or lung

C37   **Malignant neoplasm of thymus**

    EXCLUDES 1   malignant carcinoid tumor of the thymus (C7A.091)

✓4ᵗʰ C38   **Malignant neoplasm of heart, mediastinum and pleura**

    EXCLUDES 1   mesothelioma (C45.-)

   C38.0   Malignant neoplasm of heart

      Malignant neoplasm of pericardium

     EXCLUDES 1   malignant neoplasm of great vessels (C49.3)

   C38.1   Malignant neoplasm of anterior mediastinum

   C38.2   Malignant neoplasm of posterior mediastinum

   C38.3   Malignant neoplasm of mediastinum, part unspecified

   C38.4   Malignant neoplasm of pleura

   C38.8   Malignant neoplasm of overlapping sites of heart, mediastinum and pleura

✓4ᵗʰ C39   **Malignant neoplasm of other and ill-defined sites in the respiratory system and intrathoracic organs**

     Use additional code to identify:

      exposure to environmental tobacco smoke (Z77.22)

      exposure to tobacco smoke in the perinatal period (P96.81)

      history of tobacco use (Z87.891)

      occupational exposure to environmental tobacco smoke (Z57.31)

      tobacco dependence (F17.-)

      tobacco use (Z72.0)

     EXCLUDES 1   intrathoracic malignant neoplasm NOS (C76.1)

         thoracic malignant neoplasm NOS (C76.1)

   C39.0   Malignant neoplasm of upper respiratory tract, part unspecified

   C39.9   Malignant neoplasm of lower respiratory tract, part unspecified

      Malignant neoplasm of respiratory tract NOS

Malignant neoplasms of bone and articular cartilage (C40–C41)

   INCLUDES   malignant neoplasm of cartilage (articular) (joint)

         malignant neoplasm of periosteum

   EXCLUDES 1   malignant neoplasm of bone marrow NOS (C96.9)

         malignant neoplasm of synovia (C49.-)

✓4ᵗʰ C40   **Malignant neoplasm of bone and articular cartilage of limbs**

     Use additional code to identify major osseous defect, if applicable (M89.7-)

✓5ᵗʰ C40.0   Malignant neoplasm of scapula and long bones of upper limb

     C40.00   Malignant neoplasm of scapula and long bones of unspecified upper limb

     C40.01   Malignant neoplasm of scapula and long bones of right upper limb

     C40.02   Malignant neoplasm of scapula and long bones of left upper limb

✓5ᵗʰ C40.1   Malignant neoplasm of short bones of upper limb

     C40.10   Malignant neoplasm of short bones of unspecified upper limb

     C40.11   Malignant neoplasm of short bones of right upper limb

     C40.12   Malignant neoplasm of short bones of left upper limb

✓5ᵗʰ C40.2   Malignant neoplasm of long bones of lower limb

     C40.20   Malignant neoplasm of long bones of unspecified lower limb

     C40.21   Malignant neoplasm of long bones of right lower limb

     C40.22   Malignant neoplasm of long bones of left lower limb

✓5ᵗʰ C40.3   Malignant neoplasm of short bones of lower limb

     C40.30   Malignant neoplasm of short bones of unspecified lower limb

     C40.31   Malignant neoplasm of short bones of right lower limb

     C40.32   Malignant neoplasm of short bones of left lower limb

✓5ᵗʰ C40.8   Malignant neoplasm of overlapping sites of bone and articular cartilage of limb

     C40.80   Malignant neoplasm of overlapping sites of bone and articular cartilage of unspecified limb

     C40.81   Malignant neoplasm of overlapping sites of bone and articular cartilage of right limb

     C40.82   Malignant neoplasm of overlapping sites of bone and articular cartilage of left limb

✓5ᵗʰ C40.9   Malignant neoplasm of unspecified bones and articular cartilage of limb

     C40.90   Malignant neoplasm of unspecified bones and articular cartilage of unspecified limb

     C40.91   Malignant neoplasm of unspecified bones and articular cartilage of right limb

     C40.92   Malignant neoplasm of unspecified bones and articular cartilage of left limb

✓4ᵗʰ C41   **Malignant neoplasm of bone and articular cartilage of other and unspecified sites**

     EXCLUDES 1   malignant neoplasm of bones of limbs (C40.-)

         malignant neoplasm of cartilage of ear (C49.0)

         malignant neoplasm of cartilage of eyelid (C49.0)

         malignant neoplasm of cartilage of larynx (C32.3)

         malignant neoplasm of cartilage of limbs (C40.-)

         malignant neoplasm of cartilage of nose (C30.0)

   C41.0   Malignant neoplasm of bones of skull and face

      Malignant neoplasm of maxilla (superior)

      Malignant neoplasm of orbital bone

     EXCLUDES 2   carcinoma, any type except intraosseous or odontogenic of:

         maxillary sinus (C31.0)

         upper jaw (C03.0)

         malignant neoplasm of jaw bone (lower) (C41.1)

   C41.1   Malignant neoplasm of mandible

      Malignant neoplasm of inferior maxilla

      Malignant neoplasm of lower jaw bone

     EXCLUDES 2   carcinoma, any type except intraosseous or odontogenic of:

         jaw NOS (C03.9)

         lower (C03.1)

         malignant neoplasm of upper jaw bone (C41.0)

   C41.2   Malignant neoplasm of vertebral column

     EXCLUDES 1   malignant neoplasm of sacrum and coccyx (C41.4)

   C41.3   Malignant neoplasm of ribs, sternum and clavicle

   C41.4   Malignant neoplasm of pelvic bones, sacrum and coccyx

   C41.9   Malignant neoplasm of bone and articular cartilage, unspecified

Chapter 2. Neoplasms

Melanoma and other malignant neoplasms of skin (C43-C44)

✓4ᵗʰ C43   Malignant melanoma of skin

> **EXCLUDES 1**   melanoma in situ (D03.-)
> **EXCLUDES 2**   malignant melanoma of skin of genital organs (C51-C52, C60.-, C63.-)
> Merkel cell carcinoma (C4A.-)
> sites other than skin—code to malignant neoplasm of the site

C43.0   Malignant melanoma of lip

> **EXCLUDES 1**   malignant neoplasm of vermilion border of lip (C00.0-C00.2)

✓5ᵗʰ C43.1   Malignant melanoma of eyelid, including canthus

     C43.10   Malignant melanoma of unspecified eyelid, including canthus

     C43.11   Malignant melanoma of right eyelid, including canthus

     C43.12   Malignant melanoma of left eyelid, including canthus

✓5ᵗʰ C43.2   Malignant melanoma of ear and external auricular canal

     C43.20   Malignant melanoma of unspecified ear and external auricular canal

     C43.21   Malignant melanoma of right ear and external auricular canal

     C43.22   Malignant melanoma of left ear and external auricular canal

✓5ᵗʰ C43.3   Malignant melanoma of other and unspecified parts of face

     C43.30   Malignant melanoma of unspecified part of face

     C43.31   Malignant melanoma of nose

     C43.39   Malignant melanoma of other parts of face

C43.4   Malignant melanoma of scalp and neck

✓5ᵗʰ C43.5   Malignant melanoma of trunk

> **EXCLUDES 2**   malignant neoplasm of anus NOS (C21.0)
> malignant neoplasm of scrotum (C63.2)

     C43.51   Malignant melanoma of anal skin
         Malignant melanoma of anal margin
         Malignant melanoma of perianal skin

     C43.52   Malignant melanoma of skin of breast

     C43.59   Malignant melanoma of other part of trunk

✓5ᵗʰ C43.6   Malignant melanoma of upper limb, including shoulder

     C43.60   Malignant melanoma of unspecified upper limb, including shoulder

     C43.61   Malignant melanoma of right upper limb, including shoulder

     C43.62   Malignant melanoma of left upper limb, including shoulder

✓5ᵗʰ C43.7   Malignant melanoma of lower limb, including hip

     C43.70   Malignant melanoma of unspecified lower limb, including hip

     C43.71   Malignant melanoma of right lower limb, including hip

     C43.72   Malignant melanoma of left lower limb, including hip

C43.8   Malignant melanoma of overlapping sites of skin

C43.9   Malignant melanoma of skin, unspecified
     Malignant melanoma of unspecified site of skin

✓4ᵗʰ C4A   Merkel cell carcinoma

C4A.0   Merkel cell carcinoma of lip

> **EXCLUDES 1**   malignant neoplasm of vermilion border of lip (C00.0-C00.2)

✓5ᵗʰ C4A.1   Merkel cell carcinoma of eyelid, including canthus

     C4A.10   Merkel cell carcinoma of unspecified eyelid, including canthus

     C4A.11   Merkel cell carcinoma of right eyelid, including canthus

     C4A.12   Merkel cell carcinoma of left eyelid, including canthus

✓5ᵗʰ C4A.2   Merkel cell carcinoma of ear and external auricular canal

     C4A.20   Merkel cell carcinoma of unspecified ear and external auricular canal

     C4A.21   Merkel cell carcinoma of right ear and external auricular canal

     C4A.22   Merkel cell carcinoma of left ear and external auricular canal

✓5ᵗʰ C4A.3   Merkel cell carcinoma of other and unspecified parts of face

     C4A.30   Merkel cell carcinoma of unspecified part of face

     C4A.31   Merkel cell carcinoma of nose

     C4A.39   Merkel cell carcinoma of other parts of face

C4A.4   Merkel cell carcinoma of scalp and neck

✓5ᵗʰ C4A.5   Merkel cell carcinoma of trunk

> **EXCLUDES 2**   malignant neoplasm of anus NOS (C21.0)
> malignant neoplasm of scrotum (C63.2)

     C4A.51   Merkel cell carcinoma of anal skin
         Merkel cell carcinoma of anal margin
         Merkel cell carcinoma of perianal skin

     C4A.52   Merkel cell carcinoma of skin of breast

     C4A.59   Merkel cell carcinoma of other part of trunk

✓5ᵗʰ C4A.6   Merkel cell carcinoma of upper limb, including shoulder

     C4A.60   Merkel cell carcinoma of unspecified upper limb, including shoulder

     C4A.61   Merkel cell carcinoma of right upper limb, including shoulder

     C4A.62   Merkel cell carcinoma of left upper limb, including shoulder

✓5ᵗʰ C4A.7   Merkel cell carcinoma of lower limb, including hip

     C4A.70   Merkel cell carcinoma of unspecified lower limb, including hip

     C4A.71   Merkel cell carcinoma of right lower limb, including hip

     C4A.72   Merkel cell carcinoma of left lower limb, including hip

C4A.8   Merkel cell carcinoma of overlapping sites

C4A.9   Merkel cell carcinoma, unspecified
     Merkel cell carcinoma of unspecified site

✓4ᵗʰ C44   Other and unspecified malignant neoplasm of skin

> **INCLUDES**   malignant neoplasm of sebaceous glands
> malignant neoplasm of sweat glands
> **EXCLUDES 1**   Kaposi's sarcoma of skin (C46.0)
> malignant melanoma of skin (C43.-)
> malignant neoplasm of skin of genital organs (C51-C52, C60-, C63.2)
> Merkel cell carcinoma (C4A.-)

✓5ᵗʰ C44.0   Other and unspecified malignant neoplasm of skin of lip

> **EXCLUDES 1**   malignant neoplasm of lip (C00.-)

     C44.00   Unspecified malignant neoplasm of skin of lip

     C44.01   Basal cell carcinoma of skin of lip

     C44.02   Squamous cell carcinoma of skin of lip

     C44.09   Other specified malignant neoplasm of skin of lip

✓5ᵗʰ C44.1   Other and unspecified malignant neoplasm of skin of eyelid, including canthus

> **EXCLUDES 1**   connective tissue of eyelid (C49.0)

     ✓6ᵗʰ C44.10   Unspecified malignant neoplasm of skin of eyelid, including canthus

         C44.101   Unspecified malignant neoplasm of skin of unspecified eyelid, including canthus

         C44.102   Unspecified malignant neoplasm of skin of right eyelid, including canthus

         C44.109   Unspecified malignant neoplasm of skin of left eyelid, including canthus

     ✓6ᵗʰ C44.11   Basal cell carcinoma of skin of eyelid, including canthus

         C44.111   Basal cell carcinoma of skin of unspecified eyelid, including canthus

         C44.112   Basal cell carcinoma of skin of right eyelid, including canthus

         C44.119   Basal cell carcinoma of skin of left eyelid, including canthus

     ✓6ᵗʰ C44.12   Squamous cell carcinoma of skin of eyelid, including canthus

         C44.121   Squamous cell carcinoma of skin of unspecified eyelid, including canthus

         C44.122   Squamous cell carcinoma of skin of right eyelid, including canthus

         C44.129   Squamous cell carcinoma of skin of left eyelid, including canthus

     ✓6ᵗʰ C44.19   Other specified malignant neoplasm of skin of eyelid, including canthus

         C44.191   Other specified malignant neoplasm of skin of unspecified eyelid, including canthus

         C44.192   Other specified malignant neoplasm of skin of right eyelid, including canthus

---

EXCLUDES 1 Not coded here   **EXCLUDES 2** Not included here   **N** Newborn Age: 0   **P** Pediatric Age: 0-17   **M** Maternity Age: 12-55   **A** Adult Age: 15-124

452   ICD-10-CM 2016

C44.199 Other specified malignant neoplasm of skin of left eyelid, including canthus

✓5ᵗʰ **C44.2 Other and unspecified malignant neoplasm of skin of ear and external auricular canal**
    EXCLUDES 1   connective tissue of ear (C49.0)

✓6ᵗʰ **C44.20** Unspecified malignant neoplasm of skin of ear and external auricular canal

C44.201 Unspecified malignant neoplasm of skin of unspecified ear and external auricular canal

C44.202 Unspecified malignant neoplasm of skin of right ear and external auricular canal

C44.209 Unspecified malignant neoplasm of skin of left ear and external auricular canal

✓6ᵗʰ **C44.21** Basal cell carcinoma of skin of ear and external auricular canal

C44.211 Basal cell carcinoma of skin of unspecified ear and external auricular canal

C44.212 Basal cell carcinoma of skin of right ear and external auricular canal

C44.219 Basal cell carcinoma of skin of left ear and external auricular canal

✓6ᵗʰ **C44.22** Squamous cell carcinoma of skin of ear and external auricular canal

C44.221 Squamous cell carcinoma of skin of unspecified ear and external auricular canal

C44.222 Squamous cell carcinoma of skin of right ear and external auricular canal

C44.229 Squamous cell carcinoma of skin of left ear and external auricular canal

✓6ᵗʰ **C44.29** Other specified malignant neoplasm of skin of ear and external auricular canal

C44.291 Other specified malignant neoplasm of skin of unspecified ear and external auricular canal

C44.292 Other specified malignant neoplasm of skin of right ear and external auricular canal

C44.299 Other specified malignant neoplasm of skin of left ear and external auricular canal

✓5ᵗʰ **C44.3 Other and unspecified malignant neoplasm of skin of other and unspecified parts of face**

✓6ᵗʰ **C44.30** Unspecified malignant neoplasm of skin of other and unspecified parts of face

C44.300 Unspecified malignant neoplasm of skin of unspecified part of face

C44.301 Unspecified malignant neoplasm of skin of nose

C44.309 Unspecified malignant neoplasm of skin of other parts of face

✓6ᵗʰ **C44.31** Basal cell carcinoma of skin of other and unspecified parts of face

C44.310 Basal cell carcinoma of skin of unspecified parts of face

C44.311 Basal cell carcinoma of skin of nose

C44.319 Basal cell carcinoma of skin of other parts of face

✓6ᵗʰ **C44.32** Squamous cell carcinoma of skin of other and unspecified parts of face

C44.320 Squamous cell carcinoma of skin of unspecified parts of face

C44.321 Squamous cell carcinoma of skin of nose

C44.329 Squamous cell carcinoma of skin of other parts of face

✓6ᵗʰ **C44.39** Other specified malignant neoplasm of skin of other and unspecified parts of face

C44.390 Other specified malignant neoplasm of skin of unspecified parts of face

C44.391 Other specified malignant neoplasm of skin of nose

C44.399 Other specified malignant neoplasm of skin of other parts of face

✓5ᵗʰ **C44.4 Other and unspecified malignant neoplasm of skin of scalp and neck**

C44.40 Unspecified malignant neoplasm of skin of scalp and neck

C44.41 Basal cell carcinoma of skin of scalp and neck

C44.42 Squamous cell carcinoma of skin of scalp and neck

C44.49 Other specified malignant neoplasm of skin of scalp and neck

✓5ᵗʰ **C44.5 Other and unspecified malignant neoplasm of skin of trunk**
    EXCLUDES 1   anus NOS (C21.0)
                 scrotum (C63.2)

✓6ᵗʰ **C44.50** Unspecified malignant neoplasm of skin of trunk

C44.500 Unspecified malignant neoplasm of anal skin
    Unspecified malignant neoplasm of anal margin
    Unspecified malignant neoplasm of perianal skin

C44.501 Unspecified malignant neoplasm of skin of breast

C44.509 Unspecified malignant neoplasm of skin of other part of trunk

✓6ᵗʰ **C44.51** Basal cell carcinoma of skin of trunk

C44.510 Basal cell carcinoma of anal skin
    Basal cell carcinoma of anal margin
    Basal cell carcinoma of perianal skin

C44.511 Basal cell carcinoma of skin of breast

C44.519 Basal cell carcinoma of skin of other part of trunk

✓6ᵗʰ **C44.52** Squamous cell carcinoma of skin of trunk

C44.520 Squamous cell carcinoma of anal skin
    Squamous cell carcinoma of anal margin
    Squamous cell carcinoma of perianal skin

C44.521 Squamous cell carcinoma of skin of breast

C44.529 Squamous cell carcinoma of skin of other part of trunk

✓6ᵗʰ **C44.59** Other specified malignant neoplasm of skin of trunk

C44.590 Other specified malignant neoplasm of anal skin
    Other specified malignant neoplasm of anal margin
    Other specified malignant neoplasm of perianal skin

C44.591 Other specified malignant neoplasm of skin of breast

C44.599 Other specified malignant neoplasm of skin of other part of trunk

✓5ᵗʰ **C44.6 Other and unspecified malignant neoplasm of skin of upper limb, including shoulder**

✓6ᵗʰ **C44.60** Unspecified malignant neoplasm of skin of upper limb, including shoulder

C44.601 Unspecified malignant neoplasm of skin of unspecified upper limb, including shoulder

C44.602 Unspecified malignant neoplasm of skin of right upper limb, including shoulder

C44.609 Unspecified malignant neoplasm of skin of left upper limb, including shoulder

✓6ᵗʰ **C44.61** Basal cell carcinoma of skin of upper limb, including shoulder

C44.611 Basal cell carcinoma of skin of unspecified upper limb, including shoulder

C44.612 Basal cell carcinoma of skin of right upper limb, including shoulder

C44.619 Basal cell carcinoma of skin of left upper limb, including shoulder

✓6ᵗʰ **C44.62** Squamous cell carcinoma of skin of upper limb, including shoulder

C44.621 Squamous cell carcinoma of skin of unspecified upper limb, including shoulder

C44.622 Squamous cell carcinoma of skin of right upper limb, including shoulder

C44.629 Squamous cell carcinoma of skin of left upper limb, including shoulder

✓6ᵗʰ **C44.69** Other specified malignant neoplasm of skin of upper limb, including shoulder

C44.691 Other specified malignant neoplasm of skin of unspecified upper limb, including shoulder

C44.692 Other specified malignant neoplasm of skin of right upper limb, including shoulder

---

☑ Additional Character Required   ✓x7ᵗʰ Placeholder Alert   Unspecified Dx   Other Specified Dx   Manifestation   ►◄ Revised Text   ● New Code   ▲ Revised Code Title

ICD-10-CM 2016   453

C44.199–C44.692

C44.699 Other specified malignant neoplasm of skin of left upper limb, including shoulder

✓5ᵗʰ **C44.7** Other and unspecified malignant neoplasm of skin of lower limb, including hip

  ✓6ᵗʰ **C44.70** Unspecified malignant neoplasm of skin of lower limb, including hip

    C44.701 Unspecified malignant neoplasm of skin of unspecified lower limb, including hip

    C44.702 Unspecified malignant neoplasm of skin of right lower limb, including hip

    C44.709 Unspecified malignant neoplasm of skin of left lower limb, including hip

  ✓6ᵗʰ **C44.71** Basal cell carcinoma of skin of lower limb, including hip

    C44.711 Basal cell carcinoma of skin of unspecified lower limb, including hip

    C44.712 Basal cell carcinoma of skin of right lower limb, including hip

    C44.719 Basal cell carcinoma of skin of left lower limb, including hip

  ✓6ᵗʰ **C44.72** Squamous cell carcinoma of skin of lower limb, including hip

    C44.721 Squamous cell carcinoma of skin of unspecified lower limb, including hip

    C44.722 Squamous cell carcinoma of skin of right lower limb, including hip

    C44.729 Squamous cell carcinoma of skin of left lower limb, including hip

  ✓6ᵗʰ **C44.79** Other specified malignant neoplasm of skin of lower limb, including hip

    C44.791 Other specified malignant neoplasm of skin of unspecified lower limb, including hip

    C44.792 Other specified malignant neoplasm of skin of right lower limb, including hip

    C44.799 Other specified malignant neoplasm of skin of left lower limb, including hip

✓5ᵗʰ **C44.8** Other and unspecified malignant neoplasm of overlapping sites of skin

  C44.80 Unspecified malignant neoplasm of overlapping sites of skin

  C44.81 Basal cell carcinoma of overlapping sites of skin

  C44.82 Squamous cell carcinoma of overlapping sites of skin

  C44.89 Other specified malignant neoplasm of overlapping sites of skin

✓5ᵗʰ **C44.9** Other and unspecified malignant neoplasm of skin, unspecified

  C44.90 Unspecified malignant neoplasm of skin, unspecified

    Malignant neoplasm of unspecified site of skin

  C44.91 Basal cell carcinoma of skin, unspecified

  C44.92 Squamous cell carcinoma of skin, unspecified

  C44.99 Other specified malignant neoplasm of skin, unspecified

Malignant neoplasms of mesothelial and soft tissue (C45-C49)

✓4ᵗʰ **C45** Mesothelioma

  C45.0 Mesothelioma of pleura

    EXCLUDES 1 other malignant neoplasm of pleura (C38.4)

  C45.1 Mesothelioma of peritoneum

    Mesothelioma of cul-de-sac

    Mesothelioma of mesentery

    Mesothelioma of mesocolon

    Mesothelioma of omentum

    Mesothelioma of peritoneum (parietal) (pelvic)

    EXCLUDES 1 other malignant neoplasm of soft tissue of peritoneum (C48.-)

  C45.2 Mesothelioma of pericardium

    EXCLUDES 1 other malignant neoplasm of pericardium (C38.0)

  C45.7 Mesothelioma of other sites

  C45.9 Mesothelioma, unspecified

✓4ᵗʰ **C46** Kaposi's sarcoma

  Code first any human immunodeficiency virus [HIV] disease (B20)

  C46.0 Kaposi's sarcoma of skin

  C46.1 Kaposi's sarcoma of soft tissue

    Kaposi's sarcoma of blood vessel

    Kaposi's sarcoma of connective tissue

    Kaposi's sarcoma of fascia

    Kaposi's sarcoma of ligament

    Kaposi's sarcoma of lymphatic(s) NEC

    Kaposi's sarcoma of muscle

    EXCLUDES 2 Kaposi's sarcoma of lymph glands and nodes (C46.3)

  C46.2 Kaposi's sarcoma of palate

  C46.3 Kaposi's sarcoma of lymph nodes

  C46.4 Kaposi's sarcoma of gastrointestinal sites

  ✓5ᵗʰ **C46.5** Kaposi's sarcoma of lung

    C46.50 Kaposi's sarcoma of unspecified lung

    C46.51 Kaposi's sarcoma of right lung

    C46.52 Kaposi's sarcoma of left lung

  C46.7 Kaposi's sarcoma of other sites

  C46.9 Kaposi's sarcoma, unspecified

    Kaposi's sarcoma of unspecified site

✓4ᵗʰ **C47** Malignant neoplasm of peripheral nerves and autonomic nervous system

  INCLUDES malignant neoplasm of sympathetic and parasympathetic nerves and ganglia

  EXCLUDES 1 Kaposi's sarcoma of soft tissue (C46.1)

  C47.0 Malignant neoplasm of peripheral nerves of head, face and neck

    EXCLUDES 1 malignant neoplasm of peripheral nerves of orbit (C69.6-)

  ✓5ᵗʰ **C47.1** Malignant neoplasm of peripheral nerves of upper limb, including shoulder

    C47.10 Malignant neoplasm of peripheral nerves of unspecified upper limb, including shoulder

    C47.11 Malignant neoplasm of peripheral nerves of right upper limb, including shoulder

    C47.12 Malignant neoplasm of peripheral nerves of left upper limb, including shoulder

  ✓5ᵗʰ **C47.2** Malignant neoplasm of peripheral nerves of lower limb, including hip

    C47.20 Malignant neoplasm of peripheral nerves of unspecified lower limb, including hip

    C47.21 Malignant neoplasm of peripheral nerves of right lower limb, including hip

    C47.22 Malignant neoplasm of peripheral nerves of left lower limb, including hip

  C47.3 Malignant neoplasm of peripheral nerves of thorax

  C47.4 Malignant neoplasm of peripheral nerves of abdomen

  C47.5 Malignant neoplasm of peripheral nerves of pelvis

  C47.6 Malignant neoplasm of peripheral nerves of trunk, unspecified

    Malignant neoplasm of peripheral nerves of unspecified part of trunk

  C47.8 Malignant neoplasm of overlapping sites of peripheral nerves and autonomic nervous system

  C47.9 Malignant neoplasm of peripheral nerves and autonomic nervous system, unspecified

    Malignant neoplasm of unspecified site of peripheral nerves and autonomic nervous system

✓4ᵗʰ **C48** Malignant neoplasm of retroperitoneum and peritoneum

  EXCLUDES 1 Kaposi's sarcoma of connective tissue (C46.1)

    mesothelioma (C45.-)

  C48.0 Malignant neoplasm of retroperitoneum

  C48.1 Malignant neoplasm of specified parts of peritoneum

    Malignant neoplasm of cul-de-sac

    Malignant neoplasm of mesentery

    Malignant neoplasm of mesocolon

    Malignant neoplasm of omentum

    Malignant neoplasm of parietal peritoneum

    Malignant neoplasm of pelvic peritoneum

  C48.2 Malignant neoplasm of peritoneum, unspecified

  C48.8 Malignant neoplasm of overlapping sites of retroperitoneum and peritoneum

EXCLUDES 1 Not coded here   *EXCLUDES 2* Not included here   N Newborn Age: 0   P Pediatric Age: 0-17   M Maternity Age: 12-55   A Adult Age: 15-124

454

ICD-10-CM 2016

☑4ᵗʰ **C49　Malignant neoplasm of** other connective and soft tissue
　　INCLUDES　malignant neoplasm of blood vessel
　　　　　　　malignant neoplasm of bursa
　　　　　　　malignant neoplasm of cartilage
　　　　　　　malignant neoplasm of fascia
　　　　　　　malignant neoplasm of fat
　　　　　　　malignant neoplasm of ligament, except uterine
　　　　　　　malignant neoplasm of lymphatic vessel
　　　　　　　malignant neoplasm of muscle
　　　　　　　malignant neoplasm of synovia
　　　　　　　malignant neoplasm of tendon (sheath)
　　EXCLUDES 1　*malignant neoplasm of cartilage (of):*
　　　　　　　articular (C40-C41)
　　　　　　　larynx (C32.3)
　　　　　　　nose (C30.0)
　　　　　　malignant neoplasm of connective tissue of breast (C50.-)
　　EXCLUDES 2　*Kaposi's sarcoma of soft tissue (C46.1)*
　　　　　　malignant neoplasm of heart (C38.0)
　　　　　　malignant neoplasm of peripheral nerves and autonomic
　　　　　　　nervous system (C47.-)
　　　　　　malignant neoplasm of peritoneum (C48.2)
　　　　　　malignant neoplasm of retroperitoneum (C48.0)
　　　　　　malignant neoplasm of uterine ligament (C57.3)
　　　　　　mesothelioma (C45.-)

C49.0　Malignant neoplasm of connective and soft tissue of head, face and neck
　　　Malignant neoplasm of connective tissue of ear
　　　Malignant neoplasm of connective tissue of eyelid
　　　EXCLUDES 1　*connective tissue of orbit (C69.6-)*

☑5ᵗʰ **C49.1　Malignant neoplasm of connective and soft tissue of** upper limb, including shoulder
　　C49.10　Malignant neoplasm of connective and soft tissue of unspecified upper limb, including shoulder
　　C49.11　Malignant neoplasm of connective and soft tissue of right upper limb, including shoulder
　　C49.12　Malignant neoplasm of connective and soft tissue of left upper limb, including shoulder

☑5ᵗʰ **C49.2　Malignant neoplasm of connective and soft tissue of** lower limb, including hip
　　C49.20　Malignant neoplasm of connective and soft tissue of unspecified lower limb, including hip
　　C49.21　Malignant neoplasm of connective and soft tissue of right lower limb, including hip
　　C49.22　Malignant neoplasm of connective and soft tissue of left lower limb, including hip

C49.3　Malignant neoplasm of connective and soft tissue of thorax
　　　Malignant neoplasm of axilla
　　　Malignant neoplasm of diaphragm
　　　Malignant neoplasm of great vessels
　　　EXCLUDES 1　*malignant neoplasm of breast (C50.-)*
　　　　　　malignant neoplasm of heart (C38.0)
　　　　　　malignant neoplasm of mediastinum (C38.1-C38.3)
　　　　　　malignant neoplasm of thymus (C37)

C49.4　Malignant neoplasm of connective and soft tissue of abdomen
　　　Malignant neoplasm of abdominal wall
　　　Malignant neoplasm of hypochondrium

C49.5　Malignant neoplasm of connective and soft tissue of pelvis
　　　Malignant neoplasm of buttock
　　　Malignant neoplasm of groin
　　　Malignant neoplasm of perineum

C49.6　Malignant neoplasm of connective and soft tissue of trunk, unspecified
　　　Malignant neoplasm of back NOS

C49.8　Malignant neoplasm of overlapping sites **of connective and soft tissue**
　　　Primary malignant neoplasm of two or more contiguous sites of connective and soft tissue

C49.9　Malignant neoplasm of connective and soft tissue, unspecified

Malignant neoplasms of breast (C50)

☑4ᵗʰ **C50　Malignant neoplasm of** breast
　　INCLUDES　connective tissue of breast
　　　　　　　Paget's disease of breast
　　　　　　　Paget's disease of nipple
　　Use additional code to identify estrogen receptor status (Z17.0, Z17.1)
　　EXCLUDES 1　*skin of breast (C44.501, C44.511, C44.521, C44.591)*

☑5ᵗʰ **C50.0　Malignant neoplasm of** nipple and areola
　　☑6ᵗʰ **C50.01　Malignant neoplasm of nipple and areola,** female
　　　　C50.011　Malignant neoplasm of nipple and areola, right female breast　♀
　　　　C50.012　Malignant neoplasm of nipple and areola, left female breast　♀
　　　　C50.019　Malignant neoplasm of nipple and areola, unspecified female breast　♀
　　☑6ᵗʰ **C50.02　Malignant neoplasm of nipple and areola,** male
　　　　C50.021　Malignant neoplasm of nipple and areola, right male breast　♂
　　　　C50.022　Malignant neoplasm of nipple and areola, left male breast　♂
　　　　C50.029　Malignant neoplasm of nipple and areola, unspecified male breast　♂

☑5ᵗʰ **C50.1　Malignant neoplasm of** central portion of breast
　　☑6ᵗʰ **C50.11　Malignant neoplasm of central portion of breast,** female
　　　　C50.111　Malignant neoplasm of central portion of right female breast　♀
　　　　C50.112　Malignant neoplasm of central portion of left female breast　♀
　　　　C50.119　Malignant neoplasm of central portion of unspecified female breast　♀
　　☑6ᵗʰ **C50.12　Malignant neoplasm of central portion of breast,** male
　　　　C50.121　Malignant neoplasm of central portion of right male breast　♂
　　　　C50.122　Malignant neoplasm of central portion of left male breast　♂
　　　　C50.129　Malignant neoplasm of central portion of unspecified male breast　♂

☑5ᵗʰ **C50.2　Malignant neoplasm of** upper-inner quadrant of breast
　　☑6ᵗʰ **C50.21　Malignant neoplasm of upper-inner quadrant of breast,** female
　　　　C50.211　Malignant neoplasm of upper-inner quadrant of right female breast　♀
　　　　C50.212　Malignant neoplasm of upper-inner quadrant of left female breast　♀
　　　　C50.219　Malignant neoplasm of upper-inner quadrant of unspecified female breast　♀
　　☑6ᵗʰ **C50.22　Malignant neoplasm of upper-inner quadrant of breast,** male
　　　　C50.221　Malignant neoplasm of upper-inner quadrant of right male breast　♂
　　　　C50.222　Malignant neoplasm of upper-inner quadrant of left male breast　♂
　　　　C50.229　Malignant neoplasm of upper-inner quadrant of unspecified male breast　♂

☑5ᵗʰ **C50.3　Malignant neoplasm of** lower-inner quadrant of breast
　　☑6ᵗʰ **C50.31　Malignant neoplasm of lower-inner quadrant of breast,** female
　　　　C50.311　Malignant neoplasm of lower-inner quadrant of right female breast　♀
　　　　C50.312　Malignant neoplasm of lower-inner quadrant of left female breast　♀
　　　　C50.319　Malignant neoplasm of lower-inner quadrant of unspecified female breast　♀
　　☑6ᵗʰ **C50.32　Malignant neoplasm of lower-inner quadrant of breast,** male
　　　　C50.321　Malignant neoplasm of lower-inner quadrant of right male breast　♂
　　　　C50.322　Malignant neoplasm of lower-inner quadrant of left male breast　♂
　　　　C50.329　Malignant neoplasm of lower-inner quadrant of unspecified male breast　♂

☑ Additional Character Required　　☑x7ᵗʰ Placeholder Alert　　Unspecified Dx　　Other Specified Dx　　Manifestation　　▶◀ Revised Text　　● New Code　　▲ Revised Code Title

✓5ᵗʰ C50.4 Malignant neoplasm of upper-outer quadrant **of breast**

    ✓6ᵗʰ C50.41 Malignant neoplasm of upper-outer quadrant of breast, female

        C50.411 **Malignant neoplasm of upper-outer quadrant of** right **female breast** ♀

        C50.412 **Malignant neoplasm of upper-outer quadrant of** left **female breast** ♀

        C50.419 **Malignant neoplasm of upper-outer quadrant of unspecified female breast** ♀

    ✓6ᵗʰ C50.42 Malignant neoplasm of upper-outer quadrant of breast, male

        C50.421 **Malignant neoplasm of upper-outer quadrant of** right **male breast** ♂

        C50.422 **Malignant neoplasm of upper-outer quadrant of** left **male breast** ♂

        C50.429 **Malignant neoplasm of upper-outer quadrant of unspecified male breast** ♂

✓5ᵗʰ C50.5 Malignant neoplasm of lower-outer quadrant **of breast**

    ✓6ᵗʰ C50.51 Malignant neoplasm of lower-outer quadrant of breast, female

        C50.511 **Malignant neoplasm of lower-outer quadrant of** right **female breast** ♀

        C50.512 **Malignant neoplasm of lower-outer quadrant of** left **female breast** ♀

        C50.519 **Malignant neoplasm of lower-outer quadrant of unspecified female breast** ♀

    ✓6ᵗʰ C50.52 Malignant neoplasm of lower-outer quadrant of breast, male

        C50.521 **Malignant neoplasm of lower-outer quadrant of** right **male breast** ♂

        C50.522 **Malignant neoplasm of lower-outer quadrant of** left **male breast** ♂

        C50.529 **Malignant neoplasm of lower-outer quadrant of unspecified male breast** ♂

✓5ᵗʰ C50.6 Malignant neoplasm of axillary tail **of breast**

    ✓6ᵗʰ C50.61 Malignant neoplasm of axillary tail of breast, female

        C50.611 **Malignant neoplasm of axillary tail of** right **female breast** ♀

        C50.612 **Malignant neoplasm of axillary tail of** left **female breast** ♀

        C50.619 **Malignant neoplasm of axillary tail of unspecified female breast** ♀

    ✓6ᵗʰ C50.62 Malignant neoplasm of axillary tail of breast, male

        C50.621 **Malignant neoplasm of axillary tail of** right **male breast** ♂

        C50.622 **Malignant neoplasm of axillary tail of** left **male breast** ♂

        C50.629 **Malignant neoplasm of axillary tail of unspecified male breast** ♂

✓5ᵗʰ C50.8 Malignant neoplasm of overlapping sites **of breast**

    ✓6ᵗʰ C50.81 Malignant neoplasm of overlapping sites of breast, female

        C50.811 **Malignant neoplasm of overlapping sites of** right **female breast** ♀

        C50.812 **Malignant neoplasm of overlapping sites of** left **female breast** ♀

        C50.819 **Malignant neoplasm of overlapping sites of unspecified female breast** ♀

    ✓6ᵗʰ C50.82 Malignant neoplasm of overlapping sites of breast, male

        C50.821 **Malignant neoplasm of overlapping sites of** right **male breast** ♂

        C50.822 **Malignant neoplasm of overlapping sites of** left **male breast** ♂

        C50.829 **Malignant neoplasm of overlapping sites of unspecified male breast** ♂

✓5ᵗʰ C50.9 Malignant neoplasm of breast of unspecified site

    ✓6ᵗʰ C50.91 Malignant neoplasm of breast of unspecified site, female

        C50.911 **Malignant neoplasm of unspecified site of** right **female breast** ♀

        C50.912 **Malignant neoplasm of unspecified site of** left **female breast** ♀

        C50.919 **Malignant neoplasm of unspecified site of unspecified female breast** ♀

    ✓6ᵗʰ C50.92 Malignant neoplasm of breast of unspecified site, male

        C50.921 **Malignant neoplasm of unspecified site of** right **male breast** ♂

        C50.922 **Malignant neoplasm of unspecified site of** left **male breast** ♂

        C50.929 **Malignant neoplasm of unspecified site of unspecified male breast** ♂

Malignant neoplasms of female genital organs (C51-C58)

INCLUDES   malignant neoplasm of skin of female genital organs

✓4ᵗʰ C51 Malignant neoplasm of vulva

    EXCLUDES 1   carcinoma in situ of vulva (D07.1)

    C51.0 **Malignant neoplasm of** labium majus ♀
        Malignant neoplasm of Bartholin's [greater vestibular] gland

    C51.1 **Malignant neoplasm of** labium minus ♀

    C51.2 **Malignant neoplasm of** clitoris ♀

    C51.8 **Malignant neoplasm of** overlapping sites **of vulva** ♀

    C51.9 **Malignant neoplasm of vulva, unspecified** ♀
        Malignant neoplasm of external female genitalia NOS
        Malignant neoplasm of pudendum

C52 Malignant neoplasm of vagina ♀

    EXCLUDES 1   carcinoma in situ of vagina (D07.2)

✓4ᵗʰ C53 Malignant neoplasm of cervix uteri

    EXCLUDES 1   carcinoma in situ of cervix uteri (D06.-)

    C53.0 **Malignant neoplasm of** endocervix ♀

    C53.1 **Malignant neoplasm of** exocervix ♀

    C53.8 **Malignant neoplasm of** overlapping sites **of cervix uteri** ♀

    C53.9 **Malignant neoplasm of cervix uteri, unspecified** ♀

✓4ᵗʰ C54 Malignant neoplasm of corpus uteri

    C54.0 **Malignant neoplasm of** isthmus uteri ♀
        Malignant neoplasm of lower uterine segment

    C54.1 **Malignant neoplasm of** endometrium ♀

    C54.2 **Malignant neoplasm of** myometrium ♀

    C54.3 **Malignant neoplasm of** fundus uteri ♀

    C54.8 **Malignant neoplasm of** overlapping sites **of corpus uteri** ♀

    C54.9 **Malignant neoplasm of corpus uteri, unspecified** ♀

C55 Malignant neoplasm of uterus, part unspecified ♀

✓4ᵗʰ C56 Malignant neoplasm of ovary
    Use additional code to identify any functional activity

    C56.1 **Malignant neoplasm of** right **ovary** ♀

    C56.2 **Malignant neoplasm of** left **ovary** ♀

    C56.9 **Malignant neoplasm of** unspecified **ovary** ♀

✓4ᵗʰ C57 Malignant neoplasm of other and unspecified female genital organs

    ✓5ᵗʰ C57.0 Malignant neoplasm of fallopian tube
        Malignant neoplasm of oviduct
        Malignant neoplasm of uterine tube

        C57.00 **Malignant neoplasm of unspecified fallopian tube** ♀

        C57.01 **Malignant neoplasm of** right **fallopian tube** ♀

        C57.02 **Malignant neoplasm of** left **fallopian tube** ♀

    ✓5ᵗʰ C57.1 Malignant neoplasm of broad ligament

        C57.10 **Malignant neoplasm of unspecified broad ligament** ♀

        C57.11 **Malignant neoplasm of** right **broad ligament** ♀

        C57.12 **Malignant neoplasm of** left **broad ligament** ♀

    ✓5ᵗʰ C57.2 Malignant neoplasm of round ligament

        C57.20 **Malignant neoplasm of unspecified round ligament** ♀

        C57.21 **Malignant neoplasm of** right **round ligament** ♀

        C57.22 **Malignant neoplasm of** left **round ligament** ♀

    C57.3 **Malignant neoplasm of** parametrium ♀
        Malignant neoplasm of uterine ligament NOS

    C57.4 **Malignant neoplasm of** uterine adnexa, **unspecified** ♀

    C57.7 **Malignant neoplasm of other specified female genital organs** ♀
        Malignant neoplasm of wolffian body or duct

EXCLUDES 1 Not coded here   *EXCLUDES 2* Not included here   N Newborn Age: 0   P Pediatric Age: 0-17   M Maternity Age: 12-55   A Adult Age: 15-124

C57.8   **Malignant neoplasm of** overlapping sites **of female** ♀
genital organs
> Primary malignant neoplasm of two or more contiguous sites of the female genital organs whose point of origin cannot be determined
> Primary tubo-ovarian malignant neoplasm whose point of origin cannot be determined
> Primary utero-ovarian malignant neoplasm whose point of origin cannot be determined

C57.9   **Malignant neoplasm of female genital organ, unspecified** ♀
> Malignant neoplasm of female genitourinary tract NOS

C58   **Malignant neoplasm of** placenta ♀
> **INCLUDES**   choriocarcinoma NOS
> chorionepithelioma NOS
> **EXCLUDES 1**   *chorioadenoma (destruens) (D39.2)*
> *hydatidiform mole NOS (O01.9)*
> *invasive hydatidiform mole (D39.2)*
> *male choriocarcinoma NOS (C62.9-)*
> *malignant hydatidiform mole (D39.2)*

Malignant neoplasms of male genital organs (C60-C63)

> **INCLUDES**   malignant neoplasm of skin of male genital organs

✓4ᵗʰ C60   **Malignant neoplasm of** penis

C60.0   **Malignant neoplasm of** prepuce ♂
> Malignant neoplasm of foreskin

C60.1   **Malignant neoplasm of** glans **penis** ♂

C60.2   **Malignant neoplasm of** body **of penis** ♂
> Malignant neoplasm of corpus cavernosum

C60.8   **Malignant neoplasm of** overlapping sites **of penis** ♂

C60.9   **Malignant neoplasm of penis, unspecified** ♂
> Malignant neoplasm of skin of penis NOS

C61   **Malignant neoplasm of** prostate ♂
> **EXCLUDES 1**   *malignant neoplasm of seminal vesicle (C63.7)*

✓4ᵗʰ C62   **Malignant neoplasm of** testis
> Use additional code to identify any functional activity

✓5ᵗʰ C62.0   **Malignant neoplasm of** undescended **testis**
> Malignant neoplasm of ectopic testis
> Malignant neoplasm of retained testis

    C62.00   **Malignant neoplasm of unspecified undescended** ♂
testis

    C62.01   **Malignant neoplasm of undescended** right **testis** ♂

    C62.02   **Malignant neoplasm of undescended** left **testis** ♂

✓5ᵗʰ C62.1   **Malignant neoplasm of** descended **testis**
> Malignant neoplasm of scrotal testis

    C62.10   **Malignant neoplasm of unspecified descended** ♂
testis

    C62.11   **Malignant neoplasm of descended** right **testis** ♂

    C62.12   **Malignant neoplasm of descended** left **testis** ♂

✓5ᵗʰ C62.9   **Malignant neoplasm of testis,** unspecified whether
descended or undescended

    C62.90   **Malignant neoplasm of unspecified testis,** ♂
unspecified whether descended or undescended
> Malignant neoplasm of testis NOS

    C62.91   **Malignant neoplasm of** right **testis, unspecified** ♂
whether descended or undescended

    C62.92   **Malignant neoplasm of** left **testis, unspecified** ♂
whether descended or undescended

✓4ᵗʰ C63   **Malignant neoplasm of** other and unspecified male genital
organs

✓5ᵗʰ C63.0   **Malignant neoplasm of** epididymis

    C63.00   **Malignant neoplasm of unspecified epididymis** ♂

    C63.01   **Malignant neoplasm of** right **epididymis** ♂

    C63.02   **Malignant neoplasm of** left **epididymis** ♂

✓5ᵗʰ C63.1   **Malignant neoplasm of** spermatic cord

    C63.10   **Malignant neoplasm of unspecified spermatic** ♂
cord

    C63.11   **Malignant neoplasm of** right **spermatic cord** ♂

    C63.12   **Malignant neoplasm of** left **spermatic cord** ♂

C63.2   **Malignant neoplasm of** scrotum ♂
> Malignant neoplasm of skin of scrotum

C63.7   **Malignant neoplasm of other** specified **male genital** ♂
organs
> Malignant neoplasm of seminal vesicle
> Malignant neoplasm of tunica vaginalis

C63.8   **Malignant neoplasm of** overlapping sites **of male** ♂
genital organs
> Primary malignant neoplasm of two or more contiguous sites of male genital organs whose point of origin cannot be determined

C63.9   **Malignant neoplasm of male genital organ, unspecified** ♂
> Malignant neoplasm of male genitourinary tract NOS

Malignant neoplasms of urinary tract (C64-C68)

✓4ᵗʰ C64   **Malignant neoplasm of** kidney, except renal pelvis
> **EXCLUDES 1**   *malignant carcinoid tumor of the kidney (C7A.093)*
> *malignant neoplasm of renal calyces (C65.-)*
> *malignant neoplasm of renal pelvis (C65.-)*

C64.1   **Malignant neoplasm of** right **kidney, except renal pelvis**

C64.2   **Malignant neoplasm of** left **kidney, except renal pelvis**

C64.9   **Malignant neoplasm of unspecified kidney, except renal
pelvis**

✓4ᵗʰ C65   **Malignant neoplasm of** renal pelvis
> **INCLUDES**   malignant neoplasm of pelviureteric junction
> malignant neoplasm of renal calyces

C65.1   **Malignant neoplasm of** right **renal pelvis**

C65.2   **Malignant neoplasm of** left **renal pelvis**

C65.9   **Malignant neoplasm of unspecified renal pelvis**

✓4ᵗʰ C66   **Malignant neoplasm of** ureter
> **EXCLUDES 1**   *malignant neoplasm of ureteric orifice of bladder (C67.6)*

C66.1   **Malignant neoplasm of** right **ureter**

C66.2   **Malignant neoplasm of** left **ureter**

C66.9   **Malignant neoplasm of unspecified ureter**

✓4ᵗʰ C67   **Malignant neoplasm of** bladder

C67.0   **Malignant neoplasm of** trigone **of bladder**

C67.1   **Malignant neoplasm of** dome **of bladder**

C67.2   **Malignant neoplasm of** lateral wall **of bladder**

C67.3   **Malignant neoplasm of** anterior wall **of bladder**

C67.4   **Malignant neoplasm of** posterior wall **of bladder**

C67.5   **Malignant neoplasm of** bladder neck
> Malignant neoplasm of internal urethral orifice

C67.6   **Malignant neoplasm of** ureteric orifice

C67.7   **Malignant neoplasm of** urachus

C67.8   **Malignant neoplasm of** overlapping sites **of bladder**

C67.9   **Malignant neoplasm of bladder, unspecified**

✓4ᵗʰ C68   **Malignant neoplasm of** other and unspecified urinary organs
> **EXCLUDES 1**   *malignant neoplasm of female genitourinary tract NOS (C57.9)*
> *malignant neoplasm of male genitourinary tract NOS (C63.9)*

C68.0   **Malignant neoplasm of** urethra
> **EXCLUDES 1**   *malignant neoplasm of urethral orifice of bladder (C67.5)*

C68.1   **Malignant neoplasm of** paraurethral glands

C68.8   **Malignant neoplasm of** overlapping sites **of urinary organs**
> Primary malignant neoplasm of two or more contiguous sites of urinary organs whose point of origin cannot be determined

C68.9   **Malignant neoplasm of urinary organ, unspecified**
> Malignant neoplasm of urinary system NOS

Malignant neoplasms of eye, brain and other parts of central nervous system (C69-C72)

✓4ᵗʰ C69   **Malignant neoplasm of** eye and adnexa
> **EXCLUDES 1**   *malignant neoplasm of connective tissue of eyelid (C49.0)*
> *malignant neoplasm of eyelid (skin) (C43.1-, C44.1-)*
> *malignant neoplasm of optic nerve (C72.3-)*

✓5ᵗʰ C69.0   **Malignant neoplasm of** conjunctiva

    C69.00   **Malignant neoplasm of unspecified conjunctiva**

    C69.01   **Malignant neoplasm of** right **conjunctiva**

    C69.02   **Malignant neoplasm of** left **conjunctiva**

✓5ᵗʰ C69.1   **Malignant neoplasm of** cornea

    C69.10   **Malignant neoplasm of unspecified cornea**

    C69.11   **Malignant neoplasm of** right **cornea**

    C69.12   **Malignant neoplasm of** left **cornea**

☑ Additional Character Required   ✓x7ᵗʰ Placeholder Alert   Unspecified Dx   Other Specified Dx   Manifestation   ▶◀ Revised Text   ● New Code   ▲ Revised Code Title

ICD-10-CM 2016   457

Chapter 2. Neoplasms

✓5ᵗʰ **C69.2 Malignant neoplasm of retina**

    EXCLUDES 1   dark area on retina (D49.81)
           neoplasm of unspecified behavior of retina and choroid (D49.81)
           retinal freckle (D49.81)

    C69.20 Malignant neoplasm of unspecified retina
    C69.21 Malignant neoplasm of right retina
    C69.22 Malignant neoplasm of left retina

✓5ᵗʰ **C69.3 Malignant neoplasm of choroid**

    C69.30 Malignant neoplasm of unspecified choroid
    C69.31 Malignant neoplasm of right choroid
    C69.32 Malignant neoplasm of left choroid

✓5ᵗʰ **C69.4 Malignant neoplasm of ciliary body**

    C69.40 Malignant neoplasm of unspecified ciliary body
    C69.41 Malignant neoplasm of right ciliary body
    C69.42 Malignant neoplasm of left ciliary body

✓5ᵗʰ **C69.5 Malignant neoplasm of lacrimal gland and duct**

    Malignant neoplasm of lacrimal sac
    Malignant neoplasm of nasolacrimal duct

    C69.50 Malignant neoplasm of unspecified lacrimal gland and duct
    C69.51 Malignant neoplasm of right lacrimal gland and duct
    C69.52 Malignant neoplasm of left lacrimal gland and duct

✓5ᵗʰ **C69.6 Malignant neoplasm of orbit**

    Malignant neoplasm of connective tissue of orbit
    Malignant neoplasm of extraocular muscle
    Malignant neoplasm of peripheral nerves of orbit
    Malignant neoplasm of retrobulbar tissue
    Malignant neoplasm of retro-ocular tissue

    EXCLUDES 1   malignant neoplasm of orbital bone (C41.0)

    C69.60 Malignant neoplasm of unspecified orbit
    C69.61 Malignant neoplasm of right orbit
    C69.62 Malignant neoplasm of left orbit

✓5ᵗʰ **C69.8 Malignant neoplasm of overlapping sites of eye and adnexa**

    C69.80 Malignant neoplasm of overlapping sites of unspecified eye and adnexa
    C69.81 Malignant neoplasm of overlapping sites of right eye and adnexa
    C69.82 Malignant neoplasm of overlapping sites of left eye and adnexa

✓5ᵗʰ **C69.9 Malignant neoplasm of unspecified site of eye**

    Malignant neoplasm of eyeball

    C69.90 Malignant neoplasm of unspecified site of unspecified eye
    C69.91 Malignant neoplasm of unspecified site of right eye
    C69.92 Malignant neoplasm of unspecified site of left eye

✓4ᵗʰ **C70 Malignant neoplasm of meninges**

    C70.0 Malignant neoplasm of cerebral meninges
    C70.1 Malignant neoplasm of spinal meninges
    C70.9 Malignant neoplasm of meninges, unspecified

✓4ᵗʰ **C71 Malignant neoplasm of brain**

    EXCLUDES 1   malignant neoplasm of cranial nerves (C72.2-C72.5)
           retrobulbar malignant neoplasm (C69.6-)

    C71.0 Malignant neoplasm of cerebrum, except lobes and ventricles
    Malignant neoplasm of supratentorial NOS

    C71.1 Malignant neoplasm of frontal lobe
    C71.2 Malignant neoplasm of temporal lobe
    C71.3 Malignant neoplasm of parietal lobe
    C71.4 Malignant neoplasm of occipital lobe
    C71.5 Malignant neoplasm of cerebral ventricle

    EXCLUDES 1   malignant neoplasm of fourth cerebral ventricle (C71.7)

    C71.6 Malignant neoplasm of cerebellum
    C71.7 Malignant neoplasm of brain stem
    Malignant neoplasm of fourth cerebral ventricle
    Infratentorial malignant neoplasm NOS

    C71.8 Malignant neoplasm of overlapping sites of brain
    C71.9 Malignant neoplasm of brain, unspecified
    AHA: 2014, 3Q, 3

✓4ᵗʰ **C72 Malignant neoplasm of spinal cord, cranial nerves and other parts of central nervous system**

    EXCLUDES 1   malignant neoplasm of meninges (C70.-)
           malignant neoplasm of peripheral nerves and autonomic nervous system (C47.-)

    C72.0 Malignant neoplasm of spinal cord
    C72.1 Malignant neoplasm of cauda equina

✓5ᵗʰ **C72.2 Malignant neoplasm of olfactory nerve**
    Malignant neoplasm of olfactory bulb

    C72.20 Malignant neoplasm of unspecified olfactory nerve
    C72.21 Malignant neoplasm of right olfactory nerve
    C72.22 Malignant neoplasm of left olfactory nerve

✓5ᵗʰ **C72.3 Malignant neoplasm of optic nerve**

    C72.30 Malignant neoplasm of unspecified optic nerve
    C72.31 Malignant neoplasm of right optic nerve
    C72.32 Malignant neoplasm of left optic nerve

✓5ᵗʰ **C72.4 Malignant neoplasm of acoustic nerve**

    C72.40 Malignant neoplasm of unspecified acoustic nerve
    C72.41 Malignant neoplasm of right acoustic nerve
    C72.42 Malignant neoplasm of left acoustic nerve

✓5ᵗʰ **C72.5 Malignant neoplasm of other and unspecified cranial nerves**

    C72.50 Malignant neoplasm of unspecified cranial nerve
    Malignant neoplasm of cranial nerve NOS

    C72.59 Malignant neoplasm of other cranial nerves

    C72.9 Malignant neoplasm of central nervous system, unspecified
    Malignant neoplasm of unspecified site of central nervous system
    Malignant neoplasm of nervous system NOS

Malignant neoplasms of thyroid and other endocrine glands (C73-C75)

C73 Malignant neoplasm of thyroid gland
    Use additional code to identify any functional activity

✓4ᵗʰ **C74 Malignant neoplasm of adrenal gland**

✓5ᵗʰ **C74.0 Malignant neoplasm of cortex of adrenal gland**

    C74.00 Malignant neoplasm of cortex of unspecified adrenal gland
    C74.01 Malignant neoplasm of cortex of right adrenal gland
    C74.02 Malignant neoplasm of cortex of left adrenal gland

✓5ᵗʰ **C74.1 Malignant neoplasm of medulla of adrenal gland**

    C74.10 Malignant neoplasm of medulla of unspecified adrenal gland
    C74.11 Malignant neoplasm of medulla of right adrenal gland
    C74.12 Malignant neoplasm of medulla of left adrenal gland

✓5ᵗʰ **C74.9 Malignant neoplasm of unspecified part of adrenal gland**

    C74.90 Malignant neoplasm of unspecified part of unspecified adrenal gland
    C74.91 Malignant neoplasm of unspecified part of right adrenal gland
    C74.92 Malignant neoplasm of unspecified part of left adrenal gland

✓4ᵗʰ **C75 Malignant neoplasm of other endocrine glands and related structures**

    EXCLUDES 1   malignant carcinoid tumors (C7A.0-)
           malignant neoplasm of adrenal gland (C74.-)
           malignant neoplasm of endocrine pancreas (C25.4)
           malignant neoplasm of islets of Langerhans (C25.4)
           malignant neoplasm of ovary (C56.-)
           malignant neoplasm of testis (C62.-)
           malignant neoplasm of thymus (C37)
           malignant neoplasm of thyroid gland (C73)
           malignant neuroendocrine tumors (C7A.-)

    C75.0 Malignant neoplasm of parathyroid gland
    C75.1 Malignant neoplasm of pituitary gland
    C75.2 Malignant neoplasm of craniopharyngeal duct
    C75.3 Malignant neoplasm of pineal gland
    C75.4 Malignant neoplasm of carotid body
    C75.5 Malignant neoplasm of aortic body and other paraganglia
    C75.8 Malignant neoplasm with pluriglandular involvement, unspecified
    C75.9 Malignant neoplasm of endocrine gland, unspecified

EXCLUDES 1 Not coded here   EXCLUDES 2 Not included here   N Newborn Age: 0   P Pediatric Age: 0-17   M Maternity Age: 12-55   A Adult Age: 15-124

Malignant neuroendocrine tumors (C7A)

☑4th **C7A**   **Malignant** neuroendocrine tumors

Code also any associated multiple endocrine neoplasia [MEN] syndromes (E31.2-)

Use additional code to identify any associated endocrine syndrome, such as:

carcinoid syndrome (E34.0)

EXCLUDES 2   *malignant pancreatic islet cell tumors (C25.4)*
Merkel cell carcinoma (C4A.-)

☑5th **C7A.0**   **Malignant** carcinoid tumors

   C7A.00   **Malignant carcinoid tumor of unspecified site**

   ☑6th **C7A.01**   **Malignant carcinoid tumors of the** small intestine

     C7A.010   **Malignant carcinoid tumor of the** duodenum

     C7A.011   **Malignant carcinoid tumor of the** jejunum

     C7A.012   **Malignant carcinoid tumor of the** ileum

     C7A.019   **Malignant carcinoid tumor of the small intestine, unspecified portion**

   ☑6th **C7A.02**   **Malignant carcinoid tumors of the** appendix, large intestine, and rectum

     C7A.020   **Malignant carcinoid tumor of the** appendix

     C7A.021   **Malignant carcinoid tumor of the** cecum

     C7A.022   **Malignant carcinoid tumor of the** ascending colon

     C7A.023   **Malignant carcinoid tumor of the** transverse colon

     C7A.024   **Malignant carcinoid tumor of the** descending colon

     C7A.025   **Malignant carcinoid tumor of the** sigmoid colon

     C7A.026   **Malignant carcinoid tumor of the** rectum

     C7A.029   **Malignant carcinoid tumor of the large intestine, unspecified portion**

      Malignant carcinoid tumor of the colon NOS

   ☑6th **C7A.09**   **Malignant carcinoid tumors of** other sites

     C7A.090   **Malignant carcinoid tumor of the** bronchus and lung

     C7A.091   **Malignant carcinoid tumor of the** thymus

     C7A.092   **Malignant carcinoid tumor of the** stomach

     C7A.093   **Malignant carcinoid tumor of the** kidney

     C7A.094   **Malignant carcinoid tumor of the** foregut NOS

     C7A.095   **Malignant carcinoid tumor of the** midgut NOS

     C7A.096   **Malignant carcinoid tumor of the** hindgut NOS

     C7A.098   **Malignant carcinoid tumors of other sites**

C7A.1   **Malignant** poorly differentiated **neuroendocrine tumors**

High grade neuroendocrine carcinoma, any site

Malignant poorly differentiated neuroendocrine tumor NOS

Malignant poorly differentiated neuroendocrine carcinoma, any site

C7A.8   **Other malignant neuroendocrine tumors**

Secondary neuroendocrine tumors (C7B)

☑4th **C7B**   Secondary **neuroendocrine tumors**

Use additional code to identify any functional activity

☑5th **C7B.0**   **Secondary** carcinoid tumors

   C7B.00   **Secondary carcinoid tumors, unspecified site**

   C7B.01   **Secondary carcinoid tumors of** distant lymph nodes

   C7B.02   **Secondary carcinoid tumors of** liver

   C7B.03   **Secondary carcinoid tumors of** bone

   C7B.04   **Secondary carcinoid tumors of** peritoneum

     Mesentery metastasis of carcinoid tumor

   C7B.09   **Secondary carcinoid tumors of other sites**

C7B.1   **Secondary** Merkel cell carcinoma

Merkel cell carcinoma nodal presentation

Merkel cell carcinoma visceral metastatic presentation

C7B.8   **Other secondary neuroendocrine tumors**

Malignant neoplasms of ill-defined, other secondary and unspecified sites (C76-C80)

☑4th **C76**   **Malignant neoplasm of** other and ill-defined sites

EXCLUDES 1   *malignant neoplasm of female genitourinary tract NOS (C57.9)*
malignant neoplasm of male genitourinary tract NOS (C63.9)
malignant neoplasm of lymphoid, hematopoietic and related tissue (C81-C96)
malignant neoplasm of skin (C44.-)
malignant neoplasm of unspecified site NOS (C80.1)

C76.0   **Malignant neoplasm of** head, face and neck

Malignant neoplasm of cheek NOS

Malignant neoplasm of nose NOS

C76.1   **Malignant neoplasm of** thorax

Intrathoracic malignant neoplasm NOS

Malignant neoplasm of axilla NOS

Thoracic malignant neoplasm NOS

C76.2   **Malignant neoplasm of** abdomen

C76.3   **Malignant neoplasm of** pelvis

Malignant neoplasm of groin NOS

Malignant neoplasm of sites overlapping systems within the pelvis

Rectovaginal (septum) malignant neoplasm

Rectovesical (septum) malignant neoplasm

☑5th **C76.4**   **Malignant neoplasm of** upper limb

   C76.40   **Malignant neoplasm of unspecified upper limb**

   C76.41   **Malignant neoplasm of** right upper limb

   C76.42   **Malignant neoplasm of** left upper limb

☑5th **C76.5**   **Malignant neoplasm of** lower limb

   C76.50   **Malignant neoplasm of unspecified lower limb**

   C76.51   **Malignant neoplasm of** right lower limb

   C76.52   **Malignant neoplasm of** left lower limb

C76.8   **Malignant neoplasm of other** specified ill-defined sites

Malignant neoplasm of overlapping ill-defined sites

☑4th **C77**   Secondary and unspecified **malignant neoplasm of** lymph nodes

EXCLUDES 1   *malignant neoplasm of lymph nodes, specified as primary (C81-C86, C88, C96.-)*
mesentery metastasis of carcinoid tumor (C7B.04)
secondary carcinoid tumors of distant lymph nodes (C7B.01)

C77.0   **Secondary and unspecified malignant neoplasm of lymph nodes of** head, face and neck

Secondary and unspecified malignant neoplasm of supraclavicular lymph nodes

C77.1   **Secondary and unspecified malignant neoplasm of** intrathoracic **lymph nodes**

C77.2   **Secondary and unspecified malignant neoplasm of** intra-abdominal lymph nodes

C77.3   **Secondary and unspecified malignant neoplasm of** axilla and upper limb **lymph nodes**

Secondary and unspecified malignant neoplasm of pectoral lymph nodes

C77.4   **Secondary and unspecified malignant neoplasm of** inguinal and lower limb **lymph nodes**

C77.5   **Secondary and unspecified malignant neoplasm of** intrapelvic **lymph nodes**

C77.8   **Secondary and unspecified malignant neoplasm of lymph nodes of** multiple regions

C77.9   **Secondary and unspecified malignant neoplasm of lymph node, unspecified**

☑4th **C78**   Secondary **malignant neoplasm of** respiratory and digestive organs

EXCLUDES 1   *lymph node metastases (C77.0)*
secondary carcinoid tumors of liver (C7B.02)
secondary carcinoid tumors of peritoneum (C7B.04)

☑5th **C78.0**   **Secondary malignant neoplasm of** lung

   C78.00   **Secondary malignant neoplasm of unspecified lung**

   C78.01   **Secondary malignant neoplasm of** right lung

   C78.02   **Secondary malignant neoplasm of** left lung

C78.1   **Secondary malignant neoplasm of** mediastinum

C78.2   **Secondary malignant neoplasm of** pleura

☑5th **C78.3**   **Secondary malignant neoplasm of** other and unspecified respiratory organs

   C78.30   **Secondary malignant neoplasm of unspecified respiratory organ**

   C78.39   **Secondary malignant neoplasm of other respiratory organs**

☑ Additional Character Required   ✓x7th Placeholder Alert   Unspecified Dx   Other Specified Dx   Manifestation   ▶◀ Revised Text   ● New Code   ▲ Revised Code Title

ICD-10-CM 2016

459

C7A–C78.39

C78.4 **Secondary malignant neoplasm of** small intestine

C78.5 **Secondary malignant neoplasm of** large intestine and rectum

C78.6 **Secondary malignant neoplasm of** retroperitoneum and peritoneum

C78.7 **Secondary malignant neoplasm of** liver and intrahepatic bile duct

✓5th **C78.8** **Secondary malignant neoplasm of** other and unspecified digestive organs

    C78.80 **Secondary malignant neoplasm of unspecified digestive organ**

    C78.89 **Secondary malignant neoplasm of other digestive organs**

✓4th **C79** **Secondary malignant neoplasm of** other and unspecified sites

    EXCLUDES 1   *lymph node metastases (C77.0)*
          secondary carcinoid tumors (C7B.-)
          secondary neuroendocrine tumors (C7B.-)

✓5th **C79.0** **Secondary malignant neoplasm of** kidney and renal pelvis

    C79.00 **Secondary malignant neoplasm of unspecified kidney and renal pelvis**

    C79.01 **Secondary malignant neoplasm of** right **kidney and renal pelvis**

    C79.02 **Secondary malignant neoplasm of** left **kidney and renal pelvis**

✓5th **C79.1** **Secondary malignant neoplasm of** bladder and other and unspecified urinary organs

    C79.10 **Secondary malignant neoplasm of unspecified urinary organs**

    C79.11 **Secondary malignant neoplasm of** bladder

    C79.19 **Secondary malignant neoplasm of other urinary organs**

C79.2 **Secondary malignant neoplasm of** skin

    EXCLUDES 1 *secondary Merkel cell carcinoma (C7B.1)*

✓5th **C79.3** **Secondary malignant neoplasm of** brain and cerebral meninges

    C79.31 **Secondary malignant neoplasm of** brain

    C79.32 **Secondary malignant neoplasm of** cerebral meninges

✓5th **C79.4** **Secondary malignant neoplasm of** other and unspecified parts of nervous system

    C79.40 **Secondary malignant neoplasm of unspecified part of nervous system**

    C79.49 **Secondary malignant neoplasm of other parts of nervous system**

✓5th **C79.5** **Secondary malignant neoplasm of** bone and bone marrow

    EXCLUDES 1 *secondary carcinoid tumors of bone (C7B.03)*

    C79.51 **Secondary malignant neoplasm of** bone

    C79.52 **Secondary malignant neoplasm of** bone marrow

✓5th **C79.6** **Secondary malignant neoplasm of** ovary

    C79.60 **Secondary malignant neoplasm of unspecified ovary** ♀

    C79.61 **Secondary malignant neoplasm of** right ovary ♀

    C79.62 **Secondary malignant neoplasm of** left ovary ♀

✓5th **C79.7** **Secondary malignant neoplasm of** adrenal gland

    C79.70 **Secondary malignant neoplasm of unspecified adrenal gland**

    C79.71 **Secondary malignant neoplasm of** right adrenal gland

    C79.72 **Secondary malignant neoplasm of** left adrenal gland

✓5th **C79.8** **Secondary malignant neoplasm of** other specified sites

    C79.81 **Secondary malignant neoplasm of** breast

    C79.82 **Secondary malignant neoplasm of** genital organs

    C79.89 **Secondary malignant neoplasm of other specified sites**

C79.9 **Secondary malignant neoplasm of unspecified site**

    Metastatic cancer NOS
    Metastatic disease NOS

    EXCLUDES 1 *carcinomatosis NOS (C80.0)*
          generalized cancer NOS (C80.0)
          malignant (primary) neoplasm of unspecified site (C80.1)

✓4th **C80** **Malignant neoplasm without specification of site**

    EXCLUDES 1 *malignant carcinoid tumor of unspecified site (C7A.00)*
          malignant neoplasm of specified multiple sites—code to each site

C80.0 **Disseminated malignant neoplasm, unspecified**

    Carcinomatosis NOS
    Generalized cancer, unspecified site (primary) (secondary)
    Generalized malignancy, unspecified site (primary) (secondary)

C80.1 **Malignant (primary) neoplasm, unspecified**

    Cancer NOS
    Cancer unspecified site (primary)
    Carcinoma unspecified site (primary)
    Malignancy unspecified site (primary)

    EXCLUDES 1 *secondary malignant neoplasm of unspecified site (C79.9)*

C80.2 **Malignant neoplasm associated with** transplanted organ

    Code first complication of transplanted organ (T86.-)
    Use additional code to identify the specific malignancy

Malignant neoplasms of lymphoid, hematopoietic and related tissue (C81-C96)

    EXCLUDES 2 *Kaposi's sarcoma of lymph nodes (C46.3)*
          secondary and unspecified neoplasm of lymph nodes (C77.-)
          secondary neoplasm of bone marrow (C79.52)
          secondary neoplasm of spleen (C78.89)

✓4th **C81** **Hodgkin lymphoma**

    EXCLUDES 1 *personal history of Hodgkin lymphoma (Z85.71)*

✓5th **C81.0** **Nodular lymphocyte predominant** Hodgkin lymphoma

    C81.00 **Nodular lymphocyte predominant Hodgkin lymphoma, unspecified site**

    C81.01 **Nodular lymphocyte predominant Hodgkin lymphoma, lymph nodes of** head, face, and neck

    C81.02 **Nodular lymphocyte predominant Hodgkin lymphoma,** intrathoracic **lymph nodes**

    C81.03 **Nodular lymphocyte predominant Hodgkin lymphoma,** intra-abdominal **lymph nodes**

    C81.04 **Nodular lymphocyte predominant Hodgkin lymphoma, lymph nodes of** axilla and upper limb

    C81.05 **Nodular lymphocyte predominant Hodgkin lymphoma, lymph nodes of** inguinal region and lower limb

    C81.06 **Nodular lymphocyte predominant Hodgkin lymphoma,** intrapelvic **lymph nodes**

    C81.07 **Nodular lymphocyte predominant Hodgkin lymphoma,** spleen

    C81.08 **Nodular lymphocyte predominant Hodgkin lymphoma, lymph nodes of** multiple sites

    C81.09 **Nodular lymphocyte predominant Hodgkin lymphoma,** extranodal and solid organ sites

✓5th **C81.1** **Nodular sclerosis classical** Hodgkin lymphoma

    C81.10 **Nodular sclerosis classical Hodgkin lymphoma, unspecified site**

    C81.11 **Nodular sclerosis classical Hodgkin lymphoma, lymph nodes of** head, face, and neck

    C81.12 **Nodular sclerosis classical Hodgkin lymphoma,** intrathoracic **lymph nodes**

    C81.13 **Nodular sclerosis classical Hodgkin lymphoma,** intra-abdominal **lymph nodes**

    C81.14 **Nodular sclerosis classical Hodgkin lymphoma, lymph nodes of** axilla and upper limb

    C81.15 **Nodular sclerosis classical Hodgkin lymphoma, lymph nodes of** inguinal region and lower limb

    C81.16 **Nodular sclerosis classical Hodgkin lymphoma,** intrapelvic **lymph nodes**

    C81.17 **Nodular sclerosis classical Hodgkin lymphoma,** spleen

    C81.18 **Nodular sclerosis classical Hodgkin lymphoma, lymph nodes of** multiple sites

    C81.19 **Nodular sclerosis classical Hodgkin lymphoma,** extranodal and solid organ sites

✓5th **C81.2** **Mixed cellularity classical** Hodgkin lymphoma

    C81.20 **Mixed cellularity classical Hodgkin lymphoma, unspecified site**

    C81.21 **Mixed cellularity classical Hodgkin lymphoma, lymph nodes of** head, face, and neck

    C81.22 **Mixed cellularity classical Hodgkin lymphoma,** intrathoracic **lymph nodes**

EXCLUDES 1 Not coded here   EXCLUDES 2 Not included here   N Newborn Age: 0   P Pediatric Age: 0-17   M Maternity Age: 12-55   A Adult Age: 15-124

460   ICD-10-CM 2016

C81.23   **Mixed cellularity classical Hodgkin lymphoma,** intra-abdominal **lymph nodes**

C81.24   **Mixed cellularity classical Hodgkin lymphoma, lymph nodes of** axilla and upper limb

C81.25   **Mixed cellularity classical Hodgkin lymphoma, lymph nodes of** inguinal region and lower limb

C81.26   **Mixed cellularity classical Hodgkin lymphoma,** intrapelvic **lymph nodes**

C81.27   **Mixed cellularity classical Hodgkin lymphoma,** spleen

C81.28   **Mixed cellularity classical Hodgkin lymphoma, lymph nodes of** multiple sites

C81.29   **Mixed cellularity classical Hodgkin lymphoma,** extranodal and solid organ sites

✓5ᵗʰ **C81.3**   Lymphocyte-depleted classical **Hodgkin lymphoma**

C81.30   **Lymphocyte-depleted classical Hodgkin lymphoma,** unspecified **site**

C81.31   **Lymphocyte-depleted classical Hodgkin lymphoma, lymph nodes of** head, face, and neck

C81.32   **Lymphocyte-depleted classical Hodgkin lymphoma,** intrathoracic **lymph nodes**

C81.33   **Lymphocyte-depleted classical Hodgkin lymphoma,** intra-abdominal **lymph nodes**

C81.34   **Lymphocyte-depleted classical Hodgkin lymphoma, lymph nodes of** axilla and upper limb

C81.35   **Lymphocyte-depleted classical Hodgkin lymphoma, lymph nodes of** inguinal region and lower limb

C81.36   **Lymphocyte-depleted classical Hodgkin lymphoma,** intrapelvic **lymph nodes**

C81.37   **Lymphocyte-depleted classical Hodgkin lymphoma,** spleen

C81.38   **Lymphocyte-depleted classical Hodgkin lymphoma, lymph nodes of** multiple sites

C81.39   **Lymphocyte-depleted classical Hodgkin lymphoma,** extranodal and solid organ sites

✓5ᵗʰ **C81.4**   Lymphocyte-rich classical **Hodgkin lymphoma**

EXCLUDES 1   *nodular lymphocyte predominant Hodgkin lymphoma (C81.0-)*

C81.40   **Lymphocyte-rich classical Hodgkin lymphoma,** unspecified **site**

C81.41   **Lymphocyte-rich classical Hodgkin lymphoma, lymph nodes of** head, face, and neck

C81.42   **Lymphocyte-rich classical Hodgkin lymphoma,** intrathoracic **lymph nodes**

C81.43   **Lymphocyte-rich classical Hodgkin lymphoma,** intra-abdominal **lymph nodes**

C81.44   **Lymphocyte-rich classical Hodgkin lymphoma, lymph nodes of** axilla and upper limb

C81.45   **Lymphocyte-rich classical Hodgkin lymphoma, lymph nodes of** inguinal region and lower limb

C81.46   **Lymphocyte-rich classical Hodgkin lymphoma,** intrapelvic **lymph nodes**

C81.47   **Lymphocyte-rich classical Hodgkin lymphoma,** spleen

C81.48   **Lymphocyte-rich classical Hodgkin lymphoma, lymph nodes of** multiple sites

C81.49   **Lymphocyte-rich classical Hodgkin lymphoma,** extranodal and solid organ sites

✓5ᵗʰ **C81.7**   Other classical **Hodgkin lymphoma**

Classical Hodgkin lymphoma NOS

C81.70   **Other classical Hodgkin lymphoma, unspecified site**

C81.71   **Other classical Hodgkin lymphoma, lymph nodes of** head, face, and neck

C81.72   **Other classical Hodgkin lymphoma,** intrathoracic **lymph nodes**

C81.73   **Other classical Hodgkin lymphoma,** intra-abdominal **lymph nodes**

C81.74   **Other classical Hodgkin lymphoma, lymph nodes of** axilla and upper limb

C81.75   **Other classical Hodgkin lymphoma, lymph nodes of** inguinal region and lower limb

C81.76   **Other classical Hodgkin lymphoma,** intrapelvic **lymph nodes**

C81.77   **Other classical Hodgkin lymphoma,** spleen

C81.78   **Other classical Hodgkin lymphoma, lymph nodes of** multiple sites

C81.79   **Other classical Hodgkin lymphoma,** extranodal and solid organ sites

✓5ᵗʰ **C81.9**   Hodgkin lymphoma, **unspecified**

C81.90   **Hodgkin lymphoma, unspecified, unspecified site**

C81.91   **Hodgkin lymphoma, unspecified, lymph nodes of** head, face, and neck

C81.92   **Hodgkin lymphoma, unspecified,** intrathoracic **lymph nodes**

C81.93   **Hodgkin lymphoma, unspecified,** intra-abdominal **lymph nodes**

C81.94   **Hodgkin lymphoma, unspecified, lymph nodes of** axilla and upper limb

C81.95   **Hodgkin lymphoma, unspecified, lymph nodes of** inguinal region and lower limb

C81.96   **Hodgkin lymphoma, unspecified,** intrapelvic **lymph nodes**

C81.97   **Hodgkin lymphoma, unspecified,** spleen

C81.98   **Hodgkin lymphoma, unspecified, lymph nodes of** multiple sites

C81.99   **Hodgkin lymphoma, unspecified,** extranodal and solid organ sites

✓4ᵗʰ **C82**   **Follicular lymphoma**

INCLUDES   follicular lymphoma with or without diffuse areas

EXCLUDES 1   *mature T/NK-cell lymphomas (C84.-)*
personal history of non-Hodgkin lymphoma (Z85.72)

✓5ᵗʰ **C82.0**   **Follicular lymphoma** grade I

C82.00   **Follicular lymphoma grade I, unspecified site**

C82.01   **Follicular lymphoma grade I, lymph nodes of** head, face, and neck

C82.02   **Follicular lymphoma grade I,** intrathoracic **lymph nodes**

C82.03   **Follicular lymphoma grade I,** intra-abdominal **lymph nodes**

C82.04   **Follicular lymphoma grade I, lymph nodes of** axilla and upper limb

C82.05   **Follicular lymphoma grade I, lymph nodes of** inguinal region and lower limb

C82.06   **Follicular lymphoma grade I,** intrapelvic **lymph nodes**

C82.07   **Follicular lymphoma grade I,** spleen

C82.08   **Follicular lymphoma grade I, lymph nodes of** multiple sites

C82.09   **Follicular lymphoma grade I,** extranodal and solid organ sites

✓5ᵗʰ **C82.1**   **Follicular lymphoma** grade II

C82.10   **Follicular lymphoma grade II, unspecified site**

C82.11   **Follicular lymphoma grade II, lymph nodes of** head, face, and neck

C82.12   **Follicular lymphoma grade II,** intrathoracic **lymph nodes**

C82.13   **Follicular lymphoma grade II,** intra-abdominal **lymph nodes**

C82.14   **Follicular lymphoma grade II, lymph nodes of** axilla and upper limb

C82.15   **Follicular lymphoma grade II, lymph nodes of** inguinal region and lower limb

C82.16   **Follicular lymphoma grade II,** intrapelvic **lymph nodes**

C82.17   **Follicular lymphoma grade II,** spleen

C82.18   **Follicular lymphoma grade II, lymph nodes of** multiple sites

C82.19   **Follicular lymphoma grade II,** extranodal and solid organ sites

✓5ᵗʰ **C82.2**   **Follicular lymphoma** grade III, unspecified

C82.20   **Follicular lymphoma grade III, unspecified, unspecified site**

C82.21   **Follicular lymphoma grade III, unspecified, lymph nodes of** head, face, and neck

C82.22   **Follicular lymphoma grade III, unspecified,** intrathoracic **lymph nodes**

C82.23   **Follicular lymphoma grade III, unspecified,** intra-abdominal **lymph nodes**

C82.24   **Follicular lymphoma grade III, unspecified, lymph nodes of** axilla and upper limb

C82.25   **Follicular lymphoma grade III, unspecified, lymph nodes of** inguinal region and lower limb

✔ Additional Character Required   ✔x7ᵗʰ Placeholder Alert   Unspecified Dx   Other Specified Dx   Manifestation   ►◄ Revised Text   ● New Code   ▲ Revised Code Title

ICD-10-CM 2016   461

C82.26 Follicular lymphoma grade III, unspecified, intrapelvic **lymph nodes**

C82.27 Follicular lymphoma grade III, unspecified, spleen

C82.28 Follicular lymphoma grade III, unspecified, lymph nodes of multiple sites

C82.29 Follicular lymphoma grade III, unspecified, extranodal and solid organ sites

✓5th **C82.3** Follicular lymphoma grade IIIa

C82.30 Follicular lymphoma grade IIIa, unspecified site

C82.31 Follicular lymphoma grade IIIa, lymph nodes of head, face, and neck

C82.32 Follicular lymphoma grade IIIa, intrathoracic **lymph nodes**

C82.33 Follicular lymphoma grade IIIa, intra-abdominal **lymph nodes**

C82.34 Follicular lymphoma grade IIIa, lymph nodes of axilla and upper limb

C82.35 Follicular lymphoma grade IIIa, lymph nodes of inguinal region and lower limb

C82.36 Follicular lymphoma grade IIIa, intrapelvic **lymph nodes**

C82.37 Follicular lymphoma grade IIIa, spleen

C82.38 Follicular lymphoma grade IIIa, lymph nodes of multiple sites

C82.39 Follicular lymphoma grade IIIa, extranodal and solid organ sites

✓5th **C82.4** Follicular lymphoma grade IIIb

C82.40 Follicular lymphoma grade IIIb, unspecified site

C82.41 Follicular lymphoma grade IIIb, lymph nodes of head, face, and neck

C82.42 Follicular lymphoma grade IIIb, intrathoracic **lymph nodes**

C82.43 Follicular lymphoma grade IIIb, intra-abdominal **lymph nodes**

C82.44 Follicular lymphoma grade IIIb, lymph nodes of axilla and upper limb

C82.45 Follicular lymphoma grade IIIb, lymph nodes of inguinal region and lower limb

C82.46 Follicular lymphoma grade IIIb, intrapelvic **lymph nodes**

C82.47 Follicular lymphoma grade IIIb, spleen

C82.48 Follicular lymphoma grade IIIb, lymph nodes of multiple sites

C82.49 Follicular lymphoma grade IIIb, extranodal and solid organ sites

✓5th **C82.5** Diffuse follicle center **lymphoma**

C82.50 Diffuse follicle center lymphoma, unspecified site

C82.51 Diffuse follicle center lymphoma, lymph nodes of head, face, and neck

C82.52 Diffuse follicle center lymphoma, intrathoracic **lymph nodes**

C82.53 Diffuse follicle center lymphoma, intra-abdominal **lymph nodes**

C82.54 Diffuse follicle center lymphoma, lymph nodes of axilla and upper limb

C82.55 Diffuse follicle center lymphoma, lymph nodes of inguinal region and lower limb

C82.56 Diffuse follicle center lymphoma, intrapelvic **lymph nodes**

C82.57 Diffuse follicle center lymphoma, spleen

C82.58 Diffuse follicle center lymphoma, lymph nodes of multiple sites

C82.59 Diffuse follicle center lymphoma, extranodal and solid organ sites

✓5th **C82.6** Cutaneous follicle center **lymphoma**

C82.60 Cutaneous follicle center lymphoma, unspecified site

C82.61 Cutaneous follicle center lymphoma, lymph nodes of head, face, and neck

C82.62 Cutaneous follicle center lymphoma, intrathoracic **lymph nodes**

C82.63 Cutaneous follicle center lymphoma, intra-abdominal **lymph nodes**

C82.64 Cutaneous follicle center lymphoma, lymph nodes of axilla and upper limb

C82.65 Cutaneous follicle center lymphoma, lymph nodes of inguinal region and lower limb

C82.66 Cutaneous follicle center lymphoma, intrapelvic **lymph nodes**

C82.67 Cutaneous follicle center lymphoma, spleen

C82.68 Cutaneous follicle center lymphoma, lymph nodes of multiple sites

C82.69 Cutaneous follicle center lymphoma, extranodal and solid organ sites

✓5th **C82.8** Other types of follicular lymphoma

C82.80 Other types of follicular lymphoma, unspecified site

C82.81 Other types of follicular lymphoma, lymph nodes of head, face, and neck

C82.82 Other types of follicular lymphoma, intrathoracic **lymph nodes**

C82.83 Other types of follicular lymphoma, intra-abdominal **lymph nodes**

C82.84 Other types of follicular lymphoma, lymph nodes of axilla and upper limb

C82.85 Other types of follicular lymphoma, lymph nodes of inguinal region and lower limb

C82.86 Other types of follicular lymphoma, intrapelvic **lymph nodes**

C82.87 Other types of follicular lymphoma, spleen

C82.88 Other types of follicular lymphoma, lymph nodes of multiple sites

C82.89 Other types of follicular lymphoma, extranodal and solid organ sites

✓5th **C82.9** Follicular lymphoma, unspecified

C82.90 Follicular lymphoma, unspecified, unspecified site

C82.91 Follicular lymphoma, unspecified, lymph nodes of head, face, and neck

C82.92 Follicular lymphoma, unspecified, intrathoracic **lymph nodes**

C82.93 Follicular lymphoma, unspecified, intra-abdominal **lymph nodes**

C82.94 Follicular lymphoma, unspecified, lymph nodes of axilla and upper limb

C82.95 Follicular lymphoma, unspecified, lymph nodes of inguinal region and lower limb

C82.96 Follicular lymphoma, unspecified, intrapelvic **lymph nodes**

C82.97 Follicular lymphoma, unspecified, spleen

C82.98 Follicular lymphoma, unspecified, lymph nodes of multiple sites

C82.99 Follicular lymphoma, unspecified, extranodal and solid organ sites

✓4th **C83** Non-follicular **lymphoma**

EXCLUDES 1 *personal history of non-Hodgkin lymphoma (Z85.72)*

✓5th **C83.0** Small cell B-cell lymphoma

Lymphoplasmacytic lymphoma
Nodal marginal zone lymphoma
Non-leukemic variant of B-CLL
Splenic marginal zone lymphoma

EXCLUDES 1 *chronic lymphocytic leukemia (C91.1)*
mature T/NK-cell lymphomas (C84.-)
Waldenström macroglobulinemia (C88.0)

C83.00 Small cell B-cell lymphoma, unspecified site

C83.01 Small cell B-cell lymphoma, lymph nodes of head, face, and neck

C83.02 Small cell B-cell lymphoma, intrathoracic **lymph nodes**

C83.03 Small cell B-cell lymphoma, intra-abdominal **lymph nodes**

C83.04 Small cell B-cell lymphoma, lymph nodes of axilla and upper limb

C83.05 Small cell B-cell lymphoma, lymph nodes of inguinal region and lower limb

C83.06 Small cell B-cell lymphoma, intrapelvic **lymph nodes**

C83.07 Small cell B-cell lymphoma, spleen

C83.08 Small cell B-cell lymphoma, lymph nodes of multiple sites

C83.09 Small cell B-cell lymphoma, extranodal and solid organ sites

EXCLUDES 1 Not coded here   EXCLUDES 2 Not included here   N Newborn Age: 0   P Pediatric Age: 0-17   M Maternity Age: 12-55   A Adult Age: 15-124

462   ICD-10-CM 2016

Chapter 2. Neoplasms

✓5th **C83.1** **Mantle cell lymphoma**
Centrocytic lymphoma
Malignant lymphomatous polyposis

     C83.10 **Mantle cell lymphoma, unspecified site**

     C83.11 **Mantle cell lymphoma, lymph nodes of** head, face, and neck

     C83.12 **Mantle cell lymphoma, intrathoracic lymph nodes**

     C83.13 **Mantle cell lymphoma, intra-abdominal lymph nodes**

     C83.14 **Mantle cell lymphoma, lymph nodes of** axilla and upper limb

     C83.15 **Mantle cell lymphoma, lymph nodes of** inguinal region and lower limb

     C83.16 **Mantle cell lymphoma, intrapelvic lymph nodes**

     C83.17 **Mantle cell lymphoma, spleen**

     C83.18 **Mantle cell lymphoma, lymph nodes of** multiple sites

     C83.19 **Mantle cell lymphoma, extranodal and solid organ sites**

✓5th **C83.3** **Diffuse large B-cell lymphoma**
Anaplastic diffuse large B-cell lymphoma
CD30-positive diffuse large B-cell lymphoma
Centroblastic diffuse large B-cell lymphoma
Diffuse large B-cell lymphoma, subtype not specified
Immunoblastic diffuse large B-cell lymphoma
Plasmablastic diffuse large B-cell lymphoma
T-cell rich diffuse large B-cell lymphoma
     EXCLUDES 1   mature T/NK-cell lymphomas (C84.-)
               mediastinal (thymic) large B-cell lymphoma (C85.2-)

     C83.30 **Diffuse large B-cell lymphoma, unspecified site**

     C83.31 **Diffuse large B-cell lymphoma, lymph nodes of** head, face, and neck

     C83.32 **Diffuse large B-cell lymphoma, intrathoracic lymph nodes**

     C83.33 **Diffuse large B-cell lymphoma, intra-abdominal lymph nodes**

     C83.34 **Diffuse large B-cell lymphoma, lymph nodes of** axilla and upper limb

     C83.35 **Diffuse large B-cell lymphoma, lymph nodes of** inguinal region and lower limb

     C83.36 **Diffuse large B-cell lymphoma, intrapelvic lymph nodes**

     C83.37 **Diffuse large B-cell lymphoma, spleen**

     C83.38 **Diffuse large B-cell lymphoma, lymph nodes of** multiple sites

     C83.39 **Diffuse large B-cell lymphoma, extranodal and solid organ sites**

✓5th **C83.5** **Lymphoblastic (diffuse) lymphoma**
B-precursor lymphoma
Lymphoblastic B-cell lymphoma
Lymphoblastic lymphoma NOS
Lymphoblastic T-cell lymphoma
T-precursor lymphoma

     C83.50 **Lymphoblastic (diffuse) lymphoma, unspecified site**

     C83.51 **Lymphoblastic (diffuse) lymphoma, lymph nodes of** head, face, and neck

     C83.52 **Lymphoblastic (diffuse) lymphoma, intrathoracic lymph nodes**

     C83.53 **Lymphoblastic (diffuse) lymphoma, intra-abdominal lymph nodes**

     C83.54 **Lymphoblastic (diffuse) lymphoma, lymph nodes of** axilla and upper limb

     C83.55 **Lymphoblastic (diffuse) lymphoma, lymph nodes of** inguinal region and lower limb

     C83.56 **Lymphoblastic (diffuse) lymphoma, intrapelvic lymph nodes**

     C83.57 **Lymphoblastic (diffuse) lymphoma, spleen**

     C83.58 **Lymphoblastic (diffuse) lymphoma, lymph nodes of** multiple sites

     C83.59 **Lymphoblastic (diffuse) lymphoma, extranodal and solid organ sites**

✓5th **C83.7** **Burkitt lymphoma**
Atypical Burkitt lymphoma
Burkitt-like lymphoma
     EXCLUDES 1   mature B-cell leukemia Burkitt type (C91.A-)

     C83.70 **Burkitt lymphoma, unspecified site**

     C83.71 **Burkitt lymphoma, lymph nodes of** head, face, and neck

     C83.72 **Burkitt lymphoma, intrathoracic lymph nodes**

     C83.73 **Burkitt lymphoma, intra-abdominal lymph nodes**

     C83.74 **Burkitt lymphoma, lymph nodes of** axilla and upper limb

     C83.75 **Burkitt lymphoma, lymph nodes of** inguinal region and lower limb

     C83.76 **Burkitt lymphoma, intrapelvic lymph nodes**

     C83.77 **Burkitt lymphoma, spleen**

     C83.78 **Burkitt lymphoma, lymph nodes of** multiple sites

     C83.79 **Burkitt lymphoma, extranodal and solid organ sites**

✓5th **C83.8** **Other non-follicular lymphoma**
Intravascular large B-cell lymphoma
Lymphoid granulomatosis
Primary effusion B-cell lymphoma
     EXCLUDES 1   mediastinal (thymic) large B-cell lymphoma (C85.2-)
               T-cell rich B-cell lymphoma (C83.3-)

     C83.80 **Other non-follicular lymphoma, unspecified site**

     C83.81 **Other non-follicular lymphoma, lymph nodes of head, face, and neck**

     C83.82 **Other non-follicular lymphoma, intrathoracic lymph nodes**

     C83.83 **Other non-follicular lymphoma, intra-abdominal lymph nodes**

     C83.84 **Other non-follicular lymphoma, lymph nodes of axilla and upper limb**

     C83.85 **Other non-follicular lymphoma, lymph nodes of inguinal region and lower limb**

     C83.86 **Other non-follicular lymphoma, intrapelvic lymph nodes**

     C83.87 **Other non-follicular lymphoma, spleen**

     C83.88 **Other non-follicular lymphoma, lymph nodes of multiple sites**

     C83.89 **Other non-follicular lymphoma, extranodal and solid organ sites**

✓5th **C83.9** **Non-follicular (diffuse) lymphoma, unspecified**

     C83.90 **Non-follicular (diffuse) lymphoma, unspecified, unspecified site**

     C83.91 **Non-follicular (diffuse) lymphoma, unspecified, lymph nodes of head, face, and neck**

     C83.92 **Non-follicular (diffuse) lymphoma, unspecified, intrathoracic lymph nodes**

     C83.93 **Non-follicular (diffuse) lymphoma, unspecified, intra-abdominal lymph nodes**

     C83.94 **Non-follicular (diffuse) lymphoma, unspecified, lymph nodes of axilla and upper limb**

     C83.95 **Non-follicular (diffuse) lymphoma, unspecified, lymph nodes of inguinal region and lower limb**

     C83.96 **Non-follicular (diffuse) lymphoma, unspecified, intrapelvic lymph nodes**

     C83.97 **Non-follicular (diffuse) lymphoma, unspecified, spleen**

     C83.98 **Non-follicular (diffuse) lymphoma, unspecified, lymph nodes of multiple sites**

     C83.99 **Non-follicular (diffuse) lymphoma, unspecified, extranodal and solid organ sites**

✓4th **C84** **Mature T/NK-cell lymphomas**
     EXCLUDES 1   personal history of non-Hodgkin lymphoma (Z85.72)

✓5th **C84.0** **Mycosis fungoides**
     EXCLUDES 1   peripheral T-cell lymphoma, not classified (C84.4-)

     C84.00 **Mycosis fungoides, unspecified site**

     C84.01 **Mycosis fungoides, lymph nodes of** head, face, and neck

     C84.02 **Mycosis fungoides, intrathoracic lymph nodes**

     C84.03 **Mycosis fungoides, intra-abdominal lymph nodes**

     C84.04 **Mycosis fungoides, lymph nodes of** axilla and upper limb

     C84.05 **Mycosis fungoides, lymph nodes of** inguinal region and lower limb

     C84.06 **Mycosis fungoides, intrapelvic lymph nodes**

     C84.07 **Mycosis fungoides, spleen**

     C84.08 **Mycosis fungoides, lymph nodes of** multiple sites

     C84.09 **Mycosis fungoides, extranodal and solid organ sites**

✓5th **C84.1** **Sézary disease**

     C84.10 **Sézary disease, unspecified site**

     C84.11 **Sézary disease, lymph nodes of** head, face, and neck

---

✓ Additional Character Required   ✓x7th Placeholder Alert   Unspecified Dx   Other Specified Dx   Manifestation   ▶◀ Revised Text   ● New Code   ▲ Revised Code Title

C84.12   **Sézary disease**, intrathoracic **lymph nodes**

C84.13   **Sézary disease**, intra-abdominal **lymph nodes**

C84.14   **Sézary disease**, lymph nodes of axilla and upper limb

C84.15   **Sézary disease**, lymph nodes of inguinal region and lower limb

C84.16   **Sézary disease**, intrapelvic **lymph nodes**

C84.17   **Sézary disease**, spleen

C84.18   **Sézary disease**, lymph nodes of multiple sites

C84.19   **Sézary disease**, extranodal and solid organ sites

✓5ᵗʰ **C84.4**   **Peripheral T-cell lymphoma, not classified**
Lennert's lymphoma
Lymphoepithelioid lymphoma
Mature T-cell lymphoma, not elsewhere classified

C84.40   **Peripheral T-cell lymphoma, not classified, unspecified site**

C84.41   **Peripheral T-cell lymphoma, not classified, lymph nodes of** head, face, and neck

C84.42   **Peripheral T-cell lymphoma, not classified, intrathoracic lymph nodes**

C84.43   **Peripheral T-cell lymphoma, not classified, intra-abdominal lymph nodes**

C84.44   **Peripheral T-cell lymphoma, not classified, lymph nodes of** axilla and upper limb

C84.45   **Peripheral T-cell lymphoma, not classified, lymph nodes of** inguinal region and lower limb

C84.46   **Peripheral T-cell lymphoma, not classified, intrapelvic lymph nodes**

C84.47   **Peripheral T-cell lymphoma, not classified, spleen**

C84.48   **Peripheral T-cell lymphoma, not classified, lymph nodes of** multiple sites

C84.49   **Peripheral T-cell lymphoma, not classified, extranodal and solid organ sites**

✓5ᵗʰ **C84.6**   **Anaplastic large cell lymphoma,** ALK-positive
Anaplastic large cell lymphoma, CD3Ø-positive

C84.60   **Anaplastic large cell lymphoma, ALK-positive, unspecified site**

C84.61   **Anaplastic large cell lymphoma, ALK-positive, lymph nodes of** head, face, and neck

C84.62   **Anaplastic large cell lymphoma, ALK-positive, intrathoracic lymph nodes**

C84.63   **Anaplastic large cell lymphoma, ALK-positive, intra-abdominal lymph nodes**

C84.64   **Anaplastic large cell lymphoma, ALK-positive, lymph nodes of** axilla and upper limb

C84.65   **Anaplastic large cell lymphoma, ALK-positive, lymph nodes of** inguinal region and lower limb

C84.66   **Anaplastic large cell lymphoma, ALK-positive, intrapelvic lymph nodes**

C84.67   **Anaplastic large cell lymphoma, ALK-positive, spleen**

C84.68   **Anaplastic large cell lymphoma, ALK-positive, lymph nodes of** multiple sites

C84.69   **Anaplastic large cell lymphoma, ALK-positive, extranodal and solid organ sites**

✓5ᵗʰ **C84.7**   **Anaplastic large cell lymphoma,** ALK-negative

     EXCLUDES 1   *primary cutaneous CD3Ø-positive T-cell proliferations (C86.6-)*

C84.70   **Anaplastic large cell lymphoma, ALK-negative, unspecified site**

C84.71   **Anaplastic large cell lymphoma, ALK-negative, lymph nodes of** head, face, and neck

C84.72   **Anaplastic large cell lymphoma, ALK-negative, intrathoracic lymph nodes**

C84.73   **Anaplastic large cell lymphoma, ALK-negative, intra-abdominal lymph nodes**

C84.74   **Anaplastic large cell lymphoma, ALK-negative, lymph nodes of** axilla and upper limb

C84.75   **Anaplastic large cell lymphoma, ALK-negative, lymph nodes of** inguinal region and lower limb

C84.76   **Anaplastic large cell lymphoma, ALK-negative, intrapelvic lymph nodes**

C84.77   **Anaplastic large cell lymphoma, ALK-negative, spleen**

C84.78   **Anaplastic large cell lymphoma, ALK-negative, lymph nodes of** multiple sites

C84.79   **Anaplastic large cell lymphoma, ALK-negative, extranodal and solid organ sites**

✓5ᵗʰ **C84.A**   **Cutaneous T-cell lymphoma, unspecified**

C84.A0   **Cutaneous T-cell lymphoma, unspecified, unspecified site**

C84.A1   **Cutaneous T-cell lymphoma, unspecified lymph nodes of** head, face, and neck

C84.A2   **Cutaneous T-cell lymphoma, unspecified, intrathoracic lymph nodes**

C84.A3   **Cutaneous T-cell lymphoma, unspecified, intra-abdominal lymph nodes**

C84.A4   **Cutaneous T-cell lymphoma, unspecified, lymph nodes of** axilla and upper limb

C84.A5   **Cutaneous T-cell lymphoma, unspecified, lymph nodes of** inguinal region and lower limb

C84.A6   **Cutaneous T-cell lymphoma, unspecified, intrapelvic lymph nodes**

C84.A7   **Cutaneous T-cell lymphoma, unspecified,** spleen

C84.A8   **Cutaneous T-cell lymphoma, unspecified, lymph nodes of** multiple sites

C84.A9   **Cutaneous T-cell lymphoma, unspecified,** extranodal and solid organ sites

✓5ᵗʰ **C84.Z**   **Other mature T/NK-cell lymphomas**

     NOTE   If T-cell lineage or involvement is mentioned in conjunction with a specific lymphoma, code to the more specific description.

     EXCLUDES 1   *angioimmunoblastic T-cell lymphoma (C86.5)*
blastic NK-cell lymphoma (C86.4)
enteropathy-type T-cell lymphoma (C86.2)
extranodal NK-cell lymphoma, nasal type (C86.Ø)
hepatosplenic T-cell lymphoma (C86.1)
primary cutaneous CD3Ø-positive T-cell proliferations (C86.6)
subcutaneous panniculitis-like T-cell lymphoma (C86.3)
T-cell leukemia (C91.1-)

C84.Z0   **Other mature T/NK-cell lymphomas, unspecified site**

C84.Z1   **Other mature T/NK-cell lymphomas, lymph nodes of** head, face, and neck

C84.Z2   **Other mature T/NK-cell lymphomas,** intrathoracic lymph nodes

C84.Z3   **Other mature T/NK-cell lymphomas, intra-abdominal lymph nodes**

C84.Z4   **Other mature T/NK-cell lymphomas, lymph nodes of** axilla and upper limb

C84.Z5   **Other mature T/NK-cell lymphomas, lymph nodes of** inguinal region and lower limb

C84.Z6   **Other mature T/NK-cell lymphomas,** intrapelvic lymph nodes

C84.Z7   **Other mature T/NK-cell lymphomas,** spleen

C84.Z8   **Other mature T/NK-cell lymphomas, lymph nodes of** multiple sites

C84.Z9   **Other mature T/NK-cell lymphomas,** extranodal and solid organ sites

✓5ᵗʰ **C84.9**   **Mature T/NK-cell lymphomas,** unspecified
NK/T cell lymphoma NOS

     EXCLUDES 1   *mature T-cell lymphoma, not elsewhere classified (C84.4-)*

C84.90   **Mature T/NK-cell lymphomas, unspecified, unspecified site**

C84.91   **Mature T/NK-cell lymphomas, unspecified, lymph nodes of** head, face, and neck

C84.92   **Mature T/NK-cell lymphomas, unspecified, intrathoracic lymph nodes**

C84.93   **Mature T/NK-cell lymphomas, unspecified, intra-abdominal lymph nodes**

C84.94   **Mature T/NK-cell lymphomas, unspecified, lymph nodes of** axilla and upper limb

C84.95   **Mature T/NK-cell lymphomas, unspecified, lymph nodes of** inguinal region and lower limb

C84.96   **Mature T/NK-cell lymphomas, unspecified, intrapelvic lymph nodes**

C84.97   **Mature T/NK-cell lymphomas, unspecified,** spleen

C84.98   **Mature T/NK-cell lymphomas, unspecified, lymph nodes of** multiple sites

C84.99   **Mature T/NK-cell lymphomas, unspecified, extranodal and solid organ sites**

EXCLUDES 1 Not coded here   EXCLUDES 2 Not included here   N Newborn Age: 0   P Pediatric Age: 0-17   M Maternity Age: 12-55   A Adult Age: 15-124

464

ICD-10-CM 2016

☑4ᵗʰ **C85 Other specified and unspecified types of non-Hodgkin lymphoma**

EXCLUDES 1   other specified types of T/NK-cell lymphoma (C86.-)
     personal history of non-Hodgkin lymphoma (Z85.72)

☑5ᵗʰ **C85.1 Unspecified B-cell lymphoma**

     NOTE   If B-cell lineage or involvement is mentioned in conjunction with a specific lymphoma, code to the more specific description.

     C85.10 Unspecified B-cell lymphoma, unspecified site

     C85.11 Unspecified B-cell lymphoma, lymph nodes of head, face, and neck

     C85.12 Unspecified B-cell lymphoma, intrathoracic lymph nodes

     C85.13 Unspecified B-cell lymphoma, intra-abdominal lymph nodes

     C85.14 Unspecified B-cell lymphoma, lymph nodes of axilla and upper limb

     C85.15 Unspecified B-cell lymphoma, lymph nodes of inguinal region and lower limb

     C85.16 Unspecified B-cell lymphoma, intrapelvic lymph nodes

     C85.17 Unspecified B-cell lymphoma, spleen

     C85.18 Unspecified B-cell lymphoma, lymph nodes of multiple sites

     C85.19 Unspecified B-cell lymphoma, extranodal and solid organ sites

☑5ᵗʰ **C85.2 Mediastinal (thymic) large B-cell lymphoma**

     C85.20 Mediastinal (thymic) large B-cell lymphoma, unspecified site

     C85.21 Mediastinal (thymic) large B-cell lymphoma, lymph nodes of head, face, and neck

     C85.22 Mediastinal (thymic) large B-cell lymphoma, intrathoracic lymph nodes

     C85.23 Mediastinal (thymic) large B-cell lymphoma, intra-abdominal lymph nodes

     C85.24 Mediastinal (thymic) large B-cell lymphoma, lymph nodes of axilla and upper limb

     C85.25 Mediastinal (thymic) large B-cell lymphoma, lymph nodes of inguinal region and lower limb

     C85.26 Mediastinal (thymic) large B-cell lymphoma, intrapelvic lymph nodes

     C85.27 Mediastinal (thymic) large B-cell lymphoma, spleen

     C85.28 Mediastinal (thymic) large B-cell lymphoma, lymph nodes of multiple sites

     C85.29 Mediastinal (thymic) large B-cell lymphoma, extranodal and solid organ sites

☑5ᵗʰ **C85.8 Other specified types of non-Hodgkin lymphoma**

     C85.80 Other specified types of non-Hodgkin lymphoma, unspecified site

     C85.81 Other specified types of non-Hodgkin lymphoma, lymph nodes of head, face, and neck

     C85.82 Other specified types of non-Hodgkin lymphoma, intrathoracic lymph nodes

     C85.83 Other specified types of non-Hodgkin lymphoma, intra-abdominal lymph nodes

     C85.84 Other specified types of non-Hodgkin lymphoma, lymph nodes of axilla and upper limb

     C85.85 Other specified types of non-Hodgkin lymphoma, lymph nodes of inguinal region and lower limb

     C85.86 Other specified types of non-Hodgkin lymphoma, intrapelvic lymph nodes

     C85.87 Other specified types of non-Hodgkin lymphoma, spleen

     C85.88 Other specified types of non-Hodgkin lymphoma, lymph nodes of multiple sites

     C85.89 Other specified types of non-Hodgkin lymphoma, extranodal and solid organ sites

☑5ᵗʰ **C85.9 Non-Hodgkin lymphoma, unspecified**

     Lymphoma NOS
     Malignant lymphoma NOS
     Non-Hodgkin lymphoma NOS

     C85.90 Non-Hodgkin lymphoma, unspecified, unspecified site

     C85.91 Non-Hodgkin lymphoma, unspecified, lymph nodes of head, face, and neck

     C85.92 Non-Hodgkin lymphoma, unspecified, intrathoracic lymph nodes

     C85.93 Non-Hodgkin lymphoma, unspecified, intra-abdominal lymph nodes

     C85.94 Non-Hodgkin lymphoma, unspecified, lymph nodes of axilla and upper limb

     C85.95 Non-Hodgkin lymphoma, unspecified, lymph nodes of inguinal region and lower limb

     C85.96 Non-Hodgkin lymphoma, unspecified, intrapelvic lymph nodes

     C85.97 Non-Hodgkin lymphoma, unspecified, spleen

     C85.98 Non-Hodgkin lymphoma, unspecified, lymph nodes of multiple sites

     C85.99 Non-Hodgkin lymphoma, unspecified, extranodal and solid organ sites

☑4ᵗʰ **C86 Other specified types of T/NK-cell lymphoma**

EXCLUDES 1   anaplastic large cell lymphoma, ALK negative (C84.7-)
     anaplastic large cell lymphoma, ALK positive (C84.6-)
     mature T/NK-cell lymphomas (C84.-)
     other specified types of non-Hodgkin lymphoma (C85.8-)

C86.0 Extranodal NK/T-cell lymphoma, nasal type

C86.1 Hepatosplenic T-cell lymphoma
     Alpha-beta and gamma delta types

C86.2 Enteropathy-type (intestinal) T-cell lymphoma
     Enteropathy associated T-cell lymphoma

C86.3 Subcutaneous panniculitis-like T-cell lymphoma

C86.4 Blastic NK-cell lymphoma

C86.5 Angioimmunoblastic T-cell lymphoma
     Angioimmunoblastic lymphadenopathy with dysproteinemia [AILD]

C86.6 Primary cutaneous CD30-positive T-cell proliferations
     Lymphomatoid papulosis
     Primary cutaneous anaplastic large cell lymphoma
     Primary cutaneous CD30-positive large T-cell lymphoma

☑4ᵗʰ **C88 Malignant immunoproliferative diseases and certain other B-cell lymphomas**

EXCLUDES 1   B-cell lymphoma, unspecified (C85.1-)
     personal history of other malignant neoplasms of lymphoid, hematopoietic and related tissues (Z85.79)

C88.0 Waldenström macroglobulinemia
     Lymphoplasmacytic lymphoma with IgM-production
     Macroglobulinemia (idiopathic) (primary)
     EXCLUDES 1   small cell B-cell lymphoma (C83.0)

C88.2 Heavy chain disease
     Franklin disease
     Gamma heavy chain disease
     Mu heavy chain disease

C88.3 Immunoproliferative small intestinal disease
     Alpha heavy chain disease
     Mediterranean lymphoma

C88.4 Extranodal marginal zone B-cell lymphoma of mucosa-associated lymphoid tissue [MALT-lymphoma]
     Lymphoma of skin-associated lymphoid tissue [SALT-lymphoma]
     Lymphoma of bronchial-associated lymphoid tissue [BALT-lymphoma]
     EXCLUDES 1   high malignant (diffuse large B-cell) lymphoma (C83.3-)

C88.8 Other malignant immunoproliferative diseases

C88.9 Malignant immunoproliferative disease, unspecified
     Immunoproliferative disease NOS

☑4ᵗʰ **C90 Multiple myeloma and malignant plasma cell neoplasms**

EXCLUDES 1   personal history of other malignant neoplasms of lymphoid, hematopoietic and related tissues (Z85.79)

☑5ᵗʰ **C90.0 Multiple myeloma**

     Kahler's disease   Myelomatosis
     Medullary plasmacytoma   Plasma cell myeloma
     EXCLUDES 1   solitary myeloma (C90.3-)
       solitary plasmactyoma (C90.3-)

     C90.00 Multiple myeloma not having achieved remission
     Multiple myeloma with failed remission
     Multiple myeloma NOS

     C90.01 Multiple myeloma in remission

     C90.02 Multiple myeloma in relapse

☑5ᵗʰ **C90.1 Plasma cell leukemia**
     Plasmacytic leukemia

     C90.10 Plasma cell leukemia not having achieved remission
     Plasma cell leukemia with failed remission
     Plasma cell leukemia NOS

☑ Additional Character Required   ✗x7ᵗʰ Placeholder Alert   Unspecified Dx   Other Specified Dx   Manifestation   ►◄ Revised Text   ● New Code   ▲ Revised Code Title

ICD-10-CM 2016   465

C85–C90.10

Chapter 2. Neoplasms (side tab)

C90.11   **Plasma cell leukemia** in remission

C90.12   **Plasma cell leukemia** in relapse

√5th **C90.2**   **Extramedullary plasmacytoma**

     C90.20   **Extramedullary plasmacytoma** not having achieved remission

        Extramedullary plasmacytoma with failed remission
        Extramedullary plasmacytoma NOS

     C90.21   **Extramedullary plasmacytoma** in remission

     C90.22   **Extramedullary plasmacytoma** in relapse

√5th **C90.3**   **Solitary plasmacytoma**

     Localized malignant plasma cell tumor NOS
     Plasmacytoma NOS
     Solitary myeloma

     C90.30   **Solitary plasmacytoma** not having achieved remission

        Solitary plasmacytoma with failed remission
        Solitary plasmacytoma NOS

     C90.31   **Solitary plasmacytoma** in remission

     C90.32   **Solitary plasmacytoma** in relapse

√4th **C91**   **Lymphoid leukemia**

     EXCLUDES 1   personal history of leukemia (Z85.6)

√5th **C91.0**   **Acute lymphoblastic leukemia [ALL]**

     NOTE   Code C91.0 should only be used for T-cell and B-cell precursor leukemia.

     C91.00   **Acute lymphoblastic leukemia** not having achieved remission

        Acute lymphoblastic leukemia with failed remission
        Acute lymphoblastic leukemia NOS

     C91.01   **Acute lymphoblastic leukemia, in remission**

     C91.02   **Acute lymphoblastic leukemia, in relapse**

√5th **C91.1**   **Chronic lymphocytic leukemia of B-cell type**

     Lymphoplasmacytic leukemia
     Richter syndrome

     EXCLUDES 1   lymphoplasmacytic lymphoma (C83.0-)

     C91.10   **Chronic lymphocytic leukemia of B-cell type** not having achieved remission

        Chronic lymphocytic leukemia of B-cell type with failed remission
        Chronic lymphocytic leukemia of B-cell type NOS

     C91.11   **Chronic lymphocytic leukemia of B-cell type** in remission

     C91.12   **Chronic lymphocytic leukemia of B-cell type** in relapse

√5th **C91.3**   **Prolymphocytic leukemia of B-cell type**

     C91.30   **Prolymphocytic leukemia of B-cell type** not having achieved remission

        Prolymphocytic leukemia of B-cell type with failed remission
        Prolymphocytic leukemia of B-cell type NOS

     C91.31   **Prolymphocytic leukemia of B-cell type, in remission**

     C91.32   **Prolymphocytic leukemia of B-cell type, in relapse**

√5th **C91.4**   **Hairy cell leukemia**

     Leukemic reticuloendotheliosis

     C91.40   **Hairy cell leukemia** not having achieved remission
        Hairy cell leukemia with failed remission
        Hairy cell leukemia NOS

     C91.41   **Hairy cell leukemia, in remission**

     C91.42   **Hairy cell leukemia, in relapse**

√5th **C91.5**   **Adult T-cell lymphoma/leukemia (HTLV-1-associated)**

     Acute variant of adult T-cell lymphoma/leukemia (HTLV-1-associated)
     Chronic variant of adult T-cell lymphoma/leukemia (HTLV-1-associated)
     Lymphomatoid variant of adult T-cell lymphoma/leukemia (HTLV-1-associated)
     Smouldering variant of adult T-cell lymphoma/leukemia (HTLV-1-associated)

     C91.50   **Adult T-cell lymphoma/leukemia (HTLV-1-associated)** not having achieved remission   🅐
        Adult T-cell lymphoma/leukemia (HTLV-1-associated) with failed remission
        Adult T-cell lymphoma/leukemia (HTLV-1-associated) NOS

     C91.51   **Adult T-cell lymphoma/leukemia (HTLV-1-associated), in remission**   🅐

     C91.52   **Adult T-cell lymphoma/leukemia (HTLV-1-associated), in relapse**   🅐

√5th **C91.6**   **Prolymphocytic leukemia of T-cell type**

     C91.60   **Prolymphocytic leukemia of T-cell type** not having achieved remission
        Prolymphocytic leukemia of T-cell type with failed remission
        Prolymphocytic leukemia of T-cell type NOS

     C91.61   **Prolymphocytic leukemia of T-cell type, in remission**

     C91.62   **Prolymphocytic leukemia of T-cell type, in relapse**

√5th **C91.A**   **Mature B-cell leukemia Burkitt-type**

     EXCLUDES 1   Burkitt lymphoma (C83.7-)

     C91.A0   **Mature B-cell leukemia Burkitt-type** not having achieved remission
        Mature B-cell leukemia Burkitt-type with failed remission
        Mature B-cell leukemia Burkitt-type NOS

     C91.A1   **Mature B-cell leukemia Burkitt-type, in remission**

     C91.A2   **Mature B-cell leukemia Burkitt-type, in relapse**

√5th **C91.Z**   **Other lymphoid leukemia**

     T-cell large granular lymphocytic leukemia (associated with rheumatoid arthritis)

     C91.Z0   **Other lymphoid leukemia** not having achieved remission
        Other lymphoid leukemia with failed remission
        Other lymphoid leukemia NOS

     C91.Z1   **Other lymphoid leukemia, in remission**

     C91.Z2   **Other lymphoid leukemia, in relapse**

√5th **C91.9**   **Lymphoid leukemia, unspecified**

     C91.90   **Lymphoid leukemia, unspecified** not having achieved remission
        Lymphoid leukemia with failed remission
        Lymphoid leukemia NOS

     C91.91   **Lymphoid leukemia, unspecified, in remission**

     C91.92   **Lymphoid leukemia, unspecified, in relapse**

√4th **C92**   **Myeloid leukemia**

     INCLUDES   granulocytic leukemia
             myelogenous leukemia

     EXCLUDES 1   personal history of leukemia (Z85.6)

√5th **C92.0**   **Acute myeloblastic leukemia**

     Acute myeloblastic leukemia, minimal differentiation
     Acute myeloblastic leukemia (with maturation)
     Acute myeloblastic leukemia 1/ETO
     Acute myeloblastic leukemia M0
     Acute myeloblastic leukemia M1
     Acute myeloblastic leukemia M2
     Acute myeloblastic leukemia with t(8;21)
     Acute myeloblastic leukemia (without a FAB classification) NOS
     Refractory anemia with excess blasts in transformation [RAEB T]

     EXCLUDES 1   acute exacerbation of chronic myeloid leukemia (C92.10)
              refractory anemia with excess of blasts not in transformation (D46.2-)

     C92.00   **Acute myeloblastic leukemia, not having achieved remission**
        Acute myeloblastic leukemia with failed remission
        Acute myeloblastic leukemia NOS

     C92.01   **Acute myeloblastic leukemia, in remission**

     C92.02   **Acute myeloblastic leukemia, in relapse**

√5th **C92.1**   **Chronic myeloid leukemia, BCR/ABL-positive**

     Chronic myelogenous leukemia, Philadelphia chromosome (Ph1) positive
     Chronic myelogenous leukemia, t(9;22) (q34;q11)
     Chronic myelogenous leukemia with crisis of blast cells

     EXCLUDES 1   atypical chronic myeloid leukemia BCR/ABL-negative (C92.2-)
              chronic myelomonocytic leukemia (C93.1-)
              chronic myeloproliferative disease (D47.1)

     C92.10   **Chronic myeloid leukemia, BCR/ABL-positive, not having achieved remission**
        Chronic myeloid leukemia, BCR/ABL-positive with failed remission
        Chronic myeloid leukemia, BCR/ABL-positive NOS

     C92.11   **Chronic myeloid leukemia, BCR/ABL-positive, in remission**

     C92.12   **Chronic myeloid leukemia, BCR/ABL-positive, in relapse**

EXCLUDES 1 Not coded here   EXCLUDES 2 Not included here   N Newborn Age: 0   P Pediatric Age: 0-17   M Maternity Age: 12-55   🅐 Adult Age: 15-124

466   ICD-10-CM 2016

Chapter 2. Neoplasms

✓5ᵗʰ **C92.2 Atypical chronic myeloid leukemia, BCR/ABL-negative**

    C92.20 Atypical chronic myeloid leukemia, BCR/ABL-negative, not having achieved remission
        Atypical chronic myeloid leukemia, BCR/ABL-negative with failed remission
        Atypical chronic myeloid leukemia, BCR/ABL-negative NOS

    C92.21 Atypical chronic myeloid leukemia, BCR/ABL-negative, in remission

    C92.22 Atypical chronic myeloid leukemia, BCR/ABL-negative, in relapse

✓5ᵗʰ **C92.3 Myeloid sarcoma**
    A malignant tumor of immature myeloid cells
    Chloroma
    Granulocytic sarcoma

    C92.30 Myeloid sarcoma, not having achieved remission
        Myeloid sarcoma with failed remission
        Myeloid sarcoma NOS

    C92.31 Myeloid sarcoma, in remission

    C92.32 Myeloid sarcoma, in relapse

✓5ᵗʰ **C92.4 Acute promyelocytic leukemia**
    AML M3
    AML Me with t(15;17) and variants

    C92.40 Acute promyelocytic leukemia, not having achieved remission
        Acute promyelocytic leukemia with failed remission
        Acute promyelocytic leukemia NOS

    C92.41 Acute promyelocytic leukemia, in remission

    C92.42 Acute promyelocytic leukemia, in relapse

✓5ᵗʰ **C92.5 Acute myelomonocytic leukemia**
    AML M4
    AML M4 Eo with inv(16) or t(16;16)

    C92.50 Acute myelomonocytic leukemia, not having achieved remission
        Acute myelomonocytic leukemia with failed remission
        Acute myelomonocytic leukemia NOS

    C92.51 Acute myelomonocytic leukemia, in remission

    C92.52 Acute myelomonocytic leukemia, in relapse

✓5ᵗʰ **C92.6 Acute myeloid leukemia with 11q23-abnormality**
    Acute myeloid leukemia with variation of MLL-gene

    C92.60 Acute myeloid leukemia with 11q23-abnormality not having achieved remission
        Acute myeloid leukemia with 11q23-abnormality with failed remission
        Acute myeloid leukemia with 11q23-abnormality NOS

    C92.61 Acute myeloid leukemia with 11q23-abnormality in remission

    C92.62 Acute myeloid leukemia with 11q23-abnormality in relapse

✓5ᵗʰ **C92.A Acute myeloid leukemia with multilineage dysplasia**
    Acute myeloid leukemia with dysplasia of remaining hematopoesis and/or myelodysplastic disease in its history

    C92.A0 Acute myeloid leukemia with multilineage dysplasia, not having achieved remission
        Acute myeloid leukemia with multilineage dysplasia with failed remission
        Acute myeloid leukemia with multilineage dysplasia NOS

    C92.A1 Acute myeloid leukemia with multilineage dysplasia, in remission

    C92.A2 Acute myeloid leukemia with multilineage dysplasia, in relapse

✓5ᵗʰ **C92.Z Other myeloid leukemia**

    C92.Z0 Other myeloid leukemia not having achieved remission
        Myeloid leukemia NEC with failed remission
        Myeloid leukemia NEC

    C92.Z1 Other myeloid leukemia, in remission

    C92.Z2 Other myeloid leukemia, in relapse

✓5ᵗʰ **C92.9 Myeloid leukemia, unspecified**

    C92.90 Myeloid leukemia, unspecified, not having achieved remission
        Myeloid leukemia, unspecified with failed remission
        Myeloid leukemia, unspecified NOS

    C92.91 Myeloid leukemia, unspecified in remission

    C92.92 Myeloid leukemia, unspecified in relapse

✓4ᵗʰ **C93 Monocytic leukemia**
    INCLUDES monocytoid leukemia
    EXCLUDES 1 *personal history of leukemia (Z85.6)*

✓5ᵗʰ **C93.0 Acute monoblastic/monocytic leukemia**
    AML M5   AML M5b
    AML M5a

    C93.00 Acute monoblastic/monocytic leukemia, not having achieved remission
        Acute monoblastic/monocytic leukemia with failed remission
        Acute monoblastic/monocytic leukemia NOS

    C93.01 Acute monoblastic/monocytic leukemia, in remission

    C93.02 Acute monoblastic/monocytic leukemia, in relapse

✓5ᵗʰ **C93.1 Chronic myelomonocytic leukemia**
    Chronic monocytic leukemia
    CMML-1
    CMML-2
    CMML with eosinophilia

    C93.10 Chronic myelomonocytic leukemia not having achieved remission
        Chronic myelomonocytic leukemia with failed remission
        Chronic myelomonocytic leukemia NOS

    C93.11 Chronic myelomonocytic leukemia, in remission

    C93.12 Chronic myelomonocytic leukemia, in relapse

✓5ᵗʰ **C93.3 Juvenile myelomonocytic leukemia**

    C93.30 Juvenile myelomonocytic leukemia, not having achieved remission ▣
        Juvenile myelomonocytic leukemia with failed remission
        Juvenile myelomonocytic leukemia NOS

    C93.31 Juvenile myelomonocytic leukemia, in remission ▣

    C93.32 Juvenile myelomonocytic leukemia, in relapse ▣

✓5ᵗʰ **C93.Z Other monocytic leukemia**

    C93.Z0 Other monocytic leukemia, not having achieved remission
        Other monocytic leukemia NOS

    C93.Z1 Other monocytic leukemia, in remission

    C93.Z2 Other monocytic leukemia, in relapse

✓5ᵗʰ **C93.9 Monocytic leukemia, unspecified**

    C93.90 Monocytic leukemia, unspecified, not having achieved remission
        Monocytic leukemia, unspecified with failed remission
        Monocytic leukemia, unspecified NOS

    C93.91 Monocytic leukemia, unspecified in remission

    C93.92 Monocytic leukemia, unspecified in relapse

✓4ᵗʰ **C94 Other leukemias of specified cell type**
    EXCLUDES 1 *leukemic reticuloendotheliosis (C91.4-)*
        myelodysplastic syndromes (D46.-)
        personal history of leukemia (Z85.6)
        plasma cell leukemia (C90.1-)

✓5ᵗʰ **C94.0 Acute erythroid leukemia**
    Acute myeloid leukemia M6(a)(b)
    Erythroleukemia

    C94.00 Acute erythroid leukemia, not having achieved remission
        Acute erythroid leukemia with failed remission
        Acute erythroid leukemia NOS

    C94.01 Acute erythroid leukemia, in remission

    C94.02 Acute erythroid leukemia, in relapse

✓5ᵗʰ **C94.2 Acute megakaryoblastic leukemia**
    Acute myeloid leukemia M7
    Acute megakaryocytic leukemia

    C94.20 Acute megakaryoblastic leukemia not having achieved remission
        Acute megakaryoblastic leukemia with failed remission
        Acute megakaryoblastic leukemia NOS

    C94.21 Acute megakaryoblastic leukemia, in remission

    C94.22 Acute megakaryoblastic leukemia, in relapse

✓5ᵗʰ **C94.3 Mast cell leukemia**

    C94.30 Mast cell leukemia not having achieved remission
        Mast cell leukemia with failed remission
        Mast cell leukemia NOS

    C94.31 Mast cell leukemia, in remission

    C94.32 Mast cell leukemia, in relapse

☑ Additional Character Required   ✓ˣ7ᵗʰ Placeholder Alert   Unspecified Dx   Other Specified Dx   Manifestation   ▶◀ Revised Text   ● New Code   ▲ Revised Code Title

ICD-10-CM 2016   467

✓5th **C94.4　Acute panmyelosis with myelofibrosis**
Acute myelofibrosis
EXCLUDES 1　*myelofibrosis NOS (D75.81)*
secondary myelofibrosis NOS (D75.81)

　　C94.40　Acute panmyelosis with myelofibrosis not having achieved remission
Acute myelofibrosis NOS
Acute panmyelosis with myelofibrosis with failed remission
Acute panmyelosis NOS

　　C94.41　Acute panmyelosis with myelofibrosis, in remission

　　C94.42　Acute panmyelosis with myelofibrosis, in relapse

C94.6　Myelodysplastic disease, not classified
Myeloproliferative disease, not classified

✓5th **C94.8　Other specified leukemias**
Aggressive NK-cell leukemia
Acute basophilic leukemia

　　C94.80　Other specified leukemias not having achieved remission
Other specified leukemia with failed remission
Other specified leukemias NOS

　　C94.81　Other specified leukemias, in remission

　　C94.82　Other specified leukemias, in relapse

✓4th **C95　Leukemia of** unspecified cell type
EXCLUDES 1　*personal history of leukemia (Z85.6)*

✓5th **C95.0　Acute** leukemia of unspecified cell type
Acute bilineal leukemia
Acute mixed lineage leukemia
Biphenotypic acute leukemia
Stem cell leukemia of unclear lineage
EXCLUDES 1　*acute exacerbation of unspecified chronic leukemia (C95.10)*

　　C95.00　Acute leukemia of unspecified cell type not having achieved remission
Acute leukemia of unspecified cell type with failed remission
Acute leukemia NOS

　　C95.01　Acute leukemia of unspecified cell type, in remission

　　C95.02　Acute leukemia of unspecified cell type, in relapse

✓5th **C95.1　Chronic** leukemia of unspecified cell type

　　C95.10　Chronic leukemia of unspecified cell type not having achieved remission
Chronic leukemia of unspecified cell type with failed remission
Chronic leukemia NOS

　　C95.11　Chronic leukemia of unspecified cell type, in remission

　　C95.12　Chronic leukemia of unspecified cell type, in relapse

✓5th **C95.9　Leukemia,** unspecified

　　C95.90　Leukemia, unspecified not having achieved remission
Leukemia, unspecified with failed remission
Leukemia NOS

　　C95.91　Leukemia, unspecified, in remission

　　C95.92　Leukemia, unspecified, in relapse

✓4th **C96　Other and unspecified malignant neoplasms of lymphoid, hematopoietic and related tissue**
EXCLUDES 1　*personal history of other malignant neoplasms of lymphoid, hematopoietic and related tissues (Z85.79)*

C96.0　Multifocal and multisystemic (disseminated) Langerhans-cell histiocytosis
Histiocytosis X, multisystemic
Letterer-Siwe disease
EXCLUDES 1　*adult pulmonary Langerhans cell histiocytosis (J84.82)*
multifocal and unisystemic Langerhans-cell histiocytosis (C96.5)
unifocal Langerhans-cell histiocytosis (C96.6)

C96.2　Malignant mast cell tumor
Aggressive systemic mastocytosis
Mast cell sarcoma
EXCLUDES 1　*indolent mastocytosis (D47.0)*
mast cell leukemia (C94.30)
mastocytosis (congenital) (cutaneous) (Q82.2)

C96.4　Sarcoma of dendritic cells (accessory cells)
Follicular dendritic cell sarcoma
Interdigitating dendritic cell sarcoma
Langerhans cell sarcoma

C96.5　Multifocal and unisystemic Langerhans-cell histiocytosis
Hand-Schüller-Christian disease
Histiocytosis X, multifocal
EXCLUDES 1　*multifocal and multisystemic (disseminated) Langerhans-cell histiocytosis (C96.0)*
unifocal Langerhans-cell histiocytosis (C96.6)

C96.6　Unifocal Langerhans-cell histiocytosis
Eosinophilic granuloma
Histiocytosis X, unifocal
Histiocytosis X NOS
Langerhans-cell histiocytosis NOS
EXCLUDES 1　*multifocal and multisysemic (disseminated) Langerhans-cell histiocytosis (C96.0)*
multifocal and unisystemic Langerhans-cell histiocytosis (C96.5)

C96.A　Histiocytic sarcoma
Malignant histiocytosis

C96.Z　Other specified malignant neoplasms of lymphoid, hematopoietic and related tissue

C96.9　Malignant neoplasm of lymphoid, hematopoietic and related tissue, unspecified

In situ neoplasms (D00-D09)

INCLUDES　Bowen's disease
erythroplasia
grade III intraepithelial neoplasia
Queyrat's erythroplasia

✓4th **D00　Carcinoma in situ of** oral cavity, esophagus and stomach
EXCLUDES 1　*melanoma in situ (D03.-)*

✓5th **D00.0　Carcinoma in situ of** lip, oral cavity and pharynx
Use additional code to identify:
exposure to environmental tobacco smoke (Z77.22)
exposure to tobacco smoke in the perinatal period (P96.81)
history of tobacco use (Z87.891)
occupational exposure to environmental tobacco smoke (Z57.31)
tobacco dependence (F17.-)
tobacco use (Z72.0)
EXCLUDES 1　*carcinoma in situ of aryepiglottic fold or interarytenoid fold, laryngeal aspect (D02.0)*
carcinoma in situ of epiglottis NOS (D02.0)
carcinoma in situ of epiglottis suprahyoid portion (D02.0)
carcinoma in situ of skin of lip (D03.0, D04.0)

　　D00.00　Carcinoma in situ of oral cavity, unspecified site

　　D00.01　Carcinoma in situ of labial mucosa and vermilion border

　　D00.02　Carcinoma in situ of buccal mucosa

　　D00.03　Carcinoma in situ of gingiva and edentulous alveolar ridge

　　D00.04　Carcinoma in situ of soft palate

　　D00.05　Carcinoma in situ of hard palate

　　D00.06　Carcinoma in situ of floor of mouth

　　D00.07　Carcinoma in situ of tongue

　　D00.08　Carcinoma in situ of pharynx
Carcinoma in situ of aryepiglottic fold NOS
Carcinoma in situ of hypopharyngeal aspect of aryepiglottic fold
Carcinoma in situ of marginal zone of aryepiglottic fold

D00.1　Carcinoma in situ of esophagus

D00.2　Carcinoma in situ of stomach

✓4th **D01　Carcinoma in situ of** other and unspecified digestive organs
EXCLUDES 1　*melanoma in situ (D03.-)*

D01.0　Carcinoma in situ of colon
EXCLUDES 1　*carcinoma in situ of rectosigmoid junction (D01.1)*

D01.1　Carcinoma in situ of rectosigmoid junction

D01.2　Carcinoma in situ of rectum

D01.3　Carcinoma in situ of anus and anal canal
EXCLUDES 1　*carcinoma in situ of anal margin (D04.5)*
carcinoma in situ of anal skin (D04.5)
carcinoma in situ of perianal skin (D04.5)

✓5th **D01.4　Carcinoma in situ of other and unspecified parts of** intestine
EXCLUDES 1　*carcinoma in situ of ampulla of Vater (D01.5)*

　　D01.40　Carcinoma in situ of unspecified part of intestine

　　D01.49　Carcinoma in situ of other parts of intestine

EXCLUDES 1 Not coded here　　　EXCLUDES 2 Not included here　　　N Newborn Age: 0　　　P Pediatric Age: 0-17　　　M Maternity Age: 12-55　　　A Adult Age: 15-124

468　　　　　　　　　　　　　　　　　　　　　　　　　　　　　　　　　ICD-10-CM 2016

D01.5 **Carcinoma in situ of** liver, gallbladder and bile ducts
Carcinoma in situ of ampulla of Vater

D01.7 **Carcinoma in situ of other specified digestive organs**
Carcinoma in situ of pancreas

D01.9 **Carcinoma in situ of digestive organ, unspecified**

✓4ᵗʰ **D02 Carcinoma in situ of** middle ear and respiratory system
Use additional code to identify:
exposure to environmental tobacco smoke (Z77.22)
exposure to tobacco smoke in the perinatal period (P96.81)
history of tobacco use (Z87.891)
occupational exposure to environmental tobacco smoke (Z57.31)
tobacco dependence (F17.-)
tobacco use (Z72.0)
EXCLUDES 1   *melanoma in situ (D03.-)*

D02.0 **Carcinoma in situ of** larynx
Carcinoma in situ of aryepiglottic fold or interarytenoid fold,
laryngeal aspect
Carcinoma in situ of epiglottis (suprahyoid portion)
EXCLUDES 1   *carcinoma in situ of aryepiglottic fold or interarytenoid*
fold NOS (D00.08)
carcinoma in situ of hypopharyngeal aspect (D00.08)
carcinoma in situ of marginal zone (D00.08)

D02.1 **Carcinoma in situ of** trachea

✓5ᵗʰ D02.2 **Carcinoma in situ of** bronchus and lung
D02.20 **Carcinoma in situ of unspecified bronchus and lung**
D02.21 **Carcinoma in situ of** right bronchus and lung
D02.22 **Carcinoma in situ of** left bronchus and lung

D02.3 **Carcinoma in situ of other parts of respiratory system**
Carcinoma in situ of accessory sinuses
Carcinoma in situ of middle ear
Carcinoma in situ of nasal cavities
EXCLUDES 1   *carcinoma in situ of ear (external) (skin) (D04.2-)*
carcinoma in situ of nose NOS (D09.8)
carcinoma in situ of skin of nose (D04.3)

D02.4 **Carcinoma in situ of respiratory system, unspecified**

✓4ᵗʰ **D03 Melanoma in situ**

D03.0 **Melanoma in situ of** lip

✓5ᵗʰ D03.1 **Melanoma in situ of** eyelid, including canthus
D03.10 **Melanoma in situ of unspecified eyelid, including canthus**
D03.11 **Melanoma in situ of** right eyelid, including canthus
D03.12 **Melanoma in situ of** left eyelid, including canthus

✓5ᵗʰ D03.2 **Melanoma in situ of** ear and external auricular canal
D03.20 **Melanoma in situ of unspecified ear and external auricular canal**
D03.21 **Melanoma in situ of** right ear and external auricular canal
D03.22 **Melanoma in situ of** left ear and external auricular canal

✓5ᵗʰ D03.3 **Melanoma in situ of** other and unspecified parts of face
D03.30 **Melanoma in situ of unspecified part of face**
D03.39 **Melanoma in situ of other parts of face**

D03.4 **Melanoma in situ of** scalp and neck

✓5ᵗʰ D03.5 **Melanoma in situ of** trunk
D03.51 **Melanoma in situ of** anal skin
Melanoma in situ of anal margin
Melanoma in situ of perianal skin
D03.52 **Melanoma in situ of** breast (skin) (soft tissue)
D03.59 **Melanoma in situ of other part of trunk**

✓5ᵗʰ D03.6 **Melanoma in situ of** upper limb, including shoulder
D03.60 **Melanoma in situ of unspecified upper limb, including shoulder**
D03.61 **Melanoma in situ of** right upper limb, including shoulder
D03.62 **Melanoma in situ of** left upper limb, including shoulder

✓5ᵗʰ D03.7 **Melanoma in situ of** lower limb, including hip
D03.70 **Melanoma in situ of unspecified lower limb, including hip**
D03.71 **Melanoma in situ of** right lower limb, including hip
D03.72 **Melanoma in situ of** left lower limb, including hip

D03.8 **Melanoma in situ of other sites**
Melanoma in situ of scrotum
EXCLUDES 1   *carcinoma in situ of scrotum (D07.61)*

D03.9 **Melanoma in situ, unspecified**

✓4ᵗʰ **D04 Carcinoma in situ of** skin
EXCLUDES 1   *erythroplasia of Queyrat (penis) NOS (D07.4)*
melanoma in situ (D03.-)

D04.0 **Carcinoma in situ of skin of** lip
EXCLUDES 1   *carcinoma in situ of vermilion border of lip (D00.01)*

✓5ᵗʰ D04.1 **Carcinoma in situ of skin of** eyelid, including canthus
D04.10 **Carcinoma in situ of skin of unspecified eyelid, including canthus**
D04.11 **Carcinoma in situ of skin of** right eyelid, including canthus
D04.12 **Carcinoma in situ of skin of** left eyelid, including canthus

✓5ᵗʰ D04.2 **Carcinoma in situ of skin of** ear and external auricular canal
D04.20 **Carcinoma in situ of skin of unspecified ear and external auricular canal**
D04.21 **Carcinoma in situ of skin of** right ear and external auricular canal
D04.22 **Carcinoma in situ of skin of** left ear and external auricular canal

✓5ᵗʰ D04.3 **Carcinoma in situ of skin of** other and unspecified parts of face
D04.30 **Carcinoma in situ of skin of unspecified part of face**
D04.39 **Carcinoma in situ of skin of other parts of face**

D04.4 **Carcinoma in situ of skin of** scalp and neck

D04.5 **Carcinoma in situ of skin of** trunk
Carcinoma in situ of anal margin
Carcinoma in situ of anal skin
Carcinoma in situ of perianal skin
Carcinoma in situ of skin of breast
EXCLUDES 1   *carcinoma in situ of anus NOS (D01.3)*
carcinoma in situ of scrotum (D07.61)
carcinoma in situ of skin of genital organs (D07.-)

✓5ᵗʰ D04.6 **Carcinoma in situ of skin of** upper limb, including shoulder
D04.60 **Carcinoma in situ of skin of unspecified upper limb, including shoulder**
D04.61 **Carcinoma in situ of skin of** right upper limb, including shoulder
D04.62 **Carcinoma in situ of skin of** left upper limb, including shoulder

✓5ᵗʰ D04.7 **Carcinoma in situ of skin of** lower limb, including hip
D04.70 **Carcinoma in situ of skin of unspecified lower limb, including hip**
D04.71 **Carcinoma in situ of skin of** right lower limb, including hip
D04.72 **Carcinoma in situ of skin of** left lower limb, including hip

D04.8 **Carcinoma in situ of skin of other sites**
D04.9 **Carcinoma in situ of skin, unspecified**

✓4ᵗʰ **D05 Carcinoma in situ of** breast
EXCLUDES 1   *carcinoma in situ of skin of breast (D04.5)*
melanoma in situ of breast (skin) (D03.5)
Paget's disease of breast or nipple (C50.-)

✓5ᵗʰ D05.0 **Lobular** carcinoma in situ of breast
D05.00 **Lobular carcinoma in situ of unspecified breast**
D05.01 **Lobular carcinoma in situ of** right breast
D05.02 **Lobular carcinoma in situ of** left breast

✓5ᵗʰ D05.1 **Intraductal** carcinoma in situ of breast
D05.10 **Intraductal carcinoma in situ of unspecified breast**
D05.11 **Intraductal carcinoma in situ of** right breast
D05.12 **Intraductal carcinoma in situ of** left breast

✓5ᵗʰ D05.8 **Other** specified type of carcinoma in situ of breast
D05.80 **Other specified type of carcinoma in situ of unspecified breast**
D05.81 **Other specified type of carcinoma in situ of** right breast
D05.82 **Other specified type of carcinoma in situ of** left breast

✓5ᵗʰ D05.9 **Unspecified** type of carcinoma in situ of breast
D05.90 **Unspecified type of carcinoma in situ of unspecified breast**
D05.91 **Unspecified type of carcinoma in situ of** right breast
D05.92 **Unspecified type of carcinoma in situ of** left breast

---

☑ Additional Character Required   ✓₇ᵗʰ Placeholder Alert   Unspecified Dx   Other Specified Dx   Manifestation   ▶◀ Revised Text   ● New Code   ▲ Revised Code Title

✓4ᵗʰ D06 Carcinoma in situ of cervix uteri

    INCLUDES   cervical adenocarcinoma in situ
                cervical intraepithelial glandular neoplasia
                cervical intraepithelial neoplasia III [CIN III]
                severe dysplasia of cervix uteri

    EXCLUDES 1   cervical intraepithelial neoplasia II [CIN II] (N87.1)
                cytologic evidence of malignancy of cervix without histologic
                  confirmation (R87.614)
                high grade squamous intraepithelial lesion (HGSIL) of cervix
                  (R87.613)
                melanoma in situ of cervix (D03.5)
                moderate cervical dysplasia (N87.1)

    D06.0 Carcinoma in situ of endocervix   ♀
    D06.1 Carcinoma in situ of exocervix   ♀
    D06.7 Carcinoma in situ of other parts of cervix   ♀
    D06.9 Carcinoma in situ of cervix, unspecified   ♀

✓4ᵗʰ D07 Carcinoma in situ of other and unspecified genital organs

    EXCLUDES 1   melanoma in situ of trunk (D03.5)

    D07.0 Carcinoma in situ of endometrium   ♀
    D07.1 Carcinoma in situ of vulva   ♀
        Severe dysplasia of vulva
        Vulvar intraepithelial neoplasia III [VIN III]
        EXCLUDES 1   moderate dysplasia of vulva (N90.1)
                   vulvar intraepithelial neoplasia II [VIN II] (N90.1)
    D07.2 Carcinoma in situ of vagina   ♀
        Severe dysplasia of vagina
        Vaginal intraepithelial neoplasia III [VAIN III]
        EXCLUDES 1   moderate dysplasia of vagina (N89.1)
                   vaginal intraepithelial neoplasia II [VIN II] (N89.1)

    ✓5ᵗʰ D07.3 Carcinoma in situ of other and unspecified female genital organs
        D07.30 Carcinoma in situ of unspecified female genital organs   ♀
        D07.39 Carcinoma in situ of other female genital organs   ♀

    D07.4 Carcinoma in situ of penis   ♂
        Erythroplasia of Queyrat NOS
    D07.5 Carcinoma in situ of prostate   ♂
        Prostatic intraepithelial neoplasia III (PIN III)
        Severe dysplasia of prostate
        EXCLUDES 1   dysplasia (mild) (moderate) of prostate (N42.3)

    ✓5ᵗʰ D07.6 Carcinoma in situ of other and unspecified male genital organs
        D07.60 Carcinoma in situ of unspecified male genital organs   ♂
        D07.61 Carcinoma in situ of scrotum   ♂
        D07.69 Carcinoma in situ of other male genital organs   ♂

✓4ᵗʰ D09 Carcinoma in situ of other and unspecified sites

    EXCLUDES 1   melanoma in situ (D03.-)

    D09.0 Carcinoma in situ of bladder
    ✓5ᵗʰ D09.1 Carcinoma in situ of other and unspecified urinary organs
        D09.10 Carcinoma in situ of unspecified urinary organ
        D09.19 Carcinoma in situ of other urinary organs
    ✓5ᵗʰ D09.2 Carcinoma in situ of eye
        EXCLUDES 1   carcinoma in situ of skin of eyelid (D04.1-)
        D09.20 Carcinoma in situ of unspecified eye
        D09.21 Carcinoma in situ of right eye
        D09.22 Carcinoma in situ of left eye
    D09.3 Carcinoma in situ of thyroid and other endocrine glands
        EXCLUDES 1   carcinoma in situ of endocrine pancreas (D01.7)
                   carcinoma in situ of ovary (D07.39)
                   carcinoma in situ of testis (D07.69)
    D09.8 Carcinoma in situ of other specified sites
    D09.9 Carcinoma in situ, unspecified

Benign neoplasms, except benign neuroendocrine tumors (D10-D36)

✓4ᵗʰ D10 Benign neoplasm of mouth and pharynx

    D10.0 Benign neoplasm of lip
        Benign neoplasm of lip (frenulum) (inner aspect) (mucosa)
            (vermilion border)
        EXCLUDES 1   benign neoplasm of skin of lip (D22.0, D23.0)
    D10.1 Benign neoplasm of tongue
        Benign neoplasm of lingual tonsil
    D10.2 Benign neoplasm of floor of mouth

✓5ᵗʰ D10.3 Other and unspecified parts of mouth
    D10.30 Benign neoplasm of unspecified part of mouth
    D10.39 Benign neoplasm of other parts of mouth
        Benign neoplasm of minor salivary gland NOS
        EXCLUDES 1   benign odontogenic neoplasms
                   (D16.4-D16.5)
                   benign neoplasm of mucosa of lip (D10.0)
                   benign neoplasm of nasopharyngeal surface
                     of soft palate (D10.6)

    D10.4 Benign neoplasm of tonsil
        Benign neoplasm of tonsil (faucial) (palatine)
        EXCLUDES 1   benign neoplasm of lingual tonsil (D10.1)
                   benign neoplasm of pharyngeal tonsil (D10.6)
                   benign neoplasm of tonsillar fossa (D10.5)
                   benign neoplasm of tonsillar pillars (D10.5)

    D10.5 Benign neoplasm of other parts of oropharynx
        Benign neoplasm of epiglottis, anterior aspect
        Benign neoplasm of tonsillar fossa
        Benign neoplasm of tonsillar pillars
        Benign neoplasm of vallecula
        EXCLUDES 1   benign neoplasm of epiglottis NOS (D14.1)
                   benign neoplasm of epiglottis, suprahyoid portion
                   (D14.1)

    D10.6 Benign neoplasm of nasopharynx
        Benign neoplasm of pharyngeal tonsil
        Benign neoplasm of posterior margin of septum and choanae
    D10.7 Benign neoplasm of hypopharynx
    D10.9 Benign neoplasm of pharynx, unspecified

✓4ᵗʰ D11 Benign neoplasm of major salivary glands

    EXCLUDES 1   benign neoplasms of specified minor salivary glands which are
                classified according to their anatomical location
                benign neoplasms of minor salivary glands NOS (D10.39)

    D11.0 Benign neoplasm of parotid gland
    D11.7 Benign neoplasm of other major salivary glands
        Benign neoplasm of sublingual salivary gland
        Benign neoplasm of submandibular salivary gland
    D11.9 Benign neoplasm of major salivary gland, unspecified

✓4ᵗʰ D12 Benign neoplasm of colon, rectum, anus and anal canal

    EXCLUDES 1   benign carcinoid tumors of the large intestine, and rectum
                (D3A.02-)

    D12.0 Benign neoplasm of cecum
        Benign neoplasm of ileocecal valve
    D12.1 Benign neoplasm of appendix
        EXCLUDES 1   benign carcinoid tumor of the appendix (D3A.020)
    D12.2 Benign neoplasm of ascending colon
    D12.3 Benign neoplasm of transverse colon
        Benign neoplasm of hepatic flexure
        Benign neoplasm of splenic flexure
    D12.4 Benign neoplasm of descending colon
    D12.5 Benign neoplasm of sigmoid colon
    D12.6 Benign neoplasm of colon, unspecified
        Adenomatosis of colon
        Benign neoplasm of large intestine NOS
        Polyposis (hereditary) of colon
        EXCLUDES 1   inflammatory polyp of colon (K51.4-)
                   polyp of colon NOS (K63.5)
    D12.7 Benign neoplasm of rectosigmoid junction
    D12.8 Benign neoplasm of rectum
        EXCLUDES 1   benign carcinoid tumor of the rectum (D3A.026)
    D12.9 Benign neoplasm of anus and anal canal
        Benign neoplasm of anus NOS
        EXCLUDES 1   benign neoplasm of anal margin (D22.5, D23.5)
                   benign neoplasm of anal skin (D22.5, D23.5)
                   benign neoplasm of perianal skin (D22.5, D23.5)

✓4ᵗʰ D13 Benign neoplasm of other and ill-defined parts of digestive system

    EXCLUDES 1   benign stromal tumors of digestive system (D21.4)

    D13.0 Benign neoplasm of esophagus
    D13.1 Benign neoplasm of stomach
        EXCLUDES 1   benign carcinoid tumor of the stomach (D3A.092)
    D13.2 Benign neoplasm of duodenum
        EXCLUDES 1   benign carcinoid tumor of the duodenum (D3A.010)

✓5ᵗʰ **D13.3** **Benign neoplasm of other and unspecified parts of** small **intestine**

    EXCLUDES 1   *benign carcinoid tumors of the small intestine (D3A.01-)*
              benign neoplasm of ileocecal valve (D12.0)

    D13.30 **Benign neoplasm of unspecified part of small intestine**

    D13.39 **Benign neoplasm of other parts of small intestine**

D13.4 **Benign neoplasm of** liver
    Benign neoplasm of intrahepatic bile ducts

D13.5 **Benign neoplasm of** extrahepatic bile ducts

D13.6 **Benign neoplasm of** pancreas
    EXCLUDES 1   *benign neoplasm of endocrine pancreas (D13.7)*

D13.7 **Benign neoplasm of** endocrine pancreas
    Islet cell tumor
    Benign neoplasm of islets of Langerhans
    Use additional code to identify any functional activity

D13.9 **Benign neoplasm of** ill-defined sites **within the digestive system**
    Benign neoplasm of digestive system NOS
    Benign neoplasm of intestine NOS
    Benign neoplasm of spleen

✓4ᵗʰ **D14** **Benign neoplasm of** middle ear and respiratory system

D14.0 **Benign neoplasm of** middle ear, nasal cavity and accessory **sinuses**
    Benign neoplasm of cartilage of nose
    EXCLUDES 1   *benign neoplasm of auricular canal (external) (D22.2-, D23.2-)*
              benign neoplasm of bone of ear (D16.4)
              benign neoplasm of bone of nose (D16.4)
              benign neoplasm of cartilage of ear (D21.0)
              benign neoplasm of ear (external)(skin) (D22.2-, D23.2-)
              benign neoplasm of nose NOS (D36.7)
              benign neoplasm of skin of nose (D22.39, D23.39)
              benign neoplasm of olfactory bulb (D33.3)
              benign neoplasm of posterior margin of septum and choanae (D10.6)
              polyp of accessory sinus (J33.8)
              polyp of ear (middle) (H74.4)
              polyp of nasal (cavity) (J33.-)

D14.1 **Benign neoplasm of** larynx
    Adenomatous polyp of larynx
    Benign neoplasm of epiglottis (suprahyoid portion)
    EXCLUDES 1   *benign neoplasm of epiglottis, anterior aspect (D10.5)*
              polyp (nonadenomatous) of vocal cord or larynx (J38.1)

D14.2 **Benign neoplasm of** trachea

✓5ᵗʰ **D14.3** **Benign neoplasm of** bronchus and lung
    EXCLUDES 1   *benign carcinoid tumor of the bronchus and lung (D3A.090)*

    D14.30 **Benign neoplasm of unspecified bronchus and lung**
    D14.31 **Benign neoplasm of** right **bronchus and lung**
    D14.32 **Benign neoplasm of** left **bronchus and lung**

D14.4 **Benign neoplasm of respiratory system, unspecified**

✓4ᵗʰ **D15** **Benign neoplasm of** other and unspecified intrathoracic organs
    EXCLUDES 1   *benign neoplasm of mesothelial tissue (D19.-)*

D15.0 **Benign neoplasm of** thymus
    EXCLUDES 1   *benign carcinoid tumor of the thymus (D3A.091)*

D15.1 **Benign neoplasm of** heart
    EXCLUDES 1   *benign neoplasm of great vessels (D21.3)*

D15.2 **Benign neoplasm of** mediastinum

D15.7 **Benign neoplasm of other specified intrathoracic organs**

D15.9 **Benign neoplasm of intrathoracic organ, unspecified**

✓4ᵗʰ **D16** **Benign neoplasm of** bone and articular cartilage
    EXCLUDES 1   *benign neoplasm of connective tissue of ear (D21.0)*
              benign neoplasm of connective tissue of eyelid (D21.0)
              benign neoplasm of connective tissue of larynx (D14.1)
              benign neoplasm of connective tissue of nose (D14.0)
              benign neoplasm of synovia (D21.-)

✓5ᵗʰ **D16.0** **Benign neoplasm of** scapula and long bones of upper limb
    D16.00 **Benign neoplasm of scapula and long bones of unspecified upper limb**
    D16.01 **Benign neoplasm of scapula and long bones of** right **upper limb**
    D16.02 **Benign neoplasm of scapula and long bones of** left **upper limb**

✓5ᵗʰ **D16.1** **Benign neoplasm of** short bones of upper limb
    D16.10 **Benign neoplasm of short bones of unspecified upper limb**
    D16.11 **Benign neoplasm of short bones of** right **upper limb**
    D16.12 **Benign neoplasm of short bones of** left **upper limb**

✓5ᵗʰ **D16.2** **Benign neoplasm of** long bones of lower limb
    D16.20 **Benign neoplasm of long bones of unspecified lower limb**
    D16.21 **Benign neoplasm of long bones of** right **lower limb**
    D16.22 **Benign neoplasm of long bones of** left **lower limb**

✓5ᵗʰ **D16.3** **Benign neoplasm of** short bones of lower limb
    D16.30 **Benign neoplasm of short bones of unspecified lower limb**
    D16.31 **Benign neoplasm of short bones of** right **lower limb**
    D16.32 **Benign neoplasm of short bones of** left **lower limb**

D16.4 **Benign neoplasm of bones of** skull and face
    Benign neoplasm of maxilla (superior)
    Benign neoplasm of orbital bone
    Keratocyst of maxilla
    Keratocystic odontogenic tumor of maxilla
    EXCLUDES 1   *benign neoplasm of lower jaw bone (D16.5)*

D16.5 **Benign neoplasm of** lower jaw bone
    Keratocyst of mandible
    Keratocystic odontogenic tumor of mandible

D16.6 **Benign neoplasm of** vertebral column
    EXCLUDES 1   *benign neoplasm of sacrum and coccyx (D16.8)*

D16.7 **Benign neoplasm of** ribs, sternum and clavicle

D16.8 **Benign neoplasm of** pelvic bones, sacrum and coccyx

D16.9 **Benign neoplasm of bone and articular cartilage, unspecified**

✓4ᵗʰ **D17** **Benign** lipomatous neoplasm

D17.0 **Benign lipomatous neoplasm of** skin and subcutaneous tissue of head, face and neck

D17.1 **Benign lipomatous neoplasm of** skin and subcutaneous tissue of trunk

✓5ᵗʰ **D17.2** **Benign lipomatous neoplasm of** skin and subcutaneous tissue of limb
    D17.20 **Benign lipomatous neoplasm of skin and subcutaneous tissue of unspecified limb**
    D17.21 **Benign lipomatous neoplasm of skin and subcutaneous tissue of** right **arm**
    D17.22 **Benign lipomatous neoplasm of skin and subcutaneous tissue of** left **arm**
    D17.23 **Benign lipomatous neoplasm of skin and subcutaneous tissue of** right **leg**
    D17.24 **Benign lipomatous neoplasm of skin and subcutaneous tissue of** left **leg**

✓5ᵗʰ **D17.3** **Benign lipomatous neoplasm of** skin and subcutaneous tissue of other and unspecified sites
    D17.30 **Benign lipomatous neoplasm of skin and subcutaneous tissue of unspecified sites**
    D17.39 **Benign lipomatous neoplasm of skin and subcutaneous tissue of other sites**

D17.4 **Benign lipomatous neoplasm of** intrathoracic organs

D17.5 **Benign lipomatous neoplasm of** intra-abdominal organs
    EXCLUDES 1   *benign lipomatous neoplasm of peritoneum and retroperitoneum (D17.79)*

D17.6 **Benign lipomatous neoplasm of** spermatic cord   ♂

✓5ᵗʰ **D17.7** **Benign lipomatous neoplasm of** other sites
    D17.71 **Benign lipomatous neoplasm of** kidney
    D17.72 **Benign lipomatous neoplasm of other** genitourinary **organ**
    D17.79 **Benign lipomatous neoplasm of other sites**
        Benign lipomatous neoplasm of peritoneum
        Benign lipomatous neoplasm of retroperitoneum

D17.9 **Benign lipomatous neoplasm, unspecified**
    Lipoma NOS

✓4ᵗʰ **D18** **Hemangioma and lymphangioma, any site**
    EXCLUDES 1   *benign neoplasm of glomus jugulare (D35.6)*
              blue or pigmented nevus (D22.-)
              nevus NOS (D22.-)
              vascular nevus (Q82.5)

✓5ᵗʰ **D18.0** **Hemangioma**
    Angioma NOS
    Cavernous nevus
    D18.00 **Hemangioma unspecified site**

☑ Additional Character Required   ✔x7ᵗʰ Placeholder Alert   Unspecified Dx   Other Specified Dx   Manifestation   ▶◀ Revised Text   ● New Code   ▲ Revised Code Title

ICD-10-CM 2016   **471**

Chapter 2. Neoplasms

D18.01–D23.39

D18.01   **Hemangioma of** skin and subcutaneous tissue

D18.02   **Hemangioma of** intracranial structures

D18.03   **Hemangioma of** intra-abdominal structures

D18.09   **Hemangioma of other sites**

D18.1   **Lymphangioma, any site**

✓4ᵗʰ **D19**   **Benign neoplasm of** mesothelial tissue

D19.0   **Benign neoplasm of mesothelial tissue of** pleura

D19.1   **Benign neoplasm of mesothelial tissue of** peritoneum

D19.7   **Benign neoplasm of mesothelial tissue of other sites**

D19.9   **Benign neoplasm of mesothelial tissue, unspecified**
Benign mesothelioma NOS

✓4ᵗʰ **D20**   **Benign neoplasm of soft tissue of** retroperitoneum and peritoneum

     EXCLUDES 1   *benign lipomatous neoplasm of peritoneum and retroperitoneum (D17.79)*
         benign neoplasm of mesothelial tissue (D19.-)

D20.0   **Benign neoplasm of soft tissue of** retroperitoneum

D20.1   **Benign neoplasm of soft tissue of** peritoneum

✓4ᵗʰ **D21**   **Other benign neoplasms of** connective and other soft tissue

     INCLUDES   benign neoplasm of blood vessel
         benign neoplasm of bursa
         benign neoplasm of cartilage
         benign neoplasm of fascia
         benign neoplasm of fat
         benign neoplasm of ligament, except uterine
         benign neoplasm of lymphatic channel
         benign neoplasm of muscle
         benign neoplasm of synovia
         benign neoplasm of tendon (sheath)
         benign stromal tumors

     EXCLUDES 1   *benign neoplasm of articular cartilage (D16.-)*
         benign neoplasm of cartilage of larynx (D14.1)
         benign neoplasm of cartilage of nose (D14.0)
         benign neoplasm of connective tissue of breast (D24.-)
         benign neoplasm of peripheral nerves and autonomic nervous system (D36.1-)
         benign neoplasm of peritoneum (D20.1)
         benign neoplasm of retroperitoneum (D20.0)
         benign neoplasm of uterine ligament, any (D28.2)
         benign neoplasm of vascular tissue (D18.-)
         hemangioma (D18.0-)
         lipomatous neoplasm (D17.-)
         lymphangioma (D18.1)
         uterine leiomyoma (D25.-)

D21.0   **Benign neoplasm of connective and other soft tissue of** head, face and neck
Benign neoplasm of connective tissue of ear
Benign neoplasm of connective tissue of eyelid
     EXCLUDES 1   *benign neoplasm of connective tissue of orbit (D31.6-)*

✓5ᵗʰ **D21.1**   **Benign neoplasm of connective and other soft tissue of** upper limb, including shoulder

D21.10   **Benign neoplasm of connective and other soft tissue of unspecified upper limb, including shoulder**

D21.11   **Benign neoplasm of connective and other soft tissue of** right **upper limb, including shoulder**

D21.12   **Benign neoplasm of connective and other soft tissue of** left **upper limb, including shoulder**

✓5ᵗʰ **D21.2**   **Benign neoplasm of connective and other soft tissue of** lower limb, including hip

D21.20   **Benign neoplasm of connective and other soft tissue of unspecified lower limb, including hip**

D21.21   **Benign neoplasm of connective and other soft tissue of** right **lower limb, including hip**

D21.22   **Benign neoplasm of connective and other soft tissue of** left **lower limb, including hip**

D21.3   **Benign neoplasm of connective and other soft tissue of** thorax
Benign neoplasm of axilla
Benign neoplasm of diaphragm
Benign neoplasm of great vessels
     EXCLUDES 1   *benign neoplasm of heart (D15.1)*
         benign neoplasm of mediastinum (D15.2)
         benign neoplasm of thymus (D15.0)

D21.4   **Benign neoplasm of connective and other soft tissue of** abdomen
Benign stromal tumors of abdomen

D21.5   **Benign neoplasm of connective and other soft tissue of** pelvis
     EXCLUDES 1   *benign neoplasm of any uterine ligament (D28.2)*
         uterine leiomyoma (D25.-)

D21.6   **Benign neoplasm of connective and other soft tissue of trunk, unspecified**
Benign neoplasm of back NOS

D21.9   **Benign neoplasm of connective and other soft tissue, unspecified**

✓4ᵗʰ **D22**   **Melanocytic nevi**
     INCLUDES   atypical nevus
         blue hairy pigmented nevus
         nevus NOS

D22.0   **Melanocytic nevi of** lip

✓5ᵗʰ **D22.1**   **Melanocytic nevi of** eyelid, including canthus

D22.10   **Melanocytic nevi of unspecified eyelid, including canthus**

D22.11   **Melanocytic nevi of** right **eyelid, including canthus**

D22.12   **Melanocytic nevi of** left **eyelid, including canthus**

✓5ᵗʰ **D22.2**   **Melanocytic nevi of** ear and external auricular canal

D22.20   **Melanocytic nevi of unspecified ear and external auricular canal**

D22.21   **Melanocytic nevi of** right **ear and external auricular canal**

D22.22   **Melanocytic nevi of** left **ear and external auricular canal**

✓5ᵗʰ **D22.3**   **Melanocytic nevi of** other and unspecified parts of face

D22.30   **Melanocytic nevi of unspecified part of face**

D22.39   **Melanocytic nevi of other parts of face**

D22.4   **Melanocytic nevi of** scalp and neck

D22.5   **Melanocytic nevi of** trunk
Melanocytic nevi of anal margin
Melanocytic nevi of anal skin
Melanocytic nevi of perianal skin
Melanocytic nevi of skin of breast

✓5ᵗʰ **D22.6**   **Melanocytic nevi of** upper limb, including shoulder

D22.60   **Melanocytic nevi of unspecified upper limb, including shoulder**

D22.61   **Melanocytic nevi of** right **upper limb, including shoulder**

D22.62   **Melanocytic nevi of** left **upper limb, including shoulder**

✓5ᵗʰ **D22.7**   **Melanocytic nevi of** lower limb, including hip

D22.70   **Melanocytic nevi of unspecified lower limb, including hip**

D22.71   **Melanocytic nevi of** right **lower limb, including hip**

D22.72   **Melanocytic nevi of** left **lower limb, including hip**

D22.9   **Melanocytic nevi, unspecified**

✓4ᵗʰ **D23**   **Other benign neoplasms of** skin
     INCLUDES   benign neoplasm of hair follicles
         benign neoplasm of sebaceous glands
         benign neoplasm of sweat glands
     EXCLUDES 1   *benign lipomatous neoplasms of skin (D17.0-D17.3)*
         melanocytic nevi (D22.-)

D23.0   **Other benign neoplasm of skin of** lip
     EXCLUDES 1   *benign neoplasm of vermilion border of lip (D10.0)*

✓5ᵗʰ **D23.1**   **Other benign neoplasm of skin of** eyelid, including canthus

D23.10   **Other benign neoplasm of skin of unspecified eyelid, including canthus**

D23.11   **Other benign neoplasm of skin of** right **eyelid, including canthus**

D23.12   **Other benign neoplasm of skin of** left **eyelid, including canthus**

✓5ᵗʰ **D23.2**   **Other benign neoplasm of skin of** ear and external auricular canal

D23.20   **Other benign neoplasm of skin of unspecified ear and external auricular canal**

D23.21   **Other benign neoplasm of skin of** right **ear and external auricular canal**

D23.22   **Other benign neoplasm of skin of** left **ear and external auricular canal**

✓5ᵗʰ **D23.3**   **Other benign neoplasm of skin of** other and unspecified parts of face

D23.30   **Other benign neoplasm of skin of unspecified part of face**

D23.39   **Other benign neoplasm of skin of other parts of face**

EXCLUDES 1 Not coded here   *EXCLUDES 2* Not included here   N Newborn Age: 0   P Pediatric Age: 0-17   M Maternity Age: 12-55   A Adult Age: 15-124

472   ICD-10-CM 2016

D23.4 Other benign neoplasm of skin of scalp and neck

D23.5 Other benign neoplasm of skin of trunk
Other benign neoplasm of anal margin
Other benign neoplasm of anal skin
Other benign neoplasm of perianal skin
Other benign neoplasm of skin of breast
EXCLUDES 1 benign neoplasm of anus NOS (D12.9)

✓5ᵗʰ D23.6 Other benign neoplasm of skin of upper limb, including shoulder
D23.60 Other benign neoplasm of skin of unspecified upper limb, including shoulder
D23.61 Other benign neoplasm of skin of right upper limb, including shoulder
D23.62 Other benign neoplasm of skin of left upper limb, including shoulder

✓5ᵗʰ D23.7 Other benign neoplasm of skin of lower limb, including hip
D23.70 Other benign neoplasm of skin of unspecified lower limb, including hip
D23.71 Other benign neoplasm of skin of right lower limb, including hip
D23.72 Other benign neoplasm of skin of left lower limb, including hip

D23.9 Other benign neoplasm of skin, unspecified

✓4ᵗʰ D24 **Benign neoplasm of breast**
INCLUDES benign neoplasm of connective tissue of breast
benign neoplasm of soft parts of breast
fibroadenoma of breast
EXCLUDES 2 adenofibrosis of breast (N60.2)
benign cyst of breast (N60.-)
benign mammary dysplasia (N60.-)
benign neoplasm of skin of breast (D22.5, D23.5)
fibrocystic disease of breast (N60.-)

D24.1 Benign neoplasm of right breast

D24.2 Benign neoplasm of left breast

D24.9 Benign neoplasm of unspecified breast

✓4ᵗʰ D25 **Leiomyoma of uterus**
INCLUDES uterine fibroid
uterine fibromyoma
uterine myoma

D25.0 Submucous leiomyoma of uterus ♀

D25.1 Intramural leiomyoma of uterus ♀
Interstitial leiomyoma of uterus

D25.2 Subserosal leiomyoma of uterus ♀
Subperitoneal leiomyoma of uterus

D25.9 Leiomyoma of uterus, unspecified ♀

✓4ᵗʰ D26 **Other benign neoplasms of uterus**

D26.0 Other benign neoplasm of cervix uteri ♀

D26.1 Other benign neoplasm of corpus uteri ♀

D26.7 Other benign neoplasm of other parts of uterus ♀

D26.9 Other benign neoplasm of uterus, unspecified ♀

✓4ᵗʰ D27 **Benign neoplasm of ovary**
Use additional code to identify any functional activity
EXCLUDES 2 corpus albicans cyst (N83.2)
corpus luteum cyst (N83.1)
endometrial cyst (N80.1)
follicular (atretic) cyst (N83.0)
graafian follicle cyst (N83.0)
ovarian cyst NEC (N83.2)
ovarian retention cyst (N83.2)

D27.0 Benign neoplasm of right ovary ♀

D27.1 Benign neoplasm of left ovary ♀

D27.9 Benign neoplasm of unspecified ovary ♀

✓4ᵗʰ D28 **Benign neoplasm of other and unspecified female genital organs**
INCLUDES adenomatous polyp
benign neoplasm of skin of female genital organs
benign teratoma
EXCLUDES 1 epoophoron cyst (Q50.5)
fimbrial cyst (Q50.4)
Gartner's duct cyst (Q52.4)
parovarian cyst (Q50.5)

D28.0 Benign neoplasm of vulva ♀

D28.1 Benign neoplasm of vagina ♀

D28.2 Benign neoplasm of uterine tubes and ligaments ♀
Benign neoplasm of fallopian tube
Benign neoplasm of uterine ligament (broad) (round)

D28.7 Benign neoplasm of other specified female genital organs ♀

D28.9 Benign neoplasm of female genital organ, unspecified ♀

✓4ᵗʰ D29 **Benign neoplasm of male genital organs**
INCLUDES benign neoplasm of skin of male genital organs

D29.0 Benign neoplasm of penis ♂

D29.1 Benign neoplasm of prostate ♂
EXCLUDES 1 enlarged prostate (N40.-)

✓5ᵗʰ D29.2 Benign neoplasm of testis
Use additional code to identify any functional activity
D29.20 Benign neoplasm of unspecified testis ♂
D29.21 Benign neoplasm of right testis ♂
D29.22 Benign neoplasm of left testis ♂

✓5ᵗʰ D29.3 Benign neoplasm of epididymis
D29.30 Benign neoplasm of unspecified epididymis ♂
D29.31 Benign neoplasm of right epididymis ♂
D29.32 Benign neoplasm of left epididymis ♂

D29.4 Benign neoplasm of scrotum ♂
Benign neoplasm of skin of scrotum

D29.8 Benign neoplasm of other specified male genital organs ♂
Benign neoplasm of seminal vesicle
Benign neoplasm of spermatic cord
Benign neoplasm of tunica vaginalis

D29.9 Benign neoplasm of male genital organ, unspecified ♂

✓4ᵗʰ D30 **Benign neoplasm of urinary organs**

✓5ᵗʰ D30.0 Benign neoplasm of kidney
EXCLUDES 1 benign carcinoid tumor of the kidney (D3A.093)
benign neoplasm of renal calyces (D30.1-)
benign neoplasm of renal pelvis (D30.1-)
D30.00 Benign neoplasm of unspecified kidney
D30.01 Benign neoplasm of right kidney
D30.02 Benign neoplasm of left kidney

✓5ᵗʰ D30.1 Benign neoplasm of renal pelvis
D30.10 Benign neoplasm of unspecified renal pelvis
D30.11 Benign neoplasm of right renal pelvis
D30.12 Benign neoplasm of left renal pelvis

✓5ᵗʰ D30.2 Benign neoplasm of ureter
EXCLUDES 1 benign neoplasm of ureteric orifice of bladder (D30.3)
D30.20 Benign neoplasm of unspecified ureter
D30.21 Benign neoplasm of right ureter
D30.22 Benign neoplasm of left ureter

D30.3 Benign neoplasm of bladder
Benign neoplasm of ureteric orifice of bladder
Benign neoplasm of urethral orifice of bladder

D30.4 Benign neoplasm of urethra
EXCLUDES 1 benign neoplasm of urethral orifice of bladder (D30.3)

D30.8 Benign neoplasm of other specified urinary organs
Benign neoplasm of paraurethral glands

D30.9 Benign neoplasm of urinary organ, unspecified
Benign neoplasm of urinary system NOS

✓4ᵗʰ D31 **Benign neoplasm of eye and adnexa**
EXCLUDES 1 benign neoplasm of connective tissue of eyelid (D21.0)
benign neoplasm of optic nerve (D33.3)
benign neoplasm of skin of eyelid (D22.1-, D23.1-)

✓5ᵗʰ D31.0 Benign neoplasm of conjunctiva
D31.00 Benign neoplasm of unspecified conjunctiva
D31.01 Benign neoplasm of right conjunctiva
D31.02 Benign neoplasm of left conjunctiva

✓5ᵗʰ D31.1 Benign neoplasm of cornea
D31.10 Benign neoplasm of unspecified cornea
D31.11 Benign neoplasm of right cornea
D31.12 Benign neoplasm of left cornea

✓5ᵗʰ D31.2 Benign neoplasm of retina
EXCLUDES 1 dark area on retina (D49.81)
hemangioma of retina (D49.81)
neoplasm of unspecified behavior of retina and choroid (D49.81)
retinal freckle (D49.81)
D31.20 Benign neoplasm of unspecified retina
D31.21 Benign neoplasm of right retina
D31.22 Benign neoplasm of left retina

✓5ᵗʰ D31.3 Benign neoplasm of choroid
D31.30 Benign neoplasm of unspecified choroid

☑ Additional Character Required | ✓x7ᵗʰ Placeholder Alert | Unspecified Dx | Other Specified Dx | Manifestation | ▶◀ Revised Text | ● New Code | ▲ Revised Code Title

    D31.31   **Benign neoplasm of** right **choroid**

    D31.32   **Benign neoplasm of** left **choroid**

✓5ᵗʰ **D31.4**   **Benign neoplasm of** ciliary body

    D31.4Ø   **Benign neoplasm of unspecified ciliary body**

    D31.41   **Benign neoplasm of** right **ciliary body**

    D31.42   **Benign neoplasm of** left **ciliary body**

✓5ᵗʰ **D31.5**   **Benign neoplasm of** lacrimal gland and duct
    Benign neoplasm of lacrimal sac
    Benign neoplasm of nasolacrimal duct

    D31.5Ø   **Benign neoplasm of unspecified lacrimal gland and duct**

    D31.51   **Benign neoplasm of** right **lacrimal gland and duct**

    D31.52   **Benign neoplasm of** left **lacrimal gland and duct**

✓5ᵗʰ **D31.6**   **Benign neoplasm of unspecified site of** orbit
    Benign neoplasm of connective tissue of orbit
    Benign neoplasm of extraocular muscle
    Benign neoplasm of peripheral nerves of orbit
    Benign neoplasm of retrobulbar tissue
    Benign neoplasm of retro-ocular tissue
    EXCLUDES 1   benign neoplasm of orbital bone (D16.4)

    D31.6Ø   **Benign neoplasm of unspecified site of unspecified orbit**

    D31.61   **Benign neoplasm of unspecified site of** right **orbit**

    D31.62   **Benign neoplasm of unspecified site of** left **orbit**

✓5ᵗʰ **D31.9**   **Benign neoplasm of** unspecified part of eye
    Benign neoplasm of eyeball

    D31.9Ø   **Benign neoplasm of unspecified part of unspecified eye**

    D31.91   **Benign neoplasm of unspecified part of** right **eye**

    D31.92   **Benign neoplasm of unspecified part of** left **eye**

✓4ᵗʰ **D32**   **Benign neoplasm of** meninges

D32.Ø   **Benign neoplasm of** cerebral **meninges**

D32.1   **Benign neoplasm of** spinal **meninges**

D32.9   **Benign neoplasm of meninges, unspecified**
    Meningioma NOS

✓4ᵗʰ **D33**   **Benign neoplasm of** brain and other parts of central nervous system
    EXCLUDES 1   angioma (D18.Ø-)
         benign neoplasm of meninges (D32.-)
         benign neoplasm of peripheral nerves and autonomic nervous system (D36.1-)
         hemangioma (D18.Ø-)
         neurofibromatosis (Q85.Ø-)
         retro-ocular benign neoplasm (D31.6-)

D33.Ø   **Benign neoplasm of** brain, supratentorial
    Benign neoplasm of cerebral ventricle
    Benign neoplasm of cerebrum
    Benign neoplasm of frontal lobe
    Benign neoplasm of occipital lobe
    Benign neoplasm of parietal lobe
    Benign neoplasm of temporal lobe
    EXCLUDES 1   benign neoplasm of fourth ventricle (D33.1)

D33.1   **Benign neoplasm of** brain, infratentorial
    Benign neoplasm of brain stem
    Benign neoplasm of cerebellum
    Benign neoplasm of fourth ventricle

D33.2   **Benign neoplasm of brain, unspecified**

D33.3   **Benign neoplasm of** cranial nerves
    Benign neoplasm of olfactory bulb

D33.4   **Benign neoplasm of** spinal cord

D33.7   **Benign neoplasm of other specified parts of central nervous system**

D33.9   **Benign neoplasm of central nervous system, unspecified**
    Benign neoplasm of nervous system (central) NOS

D34   **Benign neoplasm of** thyroid gland
    Use additional code to identify any functional activity

✓4ᵗʰ **D35**   **Benign neoplasm of** other and unspecified endocrine glands
    Use additional code to identify any functional activity
    EXCLUDES 1   benign neoplasm of endocrine pancreas (D13.7)
         benign neoplasm of ovary (D27.-)
         benign neoplasm of testis (D29.2-)
         benign neoplasm of thymus (D15.Ø)

✓5ᵗʰ **D35.Ø**   **Benign neoplasm of** adrenal gland

    D35.ØØ   **Benign neoplasm of unspecified adrenal gland**

    D35.Ø1   **Benign neoplasm of** right **adrenal gland**

    D35.Ø2   **Benign neoplasm of** left **adrenal gland**

D35.1   **Benign neoplasm of** parathyroid gland

D35.2   **Benign neoplasm of** pituitary gland
    AHA: 2014, 3Q, 22

D35.3   **Benign neoplasm of** craniopharyngeal duct

D35.4   **Benign neoplasm of** pineal gland

D35.5   **Benign neoplasm of** carotid body

D35.6   **Benign neoplasm of** aortic body and other paraganglia
    Benign tumor of glomus jugulare

D35.7   **Benign neoplasm of other specified endocrine glands**

D35.9   **Benign neoplasm of endocrine gland, unspecified**
    Benign neoplasm of unspecified endocrine gland

✓4ᵗʰ **D36**   **Benign neoplasm of** other and unspecified sites

D36.Ø   **Benign neoplasm of** lymph nodes
    EXCLUDES 1   lymphangioma (D18.1)

✓5ᵗʰ **D36.1**   **Benign neoplasm of** peripheral nerves and autonomic nervous system
    EXCLUDES 1   benign neoplasm of peripheral nerves of orbit (D31.6-)
         neurofibromatosis (Q85.Ø-)

    D36.1Ø   **Benign neoplasm of peripheral nerves and autonomic nervous system, unspecified**

    D36.11   **Benign neoplasm of peripheral nerves and autonomic nervous system of** face, head, and neck

    D36.12   **Benign neoplasm of peripheral nerves and autonomic nervous system,** upper limb, including shoulder

    D36.13   **Benign neoplasm of peripheral nerves and autonomic nervous system of** lower limb, including hip

    D36.14   **Benign neoplasm of peripheral nerves and autonomic nervous system of** thorax

    D36.15   **Benign neoplasm of peripheral nerves and autonomic nervous system of** abdomen

    D36.16   **Benign neoplasm of peripheral nerves and autonomic nervous system of** pelvis

    D36.17   **Benign neoplasm of peripheral nerves and autonomic nervous system of** trunk, **unspecified**

D36.7   **Benign neoplasm of other specified sites**
    Benign neoplasm of nose NOS

D36.9   **Benign neoplasm, unspecified site**

Benign neuroendocrine tumors (D3A)

✓4ᵗʰ **D3A**   **Benign neuroendocrine tumors**
    Code also any associated multiple endocrine neoplasia [MEN] syndromes (E31.2-)
    Use additional code to identify any associated endocrine syndrome, such as:
         carcinoid syndrome (E34.Ø)
    EXCLUDES 2   benign pancreatic islet cell tumors (D13.7)

✓5ᵗʰ **D3A.Ø**   **Benign** carcinoid tumors

    D3A.ØØ   **Benign carcinoid tumor of unspecified site**
         Carcinoid tumor NOS

    ✓6ᵗʰ D3A.Ø1   **Benign carcinoid tumors of the** small intestine

         D3A.Ø1Ø   **Benign carcinoid tumor of the** duodenum

         D3A.Ø11   **Benign carcinoid tumor of the** jejunum

         D3A.Ø12   **Benign carcinoid tumor of the** ileum

         D3A.Ø19   **Benign carcinoid tumor of the small intestine, unspecified portion**

    ✓6ᵗʰ D3A.Ø2   **Benign carcinoid tumors of the** appendix, large intestine, and rectum

         D3A.Ø2Ø   **Benign carcinoid tumor of the** appendix

         D3A.Ø21   **Benign carcinoid tumor of the** cecum

         D3A.Ø22   **Benign carcinoid tumor of the** ascending colon

         D3A.Ø23   **Benign carcinoid tumor of the** transverse colon

         D3A.Ø24   **Benign carcinoid tumor of the** descending colon

         D3A.Ø25   **Benign carcinoid tumor of the** sigmoid colon

         D3A.Ø26   **Benign carcinoid tumor of the** rectum

         D3A.Ø29   **Benign carcinoid tumor of the large intestine, unspecified portion**
            Benign carcinoid tumor of the colon NOS

EXCLUDES 1 Not coded here   *EXCLUDES 2* Not included here   N Newborn Age: 0   P Pediatric Age: 0-17   M Maternity Age: 12-55   A Adult Age: 15-124

✓6ᵗʰ **D3A.09** **Benign carcinoid tumors of** other **sites**

    D3A.090 **Benign carcinoid tumor of the** bronchus **and lung**

    D3A.091 **Benign carcinoid tumor of the** thymus

    D3A.092 **Benign carcinoid tumor of the** stomach

    D3A.093 **Benign carcinoid tumor of the** kidney

    D3A.094 **Benign carcinoid tumor of the** foregut NOS

    D3A.095 **Benign carcinoid tumor of the** midgut NOS

    D3A.096 **Benign carcinoid tumor of the** hindgut NOS

    D3A.098 **Benign carcinoid tumors of other sites**

D3A.8 **Other benign neuroendocrine tumors**

    Neuroendocrine tumor NOS

Neoplasms of uncertain behavior, polycythemia vera and myelodysplastic syndromes (D37-D48)

NOTE   Categories D37-D44, and D48 classify by site neoplasms of uncertain behavior, i.e., histologic confirmation whether the neoplasm is malignant or benign cannot be made.

EXCLUDES 1   *neoplasms of unspecified behavior (D49.-)*

✓4ᵗʰ **D37** **Neoplasm of uncertain behavior of** oral cavity and digestive **organs**

  EXCLUDES 1   *stromal tumors of uncertain behavior of digestive system (D48.1)*

✓5ᵗʰ **D37.0** **Neoplasm of uncertain behavior of** lip, oral cavity and **pharynx**

    EXCLUDES 1   *neoplasm of uncertain behavior of aryepiglottic fold or interarytenoid fold, laryngeal aspect (D38.0)*
           neoplasm of uncertain behavior of epiglottis NOS (D38.0)
           neoplasm of uncertain behavior of skin of lip (D48.5)
           neoplasm of uncertain behavior of suprahyoid portion of epiglottis (D38.0)

    D37.01 **Neoplasm of uncertain behavior of** lip

      Neoplasm of uncertain behavior of vermilion border of lip

    D37.02 **Neoplasm of uncertain behavior of** tongue

✓6ᵗʰ   **D37.03** **Neoplasm of uncertain behavior of the** major **salivary glands**

      D37.030 **Neoplasm of uncertain behavior of the** parotid **salivary glands**

      D37.031 **Neoplasm of uncertain behavior of the** sublingual **salivary glands**

      D37.032 **Neoplasm of uncertain behavior of the** submandibular **salivary glands**

      D37.039 **Neoplasm of uncertain behavior of the major salivary glands, unspecified**

    D37.04 **Neoplasm of uncertain behavior of the** minor salivary glands

      Neoplasm of uncertain behavior of submucosal salivary glands of lip
      Neoplasm of uncertain behavior of submucosal salivary glands of cheek
      Neoplasm of uncertain behavior of submucosal salivary glands of hard palate
      Neoplasm of uncertain behavior of submucosal salivary glands of soft palate

    D37.05 **Neoplasm of uncertain behavior of** pharynx

      Neoplasm of uncertain behavior of aryepiglottic fold of pharynx NOS
      Neoplasm of uncertain behavior of hypopharyngeal aspect of aryepiglottic fold of pharynx
      Neoplasm of uncertain behavior of marginal zone of aryepiglottic fold of pharynx

    D37.09 **Neoplasm of uncertain behavior of other specified sites of the oral cavity**

D37.1 **Neoplasm of uncertain behavior of** stomach

D37.2 **Neoplasm of uncertain behavior of** small intestine

D37.3 **Neoplasm of uncertain behavior of** appendix

D37.4 **Neoplasm of uncertain behavior of** colon

D37.5 **Neoplasm of uncertain behavior of** rectum

    Neoplasm of uncertain behavior of rectosigmoid junction

D37.6 **Neoplasm of uncertain behavior of** liver, gallbladder and bile ducts

    Neoplasm of uncertain behavior of ampulla of Vater

D37.8 **Neoplasm of uncertain behavior of other specified digestive organs**

    Neoplasm of uncertain behavior of anal canal
    Neoplasm of uncertain behavior of anal sphincter
    Neoplasm of uncertain behavior of anus NOS
    Neoplasm of uncertain behavior of esophagus
    Neoplasm of uncertain behavior of intestine NOS
    Neoplasm of uncertain behavior of pancreas

    EXCLUDES 1   *neoplasm of uncertain behavior of anal margin (D48.5)*
           neoplasm of uncertain behavior of anal skin (D48.5)
           neoplasm of uncertain behavior of perianal skin (D48.5)

D37.9 **Neoplasm of uncertain behavior of digestive organ, unspecified**

✓4ᵗʰ **D38** **Neoplasm of uncertain behavior of** middle ear and respiratory and intrathoracic organs

  EXCLUDES 1   *neoplasm of uncertain behavior of heart (D48.7)*

  D38.0 **Neoplasm of uncertain behavior of** larynx

    Neoplasm of uncertain behavior of aryepiglottic fold or interarytenoid fold, laryngeal aspect
    Neoplasm of uncertain behavior of epiglottis (suprahyoid portion)

    EXCLUDES 1   *neoplasm of uncertain behavior of aryepiglottic fold or interarytenoid fold NOS (D37.05)*
           neoplasm of uncertain behavior of hypopharyngeal aspect of aryepiglottic fold (D37.05)
           neoplasm of uncertain behavior of marginal zone of aryepiglottic fold (D37.05)

  D38.1 **Neoplasm of uncertain behavior of** trachea, bronchus and lung

  D38.2 **Neoplasm of uncertain behavior of** pleura

  D38.3 **Neoplasm of uncertain behavior of** mediastinum

  D38.4 **Neoplasm of uncertain behavior of** thymus

  D38.5 **Neoplasm of uncertain behavior of other respiratory organs**

    Neoplasm of uncertain behavior of accessory sinuses
    Neoplasm of uncertain behavior of cartilage of nose
    Neoplasm of uncertain behavior of middle ear
    Neoplasm of uncertain behavior of nasal cavities

    EXCLUDES 1   *neoplasm of uncertain behavior of ear (external) (skin) (D48.5)*
           neoplasm of uncertain behavior of nose NOS (D48.7)
           neoplasm of uncertain behavior of skin of nose (D48.5)

  D38.6 **Neoplasm of uncertain behavior of respiratory organ, unspecified**

✓4ᵗʰ **D39** **Neoplasm of uncertain behavior of** female genital organs

  D39.0 **Neoplasm of uncertain behavior of** uterus   ♀

✓5ᵗʰ   **D39.1** **Neoplasm of uncertain behavior of** ovary

    Use additional code to identify any functional activity

    D39.10 **Neoplasm of uncertain behavior of unspecified ovary**   ♀

    D39.11 **Neoplasm of uncertain behavior of** right **ovary**   ♀

    D39.12 **Neoplasm of uncertain behavior of** left **ovary**   ♀

  D39.2 **Neoplasm of uncertain behavior of** placenta   ♀

    Chorioadenoma destruens
    Invasive hydatidiform mole
    Malignant hydatidiform mole

    EXCLUDES 1   *hydatidiform mole NOS (O01.9)*

  D39.8 **Neoplasm of uncertain behavior of other specified female genital organs**   ♀

    Neoplasm of uncertain behavior of skin of female genital organs

  D39.9 **Neoplasm of uncertain behavior of female genital organ, unspecified**   ♀

✓4ᵗʰ **D40** **Neoplasm of uncertain behavior of** male genital organs

  D40.0 **Neoplasm of uncertain behavior of** prostate   ♂

✓5ᵗʰ   **D40.1** **Neoplasm of uncertain behavior of** testis

    D40.10 **Neoplasm of uncertain behavior of unspecified testis**   ♂

    D40.11 **Neoplasm of uncertain behavior of** right **testis**   ♂

    D40.12 **Neoplasm of uncertain behavior of** left **testis**   ♂

  D40.8 **Neoplasm of uncertain behavior of other specified male genital organs**   ♂

    Neoplasm of uncertain behavior of skin of male genital organs

  D40.9 **Neoplasm of uncertain behavior of male genital organ, unspecified**   ♂

✓ Additional Character Required   ✓x7ᵗʰ Placeholder Alert   Unspecified Dx   Other Specified Dx   Manifestation   ▶◀ Revised Text   ● New Code   ▲ Revised Code Title

✓4ᵗʰ D41 Neoplasm of uncertain behavior of urinary organs

    ✓5ᵗʰ D41.0 Neoplasm of uncertain behavior of kidney

        EXCLUDES 1   *neoplasm of uncertain behavior of renal pelvis (D41.1-)*

        D41.00 Neoplasm of uncertain behavior of unspecified kidney

        D41.01 Neoplasm of uncertain behavior of right kidney

        D41.02 Neoplasm of uncertain behavior of left kidney

    ✓5ᵗʰ D41.1 Neoplasm of uncertain behavior of renal pelvis

        D41.10 Neoplasm of uncertain behavior of unspecified renal pelvis

        D41.11 Neoplasm of uncertain behavior of right renal pelvis

        D41.12 Neoplasm of uncertain behavior of left renal pelvis

    ✓5ᵗʰ D41.2 Neoplasm of uncertain behavior of ureter

        D41.20 Neoplasm of uncertain behavior of unspecified ureter

        D41.21 Neoplasm of uncertain behavior of right ureter

        D41.22 Neoplasm of uncertain behavior of left ureter

    D41.3 Neoplasm of uncertain behavior of urethra

    D41.4 Neoplasm of uncertain behavior of bladder

    D41.8 Neoplasm of uncertain behavior of other specified urinary organs

    D41.9 Neoplasm of uncertain behavior of unspecified urinary organ

✓4ᵗʰ D42 Neoplasm of uncertain behavior of meninges

    D42.0 Neoplasm of uncertain behavior of cerebral meninges

    D42.1 Neoplasm of uncertain behavior of spinal meninges

    D42.9 Neoplasm of uncertain behavior of meninges, unspecified

✓4ᵗʰ D43 Neoplasm of uncertain behavior of brain and central nervous system

    EXCLUDES 1   *neoplasm of uncertain behavior of peripheral nerves and autonomic nervous system (D48.2)*

    D43.0 Neoplasm of uncertain behavior of brain, supratentorial

      Neoplasm of uncertain behavior of cerebral ventricle

      Neoplasm of uncertain behavior of cerebrum

      Neoplasm of uncertain behavior of frontal lobe

      Neoplasm of uncertain behavior of occipital lobe

      Neoplasm of uncertain behavior of parietal lobe

      Neoplasm of uncertain behavior of temporal lobe

      EXCLUDES 1   *neoplasm of uncertain behavior of fourth ventricle (D43.1)*

    D43.1 Neoplasm of uncertain behavior of brain, infratentorial

      Neoplasm of uncertain behavior of brain stem

      Neoplasm of uncertain behavior of cerebellum

      Neoplasm of uncertain behavior of fourth ventricle

    D43.2 Neoplasm of uncertain behavior of brain, unspecified

    D43.3 Neoplasm of uncertain behavior of cranial nerves

    D43.4 Neoplasm of uncertain behavior of spinal cord

    D43.8 Neoplasm of uncertain behavior of other specified parts of central nervous system

    D43.9 Neoplasm of uncertain behavior of central nervous system, unspecified

      Neoplasm of uncertain behavior of nervous system (central) NOS

✓4ᵗʰ D44 Neoplasm of uncertain behavior of endocrine glands

    EXCLUDES 1   *multiple endocrine adenomatosis (E31.2-)*
          multiple endocrine neoplasia (E31.2-)
          neoplasm of uncertain behavior of endocrine pancreas (D37.8)
          neoplasm of uncertain behavior of ovary (D39.1-)
          neoplasm of uncertain behavior of testis (D40.1-)
          neoplasm of uncertain behavior of thymus (D38.4)

    D44.0 Neoplasm of uncertain behavior of thyroid gland

    ✓5ᵗʰ D44.1 Neoplasm of uncertain behavior of adrenal gland

      Use additional code to identify any functional activity

        D44.10 Neoplasm of uncertain behavior of unspecified adrenal gland

        D44.11 Neoplasm of uncertain behavior of right adrenal gland

        D44.12 Neoplasm of uncertain behavior of left adrenal gland

    D44.2 Neoplasm of uncertain behavior of parathyroid gland

    D44.3 Neoplasm of uncertain behavior of pituitary gland

      Use additional code to identify any functional activity

    D44.4 Neoplasm of uncertain behavior of craniopharyngeal duct

    D44.5 Neoplasm of uncertain behavior of pineal gland

    D44.6 Neoplasm of uncertain behavior of carotid body

    D44.7 Neoplasm of uncertain behavior of aortic body and other paraganglia

    D44.9 Neoplasm of uncertain behavior of unspecified endocrine gland

D45 Polycythemia vera

    EXCLUDES 1   *familial polycythemia (D75.0)*
          secondary polycythemia (D75.1)

✓4ᵗʰ D46 Myelodysplastic syndromes

    Use additional code for adverse effect, if applicable, to identify drug (T36-T50 with fifth or sixth character 5)

    EXCLUDES 2   *drug-induced aplastic anemia (D61.1)*

    D46.0 Refractory anemia without ring sideroblasts, so stated

      Refractory anemia without sideroblasts, without excess of blasts

    D46.1 Refractory anemia with ring sideroblasts

      RARS

    ✓5ᵗʰ D46.2 Refractory anemia with excess of blasts

        D46.20 Refractory anemia with excess of blasts, unspecified

          RAEB NOS

        D46.21 Refractory anemia with excess of blasts 1

          RAEB 1

        D46.22 Refractory anemia with excess of blasts 2

          RAEB 2

    D46.A Refractory cytopenia with multilineage dysplasia

    D46.B Refractory cytopenia with multilineage dysplasia and ring sideroblasts

      RCMD RS

    D46.C Myelodysplastic syndrome with isolated del(5q) chromosomal abnormality

      Myelodysplastic syndrome with 5q deletion

      5q minus syndrome NOS

    D46.4 Refractory anemia, unspecified

    D46.Z Other myelodysplastic syndromes

      EXCLUDES 1   *chronic myelomonocytic leukemia (C93.1-)*

    D46.9 Myelodysplastic syndrome, unspecified

      Myelodysplasia NOS

✓4ᵗʰ D47 Other neoplasms of uncertain behavior of lymphoid, hematopoietic and related tissue

    D47.0 Histiocytic and mast cell tumors of uncertain behavior

      Indolent systemic mastocytosis

      Mast cell tumor NOS

      Mastocytoma NOS

      EXCLUDES 1   *malignant mast cell tumor (C96.2)*
            mastocytosis (congenital) (cutaneous) (Q82.2)

    D47.1 Chronic myeloproliferative disease

      Chronic neutrophilic leukemia

      Myeloproliferative disease, unspecified

      EXCLUDES 1   *atypical chronic myeloid leukemia BCR/ABL-negative (C92.2-)*
            chronic myeloid leukemia BCR/ABL-positive (C92.1-)
            myelofibrosis NOS (D75.81)
            myelophthisic anemia (D61.82)
            myelophthisis (D61.82)
            secondary myelofibrosis NOS (D75.81)

    D47.2 Monoclonal gammopathy

      Monoclonal gammopathy of undetermined significance [MGUS]

    D47.3 Essential (hemorrhagic) thrombocythemia

      Essential thrombocytosis

      Idiopathic hemorrhagic thrombocythemia

    D47.4 Osteomyelofibrosis

      Chronic idiopathic myelofibrosis

      Myelofibrosis (idiopathic) (with myeloid metaplasia)

      Myelosclerosis (megakaryocytic) with myeloid metaplasia

      Secondary myelofibrosis in myeloproliferative disease

      EXCLUDES 1   *acute myelofibrosis (C94.4-)*

    ✓5ᵗʰ D47.Z Other specified neoplasms of uncertain behavior of lymphoid, hematopoietic and related tissue

        D47.Z1 Post-transplant lymphoproliferative disorder (PTLD)

          Code first complications of transplanted organs and tissue (T86.-)

        D47.Z9 Other specified neoplasms of uncertain behavior of lymphoid, hematopoietic and related tissue

          Histiocytic tumors of uncertain behavior

    D47.9 Neoplasm of uncertain behavior of lymphoid, hematopoietic and related tissue, unspecified

      Lymphoproliferative disease NOS

EXCLUDES 1 Not coded here   EXCLUDES 2 Not included here   N Newborn Age: 0   P Pediatric Age: 0-17   M Maternity Age: 12-55   A Adult Age: 15-124

476   ICD-10-CM 2016

D41–D47.9

☑4ᵗʰ **D48 Neoplasm of uncertain behavior of other and unspecified sites**
    EXCLUDES 1   neurofibromatosis (nonmalignant) (Q85.Ø-)

D48.Ø Neoplasm of uncertain behavior of bone and articular cartilage
    EXCLUDES 1   neoplasm of uncertain behavior of cartilage of ear (D48.1)
             neoplasm of uncertain behavior of cartilage of larynx (D38.Ø)
             neoplasm of uncertain behavior of cartilage of nose (D38.5)
             neoplasm of uncertain behavior of connective tissue of eyelid (D48.1)
             neoplasm of uncertain behavior of synovia (D48.1)

D48.1 Neoplasm of uncertain behavior of connective and other soft tissue
     Neoplasm of uncertain behavior of connective tissue of ear
     Neoplasm of uncertain behavior of connective tissue of eyelid
     Stromal tumors of uncertain behavior of digestive system
    EXCLUDES 1   neoplasm of uncertain behavior of articular cartilage (D48.Ø)
             neoplasm of uncertain behavior of cartilage of larynx (D38.Ø)
             neoplasm of uncertain behavior of cartilage of nose (D38.5)
             neoplasm of uncertain behavior of connective tissue of breast (D48.6-)

D48.2 Neoplasm of uncertain behavior of peripheral nerves and autonomic nervous system
    EXCLUDES 1   neoplasm of uncertain behavior of peripheral nerves of orbit (D48.7)

D48.3 Neoplasm of uncertain behavior of retroperitoneum

D48.4 Neoplasm of uncertain behavior of peritoneum

D48.5 Neoplasm of uncertain behavior of skin
     Neoplasm of uncertain behavior of anal margin
     Neoplasm of uncertain behavior of anal skin
     Neoplasm of uncertain behavior of perianal skin
     Neoplasm of uncertain behavior of skin of breast
    EXCLUDES 1   neoplasm of uncertain behavior of anus NOS (D37.8)
             neoplasm of uncertain behavior of skin of genital organs (D39.8, D4Ø.8)
             neoplasm of uncertain behavior of vermilion border of lip (D37.Ø)

☑5ᵗʰ **D48.6 Neoplasm of uncertain behavior of breast**
     Neoplasm of uncertain behavior of connective tissue of breast
     Cystosarcoma phyllodes
    EXCLUDES 1   neoplasm of uncertain behavior of skin of breast (D48.5)

     D48.6Ø Neoplasm of uncertain behavior of unspecified breast
     D48.61 Neoplasm of uncertain behavior of right breast
     D48.62 Neoplasm of uncertain behavior of left breast

D48.7 Neoplasm of uncertain behavior of other specified sites
     Neoplasm of uncertain behavior of eye
     Neoplasm of uncertain behavior of heart
     Neoplasm of uncertain behavior of peripheral nerves of orbit
    EXCLUDES 1   neoplasm of uncertain behavior of connective tissue (D48.1)
             neoplasm of uncertain behavior of skin of eyelid (D48.5)

D48.9 Neoplasm of uncertain behavior, unspecified

Neoplasms of uncertain behavior (D49)

☑4ᵗʰ **D49 Neoplasms of unspecified behavior**
    NOTE   Category D49 classifies by site neoplasms of unspecified morphology and behavior. The term "mass", unless otherwise stated, is not to be regarded as a neoplastic growth.
    INCLUDES   "growth" NOS
             neoplasm NOS
             new growth NOS
             tumor NOS
    EXCLUDES 1   neoplasms of uncertain behavior (D37-D44, D48)

D49.Ø Neoplasm of unspecified behavior of digestive system
    EXCLUDES 1   neoplasm of unspecified behavior of margin of anus (D49.2)
             neoplasm of unspecified behavior of perianal skin (D49.2)
             neoplasm of unspecified behavior of skin of anus (D49.2)

D49.1 Neoplasm of unspecified behavior of respiratory system

D49.2 Neoplasm of unspecified behavior of bone, soft tissue, and skin
    EXCLUDES 1   neoplasm of unspecified behavior of anal canal (D49.Ø)
             neoplasm of unspecified behavior of anus NOS (D49.Ø)
             neoplasm of unspecified behavior of bone marrow (D49.89)
             neoplasm of unspecified behavior of cartilage of larynx (D49.1)
             neoplasm of unspecified behavior of cartilage of nose (D49.1)
             neoplasm of unspecified behavior of connective tissue of breast (D49.3)
             neoplasm of unspecified behavior of skin of genital organs (D49.5)
             neoplasm of unspecified behavior of vermilion border of lip (D49.Ø)

D49.3 Neoplasm of unspecified behavior of breast
    EXCLUDES 1   neoplasm of unspecified behavior of skin of breast (D49.2)

D49.4 Neoplasm of unspecified behavior of bladder

D49.5 Neoplasm of unspecified behavior of other genitourinary organs

D49.6 Neoplasm of unspecified behavior of brain
    EXCLUDES 1   neoplasm of unspecified behavior of cerebral meninges (D49.7)
             neoplasm of unspecified behavior of cranial nerves (D49.7)

D49.7 Neoplasm of unspecified behavior of endocrine glands and other parts of nervous system
    EXCLUDES 1   neoplasm of unspecified behavior of peripheral, sympathetic, and parasympathetic nerves and ganglia (D49.2)

☑5ᵗʰ **D49.8 Neoplasm of unspecified behavior of other specified sites**
    EXCLUDES 1   neoplasm of unspecified behavior of eyelid (skin) (D49.2)
             neoplasm of unspecified behavior of eyelid cartilage (D49.2)
             neoplasm of unspecified behavior of great vessels (D49.2)
             neoplasm of unspecified behavior of optic nerve (D49.7)

     D49.81 Neoplasm of unspecified behavior of retina and choroid
         Dark area on retina
         Retinal freckle

     D49.89 Neoplasm of unspecified behavior of other specified sites

D49.9 Neoplasm of unspecified behavior of unspecified site

☑ Additional Character Required   ☑ₓ₇ᵗʰ Placeholder Alert   Unspecified Dx   Other Specified Dx   Manifestation   ▶◀ Revised Text   ● New Code   ▲ Revised Code Title

ICD-10-CM 2016   **477**

Chapter 3. Disease of the Blood and Blood-Forming Organs and Certain Disorders Involving the Immune Mechanism (D50–D89)

Chapter Specific Coding Guidelines and Examples
Reserved for future guideline expansion.

Chapter 3. Diseases of the Blood and Blood-forming Organs and Certain Disorders Involving the Immune Mechanism (D50-D89)

EXCLUDES 2   autoimmune disease (systemic) NOS (M35.9)
certain conditions originating in the perinatal period (P00-P96)
complications of pregnancy, childbirth and the puerperium (O00-O9A)
congenital malformations, deformations and chromosomal abnormalities (Q00-Q99)
endocrine, nutritional and metabolic diseases (E00-E88)
human immunodeficiency virus [HIV] disease (B20)
injury, poisoning and certain other consequences of external causes (S00-T88)
neoplasms (C00-D49)
symptoms, signs and abnormal clinical and laboratory findings, not elsewhere classified (R00-R94)

This chapter contains the following blocks:

D50-D53   Nutritional anemias
D55-D59   Hemolytic anemias
D60-D64   Aplastic and other anemias and other bone marrow failure syndromes
D65-D69   Coagulation defects, purpura and other hemorrhagic conditions
D70-D77   Other disorders of blood and blood-forming organs
D78   Intraoperative and postprocedural complications of the spleen
D80-D89   Certain disorders involving the immune mechanism

Nutritional anemias (D50-D53)

✓4ᵗʰ **D50   Iron deficiency anemia**
INCLUDES   asiderotic anemia
hypochromic anemia

D50.0   Iron deficiency anemia secondary to blood loss (chronic)
Posthemorrhagic anemia (chronic)
EXCLUDES 1   acute posthemorrhagic anemia (D62)
congenital anemia from fetal blood loss (P61.3)

D50.1   Sideropenic dysphagia
Kelly-Paterson syndrome
Plummer-Vinson syndrome

D50.8   Other iron deficiency anemias
Iron deficiency anemia due to inadequate dietary iron intake

D50.9   Iron deficiency anemia, unspecified

✓4ᵗʰ **D51   Vitamin B12 deficiency anemia**
EXCLUDES 1   vitamin B12 deficiency (E53.8)

D51.0   Vitamin B12 deficiency anemia due to intrinsic factor deficiency
Addison anemia
Biermer anemia
Pernicious (congenital) anemia
Congenital intrinsic factor deficiency

D51.1   Vitamin B12 deficiency anemia due to selective vitamin B12 malabsorption with proteinuria
Imerslund (Gräsbeck) syndrome
Megaloblastic hereditary anemia

D51.2   Transcobalamin II deficiency

D51.3   Other dietary vitamin B12 deficiency anemia
Vegan anemia

D51.8   Other vitamin B12 deficiency anemias

D51.9   Vitamin B12 deficiency anemia, unspecified

✓4ᵗʰ **D52   Folate deficiency anemia**
EXCLUDES 1   folate deficiency without anemia (E53.8)

D52.0   Dietary folate deficiency anemia
Nutritional megaloblastic anemia

D52.1   Drug-induced folate deficiency anemia
Use additional code for adverse effect, if applicable, to identify drug (T36-T50 with fifth or sixth character 5)

D52.8   Other folate deficiency anemias

D52.9   Folate deficiency anemia, unspecified
Folic acid deficiency anemia NOS

✓4ᵗʰ **D53   Other nutritional anemias**
INCLUDES   megaloblastic anemia unresponsive to vitamin B12 or folate therapy

D53.0   Protein deficiency anemia
Amino-acid deficiency anemia
Orotaciduric anemia
EXCLUDES 1   Lesch-Nyhan syndrome (E79.1)

D53.1   Other megaloblastic anemias, not elsewhere classified
Megaloblastic anemia NOS
EXCLUDES 1   Di Guglielmo's disease (C94.0)

D53.2   Scorbutic anemia
EXCLUDES 1   scurvy (E54)

D53.8   Other specified nutritional anemias
Anemia associated with deficiency of copper
Anemia associated with deficiency of molybdenum
Anemia associated with deficiency of zinc
EXCLUDES 1   nutritional deficiencies without anemia, such as:
copper deficiency NOS (E61.0)
molybdenum deficiency NOS (E61.5)
zinc deficiency NOS (E60)

D53.9   Nutritional anemia, unspecified
Simple chronic anemia
EXCLUDES 1   anemia NOS (D64.9)

Hemolytic anemias (D55-D59)

✓4ᵗʰ **D55   Anemia due to enzyme disorders**
EXCLUDES 1   drug-induced enzyme deficiency anemia (D59.2)

D55.0   Anemia due to glucose-6-phosphate dehydrogenase [G6PD] deficiency
Favism
G6PD deficiency anemia

D55.1   Anemia due to other disorders of glutathione metabolism
Anemia (due to) enzyme deficiencies, except G6PD, related to the hexose monophosphate [HMP] shunt pathway
Anemia (due to) hemolytic nonspherocytic (hereditary), type I

D55.2   Anemia due to disorders of glycolytic enzymes
Hemolytic nonspherocytic (hereditary) anemia, type II
Hexokinase deficiency anemia
Pyruvate kinase [PK] deficiency anemia
Triose-phosphate isomerase deficiency anemia
EXCLUDES 1   disorders of glycolysis not associated with anemia (E74.8)

D55.3   Anemia due to disorders of nucleotide metabolism

D55.8   Other anemias due to enzyme disorders

D55.9   Anemia due to enzyme disorder, unspecified

✓4ᵗʰ **D56   Thalassemia**
EXCLUDES 1   sickle-cell thalassemia (D57.4-)

D56.0   Alpha thalassemia
Alpha thalassemia major
Hemoglobin H Constant Spring
Hemoglobin H disease
Hydrops fetalis due to alpha thalassemia
Severe alpha thalassemia
Triple gene defect alpha thalassemia
Use additional code, if applicable, for hydrops fetalis due to alpha thalassemia (P56.99)
EXCLUDES 1   alpha thalassemia trait or minor (D56.3)
asymptomatic alpha thalassemia (D56.3)
hydrops fetalis due to isoimmunization (P56.0)
hydrops fetalis not due to immune hemolysis (P83.2)

D56.1   Beta thalassemia
Beta thalassemia major
Cooley's anemia
Homozygous beta thalassemia
Severe beta thalassemia
Thalassemia intermedia
Thalassemia major
EXCLUDES 1   beta thalassemia minor (D56.3)
beta thalassemia trait (D56.3)
delta-beta thalassemia (D56.2)
hemoglobin E-beta thalassemia (D56.5)
sickle-cell beta thalassemia (D57.4-)

D56.2   Delta-beta thalassemia
Homozygous delta-beta thalassemia
EXCLUDES 1   delta-beta thalassemia minor (D56.3)
delta-beta thalassemia trait (D56.3)

D56.3   Thalassemia minor
Alpha thalassemia minor
Alpha thalassemia silent carrier
Alpha thalassemia trait
Beta thalassemia minor
Beta thalassemia trait
Delta-beta thalassemia minor
Delta-beta thalassemia trait
Thalassemia trait NOS
EXCLUDES 1   alpha thalassemia (D56.0)
beta thalassemia (D56.1)
delta-beta thalassemia (D56.2)
hemoglobin E-beta thalassemia (D56.5)
sickle-cell trait (D57.3)

☑ Additional Character Required   ✓ₓ7ᵗʰ Placeholder Alert   Unspecified Dx   Other Specified Dx   Manifestation   ▶◀ Revised Text   ● New Code   ▲ Revised Code Title

D56.4   Hereditary persistence of fetal hemoglobin [HPFH]

D56.5   Hemoglobin E-beta **thalassemia**
> EXCLUDES 1   *beta thalassemia (D56.1)*
> *beta thalassemia minor (D56.3)*
> *beta thalassemia trait (D56.3)*
> *delta-beta thalassemia (D56.2)*
> *delta-beta thalassemia trait (D56.3)*
> *hemoglobin E disease (D58.2)*
> *other hemoglobinopathies (D58.2)*
> *sickle-cell beta thalassemia (D57.4-)*

D56.8   **Other thalassemias**
Dominant thalassemia
Hemoglobin C thalassemia
Mixed thalassemia
Thalassemia with other hemoglobinopathy
> EXCLUDES 1   *hemoglobin C disease (D58.2)*
> *hemoglobin E disease (D58.2)*
> *other hemoglobinopathies (D58.2)*
> *sickle-cell anemia (D57.-)*
> *sickle-cell thalassemia (D57.4)*

D56.9   **Thalassemia, unspecified**
Mediterranean anemia (with other hemoglobinopathy)

✓4th **D57**   **Sickle-cell disorders**
Use additional code for any associated fever (R50.81)
> EXCLUDES 1   *other hemoglobinopathies (D58.-)*

✓5th **D57.0**   **Hb-SS disease** with crisis
Sickle-cell disease NOS with crisis
Hb-SS disease with vasoocclusive pain

     D57.00   **Hb-SS disease with crisis, unspecified**

     D57.01   **Hb-SS disease with** acute chest syndrome

     D57.02   **Hb-SS disease with** splenic sequestration

D57.1   **Sickle-cell disease** without crisis
Hb-SS disease without crisis
Sickle-cell anemia NOS
Sickle-cell disease NOS
Sickle-cell disorder NOS

✓5th **D57.2**   **Sickle-cell/Hb-C disease**
Hb-SC disease
Hb-S/Hb-C disease

     D57.20   **Sickle-cell/Hb-C disease** without crisis

     ✓6th **D57.21**   **Sickle-cell/Hb-C disease** with crisis

         D57.211   **Sickle-cell/Hb-C disease with** acute chest syndrome

         D57.212   **Sickle-cell/Hb-C disease with** splenic sequestration

         D57.219   **Sickle-cell/Hb-C disease with crisis, unspecified**
Sickle-cell/Hb-C disease with crisis NOS

D57.3   **Sickle-cell** trait
Hb-S trait
Heterozygous hemoglobin S

✓5th **D57.4**   **Sickle-cell** thalassemia
Sickle-cell beta thalassemia
Thalassemia Hb-S disease

     D57.40   **Sickle-cell thalassemia** without crisis
Microdrepanocytosis
Sickle-cell thalassemia NOS

     ✓6th **D57.41**   **Sickle-cell thalassemia** with crisis
Sickle-cell thalassemia with vasoocclusive pain

         D57.411   **Sickle-cell thalassemia with** acute chest syndrome

         D57.412   **Sickle-cell thalassemia with** splenic sequestration

         D57.419   **Sickle-cell thalassemia with crisis, unspecified**
Sickle-cell thalassemia with crisis NOS

✓5th **D57.8**   **Other sickle-cell disorders**
Hb-SD disease
Hb-SE disease

     D57.80   **Other sickle-cell disorders** without crisis

     ✓6th **D57.81**   **Other sickle-cell disorders** with crisis

         D57.811   **Other sickle-cell disorders with** acute chest syndrome

         D57.812   **Other sickle-cell disorders with** splenic sequestration

         D57.819   **Other sickle-cell disorders with crisis, unspecified**
Other sickle-cell disorders with crisis NOS

✓4th **D58**   **Other hereditary** **hemolytic anemias**
> EXCLUDES 1   *hemolytic anemia of the newborn (P55.-)*

D58.0   **Hereditary** spherocytosis
Acholuric (familial) jaundice
Congenital (spherocytic) hemolytic icterus
Minkowski-Chauffard syndrome

D58.1   **Hereditary** elliptocytosis
Elliptocytosis (congenital)
Ovalocytosis (congenital) (hereditary)

D58.2   **Other** hemoglobinopathies
Abnormal hemoglobin NOS
Congenital Heinz body anemia
Hb-C disease
Hb-D disease
Hb-E disease
Hemoglobinopathy NOS
Unstable hemoglobin hemolytic disease
> EXCLUDES 1   *familial polycythemia (D75.0)*
> *Hb-M disease (D74.0)*
> *hemoglobin E-beta thalassemia (D56.5)*
> *hereditary persistence of fetal hemoglobin [HPFH] (D56.4)*
> *high-altitude polycythemia (D75.1)*
> *methemoglobinemia (D74.-)*
> *other hemoglobinopathies with thalassemia (D56.8)*

D58.8   **Other specified hereditary hemolytic anemias**
Stomatocytosis

D58.9   **Hereditary hemolytic anemia, unspecified**

✓4th **D59**   **Acquired** **hemolytic anemia**

D59.0   **Drug-induced autoimmune** **hemolytic anemia**
Use additional code for adverse effect, if applicable, to identify drug (T36-T50 with fifth or sixth character 5)

D59.1   **Other autoimmune** **hemolytic anemias**
Autoimmune hemolytic disease (cold type) (warm type)
Chronic cold hemagglutinin disease
Cold agglutinin disease
Cold agglutinin hemoglobinuria
Cold type (secondary) (symptomatic) hemolytic anemia
Warm type (secondary) (symptomatic) hemolytic anemia
> EXCLUDES 1   *Evans syndrome (D69.41)*
> *hemolytic disease of newborn (P55.-)*
> *paroxysmal cold hemoglobinuria (D59.6)*

D59.2   **Drug-induced nonautoimmune** **hemolytic anemia**
Drug-induced enzyme deficiency anemia
Use additional code for adverse effect, if applicable, to identify drug (T36-T50 with fifth or sixth character 5)

D59.3   **Hemolytic-uremic syndrome**
Use additional code to identify associated:
E. coli infection (B96.2-)
Pneumococcal pneumonia (J13)
Shigella dysenteriae (A03.9)

D59.4   **Other nonautoimmune** **hemolytic anemias**
Mechanical hemolytic anemia
Microangiopathic hemolytic anemia
Toxic hemolytic anemia

D59.5   **Paroxysmal nocturnal hemoglobinuria [Marchiafava-Micheli]**
> EXCLUDES 1   *hemoglobinuria NOS (R82.3)*

D59.6   **Hemoglobinuria** due to hemolysis from other external causes
Hemoglobinuria from exertion
March hemoglobinuria
Paroxysmal cold hemoglobinuria
Use additional code (Chapter 20) to identify external cause
> EXCLUDES 1   *hemoglobinuria NOS (R82.3)*

D59.8   **Other acquired hemolytic anemias**

D59.9   **Acquired hemolytic anemia, unspecified**
Idiopathic hemolytic anemia, chronic

Aplastic and other anemias and other bone marrow failure syndromes (D60-D64)

✓4th **D60**   **Acquired pure red cell aplasia [erythroblastopenia]**
> INCLUDES   red cell aplasia (acquired) (adult) (with thymoma)
> EXCLUDES 1   *congenital red cell aplasia (D61.01)*

D60.0   **Chronic** acquired pure red cell aplasia

D60.1   **Transient** acquired pure red cell aplasia

D60.8   **Other acquired pure red cell aplasias**

D60.9   **Acquired pure red cell aplasia, unspecified**

☑4ᵗʰ **D61 Other aplastic anemias and other bone marrow failure syndromes**

> *EXCLUDES 1* neutropenia (D70.-)
> AHA: 2014, 4Q, 22

☑5ᵗʰ **D61.0 Constitutional aplastic anemia**

D61.01 Constitutional (pure) red blood cell aplasia
Blackfan-Diamond syndrome
Congenital (pure) red cell aplasia
Familial hypoplastic anemia
Primary (pure) red cell aplasia
Red cell (pure) aplasia of infants
> *EXCLUDES 1* acquired red cell aplasia (D60.9)

D61.09 Other constitutional aplastic anemia
Fanconi's anemia
Pancytopenia with malformations

D61.1 Drug-induced aplastic anemia
Use additional code for adverse effect, if applicable, to identify drug (T36-T50 with fifth or sixth character 5)

D61.2 Aplastic anemia due to other external agents
Code first, if applicable, toxic effects of substances chiefly nonmedicinal as to source (T51-T65)

D61.3 Idiopathic aplastic anemia

☑5ᵗʰ **D61.8 Other specified aplastic anemias and other bone marrow failure syndromes**

☑6ᵗʰ **D61.81 Pancytopenia**
> *EXCLUDES 1* pancytopenia (due to) (with) aplastic anemia (D61.9)
> pancytopenia (due to) (with) bone marrow infiltration (D61.82)
> pancytopenia (due to) (with) congenital (pure) red cell aplasia (D61.01)
> pancytopenia (due to) (with) hairy cell leukemia (C91.4-)
> pancytopenia (due to) (with) human immunodeficiency virus disease (B20)
> pancytopenia (due to) (with) leukoerythroblastic anemia (D61.82)
> pancytopenia (due to) (with) myelodysplastic syndromes (D46.-)
> pancytopenia (due to) (with) myeloproliferative disease (D47.1)

D61.810 Antineoplastic chemotherapy induced pancytopenia
> *EXCLUDES 2* aplastic anemia due to antineoplastic chemotherapy (D61.1)

D61.811 Other drug-induced pancytopenia
> *EXCLUDES 2* aplastic anemia due to drugs (D61.1)

D61.818 Other pancytopenia

D61.82 Myelophthisis
Leukoerythroblastic anemia
Myelophthisic anemia
Panmyelophthisis
Code also the underlying disorder, such as:
malignant neoplasm of breast (C50.-)
tuberculosis (A15.-)
> *EXCLUDES 1* idiopathic myelofibrosis (D47.1)
> myelofibrosis NOS (D75.81)
> myelofibrosis with myeloid metaplasia (D47.4)
> primary myelofibrosis (D47.1)
> secondary myelofibrosis (D75.81)

D61.89 Other specified aplastic anemias and other bone marrow failure syndromes

D61.9 Aplastic anemia, unspecified
Hypoplastic anemia NOS
Medullary hypoplasia

D62 Acute posthemorrhagic anemia
> *EXCLUDES 1* anemia due to chronic blood loss (D50.0)
> blood loss anemia NOS (D50.0)
> congenital anemia from fetal blood loss (P61.3)

☑4ᵗʰ **D63 Anemia in chronic diseases classified elsewhere**

D63.0 Anemia in neoplastic disease
Code first neoplasm (C00-D49)
> *EXCLUDES 1* anemia due to antineoplastic chemotherapy (D64.81)
> aplastic anemia due to antineoplastic chemotherapy (D61.1)

D63.1 Anemia in chronic kidney disease
Erythropoietin resistant anemia (EPO resistant anemia)
Code first underlying chronic kidney disease (CKD) (N18.-)

D63.8 Anemia in other chronic diseases classified elsewhere
Code first underlying disease, such as:
diphyllobothriasis (B70.0)
hookworm disease (B76.0-B76.9)
hypothyroidism (E00.0-E03.9)
malaria (B50.0-B54)
symptomatic late syphilis (A52.79)
tuberculosis (A18.89)

☑4ᵗʰ **D64 Other anemias**
> *EXCLUDES 1* refractory anemia (D46.-)
> refractory anemia with excess blasts in transformation [RAEB T] (C92.0-)

D64.0 Hereditary sideroblastic anemia
Sex-linked hypochromic sideroblastic anemia

D64.1 Secondary sideroblastic anemia due to disease
Code first underlying disease

D64.2 Secondary sideroblastic anemia due to drugs and toxins
Code first poisoning due to drug or toxin, if applicable (T36-T65 with fifth or sixth character 1-4 or 6)
Use additional code for adverse effect, if applicable, to identify drug (T36-T50 with fifth or sixth character 5)

D64.3 Other sideroblastic anemias
Sideroblastic anemia NOS
Pyridoxine-responsive sideroblastic anemia NEC

D64.4 Congenital dyserythropoietic anemia
Dyshematopoietic anemia (congenital)
> *EXCLUDES 1* Blackfan-Diamond syndrome (D61.01)
> Di Guglielmo's disease (C94.0)

☑5ᵗʰ **D64.8 Other specified anemias**

D64.81 Anemia due to antineoplastic chemotherapy
Antineoplastic chemotherapy induced anemia
> *EXCLUDES 1* anemia in neoplastic disease (D63.0)
> aplastic anemia due to antineoplastic chemotherapy (D61.1)
> AHA: 2014, 4Q, 22

D64.89 Other specified anemias
Infantile pseudoleukemia

D64.9 Anemia, unspecified

Coagulation defects, purpura and other hemorrhagic conditions (D65-D69)

D65 Disseminated intravascular coagulation [defibrination syndrome]
Afibrinogenemia, acquired
Consumption coagulopathy
Diffuse or disseminated intravascular coagulation [DIC]
Fibrinolytic hemorrhage, acquired
Fibrinolytic purpura
Purpura fulminans
> *EXCLUDES 1* disseminated intravascular coagulation (complicating):
> abortion or ectopic or molar pregnancy (O00-O07, O08.1)
> in newborn (P60)
> pregnancy, childbirth and the puerperium (O45.0, O46.0, O67.0, O72.3)

D66 Hereditary factor VIII deficiency
Classical hemophilia
Deficiency factor VIII (with functional defect)
Hemophilia A
Hemophilia NOS
> *EXCLUDES 1* factor VIII deficiency with vascular defect (D68.0)

D67 Hereditary factor IX deficiency
Christmas disease
Factor IX deficiency (with functional defect)
Hemophilia B
Plasma thromboplastin component [PTC] deficiency

☑ Additional Character Required   ☑x7ᵗʰ Placeholder Alert   Unspecified Dx   Other Specified Dx   Manifestation   ▶◀ Revised Text   ● New Code   ▲ Revised Code Title

Chapter 3. Disease of the Blood and Blood-Forming Organs

✓4ᵗʰ D68 Other coagulation defects
> EXCLUDES 1   abnormal coagulation profile (R79.1)
> coagulation defects complicating abortion or ectopic or molar pregnancy (O00–O07, O08.1)
> coagulation defects complicating pregnancy, childbirth and the puerperium (O45.0, O46.0, O67.0, O72.3)

D68.0 Von Willebrand's disease
Angiohemophilia
Factor VIII deficiency with vascular defect
Vascular hemophilia
> EXCLUDES 1   capillary fragility (hereditary) (D69.8)
> factor VIII deficiency NOS (D66)
> factor VIII deficiency with functional defect (D66)

D68.1 Hereditary factor XI deficiency
Hemophilia C
Plasma thromboplastin antecedent [PTA] deficiency
Rosenthal's disease

D68.2 Hereditary deficiency of other clotting factors
AC globulin deficiency
Congenital afibrinogenemia
Deficiency of factor I [fibrinogen]
Deficiency of factor II [prothrombin]
Deficiency of factor V [labile]
Deficiency of factor VII [stable]
Deficiency of factor X [Stuart-Prower]
Deficiency of factor XII [Hageman]
Deficiency of factor XIII [fibrin stabilizing]
Dysfibrinogenemia (congenital)
Hypoproconvertinemia
Owren's disease
Proaccelerin deficiency

✓5ᵗʰ D68.3 Hemorrhagic disorder due to circulating anticoagulants

✓6ᵗʰ D68.31 Hemorrhagic disorder due to intrinsic circulating anticoagulants, antibodies, or inhibitors

D68.311 Acquired hemophilia
Autoimmune hemophilia
Autoimmune inhibitors to clotting factors
Secondary hemophilia

D68.312 Antiphospholipid antibody with hemorrhagic disorder
Lupus anticoagulant (LAC) with hemorrhagic disorder
Systemic lupus erythematosus [SLE] inhibitor with hemorrhagic disorder
> EXCLUDES 1   antiphospholipid antibody, finding without diagnosis (R76.0)
> antiphospholipid antibody syndrome (D68.61)
> antiphospholipid antibody with hypercoagulable state (D68.61)
> lupus anticoagulant (LAC) finding without diagnosis (R76.0)
> lupus anticoagulant (LAC) with hypercoagulable state (D68.62)
> systemic lupus erythematosus [SLE] inhibitor finding without diagnosis (R76.0)
> systemic lupus erythematosus [SLE] inhibitor with hypercoagulable state (D68.62)

D68.318 Other hemorrhagic disorder due to intrinsic circulating anticoagulants, antibodies, or inhibitors
Antithromboplastinemia
Antithromboplastinogenemia
Hemorrhagic disorder due to intrinsic increase in antithrombin
Hemorrhagic disorder due to intrinsic increase in anti-VIIIa
Hemorrhagic disorder due to intrinsic increase in anti-IXa
Hemorrhagic disorder due to intrinsic increase in anti-XIa

D68.32 Hemorrhagic disorder due to extrinsic circulating anticoagulants
Drug-induced hemorrhagic disorder
Hemorrhagic disorder due to increase in anti-IIa
Hemorrhagic disorder due to increase in anti-Xa
Hyperheparinemia
Use additional code for adverse effect, if applicable, to identify drug (T45.515, T45.525)

D68.4 Acquired coagulation factor deficiency
Deficiency of coagulation factor due to liver disease
Deficiency of coagulation factor due to vitamin K deficiency
> EXCLUDES 1   vitamin K deficiency of newborn (P53)

✓5ᵗʰ D68.5 Primary thrombophilia
Primary hypercoagulable states
> EXCLUDES 1   antiphospholipid syndrome (D68.61)
> lupus anticoagulant (D68.62)
> secondary activated protein C resistance (D68.69)
> secondary antiphospholipid antibody syndrome (D68.69)
> secondary lupus anticoagulant with hypercoagulable state (D68.69)
> secondary systemic lupus erythematosus [SLE] inhibitor with hypercoagulable state (D68.69)
> systemic lupus erythematosus [SLE] inhibitor finding without diagnosis (R76.0)
> systemic lupus erythematosus [SLE] inhibitor with hemorrhagic disorder (D68.312)
> thrombotic thrombocytopenic purpura (M31.1)

D68.51 Activated protein C resistance
Factor V Leiden mutation

D68.52 Prothrombin gene mutation

D68.59 Other primary thrombophilia
Antithrombin III deficiencyProtein C deficiency
Hypercoagulable state NOSProtein S deficiency
Primary hypercoagulable Thrombophilia NOS state NEC
Primary thrombophilia NEC

✓5ᵗʰ D68.6 Other thrombophilia
Other hypercoagulable states
> EXCLUDES 1   diffuse or disseminated intravascular coagulation [DIC] (D65)
> heparin induced thrombocytopenia (HIT) (D75.82)
> hyperhomocysteinemia (E72.11)

D68.61 Antiphospholipid syndrome
Anticardiolipin syndrome
Antiphospholipid antibody syndrome
> EXCLUDES 1   antiphospholipid antibody, finding without diagnosis (R76.0)
> antiphospholipid antibody with hemorrhagic disorder (D68.312)
> lupus anticoagulant syndrome (D68.62)

D68.62 Lupus anticoagulant syndrome
Lupus anticoagulant
Presence of systemic lupus erythematosus [SLE] inhibitor
> EXCLUDES 1   anticardiolipin syndrome (D68.61)
> antiphospholipid syndrome (D68.61)
> lupus anticoagulant (LAC) finding without diagnosis (R79.0)
> lupus anticoagulant (LAC) with hemorrhagic disorder (D68.312)

D68.69 Other thrombophilia
Hypercoagulable states NEC
Secondary hypercoagulable state NOS

D68.8 Other specified coagulation defects
> EXCLUDES 1   hemorrhagic disease of newborn (P53)

D68.9 Coagulation defect, unspecified

✓4ᵗʰ D69 Purpura and other hemorrhagic conditions
> EXCLUDES 1   benign hypergammaglobulinemic purpura (D89.0)
> cryoglobulinemic purpura (D89.1)
> essential (hemorrhagic) thrombocythemia (D47.3)
> hemorrhagic thrombocythemia (D47.3)
> purpura fulminans (D65)
> thrombotic thrombocytopenic purpura (M31.1)
> Waldenström hypergammaglobulinemic purpura (D89.0)

D69.0 Allergic purpura
Allergic vasculitis
Nonthrombocytopenic hemorrhagic purpura
Nonthrombocytopenic idiopathic purpura
Purpura anaphylactoid
Purpura Henoch(-Schönlein)
Purpura rheumatica
Vascular purpura
> EXCLUDES 1   thrombocytopenic hemorrhagic purpura (D69.3)

EXCLUDES 1 Not coded here   EXCLUDES 2 Not included here   N Newborn Age: 0   P Pediatric Age: 0-17   M Maternity Age: 12-55   A Adult Age: 15-124

482   ICD-10-CM 2016

D69.1 **Qualitative platelet defects**
Bernard-Soulier [giant platelet] syndrome
Glanzmann's disease
Grey platelet syndrome
Thromboasthenia (hemorrhagic) (hereditary)
Thrombocytopathy
EXCLUDES 1 *von Willebrand's disease (D68.0)*

D69.2 **Other nonthrombocytopenic purpura**
Purpura NOS   Senile purpura
Purpura simplex

D69.3 **Immune thrombocytopenic purpura**
Hemorrhagic (thrombocytopenic) purpura
Idiopathic thrombocytopenic purpura
Tidal platelet dysgenesis

✓5th **D69.4** **Other primary thrombocytopenia**
EXCLUDES 1 *transient neonatal thrombocytopenia (P61.0)*
Wiskott-Aldrich syndrome (D82.0)

D69.41 **Evans syndrome**

D69.42 **Congenital and hereditary thrombocytopenia purpura**
Congenital thrombocytopenia
Hereditary thrombocytopenia
Code first congenital or hereditary disorder, such as:
thrombocytopenia with absent radius (TAR syndrome) (Q87.2)

D69.49 **Other primary thrombocytopenia**
Megakaryocytic hypoplasia
Primary thrombocytopenia NOS

✓5th **D69.5** **Secondary thrombocytopenia**
EXCLUDES 1 *heparin induced thrombocytopenia (HIT) (D75.82)*
transient thrombocytopenia of newborn (P61.0)

D69.51 **Posttransfusion purpura**
Posttransfusion purpura from whole blood (fresh) or blood products
PTP

D69.59 **Other secondary thrombocytopenia**
AHA: 2014, 4Q, 22

D69.6 **Thrombocytopenia, unspecified**

D69.8 **Other specified hemorrhagic conditions**
Capillary fragility (hereditary)   Vascular pseudohemophilia

D69.9 **Hemorrhagic condition, unspecified**

Other disorders of blood and blood-forming organs (D70-D77)

✓4th **D70** **Neutropenia**
INCLUDES agranulocytosis
decreased absolute neurophile count (ANC)
Use additional code for any associated:
fever (R50.81)
mucositis (J34.81, K12.3-, K92.81, N76.81)
EXCLUDES 1 *neutropenic splenomegaly (D73.81)*
transient neonatal neutropenia (P61.5)

D70.0 **Congenital agranulocytosis**
Congenital neutropenia
Infantile genetic agranulocytosis
Kostmann's disease

D70.1 **Agranulocytosis secondary to cancer chemotherapy**
Code also underlying neoplasm
Use additional code for adverse effect, if applicable, to identify drug (T45.1X5)
AHA: 2014, 4Q, 22

D70.2 **Other drug-induced agranulocytosis**
Use additional code for adverse effect, if applicable, to identify drug (T36-T50 with fifth or sixth character 5)

D70.3 **Neutropenia due to infection**

D70.4 **Cyclic neutropenia**
Cyclic hematopoiesis
Periodic neutropenia

D70.8 **Other neutropenia**

D70.9 **Neutropenia, unspecified**

D71 **Functional disorders of polymorphonuclear neutrophils**
Cell membrane receptor complex [CR3] defect
Chronic (childhood) granulomatous disease
Congenital dysphagocytosis
Progressive septic granulomatosis

✓4th **D72** **Other disorders of white blood cells**
EXCLUDES 1 *basophilia (D72.824)*
immunity disorders (D80-D89)
neutropenia (D70)
preleukemia (syndrome) (D46.9)

D72.0 **Genetic anomalies of leukocytes**
Alder (granulation) (granulocyte) anomaly
Alder syndrome
Hereditary leukocytic hypersegmentation
Hereditary leukocytic hyposegmentation
Hereditary leukomelanopathy
May-Hegglin (granulation) (granulocyte) anomaly
May-Hegglin syndrome
Pelger-Huët (granulation) (granulocyte) anomaly
Pelger-Huët syndrome
EXCLUDES 1 *Chédiak (-Steinbrinck)-Higashi syndrome (E70.330)*

D72.1 **Eosinophilia**
Allergic eosinophilia
Hereditary eosinophilia
EXCLUDES 1 *Löffler's syndrome (J82)*
pulmonary eosinophilia (J82)

✓5th **D72.8** **Other specified disorders of white blood cells**
EXCLUDES 1 *leukemia (C91-C95)*

✓6th **D72.81** **Decreased white blood cell count**
EXCLUDES 1 *neutropenia (D70.-)*

D72.810 **Lymphocytopenia**
Decreased lymphocytes

D72.818 **Other decreased white blood cell count**
Basophilic leukopenia
Eosinophilic leukopenia
Monocytopenia
Other decreased leukocytes
Plasmacytopenia

D72.819 **Decreased white blood cell count, unspecified**
Decreased leukocytes, unspecified
Leukocytopenia, unspecified
Leukopenia
EXCLUDES 1 *malignant leukopenia (D70.9)*

✓6th **D72.82** **Elevated white blood cell count**
EXCLUDES 1 *eosinophilia (D72.1)*

D72.820 **Lymphocytosis (symptomatic)**
Elevated lymphocytes

D72.821 **Monocytosis (symptomatic)**
EXCLUDES 1 *infectious mononucleosis (B27.-)*

D72.822 **Plasmacytosis**

D72.823 **Leukemoid reaction**
Basophilic leukemoid reaction
Leukemoid reaction NOS
Lymphocytic leukemoid reaction
Monocytic leukemoid reaction
Myelocytic leukemoid reaction
Neutrophilic leukemoid reaction

D72.824 **Basophilia**

D72.825 **Bandemia**
Bandemia without diagnosis of specific infection
EXCLUDES 1 *confirmed infection—code to infection*
leukemia (C91.-, C92.-, C93.-, C94.-, C95.-)

D72.828 **Other elevated white blood cell count**

D72.829 **Elevated white blood cell count, unspecified**
Elevated leukocytes, unspecified
Leukocytosis, unspecified

D72.89 **Other specified disorders of white blood cells**
Abnormality of white blood cells NEC

D72.9 **Disorder of white blood cells, unspecified**
Abnormal leukocyte differential NOS

✓4th **D73** **Diseases of spleen**

D73.0 **Hyposplenism**
Atrophy of spleen
EXCLUDES 1 *asplenia (congenital) (Q89.01)*
postsurgical absence of spleen (Z90.81)

☑ Additional Character Required   ✓x7th Placeholder Alert   Unspecified Dx   Other Specified Dx   Manifestation   ►◄ Revised Text   ● New Code   ▲ Revised Code Title

ICD-10-CM 2016   **483**

Chapter 3. Disease of the Blood and Blood-Forming Organs

D73.1   Hypersplenism
> EXCLUDES 1   *neutropenic splenomegaly (D73.81)*
> *primary splenic neutropenia (D73.81)*
> *splenitis, splenomegaly in late syphilis (A52.79)*
> *splenitis, splenomegaly in tuberculosis (A18.85)*
> *splenomegaly NOS (R16.1)*
> *splenomegaly congenital (Q89.0)*

D73.2   Chronic congestive splenomegaly

D73.3   Abscess of spleen

D73.4   Cyst of spleen

D73.5   Infarction of spleen
Splenic rupture, nontraumatic
Torsion of spleen
> EXCLUDES 1   *rupture of spleen due to Plasmodium vivax malaria (B51.0)*
> *traumatic rupture of spleen (S36.03-)*

✓5th D73.8   Other diseases of spleen

     D73.81   Neutropenic splenomegaly
         Werner-Schultz disease

     D73.89   Other diseases of spleen
         Fibrosis of spleen NOS
         Perisplenitis
         Splenitis NOS

D73.9   Disease of spleen, unspecified

✓4th D74   Methemoglobinemia

     D74.0   Congenital methemoglobinemia
         Congenital NADH-methemoglobin reductase deficiency
         Hemoglobin-M [Hb-M] disease
         Methemoglobinemia, hereditary

     D74.8   Other methemoglobinemias
         Acquired methemoglobinemia (with sulfhemoglobinemia)
         Toxic methemoglobinemia

     D74.9   Methemoglobinemia, unspecified

✓4th D75   Other and unspecified diseases of blood and blood-forming organs
> EXCLUDES 2   *acute lymphadenitis (L04.-)*
> *chronic lymphadenitis (I88.1)*
> *enlarged lymph nodes (R59.-)*
> *hypergammaglobulinemia NOS (D89.2)*
> *lymphadenitis NOS (I88.9)*
> *mesenteric lymphadenitis (acute) (chronic) (I88.0)*

     D75.0   Familial erythrocytosis
         Benign polycythemia
         Familial polycythemia
> EXCLUDES 1   *hereditary ovalocytosis (D58.1)*

     D75.1   Secondary polycythemia
         Acquired polycythemia
         Emotional polycythemia
         Erythrocytosis NOS
         Hypoxemic polycythemia
         Nephrogenous polycythemia
         Polycythemia due to erythropoietin
         Polycythemia due to fall in plasma volume
         Polycythemia due to high altitude
         Polycythemia due to stress
         Polycythemia NOS
         Relative polycythemia
> EXCLUDES 1   *polycythemia neonatorum (P61.1)*
> *polycythemia vera (D45)*

✓5th D75.8   Other specified diseases of blood and blood-forming organs

     D75.81   Myelofibrosis
         Myelofibrosis NOS
         Secondary myelofibrosis NOS
         Code first the underlying disorder, such as:
             malignant neoplasm of breast (C50.-)
         Use additional code, if applicable, for associated therapy-related myelodysplastic syndrome (D46.-)
         Use additional code for adverse effect, if applicable, to identify drug (T45.1X5)
> EXCLUDES 1   *acute myelofibrosis (C94.4-)*
> *idiopathic myelofibrosis (D47.1)*
> *leukoerythroblastic anemia (D61.82)*
> *myelofibrosis with myeloid metaplasia (D47.4)*
> *myelophthisic anemia (D61.82)*
> *myelophthisis (D61.82)*
> *primary myelofibrosis (D47.1)*

     D75.82   Heparin induced thrombocytopenia (HIT)

D75.89   Other specified diseases of blood and blood-forming organs

D75.9   Disease of blood and blood-forming organs, unspecified

✓4th D76   Other specified diseases with participation of lymphoreticular and reticulohistiocytic tissue
> EXCLUDES 1   *(Abt-) Letterer-Siwe disease (C96.0)*
> *eosinophilic granuloma (C96.6)*
> *Hand-Schüller-Christian disease (C96.5)*
> *histiocytic sarcoma (C96.A)*
> *histiocytosis X, multifocal (C96.5)*
> *histiocytosis X, unifocal (C96.6)*
> *Langerhans-cell histiocytosis, multifocal (C96.5)*
> *Langerhans-cell histiocytosis NOS (C96.6)*
> *Langerhans-cell histiocytosis, unifocal (C96.6)*
> *leukemic reticuloendotheliosis or reticulosis (C91.4-)*
> *lipomelanotic reticuloendotheliosis or reticulosis (I89.8)*
> *malignant histiocytosis (C96.A)*

     D76.1   Hemophagocytic lymphohistiocytosis
         Familial hemophagocytic reticulosis
         Histiocytoses of mononuclear phagocytes

     D76.2   Hemophagocytic syndrome, infection-associated
         Use additional code to identify infectious agent or disease

     D76.3   Other histiocytosis syndromes
         Reticulohistiocytoma (giant-cell)
         Sinus histiocytosis with massive lymphadenopathy
         Xanthogranuloma

D77   *Other disorders of blood and blood-forming organs in diseases classified elsewhere*
Code first underlying disease, such as:
     amyloidosis (E85.-)
     congenital early syphilis (A50.0)
     echinococcosis (B67.0-B67.9)
     malaria (B50.0-B54)
     schistosomiasis [bilharziasis] (B65.0-B65.9)
     vitamin C deficiency (E54)
> EXCLUDES 1   *rupture of spleen due to Plasmodium vivax malaria (B51.0)*
> *splenitis, splenomegaly in late syphilis (A52.79)*
> *splenitis, splenomegaly in tuberculosis (A18.85)*

Intraoperative and postprocedural complications of the spleen (D78)

✓4th D78   Intraoperative and postprocedural complications of the spleen

✓5th D78.0   Intraoperative hemorrhage and hematoma of the spleen complicating a procedure
> EXCLUDES 1   *intraoperative hemorrhage and hematoma of the spleen due to accidental puncture or laceration during a procedure (D78.1-)*

     D78.01   Intraoperative hemorrhage and hematoma of the spleen complicating a procedure on the spleen

     D78.02   Intraoperative hemorrhage and hematoma of the spleen complicating other procedure

✓5th D78.1   Accidental puncture and laceration of the spleen during a procedure

     D78.11   Accidental puncture and laceration of the spleen during a procedure on the spleen

     D78.12   Accidental puncture and laceration of the spleen during other procedure

✓5th D78.2   Postprocedural hemorrhage and hematoma of the spleen following a procedure

     D78.21   Postprocedural hemorrhage and hematoma of the spleen following a procedure on the spleen

     D78.22   Postprocedural hemorrhage and hematoma of the spleen following other procedure

✓5th D78.8   Other intraoperative and postprocedural complications of the spleen
         Use additional code, if applicable, to further specify disorder

     D78.81   Other intraoperative complications of the spleen

     D78.89   Other postprocedural complications of the spleen

EXCLUDES 1 Not coded here   EXCLUDES 2 Not included here   N Newborn Age: 0   P Pediatric Age: 0-17   M Maternity Age: 12-55   A Adult Age: 15-124

484   ICD-10-CM 2016

Certain disorders involving the immune mechanism (D80-D89)

INCLUDES   defects in the complement system
immunodeficiency disorders, except human immunodeficiency virus [HIV] disease
sarcoidosis

EXCLUDES 1   autoimmune disease (systemic) NOS (M35.9)
functional disorders of polymorphonuclear neutrophils (D71)
human immunodeficiency virus [HIV] disease (B20)

✓4th **D80 Immunodeficiency with predominantly antibody defects**

D80.0 Hereditary hypogammaglobulinemia
Autosomal recessive agammaglobulinemia (Swiss type)
X-linked agammaglobulinemia [Bruton] (with growth hormone deficiency)

D80.1 Nonfamilial hypogammaglobulinemia
Agammaglobulinemia with immunoglobulin-bearing B-lymphocytes
Common variable agammaglobulinemia [CVAgamma]
Hypogammaglobulinemia NOS

D80.2 Selective deficiency of immunoglobulin A [IgA]

D80.3 Selective deficiency of immunoglobulin G [IgG] subclasses

D80.4 Selective deficiency of immunoglobulin M [IgM]

D80.5 Immunodeficiency with increased immunoglobulin M [IgM]

D80.6 Antibody deficiency with near-normal immunoglobulins or with hyperimmunoglobulinemia

D80.7 Transient hypogammaglobulinemia of infancy   N

D80.8 Other immunodeficiencies with predominantly antibody defects
Kappa light chain deficiency

D80.9 Immunodeficiency with predominantly antibody defects, unspecified

✓4th **D81 Combined immunodeficiencies**

EXCLUDES 1   autosomal recessive agammaglobulinemia (Swiss type) (D80.0)

D81.0 Severe combined immunodeficiency [SCID] with reticular dysgenesis

D81.1 Severe combined immunodeficiency [SCID] with low T- and B-cell numbers

D81.2 Severe combined immunodeficiency [SCID] with low or normal B-cell numbers

D81.3 Adenosine deaminase [ADA] deficiency

D81.4 Nezelof's syndrome

D81.5 Purine nucleoside phosphorylase [PNP] deficiency

D81.6 Major histocompatibility complex class I deficiency
Bare lymphocyte syndrome

D81.7 Major histocompatibility complex class II deficiency

✓5th **D81.8 Other combined immunodeficiencies**

✓6th **D81.81 Biotin-dependent carboxylase deficiency**
Multiple carboxylase deficiency

EXCLUDES 1   biotin-dependent carboxylase deficiency due to dietary deficiency of biotin (E53.8)

D81.810 Biotinidase deficiency

D81.818 Other biotin-dependent carboxylase deficiency
Holocarboxylase synthetase deficiency
Other multiple carboxylase deficiency

D81.819 Biotin-dependent carboxylase deficiency, unspecified
Multiple carboxylase deficiency, unspecified

D81.89 Other combined immunodeficiencies

D81.9 Combined immunodeficiency, unspecified
Severe combined immunodeficiency disorder [SCID] NOS

✓4th **D82 Immunodeficiency associated with other major defects**

EXCLUDES 1   ataxia telangiectasia [Louis-Bar] (G11.3)

D82.0 Wiskott-Aldrich syndrome
Immunodeficiency with thrombocytopenia and eczema

D82.1 Di George's syndrome
Pharyngeal pouch syndrome   Thymic aplasia or hypoplasia
Thymic alymphoplasia   with immunodeficiency

D82.2 Immunodeficiency with short-limbed stature

D82.3 Immunodeficiency following hereditary defective response to Epstein-Barr virus
X-linked lymphoproliferative disease

D82.4 Hyperimmunoglobulin E [IgE] syndrome

D82.8 Immunodeficiency associated with other specified major defects

D82.9 Immunodeficiency associated with major defect, unspecified

✓4th **D83 Common variable immunodeficiency**

D83.0 Common variable immunodeficiency with predominant abnormalities of B-cell numbers and function

D83.1 Common variable immunodeficiency with predominant immunoregulatory T-cell disorders

D83.2 Common variable immunodeficiency with autoantibodies to B- or T-cells

D83.8 Other common variable immunodeficiencies

D83.9 Common variable immunodeficiency, unspecified

✓4th **D84 Other immunodeficiencies**

D84.0 Lymphocyte function antigen-1 [LFA-1] defect

D84.1 Defects in the complement system
C1 esterase inhibitor [C1-INH] deficiency

D84.8 Other specified immunodeficiencies

D84.9 Immunodeficiency, unspecified

✓4th **D86 Sarcoidosis**

D86.0 Sarcoidosis of lung

D86.1 Sarcoidosis of lymph nodes

D86.2 Sarcoidosis of lung with sarcoidosis of lymph nodes

D86.3 Sarcoidosis of skin

✓5th **D86.8 Sarcoidosis of other sites**

D86.81 Sarcoid meningitis

D86.82 Multiple cranial nerve palsies in sarcoidosis

D86.83 Sarcoid iridocyclitis

D86.84 Sarcoid pyelonephritis
Tubulo-interstitial nephropathy in sarcoidosis

D86.85 Sarcoid myocarditis

D86.86 Sarcoid arthropathy
Polyarthritis in sarcoidosis

D86.87 Sarcoid myositis

D86.89 Sarcoidosis of other sites
Hepatic granulomaUveoparotid fever [Heerfordt]

D86.9 Sarcoidosis, unspecified

✓4th **D89 Other disorders involving the immune mechanism, not elsewhere classified**

EXCLUDES 1   hyperglobulinemia NOS (R77.1)
monoclonal gammopathy (of undetermined significance) (D47.2)

EXCLUDES 2   transplant failure and rejection (T86.-)

D89.0 Polyclonal hypergammaglobulinemia
Benign hypergammaglobulinemic purpura
Polyclonal gammopathy NOS

D89.1 Cryoglobulinemia
Cryoglobulinemic purpura   Mixed cryoglobulinemia
Cryoglobulinemic vasculitis   Primary cryoglobulinemia
Essential cryoglobulinemia   Secondary cryoglobulinemia
Idiopathic cryoglobulinemia

D89.2 Hypergammaglobulinemia, unspecified

D89.3 Immune reconstitution syndrome
Immune reconstitution inflammatory syndrome [IRIS]
Use additional code for adverse effect, if applicable, to identify drug (T36-T50 with fifth or sixth character 5)

✓5th **D89.8 Other specified disorders involving the immune mechanism, not elsewhere classified**

✓6th **D89.81 Graft-versus-host disease**
Code first underlying cause, such as:
complications of transplanted organs and tissue (T86.-)
complications of blood transfusion (T80.89)
Use additional code to identify associated manifestations, such as:
desquamative dermatitis (L30.8)
diarrhea (R19.7)
elevated bilirubin (R17)
hair loss (L65.9)

D89.810 Acute graft-versus-host disease

D89.811 Chronic graft-versus-host disease

D89.812 Acute on chronic graft-versus-host disease

D89.813 Graft-versus-host disease, unspecified

D89.82 Autoimmune lymphoproliferative syndrome [ALPS]

D89.89 Other specified disorders involving the immune mechanism, not elsewhere classified

EXCLUDES 1   human immunodeficiency virus disease (B20)

D89.9 Disorder involving the immune mechanism, unspecified
Immune disease NOS

☑ Additional Character Required   ✓x7th Placeholder Alert   Unspecified Dx   Other Specified Dx   Manifestation   ▶◀ Revised Text   ● New Code   ▲ Revised Code Title

Chapter 4. Endocrine, Nutritional, and Metabolic Diseases (E00–E89)

Chapter Specific Guidelines with Coding Examples

The chapter specific guidelines from the ICD-10-CM Official Guidelines for Coding and Reporting have been provided below. Along with these guidelines are coding examples, contained in the shaded boxes, that have been developed to help illustrate the coding and/or sequencing guidance found in these guidelines.

a. Diabetes mellitus

The diabetes mellitus codes are combination codes that include the type of diabetes mellitus, the body system affected, and the complications affecting that body system. As many codes within a particular category as are necessary to describe all of the complications of the disease may be used. They should be sequenced based on the reason for a particular encounter. Assign as many codes from categories E08–E13 as needed to identify all of the associated conditions that the patient has.

> Patient is seen for uncontrolled diabetes, type 2, with diabetic polyneuropathy and diabetic retinopathy with macular edema
>
> **E11.65**   **Type 2 diabetes mellitus with hyperglycemia**
>
> **E11.311**   **Type 2 diabetes mellitus with unspecified diabetic retinopathy with macular edema**
>
> **E11.42**   **Type 2 diabetes mellitus with diabetic polyneuropathy**
>
> *Explanation*: Use as many codes to describe the diabetic complications as needed. Many are combination codes that describe more than one condition. Code first the reason for the encounter. "Uncontrolled" is described as "with hyperglycemia."

1) Type of diabetes

The age of a patient is not the sole determining factor, though most type 1 diabetics develop the condition before reaching puberty. For this reason type 1 diabetes mellitus is also referred to as juvenile diabetes.

> A 45-year-old patient is diagnosed with Type 1 diabetes
>
> **E10.9**   **Type 1 diabetes mellitus without complications**
>
> *Explanation*: Although most type 1 diabetics are diagnosed in childhood or adolescence, it can also begin in adults.

2) Type of diabetes mellitus not documented

If the type of diabetes mellitus is not documented in the medical record the default is E11.-, Type 2 diabetes mellitus.

> Office visit lists diabetes and hypertension on patient problem list
>
> **E11.9**   **Type 2 diabetes mellitus without complications**
>
> **I10**   **Essential (primary) hypertension**
>
> *Explanation*: Since the type of diabetes was not documented and no complications were noted, the default code is E11.9.

3) Diabetes mellitus and the use of insulin

If the documentation in a medical record does not indicate the type of diabetes but does indicate that the patient uses insulin, code E11, Type 2 diabetes mellitus, should be assigned. Code Z79.4, Long-term (current) use of insulin, should also be assigned to indicate that the patient uses insulin. Code Z79.4 should not be assigned if insulin is given temporarily to bring a type 2 patient's blood sugar under control during an encounter.

> Office visit lists chronic diabetes with daily insulin use on patient problem list
>
> **E11.9**   **Type 2 diabetes mellitus without complications**
>
> **Z79.4**   **Long-term (current) use of insulin**
>
> *Explanation*: Do not assume that a patient on insulin must have type 1 diabetes. The default for diabetes without further specification defaults to type 2. Add the code for long-term use of insulin.

4) Diabetes mellitus in pregnancy and gestational diabetes

See Section I.C.15. Diabetes mellitus in pregnancy.

See Section I.C.15. Gestational (pregnancy induced) diabetes

5) Complications due to insulin pump malfunction

(a) Underdose of insulin due to insulin pump failure

An underdose of insulin due to an insulin pump failure should be assigned to a code from subcategory T85.6, Mechanical complication of other specified internal and external prosthetic devices, implants and grafts, that specifies the type of pump malfunction, as the principal or first-listed code, followed by code T38.3X6-, Underdosing of insulin and oral hypoglycemic [antidiabetic] drugs. Additional codes for the type of diabetes mellitus and any associated complications due to the underdosing should also be assigned.

> A 24-year-old type 1 diabetic male treated in ED for hyperglycemia; insulin pump found to be malfunctioning and underdosing
>
> **T85.614A**   **Breakdown (mechanical) of insulin pump, initial encounter**
>
> **T38.3X6A**   **Underdosing of insulin and oral hypoglycemic [antidiabetic] drugs, initial encounter**
>
> **E10.65**   **Type 1 diabetes mellitus with hyperglycemia**
>
> *Explanation*: The complication code for the mechanical breakdown of the pump is sequenced first, followed by the underdosing code and type of diabetes with complication. Code all other diabetic complication codes necessary to describe the patient's condition.

(b) Overdose of insulin due to insulin pump failure

The principal or first-listed code for an encounter due to an Insulin pump malfunction resulting in an overdose of insulin, should also be T85.6-, Mechanical complication of other specified internal and external prosthetic devices, implants and grafts, followed by code T38.3X1-, Poisoning by insulin and oral hypoglycemic [antidiabetic] drugs, accidental (unintentional).

> A 24-year-old type 1 diabetic male found down with diabetic coma, brought into ED and treated for hypoglycemia; insulin pump found to be malfunctioning and overdosing
>
> **T85.614A**   **Breakdown (mechanical) of insulin pump, initial encounter**
>
> **T38.3X1A**   **Poisoning by insulin and oral hypoglycemic [antidiabetic] drugs, accidental (unintentional), initial encounter**
>
> **E10.641**   **Type 1 diabetes mellitus with hypoglycemia with coma**
>
> *Explanation*: The complication code for the mechanical breakdown of the pump is sequenced first, followed by the poisoning code and type of diabetes with complication. All the characters in the combination code must be used to form a valid code and to fully describe the type of diabetes, the hypoglycemia, and the coma.

6) Secondary diabetes mellitus

Codes under categories E08, Diabetes mellitus due to underlying condition, E09, Drug or chemical induced diabetes mellitus, and E13, Other specified diabetes mellitus, identify complications/manifestations associated with secondary diabetes mellitus. Secondary diabetes is always caused by another condition or event (e.g., cystic fibrosis, malignant neoplasm of pancreas, pancreatectomy, adverse effect of drug, or poisoning).

(a) Secondary diabetes mellitus and the use of insulin

For patients who routinely use insulin, code Z79.4, Long-term (current) use of insulin, should also be assigned. Code Z79.4 should not be assigned if insulin is given temporarily to bring a patient's blood sugar under control during an encounter.

Type 2 diabetic with no complications, normally only on oral metformin, is given insulin for three days to maintain glucose control while in the hospital recovering from surgery

E11.9   **Type 2 diabetes mellitus without complications**

No code is used for insulin use

Explanation: Do not code the long term (current) use of insulin when only provided temporarily.

Type 2 diabetic with diabetic polyneuropathy on insulin

E11.42   **Type 2 diabetes mellitus with diabetic polyneuropathy**

Z79.4   **Long-term (current) use of insulin**

Explanation: Add the Z code for the long-term use of insulin because the insulin is taken chronically.

(b) Assigning and sequencing secondary diabetes codes and its causes

The sequencing of the secondary diabetes codes in relationship to codes for the cause of the diabetes is based on the Tabular List instructions for categories E08, E09 and E13.

(i) Secondary diabetes mellitus due to pancreatectomy

For postpancreatectomy diabetes mellitus (lack of insulin due to the surgical removal of all or part of the pancreas), assign code E89.1, Postprocedural hypoinsulinemia. Assign a code from category E13 and a code from subcategory Z90.41-, Acquired absence of pancreas, as additional codes.

Patient with newly diagnosed diabetes after surgical removal of part of pancreas

E89.1   **Postprocedural hypoinsulinemia**

E13.9   **Other specified diabetes mellitus without complications**

Z90.411   **Acquired partial absence of pancreas**

Explanation: Sequence the postprocedural complication of the hypoinsulinemia due to the partial removal of the pancreas as the first-listed code, followed by the other specified diabetes (NEC) with or without complications and the partial or total acquired absence of the pancreas.

(ii) Secondary diabetes due to drugs

Secondary diabetes may be caused by an adverse effect of correctly administered medications, poisoning or sequela of poisoning.

See section I.C.19.e for coding of adverse effects and poisoning, and section I.C.20 for external cause code reporting.

Initial encounter for corticosteroid-induced diabetes mellitus

E09.9   **Drug or chemical induced diabetes mellitus without complications**

T38.0X5A   **Adverse effect of glucocorticoids and synthetic analogues, initial encounter**

Explanation: If the diabetes is caused by an adverse effect of a drug, the diabetic condition is coded first. If it occurs from a poisoning or overdose, the poisoning code causing the diabetes is sequenced first.

Chapter 4. Endocrine, Nutritional and Metabolic Diseases (E00-E89)

> **NOTE**   All neoplasms, whether functionally active or not, are classified in Chapter 2. Appropriate codes in this chapter (i.e. E05.8, E07.0, E16-E31, E34-) may be used as additional codes to indicate either functional activity by neoplasms and ectopic endocrine tissue or hyperfunction and hypofunction of endocrine glands associated with neoplasms and other conditions classified elsewhere.

> *EXCLUDES 1*   *transitory endocrine and metabolic disorders specific to newborn (P70-P74)*

This chapter contains the following blocks:

E00-E07	Disorders of thyroid gland
E08-E13	Diabetes mellitus
E15-E16	Other disorders of glucose regulation and pancreatic internal secretion
E20-E35	Disorders of other endocrine glands
E36	Intraoperative complications of endocrine system
E40-E46	Malnutrition
E50-E64	Other nutritional deficiencies
E65-E68	Overweight, obesity and other hyperalimentation
E70-E88	Metabolic disorders
E89	Postprocedural endocrine and metabolic complications and disorders, not elsewhere classified

Disorders of thyroid gland (E00-E07)

✓4th E00   Congenital iodine-deficiency syndrome
Use additional code (F70-F79) to identify associated intellectual disabilities
> *EXCLUDES 1*   *subclinical iodine-deficiency hypothyroidism (E02)*

E00.0   Congenital iodine-deficiency syndrome, neurological type
Endemic cretinism, neurological type

E00.1   Congenital iodine-deficiency syndrome, myxedematous type
Endemic hypothyroid cretinism
Endemic cretinism, myxedematous type

E00.2   Congenital iodine-deficiency syndrome, mixed type
Endemic cretinism, mixed type

E00.9   Congenital iodine-deficiency syndrome, unspecified
Congenital iodine-deficiency hypothyroidism NOS
Endemic cretinism NOS

✓4th E01   Iodine-deficiency related thyroid disorders and allied conditions
> *EXCLUDES 1*   *congenital iodine-deficiency syndrome (E00.-)*
> *subclinical iodine-deficiency hypothyroidism (E02)*

E01.0   Iodine-deficiency related diffuse (endemic) goiter

E01.1   Iodine-deficiency related multinodular (endemic) goiter
Iodine-deficiency related nodular goiter

E01.2   Iodine-deficiency related (endemic) goiter, unspecified
Endemic goiter NOS

E01.8   Other iodine-deficiency related thyroid disorders and allied conditions
Acquired iodine-deficiency hypothyroidism NOS

E02   Subclinical iodine-deficiency hypothyroidism

✓4th E03   Other hypothyroidism
> *EXCLUDES 1*   *iodine-deficiency related hypothyroidism (E00-E02)*
> *postprocedural hypothyroidism (E89.0)*

E03.0   Congenital hypothyroidism with diffuse goiter
Congenital parenchymatous goiter (nontoxic)
Congenital goiter (nontoxic) NOS
> *EXCLUDES 1*   *transitory congenital goiter with normal function (P72.0)*

E03.1   Congenital hypothyroidism without goiter
Aplasia of thyroid (with myxedema)
Congenital atrophy of thyroid
Congenital hypothyroidism NOS

E03.2   Hypothyroidism due to medicaments and other exogenous substances
Code first poisoning due to drug or toxin, if applicable (T36-T65 with fifth or sixth character 1-4 or 6)
Use additional code for adverse effect, if applicable, to identify drug (T36-T50 with fifth or sixth character 5)

E03.3   Postinfectious hypothyroidism

E03.4   Atrophy of thyroid (acquired)
> *EXCLUDES 1*   *congenital atrophy of thyroid (E03.1)*

E03.5   Myxedema coma

E03.8   Other specified hypothyroidism

E03.9   Hypothyroidism, unspecified
Myxedema NOS

✓4th E04   Other nontoxic goiter
> *EXCLUDES 1*   *congenital goiter (NOS) (diffuse) (parenchymatous) (E03.0)*
> *iodine-deficiency related goiter (E00-E02)*

E04.0   Nontoxic diffuse goiter
Diffuse (colloid) nontoxic goiter
Simple nontoxic goiter

E04.1   Nontoxic single thyroid nodule
Colloid nodule (cystic) (thyroid)
Nontoxic uninodular goiter
Thyroid (cystic) nodule NOS

E04.2   Nontoxic multinodular goiter
Cystic goiter NOS
Multinodular (cystic) goiter NOS

E04.8   Other specified nontoxic goiter

E04.9   Nontoxic goiter, unspecified
Goiter NOS
Nodular goiter (nontoxic) NOS

✓4th E05   Thyrotoxicosis [hyperthyroidism]
> *EXCLUDES 1*   *chronic thyroiditis with transient thyrotoxicosis (E06.2)*
> *neonatal thyrotoxicosis (P72.1)*

✓5th E05.0   Thyrotoxicosis with diffuse goiter
Exophthalmic or toxic goiter NOS   Graves' disease   Toxic diffuse goiter

    E05.00   Thyrotoxicosis with diffuse goiter without thyrotoxic crisis or storm

    E05.01   Thyrotoxicosis with diffuse goiter with thyrotoxic crisis or storm

✓5th E05.1   Thyrotoxicosis with toxic single thyroid nodule
Thyrotoxicosis with toxic uninodular goiter

    E05.10   Thyrotoxicosis with toxic single thyroid nodule without thyrotoxic crisis or storm

    E05.11   Thyrotoxicosis with toxic single thyroid nodule with thyrotoxic crisis or storm

✓5th E05.2   Thyrotoxicosis with toxic multinodular goiter
Toxic nodular goiter NOS

    E05.20   Thyrotoxicosis with toxic multinodular goiter without thyrotoxic crisis or storm

    E05.21   Thyrotoxicosis with toxic multinodular goiter with thyrotoxic crisis or storm

✓5th E05.3   Thyrotoxicosis from ectopic thyroid tissue

    E05.30   Thyrotoxicosis from ectopic thyroid tissue without thyrotoxic crisis or storm

    E05.31   Thyrotoxicosis from ectopic thyroid tissue with thyrotoxic crisis or storm

✓5th E05.4   Thyrotoxicosis factitia

    E05.40   Thyrotoxicosis factitia without thyrotoxic crisis or storm

    E05.41   Thyrotoxicosis factitia with thyrotoxic crisis or storm

✓5th E05.8   Other thyrotoxicosis
Overproduction of thyroid-stimulating hormone

    E05.80   Other thyrotoxicosis without thyrotoxic crisis or storm

    E05.81   Other thyrotoxicosis with thyrotoxic crisis or storm

✓5th E05.9   Thyrotoxicosis, unspecified
Hyperthyroidism NOS

    E05.90   Thyrotoxicosis, unspecified without thyrotoxic crisis or storm

    E05.91   Thyrotoxicosis, unspecified with thyrotoxic crisis or storm

✓4th E06   Thyroiditis
> *EXCLUDES 1*   *postpartum thyroiditis (O90.5)*

E06.0   Acute thyroiditis
Abscess of thyroid   Suppurative thyroiditis
Pyogenic thyroiditis
Use additional code (B95-B97) to identify infectious agent

E06.1   Subacute thyroiditis
de Quervain thyroiditis   Nonsuppurative thyroiditis
Giant-cell thyroiditis   Viral thyroiditis
Granulomatous thyroiditis
> *EXCLUDES 1*   *autoimmune thyroiditis (E06.3)*

E06.2   Chronic thyroiditis with transient thyrotoxicosis
> *EXCLUDES 1*   *autoimmune thyroiditis (E06.3)*

E06.3   Autoimmune thyroiditis
Hashimoto's thyroiditis   Lymphocytic thyroiditis
Hashitoxicosis (transient)   Struma lymphomatosa
Lymphadenoid goiter

EXCLUDES 1 Not coded here   *EXCLUDES 2* Not included here   **N** Newborn Age: 0   **P** Pediatric Age: 0-17   **M** Maternity Age: 12-55   **A** Adult Age: 15-124

488   ICD-10-CM 2016

E06.4 **Drug-induced** thyroiditis
Use additional code for adverse effect, if applicable, to identify drug (T36-T50 with fifth or sixth character 5)

E06.5 Other chronic **thyroiditis**
Chronic fibrous thyroiditis　　　Ligneous thyroiditis
Chronic thyroiditis NOS　　　　Riedel thyroiditis

E06.9 **Thyroiditis, unspecified**

✓4ᵗʰ **E07** **Other disorders of thyroid**

E07.0 **Hypersecretion of calcitonin**
C-cell hyperplasia of thyroid
Hypersecretion of thyrocalcitonin

E07.1 **Dyshormogenetic goiter**
Familial dyshormogenetic goiter
Pendred's syndrome
EXCLUDES 1　transitory congenital goiter with normal function (P72.0)

✓5ᵗʰ **E07.8** **Other specified disorders of thyroid**

E07.81 **Sick-euthyroid syndrome**
Euthyroid sick-syndrome

E07.89 **Other specified disorders of thyroid**
Abnormality of thyroid-binding globulin
Hemorrhage of thyroid
Infarction of thyroid

E07.9 **Disorder of thyroid, unspecified**

Diabetes mellitus (E08-E13)

✓4ᵗʰ **E08** **Diabetes mellitus** due to underlying condition
Code first the underlying condition, such as:
congenital rubella (P35.0)
cushing's syndrome (E24.-)
cystic fibrosis (E84.-)
malignant neoplasm (C00-C96)
malnutrition (E40-E46)
pancreatitis and other diseases of the pancreas (K85.-, K86.-)
Use additional code to identify any insulin use (Z79.4)
EXCLUDES 1　drug or chemical induced diabetes mellitus (E09.-)
gestational diabetes (O24.4-)
neonatal diabetes mellitus (P70.2)
postpancreatectomy diabetes mellitus (E13.-)
postprocedural diabetes mellitus (E13.-)
secondary diabetes mellitus NEC (E13.-)
type 1 diabetes mellitus (E10.-)
type 2 diabetes mellitus (E11.-)
AHA: 2013, 4Q, 114; 2013, 3Q, 20

✓5ᵗʰ **E08.0** **Diabetes mellitus due to underlying condition with hyperosmolarity**

E08.00 **Diabetes mellitus due to underlying condition with hyperosmolarity** without nonketotic hyperglycemic-hyperosmolar coma (NKHHC)

E08.01 **Diabetes mellitus due to underlying condition with hyperosmolarity** with coma

✓5ᵗʰ **E08.1** **Diabetes mellitus due to underlying condition with ketoacidosis**

E08.10 **Diabetes mellitus due to underlying condition with ketoacidosis** without coma

E08.11 **Diabetes mellitus due to underlying condition with ketoacidosis** with coma

✓5ᵗʰ **E08.2** **Diabetes mellitus due to underlying condition with** kidney complications

E08.21 **Diabetes mellitus due to underlying condition with diabetic** nephropathy
Diabetes mellitus due to underlying condition with intercapillary glomerulosclerosis
Diabetes mellitus due to underlying condition with intracapillary glomerulonephrosis
Diabetes mellitus due to underlying condition with Kimmelstiel-Wilson disease

E08.22 **Diabetes mellitus due to underlying condition with diabetic** chronic kidney disease
Use additional code to identify stage of chronic kidney disease (N18.1-N18.6)

E08.29 **Diabetes mellitus due to underlying condition with other diabetic kidney complication**
Renal tubular degeneration in diabetes mellitus due to underlying condition

✓5ᵗʰ **E08.3** **Diabetes mellitus due to underlying condition with** ophthalmic complications

✓6ᵗʰ **E08.31** **Diabetes mellitus due to underlying condition with unspecified** diabetic retinopathy

E08.311 **Diabetes mellitus due to underlying condition with unspecified diabetic retinopathy** with macular edema

E08.319 **Diabetes mellitus due to underlying condition with unspecified diabetic retinopathy** without macular edema

✓6ᵗʰ **E08.32** **Diabetes mellitus due to underlying condition with** mild nonproliferative diabetic retinopathy
Diabetes mellitus due to underlying condition with nonproliferative diabetic retinopathy NOS

E08.321 **Diabetes mellitus due to underlying condition with mild nonproliferative diabetic retinopathy** with macular edema

E08.329 **Diabetes mellitus due to underlying condition with mild nonproliferative diabetic retinopathy** without macular edema

✓6ᵗʰ **E08.33** **Diabetes mellitus due to underlying condition with** moderate nonproliferative diabetic retinopathy

E08.331 **Diabetes mellitus due to underlying condition with moderate nonproliferative diabetic retinopathy** with macular edema

E08.339 **Diabetes mellitus due to underlying condition with moderate nonproliferative diabetic retinopathy** without macular edema

✓6ᵗʰ **E08.34** **Diabetes mellitus due to underlying condition with** severe nonproliferative diabetic retinopathy

E08.341 **Diabetes mellitus due to underlying condition with severe nonproliferative diabetic retinopathy** with macular edema

E08.349 **Diabetes mellitus due to underlying condition with severe nonproliferative diabetic retinopathy** without macular edema

✓6ᵗʰ **E08.35** **Diabetes mellitus due to underlying condition with** proliferative diabetic retinopathy

E08.351 **Diabetes mellitus due to underlying condition with proliferative diabetic retinopathy** with macular edema

E08.359 **Diabetes mellitus due to underlying condition with proliferative diabetic retinopathy** without macular edema

E08.36 **Diabetes mellitus due to underlying condition with diabetic** cataract

E08.39 **Diabetes mellitus due to underlying condition with other diabetic ophthalmic complication**
Use additional code to identify manifestation, such as:
diabetic glaucoma (H40-H42)

✓5ᵗʰ **E08.4** **Diabetes mellitus due to underlying condition with** neurological complications

E08.40 **Diabetes mellitus due to underlying condition with diabetic** neuropathy, unspecified

E08.41 **Diabetes mellitus due to underlying condition with diabetic** mononeuropathy

E08.42 **Diabetes mellitus due to underlying condition with diabetic** polyneuropathy
Diabetes mellitus due to underlying condition with diabetic neuralgia

E08.43 **Diabetes mellitus due to underlying condition with diabetic** autonomic (poly)neuropathy
Diabetes mellitus due to underlying condition with diabetic gastroparesis
AHA: 2013, 4Q, 114

E08.44 **Diabetes mellitus due to underlying condition with diabetic** amyotrophy

E08.49 **Diabetes mellitus due to underlying condition with other diabetic neurological complication**

✓5ᵗʰ **E08.5** **Diabetes mellitus due to underlying condition with** circulatory complications

E08.51 **Diabetes mellitus due to underlying condition with diabetic** peripheral angiopathy without gangrene

E08.52 **Diabetes mellitus due to underlying condition with diabetic** peripheral angiopathy with gangrene
Diabetes mellitus due to underlying condition with diabetic gangrene

E08.59 **Diabetes mellitus due to underlying condition with other circulatory complications**

☑ Additional Character Required　　✓ˣ⁷ᵗʰ Placeholder Alert　　Unspecified Dx　　Other Specified Dx　　Manifestation　　▶◀ Revised Text　　● New Code　　▲ Revised Code Title

√5ᵗʰ **E08.6** **Diabetes mellitus due to underlying condition with** other specified complications

√6ᵗʰ **E08.61** **Diabetes mellitus due to underlying condition with** diabetic arthropathy

E08.610 **Diabetes mellitus due to underlying condition with diabetic** neuropathic arthropathy
Diabetes mellitus due to underlying condition with Charcôt's joints

E08.618 **Diabetes mellitus due to underlying condition with other diabetic arthropathy**

√6ᵗʰ **E08.62** **Diabetes mellitus due to underlying condition with** skin complications

E08.620 **Diabetes mellitus due to underlying condition with** diabetic dermatitis
Diabetes mellitus due to underlying condition with diabetic necrobiosis lipoidica

E08.621 **Diabetes mellitus due to underlying condition with** foot ulcer
Use additional code to identify site of ulcer (L97.4-, L97.5-)

E08.622 **Diabetes mellitus due to underlying condition with** other skin ulcer
Use additional code to identify site of ulcer (L97.1-L97.9, L98.41-L98.49)

E08.628 **Diabetes mellitus due to underlying condition with other skin complications**

√6ᵗʰ **E08.63** **Diabetes mellitus due to underlying condition with** oral complications

E08.630 **Diabetes mellitus due to underlying condition with** periodontal disease

E08.638 **Diabetes mellitus due to underlying condition with other oral complications**

√6ᵗʰ **E08.64** **Diabetes mellitus due to underlying condition with** hypoglycemia

E08.641 **Diabetes mellitus due to underlying condition with hypoglycemia** with coma

E08.649 **Diabetes mellitus due to underlying condition with hypoglycemia** without coma

E08.65 **Diabetes mellitus due to underlying condition with** hyperglycemia

E08.69 **Diabetes mellitus due to underlying condition with other specified complication**
Use additional code to identify complication

E08.8 **Diabetes mellitus due to underlying condition** with unspecified complications

E08.9 **Diabetes mellitus due to underlying condition** without complications

√4ᵗʰ **E09** **Drug or chemical induced diabetes mellitus**
Code first poisoning due to drug or toxin, if applicable (T36-T65 with fifth or sixth character 1-4 or 6)
Use additional code for adverse effect, if applicable, to identify drug (T36-T50 with fifth or sixth character 5)
Use additional code to identify any insulin use (Z79.4)
EXCLUDES 1 *diabetes mellitus due to underlying condition (E08.-)*
gestational diabetes (O24.4-)
neonatal diabetes mellitus (P70.2)
postpancreatectomy diabetes mellitus (E13.-)
postprocedural diabetes mellitus (E13.-)
secondary diabetes mellitus NEC (E13.-)
type 1 diabetes mellitus (E10.-)
type 2 diabetes mellitus (E11.-)
AHA: 2013, 4Q, 114; 2013, 3Q, 20

√5ᵗʰ **E09.0** **Drug or chemical induced diabetes mellitus with** hyperosmolarity

E09.00 **Drug or chemical induced diabetes mellitus with hyperosmolarity** without nonketotic hyperglycemic-hyperosmolar coma **(NKHHC)**

E09.01 **Drug or chemical induced diabetes mellitus with hyperosmolarity** with coma

√5ᵗʰ **E09.1** **Drug or chemical induced diabetes mellitus with** ketoacidosis

E09.10 **Drug or chemical induced diabetes mellitus with ketoacidosis** without coma

E09.11 **Drug or chemical induced diabetes mellitus with ketoacidosis** with coma

√5ᵗʰ **E09.2** **Drug or chemical induced diabetes mellitus with** kidney complications

E09.21 **Drug or chemical induced diabetes mellitus with** diabetic nephropathy
Drug or chemical induced diabetes mellitus with intercapillary glomerulosclerosis
Drug or chemical induced diabetes mellitus with intracapillary glomerulonephrosis
Drug or chemical induced diabetes mellitus with Kimmelstiel-Wilson disease

E09.22 **Drug or chemical induced diabetes mellitus with** diabetic chronic kidney disease
Use additional code to identify stage of chronic kidney disease (N18.1-N18.6)

E09.29 **Drug or chemical induced diabetes mellitus with other diabetic kidney complication**
Drug or chemical induced diabetes mellitus with renal tubular degeneration

√5ᵗʰ **E09.3** **Drug or chemical induced diabetes mellitus with** ophthalmic complications

√6ᵗʰ **E09.31** **Drug or chemical induced diabetes mellitus with** unspecified diabetic retinopathy

E09.311 **Drug or chemical induced diabetes mellitus with unspecified diabetic retinopathy** with macular edema

E09.319 **Drug or chemical induced diabetes mellitus with unspecified diabetic retinopathy** without macular edema

√6ᵗʰ **E09.32** **Drug or chemical induced diabetes mellitus with** mild nonproliferative **diabetic retinopathy**
Drug or chemical induced diabetes mellitus with nonproliferative diabetic retinopathy NOS

E09.321 **Drug or chemical induced diabetes mellitus with mild nonproliferative diabetic retinopathy** with macular edema

E09.329 **Drug or chemical induced diabetes mellitus with mild nonproliferative diabetic retinopathy** without macular edema

√6ᵗʰ **E09.33** **Drug or chemical induced diabetes mellitus with** moderate nonproliferative **diabetic retinopathy**

E09.331 **Drug or chemical induced diabetes mellitus with moderate nonproliferative diabetic retinopathy** with macular edema

E09.339 **Drug or chemical induced diabetes mellitus with moderate nonproliferative diabetic retinopathy** without macular edema

√6ᵗʰ **E09.34** **Drug or chemical induced diabetes mellitus with** severe nonproliferative **diabetic retinopathy**

E09.341 **Drug or chemical induced diabetes mellitus with severe nonproliferative diabetic retinopathy** with macular edema

E09.349 **Drug or chemical induced diabetes mellitus with severe nonproliferative diabetic retinopathy** without macular edema

√6ᵗʰ **E09.35** **Drug or chemical induced diabetes mellitus with** proliferative **diabetic retinopathy**

E09.351 **Drug or chemical induced diabetes mellitus with proliferative diabetic retinopathy** with macular edema

E09.359 **Drug or chemical induced diabetes mellitus with proliferative diabetic retinopathy** without macular edema

E09.36 **Drug or chemical induced diabetes mellitus with** diabetic cataract

E09.39 **Drug or chemical induced diabetes mellitus with other diabetic ophthalmic complication**
Use additional code to identify manifestation, such as: diabetic glaucoma (H40-H42)

√5ᵗʰ **E09.4** **Drug or chemical induced diabetes mellitus with** neurological complications

E09.40 **Drug or chemical induced diabetes mellitus with neurological complications with diabetic neuropathy, unspecified**

E09.41 **Drug or chemical induced diabetes mellitus with** neurological complications with diabetic mononeuropathy

---

EXCLUDES 1 Not coded here   *EXCLUDES 2* Not included here   **N** Newborn Age: 0   **P** Pediatric Age: 0-17   **M** Maternity Age: 12-55   **A** Adult Age: 15-124

E09.42   Drug or chemical induced diabetes mellitus with neurological complications with diabetic **polyneuropathy**
> Drug or chemical induced diabetes mellitus with diabetic neuralgia

E09.43   Drug or chemical induced diabetes mellitus with neurological complications with diabetic **autonomic (poly)neuropathy**
> Drug or chemical induced diabetes mellitus with diabetic gastroparesis
> **AHA:** 2013, 4Q, 114

E09.44   Drug or chemical induced diabetes mellitus with neurological complications with diabetic **amyotrophy**

E09.49   Drug or chemical induced diabetes mellitus with neurological complications with other diabetic neurological complication

☑5ᵗʰ **E09.5**   Drug or chemical induced diabetes mellitus with **circulatory complications**

   E09.51   Drug or chemical induced diabetes mellitus with diabetic **peripheral angiopathy without gangrene**

   E09.52   Drug or chemical induced diabetes mellitus with diabetic **peripheral angiopathy with gangrene**
> Drug or chemical induced diabetes mellitus with diabetic gangrene

   E09.59   Drug or chemical induced diabetes mellitus with other circulatory complications

☑5ᵗʰ **E09.6**   Drug or chemical induced diabetes mellitus with **other specified complications**

  ☑6ᵗʰ **E09.61**   Drug or chemical induced diabetes mellitus with diabetic **arthropathy**

    E09.610   Drug or chemical induced diabetes mellitus with diabetic **neuropathic arthropathy**
> Drug or chemical induced diabetes mellitus with Charcôt's joints

    E09.618   Drug or chemical induced diabetes mellitus with other diabetic arthropathy

  ☑6ᵗʰ **E09.62**   Drug or chemical induced diabetes mellitus with **skin complications**

    E09.620   Drug or chemical induced diabetes mellitus with **diabetic dermatitis**
> Drug or chemical induced diabetes mellitus with diabetic necrobiosis lipoidica

    E09.621   Drug or chemical induced diabetes mellitus with **foot ulcer**
> Use additional code to identify site of ulcer (L97.4-, L97.5-)

    E09.622   Drug or chemical induced diabetes mellitus with **other skin ulcer**
> Use additional code to identify site of ulcer (L97.1-L97.9, L98.41-L98.49)

    E09.628   Drug or chemical induced diabetes mellitus with other skin complications

  ☑6ᵗʰ **E09.63**   Drug or chemical induced diabetes mellitus with **oral complications**

    E09.630   Drug or chemical induced diabetes mellitus with **periodontal disease**

    E09.638   Drug or chemical induced diabetes mellitus with other oral complications

  ☑6ᵗʰ **E09.64**   Drug or chemical induced diabetes mellitus with **hypoglycemia**

    E09.641   Drug or chemical induced diabetes mellitus with hypoglycemia **with coma**

    E09.649   Drug or chemical induced diabetes mellitus with hypoglycemia **without coma**

   E09.65   Drug or chemical induced diabetes mellitus with **hyperglycemia**

   E09.69   Drug or chemical induced diabetes mellitus with other specified complication
> Use additional code to identify complication

E09.8   Drug or chemical induced diabetes mellitus with unspecified complications

E09.9   Drug or chemical induced diabetes mellitus **without complications**

☑4ᵗʰ **E10**   **Type 1 diabetes mellitus**
> **INCLUDES**   brittle diabetes (mellitus)
> diabetes (mellitus) due to autoimmune process
> diabetes (mellitus) due to immune mediated pancreatic islet beta-cell destruction
> idiopathic diabetes (mellitus)
> juvenile onset diabetes (mellitus)
> ketosis-prone diabetes (mellitus)
>
> **EXCLUDES 1**   *diabetes mellitus due to underlying condition (E08.-)*
> *drug or chemical induced diabetes mellitus (E09.-)*
> *gestational diabetes (O24.4-)*
> *hyperglycemia NOS (R73.9)*
> *neonatal diabetes mellitus (P70.2)*
> *postpancreatectomy diabetes mellitus (E13.-)*
> *postprocedural diabetes mellitus (E13.-)*
> *secondary diabetes mellitus NEC (E13.-)*
> *type 2 diabetes mellitus (E11.-)*

  AHA: 2013, 4Q, 114; 2013, 3Q, 20

☑5ᵗʰ **E10.1**   Type 1 diabetes mellitus with **ketoacidosis**
> **AHA:** 2013, 3Q, 20

   E10.10   Type 1 diabetes mellitus with ketoacidosis **without coma**

   E10.11   Type 1 diabetes mellitus with ketoacidosis **with coma**

☑5ᵗʰ **E10.2**   Type 1 diabetes mellitus with **kidney complications**

   E10.21   Type 1 diabetes mellitus with diabetic **nephropathy**
> Type 1 diabetes mellitus with intercapillary glomerulosclerosis
> Type 1 diabetes mellitus with intracapillary glomerulonephrosis
> Type 1 diabetes mellitus with Kimmelstiel-Wilson disease

   E10.22   Type 1 diabetes mellitus with diabetic **chronic kidney disease**
> Use additional code to identify stage of chronic kidney disease (N18.1-N18.6)

   E10.29   Type 1 diabetes mellitus with other diabetic kidney complication
> Type 1 diabetes mellitus with renal tubular degeneration

☑5ᵗʰ **E10.3**   Type 1 diabetes mellitus with **ophthalmic complications**

  ☑6ᵗʰ **E10.31**   Type 1 diabetes mellitus with **unspecified diabetic retinopathy**

    E10.311   Type 1 diabetes mellitus with unspecified diabetic retinopathy **with macular edema**

    E10.319   Type 1 diabetes mellitus with unspecified diabetic retinopathy **without macular edema**

  ☑6ᵗʰ **E10.32**   Type 1 diabetes mellitus with **mild nonproliferative diabetic retinopathy**
> Type 1 diabetes mellitus with nonproliferative diabetic retinopathy NOS

    E10.321   Type 1 diabetes mellitus with mild nonproliferative diabetic retinopathy **with macular edema**

    E10.329   Type 1 diabetes mellitus with mild nonproliferative diabetic retinopathy **without macular edema**

  ☑6ᵗʰ **E10.33**   Type 1 diabetes mellitus with **moderate nonproliferative diabetic retinopathy**

    E10.331   Type 1 diabetes mellitus with moderate nonproliferative diabetic retinopathy **with macular edema**

    E10.339   Type 1 diabetes mellitus with moderate nonproliferative diabetic retinopathy **without macular edema**

  ☑6ᵗʰ **E10.34**   Type 1 diabetes mellitus with **severe nonproliferative diabetic retinopathy**

    E10.341   Type 1 diabetes mellitus with severe nonproliferative diabetic retinopathy **with macular edema**

    E10.349   Type 1 diabetes mellitus with severe nonproliferative diabetic retinopathy **without macular edema**

  ☑6ᵗʰ **E10.35**   Type 1 diabetes mellitus with **proliferative diabetic retinopathy**

    E10.351   Type 1 diabetes mellitus with proliferative diabetic retinopathy **with macular edema**

☑ Additional Character Required   ☑x7ᵗʰ Placeholder Alert   Unspecified Dx   Other Specified Dx   Manifestation   ►◄ Revised Text   ● New Code   ▲ Revised Code Title

Chapter 4. Endocrine, Nutritional, and Metabolic Diseases

E10.359–E11.36

E10.359   **Type 1 diabetes mellitus with proliferative diabetic retinopathy** without macular edema

E10.36   **Type 1 diabetes mellitus with diabetic** cataract

E10.39   **Type 1 diabetes mellitus with other diabetic ophthalmic complication**
Use additional code to identify manifestation, such as: diabetic glaucoma (H40-H42)

✓5th E10.4   **Type 1 diabetes mellitus with** neurological complications

E10.40   **Type 1 diabetes mellitus with diabetic** neuropathy, unspecified

E10.41   **Type 1 diabetes mellitus with diabetic** mononeuropathy

E10.42   **Type 1 diabetes mellitus with diabetic** polyneuropathy
Type 1 diabetes mellitus with diabetic neuralgia

E10.43   **Type 1 diabetes mellitus with diabetic** autonomic (poly)neuropathy
Type 1 diabetes mellitus with diabetic gastroparesis
AHA: 2013, 4Q, 114

E10.44   **Type 1 diabetes mellitus with diabetic** amyotrophy

E10.49   **Type 1 diabetes mellitus with other diabetic neurological complication**

✓5th E10.5   **Type 1 diabetes mellitus with** circulatory complications

E10.51   **Type 1 diabetes mellitus with diabetic** peripheral angiopathy without gangrene

E10.52   **Type 1 diabetes mellitus with diabetic** peripheral angiopathy with gangrene
Type 1 diabetes mellitus with diabetic gangrene

E10.59   **Type 1 diabetes mellitus with other circulatory complications**

✓5th E10.6   **Type 1 diabetes mellitus with** other specified complications

✓6th E10.61   **Type 1 diabetes mellitus with diabetic** arthropathy

E10.610   **Type 1 diabetes mellitus with diabetic neuropathic arthropathy**
Type 1 diabetes mellitus with Charcôt's joints

E10.618   **Type 1 diabetes mellitus with other diabetic arthropathy**

✓6th E10.62   **Type 1 diabetes mellitus with** skin complications

E10.620   **Type 1 diabetes mellitus with diabetic dermatitis**
Type 1 diabetes mellitus with diabetic necrobiosis lipoidica

E10.621   **Type 1 diabetes mellitus with** foot ulcer
Use additional code to identify site of ulcer (L97.4-, L97.5-)

E10.622   **Type 1 diabetes mellitus with** other skin ulcer
Use additional code to identify site of ulcer (L97.1-L97.9, L98.41-L98.49)

E10.628   **Type 1 diabetes mellitus with other skin complications**

✓6th E10.63   **Type 1 diabetes mellitus with** oral complications

E10.630   **Type 1 diabetes mellitus with** periodontal disease

E10.638   **Type 1 diabetes mellitus with other oral complications**

✓6th E10.64   **Type 1 diabetes mellitus with** hypoglycemia

E10.641   **Type 1 diabetes mellitus with hypoglycemia** with coma

E10.649   **Type 1 diabetes mellitus with hypoglycemia** without coma

E10.65   **Type 1 diabetes mellitus with** hyperglycemia
AHA: 2013, 3Q, 20

E10.69   **Type 1 diabetes mellitus with other specified complication**
Use additional code to identify complication

E10.8   **Type 1 diabetes mellitus with unspecified** complications

E10.9   **Type 1 diabetes mellitus** without complications

✓4th E11   **Type 2 diabetes mellitus**
INCLUDES   diabetes (mellitus) due to insulin secretory defect
diabetes NOS
insulin resistant diabetes (mellitus)
Use additional code to identify any insulin use (Z79.4)
EXCLUDES 1   *diabetes mellitus due to underlying condition (E08.-)*
drug or chemical induced diabetes mellitus (E09.-)
gestational diabetes (O24.4-)
neonatal diabetes mellitus (P70.2)
postpancreatectomy diabetes mellitus (E13.-)
postprocedural diabetes mellitus (E13.-)
secondary diabetes mellitus NEC (E13.-)
type 1 diabetes mellitus (E10.-)
AHA: 2013, 4Q, 114; 2013, 3Q, 20; 2013, 1Q, 26

✓5th E11.0   **Type 2 diabetes mellitus with** hyperosmolarity

E11.00   **Type 2 diabetes mellitus with hyperosmolarity** without nonketotic hyperglycemic-hyperosmolar coma (NKHHC)

E11.01   **Type 2 diabetes mellitus with hyperosmolarity** with coma

✓5th E11.2   **Type 2 diabetes mellitus with** kidney complications

E11.21   **Type 2 diabetes mellitus with diabetic** nephropathy
Type 2 diabetes mellitus with intercapillary glomerulosclerosis
Type 2 diabetes mellitus with intracapillary glomerulonephrosis
Type 2 diabetes mellitus with Kimmelstiel-Wilson disease

E11.22   **Type 2 diabetes mellitus with diabetic** chronic kidney disease
Use additional code to identify stage of chronic kidney disease (N18.1-N18.6)

E11.29   **Type 2 diabetes mellitus with other diabetic kidney complication**
Type 2 diabetes mellitus with renal tubular degeneration

✓5th E11.3   **Type 2 diabetes mellitus with** ophthalmic complications

✓6th E11.31   **Type 2 diabetes mellitus with unspecified** diabetic retinopathy

E11.311   **Type 2 diabetes mellitus with unspecified diabetic retinopathy** with macular edema

E11.319   **Type 2 diabetes mellitus with unspecified diabetic retinopathy** without macular edema

✓6th E11.32   **Type 2 diabetes mellitus with** mild nonproliferative **diabetic** retinopathy
Type 2 diabetes mellitus with nonproliferative diabetic retinopathy NOS

E11.321   **Type 2 diabetes mellitus with mild nonproliferative diabetic retinopathy with macular edema**

E11.329   **Type 2 diabetes mellitus with mild nonproliferative diabetic retinopathy without macular edema**

✓6th E11.33   **Type 2 diabetes mellitus with** moderate nonproliferative **diabetic** retinopathy

E11.331   **Type 2 diabetes mellitus with moderate nonproliferative diabetic retinopathy with macular edema**

E11.339   **Type 2 diabetes mellitus with moderate nonproliferative diabetic retinopathy without macular edema**

✓6th E11.34   **Type 2 diabetes mellitus with** severe nonproliferative **diabetic** retinopathy

E11.341   **Type 2 diabetes mellitus with severe nonproliferative diabetic retinopathy with macular edema**

E11.349   **Type 2 diabetes mellitus with severe nonproliferative diabetic retinopathy without macular edema**

✓6th E11.35   **Type 2 diabetes mellitus with** proliferative diabetic retinopathy

E11.351   **Type 2 diabetes mellitus with proliferative diabetic retinopathy** with macular edema

E11.359   **Type 2 diabetes mellitus with proliferative diabetic retinopathy** without macular edema

E11.36   **Type 2 diabetes mellitus with diabetic** cataract

EXCLUDES 1 Not coded here   **EXCLUDES 2** Not included here   **N** Newborn Age: 0   **P** Pediatric Age: 0-17   **M** Maternity Age: 12-55   **A** Adult Age: 15-124

492   ICD-10-CM 2016

E11.39 **Type 2 diabetes mellitus with other diabetic ophthalmic complication**
    Use additional code to identify manifestation, such as: diabetic glaucoma (H40-H42)

✓5th **E11.4** **Type 2 diabetes mellitus with neurological complications**

E11.40 **Type 2 diabetes mellitus with diabetic neuropathy, unspecified**
    AHA: 2013, 4Q, 129

E11.41 **Type 2 diabetes mellitus with diabetic mononeuropathy**

E11.42 **Type 2 diabetes mellitus with diabetic polyneuropathy**
    Type 2 diabetes mellitus with diabetic neuralgia

E11.43 **Type 2 diabetes mellitus with diabetic autonomic (poly)neuropathy**
    Type 2 diabetes mellitus with diabetic gastroparesis
    AHA: 2013, 4Q, 114

E11.44 **Type 2 diabetes mellitus with diabetic amyotrophy**

E11.49 **Type 2 diabetes mellitus with other diabetic neurological complication**

✓5th **E11.5** **Type 2 diabetes mellitus with circulatory complications**

E11.51 **Type 2 diabetes mellitus with diabetic peripheral angiopathy without gangrene**

E11.52 **Type 2 diabetes mellitus with diabetic peripheral angiopathy with gangrene**
    Type 2 diabetes mellitus with diabetic gangrene

E11.59 **Type 2 diabetes mellitus with other circulatory complications**

✓5th **E11.6** **Type 2 diabetes mellitus with other specified complications**

✓6th **E11.61** **Type 2 diabetes mellitus with diabetic arthropathy**

E11.610 **Type 2 diabetes mellitus with diabetic neuropathic arthropathy**
    Type 2 diabetes mellitus with Charcôt's joints

E11.618 **Type 2 diabetes mellitus with other diabetic arthropathy**

✓6th **E11.62** **Type 2 diabetes mellitus with skin complications**

E11.620 **Type 2 diabetes mellitus with diabetic dermatitis**
    Type 2 diabetes mellitus with diabetic necrobiosis lipoidica

E11.621 **Type 2 diabetes mellitus with foot ulcer**
    Use additional code to identify site of ulcer (L97.4-, L97.5-)

E11.622 **Type 2 diabetes mellitus with other skin ulcer**
    Use additional code to identify site of ulcer (L97.1-L97.9, L98.41-L98.49)

E11.628 **Type 2 diabetes mellitus with other skin complications**

✓6th **E11.63** **Type 2 diabetes mellitus with oral complications**

E11.630 **Type 2 diabetes mellitus with periodontal disease**

E11.638 **Type 2 diabetes mellitus with other oral complications**

✓6th **E11.64** **Type 2 diabetes mellitus with hypoglycemia**

E11.641 **Type 2 diabetes mellitus with hypoglycemia with coma**

E11.649 **Type 2 diabetes mellitus with hypoglycemia without coma**

E11.65 **Type 2 diabetes mellitus with hyperglycemia**
    AHA: 2013, 3Q, 20

E11.69 **Type 2 diabetes mellitus with other specified complication**
    Use additional code to identify complication

E11.8 **Type 2 diabetes mellitus with unspecified complications**

E11.9 **Type 2 diabetes mellitus without complications**

✓4th **E13** **Other specified diabetes mellitus**
    Diabetes mellitus due to genetic defects of beta-cell function
    Diabetes mellitus due to genetic defects in insulin action
    Postpancreatectomy diabetes mellitus
    Postprocedural diabetes mellitus
    Secondary diabetes mellitus NEC
    Use additional code to identify any insulin use (Z79.4)
    EXCLUDES 1 *diabetes (mellitus) due to autoimmune process (E10.-)*
        diabetes (mellitus) due to immune mediated pancreatic islet beta-cell destruction (E10.-)
        diabetes mellitus due to underlying condition (E08.-)
        drug or chemical induced diabetes mellitus (E09.-)
        gestational diabetes (O24.4-)
        neonatal diabetes mellitus (P70.2)
        type 2 diabetes mellitus (E11.-)
    AHA: 2013, 4Q, 114; 2013, 3Q, 20

✓5th **E13.0** **Other specified diabetes mellitus with hyperosmolarity**

E13.00 **Other specified diabetes mellitus with hyperosmolarity without nonketotic hyperglycemic-hyperosmolar coma (NKHHC)**

E13.01 **Other specified diabetes mellitus with hyperosmolarity with coma**

✓5th **E13.1** **Other specified diabetes mellitus with ketoacidosis**
    AHA: 2013, 1Q, 26

E13.10 **Other specified diabetes mellitus with ketoacidosis without coma**

E13.11 **Other specified diabetes mellitus with ketoacidosis with coma**

✓5th **E13.2** **Other specified diabetes mellitus with kidney complications**

E13.21 **Other specified diabetes mellitus with diabetic nephropathy**
    Other specified diabetes mellitus with intercapillary glomerulosclerosis
    Other specified diabetes mellitus with intracapillary glomerulonephrosis
    Other specified diabetes mellitus with Kimmelstiel-Wilson disease

E13.22 **Other specified diabetes mellitus with diabetic chronic kidney disease**
    Use additional code to identify stage of chronic kidney disease (N18.1-N18.6)

E13.29 **Other specified diabetes mellitus with other diabetic kidney complication**
    Other specified diabetes mellitus with renal tubular degeneration

✓5th **E13.3** **Other specified diabetes mellitus with ophthalmic complications**

✓6th **E13.31** **Other specified diabetes mellitus with unspecified diabetic retinopathy**

E13.311 **Other specified diabetes mellitus with unspecified diabetic retinopathy with macular edema**

E13.319 **Other specified diabetes mellitus with unspecified diabetic retinopathy without macular edema**

✓6th **E13.32** **Other specified diabetes mellitus with mild nonproliferative diabetic retinopathy**
    Other specified diabetes mellitus with nonproliferative diabetic retinopathy NOS

E13.321 **Other specified diabetes mellitus with mild nonproliferative diabetic retinopathy with macular edema**

E13.329 **Other specified diabetes mellitus with mild nonproliferative diabetic retinopathy without macular edema**

✓6th **E13.33** **Other specified diabetes mellitus with moderate nonproliferative diabetic retinopathy**

E13.331 **Other specified diabetes mellitus with moderate nonproliferative diabetic retinopathy with macular edema**

E13.339 **Other specified diabetes mellitus with moderate nonproliferative diabetic retinopathy without macular edema**

✓6th **E13.34** **Other specified diabetes mellitus with severe nonproliferative diabetic retinopathy**

E13.341 **Other specified diabetes mellitus with severe nonproliferative diabetic retinopathy with macular edema**

E13.349 **Other specified diabetes mellitus with severe nonproliferative diabetic retinopathy without macular edema**

✓ Additional Character Required   ✓x7th Placeholder Alert   Unspecified Dx   Other Specified Dx   Manifestation   ►◄ Revised Text   ● New Code   ▲ Revised Code Title

ICD-10-CM 2016   **493**

✓6th **E13.35** **Other specified diabetes mellitus with proliferative diabetic** retinopathy

E13.351 **Other specified diabetes mellitus with proliferative diabetic retinopathy** with macular edema

E13.359 **Other specified diabetes mellitus with proliferative diabetic retinopathy** without macular edema

E13.36 **Other specified diabetes mellitus with** diabetic cataract

E13.39 **Other specified diabetes mellitus with other diabetic ophthalmic complication**
Use additional code to identify manifestation, such as: diabetic glaucoma (H40-H42)

✓5th **E13.4** **Other specified diabetes mellitus with** neurological complications

E13.40 **Other specified diabetes mellitus with diabetic** neuropathy, unspecified

E13.41 **Other specified diabetes mellitus with diabetic** mononeuropathy

E13.42 **Other specified diabetes mellitus with diabetic** polyneuropathy
Other specified diabetes mellitus with diabetic neuralgia

E13.43 **Other specified diabetes mellitus with diabetic** autonomic (poly)neuropathy
Other specified diabetes mellitus with diabetic gastroparesis
AHA: 2013, 4Q, 114

E13.44 **Other specified diabetes mellitus with diabetic** amyotrophy

E13.49 **Other specified diabetes mellitus with other diabetic** neurological complication

✓5th **E13.5** **Other specified diabetes mellitus with** circulatory complications

E13.51 **Other specified diabetes mellitus with diabetic** peripheral angiopathy without gangrene

E13.52 **Other specified diabetes mellitus with diabetic** peripheral angiopathy with gangrene
Other specified diabetes mellitus with diabetic gangrene

E13.59 **Other specified diabetes mellitus with other** circulatory complications

✓5th **E13.6** **Other specified diabetes mellitus with** other specified complications

✓6th **E13.61** **Other specified diabetes mellitus with diabetic** arthropathy

E13.610 **Other specified diabetes mellitus with** diabetic neuropathic **arthropathy**
Other specified diabetes mellitus with Charcôt's joints

E13.618 **Other specified diabetes mellitus with other diabetic arthropathy**

✓6th **E13.62** **Other specified diabetes mellitus with** skin complications

E13.620 **Other specified diabetes mellitus with diabetic** dermatitis
Other specified diabetes mellitus with diabetic necrobiosis lipoidica

E13.621 **Other specified diabetes mellitus with** foot ulcer
Use additional code to identify site of ulcer (L97.4-, L97.5-)

E13.622 **Other specified diabetes mellitus with** other skin ulcer
Use additional code to identify site of ulcer (L97.1-L97.9, L98.41-L98.49)

E13.628 **Other specified diabetes mellitus with other skin complications**

✓6th **E13.63** **Other specified diabetes mellitus with** oral complications

E13.630 **Other specified diabetes mellitus with** periodontal disease

E13.638 **Other specified diabetes mellitus with** other oral complications

✓6th **E13.64** **Other specified diabetes mellitus with** hypoglycemia

E13.641 **Other specified diabetes mellitus with** hypoglycemia with coma

E13.649 **Other specified diabetes mellitus with** hypoglycemia without coma

E13.65 **Other specified diabetes mellitus with** hyperglycemia

E13.69 **Other specified diabetes mellitus with other specified complication**
Use additional code to identify complication

E13.8 **Other specified diabetes mellitus with unspecified** complications

E13.9 **Other specified diabetes mellitus** without complications

Other disorders of glucose regulation and pancreatic internal secretion (E15-E16)

E15 **Nondiabetic hypoglycemic coma**
[INCLUDES] drug-induced insulin coma in nondiabetic hyperinsulinism with hypoglycemic coma hypoglycemic coma NOS

✓4th **E16** **Other disorders of pancreatic internal secretion**

E16.0 **Drug-induced hypoglycemia without coma**
Use additional code for adverse effect, if applicable, to identify drug (T36-T50 with fifth or sixth character 5)

E16.1 **Other hypoglycemia**
Functional hyperinsulinism
Functional nonhyperinsulinemic hypoglycemia
Hyperinsulinism NOS
Hyperplasia of pancreatic islet beta cells NOS
EXCLUDES 1 *hypoglycemia in infant of diabetic mother (P70.1)*
neonatal hypoglycemia (P70.4)

E16.2 **Hypoglycemia, unspecified**

E16.3 **Increased secretion of glucagon**
Hyperplasia of pancreatic endocrine cells with glucagon excess

E16.4 **Increased secretion of gastrin**
Hypergastrinemia
Hyperplasia of pancreatic endocrine cells with gastrin excess
Zollinger-Ellison syndrome

E16.8 **Other specified disorders of pancreatic internal secretion**
Increased secretion from endocrine pancreas of growth hormone-releasing hormone
Increased secretion from endocrine pancreas of pancreatic polypeptide
Increased secretion from endocrine pancreas of somatostatin
Increased secretion from endocrine pancreas of vasoactive-intestinal polypeptide

E16.9 **Disorder of pancreatic internal secretion, unspecified**
Islet-cell hyperplasia NOS
Pancreatic endocrine cell hyperplasia NOS

Disorders of other endocrine glands (E20-E35)

EXCLUDES 1 *galactorrhea (N64.3)*
gynecomastia (N62)

✓4th **E20** **Hypoparathyroidism**
EXCLUDES 1 *Di George's syndrome (D82.1)*
postprocedural hypoparathyroidism (E89.2)
tetany NOS (R29.0)
transitory neonatal hypoparathyroidism (P71.4)

E20.0 **Idiopathic** hypoparathyroidism

E20.1 **Pseudohypoparathyroidism**

E20.8 **Other hypoparathyroidism**

E20.9 **Hypoparathyroidism, unspecified**
Parathyroid tetany

✓4th **E21** **Hyperparathyroidism and other disorders of parathyroid gland**
EXCLUDES 1 *adult osteomalacia (M83.-)*
ectopic hyperparathyroidism (E34.2)
familial hypocalciuric hypercalcemia (E83.52)
hungry bone syndrome (E83.81)
infantile and juvenile osteomalacia (E55.0)

E21.0 **Primary** hyperparathyroidism
Hyperplasia of parathyroid
Osteitis fibrosa cystica generalisata [von Recklinghausen's disease of bone]

E21.1 **Secondary** hyperparathyroidism, not elsewhere classified
EXCLUDES 1 *secondary hyperparathyroidism of renal origin (N25.81)*

E21.2 **Other** hyperparathyroidism
Tertiary hyperparathyroidism
EXCLUDES 1 *familial hypocalciuric hypercalcemia (E83.52)*

E21.3 **Hyperparathyroidism, unspecified**

E21.4 **Other specified disorders of parathyroid gland**

E21.5 **Disorder of parathyroid gland, unspecified**

✓4ᵗʰ **E22 Hyperfunction of pituitary gland**
     EXCLUDES 1   *Cushing's syndrome (E24.-)*
         Nelson's syndrome (E24.1)
         overproduction of ACTH not associated with Cushing's disease
         (E27.0)
         overproduction of pituitary ACTH (E24.0)
         overproduction of thyroid-stimulating hormone (E05.8-)

E22.0 **Acromegaly and pituitary gigantism**
     Overproduction of growth hormone
     EXCLUDES 1   *constitutional gigantism (E34.4)*
         constitutional tall stature (E34.4)
         increased secretion from endocrine pancreas of growth
         hormone-releasing hormone (E16.8)

E22.1 **Hyperprolactinemia**
     Use additional code for adverse effect, if applicable, to identify
         drug (T36-T50 with fifth or sixth character 5)

E22.2 **Syndrome of inappropriate secretion of antidiuretic hormone**

E22.8 **Other hyperfunction of pituitary gland**
     Central precocious puberty

E22.9 **Hyperfunction of pituitary gland, unspecified**

✓4ᵗʰ **E23 Hypofunction and other disorders of the pituitary gland**
     INCLUDES   the listed conditions whether the disorder is in the pituitary
         or the hypothalamus
     EXCLUDES 1   *postprocedural hypopituitarism (E89.3)*

E23.0 **Hypopituitarism**
     Fertile eunuch syndrome
     Hypogonadotropic hypogonadism
     Idiopathic growth hormone deficiency
     Isolated deficiency of gonadotropin
     Isolated deficiency of growth hormone
     Isolated deficiency of pituitary hormone
     Kallmann's syndrome
     Lorain-Levi short stature
     Necrosis of pituitary gland (postpartum)
     Panhypopituitarism
     Pituitary cachexia
     Pituitary insufficiency NOS
     Pituitary short stature
     Sheehan's syndrome
     Simmonds' disease

E23.1 **Drug-induced hypopituitarism**
     Use additional code for adverse effect, if applicable, to identify
         drug (T36-T50 with fifth or sixth character 5)

E23.2 **Diabetes insipidus**
     EXCLUDES 1   *nephrogenic diabetes insipidus (N25.1)*

E23.3 **Hypothalamic dysfunction, not elsewhere classified**
     EXCLUDES 1   *Prader-Willi syndrome (Q87.1)*
         Russell-Silver syndrome (Q87.1)

E23.6 **Other disorders of pituitary gland**
     Abscess of pituitary   Adiposogenital dystrophy

E23.7 **Disorder of pituitary gland, unspecified**

✓4ᵗʰ **E24 Cushing's syndrome**
     EXCLUDES 1   *congenital adrenal hyperplasia (E25.0)*

E24.0 **Pituitary-dependent Cushing's disease**
     Overproduction of pituitary ACTH
     Pituitary-dependent hypercorticalism

E24.1 **Nelson's syndrome**

E24.2 **Drug-induced Cushing's syndrome**
     Use additional code for adverse effect, if applicable, to identify
         drug (T36-T50 with fifth or sixth character 5)

E24.3 **Ectopic ACTH syndrome**

E24.4 **Alcohol-induced pseudo-Cushing's syndrome**

E24.8 **Other Cushing's syndrome**

E24.9 **Cushing's syndrome, unspecified**

✓4ᵗʰ **E25 Adrenogenital disorders**
     INCLUDES   adrenogenital syndromes, virilizing or feminizing, whether
         acquired or due to adrenal hyperplasia
         consequent on inborn enzyme defects in hormone synthesis
         female adrenal pseudohermaphroditism
         female heterosexual precocious pseudopuberty
         male isosexual precocious pseudopuberty
         male macrogenitosomia praecox
         male sexual precocity with adrenal hyperplasia
         male virilization (female)
     EXCLUDES 1   *indeterminate sex and pseudohermaphroditism (Q56)*
         chromosomal abnormalities (Q90-Q99)

E25.0 **Congenital adrenogenital disorders associated with enzyme
deficiency**
     Congenital adrenal hyperplasia
     21-Hydroxylase deficiency
     Salt-losing congenital adrenal hyperplasia

E25.8 **Other adrenogenital disorders**
     Idiopathic adrenogenital disorder
     Use additional code for adverse effect, if applicable, to identify
         drug (T36-T50 with fifth or sixth character 5)

E25.9 **Adrenogenital disorder, unspecified**
     Adrenogenital syndrome NOS

✓4ᵗʰ **E26 Hyperaldosteronism**

✓5ᵗʰ E26.0 **Primary hyperaldosteronism**
         E26.01 **Conn's syndrome**
             Code also adrenal adenoma (D35.0-)

         E26.02 **Glucocorticoid-remediable aldosteronism**
             Familial aldosteronism type I

         E26.09 **Other primary hyperaldosteronism**
             Primary aldosteronism due to adrenal hyperplasia
             (bilateral)

E26.1 **Secondary hyperaldosteronism**

✓5ᵗʰ E26.8 **Other hyperaldosteronism**
         E26.81 **Bartter's syndrome**
         E26.89 **Other hyperaldosteronism**

E26.9 **Hyperaldosteronism, unspecified**
     Aldosteronism NOS   Hyperaldosteronism NOS

✓4ᵗʰ **E27 Other disorders of adrenal gland**
E27.0 **Other adrenocortical overactivity**
     Overproduction of ACTH, not associated with Cushing's disease
     Premature adrenarche
     EXCLUDES 1   *Cushing's syndrome (E24.-)*

E27.1 **Primary adrenocortical insufficiency**
     Addison's disease
     Autoimmune adrenalitis
     EXCLUDES 1   *Addison only phenotype adrenoleukodystrophy*
         (E71.528)
         amyloidosis (E85.-)
         tuberculous Addison's disease (A18.7)
         Waterhouse-Friderichsen syndrome (A39.1)

E27.2 **Addisonian crisis**
     Adrenal crisis
     Adrenocortical crisis

E27.3 **Drug-induced adrenocortical insufficiency**
     Use additional code for adverse effect, if applicable, to identify
         drug (T36-T50 with fifth or sixth character 5)

✓5ᵗʰ E27.4 **Other and unspecified adrenocortical insufficiency**
     EXCLUDES 1   *adrenoleukodystrophy [Addison-Schilder] (E71.528)*
         Waterhouse-Friderichsen syndrome (A39.1)

         E27.40 **Unspecified adrenocortical insufficiency**
             Adrenocortical insufficiency NOS
             Hypoaldosteronism

         E27.49 **Other adrenocortical insufficiency**
             Adrenal hemorrhage
             Adrenal infarction

E27.5 **Adrenomedullary hyperfunction**
     Adrenomedullary hyperplasia
     Catecholamine hypersecretion

E27.8 **Other specified disorders of adrenal gland**
     Abnormality of cortisol-binding globulin

E27.9 **Disorder of adrenal gland, unspecified**

☑ Additional Character Required   ✓x7ᵗʰ Placeholder Alert   Unspecified Dx   Other Specified Dx   Manifestation   ▶◀ Revised Text   ● New Code   ▲ Revised Code Title

✓4ᵗʰ E28   Ovarian dysfunction

EXCLUDES 1   isolated gonadotropin deficiency (E23.0)
     postprocedural ovarian failure (E89.4-)

E28.0   Estrogen excess ♀
     Use additional code for adverse effect, if applicable, to identify drug (T36-T50 with fifth or sixth character 5)

E28.1   Androgen excess ♀
     Hypersecretion of ovarian androgens
     Use additional code for adverse effect, if applicable, to identify drug (T36-T50 with fifth or sixth character 5)

E28.2   Polycystic ovarian syndrome ♀
     Sclerocystic ovary syndrome
     Stein-Leventhal syndrome

✓5ᵗʰ E28.3   Primary ovarian failure

EXCLUDES 1   pure gonadal dysgenesis (Q99.1)
     Turner's syndrome (Q96.-)

✓6ᵗʰ E28.31   Premature menopause

E28.310   Symptomatic premature menopause ♀
     Symptoms such as flushing, sleeplessness, headache, lack of concentration, associated with premature menopause

E28.319   Asymptomatic premature menopause ♀
     Premature menopause NOS

E28.39   Other primary ovarian failure ♀
     Decreased estrogen
     Resistant ovary syndrome

E28.8   Other ovarian dysfunction ♀
     Ovarian hyperfunction NOS
     EXCLUDES 1   postprocedural ovarian failure (E89.4-)

E28.9   Ovarian dysfunction, unspecified ♀

✓4ᵗʰ E29   Testicular dysfunction

EXCLUDES 1   androgen insensitivity syndrome (E34.5-)
     azoospermia or oligospermia NOS (N46.0-N46.1)
     isolated gonadotropin deficiency (E23.0)
     Klinefelter's syndrome (Q98.0-Q98.2, Q98.4)

E29.0   Testicular hyperfunction ♂
     Hypersecretion of testicular hormones

E29.1   Testicular hypofunction ♂
     Defective biosynthesis of testicular androgen NOS
     5-delta-Reductase deficiency (with male pseudohermaphroditism)
     Testicular hypogonadism NOS
     Use additional code for adverse effect, if applicable, to identify drug (T36-T50 with fifth or sixth character 5)
     EXCLUDES 1   postprocedural testicular hypofunction (E89.5)

E29.8   Other testicular dysfunction ♂

E29.9   Testicular dysfunction, unspecified ♂

✓4ᵗʰ E30   Disorders of puberty, not elsewhere classified

E30.0   Delayed puberty
     Constitutional delay of puberty
     Delayed sexual development

E30.1   Precocious puberty 🅿
     Precocious menstruation
     EXCLUDES 1   Albright (-McCune) (-Sternberg) syndrome (Q78.1)
     central precocious puberty (E22.8)
     congenital adrenal hyperplasia (E25.0)
     female heterosexual precocious pseudopuberty (E25.-)
     male isosexual precocious pseudopuberty (E25.-)

E30.8   Other disorders of puberty 🅿
     Premature thelarche

E30.9   Disorder of puberty, unspecified

✓4ᵗʰ E31   Polyglandular dysfunction

EXCLUDES 1   ataxia telangiectasia [Louis-Bar] (G11.3)
     dystrophia myotonica [Steinert] (G71.11)
     pseudohypoparathyroidism (E20.1)

E31.0   Autoimmune polyglandular failure
     Schmidt's syndrome

E31.1   Polyglandular hyperfunction
     EXCLUDES 1   multiple endocrine adenomatosis (E31.2-)
     multiple endocrine neoplasia (E31.2-)

✓5ᵗʰ E31.2   Multiple endocrine neoplasia [MEN] syndromes
     Multiple endocrine adenomatosis
     Code also any associated malignancies and other conditions associated with the syndromes

E31.20   Multiple endocrine neoplasia [MEN] syndrome, unspecified
     Multiple endocrine adenomatosis NOS
     Multiple endocrine neoplasia [MEN] syndrome NOS

E31.21   Multiple endocrine neoplasia [MEN] type I
     Wermer's syndrome

E31.22   Multiple endocrine neoplasia [MEN] type IIA
     Sipple's syndrome

E31.23   Multiple endocrine neoplasia [MEN] type IIB

E31.8   Other polyglandular dysfunction

E31.9   Polyglandular dysfunction, unspecified

✓4ᵗʰ E32   Diseases of thymus

EXCLUDES 1   aplasia or hypoplasia of thymus with immunodeficiency (D82.1)
     myasthenia gravis (G70.0)

E32.0   Persistent hyperplasia of thymus
     Hypertrophy of thymus

E32.1   Abscess of thymus

E32.8   Other diseases of thymus
     EXCLUDES 1   aplasia or hypoplasia with immunodeficiency (D82.1)
     thymoma (D15.0)

E32.9   Disease of thymus, unspecified

✓4ᵗʰ E34   Other endocrine disorders

EXCLUDES 1   pseudohypoparathyroidism (E20.1)

E34.0   Carcinoid syndrome
     NOTE   May be used as an additional code to identify functional activity associated with a carcinoid tumor.

E34.1   Other hypersecretion of intestinal hormones

E34.2   Ectopic hormone secretion, not elsewhere classified
     EXCLUDES 1   ectopic ACTH syndrome (E24.3)

E34.3   Short stature due to endocrine disorder
     Constitutional short stature
     Laron-type short stature
     EXCLUDES 1   achondroplastic short stature (Q77.4)
     hypochondroplastic short stature (Q77.4)
     nutritional short stature (E45)
     pituitary short stature (E23.0)
     progeria (E34.8)
     renal short stature (N25.0)
     Russell-Silver syndrome (Q87.1)
     short-limbed stature with immunodeficiency (D82.2)
     short stature in specific dysmorphic syndromes— code to syndrome—see Alphabetical Index
     short stature NOS (R62.52)

E34.4   Constitutional tall stature
     Constitutional gigantism

✓5ᵗʰ E34.5   Androgen insensitivity syndrome

E34.50   Androgen insensitivity syndrome, unspecified
     Androgen insensitivity NOS

E34.51   Complete androgen insensitivity syndrome
     Complete androgen insensitivity
     de Quervain syndrome
     Goldberg-Maxwell syndrome

E34.52   Partial androgen insensitivity syndrome
     Partial androgen insensitivity
     Reifenstein syndrome

E34.8   Other specified endocrine disorders
     Pineal gland dysfunction
     Progeria
     EXCLUDES 2   pseudohypoparathyroidism (E20.1)

E34.9   Endocrine disorder, unspecified
     Endocrine disturbance NOS
     Hormone disturbance NOS

E35   Disorders of endocrine glands in diseases classified elsewhere

Code first underlying disease, such as:
     late congenital syphilis of thymus gland [Dubois disease] (A50.5)
Use additional code, if applicable, to identify:
     sequelae of tuberculosis of other organs (B90.8)
     EXCLUDES 1   Echinococcus granulosus infection of thyroid gland (B67.3)
     meningococcal hemorrhagic adrenalitis (A39.1)
     syphilis of endocrine gland (A52.79)
     tuberculosis of adrenal gland, except calcification (A18.7)
     tuberculosis of endocrine gland NEC (A18.82)
     tuberculosis of thyroid gland (A18.81)
     Waterhouse-Friderichsen syndrome (A39.1)

EXCLUDES 1 Not coded here   **EXCLUDES 2** Not included here   ℕ Newborn Age: 0   🅿 Pediatric Age: 0-17   Ⓜ Maternity Age: 12-55   🅰 Adult Age: 15-124

496   ICD-10-CM 2016

☑4ᵗʰ **E36 Intraoperative complications of endocrine system**
> EXCLUDES 2   *postprocedural endocrine and metabolic complications and disorders, not elsewhere classified (E89.-)*

☑5ᵗʰ **E36.0 Intraoperative hemorrhage and hematoma of an endocrine system organ or structure complicating a procedure**
> EXCLUDES 1   *intraoperative hemorrhage and hematoma of an endocrine system organ or structure due to accidental puncture or laceration during a procedure (E36.1-)*

     E36.01 Intraoperative hemorrhage and hematoma of an endocrine system organ or structure complicating an endocrine system procedure

     E36.02 Intraoperative hemorrhage and hematoma of an endocrine system organ or structure complicating other procedure

☑5ᵗʰ **E36.1 Accidental puncture and laceration of an endocrine system organ or structure during a procedure**

     E36.11 Accidental puncture and laceration of an endocrine system organ or structure during an endocrine system procedure

     E36.12 Accidental puncture and laceration of an endocrine system organ or structure during other procedure

E36.8 Other intraoperative complications of endocrine system
> Use additional code, if applicable, to further specify disorder

Malnutrition (E40-E46)

> EXCLUDES 1   *intestinal malabsorption (K90.-)*
> *sequelae of protein-calorie malnutrition (E64.0)*
> EXCLUDES 2   *nutritional anemias (D50-D53)*
> *starvation (T73.0)*

E40 Kwashiorkor
> Severe malnutrition with nutritional edema with dyspigmentation of skin and hair
> EXCLUDES 1   *marasmic kwashiorkor (E42)*

E41 Nutritional marasmus
> Severe malnutrition with marasmus
> EXCLUDES 1   *marasmic kwashiorkor (E42)*

E42 Marasmic kwashiorkor
> Intermediate form severe protein-calorie malnutrition
> Severe protein-calorie malnutrition with signs of both kwashiorkor and marasmus

E43 Unspecified severe protein-calorie malnutrition
> Starvation edema

☑4ᵗʰ **E44 Protein-calorie malnutrition of moderate and mild degree**

     E44.0 Moderate protein-calorie malnutrition

     E44.1 Mild protein-calorie malnutrition

E45 Retarded development following protein-calorie malnutrition
> Nutritional short stature
> Nutritional stunting
> Physical retardation due to malnutrition

E46 Unspecified protein-calorie malnutrition
> Malnutrition NOS
> Protein-calorie imbalance NOS
> EXCLUDES 1   *nutritional deficiency NOS (E63.9)*

Other nutritional deficiencies (E50-E64)

> EXCLUDES 2   *nutritional anemias (D50-D53)*

☑4ᵗʰ **E50 Vitamin A deficiency**
> EXCLUDES 1   *sequelae of vitamin A deficiency (E64.1)*

     E50.0 Vitamin A deficiency with conjunctival xerosis

     E50.1 Vitamin A deficiency with Bitot's spot and conjunctival xerosis
> Bitot's spot in the young child

     E50.2 Vitamin A deficiency with corneal xerosis

     E50.3 Vitamin A deficiency with corneal ulceration and xerosis

     E50.4 Vitamin A deficiency with keratomalacia

     E50.5 Vitamin A deficiency with night blindness

     E50.6 Vitamin A deficiency with xerophthalmic scars of cornea

     E50.7 Other ocular manifestations of vitamin A deficiency
> Xerophthalmia NOS

     E50.8 Other manifestations of vitamin A deficiency
> Follicular keratosis
> Xeroderma

     E50.9 Vitamin A deficiency, unspecified
> Hypovitaminosis A NOS

☑4ᵗʰ **E51 Thiamine deficiency**
> EXCLUDES 1   *sequelae of thiamine deficiency (E64.8)*

☑5ᵗʰ **E51.1 Beriberi**

     E51.11 Dry beriberi
> Beriberi NOS
> Beriberi with polyneuropathy

     E51.12 Wet beriberi
> Beriberi with cardiovascular manifestations
> Cardiovascular beriberi
> Shoshin disease

     E51.2 Wernicke's encephalopathy

     E51.8 Other manifestations of thiamine deficiency

     E51.9 Thiamine deficiency, unspecified

E52 Niacin deficiency [pellagra]
> Niacin (-tryptophan) deficiency
> Nicotinamide deficiency
> Pellagra (alcoholic)
> EXCLUDES 1   *sequelae of niacin deficiency (E64.8)*

☑4ᵗʰ **E53 Deficiency of other B group vitamins**
> EXCLUDES 1   *sequelae of vitamin B deficiency (E64.8)*

     E53.0 Riboflavin deficiency
> Ariboflavinosis
> Vitamin B2 deficiency

     E53.1 Pyridoxine deficiency
> Vitamin B6 deficiency
> EXCLUDES 1   *pyridoxine-responsive sideroblastic anemia (D64.3)*

     E53.8 Deficiency of other specified B group vitamins
> Biotin deficiency   Folic acid deficiency
> Cyanocobalamin deficiency   Pantothenic acid deficiency
> Folate deficiency   Vitamin B12 deficiency
> EXCLUDES 1   *folate deficiency anemia (D52.-)*
> *vitamin B12 deficiency anemia (D51.-)*

     E53.9 Vitamin B deficiency, unspecified

E54 Ascorbic acid deficiency
> Deficiency of vitamin C
> Scurvy
> EXCLUDES 1   *scorbutic anemia (D53.2)*
> *sequelae of vitamin C deficiency (E64.2)*

☑4ᵗʰ **E55 Vitamin D deficiency**
> EXCLUDES 1   *adult osteomalacia (M83.-)*
> *osteoporosis (M80.-)*
> *sequelae of rickets (E64.3)*

     E55.0 Rickets, active
> Infantile osteomalacia
> Juvenile osteomalacia
> EXCLUDES 1   *celiac rickets (K90.0)*
> *Crohn's rickets (K50.-)*
> *hereditary vitamin D-dependent rickets (E83.32)*
> *inactive rickets (E64.3)*
> *renal rickets (N25.0)*
> *sequelae of rickets (E64.3)*
> *vitamin D-resistant rickets (E83.31)*

     E55.9 Vitamin D deficiency, unspecified
> Avitaminosis D

☑4ᵗʰ **E56 Other vitamin deficiencies**
> EXCLUDES 1   *sequelae of other vitamin deficiencies (E64.8)*

     E56.0 Deficiency of vitamin E

     E56.1 Deficiency of vitamin K
> EXCLUDES 1   *deficiency of coagulation factor due to vitamin K deficiency (D68.4)*
> *vitamin K deficiency of newborn (P53)*

     E56.8 Deficiency of other vitamins

     E56.9 Vitamin deficiency, unspecified

E58 Dietary calcium deficiency
> EXCLUDES 1   *disorders of calcium metabolism (E83.5-)*
> *sequelae of calcium deficiency (E64.8)*

E59 Dietary selenium deficiency
> Keshan disease
> EXCLUDES 1   *sequelae of selenium deficiency (E64.8)*

E60 Dietary zinc deficiency

☑ Additional Character Required   ☑x7ᵗʰ Placeholder Alert   Unspecified Dx   Other Specified Dx   Manifestation   ▶◀ Revised Text   ● New Code   ▲ Revised Code Title

✓4th **E61** **Deficiency of other nutrient elements**
> Use additional code for adverse effect, if applicable, to identify drug (T36-T50 with fifth or sixth character 5)
> EXCLUDES 1　disorders of mineral metabolism (E83.-)
> 　　　　　　iodine deficiency related thyroid disorders (E00-E02)
> 　　　　　　sequelae of malnutrition and other nutritional deficiencies
> 　　　　　　(E64.-)

E61.0 **Copper** deficiency
E61.1 **Iron** deficiency
> EXCLUDES 1　iron deficiency anemia (D50.-)

E61.2 **Magnesium** deficiency
E61.3 **Manganese** deficiency
E61.4 **Chromium** deficiency
E61.5 **Molybdenum** deficiency
E61.6 **Vanadium** deficiency
E61.7 **Deficiency of** multiple nutrient elements
E61.8 **Deficiency of other specified nutrient elements**
E61.9 **Deficiency of nutrient element, unspecified**

✓4th **E63** **Other nutritional deficiencies**
> EXCLUDES 1　dehydration (E86.0)
> 　　　　　　failure to thrive, adult (R62.7)
> 　　　　　　failure to thrive, child (R62.51)
> 　　　　　　feeding problems in newborn (P92.-)
> 　　　　　　sequelae of malnutrition and other nutritional deficiencies
> 　　　　　　(E64.-)

E63.0 **Essential fatty acid [EFA] deficiency**
E63.1 **Imbalance of constituents of food intake**
E63.8 **Other specified nutritional deficiencies**
E63.9 **Nutritional deficiency, unspecified**

✓4th **E64** **Sequelae of malnutrition and other nutritional deficiencies**
> NOTE　This category is to be used to indicate conditions in categories E43, E44, E46, E50-E63 as the cause of sequelae, which are themselves classified elsewhere. The 'sequelae' include conditions specified as such; they also include the late effects of diseases classifiable to the above categories if the disease itself is no longer present.
> Code first condition resulting from (sequela) of malnutrition and other nutritional deficiencies

E64.0 **Sequelae of** protein-calorie **malnutrition**
> EXCLUDES 2　retarded development following protein-calorie
> 　　　　　　malnutrition (E45)

E64.1 **Sequelae of** vitamin A **deficiency**
E64.2 **Sequelae of** vitamin C **deficiency**
E64.3 **Sequelae of** rickets
E64.8 **Sequelae of other nutritional deficiencies**
E64.9 **Sequelae of unspecified nutritional deficiency**

Overweight, obesity and other hyperalimentation (E65-E68)

E65 **Localized adiposity**
> Fat pad

✓4th **E66** **Overweight and obesity**
> Code first obesity complicating pregnancy, childbirth and the puerperium, if applicable (O99.21-)
> Use additional code to identify body mass index (BMI), if known (Z68.-)
> EXCLUDES 1　adiposogenital dystrophy (E23.6)
> 　　　　　　lipomatosis NOS (E88.2)
> 　　　　　　lipomatosis dolorosa [Dercum] (E88.2)
> 　　　　　　Prader-Willi syndrome (Q87.1)

✓5th **E66.0** **Obesity** due to excess calories
　E66.01 **Morbid (severe) obesity due to excess calories**
> 　　EXCLUDES 1　morbid (severe) obesity with alveolar
> 　　　　　　　　hypoventilation (E66.2)

　E66.09 **Other** obesity due to excess calories

E66.1 **Drug-induced** obesity
> Use additional code for adverse effect, if applicable, to identify drug (T36-T50 with fifth or sixth character 5)

E66.2 Morbid (severe) **obesity with** alveolar hypoventilation
> Pickwickian syndrome

E66.3 Overweight
E66.8 **Other obesity**
E66.9 **Obesity, unspecified**
> Obesity NOS

✓4th **E67** **Other hyperalimentation**
> EXCLUDES 1　hyperalimentation NOS (R63.2)
> 　　　　　　sequelae of hyperalimentation (E68)

E67.0 **Hypervitaminosis A**
E67.1 **Hypercarotinemia**
E67.2 **Megavitamin-B6 syndrome**
E67.3 **Hypervitaminosis D**
E67.8 **Other specified hyperalimentation**

E68 **Sequelae of hyperalimentation**
> Code first condition resulting from (sequela) of hyperalimentation

Metabolic disorders (E70-E88)

> EXCLUDES 1　androgen insensitivity syndrome (E34.5-)
> 　　　　　　congenital adrenal hyperplasia (E25.0)
> 　　　　　　Ehlers-Danlos syndrome (Q79.6)
> 　　　　　　hemolytic anemias attributable to enzyme disorders (D55.-)
> 　　　　　　Marfan's syndrome (Q87.4)
> 　　　　　　5-alpha-reductase deficiency (E29.1)

✓4th **E70** **Disorders of aromatic amino-acid metabolism**
E70.0 **Classical** phenylketonuria
E70.1 **Other** hyperphenylalaninemias
✓5th **E70.2** **Disorders of** tyrosine metabolism
> 　EXCLUDES 1　transitory tyrosinemia of newborn (P74.5)

　E70.20 **Disorder of tyrosine metabolism, unspecified**
　E70.21 **Tyrosinemia**
> 　　Hypertyrosinemia

　E70.29 **Other disorders of tyrosine metabolism**
> 　　Alkaptonuria　　Ochronosis

✓5th **E70.3** Albinism
　E70.30 **Albinism, unspecified**
　✓6th **E70.31** Ocular albinism
　　E70.310 X-linked ocular albinism
　　E70.311 Autosomal recessive ocular albinism
　　E70.318 **Other ocular albinism**
　　E70.319 **Ocular albinism, unspecified**
　✓6th **E70.32** Oculocutaneous albinism
> 　　EXCLUDES 1　Chediak-Higashi syndrome (E70.330)
> 　　　　　　　　Hermansky-Pudlak syndrome (E70.331)

　　E70.320 **Tyrosinase negative oculocutaneous albinism**
> 　　　Albinism I
> 　　　Oculocutaneous albinism ty-neg

　　E70.321 **Tyrosinase positive oculocutaneous albinism**
> 　　　Albinism II
> 　　　Oculocutaneous albinism ty-pos

　　E70.328 **Other oculocutaneous albinism**
> 　　　Cross syndrome

　　E70.329 **Oculocutaneous albinism, unspecified**
　✓6th **E70.33** Albinism with hematologic abnormality
　　E70.330 Chediak-Higashi syndrome
　　E70.331 Hermansky-Pudlak syndrome
　　E70.338 **Other albinism with hematologic abnormality**
　　E70.339 **Albinism with hematologic abnormality, unspecified**
　E70.39 **Other specified albinism**
> 　　Piebaldism

✓5th **E70.4** **Disorders of** histidine metabolism
　E70.40 **Disorders of histidine metabolism, unspecified**
　E70.41 Histidinemia
　E70.49 **Other disorders of histidine metabolism**
E70.5 **Disorders of** tryptophan metabolism
E70.8 **Other disorders of aromatic amino-acid metabolism**
E70.9 **Disorder of aromatic amino-acid metabolism, unspecified**

✓4th **E71** **Disorders of branched-chain amino-acid metabolism and fatty-acid metabolism**
E71.0 Maple-syrup-urine disease
✓5th **E71.1** **Other disorders of** branched-chain amino-acid metabolism
　✓6th **E71.11** **Branched-chain** organic acidurias
　　E71.110 Isovaleric acidemia
　　E71.111 3-methylglutaconic aciduria
　　E71.118 **Other branched-chain organic acidurias**

EXCLUDES 1 Not coded here　　　　EXCLUDES 2 Not included here　　　　N Newborn Age: 0　　　P Pediatric Age: 0-17　　　M Maternity Age: 12-55　　　A Adult Age: 15-124

✓6ᵗʰ **E71.12** **Disorders of** propionate metabolism

E71.120 Methylmalonic acidemia

E71.121 Propionic acidemia

E71.128 **Other disorders of propionate metabolism**

E71.19 **Other disorders of branched-chain amino-acid metabolism**
Hyperleucine-isoleucinemia
Hypervalinemia

E71.2 **Disorder of branched-chain amino-acid metabolism, unspecified**

✓5ᵗʰ **E71.3** **Disorders of fatty-acid metabolism**
EXCLUDES 1 *peroxisomal disorders (E71.5)*
Refsum's disease (G60.1)
Schilder's disease (G37.0)
EXCLUDES 2 *carnitine deficiency due to inborn error of metabolism (E71.42)*

E71.30 **Disorder of fatty-acid metabolism, unspecified**

✓6ᵗʰ **E71.31** **Disorders of fatty-acid** oxidation

E71.310 **Long chain/very long chain acyl CoA dehydrogenase deficiency**
LCAD   VLCAD

E71.311 Medium chain **acyl CoA dehydrogenase deficiency**
MCAD

E71.312 Short chain **acyl CoA dehydrogenase deficiency**
SCAD

E71.313 Glutaric aciduria type II
Glutaric aciduria type II A
Glutaric aciduria type II B
Glutaric aciduria type II C
EXCLUDES 1 *glutaric aciduria (type 1) NOS (E72.3)*

E71.314 Muscle carnitine palmitoyltransferase deficiency

E71.318 **Other disorders of fatty-acid oxidation**

E71.32 **Disorders of** ketone metabolism

E71.39 **Other disorders of fatty-acid metabolism**

✓5ᵗʰ **E71.4** **Disorders of** carnitine metabolism
EXCLUDES 1 *muscle carnitine palmitoyltransferase deficiency (E71.314)*

E71.40 **Disorder of carnitine metabolism, unspecified**

E71.41 Primary **carnitine deficiency**

E71.42 **Carnitine deficiency due to** inborn errors of metabolism
Code also associated inborn error or metabolism

E71.43 Iatrogenic carnitine **deficiency**
Carnitine deficiency due to hemodialysis
Carnitine deficiency due to Valproic acid therapy

✓6ᵗʰ **E71.44** Other secondary **carnitine deficiency**

E71.440 **Ruvalcaba-Myhre-Smith syndrome**

E71.448 **Other secondary carnitine deficiency**

✓5ᵗʰ **E71.5** Peroxisomal disorders
EXCLUDES 1 *Schilder's disease (G37.0)*

E71.50 **Peroxisomal disorder, unspecified**

✓6ᵗʰ **E71.51** **Disorders of peroxisome** biogenesis
Group 1 peroxisomal disorders
EXCLUDES 1 *Refsum's disease (G60.1)*

E71.510 **Zellweger syndrome**

E71.511 Neonatal adrenoleukodystrophy   Ⓝ
EXCLUDES 1 *X-linked adrenoleuko- dystrophy (E71.52-)*

E71.518 **Other disorders of peroxisome biogenesis**

✓6ᵗʰ **E71.52** X-linked adrenoleukodystrophy

E71.520 Childhood cerebral **X-linked adrenoleukodystrophy**

E71.521 Adolescent **X-linked adrenoleukodystrophy**

E71.522 Adrenomyeloneuropathy

E71.528 **Other X-linked adrenoleukodystrophy**
Addison only phenotype adrenoleukodystrophy
Addison-Schilder adrenoleukodystrophy

E71.529 **X-linked adrenoleukodystrophy, unspecified type**

E71.53 **Other** group 2 **peroxisomal disorders**

✓6ᵗʰ **E71.54** Other **peroxisomal disorders**

E71.540 **Rhizomelic chondrodysplasia punctata**
EXCLUDES 1 *chondrodysplasia punctata NOS (Q77.3)*

E71.541 **Zellweger-like syndrome**

E71.542 **Other group 3 peroxisomal disorders**

E71.548 **Other peroxisomal disorders**

✓4ᵗʰ **E72** **Other disorders of amino-acid metabolism**
EXCLUDES 1 *disorders of:*
aromatic amino-acid metabolism (E70.-)
branched-chain amino-acid metabolism (E71.0-E71.2)
fatty-acid metabolism (E71.3)
purine and pyrimidine metabolism (E79.-)
gout (M1A.-, M10.-)

✓5ᵗʰ **E72.0** **Disorders of amino-acid** transport
EXCLUDES 1 *disorders of tryptophan metabolism (E70.5)*

E72.00 **Disorders of amino-acid transport, unspecified**

E72.01 **Cystinuria**

E72.02 **Hartnup's disease**

E72.03 **Lowe's syndrome**
Use additional code for associated glaucoma (H42)

E72.04 **Cystinosis**
Fanconi (-de Toni) (-Debré) syndrome with cystinosis
EXCLUDES 1 *Fanconi (-de Toni) (-Debré) syndrome without cystinosis (E72.09)*

E72.09 **Other disorders of amino-acid transport**
Fanconi (-de Toni) (-Debré) syndrome, unspecified

✓5ᵗʰ **E72.1** **Disorders of** sulfur-bearing **amino-acid metabolism**
EXCLUDES 1 *cystinosis (E72.04)*
cystinuria (E72.01)
transcobalamin II deficiency (D51.2)

E72.10 **Disorders of sulfur-bearing amino-acid metabolism, unspecified**

E72.11 **Homocystinuria**
Cystathionine synthase deficiency

E72.12 **Methylenetetrahydrofolate reductase deficiency**

E72.19 **Other disorders of sulfur-bearing amino-acid metabolism**
Cystathioninuria
Methioninemia
Sulfite oxidase deficiency

✓5ᵗʰ **E72.2** **Disorders of** urea cycle **metabolism**
EXCLUDES 1 *disorders of ornithine metabolism (E72.4)*

E72.20 **Disorder of urea cycle metabolism, unspecified**
Hyperammonemia
EXCLUDES 1 *hyperammonemia- hyperornithinemia-homocitrullinemia syndrome (E72.4)*
transient hyperammonemia of newborn (P74.6)

E72.21 **Argininemia**

E72.22 **Arginosuccinic aciduria**

E72.23 **Citrullinemia**

E72.29 **Other disorders of urea cycle metabolism**

E72.3 **Disorders of lysine and hydroxylysine metabolism**
Glutaric aciduria NOS   Hydroxylysinemia
Glutaric aciduria (type I)   Hyperlysinemia
EXCLUDES 1 *glutaric aciduria type II (E71.313)*
Refsum's disease (G60.1)
Zellweger syndrome (E71.510)

E72.4 **Disorders of ornithine metabolism**
Hyperammonemia-hyperornithinemia-homocitrullinemia syndrome
Ornithinemia (types I, II)
Ornithine transcarbamylase deficiency
EXCLUDES 1 *hereditary choroidal dystrophy (H31.2-)*

✓5ᵗʰ **E72.5** **Disorders of** glycine metabolism

E72.50 **Disorder of glycine metabolism, unspecified**

E72.51 Non-ketotic hyperglycinemia

E72.52 Trimethylaminuria

E72.53 Hyperoxaluria
Oxalosis
Oxaluria

E72.59 **Other disorders of glycine metabolism**
D-glycericacidemia
Hyperhydroxyprolinemia
Hyperprolinemia (types I, II)
Sarcosinemia

☑ Additional Character Required   ✓x7ᵗʰ Placeholder Alert   Unspecified Dx   Other Specified Dx   Manifestation   ▶◀ Revised Text   ● New Code   ▲ Revised Code Title

E72.8　Other specified disorders of amino-acid metabolism
　　Disorders of beta-amino-acid metabolism
　　Disorders of gamma-glutamyl cycle

E72.9　Disorder of amino-acid metabolism, unspecified

✓4ᵗʰ **E73　Lactose intolerance**

　E73.0　Congenital lactase deficiency

　E73.1　Secondary lactase deficiency

　E73.8　Other lactose intolerance

　E73.9　Lactose intolerance, unspecified

✓4ᵗʰ **E74　Other disorders of carbohydrate metabolism**

　　EXCLUDES 1　diabetes mellitus (E08-E13)
　　　　　hypoglycemia NOS (E16.2)
　　　　　increased secretion of glucagon (E16.3)
　　　　　mucopolysaccharidosis (E76.0-E76.3)

　✓5ᵗʰ **E74.0　Glycogen storage disease**

　　E74.00　Glycogen storage disease, unspecified

　　E74.01　von Gierke disease
　　　　Type I glycogen storage disease

　　E74.02　Pompe disease
　　　　Cardiac glycogenosis
　　　　Type II glycogen storage disease

　　E74.03　Cori disease
　　　　Forbes disease
　　　　Type III glycogen storage disease

　　E74.04　McArdle disease
　　　　Type V glycogen storage disease

　　E74.09　Other glycogen storage disease
　　　　Andersen disease
　　　　Hers disease
　　　　Tauri disease
　　　　Glycogen storage disease, types 0, IV, VI-XI
　　　　Liver phosphorylase deficiency
　　　　Muscle phosphofructokinase deficiency

　✓5ᵗʰ **E74.1　Disorders of fructose metabolism**

　　　EXCLUDES 1　muscle phosphofructokinase deficiency (E74.09)

　　E74.10　Disorder of fructose metabolism, unspecified

　　E74.11　Essential fructosuria
　　　　Fructokinase deficiency

　　E74.12　Hereditary fructose intolerance
　　　　Fructosemia

　　E74.19　Other disorders of fructose metabolism
　　　　Fructose-1, 6-diphosphatase deficiency

　✓5ᵗʰ **E74.2　Disorders of galactose metabolism**

　　E74.20　Disorders of galactose metabolism, unspecified

　　E74.21　Galactosemia

　　E74.29　Other disorders of galactose metabolism
　　　　Galactokinase deficiency

　✓5ᵗʰ **E74.3　Other disorders of intestinal carbohydrate absorption**

　　　EXCLUDES 2　lactose intolerance (E73.-)

　　E74.31　Sucrase-isomaltase deficiency

　　E74.39　Other disorders of intestinal carbohydrate absorption
　　　　Disorder of intestinal carbohydrate absorption NOS
　　　　Glucose-galactose malabsorption
　　　　Sucrase deficiency

　E74.4　Disorders of pyruvate metabolism and gluconeogenesis
　　Deficiency of phosphoenolpyruvate carboxykinase
　　Deficiency of pyruvate carboxylase
　　Deficiency of pyruvate dehydrogenase
　　　EXCLUDES 1　disorders of pyruvate metabolism and gluconeogenesis
　　　　　　with anemia (D55.-)
　　　　　　Leigh's syndrome (G31.82)

　E74.8　Other specified disorders of carbohydrate metabolism
　　Essential pentosuria
　　Renal glycosuria

　E74.9　Disorder of carbohydrate metabolism, unspecified

✓4ᵗʰ **E75　Disorders of sphingolipid metabolism and other lipid storage disorders**

　　EXCLUDES 1　mucolipidosis, types I-III (E77.0-E77.1)
　　　　　Refsum's disease (G60.1)

　✓5ᵗʰ **E75.0　GM2 gangliosidosis**

　　E75.00　GM2 gangliosidosis, unspecified

　　E75.01　Sandhoff disease

　　E75.02　Tay-Sachs disease

　　E75.09　Other GM2 gangliosidosis
　　　　Adult GM2 gangliosidosis
　　　　Juvenile GM2 gangliosidosis

　✓5ᵗʰ **E75.1　Other and unspecified gangliosidosis**

　　E75.10　Unspecified gangliosidosis
　　　　Gangliosidosis NOS

　　E75.11　Mucolipidosis IV

　　E75.19　Other gangliosidosis
　　　　GM1 gangliosidosis
　　　　GM3 gangliosidosis

　✓5ᵗʰ **E75.2　Other sphingolipidosis**

　　　EXCLUDES 1　adrenoleukodystrophy [Addison-Schilder] (E71.528)

　　E75.21　Fabry (-Anderson) disease

　　E75.22　Gaucher disease

　　E75.23　Krabbe disease

　✓6ᵗʰ　**E75.24　Niemann-Pick disease**

　　　E75.240　Niemann-Pick disease type A

　　　E75.241　Niemann-Pick disease type B

　　　E75.242　Niemann-Pick disease type C

　　　E75.243　Niemann-Pick disease type D

　　　E75.248　Other Niemann-Pick disease

　　　E75.249　Niemann-Pick disease, unspecified

　　E75.25　Metachromatic leukodystrophy

　　E75.29　Other sphingolipidosis
　　　　Farber's syndrome
　　　　Sulfatase deficiency
　　　　Sulfatide lipidosis

　E75.3　Sphingolipidosis, unspecified

　E75.4　Neuronal ceroid lipofuscinosis
　　Batten disease　　　　　　Kufs disease
　　Bielschowsky-Jansky disease　　Spielmeyer-Vogt disease

　E75.5　Other lipid storage disorders
　　Cerebrotendinous cholesterosis [van Bogaert-Scherer-Epstein]
　　Wolman's disease

　E75.6　Lipid storage disorder, unspecified

✓4ᵗʰ **E76　Disorders of glycosaminoglycan metabolism**

　✓5ᵗʰ **E76.0　Mucopolysaccharidosis, type I**

　　E76.01　Hurler's syndrome

　　E76.02　Hurler-Scheie syndrome

　　E76.03　Scheie's syndrome

　E76.1　Mucopolysaccharidosis, type II
　　Hunter's syndrome

　✓5ᵗʰ **E76.2　Other mucopolysaccharidoses**

　✓6ᵗʰ　**E76.21　Morquio mucopolysaccharidoses**

　　　E76.210　Morquio A mucopolysaccharidoses
　　　　　Classic Morquio syndrome
　　　　　Morquio syndrome A
　　　　　Mucopolysaccharidosis, type IVA

　　　E76.211　Morquio B mucopolysaccharidoses
　　　　　Morquio-like mucopolysaccharidoses
　　　　　Morquio-like syndrome
　　　　　Morquio syndrome B
　　　　　Mucopolysaccharidosis, type IVB

　　　E76.219　Morquio mucopolysaccharidoses, unspecified
　　　　　Morquio syndrome
　　　　　Mucopolysaccharidosis, type IV

　　E76.22　Sanfilippo mucopolysaccharidoses
　　　　Mucopolysaccharidosis, type III (A) (B) (C) (D)
　　　　Sanfilippo A syndrome
　　　　Sanfilippo B syndrome
　　　　Sanfilippo C syndrome
　　　　Sanfilippo D syndrome

　　E76.29　Other mucopolysaccharidoses
　　　　beta-Glucuronidase deficiency
　　　　Maroteaux-Lamy (mild) (severe) syndrome
　　　　Mucopolysaccharidosis, types VI, VII

　E76.3　Mucopolysaccharidosis, unspecified

　E76.8　Other disorders of glucosaminoglycan metabolism

　E76.9　Glucosaminoglycan metabolism disorder, unspecified

✓4ᵗʰ **E77　Disorders of glycoprotein metabolism**

　E77.0　Defects in post-translational modification of lysosomal enzymes
　　Mucolipidosis II [I-cell disease]
　　Mucolipidosis III [pseudo-Hurler polydystrophy]

EXCLUDES 1 Not coded here　　EXCLUDES 2 Not included here　　N Newborn Age: 0　　P Pediatric Age: 0-17　　M Maternity Age: 12-55　　A Adult Age: 15-124

500　　　　　　　　　　　　　　　　　　　　　　　　　　　ICD-10-CM 2016

E77.1   **Defects in glycoprotein degradation**
       Aspartylglucosaminuria
       Fucosidosis
       Mannosidosis
       Sialidosis [mucolipidosis I]

E77.8   **Other disorders of glycoprotein metabolism**

E77.9   **Disorder of glycoprotein metabolism, unspecified**

✓4ᵗʰ **E78**   **Disorders of lipoprotein metabolism and other lipidemias**
     EXCLUDES 1   *sphingolipidosis (E75.0-E75.3)*

   E78.0   **Pure hypercholesterolemia**
       Familial hypercholesterolemia
       Fredrickson's hyperlipoproteinemia, type IIa
       Hyperbetalipoproteinemia
       Hyperlipidemia, Group A
       Low-density-lipoprotein-type [LDL] hyperlipoproteinemia

   E78.1   **Pure hyperglyceridemia**
       Elevated fasting triglycerides
       Endogenous hyperglyceridemia
       Fredrickson's hyperlipoproteinemia, type IV
       Hyperlipidemia, group B
       Hyperprebetalipoproteinemia
       Very-low-density-lipoprotein-type [VLDL] hyperlipoproteinemia

   E78.2   **Mixed hyperlipidemia**
       Broad- or floating-betalipoproteinemia
       Combined hyperlipidemia NOS
       Elevated cholesterol with elevated triglycerides NEC
       Fredrickson's hyperlipoproteinemia, type IIb or III
       Hyperbetalipoproteinemia with prebetalipoproteinemia
       Hypercholesteremia with endogenous hyperglyceridemia
       Hyperlipidemia, group C
       Tubo-eruptive xanthoma
       Xanthoma tuberosum
       EXCLUDES 1   *cerebrotendinous cholesterosis [van Bogaert-Scherer-Epstein] (E75.5)*
             familial combined hyperlipidemia (E78.4)

   E78.3   **Hyperchylomicronemia**
       Chylomicron retention disease
       Fredrickson's hyperlipoproteinemia, type I or V
       Hyperlipidemia, group D
       Mixed hyperglyceridemia

   E78.4   **Other hyperlipidemia**
       Familial combined hyperlipidemia

   E78.5   **Hyperlipidemia, unspecified**

   E78.6   **Lipoprotein deficiency**
       Abetalipoproteinemia
       Depressed HDL cholesterol
       High-density lipoprotein deficiency
       Hypoalphalipoproteinemia
       Hypobetalipoproteinemia (familial)
       Lecithin cholesterol acyltransferase deficiency
       Tangier disease

✓5ᵗʰ   **E78.7**   **Disorders of bile acid and cholesterol metabolism**
       EXCLUDES 1   *Niemann-Pick disease type C (E75.242)*

     E78.70   **Disorder of bile acid and cholesterol metabolism, unspecified**

     E78.71   **Barth syndrome**

     E78.72   **Smith-Lemli-Opitz syndrome**

     E78.79   **Other disorders of bile acid and cholesterol metabolism**

✓5ᵗʰ   **E78.8**   **Other disorders of lipoprotein metabolism**

     E78.81   **Lipoid dermatoarthritis**

     E78.89   **Other lipoprotein metabolism disorders**

   E78.9   **Disorder of lipoprotein metabolism, unspecified**

✓4ᵗʰ **E79**   **Disorders of purine and pyrimidine metabolism**
     EXCLUDES 1   *Ataxia-telangiectasia (Q87.1)*
             Bloom's syndrome (Q82.8)
             Cockayne's syndrome (Q87.1)
             calculus of kidney (N20.0)
             combined immunodeficiency disorders (D81.-)
             Fanconi's anemia (D61.09)
             gout (M1A.-, M10.-)
             orotaciduric anemia (D53.0)
             progeria (E34.8)
             Werner's syndrome (E34.8)
             xeroderma pigmentosum (Q82.1)

   E79.0   **Hyperuricemia without signs of inflammatory arthritis and tophaceous disease**
       Asymptomatic hyperuricemia

   E79.1   **Lesch-Nyhan syndrome**
       HGPRT deficiency

   E79.2   **Myoadenylate deaminase deficiency**

   E79.8   **Other disorders of purine and pyrimidine metabolism**
       Hereditary xanthinuria

   E79.9   **Disorder of purine and pyrimidine metabolism, unspecified**

✓4ᵗʰ **E80**   **Disorders of porphyrin and bilirubin metabolism**
     INCLUDES   defects of catalase and peroxidase

   E80.0   **Hereditary erythropoietic porphyria**
       Congenital erythropoietic porphyria
       Erythropoietic protoporphyria

   E80.1   **Porphyria cutanea tarda**

✓5ᵗʰ   **E80.2**   **Other and unspecified porphyria**

     E80.20   **Unspecified porphyria**
         Porphyria NOS

     E80.21   **Acute intermittent (hepatic) porphyria**

     E80.29   **Other porphyria**
         Hereditary coproporphyria

   E80.3   **Defects of catalase and peroxidase**
       Acatalasia [Takahara]

   E80.4   **Gilbert syndrome**

   E80.5   **Crigler-Najjar syndrome**

   E80.6   **Other disorders of bilirubin metabolism**
       Dubin-Johnson syndrome
       Rotor's syndrome

   E80.7   **Disorder of bilirubin metabolism, unspecified**

✓4ᵗʰ **E83**   **Disorders of mineral metabolism**
     EXCLUDES 1   *dietary mineral deficiency (E58-E61)*
             parathyroid disorders (E20-E21)
             vitamin D deficiency (E55.-)

✓5ᵗʰ   **E83.0**   **Disorders of copper metabolism**

     E83.00   **Disorder of copper metabolism, unspecified**

     E83.01   **Wilson's disease**
         Code also associated Kayser Fleischer ring (H18.04-)

     E83.09   **Other disorders of copper metabolism**
         Menkes' (kinky hair) (steely hair) disease

✓5ᵗʰ   **E83.1**   **Disorders of iron metabolism**
     EXCLUDES 1   *iron deficiency anemia (D50.-)*
             sideroblastic anemia (D64.0-D64.3)

     E83.10   **Disorder of iron metabolism, unspecified**

✓6ᵗʰ   **E83.11**   **Hemochromatosis**

       E83.110   **Hereditary hemochromatosis**
           Bronzed diabetes
           Pigmentary cirrhosis (of liver)
           Primary (hereditary) hemochromatosis

       E83.111   **Hemochromatosis due to repeated red blood cell transfusions**
           Iron overload due to repeated red blood cell transfusions
           Transfusion (red blood cell) associated hemochromatosis

       E83.118   **Other hemochromatosis**

       E83.119   **Hemochromatosis, unspecified**

     E83.19   **Other disorders of iron metabolism**
         Use additional code, if applicable, for idiopathic pulmonary hemosiderosis (J84.03)

   E83.2   **Disorders of zinc metabolism**
       Acrodermatitis enteropathica

✓5ᵗʰ   **E83.3**   **Disorders of phosphorus metabolism and phosphatases**
     EXCLUDES 1   *adult osteomalacia (M83.-)*
             osteoporosis (M80.-)

     E83.30   **Disorder of phosphorus metabolism, unspecified**

     E83.31   **Familial hypophosphatemia**
         Vitamin D-resistant osteomalacia
         Vitamin D-resistant rickets
         EXCLUDES 1   *vitamin D-deficiency rickets (E55.0)*

     E83.32   **Hereditary vitamin D-dependent rickets (type 1) (type 2)**
         25-hydroxyvitamin D 1-alpha-hydroxylase deficiency
         Pseudovitamin D deficiency
         Vitamin D receptor defect

     E83.39   **Other disorders of phosphorus metabolism**
         Acid phosphatase deficiency
         Hypophosphatasia

✓5ᵗʰ   **E83.4**   **Disorders of magnesium metabolism**

     E83.40   **Disorders of magnesium metabolism, unspecified**

     E83.41   **Hypermagnesemia**

     E83.42   **Hypomagnesemia**

☑ Additional Character Required   x7ᵗʰ Placeholder Alert   Unspecified Dx   Other Specified Dx   Manifestation   ▶◀ Revised Text   ● New Code   ▲ Revised Code Title

E83.49   **Other disorders of magnesium metabolism**

✓5th **E83.5**   **Disorders of calcium metabolism**
     EXCLUDES1   *chondrocalcinosis (M11.1-M11.2)*
               hungry bone syndrome (E83.81)
               hyperparathyroidism (E21.0-E21.3)

     E83.50   **Unspecified disorder of calcium metabolism**

     E83.51   **Hypocalcemia**

     E83.52   **Hypercalcemia**
            Familial hypocalciuric hypercalcemia

     E83.59   **Other disorders of calcium metabolism**
            Idiopathic hypercalciuria

✓5th **E83.8**   **Other disorders of mineral metabolism**

     E83.81   **Hungry bone syndrome**

     E83.89   **Other disorders of mineral metabolism**

E83.9   **Disorder of mineral metabolism, unspecified**

✓4th **E84**   **Cystic fibrosis**
     INCLUDES   mucoviscidosis

     E84.0   **Cystic fibrosis with pulmonary manifestations**
         Use additional code to identify any infectious organism present, such as:
         Pseudomonas (B96.5)

✓5th **E84.1**   **Cystic fibrosis with intestinal manifestations**

     E84.11   **Meconium ileus in cystic fibrosis**   N
         EXCLUDES1   *meconium ileus not due to cystic fibrosis (P76.0)*

     E84.19   **Cystic fibrosis with other intestinal manifestations**
         Distal intestinal obstruction syndrome

     E84.8   **Cystic fibrosis with other manifestations**

     E84.9   **Cystic fibrosis, unspecified**

✓4th **E85**   **Amyloidosis**
     EXCLUDES1   *Alzheimer's disease (G30.0-)*

     E85.0   **Non-neuropathic heredofamilial amyloidosis**
         Familial Mediterranean fever
         Hereditary amyloid nephropathy

     E85.1   **Neuropathic heredofamilial amyloidosis**
         Amyloid polyneuropathy (Portuguese)
         AHA: 2012, 4Q, 99

     E85.2   **Heredofamilial amyloidosis, unspecified**

     E85.3   **Secondary systemic amyloidosis**
         Hemodialysis-associated amyloidosis

     E85.4   **Organ-limited amyloidosis**
         Localized amyloidosis

     E85.8   **Other amyloidosis**

     E85.9   **Amyloidosis, unspecified**

✓4th **E86**   **Volume depletion**
     EXCLUDES1   *dehydration of newborn (P74.1)*
               hypovolemic shock NOS (R57.1)
               postprocedural hypovolemic shock (T81.19)
               traumatic hypovolemic shock (T79.4)

     E86.0   **Dehydration**
         AHA: 2014, 1Q, 7

     E86.1   **Hypovolemia**
         Depletion of volume of plasma

     E86.9   **Volume depletion, unspecified**

✓4th **E87**   **Other disorders of fluid, electrolyte and acid-base balance**
     EXCLUDES1   *diabetes insipidus (E23.2)*
               electrolyte imbalance associated with hyperemesis gravidarum (O21.1)
               electrolyte imbalance following ectopic or molar pregnancy (O08.5)
               familial periodic paralysis (G72.3)

     E87.0   **Hyperosmolality and hypernatremia**
         Sodium [Na] excess
         Sodium [Na] overload
         AHA: 2014, 1Q, 7

     E87.1   **Hypo-osmolality and hyponatremia**
         Sodium [Na] deficiency
         EXCLUDES1   *syndrome of inappropriate secretion of antidiuretic hormone (E22.2)*
         AHA: 2014, 1Q, 7

     E87.2   **Acidosis**
         Acidosis NOS   Metabolic acidosis
         Lactic acidosis   Respiratory acidosis
         EXCLUDES1   *diabetic acidosis—see categories E08-E10, E13 with ketoacidosis*

E87.3   **Alkalosis**
     Alkalosis NOS   Respiratory alkalosis
     Metabolic alkalosis

E87.4   **Mixed disorder of acid-base balance**

E87.5   **Hyperkalemia**
     Potassium [K] excess   Potassium [K] overload

E87.6   **Hypokalemia**
     Potassium [K] deficiency

✓5th **E87.7**   **Fluid overload**
     EXCLUDES1   *edema NOS (R60.9)*
               fluid retention (R60.9)

     E87.70   **Fluid overload, unspecified**

     E87.71   **Transfusion associated circulatory overload**
         Fluid overload due to transfusion (blood) (blood components)
         TACO

     E87.79   **Other fluid overload**

E87.8   **Other disorders of electrolyte and fluid balance, not elsewhere classified**
     Electrolyte imbalance NOS
     Hyperchloremia
     Hypochloremia

✓4th **E88**   **Other and unspecified metabolic disorders**
     Use additional codes for associated conditions
     EXCLUDES1   *histiocytosis X (chronic) (C96.6)*

✓5th **E88.0**   **Disorders of plasma-protein metabolism, not elsewhere classified**
     EXCLUDES1   *disorder of lipoprotein metabolism (E78.-)*
               monoclonal gammopathy (of undetermined significance) (D47.2)
               polyclonal hypergammaglobulinemia (D89.0)
               Waldenström's macroglobulinemia (C88.0)

     E88.01   **Alpha-1-antitrypsin deficiency**
         AAT deficiency

     E88.09   **Other disorders of plasma-protein metabolism, not elsewhere classified**
         Bisalbuminemia

E88.1   **Lipodystrophy, not elsewhere classified**
     Lipodystrophy NOS
     EXCLUDES1   *Whipple's disease (K90.81)*

E88.2   **Lipomatosis, not elsewhere classified**
     Lipomatosis NOS
     Lipomatosis (Check) dolorosa [Dercum]

E88.3   **Tumor lysis syndrome**
     Tumor lysis syndrome (spontaneous)
     Tumor lysis syndrome following antineoplastic drug chemotherapy
     Use additional code for adverse effect, if applicable, to identify drug (T45.1X5)

✓5th **E88.4**   **Mitochondrial metabolism disorders**
     EXCLUDES1   *disorders of pyruvate metabolism (E74.4)*
               Kearns-Sayre syndrome (H49.81)
               Leber's disease (H47.22)
               Leigh's encephalopathy (G31.82)
               Mitochondrial myopathy, NEC (G71.3)
               Reye's syndrome (G93.7)

     E88.40   **Mitochondrial metabolism disorder, unspecified**

     E88.41   **MELAS syndrome**
         Mitochondrial myopathy, encephalopathy, lactic acidosis and stroke-like episodes

     E88.42   **MERRF syndrome**
         Myoclonic epilepsy associated with ragged-red fibers
         Code also myoclonic epilepsy (G40.3-)

     E88.49   **Other mitochondrial metabolism disorders**

✓5th **E88.8**   **Other specified metabolic disorders**

     E88.81   **Metabolic syndrome**
         Dysmetabolic syndrome X
         Use additional codes for associated manifestations, such as:
         obesity (E66.-)

     E88.89   **Other specified metabolic disorders**
         Launois-Bensaude adenolipomatosis
         EXCLUDES1   *adult pulmonary Langerhans cell histiocytosis (J84.82)*

E88.9   **Metabolic disorder, unspecified**

EXCLUDES1 Not coded here   EXCLUDES2 Not included here   N Newborn Age: 0   P Pediatric Age: 0-17   M Maternity Age: 12-55   A Adult Age: 15-124

☑4ᵗʰ E89 Postprocedural endocrine and metabolic complications and disorders, not elsewhere classified

> EXCLUDES 2 *intraoperative complications of endocrine system organ or structure (E36.0-, E36.1-, E36.8)*

E89.0 Postprocedural hypothyroidism
Postirradiation hypothyroidism
Postsurgical hypothyroidism

E89.1 Postprocedural hypoinsulinemia
Postpancreatectomy hyperglycemia
Postsurgical hypoinsulinemia
Use additional code, if applicable, to identify:
acquired absence of pancreas (Z90.41-)
diabetes mellitus (postpancreatectomy) (postprocedural) (E13.-)
insulin use (Z79.4)

> EXCLUDES 1 *transient postprocedural hyperglycemia (R73.9)*
> *transient postprocedural hypoglycemia (E16.2)*

E89.2 Postprocedural hypoparathyroidism
Parathyroprival tetany

E89.3 Postprocedural hypopituitarism
Postirradiation hypopituitarism

☑5ᵗʰ E89.4 Postprocedural ovarian failure

E89.40 Asymptomatic postprocedural ovarian failure ♀
Postprocedural ovarian failure NOS

E89.41 Symptomatic postprocedural ovarian failure ♀
Symptoms such as flushing, sleeplessness, headache, lack of concentration, associated with postprocedural menopause

E89.5 Postprocedural testicular hypofunction ♂

E89.6 Postprocedural adrenocortical (-medullary) hypofunction

☑5ᵗʰ E89.8 Other postprocedural endocrine and metabolic complications and disorders

☑6ᵗʰ E89.81 Postprocedural hemorrhage and hematoma of an endocrine system organ or structure following a procedure

E89.810 Postprocedural hemorrhage and hematoma of an endocrine system organ or structure following an endocrine system procedure

E89.811 Postprocedural hemorrhage and hematoma of an endocrine system organ or structure following other procedure

E89.89 Other postprocedural endocrine and metabolic complications and disorders
Use additional code, if applicable, to further specify disorder

☑ Additional Character Required   ☑x7ᵗʰ Placeholder Alert   Unspecified Dx   Other Specified Dx   Manifestation   ►◄ Revised Text   ● New Code   ▲ Revised Code Title

ICD-10-CM 2016   503

Chapter 5. Mental, Behavioral and Neurodevelopmental Disorders

Chapter 5. Mental, Behavioral and Neurodevelopmental Disorders (F01–F99)

Chapter Specific Guidelines with Coding Examples

The chapter specific guidelines from the ICD-10-CM Official Guidelines for Coding and Reporting have been provided below. Along with these guidelines are coding examples, contained in the shaded boxes, that have been developed to help illustrate the coding and/or sequencing guidance found in these guidelines.

a. Pain disorders related to psychological factors

Assign code F45.41, for pain that is exclusively related to psychological disorders. As indicated by the Excludes 1 note under category G89, a code from category G89 should not be assigned with code F45.41.

> Perceived abdominal pain determined to be persistent somatoform pain disorder
>
> **F45.41   Pain disorder exclusively related to psychological factors**
>
> *Explanation*: This pain was diagnosed as being exclusively psychological; therefore, no code from category G89 is added.

Code F45.42, Pain disorders with related psychological factors, should be used with a code from category G89, Pain, not elsewhere classified, if there is documentation of a psychological component for a patient with acute or chronic pain.
See Section I.C.6. Pain

b. Mental and behavioral disorders due to psychoactive substance use

1) In remission

Selection of codes for "in remission" for categories F10-F19, Mental and behavioral disorders due to psychoactive substance use (categories F10-F19 with -.21) requires the provider's clinical judgment. The appropriate codes for "in remission" are assigned only on the basis of provider documentation (as defined in the Official Guidelines for Coding and Reporting).

> Medical history: Opioid dependence in remission
>
> **F11.21   Opioid dependence, in remission**
>
> *Explanation*: The "in remission" codes are assigned when the provider documents the remission.

2) Psychoactive substance use, abuse and dependence

When the provider documentation refers to use, abuse and dependence of the same substance (e.g. alcohol, opioid, cannabis, etc.), only one code should be assigned to identify the pattern of use based on the following hierarchy:

- If both use and abuse are documented, assign only the code for abuse
- If both abuse and dependence are documented, assign only the code for dependence
- If use, abuse and dependence are all documented, assign only the code for dependence
- If both use and dependence are documented, assign only the code for dependence.

> History and physical notes cannabis dependence; progress note says cannabis abuse
>
> **F12.20   Cannabis dependence, uncomplicated**
>
> *Explanation*: In the hierarchy, the dependence code is used if both abuse and dependence are documented.

> Discharge summary says cocaine abuse; progress notes list cocaine use
>
> **F14.10   Cocaine abuse, uncomplicated**
>
> *Explanation*: In the hierarchy, the abuse code is used if both abuse and use are documented.

3) Psychoactive Substance Use

As with all other diagnoses, the codes for psychoactive substance use (F10.9-, F11.9-, F12.9-, F13.9-, F14.9-, F15.9-, F16.9-) should only be assigned based on provider documentation and when they meet the definition of a reportable diagnosis (see Section III, Reporting Additional Diagnoses). The codes are to be used only when the psychoactive substance use is associated with a mental or behavioral disorder, and such a relationship is documented by the provider.

> ED reports that a 27-year-old female tripped and broke her right ankle. Her friends reported that they were drinking and dancing at a nightclub.
>
> **S82.891A   Other fracture of right lower leg, initial encounter for closed fracture**
>
> **W01.0XXA   Fall on same level from slipping, tripping and stumbling, initial encounter**
>
> **Y92.252   Music hall as the place of occurrence of the external cause**
>
> **Y93.41   Activity, dancing**
>
> *Explanation*: Note that no code was added for alcohol use or abuse. Unless it is specifically associated with a diagnosis by provider documentation and meets the definition of a reportable diagnosis, it is not assigned. However, if the documentation from the provider stated: "The patient tripped, fell and fractured her right ankle while dancing due to her elevated blood alcohol, consistent with her ongoing alcohol abuse," the following code would be added:
>
> **F10.10   Alcohol abuse, uncomplicated**

Chapter 5. Mental, Behavioral, and Neurodevelopmental Disorders (F01-F99)

> **INCLUDES**   disorders of psychological development
> **EXCLUDES 2**   *symptoms, signs and abnormal clinical laboratory findings, not elsewhere classified (R00-R99)*

This chapter contains the following blocks:

F01-F09	Mental disorders due to known physiological conditions
F10-F19	Mental and behavioral disorders due to psychoactive substance use
F20-F29	Schizophrenia, schizotypal, delusional, and other non-mood psychotic disorders
F30-F39	Mood [affective] disorders
F40-F48	Anxiety, dissociative, stress-related, somatoform and other nonpsychotic mental disorders
F50-F59	Behavioral syndromes associated with physiological disturbances and physical factors
F60-F69	Disorders of adult personality and behavior
F70-F79	Intellectual disabilities
F80-F89	Pervasive and specific developmental disorders
F90-F98	Behavioral and emotional disorders with onset usually occurring in childhood and adolescence
F99	Unspecified mental disorder

Mental disorders due to known physiological conditions (F01-F09)

> **NOTE**   This block comprises a range of mental disorders grouped together on the basis of their having in common a demonstrable etiology in cerebral disease, brain injury, or other insult leading to cerebral dysfunction. The dysfunction may be primary, as in diseases, injuries, and insults that affect the brain directly and selectively; or secondary, as in systemic diseases and disorders that attack the brain only as one of the multiple organs or systems of the body that are involved.

✓4ᵗʰ F01 Vascular dementia

Vascular dementia as a result of infarction of the brain due to vascular disease, including hypertensive cerebrovascular disease.
> **INCLUDES**   arteriosclerotic dementia

Code first the underlying physiological condition or sequelae of cerebrovascular disease.

✓5ᵗʰ F01.5 Vascular dementia

F01.50   **Vascular dementia** without behavioral disturbance   🅰

F01.51   **Vascular dementia** with behavioral disturbance   🅰
Vascular dementia with aggressive behavior
Vascular dementia with combative behavior
Vascular dementia with violent behavior
Use additional code, if applicable, to identify wandering in vascular dementia (Z91.83)

✓4ᵗʰ F02 Dementia in other diseases classified elsewhere

Code first the underlying physiological condition, such as:
Alzheimer's (G30.-)
cerebral lipidosis (E75.4)
Creutzfeldt-Jakob disease (A81.0-)
dementia with Lewy bodies (G31.83)
epilepsy and recurrent seizures (G40.-)
frontotemporal dementia (G31.09)
hepatolenticular degeneration (E83.0)
human immunodeficiency virus [HIV] disease (B20)
hypercalcemia (E83.52)
hypothyroidism, acquired (E00-E03.-)
intoxications (T36-T65)
Jakob-Creutzfeldt disease (A81.0-)
multiple sclerosis (G35)
neurosyphilis (A52.17)
niacin deficiency [pellagra] (E52)
Parkinson's disease (G20)
Pick's disease (G31.01)
polyarteritis nodosa (M30.0)
systemic lupus erythematosus (M32.-)
trypanosomiasis (B56.-, B57.-)
vitamin B deficiency (E53.8)
> **EXCLUDES 1**   *dementia with Parkinsonism (G31.83)*
> **EXCLUDES 2**   *dementia in alcohol and psychoactive substance disorders (F10-F19, with .17, .27, .97)*
> *vascular dementia (F01.5-)*

✓5ᵗʰ F02.8 Dementia in other diseases classified elsewhere

F02.80   *Dementia in other diseases classified elsewhere without behavioral disturbance*
Dementia in other diseases classified elsewhere NOS

F02.81   *Dementia in other diseases classified elsewhere with behavioral disturbance*
Dementia in other diseases classified elsewhere with aggressive behavior
Dementia in other diseases classified elsewhere with combative behavior
Dementia in other diseases classified elsewhere with violent behavior
Use additional code, if applicable, to identify wandering in dementia in conditions classified elsewhere (Z91.83)

✓4ᵗʰ F03 Unspecified dementia

Presenile dementia NOS
Presenile psychosis NOS
Primary degenerative dementia NOS
Senile dementia NOS
Senile dementia depressed or paranoid type
Senile psychosis NOS
> **EXCLUDES 1**   *senility NOS (R41.81)*
> **EXCLUDES 2**   *mild memory disturbance due to known physiological condition (F06.8)*
> *senile dementia with delirium or acute confusional state (F05)*

✓5ᵗʰ F03.9 Unspecified dementia

F03.90   **Unspecified dementia** without behavioral disturbance   🅰
Dementia NOS
AHA: 2012, 4Q, 92

F03.91   **Unspecified dementia** with behavioral disturbance   🅰
Unspecified dementia with aggressive behavior
Unspecified dementia with combative behavior
Unspecified dementia with violent behavior
Use additional code, if applicable, to identify wandering in unspecified dementia (Z91.83)

F04 Amnestic disorder due to known physiological condition

Korsakov's psychosis or syndrome, nonalcoholic
Code first the underlying physiological condition
> **EXCLUDES 1**   *amnesia NOS (R41.3)*
> *anterograde amnesia (R41.1)*
> *dissociative amnesia (F44.0)*
> *retrograde amnesia (R41.2)*
> **EXCLUDES 2**   *alcohol-induced or unspecified Korsakov's syndrome (F10.26, F10.96)*
> *Korsakov's syndrome induced by other psychoactive substances (F13.26, F13.96, F19.16, F19.26, F19.96)*

F05 Delirium due to known physiological condition

Acute or subacute brain syndrome
Acute or subacute confusional state (nonalcoholic)
Acute or subacute infective psychosis
Acute or subacute organic reaction
Acute or subacute psycho-organic syndrome
Delirium of mixed etiology
Delirium superimposed on dementia
Sundowning
Code first the underlying physiological condition
> **EXCLUDES 1**   *delirium NOS (R41.0)*
> **EXCLUDES 2**   *delirium tremens alcohol-induced or unspecified (F10.231, F10.921)*

✓4ᵗʰ F06 Other mental disorders due to known physiological condition

> **INCLUDES**   mental disorders due to endocrine disorder
> mental disorders due to exogenous hormone
> mental disorders due to exogenous toxic substance
> mental disorders due to primary cerebral disease
> mental disorders due to somatic illness
> mental disorders due to systemic disease affecting the brain

Code first the underlying physiological condition
> **EXCLUDES 1**   *unspecified dementia (F03)*
> **EXCLUDES 2**   *delirium due to known physiological condition (F05)*
> *dementia as classified in F01-F02*
> *other mental disorders associated with alcohol and other psychoactive substances (F10-F19)*

F06.0   **Psychotic disorder** with hallucinations **due to known physiological condition**
Organic hallucinatory state (nonalcoholic)
> **EXCLUDES 2**   *hallucinations and perceptual disturbance induced by alcohol and other psychoactive substances (F10-F19 with .151, .251, .951)*
> *schizophrenia (F20.-)*

☑ Additional Character Required   ✓7ᵗʰ Placeholder Alert   Unspecified Dx   Other Specified Dx   Manifestation   ▶◀ Revised Text   ● New Code   ▲ Revised Code Title

Chapter 5. Mental, Behavioral and Neurodevelopmental Disorders

F06.1   Catatonic disorder due to known physiological condition
> *EXCLUDES 1*   catatonic stupor (R40.1)
> stupor NOS (R40.1)
> *EXCLUDES 2*   catatonic schizophrenia (F20.2)
> dissociative stupor (F44.2)

F06.2   Psychotic disorder with delusions due to known physiological condition
Paranoid and paranoid-hallucinatory organic states
Schizophrenia-like psychosis in epilepsy
> *EXCLUDES 2*   alcohol and drug-induced psychotic disorder (F10-F19
> with .150, .250, .950)
> brief psychotic disorder (F23)
> delusional disorder (F22)
> schizophrenia (F20.-)

√5ᵗʰ F06.3   Mood disorder due to known physiological condition
> *EXCLUDES 2*   mood disorders due to alcohol and other psychoactive
> substances (F10-F19 with .14, .24, .94)
> mood disorders, not due to known physiological
> condition or unspecified (F30-F39)

    F06.30   Mood disorder due to known physiological condition, unspecified

    F06.31   Mood disorder due to known physiological condition with depressive features

    F06.32   Mood disorder due to known physiological condition with major depressive-like episode

    F06.33   Mood disorder due to known physiological condition with manic features

    F06.34   Mood disorder due to known physiological condition with mixed features

F06.4   Anxiety disorder due to known physiological condition
> *EXCLUDES 2*   anxiety disorders due to alcohol and other psychoactive
> substances (F10-F19 with .180, .280, .980)
> anxiety disorders, not due to known physiological
> condition or unspecified (F40.-, F41.-)

F06.8   Other specified mental disorders due to known physiological condition
Epileptic psychosis NOS
Organic dissociative disorder
Organic emotionally labile [asthenic] disorder

√4ᵗʰ F07   Personality and behavioral disorders due to known physiological condition
Code first the underlying physiological condition

F07.0   Personality change due to known physiological condition
Frontal lobe syndrome
Limbic epilepsy personality syndrome
Lobotomy syndrome
Organic personality disorder
Organic pseudopsychopathic personality
Organic pseudoretarded personality
Postleucotomy syndrome
Code first underlying physiological condition
> *EXCLUDES 1*   mild cognitive impairment (G31.84)
> postconcussional syndrome (F07.81)
> postencephalitic syndrome (F07.89)
> signs and symptoms involving emotional state (R45.-)
> *EXCLUDES 2*   specific personality disorder (F60.-)

√5ᵗʰ F07.8   Other personality and behavioral disorders due to known physiological condition

    F07.81   Postconcussional syndrome
Postcontusional syndrome (encephalopathy)
Post-traumatic brain syndrome, nonpsychotic
Use additional code to identify associated
post-traumatic headache, if applicable (G44.3-)
> *EXCLUDES 1*   current concussion (brain) (S06.0-)
> postencephalitic syndrome (F07.89)

    F07.89   Other personality and behavioral disorders due to known physiological condition
Postencephalitic syndrome
Right hemispheric organic affective disorder

F07.9   Unspecified personality and behavioral disorder due to known physiological condition
Organic psychosyndrome

F09   Unspecified mental disorder due to known physiological condition
Mental disorder NOS due to known physiological condition
Organic brain syndrome NOS
Organic mental disorder NOS
Organic psychosis NOS
Symptomatic psychosis NOS
Code first the underlying physiological condition
> *EXCLUDES 1*   psychosis NOS (F29)

Mental and behavioral disorders due to psychoactive substance use (F10-F19)

√4ᵗʰ F10   Alcohol related disorders
Use additional code for blood alcohol level, if applicable (Y90.-)

√5ᵗʰ F10.1   Alcohol abuse
> *EXCLUDES 1*   alcohol dependence (F10.2-)
> alcohol use, unspecified (F10.9-)

    F10.10   Alcohol abuse, uncomplicated

    √6ᵗʰ F10.12   Alcohol abuse with intoxication

        F10.120   Alcohol abuse with intoxication, uncomplicated

        F10.121   Alcohol abuse with intoxication delirium

        F10.129   Alcohol abuse with intoxication, unspecified

    F10.14   Alcohol abuse with alcohol-induced mood disorder

    √6ᵗʰ F10.15   Alcohol abuse with alcohol-induced psychotic disorder

        F10.150   Alcohol abuse with alcohol-induced psychotic disorder with delusions

        F10.151   Alcohol abuse with alcohol-induced psychotic disorder with hallucinations

        F10.159   Alcohol abuse with alcohol-induced psychotic disorder, unspecified

    √6ᵗʰ F10.18   Alcohol abuse with other alcohol-induced disorders

        F10.180   Alcohol abuse with alcohol-induced anxiety disorder

        F10.181   Alcohol abuse with alcohol-induced sexual dysfunction

        F10.182   Alcohol abuse with alcohol-induced sleep disorder

        F10.188   Alcohol abuse with other alcohol-induced disorder

    F10.19   Alcohol abuse with unspecified alcohol-induced disorder

√5ᵗʰ F10.2   Alcohol dependence
> *EXCLUDES 1*   alcohol abuse (F10.1-)
> alcohol use, unspecified (F10.9-)
> *EXCLUDES 2*   toxic effect of alcohol (T51.0-)

    F10.20   Alcohol dependence, uncomplicated

    F10.21   Alcohol dependence, in remission

    √6ᵗʰ F10.22   Alcohol dependence with intoxication
Acute drunkenness (in alcoholism)
> *EXCLUDES 1*   alcohol dependence with withdrawal
> (F10.23-)

        F10.220   Alcohol dependence with intoxication, uncomplicated

        F10.221   Alcohol dependence with intoxication delirium

        F10.229   Alcohol dependence with intoxication, unspecified

    √6ᵗʰ F10.23   Alcohol dependence with withdrawal
> *EXCLUDES 1*   Alcohol dependence with intoxication
> (F10.22-)

        F10.230   Alcohol dependence with withdrawal, uncomplicated

        F10.231   Alcohol dependence with withdrawal delirium

        F10.232   Alcohol dependence with withdrawal with perceptual disturbance

        F10.239   Alcohol dependence with withdrawal, unspecified

    F10.24   Alcohol dependence with alcohol-induced mood disorder

    √6ᵗʰ F10.25   Alcohol dependence with alcohol-induced psychotic disorder

        F10.250   Alcohol dependence with alcohol-induced psychotic disorder with delusions

        F10.251   Alcohol dependence with alcohol-induced psychotic disorder with hallucinations

        F10.259   Alcohol dependence with alcohol-induced psychotic disorder, unspecified

    F10.26   Alcohol dependence with alcohol-induced persisting amnestic disorder

    F10.27   Alcohol dependence with alcohol-induced persisting dementia

---

EXCLUDES 1 Not coded here   *EXCLUDES 2* Not included here   **N** Newborn Age: 0   **P** Pediatric Age: 0-17   **M** Maternity Age: 12-55   **A** Adult Age: 15-124

☑6ᵗʰ **F10.28 Alcohol dependence with** other **alcohol-induced disorders**

     F10.280 Alcohol dependence with alcohol-induced anxiety disorder

     F10.281 Alcohol dependence with alcohol-induced sexual dysfunction

     F10.282 Alcohol dependence with alcohol-induced sleep disorder

     F10.288 Alcohol dependence with other alcohol-induced disorder

   F10.29 Alcohol dependence with unspecified alcohol-induced disorder

☑5ᵗʰ **F10.9 Alcohol** use, unspecified

     EXCLUDES 1   *alcohol abuse (F10.1-)*
                 alcohol dependence (F10.2-)

   ☑6ᵗʰ **F10.92 Alcohol use, unspecified with** intoxication

     F10.920 Alcohol use, unspecified with intoxication, uncomplicated

     F10.921 Alcohol use, unspecified with intoxication delirium

     F10.929 Alcohol use, unspecified with intoxication, unspecified

   F10.94 Alcohol use, unspecified with alcohol-induced mood disorder

   ☑6ᵗʰ **F10.95 Alcohol use, unspecified with alcohol-induced** psychotic disorder

     F10.950 Alcohol use, unspecified with alcohol-induced psychotic disorder with delusions

     F10.951 Alcohol use, unspecified with alcohol-induced psychotic disorder with hallucinations

     F10.959 Alcohol use, unspecified with alcohol-induced psychotic disorder, unspecified

   F10.96 Alcohol use, unspecified with alcohol-induced persisting amnestic disorder

   F10.97 Alcohol use, unspecified with alcohol-induced persisting dementia

   ☑6ᵗʰ **F10.98 Alcohol use,** unspecified **with other alcohol-induced disorders**

     F10.980 Alcohol use, unspecified with alcohol-induced anxiety disorder

     F10.981 Alcohol use, unspecified with alcohol-induced sexual dysfunction

     F10.982 Alcohol use, unspecified with alcohol-induced sleep disorder

     F10.988 Alcohol use, unspecified with other alcohol-induced disorder

   F10.99 Alcohol use, unspecified with unspecified alcohol-induced disorder

☑4ᵗʰ **F11 Opioid** related disorders

   ☑5ᵗʰ **F11.1 Opioid** abuse

     EXCLUDES 1   *opioid dependence (F11.2-)*
                 opioid use, unspecified (F11.9-)

   F11.10 Opioid abuse, uncomplicated

   ☑6ᵗʰ **F11.12 Opioid abuse with** intoxication

     F11.120 Opioid abuse with intoxication, uncomplicated

     F11.121 Opioid abuse with intoxication delirium

     F11.122 Opioid abuse with intoxication with perceptual disturbance

     F11.129 Opioid abuse with intoxication, unspecified

   F11.14 Opioid abuse with opioid-induced mood disorder

   ☑6ᵗʰ **F11.15 Opioid abuse with opioid-induced** psychotic disorder

     F11.150 Opioid abuse with opioid-induced psychotic disorder with delusions

     F11.151 Opioid abuse with opioid-induced psychotic disorder with hallucinations

     F11.159 Opioid abuse with opioid-induced psychotic disorder, unspecified

   ☑6ᵗʰ **F11.18 Opioid abuse with** other **opioid-induced disorder**

     F11.181 Opioid abuse with opioid-induced sexual dysfunction

     F11.182 Opioid abuse with opioid-induced sleep disorder

     F11.188 Opioid abuse with other opioid-induced disorder

   F11.19 Opioid abuse with unspecified opioid-induced disorder

☑5ᵗʰ **F11.2 Opioid** dependence

     EXCLUDES 1   *opioid abuse (F11.1-)*
                 opioid use, unspecified (F11.9-)
     EXCLUDES 2   *opioid poisoning (T40.0-T40.2-)*

   F11.20 Opioid dependence, uncomplicated

   F11.21 Opioid dependence, in remission

   ☑6ᵗʰ **F11.22 Opioid dependence with** intoxication

     EXCLUDES 1   *opioid dependence with withdrawal (F11.23)*

     F11.220 Opioid dependence with intoxication, uncomplicated

     F11.221 Opioid dependence with intoxication delirium

     F11.222 Opioid dependence with intoxication with perceptual disturbance

     F11.229 Opioid dependence with intoxication, unspecified

   F11.23 Opioid dependence with withdrawal

     EXCLUDES 1   *opioid dependence with intoxication (F11.22-)*

   F11.24 Opioid dependence with opioid-induced mood disorder

   ☑6ᵗʰ **F11.25 Opioid dependence with opioid-induced** psychotic disorder

     F11.250 Opioid dependence with opioid-induced psychotic disorder with delusions

     F11.251 Opioid dependence with opioid-induced psychotic disorder with hallucinations

     F11.259 Opioid dependence with opioid-induced psychotic disorder, unspecified

   ☑6ᵗʰ **F11.28 Opioid dependence with** other **opioid-induced disorder**

     F11.281 Opioid dependence with opioid-induced sexual dysfunction

     F11.282 Opioid dependence with opioid-induced sleep disorder

     F11.288 Opioid dependence with other opioid-induced disorder

   F11.29 Opioid dependence with unspecified opioid-induced disorder

☑5ᵗʰ **F11.9 Opioid use,** unspecified

     EXCLUDES 1   *opioid abuse (F11.1-)*
                 opioid dependence (F11.2-)

   F11.90 Opioid use, unspecified, uncomplicated

   ☑6ᵗʰ **F11.92 Opioid use, unspecified with** intoxication

     EXCLUDES 1   *opioid use, unspecified with withdrawal (F11.93)*

     F11.920 Opioid use, unspecified with intoxication, uncomplicated

     F11.921 Opioid use, unspecified with intoxication delirium

     F11.922 Opioid use, unspecified with intoxication with perceptual disturbance

     F11.929 Opioid use, unspecified with intoxication, unspecified

   F11.93 Opioid use, unspecified with withdrawal

     EXCLUDES 1   *opioid use, unspecified with intoxication (F11.92-)*

   F11.94 Opioid use, unspecified with opioid-induced mood disorder

   ☑6ᵗʰ **F11.95 Opioid use, unspecified with opioid-induced** psychotic disorder

     F11.950 Opioid use, unspecified with opioid-induced psychotic disorder with delusions

     F11.951 Opioid use, unspecified with opioid-induced psychotic disorder with hallucinations

     F11.959 Opioid use, unspecified with opioid-induced psychotic disorder, unspecified

---

☑ Additional Character Required   ✓×7ᵗʰ Placeholder Alert   Unspecified Dx   Other Specified Dx   Manifestation   ▶◀ Revised Text   ● New Code   ▲ Revised Code Title

✓6ᵗʰ **F11.98** **Opioid use, unspecified with** other **specified opioid-induced disorder**

     F11.981 **Opioid use, unspecified with opioid-induced** sexual dysfunction

     F11.982 **Opioid use, unspecified with opioid-induced** sleep disorder

     F11.988 **Opioid use, unspecified with other opioid-induced disorder**

     F11.99 **Opioid use, unspecified with unspecified opioid-induced disorder**

✓4ᵗʰ **F12** **Cannabis related disorders**

     INCLUDES   marijuana

✓5ᵗʰ **F12.1** **Cannabis abuse**

     EXCLUDES 1   cannabis dependence (F12.2-)
                cannabis use, unspecified (F12.9-)

     F12.10 **Cannabis abuse,** uncomplicated

✓6ᵗʰ **F12.12** **Cannabis abuse with** intoxication

     F12.120 **Cannabis abuse with intoxication,** uncomplicated

     F12.121 **Cannabis abuse with intoxication** delirium

     F12.122 **Cannabis abuse with intoxication with** perceptual disturbance

     F12.129 **Cannabis abuse with intoxication, unspecified**

✓6ᵗʰ **F12.15** **Cannabis abuse with** psychotic disorder

     F12.150 **Cannabis abuse with psychotic disorder with** delusions

     F12.151 **Cannabis abuse with psychotic disorder with** hallucinations

     F12.159 **Cannabis abuse with psychotic disorder, unspecified**

✓6ᵗʰ **F12.18** **Cannabis abuse with** other **cannabis-induced disorder**

     F12.180 **Cannabis abuse with cannabis-induced** anxiety disorder

     F12.188 **Cannabis abuse with other cannabis-induced disorder**

     F12.19 **Cannabis abuse with unspecified cannabis-induced disorder**

✓5ᵗʰ **F12.2** **Cannabis dependence**

     EXCLUDES 1   cannabis abuse (F12.1-)
                cannabis use, unspecified (F12.9-)
     EXCLUDES 2   cannabis poisoning (T40.7-)

     F12.20 **Cannabis dependence,** uncomplicated

     F12.21 **Cannabis dependence,** in remission

✓6ᵗʰ **F12.22** **Cannabis dependence with** intoxication

     F12.220 **Cannabis dependence with intoxication,** uncomplicated

     F12.221 **Cannabis dependence with intoxication delirium**

     F12.222 **Cannabis dependence with intoxication with** perceptual disturbance

     F12.229 **Cannabis dependence with intoxication, unspecified**

✓6ᵗʰ **F12.25** **Cannabis dependence with** psychotic disorder

     F12.250 **Cannabis dependence with psychotic disorder with** delusions

     F12.251 **Cannabis dependence with psychotic disorder with** hallucinations

     F12.259 **Cannabis dependence with psychotic disorder, unspecified**

✓6ᵗʰ **F12.28** **Cannabis dependence with** other **cannabis-induced disorder**

     F12.280 **Cannabis dependence with cannabis-induced** anxiety disorder

     F12.288 **Cannabis dependence with other cannabis-induced disorder**

     F12.29 **Cannabis dependence with unspecified cannabis-induced disorder**

✓5ᵗʰ **F12.9** **Cannabis use,** unspecified

     EXCLUDES 1   cannabis abuse (F12.1-)
                cannabis dependence (F12.2-)

     F12.90 **Cannabis use, unspecified,** uncomplicated

✓6ᵗʰ **F12.92** **Cannabis use, unspecified with** intoxication

     F12.920 **Cannabis use, unspecified with intoxication,** uncomplicated

     F12.921 **Cannabis use, unspecified with intoxication** delirium

     F12.922 **Cannabis use, unspecified with intoxication with** perceptual disturbance

     F12.929 **Cannabis use, unspecified with intoxication, unspecified**

✓6ᵗʰ **F12.95** **Cannabis use, unspecified with** psychotic disorder

     F12.950 **Cannabis use, unspecified with psychotic disorder with** delusions

     F12.951 **Cannabis use, unspecified with psychotic disorder with** hallucinations

     F12.959 **Cannabis use, unspecified with psychotic disorder, unspecified**

✓6ᵗʰ **F12.98** **Cannabis use, unspecified with** other **cannabis-induced disorder**

     F12.980 **Cannabis use, unspecified with** anxiety disorder

     F12.988 **Cannabis use, unspecified with other cannabis-induced disorder**

     F12.99 **Cannabis use, unspecified with unspecified cannabis-induced disorder**

✓4ᵗʰ **F13** **Sedative, hypnotic, or anxiolytic related disorders**

✓5ᵗʰ **F13.1** **Sedative, hypnotic or anxiolytic-related** abuse

     EXCLUDES 1   sedative, hypnotic or anxiolytic-related dependence (F13.2-)
                sedative, hypnotic, or anxiolytic use, unspecified (F13.9-)

     F13.10 **Sedative, hypnotic or anxiolytic abuse,** uncomplicated

✓6ᵗʰ **F13.12** **Sedative, hypnotic or anxiolytic abuse with** intoxication

     F13.120 **Sedative, hypnotic or anxiolytic abuse with intoxication,** uncomplicated

     F13.121 **Sedative, hypnotic or anxiolytic abuse with intoxication** delirium

     F13.129 **Sedative, hypnotic or anxiolytic abuse with intoxication, unspecified**

     F13.14 **Sedative, hypnotic or anxiolytic abuse with sedative, hypnotic or anxiolytic-induced** mood disorder

✓6ᵗʰ **F13.15** **Sedative, hypnotic or anxiolytic abuse with sedative, hypnotic or anxiolytic-induced** psychotic disorder

     F13.150 **Sedative, hypnotic or anxiolytic abuse with sedative, hypnotic or anxiolytic-induced psychotic disorder with** delusions

     F13.151 **Sedative, hypnotic or anxiolytic abuse with sedative, hypnotic or anxiolytic-induced psychotic disorder with** hallucinations

     F13.159 **Sedative, hypnotic or anxiolytic abuse with sedative, hypnotic or anxiolytic-induced psychotic disorder, unspecified**

✓6ᵗʰ **F13.18** **Sedative, hypnotic or anxiolytic abuse with** other **sedative, hypnotic or anxiolytic-induced disorders**

     F13.180 **Sedative, hypnotic or anxiolytic abuse with sedative, hypnotic or anxiolytic-induced** anxiety disorder

     F13.181 **Sedative, hypnotic or anxiolytic abuse with sedative, hypnotic or anxiolytic-induced** sexual dysfunction

     F13.182 **Sedative, hypnotic or anxiolytic abuse with sedative, hypnotic or anxiolytic-induced** sleep disorder

     F13.188 **Sedative, hypnotic or anxiolytic abuse with other sedative, hypnotic or anxiolytic-induced disorder**

     F13.19 **Sedative, hypnotic or anxiolytic abuse with unspecified sedative, hypnotic or anxiolytic-induced disorder**

✓5ᵗʰ **F13.2** **Sedative, hypnotic or anxiolytic-related** dependence

     EXCLUDES 1   sedative, hypnotic or anxiolytic-related abuse (F13.1-)
                sedative, hypnotic, or anxiolytic use, unspecified (F13.9-)
     EXCLUDES 2   sedative, hypnotic, or anxiolytic poisoning (T42.-)

     F13.20 **Sedative, hypnotic or anxiolytic dependence,** uncomplicated

     F13.21 **Sedative, hypnotic or anxiolytic dependence,** in remission

---

EXCLUDES 1 Not coded here   EXCLUDES 2 Not included here   N Newborn Age: 0   P Pediatric Age: 0-17   M Maternity Age: 12-55   A Adult Age: 15-124

508   ICD-10-CM 2016

✓6ᵗʰ **F13.22** **Sedative, hypnotic or anxiolytic dependence with intoxication**
> EXCLUDES 1   *sedative, hypnotic or anxiolytic dependence with withdrawal (F13.23-)*

    F13.220 **Sedative, hypnotic or anxiolytic dependence with intoxication, uncomplicated**

    F13.221 **Sedative, hypnotic or anxiolytic dependence with intoxication** delirium

    F13.229 **Sedative, hypnotic or anxiolytic dependence with intoxication, unspecified**

✓6ᵗʰ **F13.23** **Sedative, hypnotic or anxiolytic dependence with withdrawal**
> EXCLUDES 1   *sedative, hypnotic or anxiolytic dependence with intoxication (F13.22-)*

    F13.230 **Sedative, hypnotic or anxiolytic dependence with withdrawal, uncomplicated**

    F13.231 **Sedative, hypnotic or anxiolytic dependence with withdrawal** delirium

    F13.232 **Sedative, hypnotic or anxiolytic dependence with withdrawal with perceptual disturbance**

    F13.239 **Sedative, hypnotic or anxiolytic dependence with withdrawal, unspecified**

F13.24 **Sedative, hypnotic or anxiolytic dependence with sedative, hypnotic or anxiolytic-induced** mood disorder

✓6ᵗʰ **F13.25** **Sedative, hypnotic or anxiolytic dependence with sedative, hypnotic or anxiolytic-induced** psychotic disorder

    F13.250 **Sedative, hypnotic or anxiolytic dependence with sedative, hypnotic or anxiolytic-induced psychotic disorder with** delusions

    F13.251 **Sedative, hypnotic or anxiolytic dependence with sedative, hypnotic or anxiolytic-induced psychotic disorder with** hallucinations

    F13.259 **Sedative, hypnotic or anxiolytic dependence with sedative, hypnotic or anxiolytic-induced psychotic disorder, unspecified**

F13.26 **Sedative, hypnotic or anxiolytic dependence with sedative, hypnotic or anxiolytic-induced** persisting amnestic disorder

F13.27 **Sedative, hypnotic or anxiolytic dependence with sedative, hypnotic or anxiolytic-induced** persisting dementia

✓6ᵗʰ **F13.28** **Sedative, hypnotic or anxiolytic dependence with** other **sedative, hypnotic or anxiolytic-induced disorders**

    F13.280 **Sedative, hypnotic or anxiolytic dependence with sedative, hypnotic or anxiolytic-induced** anxiety disorder

    F13.281 **Sedative, hypnotic or anxiolytic dependence with sedative, hypnotic or anxiolytic-induced** sexual dysfunction

    F13.282 **Sedative, hypnotic or anxiolytic dependence with sedative, hypnotic or anxiolytic-induced** sleep disorder

    F13.288 **Sedative, hypnotic or anxiolytic dependence with other sedative, hypnotic or anxiolytic-induced disorder**

F13.29 **Sedative, hypnotic or anxiolytic dependence with unspecified sedative, hypnotic or anxiolytic-induced disorder**

✓5ᵗʰ **F13.9** **Sedative, hypnotic or anxiolytic-related use,** unspecified
> EXCLUDES 1   *sedative, hypnotic or anxiolytic-related abuse (F13.1-)*
> *sedative, hypnotic or anxiolytic-related dependence (F13.2-)*

    F13.90 **Sedative, hypnotic, or anxiolytic use, unspecified, uncomplicated**

✓6ᵗʰ **F13.92** **Sedative, hypnotic or anxiolytic use, unspecified with** intoxication
> EXCLUDES 1   *sedative, hypnotic or anxiolytic use, unspecified with withdrawal (F13.93-)*

    F13.920 **Sedative, hypnotic or anxiolytic use, unspecified with intoxication, uncomplicated**

    F13.921 **Sedative, hypnotic or anxiolytic use, unspecified with intoxication** delirium

    F13.929 **Sedative, hypnotic or anxiolytic use, unspecified with intoxication, unspecified**

✓6ᵗʰ **F13.93** **Sedative, hypnotic or anxiolytic use, unspecified with** withdrawal
> EXCLUDES 1   *sedative, hypnotic or anxiolytic use, unspecified with intoxication (F13.92-)*

    F13.930 **Sedative, hypnotic or anxiolytic use, unspecified with withdrawal, uncomplicated**

    F13.931 **Sedative, hypnotic or anxiolytic use, unspecified with withdrawal** delirium

    F13.932 **Sedative, hypnotic or anxiolytic use, unspecified with withdrawal with** perceptual disturbances

    F13.939 **Sedative, hypnotic or anxiolytic use, unspecified with withdrawal, unspecified**

F13.94 **Sedative, hypnotic or anxiolytic use, unspecified with sedative, hypnotic or anxiolytic-induced** mood disorder

✓6ᵗʰ **F13.95** **Sedative, hypnotic or anxiolytic use, unspecified with sedative, hypnotic or anxiolytic-induced** psychotic disorder

    F13.950 **Sedative, hypnotic or anxiolytic use, unspecified with sedative, hypnotic or anxiolytic-induced psychotic disorder with** delusions

    F13.951 **Sedative, hypnotic or anxiolytic use, unspecified with sedative, hypnotic or anxiolytic-induced psychotic disorder with** hallucinations

    F13.959 **Sedative, hypnotic or anxiolytic use, unspecified with sedative, hypnotic or anxiolytic-induced psychotic disorder, unspecified**

F13.96 **Sedative, hypnotic or anxiolytic use, unspecified with sedative, hypnotic or anxiolytic-induced** persisting amnestic disorder

F13.97 **Sedative, hypnotic or anxiolytic use, unspecified with sedative, hypnotic or anxiolytic-induced** persisting dementia

✓6ᵗʰ **F13.98** **Sedative, hypnotic or anxiolytic use, unspecified with** other **sedative, hypnotic or anxiolytic-induced disorders**

    F13.980 **Sedative, hypnotic or anxiolytic use, unspecified with sedative, hypnotic or anxiolytic-induced** anxiety disorder

    F13.981 **Sedative, hypnotic or anxiolytic use, unspecified with sedative, hypnotic or anxiolytic-induced** sexual dysfunction

    F13.982 **Sedative, hypnotic or anxiolytic use, unspecified with sedative, hypnotic or anxiolytic-induced** sleep disorder

    F13.988 **Sedative, hypnotic or anxiolytic use, unspecified with other sedative, hypnotic or anxiolytic-induced disorder**

F13.99 **Sedative, hypnotic or anxiolytic use, unspecified with unspecified sedative, hypnotic or anxiolytic-induced disorder**

✓4ᵗʰ **F14** **Cocaine related disorders**
> EXCLUDES 2   *other stimulant-related disorders (F15.-)*

✓5ᵗʰ **F14.1** **Cocaine** abuse
> EXCLUDES 1   *cocaine dependence (F14.2-)*
> *cocaine use, unspecified (F14.9-)*

    F14.10 **Cocaine abuse,** uncomplicated

✓6ᵗʰ **F14.12** **Cocaine abuse with** intoxication

    F14.120 **Cocaine abuse with intoxication, uncomplicated**

    F14.121 **Cocaine abuse with intoxication with** delirium

---

☑ Additional Character Required   ✓x7ᵗʰ Placeholder Alert   Unspecified Dx   Other Specified Dx   Manifestation   ▶◀ Revised Text   ● New Code   ▲ Revised Code Title

F14.122 Cocaine abuse with intoxication with perceptual disturbance

F14.129 Cocaine abuse with intoxication, unspecified

F14.14 Cocaine abuse with cocaine-induced mood disorder

√6th F14.15 Cocaine abuse with cocaine-induced psychotic disorder

F14.150 Cocaine abuse with cocaine-induced psychotic disorder with delusions

F14.151 Cocaine abuse with cocaine-induced psychotic disorder with hallucinations

F14.159 Cocaine abuse with cocaine-induced psychotic disorder, unspecified

√6th F14.18 Cocaine abuse with other cocaine-induced disorder

F14.180 Cocaine abuse with cocaine-induced anxiety disorder

F14.181 Cocaine abuse with cocaine-induced sexual dysfunction

F14.182 Cocaine abuse with cocaine-induced sleep disorder

F14.188 Cocaine abuse with other cocaine-induced disorder

F14.19 Cocaine abuse with unspecified cocaine-induced disorder

√5th F14.2 Cocaine dependence

EXCLUDES 1   cocaine abuse (F14.1-)
cocaine use, unspecified (F14.9-)
EXCLUDES 2   cocaine poisoning (T40.5-)

F14.20 Cocaine dependence, uncomplicated

F14.21 Cocaine dependence, in remission

√6th F14.22 Cocaine dependence with intoxication

EXCLUDES 1   cocaine dependence with withdrawal (F14.23)

F14.220 Cocaine dependence with intoxication, uncomplicated

F14.221 Cocaine dependence with intoxication delirium

F14.222 Cocaine dependence with intoxication with perceptual disturbance

F14.229 Cocaine dependence with intoxication, unspecified

F14.23 Cocaine dependence with withdrawal

EXCLUDES 1   cocaine dependence with intoxication (F14.22-)

F14.24 Cocaine dependence with cocaine-induced mood disorder

√6th F14.25 Cocaine dependence with cocaine-induced psychotic disorder

F14.250 Cocaine dependence with cocaine-induced psychotic disorder with delusions

F14.251 Cocaine dependence with cocaine-induced psychotic disorder with hallucinations

F14.259 Cocaine dependence with cocaine-induced psychotic disorder, unspecified

√6th F14.28 Cocaine dependence with other cocaine-induced disorder

F14.280 Cocaine dependence with cocaine-induced anxiety disorder

F14.281 Cocaine dependence with cocaine-induced sexual dysfunction

F14.282 Cocaine dependence with cocaine-induced sleep disorder

F14.288 Cocaine dependence with other cocaine-induced disorder

F14.29 Cocaine dependence with unspecified cocaine-induced disorder

√5th F14.9 Cocaine use, unspecified

EXCLUDES 1   cocaine abuse (F14.1-)
cocaine dependence (F14.2-)

F14.90 Cocaine use, unspecified, uncomplicated

√6th F14.92 Cocaine use, unspecified with intoxication

F14.920 Cocaine use, unspecified with intoxication, uncomplicated

F14.921 Cocaine use, unspecified with intoxication delirium

F14.922 Cocaine use, unspecified with intoxication with perceptual disturbance

F14.929 Cocaine use, unspecified with intoxication, unspecified

F14.94 Cocaine use, unspecified with cocaine-induced mood disorder

√6th F14.95 Cocaine use, unspecified with cocaine-induced psychotic disorder

F14.950 Cocaine use, unspecified with cocaine-induced psychotic disorder with delusions

F14.951 Cocaine use, unspecified with cocaine-induced psychotic disorder with hallucinations

F14.959 Cocaine use, unspecified with cocaine-induced psychotic disorder, unspecified

√6th F14.98 Cocaine use, unspecified with other specified cocaine-induced disorder

F14.980 Cocaine use, unspecified with cocaine-induced anxiety disorder

F14.981 Cocaine use, unspecified with cocaine-induced sexual dysfunction

F14.982 Cocaine use, unspecified with cocaine-induced sleep disorder

F14.988 Cocaine use, unspecified with other cocaine-induced disorder

F14.99 Cocaine use, unspecified with unspecified cocaine-induced disorder

√4th F15 Other stimulant related disorders

INCLUDES   amphetamine-related disorders
caffeine
EXCLUDES 2   cocaine-related disorders (F14.-)

√5th F15.1 Other stimulant abuse

EXCLUDES 1   other stimulant dependence (F15.2-)
other stimulant use, unspecified (F15.9-)

F15.10 Other stimulant abuse, uncomplicated

√6th F15.12 Other stimulant abuse with intoxication

F15.120 Other stimulant abuse with intoxication, uncomplicated

F15.121 Other stimulant abuse with intoxication delirium

F15.122 Other stimulant abuse with intoxication with perceptual disturbance

F15.129 Other stimulant abuse with intoxication, unspecified

F15.14 Other stimulant abuse with stimulant-induced mood disorder

√6th F15.15 Other stimulant abuse with stimulant-induced psychotic disorder

F15.150 Other stimulant abuse with stimulant-induced psychotic disorder with delusions

F15.151 Other stimulant abuse with stimulant-induced psychotic disorder with hallucinations

F15.159 Other stimulant abuse with stimulant-induced psychotic disorder, unspecified

√6th F15.18 Other stimulant abuse with other stimulant-induced disorder

F15.180 Other stimulant abuse with stimulant-induced anxiety disorder

F15.181 Other stimulant abuse with stimulant-induced sexual dysfunction

F15.182 Other stimulant abuse with stimulant-induced sleep disorder

F15.188 Other stimulant abuse with other stimulant-induced disorder

F15.19 Other stimulant abuse with unspecified stimulant-induced disorder

√5th F15.2 Other stimulant dependence

EXCLUDES 1   other stimulant abuse (F15.1-)
other stimulant use, unspecified (F15.9-)

F15.20 Other stimulant dependence, uncomplicated

F15.21 Other stimulant dependence, in remission

EXCLUDES 1 Not coded here   EXCLUDES 2 Not included here   N Newborn Age: 0   P Pediatric Age: 0-17   M Maternity Age: 12-55   A Adult Age: 15-124

510

ICD-10-CM 2016

✓6ᵗʰ **F15.22** **Other stimulant dependence with** intoxication
    EXCLUDES 1   *other stimulant dependence with withdrawal (F15.23)*

    F15.220 **Other stimulant dependence with intoxication,** uncomplicated

    F15.221 **Other stimulant dependence with intoxication** delirium

    F15.222 **Other stimulant dependence with intoxication with** perceptual disturbance

    F15.229 **Other stimulant dependence with intoxication,** unspecified

F15.23 **Other stimulant dependence with** withdrawal
    EXCLUDES 1   *other stimulant dependence with intoxication (F15.22-)*

F15.24 **Other stimulant dependence with stimulant-induced** mood disorder

✓6ᵗʰ **F15.25** **Other stimulant dependence with stimulant-induced** psychotic disorder

    F15.250 **Other stimulant dependence with stimulant-induced psychotic disorder with** delusions

    F15.251 **Other stimulant dependence with stimulant-induced psychotic disorder with** hallucinations

    F15.259 **Other stimulant dependence with stimulant-induced psychotic disorder,** unspecified

✓6ᵗʰ **F15.28** **Other stimulant dependence with** other stimulant-induced disorder

    F15.280 **Other stimulant dependence with stimulant-induced** anxiety disorder

    F15.281 **Other stimulant dependence with stimulant-induced** sexual dysfunction

    F15.282 **Other stimulant dependence with stimulant-induced** sleep disorder

    F15.288 **Other stimulant dependence with other stimulant-induced disorder**

F15.29 **Other stimulant depe ndence with unspecified stimulant-induced disorder**

✓5ᵗʰ **F15.9** **Other stimulant use,** unspecified
    EXCLUDES 1   *other stimulant abuse (F15.1-)*
               other stimulant dependence (F15.2-)

F15.90 **Other stimulant use, unspecified,** uncomplicated

✓6ᵗʰ **F15.92** **Other stimulant use, unspecified with intoxication**
    EXCLUDES 1   *other stimulant use, unspecified with withdrawal (F15.93)*

    F15.920 **Other stimulant use, unspecified with intoxication,** uncomplicated

    F15.921 **Other stimulant use, unspecified with intoxication** delirium

    F15.922 **Other stimulant use, unspecified with intoxication with** perceptual disturbance

    F15.929 **Other stimulant use, unspecified with intoxication,** unspecified

F15.93 **Other stimulant use, unspecified with** withdrawal
    EXCLUDES 1   *other stimulant use, unspecified with intoxication (F15.92-)*

F15.94 **Other stimulant use, unspecified with stimulant-induced** mood disorder

✓6ᵗʰ **F15.95** **Other stimulant use, unspecified with stimulant-induced** psychotic disorder

    F15.950 **Other stimulant use, unspecified with stimulant-induced p sychotic disorder with** delusions

    F15.951 **Other stimulant use, unspecified with stimulant-induced p sychotic disorder with** hallucinations

    F15.959 **Other stimulant use, unspecified with stimulant-induced psychotic disorder,** unspecified

✓6ᵗʰ **F15.98** **Other stimulant use, unspecified with** other stimulant-induced disorder

    F15.980 **Other stimulant use, unspecified with stimulant-induced** anxiety disorder

    F15.981 **Other stimulant use, unspecified with stimulant-induced** sexual dysfunction

    F15.982 **Other stimulant use, unspecified with stimulant-induced** sleep disorder

    F15.988 **Other stimulant use, unspecified with other stimulant-induced disorder**

F15.99 **Other stimulant use, unspecified with unspecified stimulant-induced disorder**

✓4ᵗʰ **F16** **Hallucinogen related disorders**
    INCLUDES   ecstasy
               PCP
               phencyclidine

✓5ᵗʰ **F16.1** **Hallucinogen** abuse
    EXCLUDES 1   *hallucinogen dependence (F16.2-)*
               hallucinogen use, unspecified (F16.9-)

F16.10 **Hallucinogen abuse,** uncomplicated

✓6ᵗʰ **F16.12** **Hallucinogen abuse with** intoxication

    F16.120 **Hallucinogen abuse with intoxication,** uncomplicated

    F16.121 **Hallucinogen abuse with intoxication with** delirium

    F16.122 **Hallucinogen abuse with intoxication with** perceptual disturbance

    F16.129 **Hallucinogen abuse with intoxication,** unspecified

F16.14 **Hallucinogen abuse with hallucinogen-induced** mood disorder

✓6ᵗʰ **F16.15** **Hallucinogen abuse with hallucinogen-induced** psychotic disorder

    F16.150 **Hallucinogen abuse with hallucinogen-induced psychotic disorder with** delusions

    F16.151 **Hallucinogen abuse with hallucinogen-induced psychotic disorder with** hallucinations

    F16.159 **Hallucinogen abuse with hallucinogen-induced psychotic disorder,** unspecified

✓6ᵗʰ **F16.18** **Hallucinogen abuse with** other hallucinogen-induced disorder

    F16.180 **Hallucinogen abuse with hallucinogen-induced** anxiety disorder

    F16.183 **Hallucinogen abuse with hallucinogen persisting perception disorder (flashbacks)**

    F16.188 **Hallucinogen abuse with other hallucinogen-induced disorder**

F16.19 **Hallucinogen abuse with unspecified hallucinogen-induced disorder**

✓5ᵗʰ **F16.2** **Hallucinogen** dependence
    EXCLUDES 1   *hallucinogen abuse (F16.1-)*
               hallucinogen use, unspecified (F16.9-)

F16.20 **Hallucinogen dependence,** uncomplicated

F16.21 **Hallucinogen dependence,** in remission

✓6ᵗʰ **F16.22** **Hallucinogen dependence with** intoxication

    F16.220 **Hallucinogen dependence with intoxication,** uncomplicated

    F16.221 **Hallucinogen dependence with intoxication with** delirium

    F16.229 **Hallucinogen dependence with intoxication,** unspecified

F16.24 **Hallucinogen dependence with hallucinogen-induced** mood disorder

✓6ᵗʰ **F16.25** **Hallucinogen dependence with hallucinogen-induced** psychotic disorder

    F16.250 **Hallucinogen dependence with hallucinogen-induced psychotic disorder with** delusions

    F16.251 **Hallucinogen dependence with hallucinogen-induced psychotic disorder with** hallucinations

    F16.259 **Hallucinogen dependence with hallucinogen-induced psychotic disorder,** unspecified

✓6ᵗʰ **F16.28** **Hallucinogen dependence with** other hallucinogen-induced disorder

    F16.280 **Hallucinogen dependence with hallucinogen-induced** anxiety disorder

    F16.283 **Hallucinogen dependence with hallucinogen** persisting perception disorder (flashbacks)

☑ Additional Character Required   ᵛˣᵗ Placeholder Alert   Unspecified Dx   Other Specified Dx   Manifestation   ▶◀ Revised Text   ● New Code   ▲ Revised Code Title

F16.288 Hallucinogen dependence with other hallucinogen-induced disorder

F16.29 Hallucinogen dependence with unspecified hallucinogen-induced disorder

✓5th **F16.9** Hallucinogen use, unspecified
> EXCLUDES 1   hallucinogen abuse (F16.1-)
> hallucinogen dependence (F16.2-)

F16.90 Hallucinogen use, unspecified, uncomplicated

✓6th **F16.92** Hallucinogen use, unspecified with intoxication

F16.920 Hallucinogen use, unspecified with intoxication, uncomplicated

F16.921 Hallucinogen use, unspecified with intoxication with delirium

F16.929 Hallucinogen use, unspecified with intoxication, unspecified

F16.94 Hallucinogen use, unspecified with hallucinogen-induced mood disorder

✓6th **F16.95** Hallucinogen use, unspecified with hallucinogen-induced psychotic disorder

F16.950 Hallucinogen use, unspecified with hallucinogen-induced psychotic disorder with delusions

F16.951 Hallucinogen use, unspecified with hallucinogen-induced psychotic disorder with hallucinations

F16.959 Hallucinogen use, unspecified with hallucinogen-induced psychotic disorder, unspecified

✓6th **F16.98** Hallucinogen use, unspecified with other specified hallucinogen-induced disorder

F16.980 Hallucinogen use, unspecified with hallucinogen-induced anxiety disorder

F16.983 Hallucinogen use, unspecified with hallucinogen persisting perception disorder (flashbacks)

F16.988 Hallucinogen use, unspecified with other hallucinogen-induced disorder

F16.99 Hallucinogen use, unspecified with unspecified hallucinogen-induced disorder

✓4th **F17** Nicotine dependence
> EXCLUDES 1   history of tobacco dependence (Z87.891)
> tobacco use NOS (Z72.0)
>
> EXCLUDES 2   tobacco use (smoking) during pregnancy, childbirth and the puerperium (O99.33-)
> toxic effect of nicotine (T65.2-)

AHA: 2013, 4Q, 108-109

✓5th **F17.2** Nicotine dependence

✓6th **F17.20** Nicotine dependence, unspecified

F17.200 Nicotine dependence, unspecified, uncomplicated

F17.201 Nicotine dependence, unspecified, in remission

F17.203 Nicotine dependence unspecified, with withdrawal

F17.208 Nicotine dependence, unspecified, with other nicotine-induced disorders

F17.209 Nicotine dependence, unspecified, with unspecified nicotine-induced disorders

✓6th **F17.21** Nicotine dependence, cigarettes

F17.210 Nicotine dependence, cigarettes, uncomplicated

F17.211 Nicotine dependence, cigarettes, in remission

F17.213 Nicotine dependence, cigarettes, with withdrawal

F17.218 Nicotine dependence, cigarettes, with other nicotine-induced disorders

F17.219 Nicotine dependence, cigarettes, with unspecified nicotine-induced disorders

✓6th **F17.22** Nicotine dependence, chewing tobacco

F17.220 Nicotine dependence, chewing tobacco, uncomplicated

F17.221 Nicotine dependence, chewing tobacco, in remission

F17.223 Nicotine dependence, chewing tobacco, with withdrawal

F17.228 Nicotine dependence, chewing tobacco, with other nicotine-induced disorders

F17.229 Nicotine dependence, chewing tobacco, with unspecified nicotine-induced disorders

✓6th **F17.29** Nicotine dependence, other tobacco product

F17.290 Nicotine dependence, other tobacco product, uncomplicated

F17.291 Nicotine dependence, other tobacco product, in remission

F17.293 Nicotine dependence, other tobacco product, with withdrawal

F17.298 Nicotine dependence, other tobacco product, with other nicotine-induced disorders

F17.299 Nicotine dependence, other tobacco product, with unspecified nicotine-induced disorders

✓4th **F18** Inhalant related disorders
> INCLUDES   volatile solvents

✓5th **F18.1** Inhalant abuse
> EXCLUDES 1   inhalant dependence (F18.2-)
> inhalant use, unspecified (F18.9-)

F18.10 Inhalant abuse, uncomplicated

✓6th **F18.12** Inhalant abuse with intoxication

F18.120 Inhalant abuse with intoxication, uncomplicated

F18.121 Inhalant abuse with intoxication delirium

F18.129 Inhalant abuse with intoxication, unspecified

F18.14 Inhalant abuse with inhalant-induced mood disorder

✓6th **F18.15** Inhalant abuse with inhalant-induced psychotic disorder

F18.150 Inhalant abuse with inhalant-induced psychotic disorder with delusions

F18.151 Inhalant abuse with inhalant-induced psychotic disorder with hallucinations

F18.159 Inhalant abuse with inhalant-induced psychotic disorder, unspecified

F18.17 Inhalant abuse with inhalant-induced dementia

✓6th **F18.18** Inhalant abuse with other inhalant-induced disorders

F18.180 Inhalant abuse with inhalant-induced anxiety disorder

F18.188 Inhalant abuse with other inhalant-induced disorder

F18.19 Inhalant abuse with unspecified inhalant-induced disorder

✓5th **F18.2** Inhalant dependence
> EXCLUDES 1   inhalant abuse (F18.1-)
> inhalant use, unspecified (F18.9-)

F18.20 Inhalant dependence, uncomplicated

F18.21 Inhalant dependence, in remission

✓6th **F18.22** Inhalant dependence with intoxication

F18.220 Inhalant dependence with intoxication, uncomplicated

F18.221 Inhalant dependence with intoxication delirium

F18.229 Inhalant dependence with intoxication, unspecified

F18.24 Inhalant dependence with inhalant-induced mood disorder

✓6th **F18.25** Inhalant dependence with inhalant-induced psychotic disorder

F18.250 Inhalant dependence with inhalant-induced psychotic disorder with delusions

F18.251 Inhalant dependence with inhalant-induced psychotic disorder with hallucinations

F18.259 Inhalant dependence with inhalant-induced psychotic disorder, unspecified

F18.27 Inhalant dependence with inhalant-induced dementia

EXCLUDES 1   Not coded here   EXCLUDES 2   Not included here   N Newborn Age: 0   P Pediatric Age: 0-17   M Maternity Age: 12-55   A Adult Age: 15-124

✓6ᵗʰ **F18.28** **Inhalant dependence with** other inhalant-induced disorders

    F18.280 **Inhalant dependence with inhalant-induced** anxiety disorder

    F18.288 **Inhalant dependence with other inhalant-induced disorder**

  F18.29 **Inhalant dependence with unspecified inhalant-induced disorder**

✓5ᵗʰ **F18.9** **Inhalant use,** unspecified

    EXCLUDES 1 *inhalant abuse (F18.1-)*
               inhalant dependence (F18.2-)

  F18.90 **Inhalant use, unspecified,** uncomplicated

✓6ᵗʰ **F18.92** **Inhalant use, unspecified with** intoxication

    F18.920 **Inhalant use, unspecified with intoxication,** uncomplicated

    F18.921 **Inhalant use, unspecified with intoxication with** delirium

    F18.929 **Inhalant use, unspecified with intoxication, unspecified**

  F18.94 **Inhalant use, unspecified with inhalant-induced** mood disorder

✓6ᵗʰ **F18.95** **Inhalant use, unspecified with inhalant-induced** psychotic disorder

    F18.950 **Inhalant use, unspecified with inhalant-induced psychotic disorder with** delusions

    F18.951 **Inhalant use, unspecified with inhalant-induced psychotic disorder with** hallucinations

    F18.959 **Inhalant use, unspecified with inhalant-induced psychotic disorder, unspecified**

  F18.97 **Inhalant use, unspecified with inhalant-induced** persisting dementia

✓6ᵗʰ **F18.98** **Inhalant use, unspecified with** other inhalant-induced disorders

    F18.980 **Inhalant use, unspecified with inhalant-induced** anxiety disorder

    F18.988 **Inhalant use, unspecified with other inhalant-induced disorder**

  F18.99 **Inhalant use, unspecified with unspecified inhalant-induced disorder**

✓4ᵗʰ **F19** Other psychoactive **substance related disorders**

  INCLUDES polysubstance drug use (indiscriminate drug use)

✓5ᵗʰ **F19.1** **Other psychoactive substance** abuse

    EXCLUDES 1 *other psychoactive substance dependence (F19.2-)*
               other psychoactive substance use, unspecified (F19.9-)

  F19.10 **Other psychoactive substance abuse,** uncomplicated

✓6ᵗʰ **F19.12** **Other psychoactive substance abuse with** intoxication

    F19.120 **Other psychoactive substance abuse with intoxication,** uncomplicated

    F19.121 **Other psychoactive substance abuse with intoxication** delirium

    F19.122 **Other psychoactive substance abuse with intoxication with** perceptual disturbances

    F19.129 **Other psychoactive substance abuse with intoxication, unspecified**

  F19.14 **Other psychoactive substance abuse with psychoactive substance-induced** mood disorder

✓6ᵗʰ **F19.15** **Other psychoactive substance abuse with psychoactive substance-induced** psychotic disorder

    F19.150 **Other psychoactive substance abuse with psychoactive substance-induced psychotic disorder with** delusions

    F19.151 **Other psychoactive substance abuse with psychoactive substance-induced psychotic disorder with** hallucinations

    F19.159 **Other psychoactive substance abuse with psychoactive substance-induced psychotic disorder, unspecified**

  F19.16 **Other psychoactive substance abuse with psychoactive substance-induced** persisting amnestic disorder

  F19.17 **Other psychoactive substance abuse with psychoactive substance-induced** persisting dementia

✓6ᵗʰ **F19.18** **Other psychoactive substance abuse with** other psychoactive substance-induced disorders

    F19.180 **Other psychoactive substance abuse with psychoactive substance-induced** anxiety disorder

    F19.181 **Other psychoactive substance abuse with psychoactive substance-induced** sexual dysfunction

    F19.182 **Other psychoactive substance abuse with psychoactive substance-induced** sleep disorder

    F19.188 **Other psychoactive substance abuse with other psychoactive substance-induced disorder**

  F19.19 **Other psychoactive substance abuse with unspecified psychoactive substance-induced disorder**

✓5ᵗʰ **F19.2** **Other psychoactive substance** dependence

    EXCLUDES 1 *other psychoactive substance abuse (F19.1-)*
               other psychoactive substance use, unspecified (F19.9-)

  F19.20 **Other psychoactive substance dependence,** uncomplicated

  F19.21 **Other psychoactive substance dependence,** in remission

✓6ᵗʰ **F19.22** **Other psychoactive substance dependence with** intoxication

    EXCLUDES 1 *other psychoactive substance dependence with withdrawal (F19.23-)*

    F19.220 **Other psychoactive substance dependence with intoxication,** uncomplicated

    F19.221 **Other psychoactive substance dependence with intoxication** delirium

    F19.222 **Other psychoactive substance dependence with intoxication with** perceptual disturbance

    F19.229 **Other psychoactive substance dependencewith intoxication, unspecified**

✓6ᵗʰ **F19.23** **Other psychoactive substance dependence with** withdrawal

    EXCLUDES 1 *other psychoactive substance dependence with intoxication (F19.22-)*

    F19.230 **Other psychoactive substance dependence with withdrawal,** uncomplicated

    F19.231 **Other psychoactive substance dependence with withdrawal** delirium

    F19.232 **Other psychoactive substance dependence with withdrawal with** perceptual disturbance

    F19.239 **Other psychoactive substance dependence with withdrawal, unspecified**

  F19.24 **Other psychoactive substance dependence with psychoactive substance-induced** mood disorder

✓6ᵗʰ **F19.25** **Other psychoactive substance dependence with psychoactive substance-induced** psychotic disorder

    F19.250 **Other psychoactive substance dependence with psychoactive substance-induced psychotic disorder with** delusions

    F19.251 **Other psychoactive substance dependence with psychoactive substance-induced psychotic disorder with** hallucinations

    F19.259 **Other psychoactive substance dependence with psychoactive substance-induced psychotic disorder, unspecified**

  F19.26 **Other psychoactive substance dependence with psychoactive substance-induced** persisting amnestic disorder

  F19.27 **Other psychoactive substance dependence with psychoactive substance-induced** persisting dementia

✓6ᵗʰ **F19.28** **Other psychoactive substance dependence with** other psychoactive substance-induced disorders

    F19.280 **Other psychoactive substance dependence with psychoactive substance-induced** anxiety disorder

☑ Additional Character Required ✓×7ᵗʰ Placeholder Alert Unspecified Dx Other Specified Dx Manifestation ▶◀ Revised Text ● New Code ▲ Revised Code Title

ICD-10-CM 2016   513

F19.281   Other psychoactive substance dependence with psychoactive substance-induced sexual dysfunction

F19.282   Other psychoactive substance dependence with psychoactive substance-induced sleep disorder

F19.288   Other psychoactive substance dependence with other psychoactive substance-induced disorder

F19.29   Other psychoactive substance dependence with unspecified psychoactive substance-induced disorder

✓5ᵗʰ F19.9   Other psychoactive substance use, unspecified
> EXCLUDES 1   *other psychoactive substance abuse (F19.1-)*
> *other psychoactive substance dependence (F19.2-)*

F19.90   Other psychoactive substance use, unspecified, uncomplicated

✓6ᵗʰ F19.92   Other psychoactive substance use, unspecified with intoxication
> EXCLUDES 1   *other psychoactive substance use, unspecified with withdrawal (F19.93)*

F19.920   Other psychoactive substance use, unspecified with intoxication, uncomplicated

F19.921   Other psychoactive substance use, unspecified with intoxication with delirium

F19.922   Other psychoactive substance use, unspecified with intoxication with perceptual disturbance

F19.929   Other psychoactive substance use, unspecified with intoxication, unspecified

✓6ᵗʰ F19.93   Other psychoactive substance use, unspecified with withdrawal
> EXCLUDES 1   *other psychoactive substance use, unspecified with intoxication (F19.92-)*

F19.930   Other psychoactive substance use, unspecified with withdrawal, uncomplicated

F19.931   Other psychoactive substance use, unspecified with withdrawal delirium

F19.932   Other psychoactive substance use, unspecified with withdrawal with perceptual disturbance

F19.939   Other psychoactive substance use, unspecified with withdrawal, unspecified

F19.94   Other psychoactive substance use, unspecified with psychoactive substance-induced mood disorder

✓6ᵗʰ F19.95   Other psychoactive substance use, unspecified with psychoactive substance-induced psychotic disorder

F19.950   Other psychoactive substance use, unspecified with psychoactive substance-induced psychotic disorder with delusions

F19.951   Other psychoactive substance use, unspecified with psychoactive substance-induced psychotic disorder with hallucinations

F19.959   Other psychoactive substance use, unspecified with psychoactive substance-induced psychotic disorder, unspecified

F19.96   Other psychoactive substance use, unspecified with psychoactive substance-induced persisting amnestic disorder

F19.97   Other psychoactive substance use, unspecified with psychoactive substance-induced persisting dementia

✓6ᵗʰ F19.98   Other psychoactive substance use, unspecified with other psychoactive substance-induced disorders

F19.980   Other psychoactive substance use, unspecified with psychoactive substance-induced anxiety disorder

F19.981   Other psychoactive substance use, unspecified with psychoactive substance-induced sexual dysfunction

F19.982   Other psychoactive substance use, unspecified with psychoactive substance-induced sleep disorder

F19.988   Other psychoactive substance use, unspecified with other psychoactive substance-induced disorder

F19.99   Other psychoactive substance use, unspecified with unspecified psychoactive substance-induced disorder

Schizophrenia, schizotypal, delusional, and other non-mood psychotic disorders (F20-F29)

✓4ᵗʰ F20   **Schizophrenia**
> EXCLUDES 1   *brief psychotic disorder (F23)*
> *cyclic schizophrenia (F25.0)*
> *mood [affective] disorders with psychotic symptoms (F30.2, F31.2, F31.5, F31.64, F32.3, F33.3)*
> *schizoaffective disorder (F25.-)*
> *schizophrenic reaction NOS (F23)*
>
> EXCLUDES 2   *schizophrenic reaction in:*
> *alcoholism (F10.15-, F10.25-, F10.95-)*
> *brain disease (F06.2)*
> *epilepsy (F06.2)*
> *psychoactive drug use (F11-F19 with .15, .25, .95)*
> *schizotypal disorder (F21)*

F20.0   **Paranoid schizophrenia**
Paraphrenic schizophrenia
> EXCLUDES 1   *involutional paranoid state (F22)*
> *paranoia (F22)*

F20.1   **Disorganized schizophrenia**
Hebephrenic schizophrenia
Hebephrenia

F20.2   **Catatonic schizophrenia**
Schizophrenic catalepsy
Schizophrenic catatonia
Schizophrenic flexibilitas cerea
> EXCLUDES 1   *catatonic stupor (R40.1)*

F20.3   **Undifferentiated schizophrenia**
Atypical schizophrenia
> EXCLUDES 1   *acute schizophrenia-like psychotic disorder (F23)*
> EXCLUDES 2   *post-schizophrenic depression (F32.8)*

F20.5   **Residual schizophrenia**
Restzustand (schizophrenic)
Schizophrenic residual state

✓5ᵗʰ F20.8   **Other schizophrenia**

F20.81   **Schizophreniform disorder**
Schizophreniform psychosis NOS

F20.89   **Other schizophrenia**
Cenesthopathic schizophrenia
Simple schizophrenia

F20.9   **Schizophrenia, unspecified**

F21   **Schizotypal disorder**
Borderline schizophrenia
Latent schizophrenia
Latent schizophrenic reaction
Prepsychotic schizophrenia
Prodromal schizophrenia
Pseudoneurotic schizophrenia
Pseudopsychopathic schizophrenia
Schizotypal personality disorder
> EXCLUDES 2   *Asperger's syndrome (F84.5)*
> *schizoid personality disorder (F60.1)*

F22   **Delusional disorders**
Delusional dysmorphophobia
Involutional paranoid state
Paranoia
Paranoia querulans
Paranoid psychosis
Paranoid state
Paraphrenia (late)
Sensitiver Beziehungswahn
> EXCLUDES 1   *mood [affective] disorders with psychotic symptoms (F30.2, F31.2, F31.5, F31.64, F32.3, F33.3)*
> *paranoid schizophrenia (F20.0)*
> EXCLUDES 2   *paranoid personality disorder (F60.0)*
> *paranoid psychosis, psychogenic (F23)*
> *paranoid reaction (F23)*

F23   **Brief psychotic disorder**
Paranoid reaction
Psychogenic paranoid psychosis
> EXCLUDES 2   *mood [affective] disorders with psychotic symptoms (F30.2, F31.2, F31.5, F31.64, F32.3, F33.3)*

F24   **Shared psychotic disorder**
Folie à deux
Induced paranoid disorder
Induced psychotic disorder

EXCLUDES 1 Not coded here   EXCLUDES 2 Not included here   N Newborn Age: 0   P Pediatric Age: 0-17   M Maternity Age: 12-55   A Adult Age: 15-124

514   ICD-10-CM 2016

✓4ᵗʰ **F25 Schizoaffective disorders**

> EXCLUDES 1   *mood [affective] disorders with psychotic symptoms (F30.2, F31.2, F31.5, F31.64, F32.3, F33.3)*
> *schizophrenia (F20.-)*

F25.0 Schizoaffective disorder, bipolar type
> Cyclic schizophrenia
> Schizoaffective disorder, manic type
> Schizoaffective disorder, mixed type
> Schizoaffective psychosis, bipolar type
> Schizophreniform psychosis, manic type

F25.1 Schizoaffective disorder, depressive type
> Schizoaffective psychosis, depressive type
> Schizophreniform psychosis, depressive type

F25.8 Other schizoaffective disorders

F25.9 Schizoaffective disorder, unspecified
> Schizoaffective psychosis NOS

F28 Other psychotic disorder not due to a substance or known physiological condition
> Chronic hallucinatory psychosis

F29 Unspecified psychosis not due to a substance or known physiological condition
> Psychosis NOS
> EXCLUDES 1   *mental disorder NOS (F99)*
> *unspecified mental disorder due to known physiological condition (F09)*

Mood [affective] disorders (F30-F39)

✓4ᵗʰ **F30 Manic episode**
> INCLUDES   bipolar disorder, single manic episode
> mixed affective episode
> EXCLUDES 1   *bipolar disorder (F31.-)*
> *major depressive disorder, recurrent (F33.-)*
> *major depressive disorder, single episode (F32.-)*

✓5ᵗʰ **F30.1 Manic episode** without psychotic symptoms

> **F30.10 Manic episode without psychotic symptoms, unspecified**

> **F30.11 Manic episode without psychotic symptoms,** mild

> **F30.12 Manic episode without psychotic symptoms, moderate**

> **F30.13 Manic episode,** severe, **without psychotic symptoms**

F30.2 Manic episode, severe with psychotic symptoms
> Manic stupor
> Mania with mood-congruent psychotic symptoms
> Mania with mood-incongruent psychotic symptoms

F30.3 Manic episode in partial remission

F30.4 Manic episode in full remission

F30.8 Other manic episodes
> Hypomania

F30.9 Manic episode, unspecified
> Mania NOS

✓4ᵗʰ **F31 Bipolar disorder**
> INCLUDES   manic-depressive illness
> manic-depressive psychosis
> manic-depressive reaction
> EXCLUDES 1   *bipolar disorder, single manic episode (F30.-)*
> *major depressive disorder, single episode (F32.-)*
> *major depressive disorder, recurrent (F33.-)*
> EXCLUDES 2   *cyclothymia (F34.0)*

F31.0 Bipolar disorder, current episode hypomanic

✓5ᵗʰ **F31.1 Bipolar disorder, current episode** manic without psychotic features

> **F31.10 Bipolar disorder, current episode manic without psychotic features, unspecified**

> **F31.11 Bipolar disorder, current episode manic without psychotic features,** mild

> **F31.12 Bipolar disorder, current episode manic without psychotic features,** moderate

> **F31.13 Bipolar disorder, current episode manic without psychotic features,** severe

F31.2 Bipolar disorder, current episode manic severe with psychotic features
> Bipolar disorder, current episode manic with mood-congruent psychotic symptoms
> Bipolar disorder, current episode manic with mood-incongruent psychotic symptoms

✓5ᵗʰ **F31.3 Bipolar disorder, current episode** depressed, mild or moderate severity

> **F31.30 Bipolar disorder, current episode depressed, mild or moderate severity, unspecified**

> **F31.31 Bipolar disorder, current episode depressed,** mild

> **F31.32 Bipolar disorder, current episode depressed, moderate**

F31.4 Bipolar disorder, current episode depressed, severe, without psychotic features

F31.5 Bipolar disorder, current episode depressed, severe, with psychotic features
> Bipolar disorder, current episode depressed with mood-incongruent psychotic symptoms
> Bipolar disorder, current episode depressed with mood-congruent psychotic symptoms

✓5ᵗʰ **F31.6 Bipolar disorder, current episode** mixed

> **F31.60 Bipolar disorder, current episode mixed, unspecified**

> **F31.61 Bipolar disorder, current episode mixed,** mild

> **F31.62 Bipolar disorder, current episode mixed,** moderate

> **F31.63 Bipolar disorder, current episode mixed,** severe, without psychotic features

> **F31.64 Bipolar disorder, current episode mixed,** severe, with psychotic features
> > Bipolar disorder, current episode mixed with mood-congruent psychotic symptoms
> > Bipolar disorder, current episode mixed with mood-incongruent psychotic symptoms

✓5ᵗʰ **F31.7 Bipolar disorder, currently** in remission

> **F31.70 Bipolar disorder, currently in remission, most recent episode unspecified**

> **F31.71 Bipolar disorder, in partial remission, most recent episode** hypomanic

> **F31.72 Bipolar disorder, in full remission, most recent episode** hypomanic

> **F31.73 Bipolar disorder, in partial remission, most recent episode** manic

> **F31.74 Bipolar disorder, in full remission, most recent episode** manic

> **F31.75 Bipolar disorder, in partial remission, most recent episode** depressed

> **F31.76 Bipolar disorder, in full remission, most recent episode** depressed

> **F31.77 Bipolar disorder, in partial remission, most recent episode** mixed

> **F31.78 Bipolar disorder, in full remission, most recent episode** mixed

✓5ᵗʰ **F31.8 Other bipolar disorders**

> **F31.81 Bipolar II disorder**

> **F31.89 Other bipolar disorder**
> > Recurrent manic episodes NOS

F31.9 Bipolar disorder, unspecified

✓4ᵗʰ **F32 Major depressive disorder,** single episode
> INCLUDES   single episode of agitated depression
> single episode of depressive reaction
> single episode of major depression
> single episode of psychogenic depression
> single episode of reactive depression
> single episode of vital depression
> EXCLUDES 1   *bipolar disorder (F31.-)*
> *manic episode (F30.-)*
> *recurrent depressive disorder (F33.-)*
> EXCLUDES 2   *adjustment disorder (F43.2)*

F32.0 Major depressive disorder, single episode, mild

F32.1 Major depressive disorder, single episode, moderate

F32.2 Major depressive disorder, single episode, severe without psychotic features

F32.3 Major depressive disorder, single episode, severe with psychotic features
> Single episode of major depression with mood-congruent psychotic symptoms
> Single episode of major depression with mood-incongruent psychotic symptoms
> Single episode of major depression with psychotic symptoms
> Single episode of psychogenic depressive psychosis
> Single episode of psychotic depression
> Single episode of reactive depressive psychosis

F32.4 Major depressive disorder, single episode, in partial remission

---

✓ Additional Character Required   ✗7ᵗʰ Placeholder Alert   Unspecified Dx   Other Specified Dx   Manifestation   ►◄ Revised Text   ● New Code   ▲ Revised Code Title

F32.5   **Major depressive disorder, single episode,** in full remission

F32.8   **Other depressive episodes**
Atypical depression
Post-schizophrenic depression
Single episode of 'masked' depression NOS

F32.9   **Major depressive disorder, single episode, unspecified**
Depression NOS
Depressive disorder NOS
Major depression NOS
AHA: 2013, 4Q, 107

✓4th **F33   Major depressive disorder, recurrent**
Recurrent episodes of depressive reaction
Recurrent episodes of endogenous depression
Recurrent episodes of major depression
Recurrent episodes of psychogenic depression
Recurrent episodes of reactive depression
Recurrent episodes of seasonal depressive disorder
Recurrent episodes of vital depression
EXCLUDES 1   bipolar disorder (F31.-)
manic episode (F30.-)

F33.0   **Major depressive disorder, recurrent,** mild

F33.1   **Major depressive disorder, recurrent,** moderate

F33.2   **Major depressive disorder, recurrent,** severe without psychotic features

F33.3   **Major depressive disorder, recurrent,** severe with psychotic symptoms
Endogenous depression with psychotic symptoms
Recurrent severe episodes of major depression with mood-congruent psychotic symptoms
Recurrent severe episodes of major depression with mood-incongruent psychotic symptoms
Recurrent severe episodes of major depression with psychotic symptoms
Recurrent severe episodes of psychogenic depressive psychosis
Recurrent severe episodes of psychotic depression
Recurrent severe episodes of reactive depressive psychosis

✓5th F33.4   **Major depressive disorder, recurrent,** in remission
F33.40   **Major depressive disorder, recurrent,** in remission, unspecified
F33.41   **Major depressive disorder, recurrent,** in partial remission
F33.42   **Major depressive disorder, recurrent,** in full remission

F33.8   **Other recurrent depressive disorders**
Recurrent brief depressive episodes

F33.9   **Major depressive disorder, recurrent, unspecified**
Monopolar depression NOS

✓4th **F34   Persistent mood [affective] disorders**
F34.0   **Cyclothymic disorder**
Affective personality disorder
Cycloid personality
Cyclothymia
Cyclothymic personality

F34.1   **Dysthymic disorder**
Depressive neurosis
Depressive personality disorder
Dysthymia
Neurotic depression
Persistent anxiety depression
EXCLUDES 2   anxiety depression (mild or not persistent) (F41.8)

F34.8   **Other persistent mood [affective] disorders**

F34.9   **Persistent mood [affective] disorder, unspecified**

F39   Unspecified mood [affective] disorder
Affective psychosis NOS

Anxiety, dissociative, stress-related, somatoform and other nonpsychotic mental disorders (F40-F48)

✓4th **F40   Phobic anxiety disorders**
✓5th F40.0   **Agoraphobia**
F40.00   **Agoraphobia, unspecified**
F40.01   **Agoraphobia** with panic disorder
Panic disorder with agoraphobia
EXCLUDES 1   panic disorder without agoraphobia (F41.0)
F40.02   **Agoraphobia** without panic disorder

✓5th F40.1   **Social phobias**
Anthropophobia
Social anxiety disorder of childhood
Social neurosis
F40.10   **Social phobia, unspecified**
F40.11   **Social phobia,** generalized

✓5th F40.2   **Specific (isolated) phobias**
EXCLUDES 2   dysmorphophobia (nondelusional) (F45.22)
nosophobia (F45.22)

✓6th F40.21   **Animal type phobia**
F40.210   **Arachnophobia**
Fear of spiders
F40.218   **Other animal type phobia**

✓6th F40.22   **Natural environment type phobia**
F40.220   **Fear of thunderstorms**
F40.228   **Other natural environment type phobia**

✓6th F40.23   **Blood, injection, injury type phobia**
F40.230   **Fear of blood**
F40.231   **Fear of injections and transfusions**
F40.232   **Fear of other medical care**
F40.233   **Fear of injury**

✓6th F40.24   **Situational type phobia**
F40.240   **Claustrophobia**
F40.241   **Acrophobia**
F40.242   **Fear of bridges**
F40.243   **Fear of flying**
F40.248   **Other situational type phobia**

✓6th F40.29   **Other specified phobia**
F40.290   **Androphobia**
Fear of men
F40.291   **Gynephobia**
Fear of women
F40.298   **Other specified phobia**

F40.8   **Other phobic anxiety disorders**
Phobic anxiety disorder of childhood

F40.9   **Phobic anxiety disorder, unspecified**
Phobia NOS
Phobic state NOS

✓4th **F41   Other anxiety disorders**
EXCLUDES 2   anxiety in:
acute stress reaction (F43.0)
transient adjustment reaction (F43.2)
neurasthenia (F48.8)
psychophysiologic disorders (F45.-)
separation anxiety (F93.0)

F41.0   **Panic disorder [episodic paroxysmal anxiety]** without agoraphobia
Panic attack   Panic state
EXCLUDES 1   panic disorder with agoraphobia (F40.01)

F41.1   **Generalized anxiety disorder**
Anxiety neurosis   Anxiety state
Anxiety reaction   Overanxious disorder
EXCLUDES 2   neurasthenia (F48.8)

F41.3   **Other mixed anxiety disorders**

F41.8   **Other specified anxiety disorders**
Anxiety depression (mild or not persistent)
Anxiety hysteria
Mixed anxiety and depressive disorder

F41.9   **Anxiety disorder, unspecified**
Anxiety NOS

F42   Obsessive-compulsive disorder
Anancastic neurosis
Obsessive-compulsive neurosis
EXCLUDES 2   obsessive-compulsive personality (disorder) (F60.5)
obsessive-compulsive symptoms occurring in depression (F32-F33)
obsessive-compulsive symptoms occurring in schizophrenia (F20.-)

EXCLUDES 1   Not coded here   EXCLUDES 2   Not included here   N Newborn Age: 0   P Pediatric Age: 0-17   M Maternity Age: 12-55   A Adult Age: 15-124

516   ICD-10-CM 2016

Chapter 5. Mental, Behavioral and Neurodevelopmental Disorders

☑4th F43 Reaction to severe stress, and adjustment disorders

F43.0 Acute stress reaction
Acute crisis reaction
Acute reaction to stress
Combat and operational stress reaction
Combat fatigue
Crisis state
Psychic shock

☑5th F43.1 Post-traumatic stress disorder (PTSD)
Traumatic neurosis

     F43.10 Post-traumatic stress disorder, unspecified

     F43.11 Post-traumatic stress disorder, acute

     F43.12 Post-traumatic stress disorder, chronic

☑5th F43.2 Adjustment disorders
Culture shock
Grief reaction
Hospitalism in children
EXCLUDES 2   *separation anxiety disorder of childhood (F93.0)*

     F43.20 Adjustment disorder, unspecified

     F43.21 Adjustment disorder with depressed mood
        AHA: 2014, 1Q, 25

     F43.22 Adjustment disorder with anxiety

     F43.23 Adjustment disorder with mixed anxiety and depressed mood

     F43.24 Adjustment disorder with disturbance of conduct

     F43.25 Adjustment disorder with mixed disturbance of emotions and conduct

     F43.29 Adjustment disorder with other symptoms

F43.8 Other reactions to severe stress

F43.9 Reaction to severe stress, unspecified

☑4th F44 Dissociative and conversion disorders
INCLUDES   conversion hysteria
          conversion reaction
          hysteria
          hysterical psychosis
EXCLUDES 2   *malingering [conscious simulation] (Z76.5)*

F44.0 Dissociative amnesia
EXCLUDES 1   *amnesia NOS (R41.3)*
          anterograde amnesia (R41.1)
          retrograde amnesia (R41.2)
EXCLUDES 2   *alcohol- or other psychoactive substance-induced amnestic disorder (F10, F13, F19 with .26, .96)*
          amnestic disorder due to known physiological condition (F04)
          postictal amnesia in epilepsy (G40.-)

F44.1 Dissociative fugue
EXCLUDES 2   *postictal fugue in epilepsy (G40.-)*

F44.2 Dissociative stupor
EXCLUDES 1   *catatonic stupor (R40.1)*
          stupor NOS (R40.1)
EXCLUDES 2   *catatonic disorder due to known physiological condition (F06.1)*
          depressive stupor (F32, F33)
          manic stupor (F30, F31)

F44.4 Conversion disorder with motor symptom or deficit
Dissociative motor disorders
Psychogenic aphonia
Psychogenic dysphonia

F44.5 Conversion disorder with seizures or convulsions
Dissociative convulsions

F44.6 Conversion disorder with sensory symptom or deficit
Dissociative anesthesia and sensory loss
Psychogenic deafness

F44.7 Conversion disorder with mixed symptom presentation

☑5th F44.8 Other dissociative and conversion disorders

     F44.81 Dissociative identity disorder
        Multiple personality disorder

     F44.89 Other dissociative and conversion disorders
        Ganser's syndrome
        Psychogenic confusion
        Psychogenic twilight state
        Trance and possession disorders

F44.9 Dissociative and conversion disorder, unspecified
Dissociative disorder NOS

☑4th F45 Somatoform disorders
EXCLUDES 2   *dissociative and conversion disorders (F44.-)*
          factitious disorders (F68.1-)
          hair-plucking (F63.3)
          lalling (F80.0)
          lisping (F80.0)
          malingering [conscious simulation] (Z76.5)
          nail-biting (F98.8)
          psychological or behavioral factors associated with disorders or diseases classified elsewhere (F54)
          sexual dysfunction, not due to a substance or known physiological condition (F52.-)
          thumb-sucking (F98.8)
          tic disorders (in childhood and adolescence) (F95.-)
          Tourette's syndrome (F95.2)
          trichotillomania (F63.3)

F45.0 Somatization disorder
Briquet's disorder
Multiple psychosomatic disorder

F45.1 Undifferentiated somatoform disorder
Undifferentiated psychosomatic disorder

☑5th F45.2 Hypochondriacal disorders
EXCLUDES 2   *delusional dysmorphophobia (F22)*
          fixed delusions about bodily functions or shape (F22)

     F45.20 Hypochondriacal disorder, unspecified

     F45.21 Hypochondriasis
        Hypochondriacal neurosis

     F45.22 Body dysmorphic disorder
        Dysmorphophobia (nondelusional)
        Nosophobia

     F45.29 Other hypochondriacal disorders

☑5th F45.4 Pain disorders related to psychological factors
EXCLUDES 1   *pain NOS (R52)*

     F45.41 Pain disorder exclusively related to psychological factors
        Somatoform pain disorder (persistent)

     F45.42 Pain disorder with related psychological factors
        Code also associated acute or chronic pain (G89.-)

F45.8 Other somatoform disorders
Psychogenic dysmenorrhea
Psychogenic dysphagia, including "globus hystericus"
Psychogenic pruritus
Psychogenic torticollis
Somatoform autonomic dysfunction
Teeth grinding
EXCLUDES 1   *sleep related teeth grinding (G47.63)*

F45.9 Somatoform disorder, unspecified
Psychosomatic disorder NOS

☑4th F48 Other nonpsychotic mental disorders

F48.1 Depersonalization-derealization syndrome

F48.2 Pseudobulbar affect
Involuntary emotional expression disorder
Code first underlying cause, if known, such as:
     amyotrophic lateral sclerosis (G12.21)
     multiple sclerosis (G35)
     sequelae of cerebrovascular disease (I69.-)
     sequelae of traumatic intracranial injury (S06.-)

F48.8 Other specified nonpsychotic mental disorders
Dhat syndrome
Neurasthenia
Occupational neurosis, including writer's cramp
Psychasthenia
Psychasthenic neurosis
Psychogenic syncope

F48.9 Nonpsychotic mental disorder, unspecified
Neurosis NOS

Behavioral syndromes associated with physiological disturbances and physical factors (F50-F59)

☑4th F50 Eating disorders
EXCLUDES 1   *anorexia NOS (R63.0)*
          feeding difficulties (R63.3)
          polyphagia (R63.2)
EXCLUDES 2   *feeding disorder in infancy or childhood (F98.2-)*

☑5th F50.0 Anorexia nervosa
EXCLUDES 1   *loss of appetite (R63.0)*
          psychogenic loss of appetite (F50.8)

     F50.00 Anorexia nervosa, unspecified

     F50.01 Anorexia nervosa, restricting type

☑ Additional Character Required   ✓x7th Placeholder Alert   Unspecified Dx   Other Specified Dx   Manifestation   ▶◀ Revised Text   ● New Code   ▲ Revised Code Title

F50.02   **Anorexia nervosa,** binge eating/purging type
> EXCLUDES 1   *bulimia nervosa (F50.2)*

F50.2   **Bulimia nervosa**
Bulimia NOS
Hyperorexia nervosa
> EXCLUDES 1   *anorexia nervosa, binge eating/purging type (F50.02)*

F50.8   **Other eating disorders**
Pica in adults
Psychogenic loss of appetite
> EXCLUDES 2   *pica of infancy and childhood (F98.3)*

F50.9   **Eating disorder, unspecified**
Atypical anorexia nervosa
Atypical bulimia nervosa

✓4ᵗʰ **F51   Sleep disorders not due to a substance or known physiological condition**
> EXCLUDES 2   *organic sleep disorders (G47.-)*

✓5ᵗʰ   **F51.0   Insomnia not due to a substance or known physiological condition**
> EXCLUDES 2   *alcohol related insomnia (F10.182, F10.282, F10.982)*
> *drug-related insomnia (F11.182, F11.282, F11.982, F13.182, F13.282, F13.982, F14.182, F14.282, F14.982, F15.182, F15.282, F15.982, F19.182, F19.282, F19.982)*
> *insomnia NOS (G47.0-)*
> *insomnia due to known physiological condition (G47.0-)*
> *organic insomnia (G47.0-)*
> *sleep deprivation (Z72.820)*

F51.01   **Primary insomnia**
Idiopathic insomnia

F51.02   **Adjustment insomnia**

F51.03   **Paradoxical insomnia**

F51.04   **Psychophysiologic insomnia**

F51.05   **Insomnia due to** other mental disorder
Code also associated mental disorder

F51.09   **Other insomnia not due to a substance or known physiological condition**

✓5ᵗʰ   **F51.1   Hypersomnia not due to a substance or known physiological condition**
> EXCLUDES 2   *alcohol related hypersomnia (F10.182, F10.282, F10.982)*
> *drug-related hypersomnia (F11.182, F11.282, F11.982, F13.182, F13.282, F13.982, F14.182, F14.282, F14.982, F15.182, F15.282, F15.982, F19.182, F19.282, F19.982)*
> *hypersomnia NOS (G47.10)*
> *hypersomnia due to known physiological condition (G47.10)*
> *idiopathic hypersomnia (G47.11, G47.12)*
> *narcolepsy (G47.4-)*

F51.11   **Primary hypersomnia**

F51.12   **Insufficient sleep syndrome**
> EXCLUDES 1   *sleep deprivation (Z72.820)*

F51.13   **Hypersomnia due to** other mental disorder
Code also associated mental disorder

F51.19   **Other hypersomnia not due to a substance or known physiological condition**

F51.3   **Sleepwalking [somnambulism]**

F51.4   **Sleep terrors [night terrors]**

F51.5   **Nightmare disorder**
Dream anxiety disorder

F51.8   **Other sleep disorders not due to a substance or known physiological condition**

F51.9   **Sleep disorder not due to a substance or known physiological condition, unspecified**
Emotional sleep disorder NOS

✓4ᵗʰ **F52   Sexual dysfunction not due to a substance or known physiological condition**
> EXCLUDES 2   *Dhat syndrome (F48.8)*

F52.0   **Hypoactive sexual desire disorder**
Anhedonia (sexual)
Lack or loss of sexual desire
> EXCLUDES 1   *decreased libido (R68.82)*

F52.1   **Sexual aversion disorder**
Sexual aversion and lack of sexual enjoyment

✓5ᵗʰ   **F52.2   Sexual arousal disorders**
Failure of genital response

F52.21   **Male erectile disorder** ♂
Psychogenic impotence
> EXCLUDES 1   *impotence of organic origin (N52.-)*
> *impotence NOS (N52.-)*

F52.22   **Female sexual arousal disorder** ♀
Frigidity

✓5ᵗʰ   **F52.3   Orgasmic disorder**
Inhibited orgasm
Psychogenic anorgasmy

F52.31   **Female orgasmic disorder** ♀

F52.32   **Male orgasmic disorder** ♂

F52.4   **Premature ejaculation** ♂

F52.5   **Vaginismus not due to a substance or known physiological condition** ♀
Psychogenic vaginismus
> EXCLUDES 2   *vaginismus (due to a known physiological condition) (N94.2)*

F52.6   **Dyspareunia not due to a substance or known physiological condition** ♀
Psychogenic dyspareunia
> EXCLUDES 2   *dyspareunia (due to a known physiological condition) (N94.1)*

F52.8   **Other sexual dysfunction not due to a substance or known physiological condition**
Excessive sexual drive
Nymphomania
Satyriasis

F52.9   **Unspecified sexual dysfunction not due to a substance or known physiological condition**
Sexual dysfunction NOS

F53   **Puerperal psychosis** ♀
Postpartum depression
> EXCLUDES 1   *mood disorders with psychotic features (F30.2, F31.2, F31.5, F31.64, F32.3, F33.3)*
> *postpartum dysphoria (O90.6)*
> *psychosis in schizophrenia, schizotypal, delusional, and other psychotic disorders (F20-F29)*

F54   *Psychological and behavioral factors associated with disorders or diseases classified elsewhere*
Psychological factors affecting physical conditions
Code first the associated physical disorder, such as:
    asthma (J45.-)
    dermatitis (L23-L25)
    gastric ulcer (K25.-)
    mucous colitis (K58.-)
    ulcerative colitis (K51.-)
    urticaria (L50.-)
> EXCLUDES 2   *tension-type headache (G44.2)*

✓4ᵗʰ **F55   Abuse of non-psychoactive substances**
> EXCLUDES 2   *abuse of psychoactive substances (F10-F19)*

F55.0   **Abuse of antacids**

F55.1   **Abuse of herbal or folk remedies**

F55.2   **Abuse of laxatives**

F55.3   **Abuse of steroids or hormones**

F55.4   **Abuse of vitamins**

F55.8   **Abuse of other non-psychoactive substances**

F59   **Unspecified behavioral syndromes associated with physiological disturbances and physical factors**
Psychogenic physiological dysfunction NOS

Disorders of adult personality and behavior (F60-F69)

✓4ᵗʰ **F60   Specific personality disorders**

F60.0   **Paranoid personality disorder**
Expansive paranoid personality (disorder)
Fanatic personality (disorder)
Paranoid personality (disorder)
Querulant personality (disorder)
Sensitive paranoid personality (disorder)
> EXCLUDES 2   *paranoia (F22)*
> *paranoia querulans (F22)*
> *paranoid psychosis (F22)*
> *paranoid schizophrenia (F20.0)*
> *paranoid state (F22)*

EXCLUDES 1 Not coded here   EXCLUDES 2 Not included here   N Newborn Age: 0   P Pediatric Age: 0-17   M Maternity Age: 12-55   A Adult Age: 15-124

518   ICD-10-CM 2016

F60.1 Schizoid personality disorder
- EXCLUDES 2 *Asperger's syndrome (F84.5)*
  - *delusional disorder (F22)*
  - *schizoid disorder of childhood (F84.5)*
  - *schizophrenia (F20.-)*
  - *schizotypal disorder (F21)*

F60.2 Antisocial personality disorder
- Amoral personality (disorder)
- Asocial personality (disorder)
- Dissocial personality disorder
- Psychopathic personality (disorder)
- Sociopathic personality (disorder)
- EXCLUDES 1 *conduct disorders (F91.-)*
- EXCLUDES 2 *borderline personality disorder (F60.3)*

F60.3 Borderline personality disorder
- Aggressive personality (disorder)
- Emotionally unstable personality disorder
- Explosive personality (disorder)
- EXCLUDES 2 *antisocial personality disorder (F60.2)*

F60.4 Histrionic personality disorder
- Hysterical personality (disorder)
- Psychoinfantile personality (disorder)

F60.5 Obsessive-compulsive personality disorder
- Anankastic personality (disorder)
- Compulsive personality (disorder)
- Obsessional personality (disorder)
- EXCLUDES 2 *obsessive-compulsive disorder (F42)*

F60.6 Avoidant personality disorder
- Anxious personality disorder

F60.7 Dependent personality disorder
- Asthenic personality (disorder)
- Inadequate personality (disorder)
- Passive personality (disorder)

✓5th **F60.8 Other specific personality disorders**
- **F60.81 Narcissistic personality disorder**
- **F60.89 Other specific personality disorders**
  - Eccentric personality disorder
  - "Haltlose" type personality disorder
  - Immature personality disorder
  - Passive-aggressive personality disorder
  - Psychoneurotic personality disorder
  - Self-defeating personality disorder

F60.9 Personality disorder, unspecified
- Character disorder NOS
- Character neurosis NOS
- Pathological personality NOS

✓4th **F63 Impulse disorders**
- EXCLUDES 2 *habitual excessive use of alcohol or psychoactive substances (F10-F19)*
  - *impulse disorders involving sexual behavior (F65.-)*

F63.0 Pathological gambling
- Compulsive gambling
- EXCLUDES 1 *gambling and betting NOS (Z72.6)*
- EXCLUDES 2 *excessive gambling by manic patients (F30, F31)*
  - *gambling in antisocial personality disorder (F60.2)*

F63.1 Pyromania
- Pathological fire-setting
- EXCLUDES 2 *fire-setting (by) (in):*
  - *adult with antisocial personality disorder (F60.2)*
  - *alcohol or psychoactive substance intoxication (F10-F19)*
  - *conduct disorders (F91.-)*
  - *mental disorders due to known physiological condition (F01-F09)*
  - *schizophrenia (F20.-)*

F63.2 Kleptomania
- Pathological stealing
- EXCLUDES 1 *shoplifting as the reason for observation for suspected mental disorder (Z03.8)*
- EXCLUDES 2 *depressive disorder with stealing (F31-F33)*
  - *stealing due to underlying mental condition—code to mental condition*
  - *stealing in mental disorders due to known physiological condition (F01-F09)*

F63.3 Trichotillomania
- Hair plucking
- EXCLUDES 2 *other stereotyped movement disorder (F98.4)*

✓5th **F63.8 Other impulse disorders**
- **F63.81 Intermittent explosive disorder**
- **F63.89 Other impulse disorders**

F63.9 Impulse disorder, unspecified
- Impulse control disorder NOS

✓4th **F64 Gender identity disorders**
- **F64.1 Gender identity disorder in adolescence and adulthood**
  - Dual role transvestism
  - Transsexualism
  - Use additional code to identify sex reassignment status (Z87.890)
  - EXCLUDES 1 *gender identity disorder in childhood (F64.2)*
  - EXCLUDES 2 *fetishistic transvestism (F65.1)*
- **F64.2 Gender identity disorder of childhood**   P
  - EXCLUDES 1 *gender identity disorder in adolescence and adulthood (F64.1)*
  - EXCLUDES 2 *sexual maturation disorder (F66)*
- **F64.8 Other gender identity disorders**
- **F64.9 Gender identity disorder, unspecified**
  - Gender-role disorder NOS

✓4th **F65 Paraphilias**
- **F65.0 Fetishism**
- **F65.1 Transvestic fetishism**
  - Fetishistic transvestism
- **F65.2 Exhibitionism**
- **F65.3 Voyeurism**
- **F65.4 Pedophilia**
- ✓5th **F65.5 Sadomasochism**
  - **F65.50 Sadomasochism, unspecified**
  - **F65.51 Sexual masochism**
  - **F65.52 Sexual sadism**
- ✓5th **F65.8 Other paraphilias**
  - **F65.81 Frotteurism**
  - **F65.89 Other paraphilias**
    - Necrophilia
- **F65.9 Paraphilia, unspecified**
  - Sexual deviation NOS

F66 Other sexual disorders
- Sexual maturation disorder
- Sexual relationship disorder

✓4th **F68 Other disorders of adult personality and behavior**
- ✓5th **F68.1 Factitious disorder**
  - Compensation neurosis
  - Elaboration of physical symptoms for psychological reasons
  - Hospital hopper syndrome
  - Münchhausen's syndrome
  - Peregrinating patient
  - EXCLUDES 2 *factitial dermatitis (L98.1)*
    - *person feigning illness (with obvious motivation) (Z76.5)*
  - **F68.10 Factitious disorder, unspecified**
  - **F68.11 Factitious disorder with predominantly psychological signs and symptoms**
  - **F68.12 Factitious disorder with predominantly physical signs and symptoms**
  - **F68.13 Factitious disorder with combined psychological and physical signs and symptoms**
- **F68.8 Other specified disorders of adult personality and behavior**

F69 Unspecified disorder of adult personality and behavior   A

Intellectual Disabilities (F70-F79)

Code first any associated physical or developmental disorders
- EXCLUDES 1 *borderline intellectual functioning, IQ above 70 to 84 (R41.83)*

F70 Mild intellectual disabilities
- IQ level 50-55 to approximately 70
- Mild mental subnormality

F71 Moderate intellectual disabilities
- IQ level 35-40 to 50-55
- Moderate mental subnormality

F72 Severe intellectual disabilities
- IQ 20-25 to 35-40
- Severe mental subnormality

F73 Profound intellectual disabilities
- IQ level below 20-25
- Profound mental subnormality

☑ Additional Character Required   ✓x7th Placeholder Alert   Unspecified Dx   Other Specified Dx   Manifestation   ▶◀ Revised Text   ● New Code   ▲ Revised Code Title

F78 **Other intellectual disabilities**

F79 **Unspecified intellectual disabilities**
Mental deficiency NOS
Mental subnormality NOS

Pervasive and specific developmental disorders (F80-F89)

✅4ᵗʰ **F80** **Specific developmental disorders of speech and language**

F80.0 **Phonological disorder**
Dyslalia
Functional speech articulation disorder
Lalling
Lisping
Phonological developmental disorder
Speech articulation developmental disorder
EXCLUDES 1 *speech articulation impairment due to aphasia NOS (R47.01)*
speech articulation impairment due to apraxia (R48.2)
EXCLUDES 2 *speech articulation impairment due to hearing loss (F80.4)*
speech articulation impairment due to intellectual disabilities (F70-F79)
speech articulation impairment with expressive language developmental disorder (F80.1)
speech articulation impairment with mixed receptive expressive language developmental disorder (F80.2)

F80.1 **Expressive language disorder**
Developmental dysphasia or aphasia, expressive type
EXCLUDES 1 *dysphasia and aphasia NOS (R47.-)*
mixed receptive-expressive language disorder (F80.2)
EXCLUDES 2 *acquired aphasia with epilepsy [Landau-Kleffner] (G40.80-)*
intellectual disabilities (F70-F79)
pervasive developmental disorders (F84.-)
selective mutism (F94.0)

F80.2 **Mixed receptive-expressive language disorder**
Developmental dysphasia or aphasia, receptive type
Developmental Wernicke's aphasia
EXCLUDES 1 *central auditory processing disorder (H93.25)*
dysphasia or aphasia NOS (R47.-)
expressive language disorder (F80.1)
expressive type dysphasia or aphasia (F80.1)
word deafness (H93.25)
EXCLUDES 2 *acquired aphasia with epilepsy [Landau-Kleffner] (G40.80-)*
intellectual disabilities (F70-F79)
pervasive developmental disorders (F84.-)
selective mutism (F94.0)

F80.4 **Speech and language development delay due to hearing loss**
Code also type of hearing loss (H90.-, H91.-)

✅5ᵗʰ **F80.8** **Other developmental disorders of speech and language**

F80.81 **Childhood onset fluency disorder**
Cluttering NOS
Stuttering NOS
EXCLUDES 1 *adult onset fluency disorder (F98.5)*
fluency disorder in conditions classified elsewhere (R47.82)
fluency disorder (stuttering) following cerebrovascular disease (I69. with final characters-23)

F80.89 **Other developmental disorders of speech and language**

F80.9 **Developmental disorder of speech and language, unspecified**
Communication disorder NOS
Language disorder NOS

✅4ᵗʰ **F81** **Specific developmental disorders of scholastic skills**

F81.0 **Specific reading disorder**
"Backward reading"
Developmental dyslexia
Specific reading retardation
EXCLUDES 1 *alexia NOS (R48.0)*
dyslexia NOS (R48.0)

F81.2 **Mathematics disorder**
Developmental acalculia
Developmental arithmetical disorder
Developmental Gerstmann's syndrome
EXCLUDES 1 *acalculia NOS (R48.8)*
EXCLUDES 2 *arithmetical difficulties associated with a reading disorder (F81.0)*
arithmetical difficulties associated with a spelling disorder (F81.81)
arithmetical difficulties due to inadequate teaching (Z55.8)

✅5ᵗʰ **F81.8** **Other developmental disorders of scholastic skills**

F81.81 **Disorder of written expression**
Specific spelling disorder

F81.89 **Other developmental disorders of scholastic skills**

F81.9 **Developmental disorder of scholastic skills, unspecified**
Knowledge acquisition disability NOS
Learning disability NOS
Learning disorder NOS

F82 **Specific developmental disorder of motor function**
Clumsy child syndrome
Developmental coordination disorder
Developmental dyspraxia
EXCLUDES 1 *abnormalities of gait and mobility (R26.-)*
lack of coordination (R27.-)
EXCLUDES 2 *lack of coordination secondary to intellectual disabilities (F70-F79)*

✅4ᵗʰ **F84** **Pervasive developmental disorders**
Use additional code to identify any associated medical condition and intellectual disabilities

F84.0 **Autistic disorder**
Infantile autism
Infantile psychosis
Kanner's syndrome
EXCLUDES 1 *Asperger's syndrome (F84.5)*

F84.2 **Rett's syndrome**
EXCLUDES 1 *Asperger's syndrome (F84.5)*
Autistic disorder (F84.0)
Other childhood disintegrative disorder (F84.3)

F84.3 **Other childhood disintegrative disorder** P
Dementia infantilis
Disintegrative psychosis
Heller's syndrome
Symbiotic psychosis
Use additional code to identify any associated neurological condition
EXCLUDES 1 *Asperger's syndrome (F84.5)*
Autistic disorder (F84.0)
Rett's syndrome (F84.2)

F84.5 **Asperger's syndrome**
Asperger's disorder
Autistic psychopathy
Schizoid disorder of childhood

F84.8 **Other pervasive developmental disorders**
Overactive disorder associated with intellectual disabilities and stereotyped movements

F84.9 **Pervasive developmental disorder, unspecified**
Atypical autism

F88 **Other disorders of psychological development**
Developmental agnosia

F89 **Unspecified disorder of psychological development**
Developmental disorder NOS

Behavioral and emotional disorders with onset usually occurring in childhood and adolescence (F90-F98)

NOTE Codes within categories F90-F98 may be used regardless of the age of a patient. These disorders generally have onset within the childhood or adolescent years, but may continue throughout life or not be diagnosed until adulthood.

✅4ᵗʰ **F90** **Attention-deficit hyperactivity disorders**
INCLUDES attention deficit disorder with hyperactivity
attention deficit syndrome with hyperactivity
EXCLUDES 2 *anxiety disorders (F40.-, F41.-)*
mood [affective] disorders (F30-F39)
pervasive developmental disorders (F84.-)
schizophrenia (F20.-)

F90.0 **Attention-deficit hyperactivity disorder, predominantly inattentive type**

EXCLUDES 1 Not coded here   EXCLUDES 2 Not included here   N Newborn Age: 0   P Pediatric Age: 0-17   M Maternity Age: 12-55   A Adult Age: 15-124

F90.1   **Attention-deficit hyperactivity disorder, predominantly hyperactive type**

F90.2   **Attention-deficit hyperactivity disorder, combined type**

F90.8   **Attention-deficit hyperactivity disorder, other type**

F90.9   **Attention-deficit hyperactivity disorder, unspecified type**
     Attention-deficit hyperactivity disorder of childhood or adolescence NOS
     Attention-deficit hyperactivity disorder NOS

✓4ᵗʰ **F91**   **Conduct disorders**
     EXCLUDES 1   *antisocial behavior (Z72.81-)*
         antisocial personality disorder (F60.2)
     EXCLUDES 2   *conduct problems associated with attention-deficit hyperactivity disorder (F90.-)*
         mood [affective] disorders (F30-F39)
         pervasive developmental disorders (F84.-)
         schizophrenia (F20.-)

F91.0   **Conduct disorder confined to family context**

F91.1   **Conduct disorder, childhood-onset type**
     Unsocialized conduct disorder
     Conduct disorder, solitary aggressive type
     Unsocialized aggressive disorder

F91.2   **Conduct disorder, adolescent-onset type**
     Socialized conduct disorder
     Conduct disorder, group type

F91.3   **Oppositional defiant disorder**

F91.8   **Other conduct disorders**

F91.9   **Conduct disorder, unspecified**
     Behavioral disorder NOS
     Conduct disorder NOS
     Disruptive behavior disorder NOS

✓4ᵗʰ **F93**   **Emotional disorders with onset specific to childhood**

F93.0   **Separation anxiety disorder of childhood**   P
     EXCLUDES 2   *mood [affective] disorders (F30-F39)*
         nonpsychotic mental disorders (F40-F48)
         phobic anxiety disorder of childhood (F40.8)
         social phobia (F40.1)

F93.8   **Other childhood emotional disorders**   P
     Identity disorder
     EXCLUDES 2   *gender identity disorder of childhood (F64.2)*

F93.9   **Childhood emotional disorder, unspecified**   P

✓4ᵗʰ **F94**   **Disorders of social functioning with onset specific to childhood and adolescence**

F94.0   **Selective mutism**
     Elective mutism
     EXCLUDES 2   *pervasive developmental disorders (F84.-)*
         schizophrenia (F20.-)
         specific developmental disorders of speech and language (F80.-)
         transient mutism as part of separation anxiety in young children (F93.0)

F94.1   **Reactive attachment disorder of childhood**   P
     Use additional code to identify any associated failure to thrive or growth retardation
     EXCLUDES 1   *disinhibited attachment disorder of childhood (F94.1)*
         normal variation in pattern of selective attachment
     EXCLUDES 2   *Asperger's syndrome (F84.5)*
         maltreatment syndromes (T74.-)
         sexual or physical abuse in childhood, resulting in psychosocial problems (Z62.81-)

F94.2   **Disinhibited attachment disorder of childhood**   P
     Affectionless psychopathy
     Institutional syndrome
     EXCLUDES 1   *reactive attachment disorder of childhood (F94.1)*
     EXCLUDES 2   *Asperger's syndrome (F84.5)*
         attention-deficit hyperactivity disorders (F90.-)
         hospitalism in children (F43.2-)

F94.8   **Other childhood disorders of social functioning**   P

F94.9   **Childhood disorder of social functioning, unspecified**   P

✓4ᵗʰ **F95**   **Tic disorder**

F95.0   **Transient tic disorder**

F95.1   **Chronic motor or vocal tic disorder**

F95.2   **Tourette's disorder**
     Combined vocal and multiple motor tic disorder [de la Tourette]
     Tourette's syndrome

F95.8   **Other tic disorders**

F95.9   **Tic disorder, unspecified**
     Tic NOS

✓4ᵗʰ **F98**   **Other behavioral and emotional disorders with onset usually occurring in childhood and adolescence**
     EXCLUDES 2   *breath-holding spells (R06.89)*
         gender identity disorder of childhood (F64.2)
         Kleine-Levin syndrome (G47.13)
         obsessive-compulsive disorder (F42)
         sleep disorders not due to a substance or known physiological condition (F51.-)

F98.0   **Enuresis not due to a substance or known physiological condition**
     Enuresis (primary) (secondary) of nonorganic origin
     Functional enuresis
     Psychogenic enuresis
     Urinary incontinence of nonorganic origin
     EXCLUDES 1   *enuresis NOS (R32)*

F98.1   **Encopresis not due to a substance or known physiological condition**
     Functional encopresis
     Incontinence of feces of nonorganic origin
     Psychogenic encopresis
     Use additional code to identify the cause of any coexisting constipation
     EXCLUDES 1   *encopresis NOS (R15.-)*

✓5ᵗʰ **F98.2**   **Other feeding disorders of infancy and childhood**
     EXCLUDES 1   *feeding difficulties (R63.3)*
     EXCLUDES 2   *anorexia nervosa and other eating disorders (F50.-)*
         feeding problems of newborn (P92.-)
         pica of infancy or childhood (F98.3)

     F98.21   **Rumination disorder of infancy**   P

     F98.29   **Other feeding disorders of infancy and early childhood**   P

F98.3   **Pica of infancy and childhood**   P

F98.4   **Stereotyped movement disorders**
     Stereotype/habit disorder
     EXCLUDES 1   *abnormal involuntary movements (R25.-)*
     EXCLUDES 2   *compulsions in obsessive-compulsive disorder (F42)*
         hair plucking (F63.3)
         movement disorders of organic origin (G20-G25)
         nail-biting (F98.8)
         nose-picking (F98.8)
         stereotypies that are part of a broader psychiatric condition (F01-F95)
         thumb-sucking (F98.8)
         tic disorders (F95.-)
         trichotillomania (F63.3)

F98.5   **Adult onset fluency disorder**
     EXCLUDES 1   *childhood onset fluency disorder (F80.81)*
         dysphasia (R47.02)
         fluency disorder in conditions classified elsewhere (R47.82)
         fluency disorder (stuttering) following cerebrovascular disease (I69. with final characters -23)
         tic disorders (F95.-)

F98.8   **Other specified behavioral and emotional disorders with onset usually occurring in childhood and adolescence**   P
     Excessive masturbation
     Nail-biting
     Nose-picking
     Thumb-sucking

F98.9   **Unspecified behavioral and emotional disorders with onset usually occurring in childhood and adolescence**   P

Unspecified mental disorder (F99)

F99   **Mental disorder, not otherwise specified**
     Mental illness NOS
     EXCLUDES 1   *unspecified mental disorder due to known physiological condition (F09)*

☑ Additional Character Required   ✓×7ᵗʰ Placeholder Alert   Unspecified Dx   Other Specified Dx   Manifestation   ▶◀ Revised Text   ● New Code   ▲ Revised Code Title

Chapter 6. Diseases of the Nervous System (G00-G99)

Chapter Specific Guidelines with Coding Examples

The chapter specific guidelines from the ICD-10-CM Official Guidelines for Coding and Reporting have been provided below. Along with these guidelines are coding examples, contained in the shaded boxes, that have been developed to help illustrate the coding and/or sequencing guidance found in these guidelines.

a. Dominant/nondominant side

Codes from category G81, Hemiplegia and hemiparesis, and subcategories G83.1, Monoplegia of lower limb, G83.2, Monoplegia of upper limb, and G83.3, Monoplegia, unspecified, identify whether the dominant or nondominant side is affected. Should the affected side be documented, but not specified as dominant or nondominant, and the classification system does not indicate a default, code selection is as follows:

- For ambidextrous patients, the default should be dominant.
- If the left side is affected, the default is non-dominant.
- If the right side is affected, the default is dominant.

Hemiplegia affecting left side of ambidextrous patient

G81.92   Hemiplegia, unspecified affecting left dominant side

Explanation: Documentation states that the left side is affected and dominant is used for ambidextrous persons.

Right spastic hemiplegia, unknown whether patient is right- or left-handed

G81.11   Spastic hemiplegia affecting right dominant side

Explanation: Since it is unknown whether the patient is right- or left-handed, if the right side is affected, the default is dominant.

---

b. Pain—Category G89

1) General coding information

Codes in category G89, Pain, not elsewhere classified, may be used in conjunction with codes from other categories and chapters to provide more detail about acute or chronic pain and neoplasm-related pain, unless otherwise indicated below.

If the pain is not specified as acute or chronic, post-thoracotomy, postprocedural, or neoplasm-related, do not assign codes from category G89.

A code from category G89 should not be assigned if the underlying (definitive) diagnosis is known, unless the reason for the encounter is pain control/ management and not management of the underlying condition.

When an admission or encounter is for a procedure aimed at treating the underlying condition (e.g., spinal fusion, kyphoplasty), a code for the underlying condition (e.g., vertebral fracture, spinal stenosis) should be assigned as the principal diagnosis. No code from category G89 should be assigned.

Elderly patient with back pain is admitted for outpatient kyphoplasty for age-related osteopathic compression fracture at vertebra T3

M80.08XA   Age-related osteoporosis with current pathological fracture, vertebra(e), initial encounter

Explanation: No code is assigned for the pain as it is inherent in the underlying condition being treated.

(a) Category G89 codes as principal or first-listed diagnosis

Category G89 codes are acceptable as principal diagnosis or the first-listed code:

- When pain control or pain management is the reason for the admission/encounter (e.g., a patient with displaced intervertebral disc, nerve impingement and severe back pain presents for injection of steroid into the spinal canal). The underlying cause of the pain should be reported as an additional diagnosis, if known.

Patient presents for a steroid injection for control of pain of chronic right knee due to primary degenerative joint disease

G89.29   Other chronic pain

M17.11   Unilateral primary osteoarthritis, right knee

Explanation: Since the encounter is for control of pain, not treating the underlying condition, the pain code is sequenced first followed by the underlying condition. The M25 pain code is not necessary as the underlying condition code represents the specific site.

- When a patient is admitted for the insertion of a neurostimulator for pain control, assign the appropriate pain code as the principal or first-listed diagnosis. When an admission or encounter is for a procedure aimed at treating the underlying condition and a neurostimulator is inserted for pain control during the same admission/encounter, a code for the underlying condition should be assigned as the principal diagnosis and the appropriate pain code should be assigned as a secondary diagnosis.

(b) Use of category G89 codes in conjunction with site specific pain codes

(i) Assigning category G89 and site-specific pain codes

Codes from category G89 may be used in conjunction with codes that identify the site of pain (including codes from chapter 18) if the category G89 code provides additional information. For example, if the code describes the site of the pain, but does not fully describe whether the pain is acute or chronic, then both codes should be assigned.

Patient is seen to evaluate chronic left shoulder pain

M25.512   Pain in left shoulder

G89.29   Other chronic pain

Explanation: No underlying condition has been determined yet so the pain would be the reason for the visit. The M25 pain code in this instance does not fully describe the condition as it does not represent that the pain is chronic. The G89 chronic pain code is assigned to provide specificity.

(ii) Sequencing of category G89 codes with site-specific pain codes

The sequencing of category G89 codes with site-specific pain codes (including chapter 18 codes), is dependent on the circumstances of the encounter/admission as follows:

- If the encounter is for pain control or pain management, assign the code from category G89 followed by the code identifying the specific site of pain (e.g., encounter for pain management for acute neck pain from trauma is assigned code G89.11, Acute pain due to trauma, followed by code M54.2, Cervicalgia, to identify the site of pain).

Management of acute, traumatic right knee pain

G89.11   Acute pain due to trauma

M25.561   Pain in right knee

Explanation: The reason for the encounter is to manage or control the pain, not to treat or evaluate an underlying condition. The G89 pain code is assigned as the principal diagnosis but in this instance does not fully describe the condition as it does not include the site and laterality. The M25 pain code is added to provide this information.

- If the encounter is for any other reason except pain control or pain management, and a related definitive diagnosis has not been established (confirmed) by the provider, assign the code for the specific site of pain first, followed by the appropriate code from category G89.

Tests are performed to investigate the source of the patient's chronic epigastric abdominal pain

R10.13	Epigastric pain
G89.29	Other chronic pain

Explanation: In this instance the patient's epigastric pain is not being treated; rather the source of the pain is being investigated. A code from chapter 18 for epigastric pain is sequenced before the additional specificity of the G89 code for the chronic pain.

2) Pain due to devices, implants and grafts

See Section I.C.19. Pain due to medical devices

3) Postoperative Pain

The provider's documentation should be used to guide the coding of postoperative pain, as well as *Section III. Reporting Additional Diagnoses* and *Section IV. Diagnostic Coding and Reporting in the Outpatient Setting*.

The default for post-thoracotomy and other postoperative pain not specified as acute or chronic is the code for the acute form.

Routine or expected postoperative pain immediately after surgery should not be coded.

Pain pump dose is increased for the patient's unexpected, extreme pain post-thoracotomy

G89.12	Acute post-thoracotomy pain

Explanation: When acute or chronic is not documented, default to acute. The use of "unexpected, extreme" and the increase of medication dosage indicate that the pain was more than routine or expected.

(a) Postoperative pain not associated with specific postoperative complication

Postoperative pain not associated with a specific postoperative complication is assigned to the appropriate postoperative pain code in category G89.

(b) Postoperative pain associated with specific postoperative complication

Postoperative pain associated with a specific postoperative complication (such as painful wire sutures) is assigned to the appropriate code(s) found in Chapter 19, Injury, poisoning, and certain other consequences of external causes. If appropriate, use additional code(s) from category G89 to identify acute or chronic pain (G89.18 or G89.28).

4) Chronic pain

Chronic pain is classified to subcategory G89.2. There is no time frame defining when pain becomes chronic pain. The provider's documentation should be used to guide use of these codes.

5) Neoplasm related pain

Code G89.3 is assigned to pain documented as being related, associated or due to cancer, primary or secondary malignancy, or tumor. This code is assigned regardless of whether the pain is acute or chronic.

This code may be assigned as the principal or first-listed code when the stated reason for the admission/encounter is documented as pain control/pain management. The underlying neoplasm should be reported as an additional diagnosis.

Pain medication adjustment for chronic pain from bone metastasis

G89.3	Neoplasm related pain (acute)(chronic)
C79.51	Secondary malignant neoplasm of bone

Explanation: Since the encounter was for pain medication management, the pain, rather than the neoplasm, was the reason for the encounter and is sequenced first. This "neoplasm-related pain" code includes both acute and chronic pain.

When the reason for the admission/encounter is management of the neoplasm and the pain associated with the neoplasm is also documented, code G89.3 may be assigned as an additional diagnosis. It is not necessary to assign an additional code for the site of the pain.

See Section I.C.2 for instructions on the sequencing of neoplasms for all other stated reasons for the admission/encounter (except for pain control/pain management).

Patient with lung cancer presents with acute hip pain and is evaluated and found to have iliac bone metastasis

C79.51	Secondary malignant neoplasm of bone
C34.90	Malignant neoplasm of unspecified part of unspecified bronchus or lung
G89.3	Neoplasm related pain (acute)(chronic)

Explanation: The reason for the encounter was the evaluation and diagnosis of the bone metastasis, whose code would be assigned as first-listed, followed by codes for the primary neoplasm and the pain due to the iliac bone metastasis.

6) Chronic pain syndrome

Central pain syndrome (G89.0) and chronic pain syndrome (G89.4) are different than the term "chronic pain," and therefore codes should only be used when the provider has specifically documented this condition.

See Section I.C.5. Pain disorders related to psychological factors

Chapter 6. Diseases of the Nervous System (G00-G99)

> EXCLUDES 2   *certain conditions originating in the perinatal period (P04-P96)*
> *certain infectious and parasitic diseases (A00-B99)*
> *complications of pregnancy, childbirth and the puerperium (O00-O9A)*
> *congenital malformations, deformations, and chromosomal abnormalities (Q00-Q99)*
> *endocrine, nutritional and metabolic diseases (E00-E88)*
> *injury, poisoning and certain other consequences of external causes (S00-T88)*
> *neoplasms (C00-D49)*
> *symptoms, signs and abnormal clinical and laboratory findings, not elsewhere classified (R00-R94)*

This chapter contains the following blocks:

G00-G09	Inflammatory diseases of the central nervous system
G10-G14	Systemic atrophies primarily affecting the central nervous system
G20-G26	Extrapyramidal and movement disorders
G30-G32	Other degenerative diseases of the nervous system
G35-G37	Demyelinating diseases of the central nervous system
G40-G47	Episodic and paroxysmal disorders
G50-G59	Nerve, nerve root and plexus disorders
G60-G65	Polyneuropathies and other disorders of the peripheral nervous system
G70-G73	Diseases of myoneural junction and muscle
G80-G83	Cerebral palsy and other paralytic syndromes
G89-G99	Other disorders of the nervous system

Inflammatory diseases of the central nervous system (G00-G09)

✓4ᵗʰ **G00**   **Bacterial meningitis, not elsewhere classified**

> INCLUDES   bacterial arachnoiditis
> bacterial leptomeningitis
> bacterial meningitis
> bacterial pachymeningitis

> EXCLUDES 1   *bacterial:*
> *meningoencephalitis (G04.2)*
> *meningomyelitis (G04.2)*

G00.0   **Hemophilus meningitis**
Meningitis due to Hemophilus influenzae

G00.1   **Pneumococcal meningitis**

G00.2   **Streptococcal meningitis**
Use additional code to further identify organism (B95.0-B95.5)

G00.3   **Staphylococcal meningitis**
Use additional code to further identify organism (B95.61-B95.8)

G00.8   **Other bacterial meningitis**
Meningitis due to Escherichia coli
Meningitis due to Friedländer's bacillus
Meningitis due to Klebsiella
Use additional code to further identify organism (B96.-)

G00.9   **Bacterial meningitis, unspecified**
Meningitis due to gram-negative bacteria, unspecified
Purulent meningitis NOS
Pyogenic meningitis NOS
Suppurative meningitis NOS

G01   *Meningitis in bacterial diseases classified elsewhere*

> Code first underlying disease
> EXCLUDES 1   *meningitis (in):*
> *gonococcal (A54.81)*
> *leptospirosis (A27.81)*
> *listeriosis (A32.11)*
> *Lyme disease (A69.21)*
> *meningococcal (A39.0)*
> *neurosyphilis (A52.13)*
> *tuberculosis (A17.0)*
> *meningoencephalitis and meningomyelitis in bacterial diseases classified elsewhere (G05)*

G02   *Meningitis in other infectious and parasitic diseases classified elsewhere*

> Code first underlying disease, such as:
> African trypanosomiasis (B56.-)
> poliovirus infection (A80.-)
> EXCLUDES 1   *candidal meningitis (B37.5)*
> *coccidioidomycosis meningitis (B38.4)*
> *cryptococcal meningitis (B45.1)*
> *herpesviral [herpes simplex] meningitis (B00.3)*
> *infectious mononucleosis complicated by meningitis (B27.- with fourth character 2)*
> *measles complicated by meningitis (B05.1)*
> *meningoencephalitis and meningomyelitis in other infectious and parasitic diseases classified elsewhere (G05)*
> *mumps meningitis (B26.1)*
> *rubella meningitis (B06.02)*
> *varicella [chickenpox] meningitis (B01.0)*
> *zoster meningitis (B02.1)*

✓4ᵗʰ **G03**   **Meningitis due to other and unspecified causes**

> INCLUDES   arachnoiditis NOS
> leptomeningitis NOS
> meningitis NOS
> pachymeningitis NOS

> EXCLUDES 1   *meningoencephalitis (G04.-)*
> *meningomyelitis (G04.-)*

G03.0   **Nonpyogenic meningitis**
Aseptic meningitis
Nonbacterial meningitis

G03.1   **Chronic meningitis**

G03.2   **Benign recurrent meningitis [Mollaret]**

G03.8   **Meningitis due to other specified causes**

G03.9   **Meningitis, unspecified**
Arachnoiditis (spinal) NOS

✓4ᵗʰ **G04**   **Encephalitis, myelitis and encephalomyelitis**

> INCLUDES   acute ascending myelitis
> meningoencephalitis
> meningomyelitis

> EXCLUDES 1   *encephalopathy NOS (G93.40)*
> EXCLUDES 2   *acute transverse myelitis (G37.3-)*
> *alcoholic encephalopathy (G31.2)*
> *benign myalgic encephalomyelitis (G93.3)*
> *multiple sclerosis (G35)*
> *subacute necrotizing myelitis (G37.4)*
> *toxic encephalitis (G92)*
> *toxic encephalopathy (G92)*

✓5ᵗʰ **G04.0**   **Acute disseminated encephalitis and encephalomyelitis (ADEM)**

> EXCLUDES 1   *acute necrotizing hemorrhagic encephalopathy (G04.3-)*
> *other noninfectious acute disseminated encephalomyelitis (noninfectious ADEM) (G04.81)*

G04.00   **Acute disseminated encephalitis and encephalomyelitis, unspecified**

G04.01   **Postinfectious acute disseminated encephalitis and encephalomyelitis (postinfectious ADEM)**

> EXCLUDES 1   *post chickenpox encephalitis (B01.1)*
> *post measles encephalitis (B05.0)*
> *post measles myelitis (B05.1)*

G04.02   **Postimmunization acute disseminated encephalitis, myelitis and encephalomyelitis**
Encephalitis, postimmunization
Encephalomyelitis, postimmunization
Use additional code to identify the vaccine (T50.A-, T50.B-, T50.Z-)

G04.1   **Tropical spastic paraplegia**

G04.2   **Bacterial meningoencephalitis and meningomyelitis, not elsewhere classified**

✓5ᵗʰ **G04.3**   **Acute necrotizing hemorrhagic encephalopathy**

> EXCLUDES 1   *acute disseminated encephalitis and encephalomyelitis (G04.0-)*

G04.30   **Acute necrotizing hemorrhagic encephalopathy, unspecified**

G04.31   **Postinfectious acute necrotizing hemorrhagic encephalopathy**

G04.32   **Postimmunization acute necrotizing hemorrhagic encephalopathy**
Use additional code to identify the vaccine (T50.A-, T50.B-, T50.Z-)

EXCLUDES 1 Not coded here   EXCLUDES 2 Not included here   N Newborn Age: 0   P Pediatric Age: 0-17   M Maternity Age: 12-55   A Adult Age: 15-124

524   ICD-10-CM 2016

G04.39 Other acute necrotizing hemorrhagic encephalopathy
>> Code also underlying etiology, if applicable

✓5ᵗʰ **G04.8 Other encephalitis, myelitis and encephalomyelitis**
> Code also any associated seizure (G40.-, R56.9)

G04.81 Other encephalitis and encephalomyelitis
>> Noninfectious acute disseminated encephalomyelitis (noninfectious ADEM)

G04.89 Other myelitis

✓5ᵗʰ **G04.9 Encephalitis, myelitis and encephalomyelitis, unspecified**

G04.90 Encephalitis and encephalomyelitis, unspecified
>> Ventriculitis (cerebral) NOS

G04.91 Myelitis, unspecified

✓4ᵗʰ **G05 Encephalitis, myelitis and encephalomyelitis in diseases classified elsewhere**
> *Code first underlying disease, such as:*
> *human immunodeficiency virus [HIV] disease (B20)*
> *poliovirus (A80.-)*
> *suppurative otitis media (H66.01-H66.4)*
> *trichinellosis (B75)*
>> EXCLUDES 1   *adenoviral encephalitis, myelitis and encephalomyelitis (A85.1)*
>> *congenital toxoplasmosis encephalitis, myelitis and encephalomyelitis (P37.1)*
>> *cytomegaloviral encephalitis, myelitis and encephalomyelitis (B25.8)*
>> *encephalitis, myelitis and encephalomyelitis (in) measles (B05.0)*
>> *encephalitis, myelitis and encephalomyelitis (in) systemic lupus erythematosus (M32.19)*
>> *enteroviral encephalitis, myelitis and encephalomyelitis (A85.0)*
>> *eosinophilic meningoencephalitis (B83.2)*
>> *herpesviral [herpes simplex] encephalitis, myelitis and encephalomyelitis (B00.4)*
>> *listerial encephalitis, myelitis and encephalomyelitis (A32.12)*
>> *meningococcal encephalitis, myelitis and encephalomyelitis (A39.81)*
>> *mumps encephalitis, myelitis and encephalomyelitis (B26.2)*
>> *postchickenpox encephalitis, myelitis and encephalomyelitis (B01.1-)*
>> *rubella encephalitis, myelitis and encephalomyelitis (B06.01)*
>> *toxoplasmosis encephalitis, myelitis and encephalomyelitis (B58.2)*
>> *zoster encephalitis, myelitis and encephalomyelitis (B02.0)*

G05.3 Encephalitis and encephalomyelitis in diseases classified elsewhere
>> Meningoencephalitis in diseases classified elsewhere

G05.4 Myelitis in diseases classified elsewhere
>> Meningomyelitis in diseases classified elsewhere

✓4ᵗʰ **G06 Intracranial and intraspinal abscess and granuloma**
> Use additional code (B95-B97) to identify infectious agent

G06.0 Intracranial abscess and granuloma
>> Brain [any part] abscess (embolic)
>> Cerebellar abscess (embolic)
>> Cerebral abscess (embolic)
>> Intracranial epidural abscess or granuloma
>> Intracranial extradural abscess or granuloma
>> Intracranial subdural abscess or granuloma
>> Otogenic abscess (embolic)
>> EXCLUDES 1   *tuberculous intracranial abscess and granuloma (A17.81)*

G06.1 Intraspinal abscess and granuloma
>> Abscess (embolic) of spinal cord [any part]
>> Intraspinal epidural abscess or granuloma
>> Intraspinal extradural abscess or granuloma
>> Intraspinal subdural abscess or granuloma
>> EXCLUDES 1   *tuberculous intraspinal abscess and granuloma (A17.81)*

G06.2 Extradural and subdural abscess, unspecified

G07 Intracranial and intraspinal abscess and granuloma in diseases classified elsewhere
> *Code first underlying disease, such as:*
> *schistosomiasis granuloma of brain (B65.-)*
>> EXCLUDES 1   *abscess of brain:*
>> *amebic (A06.6)*
>> *chromomycotic (B43.1)*
>> *gonococcal (A54.82)*
>> *tuberculous (A17.81)*
>> *tuberculoma of meninges (A17.1)*

G08 Intracranial and intraspinal phlebitis and thrombophlebitis
> Septic embolism of intracranial or intraspinal venous sinuses and veins
> Septic endophlebitis of intracranial or intraspinal venous sinuses and veins
> Septic phlebitis of intracranial or intraspinal venous sinuses and veins
> Septic thrombophlebitis of intracranial or intraspinal venous sinuses and veins
> Septic thrombosis of intracranial or intraspinal venous sinuses and veins
>> EXCLUDES 1   *intracranial phlebitis and thrombophlebitis complicating:*
>> *abortion, ectopic or molar pregnancy (O00-O07, O08.7)*
>> *pregnancy, childbirth and the puerperium (O22.5, O87.3)*
>> *nonpyogenic intracranial phlebitis and thrombophlebitis (I67.6)*
>> EXCLUDES 2   *intracranial phlebitis and thrombophlebitis complicating nonpyogenic intraspinal phlebitis and thrombophlebitis (G95.1)*

G09 Sequelae of inflammatory diseases of central nervous system
>> NOTE   Category G09 is to be used to indicate conditions whose primary classification is to G00-G08 as the cause of sequelae, themselves classifiable elsewhere. The "sequelae" include conditions specified as residuals.
> Code first condition resulting from (sequela) of inflammatory diseases of central nervous system

Systemic atrophies primarily affecting the central nervous system (G10-G14)

G10 Huntington's disease
> Huntington's chorea
> Huntington's dementia

✓4ᵗʰ **G11 Hereditary ataxia**
>> EXCLUDES 2   *cerebral palsy (G80.-)*
>> *hereditary and idiopathic neuropathy (G60.-)*
>> *metabolic disorders (E70-E88)*

G11.0 Congenital nonprogressive ataxia

G11.1 Early-onset cerebellar ataxia
>> Early-onset cerebellar ataxia with essential tremor
>> Early-onset cerebellar ataxia with myoclonus [Hunt's ataxia]
>> Early-onset cerebellar ataxia with retained tendon reflexes
>> Friedreich's ataxia (autosomal recessive)
>> X-linked recessive spinocerebellar ataxia

G11.2 Late-onset cerebellar ataxia   🄰

G11.3 Cerebellar ataxia with defective DNA repair
>> Ataxia telangiectasia [Louis-Bar]
>> EXCLUDES 2   *Cockayne's syndrome (Q87.1)*
>> *other disorders of purine and pyrimidine metabolism (E79.-)*
>> *xeroderma pigmentosum (Q82.1)*

G11.4 Hereditary spastic paraplegia

G11.8 Other hereditary ataxias

G11.9 Hereditary ataxia, unspecified
>> Hereditary cerebellar ataxia NOS
>> Hereditary cerebellar degeneration
>> Hereditary cerebellar disease
>> Hereditary cerebellar syndrome

✓4ᵗʰ **G12 Spinal muscular atrophy and related syndromes**

G12.0 Infantile spinal muscular atrophy, type I [Werdnig-Hoffman]

G12.1 Other inherited spinal muscular atrophy
>> Adult form spinal muscular atrophy
>> Childhood form, type II spinal muscular atrophy
>> Distal spinal muscular atrophy
>> Juvenile form, type III spinal muscular atrophy [Kugelberg-Welander]
>> Progressive bulbar palsy of childhood [Fazio-Londe]
>> Scapuloperoneal form spinal muscular atrophy

✓5ᵗʰ **G12.2 Motor neuron disease**

G12.20 Motor neuron disease, unspecified

G12.21 Amyotrophic lateral sclerosis   🄰
>> Progressive spinal muscle atrophy

G12.22 Progressive bulbar palsy

G12.29 Other motor neuron disease
>> Familial motor neuron disease
>> Primary lateral sclerosis

G12.8 Other spinal muscular atrophies and related syndromes

G12.9 Spinal muscular atrophy, unspecified

✓ Additional Character Required   ✓ₓ7ᵗʰ Placeholder Alert   Unspecified Dx   Other Specified Dx   Manifestation   ►◄ Revised Text   ● New Code   ▲ Revised Code Title

ICD-10-CM 2016   525

Chapter 6. Diseases of the Nervous System

✓4ᵗʰ **G13 Systemic atrophies primarily affecting central nervous system in diseases classified elsewhere**

G13.0 *Paraneoplastic neuromyopathy and neuropathy*
Carcinomatous neuromyopathy
Sensorial paraneoplastic neuropathy [Denny Brown]
Code first underlying neoplasm (C00-D49)

G13.1 *Other systemic atrophy primarily affecting central nervous system in neoplastic disease*
Paraneoplastic limbic encephalopathy
Code first underlying neoplasm (C00-D49)

G13.2 *Systemic atrophy primarily affecting the central nervous system in myxedema*
Code first underlying disease, such as:
hypothyroidism (E03.-)
myxedematous congenital iodine deficiency (E00.1)

G13.8 *Systemic atrophy primarily affecting central nervous system in other diseases classified elsewhere*
Code first underlying disease

G14 Postpolio syndrome
Postpolio myelitic syndrome
EXCLUDES 1 *sequelae of poliomyelitis (B91)*

Extrapyramidal and movement disorders (G20-G26)

G20 Parkinson's disease
Hemiparkinsonism
Idiopathic Parkinsonism or Parkinson's disease
Paralysis agitans
Parkinsonism or Parkinson's disease NOS
Primary Parkinsonism or Parkinson's disease
EXCLUDES 1 *dementia with Parkinsonism (G31.83)*

✓4ᵗʰ **G21 Secondary parkinsonism**
EXCLUDES 1 *dementia with Parkinsonism (G31.83)*
Huntington's disease (G10)
Shy-Drager syndrome (G90.3)
syphilitic Parkinsonism (A52.19)

G21.0 Malignant neuroleptic syndrome
Use additional code for adverse effect, if applicable, to identify drug (T43.3X5, T43.4X5, T43.505, T43.595)
EXCLUDES 1 *neuroleptic induced parkinsonism (G21.11)*

✓5ᵗʰ **G21.1 Other drug-induced secondary parkinsonism**

G21.11 Neuroleptic induced parkinsonism
Use additional code for adverse effect, if applicable, to identify drug (T43.3X5, T43.4X5, T43.505, T43.595)
EXCLUDES 1 *malignant neuroleptic syndrome (G21.0)*

G21.19 Other drug induced secondary parkinsonism
Use additional code for adverse effect, if applicable, to identify drug (T36-T50 with fifth or sixth character 5)

G21.2 Secondary parkinsonism due to other external agents
Code first (T51-T65) to identify external agent

G21.3 Postencephalitic parkinsonism

G21.4 Vascular parkinsonism

G21.8 Other secondary parkinsonism

G21.9 Secondary parkinsonism, unspecified

✓4ᵗʰ **G23 Other degenerative diseases of basal ganglia**
EXCLUDES 2 *multi-system degeneration of the autonomic nervous system (G90.3)*

G23.0 Hallervorden-Spatz disease
Pigmentary pallidal degeneration

G23.1 Progressive supranuclear ophthalmoplegia [Steele-Richardson-Olszewski]
Progressive supranuclear palsy

G23.2 Striatonigral degeneration

G23.8 Other specified degenerative diseases of basal ganglia
Calcification of basal ganglia

G23.9 Degenerative disease of basal ganglia, unspecified

✓4ᵗʰ **G24 Dystonia**
INCLUDES dyskinesia
EXCLUDES 2 *athetoid cerebral palsy (G80.3)*

✓5ᵗʰ **G24.0 Drug induced dystonia**
Use additional code for adverse effect, if applicable, to identify drug (T36-T50 with fifth or sixth character5)

G24.01 Drug induced subacute dyskinesia
Drug induced blepharospasm
Drug induced orofacial dyskinesia
Neuroleptic induced tardive dyskinesia
Tardive dyskinesia

G24.02 Drug induced acute dystonia
Acute dystonic reaction to drugs
Neuroleptic induced acute dystonia

G24.09 Other drug induced dystonia

G24.1 Genetic torsion dystonia
Dystonia deformans progressiva
Dystonia musculorum deformans
Familial torsion dystonia
Idiopathic familial dystonia
Idiopathic (torsion) dystonia NOS
(Schwalbe-) Ziehen-Oppenheim disease

G24.2 Idiopathic nonfamilial dystonia

G24.3 Spasmodic torticollis
EXCLUDES 1 *congenital torticollis (Q68.0)*
hysterical torticollis (F44.4)
ocular torticollis (R29.891)
psychogenic torticollis (F45.8)
torticollis NOS (M43.6)
traumatic recurrent torticollis (S13.4)

G24.4 Idiopathic orofacial dystonia
Orofacial dyskinesia
EXCLUDES 1 *drug induced orofacial dyskinesia (G24.01)*

G24.5 Blepharospasm
EXCLUDES 1 *drug induced blepharospasm (G24.01)*

G24.8 Other dystonia
Acquired torsion dystonia NOS

G24.9 Dystonia, unspecified
Dyskinesia NOS

✓4ᵗʰ **G25 Other extrapyramidal and movement disorders**
EXCLUDES 2 *sleep related movement disorders (G47.6-)*

G25.0 Essential tremor
Familial tremor
EXCLUDES 1 *tremor NOS (R25.1)*

G25.1 Drug-induced tremor
Use additional code for adverse effect, if applicable, to identify drug (T36-T50 with fifth or sixth character 5)

G25.2 Other specified forms of tremor
Intention tremor

G25.3 Myoclonus
Drug-induced myoclonus
Palatal myoclonus
Use additional code for adverse effect, if applicable, to identify drug (T36-T50 with fifth or sixth character 5)
EXCLUDES 1 *facial myokymia (G51.4)*
myoclonic epilepsy (G40.-)

G25.4 Drug-induced chorea
Use additional code for adverse effect, if applicable, to identify drug (T36-T50 with fifth or sixth character 5)

G25.5 Other chorea
Chorea NOS
EXCLUDES 1 *chorea NOS with heart involvement (I02.0)*
Huntington's chorea (G10)
rheumatic chorea (I02.-)
Sydenham's chorea (I02.-)

✓5ᵗʰ **G25.6 Drug induced tics and other tics of organic origin**

G25.61 Drug induced tics
Use additional code for adverse effect, if applicable, to identify drug (T36-T50 with fifth or sixth character 5)

G25.69 Other tics of organic origin
EXCLUDES 1 *habit spasm (F95.9)*
tic NOS (F95.9)
Tourette's syndrome (F95.2)

✓5ᵗʰ **G25.7 Other and unspecified drug induced movement disorders**
Use additional code for adverse effect, if applicable, to identify drug (T36-T50 with fifth or sixth character 5)

G25.70 Drug induced movement disorder, unspecified

EXCLUDES 1 Not coded here   EXCLUDES 2 Not included here   N Newborn Age: 0   P Pediatric Age: 0-17   M Maternity Age: 12-55   A Adult Age: 15-124

526   ICD-10-CM 2016

G25.71   Drug induced akathisia
Drug induced acathisia
Neuroleptic induced acute akathisia

G25.79   Other drug induced movement disorders

☑5ᵗʰ **G25.8   Other specified extrapyramidal and movement disorders**

G25.81   Restless legs syndrome

G25.82   Stiff-man syndrome

G25.83   Benign shuddering attacks

G25.89   Other specified extrapyramidal and movement disorders

G25.9   Extrapyramidal and movement disorder, unspecified

G26   Extrapyramidal and movement disorders in diseases classified elsewhere
Code first underlying disease

Other degenerative diseases of the nervous system (G30-G32)

☑4ᵗʰ **G30   Alzheimer's disease**
INCLUDES   Alzheimer's dementia senile and presenile forms
Use additional code to identify:
delirium, if applicable (F05)
dementia with behavioral disturbance (F02.81)
dementia without behavioral disturbance (F02.80)
EXCLUDES 1   *senile degeneration of brain NEC (G31.1)*
senile dementia NOS (F03)
senility NOS (R41.81)

G30.0   Alzheimer's disease with early onset

G30.1   Alzheimer's disease with late onset   ▲

G30.8   Other Alzheimer's disease

G30.9   Alzheimer's disease, unspecified
AHA: 2012, 4Q, 95

☑4ᵗʰ **G31   Other degenerative diseases of nervous system, not elsewhere classified**
Use additional code to identify:
dementia with behavioral disturbance (F02.81)
dementia without behavioral disturbance (F02.80)
EXCLUDES 2   *Reye's syndrome (G93.7)*

☑5ᵗʰ **G31.0   Frontotemporal dementia**

G31.01   Pick's disease
Primary progressive aphasia
Progressive isolated aphasia

G31.09   Other frontotemporal dementia
Frontal dementia

G31.1   Senile degeneration of brain, not elsewhere classified
EXCLUDES 1   *Alzheimer's disease (G30.-)*
senility NOS (R41.81)

G31.2   Degeneration of nervous system due to alcohol
Alcoholic cerebellar ataxia
Alcoholic cerebellar degeneration
Alcoholic cerebral degeneration
Alcoholic encephalopathy
Dysfunction of the autonomic nervous system due to alcohol
Code also associated alcoholism (F10.-)

☑5ᵗʰ **G31.8   Other specified degenerative diseases of nervous system**

G31.81   Alpers disease
Grey-matter degeneration

G31.82   Leigh's disease
Subacute necrotizing encephalopathy

G31.83   Dementia with Lewy bodies
Dementia with Parkinsonism
Lewy body dementia
Lewy body disease

G31.84   Mild cognitive impairment, so stated
EXCLUDES 1   *age related cognitive decline (R41.81)*
altered mental status (R41.82)
cerebral degeneration (G31.9)
change in mental status (R41.82)
cognitive deficits following (sequelae of) cerebral hemorrhage or infarction (I69.01, I69.11, I69.21, I69.31, I69.81, I69.91)
cognitive impairment due to intracranial or head injury (S06.-)
dementia (F01.-, F02.-, F03)
mild memory disturbance (F06.8)
neurologic neglect syndrome (R41.4)
personality change, nonpsychotic (F68.8)

G31.85   Corticobasal degeneration

G31.89   Other specified degenerative diseases of nervous system

G31.9   Degenerative disease of nervous system, unspecified

☑4ᵗʰ **G32   Other degenerative disorders of nervous system in diseases classified elsewhere**

G32.0   Subacute combined degeneration of spinal cord in diseases classified elsewhere
Dana-Putnam syndrome
Sclerosis of spinal cord (combined) (dorsolateral) (posterolateral)
Code first underlying disease, such as:
vitamin B12 deficiency (E53.8)
vitamin B12 deficiency:
anemia (D51.9)
dietary (D51.3)
pernicious (D51.0)
EXCLUDES 1   *syphilitic combined degeneration of spinal cord (A52.11)*

☑5ᵗʰ **G32.8   Other specified degenerative disorders of nervous system in diseases classified elsewhere**
Code first underlying disease, such as:
amyloidosis cerebral degeneration (E85.-)
cerebral degeneration (due to) hypothyroidism (E00.0-E03.9)
cerebral degeneration (due to) neoplasm (C00-D49)
cerebral degeneration (due to) vitamin B deficiency, except thiamine (E52-E53.-)
EXCLUDES 1   *superior hemorrhagic polioencephalitis [Wernicke's encephalopathy] (E51.2)*

G32.81   Cerebellar ataxia in diseases classified elsewhere
Code first underlying disease, such as:
celiac disease (with gluten ataxia) (K90.0)
cerebellar ataxia (in) neoplastic disease (paraneoplastic cerebellar degeneration) (C00-D49)
non-celiac gluten ataxia (M35.9)
EXCLUDES 1   *systemic atrophy primarily affecting the central nervous system in alcoholic cerebellar ataxia (G31.2)*
systemic atrophy primarily affecting the central nervous system in myxedema (G13.2)

G32.89   Other specified degenerative disorders of nervous system in diseases classified elsewhere
Degenerative encephalopathy in diseases classified elsewhere

Demyelinating diseases of the central nervous system (G35-G37)

G35   Multiple sclerosis
Disseminated multiple sclerosis
Generalized multiple sclerosis
Multiple sclerosis NOS
Multiple sclerosis of brain stem
Multiple sclerosis of cord

☑4ᵗʰ **G36   Other acute disseminated demyelination**
EXCLUDES 1   *postinfectious encephalitis and encephalomyelitis NOS (G04.01)*

G36.0   Neuromyelitis optica [Devic]
Demyelination in optic neuritis
EXCLUDES 1   *optic neuritis NOS (H46)*

G36.1   Acute and subacute hemorrhagic leukoencephalitis [Hurst]

G36.8   Other specified acute disseminated demyelination

G36.9   Acute disseminated demyelination, unspecified

☑4ᵗʰ **G37   Other demyelinating diseases of central nervous system**

G37.0   Diffuse sclerosis of central nervous system
Periaxial encephalitis
Schilder's disease
EXCLUDES 1   *X linked adrenoleukodystrophy (E71.52-)*

G37.1   Central demyelination of corpus callosum

G37.2   Central pontine myelinolysis

G37.3   Acute transverse myelitis in demyelinating disease of central nervous system
Acute transverse myelitis NOS
Acute transverse myelopathy
EXCLUDES 1   *multiple sclerosis (G35)*
neuromyelitis optica [Devic] (G36.0)

G37.4   Subacute necrotizing myelitis of central nervous system

G37.5   Concentric sclerosis [Balo] of central nervous system

G37.8   Other specified demyelinating diseases of central nervous system

---

☑ Additional Character Required   ᵛˣ⁷ᵗʰ Placeholder Alert   Unspecified Dx   Other Specified Dx   Manifestation   ▶◀ Revised Text   ● New Code   ▲ Revised Code Title

Chapter 6. Diseases of the Nervous System

G37.9   Demyelinating disease of central nervous system, unspecified

Episodic and paroxysmal disorders (G40-G47)

✓4th **G40   Epilepsy and recurrent seizures**

> **NOTE**   The following terms are to be considered equivalent to intractable: pharmacoresistant (pharmacologically resistant), treatment resistant, refractory (medically) and poorly controlled

> **EXCLUDES 1**   conversion disorder with seizures (F44.5)
> convulsions NOS (R56.9)
> hippocampal sclerosis (G93.81)
> mesial temporal sclerosis (G93.81)
> post traumatic seizures (R56.1)
> seizure (convulsive) NOS (R56.9)
> seizure of newborn (P90)
> temporal sclerosis (G93.81)
> Todd's paralysis (G83.8)

✓5th **G40.0   Localization-related (focal) (partial) idiopathic epilepsy and epileptic syndromes with** seizures of localized onset
> Benign childhood epilepsy with centrotemporal EEG spikes
> Childhood epilepsy with occipital EEG paroxysms
> **EXCLUDES 1**   adult onset localization-related epilepsy (G40.1-, G40.2-)

✓6th **G40.00   Localization-related (focal) (partial) idiopathic epilepsy and epileptic syndromes with seizures of localized onset,** not intractable
> Localization-related (focal) (partial) idiopathic epilepsy and epileptic syndromes with seizures of localized onset without intractability

     G40.001   Localization-related (focal) (partial) idiopathic epilepsy and epileptic syndromes with seizures of localized onset, not intractable, with status epilepticus

     G40.009   Localization-related (focal) (partial) idiopathic epilepsy and epileptic syndromes with seizures of localized onset, not intractable, without status epilepticus
> Localization-related (focal) (partial) idiopathic epilepsy and epileptic syndromes with seizures of localized onset NOS

✓6th **G40.01   Localization-related (focal) (partial) idiopathic epilepsy and epileptic syndromes with seizures of localized onset,** intractable

     G40.011   Localization-related (focal) (partial) idiopathic epilepsy and epileptic syndromes with seizures of localized onset, intractable, with status epilepticus

     G40.019   Localization-related (focal) (partial) idiopathic epilepsy and epileptic syndromes with seizures of localized onset, intractable, without status epilepticus

✓5th **G40.1   Localization-related (focal) (partial) symptomatic epilepsy and epileptic syndromes with** simple partial seizures
> Attacks without alteration of consciousness
> Epilepsia partialis continua [Kozhevnikof]
> Simple partial seizures developing into secondarily generalized seizures

✓6th **G40.10   Localization-related (focal) (partial) symptomatic epilepsy and epileptic syndromes with simple partial seizures,** not intractable
> Localization-related (focal) (partial) symptomatic epilepsy and epileptic syndromes with simple partial seizures without intractability

     G40.101   Localization-related (focal) (partial) symptomatic epilepsy and epileptic syndromes with simple partial seizures, not intractable, with status epilepticus

     G40.109   Localization-related (focal) (partial) symptomatic epilepsy and epileptic syndromes with simple partial seizures, not intractable, without status epilepticus
> Localization-related (focal) (partial) symptomatic epilepsy and epileptic syndromes with simple partial seizures NOS

✓6th **G40.11   Localization-related (focal) (partial) symptomatic epilepsy and epileptic syndromes with simple partial seizures,** intractable

     G40.111   Localization-related (focal) (partial) symptomatic epilepsy and epileptic syndromes with simple partial seizures, intractable, with status epilepticus

     G40.119   Localization-related (focal) (partial) symptomatic epilepsy and epileptic syndromes with simple partial seizures, intractable, without status epilepticus

✓5th **G40.2   Localization-related (focal) (partial) symptomatic epilepsy and epileptic syndromes** with complex partial seizures
> Attacks with alteration of consciousness, often with automatisms
> Complex partial seizures developing into secondarily generalized seizures

✓6th **G40.20   Localization-related (focal) (partial) symptomatic epilepsy and epileptic syndromes with complex partial seizures,** not intractable
> Localization-related (focal) (partial) symptomatic epilepsy and epileptic syndromes with complex partial seizures without intractability

     G40.201   Localization-related (focal) (partial) symptomatic epilepsy and epileptic syndromes with complex partial seizures, not intractable, with status epilepticus

     G40.209   Localization-related (focal) (partial) symptomatic epilepsy and epileptic syndromes with complex partial seizures, not intractable, without status epilepticus
> Localization-related (focal) (partial) symptomatic epilepsy and epileptic syndromes with complex partial seizures NOS

✓6th **G40.21   Localization-related (focal) (partial) symptomatic epilepsy and epileptic syndromes with complex partial seizures,** intractable

     G40.211   Localization-related (focal) (partial) symptomatic epilepsy and epileptic syndromes with complex partial seizures, intractable, with status epilepticus

     G40.219   Localization-related (focal) (partial) symptomatic epilepsy and epileptic syndromes with complex partial seizures, intractable, without status epilepticus

✓5th **G40.3   Generalized idiopathic epilepsy and epileptic syndromes**
> Code also MERRF syndrome, if applicable (E88.42)

✓6th **G40.30   Generalized idiopathic epilepsy and epileptic syndromes,** not intractable
> Generalized idiopathic epilepsy and epileptic syndromes without intractability

     G40.301   Generalized idiopathic epilepsy and epileptic syndromes, not intractable, with status epilepticus

     G40.309   Generalized idiopathic epilepsy and epileptic syndromes, not intractable, without status epilepticus
> Generalized idiopathic epilepsy and epileptic syndromes NOS

✓6th **G40.31   Generalized idiopathic epilepsy and epileptic syndromes,** intractable

     G40.311   Generalized idiopathic epilepsy and epileptic syndromes, intractable, with status epilepticus

     G40.319   Generalized idiopathic epilepsy and epileptic syndromes, intractable, without status epilepticus

✓5th **G40.A   Absence epileptic syndrome**
> Childhood absence epilepsy [pyknolepsy]
> Juvenile absence epilepsy
> Absence epileptic syndrome, NOS

✓6th **G40.A0   Absence epileptic syndrome,** not intractable

     G40.A01   Absence epileptic syndrome, not intractable, with status epilepticus

     G40.A09   Absence epileptic syndrome, not intractable, without status epilepticus

✓6th **G40.A1   Absence epileptic syndrome,** intractable

     G40.A11   Absence epileptic syndrome, intractable, with status epilepticus

EXCLUDES 1 Not coded here   **EXCLUDES 2** Not included here   **N** Newborn Age: 0   **P** Pediatric Age: 0-17   **M** Maternity Age: 12-55   **A** Adult Age: 15-124

528   ICD-10-CM 2016

G40.A19   **Absence epileptic syndrome, intractable, without status epilepticus**

✓5ᵗʰ **G40.B** Juvenile myoclonic epilepsy [impulsive petit mal]

  ✓6ᵗʰ **G40.B0** Juvenile myoclonic epilepsy, not intractable

     G40.B01 **Juvenile myoclonic epilepsy, not intractable, with status epilepticus**

     G40.B09 **Juvenile myoclonic epilepsy, not intractable, without status epilepticus**

  ✓6ᵗʰ **G40.B1** Juvenile myoclonic epilepsy, intractable

     G40.B11 **Juvenile myoclonic epilepsy, intractable, with status epilepticus**

     G40.B19 **Juvenile myoclonic epilepsy, intractable, without status epilepticus**

✓5ᵗʰ **G40.4** Other generalized **epilepsy and epileptic syndromes**
  Epilepsy with grand mal seizures on awakening
  Epilepsy with myoclonic absences
  Epilepsy with myoclonic-astatic seizures
  Grand mal seizure NOS
  Nonspecific atonic epileptic seizures
  Nonspecific clonic epileptic seizures
  Nonspecific myoclonic epileptic seizures
  Nonspecific tonic epileptic seizures
  Nonspecific tonic-clonic epileptic seizures
  Symptomatic early myoclonic encephalopathy

  ✓6ᵗʰ **G40.40** **Other generalized epilepsy and epileptic syndromes, not intractable**
    Other generalized epilepsy and epileptic syndromes without intractability
    Other generalized epilepsy and epileptic syndromes NOS

     G40.401 **Other generalized epilepsy and epileptic syndromes, not intractable, with status epilepticus**

     G40.409 **Other generalized epilepsy and epileptic syndromes, not intractable, without status epilepticus**

  ✓6ᵗʰ **G40.41** **Other generalized epilepsy and epileptic syndromes, intractable**

     G40.411 **Other generalized epilepsy and epileptic syndromes, intractable, with status epilepticus**

     G40.419 **Other generalized epilepsy and epileptic syndromes, intractable, without status epilepticus**

✓5ᵗʰ **G40.5** **Epileptic seizures related to** external causes
  Epileptic seizures related to alcohol
  Epileptic seizures related to drugs
  Epileptic seizures related to hormonal changes
  Epileptic seizures related to sleep deprivation
  Epileptic seizures related to stress
  Code also, if applicable, associated epilepsy and recurrent seizures (G40.-)
  Use additional code for adverse effect, if applicable, to identify drug (T36-T50 with fifth or sixth character 5)

  ✓6ᵗʰ **G40.50** **Epileptic seizures related to external causes,** not intractable

     G40.501 **Epileptic seizures related to external causes, not intractable, with status epilepticus**

     G40.509 **Epileptic seizures related to external causes, not intractable, without status epilepticus**
      Epileptic seizures related to external causes, NOS

✓5ᵗʰ **G40.8** **Other epilepsy and recurrent seizures**
  Epilepsies and epileptic syndromes undetermined as to whether they are focal or generalized
  Landau-Kleffner syndrome

  ✓6ᵗʰ **G40.80** **Other epilepsy**

     G40.801 **Other epilepsy, not intractable, with status epilepticus**
      Other epilepsy without intractability with status epilepticus

     G40.802 **Other epilepsy, not intractable, without status epilepticus**
      Other epilepsy without intractability without status epilepticus

     G40.803 **Other epilepsy, intractable, with status epilepticus**

     G40.804 **Other epilepsy, intractable, without status epilepticus**

  ✓6ᵗʰ **G40.81** **Lennox-Gastaut syndrome**

     G40.811 **Lennox-Gastaut syndrome,** not intractable, with status epilepticus

     G40.812 **Lennox-Gastaut syndrome,** not intractable, without status epilepticus

     G40.813 **Lennox-Gastaut syndrome, intractable, with status epilepticus**

     G40.814 **Lennox-Gastaut syndrome, intractable, without status epilepticus**

  ✓6ᵗʰ **G40.82** **Epileptic spasms**
    Infantile spasms
    Salaam attacks
    West's syndrome

     G40.821 **Epileptic spasms, not intractable, with status epilepticus**

     G40.822 **Epileptic spasms, not intractable, without status epilepticus**

     G40.823 **Epileptic spasms, intractable, with status epilepticus**

     G40.824 **Epileptic spasms, intractable, without status epilepticus**

   G40.89 **Other seizures**
    EXCLUDES 1   *post traumatic seizures (R56.1)*
     recurrent seizures NOS (G40.909)
     seizure NOS (R56.9)

✓5ᵗʰ **G40.9** **Epilepsy,** unspecified

  ✓6ᵗʰ **G40.90** **Epilepsy, unspecified,** not intractable
    Epilepsy, unspecified, without intractability

     G40.901 **Epilepsy, unspecified, not intractable, with status epilepticus**

     G40.909 **Epilepsy, unspecified, not intractable, without status epilepticus**
      Epilepsy NOS
      Epileptic convulsions NOS
      Epileptic fits NOS
      Epileptic seizures NOS
      Recurrent seizures NOS
      Seizure disorder NOS

  ✓6ᵗʰ **G40.91** **Epilepsy, unspecified,** intractable
    Intractable seizure disorder NOS

     G40.911 **Epilepsy, unspecified, intractable, with status epilepticus**

     G40.919 **Epilepsy, unspecified, intractable, without status epilepticus**

✓4ᵗʰ **G43** **Migraine**
  NOTE   The following terms are to be considered equivalent to intractable: pharmacoresistant (pharmacologically resistant), treatment resistant, refractory (medically) and poorly controlled.
  Use additional code for adverse effect, if applicable, to identify drug (T36-T50 with fifth or sixth character 5)
  EXCLUDES 1   *headache NOS (R51)*
    lower half migraine (G44.00)
  EXCLUDES 2   *headache syndromes (G44.-)*

✓5ᵗʰ **G43.0** **Migraine** without aura
  Common migraine
  EXCLUDES 1   *chronic migraine without aura (G43.7-)*

  ✓6ᵗʰ **G43.00** **Migraine without aura,** not intractable
    Migraine without aura without mention of refractory migraine

     G43.001 **Migraine without aura, not intractable, with status migrainosus**

     G43.009 **Migraine without aura, not intractable, without status migrainosus**
      Migraine without aura NOS

  ✓6ᵗʰ **G43.01** **Migraine without aura,** intractable
    Migraine without aura with refractory migraine

     G43.011 **Migraine without aura, intractable, with status migrainosus**

     G43.019 **Migraine without aura, intractable, without status migrainosus**

✔ Additional Character Required   ✓ˣ7ᵗʰ Placeholder Alert   Unspecified Dx   Other Specified Dx   Manifestation   ▶◀ Revised Text   ● New Code   ▲ Revised Code Title

Chapter 6. Diseases of the Nervous System

G43.1–G43.821

✓5ᵗʰ **G43.1** **Migraine** with aura
Basilar migraine
Classical migraine
Migraine equivalents
Migraine preceded or accompanied by transient focal neurological phenomena
Migraine triggered seizures
Migraine with acute-onset aura
Migraine with aura without headache (migraine equivalents)
Migraine with prolonged aura
Migraine with typical aura
Retinal migraine
Code also any associated seizure (G40.-, R56.9)
EXCLUDES 1   *persistent migraine aura (G43.5-, G43.6-)*

    ✓6ᵗʰ **G43.10** **Migraine with aura,** not intractable
Migraine with aura without mention of refractory migraine

       G43.101 **Migraine with aura, not intractable,** with status migrainosus

       G43.109 **Migraine with aura, not intractable,** without status migrainosus
Migraine with aura NOS

    ✓6ᵗʰ **G43.11** **Migraine with aura,** intractable
Migraine with aura with refractory migraine

       G43.111 **Migraine with aura, intractable,** with status migrainosus

       G43.119 **Migraine with aura, intractable,** without status migrainosus

✓5ᵗʰ **G43.4** **Hemiplegic** migraine
Familial migraine
Sporadic migraine

    ✓6ᵗʰ **G43.40** **Hemiplegic migraine,** not intractable
Hemiplegic migraine without refractory migraine

       G43.401 **Hemiplegic migraine, not intractable,** with status migrainosus

       G43.409 **Hemiplegic migraine, not intractable,** without status migrainosus
Hemiplegic migraine NOS

    ✓6ᵗʰ **G43.41** **Hemiplegic migraine,** intractable
Hemiplegic migraine with refractory migraine

       G43.411 **Hemiplegic migraine, intractable,** with status migrainosus

       G43.419 **Hemiplegic migraine, intractable,** without status migrainosus

✓5ᵗʰ **G43.5** **Persistent** migraine aura without cerebral infarction

    ✓6ᵗʰ **G43.50** **Persistent migraine aura without cerebral infarction,** not intractable
Persistent migraine aura without cerebral infarction, without refractory migraine

       G43.501 **Persistent migraine aura without cerebral infarction, not intractable,** with status migrainosus

       G43.509 **Persistent migraine aura without cerebral infarction, not intractable,** without status migrainosus
Persistent migraine aura NOS

    ✓6ᵗʰ **G43.51** **Persistent migraine aura without cerebral infarction,** intractable
Persistent migraine aura without cerebral infarction, with refractory migraine

       G43.511 **Persistent migraine aura without cerebral infarction, intractable,** with status migrainosus

       G43.519 **Persistent migraine aura without cerebral infarction, intractable,** without status migrainosus

✓5ᵗʰ **G43.6** **Persistent** migraine aura with cerebral infarction
Code also the type of cerebral infarction (I63.-)

    ✓6ᵗʰ **G43.60** **Persistent migraine aura with cerebral infarction,** not intractable
Persistent migraine aura with cerebral infarction, without refractory migraine

       G43.601 **Persistent migraine aura with cerebral infarction, not intractable,** with status migrainosus

       G43.609 **Persistent migraine aura with cerebral infarction, not intractable,** without status migrainosus

    ✓6ᵗʰ **G43.61** **Persistent migraine aura with cerebral infarction,** intractable
Persistent migraine aura with cerebral infarction, with refractory migraine

       G43.611 **Persistent migraine aura with cerebral infarction, intractable,** with status migrainosus

       G43.619 **Persistent migraine aura with cerebral infarction, intractable,** without status migrainosus

✓5ᵗʰ **G43.7** **Chronic** migraine without aura
Transformed migraine
EXCLUDES 1   *migraine without aura (G43.0-)*

    ✓6ᵗʰ **G43.70** **Chronic migraine without aura,** not intractable
Chronic migraine without aura, without refractory migraine

       G43.701 **Chronic migraine without aura, not intractable,** with status migrainosus

       G43.709 **Chronic migraine without aura, not intractable,** without status migrainosus
Chronic migraine without aura NOS

    ✓6ᵗʰ **G43.71** **Chronic migraine without aura,** intractable
Chronic migraine without aura, with refractory migraine

       G43.711 **Chronic migraine without aura, intractable,** with status migrainosus

       G43.719 **Chronic migraine without aura,** intractable, without status migrainosus

✓5ᵗʰ **G43.A** **Cyclical** vomiting

    G43.A0 **Cyclical vomiting,** not intractable
Cyclical vomiting, without refractory migraine

    G43.A1 **Cyclical vomiting,** intractable
Cyclical vomiting, with refractory migraine

✓5ᵗʰ **G43.B** **Ophthalmoplegic** migraine

    G43.B0 **Ophthalmoplegic migraine,** not intractable
Ophthalmoplegic migraine, without refractory migraine

    G43.B1 **Ophthalmoplegic migraine,** intractable
Ophthalmoplegic migraine, with refractory migraine

✓5ᵗʰ **G43.C** **Periodic headache** syndromes in child or adult

    G43.C0 **Periodic headache syndromes in child or adult,** not intractable
Periodic headache syndromes in child or adult, without refractory migraine

    G43.C1 **Periodic headache syndromes in child or adult,** intractable
Periodic headache syndromes in child or adult, with refractory migraine

✓5ᵗʰ **G43.D** **Abdominal** migraine

    G43.D0 **Abdominal migraine,** not intractable
Abdominal migraine, without refractory migraine

    G43.D1 **Abdominal migraine,** intractable
Abdominal migraine, with refractory migraine

✓5ᵗʰ **G43.8** **Other** migraine

    ✓6ᵗʰ **G43.80** **Other migraine,** not intractable
Other migraine, without refractory migraine

       G43.801 **Other migraine, not intractable, with status migrainosus**

       G43.809 **Other migraine, not intractable, without status migrainosus**

    ✓6ᵗʰ **G43.81** **Other migraine,** intractable
Other migraine, with refractory migraine

       G43.811 **Other migraine, intractable, with status migrainosus**

       G43.819 **Other migraine, intractable, without status migrainosus**

    ✓6ᵗʰ **G43.82** **Menstrual** migraine, not intractable
Menstrual headache, not intractable
Menstrual migraine, without refractory migraine
Menstrually related migraine, not intractable
Pre-menstrual headache, not intractable
Pre-menstrual migraine, not intractable
Pure menstrual migraine, not intractable
Code also associated premenstrual tension syndrome (N94.3)

       G43.821 **Menstrual migraine, not intractable, with status migrainosus** ♀

EXCLUDES 1 Not coded here   EXCLUDES 2 Not included here   N Newborn Age: 0   P Pediatric Age: 0-17   M Maternity Age: 12-55   A Adult Age: 15-124

530   ICD-10-CM 2016

G43.829   Menstrual migraine, not intractable, ♀
without status migrainosus
    Menstrual migraine NOS

✓6ᵗʰ **G43.83**   Menstrual **migraine, intractable**
    Menstrual headache, intractable
    Menstrual migraine, with refractory migraine
    Menstrually related migraine, intractable
    Pre-menstrual headache, intractable
    Pre-menstrual migraine, intractable
    Pure menstrual migraine, intractable
    Code also associated premenstrual tension syndrome
      (N94.3)

G43.831   Menstrual migraine, intractable, with ♀
status migrainosus

G43.839   Menstrual migraine, intractable, ♀
without status migrainosus

✓5ᵗʰ **G43.9**   **Migraine,** unspecified

✓6ᵗʰ **G43.90**   **Migraine, unspecified,** not intractable
    Migraine, unspecified, without refractory migraine

G43.901   Migraine, unspecified, not intractable,
with status migrainosus
    Status migrainosus NOS

G43.909   Migraine, unspecified, not intractable,
without status migrainosus
    Migraine NOS

✓6ᵗʰ **G43.91**   Migraine, unspecified, intractable
    Migraine, unspecified, with refractory migraine

G43.911   Migraine, unspecified, intractable,
with status migrainosus

G43.919   Migraine, unspecified, intractable,
without status migrainosus

✓4ᵗʰ **G44**   **Other headache syndrome**
   EXCLUDES 1   headache NOS (R51)
   EXCLUDES 2   atypical facial pain (G50.1)
         headache due to lumbar puncture (G97.1)
         migraines (G43.-)
         trigeminal neuralgia (G50.0)

✓5ᵗʰ **G44.0**   **Cluster headaches and other trigeminal autonomic
cephalgias (TAC)**

✓6ᵗʰ **G44.00**   **Cluster headache syndrome,** unspecified
    Ciliary neuralgia
    Cluster headache NOS
    Histamine cephalgia
    Lower half migraine
    Migrainous neuralgia

G44.001   Cluster headache syndrome, unspecified,
intractable

G44.009   Cluster headache syndrome, unspecified,
not intractable
    Cluster headache syndrome NOS

✓6ᵗʰ **G44.01**   Episodic **cluster headache**

G44.011   Episodic cluster headache, intractable

G44.019   Episodic cluster headache, not intractable
    Episodic cluster headache NOS

✓6ᵗʰ **G44.02**   Chronic **cluster headache**

G44.021   Chronic cluster headache, intractable

G44.029   Chronic cluster headache, not intractable
    Chronic cluster headache NOS

✓6ᵗʰ **G44.03**   Episodic **paroxysmal hemicrania**
    Paroxysmal hemicrania NOS

G44.031   Episodic paroxysmal hemicrania,
intractable

G44.039   Episodic paroxysmal hemicrania, not
intractable
    Episodic paroxysmal hemicrania NOS

✓6ᵗʰ **G44.04**   Chronic **paroxysmal hemicrania**

G44.041   Chronic paroxysmal hemicrania,
intractable

G44.049   Chronic paroxysmal hemicrania, not
intractable
    Chronic paroxysmal hemicrania NOS

✓6ᵗʰ **G44.05**   Short lasting unilateral **neuralgiform headache with
conjunctival injection and tearing (SUNCT)**

G44.051   Short lasting unilateral neuralgiform
headache with conjunctival injection and
tearing (SUNCT), intractable

G44.059   Short lasting unilateral neuralgiform
headache with conjunctival injection and
tearing (SUNCT), not intractable
    Short lasting unilateral neuralgiform
headache with conjunctival injection
and tearing (SUNCT) NOS

✓6ᵗʰ **G44.09**   Other **trigeminal autonomic cephalgias (TAC)**

G44.091   Other trigeminal autonomic cephalgias
(TAC), intractable

G44.099   Other trigeminal autonomic cephalgias
syndrome (TAC), not intractable

G44.1   Vascular **headache, not elsewhere classified**
   EXCLUDES 2   cluster headache (G44.0)
         complicated headache syndromes (G44.5-)
         drug-induced headache (G44.4-)
         migraine (G43.-)
         other specified headache syndromes (G44.8-)
         post-traumatic headache (G44.3-)
         tension-type headache (G44.2-)

✓5ᵗʰ **G44.2**   **Tension-type headache**

✓6ᵗʰ **G44.20**   **Tension-type headache,** unspecified

G44.201   Tension-type headache, unspecified,
intractable

G44.209   Tension-type headache, unspecified,
not intractable
    Tension headache NOS

✓6ᵗʰ **G44.21**   Episodic **tension-type headache**

G44.211   Episodic tension-type headache,
intractable

G44.219   Episodic tension-type headache, not
intractable
    Episodic tension-type headache NOS

✓6ᵗʰ **G44.22**   Chronic **tension-type headache**

G44.221   Chronic tension-type headache,
intractable

G44.229   Chronic tension-type headache, not
intractable
    Chronic tension-type headache NOS

✓5ᵗʰ **G44.3**   **Post-traumatic headache**

✓6ᵗʰ **G44.30**   **Post-traumatic headache,** unspecified

G44.301   Post-traumatic headache, unspecified,
intractable

G44.309   Post-traumatic headache, unspecified,
not intractable
    Post-traumatic headache NOS

✓6ᵗʰ **G44.31**   Acute **post-traumatic headache**

G44.311   Acute post-traumatic headache,
intractable

G44.319   Acute post-traumatic headache, not
intractable
    Acute post-traumatic headache NOS

✓6ᵗʰ **G44.32**   Chronic **post-traumatic headache**

G44.321   Chronic post-traumatic headache,
intractable

G44.329   Chronic post-traumatic headache, not
intractable
    Chronic post-traumatic headache NOS

✓5ᵗʰ **G44.4**   **Drug-induced headache, not elsewhere classified**
    Medication overuse headache
    Use additional code for adverse effect, if applicable, to identify
      drug (T36-T50 with fifth or sixth character 5)

G44.40   Drug-induced headache, not elsewhere classified,
not intractable

G44.41   Drug-induced headache, not elsewhere classified,
intractable

✓5ᵗʰ **G44.5**   **Complicated headache syndromes**

G44.51   Hemicrania continua

G44.52   New daily persistent headache (NDPH)

G44.53   Primary thunderclap **headache**

G44.59   Other complicated **headache syndrome**

✓5ᵗʰ **G44.8**   Other specified **headache syndromes**

G44.81   Hypnic **headache**

G44.82   **Headache associated with** sexual activity
    Orgasmic headache
    Preorgasmic headache

G44.83   Primary cough **headache**

G44.84   Primary exertional **headache**

✓ Additional Character Required   ✓ˣ⁷ᵗʰ Placeholder Alert   Unspecified Dx   Other Specified Dx   Manifestation   ►◄ Revised Text   ● New Code   ▲ Revised Code Title

G44.85   **Primary** stabbing **headache**

G44.89   **Other headache syndrome**

✓4ᵗʰ **G45**   **Transient cerebral ischemic attacks and related syndromes**

    EXCLUDES 1   *neonatal cerebral ischemia (P91.0)*
                 transient retinal artery occlusion (H34.0-)

G45.0   **Vertebro-basilar artery syndrome**

G45.1   **Carotid artery syndrome (hemispheric)**   Ⓐ

G45.2   **Multiple and bilateral precerebral artery syndromes**   Ⓐ

G45.3   **Amaurosis fugax**

G45.4   **Transient global amnesia**

    EXCLUDES 1   *amnesia NOS (R41.3)*

G45.8   **Other transient cerebral ischemic attacks and related syndromes**   Ⓐ

G45.9   **Transient cerebral ischemic attack, unspecified**   Ⓐ
     Spasm of cerebral artery
     TIA
     Transient cerebral ischemia NOS

✓4ᵗʰ **G46**   **Vascular syndromes of brain in cerebrovascular diseases**
     Code first underlying cerebrovascular disease (I60-I69)

G46.0   **Middle** cerebral artery **syndrome**   Ⓐ

G46.1   **Anterior** cerebral artery **syndrome**   Ⓐ

G46.2   **Posterior** cerebral artery **syndrome**   Ⓐ

G46.3   **Brain stem stroke syndrome**
     Benedikt syndrome
     Claude syndrome
     Foville syndrome
     Millard-Gubler syndrome
     Wallenberg syndrome
     Weber syndrome

G46.4   **Cerebellar stroke syndrome**

G46.5   **Pure motor lacunar syndrome**

G46.6   **Pure sensory lacunar syndrome**

G46.7   **Other lacunar syndromes**

G46.8   **Other vascular syndromes of brain in cerebrovascular diseases**

✓4ᵗʰ **G47**   **Sleep disorders**

    EXCLUDES 2   *nightmares (F51.5)*
                 nonorganic sleep disorders (F51.-)
                 sleep terrors (F51.4)
                 sleepwalking (F51.3)

✓5ᵗʰ **G47.0**   **Insomnia**

    EXCLUDES 2   *alcohol related insomnia (F10.182, F10.282, F10.982)*
                 drug-related insomnia (F11.182, F11.282, F11.982,
                       F13.182, F13.282, F13.982, F14.182,
                       F14.282,F14.982, F15.182, F15.282, F15.982,
                       F19.182, F19.282, F19.982)
                 idiopathic insomnia (F51.01)
                 insomnia due to a mental disorder (F51.05)
                 insomnia not due to a substance or known
                       physiological condition (F51.0-)
                 nonorganic insomnia (F51.0-)
                 primary insomnia (F51.01)
                 sleep apnea (G47.3-)

G47.00   **Insomnia, unspecified**
     Insomnia NOS

G47.01   **Insomnia** due to medical condition
     Code also associated medical condition

G47.09   **Other insomnia**

✓5ᵗʰ **G47.1**   **Hypersomnia**

    EXCLUDES 2   *alcohol-related hypersomnia (F10.182, F10.282, F10.982)*
                 drug-related hypersomnia (F11.182, F11.282, F11.982,
                       F13.182, F13.282, F13.982, F14.182,F14.282,
                       F14.982, F15.182, F15.282, F15.982, F19.182,
                       F19.282, F19.982)
                 hypersomnia due to a mental disorder (F51.13)
                 hypersomnia not due to a substance or known
                       physiological condition (F51.1-)
                 primary hypersomnia (F51.11)
                 sleep apnea (G47.3-)

G47.10   **Hypersomnia, unspecified**
     Hypersomnia NOS

G47.11   **Idiopathic** hypersomnia with long sleep time
     Idiopathic hypersomnia NOS

G47.12   **Idiopathic** hypersomnia without long sleep time

G47.13   **Recurrent** hypersomnia
     Kleine-Levin syndrome
     Menstrual related hypersomnia

G47.14   **Hypersomnia** due to medical condition
     Code also associated medical condition

G47.19   **Other hypersomnia**

✓5ᵗʰ **G47.2**   **Circadian rhythm sleep disorders**
     Disorders of the sleep wake schedule
     Inversion of nyctohemeral rhythm
     Inversion of sleep rhythm

G47.20   **Circadian rhythm sleep disorder, unspecified type**
     Sleep wake schedule disorder NOS

G47.21   **Circadian rhythm sleep disorder,** delayed sleep phase **type**
     Delayed sleep phase syndrome

G47.22   **Circadian rhythm sleep disorder,** advanced sleep phase **type**

G47.23   **Circadian rhythm sleep disorder,** irregular sleep wake **type**
     Irregular sleep-wake pattern

G47.24   **Circadian rhythm sleep disorder,** free running **type**

G47.25   **Circadian rhythm sleep disorder,** jet lag **type**

G47.26   **Circadian rhythm sleep disorder,** shift work **type**

G47.27   *Circadian rhythm sleep disorder in conditions classified elsewhere*
     Code first underlying condition

G47.29   **Other circadian rhythm sleep disorder**

✓5ᵗʰ **G47.3**   **Sleep apnea**
     Code also any associated underlying condition

    EXCLUDES 1   *apnea NOS (R06.81)*
                 Cheyne-Stokes breathing (R06.3)
                 pickwickian syndrome (E66.2)
                 sleep apnea of newborn (P28.3)

G47.30   **Sleep apnea, unspecified**
     Sleep apnea NOS

G47.31   **Primary central sleep apnea**

G47.32   **High altitude periodic breathing**

G47.33   **Obstructive sleep apnea** (adult) (pediatric)

    EXCLUDES 1   *obstructive sleep apnea of newborn (P28.3)*

G47.34   **Idiopathic sleep related nonobstructive alveolar hypoventilation**
     Sleep related hypoxia

G47.35   **Congenital central alveolar hypoventilation syndrome**

G47.36   *Sleep related hypoventilation in conditions classified elsewhere*
     Sleep related hypoxemia in conditions classified elsewhere
     Code first underlying condition

G47.37   *Central sleep apnea in conditions classified elsewhere*
     Code first underlying condition

G47.39   **Other sleep apnea**

✓5ᵗʰ **G47.4**   **Narcolepsy and cataplexy**

✓6ᵗʰ **G47.41**   **Narcolepsy**

G47.411   **Narcolepsy** with cataplexy

G47.419   **Narcolepsy** without cataplexy
     Narcolepsy NOS

✓6ᵗʰ **G47.42**   **Narcolepsy in conditions classified elsewhere**
     Code first underlying condition

G47.421   *Narcolepsy in conditions classified elsewhere with cataplexy*

G47.429   *Narcolepsy in conditions classified elsewhere without cataplexy*

✓5ᵗʰ **G47.5**   **Parasomnia**

    EXCLUDES 1   *alcohol induced parasomnia (F10.182, F10.282, F10.982)*
                 drug induced parasomnia (F11.182, F11.282, F11.982,
                     F13.182, F13.282, F13.982, F14.182, F14.282,
                     F14.982, F15.182, F15.282, F15.982, F19.182,
                     F19.282, F19.982)
                 parasomnia not due to a substance or known
                     physiological condition (F51.8)

G47.50   **Parasomnia, unspecified**
     Parasomnia NOS

G47.51   **Confusional arousals**

G47.52   **REM sleep behavior disorder**

G47.53   **Recurrent isolated sleep paralysis**

EXCLUDES 1 Not coded here   EXCLUDES 2 Not included here   Ⓝ Newborn Age: 0   Ⓟ Pediatric Age: 0-17   Ⓜ Maternity Age: 12-55   Ⓐ Adult Age: 15-124

G47.54   *Parasomnia in conditions classified elsewhere*
Code first underlying condition

G47.59   **Other parasomnia**

✓5ᵗʰ **G47.6**   **Sleep related movement disorders**
EXCLUDES 2   *restless legs syndrome (G25.81)*

G47.61   **Periodic limb movement disorder**

G47.62   **Sleep related leg cramps**

G47.63   **Sleep related bruxism**
EXCLUDES 1   *psychogenic bruxism (F45.8)*

G47.69   **Other sleep related movement disorders**

G47.8   **Other sleep disorders**

G47.9   **Sleep disorder, unspecified**
Sleep disorder NOS

Nerve, nerve root and plexus disorders (G50-G59)

EXCLUDES 1   *current traumatic nerve, nerve root and plexus disorders—see Injury, nerve by body region*
neuralgia NOS (M79.2)
neuritis NOS (M79.2)
peripheral neuritis in pregnancy (O26.82-)
radiculitis NOS (M54.1-)

✓4ᵗʰ **G50**   **Disorders of trigeminal nerve**
INCLUDES   disorders of 5th cranial nerve

G50.0   **Trigeminal neuralgia**
Syndrome of paroxysmal facial pain
Tic douloureux

G50.1   **Atypical facial pain**

G50.8   **Other disorders of trigeminal nerve**

G50.9   **Disorder of trigeminal nerve, unspecified**

✓4ᵗʰ **G51**   **Facial nerve disorders**
INCLUDES   disorders of 7th cranial nerve

G51.0   **Bell's palsy**
Facial palsy

G51.1   **Geniculate ganglionitis**
EXCLUDES 1   *postherpetic geniculate ganglionitis (B02.21)*

G51.2   **Melkersson's syndrome**
Melkersson-Rosenthal syndrome

G51.3   **Clonic hemifacial spasm**

G51.4   **Facial myokymia**

G51.8   **Other disorders of facial nerve**

G51.9   **Disorder of facial nerve, unspecified**

✓4ᵗʰ **G52**   **Disorders of other cranial nerves**
EXCLUDES 2   *disorders of acoustic [8th] nerve (H93.3)*
disorders of optic [2nd] nerve (H46, H47.0)
paralytic strabismus due to nerve palsy (H49.0-H49.2)

G52.0   **Disorders of olfactory nerve**
Disorders of 1st cranial nerve

G52.1   **Disorders of glossopharyngeal nerve**
Disorder of 9th cranial nerve
Glossopharyngeal neuralgia

G52.2   **Disorders of vagus nerve**
Disorders of pneumogastric [10th] nerve

G52.3   **Disorders of hypoglossal nerve**
Disorders of 12th cranial nerve

G52.7   **Disorders of multiple cranial nerves**
Polyneuritis cranialis

G52.8   **Disorders of other specified cranial nerves**

G52.9   **Cranial nerve disorder, unspecified**

G53   *Cranial nerve disorders in diseases classified elsewhere*
Code first underlying disease, such as:
neoplasm (C00-D49)
EXCLUDES 1   *multiple cranial nerve palsy in sarcoidosis (D86.82)*
multiple cranial nerve palsy in syphilis (A52.15)
postherpetic geniculate ganglionitis (B02.21)
postherpetic trigeminal neuralgia (B02.22)

✓4ᵗʰ **G54**   **Nerve root and plexus disorders**
EXCLUDES 1   *current traumatic nerve root and plexus disorders—see nerve injury by body region*
intervertebral disc disorders (M50-M51)
neuralgia or neuritis NOS (M79.2)
neuritis or radiculitis brachial NOS (M54.13)
neuritis or radiculitis lumbar NOS (M54.16)
neuritis or radiculitis lumbosacral NOS (M54.17)
neuritis or radiculitis thoracic NOS (M54.14)
radiculitis NOS (M54.10)
radiculopathy NOS (M54.10)
spondylosis (M47.-)

G54.0   **Brachial plexus disorders**
Thoracic outlet syndrome

G54.1   **Lumbosacral plexus disorders**

G54.2   **Cervical root disorders, not elsewhere classified**

G54.3   **Thoracic root disorders, not elsewhere classified**

G54.4   **Lumbosacral root disorders, not elsewhere classified**

G54.5   **Neuralgic amyotrophy**
Parsonage-Aldren-Turner syndrome
Shoulder-girdle neuritis
EXCLUDES 1   *neuralgic amyotrophy in diabetes mellitus (E08-E13 with .44)*

G54.6   **Phantom limb syndrome with pain**

G54.7   **Phantom limb syndrome without pain**
Phantom limb syndrome NOS

G54.8   **Other nerve root and plexus disorders**

G54.9   **Nerve root and plexus disorder, unspecified**

G55   *Nerve root and plexus compressions in diseases classified elsewhere*
Code first underlying disease, such as:
neoplasm (C00-D49)
EXCLUDES 1   *nerve root compression (due to) (in) ankylosing spondylitis (M45.-)*
nerve root compression (due to) (in) dorsopathies (M53.-, M54.-)
nerve root compression (due to) (in) intervertebral disc disorders (M50.1-, M51.1-)
nerve root compression (due to) (in) spondylopathies (M46.-, M48.-)

✓4ᵗʰ **G56**   **Mononeuropathies of upper limb**
EXCLUDES 1   *current traumatic nerve disorder—see nerve injury by body region*

✓5ᵗʰ **G56.0**   **Carpal tunnel syndrome**

G56.00   **Carpal tunnel syndrome, unspecified upper limb**

G56.01   **Carpal tunnel syndrome, right upper limb**

G56.02   **Carpal tunnel syndrome, left upper limb**

✓5ᵗʰ **G56.1**   **Other lesions of median nerve**

G56.10   **Other lesions of median nerve, unspecified upper limb**

G56.11   **Other lesions of median nerve, right upper limb**

G56.12   **Other lesions of median nerve, left upper limb**

✓5ᵗʰ **G56.2**   **Lesion of ulnar nerve**
Tardy ulnar nerve palsy

G56.20   **Lesion of ulnar nerve, unspecified upper limb**

G56.21   **Lesion of ulnar nerve, right upper limb**

G56.22   **Lesion of ulnar nerve, left upper limb**

✓5ᵗʰ **G56.3**   **Lesion of radial nerve**

G56.30   **Lesion of radial nerve, unspecified upper limb**

G56.31   **Lesion of radial nerve, right upper limb**

G56.32   **Lesion of radial nerve, left upper limb**

✓5ᵗʰ **G56.4**   **Causalgia of upper limb**
Complex regional pain syndrome II of upper limb
EXCLUDES 1   *complex regional pain syndrome I of lower limb (G90.52-)*
complex regional pain syndrome I of upper limb (G90.51-)
complex regional pain syndrome II of lower limb (G57.7-)
reflex sympathetic dystrophy of lower limb (G90.52-)
reflex sympathetic dystrophy of upper limb (G90.51-)

G56.40   **Causalgia of unspecified upper limb**

G56.41   **Causalgia of right upper limb**

G56.42   **Causalgia of left upper limb**

☑ Additional Character Required   ✓x7ᵗʰ Placeholder Alert   Unspecified Dx   Other Specified Dx   Manifestation   ▶◀ Revised Text   ● New Code   ▲ Revised Code Title

✓5ᵗʰ **G56.8** Other **specified mononeuropathies of upper limb**
Interdigital neuroma of upper limb

G56.80 **Other specified mononeuropathies of unspecified upper limb**

G56.81 **Other specified mononeuropathies of** right **upper limb**

G56.82 **Other specified mononeuropathies of** left **upper limb**

✓5ᵗʰ **G56.9** Unspecified **mononeuropathy of upper limb**

G56.90 **Unspecified mononeuropathy of unspecified upper limb**

G56.91 **Unspecified mononeuropathy of** right **upper limb**

G56.92 **Unspecified mononeuropathy of** left **upper limb**

✓4ᵗʰ **G57** **Mononeuropathies of** lower limb

EXCLUDES 1　current traumatic nerve disorder—see nerve injury by body region

✓5ᵗʰ **G57.0** **Lesion of** sciatic nerve

EXCLUDES 1　sciatica NOS (M54.3-)

EXCLUDES 2　sciatica attributed to intervertebral disc disorder (M51.1-)

G57.00 **Lesion of sciatic nerve, unspecified lower limb**

G57.01 **Lesion of sciatic nerve,** right **lower limb**

G57.02 **Lesion of sciatic nerve,** left **lower limb**

✓5ᵗʰ **G57.1** Meralgia paresthetica
Lateral cutaneous nerve of thigh syndrome

G57.10 **Meralgia paresthetica, unspecified lower limb**

G57.11 **Meralgia paresthetica,** right **lower limb**

G57.12 **Meralgia paresthetica,** right **lower limb**

✓5ᵗʰ **G57.2** **Lesion of** femoral nerve

G57.20 **Lesion of femoral nerve, unspecified lower limb**

G57.21 **Lesion of femoral nerve,** right **lower limb**

G57.22 **Lesion of femoral nerve,** left **lower limb**

✓5ᵗʰ **G57.3** **Lesion of** lateral popliteal nerve
Peroneal nerve palsy

G57.30 **Lesion of lateral popliteal nerve, unspecified lower limb**

G57.31 **Lesion of lateral popliteal nerve,** right **lower limb**

G57.32 **Lesion of lateral popliteal nerve,** left **lower limb**

✓5ᵗʰ **G57.4** **Lesion of** medial popliteal nerve

G57.40 **Lesion of medial popliteal nerve, unspecified lower limb**

G57.41 **Lesion of medial popliteal nerve,** right **lower limb**

G57.42 **Lesion of medial popliteal nerve,** left **lower limb**

✓5ᵗʰ **G57.5** Tarsal tunnel syndrome

G57.50 **Tarsal tunnel syndrome, unspecified lower limb**

G57.51 **Tarsal tunnel syndrome, right** lower limb

G57.52 **Tarsal tunnel syndrome, left** lower limb

✓5ᵗʰ **G57.6** **Lesion of** plantar nerve
Morton's metatarsalgia

G57.60 **Lesion of plantar nerve, unspecified lower limb**

G57.61 **Lesion of plantar nerve,** right **lower limb**

G57.62 **Lesion of plantar nerve,** left **lower limb**

✓5ᵗʰ **G57.7** Causalgia **of** lower limb
Complex regional pain syndrome II of lower limb

EXCLUDES 1　complex regional pain syndrome I of lower limb (G90.52-)
complex regional pain syndrome I of upper limb (G90.51-)
complex regional pain syndrome II of upper limb (G56.4-)
reflex sympathetic dystrophy of lower limb (G90.52-)
reflex sympathetic dystrophy of upper limb (G90.51-)

G57.70 **Causalgia of unspecified lower limb**

G57.71 **Causalgia of** right **lower limb**

G57.72 **Causalgia of** left **lower limb**

✓5ᵗʰ **G57.8** Other **specified mononeuropathies of lower limb**
Interdigital neuroma of lower limb

G57.80 **Other specified mononeuropathies of unspecified lower limb**

G57.81 **Other specified mononeuropathies of** right **lower limb**

G57.82 **Other specified mononeuropathies of** left **lower limb**

✓5ᵗʰ **G57.9** Unspecified **mononeuropathy of lower limb**

G57.90 **Unspecified mononeuropathy of unspecified lower limb**

G57.91 **Unspecified mononeuropathy of** right **lower limb**

G57.92 **Unspecified mononeuropathy of** left **lower limb**

✓4ᵗʰ **G58** **Other mononeuropathies**

G58.0 **Intercostal neuropathy**

G58.7 **Mononeuritis multiplex**

G58.8 **Other specified mononeuropathies**

G58.9 **Mononeuropathy, unspecified**

G59 *Mononeuropathy in diseases classified elsewhere*
Code first underlying disease

EXCLUDES 1　diabetic mononeuropathy (E08-E13 with .41)
syphilitic nerve paralysis (A52.19)
syphilitic neuritis (A52.15)
tuberculous mononeuropathy (A17.83)

Polyneuropathies and other disorders of the peripheral nervous system (G60-G65)

EXCLUDES 1　neuralgia NOS (M79.2)
neuritis NOS (M79.2)
peripheral neuritis in pregnancy (O26.82-)
radiculitis NOS (M54.10)

✓4ᵗʰ **G60** **Hereditary and idiopathic** neuropathy

G60.0 **Hereditary** motor and sensory **neuropathy**
Charcôt-Marie-Tooth disease
Déjérine-Sottas disease
Hereditary motor and sensory neuropathy, types I-IV
Hypertrophic neuropathy of infancy
Peroneal muscular atrophy (axonal type) (hypertrophic type)
Roussy-Levy syndrome

G60.1 **Refsum's disease**
Infantile Refsum disease

G60.2 **Neuropathy** in association with hereditary ataxia

G60.3 **Idiopathic** progressive **neuropathy**

G60.8 **Other hereditary and idiopathic neuropathies**
Dominantly inherited sensory neuropathy
Morvan's disease
Nelaton's syndrome
Recessively inherited sensory neuropathy

G60.9 **Hereditary and idiopathic neuropathy, unspecified**

✓4ᵗʰ **G61** **Inflammatory** polyneuropathy

G61.0 **Guillain-Barre syndrome**
Acute (post-)infective polyneuritis
Miller Fisher syndrome
AHA: 2014, 2Q, 4

G61.1 **Serum** neuropathy
Use additional code for adverse effect, if applicable, to identify serum (T50.-)

✓5ᵗʰ **G61.8** **Other inflammatory polyneuropathies**

G61.81 **Chronic inflammatory demyelinating polyneuritis**

G61.89 **Other inflammatory polyneuropathies**

G61.9 **Inflammatory polyneuropathy, unspecified**

✓4ᵗʰ **G62** **Other and unspecified polyneuropathies**

G62.0 **Drug-induced polyneuropathy**
Use additional code for adverse effect, if applicable, to identify drug (T36-T50 with fifth or sixth character 5)

G62.1 **Alcoholic polyneuropathy**

G62.2 **Polyneuropathy due to other toxic agents**
Code first (T51-T65) to identify toxic agent

✓5ᵗʰ **G62.8** **Other specified polyneuropathies**

G62.81 **Critical illness polyneuropathy**
Acute motor neuropathy

G62.82 **Radiation-induced polyneuropathy**
Use additional external cause code (W88-W90, X39.0-) to identify cause

G62.89 **Other specified polyneuropathies**

G62.9 **Polyneuropathy, unspecified**
Neuropathy NOS

EXCLUDES 1　Not coded here　　EXCLUDES 2　Not included here　　N Newborn Age: 0　　P Pediatric Age: 0-17　　M Maternity Age: 12-55　　A Adult Age: 15-124

534
ICD-10-CM 2016

G63   *Polyneuropathy in diseases classified elsewhere*
> *Code first underlying disease, such as:*
>   *amyloidosis (E85.-)*
>   *endocrine disease, except diabetes (E00-E07, E15-E16, E20-E34)*
>   *metabolic diseases (E70-E88)*
>   *neoplasm (C00-D49)*
>   *nutritional deficiency (E40-E64)*
> **EXCLUDES 1**   *polyneuropathy (in):*
>   *diabetes mellitus (E08-E13 with .42)*
>   *diphtheria (A36.83)*
>   *infectious mononucleosis (B27.0-B27.9 with 1)*
>   *Lyme disease (A69.22)*
>   *mumps (B26.84)*
>   *postherpetic (B02.23)*
>   *rheumatoid arthritis (M05.33)*
>   *scleroderma (M34.83)*
>   *systemic lupus erythematosus (M32.19)*
> **AHA:** 2012, 4Q, 99

G64   **Other disorders of peripheral nervous system**
> Disorder of peripheral nervous system NOS

☑4ᵗʰ **G65**   **Sequelae of inflammatory and toxic polyneuropathies**
> Code first condition resulting from (sequela) of inflammatory and toxic polyneuropathies

    G65.0   **Sequelae of Guillain-Barré syndrome**

    G65.1   **Sequelae of other inflammatory polyneuropathy**

    G65.2   **Sequelae of toxic polyneuropathy**

Diseases of myoneural junction and muscle (G70-G73)

☑4ᵗʰ **G70**   **Myasthenia gravis and other myoneural disorders**
> **EXCLUDES 1**   *botulism (A05.1, A48.51-A48.52)*
>   *transient neonatal myasthenia gravis (P94.0)*

    ☑5ᵗʰ **G70.0**   **Myasthenia gravis**

       G70.00   **Myasthenia gravis without (acute) exacerbation**
> Myasthenia gravis NOS

       G70.01   **Myasthenia gravis with (acute) exacerbation**
> Myasthenia gravis in crisis

    G70.1   **Toxic myoneural disorders**
> Code first (T51-T65) to identify toxic agent

    G70.2   **Congenital and developmental myasthenia**

    ☑5ᵗʰ **G70.8**   **Other specified myoneural disorders**

       G70.80   **Lambert-Eaton syndrome, unspecified**
> Lambert-Eaton syndrome NOS

       G70.81   *Lambert-Eaton syndrome in disease classified elsewhere*
> *Code first underlying disease*
> **EXCLUDES 1**   *Lambert-Eaton syndrome in neoplastic disease (G73.1)*

       G70.89   **Other specified myoneural disorders**

    G70.9   **Myoneural disorder, unspecified**

☑4ᵗʰ **G71**   **Primary disorders of muscles**
> **EXCLUDES 2**   *arthrogryposis multiplex congenita (Q74.3)*
>   *metabolic disorders (E70-E88)*
>   *myositis (M60.-)*

    G71.0   **Muscular dystrophy**
> Autosomal recessive, childhood type, muscular dystrophy resembling Duchenne or Becker muscular dystrophy
> Benign [Becker] muscular dystrophy
> Benign scapuloperoneal muscular dystrophy with early contractures [Emery-Dreifuss]
> Congenital muscular dystrophy NOS
> Congenital muscular dystrophy with specific morphological abnormalities of the muscle fiber
> Distal muscular dystrophy
> Facioscapulohumeral muscular dystrophy
> Limb-girdle muscular dystrophy
> Ocular muscular dystrophy
> Oculopharyngeal muscular dystrophy
> Scapuloperoneal muscular dystrophy
> Severe [Duchenne] muscular dystrophy

    ☑5ᵗʰ **G71.1**   **Myotonic disorders**

       G71.11   **Myotonic muscular dystrophy**
> Dystrophia myotonica [Steinert]
> Myotonia atrophica
> Myotonic dystrophy
> Proximal myotonic myopathy (PROMM)
> Steinert disease

       G71.12   **Myotonia congenita**
> Acetazolamide responsive myotonia congenita
> Dominant myotonia congenita [Thomsen disease]
> Myotonia levior
> Recessive myotonia congenita [Becker disease]

       G71.13   **Myotonic chondrodystrophy**
> Chondrodystrophic myotonia
> Congenital myotonic chondrodystrophy
> Schwartz-Jampel disease

       G71.14   **Drug induced myotonia**
> Use additional code for adverse effect, if applicable, to identify drug (T36-T50 with fifth or sixth character 5)

       G71.19   **Other specified myotonic disorders**
> Myotonia fluctuans
> Myotonia permanens
> Neuromyotonia [Isaacs]
> Paramyotonia congenita (of von Eulenburg)
> Pseudomyotonia
> Symptomatic myotonia

    G71.2   **Congenital myopathies**
> Central core disease
> Fiber-type disproportion
> Minicore disease
> Multicore disease
> Myotubular (centronuclear) myopathy
> Nemaline myopathy
> **EXCLUDES 1**   *arthrogryposis multiplex congenita (Q74.3)*

    G71.3   **Mitochondrial myopathy, not elsewhere classified**
> **EXCLUDES 1**   *Kearns-Sayre syndrome (H49.81)*
>   *Leber's disease (H47.21)*
>   *Leigh's encephalopathy (G31.82)*
>   *mitochondrial metabolism disorders (E88.4-)*
>   *Reye's syndrome (G93.7)*

    G71.8   **Other primary disorders of muscles**

    G71.9   **Primary disorder of muscle, unspecified**
> Hereditary myopathy NOS

☑4ᵗʰ **G72**   **Other and unspecified myopathies**
> **EXCLUDES 1**   *arthrogryposis multiplex congenita (Q74.3)*
>   *dermatopolymyositis (M33.-)*
>   *ischemic infarction of muscle (M62.2-)*
>   *myositis (M60.-)*
>   *polymyositis (M33.2-)*

    G72.0   **Drug-induced myopathy**
> Use additional code for adverse effect, if applicable, to identify drug (T36-T50 with fifth or sixth character 5)

    G72.1   **Alcoholic myopathy**
> Use additional code to identify alcoholism (F10.-)

    G72.2   **Myopathy due to other toxic agents**
> Code first (T51-T65) to identify toxic agent

    G72.3   **Periodic paralysis**
> Familial periodic paralysis
> Hyperkalemic periodic paralysis (familial)
> Hypokalemic periodic paralysis (familial)
> Myotonic periodic paralysis (familial)
> Normokalemic paralysis (familial)
> Potassium sensitive periodic paralysis
> **EXCLUDES 1**   *paramyotonia congenita (of von Eulenburg) (G71.19)*

    ☑5ᵗʰ **G72.4**   **Inflammatory and immune myopathies, not elsewhere classified**

       G72.41   **Inclusion body myositis [IBM]**

       G72.49   **Other inflammatory and immune myopathies, not elsewhere classified**
> Inflammatory myopathy NOS

    ☑5ᵗʰ **G72.8**   **Other specified myopathies**

       G72.81   **Critical illness myopathy**
> Acute necrotizing myopathy
> Acute quadriplegic myopathy
> Intensive care (ICU) myopathy
> Myopathy of critical illness

       G72.89   **Other specified myopathies**

    G72.9   **Myopathy, unspecified**

☑4ᵗʰ **G73**   **Disorders of myoneural junction and muscle in diseases classified elsewhere**

    G73.1   *Lambert-Eaton syndrome in neoplastic disease*
> *Code first underlying neoplasm (C00-D49)*
> **EXCLUDES 1**   *Lambert-Eaton syndrome not associated with neoplasm (G70.80-G70.81)*

☑ Additional Character Required   ✕7ᵗʰ Placeholder Alert   Unspecified Dx   Other Specified Dx   Manifestation   ▶◀ Revised Text   ● New Code   ▲ Revised Code Title

Chapter 6. Diseases of the Nervous System

G73.3 Myasthenic syndromes in other diseases classified elsewhere
Code first underlying disease, such as:
neoplasm (C00-D49)
thyrotoxicosis (E05.-)

G73.7 Myopathy in diseases classified elsewhere
Code first underlying disease, such as:
hyperparathyroidism (E21.0, E21.3)
hypoparathyroidism (E20.-)
glycogen storage disease (E74.0)
lipid storage disorders (E75.-)
EXCLUDES 1 myopathy in:
rheumatoid arthritis (M05.4-)
sarcoidosis (D86.87)
scleroderma (M34.82)
sicca syndrome [Sjögren] (M35.03)
systemic lupus erythematosus (M32.19)

Cerebral palsy and other paralytic syndromes (G80-G83)

✓4th **G80 Cerebral palsy**
EXCLUDES 1 hereditary spastic paraplegia (G11.4)

G80.0 Spastic quadriplegic cerebral palsy
Congenital spastic paralysis (cerebral)

G80.1 Spastic diplegic cerebral palsy
Spastic cerebral palsy NOS

G80.2 Spastic hemiplegic cerebral palsy

G80.3 Athetoid cerebral palsy
Double athetosis (syndrome)
Dyskinetic cerebral palsy
Dystonic cerebral palsy
Vogt disease

G80.4 Ataxic cerebral palsy

G80.8 Other cerebral palsy
Mixed cerebral palsy syndromes

G80.9 Cerebral palsy, unspecified
Cerebral palsy NOS

✓4th **G81 Hemiplegia and hemiparesis**
NOTE This category is to be used only when hemiplegia (complete)(incomplete) is reported without further specification, or is stated to be old or longstanding but of unspecified cause. The category is also for use in multiple coding to identify these types of hemiplegia resulting from any cause.
EXCLUDES 1 congenital cerebral palsy (G80.-)
hemiplegia and hemiparesis due to sequela of cerebrovascular disease (I69.05-, I69.15-, I69.25-, I69.35-, I69.85-, I69.95-)
AHA: 2015, 1Q, 25

✓5th **G81.0 Flaccid hemiplegia**
G81.00 Flaccid hemiplegia affecting unspecified side
G81.01 Flaccid hemiplegia affecting right dominant side
G81.02 Flaccid hemiplegia affecting left dominant side
G81.03 Flaccid hemiplegia affecting right nondominant side
G81.04 Flaccid hemiplegia affecting left nondominant side

✓5th **G81.1 Spastic hemiplegia**
G81.10 Spastic hemiplegia affecting unspecified side
G81.11 Spastic hemiplegia affecting right dominant side
G81.12 Spastic hemiplegia affecting left dominant side
G81.13 Spastic hemiplegia affecting right nondominant side
G81.14 Spastic hemiplegia affecting left nondominant side

✓5th **G81.9 Hemiplegia, unspecified**
AHA: 2014, 1Q, 23
G81.90 Hemiplegia, unspecified affecting unspecified side
G81.91 Hemiplegia, unspecified affecting right dominant side
G81.92 Hemiplegia, unspecified affecting left dominant side
G81.93 Hemiplegia, unspecified affecting right nondominant side
G81.94 Hemiplegia, unspecified affecting left nondominant side

✓4th **G82 Paraplegia (paraparesis) and quadriplegia (quadriparesis)**
NOTE This category is to be used only when the listed conditions are reported without further specification, or are stated to be old or longstanding but of unspecified cause. The category is also for use in multiple coding to identify these conditions resulting from any cause
EXCLUDES 1 congenital cerebral palsy (G80.-)
functional quadriplegia (R53.2)
hysterical paralysis (F44.4)

✓5th **G82.2 Paraplegia**
Paralysis of both lower limbs NOS
Paraparesis (lower) NOS
Paraplegia (lower) NOS
G82.20 Paraplegia, unspecified
G82.21 Paraplegia, complete
G82.22 Paraplegia, incomplete

✓5th **G82.5 Quadriplegia**
G82.50 Quadriplegia, unspecified
G82.51 Quadriplegia, C1-C4 complete
G82.52 Quadriplegia, C1-C4 incomplete
G82.53 Quadriplegia, C5-C7 complete
G82.54 Quadriplegia, C5-C7 incomplete

✓4th **G83 Other paralytic syndromes**
NOTE This category is to be used only when the listed conditions are reported without further specification, or are stated to be old or longstanding but of unspecified cause. The category is also for use in multiple coding to identify these conditions resulting from any cause.
INCLUDES paralysis (complete) (incomplete), except as in G80-G82

G83.0 Diplegia of upper limbs
Diplegia (upper)
Paralysis of both upper limbs

✓5th **G83.1 Monoplegia of lower limb**
Paralysis of lower limb
EXCLUDES 1 monoplegia of lower limbs due to sequela of cerebrovascular disease (I69.04-, I69.14-, I69.24-, I69.34-, I69.84-, I69.94-)
G83.10 Monoplegia of lower limb affecting unspecified side
G83.11 Monoplegia of lower limb affecting right dominant side
G83.12 Monoplegia of lower limb affecting left dominant side
G83.13 Monoplegia of lower limb affecting right nondominant side
G83.14 Monoplegia of lower limb affecting left nondominant side

✓5th **G83.2 Monoplegia of upper limb**
Paralysis of upper limb
EXCLUDES 1 monoplegia of upper limbs due to sequela of cerebrovascular disease (I69.03-, I69.13-, I69.23-, I69.33-, I69.83-, I69.93-)
G83.20 Monoplegia of upper limb affecting unspecified side
G83.21 Monoplegia of upper limb affecting right dominant side
G83.22 Monoplegia of upper limb affecting left dominant side
G83.23 Monoplegia of upper limb affecting right nondominant side
G83.24 Monoplegia of upper limb affecting left nondominant side

✓5th **G83.3 Monoplegia, unspecified**
G83.30 Monoplegia, unspecified affecting unspecified side
G83.31 Monoplegia, unspecified affecting right dominant side
G83.32 Monoplegia, unspecified affecting left dominant side
G83.33 Monoplegia, unspecified affecting right nondominant side
G83.34 Monoplegia, unspecified affecting left nondominant side

G83.4 Cauda equina syndrome
Neurogenic bladder due to cauda equina syndrome
EXCLUDES 1 cord bladder NOS (G95.89)
neurogenic bladder NOS (N31.9)

G83.5 Locked-in state

EXCLUDES 1 Not coded here   EXCLUDES 2 Not included here   N Newborn Age: 0   P Pediatric Age: 0-17   M Maternity Age: 12-55   A Adult Age: 15-124

536   ICD-10-CM 2016

☑5ᵗʰ **G83.8 Other specified paralytic syndromes**
> *EXCLUDES 1* *paralytic syndromes due to current spinal cord injury—code to spinal cord injury (S14, S24, S34)*

    G83.81 Brown-Séquard syndrome

    G83.82 Anterior cord syndrome

    G83.83 Posterior cord syndrome

    G83.84 Todd's paralysis (postepileptic)

    G83.89 Other specified paralytic syndromes

G83.9 Paralytic syndrome, unspecified

Other disorders of the nervous system (G89-G99)

☑4ᵗʰ **G89 Pain, not elsewhere classified**
> Code also related psychological factors associated with pain (F45.42)
> *EXCLUDES 1* *generalized pain NOS (R52)*
> *pain disorders exclusively related to psychological factors (F45.41)*
> *pain NOS (R52)*
> *EXCLUDES 2* *atypical face pain (G50.1)*
> *headache syndromes (G44.-)*
> *localized pain, unspecified type—code to pain by site, such as:*
>   *abdomen pain (R10.-)*
>   *back pain (M54.9)*
>   *breast pain (N64.4)*
>   *chest pain (R07.1-R07.9)*
>   *ear pain (H92.0-)*
>   *eye pain (H57.1)*
>   *headache (R51)*
>   *joint pain (M25.5-)*
>   *limb pain (M79.6-)*
>   *lumbar region pain (M54.5)*
>   *painful urination (R30.9)*
>   *pelvic and perineal pain (R10.2)*
>   *renal colic (N23)*
>   *shoulder pain (M25.51-)*
>   *spine pain (M54.-)*
>   *throat pain (R07.0)*
>   *tongue pain (K14.6)*
>   *tooth pain (K08.8)*
> *migraines (G43.-)*
> *myalgia (M79.1)*
> *pain from prosthetic devices, implants, and grafts (T82.84, T83.84, T84.84, T85.84)*
> *phantom limb syndrome with pain (G54.6)*
> *vulvar vestibulitis (N94.810)*
> *vulvodynia (N94.81-)*

G89.0 Central pain syndrome
> Déjérine-Roussy syndrome
> Myelopathic pain syndrome
> Thalamic pain syndrome (hyperesthetic)

☑5ᵗʰ **G89.1 Acute pain, not elsewhere classified**

    G89.11 Acute pain due to trauma

    G89.12 Acute post-thoracotomy pain
>   Post-thoracotomy pain NOS

    G89.18 Other acute postprocedural pain
>   Postoperative pain NOS
>   Postprocedural pain NOS

☑5ᵗʰ **G89.2 Chronic pain, not elsewhere classified**
> *EXCLUDES 1* *causalgia, lower limb (G57.7-)*
> *causalgia, upper limb (G56.4-)*
> *central pain syndrome (G89.0)*
> *chronic pain syndrome (G89.4)*
> *complex regional pain syndrome II, lower limb (G57.7-)*
> *complex regional pain syndrome II, upper limb (G56.4-)*
> *neoplasm related chronic pain (G89.3)*
> *reflex sympathetic dystrophy (G90.5-)*

    G89.21 Chronic pain due to trauma

    G89.22 Chronic post-thoracotomy pain

    G89.28 Other chronic postprocedural pain
>   Other chronic postoperative pain

    G89.29 Other chronic pain

G89.3 Neoplasm related pain (acute) (chronic)
> Cancer associated pain
> Pain due to malignancy (primary) (secondary)
> Tumor associated pain

G89.4 Chronic pain syndrome
> Chronic pain associated with significant psychosocial dysfunction

☑4ᵗʰ **G90 Disorders of autonomic nervous system**
> *EXCLUDES 1* *dysfunction of the autonomic nervous system due to alcohol (G31.2)*

☑5ᵗʰ **G90.0 Idiopathic peripheral autonomic neuropathy**

    G90.01 Carotid sinus syncope
>   Carotid sinus syndrome

    G90.09 Other idiopathic peripheral autonomic neuropathy
>   Idiopathic peripheral autonomic neuropathy NOS

G90.1 Familial dysautonomia [Riley-Day]

G90.2 Horner's syndrome
> Bernard(-Horner) syndrome
> Cervical sympathetic dystrophy or paralysis

G90.3 Multi-system degeneration of the autonomic nervous system
> Neurogenic orthostatic hypotension [Shy-Drager]
> *EXCLUDES 1* *orthostatic hypotension NOS (I95.1)*

G90.4 Autonomic dysreflexia
> Use additional code to identify the cause, such as:
>   fecal impaction (K56.41)
>   pressure ulcer (pressure area) (L89.-)
>   urinary tract infection (N39.0)

☑5ᵗʰ **G90.5 Complex regional pain syndrome I (CRPS I)**
> Reflex sympathetic dystrophy
> *EXCLUDES 1* *causalgia of lower limb (G57.7-)*
> *causalgia of upper limb (G56.4-)*
> *complex regional pain syndrome II of lower limb (G57.7-)*
> *complex regional pain syndrome II of upper limb (G56.4-)*

    G90.50 Complex regional pain syndrome I, unspecified

☑6ᵗʰ **G90.51 Complex regional pain syndrome I of upper limb**

    G90.511 Complex regional pain syndrome I of right upper limb

    G90.512 Complex regional pain syndrome I of left upper limb

    G90.513 Complex regional pain syndrome I of upper limb, bilateral

    G90.519 Complex regional pain syndrome I of unspecified upper limb

☑6ᵗʰ **G90.52 Complex regional pain syndrome I of lower limb**

    G90.521 Complex regional pain syndrome I of right lower limb

    G90.522 Complex regional pain syndrome I of left lower limb

    G90.523 Complex regional pain syndrome I of lower limb, bilateral

    G90.529 Complex regional pain syndrome I of unspecified lower limb

    G90.59 Complex regional pain syndrome I of other specified site

G90.8 Other disorders of autonomic nervous system

G90.9 Disorder of the autonomic nervous system, unspecified

☑4ᵗʰ **G91 Hydrocephalus**
> *INCLUDES* acquired hydrocephalus
> *EXCLUDES 1* *Arnold-Chiari syndrome with hydrocephalus (Q07.-)*
> *congenital hydrocephalus (Q03.-)*
> *spina bifida with hydrocephalus (Q05.-)*

G91.0 Communicating hydrocephalus
> Secondary normal pressure hydrocephalus

G91.1 Obstructive hydrocephalus

G91.2 (Idiopathic) normal pressure hydrocephalus
> Normal pressure hydrocephalus NOS

G91.3 Post-traumatic hydrocephalus, unspecified

G91.4 Hydrocephalus in diseases classified elsewhere
> Code first underlying condition, such as:
>   congenital syphilis (A50.4-)
>   neoplasm (C00-D49)
> *EXCLUDES 1* *hydrocephalus due to congenital toxoplasmosis (P37.1)*
> **AHA:** 2014, 3Q, 3

G91.8 Other hydrocephalus

G91.9 Hydrocephalus, unspecified

G92 Toxic encephalopathy
> Toxic encephalitis
> Toxic metabolic encephalopathy
> Code first (T51-T65) to identify toxic agent

☑ Additional Character Required   ✗ᵗʰ Placeholder Alert   Unspecified Dx   Other Specified Dx   Manifestation   ▶◀ Revised Text   ● New Code   ▲ Revised Code Title

Chapter 6. Diseases of the Nervous System

✓4th **G93 Other disorders of brain**

G93.0 Cerebral cysts
Arachnoid cyst
Porencephalic cyst, acquired
EXCLUDES 1   acquired periventricular cysts of newborn (P91.1)
      congenital cerebral cysts (Q04.6)

G93.1 Anoxic brain damage, not elsewhere classified
EXCLUDES 1   cerebral anoxia due to anesthesia during labor and
      delivery (O74.3)
      cerebral anoxia due to anesthesia during the
      puerperium (O89.2)
      neonatal anoxia (P84)

G93.2 Benign intracranial hypertension
EXCLUDES 1   hypertensive encephalopathy (I67.4)

G93.3 Postviral fatigue syndrome
Benign myalgic encephalomyelitis
EXCLUDES 1   chronic fatigue syndrome NOS (R53.82)

✓5th **G93.4 Other and unspecified encephalopathy**
EXCLUDES 1   alcoholic encephalopathy (G31.2)
      encephalopathy in diseases classified elsewhere (G94)
      hypertensive encephalopathy (I67.4)
      toxic (metabolic) encephalopathy (G92)

     G93.40 Encephalopathy, unspecified

     G93.41 Metabolic encephalopathy
        Septic encephalopathy

     G93.49 Other encephalopathy
        Encephalopathy NEC

G93.5 Compression of brain
Arnold-Chiari type 1 compression of brain
Compression of brain (stem)
Herniation of brain (stem)
EXCLUDES 1   diffuse traumatic compression of brain (S06.2-)
      focal traumatic compression of brain (S06.3-)

G93.6 Cerebral edema
EXCLUDES 1   cerebral edema due to birth injury (P11.0)
      traumatic cerebral edema (S06.1-)

G93.7 Reye's syndrome   P
Code first (T39.0-), if salicylates-induced

✓5th **G93.8 Other specified disorders of brain**

     G93.81 Temporal sclerosis
        Hippocampal sclerosis
        Mesial temporal sclerosis

     G93.82 Brain death

     G93.89 Other specified disorders of brain
        Postradiation encephalopathy

G93.9 Disorder of brain, unspecified

G94 Other disorders of brain in diseases classified elsewhere
Code first underlying disease
EXCLUDES 1   encephalopathy in congenital syphilis (A50.49)
      encephalopathy in influenza (J09.X9, J10.81, J11.81)
      encephalopathy in syphilis (A52.19)
      hydrocephalus in diseases classified elsewhere (G91.4)

✓4th **G95 Other and unspecified diseases of spinal cord**
EXCLUDES 2   myelitis (G04.-)

G95.0 Syringomyelia and syringobulbia

✓5th **G95.1 Vascular myelopathies**
EXCLUDES 2   intraspinal phlebitis and thrombophlebitis, except
      non-pyogenic (G08)

     **G95.11 Acute infarction of spinal cord (embolic)
        (nonembolic)**
        Anoxia of spinal cord
        Arterial thrombosis of spinal cord

     G95.19 Other vascular myelopathies
        Edema of spinal cord
        Hematomyelia
        Nonpyogenic intraspinal phlebitis and
          thrombophlebitis
        Subacute necrotic myelopathy

✓5th **G95.2 Other and unspecified cord compression**

     G95.20 Unspecified cord compression

     G95.29 Other cord compression

✓5th **G95.8 Other specified diseases of spinal cord**
EXCLUDES 1   neurogenic bladder NOS (N31.9)
      neurogenic bladder due to cauda equina syndrome
        (G83.4)
      neuromuscular dysfunction of bladder without spinal
        cord lesion (N31.-)

     G95.81 Conus medullaris syndrome

     G95.89 Other specified diseases of spinal cord
        Cord bladder NOS
        Drug-induced myelopathy
        Radiation-induced myelopathy
        EXCLUDES 1   myelopathy NOS (G95.9)

G95.9 Disease of spinal cord, unspecified
Myelopathy NOS

✓4th **G96 Other disorders of central nervous system**

G96.0 Cerebrospinal fluid leak
EXCLUDES 1   cerebrospinal fluid leak from spinal puncture (G97.0)

✓5th **G96.1 Disorders of meninges, not elsewhere classified**

     G96.11 Dural tear
        EXCLUDES 1   accidental puncture or laceration of dura
            during a procedure (G97.41)
        AHA: 2014, 4Q, 24

     G96.12 Meningeal adhesions (cerebral) (spinal)

     **G96.19 Other disorders of meninges, not elsewhere
        classified**

G96.8 Other specified disorders of central nervous system

G96.9 Disorder of central nervous system, unspecified

✓4th **G97 Intraoperative and postprocedural complications and disorders
of nervous system, not elsewhere classified**
EXCLUDES 2   intraoperative and postprocedural cerebrovascular infarction
      (I97.81-, I97.82-)

G97.0 Cerebrospinal fluid leak from spinal puncture

G97.1 Other reaction to spinal and lumbar puncture
Headache due to lumbar puncture

G97.2 Intracranial hypotension following ventricular shunting

✓5th **G97.3 Intraoperative hemorrhage and hematoma of a nervous
system organ or structure complicating a procedure**
EXCLUDES 1   intraoperative hemorrhage and hematoma of a
      nervous system organ or structure due to
      accidental puncture and laceration during a
      procedure (G97.4-)

     **G97.31 Intraoperative hemorrhage and hematoma of a
        nervous system organ or structure complicating a
        nervous system procedure**

     **G97.32 Intraoperative hemorrhage and hematoma of a
        nervous system organ or structure complicating
        other procedure**

✓5th **G97.4 Accidental puncture and laceration of a nervous system organ
or structure during a procedure**

     **G97.41 Accidental puncture or laceration of dura during a
        procedure**
        Incidental (inadvertent) durotomy
        AHA: 2014, 4Q, 24

     **G97.48 Accidental puncture and laceration of other nervous
        system organ or structure during a nervous system
        procedure**

     **G97.49 Accidental puncture and laceration of other nervous
        system organ or structure during other procedure**

✓5th **G97.5 Postprocedural hemorrhage and hematoma of a nervous
system organ or structure following a procedure**

     **G97.51 Postprocedural hemorrhage and hematoma of a
        nervous system organ or structure following a
        nervous system procedure**

     **G97.52 Postprocedural hemorrhage and hematoma of a
        nervous system organ or structure following other
        procedure**

✓5th **G97.8 Other intraoperative and postprocedural complications and
disorders of nervous system**
Use additional code to further specify disorder

     **G97.81 Other intraoperative complications of nervous
        system**

     **G97.82 Other postprocedural complications and disorders
        of nervous system**

EXCLUDES 1 Not coded here   EXCLUDES 2 Not included here   N Newborn Age: 0   P Pediatric Age: 0-17   M Maternity Age: 12-55   A Adult Age: 15-124

538   ICD-10-CM 2016

☑4ᵗʰ **G98** **Other disorders of nervous system not elsewhere classified**

     INCLUDES   nervous system disorder NOS

    G98.0 **Neurogenic arthritis, not elsewhere classified**

        Nonsyphilitic neurogenic arthropathy NEC

        Nonsyphilitic neurogenic spondylopathy NEC

        EXCLUDES 1   spondylopathy (in):

                syringomyelia and syringobulbia (G95.0)

                tabes dorsalis (A52.11)

    G98.8 **Other disorders of nervous system**

        Nervous system disorder NOS

☑4ᵗʰ **G99** **Other disorders of nervous system in diseases classified elsewhere**

    G99.0 *Autonomic neuropathy in diseases classified elsewhere*

        Code first underlying disease, such as:

          amyloidosis (E85.-)

          gout (M1A.-, M10.-)

          hyperthyroidism (E05.-)

        EXCLUDES 1   *diabetic autonomic neuropathy (E08-E13 with .43)*

    G99.2 *Myelopathy in diseases classified elsewhere*

        Code first underlying disease, such as:

          neoplasm (C00-D49)

        EXCLUDES 1   *myelopathy in:*

              intervertebral disease (M50.0-, M51.0-)

              spondylosis (M47.0-, M47.1-)

    G99.8 *Other specified disorders of nervous system in diseases classified elsewhere*

        Code first underlying disorder, such as:

          amyloidosis (E85.-)

          avitaminosis (E56.9)

        EXCLUDES 1   *nervous system involvement in:*

              cysticercosis (B69.0)

              rubella (B06.0-)

              syphilis (A52.1-)

☑ Additional Character Required   ☑x7ᵗʰ Placeholder Alert   Unspecified Dx   Other Specified Dx   Manifestation   ►◄ Revised Text   ● New Code   ▲ Revised Code Title

Chapter 7. Diseases of the Eye and Adnexa (H00–H59)

Chapter Specific Guidelines with Coding Examples

The chapter specific guidelines from the ICD-10-CM Official Guidelines for Coding and Reporting have been provided below. Along with these guidelines are coding examples, contained in the shaded boxes, that have been developed to help illustrate the coding and/or sequencing guidance found in these guidelines.

a. Glaucoma

1) Assigning glaucoma codes

Assign as many codes from category H40, Glaucoma, as needed to identify the type of glaucoma, the affected eye, and the glaucoma stage.

2) Bilateral glaucoma with same type and stage

When a patient has bilateral glaucoma and both eyes are documented as being the same type and stage, and there is a code for bilateral glaucoma, report only the code for the type of glaucoma, bilateral, with the seventh character for the stage.

> Bilateral severe stage pigmentary glaucoma
>
> **H40.1333   Pigmentary glaucoma, bilateral, severe stage**
>
> *Explanation*: In this scenario, the patient has the same type and stage of glaucoma in both eyes. As this type of glaucoma has a code for bilateral, assign only the code for the bilateral glaucoma with the seventh character for the stage.

When a patient has bilateral glaucoma and both eyes are documented as being the same type and stage, and the classification does not provide a code for bilateral glaucoma (i.e. subcategories H40.10, H40.11 and H40.20) report only one code for the type of glaucoma with the appropriate seventh character for the stage.

> Bilateral, mild stage, primary open-angle glaucoma
>
> **H40.11X1   Primary open-angle glaucoma, mild stage**
>
> *Explanation*: In this scenario, the patient has glaucoma of the same type and stage of both eyes, but there is no code specifically for bilateral glaucoma. Only one code is assigned with the appropriate seventh character for the stage.

3) Bilateral glaucoma stage with different types or stages

When a patient has bilateral glaucoma and each eye is documented as having a different type or stage, and the classification distinguishes laterality, assign the appropriate code for each eye rather than the code for bilateral glaucoma.

> Bilateral chronic angle-closure glaucoma; right eye is documented as mild stage and left eye as moderate stage
>
> **H40.2211   Chronic angle-closure glaucoma, right eye, mild stage**
>
> **H40.2222   Chronic angle-closure glaucoma, left eye, moderate stage**
>
> *Explanation*: In this scenario the patient has the same type of glaucoma in both eyes, but each eye is at a different stage. Because the subcategory for this condition identifies laterality, one code is assigned for the right eye and one code is assigned for the left eye, each with the appropriate seventh character for the stage appended.

When a patient has bilateral glaucoma and each eye is documented as having a different type, and the classification does not distinguish laterality (i.e. subcategories H40.10, H40.11 and H40.20), assign one code for each type of glaucoma with the appropriate seventh character for the stage.

> Documentation relates mild, unspecified primary angle-closure glaucoma of the left eye with mild primary open-angle glaucoma of the right eye
>
> **H40.20X1   Unspecified primary angle-closure glaucoma, mild stage**
>
> **H40.11X1   Primary open-angle glaucoma, mild stage**
>
> *Explanation*: In this scenario the patient has a different type of glaucoma in each eye and the classification does not distinguish laterality. A code for each type of glaucoma is assigned, each with the appropriate seventh character for the stage.

When a patient has bilateral glaucoma and each eye is documented as having the same type, but different stage, and the classification does not distinguish laterality (i.e. subcategories H40.10, H40.11 and H40.20), assign a code for the type of glaucoma for each eye with the seventh character for the specific glaucoma stage documented for each eye.

> Bilateral primary open-angle glaucoma; the right eye is documented to be in mild stage and the left eye as being in moderate stage
>
> **H40.11X2   Primary open-angle glaucoma, moderate stage**
>
> **H40.11X1   Primary open-angle glaucoma, mild stage**
>
> *Explanation*: In this scenario the patient has the same type of glaucoma in each eye but each eye is at a different stage, and the classification does not distinguish laterality at this subcategory level. Two codes are assigned; both codes represent the same type of glaucoma but each has a different seventh character identifying the appropriate stage for each eye.

4) Patient admitted with glaucoma and stage evolves during the admission

If a patient is admitted with glaucoma and the stage progresses during the admission, assign the code for highest stage documented.

> Patient admitted with mild low-tension glaucoma of the right eye, which progresses to moderate stage during the patient's stay
>
> **H40.1212   Low-tension glaucoma, right eye, moderate stage**
>
> *Explanation*: When the glaucoma stage progresses during an admission, assign only the code for the highest stage documented.

5) Indeterminate stage glaucoma

Assignment of the seventh character "4" for "indeterminate stage" should be based on the clinical documentation. The seventh character "4" is used for glaucomas whose stage cannot be clinically determined. This seventh character should not be confused with the seventh character "0", unspecified, which should be assigned when there is no documentation regarding the stage of the glaucoma.

Chapter 7. Diseases of the Eye and Adnexa (H00-H59)

NOTE Use an external cause code following the code for the eye condition, if applicable, to identify the cause of the eye condition.

EXCLUDES 2 *certain conditions originating in the perinatal period (P04-P96)*
certain infectious and parasitic diseases (A00-B99)
complications of pregnancy, childbirth and the puerperium (O00-O9A)
congenital malformations, deformations, and chromosomal abnormalities (Q00-Q99)
diabetes mellitus related eye conditions (E09.3-, E10.3-, E11.3-, E13.3-)
endocrine, nutritional and metabolic diseases (E00-E88)
injury (trauma) of eye and orbit (S05.-)
injury, poisoning and certain other consequences of external causes (S00-T88)
neoplasms (C00-D49)
symptoms, signs and abnormal clinical and laboratory findings, not elsewhere classified (R00-R94)
syphilis related eye disorders (A50.01, A50.3-, A51.43, A52.71)

This chapter contains the following blocks:

H00-H05   Disorders of eyelid, lacrimal system and orbit
H10-H11   Disorders of conjunctiva
H15-H22   Disorders of sclera, cornea, iris and ciliary body
H25-H28   Disorders of lens
H30-H36   Disorders of choroid and retina
H40-H42   Glaucoma
H43-H44   Disorders of vitreous body and globe
H46-H47   Disorders of optic nerve and visual pathways
H49-H52   Disorders of ocular muscles, binocular movement, accommodation and refraction
H53-H54   Visual disturbances and blindness
H55-H57   Other disorders of eye and adnexa
H59   Intraoperative and postprocedural complications and disorders of eye and adnexa, not elsewhere classified

Disorders of eyelid, lacrimal system and orbit (H00-H05)

EXCLUDES 2 *open wound of eyelid (S01.1-)*
superficial injury of eyelid (S00.1-, S00.2-)

✓4th H00 Hordeolum and chalazion

✓5th H00.0 Hordeolum (externum) (internum) of eyelid

     ✓6th H00.01 Hordeolum externum
        Hordeolum NOS
        Stye
        H00.011 Hordeolum externum right upper **eyelid**
        H00.012 Hordeolum externum right lower **eyelid**
        H00.013 Hordeolum externum right eye, unspecified eyelid
        H00.014 Hordeolum externum left upper **eyelid**
        H00.015 Hordeolum externum left lower **eyelid**
        H00.016 Hordeolum externum left eye, unspecified eyelid
        H00.019 Hordeolum externum unspecified eye, unspecified eyelid

     ✓6th H00.02 Hordeolum internum
        Infection of meibomian gland
        H00.021 Hordeolum internum right upper **eyelid**
        H00.022 Hordeolum internum right lower **eyelid**
        H00.023 Hordeolum internum right eye, unspecified eyelid
        H00.024 Hordeolum internum left upper **eyelid**
        H00.025 Hordeolum internum left lower **eyelid**
        H00.026 Hordeolum internum left eye, unspecified eyelid
        H00.029 Hordeolum internum unspecified eye, unspecified eyelid

     ✓6th H00.03 Abscess of eyelid
        Furuncle of eyelid
        H00.031 Abscess of right upper **eyelid**
        H00.032 Abscess of right lower **eyelid**
        H00.033 Abscess of eyelid right eye, unspecified eyelid
        H00.034 Abscess of left upper **eyelid**
        H00.035 Abscess of left lower **eyelid**
        H00.036 Abscess of eyelid left eye, unspecified eyelid
        H00.039 Abscess of eyelid unspecified eye, unspecified eyelid

✓5th H00.1 Chalazion
    Meibomian (gland) cyst
     EXCLUDES 2 *infected meibomian gland (H00.02-)*
    H00.11 Chalazion right upper **eyelid**
    H00.12 Chalazion right lower **eyelid**
    H00.13 Chalazion right eye, unspecified eyelid
    H00.14 Chalazion left upper **eyelid**
    H00.15 Chalazion left lower **eyelid**
    H00.16 Chalazion left eye, unspecified eyelid
    H00.19 Chalazion unspecified eye, unspecified eyelid

✓4th H01 Other inflammation of eyelid

✓5th H01.0 Blepharitis
     EXCLUDES 1 *blepharoconjunctivitis (H10.5-)*

     ✓6th H01.00 Unspecified blepharitis
        H01.001 Unspecified blepharitis right upper **eyelid**
        H01.002 Unspecified blepharitis right lower **eyelid**
        H01.003 Unspecified blepharitis right eye, unspecified eyelid
        H01.004 Unspecified blepharitis left upper **eyelid**
        H01.005 Unspecified blepharitis left lower **eyelid**
        H01.006 Unspecified blepharitis left eye, unspecified eyelid
        H01.009 Unspecified blepharitis unspecified eye, unspecified eyelid

     ✓6th H01.01 Ulcerative blepharitis
        H01.011 Ulcerative blepharitis right upper **eyelid**
        H01.012 Ulcerative blepharitis right lower **eyelid**
        H01.013 Ulcerative blepharitis right eye, unspecified eyelid
        H01.014 Ulcerative blepharitis left upper **eyelid**
        H01.015 Ulcerative blepharitis left lower **eyelid**
        H01.016 Ulcerative blepharitis left eye, unspecified eyelid
        H01.019 Ulcerative blepharitis unspecified eye, unspecified eyelid

     ✓6th H01.02 Squamous blepharitis
        H01.021 Squamous blepharitis right upper **eyelid**
        H01.022 Squamous blepharitis right lower **eyelid**
        H01.023 Squamous blepharitis right eye, unspecified eyelid
        H01.024 Squamous blepharitis left upper **eyelid**
        H01.025 Squamous blepharitis left lower **eyelid**
        H01.026 Squamous blepharitis left eye, unspecified eyelid
        H01.029 Squamous blepharitis unspecified eye, unspecified eyelid

✓5th H01.1 Noninfectious dermatoses of eyelid

     ✓6th H01.11 Allergic dermatitis of eyelid
        Contact dermatitis of eyelid
        H01.111 Allergic dermatitis of right upper **eyelid**
        H01.112 Allergic dermatitis of right lower **eyelid**
        H01.113 Allergic dermatitis of right eye, unspecified eyelid
        H01.114 Allergic dermatitis of left upper **eyelid**
        H01.115 Allergic dermatitis of left lower **eyelid**
        H01.116 Allergic dermatitis of left eye, unspecified eyelid
        H01.119 Allergic dermatitis of unspecified eye, unspecified eyelid

     ✓6th H01.12 Discoid lupus erythematosus of eyelid
        H01.121 Discoid lupus erythematosus of right upper **eyelid**
        H01.122 Discoid lupus erythematosus of right lower **eyelid**
        H01.123 Discoid lupus erythematosus of right eye, unspecified eyelid
        H01.124 Discoid lupus erythematosus of left upper **eyelid**
        H01.125 Discoid lupus erythematosus of left lower **eyelid**
        H01.126 Discoid lupus erythematosus of left eye, unspecified eyelid
        H01.129 Discoid lupus erythematosus of unspecified eye, unspecified eyelid

---

✓ Additional Character Required   ✓x7th Placeholder Alert   Unspecified Dx   Other Specified Dx   Manifestation   ►◄ Revised Text   ● New Code   ▲ Revised Code Title

Chapter 7. Diseases of the Eye and Adnexa

H01.13–H02.142

✓6ᵗʰ **H01.13 Eczematous dermatitis of eyelid**
- H01.131 **Eczematous dermatitis of right upper eyelid**
- H01.132 **Eczematous dermatitis of right lower eyelid**
- H01.133 **Eczematous dermatitis of right eye, unspecified eyelid**
- H01.134 **Eczematous dermatitis of left upper eyelid**
- H01.135 **Eczematous dermatitis of left lower eyelid**
- H01.136 **Eczematous dermatitis of left eye, unspecified eyelid**
- H01.139 **Eczematous dermatitis of unspecified eye, unspecified eyelid**

✓6ᵗʰ **H01.14 Xeroderma of eyelid**
- H01.141 **Xeroderma of right upper eyelid**
- H01.142 **Xeroderma of right lower eyelid**
- H01.143 **Xeroderma of right eye, unspecified eyelid**
- H01.144 **Xeroderma of left upper eyelid**
- H01.145 **Xeroderma of left lower eyelid**
- H01.146 **Xeroderma of left eye, unspecified eyelid**
- H01.149 **Xeroderma of unspecified eye, unspecified eyelid**

H01.8 Other specified inflammations of eyelid

H01.9 Unspecified inflammation of eyelid
     Inflammation of eyelid NOS

✓4ᵗʰ **H02 Other disorders of eyelid**
     EXCLUDES 1   *congenital malformations of eyelid (Q10.0-Q10.3)*

✓5ᵗʰ **H02.0 Entropion and trichiasis of eyelid**

✓6ᵗʰ **H02.00 Unspecified entropion of eyelid**
- H02.001 **Unspecified entropion of right upper eyelid**
- H02.002 **Unspecified entropion of right lower eyelid**
- H02.003 **Unspecified entropion of right eye, unspecified eyelid**
- H02.004 **Unspecified entropion of left upper eyelid**
- H02.005 **Unspecified entropion of left lower eyelid**
- H02.006 **Unspecified entropion of left eye, unspecified eyelid**
- H02.009 **Unspecified entropion of unspecified eye, unspecified eyelid**

✓6ᵗʰ **H02.01 Cicatricial entropion of eyelid**
- H02.011 **Cicatricial entropion of right upper eyelid**
- H02.012 **Cicatricial entropion of right lower eyelid**
- H02.013 **Cicatricial entropion of right eye, unspecified eyelid**
- H02.014 **Cicatricial entropion of left upper eyelid**
- H02.015 **Cicatricial entropion of left lower eyelid**
- H02.016 **Cicatricial entropion of left eye, unspecified eyelid**
- H02.019 **Cicatricial entropion of unspecified eye, unspecified eyelid**

✓6ᵗʰ **H02.02 Mechanical entropion of eyelid**
- H02.021 **Mechanical entropion of right upper eyelid**
- H02.022 **Mechanical entropion of right lower eyelid**
- H02.023 **Mechanical entropion of right eye, unspecified eyelid**
- H02.024 **Mechanical entropion of left upper eyelid**
- H02.025 **Mechanical entropion of left lower eyelid**
- H02.026 **Mechanical entropion of left eye, unspecified eyelid**
- H02.029 **Mechanical entropion of unspecified eye, unspecified eyelid**

✓6ᵗʰ **H02.03 Senile entropion of eyelid**
- H02.031 **Senile entropion of right upper eyelid** Ⓐ
- H02.032 **Senile entropion of right lower eyelid** Ⓐ
- H02.033 **Senile entropion of right eye, unspecified eyelid** Ⓐ
- H02.034 **Senile entropion of left upper eyelid** Ⓐ
- H02.035 **Senile entropion of left lower eyelid** Ⓐ
- H02.036 **Senile entropion of left eye, unspecified eyelid** Ⓐ
- H02.039 **Senile entropion of unspecified eye, unspecified eyelid** Ⓐ

✓6ᵗʰ **H02.04 Spastic entropion of eyelid**
- H02.041 **Spastic entropion of right upper eyelid**
- H02.042 **Spastic entropion of right lower eyelid**
- H02.043 **Spastic entropion of right eye, unspecified eyelid**
- H02.044 **Spastic entropion of left upper eyelid**
- H02.045 **Spastic entropion of left lower eyelid**
- H02.046 **Spastic entropion of left eye, unspecified eyelid**
- H02.049 **Spastic entropion of unspecified eye, unspecified eyelid**

✓6ᵗʰ **H02.05 Trichiasis without entropian**
- H02.051 **Trichiasis without entropian right upper eyelid**
- H02.052 **Trichiasis without entropian right lower eyelid**
- H02.053 **Trichiasis without entropian right eye, unspecified eyelid**
- H02.054 **Trichiasis without entropian left upper eyelid**
- H02.055 **Trichiasis without entropian left lower eyelid**
- H02.056 **Trichiasis without entropian left eye, unspecified eyelid**
- H02.059 **Trichiasis without entropian unspecified eye, unspecified eyelid**

✓5ᵗʰ **H02.1 Ectropion of eyelid**

✓6ᵗʰ **H02.10 Unspecified ectropion of eyelid**
- H02.101 **Unspecified ectropion of right upper eyelid**
- H02.102 **Unspecified ectropion of right lower eyelid**
- H02.103 **Unspecified ectropion of right eye, unspecified eyelid**
- H02.104 **Unspecified ectropion of left upper eyelid**
- H02.105 **Unspecified ectropion of left lower eyelid**
- H02.106 **Unspecified ectropion of left eye, unspecified eyelid**
- H02.109 **Unspecified ectropion of unspecified eye, unspecified eyelid**

✓6ᵗʰ **H02.11 Cicatricial ectropion of eyelid**
- H02.111 **Cicatricial ectropion of right upper eyelid**
- H02.112 **Cicatricial ectropion of right lower eyelid**
- H02.113 **Cicatricial ectropion of right eye, unspecified eyelid**
- H02.114 **Cicatricial ectropion of left upper eyelid**
- H02.115 **Cicatricial ectropion of left lower eyelid**
- H02.116 **Cicatricial ectropion of left eye, unspecified eyelid**
- H02.119 **Cicatricial ectropion of unspecified eye, unspecified eyelid**

✓6ᵗʰ **H02.12 Mechanical ectropion of eyelid**
- H02.121 **Mechanical ectropion of right upper eyelid**
- H02.122 **Mechanical ectropion of right lower eyelid**
- H02.123 **Mechanical ectropion of right eye, unspecified eyelid**
- H02.124 **Mechanical ectropion of left upper eyelid**
- H02.125 **Mechanical ectropion of left lower eyelid**
- H02.126 **Mechanical ectropion of left eye, unspecified eyelid**
- H02.129 **Mechanical ectropion of unspecified eye, unspecified eyelid**

✓6ᵗʰ **H02.13 Senile ectropion of eyelid**
- H02.131 **Senile ectropion of right upper eyelid** Ⓐ
- H02.132 **Senile ectropion of right lower eyelid** Ⓐ
- H02.133 **Senile ectropion of right eye, unspecified eyelid** Ⓐ
- H02.134 **Senile ectropion of left upper eyelid** Ⓐ
- H02.135 **Senile ectropion of left lower eyelid** Ⓐ
- H02.136 **Senile ectropion of left eye, unspecified eyelid** Ⓐ
- H02.139 **Senile ectropion of unspecified eye, unspecified eyelid** Ⓐ

✓6ᵗʰ **H02.14 Spastic ectropion of eyelid**
- H02.141 **Spastic ectropion of right upper eyelid**
- H02.142 **Spastic ectropion of right lower eyelid**

| EXCLUDES 1 Not coded here | EXCLUDES 2 Not included here | Ⓝ Newborn Age: 0 | Ⓟ Pediatric Age: 0-17 | Ⓜ Maternity Age: 12-55 | Ⓐ Adult Age: 15-124 |

542   **ICD-10-CM 2016**

H02.143   **Spastic ectropion of** right eye, unspecified eyelid
H02.144   **Spastic ectropion of** left upper **eyelid**
H02.145   **Spastic ectropion of** left lower **eyelid**
H02.146   **Spastic ectropion of** left eye, unspecified eyelid
H02.149   **Spastic ectropion of unspecified eye, unspecified eyelid**

✓5ᵗʰ   **H02.2   Lagophthalmos**

     ✓6ᵗʰ   **H02.20   Unspecified lagophthalmos**

         H02.201   **Unspecified lagophthalmos** right upper **eyelid**
         H02.202   **Unspecified lagophthalmos** right lower **eyelid**
         H02.203   **Unspecified lagophthalmos** right eye, unspecified eyelid
         H02.204   **Unspecified lagophthalmos** left upper **eyelid**
         H02.205   **Unspecified lagophthalmos** left lower **eyelid**
         H02.206   **Unspecified lagophthalmos** left eye, unspecified eyelid
         H02.209   **Unspecified lagophthalmos unspecified eye, unspecified eyelid**

     ✓6ᵗʰ   **H02.21   Cicatricial lagophthalmos**

         H02.211   **Cicatricial lagophthalmos** right upper **eyelid**
         H02.212   **Cicatricial lagophthalmos** right lower **eyelid**
         H02.213   **Cicatricial lagophthalmos** right eye, unspecified eyelid
         H02.214   **Cicatricial lagophthalmos** left upper **eyelid**
         H02.215   **Cicatricial lagophthalmos** left lower **eyelid**
         H02.216   **Cicatricial lagophthalmos** left eye, unspecified eyelid
         H02.219   **Cicatricial lagophthalmos unspecified eye, unspecified eyelid**

     ✓6ᵗʰ   **H02.22   Mechanical lagophthalmos**

         H02.221   **Mechanical lagophthalmos** right upper **eyelid**
         H02.222   **Mechanical lagophthalmos** right lower **eyelid**
         H02.223   **Mechanical lagophthalmos** right eye, unspecified eyelid
         H02.224   **Mechanical lagophthalmos** left upper **eyelid**
         H02.225   **Mechanical lagophthalmos** left lower **eyelid**
         H02.226   **Mechanical lagophthalmos** left eye, unspecified eyelid
         H02.229   **Mechanical lagophthalmos unspecified eye, unspecified eyelid**

     ✓6ᵗʰ   **H02.23   Paralytic lagophthalmos**

         H02.231   **Paralytic lagophthalmos** right upper **eyelid**
         H02.232   **Paralytic lagophthalmos** right lower **eyelid**
         H02.233   **Paralytic lagophthalmos** right eye, unspecified eyelid
         H02.234   **Paralytic lagophthalmos** left upper **eyelid**
         H02.235   **Paralytic lagophthalmos** left lower **eyelid**
         H02.236   **Paralytic lagophthalmos** left eye, unspecified eyelid
         H02.239   **Paralytic lagophthalmos unspecified eye, unspecified eyelid**

✓5ᵗʰ   **H02.3   Blepharochalasis**
         Pseudoptosis

     H02.30   **Blepharochalasis unspecified eye, unspecified eyelid**
     H02.31   **Blepharochalasis** right upper **eyelid**
     H02.32   **Blepharochalasis** right lower **eyelid**
     H02.33   **Blepharochalasis** right eye, unspecified eyelid
     H02.34   **Blepharochalasis** left upper **eyelid**
     H02.35   **Blepharochalasis** left lower **eyelid**
     H02.36   **Blepharochalasis** left eye, unspecified eyelid

---

✓5ᵗʰ   **H02.4   Ptosis of eyelid**

     ✓6ᵗʰ   **H02.40   Unspecified ptosis of eyelid**

         H02.401   **Unspecified ptosis of** right **eyelid**
         H02.402   **Unspecified ptosis of** left **eyelid**
         H02.403   **Unspecified ptosis of** bilateral **eyelids**
         H02.409   **Unspecified ptosis of unspecified eyelid**

     ✓6ᵗʰ   **H02.41   Mechanical ptosis of eyelid**

         H02.411   **Mechanical ptosis of** right **eyelid**
         H02.412   **Mechanical ptosis of** left **eyelid**
         H02.413   **Mechanical ptosis of** bilateral **eyelids**
         H02.419   **Mechanical ptosis of unspecified eyelid**

     ✓6ᵗʰ   **H02.42   Myogenic ptosis of eyelid**

         H02.421   **Myogenic ptosis of** right **eyelid**
         H02.422   **Myogenic ptosis of** left **eyelid**
         H02.423   **Myogenic ptosis of** bilateral **eyelids**
         H02.429   **Myogenic ptosis of unspecified eyelid**

     ✓6ᵗʰ   **H02.43   Paralytic ptosis of eyelid**
         Neurogenic ptosis of eyelid

         H02.431   **Paralytic ptosis of** right **eyelid**
         H02.432   **Paralytic ptosis of** left **eyelid**
         H02.433   **Paralytic ptosis of** bilateral **eyelids**
         H02.439   **Paralytic ptosis unspecified eyelid**

✓5ᵗʰ   **H02.5   Other disorders affecting eyelid function**

     EXCLUDES 2   blepharospasm (G24.5)
                 organic tic (G25.69)
                 psychogenic tic (F95.-)

     ✓6ᵗʰ   **H02.51   Abnormal innervation syndrome**

         H02.511   **Abnormal innervation syndrome** right upper **eyelid**
         H02.512   **Abnormal innervation syndrome** right lower **eyelid**
         H02.513   **Abnormal innervation syndrome** right eye, unspecified eyelid
         H02.514   **Abnormal innervation syndrome** left upper **eyelid**
         H02.515   **Abnormal innervation syndrome** left lower **eyelid**
         H02.516   **Abnormal innervation syndrome** left eye, unspecified eyelid
         H02.519   **Abnormal innervation syndrome unspecified eye, unspecified eyelid**

     ✓6ᵗʰ   **H02.52   Blepharophimosis**
         Ankyloblepharon

         H02.521   **Blepharophimosis** right upper **eyelid**
         H02.522   **Blepharophimosis** right lower **eyelid**
         H02.523   **Blepharophimosis** right eye, unspecified eyelid
         H02.524   **Blepharophimosis** left upper **eyelid**
         H02.525   **Blepharophimosis** left lower **eyelid**
         H02.526   **Blepharophimosis** left eye, unspecified eyelid
         H02.529   **Blepharophimosis unspecified eye, unspecified lid**

     ✓6ᵗʰ   **H02.53   Eyelid retraction**
         Eyelid lag

         H02.531   **Eyelid retraction** right upper **eyelid**
         H02.532   **Eyelid retraction** right lower **eyelid**
         H02.533   **Eyelid retraction** right eye, unspecified eyelid
         H02.534   **Eyelid retraction** left upper **eyelid**
         H02.535   **Eyelid retraction** left lower **eyelid**
         H02.536   **Eyelid retraction** left eye, unspecified eyelid
         H02.539   **Eyelid retraction unspecified eye, unspecified lid**

     H02.59   **Other disorders affecting eyelid function**
         Deficient blink reflex
         Sensory disorders

✓5ᵗʰ   **H02.6   Xanthelasma of eyelid**

     H02.60   **Xanthelasma of unspecified eye, unspecified eyelid**
     H02.61   **Xanthelasma of** right upper **eyelid**
     H02.62   **Xanthelasma of** right lower **eyelid**
     H02.63   **Xanthelasma of** right eye, unspecified eyelid
     H02.64   **Xanthelasma of** left upper **eyelid**
     H02.65   **Xanthelasma of** left lower **eyelid**

☑ Additional Character Required   ✓ˣ⁷ᵗʰ Placeholder Alert   Unspecified Dx   Other Specified Dx   Manifestation   ►◄ Revised Text   ● New Code   ▲ Revised Code Title

ICD-10-CM 2016   543

H02.66 **Xanthelasma of** left eye, **unspecified eyelid**

√5ᵗʰ H02.7 **Other and unspecified degenerative disorders of eyelid and periocular area**

   H02.70 **Unspecified degenerative disorders of eyelid and periocular area**

  √6ᵗʰ H02.71 **Chloasma of eyelid and periocular area**
    Dyspigmentation of eyelid
    Hyperpigmentation of eyelid

    H02.711 **Chloasma of** right upper **eyelid and periocular area**

    H02.712 **Chloasma of** right lower **eyelid and periocular area**

    H02.713 **Chloasma of** right eye, **unspecified eyelid and periocular area**

    H02.714 **Chloasma of** left upper **eyelid and periocular area**

    H02.715 **Chloasma of** left lower **eyelid and periocular area**

    H02.716 **Chloasma of** left eye, **unspecified eyelid and periocular area**

    H02.719 **Chloasma of unspecified eye, unspecified eyelid and periocular area**

  √6ᵗʰ H02.72 **Madarosis of eyelid and periocular area**
    Hypotrichosis of eyelid

    H02.721 **Madarosis of** right upper **eyelid and periocular area**

    H02.722 **Madarosis of** right lower **eyelid and periocular area**

    H02.723 **Madarosis of** right eye, **unspecified eyelid and periocular area**

    H02.724 **Madarosis of** left upper **eyelid and periocular area**

    H02.725 **Madarosis of** left lower **eyelid and periocular area**

    H02.726 **Madarosis of** left eye, **unspecified eyelid and periocular area**

    H02.729 **Madarosis of unspecified eye, unspecified eyelid and periocular area**

  √6ᵗʰ H02.73 **Vitiligo of eyelid and periocular area**
    Hypopigmentation of eyelid

    H02.731 **Vitiligo of** right upper **eyelid and periocular area**

    H02.732 **Vitiligo of** right lower **eyelid and periocular area**

    H02.733 **Vitiligo of** right eye, **unspecified eyelid and periocular area**

    H02.734 **Vitiligo of** left upper **eyelid and periocular area**

    H02.735 **Vitiligo of** left lower **eyelid and periocular area**

    H02.736 **Vitiligo of** left eye, **unspecified eyelid and periocular area**

    H02.739 **Vitiligo of unspecified eye, unspecified eyelid and periocular area**

   H02.79 **Other degenerative disorders of eyelid and periocular area**

√5ᵗʰ H02.8 **Other specified disorders of eyelid**

  √6ᵗʰ H02.81 **Retained foreign body in eyelid**
    Use additional code to identify the type of retained foreign body (Z18.-)

    EXCLUDES 1 *laceration of eyelid with foreign body (S01.12-)*
       retained intraocular foreign body (H44.6-, H44.7-)
       superficial foreign body of eyelid and periocular area (S00.25-)

    H02.811 **Retained foreign body in** right upper **eyelid**

    H02.812 **Retained foreign body in** right lower **eyelid**

    H02.813 **Retained foreign body in** right eye, **unspecified eyelid**

    H02.814 **Retained foreign body in** left upper **eyelid**

    H02.815 **Retained foreign body in** left lower **eyelid**

    H02.816 **Retained foreign body in** left eye, **unspecified eyelid**

    H02.819 **Retained foreign body in unspecified eye, unspecified eyelid**

  √6ᵗʰ H02.82 **Cysts of eyelid**
    Sebaceous cyst of eyelid

    H02.821 **Cysts of** right upper **eyelid**

    H02.822 **Cysts of** right lower **eyelid**

    H02.823 **Cysts of** right eye, **unspecified eyelid**

    H02.824 **Cysts of** left upper **eyelid**

    H02.825 **Cysts of** left lower **eyelid**

    H02.826 **Cysts of** left eye, **unspecified eyelid**

    H02.829 **Cysts of unspecified eye, unspecified eyelid**

  √6ᵗʰ H02.83 **Dermatochalasis of eyelid**

    H02.831 **Dermatochalasis of** right upper **eyelid**

    H02.832 **Dermatochalasis of** right lower **eyelid**

    H02.833 **Dermatochalasis of** right eye, **unspecified eyelid**

    H02.834 **Dermatochalasis of** left upper **eyelid**

    H02.835 **Dermatochalasis of** left lower **eyelid**

    H02.836 **Dermatochalasis of** left eye, **unspecified eyelid**

    H02.839 **Dermatochalasis of unspecified eye, unspecified eyelid**

  √6ᵗʰ H02.84 **Edema of eyelid**
    Hyperemia of eyelid

    H02.841 **Edema of** right upper **eyelid**

    H02.842 **Edema of** right lower **eyelid**

    H02.843 **Edema of** right eye, **unspecified eyelid**

    H02.844 **Edema of** left upper **eyelid**

    H02.845 **Edema of** left lower **eyelid**

    H02.846 **Edema of** left eye, **unspecified eyelid**

    H02.849 **Edema of unspecified eye, unspecified eyelid**

  √6ᵗʰ H02.85 **Elephantiasis of eyelid**

    H02.851 **Elephantiasis of** right upper **eyelid**

    H02.852 **Elephantiasis of** right lower **eyelid**

    H02.853 **Elephantiasis of** right eye, **unspecified eyelid**

    H02.854 **Elephantiasis of** left upper **eyelid**

    H02.855 **Elephantiasis of** left lower **eyelid**

    H02.856 **Elephantiasis of** left eye, **unspecified eyelid**

    H02.859 **Elephantiasis of unspecified eye, unspecified eyelid**

  √6ᵗʰ H02.86 **Hypertrichosis of eyelid**

    H02.861 **Hypertrichosis of** right upper **eyelid**

    H02.862 **Hypertrichosis of** right lower **eyelid**

    H02.863 **Hypertrichosis of** right eye, **unspecified eyelid**

    H02.864 **Hypertrichosis of** left upper **eyelid**

    H02.865 **Hypertrichosis of** left lower **eyelid**

    H02.866 **Hypertrichosis of** left eye, **unspecified eyelid**

    H02.869 **Hypertrichosis of unspecified eye, unspecified eyelid**

  √6ᵗʰ H02.87 **Vascular anomalies of eyelid**

    H02.871 **Vascular anomalies of** right upper **eyelid**

    H02.872 **Vascular anomalies of** right lower **eyelid**

    H02.873 **Vascular anomalies of** right eye, **unspecified eyelid**

    H02.874 **Vascular anomalies of** left upper **eyelid**

    H02.875 **Vascular anomalies of** left lower **eyelid**

    H02.876 **Vascular anomalies of** left eye, **unspecified eyelid**

    H02.879 **Vascular anomalies of unspecified eye, unspecified eyelid**

   H02.89 **Other specified disorders of eyelid**
    Hemorrhage of eyelid

  H02.9 **Unspecified disorder of eyelid**
    Disorder of eyelid NOS

√4ᵗʰ **H04 Disorders of lacrimal system**
    EXCLUDES 1 *congenital malformations of lacrimal system (Q10.4-Q10.6)*

  √5ᵗʰ H04.0 **Dacryoadenitis**

   √6ᵗʰ H04.00 **Unspecified dacryoadenitis**

    H04.001 **Unspecified dacryoadenitis,** right **lacrimal gland**

EXCLUDES 1 Not coded here   *EXCLUDES 2* Not included here   N Newborn Age: 0   P Pediatric Age: 0-17   M Maternity Age: 12-55   A Adult Age: 15-124

544   ICD-10-CM 2016

H04.002 **Unspecified dacryoadenitis, left lacrimal gland**

H04.003 **Unspecified dacryoadenitis, bilateral lacrimal glands**

H04.009 **Unspecified dacryoadenitis, unspecified lacrimal gland**

✓6th **H04.01 Acute dacryoadenitis**

H04.011 **Acute dacryoadenitis, right lacrimal gland**

H04.012 **Acute dacryoadenitis, left lacrimal gland**

H04.013 **Acute dacryoadenitis, bilateral lacrimal glands**

H04.019 **Acute dacryoadenitis, unspecified lacrimal gland**

✓6th **H04.02 Chronic dacryoadenitis**

H04.021 **Chronic dacryoadenitis, right lacrimal gland**

H04.022 **Chronic dacryoadenitis, left lacrimal gland**

H04.023 **Chronic dacryoadenitis, bilateral lacrimal glands**

H04.029 **Chronic dacryoadenitis, unspecified lacrimal gland**

✓6th **H04.03 Chronic enlargement of lacrimal gland**

H04.031 **Chronic enlargement of right lacrimal gland**

H04.032 **Chronic enlargement of left lacrimal gland**

H04.033 **Chronic enlargement of bilateral lacrimal glands**

H04.039 **Chronic enlargement of unspecified lacrimal gland**

✓5th **H04.1 Other disorders of lacrimal gland**

✓6th **H04.11 Dacryops**

H04.111 **Dacryops of right lacrimal gland**

H04.112 **Dacryops of left lacrimal gland**

H04.113 **Dacryops of bilateral lacrimal glands**

H04.119 **Dacryops of unspecified lacrimal gland**

✓6th **H04.12 Dry eye syndrome**
Tear film insufficiency, NOS

H04.121 **Dry eye syndrome of right lacrimal gland**

H04.122 **Dry eye syndrome of left lacrimal gland**

H04.123 **Dry eye syndrome of bilateral lacrimal glands**

H04.129 **Dry eye syndrome of unspecified lacrimal gland**

✓6th **H04.13 Lacrimal cyst**
Lacrimal cystic degeneration

H04.131 **Lacrimal cyst, right lacrimal gland**

H04.132 **Lacrimal cyst, left lacrimal gland**

H04.133 **Lacrimal cyst, bilateral lacrimal glands**

H04.139 **Lacrimal cyst, unspecified lacrimal gland**

✓6th **H04.14 Primary lacrimal gland atrophy**

H04.141 **Primary lacrimal gland atrophy, right lacrimal gland**

H04.142 **Primary lacrimal gland atrophy, left lacrimal gland**

H04.143 **Primary lacrimal gland atrophy, bilateral lacrimal glands**

H04.149 **Primary lacrimal gland atrophy, unspecified lacrimal gland**

✓6th **H04.15 Secondary lacrimal gland atrophy**

H04.151 **Secondary lacrimal gland atrophy, right lacrimal gland**

H04.152 **Secondary lacrimal gland atrophy, left lacrimal gland**

H04.153 **Secondary lacrimal gland atrophy, bilateral lacrimal glands**

H04.159 **Secondary lacrimal gland atrophy, unspecified lacrimal gland**

✓6th **H04.16 Lacrimal gland dislocation**

H04.161 **Lacrimal gland dislocation, right lacrimal gland**

H04.162 **Lacrimal gland dislocation, left lacrimal gland**

H04.163 **Lacrimal gland dislocation, bilateral lacrimal glands**

H04.169 **Lacrimal gland dislocation, unspecified lacrimal gland**

H04.19 **Other specified disorders of lacrimal gland**

✓5th **H04.2 Epiphora**

✓6th **H04.20 Unspecified epiphora**

H04.201 **Unspecified epiphora, right lacrimal gland**

H04.202 **Unspecified epiphora, left lacrimal gland**

H04.203 **Unspecified epiphora, bilateral lacrimal glands**

H04.209 **Unspecified epiphora, unspecified lacrimal gland**

✓6th **H04.21 Epiphora due to excess lacrimation**

H04.211 **Epiphora due to excess lacrimation, right lacrimal gland**

H04.212 **Epiphora due to excess lacrimation, left lacrimal gland**

H04.213 **Epiphora due to excess lacrimation, bilateral lacrimal glands**

H04.219 **Epiphora due to excess lacrimation, unspecified lacrimal gland**

✓6th **H04.22 Epiphora due to insufficient drainage**

H04.221 **Epiphora due to insufficient drainage, right lacrimal gland**

H04.222 **Epiphora due to insufficient drainage, left lacrimal gland**

H04.223 **Epiphora due to insufficient drainage, bilateral lacrimal glands**

H04.229 **Epiphora due to insufficient drainage, unspecified lacrimal gland**

✓5th **H04.3 Acute and unspecified inflammation of lacrimal passages**
EXCLUDES 1 *neonatal dacryocystitis (P39.1)*

✓6th **H04.30 Unspecified dacryocystitis**

H04.301 **Unspecified dacryocystitis of right lacrimal passage**

H04.302 **Unspecified dacryocystitis of left lacrimal passage**

H04.303 **Unspecified dacryocystitis of bilateral lacrimal passages**

H04.309 **Unspecified dacryocystitis of unspecified lacrimal passage**

✓6th **H04.31 Phlegmonous dacryocystitis**

H04.311 **Phlegmonous dacryocystitis of right lacrimal passage**

H04.312 **Phlegmonous dacryocystitis of left lacrimal passage**

H04.313 **Phlegmonous dacryocystitis of bilateral lacrimal passages**

H04.319 **Phlegmonous dacryocystitis of unspecified lacrimal passage**

✓6th **H04.32 Acute dacryocystitis**
Acute dacryopericystitis

H04.321 **Acute dacryocystitis of right lacrimal passage**

H04.322 **Acute dacryocystitis of left lacrimal passage**

H04.323 **Acute dacryocystitis of bilateral lacrimal passages**

H04.329 **Acute dacryocystitis of unspecified lacrimal passage**

✓6th **H04.33 Acute lacrimal canaliculitis**

H04.331 **Acute lacrimal canaliculitis of right lacrimal passage**

H04.332 **Acute lacrimal canaliculitis of left lacrimal passage**

H04.333 **Acute lacrimal canaliculitis of bilateral lacrimal passages**

H04.339 **Acute lacrimal canaliculitis of unspecified lacrimal passage**

✓5th **H04.4 Chronic inflammation of lacrimal passages**

✓6th **H04.41 Chronic dacryocystitis**

H04.411 **Chronic dacryocystitis of right lacrimal passage**

H04.412 **Chronic dacryocystitis of left lacrimal passage**

H04.413 **Chronic dacryocystitis of bilateral lacrimal passages**

H04.419 **Chronic dacryocystitis of unspecified lacrimal passage**

✓ Additional Character Required ✓x7th Placeholder Alert Unspecified Dx Other Specified Dx Manifestation ▶◀ Revised Text ● New Code ▲ Revised Code Title

Chapter 7. Diseases of the Eye and Adnexa

√6ᵗʰ H04.42 Chronic lacrimal canaliculitis
- **H04.421** Chronic lacrimal canaliculitis of right lacrimal passage
- **H04.422** Chronic lacrimal canaliculitis of left lacrimal passage
- **H04.423** Chronic lacrimal canaliculitis of bilateral lacrimal passages
- **H04.429** Chronic lacrimal canaliculitis of unspecified lacrimal passage

√6ᵗʰ H04.43 Chronic lacrimal mucocele
- **H04.431** Chronic lacrimal mucocele of right lacrimal passage
- **H04.432** Chronic lacrimal mucocele of left lacrimal passage
- **H04.433** Chronic lacrimal mucocele of bilateral lacrimal passages
- **H04.439** Chronic lacrimal mucocele of unspecified lacrimal passage

√5ᵗʰ H04.5 Stenosis and insufficiency of lacrimal passages
√6ᵗʰ H04.51 Dacryolith
- **H04.511** Dacryolith of right lacrimal passage
- **H04.512** Dacryolith of left lacrimal passage
- **H04.513** Dacryolith of bilateral lacrimal passages
- **H04.519** Dacryolith of unspecified lacrimal passage

√6ᵗʰ H04.52 Eversion of lacrimal punctum
- **H04.521** Eversion of right lacrimal punctum
- **H04.522** Eversion of left lacrimal punctum
- **H04.523** Eversion of bilateral lacrimal punctum
- **H04.529** Eversion of unspecified lacrimal punctum

√6ᵗʰ H04.53 Neonatal obstruction of nasolacrimal duct
> EXCLUDES 1   congenital stenosis and stricture of lacrimal duct (Q10.5)
- **H04.531** Neonatal obstruction of right nasolacrimal duct   N
- **H04.532** Neonatal obstruction of left nasolacrimal duct   N
- **H04.533** Neonatal obstruction of bilateral nasolacrimal duct   N
- **H04.539** Neonatal obstruction of unspecified nasolacrimal duct   N

√6ᵗʰ H04.54 Stenosis of lacrimal canaliculi
- **H04.541** Stenosis of right lacrimal canaliculi
- **H04.542** Stenosis of left lacrimal canaliculi
- **H04.543** Stenosis of bilateral lacrimal canaliculi
- **H04.549** Stenosis of unspecified lacrimal canaliculi

√6ᵗʰ H04.55 Acquired stenosis of nasolacrimal duct
- **H04.551** Acquired stenosis of right nasolacrimal duct
- **H04.552** Acquired stenosis of left nasolacrimal duct
- **H04.553** Acquired stenosis of bilateral nasolacrimal duct
- **H04.559** Acquired stenosis of unspecified nasolacrimal duct

√6ᵗʰ H04.56 Stenosis of lacrimal punctum
- **H04.561** Stenosis of right lacrimal punctum
- **H04.562** Stenosis of left lacrimal punctum
- **H04.563** Stenosis of bilateral lacrimal punctum
- **H04.569** Stenosis of unspecified lacrimal punctum

√6ᵗʰ H04.57 Stenosis of lacrimal sac
- **H04.571** Stenosis of right lacrimal sac
- **H04.572** Stenosis of left lacrimal sac
- **H04.573** Stenosis of bilateral lacrimal sac
- **H04.579** Stenosis of unspecified lacrimal sac

√5ᵗʰ H04.6 Other changes of lacrimal passages
√6ᵗʰ H04.61 Lacrimal fistula
- **H04.611** Lacrimal fistula right lacrimal passage
- **H04.612** Lacrimal fistula left lacrimal passage
- **H04.613** Lacrimal fistula bilateral lacrimal passages
- **H04.619** Lacrimal fistula unspecified lacrimal passage
- **H04.69** Other changes of lacrimal passages

√5ᵗʰ H04.8 Other disorders of lacrimal system
√6ᵗʰ H04.81 Granuloma of lacrimal passages
- **H04.811** Granuloma of right lacrimal passage

- **H04.812** Granuloma of left lacrimal passage
- **H04.813** Granuloma of bilateral lacrimal passages
- **H04.819** Granuloma of unspecified lacrimal passage
- **H04.89** Other disorders of lacrimal system
- **H04.9** Disorder of lacrimal system, unspecified

√4ᵗʰ H05 Disorders of orbit
> EXCLUDES 1   congenital malformation of orbit (Q10.7)

√5ᵗʰ H05.0 Acute inflammation of orbit
- **H05.00** Unspecified acute inflammation of orbit
√6ᵗʰ H05.01 Cellulitis of orbit
   Abscess of orbit
- **H05.011** Cellulitis of right orbit
- **H05.012** Cellulitis of left orbit
- **H05.013** Cellulitis of bilateral orbits
- **H05.019** Cellulitis of unspecified orbit

√6ᵗʰ H05.02 Osteomyelitis of orbit
- **H05.021** Osteomyelitis of right orbit
- **H05.022** Osteomyelitis of left orbit
- **H05.023** Osteomyelitis of bilateral orbits
- **H05.029** Osteomyelitis of unspecified orbit

√6ᵗʰ H05.03 Periostitis of orbit
- **H05.031** Periostitis of right orbit
- **H05.032** Periostitis of left orbit
- **H05.033** Periostitis of bilateral orbits
- **H05.039** Periostitis of unspecified orbit

√6ᵗʰ H05.04 Tenonitis of orbit
- **H05.041** Tenonitis of right orbit
- **H05.042** Tenonitis of left orbit
- **H05.043** Tenonitis of bilateral orbits
- **H05.049** Tenonitis of unspecified orbit

√5ᵗʰ H05.1 Chronic inflammatory disorders of orbit
- **H05.10** Unspecified chronic inflammatory disorders of orbit
√6ᵗʰ H05.11 Granuloma of orbit
   Pseudotumor (inflammatory) of orbit
- **H05.111** Granuloma of right orbit
- **H05.112** Granuloma of left orbit
- **H05.113** Granuloma of bilateral orbits
- **H05.119** Granuloma of unspecified orbit

√6ᵗʰ H05.12 Orbital myositis
- **H05.121** Orbital myositis, right orbit
- **H05.122** Orbital myositis, left orbit
- **H05.123** Orbital myositis, bilateral
- **H05.129** Orbital myositis, unspecified orbit

√5ᵗʰ H05.2 Exophthalmic conditions
- **H05.20** Unspecified exophthalmos
√6ᵗʰ H05.21 Displacement (lateral) of globe
- **H05.211** Displacement (lateral) of globe, right eye
- **H05.212** Displacement (lateral) of globe, left eye
- **H05.213** Displacement (lateral) of globe, bilateral
- **H05.219** Displacement (lateral) of globe, unspecified eye

√6ᵗʰ H05.22 Edema of orbit
   Orbital congestion
- **H05.221** Edema of right orbit
- **H05.222** Edema of left orbit
- **H05.223** Edema of bilateral orbit
- **H05.229** Edema of unspecified orbit

√6ᵗʰ H05.23 Hemorrhage of orbit
- **H05.231** Hemorrhage of right orbit
- **H05.232** Hemorrhage of left orbit
- **H05.233** Hemorrhage of bilateral orbit
- **H05.239** Hemorrhage of unspecified orbit

√6ᵗʰ H05.24 Constant exophthalmos
- **H05.241** Constant exophthalmos, right eye
- **H05.242** Constant exophthalmos, left eye
- **H05.243** Constant exophthalmos, bilateral
- **H05.249** Constant exophthalmos, unspecified eye

√6ᵗʰ H05.25 Intermittent exophthalmos
- **H05.251** Intermittent exophthalmos, right eye
- **H05.252** Intermittent exophthalmos, left eye

EXCLUDES 1 Not coded here   **EXCLUDES 2** Not included here   N Newborn Age: 0   P Pediatric Age: 0-17   M Maternity Age: 12-55   A Adult Age: 15-124

H05.253   **Intermittent exophthalmos**, bilateral

H05.259   **Intermittent exophthalmos, unspecified eye**

✓6ᵗʰ   **H05.26**   Pulsating **exophthalmos**

H05.261   **Pulsating exophthalmos**, right **eye**

H05.262   **Pulsating exophthalmos**, left **eye**

H05.263   **Pulsating exophthalmos**, bilateral

H05.269   **Pulsating exophthalmos, unspecified eye**

✓5ᵗʰ   **H05.3**   **Deformity of orbit**

> EXCLUDES 1   *congenital deformity of orbit (Q10.7)*
> *hypertelorism (Q75.2)*

H05.30   **Unspecified deformity of orbit**

✓6ᵗʰ   **H05.31**   Atrophy **of orbit**

H05.311   **Atrophy of** right **orbit**

H05.312   **Atrophy of** left **orbit**

H05.313   **Atrophy of** bilateral **orbit**

H05.319   **Atrophy of unspecified orbit**

✓6ᵗʰ   **H05.32**   Deformity of orbit due to bone disease

> Code also associated bone disease

H05.321   **Deformity of** right **orbit due to bone disease**

H05.322   **Deformity of** left **orbit due to bone disease**

H05.323   **Deformity of** bilateral **orbits due to bone disease**

H05.329   **Deformity of unspecified orbit due to bone disease**

✓6ᵗʰ   **H05.33**   Deformity of orbit due to trauma or surgery

H05.331   **Deformity of** right **orbit due to trauma or surgery**

H05.332   **Deformity of** left **orbit due to trauma or surgery**

H05.333   **Deformity of** bilateral **orbits due to trauma or surgery**

H05.339   **Deformity of unspecified orbit due to trauma or surgery**

✓6ᵗʰ   **H05.34**   Enlargement **of orbit**

H05.341   **Enlargement of** right **orbit**

H05.342   **Enlargement of** left **orbit**

H05.343   **Enlargement of** bilateral **orbits**

H05.349   **Enlargement of unspecified orbit**

✓6ᵗʰ   **H05.35**   Exostosis **of orbit**

H05.351   **Exostosis of** right **orbit**

H05.352   **Exostosis of** left **orbit**

H05.353   **Exostosis of** bilateral **orbits**

H05.359   **Exostosis of unspecified orbit**

✓5ᵗʰ   **H05.4**   Enophthalmos

✓6ᵗʰ   **H05.40**   Unspecified **enophthalmos**

H05.401   **Unspecified enophthalmos**, right **eye**

H05.402   **Unspecified enophthalmos**, left **eye**

H05.403   **Unspecified enophthalmos**, bilateral

H05.409   **Unspecified enophthalmos, unspecified eye**

✓6ᵗʰ   **H05.41**   Enophthalmos due to atrophy of orbital tissue

H05.411   **Enophthalmos due to atrophy of orbital tissue**, right **eye**

H05.412   **Enophthalmos due to atrophy of orbital tissue**, left **eye**

H05.413   **Enophthalmos due to atrophy of orbital tissue**, bilateral

H05.419   **Enophthalmos due to atrophy of orbital tissue, unspecified eye**

✓6ᵗʰ   **H05.42**   Enophthalmos due to trauma or surgery

H05.421   **Enophthalmos due to trauma or surgery**, right **eye**

H05.422   **Enophthalmos due to trauma or surgery**, left **eye**

H05.423   **Enophthalmos due to trauma or surgery**, bilateral

H05.429   **Enophthalmos due to trauma or surgery, unspecified eye**

✓5ᵗʰ   **H05.5**   **Retained (old) foreign body following penetrating wound of orbit**

> Retrobulbar foreign body
> Use additional code to identify the type of retained foreign body (Z18.-)
> > EXCLUDES 1   *current penetrating wound of orbit (S05.4-)*
> > EXCLUDES 2   *retained foreign body of eyelid (H02.81-)*
> > *retained intraocular foreign body (H44.6-, H44.7-)*

H05.50   **Retained (old) foreign body following penetrating wound of unspecified orbit**

H05.51   **Retained (old) foreign body following penetrating wound of** right **orbit**

H05.52   **Retained (old) foreign body following penetrating wound of** left **orbit**

H05.53   **Retained (old) foreign body following penetrating wound of** bilateral **orbits**

✓5ᵗʰ   **H05.8**   **Other disorders of orbit**

✓6ᵗʰ   **H05.81**   Cyst **of orbit**

> Encephalocele of orbit

H05.811   **Cyst of** right **orbit**

H05.812   **Cyst of** left **orbit**

H05.813   **Cyst of** bilateral **orbits**

H05.819   **Cyst of unspecified orbit**

✓6ᵗʰ   **H05.82**   Myopathy of extraocular muscles

H05.821   **Myopathy of extraocular muscles**, right **orbit**

H05.822   **Myopathy of extraocular muscles**, left **orbit**

H05.823   **Myopathy of extraocular muscles**, bilateral

H05.829   **Myopathy of extraocular muscles, unspecified orbit**

H05.89   **Other disorders of orbit**

H05.9   **Unspecified disorder of orbit**

Disorders of conjunctiva (H10-H11)

✓4ᵗʰ   **H10**   **Conjunctivitis**

> EXCLUDES 1   *keratoconjunctivitis (H16.2-)*

✓5ᵗʰ   **H10.0**   Mucopurulent **conjunctivitis**

✓6ᵗʰ   **H10.01**   **Acute follicular conjunctivitis**

H10.011   **Acute follicular conjunctivitis**, right **eye**

H10.012   **Acute follicular conjunctivitis**, left **eye**

H10.013   **Acute follicular conjunctivitis**, bilateral

H10.019   **Acute follicular conjunctivitis, unspecified eye**

✓6ᵗʰ   **H10.02**   **Other mucopurulent conjunctivitis**

H10.021   **Other mucopurulent conjunctivitis, right eye**

H10.022   **Other mucopurulent conjunctivitis, left eye**

H10.023   **Other mucopurulent conjunctivitis, bilateral**

H10.029   **Other mucopurulent conjunctivitis, unspecified eye**

✓5ᵗʰ   **H10.1**   Acute atopic **conjunctivitis**

> Acute papillary conjunctivitis

H10.10   **Acute atopic conjunctivitis, unspecified eye**

H10.11   **Acute atopic conjunctivitis**, right **eye**

H10.12   **Acute atopic conjunctivitis**, left **eye**

H10.13   **Acute atopic conjunctivitis**, bilateral

✓5ᵗʰ   **H10.2**   Other acute **conjunctivitis**

✓6ᵗʰ   **H10.21**   Acute toxic **conjunctivitis**

> Acute chemical conjunctivitis
> Code first (T51-T65) to identify chemical and intent
> > EXCLUDES 1   *burn and corrosion of eye and adnexa (T26.-)*

H10.211   **Acute toxic conjunctivitis**, right **eye**

H10.212   **Acute toxic conjunctivitis**, left **eye**

H10.213   **Acute toxic conjunctivitis**, bilateral

H10.219   **Acute toxic conjunctivitis, unspecified eye**

✓6ᵗʰ   **H10.22**   Pseudomembranous **conjunctivitis**

H10.221   **Pseudomembranous conjunctivitis**, right **eye**

H10.222   **Pseudomembranous conjunctivitis**, left **eye**

✓ Additional Character Required   ✓x7ᵗʰ Placeholder Alert   Unspecified Dx   Other Specified Dx   Manifestation   ▶◀ Revised Text   ● New Code   ▲ Revised Code Title

H10.223　Pseudomembranous conjunctivitis, bilateral

H10.229　Pseudomembranous conjunctivitis, unspecified eye

✓6ᵗʰ **H10.23　Serous conjunctivitis, except viral**
　　EXCLUDES 1　viral conjunctivitis (B30.-)

H10.231　Serous conjunctivitis, except viral, right eye

H10.232　Serous conjunctivitis, except viral, left eye

H10.233　Serous conjunctivitis, except viral, bilateral

H10.239　Serous conjunctivitis, except viral, unspecified eye

✓5ᵗʰ **H10.3　Unspecified acute conjunctivitis**
　　EXCLUDES 1　ophthalmia neonatorum NOS (P39.1)

H10.30　Unspecified acute conjunctivitis, unspecified eye

H10.31　Unspecified acute conjunctivitis, right eye

H10.32　Unspecified acute conjunctivitis, left eye

H10.33　Unspecified acute conjunctivitis, bilateral

✓5ᵗʰ **H10.4　Chronic conjunctivitis**

✓6ᵗʰ **H10.40　Unspecified chronic conjunctivitis**

H10.401　Unspecified chronic conjunctivitis, right eye

H10.402　Unspecified chronic conjunctivitis, left eye

H10.403　Unspecified chronic conjunctivitis, bilateral

H10.409　Unspecified chronic conjunctivitis, unspecified eye

✓6ᵗʰ **H10.41　Chronic giant papillary conjunctivitis**

H10.411　Chronic giant papillary conjunctivitis, right eye

H10.412　Chronic giant papillary conjunctivitis, left eye

H10.413　Chronic giant papillary conjunctivitis, bilateral

H10.419　Chronic giant papillary conjunctivitis, unspecified eye

✓6ᵗʰ **H10.42　Simple chronic conjunctivitis**

H10.421　Simple chronic conjunctivitis, right eye

H10.422　Simple chronic conjunctivitis, left eye

H10.423　Simple chronic conjunctivitis, bilateral

H10.429　Simple chronic conjunctivitis, unspecified eye

✓6ᵗʰ **H10.43　Chronic follicular conjunctivitis**

H10.431　Chronic follicular conjunctivitis, right eye

H10.432　Chronic follicular conjunctivitis, left eye

H10.433　Chronic follicular conjunctivitis, bilateral

H10.439　Chronic follicular conjunctivitis, unspecified eye

H10.44　Vernal conjunctivitis
　　EXCLUDES 1　vernal keratoconjunctivitis with limbar and corneal involvement (H16.26-)

H10.45　Other chronic allergic conjunctivitis

✓5ᵗʰ **H10.5　Blepharoconjunctivitis**

✓6ᵗʰ **H10.50　Unspecified blepharoconjunctivitis**

H10.501　Unspecified blepharoconjunctivitis, right eye

H10.502　Unspecified blepharoconjunctivitis, left eye

H10.503　Unspecified blepharoconjunctivitis, bilateral

H10.509　Unspecified blepharoconjunctivitis, unspecified eye

✓6ᵗʰ **H10.51　Ligneous conjunctivitis**

H10.511　Ligneous conjunctivitis, right eye

H10.512　Ligneous conjunctivitis, left eye

H10.513　Ligneous conjunctivitis, bilateral

H10.519　Ligneous conjunctivitis, unspecified eye

✓6ᵗʰ **H10.52　Angular blepharoconjunctivitis**

H10.521　Angular blepharoconjunctivitis, right eye

H10.522　Angular blepharoconjunctivitis, left eye

H10.523　Angular blepharoconjunctivitis, bilateral

H10.529　Angular blepharoconjunctivitis, unspecified eye

✓6ᵗʰ **H10.53　Contact blepharoconjunctivitis**

H10.531　Contact blepharoconjunctivitis, right eye

H10.532　Contact blepharoconjunctivitis, left eye

H10.533　Contact blepharoconjunctivitis, bilateral

H10.539　Contact blepharoconjunctivitis, unspecified eye

✓5ᵗʰ **H10.8　Other conjunctivitis**

✓6ᵗʰ **H10.81　Pingueculitis**
　　EXCLUDES 1　pinguecula (H11.15-)

H10.811　Pingueculitis, right eye

H10.812　Pingueculitis, left eye

H10.813　Pingueculitis, bilateral

H10.819　Pingueculitis, unspecified eye

H10.89　Other conjunctivitis

H10.9　Unspecified conjunctivitis

✓4ᵗʰ **H11　Other disorders of conjunctiva**
　　EXCLUDES 1　keratoconjunctivitis (H16.2-)

✓5ᵗʰ **H11.0　Pterygium of eye**
　　EXCLUDES 1　pseudopterygium (H11.81-)

✓6ᵗʰ **H11.00　Unspecified pterygium**

H11.001　Unspecified pterygium of right eye

H11.002　Unspecified pterygium of left eye

H11.003　Unspecified pterygium of eye, bilateral

H11.009　Unspecified pterygium of unspecified eye

✓6ᵗʰ **H11.01　Amyloid pterygium**

H11.011　Amyloid pterygium of right eye

H11.012　Amyloid pterygium of left eye

H11.013　Amyloid pterygium of eye, bilateral

H11.019　Amyloid pterygium of unspecified eye

✓6ᵗʰ **H11.02　Central pterygium of eye**

H11.021　Central pterygium of right eye

H11.022　Central pterygium of left eye

H11.023　Central pterygium of eye, bilateral

H11.029　Central pterygium of unspecified eye

✓6ᵗʰ **H11.03　Double pterygium of eye**

H11.031　Double pterygium of right eye

H11.032　Double pterygium of left eye

H11.033　Double pterygium of eye, bilateral

H11.039　Double pterygium of unspecified eye

✓6ᵗʰ **H11.04　Peripheral pterygium of eye, stationary**

H11.041　Peripheral pterygium, stationary, right eye

H11.042　Peripheral pterygium, stationary, left eye

H11.043　Peripheral pterygium, stationary, bilateral

H11.049　Peripheral pterygium, stationary, unspecified eye

✓6ᵗʰ **H11.05　Peripheral pterygium of eye, progressive**

H11.051　Peripheral pterygium, progressive, right eye

H11.052　Peripheral pterygium, progressive, left eye

H11.053　Peripheral pterygium, progressive, bilateral

H11.059　Peripheral pterygium, progressive, unspecified eye

✓6ᵗʰ **H11.06　Recurrent pterygium of eye**

H11.061　Recurrent pterygium of right eye

H11.062　Recurrent pterygium of left eye

H11.063　Recurrent pterygium of eye, bilateral

H11.069　Recurrent pterygium of unspecified eye

✓5ᵗʰ **H11.1　Conjunctival degenerations and deposits**
　　EXCLUDES 2　pseudopterygium (H11.81)

H11.10　Unspecified conjunctival degenerations

✓6ᵗʰ **H11.11　Conjunctival deposits**

H11.111　Conjunctival deposits, right eye

H11.112　Conjunctival deposits, left eye

H11.113　Conjunctival deposits, bilateral

H11.119　Conjunctival deposits, unspecified eye

✓6ᵗʰ **H11.12　Conjunctival concretions**

H11.121　Conjunctival concretions, right eye

H11.122　Conjunctival concretions, left eye

H11.123　Conjunctival concretions, bilateral

EXCLUDES 1 Not coded here　　*EXCLUDES 2* Not included here　　N Newborn Age: 0　　P Pediatric Age: 0-17　　M Maternity Age: 12-55　　A Adult Age: 15-124

548　　ICD-10-CM 2016

H11.129   **Conjunctival concretions, unspecified eye**

☑6ᵗʰ **H11.13**   **Conjunctival** pigmentations
Conjunctival argyrosis [argyria]

H11.131   **Conjunctival pigmentations, right eye**

H11.132   **Conjunctival pigmentations, left eye**

H11.133   **Conjunctival pigmentations, bilateral**

H11.139   **Conjunctival pigmentations, unspecified eye**

☑6ᵗʰ **H11.14**   **Conjunctival xerosis, unspecified**
EXCLUDES 1   xerosis of conjunctiva due to vitamin A deficiency (E50.0, E50.1)

H11.141   **Conjunctival xerosis, unspecified, right eye**

H11.142   **Conjunctival xerosis , unspecified, left eye**

H11.143   **Conjunctival xerosis, unspecified, bilateral**

H11.149   **Conjunctival xerosis, unspecified, unspecified eye**

☑6ᵗʰ **H11.15**   Pinguecula
EXCLUDES 1   pingueculitis (H10.81-)

H11.151   **Pinguecula, right eye**

H11.152   **Pinguecula, left eye**

H11.153   **Pinguecula, bilateral**

H11.159   **Pinguecula, unspecified eye**

☑5ᵗʰ **H11.2**   **Conjunctival scars**

☑6ᵗʰ **H11.21**   **Conjunctival** adhesions and strands (localized)

H11.211   **Conjunctival adhesions and strands (localized), right eye**

H11.212   **Conjunctival adhesions and strands (localized), left eye**

H11.213   **Conjunctival adhesions and strands (localized), bilateral**

H11.219   **Conjunctival adhesions and strands (localized), unspecified eye**

☑6ᵗʰ **H11.22**   **Conjunctival** granuloma

H11.221   **Conjunctival granuloma, right eye**

H11.222   **Conjunctival granuloma, left eye**

H11.223   **Conjunctival granuloma, bilateral**

H11.229   **Conjunctival granuloma, unspecified**

☑6ᵗʰ **H11.23**   Symblepharon

H11.231   **Symblepharon, right eye**

H11.232   **Symblepharon, left eye**

H11.233   **Symblepharon, bilateral**

H11.239   **Symblepharon, unspecified eye**

☑6ᵗʰ **H11.24**   Scarring of conjunctiva

H11.241   **Scarring of conjunctiva, right eye**

H11.242   **Scarring of conjunctiva, left eye**

H11.243   **Scarring of conjunctiva, bilateral**

H11.249   **Scarring of conjunctiva, unspecified eye**

☑5ᵗʰ **H11.3**   **Conjunctival hemorrhage**
Subconjunctival hemorrhage

H11.30   **Conjunctival hemorrhage, unspecified eye**

H11.31   **Conjunctival hemorrhage, right eye**

H11.32   **Conjunctival hemorrhage, left eye**

H11.33   **Conjunctival hemorrhage, bilateral**

☑5ᵗʰ **H11.4**   **Other conjunctival vascular disorders and cysts**

☑6ᵗʰ **H11.41**   **Vascular abnormalities** of conjunctiva
Conjunctival aneurysm

H11.411   **Vascular abnormalities of conjunctiva, right eye**

H11.412   **Vascular abnormalities of conjunctiva, left eye**

H11.413   **Vascular abnormalities of conjunctiva, bilateral**

H11.419   **Vascular abnormalities of conjunctiva, unspecified eye**

☑6ᵗʰ **H11.42**   **Conjunctival** edema

H11.421   **Conjunctival edema, right eye**

H11.422   **Conjunctival edema, left eye**

H11.423   **Conjunctival edema, bilateral**

H11.429   **Conjunctival edema, unspecified eye**

☑6ᵗʰ **H11.43**   **Conjunctival** hyperemia

H11.431   **Conjunctival hyperemia, right eye**

H11.432   **Conjunctival hyperemia, left eye**

H11.433   **Conjunctival hyperemia, bilateral**

H11.439   **Conjunctival hyperemia, unspecified eye**

☑6ᵗʰ **H11.44**   **Conjunctival** cysts

H11.441   **Conjunctival cysts, right eye**

H11.442   **Conjunctival cysts, left eye**

H11.443   **Conjunctival cysts, bilateral**

H11.449   **Conjunctival cysts, unspecified eye**

☑5ᵗʰ **H11.8**   **Other specified disorders of conjunctiva**

☑6ᵗʰ **H11.81**   **Pseudopterygium of conjunctiva**

H11.811   **Pseudopterygium of conjunctiva, right eye**

H11.812   **Pseudopterygium of conjunctiva, left eye**

H11.813   **Pseudopterygium of conjunctiva, bilateral**

H11.819   **Pseudopterygium of conjunctiva, unspecified eye**

☑6ᵗʰ **H11.82**   **Conjunctivochalasis**

H11.821   **Conjunctivochalasis, right eye**

H11.822   **Conjunctivochalasis, left eye**

H11.823   **Conjunctivochalasis, bilateral**

H11.829   **Conjunctivochalasis, unspecified eye**

H11.89   **Other specified disorders of conjunctiva**

H11.9   **Unspecified disorder of conjunctiva**

Disorders of sclera, cornea, iris and ciliary body (H15-H22)

☑4ᵗʰ **H15**   **Disorders of sclera**

☑5ᵗʰ **H15.0**   **Scleritis**

☑6ᵗʰ **H15.00**   Unspecified scleritis

H15.001   **Unspecified scleritis, right eye**

H15.002   **Unspecified scleritis, left eye**

H15.003   **Unspecified scleritis, bilateral**

H15.009   **Unspecified scleritis, unspecified eye**

☑6ᵗʰ **H15.01**   Anterior scleritis

H15.011   **Anterior scleritis, right eye**

H15.012   **Anterior scleritis, left eye**

H15.013   **Anterior scleritis, bilateral**

H15.019   **Anterior scleritis, unspecified eye**

☑6ᵗʰ **H15.02**   Brawny scleritis

H15.021   **Brawny scleritis, right eye**

H15.022   **Brawny scleritis, left eye**

H15.023   **Brawny scleritis, bilateral**

H15.029   **Brawny scleritis, unspecified eye**

☑6ᵗʰ **H15.03**   Posterior scleritis
Sclerotenonitis

H15.031   **Posterior scleritis, right eye**

H15.032   **Posterior scleritis, left eye**

H15.033   **Posterior scleritis, bilateral**

H15.039   **Posterior scleritis, unspecified eye**

☑6ᵗʰ **H15.04**   Scleritis with corneal involvement

H15.041   **Scleritis with corneal involvement, right eye**

H15.042   **Scleritis with corneal involvement, left eye**

H15.043   **Scleritis with corneal involvement, bilateral**

H15.049   **Scleritis with corneal involvement, unspecified eye**

☑6ᵗʰ **H15.05**   Scleromalacia perforans

H15.051   **Scleromalacia perforans, right eye**

H15.052   **Scleromalacia perforans, left eye**

H15.053   **Scleromalacia perforans, bilateral**

H15.059   **Scleromalacia perforans, unspecified eye**

☑6ᵗʰ **H15.09**   Other scleritis
Scleral abscess

H15.091   **Other scleritis, right eye**

H15.092   **Other scleritis, left eye**

H15.093   **Other scleritis, bilateral**

H15.099   **Other scleritis, unspecified eye**

☑5ᵗʰ **H15.1**   **Episcleritis**

☑6ᵗʰ **H15.10**   Unspecified episcleritis

H15.101   **Unspecified episcleritis, right eye**

H15.102   **Unspecified episcleritis, left eye**

H15.103   **Unspecified episcleritis, bilateral**

H15.109   **Unspecified episcleritis, unspecified eye**

☑ Additional Character Required   ☑ₓ7ᵗʰ Placeholder Alert   Unspecified Dx   Other Specified Dx   Manifestation   ▶◀ Revised Text   ● New Code   ▲ Revised Code Title

√6th H15.11 Episcleritis periodica fugax
   H15.111 Episcleritis periodica fugax, **right eye**
   H15.112 Episcleritis periodica fugax, **left eye**
   H15.113 Episcleritis periodica fugax, **bilateral**
   H15.119 **Episcleritis periodica fugax, unspecified eye**

√6th H15.12 Nodular episcleritis
   H15.121 Nodular episcleritis, **right eye**
   H15.122 Nodular episcleritis, **left eye**
   H15.123 Nodular episcleritis, **bilateral**
   H15.129 **Nodular episcleritis, unspecified eye**

√5th H15.8 Other disorders of sclera
   EXCLUDES 2 blue sclera (Q13.5)
             degenerative myopia (H44.2-)

√6th H15.81 Equatorial staphyloma
   H15.811 Equatorial staphyloma, **right eye**
   H15.812 Equatorial staphyloma, **left eye**
   H15.813 Equatorial staphyloma, **bilateral**
   H15.819 **Equatorial staphyloma, unspecified eye**

√6th H15.82 Localized anterior staphyloma
   H15.821 Localized anterior staphyloma, **right eye**
   H15.822 Localized anterior staphyloma, **left eye**
   H15.823 Localized anterior staphyloma, **bilateral**
   H15.829 **Localized anterior staphyloma, unspecified eye**

√6th H15.83 Staphyloma posticum
   H15.831 Staphyloma posticum, **right eye**
   H15.832 Staphyloma posticum, **left eye**
   H15.833 Staphyloma posticum, **bilateral**
   H15.839 **Staphyloma posticum, unspecified eye**

√6th H15.84 Scleral ectasia
   H15.841 Scleral ectasia, **right eye**
   H15.842 Scleral ectasia, **left eye**
   H15.843 Scleral ectasia, **bilateral**
   H15.849 **Scleral ectasia, unspecified eye**

√6th H15.85 Ring staphyloma
   H15.851 Ring staphyloma, **right eye**
   H15.852 Ring staphyloma, **left eye**
   H15.853 Ring staphyloma, **bilateral**
   H15.859 **Ring staphyloma, unspecified eye**

   H15.89 **Other disorders of sclera**

   H15.9 **Unspecified disorder of sclera**

√4th H16 Keratitis

√5th H16.0 Corneal ulcer

√6th H16.00 Unspecified corneal ulcer
   H16.001 **Unspecified corneal ulcer, right eye**
   H16.002 **Unspecified corneal ulcer, left eye**
   H16.003 **Unspecified corneal ulcer, bilateral**
   H16.009 **Unspecified corneal ulcer, unspecified eye**

√6th H16.01 Central corneal ulcer
   H16.011 Central corneal ulcer, **right eye**
   H16.012 Central corneal ulcer, **left eye**
   H16.013 Central corneal ulcer, **bilateral**
   H16.019 **Central corneal ulcer, unspecified eye**

√6th H16.02 Ring corneal ulcer
   H16.021 Ring corneal ulcer, **right eye**
   H16.022 Ring corneal ulcer, **left eye**
   H16.023 Ring corneal ulcer, **bilateral**
   H16.029 **Ring corneal ulcer, unspecified eye**

√6th H16.03 Corneal ulcer with hypopyon
   H16.031 Corneal ulcer with hypopyon, **right eye**
   H16.032 Corneal ulcer with hypopyon, **left eye**
   H16.033 Corneal ulcer with hypopyon, **bilateral**
   H16.039 **Corneal ulcer with hypopyon, unspecified eye**

√6th H16.04 Marginal corneal ulcer
   H16.041 Marginal corneal ulcer, **right eye**
   H16.042 Marginal corneal ulcer, **left eye**
   H16.043 Marginal corneal ulcer, **bilateral**
   H16.049 **Marginal corneal ulcer, unspecified eye**

√6th H16.05 Mooren's corneal ulcer
   H16.051 Mooren's corneal ulcer, **right eye**
   H16.052 Mooren's corneal ulcer, **left eye**
   H16.053 Mooren's corneal ulcer, **bilateral**
   H16.059 **Mooren's corneal ulcer, unspecified eye**

√6th H16.06 Mycotic corneal ulcer
   H16.061 Mycotic corneal ulcer, **right eye**
   H16.062 Mycotic corneal ulcer, **left eye**
   H16.063 Mycotic corneal ulcer, **bilateral**
   H16.069 **Mycotic corneal ulcer, unspecified eye**

√6th H16.07 Perforated corneal ulcer
   H16.071 Perforated corneal ulcer, **right eye**
   H16.072 Perforated corneal ulcer, **left eye**
   H16.073 Perforated corneal ulcer, **bilateral**
   H16.079 **Perforated corneal ulcer, unspecified eye**

√5th H16.1 Other and unspecified superficial keratitis without conjunctivitis

√6th H16.10 Unspecified superficial keratitis
   H16.101 **Unspecified superficial keratitis, right eye**
   H16.102 **Unspecified superficial keratitis, left eye**
   H16.103 **Unspecified superficial keratitis, bilateral**
   H16.109 **Unspecified superficial keratitis, unspecified eye**

√6th H16.11 Macular keratitis
   Areolar keratitis
   Nummular keratitis
   Stellate keratitis
   Striate keratitis
   H16.111 Macular keratitis, **right eye**
   H16.112 Macular keratitis, **left eye**
   H16.113 Macular keratitis, **bilateral**
   H16.119 **Macular keratitis, unspecified eye**

√6th H16.12 Filamentary keratitis
   H16.121 Filamentary keratitis, **right eye**
   H16.122 Filamentary keratitis, **left eye**
   H16.123 Filamentary keratitis, **bilateral**
   H16.129 **Filamentary keratitis, unspecified eye**

√6th H16.13 Photokeratitis
   Snow blindness
   Welders keratitis
   H16.131 Photokeratitis, **right eye**
   H16.132 Photokeratitis, **left eye**
   H16.133 Photokeratitis, **bilateral**
   H16.139 **Photokeratitis, unspecified eye**

√6th H16.14 Punctate keratitis
   H16.141 Punctate keratitis, **right eye**
   H16.142 Punctate keratitis, **left eye**
   H16.143 Punctate keratitis, **bilateral**
   H16.149 **Punctate keratitis, unspecified eye**

√5th H16.2 Keratoconjunctivitis

√6th H16.20 Unspecified keratoconjunctivitis
   Superficial keratitis with conjunctivitis NOS
   H16.201 **Unspecified keratoconjunctivitis, right eye**
   H16.202 **Unspecified keratoconjunctivitis, left eye**
   H16.203 **Unspecified keratoconjunctivitis, bilateral**
   H16.209 **Unspecified keratoconjunctivitis, unspecified eye**

√6th H16.21 Exposure keratoconjunctivitis
   H16.211 Exposure keratoconjunctivitis, **right eye**
   H16.212 Exposure keratoconjunctivitis, **left eye**
   H16.213 Exposure keratoconjunctivitis, **bilateral**
   H16.219 **Exposure keratoconjunctivitis, unspecified eye**

√6th H16.22 Keratoconjunctivitis sicca, not specified as Sjögren's
   EXCLUDES 1 Sjögren's syndrome (M35.01)
   H16.221 **Keratoconjunctivitis sicca, not specified as Sjögren's, right eye**
   H16.222 **Keratoconjunctivitis sicca, not specified as Sjögren's, left eye**
   H16.223 **Keratoconjunctivitis sicca, not specified as Sjögren's, bilateral**
   H16.229 **Keratoconjunctivitis sicca, not specified as Sjögren's, unspecified eye**

EXCLUDES 1 Not coded here   EXCLUDES 2 Not included here   N Newborn Age: 0   P Pediatric Age: 0-17   M Maternity Age: 12-55   A Adult Age: 15-124

550   ICD-10-CM 2016

✓6th **H16.23** Neurotrophic **keratoconjunctivitis**
- **H16.231** Neurotrophic keratoconjunctivitis, right eye
- **H16.232** Neurotrophic keratoconjunctivitis, left eye
- **H16.233** Neurotrophic keratoconjunctivitis, bilateral
- **H16.239** Neurotrophic keratoconjunctivitis, unspecified eye

✓6th **H16.24** Ophthalmia nodosa
- **H16.241** Ophthalmia nodosa, right eye
- **H16.242** Ophthalmia nodosa, left eye
- **H16.243** Ophthalmia nodosa, bilateral
- **H16.249** Ophthalmia nodosa, unspecified eye

✓6th **H16.25** Phlyctenular **keratoconjunctivitis**
- **H16.251** Phlyctenular keratoconjunctivitis, right eye
- **H16.252** Phlyctenular keratoconjunctivitis, left eye
- **H16.253** Phlyctenular keratoconjunctivitis, bilateral
- **H16.259** Phlyctenular keratoconjunctivitis, unspecified eye

✓6th **H16.26** Vernal **keratoconjunctivitis, with** limbar and corneal involvement
> EXCLUDES 1   *vernal conjunctivitis without limbar and corneal involvement (H10.44)*
- **H16.261** Vernal keratoconjunctivitis, with limbar and corneal involvement, right eye
- **H16.262** Vernal keratoconjunctivitis, with limbar and corneal involvement, left eye
- **H16.263** Vernal keratoconjunctivitis, with limbar and corneal involvement, bilateral
- **H16.269** Vernal keratoconjunctivitis, with limbar and corneal involvement, unspecified eye

✓6th **H16.29** Other **keratoconjunctivitis**
- **H16.291** Other keratoconjunctivitis, right eye
- **H16.292** Other keratoconjunctivitis, left eye
- **H16.293** Other keratoconjunctivitis, bilateral
- **H16.299** Other keratoconjunctivitis, unspecified eye

✓5th **H16.3** Interstitial and deep keratitis

✓6th **H16.30** Unspecified **interstitial keratitis**
- **H16.301** Unspecified interstitial keratitis, right eye
- **H16.302** Unspecified interstitial keratitis, left eye
- **H16.303** Unspecified interstitial keratitis, bilateral
- **H16.309** Unspecified interstitial keratitis, unspecified eye

✓6th **H16.31** Corneal **abscess**
- **H16.311** Corneal abscess, right eye
- **H16.312** Corneal abscess, left eye
- **H16.313** Corneal abscess, bilateral
- **H16.319** Corneal abscess, unspecified eye

✓6th **H16.32** Diffuse **interstitial keratitis**
> Cogan's syndrome
- **H16.321** Diffuse interstitial keratitis, right eye
- **H16.322** Diffuse interstitial keratitis, left eye
- **H16.323** Diffuse interstitial keratitis, bilateral
- **H16.329** Diffuse interstitial keratitis, unspecified eye

✓6th **H16.33** Sclerosing **keratitis**
- **H16.331** Sclerosing keratitis, right eye
- **H16.332** Sclerosing keratitis, left eye
- **H16.333** Sclerosing keratitis, bilateral
- **H16.339** Sclerosing keratitis, unspecified eye

✓6th **H16.39** Other **interstitial and deep keratitis**
- **H16.391** Other interstitial and deep keratitis, right eye
- **H16.392** Other interstitial and deep keratitis, left eye
- **H16.393** Other interstitial and deep keratitis, bilateral
- **H16.399** Other interstitial and deep keratitis, unspecified eye

✓5th **H16.4** Corneal neovascularization

✓6th **H16.40** Unspecified corneal neovascularization
- **H16.401** Unspecified corneal neovascularization, right eye
- **H16.402** Unspecified corneal neovascularization, left eye
- **H16.403** Unspecified corneal neovascularization, bilateral
- **H16.409** Unspecified corneal neovascularization, unspecified eye

✓6th **H16.41** Ghost vessels (corneal)
- **H16.411** Ghost vessels (corneal), right eye
- **H16.412** Ghost vessels (corneal), left eye
- **H16.413** Ghost vessels (corneal), bilateral
- **H16.419** Ghost vessels (corneal), unspecified eye

✓6th **H16.42** Pannus (corneal)
- **H16.421** Pannus (corneal), right eye
- **H16.422** Pannus (corneal), left eye
- **H16.423** Pannus (corneal), bilateral
- **H16.429** Pannus (corneal), unspecified eye

✓6th **H16.43** Localized vascularization of cornea
- **H16.431** Localized vascularization of cornea, right eye
- **H16.432** Localized vascularization of cornea, left eye
- **H16.433** Localized vascularization of cornea, bilateral
- **H16.439** Localized vascularization of cornea, unspecified eye

✓6th **H16.44** Deep vascularization of cornea
- **H16.441** Deep vascularization of cornea, right eye
- **H16.442** Deep vascularization of cornea, left eye
- **H16.443** Deep vascularization of cornea, bilateral
- **H16.449** Deep vascularization of cornea, unspecified eye

H16.8 Other keratitis

H16.9 Unspecified keratitis

✓4th **H17** Corneal scars and opacities

✓5th **H17.0** Adherent leukoma
- **H17.00** Adherent leukoma, unspecified eye
- **H17.01** Adherent leukoma, right eye
- **H17.02** Adherent leukoma, left eye
- **H17.03** Adherent leukoma, bilateral

✓5th **H17.1** Central corneal opacity
- **H17.10** Central corneal opacity, unspecified eye
- **H17.11** Central corneal opacity, right eye
- **H17.12** Central corneal opacity, left eye
- **H17.13** Central corneal opacity, bilateral

✓5th **H17.8** Other corneal scars and opacities

✓6th **H17.81** Minor opacity of cornea
> Corneal nebula
- **H17.811** Minor opacity of cornea, right eye
- **H17.812** Minor opacity of cornea, left eye
- **H17.813** Minor opacity of cornea, bilateral
- **H17.819** Minor opacity of cornea, unspecified eye

✓6th **H17.82** Peripheral opacity of cornea
- **H17.821** Peripheral opacity of cornea, right eye
- **H17.822** Peripheral opacity of cornea, left eye
- **H17.823** Peripheral opacity of cornea, bilateral
- **H17.829** Peripheral opacity of cornea, unspecified eye

H17.89 Other corneal scars and opacities

H17.9 Unspecified corneal scar and opacity

✓4th **H18** Other disorders of cornea

✓5th **H18.0** Corneal pigmentations and deposits

✓6th **H18.00** Unspecified corneal deposit
- **H18.001** Unspecified corneal deposit, right eye
- **H18.002** Unspecified corneal deposit, left eye
- **H18.003** Unspecified corneal deposit, bilateral
- **H18.009** Unspecified corneal deposit, unspecified eye

☑ Additional Character Required   ✓x7th Placeholder Alert   Unspecified Dx   Other Specified Dx   Manifestation   ▶◀ Revised Text   ● New Code   ▲ Revised Code Title

ICD-10-CM 2016   551

Chapter 7. Diseases of the Eye and Adnexa

√6ᵗʰ **H18.01** **Anterior** corneal pigmentations
Staehli's line
  H18.011 **Anterior corneal pigmentations, right** eye
  H18.012 **Anterior corneal pigmentations, left** eye
  H18.013 **Anterior corneal pigmentations, bilateral**
  H18.019 **Anterior corneal pigmentations, unspecified eye**

√6ᵗʰ **H18.02** **Argentous** corneal deposits
  H18.021 **Argentous corneal deposits, right** eye
  H18.022 **Argentous corneal deposits, left** eye
  H18.023 **Argentous corneal deposits, bilateral**
  H18.029 **Argentous corneal deposits, unspecified eye**

√6ᵗʰ **H18.03** **Corneal deposits in** metabolic disorders
Code also associated metabolic disorder
  H18.031 **Corneal deposits in metabolic disorders, right eye**
  H18.032 **Corneal deposits in metabolic disorders, left eye**
  H18.033 **Corneal deposits in metabolic disorders, bilateral**
  H18.039 **Corneal deposits in metabolic disorders, unspecified eye**

√6ᵗʰ **H18.04** **Kayser-Fleischer ring**
Code also associated Wilson's disease (E83.01)
  H18.041 **Kayser-Fleischer ring, right** eye
  H18.042 **Kayser-Fleischer ring, left** eye
  H18.043 **Kayser-Fleischer ring, bilateral**
  H18.049 **Kayser-Fleischer ring, unspecified eye**

√6ᵗʰ **H18.05** **Posterior** corneal pigmentations
Krukenberg's spindle
  H18.051 **Posterior corneal pigmentations, right** eye
  H18.052 **Posterior corneal pigmentations, left** eye
  H18.053 **Posterior corneal pigmentations, bilateral**
  H18.059 **Posterior corneal pigmentations, unspecified eye**

√6ᵗʰ **H18.06** **Stromal** corneal pigmentations
Hematocornea
  H18.061 **Stromal corneal pigmentations, right** eye
  H18.062 **Stromal corneal pigmentations, left** eye
  H18.063 **Stromal corneal pigmentations, bilateral**
  H18.069 **Stromal corneal pigmentations, unspecified eye**

√5ᵗʰ **H18.1** **Bullous keratopathy**
  H18.10 **Bullous keratopathy, unspecified eye**
  H18.11 **Bullous keratopathy, right** eye
  H18.12 **Bullous keratopathy, left** eye
  H18.13 **Bullous keratopathy, bilateral**

√5ᵗʰ **H18.2** **Other and unspecified corneal edema**
  H18.20 **Unspecified corneal edema**

√6ᵗʰ **H18.21** **Corneal edema** secondary to contact lens
  EXCLUDES 2 other corneal disorders due to contact lens (H18.82-)
  H18.211 **Corneal edema secondary to contact lens, right eye**
  H18.212 **Corneal edema secondary to contact lens, left eye**
  H18.213 **Corneal edema secondary to contact lens, bilateral**
  H18.219 **Corneal edema secondary to contact lens, unspecified eye**

√6ᵗʰ **H18.22** **Idiopathic** corneal edema
  H18.221 **Idiopathic corneal edema, right** eye
  H18.222 **Idiopathic corneal edema, left** eye
  H18.223 **Idiopathic corneal edema, bilateral**
  H18.229 **Idiopathic corneal edema, unspecified eye**

√6ᵗʰ **H18.23** **Secondary** corneal edema
  H18.231 **Secondary corneal edema, right** eye
  H18.232 **Secondary corneal edema, left** eye
  H18.233 **Secondary corneal edema, bilateral**
  H18.239 **Secondary corneal edema, unspecified eye**

√5ᵗʰ **H18.3** **Changes of corneal membranes**
  H18.30 **Unspecified corneal membrane change**

√6ᵗʰ **H18.31** **Folds and rupture in** Bowman's membrane
  H18.311 **Folds and rupture in Bowman's membrane, right** eye
  H18.312 **Folds and rupture in Bowman's membrane, left** eye
  H18.313 **Folds and rupture in Bowman's membrane, bilateral**
  H18.319 **Folds and rupture in Bowman's membrane, unspecified eye**

√6ᵗʰ **H18.32** **Folds in** Descemet's membrane
  H18.321 **Folds in Descemet's membrane, right** eye
  H18.322 **Folds in Descemet's membrane, left** eye
  H18.323 **Folds in Descemet's membrane, bilateral**
  H18.329 **Folds in Descemet's membrane, unspecified eye**

√6ᵗʰ **H18.33** **Rupture in** Descemet's membrane
  H18.331 **Rupture in Descemet's membrane, right** eye
  H18.332 **Rupture in Descemet's membrane, left** eye
  H18.333 **Rupture in Descemet's membrane, bilateral**
  H18.339 **Rupture in Descemet's membrane, unspecified eye**

√5ᵗʰ **H18.4** **Corneal degeneration**
  EXCLUDES 1 Mooren's ulcer (H16.0-)
  recurrent erosion of cornea (H18.83-)
  H18.40 **Unspecified corneal degeneration**

√6ᵗʰ **H18.41** **Arcus senilis**
Senile corneal changes
  H18.411 **Arcus senilis, right** eye
  H18.412 **Arcus senilis, left** eye
  H18.413 **Arcus senilis, bilateral**
  H18.419 **Arcus senilis, unspecified eye**

√6ᵗʰ **H18.42** **Band** keratopathy
  H18.421 **Band keratopathy, right** eye
  H18.422 **Band keratopathy, left** eye
  H18.423 **Band keratopathy, bilateral**
  H18.429 **Band keratopathy, unspecified eye**

  H18.43 **Other calcerous corneal degeneration**

√6ᵗʰ **H18.44** **Keratomalacia**
  EXCLUDES 1 keratomalacia due to vitamin A deficiency (E50.4)
  H18.441 **Keratomalacia, right** eye
  H18.442 **Keratomalacia, left** eye
  H18.443 **Keratomalacia, bilateral**
  H18.449 **Keratomalacia, unspecified eye**

√6ᵗʰ **H18.45** **Nodular** corneal degeneration
  H18.451 **Nodular corneal degeneration, right** eye
  H18.452 **Nodular corneal degeneration, left** eye
  H18.453 **Nodular corneal degeneration, bilateral**
  H18.459 **Nodular corneal degeneration, unspecified eye**

√6ᵗʰ **H18.46** **Peripheral** corneal degeneration
  H18.461 **Peripheral corneal degeneration, right** eye
  H18.462 **Peripheral corneal degeneration, left** eye
  H18.463 **Peripheral corneal degeneration, bilateral**
  H18.469 **Peripheral corneal degeneration, unspecified eye**

  H18.49 **Other corneal degeneration**

√5ᵗʰ **H18.5** **Hereditary corneal dystrophies**
  H18.50 **Unspecified hereditary corneal dystrophies**
  H18.51 **Endothelial** corneal dystrophy
Fuchs' dystrophy
  H18.52 **Epithelial (juvenile) corneal dystrophy**
  H18.53 **Granular** corneal dystrophy
  H18.54 **Lattice** corneal dystrophy
  H18.55 **Macular** corneal dystrophy
  H18.59 **Other hereditary corneal dystrophies**

√5ᵗʰ **H18.6** **Keratoconus**
√6ᵗʰ **H18.60** **Keratoconus,** unspecified
  H18.601 **Keratoconus, unspecified, right** eye
  H18.602 **Keratoconus, unspecified, left** eye

EXCLUDES 1 Not coded here   EXCLUDES 2 Not included here   N Newborn Age: 0   P Pediatric Age: 0-17   M Maternity Age: 12-55   A Adult Age: 15-124

552   ICD-10-CM 2016

     H18.603   **Keratoconus, unspecified,** bilateral
     H18.609   **Keratoconus, unspecified, unspecified eye**

√6ᵗʰ **H18.61**   **Keratoconus,** stable
     H18.611   **Keratoconus, stable,** right **eye**
     H18.612   **Keratoconus, stable,** left **eye**
     H18.613   **Keratoconus, stable,** bilateral
     H18.619   **Keratoconus, stable, unspecified eye**

√6ᵗʰ **H18.62**   **Keratoconus,** unstable
     Acute hydrops
     H18.621   **Keratoconus, unstable,** right **eye**
     H18.622   **Keratoconus, unstable,** left **eye**
     H18.623   **Keratoconus, unstable,** bilateral
     H18.629   **Keratoconus, unstable, unspecified eye**

√5ᵗʰ **H18.7**   **Other and unspecified corneal deformities**
     EXCLUDES 1   *congenital malformations of cornea (Q13.3-Q13.4)*

     H18.70   **Unspecified corneal deformity**

√6ᵗʰ **H18.71**   **Corneal** ectasia
     H18.711   **Corneal ectasia,** right **eye**
     H18.712   **Corneal ectasia,** left **eye**
     H18.713   **Corneal ectasia,** bilateral
     H18.719   **Corneal ectasia, unspecified eye**

√6ᵗʰ **H18.72**   **Corneal** staphyloma
     H18.721   **Corneal staphyloma,** right **eye**
     H18.722   **Corneal staphyloma,** left **eye**
     H18.723   **Corneal staphyloma,** bilateral
     H18.729   **Corneal staphyloma, unspecified eye**

√6ᵗʰ **H18.73**   Descemetocele
     H18.731   **Descemetocele,** right **eye**
     H18.732   **Descemetocele,** left **eye**
     H18.733   **Descemetocele,** bilateral
     H18.739   **Descemetocele, unspecified eye**

√6ᵗʰ **H18.79**   Other corneal deformities
     H18.791   **Other corneal deformities,** right **eye**
     H18.792   **Other corneal deformities,** left **eye**
     H18.793   **Other corneal deformities,** bilateral
     H18.799   **Other corneal deformities, unspecified eye**

√5ᵗʰ **H18.8**   **Other specified disorders of cornea**

√6ᵗʰ **H18.81**   **Anesthesia and hypoesthesia of cornea**
     H18.811   **Anesthesia and hypoesthesia of cornea,** right **eye**
     H18.812   **Anesthesia and hypoesthesia of cornea,** left **eye**
     H18.813   **Anesthesia and hypoesthesia of cornea,** bilateral
     H18.819   **Anesthesia and hypoesthesia of cornea, unspecified eye**

√6ᵗʰ **H18.82**   **Corneal disorder due to contact lens**
     EXCLUDES 2   *corneal edema due to contact lens (H18.21-)*
     H18.821   **Corneal disorder due to contact lens,** right **eye**
     H18.822   **Corneal disorder due to contact lens,** left **eye**
     H18.823   **Corneal disorder due to contact lens,** bilateral
     H18.829   **Corneal disorder due to contact lens, unspecified eye**

√6ᵗʰ **H18.83**   **Recurrent erosion of cornea**
     H18.831   **Recurrent erosion of cornea,** right **eye**
     H18.832   **Recurrent erosion of cornea,** left **eye**
     H18.833   **Recurrent erosion of cornea,** bilateral
     H18.839   **Recurrent erosion of cornea, unspecified eye**

√6ᵗʰ **H18.89**   **Other specified disorders of cornea**
     H18.891   **Other specified disorders of cornea,** right **eye**
     H18.892   **Other specified disorders of cornea,** left **eye**
     H18.893   **Other specified disorders of cornea,** bilateral
     H18.899   **Other specified disorders of cornea, unspecified eye**

     H18.9   **Unspecified disorder of cornea**

√4ᵗʰ **H20**   **Iridocyclitis**

√5ᵗʰ **H20.0**   **Acute** and subacute **iridocyclitis**
     Acute anterior uveitis
     Acute cyclitis
     Acute iritis
     Subacute anterior uveitis
     Subacute cyclitis
     Subacute iritis
     EXCLUDES 1   *iridocyclitis, iritis, uveitis (due to) (in) diabetes mellitus (E08-E13 with .39)*
     iridocyclitis, iritis, uveitis (due to) (in) diphtheria (A36.89)
     iridocyclitis, iritis, uveitis (due to) (in) gonococcal (A54.32)
     iridocyclitis, iritis, uveitis (due to) (in) herpes (simplex) (B00.51)
     iridocyclitis, iritis, uveitis (due to) (in) herpes zoster (B02.32)
     iridocyclitis, iritis, uveitis (due to) (in) late congenital syphilis (A50.39)
     iridocyclitis, iritis, uveitis (due to) (in) late syphilis (A52.71)
     iridocyclitis, iritis, uveitis (due to) (in) sarcoidosis (D86.83)
     iridocyclitis, iritis, uveitis (due to) (in) syphilis (A51.43)
     iridocyclitis, iritis, uveitis (due to) (in) toxoplasmosis (B58.09)
     iridocyclitis, iritis, uveitis (due to) (in) tuberculosis (A18.54)

     H20.00   **Unspecified acute and subacute iridocyclitis**

√6ᵗʰ **H20.01**   Primary **iridocyclitis**
     H20.011   **Primary iridocyclitis,** right **eye**
     H20.012   **Primary iridocyclitis,** left **eye**
     H20.013   **Primary iridocyclitis,** bilateral
     H20.019   **Primary iridocyclitis, unspecified eye**

√6ᵗʰ **H20.02**   **Recurrent acute iridocyclitis**
     H20.021   **Recurrent acute iridocyclitis,** right **eye**
     H20.022   **Recurrent acute iridocyclitis,** left **eye**
     H20.023   **Recurrent acute iridocyclitis,** bilateral
     H20.029   **Recurrent acute iridocyclitis, unspecified eye**

√6ᵗʰ **H20.03**   **Secondary infectious iridocyclitis**
     H20.031   **Secondary infectious iridocyclitis,** right **eye**
     H20.032   **Secondary infectious iridocyclitis,** left **eye**
     H20.033   **Secondary infectious iridocyclitis,** bilateral
     H20.039   **Secondary infectious iridocyclitis, unspecified eye**

√6ᵗʰ **H20.04**   **Secondary noninfectious iridocyclitis**
     H20.041   **Secondary noninfectious iridocyclitis,** right **eye**
     H20.042   **Secondary noninfectious iridocyclitis,** left **eye**
     H20.043   **Secondary noninfectious iridocyclitis,** bilateral
     H20.049   **Secondary noninfectious iridocyclitis, unspecified eye**

√6ᵗʰ **H20.05**   **Hypopyon**
     H20.051   **Hypopyon,** right **eye**
     H20.052   **Hypopyon,** left **eye**
     H20.053   **Hypopyon,** bilateral
     H20.059   **Hypopyon, unspecified eye**

√5ᵗʰ **H20.1**   Chronic **iridocyclitis**
     Use additional code for any associated cataract (H26.21-)
     EXCLUDES 2   *posterior cyclitis (H30.2-)*
     H20.10   **Chronic iridocyclitis, unspecified eye**
     H20.11   **Chronic iridocyclitis,** right **eye**
     H20.12   **Chronic iridocyclitis,** left **eye**
     H20.13   **Chronic iridocyclitis,** bilateral

√5ᵗʰ **H20.2**   **Lens-induced iridocyclitis**
     H20.20   **Lens-induced iridocyclitis, unspecified eye**
     H20.21   **Lens-induced iridocyclitis,** right **eye**
     H20.22   **Lens-induced iridocyclitis,** left **eye**
     H20.23   **Lens-induced iridocyclitis,** bilateral

☑ Additional Character Required   √x7ᵗʰ Placeholder Alert   Unspecified Dx   Other Specified Dx   Manifestation   ▶◀ Revised Text   ● New Code   ▲ Revised Code Title

✓5ᵗʰ **H20.8** **Other iridocyclitis**
EXCLUDES 2 glaucomatocyclitis crises (H40.4-)
posterior cyclitis (H30.2-)
sympathetic uveitis (H44.13-)

✓6ᵗʰ **H20.81** **Fuchs' heterochromic cyclitis**
H20.811 **Fuchs' heterochromic cyclitis, right eye**
H20.812 **Fuchs' heterochromic cyclitis, left eye**
H20.813 **Fuchs' heterochromic cyclitis, bilateral**
H20.819 **Fuchs' heterochromic cyclitis, unspecified eye**

✓6ᵗʰ **H20.82** **Vogt-Koyanagi syndrome**
H20.821 **Vogt-Koyanagi syndrome, right eye**
H20.822 **Vogt-Koyanagi syndrome, left eye**
H20.823 **Vogt-Koyanagi syndrome, bilateral**
H20.829 **Vogt-Koyanagi syndrome, unspecified eye**

H20.9 **Unspecified iridocyclitis**
Uveitis NOS

✓4ᵗʰ **H21** **Other disorders of iris and ciliary body**
EXCLUDES 2 sympathetic uveitis (H44.1-)

✓5ᵗʰ **H21.0** **Hyphema**
EXCLUDES 1 traumatic hyphema (S05.1-)
H21.00 **Hyphema, unspecified eye**
H21.01 **Hyphema, right eye**
H21.02 **Hyphema, left eye**
H21.03 **Hyphema, bilateral**

✓5ᵗʰ **H21.1** **Other vascular disorders of iris and ciliary body**
Neovascularization of iris or ciliary body
Rubeosis iridis
Rubeosis of iris

✓6ᵗʰ **H21.1X** **Other vascular disorders of iris and ciliary body**
H21.1X1 **Other vascular disorders of iris and ciliary body, right eye**
H21.1X2 **Other vascular disorders of iris and ciliary body, left eye**
H21.1X3 **Other vascular disorders of iris and ciliary body, bilateral**
H21.1X9 **Other vascular disorders of iris and ciliary body, unspecified eye**

✓5ᵗʰ **H21.2** **Degeneration of iris and ciliary body**
✓6ᵗʰ **H21.21** **Degeneration of chamber angle**
H21.211 **Degeneration of chamber angle, right eye**
H21.212 **Degeneration of chamber angle, left eye**
H21.213 **Degeneration of chamber angle, bilateral**
H21.219 **Degeneration of chamber angle, unspecified eye**

✓6ᵗʰ **H21.22** **Degeneration of ciliary body**
H21.221 **Degeneration of ciliary body, right eye**
H21.222 **Degeneration of ciliary body, left eye**
H21.223 **Degeneration of ciliary body, bilateral**
H21.229 **Degeneration of ciliary body, unspecified eye**

✓6ᵗʰ **H21.23** **Degeneration of iris (pigmentary)**
Translucency of iris
H21.231 **Degeneration of iris (pigmentary), right eye**
H21.232 **Degeneration of iris (pigmentary), left eye**
H21.233 **Degeneration of iris (pigmentary), bilateral**
H21.239 **Degeneration of iris (pigmentary), unspecified eye**

✓6ᵗʰ **H21.24** **Degeneration of pupillary margin**
H21.241 **Degeneration of pupillary margin, right eye**
H21.242 **Degeneration of pupillary margin, left eye**
H21.243 **Degeneration of pupillary margin, bilateral**
H21.249 **Degeneration of pupillary margin, unspecified eye**

✓6ᵗʰ **H21.25** **Iridoschisis**
H21.251 **Iridoschisis, right eye**
H21.252 **Iridoschisis, left eye**
H21.253 **Iridoschisis, bilateral**
H21.259 **Iridoschisis, unspecified eye**

✓6ᵗʰ **H21.26** **Iris atrophy (essential) (progressive)**
H21.261 **Iris atrophy (essential) (progressive), right eye**
H21.262 **Iris atrophy (essential) (progressive), left eye**
H21.263 **Iris atrophy (essential) (progressive), bilateral**
H21.269 **Iris atrophy (essential) (progressive), unspecified eye**

✓6ᵗʰ **H21.27** **Miotic pupillary cyst**
H21.271 **Miotic pupillary cyst, right eye**
H21.272 **Miotic pupillary cyst, left eye**
H21.273 **Miotic pupillary cyst, bilateral**
H21.279 **Miotic pupillary cyst, unspecified eye**

H21.29 **Other iris atrophy**

✓5ᵗʰ **H21.3** **Cyst of iris, ciliary body and anterior chamber**
EXCLUDES 2 miotic pupillary cyst (H21.27-)

✓6ᵗʰ **H21.30** **Idiopathic cysts of iris, ciliary body or anterior chamber**
Cyst of iris, ciliary body or anterior chamber NOS
H21.301 **Idiopathic cysts of iris, ciliary body or anterior chamber, right eye**
H21.302 **Idiopathic cysts of iris, ciliary body or anterior chamber, left eye**
H21.303 **Idiopathic cysts of iris, ciliary body or anterior chamber, bilateral**
H21.309 **Idiopathic cysts of iris, ciliary body or anterior chamber, unspecified eye**

✓6ᵗʰ **H21.31** **Exudative cysts of iris or anterior chamber**
H21.311 **Exudative cysts of iris or anterior chamber, right eye**
H21.312 **Exudative cysts of iris or anterior chamber, left eye**
H21.313 **Exudative cysts of iris or anterior chamber, bilateral**
H21.319 **Exudative cysts of iris or anterior chamber, unspecified eye**

✓6ᵗʰ **H21.32** **Implantation cysts of iris, ciliary body or anterior chamber**
H21.321 **Implantation cysts of iris, ciliary body or anterior chamber, right eye**
H21.322 **Implantation cysts of iris, ciliary body or anterior chamber, left eye**
H21.323 **Implantation cysts of iris, ciliary body or anterior chamber, bilateral**
H21.329 **Implantation cysts of iris, ciliary body or anterior chamber, unspecified eye**

✓6ᵗʰ **H21.33** **Parasitic cyst of iris, ciliary body or anterior chamber**
H21.331 **Parasitic cyst of iris, ciliary body or anterior chamber, right eye**
H21.332 **Parasitic cyst of iris, ciliary body or anterior chamber, left eye**
H21.333 **Parasitic cyst of iris, ciliary body or anterior chamber, bilateral**
H21.339 **Parasitic cyst of iris, ciliary body or anterior chamber, unspecified eye**

✓6ᵗʰ **H21.34** **Primary cyst of pars plana**
H21.341 **Primary cyst of pars plana, right eye**
H21.342 **Primary cyst of pars plana, left eye**
H21.343 **Primary cyst of pars plana, bilateral**
H21.349 **Primary cyst of pars plana, unspecified eye**

✓6ᵗʰ **H21.35** **Exudative cyst of pars plana**
H21.351 **Exudative cyst of pars plana, right eye**
H21.352 **Exudative cyst of pars plana, left eye**
H21.353 **Exudative cyst of pars plana, bilateral**
H21.359 **Exudative cyst of pars plana, unspecified eye**

✓5ᵗʰ **H21.4** **Pupillary membranes**
Iris bombé   Pupillary seclusion
Pupillary occlusion
EXCLUDES 1 congenital pupillary membranes (Q13.8)
H21.40 **Pupillary membranes, unspecified eye**
H21.41 **Pupillary membranes, right eye**
H21.42 **Pupillary membranes, left eye**
H21.43 **Pupillary membranes, bilateral**

EXCLUDES 1 Not coded here   EXCLUDES 2 Not included here   N Newborn Age: 0   P Pediatric Age: 0-17   M Maternity Age: 12-55   A Adult Age: 15-124

554

ICD-10-CM 2016

✓5ᵗʰ H21.5 Other and unspecified adhesions and disruptions of iris and ciliary body
EXCLUDES 1   *corectopia (Q13.2)*

  ✓6ᵗʰ H21.50 Unspecified adhesions of iris
    Synechia (iris) NOS
    H21.501   Unspecified adhesions of iris, right eye
    H21.502   Unspecified adhesions of iris, left eye
    H21.503   Unspecified adhesions of iris, bilateral
    H21.509   Unspecified adhesions of iris and ciliary body, unspecified eye

  ✓6ᵗʰ H21.51 Anterior synechiae (iris)
    H21.511   Anterior synechiae (iris), right eye
    H21.512   Anterior synechiae (iris), left eye
    H21.513   Anterior synechiae (iris), bilateral
    H21.519   Anterior synechiae (iris), unspecified eye

  ✓6ᵗʰ H21.52 Goniosynechiae
    H21.521   Goniosynechiae, right eye
    H21.522   Goniosynechiae, left eye
    H21.523   Goniosynechiae, bilateral
    H21.529   Goniosynechiae, unspecified eye

  ✓6ᵗʰ H21.53 Iridodialysis
    H21.531   Iridodialysis, right eye
    H21.532   Iridodialysis, left eye
    H21.533   Iridodialysis, bilateral
    H21.539   Iridodialysis, unspecified eye

  ✓6ᵗʰ H21.54 Posterior synechiae (iris)
    H21.541   Posterior synechiae (iris), right eye
    H21.542   Posterior synechiae (iris), left eye
    H21.543   Posterior synechiae (iris), bilateral
    H21.549   Posterior synechiae (iris), unspecified eye

  ✓6ᵗʰ H21.55 Recession of chamber angle
    H21.551   Recession of chamber angle, right eye
    H21.552   Recession of chamber angle, left eye
    H21.553   Recession of chamber angle, bilateral
    H21.559   Recession of chamber angle, unspecified eye

  ✓6ᵗʰ H21.56 Pupillary abnormalities
    Deformed pupil
    Ectopic pupil
    Rupture of sphincter, pupil
    EXCLUDES 1   *congenital deformity of pupil (Q13.2-)*
    H21.561   Pupillary abnormality, right eye
    H21.562   Pupillary abnormality, left eye
    H21.563   Pupillary abnormality, bilateral
    H21.569   Pupillary abnormality, unspecified eye

✓5ᵗʰ H21.8 Other specified disorders of iris and ciliary body
  H21.81 Floppy iris syndrome
    Intraoperative floppy iris syndrome (IFIS)
    Use additional code for adverse effect, if applicable, to identify drug (T36-T50 with fifth or sixth character 5)
  H21.82 Plateau iris syndrome (post-iridectomy) (postprocedural)
  H21.89 Other specified disorders of iris and ciliary body

H21.9 Unspecified disorder of iris and ciliary body

H22 Disorders of iris and ciliary body in diseases classified elsewhere
Code first underlying disease, such as:
  gout (M1A.-, M10.-)
  leprosy (A30.-)
  parasitic disease (B89)

Disorders of lens (H25-H28)

✓4ᵗʰ H25 Age-related cataract
Senile cataract
EXCLUDES 2   *capsular glaucoma with pseudoexfoliation of lens (H40.1-)*

✓5ᵗʰ H25.0 Age-related incipient cataract
  ✓6ᵗʰ H25.01 Cortical age-related cataract
    H25.011   Cortical age-related cataract, right eye   A
    H25.012   Cortical age-related cataract, left eye   A
    H25.013   Cortical age-related cataract, bilateral   A
    H25.019   Cortical age-related cataract, unspecified eye   A

  ✓6ᵗʰ H25.03 Anterior subcapsular polar age-related cataract
    H25.031   Anterior subcapsular polar age-related cataract, right eye   A
    H25.032   Anterior subcapsular polar age-related cataract, left eye   A
    H25.033   Anterior subcapsular polar age-related cataract, bilateral   A
    H25.039   Anterior subcapsular polar age-related cataract, unspecified eye   A

  ✓6ᵗʰ H25.04 Posterior subcapsular polar age-related cataract
    H25.041   Posterior subcapsular polar age-related cataract, right eye   A
    H25.042   Posterior subcapsular polar age-related cataract, left eye   A
    H25.043   Posterior subcapsular polar age-related cataract, bilateral   A
    H25.049   Posterior subcapsular polar age-related cataract, unspecified eye   A

  ✓6ᵗʰ H25.09 Other age-related incipient cataract
    Coronary age-related cataract
    Punctate age-related cataract
    Water clefts
    H25.091   Other age-related incipient cataract, right eye   A
    H25.092   Other age-related incipient cataract, left eye   A
    H25.093   Other age-related incipient cataract, bilateral   A
    H25.099   Other age-related incipient cataract, unspecified eye   A

✓5ᵗʰ H25.1 Age-related nuclear cataract
Cataracta brunescens
Nuclear sclerosis cataract
  H25.10   Age-related nuclear cataract, unspecified eye   A
  H25.11   Age-related nuclear cataract, right eye   A
  H25.12   Age-related nuclear cataract, left eye   A
  H25.13   Age-related nuclear cataract, bilateral   A

✓5ᵗʰ H25.2 Age-related cataract, morgagnian type
Age-related hypermature cataract
  H25.20   Age-related cataract, morgagnian type, unspecified eye   A
  H25.21   Age-related cataract, morgagnian type, right eye   A
  H25.22   Age-related cataract, morgagnian type, left eye   A
  H25.23   Age-related cataract, morgagnian type, bilateral   A

✓5ᵗʰ H25.8 Other age-related cataract
  ✓6ᵗʰ H25.81 Combined forms of age-related cataract
    H25.811   Combined forms of age-related cataract, right eye   A
    H25.812   Combined forms of age-related cataract, left eye   A
    H25.813   Combined forms of age-related cataract, bilateral   A
    H25.819   Combined forms of age-related cataract, unspecified eye   A
  H25.89 Other age-related cataract   A

H25.9 Unspecified age-related cataract   A

✓4ᵗʰ H26 Other cataract
EXCLUDES 1   *congenital cataract (Q12.0)*

✓5ᵗʰ H26.0 Infantile and juvenile cataract
  ✓6ᵗʰ H26.00 Unspecified infantile and juvenile cataract
    H26.001   Unspecified infantile and juvenile cataract, right eye   P
    H26.002   Unspecified infantile and juvenile cataract, left eye   P
    H26.003   Unspecified infantile and juvenile cataract, bilateral   P
    H26.009   Unspecified infantile and juvenile cataract, unspecified eye   P

  ✓6ᵗʰ H26.01 Infantile and juvenile cortical, lamellar, or zonular cataract
    H26.011   Infantile and juvenile cortical, lamellar, or zonular cataract, right eye   P
    H26.012   Infantile and juvenile cortical, lamellar, or zonular cataract, left eye   P

☑ Additional Character Required   ✓x7ᵗʰ Placeholder Alert   Unspecified Dx   Other Specified Dx   Manifestation   ▶◀ Revised Text   ● New Code   ▲ Revised Code Title

Chapter 7. Diseases of the Eye and Adnexa

H26.013   Infantile and juvenile cortical, lamellar, or zonular cataract, **bilateral** ℙ

H26.019   Infantile and juvenile cortical, lamellar, or zonular cataract, **unspecified eye** ℙ

✓6ᵗʰ **H26.03**   Infantile and juvenile **nuclear** cataract

H26.031   Infantile and juvenile nuclear cataract, **right** eye ℙ

H26.032   Infantile and juvenile nuclear cataract, **left** eye ℙ

H26.033   Infantile and juvenile nuclear cataract, **bilateral** ℙ

H26.039   Infantile and juvenile nuclear cataract, **unspecified eye** ℙ

✓6ᵗʰ **H26.04**   Anterior subcapsular polar infantile and juvenile cataract

H26.041   Anterior subcapsular polar infantile and juvenile cataract, **right** eye ℙ

H26.042   Anterior subcapsular polar infantile and juvenile cataract, **left** eye ℙ

H26.043   Anterior subcapsular polar infantile and juvenile cataract, **bilateral** ℙ

H26.049   Anterior subcapsular polar infantile and juvenile cataract, **unspecified eye** ℙ

✓6ᵗʰ **H26.05**   Posterior subcapsular polar infantile and juvenile cataract

H26.051   Posterior subcapsular polar infantile and juvenile cataract, **right** eye ℙ

H26.052   Posterior subcapsular polar infantile and juvenile cataract, **left** eye ℙ

H26.053   Posterior subcapsular polar infantile and juvenile cataract, **bilateral** ℙ

H26.059   Posterior subcapsular polar infantile and juvenile cataract, **unspecified eye** ℙ

✓6ᵗʰ **H26.06**   Combined forms of infantile and juvenile cataract

H26.061   Combined forms of infantile and juvenile cataract, **right** eye ℙ

H26.062   Combined forms of infantile and juvenile cataract, **left** eye ℙ

H26.063   Combined forms of infantile and juvenile cataract, **bilateral** ℙ

H26.069   Combined forms of infantile and juvenile cataract, **unspecified eye** ℙ

H26.09   Other infantile and juvenile cataract ℙ

✓5ᵗʰ **H26.1**   Traumatic **cataract**
Use additional code (Chapter 20) to identify external cause

✓6ᵗʰ **H26.10**   Unspecified traumatic cataract

H26.101   Unspecified traumatic cataract, **right eye**

H26.102   Unspecified traumatic cataract, **left eye**

H26.103   Unspecified traumatic cataract, **bilateral**

H26.109   Unspecified traumatic cataract, **unspecified eye**

✓6ᵗʰ **H26.11**   Localized traumatic opacities

H26.111   Localized traumatic opacities, **right eye**

H26.112   Localized traumatic opacities, **left eye**

H26.113   Localized traumatic opacities, **bilateral**

H26.119   Localized traumatic opacities, **unspecified eye**

✓6ᵗʰ **H26.12**   Partially resolved traumatic cataract

H26.121   Partially resolved traumatic cataract, **right eye**

H26.122   Partially resolved traumatic cataract, **left eye**

H26.123   Partially resolved traumatic cataract, **bilateral**

H26.129   Partially resolved traumatic cataract, **unspecified eye**

✓6ᵗʰ **H26.13**   Total traumatic cataract

H26.131   Total traumatic cataract, **right eye**

H26.132   Total traumatic cataract, **left eye**

H26.133   Total traumatic cataract, **bilateral**

H26.139   Total traumatic cataract, **unspecified eye**

✓5ᵗʰ **H26.2**   Complicated **cataract**

H26.20   Unspecified complicated cataract
Cataracta complicata NOS

✓6ᵗʰ **H26.21**   Cataract **with neovascularization**
Code also associated condition, such as:
chronic iridocyclitis (H20.1-)

H26.211   Cataract with neovascularization, **right eye**

H26.212   Cataract with neovascularization, **left eye**

H26.213   Cataract with neovascularization, **bilateral**

H26.219   Cataract with neovascularization, **unspecified eye**

✓6ᵗʰ **H26.22**   Cataract **secondary to ocular disorders (degenerative) (inflammatory)**
Code also associated ocular disorder

H26.221   Cataract secondary to ocular disorders (degenerative) (inflammatory), **right eye**

H26.222   Cataract secondary to ocular disorders (degenerative) (inflammatory), **left eye**

H26.223   Cataract secondary to ocular disorders (degenerative) (inflammatory), **bilateral**

H26.229   Cataract secondary to ocular disorders (degenerative) (inflammatory), **unspecified eye**

✓6ᵗʰ **H26.23**   Glaucomatous flecks (subcapsular)
Code first underlying glaucoma (H40-H42)

H26.231   Glaucomatous flecks (subcapsular), **right eye**

H26.232   Glaucomatous flecks (subcapsular), **left eye**

H26.233   Glaucomatous flecks (subcapsular), **bilateral**

H26.239   Glaucomatous flecks (subcapsular), **unspecified eye**

✓5ᵗʰ **H26.3**   Drug-induced **cataract**
Toxic cataract
Use additional code for adverse effect, if applicable, to identify drug (T36-T50 with fifth or sixth character 5)

H26.30   Drug-induced cataract, **unspecified eye**

H26.31   Drug-induced cataract, **right eye**

H26.32   Drug-induced cataract, **left eye**

H26.33   Drug-induced cataract, **bilateral**

✓5ᵗʰ **H26.4**   Secondary **cataract**

H26.40   Unspecified secondary cataract

✓6ᵗʰ **H26.41**   Soemmering's ring

H26.411   Soemmering's ring, **right** eye

H26.412   Soemmering's ring, **left** eye

H26.413   Soemmering's ring, **bilateral**

H26.419   Soemmering's ring, **unspecified eye**

✓6ᵗʰ **H26.49**   Other secondary cataract

H26.491   Other secondary cataract, **right eye**

H26.492   Other secondary cataract, **left eye**

H26.493   Other secondary cataract, **bilateral**

H26.499   Other secondary cataract, **unspecified eye**

H26.8   Other specified **cataract**

H26.9   Unspecified **cataract**

✓4ᵗʰ **H27**   **Other disorders of lens**
EXCLUDES 1   *congenital lens malformations (Q12.-)*
mechanical complications of intraocular lens implant (T85.2)
pseudophakia (Z96.1)

✓5ᵗʰ **H27.0**   Aphakia
Acquired absence of lens
Acquired aphakia
Aphakia due to trauma
EXCLUDES 1   *cataract extraction status (Z98.4-)*
congenital absence of lens (Q12.3)
congenital aphakia (Q12.3)

H27.00   Aphakia, **unspecified eye**

H27.01   Aphakia, **right eye**

H27.02   Aphakia, **left eye**

H27.03   Aphakia, **bilateral**

✓5ᵗʰ **H27.1**   Dislocation of **lens**

H27.10   Unspecified dislocation of lens

✓6ᵗʰ **H27.11**   Subluxation of lens

H27.111   Subluxation of lens, **right eye**

H27.112   Subluxation of lens, **left eye**

H27.113   Subluxation of lens, **bilateral**

H27.119   Subluxation of lens, **unspecified eye**

EXCLUDES 1 Not coded here   **EXCLUDES 2** Not included here   Ⓝ Newborn Age: 0   ℙ Pediatric Age: 0-17   Ⓜ Maternity Age: 12-55   Ⓐ Adult Age: 15-124

556

ICD-10-CM 2016

☑6ᵗʰ **H27.12** **Anterior dislocation of lens**
    H27.121 Anterior dislocation of lens, right eye
    H27.122 Anterior dislocation of lens, left eye
    H27.123 Anterior dislocation of lens, bilateral
    H27.129 Anterior dislocation of lens, unspecified eye

☑6ᵗʰ **H27.13** **Posterior dislocation of lens**
    H27.131 Posterior dislocation of lens, right eye
    H27.132 Posterior dislocation of lens, left eye
    H27.133 Posterior dislocation of lens, bilateral
    H27.139 Posterior dislocation of lens, unspecified eye

H27.8 **Other specified disorders of lens**

H27.9 **Unspecified disorder of lens**

H28 *Cataract in diseases classified elsewhere*
    Code first underlying disease, such as:
      hypoparathyroidism (E20.-)
      myotonia (G71.1-)
      myxedema (E03.-)
      protein-calorie malnutrition (E40-E46)
    EXCLUDES 1 *cataract in diabetes mellitus (E08.36, E09.36, E10.36, E11.36, E13.36)*

Disorders of choroid and retina (H30-H36)

☑4ᵗʰ **H30** **Chorioretinal inflammation**

☑5ᵗʰ **H30.0** **Focal chorioretinal inflammation**
    Focal chorioretinitis
    Focal choroiditis
    Focal retinitis
    Focal retinochoroiditis

☑6ᵗʰ **H30.00** **Unspecified focal chorioretinal inflammation**
    Focal chorioretinitis NOS
    Focal choroiditis NOS
    Focal retinitis NOS
    Focal retinochoroiditis NOS
    H30.001 Unspecified focal chorioretinal inflammation, right eye
    H30.002 Unspecified focal chorioretinal inflammation, left eye
    H30.003 Unspecified focal chorioretinal inflammation, bilateral
    H30.009 Unspecified focal chorioretinal inflammation, unspecified eye

☑6ᵗʰ **H30.01** **Focal chorioretinal inflammation, juxtapapillary**
    H30.011 Focal chorioretinal inflammation, juxtapapillary, right eye
    H30.012 Focal chorioretinal inflammation, juxtapapillary, left eye
    H30.013 Focal chorioretinal inflammation, juxtapapillary, bilateral
    H30.019 Focal chorioretinal inflammation, juxtapapillary, unspecified eye

☑6ᵗʰ **H30.02** **Focal chorioretinal inflammation of posterior pole**
    H30.021 Focal chorioretinal inflammation of posterior pole, right eye
    H30.022 Focal chorioretinal inflammation of posterior pole, left eye
    H30.023 Focal chorioretinal inflammation of posterior pole, bilateral
    H30.029 Focal chorioretinal inflammation of posterior pole, unspecified eye

☑6ᵗʰ **H30.03** **Focal chorioretinal inflammation, peripheral**
    H30.031 Focal chorioretinal inflammation, peripheral, right eye
    H30.032 Focal chorioretinal inflammation, peripheral, left eye
    H30.033 Focal chorioretinal inflammation, peripheral, bilateral
    H30.039 Focal chorioretinal inflammation, peripheral, unspecified eye

☑6ᵗʰ **H30.04** **Focal chorioretinal inflammation, macular or paramacular**
    H30.041 Focal chorioretinal inflammation, macular or paramacular, right eye
    H30.042 Focal chorioretinal inflammation, macular or paramacular, left eye

    H30.043 Focal chorioretinal inflammation, macular or paramacular, bilateral
    H30.049 Focal chorioretinal inflammation, macular or paramacular, unspecified eye

☑5ᵗʰ **H30.1** **Disseminated chorioretinal inflammation**
    Disseminated chorioretinitis
    Disseminated choroiditis
    Disseminated retinitis
    Disseminated retinochoroiditis
    EXCLUDES 2 *exudative retinopathy (H35.02-)*

☑6ᵗʰ **H30.10** **Unspecified disseminated chorioretinal inflammation**
    Disseminated chorioretinitis NOS
    Disseminated choroiditis NOS
    Disseminated retinitis NOS
    Disseminated retinochoroiditis NOS
    H30.101 Unspecified disseminated chorioretinal inflammation, right eye
    H30.102 Unspecified disseminated chorioretinal inflammation, left eye
    H30.103 Unspecified disseminated chorioretinal inflammation, bilateral
    H30.109 Unspecified disseminated chorioretinal inflammation, unspecified eye

☑6ᵗʰ **H30.11** **Disseminated chorioretinal inflammation of posterior pole**
    H30.111 Disseminated chorioretinal inflammation of posterior pole, right eye
    H30.112 Disseminated chorioretinal inflammation of posterior pole, left eye
    H30.113 Disseminated chorioretinal inflammation of posterior pole, bilateral
    H30.119 Disseminated chorioretinal inflammation of posterior pole, unspecified eye

☑6ᵗʰ **H30.12** **Disseminated chorioretinal inflammation, peripheral**
    H30.121 Disseminated chorioretinal inflammation, peripheral right eye
    H30.122 Disseminated chorioretinal inflammation, peripheral, left eye
    H30.123 Disseminated chorioretinal inflammation, peripheral, bilateral
    H30.129 Disseminated chorioretinal inflammation, peripheral, unspecified eye

☑6ᵗʰ **H30.13** **Disseminated chorioretinal inflammation, generalized**
    H30.131 Disseminated chorioretinal inflammation, generalized, right eye
    H30.132 Disseminated chorioretinal inflammation, generalized, left eye
    H30.133 Disseminated chorioretinal inflammation, generalized, bilateral
    H30.139 Disseminated chorioretinal inflammation, generalized, unspecified eye

☑6ᵗʰ **H30.14** **Acute posterior multifocal placoid pigment epitheliopathy**
    H30.141 Acute posterior multifocal placoid pigment epitheliopathy, right eye
    H30.142 Acute posterior multifocal placoid pigment epitheliopathy, left eye
    H30.143 Acute posterior multifocal placoid pigment epitheliopathy, bilateral
    H30.149 Acute posterior multifocal placoid pigment epitheliopathy, unspecified eye

☑5ᵗʰ **H30.2** **Posterior cyclitis**
    Pars planitis
    H30.20 Posterior cyclitis, unspecified eye
    H30.21 Posterior cyclitis, right eye
    H30.22 Posterior cyclitis, left eye
    H30.23 Posterior cyclitis, bilateral

☑5ᵗʰ **H30.8** **Other chorioretinal inflammations**

☑6ᵗʰ **H30.81** **Harada's disease**
    H30.811 Harada's disease, right eye
    H30.812 Harada's disease, left eye
    H30.813 Harada's disease, bilateral
    H30.819 Harada's disease, unspecified eye

☑ Additional Character Required   ☑x7ᵗʰ Placeholder Alert   Unspecified Dx   Other Specified Dx   Manifestation   ►◄ Revised Text   ● New Code   ▲ Revised Code Title

✓6th **H30.89** Other chorioretinal inflammations
- **H30.891** Other chorioretinal inflammations, right eye
- **H30.892** Other chorioretinal inflammations, left eye
- **H30.893** Other chorioretinal inflammations, bilateral
- **H30.899** Other chorioretinal inflammations, unspecified eye

✓5th **H30.9** Unspecified chorioretinal inflammation
Chorioretinitis NOS   Retinitis NOS
Choroiditis NOS   Retinochoroiditis NOS
Neuroretinitis NOS
- **H30.90** Unspecified chorioretinal inflammation, unspecified eye
- **H30.91** Unspecified chorioretinal inflammation, right eye
- **H30.92** Unspecified chorioretinal inflammation, left eye
- **H30.93** Unspecified chorioretinal inflammation, bilateral

✓4th **H31** Other disorders of choroid

✓5th **H31.0** Chorioretinal scars
  EXCLUDES 2   postsurgical chorioretinal scars (H59.81-)

  ✓6th **H31.00** Unspecified chorioretinal scars
  - **H31.001** Unspecified chorioretinal scars, right eye
  - **H31.002** Unspecified chorioretinal scars, left eye
  - **H31.003** Unspecified chorioretinal scars, bilateral
  - **H31.009** Unspecified chorioretinal scars, unspecified eye

  ✓6th **H31.01** Macula scars of posterior pole (postinflammatory) (post-traumatic)
    EXCLUDES 1   postprocedural chorioretinal scar (H59.81-)
  - **H31.011** Macula scars of posterior pole (postinflammatory) (post-traumatic), right eye
  - **H31.012** Macula scars of posterior pole (postinflammatory) (post-traumatic), left eye
  - **H31.013** Macula scars of posterior pole (postinflammatory) (post-traumatic), bilateral
  - **H31.019** Macula scars of posterior pole (postinflammatory) (post-traumatic), unspecified eye

  ✓6th **H31.02** Solar retinopathy
  - **H31.021** Solar retinopathy, right eye
  - **H31.022** Solar retinopathy, left eye
  - **H31.023** Solar retinopathy, bilateral
  - **H31.029** Solar retinopathy, unspecified eye

  ✓6th **H31.09** Other chorioretinal scars
  - **H31.091** Other chorioretinal scars, right eye
  - **H31.092** Other chorioretinal scars, left eye
  - **H31.093** Other chorioretinal scars, bilateral
  - **H31.099** Other chorioretinal scars, unspecified eye

✓5th **H31.1** Choroidal degeneration
  EXCLUDES 2   angioid streaks of macula (H35.33)

  ✓6th **H31.10** Unspecified choroidal degeneration
  Choroidal sclerosis NOS
  - **H31.101** Choroidal degeneration, unspecified, right eye
  - **H31.102** Choroidal degeneration, unspecified, left eye
  - **H31.103** Choroidal degeneration, unspecified, bilateral
  - **H31.109** Choroidal degeneration, unspecified, unspecified eye

  ✓6th **H31.11** Age-related choroidal atrophy
  - **H31.111** Age-related choroidal atrophy, right eye Ⓐ
  - **H31.112** Age-related choroidal atrophy, left eye Ⓐ
  - **H31.113** Age-related choroidal atrophy, bilateral Ⓐ
  - **H31.119** Age-related choroidal atrophy, unspecified eye Ⓐ

  ✓6th **H31.12** Diffuse secondary atrophy of choroid
  - **H31.121** Diffuse secondary atrophy of choroid, right eye

- **H31.122** Diffuse secondary atrophy of choroid, left eye
- **H31.123** Diffuse secondary atrophy of choroid, bilateral
- **H31.129** Diffuse secondary atrophy of choroid, unspecified eye

✓5th **H31.2** Hereditary choroidal dystrophy
  EXCLUDES 2   hyperornithinemia (E72.4)
               ornithinemia (E72.4)
- **H31.20** Hereditary choroidal dystrophy, unspecified
- **H31.21** Choroideremia
- **H31.22** Choroidal dystrophy (central areolar) (generalized) (peripapillary)
- **H31.23** Gyrate atrophy, choroid
- **H31.29** Other hereditary choroidal dystrophy

✓5th **H31.3** Choroidal hemorrhage and rupture

  ✓6th **H31.30** Unspecified choroidal hemorrhage
  - **H31.301** Unspecified choroidal hemorrhage, right eye
  - **H31.302** Unspecified choroidal hemorrhage, left eye
  - **H31.303** Unspecified choroidal hemorrhage, bilateral
  - **H31.309** Unspecified choroidal hemorrhage, unspecified eye

  ✓6th **H31.31** Expulsive choroidal hemorrhage
  - **H31.311** Expulsive choroidal hemorrhage, right eye
  - **H31.312** Expulsive choroidal hemorrhage, left eye
  - **H31.313** Expulsive choroidal hemorrhage, bilateral
  - **H31.319** Expulsive choroidal hemorrhage, unspecified eye

  ✓6th **H31.32** Choroidal rupture
  - **H31.321** Choroidal rupture, right eye
  - **H31.322** Choroidal rupture, left eye
  - **H31.323** Choroidal rupture, bilateral
  - **H31.329** Choroidal rupture, unspecified eye

✓5th **H31.4** Choroidal detachment

  ✓6th **H31.40** Unspecified choroidal detachment
  - **H31.401** Unspecified choroidal detachment, right eye
  - **H31.402** Unspecified choroidal detachment, left eye
  - **H31.403** Unspecified choroidal detachment, bilateral
  - **H31.409** Unspecified choroidal detachment, unspecified eye

  ✓6th **H31.41** Hemorrhagic choroidal detachment
  - **H31.411** Hemorrhagic choroidal detachment, right eye
  - **H31.412** Hemorrhagic choroidal detachment, left eye
  - **H31.413** Hemorrhagic choroidal detachment, bilateral
  - **H31.419** Hemorrhagic choroidal detachment, unspecified eye

  ✓6th **H31.42** Serous choroidal detachment
  - **H31.421** Serous choroidal detachment, right eye
  - **H31.422** Serous choroidal detachment, left eye
  - **H31.423** Serous choroidal detachment, bilateral
  - **H31.429** Serous choroidal detachment, unspecified eye

H31.8 Other specified disorders of choroid

H31.9 Unspecified disorder of choroid

H32 *Chorioretinal disorders in diseases classified elsewhere*
Code first underlying disease, such as:
  congenital toxoplasmosis (P37.1)
  histoplasmosis (B39.-)
  leprosy (A30.-)
  EXCLUDES 1   chorioretinitis (in):
               toxoplasmosis (acquired) (B58.01)
               tuberculosis (A18.53)

☑4th H33   Retinal detachments and breaks
     EXCLUDES 1   detachment of retinal pigment epithelium (H35.72-, H35.73-)

   ☑5th H33.0   Retinal detachment with retinal break
       Rhegmatogenous retinal detachment
       EXCLUDES 1   serous retinal detachment (without retinal break) (H33.2-)

     ☑6th H33.00   Unspecified retinal detachment with retinal break
         H33.001   **Unspecified retinal detachment with retinal break, right eye**
         H33.002   **Unspecified retinal detachment with retinal break, left eye**
         H33.003   **Unspecified retinal detachment with retinal break, bilateral**
         H33.009   **Unspecified retinal detachment with retinal break, unspecified eye**

     ☑6th H33.01   Retinal detachment with single break
         H33.011   **Retinal detachment with single break, right eye**
         H33.012   **Retinal detachment with single break, left eye**
         H33.013   **Retinal detachment with single break, bilateral**
         H33.019   **Retinal detachment with single break, unspecified eye**

     ☑6th H33.02   Retinal detachment with multiple breaks
         H33.021   **Retinal detachment with multiple breaks, right eye**
         H33.022   **Retinal detachment with multiple breaks, left eye**
         H33.023   **Retinal detachment with multiple breaks, bilateral**
         H33.029   **Retinal detachment with multiple breaks, unspecified eye**

     ☑6th H33.03   Retinal detachment with giant retinal tear
         H33.031   **Retinal detachment with giant retinal tear, right eye**
         H33.032   **Retinal detachment with giant retinal tear, left eye**
         H33.033   **Retinal detachment with giant retinal tear, bilateral**
         H33.039   **Retinal detachment with giant retinal tear, unspecified eye**

     ☑6th H33.04   Retinal detachment with retinal dialysis
         H33.041   **Retinal detachment with retinal dialysis, right eye**
         H33.042   **Retinal detachment with retinal dialysis, left eye**
         H33.043   **Retinal detachment with retinal dialysis, bilateral**
         H33.049   **Retinal detachment with retinal dialysis, unspecified eye**

     ☑6th H33.05   Total retinal detachment
         H33.051   **Total retinal detachment, right eye**
         H33.052   **Total retinal detachment, left eye**
         H33.053   **Total retinal detachment, bilateral**
         H33.059   **Total retinal detachment, unspecified eye**

   ☑5th H33.1   Retinoschisis and retinal cysts
       EXCLUDES 1   congenital retinoschisis (Q14.1)
                   microcystoid degeneration of retina (H35.42-)

     ☑6th H33.10   Unspecified retinoschisis
         H33.101   **Unspecified retinoschisis, right eye**
         H33.102   **Unspecified retinoschisis, left eye**
         H33.103   **Unspecified retinoschisis, bilateral**
         H33.109   **Unspecified retinoschisis, unspecified eye**

     ☑6th H33.11   Cyst of ora serrata
         H33.111   **Cyst of ora serrata, right eye**
         H33.112   **Cyst of ora serrata, left eye**
         H33.113   **Cyst of ora serrata, bilateral**
         H33.119   **Cyst of ora serrata, unspecified eye**

     ☑6th H33.12   Parasitic cyst of retina
         H33.121   **Parasitic cyst of retina, right eye**
         H33.122   **Parasitic cyst of retina, left eye**
         H33.123   **Parasitic cyst of retina, bilateral**
         H33.129   **Parasitic cyst of retina, unspecified eye**

     ☑6th H33.19   Other retinoschisis and retinal cysts
         Pseudocyst of retina
         H33.191   **Other retinoschisis and retinal cysts, right eye**
         H33.192   **Other retinoschisis and retinal cysts, left eye**
         H33.193   **Other retinoschisis and retinal cysts, bilateral**
         H33.199   **Other retinoschisis and retinal cysts, unspecified eye**

   ☑5th H33.2   Serous retinal detachment
       Retinal detachment NOS
       Retinal detachment without retinal break
       EXCLUDES 1   central serous chorioretinopathy (H35.71-)
     H33.20   **Serous retinal detachment, unspecified eye**
     H33.21   **Serous retinal detachment, right eye**
     H33.22   **Serous retinal detachment, left eye**
     H33.23   **Serous retinal detachment, bilateral**

   ☑5th H33.3   Retinal breaks without detachment
       EXCLUDES 1   chorioretinal scars after surgery for detachment (H59.81-)
                   peripheral retinal degeneration without break (H35.4-)

     ☑6th H33.30   Unspecified retinal break
         H33.301   **Unspecified retinal break, right eye**
         H33.302   **Unspecified retinal break, left eye**
         H33.303   **Unspecified retinal break, bilateral**
         H33.309   **Unspecified retinal break, unspecified eye**

     ☑6th H33.31   Horseshoe tear of retina without detachment
         Operculum of retina without detachment
         H33.311   **Horseshoe tear of retina without detachment, right eye**
         H33.312   **Horseshoe tear of retina without detachment, left eye**
         H33.313   **Horseshoe tear of retina without detachment, bilateral**
         H33.319   **Horseshoe tear of retina without detachment, unspecified eye**

     ☑6th H33.32   Round hole of retina without detachment
         H33.321   **Round hole, right eye**
         H33.322   **Round hole, left eye**
         H33.323   **Round hole, bilateral**
         H33.329   **Round hole, unspecified eye**

     ☑6th H33.33   Multiple defects of retina without detachment
         H33.331   **Multiple defects of retina without detachment, right eye**
         H33.332   **Multiple defects of retina without detachment, left eye**
         H33.333   **Multiple defects of retina without detachment, bilateral**
         H33.339   **Multiple defects of retina without detachment, unspecified eye**

   ☑5th H33.4   Traction detachment of retina
       Proliferative vitreo-retinopathy with retinal detachment
     H33.40   **Traction detachment of retina, unspecified eye**
     H33.41   **Traction detachment of retina, right eye**
     H33.42   **Traction detachment of retina, left eye**
     H33.43   **Traction detachment of retina, bilateral**

     H33.8   **Other retinal detachments**

☑4th H34   Retinal vascular occlusions
     EXCLUDES 1   amaurosis fugax (G45.3)

   ☑5th H34.0   Transient retinal artery occlusion
     H34.00   **Transient retinal artery occlusion, unspecified eye**
     H34.01   **Transient retinal artery occlusion, right eye**
     H34.02   **Transient retinal artery occlusion, left eye**
     H34.03   **Transient retinal artery occlusion, bilateral**

   ☑5th H34.1   Central retinal artery occlusion
     H34.10   **Central retinal artery occlusion, unspecified eye**
     H34.11   **Central retinal artery occlusion, right eye**
     H34.12   **Central retinal artery occlusion, left eye**
     H34.13   **Central retinal artery occlusion, bilateral**

Chapter 7. Diseases of the Eye and Adnexa

H33–H34.13

☑ Additional Character Required   ☑7th Placeholder Alert   Unspecified Dx   Other Specified Dx   Manifestation   ▶◀ Revised Text   ● New Code   ▲ Revised Code Title

ICD-10-CM 2016   559

✓5th **H34.2** **Other retinal artery occlusions**
- ✓6th **H34.21** **Partial retinal artery occlusion**
  Hollenhorst's plaque
  Retinal microembolism
  - **H34.211** **Partial retinal artery occlusion, right eye**
  - **H34.212** **Partial retinal artery occlusion, left eye**
  - **H34.213** **Partial retinal artery occlusion, bilateral**
  - **H34.219** **Partial retinal artery occlusion, unspecified eye**
- ✓6th **H34.23** **Retinal artery branch occlusion**
  - **H34.231** **Retinal artery branch occlusion, right eye**
  - **H34.232** **Retinal artery branch occlusion, left eye**
  - **H34.233** **Retinal artery branch occlusion, bilateral**
  - **H34.239** **Retinal artery branch occlusion, unspecified eye**

✓5th **H34.8** **Other retinal vascular occlusions**
- ✓6th **H34.81** **Central retinal vein occlusion**
  - **H34.811** **Central retinal vein occlusion, right eye**
  - **H34.812** **Central retinal vein occlusion, left eye**
  - **H34.813** **Central retinal vein occlusion, bilateral**
  - **H34.819** **Central retinal vein occlusion, unspecified eye**
- ✓6th **H34.82** **Venous engorgement**
  Incipient retinal vein occlusion
  Partial retinal vein occlusion
  - **H34.821** **Venous engorgement, right eye**
  - **H34.822** **Venous engorgement, left eye**
  - **H34.823** **Venous engorgement, bilateral**
  - **H34.829** **Venous engorgement, unspecified eye**
- ✓6th **H34.83** **Tributary (branch) retinal vein occlusion**
  - **H34.831** **Tributary (branch) retinal vein occlusion, right eye**
  - **H34.832** **Tributary (branch) retinal vein occlusion, left eye**
  - **H34.833** **Tributary (branch) retinal vein occlusion, bilateral**
  - **H34.839** **Tributary (branch) retinal vein occlusion, unspecified eye**

H34.9 **Unspecified retinal vascular occlusion**

✓4th **H35** **Other retinal disorders**
EXCLUDES 2 *diabetic retinal disorders (E08.311- E08.359, E09.311- E09.359, E10.311- E10.359, E11.311- E11.359, E13.311- E13.359)*

✓5th **H35.0** **Background retinopathy and retinal vascular changes**
  Code also any associated hypertension (I10.-)
- **H35.00** **Unspecified background retinopathy**
- ✓6th **H35.01** **Changes in retinal vascular appearance**
  Retinal vascular sheathing
  - **H35.011** **Changes in retinal vascular appearance, right eye**
  - **H35.012** **Changes in retinal vascular appearance, left eye**
  - **H35.013** **Changes in retinal vascular appearance, bilateral**
  - **H35.019** **Changes in retinal vascular appearance, unspecified eye**
- ✓6th **H35.02** **Exudative retinopathy**
  Coats retinopathy
  - **H35.021** **Exudative retinopathy, right eye**
  - **H35.022** **Exudative retinopathy, left eye**
  - **H35.023** **Exudative retinopathy, bilateral**
  - **H35.029** **Exudative retinopathy, unspecified eye**
- ✓6th **H35.03** **Hypertensive retinopathy**
  - **H35.031** **Hypertensive retinopathy, right eye**
  - **H35.032** **Hypertensive retinopathy, left eye**
  - **H35.033** **Hypertensive retinopathy, bilateral**
  - **H35.039** **Hypertensive retinopathy, unspecified eye**
- ✓6th **H35.04** **Retinal micro-aneurysms, unspecified**
  - **H35.041** **Retinal micro-aneurysms, unspecified, right eye**
  - **H35.042** **Retinal micro-aneurysms, unspecified, left eye**
  - **H35.043** **Retinal micro-aneurysms, unspecified, bilateral**
  - **H35.049** **Retinal micro-aneurysms, unspecified, unspecified eye**
- ✓6th **H35.05** **Retinal neovascularization, unspecified**
  - **H35.051** **Retinal neovascularization, unspecified, right eye**
  - **H35.052** **Retinal neovascularization, unspecified, left eye**
  - **H35.053** **Retinal neovascularization, unspecified, bilateral**
  - **H35.059** **Retinal neovascularization, unspecified, unspecified eye**
- ✓6th **H35.06** **Retinal vasculitis**
  Eales diseaseRetinal perivasculitis
  - **H35.061** **Retinal vasculitis, right eye**
  - **H35.062** **Retinal vasculitis, left eye**
  - **H35.063** **Retinal vasculitis, bilateral**
  - **H35.069** **Retinal vasculitis, unspecified eye**
- ✓6th **H35.07** **Retinal telangiectasis**
  - **H35.071** **Retinal telangiectasis, right eye**
  - **H35.072** **Retinal telangiectasis, left eye**
  - **H35.073** **Retinal telangiectasis, bilateral**
  - **H35.079** **Retinal telangiectasis, unspecified eye**
- **H35.09** **Other intraretinal microvascular abnormalities**
  Retinal varices

✓5th **H35.1** **Retinopathy of prematurity**
- ✓6th **H35.10** **Retinopathy of prematurity, unspecified**
  Retinopathy of prematurity NOS
  - **H35.101** **Retinopathy of prematurity, unspecified, right eye**
  - **H35.102** **Retinopathy of prematurity, unspecified, left eye**
  - **H35.103** **Retinopathy of prematurity, unspecified, bilateral**
  - **H35.109** **Retinopathy of prematurity, unspecified, unspecified eye**
- ✓6th **H35.11** **Retinopathy of prematurity, stage 0**
  - **H35.111** **Retinopathy of prematurity, stage 0, right eye**
  - **H35.112** **Retinopathy of prematurity, stage 0, left eye**
  - **H35.113** **Retinopathy of prematurity, stage 0, bilateral**
  - **H35.119** **Retinopathy of prematurity, stage 0, unspecified eye**
- ✓6th **H35.12** **Retinopathy of prematurity, stage 1**
  - **H35.121** **Retinopathy of prematurity, stage 1, right eye**
  - **H35.122** **Retinopathy of prematurity, stage 1, left eye**
  - **H35.123** **Retinopathy of prematurity, stage 1, bilateral**
  - **H35.129** **Retinopathy of prematurity, stage 1, unspecified eye**
- ✓6th **H35.13** **Retinopathy of prematurity, stage 2**
  - **H35.131** **Retinopathy of prematurity, stage 2, right eye**
  - **H35.132** **Retinopathy of prematurity, stage 2, left eye**
  - **H35.133** **Retinopathy of prematurity, stage 2, bilateral**
  - **H35.139** **Retinopathy of prematurity, stage 2, unspecified eye**
- ✓6th **H35.14** **Retinopathy of prematurity, stage 3**
  - **H35.141** **Retinopathy of prematurity, stage 3, right eye**
  - **H35.142** **Retinopathy of prematurity, stage 3, left eye**
  - **H35.143** **Retinopathy of prematurity, stage 3, bilateral**
  - **H35.149** **Retinopathy of prematurity, stage 3, unspecified eye**
- ✓6th **H35.15** **Retinopathy of prematurity, stage 4**
  - **H35.151** **Retinopathy of prematurity, stage 4, right eye**
  - **H35.152** **Retinopathy of prematurity, stage 4, left eye**

EXCLUDES 1 Not coded here   EXCLUDES 2 Not included here   N Newborn Age: 0   P Pediatric Age: 0-17   M Maternity Age: 12-55   A Adult Age: 15-124

560   ICD-10-CM 2016

H35.153　Retinopathy of prematurity, stage 4, bilateral

H35.159　Retinopathy of prematurity, stage 4, unspecified eye

✓6ᵗʰ　**H35.16　Retinopathy of prematurity, stage 5**

H35.161　Retinopathy of prematurity, stage 5, right eye

H35.162　Retinopathy of prematurity, stage 5, left eye

H35.163　Retinopathy of prematurity, stage 5, bilateral

H35.169　Retinopathy of prematurity, stage 5, unspecified eye

✓6ᵗʰ　**H35.17　Retrolental fibroplasia**

H35.171　Retrolental fibroplasia, right eye

H35.172　Retrolental fibroplasia, left eye

H35.173　Retrolental fibroplasia, bilateral

H35.179　Retrolental fibroplasia, unspecified eye

✓5ᵗʰ　**H35.2　Other non-diabetic proliferative retinopathy**
Proliferative vitreo-retinopathy

　　EXCLUDES 1　_proliferative vitreo-retinopathy with retinal detachment (H33.4-)_

H35.20　**Other non-diabetic proliferative retinopathy, unspecified eye**

H35.21　**Other non-diabetic proliferative retinopathy, right eye**

H35.22　**Other non-diabetic proliferative retinopathy, left eye**

H35.23　**Other non-diabetic proliferative retinopathy, bilateral**

✓5ᵗʰ　**H35.3　Degeneration of macula and posterior pole**

H35.30　**Unspecified macular degeneration**　　Ⓐ
Age-related macular degeneration

H35.31　Nonexudative age-related **macular degeneration**　Ⓐ
Atrophic age-related macular degeneration

H35.32　Exudative age-related **macular degeneration**　Ⓐ

H35.33　Angioid streaks **of macula**

✓6ᵗʰ　**H35.34　Macular cyst, hole, or pseudohole**

H35.341　Macular cyst, hole, or pseudohole, **right eye**

H35.342　Macular cyst, hole, or pseudohole, **left eye**

H35.343　Macular cyst, hole, or pseudohole, **bilateral**

H35.349　**Macular cyst, hole, or pseudohole, unspecified eye**

✓6ᵗʰ　**H35.35　Cystoid macular degeneration**

　　EXCLUDES 1　_cystoid macular edema following cataract surgery (H59.03-)_

H35.351　Cystoid macular degeneration, **right eye**

H35.352　Cystoid macular degeneration, **left eye**

H35.353　Cystoid macular degeneration, **bilateral**

H35.359　**Cystoid macular degeneration, unspecified eye**

✓6ᵗʰ　**H35.36　Drusen (degenerative) of macula**

H35.361　Drusen (degenerative) of macula, **right eye**

H35.362　Drusen (degenerative) of macula, **left eye**

H35.363　Drusen (degenerative) of macula, **bilateral**

H35.369　**Drusen (degenerative) of macula, unspecified eye**

✓6ᵗʰ　**H35.37　Puckering of macula**

H35.371　Puckering of macula, **right eye**

H35.372　Puckering of macula, **left eye**

H35.373　Puckering of macula, **bilateral**

H35.379　**Puckering of macula, unspecified eye**

✓6ᵗʰ　**H35.38　Toxic maculopathy**
Code first poisoning due to drug or toxin, if applicable (T36-T65 with fifth or sixth character 1-4 or 6)
Use additional code for adverse effect, if applicable, to identify drug (T36-T50 with fifth or sixth character 5)

H35.381　Toxic maculopathy, **right eye**

H35.382　Toxic maculopathy, **left eye**

H35.383　Toxic maculopathy, **bilateral**

H35.389　**Toxic maculopathy, unspecified eye**

✓5ᵗʰ　**H35.4　Peripheral retinal degeneration**

　　EXCLUDES 1　_hereditary retinal degeneration (dystrophy) (H35.5-)_
peripheral retinal degeneration with retinal break (H33.3-)

H35.40　**Unspecified peripheral retinal degeneration**

✓6ᵗʰ　**H35.41　Lattice degeneration of retina**
Palisade degeneration of retina

H35.411　Lattice degeneration of retina, **right eye**

H35.412　Lattice degeneration of retina, **left eye**

H35.413　Lattice degeneration of retina, **bilateral**

H35.419　**Lattice degeneration of retina, unspecified eye**

✓6ᵗʰ　**H35.42　Microcystoid degeneration of retina**

H35.421　Microcystoid degeneration of retina, **right eye**

H35.422　Microcystoid degeneration of retina, **left eye**

H35.423　Microcystoid degeneration of retina, **bilateral**

H35.429　**Microcystoid degeneration of retina, unspecified eye**

✓6ᵗʰ　**H35.43　Paving stone degeneration of retina**

H35.431　Paving stone degeneration of retina, **right eye**

H35.432　Paving stone degeneration of retina, **left eye**

H35.433　Paving stone degeneration of retina, **bilateral**

H35.439　**Paving stone degeneration of retina, unspecified eye**

✓6ᵗʰ　**H35.44　Age-related reticular degeneration of retina**

H35.441　**Age-related reticular degeneration of** Ⓐ **retina, right eye**

H35.442　**Age-related reticular degeneration of** Ⓐ **retina, left eye**

H35.443　**Age-related reticular degeneration of** Ⓐ **retina, bilateral**

H35.449　**Age-related reticular degeneration of** Ⓐ **retina, unspecified eye**

✓6ᵗʰ　**H35.45　Secondary pigmentary degeneration**

H35.451　Secondary pigmentary degeneration, **right eye**

H35.452　Secondary pigmentary degeneration, **left eye**

H35.453　Secondary pigmentary degeneration, **bilateral**

H35.459　**Secondary pigmentary degeneration, unspecified eye**

✓6ᵗʰ　**H35.46　Secondary vitreoretinal degeneration**

H35.461　Secondary vitreoretinal degeneration, **right eye**

H35.462　Secondary vitreoretinal degeneration, **left eye**

H35.463　Secondary vitreoretinal degeneration, **bilateral**

H35.469　**Secondary vitreoretinal degeneration, unspecified eye**

✓5ᵗʰ　**H35.5　Hereditary retinal dystrophy**

　　EXCLUDES 1　_dystrophies primarily involving Bruch's membrane (H31.1-)_

H35.50　**Unspecified hereditary retinal dystrophy**

H35.51　**Vitreoretinal dystrophy**

H35.52　**Pigmentary retinal dystrophy**
Albipunctate retinal dystrophy
Retinitis pigmentosa
Tapetoretinal dystrophy

H35.53　**Other dystrophies primarily involving the sensory retina**
Stargardt's disease

H35.54　**Dystrophies primarily involving the retinal pigment epithelium**
Vitelliform retinal dystrophy

✓5ᵗʰ　**H35.6　Retinal hemorrhage**

H35.60　**Retinal hemorrhage, unspecified eye**

H35.61　**Retinal hemorrhage, right eye**

H35.62　**Retinal hemorrhage, left eye**

H35.63　**Retinal hemorrhage, bilateral**

☑ Additional Character Required　　✓x7ᵗʰ Placeholder Alert　　Unspecified Dx　　Other Specified Dx　　Manifestation　　►◄ Revised Text　　● New Code　　▲ Revised Code Title

✓5th **H35.7** **Separation of retinal layers**
> EXCLUDES 1   *retinal detachment (serous) (H33.2-)*
> *rhegmatogenous retinal detachment (H33.0-)*

H35.70 **Unspecified separation of retinal layers**

✓6th **H35.71** **Central serous chorioretinopathy**
- **H35.711** **Central serous chorioretinopathy, right eye**
- **H35.712** **Central serous chorioretinopathy, left eye**
- **H35.713** **Central serous chorioretinopathy, bilateral**
- **H35.719** **Central serous chorioretinopathy, unspecified eye**

✓6th **H35.72** **Serous detachment of retinal pigment epithelium**
- **H35.721** **Serous detachment of retinal pigment epithelium, right eye**
- **H35.722** **Serous detachment of retinal pigment epithelium, left eye**
- **H35.723** **Serous detachment of retinal pigment epithelium, bilateral**
- **H35.729** **Serous detachment of retinal pigment epithelium, unspecified eye**

✓6th **H35.73** **Hemorrhagic detachment of retinal pigment epithelium**
- **H35.731** **Hemorrhagic detachment of retinal pigment epithelium, right eye**
- **H35.732** **Hemorrhagic detachment of retinal pigment epithelium, left eye**
- **H35.733** **Hemorrhagic detachment of retinal pigment epithelium, bilateral**
- **H35.739** **Hemorrhagic detachment of retinal pigment epithelium, unspecified eye**

✓5th **H35.8** **Other specified retinal disorders**
> EXCLUDES 2   *retinal hemorrhage (H35.6-)*

H35.81 **Retinal edema**
> Retinal cotton wool spots

H35.82 **Retinal ischemia**

H35.89 **Other specified retinal disorders**

H35.9 **Unspecified retinal disorder**

H36 ***Retinal disorders in diseases classified elsewhere***
> *Code first underlying disease, such as:*
> *lipid storage disorders (E75.-)*
> *sickle-cell disorders (D57.-)*
> EXCLUDES 1   *arteriosclerotic retinopathy (H35.0-)*
> *diabetic retinopathy (E08.3-, E09.3-, E10.3-, E11.3-, E13.3-)*

Glaucoma (H40-H42)

✓4th **H40** **Glaucoma**
> EXCLUDES 1   *absolute glaucoma (H44.51-)*
> *congenital glaucoma (Q15.0)*
> *traumatic glaucoma due to birth injury (P15.3)*

✓5th **H40.0** **Glaucoma suspect**

✓6th **H40.00** **Preglaucoma, unspecified**
- **H40.001** **Preglaucoma, unspecified, right eye**
- **H40.002** **Preglaucoma, unspecified, left eye**
- **H40.003** **Preglaucoma, unspecified, bilateral**
- **H40.009** **Preglaucoma, unspecified, unspecified eye**

✓6th **H40.01** **Open angle with borderline findings, low risk**
> Open angle, low risk
- **H40.011** **Open angle with borderline findings, low risk, right eye**
- **H40.012** **Open angle with borderline findings, low risk, left eye**
- **H40.013** **Open angle with borderline findings, low risk, bilateral**
- **H40.019** **Open angle with borderline findings, low risk, unspecified eye**

✓6th **H40.02** **Open angle with borderline findings, high risk**
> Open angle, high risk
- **H40.021** **Open angle with borderline findings, high risk, right eye**
- **H40.022** **Open angle with borderline findings, high risk, left eye**
- **H40.023** **Open angle with borderline findings, high risk, bilateral**

- **H40.029** **Open angle with borderline findings, high risk, unspecified eye**

✓6th **H40.03** **Anatomical narrow angle**
> Primary angle closure suspect
- **H40.031** **Anatomical narrow angle, right eye**
- **H40.032** **Anatomical narrow angle, left eye**
- **H40.033** **Anatomical narrow angle, bilateral**
- **H40.039** **Anatomical narrow angle, unspecified eye**

✓6th **H40.04** **Steroid responder**
- **H40.041** **Steroid responder, right eye**
- **H40.042** **Steroid responder, left eye**
- **H40.043** **Steroid responder, bilateral**
- **H40.049** **Steroid responder, unspecified eye**

✓6th **H40.05** **Ocular hypertension**
- **H40.051** **Ocular hypertension, right eye**
- **H40.052** **Ocular hypertension, left eye**
- **H40.053** **Ocular hypertension, bilateral**
- **H40.059** **Ocular hypertension, unspecified eye**

✓6th **H40.06** **Primary angle closure without glaucoma damage**
- **H40.061** **Primary angle closure without glaucoma damage, right eye**
- **H40.062** **Primary angle closure without glaucoma damage, left eye**
- **H40.063** **Primary angle closure without glaucoma damage, bilateral**
- **H40.069** **Primary angle closure without glaucoma damage, unspecified eye**

✓5th **H40.1** **Open-angle glaucoma**

> One of the following 7th characters is to be assigned to each code in subcategories H40.10, H40.11, H40.12-, H40.13-, and H40.14- to designate the stage of glaucoma.
> 0   stage unspecified
> 1   mild stage
> 2   moderate stage
> 3   severe stage
> 4   indeterminate stage

✓x7th **H40.10** **Unspecified open-angle glaucoma**

✓x7th **H40.11** **Primary open-angle glaucoma**
> Chronic simple glaucoma

✓6th **H40.12** **Low-tension glaucoma**
- ✓7th **H40.121** **Low-tension glaucoma, right eye**
- ✓7th **H40.122** **Low-tension glaucoma, left eye**
- ✓7th **H40.123** **Low-tension glaucoma, bilateral**
- ✓7th **H40.129** **Low-tension glaucoma, unspecified eye**

✓6th **H40.13** **Pigmentary glaucoma**
- ✓7th **H40.131** **Pigmentary glaucoma, right eye**
- ✓7th **H40.132** **Pigmentary glaucoma, left eye**
- ✓7th **H40.133** **Pigmentary glaucoma, bilateral**
- ✓7th **H40.139** **Pigmentary glaucoma, unspecified eye**

✓6th **H40.14** **Capsular glaucoma with pseudoexfoliation of lens**
- ✓7th **H40.141** **Capsular glaucoma with pseudoexfoliation of lens, right eye**
- ✓7th **H40.142** **Capsular glaucoma with pseudoexfoliation of lens, left eye**
- ✓7th **H40.143** **Capsular glaucoma with pseudoexfoliation of lens, bilateral**
- ✓7th **H40.149** **Capsular glaucoma with pseudoexfoliation of lens, unspecified eye**

✓6th **H40.15** **Residual stage of open-angle glaucoma**
- **H40.151** **Residual stage of open-angle glaucoma, right eye**
- **H40.152** **Residual stage of open-angle glaucoma, left eye**
- **H40.153** **Residual stage of open-angle glaucoma, bilateral**
- **H40.159** **Residual stage of open-angle glaucoma, unspecified eye**

EXCLUDES 1 Not coded here   EXCLUDES 2 Not included here   N Newborn Age: 0   P Pediatric Age: 0-17   M Maternity Age: 12-55   A Adult Age: 15-124

562

ICD-10-CM 2016

☑5ᵗʰ **H40.2 Primary angle-closure glaucoma**
    EXCLUDES 1 *aqueous misdirection (H40.83-)*
           malignant glaucoma (H40.83-)

One of the following 7th characters is to be assigned to each code in subcategories H40.20 and H40.22- to designate the stage of glaucoma.
0   stage unspecified
1   mild stage
2   moderate stage
3   severe stage
4   indeterminate stage

  ☑x7ᵗʰ **H40.20 Unspecified primary angle-closure glaucoma**

  ☑6ᵗʰ **H40.21 Acute angle-closure glaucoma**
      Acute angle-closure glaucoma attack
      Acute angle-closure glaucoma crisis
      H40.211 Acute angle-closure glaucoma, right eye
      H40.212 Acute angle-closure glaucoma, left eye
      H40.213 Acute angle-closure glaucoma, bilateral
      H40.219 Acute angle-closure glaucoma, unspecified eye

  ☑6ᵗʰ **H40.22 Chronic angle-closure glaucoma**
      Chronic primary angle-closure glaucoma
    ☑7ᵗʰ **H40.221 Chronic angle-closure glaucoma, right eye**
    ☑7ᵗʰ **H40.222 Chronic angle-closure glaucoma, left eye**
    ☑7ᵗʰ **H40.223 Chronic angle-closure glaucoma, bilateral**
    ☑7ᵗʰ **H40.229 Chronic angle-closure glaucoma, unspecified eye**

  ☑6ᵗʰ **H40.23 Intermittent angle-closure glaucoma**
      H40.231 Intermittent angle-closure glaucoma, right eye
      H40.232 Intermittent angle-closure glaucoma, left eye
      H40.233 Intermittent angle-closure glaucoma, bilateral
      H40.239 Intermittent angle-closure glaucoma, unspecified eye

  ☑6ᵗʰ **H40.24 Residual stage of angle-closure glaucoma**
      H40.241 Residual stage of angle-closure glaucoma, right eye
      H40.242 Residual stage of angle-closure glaucoma, left eye
      H40.243 Residual stage of angle-closure glaucoma, bilateral
      H40.249 Residual stage of angle-closure glaucoma, unspecified eye

☑5ᵗʰ **H40.3 Glaucoma secondary to eye trauma**
    Code also underlying condition

One of the following 7th characters is to be assigned to each code in subcategory H40.3- to designate the stage of glaucoma.
0   stage unspecified
1   mild stage
2   moderate stage
3   severe stage
4   indeterminate stage

  ☑x7ᵗʰ **H40.30 Glaucoma secondary to eye trauma, unspecified eye**
  ☑x7ᵗʰ **H40.31 Glaucoma secondary to eye trauma, right eye**
  ☑x7ᵗʰ **H40.32 Glaucoma secondary to eye trauma, left eye**
  ☑x7ᵗʰ **H40.33 Glaucoma secondary to eye trauma, bilateral**

☑5ᵗʰ **H40.4 Glaucoma secondary to eye inflammation**
    Code also underlying condition

One of the following 7th characters is to be assigned to each code in subcategory H40.4- to designate the stage of glaucoma.
0   stage unspecified
1   mild stage
2   moderate stage
3   severe stage
4   indeterminate stage

  ☑x7ᵗʰ **H40.40 Glaucoma secondary to eye inflammation, unspecified eye**
  ☑x7ᵗʰ **H40.41 Glaucoma secondary to eye inflammation, right eye**
  ☑x7ᵗʰ **H40.42 Glaucoma secondary to eye inflammation, left eye**
  ☑x7ᵗʰ **H40.43 Glaucoma secondary to eye inflammation, bilateral**

☑5ᵗʰ **H40.5 Glaucoma secondary to other eye disorders**
    Code also underlying eye disorder

One of the following 7th characters is to be assigned to each code in subcategory H40.5- to designate the stage of glaucoma.
0   stage unspecified
1   mild stage
2   moderate stage
3   severe stage
4   indeterminate stage

  ☑x7ᵗʰ **H40.50 Glaucoma secondary to other eye disorders, unspecified eye**
  ☑x7ᵗʰ **H40.51 Glaucoma secondary to other eye disorders, right eye**
  ☑x7ᵗʰ **H40.52 Glaucoma secondary to other eye disorders, left eye**
  ☑x7ᵗʰ **H40.53 Glaucoma secondary to other eye disorders, bilateral**

☑5ᵗʰ **H40.6 Glaucoma secondary to drugs**
    Use additional code for adverse effect, if applicable, to identify drug (T36-T50 with fifth or sixth character 5)

One of the following 7th characters is to be assigned to each code in subcategory H40.6- to designate the stage of glaucoma.
0   stage unspecified
1   mild stage
2   moderate stage
3   severe stage
4   indeterminate stage

  ☑x7ᵗʰ **H40.60 Glaucoma secondary to drugs, unspecified eye**
  ☑x7ᵗʰ **H40.61 Glaucoma secondary to drugs, right eye**
  ☑x7ᵗʰ **H40.62 Glaucoma secondary to drugs, left eye**
  ☑x7ᵗʰ **H40.63 Glaucoma secondary to drugs, bilateral**

☑5ᵗʰ **H40.8 Other glaucoma**
  ☑6ᵗʰ **H40.81 Glaucoma with increased episcleral venous pressure**
      H40.811 Glaucoma with increased episcleral venous pressure, right eye
      H40.812 Glaucoma with increased episcleral venous pressure, left eye
      H40.813 Glaucoma with increased episcleral venous pressure, bilateral
      H40.819 Glaucoma with increased episcleral venous pressure, unspecified eye

  ☑6ᵗʰ **H40.82 Hypersecretion glaucoma**
      H40.821 Hypersecretion glaucoma, right eye
      H40.822 Hypersecretion glaucoma, left eye
      H40.823 Hypersecretion glaucoma, bilateral
      H40.829 Hypersecretion glaucoma, unspecified eye

  ☑6ᵗʰ **H40.83 Aqueous misdirection**
      Malignant glaucoma
      H40.831 Aqueous misdirection, right eye
      H40.832 Aqueous misdirection, left eye
      H40.833 Aqueous misdirection, bilateral
      H40.839 Aqueous misdirection, unspecified eye

      H40.89 Other specified glaucoma

    H40.9 Unspecified glaucoma

H42 Glaucoma in diseases classified elsewhere
    Code first underlying condition, such as:
      amyloidosis (E85.-)
      aniridia (Q13.1)
      Lowe's syndrome (E72.03)
      Reiger's anomaly (Q13.81)
      specified metabolic disorder (E70-E88)
    EXCLUDES 1 *glaucoma (in):*
        diabetes mellitus (E08.39, E09.39, E10.39, E11.39, E13.39)
        onchocerciasis (B73.02)
        syphilis (A52.71)
        tuberculous (A18.59)

Disorders of vitreous body and globe (H43-H44)

☑4ᵗʰ **H43 Disorders of vitreous body**
  ☑5ᵗʰ **H43.0 Vitreous prolapse**
      EXCLUDES 1 *traumatic vitreous prolapse (S05.2-)*
           vitreous syndrome following cataract surgery (H59.0-)
      H43.00 Vitreous prolapse, unspecified eye
      H43.01 Vitreous prolapse, right eye

☑ Additional Character Required   x7ᵗʰ Placeholder Alert   Unspecified Dx   Other Specified Dx   Manifestation   ►◄ Revised Text   ● New Code   ▲ Revised Code Title

ICD-10-CM 2016   **563**

H43.02 Vitreous prolapse, left eye

H43.03 Vitreous prolapse, bilateral

√5th **H43.1** Vitreous hemorrhage

H43.10 Vitreous hemorrhage, unspecified eye

H43.11 Vitreous hemorrhage, right eye

H43.12 Vitreous hemorrhage, left eye

H43.13 Vitreous hemorrhage, bilateral

√5th **H43.2** Crystalline deposits in vitreous body

H43.20 Crystalline deposits in vitreous body, unspecified eye

H43.21 Crystalline deposits in vitreous body, right eye

H43.22 Crystalline deposits in vitreous body, left eye

H43.23 Crystalline deposits in vitreous body, bilateral

√5th **H43.3** Other vitreous opacities

√6th **H43.31** Vitreous membranes and strands

H43.311 Vitreous membranes and strands, right eye

H43.312 Vitreous membranes and strands, left eye

H43.313 Vitreous membranes and strands, bilateral

H43.319 Vitreous membranes and strands, unspecified eye

√6th **H43.39** Other vitreous opacities
Vitreous floaters

H43.391 Other vitreous opacities, right eye

H43.392 Other vitreous opacities, left eye

H43.393 Other vitreous opacities, bilateral

H43.399 Other vitreous opacities, unspecified eye

√5th **H43.8** Other disorders of vitreous body

EXCLUDES 1 proliferative vitreo-retinopathy with retinal detachment (H33.4-)

EXCLUDES 2 vitreous abscess (H44.02-)

√6th **H43.81** Vitreous degeneration
Vitreous detachment

H43.811 Vitreous degeneration, right eye

H43.812 Vitreous degeneration, left eye

H43.813 Vitreous degeneration, bilateral

H43.819 Vitreous degeneration, unspecified eye

√6th **H43.82** Vitreomacular adhesion
Vitreomacular traction

H43.821 Vitreomacular adhesion, right eye A

H43.822 Vitreomacular adhesion, left eye A

H43.823 Vitreomacular adhesion, bilateral A

H43.829 Vitreomacular adhesion, unspecified eye A

H43.89 Other disorders of vitreous body

H43.9 Unspecified disorder of vitreous body

√4th **H44** Disorders of globe
INCLUDES disorders affecting multiple structures of eye

√5th **H44.0** Purulent endophthalmitis
Use additional code to identify organism

EXCLUDES 1 bleb associated endophthalmitis (H59.4-)

√6th **H44.00** Unspecified purulent endophthalmitis

H44.001 Unspecified purulent endophthalmitis, right eye

H44.002 Unspecified purulent endophthalmitis, left eye

H44.003 Unspecified purulent endophthalmitis, bilateral

H44.009 Unspecified purulent endophthalmitis, unspecified eye

√6th **H44.01** Panophthalmitis (acute)

H44.011 Panophthalmitis (acute), right eye

H44.012 Panophthalmitis (acute), left eye

H44.013 Panophthalmitis (acute), bilateral

H44.019 Panophthalmitis (acute), unspecified eye

√6th **H44.02** Vitreous abscess (chronic)

H44.021 Vitreous abscess (chronic), right eye

H44.022 Vitreous abscess (chronic), left eye

H44.023 Vitreous abscess (chronic), bilateral

H44.029 Vitreous abscess (chronic), unspecified eye

√5th **H44.1** Other endophthalmitis

EXCLUDES 1 bleb associated endophthalmitis (H59.4-)

EXCLUDES 2 ophthalmia nodosa (H16.2-)

√6th **H44.11** Panuveitis

H44.111 Panuveitis, right eye

H44.112 Panuveitis, left eye

H44.113 Panuveitis, bilateral

H44.119 Panuveitis, unspecified eye

√6th **H44.12** Parasitic endophthalmitis, unspecified

H44.121 Parasitic endophthalmitis, unspecified, right eye

H44.122 Parasitic endophthalmitis, unspecified, left eye

H44.123 Parasitic endophthalmitis, unspecified, bilateral

H44.129 Parasitic endophthalmitis, unspecified, unspecified eye

√6th **H44.13** Sympathetic uveitis

H44.131 Sympathetic uveitis, right eye

H44.132 Sympathetic uveitis, left eye

H44.133 Sympathetic uveitis, bilateral

H44.139 Sympathetic uveitis, unspecified eye

H44.19 Other endophthalmitis

√5th **H44.2** Degenerative myopia
Malignant myopia

H44.20 Degenerative myopia, unspecified eye

H44.21 Degenerative myopia, right eye

H44.22 Degenerative myopia, left eye

H44.23 Degenerative myopia, bilateral

√5th **H44.3** Other and unspecified degenerative disorders of globe

H44.30 Unspecified degenerative disorder of globe

√6th **H44.31** Chalcosis

H44.311 Chalcosis, right eye

H44.312 Chalcosis, left eye

H44.313 Chalcosis, bilateral

H44.319 Chalcosis, unspecified eye

√6th **H44.32** Siderosis of eye

H44.321 Siderosis of eye, right eye

H44.322 Siderosis of eye, left eye

H44.323 Siderosis of eye, bilateral

H44.329 Siderosis of eye, unspecified eye

√6th **H44.39** Other degenerative disorders of globe

H44.391 Other degenerative disorders of globe, right eye

H44.392 Other degenerative disorders of globe, left eye

H44.393 Other degenerative disorders of globe, bilateral

H44.399 Other degenerative disorders of globe, unspecified eye

√5th **H44.4** Hypotony of eye

H44.40 Unspecified hypotony of eye

√6th **H44.41** Flat anterior chamber hypotony of eye

H44.411 Flat anterior chamber hypotony of right eye

H44.412 Flat anterior chamber hypotony of left eye

H44.413 Flat anterior chamber hypotony of eye, bilateral

H44.419 Flat anterior chamber hypotony of unspecified eye

√6th **H44.42** Hypotony of eye due to ocular fistula

H44.421 Hypotony of right eye due to ocular fistula

H44.422 Hypotony of left eye due to ocular fistula

H44.423 Hypotony of eye due to ocular fistula, bilateral

H44.429 Hypotony of unspecified eye due to ocular fistula

√6th **H44.43** Hypotony of eye due to other ocular disorders

H44.431 Hypotony of eye due to other ocular disorders, right eye

H44.432 Hypotony of eye due to other ocular disorders, left eye

H44.433 Hypotony of eye due to other ocular disorders, bilateral

EXCLUDES 1 Not coded here   EXCLUDES 2 Not included here   N Newborn Age: 0   P Pediatric Age: 0-17   M Maternity Age: 12-55   A Adult Age: 15-124

564

ICD-10-CM 2016

H44.439   **Hypotony of eye due to other ocular disorders, unspecified eye**

✓6ᵗʰ H44.44   Primary **hypotony of eye**
　　H44.441   **Primary hypotony of** right **eye**
　　H44.442   **Primary hypotony of** left **eye**
　　H44.443   **Primary hypotony of eye,** bilateral
　　H44.449   **Primary hypotony of unspecified eye**

✓5ᵗʰ H44.5   **Degenerated conditions of globe**
　　H44.50   **Unspecified degenerated conditions of globe**

✓6ᵗʰ H44.51   **Absolute glaucoma**
　　H44.511   **Absolute glaucoma,** right **eye**
　　H44.512   **Absolute glaucoma,** left **eye**
　　H44.513   **Absolute glaucoma,** bilateral
　　H44.519   **Absolute glaucoma, unspecified eye**

✓6ᵗʰ H44.52   **Atrophy of globe**
　　　　　Phthisis bulbi
　　H44.521   **Atrophy of globe,** right **eye**
　　H44.522   **Atrophy of globe,** left **eye**
　　H44.523   **Atrophy of globe,** bilateral
　　H44.529   **Atrophy of globe, unspecified eye**

✓6ᵗʰ H44.53   **Leucocoria**
　　H44.531   **Leucocoria,** right **eye**
　　H44.532   **Leucocoria,** left **eye**
　　H44.533   **Leucocoria,** bilateral
　　H44.539   **Leucocoria, unspecified eye**

✓5ᵗʰ H44.6   **Retained (old) intraocular foreign body,** magnetic
　　Use additional code to identify magnetic foreign body (Z18.11)
　　EXCLUDES 1   *current intraocular foreign body (S05.-)*
　　EXCLUDES 2   *retained foreign body in eyelid (H02.81-)*
　　　　　retained (old) foreign body following penetrating wound of orbit (H05.5-)
　　　　　retained (old) intraocular foreign body, nonmagnetic (H44.7-)

✓6ᵗʰ H44.60   Unspecified **retained (old) intraocular foreign body,** magnetic
　　H44.601   **Unspecified retained (old) intraocular foreign body, magnetic,** right **eye**
　　H44.602   **Unspecified retained (old) intraocular foreign body, magnetic,** left **eye**
　　H44.603   **Unspecified retained (old) intraocular foreign body, magnetic,** bilateral
　　H44.609   **Unspecified retained (old) intraocular foreign body, magnetic, unspecified eye**

✓6ᵗʰ H44.61   **Retained (old) magnetic foreign body in** anterior chamber
　　H44.611   **Retained (old) magnetic foreign body in anterior chamber,** right **eye**
　　H44.612   **Retained (old) magnetic foreign body in anterior chamber,** left **eye**
　　H44.613   **Retained (old) magnetic foreign body in anterior chamber,** bilateral
　　H44.619   **Retained (old) magnetic foreign body in anterior chamber, unspecified eye**

✓6ᵗʰ H44.62   **Retained (old) magnetic foreign body in** iris or ciliary body
　　H44.621   **Retained (old) magnetic foreign body in iris or ciliary body,** right **eye**
　　H44.622   **Retained (old) magnetic foreign body in iris or ciliary body,** left **eye**
　　H44.623   **Retained (old) magnetic foreign body in iris or ciliary body,** bilateral
　　H44.629   **Retained (old) magnetic foreign body in iris or ciliary body, unspecified eye**

✓6ᵗʰ H44.63   **Retained (old) magnetic foreign body in** lens
　　H44.631   **Retained (old) magnetic foreign body in lens,** right **eye**
　　H44.632   **Retained (old) magnetic foreign body in lens,** left **eye**
　　H44.633   **Retained (old) magnetic foreign body in lens,** bilateral
　　H44.639   **Retained (old) magnetic foreign body in lens, unspecified eye**

✓6ᵗʰ H44.64   **Retained (old) magnetic foreign body in** posterior wall of globe
　　H44.641   **Retained (old) magnetic foreign body in posterior wall of globe,** right **eye**

H44.642   **Retained (old) magnetic foreign body in posterior wall of globe,** left **eye**
H44.643   **Retained (old) magnetic foreign body in posterior wall of globe,** bilateral
H44.649   **Retained (old) magnetic foreign body in posterior wall of globe, unspecified eye**

✓6ᵗʰ H44.65   **Retained (old) magnetic foreign body in** vitreous body
　　H44.651   **Retained (old) magnetic foreign body in vitreous body,** right **eye**
　　H44.652   **Retained (old) magnetic foreign body in vitreous body,** left **eye**
　　H44.653   **Retained (old) magnetic foreign body in vitreous body,** bilateral
　　H44.659   **Retained (old) magnetic foreign body in vitreous body, unspecified eye**

✓6ᵗʰ H44.69   **Retained (old) intraocular foreign body, magnetic, in** other or multiple sites
　　H44.691   **Retained (old) intraocular foreign body, magnetic, in other or multiple sites,** right **eye**
　　H44.692   **Retained (old) intraocular foreign body, magnetic, in other or multiple sites,** left **eye**
　　H44.693   **Retained (old) intraocular foreign body, magnetic, in other or multiple sites,** bilateral
　　H44.699   **Retained (old) intraocular foreign body, magnetic, in other or multiple sites, unspecified eye**

✓5ᵗʰ H44.7   **Retained (old) intraocular foreign body,** nonmagnetic
　　Use additional code to identify nonmagnetic foreign body (Z18.01-Z18.10, Z18.12, Z18.2-Z18.9)
　　EXCLUDES 1   *current intraocular foreign body (S05.-)*
　　EXCLUDES 2   *retained foreign body in eyelid (H02.81-)*
　　　　　retained (old) foreign body following penetrating wound of orbit (H05.5-)
　　　　　retained (old) intraocular foreign body, magnetic (H44.6-)

✓6ᵗʰ H44.70   Unspecified **retained (old) intraocular foreign body,** nonmagnetic
　　H44.701   **Unspecified retained (old) intraocular foreign body, nonmagnetic,** right **eye**
　　H44.702   **Unspecified retained (old) intraocular foreign body, nonmagnetic,** left **eye**
　　H44.703   **Unspecified retained (old) intraocular foreign body, nonmagnetic,** bilateral
　　H44.709   **Unspecified retained (old) intraocular foreign body, nonmagnetic, unspecified eye**
　　　　　Retained (old) intraocular foreign body NOS

✓6ᵗʰ H44.71   **Retained (nonmagnetic) (old) foreign body in** anterior chamber
　　H44.711   **Retained (nonmagnetic) (old) foreign body in anterior chamber,** right **eye**
　　H44.712   **Retained (nonmagnetic) (old) foreign body in anterior chamber,** left **eye**
　　H44.713   **Retained (nonmagnetic) (old) foreign body in anterior chamber,** bilateral
　　H44.719   **Retained (nonmagnetic) (old) foreign body in anterior chamber, unspecified eye**

✓6ᵗʰ H44.72   **Retained (nonmagnetic) (old) foreign body in** iris or ciliary body
　　H44.721   **Retained (nonmagnetic) (old) foreign body in iris or ciliary body,** right **eye**
　　H44.722   **Retained (nonmagnetic) (old) foreign body in iris or ciliary body,** left **eye**
　　H44.723   **Retained (nonmagnetic) (old) foreign body in iris or ciliary body,** bilateral
　　H44.729   **Retained (nonmagnetic) (old) foreign body in iris or ciliary body, unspecified eye**

✓6ᵗʰ H44.73   **Retained (nonmagnetic) (old) foreign body in** lens
　　H44.731   **Retained (nonmagnetic) (old) foreign body in lens,** right **eye**
　　H44.732   **Retained (nonmagnetic) (old) foreign body in lens,** left **eye**
　　H44.733   **Retained (nonmagnetic) (old) foreign body in lens,** bilateral

---

✓ Additional Character Required   ✓x7ᵗʰ Placeholder Alert   Unspecified Dx   Other Specified Dx   Manifestation   ▶◀ Revised Text   ● New Code   ▲ Revised Code Title

   H44.739   Retained (nonmagnetic) (old) foreign body in lens, unspecified eye

✓6ᵗʰ H44.74   Retained (nonmagnetic) (old) foreign body in posterior wall of globe
   H44.741   Retained (nonmagnetic) (old) foreign body in posterior wall of globe, right eye
   H44.742   Retained (nonmagnetic) (old) foreign body in posterior wall of globe, left eye
   H44.743   Retained (nonmagnetic) (old) foreign body in posterior wall of globe, bilateral
   H44.749   Retained (nonmagnetic) (old) foreign body in posterior wall of globe, unspecified eye

✓6ᵗʰ H44.75   Retained (nonmagnetic) (old) foreign body in vitreous body
   H44.751   Retained (nonmagnetic) (old) foreign body in vitreous body, right eye
   H44.752   Retained (nonmagnetic) (old) foreign body in vitreous body, left eye
   H44.753   Retained (nonmagnetic) (old) foreign body in vitreous body, bilateral
   H44.759   Retained (nonmagnetic) (old) foreign body in vitreous body, unspecified eye

✓6ᵗʰ H44.79   Retained (old) intraocular foreign body, nonmagnetic, in other or multiple sites
   H44.791   Retained (old) intraocular foreign body, nonmagnetic, in other or multiple sites, right eye
   H44.792   Retained (old) intraocular foreign body, nonmagnetic, in other or multiple sites, left eye
   H44.793   Retained (old) intraocular foreign body, nonmagnetic, in other or multiple sites, bilateral
   H44.799   Retained (old) intraocular foreign body, nonmagnetic, in other or multiple sites, unspecified eye

✓5ᵗʰ H44.8   Other disorders of globe
 ✓6ᵗʰ H44.81   Hemophthalmos
   H44.811   Hemophthalmos, right eye
   H44.812   Hemophthalmos, left eye
   H44.813   Hemophthalmos, bilateral
   H44.819   Hemophthalmos, unspecified eye
 ✓6ᵗʰ H44.82   Luxation of globe
   H44.821   Luxation of globe, right eye
   H44.822   Luxation of globe, left eye
   H44.823   Luxation of globe, bilateral
   H44.829   Luxation of globe, unspecified eye
 H44.89   Other disorders of globe
H44.9   Unspecified disorder of globe

Disorders of optic nerve and visual pathways (H46-H47)

✓4ᵗʰ H46   Optic neuritis
 EXCLUDES 2   ischemic optic neuropathy (H47.01-)
       neuromyelitis optica [Devic] (G36.0)

✓5ᵗʰ H46.0   Optic papillitis
 H46.00   Optic papillitis, unspecified eye
 H46.01   Optic papillitis, right eye
 H46.02   Optic papillitis, left eye
 H46.03   Optic papillitis, bilateral

✓5ᵗʰ H46.1   Retrobulbar neuritis
 Retrobulbar neuritis NOS
  EXCLUDES 1   syphilitic retrobulbar neuritis (A52.15)
 H46.10   Retrobulbar neuritis, unspecified eye
 H46.11   Retrobulbar neuritis, right eye
 H46.12   Retrobulbar neuritis, left eye
 H46.13   Retrobulbar neuritis, bilateral
H46.2   Nutritional optic neuropathy
H46.3   Toxic optic neuropathy
 Code first (T51-T65) to identify cause
H46.8   Other optic neuritis
H46.9   Unspecified optic neuritis

✓4ᵗʰ H47   Other disorders of optic [2nd] nerve and visual pathways
✓5ᵗʰ H47.0   Disorders of optic nerve, not elsewhere classified
 ✓6ᵗʰ H47.01   Ischemic optic neuropathy
   H47.011   Ischemic optic neuropathy, right eye
   H47.012   Ischemic optic neuropathy, left eye
   H47.013   Ischemic optic neuropathy, bilateral
   H47.019   Ischemic optic neuropathy, unspecified eye
 ✓6ᵗʰ H47.02   Hemorrhage in optic nerve sheath
   H47.021   Hemorrhage in optic nerve sheath, right eye
   H47.022   Hemorrhage in optic nerve sheath, left eye
   H47.023   Hemorrhage in optic nerve sheath, bilateral
   H47.029   Hemorrhage in optic nerve sheath, unspecified eye
 ✓6ᵗʰ H47.03   Optic nerve hypoplasia
   H47.031   Optic nerve hypoplasia, right eye
   H47.032   Optic nerve hypoplasia, left eye
   H47.033   Optic nerve hypoplasia, bilateral
   H47.039   Optic nerve hypoplasia, unspecified eye
 ✓6ᵗʰ H47.09   Other disorders of optic nerve, not elsewhere classified
  Compression of optic nerve
   H47.091   Other disorders of optic nerve, not elsewhere classified, right eye
   H47.092   Other disorders of optic nerve, not elsewhere classified, left eye
   H47.093   Other disorders of optic nerve, not elsewhere classified, bilateral
   H47.099   Other disorders of optic nerve, not elsewhere classified, unspecified eye

✓5ᵗʰ H47.1   Papilledema
 H47.10   Unspecified papilledema
 H47.11   Papilledema associated with increased intracranial pressure
 H47.12   Papilledema associated with decreased ocular pressure
 H47.13   Papilledema associated with retinal disorder
 ✓6ᵗʰ H47.14   Foster-Kennedy syndrome
   H47.141   Foster-Kennedy syndrome, right eye
   H47.142   Foster-Kennedy syndrome, left eye
   H47.143   Foster-Kennedy syndrome, bilateral
   H47.149   Foster-Kennedy syndrome, unspecified eye

✓5ᵗʰ H47.2   Optic atrophy
 H47.20   Unspecified optic atrophy
 ✓6ᵗʰ H47.21   Primary optic atrophy
   H47.211   Primary optic atrophy, right eye
   H47.212   Primary optic atrophy, left eye
   H47.213   Primary optic atrophy, bilateral
   H47.219   Primary optic atrophy, unspecified eye
 H47.22   Hereditary optic atrophy
  Leber's optic atrophy
 ✓6ᵗʰ H47.23   Glaucomatous optic atrophy
   H47.231   Glaucomatous optic atrophy, right eye
   H47.232   Glaucomatous optic atrophy, left eye
   H47.233   Glaucomatous optic atrophy, bilateral
   H47.239   Glaucomatous optic atrophy, unspecified eye
 ✓6ᵗʰ H47.29   Other optic atrophy
  Temporal pallor of optic disc
   H47.291   Other optic atrophy, right eye
   H47.292   Other optic atrophy, left eye
   H47.293   Other optic atrophy, bilateral
   H47.299   Other optic atrophy, unspecified eye

✓5ᵗʰ H47.3   Other disorders of optic disc
 ✓6ᵗʰ H47.31   Coloboma of optic disc
   H47.311   Coloboma of optic disc, right eye
   H47.312   Coloboma of optic disc, left eye
   H47.313   Coloboma of optic disc, bilateral
   H47.319   Coloboma of optic disc, unspecified eye

EXCLUDES 1 Not coded here   EXCLUDES 2 Not included here   N Newborn Age: 0   P Pediatric Age: 0-17   M Maternity Age: 12-55   A Adult Age: 15-124

566   ICD-10-CM 2016

✓6th **H47.32** Drusen of optic disc
- **H47.321** Drusen of optic disc, **right** eye
- **H47.322** Drusen of optic disc, **left** eye
- **H47.323** Drusen of optic disc, **bilateral**
- **H47.329** Drusen of optic disc, **unspecified** eye

✓6th **H47.33** Pseudopapilledema of optic disc
- **H47.331** Pseudopapilledema of optic disc, **right** eye
- **H47.332** Pseudopapilledema of optic disc, **left** eye
- **H47.333** Pseudopapilledema of optic disc, **bilateral**
- **H47.339** Pseudopapilledema of optic disc, **unspecified** eye

✓6th **H47.39** Other disorders of optic disc
- **H47.391** Other disorders of optic disc, **right** eye
- **H47.392** Other disorders of optic disc, **left** eye
- **H47.393** Other disorders of optic disc, **bilateral**
- **H47.399** Other disorders of optic disc, **unspecified** eye

✓5th **H47.4** **Disorders of optic chiasm**
Code also underlying condition
- **H47.41** Disorders of optic chiasm in (due to) inflammatory disorders
- **H47.42** Disorders of optic chiasm in (due to) neoplasm
- **H47.43** Disorders of optic chiasm in (due to) vascular disorders
- **H47.49** Disorders of optic chiasm in (due to) other disorders

✓5th **H47.5** **Disorders of other visual pathways**
Disorders of optic tracts, geniculate nuclei and optic radiations
Code also underlying condition

✓6th **H47.51** Disorders of visual pathways in (due to) inflammatory disorders
- **H47.511** Disorders of visual pathways in (due to) inflammatory disorders, **right** side
- **H47.512** Disorders of visual pathways in (due to) inflammatory disorders, **left** side
- **H47.519** Disorders of visual pathways in (due to) inflammatory disorders, **unspecified** side

✓6th **H47.52** Disorders of visual pathways in (due to) neoplasm
- **H47.521** Disorders of visual pathways in (due to) neoplasm, **right** side
- **H47.522** Disorders of visual pathways in (due to) neoplasm, **left** side
- **H47.529** Disorders of visual pathways in (due to) neoplasm, **unspecified** side

✓6th **H47.53** Disorders of visual pathways in (due to) vascular disorders
- **H47.531** Disorders of visual pathways in (due to) vascular disorders, **right** side
- **H47.532** Disorders of visual pathways in (due to) vascular disorders, **left** side
- **H47.539** Disorders of visual pathways in (due to) vascular disorders, **unspecified** side

✓5th **H47.6** **Disorders of visual cortex**
Code also underlying condition
EXCLUDES 1 injury to visual cortex S04.04

✓6th **H47.61** Cortical blindness
- **H47.611** Cortical blindness, **right** side of brain
- **H47.612** Cortical blindness, **left** side of brain
- **H47.619** Cortical blindness, **unspecified** side of brain

✓6th **H47.62** Disorders of visual cortex in (due to) inflammatory disorders
- **H47.621** Disorders of visual cortex in (due to) inflammatory disorders, **right** side of brain
- **H47.622** Disorders of visual cortex in (due to) inflammatory disorders, **left** side of brain
- **H47.629** Disorders of visual cortex in (due to) inflammatory disorders, **unspecified** side of brain

✓6th **H47.63** Disorders of visual cortex in (due to) neoplasm
- **H47.631** Disorders of visual cortex in (due to) neoplasm, **right** side of brain
- **H47.632** Disorders of visual cortex in (due to) neoplasm, **left** side of brain
- **H47.639** Disorders of visual cortex in (due to) neoplasm, **unspecified** side of brain

✓6th **H47.64** Disorders of visual cortex in (due to) vascular disorders
- **H47.641** Disorders of visual cortex in (due to) vascular disorders, **right** side of brain
- **H47.642** Disorders of visual cortex in (due to) vascular disorders, **left** side of brain
- **H47.649** Disorders of visual cortex in (due to) vascular disorders, **unspecified** side of brain

H47.9 Unspecified disorder of visual pathways

Disorders of ocular muscles, binocular movement, accommodation and refraction (H49-H52)

EXCLUDES 2 *nystagmus and other irregular eye movements (H55)*

✓4th **H49** **Paralytic strabismus**
EXCLUDES 2 *internal ophthalmoplegia (H52.51-)*
internuclear ophthalmoplegia (H51.2-)
progressive supranuclear ophthalmoplegia (G23.1)

✓5th **H49.0** Third [oculomotor] nerve palsy
- **H49.00** **Third [oculomotor] nerve palsy, unspecified eye**
- **H49.01** **Third [oculomotor] nerve palsy, right eye**
- **H49.02** **Third [oculomotor] nerve palsy, left eye**
- **H49.03** **Third [oculomotor] nerve palsy, bilateral**

✓5th **H49.1** Fourth [trochlear] nerve palsy
- **H49.10** **Fourth [trochlear] nerve palsy, unspecified eye**
- **H49.11** **Fourth [trochlear] nerve palsy, right eye**
- **H49.12** **Fourth [trochlear] nerve palsy, left eye**
- **H49.13** **Fourth [trochlear] nerve palsy, bilateral**

✓5th **H49.2** Sixth [abducent] nerve palsy
- **H49.20** **Sixth [abducent] nerve palsy, unspecified eye**
- **H49.21** **Sixth [abducent] nerve palsy, right eye**
- **H49.22** **Sixth [abducent] nerve palsy, left eye**
- **H49.23** **Sixth [abducent] nerve palsy, bilateral**

✓5th **H49.3** Total (external) ophthalmoplegia
- **H49.30** **Total (external) ophthalmoplegia, unspecified eye**
- **H49.31** **Total (external) ophthalmoplegia, right eye**
- **H49.32** **Total (external) ophthalmoplegia, left eye**
- **H49.33** **Total (external) ophthalmoplegia, bilateral**

✓5th **H49.4** Progressive external ophthalmoplegia
EXCLUDES 1 *Kearns-Sayre syndrome (H49.81-)*
- **H49.40** **Progressive external ophthalmoplegia, unspecified eye**
- **H49.41** **Progressive external ophthalmoplegia, right eye**
- **H49.42** **Progressive external ophthalmoplegia, left eye**
- **H49.43** **Progressive external ophthalmoplegia, bilateral**

✓5th **H49.8** Other paralytic strabismus

✓6th **H49.81** Kearns-Sayre syndrome
Progressive external ophthalmoplegia with pigmentary retinopathy
Use additional code for other manifestation, such as: heart block (I45.9)
- **H49.811** **Kearns-Sayre syndrome, right eye**
- **H49.812** **Kearns-Sayre syndrome, left eye**
- **H49.813** **Kearns-Sayre syndrome, bilateral**
- **H49.819** **Kearns-Sayre syndrome, unspecified eye**

✓6th **H49.88** Other paralytic strabismus
External ophthalmoplegia NOS
- **H49.881** Other paralytic strabismus, **right** eye
- **H49.882** Other paralytic strabismus, **left** eye
- **H49.883** Other paralytic strabismus, **bilateral**
- **H49.889** Other paralytic strabismus, **unspecified** eye

H49.9 Unspecified paralytic strabismus

✓4th **H50** **Other strabismus**

✓5th **H50.0** Esotropia
Convergent concomitant strabismus
EXCLUDES 1 *intermittent esotropia (H50.31-, H50.32)*
- **H50.00** **Unspecified esotropia**

✓6th **H50.01** Monocular esotropia
- **H50.011** Monocular esotropia, **right** eye
- **H50.012** Monocular esotropia, **left** eye

✓ Additional Character Required   ✓x7th Placeholder Alert   Unspecified Dx   Other Specified Dx   Manifestation   ▶◀ Revised Text   ● New Code   ▲ Revised Code Title

ICD-10-CM 2016   567

✓6ᵗʰ **H50.02** **Monocular esotropia with** A pattern
     H50.021 **Monocular esotropia with A pattern, right** eye
     H50.022 **Monocular esotropia with A pattern, left** eye

✓6ᵗʰ **H50.03** **Monocular esotropia with** V pattern
     H50.031 **Monocular esotropia with V pattern, right** eye
     H50.032 **Monocular esotropia with V pattern, left** eye

✓6ᵗʰ **H50.04** **Monocular esotropia with** other noncomitancies
     H50.041 **Monocular esotropia with other noncomitancies, right** eye
     H50.042 **Monocular esotropia with other noncomitancies, left** eye

H50.05 Alternating **esotropia**

H50.06 Alternating **esotropia with** A pattern

H50.07 Alternating **esotropia with** V pattern

H50.08 Alternating **esotropia with other** noncomitancies

✓5ᵗʰ **H50.1** **Exotropia**
     Divergent concomitant strabismus
     EXCLUDES 1   *intermittent exotropia (H50.33-, H50.34)*

     H50.10 **Unspecified exotropia**

✓6ᵗʰ **H50.11** Monocular **exotropia**
     H50.111 **Monocular exotropia, right** eye
     H50.112 **Monocular exotropia, left** eye

✓6ᵗʰ **H50.12** **Monocular exotropia with** A pattern
     H50.121 **Monocular exotropia with A pattern, right** eye
     H50.122 **Monocular exotropia with A pattern, left** eye

✓6ᵗʰ **H50.13** **Monocular exotropia with** V pattern
     H50.131 **Monocular exotropia with V pattern, right** eye
     H50.132 **Monocular exotropia with V pattern, left** eye

✓6ᵗʰ **H50.14** **Monocular exotropia with** other noncomitancies
     H50.141 **Monocular exotropia with other noncomitancies, right** eye
     H50.142 **Monocular exotropia with other noncomitancies, left** eye

H50.15 Alternating **exotropia**

H50.16 Alternating **exotropia with** A pattern

H50.17 Alternating **exotropia with** V pattern

H50.18 Alternating **exotropia with other** noncomitancies

✓5ᵗʰ **H50.2** **Vertical strabismus**
     Hypertropia
     H50.21 **Vertical strabismus, right** eye
     H50.22 **Vertical strabismus, left** eye

✓5ᵗʰ **H50.3** **Intermittent heterotropia**
     H50.30 **Unspecified intermittent heterotropia**

✓6ᵗʰ **H50.31** **Intermittent** monocular esotropia
     H50.311 **Intermittent monocular esotropia, right** eye
     H50.312 **Intermittent monocular esotropia, left** eye

     H50.32 **Intermittent** alternating **esotropia**

✓6ᵗʰ **H50.33** **Intermittent** monocular **exotropia**
     H50.331 **Intermittent monocular exotropia, right** eye
     H50.332 **Intermittent monocular exotropia, left** eye

     H50.34 **Intermittent** alternating **exotropia**

✓5ᵗʰ **H50.4** **Other and unspecified heterotropia**
     H50.40 **Unspecified heterotropia**

✓6ᵗʰ **H50.41** Cyclotropia
     H50.411 **Cyclotropia, right** eye
     H50.412 **Cyclotropia, left** eye

     H50.42 **Monofixation** syndrome

     H50.43 **Accommodative component in esotropia**

✓5ᵗʰ **H50.5** **Heterophoria**
     H50.50 **Unspecified heterophoria**

     H50.51 **Esophoria**

     H50.52 **Exophoria**

     H50.53 Vertical **heterophoria**

H50.54 Cyclophoria

H50.55 Alternating heterophoria

✓5ᵗʰ **H50.6** **Mechanical strabismus**
     H50.60 **Mechanical strabismus, unspecified**

✓6ᵗʰ **H50.61** Brown's sheath **syndrome**
     H50.611 **Brown's sheath syndrome, right** eye
     H50.612 **Brown's sheath syndrome, left** eye

     H50.69 **Other mechanical strabismus**
         Strabismus due to adhesions
         Traumatic limitation of duction of eye muscle

✓5ᵗʰ **H50.8** **Other specified strabismus**

✓6ᵗʰ **H50.81** Duane's **syndrome**
     H50.811 **Duane's syndrome, right** eye
     H50.812 **Duane's syndrome, left** eye

     H50.89 **Other specified strabismus**

H50.9 **Unspecified strabismus**

✓4ᵗʰ **H51** **Other disorders of binocular movement**

H51.0 **Palsy (spasm) of conjugate gaze**

✓5ᵗʰ **H51.1** **Convergence insufficiency and excess**
     H51.11 **Convergence** insufficiency
     H51.12 **Convergence** excess

✓5ᵗʰ **H51.2** **Internuclear ophthalmoplegia**
     H51.20 **Internuclear ophthalmoplegia, unspecified eye**
     H51.21 **Internuclear ophthalmoplegia, right** eye
     H51.22 **Internuclear ophthalmoplegia, left** eye
     H51.23 **Internuclear ophthalmoplegia, bilateral**

H51.8 **Other specified disorders of binocular movement**

H51.9 **Unspecified disorder of binocular movement**

✓4ᵗʰ **H52** **Disorders of refraction and accommodation**

✓5ᵗʰ **H52.0** **Hypermetropia**
     H52.00 **Hypermetropia, unspecified eye**
     H52.01 **Hypermetropia, right** eye
     H52.02 **Hypermetropia, left** eye
     H52.03 **Hypermetropia, bilateral**

✓5ᵗʰ **H52.1** **Myopia**
     EXCLUDES 1   *degenerative myopia (H44.2-)*
     H52.10 **Myopia, unspecified eye**
     H52.11 **Myopia, right** eye
     H52.12 **Myopia, left** eye
     H52.13 **Myopia, bilateral**

✓5ᵗʰ **H52.2** **Astigmatism**

✓6ᵗʰ **H52.20** Unspecified **astigmatism**
     H52.201 **Unspecified astigmatism, right** eye
     H52.202 **Unspecified astigmatism, left** eye
     H52.203 **Unspecified astigmatism, bilateral**
     H52.209 **Unspecified astigmatism, unspecified eye**

✓6ᵗʰ **H52.21** Irregular **astigmatism**
     H52.211 **Irregular astigmatism, right** eye
     H52.212 **Irregular astigmatism, left** eye
     H52.213 **Irregular astigmatism, bilateral**
     H52.219 **Irregular astigmatism, unspecified eye**

✓6ᵗʰ **H52.22** Regular **astigmatism**
     H52.221 **Regular astigmatism, right** eye
     H52.222 **Regular astigmatism, left** eye
     H52.223 **Regular astigmatism, bilateral**
     H52.229 **Regular astigmatism, unspecified eye**

✓5ᵗʰ **H52.3** **Anisometropia and aniseikonia**
     H52.31 **Anisometropia**
     H52.32 **Aniseikonia**

H52.4 **Presbyopia**

✓5ᵗʰ **H52.5** **Disorders of accommodation**

✓6ᵗʰ **H52.51** Internal ophthalmoplegia (complete) (total)
     H52.511 **Internal ophthalmoplegia (complete) (total), right** eye
     H52.512 **Internal ophthalmoplegia (complete) (total), left** eye
     H52.513 **Internal ophthalmoplegia (complete) (total), bilateral**
     H52.519 **Internal ophthalmoplegia (complete) (total), unspecified eye**

EXCLUDES 1 Not coded here   *EXCLUDES 2* Not included here   N Newborn Age: 0   P Pediatric Age: 0-17   M Maternity Age: 12-55   A Adult Age: 15-124

✓6ᵗʰ **H52.52 Paresis of accommodation**
     H52.521   Paresis of accommodation, right eye
     H52.522   Paresis of accommodation, left eye
     H52.523   Paresis of accommodation, bilateral
     H52.529   Paresis of accommodation, unspecified eye

✓6ᵗʰ **H52.53 Spasm of accommodation**
     H52.531   Spasm of accommodation, right eye
     H52.532   Spasm of accommodation, left eye
     H52.533   Spasm of accommodation, bilateral
     H52.539   Spasm of accommodation, unspecified eye

H52.6 Other disorders of refraction
H52.7 Unspecified disorder of refraction

Visual disturbances and blindness (H53-H54)

✓4ᵗʰ **H53 Visual disturbances**
✓5ᵗʰ **H53.0 Amblyopia ex anopsia**
     EXCLUDES 1   *amblyopia due to vitamin A deficiency (E50.5)*

✓6ᵗʰ **H53.00 Unspecified amblyopia**
     H53.001   Unspecified amblyopia, right eye
     H53.002   Unspecified amblyopia, left eye
     H53.003   Unspecified amblyopia, bilateral
     H53.009   Unspecified amblyopia, unspecified eye

✓6ᵗʰ **H53.01 Deprivation amblyopia**
     H53.011   Deprivation amblyopia, right eye
     H53.012   Deprivation amblyopia, left eye
     H53.013   Deprivation amblyopia, bilateral
     H53.019   Deprivation amblyopia, unspecified eye

✓6ᵗʰ **H53.02 Refractive amblyopia**
     H53.021   Refractive amblyopia, right eye
     H53.022   Refractive amblyopia, left eye
     H53.023   Refractive amblyopia, bilateral
     H53.029   Refractive amblyopia, unspecified eye

✓6ᵗʰ **H53.03 Strabismic amblyopia**
     EXCLUDES 1   *strabismus (H50.-)*
     H53.031   Strabismic amblyopia, right eye
     H53.032   Strabismic amblyopia, left eye
     H53.033   Strabismic amblyopia, bilateral
     H53.039   Strabismic amblyopia, unspecified eye

✓5ᵗʰ **H53.1 Subjective visual disturbances**
     EXCLUDES 1   *subjective visual disturbances due to vitamin A deficiency (E50.5)*
              visual hallucinations (R44.1)

     H53.10 Unspecified subjective visual disturbances
     H53.11 Day blindness
         Hemeralopia

✓6ᵗʰ **H53.12 Transient visual loss**
     Scintillating scotoma
     EXCLUDES 1   *amaurosis fugax (G45.3-)*
              transient retinal artery occlusion (H34.0-)
     H53.121   Transient visual loss, right eye
     H53.122   Transient visual loss, left eye
     H53.123   Transient visual loss, bilateral
     H53.129   Transient visual loss, unspecified eye

✓6ᵗʰ **H53.13 Sudden visual loss**
     H53.131   Sudden visual loss, right eye
     H53.132   Sudden visual loss, left eye
     H53.133   Sudden visual loss, bilateral
     H53.139   Sudden visual loss, unspecified eye

✓6ᵗʰ **H53.14 Visual discomfort**
     Asthenopia   Photophobia
     H53.141   Visual discomfort, right eye
     H53.142   Visual discomfort, left eye
     H53.143   Visual discomfort, bilateral
     H53.149   Visual discomfort, unspecified

     H53.15 Visual distortions of shape and size
         Metamorphopsia
     H53.16 Psychophysical visual disturbances
     H53.19 Other subjective visual disturbances
         Visual halos

H53.2 Diplopia
     Double vision

✓5ᵗʰ **H53.3 Other and unspecified disorders of binocular vision**
     H53.30 Unspecified disorder of binocular vision
     H53.31 Abnormal retinal correspondence
     H53.32 Fusion with defective stereopsis
     H53.33 Simultaneous visual perception without fusion
     H53.34 Suppression of binocular vision

✓5ᵗʰ **H53.4 Visual field defects**
     H53.40 Unspecified visual field defects

✓6ᵗʰ **H53.41 Scotoma involving central area**
     Central scotoma
     H53.411   Scotoma involving central area, right eye
     H53.412   Scotoma involving central area, left eye
     H53.413   Scotoma involving central area, bilateral
     H53.419   Scotoma involving central area, unspecified eye

✓6ᵗʰ **H53.42 Scotoma of blind spot area**
     Enlarged blind spot
     H53.421   Scotoma of blind spot area, right eye
     H53.422   Scotoma of blind spot area, left eye
     H53.423   Scotoma of blind spot area, bilateral
     H53.429   Scotoma of blind spot area, unspecified eye

✓6ᵗʰ **H53.43 Sector or arcuate defects**
     Arcuate scotoma   Bjerrum scotoma
     H53.431   Sector or arcuate defects, right eye
     H53.432   Sector or arcuate defects, left eye
     H53.433   Sector or arcuate defects, bilateral
     H53.439   Sector or arcuate defects, unspecified eye

✓6ᵗʰ **H53.45 Other localized visual field defect**
     Peripheral visual field defect
     Ring scotoma NOS
     Scotoma NOS
     H53.451   Other localized visual field defect, right eye
     H53.452   Other localized visual field defect, left eye
     H53.453   Other localized visual field defect, bilateral
     H53.459   Other localized visual field defect, unspecified eye

✓6ᵗʰ **H53.46 Homonymous bilateral field defects**
     Homonymous hemianopia
     Homonymous hemianopsia
     Quadrant anopia
     Quadrant anopsia
     H53.461   Homonymous bilateral field defects, right side
     H53.462   Homonymous bilateral field defects, left side
     H53.469   Homonymous bilateral field defects, unspecified side
         Homonymous bilateral field defects NOS

     H53.47 Heteronymous bilateral field defects
         Heteronymous hemianop(s)ia

✓6ᵗʰ **H53.48 Generalized contraction of visual field**
     H53.481   Generalized contraction of visual field, right eye
     H53.482   Generalized contraction of visual field, left eye
     H53.483   Generalized contraction of visual field, bilateral
     H53.489   Generalized contraction of visual field, unspecified eye

✓5ᵗʰ **H53.5 Color vision deficiencies**
     Color blindness
     EXCLUDES 2   *day blindness (H53.11)*
     H53.50 Unspecified color vision deficiencies
         Color blindness NOS
     H53.51 Achromatopsia
     H53.52 Acquired color vision deficiency
     H53.53 Deuteranomaly
         Deuteranopia
     H53.54 Protanomaly
         Protanopia
     H53.55 Tritanomaly
         Tritanopia
     H53.59 Other color vision deficiencies

✓ Additional Character Required   ✓×7ᵗʰ Placeholder Alert   Unspecified Dx   Other Specified Dx   Manifestation   ▶◀ Revised Text   ● New Code   ▲ Revised Code Title

✓5ᵗʰ H53.6 Night blindness
> EXCLUDES 1 *night blindness due to vitamin A deficiency (E50.5)*

    H53.60 Unspecified night blindness
    H53.61 Abnormal dark adaptation curve
    H53.62 Acquired night blindness
    H53.63 Congenital night blindness
    H53.69 Other night blindness

✓5ᵗʰ H53.7 Vision sensitivity deficiencies
    H53.71 Glare sensitivity
    H53.72 Impaired contrast sensitivity

H53.8 Other visual disturbances
H53.9 Unspecified visual disturbance

✓4ᵗʰ H54 Blindness and low vision
> NOTE For definition of visual impairment categories see table below

Code first any associated underlying cause of the blindness
> EXCLUDES 1 *amaurosis fugax (G45.3)*

H54.0 Blindness, both eyes
> Visual impairment categories 3, 4, 5 in both eyes.

✓5ᵗʰ H54.1 Blindness, one eye, low vision other eye
> Visual impairment categories 3, 4, 5 in one eye, with categories 1 or 2 in the other eye.

    H54.10 Blindness, one eye, low vision other eye, unspecified eyes
    H54.11 Blindness, right eye, low vision left eye
    H54.12 Blindness, left eye, low vision right eye

H54.2 Low vision, both eyes
> Visual impairment categories 1 or 2 in both eyes.

H54.3 Unqualified visual loss, both eyes
> Visual impairment category 9 in both eyes.

✓5ᵗʰ H54.4 Blindness, one eye
> Visual impairment categories 3, 4, 5 in one eye [normal vision in other eye]

    H54.40 Blindness, one eye, unspecified eye
    H54.41 Blindness, right eye, normal vision left eye
    H54.42 Blindness, left eye, normal vision right eye

✓5ᵗʰ H54.5 Low vision, one eye
> Visual impairment categories 1 or 2 in one eye [normal vision in other eye].

    H54.50 Low vision, one eye, unspecified eye
    H54.51 Low vision, right eye, normal vision left eye
    H54.52 Low vision, left eye, normal vision right eye

✓5ᵗʰ H54.6 Unqualified visual loss, one eye
> Visual impairment category 9 in one eye [normal vision in other eye].

    H54.60 Unqualified visual loss, one eye, unspecified
    H54.61 Unqualified visual loss, right eye, normal vision left eye
    H54.62 Unqualified visual loss, left eye, normal vision right eye

H54.7 Unspecified visual loss
> Visual impairment category 9 NOS

H54.8 Legal blindness, as defined in USA
> Blindness NOS according to USA definition
> EXCLUDES 1 *legal blindness with specification of impairment level (H54.0-H54.7)*

> NOTE The following table gives a classification of severity of visual impairment recommended by a WHO Study Group on the Prevention of Blindness, Geneva, 6-10 November l972.
>
> The term "low vision" in category H54 comprises categories 1 and 2 of the table, the term "blindness" categories 3, 4 and 5, and the term "unqualified visual loss" category 9.
>
> If the extent of the visual field is taken into account, patients with a field no greater than 10 but greater than 5 around central fixation should be placed in category 3 and patients with a field no greater than 5 around central fixation should be placed in 4, even if the central acuity is not impaired.

Category of visual impairment	Visual acuity with best possible correction	
	Maximum less than:	**Minimum equal to or better than:**
1	6/18 3/10 (0.3) 20/70	6/60 1/10 (0.1) 20/200
2	6/60 1/10 (0.1) 20/200	3/60 1/20 (0.5) 20/400
3	3/60 1/20 (0.05) 20/400	1/60 (finger counting at one meter) 1/50 (0.02) 5/300 (20/1200)
4	1/60 (finger counting at one meter) 1/50 (0.02) 5/300	Light perception
5	No light perception	
9	Undetermined or unspecified	

Other disorders of eye and adnexa (H55-H59)

✓4ᵗʰ H55 Nystagmus and other irregular eye movements
  ✓5ᵗʰ H55.0 Nystagmus
    H55.00 Unspecified nystagmus
    H55.01 Congenital nystagmus
    H55.02 Latent nystagmus
    H55.03 Visual deprivation nystagmus
    H55.04 Dissociated nystagmus
    H55.09 Other forms of nystagmus

  ✓5ᵗʰ H55.8 Other irregular eye movements
    H55.81 Saccadic eye movements
    H55.89 Other irregular eye movements

✓4ᵗʰ H57 Other disorders of eye and adnexa
  ✓5ᵗʰ H57.0 Anomalies of pupillary function
    H57.00 Unspecified anomaly of pupillary function
    H57.01 Argyll Robertson pupil, atypical
> EXCLUDES 1 *syphilitic Argyll Robertson pupil (A52.19)*

    H57.02 Anisocoria
    H57.03 Miosis
    H57.04 Mydriasis
  ✓6ᵗʰ H57.05 Tonic pupil
    H57.051 Tonic pupil, right eye
    H57.052 Tonic pupil, left eye
    H57.053 Tonic pupil, bilateral
    H57.059 Tonic pupil, unspecified eye
    H57.09 Other anomalies of pupillary function

  ✓5ᵗʰ H57.1 Ocular pain
    H57.10 Ocular pain, unspecified eye
    H57.11 Ocular pain, right eye
    H57.12 Ocular pain, left eye
    H57.13 Ocular pain, bilateral

H57.8 Other specified disorders of eye and adnexa
H57.9 Unspecified disorder of eye and adnexa

✓4ᵗʰ H59 Intraoperative and postprocedural complications and disorders of eye and adnexa, not elsewhere classified
> EXCLUDES 1 *mechanical complication of intraocular lens (T85.2)*
> *mechanical complication of other ocular prosthetic devices, implants and grafts (T85.3)*
> *pseudophakia (Z96.1)*
> *secondary cataracts (H26.4-)*

  ✓5ᵗʰ H59.0 Disorders of the eye following cataract surgery
  ✓6ᵗʰ H59.01 Keratopathy (bullous aphakic) following cataract surgery
> Vitreal corneal syndrome
> Vitreous (touch) syndrome

    H59.011 Keratopathy (bullous aphakic) following cataract surgery, right eye
    H59.012 Keratopathy (bullous aphakic) following cataract surgery, left eye

EXCLUDES 1 Not coded here   EXCLUDES 2 Not included here   N Newborn Age: 0   P Pediatric Age: 0-17   M Maternity Age: 12-55   A Adult Age: 15-124

570   ICD-10-CM 2016

H59.013 **Keratopathy (bullous aphakic) following cataract surgery, bilateral**

H59.019 **Keratopathy (bullous aphakic) following cataract surgery, unspecified eye**

✓6ᵗʰ **H59.02** Cataract **(lens) fragments** in eye following cataract surgery

H59.021 **Cataract (lens) fragments in eye following cataract surgery, right eye**

H59.022 **Cataract (lens) fragments in eye following cataract surgery, left eye**

H59.023 **Cataract (lens) fragments in eye following cataract surgery, bilateral**

H59.029 **Cataract (lens) fragments in eye following cataract surgery, unspecified eye**

✓6ᵗʰ **H59.03** Cystoid macular edema **following cataract surgery**

H59.031 **Cystoid macular edema following cataract surgery, right eye**

H59.032 **Cystoid macular edema following cataract surgery, left eye**

H59.033 **Cystoid macular edema following cataract surgery, bilateral**

H59.039 **Cystoid macular edema following cataract surgery, unspecified eye**

✓6ᵗʰ **H59.09** Other disorders of the eye following cataract surgery

H59.091 **Other disorders of the right eye following cataract surgery**

H59.092 **Other disorders of the left eye following cataract surgery**

H59.093 **Other disorders of the eye following cataract surgery, bilateral**

H59.099 **Other disorders of unspecified eye following cataract surgery**

✓5ᵗʰ **H59.1** Intraoperative hemorrhage and hematoma **of eye and adnexa complicating a procedure**

> EXCLUDES 1 *intraoperative hemorrhage and hematoma of eye and adnexa due to accidental puncture or laceration during a procedure (H59.2-)*

✓6ᵗʰ **H59.11** Intraoperative hemorrhage and hematoma of eye and adnexa complicating an ophthalmic procedure

H59.111 **Intraoperative hemorrhage and hematoma of right eye and adnexa complicating an ophthalmic procedure**

H59.112 **Intraoperative hemorrhage and hematoma of left eye and adnexa complicating an ophthalmic procedure**

H59.113 **Intraoperative hemorrhage and hematoma of eye and adnexa complicating an ophthalmic procedure, bilateral**

H59.119 **Intraoperative hemorrhage and hematoma of unspecified eye and adnexa complicating an ophthalmic procedure**

✓6ᵗʰ **H59.12** Intraoperative hemorrhage and hematoma of eye and adnexa complicating other procedure

H59.121 **Intraoperative hemorrhage and hematoma of right eye and adnexa complicating other procedure**

H59.122 **Intraoperative hemorrhage and hematoma of left eye and adnexa complicating other procedure**

H59.123 **Intraoperative hemorrhage and hematoma of eye and adnexa complicating other procedure, bilateral**

H59.129 **Intraoperative hemorrhage and hematoma of unspecified eye and adnexa complicating other procedure**

✓5ᵗʰ **H59.2** Accidental puncture and laceration **of eye and adnexa during a procedure**

✓6ᵗʰ **H59.21** Accidental puncture and laceration of eye and adnexa during an ophthalmic procedure

H59.211 **Accidental puncture and laceration of right eye and adnexa during an ophthalmic procedure**

H59.212 **Accidental puncture and laceration of left eye and adnexa during an ophthalmic procedure**

H59.213 **Accidental puncture and laceration of eye and adnexa during an ophthalmic procedure, bilateral**

H59.219 **Accidental puncture and laceration of unspecified eye and adnexa during an ophthalmic procedure**

✓6ᵗʰ **H59.22** Accidental puncture and laceration of eye and adnexa during other procedure

H59.221 **Accidental puncture and laceration of right eye and adnexa during other procedure**

H59.222 **Accidental puncture and laceration of left eye and adnexa during other procedure**

H59.223 **Accidental puncture and laceration of eye and adnexa during other procedure, bilateral**

H59.229 **Accidental puncture and laceration of unspecified eye and adnexa during other procedure**

✓5ᵗʰ **H59.3** Postprocedural hemorrhage and hematoma **of eye and adnexa following a procedure**

✓6ᵗʰ **H59.31** Postprocedural hemorrhage and hematoma of eye and adnexa following an ophthalmic procedure

H59.311 **Postprocedural hemorrhage and hematoma of right eye and adnexa following an ophthalmic procedure**

H59.312 **Postprocedural hemorrhage and hematoma of left eye and adnexa following an ophthalmic procedure**

H59.313 **Postprocedural hemorrhage and hematoma of eye and adnexa following an ophthalmic procedure, bilateral**

H59.319 **Postprocedural hemorrhage and hematoma of unspecified eye and adnexa following an ophthalmic procedure**

✓6ᵗʰ **H59.32** Postprocedural hemorrhage and hematoma of eye and adnexa following other procedure

H59.321 **Postprocedural hemorrhage and hematoma of right eye and adnexa following other procedure**

H59.322 **Postprocedural hemorrhage and hematoma of left eye and adnexa following other procedure**

H59.323 **Postprocedural hemorrhage and hematoma of eye and adnexa following other procedure, bilateral**

H59.329 **Postprocedural hemorrhage and hematoma of unspecified eye and adnexa following other procedure**

✓5ᵗʰ **H59.4** Inflammation (infection) of postprocedural bleb
Postprocedural blebitis

> EXCLUDES 1 *filtering (vitreous) bleb after glaucoma surgery status (Z98.83)*

H59.40 **Inflammation (infection) of postprocedural bleb, unspecified**

H59.41 **Inflammation (infection) of postprocedural bleb, stage 1**

H59.42 **Inflammation (infection) of postprocedural bleb, stage 2**

H59.43 **Inflammation (infection) of postprocedural bleb, stage 3**
Bleb endophthalmitis

✓5ᵗʰ **H59.8** Other intraoperative and postprocedural complications and disorders of eye and adnexa, not elsewhere classified

✓6ᵗʰ **H59.81** Chorioretinal scars after surgery for detachment

H59.811 **Chorioretinal scars after surgery for detachment, right eye**

H59.812 **Chorioretinal scars after surgery for detachment, left eye**

H59.813 **Chorioretinal scars after surgery for detachment, bilateral**

H59.819 **Chorioretinal scars after surgery for detachment, unspecified eye**

H59.88 **Other intraoperative complications of eye and adnexa, not elsewhere classified**

H59.89 **Other postprocedural complications and disorders of eye and adnexa, not elsewhere classified**

☑ Additional Character Required   ✓x7ᵗʰ Placeholder Alert   Unspecified Dx   Other Specified Dx   Manifestation   ▶◀ Revised Text   ● New Code   ▲ Revised Code Title

Chapter 8. Diseases of the Ear and Mastoid Process (H60–H95)

Chapter Specific Coding Guidelines and Examples
Reserved for future guideline expansion.

Chapter 8. Diseases of the Ear and Mastoid Process (H60-H95)

NOTE Use an external cause code following the code for the ear condition, if applicable, to identify the cause of the ear condition.

EXCLUDES 2 *certain conditions originating in the perinatal period (P04-P96)*
certain infectious and parasitic diseases (A00-B99)
complications of pregnancy, childbirth and the puerperium (O00-O9A)
congenital malformations, deformations and chromosomal abnormalities (Q00-Q99)
endocrine, nutritional and metabolic diseases (E00-E88)
injury, poisoning and certain other consequences of external causes (S00-T88)
neoplasms (C00-D49)
symptoms, signs and abnormal clinical and laboratory findings, not elsewhere classified (R00-R94)

This chapter contains the following blocks:

H60-H62   Diseases of external ear
H65-H75   Diseases of middle ear and mastoid
H80-H83   Diseases of inner ear
H90-H94   Other disorders of ear
H95   Intraoperative and postprocedural complications and disorders of ear and mastoid process, not elsewhere classified

Diseases of external ear (H60-H62)

✓4ᵗʰ **H60**   **Otitis externa**

   ✓5ᵗʰ **H60.0**   Abscess of external ear
         Boil of external ear
         Carbuncle of auricle or external auditory canal
         Furuncle of external ear
       H60.00   **Abscess of external ear, unspecified ear**
       H60.01   **Abscess of right external ear**
       H60.02   **Abscess of left external ear**
       H60.03   **Abscess of external ear, bilateral**

   ✓5ᵗʰ **H60.1**   Cellulitis of external ear
         Cellulitis of auricle
         Cellulitis of external auditory canal
       H60.10   **Cellulitis of external ear, unspecified ear**
       H60.11   **Cellulitis of right external ear**
       H60.12   **Cellulitis of left external ear**
       H60.13   **Cellulitis of external ear, bilateral**

   ✓5ᵗʰ **H60.2**   Malignant otitis externa
       H60.20   **Malignant otitis externa, unspecified ear**
       H60.21   **Malignant otitis externa, right ear**
       H60.22   **Malignant otitis externa, left ear**
       H60.23   **Malignant otitis externa, bilateral**

   ✓5ᵗʰ **H60.3**   Other infective otitis externa
      ✓6ᵗʰ **H60.31**   Diffuse otitis externa
         H60.311   **Diffuse otitis externa, right ear**
         H60.312   **Diffuse otitis externa, left ear**
         H60.313   **Diffuse otitis externa, bilateral**
         H60.319   **Diffuse otitis externa, unspecified ear**
      ✓6ᵗʰ **H60.32**   Hemorrhagic otitis externa
         H60.321   **Hemorrhagic otitis externa, right ear**
         H60.322   **Hemorrhagic otitis externa, left ear**
         H60.323   **Hemorrhagic otitis externa, bilateral**
         H60.329   **Hemorrhagic otitis externa, unspecified ear**
      ✓6ᵗʰ **H60.33**   Swimmer's ear
         H60.331   **Swimmer's ear, right ear**
         H60.332   **Swimmer's ear, left ear**
         H60.333   **Swimmer's ear, bilateral**
         H60.339   **Swimmer's ear, unspecified ear**
      ✓6ᵗʰ **H60.39**   Other infective otitis externa
         H60.391   **Other infective otitis externa, right ear**
         H60.392   **Other infective otitis externa, left ear**
         H60.393   **Other infective otitis externa, bilateral**
         H60.399   **Other infective otitis externa, unspecified ear**

   ✓5ᵗʰ **H60.4**   Cholesteatoma of external ear
         Keratosis obturans of external ear (canal)
         EXCLUDES 2 *cholesteatoma of middle ear (H71.-)*
                 recurrent cholesteatoma of postmastoidectomy cavity (H95.0-)
       H60.40   **Cholesteatoma of external ear, unspecified ear**

       H60.41   **Cholesteatoma of right external ear**
       H60.42   **Cholesteatoma of left external ear**
       H60.43   **Cholesteatoma of external ear, bilateral**

   ✓5ᵗʰ **H60.5**   Acute noninfective otitis externa
      ✓6ᵗʰ **H60.50**   Unspecified acute noninfective otitis externa
                 Acute otitis externa NOS
         H60.501   **Unspecified acute noninfective otitis externa, right ear**
         H60.502   **Unspecified acute noninfective otitis externa, left ear**
         H60.503   **Unspecified acute noninfective otitis externa, bilateral**
         H60.509   **Unspecified acute noninfective otitis externa, unspecified ear**
      ✓6ᵗʰ **H60.51**   Acute actinic otitis externa
         H60.511   **Acute actinic otitis externa, right ear**
         H60.512   **Acute actinic otitis externa, left ear**
         H60.513   **Acute actinic otitis externa, bilateral**
         H60.519   **Acute actinic otitis externa, unspecified ear**
      ✓6ᵗʰ **H60.52**   Acute chemical otitis externa
         H60.521   **Acute chemical otitis externa, right ear**
         H60.522   **Acute chemical otitis externa, left ear**
         H60.523   **Acute chemical otitis externa, bilateral**
         H60.529   **Acute chemical otitis externa, unspecified ear**
      ✓6ᵗʰ **H60.53**   Acute contact otitis externa
         H60.531   **Acute contact otitis externa, right ear**
         H60.532   **Acute contact otitis externa, left ear**
         H60.533   **Acute contact otitis externa, bilateral**
         H60.539   **Acute contact otitis externa, unspecified ear**
      ✓6ᵗʰ **H60.54**   Acute eczematoid otitis externa
         H60.541   **Acute eczematoid otitis externa, right ear**
         H60.542   **Acute eczematoid otitis externa, left ear**
         H60.543   **Acute eczematoid otitis externa, bilateral**
         H60.549   **Acute eczematoid otitis externa, unspecified ear**
      ✓6ᵗʰ **H60.55**   Acute reactive otitis externa
         H60.551   **Acute reactive otitis externa, right ear**
         H60.552   **Acute reactive otitis externa, left ear**
         H60.553   **Acute reactive otitis externa, bilateral**
         H60.559   **Acute reactive otitis externa, unspecified ear**
      ✓6ᵗʰ **H60.59**   Other noninfective acute otitis externa
         H60.591   **Other noninfective acute otitis externa, right ear**
         H60.592   **Other noninfective acute otitis externa, left ear**
         H60.593   **Other noninfective acute otitis externa, bilateral**
         H60.599   **Other noninfective acute otitis externa, unspecified ear**

   ✓5ᵗʰ **H60.6**   Unspecified chronic otitis externa
       H60.60   **Unspecified chronic otitis externa, unspecified ear**
       H60.61   **Unspecified chronic otitis externa, right ear**
       H60.62   **Unspecified chronic otitis externa, left ear**
       H60.63   **Unspecified chronic otitis externa, bilateral**

   ✓5ᵗʰ **H60.8**   Other otitis externa
      ✓6ᵗʰ **H60.8X**   Other otitis externa
         H60.8X1   **Other otitis externa, right ear**
         H60.8X2   **Other otitis externa, left ear**
         H60.8X3   **Other otitis externa, bilateral**
         H60.8X9   **Other otitis externa, unspecified ear**

   ✓5ᵗʰ **H60.9**   Unspecified otitis externa
       H60.90   **Unspecified otitis externa, unspecified ear**
       H60.91   **Unspecified otitis externa, right ear**
       H60.92   **Unspecified otitis externa, left ear**
       H60.93   **Unspecified otitis externa, bilateral**

✓ Additional Character Required   ✓x7ᵗʰ Placeholder Alert   Unspecified Dx   Other Specified Dx   Manifestation   ▶◀ Revised Text   ● New Code   ▲ Revised Code Title

✓4ᵗʰ **H61** **Other disorders of external ear**

✓5ᵗʰ **H61.0** **Chondritis and perichondritis of external ear**
Chondrodermatitis nodularis chronica helicis
Perichondritis of auricle
Perichondritis of pinna

✓6ᵗʰ **H61.00** **Unspecified perichondritis of external ear**
H61.001 **Unspecified perichondritis of right external ear**
H61.002 **Unspecified perichondritis of left external ear**
H61.003 **Unspecified perichondritis of external ear, bilateral**
H61.009 **Unspecified perichondritis of external ear, unspecified ear**

✓6ᵗʰ **H61.01** **Acute perichondritis of external ear**
H61.011 **Acute perichondritis of right external ear**
H61.012 **Acute perichondritis of left external ear**
H61.013 **Acute perichondritis of external ear, bilateral**
H61.019 **Acute perichondritis of external ear, unspecified ear**

✓6ᵗʰ **H61.02** **Chronic perichondritis of external ear**
H61.021 **Chronic perichondritis of right external ear**
H61.022 **Chronic perichondritis of left external ear**
H61.023 **Chronic perichondritis of external ear, bilateral**
H61.029 **Chronic perichondritis of external ear, unspecified ear**

✓6ᵗʰ **H61.03** **Chondritis of external ear**
Chondritis of auricle
Chondritis of pinna
AHA: 2015, 1Q, 18
H61.031 **Chondritis of right external ear**
H61.032 **Chondritis of left external ear**
H61.033 **Chondritis of external ear, bilateral**
H61.039 **Chondritis of external ear, unspecified ear**

✓5ᵗʰ **H61.1** **Noninfective disorders of pinna**
EXCLUDES 2 *cauliflower ear (M95.1-)*
gouty tophi of ear (M1A.-)

✓6ᵗʰ **H61.10** **Unspecified noninfective disorders of pinna**
Disorder of pinna NOS
H61.101 **Unspecified noninfective disorders of pinna, right ear**
H61.102 **Unspecified noninfective disorders of pinna, left ear**
H61.103 **Unspecified noninfective disorders of pinna, bilateral**
H61.109 **Unspecified noninfective disorders of pinna, unspecified ear**

✓6ᵗʰ **H61.11** **Acquired deformity of pinna**
Acquired deformity of auricle
EXCLUDES 2 *cauliflower ear (M95.1-)*
H61.111 **Acquired deformity of pinna, right ear**
H61.112 **Acquired deformity of pinna, left ear**
H61.113 **Acquired deformity of pinna, bilateral**
H61.119 **Acquired deformity of pinna, unspecified ear**

✓6ᵗʰ **H61.12** **Hematoma of pinna**
Hematoma of auricle
H61.121 **Hematoma of pinna, right ear**
H61.122 **Hematoma of pinna, left ear**
H61.123 **Hematoma of pinna, bilateral**
H61.129 **Hematoma of pinna, unspecified ear**

✓6ᵗʰ **H61.19** **Other noninfective disorders of pinna**
H61.191 **Noninfective disorders of pinna, right ear**
H61.192 **Noninfective disorders of pinna, left ear**
H61.193 **Noninfective disorders of pinna, bilateral**
H61.199 **Noninfective disorders of pinna, unspecified ear**

✓5ᵗʰ **H61.2** **Impacted cerumen**
Wax in ear
H61.20 **Impacted cerumen, unspecified ear**
H61.21 **Impacted cerumen, right ear**
H61.22 **Impacted cerumen, left ear**
H61.23 **Impacted cerumen, bilateral**

✓5ᵗʰ **H61.3** **Acquired stenosis of external ear canal**
Collapse of external ear canal
EXCLUDES 1 *postprocedural stenosis of external ear canal (H95.81-)*

✓6ᵗʰ **H61.30** **Acquired stenosis of external ear canal, unspecified**
H61.301 **Acquired stenosis of right external ear canal, unspecified**
H61.302 **Acquired stenosis of left external ear canal, unspecified**
H61.303 **Acquired stenosis of external ear canal, unspecified, bilateral**
H61.309 **Acquired stenosis of external ear canal, unspecified, unspecified ear**

✓6ᵗʰ **H61.31** **Acquired stenosis of external ear canal secondary to trauma**
H61.311 **Acquired stenosis of right external ear canal secondary to trauma**
H61.312 **Acquired stenosis of left external ear canal secondary to trauma**
H61.313 **Acquired stenosis of external ear canal secondary to trauma, bilateral**
H61.319 **Acquired stenosis of external ear canal secondary to trauma, unspecified ear**

✓6ᵗʰ **H61.32** **Acquired stenosis of external ear canal secondary to inflammation and infection**
H61.321 **Acquired stenosis of right external ear canal secondary to inflammation and infection**
H61.322 **Acquired stenosis of left external ear canal secondary to inflammation and infection**
H61.323 **Acquired stenosis of external ear canal secondary to inflammation and infection, bilateral**
H61.329 **Acquired stenosis of external ear canal secondary to inflammation and infection, unspecified ear**

✓6ᵗʰ **H61.39** **Other acquired stenosis of external ear canal**
H61.391 **Other acquired stenosis of right external ear canal**
H61.392 **Other acquired stenosis of left external ear canal**
H61.393 **Other acquired stenosis of external ear canal, bilateral**
H61.399 **Other acquired stenosis of external ear canal, unspecified ear**

✓5ᵗʰ **H61.8** **Other specified disorders of external ear**

✓6ᵗʰ **H61.81** **Exostosis of external canal**
H61.811 **Exostosis of right external canal**
H61.812 **Exostosis of left external canal**
H61.813 **Exostosis of external canal, bilateral**
H61.819 **Exostosis of external canal, unspecified ear**

✓6ᵗʰ **H61.89** **Other specified disorders of external ear**
H61.891 **Other specified disorders of right external ear**
H61.892 **Other specified disorders of left external ear**
H61.893 **Other specified disorders of external ear, bilateral**
H61.899 **Other specified disorders of external ear, unspecified ear**

✓5ᵗʰ **H61.9** **Disorder of external ear, unspecified**
H61.90 **Disorder of external ear, unspecified, unspecified ear**
H61.91 **Disorder of right external ear, unspecified**
H61.92 **Disorder of left external ear, unspecified**
H61.93 **Disorder of external ear, unspecified, bilateral**

✓4ᵗʰ **H62** **Disorders of external ear in diseases classified elsewhere**

✓5ᵗʰ **H62.4** **Otitis externa in other diseases classified elsewhere**
Code first underlying disease, such as:
erysipelas (A46)
impetigo (L01.0)
EXCLUDES 1 *otitis externa (in):*
candidiasis (B37.84)
herpes viral [herpes simplex] (B00.1)
herpes zoster (B02.8)

H62.40 *Otitis externa in other diseases classified elsewhere, unspecified ear*

EXCLUDES 1 Not coded here   EXCLUDES 2 Not included here   N Newborn Age: 0   P Pediatric Age: 0-17   M Maternity Age: 12-55   A Adult Age: 15-124

574   ICD-10-CM 2016

H62.41 *Otitis externa in other diseases classified elsewhere, right ear*

H62.42 *Otitis externa in other diseases classified elsewhere, left ear*

H62.43 *Otitis externa in other diseases classified elsewhere, bilateral*

✓5ᵗʰ **H62.8 Other disorders of external ear in diseases classified elsewhere**

Code first underlying disease, such as:
gout (M1A.-, M10.-)

✓6ᵗʰ **H62.8X Other disorders of external ear in diseases classified elsewhere**

H62.8X1 *Other disorders of right external ear in diseases classified elsewhere*

H62.8X2 *Other disorders of left external ear in diseases classified elsewhere*

H62.8X3 *Other disorders of external ear in diseases classified elsewhere, bilateral*

H62.8X9 *Other disorders of external ear in diseases classified elsewhere, unspecified ear*

Diseases of middle ear and mastoid (H65-H75)

✓4ᵗʰ **H65 Nonsuppurative otitis media**

INCLUDES nonsuppurative otitis media with myringitis

Use additional code for any associated perforated tympanic membrane (H72.-)

Use additional code to identify:
exposure to environmental tobacco smoke (Z77.22)
exposure to tobacco smoke in the perinatal period (P96.81)
history of tobacco use (Z87.891)
occupational exposure to environmental tobacco smoke (Z57.31)
tobacco dependence (F17.-)
tobacco use (Z72.0)

✓5ᵗʰ **H65.0 Acute serous otitis media**

Acute and subacute secretory otitis

H65.00 Acute serous otitis media, unspecified ear

H65.01 Acute serous otitis media, right ear

H65.02 Acute serous otitis media, left ear

H65.03 Acute serous otitis media, bilateral

H65.04 Acute serous otitis media, recurrent, right ear

H65.05 Acute serous otitis media, recurrent, left ear

H65.06 Acute serous otitis media, recurrent, bilateral

H65.07 Acute serous otitis media, recurrent, unspecified ear

✓5ᵗʰ **H65.1 Other acute nonsuppurative otitis media**

EXCLUDES 1 *otitic barotrauma (T70.0)*
otitis media (acute) NOS (H66.9)

✓6ᵗʰ **H65.11 Acute and subacute allergic otitis media (mucoid) (sanguinous) (serous)**

H65.111 Acute and subacute allergic otitis media (mucoid) (sanguinous) (serous), right ear

H65.112 Acute and subacute allergic otitis media (mucoid) (sanguinous) (serous), left ear

H65.113 Acute and subacute allergic otitis media (mucoid) (sanguinous) (serous), bilateral

H65.114 Acute and subacute allergic otitis media (mucoid) (sanguinous) (serous), recurrent, right ear

H65.115 Acute and subacute allergic otitis media (mucoid) (sanguinous) (serous), recurrent, left ear

H65.116 Acute and subacute allergic otitis media (mucoid) (sanguinous) (serous), recurrent, bilateral

H65.117 Acute and subacute allergic otitis media (mucoid) (sanguinous) (serous), recurrent, unspecified ear

H65.119 Acute and subacute allergic otitis media (mucoid) (sanguinous) (serous), unspecified ear

✓6ᵗʰ **H65.19 Other acute nonsuppurative otitis media**

Acute and subacute mucoid otitis media
Acute and subacute nonsuppurative otitis media NOS
Acute and subacute sanguinous otitis media
Acute and subacute seromucinous otitis media

H65.191 Other acute nonsuppurative otitis media, right ear

H65.192 Other acute nonsuppurative otitis media, left ear

H65.193 Other acute nonsuppurative otitis media, bilateral

H65.194 Other acute nonsuppurative otitis media, recurrent, right ear

H65.195 Other acute nonsuppurative otitis media, recurrent, left ear

H65.196 Other acute nonsuppurative otitis media, recurrent, bilateral

H65.197 Other acute nonsuppurative otitis media recurrent, unspecified ear

H65.199 Other acute nonsuppurative otitis media, unspecified ear

✓5ᵗʰ **H65.2 Chronic serous otitis media**

Chronic tubotympanal catarrh

H65.20 Chronic serous otitis media, unspecified ear

H65.21 Chronic serous otitis media, right ear

H65.22 Chronic serous otitis media, left ear

H65.23 Chronic serous otitis media, bilateral

✓5ᵗʰ **H65.3 Chronic mucoid otitis media**

Chronic mucinous otitis media
Chronic secretory otitis media
Glue ear
Chronic transudative otitis media
EXCLUDES 1 *adhesive middle ear disease (H74.1)*

H65.30 Chronic mucoid otitis media, unspecified ear

H65.31 Chronic mucoid otitis media, right ear

H65.32 Chronic mucoid otitis media, left ear

H65.33 Chronic mucoid otitis media, bilateral

✓5ᵗʰ **H65.4 Other chronic nonsuppurative otitis media**

✓6ᵗʰ **H65.41 Chronic allergic otitis media**

H65.411 Chronic allergic otitis media, right ear

H65.412 Chronic allergic otitis media, left ear

H65.413 Chronic allergic otitis media, bilateral

H65.419 Chronic allergic otitis media, unspecified ear

✓6ᵗʰ **H65.49 Other chronic nonsuppurative otitis media**

Chronic exudative otitis media
Chronic nonsuppurative otitis media NOS
Chronic otitis media with effusion (nonpurulent)
Chronic seromucinous otitis media

H65.491 Other chronic nonsuppurative otitis media, right ear

H65.492 Other chronic nonsuppurative otitis media, left ear

H65.493 Other chronic nonsuppurative otitis media, bilateral

H65.499 Other chronic nonsuppurative otitis media, unspecified ear

✓5ᵗʰ **H65.9 Unspecified nonsuppurative otitis media**

Allergic otitis media NOS
Catarrhal otitis media NOS
Exudative otitis media NOS
Mucoid otitis media NOS
Otitis media with effusion (nonpurulent) NOS
Secretory otitis media NOS
Seromucinous otitis media NOS
Serous otitis media NOS
Transudative otitis media NOS

H65.90 Unspecified nonsuppurative otitis media, unspecified ear

H65.91 Unspecified nonsuppurative otitis media, right ear

H65.92 Unspecified nonsuppurative otitis media, left ear

H65.93 Unspecified nonsuppurative otitis media, bilateral

✓4ᵗʰ **H66 Suppurative and unspecified otitis media**

INCLUDES suppurative and unspecified otitis media with myringitis
Use additional code to identify:
exposure to environmental tobacco smoke (Z77.22)
exposure to tobacco smoke in the perinatal period (P96.81)
history of tobacco use (Z87.891)
occupational exposure to environmental tobacco smoke (Z57.31)
tobacco dependence (F17.-)
tobacco use (Z72.0)

✓5ᵗʰ **H66.0 Acute suppurative otitis media**

✓6ᵗʰ **H66.00 Acute suppurative otitis media without spontaneous rupture of ear drum**

H66.001 Acute suppurative otitis media without spontaneous rupture of ear drum, right ear

☑ Additional Character Required   ✓ʇᵗʰ Placeholder Alert   Unspecified Dx   Other Specified Dx   Manifestation   ▶◀ Revised Text   ● New Code   ▲ Revised Code Title

ICD-10-CM 2016   575

H66.002   **Acute suppurative otitis media without spontaneous rupture of ear drum, left ear**

H66.003   **Acute suppurative otitis media without spontaneous rupture of ear drum, bilateral**

H66.004   **Acute suppurative otitis media without spontaneous rupture of ear drum, recurrent, right ear**

H66.005   **Acute suppurative otitis media without spontaneous rupture of ear drum, recurrent, left ear**

H66.006   **Acute suppurative otitis media without spontaneous rupture of ear drum, recurrent, bilateral**

H66.007   **Acute suppurative otitis media without spontaneous rupture of ear drum, recurrent, unspecified ear**

H66.009   **Acute suppurative otitis media without spontaneous rupture of ear drum, unspecified ear**

✓6th **H66.01   Acute suppurative otitis media with spontaneous rupture of ear drum**

H66.011   **Acute suppurative otitis media with spontaneous rupture of ear drum, right ear**

H66.012   **Acute suppurative otitis media with spontaneous rupture of ear drum, left ear**

H66.013   **Acute suppurative otitis media with spontaneous rupture of ear drum, bilateral**

H66.014   **Acute suppurative otitis media with spontaneous rupture of ear drum, recurrent, right ear**

H66.015   **Acute suppurative otitis media with spontaneous rupture of ear drum, recurrent, left ear**

H66.016   **Acute suppurative otitis media with spontaneous rupture of ear drum, recurrent, bilateral**

H66.017   **Acute suppurative otitis media with spontaneous rupture of ear drum, recurrent, unspecified ear**

H66.019   **Acute suppurative otitis media with spontaneous rupture of ear drum, unspecified ear**

✓5th **H66.1   Chronic tubotympanic suppurative otitis media**
Benign chronic suppurative otitis media
Chronic tubotympanic disease
Use additional code for any associated perforated tympanic membrane (H72.-)

H66.10   **Chronic tubotympanic suppurative otitis media, unspecified**

H66.11   **Chronic tubotympanic suppurative otitis media, right ear**

H66.12   **Chronic tubotympanic suppurative otitis media, left ear**

H66.13   **Chronic tubotympanic suppurative otitis media, bilateral**

✓5th **H66.2   Chronic atticoantral suppurative otitis media**
Chronic atticoantral disease
Use additional code for any associated perforated tympanic membrane (H72.-)

H66.20   **Chronic atticoantral suppurative otitis media, unspecified ear**

H66.21   **Chronic atticoantral suppurative otitis media, right ear**

H66.22   **Chronic atticoantral suppurative otitis media, left ear**

H66.23   **Chronic atticoantral suppurative otitis media, bilateral**

✓5th **H66.3   Other chronic suppurative otitis media**
Chronic suppurative otitis media NOS
Use additional code for any associated perforated tympanic membrane (H72.-)
EXCLUDES 1   tuberculous otitis media (A18.6)

✓6th **H66.3X   Other chronic suppurative otitis media**

H66.3X1   **Other chronic suppurative otitis media, right ear**

H66.3X2   **Other chronic suppurative otitis media, left ear**

H66.3X3   **Other chronic suppurative otitis media, bilateral**

H66.3X9   **Other chronic suppurative otitis media, unspecified ear**

✓5th **H66.4   Suppurative otitis media, unspecified**
Purulent otitis media NOS
Use additional code for any associated perforated tympanic membrane (H72.-)

H66.40   **Suppurative otitis media, unspecified, unspecified ear**

H66.41   **Suppurative otitis media, unspecified, right ear**

H66.42   **Suppurative otitis media, unspecified, left ear**

H66.43   **Suppurative otitis media, unspecified, bilateral**

✓5th **H66.9   Otitis media, unspecified**
Otitis media NOS
Acute otitis media NOS
Chronic otitis media NOS
Use additional code for any associated perforated tympanic membrane (H72.-)

H66.90   **Otitis media, unspecified, unspecified ear**

H66.91   **Otitis media, unspecified, right ear**

H66.92   **Otitis media, unspecified, left ear**

H66.93   **Otitis media, unspecified, bilateral**

✓4th **H67   Otitis media in diseases classified elsewhere**
Code first underlying disease, such as:
viral disease NEC (B00-B34)
Use additional code for any associated perforated tympanic membrane (H72.-)
EXCLUDES 1   otitis media in:
    influenza (J09.X9, J10.83, J11.83)
    measles (B05.3)
    scarlet fever (A38.0)
    tuberculosis (A18.6)

H67.1   *Otitis media in diseases classified elsewhere, right ear*

H67.2   *Otitis media in diseases classified elsewhere, left ear*

H67.3   *Otitis media in diseases classified elsewhere, bilateral*

H67.9   *Otitis media in diseases classified elsewhere, unspecified ear*

✓4th **H68   Eustachian salpingitis and obstruction**

✓5th **H68.0   Eustachian salpingitis**

✓6th **H68.00   Unspecified Eustachian salpingitis**

H68.001   **Unspecified Eustachian salpingitis, right ear**

H68.002   **Unspecified Eustachian salpingitis, left ear**

H68.003   **Unspecified Eustachian salpingitis, bilateral**

H68.009   **Unspecified Eustachian salpingitis, unspecified ear**

✓6th **H68.01   Acute Eustachian salpingitis**

H68.011   **Acute Eustachian salpingitis, right ear**

H68.012   **Acute Eustachian salpingitis, left ear**

H68.013   **Acute Eustachian salpingitis, bilateral**

H68.019   **Acute Eustachian salpingitis, unspecified ear**

✓6th **H68.02   Chronic Eustachian salpingitis**

H68.021   **Chronic Eustachian salpingitis, right ear**

H68.022   **Chronic Eustachian salpingitis, left ear**

H68.023   **Chronic Eustachian salpingitis, bilateral**

H68.029   **Chronic Eustachian salpingitis, unspecified ear**

✓5th **H68.1   Obstruction of Eustachian tube**
Stenosis of Eustachian tube   Stricture of Eustachian tube

✓6th **H68.10   Unspecified obstruction of Eustachian tube**

H68.101   **Unspecified obstruction of Eustachian tube, right ear**

H68.102   **Unspecified obstruction of Eustachian tube, left ear**

H68.103   **Unspecified obstruction of Eustachian tube, bilateral**

H68.109   **Unspecified obstruction of Eustachian tube, unspecified ear**

✓6th **H68.11   Osseous obstruction of Eustachian tube**

H68.111   **Osseous obstruction of Eustachian tube, right ear**

H68.112   **Osseous obstruction of Eustachian tube, left ear**

EXCLUDES 1 Not coded here   *EXCLUDES 2* Not included here   N Newborn Age: 0   P Pediatric Age: 0-17   M Maternity Age: 12-55   A Adult Age: 15-124

576   ICD-10-CM 2016

H66.002–H68.112

H68.113　**Osseous obstruction of Eustachian tube,** bilateral

H68.119　**Osseous obstruction of Eustachian tube, unspecified ear**

✓6ᵗʰ　H68.12　Intrinsic cartilagenous **obstruction of Eustachian tube**

H68.121　**Intrinsic cartilagenous obstruction of Eustachian tube,** right ear

H68.122　**Intrinsic cartilagenous obstruction of Eustachian tube,** left ear

H68.123　**Intrinsic cartilagenous obstruction of Eustachian tube,** bilateral

H68.129　**Intrinsic cartilagenous obstruction of Eustachian tube, unspecified ear**

✓6ᵗʰ　H68.13　Extrinsic cartilagenous **obstruction of Eustachian tube**

Compression of Eustachian tube

H68.131　**Extrinsic cartilagenous obstruction of Eustachian tube,** right ear

H68.132　**Extrinsic cartilagenous obstruction of Eustachian tube,** left ear

H68.133　**Extrinsic cartilagenous obstruction of Eustachian tube,** bilateral

H68.139　**Extrinsic cartilagenous obstruction of Eustachian tube, unspecified ear**

✓4ᵗʰ　**H69　Other and unspecified disorders of Eustachian tube**

✓5ᵗʰ　H69.0　Patulous **Eustachian tube**

H69.00　**Patulous Eustachian tube, unspecified ear**

H69.01　**Patulous Eustachian tube,** right ear

H69.02　**Patulous Eustachian tube,** left ear

H69.03　**Patulous Eustachian tube,** bilateral

✓5ᵗʰ　H69.8　Other specified **disorders of Eustachian tube**

H69.80　**Other specified disorders of Eustachian tube, unspecified ear**

H69.81　**Other specified disorders of Eustachian tube,** right ear

H69.82　**Other specified disorders of Eustachian tube,** left ear

H69.83　**Other specified disorders of Eustachian tube,** bilateral

✓5ᵗʰ　H69.9　Unspecified **Eustachian tube disorder**

H69.90　**Unspecified Eustachian tube disorder, unspecified ear**

H69.91　**Unspecified Eustachian tube disorder,** right ear

H69.92　**Unspecified Eustachian tube disorder,** left ear

H69.93　**Unspecified Eustachian tube disorder,** bilateral

✓4ᵗʰ　**H70　Mastoiditis and related conditions**

✓5ᵗʰ　H70.0　Acute **mastoiditis**

Abscess of mastoid
Empyema of mastoid

✓6ᵗʰ　H70.00　**Acute mastoiditis** without complications

H70.001　**Acute mastoiditis without complications,** right ear

H70.002　**Acute mastoiditis without complications,** left ear

H70.003　**Acute mastoiditis without complications,** bilateral

H70.009　**Acute mastoiditis without complications, unspecified ear**

✓6ᵗʰ　H70.01　Subperiosteal abscess **of mastoid**

H70.011　**Subperiosteal abscess of mastoid,** right ear

H70.012　**Subperiosteal abscess of mastoid,** left ear

H70.013　**Subperiosteal abscess of mastoid,** bilateral

H70.019　**Subperiosteal abscess of mastoid, unspecified ear**

✓6ᵗʰ　H70.09　Acute **mastoiditis** with other complications

H70.091　**Acute mastoiditis with other complications,** right ear

H70.092　**Acute mastoiditis with other complications,** left ear

H70.093　**Acute mastoiditis with other complications,** bilateral

H70.099　**Acute mastoiditis with other complications, unspecified ear**

✓5ᵗʰ　H70.1　Chronic **mastoiditis**

Caries of mastoid
Fistula of mastoid

EXCLUDES 1　*tuberculous mastoiditis (A18.03)*

H70.10　**Chronic mastoiditis, unspecified ear**

H70.11　**Chronic mastoiditis,** right ear

H70.12　**Chronic mastoiditis,** left ear

H70.13　**Chronic mastoiditis,** bilateral

✓5ᵗʰ　H70.2　Petrositis

Inflammation of petrous bone

✓6ᵗʰ　H70.20　Unspecified **petrositis**

H70.201　**Unspecified petrositis,** right ear

H70.202　**Unspecified petrositis,** left ear

H70.203　**Unspecified petrositis,** bilateral

H70.209　**Unspecified petrositis, unspecified ear**

✓6ᵗʰ　H70.21　Acute **petrositis**

H70.211　**Acute petrositis,** right ear

H70.212　**Acute petrositis,** left ear

H70.213　**Acute petrositis,** bilateral

H70.219　**Acute petrositis, unspecified ear**

✓6ᵗʰ　H70.22　Chronic **petrositis**

H70.221　**Chronic petrositis,** right ear

H70.222　**Chronic petrositis,** left ear

H70.223　**Chronic petrositis,** bilateral

H70.229　**Chronic petrositis, unspecified ear**

✓5ᵗʰ　H70.8　**Other mastoiditis and related conditions**

EXCLUDES 1　*preauricular sinus and cyst (Q18.1)*
sinus, fistula, and cyst of branchial cleft (Q18.0)

✓6ᵗʰ　H70.81　Postauricular **fistula**

H70.811　**Postauricular fistula,** right ear

H70.812　**Postauricular fistula,** left ear

H70.813　**Postauricular fistula,** bilateral

H70.819　**Postauricular fistula, unspecified ear**

✓6ᵗʰ　H70.89　Other **mastoiditis and related conditions**

H70.891　**Other mastoiditis and related conditions,** right ear

H70.892　**Other mastoiditis and related conditions,** left ear

H70.893　**Other mastoiditis and related conditions,** bilateral

H70.899　**Other mastoiditis and related conditions, unspecified ear**

✓5ᵗʰ　H70.9　Unspecified **mastoiditis**

H70.90　**Unspecified mastoiditis, unspecified ear**

H70.91　**Unspecified mastoiditis,** right ear

H70.92　**Unspecified mastoiditis,** left ear

H70.93　**Unspecified mastoiditis,** bilateral

✓4ᵗʰ　**H71　Cholesteatoma of middle ear**

EXCLUDES 2　*cholesteatoma of external ear (H60.4-)*
recurrent cholesteatoma of postmastoidectomy cavity (H95.0-)

✓5ᵗʰ　H71.0　Cholesteatoma of attic

H71.00　**Cholesteatoma of attic, unspecified ear**

H71.01　**Cholesteatoma of attic,** right ear

H71.02　**Cholesteatoma of attic,** left ear

H71.03　**Cholesteatoma of attic,** bilateral

✓5ᵗʰ　H71.1　Cholesteatoma of tympanum

H71.10　**Cholesteatoma of tympanum, unspecified ear**

H71.11　**Cholesteatoma of tympanum,** right ear

H71.12　**Cholesteatoma of tympanum,** left ear

H71.13　**Cholesteatoma of tympanum,** bilateral

✓5ᵗʰ　H71.2　Cholesteatoma of mastoid

H71.20　**Cholesteatoma of mastoid, unspecified ear**

H71.21　**Cholesteatoma of mastoid,** right ear

H71.22　**Cholesteatoma of mastoid,** left ear

H71.23　**Cholesteatoma of mastoid,** bilateral

✓5ᵗʰ　H71.3　Diffuse cholesteatosis

H71.30　**Diffuse cholesteatosis, unspecified ear**

H71.31　**Diffuse cholesteatosis,** right ear

H71.32　**Diffuse cholesteatosis,** left ear

H71.33　**Diffuse cholesteatosis,** bilateral

✓ Additional Character Required　　✓x7ᵗʰ Placeholder Alert　　Unspecified Dx　　Other Specified Dx　　Manifestation　　►◄ Revised Text　　● New Code　　▲ Revised Code Title

✓5ᵗʰ **H71.9** Unspecified **cholesteatoma**

    H71.90 **Unspecified cholesteatoma, unspecified ear**

    H71.91 **Unspecified cholesteatoma, right ear**

    H71.92 **Unspecified cholesteatoma, left ear**

    H71.93 **Unspecified cholesteatoma, bilateral**

✓4ᵗʰ **H72** **Perforation of tympanic membrane**

    INCLUDES persistent post-traumatic perforation of ear drum
          postinflammatory perforation of ear drum

    Code first any associated otitis media (H65.-, H66.1-, H66.2-, H66.3-, H66.4-, H66.9-, H67.-)

    EXCLUDES 1 *acute suppurative otitis media with rupture of the tympanic membrane (H66.01-)*
            traumatic rupture of ear drum (S09.2-)

  ✓5ᵗʰ **H72.0** **Central** perforation of tympanic membrane

    H72.00 **Central perforation of tympanic membrane, unspecified ear**

    H72.01 **Central perforation of tympanic membrane, right ear**

    H72.02 **Central perforation of tympanic membrane, left ear**

    H72.03 **Central perforation of tympanic membrane, bilateral**

  ✓5ᵗʰ **H72.1** **Attic** perforation of tympanic membrane
    Perforation of pars flaccida

    H72.10 **Attic perforation of tympanic membrane, unspecified ear**

    H72.11 **Attic perforation of tympanic membrane, right ear**

    H72.12 **Attic perforation of tympanic membrane, left ear**

    H72.13 **Attic perforation of tympanic membrane, bilateral**

  ✓5ᵗʰ **H72.2** Other marginal perforations of tympanic membrane

    ✓6ᵗʰ **H72.2X** **Other marginal** perforations of tympanic membrane

      H72.2X1 **Other marginal perforations of tympanic membrane, right ear**

      H72.2X2 **Other marginal perforations of tympanic membrane, left ear**

      H72.2X3 **Other marginal perforations of tympanic membrane, bilateral**

      H72.2X9 **Other marginal perforations of tympanic membrane, unspecified ear**

  ✓5ᵗʰ **H72.8** **Other** perforations of tympanic membrane

    ✓6ᵗʰ **H72.81** **Multiple** perforations of tympanic membrane

      H72.811 **Multiple perforations of tympanic membrane, right ear**

      H72.812 **Multiple perforations of tympanic membrane, left ear**

      H72.813 **Multiple perforations of tympanic membrane, bilateral**

      H72.819 **Multiple perforations of tympanic membrane, unspecified ear**

    ✓6ᵗʰ **H72.82** **Total** perforations of tympanic membrane

      H72.821 **Total perforations of tympanic membrane, right ear**

      H72.822 **Total perforations of tympanic membrane, left ear**

      H72.823 **Total perforations of tympanic membrane, bilateral**

      H72.829 **Total perforations of tympanic membrane, unspecified ear**

  ✓5ᵗʰ **H72.9** Unspecified perforation of tympanic membrane

    H72.90 **Unspecified perforation of tympanic membrane, unspecified ear**

    H72.91 **Unspecified perforation of tympanic membrane, right ear**

    H72.92 **Unspecified perforation of tympanic membrane, left ear**

    H72.93 **Unspecified perforation of tympanic membrane, bilateral**

✓4ᵗʰ **H73** **Other disorders of tympanic membrane**

  ✓5ᵗʰ **H73.0** **Acute myringitis**

    EXCLUDES 1 *acute myringitis with otitis media (H65, H66)*

    ✓6ᵗʰ **H73.00** Unspecified **acute myringitis**
      Acute tympanitis NOS

      H73.001 **Acute myringitis, right ear**

      H73.002 **Acute myringitis, left ear**

      H73.003 **Acute myringitis, bilateral**

      H73.009 **Acute myringitis, unspecified ear**

    ✓6ᵗʰ **H73.01** **Bullous** myringitis

      H73.011 **Bullous myringitis, right ear**

      H73.012 **Bullous myringitis, left ear**

      H73.013 **Bullous myringitis, bilateral**

      H73.019 **Bullous myringitis, unspecified ear**

    ✓6ᵗʰ **H73.09** Other acute **myringitis**

      H73.091 **Other acute myringitis, right ear**

      H73.092 **Other acute myringitis, left ear**

      H73.093 **Other acute myringitis, bilateral**

      H73.099 **Other acute myringitis, unspecified ear**

  ✓5ᵗʰ **H73.1** Chronic **myringitis**
    Chronic tympanitis

    EXCLUDES 1 *chronic myringitis with otitis media (H65, H66)*

    H73.10 **Chronic myringitis, unspecified ear**

    H73.11 **Chronic myringitis, right ear**

    H73.12 **Chronic myringitis, left ear**

    H73.13 **Chronic myringitis, bilateral**

  ✓5ᵗʰ **H73.2** Unspecified **myringitis**

    H73.20 **Unspecified myringitis, unspecified ear**

    H73.21 **Unspecified myringitis, right ear**

    H73.22 **Unspecified myringitis, left ear**

    H73.23 **Unspecified myringitis, bilateral**

  ✓5ᵗʰ **H73.8** Other specified disorders of tympanic membrane

    ✓6ᵗʰ **H73.81** **Atrophic flaccid** tympanic membrane

      H73.811 **Atrophic flaccid tympanic membrane, right ear**

      H73.812 **Atrophic flaccid tympanic membrane, left ear**

      H73.813 **Atrophic flaccid tympanic membrane, bilateral**

      H73.819 **Atrophic flaccid tympanic membrane, unspecified ear**

    ✓6ᵗʰ **H73.82** **Atrophic nonflaccid** tympanic membrane

      H73.821 **Atrophic nonflaccid tympanic membrane, right ear**

      H73.822 **Atrophic nonflaccid tympanic membrane, left ear**

      H73.823 **Atrophic nonflaccid tympanic membrane, bilateral**

      H73.829 **Atrophic nonflaccid tympanic membrane, unspecified ear**

    ✓6ᵗʰ **H73.89** Other **specified** disorders of tympanic membrane

      H73.891 **Other specified disorders of tympanic membrane, right ear**

      H73.892 **Other specified disorders of tympanic membrane, left ear**

      H73.893 **Other specified disorders of tympanic membrane, bilateral**

      H73.899 **Other specified disorders of tympanic membrane, unspecified ear**

  ✓5ᵗʰ **H73.9** Unspecified disorder of tympanic membrane

    H73.90 **Unspecified disorder of tympanic membrane, unspecified ear**

    H73.91 **Unspecified disorder of tympanic membrane, right ear**

    H73.92 **Unspecified disorder of tympanic membrane, left ear**

    H73.93 **Unspecified disorder of tympanic membrane, bilateral**

✓4ᵗʰ **H74** **Other disorders of middle ear mastoid**

    EXCLUDES 2 *mastoiditis (H70.-)*

  ✓5ᵗʰ **H74.0** Tympanosclerosis

    H74.01 **Tympanosclerosis, right ear**

    H74.02 **Tympanosclerosis, left ear**

    H74.03 **Tympanosclerosis, bilateral**

    H74.09 **Tympanosclerosis, unspecified ear**

  ✓5ᵗʰ **H74.1** Adhesive middle ear disease
    Adhesive otitis

    EXCLUDES 1 *glue ear (H65.3-)*

    H74.11 **Adhesive right middle ear disease**

    H74.12 **Adhesive left middle ear disease**

    H74.13 **Adhesive middle ear disease, bilateral**

    H74.19 **Adhesive middle ear disease, unspecified ear**

EXCLUDES 1 Not coded here   EXCLUDES 2 Not included here   N Newborn Age: 0   P Pediatric Age: 0-17   M Maternity Age: 12-55   A Adult Age: 15-124

578   ICD-10-CM 2016

✓5ᵗʰ H74.2 Discontinuity and dislocation of ear ossicles
- **H74.20 Discontinuity and dislocation of ear ossicles, unspecified ear**
- **H74.21 Discontinuity and dislocation of right ear ossicles**
- **H74.22 Discontinuity and dislocation of left ear ossicles**
- **H74.23 Discontinuity and dislocation of ear ossicles, bilateral**

✓5ᵗʰ H74.3 Other acquired abnormalities of ear ossicles
- **✓6ᵗʰ H74.31 Ankylosis of ear ossicles**
  - **H74.311 Ankylosis of ear ossicles, right ear**
  - **H74.312 Ankylosis of ear ossicles, left ear**
  - **H74.313 Ankylosis of ear ossicles, bilateral**
  - **H74.319 Ankylosis of ear ossicles, unspecified ear**
- **✓6ᵗʰ H74.32 Partial loss of ear ossicles**
  - **H74.321 Partial loss of ear ossicles, right ear**
  - **H74.322 Partial loss of ear ossicles, left ear**
  - **H74.323 Partial loss of ear ossicles, bilateral**
  - **H74.329 Partial loss of ear ossicles, unspecified ear**
- **✓6ᵗʰ H74.39 Other acquired abnormalities of ear ossicles**
  - **H74.391 Other acquired abnormalities of right ear ossicles**
  - **H74.392 Other acquired abnormalities of left ear ossicles**
  - **H74.393 Other acquired abnormalities of ear ossicles, bilateral**
  - **H74.399 Other acquired abnormalities of ear ossicles, unspecified ear**

✓5ᵗʰ H74.4 Polyp of middle ear
- **H74.40 Polyp of middle ear, unspecified ear**
- **H74.41 Polyp of right middle ear**
- **H74.42 Polyp of left middle ear**
- **H74.43 Polyp of middle ear, bilateral**

✓5ᵗʰ H74.8 Other specified disorders of middle ear and mastoid
- **✓6ᵗʰ H74.8X Other specified disorders of middle ear and mastoid**
  - **H74.8X1 Other specified disorders of right middle ear and mastoid**
  - **H74.8X2 Other specified disorders of left middle ear and mastoid**
  - **H74.8X3 Other specified disorders of middle ear and mastoid, bilateral**
  - **H74.8X9 Other specified disorders of middle ear and mastoid, unspecified ear**

✓5ᵗʰ H74.9 Unspecified disorder of middle ear and mastoid
- **H74.90 Unspecified disorder of middle ear and mastoid, unspecified ear**
- **H74.91 Unspecified disorder of right middle ear and mastoid**
- **H74.92 Unspecified disorder of left middle ear and mastoid**
- **H74.93 Unspecified disorder of middle ear and mastoid, bilateral**

✓4ᵗʰ H75 Other disorders of middle ear and mastoid in diseases classified elsewhere

Code first underlying disease

✓5ᵗʰ H75.0 Mastoiditis in infectious and parasitic diseases classified elsewhere

> **EXCLUDES 1** mastoiditis (in):
> syphilis (A52.77)
> tuberculosis (A18.03)

- *H75.00 Mastoiditis in infectious and parasitic diseases classified elsewhere, unspecified ear*
- *H75.01 Mastoiditis in infectious and parasitic diseases classified elsewhere, right ear*
- *H75.02 Mastoiditis in infectious and parasitic diseases classified elsewhere, left ear*
- *H75.03 Mastoiditis in infectious and parasitic diseases classified elsewhere, bilateral*

✓5ᵗʰ H75.8 Other specified disorders of middle ear and mastoid in diseases classified elsewhere
- *H75.80 Other specified disorders of middle ear and mastoid in diseases classified elsewhere, unspecified ear*
- *H75.81 Other specified disorders of right middle ear and mastoid in diseases classified elsewhere*
- *H75.82 Other specified disorders of left middle ear and mastoid in diseases classified elsewhere*

- *H75.83 Other specified disorders of middle ear and mastoid in diseases classified elsewhere, bilateral*

Diseases of inner ear (H80-H83)

✓4ᵗʰ H80 Otosclerosis

> **INCLUDES** Otospongiosis

✓5ᵗʰ H80.0 Otosclerosis involving oval window, nonobliterative
- **H80.00 Otosclerosis involving oval window, nonobliterative, unspecified ear**
- **H80.01 Otosclerosis involving oval window, nonobliterative, right ear**
- **H80.02 Otosclerosis involving oval window, nonobliterative, left ear**
- **H80.03 Otosclerosis involving oval window, nonobliterative, bilateral**

✓5ᵗʰ H80.1 Otosclerosis involving oval window, obliterative
- **H80.10 Otosclerosis involving oval window, obliterative, unspecified ear**
- **H80.11 Otosclerosis involving oval window, obliterative, right ear**
- **H80.12 Otosclerosis involving oval window, obliterative, left ear**
- **H80.13 Otosclerosis involving oval window, obliterative, bilateral**

✓5ᵗʰ H80.2 Cochlear otosclerosis

> Otosclerosis involving otic capsule
> Otosclerosis involving round window

- **H80.20 Cochlear otosclerosis, unspecified ear**
- **H80.21 Cochlear otosclerosis, right ear**
- **H80.22 Cochlear otosclerosis, left ear**
- **H80.23 Cochlear otosclerosis, bilateral**

✓5ᵗʰ H80.8 Other otosclerosis
- **H80.80 Other otosclerosis, unspecified ear**
- **H80.81 Other otosclerosis, right ear**
- **H80.82 Other otosclerosis, left ear**
- **H80.83 Other otosclerosis, bilateral**

✓5ᵗʰ H80.9 Unspecified otosclerosis
- **H80.90 Unspecified otosclerosis, unspecified ear**
- **H80.91 Unspecified otosclerosis, right ear**
- **H80.92 Unspecified otosclerosis, left ear**
- **H80.93 Unspecified otosclerosis, bilateral**

✓4ᵗʰ H81 Disorders of vestibular function

> **EXCLUDES 1** epidemic vertigo (A88.1)
> vertigo NOS (R42)

✓5ᵗʰ H81.0 Ménière's disease

> Labyrinthine hydrops
> Ménière's syndrome or vertigo

- **H81.01 Ménière's disease, right ear**
- **H81.02 Ménière's disease, left ear**
- **H81.03 Ménière's disease, bilateral**
- **H81.09 Ménière's disease, unspecified ear**

✓5ᵗʰ H81.1 Benign paroxysmal vertigo
- **H81.10 Benign paroxysmal vertigo, unspecified ear**
- **H81.11 Benign paroxysmal vertigo, right ear**
- **H81.12 Benign paroxysmal vertigo, left ear**
- **H81.13 Benign paroxysmal vertigo, bilateral**

✓5ᵗʰ H81.2 Vestibular neuronitis
- **H81.20 Vestibular neuronitis, unspecified ear**
- **H81.21 Vestibular neuronitis, right ear**
- **H81.22 Vestibular neuronitis, left ear**
- **H81.23 Vestibular neuronitis, bilateral**

✓5ᵗʰ H81.3 Other peripheral vertigo
- **✓6ᵗʰ H81.31 Aural vertigo**
  - **H81.311 Aural vertigo, right ear**
  - **H81.312 Aural vertigo, left ear**
  - **H81.313 Aural vertigo, bilateral**
  - **H81.319 Aural vertigo, unspecified ear**
- **✓6ᵗʰ H81.39 Other peripheral vertigo**
  - Lermoyez' syndrome
  - Otogenic vertigo
  - Peripheral vertigo NOS
  - **H81.391 Other peripheral vertigo, right ear**

✓ Additional Character Required   ✗x7ᵗʰ Placeholder Alert   Unspecified Dx   Other Specified Dx   Manifestation   ▶◀ Revised Text   ● New Code   ▲ Revised Code Title

Chapter 8. Diseases of the Ear and Mastoid Process

         H81.392   **Other peripheral vertigo, left ear**
         H81.393   **Other peripheral vertigo, bilateral**
         H81.399   **Other peripheral vertigo, unspecified ear**

✓5th H81.4   **Vertigo of central origin**
     Central positional nystagmus
     H81.41   **Vertigo of central origin, right ear**
     H81.42   **Vertigo of central origin, left ear**
     H81.43   **Vertigo of central origin, bilateral**
     H81.49   **Vertigo of central origin, unspecified ear**

✓5th H81.8   **Other disorders of vestibular function**
     ✓6th H81.8X   **Other disorders of vestibular function**
         H81.8X1   **Other disorders of vestibular function, right ear**
         H81.8X2   **Other disorders of vestibular function, left ear**
         H81.8X3   **Other disorders of vestibular function, bilateral**
         H81.8X9   **Other disorders of vestibular function, unspecified ear**

✓5th H81.9   **Unspecified disorder of vestibular function**
     Vertiginous syndrome NOS
     H81.90   **Unspecified disorder of vestibular function, unspecified ear**
     H81.91   **Unspecified disorder of vestibular function, right ear**
     H81.92   **Unspecified disorder of vestibular function, left ear**
     H81.93   **Unspecified disorder of vestibular function, bilateral**

✓4th H82   **Vertiginous syndromes in diseases classified elsewhere**
     Code first underlying disease
     EXCLUDES 1   *epidemic vertigo (A88.1)*

     H82.1   *Vertiginous syndromes in diseases classified elsewhere, right ear*
     H82.2   *Vertiginous syndromes in diseases classified elsewhere, left ear*
     H82.3   *Vertiginous syndromes in diseases classified elsewhere, bilateral*
     H82.9   *Vertiginous syndromes in diseases classified elsewhere, unspecified ear*

✓4th H83   **Other diseases of inner ear**
     ✓5th H83.0   **Labyrinthitis**
         H83.01   **Labyrinthitis, right ear**
         H83.02   **Labyrinthitis, left ear**
         H83.03   **Labyrinthitis, bilateral**
         H83.09   **Labyrinthitis, unspecified ear**

     ✓5th H83.1   **Labyrinthine fistula**
         H83.11   **Labyrinthine fistula, right ear**
         H83.12   **Labyrinthine fistula, left ear**
         H83.13   **Labyrinthine fistula, bilateral**
         H83.19   **Labyrinthine fistula, unspecified ear**

     ✓5th H83.2   **Labyrinthine dysfunction**
     Labyrinthine hypersensitivity
     Labyrinthine hypofunction
     Labyrinthine loss of function
     ✓6th H83.2X   **Labyrinthine dysfunction**
         H83.2X1   **Labyrinthine dysfunction, right ear**
         H83.2X2   **Labyrinthine dysfunction, left ear**
         H83.2X3   **Labyrinthine dysfunction, bilateral**
         H83.2X9   **Labyrinthine dysfunction, unspecified ear**

     ✓5th H83.3   **Noise effects on inner ear**
     Acoustic trauma of inner ear
     Noise-induced hearing loss of inner ear
     ✓6th H83.3X   **Noise effects on inner ear**
         H83.3X1   **Noise effects on right inner ear**
         H83.3X2   **Noise effects on left inner ear**
         H83.3X3   **Noise effects on inner ear, bilateral**
         H83.3X9   **Noise effects on inner ear, unspecified ear**

     ✓5th H83.8   **Other specified diseases of inner ear**
     ✓6th H83.8X   **Other specified diseases of inner ear**
         H83.8X1   **Other specified diseases of right inner ear**
         H83.8X2   **Other specified diseases of left inner ear**
         H83.8X3   **Other specified diseases of inner ear, bilateral**
         H83.8X9   **Other specified diseases of inner ear, unspecified ear**

✓5th H83.9   **Unspecified disease of inner ear**
     H83.90   **Unspecified disease of inner ear, unspecified ear**
     H83.91   **Unspecified disease of right inner ear**
     H83.92   **Unspecified disease of left inner ear**
     H83.93   **Unspecified disease of inner ear, bilateral**

Other disorders of ear (H90-H94)

✓4th H90   **Conductive and sensorineural hearing loss**
     EXCLUDES 1   *deaf nonspeaking NEC (H91.3)*
         deafness NOS (H91.9-)
         hearing loss NOS (H91.9-)
         noise-induced hearing loss (H83.3-)
         ototoxic hearing loss (H91.0-)
         sudden (idiopathic) hearing loss (H91.2-)

     H90.0   **Conductive hearing loss, bilateral**

     ✓5th H90.1   **Conductive hearing loss, unilateral with unrestricted hearing on the contralateral side**
         H90.11   **Conductive hearing loss, unilateral, right ear, with unrestricted hearing on the contralateral side**
         H90.12   **Conductive hearing loss, unilateral, left ear, with unrestricted hearing on the contralateral side**

     H90.2   **Conductive hearing loss, unspecified**
     Conductive deafness NOS

     H90.3   **Sensorineural hearing loss, bilateral**

     ✓5th H90.4   **Sensorineural hearing loss, unilateral with unrestricted hearing on the contralateral side**
         H90.41   **Sensorineural hearing loss, unilateral, right ear, with unrestricted hearing on the contralateral side**
         H90.42   **Sensorineural hearing loss, unilateral, left ear, with unrestricted hearing on the contralateral side**

     H90.5   **Unspecified sensorineural hearing loss**
     Central hearing loss NOS
     Congenital deafness NOS
     Neural hearing loss NOS
     Perceptive hearing loss NOS
     Sensorineural deafness NOS
     Sensory hearing loss NOS
     EXCLUDES 1   *abnormal auditory perception (H93.2-)*
         psychogenic deafness (F44.6)

     H90.6   **Mixed conductive and sensorineural hearing loss, bilateral**

     ✓5th H90.7   **Mixed conductive and sensorineural hearing loss, unilateral with unrestricted hearing on the contralateral side**
         H90.71   **Mixed conductive and sensorineural hearing loss, unilateral, right ear, with unrestricted hearing on the contralateral side**
         H90.72   **Mixed conductive and sensorineural hearing loss, unilateral, left ear, with unrestricted hearing on the contralateral side**

     H90.8   **Mixed conductive and sensorineural hearing loss, unspecified**

✓4th H91   **Other and unspecified hearing loss**
     EXCLUDES 1   *abnormal auditory perception (H93.2-)*
         hearing loss as classified in H90-
         impacted cerumen (H61.2-)
         noise-induced hearing loss (H83.3-)
         psychogenic deafness (F44.6)
         transient ischemic deafness (H93.01-)

     ✓5th H91.0   **Ototoxic hearing loss**
     Code first poisoning due to drug or toxin, if applicable (T36-T65 with fifth or sixth character 1-4 or 6)
     Use additional code for adverse effect, if applicable, to identify drug (T36-T50 with fifth or sixth character 5)
         H91.01   **Ototoxic hearing loss, right ear**
         H91.02   **Ototoxic hearing loss, left ear**
         H91.03   **Ototoxic hearing loss, bilateral**
         H91.09   **Ototoxic hearing loss, unspecified ear**

     ✓5th H91.1   **Presbycusis**
     Presbyacusia
         H91.10   **Presbycusis, unspecified ear**
         H91.11   **Presbycusis, right ear**
         H91.12   **Presbycusis, left ear**
         H91.13   **Presbycusis, bilateral**

     ✓5th H91.2   **Sudden idiopathic hearing loss**
     Sudden hearing loss NOS
         H91.20   **Sudden idiopathic hearing loss, unspecified ear**
         H91.21   **Sudden idiopathic hearing loss, right ear**
         H91.22   **Sudden idiopathic hearing loss, left ear**

EXCLUDES 1 Not coded here   EXCLUDES 2 Not included here   N Newborn Age: 0   P Pediatric Age: 0-17   M Maternity Age: 12-55   A Adult Age: 15-124

580   ICD-10-CM 2016

H81.392–H91.22

H91.23 **Sudden idiopathic hearing loss,** bilateral

H91.3 **Deaf nonspeaking, not elsewhere classified**

✓5ᵗʰ H91.8 **Other specified hearing loss**

   ✓6ᵗʰ H91.8X **Other specified hearing loss**

      H91.8X1 **Other specified hearing loss,** right **ear**

      H91.8X2 **Other specified hearing loss,** left **ear**

      H91.8X3 **Other specified hearing loss,** bilateral

      H91.8X9 **Other specified hearing loss, unspecified ear**

✓5ᵗʰ H91.9 **Unspecified hearing loss**
Deafness NOS
High frequency deafness
Low frequency deafness

   H91.90 **Unspecified hearing loss, unspecified ear**

   H91.91 **Unspecified hearing loss,** right **ear**

   H91.92 **Unspecified hearing loss,** left **ear**

   H91.93 **Unspecified hearing loss,** bilateral

✓4ᵗʰ **H92 Otalgia and effusion of ear**

✓5ᵗʰ H92.0 Otalgia

   H92.01 **Otalgia,** right **ear**

   H92.02 **Otalgia,** left **ear**

   H92.03 **Otalgia,** bilateral

   H92.09 **Otalgia, unspecified ear**

✓5ᵗʰ H92.1 Otorrhea
   EXCLUDES 1 *leakage of cerebrospinal fluid through ear (G96.0)*

   H92.10 **Otorrhea, unspecified ear**

   H92.11 **Otorrhea,** right **ear**

   H92.12 **Otorrhea,** left **ear**

   H92.13 **Otorrhea,** bilateral

✓5ᵗʰ H92.2 Otorrhagia
   EXCLUDES 1 *traumatic otorrhagia—code to injury*

   H92.20 **Otorrhagia, unspecified ear**

   H92.21 **Otorrhagia,** right **ear**

   H92.22 **Otorrhagia,** left **ear**

   H92.23 **Otorrhagia,** bilateral

✓4ᵗʰ **H93 Other disorders of ear, not elsewhere classified**

✓5ᵗʰ H93.0 **Degenerative and vascular disorders of ear**
   EXCLUDES 1 *presbycusis (H91.1)*

   ✓6ᵗʰ H93.01 **Transient ischemic deafness**

      H93.011 **Transient ischemic deafness,** right **ear**

      H93.012 **Transient ischemic deafness,** left **ear**

      H93.013 **Transient ischemic deafness,** bilateral

      H93.019 **Transient ischemic deafness, unspecified ear**

   ✓6ᵗʰ H93.09 **Unspecified degenerative and vascular disorders of ear**

      H93.091 **Unspecified degenerative and vascular disorders of** right **ear**

      H93.092 **Unspecified degenerative and vascular disorders of** left **ear**

      H93.093 **Unspecified degenerative and vascular disorders of ear,** bilateral

      H93.099 **Unspecified degenerative and vascular disorders of unspecified ear**

✓5ᵗʰ H93.1 **Tinnitus**

   H93.11 **Tinnitus,** right **ear**

   H93.12 **Tinnitus,** left **ear**

   H93.13 **Tinnitus,** bilateral

   H93.19 **Tinnitus, unspecified ear**

✓5ᵗʰ H93.2 **Other abnormal auditory perceptions**
   EXCLUDES 2 *auditory hallucinations (R44.0)*

   ✓6ᵗʰ H93.21 **Auditory recruitment**

      H93.211 **Auditory recruitment,** right **ear**

      H93.212 **Auditory recruitment,** left **ear**

      H93.213 **Auditory recruitment,** bilateral

      H93.219 **Auditory recruitment, unspecified ear**

   ✓6ᵗʰ H93.22 **Diplacusis**

      H93.221 **Diplacusis,** right **ear**

      H93.222 **Diplacusis,** left **ear**

      H93.223 **Diplacusis,** bilateral

      H93.229 **Diplacusis, unspecified ear**

   ✓6ᵗʰ H93.23 **Hyperacusis**

      H93.231 **Hyperacusis,** right **ear**

      H93.232 **Hyperacusis,** left **ear**

      H93.233 **Hyperacusis,** bilateral

      H93.239 **Hyperacusis, unspecified ear**

   ✓6ᵗʰ H93.24 **Temporary auditory threshold shift**

      H93.241 **Temporary auditory threshold shift,** right **ear**

      H93.242 **Temporary auditory threshold shift,** left **ear**

      H93.243 **Temporary auditory threshold shift,** bilateral

      H93.249 **Temporary auditory threshold shift, unspecified ear**

   H93.25 **Central auditory processing disorder**
Congenital auditory imperception
Word deafness
   EXCLUDES 1 *mixed receptive-expressive language disorder (F80.2)*

   ✓6ᵗʰ H93.29 **Other abnormal auditory perceptions**

      H93.291 **Other abnormal auditory perceptions,** right **ear**

      H93.292 **Other abnormal auditory perceptions,** left **ear**

      H93.293 **Other abnormal auditory perceptions,** bilateral

      H93.299 **Other abnormal auditory perceptions, unspecified ear**

✓5ᵗʰ H93.3 **Disorders of acoustic nerve**
Disorder of 8th cranial nerve
   EXCLUDES 1 *acoustic neuroma (D33.3)*
           syphilitic acoustic neuritis (A52.15)

   ✓6ᵗʰ H93.3X **Disorders of acoustic nerve**

      H93.3X1 **Disorders of** right **acoustic nerve**

      H93.3X2 **Disorders of** left **acoustic nerve**

      H93.3X3 **Disorders of** bilateral **acoustic nerves**

      H93.3X9 **Disorders of unspecified acoustic nerve**

✓5ᵗʰ H93.8 **Other specified disorders of ear**

   ✓6ᵗʰ H93.8X **Other specified disorders of ear**

      H93.8X1 **Other specified disorders of** right **ear**

      H93.8X2 **Other specified disorders of** left **ear**

      H93.8X3 **Other specified disorders of ear,** bilateral

      H93.8X9 **Other specified disorders of ear, unspecified ear**

✓5ᵗʰ H93.9 **Unspecified disorder of ear**

   H93.90 **Unspecified disorder of ear, unspecified ear**

   H93.91 **Unspecified disorder of** right **ear**

   H93.92 **Unspecified disorder of** left **ear**

   H93.93 **Unspecified disorder of ear,** bilateral

✓4ᵗʰ **H94 Other disorders of ear in diseases classified elsewhere**

✓5ᵗʰ H94.0 **Acoustic neuritis in infectious and parasitic diseases classified elsewhere**
Code first underlying disease, such as:
   parasitic disease (B65-B89)
   EXCLUDES 1 *acoustic neuritis (in):*
           herpes zoster (B02.29)
           syphilis (A52.15)

   H94.00 *Acoustic neuritis in infectious and parasitic diseases classified elsewhere, unspecified ear*

   H94.01 *Acoustic neuritis in infectious and parasitic diseases classified elsewhere, right ear*

   H94.02 *Acoustic neuritis in infectious and parasitic diseases classified elsewhere, left ear*

   H94.03 *Acoustic neuritis in infectious and parasitic diseases classified elsewhere, bilateral*

✓5ᵗʰ H94.8 **Other specified disorders of ear in diseases classified elsewhere**
Code first underlying disease, such as:
   congenital syphilis (A50.0)
   EXCLUDES 1 *aural myiasis (B87.4)*
           syphilitic labyrinthitis (A52.79)

   H94.80 *Other specified disorders of ear in diseases classified elsewhere, unspecified ear*

   H94.81 *Other specified disorders of right ear in diseases classified elsewhere*

✓ Additional Character Required   ✓ˣ⁷ᵗʰ Placeholder Alert   Unspecified Dx   Other Specified Dx   Manifestation   ▶◀ Revised Text   ● New Code   ▲ Revised Code Title

Chapter 8. Diseases of the Ear and Mastoid Process

H94.82–H95.89

H94.82   *Other specified disorders of left ear in diseases classified elsewhere*

H94.83   *Other specified disorders of ear in diseases classified elsewhere, bilateral*

Intraoperative and postprocedural complications and disorders of ear and mastoid process, not elsewhere classified (H95)

✓4ᵗʰ **H95**   **Intraoperative and postprocedural complications and disorders of ear and mastoid process, not elsewhere classified**

   ✓5ᵗʰ **H95.0**   **Recurrent cholesteatoma of postmastoidectomy cavity**

     H95.00   **Recurrent cholesteatoma of postmastoidectomy cavity, unspecified ear**

     H95.01   **Recurrent cholesteatoma of postmastoidectomy cavity, right ear**

     H95.02   **Recurrent cholesteatoma of postmastoidectomy cavity, left ear**

     H95.03   **Recurrent cholesteatoma of postmastoidectomy cavity, bilateral ears**

   ✓5ᵗʰ **H95.1**   **Other disorders of ear and mastoid process following mastoidectomy**

     ✓6ᵗʰ **H95.11**   **Chronic inflammation of postmastoidectomy cavity**

       H95.111   **Chronic inflammation of postmastoidectomy cavity, right ear**

       H95.112   **Chronic inflammation of postmastoidectomy cavity, left ear**

       H95.113   **Chronic inflammation of postmastoidectomy cavity, bilateral ears**

       H95.119   **Chronic inflammation of postmastoidectomy cavity, unspecified ear**

     ✓6ᵗʰ **H95.12**   **Granulation of postmastoidectomy cavity**

       H95.121   **Granulation of postmastoidectomy cavity, right ear**

       H95.122   **Granulation of postmastoidectomy cavity, left ear**

       H95.123   **Granulation of postmastoidectomy cavity, bilateral ears**

       H95.129   **Granulation of postmastoidectomy cavity, unspecified ear**

     ✓6ᵗʰ **H95.13**   **Mucosal cyst of postmastoidectomy cavity**

       H95.131   **Mucosal cyst of postmastoidectomy cavity, right ear**

       H95.132   **Mucosal cyst of postmastoidectomy cavity, left ear**

       H95.133   **Mucosal cyst of postmastoidectomy cavity, bilateral ears**

       H95.139   **Mucosal cyst of postmastoidectomy cavity, unspecified ear**

     ✓6ᵗʰ **H95.19**   **Other disorders following mastoidectomy**

       H95.191   **Other disorders following mastoidectomy, right ear**

       H95.192   **Other disorders following mastoidectomy, left ear**

       H95.193   **Other disorders following mastoidectomy, bilateral ears**

       H95.199   **Other disorders following mastoidectomy, unspecified ear**

   ✓5ᵗʰ **H95.2**   **Intraoperative hemorrhage and hematoma of ear and mastoid process complicating a procedure**

     EXCLUDES 1   *intraoperative hemorrhage and hematoma of ear and mastoid process due to accidental puncture or laceration during a procedure (H95.3-)*

     H95.21   **Intraoperative hemorrhage and hematoma of ear and mastoid process complicating a procedure** on the ear and mastoid process

     H95.22   **Intraoperative hemorrhage and hematoma of ear and mastoid process complicating** other procedure

   ✓5ᵗʰ **H95.3**   **Accidental puncture and laceration of ear and mastoid process during a procedure**

     H95.31   **Accidental puncture and laceration of the ear and mastoid process** during a procedure on the ear and mastoid process

     H95.32   **Accidental puncture and laceration of the ear and mastoid process during** other procedure

   ✓5ᵗʰ **H95.4**   **Postprocedural hemorrhage and hematoma of ear and mastoid process following a procedure**

     H95.41   **Postprocedural hemorrhage and hematoma of ear and mastoid process following a** procedure on the ear and mastoid process

     H95.42   **Postprocedural hemorrhage and hematoma of ear and mastoid process following** other procedure

   ✓5ᵗʰ **H95.8**   **Other** intraoperative and postprocedural complications and disorders of the ear and mastoid process, not elsewhere classified

     EXCLUDES 2   *postprocedural complications and disorders following mastoidectomy (H95.0-, H95.1-)*

     ✓6ᵗʰ **H95.81**   Postprocedural stenosis of external ear canal

       H95.811   **Postprocedural stenosis of** right **external ear canal**

       H95.812   **Postprocedural stenosis of** left **external ear canal**

       H95.813   **Postprocedural stenosis of external ear canal,** bilateral

       H95.819   **Postprocedural stenosis of unspecified external ear canal**

     H95.88   **Other** intraoperative **complications and disorders of the ear and mastoid process, not elsewhere classified**

       Use additional code, if applicable, to further specify disorder

     H95.89   **Other** postprocedural **complications and disorders of the ear and mastoid process, not elsewhere classified**

       Use additional code, if applicable, to further specify disorder

EXCLUDES 1 Not coded here   **EXCLUDES 2** Not included here   **N** Newborn Age: 0   **P** Pediatric Age: 0-17   **M** Maternity Age: 12-55   **A** Adult Age: 15-124

582

ICD-10-CM 2016

Chapter 9. Diseases of the Circulatory System (I00–I99)

Chapter Specific Guidelines with Coding Examples

The chapter specific guidelines from the ICD-10-CM Official Guidelines for Coding and Reporting have been provided below. Along with these guidelines are coding examples, contained in the shaded boxes, that have been developed to help illustrate the coding and/or sequencing guidance found in these guidelines.

a. Hypertension

1) Hypertension with heart disease

Heart conditions classified to I50.- or I51.4-I51.9, are assigned to a code from category I11, Hypertensive heart disease, when a causal relationship is stated (due to hypertension) or implied (hypertensive). Use an additional code from category I50, Heart failure, to identify the type of heart failure in those patients with heart failure.

The same heart conditions (I50.-, I51.4-I51.9) with hypertension, but without a stated causal relationship, are coded separately. Sequence according to the circumstances of the admission/encounter.

Hypertensive heart disease with left heart failure

I11.0	**Hypertensive heart disease with heart failure**
I50.1	**Left ventricular failure**

Explanation: A causal relationship between hypertension and heart disease must be stated or implied to report codes from category I11 Hypertensive heart disease. Use an additional code to identify type of heart failure (I50.-).

---

2) Hypertensive chronic kidney disease

Assign codes from category I12, Hypertensive chronic kidney disease, when both hypertension and a condition classifiable to category N18, Chronic kidney disease (CKD), are present. Unlike hypertension with heart disease, ICD-10-CM presumes a cause-and-effect relationship and classifies chronic kidney disease with hypertension as hypertensive chronic kidney disease.

The appropriate code from category N18 should be used as a secondary code with a code from category I12 to identify the stage of chronic kidney disease.

See Section I.C.14. Chronic kidney disease.

If a patient has hypertensive chronic kidney disease and acute renal failure, an additional code for the acute renal failure is required.

Patient is admitted with stage IV chronic kidney disease (CKD). The physician has also documented hypertension for this patient.

I12.9	**Hypertensive chronic kidney disease with stage 1 through stage 4 chronic kidney disease, or unspecified chronic kidney disease**
N18.4	**Chronic kidney disease, stage 4 (severe)**

Explanation: A causal relationship between hypertension and chronic kidney disease (CKD) is **assumed** unless otherwise documented. Use an additional code to identify the stage of chronic kidney disease.

---

3) Hypertensive heart and chronic kidney disease

Assign codes from combination category I13, Hypertensive heart and chronic kidney disease, when both hypertensive kidney disease and hypertensive heart disease are stated in the diagnosis. Assume a relationship between the hypertension and the chronic kidney disease, whether or not the condition is so designated. If heart failure is present, assign an additional code from category I50 to identify the type of heart failure.

The appropriate code from category N18, Chronic kidney disease, should be used as a secondary code with a code from category I13 to identify the stage of chronic kidney disease.

See Section I.C.14. Chronic kidney disease.

The codes in category I13, Hypertensive heart and chronic kidney disease, are combination codes that include hypertension, heart disease and chronic kidney disease. The Includes note at I13 specifies that the conditions included at I11 and I12 are included together in I13. If a patient has hypertension, heart disease and chronic kidney disease then a code from I13 should be used, not individual codes for hypertension, heart disease and chronic kidney disease, or codes from I11 or I12.

For patients with both acute renal failure and chronic kidney disease an additional code for acute renal failure is required.

Hypertensive heart and kidney disease with congestive heart failure and stage 2 chronic kidney disease

I13.0	**Hypertensive heart and chronic kidney disease with heart failure and stage 1 through stage 4 chronic kidney disease, or unspecified chronic kidney disease**
I50.9	**Heart failure, unspecified**
N18.2	**Chronic kidney disease, stage 2 (mild)**

Explanation: Combination codes in category I13 are used to report conditions classifiable to *both* categories I11 and I12. Do not report conditions classifiable to I11 and I12 separately. Use additional codes to report type of heart failure and stage of CKD.

---

4) Hypertensive cerebrovascular disease

For hypertensive cerebrovascular disease, first assign the appropriate code from categories I60-I69, followed by the appropriate hypertension code.

Rupture of cerebral aneurysm caused by malignant hypertension

I60.8	**Other nontraumatic subarachnoid hemorrhage**
I10	**Essential (primary) hypertension**

Explanation: Hypertensive cerebrovascular disease requires two codes: the appropriate I60–I69 code followed by the appropriate hypertension code.

---

5) Hypertensive retinopathy

Subcategory H35.0, Background retinopathy and retinal vascular changes, should be used with a code from category I10 – I15, Hypertensive disease to include the systemic hypertension. The sequencing is based on the reason for the encounter.

Hypertensive retinopathy of the right eye

H35.031	**Hypertensive retinopathy, right eye**
I10	**Essential (primary) hypertension**

Explanation: Hypertensive retinopathy requires two codes: the appropriate subcategory H35.0 code and a code for the hypertension.

---

6) Hypertension, secondary

Secondary hypertension is due to an underlying condition. Two codes are required: one to identify the underlying etiology and one from category I15 to identify the hypertension. Sequencing of codes is determined by the reason for admission/encounter.

Renovascular hypertension due to renal artery atherosclerosis

I15.0	**Renovascular hypertension**
I70.1	**Atherosclerosis of renal artery**

Explanation: Secondary hypertension requires two codes: a code to identify the etiology and the appropriate I15 code.

---

7) Hypertension, transient

Assign code R03.0, Elevated blood pressure reading without diagnosis of hypertension, unless patient has an established diagnosis of hypertension. Assign code O13.-, Gestational [pregnancy-induced] hypertension without significant proteinuria, or O14.-, Pre-eclampsia, for transient hypertension of pregnancy.

8) Hypertension, controlled

This diagnostic statement usually refers to an existing state of hypertension under control by therapy. Assign the appropriate code from categories I10-I15, Hypertensive diseases.

9) Hypertension, uncontrolled

Uncontrolled hypertension may refer to untreated hypertension or hypertension not responding to current therapeutic regimen. In either case, assign the appropriate code from categories I10-I15, Hypertensive diseases.

b. Atherosclerotic coronary artery disease and angina

ICD-10-CM has combination codes for atherosclerotic heart disease with angina pectoris. The subcategories for these codes are I25.11, Atherosclerotic heart disease of native coronary artery with angina pectoris and I25.7,

Atherosclerosis of coronary artery bypass graft(s) and coronary artery of transplanted heart with angina pectoris.

When using one of these combination codes it is not necessary to use an additional code for angina pectoris. A causal relationship can be assumed in a patient with both atherosclerosis and angina pectoris, unless the documentation indicates the angina is due to something other than the atherosclerosis.

If a patient with coronary artery disease is admitted due to an acute myocardial infarction (AMI), the AMI should be sequenced before the coronary artery disease.

See Section I.C.9. Acute myocardial infarction (AMI)

> Patient is being seen for spastic angina pectoris. She also has a documented history of progressive coronary artery disease of the native vessels.
>
> **I25.111**   **Atherosclerotic heart disease of native coronary artery with angina pectoris with documented spasm**
>
> *Explanation*: Report the combination code for atherosclerotic heart disease (coronary artery disease) with angina pectoris. A causal relationship is assumed in a patient with both atherosclerosis and angina pectoris, unless the documentation indicates the angina is due to something other than the atherosclerosis. When using one of these combination codes, it is not necessary to use an additional code for angina pectoris.

c. Intraoperative and postprocedural cerebrovascular accident

Medical record documentation should clearly specify the cause- and- effect relationship between the medical intervention and the cerebrovascular accident in order to assign a code for intraoperative or postprocedural cerebrovascular accident.

Proper code assignment depends on whether it was an infarction or hemorrhage and whether it occurred intraoperatively or postoperatively. If it was a cerebral hemorrhage, code assignment depends on the type of procedure performed.

> Embolic cerebral infarction of the right middle cerebral artery that occurred during hip replacement surgery. The surgeon documented as due to the surgery.
>
> **I97.811**   **Intraoperative cerebrovascular infarction during other surgery**
>
> **I63.411**   **Cerebral infarction due to embolism of right middle cerebral artery**
>
> *Explanation*: Code assignment for intraoperative or postprocedural cerebrovascular accident is based on the provider's documentation of a cause-and-effect relationship between the condition and the procedure. Proper code assignment also depends on whether the cerebrovascular accident was an infarction or hemorrhage, occurred intraoperatively or postoperatively, and the type of procedure performed.

d. Sequelae of cerebrovascular disease

1) Category I69, Sequelae of cerebrovascular disease

Category I69 is used to indicate conditions classifiable to categories I60–I67 as the causes of sequela (neurologic deficits), themselves classified elsewhere. These "late effects" include neurologic deficits that persist after initial onset of conditions classifiable to categories I60–I67. The neurologic deficits caused by cerebrovascular disease may be present from the onset or may arise at any time after the onset of the condition classifiable to categories I60–I67.

Codes from category I69, Sequelae of cerebrovascular disease, that specify hemiplegia, hemiparesis and monoplegia identify whether the dominant or nondominant side is affected. Should the affected side be documented, but not specified as dominant or nondominant, and the classification system does not indicate a default, code selection is as follows:

- For ambidextrous patients, the default should be dominant.
- If the left side is affected, the default is non-dominant.
- If the right side is affected, the default is dominant.

2) Codes from category I69 with codes from I60–I67

Codes from category I69 may be assigned on a health care record with codes from I60–I67, if the patient has a current cerebrovascular disease and deficits from an old cerebrovascular disease.

3) Codes from category I69 and Personal history of transient ischemic attack (TIA) and cerebral infarction (Z86.73)

Codes from category I69 should not be assigned if the patient does not have neurologic deficits.

See Section I.C.21. 4. History (of) for use of personal history codes

Flaccid hemiparesis of the right side due to old cerebral infarction

> **I69.351**   **Hemiplegia and hemiparesis following cerebral infarction affecting right dominant side**
>
> *Explanation*: Sequela codes specify the residual effect that remains after the acute phase of a previous illness or injury (I60–I67). The "sequelae" include conditions specified as such or as residuals, which may occur at any time, even months or years, after the onset of the causal condition. There is no time limit restricting the reporting of sequela (late effect) codes. For this scenario, the documentation indicates that the right side is affected but does not note which side is the patient's dominant side, e.g., right or left. The default is to assume the right side is the dominant side.

e. Acute myocardial infarction (AMI)

1) ST elevation myocardial infarction (STEMI) and non ST elevation myocardial infarction (NSTEMI)

The ICD-10-CM codes for acute myocardial infarction (AMI) identify the site, such as anterolateral wall or true posterior wall. Subcategories I21.0-I21.2 and code I21.3 are used for ST elevation myocardial infarction (STEMI). Code I21.4, Non-ST elevation (NSTEMI) myocardial infarction, is used for non ST elevation myocardial infarction (NSTEMI) and nontransmural MIs.

If NSTEMI evolves to STEMI, assign the STEMI code. If STEMI converts to NSTEMI due to thrombolytic therapy, it is still coded as STEMI.

For encounters occurring while the myocardial infarction is equal to, or less than, four weeks old, including transfers to another acute setting or a postacute setting, and the patient requires continued care for the myocardial infarction, codes from category I21 may continue to be reported. For encounters after the 4 week time frame and the patient is still receiving care related to the myocardial infarction, the appropriate aftercare code should be assigned, rather than a code from category I21. For old or healed myocardial infarctions not requiring further care, code I25.2, Old myocardial infarction, may be assigned.

> Acute inferior NSTEMI evolved into STEMI
>
> **I21.19**   **ST elevation (STEMI) myocardial infarction involving other coronary artery of inferior wall**
>
> *Explanation*: If an NSTEMI converts to a STEMI, report only the STEMI code.

2) Acute myocardial infarction, unspecified

Code I21.3, ST elevation (STEMI) myocardial infarction of unspecified site, is the default for unspecified acute myocardial infarction. If only STEMI or transmural MI without the site is documented, assign code I21.3.

3) AMI documented as nontransmural or subendocardial but site provided

If an AMI is documented as nontransmural or subendocardial, but the site is provided, it is still coded as a subendocardial AMI.

See Section I.C.21.3 for information on coding status post administration of tPA in a different facility within the last 24 hours.

> Acute inferior subendocardial myocardial infarction (NSTEMI)
>
> **I21.4**   **Non-ST elevation (NSTEMI) myocardial infarction**
>
> *Explanation*: An AMI documented as subendocardial or nontransmural is coded as such (I21.4, I22.2), even if the site of infarction is specified.

4) Subsequent acute myocardial infarction

A code from category I22, Subsequent ST elevation (STEMI) and non ST elevation (NSTEMI) myocardial infarction, is to be used when a patient who has suffered an AMI has a new AMI within the 4 week time frame of the initial AMI. A code from category I22 must be used in conjunction with a code from category I21. The sequencing of the I22 and I21 codes depends on the circumstances of the encounter.

> Acute inferior STEMI status post acute NSTEMI two weeks ago.
>
> **I22.1**   **Subsequent ST elevation (STEMI) myocardial infarction of inferior wall**
>
> **I21.4**   **Non-ST elevation (NSTEMI) myocardial infarction**
>
> *Explanation*: A code from I22 must be used in conjunction with a code from I21 when a patient who has suffered an AMI has a new AMI within four weeks of the initial one. Category I22 is never reported alone. The guidelines for assigning the correct I22 code are the same as those for reporting the initial MI (I21). Sequencing is determined by the circumstances of the encounter.

Chapter 9. Diseases of the Circulatory System (I00–I99)

EXCLUDES 2   certain conditions originating in the perinatal period (P04-P96)
certain infectious and parasitic diseases (A00-B99)
complications of pregnancy, childbirth and the puerperium (O00-O9A)
congenital malformations, deformations, and chromosomal abnormalities (Q00-Q99)
endocrine, nutritional and metabolic diseases (E00-E88)
injury, poisoning and certain other consequences of external causes (S00-T88)
neoplasms (C00-D49)
symptoms, signs and abnormal clinical and laboratory findings, not elsewhere classified (R00-R94)
systemic connective tissue disorders (M30-M36)
transient cerebral ischemic attacks and related syndromes (G45.-)

This chapter contains the following blocks:

I00-I02	Acute rheumatic fever
I05-I09	Chronic rheumatic heart diseases
I10-I15	Hypertensive diseases
I20-I25	Ischemic heart diseases
I26-I28	Pulmonary heart disease and diseases of pulmonary circulation
I30-I52	Other forms of heart disease
I60-I69	Cerebrovascular diseases
I70-I79	Diseases of arteries, arterioles and capillaries
I80-I89	Diseases of veins, lymphatic vessels and lymph nodes, not elsewhere classified
I95-I99	Other and unspecified disorders of the circulatory system

Acute rheumatic fever (I00-I02)

I00   **Rheumatic fever without heart involvement**
INCLUDES   arthritis, rheumatic, acute or subacute
EXCLUDES 1   rheumatic fever with heart involvement (I01.0-I01.9)

✓4ᵗʰ I01   **Rheumatic fever with heart involvement**
EXCLUDES 1   chronic diseases of rheumatic origin (I05-I09) unless rheumatic fever is also present or there is evidence of reactivation or activity of the rheumatic process.

I01.0   **Acute rheumatic pericarditis**
Any condition in I00 with pericarditis
Rheumatic pericarditis (acute)
EXCLUDES 1   acute pericarditis not specified as rheumatic (I30.-)

I01.1   **Acute rheumatic endocarditis**
Any condition in I00 with endocarditis or valvulitis
Acute rheumatic valvulitis

I01.2   **Acute rheumatic myocarditis**
Any condition in I00 with myocarditis

I01.8   **Other acute rheumatic heart disease**
Any condition in I00 with other or multiple types of heart involvement
Acute rheumatic pancarditis

I01.9   **Acute rheumatic heart disease, unspecified**
Any condition in I00 with unspecified type of heart involvement
Rheumatic carditis, acute
Rheumatic heart disease, active or acute

✓4ᵗʰ I02   **Rheumatic chorea**
INCLUDES   Sydenham's chorea
EXCLUDES 1   chorea NOS (G25.5)
Huntington's chorea (G10)

I02.0   **Rheumatic chorea with heart involvement**
Chorea NOS with heart involvement
Rheumatic chorea with heart involvement of any type classifiable under I01-

I02.9   **Rheumatic chorea without heart involvement**
Rheumatic chorea NOS

Chronic rheumatic heart diseases (I05-I09)

✓4ᵗʰ I05   **Rheumatic mitral valve diseases**
INCLUDES   conditions classifiable to both I05.0 and I05.2-I05.9, whether specified as rheumatic or not
EXCLUDES 1   mitral valve disease specified as nonrheumatic (I34.-)
mitral valve disease with aortic and/or tricuspid valve involvement (I08.-)

I05.0   **Rheumatic mitral stenosis**
Mitral (valve) obstruction (rheumatic)

I05.1   **Rheumatic mitral insufficiency**
Rheumatic mitral incompetence
Rheumatic mitral regurgitation
EXCLUDES 1   mitral insufficiency not specified as rheumatic (I34.0)

I05.2   **Rheumatic mitral stenosis with insufficiency**
Rheumatic mitral stenosis with incompetence or regurgitation

I05.8   **Other rheumatic mitral valve diseases**
Rheumatic mitral (valve) failure

I05.9   **Rheumatic mitral valve disease, unspecified**
Rheumatic mitral (valve) disorder (chronic) NOS

✓4ᵗʰ I06   **Rheumatic aortic valve diseases**
EXCLUDES 1   aortic valve disease not specified as rheumatic (I35.-)
aortic valve disease with mitral and/or tricuspid valve involvement (I08.-)

I06.0   **Rheumatic aortic stenosis**
Rheumatic aortic (valve) obstruction

I06.1   **Rheumatic aortic insufficiency**
Rheumatic aortic incompetence
Rheumatic aortic regurgitation

I06.2   **Rheumatic aortic stenosis with insufficiency**
Rheumatic aortic stenosis with incompetence or regurgitation

I06.8   **Other rheumatic aortic valve diseases**

I06.9   **Rheumatic aortic valve disease, unspecified**
Rheumatic aortic (valve) disease NOS

✓4ᵗʰ I07   **Rheumatic tricuspid valve diseases**
INCLUDES   rheumatic tricuspid valve diseases specified as rheumatic or unspecified
EXCLUDES 1   tricuspid valve disease specified as nonrheumatic (I36.-)
tricuspid valve disease with aortic and/or mitral valve involvement (I08.-)

I07.0   **Rheumatic tricuspid stenosis**
Tricuspid (valve) stenosis (rheumatic)

I07.1   **Rheumatic tricuspid insufficiency**
Tricuspid (valve) insufficiency (rheumatic)

I07.2   **Rheumatic tricuspid stenosis and insufficiency**

I07.8   **Other rheumatic tricuspid valve diseases**

I07.9   **Rheumatic tricuspid valve disease, unspecified**
Rheumatic tricuspid valve disorder NOS

✓4ᵗʰ I08   **Multiple valve diseases**
INCLUDES   multiple valve diseases specified as rheumatic or unspecified
EXCLUDES 1   endocarditis, valve unspecified (I38)
multiple valve disease specified a nonrheumatic (I34.-, I35.-, I36.-, I37.-, I38.-, Q22.-, Q23.-, Q24.8-)
rheumatic valve disease NOS (I09.1)

I08.0   **Rheumatic disorders of both mitral and aortic valves**
Involvement of both mitral and aortic valves specified as rheumatic or unspecified

I08.1   **Rheumatic disorders of both mitral and tricuspid valves**

I08.2   **Rheumatic disorders of both aortic and tricuspid valves**

I08.3   **Combined rheumatic disorders of mitral, aortic and tricuspid valves**

I08.8   **Other rheumatic multiple valve diseases**

I08.9   **Rheumatic multiple valve disease, unspecified**

✓4ᵗʰ I09   **Other rheumatic heart diseases**

I09.0   **Rheumatic myocarditis**
EXCLUDES 1   myocarditis not specified as rheumatic (I51.4)

I09.1   **Rheumatic diseases of endocardium, valve unspecified**
Rheumatic endocarditis (chronic)
Rheumatic valvulitis (chronic)
EXCLUDES 1   endocarditis, valve unspecified (I38)

I09.2   **Chronic rheumatic pericarditis**
Adherent pericardium, rheumatic
Chronic rheumatic mediastinopericarditis
Chronic rheumatic myopericarditis
EXCLUDES 1   chronic pericarditis not specified as rheumatic (I31.-)

✓5ᵗʰ I09.8   **Other specified rheumatic heart diseases**

I09.81   **Rheumatic heart failure**
Use additional code to identify type of heart failure (I50.-)

I09.89   **Other specified rheumatic heart diseases**
Rheumatic disease of pulmonary valve

I09.9   **Rheumatic heart disease, unspecified**
Rheumatic carditis
EXCLUDES 1   rheumatoid carditis (M05.31)

☑ Additional Character Required   ✓x7ᵗʰ Placeholder Alert   Unspecified Dx   Other Specified Dx   Manifestation   ►◄ Revised Text   ● New Code   ▲ Revised Code Title

Chapter 9. Diseases of the Circulatory System

Hypertensive diseases (I10-I15)

Use additional code to identify:
  exposure to environmental tobacco smoke (Z77.22)
  history of tobacco use (Z87.891)
  occupational exposure to environmental tobacco smoke (Z57.31)
  tobacco dependence (F17.-)
  tobacco use (Z72.0)
    EXCLUDES1   *hypertensive disease complicating pregnancy, childbirth and the puerperium (O10-O11, O13-O16)*
        neonatal hypertension (P29.2)
        primary pulmonary hypertension (I27.0)

I10   **Essential (primary) hypertension**
    INCLUDES   high blood pressure
        hypertension (arterial) (benign) (essential) (malignant) (primary) (systemic)
    EXCLUDES1   *hypertensive disease complicating pregnancy, childbirth and the puerperium (O10-O11, O13-O16)*
    EXCLUDES2   *essential (primary) hypertension involving vessels of brain (I60-I69)*
        essential (primary) hypertension involving vessels of eye (H35.0-)

✓4ᵗʰ I11   **Hypertensive heart disease**
    INCLUDES   any condition in I51.4-I51.9 due to hypertension

  I11.0   **Hypertensive heart disease with heart failure**
    Hypertensive heart failure
    Use additional code to identify type of heart failure (I50.-)

  I11.9   **Hypertensive heart disease without heart failure**
    Hypertensive heart disease NOS

✓4ᵗʰ I12   **Hypertensive chronic kidney disease**
    INCLUDES   any condition in N18- and N26- due to hypertension
        arteriosclerosis of kidney
        arteriosclerotic nephritis (chronic) (interstitial)
        hypertensive nephropathy
        nephrosclerosis
    EXCLUDES1   *hypertension due to kidney disease (I15.0, I15.1)*
        renovascular hypertension (I15.0)
        secondary hypertension (I15.-)
    EXCLUDES2   *acute kidney failure (N17.-)*

  I12.0   **Hypertensive chronic kidney disease with stage 5 chronic kidney disease or end stage renal disease**
    Use additional code to identify the stage of chronic kidney disease (N18.5, N18.6)

  I12.9   **Hypertensive chronic kidney disease with stage 1 through stage 4 chronic kidney disease, or unspecified chronic kidney disease**
    Hypertensive chronic kidney disease NOS
    Hypertensive renal disease NOS
    Use additional code to identify the stage of chronic kidney disease (N18.1-N18.4, N18.9)

✓4ᵗʰ I13   **Hypertensive heart and chronic kidney disease**
    INCLUDES   any condition in I11- with any condition in I12-
        cardiorenal disease
        cardiovascular renal disease

  I13.0   **Hypertensive heart and chronic kidney disease with heart failure and stage 1 through stage 4 chronic kidney disease, or unspecified chronic kidney disease**
    Use additional code to identify type of heart failure (I50.-)
    Use additional code to identify stage of chronic kidney disease (N18.1-N18.4, N18.9)

  ✓5ᵗʰ I13.1   **Hypertensive heart and chronic kidney disease without heart failure**

    I13.10   **Hypertensive heart and chronic kidney disease without heart failure, with stage 1 through stage 4 chronic kidney disease, or unspecified chronic kidney disease**
      Hypertensive heart disease and hypertensive chronic kidney disease NOS
      Use additional code to identify the stage of chronic kidney disease (N18.1-N18.4, N18.9)

    I13.11   **Hypertensive heart and chronic kidney disease without heart failure, with stage 5 chronic kidney disease, or end stage renal disease**
      Use additional code to identify the stage of chronic kidney disease (N18.5, N18.6)

  I13.2   **Hypertensive heart and chronic kidney disease with heart failure and with stage 5 chronic kidney disease, or end stage renal disease**
    Use additional code to identify type of heart failure (I50.-)
    Use additional code to identify the stage of chronic kidney disease (N18.5, N18.6)

✓4ᵗʰ I15   **Secondary hypertension**
    Code also underlying condition
    EXCLUDES1   *postprocedural hypertension (I97.3)*
    EXCLUDES2   *secondary hypertension involving vessels of brain (I60-I69)*
        secondary hypertension involving vessels of eye (H35.0-)

  I15.0   **Renovascular hypertension**
  I15.1   **Hypertension secondary to other renal disorders**
  I15.2   **Hypertension secondary to endocrine disorders**
  I15.8   **Other secondary hypertension**
  I15.9   **Secondary hypertension, unspecified**

Ischemic heart diseases (I20-I25)

Use additional code to identify presence of hypertension (I10-I15)

✓4ᵗʰ I20   **Angina pectoris**
    Use additional code to identify:
      exposure to environmental tobacco smoke (Z77.22)
      history of tobacco use (Z87.891)
      occupational exposure to environmental tobacco smoke (Z57.31)
      tobacco dependence (F17.-)
      tobacco use (Z72.0)
    EXCLUDES1   *angina pectoris with atherosclerotic heart disease of native coronary arteries (I25.1-)*
        atherosclerosis of coronary artery bypass graft(s) and coronary artery of transplanted heart with angina pectoris (I25.7-)
        postinfarction angina (I23.7)

  I20.0   **Unstable angina**   🅐
    Accelerated angina
    Crescendo angina
    De novo effort angina
    Intermediate coronary syndrome
    Preinfarction syndrome
    Worsening effort angina

  I20.1   **Angina pectoris with documented spasm**   🅐
    Angiospastic angina
    Prinzmetal angina
    Spasm-induced angina
    Variant angina

  I20.8   **Other forms of angina pectoris**   🅐
    Angina equivalent
    Angina of effort
    Coronary slow flow syndrome
    Stenocardia
    Use additional code(s) for symptoms associated with angina equivalent

  I20.9   **Angina pectoris, unspecified**   🅐
    Angina NOS
    Anginal syndrome
    Cardiac angina
    Ischemic chest pain

✓4ᵗʰ I21   **ST elevation (STEMI) and non-ST elevation (NSTEMI) myocardial infarction**
    INCLUDES   cardiac infarction
        coronary (artery) embolism
        coronary (artery) occlusion
        coronary (artery) rupture
        coronary (artery) thrombosis
        infarction of heart, myocardium, or ventricle
        myocardial infarction specified as acute or with a stated duration of 4 weeks (28 days) or less from onset
    Use additional code, if applicable, to identify:
      exposure to environmental tobacco smoke (Z77.22)
      history of tobacco use (Z87.891)
      occupational exposure to environmental tobacco smoke (Z57.31)
      status post administration of tPA (rtPA) in a different facility within the last 24 hours prior to admission to current facility (Z92.82)
      tobacco dependence (F17.-)
      tobacco use (Z72.0)
    EXCLUDES2   *old myocardial infarction (I25.2)*
        postmyocardial infarction syndrome (I24.1)
        subsequent myocardial infarction (I22.-)
    AHA: 2013, 1Q, 25; 2012, 4Q, 96, 102-103

  ✓5ᵗʰ I21.0   **ST elevation (STEMI) myocardial infarction of anterior wall**

    I21.01   **ST elevation (STEMI) myocardial infarction involving left main coronary artery**   🅐

    I21.02   **ST elevation (STEMI) myocardial infarction involving left anterior descending coronary artery**   🅐
      ST elevation (STEMI) myocardial infarction involving diagonal coronary artery
      AHA: 2013, 1Q, 25

EXCLUDES1 Not coded here   EXCLUDES2 Not included here   🅝 Newborn Age: 0   🅟 Pediatric Age: 0-17   🅜 Maternity Age: 12-55   🅐 Adult Age: 15-124

I21.Ø9   **ST elevation (STEMI) myocardial infarction involving other coronary artery of anterior wall**   Ⓐ
Acute transmural myocardial infarction of anterior wall
Anteroapical transmural (Q wave) infarction (acute)
Anterolateral transmural (Q wave) infarction (acute)
Anteroseptal transmural (Q wave) infarction (acute)
Transmural (Q wave) infarction (acute) (of) anterior (wall) NOS
AHA: 2012, 4Q, 102-103

✓5th **I21.1**   **ST elevation (STEMI) myocardial infarction of inferior wall**

I21.11   **ST elevation (STEMI) myocardial infarction involving right coronary artery**   Ⓐ
Inferoposterior transmural (Q wave) infarction (acute)

I21.19   **ST elevation (STEMI) myocardial infarction involving other coronary artery of inferior wall**   Ⓐ
Acute transmural myocardial infarction of inferior wall
Inferolateral transmural (Q wave) infarction (acute)
Transmural (Q wave) infarction (acute) (of) diaphragmatic wall
Transmural (Q wave) infarction (acute) (of) inferior (wall) NOS
EXCLUDES 2 *ST elevation (STEMI) myocardial infarction involving left circumflex coronary artery (I21.21)*
AHA: 2012, 4Q, 96

✓5th **I21.2**   **ST elevation (STEMI) myocardial infarction of other sites**

I21.21   **ST elevation (STEMI) myocardial infarction involving left circumflex coronary artery**   Ⓐ
ST elevation (STEMI) myocardial infarction involving oblique marginal coronary artery

I21.29   **ST elevation (STEMI) myocardial infarction involving other sites**   Ⓐ
Acute transmural myocardial infarction of other sites
Apical-lateral transmural (Q wave) infarction (acute)
Basal-lateral transmural (Q wave) infarction (acute)
High lateral transmural (Q wave) infarction (acute)
Lateral (wall) NOS transmural (Q wave) infarction (acute)
Posterior (true) transmural (Q wave) infarction (acute)
Posterobasal transmural (Q wave) infarction (acute)
Posterolateral transmural (Q wave) infarction (acute)
Posteroseptal transmural (Q wave) infarction (acute)
Septal transmural (Q wave) infarction (acute) NOS

I21.3   **ST elevation (STEMI) myocardial infarction of unspecified site**   Ⓐ
Acute transmural myocardial infarction of unspecified site
Myocardial infarction (acute) NOS
Transmural (Q wave) myocardial infarction NOS

I21.4   **Non-ST elevation (NSTEMI) myocardial infarction**   Ⓐ
Acute subendocardial myocardial infarction
Non-Q wave myocardial infarction NOS
Nontransmural myocardial infarction NOS

✓4th **I22**   **Subsequent ST elevation (STEMI) and non-ST elevation (NSTEMI) myocardial infarction**
INCLUDES   acute myocardial infarction occurring within four weeks (28 days) of a previous acute myocardial infarction, regardless of site
cardiac infarction
coronary (artery) embolism
coronary (artery) occlusion
coronary (artery) rupture
coronary (artery) thrombosis
infarction of heart, myocardium, or ventricle
recurrent myocardial infarction
reinfarction of myocardium
rupture of heart, myocardium, or ventricle
Use additional code, if applicable, to identify:
exposure to environmental tobacco smoke (Z77.22)
history of tobacco use (Z87.891)
occupational exposure to environmental tobacco smoke (Z57.31)
status post administration of tPA (rtPA) in a different facility within the last 24 hours prior to admission to current facility (Z92.82)
tobacco dependence (F17.-)
tobacco use (Z72.Ø)
AHA: 2013, 1Q, 25; 2012, 4Q, 97, 102-103

I22.Ø   **Subsequent ST elevation (STEMI) myocardial infarction of anterior wall**   Ⓐ
Subsequent acute transmural myocardial infarction of anterior wall
Subsequent transmural (Q wave) infarction (acute)(of) anterior (wall) NOS
Subsequent anteroapical transmural (Q wave) infarction (acute)
Subsequent anterolateral transmural (Q wave) infarction (acute)
Subsequent anteroseptal transmural (Q wave) infarction (acute)

I22.1   **Subsequent ST elevation (STEMI) myocardial infarction of inferior wall**   Ⓐ
Subsequent acute transmural myocardial infarction of inferior wall
Subsequent transmural (Q wave) infarction (acute)(of) diaphragmatic wall
Subsequent transmural (Q wave) infarction (acute)(of) inferior (wall) NOS
Subsequent inferolateral transmural (Q wave) infarction (acute)
Subsequent inferoposterior transmural (Q wave) infarction (acute)
AHA: 2012, 4Q, 102

I22.2   **Subsequent non-ST elevation (NSTEMI) myocardial infarction**   Ⓐ
Subsequent acute subendocardial myocardial infarction
Subsequent non-Q wave myocardial infarction NOS
Subsequent nontransmural myocardial infarction NOS

I22.8   **Subsequent ST elevation (STEMI) myocardial infarction of other sites**   Ⓐ
Subsequent acute transmural myocardial infarction of other sites
Subsequent apical-lateral transmural (Q wave) myocardial infarction (acute)
Subsequent basal-lateral transmural (Q wave) myocardial infarction (acute)
Subsequent high lateral transmural (Q wave) myocardial infarction (acute)
Subsequent transmural (Q wave) myocardial infarction (acute)(of) lateral (wall) NOS
Subsequent posterior (true)transmural (Q wave) myocardial infarction (acute)
Subsequent posterobasal transmural (Q wave) myocardial infarction (acute)
Subsequent posterolateral transmural (Q wave) myocardial infarction (acute)
Subsequent posteroseptal transmural (Q wave) myocardial infarction (acute)
Subsequent septal NOS transmural (Q wave) myocardial infarction (acute)

I22.9   **Subsequent ST elevation (STEMI) myocardial infarction of unspecified site**   Ⓐ
Subsequent acute myocardial infarction of unspecified site
Subsequent myocardial infarction (acute) NOS

✓4th **I23**   **Certain current complications following ST elevation (STEMI) and non-ST elevation (NSTEMI) myocardial infarction (within the 28 day period)**

I23.Ø   **Hemopericardium as current complication following acute myocardial infarction**   Ⓐ
EXCLUDES 1 *hemopericardium not specified as current complication following acute myocardial infarction (I31.2)*

I23.1   **Atrial septal defect as current complication following acute myocardial infarction**   Ⓐ
EXCLUDES 1 *acquired atrial septal defect not specified as current complication following acute myocardial infarction (I51.Ø)*

I23.2   **Ventricular septal defect as current complication following acute myocardial infarction**   Ⓐ
EXCLUDES 1 *acquired ventricular septal defect not specified as current complication following acute myocardial infarction (I51.Ø)*

I23.3   **Rupture of cardiac wall without hemopericardium as current complication following acute myocardial infarction**   Ⓐ

I23.4   **Rupture of chordae tendineae as current complication following acute myocardial infarction**   Ⓐ
EXCLUDES 1 *rupture of chordae tendineae not specified as current complication following acute myocardial infarction (I51.1)*

I23.5   **Rupture of papillary muscle as current complication following acute myocardial infarction**   Ⓐ
EXCLUDES 1 *rupture of papillary muscle not specified as current complication following acute myocardial infarction (I51.2)*

I23.6   **Thrombosis of atrium, auricular appendage, and ventricle as current complications following acute myocardial infarction**   Ⓐ
EXCLUDES 1 *thrombosis of atrium, auricular appendage, and ventricle not specified as current complication following acute myocardial infarction (I51.3)*

I23.7   **Postinfarction angina**   Ⓐ

I23.8   **Other current complications following acute myocardial infarction**   Ⓐ

✓ Additional Character Required   ✓x7th Placeholder Alert   Unspecified Dx   Other Specified Dx   Manifestation   ▶◀ Revised Text   ● New Code   ▲ Revised Code Title

✓4th **I24** **Other acute ischemic heart diseases**
    EXCLUDES 1   *angina pectoris (I20.-)*
           transient myocardial ischemia in newborn (P29.4)

   I24.0 **Acute coronary thrombosis not resulting in myocardial** A
       infarction
       Acute coronary (artery) (vein) embolism not resulting in
          myocardial infarction
       Acute coronary (artery) (vein) occlusion not resulting in
          myocardial infarction
       Acute coronary (artery) (vein) thromboembolism not resulting in
          myocardial infarction
       EXCLUDES 1   *atherosclerotic heart disease (I25.1-)*
       AHA: 2013, 1Q, 24

   I24.1 **Dressler's syndrome** A
       Postmyocardial infarction syndrome
       EXCLUDES 1   *postinfarction angina (I23.7)*

   I24.8 **Other forms of acute ischemic heart disease** A

   I24.9 **Acute ischemic heart disease, unspecified** A
       EXCLUDES 1   *ischemic heart disease (chronic) NOS (I25.9)*

✓4th **I25** **Chronic ischemic heart disease**
   Use additional code to identify:
     chronic total occlusion of coronary artery (I25.82)
     exposure to environmental tobacco smoke (Z77.22)
     history of tobacco use (Z87.891)
     occupational exposure to environmental tobacco smoke (Z57.31)
     tobacco dependence (F17.-)
     tobacco use (Z72.0)

   I25.1 **Atherosclerotic heart disease of native coronary artery**
       Atherosclerotic cardiovascular disease
       Coronary (artery) atheroma
       Coronary (artery) atherosclerosis
       Coronary (artery) disease
       Coronary (artery) sclerosis
       Use additional code, if applicable, to identify:
         coronary atherosclerosis due to calcified coronary lesion
           (I25.84)
         coronary atherosclerosis due to lipid rich plaque (I25.83)
       EXCLUDES 2   *atheroembolism (I75.-)*
            atherosclerosis of coronary artery bypass graft(s) and
              transplanted heart (I25.7-)

     I25.10 **Atherosclerotic heart disease of native coronary** A
         artery without angina pectoris
         Atherosclerotic heart disease NOS
         AHA: 2012, 4Q, 92

   ✓6th **I25.11** **Atherosclerotic heart disease of native coronary**
         artery with angina pectoris

       I25.110 **Atherosclerotic heart disease of native** A
           coronary artery with unstable angina
           pectoris
           EXCLUDES 1   *unstable angina without*
                atherosclerotic heart disease
                (I20.0)

       I25.111 **Atherosclerotic heart disease of native** A
           coronary artery with angina pectoris
           with documented spasm
           EXCLUDES 1   *angina pectoris with documented*
                spasm without
                atherosclerotic heart disease
                (I20.1)

       I25.118 **Atherosclerotic heart disease of native** A
           coronary artery with other forms of
           angina pectoris
           EXCLUDES 1   *other forms of angina pectoris*
                without atherosclerotic
                heart disease (I20.8)

       I25.119 **Atherosclerotic heart disease of native** A
           coronary artery with unspecified angina
           pectoris
           Atherosclerotic heart disease with angina
             NOS
           Atherosclerotic heart disease with ischemic
             chest pain
           EXCLUDES 1   *unspecified angina pectoris*
                without atherosclerotic
                heart disease (I20.9)

   I25.2 **Old myocardial infarction** A
       Healed myocardial infarction
       Past myocardial infarction diagnosed by ECG or other
          investigation, but currently presenting no symptoms

   I25.3 **Aneurysm of heart**
       Mural aneurysm
       Ventricular aneurysm

✓5th **I25.4** **Coronary artery aneurysm and dissection**

   I25.41 **Coronary artery aneurysm**
       Coronary arteriovenous fistula, acquired
       EXCLUDES 1   *congenital coronary (artery) aneurysm*
             (Q24.5)

   I25.42 **Coronary artery dissection**

   I25.5 **Ischemic cardiomyopathy**
       EXCLUDES 2   *coronary atherosclerosis (I25.1-, I25.7-)*

   I25.6 **Silent myocardial ischemia**

✓5th **I25.7** **Atherosclerosis of coronary artery bypass graft(s) and**
       coronary artery of transplanted heart with angina pectoris
       Use additional code, if applicable, to identify:
         coronary atherosclerosis due to calcified coronary lesion
           (I25.84)
         coronary atherosclerosis due to lipid rich plaque (I25.83)
       EXCLUDES 1   *atherosclerosis of bypass graft(s) of transplanted heart*
            without angina pectoris (I25.812)
            atherosclerosis of coronary artery bypass graft(s)
              without angina pectoris (I25.810)
            atherosclerosis of native coronary artery of
              transplanted heart without angina pectoris
              (I25.811)
            embolism or thrombus of coronary artery bypass
              graft(s) (T82.8-)

   ✓6th **I25.70** **Atherosclerosis of coronary artery bypass graft(s),**
         unspecified, with angina pectoris

       I25.700 **Atherosclerosis of coronary artery** A
           bypass graft(s), unspecified, with
           unstable angina pectoris
           EXCLUDES 1   *unstable angina pectoris without*
                atherosclerosis of coronary
                artery bypass graft (I20.0)

       I25.701 **Atherosclerosis of coronary artery** A
           bypass graft(s), unspecified, with
           angina pectoris with documented spasm
           EXCLUDES 1   *angina pectoris with documented*
                spasm without
                atherosclerosis of coronary
                artery bypass graft (I20.1)

       I25.708 **Atherosclerosis of coronary artery** A
           bypass graft(s), unspecified, with
           other forms of angina pectoris
           EXCLUDES 1   *other forms of angina pectoris*
                without atherosclerosis of
                coronary artery bypass graft
                (I20.8)

       I25.709 **Atherosclerosis of coronary artery** A
           bypass graft(s), unspecified, with
           unspecified angina pectoris
           EXCLUDES 1   *unspecified angina pectoris*
                without atherosclerosis of
                coronary artery bypass graft
                (I20.9)

   ✓6th **I25.71** **Atherosclerosis of autologous vein coronary artery**
         bypass graft(s) with angina pectoris

       I25.710 **Atherosclerosis of autologous vein** A
           coronary artery bypass graft(s) with
           unstable angina pectoris
           EXCLUDES 1   *unstable angina without*
                atherosclerosis of
                autologous vein coronary
                artery bypass graft(s) (I20.0)

       I25.711 **Atherosclerosis of autologous vein** A
           coronary artery bypass graft(s) with
           angina pectoris with documented spasm
           EXCLUDES 1   *angina pectoris with documented*
                spasm without
                atherosclerosis of
                autologous vein coronary
                artery bypass graft(s) (I20.1)

       I25.718 **Atherosclerosis of autologous vein** A
           coronary artery bypass graft(s) with
           other forms of angina pectoris
           EXCLUDES 1   *other forms of angina pectoris*
                without atherosclerosis of
                autologous vein coronary
                artery bypass graft(s) (I20.8)

EXCLUDES 1 Not coded here   *EXCLUDES 2* Not included here   N Newborn Age: 0   P Pediatric Age: 0-17   M Maternity Age: 12-55   A Adult Age: 15-124

I25.719   **Atherosclerosis of autologous vein coronary artery bypass graft(s) with unspecified angina pectoris**   A
> *EXCLUDES 1*   *unspecified angina pectoris without atherosclerosis of autologous vein coronary artery bypass graft(s) (I20.9)*

✓6ᵗʰ   I25.72   **Atherosclerosis of autologous artery coronary artery bypass graft(s) with angina pectoris**
Atherosclerosis of internal mammary artery graft with angina pectoris

I25.720   **Atherosclerosis of autologous artery coronary artery bypass graft(s) with unstable angina pectoris**   A
> *EXCLUDES 1*   *unstable angina without atherosclerosis of autologous artery coronary artery bypass graft(s) (I20.0)*

I25.721   **Atherosclerosis of autologous artery coronary artery bypass graft(s) with angina pectoris with documented spasm**   A
> *EXCLUDES 1*   *angina pectoris with documented spasm without atherosclerosis of autologous artery coronary artery bypass graft(s) (I20.1)*

I25.728   **Atherosclerosis of autologous artery coronary artery bypass graft(s) with other forms of angina pectoris**   A
> *EXCLUDES 1*   *other forms of angina pectoris without atherosclerosis of autologous artery coronary artery bypass graft(s) (I20.8)*

I25.729   **Atherosclerosis of autologous artery coronary artery bypass graft(s) with unspecified angina pectoris**   A
> *EXCLUDES 1*   *unspecified angina pectoris without atherosclerosis of autologous artery coronary artery bypass graft(s) (I20.9)*

✓6ᵗʰ   I25.73   **Atherosclerosis of nonautologous biological coronary artery bypass graft(s) with angina pectoris**

I25.730   **Atherosclerosis of nonautologous biological coronary artery bypass graft(s) with unstable angina pectoris**   A
> *EXCLUDES 1*   *unstable angina without atherosclerosis of nonautologous biological coronary artery bypass graft(s) (I20.0)*

I25.731   **Atherosclerosis of nonautologous biological coronary artery bypass graft(s) with angina pectoris with documented spasm**   A
> *EXCLUDES 1*   *angina pectoris with documented spasm without atherosclerosis of nonautologous biological coronary artery bypass graft(s) (I20.1)*

I25.738   **Atherosclerosis of nonautologous biological coronary artery bypass graft(s) with other forms of angina pectoris**   A
> *EXCLUDES 1*   *other forms of angina pectoris without atherosclerosis of nonautologous biological coronary artery bypass graft(s) (I20.8)*

I25.739   **Atherosclerosis of nonautologous biological coronary artery bypass graft(s) with unspecified angina pectoris**   A
> *EXCLUDES 1*   *unspecified angina pectoris without atherosclerosis of nonautologous biological coronary artery bypass graft(s) (I20.9)*

✓6ᵗʰ   I25.75   **Atherosclerosis of native coronary artery of transplanted heart with angina pectoris**
> *EXCLUDES 1*   *atherosclerosis of native coronary artery of transplanted heart without angina pectoris (I25.811)*

I25.750   **Atherosclerosis of native coronary artery of transplanted heart with unstable angina**   A

I25.751   **Atherosclerosis of native coronary artery of transplanted heart with angina pectoris with documented spasm**   A

I25.758   **Atherosclerosis of native coronary artery of transplanted heart with other forms of angina pectoris**   A

I25.759   **Atherosclerosis of native coronary artery of transplanted heart with unspecified angina pectoris**   A

✓6ᵗʰ   I25.76   **Atherosclerosis of bypass graft of coronary artery of transplanted heart with angina pectoris**
> *EXCLUDES 1*   *atherosclerosis of bypass graft of coronary artery of transplanted heart without angina pectoris (I25.812)*

I25.760   **Atherosclerosis of bypass graft of coronary artery of transplanted heart with unstable angina**   A

I25.761   **Atherosclerosis of bypass graft of coronary artery of transplanted heart with angina pectoris with documented spasm**   A

I25.768   **Atherosclerosis of bypass graft of coronary artery of transplanted heart with other forms of angina pectoris**   A

I25.769   **Atherosclerosis of bypass graft of coronary artery of transplanted heart with unspecified angina pectoris**   A

✓6ᵗʰ   I25.79   **Atherosclerosis of other coronary artery bypass graft(s) with angina pectoris**

I25.790   **Atherosclerosis of other coronary artery bypass graft(s) with unstable angina pectoris**   A
> *EXCLUDES 1*   *unstable angina without atherosclerosis of other coronary artery bypass graft(s) (I20.0)*

I25.791   **Atherosclerosis of other coronary artery bypass graft(s) with angina pectoris with documented spasm**   A
> *EXCLUDES 1*   *angina pectoris with documented spasm without atherosclerosis of other coronary artery bypass graft(s) (I20.1)*

I25.798   **Atherosclerosis of other coronary artery bypass graft(s) with other forms of angina pectoris**   A
> *EXCLUDES 1*   *other forms of angina pectoris without atherosclerosis of other coronary artery bypass graft(s) (I20.8)*

I25.799   **Atherosclerosis of other coronary artery bypass graft(s) with unspecified angina pectoris**   A
> *EXCLUDES 1*   *unspecified angina pectoris without atherosclerosis of other coronary artery bypass graft(s) (I20.9)*

✓5ᵗʰ   I25.8   **Other forms of chronic ischemic heart disease**

✓6ᵗʰ   I25.81   **Atherosclerosis of other coronary vessels without angina pectoris**
Use additional code, if applicable, to identify:
     coronary atherosclerosis due to calcified coronary lesion (I25.84)
     coronary atherosclerosis due to lipid rich plaque (I25.83)
> *EXCLUDES 1*   *atherosclerotic heart disease of native coronary artery without angina pectoris (I25.10)*

I25.810   **Atherosclerosis of coronary artery bypass graft(s) without angina pectoris**   A
Atherosclerosis of coronary artery bypass graft NOS
> *EXCLUDES 1*   *atherosclerosis of coronary bypass graft(s) with angina pectoris (I25.70--I25.73-, I25.79-)*

☑ Additional Character Required   ✓x7ᵗʰ Placeholder Alert   Unspecified Dx   Other Specified Dx   Manifestation   ▶◀ Revised Text   ● New Code   ▲ Revised Code Title

I25.811 Atherosclerosis of native coronary artery of transplanted heart without angina pectoris   A

Atherosclerosis of native coronary artery of transplanted heart NOS

EXCLUDES 1   *atherosclerosis of native coronary artery of transplanted heart with angina pectoris (I25.75-)*

I25.812 Atherosclerosis of bypass graft of coronary artery of transplanted heart without angina pectoris   A

Atherosclerosis of bypass graft of transplanted heart NOS

EXCLUDES 1   *atherosclerosis of bypass graft of transplanted heart with angina pectoris (I25.76)*

I25.82 Chronic total occlusion of coronary artery

Complete occlusion of coronary artery

Total occlusion of coronary artery

Code first coronary atherosclerosis (I25.1-, I25.7-, I25.81-)

EXCLUDES 1   *acute coronary occlusion with myocardial infarction (I21.-, I22.-)*

acute coronary occlusion without myocardial infarction (I24.0)

I25.83 Coronary atherosclerosis due to lipid rich plaque   A

Code first coronary atherosclerosis (I25.1-, I25.7-, I25.81-)

I25.84 Coronary atherosclerosis due to calcified coronary lesion

Coronary atherosclerosis due to severely calcified coronary lesion

Code first coronary atherosclerosis (I25.1-, I25.7-, I25.81-)

I25.89 Other forms of chronic ischemic heart disease

I25.9 Chronic ischemic heart disease, unspecified

Ischemic heart disease (chronic) NOS

Pulmonary heart disease and diseases of pulmonary circulation (I26-I28)

✓4ᵗʰ **I26 Pulmonary embolism**

Pulmonary (acute) (artery)(vein) infarction

Pulmonary (acute) (artery)(vein) thromboembolism

Pulmonary (acute) (artery)(vein) thrombosis

EXCLUDES 2   *chronic pulmonary embolism (I27.82)*

personal history of pulmonary embolism (Z86.711)

pulmonary embolism due to trauma (T79.0, T79.1)

pulmonary embolism due to complications of surgical and medical care (T80.0, T81.7-, T82.8-)

pulmonary embolism complicating abortion, ectopic or molar pregnancy (O00-O07, O08.2)

pulmonary embolism complicating pregnancy, childbirth and the puerperium (O88.-)

septic (non-pulmonary) arterial embolism (I76)

✓5ᵗʰ **I26.0 Pulmonary embolism with acute cor pulmonale**

I26.01 Septic pulmonary embolism with acute cor pulmonale

Code first underlying infection

I26.02 Saddle embolus of pulmonary artery with acute cor pulmonale

I26.09 Other pulmonary embolism with acute cor pulmonale

Acute cor pulmonale NOS

AHA: 2014, 4Q, 21

✓5ᵗʰ **I26.9 Pulmonary embolism without acute cor pulmonale**

I26.90 Septic pulmonary embolism without acute cor pulmonale

Code first underlying infection

I26.92 Saddle embolus of pulmonary artery without acute cor pulmonale

I26.99 Other pulmonary embolism without acute cor pulmonale

Acute pulmonary embolism NOS

Pulmonary embolism NOS

✓4ᵗʰ **I27 Other pulmonary heart diseases**

I27.0 Primary pulmonary hypertension

EXCLUDES 1   *pulmonary hypertension NOS (I27.2)*

secondary pulmonary hypertension (I27.2)

I27.1 Kyphoscoliotic heart disease

I27.2 Other secondary pulmonary hypertension

Pulmonary hypertension NOS

Code also associated underlying condition

AHA: 2014, 4Q, 21

✓5ᵗʰ **I27.8 Other specified pulmonary heart diseases**

I27.81 Cor pulmonale (chronic)

Cor pulmonale NOS

EXCLUDES 1   *acute cor pulmonale (I26.0-)*

AHA: 2014, 4Q, 21

I27.82 Chronic pulmonary embolism

Use additional code, if applicable, for associated long-term (current) use of anticoagulants (Z79.01)

EXCLUDES 1   *personal history of pulmonary embolism (Z86.711)*

I27.89 Other specified pulmonary heart diseases

Eisenmenger's complex

Eisenmenger's syndrome

EXCLUDES 1   *Eisenmenger's defect (Q21.8)*

I27.9 Pulmonary heart disease, unspecified

Chronic cardiopulmonary disease

✓4ᵗʰ **I28 Other diseases of pulmonary vessels**

I28.0 Arteriovenous fistula of pulmonary vessels

EXCLUDES 1   *congenital arteriovenous fistula (Q25.72)*

I28.1 Aneurysm of pulmonary artery

EXCLUDES 1   *congenital aneurysm (Q25.79)*

congenital arteriovenous aneurysm (Q25.72)

I28.8 Other diseases of pulmonary vessels

Pulmonary arteritis

Pulmonary endarteritis

Rupture of pulmonary vessels

Stenosis of pulmonary vessels

Stricture of pulmonary vessels

I28.9 Disease of pulmonary vessels, unspecified

Other forms of heart disease (I30-I52)

✓4ᵗʰ **I30 Acute pericarditis**

INCLUDES   acute mediastinopericarditis

acute myopericarditis

acute pericardial effusion

acute pleuropericarditis

acute pneumopericarditis

EXCLUDES 1   *Dressler's syndrome (I24.1)*

rheumatic pericarditis (acute) (I01.0)

I30.0 Acute nonspecific idiopathic pericarditis

I30.1 Infective pericarditis

Pneumococcal pericarditis

Pneumopyopericardium

Purulent pericarditis

Pyopericarditis

Pyopericardium

Pyopneumopericardium

Staphylococcal pericarditis

Streptococcal pericarditis

Suppurative pericarditis

Viral pericarditis

Use additional code (B95-B97) to identify infectious agent

I30.8 Other forms of acute pericarditis

I30.9 Acute pericarditis, unspecified

✓4ᵗʰ **I31 Other diseases of pericardium**

EXCLUDES 1   *diseases of pericardium specified as rheumatic (I09.2)*

postcardiotomy syndrome (I97.0)

traumatic injury to pericardium (S26.-)

I31.0 Chronic adhesive pericarditis

Accretio cordis

Adherent pericardium

Adhesive mediastinopericarditis

I31.1 Chronic constrictive pericarditis

Concretio cordis

Pericardial calcification

I31.2 Hemopericardium, not elsewhere classified

EXCLUDES 1   *hemopericardium as current complication following acute myocardial infarction (I23.0)*

I31.3 Pericardial effusion (noninflammatory)

Chylopericardium

EXCLUDES 1   *acute pericardial effusion (I30.9)*

I31.4 Cardiac tamponade

Code first underlying cause

EXCLUDES 1   Not coded here   EXCLUDES 2   Not included here   N Newborn Age: 0   P Pediatric Age: 0-17   M Maternity Age: 12-55   A Adult Age: 15-124

590   ICD-10-CM 2016

I31.8 Other specified diseases of pericardium
Epicardial plaques
Focal pericardial adhesions

I31.9 Disease of pericardium, unspecified
Pericardial (chronic) NOS

I32 Pericarditis in diseases classified elsewhere
Code first underlying disease
EXCLUDES 1   pericarditis (in):
     coxsackie (virus) (B33.23)
     gonococcal (A54.83)
     meningococcal (A39.53)
     rheumatoid (arthritis) (M05.31)
     syphilitic (A52.06)
     systemic lupus erythematosus (M32.12)
     tuberculosis (A18.84)

✓4th I33 Acute and subacute endocarditis
EXCLUDES 1   acute rheumatic endocarditis (I01.1)
     endocarditis NOS (I38)

I33.0 Acute and subacute infective endocarditis
Bacterial endocarditis (acute) (subacute)
Infective endocarditis (acute) (subacute) NOS
Endocarditis lenta (acute) (subacute)
Malignant endocarditis (acute) (subacute)
Purulent endocarditis (acute) (subacute)
Septic endocarditis (acute) (subacute)
Ulcerative endocarditis (acute) (subacute)
Vegetative endocarditis (acute) (subacute)
Use additional code (B95-B97) to identify infectious agent

I33.9 Acute and subacute endocarditis, unspecified
Acute endocarditis NOS
Acute myoendocarditis NOS
Acute periendocarditis NOS
Subacute endocarditis NOS
Subacute myoendocarditis NOS
Subacute periendocarditis NOS

✓4th I34 Nonrheumatic mitral valve disorders
EXCLUDES 1   mitral valve disease (I05.9)
     mitral valve failure (I05.8)
     mitral valve stenosis (I05.0)
     mitral valve disorder of unspecified cause with diseases of aortic
       and/or tricuspid valve(s) (I08.-)
     mitral valve disorder of unspecified cause with mitral stenosis or
       obstruction (I05.0)
     mitral valve disorder specified as congenital (Q23.2, Q23.3)
     mitral valve disorder specified as rheumatic (I05.-)

I34.0 Nonrheumatic mitral (valve) insufficiency
Nonrheumatic mitral (valve) incompetence NOS
Nonrheumatic mitral (valve) regurgitation NOS

I34.1 Nonrheumatic mitral (valve) prolapse
Floppy nonrheumatic mitral valve syndrome
EXCLUDES 1   Marfan's syndrome (Q87.4-)

I34.2 Nonrheumatic mitral (valve) stenosis

I34.8 Other nonrheumatic mitral valve disorders

I34.9 Nonrheumatic mitral valve disorder, unspecified

✓4th I35 Nonrheumatic aortic valve disorders
EXCLUDES 1   aortic valve disorder of unspecified cause but with diseases of
       mitral and/or tricuspid valve(s) (I08.-)
     aortic valve disorder specified as congenital (Q23.0, Q23.1)
     aortic valve disorder specified as rheumatic (I06.-)
     hypertrophic subaortic stenosis (I42.1)

I35.0 Nonrheumatic aortic (valve) stenosis

I35.1 Nonrheumatic aortic (valve) insufficiency
Nonrheumatic aortic (valve) incompetence NOS
Nonrheumatic aortic (valve) regurgitation NOS

I35.2 Nonrheumatic aortic (valve) stenosis with insufficiency

I35.8 Other nonrheumatic aortic valve disorders

I35.9 Nonrheumatic aortic valve disorder, unspecified

✓4th I36 Nonrheumatic tricuspid valve disorders
EXCLUDES 1   tricuspid valve disorders of unspecified cause (I07.-)
     tricuspid valve disorders specified as congenital (Q22.4, Q22.8,
       Q22.9)
     tricuspid valve disorders specified as rheumatic (I07.-)
     tricuspid valve disorders with aortic and/or mitral valve
       involvement (I08.-)

I36.0 Nonrheumatic tricuspid (valve) stenosis

I36.1 Nonrheumatic tricuspid (valve) insufficiency
Nonrheumatic tricuspid (valve) incompetence
Nonrheumatic tricuspid (valve) regurgitation

I36.2 Nonrheumatic tricuspid (valve) stenosis with insufficiency

I36.8 Other nonrheumatic tricuspid valve disorders

I36.9 Nonrheumatic tricuspid valve disorder, unspecified

✓4th I37 Nonrheumatic pulmonary valve disorders
EXCLUDES 1   pulmonary valve disorder specified as congenital (Q22.1, Q22.2,
       Q22.3)
     pulmonary valve disorder specified as rheumatic (I09.89)

I37.0 Nonrheumatic pulmonary valve stenosis

I37.1 Nonrheumatic pulmonary valve insufficiency
Nonrheumatic pulmonary valve incompetence
Nonrheumatic pulmonary valve regurgitation

I37.2 Nonrheumatic pulmonary valve stenosis with insufficiency

I37.8 Other nonrheumatic pulmonary valve disorders

I37.9 Nonrheumatic pulmonary valve disorder, unspecified

I38 Endocarditis, valve unspecified
INCLUDES   endocarditis (chronic) NOS
     valvular incompetence NOS
     valvular insufficiency NOS
     valvular regurgitation NOS
     valvular stenosis NOS
     valvulitis (chronic) NOS
EXCLUDES 1   congenital insufficiency of cardiac valve NOS (Q24.8)
     congenital stenosis of cardiac valve NOS (Q24.8)
     endocardial fibroelastosis (I42.4)
     endocarditis specified as rheumatic (I09.1)

I39 Endocarditis and heart valve disorders in diseases classified elsewhere
Code first underlying disease, such as:
     Q fever (A78)
EXCLUDES 1   endocardial involvement in:
     candidiasis (B37.6)
     gonococcal infection (A54.83)
     Libman-Sacks disease (M32.11)
     listerosis (A32.82)
     meningococcal infection (A39.51)
     rheumatoid arthritis (M05.31)
     syphilis (A52.03)
     tuberculosis (A18.84)
     typhoid fever (A01.02)

✓4th I40 Acute myocarditis
INCLUDES   subacute myocarditis
EXCLUDES 1   acute rheumatic myocarditis (I01.2)

I40.0 Infective myocarditis
Septic myocarditis
Use additional code (B95-B97) to identify infectious agent

I40.1 Isolated myocarditis
Fiedler's myocarditis
Giant cell myocarditis
Idiopathic myocarditis

I40.8 Other acute myocarditis

I40.9 Acute myocarditis, unspecified

I41 Myocarditis in diseases classified elsewhere
Code first underlying disease, such as:
     typhus (A75.0-A75.9)
EXCLUDES 1   myocarditis (in):
     Chagas' disease (chronic) (B57.2)
       acute (B57.0)
     coxsackie (virus) infection (B33.22)
     diphtheritic (A36.81)
     gonococcal (A54.83)
     influenzal (J09.X9, J10.82, J11.82)
     meningococcal (A39.52)
     mumps (B26.82)
     rheumatoid arthritis (M05.31)
     sarcoid (D86.85)
     syphilis (A52.06)
     toxoplasmosis (B58.81)
     tuberculous (A18.84)

✓4th I42 Cardiomyopathy
INCLUDES   myocardiopathy
Code first pre-existing cardiomyopathy complicating pregnancy and
     puerperium (O99.4)
EXCLUDES 1   ischemic cardiomyopathy (I25.5)
     peripartum cardiomyopathy (O90.3)
EXCLUDES 2   ventricular hypertrophy (I51.7)

I42.0 Dilated cardiomyopathy
Congestive cardiomyopathy

I42.1 Obstructive hypertrophic cardiomyopathy
Hypertrophic subaortic stenosis (idiopathic)

☑ Additional Character Required   ✓x7th Placeholder Alert   Unspecified Dx   Other Specified Dx   Manifestation   ►◄ Revised Text   ● New Code   ▲ Revised Code Title

Chapter 9. Diseases of the Circulatory System

I42.2   **Other hypertrophic cardiomyopathy**
Nonobstructive hypertrophic cardiomyopathy

I42.3   **Endomyocardial (eosinophilic) disease**
Endomyocardial (tropical) fibrosis
Löffler's endocarditis

I42.4   **Endocardial fibroelastosis**
Congenital cardiomyopathy
Elastomyofibrosis

I42.5   **Other restrictive cardiomyopathy**
Constrictive cardiomyopathy NOS

I42.6   **Alcoholic cardiomyopathy**
Code also presence of alcoholism (F10.-)

I42.7   **Cardiomyopathy due to drug and external agent**
Code first poisoning due to drug or toxin, if applicable (T36-T65 with fifth or sixth character 1-4 or 6)
Use additional code for adverse effect, if applicable, to identify drug (T36-T50 with fifth or sixth character 5)

I42.8   **Other cardiomyopathies**

I42.9   **Cardiomyopathy, unspecified**
Cardiomyopathy (primary) (secondary) NOS

I43   *Cardiomyopathy in diseases classified elsewhere*
Code first underlying disease, such as:
amyloidosis (E85.-)
glycogen storage disease (E74.0)
gout (M10.0-)
thyrotoxicosis (E05.0-E05.9-)
EXCLUDES 1   *cardiomyopathy (in):*
coxsackie (virus) (B33.24)
diphtheria (A36.81)
sarcoidosis (D86.85)
tuberculosis (A18.84)

✓4ᵗʰ **I44**   **Atrioventricular and left bundle-branch block**

I44.0   **Atrioventricular block, first degree**

I44.1   **Atrioventricular block, second degree**
Atrioventricular block, type I and II
Möbitz block, type I and II
Second degree block, type I and II
Wenckebach's block

I44.2   **Atrioventricular block, complete**
Complete heart block NOS
Third degree block

✓5ᵗʰ **I44.3**   **Other and unspecified atrioventricular block**
Atrioventricular block NOS

     I44.30   **Unspecified atrioventricular block**

     I44.39   **Other atrioventricular block**

I44.4   **Left anterior fascicular block**

I44.5   **Left posterior fascicular block**

✓5ᵗʰ **I44.6**   **Other and unspecified fascicular block**

     I44.60   **Unspecified fascicular block**
Left bundle-branch hemiblock NOS

     I44.69   **Other fascicular block**

I44.7   **Left bundle-branch block, unspecified**

✓4ᵗʰ **I45**   **Other conduction disorders**

I45.0   **Right fascicular block**

✓5ᵗʰ **I45.1**   **Other and unspecified right bundle-branch block**

     I45.10   **Unspecified right bundle-branch block**
Right bundle-branch block NOS

     I45.19   **Other right bundle-branch block**

I45.2   **Bifascicular block**

I45.3   **Trifascicular block**

I45.4   **Nonspecific intraventricular block**
Bundle-branch block NOS

I45.5   **Other specified heart block**
Sinoatrial block
Sinoauricular block
EXCLUDES 1   *heart block NOS (I45.9)*

I45.6   **Pre-excitation syndrome**
Accelerated atrioventricular conduction
Accessory atrioventricular conduction
Anomalous atrioventricular excitation
Lown-Ganong-Levine syndrome
Pre-excitation atrioventricular conduction
Wolff-Parkinson-White syndrome

✓5ᵗʰ **I45.8**   **Other specified conduction disorders**

     I45.81   **Long QT syndrome**

     I45.89   **Other specified conduction disorders**
Atrioventricular [AV] dissociation
Interference dissociation
Isorhythmic dissociation
Nonparoxysmal AV nodal tachycardia
AHA: 2013, 2Q, 31

I45.9   **Conduction disorder, unspecified**
Heart block NOS
Stokes-Adams syndrome

✓4ᵗʰ **I46**   **Cardiac arrest**
EXCLUDES 1   *cardiogenic shock (R57.0)*

I46.2   **Cardiac arrest due to underlying cardiac condition**
Code first underlying cardiac condition

I46.8   **Cardiac arrest due to other underlying condition**
Code first underlying condition

I46.9   **Cardiac arrest, cause unspecified**

✓4ᵗʰ **I47**   **Paroxysmal tachycardia**
Code first tachycardia complicating:
abortion or ectopic or molar pregnancy (O00-O07, O08.8)
obstetric surgery and procedures (O75.4)
EXCLUDES 1   *tachycardia NOS (R00.0)*
sinoauricular tachycardia NOS (R00.0)
sinus [sinusal] tachycardia NOS (R00.0)

I47.0   **Re-entry ventricular arrhythmia**

I47.1   **Supraventricular tachycardia**
Atrial (paroxysmal) tachycardia
Atrioventricular [AV] (paroxysmal) tachycardia
Atrioventricular re-entrant (nodal) tachycardia [AVNRT] [AVRT]
Junctional (paroxysmal) tachycardia
Nodal (paroxysmal) tachycardia

I47.2   **Ventricular tachycardia**
AHA: 2013, 3Q, 23

I47.9   **Paroxysmal tachycardia, unspecified**
Bouveret (-Hoffman) syndrome

✓4ᵗʰ **I48**   **Atrial fibrillation and flutter**

I48.0   **Paroxysmal atrial fibrillation**

I48.1   **Persistent atrial fibrillation**

I48.2   **Chronic atrial fibrillation**
Permanent atrial fibrillation

I48.3   **Typical atrial flutter**
Type I atrial flutter

I48.4   **Atypical atrial flutter**
Type II atrial flutter

✓5ᵗʰ **I48.9**   **Unspecified atrial fibrillation and atrial flutter**

     I48.91   **Unspecified atrial fibrillation**

     I48.92   **Unspecified atrial flutter**

✓4ᵗʰ **I49**   **Other cardiac arrhythmias**
Code first cardiac arrhythmia complicating:
abortion or ectopic or molar pregnancy (O00-O07, O08.8)
obstetric surgery and procedures (O75.4)
EXCLUDES 1   *bradycardia NOS (R00.1)*
neonatal dysrhythmia (P29.1-)
sinoatrial bradycardia (R00.1)
sinus bradycardia (R00.1)
vagal bradycardia (R00.1)

✓5ᵗʰ **I49.0**   **Ventricular fibrillation and flutter**

     I49.01   **Ventricular fibrillation**

     I49.02   **Ventricular flutter**

I49.1   **Atrial premature depolarization**
Atrial premature beats

I49.2   **Junctional premature depolarization**

I49.3   **Ventricular premature depolarization**

✓5ᵗʰ **I49.4**   **Other and unspecified premature depolarization**

     I49.40   **Unspecified premature depolarization**
Premature beats NOS

     I49.49   **Other premature depolarization**
Ectopic beatsExtrasystolic arrhythmias
ExtrasystolesPremature contractions

I49.5   **Sick sinus syndrome**
Tachycardia-bradycardia syndrome

I49.8   **Other specified cardiac arrhythmias**
Coronary sinus rhythm disorder
Ectopic rhythm disorder
Nodal rhythm disorder

I49.9   **Cardiac arrhythmia, unspecified**
Arrhythmia (cardiac) NOS

EXCLUDES 1 Not coded here   EXCLUDES 2 Not included here   N Newborn Age: 0   P Pediatric Age: 0-17   M Maternity Age: 12-55   A Adult Age: 15-124

Chapter 9. Diseases of the Circulatory System

✓4th **I50 Heart failure**
Code first:
heart failure complicating abortion or ectopic or molar pregnancy (O00-O07, O08.8)
heart failure following surgery (I97.13-)
heart failure due to hypertension (I11.0)
heart failure due to hypertension with chronic kidney disease (I13.-)
obstetric surgery and procedures (O75.4)
rheumatic heart failure (I09.81)
EXCLUDES 1   cardiac arrest (I46.-)
neonatal cardiac failure (P29.0)
AHA: 2014, 1Q, 25; 2013, 2Q, 33

I50.1 Left ventricular failure
Cardiac asthma
Edema of lung with heart disease NOS
Edema of lung with heart failure
Left heart failure
Pulmonary edema with heart disease NOS
Pulmonary edema with heart failure
EXCLUDES 1   edema of lung without heart disease or heart failure (J81.-)
pulmonary edema without heart disease or failure (J81.-)

✓5th **I50.2 Systolic (congestive) heart failure**
EXCLUDES 1   combined systolic (congestive) and diastolic (congestive) heart failure (I50.4-)

I50.20 **Unspecified systolic (congestive) heart failure**
I50.21 **Acute systolic (congestive) heart failure**
I50.22 **Chronic systolic (congestive) heart failure**
I50.23 **Acute on chronic systolic (congestive) heart failure**

✓5th **I50.3 Diastolic (congestive) heart failure**
EXCLUDES 1   combined systolic (congestive) and diastolic (congestive) heart failure (I50.4-)

I50.30 **Unspecified diastolic (congestive) heart failure**
I50.31 **Acute diastolic (congestive) heart failure**
I50.32 **Chronic diastolic (congestive) heart failure**
I50.33 **Acute on chronic diastolic (congestive) heart failure**

✓5th **I50.4 Combined systolic (congestive) and diastolic (congestive) heart failure**
I50.40 **Unspecified combined systolic (congestive) and diastolic (congestive) heart failure**
I50.41 **Acute combined systolic (congestive) and diastolic (congestive) heart failure**
I50.42 **Chronic combined systolic (congestive) and diastolic (congestive) heart failure**
I50.43 **Acute on chronic combined systolic (congestive) and diastolic (congestive) heart failure**

I50.9 Heart failure, unspecified
Biventricular (heart) failure NOS
Cardiac, heart or myocardial failure NOS
Congestive heart disease
Congestive heart failure NOS
Right ventricular failure (secondary to left heart failure)
EXCLUDES 1   fluid overload (E87.70)
AHA: 2014, 4Q, 21; 2012, 4Q, 92

✓4th **I51 Complications and ill-defined descriptions of heart disease**
EXCLUDES 1   any condition in I51.4-I51.9 due to hypertension (I11.-)
any condition in I51.4-I51.9 due to hypertension and chronic kidney disease (I13.-)
heart disease specified as rheumatic (I00-I09)

I51.0 Cardiac septal defect, acquired   A
Acquired septal atrial defect (old)
Acquired septal auricular defect (old)
Acquired septal ventricular defect (old)
EXCLUDES 1   cardiac septal defect as current complication following acute myocardial infarction (I23.1, I23.2)

I51.1 Rupture of chordae tendineae, not elsewhere classified
EXCLUDES 1   rupture of chordae tendineae as current complication following acute myocardial infarction (I23.4)

I51.2 Rupture of papillary muscle, not elsewhere classified
EXCLUDES 1   rupture of papillary muscle as current complication following acute myocardial infarction (I23.5)

I51.3 Intracardiac thrombosis, not elsewhere classified
Apical thrombosis (old)   Mural thrombosis (old)
Atrial thrombosis (old)   Ventricular thrombosis (old)
Auricular thrombosis (old)
EXCLUDES 1   intracardiac thrombosis as current complication following acute myocardial infarction (I23.6)
AHA: 2013, 1Q, 24

I51.4 Myocarditis, unspecified
Chronic (interstitial) myocarditis
Myocardial fibrosis
Myocarditis NOS
EXCLUDES 1   acute or subacute myocarditis (I40.-)

I51.5 Myocardial degeneration
Fatty degeneration of heart or myocardium
Myocardial disease
Senile degeneration of heart or myocardium

I51.7 Cardiomegaly
Cardiac dilatation
Cardiac hypertrophy
Ventricular dilatation

✓5th **I51.8 Other ill-defined heart diseases**
I51.81 Takotsubo syndrome
Reversible left ventricular dysfunction following sudden emotional stress
Stress induced cardiomyopathy
Takotsubo cardiomyopathy
Transient left ventricular apical ballooning syndrome

I51.89 Other ill-defined heart diseases
Carditis (acute)(chronic)
Pancarditis (acute)(chronic)

I51.9 Heart disease, unspecified

I52 Other heart disorders in diseases classified elsewhere
Code first underlying disease, such as:
congenital syphilis (A50.5)
mucopolysaccharidosis (E76.3)
schistosomiasis (B65.0-B65.9)
EXCLUDES 1   heart disease (in):
gonococcal infection (A54.83)
meningococcal infection (A39.50)
rheumatoid arthritis (M05.31)
syphilis (A52.06)

Cerebrovascular diseases (I60-I69)

Use additional code to identify presence of:
alcohol abuse and dependence (F10.-)
exposure to environmental tobacco smoke (Z77.22)
history of tobacco use (Z87.891)
hypertension (I10-I15)
occupational exposure to environmental tobacco smoke (Z57.31)
tobacco dependence (F17.-)
tobacco use (Z72.0)
EXCLUDES 1   transient cerebral ischemic attacks and related syndromes (G45.-)
traumatic intracranial hemorrhage (S06.-)
AHA: 2014, 3Q, 5; 2012, 4Q, 91-92

✓4th **I60 Nontraumatic subarachnoid hemorrhage**
INCLUDES   ruptured cerebral aneurysm
EXCLUDES 1   sequelae of subarachnoid hemorrhage (I69.0-)
syphilitic ruptured cerebral aneurysm (A52.05)

✓5th **I60.0 Nontraumatic subarachnoid hemorrhage from carotid siphon and bifurcation**
I60.00 **Nontraumatic subarachnoid hemorrhage from unspecified carotid siphon and bifurcation**
I60.01 **Nontraumatic subarachnoid hemorrhage from right carotid siphon and bifurcation**
I60.02 **Nontraumatic subarachnoid hemorrhage from left carotid siphon and bifurcation**

✓5th **I60.1 Nontraumatic subarachnoid hemorrhage from middle cerebral artery**
I60.10 **Nontraumatic subarachnoid hemorrhage from unspecified middle cerebral artery**
I60.11 **Nontraumatic subarachnoid hemorrhage from right middle cerebral artery**
I60.12 **Nontraumatic subarachnoid hemorrhage from left middle cerebral artery**

✓5th **I60.2 Nontraumatic subarachnoid hemorrhage from anterior communicating artery**
I60.20 **Nontraumatic subarachnoid hemorrhage from unspecified anterior communicating artery**
I60.21 **Nontraumatic subarachnoid hemorrhage from right anterior communicating artery**
I60.22 **Nontraumatic subarachnoid hemorrhage from left anterior communicating artery**

✓5th **I60.3 Nontraumatic subarachnoid hemorrhage from posterior communicating artery**
I60.30 **Nontraumatic subarachnoid hemorrhage from unspecified posterior communicating artery**

✓ Additional Character Required   ✓x7th Placeholder Alert   Unspecified Dx   Other Specified Dx   Manifestation   ►◄ Revised Text   ● New Code   ▲ Revised Code Title

I60.31 Nontraumatic subarachnoid hemorrhage from right posterior communicating artery

I60.32 Nontraumatic subarachnoid hemorrhage from left posterior communicating artery

I60.4 Nontraumatic subarachnoid hemorrhage from basilar artery

✓5th **I60.5** Nontraumatic subarachnoid hemorrhage from vertebral artery

    I60.50 Nontraumatic subarachnoid hemorrhage from unspecified vertebral artery

    I60.51 Nontraumatic subarachnoid hemorrhage from right vertebral artery

    I60.52 Nontraumatic subarachnoid hemorrhage from left vertebral artery

I60.6 Nontraumatic subarachnoid hemorrhage from other intracranial arteries

I60.7 Nontraumatic subarachnoid hemorrhage from unspecified intracranial artery

    Ruptured (congenital) berry aneurysm
    Ruptured (congenital) cerebral aneurysm
    Subarachnoid hemorrhage (nontraumatic) from cerebral artery NOS
    Subarachnoid hemorrhage (nontraumatic) from communicating artery NOS

    EXCLUDES 1 berry aneurysm, nonruptured (I67.1)

I60.8 Other nontraumatic subarachnoid hemorrhage
    Meningeal hemorrhage
    Rupture of cerebral arteriovenous malformation

I60.9 Nontraumatic subarachnoid hemorrhage, unspecified

✓4th **I61** Nontraumatic intracerebral **hemorrhage**
    EXCLUDES 1 sequelae of intracerebral hemorrhage (I69.1-)

I61.0 Nontraumatic intracerebral hemorrhage in hemisphere, subcortical
    Deep intracerebral hemorrhage (nontraumatic)

I61.1 Nontraumatic intracerebral hemorrhage in hemisphere, cortical
    Cerebral lobe hemorrhage (nontraumatic)
    Superficial intracerebral hemorrhage (nontraumatic)

I61.2 Nontraumatic intracerebral hemorrhage in hemisphere, unspecified

I61.3 Nontraumatic intracerebral hemorrhage in brain stem

I61.4 Nontraumatic intracerebral hemorrhage in cerebellum

I61.5 Nontraumatic intracerebral hemorrhage, intraventricular

I61.6 Nontraumatic intracerebral hemorrhage, multiple localized

I61.8 Other nontraumatic intracerebral hemorrhage

I61.9 Nontraumatic intracerebral hemorrhage, unspecified

✓4th **I62** Other and unspecified nontraumatic intracranial **hemorrhage**
    EXCLUDES 1 sequelae of intracranial hemorrhage (I69.2)

✓5th **I62.0** Nontraumatic subdural hemorrhage

    I62.00 Nontraumatic subdural hemorrhage, unspecified

    I62.01 Nontraumatic acute subdural hemorrhage

    I62.02 Nontraumatic subacute subdural hemorrhage

    I62.03 Nontraumatic chronic subdural hemorrhage

I62.1 Nontraumatic extradural hemorrhage
    Nontraumatic epidural hemorrhage

I62.9 Nontraumatic intracranial hemorrhage, unspecified

✓4th **I63** Cerebral infarction
    INCLUDES occlusion and stenosis of cerebral and precerebral arteries, resulting in cerebral infarction
    Use additional code, if applicable, to identify status post administration of tPA (rtPA) in a different facility within the last 24 hours prior to admission to current facility (Z92.82)
    EXCLUDES 1 sequelae of cerebral infarction (I69.3-)
    AHA: 2014, 1Q, 23

✓5th **I63.0** Cerebral infarction due to thrombosis of precerebral arteries

    I63.00 Cerebral infarction due to thrombosis of unspecified precerebral artery

    ✓6th **I63.01** Cerebral infarction due to thrombosis of vertebral artery

        I63.011 Cerebral infarction due to thrombosis of right vertebral artery **A**

        I63.012 Cerebral infarction due to thrombosis of left vertebral artery **A**

        I63.019 Cerebral infarction due to thrombosis of unspecified vertebral artery **A**

    I63.02 Cerebral infarction due to thrombosis of basilar artery **A**

✓6th **I63.03** Cerebral infarction due to thrombosis of carotid artery

    I63.031 Cerebral infarction due to thrombosis of right carotid artery

    I63.032 Cerebral infarction due to thrombosis of left carotid artery

    I63.039 Cerebral infarction due to thrombosis of unspecified carotid artery

I63.09 Cerebral infarction due to thrombosis of other precerebral artery

✓5th **I63.1** Cerebral infarction due to embolism of precerebral arteries

    I63.10 Cerebral infarction due to embolism of unspecified precerebral artery

    ✓6th **I63.11** Cerebral infarction due to embolism of vertebral artery

        I63.111 Cerebral infarction due to embolism of right vertebral artery **A**

        I63.112 Cerebral infarction due to embolism of left vertebral artery **A**

        I63.119 Cerebral infarction due to embolism of unspecified vertebral artery **A**

    I63.12 Cerebral infarction due to embolism of basilar artery **A**

    ✓6th **I63.13** Cerebral infarction due to embolism of carotid artery

        I63.131 Cerebral infarction due to embolism of right carotid artery

        I63.132 Cerebral infarction due to embolism of left carotid artery

        I63.139 Cerebral infarction due to embolism of unspecified carotid artery

    I63.19 Cerebral infarction due to embolism of other precerebral artery

✓5th **I63.2** Cerebral infarction due to unspecified occlusion or stenosis of precerebral arteries

    I63.20 Cerebral infarction due to unspecified occlusion or stenosis of unspecified precerebral arteries

    ✓6th **I63.21** Cerebral infarction due to unspecified occlusion or stenosis of vertebral arteries

        I63.211 Cerebral infarction due to unspecified occlusion or stenosis of right vertebral arteries **A**

        I63.212 Cerebral infarction due to unspecified occlusion or stenosis of left vertebral arteries **A**

        I63.219 Cerebral infarction due to unspecified occlusion or stenosis of unspecified vertebral arteries **A**

    I63.22 Cerebral infarction due to unspecified occlusion or stenosis of basilar arteries **A**

    ✓6th **I63.23** Cerebral infarction due to unspecified occlusion or stenosis of carotid arteries

        I63.231 Cerebral infarction due to unspecified occlusion or stenosis of right carotid arteries

        I63.232 Cerebral infarction due to unspecified occlusion or stenosis of left carotid arteries

        I63.239 Cerebral infarction due to unspecified occlusion or stenosis of unspecified carotid arteries

    I63.29 Cerebral infarction due to unspecified occlusion or stenosis of other precerebral arteries

✓5th **I63.3** Cerebral infarction due to thrombosis of cerebral arteries

    I63.30 Cerebral infarction due to thrombosis of unspecified cerebral artery **A**

    ✓6th **I63.31** Cerebral infarction due to thrombosis of middle cerebral artery

        I63.311 Cerebral infarction due to thrombosis of right middle cerebral artery **A**

        I63.312 Cerebral infarction due to thrombosis of left middle cerebral artery **A**

        I63.319 Cerebral infarction due to thrombosis of unspecified middle cerebral artery **A**

    ✓6th **I63.32** Cerebral infarction due to thrombosis of anterior cerebral artery

        I63.321 Cerebral infarction due to thrombosis of right anterior cerebral artery **A**

EXCLUDES 1 Not coded here   **EXCLUDES 2** Not included here   **N** Newborn Age: 0   **P** Pediatric Age: 0-17   **M** Maternity Age: 12-55   **A** Adult Age: 15-124

594

ICD-10-CM 2016

I63.322 Cerebral infarction due to thrombosis of left anterior cerebral artery ◰

I63.329 Cerebral infarction due to thrombosis of unspecified anterior cerebral artery ◰

✓6ᵗʰ **I63.33** Cerebral infarction due to thrombosis of posterior cerebral artery

I63.331 Cerebral infarction due to thrombosis of right posterior cerebral artery ◰

I63.332 Cerebral infarction due to thrombosis of left posterior cerebral artery ◰

I63.339 Cerebral infarction due to thrombosis of unspecified posterior cerebral artery ◰

✓6ᵗʰ **I63.34** Cerebral infarction due to thrombosis of cerebellar artery

I63.341 Cerebral infarction due to thrombosis of right cerebellar artery ◰

I63.342 Cerebral infarction due to thrombosis of left cerebellar artery ◰

I63.349 Cerebral infarction due to thrombosis of unspecified cerebellar artery ◰

I63.39 Cerebral infarction due to thrombosis of other cerebral artery ◰

✓5ᵗʰ **I63.4** Cerebral infarction due to embolism of cerebral arteries

I63.40 Cerebral infarction due to embolism of unspecified cerebral artery ◰

✓6ᵗʰ **I63.41** Cerebral infarction due to embolism of middle cerebral artery

I63.411 Cerebral infarction due to embolism of right middle cerebral artery ◰

I63.412 Cerebral infarction due to embolism of left middle cerebral artery ◰

I63.419 Cerebral infarction due to embolism of unspecified middle cerebral artery ◰

✓6ᵗʰ **I63.42** Cerebral infarction due to embolism of anterior cerebral artery

I63.421 Cerebral infarction due to embolism of right anterior cerebral artery ◰

I63.422 Cerebral infarction due to embolism of left anterior cerebral artery ◰

I63.429 Cerebral infarction due to embolism of unspecified anterior cerebral artery ◰

✓6ᵗʰ **I63.43** Cerebral infarction due to embolism of posterior cerebral artery

I63.431 Cerebral infarction due to embolism of right posterior cerebral artery ◰

I63.432 Cerebral infarction due to embolism of left posterior cerebral artery ◰

I63.439 Cerebral infarction due to embolism of unspecified posterior cerebral artery ◰

✓6ᵗʰ **I63.44** Cerebral infarction due to embolism of cerebellar artery

I63.441 Cerebral infarction due to embolism of right cerebellar artery ◰

I63.442 Cerebral infarction due to embolism of left cerebellar artery ◰

I63.449 Cerebral infarction due to embolism of unspecified cerebellar artery ◰

I63.49 Cerebral infarction due to embolism of other cerebral artery ◰

✓5ᵗʰ **I63.5** Cerebral infarction due to unspecified occlusion or stenosis of cerebral arteries

I63.50 Cerebral infarction due to unspecified occlusion or stenosis of unspecified cerebral artery

✓6ᵗʰ **I63.51** Cerebral infarction due to unspecified occlusion or stenosis of middle cerebral artery

I63.511 Cerebral infarction due to unspecified occlusion or stenosis of right middle cerebral artery

I63.512 Cerebral infarction due to unspecified occlusion or stenosis of left middle cerebral artery

I63.519 Cerebral infarction due to unspecified occlusion or stenosis of unspecified middle cerebral artery

✓6ᵗʰ **I63.52** Cerebral infarction due to unspecified occlusion or stenosis of anterior cerebral artery

I63.521 Cerebral infarction due to unspecified occlusion or stenosis of right anterior cerebral artery

I63.522 Cerebral infarction due to unspecified occlusion or stenosis of left anterior cerebral artery

I63.529 Cerebral infarction due to unspecified occlusion or stenosis of unspecified anterior cerebral artery

✓6ᵗʰ **I63.53** Cerebral infarction due to unspecified occlusion or stenosis of posterior cerebral artery

I63.531 Cerebral infarction due to unspecified occlusion or stenosis of right posterior cerebral artery

I63.532 Cerebral infarction due to unspecified occlusion or stenosis of left posterior cerebral artery

I63.539 Cerebral infarction due to unspecified occlusion or stenosis of unspecified posterior cerebral artery

✓6ᵗʰ **I63.54** Cerebral infarction due to unspecified occlusion or stenosis of cerebellar artery

I63.541 Cerebral infarction due to unspecified occlusion or stenosis of right cerebellar artery

I63.542 Cerebral infarction due to unspecified occlusion or stenosis of left cerebellar artery

I63.549 Cerebral infarction due to unspecified occlusion or stenosis of unspecified cerebellar artery

I63.59 Cerebral infarction due to unspecified occlusion or stenosis of other cerebral artery

I63.6 Cerebral infarction due to cerebral venous thrombosis, nonpyogenic ◰

I63.8 Other cerebral infarction

I63.9 Cerebral infarction, unspecified
Stroke NOS
AHA: 2015, 1Q, 25

✓4ᵗʰ **I65** Occlusion and stenosis of precerebral arteries, not resulting in cerebral infarction

INCLUDES   embolism of precerebral artery
narrowing of precerebral artery
obstruction (complete) (partial) of precerebral artery
thrombosis of precerebral artery

EXCLUDES 1   *insufficiency, NOS, of precerebral artery (G45.-)*
insufficiency of precerebral arteries causing cerebral infarction (I63.0-I63.2)

✓5ᵗʰ **I65.0** Occlusion and stenosis of vertebral artery

I65.01 Occlusion and stenosis of right vertebral artery ◰

I65.02 Occlusion and stenosis of left vertebral artery ◰

I65.03 Occlusion and stenosis of bilateral vertebral arteries ◰

I65.09 Occlusion and stenosis of unspecified vertebral artery ◰

I65.1 Occlusion and stenosis of basilar artery ◰

✓5ᵗʰ **I65.2** Occlusion and stenosis of carotid artery

I65.21 Occlusion and stenosis of right carotid artery ◰

I65.22 Occlusion and stenosis of left carotid artery ◰

I65.23 Occlusion and stenosis of bilateral carotid arteries ◰

I65.29 Occlusion and stenosis of unspecified carotid artery ◰

I65.8 Occlusion and stenosis of other precerebral arteries ◰

I65.9 Occlusion and stenosis of unspecified precerebral artery ◰
Occlusion and stenosis of precerebral artery NOS

☑ Additional Character Required   ✓ₓ7ᵗʰ Placeholder Alert   Unspecified Dx   Other Specified Dx   Manifestation   ▶◀ Revised Text   ● New Code   ▲ Revised Code Title

Chapter 9. Diseases of the Circulatory System *(left margin vertical text)*

✓4th **I66** **Occlusion and stenosis of cerebral arteries, not resulting in cerebral infarction**

> INCLUDES   embolism of cerebral artery
> narrowing of cerebral artery
> obstruction (complete) (partial) of cerebral artery
> thrombosis of cerebral artery
>
> EXCLUDES 1   occlusion and stenosis of cerebral artery causing cerebral infarction (I63.3-I63.5)

✓5th **I66.0** **Occlusion and stenosis of middle cerebral artery**

     I66.01 **Occlusion and stenosis of right middle cerebral artery** 🄰

     I66.02 **Occlusion and stenosis of left middle cerebral artery** 🄰

     I66.03 **Occlusion and stenosis of bilateral middle cerebral arteries** 🄰

     I66.09 **Occlusion and stenosis of unspecified middle cerebral artery** 🄰

✓5th **I66.1** **Occlusion and stenosis of anterior cerebral artery**

     I66.11 **Occlusion and stenosis of right anterior cerebral artery** 🄰

     I66.12 **Occlusion and stenosis of left anterior cerebral artery** 🄰

     I66.13 **Occlusion and stenosis of bilateral anterior cerebral arteries** 🄰

     I66.19 **Occlusion and stenosis of unspecified anterior cerebral artery** 🄰

✓5th **I66.2** **Occlusion and stenosis of posterior cerebral artery**

     I66.21 **Occlusion and stenosis of right posterior cerebral artery** 🄰

     I66.22 **Occlusion and stenosis of left posterior cerebral artery** 🄰

     I66.23 **Occlusion and stenosis of bilateral posterior cerebral arteries** 🄰

     I66.29 **Occlusion and stenosis of unspecified posterior cerebral artery** 🄰

     I66.3 **Occlusion and stenosis of cerebellar arteries** 🄰

     I66.8 **Occlusion and stenosis of other cerebral arteries** 🄰
> Occlusion and stenosis of perforating arteries

     I66.9 **Occlusion and stenosis of unspecified cerebral artery** 🄰

✓4th **I67** **Other cerebrovascular diseases**

> EXCLUDES 1   sequelae of the listed conditions (I69.8)

     I67.0 **Dissection of cerebral arteries, nonruptured**
> EXCLUDES 1   ruptured cerebral arteries (I60.7)

     I67.1 **Cerebral aneurysm, nonruptured**
> Cerebral aneurysm NOS
> Cerebral arteriovenous fistula, acquired
> Internal carotid artery aneurysm, intracranial portion
> Internal carotid artery aneurysm, NOS
> EXCLUDES 1   congenital cerebral aneurysm, nonruptured (Q28.-)
> ruptured cerebral aneurysm (I60.7)

     I67.2 **Cerebral atherosclerosis** 🄰
> Atheroma of cerebral and precerebral arteries

     I67.3 **Progressive vascular leukoencephalopathy**
> Binswanger's disease

     I67.4 **Hypertensive encephalopathy**

     I67.5 **Moyamoya disease**

     I67.6 **Nonpyogenic thrombosis of intracranial venous system**
> Nonpyogenic thrombosis of cerebral vein
> Nonpyogenic thrombosis of intracranial venous sinus
> EXCLUDES 1   nonpyogenic thrombosis of intracranial venous system causing infarction (I63.6)

     I67.7 **Cerebral arteritis, not elsewhere classified**
> Granulomatous angiitis of the nervous system
> EXCLUDES 1   allergic granulomatous angiitis (M30.1)

✓5th **I67.8** **Other specified cerebrovascular diseases**

     I67.81 **Acute cerebrovascular insufficiency**
> Acute cerebrovascular insufficiency unspecified as to location or reversibility

     I67.82 **Cerebral ischemia**
> Chronic cerebral ischemia

     I67.83 **Posterior reversible encephalopathy syndrome**
> PRES

✓6th **I67.84** **Cerebral vasospasm and vasoconstriction**

     I67.841 **Reversible cerebrovascular vasoconstriction syndrome** 🄰
> Call-Fleming syndrome
> Code first underlying condition, if applicable, such as eclampsia (O15.00-O15.9)

     I67.848 **Other cerebrovascular vasospasm and vasoconstriction** 🄰

     I67.89 **Other cerebrovascular disease**

     I67.9 **Cerebrovascular disease, unspecified**

✓4th **I68** **Cerebrovascular disorders in diseases classified elsewhere**

     I68.0 *Cerebral amyloid angiopathy*
> *Code first underlying amyloidosis (E85.-)*

     I68.2 *Cerebral arteritis in other diseases classified elsewhere*
> *Code first underlying disease*
> EXCLUDES 1   cerebral arteritis (in):
> listerosis (A32.89)
> systemic lupus erythematosus (M32.19)
> syphilis (A52.04)
> tuberculosis (A18.89)

     I68.8 *Other cerebrovascular disorders in diseases classified elsewhere*
> *Code first underlying disease*
> EXCLUDES 1   syphilitic cerebral aneurysm (A52.05)

✓4th **I69** **Sequelae of cerebrovascular disease**

> NOTE   Category I69 is to be used to indicate conditions in I60-I67 as the cause of sequelae. The "sequelae" include conditions specified as such or as residuals which may occur at any time after the onset of the causal condition
>
> EXCLUDES 1   personal history of cerebral infarction without residual deficit (Z86.73)
> personal history of prolonged reversible ischemic neurologic deficit (PRIND) (Z86.73)
> personal history of reversible ischemic neurologcial deficit (RIND) (Z86.73)
> sequelae of traumatic intracranial injury (S06.-)
> transient ischemic attack (TIA) (G45.9)

AHA: 2012, 4Q, 106

✓5th **I69.0** **Sequelae of nontraumatic subarachnoid hemorrhage**

     I69.00 **Unspecified sequelae of nontraumatic subarachnoid hemorrhage**

     I69.01 **Cognitive deficits following nontraumatic subarachnoid hemorrhage**

✓6th **I69.02** **Speech and language deficits following nontraumatic subarachnoid hemorrhage**

     I69.020 **Aphasia following nontraumatic subarachnoid hemorrhage**

     I69.021 **Dysphasia following nontraumatic subarachnoid hemorrhage**

     I69.022 **Dysarthria following nontraumatic subarachnoid hemorrhage**

     I69.023 **Fluency disorder following nontraumatic subarachnoid hemorrhage**
> Stuttering following nontraumatic subarachnoid hemorrhage

     I69.028 **Other speech and language deficits following nontraumatic subarachnoid hemorrhage**

✓6th **I69.03** **Monoplegia of upper limb following nontraumatic subarachnoid hemorrhage**

     I69.031 **Monoplegia of upper limb following nontraumatic subarachnoid hemorrhage affecting right dominant side**

     I69.032 **Monoplegia of upper limb following nontraumatic subarachnoid hemorrhage affecting left dominant side**

     I69.033 **Monoplegia of upper limb following nontraumatic subarachnoid hemorrhage affecting right non-dominant side**

     I69.034 **Monoplegia of upper limb following nontraumatic subarachnoid hemorrhage affecting left non-dominant side**

     I69.039 **Monoplegia of upper limb following nontraumatic subarachnoid hemorrhage affecting unspecified side**

EXCLUDES 1 Not coded here   EXCLUDES 2 Not included here   🄽 Newborn Age: 0   🄿 Pediatric Age: 0-17   🄼 Maternity Age: 12-55   🄰 Adult Age: 15-124

√6th I69.04 Monoplegia of lower limb following nontraumatic subarachnoid hemorrhage

I69.041 Monoplegia of lower limb following nontraumatic subarachnoid hemorrhage affecting right dominant side

I69.042 Monoplegia of lower limb following nontraumatic subarachnoid hemorrhage affecting left dominant side

I69.043 Monoplegia of lower limb following nontraumatic subarachnoid hemorrhage affecting right non-dominant side

I69.044 Monoplegia of lower limb following nontraumatic subarachnoid hemorrhage affecting left non-dominant side

I69.049 Monoplegia of lower limb following nontraumatic subarachnoid hemorrhage affecting unspecified side

√6th I69.05 Hemiplegia and hemiparesis following nontraumatic subarachnoid hemorrhage
    AHA: 2015, 1Q, 25

I69.051 Hemiplegia and hemiparesis following nontraumatic subarachnoid hemorrhage affecting right dominant side

I69.052 Hemiplegia and hemiparesis following nontraumatic subarachnoid hemorrhage affecting left dominant side

I69.053 Hemiplegia and hemiparesis following nontraumatic subarachnoid hemorrhage affecting right non-dominant side

I69.054 Hemiplegia and hemiparesis following nontraumatic subarachnoid hemorrhage affecting left non-dominant side

I69.059 Hemiplegia and hemiparesis following nontraumatic subarachnoid hemorrhage affecting unspecified side

√6th I69.06 Other paralytic syndrome following nontraumatic subarachnoid hemorrhage
Use additional code to identify type of paralytic syndrome, such as:
   locked-in state (G83.5)
   quadriplegia (G82.5-)
   EXCLUDES 1   *hemiplegia/hemiparesis following nontraumatic subarachnoid hemorrhage (I69.05-)*
      monoplegia of lower limb following nontraumatic subarachnoid hemorrhage (I69.04-)
      monoplegia of upper limb following nontraumatic subarachnoid hemorrhage (I69.03-)

I69.061 Other paralytic syndrome following nontraumatic subarachnoid hemorrhage affecting right dominant side

I69.062 Other paralytic syndrome following nontraumatic subarachnoid hemorrhage affecting left dominant side

I69.063 Other paralytic syndrome following nontraumatic subarachnoid hemorrhage affecting right non-dominant side

I69.064 Other paralytic syndrome following nontraumatic subarachnoid hemorrhage affecting left non-dominant side

I69.065 Other paralytic syndrome following nontraumatic subarachnoid hemorrhage, bilateral

I69.069 Other paralytic syndrome following nontraumatic subarachnoid hemorrhage affecting unspecified side

√6th I69.09 Other sequelae of nontraumatic subarachnoid hemorrhage

I69.090 Apraxia following nontraumatic subarachnoid hemorrhage

I69.091 Dysphagia following nontraumatic subarachnoid hemorrhage
Use additional code to identify the type of dysphagia, if known (R13.1-)

I69.092 Facial weakness following nontraumatic subarachnoid hemorrhage
Facial droop following nontraumatic subarachnoid hemorrhage

I69.093 Ataxia following nontraumatic subarachnoid hemorrhage

I69.098 Other sequelae following nontraumatic subarachnoid hemorrhage
Alterations of sensation following nontraumatic subarachnoid hemorrhage
Disturbance of vision following nontraumatic subarachnoid hemorrhage
Use additional code to identify the sequelae

√5th I69.1 Sequelae of nontraumatic intracerebral hemorrhage

I69.10 Unspecified sequelae of nontraumatic intracerebral hemorrhage

I69.11 Cognitive deficits following nontraumatic intracerebral hemorrhage

√6th I69.12 Speech and language deficits following nontraumatic intracerebral hemorrhage

I69.120 Aphasia following nontraumatic intracerebral hemorrhage

I69.121 Dysphasia following nontraumatic intracerebral hemorrhage

I69.122 Dysarthria following nontraumatic intracerebral hemorrhage

I69.123 Fluency disorder following nontraumatic intracerebral hemorrhage
Stuttering following nontraumatic subarachnoid hemorrhage

I69.128 Other speech and language deficits following nontraumatic intracerebral hemorrhage

√6th I69.13 Monoplegia of upper limb following nontraumatic intracerebral hemorrhage

I69.131 Monoplegia of upper limb following nontraumatic intracerebral hemorrhage affecting right dominant side

I69.132 Monoplegia of upper limb following nontraumatic intracerebral hemorrhage affecting left dominant side

I69.133 Monoplegia of upper limb following nontraumatic intracerebral hemorrhage affecting right non-dominant side

I69.134 Monoplegia of upper limb following nontraumatic intracerebral hemorrhage affecting left non-dominant side

I69.139 Monoplegia of upper limb following nontraumatic intracerebral hemorrhage affecting unspecified side

√6th I69.14 Monoplegia of lower limb following nontraumatic intracerebral hemorrhage

I69.141 Monoplegia of lower limb following nontraumatic intracerebral hemorrhage affecting right dominant side

I69.142 Monoplegia of lower limb following nontraumatic intracerebral hemorrhage affecting left dominant side

I69.143 Monoplegia of lower limb following nontraumatic intracerebral hemorrhage affecting right non-dominant side

I69.144 Monoplegia of lower limb following nontraumatic intracerebral hemorrhage affecting left non-dominant side

I69.149 Monoplegia of lower limb following nontraumatic intracerebral hemorrhage affecting unspecified side

√6th I69.15 Hemiplegia and hemiparesis following nontraumatic intracerebral hemorrhage
    AHA: 2015, 1Q, 25

I69.151 Hemiplegia and hemiparesis following nontraumatic intracerebral hemorrhage affecting right dominant side

I69.152 Hemiplegia and hemiparesis following nontraumatic intracerebral hemorrhage affecting left dominant side

I69.153 Hemiplegia and hemiparesis following nontraumatic intracerebral hemorrhage affecting right non-dominant side

I69.154 Hemiplegia and hemiparesis following nontraumatic intracerebral hemorrhage affecting left non-dominant side

I69.159 Hemiplegia and hemiparesis following nontraumatic intracerebral hemorrhage affecting unspecified side

---

☑ Additional Character Required   √×7th Placeholder Alert   Unspecified Dx   Other Specified Dx   Manifestation   ▶◀ Revised Text   ● New Code   ▲ Revised Code Title

✓6ᵗʰ I69.16   **Other paralytic syndrome following nontraumatic intracerebral hemorrhage**

Use additional code to identify type of paralytic syndrome, such as:
locked-in state (G83.5)
quadriplegia (G82.5-)

EXCLUDES 1   hemiplegia/hemiparesis following nontraumatic intracerebral hemorrhage (I69.15-)
monoplegia of lower limb following nontraumatic intracerebral hemorrhage (I69.14-)
monoplegia of upper limb following nontraumatic intracerebral hemorrhage (I69.13-)

I69.161   **Other paralytic syndrome following nontraumatic intracerebral hemorrhage affecting right dominant side**

I69.162   **Other paralytic syndrome following nontraumatic intracerebral hemorrhage affecting left dominant side**

I69.163   **Other paralytic syndrome following nontraumatic intracerebral hemorrhage affecting right non-dominant side**

I69.164   **Other paralytic syndrome following nontraumatic intracerebral hemorrhage affecting left non-dominant side**

I69.165   **Other paralytic syndrome following nontraumatic intracerebral hemorrhage, bilateral**

I69.169   **Other paralytic syndrome following nontraumatic intracerebral hemorrhage affecting unspecified side**

✓6ᵗʰ I69.19   **Other sequelae of nontraumatic intracerebral hemorrhage**

I69.190   **Apraxia following nontraumatic intracerebral hemorrhage**

I69.191   **Dysphagia following nontraumatic intracerebral hemorrhage**
Use additional code to identify the type of dysphagia, if known (R13.1-)

I69.192   **Facial weakness following nontraumatic intracerebral hemorrhage**
Facial droop following nontraumatic intracerebral hemorrhage

I69.193   **Ataxia following nontraumatic intracerebral hemorrhage**

I69.198   **Other sequelae of nontraumatic intracerebral hemorrhage**
Alteration of sensations following nontraumatic intracerebral hemorrhage
Disturbance of vision following nontraumatic intracerebral hemorrhage
Use additional code to identify the sequelae

✓5ᵗʰ I69.2   **Sequelae of other nontraumatic intracranial hemorrhage**

I69.20   **Unspecified sequelae of other nontraumatic intracranial hemorrhage**

I69.21   **Cognitive deficits following other nontraumatic intracranial hemorrhage**

✓6ᵗʰ I69.22   **Speech and language deficits following other nontraumatic intracranial hemorrhage**

I69.220   **Aphasia following other nontraumatic intracranial hemorrhage**

I69.221   **Dysphasia following other nontraumatic intracranial hemorrhage**

I69.222   **Dysarthria following other nontraumatic intracranial hemorrhage**

I69.223   **Fluency disorder following other nontraumatic intracranial hemorrhage**
Stuttering following nontraumatic subarachnoid hemorrhage

I69.228   **Other speech and language deficits following other nontraumatic intracranial hemorrhage**

✓6ᵗʰ I69.23   **Monoplegia of upper limb following other nontraumatic intracranial hemorrhage**

I69.231   **Monoplegia of upper limb following other nontraumatic intracranial hemorrhage affecting right dominant side**

I69.232   **Monoplegia of upper limb following other nontraumatic intracranial hemorrhage affecting left dominant side**

I69.233   **Monoplegia of upper limb following other nontraumatic intracranial hemorrhage affecting right non-dominant side**

I69.234   **Monoplegia of upper limb following other nontraumatic intracranial hemorrhage affecting left non-dominant side**

I69.239   **Monoplegia of upper limb following other nontraumatic intracranial hemorrhage affecting unspecified side**

✓6ᵗʰ I69.24   **Monoplegia of lower limb following other nontraumatic intracranial hemorrhage**

I69.241   **Monoplegia of lower limb following other nontraumatic intracranial hemorrhage affecting right dominant side**

I69.242   **Monoplegia of lower limb following other nontraumatic intracranial hemorrhage affecting left dominant side**

I69.243   **Monoplegia of lower limb following other nontraumatic intracranial hemorrhage affecting right non-dominant side**

I69.244   **Monoplegia of lower limb following other nontraumatic intracranial hemorrhage affecting left non-dominant side**

I69.249   **Monoplegia of lower limb following other nontraumatic intracranial hemorrhage affecting unspecified side**

✓6ᵗʰ I69.25   **Hemiplegia and hemiparesis following other nontraumatic intracranial hemorrhage**
AHA: 2015, 1Q, 25

I69.251   **Hemiplegia and hemiparesis following other nontraumatic intracranial hemorrhage affecting right dominant side**

I69.252   **Hemiplegia and hemiparesis following other nontraumatic intracranial hemorrhage affecting left dominant side**

I69.253   **Hemiplegia and hemiparesis following other nontraumatic intracranial hemorrhage affecting right non-dominant side**

I69.254   **Hemiplegia and hemiparesis following other nontraumatic intracranial hemorrhage affecting left non-dominant side**

I69.259   **Hemiplegia and hemiparesis following other nontraumatic intracranial hemorrhage affecting unspecified side**

✓6ᵗʰ I69.26   **Other paralytic syndrome following other nontraumatic intracranial hemorrhage**

Use additional code to identify type of paralytic syndrome, such as:
locked-in state (G83.5)
quadriplegia (G82.5-)

EXCLUDES 1   hemiplegia/hemiparesis following other nontraumatic intracranial hemorrhage (I69.25-)
monoplegia of lower limb following other nontraumatic intracranial hemorrhage (I69.24-)
monoplegia of upper limb following other nontraumatic intracranial hemorrhage (I69.23-)

I69.261   **Other paralytic syndrome following other nontraumatic intracranial hemorrhage affecting right dominant side**

I69.262   **Other paralytic syndrome following other nontraumatic intracranial hemorrhage affecting left dominant side**

I69.263   **Other paralytic syndrome following other nontraumatic intracranial hemorrhage affecting right non-dominant side**

I69.264   **Other paralytic syndrome following other nontraumatic intracranial hemorrhage affecting left non-dominant side**

EXCLUDES 1 Not coded here   *EXCLUDES 2* Not included here   **N** Newborn Age: 0   **P** Pediatric Age: 0-17   **M** Maternity Age: 12-55   **A** Adult Age: 15-124

I69.265 **Other paralytic syndrome following other nontraumatic intracranial hemorrhage, bilateral**

I69.269 **Other paralytic syndrome following other nontraumatic intracranial hemorrhage affecting unspecified side**

✓6ᵗʰ **I69.29** Other sequelae of other nontraumatic intracranial hemorrhage

     I69.290 **Apraxia following other nontraumatic intracranial hemorrhage**

     I69.291 **Dysphagia following other nontraumatic intracranial hemorrhage**
         Use additional code to identify the type of dysphagia, if known (R13.1-)

     I69.292 **Facial weakness following other nontraumatic intracranial hemorrhage**
         Facial droop following other nontraumatic intracranial hemorrhage

     I69.293 **Ataxia following other nontraumatic intracranial hemorrhage**

     I69.298 **Other sequelae of other nontraumatic intracranial hemorrhage**
         Alteration of sensation following other nontraumatic intracranial hemorrhage
         Disturbance of vision following other nontraumatic intracranial hemorrhage
         Use additional code to identify the sequelae

✓5ᵗʰ **I69.3** **Sequelae of** cerebral infarction
     Sequelae of stroke NOS
     AHA: 2013, 4Q, 127-128; 2012, 4Q, 92, 94

     I69.30 **Unspecified sequelae of cerebral infarction**

     I69.31 **Cognitive deficits following cerebral infarction**

✓6ᵗʰ **I69.32** **Speech and** language deficits **following cerebral infarction**

     I69.320 **Aphasia following cerebral infarction**

     I69.321 **Dysphasia following cerebral infarction**
         AHA: 2012, 4Q, 91

     I69.322 **Dysarthria following cerebral infarction**

     I69.323 **Fluency disorder following cerebral infarction**
         Stuttering following nontraumatic subarachnoid hemorrhage

     I69.328 **Other speech and language deficits following cerebral infarction**

✓6ᵗʰ **I69.33** **Monoplegia** of upper limb **following cerebral infarction**

     I69.331 **Monoplegia of upper limb following cerebral infarction affecting** right dominant **side**

     I69.332 **Monoplegia of upper limb following cerebral infarction affecting** left dominant **side**

     I69.333 **Monoplegia of upper limb following cerebral infarction affecting** right non-dominant **side**

     I69.334 **Monoplegia of upper limb following cerebral infarction affecting** left non-dominant **side**

     I69.339 **Monoplegia of upper limb following cerebral infarction affecting unspecified side**

✓6ᵗʰ **I69.34** **Monoplegia** of lower limb **following cerebral infarction**

     I69.341 **Monoplegia of lower limb following cerebral infarction affecting** right dominant **side**

     I69.342 **Monoplegia of lower limb following cerebral infarction affecting** left dominant **side**

     I69.343 **Monoplegia of lower limb following cerebral infarction affecting** right non-dominant **side**

     I69.344 **Monoplegia of lower limb following cerebral infarction affecting** left non-dominant **side**

     I69.349 **Monoplegia of lower limb following cerebral infarction affecting unspecified side**

✓6ᵗʰ **I69.35** Hemiplegia **and** hemiparesis **following cerebral infarction**
     AHA: 2015, 1Q, 25

     I69.351 **Hemiplegia and hemiparesis following cerebral infarction affecting** right dominant **side**

     I69.352 **Hemiplegia and hemiparesis following cerebral infarction affecting** left dominant **side**

     I69.353 **Hemiplegia and hemiparesis following cerebral infarction affecting** right non-dominant **side**

     I69.354 **Hemiplegia and hemiparesis following cerebral infarction affecting** left non-dominant **side**
         AHA: 2012, 4Q, 91

     I69.359 **Hemiplegia and hemiparesis following cerebral infarction affecting unspecified side**

✓6ᵗʰ **I69.36** **Other paralytic syndrome following cerebral infarction**
     Use additional code to identify type of paralytic syndrome, such as:
         locked-in state (G83.5)
         quadriplegia (G82.5-)
     EXCLUDES 1 *hemiplegia/hemiparesis following cerebral infarction (I69.35-)*
         monoplegia of lower limb following cerebral infarction (I69.34-)
         monoplegia of upper limb following cerebral infarction (I69.33-)

     I69.361 **Other paralytic syndrome following cerebral infarction affecting** right dominant **side**

     I69.362 **Other paralytic syndrome following cerebral infarction affecting** left dominant **side**

     I69.363 **Other paralytic syndrome following cerebral infarction affecting** right non-dominant **side**

     I69.364 **Other paralytic syndrome following cerebral infarction affecting** left non-dominant **side**

     I69.365 **Other paralytic syndrome following cerebral infarction, bilateral**

     I69.369 **Other paralytic syndrome following cerebral infarction affecting unspecified side**

✓6ᵗʰ **I69.39** Other sequelae of cerebral infarction

     I69.390 **Apraxia following cerebral infarction**

     I69.391 **Dysphagia following cerebral infarction**
         Use additional code to identify the type of dysphagia, if known (R13.1-)

     I69.392 **Facial weakness following cerebral infarction**
         Facial droop following cerebral infarction

     I69.393 **Ataxia following cerebral infarction**

     I69.398 **Other sequelae of cerebral infarction**
         Alteration of sensation following cerebral infarction
         Disturbance of vision following cerebral infarction
         Use additional code to identify the sequelae

✓5ᵗʰ **I69.8** **Sequelae of** other cerebrovascular diseases
     EXCLUDES 1 *sequelae of traumatic intracranial injury (S06.-)*

     I69.80 **Unspecified sequelae of other cerebrovascular disease**

     I69.81 **Cognitive deficits following other cerebrovascular disease**

✓6ᵗʰ **I69.82** **Speech and** language deficits **following other cerebrovascular disease**

     I69.820 **Aphasia following other cerebrovascular disease**

     I69.821 **Dysphasia following other cerebrovascular disease**

     I69.822 **Dysarthria following other cerebrovascular disease**

☑ Additional Character Required   ✓x7ᵗʰ Placeholder Alert   Unspecified Dx   Other Specified Dx   Manifestation   ▶◀ Revised Text   ● New Code   ▲ Revised Code Title

I69.823   **Fluency** disorder following other cerebrovascular disease
> Stuttering following nontraumatic subarachnoid hemorrhage

I69.828   **Other speech and language deficits following other cerebrovascular disease**

✓6ᵗʰ   **I69.83**   Monoplegia of upper limb following other cerebrovascular disease

I69.831   **Monoplegia of upper limb following other cerebrovascular disease affecting** right **dominant** side

I69.832   **Monoplegia of upper limb following other cerebrovascular disease affecting** left **dominant** side

I69.833   **Monoplegia of upper limb following other cerebrovascular disease affecting** right **non-dominant** side

I69.834   **Monoplegia of upper limb following other cerebrovascular disease affecting** left **non-dominant** side

I69.839   **Monoplegia of upper limb following other cerebrovascular disease affecting unspecified side**

✓6ᵗʰ   **I69.84**   Monoplegia of lower limb following other cerebrovascular disease

I69.841   **Monoplegia of lower limb following other cerebrovascular disease affecting** right **dominant** side

I69.842   **Monoplegia of lower limb following other cerebrovascular disease affecting** left **dominant** side

I69.843   **Monoplegia of lower limb following other cerebrovascular disease affecting** right **non-dominant** side

I69.844   **Monoplegia of lower limb following other cerebrovascular disease affecting** left **non-dominant** side

I69.849   **Monoplegia of lower limb following other cerebrovascular disease affecting unspecified side**

✓6ᵗʰ   **I69.85**   Hemiplegia and hemiparesis following other cerebrovascular disease
> **AHA:** 2015, 1Q, 25

I69.851   **Hemiplegia and hemiparesis following other cerebrovascular disease affecting right dominant** side

I69.852   **Hemiplegia and hemiparesis following other cerebrovascular disease affecting left dominant** side

I69.853   **Hemiplegia and hemiparesis following other cerebrovascular disease affecting right non-dominant** side

I69.854   **Hemiplegia and hemiparesis following other cerebrovascular disease affecting left non-dominant** side

I69.859   **Hemiplegia and hemiparesis following other cerebrovascular disease affecting unspecified side**

✓6ᵗʰ   **I69.86**   Other paralytic syndrome following other cerebrovascular disease
> Use additional code to identify type of paralytic syndrome, such as:
> locked-in state (G83.5)
> quadriplegia (G82.5-)
> EXCLUDES 1   *hemiplegia/hemiparesis following other cerebrovascular disease (I69.85-)*
> *monoplegia of lower limb following other cerebrovascular disease (I69.84-)*
> *monoplegia of upper limb following other cerebrovascular disease (I69.83-)*

I69.861   **Other paralytic syndrome following other cerebrovascular disease affecting** right **dominant** side

I69.862   **Other paralytic syndrome following other cerebrovascular disease affecting** left **dominant** side

I69.863   **Other paralytic syndrome following other cerebrovascular disease affecting** right **non-dominant** side

I69.864   **Other paralytic syndrome following other cerebrovascular disease affecting** left **non-dominant** side

I69.865   **Other paralytic syndrome following other cerebrovascular disease, bilateral**

I69.869   **Other paralytic syndrome following other cerebrovascular disease affecting unspecified side**

✓6ᵗʰ   **I69.89**   Other sequelae of other cerebrovascular disease

I69.890   **Apraxia following other cerebrovascular disease**

I69.891   **Dysphagia following other cerebrovascular disease**
> Use additional code to identify the type of dysphagia, if known (R13.1-)

I69.892   **Facial weakness following other cerebrovascular disease**
> Facial droop following other cerebrovascular disease

I69.893   **Ataxia following other cerebrovascular disease**

I69.898   **Other sequelae of other cerebrovascular disease**
> Alteration of sensation following other cerebrovascular disease
> Disturbance of vision following other cerebrovascular disease
> Use additional code to identify the sequelae

✓5ᵗʰ   **I69.9**   **Sequelae of** unspecified cerebrovascular diseases
> EXCLUDES 1   *sequelae of stroke (I69.3)*
> *sequelae of traumatic intracranial injury (S06.-)*

I69.90   **Unspecified sequelae of unspecified cerebrovascular disease**

I69.91   **Cognitive deficits following unspecified cerebrovascular disease**

✓6ᵗʰ   **I69.92**   Speech and language deficits following unspecified cerebrovascular disease

I69.920   **Aphasia following unspecified cerebrovascular disease**

I69.921   **Dysphasia following unspecified cerebrovascular disease**

I69.922   **Dysarthria following unspecified cerebrovascular disease**

I69.923   **Fluency disorder following unspecified cerebrovascular disease**
> Stuttering following nontraumatic subarachnoid hemorrhage

I69.928   **Other speech and language deficits following unspecified cerebrovascular disease**

✓6ᵗʰ   **I69.93**   Monoplegia of upper limb following unspecified cerebrovascular disease

I69.931   **Monoplegia of upper limb following unspecified cerebrovascular disease affecting** right dominant **side**

I69.932   **Monoplegia of upper limb following unspecified cerebrovascular disease affecting** left dominant **side**

I69.933   **Monoplegia of upper limb following unspecified cerebrovascular disease affecting** right non-dominant **side**

I69.934   **Monoplegia of upper limb following unspecified cerebrovascular disease affecting** left non-dominant **side**

I69.939   **Monoplegia of upper limb following unspecified cerebrovascular disease affecting unspecified side**

✓6ᵗʰ   **I69.94**   Monoplegia of lower limb following unspecified cerebrovascular disease

I69.941   **Monoplegia of lower limb following unspecified cerebrovascular disease affecting** right dominant **side**

I69.942   **Monoplegia of lower limb following unspecified cerebrovascular disease affecting** left dominant **side**

I69.943   **Monoplegia of lower limb following unspecified cerebrovascular disease affecting** right non-dominant **side**

I69.944   **Monoplegia of lower limb following unspecified cerebrovascular disease affecting** left non-dominant **side**

EXCLUDES 1   Not coded here   EXCLUDES 2   Not included here   N Newborn Age: 0   P Pediatric Age: 0-17   M Maternity Age: 12-55   A Adult Age: 15-124

I69.949   **Monoplegia of lower limb following unspecified cerebrovascular disease affecting unspecified side**

✓6th **I69.95**   **Hemiplegia and hemiparesis following unspecified cerebrovascular disease**
    AHA: 2015, 1Q, 25

I69.951   **Hemiplegia and hemiparesis following unspecified cerebrovascular disease affecting right dominant side**

I69.952   **Hemiplegia and hemiparesis following unspecified cerebrovascular disease affecting left dominant side**

I69.953   **Hemiplegia and hemiparesis following unspecified cerebrovascular disease affecting right non-dominant side**

I69.954   **Hemiplegia and hemiparesis following unspecified cerebrovascular disease affecting left non-dominant side**

I69.959   **Hemiplegia and hemiparesis following unspecified cerebrovascular disease affecting unspecified side**

✓6th **I69.96**   **Other paralytic syndrome following unspecified cerebrovascular disease**
    Use additional code to identify type of paralytic syndrome, such as:
        locked-in state (G83.5)
        quadriplegia (G82.5-)
    EXCLUDES 1   *hemiplegia/hemiparesis following unspecified cerebrovascular disease (I69.95-)*
           monoplegia of lower limb following unspecified cerebrovascular disease (I69.94-)
           monoplegia of upper limb following unspecified cerebrovascular disease (I69.93-)

I69.961   **Other paralytic syndrome following unspecified cerebrovascular disease affecting right dominant side**

I69.962   **Other paralytic syndrome following unspecified cerebrovascular disease affecting left dominant side**

I69.963   **Other paralytic syndrome following unspecified cerebrovascular disease affecting right non-dominant side**

I69.964   **Other paralytic syndrome following unspecified cerebrovascular disease affecting left non-dominant side**

I69.965   **Other paralytic syndrome following unspecified cerebrovascular disease, bilateral**

I69.969   **Other paralytic syndrome following unspecified cerebrovascular disease affecting unspecified side**

✓6th **I69.99**   **Other sequelae of unspecified cerebrovascular disease**

I69.990   **Apraxia following unspecified cerebrovascular disease**

I69.991   **Dysphagia following unspecified cerebrovascular disease**
    Use additional code to identify the type of dysphagia, if known (R13.1-)

I69.992   **Facial weakness following unspecified cerebrovascular disease**
    Facial droop following unspecified cerebrovascular disease

I69.993   **Ataxia following unspecified cerebrovascular disease**

I69.998   **Other sequelae following unspecified cerebrovascular disease**
    Alteration in sensation following unspecified cerebrovascular disease
    Disturbance of vision following unspecified cerebrovascular disease
    Use additional code to identify the sequelae

Diseases of arteries, arterioles and capillaries (I70-I79)

✓4th **I70**   **Atherosclerosis**
    INCLUDES   arteriolosclerosis
              arterial degeneration
              arteriosclerosis
              arteriosclerotic vascular disease
              arteriovascular degeneration
              atheroma
              endarteritis deformans or obliterans
              senile arteritis
              senile endarteritis
              vascular degeneration
    Use additional code to identify:
        exposure to environmental tobacco smoke (Z77.22)
        history of tobacco use (Z87.891)
        occupational exposure to environmental tobacco smoke (Z57.31)
        tobacco dependence (F17.-)
        tobacco use (Z72.0)
    EXCLUDES 2   *arteriosclerotic cardiovascular disease (I25.1-)*
           arteriosclerotic heart disease (I25.1-)
           atheroembolism (I75.-)
           cerebral atherosclerosis (I67.2)
           coronary atherosclerosis (I25.1-)
           mesenteric atherosclerosis (K55.1)
           precerebral atherosclerosis (I67.2)
           primary pulmonary atherosclerosis (I27.0)

I70.0   **Atherosclerosis of aorta**   A

I70.1   **Atherosclerosis of renal artery**   A
    Goldblatt's kidney
    EXCLUDES 2   *atherosclerosis of renal arterioles (I12.-)*

✓5th **I70.2**   **Atherosclerosis of native arteries of the extremities**
    Mönckeberg's (medial) sclerosis
    Use additional code, if applicable, to identify chronic total occlusion of artery of extremity (I70.92)
    EXCLUDES 2   *atherosclerosis of bypass graft of extremities (I70.30-I70.79)*

✓6th **I70.20**   **Unspecified atherosclerosis of native arteries of extremities**

I70.201   **Unspecified atherosclerosis of native arteries of extremities, right leg**   A

I70.202   **Unspecified atherosclerosis of native arteries of extremities, left leg**   A

I70.203   **Unspecified atherosclerosis of native arteries of extremities, bilateral legs**   A

I70.208   **Unspecified atherosclerosis of native arteries of extremities, other extremity**   A

I70.209   **Unspecified atherosclerosis of native arteries of extremities, unspecified extremity**   A

✓6th **I70.21**   **Atherosclerosis of native arteries of extremities with intermittent claudication**

I70.211   **Atherosclerosis of native arteries of extremities with intermittent claudication, right leg**   A

I70.212   **Atherosclerosis of native arteries of extremities with intermittent claudication, left leg**   A

I70.213   **Atherosclerosis of native arteries of extremities with intermittent claudication, bilateral legs**   A

I70.218   **Atherosclerosis of native arteries of extremities with intermittent claudication, other extremity**   A

I70.219   **Atherosclerosis of native arteries of extremities with intermittent claudication, unspecified extremity**   A

✓6th **I70.22**   **Atherosclerosis of native arteries of extremities with rest pain**
    INCLUDES   any condition classifiable to I70.21-

I70.221   **Atherosclerosis of native arteries of extremities with rest pain, right leg**   A

I70.222   **Atherosclerosis of native arteries of extremities with rest pain, left leg**   A

I70.223   **Atherosclerosis of native arteries of extremities with rest pain, bilateral legs**   A

I70.228   **Atherosclerosis of native arteries of extremities with rest pain, other extremity**   A

✓ Additional Character Required   ✓x7th Placeholder Alert   Unspecified Dx   Other Specified Dx   Manifestation   ▶◀ Revised Text   ● New Code   ▲ Revised Code Title

ICD-10-CM 2016   601

I70.229 Atherosclerosis of native arteries of extremities with rest pain, unspecified extremity ▲

✓6th **I70.23** Atherosclerosis of native arteries of right leg with ulceration
> INCLUDES　any condition classifiable to I70.211 and I70.221
> Use additional code to identify severity of ulcer (L97.-)

　I70.231 Atherosclerosis of native arteries of right leg with ulceration of thigh ▲

　I70.232 Atherosclerosis of native arteries of right leg with ulceration of calf ▲

　I70.233 Atherosclerosis of native arteries of right leg with ulceration of ankle ▲

　I70.234 Atherosclerosis of native arteries of right leg with ulceration of heel and midfoot ▲
> Atherosclerosis of native arteries of right leg with ulceration of plantar surface of midfoot

　I70.235 Atherosclerosis of native arteries of right leg with ulceration of other part of foot ▲
> Atherosclerosis of native arteries of right leg extremities with ulceration of toe

　I70.238 Atherosclerosis of native arteries of right leg with ulceration of other part of lower right leg ▲

　I70.239 Atherosclerosis of native arteries of right leg with ulceration of unspecified site ▲

✓6th **I70.24** Atherosclerosis of native arteries of left leg with ulceration
> INCLUDES　any condition classifiable to I70.212 and I70.222
> Use additional code to identify severity of ulcer (L97.-)

　I70.241 Atherosclerosis of native arteries of left leg with ulceration of thigh ▲

　I70.242 Atherosclerosis of native arteries of left leg with ulceration of calf ▲

　I70.243 Atherosclerosis of native arteries of left leg with ulceration of ankle ▲

　I70.244 Atherosclerosis of native arteries of left leg with ulceration of heel and midfoot ▲
> Atherosclerosis of native arteries of left leg with ulceration of plantar surface of midfoot

　I70.245 Atherosclerosis of native arteries of left leg with ulceration of other part of foot ▲
> Atherosclerosis of native arteries of left leg extremities with ulceration of toe

　I70.248 Atherosclerosis of native arteries of left leg with ulceration of other part of lower left leg ▲

　I70.249 Atherosclerosis of native arteries of left leg with ulceration of unspecified site ▲

I70.25 Atherosclerosis of native arteries of other extremities with ulceration ▲
> INCLUDES　any condition classifiable to I70.218 and I70.228
> Use additional code to identify the severity of the ulcer (L98.49-)

✓6th **I70.26** Atherosclerosis of native arteries of extremities with gangrene
> INCLUDES　any condition classifiable to I70.21-, I70.22-, I70.23-, I70.24-, and I70.25-
> Use additional code to identify the severity of any ulcer (L97.-, L98.49-), if applicable

　I70.261 Atherosclerosis of native arteries of extremities with gangrene, right leg ▲

　I70.262 Atherosclerosis of native arteries of extremities with gangrene, left leg ▲

　I70.263 Atherosclerosis of native arteries of extremities with gangrene, bilateral legs ▲

　I70.268 Atherosclerosis of native arteries of extremities with gangrene, other extremity ▲

　I70.269 Atherosclerosis of native arteries of extremities with gangrene, unspecified extremity ▲

✓6th **I70.29** Other atherosclerosis of native arteries of extremities

　I70.291 Other atherosclerosis of native arteries of extremities, right leg ▲

　I70.292 Other atherosclerosis of native arteries of extremities, left leg ▲

　I70.293 Other atherosclerosis of native arteries of extremities, bilateral legs ▲

　I70.298 Other atherosclerosis of native arteries of extremities, other extremity ▲

　I70.299 Other atherosclerosis of native arteries of extremities, unspecified extremity ▲

✓5th **I70.3** Atherosclerosis of unspecified type of bypass graft(s) of the extremities
> Use additional code, if applicable, to identify chronic total occlusion of artery of extremity (I70.92)
> EXCLUDES 1　embolism or thrombus of bypass graft(s) of extremities (T82.8-)

✓6th **I70.30** Unspecified atherosclerosis of unspecified type of bypass graft(s) of the extremities

　I70.301 Unspecified atherosclerosis of unspecified type of bypass graft(s) of the extremities, right leg ▲

　I70.302 Unspecified atherosclerosis of unspecified type of bypass graft(s) of the extremities, left leg ▲

　I70.303 Unspecified atherosclerosis of unspecified type of bypass graft(s) of the extremities, bilateral legs ▲

　I70.308 Unspecified atherosclerosis of unspecified type of bypass graft(s) of the extremities, other extremity ▲

　I70.309 Unspecified atherosclerosis of unspecified type of bypass graft(s) of the extremities, unspecified extremity ▲

✓6th **I70.31** Atherosclerosis of unspecified type of bypass graft(s) of the extremities with intermittent claudication

　I70.311 Atherosclerosis of unspecified type of bypass graft(s) of the extremities with intermittent claudication, right leg ▲

　I70.312 Atherosclerosis of unspecified type of bypass graft(s) of the extremities with intermittent claudication, left leg ▲

　I70.313 Atherosclerosis of unspecified type of bypass graft(s) of the extremities with intermittent claudication, bilateral legs ▲

　I70.318 Atherosclerosis of unspecified type of bypass graft(s) of the extremities with intermittent claudication, other extremity ▲

　I70.319 Atherosclerosis of unspecified type of bypass graft(s) of the extremities with intermittent claudication, unspecified extremity ▲

✓6th **I70.32** Atherosclerosis of unspecified type of bypass graft(s) of the extremities with rest pain
> INCLUDES　any condition classifiable to I70.31-

　I70.321 Atherosclerosis of unspecified type of bypass graft(s) of the extremities with rest pain, right leg ▲

　I70.322 Atherosclerosis of unspecified type of bypass graft(s) of the extremities with rest pain, left leg ▲

　I70.323 Atherosclerosis of unspecified type of bypass graft(s) of the extremities with rest pain, bilateral legs ▲

　I70.328 Atherosclerosis of unspecified type of bypass graft(s) of the extremities with rest pain, other extremity ▲

　I70.329 Atherosclerosis of unspecified type of bypass graft(s) of the extremities with rest pain, unspecified extremity ▲

✓6th **I70.33** Atherosclerosis of unspecified type of bypass graft(s) of the right leg with ulceration
> INCLUDES　any condition classifiable to I70.311 and I70.321
> Use additional code to identify severity of ulcer (L97.-)

　I70.331 Atherosclerosis of unspecified type of bypass graft(s) of the right leg with ulceration of thigh ▲

EXCLUDES 1 Not coded here　　　EXCLUDES 2 Not included here　　　N Newborn Age: 0　　　P Pediatric Age: 0-17　　　M Maternity Age: 12-55　　　A Adult Age: 15-124

602　　　　　　ICD-10-CM 2016

I70.332   Atherosclerosis of unspecified type of bypass graft(s) of the right leg with ulceration of calf   **A**

I70.333   Atherosclerosis of unspecified type of bypass graft(s) of the right leg with ulceration of ankle   **A**

I70.334   Atherosclerosis of unspecified type of bypass graft(s) of the right leg with ulceration of heel and midfoot   **A**
Atherosclerosis of unspecified type of bypass graft(s) of right leg with ulceration of plantar surface of midfoot

I70.335   Atherosclerosis of unspecified type of bypass graft(s) of the right leg with ulceration of other part of foot   **A**
Atherosclerosis of unspecified type of bypass graft(s) of the right leg with ulceration of toe

I70.338   Atherosclerosis of unspecified type of bypass graft(s) of the right leg with ulceration of other part of lower leg   **A**

I70.339   Atherosclerosis of unspecified type of bypass graft(s) of the right leg with ulceration of unspecified site   **A**

✓6ᵗʰ **I70.34**   **Atherosclerosis of unspecified type of bypass graft(s) of the left leg with ulceration**
INCLUDES   any condition classifiable to I70.312 and I70.322
Use additional code to identify severity of ulcer (L97.-)

I70.341   Atherosclerosis of unspecified type of bypass graft(s) of the left leg with ulceration of thigh   **A**

I70.342   Atherosclerosis of unspecified type of bypass graft(s) of the left leg with ulceration of calf   **A**

I70.343   Atherosclerosis of unspecified type of bypass graft(s) of the left leg with ulceration of ankle   **A**

I70.344   Atherosclerosis of unspecified type of bypass graft(s) of the left leg with ulceration of heel and midfoot   **A**
Atherosclerosis of unspecified type of bypass graft(s) of left leg with ulceration of plantar surface of midfoot

I70.345   Atherosclerosis of unspecified type of bypass graft(s) of the left leg with ulceration of other part of foot   **A**
Atherosclerosis of unspecified type of bypass graft(s) of the left leg with ulceration of toe

I70.348   Atherosclerosis of unspecified type of bypass graft(s) of the left leg with ulceration of other part of lower leg   **A**

I70.349   Atherosclerosis of unspecified type of bypass graft(s) of the left leg with ulceration of unspecified site   **A**

I70.35   Atherosclerosis of unspecified type of bypass graft(s) of other extremity with ulceration   **A**
INCLUDES   any condition classifiable to I70.318 and I70.328
Use additional code to identify severity of ulcer (L98.49-)

✓6ᵗʰ **I70.36**   **Atherosclerosis of unspecified type of bypass graft(s) of the extremities with gangrene**
INCLUDES   any condition classifiable to I70.31-, I70.32-, I70.33-, I70.34-, I70.35
Use additional code to identify the severity of any ulcer (L97.-, L98.49-), if applicable

I70.361   Atherosclerosis of unspecified type of bypass graft(s) of the extremities with gangrene, right leg   **A**

I70.362   Atherosclerosis of unspecified type of bypass graft(s) of the extremities with gangrene, left leg   **A**

I70.363   Atherosclerosis of unspecified type of bypass graft(s) of the extremities with gangrene, bilateral legs   **A**

I70.368   Atherosclerosis of unspecified type of bypass graft(s) of the extremities with gangrene, other extremity   **A**

I70.369   Atherosclerosis of unspecified type of bypass graft(s) of the extremities with gangrene, unspecified extremity   **A**

✓6ᵗʰ **I70.39**   **Other atherosclerosis of unspecified type of bypass graft(s) of the extremities**

I70.391   Other atherosclerosis of unspecified type of bypass graft(s) of the extremities, right leg   **A**

I70.392   Other atherosclerosis of unspecified type of bypass graft(s) of the extremities, left leg   **A**

I70.393   Other atherosclerosis of unspecified type of bypass graft(s) of the extremities, bilateral legs   **A**

I70.398   Other atherosclerosis of unspecified type of bypass graft(s) of the extremities, other extremity   **A**

I70.399   Other atherosclerosis of unspecified type of bypass graft(s) of the extremities, unspecified extremity   **A**

✓5ᵗʰ **I70.4**   **Atherosclerosis of autologous vein bypass graft(s) of the extremities**
Use additional code, if applicable, to identify chronic total occlusion of artery of extremity (I70.92)

✓6ᵗʰ **I70.40**   **Unspecified atherosclerosis of autologous vein bypass graft(s) of the extremities**

I70.401   Unspecified atherosclerosis of autologous vein bypass graft(s) of the extremities, right leg   **A**

I70.402   Unspecified atherosclerosis of autologous vein bypass graft(s) of the extremities, left leg   **A**

I70.403   Unspecified atherosclerosis of autologous vein bypass graft(s) of the extremities, bilateral legs   **A**

I70.408   Unspecified atherosclerosis of autologous vein bypass graft(s) of the extremities, other extremity   **A**

I70.409   Unspecified atherosclerosis of autologous vein bypass graft(s) of the extremities, unspecified extremity   **A**

✓6ᵗʰ **I70.41**   **Atherosclerosis of autologous vein bypass graft(s) of the extremities with intermittent claudication**

I70.411   Atherosclerosis of autologous vein bypass graft(s) of the extremities with intermittent claudication, right leg   **A**

I70.412   Atherosclerosis of autologous vein bypass graft(s) of the extremities with intermittent claudication, left leg   **A**

I70.413   Atherosclerosis of autologous vein bypass graft(s) of the extremities with intermittent claudication, bilateral legs   **A**

I70.418   Atherosclerosis of autologous vein bypass graft(s) of the extremities with intermittent claudication, other extremity   **A**

I70.419   Atherosclerosis of autologous vein bypass graft(s) of the extremities with intermittent claudication, unspecified extremity   **A**

✓6ᵗʰ **I70.42**   **Atherosclerosis of autologous vein bypass graft(s) of the extremities with rest pain**
INCLUDES   any condition classifiable to I70.41-

I70.421   Atherosclerosis of autologous vein bypass graft(s) of the extremities with rest pain, right leg   **A**

I70.422   Atherosclerosis of autologous vein bypass graft(s) of the extremities with rest pain, left leg   **A**

I70.423   Atherosclerosis of autologous vein bypass graft(s) of the extremities with rest pain, bilateral legs   **A**

I70.428   Atherosclerosis of autologous vein bypass graft(s) of the extremities with rest pain, other extremity   **A**

I70.429   Atherosclerosis of autologous vein bypass graft(s) of the extremities with rest pain, unspecified extremity   **A**

✔ Additional Character Required   ✗x7ᵗʰ Placeholder Alert   Unspecified Dx   Other Specified Dx   Manifestation   ▶◀ Revised Text   ● New Code   ▲ Revised Code Title

ICD-10-CM 2016   603

✓6th **I70.43** **Atherosclerosis of autologous vein bypass graft(s) of the right leg with ulceration**
> INCLUDES   any condition classifiable to I70.411 and I70.421
> Use additional code to identify severity of ulcer (L97.-)

- **I70.431** **Atherosclerosis of autologous vein bypass graft(s) of the right leg with ulceration of thigh**   A
- **I70.432** **Atherosclerosis of autologous vein bypass graft(s) of the right leg with ulceration of calf**   A
- **I70.433** **Atherosclerosis of autologous vein bypass graft(s) of the right leg with ulceration of ankle**   A
- **I70.434** **Atherosclerosis of autologous vein bypass graft(s) of the right leg with ulceration of heel and midfoot**   A
  > Atherosclerosis of autologous vein bypass graft(s) of right leg with ulceration of plantar surface of midfoot
- **I70.435** **Atherosclerosis of autologous vein bypass graft(s) of the right leg with ulceration of other part of foot**   A
  > Atherosclerosis of autologous vein bypass graft(s) of right leg with ulceration of toe
- **I70.438** **Atherosclerosis of autologous vein bypass graft(s) of the right leg with ulceration of other part of lower leg**   A
- **I70.439** **Atherosclerosis of autologous vein bypass graft(s) of the right leg with ulceration of unspecified site**   A

✓6th **I70.44** **Atherosclerosis of autologous vein bypass graft(s) of the left leg with ulceration**
> INCLUDES   any condition classifiable to I70.412 and I70.422
> Use additional code to identify severity of ulcer (L97.-)

- **I70.441** **Atherosclerosis of autologous vein bypass graft(s) of the left leg with ulceration of thigh**   A
- **I70.442** **Atherosclerosis of autologous vein bypass graft(s) of the left leg with ulceration of calf**   A
- **I70.443** **Atherosclerosis of autologous vein bypass graft(s) of the left leg with ulceration of ankle**   A
- **I70.444** **Atherosclerosis of autologous vein bypass graft(s) of the left leg with ulceration of heel and midfoot**   A
  > Atherosclerosis of autologous vein bypass graft(s) of left leg with ulceration of plantar surface of midfoot
- **I70.445** **Atherosclerosis of autologous vein bypass graft(s) of the left leg with ulceration of other part of foot**   A
  > Atherosclerosis of autologous vein bypass graft(s) of left leg with ulceration of toe
- **I70.448** **Atherosclerosis of autologous vein bypass graft(s) of the left leg with ulceration of other part of lower leg**   A
- **I70.449** **Atherosclerosis of autologous vein bypass graft(s) of the left leg with ulceration of unspecified site**   A

I70.45 **Atherosclerosis of autologous vein bypass graft(s) of other extremity with ulceration**   A
> INCLUDES   any condition classifiable to I70.418, I70.428, and I70.438
> Use additional code to identify severity of ulcer (L98.49)

✓6th **I70.46** **Atherosclerosis of autologous vein bypass graft(s) of the extremities with gangrene**
> INCLUDES   any condition classifiable to I70.41-, I70.42-, and I70.43-, I70.44-, I70.45
> Use additional code to identify the severity of any ulcer (L97.-, L98.49-), if applicable

- **I70.461** **Atherosclerosis of autologous vein bypass graft(s) of the extremities with gangrene, right leg**   A
- **I70.462** **Atherosclerosis of autologous vein bypass graft(s) of the extremities with gangrene, left leg**   A
- **I70.463** **Atherosclerosis of autologous vein bypass graft(s) of the extremities with gangrene, bilateral legs**   A
- **I70.468** **Atherosclerosis of autologous vein bypass graft(s) of the extremities with gangrene, other extremity**   A
- **I70.469** **Atherosclerosis of autologous vein bypass graft(s) of the extremities with gangrene, unspecified extremity**   A

✓6th **I70.49** **Other atherosclerosis of autologous vein bypass graft(s) of the extremities**

- **I70.491** **Other atherosclerosis of autologous vein bypass graft(s) of the extremities, right leg**   A
- **I70.492** **Other atherosclerosis of autologous vein bypass graft(s) of the extremities, left leg**   A
- **I70.493** **Other atherosclerosis of autologous vein bypass graft(s) of the extremities, bilateral legs**   A
- **I70.498** **Other atherosclerosis of autologous vein bypass graft(s) of the extremities, other extremity**   A
- **I70.499** **Other atherosclerosis of autologous vein bypass graft(s) of the extremities, unspecified extremity**   A

✓5th **I70.5** **Atherosclerosis of nonautologous biological bypass graft(s) of the extremities**
> Use additional code, if applicable, to identify chronic total occlusion of artery of extremity (I70.92)

✓6th **I70.50** **Unspecified atherosclerosis of nonautologous biological bypass graft(s) of the extremities**

- **I70.501** **Unspecified atherosclerosis of nonautologous biological bypass graft(s) of the extremities, right leg**   A
- **I70.502** **Unspecified atherosclerosis of nonautologous biological bypass graft(s) of the extremities, left leg**   A
- **I70.503** **Unspecified atherosclerosis of nonautologous biological bypass graft(s) of the extremities, bilateral legs**   A
- **I70.508** **Unspecified atherosclerosis of nonautologous biological bypass graft(s) of the extremities, other extremity**   A
- **I70.509** **Unspecified atherosclerosis of nonautologous biological bypass graft(s) of the extremities, unspecified extremity**   A

✓6th **I70.51** **Atherosclerosis of nonautologous biological bypass graft(s) of the extremities with intermittent claudication**

- **I70.511** **Atherosclerosis of nonautologous biological bypass graft(s) of the extremities with intermittent claudication, right leg**   A
- **I70.512** **Atherosclerosis of nonautologous biological bypass graft(s) of the extremities with intermittent claudication, left leg**   A
- **I70.513** **Atherosclerosis of nonautologous biological bypass graft(s) of the extremities with intermittent claudication, bilateral legs**   A
- **I70.518** **Atherosclerosis of nonautologous biological bypass graft(s) of the extremities with intermittent claudication, other extremity**   A
- **I70.519** **Atherosclerosis of nonautologous biological bypass graft(s) of the extremities with intermittent claudication, unspecified extremity**   A

✓6th **I70.52** **Atherosclerosis of nonautologous biological bypass graft(s) of the extremities with rest pain**
> INCLUDES   any condition classifiable to I70.51-

- **I70.521** **Atherosclerosis of nonautologous biological bypass graft(s) of the extremities with rest pain, right leg**   A
- **I70.522** **Atherosclerosis of nonautologous biological bypass graft(s) of the extremities with rest pain, left leg**   A

EXCLUDES 1 Not coded here   EXCLUDES 2 Not included here   N Newborn Age: 0   P Pediatric Age: 0-17   M Maternity Age: 12-55   A Adult Age: 15-124

604   ICD-10-CM 2016

I70.523   Atherosclerosis of nonautologous biological bypass graft(s) of the extremities with rest pain, bilateral legs   Ⓐ

I70.528   Atherosclerosis of nonautologous biological bypass graft(s) of the extremities with rest pain, other extremity   Ⓐ

I70.529   Atherosclerosis of nonautologous biological bypass graft(s) of the extremities with rest pain, unspecified extremity   Ⓐ

✓6ᵗʰ **I70.53**   Atherosclerosis of nonautologous biological bypass graft(s) of the right leg with ulceration
   INCLUDES   any condition classifiable to I70.511 and I70.521
   Use additional code to identify severity of ulcer (L97.-)

I70.531   Atherosclerosis of nonautologous biological bypass graft(s) of the right leg with ulceration of thigh   Ⓐ

I70.532   Atherosclerosis of nonautologous biological bypass graft(s) of the right leg with ulceration of calf   Ⓐ

I70.533   Atherosclerosis of nonautologous biological bypass graft(s) of the right leg with ulceration of ankle   Ⓐ

I70.534   Atherosclerosis of nonautologous biological bypass graft(s) of the right leg with ulceration of heel and midfoot   Ⓐ
   Atherosclerosis of nonautologous biological bypass graft(s) of right leg with ulceration of plantar surface of midfoot

I70.535   Atherosclerosis of nonautologous biological bypass graft(s) of the right leg with ulceration of other part of foot   Ⓐ
   Atherosclerosis of nonautologous biological bypass graft(s) of the right leg with ulceration of toe

I70.538   Atherosclerosis of nonautologous biological bypass graft(s) of the right leg with ulceration of other part of lower leg   Ⓐ

I70.539   Atherosclerosis of nonautologous biological bypass graft(s) of the right leg with ulceration of unspecified site   Ⓐ

✓6ᵗʰ **I70.54**   Atherosclerosis of nonautologous biological bypass graft(s) of the left leg with ulceration
   INCLUDES   any condition classifiable to I70.512 and I70.522
   Use additional code to identify severity of ulcer (L97.-)

I70.541   Atherosclerosis of nonautologous biological bypass graft(s) of the left leg with ulceration of thigh   Ⓐ

I70.542   Atherosclerosis of nonautologous biological bypass graft(s) of the left leg with ulceration of calf   Ⓐ

I70.543   Atherosclerosis of nonautologous biological bypass graft(s) of the left leg with ulceration of ankle   Ⓐ

I70.544   Atherosclerosis of nonautologous biological bypass graft(s) of the left leg with ulceration of heel and midfoot   Ⓐ
   Atherosclerosis of nonautologous biological bypass graft(s) of left leg with ulceration of plantar surface of midfoot

I70.545   Atherosclerosis of nonautologous biological bypass graft(s) of the left leg with ulceration of other part of foot   Ⓐ
   Atherosclerosis of nonautologous biological bypass graft(s) of the left leg with ulceration of toe

I70.548   Atherosclerosis of nonautologous biological bypass graft(s) of the left leg with ulceration of other part of lower leg   Ⓐ

I70.549   Atherosclerosis of nonautologous biological bypass graft(s) of the left leg with ulceration of unspecified site   Ⓐ

I70.55   Atherosclerosis of nonautologous biological bypass graft(s) of other extremity with ulceration   Ⓐ
   INCLUDES   any condition classifiable to I70.518, I70.528, and I70.538
   Use additional code to identify severity of ulcer (L98.49)

✓6ᵗʰ **I70.56**   Atherosclerosis of nonautologous biological bypass graft(s) of the extremities with gangrene
   INCLUDES   any condition classifiable to I70.51-, I70.52-, and I70.53-, I70.54-, I70.55
   Use additional code to identify the severity of any ulcer (L97.-, L98.49-), if applicable

I70.561   Atherosclerosis of nonautologous biological bypass graft(s) of the extremities with gangrene, right leg   Ⓐ

I70.562   Atherosclerosis of nonautologous biological bypass graft(s) of the extremities with gangrene, left leg   Ⓐ

I70.563   Atherosclerosis of nonautologous biological bypass graft(s) of the extremities with gangrene, bilateral legs   Ⓐ

I70.568   Atherosclerosis of nonautologous biological bypass graft(s) of the extremities with gangrene, other extremity   Ⓐ

I70.569   Atherosclerosis of nonautologous biological bypass graft(s) of the extremities with gangrene, unspecified extremity   Ⓐ

✓6ᵗʰ **I70.59**   Other atherosclerosis of nonautologous biological bypass graft(s) of the extremities

I70.591   Other atherosclerosis of nonautologous biological bypass graft(s) of the extremities, right leg   Ⓐ

I70.592   Other atherosclerosis of nonautologous biological bypass graft(s) of the extremities, left leg   Ⓐ

I70.593   Other atherosclerosis of nonautologous biological bypass graft(s) of the extremities, bilateral legs   Ⓐ

I70.598   Other atherosclerosis of nonautologous biological bypass graft(s) of the extremities, other extremity   Ⓐ

I70.599   Other atherosclerosis of nonautologous biological bypass graft(s) of the extremities, unspecified extremity   Ⓐ

✓5ᵗʰ **I70.6**   Atherosclerosis of nonbiological bypass graft(s) of the extremities
   Use additional code, if applicable, to identify chronic total occlusion of artery of extremity (I70.92)

✓6ᵗʰ **I70.60**   Unspecified atherosclerosis of nonbiological bypass graft(s) of the extremities

I70.601   Unspecified atherosclerosis of nonbiological bypass graft(s) of the extremities, right leg   Ⓐ

I70.602   Unspecified atherosclerosis of nonbiological bypass graft(s) of the extremities, left leg   Ⓐ

I70.603   Unspecified atherosclerosis of nonbiological bypass graft(s) of the extremities, bilateral legs   Ⓐ

I70.608   Unspecified atherosclerosis of nonbiological bypass graft(s) of the extremities, other extremity   Ⓐ

I70.609   Unspecified atherosclerosis of nonbiological bypass graft(s) of the extremities, unspecified extremity   Ⓐ

✓6ᵗʰ **I70.61**   Atherosclerosis of nonbiological bypass graft(s) of the extremities with intermittent claudication

I70.611   Atherosclerosis of nonbiological bypass graft(s) of the extremities with intermittent claudication, right leg   Ⓐ

I70.612   Atherosclerosis of nonbiological bypass graft(s) of the extremities with intermittent claudication, left leg   Ⓐ

I70.613   Atherosclerosis of nonbiological bypass graft(s) of the extremities with intermittent claudication, bilateral legs   Ⓐ

I70.618   Atherosclerosis of nonbiological bypass graft(s) of the extremities with intermittent claudication, other extremity   Ⓐ

I70.619   Atherosclerosis of nonbiological bypass graft(s) of the extremities with intermittent claudication, unspecified extremity   Ⓐ

☑ Additional Character Required   ✓ₓ7ᵗʰ Placeholder Alert   Unspecified Dx   Other Specified Dx   Manifestation   ▶◀ Revised Text   ● New Code   ▲ Revised Code Title

ICD-10-CM 2016   **605**

Chapter 9. Diseases of the Circulatory System

✓6th **I70.62** **Atherosclerosis of nonbiological bypass graft(s) of the extremities with** rest pain 🅐
> INCLUDES   any condition classifiable to I70.61-

    I70.621   **Atherosclerosis of nonbiological bypass graft(s) of the extremities with rest pain,** right leg 🅐

    I70.622   **Atherosclerosis of nonbiological bypass graft(s) of the extremities with rest pain,** left leg 🅐

    I70.623   **Atherosclerosis of nonbiological bypass graft(s) of the extremities with rest pain,** bilateral legs 🅐

    I70.628   **Atherosclerosis of nonbiological bypass graft(s) of the extremities with rest pain, other extremity** 🅐

    I70.629   **Atherosclerosis of nonbiological bypass graft(s) of the extremities with rest pain, unspecified extremity** 🅐

✓6th **I70.63** **Atherosclerosis of nonbiological bypass graft(s) of the** right leg with ulceration
> INCLUDES   any condition classifiable to I70.611 and I70.621
Use additional code to identify severity of ulcer (L97.-)

    I70.631   **Atherosclerosis of nonbiological bypass graft(s) of the right leg with ulceration of** thigh 🅐

    I70.632   **Atherosclerosis of nonbiological bypass graft(s) of the right leg with ulceration of** calf 🅐

    I70.633   **Atherosclerosis of nonbiological bypass graft(s) of the right leg with ulceration of** ankle 🅐

    I70.634   **Atherosclerosis of nonbiological bypass graft(s) of the right leg with ulceration of** heel and midfoot 🅐
> Atherosclerosis of nonbiological bypass graft(s) of right leg with ulceration of plantar surface of midfoot

    I70.635   **Atherosclerosis of nonbiological bypass graft(s) of the right leg with ulceration of other** part of foot 🅐
> Atherosclerosis of nonbiological bypass graft(s) of the right leg with ulceration of toe

    I70.638   **Atherosclerosis of nonbiological bypass graft(s) of the right leg with ulceration of other** part of lower leg 🅐

    I70.639   **Atherosclerosis of nonbiological bypass graft(s) of the right leg with ulceration of unspecified site** 🅐

✓6th **I70.64** **Atherosclerosis of nonbiological bypass graft(s) of the** left leg with ulceration
> INCLUDES   any condition classifiable to I70.612 and I70.622
Use additional code to identify severity of ulcer (L97.-)

    I70.641   **Atherosclerosis of nonbiological bypass graft(s) of the left leg with ulceration of** thigh 🅐

    I70.642   **Atherosclerosis of nonbiological bypass graft(s) of the left leg with ulceration of** calf 🅐

    I70.643   **Atherosclerosis of nonbiological bypass graft(s) of the left leg with ulceration of** ankle 🅐

    I70.644   **Atherosclerosis of nonbiological bypass graft(s) of the left leg with ulceration of** heel and midfoot 🅐
> Atherosclerosis of nonbiological bypass graft(s) of left leg with ulceration of plantar surface of midfoot

    I70.645   **Atherosclerosis of nonbiological bypassgraft(s) of the left leg with ulceration of other** part of foot 🅐
> Atherosclerosis of nonbiological bypass graft(s) of the left leg with ulceration of toe

    I70.648   **Atherosclerosis of nonbiological bypass graft(s) of the left leg with ulceration of other** part of lower leg 🅐

    I70.649   **Atherosclerosis of nonbiological bypass graft(s) of the left leg with ulceration of unspecified site** 🅐

I70.65   **Atherosclerosis of nonbiological bypass graft(s) of other extremity with** ulceration 🅐
> INCLUDES   any condition classifiable to I70.618 and I70.628
Use additional code to identify severity of ulcer (L98.49)

✓6th **I70.66** **Atherosclerosis of nonbiological bypass graft(s) of the extremities with** gangrene
> INCLUDES   any condition classifiable to I70.61-, I70.62-, I70.63-, I70.64-, I70.65
Use additional code to identify the severity of any ulcer (L97.-, L98.49-), if applicable

    I70.661   **Atherosclerosis of nonbiological bypass graft(s) of the extremities with gangrene, right leg** 🅐

    I70.662   **Atherosclerosis of nonbiological bypass graft(s) of the extremities with gangrene, left leg** 🅐

    I70.663   **Atherosclerosis of nonbiological bypass graft(s) of the extremities with gangrene, bilateral legs** 🅐

    I70.668   **Atherosclerosis of nonbiological bypass graft(s) of the extremities with gangrene, other extremity** 🅐

    I70.669   **Atherosclerosis of nonbiological bypass graft(s) of the extremities with gangrene, unspecified extremity** 🅐

✓6th **I70.69** Other **atherosclerosis of nonbiological bypass graft(s) of the extremities**

    I70.691   **Other atherosclerosis of nonbiological bypass graft(s) of the extremities,** right leg 🅐

    I70.692   **Other atherosclerosis of nonbiological bypass graft(s) of the extremities,** left leg 🅐

    I70.693   **Other atherosclerosis of nonbiological bypass graft(s) of the extremities,** bilateral legs 🅐

    I70.698   **Other atherosclerosis of nonbiological bypass graft(s) of the extremities, other extremity** 🅐

    I70.699   **Other atherosclerosis of nonbiological bypass graft(s) of the extremities, unspecified extremity** 🅐

✓5th **I70.7** **Atherosclerosis of** other type of **bypass graft(s) of the extremities**
> Use additional code, if applicable, to identify chronic total occlusion of artery of extremity (I70.92)

✓6th **I70.70** Unspecified **atherosclerosis of other type of bypass graft(s) of the extremities**

    I70.701   **Unspecified atherosclerosis of other type of bypass graft(s) of the extremities,** right leg 🅐

    I70.702   **Unspecified atherosclerosis of other type of bypass graft(s) of the extremities,** left leg 🅐

    I70.703   **Unspecified atherosclerosis of other type of bypass graft(s) of the extremities,** bilateral legs 🅐

    I70.708   **Unspecified atherosclerosis of other type of bypass graft(s) of the extremities, other extremity** 🅐

    I70.709   **Unspecified atherosclerosis of other type of bypass graft(s) of the extremities, unspecified extremity** 🅐

✓6th **I70.71** **Atherosclerosis of other type of bypass graft(s) of the extremities with** intermittent claudication

    I70.711   **Atherosclerosis of other type of bypass graft(s) of the extremities with intermittent claudication,** right leg 🅐

    I70.712   **Atherosclerosis of other type of bypass graft(s) of the extremities with intermittent claudication,** left leg 🅐

    I70.713   **Atherosclerosis of other type of bypass graft(s) of the extremities with intermittent claudication,** bilateral legs 🅐

    I70.718   **Atherosclerosis of other type of bypass graft(s) of the extremities with intermittent claudication, other extremity** 🅐

EXCLUDES 1 Not coded here   EXCLUDES 2 Not included here   N Newborn Age: 0   P Pediatric Age: 0-17   M Maternity Age: 12-55   A Adult Age: 15-124

606   ICD-10-CM 2016

I70.719   Atherosclerosis of other type of bypass graft(s) of the extremities with intermittent claudication, unspecified extremity   Ⓐ

✓6ᵗʰ **I70.72**   Atherosclerosis of other type of bypass graft(s) of the extremities with rest pain
INCLUDES   any condition classifiable to I70.71-

I70.721   Atherosclerosis of other type of bypass graft(s) of the extremities with rest pain, right leg   Ⓐ

I70.722   Atherosclerosis of other type of bypass graft(s) of the extremities with rest pain, left leg   Ⓐ

I70.723   Atherosclerosis of other type of bypass graft(s) of the extremities with rest pain, bilateral legs   Ⓐ

I70.728   Atherosclerosis of other type of bypass graft(s) of the extremities with rest pain, other extremity   Ⓐ

I70.729   Atherosclerosis of other type of bypass graft(s) of the extremities with rest pain, unspecified extremity   Ⓐ

✓6ᵗʰ **I70.73**   Atherosclerosis of other type of bypass graft(s) of the right leg with ulceration
INCLUDES   any condition classifiable to I70.711 and I70.721
Use additional code to identify severity of ulcer (L97.-)

I70.731   Atherosclerosis of other type of bypass graft(s) of the right leg with ulceration of thigh   Ⓐ

I70.732   Atherosclerosis of other type of bypass graft(s) of the right leg with ulceration of calf   Ⓐ

I70.733   Atherosclerosis of other type of bypass graft(s) of the right leg with ulceration of ankle   Ⓐ

I70.734   Atherosclerosis of other type of bypass graft(s) of the right leg with ulceration of heel and midfoot   Ⓐ
Atherosclerosis of other type of bypass graft(s) of right leg with ulceration of plantar surface of midfoot

I70.735   Atherosclerosis of other type of bypass graft(s) of the right leg with ulceration of other part of foot   Ⓐ
Atherosclerosis of other type of bypass graft(s) of right leg with ulceration of toe

I70.738   Atherosclerosis of other type of bypass graft(s) of the right leg with ulceration of other part of lower leg   Ⓐ

I70.739   Atherosclerosis of other type of bypass graft(s) of the right leg with ulceration of unspecified site   Ⓐ

✓6ᵗʰ **I70.74**   Atherosclerosis of other type of bypass graft(s) of the left leg with ulceration
INCLUDES   any condition classifiable to I70.712 and I70.722
Use additional code to identify severity of ulcer (L97.-)

I70.741   Atherosclerosis of other type of bypass graft(s) of the left leg with ulceration of thigh   Ⓐ

I70.742   Atherosclerosis of other type of bypass graft(s) of the left leg with ulceration of calf   Ⓐ

I70.743   Atherosclerosis of other type of bypass raft(s) of the left leg with ulceration of ankle   Ⓐ

I70.744   Atherosclerosis of other type of bypass graft(s) of the left leg with ulceration of heel and midfoot   Ⓐ
Atherosclerosis of other type of bypass graft(s) of left leg with ulceration of plantar surface of midfoot

I70.745   Atherosclerosis of other type of bypass graft(s) of the left leg with ulceration of other part of foot   Ⓐ
Atherosclerosis of other type of bypass graft(s) of left leg with ulceration of toe

I70.748   Atherosclerosis of other type of bypass graft(s) of the left leg with ulceration of other part of lower leg   Ⓐ

I70.749   Atherosclerosis of other type of bypass graft(s) of the left leg with ulceration of unspecified site   Ⓐ

I70.75   Atherosclerosis of other type of bypass graft(s) of other extremity with ulceration   Ⓐ
INCLUDES   any condition classifiable to I70.718 and I70.728
Use additional code to identify severity of ulcer (L98.49)

✓6ᵗʰ **I70.76**   Atherosclerosis of other type of bypass graft(s) of the extremities with gangrene
INCLUDES   any condition classifiable to I70.71-, I70.72-, I70.73-, I70.74-, I70.75
Use additional code to identify the severity of any ulcer (L97.-, L98.49-), if applicable

I70.761   Atherosclerosis of other type of bypass graft(s) of the extremities with gangrene, right leg   Ⓐ

I70.762   Atherosclerosis of other type of bypass graft(s) of the extremities with gangrene, left leg   Ⓐ

I70.763   Atherosclerosis of other type of bypass graft(s) of the extremities with gangrene, bilateral legs   Ⓐ

I70.768   Atherosclerosis of other type of bypass graft(s) of the extremities with gangrene, other extremity   Ⓐ

I70.769   Atherosclerosis of other type of bypass graft(s) of the extremities with gangrene, unspecified extremity   Ⓐ

✓6ᵗʰ **I70.79**   Other atherosclerosis of other type of bypass graft(s) of the extremities

I70.791   Other atherosclerosis of other type of bypass graft(s) of the extremities, right leg   Ⓐ

I70.792   Other atherosclerosis of other type of bypass graft(s) of the extremities, left leg   Ⓐ

I70.793   Other atherosclerosis of other type of bypass graft(s) of the extremities, bilateral legs   Ⓐ

I70.798   Other atherosclerosis of other type of bypass graft(s) of the extremities, other extremity   Ⓐ

I70.799   Other atherosclerosis of other type of bypass graft(s) of the extremities, unspecified extremity   Ⓐ

I70.8   Atherosclerosis of other arteries   Ⓐ

✓5ᵗʰ **I70.9**   Other and unspecified atherosclerosis

I70.90   Unspecified atherosclerosis   Ⓐ

I70.91   Generalized atherosclerosis   Ⓐ

I70.92   Chronic total occlusion of artery of the extremities   Ⓐ
Complete occlusion of artery of the extremities
Total occlusion of artery of the extremities
Code first atherosclerosis of arteries of the extremities (I70.2-, I70.3-, I70.4-, I70.5-, I70.6-, I70.7-)

✓4ᵗʰ **I71**   **Aortic aneurysm and dissection**
EXCLUDES 1   aortic ectasia (I77.81-)
syphilitic aortic aneurysm (A52.01)
traumatic aortic aneurysm (S25.09, S35.09)

✓5ᵗʰ **I71.0**   Dissection of aorta

I71.00   Dissection of unspecified site of aorta   Ⓐ

I71.01   Dissection of thoracic aorta   Ⓐ

I71.02   Dissection of abdominal aorta   Ⓐ

I71.03   Dissection of thoracoabdominal aorta   Ⓐ

I71.1   Thoracic aortic aneurysm, ruptured   Ⓐ

I71.2   Thoracic aortic aneurysm, without rupture   Ⓐ

I71.3   Abdominal aortic aneurysm, ruptured   Ⓐ

I71.4   Abdominal aortic aneurysm, without rupture   Ⓐ

I71.5   Thoracoabdominal aortic aneurysm, ruptured   Ⓐ

I71.6   Thoracoabdominal aortic aneurysm, without rupture   Ⓐ

I71.8   Aortic aneurysm of unspecified site, ruptured   Ⓐ
Rupture of aorta NOS

☑ Additional Character Required   ✓x7ᵗʰ Placeholder Alert   Unspecified Dx   Other Specified Dx   Manifestation   ▶◀ Revised Text   ● New Code   ▲ Revised Code Title

I71.9   **Aortic aneurysm of unspecified site,** without rupture   A
     Aneurysm of aorta
     Dilatation of aorta
     Hyaline necrosis of aorta

✓4ᵗʰ **I72**   **Other aneurysm**
     INCLUDES   aneurysm (cirsoid) (false) (ruptured)
     EXCLUDES 2   acquired aneurysm (I77.0)
         aneurysm (of) aorta (I71.-)
         aneurysm (of) arteriovenous NOS (Q27.3-)
         carotid artery dissection (I77.71)
         cerebral (nonruptured) aneurysm (I67.1)
         coronary aneurysm (I25.4)
         coronary artery dissection (I25.42)
         dissection of artery NEC (I77.79)
         heart aneurysm (I25.3)
         iliac artery dissection (I77.72)
         pulmonary artery aneurysm (I28.1)
         renal artery dissection (I77.73)
         retinal aneurysm (H35.0)
         ruptured cerebral aneurysm (I60.7)
         varicose aneurysm (I77.0)
         vertebral artery dissection (I77.74)

I72.0   **Aneurysm of** carotid artery   A
     Aneurysm of common carotid artery
     Aneurysm of external carotid artery
     Aneurysm of internal carotid artery, extracranial portion
     EXCLUDES 1   aneurysm of internal carotid artery, intracranial portion (I67.1)
         aneurysm of internal carotid artery NOS (I67.1)

I72.1   **Aneurysm of artery of** upper extremity   A
I72.2   **Aneurysm of** renal artery   A
I72.3   **Aneurysm of** iliac artery   A
I72.4   **Aneurysm of artery of** lower extremity   A
I72.8   **Aneurysm of other specified arteries**   A
I72.9   **Aneurysm of unspecified site**   A

✓4ᵗʰ **I73**   **Other peripheral vascular diseases**
     EXCLUDES 2   chilblains (T69.1)
         frostbite (T33- T34)
         immersion hand or foot (T69.0-)
         spasm of cerebral artery (G45.9)

✓5ᵗʰ **I73.0**   **Raynaud's syndrome**
     Raynaud's disease
     Raynaud's phenomenon (secondary)
     I73.00   **Raynaud's syndrome** without gangrene
     I73.01   **Raynaud's syndrome** with gangrene

I73.1   **Thromboangiitis obliterans [Buerger's disease]**

✓5ᵗʰ **I73.8**   **Other specified peripheral vascular diseases**
     EXCLUDES 1   diabetic (peripheral) angiopathy (E08-E13 with .51-.52)
     I73.81   **Erythromelalgia**
     I73.89   **Other specified peripheral vascular diseases**
         Acrocyanosis
         Erythrocyanosis
         Simple acroparesthesia [Schultze's type]
         Vasomotor acroparesthesia [Nothnagel's type]

I73.9   **Peripheral vascular disease, unspecified**
     Intermittent claudication
     Peripheral angiopathy NOS
     Spasm of artery
     EXCLUDES 1   atherosclerosis of the extremities (I70.2--I70.7-)

✓4ᵗʰ **I74**   **Arterial embolism and thrombosis**
     Embolic infarction
     Embolic occlusion
     Thrombotic infarction
     Thrombotic occlusion
     Code first:
         embolism and thrombosis complicating abortion or ectopic or molar pregnancy (O00-O07, O08.2)
         embolism and thrombosis complicating pregnancy, childbirth and the puerperium (O88.-)
     EXCLUDES 2   atheroembolism (I75.-)
         basilar embolism and thrombosis (I63.0-I63.2, I65.1)
         carotid embolism and thrombosis (I63.0-I63.2, I65.2)
         cerebral embolism and thrombosis (I63.3-I63.5, I66-)
         coronary embolism and thrombosis (I21-I25)
         mesenteric embolism and thrombosis (K55.0)
         ophthalmic embolism and thrombosis (H34.-)
         precerebral embolism and thrombosis NOS (I63.0-I63.2, I65.9)
         pulmonary embolism and thrombosIs (I26.-)
         renal embolism and thrombosis (N28.0)
         retinal embolism and thrombosis (H34.-)
         septic embolism and thrombosis (I76)
         vertebral embolism and thrombosis (I63.0-I63.2, I65.0)

✓5ᵗʰ **I74.0**   **Embolism and thrombosis of** abdominal aorta
     I74.01   **Saddle embolus of abdominal aorta**
     I74.09   **Other** arterial **embolism and thrombosis of abdominal aorta**
         Aortic bifurcation syndrome
         Aortoiliac obstruction
         Leriche's syndrome

✓5ᵗʰ **I74.1**   **Embolism and thrombosis of** other and unspecified parts **of aorta**
     I74.10   **Embolism and thrombosis of unspecified parts of aorta**
     I74.11   **Embolism and thrombosis of** thoracic **aorta**
     I74.19   **Embolism and thrombosis of other** parts of aorta

I74.2   **Embolism and thrombosis of arteries of the** upper extremities
I74.3   **Embolism and thrombosis of arteries of the** lower extremities
I74.4   **Embolism and thrombosis of arteries of extremities, unspecified**
     Peripheral arterial embolism NOS
I74.5   **Embolism and thrombosis of** iliac **artery**
I74.8   **Embolism and thrombosis of other arteries**
I74.9   **Embolism and thrombosis of unspecified artery**

✓4ᵗʰ **I75**   **Atheroembolism**
     Atherothrombotic microembolism
     Cholesterol embolism

✓5ᵗʰ **I75.0**   **Atheroembolism of** extremities
     ✓6ᵗʰ **I75.01**   **Atheroembolism of** upper **extremity**
         I75.011   **Atheroembolism of** right **upper extremity**
         I75.012   **Atheroembolism of** left **upper extremity**
         I75.013   **Atheroembolism of** bilateral **upper extremities**
         I75.019   **Atheroembolism of unspecified upper extremity**
     ✓6ᵗʰ **I75.02**   **Atheroembolism of** lower **extremity**
         I75.021   **Atheroembolism of** right **lower extremity**
         I75.022   **Atheroembolism of** left **lower extremity**
         I75.023   **Atheroembolism of** bilateral **lower extremities**
         I75.029   **Atheroembolism of unspecified lower extremity**

✓5ᵗʰ **I75.8**   **Atheroembolism of** other sites
     I75.81   **Atheroembolism of** kidney
         Use additional code for any associated acute kidney failure and chronic kidney disease (N17.-, N18.-)
     I75.89   **Atheroembolism of other site**

I76   **Septic arterial embolism**
     Code first underlying infection, such as:
         infective endocarditis (I33.0)
         lung abscess (J85.-)
     Use additional code to identify the site of the embolism (I74.-)
     EXCLUDES 2   septic pulmonary embolism (I26.01, I26.90)

EXCLUDES 1 Not coded here   EXCLUDES 2 Not included here   N Newborn Age: 0   P Pediatric Age: 0-17   M Maternity Age: 12-55   A Adult Age: 15-124

✓4th **I77   Other disorders of arteries and arterioles**
> EXCLUDES 2   *collagen (vascular) diseases (M30-M36)*
> *hypersensitivity angiitis (M31.0)*
> *pulmonary artery (I28.-)*

I77.0   Arteriovenous fistula, acquired
> Aneurysmal varix
> Arteriovenous aneurysm, acquired
> > EXCLUDES 1   *arteriovenous aneurysm NOS (Q27.3-)*
> > *presence of arteriovenous shunt (fistula) for dialysis (Z99.2)*
> > *traumatic—see injury of blood vessel by body region*
> > EXCLUDES 2   *cerebral (I67.1)*
> > *coronary (I25.4)*

I77.1   Stricture of artery
> Narrowing of artery

I77.2   Rupture of artery
> Erosion of artery
> Fistula of artery
> Ulcer of artery
> > EXCLUDES 1   *traumatic rupture of artery—see injury of blood vessel by body region*

I77.3   Arterial fibromuscular dysplasia
> Fibromuscular hyperplasia (of) carotid artery
> Fibromuscular hyperplasia (of) renal artery

I77.4   Celiac artery compression syndrome

I77.5   Necrosis of artery

I77.6   Arteritis, unspecified
> Aortitis NOS
> Endarteritis NOS
> > EXCLUDES 1   *arteritis or endarteritis:*
> > *aortic arch (M31.4)*
> > *cerebral NEC (I67.7)*
> > *coronary (I25.89)*
> > *deformans (I70.-)*
> > *giant cell (M31.5., M31.6)*
> > *obliterans (I70.-)*
> > *senile (I70.-)*

✓5th **I77.7   Other arterial dissection**
> > EXCLUDES 2   *dissection of aorta (I71.0-)*
> > *dissection of coronary artery (I25.42)*

> **I77.71   Dissection of carotid artery**
> **I77.72   Dissection of iliac artery**
> **I77.73   Dissection of renal artery**
> **I77.74   Dissection of vertebral artery**
> **I77.79   Dissection of other artery**

✓5th **I77.8   Other specified disorders of arteries and arterioles**
> ✓6th **I77.81   Aortic ectasia**
> > Ectasis aorta
> > > EXCLUDES 1   *aortic aneurysm and dissection (I71.0-)*
> > **I77.810   Thoracic aortic ectasia**
> > **I77.811   Abdominal aortic ectasia**
> > **I77.812   Thoracoabdominal aortic ectasia**
> > **I77.819   Aortic ectasia, unspecified site**
> **I77.89   Other specified disorders of arteries and arterioles**

I77.9   Disorder of arteries and arterioles, unspecified

✓4th **I78   Diseases of capillaries**
I78.0   Hereditary hemorrhagic telangiectasia
> Rendu-Osler-Weber disease

I78.1   Nevus, non-neoplastic
> Araneus nevus
> Senile nevus
> Spider nevus
> Stellar nevus
> > EXCLUDES 1   *nevus NOS (D22.-)*
> > *vascular NOS (Q82.5)*
> > EXCLUDES 2   *blue nevus (D22.-)*
> > *flammeus nevus (Q82.5)*
> > *hairy nevus (D22.-)*
> > *melanocytic nevus (D22.-)*
> > *pigmented nevus (D22.-)*
> > *portwine nevus (Q82.5)*
> > *sanguineous nevus (Q82.5)*
> > *strawberry nevus (Q82.5)*
> > *verrucous nevus (Q82.5)*

I78.8   Other diseases of capillaries
I78.9   Disease of capillaries, unspecified

✓4th **I79   Disorders of arteries, arterioles and capillaries in diseases classified elsewhere**

I79.0   Aneurysm of aorta in diseases classified elsewhere   ▲
> Code first underlying disease
> > EXCLUDES 1   *syphilitic aneurysm (A52.01)*

I79.1   Aortitis in diseases classified elsewhere
> Code first underlying disease
> > EXCLUDES 1   *syphilitic aortitis (A52.02)*

I79.8   Other disorders of arteries, arterioles and capillaries in diseases classified elsewhere
> Code first underlying disease, such as:
> amyloidosis (E85.-)
> > EXCLUDES 1   *diabetic (peripheral) angiopathy (E08-E13 with .51-.52)*
> > *syphilitic endarteritis (A52.09)*
> > *tuberculous endarteritis (A18.89)*

Diseases of veins, lymphatic vessels and lymph nodes, not elsewhere classified (I80-I89)

✓4th **I80   Phlebitis and thrombophlebitis**
> INCLUDES   endophlebitis
> inflammation, vein
> periphlebitis
> suppurative phlebitis

Code first:
> phlebitis and thrombophlebitis complicating abortion, ectopic or molar pregnancy (O00-O07, O08.7)
> phlebitis and thrombophlebitis complicating pregnancy, childbirth and the puerperium (O22.-, O87.-)
> > EXCLUDES 1   *venous embolism and thrombosis of lower extremities ((I82.4-, I82.5-, I82.81-)*

✓5th **I80.0   Phlebitis and thrombophlebitis of superficial vessels of lower extremities**
> Phlebitis and thrombophlebitis of femoropopliteal vein
> > **I80.00   Phlebitis and thrombophlebitis of superficial vessels of unspecified lower extremity**
> > **I80.01   Phlebitis and thrombophlebitis of superficial vessels of right lower extremity**
> > **I80.02   Phlebitis and thrombophlebitis of superficial vessels of left lower extremity**
> > **I80.03   Phlebitis and thrombophlebitis of superficial vessels of lower extremities, bilateral**

✓5th **I80.1   Phlebitis and thrombophlebitis of femoral vein**
> **I80.10   Phlebitis and thrombophlebitis of unspecified femoral vein**
> **I80.11   Phlebitis and thrombophlebitis of right femoral vein**
> **I80.12   Phlebitis and thrombophlebitis of left femoral vein**
> **I80.13   Phlebitis and thrombophlebitis of femoral vein, bilateral**

✓5th **I80.2   Phlebitis and thrombophlebitis of other and unspecified deep vessels of lower extremities**
> ✓6th **I80.20   Phlebitis and thrombophlebitis of unspecified deep vessels of lower extremities**
> > **I80.201   Phlebitis and thrombophlebitis of unspecified deep vessels of right lower extremity**
> > **I80.202   Phlebitis and thrombophlebitis of unspecified deep vessels of left lower extremity**
> > **I80.203   Phlebitis and thrombophlebitis of unspecified deep vessels of lower extremities, bilateral**
> > **I80.209   Phlebitis and thrombophlebitis of unspecified deep vessels of unspecified lower extremity**
> ✓6th **I80.21   Phlebitis and thrombophlebitis of iliac vein**
> > **I80.211   Phlebitis and thrombophlebitis of right iliac vein**
> > **I80.212   Phlebitis and thrombophlebitis of left iliac vein**
> > **I80.213   Phlebitis and thrombophlebitis of iliac vein, bilateral**
> > **I80.219   Phlebitis and thrombophlebitis of unspecified iliac vein**
> ✓6th **I80.22   Phlebitis and thrombophlebitis of popliteal vein**
> > **I80.221   Phlebitis and thrombophlebitis of right popliteal vein**

☑ Additional Character Required   ✓x7th Placeholder Alert   Unspecified Dx   Other Specified Dx   Manifestation   ▶◀ Revised Text   ● New Code   ▲ Revised Code Title

     I80.222   **Phlebitis and thrombophlebitis of** left **popliteal vein**

     I80.223   **Phlebitis and thrombophlebitis of popliteal vein,** bilateral

     I80.229   **Phlebitis and thrombophlebitis of unspecified popliteal vein**

    ✓6ᵗʰ **I80.23**   **Phlebitis and thrombophlebitis of** tibial **vein**

     I80.231   **Phlebitis and thrombophlebitis of** right **tibial vein**

     I80.232   **Phlebitis and thrombophlebitis of** left **tibial vein**

     I80.233   **Phlebitis and thrombophlebitis of tibial vein,** bilateral

     I80.239   **Phlebitis and thrombophlebitis of unspecified tibial vein**

    ✓6ᵗʰ **I80.29**   **Phlebitis and thrombophlebitis of** other **deep vessels of lower extremities**

     I80.291   **Phlebitis and thrombophlebitis of other deep vessels of** right **lower extremity**

     I80.292   **Phlebitis and thrombophlebitis of other deep vessels of** left **lower extremity**

     I80.293   **Phlebitis and thrombophlebitis of other deep vessels of lower extremity,** bilateral

     I80.299   **Phlebitis and thrombophlebitis of other deep vessels of unspecified lower extremity**

   I80.3   **Phlebitis and thrombophlebitis of lower extremities, unspecified**

   I80.8   **Phlebitis and thrombophlebitis of other sites**

   I80.9   **Phlebitis and thrombophlebitis of unspecified site**

I81   **Portal vein thrombosis**
Portal (vein) obstruction
   EXCLUDES 2   *hepatic vein thrombosis (I82.0)*
          phlebitis of portal vein (K75.1)

✓4ᵗʰ **I82**   **Other venous embolism and thrombosis**
Code first venous embolism and thrombosis complicating:
   abortion, ectopic or molar pregnancy (O00-O07, O08.7)
   pregnancy, childbirth and the puerperium (O22.-, O87.-)
   EXCLUDES 2   *venous embolism and thrombosis (of):*
          cerebral (I63.6, I67.6)
          coronary (I21-I25)
          intracranial and intraspinal, septic or NOS (G08)
          intracranial, nonpyogenic (I67.6)
          intraspinal, nonpyogenic (G95.1)
          mesenteric (K55.0)
          portal (I81)
          pulmonary (I26.-)

   I82.0   **Budd-Chiari syndrome**
     Hepatic vein thrombosis

   I82.1   **Thrombophlebitis migrans**

✓5ᵗʰ **I82.2**   **Embolism and thrombosis of** vena cava and other thoracic **veins**

    ✓6ᵗʰ **I82.21**   **Embolism and thrombosis of** superior vena cava

     I82.210   **Acute embolism and thrombosis of superior vena cava**
          Embolism and thrombosis of superior vena cava NOS

     I82.211   **Chronic embolism and thrombosis of superior vena cava**

    ✓6ᵗʰ **I82.22**   **Embolism and thrombosis of** inferior vena cava

     I82.220   **Acute embolism and thrombosis of inferior vena cava**
          Embolism and thrombosis of inferior vena cava NOS

     I82.221   **Chronic embolism and thrombosis of inferior vena cava**

    ✓6ᵗʰ **I82.29**   **Embolism and thrombosis of** other thoracic veins
     Embolism and thrombosis of brachiocephalic (innominate) vein

     I82.290   **Acute embolism and thrombosis of other thoracic veins**

     I82.291   **Chronic embolism and thrombosis of other thoracic veins**

   I82.3   **Embolism and thrombosis of** renal vein

✓5ᵗʰ **I82.4**   **Acute embolism and thrombosis of deep veins of lower extremity**

    ✓6ᵗʰ **I82.40**   **Acute embolism and thrombosis of unspecified deep veins of lower extremity**
     Deep vein thrombosis NOS
     DVT NOS
     EXCLUDES 1   *acute embolism and thrombosis of unspecified deep veins of distal lower extremity (I82.4Z-)*
          acute embolism and thrombosis of unspecified deep veins of proximal lower extremity (I82.4Y-)

     I82.401   **Acute embolism and thrombosis of unspecified deep veins of** right **lower extremity**

     I82.402   **Acute embolism and thrombosis of unspecified deep veins of** left **lower extremity**

     I82.403   **Acute embolism and thrombosis of unspecified deep veins of lower extremity, bilateral**

     I82.409   **Acute embolism and thrombosis of unspecified deep veins of unspecified lower extremity**

    ✓6ᵗʰ **I82.41**   **Acute embolism and thrombosis of** femoral vein

     I82.411   **Acute embolism and thrombosis of** right **femoral vein**

     I82.412   **Acute embolism and thrombosis of** left **femoral vein**

     I82.413   **Acute embolism and thrombosis of femoral vein,** bilateral

     I82.419   **Acute embolism and thrombosis of unspecified femoral vein**

    ✓6ᵗʰ **I82.42**   **Acute embolism and thrombosis of** iliac vein

     I82.421   **Acute embolism and thrombosis of** right **iliac vein**

     I82.422   **Acute embolism and thrombosis of** left **iliac vein**

     I82.423   **Acute embolism and thrombosis of iliac vein,** bilateral

     I82.429   **Acute embolism and thrombosis of unspecified iliac vein**

    ✓6ᵗʰ **I82.43**   **Acute embolism and thrombosis of** popliteal vein

     I82.431   **Acute embolism and thrombosis of** right **popliteal vein**

     I82.432   **Acute embolism and thrombosis of** left **popliteal vein**

     I82.433   **Acute embolism and thrombosis of popliteal vein,** bilateral

     I82.439   **Acute embolism and thrombosis of unspecified popliteal vein**

    ✓6ᵗʰ **I82.44**   **Acute embolism and thrombosis of** tibial vein

     I82.441   **Acute embolism and thrombosis of** right **tibial vein**

     I82.442   **Acute embolism and thrombosis of** left **tibial vein**

     I82.443   **Acute embolism and thrombosis of tibial vein,** bilateral

     I82.449   **Acute embolism and thrombosis of unspecified tibial vein**

    ✓6ᵗʰ **I82.49**   **Acute embolism and thrombosis of** other specified deep vein of lower extremity

     I82.491   **Acute embolism and thrombosis of other specified deep vein of** right **lower extremity**

     I82.492   **Acute embolism and thrombosis of other specified deep vein of** left **lower extremity**

     I82.493   **Acute embolism and thrombosis of other specified deep vein of lower extremity, bilateral**

     I82.499   **Acute embolism and thrombosis of other specified deep vein of unspecified lower extremity**

EXCLUDES 1 Not coded here   EXCLUDES 2 Not included here   N Newborn Age: 0   P Pediatric Age: 0-17   M Maternity Age: 12-55   A Adult Age: 15-124

610   ICD-10-CM 2016

√6ᵗʰ **I82.4Y** **Acute embolism and thrombosis of unspecified deep veins of proximal lower extremity**
Acute embolism and thrombosis of deep vein of thigh NOS
Acute embolism and thrombosis of deep vein of upper leg NOS

  I82.4Y1 **Acute embolism and thrombosis of unspecified deep veins of right proximal lower extremity**

  I82.4Y2 **Acute embolism and thrombosis of unspecified deep veins of left proximal lower extremity**

  I82.4Y3 **Acute embolism and thrombosis of unspecified deep veins of proximal lower extremity, bilateral**

  I82.4Y9 **Acute embolism and thrombosis of unspecified deep veins of unspecified proximal lower extremity**

√6ᵗʰ **I82.4Z** **Acute embolism and thrombosis of unspecified deep veins of distal lower extremity**
Acute embolism and thrombosis of deep vein of calf NOS
Acute embolism and thrombosis of deep vein of lower leg NOS

  I82.4Z1 **Acute embolism and thrombosis of unspecified deep veins of right distal lower extremity**

  I82.4Z2 **Acute embolism and thrombosis of unspecified deep veins of left distal lower extremity**

  I82.4Z3 **Acute embolism and thrombosis of unspecified deep veins of distal lower extremity, bilateral**

  I82.4Z9 **Acute embolism and thrombosis of unspecified deep veins of unspecified distal lower extremity**

√5ᵗʰ **I82.5** **Chronic embolism and thrombosis of deep veins of lower extremity**
Use additional code, if applicable, for associated long-term (current) use of anticoagulants (Z79.01)
EXCLUDES 1 personal history of venous embolism and thrombosis (Z86.718)

√6ᵗʰ **I82.50** **Chronic embolism and thrombosis of unspecified deep veins of lower extremity**
EXCLUDES 1 chronic embolism and thrombosis of unspecified deep veins of distal lower extremity (I82.5Z-)
chronic embolism and thrombosis of unspecified deep veins of proximal lower extremity (I82.5Y-)

  I82.501 **Chronic embolism and thrombosis of unspecified deep veins of right lower extremity**

  I82.502 **Chronic embolism and thrombosis of unspecified deep veins of left lower extremity**

  I82.503 **Chronic embolism and thrombosis of unspecified deep veins of lower extremity, bilateral**

  I82.509 **Chronic embolism and thrombosis of unspecified deep veins of unspecified lower extremity**

√6ᵗʰ **I82.51** **Chronic embolism and thrombosis of femoral vein**

  I82.511 **Chronic embolism and thrombosis of right femoral vein**

  I82.512 **Chronic embolism and thrombosis of left femoral vein**

  I82.513 **Chronic embolism and thrombosis of femoral vein, bilateral**

  I82.519 **Chronic embolism and thrombosis of unspecified femoral vein**

√6ᵗʰ **I82.52** **Chronic embolism and thrombosis of iliac vein**

  I82.521 **Chronic embolism and thrombosis of right iliac vein**

  I82.522 **Chronic embolism and thrombosis of left iliac vein**

  I82.523 **Chronic embolism and thrombosis of iliac vein, bilateral**

  I82.529 **Chronic embolism and thrombosis of unspecified iliac vein**

√6ᵗʰ **I82.53** **Chronic embolism and thrombosis of popliteal vein**

  I82.531 **Chronic embolism and thrombosis of right popliteal vein**

  I82.532 **Chronic embolism and thrombosis of left popliteal vein**

  I82.533 **Chronic embolism and thrombosis of popliteal vein, bilateral**

  I82.539 **Chronic embolism and thrombosis of unspecified popliteal vein**

√6ᵗʰ **I82.54** **Chronic embolism and thrombosis of tibial vein**

  I82.541 **Chronic embolism and thrombosis of right tibial vein**

  I82.542 **Chronic embolism and thrombosis of left tibial vein**

  I82.543 **Chronic embolism and thrombosis of tibial vein, bilateral**

  I82.549 **Chronic embolism and thrombosis of unspecified tibial vein**

√6ᵗʰ **I82.59** **Chronic embolism and thrombosis of other specified deep vein of lower extremity**

  I82.591 **Chronic embolism and thrombosis of other specified deep vein of right lower extremity**

  I82.592 **Chronic embolism and thrombosis of other specified deep vein of left lower extremity**

  I82.593 **Chronic embolism and thrombosis of other specified deep vein of lower extremity, bilateral**

  I82.599 **Chronic embolism and thrombosis of other specified deep vein of unspecified lower extremity**

√6ᵗʰ **I82.5Y** **Chronic embolism and thrombosis of unspecified deep veins of proximal lower extremity**
Chronic embolism and thrombosis of deep veins of thigh NOS
Chronic embolism and thrombosis of deep veins of upper leg NOS

  I82.5Y1 **Chronic embolism and thrombosis of unspecified deep veins of right proximal lower extremity**

  I82.5Y2 **Chronic embolism and thrombosis of unspecified deep veins of left proximal lower extremity**

  I82.5Y3 **Chronic embolism and thrombosis of unspecified deep veins of proximal lower extremity, bilateral**

  I82.5Y9 **Chronic embolism and thrombosis of unspecified deep veins of unspecified proximal lower extremity**

√6ᵗʰ **I82.5Z** **Chronic embolism and thrombosis of unspecified deep veins of distal lower extremity**
Chronic embolism and thrombosis of deep veins of calf NOS
Chronic embolism and thrombosis of deep veins of lower leg NOS

  I82.5Z1 **Chronic embolism and thrombosis of unspecified deep veins of right distal lower extremity**

  I82.5Z2 **Chronic embolism and thrombosis of unspecified deep veins of left distal lower extremity**

  I82.5Z3 **Chronic embolism and thrombosis of unspecified deep veins of distal lower extremity, bilateral**

  I82.5Z9 **Chronic embolism and thrombosis of unspecified deep veins of unspecified distal lower extremity**

√5ᵗʰ **I82.6** **Acute embolism and thrombosis of veins of upper extremity**

√6ᵗʰ **I82.60** **Acute embolism and thrombosis of unspecified veins of upper extremity**

  I82.601 **Acute embolism and thrombosis of unspecified veins of right upper extremity**

  I82.602 **Acute embolism and thrombosis of unspecified veins of left upper extremity**

  I82.603 **Acute embolism and thrombosis of unspecified veins of upper extremity, bilateral**

☑ Additional Character Required   √ₓ7ᵗʰ Placeholder Alert   Unspecified Dx   Other Specified Dx   Manifestation   ►◄ Revised Text   ● New Code   ▲ Revised Code Title

ICD-10-CM 2016   611

I82.609   **Acute embolism and thrombosis of unspecified veins of unspecified upper extremity**

√6ᵗʰ I82.61   **Acute embolism and thrombosis of superficial veins of upper extremity**
Acute embolism and thrombosis of antecubital vein
Acute embolism and thrombosis of basilic vein
Acute embolism and thrombosis of cephalic vein

I82.611   **Acute embolism and thrombosis of superficial veins of right upper extremity**

I82.612   **Acute embolism and thrombosis of superficial veins of left upper extremity**

I82.613   **Acute embolism and thrombosis of superficial veins of upper extremity, bilateral**

I82.619   **Acute embolism and thrombosis of superficial veins of unspecified upper extremity**

√6ᵗʰ I82.62   **Acute embolism and thrombosis of deep veins of upper extremity**
Acute embolism and thrombosis of brachial vein
Acute embolism and thrombosis of radial vein
Acute embolism and thrombosis of ulnar vein

I82.621   **Acute embolism and thrombosis of deep veins of right upper extremity**

I82.622   **Acute embolism and thrombosis of deep veins of left upper extremity**

I82.623   **Acute embolism and thrombosis of deep veins of upper extremity, bilateral**

I82.629   **Acute embolism and thrombosis of deep veins of unspecified upper extremity**

√5ᵗʰ I82.7   **Chronic embolism and thrombosis of veins of upper extremity**
Use additional code, if applicable, for associated long-term (current) use of anticoagulants (Z79.01)
EXCLUDES 1   personal history of venous embolism and thrombosis (Z86.718)

√6ᵗʰ I82.70   **Chronic embolism and thrombosis of unspecified veins of upper extremity**

I82.701   **Chronic embolism and thrombosis of unspecified veins of right upper extremity**

I82.702   **Chronic embolism and thrombosis of unspecified veins of left upper extremity**

I82.703   **Chronic embolism and thrombosis of unspecified veins of upper extremity, bilateral**

I82.709   **Chronic embolism and thrombosis of unspecified veins of unspecified upper extremity**

√6ᵗʰ I82.71   **Chronic embolism and thrombosis of superficial veins of upper extremity**
Chronic embolism and thrombosis of antecubital vein
Chronic embolism and thrombosis of basilic vein
Chronic embolism and thrombosis of cephalic vein

I82.711   **Chronic embolism and thrombosis of superficial veins of right upper extremity**

I82.712   **Chronic embolism and thrombosis of superficial veins of left upper extremity**

I82.713   **Chronic embolism and thrombosis of superficial veins of upper extremity, bilateral**

I82.719   **Chronic embolism and thrombosis of superficial veins of unspecified upper extremity**

√6ᵗʰ I82.72   **Chronic embolism and thrombosis of deep veins of upper extremity**
Chronic embolism and thrombosis of brachial vein
Chronic embolism and thrombosis of radial vein
Chronic embolism and thrombosis of ulnar vein

I82.721   **Chronic embolism and thrombosis of deep veins of right upper extremity**

I82.722   **Chronic embolism and thrombosis of deep veins of left upper extremity**

I82.723   **Chronic embolism and thrombosis of deep veins of upper extremity, bilateral**

I82.729   **Chronic embolism and thrombosis of deep veins of unspecified upper extremity**

√5ᵗʰ I82.A   **Embolism and thrombosis of axillary vein**

√6ᵗʰ I82.A1   **Acute embolism and thrombosis of axillary vein**

I82.A11   **Acute embolism and thrombosis of right axillary vein**

I82.A12   **Acute embolism and thrombosis of left axillary vein**

I82.A13   **Acute embolism and thrombosis of axillary vein, bilateral**

I82.A19   **Acute embolism and thrombosis of unspecified axillary vein**

√6ᵗʰ I82.A2   **Chronic embolism and thrombosis of axillary vein**

I82.A21   **Chronic embolism and thrombosis of right axillary vein**

I82.A22   **Chronic embolism and thrombosis of left axillary vein**

I82.A23   **Chronic embolism and thrombosis of axillary vein, bilateral**

I82.A29   **Chronic embolism and thrombosis of unspecified axillary vein**

√5ᵗʰ I82.B   **Embolism and thrombosis of subclavian vein**

√6ᵗʰ I82.B1   **Acute embolism and thrombosis of subclavian vein**

I82.B11   **Acute embolism and thrombosis of right subclavian vein**

I82.B12   **Acute embolism and thrombosis of left subclavian vein**

I82.B13   **Acute embolism and thrombosis of subclavian vein, bilateral**

I82.B19   **Acute embolism and thrombosis of unspecified subclavian vein**

√6ᵗʰ I82.B2   **Chronic embolism and thrombosis of subclavian vein**

I82.B21   **Chronic embolism and thrombosis of right subclavian vein**

I82.B22   **Chronic embolism and thrombosis of left subclavian vein**

I82.B23   **Chronic embolism and thrombosis of subclavian vein, bilateral**

I82.B29   **Chronic embolism and thrombosis of unspecified subclavian vein**

√5ᵗʰ I82.C   **Embolism and thrombosis of internal jugular vein**

√6ᵗʰ I82.C1   **Acute embolism and thrombosis of internal jugular vein**

I82.C11   **Acute embolism and thrombosis of right internal jugular vein**

I82.C12   **Acute embolism and thrombosis of left internal jugular vein**

I82.C13   **Acute embolism and thrombosis of internal jugular vein, bilateral**

I82.C19   **Acute embolism and thrombosis of unspecified internal jugular vein**

√6ᵗʰ I82.C2   **Chronic embolism and thrombosis of internal jugular vein**

I82.C21   **Chronic embolism and thrombosis of right internal jugular vein**

I82.C22   **Chronic embolism and thrombosis of left internal jugular vein**

I82.C23   **Chronic embolism and thrombosis of internal jugular vein, bilateral**

I82.C29   **Chronic embolism and thrombosis of unspecified internal jugular vein**

√5ᵗʰ I82.8   **Embolism and thrombosis of other specified veins**
Use additional code, if applicable, for associated long-term (current) use of anticoagulants (Z79.01)

√6ᵗʰ I82.81   **Embolism and thrombosis of superficial veins of lower extremities**
Embolism and thrombosis of saphenous vein (greater) (lesser)

I82.811   **Embolism and thrombosis of superficial veins of right lower extremities**

I82.812   **Embolism and thrombosis of superficial veins of left lower extremities**

I82.813   **Embolism and thrombosis of superficial veins of lower extremities, bilateral**

I82.819   **Embolism and thrombosis of superficial veins of unspecified lower extremities**

√6ᵗʰ I82.89   **Embolism and thrombosis of other specified veins**

I82.890   **Acute embolism and thrombosis of other specified veins**

I82.891   **Chronic embolism and thrombosis of other specified veins**

EXCLUDES 1 Not coded here   EXCLUDES 2 Not included here   N Newborn Age: 0   P Pediatric Age: 0-17   M Maternity Age: 12-55   A Adult Age: 15-124

612   ICD-10-CM 2016

✓5ᵗʰ I82.9   Embolism and thrombosis of unspecified **vein**

     I82.90   Acute embolism and thrombosis of unspecified vein
         Embolism of vein NOS
         Thrombosis (vein) NOS

     I82.91   Chronic embolism and thrombosis of unspecified vein

✓4ᵗʰ I83   Varicose veins of lower extremities
     EXCLUDES 1   *varicose veins complicating pregnancy (O22.0-)*
                   varicose veins complicating the puerperium (O87.4)

✓5ᵗʰ I83.0   Varicose veins of lower extremities with ulcer
     Use additional code to identify severity of ulcer (L97.-)

     ✓6ᵗʰ I83.00   Varicose veins of unspecified **lower extremity with ulcer**

         I83.001   Varicose veins of unspecified lower extremity with ulcer of thigh

         I83.002   Varicose veins of unspecified lower extremity with ulcer of calf

         I83.003   Varicose veins of unspecified lower extremity with ulcer of ankle

         I83.004   Varicose veins of unspecified lower extremity with ulcer of heel and midfoot
             Varicose veins of unspecified lower extremity with ulcer of plantar surface of midfoot

         I83.005   Varicose veins of unspecified lower extremity with ulcer other part of foot
             Varicose veins of unspecified lower extremity with ulcer of toe

         I83.008   Varicose veins of unspecified lower extremity with ulcer other part of lower leg

         I83.009   Varicose veins of unspecified lower extremity with ulcer of unspecified site

     ✓6ᵗʰ I83.01   Varicose veins of right **lower extremity with ulcer**

         I83.011   Varicose veins of right lower extremity with ulcer of thigh

         I83.012   Varicose veins of right lower extremity with ulcer of calf

         I83.013   Varicose veins of right lower extremity with ulcer of ankle

         I83.014   Varicose veins of right lower extremity with ulcer of heel and midfoot
             Varicose veins of right lower extremity with ulcer of plantar surface of midfoot

         I83.015   Varicose veins of right lower extremity with ulcer other part of foot
             Varicose veins of right lower extremity with ulcer of toe

         I83.018   Varicose veins of right lower extremity with ulcer other part of lower leg

         I83.019   Varicose veins of right lower extremity with ulcer of unspecified site

     ✓6ᵗʰ I83.02   Varicose veins of left **lower extremity with ulcer**

         I83.021   Varicose veins of left lower extremity with ulcer of thigh

         I83.022   Varicose veins of left lower extremity with ulcer of calf

         I83.023   Varicose veins of left lower extremity with ulcer of ankle

         I83.024   Varicose veins of left lower extremity with ulcer of heel and midfoot
             Varicose veins of left lower extremity with ulcer of plantar surface of midfoot

         I83.025   Varicose veins of left lower extremity with ulcer other part of foot
             Varicose veins of left lower extremity with ulcer of toe

         I83.028   Varicose veins of left lower extremity with ulcer other part of lower leg

         I83.029   Varicose veins of left lower extremity with ulcer of unspecified site

✓5ᵗʰ I83.1   Varicose veins of lower extremities with inflammation
     Stasis dermatitis

     I83.10   Varicose veins of unspecified lower extremity with inflammation

     I83.11   Varicose veins of right **lower extremity with inflammation**

     I83.12   Varicose veins of left **lower extremity with inflammation**

✓5ᵗʰ I83.2   Varicose veins of lower extremities with both ulcer and inflammation
     Use additional code to identify severity of ulcer (L97.-)

     ✓6ᵗʰ I83.20   Varicose veins of unspecified **lower extremity with both ulcer and inflammation**

         I83.201   Varicose veins of unspecified lower extremity with both ulcer of thigh **and inflammation**

         I83.202   Varicose veins of unspecified lower extremity with both ulcer of calf **and inflammation**

         I83.203   Varicose veins of unspecified lower extremity with both ulcer of ankle **and inflammation**

         I83.204   Varicose veins of unspecified lower extremity with both ulcer of heel and midfoot **and inflammation**
             Varicose veins of unspecified lower extremity with both ulcer of plantar surface of midfoot and inflammation

         I83.205   Varicose veins of unspecified lower extremity with both ulcer of other part of foot **and inflammation**
             Varicose veins of unspecified lower extremity with both ulcer of toe and inflammation

         I83.208   Varicose veins of unspecified lower extremity with both ulcer of other part of lower extremity **and inflammation**

         I83.209   Varicose veins of unspecified lower extremity with both ulcer of unspecified site and inflammation

     ✓6ᵗʰ I83.21   Varicose veins of right **lower extremity with both ulcer and inflammation**

         I83.211   Varicose veins of right lower extremity with both ulcer of thigh **and inflammation**

         I83.212   Varicose veins of right lower extremity with both ulcer of calf **and inflammation**

         I83.213   Varicose veins of right lower extremity with both ulcer of ankle **and inflammation**

         I83.214   Varicose veins of right lower extremity with both ulcer of heel and midfoot **and inflammation**
             Varicose veins of right lower extremity with both ulcer of plantar surface of midfoot and inflammation

         I83.215   Varicose veins of right lower extremity with both ulcer other part of foot **and inflammation**
             Varicose veins of right lower extremity with both ulcer of toe and inflammation

         I83.218   Varicose veins of right lower extremity with both ulcer of other part of lower extremity **and inflammation**

         I83.219   Varicose veins of right lower extremity with both ulcer of unspecified site and inflammation

     ✓6ᵗʰ I83.22   Varicose veins of left **lower extremity with both ulcer and inflammation**

         I83.221   Varicose veins of left lower extremity with both ulcer of thigh **and inflammation**

         I83.222   Varicose veins of left lower extremity with both ulcer of calf **and inflammation**

         I83.223   Varicose veins of left lower extremity with both ulcer of ankle **and inflammation**

         I83.224   Varicose veins of left lower extremity with both ulcer of heel and midfoot **and inflammation**
             Varicose veins of left lower extremity with both ulcer of plantar surface of midfoot and inflammation

         I83.225   Varicose veins of left lower extremity with both ulcer other part of foot **and inflammation**
             Varicose veins of left lower extremity with both ulcer of toe and inflammation

         I83.228   Varicose veins of left lower extremity with both ulcer of other part of lower extremity **and inflammation**

         I83.229   Varicose veins of left lower extremity with both ulcer of unspecified site and inflammation

---

☑ Additional Character Required   ✓x7ᵗʰ Placeholder Alert   Unspecified Dx   Other Specified Dx   Manifestation   ▶◀ Revised Text   ● New Code   ▲ Revised Code Title

✓5ᵗʰ **I83.8 Varicose veins of lower extremities with** other complications

  ✓6ᵗʰ **I83.81 Varicose veins of lower extremities with** pain

    I83.811 Varicose veins of right lower extremities with pain   🄰

    I83.812 Varicose veins of left lower extremities with pain   🄰

    I83.813 Varicose veins of bilateral lower extremities with pain   🄰

    I83.819 Varicose veins of unspecified lower extremities with pain   🄰

  ✓6ᵗʰ **I83.89 Varicose veins of lower extremities with** other complications

    Varicose veins of lower extremities with edema
    Varicose veins of lower extremities with swelling

    I83.891 Varicose veins of right lower extremities with other complications   🄰

    I83.892 Varicose veins of left lower extremities with other complications   🄰

    I83.893 Varicose veins of bilateral lower extremities with other complications   🄰

    I83.899 Varicose veins of unspecified lower extremities with other complications   🄰

✓5ᵗʰ **I83.9 Asymptomatic varicose veins of lower extremities**

  Phlebectasia of lower extremities
  Varicose veins of lower extremities
  Varix of lower extremities

  I83.90 Asymptomatic varicose veins of unspecified lower extremity   🄰

    Varicose veins NOS

  I83.91 Asymptomatic varicose veins of right lower extremity   🄰

  I83.92 Asymptomatic varicose veins of left lower extremity   🄰

  I83.93 Asymptomatic varicose veins of bilateral lower extremities   🄰

✓4ᵗʰ **I85 Esophageal varices**

  Use additional code to identify:
  alcohol abuse and dependence (F1Ø.-)

  ✓5ᵗʰ **I85.Ø Esophageal varices**

    Idiopathic esophageal varices
    Primary esophageal varices

    I85.ØØ Esophageal varices without bleeding
      Esophageal varices NOS

    I85.Ø1 Esophageal varices with bleeding

  ✓5ᵗʰ **I85.1 Secondary esophageal varices**

    Esophageal varices secondary to alcoholic liver disease
    Esophageal varices secondary to cirrhosis of liver
    Esophageal varices secondary to schistosomiasis
    Esophageal varices secondary to toxic liver disease
    Code first underlying disease

    I85.1Ø Secondary esophageal varices without bleeding

    I85.11 Secondary esophageal varices with bleeding

✓4ᵗʰ **I86 Varicose veins of other sites**

  EXCLUDES 1   varicose veins of unspecified site (I83.9-)
  EXCLUDES 2   retinal varices (H35.Ø-)

  I86.Ø Sublingual varices

  I86.1 Scrotal varices   ♂
    Varicocele

  I86.2 Pelvic varices

  I86.3 Vulval varices   🄰♀
    EXCLUDES 1   vulval varices complicating childbirth and the puerperium (O87.8)
       vulval varices complicating pregnancy (O22.1-)

  I86.4 Gastric varices

  I86.8 Varicose veins of other specified sites   🄰
    Varicose ulcer of nasal septum

✓4ᵗʰ **I87 Other disorders of veins**

  ✓5ᵗʰ **I87.Ø Postthrombotic syndrome**
    Chronic venous hypertension due to deep vein thrombosis
    Postphlebitic syndrome
    EXCLUDES 1   chronic venous hypertension without deep vein thrombosis (I87.3-)

    ✓6ᵗʰ **I87.ØØ Postthrombotic syndrome** without complications
      Asymptomatic postthrombotic syndrome

      I87.ØØ1 Postthrombotic syndrome without complications of right lower **extremity**

      I87.ØØ2 Postthrombotic syndrome without complications of left lower **extremity**

      I87.ØØ3 Postthrombotic syndrome without complications of bilateral lower **extremity**

      I87.ØØ9 Postthrombotic syndrome without complications of unspecified extremity
        Postthrombotic syndrome NOS

    ✓6ᵗʰ **I87.Ø1 Postthrombotic syndrome with** ulcer
      Use additional code to specify site and severity of ulcer (L97.-)

      I87.Ø11 Postthrombotic syndrome with ulcer of right lower **extremity**

      I87.Ø12 Postthrombotic syndrome with ulcer of left lower **extremity**

      I87.Ø13 Postthrombotic syndrome with ulcer of bilateral lower **extremity**

      I87.Ø19 Postthrombotic syndrome with ulcer of unspecified lower extremity

    ✓6ᵗʰ **I87.Ø2 Postthrombotic syndrome with** inflammation

      I87.Ø21 Postthrombotic syndrome with inflammation of right lower **extremity**

      I87.Ø22 Postthrombotic syndrome with inflammation of left lower **extremity**

      I87.Ø23 Postthrombotic syndrome with inflammation of bilateral lower **extremity**

      I87.Ø29 Postthrombotic syndrome with inflammation of unspecified lower extremity

    ✓6ᵗʰ **I87.Ø3 Postthrombotic syndrome with** ulcer and inflammation
      Use additional code to specify site and severity of ulcer (L97.-)

      I87.Ø31 Postthrombotic syndrome with ulcer and inflammation of right lower **extremity**

      I87.Ø32 Postthrombotic syndrome with ulcer and inflammation of left lower **extremity**

      I87.Ø33 Postthrombotic syndrome with ulcer and inflammation of bilateral lower **extremity**

      I87.Ø39 Postthrombotic syndrome with ulcer and inflammation of unspecified lower extremity

    ✓6ᵗʰ **I87.Ø9 Postthrombotic syndrome with** other complications

      I87.Ø91 Postthrombotic syndrome with other complications of right lower **extremity**

      I87.Ø92 Postthrombotic syndrome with other complications of left lower **extremity**

      I87.Ø93 Postthrombotic syndrome with other complications of bilateral lower **extremity**

      I87.Ø99 Postthrombotic syndrome with other complications of unspecified lower extremity

  I87.1 Compression of vein
    Stricture of vein
    Vena cava syndrome (inferior) (superior)
    EXCLUDES 2   compression of pulmonary vein (I28.8)

  I87.2 Venous insufficiency (chronic) (peripheral)

  ✓5ᵗʰ **I87.3 Chronic venous hypertension (idiopathic)**
    Stasis edema
    EXCLUDES 1   chronic venous hypertension due to deep vein thrombosis (I87.Ø-)
       varicose veins of lower extremities (I83.-)

    ✓6ᵗʰ **I87.3Ø Chronic venous hypertension (idiopathic)** without complications
      Asymptomatic chronic venous hypertension (idiopathic)

      I87.3Ø1 Chronic venous hypertension (idiopathic) without complications of right lower **extremity**

      I87.3Ø2 Chronic venous hypertension (idiopathic) without complications of left lower **extremity**

      I87.3Ø3 Chronic venous hypertension (idiopathic) without complications of bilateral lower **extremity**

      I87.3Ø9 Chronic venous hypertension (idiopathic) without complications of unspecified lower extremity
        Chronic venous hypertension NOS

EXCLUDES 1 Not coded here   EXCLUDES 2 Not included here   🅽 Newborn Age: 0   🅿 Pediatric Age: 0-17   🅼 Maternity Age: 12-55   🄰 Adult Age: 15-124

☑6ᵗʰ **I87.31   Chronic venous hypertension (idiopathic) with ulcer**
Use additional code to specify site and severity of ulcer (L97.-)

     I87.311   Chronic venous hypertension (idiopathic) with ulcer of right lower extremity

     I87.312   Chronic venous hypertension (idiopathic) with ulcer of left lower extremity

     I87.313   Chronic venous hypertension (idiopathic) with ulcer of bilateral lower extremity

     I87.319   Chronic venous hypertension (idiopathic) with ulcer of unspecified lower extremity

☑6ᵗʰ **I87.32   Chronic venous hypertension (idiopathic) with inflammation**

     I87.321   Chronic venous hypertension (idiopathic) with inflammation of right lower extremity

     I87.322   Chronic venous hypertension (idiopathic) with inflammation of left lower extremity

     I87.323   Chronic venous hypertension (idiopathic) with inflammation of bilateral lower extremity

     I87.329   Chronic venous hypertension (idiopathic) with inflammation of unspecified lower extremity

☑6ᵗʰ **I87.33   Chronic venous hypertension (idiopathic) with ulcer and inflammation**
Use additional code to specify site and severity of ulcer (L97.-)

     I87.331   Chronic venous hypertension (idiopathic) with ulcer and inflammation of right lower extremity

     I87.332   Chronic venous hypertension (idiopathic) with ulcer and inflammation of left lower extremity

     I87.333   Chronic venous hypertension (idiopathic) with ulcer and inflammation of bilateral lower extremity

     I87.339   Chronic venous hypertension (idiopathic) with ulcer and inflammation of unspecified lower extremity

☑6ᵗʰ **I87.39   Chronic venous hypertension (idiopathic) with other complications**

     I87.391   Chronic venous hypertension (idiopathic) with other complications of right lower extremity

     I87.392   Chronic venous hypertension (idiopathic) with other complications of left lower extremity

     I87.393   Chronic venous hypertension (idiopathic) with other complications of bilateral lower extremity

     I87.399   Chronic venous hypertension (idiopathic) with other complications of unspecified lower extremity

I87.8   Other specified disorders of veins
Phlebosclerosis
Venofibrosis

I87.9   Disorder of vein, unspecified

☑4ᵗʰ **I88   Nonspecific lymphadenitis**
EXCLUDES 1   acute lymphadenitis, except mesenteric (L04.-)
enlarged lymph nodes NOS (R59.-)
human immunodeficiency virus [HIV] disease resulting in generalized lymphadenopathy (B20)

I88.0   Nonspecific mesenteric lymphadenitis
Mesenteric lymphadenitis (acute)(chronic)

I88.1   Chronic lymphadenitis, except mesenteric
Adenitis
Lymphadenitis

I88.8   Other nonspecific lymphadenitis

I88.9   Nonspecific lymphadenitis, unspecified
Lymphadenitis NOS

☑4ᵗʰ **I89   Other noninfective disorders of lymphatic vessels and lymph nodes**
EXCLUDES 1   chylocele, tunica vaginalis (nonfilarial) NOS (N50.8)
enlarged lymph nodes NOS (R59.-)
filarial chylocele (B74.-)
hereditary lymphedema (Q82.0)

I89.0   Lymphedema, not elsewhere classified
Elephantiasis (nonfilarial) NOS
Lymphangiectasis
Obliteration, lymphatic vessel
Praecox lymphedema
Secondary lymphedema
EXCLUDES 1   postmastectomy lymphedema (I97.2)

I89.1   Lymphangitis
Chronic lymphangitis
Lymphangitis NOS
Subacute lymphangitis
EXCLUDES 1   acute lymphangitis (L03.-)

I89.8   Other specified noninfective disorders of lymphatic vessels and lymph nodes
Chylocele (nonfilarial)
Chylous ascites
Chylous cyst
Lipomelanotic reticulosis
Lymph node or vessel fistula
Lymph node or vessel infarction
Lymph node or vessel rupture

I89.9   Noninfective disorder of lymphatic vessels and lymph nodes, unspecified
Disease of lymphatic vessels NOS

Other and unspecified disorders of the circulatory system (I95-I99)

☑4ᵗʰ **I95   Hypotension**
EXCLUDES 1   cardiovascular collapse (R57.9)
maternal hypotension syndrome (O26.5-)
nonspecific low blood pressure reading NOS (R03.1)

I95.0   Idiopathic hypotension

I95.1   Orthostatic hypotension
Hypotension, postural
EXCLUDES 1   neurogenic orthostatic hypotension [Shy-Drager] (G90.3)
orthostatic hypotension due to drugs (I95.2)

I95.2   Hypotension due to drugs
Orthostatic hypotension due to drugs
Use additional code for adverse effect, if applicable, to identify drug (T36-T50 with fifth or sixth character 5)

I95.3   Hypotension of hemodialysis
Intra-dialytic hypotension

☑5ᵗʰ **I95.8   Other hypotension**

     I95.81   Postprocedural hypotension

     I95.89   Other hypotension
Chronic hypotension

I95.9   Hypotension, unspecified

I96   Gangrene, not elsewhere classified
Gangrenous cellulitis
EXCLUDES 1   gangrene in atherosclerosis of native arteries of the extremities (I70.26)
gangrene in diabetes mellitus (E08-E13)
gangrene in hernia (K40.1, K40.4, K41.1, K41.4, K42.1, K43.1-, K44.1, K45.1, K46.1)
gangrene in other peripheral vascular diseases (I73.-)
gangrene of certain specified sites—see Alphabetical Index
gas gangrene (A48.0)
pyoderma gangrenosum (L88)
AHA: 2013, 2Q, 34

☑4ᵗʰ **I97   Intraoperative and postprocedural complications and disorders of circulatory system, not elsewhere classified**
EXCLUDES 2   postprocedural shock (T81.1-)

I97.0   Postcardiotomy syndrome

☑5ᵗʰ **I97.1   Other postprocedural cardiac functional disturbances**
EXCLUDES 2   acute pulmonary insufficiency following thoracic surgery (J95.1)
intraoperative cardiac functional disturbances (I97.7-)

     ☑6ᵗʰ **I97.11   Postprocedural cardiac insufficiency**

         I97.110   Postprocedural cardiac insufficiency following cardiac surgery

         I97.111   Postprocedural cardiac insufficiency following other surgery

☑ Additional Character Required   ☑x7ᵗʰ Placeholder Alert   Unspecified Dx   Other Specified Dx   Manifestation   ►◄ Revised Text   ● New Code   ▲ Revised Code Title

ICD-10-CM 2016   615

Chapter 9. Diseases of the Circulatory System

I97.12–I99.9

✓6th **I97.12** **Postprocedural** cardiac arrest

    I97.120 **Postprocedural cardiac arrest following cardiac surgery**

    I97.121 **Postprocedural cardiac arrest following other surgery**

✓6th **I97.13** **Postprocedural** heart failure

    Use additional code to identify the heart failure (I50.-)

    I97.130 **Postprocedural heart failure following cardiac surgery**

    I97.131 **Postprocedural heart failure following other surgery**

✓6th **I97.19** **Other postprocedural cardiac** functional disturbances

    Use additional code, if applicable, to further specify disorder

    I97.190 **Other postprocedural cardiac functional disturbances following** cardiac surgery

    I97.191 **Other postprocedural cardiac functional disturbances following** other surgery

I97.2 **Postmastectomy lymphedema syndrome** 🅰

    Elephantiasis due to mastectomy
    Obliteration of lymphatic vessels

I97.3 **Postprocedural hypertension**

✓5th **I97.4** **Intraoperative hemorrhage and hematoma of a circulatory system organ or structure complicating a procedure**

    EXCLUDES 1   intraoperative hemorrhage and hematoma of a circulatory system organ or structure due to accidental puncture and laceration during a procedure (I97.5-)

    EXCLUDES 2   intraoperative cerebrovascular hemorrhage complicating a procedure (G97.3-)

✓6th **I97.41** **Intraoperative hemorrhage and hematoma of a circulatory system organ or structure complicating a circulatory system procedure**

    I97.410 **Intraoperative hemorrhage and hematoma of a circulatory system organ or structure complicating a** cardiac catheterization

    I97.411 **Intraoperative hemorrhage and hematoma of a circulatory system organ or structure complicating a** cardiac bypass

    I97.418 **Intraoperative hemorrhage and hematoma of a circulatory system organ or structure complicating** other circulatory system procedure

I97.42 **Intraoperative hemorrhage and hematoma of a circulatory system organ or structure complicating other procedure**

✓5th **I97.5** **Accidental puncture and laceration of a circulatory system organ or structure during a procedure**

    EXCLUDES 2   accidental puncture and laceration of brain during a procedure (G97.4-)

I97.51 **Accidental puncture and laceration of a circulatory system organ or structure during a** circulatory system procedure

I97.52 **Accidental puncture and laceration of a circulatory system organ or structure during** other procedure

✓5th **I97.6** **Postprocedural hemorrhage and hematoma of a circulatory system organ or structure following a procedure**

    EXCLUDES 2   postprocedural cerebrovascular hemorrhage complicating a procedure (G97.5-)

✓6th **I97.61** **Postprocedural hemorrhage and hematoma of a circulatory system organ or structure following a circulatory system procedure**

    I97.610 **Postprocedural hemorrhage and hematoma of a circulatory system organ or structure following a** cardiac catheterization

    I97.611 **Postprocedural hemorrhage and hematoma of a circulatory system organ or structure following** cardiac bypass

    I97.618 **Postprocedural hemorrhage and hematoma of a circulatory system organ or structure following** other circulatory system procedure

I97.62 **Postprocedural hemorrhage and hematoma of a circulatory system organ or structure following other procedure**

✓5th **I97.7** **Intraoperative** cardiac functional disturbances

    EXCLUDES 2   acute pulmonary insufficiency following thoracic surgery (J95.1)
    postprocedural cardiac functional disturbances (I97.1-)

✓6th **I97.71** **Intraoperative** cardiac arrest

    I97.710 **Intraoperative cardiac arrest during** cardiac surgery

    I97.711 **Intraoperative cardiac arrest during other surgery**

✓6th **I97.79** **Other intraoperative cardiac functional disturbances**

    Use additional code, if applicable, to further specify disorder

    I97.790 **Other intraoperative cardiac functional disturbances during** cardiac surgery

    I97.791 **Other intraoperative cardiac functional disturbances during** other surgery

✓5th **I97.8** **Other intraoperative and postprocedural complications and disorders of the circulatory system, not elsewhere classified**

    Use additional code, if applicable, to further specify disorder

✓6th **I97.81** **Intraoperative** cerebrovascular infarction

    I97.810 **Intraoperative cerebrovascular infarction during** cardiac surgery

    I97.811 **Intraoperative cerebrovascular infarction during** other surgery

✓6th **I97.82** **Postprocedural** cerebrovascular infarction

    I97.820 **Postprocedural cerebrovascular infarction during** cardiac surgery

    I97.821 **Postprocedural cerebrovascular infarction during** other surgery

    I97.88 **Other** intraoperative **complications of the circulatory system, not elsewhere classified**

    I97.89 **Other** postprocedural **complications and disorders of the circulatory system, not elsewhere classified**

✓4th **I99** **Other and unspecified disorders of circulatory system**

    I99.8 **Other disorder of circulatory system**

    I99.9 **Unspecified disorder of circulatory system**

EXCLUDES 1 Not coded here   EXCLUDES 2 Not included here   🅝 Newborn Age: 0   🅟 Pediatric Age: 0-17   🅜 Maternity Age: 12-55   🅐 Adult Age: 15-124

616   ICD-10-CM 2016

Chapter 10. Diseases of the Respiratory System (J00–J99)

Chapter Specific Guidelines with Coding Examples

The chapter specific guidelines from the ICD-10-CM Official Guidelines for Coding and Reporting have been provided below. Along with these guidelines are coding examples, contained in the shaded boxes, that have been developed to help illustrate the coding and/or sequencing guidance found in these guidelines.

a. Chronic obstructive pulmonary disease [COPD] and asthma

1) Acute exacerbation of chronic obstructive bronchitis and asthma

The codes in categories J44 and J45 distinguish between uncomplicated cases and those in acute exacerbation. An acute exacerbation is a worsening or a decompensation of a chronic condition. An acute exacerbation is not equivalent to an infection superimposed on a chronic condition, though an exacerbation may be triggered by an infection.

Acute streptococcal bronchitis with acute exacerbation of COPD

J20.2	**Acute bronchitis due to streptococcus**
J44.0	**Chronic obstructive pulmonary disease with acute lower respiratory infection**
J44.1	**Chronic obstructive pulmonary disease with (acute) exacerbation**

Explanation: ICD-10-CM uses combination codes to create organism-specific classifications for acute bronchitis. Category J44 codes include combination codes with severity components, which differentiate between COPD with acute lower respiratory infection (acute bronchitis), COPD with acute exacerbation, and COPD without mention of a complication (unspecified).

An acute exacerbation is a worsening or a decompensation of a chronic condition. An acute exacerbation is not equivalent to an infection superimposed on a chronic condition, though an exacerbation may be triggered by an infection, as in this example.

Exacerbation of moderate persistent asthma with status asthmaticus

J45.42	**Moderate persistent asthma with status asthmaticus**

Explanation: Category J45 Asthma includes severity-specific subcategories and fifth-character codes to distinguish between uncomplicated cases, those in acute exacerbation, and those with status asthmaticus.

---

b. Acute respiratory failure

1) Acute respiratory failure as principal diagnosis

A code from subcategory J96.0, Acute respiratory failure, or subcategory J96.2, Acute and chronic respiratory failure, may be assigned as a principal diagnosis when it is the condition established after study to be chiefly responsible for occasioning the admission to the hospital, and the selection is supported by the Alphabetic Index and Tabular List. However, chapter-specific coding guidelines (such as obstetrics, poisoning, HIV, newborn) that provide sequencing direction take precedence.

Acute hypoxic respiratory failure due to COPD exacerbation

J96.01	**Acute respiratory failure with hypoxia**
J44.1	**Chronic obstructive pulmonary disease with (acute) exacerbation**

Explanation: Category J96 classifies respiratory failure with combination codes that designate the severity and the presence of hypoxia and hypercapnia. Code J96.01 is sequenced as the first-listed diagnosis, as the reason for the admission. Respiratory failure may be assigned as a principal diagnosis when it is the condition established after study to be chiefly responsible for occasioning the admission to the hospital and the selection is supported by the Alphabetic Index and Tabular List.

---

2) Acute respiratory failure as secondary diagnosis

Respiratory failure may be listed as a secondary diagnosis if it occurs after admission, or if it is present on admission, but does not meet the definition of principal diagnosis.

Acute respiratory failure due to accidental oxycodone overdose

T40.2X1A	**Poisoning by other opioids, accidental (unintentional), initial encounter**
J96.00	**Acute respiratory failure, unspecified whether with hypoxia or hypercapnia**

Explanation: Respiratory failure may be assigned as a principal diagnosis when it is the condition established after study to be chiefly responsible for occasioning the admission to the hospital, and the selection is supported by the Alphabetic Index and Tabular List. However, chapter-specific coding guidelines, such as poisoning, that provide sequencing direction take precedence. When coding a poisoning or reaction to the improper use of a medication (e.g. overdose, wrong substance given or taken in error, wrong route of administration), first assign the appropriate code from categories T36–T50. Use additional code(s) for all manifestations of the poisoning. In this instance, the respiratory failure is a manifestation of the poisoning and is sequenced as a secondary diagnosis.

Acute pneumococcal pneumonia with subsequent development of acute respiratory failure

J13	**Pneumonia due to Streptococcus pneumoniae**
J96.00	**Acute respiratory failure, unspecified whether with hypoxia or hypercapnia**

Explanation: Acute respiratory failure may be listed as a secondary diagnosis if it occurs after admission, or if it is present on admission but does not meet the definition of principal diagnosis.

---

3) Sequencing of acute respiratory failure and another acute condition

When a patient is admitted with respiratory failure and another acute condition, (e.g., myocardial infarction, cerebrovascular accident, aspiration pneumonia), the principal diagnosis will not be the same in every situation. This applies whether the other acute condition is a respiratory or nonrespiratory condition. Selection of the principal diagnosis will be dependent on the circumstances of admission. If both the respiratory failure and the other acute condition are equally responsible for occasioning the admission to the hospital, and there are no chapter-specific sequencing rules, the guideline regarding two or more diagnoses that equally meet the definition for principal diagnosis (Section II, C.) may be applied in these situations.

If the documentation is not clear as to whether acute respiratory failure and another condition are equally responsible for occasioning the admission, query the provider for clarification.

Acute pneumococcal pneumonia and acute respiratory failure, both present on admission

J96.00	**Acute respiratory failure, unspecified whether with hypoxia or hypercapnia**
J13	**Pneumonia due to Streptococcus pneumoniae**

Explanation: When a patient is admitted with respiratory failure and another acute condition, such as a bacterial pneumonia, the principal diagnosis is not the same in every situation. This applies whether the other acute condition is a respiratory or nonrespiratory condition. The principal diagnosis depends on the circumstances of admission.

---

c. Influenza due to certain identified influenza viruses

Code only confirmed cases of influenza due to certain identified influenza viruses (category J09), and due to other identified influenza virus (category J10). This is an exception to the hospital inpatient guideline Section II, H. (Uncertain Diagnosis).

In this context, "confirmation" does not require documentation of positive laboratory testing specific for avian or other novel influenza A or other identified influenza virus. However, coding should be based on the provider's diagnostic statement that the patient has avian influenza, or other novel influenza A, for category J09, or has another particular identified strain of influenza, such as H1N1 or H3N2, but not identified as novel or variant, for category J10.

Chapter 10. Diseases of the Respiratory System

If the provider records "suspected" or "possible" or "probable" avian influenza, or novel influenza, or other identified influenza, then the appropriate influenza code from category J11, Influenza due to unidentified influenza virus, should be assigned. A code from category J09, Influenza due to certain identified influenza viruses, should not be assigned nor should a code from category J10, Influenza due to other identified influenza virus.

Influenza due to avian influenza virus with pneumonia

J09.X1   **Influenza due to identified novel influenza A virus with pneumonia**

Explanation: Codes in category J09 Influenza due to certain identified influenza viruses should be assigned only for confirmed cases. "Confirmation" does not require positive laboratory testing of a specific influenza virus but does need to be based on the provider's diagnostic statement, which should not include terms such as "possible," "probable," or "suspected."

d. Ventilator associated pneumonia

1) Documentation of ventilator associated pneumonia

As with all procedural or postprocedural complications, code assignment is based on the provider's documentation of the relationship between the condition and the procedure.

Code J95.851, Ventilator associated pneumonia, should be assigned only when the provider has documented ventilator associated pneumonia (VAP). An additional code to identify the organism (e.g., Pseudomonas aeruginosa, code B96.5) should also be assigned. Do not assign an additional code from categories J12-J18 to identify the type of pneumonia.

Code J95.851 should not be assigned for cases where the patient has pneumonia and is on a mechanical ventilator and the provider has not specifically stated that the pneumonia is ventilator-associated pneumonia. If the documentation is unclear as to whether the patient has a pneumonia that is a complication attributable to the mechanical ventilator, query the provider.

2) Ventilator associated pneumonia develops after admission

A patient may be admitted with one type of pneumonia (e.g., code J13, Pneumonia due to Streptococcus pneumonia) and subsequently develop VAP. In this instance, the principal diagnosis would be the appropriate code from categories J12-J18 for the pneumonia diagnosed at the time of admission. Code J95.851, Ventilator associated pneumonia, would be assigned as an additional diagnosis when the provider has also documented the presence of ventilator associated pneumonia.

Patient with pneumonia due to *Klebsiella pneumoniae* develops superimposed MRSA ventilator-associated pneumonia

J15.0   **Pneumonia due to Klebsiella pneumoniae**

J95.851   **Ventilator associated pneumonia**

B95.62   **Methicillin resistant Staphylococcus aureus infection as the cause of diseases classified elsewhere**

Explanation: Code assignment for ventilator associated pneumonia is based on the provider's documentation of the relationship between the condition and the procedure and is reported only when the provider has documented ventilator-associated pneumonia (VAP).

A patient may be admitted with one type of pneumonia and subsequently develop VAP. In this example, the principal diagnosis code describes the pneumonia diagnosed at the time of admission, with code J95.851 Ventilator associated pneumonia, assigned as secondary.

Chapter 10. Diseases of the Respiratory System (J00-J99)

NOTE   When a respiratory condition is described as occurring in more than one site and is not specifically indexed, it should be classified to the lower anatomic site (e.g. tracheobronchitis to bronchitis in J40).

Use additional code, where applicable, to identify:
exposure to environmental tobacco smoke (Z77.22)
exposure to tobacco smoke in the perinatal period (P96.81)
history of tobacco use (Z87.891)
occupational exposure to environmental tobacco smoke (Z57.31)
tobacco dependence (F17.-)
tobacco use (Z72.0)

EXCLUDES 2   *certain conditions originating in the perinatal period (P04-P96)*
certain infectious and parasitic diseases (A00-B99)
complications of pregnancy, childbirth and the puerperium (O00-O9A)
congenital malformations, deformations and chromosomal abnormalities (Q00-Q99)
endocrine, nutritional and metabolic diseases (E00-E88)
injury, poisoning and certain other consequences of external causes (S00-T88)
neoplasms (C00-D49)
smoke inhalation (T59.81-)
symptoms, signs and abnormal clinical and laboratory findings, not elsewhere classified (R00-R94)

This chapter contains the following blocks:
J00-J06   Acute upper respiratory infections
J09-J18   Influenza and pneumonia
J20-J22   Other acute lower respiratory infections
J30-J39   Other diseases of upper respiratory tract
J40-J47   Chronic lower respiratory diseases
J60-J70   Lung diseases due to external agents
J80-J84   Other respiratory diseases principally affecting the interstitium
J85-J86   Suppurative and necrotic conditions of the lower respiratory tract
J90-J94   Other diseases of the pleura
J95   Intraoperative and postprocedural complications and disorders of respiratory system, not elsewhere classified
J96-J99   Other diseases of the respiratory system

Acute upper respiratory infections (J00-J06)

EXCLUDES 1   *influenza virus with other respiratory manifestations (J09.X2, J10.1, J11.1)*

EXCLUDES 2   *chronic obstructive pulmonary disease with acute lower respiratory infection (J44.0)*

J00   Acute nasopharyngitis (common cold)
Acute rhinitis
Coryza (acute)
Infective nasopharyngitis NOS
Infective rhinitis
Nasal catarrh, acute
Nasopharyngitis NOS
EXCLUDES 1   *acute pharyngitis (J02.-)*
acute sore throat NOS (J02.9)
pharyngitis NOS (J02.9)
rhinitis NOS (J31.0)
sore throat NOS (J02.9)
EXCLUDES 2   *allergic rhinitis (J30.1-J30.9)*
chronic pharyngitis (J31.2)
chronic rhinitis (J31.0)
chronic sore throat (J31.2)
nasopharyngitis, chronic (J31.1)
vasomotor rhinitis (J30.0)

☑4ᵗʰ J01   Acute sinusitis
INCLUDES   acute abscess of sinus
acute empyema of sinus
acute infection of sinus
acute inflammation of sinus
acute suppuration of sinus
Use additional code (B95-B97) to identify infectious agent
EXCLUDES 1   *sinusitis NOS (J32.9)*
EXCLUDES 2   *chronic sinusitis (J32.0-J32.8)*

   ☑5ᵗʰ J01.0   Acute maxillary sinusitis
Acute antritis
     J01.00   Acute maxillary sinusitis, unspecified
     J01.01   Acute recurrent maxillary sinusitis

   ☑5ᵗʰ J01.1   Acute frontal sinusitis
     J01.10   Acute frontal sinusitis, unspecified
     J01.11   Acute recurrent frontal sinusitis

   ☑5ᵗʰ J01.2   Acute ethmoidal sinusitis
     J01.20   Acute ethmoidal sinusitis, unspecified
     J01.21   Acute recurrent ethmoidal sinusitis

   ☑5ᵗʰ J01.3   Acute sphenoidal sinusitis
     J01.30   Acute sphenoidal sinusitis, unspecified
     J01.31   Acute recurrent sphenoidal sinusitis

   ☑5ᵗʰ J01.4   Acute pansinusitis
     J01.40   Acute pansinusitis, unspecified
     J01.41   Acute recurrent pansinusitis

   ☑5ᵗʰ J01.8   Other acute sinusitis
     J01.80   Other acute sinusitis
       Acute sinusitis involving more than one sinus but not pansinusitis
     J01.81   Other acute recurrent sinusitis
       Acute recurrent sinusitis involving more than one sinus but not pansinusitis

   ☑5ᵗʰ J01.9   Acute sinusitis, unspecified
     J01.90   Acute sinusitis, unspecified
     J01.91   Acute recurrent sinusitis, unspecified

☑4ᵗʰ J02   Acute pharyngitis
INCLUDES   acute sore throat
EXCLUDES 1   *acute laryngopharyngitis (J06.0)*
peritonsillar abscess (J36)
pharyngeal abscess (J39.1)
retropharyngeal abscess (J39.0)
EXCLUDES 2   *chronic pharyngitis (J31.2)*

   J02.0   Streptococcal pharyngitis
Septic pharyngitis
Streptococcal sore throat
EXCLUDES 2   *scarlet fever (A38.-)*

   J02.8   Acute pharyngitis due to other specified organisms
Use additional code (B95-B97) to identify infectious agent
EXCLUDES 1   *acute pharyngitis due to coxsackie virus (B08.5)*
acute pharyngitis due to gonococcus (A54.5)
acute pharyngitis due to herpes [simplex] virus (B00.2)
acute pharyngitis due to infectious mononucleosis (B27.-)
enteroviral vesicular pharyngitis (B08.5)

   J02.9   Acute pharyngitis, unspecified
Gangrenous pharyngitis (acute)
Infective pharyngitis (acute) NOS
Pharyngitis (acute) NOS
Sore throat (acute) NOS
Suppurative pharyngitis (acute)
Ulcerative pharyngitis (acute)

☑4ᵗʰ J03   Acute tonsillitis
EXCLUDES 1   *acute sore throat (J02.-)*
hypertrophy of tonsils (J35.1)
peritonsillar abscess (J36)
sore throat NOS (J02.9)
streptococcal sore throat (J02.0)
EXCLUDES 2   *chronic tonsillitis (J35.0)*

   ☑5ᵗʰ J03.0   Streptococcal tonsillitis
     J03.00   Acute streptococcal tonsillitis, unspecified
     J03.01   Acute recurrent streptococcal tonsillitis

   ☑5ᵗʰ J03.8   Acute tonsillitis due to other specified organisms
Use additional code (B95-B97) to identify infectious agent
EXCLUDES 1   *diphtheritic tonsillitis (A36.0)*
herpesviral pharyngotonsillitis (B00.2)
streptococcal tonsillitis (J03.0)
tuberculous tonsillitis (A15.8)
Vincent's tonsillitis (A69.1)
     J03.80   Acute tonsillitis due to other specified organisms
     J03.81   Acute recurrent tonsillitis due to other specified organisms

   ☑5ᵗʰ J03.9   Acute tonsillitis, unspecified
Follicular tonsillitis (acute)
Gangrenous tonsillitis (acute)
Infective tonsillitis (acute)
Tonsillitis (acute) NOS
Ulcerative tonsillitis (acute)
     J03.90   Acute tonsillitis, unspecified
     J03.91   Acute recurrent tonsillitis, unspecified

☑ Additional Character Required   ✔x7ᵗʰ Placeholder Alert   Unspecified Dx   Other Specified Dx   Manifestation   ▶◀ Revised Text   ● New Code   ▲ Revised Code Title

ICD-10-CM 2016   619

✓4ᵗʰ J04 Acute laryngitis and tracheitis
Use additional code (B95-B97) to identify infectious agent
EXCLUDES 1   *acute obstructive laryngitis [croup] and epiglottitis (J05.-)*
EXCLUDES 2   *laryngismus (stridulus) (J38.5)*

    J04.0 Acute laryngitis
        Edematous laryngitis (acute)
        Laryngitis (acute) NOS
        Subglottic laryngitis (acute)
        Suppurative laryngitis (acute)
        Ulcerative laryngitis (acute)
        EXCLUDES 1   *acute obstructive laryngitis (J05.0)*
        EXCLUDES 2   *chronic laryngitis (J37.0)*

    ✓5ᵗʰ J04.1 Acute tracheitis
        Acute viral tracheitis
        Catarrhal tracheitis (acute)
        Tracheitis (acute) NOS
        EXCLUDES 2   *chronic tracheitis (J42)*

        J04.10 Acute tracheitis without obstruction
        J04.11 Acute tracheitis with obstruction

    J04.2 Acute laryngotracheitis
        Laryngotracheitis NOS
        Tracheitis (acute) with laryngitis (acute)
        EXCLUDES 1   *acute obstructive laryngotracheitis (J05.0)*
        EXCLUDES 2   *chronic laryngotracheitis (J37.1)*

    ✓5ᵗʰ J04.3 Supraglottitis, unspecified
        J04.30 Supraglottitis, unspecified, without obstruction
        J04.31 Supraglottitis, unspecified, with obstruction

✓4ᵗʰ J05 Acute obstructive laryngitis [croup] and epiglottitis
Use additional code (B95-B97) to identify infectious agent

    J05.0 Acute obstructive laryngitis [croup]
        Obstructive laryngitis (acute) NOS
        Obstructive laryngotracheitis NOS

    ✓5ᵗʰ J05.1 Acute epiglottitis
        EXCLUDES 2   *epiglottitis, chronic (J37.0)*

        J05.10 Acute epiglottitis without obstruction
            Epiglottitis NOS
        J05.11 Acute epiglottitis with obstruction

✓4ᵗʰ J06 Acute upper respiratory infections of multiple and unspecified sites
    EXCLUDES 1   *acute respiratory infection NOS (J22)*
           streptococcal pharyngitis (J02.0)3

    J06.0 Acute laryngopharyngitis

    J06.9 Acute upper respiratory infection, unspecified
        Upper respiratory disease, acute
        Upper respiratory infection NOS

Influenza and pneumonia (J09-J18)

EXCLUDES 2   *allergic or eosinophilic pneumonia (J82)*
           aspiration pneumonia NOS (J69.0)
           congenital pneumonia (P23.9)
           lipid pneumonia (J69.1)
           meconium pneumonia (P24.01)
           neonatal aspiration pneumonia (P24.-)
           pneumonia due to solids and liquids (J69.-)
           rheumatic pneumonia (I00)
           ventilator associated pneumonia (J95.851)

✓4ᵗʰ J09 Influenza due to certain identified influenza viruses
    EXCLUDES 1   *seasonal influenza due to other identified influenza virus (J10.-)*
           seasonal influenza due to unidentified influenza virus (J11.-)

    ✓5ᵗʰ J09.X Influenza due to identified novel influenza A virus
        Avian influenza
        Bird influenza
        Influenza A/H5N1
        Influenza of other animal origin, not bird or swine
        Swine influenza virus (viruses that normally cause infections in pigs)

        J09.X1 Influenza due to identified novel influenza A virus with pneumonia
            Code also, if applicable, associated:
                lung abscess (J85.1)
                other specified type of pneumonia

        J09.X2 Influenza due to identified novel influenza A virus with other respiratory manifestations
            Influenza due to identified novel influenza A virus NOS
            Influenza due to identified novel influenza A virus with laryngitis
            Influenza due to identified novel influenza A virus with pharyngitis
            Influenza due to identified novel influenza A virus with upper respiratory symptoms
            Use additional code, if applicable, for associated:
                pleural effusion (J91.8)
                sinusitis (J01.-)

        J09.X3 Influenza due to identified novel influenza A virus with gastrointestinal manifestations
            Influenza due to identified novel influenza A virus gastroenteritis
            EXCLUDES 1   *'intestinal flu' [viral gastroenteritis] (A08.-)*

        J09.X9 Influenza due to identified novel influenza A virus with other manifestations
            Influenza due to identified novel influenza A virus with encephalopathy
            Influenza due to identified novel influenza A virus with myocarditis
            Influenza due to identified novel influenza A virus with otitis media
            Use additional code to identify manifestation

✓4ᵗʰ J10 Influenza due to other identified influenza virus
    EXCLUDES 1   *influenza due to avian influenza virus (J09.X-)*
           influenza due to swine flu (J09.X-)
           influenza due to unidentifed influenza virus (J11.-)

    ✓5ᵗʰ J10.0 Influenza due to other identified influenza virus with pneumonia
        Code also associated lung abscess, if applicable (J85.1)

        J10.00 Influenza due to other identified influenza virus with unspecified type of pneumonia
        J10.01 Influenza due to other identified influenza virus with the same other identified influenza virus pneumonia
        J10.08 Influenza due to other identified influenza virus with other specified pneumonia
            Code also other specified type of pneumonia

    J10.1 Influenza due to other identified influenza virus with other respiratory manifestations
        Influenza due to other identified influenza virus NOS
        Influenza due to other identified influenza virus with laryngitis
        Influenza due to other identified influenza virus with pharyngitis
        Influenza due to other identified influenza virus with upper respiratory symptoms
        Use additional code for associated pleural effusion, if applicable (J91.8)
        Use additional code for associated sinusitis, if applicable (J01.-)

    J10.2 Influenza due to other identified influenza virus with gastrointestinal manifestations
        Influenza due to other identified influenza virus gastroenteritis
        EXCLUDES 1   *'intestinal flu' [viral gastroenteritis] (A08.-)*

    ✓5ᵗʰ J10.8 Influenza due to other identified influenza virus with other manifestations
        J10.81 Influenza due to other identified influenza virus with encephalopathy
        J10.82 Influenza due to other identified influenza virus with myocarditis
        J10.83 Influenza due to other identified influenza virus with otitis media
            Use additional code for any associated perforated tympanic membrane (H72.-)
        J10.89 Influenza due to other identified influenza virus with other manifestations
            Use additional codes to identify the manifestations

✓4ᵗʰ J11 Influenza due to unidentified influenza virus
    ✓5ᵗʰ J11.0 Influenza due to unidentified influenza virus with pneumonia
        Code also associated lung abscess, if applicable (J85.1)

        J11.00 Influenza due to unidentified influenza virus with unspecified type of pneumonia
            Influenza with pneumonia NOS

        J11.08 Influenza due to unidentified influenza virus with specified pneumonia
            Code also other specified type of pneumonia

J11.1 Influenza due to unidentified influenza virus with other respiratory manifestations
Influenza NOS
Influenzal laryngitis NOS
Influenzal pharyngitis NOS
Influenza with upper respiratory symptoms NOS
Use additional code for associated pleural effusion, if applicable (J91.8)
Use additional code for associated sinusitis, if applicable (J01.-)

J11.2 Influenza due to unidentified influenza virus with gastrointestinal manifestations
Influenza gastroenteritis NOS
EXCLUDES 1   *'intestinal flu' [viral gastroenteritis] (A08.-)*

✓5th **J11.8 Influenza due to unidentified influenza virus with other manifestations**

    J11.81 Influenza due to unidentified influenza virus with encephalopathy
      Influenzal encephalopathy NOS

    J11.82 Influenza due to unidentified influenza virus with myocarditis
      Influenzal myocarditis NOS

    J11.83 Influenza due to unidentified influenza virus with otitis media
      Influenzal otitis media NOS
      Use additional code for any associated perforated tympanic membrane (H72.-)

    J11.89 Influenza due to unidentified influenza virus with other manifestations
      Use additional codes to identify the manifestations

✓4th **J12 Viral pneumonia, not elsewhere classified**
   INCLUDES   bronchopneumonia due to viruses other than influenza viruses
Code first associated influenza, if applicable (J09.X1, J10.0-, J11.0-)
Code also associated abscess, if applicable (J85.1)
EXCLUDES 1   *aspiration pneumonia due to anesthesia during labor and delivery (O74.0)*
      aspiration pneumonia due to anesthesia during pregnancy (O29)
      aspiration pneumonia due to anesthesia during puerperium (O89.0)
      aspiration pneumonia due to solids and liquids (J69.-)
      aspiration pneumonia NOS (J69.0)
      congenital pneumonia (P23.0)
      congenital rubella pneumonitis (P35.0)
      interstitial pneumonia NOS (J84.9)
      lipid pneumonia (J69.1)
      neonatal aspiration pneumonia (P24.-)
   AHA: 2013, 4Q, 118

J12.0 Adenoviral pneumonia

J12.1 Respiratory syncytial virus pneumonia

J12.2 Parainfluenza virus pneumonia

J12.3 Human metapneumovirus pneumonia

✓5th **J12.8 Other viral pneumonia**

    J12.81 Pneumonia due to SARS-associated coronavirus
      Severe acute respiratory syndrome NOS

    J12.89 Other viral pneumonia

J12.9 Viral pneumonia, unspecified

J13 Pneumonia due to Streptococcus pneumoniae
Bronchopneumonia due to S. pneumoniae
Code first associated influenza, if applicable (J09.X1, J10.0-, J11.0-)
Code also associated lung abscess, if applicable (J85.1)
EXCLUDES 1   *congenital pneumonia due to S. pneumoniae (P23.6)*
      lobar pneumonia, unspecified organism (J18.1)
      pneumonia due to other streptococci (J15.3-J15.4)
   AHA: 2013, 4Q, 118

J14 Pneumonia due to Hemophilus influenzae
Bronchopneumonia due to H. influenzae
Code first associated influenza, if applicable (J09.X1, J10.0-, J11.0-)
Code also associated lung abscess, if applicable (J85.1)
EXCLUDES 1   *congenital pneumonia due to H. influenzae (P23.6)*
   AHA: 2013, 4Q, 118

✓4th **J15 Bacterial pneumonia, not elsewhere classified**
Bronchopneumonia due to bacteria other than S. pneumoniae and H. influenzae
Code first associated influenza, if applicable (J09.X1, J10.0-, J11.0-)
Code also associated lung abscess, if applicable (J85.1)
EXCLUDES 1   *chlamydial pneumonia (J16.0)*
      congenital pneumonia (P23.-)
      Legionnaires' disease (A48.1)
      spirochetal pneumonia (A69.8)
   AHA: 2013, 4Q, 118

J15.0 Pneumonia due to Klebsiella pneumoniae

J15.1 Pneumonia due to Pseudomonas

✓5th **J15.2 Pneumonia due to staphylococcus**

    J15.20 Pneumonia due to staphylococcus, unspecified

    ✓6th **J15.21 Pneumonia due to Staphylococcus aureus**

      J15.211 Pneumonia due to methicillin susceptible Staphylococcus aureus
        MSSA pneumonia
        Pneumonia due to Staphylococcus aureus NOS

      J15.212 Pneumonia due to methicillin resistant Staphylococcus aureus

    J15.29 Pneumonia due to other staphylococcus

J15.3 Pneumonia due to streptococcus, group B

J15.4 Pneumonia due to other streptococci
EXCLUDES 1   *pneumonia due to streptococcus, group B (J15.3)*
      pneumonia due to Streptococcus pneumoniae (J13)

J15.5 Pneumonia due to Escherichia coli

J15.6 Pneumonia due to other aerobic Gram-negative bacteria
Pneumonia due to Serratia marcescens

J15.7 Pneumonia due to Mycoplasma pneumoniae

J15.8 Pneumonia due to other specified bacteria

J15.9 Unspecified bacterial pneumonia
Pneumonia due to gram-positive bacteria

✓4th **J16 Pneumonia due to other infectious organisms, not elsewhere classified**
Code first associated influenza, if applicable (J09.X1, J10.0-, J11.0-)
Code also associated lung abscess, if applicable (J85.1)
EXCLUDES 1   *congenital pneumonia (P23.-)*
      ornithosis (A70)
      pneumocystosis (B59)
      pneumonia NOS (J18.9)
   AHA: 2013, 4Q, 118

J16.0 Chlamydial pneumonia

J16.8 Pneumonia due to other specified infectious organisms

J17 Pneumonia in diseases classified elsewhere
Code first underlying disease, such as:
   Q fever (A78)
   rheumatic fever (I00)
   schistosomiasis (B65.0-B65.9)
EXCLUDES 1   *candidial pneumonia (B37.1)*
      chlamydial pneumonia (J16.0)
      gonorrheal pneumonia (A54.84)
      histoplasmosis pneumonia (B39.0-B39.2)
      measles pneumonia (B05.2)
      nocardiosis pneumonia (A43.0)
      pneumocystosis (B59)
      pneumonia due to Pneumocystis carinii (B59)
      pneumonia due to Pneumocystis jiroveci (B59)
      pneumonia in actinomycosis (A42.0)
      pneumonia in anthrax (A22.1)
      pneumonia in ascariasis (B77.81)
      pneumonia in aspergillosis (B44.0-B44.1)
      pneumonia in coccidioidomycosis (B38.0-B38.2)
      pneumonia in cytomegalovirus disease (B25.0)
      pneumonia in toxoplasmosis (B58.3)
      rubella pneumonia (B06.81)
      salmonella pneumonia (A02.22)
      spirochetal infection NEC with pneumonia (A69.8)
      tularemia pneumonia (A21.2)
      typhoid fever with pneumonia (A01.03)
      varicella pneumonia (B01.2)
      whooping cough with pneumonia (A37 with fifth-character 1)
   AHA: 2013, 4Q, 118

☑ Additional Character Required   ✓7th Placeholder Alert   Unspecified Dx   Other Specified Dx   Manifestation   ►◄ Revised Text   ● New Code   ▲ Revised Code Title

✓4ᵗʰ **J18 Pneumonia, unspecified organism**

Code first associated influenza, if applicable (J09.X1, J10.0-, J11.0-)

EXCLUDES 1 abscess of lung with pneumonia (J85.1)

aspiration pneumonia due to anesthesia during labor and delivery (O74.0)

aspiration pneumonia due to anesthesia during pregnancy (O29)

aspiration pneumonia due to anesthesia during puerperium (O89.0)

aspiration pneumonia due to solids and liquids (J69.-)

aspiration pneumonia NOS (J69.0)

congenital pneumonia (P23.0)

drug-induced interstitial lung disorder (J70.2-J70.4)

interstitial pneumonia NOS (J84.9)

lipid pneumonia (J69.1)

neonatal aspiration pneumonia (P24.-)

pneumonitis due to external agents (J67-J70)

pneumonitis due to fumes and vapors (J68.0)

usual interstitial pneumonia (J84.17)

AHA: 2013, 4Q, 118

J18.0 Bronchopneumonia, unspecified organism

EXCLUDES 1 hypostatic bronchopneumonia (J18.2)

lipid pneumonia (J69.1)

EXCLUDES 2 acute bronchiolitis (J21.-)

chronic bronchiolitis (J44.9)

J18.1 Lobar pneumonia, unspecified organism

J18.2 Hypostatic pneumonia, unspecified organism

Hypostatic bronchopneumonia

Passive pneumonia

J18.8 Other pneumonia, unspecified organism

J18.9 Pneumonia, unspecified organism

AHA: 2014, 3Q, 4; 2013, 4Q, 119; 2012, 4Q, 94

Other acute lower respiratory infections (J20-J22)

EXCLUDES 2 chronic obstructive pulmonary disease with acute lower respiratory infection (J44.0)

✓4ᵗʰ **J20 Acute bronchitis**

INCLUDES acute and subacute bronchitis (with) bronchospasm

acute and subacute bronchitis (with) tracheitis

acute and subacute bronchitis (with) tracheobronchitis, acute

acute and subacute fibrinous bronchitis

acute and subacute membranous bronchitis

acute and subacute purulent bronchitis

acute and subacute septic bronchitis

EXCLUDES 1 bronchitis NOS (J40)

tracheobronchitis NOS (J40)

EXCLUDES 2 acute bronchitis with bronchiectasis (J47.0)

acute bronchitis with chronic obstructive asthma (J44.0)

acute bronchitis with chronic obstructive pulmonary disease (J44.0)

allergic bronchitis NOS (J45.909)

bronchitis due to chemicals, fumes and vapors (J68.0)

chronic bronchitis NOS (J42)

chronic mucopurulent bronchitis (J41.1)

chronic obstructive bronchitis (J44.-)

chronic obstructive tracheobronchitis (J44.-)

chronic simple bronchitis (J41.0)

chronic tracheobronchitis (J42)

J20.0 Acute bronchitis due to Mycoplasma pneumoniae

J20.1 Acute bronchitis due to Hemophilus influenzae

J20.2 Acute bronchitis due to streptococcus

J20.3 Acute bronchitis due to coxsackievirus

J20.4 Acute bronchitis due to parainfluenza virus

J20.5 Acute bronchitis due to respiratory syncytial virus

J20.6 Acute bronchitis due to rhinovirus

J20.7 Acute bronchitis due to echovirus

J20.8 Acute bronchitis due to other specified organisms

J20.9 Acute bronchitis, unspecified

✓4ᵗʰ **J21 Acute bronchiolitis**

Acute bronchiolitis with bronchospasm

EXCLUDES 2 respiratory bronchiolitis interstitial lung disease (J84.115)

J21.0 Acute bronchiolitis due to respiratory syncytial virus

J21.1 Acute bronchiolitis due to human metapneumovirus

J21.8 Acute bronchiolitis due to other specified organisms

J21.9 Acute bronchiolitis, unspecified

Bronchiolitis (acute)

EXCLUDES 1 chronic bronchiolitis (J44.-)

J22 Unspecified acute lower respiratory infection

Acute (lower) respiratory (tract) infection NOS

EXCLUDES 1 upper respiratory infection (acute) (J06.9)

Other diseases of upper respiratory tract (J30-J39)

✓4ᵗʰ **J30 Vasomotor and allergic rhinitis**

INCLUDES spasmodic rhinorrhea

EXCLUDES 1 allergic rhinitis with asthma (bronchial) (J45.909)

rhinitis NOS (J31.0)

J30.0 Vasomotor rhinitis

J30.1 Allergic rhinitis due to pollen

Allergy NOS due to pollen

Hay fever

Pollinosis

J30.2 Other seasonal allergic rhinitis

J30.5 Allergic rhinitis due to food

✓5ᵗʰ **J30.8 Other allergic rhinitis**

J30.81 Allergic rhinitis due to animal (cat) (dog) hair and dander

J30.89 Other allergic rhinitis

Perennial allergic rhinitis

J30.9 Allergic rhinitis, unspecified

✓4ᵗʰ **J31 Chronic rhinitis, nasopharyngitis and pharyngitis**

Use additional code to identify:

exposure to environmental tobacco smoke (Z77.22)

exposure to tobacco smoke in the perinatal period (P96.81)

history of tobacco use (Z87.891)

occupational exposure to environmental tobacco smoke (Z57.31)

tobacco dependence (F17.-)

tobacco use (Z72.0)

J31.0 Chronic rhinitis

Atrophic rhinitis (chronic)

Granulomatous rhinitis (chronic)

Hypertrophic rhinitis (chronic)

Obstructive rhinitis (chronic)

Ozena

Purulent rhinitis (chronic)

Rhinitis (chronic) NOS

Ulcerative rhinitis (chronic)

EXCLUDES 1 allergic rhinitis (J30.1-J30.9)

vasomotor rhinitis (J30.0)

J31.1 Chronic nasopharyngitis

EXCLUDES 2 acute nasopharyngitis (J00)

J31.2 Chronic pharyngitis

Atrophic pharyngitis (chronic)

Chronic sore throat

Granular pharyngitis (chronic)

Hypertrophic pharyngitis (chronic)

EXCLUDES 2 acute pharyngitis (J02.9)

✓4ᵗʰ **J32 Chronic sinusitis**

INCLUDES sinus abscess

sinus empyema

sinus infection

sinus suppuration

Use additional code to identify:

exposure to environmental tobacco smoke (Z77.22)

exposure to tobacco smoke in the perinatal period (P96.81)

history of tobacco use (Z87.891)

infectious agent (B95-B97)

occupational exposure to environmental tobacco smoke (Z57.31)

tobacco dependence (F17.-)

tobacco use (Z72.0)

EXCLUDES 2 acute sinusitis (J01.-)

J32.0 Chronic maxillary sinusitis

Antritis (chronic)

Maxillary sinusitis NOS

J32.1 Chronic frontal sinusitis

Frontal sinusitis NOS

J32.2 Chronic ethmoidal sinusitis

Ethmoidal sinusitis NOS

EXCLUDES 1 Woakes' ethmoiditis (J33.1)

J32.3 Chronic sphenoidal sinusitis

Sphenoidal sinusitis NOS

J32.4 Chronic pansinusitis

Pansinusitis NOS

J32.8 Other chronic sinusitis

Sinusitis (chronic) involving more than one sinus but not pansinusitis

EXCLUDES 1 Not coded here   EXCLUDES 2 Not included here   N Newborn Age: 0   P Pediatric Age: 0-17   M Maternity Age: 12-55   A Adult Age: 15-124

622

ICD-10-CM 2016

J32.9   Chronic sinusitis, unspecified
Sinusitis (chronic) NOS

✓4ᵗʰ **J33   Nasal polyp**
Use additional code to identify:
exposure to environmental tobacco smoke (Z77.22)
exposure to tobacco smoke in the perinatal period (P96.81)
history of tobacco use (Z87.891)
occupational exposure to environmental tobacco smoke (Z57.31)
tobacco dependence (F17.-)
tobacco use (Z72.0)
EXCLUDES 1   adenomatous polyps (D14.0)

J33.0   Polyp of nasal cavity
Choanal polyp
Nasopharyngeal polyp

J33.1   Polypoid sinus degeneration
Woakes' syndrome or ethmoiditis

J33.8   Other polyp of sinus
Accessory polyp of sinus
Ethmoidal polyp of sinus
Maxillary polyp of sinus
Sphenoidal polyp of sinus

J33.9   Nasal polyp, unspecified

✓4ᵗʰ **J34   Other and unspecified disorders of nose and nasal sinuses**
EXCLUDES 2   varicose ulcer of nasal septum (I86.8)

J34.0   Abscess, furuncle and carbuncle of nose
Cellulitis of nose
Necrosis of nose
Ulceration of nose

J34.1   Cyst and mucocele of nose and nasal sinus

J34.2   Deviated nasal septum
Deflection or deviation of septum (nasal) (acquired)
EXCLUDES 1   congenital deviated nasal septum (Q67.4)

J34.3   Hypertrophy of nasal turbinates

✓5ᵗʰ **J34.8   Other specified disorders of nose and nasal sinuses**

J34.81   Nasal mucositis (ulcerative)
Code also type of associated therapy, such as:
antineoplastic and immunosuppressive drugs
(T45.1X-)
radiological procedure and radiotherapy (Y84.2)
EXCLUDES 2   gastrointestinal mucositis (ulcerative)
(K92.81)
mucositis (ulcerative) of vagina and vulva
(N76.81)
oral mucositis (ulcerative) (K12.3-)

J34.89   Other specified disorders of nose and nasal sinuses
Perforation of nasal septum NOS
Rhinolith

J34.9   Unspecified disorder of nose and nasal sinuses

✓4ᵗʰ **J35   Chronic diseases of tonsils and adenoids**
Use additional code to identify:
exposure to environmental tobacco smoke (Z77.22)
exposure to tobacco smoke in the perinatal period (P96.81)
history of tobacco use (Z87.891)
occupational exposure to environmental tobacco smoke (Z57.31)
tobacco dependence (F17.-)
tobacco use (Z72.0)

✓5ᵗʰ **J35.0   Chronic tonsillitis and adenoiditis**
EXCLUDES 2   acute tonsillitis (J03.-)

J35.01   Chronic tonsillitis

J35.02   Chronic adenoiditis

J35.03   Chronic tonsillitis and adenoiditis

J35.1   Hypertrophy of tonsils
Enlargement of tonsils
EXCLUDES 1   hypertrophy of tonsils with tonsillitis (J35.0-)

J35.2   Hypertrophy of adenoids
Enlargement of adenoids
EXCLUDES 1   hypertrophy of adenoids with adenoiditis (J35.0-)

J35.3   Hypertrophy of tonsils with hypertrophy of adenoids
EXCLUDES 1   hypertrophy of tonsils and adenoids with tonsillitis and
adenoiditis (J35.03)

J35.8   Other chronic diseases of tonsils and adenoids
Adenoid vegetations
Amygdalolith
Calculus, tonsil
Cicatrix of tonsil (and adenoid)
Tonsillar tag
Ulcer of tonsil

J35.9   Chronic disease of tonsils and adenoids, unspecified
Disease (chronic) of tonsils and adenoids NOS

J36   Peritonsillar abscess
INCLUDES   abscess of tonsil
peritonsillar cellulitis
quinsy
Use additional code (B95-B97) to identify infectious agent
EXCLUDES 1   acute tonsillitis (J03.-)
chronic tonsillitis (J35.0)
retropharyngeal abscess (J39.0)
tonsillitis NOS (J03.9-)

✓4ᵗʰ **J37   Chronic laryngitis and laryngotracheitis**
Use additional code to identify:
exposure to environmental tobacco smoke (Z77.22)
exposure to tobacco smoke in the perinatal period (P96.81)
history of tobacco use (Z87.891)
infectious agent (B95-B97)
occupational exposure to environmental tobacco smoke (Z57.31)
tobacco dependence (F17.-)
tobacco use (Z72.0)

J37.0   Chronic laryngitis
Catarrhal laryngitis
Hypertrophic laryngitis
Sicca laryngitis
EXCLUDES 2   acute laryngitis (J04.0)
obstructive (acute) laryngitis (J05.0)

J37.1   Chronic laryngotracheitis
Laryngitis, chronic, with tracheitis (chronic)
Tracheitis, chronic, with laryngitis
EXCLUDES 1   chronic tracheitis (J42)
EXCLUDES 2   acute laryngotracheitis (J04.2)
acute tracheitis (J04.1)

✓4ᵗʰ **J38   Diseases of vocal cords and larynx, not elsewhere classified**
Use additional code to identify:
exposure to environmental tobacco smoke (Z77.22)
exposure to tobacco smoke in the perinatal period (P96.81)
history of tobacco use (Z87.891)
occupational exposure to environmental tobacco smoke (Z57.31)
tobacco dependence (F17.-)
tobacco use (Z72.0)
EXCLUDES 1   congenital laryngeal stridor (P28.89)
obstructive laryngitis (acute) (J05.0)
postprocedural subglottic stenosis (J95.5)
stridor (R06.1)
ulcerative laryngitis (J04.0)

✓5ᵗʰ **J38.0   Paralysis of vocal cords and larynx**
Laryngoplegia
Paralysis of glottis

J38.00   Paralysis of vocal cords and larynx, unspecified

J38.01   Paralysis of vocal cords and larynx, unilateral

J38.02   Paralysis of vocal cords and larynx, bilateral

J38.1   Polyp of vocal cord and larynx
EXCLUDES 1   adenomatous polyps (D14.1)

J38.2   Nodules of vocal cords
Chorditis (fibrinous)(nodosa)(tuberosa)
Singer's nodes
Teacher's nodes

J38.3   Other diseases of vocal cords
Abscess of vocal cords
Cellulitis of vocal cords
Granuloma of vocal cords
Leukokeratosis of vocal cords
Leukoplakia of vocal cords

J38.4   Edema of larynx
Edema (of) glottis
Subglottic edema
Supraglottic edema
EXCLUDES 1   acute obstructive laryngitis [croup] (J05.0)
edematous laryngitis (J04.0)

J38.5   Laryngeal spasm
Laryngismus (stridulus)

J38.6   Stenosis of larynx

J38.7   Other diseases of larynx

Abscess of larynx	Pachyderma of larynx
Cellulitis of larynx	Perichondritis of larynx
Disease of larynx NOS	Ulcer of larynx
Necrosis of larynx	

✓4ᵗʰ **J39** **Other diseases of upper respiratory tract**
- EXCLUDES 1   *acute respiratory infection NOS (J22)*
  acute upper respiratory infection (J06.9)
  upper respiratory inflammation due to chemicals, gases, fumes or vapors (J68.2)

J39.0 **Retropharyngeal and parapharyngeal abscess**
  Peripharyngeal abscess
  - EXCLUDES 1   *peritonsillar abscess (J36)*

J39.1 **Other abscess of pharynx**
  Cellulitis of pharynx
  Nasopharyngeal abscess

J39.2 **Other diseases of pharynx**
  Cyst of pharynx
  Edema of pharynx
  - EXCLUDES 2   *chronic pharyngitis (J31.2)*
    ulcerative pharyngitis (J02.9)

J39.3 **Upper respiratory tract hypersensitivity reaction, site unspecified**
  - EXCLUDES 1   *hypersensitivity reaction of upper respiratory tract, such as:*
    extrinsic allergic alveolitis (J67.9)
    pneumoconiosis (J60-J67.9)

J39.8 **Other specified diseases of upper respiratory tract**

J39.9 **Disease of upper respiratory tract, unspecified**

Chronic lower respiratory diseases (J40-J47)

- EXCLUDES 1   *bronchitis due to chemicals, gases, fumes and vapors (J68.0)*
- EXCLUDES 2   *cystic fibrosis (E84.-)*

J40 **Bronchitis, not specified as acute or chronic**
  Bronchitis NOS
  Bronchitis with tracheitis NOS
  Catarrhal bronchitis
  Tracheobronchitis NOS
  Use additional code to identify:
     exposure to environmental tobacco smoke (Z77.22)
     exposure to tobacco smoke in the perinatal period (P96.81)
     history of tobacco use (Z87.891)
     occupational exposure to environmental tobacco smoke (Z57.31)
     tobacco dependence (F17.-)
     tobacco use (Z72.0)
  - EXCLUDES 1   *acute bronchitis (J20.-)*
    allergic bronchitis NOS (J45.909)
    asthmatic bronchitis NOS (J45.9-)
    bronchitis due to chemicals, gases, fumes and vapors (J68.0)

✓4ᵗʰ **J41** **Simple and mucopurulent chronic bronchitis**
  Use additional code to identify:
     exposure to environmental tobacco smoke (Z77.22)
     exposure to tobacco smoke in the perinatal period (P96.81)
     history of tobacco use (Z87.891)
     occupational exposure to environmental tobacco smoke (Z57.31)
     tobacco dependence (F17.-)
     tobacco use (Z72.0)
  - EXCLUDES 1   *chronic bronchitis NOS (J42)*
    chronic obstructive bronchitis (J44.-)

J41.0 **Simple chronic bronchitis**

J41.1 **Mucopurulent chronic bronchitis**

J41.8 **Mixed simple and mucopurulent chronic bronchitis**

J42 **Unspecified chronic bronchitis**
  Chronic bronchitis NOS
  Chronic tracheitis
  Chronic tracheobronchitis
  Use additional code to identify:
     exposure to environmental tobacco smoke (Z77.22)
     exposure to tobacco smoke in the perinatal period (P96.81)
     history of tobacco use (Z87.891)
     occupational exposure to environmental tobacco smoke (Z57.31)
     tobacco dependence (F17.-)
     tobacco use (Z72.0)
  - EXCLUDES 1   *chronic asthmatic bronchitis (J44.-)*
    chronic bronchitis with airways obstruction (J44.-)
    chronic emphysematous bronchitis (J44.-)
    chronic obstructive pulmonary disease NOS (J44.9)
    simple and mucopurulent chronic bronchitis (J41.-)

✓4ᵗʰ **J43** **Emphysema**
  Use additional code to identify:
     exposure to environmental tobacco smoke (Z77.22)
     history of tobacco use (Z87.891)
     occupational exposure to environmental tobacco smoke (Z57.31)
     tobacco dependence (F17.-)
     tobacco use (Z72.0)
  - EXCLUDES 1   *compensatory emphysema (J98.3)*
    emphysema due to inhalation of chemicals, gases, fumes or vapors (J68.4)
    emphysema with chronic (obstructive) bronchitis (J44.-)
    emphysematous (obstructive) bronchitis (J44.-)
    interstitial emphysema (J98.2)
    mediastinal emphysema (J98.2)
    neonatal interstitial emphysema (P25.0)
    surgical (subcutaneous) emphysema (T81.82)
    traumatic subcutaneous emphysema (T79.7)

J43.0 **Unilateral pulmonary emphysema [MacLeod's syndrome]**
  Swyer-James syndrome
  Unilateral emphysema
  Unilateral hyperlucent lung
  Unilateral pulmonary artery functional hypoplasia
  Unilateral transparency of lung

J43.1 **Panlobular emphysema**
  Panacinar emphysema

J43.2 **Centrilobular emphysema**

J43.8 **Other emphysema**

J43.9 **Emphysema, unspecified**
  Bullous emphysema (lung)(pulmonary)
  Emphysema (lung)(pulmonary) NOS
  Emphysematous bleb
  Vesicular emphysema (lung)(pulmonary)

✓4ᵗʰ **J44** **Other chronic obstructive pulmonary disease**
  - INCLUDES   asthma with chronic obstructive pulmonary disease
    chronic asthmatic (obstructive) bronchitis
    chronic bronchitis with airways obstruction
    chronic bronchitis with emphysema
    chronic emphysematous bronchitis
    chronic obstructive asthma
    chronic obstructive bronchitis
    chronic obstructive tracheobronchitis
  Code also type of asthma, if applicable (J45.-)
  Use additional code to identify:
     exposure to environmental tobacco smoke (Z77.22)
     history of tobacco use (Z87.891)
     occupational exposure to environmental tobacco smoke (Z57.31)
     tobacco dependence (F17.-)
     tobacco use (Z72.0)
  - EXCLUDES 1   *bronchiectasis (J47.-)*
    chronic bronchitis NOS (J42)
    chronic simple and mucopurulent bronchitis (J41.-)
    chronic tracheitis (J42)
    chronic tracheobronchitis (J42)
    emphysema without chronic bronchitis (J43.-)
    lung diseases due to external agents (J60-J70)
  AHA: 2013, 4Q, 109

J44.0 **Chronic obstructive pulmonary disease with acute lower respiratory infection**
  Use additional code to identify the infection

J44.1 **Chronic obstructive pulmonary disease with (acute) exacerbation**
  Decompensated COPD
  Decompensated COPD with (acute) exacerbation
  - EXCLUDES 2   *chronic obstructive pulmonary disease [COPD] with acute bronchitis (J44.0)*

J44.9 **Chronic obstructive pulmonary disease, unspecified**
  Chronic obstructive airway disease NOS
  Chronic obstructive lung disease NOS
  AHA: 2014, 4Q, 21; 2013, 4Q, 129

EXCLUDES 1 Not coded here   EXCLUDES 2 Not included here   N Newborn Age: 0   P Pediatric Age: 0-17   M Maternity Age: 12-55   A Adult Age: 15-124

624   ICD-10-CM 2016

✓4ᵗʰ J45 Asthma

INCLUDES allergic (predominantly) asthma
allergic bronchitis nos
allergic rhinitis with asthma
atopic asthma
extrinsic allergic asthma
hay fever with asthma
idiosyncratic asthma
intrinsic nonallergic asthma
nonallergic asthma

Use additional code to identify:
exposure to environmental tobacco smoke (Z77.22)
exposure to tobacco smoke in the perinatal period (P96.81)
history of tobacco use (Z87.891)
occupational exposure to environmental tobacco smoke (Z57.31)
tobacco dependence (F17.-)
tobacco use (Z72.0)

EXCLUDES 1 detergent asthma (J69.8)
eosinophilic asthma (J82)
lung diseases due to external agents (J60-J70)
miner's asthma (J60)
wheezing NOS (R06.2)
wood asthma (J67.8)

EXCLUDES 2 asthma with chronic obstructive pulmonary disease (J44.9)
chronic asthmatic (obstructive) bronchitis (J44.9)
chronic obstructive asthma (J44.9)

✓5ᵗʰ J45.2 Mild intermittent asthma

J45.20 Mild intermittent asthma, uncomplicated
Mild intermittent asthma NOS

J45.21 Mild intermittent asthma with (acute) exacerbation

J45.22 Mild intermittent asthma with status asthmaticus

✓5ᵗʰ J45.3 Mild persistent asthma

J45.30 Mild persistent asthma, uncomplicated
Mild persistent asthma NOS

J45.31 Mild persistent asthma with (acute) exacerbation

J45.32 Mild persistent asthma with status asthmaticus

✓5ᵗʰ J45.4 Moderate persistent asthma

J45.40 Moderate persistent asthma, uncomplicated
Moderate persistent asthma NOS

J45.41 Moderate persistent asthma with (acute) exacerbation

J45.42 Moderate persistent asthma with status asthmaticus

✓5ᵗʰ J45.5 Severe persistent asthma

J45.50 Severe persistent asthma, uncomplicated
Severe persistent asthma NOS

J45.51 Severe persistent asthma with (acute) exacerbation

J45.52 Severe persistent asthma with status asthmaticus

✓5ᵗʰ J45.9 Other and unspecified asthma

✓6ᵗʰ J45.90 Unspecified asthma
Asthmatic bronchitis NOS
Childhood asthma NOS
Late onset asthma

J45.901 Unspecified asthma with (acute) exacerbation

J45.902 Unspecified asthma with status asthmaticus

J45.909 Unspecified asthma, uncomplicated
Asthma NOS

✓6ᵗʰ J45.99 Other asthma

J45.990 Exercise induced bronchospasm

J45.991 Cough variant asthma

J45.998 Other asthma

✓4ᵗʰ J47 Bronchiectasis

INCLUDES bronchiolectasis

Use additional code to identify:
exposure to environmental tobacco smoke (Z77.22)
exposure to tobacco smoke in the perinatal period (P96.81)
history of tobacco use (Z87.891)
occupational exposure to environmental tobacco smoke (Z57.31)
tobacco dependence (F17.-)
tobacco use (Z72.0)

EXCLUDES 1 congenital bronchiectasis (Q33.4)
tuberculous bronchiectasis (current disease) (A15.0)

J47.0 Bronchiectasis with acute lower respiratory infection
Bronchiectasis with acute bronchitis

J47.1 Bronchiectasis with (acute) exacerbation

J47.9 Bronchiectasis, uncomplicated
Bronchiectasis NOS

Lung diseases due to external agents (J60-J70)

EXCLUDES 2 asthma (J45.-)
malignant neoplasm of bronchus and lung (C34.-)

J60 Coalworker's pneumoconiosis   A
Anthracosilicosis   Black lung disease
Anthracosis   Coalworker's lung

EXCLUDES 1 coalworker pneumoconiosis with tuberculosis, any type in A15 (J65)

J61 Pneumoconiosis due to asbestos and other mineral fibers   A
Asbestosis

EXCLUDES 1 pleural plaque with asbestosis (J92.0)
pneumoconiosis with tuberculosis, any type in A15 (J65)

✓4ᵗʰ J62 Pneumoconiosis due to dust containing silica

INCLUDES silicotic fibrosis (massive) of lung

EXCLUDES 1 pneumoconiosis with tuberculosis, any type in A15 (J65)

J62.0 Pneumoconiosis due to talc dust

J62.8 Pneumoconiosis due to other dust containing silica
Silicosis NOS

✓4ᵗʰ J63 Pneumoconiosis due to other inorganic dusts

EXCLUDES 1 pneumoconiosis with tuberculosis, any type in A15 (J65)

J63.0 Aluminosis (of lung)

J63.1 Bauxite fibrosis (of lung)

J63.2 Berylliosis

J63.3 Graphite fibrosis (of lung)

J63.4 Siderosis

J63.5 Stannosis

J63.6 Pneumoconiosis due to other specified inorganic dusts

J64 Unspecified pneumoconiosis

EXCLUDES 1 pneumonoconiosis with tuberculosis, any type in A15 (J65)

J65 Pneumoconiosis associated with tuberculosis
Any condition in J60-J64 with tuberculosis, any type in A15
Silicotuberculosis

✓4ᵗʰ J66 Airway disease due to specific organic dust

EXCLUDES 2 allergic alveolitis (J67.-)
asbestosis (J61)
bagassosis (J67.1)
farmer's lung (J67.0)
hypersensitivity pneumonitis due to organic dust (J67.-)
reactive airways dysfunction syndrome (J68.3)

J66.0 Byssinosis
Airway disease due to cotton dust

J66.1 Flax-dressers' disease

J66.2 Cannabinosis

J66.8 Airway disease due to other specific organic dusts

✓4ᵗʰ J67 Hypersensitivity pneumonitis due to organic dust

INCLUDES allergic alveolitis and pneumonitis due to inhaled organic dust and particles of fungal, actinomycetic or other origin

EXCLUDES 1 pneumonitis due to inhalation of chemicals, gases, fumes or vapors (J68.0)

J67.0 Farmer's lung
Harvester's lung   Moldy hay disease
Haymaker's lung

J67.1 Bagassosis
Bagasse disease   Bagasse pneumonitis

J67.2 Bird fancier's lung
Budgerigar fancier's disease or lung
Pigeon fancier's disease or lung

J67.3 Suberosis
Corkhandler's disease or lung
Corkworker's disease or lung

J67.4 Maltworker's lung
Alveolitis due to Aspergillus clavatus

J67.5 Mushroom-worker's lung

J67.6 Maple-bark-stripper's lung
Alveolitis due to Cryptostroma corticale
Cryptostromosis

J67.7 Air conditioner and humidifier lung
Allergic alveolitis due to fungal, thermophilic actinomycetes and other organisms growing in ventilation [air conditioning] systems

J67.8 Hypersensitivity pneumonitis due to other organic dusts
Cheese-washer's lung   Furrier's lung
Coffee-worker's lung   Sequoiosis
Fish-meal worker's lung

✓ Additional Character Required   ✓x7ᵗʰ Placeholder Alert   Unspecified Dx   Other Specified Dx   Manifestation   ►◄ Revised Text   ● New Code   ▲ Revised Code Title

Chapter 10. Diseases of the Respiratory System

J67.9   **Hypersensitivity pneumonitis due to unspecified organic dust**
Allergic alveolitis (extrinsic) NOS
Hypersensitivity pneumonitis NOS

✓4ᵗʰ **J68**   **Respiratory conditions due to inhalation of chemicals, gases, fumes and vapors**
Code first (T51-T65) to identify cause
Use additional code to identify associated respiratory conditions, such as:
    acute respiratory failure (J96.Ø-)

J68.Ø   **Bronchitis and pneumonitis due to chemicals, gases, fumes and vapors**
Chemical bronchitis (acute)

J68.1   **Pulmonary edema due to chemicals, gases, fumes and vapors**
Chemical pulmonary edema (acute) (chronic)
EXCLUDES 1   *pulmonary edema (acute) (chronic) NOS (J81.-)*

J68.2   **Upper respiratory inflammation due to chemicals, gases, fumes and vapors, not elsewhere classified**

J68.3   **Other acute and subacute respiratory conditions due to chemicals, gases, fumes and vapors**
Reactive airways dysfunction syndrome

J68.4   **Chronic respiratory conditions due to chemicals, gases, fumes and vapors**
Emphysema (diffuse) (chronic) due to inhalation of chemicals, gases, fumes and vapors
Obliterative bronchiolitis (chronic) (subacute) due to inhalation of chemicals, gases, fumes and vapors
Pulmonary fibrosis (chronic) due to inhalation of chemicals, gases, fumes and vapors
EXCLUDES 1   *chronic pulmonary edema due to chemicals, gases, fumes and vapors (J68.1)*

J68.8   **Other respiratory conditions due to chemicals, gases, fumes and vapors**

J68.9   **Unspecified respiratory condition due to chemicals, gases, fumes and vapors**

✓4ᵗʰ **J69**   **Pneumonitis due to solids and liquids**
EXCLUDES 1   *neonatal aspiration syndromes (P24.-)*
    postprocedural pneumonitis (J95.4)

J69.Ø   **Pneumonitis due to inhalation of food and vomit**
Aspiration pneumonia NOS
Aspiration pneumonia (due to) food (regurgitated)
Aspiration pneumonia (due to) gastric secretions
Aspiration pneumonia (due to) milk
Aspiration pneumonia (due to) vomit
Code also any associated foreign body in respiratory tract (T17.-)
EXCLUDES 1   *chemical pneumonitis due to anesthesia (J95.4)*
    obstetric aspiration pneumonitis (O74.Ø)

J69.1   **Pneumonitis due to inhalation of oils and essences**
Exogenous lipoid pneumonia
Lipid pneumonia NOS
Code first (T51-T65) to identify substance
EXCLUDES 1   *endogenous lipoid pneumonia (J84.89)*

J69.8   **Pneumonitis due to inhalation of other solids and liquids**
Pneumonitis due to aspiration of blood
Pneumonitis due to aspiration of detergent
Code first (T51-T65) to identify substance

✓4ᵗʰ **J70**   **Respiratory conditions due to other external agents**

J70.Ø   **Acute pulmonary manifestations due to radiation**
Radiation pneumonitis
Use additional code (W88-W90, X39.Ø-) to identify the external cause

J70.1   **Chronic and other pulmonary manifestations due to radiation**
Fibrosis of lung following radiation
Use additional code (W88-W90, X39.Ø-) to identify the external cause

J70.2   **Acute drug-induced interstitial lung disorders**
Use additional code for adverse effect, if applicable, to identify drug (T36-T5Ø with fifth or sixth character 5)
EXCLUDES 1   *interstitial pneumonia NOS (J84.9)*
    lymphoid interstitial pneumonia (J84.2)

J70.3   **Chronic drug-induced interstitial lung disorders**
Use additional code for adverse effect, if applicable, to identify drug (T36-T5Ø with fifth or sixth character 5)
EXCLUDES 1   *interstitial pneumonia NOS (J84.9)*
    lymphoid interstitial pneumonia (J84.2)

J70.4   **Drug-induced interstitial lung disorders, unspecified**
Use additional code for adverse effect, if applicable, to identify drug (T36-T5Ø with fifth or sixth character 5)
EXCLUDES 1   *interstitial pneumonia NOS (J84.9)*
    lymphoid interstitial pneumonia (J84.2)

J70.5   **Respiratory conditions due to smoke inhalation**
Smoke inhalation NOS
EXCLUDES 1   *smoke inhalation due to chemicals, gases, fumes and vapors (J68.9)*
AHA: 2013, 4Q, 121

J70.8   **Respiratory conditions due to other specified external agents**
Code first (T51-T65) to identify the external agent

J70.9   **Respiratory conditions due to unspecified external agent**
Code first (T51-T65) to identify the external agent

Other respiratory diseases principally affecting the interstitium (J8Ø-J84)

J80   **Acute respiratory distress syndrome**
Acute respiratory distress syndrome in adult or child
Adult hyaline membrane disease
EXCLUDES 1   *respiratory distress syndrome in newborn (perinatal) (P22.Ø)*

✓4ᵗʰ **J81**   **Pulmonary edema**
Use additional code to identify:
    exposure to environmental tobacco smoke (Z77.22)
    history of tobacco use (Z87.891)
    occupational exposure to environmental tobacco smoke (Z57.31)
    tobacco dependence (F17.-)
    tobacco use (Z72.Ø)
EXCLUDES 1   *chemical (acute) pulmonary edema (J68.1)*
    hypostatic pneumonia (J18.2)
    passive pneumonia (J18.2)
    pulmonary edema due to external agents (J6Ø-J70)
    pulmonary edema with heart disease NOS (I5Ø.1)
    pulmonary edema with heart failure (I5Ø.1)

J81.Ø   **Acute pulmonary edema**
Acute edema of lung

J81.1   **Chronic pulmonary edema**
Pulmonary congestion (chronic) (passive)
Pulmonary edema NOS

J82   **Pulmonary eosinophilia, not elsewhere classified**
Allergic pneumonia
Eosinophilic asthma
Eosinophilic pneumonia
Löffler's pneumonia
Tropical (pulmonary) eosinophilia NOS
EXCLUDES 1   *pulmonary eosinophilia due to aspergillosis (B44.-)*
    pulmonary eosinophilia due to drugs (J70.2-J70.4)
    pulmonary eosinophilia due to specified parasitic infection (B5Ø-B83)
    pulmonary eosinophilia due to systemic connective tissue disorders (M3Ø-M36)
    pulmonary infiltrate NOS (R91.8)

✓4ᵗʰ **J84**   **Other interstitial pulmonary diseases**
EXCLUDES 1   *drug-induced interstitial lung disorders (J70.2-J70.4)*
    interstitial emphysema (J98.2)
    lung diseases due to external agents (J6Ø-J70)

✓5ᵗʰ **J84.Ø**   **Alveolar and parieto-alveolar conditions**

J84.Ø1   **Alveolar proteinosis**

J84.Ø2   **Pulmonary alveolar microlithiasis**

J84.Ø3   ***Idiopathic pulmonary hemosiderosis***
Essential brown induration of lung
Code first underlying disease, such as:
    disorders of iron metabolism (E83.1-)
EXCLUDES 1   *acute idiopathic pulmonary hemorrhage in infants [AIPHI] (RØ4.81)*

J84.Ø9   **Other alveolar and parieto-alveolar conditions**

✓5ᵗʰ **J84.1**   **Other interstitial pulmonary diseases with fibrosis**
EXCLUDES 1   *pulmonary fibrosis (chronic) due to inhalation of chemicals, gases, fumes or vapors (J68.4)*
    pulmonary fibrosis (chronic) following radiation (J70.1)

J84.10   **Pulmonary fibrosis, unspecified**
Capillary fibrosis of lung
Cirrhosis of lung (chronic) NOS
Fibrosis of lung (atrophic) (chronic) (confluent) (massive) (perialveolar) (peribronchial) NOS
Induration of lung (chronic) NOS
Postinflammatory pulmonary fibrosis

✓6ᵗʰ **J84.11**   **Idiopathic interstitial pneumonia**
EXCLUDES 1   *lymphoid interstitial pneumonia (J84.2)*
    pneumocystis pneumonia (B59)

J84.111   **Idiopathic interstitial pneumonia, not otherwise specified**

EXCLUDES 1 Not coded here   *EXCLUDES 2* Not included here   N Newborn Age: 0   P Pediatric Age: 0-17   M Maternity Age: 12-55   A Adult Age: 15-124

626   ICD-10-CM 2016

J84.112 **Idiopathic pulmonary fibrosis**
    Cryptogenic fibrosing alveolitis
    Idiopathic fibrosing alveolitis

J84.113 **Idiopathic non-specific interstitial pneumonitis**
    EXCLUDES 1 *non-specific interstitial pneumonia NOS, or due to known underlying cause (J84.89)*

J84.114 **Acute interstitial pneumonitis**
    Hamman-Rich syndrome
    EXCLUDES 1 *pneumocystis pneumonia (B59)*

J84.115 **Respiratory bronchiolitis interstitial lung disease**

J84.116 **Cryptogenic organizing pneumonia**
    EXCLUDES 1 *organizing pneumonia NOS, or due to known underlying cause (J84.89)*

J84.117 **Desquamative interstitial pneumonia**

J84.17 *Other interstitial pulmonary diseases with fibrosis in diseases classified elsewhere*
    Interstitial pneumonia (nonspecific) (usual) due to collagen vascular disease
    Interstitial pneumonia (nonspecific) (usual) in diseases classified elsewhere
    Organizing pneumonia due to collagen vascular disease
    Organizing pneumonia in diseases classified elsewhere
    Code first underlying disease, such as:
      progressive systemic sclerosis (M34.0)
      rheumatoid arthritis (M05.00-M06.9)
      systemic lupus erythematosis (M32.0-M32.9)

J84.2 **Lymphoid interstitial pneumonia**
    Lymphoid interstitial pneumonitis

✓5ᵗʰ **J84.8** **Other specified interstitial pulmonary diseases**
    EXCLUDES 1 *exogenous lipoid pneumonia (J69.1)*
               unspecified lipoid pneumonia (J69.1)

J84.81 **Lymphangioleiomyomatosis** ♀
    Lymphangiomyomatosis

J84.82 **Adult pulmonary Langerhans cell histiocytosis** Ⓐ
    Adult PLCH

J84.83 **Surfactant mutations of the lung**

✓6ᵗʰ **J84.84** **Other interstitial lung diseases of childhood**

J84.841 **Neuroendocrine cell hyperplasia of infancy**

J84.842 **Pulmonary interstitial glycogenosis**

J84.843 **Alveolar capillary dysplasia with vein misalignment**

J84.848 **Other interstitial lung diseases of childhood** Ⓟ

J84.89 **Other specified interstitial pulmonary diseases**
    Endogenous lipoid pneumonia
    Interstitial pneumonitis
    Non-specific interstitial pneumonitis NOS
    Organizing pneumonia due to known underlying cause
    Organizing pneumonia NOS
    Code first, if applicable:
      poisoning due to drug or toxin (T51-T65 with fifth or sixth character to indicate intent), for toxic pneumonopathy
    underlying cause of pneumonopathy, if known
    Use additional code, for adverse effect, to identify drug (T36-T50 with fifth or sixth character 5), if drug-induced
    EXCLUDES 1 *cryptogenic organizing pneumonia (J84.116)*
               idiopathic non-specific interstitial pneumonitis (J84.113)
               lipoid pneumonia, exogenous or unspecified (J69.1)
               lymphoid interstitial pneumonia (J84.2)

J84.9 **Interstitial pulmonary disease, unspecified**
    Interstitial pneumonia NOS

Suppurative and necrotic conditions of the lower respiratory tract (J85-J86)

✓4ᵗʰ **J85** **Abscess of lung and mediastinum**
    Use additional code (B95-B97) to identify infectious agent.

J85.0 **Gangrene and necrosis of lung**

J85.1 **Abscess of lung with pneumonia**
    Code also the type of pneumonia

J85.2 **Abscess of lung without pneumonia**
    Abscess of lung NOS

J85.3 **Abscess of mediastinum**

✓4ᵗʰ **J86** **Pyothorax**
    Use additional code (B95-B97) to identify infectious agent
    EXCLUDES 1 *abscess of lung (J85.-)*
               pyothorax due to tuberculosis (A15.6)

J86.0 **Pyothorax with fistula**
    Bronchocutaneous fistula
    Bronchopleural fistula
    Hepatopleural fistula
    Mediastinal fistula
    Pleural fistula
    Thoracic fistula
    Any condition classifiable to J86.9 with fistula

J86.9 **Pyothorax without fistula**
    Abscess of pleura
    Abscess of thorax
    Empyema (chest) (lung) (pleura)
    Fibrinopurulent pleurisy
    Purulent pleurisy
    Pyopneumothorax
    Septic pleurisy
    Seropurulent pleurisy
    Suppurative pleurisy

Other diseases of the pleura (J90-J94)

J90 **Pleural effusion, not elsewhere classified**
    Encysted pleurisy
    Pleural effusion NOS
    Pleurisy with effusion (exudative) (serous)
    EXCLUDES 1 *chylous (pleural) effusion (J94.0)*
               malignant pleural effusion (J91.0))
               pleurisy NOS (R09.1)
               tuberculous pleural effusion (A15.6)

✓4ᵗʰ **J91** **Pleural effusion in conditions classified elsewhere**
    EXCLUDES 2 *pleural effusion in heart failure (I50.-)*
               pleural effusion in systemic lupus erythematosus (M32.13)

J91.0 *Malignant pleural effusion*
    Code first underlying neoplasm

J91.8 *Pleural effusion in other conditions classified elsewhere*
    Code first underlying disease, such as:
      filariasis (B74.0-B74.9)
      influenza (J09.X2, J10.1, J11.1)

✓4ᵗʰ **J92** **Pleural plaque**
    INCLUDES pleural thickening

J92.0 **Pleural plaque with presence of asbestos**

J92.9 **Pleural plaque without asbestos**
    Pleural plaque NOS

✓4ᵗʰ **J93** **Pneumothorax and air leak**
    EXCLUDES 1 *congenital or perinatal pneumothorax (P25.1)*
               postprocedural air leak (J95.812)
               postprocedural pneumothorax (J95.811)
               traumatic pneumothorax (S27.0)
               tuberculous (current disease) pneumothorax (A15.-)
               pyopneumothorax (J86.-)

J93.0 **Spontaneous tension pneumothorax**

✓5ᵗʰ **J93.1** **Other spontaneous pneumothorax**

J93.11 **Primary spontaneous pneumothorax**

J93.12 **Secondary spontaneous pneumothorax**
    Code first underlying condition, such as:
      catamenial pneumothorax due to endometriosis (N80.8)
      cystic fibrosis (E84.-)
      eosinophilic pneumonia (J82)
      lymphangioleiomyomatosis (J84.81)
      malignant neoplasm of bronchus and lung (C34.-)
      Marfan's syndrome (Q87.4)
      pneumonia due to Pneumocystis carinii (B59)
      secondary malignant neoplasm of lung (C78.0-)
      spontaneous rupture of the esophagus (K22.3)

☑ Additional Character Required   ✓x7ᵗʰ Placeholder Alert   Unspecified Dx   Other Specified Dx   Manifestation   ▶◀ Revised Text   ● New Code   ▲ Revised Code Title

Chapter 10. Diseases of the Respiratory System

J93.8–J96.11

✓5ᵗʰ **J93.8**   Other pneumothorax and air leak

   J93.81   Chronic pneumothorax

   J93.82   Other air leak
       Persistent air leak

   J93.83   Other pneumothorax
       Acute pneumothorax
       Spontaneous pneumothorax NOS

J93.9   Pneumothorax, unspecified
       Pneumothorax NOS

✓4ᵗʰ **J94**   **Other pleural conditions**
   EXCLUDES 1   pleurisy NOS (R09.1)
       traumatic hemopneumothorax (S27.2)
       traumatic hemothorax (S27.1)
       tuberculous pleural conditions (current disease) (A15.-)

J94.0   Chylous effusion
       Chyliform effusion

J94.1   Fibrothorax

J94.2   Hemothorax
       Hemopneumothorax

J94.8   Other specified pleural conditions
       Hydropneumothorax
       Hydrothorax

J94.9   Pleural condition, unspecified

Intraoperative and postprocedural complications and disorders of respiratory system, not elsewhere classified (J95)

✓4ᵗʰ **J95**   **Intraoperative and postprocedural complications and disorders of respiratory system, not elsewhere classified**
   EXCLUDES 2   aspiration pneumonia (J69.-)
       emphysema (subcutaneous) resulting from a procedure (T81.82)
       hypostatic pneumonia (J18.2)
       pulmonary manifestations due to radiation (J70.0- J70.1)

✓5ᵗʰ **J95.0**   Tracheostomy complications

   J95.00   Unspecified tracheostomy complication

   J95.01   Hemorrhage from tracheostomy stoma

   J95.02   Infection of tracheostomy stoma
       Use additional code to identify type of infection, such as:
         cellulitis of neck (L03.8)
         sepsis (A40, A41-)

   J95.03   Malfunction of tracheostomy stoma
       Mechanical complication of tracheostomy stoma
       Obstruction of tracheostomy airway
       Tracheal stenosis due to tracheostomy

   J95.04   Tracheo-esophageal fistula following tracheostomy

   J95.09   Other tracheostomy complication

J95.1   Acute pulmonary insufficiency following thoracic surgery
   EXCLUDES 2   functional disturbances following cardiac surgery (I97.0, I97.1-)

J95.2   Acute pulmonary insufficiency following nonthoracic surgery
   EXCLUDES 2   functional disturbances following cardiac surgery (I97.0, I97.1-)

J95.3   Chronic pulmonary insufficiency following surgery
   EXCLUDES 2   functional disturbances following cardiac surgery (I97.0, I97.1-)

J95.4   Chemical pneumonitis due to anesthesia
       Mendelson's syndrome
       Postprocedural aspiration pneumonia
       Use additional code for adverse effect, if applicable, to identify drug (T41.- with fifth or sixth character 5)
   EXCLUDES 1   aspiration pneumonitis due to anesthesia complicating labor and delivery (O74.0)
       aspiration pneumonitis due to anesthesia complicating pregnancy (O29)
       aspiration pneumonitis due to anesthesia complicating the puerperium (O89.01)

J95.5   Postprocedural subglottic stenosis

✓5ᵗʰ **J95.6**   Intraoperative hemorrhage and hematoma of a respiratory system organ or structure complicating a procedure
   EXCLUDES 1   intraoperative hemorrhage and hematoma of a respiratory system organ or structure due to accidental puncture and laceration during procedure (J95.7-)

   J95.61   Intraoperative hemorrhage and hematoma of a respiratory system organ or structure complicating a respiratory system procedure

   J95.62   Intraoperative hemorrhage and hematoma of a respiratory system organ or structure complicating other procedure

✓5ᵗʰ **J95.7**   Accidental puncture and laceration of a respiratory system organ or structure during a procedure
   EXCLUDES 2   postprocedural pneumothorax (J95.811)

   J95.71   Accidental puncture and laceration of a respiratory system organ or structure during a respiratory system procedure

   J95.72   Accidental puncture and laceration of a respiratory system organ or structure during other procedure

✓5ᵗʰ **J95.8**   Other intraoperative and postprocedural complications and disorders of respiratory system, not elsewhere classified

  ✓6ᵗʰ **J95.81**   Postprocedural pneumothorax and air leak

     J95.811   Postprocedural pneumothorax

     J95.812   Postprocedural air leak

  ✓6ᵗʰ **J95.82**   Postprocedural respiratory failure
     EXCLUDES 1   respiratory failure in other conditions (J96.-)

     J95.821   Acute postprocedural respiratory failure
        Postprocedural respiratory failure NOS

     J95.822   Acute and chronic postprocedural respiratory failure

  ✓6ᵗʰ **J95.83**   Postprocedural hemorrhage and hematoma of a respiratory system organ or structure following a procedure

     J95.830   Postprocedural hemorrhage and hematoma of a respiratory system organ or structure following a respiratory system procedure

     J95.831   Postprocedural hemorrhage and hematoma of a respiratory system organ or structure following other procedure

   J95.84   Transfusion-related acute lung injury (TRALI)

  ✓6ᵗʰ **J95.85**   Complication of respirator [ventilator]

     J95.850   Mechanical complication of respirator
       EXCLUDES 1   encounter for respirator [ventilator] dependence during power failure (Z99.12)

     J95.851   Ventilator associated pneumonia
       Ventilator associated pneumonitis
       Use additional code to identify the organism, if known (B95.-, B96.-, B97.-)
       EXCLUDES 1   ventilator lung in newborn (P27.8)

     J95.859   Other complication of respirator [ventilator]

   J95.88   Other intraoperative complications of respiratory system, not elsewhere classified

   J95.89   Other postprocedural complications and disorders of respiratory system, not elsewhere classified
       Use additional code to identify disorder, such as:
         aspiration pneumonia (J69.-)
         bacterial or viral pneumonia (J12-J18)
       EXCLUDES 2   acute pulmonary insufficiency following thoracic surgery (J95.1)
         postprocedural subglottic stenosis (J95.5)

Other diseases of the respiratory system (J96-J99)

✓4ᵗʰ **J96**   **Respiratory failure, not elsewhere classified**
   EXCLUDES 1   acute respiratory distress syndrome (J80)
       cardiorespiratory failure (R09.2)
       newborn respiratory distress syndrome (P22.0)
       postprocedural respiratory failure (J95.82-)
       respiratory arrest (R09.2)
       respiratory arrest of newborn (P28.81)
       respiratory failure of newborn (P28.5)

✓5ᵗʰ **J96.0**   Acute respiratory failure

   J96.00   Acute respiratory failure, unspecified whether with hypoxia or hypercapnia
       AHA: 2013, 4Q, 121

   J96.01   Acute respiratory failure with hypoxia

   J96.02   Acute respiratory failure with hypercapnia

✓5ᵗʰ **J96.1**   Chronic respiratory failure

   J96.10   Chronic respiratory failure, unspecified whether with hypoxia or hypercapnia
       AHA: 2015, 1Q, 21

   J96.11   Chronic respiratory failure with hypoxia
       AHA: 2013, 4Q, 129

EXCLUDES 1 Not coded here   *EXCLUDES 2* Not included here   N Newborn Age: 0   P Pediatric Age: 0-17   M Maternity Age: 12-55   A Adult Age: 15-124

628   ICD-10-CM 2016

    J96.12   **Chronic respiratory failure with** hypercapnia

☑5ᵗʰ **J96.2** Acute and chronic **respiratory failure**
    Acute on chronic respiratory failure

    J96.20   **Acute and chronic respiratory failure,** unspecified
          whether with hypoxia or hypercapnia

    J96.21   **Acute and chronic respiratory failure with** hypoxia

    J96.22   **Acute and chronic respiratory failure with**
          hypercapnia

☑5ᵗʰ **J96.9** **Respiratory failure,** unspecified

    J96.90   **Respiratory failure, unspecified,** unspecified
          whether with hypoxia or hypercapnia

    J96.91   **Respiratory failure, unspecified with** hypoxia

    J96.92   **Respiratory failure, unspecified with** hypercapnia

☑4ᵗʰ **J98** **Other respiratory disorders**
    Use additional code to identify:
      exposure to environmental tobacco smoke (Z77.22)
      exposure to tobacco smoke in the perinatal period (P96.81)
      history of tobacco use (Z87.891)
      occupational exposure to environmental tobacco smoke (Z57.31)
      tobacco dependence (F17.-)
      tobacco use (Z72.0)
    EXCLUDES 1   *newborn apnea (P28.4)*
          newborn sleep apnea (P28.3)
    EXCLUDES 2   *apnea NOS (R06.81)*
          sleep apnea (G47.3-)

☑5ᵗʰ **J98.0** **Diseases of bronchus, not elsewhere classified**

    J98.01   **Acute bronchospasm**
        EXCLUDES 1   *acute bronchiolitis with bronchospasm*
             (J21.-)
            acute bronchitis with bronchospasm (J20.-)
            asthma (J45.-)
            exercise induced bronchospasm (J45.990)

    J98.09   **Other diseases of bronchus, not elsewhere classified**
        Broncholithiasis
        Calcification of bronchus
        Stenosis of bronchus
        Tracheobronchial collapse
        Tracheobronchial dyskinesia
        Ulcer of bronchus

☑5ᵗʰ **J98.1** **Pulmonary collapse**
    EXCLUDES 1   *therapeutic collapse of lung status (Z98.3)*

    J98.11   **Atelectasis**
        EXCLUDES 1   *newborn atelectasis*
             tuberculous atelectasis (current disease)
               (A15)

    J98.19   **Other pulmonary collapse**

  J98.2 **Interstitial emphysema**
    Mediastinal emphysema
    EXCLUDES 1   *emphysema NOS (J43.9)*
          emphysema in newborn (P25.0)
          surgical emphysema (subcutaneous) (T81.82)
          traumatic subcutaneous emphysema (T79.7)

  J98.3 **Compensatory emphysema**

  J98.4 **Other disorders of lung**
    Calcification of lung
    Cystic lung disease (acquired)
    Lung disease NOS
    Pulmolithiasis
    EXCLUDES 1   *acute interstitial pneumonitis (J84.114)*
          pulmonary insufficiency following surgery (J95.1-J95.2)

  J98.5 **Diseases of mediastinum, not elsewhere classified**
    Fibrosis of mediastinum
    Hernia of mediastinum
    Retraction of mediastinum
    Mediastinitis
    EXCLUDES 2   *abscess of mediastinum (J85.3)*

  J98.6 **Disorders of diaphragm**
    Diaphragmatitis
    Paralysis of diaphragm
    Relaxation of diaphragm
    EXCLUDES 1   *congenital malformation of diaphragm NEC (Q79.1)*
          congenital diaphragmatic hernia (Q79.0)
    EXCLUDES 2   *diaphragmatic hernia (K44.-)*

  J98.8 **Other specified respiratory disorders**

  J98.9 **Respiratory disorder, unspecified**
    Respiratory disease (chronic) NOS

J99 *Respiratory disorders in diseases classified elsewhere*
    Code first underlying disease, such as:
      amyloidosis (E85.-)
      ankylosing spondylitis (M45)
      congenital syphilis (A50.5)
      cryoglobulinemia (D89.1)
      early congenital syphilis (A50.0)
      schistosomiasis (B65.0-B65.9)
    EXCLUDES 1   *respiratory disorders in:*
        amebiasis (A06.5)
        blastomycosis (B40.0-B40.2)
        candidiasis (B37.1)
        coccidioidomycosis (B38.0-B38.2)
        cystic fibrosis with pulmonary manifestations (E84.0)
        dermatomyositis (M33.01, M33.11)
        histoplasmosis (B39.0-B39.2)
        late syphilis (A52.72, A52.73)
        polymyositis (M33.21)
        sicca syndrome (M35.02)
        systemic lupus erythematosus (M32.13)
        systemic sclerosis (M34.81)
        Wegener's granulomatosis (M31.30-M31.31)

☑ Additional Character Required   ☑x7ᵗʰ Placeholder Alert   Unspecified Dx   Other Specified Dx   Manifestation   ▶◀ Revised Text   ● New Code   ▲ Revised Code Title

Chapter 11. Diseases of the Digestive System (KØØ–K95)

Chapter Specific Coding Guidelines and Examples
Reserved for future guideline expansion.

Chapter 11. Diseases of the Digestive System (K00-K95)

> EXCLUDES 2   *certain conditions originating in the perinatal period (P04-P96)*
> *certain infectious and parasitic diseases (A00-B99)*
> *complications of pregnancy, childbirth and the puerperium (O00-O9A)*
> *congenital malformations, deformations and chromosomal abnormalities (Q00-Q99)*
> *endocrine, nutritional and metabolic diseases (E00-E88)*
> *injury, poisoning and certain other consequences of external causes (S00-T88)*
> *neoplasms (C00-D49)*
> *symptoms, signs and abnormal clinical and laboratory findings, not elsewhere classified (R00-R94)*

This chapter contains the following blocks:

K00-K14	Diseases of oral cavity and salivary glands
K20-K31	Diseases of esophagus, stomach and duodenum
K35-K38	Diseases of appendix
K40-K46	Hernia
K50-K52	Noninfective enteritis and colitis
K55-K64	Other diseases of intestines
K65-K68	Diseases of peritoneum and retroperitoneum
K70-K77	Diseases of liver
K80-K87	Disorders of gallbladder, biliary tract and pancreas
K90-K95	Other diseases of the digestive system

Diseases of oral cavity and salivary glands (K00-K14)

☑4ᵗʰ **K00**   **Disorders of tooth development and eruption**
> EXCLUDES 2   *embedded and impacted teeth (K01.-)*

K00.0   **Anodontia**
Hypodontia
Oligodontia
> EXCLUDES 1   *acquired absence of teeth (K08.1-)*

K00.1   **Supernumerary teeth**
Distomolar
Fourth molar
Mesiodens
Paramolar
Supplementary teeth
> EXCLUDES 2   *supernumerary roots (K00.2)*

K00.2   **Abnormalities of size and form of teeth**
Concrescence of teeth
Dens evaginatus
Dens in dente
Dens invaginatus
Enamel pearls
Fusion of teeth
Gemination of teeth
Macrodontia
Microdontia
Peg-shaped [conical] teeth
Supernumerary roots
Taurodontism
Tuberculum paramolare
> EXCLUDES 1   *abnormalities of teeth due to congenital syphilis (A50.5)*
> *tuberculum Carabelli, which is regarded as a normal variation and should not be coded*

K00.3   **Mottled teeth**
Dental fluorosis
Mottling of enamel
Nonfluoride enamel opacities
> EXCLUDES 2   *deposits [accretions] on teeth (K03.6)*

K00.4   **Disturbances in tooth formation**
Aplasia and hypoplasia of cementum
Dilaceration of tooth
Enamel hypoplasia (neonatal) (postnatal) (prenatal)
Regional odontodysplasia
Turner's tooth
> EXCLUDES 1   *Hutchinson's teeth and mulberry molars in congenital syphilis (A50.5)*
> EXCLUDES 2   *mottled teeth (K00.3)*

K00.5   **Hereditary disturbances in tooth structure, not elsewhere classified**
Amelogenesis imperfecta
Dentinogenesis imperfecta
Odontogenesis imperfecta
Dentinal dysplasia
Shell teeth

K00.6   **Disturbances in tooth eruption**
Dentia praecox
Natal tooth
Neonatal tooth
Premature eruption of tooth
Premature shedding of primary [deciduous] tooth
Prenatal teeth
Retained [persistent] primary tooth
> EXCLUDES 2   *embedded and impacted teeth (K01.-)*

K00.7   **Teething syndrome**

K00.8   **Other disorders of tooth development**
Color changes during tooth formation
Intrinsic staining of teeth NOS
> EXCLUDES 2   *posteruptive color changes (K03.7)*

K00.9   **Disorder of tooth development, unspecified**
Disorder of odontogenesis NOS

☑4ᵗʰ **K01**   **Embedded and impacted teeth**
> EXCLUDES 1   *abnormal position of fully erupted teeth (M26.3-)*

K01.0   **Embedded teeth**

K01.1   **Impacted teeth**

☑4ᵗʰ **K02**   **Dental caries**
Dental cavities
Tooth decay

K02.3   **Arrested dental caries**
Arrested coronal and root caries

☑5ᵗʰ **K02.5**   **Dental caries on pit and fissure surface**
Dental caries on chewing surface of tooth

     K02.51   **Dental caries on pit and fissure surface limited to enamel**
White spot lesions [initial caries] on pit and fissure surface of tooth

     K02.52   **Dental caries on pit and fissure surface penetrating into dentin**

     K02.53   **Dental caries on pit and fissure surface penetrating into pulp**

☑5ᵗʰ **K02.6**   **Dental caries on smooth surface**

     K02.61   **Dental caries on smooth surface limited to enamel**
White spot lesions [initial caries] on smooth surface of tooth

     K02.62   **Dental caries on smooth surface penetrating into dentin**

     K02.63   **Dental caries on smooth surface penetrating into pulp**

K02.7   **Dental root caries**

K02.9   **Dental caries, unspecified**

☑4ᵗʰ **K03**   **Other diseases of hard tissues of teeth**
> EXCLUDES 2   *bruxism (F45.8)*
> *dental caries (K02.-)*
> *teeth-grinding NOS (F45.8)*

K03.0   **Excessive attrition of teeth**
Approximal wear of teeth
Occlusal wear of teeth

K03.1   **Abrasion of teeth**
Dentifrice abrasion of teeth
Habitual abrasion of teeth
Occupational abrasion of teeth
Ritual abrasion of teeth
Traditional abrasion of teeth
Wedge defect NOS

K03.2   **Erosion of teeth**
Erosion of teeth due to diet
Erosion of teeth due to drugs and medicaments
Erosion of teeth due to persistent vomiting
Erosion of teeth NOS
Idiopathic erosion of teeth
Occupational erosion of teeth

K03.3   **Pathological resorption of teeth**
Internal granuloma of pulp
Resorption of teeth (external)

K03.4   **Hypercementosis**
Cementation hyperplasia

K03.5   **Ankylosis of teeth**

☑ Additional Character Required   ✓ₓ7ᵗʰ Placeholder Alert   Unspecified Dx   Other Specified Dx   Manifestation   ▶◀ Revised Text   ● New Code   ▲ Revised Code Title

Chapter 11. Diseases of the Digestive System

K03.6   **Deposits [accretions] on teeth**
Betel deposits [accretions] on teeth
Black deposits [accretions] on teeth
Extrinsic staining of teeth NOS
Green deposits [accretions] on teeth
Materia alba deposits [accretions] on teeth
Orange deposits [accretions] on teeth
Staining of teeth NOS
Subgingival dental calculus
Supragingival dental calculus
Tobacco deposits [accretions] on teeth

K03.7   **Posteruptive color changes of dental hard tissues**
EXCLUDES 2   deposits [accretions] on teeth (K03.6)

✓5ᵗʰ **K03.8**   **Other specified diseases of hard tissues of teeth**

     K03.81   **Cracked tooth**
       EXCLUDES 1   asymptomatic craze lines in enamel—omit code
         broken or fractured tooth due to trauma (S02.5)

     K03.89   **Other specified diseases of hard tissues of teeth**

K03.9   **Disease of hard tissues of teeth, unspecified**

✓4ᵗʰ **K04**   **Diseases of pulp and periapical tissues**

K04.0   **Pulpitis**
Acute pulpitis
Chronic (hyperplastic) (ulcerative) pulpitis
Irreversible pulpitis
Reversible pulpitis

K04.1   **Necrosis of pulp**
Pulpal gangrene

K04.2   **Pulp degeneration**
Denticles
Pulpal calcifications
Pulpal stones

K04.3   **Abnormal hard tissue formation in pulp**
Secondary or irregular dentine

K04.4   **Acute apical periodontitis of pulpal origin**
Acute apical periodontitis NOS
EXCLUDES 1   acute periodontitis (K05.2-)

K04.5   **Chronic apical periodontitis**
Apical or periapical granuloma
Apical periodontitis NOS
EXCLUDES 1   chronic periodontitis (K05.3-)

K04.6   **Periapical abscess with sinus**
Dental abscess with sinus
Dentoalveolar abscess with sinus

K04.7   **Periapical abscess without sinus**
Dental abscess without sinus
Dentoalveolar abscess without sinus
Periapical abscess without sinus

K04.8   **Radicular cyst**
Apical (periodontal) cyst
Periapical cyst
Residual radicular cyst
EXCLUDES 2   lateral periodontal cyst (K09.0)

✓5ᵗʰ **K04.9**   **Other and unspecified diseases of pulp and periapical tissues**

     K04.90   **Unspecified diseases of pulp and periapical tissues**

     K04.99   **Other diseases of pulp and periapical tissues**

✓4ᵗʰ **K05**   **Gingivitis and periodontal diseases**
Use additional code to identify:
alcohol abuse and dependence (F10.-)
exposure to environmental tobacco smoke (Z77.22)
exposure to tobacco smoke in the perinatal period (P96.81)
history of tobacco use (Z87.891)
occupational exposure to environmental tobacco smoke (Z57.31)
tobacco dependence (F17.-)
tobacco use (Z72.0)

✓5ᵗʰ **K05.0**   **Acute gingivitis**
EXCLUDES 1   acute necrotizing ulcerative gingivitis (A69.1)
         herpesviral [herpes simplex] gingivostomatitis (B00.2)

     K05.00   **Acute gingivitis, plaque induced**
       Acute gingivitis NOS

     K05.01   **Acute gingivitis, non-plaque induced**

✓5ᵗʰ **K05.1**   **Chronic gingivitis**
Desquamative gingivitis (chronic)
Gingivitis (chronic) NOS
Hyperplastic gingivitis (chronic)
Simple marginal gingivitis (chronic)
Ulcerative gingivitis (chronic)

     K05.10   **Chronic gingivitis, plaque induced**
       Chronic gingivitis NOS
       Gingivitis NOS

     K05.11   **Chronic gingivitis, non-plaque induced**

✓5ᵗʰ **K05.2**   **Aggressive periodontitis**
Acute pericoronitis
EXCLUDES 1   acute apical periodontitis (K04.4)
         periapical abscess (K04.7)
         periapical abscess with sinus (K04.6)

     K05.20   **Aggressive periodontitis, unspecified**

     K05.21   **Aggressive periodontitis, localized**
       Periodontal abscess

     K05.22   **Aggressive periodontitis, generalized**

✓5ᵗʰ **K05.3**   **Chronic periodontitis**
Chronic pericoronitis
Complex periodontitis
Periodontitis NOS
Simplex periodontitis
EXCLUDES 1   chronic apical periodontitis (K04.5)

     K05.30   **Chronic periodontitis, unspecified**

     K05.31   **Chronic periodontitis, localized**

     K05.32   **Chronic periodontitis, generalized**

K05.4   **Periodontosis**
Juvenile periodontosis

K05.5   **Other periodontal diseases**
EXCLUDES 2   leukoplakia of gingiva (K13.21)

K05.6   **Periodontal disease, unspecified**

✓4ᵗʰ **K06**   **Other disorders of gingiva and edentulous alveolar ridge**
EXCLUDES 2   acute gingivitis (K05.0)
         atrophy of edentulous alveolar ridge (K08.2)
         chronic gingivitis (K05.1)
         gingivitis NOS (K05.1)

K06.0   **Gingival recession**
Gingival recession (generalized) (localized) (postinfective) (postprocedural)

K06.1   **Gingival enlargement**
Gingival fibromatosis

K06.2   **Gingival and edentulous alveolar ridge lesions associated with trauma**
Irritative hyperplasia of edentulous ridge [denture hyperplasia]
Use additional code (Chapter 20) to identify external cause or denture status (Z97.2)

K06.8   **Other specified disorders of gingiva and edentulous alveolar ridge**
Fibrous epulis
Flabby alveolar ridge
Giant cell epulis
Peripheral giant cell granuloma of gingiva
Pyogenic granuloma of gingiva
EXCLUDES 2   gingival cyst (K09.0)

K06.9   **Disorder of gingiva and edentulous alveolar ridge, unspecified**

✓4ᵗʰ **K08**   **Other disorders of teeth and supporting structures**
EXCLUDES 2   dentofacial anomalies [including malocclusion] (M26.-)
         disorders of jaw (M27.-)

K08.0   **Exfoliation of teeth due to systemic causes**
Code also underlying systemic condition

✓5ᵗʰ **K08.1**   **Complete loss of teeth**
Acquired loss of teeth, complete
EXCLUDES 1   congenital absence of teeth (K00.0)
         exfoliation of teeth due to systemic causes (K08.0)
         partial loss of teeth (K08.4-)

     ✓6ᵗʰ **K08.10**   **Complete loss of teeth, unspecified cause**

         K08.101   **Complete loss of teeth, unspecified cause, class I**

         K08.102   **Complete loss of teeth, unspecified cause, class II**

         K08.103   **Complete loss of teeth, unspecified cause, class III**

         K08.104   **Complete loss of teeth, unspecified cause, class IV**

EXCLUDES 1 Not coded here   *EXCLUDES 2* Not included here   **N** Newborn Age: 0   **P** Pediatric Age: 0-17   **M** Maternity Age: 12-55   **A** Adult Age: 15-124

632   ICD-10-CM 2016

K08.109   **Complete loss of teeth, unspecified cause, unspecified class**
     Edentulism NOS

✓6ᵗʰ **K08.11**   **Complete loss of teeth** due to trauma

K08.111   **Complete loss of teeth due to trauma, class I**

K08.112   **Complete loss of teeth due to trauma, class II**

K08.113   **Complete loss of teeth due to trauma, class III**

K08.114   **Complete loss of teeth due to trauma, class IV**

K08.119   **Complete loss of teeth due to trauma, unspecified class**

✓6ᵗʰ **K08.12**   **Complete loss of teeth due to** periodontal diseases

K08.121   **Complete loss of teeth due to periodontal diseases, class I**

K08.122   **Complete loss of teeth due to periodontal diseases, class II**

K08.123   **Complete loss of teeth due to periodontal diseases, class III**

K08.124   **Complete loss of teeth due to periodontal diseases, class IV**

K08.129   **Complete loss of teeth due to periodontal diseases, unspecified class**

✓6ᵗʰ **K08.13**   **Complete loss of teeth due to** caries

K08.131   **Complete loss of teeth due to caries, class I**

K08.132   **Complete loss of teeth due to caries, class II**

K08.133   **Complete loss of teeth due to caries, class III**

K08.134   **Complete loss of teeth due to caries, class IV**

K08.139   **Complete loss of teeth due to caries, unspecified class**

✓6ᵗʰ **K08.19**   **Complete loss of teeth due to** other specified cause

K08.191   **Complete loss of teeth due to other specified cause, class I**

K08.192   **Complete loss of teeth due to other specified cause, class II**

K08.193   **Complete loss of teeth due to other specified cause, class III**

K08.194   **Complete loss of teeth due to other specified cause, class IV**

K08.199   **Complete loss of teeth due to other specified cause, unspecified class**

✓5ᵗʰ **K08.2**   **Atrophy of edentulous alveolar ridge**

K08.20   **Unspecified atrophy of edentulous alveolar ridge**
     Atrophy of the mandible NOS
     Atrophy of the maxilla NOS

K08.21   **Minimal atrophy of the mandible**
     Minimal atrophy of the edentulous mandible

K08.22   **Moderate atrophy of the mandible**
     Moderate atrophy of the edentulous mandible

K08.23   **Severe atrophy of the mandible**
     Severe atrophy of the edentulous mandible

K08.24   **Minimal atrophy of maxilla**
     Minimal atrophy of the edentulous maxilla

K08.25   **Moderate atrophy of the maxilla**
     Moderate atrophy of the edentulous maxilla

K08.26   **Severe atrophy of the maxilla**
     Severe atrophy of the edentulous maxilla

K08.3   **Retained dental root**

✓5ᵗʰ **K08.4**   **Partial loss of teeth**
     Acquired loss of teeth, partial
     EXCLUDES 1   complete loss of teeth (K08.1-)
         congenital absence of teeth (K00.0)
     EXCLUDES 2   exfoliation of teeth due to systemic causes (K08.0)

✓6ᵗʰ **K08.40**   **Partial loss of teeth,** unspecified cause

K08.401   **Partial loss of teeth, unspecified cause, class I**

K08.402   **Partial loss of teeth, unspecified cause, class II**

K08.403   **Partial loss of teeth, unspecified cause, class III**

K08.404   **Partial loss of teeth, unspecified cause, class IV**

K08.409   **Partial loss of teeth, unspecified cause, unspecified class**
     Tooth extraction status NOS

✓6ᵗʰ **K08.41**   **Partial loss of teeth due to** trauma

K08.411   **Partial loss of teeth due to trauma, class I**

K08.412   **Partial loss of teeth due to trauma, class II**

K08.413   **Partial loss of teeth due to trauma, class III**

K08.414   **Partial loss of teeth due to trauma, class IV**

K08.419   **Partial loss of teeth due to trauma, unspecified class**

✓6ᵗʰ **K08.42**   **Partial loss of teeth due to** periodontal diseases

K08.421   **Partial loss of teeth due to periodontal diseases, class I**

K08.422   **Partial loss of teeth due to periodontal diseases, class II**

K08.423   **Partial loss of teeth due to periodontal diseases, class III**

K08.424   **Partial loss of teeth due to periodontal diseases, class IV**

K08.429   **Partial loss of teeth due to periodontal diseases, unspecified class**

✓6ᵗʰ **K08.43**   **Partial loss of teeth due to** caries

K08.431   **Partial loss of teeth due to caries, class I**

K08.432   **Partial loss of teeth due to caries, class II**

K08.433   **Partial loss of teeth due to caries, class III**

K08.434   **Partial loss of teeth due to caries, class IV**

K08.439   **Partial loss of teeth due to caries, unspecified class**

✓6ᵗʰ **K08.49**   **Partial loss of teeth due to** other specified cause

K08.491   **Partial loss of teeth due to other specified cause, class I**

K08.492   **Partial loss of teeth due to other specified cause, class II**

K08.493   **Partial loss of teeth due to other specified cause, class III**

K08.494   **Partial loss of teeth due to other specified cause, class IV**

K08.499   **Partial loss of teeth due to other specified cause, unspecified class**

✓5ᵗʰ **K08.5**   **Unsatisfactory restoration of tooth**
     Defective bridge, crown, filling
     Defective dental restoration
     EXCLUDES 1   dental restoration status (Z98.811)
     EXCLUDES 2   endosseous dental implant failure (M27.6-)
         unsatisfactory endodontic treatment (M27.5-)

K08.50   **Unsatisfactory restoration of tooth, unspecified**
     Defective dental restoration NOS

K08.51   **Open restoration margins of tooth**
     Dental restoration failure of marginal integrity
     Open margin on tooth restoration
     Poor gingival margin to tooth restoration

K08.52   **Unrepairable overhanging of dental restorative materials**
     Overhanging of tooth restoration

✓6ᵗʰ **K08.53**   **Fractured dental restorative material**
     EXCLUDES 1   cracked tooth (K03.81)
         traumatic fracture of tooth (S02.5)

K08.530   **Fractured dental restorative material without loss of material**

K08.531   **Fractured dental restorative material with loss of material**

K08.539   **Fractured dental restorative material, unspecified**

K08.54   **Contour of existing restoration of tooth biologically incompatible with oral health**
     Dental restoration failure of periodontal anatomical integrity
     Unacceptable contours of existing restoration of tooth
     Unacceptable morphology of existing restoration of tooth

K08.55   **Allergy to existing dental restorative material**
     Use additional code to identify the specific type of allergy

K08.56   **Poor aesthetic of existing restoration of tooth**
     Dental restoration aesthetically inadequate or displeasing

K08.59   **Other unsatisfactory restoration of tooth**
     Other defective dental restoration

✓ Additional Character Required   ✓x7ᵗʰ Placeholder Alert   Unspecified Dx   Other Specified Dx   Manifestation   ►◄ Revised Text   ● New Code   ▲ Revised Code Title

Chapter 11. Diseases of the Digestive System

K08.8   **Other specified disorders of teeth and supporting structures**
Enlargement of alveolar ridge NOS
Irregular alveolar process
Toothache NOS

K08.9   **Disorder of teeth and supporting structures, unspecified**

✓4th **K09**   **Cysts of oral region, not elsewhere classified**
    INCLUDES   lesions showing histological features both of aneurysmal cyst
            and of another fibro-osseous lesion
    EXCLUDES 2   cysts of jaw (M27.0-, M27.4-)
             radicular cyst (K04.8)

K09.0   **Developmental odontogenic cysts**
Dentigerous cyst
Eruption cyst
Follicular cyst
Gingival cyst
Lateral periodontal cyst
Primordial cyst
    EXCLUDES 2   keratocysts (D16.4, D16.5)
             odontogenic keratocystic tumors (D16.4, D16.5)

K09.1   **Developmental (nonodontogenic) cysts of oral region**
Cyst (of) incisive canal
Cyst (of) palatine of papilla
Globulomaxillary cyst
Median palatal cyst
Nasoalveolar cyst
Nasolabial cyst
Nasopalatine duct cyst

K09.8   **Other cysts of oral region, not elsewhere classified**
Dermoid cyst
Epidermoid cyst
Lymphoepithelial cyst
Epstein's pearl

K09.9   **Cyst of oral region, unspecified**

✓4th **K11**   **Diseases of salivary glands**
Use additional code to identify:
    alcohol abuse and dependence (F10.-)
    exposure to environmental tobacco smoke (Z77.22)
    exposure to tobacco smoke in the perinatal period (P96.81)
    history of tobacco use (Z87.891)
    occupational exposure to environmental tobacco smoke (Z57.31)
    tobacco dependence (F17.-)
    tobacco use (Z72.0)

K11.0   **Atrophy of salivary gland**

K11.1   **Hypertrophy of salivary gland**

✓5th **K11.2**   **Sialoadenitis**
Parotitis
    EXCLUDES 1   epidemic parotitis (B26.-)
             mumps (B26.-)
             uveoparotid fever [Heerfordt] (D86.89)

K11.20   **Sialoadenitis, unspecified**

K11.21   **Acute sialoadenitis**
    EXCLUDES 1   acute recurrent sialoadenitis (K11.22)

K11.22   **Acute recurrent sialoadenitis**

K11.23   **Chronic sialoadenitis**

K11.3   **Abscess of salivary gland**

K11.4   **Fistula of salivary gland**
    EXCLUDES 1   congenital fistula of salivary gland (Q38.4)

K11.5   **Sialolithiasis**
Calculus of salivary gland or duct
Stone of salivary gland or duct

K11.6   **Mucocele of salivary gland**
Mucous extravasation cyst of salivary gland
Mucous retention cyst of salivary gland
Ranula

K11.7   **Disturbances of salivary secretion**
Hypoptyalism
Ptyalism
Xerostomia
    EXCLUDES 2   dry mouth NOS (R68.2)

K11.8   **Other diseases of salivary glands**
Benign lymphoepithelial lesion of salivary gland
Mikulicz' disease
Necrotizing sialometaplasia
Sialectasia
Stenosis of salivary duct
Stricture of salivary duct
    EXCLUDES 1   sicca syndrome [Sjögren] (M35.0-)

K11.9   **Disease of salivary gland, unspecified**
Sialoadenopathy NOS

✓4th **K12**   **Stomatitis and related lesions**
Use additional code to identify:
    alcohol abuse and dependence (F10.-)
    exposure to environmental tobacco smoke (Z77.22)
    exposure to tobacco smoke in the perinatal period (P96.81)
    history of tobacco use (Z87.891)
    occupational exposure to environmental tobacco smoke (Z57.31)
    tobacco dependence (F17.-)
    tobacco use (Z72.0)
    EXCLUDES 1   cancrum oris (A69.0)
             cheilitis (K13.0)
             gangrenous stomatitis (A69.0)
             herpesviral [herpes simplex] gingivostomatitis (B00.2)
             noma (A69.0)

K12.0   **Recurrent oral aphthae**
Aphthous stomatitis (major) (minor)
Bednar's aphthae
Periadenitis mucosa necrotica recurrens
Recurrent aphthous ulcer
Stomatitis herpetiformis

K12.1   **Other forms of stomatitis**
Stomatitis NOS   Ulcerative stomatitis
Denture stomatitis   Vesicular stomatitis
    EXCLUDES 1   acute necrotizing ulcerative stomatitis (A69.1)
             Vincent's stomatitis (A69.1)

K12.2   **Cellulitis and abscess of mouth**
Cellulitis of mouth (floor)
Submandibular abscess
    EXCLUDES 2   abscess of salivary gland (K11.3)
             abscess of tongue (K14.0)
             periapical abscess (K04.6-K04.7)
             periodontal abscess (K05.21)
             peritonsillar abscess (J36)

✓5th **K12.3**   **Oral mucositis (ulcerative)**
Mucositis (oral) (oropharyneal)
    EXCLUDES 2   gastrointestinal mucositis (ulcerative) (K92.81)
             mucositis (ulcerative) of vagina and vulva (N76.81)
             nasal mucositis (ulcerative) (J34.81)

K12.30   **Oral mucositis (ulcerative), unspecified**

K12.31   **Oral mucositis (ulcerative) due to antineoplastic therapy**
Use additional code for adverse effect, if applicable, to identify antineoplastic and immunosuppressive drugs (T45.1X5)
Use additional code for other antineoplastic therapy, such as:
    radiological procedure and radiotherapy (Y84.2)

K12.32   **Oral mucositis (ulcerative) due to other drugs**
Use additional code for adverse effect, if applicable, to identify drug (T36-T50 with fifth or sixth character 5)

K12.33   **Oral mucositis (ulcerative) due to radiation**
Use additional external cause code (W88-W90, X39.0-) to identify cause

K12.39   **Other oral mucositis (ulcerative)**
Viral oral mucositis (ulcerative)

EXCLUDES 1 Not coded here   EXCLUDES 2 Not included here   N Newborn Age: 0   P Pediatric Age: 0-17   M Maternity Age: 12-55   A Adult Age: 15-124

634   ICD-10-CM 2016

✓4ᵗʰ **K13 Other diseases of lip and oral mucosa**
    INCLUDES   epithelial disturbances of tongue
    Use additional code to identify:
      alcohol abuse and dependence (F10.-)
      exposure to environmental tobacco smoke (Z77.22)
      exposure to tobacco smoke in the perinatal period (P96.81)
      history of tobacco use (Z87.891)
      occupational exposure to environmental tobacco smoke (Z57.31)
      tobacco dependence (F17.-)
      tobacco use (Z72.0)
    EXCLUDES 2   certain disorders of gingiva and edentulous alveolar ridge
        (K05-K06)
        cysts of oral region (K09.-)
        diseases of tongue (K14.-)
        stomatitis and related lesions (K12.-)

    K13.0 Diseases of lips

Abscess of lips	Exfoliative cheilitis
Angular cheilitis	Fistula of lips
Cellulitis of lips	Glandular cheilitis
Cheilitis NOS	Hypertrophy of lips
Cheilodynia	Perlèche NEC
Cheilosis	

      EXCLUDES 1   *ariboflavinosis (E53.0)*
         cheilitis due to radiation-related disorders (L55-L59)
         congenital fistula of lips (Q38.0)
         congenital hypertrophy of lips (Q18.6)
         Perlèche due to candidiasis (B37.83)
         Perlèche due to riboflavin deficiency (E53.0)

    K13.1 Cheek and lip biting

✓5ᵗʰ   **K13.2 Leukoplakia and other disturbances of oral epithelium, including tongue**
      EXCLUDES 1   *carcinoma in situ of oral epithelium (D00.0-)*
         hairy leukoplakia (K13.3)

      K13.21 Leukoplakia of oral mucosa, including tongue
         Leukokeratosis of oral mucosa
         Leukoplakia of gingiva, lips, tongue
         EXCLUDES 1   *hairy leukoplakia (K13.3)*
             leukokeratosis nicotina palati (K13.24)

      K13.22 Minimal keratinized residual ridge mucosa
         Minimal keratinization of alveolar ridge mucosa

      K13.23 Excessive keratinized residual ridge mucosa
         Excessive keratinization of alveolar ridge mucosa

      K13.24 Leukokeratosis nicotina palati
         Smoker's palate

      K13.29 Other disturbances of oral epithelium, including tongue
         Erythroplakia of mouth or tongue
         Focal epithelial hyperplasia of mouth or tongue
         Leukoedema of mouth or tongue
         Other oral epithelium disturbances

    K13.3 Hairy leukoplakia

    K13.4 Granuloma and granuloma-like lesions of oral mucosa

Eosinophilic granuloma	Verrucous xanthoma
Granuloma pyogenicum	

    K13.5 Oral submucous fibrosis
      Submucous fibrosis of tongue

    K13.6 Irritative hyperplasia of oral mucosa
      EXCLUDES 2   *irritative hyperplasia of edentulous ridge [denture*
            hyperplasia] (K06.2)

✓5ᵗʰ   **K13.7 Other and unspecified lesions of oral mucosa**
      K13.70 Unspecified lesions of oral mucosa

      K13.79 Other lesions of oral mucosa
         Focal oral mucinosis

✓4ᵗʰ **K14 Diseases of tongue**
    Use additional code to identify:
      alcohol abuse and dependence (F10.-)
      exposure to environmental tobacco smoke (Z77.22)
      history of tobacco use (Z87.891)
      occupational exposure to environmental tobacco smoke (Z57.31)
      tobacco dependence (F17.-)
      tobacco use (Z72.0)
    EXCLUDES 2   *erythroplakia (K13.29)*
        focal epithelial hyperplasia (K13.29)
        leukedema of tongue (K13.29)
        leukoplakia of tongue (K13.21)
        hairy leukoplakia (K13.3)
        macroglossia (congenital) (Q38.2)
        submucous fibrosis of tongue (K13.5)

    K14.0 Glossitis

Abscess of tongue	Ulceration (traumatic) of tongue

      EXCLUDES 1   *atrophic glossitis (K14.4)*

    K14.1 Geographic tongue
      Benign migratory glossitis
      Glossitis areata exfoliativa

    K14.2 Median rhomboid glossitis

    K14.3 Hypertrophy of tongue papillae
      Black hairy tongue
      Coated tongue
      Hypertrophy of foliate papillae
      Lingua villosa nigra

    K14.4 Atrophy of tongue papillae
      Atrophic glossitis

    K14.5 Plicated tongue
      Fissured tongue
      Furrowed tongue
      Scrotal tongue
      EXCLUDES 1   *fissured tongue, congenital (Q38.3)*

    K14.6 Glossodynia
      Glossopyrosis
      Painful tongue

    K14.8 Other diseases of tongue
      Atrophy of tongue
      Crenated tongue
      Enlargement of tongue
      Glossocele
      Glossoptosis
      Hypertrophy of tongue

    K14.9 Disease of tongue, unspecified
      Glossopathy NOS

Diseases of esophagus, stomach and duodenum (K20-K31)

    EXCLUDES 2   *hiatus hernia (K44.-)*

✓4ᵗʰ **K20 Esophagitis**
    Use additional code to identify:
      alcohol abuse and dependence (F10.-)
    EXCLUDES 1   *erosion of esophagus (K22.1-)*
        esophagitis with gastro-esophageal reflux disease (K21.0)
        reflux esophagitis (K21.0)
        ulcerative esophagitis (K22.1-)
    EXCLUDES 2   *eosinophilic gastritis or gastroenteritis (K52.81)*

    K20.0 Eosinophilic esophagitis

    K20.8 Other esophagitis
      Abscess of esophagus

    K20.9 Esophagitis, unspecified
      Esophagitis NOS

✓4ᵗʰ **K21 Gastro-esophageal reflux disease**
    EXCLUDES 1   *newborn esophageal reflux (P78.83)*

    K21.0 Gastro-esophageal reflux disease with esophagitis
      Reflux esophagitis

    K21.9 Gastro-esophageal reflux disease without esophagitis
      Esophageal reflux NOS

✓4ᵗʰ **K22 Other diseases of esophagus**
    EXCLUDES 2   *esophageal varices (I85.-)*

    K22.0 Achalasia of cardia
      Achalasia NOS
      Cardiospasm
      EXCLUDES 1   *congenital cardiospasm (Q39.5)*

✓5ᵗʰ   **K22.1 Ulcer of esophagus**
      Barrett's ulcer
      Erosion of esophagus
      Fungal ulcer of esophagus
      Peptic ulcer of esophagus
      Ulcer of esophagus due to ingestion of chemicals
      Ulcer of esophagus due to ingestion of drugs and medicaments
      Ulcerative esophagitis
      Code first poisoning due to drug or toxin, if applicable (T36-T65
        with fifth or sixth character 1-4 or 6)
      Use additional code for adverse effect, if applicable, to identify
        drug (T36-T50 with fifth or sixth character 5)
      EXCLUDES 1   *Barrett's esophagus (K22.7-)*

      K22.10 Ulcer of esophagus without bleeding
         Ulcer of esophagus NOS

      K22.11 Ulcer of esophagus with bleeding
         EXCLUDES 1   *bleeding esophageal varices (I85.01, I85.11)*

    K22.2 Esophageal obstruction
      Compression of esophagus
      Constriction of esophagus
      Stenosis of esophagus
      Stricture of esophagus
      EXCLUDES 1   *congenital stenosis or stricture of esophagus (Q39.3)*

✓ Additional Character Required   ✓x7ᵗʰ Placeholder Alert   **Unspecified Dx**   Other Specified Dx   Manifestation   ▶◀ Revised Text   ● New Code   ▲ Revised Code Title

K22.3 Perforation of esophagus
Rupture of esophagus
> *EXCLUDES 1* *traumatic perforation of (thoracic) esophagus (S27.8-)*

K22.4 Dyskinesia of esophagus
Corkscrew esophagus
Diffuse esophageal spasm
Spasm of esophagus
> *EXCLUDES 1* *cardiospasm (K22.0)*

K22.5 Diverticulum of esophagus, acquired
Esophageal pouch, acquired
> *EXCLUDES 1* *diverticulum of esophagus (congenital) (Q39.6)*

K22.6 Gastro-esophageal laceration-hemorrhage syndrome
Mallory-Weiss syndrome

✓5ᵗʰ **K22.7 Barrett's esophagus**
Barrett's disease
Barrett's syndrome
> *EXCLUDES 1* *Barrett's ulcer (K22.1)*
> *malignant neoplasm of esophagus (C15.-)*

K22.70 Barrett's esophagus without dysplasia
Barrett's esophagus NOS

✓6ᵗʰ **K22.71 Barrett's esophagus with dysplasia**

K22.710 Barrett's esophagus with low grade dysplasia

K22.711 Barrett's esophagus with high grade dysplasia

K22.719 Barrett's esophagus with dysplasia, unspecified

K22.8 Other specified diseases of esophagus
Hemorrhage of esophagus NOS
> *EXCLUDES 2* *esophageal varices (I85.-)*
> *Paterson-Kelly syndrome (D50.1)*

K22.9 Disease of esophagus, unspecified

K23 Disorders of esophagus in diseases classified elsewhere
Code first underlying disease, such as:
congenital syphilis (A50.5)
> *EXCLUDES 1* *late syphilis (A52.79)*
> *megaesophagus due to Chagas' disease (B57.31)*
> *tuberculosis (A18.83)*

✓4ᵗʰ **K25 Gastric ulcer**
> INCLUDES erosion (acute) of stomach
> pylorus ulcer (peptic)
> stomach ulcer (peptic)

Use additional code to identify:
alcohol abuse and dependence (F10.-)
> *EXCLUDES 1* *acute gastritis (K29.0-)*
> *peptic ulcer NOS (K27.-)*

K25.0 Acute gastric ulcer with hemorrhage
K25.1 Acute gastric ulcer with perforation
K25.2 Acute gastric ulcer with both hemorrhage and perforation
K25.3 Acute gastric ulcer without hemorrhage or perforation
K25.4 Chronic or unspecified gastric ulcer with hemorrhage
K25.5 Chronic or unspecified gastric ulcer with perforation
K25.6 Chronic or unspecified gastric ulcer with both hemorrhage and perforation
K25.7 Chronic gastric ulcer without hemorrhage or perforation
K25.9 Gastric ulcer, unspecified as acute or chronic, without hemorrhage or perforation

✓4ᵗʰ **K26 Duodenal ulcer**
> INCLUDES erosion (acute) of duodenum
> duodenum ulcer (peptic)
> postpyloric ulcer (peptic)

Use additional code to identify:
alcohol abuse and dependence (F10.-)
> *EXCLUDES 1* *peptic ulcer NOS (K27.-)*

K26.0 Acute duodenal ulcer with hemorrhage
K26.1 Acute duodenal ulcer with perforation
K26.2 Acute duodenal ulcer with both hemorrhage and perforation
K26.3 Acute duodenal ulcer without hemorrhage or perforation
K26.4 Chronic or unspecified duodenal ulcer with hemorrhage
K26.5 Chronic or unspecified duodenal ulcer with perforation
K26.6 Chronic or unspecified duodenal ulcer with both hemorrhage and perforation
K26.7 Chronic duodenal ulcer without hemorrhage or perforation
K26.9 Duodenal ulcer, unspecified as acute or chronic, without hemorrhage or perforation

✓4ᵗʰ **K27 Peptic ulcer, site unspecified**
> INCLUDES gastroduodenal ulcer NOS
> peptic ulcer NOS

Use additional code to identify:
alcohol abuse and dependence (F10.-)
> *EXCLUDES 1* *peptic ulcer of newborn (P78.82)*

K27.0 Acute peptic ulcer, site unspecified, with hemorrhage
K27.1 Acute peptic ulcer, site unspecified, with perforation
K27.2 Acute peptic ulcer, site unspecified, with both hemorrhage and perforation
K27.3 Acute peptic ulcer, site unspecified, without hemorrhage or perforation
K27.4 Chronic or unspecified peptic ulcer, site unspecified, with hemorrhage
K27.5 Chronic or unspecified peptic ulcer, site unspecified, with perforation
K27.6 Chronic or unspecified peptic ulcer, site unspecified, with both hemorrhage and perforation
K27.7 Chronic peptic ulcer, site unspecified, without hemorrhage or perforation
K27.9 Peptic ulcer, site unspecified, unspecified as acute or chronic, without hemorrhage or perforation

✓4ᵗʰ **K28 Gastrojejunal ulcer**
> INCLUDES anastomotic ulcer (peptic) or erosion
> gastrocolic ulcer (peptic) or erosion
> gastrointestinal ulcer (peptic) or erosion
> gastrojejunal ulcer (peptic) or erosion
> jejunal ulcer (peptic) or erosion
> marginal ulcer (peptic) or erosion
> stomal ulcer (peptic) or erosion

Use additional code to identify:
alcohol abuse and dependence (F10.-)
> *EXCLUDES 1* *primary ulcer of small intestine (K63.3)*

K28.0 Acute gastrojejunal ulcer with hemorrhage
K28.1 Acute gastrojejunal ulcer with perforation
K28.2 Acute gastrojejunal ulcer with both hemorrhage and perforation
K28.3 Acute gastrojejunal ulcer without hemorrhage or perforation
K28.4 Chronic or unspecified gastrojejunal ulcer with hemorrhage
K28.5 Chronic or unspecified gastrojejunal ulcer with perforation
K28.6 Chronic or unspecified gastrojejunal ulcer with both hemorrhage and perforation
K28.7 Chronic gastrojejunal ulcer without hemorrhage or perforation
K28.9 Gastrojejunal ulcer, unspecified as acute or chronic, without hemorrhage or perforation

✓4ᵗʰ **K29 Gastritis and duodenitis**
> *EXCLUDES 1* *eosinophilic gastritis or gastroenteritis (K52.81)*
> *Zollinger-Ellison syndrome (E16.4)*

✓5ᵗʰ **K29.0 Acute gastritis**
Use additional code to identify:
alcohol abuse and dependence (F10.-)
> *EXCLUDES 1* *erosion (acute) of stomach (K25.-)*

K29.00 Acute gastritis without bleeding
K29.01 Acute gastritis with bleeding

✓5ᵗʰ **K29.2 Alcoholic gastritis**
Use additional code to identify:
alcohol abuse and dependence (F10.-)

K29.20 Alcoholic gastritis without bleeding
K29.21 Alcoholic gastritis with bleeding

✓5ᵗʰ **K29.3 Chronic superficial gastritis**

K29.30 Chronic superficial gastritis without bleeding
K29.31 Chronic superficial gastritis with bleeding

✓5ᵗʰ **K29.4 Chronic atrophic gastritis**
Gastric atrophy

K29.40 Chronic atrophic gastritis without bleeding
K29.41 Chronic atrophic gastritis with bleeding

✓5ᵗʰ **K29.5 Unspecified chronic gastritis**
Chronic antral gastritis
Chronic fundal gastritis

K29.50 Unspecified chronic gastritis without bleeding
K29.51 Unspecified chronic gastritis with bleeding

EXCLUDES 1 Not coded here   *EXCLUDES 2* Not included here   N Newborn Age: 0   P Pediatric Age: 0-17   M Maternity Age: 12-55   A Adult Age: 15-124

636   ICD-10-CM 2016

✓5ᵗʰ **K29.6** **Other gastritis**
　　Giant hypertrophic gastritis
　　Granulomatous gastritis
　　Ménétrier's disease
　　K29.60 **Other gastritis without bleeding**
　　K29.61 **Other gastritis with bleeding**

✓5ᵗʰ **K29.7** **Gastritis, unspecified**
　　K29.70 **Gastritis, unspecified, without bleeding**
　　K29.71 **Gastritis, unspecified, with bleeding**

✓5ᵗʰ **K29.8** **Duodenitis**
　　K29.80 **Duodenitis without bleeding**
　　K29.81 **Duodenitis with bleeding**

✓5ᵗʰ **K29.9** **Gastroduodenitis, unspecified**
　　K29.90 **Gastroduodenitis, unspecified, without bleeding**
　　K29.91 **Gastroduodenitis, unspecified, with bleeding**

K30 **Functional dyspepsia**
　　Indigestion
　　EXCLUDES 1　*dyspepsia NOS (R10.13)*
　　　　　　　heartburn (R12)
　　　　　　　nervous dyspepsia (F45.8)
　　　　　　　neurotic dyspepsia (F45.8)
　　　　　　　psychogenic dyspepsia (F45.8)

✓4ᵗʰ **K31** **Other diseases of stomach and duodenum**
　　INCLUDES　functional disorders of stomach
　　EXCLUDES 2　*diabetic gastroparesis (E08.43, E09.43, E10.43, E11.43, E13.43)*
　　　　　　　diverticulum of duodenum (K57.00-K57.13)

　　K31.0 **Acute dilatation of stomach**
　　　　Acute distention of stomach

　　K31.1 **Adult hypertrophic pyloric stenosis**　　　　　Ⓐ
　　　　Pyloric stenosis NOS
　　　　EXCLUDES 1　*congenital or infantile pyloric stenosis (Q40.0)*

　　K31.2 **Hourglass stricture and stenosis of stomach**
　　　　EXCLUDES 1　*congenital hourglass stomach (Q40.2)*
　　　　　　　　hourglass contraction of stomach (K31.89)

　　K31.3 **Pylorospasm, not elsewhere classified**
　　　　EXCLUDES 1　*congenital or infantile pylorospasm (Q40.0)*
　　　　　　　　neurotic pylorospasm (F45.8)
　　　　　　　　psychogenic pylorospasm (F45.8)

　　K31.4 **Gastric diverticulum**
　　　　EXCLUDES 1　*congenital diverticulum of stomach (Q40.2)*

　　K31.5 **Obstruction of duodenum**
　　　　Constriction of duodenum
　　　　Duodenal ileus (chronic)
　　　　Stenosis of duodenum
　　　　Stricture of duodenum
　　　　Volvulus of duodenum
　　　　EXCLUDES 1　*congenital stenosis of duodenum (Q41.0)*

　　K31.6 **Fistula of stomach and duodenum**
　　　　Gastrocolic fistula
　　　　Gastrojejunocolic fistula

　　K31.7 **Polyp of stomach and duodenum**
　　　　EXCLUDES 1　*adenomatous polyp of stomach (D13.1)*

✓5ᵗʰ **K31.8** **Other specified diseases of stomach and duodenum**
　　✓6ᵗʰ **K31.81** **Angiodysplasia of stomach and duodenum**
　　　　K31.811 **Angiodysplasia of stomach and duodenum with bleeding**
　　　　K31.819 **Angiodysplasia of stomach and duodenum without bleeding**
　　　　　　Angiodysplasia of stomach and duodenum NOS

　　　K31.82 **Dieulafoy lesion (hemorrhagic) of stomach and duodenum**
　　　　　EXCLUDES 2　*Dieulafoy lesion of intestine (K63.81)*

　　　K31.83 **Achlorhydria**

　　　K31.84 **Gastroparesis**
　　　　　Gastroparalysis
　　　　　Code first underlying disease, if known, such as:
　　　　　　anorexia nervosa (F50.0-)
　　　　　　diabetes mellitus (E08.43, E09.43, E10.43, E11.43, E13.43)
　　　　　　scleroderma (M34.-)
　　　　　AHA: 2013, 4Q, 114

　　　K31.89 **Other diseases of stomach and duodenum**
　　K31.9 **Disease of stomach and duodenum, unspecified**

Diseases of appendix (K35-K38)

✓4ᵗʰ **K35** **Acute appendicitis**
　　K35.2 **Acute appendicitis with generalized peritonitis**
　　　　Appendicitis (acute) with generalized (diffuse) peritonitis following rupture or perforation of appendix
　　　　Perforated appendix NOS
　　　　Ruptured appendix NOS

　　K35.3 **Acute appendicitis with localized peritonitis**
　　　　Acute appendicitis with or without perforation or rupture NOS
　　　　Acute appendicitis with or without perforation or rupture with localized peritonitis
　　　　Acute appendicitis with peritoneal abscess

　✓5ᵗʰ **K35.8** **Other and unspecified acute appendicitis**
　　　K35.80 **Unspecified acute appendicitis**
　　　　　Acute appendicitis NOS
　　　　　Acute appendicitis without (localized) (generalized) peritonitis

　　　K35.89 **Other acute appendicitis**

K36 **Other appendicitis**
　　Chronic appendicitis
　　Recurrent appendicitis

K37 **Unspecified appendicitis**
　　EXCLUDES 1　*unspecified appendicitis with peritonitis (K35.2-K35.3)*

✓4ᵗʰ **K38** **Other diseases of appendix**
　　K38.0 **Hyperplasia of appendix**
　　K38.1 **Appendicular concretions**
　　　　Fecalith of appendix
　　　　Stercolith of appendix
　　K38.2 **Diverticulum of appendix**
　　K38.3 **Fistula of appendix**
　　K38.8 **Other specified diseases of appendix**
　　　　Intussusception of appendix
　　K38.9 **Disease of appendix, unspecified**

Hernia (K40-K46)

NOTE　Hernia with both gangrene and obstruction is classified to hernia with gangrene.
INCLUDES　acquired hernia
　　　　congenital [except diaphragmatic or hiatus] hernia
　　　　recurrent hernia

✓4ᵗʰ **K40** **Inguinal hernia**
　　INCLUDES　bubonocele
　　　　　direct inguinal hernia
　　　　　double inguinal hernia
　　　　　indirect inguinal hernia
　　　　　inguinal hernia NOS
　　　　　oblique inguinal hernia
　　　　　scrotal hernia

　✓5ᵗʰ **K40.0** **Bilateral inguinal hernia, with obstruction, without gangrene**
　　　Inguinal hernia (bilateral) causing obstruction without gangrene
　　　Incarcerated inguinal hernia (bilateral) without gangrene
　　　Irreducible inguinal hernia (bilateral) without gangrene
　　　Strangulated inguinal hernia (bilateral) without gangrene

　　　K40.00 **Bilateral inguinal hernia, with obstruction, without gangrene, not specified as recurrent**
　　　　　Bilateral inguinal hernia, with obstruction, without gangrene NOS

　　　K40.01 **Bilateral inguinal hernia, with obstruction, without gangrene, recurrent**

　✓5ᵗʰ **K40.1** **Bilateral inguinal hernia, with gangrene**
　　　K40.10 **Bilateral inguinal hernia, with gangrene, not specified as recurrent**
　　　　　Bilateral inguinal hernia, with gangrene NOS

　　　K40.11 **Bilateral inguinal hernia, with gangrene, recurrent**

　✓5ᵗʰ **K40.2** **Bilateral inguinal hernia, without obstruction or gangrene**
　　　K40.20 **Bilateral inguinal hernia, without obstruction or gangrene, not specified as recurrent**
　　　　　Bilateral inguinal hernia NOS

　　　K40.21 **Bilateral inguinal hernia, without obstruction or gangrene, recurrent**

✓ Additional Character Required　　✓x7ᵗʰ Placeholder Alert　　Unspecified Dx　　Other Specified Dx　　Manifestation　　▶◀ Revised Text　　● New Code　　▲ Revised Code Title

Chapter 11. Diseases of the Digestive System

☑5ᵗʰ K40.3 **Unilateral inguinal hernia, with obstruction, without gangrene**
    Inguinal hernia (unilateral) causing obstruction without gangrene
    Incarcerated inguinal hernia (unilateral) without gangrene
    Irreducible inguinal hernia (unilateral) without gangrene
    Strangulated inguinal hernia (unilateral) without gangrene

    K40.30 **Unilateral inguinal hernia, with obstruction, without gangrene, not specified as recurrent**
        Inguinal hernia, with obstruction NOS
        Unilateral inguinal hernia, with obstruction, without gangrene NOS

    K40.31 **Unilateral inguinal hernia, with obstruction, without gangrene, recurrent**

☑5ᵗʰ K40.4 **Unilateral inguinal hernia, with gangrene**
    K40.40 **Unilateral inguinal hernia, with gangrene, not specified as recurrent**
        Inguinal hernia with gangrene NOS
        Unilateral inguinal hernia with gangrene NOS

    K40.41 **Unilateral inguinal hernia, with gangrene, recurrent**

☑5ᵗʰ K40.9 **Unilateral inguinal hernia, without obstruction or gangrene**
    K40.90 **Unilateral inguinal hernia, without obstruction or gangrene, not specified as recurrent**
        Inguinal hernia NOS
        Unilateral inguinal hernia NOS

    K40.91 **Unilateral inguinal hernia, without obstruction or gangrene, recurrent**

☑4ᵗʰ K41 **Femoral hernia**

☑5ᵗʰ K41.0 **Bilateral femoral hernia, with obstruction, without gangrene**
    Femoral hernia (bilateral) causing obstruction, without gangrene
    Incarcerated femoral hernia (bilateral), without gangrene
    Irreducible femoral hernia (bilateral), without gangrene
    Strangulated femoral hernia (bilateral), without gangrene

    K41.00 **Bilateral femoral hernia, with obstruction, without gangrene, not specified as recurrent**
        Bilateral femoral hernia, with obstruction, without gangrene NOS

    K41.01 **Bilateral femoral hernia, with obstruction, without gangrene, recurrent**

☑5ᵗʰ K41.1 **Bilateral femoral hernia, with gangrene**
    K41.10 **Bilateral femoral hernia, with gangrene, not specified as recurrent**
        Bilateral femoral hernia, with gangrene NOS

    K41.11 **Bilateral femoral hernia, with gangrene, recurrent**

☑5ᵗʰ K41.2 **Bilateral femoral hernia, without obstruction or gangrene**
    K41.20 **Bilateral femoral hernia, without obstruction or gangrene, not specified as recurrent**
        Bilateral femoral hernia NOS

    K41.21 **Bilateral femoral hernia, without obstruction or gangrene, recurrent**

☑5ᵗʰ K41.3 **Unilateral femoral hernia, with obstruction, without gangrene**
    Femoral hernia (unilateral) causing obstruction, without gangrene
    Incarcerated femoral hernia (unilateral), without gangrene
    Irreducible femoral hernia (unilateral), without gangrene
    Strangulated femoral hernia (unilateral), without gangrene

    K41.30 **Unilateral femoral hernia, with obstruction, without gangrene, not specified as recurrent**
        Femoral hernia, with obstruction NOS
        Unilateral femoral hernia, with obstruction NOS

    K41.31 **Unilateral femoral hernia, with obstruction, without gangrene, recurrent**

☑5ᵗʰ K41.4 **Unilateral femoral hernia, with gangrene**
    K41.40 **Unilateral femoral hernia, with gangrene, not specified as recurrent**
        Femoral hernia, with gangrene NOS
        Unilateral femoral hernia, with gangrene NOS

    K41.41 **Unilateral femoral hernia, with gangrene, recurrent**

☑5ᵗʰ K41.9 **Unilateral femoral hernia, without obstruction or gangrene**
    K41.90 **Unilateral femoral hernia, without obstruction or gangrene, not specified as recurrent**
        Femoral hernia NOS
        Unilateral femoral hernia NOS

    K41.91 **Unilateral femoral hernia, without obstruction or gangrene, recurrent**

☑4ᵗʰ K42 **Umbilical hernia**
    INCLUDES paraumbilical hernia
    EXCLUDES 1 *omphalocele (Q79.2)*

    K42.0 **Umbilical hernia with obstruction, without gangrene**
        Umbilical hernia causing obstruction, without gangrene
        Incarcerated umbilical hernia, without gangrene
        Irreducible umbilical hernia, without gangrene
        Strangulated umbilical hernia, without gangrene

    K42.1 **Umbilical hernia with gangrene**
        Gangrenous umbilical hernia

    K42.9 **Umbilical hernia without obstruction or gangrene**
        Umbilical hernia NOS

☑4ᵗʰ K43 **Ventral hernia**

    K43.0 **Incisional hernia with obstruction, without gangrene**
        Incisional hernia causing obstruction, without gangrene
        Incarcerated incisional hernia, without gangrene
        Irreducible incisional hernia, without gangrene
        Strangulated incisional hernia, without gangrene

    K43.1 **Incisional hernia with gangrene**
        Gangrenous incisional hernia

    K43.2 **Incisional hernia without obstruction or gangrene**
        Incisional hernia NOS

    K43.3 **Parastomal hernia with obstruction, without gangrene**
        Incarcerated parastomal hernia, without gangrene
        Irreducible parastomal hernia, without gangrene
        Parastomal hernia causing obstruction, without gangrene
        Strangulated parastomal hernia, without gangrene

    K43.4 **Parastomal hernia with gangrene**
        Gangrenous parastomal hernia

    K43.5 **Parastomal hernia without obstruction or gangrene**
        Parastomal hernia NOS

    K43.6 **Other and unspecified ventral hernia with obstruction, without gangrene**
        Epigastric hernia causing obstruction, without gangrene
        Hypogastric hernia causing obstruction, without gangrene
        Incarcerated epigastric hernia without gangrene
        Incarcerated hypogastric hernia without gangrene
        Incarcerated midline hernia without gangrene
        Incarcerated spigelian hernia without gangrene
        Incarcerated subxiphoid hernia without gangrene
        Irreducible epigastric hernia without gangrene
        Irreducible hypogastric hernia without gangrene
        Irreducible midline hernia without gangrene
        Irreducible spigelian hernia without gangrene
        Irreducible subxiphoid hernia without gangrene
        Midline hernia causing obstruction, without gangrene
        Spigelian hernia causing obstruction, without gangrene
        Strangulated epigastric hernia without gangrene
        Strangulated hypogastric hernia without gangrene
        Strangulated midline hernia without gangrene
        Strangulated spigelian hernia without gangrene
        Strangulated subxiphoid hernia without gangrene
        Subxiphoid hernia causing obstruction, without gangrene

    K43.7 **Other and unspecified ventral hernia with gangrene**
        Any condition listed under K43.6 specified as gangrenous

    K43.9 **Ventral hernia without obstruction or gangrene**
        Epigastric hernia
        Ventral hernia NOS

☑4ᵗʰ K44 **Diaphragmatic hernia**
    INCLUDES hiatus hernia (esophageal) (sliding)
             paraesophageal hernia
    EXCLUDES 1 *congenital diaphragmatic hernia (Q79.0)*
             congenital hiatus hernia (Q40.1)

    K44.0 **Diaphragmatic hernia with obstruction, without gangrene**
        Diaphragmatic hernia causing obstruction
        Incarcerated diaphragmatic hernia
        Irreducible diaphragmatic hernia
        Strangulated diaphragmatic hernia

    K44.1 **Diaphragmatic hernia with gangrene**
        Gangrenous diaphragmatic hernia

    K44.9 **Diaphragmatic hernia without obstruction or gangrene**
        Diaphragmatic hernia NOS

EXCLUDES 1 Not coded here   **EXCLUDES 2** Not included here   **N** Newborn Age: 0   **P** Pediatric Age: 0-17   **M** Maternity Age: 12-55   **A** Adult Age: 15-124

638   ICD-10-CM 2016

☑4ᵗʰ **K45** **Other abdominal hernia**
    INCLUDES abdominal hernia, specified site NEC
              lumbar hernia
              obturator hernia
              pudendal hernia
              retroperitoneal hernia
              sciatic hernia

    K45.0 **Other specified abdominal hernia** with obstruction, without gangrene
        Other specified abdominal hernia causing obstruction
        Other specified incarcerated abdominal hernia
        Other specified irreducible abdominal hernia
        Other specified strangulated abdominal hernia

    K45.1 **Other specified abdominal hernia** with gangrene
        Any condition listed under K45 specified as gangrenous

    K45.8 **Other specified abdominal hernia** without obstruction or gangrene

☑4ᵗʰ **K46** **Unspecified abdominal hernia**
    INCLUDES enterocele
              epiplocele
              hernia NOS
              interstitial hernia
              intestinal hernia
              intra-abdominal hernia
    EXCLUDES 1 *vaginal enterocele (N81.5)*

    K46.0 **Unspecified abdominal hernia** with obstruction, without gangrene
        Unspecified abdominal hernia causing obstruction
        Unspecified incarcerated abdominal hernia
        Unspecified irreducible abdominal hernia
        Unspecified strangulated abdominal hernia

    K46.1 **Unspecified abdominal hernia** with gangrene
        Any condition listed under K46 specified as gangrenous

    K46.9 **Unspecified abdominal hernia** without obstruction or gangrene
        Abdominal hernia NOS

Noninfective enteritis and colitis (K50-K52)

    INCLUDES noninfective inflammatory bowel disease
    EXCLUDES 1 *irritable bowel syndrome (K58.-)*
              megacolon (K59.3)

☑4ᵗʰ **K50** **Crohn's disease [regional enteritis]**
    INCLUDES granulomatous enteritis
    Use additional code to identify manifestations, such as:
        pyoderma gangrenosum (L88)
    EXCLUDES 1 *ulcerative colitis (K51.-)*
    AHA: 2012, 4Q, 104

  ☑5ᵗʰ **K50.0** **Crohn's disease of** small intestine
        Crohn's disease [regional enteritis] of duodenum
        Crohn's disease [regional enteritis] of ileum
        Crohn's disease [regional enteritis] of jejunum
        Regional ileitis
        Terminal ileitis
        EXCLUDES 1 *Crohn's disease of both small and large intestine (K50.8-)*

    K50.00 **Crohn's disease of small intestine** without complications

  ☑6ᵗʰ **K50.01** **Crohn's disease of small intestine** with complications
      K50.011 **Crohn's disease of small intestine with** rectal bleeding
      K50.012 **Crohn's disease of small intestine with** intestinal obstruction
      K50.013 **Crohn's disease of small intestine with** fistula
      K50.014 **Crohn's disease of small intestine with** abscess
          AHA: 2012, 4Q, 104
      K50.018 **Crohn's disease of small intestine with other complication**
      K50.019 **Crohn's disease of small intestine with unspecified complications**

  ☑5ᵗʰ **K50.1** **Crohn's disease of** large intestine
        Crohn's disease [regional enteritis] of colon
        Crohn's disease [regional enteritis] of large bowel
        Crohn's disease [regional enteritis] of rectum
        Granulomatous colitis
        Regional colitis
        EXCLUDES 1 *Crohn's disease of both small and large intestine (K50.8)*

    K50.10 **Crohn's disease of large intestine** without complications

  ☑6ᵗʰ **K50.11** **Crohn's disease of large intestine** with complications
      K50.111 **Crohn's disease of large intestine with** rectal bleeding
      K50.112 **Crohn's disease of large intestine with** intestinal obstruction
      K50.113 **Crohn's disease of large intestine with** fistula
      K50.114 **Crohn's disease of large intestine with** abscess
      K50.118 **Crohn's disease of large intestine with other complication**
      K50.119 **Crohn's disease of large intestine with unspecified complications**

  ☑5ᵗʰ **K50.8** **Crohn's disease of** both small and large intestine
    K50.80 **Crohn's disease of both small and large intestine** without complications

  ☑6ᵗʰ **K50.81** **Crohn's disease of both small and large intestine** with complications
      K50.811 **Crohn's disease of both small and large intestine with** rectal bleeding
      K50.812 **Crohn's disease of both small and large intestine with** intestinal obstruction
      K50.813 **Crohn's disease of both small and large intestine with** fistula
      K50.814 **Crohn's disease of both small and large intestine with** abscess
      K50.818 **Crohn's disease of both small and large intestine with other complication**
      K50.819 **Crohn's disease of both small and large intestine with unspecified complications**

  ☑5ᵗʰ **K50.9** **Crohn's disease,** unspecified
    K50.90 **Crohn's disease, unspecified,** without complications
        Crohn's disease NOS
        Regional enteritis NOS

  ☑6ᵗʰ **K50.91** **Crohn's disease, unspecified,** with complications
      K50.911 **Crohn's disease, unspecified, with** rectal bleeding
      K50.912 **Crohn's disease, unspecified, with** intestinal obstruction
      K50.913 **Crohn's disease, unspecified, with** fistula
      K50.914 **Crohn's disease, unspecified, with** abscess
      K50.918 **Crohn's disease, unspecified, with other complication**
      K50.919 **Crohn's disease, unspecified, with unspecified complications**

☑4ᵗʰ **K51** **Ulcerative colitis**
    Use additional code to identify manifestations, such as:
        pyoderma gangrenosum (L88)
    EXCLUDES 1 *Crohn's disease [regional enteritis] (K50.-)*

  ☑5ᵗʰ **K51.0** **Ulcerative (chronic)** pancolitis
        Backwash ileitis

    K51.00 **Ulcerative (chronic) pancolitis** without complications
        Ulcerative (chronic) pancolitis NOS

  ☑6ᵗʰ **K51.01** **Ulcerative (chronic) pancolitis** with complications
      K51.011 **Ulcerative (chronic) pancolitis with** rectal bleeding
      K51.012 **Ulcerative (chronic) pancolitis with** intestinal obstruction
      K51.013 **Ulcerative (chronic) pancolitis with** fistula
      K51.014 **Ulcerative (chronic) pancolitis with** abscess
      K51.018 **Ulcerative (chronic) pancolitis with other complication**
      K51.019 **Ulcerative (chronic) pancolitis with unspecified complications**

  ☑5ᵗʰ **K51.2** **Ulcerative (chronic)** proctitis
    K51.20 **Ulcerative (chronic) proctitis** without complications
        Ulcerative (chronic) proctitis NOS

  ☑6ᵗʰ **K51.21** **Ulcerative (chronic) proctitis** with complications
      K51.211 **Ulcerative (chronic) proctitis with** rectal bleeding
      K51.212 **Ulcerative (chronic) proctitis with** intestinal obstruction
      K51.213 **Ulcerative (chronic) proctitis with** fistula
      K51.214 **Ulcerative (chronic) proctitis with** abscess

---

☑ Additional Character Required   ✓7ᵗʰ Placeholder Alert   Unspecified Dx   Other Specified Dx   Manifestation   ▶◀ Revised Text   ● New Code   ▲ Revised Code Title

    K51.218   Ulcerative (chronic) proctitis with other complication

    K51.219   Ulcerative (chronic) proctitis with unspecified complications

✓5ᵗʰ **K51.3**   Ulcerative (chronic) rectosigmoiditis

    K51.30   Ulcerative (chronic) rectosigmoiditis without complications
         Ulcerative (chronic) rectosigmoiditis NOS

    ✓6ᵗʰ **K51.31**   Ulcerative (chronic) rectosigmoiditis with complications

        K51.311   Ulcerative (chronic) rectosigmoiditis with rectal bleeding

        K51.312   Ulcerative (chronic) rectosigmoiditis with intestinal obstruction

        K51.313   Ulcerative (chronic) rectosigmoiditis with fistula

        K51.314   Ulcerative (chronic) rectosigmoiditis with abscess

        K51.318   Ulcerative (chronic) rectosigmoiditis with other complication

        K51.319   Ulcerative (chronic) rectosigmoiditis with unspecified complications

✓5ᵗʰ **K51.4**   Inflammatory polyps of colon

    EXCLUDES 1   adenomatous polyp of colon (D12.6)
         polyposis of colon (D12.6)
         polyps of colon NOS (K63.5)

    K51.40   Inflammatory polyps of colon without complications
         Inflammatory polyps of colon NOS

    ✓6ᵗʰ **K51.41**   Inflammatory polyps of colon with complications

        K51.411   Inflammatory polyps of colon with rectal bleeding

        K51.412   Inflammatory polyps of colon with intestinal obstruction

        K51.413   Inflammatory polyps of colon with fistula

        K51.414   Inflammatory polyps of colon with abscess

        K51.418   Inflammatory polyps of colon with other complication

        K51.419   Inflammatory polyps of colon with unspecified complications

✓5ᵗʰ **K51.5**   Left sided colitis
     Left hemicolitis

    K51.50   Left sided colitis without complications
         Left sided colitis NOS

    ✓6ᵗʰ **K51.51**   Left sided colitis with complications

        K51.511   Left sided colitis with rectal bleeding

        K51.512   Left sided colitis with intestinal obstruction

        K51.513   Left sided colitis with fistula

        K51.514   Left sided colitis with abscess

        K51.518   Left sided colitis with other complication

        K51.519   Left sided colitis with unspecified complications

✓5ᵗʰ **K51.8**   Other ulcerative colitis

    K51.80   Other ulcerative colitis without complications

    ✓6ᵗʰ **K51.81**   Other ulcerative colitis with complications

        K51.811   Other ulcerative colitis with rectal bleeding

        K51.812   Other ulcerative colitis with intestinal obstruction

        K51.813   Other ulcerative colitis with fistula

        K51.814   Other ulcerative colitis with abscess

        K51.818   Other ulcerative colitis with other complication

        K51.819   Other ulcerative colitis with unspecified complications

✓5ᵗʰ **K51.9**   Ulcerative colitis, unspecified

    K51.90   Ulcerative colitis, unspecified, without complications

    ✓6ᵗʰ **K51.91**   Ulcerative colitis, unspecified, with complications

        K51.911   Ulcerative colitis, unspecified with rectal bleeding

        K51.912   Ulcerative colitis, unspecified with intestinal obstruction

        K51.913   Ulcerative colitis, unspecified with fistula

        K51.914   Ulcerative colitis, unspecified with abscess

    K51.918   Ulcerative colitis, unspecified with other complication

    K51.919   Ulcerative colitis, unspecified with unspecified complications

✓4ᵗʰ **K52**   **Other and unspecified noninfective gastroenteritis and colitis**

    K52.0   Gastroenteritis and colitis due to radiation

    K52.1   Toxic gastroenteritis and colitis
         Drug-induced gastroenteritis and colitis
         Code first (T51-T65) to identify toxic agent
         Use additional code for adverse effect, if applicable, to identify drug (T36-T50 with fifth or sixth character 5)

    K52.2   Allergic and dietetic gastroenteritis and colitis
         Food hypersensitivity gastroenteritis or colitis
         Use additional code to identify type of food allergy (Z91.01-, Z91.02-)

    ✓5ᵗʰ **K52.8**   Other specified noninfective gastroenteritis and colitis

        K52.81   Eosinophilic gastritis or gastroenteritis
             Eosinophilic enteritis
             EXCLUDES 1   eosinophilic esophagitis (K20.0)

        K52.82   Eosinophilic colitis

        K52.89   Other specified noninfective gastroenteritis and colitis
             Collagenous colitis
             Lymphocytic colitis
             Microscopic colitis (collagenous or lymphocytic)

    K52.9   Noninfective gastroenteritis and colitis, unspecified

Colitis NOS	Ileitis NOS
Enteritis NOS	Jejunitis NOS
Gastroenteritis NOS	Sigmoiditis NOS

         EXCLUDES 1   diarrhea NOS (R19.7)
             functional diarrhea (K59.1)
             infectious gastroenteritis and colitis NOS (A09)
             neonatal diarrhea (noninfective) (P78.3)
             psychogenic diarrhea (F45.8)

Other diseases of intestines (K55-K64)

✓4ᵗʰ **K55**   **Vascular disorders of intestine**
    EXCLUDES 1   necrotizing enterocolitis of newborn (P77.-)

    K55.0   Acute vascular disorders of intestine
         Acute fulminant ischemic colitis
         Acute intestinal infarction
         Acute small intestine ischemia
         Infarction of appendices epiploicae
         Mesenteric (artery) (vein) embolism
         Mesenteric (artery) (vein) infarction
         Mesenteric (artery) (vein) thrombosis
         Necrosis of intestine
         Subacute ischemic colitis

    K55.1   Chronic vascular disorders of intestine

Chronic ischemic colitis	Mesenteric atherosclerosis
Chronic ischemic enteritis	Mesenteric vascular
Chronic ischemic enterocolitis	insufficiency
Ischemic stricture of intestine	

    ✓5ᵗʰ **K55.2**   Angiodysplasia of colon

        K55.20   Angiodysplasia of colon without hemorrhage

        K55.21   Angiodysplasia of colon with hemorrhage

    K55.8   Other vascular disorders of intestine

    K55.9   Vascular disorder of intestine, unspecified
         Ischemic colitis
         Ischemic enteritis
         Ischemic enterocolitis

✓4ᵗʰ **K56**   **Paralytic ileus and intestinal obstruction without hernia**
    EXCLUDES 1   congenital stricture or stenosis of intestine (Q41-Q42)
         cystic fibrosis with meconium ileus (E84.11)
         intestinal obstruction with hernia (K40-K46)
         ischemic stricture of intestine (K55.1)
         meconium ileus NOS (P76.0)
         neonatal intestinal obstructions classifiable to P76-
         obstruction of duodenum (K31.5)
         postprocedural intestinal obstruction (K91.3)
         stenosis of anus or rectum (K62.4)

    K56.0   Paralytic ileus
         Paralysis of bowel
         Paralysis of colon
         Paralysis of intestine
         EXCLUDES 1   gallstone ileus (K56.3)
             ileus NOS (K56.7)
             obstructive ileus NOS (K56.69)

EXCLUDES 1 Not coded here   *EXCLUDES 2* Not included here   N Newborn Age: 0   P Pediatric Age: 0-17   M Maternity Age: 12-55   A Adult Age: 15-124

640   ICD-10-CM 2016

K56.1 Intussusception
Intussusception or invagination of bowel
Intussusception or invagination of colon
Intussusception or invagination of intestine
Intussusception or invagination of rectum
EXCLUDES 2 intussusception of appendix (K38.8)

K56.2 Volvulus
Strangulation of colon or intestine
Torsion of colon or intestine
Twist of colon or intestine
EXCLUDES 2 volvulus of duodenum (K31.5)

K56.3 Gallstone ileus
Obstruction of intestine by gallstone

✓5ᵗʰ K56.4 Other impaction of intestine
K56.41 Fecal impaction
EXCLUDES 1 constipation (K59.0-)
incomplete defecation (R15.0)

K56.49 Other impaction of intestine

K56.5 Intestinal adhesions [bands] with obstruction (postprocedural) (postinfection)
Abdominal hernia due to adhesions with obstruction
Peritoneal adhesions [bands] with intestinal obstruction (postprocedural) (postinfection)

✓5ᵗʰ K56.6 Other and unspecified intestinal obstruction
K56.60 Unspecified intestinal obstruction
Intestinal obstruction NOS
EXCLUDES 1 intestinal obstruction due to specified condition—code to condition

K56.69 Other intestinal obstruction
Enterostenosis NOS
Obstructive ileus NOS
Occlusion of colon or intestine NOS
Stenosis of colon or intestine NOS
Stricture of colon or intestine NOS
EXCLUDES 1 intestinal obstruction due to specified condition—code to condition

K56.7 Ileus, unspecified
EXCLUDES 1 obstructive ileus (K56.69)

✓4ᵗʰ K57 Diverticular disease of intestine
EXCLUDES 1 congenital diverticulum of intestine (Q43.8)
Meckel's diverticulum (Q43.0)
EXCLUDES 2 diverticulum of appendix (K38.2)

✓5ᵗʰ K57.0 Diverticulitis of small intestine with perforation and abscess
Diverticulitis of small intestine with peritonitis
EXCLUDES 1 diverticulitis of both small and large intestine with perforation and abscess (K57.4-)

K57.00 Diverticulitis of small intestine with perforation and abscess without bleeding

K57.01 Diverticulitis of small intestine with perforation and abscess with bleeding

✓5ᵗʰ K57.1 Diverticular disease of small intestine without perforation or abscess
EXCLUDES 1 diverticular disease of both small and large intestine without perforation or abscess (K57.5-)

K57.10 Diverticulosis of small intestine without perforation or abscess without bleeding
Diverticular disease of small intestine NOS

K57.11 Diverticulosis of small intestine without perforation or abscess with bleeding

K57.12 Diverticulitis of small intestine without perforation or abscess without bleeding

K57.13 Diverticulitis of small intestine without perforation or abscess with bleeding

✓5ᵗʰ K57.2 Diverticulitis of large intestine with perforation and abscess
Diverticulitis of colon with peritonitis
EXCLUDES 1 diverticulitis of both small and large intestine with perforation and abscess (K57.4-)

K57.20 Diverticulitis of large intestine with perforation and abscess without bleeding

K57.21 Diverticulitis of large intestine with perforation and abscess with bleeding

✓5ᵗʰ K57.3 Diverticular disease of large intestine without perforation or abscess
EXCLUDES 1 diverticular disease of both small and large intestine without perforation or abscess (K57.5-)

K57.30 Diverticulosis of large intestine without perforation or abscess without bleeding
Diverticular disease of colon NOS

K57.31 Diverticulosis of large intestine without perforation or abscess with bleeding

K57.32 Diverticulitis of large intestine without perforation or abscess without bleeding

K57.33 Diverticulitis of large intestine without perforation or abscess with bleeding

✓5ᵗʰ K57.4 Diverticulitis of both small and large intestine with perforation and abscess
Diverticulitis of both small and large intestine with peritonitis

K57.40 Diverticulitis of both small and large intestine with perforation and abscess without bleeding

K57.41 Diverticulitis of both small and large intestine with perforation and abscess with bleeding

✓5ᵗʰ K57.5 Diverticular disease of both small and large intestine without perforation or abscess
K57.50 Diverticulosis of both small and large intestine without perforation or abscess without bleeding
Diverticular disease of both small and large intestine NOS

K57.51 Diverticulosis of both small and large intestine without perforation or abscess with bleeding

K57.52 Diverticulitis of both small and large intestine without perforation or abscess without bleeding

K57.53 Diverticulitis of both small and large intestine without perforation or abscess with bleeding

✓5ᵗʰ K57.8 Diverticulitis of intestine, part unspecified, with perforation and abscess
Diverticulitis of intestine NOS with peritonitis

K57.80 Diverticulitis of intestine, part unspecified, with perforation and abscess without bleeding

K57.81 Diverticulitis of intestine, part unspecified, with perforation and abscess with bleeding

✓5ᵗʰ K57.9 Diverticular disease of intestine, part unspecified, without perforation or abscess
K57.90 Diverticulosis of intestine, part unspecified, without perforation or abscess without bleeding
Diverticular disease of intestine NOS

K57.91 Diverticulosis of intestine, part unspecified, without perforation or abscess with bleeding

K57.92 Diverticulitis of intestine, part unspecified, without perforation or abscess without bleeding

K57.93 Diverticulitis of intestine, part unspecified, without perforation or abscess with bleeding

✓4ᵗʰ K58 Irritable bowel syndrome
INCLUDES irritable colon
spastic colon

K58.0 Irritable bowel syndrome with diarrhea

K58.9 Irritable bowel syndrome without diarrhea
Irritable bowel syndrome NOS

✓4ᵗʰ K59 Other functional intestinal disorders
EXCLUDES 1 change in bowel habit NOS (R19.4)
intestinal malabsorption (K90.-)
psychogenic intestinal disorders (F45.8)
EXCLUDES 2 functional disorders of stomach (K31.-)

✓5ᵗʰ K59.0 Constipation
EXCLUDES 1 fecal impaction (K56.41)
incomplete defecation (R15.0)

K59.00 Constipation, unspecified
K59.01 Slow transit constipation
K59.02 Outlet dysfunction constipation
K59.09 Other constipation

K59.1 Functional diarrhea
EXCLUDES 1 diarrhea NOS (R19.7)
irritable bowel syndrome with diarrhea (K58.0)

K59.2 Neurogenic bowel, not elsewhere classified

K59.3 Megacolon, not elsewhere classified
Dilatation of colon
Toxic megacolon
Code first (T51-T65) to identify toxic agent
EXCLUDES 1 congenital megacolon (aganglionic) (Q43.1)
megacolon (due to) (in) Chagas' disease (B57.32)
megacolon (due to) (in) Clostridium difficile (A04.7)
megacolon (due to) (in) Hirschsprung's disease (Q43.1)

K59.4 Anal spasm
Proctalgia fugax

☑ Additional Character Required · ✓ₓ7ᵗʰ Placeholder Alert · Unspecified Dx · Other Specified Dx · Manifestation · ►◄ Revised Text · ● New Code · ▲ Revised Code Title

Chapter 11. Diseases of the Digestive System

K59.8   **Other specified functional intestinal disorders**
Atony of colon
Pseudo-obstruction (acute) (chronic) of intestine

K59.9   **Functional intestinal disorder, unspecified**

✓4ᵗʰ **K60**   **Fissure and fistula of anal and rectal regions**
> EXCLUDES 1   *fissure and fistula of anal and rectal regions with abscess or cellulitis (K61.-)*
> EXCLUDES 2   *anal sphincter tear (healed) (nontraumatic) (old) (K62.81)*

K60.0   **Acute anal fissure**

K60.1   **Chronic anal fissure**

K60.2   **Anal fissure, unspecified**

K60.3   **Anal fistula**

K60.4   **Rectal fistula**
Fistula of rectum to skin
> EXCLUDES 1   *rectovaginal fistula (N82.3)*
> *vesicorectal fistual (N32.1)*

K60.5   **Anorectal fistula**

✓4ᵗʰ **K61**   **Abscess of anal and rectal regions**
> INCLUDES   abscess of anal and rectal regions
> cellulitis of anal and rectal regions

K61.0   **Anal abscess**
Perianal abscess
> EXCLUDES 1   *intrasphincteric abscess (K61.4)*

K61.1   **Rectal abscess**
Perirectal abscess
> EXCLUDES 1   *ischiorectal abscess (K61.3)*
> **AHA:** 2012, 4Q, 104

K61.2   **Anorectal abscess**

K61.3   **Ischiorectal abscess**
Abscess of ischiorectal fossa

K61.4   **Intrasphincteric abscess**

✓4ᵗʰ **K62**   **Other diseases of anus and rectum**
> INCLUDES   anal canal
> EXCLUDES 2   *colostomy and enterostomy malfunction (K94.0-, K94.1-)*
> *fecal incontinence (R15.-)*
> *hemorrhoids (K64.-)*

K62.0   **Anal polyp**

K62.1   **Rectal polyp**
> EXCLUDES 1   *adenomatous polyp (D12.8)*

K62.2   **Anal prolapse**
Prolapse of anal canal

K62.3   **Rectal prolapse**
Prolapse of rectal mucosa

K62.4   **Stenosis of anus and rectum**
Stricture of anus (sphincter)

K62.5   **Hemorrhage of anus and rectum**
> EXCLUDES 1   *gastrointestinal bleeding NOS (K92.2)*
> *melena (K92.1)*
> *neonatal rectal hemorrhage (P54.2)*

K62.6   **Ulcer of anus and rectum**
Solitary ulcer of anus and rectum
Stercoral ulcer of anus and rectum
> EXCLUDES 1   *fissure and fistula of anus and rectum (K60.-)*
> *ulcerative colitis (K51.-)*

K62.7   **Radiation proctitis**
Use additional code to identify the type of radiation (W90.-)

✓5ᵗʰ **K62.8**   **Other specified diseases of anus and rectum**
> EXCLUDES 2   *ulcerative proctitis (K51.2)*

K62.81   **Anal sphincter tear (healed) (nontraumatic) (old)**
Tear of anus, nontraumatic
Use additional code for any associated fecal incontinence (R15.-)
> EXCLUDES 2   *anal fissure (K60.-)*
> *anal sphincter tear (healed) (old) complicating delivery (O34.7-)*
> *traumatic tear of anal sphincter (S31.831)*

K62.82   **Dysplasia of anus**
Anal intraepithelial neoplasia I and II (AIN I and II) (histologically confirmed)
Dysplasia of anus NOS
Mild and moderate dysplasia of anus (histologically confirmed)
> EXCLUDES 1   *abnormal results from anal cytologic examination without histologic confirmation (R85.61-)*
> *anal intraepithelial neoplasia III (D01.3)*
> *carcinoma in situ of anus (D01.3)*
> *HGSIL of anus (R85.613)*
> *severe dysplasia of anus (D01.3)*

K62.89   **Other specified diseases of anus and rectum**
Proctitis NOS
Use additional code for any associated fecal incontinence (R15.-)

K62.9   **Disease of anus and rectum, unspecified**

✓4ᵗʰ **K63**   **Other diseases of intestine**

K63.0   **Abscess of intestine**
> EXCLUDES 1   *abscess of intestine with Crohn's disease (K50.014, K50.114, K50.814, K50.914)*
> *abscess of intestine with diverticular disease (K57.0, K57.2, K57.4, K57.8)*
> *abscess of intestine with ulcerative colitis (K51.014, K51.214, K51.314, K51.414, K51.514, K51.814, K51.914)*
> EXCLUDES 2   *abscess of anal and rectal regions (K61.-)*
> *abscess of appendix (K35.3)*

K63.1   **Perforation of intestine (nontraumatic)**
Perforation (nontraumatic) of rectum
> EXCLUDES 1   *perforation (nontraumatic) of duodenum (K26.-)*
> *perforation (nontraumatic) of intestine with diverticular disease (K57.0, K57.2, K57.4, K57.8)*
> EXCLUDES 2   *perforation (nontraumatic) of appendix (K35.2, K35.3)*

K63.2   **Fistula of intestine**
> EXCLUDES 1   *fistula of duodenum (K31.6)*
> *fistula of intestine with Crohn's disease (K50.013, K50.113, K50.813, K50.913)*
> *fistula of intestine with ulcerative colitis (K51.013, K51.213, K51.313, K51.413, K51.513, K51.813, K51.913)*
> EXCLUDES 2   *fistula of anal and rectal regions (K60.-)*
> *fistula of appendix (K38.3)*
> *intestinal-genital fistula, female (N82.2-N82.4)*
> *vesicointestinal fistula (N32.1)*

K63.3   **Ulcer of intestine**
Primary ulcer of small intestine
> EXCLUDES 1   *duodenal ulcer (K26.-)*
> *gastrointestinal ulcer (K28.-)*
> *gastrojejunal ulcer (K28.-)*
> *jejunal ulcer (K28.-)*
> *peptic ulcer, site unspecified (K27.-)*
> *ulcer of intestine with perforation (K63.1)*
> *ulcer of anus or rectum (K62.6)*
> *ulcerative colitis (K51.-)*

K63.4   **Enteroptosis**

K63.5   **Polyp of colon**
> EXCLUDES 1   *adenomatous polyp of colon (D12.6)*
> *inflammatory polyp of colon (K51.4-)*
> *polyposis of colon (D12.6)*

✓5ᵗʰ **K63.8**   **Other specified diseases of intestine**

K63.81   **Dieulafoy lesion of intestine**
> EXCLUDES 2   *Dieulafoy lesion of stomach and duodenum (K31.82)*

K63.89   **Other specified diseases of intestine**
> **AHA:** 2013, 2Q, 31

K63.9   **Disease of intestine, unspecified**

✓4ᵗʰ **K64**   **Hemorrhoids and perianal venous thrombosis**
> INCLUDES   piles
> EXCLUDES 1   *hemorrhoids complicating childbirth and the puerperium (O87.2)*
> *hemorrhoids complicating pregnancy (O22.4)*

K64.0   **First degree hemorrhoids**
Grade/stage I hemorrhoids
Hemorrhoids (bleeding) without prolapse outside of anal canal

K64.1   **Second degree hemorrhoids**
Grade/stage II hemorrhoids
Hemorrhoids (bleeding) that prolapse with straining, but retract spontaneously

---

EXCLUDES 1 Not coded here   EXCLUDES 2 Not included here   N Newborn Age: 0   P Pediatric Age: 0-17   M Maternity Age: 12-55   A Adult Age: 15-124

642   ICD-10-CM 2016

K64.2   **Third degree hemorrhoids**
Grade/stage III hemorrhoids
Hemorrhoids (bleeding) that prolapse with straining and require manual replacement back inside anal canal

K64.3   **Fourth degree hemorrhoids**
Grade/stage IV hemorrhoids
Hemorrhoids (bleeding) with prolapsed tissue that cannot be manually replaced

K64.4   **Residual hemorrhoidal skin tags**
External hemorrhoids, NOS
Skin tags of anus

K64.5   **Perianal venous thrombosis**
External hemorrhoids with thrombosis
Perianal hematoma
Thrombosed hemorrhoids NOS

K64.8   **Other hemorrhoids**
Internal hemorrhoids, without mention of degree
Prolapsed hemorrhoids, degree not specified

K64.9   **Unspecified hemorrhoids**
Hemorrhoids (bleeding) NOS
Hemorrhoids (bleeding) without mention of degree

Diseases of peritoneum and retroperitoneum (K65-K68)

✓4th   **K65**   **Peritonitis**
Use additional code (B95-B97), to identify infectious agent
EXCLUDES 1   acute appendicitis with generalized peritonitis (K35.2)
aseptic peritonitis (T81.6)
benign paroxysmal peritonitis (E85.0)
chemical peritonitis (T81.6)
diverticulitis of both small and large intestine with peritonitis (K57.4-)
diverticulitis of colon with peritonitis (K57.2-)
diverticulitis of intestine, NOS, with peritonitis (K57.8-)
diverticulitis of small intestine with peritonitis (K57.0-)
gonococcal peritonitis (A54.85)
neonatal peritonitis (P78.0-P78.1)
pelvic peritonitis, female (N73.3-N73.5)
periodic familial peritonitis (E85.0)
peritonitis due to talc or other foreign substance (T81.6)
peritonitis in chlamydia (A74.81)
peritonitis in diphtheria (A36.89)
peritonitis in syphilis (late) (A52.74)
peritonitis in tuberculosis (A18.31)
peritonitis with or following abortion or ectopic or molar pregnancy (O00-O07, O08.0)
peritonitis with or following appendicitis (K35.-)
peritonitis with or following diverticular disease of intestine (K57.-)
puerperal peritonitis (O85)
retroperitoneal infections (K68.-)

K65.0   **Generalized (acute) peritonitis**
Pelvic peritonitis (acute), male
Subphrenic peritonitis (acute)
Suppurative peritonitis (acute)

K65.1   **Peritoneal abscess**
Abdominopelvic abscess   Subdiaphragmatic abscess
Abscess (of) omentum   Subhepatic abscess
Abscess (of) peritoneum   Subphrenic abscess
Mesenteric abscess
Retrocecal abscess

K65.2   **Spontaneous bacterial peritonitis**
EXCLUDES 1   bacterial peritonitis NOS (K65.9)

K65.3   **Choleperitonitis**
Peritonitis due to bile

K65.4   **Sclerosing mesenteritis**
Fat necrosis of peritoneum
(Idiopathic) sclerosing mesenteric fibrosis
Mesenteric lipodystrophy
Mesenteric panniculitis
Retractile mesenteritis

K65.8   **Other peritonitis**
Chronic proliferative peritonitis
Peritonitis due to urine

K65.9   **Peritonitis, unspecified**
Bacterial peritonitis NOS
AHA: 2013, 2Q, 31

✓4th   **K66**   **Other disorders of peritoneum**
EXCLUDES 2   ascites (R18.-)
peritoneal effusion (chronic) (R18.8)

K66.0   **Peritoneal adhesions (postprocedural) (postinfection)**
Adhesions (of) abdominal (wall)   Adhesions (of) omentum
Adhesions (of) diaphragm   Adhesions (of) stomach
Adhesions (of) intestine   Adhesive bands
Adhesions (of) male pelvis   Mesenteric adhesions
EXCLUDES 1   female pelvic adhesions [bands] (N73.6)
peritoneal adhesions with intestinal obstruction (K56.5)

K66.1   **Hemoperitoneum**
EXCLUDES 1   traumatic hemoperitoneum (S36.8-)

K66.8   **Other specified disorders of peritoneum**

K66.9   **Disorder of peritoneum, unspecified**

K67   *Disorders of peritoneum in infectious diseases classified elsewhere*
Code first underlying disease, such as:
congenital syphilis (A50.0)
helminthiasis (B65.0-B83.9)
EXCLUDES 1   peritonitis in chlamydia (A74.81)
peritonitis in diphtheria (A36.89)
peritonitis in gonococcal (A54.85)
peritonitis in syphilis (late) (A52.74)
peritonitis in tuberculosis (A18.31)

✓4th   **K68**   **Disorders of retroperitoneum**

✓5th   **K68.1**   **Retroperitoneal abscess**

K68.11   **Postprocedural retroperitoneal abscess**

K68.12   **Psoas muscle abscess**

K68.19   **Other retroperitoneal abscess**

K68.9   **Other disorders of retroperitoneum**

Diseases of liver (K70-K77)

EXCLUDES 1   jaundice NOS (R17)
EXCLUDES 2   hemochromatosis (E83.11-)
Reye's syndrome (G93.7)
viral hepatitis (B15-B19)
Wilson's disease (E83.0)

✓4th   **K70**   **Alcoholic liver disease**
Use additional code to identify:
alcohol abuse and dependence (F10.-)

K70.0   **Alcoholic fatty liver**   Ⓐ

✓5th   **K70.1**   **Alcoholic hepatitis**

K70.10   **Alcoholic hepatitis without ascites**   Ⓐ

K70.11   **Alcoholic hepatitis with ascites**   Ⓐ

K70.2   **Alcoholic fibrosis and sclerosis of liver**   Ⓐ

✓5th   **K70.3**   **Alcoholic cirrhosis of liver**
Alcoholic cirrhosis NOS

K70.30   **Alcoholic cirrhosis of liver without ascites**   Ⓐ

K70.31   **Alcoholic cirrhosis of liver with ascites**   Ⓐ

✓5th   **K70.4**   **Alcoholic hepatic failure**
Acute alcoholic hepatic failure
Alcoholic hepatic failure NOS
Chronic alcoholic hepatic failure
Subacute alcoholic hepatic failure

K70.40   **Alcoholic hepatic failure without coma**   Ⓐ

K70.41   **Alcoholic hepatic failure with coma**   Ⓐ

K70.9   **Alcoholic liver disease, unspecified**   Ⓐ

✓4th   **K71**   **Toxic liver disease**
INCLUDES   drug-induced idiosyncratic (unpredictable) liver disease
drug-induced toxic (predictable) liver disease
Code first poisoning due to drug or toxin, if applicable (T36-T65 with fifth or sixth character 1-4 or 6)
Use additional code for adverse effect, if applicable, to identify drug (T36-T50 with fifth or sixth character 5)
EXCLUDES 2   alcoholic liver disease (K70.-)
Budd-Chiari syndrome (I82.0)

K71.0   **Toxic liver disease with cholestasis**
Cholestasis with hepatocyte injury
"Pure" cholestasis

✓5th   **K71.1**   **Toxic liver disease with hepatic necrosis**
Hepatic failure (acute) (chronic) due to drugs

K71.10   **Toxic liver disease with hepatic necrosis, without coma**

K71.11   **Toxic liver disease with hepatic necrosis, with coma**

K71.2   **Toxic liver disease with acute hepatitis**

K71.3   **Toxic liver disease with chronic persistent hepatitis**

☑ Additional Character Required   ✗x7th Placeholder Alert   Unspecified Dx   Other Specified Dx   Manifestation   ►◄ Revised Text   ● New Code   ▲ Revised Code Title

ICD-10-CM 2016   643

K71.4 Toxic liver disease with chronic lobular hepatitis

✓5ᵗʰ **K71.5** Toxic liver disease with chronic active hepatitis
Toxic liver disease with lupoid hepatitis

   K71.50 Toxic liver disease with chronic active hepatitis without ascites

   K71.51 Toxic liver disease with chronic active hepatitis with ascites

K71.6 Toxic liver disease with hepatitis, not elsewhere classified

K71.7 Toxic liver disease with fibrosis and cirrhosis of liver

K71.8 Toxic liver disease with other disorders of liver
Toxic liver disease with focal nodular hyperplasia
Toxic liver disease with hepatic granulomas
Toxic liver disease with peliosis hepatis
Toxic liver disease with veno-occlusive disease of liver

K71.9 Toxic liver disease, unspecified

✓4ᵗʰ **K72** Hepatic failure, not elsewhere classified
INCLUDES acute hepatitis NEC, with hepatic failure
fulminant hepatitis NEC, with hepatic failure
hepatic encephalopathy NOS
liver (cell) necrosis with hepatic failure
malignant hepatitis NEC, with hepatic failure
yellow liver atrophy or dystrophy
EXCLUDES 1 alcoholic hepatic failure (K70.4)
hepatic failure with toxic liver disease (K71.1-)
icterus of newborn (P55-P59)
postprocedural hepatic failure (K91.82)
viral hepatitis with hepatic coma (B15-B19)
EXCLUDES 2 hepatic failure complicating abortion or ectopic or molar pregnancy (O00-O07, O08.8)
hepatic failure complicating pregnancy, childbirth and the puerperium (O26.6-)

✓5ᵗʰ **K72.0** Acute and subacute hepatic failure
AHA: 2014, 2Q, 13

   K72.00 Acute and subacute hepatic failure without coma

   K72.01 Acute and subacute hepatic failure with coma

✓5ᵗʰ **K72.1** Chronic hepatic failure

   K72.10 Chronic hepatic failure without coma

   K72.11 Chronic hepatic failure with coma

✓5ᵗʰ **K72.9** Hepatic failure, unspecified

   K72.90 Hepatic failure, unspecified without coma

   K72.91 Hepatic failure, unspecified with coma
Hepatic coma NOS

✓4ᵗʰ **K73** Chronic hepatitis, not elsewhere classified
EXCLUDES 1 alcoholic hepatitis (chronic) (K70.1-)
drug-induced hepatitis (chronic) (K71.-)
granulomatous hepatitis (chronic) NEC (K75.3)
reactive, nonspecific hepatitis (chronic) (K75.2)
viral hepatitis (chronic) (B15-B19)

K73.0 Chronic persistent hepatitis, not elsewhere classified

K73.1 Chronic lobular hepatitis, not elsewhere classified

K73.2 Chronic active hepatitis, not elsewhere classified

K73.8 Other chronic hepatitis, not elsewhere classified

K73.9 Chronic hepatitis, unspecified

✓4ᵗʰ **K74** Fibrosis and cirrhosis of liver
Code also, if applicable, viral hepatitis (acute) (chronic) (B15-B19)
EXCLUDES 1 alcoholic cirrhosis (of liver) (K70.3)
alcoholic fibrosis of liver (K70.2)
cardiac sclerosis of liver (K76.1)
cirrhosis (of liver) with toxic liver disease (K71.7)
congenital cirrhosis (of liver) (P78.81)
pigmentary cirrhosis (of liver) (E83.110)

K74.0 Hepatic fibrosis

K74.1 Hepatic sclerosis

K74.2 Hepatic fibrosis with hepatic sclerosis

K74.3 Primary biliary cirrhosis
Chronic nonsuppurative destructive cholangitis

K74.4 Secondary biliary cirrhosis

K74.5 Biliary cirrhosis, unspecified

✓5ᵗʰ **K74.6** Other and unspecified cirrhosis of liver

   K74.60 Unspecified cirrhosis of liver
Cirrhosis (of liver) NOS

   K74.69 Other cirrhosis of liver
Cryptogenic cirrhosis (of liver)
Macronodular cirrhosis (of liver)
Micronodular cirrhosis (of liver)
Mixed type cirrhosis (of liver)
Portal cirrhosis (of liver)
Postnecrotic cirrhosis (of liver)

✓4ᵗʰ **K75** Other inflammatory liver diseases
EXCLUDES 2 toxic liver disease (K71.-)

K75.0 Abscess of liver
Cholangitic hepatic abscess
Hematogenic hepatic abscess
Hepatic abscess NOS
Lymphogenic hepatic abscess
Pylephlebitic hepatic abscess
EXCLUDES 1 amebic liver abscess (A06.4)
cholangitis without liver abscess (K83.0)
pylephlebitis without liver abscess (K75.1)

K75.1 Phlebitis of portal vein
Pylephlebitis
EXCLUDES 1 pylephlebitic liver abscess (K75.0)

K75.2 Nonspecific reactive hepatitis
EXCLUDES 1 acute or subacute hepatitis (K72.0-)
chronic hepatitis NEC (K73.-)
viral hepatitis (B15-B19)

K75.3 Granulomatous hepatitis, not elsewhere classified
EXCLUDES 1 acute or subacute hepatitis (K72.0-)
chronic hepatitis NEC (K73.-)
viral hepatitis (B15-B19)

K75.4 Autoimmune hepatitis
Lupoid hepatitis NEC

✓5ᵗʰ **K75.8** Other specified inflammatory liver diseases

   K75.81 Nonalcoholic steatohepatitis (NASH)

   K75.89 Other specified inflammatory liver diseases

K75.9 Inflammatory liver disease, unspecified
Hepatitis NOS
EXCLUDES 1 acute or subacute hepatitis (K72.0-)
chronic hepatitis NEC (K73.-)
viral hepatitis (B15-B19)

✓4ᵗʰ **K76** Other diseases of liver
EXCLUDES 2 alcoholic liver disease (K70.-)
amyloid degeneration of liver (E85.-)
cystic disease of liver (congenital) (Q44.6)
hepatic vein thrombosis (I82.0)
hepatomegaly NOS (R16.0)
pigmentary cirrhosis (of liver) (E83.110)
portal vein thrombosis (I81)
toxic liver disease (K71.-)

K76.0 Fatty (change of) liver, not elsewhere classified
Nonalcoholic fatty liver disease (NAFLD)
EXCLUDES 1 nonalcoholic steatohepatitis (NASH) (K75.81)

K76.1 Chronic passive congestion of liver
Cardiac cirrhosis
Cardiac sclerosis

K76.2 Central hemorrhagic necrosis of liver
EXCLUDES 1 liver necrosis with hepatic failure (K72.-)

K76.3 Infarction of liver

K76.4 Peliosis hepatis
Hepatic angiomatosis

K76.5 Hepatic veno-occlusive disease
EXCLUDES 1 Budd-Chiari syndrome (I82.0)

K76.6 Portal hypertension
Use additional code for any associated complications, such as:
portal hypertensive gastropathy (K31.89)

K76.7 Hepatorenal syndrome
EXCLUDES 1 hepatorenal syndrome following labor and delivery (O90.4)
postprocedural hepatorenal syndrome (K91.82)

✓5ᵗʰ **K76.8** Other specified diseases of liver

   K76.81 Hepatopulmonary syndrome
Code first underlying liver disease, such as:
alcoholic cirrhosis of liver (K70.3-)
cirrhosis of liver without mention of alcohol (K74.6-)

   K76.89 Other specified diseases of liver
Cyst (simple) of liver
Focal nodular hyperplasia of liver
Hepatoptosis

K76.9 Liver disease, unspecified

EXCLUDES 1 Not coded here   EXCLUDES 2 Not included here   N Newborn Age: 0   P Pediatric Age: 0-17   M Maternity Age: 12-55   A Adult Age: 15-124

644   ICD-10-CM 2016

K77 *Liver disorders in diseases classified elsewhere*
    Code first underlying disease, such as:
      amyloidosis (E85.-)
      congenital syphilis (A50.0, A50.5)
      congenital toxoplasmosis (P37.1)
      schistosomiasis (B65.0-B65.9)
    EXCLUDES 1 *alcoholic hepatitis (K70.1-)*
        alcoholic liver disease (K70-.)
        cytomegaloviral hepatitis (B25.1)
        herpesviral [herpes simplex] hepatitis (B00.81)
        infectious mononucleosis with liver disease
          (B27.0-B27.9 with .9)
        mumps hepatitis (B26.81)
        sarcoidosis with liver disease (D86.89)
        secondary syphilis with liver disease (A51.45)
        syphilis (late) with liver disease (A52.74)
        toxoplasmosis (acquired) hepatitis (B58.1)
        tuberculosis with liver disease (A18.83)

Disorders of gallbladder, biliary tract and pancreas (K80-K87)

☑4th **K80** **Cholelithiasis**
    EXCLUDES 1 *retained cholelithiasis following cholecystectomy (K91.86)*

☑5th **K80.0** **Calculus of gallbladder with acute cholecystitis**
    Any condition listed in K80.2 with acute cholecystitis

    K80.00 **Calculus of gallbladder with acute cholecystitis without obstruction**

    K80.01 **Calculus of gallbladder with acute cholecystitis with obstruction**

☑5th **K80.1** **Calculus of gallbladder with other cholecystitis**

    K80.10 **Calculus of gallbladder with chronic cholecystitis without obstruction**
        Cholelithiasis with cholecystitis NOS

    K80.11 **Calculus of gallbladder with chronic cholecystitis with obstruction**

    K80.12 **Calculus of gallbladder with acute and chronic cholecystitis without obstruction**

    K80.13 **Calculus of gallbladder with acute and chronic cholecystitis with obstruction**

    K80.18 **Calculus of gallbladder with other cholecystitis without obstruction**

    K80.19 **Calculus of gallbladder with other cholecystitis with obstruction**

☑5th **K80.2** **Calculus of gallbladder without cholecystitis**
    Cholecystolithiasis without cholecystitis
    Cholelithiasis (without cholecystitis)
    Colic (recurrent) of gallbladder (without cholecystitis)
    Gallstone (impacted) of cystic duct (without cholecystitis)
    Gallstone (impacted) of gallbladder (without cholecystitis)

    K80.20 **Calculus of gallbladder without cholecystitis without obstruction**

    K80.21 **Calculus of gallbladder without cholecystitis with obstruction**

☑5th **K80.3** **Calculus of bile duct with cholangitis**
    Any condition listed in K80.5 with cholangitis

    K80.30 **Calculus of bile duct with cholangitis, unspecified, without obstruction**

    K80.31 **Calculus of bile duct with cholangitis, unspecified, with obstruction**

    K80.32 **Calculus of bile duct with acute cholangitis without obstruction**

    K80.33 **Calculus of bile duct with acute cholangitis with obstruction**

    K80.34 **Calculus of bile duct with chronic cholangitis without obstruction**

    K80.35 **Calculus of bile duct with chronic cholangitis with obstruction**

    K80.36 **Calculus of bile duct with acute and chronic cholangitis without obstruction**

    K80.37 **Calculus of bile duct with acute and chronic cholangitis with obstruction**

☑5th **K80.4** **Calculus of bile duct with cholecystitis**
    Any condition listed in K80.5 with cholecystitis (with cholangitis)

    K80.40 **Calculus of bile duct with cholecystitis, unspecified, without obstruction**

    K80.41 **Calculus of bile duct with cholecystitis, unspecified, with obstruction**

    K80.42 **Calculus of bile duct with acute cholecystitis without obstruction**

    K80.43 **Calculus of bile duct with acute cholecystitis with obstruction**

    K80.44 **Calculus of bile duct with chronic cholecystitis without obstruction**

    K80.45 **Calculus of bile duct with chronic cholecystitis with obstruction**

    K80.46 **Calculus of bile duct with acute and chronic cholecystitis without obstruction**

    K80.47 **Calculus of bile duct with acute and chronic cholecystitis with obstruction**

☑5th **K80.5** **Calculus of bile duct without cholangitis or cholecystitis**
    Choledocholithiasis (without cholangitis or cholecystitis)
    Gallstone (impacted) of bile duct NOS (without cholangitis or cholecystitis)
    Gallstone (impacted) of common duct (without cholangitis or cholecystitis)
    Gallstone (impacted) of hepatic duct (without cholangitis or cholecystitis)
    Hepatic cholelithiasis (without cholangitis or cholecystitis)
    Hepatic colic (recurrent) (without cholangitis or cholecystitis)

    K80.50 **Calculus of bile duct without cholangitis or cholecystitis without obstruction**

    K80.51 **Calculus of bile duct without cholangitis or cholecystitis with obstruction**

☑5th **K80.6** **Calculus of gallbladder and bile duct with cholecystitis**

    K80.60 **Calculus of gallbladder and bile duct with cholecystitis, unspecified, without obstruction**

    K80.61 **Calculus of gallbladder and bile duct with cholecystitis, unspecified, with obstruction**

    K80.62 **Calculus of gallbladder and bile duct with acute cholecystitis without obstruction**

    K80.63 **Calculus of gallbladder and bile duct with acute cholecystitis with obstruction**

    K80.64 **Calculus of gallbladder and bile duct with chronic cholecystitis without obstruction**

    K80.65 **Calculus of gallbladder and bile duct with chronic cholecystitis with obstruction**

    K80.66 **Calculus of gallbladder and bile duct with acute and chronic cholecystitis without obstruction**

    K80.67 **Calculus of gallbladder and bile duct with acute and chronic cholecystitis with obstruction**

☑5th **K80.7** **Calculus of gallbladder and bile duct without cholecystitis**

    K80.70 **Calculus of gallbladder and bile duct without cholecystitis without obstruction**

    K80.71 **Calculus of gallbladder and bile duct without cholecystitis with obstruction**

☑5th **K80.8** **Other cholelithiasis**

    K80.80 **Other cholelithiasis without obstruction**

    K80.81 **Other cholelithiasis with obstruction**

☑4th **K81** **Cholecystitis**
    EXCLUDES 1 *cholecystitis with cholelithiasis (K80.-)*

    K81.0 **Acute cholecystitis**
        Abscess of gallbladder
        Angiocholecystitis
        Emphysematous (acute) cholecystitis
        Empyema of gallbladder
        Gangrene of gallbladder
        Gangrenous cholecystitis
        Suppurative cholecystitis

    K81.1 **Chronic cholecystitis**

    K81.2 **Acute cholecystitis with chronic cholecystitis**

    K81.9 **Cholecystitis, unspecified**

☑4th **K82** **Other diseases of gallbladder**
    EXCLUDES 1 *nonvisualization of gallbladder (R93.2)*
        postcholecystectomy syndrome (K91.5)

    K82.0 **Obstruction of gallbladder**
        Occlusion of cystic duct or gallbladder without cholelithiasis
        Stenosis of cystic duct or gallbladder without cholelithiasis
        Stricture of cystic duct or gallbladder without cholelithiasis
        EXCLUDES 1 *obstruction of gallbladder with cholelithiasis (K80.-)*

    K82.1 **Hydrops of gallbladder**
        Mucocele of gallbladder

    K82.2 **Perforation of gallbladder**
        Rupture of cystic duct or gallbladder

    K82.3 **Fistula of gallbladder**
        Cholecystocolic fistula
        Cholecystoduodenal fistula

☑ Additional Character Required   **v1 7th** Placeholder Alert   Unspecified Dx   Other Specified Dx   Manifestation   ►◄ Revised Text   ● New Code   ▲ Revised Code Title

K82.4　Cholesterolosis of gallbladder
Strawberry gallbladder
EXCLUDES 1　*cholesterolosis of gallbladder with cholecystitis (K81.-)*
cholesterolosis of gallbladder with cholelithiasis (K80.-)

K82.8　Other specified diseases of gallbladder
Adhesions of cystic duct or gallbladder
Atrophy of cystic duct or gallbladder
Cyst of cystic duct or gallbladder
Dyskinesia of cystic duct or gallbladder
Hypertrophy of cystic duct or gallbladder
Nonfunctioning of cystic duct or gallbladder
Ulcer of cystic duct or gallbladder

K82.9　Disease of gallbladder, unspecified

✓4ᵗʰ **K83　Other diseases of biliary tract**
EXCLUDES 1　*postcholecystectomy syndrome (K91.5)*
EXCLUDES 2　*conditions involving the gallbladder (K81-K82)*
conditions involving the cystic duct (K81-K82)

K83.0　Cholangitis
Ascending cholangitis
Cholangitis NOS
Primary cholangitis
Recurrent cholangitis
Sclerosing cholangitis
Secondary cholangitis
Stenosing cholangitis
Suppurative cholangitis
EXCLUDES 1　*cholangitic liver abscess (K75.0)*
cholangitis with choledocholithiasis (K80.3-, K80.4-)
chronic nonsuppurative destructive cholangitis (K74.3)

K83.1　Obstruction of bile duct
Occlusion of bile duct without cholelithiasis
Stenosis of bile duct without cholelithiasis
Stricture of bile duct without cholelithiasis
EXCLUDES 1　*congenital obstruction of bile duct (Q44.3)*
obstruction of bile duct with cholelithiasis (K80.-)

K83.2　Perforation of bile duct
Rupture of bile duct

K83.3　Fistula of bile duct
Choledochoduodenal fistula

K83.4　Spasm of sphincter of Oddi

K83.5　Biliary cyst

K83.8　Other specified diseases of biliary tract
Adhesions of biliary tract
Atrophy of biliary tract
Hypertrophy of biliary tract
Ulcer of biliary tract

K83.9　Disease of biliary tract, unspecified

✓4ᵗʰ **K85　Acute pancreatitis**
Abscess of pancreas
Acute necrosis of pancreas
Acute (recurrent) pancreatitis
Gangrene of (gangrenous) pancreas
Hemorrhagic pancreatitis
Infective necrosis of pancreas
Subacute pancreatitis
Suppurative pancreatitis

K85.0　Idiopathic acute pancreatitis

K85.1　Biliary acute pancreatitis
Gallstone pancreatitis

K85.2　Alcohol induced acute pancreatitis
EXCLUDES 2　*alcohol induced chronic pancreatitis (K86.0)*

K85.3　Drug induced acute pancreatitis
Use additional code for adverse effect, if applicable, to identify drug (T36-T50 with fifth or sixth character 5)
Use additional code to identify drug abuse and dependence (F11.- F17.-)

K85.8　Other acute pancreatitis

K85.9　Acute pancreatitis, unspecified
Pancreatitis NOS

✓4ᵗʰ **K86　Other diseases of pancreas**
EXCLUDES 2　*fibrocystic disease of pancreas (E84.-)*
islet cell tumor (of pancreas) (D13.7)
pancreatic steatorrhea (K90.3)

K86.0　Alcohol-induced chronic pancreatitis
Use additional code to identify:
alcohol abuse and dependence (F10.-)
EXCLUDES 2　*alcohol induced acute pancreatitis (K85.2)*

K86.1　Other chronic pancreatitis
Chronic pancreatitis NOS
Infectious chronic pancreatitis
Recurrent chronic pancreatitis
Relapsing chronic pancreatitis

K86.2　Cyst of pancreas

K86.3　Pseudocyst of pancreas

K86.8　Other specified diseases of pancreas
Aseptic pancreatic necrosis
Atrophy of pancreas
Calculus of pancreas
Cirrhosis of pancreas
Fibrosis of pancreas
Pancreatic fat necrosis
Pancreatic infantilism
Pancreatic necrosis NOS

K86.9　Disease of pancreas, unspecified

K87　Disorders of gallbladder, biliary tract and pancreas in diseases classified elsewhere
Code first underlying disease
EXCLUDES 1　*cytomegaloviral pancreatitis (B25.2)*
mumps pancreatitis (B26.3)
syphilitic gallbladder (A52.74)
syphilitic pancreas (A52.74)
tuberculosis of gallbladder (A18.83)
tuberculosis of pancreas (A18.83)

Other diseases of the digestive system (K90-K95)

✓4ᵗʰ **K90　Intestinal malabsorption**
EXCLUDES 1　*intestinal malabsorption following gastrointestinal surgery (K91.2)*

K90.0　Celiac disease
Gluten-sensitive enteropathy
Idiopathic steatorrhea
Nontropical sprue
Use additional code for associated disorders including:
dermatitis herpetiformis (L13.0)
gluten ataxia (G32.81)

K90.1　Tropical sprue
Sprue NOS
Tropical steatorrhea

K90.2　Blind loop syndrome, not elsewhere classified
Blind loop syndrome NOS
EXCLUDES 1　*congenital blind loop syndrome (Q43.8)*
postsurgical blind loop syndrome (K91.2)

K90.3　Pancreatic steatorrhea

K90.4　Malabsorption due to intolerance, not elsewhere classified
Malabsorption due to intolerance to carbohydrate
Malabsorption due to intolerance to fat
Malabsorption due to intolerance to protein
Malabsorption due to intolerance to starch
EXCLUDES 2　*gluten-sensitive enteropathy (K90.0)*
lactose intolerance (E73.-)

✓5ᵗʰ **K90.8　Other intestinal malabsorption**

K90.81　Whipple's disease

K90.89　Other intestinal malabsorption

K90.9　Intestinal malabsorption, unspecified

✓4ᵗʰ **K91　Intraoperative and postprocedural complications and disorders of digestive system, not elsewhere classified**
EXCLUDES 2　*complications of artificial opening of digestive system (K94.-)*
complications of bariatric procedures (K95.-)
gastrojejunal ulcer (K28.-)
postprocedural (radiation) retroperitoneal abscess (K68.11)
radiation colitis (K52.0)
radiation gastroenteritis (K52.0)
radiation proctitis (K62.7)

K91.0　Vomiting following gastrointestinal surgery

K91.1　Postgastric surgery syndromes
Dumping syndrome
Postgastrectomy syndrome
Postvagotomy syndrome

K91.2　Postsurgical malabsorption, not elsewhere classified
Postsurgical blind loop syndrome
EXCLUDES 1　*malabsorption osteomalacia in adults (M83.2)*
malabsorption osteoporosis, postsurgical (M80.8-, M81.8)

K91.3　Postprocedural intestinal obstruction

K91.5　Postcholecystectomy syndrome

EXCLUDES 1 Not coded here　　　EXCLUDES 2 Not included here　　　N Newborn Age: 0　　　P Pediatric Age: 0-17　　　M Maternity Age: 12-55　　　A Adult Age: 15-124

646

ICD-10-CM 2016

✓5ᵗʰ **K91.6** Intraoperative hemorrhage and hematoma of a digestive system organ or structure complicating a procedure

> EXCLUDES 1 *intraoperative hemorrhage and hematoma of a digestive system organ or structure due to accidental puncture and laceration during a procedure (K91.7-)*

K91.61 Intraoperative hemorrhage and hematoma of a digestive system organ or structure complicating a digestive sytem procedure

K91.62 Intraoperative hemorrhage and hematoma of a digestive system organ or structure complicating other procedure

✓5ᵗʰ **K91.7** Accidental puncture and laceration of a digestive system organ or structure during a procedure

K91.71 Accidental puncture and laceration of a digestive system organ or structure during a digestive system procedure

K91.72 Accidental puncture and laceration of a digestive system organ or structure during other procedure

✓5ᵗʰ **K91.8** Other intraoperative and postprocedural complications and disorders of digestive system

K91.81 Other intraoperative complications of digestive system

K91.82 Postprocedural hepatic failure

K91.83 Postprocedural hepatorenal syndrome

✓6ᵗʰ **K91.84** Postprocedural hemorrhage and hematoma of a digestive system organ or structure following a procedure

K91.840 Postprocedural hemorrhage and hematoma of a digestive system organ or structure following a digestive system procedure

K91.841 Postprocedural hemorrhage and hematoma of a digestive system organ or structure following other procedure

✓6ᵗʰ **K91.85** Complications of intestinal pouch

K91.850 Pouchitis
Inflammation of internal ileoanal pouch

K91.858 Other complications of intestinal pouch

K91.86 Retained cholelithiasis following cholecystectomy

K91.89 Other postprocedural complications and disorders of digestive system
Use additional code, if applicable, to further specify disorder
> EXCLUDES 2 *postprocedural retroperitoneal abscess (K68.11)*

✓4ᵗʰ **K92** Other diseases of digestive system

> EXCLUDES 1 *neonatal gastrointestinal hemorrhage (P54.0-P54.3)*

K92.0 Hematemesis

K92.1 Melena
> EXCLUDES 1 *occult blood in feces (R19.5)*

K92.2 Gastrointestinal hemorrhage, unspecified
Gastric hemorrhage NOS
Intestinal hemorrhage NOS
> EXCLUDES 1 *acute hemorrhagic gastritis (K29.01)*
> *hemorrhage of anus and rectum (K62.5)*
> *angiodysplasia of stomach with hemorrhage (K31.811)*
> *diverticular disease with hemorrhage (K57.-)*
> *gastritis and duodenitis with hemorrhage (K29.-)*
> *peptic ulcer with hemorrhage (K25-K28)*

✓5ᵗʰ **K92.8** Other specified diseases of the digestive system

K92.81 Gastrointestinal mucositis (ulcerative)
Code also type of associated therapy, such as:
antineoplastic and immunosuppressive drugs (T45.1X-)
radiological procedure and radiotherapy (Y84.2)
> EXCLUDES 2 *mucositis (ulcerative) of vagina and vulva (N76.81)*
> *nasal mucositis (ulcerative) (J34.81)*
> *oral mucositis (ulcerative) (K12.3-)*

K92.89 Other specified diseases of the digestive system

K92.9 Disease of digestive system, unspecified

✓4ᵗʰ **K94** Complications of artificial openings of the digestive system

✓5ᵗʰ **K94.0** Colostomy complications

K94.00 Colostomy complication, unspecified

K94.01 Colostomy hemorrhage

K94.02 Colostomy infection
Use additional code to specify type of infection, such as:
cellulitis of abdominal wall (L03.311)
sepsis (A40-, A41-)

K94.03 Colostomy malfunction
Mechanical complication of colostomy

K94.09 Other complications of colostomy

✓5ᵗʰ **K94.1** Enterostomy complications

K94.10 Enterostomy complication, unspecified

K94.11 Enterostomy hemorrhage

K94.12 Enterostomy infection
Use additional code to specify type of infection, such as:
cellulitis of abdominal wall (L03.311)
sepsis (A40-, A41-)

K94.13 Enterostomy malfunction
Mechanical complication of enterostomy

K94.19 Other complications of enterostomy

✓5ᵗʰ **K94.2** Gastrostomy complications

K94.20 Gastrostomy complication, unspecified

K94.21 Gastrostomy hemorrhage

K94.22 Gastrostomy infection
Use additional code to specify type of infection, such as:
cellulitis of abdominal wall (L03.311)
sepsis (A40-, A41-)

K94.23 Gastrostomy malfunction
Mechanical complication of gastrostomy

K94.29 Other complications of gastrostomy

✓5ᵗʰ **K94.3** Esophagostomy complications

K94.30 Esophagostomy complications, unspecified

K94.31 Esophagostomy hemorrhage

K94.32 Esophagostomy infection
Use additional code to identify the infection

K94.33 Esophagostomy malfunction
Mechanical complication of esophagostomy

K94.39 Other complications of esophagostom

✓4ᵗʰ **K95** Complications of bariatric procedures

✓5ᵗʰ **K95.0** Complications of gastric band procedure

K95.01 Infection due to gastric band procedure
Use additional code to specify type of infection or organism, such as:
bacterial and viral infectious agents (B95.-, B96.-)
cellulitis of abdominal wall (L03.311)
sepsis (A40.-, A41.-)

K95.09 Other complications of gastric band procedure
Use additional code, if applicable, to further specify complication

✓5ᵗʰ **K95.8** Complications of other bariatric procedure
> EXCLUDES 1 *complications of gastric band surgery (K95.0-)*

K95.81 Infection due to other bariatric procedure
Use additional code to specify type of infection or organism, such as:
bacterial and viral infectious agents (B95.-, B96.-)
cellulitis of abdominal wall (L03.311)
sepsis (A40.-, A41.-)

K95.89 Other complications of other bariatric procedure
Use additional code, if applicable, to further specify complication

---

☑ Additional Character Required   ✗x7ᵗʰ Placeholder Alert   Unspecified Dx   Other Specified Dx   Manifestation   ►◄ Revised Text   ● New Code   ▲ Revised Code Title

Chapter 12. Diseases of the Skin and Subcutaneous Tissue (L00–L99)

Chapter Specific Guidelines with Coding Examples

The chapter specific guidelines from the ICD-10-CM Official Guidelines for Coding and Reporting have been provided below. Along with these guidelines are coding examples, contained in the shaded boxes, that have been developed to help illustrate the coding and/or sequencing guidance found in these guidelines.

a. Pressure ulcer stage codes

1) Pressure ulcer stages

Codes from category L89, Pressure ulcer, are combination codes that identify the site of the pressure ulcer as well as the stage of the ulcer.

The ICD-10-CM classifies pressure ulcer stages based on severity, which is designated by stages 1-4, unspecified stage and unstageable.

Assign as many codes from category L89 as needed to identify all the pressure ulcers the patient has, if applicable.

> Stage 4 pressure ulcer right heel, 9 x 10 cm that invades the muscle and fascia; stage 2 pressure ulcer of left elbow
>
> **L89.614**   **Pressure ulcer of right heel, stage 4**
>
> **L89.022**   **Pressure ulcer of left elbow, stage 2**
>
> *Explanation:* Patient has a right heel pressure ulcer documented as stage 4 and a left elbow pressure ulcer documented as stage 2. Combination codes from category L89 Pressure ulcer, identify the site of the pressure ulcer as well as the stage. Assign as many codes from category L89 as needed to identify all the pressure ulcers the patient has.

2) Unstageable pressure ulcers

Assignment of the code for unstageable pressure ulcer (L89.--0) should be based on the clinical documentation. These codes are used for pressure ulcers whose stage cannot be clinically determined (e.g., the ulcer is covered by eschar or has been treated with a skin or muscle graft) and pressure ulcers that are documented as deep tissue injury but not documented as due to trauma. This code should not be confused with the codes for unspecified stage (L89.--9). When there is no documentation regarding the stage of the pressure ulcer, assign the appropriate code for unspecified stage (L89.--9).

> Pressure ulcer of the right lower back documented as unstageable due to the presence of thick eschar covering the ulcer
>
> **L89.130**   **Pressure ulcer of right lower back, unstageable**
>
> *Explanation:* Codes for unstageable pressure ulcers are assigned when the stage cannot be clinically determined (e.g., the ulcer is covered by eschar or has been treated with a skin or muscle graft).

3) Documented pressure ulcer stage

Assignment of the pressure ulcer stage code should be guided by clinical documentation of the stage or documentation of the terms found in the Alphabetic Index. For clinical terms describing the stage that are not found in the Alphabetic Index, and there is no documentation of the stage, the provider should be queried.

> Left heel pressure ulcer with partial thickness skin loss involving the dermis
>
> **L89.622**   **Pressure ulcer of left heel, stage 2**
>
> *Explanation:* Code assignment for the pressure ulcer stage should be guided by either the clinical documentation of the stage or the documentation of terms found in the Alphabetic Index. The clinical documentation describing the left heel pressure ulcer "partial thickness skin loss involving the dermis" matches the ICD-10-CM index parenthetical description for stage 2 "(abrasion, blister, partial thickness skin loss involving epidermis and/or dermis)."

4) Patients admitted with pressure ulcers documented as healed

No code is assigned if the documentation states that the pressure ulcer is completely healed.

> Patient receiving follow-up examination of a completely healed pressure ulcer of the foot
>
> **Z09**   **Encounter for follow-up examination after completed treatment for conditions other than malignant neoplasm**
>
> **Z87.2**   **Personal history of diseases of the skin and subcutaneous tissue**
>
> *Explanation:* Assign only codes for the reason for the encounter and the personal history of the pressure ulcer. Personal history code Z87.2 includes conditions classifiable to L00–L99 such as pressure ulcer. No code is assigned for a pressure ulcer documented as completely healed.

5) Patients admitted with pressure ulcers documented as healing

Pressure ulcers described as healing should be assigned the appropriate pressure ulcer stage code based on the documentation in the medical record. If the documentation does not provide information about the stage of the healing pressure ulcer, assign the appropriate code for unspecified stage.

If the documentation is unclear as to whether the patient has a current (new) pressure ulcer or if the patient is being treated for a healing pressure ulcer, query the provider.

> Healing stage 2 sacral pressure ulcer
>
> **L89.152**   **Pressure ulcer of sacral region, stage 2**
>
> *Explanation:* Pressure ulcers described as healing should be assigned the appropriate code for the pressure ulcer stage as documented.

6) Patient admitted with pressure ulcer evolving into another stage during the admission

If a patient is admitted with a pressure ulcer at one stage and it progresses to a higher stage, assign the code for the highest stage reported for that site.

> Stage 3 right hip pressure ulcer worsened during admission to a stage 4 pressure ulcer
>
> **L89.214**   **Pressure ulcer of right hip, stage 4**
>
> *Explanation:* A pressure ulcer that progresses from a lower stage to a higher stage is assigned only the code for the highest stage reported for that site.

Chapter 12. Diseases of the Skin and Subcutaneous Tissue (L00-L99)

EXCLUDES 2
certain conditions originating in the perinatal period (P04-P96)
certain infectious and parasitic diseases (A00-B99)
complications of pregnancy, childbirth and the puerperium (O00-O9A)
congenital malformations, deformations, and chromosomal abnormalities (Q00-Q99)
endocrine, nutritional and metabolic diseases (E00-E88)
lipomelanotic reticulosis (I89.8)
neoplasms (C00-D49)
symptoms, signs and abnormal clinical and laboratory findings, not elsewhere classified (R00-R94)
systemic connective tissue disorders (M30-M36)
viral warts (B07.-)

This chapter contains the following blocks:

L00-L08   Infections of the skin and subcutaneous tissue
L10-L14   Bullous disorders
L20-L30   Dermatitis and eczema
L40-L45   Papulosquamous disorders
L49-L54   Urticaria and erythema
L55-L59   Radiation-related disorders of the skin and subcutaneous tissue
L60-L75   Disorders of skin appendages
L76   Intraoperative and postprocedural complications of skin and subcutaneous tissue
L80-L99   Other disorders of the skin and subcutaneous tissue

Infections of the skin and subcutaneous tissue (L00-L08)

Use additional code (B95-B97) to identify infectious agent

EXCLUDES 2
hordeolum (H00.0)
infective dermatitis (L30.3)
local infections of skin classified in Chapter 1
lupus panniculitis (L93.2)
panniculitis NOS (M79.3)
panniculitis of neck and back (M54.0-)
Perlèche NOS (K13.0)
Perlèche due to candidiasis (B37.0)
Perlèche due to riboflavin deficiency (E53.0)
pyogenic granuloma (L98.0)
relapsing panniculitis [Weber-Christian] (M35.6)
viral warts (B07.-)
zoster (B02.-)

L00   Staphylococcal scalded skin syndrome
Ritter's disease
Use additional code to identify percentage of skin exfoliation (L49.-)

EXCLUDES 1
bullous impetigo (L01.03)
pemphigus neonatorum (L01.03)
toxic epidermal necrolysis [Lyell] (L51.2)

✔4th **L01   Impetigo**
EXCLUDES 1   impetigo herpetiformis (L40.1)

✔5th **L01.0   Impetigo**
Impetigo contagiosa   Impetigo vulgaris

L01.00   Impetigo, unspecified
Impetigo NOS

L01.01   Non-bullous impetigo

L01.02   Bockhart's impetigo
Impetigo follicularis   Superficial pustular
Perifolliculitis NOS   perifolliculitis

L01.03   Bullous impetigo
Impetigo neonatorum Pemphigus neonatorum

L01.09   Other impetigo
Ulcerative impetigo

L01.1   Impetiginization of other dermatoses

✔4th **L02   Cutaneous abscess, furuncle and carbuncle**
Use additional code to identify organism (B95-B96)

EXCLUDES 2
abscess of anus and rectal regions (K61.-)
abscess of female genital organs (external) (N76.4)
abscess of male genital organs (external) (N48.2, N49-)

✔5th **L02.0   Cutaneous abscess, furuncle and carbuncle of face**

EXCLUDES 2
abscess of ear, external (H60.0)
abscess of eyelid (H00.0)
abscess of head [any part, except face] (L02.8)
abscess of lacrimal gland (H04.0)
abscess of lacrimal passages (H04.3)
abscess of mouth (K12.2)
abscess of nose (J34.0)
abscess of orbit (H05.0)
submandibular abscess (K12.2)

L02.01   Cutaneous abscess of face

L02.02   Furuncle of face
Boil of face
Folliculitis of face

L02.03   Carbuncle of face

✔5th **L02.1   Cutaneous abscess, furuncle and carbuncle of neck**

L02.11   Cutaneous abscess of neck

L02.12   Furuncle of neck
Boil of neck
Folliculitis of neck

L02.13   Carbuncle of neck

✔5th **L02.2   Cutaneous abscess, furuncle and carbuncle of trunk**

EXCLUDES 1
non-newborn omphalitis (L08.82)
omphalitis of newborn (P38.-)

EXCLUDES 2
abscess of breast (N61)
abscess of buttocks (L02.3)
abscess of female external genital organs (N76.4)
abscess of hip (L02.4)
abscess of male external genital organs (N48.2, N49-)

✔6th **L02.21   Cutaneous abscess of trunk**

L02.211   Cutaneous abscess of abdominal wall

L02.212   Cutaneous abscess of back [any part, except buttock]

L02.213   Cutaneous abscess of chest wall

L02.214   Cutaneous abscess of groin

L02.215   Cutaneous abscess of perineum

L02.216   Cutaneous abscess of umbilicus

L02.219   Cutaneous abscess of trunk, unspecified

✔6th **L02.22   Furuncle of trunk**
Boil of trunk
Folliculitis of trunk

L02.221   Furuncle of abdominal wall

L02.222   Furuncle of back [any part, except buttock]

L02.223   Furuncle of chest wall

L02.224   Furuncle of groin

L02.225   Furuncle of perineum

L02.226   Furuncle of umbilicus

L02.229   Furuncle of trunk, unspecified

✔6th **L02.23   Carbuncle of trunk**

L02.231   Carbuncle of abdominal wall

L02.232   Carbuncle of back [any part, except buttock]

L02.233   Carbuncle of chest wall

L02.234   Carbuncle of groin

L02.235   Carbuncle of perineum

L02.236   Carbuncle of umbilicus

L02.239   Carbuncle of trunk, unspecified

✔5th **L02.3   Cutaneous abscess, furuncle and carbuncle of buttock**
EXCLUDES 1   pilonidal cyst with abscess (L05.01)

L02.31   Cutaneous abscess of buttock
Cutaneous abscess of gluteal region

L02.32   Furuncle of buttock
Boil of buttock
Folliculitis of buttock
Furuncle of gluteal region

L02.33   Carbuncle of buttock
Carbuncle of gluteal region

✔5th **L02.4   Cutaneous abscess, furuncle and carbuncle of limb**

EXCLUDES 2
cutaneous abscess, furuncle and carbuncle of groin (L02.214, L02.224, L02.234)
cutaneous abscess, furuncle and carbuncle of hand (L02.5-)
cutaneous abscess, furuncle and carbuncle of foot (L02.6-)

✔6th **L02.41   Cutaneous abscess of limb**

L02.411   Cutaneous abscess of right axilla

L02.412   Cutaneous abscess of left axilla

L02.413   Cutaneous abscess of right upper limb

L02.414   Cutaneous abscess of left upper limb

L02.415   Cutaneous abscess of right lower limb

L02.416   Cutaneous abscess of left lower limb

L02.419   Cutaneous abscess of limb, unspecified

✔6th **L02.42   Furuncle of limb**
Boil of limb
Folliculitis of limb

L02.421   Furuncle of right axilla

☑ Additional Character Required   ✔x7th Placeholder Alert   Unspecified Dx   Other Specified Dx   Manifestation   ▶◀ Revised Text   ● New Code   ▲ Revised Code Title

L02.422   Furuncle of left axilla
L02.423   Furuncle of right upper limb
L02.424   Furuncle of left upper limb
L02.425   Furuncle of right lower limb
L02.426   Furuncle of left lower limb
L02.429   **Furuncle of limb, unspecified**

✓6th L02.43   Carbuncle of limb
L02.431   Carbuncle of right axilla
L02.432   Carbuncle of left axilla
L02.433   Carbuncle of right upper limb
L02.434   Carbuncle of left upper limb
L02.435   Carbuncle of right lower limb
L02.436   Carbuncle of left lower limb
L02.439   **Carbuncle of limb, unspecified**

✓5th L02.5   Cutaneous abscess, furuncle and carbuncle of hand
✓6th L02.51   Cutaneous abscess of hand
L02.511   Cutaneous abscess of right hand
L02.512   Cutaneous abscess of left hand
L02.519   **Cutaneous abscess of unspecified hand**

✓6th L02.52   Furuncle hand
Boil of hand
Folliculitis of hand
L02.521   Furuncle right hand
L02.522   Furuncle left hand
L02.529   **Furuncle unspecified hand**

✓6th L02.53   Carbuncle of hand
L02.531   Carbuncle of right hand
L02.532   Carbuncle of left hand
L02.539   **Carbuncle of unspecified hand**

✓5th L02.6   Cutaneous abscess, furuncle and carbuncle of foot
✓6th L02.61   Cutaneous abscess of foot
L02.611   Cutaneous abscess of right foot
L02.612   Cutaneous abscess of left foot
L02.619   **Cutaneous abscess of unspecified foot**

✓6th L02.62   Furuncle of foot
Boil of foot
Folliculitis of foot
L02.621   Furuncle of right foot
L02.622   Furuncle of left foot
L02.629   **Furuncle of unspecified foot**

✓6th L02.63   Carbuncle of foot
L02.631   Carbuncle of right foot
L02.632   Carbuncle of left foot
L02.639   **Carbuncle of unspecified foot**

✓5th L02.8   Cutaneous abscess, furuncle and carbuncle of other sites
✓6th L02.81   Cutaneous abscess of other sites
L02.811   Cutaneous abscess of head [any part, except face]
L02.818   **Cutaneous abscess of other sites**

✓6th L02.82   Furuncle of other sites
Boil of other sites
Folliculitis of other sites
L02.821   Furuncle of head [any part, except face]
L02.828   **Furuncle of other sites**

✓6th L02.83   Carbuncle of other sites
L02.831   Carbuncle of head [any part, except face]
L02.838   **Carbuncle of other sites**

✓5th L02.9   Cutaneous abscess, furuncle and carbuncle, unspecified
L02.91   Cutaneous abscess, unspecified
L02.92   Furuncle, unspecified
Boil NOS
Furunculosis NOS
L02.93   Carbuncle, unspecified

✓4th **L03**   **Cellulitis and acute lymphangitis**
EXCLUDES 2   *cellulitis of anal and rectal region (K61.-)*
cellulitis of external auditory canal (H60.1)
cellulitis of eyelid (H00.03-)
cellulitis of female external genital organs (N76.4)
cellulitis of lacrimal apparatus (H04.3)
cellulitis of male external genital organs (N48.2, N49-)
cellulitis of mouth (K12.2)
cellulitis of nose (J34.0)
eosinophilic cellulitis [Wells] (L98.3)
febrile neutrophilic dermatosis [Sweet] (L98.2)
lymphangitis (chronic) (subacute) (I89.1)

✓5th **L03.0**   **Cellulitis and acute lymphangitis of finger and toe**
Infection of nail
Onychia
Paronychia
Perionychia

✓6th L03.01   Cellulitis of finger
Felon
Whitlow
EXCLUDES 1   *herpetic whitlow (B00.89)*
L03.011   Cellulitis of right finger
L03.012   Cellulitis of left finger
L03.019   **Cellulitis of unspecified finger**

✓6th L03.02   Acute lymphangitis of finger
Hangnail with lymphangitis of finger
L03.021   Acute lymphangitis of right finger
L03.022   Acute lymphangitis of left finger
L03.029   **Acute lymphangitis of unspecified finger**

✓6th L03.03   Cellulitis of toe
L03.031   Cellulitis of right toe
L03.032   Cellulitis of left toe
L03.039   **Cellulitis of unspecified toe**

✓6th L03.04   Acute lymphangitis of toe
Hangnail with lymphangitis of toe
L03.041   Acute lymphangitis of right toe
L03.042   Acute lymphangitis of left toe
L03.049   **Acute lymphangitis of unspecified toe**

✓5th **L03.1**   **Cellulitis and acute lymphangitis of other parts of limb**
✓6th L03.11   Cellulitis of other parts of limb
EXCLUDES 2   *cellulitis of fingers (L03.01-)*
cellulitis of toes (L03.03-)
groin (L03.314)
L03.111   Cellulitis of right axilla
L03.112   Cellulitis of left axilla
L03.113   Cellulitis of right upper limb
L03.114   Cellulitis of left upper limb
L03.115   Cellulitis of right lower limb
L03.116   Cellulitis of left lower limb
L03.119   **Cellulitis of unspecified part of limb**

✓6th L03.12   Acute lymphangitis of other parts of limb
EXCLUDES 2   *acute lymphangitis of fingers (L03.02-)*
acute lymphangitis of groin (L03.324)
acute lymphangitis of toes (L03.04-)
L03.121   Acute lymphangitis of right axilla
L03.122   Acute lymphangitis of left axilla
L03.123   Acute lymphangitis of right upper limb
L03.124   Acute lymphangitis of left upper limb
L03.125   Acute lymphangitis of right lower limb
L03.126   Acute lymphangitis of left lower limb
L03.129   **Acute lymphangitis of unspecified part of limb**

✓5th **L03.2**   **Cellulitis and acute lymphangitis of face and neck**
✓6th L03.21   Cellulitis and acute lymphangitis of face
L03.211   Cellulitis of face
EXCLUDES 2   *cellulitis of ear (H60.1-)*
cellulitis of eyelid (H00.03-)
cellulitis of head (L03.811)
cellulitis of lacrimal apparatus (H04.3)
cellulitis of lip (K13.0)
cellulitis of mouth (K12.2)
cellulitis of nose (internal) (J34.0)
cellulitis of orbit (H05.0)
cellulitis of scalp (L03.811)
AHA: 2013, 4Q, 123
L03.212   Acute lymphangitis of face

☑6ᵗʰ **L03.22 Cellulitis and acute lymphangitis of neck**
    L03.221 Cellulitis of neck
    L03.222 Acute lymphangitis of neck

☑5ᵗʰ **L03.3 Cellulitis and acute lymphangitis of trunk**
  ☑6ᵗʰ **L03.31 Cellulitis of trunk**
     EXCLUDES 2 *cellulitis of anal and rectal regions (K61.-)*
       cellulitis of breast NOS (N61)
       cellulitis of female external genital organs
         (N76.4)
       cellulitis of male external genital organs
         (N48.2, N49-)
       omphalitis of newborn (P38.-)
       puerperal cellulitis of breast (O91.2)
    L03.311 Cellulitis of abdominal wall
      EXCLUDES 2 *cellulitis of umbilicus (L03.316)*
         cellulitis of groin (L03.314)
    L03.312 Cellulitis of back [any part except buttock]
    L03.313 Cellulitis of chest wall
    L03.314 Cellulitis of groin
    L03.315 Cellulitis of perineum
    L03.316 Cellulitis of umbilicus
    L03.317 Cellulitis of buttock
    L03.319 Cellulitis of trunk, unspecified
  ☑6ᵗʰ **L03.32 Acute lymphangitis of trunk**
    L03.321 Acute lymphangitis of abdominal wall
    L03.322 Acute lymphangitis of back [any part except buttock]
    L03.323 Acute lymphangitis of chest wall
    L03.324 Acute lymphangitis of groin
    L03.325 Acute lymphangitis of perineum
    L03.326 Acute lymphangitis of umbilicus
    L03.327 Acute lymphangitis of buttock
    L03.329 Acute lymphangitis of trunk, unspecified

☑5ᵗʰ **L03.8 Cellulitis and acute lymphangitis of other sites**
  ☑6ᵗʰ **L03.81 Cellulitis of other sites**
    L03.811 Cellulitis of head [any part, except face]
      Cellulitis of scalp
      EXCLUDES 2 *cellulitis of face (L03.211)*
    L03.818 Cellulitis of other sites
  ☑6ᵗʰ **L03.89 Acute lymphangitis of other sites**
    L03.891 Acute lymphangitis of head [any part, except face]
    L03.898 Acute lymphangitis of other sites

☑5ᵗʰ **L03.9 Cellulitis and acute lymphangitis, unspecified**
    L03.90 Cellulitis, unspecified
    L03.91 Acute lymphangitis, unspecified
      EXCLUDES 1 *lymphangitis NOS (I89.1)*

☑4ᵗʰ **L04 Acute lymphadenitis**
  INCLUDES abscess (acute) of lymph nodes, except mesenteric
      acute lymphadenitis, except mesenteric
  EXCLUDES 1 *chronic or subacute lymphadenitis, except mesenteric (I88.1)*
      enlarged lymph nodes (R59.-)
      human immunodeficiency virus [HIV] disease resulting in
        generalized lymphadenopathy (B20)
      lymphadenitis NOS (I88.9)
      nonspecific mesenteric lymphadenitis (I88.0)
  L04.0 Acute lymphadenitis of face, head and neck
  L04.1 Acute lymphadenitis of trunk
  L04.2 Acute lymphadenitis of upper limb
    Acute lymphadenitis of axilla
    Acute lymphadenitis of shoulder
  L04.3 Acute lymphadenitis of lower limb
    Acute lymphadenitis of hip
    EXCLUDES 2 *acute lymphadenitis of groin (L04.1)*
  L04.8 Acute lymphadenitis of other sites
  L04.9 Acute lymphadenitis, unspecified

☑4ᵗʰ **L05 Pilonidal cyst and sinus**
  ☑5ᵗʰ **L05.0 Pilonidal cyst and sinus with abscess**
    L05.01 Pilonidal cyst with abscess
      Parasacral dimple with abscess
      Pilonidal abscess
      Pilonidal dimple with abscess
      Postanal dimple with abscess

    L05.02 Pilonidal sinus with abscess
      Coccygeal fistula with abscess
      Coccygeal sinus with abscess
      Pilonidal fistula with abscess
  ☑5ᵗʰ **L05.9 Pilonidal cyst and sinus without abscess**
    L05.91 Pilonidal cyst without abscess
      Parasacral dimple
      Pilonidal dimple
      Postanal dimple
      Pilonidal cyst NOS
    L05.92 Pilonidal sinus without abscess
      Coccygeal fistula
      Coccygeal sinus without abscess
      Pilonidal fistula

☑4ᵗʰ **L08 Other local infections of skin and subcutaneous tissue**
  L08.0 Pyoderma
    Dermatitis gangrenosa
    Purulent dermatitis
    Septic dermatitis
    Suppurative dermatitis
    EXCLUDES 1 *pyoderma gangrenosum (L88)*
      pyoderma vegetans (L08.81)
  L08.1 Erythrasma
  ☑5ᵗʰ **L08.8 Other specified local infections of the skin and subcutaneous tissue**
    L08.81 Pyoderma vegetans
      EXCLUDES 1 *pyoderma gangrenosum (L88)*
      pyoderma NOS (L08.0)
    L08.82 Omphalitis not of newborn
      EXCLUDES 1 *omphalitis of newborn (P38.-)*
    L08.89 Other specified local infections of the skin and subcutaneous tissue
  L08.9 Local infection of the skin and subcutaneous tissue, unspecified

Bullous disorders (L10-L14)

EXCLUDES 1 *benign familial pemphigus [Hailey-Hailey] (Q82.8)*
    staphylococcal scalded skin syndrome (L00)
    toxic epidermal necrolysis [Lyell] (L51.2)

☑4ᵗʰ **L10 Pemphigus**
  EXCLUDES 1 *pemphigus neonatorum (L01.03)*
  L10.0 Pemphigus vulgaris
  L10.1 Pemphigus vegetans
  L10.2 Pemphigus foliaceous
  L10.3 Brazilian pemphigus [fogo selvagem]
  L10.4 Pemphigus erythematosus
    Senear-Usher syndrome
  L10.5 Drug-induced pemphigus
    Use additional code for adverse effect, if applicable, to identify drug (T36-T50 with fifth or sixth character 5)
  ☑5ᵗʰ **L10.8 Other pemphigus**
    L10.81 Paraneoplastic pemphigus
    L10.89 Other pemphigus
  L10.9 Pemphigus, unspecified

☑4ᵗʰ **L11 Other acantholytic disorders**
  L11.0 Acquired keratosis follicularis
    EXCLUDES 1 *keratosis follicularis (congenital) [Darier-White] (Q82.8)*
  L11.1 Transient acantholytic dermatosis [Grover]
  L11.8 Other specified acantholytic disorders
  L11.9 Acantholytic disorder, unspecified

☑4ᵗʰ **L12 Pemphigoid**
  EXCLUDES 1 *herpes gestationis (O26.4-)*
    impetigo herpetiformis (L40.1)
  L12.0 Bullous pemphigoid
  L12.1 Cicatricial pemphigoid
    Benign mucous membrane pemphigoid
  L12.2 Chronic bullous disease of childhood ℗
    Juvenile dermatitis herpetiformis
  ☑5ᵗʰ **L12.3 Acquired epidermolysis bullosa**
    EXCLUDES 1 *epidermolysis bullosa (congenital) (Q81.-)*
    L12.30 Acquired epidermolysis bullosa, unspecified
    L12.31 Epidermolysis bullosa due to drug
      Use additional code for adverse effect, if applicable, to identify drug (T36-T50 with fifth or sixth character 5)

☑ Additional Character Required   ☑ₓ7 Placeholder Alert   Unspecified Dx   Other Specified Dx   Manifestation   ►◄ Revised Text   ● New Code   ▲ Revised Code Title

L12.35   Other acquired epidermolysis bullosa

L12.8   Other pemphigoid

L12.9   Pemphigoid, unspecified

✓4ᵗʰ **L13**   Other bullous disorders

     L13.0   Dermatitis herpetiformis
         Duhring's disease
         Hydroa herpetiformis
         EXCLUDES 1   *juvenile dermatitis herpetiformis (L12.2)*
                 senile dermatitis herpetiformis (L12.0)

     L13.1   Subcorneal pustular dermatitis
         Sneddon-Wilkinson disease

     L13.8   Other specified bullous disorders

     L13.9   Bullous disorder, unspecified

L14   *Bullous disorders in diseases classified elsewhere*
     Code first underlying disease

Dermatitis and eczema (L20-L30)

NOTE   In this block the terms dermatitis and eczema are used synonymously and interchangeably.

EXCLUDES 2   *chronic (childhood) granulomatous disease (D71)*
         dermatitis gangrenosa (L08.0)
         dermatitis herpetiformis (L13.0)
         dry skin dermatitis (L85.3)
         factitial dermatitis (L98.1)
         perioral dermatitis (L71.0)
         radiation-related disorders of the skin and subcutaneous tissue (L55-L59)
         stasis dermatitis (I83.1-I83.2)

✓4ᵗʰ **L20**   Atopic dermatitis

     L20.0   Besnier's prurigo

✓5ᵗʰ   **L20.8**   Other atopic dermatitis
         EXCLUDES 2   *circumscribed neurodermatitis (L28.0)*

         L20.81   Atopic neurodermatitis
                 Diffuse neurodermatitis

         L20.82   Flexural eczema

         L20.83   Infantile (acute) (chronic) eczema   P

         L20.84   Intrinsic (allergic) eczema

         L20.89   Other atopic dermatitis

     L20.9   Atopic dermatitis, unspecified

✓4ᵗʰ **L21**   Seborrheic dermatitis
     EXCLUDES 2   *infective dermatitis (L30.3)*
              seborrheic keratosis (L82.-)

     L21.0   Seborrhea capitis   P
         Cradle cap

     L21.1   Seborrheic infantile dermatitis   P

     L21.8   Other seborrheic dermatitis

     L21.9   Seborrheic dermatitis, unspecified
         Seborrhea NOS

L22   Diaper dermatitis
     Diaper erythema
     Diaper rash
     Psoriasiform diaper rash

✓4ᵗʰ **L23**   Allergic contact dermatitis
     EXCLUDES 1   *allergy NOS (T78.40)*
              contact dermatitis NOS (L25.9)
              dermatitis NOS (L30.9)
     EXCLUDES 2   *dermatitis due to substances taken internally (L27.-)*
              dermatitis of eyelid (H01.1-)
              diaper dermatitis (L22)
              eczema of external ear (H60.5-)
              irritant contact dermatitis (L24.-)
              perioral dermatitis (L71.0)
              radiation-related disorders of the skin and subcutaneous tissue (L55-L59)

     L23.0   Allergic contact dermatitis due to metals
         Allergic contact dermatitis due to chromium
         Allergic contact dermatitis due to nickel

     L23.1   Allergic contact dermatitis due to adhesives

     L23.2   Allergic contact dermatitis due to cosmetics

     L23.3   Allergic contact dermatitis due to drugs in contact with skin
         Use additional code for adverse effect, if applicable, to identify drug (T36-T50 with fifth or sixth character 5)
         EXCLUDES 2   *dermatitis due to ingested drugs and medicaments (L27.0-L27.1)*

     L23.4   Allergic contact dermatitis due to dyes

     L23.5   Allergic contact dermatitis due to other chemical products
         Allergic contact dermatitis due to cement
         Allergic contact dermatitis due to insecticide
         Allergic contact dermatitis due to plastic
         Allergic contact dermatitis due to rubber

     L23.6   Allergic contact dermatitis due to food in contact with the skin
         EXCLUDES 2   *dermatitis due to ingested food (L27.2)*

     L23.7   Allergic contact dermatitis due to plants, except food
         EXCLUDES 2   *allergy NOS due to pollen (J30.1)*

✓5ᵗʰ   **L23.8**   Allergic contact dermatitis due to other agents

         L23.81   Allergic contact dermatitis due to animal (cat) (dog) dander
                 Allergic contact dermatitis due to animal (cat) (dog) hair

         L23.89   Allergic contact dermatitis due to other agents

     L23.9   Allergic contact dermatitis, unspecified cause
         Allergic contact eczema NOS

✓4ᵗʰ **L24**   Irritant contact dermatitis
     EXCLUDES 1   *allergy NOS (T78.40)*
              contact dermatitis NOS (L25.9)
              dermatitis NOS (L30.9)
     EXCLUDES 2   *allergic contact dermatitis (L23.-)*
              dermatitis due to substances taken internally (L27.-)
              dermatitis of eyelid (H01.1-)
              diaper dermatitis (L22)
              eczema of external ear (H60.5-)
              perioral dermatitis (L71.0)
              radiation-related disorders of the skin and subcutaneous tissue (L55-L59)

     L24.0   Irritant contact dermatitis due to detergents

     L24.1   Irritant contact dermatitis due to oils and greases

     L24.2   Irritant contact dermatitis due to solvents
         Irritant contact dermatitis due to chlorocompound
         Irritant contact dermatitis due to cyclohexane
         Irritant contact dermatitis due to ester
         Irritant contact dermatitis due to glycol
         Irritant contact dermatitis due to hydrocarbon
         Irritant contact dermatitis due to ketone

     L24.3   Irritant contact dermatitis due to cosmetics

     L24.4   Irritant contact dermatitis due to drugs in contact with skin
         Use additional code for adverse effect, if applicable, to identify drug (T36-T50 with fifth or sixth character 5)

     L24.5   Irritant contact dermatitis due to other chemical products
         Irritant contact dermatitis due to cement
         Irritant contact dermatitis due to insecticide
         Irritant contact dermatitis due to plastic
         Irritant contact dermatitis due to rubber

     L24.6   Irritant contact dermatitis due to food in contact with skin
         EXCLUDES 2   *dermatitis due to ingested food (L27.2)*

     L24.7   Irritant contact dermatitis due to plants, except food
         EXCLUDES 2   *allergy NOS to pollen (J30.1)*

✓5ᵗʰ   **L24.8**   Irritant contact dermatitis due to other agents

         L24.81   Irritant contact dermatitis due to metals
                 Irritant contact dermatitis due to chromium
                 Irritant contact dermatitis due to nickel

         L24.89   Irritant contact dermatitis due to other agents
                 Irritant contact dermatitis due to dyes

     L24.9   Irritant contact dermatitis, unspecified cause
         Irritant contact eczema NOS

✓4ᵗʰ **L25**   Unspecified contact dermatitis
     EXCLUDES 1   *allergic contact dermatitis (L23.-)*
              allergy NOS (T78.40)
              dermatitis NOS (L30.9)
              irritant contact dermatitis (L24.-)
     EXCLUDES 2   *dermatitis due to ingested substances (L27.-)*
              dermatitis of eyelid (H01.1-)
              eczema of external ear (H60.5-)
              perioral dermatitis (L71.0)
              radiation-related disorders of the skin and subcutaneous tissue (L55-L59)

     L25.0   Unspecified contact dermatitis due to cosmetics

     L25.1   Unspecified contact dermatitis due to drugs in contact with skin
         Use additional code for adverse effect, if applicable, to identify drug (T36-T50 with fifth or sixth character 5)
         EXCLUDES 2   *dermatitis due to ingested drugs and medicaments (L27.0-L27.1)*

     L25.2   Unspecified contact dermatitis due to dyes

EXCLUDES1 Not coded here   EXCLUDES2 Not included here   N Newborn Age: 0   P Pediatric Age: 0-17   M Maternity Age: 12-55   A Adult Age: 15-124

652   ICD-10-CM 2016

L25.3   **Unspecified contact dermatitis due to** other chemical products
    Unspecified contact dermatitis due to cement
    Unspecified contact dermatitis due to insecticide

L25.4   **Unspecified contact dermatitis due to** food in contact with skin
    EXCLUDES 2   *dermatitis due to ingested food (L27.2)*

L25.5   **Unspecified contact dermatitis due to** plants, except food
    EXCLUDES 1   *nettle rash (L50.9)*
    EXCLUDES 2   *allergy NOS due to pollen (J30.1)*

L25.8   **Unspecified contact dermatitis due to other** agents

L25.9   **Unspecified contact dermatitis, unspecified cause**
    Contact dermatitis (occupational) NOS
    Contact eczema (occupational) NOS

L26   **Exfoliative dermatitis**
    Hebra's pityriasis
    EXCLUDES 1   *Ritter's disease (L00)*

☑4ᵗʰ **L27**   **Dermatitis due to substances taken internally**
    EXCLUDES 1   *allergy NOS (T78.40)*
    EXCLUDES 2   *adverse food reaction, except dermatitis (T78.0-T78.1)*
          contact dermatitis (L23-L25)
          drug photoallergic response (L56.1)
          drug phototoxic response (L56.0)
          urticaria (L50.-)

L27.0   **Generalized skin eruption due to** drugs and medicaments **taken internally**
    Use additional code for adverse effect, if applicable, to identify drug (T36-T50 with fifth or sixth character 5)

L27.1   **Localized skin eruption due to** drugs and medicaments **taken internally**
    Use additional code for adverse effect, if applicable, to identify drug (T36-T50 with fifth or sixth character 5)

L27.2   **Dermatitis due to ingested** food
    EXCLUDES 2   *dermatitis due to food in contact with skin (L23.6, L24.6, L25.4)*

L27.8   **Dermatitis due to other substances taken internally**

L27.9   **Dermatitis due to unspecified substance taken internally**

☑4ᵗʰ **L28**   **Lichen simplex chronicus and prurigo**

L28.0   **Lichen simplex chronicus**
    Circumscribed neurodermatitis
    Lichen NOS

L28.1   **Prurigo nodularis**

L28.2   **Other prurigo**
    Prurigo NOS
    Prurigo Hebra
    Prurigo mitis
    Urticaria papulosa

☑4ᵗʰ **L29**   **Pruritus**
    EXCLUDES 1   *neurotic excoriation (L98.1)*
          psychogenic pruritus (F45.8)

L29.0   **Pruritus ani**

L29.1   **Pruritus scroti**   ♂

L29.2   **Pruritus vulvae**   ♀

L29.3   **Anogenital pruritus, unspecified**

L29.8   **Other pruritus**

L29.9   **Pruritus, unspecified**
    Itch NOS

☑4ᵗʰ **L30**   **Other and unspecified dermatitis**
    EXCLUDES 2   *contact dermatitis (L23-L25)*
          dry skin dermatitis (L85.3)
          small plaque parapsoriasis (L41.3)
          stasis dermatitis (I83.1-.2)

L30.0   **Nummular dermatitis**

L30.1   **Dyshidrosis [pompholyx]**

L30.2   **Cutaneous autosensitization**
    Candidid [levurid]
    Dermatophytid
    Eczematid

L30.3   **Infective dermatitis**
    Infectious eczematoid dermatitis

L30.4   **Erythema intertrigo**

L30.5   **Pityriasis alba**

L30.8   **Other specified dermatitis**

L30.9   **Dermatitis, unspecified**
    Eczema NOS

Papulosquamous disorders (L40-L45)

☑4ᵗʰ **L40**   **Psoriasis**

L40.0   **Psoriasis vulgaris**
    Nummular psoriasis
    Plaque psoriasis

L40.1   **Generalized pustular psoriasis**
    Impetigo herpetiformis
    Von Zumbusch's disease

L40.2   **Acrodermatitis continua**

L40.3   **Pustulosis palmaris et plantaris**

L40.4   **Guttate psoriasis**

☑5ᵗʰ **L40.5**   **Arthropathic psoriasis**

    L40.50   **Arthropathic psoriasis, unspecified**

    L40.51   **Distal interphalangeal psoriatic arthropathy**

    L40.52   **Psoriatic arthritis mutilans**

    L40.53   **Psoriatic spondylitis**

    L40.54   **Psoriatic juvenile arthropathy**

    L40.59   **Other psoriatic arthropathy**

L40.8   **Other psoriasis**
    Flexural psoriasis

L40.9   **Psoriasis, unspecified**

☑4ᵗʰ **L41**   **Parapsoriasis**
    EXCLUDES 1   *poikiloderma vasculare atrophicans (L94.5)*

L41.0   **Pityriasis lichenoides et varioliformis acuta**
    Mucha-Habermann disease

L41.1   **Pityriasis lichenoides chronica**

L41.3   **Small plaque parapsoriasis**

L41.4   **Large plaque parapsoriasis**

L41.5   **Retiform parapsoriasis**

L41.8   **Other parapsoriasis**

L41.9   **Parapsoriasis, unspecified**

L42   **Pityriasis rosea**

☑4ᵗʰ **L43**   **Lichen planus**
    EXCLUDES 1   *lichen planopilaris (L66.1)*

L43.0   **Hypertrophic lichen planus**

L43.1   **Bullous lichen planus**

L43.2   **Lichenoid drug reaction**
    Use additional code for adverse effect, if applicable, to identify drug (T36-T50 with fifth or sixth character 5)

L43.3   **Subacute (active) lichen planus**
    Lichen planus tropicus

L43.8   **Other lichen planus**

L43.9   **Lichen planus, unspecified**

☑4ᵗʰ **L44**   **Other papulosquamous disorders**

L44.0   **Pityriasis rubra pilaris**

L44.1   **Lichen nitidus**

L44.2   **Lichen striatus**

L44.3   **Lichen ruber moniliformis**

L44.4   **Infantile papular acrodermatitis [Gianotti-Crosti]**   ℙ

L44.8   **Other specified papulosquamous disorders**

L44.9   **Papulosquamous disorder, unspecified**

L45   ***Papulosquamous disorders in diseases classified elsewhere***
    Code first underlying disease

Urticaria and erythema (L49-L54)

    EXCLUDES 1   *Lyme disease (A69.2-)*
          rosacea (L71.-)

☑4ᵗʰ **L49**   **Exfoliation due to erythematous conditions according to extent of body surface involved**
    Code first erythematous condition causing exfoliation, such as:
      Ritter's disease (L00)
      (Staphylococcal) scalded skin syndrom (L00)
      Stevens-Johnson syndrome (L51.1)
      Stevens-Johnson syndrome-toxic epidermal necrolysis overlap syndrome (L51.3)
      toxic epidermal necrolysis (L51.2)

L49.0   **Exfoliation due to erythematous condition involving** less than 10 percent **of body surface**
    Exfoliation due to erythematous condition NOS

L49.1   **Exfoliation due to erythematous condition involving** 10-19 percent **of body surface**

☑ Additional Character Required   ✓ˣ7ᵗʰ Placeholder Alert   Unspecified Dx   Other Specified Dx   Manifestation   ▶◀ Revised Text   ● New Code   ▲ Revised Code Title

L49.2 **Exfoliation due to erythematous condition involving** 20-29 **percent of body surface**

L49.3 **Exfoliation due to erythematous condition involving** 30-39 **percent of body surface**

L49.4 **Exfoliation due to erythematous condition involving** 40-49 **percent of body surface**

L49.5 **Exfoliation due to erythematous condition involving** 50-59 **percent of body surface**

L49.6 **Exfoliation due to erythematous condition involving** 60-69 **percent of body surface**

L49.7 **Exfoliation due to erythematous condition involving** 70-79 **percent of body surface**

L49.8 **Exfoliation due to erythematous condition involving** 80-89 **percent of body surface**

L49.9 **Exfoliation due to erythematous condition involving** 90 or **more percent of body surface**

✓4ᵗʰ **L50** **Urticaria**

> EXCLUDES 1   allergic contact dermatitis (L23.-)
> angioneurotic edema (T78.3)
> giant urticaria (T78.3)
> hereditary angio-edema (D84.1)
> Quincke's edema (T78.3)
> serum urticaria (T80.6-)
> solar urticaria (L56.3)
> urticaria neonatorum (P83.8)
> urticaria papulosa (L28.2)
> urticaria pigmentosa (Q82.2)

L50.0 **Allergic urticaria**

L50.1 **Idiopathic urticaria**

L50.2 **Urticaria due to cold and heat**

L50.3 **Dermatographic urticaria**

L50.4 **Vibratory urticaria**

L50.5 **Cholinergic urticaria**

L50.6 **Contact urticaria**

L50.8 **Other urticaria**
> Chronic urticaria
> Recurrent periodic urticaria

L50.9 **Urticaria, unspecified**

✓4ᵗʰ **L51** **Erythema multiforme**

Use additional code for adverse effect, if applicable, to identify drug (T36-T50 with fifth or sixth character 5)

Use additional code to identify associated manifestations, such as:
> arthropathy associated with dermatological disorders (M14.8-)
> conjunctival edema (H11.42)
> conjunctivitis (H10.22-)
> corneal scars and opacities (H17.-)
> corneal ulcer (H16.0-)
> edema of eyelid (H02.84)
> inflammation of eyelid (H01.8)
> keratoconjunctivitis sicca (H16.22-)
> mechanical lagophthalmos (H02.22-)
> stomatitis (K12.-)
> symblepharon (H11.23-)

Use additional code to identify percentage of skin exfoliation (L49.-)

> EXCLUDES 1   staphylococcal scalded skin syndrome (L00)
> Ritter's disease (L00)

L51.0 **Nonbullous erythema multiforme**

L51.1 **Stevens-Johnson syndrome**

L51.2 **Toxic epidermal necrolysis [Lyell]**

L51.3 **Stevens-Johnson syndrome-toxic epidermal necrolysis overlap syndrome**
> SJS-TEN overlap syndrome

L51.8 **Other erythema multiforme**

L51.9 **Erythema multiforme, unspecified**
> Erythema iris
> Erythema multiforme major NOS
> Erythema multiforme minor NOS
> Herpes iris

L52 **Erythema nodosum**
> EXCLUDES 1   tuberculous erythema nodosum (A18.4)

✓4ᵗʰ **L53** **Other erythematous conditions**

> EXCLUDES 1   erythema ab igne (L59.0)
> erythema due to external agents in contact with skin (L23-L25)
> erythema intertrigo (L30.4)

L53.0 **Toxic erythema**
> Code first poisoning due to drug or toxin, if applicable (T36-T65 with fifth or sixth character 1-4 or 6)
> Use additional code for adverse effect, if applicable, to identify drug (T36-T50 with fifth or sixth character 5)
>> EXCLUDES 1   neonatal erythema toxicum (P83.1)

L53.1 **Erythema annulare centrifugum**

L53.2 **Erythema marginatum**

L53.3 **Other chronic figurate erythema**

L53.8 **Other specified erythematous conditions**

L53.9 **Erythematous condition, unspecified**
> Erythema NOS
> Erythroderma NOS

L54 **Erythema in diseases classified elsewhere**
> Code first underlying disease

Radiation-related disorders of the skin and subcutaneous tissue (L55-L59)

✓4ᵗʰ **L55** **Sunburn**

L55.0 **Sunburn of first degree**

L55.1 **Sunburn of second degree**

L55.2 **Sunburn of third degree**

L55.9 **Sunburn, unspecified**

✓4ᵗʰ **L56** **Other acute skin changes due to ultraviolet radiation**
> Use additional code to identify the source of the ultraviolet radiation (W89, X32)

L56.0 **Drug phototoxic response**
> Use additional code for adverse effect, if applicable, to identify drug (T36-T50 with fifth or sixth character 5)

L56.1 **Drug photoallergic response**
> Use additional code for adverse effect, if applicable, to identify drug (T36-T50 with fifth or sixth character 5)

L56.2 **Photocontact dermatitis [berloque dermatitis]**

L56.3 **Solar urticaria**

L56.4 **Polymorphous light eruption**

L56.5 **Disseminated superficial actinic porokeratosis (DSAP)**

L56.8 **Other specified acute skin changes due to ultraviolet radiation**

L56.9 **Acute skin change due to ultraviolet radiation, unspecified**

✓4ᵗʰ **L57** **Skin changes due to chronic exposure to nonionizing radiation**
> Use additional code to identify the source of the ultraviolet radiation (W89, X32)

L57.0 **Actinic keratosis**
> Keratosis NOS
> Senile keratosis
> Solar keratosis

L57.1 **Actinic reticuloid**

L57.2 **Cutis rhomboidalis nuchae**

L57.3 **Poikiloderma of Civatte**

L57.4 **Cutis laxa senilis**
> Elastosis senilis

L57.5 **Actinic granuloma**

L57.8 **Other skin changes due to chronic exposure to nonionizing radiation**
> Farmer's skin
> Sailor's skin
> Solar dermatitis

L57.9 **Skin changes due to chronic exposure to nonionizing radiation, unspecified**

✓4ᵗʰ **L58** **Radiodermatitis**
> Use additional code to identify the source of the radiation (W88, W90)

L58.0 **Acute radiodermatitis**

L58.1 **Chronic radiodermatitis**

L58.9 **Radiodermatitis, unspecified**

✓4ᵗʰ **L59** **Other disorders of skin and subcutaneous tissue related to radiation**

L59.0 **Erythema ab igne [dermatitis ab igne]**

L59.8 **Other specified disorders of the skin and subcutaneous tissue related to radiation**

EXCLUDES 1 Not coded here   EXCLUDES 2 Not included here   N Newborn Age: 0   P Pediatric Age: 0-17   M Maternity Age: 12-55   A Adult Age: 15-124

654   ICD-10-CM 2016

L59.9   **Disorder of the skin and subcutaneous tissue related to radiation, unspecified**

Disorders of skin appendages (L60-L75)

EXCLUDES 1   *congenital malformations of integument (Q84.-)*

✓4ᵗʰ **L60   Nail disorders**
> EXCLUDES 2   *clubbing of nails (R68.3)*
> *onychia and paronychia (L03.0-)*

L60.0   **Ingrowing nail**

L60.1   **Onycholysis**

L60.2   **Onychogryphosis**

L60.3   **Nail dystrophy**

L60.4   **Beau's lines**

L60.5   **Yellow nail syndrome**

L60.8   **Other nail disorders**

L60.9   **Nail disorder, unspecified**

L62   Nail disorders in diseases classified elsewhere
> *Code first underlying disease, such as:*
> *pachydermoperiostosis (M89.4-)*

✓4ᵗʰ **L63   Alopecia areata**

L63.0   **Alopecia (capitis)** totalis

L63.1   **Alopecia** universalis

L63.2   **Ophiasis**

L63.8   **Other alopecia areata**

L63.9   **Alopecia areata, unspecified**

✓4ᵗʰ **L64   Androgenic alopecia**
> INCLUDES   male-pattern baldness

L64.0   **Drug-induced androgenic alopecia**
> Use additional code for adverse effect, if applicable, to identify drug (T36-T50 with fifth or sixth character 5)

L64.8   **Other androgenic alopecia**

L64.9   **Androgenic alopecia, unspecified**

✓4ᵗʰ **L65   Other nonscarring hair loss**
> Use additional code for adverse effect, if applicable, to identify drug (T36-T50 with fifth or sixth character 5)
> EXCLUDES 1   *trichotillomania (F63.3)*

L65.0   **Telogen effluvium**

L65.1   **Anagen effluvium**

L65.2   **Alopecia mucinosa**

L65.8   **Other specified nonscarring hair loss**

L65.9   **Nonscarring hair loss, unspecified**
> Alopecia NOS

✓4ᵗʰ **L66   Cicatricial alopecia [scarring hair loss]**

L66.0   **Pseudopelade**

L66.1   **Lichen planopilaris**
> Follicular lichen planus

L66.2   **Folliculitis decalvans**

L66.3   **Perifolliculitis capitis abscedens**

L66.4   **Folliculitis ulerythematosa reticulata**

L66.8   **Other cicatricial alopecia**
> **AHA:** 2015, 1Q, 19

L66.9   **Cicatricial alopecia, unspecified**

✓4ᵗʰ **L67   Hair color and hair shaft abnormalities**
> EXCLUDES 1   *monilethrix (Q84.1)*
> *pili annulati (Q84.1)*
> *telogen effluvium (L65.0)*

L67.0   **Trichorrhexis nodosa**

L67.1   **Variations in hair color**
> Canities
> Greyness, hair (premature)
> Heterochromia of hair
> Poliosis circumscripta, acquired
> Poliosis NOS

L67.8   **Other hair color and hair shaft abnormalities**
> Fragilitas crinium

L67.9   **Hair color and hair shaft abnormality, unspecified**

✓4ᵗʰ **L68   Hypertrichosis**
> INCLUDES   excess hair
> EXCLUDES 1   *congenital hypertrichosis (Q84.2)*
> *persistent lanugo (Q84.2)*

L68.0   **Hirsutism**

L68.1   **Acquired hypertrichosis lanuginosa**

L68.2   **Localized hypertrichosis**

L68.3   **Polytrichia**

L68.8   **Other hypertrichosis**

L68.9   **Hypertrichosis, unspecified**

✓4ᵗʰ **L70   Acne**
> EXCLUDES 2   *acne keloid (L73.0)*

L70.0   **Acne** vulgaris

L70.1   **Acne** conglobata

L70.2   **Acne** varioliformis
> Acne necrotica miliaris

L70.3   **Acne** tropica

L70.4   **Infantile acne**   P

L70.5   **Acné** excoriée des jeunes filles
> Picker's acne

L70.8   **Other acne**

L70.9   **Acne, unspecified**

✓4ᵗʰ **L71   Rosacea**
> Use additional code for adverse effect, if applicable, to identify drug (T36-T50 with fifth or sixth character 5)

L71.0   **Perioral dermatitis**

L71.1   **Rhinophyma**

L71.8   **Other rosacea**

L71.9   **Rosacea, unspecified**

✓4ᵗʰ **L72   Follicular cysts of skin and subcutaneous tissue**

L72.0   **Epidermal cyst**

✓5ᵗʰ   L72.1   **Pilar and trichodermal cyst**

L72.11   **Pilar cyst**

L72.12   **Trichodermal cyst**
> Trichilemmal (proliferating) cyst

L72.2   **Steatocystoma multiplex**

L72.3   **Sebaceous cyst**
> EXCLUDES 2   *pilar cyst (L72.11)*
> *trichilemmal (proliferating) cyst (L72.12)*

L72.8   **Other follicular cysts of the skin and subcutaneous tissue**

L72.9   **Follicular cyst of the skin and subcutaneous tissue, unspecified**

✓4ᵗʰ **L73   Other follicular disorders**

L73.0   **Acne keloid**

L73.1   **Pseudofolliculitis barbae**

L73.2   **Hidradenitis suppurativa**

L73.8   **Other specified follicular disorders**
> Sycosis barbae

L73.9   **Follicular disorder, unspecified**

✓4ᵗʰ **L74   Eccrine sweat disorders**
> EXCLUDES 2   *generalized hyperhidrosis (R61)*

L74.0   **Miliaria** rubra

L74.1   **Miliaria** crystallina

L74.2   **Miliaria** profunda
> Miliaria tropicalis

L74.3   **Miliaria, unspecified**

L74.4   **Anhidrosis**
> Hypohidrosis

✓5ᵗʰ   L74.5   **Focal hyperhidrosis**

✓6ᵗʰ   L74.51   **Primary focal hyperhidrosis**

L74.510   **Primary focal hyperhidrosis, axilla**

L74.511   **Primary focal hyperhidrosis, face**

L74.512   **Primary focal hyperhidrosis, palms**

L74.513   **Primary focal hyperhidrosis, soles**

L74.519   **Primary focal hyperhidrosis, unspecified**

L74.52   **Secondary focal hyperhidrosis**
> Frey's syndrome

L74.8   **Other eccrine sweat disorders**

L74.9   **Eccrine sweat disorder, unspecified**
> Sweat gland disorder NOS

✓4ᵗʰ **L75   Apocrine sweat disorders**
> EXCLUDES 1   *dyshidrosis (L30.1)*
> *hidradenitis suppurativa (L73.2)*

L75.0   **Bromhidrosis**

L75.1   **Chromhidrosis**

L75.2   **Apocrine miliaria**
> Fox-Fordyce disease

✓ Additional Character Required   ✓x7ᵗʰ Placeholder Alert   Unspecified Dx   Other Specified Dx   Manifestation   ►◄ Revised Text   ● New Code   ▲ Revised Code Title

L75.8 Other apocrine sweat disorders

L75.9 Apocrine sweat disorder, unspecified

Intraoperative and postprocedural complications of skin and subcutaneous tissue (L76)

✓4ᵗʰ **L76 Intraoperative and postprocedural complications of skin and subcutaneous tissue**

  ✓5ᵗʰ **L76.0 Intraoperative hemorrhage and hematoma of skin and subcutaneous tissue complicating a procedure**

    EXCLUDES 1   *intraoperative hemorrhage and hematoma of skin and subcutaneous tissue due to accidental puncture and laceration during a procedure (L76.1-)*

    L76.01 Intraoperative hemorrhage and hematoma of skin and subcutaneous tissue complicating a dermatologic procedure

    L76.02 Intraoperative hemorrhage and hematoma of skin and subcutaneous tissue complicating other procedure

  ✓5ᵗʰ **L76.1 Accidental puncture and laceration of skin and subcutaneous tissue during a procedure**

    L76.11 Accidental puncture and laceration of skin and subcutaneous tissue during a dermatologic procedure

    L76.12 Accidental puncture and laceration of skin and subcutaneous tissue during other procedure

  ✓5ᵗʰ **L76.2 Postprocedural hemorrhage and hematoma of skin and subcutaneous tissue following a procedure**

    L76.21 Postprocedural hemorrhage and hematoma of skin and subcutaneous tissue following a dermatologic procedure

    L76.22 Postprocedural hemorrhage and hematoma of skin and subcutaneous tissue following other procedure

  ✓5ᵗʰ **L76.8 Other intraoperative and postprocedural complications of skin and subcutaneous tissue**

    Use additional code, if applicable, to further specify disorder

    L76.81 Other intraoperative complications of skin and subcutaneous tissue

    L76.82 Other postprocedural complications of skin and subcutaneous tissue

Other disorders of the skin and subcutaneous tissue (L80-L99)

L80 Vitiligo

  EXCLUDES 2   *vitiligo of eyelids (H02.73-)*
         vitiligo of vulva (N90.89)

✓4ᵗʰ **L81 Other disorders of pigmentation**

  EXCLUDES 1   *birthmark NOS (Q82.5)*
         Peutz-Jeghers syndrome (Q85.8)
  EXCLUDES 2   *nevus—see Alphabetical Index*

  L81.0 Postinflammatory hyperpigmentation

  L81.1 Chloasma

  L81.2 Freckles

  L81.3 Café au lait spots

  L81.4 Other melanin hyperpigmentation
    Lentigo

  L81.5 Leukoderma, not elsewhere classified

  L81.6 Other disorders of diminished melanin formation

  L81.7 Pigmented purpuric dermatosis
    Angioma serpiginosum

  L81.8 Other specified disorders of pigmentation
    Iron pigmentation
    Tattoo pigmentation

  L81.9 Disorder of pigmentation, unspecified

✓4ᵗʰ **L82 Seborrheic keratosis**

  INCLUDES   dermatosis papulosa nigra
         Leser-Trélat disease
  EXCLUDES 2   *seborrheic dermatitis (L21.-)*

  L82.0 Inflamed seborrheic keratosis

  L82.1 Other seborrheic keratosis
    Seborrheic keratosis NOS

L83 Acanthosis nigricans
  Confluent and reticulated papillomatosis

L84 Corns and callosities
  Callus
  Clavus

✓4ᵗʰ **L85 Other epidermal thickening**

  EXCLUDES 2   *hypertrophic disorders of the skin (L91.-)*

  L85.0 Acquired ichthyosis
    EXCLUDES 1   *congenital ichthyosis (Q80.-)*

  L85.1 Acquired keratosis [keratoderma] palmaris et plantaris
    EXCLUDES 1   *inherited keratosis palmaris et plantaris (Q82.8)*

  L85.2 Keratosis punctata (palmaris et plantaris)

  L85.3 Xerosis cutis
    Dry skin dermatitis

  L85.8 Other specified epidermal thickening
    Cutaneous horn

  L85.9 Epidermal thickening, unspecified

L86 Keratoderma in diseases classified elsewhere
  Code first underlying disease, such as:
    Reiter's disease (M02.3-)
  EXCLUDES 1   *gonococcal keratoderma (A54.89)*
         gonococcal keratosis (A54.89)
         keratoderma due to vitamin A deficiency (E50.8)
         keratosis due to vitamin A deficiency (E50.8)
         xeroderma due to vitamin A deficiency (E50.8)

✓4ᵗʰ **L87 Transepidermal elimination disorders**

  EXCLUDES 1   *granuloma annulare (perforating) (L92.0)*

  L87.0 Keratosis follicularis et parafollicularis in cutem penetrans
    Hyperkeratosis follicularis penetrans
    Kyrle disease

  L87.1 Reactive perforating collagenosis

  L87.2 Elastosis perforans serpiginosa

  L87.8 Other transepidermal elimination disorders

  L87.9 Transepidermal elimination disorder, unspecified

L88 Pyoderma gangrenosum
  Phagedenic pyoderma
  EXCLUDES 1   *dermatitis gangrenosa (L08.0)*

✓4ᵗʰ **L89 Pressure ulcer**
  Bed sore
  Decubitus ulcer
  Plaster ulcer
  Pressure area
  Pressure sore
  Code first any associated gangrene (I96)
  EXCLUDES 2   *decubitus (trophic) ulcer of cervix (uteri) (N86)*
         diabetic ulcers (E08.621, E08.622, E09.621, E09.622, E10.621, E10.622, E11.621, E11.622, E13.621, E13.622)
         non-pressure chronic ulcer of skin (L97.-)
         skin infections (L00-L08)
         varicose ulcer (I83.0, I83.2)

  ✓5ᵗʰ **L89.0 Pressure ulcer of elbow**

    ✓6ᵗʰ **L89.00 Pressure ulcer of unspecified elbow**

      L89.000 Pressure ulcer of unspecified elbow, unstageable

      L89.001 Pressure ulcer of unspecified elbow, stage 1
        Healing pressure ulcer of unspecified elbow, stage 1
        Pressure pre-ulcer skin changes limited to persistent focal edema, unspecified elbow

      L89.002 Pressure ulcer of unspecified elbow, stage 2
        Healing pressure ulcer of unspecified elbow, stage 2
        Pressure ulcer with abrasion, blister, partial thickness skin loss involving epidermis and/or dermis, unspecified elbow

      L89.003 Pressure ulcer of unspecified elbow, stage 3
        Healing pressure ulcer of unspecified elbow, stage 3
        Pressure ulcer with full thickness skin loss involving damage or necrosis of subcutaneous tissue, unspecified elbow

      L89.004 Pressure ulcer of unspecified elbow, stage 4
        Healing pressure ulcer of unspecified elbow, stage 4
        Pressure ulcer with necrosis of soft tissues through to underlying muscle, tendon, or bone, unspecified elbow

EXCLUDES 1 Not coded here   EXCLUDES 2 Not included here   N Newborn Age: 0   P Pediatric Age: 0-17   M Maternity Age: 12-55   A Adult Age: 15-124

656   ICD-10-CM 2016

L89.009 **Pressure ulcer of unspecified elbow, unspecified stage**
    Healing pressure ulcer of elbow NOS
    Healing pressure ulcer of unspecified elbow, unspecified stage

☑6ᵗʰ **L89.01** **Pressure ulcer of** right elbow

L89.010 **Pressure ulcer of right elbow, unstageable**

L89.011 **Pressure ulcer of right elbow, stage 1**
    Healing pressure ulcer of right elbow, stage 1
    Pressure pre-ulcer skin changes limited to persistent focal edema, right elbow

L89.012 **Pressure ulcer of right elbow, stage 2**
    Healing pressure ulcer of right elbow, stage 2
    Pressure ulcer with abrasion, blister, partial thickness skin loss involving epidermis and/or dermis, right elbow

L89.013 **Pressure ulcer of right elbow, stage 3**
    Healing pressure ulcer of right elbow, stage 3
    Pressure ulcer with full thickness skin loss involving damage or necrosis of subcutaneous tissue, right elbow

L89.014 **Pressure ulcer of right elbow, stage 4**
    Healing pressure ulcer of right elbow, stage 4
    Pressure ulcer with necrosis of soft tissues through to underlying muscle, tendon, or bone, right elbow

L89.019 **Pressure ulcer of right elbow, unspecified stage**
    Healing pressure right of elbow NOS
    Healing pressure ulcer of unspecified elbow, unspecified stage

☑6ᵗʰ **L89.02** **Pressure ulcer of** left elbow

L89.020 **Pressure ulcer of left elbow, unstageable**

L89.021 **Pressure ulcer of left elbow, stage 1**
    Healing pressure ulcer of left elbow, stage 1
    Pressure pre-ulcer skin changes limited to persistent focal edema, left elbow

L89.022 **Pressure ulcer of left elbow, stage 2**
    Healing pressure ulcer of left elbow, stage 2
    Pressure ulcer with abrasion, blister, partial thickness skin loss involving epidermis and/or dermis, left elbow

L89.023 **Pressure ulcer of left elbow, stage 3**
    Healing pressure ulcer of left elbow, stage 3
    Pressure ulcer with full thickness skin loss involving damage or necrosis of subcutaneous tissue, left elbow

L89.024 **Pressure ulcer of left elbow, stage 4**
    Healing pressure ulcer of left elbow, stage 4
    Pressure ulcer with necrosis of soft tissues through to underlying muscle, tendon, or bone, left elbow

L89.029 **Pressure ulcer of left elbow, unspecified stage**
    Healing pressure ulcer of left of elbow NOS
    Healing pressure ulcer of unspecified elbow, unspecified stage

☑5ᵗʰ **L89.1** **Pressure ulcer of** back

☑6ᵗʰ **L89.10** **Pressure ulcer of** unspecified part of back

L89.100 **Pressure ulcer of unspecified part of back, unstageable**

L89.101 **Pressure ulcer of unspecified part of back, stage 1**
    Healing pressure ulcer of unspecified part of back, stage 1
    Pressure pre-ulcer skin changes limited to persistent focal edema, unspecified part of back

L89.102 **Pressure ulcer of unspecified part of back, stage 2**
    Healing pressure ulcer of unspecified part of back, stage 2
    Pressure ulcer with abrasion, blister, partial thickness skin loss involving epidermis and/or dermis, unspecified part of back

L89.103 **Pressure ulcer of unspecified part of back, stage 3**
    Healing pressure ulcer of unspecified part of back, stage 3
    Pressure ulcer with full thickness skin loss involving damage or necrosis of subcutaneous tissue, unspecified part of back

L89.104 **Pressure ulcer of unspecified part of back, stage 4**
    Healing pressure ulcer of unspecified part of back, stage 4
    Pressure ulcer with necrosis of soft tissues through to underlying muscle, tendon, or bone, unspecified part of back

L89.109 **Pressure ulcer of unspecified part of back, unspecified stage**
    Healing pressure ulcer of unspecified part of back NOS
    Healing pressure ulcer of unspecified part of back, unspecified stage

☑6ᵗʰ **L89.11** **Pressure ulcer of** right upper back
    Pressure ulcer of right shoulder blade

L89.110 **Pressure ulcer of right upper back, unstageable**

L89.111 **Pressure ulcer of right upper back, stage 1**
    Healing pressure ulcer of right upper back, stage 1
    Pressure pre-ulcer skin changes limited to persistent focal edema, right upper back

L89.112 **Pressure ulcer of right upper back, stage 2**
    Healing pressure ulcer of right upper back, stage 2
    Pressure ulcer with abrasion, blister, partial thickness skin loss involving epidermis and/or dermis, right upper back

L89.113 **Pressure ulcer of right upper back, stage 3**
    Healing pressure ulcer of right upper back, stage 3
    Pressure ulcer with full thickness skin loss involving damage or necrosis of subcutaneous tissue, right upper back

L89.114 **Pressure ulcer of right upper back, stage 4**
    Healing pressure ulcer of right upper back, stage 4
    Pressure ulcer with necrosis of soft tissues through to underlying muscle, tendon, or bone, right upper back

L89.119 **Pressure ulcer of right upper back, unspecified stage**
    Healing pressure ulcer of right upper back NOS
    Healing pressure ulcer of right upper back, unspecified stage

☑6ᵗʰ **L89.12** **Pressure ulcer of** left upper back
    Pressure ulcer of left shoulder blade

L89.120 **Pressure ulcer of left upper back, unstageable**

L89.121 **Pressure ulcer of left upper back, stage 1**
    Healing pressure ulcer of left upper back, stage 1
    Pressure pre-ulcer skin changes limited to persistent focal edema, left upper back

L89.122 **Pressure ulcer of left upper back, stage 2**
    Healing pressure ulcer of left upper back, stage 2
    Pressure ulcer with abrasion, blister, partial thickness skin loss involving epidermis and/or dermis, left upper back

L89.123 **Pressure ulcer of left upper back, stage 3**
    Healing pressure ulcer of left upper back, stage 3
    Pressure ulcer with full thickness skin loss involving damage or necrosis of subcutaneous tissue, left upper back

L89.124 **Pressure ulcer of left upper back, stage 4**
    Healing pressure ulcer of left upper back, stage 4
    Pressure ulcer with necrosis of soft tissues through to underlying muscle, tendon, or bone, left upper back

---

☑ Additional Character Required   ☑x7ᵗʰ Placeholder Alert   Unspecified Dx   Other Specified Dx   Manifestation   ▶◀ Revised Text   ● New Code   ▲ Revised Code Title

L89.129   **Pressure ulcer of left upper back, unspecified stage**
  Healing pressure ulcer of left upper back NOS
  Healing pressure ulcer of left upper back, unspecified stage

✓6ᵗʰ   **L89.13**   **Pressure ulcer of** right lower back

L89.130   **Pressure ulcer of right lower back, unstageable**

L89.131   **Pressure ulcer of right lower back, stage 1**
  Healing pressure ulcer of right lower back, stage 1
  Pressure pre-ulcer skin changes limited to persistent focal edema, right lower back

L89.132   **Pressure ulcer of right lower back, stage 2**
  Healing pressure ulcer of right lower back, stage 2
  Pressure ulcer with abrasion, blister, partial thickness skin loss involving epidermis and/or dermis, right lower back

L89.133   **Pressure ulcer of right lower back, stage 3**
  Healing pressure ulcer of right lower back, stage 3
  Pressure ulcer with full thickness skin loss involving damage or necrosis of subcutaneous tissue, right lower back

L89.134   **Pressure ulcer of right lower back, stage 4**
  Healing pressure ulcer of right lower back, stage 4
  Pressure ulcer with necrosis of soft tissues through to underlying muscle, tendon, or bone, right lower back

L89.139   **Pressure ulcer of right lower back, unspecified stage**
  Healing pressure ulcer of right lower back NOS
  Healing pressure ulcer of right lower back, unspecified stage

✓6ᵗʰ   **L89.14**   **Pressure ulcer of** left lower back

L89.140   **Pressure ulcer of left lower back, unstageable**

L89.141   **Pressure ulcer of left lower back, stage 1**
  Healing pressure ulcer of left lower back, stage 1
  Pressure pre-ulcer skin changes limited to persistent focal edema, left lower back

L89.142   **Pressure ulcer of left lower back, stage 2**
  Healing pressure ulcer of left lower back, stage 2
  Pressure ulcer with abrasion, blister, partial thickness skin loss involving epidermis and/or dermis, left lower back

L89.143   **Pressure ulcer of left lower back, stage 3**
  Healing pressure ulcer of left lower back, stage 3
  Pressure ulcer with full thickness skin loss involving damage or necrosis of subcutaneous tissue, left lower back

L89.144   **Pressure ulcer of left lower back, stage 4**
  Healing pressure ulcer of left lower back, stage 4
  Pressure ulcer with necrosis of soft tissues through to underlying muscle, tendon, or bone, left lower back

L89.149   **Pressure ulcer of left lower back, unspecified stage**
  Healing pressure ulcer of left lower back NOS
  Healing pressure ulcer of left lower back, unspecified stage

✓6ᵗʰ   **L89.15**   **Pressure ulcer of** sacral region
  Pressure ulcer of coccyx
  Pressure ulcer of tailbone

L89.150   **Pressure ulcer of sacral region, unstageable**

L89.151   **Pressure ulcer of sacral region, stage 1**
  Healing pressure ulcer of sacral region, stage 1
  Pressure pre-ulcer skin changes limited to persistent focal edema, sacral region

L89.152   **Pressure ulcer of sacral region, stage 2**
  Healing pressure ulcer of sacral region, stage 2
  Pressure ulcer with abrasion, blister, partial thickness skin loss involving epidermis and/or dermis, sacral region

L89.153   **Pressure ulcer of sacral region, stage 3**
  Healing pressure ulcer of sacral region, stage 3
  Pressure ulcer with full thickness skin loss involving damage or necrosis of subcutaneous tissue, sacral region

L89.154   **Pressure ulcer of sacral region, stage 4**
  Healing pressure ulcer of sacral region, stage 4
  Pressure ulcer with necrosis of soft tissues through to underlying muscle, tendon, or bone, sacral region

L89.159   **Pressure ulcer of sacral region, unspecified stage**
  Healing pressure ulcer of sacral region NOS
  Healing pressure ulcer of sacral region, unspecified stage

✓5ᵗʰ   **L89.2**   **Pressure ulcer of** hip

✓6ᵗʰ   **L89.20**   **Pressure ulcer of** unspecified hip

L89.200   **Pressure ulcer of unspecified hip, unstageable**

L89.201   **Pressure ulcer of unspecified hip, stage 1**
  Healing pressure ulcer of unspecified hip, stage 1
  Pressure pre-ulcer skin changes limited to persistent focal edema, unspecified hip

L89.202   **Pressure ulcer of unspecified hip, stage 2**
  Healing pressure ulcer of unspecified hip, stage 2
  Pressure ulcer with abrasion, blister, partial thickness skin loss involving epidermis and/or dermis, unspecified hip

L89.203   **Pressure ulcer of unspecified hip, stage 3**
  Healing pressure ulcer of unspecified hip, stage 3
  Pressure ulcer with full thickness skin loss involving damage or necrosis of subcutaneous tissue, unspecified hip

L89.204   **Pressure ulcer of unspecified hip, stage 4**
  Healing pressure ulcer of unspecified hip, stage 4
  Pressure ulcer with necrosis of soft tissues through to underlying muscle, tendon, or bone, unspecified hip

L89.209   **Pressure ulcer of unspecified hip, unspecified stage**
  Healing pressure ulcer of unspecified hip NOS
  Healing pressure ulcer of unspecified hip, unspecified stage

✓6ᵗʰ   **L89.21**   **Pressure ulcer of** right hip

L89.210   **Pressure ulcer of right hip, unstageable**

L89.211   **Pressure ulcer of right hip, stage 1**
  Healing pressure ulcer of right hip, stage 1
  Pressure pre-ulcer skin changes limited to persistent focal edema, right hip

L89.212   **Pressure ulcer of right hip, stage 2**
  Healing pressure ulcer of right hip, stage 2
  Pressure ulcer with abrasion, blister, partial thickness skin loss involving epidermis and/or dermis, right hip

L89.213   **Pressure ulcer of right hip, stage 3**
  Healing pressure ulcer of right hip, stage 3
  Pressure ulcer with full thickness skin loss involving damage or necrosis of subcutaneous tissue, right hip

L89.214   **Pressure ulcer of right hip, stage 4**
  Healing pressure ulcer of right hip, stage 4
  Pressure ulcer with necrosis of soft tissues through to underlying muscle, tendon, or bone, right hip

EXCLUDES 1 Not coded here   **EXCLUDES 2** Not included here   **N** Newborn Age: 0   **P** Pediatric Age: 0-17   **M** Maternity Age: 12-55   **A** Adult Age: 15-124

658   ICD-10-CM 2016

L89.219 **Pressure ulcer of right hip, unspecified stage**
    Healing pressure ulcer of right hip NOS
    Healing pressure ulcer of right hip, unspecified stage

✓6ᵗʰ **L89.22** **Pressure ulcer of** left hip

  L89.220 **Pressure ulcer of left hip,** unstageable

  L89.221 **Pressure ulcer of left hip,** stage 1
    Healing pressure ulcer of left hip, stage 1
    Pressure pre-ulcer skin changes limited to persistent focal edema, left hip

  L89.222 **Pressure ulcer of left hip,** stage 2
    Healing pressure ulcer of left hip, stage 2
    Pressure ulcer with abrasion, blister, partial thickness skin loss involving epidermis and/or dermis, left hip

  L89.223 **Pressure ulcer of left hip,** stage 3
    Healing pressure ulcer of left hip, stage 3
    Pressure ulcer with full thickness skin loss involving damage or necrosis of subcutaneous tissue, left hip

  L89.224 **Pressure ulcer of left hip,** stage 4
    Healing pressure ulcer of left hip, stage 4
    Pressure ulcer with necrosis of soft tissues through to underlying muscle, tendon, or bone, left hip

  L89.229 **Pressure ulcer of left hip, unspecified stage**
    Healing pressure ulcer of left hip NOS
    Healing pressure ulcer of left hip, unspecified stage

✓5ᵗʰ **L89.3** **Pressure ulcer of** buttock

  ✓6ᵗʰ **L89.30** **Pressure ulcer of** unspecified buttock

    L89.300 **Pressure ulcer of unspecified buttock, unstageable**

    L89.301 **Pressure ulcer of unspecified buttock, stage 1**
      Healing pressure ulcer of unspecified buttock, stage 1
      Pressure pre-ulcer skin changes limited to persistent focal edema, unspecified buttock

    L89.302 **Pressure ulcer of unspecified buttock, stage 2**
      Healing pressure ulcer of unspecified buttock, stage 2
      Pressure ulcer with abrasion, blister, partial thickness skin loss involving epidermis and/or dermis, unspecified buttock

    L89.303 **Pressure ulcer of unspecified buttock, stage 3**
      Healing pressure ulcer of unspecified buttock, stage 3
      Pressure ulcer with full thickness skin loss involving damage or necrosis of subcutaneous tissue, unspecified buttock

    L89.304 **Pressure ulcer of unspecified buttock, stage 4**
      Healing pressure ulcer of unspecified buttock, stage 4
      Pressure ulcer with necrosis of soft tissues through to underlying muscle, tendon, or bone, unspecified buttock

    L89.309 **Pressure ulcer of unspecified buttock, unspecified stage**
      Healing pressure ulcer of unspecified buttock NOS
      Healing pressure ulcer of unspecified buttock, unspecified stage

  ✓6ᵗʰ **L89.31** **Pressure ulcer of** right buttock

    L89.310 **Pressure ulcer of right buttock, unstageable**

    L89.311 **Pressure ulcer of right buttock,** stage 1
      Healing pressure ulcer of right buttock, stage 1
      Pressure pre-ulcer skin changes limited to persistent focal edema, right buttock

    L89.312 **Pressure ulcer of right buttock,** stage 2
      Healing pressure ulcer of right buttock, stage 2
      Pressure ulcer with abrasion, blister, partial thickness skin loss involving epidermis and/or dermis, right buttock

    L89.313 **Pressure ulcer of right buttock,** stage 3
      Healing pressure ulcer of right buttock, stage 3
      Pressure ulcer with full thickness skin loss involving damage or necrosis of subcutaneous tissue, right buttock

    L89.314 **Pressure ulcer of right buttock,** stage 4
      Healing pressure ulcer of right buttock, stage 4
      Pressure ulcer with necrosis of soft tissues through to underlying muscle, tendon, or bone, right buttock

    L89.319 **Pressure ulcer of right buttock, unspecified stage**
      Healing pressure ulcer of right buttock NOS
      Healing pressure ulcer of right buttock, unspecified stage

  ✓6ᵗʰ **L89.32** **Pressure ulcer of** left buttock

    L89.320 **Pressure ulcer of left buttock,** unstageable

    L89.321 **Pressure ulcer of left buttock,** stage 1
      Healing pressure ulcer of left buttock, stage 1
      Pressure pre-ulcer skin changes limited to persistent focal edema, left buttock

    L89.322 **Pressure ulcer of left buttock,** stage 2
      Healing pressure ulcer of left buttock, stage 2
      Pressure ulcer with abrasion, blister, partial thickness skin loss involving epidermis and/or dermis, left buttock

    L89.323 **Pressure ulcer of left buttock,** stage 3
      Healing pressure ulcer of left buttock, stage 3
      Pressure ulcer with full thickness skin loss involving damage or necrosis of subcutaneous tissue, left buttock

    L89.324 **Pressure ulcer of left buttock,** stage 4
      Healing pressure ulcer of left buttock, stage 4
      Pressure ulcer with necrosis of soft tissues through to underlying muscle, tendon, or bone, left buttock

    L89.329 **Pressure ulcer of left buttock, unspecified stage**
      Healing pressure ulcer of left buttock NOS
      Healing pressure ulcer of left buttock, unspecified stage

✓5ᵗʰ **L89.4** **Pressure ulcer of contiguous site of** back, buttock and hip

  L89.40 **Pressure ulcer of contiguous site of back, buttock and hip, unspecified stage**
    Healing pressure ulcer of contiguous site of back, buttock and hip NOS
    Healing pressure ulcer of contiguous site of back, buttock and hip, unspecified stage

  L89.41 **Pressure ulcer of contiguous site of back, buttock and hip,** stage 1
    Healing pressure ulcer of contiguous site of back, buttock and hip, stage 1
    Pressure pre-ulcer skin changes limited to persistent focal edema, contiguous site of back, buttock and hip

  L89.42 **Pressure ulcer of contiguous site of back, buttock and hip,** stage 2
    Healing pressure ulcer of contiguous site of back, buttock and hip, stage 2
    Pressure ulcer with abrasion, blister, partial thickness skin loss involving epidermis and/or dermis, contiguous site of back, buttock and hip

  L89.43 **Pressure ulcer of contiguous site of back, buttock and hip,** stage 3
    Healing pressure ulcer of contiguous site of back, buttock and hip, stage 3
    Pressure ulcer with full thickness skin loss involving damage or necrosis of subcutaneous tissue, contiguous site of back, buttock and hip

---

☑ Additional Character Required   ✓x7ᵗʰ Placeholder Alert   Unspecified Dx   Other Specified Dx   Manifestation   ▶◀ Revised Text   ● New Code   ▲ Revised Code Title

ICD-10-CM 2016   **659**

Chapter 12. Diseases of the Skin and Subcutaneous Tissue

L89.219–L89.43

L89.44 **Pressure ulcer of contiguous site of back, buttock and hip, stage 4**

Healing pressure ulcer of contiguous site of back, buttock and hip, stage 4

Pressure ulcer with necrosis of soft tissues through to underlying muscle, tendon, or bone, contiguous site of back, buttock and hip

L89.45 **Pressure ulcer of contiguous site of back, buttock and hip, unstageable**

✓5th **L89.5** **Pressure ulcer of ankle**

  ✓6th **L89.50** **Pressure ulcer of unspecified ankle**

L89.500 **Pressure ulcer of unspecified ankle, unstageable**

L89.501 **Pressure ulcer of unspecified ankle, stage 1**

Healing pressure ulcer of unspecified ankle, stage 1

Pressure pre-ulcer skin changes limited to persistent focal edema, unspecified ankle

L89.502 **Pressure ulcer of unspecified ankle, stage 2**

Healing pressure ulcer of unspecified ankle, stage 2

Pressure ulcer with abrasion, blister, partial thickness skin loss involving epidermis and/or dermis, unspecified ankle

L89.503 **Pressure ulcer of unspecified ankle, stage 3**

Healing pressure ulcer of unspecified ankle, stage 3

Pressure ulcer with full thickness skin loss involving damage or necrosis of subcutaneous tissue, unspecified ankle

L89.504 **Pressure ulcer of unspecified ankle, stage 4**

Healing pressure ulcer of unspecified ankle, stage 4

Pressure ulcer with necrosis of soft tissues through to underlying muscle, tendon, or bone, unspecified ankle

L89.509 **Pressure ulcer of unspecified ankle, unspecified stage**

Healing pressure ulcer of unspecified ankle NOS

Healing pressure ulcer of unspecified ankle, unspecified stage

  ✓6th **L89.51** **Pressure ulcer of right ankle**

L89.510 **Pressure ulcer of right ankle, unstageable**

L89.511 **Pressure ulcer of right ankle, stage 1**

Healing pressure ulcer of right ankle, stage 1

Pressure pre-ulcer skin changes limited to persistent focal edema, right ankle

L89.512 **Pressure ulcer of right ankle, stage 2**

Healing pressure ulcer of right ankle, stage 2

Pressure ulcer with abrasion, blister, partial thickness skin loss involving epidermis and/or dermis, right ankle

L89.513 **Pressure ulcer of right ankle, stage 3**

Healing pressure ulcer of right ankle, stage 3

Pressure ulcer with full thickness skin loss involving damage or necrosis of subcutaneous tissue, right ankle

L89.514 **Pressure ulcer of right ankle, stage 4**

Healing pressure ulcer of right ankle, stage 4

Pressure ulcer with necrosis of soft tissues through to underlying muscle, tendon, or bone, right ankle

L89.519 **Pressure ulcer of right ankle, unspecified stage**

Healing pressure ulcer of right ankle NOS

Healing pressure ulcer of right ankle, unspecified stage

  ✓6th **L89.52** **Pressure ulcer of left ankle**

L89.520 **Pressure ulcer of left ankle, unstageable**

L89.521 **Pressure ulcer of left ankle, stage 1**

Healing pressure ulcer of left ankle, stage 1

Pressure pre-ulcer skin changes limited to persistnt focal edema, left ankle

L89.522 **Pressure ulcer of left ankle, stage 2**

Healing pressure ulcer of left ankle, stage 2

Pressure ulcer with abrasion, blister, partial thickness skin loss involving epidermis and/or dermis, left ankle

L89.523 **Pressure ulcer of left ankle, stage 3**

Healing pressure ulcer of left ankle, stage 3

Pressure ulcer with full thickness skin loss involving damage or necrosis of subcutaneous tissue, left ankle

L89.524 **Pressure ulcer of left ankle, stage 4**

Healing pressure ulcer of left ankle, stage 4

Pressure ulcer with necrosis of soft tissues through to underlying muscle, tendon, or bone, left ankle

L89.529 **Pressure ulcer of left ankle, unspecified stage**

Healing pressure ulcer of left ankle NOS

Healing pressure ulcer of left ankle, unspecified stage

✓5th **L89.6** **Pressure ulcer of heel**

  ✓6th **L89.60** **Pressure ulcer of unspecified heel**

L89.600 **Pressure ulcer of unspecified heel, unstageable**

L89.601 **Pressure ulcer of unspecified heel, stage 1**

Healing pressure ulcer of unspecified heel, stage 1

Pressure pre-ulcer skin changes limited to persistent focal edema, unspecified heel

L89.602 **Pressure ulcer of unspecified heel, stage 2**

Healing pressure ulcer of unspecified heel, stage 2

Pressure ulcer with abrasion, blister, partial thickness skin loss involving epidermis and/or dermis, unspecified heel

L89.603 **Pressure ulcer of unspecified heel, stage 3**

Healing pressure ulcer of unspecified heel, stage 3

Pressure ulcer with full thickness skin loss involving damage or necrosis of subcutaneous tissue, unspecified heel

L89.604 **Pressure ulcer of unspecified heel, stage 4**

Healing pressure ulcer of unspecified heel, stage 4

Pressure ulcer with necrosis of soft tissues through to underlying muscle, tendon, or bone, unspecified heel

L89.609 **Pressure ulcer of unspecified heel, unspecified stage**

Healing pressure ulcer of unspecified heel NOS

Healing pressure ulcer of unspecified heel, unspecified stage

  ✓6th **L89.61** **Pressure ulcer of right heel**

L89.610 **Pressure ulcer of right heel, unstageable**

L89.611 **Pressure ulcer of right heel, stage 1**

Healing pressure ulcer of right heel, stage 1

Pressure pre-ulcer skin changes limited to persistent focal edema, right heel

L89.612 **Pressure ulcer of right heel, stage 2**

Healing pressure ulcer of right heel, stage 2

Pressure ulcer with abrasion, blister, partial thickness skin loss involving epidermis and/or dermis, right heel

L89.613 **Pressure ulcer of right heel, stage 3**

Healing pressure ulcer of right heel, stage 3

Pressure ulcer with full thickness skin loss involving damage or necrosis of subcutaneous tissue, right heel

EXCLUDES 1 Not coded here   EXCLUDES 2 Not included here   N Newborn Age: 0   P Pediatric Age: 0-17   M Maternity Age: 12-55   A Adult Age: 15-124

660

ICD-10-CM 2016

L89.614   **Pressure ulcer of right heel, stage 4**
Healing pressure ulcer of right heel, stage 4
Pressure ulcer with necrosis of soft tissues through to underlying muscle, tendon, or bone, right heel

L89.619   **Pressure ulcer of right heel, unspecified stage**
Healing pressure ulcer of right heel NOS
Healing pressure ulcer of unspecified heel, right stage

√6ᵗʰ **L89.62**   **Pressure ulcer of left heel**

L89.620   **Pressure ulcer of left heel, unstageable**

L89.621   **Pressure ulcer of left heel, stage 1**
Healing pressure ulcer of left heel, stage 1
Pressure pre-ulcer skin changes limited to persistent focal edema, left heel

L89.622   **Pressure ulcer of left heel, stage 2**
Healing pressure ulcer of left heel, stage 2
Pressure ulcer with abrasion, blister, partial thickness skin loss involving epidermis and/or dermis, left heel

L89.623   **Pressure ulcer of left heel, stage 3**
Healing pressure ulcer of left heel, stage 3
Pressure ulcer with full thickness skin loss involving damage or necrosis of subcutaneous tissue, left heel

L89.624   **Pressure ulcer of left heel, stage 4**
Healing pressure ulcer of left heel, stage 4
Pressure ulcer with necrosis of soft tissues through to underlying muscle, tendon, or bone, left heel

L89.629   **Pressure ulcer of left heel, unspecified stage**
Healing pressure ulcer of left heel NOS
Healing pressure ulcer of left heel, unspecified stage

√5ᵗʰ **L89.8**   **Pressure ulcer of other site**

√6ᵗʰ **L89.81**   **Pressure ulcer of head**
Pressure ulcer of face

L89.810   **Pressure ulcer of head, unstageable**

L89.811   **Pressure ulcer of head, stage 1**
Healing pressure ulcer of head, stage 1
Pressure pre-ulcer skin changes limited to persistent focal edema, head

L89.812   **Pressure ulcer of head, stage 2**
Healing pressure ulcer of head, stage 2
Pressure ulcer with abrasion, blister, partial thickness skin loss involving epidermis and/or dermis, head

L89.813   **Pressure ulcer of head, stage 3**
Healing pressure ulcer of head, stage 3
Pressure ulcer with full thickness skin loss involving damage or necrosis of subcutaneous tissue, head

L89.814   **Pressure ulcer of head, stage 4**
Healing pressure ulcer of head, stage 4
Pressure ulcer with necrosis of soft tissues through to underlying muscle, tendon, or bone, head

L89.819   **Pressure ulcer of head, unspecified stage**
Healing pressure ulcer of head NOS
Healing pressure ulcer of head, unspecified stage

√6ᵗʰ **L89.89**   **Pressure ulcer of other site**

L89.890   **Pressure ulcer of other site, unstageable**

L89.891   **Pressure ulcer of other site, stage 1**
Healing pressure ulcer of other site, stage 1
Pressure pre-ulcer skin changes limited to persistent focal edema, other site

L89.892   **Pressure ulcer of other site, stage 2**
Healing pressure ulcer of other site, stage 2
Pressure ulcer with abrasion, blister, partial thickness skin loss involving epidermis and/or dermis, other site

L89.893   **Pressure ulcer of other site, stage 3**
Healing pressure ulcer of other site, stage 3
Pressure ulcer with full thickness skin loss involving damage or necrosis of subcutaneous tissue, other site

L89.894   **Pressure ulcer of other site, stage 4**
Healing pressure ulcer of other site, stage 4
Pressure ulcer with necrosis of soft tissues through to underlying muscle, tendon, or bone, other site

L89.899   **Pressure ulcer of other site, unspecified stage**
Healing pressure ulcer of other site NOS
Healing pressure ulcer of other site, unspecified stage

√5ᵗʰ **L89.9**   **Pressure ulcer of unspecified site**

L89.90   **Pressure ulcer of unspecified site, unspecified stage**
Healing pressure ulcer of unspecified site NOS
Healing pressure ulcer of unspecified site, unspecified stage

L89.91   **Pressure ulcer of unspecified site, stage 1**
Healing pressure ulcer of unspecified site, stage 1
Pressure pre-ulcer skin changes limited to persistent focal edema, unspecified site

L89.92   **Pressure ulcer of unspecified site, stage 2**
Healing pressure ulcer of unspecified site, stage 2
Pressure ulcer with abrasion, blister, partial thickness skin loss involving epidermis and/or dermis, unspecified site

L89.93   **Pressure ulcer of unspecified site, stage 3**
Healing pressure ulcer of unspecified site, stage 3
Pressure ulcer with full thickness skin loss involving damage or necrosis of subcutaneous tissue, unspecified site

L89.94   **Pressure ulcer of unspecified site, stage 4**
Healing pressure ulcer of unspecified site, stage 4
Pressure ulcer with necrosis of soft tissues through to underlying muscle, tendon, or bone, unspecified site

L89.95   **Pressure ulcer of unspecified site, unstageable**

√4ᵗʰ **L90**   **Atrophic disorders of skin**

L90.0   **Lichen sclerosus et atrophicus**
EXCLUDES 2   *lichen sclerosus of external female genital organs (N90.4)*
lichen sclerosus of external male genital organs (N48.0)

L90.1   **Anetoderma of Schweninger-Buzzi**

L90.2   **Anetoderma of Jadassohn-Pellizzari**

L90.3   **Atrophoderma of Pasini and Pierini**

L90.4   **Acrodermatitis chronica atrophicans**

L90.5   **Scar conditions and fibrosis of skin**
Adherent scar (skin)
Cicatrix
Disfigurement of skin due to scar
Fibrosis of skin NOS
Scar NOS
EXCLUDES 2   *hypertrophic scar (L91.0)*
keloid scar (L91.0)
AHA: 2015, 1Q, 19

L90.6   **Striae atrophicae**

L90.8   **Other atrophic disorders of skin**

L90.9   **Atrophic disorder of skin, unspecified**

√4ᵗʰ **L91**   **Hypertrophic disorders of skin**

L91.0   **Hypertrophic scar**
Keloid
Keloid scar
EXCLUDES 2   *acne keloid (L73.0)*
scar NOS (L90.5)

L91.8   **Other hypertrophic disorders of the skin**

L91.9   **Hypertrophic disorder of the skin, unspecified**

√4ᵗʰ **L92**   **Granulomatous disorders of skin and subcutaneous tissue**
EXCLUDES 2   *actinic granuloma (L57.5)*

L92.0   **Granuloma annulare**
Perforating granuloma annulare

L92.1   **Necrobiosis lipoidica, not elsewhere classified**
EXCLUDES 1   *necrobiosis lipoidica associated with diabetes mellitus (E08-E13 with .620)*

☑ Additional Character Required   √x7ᵗʰ Placeholder Alert   Unspecified Dx   Other Specified Dx   Manifestation   ▶◀ Revised Text   ● New Code   ▲ Revised Code Title

L92.2   Granuloma faciale [eosinophilic granuloma of skin]

L92.3   Foreign body granuloma of the skin and subcutaneous tissue
Use additional code to identify the type of retained foreign body (Z18.-)

L92.8   Other granulomatous disorders of the skin and subcutaneous tissue

L92.9   Granulomatous disorder of the skin and subcutaneous tissue, unspecified

✓4ᵗʰ L93   Lupus erythematosus
Use additional code for adverse effect, if applicable, to identify drug (T36-T50 with fifth or sixth character 5)

> EXCLUDES 1   lupus exedens (A18.4)
> lupus vulgaris (A18.4)
> scleroderma (M34.-)
> systemic lupus erythematosus (M32.-)

L93.0   Discoid lupus erythematosus
Lupus erythematosus NOS

L93.1   Subacute cutaneous lupus erythematosus

L93.2   Other local lupus erythematosus
Lupus erythematosus profundus
Lupus panniculitis

✓4ᵗʰ L94   Other localized connective tissue disorders
> EXCLUDES 1   systemic connective tissue disorders (M30-M36)

L94.0   Localized scleroderma [morphea]
Circumscribed scleroderma

L94.1   Linear scleroderma
En coup de sabre lesion

L94.2   Calcinosis cutis

L94.3   Sclerodactyly

L94.4   Gottron's papules

L94.5   Poikiloderma vasculare atrophicans

L94.6   Ainhum

L94.8   Other specified localized connective tissue disorders

L94.9   Localized connective tissue disorder, unspecified

✓4ᵗʰ L95   Vasculitis limited to skin, not elsewhere classified
> EXCLUDES 1   angioma serpiginosum (L81.7)
> Henoch(-Schönlein) purpura (D69.0)
> hypersensitivity angiitis (M31.0)
> lupus panniculitis (L93.2)
> panniculitis NOS (M79.3)
> panniculitis of neck and back (M54.0-)
> polyarteritis nodosa (M30.0)
> relapsing panniculitis (M35.6)
> rheumatoid vasculitis (M05.2)
> serum sickness (T80.6-)
> urticaria (L50.-)
> Wegener's granulomatosis (M31.3-)

L95.0   Livedoid vasculitis
Atrophie blanche (en plaque)

L95.1   Erythema elevatum diutinum

L95.8   Other vasculitis limited to the skin

L95.9   Vasculitis limited to the skin, unspecified

✓4ᵗʰ L97   Non-pressure chronic ulcer of lower limb, not elsewhere classified
> INCLUDES   chronic ulcer of skin of lower limb NOS
> non-healing ulcer of skin
> non-infected sinus of skin
> trophic ulcer NOS
> tropical ulcer NOS
> ulcer of skin of lower limb NOS

Code first any associated underlying condition, such as:
atherosclerosis of the lower extremities (I70.23-, I70.24-, I70.33-, I70.34-, I70.43-, I70.44-, I70.53-, I70.54-, I70.63-, I70.64-, I70.73-, I70.74-)
chronic venous hypertension (I87.31-, I87.33-)
diabetic ulcers (E08.621, E08.622, E09.621, E09.622, E10.621, E10.622, E11.621, E11.622, E13.621, E13.622)
postphlebitic syndrome (I87.01-, I87.03-)
postthrombotic syndrome (I87.01-, I87.03-)
varicose ulcer (I83.0-, I83.2-)
Code first any associated gangrene (I96)

> EXCLUDES 2   pressure ulcer (pressure area) (L89.-)
> skin infections (L00-L08)
> specific infections classified to A00-B99

✓5ᵗʰ L97.1   Non-pressure chronic ulcer of thigh

✓6ᵗʰ L97.10   Non-pressure chronic ulcer of unspecified thigh

L97.101   Non-pressure chronic ulcer of unspecified thigh limited to breakdown of skin

L97.102   Non-pressure chronic ulcer of unspecified thigh with fat layer exposed

L97.103   Non-pressure chronic ulcer of unspecified thigh with necrosis of muscle

L97.104   Non-pressure chronic ulcer of unspecified thigh with necrosis of bone

L97.109   Non-pressure chronic ulcer of unspecified thigh with unspecified severity

✓6ᵗʰ L97.11   Non-pressure chronic ulcer of right thigh

L97.111   Non-pressure chronic ulcer of right thigh limited to breakdown of skin

L97.112   Non-pressure chronic ulcer of right thigh with fat layer exposed

L97.113   Non-pressure chronic ulcer of right thigh with necrosis of muscle

L97.114   Non-pressure chronic ulcer of right thigh with necrosis of bone

L97.119   Non-pressure chronic ulcer of right thigh with unspecified severity

✓6ᵗʰ L97.12   Non-pressure chronic ulcer of left thigh

L97.121   Non-pressure chronic ulcer of left thigh limited to breakdown of skin

L97.122   Non-pressure chronic ulcer of left thigh with fat layer exposed

L97.123   Non-pressure chronic ulcer of left thigh with necrosis of muscle

L97.124   Non-pressure chronic ulcer of left thigh with necrosis of bone

L97.129   Non-pressure chronic ulcer of left thigh with unspecified severity

✓5ᵗʰ L97.2   Non-pressure chronic ulcer of calf

✓6ᵗʰ L97.20   Non-pressure chronic ulcer of unspecified calf

L97.201   Non-pressure chronic ulcer of unspecified calf limited to breakdown of skin

L97.202   Non-pressure chronic ulcer of unspecified calf with fat layer exposed

L97.203   Non-pressure chronic ulcer of unspecified calf with necrosis of muscle

L97.204   Non-pressure chronic ulcer of unspecified calf with necrosis of bone

L97.209   Non-pressure chronic ulcer of unspecified calf with unspecified severity

✓6ᵗʰ L97.21   Non-pressure chronic ulcer of right calf

L97.211   Non-pressure chronic ulcer of right calf limited to breakdown of skin

L97.212   Non-pressure chronic ulcer of right calf with fat layer exposed

L97.213   Non-pressure chronic ulcer of right calf with necrosis of muscle

L97.214   Non-pressure chronic ulcer of right calf with necrosis of bone

L97.219   Non-pressure chronic ulcer of right calf with unspecified severity

✓6ᵗʰ L97.22   Non-pressure chronic ulcer of left calf

L97.221   Non-pressure chronic ulcer of left calf limited to breakdown of skin

L97.222   Non-pressure chronic ulcer of left calf with fat layer exposed

L97.223   Non-pressure chronic ulcer of left calf with necrosis of muscle

L97.224   Non-pressure chronic ulcer of left calf with necrosis of bone

L97.229   Non-pressure chronic ulcer of left calf with unspecified severity

✓5ᵗʰ L97.3   Non-pressure chronic ulcer of ankle

✓6ᵗʰ L97.30   Non-pressure chronic ulcer of unspecified ankle

L97.301   Non-pressure chronic ulcer of unspecified ankle limited to breakdown of skin

L97.302   Non-pressure chronic ulcer of unspecified ankle with fat layer exposed

L97.303   Non-pressure chronic ulcer of unspecified ankle with necrosis of muscle

L97.304   Non-pressure chronic ulcer of unspecified ankle with necrosis of bone

L97.309   Non-pressure chronic ulcer of unspecified ankle with unspecified severity

---

EXCLUDES 1 Not coded here   EXCLUDES 2 Not included here   N Newborn Age: 0   P Pediatric Age: 0-17   M Maternity Age: 12-55   A Adult Age: 15-124

662

ICD-10-CM 2016

☑6ᵗʰ **L97.31** Non-pressure chronic ulcer of right ankle
  L97.311 Non-pressure chronic ulcer of right ankle limited to breakdown of skin
  L97.312 Non-pressure chronic ulcer of right ankle with fat layer exposed
  L97.313 Non-pressure chronic ulcer of right ankle with necrosis of muscle
  L97.314 Non-pressure chronic ulcer of right ankle with necrosis of bone
  L97.319 Non-pressure chronic ulcer of right ankle with unspecified severity

☑6ᵗʰ **L97.32** Non-pressure chronic ulcer of left ankle
  L97.321 Non-pressure chronic ulcer of left ankle limited to breakdown of skin
  L97.322 Non-pressure chronic ulcer of left ankle with fat layer exposed
  L97.323 Non-pressure chronic ulcer of left ankle with necrosis of muscle
  L97.324 Non-pressure chronic ulcer of left ankle with necrosis of bone
  L97.329 Non-pressure chronic ulcer of left ankle with unspecified severity

☑5ᵗʰ **L97.4** Non-pressure chronic ulcer of heel and midfoot
  Non-pressure chronic ulcer of plantar surface of midfoot

☑6ᵗʰ **L97.40** Non-pressure chronic ulcer of unspecified heel and midfoot
  L97.401 Non-pressure chronic ulcer of unspecified heel and midfoot limited to breakdown of skin
  L97.402 Non-pressure chronic ulcer of unspecified heel and midfoot with fat layer exposed
  L97.403 Non-pressure chronic ulcer of unspecified heel and midfoot with necrosis of muscle
  L97.404 Non-pressure chronic ulcer of unspecified heel and midfoot with necrosis of bone
  L97.409 Non-pressure chronic ulcer of unspecified heel and midfoot with unspecified severity

☑6ᵗʰ **L97.41** Non-pressure chronic ulcer of right heel and midfoot
  L97.411 Non-pressure chronic ulcer of right heel and midfoot limited to breakdown of skin
  L97.412 Non-pressure chronic ulcer of right heel and midfoot with fat layer exposed
  L97.413 Non-pressure chronic ulcer of right heel and midfoot with necrosis of muscle
  L97.414 Non-pressure chronic ulcer of right heel and midfoot with necrosis of bone
  L97.419 Non-pressure chronic ulcer of right heel and midfoot with unspecified severity

☑6ᵗʰ **L97.42** Non-pressure chronic ulcer of left heel and midfoot
  L97.421 Non-pressure chronic ulcer of left heel and midfoot limited to breakdown of skin
  L97.422 Non-pressure chronic ulcer of left heel and midfoot with fat layer exposed
  L97.423 Non-pressure chronic ulcer of left heel and midfoot with necrosis of muscle
  L97.424 Non-pressure chronic ulcer of left heel and midfoot with necrosis of bone
  L97.429 Non-pressure chronic ulcer of left heel and midfoot with unspecified severity

☑5ᵗʰ **L97.5** Non-pressure chronic ulcer of other part of foot
  Non-pressure chronic ulcer of toe

☑6ᵗʰ **L97.50** Non-pressure chronic ulcer of other part of unspecified foot
  L97.501 Non-pressure chronic ulcer of other part of unspecified foot limited to breakdown of skin
  L97.502 Non-pressure chronic ulcer of other part of unspecified foot with fat layer exposed
  L97.503 Non-pressure chronic ulcer of other part of unspecified foot with necrosis of muscle
  L97.504 Non-pressure chronic ulcer of other part of unspecified foot with necrosis of bone
  L97.509 Non-pressure chronic ulcer of other part of unspecified foot with unspecified severity

☑6ᵗʰ **L97.51** Non-pressure chronic ulcer of other part of right foot
  L97.511 Non-pressure chronic ulcer of other part of right foot limited to breakdown of skin
  L97.512 Non-pressure chronic ulcer of other part of right foot with fat layer exposed
  L97.513 Non-pressure chronic ulcer of other part of right foot with necrosis of muscle
  L97.514 Non-pressure chronic ulcer of other part of right foot with necrosis of bone
  L97.519 Non-pressure chronic ulcer of other part of right foot with unspecified severity

☑6ᵗʰ **L97.52** Non-pressure chronic ulcer of other part of left foot
  L97.521 Non-pressure chronic ulcer of other part of left foot limited to breakdown of skin
  L97.522 Non-pressure chronic ulcer of other part of left foot with fat layer exposed
  L97.523 Non-pressure chronic ulcer of other part of left foot with necrosis of muscle
  L97.524 Non-pressure chronic ulcer of other part of left foot with necrosis of bone
  L97.529 Non-pressure chronic ulcer of other part of left foot with unspecified severity

☑5ᵗʰ **L97.8** Non-pressure chronic ulcer of other part of lower leg

☑6ᵗʰ **L97.80** Non-pressure chronic ulcer of other part of unspecified lower leg
  L97.801 Non-pressure chronic ulcer of other part of unspecified lower leg limited to breakdown of skin
  L97.802 Non-pressure chronic ulcer of other part of unspecified lower leg with fat layer exposed
  L97.803 Non-pressure chronic ulcer of other part of unspecified lower leg with necrosis of muscle
  L97.804 Non-pressure chronic ulcer of other part of unspecified lower leg with necrosis of bone
  L97.809 Non-pressure chronic ulcer of other part of unspecified lower leg with unspecified severity

☑6ᵗʰ **L97.81** Non-pressure chronic ulcer of other part of right lower leg
  L97.811 Non-pressure chronic ulcer of other part of right lower leg limited to breakdown of skin
  L97.812 Non-pressure chronic ulcer of other part of right lower leg with fat layer exposed
  L97.813 Non-pressure chronic ulcer of other part of right lower leg with necrosis of muscle
  L97.814 Non-pressure chronic ulcer of other part of right lower leg with necrosis of bone
  L97.819 Non-pressure chronic ulcer of other part of right lower leg with unspecified severity

☑6ᵗʰ **L97.82** Non-pressure chronic ulcer of other part of left lower leg
  L97.821 Non-pressure chronic ulcer of other part of left lower leg limited to breakdown of skin
  L97.822 Non-pressure chronic ulcer of other part of left lower leg with fat layer exposed
  L97.823 Non-pressure chronic ulcer of other part of left lower leg with necrosis of muscle
  L97.824 Non-pressure chronic ulcer of other part of left lower leg with necrosis of bone
  L97.829 Non-pressure chronic ulcer of other part of left lower leg with unspecified severity

☑5ᵗʰ **L97.9** Non-pressure chronic ulcer of unspecified part of lower leg

☑6ᵗʰ **L97.90** Non-pressure chronic ulcer of unspecified part of unspecified lower leg
  L97.901 Non-pressure chronic ulcer of unspecified part of unspecified lower leg limited to breakdown of skin
  L97.902 Non-pressure chronic ulcer of unspecified part of unspecified lower leg with fat layer exposed
  L97.903 Non-pressure chronic ulcer of unspecified part of unspecified lower leg with necrosis of muscle
  L97.904 Non-pressure chronic ulcer of unspecified part of unspecified lower leg with necrosis of bone

---

☑ Additional Character Required   ✓7ᵗʰ Placeholder Alert   Unspecified Dx   Other Specified Dx   Manifestation   ▶◀ Revised Text   ● New Code   ▲ Revised Code Title

     L97.909   Non-pressure chronic ulcer of unspecified part of unspecified lower leg with unspecified severity

✓6ᵗʰ **L97.91**   Non-pressure chronic ulcer of unspecified part of right lower leg

     L97.911   Non-pressure chronic ulcer of unspecified part of right lower leg limited to breakdown of skin

     L97.912   Non-pressure chronic ulcer of unspecified part of right lower leg with fat layer exposed

     L97.913   Non-pressure chronic ulcer of unspecified part of right lower leg with necrosis of muscle

     L97.914   Non-pressure chronic ulcer of unspecified part of right lower leg with necrosis of bone

     L97.919   Non-pressure chronic ulcer of unspecified part of right lower leg with unspecified severity

✓6ᵗʰ **L97.92**   Non-pressure chronic ulcer of unspecified part of left lower leg

     L97.921   Non-pressure chronic ulcer of unspecified part of left lower leg limited to breakdown of skin

     L97.922   Non-pressure chronic ulcer of unspecified part of left lower leg with fat layer exposed

     L97.923   Non-pressure chronic ulcer of unspecified part of left lower leg with necrosis of muscle

     L97.924   Non-pressure chronic ulcer of unspecified part of left lower leg with necrosis of bone

     L97.929   Non-pressure chronic ulcer of unspecified part of left lower leg with unspecified severity

✓4ᵗʰ **L98**   **Other disorders of skin and subcutaneous tissue, not elsewhere classified**

L98.0   **Pyogenic granuloma**

     EXCLUDES 2   pyogenic granuloma of gingiva (K06.8)
     pyogenic granuloma of maxillary alveolar ridge (K04.5)
     pyogenic granuloma of oral mucosa (K13.4)

L98.1   **Factitial dermatitis**
     Neurotic excoriation

L98.2   **Febrile neutrophilic dermatosis [Sweet]**

L98.3   **Eosinophilic cellulitis [Wells]**

✓5ᵗʰ **L98.4**   **Non-pressure chronic ulcer of skin, not elsewhere classified**
     Chronic ulcer of skin NOS
     Tropical ulcer NOS
     Ulcer of skin NOS

     EXCLUDES 2   pressure ulcer (pressure area) (L89.-)
     gangrene (I96)
     skin infections (L00-L08)
     specific infections classified to A00-B99
     ulcer of lower limb NEC (L97.-)
     varicose ulcer (I83.0-I82.2)

✓6ᵗʰ **L98.41**   **Non-pressure chronic ulcer of buttock**

     L98.411   Non-pressure chronic ulcer of buttock limited to breakdown of skin

     L98.412   Non-pressure chronic ulcer of buttock with fat layer exposed

     L98.413   Non-pressure chronic ulcer of buttock with necrosis of muscle

     L98.414   Non-pressure chronic ulcer of buttock with necrosis of bone

     L98.419   Non-pressure chronic ulcer of buttock with unspecified severity

✓6ᵗʰ **L98.42**   **Non-pressure chronic ulcer of back**

     L98.421   Non-pressure chronic ulcer of back limited to breakdown of skin

     L98.422   Non-pressure chronic ulcer of back with fat layer exposed

     L98.423   Non-pressure chronic ulcer of back with necrosis of muscle

     L98.424   Non-pressure chronic ulcer of back with necrosis of bone

     L98.429   Non-pressure chronic ulcer of back with unspecified severity

✓6ᵗʰ **L98.49**   **Non-pressure chronic ulcer of skin of other sites**
     Non-pressure chronic ulcer of skin NOS

     L98.491   Non-pressure chronic ulcer of skin of other sites limited to breakdown of skin

     L98.492   Non-pressure chronic ulcer of skin of other sites with fat layer exposed

     L98.493   Non-pressure chronic ulcer of skin of other sites with necrosis of muscle

     L98.494   Non-pressure chronic ulcer of skin of other sites with necrosis of bone

     L98.499   Non-pressure chronic ulcer of skin of other sites with unspecified severity

L98.5   **Mucinosis of the skin**
     Focal mucinosis
     Lichen myxedematosus
     Reticular erythematous mucinosis

     EXCLUDES 1   focal oral mucinosis (K13.79)
     myxedema (E03.9)

L98.6   **Other infiltrative disorders of the skin and subcutaneous tissue**

     EXCLUDES 1   hyalinosis cutis et mucosae (E78.89)

L98.8   **Other specified disorders of the skin and subcutaneous tissue**
     AHA: 2013, 2Q, 32

L98.9   **Disorder of the skin and subcutaneous tissue, unspecified**

L99   ***Other disorders of skin and subcutaneous tissue in diseases classified elsewhere***

     Code first underlying disease, such as:
     amyloidosis (E85.-)

     EXCLUDES 1   skin disorders in diabetes (E08-E13 with .62)
     skin disorders in gonorrhea (A54.89)
     skin disorders in syphilis (A51.31, A52.79)

EXCLUDES 1 Not coded here   EXCLUDES 2 Not included here   N Newborn Age: 0   P Pediatric Age: 0-17   M Maternity Age: 12-55   A Adult Age: 15-124

664   ICD-10-CM 2016

Chapter 13. Diseases of the Musculoskeletal System and Connective Tissue (M00–M99)

Chapter Specific Guidelines with Coding Examples

The chapter specific guidelines from the ICD-10-CM Official Guidelines for Coding and Reporting have been provided below. Along with these guidelines are coding examples, contained in the shaded boxes, that have been developed to help illustrate the coding and/or sequencing guidance found in these guidelines.

a. Site and laterality

Most of the codes within Chapter 13 have site and laterality designations. The site represents the bone, joint or the muscle involved. For some conditions where more than one bone, joint or muscle is usually involved, such as osteoarthritis, there is a "multiple sites" code available. For categories where no multiple site code is provided and more than one bone, joint or muscle is involved, multiple codes should be used to indicate the different sites involved.

Right elbow infective bursitis

M71.121   Other infective bursitis, right elbow

Explanation: Most of the codes within chapter 13 have site and laterality designations. The site represents the bone, joint, or the muscle involved.

Rheumatoid arthritis of multiple sites without rheumatoid factor

M06.09   Rheumatoid arthritis without rheumatoid factor, multiple sites

Explanation: For some conditions where more than one bone, joint or muscle is usually involved, such as osteoarthritis, there is a "multiple sites" code available.

Osteomyelitis of the fourth thoracic and second lumbar vertebrae

M46.24   Osteomyelitis of vertebra, thoracic region

M46.26   Osteomyelitis of vertebra, lumbar region

Explanation: For categories without a multiple site code and more than one bone, joint, or muscle is involved, multiple codes should be used to indicate the different sites involved.

1) Bone versus joint

For certain conditions, the bone may be affected at the upper or lower end, (e.g., avascular necrosis of bone, M87, Osteoporosis, M80, M81). Though the portion of the bone affected may be at the joint, the site designation will be the bone, not the joint.

Idiopathic avascular necrosis of the femoral head of the left hip joint

M87.052   Idiopathic aseptic necrosis of left femur

Explanation: For certain conditions such as avascular necrosis, the bone may be affected at the joint, but the site designation is the bone, not the joint.

b. Acute traumatic versus chronic or recurrent musculoskeletal conditions

Many musculoskeletal conditions are a result of previous injury or trauma to a site, or are recurrent conditions. Bone, joint or muscle conditions that are the result of a healed injury are usually found in chapter 13. Recurrent bone, joint or muscle conditions are also usually found in chapter 13. Any current, acute injury should be coded to the appropriate injury code from chapter 19. Chronic or recurrent conditions should generally be coded with a code from chapter 13. If it is difficult to determine from the documentation in the record which code is best to describe a condition, query the provider.

Acute traumatic bucket handle tear of right medial meniscus

S83.211A   Bucket-handle tear of medial meniscus, current injury, right knee, initial encounter

Explanation: Any current, acute injury is not coded in chapter 13. It should instead be coded to the appropriate injury code from chapter 19.

Old bucket handle tear of right medial meniscus

M23.203   Derangement of unspecified medial meniscus due to old tear or injury, right knee

Explanation: Chronic or recurrent conditions should generally be coded with a code from chapter 13.

c. Coding of Pathologic Fractures

7th character A is for use as long as the patient is receiving active treatment for the fracture. Examples of active treatment are: surgical treatment, emergency department encounter, evaluation and

continuing treatment by the same or a different physician. While the patient may be seen by a new or different provider over the course of treatment for a pathological fracture, assignment of the 7th character is based on whether the patient is undergoing active treatment and not whether the provider is seeing the patient for the first time.

7th character, D is to be used for encounters after the patient has completed active treatment. The other 7th characters, listed under each subcategory in the Tabular List, are to be used for subsequent encounters for treatment of problems associated with the healing, such as malunions, nonunions, and sequelae.

Care for complications of surgical treatment for fracture repairs during the healing or recovery phase should be coded with the appropriate complication codes.

See Section I.C.19. Coding of traumatic fractures.

Pathologic fracture of left foot, unknown cause, currently under active treatment by a follow-up provider

M84.475A   Pathological fracture, left foot, initial encounter for fracture

Explanation: Seventh character A is for use as long as the patient is receiving active treatment for a pathologic fracture. Examples of active treatment are surgical treatment, emergency department encounter, evaluation, and continuing treatment by the same or a different physician.

The seventh character is based on whether the patient is undergoing active treatment and not whether the provider is seeing the patient for the first time.

d. Osteoporosis

Osteoporosis is a systemic condition, meaning that all bones of the musculoskeletal system are affected. Therefore, site is not a component of the codes under category M81, Osteoporosis without current pathological fracture. The site codes under category M80, Osteoporosis with current pathological fracture, identify the site of the fracture, not the osteoporosis.

1) Osteoporosis without pathological fracture

Category M81, Osteoporosis without current pathological fracture, is for use for patients with osteoporosis who do not currently have a pathologic fracture due to the osteoporosis, even if they have had a fracture in the past. For patients with a history of osteoporosis fractures, status code Z87.310, Personal history of (healed) osteoporosis fracture, should follow the code from M81.

Age-related osteoporosis with healed osteoporotic fracture of the lumbar vertebra

M81.0   Age-related osteoporosis without current pathological fracture

Z87.310   Personal history of (healed) osteoporosis fracture

Explanation: Category M81 is used for patients with osteoporosis who do not currently have a pathologic fracture due to the osteoporosis. To report a previous (healed) fracture, status code Z87.310 Personal history of (healed) osteoporosis fracture, should follow the code from M81.

2) Osteoporosis with current pathological fracture

Category M80, Osteoporosis with current pathological fracture, is for patients who have a current pathologic fracture at the time of an encounter. The codes under M80 identify the site of the fracture. A code from category M80, not a traumatic fracture code, should be used for any patient with known osteoporosis who suffers a fracture, even if the patient had a minor fall or trauma, if that fall or trauma would not usually break a normal, healthy bone.

Disuse osteoporosis with current fracture of right shoulder sustained lifting a grocery bag, initial encounter

M80.811A   Other osteoporosis with current pathological fracture, right shoulder, initial encounter for fracture

Explanation: A code from category M80, not a traumatic fracture code, should be used for any patient with known osteoporosis who suffers a fracture, even if the patient had a minor fall or trauma, if that fall or trauma would not usually break a normal, healthy bone.

Muscle/Tendon Table

ICD-10-CM categorizes certain muscles and tendons in the upper and lower extremities by their action (e.g., extension, flexion), their anatomical location (e.g., posterior, anterior), and/or whether they are intrinsic or extrinsic to a certain anatomical area. The Muscle/Tendon Table is provided at the beginning of chapters 13 and 19 as a resource to help users when code selection depends on one or more of these characteristics. The categories and/or subcategories that relate to this table are identified by the icon ✦. Please note that this table is not all-inclusive, and proper code assignment should be based on the provider's documentation.

Body Region	Muscle	Extensor Tendon	Flexor Tendon	Other Tendon
Shoulder				
	Deltoid	Posterior deltoid	Anterior deltoid	
	Rotator cuff			
	Infraspinatus			Infraspinatus
	Subscapularis			Subscapularis
	Supraspinatus			Supraspinatus
	Teres minor			Teres minor
	Teres major	Teres major		
Upper arm				
	Anterior muscles			
	Biceps brachii — long head		Biceps brachii — long head	
	Biceps brachii — short head		Biceps brachii — short head	
	Brachialis		Brachialis	
	Coracobrachialis		Coracobrachialis	
	Posterior muscles			
	Triceps brachii	Triceps brachii		
Forearm				
	Anterior muscles			
	Flexors			
	Deep			
	Flexor digitorum profundus		Flexor digitorum profundus	
	Flexor pollicis longus		Flexor pollicis longus	
	Intermediate			
	Flexor digitorum superficialis		Flexor digitorum superficialis	
	Superficial			
	Flexor carpi radialis		Flexor carpi radialis	
	Flexor carpi ulnaris		Flexor carpi ulnaris	
	Palmaris longus		Palmaris longus	
	Pronators			
	Pronator quadratus			Pronator quadratus
	Pronator teres			Pronator teres
	Posterior muscles			
	Extensors			
	Deep			
	Abductor pollicis longus			Abductor pollicis longus
	Extensor indicis	Extensor indicis		
	Extensor pollicis brevis	Extensor pollicis brevis		
	Extensor pollicis longus	Extensor pollicis longus		
	Superficial			
	Brachioradialis			Brachioradialis
	Extensor carpi radialis brevis	Extensor carpi radialis brevis		
	Extensor carpi radialis longus	Extensor carpi radialis longus		
	Extensor carpi ulnaris	Extensor carpi ulnaris		
	Extensor digiti minimi	Extensor digiti minimi		
	Extensor digitorum	Extensor digitorum		
	Anconeus	Anconeus		
	Supinator			Supinator

Body Region	Muscle	Extensor Tendon	Flexor Tendon	Other Tendon
Hand				
Extrinsic — attach to a site in the forearm as well as a site in the hand with action related to hand movement at the wrist				
	Extensor carpi radialis brevis	Extensor carpi radialis brevis		
	Extensor carpi radialis longus	Extensor carpie radialis longus		
	Extensor carpi ulnaris	Extensor carpi ulnaris		
	Flexor carpi radialis		Flexor carpi radialis	
	Flexor carpi ulnaris		Flexor carpi ulnaris	
	Flexor digitorum superficialis		Flexor digitorum superficialis	
	Palmaris longus		Palmaris longus	
Extrinsic — attach to a site in the forearm as well as a site in the hand with action in the hand related to finger movement				
	Adductor pollicis longus			Adductor pollicis longus
	Extensor digiti minimi	Extensor digiti minimi		
	Extensor digitorum	Extensor digitorum		
	Extensor indicis	Extensor indicis		
	Flexor digitorum profundus		Flexor digitorum profundus	
	Flexor digitorum superficialis		Flexor digitorum superficialis	
Extrinsic — attach to a site in the forearm as well as a site in the hand with action in the hand related to thumb movement				
	Extensor pollicis brevis	Extensor pollicis brevis		
	Extensor pollicis longus	Extensor pollicis longus		
	Flexor pollicis longus		Flexor pollicis longus	
Intrinsic — found within the hand only				
	Adductor pollicis			Adductor pollicis
	Dorsal interossei	Dorsal interossei	Dorsal interossei	
	Lumbricals	Lumbricals	Lumbricals	
	Palmaris brevis			Palmaris brevis
	Palmar interossei	Palmar interossei	Palmar interossei	
	Hypothenar muscles			
	Abductor digiti minimi			Abductor digiti minimi
	Flexor digiti minimi brevis		Flexor digiti minimi brevis	
	Oppenens digiti minimi		Oppenens digiti minimi	
	Thenar muscles			
	Abductor pollicis brevis			Abductor pollicis brevis
	Flexor pollicis brevis		Flexor pollicis brevis	
	Oppenens pollicis		Oppenens pollicis	
Thigh				
	Anterior muscles			
	Iliopsoas		Iliopsoas	
	Pectineus		Pectineus	
	Quadriceps	Quadriceps		
	Rectus femoris	Rectus femoris — Extends knee	Rectus femoris — Flexes hip	
	Vastus intermedius	Vastus intermedius		
	Vastus lateralis	Vastus lateralis		
	Vastus medialis	Vastus medialis		
	Sartorius		Sartorius	
	Medial muscles			
	Adductor brevis			Adductor brevis
	Adductor longus			Adductor longus
	Adductor magnus			Adductor magnus
	Gracilis			Gracilis
	Obturator externus			Obturator externus
	Posterior muscles			
	Hamstring	Hamstring — Extends hip	Hamstring — Flexes knee	
	Biceps femoris	Biceps femoris	Biceps femoris	
	Semimembranosus	Semimembranosus	Semimembranosus	
	Semitendinosus	Semitendinosus	Semitendinosus	

Body Region	Muscle	Extensor Tendon	Flexor Tendon	Other Tendon
Lower leg				
	Anterior muscles			
	Extensor digitorum longus	Extensor digitorum longus		
	Extensor hallucis longus	Extensor hallucis longus		
	Fibularis (peroneus) tertius	Fibularis (peroneus) tertius		
	Tibialis anterior	Tibialis anterior		Tibialis anterior
	Lateral muscles			
	Fibularis (peroneus) brevis		Fibularis (peroneus) brevis	
	Fibularis (peroneus) longus		Fibularis (peroneus) longus	
	Posterior muscles			
	Deep			
	Flexor digitorum longus		Flexor digitorum longus	
	Flexor hallucis longus		Flexor hallucis longus	
	Popliteus		Popliteus	
	Tibialis posterior		Tibialis posterior	
	Superficial			
	Gastrocnemius		Gastrocnemius	
	Plantaris		Plantaris	
	Soleus		Soleus	
				Calcaneal (Achilles)
Ankle/Foot				
Extrinsic — attach to a site in the lower leg as well as a site in the foot with action related to foot movement at the ankle				
	Plantaris		Plantaris	
	Soleus		Soleus	
	Tibialis anterior	Tibialis anterior		
	Tibialis posterior		Tibialis posterior	
Extrinsic — attach to a site in the lower leg as well as a site in the foot with action in the foot related to toe movement				
	Extensor digitorum longus	Extensor digitorum longus		
	Extensor hallicus longus	Extensor hallicus longus		
	Flexor digitorum longus		Flexor digitorum longus	
	Flexor hallucis longus		Flexor hallucis longus	
Intrinsic — found within the ankle/foot only				
	Dorsal muscles			
	Extensor digitorum brevis	Extensor digitorum brevis		
	Extensor hallucis brevis	Extensor hallucis brevis		
	Plantar muscles			
	Abductor digiti minimi		Abductor digiti minimi	
	Abductor hallucis		Abductor hallucis	
	Dorsal interossei	Dorsal interossei	Dorsal interossei	
	Flexor digiti minimi brevis		Flexor digiti minimi brevis	
	Flexor digitorum brevis		Flexor digitorum brevis	
	Flexor hallucis brevis		Flexor hallucis brevis	
	Lumbricals	Lumbricals	Lumbricals	
	Quadratus plantae		Quadratus plantae	
	Plantar interossei	Plantar interossei	Plantar interossei	

Chapter 13. Diseases of the Musculoskeletal System and Connective Tissue (M00-M99)

NOTE   Use an external cause code following the code for the musculoskeletal condition, if applicable, to identify the cause of the musculoskeletal condition.

EXCLUDES 2   *arthropathic psoriasis (L40.5-)*
certain conditions originating in the perinatal period (P04-P96)
certain infectious and parasitic diseases (A00-B99)
compartment syndrome (traumatic) (T79.A-)
complications of pregnancy, childbirth and the puerperium (O00-O9A)
congenital malformations, deformations, and chromosomal abnormalities (Q00-Q99)
endocrine, nutritional and metabolic diseases (E00-E88)
injury, poisoning and certain other consequences of external causes (S00-T88)
neoplasms (C00-D49)
symptoms, signs and abnormal clinical and laboratory findings, not elsewhere classified (R00-R94)

This chapter contains the following blocks:

M00-M02	Infectious arthropathies
M05-M14	Inflammatory polyarthropathies
M15-M19	Osteoarthritis
M20-M25	Other joint disorders
M26-M27	Dentofacial anomalies [including malocclusion] and other disorders of jaw
M30-M36	Systemic connective tissue disorders
M40-M43	Deforming dorsopathies
M45-M49	Spondylopathies
M50-M54	Other dorsopathies
M60-M63	Disorders of muscles
M65-M67	Disorders of synovium and tendon
M70-M79	Other soft tissue disorders
M80-M85	Disorders of bone density and structure
M86-M90	Other osteopathies
M91-M94	Chondropathies
M95	Other disorders of the musculoskeletal system and connective tissue
M96	Intraoperative and postprocedural complications and disorders of musculoskeletal system, not elsewhere classified
M99	Biomechanical lesions, not elsewhere classified

ARTHROPATHIES (M00-M25)

INCLUDES   disorders affecting predominantly peripheral (limb) joints

Infectious arthropathies (M00-M02)

NOTE   This block comprises arthropathies due to microbiological agents. Distinction is made between the following types of etiological relationship:

a) direct infection of joint, where organisms invade synovial tissue and microbial antigen is present in the joint;

b) indirect infection, which may be of two types: a reactive arthropathy, where microbial infection of the body is established but neither organisms nor antigens can be identified in the joint, and a postinfective arthropathy, where microbial antigen is present but recovery of an organism is inconstant and evidence of local multiplication is lacking.

✓4ᵗʰ M00 Pyogenic arthritis

   ✓5ᵗʰ M00.0 Staphylococcal arthritis and polyarthritis
     Use additional code (B95.61-B95.8) to identify bacterial agent
     EXCLUDES 2   *infection and inflammatory reaction due to internal joint prosthesis (T84.5-)*

     M00.00   Staphylococcal arthritis, unspecified joint
     ✓6ᵗʰ M00.01   Staphylococcal arthritis, shoulder
       M00.011   Staphylococcal arthritis, right shoulder
       M00.012   Staphylococcal arthritis, left shoulder
       M00.019   Staphylococcal arthritis, unspecified shoulder
     ✓6ᵗʰ M00.02   Staphylococcal arthritis, elbow
       M00.021   Staphylococcal arthritis, right elbow
       M00.022   Staphylococcal arthritis, left elbow
       M00.029   Staphylococcal arthritis, unspecified elbow
     ✓6ᵗʰ M00.03   Staphylococcal arthritis, wrist
       Staphylococcal arthritis of carpal bones
       M00.031   Staphylococcal arthritis, right wrist
       M00.032   Staphylococcal arthritis, left wrist
       M00.039   Staphylococcal arthritis, unspecified wrist

     ✓6ᵗʰ M00.04   Staphylococcal arthritis, hand
       Staphylococcal arthritis of metacarpus and phalanges
       M00.041   Staphylococcal arthritis, right hand
       M00.042   Staphylococcal arthritis, left hand
       M00.049   Staphylococcal arthritis, unspecified hand
     ✓6ᵗʰ M00.05   Staphylococcal arthritis, hip
       M00.051   Staphylococcal arthritis, right hip
       M00.052   Staphylococcal arthritis, left hip
       M00.059   Staphylococcal arthritis, unspecified hip
     ✓6ᵗʰ M00.06   Staphylococcal arthritis, knee
       M00.061   Staphylococcal arthritis, right knee
       M00.062   Staphylococcal arthritis, left knee
       M00.069   Staphylococcal arthritis, unspecified knee
     ✓6ᵗʰ M00.07   Staphylococcal arthritis, ankle and foot
       Staphylococcal arthritis, tarsus, metatarsus and phalanges
       M00.071   Staphylococcal arthritis, right ankle and foot
       M00.072   Staphylococcal arthritis, left ankle and foot
       M00.079   Staphylococcal arthritis, unspecified ankle and foot
     M00.08   Staphylococcal arthritis, vertebrae
     M00.09   Staphylococcal polyarthritis

   ✓5ᵗʰ M00.1 Pneumococcal arthritis and polyarthritis
     M00.10   Pneumococcal arthritis, unspecified joint
     ✓6ᵗʰ M00.11   Pneumococcal arthritis, shoulder
       M00.111   Pneumococcal arthritis, right shoulder
       M00.112   Pneumococcal arthritis, left shoulder
       M00.119   Pneumococcal arthritis, unspecified shoulder
     ✓6ᵗʰ M00.12   Pneumococcal arthritis, elbow
       M00.121   Pneumococcal arthritis, right elbow
       M00.122   Pneumococcal arthritis, left elbow
       M00.129   Pneumococcal arthritis, unspecified elbow
     ✓6ᵗʰ M00.13   Pneumococcal arthritis, wrist
       Pneumococcal arthritis of carpal bones
       M00.131   Pneumococcal arthritis, right wrist
       M00.132   Pneumococcal arthritis, left wrist
       M00.139   Pneumococcal arthritis, unspecified wrist
     ✓6ᵗʰ M00.14   Pneumococcal arthritis, hand
       Pneumococcal arthritis of metacarpus and phalanges
       M00.141   Pneumococcal arthritis, right hand
       M00.142   Pneumococcal arthritis, left hand
       M00.149   Pneumococcal arthritis, unspecified hand
     ✓6ᵗʰ M00.15   Pneumococcal arthritis, hip
       M00.151   Pneumococcal arthritis, right hip
       M00.152   Pneumococcal arthritis, left hip
       M00.159   Pneumococcal arthritis, unspecified hip
     ✓6ᵗʰ M00.16   Pneumococcal arthritis, knee
       M00.161   Pneumococcal arthritis, right knee
       M00.162   Pneumococcal arthritis, left knee
       M00.169   Pneumococcal arthritis, unspecified knee
     ✓6ᵗʰ M00.17   Pneumococcal arthritis, ankle and foot
       Pneumococcal arthritis, tarsus, metatarsus and phalanges
       M00.171   Pneumococcal arthritis, right ankle and foot
       M00.172   Pneumococcal arthritis, left ankle and foot
       M00.179   Pneumococcal arthritis, unspecified ankle and foot
     M00.18   Pneumococcal arthritis, vertebrae
     M00.19   Pneumococcal polyarthritis

   ✓5ᵗʰ M00.2 Other streptococcal arthritis and polyarthritis
     Use additional code (B95.0-B95.2, B95.4-B95.5) to identify bacterial agent
     M00.20   Other streptococcal arthritis, unspecified joint
     ✓6ᵗʰ M00.21   Other streptococcal arthritis, shoulder
       M00.211   Other streptococcal arthritis, right shoulder
       M00.212   Other streptococcal arthritis, left shoulder
       M00.219   Other streptococcal arthritis, unspecified shoulder

---

✔ Additional Character Required   ✔x7ᵗʰ Placeholder Alert   Unspecified Dx   Other Specified Dx   Manifestation   ▶◀ Revised Text   ● New Code   ▲ Revised Code Title

√6ᵗʰ **M00.22 Other streptococcal arthritis,** elbow
     M00.221 Other streptococcal arthritis, right **elbow**
     M00.222 Other streptococcal arthritis, left **elbow**
     M00.229 Other streptococcal arthritis, unspecified elbow

√6ᵗʰ **M00.23 Other streptococcal arthritis,** wrist
     Other streptococcal arthritis of carpal bones
     M00.231 Other streptococcal arthritis, right **wrist**
     M00.232 Other streptococcal arthritis, left **wrist**
     M00.239 Other streptococcal arthritis, unspecified wrist

√6ᵗʰ **M00.24 Other streptococcal arthritis,** hand
     Other streptococcal arthritis metacarpus and phalanges
     M00.241 Other streptococcal arthritis, right **hand**
     M00.242 Other streptococcal arthritis, left **hand**
     M00.249 Other streptococcal arthritis, unspecified hand

√6ᵗʰ **M00.25 Other streptococcal arthritis,** hip
     M00.251 Other streptococcal arthritis, right **hip**
     M00.252 Other streptococcal arthritis, left **hip**
     M00.259 Other streptococcal arthritis, unspecified hip

√6ᵗʰ **M00.26 Other streptococcal arthritis,** knee
     M00.261 Other streptococcal arthritis, right **knee**
     M00.262 Other streptococcal arthritis, left **knee**
     M00.269 Other streptococcal arthritis, unspecified knee

√6ᵗʰ **M00.27 Other streptococcal arthritis,** ankle and foot
     Other streptococcal arthritis, tarsus, metatarsus and phalanges
     M00.271 Other streptococcal arthritis, right **ankle and foot**
     M00.272 Other streptococcal arthritis, left **ankle and foot**
     M00.279 Other streptococcal arthritis, unspecified ankle and foot

     M00.28 Other streptococcal arthritis, vertebrae
     M00.29 Other streptococcal polyarthritis

√5ᵗʰ **M00.8 Arthritis and polyarthritis due to other bacteria**
     Use additional code (B96) to identify bacteria
     M00.80 Arthritis due to other bacteria, unspecified joint

√6ᵗʰ **M00.81 Arthritis due to other bacteria,** shoulder
     M00.811 Arthritis due to other bacteria, right **shoulder**
     M00.812 Arthritis due to other bacteria, left **shoulder**
     M00.819 Arthritis due to other bacteria, unspecified shoulder

√6ᵗʰ **M00.82 Arthritis due to other bacteria,** elbow
     M00.821 Arthritis due to other bacteria, right **elbow**
     M00.822 Arthritis due to other bacteria, left **elbow**
     M00.829 Arthritis due to other bacteria, unspecified elbow

√6ᵗʰ **M00.83 Arthritis due to other bacteria,** wrist
     Arthritis due to other bacteria, carpal bones
     M00.831 Arthritis due to other bacteria, right **wrist**
     M00.832 Arthritis due to other bacteria, left **wrist**
     M00.839 Arthritis due to other bacteria, unspecified wrist

√6ᵗʰ **M00.84 Arthritis due to other bacteria,** hand
     Arthritis due to other bacteria, metacarpus and phalanges
     M00.841 Arthritis due to other bacteria, right **hand**
     M00.842 Arthritis due to other bacteria, left **hand**
     M00.849 Arthritis due to other bacteria, unspecified hand

√6ᵗʰ **M00.85 Arthritis due to other bacteria,** hip
     M00.851 Arthritis due to other bacteria, right **hip**
     M00.852 Arthritis due to other bacteria, left **hip**
     M00.859 Arthritis due to other bacteria, unspecified hip

√6ᵗʰ **M00.86 Arthritis due to other bacteria,** knee
     M00.861 Arthritis due to other bacteria, right **knee**
     M00.862 Arthritis due to other bacteria, left **knee**

     M00.869 Arthritis due to other bacteria, unspecified knee

√6ᵗʰ **M00.87 Arthritis due to other bacteria,** ankle and foot
     Arthritis due to other bacteria, tarsus, metatarsus, and phalanges
     M00.871 Arthritis due to other bacteria, right **ankle and foot**
     M00.872 Arthritis due to other bacteria, left **ankle and foot**
     M00.879 Arthritis due to other bacteria, unspecified ankle and foot

     M00.88 Arthritis due to other bacteria, vertebrae
     M00.89 Polyarthritis due to other bacteria

M00.9 Pyogenic arthritis, unspecified
     Infective arthritis NOS

√4ᵗʰ **M01 Direct infections of joint in infectious and parasitic diseases classified elsewhere**
     Code first underlying disease, such as:
     leprosy [Hansen's disease] (A30.-)
     mycoses (B35-B49)
     O'nyong-nyong fever (A92.1)
     paratyphoid fever (A01.1-A01.4)
     EXCLUDES 1   *arthropathy in Lyme disease (A69.23)*
         gonococcal arthritis (A54.42)
         meningococcal arthritis (A39.83)
         mumps arthritis (B26.85)
         postinfective arthropathy (M02.-)
         postmeningococcal arthritis (A39.84)
         reactive arthritis (M02.3)
         rubella arthritis (B06.82)
         sarcoidosis arthritis (D86.86)
         typhoid fever arthritis (A01.04)
         tuberculosis arthritis (A18.01-A18.02)

√5ᵗʰ **M01.X Direct infection of joint in infectious and parasitic diseases classified elsewhere**
     M01.X0 Direct infection of** unspecified joint **in infectious and parasitic diseases classified elsewhere

√6ᵗʰ **M01.X1 Direct infection of** shoulder **joint in infectious and parasitic diseases classified elsewhere**
     M01.X11 Direct infection of** right shoulder **in infectious and parasitic diseases classified elsewhere
     M01.X12 Direct infection of** left shoulder **in infectious and parasitic diseases classified elsewhere
     M01.X19 Direct infection of** unspecified shoulder **in infectious and parasitic diseases classified elsewhere

√6ᵗʰ **M01.X2 Direct infection of** elbow **in infectious and parasitic diseases classified elsewhere**
     M01.X21 Direct infection of** right elbow **in infectious and parasitic diseases classified elsewhere
     M01.X22 Direct infection of** left elbow **in infectious and parasitic diseases classified elsewhere
     M01.X29 Direct infection of** unspecified elbow **in infectious and parasitic diseases classified elsewhere

√6ᵗʰ **M01.X3 Direct infection of** wrist **in infectious and parasitic diseases classified elsewhere**
     Direct infection of carpal bones in infectious and parasitic diseases classified elsewhere
     M01.X31 Direct infection of** right wrist **in infectious and parasitic diseases classified elsewhere
     M01.X32 Direct infection of** left wrist **in infectious and parasitic diseases classified elsewhere
     M01.X39 Direct infection of** unspecified wrist **in infectious and parasitic diseases classified elsewhere

√6ᵗʰ **M01.X4 Direct infection of** hand **in infectious and parasitic diseases classified elsewhere**
     Direct infection of metacarpus and phalanges in infectious and parasitic diseases classified elsewhere
     M01.X41 Direct infection of** right hand **in infectious and parasitic diseases classified elsewhere
     M01.X42 Direct infection of** left hand **in infectious and parasitic diseases classified elsewhere
     M01.X49 Direct infection of** unspecified hand **in infectious and parasitic diseases classified elsewhere

---

EXCLUDES 1 Not coded here   EXCLUDES 2 Not included here   N Newborn Age: 0   P Pediatric Age: 0-17   M Maternity Age: 12-55   A Adult Age: 15-124

670   ICD-10-CM 2016

☑6ᵗʰ **M01.X5** **Direct infection of hip in infectious and parasitic diseases classified elsewhere**

M01.X51   *Direct infection of right hip in infectious and parasitic diseases classified elsewhere*

M01.X52   *Direct infection of left hip in infectious and parasitic diseases classified elsewhere*

M01.X59   *Direct infection of unspecified hip in infectious and parasitic diseases classified elsewhere*

☑6ᵗʰ **M01.X6** **Direct infection of knee in infectious and parasitic diseases classified elsewhere**

M01.X61   *Direct infection of right knee in infectious and parasitic diseases classified elsewhere*

M01.X62   *Direct infection of left knee in infectious and parasitic diseases classified elsewhere*

M01.X69   *Direct infection of unspecified knee in infectious and parasitic diseases classified elsewhere*

☑6ᵗʰ **M01.X7** **Direct infection of ankle and foot in infectious and parasitic diseases classified elsewhere**

Direct infection of tarsus, metatarsus and phalanges in infectious and parasitic diseases classified elsewhere

M01.X71   *Direct infection of right ankle and foot in infectious and parasitic diseases classified elsewhere*

M01.X72   *Direct infection of left ankle and foot in infectious and parasitic diseases classified elsewhere*

M01.X79   *Direct infection of unspecified ankle and foot in infectious and parasitic diseases classified elsewhere*

M01.X8   *Direct infection of vertebrae in infectious and parasitic diseases classified elsewhere*

M01.X9   *Direct infection of multiple joints in infectious and parasitic diseases classified elsewhere*

☑4ᵗʰ **M02** **Postinfective and reactive arthropathies**

Code first underlying disease, such as:
    congenital syphilis [Clutton's joints] (A50.5)
    enteritis due to Yersinia enterocolitica (A04.6)
    infective endocarditis (I33.0)
    viral hepatitis (B15-B19)

EXCLUDES 1   *Behçet's disease (M35.2)*
    direct infections of joint in infectious and parasitic diseases classified elsewhere (M01.-)
    postmeningococcal arthritis (A39.84)
    mumps arthritis (B26.85)
    rheumatic fever (I00)
    rubella arthritis (B06.82)
    syphilis arthritis (late) (A52.77)
    tabetic arthropathy [Charcôt's] (A52.16)

☑5ᵗʰ **M02.0** **Arthropathy following intestinal bypass**

M02.00 **Arthropathy following intestinal bypass, unspecified site**

☑6ᵗʰ **M02.01** **Arthropathy following intestinal bypass, shoulder**

M02.011 **Arthropathy following intestinal bypass, right shoulder**

M02.012 **Arthropathy following intestinal bypass, left shoulder**

M02.019 **Arthropathy following intestinal bypass, unspecified shoulder**

☑6ᵗʰ **M02.02** **Arthropathy following intestinal bypass, elbow**

M02.021 **Arthropathy following intestinal bypass, right elbow**

M02.022 **Arthropathy following intestinal bypass, left elbow**

M02.029 **Arthropathy following intestinal bypass, unspecified elbow**

☑6ᵗʰ **M02.03** **Arthropathy following intestinal bypass, wrist**

Arthropathy following intestinal bypass, carpal bones

M02.031 **Arthropathy following intestinal bypass, right wrist**

M02.032 **Arthropathy following intestinal bypass, left wrist**

M02.039 **Arthropathy following intestinal bypass, unspecified wrist**

☑6ᵗʰ **M02.04** **Arthropathy following intestinal bypass, hand**

Arthropathy following intestinal bypass, metacarpals and phalanges

M02.041 **Arthropathy following intestinal bypass, right hand**

M02.042 **Arthropathy following intestinal bypass, left hand**

M02.049 **Arthropathy following intestinal bypass, unspecified hand**

☑6ᵗʰ **M02.05** **Arthropathy following intestinal bypass, hip**

M02.051 **Arthropathy following intestinal bypass, right hip**

M02.052 **Arthropathy following intestinal bypass, left hip**

M02.059 **Arthropathy following intestinal bypass, unspecified hip**

☑6ᵗʰ **M02.06** **Arthropathy following intestinal bypass, knee**

M02.061 **Arthropathy following intestinal bypass, right knee**

M02.062 **Arthropathy following intestinal bypass, left knee**

M02.069 **Arthropathy following intestinal bypass, unspecified knee**

☑6ᵗʰ **M02.07** **Arthropathy following intestinal bypass, ankle and foot**

Arthropathy following intestinal bypass, tarsus, metatarsus and phalanges

M02.071 **Arthropathy following intestinal bypass, right ankle and foot**

M02.072 **Arthropathy following intestinal bypass, left ankle and foot**

M02.079 **Arthropathy following intestinal bypass, unspecified ankle and foot**

M02.08 **Arthropathy following intestinal bypass, vertebrae**

M02.09 **Arthropathy following intestinal bypass, multiple sites**

☑5ᵗʰ **M02.1** **Postdysenteric arthropathy**

M02.10 **Postdysenteric arthropathy, unspecified site**

☑6ᵗʰ **M02.11** **Postdysenteric arthropathy, shoulder**

M02.111 **Postdysenteric arthropathy, right shoulder**

M02.112 **Postdysenteric arthropathy, left shoulder**

M02.119 **Postdysenteric arthropathy, unspecified shoulder**

☑6ᵗʰ **M02.12** **Postdysenteric arthropathy, elbow**

M02.121 **Postdysenteric arthropathy, right elbow**

M02.122 **Postdysenteric arthropathy, left elbow**

M02.129 **Postdysenteric arthropathy, unspecified elbow**

☑6ᵗʰ **M02.13** **Postdysenteric arthropathy, wrist**

Postdysenteric arthropathy, carpal bones

M02.131 **Postdysenteric arthropathy, right wrist**

M02.132 **Postdysenteric arthropathy, left wrist**

M02.139 **Postdysenteric arthropathy, unspecified wrist**

☑6ᵗʰ **M02.14** **Postdysenteric arthropathy, hand**

Postdysenteric arthropathy, metacarpus and phalanges

M02.141 **Postdysenteric arthropathy, right hand**

M02.142 **Postdysenteric arthropathy, left hand**

M02.149 **Postdysenteric arthropathy, unspecified hand**

☑6ᵗʰ **M02.15** **Postdysenteric arthropathy, hip**

M02.151 **Postdysenteric arthropathy, right hip**

M02.152 **Postdysenteric arthropathy, left hip**

M02.159 **Postdysenteric arthropathy, unspecified hip**

☑6ᵗʰ **M02.16** **Postdysenteric arthropathy, knee**

M02.161 **Postdysenteric arthropathy, right knee**

M02.162 **Postdysenteric arthropathy, left knee**

M02.169 **Postdysenteric arthropathy, unspecified knee**

☑ Additional Character Required   ☑×7ᵗʰ Placeholder Alert   Unspecified Dx   Other Specified Dx   Manifestation   ►◄ Revised Text   ● New Code   ▲ Revised Code Title

✓6ᵗʰ **M02.17 Postdysenteric arthropathy,** ankle and foot
    Postdysenteric arthropathy, tarsus, metatarsus and phalanges
    M02.171 Postdysenteric arthropathy, right **ankle and foot**
    M02.172 Postdysenteric arthropathy, left **ankle and foot**
    M02.179 Postdysenteric arthropathy, unspecified ankle and foot

    M02.18 Postdysenteric arthropathy, vertebrae
    M02.19 Postdysenteric arthropathy, multiple sites

✓5ᵗʰ **M02.2 Postimmunization arthropathy**
    M02.20 Postimmunization arthropathy, unspecified site
✓6ᵗʰ **M02.21 Postimmunization arthropathy,** shoulder
    M02.211 Postimmunization arthropathy, right **shoulder**
    M02.212 Postimmunization arthropathy, left **shoulder**
    M02.219 Postimmunization arthropathy, unspecified shoulder

✓6ᵗʰ **M02.22 Postimmunization arthropathy,** elbow
    M02.221 Postimmunization arthropathy, right **elbow**
    M02.222 Postimmunization arthropathy, left **elbow**
    M02.229 Postimmunization arthropathy, unspecified elbow

✓6ᵗʰ **M02.23 Postimmunization arthropathy,** wrist
    Postimmunization arthropathy, carpal bones
    M02.231 Postimmunization arthropathy, right **wrist**
    M02.232 Postimmunization arthropathy, left **wrist**
    M02.239 Postimmunization arthropathy, unspecified wrist

✓6ᵗʰ **M02.24 Postimmunization arthropathy,** hand
    Postimmunization arthropathy, metacarpus and phalanges
    M02.241 Postimmunization arthropathy, right **hand**
    M02.242 Postimmunization arthropathy, left **hand**
    M02.249 Postimmunization arthropathy, unspecified hand

✓6ᵗʰ **M02.25 Postimmunization arthropathy,** hip
    M02.251 Postimmunization arthropathy, right **hip**
    M02.252 Postimmunization arthropathy, left **hip**
    M02.259 Postimmunization arthropathy, unspecified hip

✓6ᵗʰ **M02.26 Postimmunization arthropathy,** knee
    M02.261 Postimmunization arthropathy, right **knee**
    M02.262 Postimmunization arthropathy, left **knee**
    M02.269 Postimmunization arthropathy, unspecified knee

✓6ᵗʰ **M02.27 Postimmunization arthropathy,** ankle and foot
    Postimmunization arthropathy, tarsus, metatarsus and phalanges
    M02.271 Postimmunization arthropathy, right **ankle and foot**
    M02.272 Postimmunization arthropathy, left **ankle and foot**
    M02.279 Postimmunization arthropathy, unspecified ankle and foot

    M02.28 Postimmunization arthropathy, vertebrae
    M02.29 Postimmunization arthropathy, multiple sites

✓5ᵗʰ **M02.3 Reiter's disease**
    Reactive arthritis
    M02.30 Reiter's disease, unspecified site
✓6ᵗʰ **M02.31 Reiter's disease,** shoulder
    M02.311 Reiter's disease, right **shoulder**
    M02.312 Reiter's disease, left **shoulder**
    M02.319 Reiter's disease, unspecified shoulder

✓6ᵗʰ **M02.32 Reiter's disease,** elbow
    M02.321 Reiter's disease, right **elbow**
    M02.322 Reiter's disease, left **elbow**
    M02.329 Reiter's disease, unspecified elbow

✓6ᵗʰ **M02.33 Reiter's disease,** wrist
    Reiter's disease, carpal bones
    M02.331 Reiter's disease, right **wrist**
    M02.332 Reiter's disease, left **wrist**
    M02.339 Reiter's disease, unspecified wrist

✓6ᵗʰ **M02.34 Reiter's disease,** hand
    Reiter's disease, metacarpus and phalanges
    M02.341 Reiter's disease, right **hand**
    M02.342 Reiter's disease, left **hand**
    M02.349 Reiter's disease, unspecified hand

✓6ᵗʰ **M02.35 Reiter's disease,** hip
    M02.351 Reiter's disease, right **hip**
    M02.352 Reiter's disease, left **hip**
    M02.359 Reiter's disease, unspecified hip

✓6ᵗʰ **M02.36 Reiter's disease,** knee
    M02.361 Reiter's disease, right **knee**
    M02.362 Reiter's disease, left **knee**
    M02.369 Reiter's disease, unspecified knee

✓6ᵗʰ **M02.37 Reiter's disease,** ankle and foot
    Reiter's disease, tarsus, metatarsus and phalanges
    M02.371 Reiter's disease, right **ankle and foot**
    M02.372 Reiter's disease, left **ankle and foot**
    M02.379 Reiter's disease, unspecified ankle and foot

    M02.38 Reiter's disease, vertebrae
    M02.39 Reiter's disease, multiple sites

✓5ᵗʰ **M02.8 Other reactive arthropathies**
    M02.80 Other reactive arthropathies, unspecified site
✓6ᵗʰ **M02.81 Other reactive arthropathies,** shoulder
    M02.811 Other reactive arthropathies, right **shoulder**
    M02.812 Other reactive arthropathies, left **shoulder**
    M02.819 Other reactive arthropathies, unspecified shoulder

✓6ᵗʰ **M02.82 Other reactive arthropathies,** elbow
    M02.821 Other reactive arthropathies, right **elbow**
    M02.822 Other reactive arthropathies, left **elbow**
    M02.829 Other reactive arthropathies, unspecified elbow

✓6ᵗʰ **M02.83 Other reactive arthropathies,** wrist
    Other reactive arthropathies, carpal bones
    M02.831 Other reactive arthropathies, right **wrist**
    M02.832 Other reactive arthropathies, left **wrist**
    M02.839 Other reactive arthropathies, unspecified wrist

✓6ᵗʰ **M02.84 Other reactive arthropathies,** hand
    Other reactive arthropathies, metacarpus and phalanges
    M02.841 Other reactive arthropathies, right **hand**
    M02.842 Other reactive arthropathies, left **hand**
    M02.849 Other reactive arthropathies, unspecified hand

✓6ᵗʰ **M02.85 Other reactive arthropathies,** hip
    M02.851 Other reactive arthropathies, right **hip**
    M02.852 Other reactive arthropathies, left **hip**
    M02.859 Other reactive arthropathies, unspecified hip

✓6ᵗʰ **M02.86 Other reactive arthropathies,** knee
    M02.861 Other reactive arthropathies, right **knee**
    M02.862 Other reactive arthropathies, left **knee**
    M02.869 Other reactive arthropathies, unspecified knee

✓6ᵗʰ **M02.87 Other reactive arthropathies,** ankle and foot
    Other reactive arthropathies, tarsus, metatarsus and phalanges
    M02.871 Other reactive arthropathies, right **ankle and foot**
    M02.872 Other reactive arthropathies, left **ankle and foot**
    M02.879 Other reactive arthropathies, unspecified ankle and foot

    M02.88 Other reactive arthropathies, vertebrae
    M02.89 Other reactive arthropathies, multiple sites
    M02.9 Reactive arthropathy, unspecified

EXCLUDES 1 Not coded here   **EXCLUDES 2** Not included here   **N** Newborn Age: 0   **P** Pediatric Age: 0-17   **M** Maternity Age: 12-55   **A** Adult Age: 15-124

672   ICD-10-CM 2016

Inflammatory polyarthropathies (M05-M14)

✓4ᵗʰ **M05 Rheumatoid arthritis with rheumatoid factor**

     EXCLUDES 1   rheumatic fever (I00)
                     juvenile rheumatoid arthritis (M08.-)
                     rheumatoid arthritis of spine (M45.-)

✓5ᵗʰ **M05.0 Felty's syndrome**
           Rheumatoid arthritis with splenoadenomegaly and leukopenia

     M05.00 Felty's syndrome, unspecified site

   ✓6ᵗʰ **M05.01 Felty's syndrome, shoulder**
       M05.011 Felty's syndrome, right shoulder
       M05.012 Felty's syndrome, left shoulder
       M05.019 Felty's syndrome, unspecified shoulder

   ✓6ᵗʰ **M05.02 Felty's syndrome, elbow**
       M05.021 Felty's syndrome, right elbow
       M05.022 Felty's syndrome, left elbow
       M05.029 Felty's syndrome, unspecified elbow

   ✓6ᵗʰ **M05.03 Felty's syndrome, wrist**
          Felty's syndrome, carpal bones
       M05.031 Felty's syndrome, right wrist
       M05.032 Felty's syndrome, left wrist
       M05.039 Felty's syndrome, unspecified wrist

   ✓6ᵗʰ **M05.04 Felty's syndrome, hand**
          Felty's syndrome, metacarpus and phalanges
       M05.041 Felty's syndrome, right hand
       M05.042 Felty's syndrome, left hand
       M05.049 Felty's syndrome, unspecified hand

   ✓6ᵗʰ **M05.05 Felty's syndrome, hip**
       M05.051 Felty's syndrome, right hip
       M05.052 Felty's syndrome, left hip
       M05.059 Felty's syndrome, unspecified hip

   ✓6ᵗʰ **M05.06 Felty's syndrome, knee**
       M05.061 Felty's syndrome, right knee
       M05.062 Felty's syndrome, left knee
       M05.069 Felty's syndrome, unspecified knee

   ✓6ᵗʰ **M05.07 Felty's syndrome, ankle and foot**
          Felty's syndrome, tarsus, metatarsus and phalanges
       M05.071 Felty's syndrome, right ankle and foot
       M05.072 Felty's syndrome, left ankle and foot
       M05.079 Felty's syndrome, unspecified ankle and foot

     M05.09 Felty's syndrome, multiple sites

✓5ᵗʰ **M05.1 Rheumatoid lung disease with rheumatoid arthritis**

     M05.10 Rheumatoid lung disease with rheumatoid arthritis of unspecified site

   ✓6ᵗʰ **M05.11 Rheumatoid lung disease with rheumatoid arthritis of shoulder**
       M05.111 Rheumatoid lung disease with rheumatoid arthritis of right shoulder
       M05.112 Rheumatoid lung disease with rheumatoid arthritis of left shoulder
       M05.119 Rheumatoid lung disease with rheumatoid arthritis of unspecified shoulder

   ✓6ᵗʰ **M05.12 Rheumatoid lung disease with rheumatoid arthritis of elbow**
       M05.121 Rheumatoid lung disease with rheumatoid arthritis of right elbow
       M05.122 Rheumatoid lung disease with rheumatoid arthritis of left elbow
       M05.129 Rheumatoid lung disease with rheumatoid arthritis of unspecified elbow

   ✓6ᵗʰ **M05.13 Rheumatoid lung disease with rheumatoid arthritis of wrist**
          Rheumatoid lung disease with rheumatoid arthritis, carpal bones
       M05.131 Rheumatoid lung disease with rheumatoid arthritis of right wrist
       M05.132 Rheumatoid lung disease with rheumatoid arthritis of left wrist
       M05.139 Rheumatoid lung disease with rheumatoid arthritis of unspecified wrist

   ✓6ᵗʰ **M05.14 Rheumatoid lung disease with rheumatoid arthritis of hand**
          Rheumatoid lung disease with rheumatoid arthritis, metacarpus and phalanges
       M05.141 Rheumatoid lung disease with rheumatoid arthritis of right hand
       M05.142 Rheumatoid lung disease with rheumatoid arthritis of left hand
       M05.149 Rheumatoid lung disease with rheumatoid arthritis of unspecified hand

   ✓6ᵗʰ **M05.15 Rheumatoid lung disease with rheumatoid arthritis of hip**
       M05.151 Rheumatoid lung disease with rheumatoid arthritis of right hip
       M05.152 Rheumatoid lung disease with rheumatoid arthritis of left hip
       M05.159 Rheumatoid lung disease with rheumatoid arthritis of unspecified hip

   ✓6ᵗʰ **M05.16 Rheumatoid lung disease with rheumatoid arthritis of knee**
       M05.161 Rheumatoid lung disease with rheumatoid arthritis of right knee
       M05.162 Rheumatoid lung disease with rheumatoid arthritis of left knee
       M05.169 Rheumatoid lung disease with rheumatoid arthritis of unspecified knee

   ✓6ᵗʰ **M05.17 Rheumatoid lung disease with rheumatoid arthritis of ankle and foot**
          Rheumatoid lung disease with rheumatoid arthritis, tarsus, metatarsus and phalanges
       M05.171 Rheumatoid lung disease with rheumatoid arthritis of right ankle and foot
       M05.172 Rheumatoid lung disease with rheumatoid arthritis of left ankle and foot
       M05.179 Rheumatoid lung disease with rheumatoid arthritis of unspecified ankle and foot

     M05.19 Rheumatoid lung disease with rheumatoid arthritis of multiple sites

✓5ᵗʰ **M05.2 Rheumatoid vasculitis with rheumatoid arthritis**

     M05.20 Rheumatoid vasculitis with rheumatoid arthritis of unspecified site

   ✓6ᵗʰ **M05.21 Rheumatoid vasculitis with rheumatoid arthritis of shoulder**
       M05.211 Rheumatoid vasculitis with rheumatoid arthritis of right shoulder
       M05.212 Rheumatoid vasculitis with rheumatoid arthritis of left shoulder
       M05.219 Rheumatoid vasculitis with rheumatoid arthritis of unspecified shoulder

   ✓6ᵗʰ **M05.22 Rheumatoid vasculitis with rheumatoid arthritis of elbow**
       M05.221 Rheumatoid vasculitis with rheumatoid arthritis of right elbow
       M05.222 Rheumatoid vasculitis with rheumatoid arthritis of left elbow
       M05.229 Rheumatoid vasculitis with rheumatoid arthritis of unspecified elbow

   ✓6ᵗʰ **M05.23 Rheumatoid vasculitis with rheumatoid arthritis of wrist**
          Rheumatoid vasculitis with rheumatoid arthritis, carpal bones
       M05.231 Rheumatoid vasculitis with rheumatoid arthritis of right wrist
       M05.232 Rheumatoid vasculitis with rheumatoid arthritis of left wrist
       M05.239 Rheumatoid vasculitis with rheumatoid arthritis of unspecified wrist

   ✓6ᵗʰ **M05.24 Rheumatoid vasculitis with rheumatoid arthritis of hand**
          Rheumatoid vasculitis with rheumatoid arthritis, metacarpus and phalanges
       M05.241 Rheumatoid vasculitis with rheumatoid arthritis of right hand
       M05.242 Rheumatoid vasculitis with rheumatoid arthritis of left hand
       M05.249 Rheumatoid vasculitis with rheumatoid arthritis of unspecified hand

---

✓ Additional Character Required   ✓ₓ7ᵗʰ Placeholder Alert   Unspecified Dx   Other Specified Dx   Manifestation   ►◄ Revised Text   ● New Code   ▲ Revised Code Title

✓6ᵗʰ **M05.25** **Rheumatoid vasculitis with rheumatoid arthritis of hip**
    M05.251 **Rheumatoid vasculitis with rheumatoid arthritis of right hip**
    M05.252 **Rheumatoid vasculitis with rheumatoid arthritis of left hip**
    M05.259 **Rheumatoid vasculitis with rheumatoid arthritis of unspecified hip**

✓6ᵗʰ **M05.26** **Rheumatoid vasculitis with rheumatoid arthritis of knee**
    M05.261 **Rheumatoid vasculitis with rheumatoid arthritis of right knee**
    M05.262 **Rheumatoid vasculitis with rheumatoid arthritis of left knee**
    M05.269 **Rheumatoid vasculitis with rheumatoid arthritis of unspecified knee**

✓6ᵗʰ **M05.27** **Rheumatoid vasculitis with rheumatoid arthritis of ankle and foot**
    Rheumatoid vasculitis with rheumatoid arthritis, tarsus, metatarsus and phalanges
    M05.271 **Rheumatoid vasculitis with rheumatoid arthritis of right ankle and foot**
    M05.272 **Rheumatoid vasculitis with rheumatoid arthritis of left ankle and foot**
    M05.279 **Rheumatoid vasculitis with rheumatoid arthritis of unspecified ankle and foot**

M05.29 **Rheumatoid vasculitis with rheumatoid arthritis of multiple sites**

✓5ᵗʰ **M05.3** **Rheumatoid heart disease with rheumatoid arthritis**
    Rheumatoid carditis   Rheumatoid myocarditis
    Rheumatoid endocarditis   Rheumatoid pericarditis
    M05.30 **Rheumatoid heart disease with rheumatoid arthritis of unspecified site**

✓6ᵗʰ **M05.31** **Rheumatoid heart disease with rheumatoid arthritis of shoulder**
    M05.311 **Rheumatoid heart disease with rheumatoid arthritis of right shoulder**
    M05.312 **Rheumatoid heart disease with rheumatoid arthritis of left shoulder**
    M05.319 **Rheumatoid heart disease with rheumatoid arthritis of unspecified shoulder**

✓6ᵗʰ **M05.32** **Rheumatoid heart disease with rheumatoid arthritis of elbow**
    M05.321 **Rheumatoid heart disease with rheumatoid arthritis of right elbow**
    M05.322 **Rheumatoid heart disease with rheumatoid arthritis of left elbow**
    M05.329 **Rheumatoid heart disease with rheumatoid arthritis of unspecified elbow**

✓6ᵗʰ **M05.33** **Rheumatoid heart disease with rheumatoid arthritis of wrist**
    Rheumatoid heart disease with rheumatoid arthritis, carpal bones
    M05.331 **Rheumatoid heart disease with rheumatoid arthritis of right wrist**
    M05.332 **Rheumatoid heart disease with rheumatoid arthritis of left wrist**
    M05.339 **Rheumatoid heart disease with rheumatoid arthritis of unspecified wrist**

✓6ᵗʰ **M05.34** **Rheumatoid heart disease with rheumatoid arthritis of hand**
    Rheumatoid heart disease with rheumatoid arthritis, metacarpus and phalanges
    M05.341 **Rheumatoid heart disease with rheumatoid arthritis of right hand**
    M05.342 **Rheumatoid heart disease with rheumatoid arthritis of left hand**
    M05.349 **Rheumatoid heart disease with rheumatoid arthritis of unspecified hand**

✓6ᵗʰ **M05.35** **Rheumatoid heart disease with rheumatoid arthritis of hip**
    M05.351 **Rheumatoid heart disease with rheumatoid arthritis of right hip**
    M05.352 **Rheumatoid heart disease with rheumatoid arthritis of left hip**
    M05.359 **Rheumatoid heart disease with rheumatoid arthritis of unspecified hip**

✓6ᵗʰ **M05.36** **Rheumatoid heart disease with rheumatoid arthritis of knee**
    M05.361 **Rheumatoid heart disease with rheumatoid arthritis of right knee**
    M05.362 **Rheumatoid heart disease with rheumatoid arthritis of left knee**
    M05.369 **Rheumatoid heart disease with rheumatoid arthritis of unspecified knee**

✓6ᵗʰ **M05.37** **Rheumatoid heart disease with rheumatoid arthritis of ankle and foot**
    Rheumatoid heart disease with rheumatoid arthritis, tarsus, metatarsus and phalanges
    M05.371 **Rheumatoid heart disease with rheumatoid arthritis of right ankle and foot**
    M05.372 **Rheumatoid heart disease with rheumatoid arthritis of left ankle and foot**
    M05.379 **Rheumatoid heart disease with rheumatoid arthritis of unspecified ankle and foot**

M05.39 **Rheumatoid heart disease with rheumatoid arthritis of multiple sites**

✓5ᵗʰ **M05.4** **Rheumatoid myopathy with rheumatoid arthritis**
    M05.40 **Rheumatoid myopathy with rheumatoid arthritis of unspecified site**

✓6ᵗʰ **M05.41** **Rheumatoid myopathy with rheumatoid arthritis of shoulder**
    M05.411 **Rheumatoid myopathy with rheumatoid arthritis of right shoulder**
    M05.412 **Rheumatoid myopathy with rheumatoid arthritis of left shoulder**
    M05.419 **Rheumatoid myopathy with rheumatoid arthritis of unspecified shoulder**

✓6ᵗʰ **M05.42** **Rheumatoid myopathy with rheumatoid arthritis of elbow**
    M05.421 **Rheumatoid myopathy with rheumatoid arthritis of right elbow**
    M05.422 **Rheumatoid myopathy with rheumatoid arthritis of left elbow**
    M05.429 **Rheumatoid myopathy with rheumatoid arthritis of unspecified elbow**

✓6ᵗʰ **M05.43** **Rheumatoid myopathy with rheumatoid arthritis of wrist**
    Rheumatoid myopathy with rheumatoid arthritis, carpal bones
    M05.431 **Rheumatoid myopathy with rheumatoid arthritis of right wrist**
    M05.432 **Rheumatoid myopathy with rheumatoid arthritis of left wrist**
    M05.439 **Rheumatoid myopathy with rheumatoid arthritis of unspecified wrist**

✓6ᵗʰ **M05.44** **Rheumatoid myopathy with rheumatoid arthritis of hand**
    Rheumatoid myopathy with rheumatoid arthritis, metacarpus and phalanges
    M05.441 **Rheumatoid myopathy with rheumatoid arthritis of right hand**
    M05.442 **Rheumatoid myopathy with rheumatoid arthritis of left hand**
    M05.449 **Rheumatoid myopathy with rheumatoid arthritis of unspecified hand**

✓6ᵗʰ **M05.45** **Rheumatoid myopathy with rheumatoid arthritis of hip**
    M05.451 **Rheumatoid myopathy with rheumatoid arthritis of right hip**
    M05.452 **Rheumatoid myopathy with rheumatoid arthritis of left hip**
    M05.459 **Rheumatoid myopathy with rheumatoid arthritis of unspecified hip**

✓6ᵗʰ **M05.46** **Rheumatoid myopathy with rheumatoid arthritis of knee**
    M05.461 **Rheumatoid myopathy with rheumatoid arthritis of right knee**
    M05.462 **Rheumatoid myopathy with rheumatoid arthritis of left knee**
    M05.469 **Rheumatoid myopathy with rheumatoid arthritis of unspecified knee**

✓6ᵗʰ **M05.47 Rheumatoid myopathy with rheumatoid arthritis of ankle and foot**
     Rheumatoid myopathy with rheumatoid arthritis, tarsus, metatarsus and phalanges

     M05.471 Rheumatoid myopathy with rheumatoid arthritis of right ankle and foot

     M05.472 Rheumatoid myopathy with rheumatoid arthritis of left ankle and foot

     M05.479 Rheumatoid myopathy with rheumatoid arthritis of unspecified ankle and foot

     M05.49 Rheumatoid myopathy with rheumatoid arthritis of multiple sites

✓5ᵗʰ **M05.5 Rheumatoid polyneuropathy with rheumatoid arthritis**

     M05.50 Rheumatoid polyneuropathy with rheumatoid arthritis of unspecified site

✓6ᵗʰ **M05.51 Rheumatoid polyneuropathy with rheumatoid arthritis of shoulder**

     M05.511 Rheumatoid polyneuropathy with rheumatoid arthritis of right shoulder

     M05.512 Rheumatoid polyneuropathy with rheumatoid arthritis of left shoulder

     M05.519 Rheumatoid polyneuropathy with rheumatoid arthritis of unspecified shoulder

✓6ᵗʰ **M05.52 Rheumatoid polyneuropathy with rheumatoid arthritis of elbow**

     M05.521 Rheumatoid polyneuropathy with rheumatoid arthritis of right elbow

     M05.522 Rheumatoid polyneuropathy with rheumatoid arthritis of left elbow

     M05.529 Rheumatoid polyneuropathy with rheumatoid arthritis of unspecified elbow

✓6ᵗʰ **M05.53 Rheumatoid polyneuropathy with rheumatoid arthritis of wrist**
     Rheumatoid polyneuropathy with rheumatoid arthritis, carpal bones

     M05.531 Rheumatoid polyneuropathy with rheumatoid arthritis of right wrist

     M05.532 Rheumatoid polyneuropathy with rheumatoid arthritis of left wrist

     M05.539 Rheumatoid polyneuropathy with rheumatoid arthritis of unspecified wrist

✓6ᵗʰ **M05.54 Rheumatoid polyneuropathy with rheumatoid arthritis of hand**
     Rheumatoid polyneuropathy with rheumatoid arthritis, metacarpus and phalanges

     M05.541 Rheumatoid polyneuropathy with rheumatoid arthritis of right hand

     M05.542 Rheumatoid polyneuropathy with rheumatoid arthritis of left hand

     M05.549 Rheumatoid polyneuropathy with rheumatoid arthritis of unspecified hand

✓6ᵗʰ **M05.55 Rheumatoid polyneuropathy with rheumatoid arthritis of hip**

     M05.551 Rheumatoid polyneuropathy with rheumatoid arthritis of right hip

     M05.552 Rheumatoid polyneuropathy with rheumatoid arthritis of left hip

     M05.559 Rheumatoid polyneuropathy with rheumatoid arthritis of unspecified hip

✓6ᵗʰ **M05.56 Rheumatoid polyneuropathy with rheumatoid arthritis of knee**

     M05.561 Rheumatoid polyneuropathy with rheumatoid arthritis of right knee

     M05.562 Rheumatoid polyneuropathy with rheumatoid arthritis of left knee

     M05.569 Rheumatoid polyneuropathy with rheumatoid arthritis of unspecified knee

✓6ᵗʰ **M05.57 Rheumatoid polyneuropathy with rheumatoid arthritis of ankle and foot**
     Rheumatoid polyneuropathy with rheumatoid arthritis, tarsus, metatarsus and phalanges

     M05.571 Rheumatoid polyneuropathy with rheumatoid arthritis of right ankle and foot

     M05.572 Rheumatoid polyneuropathy with rheumatoid arthritis of left ankle and foot

     M05.579 Rheumatoid polyneuropathy with rheumatoid arthritis of unspecified ankle and foot

     M05.59 Rheumatoid polyneuropathy with rheumatoid arthritis of multiple sites

✓5ᵗʰ **M05.6 Rheumatoid arthritis with involvement of other organs and systems**

     M05.60 Rheumatoid arthritis of unspecified site with involvement of other organs and systems

✓6ᵗʰ **M05.61 Rheumatoid arthritis of shoulder with involvement of other organs and systems**

     M05.611 Rheumatoid arthritis of right shoulder with involvement of other organs and systems

     M05.612 Rheumatoid arthritis of left shoulder with involvement of other organs and systems

     M05.619 Rheumatoid arthritis of unspecified shoulder with involvement of other organs and systems

✓6ᵗʰ **M05.62 Rheumatoid arthritis of elbow with involvement of other organs and systems**

     M05.621 Rheumatoid arthritis of right elbow with involvement of other organs and systems

     M05.622 Rheumatoid arthritis of left elbow with involvement of other organs and systems

     M05.629 Rheumatoid arthritis of unspecified elbow with involvement of other organs and systems

✓6ᵗʰ **M05.63 Rheumatoid arthritis of wrist with involvement of other organs and systems**
     Rheumatoid arthritis of carpal bones with involvement of other organs and systems

     M05.631 Rheumatoid arthritis of right wrist with involvement of other organs and systems

     M05.632 Rheumatoid arthritis of left wrist with involvement of other organs and systems

     M05.639 Rheumatoid arthritis of unspecified wrist with involvement of other organs and systems

✓6ᵗʰ **M05.64 Rheumatoid arthritis of hand with involvement of other organs and systems**
     Rheumatoid arthritis of metacarpus and phalanges with involvement of other organs and systems

     M05.641 Rheumatoid arthritis of right hand with involvement of other organs and systems

     M05.642 Rheumatoid arthritis of left hand with involvement of other organs and systems

     M05.649 Rheumatoid arthritis of unspecified hand with involvement of other organs and systems

✓6ᵗʰ **M05.65 Rheumatoid arthritis of hip with involvement of other organs and systems**

     M05.651 Rheumatoid arthritis of right hip with involvement of other organs and systems

     M05.652 Rheumatoid arthritis of left hip with involvement of other organs and systems

     M05.659 Rheumatoid arthritis of unspecified hip with involvement of other organs and systems

✓6ᵗʰ **M05.66 Rheumatoid arthritis of knee with involvement of other organs and systems**

     M05.661 Rheumatoid arthritis of right knee with involvement of other organs and systems

     M05.662 Rheumatoid arthritis of left knee with involvement of other organs and systems

     M05.669 Rheumatoid arthritis of unspecified knee with involvement of other organs and systems

✓6ᵗʰ **M05.67 Rheumatoid arthritis of ankle and foot with involvement of other organs and systems**
     Rheumatoid arthritis of tarsus, metatarsus and phalanges with involvement of other organs and systems

     M05.671 Rheumatoid arthritis of right ankle and foot with involvement of other organs and systems

     M05.672 Rheumatoid arthritis of left ankle and foot with involvement of other organs and systems

---

✓ Additional Character Required   ✗7ᵗʰ Placeholder Alert   Unspecified Dx   Other Specified Dx   Manifestation   ►◄ Revised Text   ● New Code   ▲ Revised Code Title

        M05.679   Rheumatoid arthritis of unspecified ankle and foot with involvement of other organs and systems

   M05.69   Rheumatoid arthritis of multiple sites with involvement of other organs and systems

✓5ᵗʰ   **M05.7**   Rheumatoid arthritis with rheumatoid factor without organ or systems involvement

   M05.70   Rheumatoid arthritis with rheumatoid factor of unspecified site without organ or systems involvement

   ✓6ᵗʰ   M05.71   Rheumatoid arthritis with rheumatoid factor of shoulder without organ or systems involvement

        M05.711   Rheumatoid arthritis with rheumatoid factor of right shoulder without organ or systems involvement

        M05.712   Rheumatoid arthritis with rheumatoid factor of left shoulder without organ or systems involvement

        M05.719   Rheumatoid arthritis with rheumatoid factor of unspecified shoulder without organ or systems involvement

   ✓6ᵗʰ   M05.72   Rheumatoid arthritis with rheumatoid factor of elbow without organ or systems involvement

        M05.721   Rheumatoid arthritis with rheumatoid factor of right elbow without organ or systems involvement

        M05.722   Rheumatoid arthritis with rheumatoid factor of left elbow without organ or systems involvement

        M05.729   Rheumatoid arthritis with rheumatoid factor of unspecified elbow without organ or systems involvement

   ✓6ᵗʰ   M05.73   Rheumatoid arthritis with rheumatoid factor of wrist without organ or systems involvement

        M05.731   Rheumatoid arthritis with rheumatoid factor of right wrist without organ or systems involvement

        M05.732   Rheumatoid arthritis with rheumatoid factor of left wrist without organ or systems involvement

        M05.739   Rheumatoid arthritis with rheumatoid factor of unspecified wrist without organ or systems involvement

   ✓6ᵗʰ   M05.74   Rheumatoid arthritis with rheumatoid factor of hand without organ or systems involvement

        M05.741   Rheumatoid arthritis with rheumatoid factor of right hand without organ or systems involvement

        M05.742   Rheumatoid arthritis with rheumatoid factor of left hand without organ or systems involvement

        M05.749   Rheumatoid arthritis with rheumatoid factor of unspecified hand without organ or systems involvement

   ✓6ᵗʰ   M05.75   Rheumatoid arthritis with rheumatoid factor of hip without organ or systems involvement

        M05.751   Rheumatoid arthritis with rheumatoid factor of right hip without organ or systems involvement

        M05.752   Rheumatoid arthritis with rheumatoid factor of left hip without organ or systems involvement

        M05.759   Rheumatoid arthritis with rheumatoid factor of unspecified hip without organ or systems involvement

   ✓6ᵗʰ   M05.76   Rheumatoid arthritis with rheumatoid factor of knee without organ or systems involvement

        M05.761   Rheumatoid arthritis with rheumatoid factor of right knee without organ or systems involvement

        M05.762   Rheumatoid arthritis with rheumatoid factor of left knee without organ or systems involvement

        M05.769   Rheumatoid arthritis with rheumatoid factor of unspecified knee without organ or systems involvement

   ✓6ᵗʰ   M05.77   Rheumatoid arthritis with rheumatoid factor of ankle and foot without organ or systems involvement

        M05.771   Rheumatoid arthritis with rheumatoid factor of right ankle and foot without organ or systems involvement

        M05.772   Rheumatoid arthritis with rheumatoid factor of left ankle and foot without organ or systems involvement

        M05.779   Rheumatoid arthritis with rheumatoid factor of unspecified ankle and foot without organ or systems involvement

   M05.79   Rheumatoid arthritis with rheumatoid factor of multiple sites without organ or systems involvement

✓5ᵗʰ   **M05.8**   Other rheumatoid arthritis with rheumatoid factor

   M05.80   Other rheumatoid arthritis with rheumatoid factor of unspecified site

   ✓6ᵗʰ   M05.81   Other rheumatoid arthritis with rheumatoid factor of shoulder

        M05.811   Other rheumatoid arthritis with rheumatoid factor of right shoulder

        M05.812   Other rheumatoid arthritis with rheumatoid factor of left shoulder

        M05.819   Other rheumatoid arthritis with rheumatoid factor of unspecified shoulder

   ✓6ᵗʰ   M05.82   Other rheumatoid arthritis with rheumatoid factor of elbow

        M05.821   Other rheumatoid arthritis with rheumatoid factor of right elbow

        M05.822   Other rheumatoid arthritis with rheumatoid factor of left elbow

        M05.829   Other rheumatoid arthritis with rheumatoid factor of unspecified elbow

   ✓6ᵗʰ   M05.83   Other rheumatoid arthritis with rheumatoid factor of wrist

        M05.831   Other rheumatoid arthritis with rheumatoid factor of right wrist

        M05.832   Other rheumatoid arthritis with rheumatoid factor of left wrist

        M05.839   Other rheumatoid arthritis with rheumatoid factor of unspecified wrist

   ✓6ᵗʰ   M05.84   Other rheumatoid arthritis with rheumatoid factor of hand

        M05.841   Other rheumatoid arthritis with rheumatoid factor of right hand

        M05.842   Other rheumatoid arthritis with rheumatoid factor of left hand

        M05.849   Other rheumatoid arthritis with rheumatoid factor of unspecified hand

   ✓6ᵗʰ   M05.85   Other rheumatoid arthritis with rheumatoid factor of hip

        M05.851   Other rheumatoid arthritis with rheumatoid factor of right hip

        M05.852   Other rheumatoid arthritis with rheumatoid factor of left hip

        M05.859   Other rheumatoid arthritis with rheumatoid factor of unspecified hip

   ✓6ᵗʰ   M05.86   Other rheumatoid arthritis with rheumatoid factor of knee

        M05.861   Other rheumatoid arthritis with rheumatoid factor of right knee

        M05.862   Other rheumatoid arthritis with rheumatoid factor of left knee

        M05.869   Other rheumatoid arthritis with rheumatoid factor of unspecified knee

   ✓6ᵗʰ   M05.87   Other rheumatoid arthritis with rheumatoid factor of ankle and foot

        M05.871   Other rheumatoid arthritis with rheumatoid factor of right ankle and foot

        M05.872   Other rheumatoid arthritis with rheumatoid factor of left ankle and foot

        M05.879   Other rheumatoid arthritis with rheumatoid factor of unspecified ankle and foot

   M05.89   Other rheumatoid arthritis with rheumatoid factor of multiple sites

 M05.9   Rheumatoid arthritis with rheumatoid factor, unspecified

---

EXCLUDES 1 Not coded here   EXCLUDES 2 Not included here   N Newborn Age: 0   P Pediatric Age: 0-17   M Maternity Age: 12-55   A Adult Age: 15-124

✓4ᵗʰ **M06 Other rheumatoid arthritis**

  ✓5ᵗʰ **M06.0 Rheumatoid arthritis** without rheumatoid factor

    M06.00 Rheumatoid arthritis without rheumatoid factor, unspecified site

    ✓6ᵗʰ **M06.01 Rheumatoid arthritis without rheumatoid factor, shoulder**

      M06.011 Rheumatoid arthritis without rheumatoid factor, right shoulder

      M06.012 Rheumatoid arthritis without rheumatoid factor, left shoulder

      M06.019 Rheumatoid arthritis without rheumatoid factor, unspecified shoulder

    ✓6ᵗʰ **M06.02 Rheumatoid arthritis without rheumatoid factor, elbow**

      M06.021 Rheumatoid arthritis without rheumatoid factor, right elbow

      M06.022 Rheumatoid arthritis without rheumatoid factor, left elbow

      M06.029 Rheumatoid arthritis without rheumatoid factor, unspecified elbow

    ✓6ᵗʰ **M06.03 Rheumatoid arthritis without rheumatoid factor, wrist**

      M06.031 Rheumatoid arthritis without rheumatoid factor, right wrist

      M06.032 Rheumatoid arthritis without rheumatoid factor, left wrist

      M06.039 Rheumatoid arthritis without rheumatoid factor, unspecified wrist

    ✓6ᵗʰ **M06.04 Rheumatoid arthritis without rheumatoid factor, hand**

      M06.041 Rheumatoid arthritis without rheumatoid factor, right hand

      M06.042 Rheumatoid arthritis without rheumatoid factor, left hand

      M06.049 Rheumatoid arthritis without rheumatoid factor, unspecified hand

    ✓6ᵗʰ **M06.05 Rheumatoid arthritis without rheumatoid factor, hip**

      M06.051 Rheumatoid arthritis without rheumatoid factor, right hip

      M06.052 Rheumatoid arthritis without rheumatoid factor, left hip

      M06.059 Rheumatoid arthritis without rheumatoid factor, unspecified hip

    ✓6ᵗʰ **M06.06 Rheumatoid arthritis without rheumatoid factor, knee**

      M06.061 Rheumatoid arthritis without rheumatoid factor, right knee

      M06.062 Rheumatoid arthritis without rheumatoid factor, left knee

      M06.069 Rheumatoid arthritis without rheumatoid factor, unspecified knee

    ✓6ᵗʰ **M06.07 Rheumatoid arthritis without rheumatoid factor, ankle and foot**

      M06.071 Rheumatoid arthritis without rheumatoid factor, right ankle and foot

      M06.072 Rheumatoid arthritis without rheumatoid factor, left ankle and foot

      M06.079 Rheumatoid arthritis without rheumatoid factor, unspecified ankle and foot

    M06.08 Rheumatoid arthritis without rheumatoid factor, vertebrae

    M06.09 Rheumatoid arthritis without rheumatoid factor, multiple sites

  M06.1 Adult-onset Still's disease 🅐

    EXCLUDES 1 Still's disease NOS (M08.2-)

  ✓5ᵗʰ **M06.2 Rheumatoid bursitis**

    M06.20 Rheumatoid bursitis, unspecified site

    ✓6ᵗʰ **M06.21 Rheumatoid bursitis, shoulder**

      M06.211 Rheumatoid bursitis, right shoulder

      M06.212 Rheumatoid bursitis, left shoulder

      M06.219 Rheumatoid bursitis, unspecified shoulder

    ✓6ᵗʰ **M06.22 Rheumatoid bursitis, elbow**

      M06.221 Rheumatoid bursitis, right elbow

      M06.222 Rheumatoid bursitis, left elbow

      M06.229 Rheumatoid bursitis, unspecified elbow

    ✓6ᵗʰ **M06.23 Rheumatoid bursitis, wrist**

      M06.231 Rheumatoid bursitis, right wrist

      M06.232 Rheumatoid bursitis, left wrist

      M06.239 Rheumatoid bursitis, unspecified wrist

    ✓6ᵗʰ **M06.24 Rheumatoid bursitis, hand**

      M06.241 Rheumatoid bursitis, right hand

      M06.242 Rheumatoid bursitis, left hand

      M06.249 Rheumatoid bursitis, unspecified hand

    ✓6ᵗʰ **M06.25 Rheumatoid bursitis, hip**

      M06.251 Rheumatoid bursitis, right hip

      M06.252 Rheumatoid bursitis, left hip

      M06.259 Rheumatoid bursitis, unspecified hip

    ✓6ᵗʰ **M06.26 Rheumatoid bursitis, knee**

      M06.261 Rheumatoid bursitis, right knee

      M06.262 Rheumatoid bursitis, left knee

      M06.269 Rheumatoid bursitis, unspecified knee

    ✓6ᵗʰ **M06.27 Rheumatoid bursitis, ankle and foot**

      M06.271 Rheumatoid bursitis, right ankle and foot

      M06.272 Rheumatoid bursitis, left ankle and foot

      M06.279 Rheumatoid bursitis, unspecified ankle and foot

    M06.28 Rheumatoid bursitis, vertebrae

    M06.29 Rheumatoid bursitis, multiple sites

  ✓5ᵗʰ **M06.3 Rheumatoid nodule**

    M06.30 Rheumatoid nodule, unspecified site

    ✓6ᵗʰ **M06.31 Rheumatoid nodule, shoulder**

      M06.311 Rheumatoid nodule, right shoulder

      M06.312 Rheumatoid nodule, left shoulder

      M06.319 Rheumatoid nodule, unspecified shoulder

    ✓6ᵗʰ **M06.32 Rheumatoid nodule, elbow**

      M06.321 Rheumatoid nodule, right elbow

      M06.322 Rheumatoid nodule, left elbow

      M06.329 Rheumatoid nodule, unspecified elbow

    ✓6ᵗʰ **M06.33 Rheumatoid nodule, wrist**

      M06.331 Rheumatoid nodule, right wrist

      M06.332 Rheumatoid nodule, left wrist

      M06.339 Rheumatoid nodule, unspecified wrist

    ✓6ᵗʰ **M06.34 Rheumatoid nodule, hand**

      M06.341 Rheumatoid nodule, right hand

      M06.342 Rheumatoid nodule, left hand

      M06.349 Rheumatoid nodule, unspecified hand

    ✓6ᵗʰ **M06.35 Rheumatoid nodule, hip**

      M06.351 Rheumatoid nodule, right hip

      M06.352 Rheumatoid nodule, left hip

      M06.359 Rheumatoid nodule, unspecified hip

    ✓6ᵗʰ **M06.36 Rheumatoid nodule, knee**

      M06.361 Rheumatoid nodule, right knee

      M06.362 Rheumatoid nodule, left knee

      M06.369 Rheumatoid nodule, unspecified knee

    ✓6ᵗʰ **M06.37 Rheumatoid nodule, ankle and foot**

      M06.371 Rheumatoid nodule, right ankle and foot

      M06.372 Rheumatoid nodule, left ankle and foot

      M06.379 Rheumatoid nodule, unspecified ankle and foot

    M06.38 Rheumatoid nodule, vertebrae

    M06.39 Rheumatoid nodule, multiple sites

  M06.4 Inflammatory polyarthropathy

    EXCLUDES 1 polyarthritis NOS (M13.0)

  ✓5ᵗʰ **M06.8 Other specified rheumatoid arthritis**

    ✓6ᵗʰ **M06.80 Other specified rheumatoid arthritis, unspecified site**

    ✓6ᵗʰ **M06.81 Other specified rheumatoid arthritis, shoulder**

      M06.811 Other specified rheumatoid arthritis, right shoulder

      M06.812 Other specified rheumatoid arthritis, left shoulder

      M06.819 Other specified rheumatoid arthritis, unspecified shoulder

    ✓6ᵗʰ **M06.82 Other specified rheumatoid arthritis, elbow**

      M06.821 Other specified rheumatoid arthritis, right elbow

☑ Additional Character Required   ✓x7ᵗʰ Placeholder Alert   Unspecified Dx   Other Specified Dx   Manifestation   ►◄ Revised Text   ● New Code   ▲ Revised Code Title

ICD-10-CM 2016   677

M06.822 **Other specified rheumatoid arthritis, left** elbow

M06.829 **Other specified rheumatoid arthritis,** unspecified elbow

✓6th M06.83 **Other specified rheumatoid arthritis, wrist**

M06.831 **Other specified rheumatoid arthritis, right wrist**

M06.832 **Other specified rheumatoid arthritis, left wrist**

M06.839 **Other specified rheumatoid arthritis, unspecified wrist**

✓6th M06.84 **Other specified rheumatoid arthritis, hand**

M06.841 **Other specified rheumatoid arthritis, right hand**

M06.842 **Other specified rheumatoid arthritis, left hand**

M06.849 **Other specified rheumatoid arthritis, unspecified hand**

✓6th M06.85 **Other specified rheumatoid arthritis, hip**

M06.851 **Other specified rheumatoid arthritis, right hip**

M06.852 **Other specified rheumatoid arthritis, left hip**

M06.859 **Other specified rheumatoid arthritis, unspecified hip**

✓6th M06.86 **Other specified rheumatoid arthritis, knee**

M06.861 **Other specified rheumatoid arthritis, right knee**

M06.862 **Other specified rheumatoid arthritis, left knee**

M06.869 **Other specified rheumatoid arthritis, unspecified knee**

✓6th M06.87 **Other specified rheumatoid arthritis, ankle and foot**

M06.871 **Other specified rheumatoid arthritis, right ankle and foot**

M06.872 **Other specified rheumatoid arthritis, left ankle and foot**

M06.879 **Other specified rheumatoid arthritis, unspecified ankle and foot**

M06.88 **Other specified rheumatoid arthritis, vertebrae**

M06.89 **Other specified rheumatoid arthritis, multiple sites**

M06.9 **Rheumatoid arthritis, unspecified**

✓4th **M07 Enteropathic arthropathies**

Code also associated enteropathy, such as:
regional enteritis [Crohn's disease] (K50.-)
ulcerative colitis (K51.-)

EXCLUDES 1   psoriatic arthropathies (L40.5-)

✓5th **M07.6 Enteropathic arthropathies**

M07.60 **Enteropathic arthropathies, unspecified site**

✓6th M07.61 **Enteropathic arthropathies, shoulder**

M07.611 **Enteropathic arthropathies, right shoulder**

M07.612 **Enteropathic arthropathies, left shoulder**

M07.619 **Enteropathic arthropathies, unspecified shoulder**

✓6th M07.62 **Enteropathic arthropathies, elbow**

M07.621 **Enteropathic arthropathies, right elbow**

M07.622 **Enteropathic arthropathies, left elbow**

M07.629 **Enteropathic arthropathies, unspecified elbow**

✓6th M07.63 **Enteropathic arthropathies, wrist**

M07.631 **Enteropathic arthropathies, right wrist**

M07.632 **Enteropathic arthropathies, left wrist**

M07.639 **Enteropathic arthropathies, unspecified wrist**

✓6th M07.64 **Enteropathic arthropathies, hand**

M07.641 **Enteropathic arthropathies, right hand**

M07.642 **Enteropathic arthropathies, left hand**

M07.649 **Enteropathic arthropathies, unspecified hand**

✓6th M07.65 **Enteropathic arthropathies, hip**

M07.651 **Enteropathic arthropathies, right hip**

M07.652 **Enteropathic arthropathies, left hip**

M07.659 **Enteropathic arthropathies, unspecified hip**

✓6th M07.66 **Enteropathic arthropathies, knee**

M07.661 **Enteropathic arthropathies, right knee**

M07.662 **Enteropathic arthropathies, left knee**

M07.669 **Enteropathic arthropathies, unspecified knee**

✓6th M07.67 **Enteropathic arthropathies, ankle and foot**

M07.671 **Enteropathic arthropathies, right ankle and foot**

M07.672 **Enteropathic arthropathies, left ankle and foot**

M07.679 **Enteropathic arthropathies, unspecified ankle and foot**

M07.68 **Enteropathic arthropathies, vertebrae**

M07.69 **Enteropathic arthropathies, multiple sites**

✓4th **M08 Juvenile arthritis**

Code also any associated underlying condition, such as:
regional enteritis [Crohn's disease] (K50.-)
ulcerative colitis (K51.-)

EXCLUDES 1   arthropathy in Whipple's disease (M14.8)
Felty's syndrome (M05.0)
juvenile dermatomyositis (M33.0-)
psoriatic juvenile arthropathy (L40.54)

✓5th **M08.0 Unspecified juvenile rheumatoid arthritis**

Juvenile rheumatoid arthritis with or without rheumatoid factor

M08.00 **Unspecified juvenile rheumatoid arthritis of unspecified site**

✓6th M08.01 **Unspecified juvenile rheumatoid arthritis, shoulder**

M08.011 **Unspecified juvenile rheumatoid arthritis, right shoulder**

M08.012 **Unspecified juvenile rheumatoid arthritis, left shoulder**

M08.019 **Unspecified juvenile rheumatoid arthritis, unspecified shoulder**

✓6th M08.02 **Unspecified juvenile rheumatoid arthritis of elbow**

M08.021 **Unspecified juvenile rheumatoid arthritis, right elbow**

M08.022 **Unspecified juvenile rheumatoid arthritis, left elbow**

M08.029 **Unspecified juvenile rheumatoid arthritis, unspecified elbow**

✓6th M08.03 **Unspecified juvenile rheumatoid arthritis, wrist**

M08.031 **Unspecified juvenile rheumatoid arthritis, right wrist**

M08.032 **Unspecified juvenile rheumatoid arthritis, left wrist**

M08.039 **Unspecified juvenile rheumatoid arthritis, unspecified wrist**

✓6th M08.04 **Unspecified juvenile rheumatoid arthritis, hand**

M08.041 **Unspecified juvenile rheumatoid arthritis, right hand**

M08.042 **Unspecified juvenile rheumatoid arthritis, left hand**

M08.049 **Unspecified juvenile rheumatoid arthritis, unspecified hand**

✓6th M08.05 **Unspecified juvenile rheumatoid arthritis, hip**

M08.051 **Unspecified juvenile rheumatoid arthritis, right hip**

M08.052 **Unspecified juvenile rheumatoid arthritis, left hip**

M08.059 **Unspecified juvenile rheumatoid arthritis, unspecified hip**

✓6th M08.06 **Unspecified juvenile rheumatoid arthritis, knee**

M08.061 **Unspecified juvenile rheumatoid arthritis, right knee**

M08.062 **Unspecified juvenile rheumatoid arthritis, left knee**

M08.069 **Unspecified juvenile rheumatoid arthritis, unspecified knee**

✓6th M08.07 **Unspecified juvenile rheumatoid arthritis, ankle and foot**

M08.071 **Unspecified juvenile rheumatoid arthritis, right ankle and foot**

M08.072 **Unspecified juvenile rheumatoid arthritis, left ankle and foot**

M08.079 **Unspecified juvenile rheumatoid arthritis, unspecified ankle and foot**

M08.08 **Unspecified juvenile rheumatoid arthritis, vertebrae**

EXCLUDES 1 Not coded here   EXCLUDES 2 Not included here   N Newborn Age: 0   P Pediatric Age: 0-17   M Maternity Age: 12-55   A Adult Age: 15-124

M08.09 Unspecified juvenile rheumatoid arthritis, multiple sites

M08.1 Juvenile ankylosing spondylitis
> EXCLUDES 1 ankylosing spondylitis in adults (M45.0-)

✓5ᵗʰ M08.2 Juvenile rheumatoid arthritis with systemic onset
> Still's disease NOS
> EXCLUDES 1 adult-onset Still's disease (M06.1-)

M08.20 Juvenile rheumatoid arthritis with systemic onset, unspecified site

✓6ᵗʰ M08.21 Juvenile rheumatoid arthritis with systemic onset, shoulder
> **M08.211** Juvenile rheumatoid arthritis with systemic onset, right shoulder
> **M08.212** Juvenile rheumatoid arthritis with systemic onset, left shoulder
> **M08.219** Juvenile rheumatoid arthritis with systemic onset, unspecified shoulder

✓6ᵗʰ M08.22 Juvenile rheumatoid arthritis with systemic onset, elbow
> **M08.221** Juvenile rheumatoid arthritis with systemic onset, right elbow
> **M08.222** Juvenile rheumatoid arthritis with systemic onset, left elbow
> **M08.229** Juvenile rheumatoid arthritis with systemic onset, unspecified elbow

✓6ᵗʰ M08.23 Juvenile rheumatoid arthritis with systemic onset, wrist
> **M08.231** Juvenile rheumatoid arthritis with systemic onset, right wrist
> **M08.232** Juvenile rheumatoid arthritis with systemic onset, left wrist
> **M08.239** Juvenile rheumatoid arthritis with systemic onset, unspecified wrist

✓6ᵗʰ M08.24 Juvenile rheumatoid arthritis with systemic onset, hand
> **M08.241** Juvenile rheumatoid arthritis with systemic onset, right hand
> **M08.242** Juvenile rheumatoid arthritis with systemic onset, left hand
> **M08.249** Juvenile rheumatoid arthritis with systemic onset, unspecified hand

✓6ᵗʰ M08.25 Juvenile rheumatoid arthritis with systemic onset, hip
> **M08.251** Juvenile rheumatoid arthritis with systemic onset, right hip
> **M08.252** Juvenile rheumatoid arthritis with systemic onset, left hip
> **M08.259** Juvenile rheumatoid arthritis with systemic onset, unspecified hip

✓6ᵗʰ M08.26 Juvenile rheumatoid arthritis with systemic onset, knee
> **M08.261** Juvenile rheumatoid arthritis with systemic onset, right knee
> **M08.262** Juvenile rheumatoid arthritis with systemic onset, left knee
> **M08.269** Juvenile rheumatoid arthritis with systemic onset, unspecified knee

✓6ᵗʰ M08.27 Juvenile rheumatoid arthritis with systemic onset, ankle and foot
> **M08.271** Juvenile rheumatoid arthritis with systemic onset, right ankle and foot
> **M08.272** Juvenile rheumatoid arthritis with systemic onset, left ankle and foot
> **M08.279** Juvenile rheumatoid arthritis with systemic onset, unspecified ankle and foot

M08.28 Juvenile rheumatoid arthritis with systemic onset, vertebrae

M08.29 Juvenile rheumatoid arthritis with systemic onset, multiple sites

M08.3 Juvenile rheumatoid polyarthritis (seronegative)

✓5ᵗʰ M08.4 Pauciarticular juvenile rheumatoid arthritis

M08.40 Pauciarticular juvenile rheumatoid arthritis, unspecified site

✓6ᵗʰ M08.41 Pauciarticular juvenile rheumatoid arthritis, shoulder
> **M08.411** Pauciarticular juvenile rheumatoid arthritis, right shoulder

> **M08.412** Pauciarticular juvenile rheumatoid arthritis, left shoulder
> **M08.419** Pauciarticular juvenile rheumatoid arthritis, unspecified shoulder

✓6ᵗʰ M08.42 Pauciarticular juvenile rheumatoid arthritis, elbow
> **M08.421** Pauciarticular juvenile rheumatoid arthritis, right elbow
> **M08.422** Pauciarticular juvenile rheumatoid arthritis, left elbow
> **M08.429** Pauciarticular juvenile rheumatoid arthritis, unspecified elbow

✓6ᵗʰ M08.43 Pauciarticular juvenile rheumatoid arthritis, wrist
> **M08.431** Pauciarticular juvenile rheumatoid arthritis, right wrist
> **M08.432** Pauciarticular juvenile rheumatoid arthritis, left wrist
> **M08.439** Pauciarticular juvenile rheumatoid arthritis, unspecified wrist

✓6ᵗʰ M08.44 Pauciarticular juvenile rheumatoid arthritis, hand
> **M08.441** Pauciarticular juvenile rheumatoid arthritis, right hand
> **M08.442** Pauciarticular juvenile rheumatoid arthritis, left hand
> **M08.449** Pauciarticular juvenile rheumatoid arthritis, unspecified hand

✓6ᵗʰ M08.45 Pauciarticular juvenile rheumatoid arthritis, hip
> **M08.451** Pauciarticular juvenile rheumatoid arthritis, right hip
> **M08.452** Pauciarticular juvenile rheumatoid arthritis, left hip
> **M08.459** Pauciarticular juvenile rheumatoid arthritis, unspecified hip

✓6ᵗʰ M08.46 Pauciarticular juvenile rheumatoid arthritis, knee
> **M08.461** Pauciarticular juvenile rheumatoid arthritis, right knee
> **M08.462** Pauciarticular juvenile rheumatoid arthritis, left knee
> **M08.469** Pauciarticular juvenile rheumatoid arthritis, unspecified knee

✓6ᵗʰ M08.47 Pauciarticular juvenile rheumatoid arthritis, ankle and foot
> **M08.471** Pauciarticular juvenile rheumatoid arthritis, right ankle and foot
> **M08.472** Pauciarticular juvenile rheumatoid arthritis, left ankle and foot
> **M08.479** Pauciarticular juvenile rheumatoid arthritis, unspecified ankle and foot

M08.48 Pauciarticular juvenile rheumatoid arthritis, vertebrae

✓5ᵗʰ M08.8 Other juvenile arthritis

M08.80 Other juvenile arthritis, unspecified site

✓6ᵗʰ M08.81 Other juvenile arthritis, shoulder
> **M08.811** Other juvenile arthritis, right shoulder
> **M08.812** Other juvenile arthritis, left shoulder
> **M08.819** Other juvenile arthritis, unspecified shoulder

✓6ᵗʰ M08.82 Other juvenile arthritis, elbow
> **M08.821** Other juvenile arthritis, right elbow
> **M08.822** Other juvenile arthritis, left elbow
> **M08.829** Other juvenile arthritis, unspecified elbow

✓6ᵗʰ M08.83 Other juvenile arthritis, wrist
> **M08.831** Other juvenile arthritis, right wrist
> **M08.832** Other juvenile arthritis, left wrist
> **M08.839** Other juvenile arthritis, unspecified wrist

✓6ᵗʰ M08.84 Other juvenile arthritis, hand
> **M08.841** Other juvenile arthritis, right hand
> **M08.842** Other juvenile arthritis, left hand
> **M08.849** Other juvenile arthritis, unspecified hand

✓6ᵗʰ M08.85 Other juvenile arthritis, hip
> **M08.851** Other juvenile arthritis, right hip
> **M08.852** Other juvenile arthritis, left hip
> **M08.859** Other juvenile arthritis, unspecified hip

✓6ᵗʰ M08.86 Other juvenile arthritis, knee
> **M08.861** Other juvenile arthritis, right knee
> **M08.862** Other juvenile arthritis, left knee

☑ Additional Character Required   ✓x7ᵗʰ Placeholder Alert   Unspecified Dx   Other Specified Dx   Manifestation   ▶◀ Revised Text   ● New Code   ▲ Revised Code Title

M08.869   **Other juvenile arthritis, unspecified knee**

✓6ᵗʰ   M08.87   **Other juvenile arthritis, ankle and foot**

    M08.871   **Other juvenile arthritis, right ankle and foot**

    M08.872   **Other juvenile arthritis, left ankle and foot**

    M08.879   **Other juvenile arthritis, unspecified ankle and foot**

   M08.88   **Other juvenile arthritis, other specified site**
        Other juvenile arthritis, vertebrae

   M08.89   **Other juvenile arthritis, multiple sites**

✓5ᵗʰ   **M08.9   Juvenile arthritis, unspecified**

    EXCLUDES 1   *juvenile rheumatoid arthritis, unspecified (M08.0-)*

   M08.90   **Juvenile arthritis, unspecified, unspecified site**

✓6ᵗʰ   M08.91   **Juvenile arthritis, unspecified, shoulder**

    M08.911   **Juvenile arthritis, unspecified, right shoulder**

    M08.912   **Juvenile arthritis, unspecified, left shoulder**

    M08.919   **Juvenile arthritis, unspecified, unspecified shoulder**

✓6ᵗʰ   M08.92   **Juvenile arthritis, unspecified, elbow**

    M08.921   **Juvenile arthritis, unspecified, right elbow**

    M08.922   **Juvenile arthritis, unspecified, left elbow**

    M08.929   **Juvenile arthritis, unspecified, unspecified elbow**

✓6ᵗʰ   M08.93   **Juvenile arthritis, unspecified, wrist**

    M08.931   **Juvenile arthritis, unspecified, right wrist**

    M08.932   **Juvenile arthritis, unspecified, left wrist**

    M08.939   **Juvenile arthritis, unspecified, unspecified wrist**

✓6ᵗʰ   M08.94   **Juvenile arthritis, unspecified, hand**

    M08.941   **Juvenile arthritis, unspecified, right hand**

    M08.942   **Juvenile arthritis, unspecified, left hand**

    M08.949   **Juvenile arthritis, unspecified, unspecified hand**

✓6ᵗʰ   M08.95   **Juvenile arthritis, unspecified, hip**

    M08.951   **Juvenile arthritis, unspecified, right hip**

    M08.952   **Juvenile arthritis, unspecified, left hip**

    M08.959   **Juvenile arthritis, unspecified, unspecified hip**

✓6ᵗʰ   M08.96   **Juvenile arthritis, unspecified, knee**

    M08.961   **Juvenile arthritis, unspecified, right knee**

    M08.962   **Juvenile arthritis, unspecified, left knee**

    M08.969   **Juvenile arthritis, unspecified, unspecified knee**

✓6ᵗʰ   M08.97   **Juvenile arthritis, unspecified, ankle and foot**

    M08.971   **Juvenile arthritis, unspecified, right ankle and foot**

    M08.972   **Juvenile arthritis, unspecified, left ankle and foot**

    M08.979   **Juvenile arthritis, unspecified, unspecified ankle and foot**

   M08.98   **Juvenile arthritis, unspecified, vertebrae**

   M08.99   **Juvenile arthritis, unspecified, multiple sites**

✓4ᵗʰ   **M1A   Chronic gout**

    Use additional code to identify:
       autonomic neuropathy in diseases classified elsewhere (G99.0)
       calculus of urinary tract in diseases classified elsewhere (N22)
       cardiomyopathy in diseases classified elsewhere (I43)
       disorders of external ear in diseases classified elsewhere (H61.1-, H62.8-)
       disorders of iris and ciliary body in diseases classified elsewhere (H22)
       glomerular disorders in diseases classified elsewhere (N08)

    EXCLUDES 1   *acute gout (M10.-)*
             gout NOS (M10.-)

    The appropriate 7th character is to be added to each code from category M1A.
    0   without tophus (tophi)
    1   with tophus (tophi)

✓5ᵗʰ   **M1A.0   Idiopathic chronic gout**
     Chronic gouty bursitis   Primary chronic gout

   ✓×7ᵗʰ   M1A.00   **Idiopathic chronic gout, unspecified site**

   ✓6ᵗʰ   M1A.01   **Idiopathic chronic gout, shoulder**

     ✓7ᵗʰ   M1A.011   **Idiopathic chronic gout, right shoulder**

     ✓7ᵗʰ   M1A.012   **Idiopathic chronic gout, left shoulder**

     ✓7ᵗʰ   M1A.019   **Idiopathic chronic gout, unspecified shoulder**

   ✓6ᵗʰ   M1A.02   **Idiopathic chronic gout, elbow**

     ✓7ᵗʰ   M1A.021   **Idiopathic chronic gout, right elbow**

     ✓7ᵗʰ   M1A.022   **Idiopathic chronic gout, left elbow**

     ✓7ᵗʰ   M1A.029   **Idiopathic chronic gout, unspecified elbow**

   ✓6ᵗʰ   M1A.03   **Idiopathic chronic gout, wrist**

     ✓7ᵗʰ   M1A.031   **Idiopathic chronic gout, right wrist**

     ✓7ᵗʰ   M1A.032   **Idiopathic chronic gout, left wrist**

     ✓7ᵗʰ   M1A.039   **Idiopathic chronic gout, unspecified wrist**

   ✓6ᵗʰ   M1A.04   **Idiopathic chronic gout, hand**

     ✓7ᵗʰ   M1A.041   **Idiopathic chronic gout, right hand**

     ✓7ᵗʰ   M1A.042   **Idiopathic chronic gout, left hand**

     ✓7ᵗʰ   M1A.049   **Idiopathic chronic gout, unspecified hand**

   ✓6ᵗʰ   M1A.05   **Idiopathic chronic gout, hip**

     ✓7ᵗʰ   M1A.051   **Idiopathic chronic gout, right hip**

     ✓7ᵗʰ   M1A.052   **Idiopathic chronic gout, left hip**

     ✓7ᵗʰ   M1A.059   **Idiopathic chronic gout, unspecified hip**

   ✓6ᵗʰ   M1A.06   **Idiopathic chronic gout, knee**

     ✓7ᵗʰ   M1A.061   **Idiopathic chronic gout, right knee**

     ✓7ᵗʰ   M1A.062   **Idiopathic chronic gout, left knee**

     ✓7ᵗʰ   M1A.069   **Idiopathic chronic gout, unspecified knee**

   ✓6ᵗʰ   M1A.07   **Idiopathic chronic gout, ankle and foot**

     ✓7ᵗʰ   M1A.071   **Idiopathic chronic gout, right ankle and foot**

     ✓7ᵗʰ   M1A.072   **Idiopathic chronic gout, left ankle and foot**

     ✓7ᵗʰ   M1A.079   **Idiopathic chronic gout, unspecified ankle and foot**

   ✓×7ᵗʰ   M1A.08   **Idiopathic chronic gout, vertebrae**

   ✓×7ᵗʰ   M1A.09   **Idiopathic chronic gout, multiple sites**

✓5ᵗʰ   **M1A.1   Lead-induced chronic gout**
     Code first toxic effects of lead and its compounds (T56.0-)

   ✓×7ᵗʰ   M1A.10   **Lead-induced chronic gout, unspecified site**

   ✓6ᵗʰ   M1A.11   **Lead-induced chronic gout, shoulder**

     ✓7ᵗʰ   M1A.111   **Lead-induced chronic gout, right shoulder**

     ✓7ᵗʰ   M1A.112   **Lead-induced chronic gout, left shoulder**

     ✓7ᵗʰ   M1A.119   **Lead-induced chronic gout, unspecified shoulder**

   ✓6ᵗʰ   M1A.12   **Lead-induced chronic gout, elbow**

     ✓7ᵗʰ   M1A.121   **Lead-induced chronic gout, right elbow**

     ✓7ᵗʰ   M1A.122   **Lead-induced chronic gout, left elbow**

     ✓7ᵗʰ   M1A.129   **Lead-induced chronic gout, unspecified elbow**

   ✓6ᵗʰ   M1A.13   **Lead-induced chronic gout, wrist**

     ✓7ᵗʰ   M1A.131   **Lead-induced chronic gout, right wrist**

     ✓7ᵗʰ   M1A.132   **Lead-induced chronic gout, left wrist**

     ✓7ᵗʰ   M1A.139   **Lead-induced chronic gout, unspecified wrist**

   ✓6ᵗʰ   M1A.14   **Lead-induced chronic gout, hand**

     ✓7ᵗʰ   M1A.141   **Lead-induced chronic gout, right hand**

     ✓7ᵗʰ   M1A.142   **Lead-induced chronic gout, left hand**

     ✓7ᵗʰ   M1A.149   **Lead-induced chronic gout, unspecified hand**

   ✓6ᵗʰ   M1A.15   **Lead-induced chronic gout, hip**

     ✓7ᵗʰ   M1A.151   **Lead-induced chronic gout, right hip**

     ✓7ᵗʰ   M1A.152   **Lead-induced chronic gout, left hip**

     ✓7ᵗʰ   M1A.159   **Lead-induced chronic gout, unspecified hip**

   ✓6ᵗʰ   M1A.16   **Lead-induced chronic gout, knee**

     ✓7ᵗʰ   M1A.161   **Lead-induced chronic gout, right knee**

     ✓7ᵗʰ   M1A.162   **Lead-induced chronic gout, left knee**

     ✓7ᵗʰ   M1A.169   **Lead-induced chronic gout, unspecified knee**

   ✓6ᵗʰ   M1A.17   **Lead-induced chronic gout, ankle and foot**

     ✓7ᵗʰ   M1A.171   **Lead-induced chronic gout, right ankle and foot**

EXCLUDES 1 Not coded here   *EXCLUDES 2* Not included here   **N** Newborn Age: 0   **P** Pediatric Age: 0-17   **M** Maternity Age: 12-55   **A** Adult Age: 15-124

680   ICD-10-CM 2016

✓7ᵗʰ **M1A.172** **Lead-induced chronic gout,** left **ankle and foot**

✓7ᵗʰ **M1A.179** Lead-induced chronic gout, unspecified ankle and foot

✓x7ᵗʰ **M1A.18** **Lead-induced chronic gout,** vertebrae

✓x7ᵗʰ **M1A.19** **Lead-induced chronic gout,** multiple sites

✓5ᵗʰ **M1A.2** **Drug-induced** chronic gout

Use additional code for adverse effect, if applicable, to identify drug (T36-T50 with fifth or sixth character 5)

✓x7ᵗʰ **M1A.20** Drug-induced chronic gout, unspecified site

✓6ᵗʰ **M1A.21** **Drug-induced chronic gout,** shoulder

✓7ᵗʰ **M1A.211** **Drug-induced chronic gout,** right **shoulder**

✓7ᵗʰ **M1A.212** **Drug-induced chronic gout,** left **shoulder**

✓7ᵗʰ **M1A.219** Drug-induced chronic gout, unspecified shoulder

✓6ᵗʰ **M1A.22** **Drug-induced chronic gout,** elbow

✓7ᵗʰ **M1A.221** **Drug-induced chronic gout,** right **elbow**

✓7ᵗʰ **M1A.222** **Drug-induced chronic gout,** left **elbow**

✓7ᵗʰ **M1A.229** Drug-induced chronic gout, unspecified elbow

✓6ᵗʰ **M1A.23** **Drug-induced chronic gout,** wrist

✓7ᵗʰ **M1A.231** **Drug-induced chronic gout,** right **wrist**

✓7ᵗʰ **M1A.232** **Drug-induced chronic gout,** left **wrist**

✓7ᵗʰ **M1A.239** Drug-induced chronic gout, unspecified wrist

✓6ᵗʰ **M1A.24** **Drug-induced chronic gout,** hand

✓7ᵗʰ **M1A.241** **Drug-induced chronic gout,** right **hand**

✓7ᵗʰ **M1A.242** **Drug-induced chronic gout,** left **hand**

✓7ᵗʰ **M1A.249** Drug-induced chronic gout, unspecified hand

✓6ᵗʰ **M1A.25** **Drug-induced chronic gout,** hip

✓7ᵗʰ **M1A.251** **Drug-induced chronic gout,** right **hip**

✓7ᵗʰ **M1A.252** **Drug-induced chronic gout,** left **hip**

✓7ᵗʰ **M1A.259** Drug-induced chronic gout, unspecified hip

✓6ᵗʰ **M1A.26** **Drug-induced chronic gout,** knee

✓7ᵗʰ **M1A.261** **Drug-induced chronic gout,** right **knee**

✓7ᵗʰ **M1A.262** **Drug-induced chronic gout,** left **knee**

✓7ᵗʰ **M1A.269** Drug-induced chronic gout, unspecified knee

✓6ᵗʰ **M1A.27** **Drug-induced chronic gout,** ankle and foot

✓7ᵗʰ **M1A.271** **Drug-induced chronic gout,** right **ankle and foot**

✓7ᵗʰ **M1A.272** **Drug-induced chronic gout,** left **ankle and foot**

✓7ᵗʰ **M1A.279** Drug-induced chronic gout, unspecified ankle and foot

✓x7ᵗʰ **M1A.28** **Drug-induced chronic gout,** vertebrae

✓x7ᵗʰ **M1A.29** **Drug-induced chronic gout,** multiple sites

✓5ᵗʰ **M1A.3** **Chronic gout** due to renal impairment

Code first associated renal disease

✓x7ᵗʰ **M1A.30** Chronic gout due to renal impairment, unspecified site

✓6ᵗʰ **M1A.31** **Chronic gout due to renal impairment,** shoulder

✓7ᵗʰ **M1A.311** **Chronic gout due to renal impairment,** right **shoulder**

✓7ᵗʰ **M1A.312** **Chronic gout due to renal impairment,** left **shoulder**

✓7ᵗʰ **M1A.319** Chronic gout due to renal impairment, unspecified shoulder

✓6ᵗʰ **M1A.32** **Chronic gout due to renal impairment,** elbow

✓7ᵗʰ **M1A.321** **Chronic gout due to renal impairment,** right **elbow**

✓7ᵗʰ **M1A.322** **Chronic gout due to renal impairment,** left **elbow**

✓7ᵗʰ **M1A.329** Chronic gout due to renal impairment, unspecified elbow

✓6ᵗʰ **M1A.33** **Chronic gout due to renal impairment,** wrist

✓7ᵗʰ **M1A.331** **Chronic gout due to renal impairment,** right **wrist**

✓7ᵗʰ **M1A.332** **Chronic gout due to renal impairment,** left **wrist**

✓7ᵗʰ **M1A.339** Chronic gout due to renal impairment, unspecified wrist

✓6ᵗʰ **M1A.34** **Chronic gout due to renal impairment,** hand

✓7ᵗʰ **M1A.341** **Chronic gout due to renal impairment,** right **hand**

✓7ᵗʰ **M1A.342** **Chronic gout due to renal impairment,** left **hand**

✓7ᵗʰ **M1A.349** Chronic gout due to renal impairment, unspecified hand

✓6ᵗʰ **M1A.35** **Chronic gout due to renal impairment,** hip

✓7ᵗʰ **M1A.351** **Chronic gout due to renal impairment,** right **hip**

✓7ᵗʰ **M1A.352** **Chronic gout due to renal impairment,** left **hip**

✓7ᵗʰ **M1A.359** Chronic gout due to renal impairment, unspecified hip

✓6ᵗʰ **M1A.36** **Chronic gout due to renal impairment,** knee

✓7ᵗʰ **M1A.361** **Chronic gout due to renal impairment,** right **knee**

✓7ᵗʰ **M1A.362** **Chronic gout due to renal impairment,** left **knee**

✓7ᵗʰ **M1A.369** Chronic gout due to renal impairment, unspecified knee

✓6ᵗʰ **M1A.37** **Chronic gout due to renal impairment,** ankle and foot

✓7ᵗʰ **M1A.371** **Chronic gout due to renal impairment,** right **ankle and foot**

✓7ᵗʰ **M1A.372** **Chronic gout due to renal impairment,** left **ankle and foot**

✓7ᵗʰ **M1A.379** Chronic gout due to renal impairment, unspecified ankle and foot

✓x7ᵗʰ **M1A.38** **Chronic gout due to renal impairment,** vertebrae

✓x7ᵗʰ **M1A.39** **Chronic gout due to renal impairment,** multiple sites

✓5ᵗʰ **M1A.4** **Other secondary** chronic gout

Code first associated condition

✓x7ᵗʰ **M1A.40** Other secondary chronic gout, unspecified site

✓6ᵗʰ **M1A.41** **Other secondary chronic gout,** shoulder

✓7ᵗʰ **M1A.411** Other secondary chronic gout, right shoulder

✓7ᵗʰ **M1A.412** Other secondary chronic gout, left shoulder

✓7ᵗʰ **M1A.419** Other secondary chronic gout, unspecified shoulder

✓6ᵗʰ **M1A.42** **Other secondary chronic gout,** elbow

✓7ᵗʰ **M1A.421** Other secondary chronic gout, right elbow

✓7ᵗʰ **M1A.422** Other secondary chronic gout, left elbow

✓7ᵗʰ **M1A.429** Other secondary chronic gout, unspecified elbow

✓6ᵗʰ **M1A.43** **Other secondary chronic gout,** wrist

✓7ᵗʰ **M1A.431** Other secondary chronic gout, right wrist

✓7ᵗʰ **M1A.432** Other secondary chronic gout, left wrist

✓7ᵗʰ **M1A.439** Other secondary chronic gout, unspecified wrist

✓6ᵗʰ **M1A.44** **Other secondary chronic gout,** hand

✓7ᵗʰ **M1A.441** Other secondary chronic gout, right hand

✓7ᵗʰ **M1A.442** Other secondary chronic gout, left hand

✓7ᵗʰ **M1A.449** Other secondary chronic gout, unspecified hand

✓6ᵗʰ **M1A.45** **Other secondary chronic gout,** hip

✓7ᵗʰ **M1A.451** Other secondary chronic gout, right hip

✓7ᵗʰ **M1A.452** Other secondary chronic gout, left hip

✓7ᵗʰ **M1A.459** Other secondary chronic gout, unspecified hip

✓6ᵗʰ **M1A.46** **Other secondary chronic gout,** knee

✓7ᵗʰ **M1A.461** Other secondary chronic gout, right knee

✓7ᵗʰ **M1A.462** Other secondary chronic gout, left knee

✓7ᵗʰ **M1A.469** Other secondary chronic gout, unspecified knee

---

✓ Additional Character Required   ✓x7ᵗʰ Placeholder Alert   Unspecified Dx   Other Specified Dx   Manifestation   ▶◀ Revised Text   ● New Code   ▲ Revised Code Title

ICD-10-CM 2016   681

√6ᵗʰ **M1A.47** Other secondary chronic gout, ankle and foot

√7ᵗʰ   **M1A.471** **Other secondary chronic gout, right ankle and foot**

√7ᵗʰ   **M1A.472** **Other secondary chronic gout, left ankle and foot**

√7ᵗʰ   **M1A.479** **Other secondary chronic gout, unspecified ankle and foot**

√x7ᵗʰ **M1A.48** **Other secondary chronic gout, vertebrae**

√x7ᵗʰ **M1A.49** **Other secondary chronic gout, multiple sites**

√x7ᵗʰ **M1A.9** **Chronic gout, unspecified**

√4ᵗʰ **M10 Gout**

Acute gout   Gout NOS
Gout attack   Podagra
Gout flare
Use additional code to identify:
    autonomic neuropathy in diseases classified elsewhere (G99.0)
    calculus of urinary tract in diseases classified elsewhere (N22)
    cardiomyopathy in diseases classified elsewhere (I43)
    disorders of external ear in diseases classified elsewhere (H61.1-, H62.8-)
    disorders of iris and ciliary body in diseases classified elsewhere (H22)
    glomerular disorders in diseases classified elsewhere (N08)

EXCLUDES 1   chronic gout (M1A.-)

√5ᵗʰ **M10.0** **Idiopathic gout**
Gouty bursitis
Primary gout

M10.00 **Idiopathic gout, unspecified site**

√6ᵗʰ **M10.01** **Idiopathic gout, shoulder**
   M10.011 **Idiopathic gout, right shoulder**
   M10.012 **Idiopathic gout, left shoulder**
   M10.019 **Idiopathic gout, unspecified shoulder**

√6ᵗʰ **M10.02** **Idiopathic gout, elbow**
   M10.021 **Idiopathic gout, right elbow**
   M10.022 **Idiopathic gout, left elbow**
   M10.029 **Idiopathic gout, unspecified elbow**

√6ᵗʰ **M10.03** **Idiopathic gout, wrist**
   M10.031 **Idiopathic gout, right wrist**
   M10.032 **Idiopathic gout, left wrist**
   M10.039 **Idiopathic gout, unspecified wrist**

√6ᵗʰ **M10.04** **Idiopathic gout, hand**
   M10.041 **Idiopathic gout, right hand**
   M10.042 **Idiopathic gout, left hand**
   M10.049 **Idiopathic gout, unspecified hand**

√6ᵗʰ **M10.05** **Idiopathic gout, hip**
   M10.051 **Idiopathic gout, right hip**
   M10.052 **Idiopathic gout, left hip**
   M10.059 **Idiopathic gout, unspecified hip**

√6ᵗʰ **M10.06** **Idiopathic gout, knee**
   M10.061 **Idiopathic gout, right knee**
   M10.062 **Idiopathic gout, left knee**
   M10.069 **Idiopathic gout, unspecified knee**

√6ᵗʰ **M10.07** **Idiopathic gout, ankle and foot**
   M10.071 **Idiopathic gout, right ankle and foot**
   M10.072 **Idiopathic gout, left ankle and foot**
   M10.079 **Idiopathic gout, unspecified ankle and foot**

M10.08 **Idiopathic gout, vertebrae**

M10.09 **Idiopathic gout, multiple sites**

√5ᵗʰ **M10.1** **Lead-induced gout**
Code first toxic effects of lead and its compounds (T56.0-)

M10.10 **Lead-induced gout, unspecified site**

√6ᵗʰ **M10.11** **Lead-induced gout, shoulder**
   M10.111 **Lead-induced gout, right shoulder**
   M10.112 **Lead-induced gout, left shoulder**
   M10.119 **Lead-induced gout, unspecified shoulder**

√6ᵗʰ **M10.12** **Lead-induced gout, elbow**
   M10.121 **Lead-induced gout, right elbow**
   M10.122 **Lead-induced gout, left elbow**
   M10.129 **Lead-induced gout, unspecified elbow**

√6ᵗʰ **M10.13** **Lead-induced gout, wrist**
   M10.131 **Lead-induced gout, right wrist**
   M10.132 **Lead-induced gout, left wrist**
   M10.139 **Lead-induced gout, unspecified wrist**

√6ᵗʰ **M10.14** **Lead-induced gout, hand**
   M10.141 **Lead-induced gout, right hand**
   M10.142 **Lead-induced gout, left hand**
   M10.149 **Lead-induced gout, unspecified hand**

√6ᵗʰ **M10.15** **Lead-induced gout, hip**
   M10.151 **Lead-induced gout, right hip**
   M10.152 **Lead-induced gout, left hip**
   M10.159 **Lead-induced gout, unspecified hip**

√6ᵗʰ **M10.16** **Lead-induced gout, knee**
   M10.161 **Lead-induced gout, right knee**
   M10.162 **Lead-induced gout, left knee**
   M10.169 **Lead-induced gout, unspecified knee**

√6ᵗʰ **M10.17** **Lead-induced gout, ankle and foot**
   M10.171 **Lead-induced gout, right ankle and foot**
   M10.172 **Lead-induced gout, left ankle and foot**
   M10.179 **Lead-induced gout, unspecified ankle and foot**

M10.18 **Lead-induced gout, vertebrae**

M10.19 **Lead-induced gout, multiple sites**

√5ᵗʰ **M10.2** **Drug-induced gout**
Use additional code for adverse effect, if applicable, to identify drug (T36-T50 with fifth or sixth character 5)

M10.20 **Drug-induced gout, unspecified site**

√6ᵗʰ **M10.21** **Drug-induced gout, shoulder**
   M10.211 **Drug-induced gout, right shoulder**
   M10.212 **Drug-induced gout, left shoulder**
   M10.219 **Drug-induced gout, unspecified shoulder**

√6ᵗʰ **M10.22** **Drug-induced gout, elbow**
   M10.221 **Drug-induced gout, right elbow**
   M10.222 **Drug-induced gout, left elbow**
   M10.229 **Drug-induced gout, unspecified elbow**

√6ᵗʰ **M10.23** **Drug-induced gout, wrist**
   M10.231 **Drug-induced gout, right wrist**
   M10.232 **Drug-induced gout, left wrist**
   M10.239 **Drug-induced gout, unspecified wrist**

√6ᵗʰ **M10.24** **Drug-induced gout, hand**
   M10.241 **Drug-induced gout, right hand**
   M10.242 **Drug-induced gout, left hand**
   M10.249 **Drug-induced gout, unspecified hand**

√6ᵗʰ **M10.25** **Drug-induced gout, hip**
   M10.251 **Drug-induced gout, right hip**
   M10.252 **Drug-induced gout, left hip**
   M10.259 **Drug-induced gout, unspecified hip**

√6ᵗʰ **M10.26** **Drug-induced gout, knee**
   M10.261 **Drug-induced gout, right knee**
   M10.262 **Drug-induced gout, left knee**
   M10.269 **Drug-induced gout, unspecified knee**

√6ᵗʰ **M10.27** **Drug-induced gout, ankle and foot**
   M10.271 **Drug-induced gout, right ankle and foot**
   M10.272 **Drug-induced gout, left ankle and foot**
   M10.279 **Drug-induced gout, unspecified ankle and foot**

M10.28 **Drug-induced gout, vertebrae**

M10.29 **Drug-induced gout, multiple sites**

√5ᵗʰ **M10.3** **Gout due to renal impairment**
Code first associated renal disease

M10.30 **Gout due to renal impairment, unspecified site**

√6ᵗʰ **M10.31** **Gout due to renal impairment, shoulder**
   M10.311 **Gout due to renal impairment, right shoulder**
   M10.312 **Gout due to renal impairment, left shoulder**
   M10.319 **Gout due to renal impairment, unspecified shoulder**

√6ᵗʰ **M10.32** **Gout due to renal impairment, elbow**
   M10.321 **Gout due to renal impairment, right elbow**
   M10.322 **Gout due to renal impairment, left elbow**
   M10.329 **Gout due to renal impairment, unspecified elbow**

√6ᵗʰ **M10.33** **Gout due to renal impairment, wrist**
   M10.331 **Gout due to renal impairment, right wrist**
   M10.332 **Gout due to renal impairment, left wrist**

EXCLUDES 1 Not coded here   EXCLUDES 2 Not included here   N Newborn Age: 0   P Pediatric Age: 0-17   M Maternity Age: 12-55   A Adult Age: 15-124

682

ICD-10-CM 2016

M10.339 Gout due to renal impairment, unspecified wrist

✓6ᵗʰ M10.34 Gout due to renal impairment, hand
    M10.341 Gout due to renal impairment, right hand
    M10.342 Gout due to renal impairment, left hand
    M10.349 Gout due to renal impairment, unspecified hand

✓6ᵗʰ M10.35 Gout due to renal impairment, hip
    M10.351 Gout due to renal impairment, right hip
    M10.352 Gout due to renal impairment, left hip
    M10.359 Gout due to renal impairment, unspecified hip

✓6ᵗʰ M10.36 Gout due to renal impairment, knee
    M10.361 Gout due to renal impairment, right knee
    M10.362 Gout due to renal impairment, left knee
    M10.369 Gout due to renal impairment, unspecified knee

✓6ᵗʰ M10.37 Gout due to renal impairment, ankle and foot
    M10.371 Gout due to renal impairment, right ankle and foot
    M10.372 Gout due to renal impairment, left ankle and foot
    M10.379 Gout due to renal impairment, unspecified ankle and foot

M10.38 Gout due to renal impairment, vertebrae
M10.39 Gout due to renal impairment, multiple sites

✓5ᵗʰ M10.4 Other secondary gout
    Code first associated condition
    M10.40 Other secondary gout, unspecified site

✓6ᵗʰ M10.41 Other secondary gout, shoulder
    M10.411 Other secondary gout, right shoulder
    M10.412 Other secondary gout, left shoulder
    M10.419 Other secondary gout, unspecified shoulder

✓6ᵗʰ M10.42 Other secondary gout, elbow
    M10.421 Other secondary gout, right elbow
    M10.422 Other secondary gout, left elbow
    M10.429 Other secondary gout, unspecified elbow

✓6ᵗʰ M10.43 Other secondary gout, wrist
    M10.431 Other secondary gout, right wrist
    M10.432 Other secondary gout, left wrist
    M10.439 Other secondary gout, unspecified wrist

✓6ᵗʰ M10.44 Other secondary gout, hand
    M10.441 Other secondary gout, right hand
    M10.442 Other secondary gout, left hand
    M10.449 Other secondary gout, unspecified hand

✓6ᵗʰ M10.45 Other secondary gout, hip
    M10.451 Other secondary gout, right hip
    M10.452 Other secondary gout, left hip
    M10.459 Other secondary gout, unspecified hip

✓6ᵗʰ M10.46 Other secondary gout, knee
    M10.461 Other secondary gout, right knee
    M10.462 Other secondary gout, left knee
    M10.469 Other secondary gout, unspecified knee

✓6ᵗʰ M10.47 Other secondary gout, ankle and foot
    M10.471 Other secondary gout, right ankle and foot
    M10.472 Other secondary gout, left ankle and foot
    M10.479 Other secondary gout, unspecified ankle and foot

M10.48 Other secondary gout, vertebrae
M10.49 Other secondary gout, multiple sites

M10.9 Gout, unspecified
    Gout NOS

✓4ᵗʰ **M11 Other crystal arthropathies**

✓5ᵗʰ M11.0 Hydroxyapatite deposition disease
    M11.00 Hydroxyapatite deposition disease, unspecified site

✓6ᵗʰ M11.01 Hydroxyapatite deposition disease, shoulder
    M11.011 Hydroxyapatite deposition disease, right shoulder
    M11.012 Hydroxyapatite deposition disease, left shoulder

M11.019 Hydroxyapatite deposition disease, unspecified shoulder

✓6ᵗʰ M11.02 Hydroxyapatite deposition disease, elbow
    M11.021 Hydroxyapatite deposition disease, right elbow
    M11.022 Hydroxyapatite deposition disease, left elbow
    M11.029 Hydroxyapatite deposition disease, unspecified elbow

✓6ᵗʰ M11.03 Hydroxyapatite deposition disease, wrist
    M11.031 Hydroxyapatite deposition disease, right wrist
    M11.032 Hydroxyapatite deposition disease, left wrist
    M11.039 Hydroxyapatite deposition disease, unspecified wrist

✓6ᵗʰ M11.04 Hydroxyapatite deposition disease, hand
    M11.041 Hydroxyapatite deposition disease, right hand
    M11.042 Hydroxyapatite deposition disease, left hand
    M11.049 Hydroxyapatite deposition disease, unspecified hand

✓6ᵗʰ M11.05 Hydroxyapatite deposition disease, hip
    M11.051 Hydroxyapatite deposition disease, right hip
    M11.052 Hydroxyapatite deposition disease, left hip
    M11.059 Hydroxyapatite deposition disease, unspecified hip

✓6ᵗʰ M11.06 Hydroxyapatite deposition disease, knee
    M11.061 Hydroxyapatite deposition disease, right knee
    M11.062 Hydroxyapatite deposition disease, left knee
    M11.069 Hydroxyapatite deposition disease, unspecified knee

✓6ᵗʰ M11.07 Hydroxyapatite deposition disease, ankle and foot
    M11.071 Hydroxyapatite deposition disease, right ankle and foot
    M11.072 Hydroxyapatite deposition disease, left ankle and foot
    M11.079 Hydroxyapatite deposition disease, unspecified ankle and foot

M11.08 Hydroxyapatite deposition disease, vertebrae
M11.09 Hydroxyapatite deposition disease, multiple sites

✓5ᵗʰ M11.1 Familial chondrocalcinosis
    M11.10 Familial chondrocalcinosis, unspecified site

✓6ᵗʰ M11.11 Familial chondrocalcinosis, shoulder
    M11.111 Familial chondrocalcinosis, right shoulder
    M11.112 Familial chondrocalcinosis, left shoulder
    M11.119 Familial chondrocalcinosis, unspecified shoulder

✓6ᵗʰ M11.12 Familial chondrocalcinosis, elbow
    M11.121 Familial chondrocalcinosis, right elbow
    M11.122 Familial chondrocalcinosis, left elbow
    M11.129 Familial chondrocalcinosis, unspecified elbow

✓6ᵗʰ M11.13 Familial chondrocalcinosis, wrist
    M11.131 Familial chondrocalcinosis, right wrist
    M11.132 Familial chondrocalcinosis, left wrist
    M11.139 Familial chondrocalcinosis, unspecified wrist

✓6ᵗʰ M11.14 Familial chondrocalcinosis, hand
    M11.141 Familial chondrocalcinosis, right hand
    M11.142 Familial chondrocalcinosis, left hand
    M11.149 Familial chondrocalcinosis, unspecified hand

✓6ᵗʰ M11.15 Familial chondrocalcinosis, hip
    M11.151 Familial chondrocalcinosis, right hip
    M11.152 Familial chondrocalcinosis, left hip
    M11.159 Familial chondrocalcinosis, unspecified hip

✓ Additional Character Required   ✓x7ᵗʰ Placeholder Alert   Unspecified Dx   Other Specified Dx   Manifestation   ►◄ Revised Text   ● New Code   ▲ Revised Code Title

✓6ᵗʰ M11.16 Familial chondrocalcinosis, knee
    M11.161 Familial chondrocalcinosis, right knee
    M11.162 Familial chondrocalcinosis, left knee
    M11.169 Familial chondrocalcinosis, unspecified knee

✓6ᵗʰ M11.17 Familial chondrocalcinosis, ankle and foot
    M11.171 Familial chondrocalcinosis, right ankle and foot
    M11.172 Familial chondrocalcinosis, left ankle and foot
    M11.179 Familial chondrocalcinosis, unspecified ankle and foot

M11.18 Familial chondrocalcinosis, vertebrae
M11.19 Familial chondrocalcinosis, multiple sites

✓5ᵗʰ M11.2 Other chondrocalcinosis
    Chondrocalcinosis NOS

M11.20 Other chondrocalcinosis, unspecified site

✓6ᵗʰ M11.21 Other chondrocalcinosis, shoulder
    M11.211 Other chondrocalcinosis, right shoulder
    M11.212 Other chondrocalcinosis, left shoulder
    M11.219 Other chondrocalcinosis, unspecified shoulder

✓6ᵗʰ M11.22 Other chondrocalcinosis, elbow
    M11.221 Other chondrocalcinosis, right elbow
    M11.222 Other chondrocalcinosis, left elbow
    M11.229 Other chondrocalcinosis, unspecified elbow

✓6ᵗʰ M11.23 Other chondrocalcinosis, wrist
    M11.231 Other chondrocalcinosis, right wrist
    M11.232 Other chondrocalcinosis, left wrist
    M11.239 Other chondrocalcinosis, unspecified wrist

✓6ᵗʰ M11.24 Other chondrocalcinosis, hand
    M11.241 Other chondrocalcinosis, right hand
    M11.242 Other chondrocalcinosis, left hand
    M11.249 Other chondrocalcinosis, unspecified hand

✓6ᵗʰ M11.25 Other chondrocalcinosis, hip
    M11.251 Other chondrocalcinosis, right hip
    M11.252 Other chondrocalcinosis, left hip
    M11.259 Other chondrocalcinosis, unspecified hip

✓6ᵗʰ M11.26 Other chondrocalcinosis, knee
    M11.261 Other chondrocalcinosis, right knee
    M11.262 Other chondrocalcinosis, left knee
    M11.269 Other chondrocalcinosis, unspecified knee

✓6ᵗʰ M11.27 Other chondrocalcinosis, ankle and foot
    M11.271 Other chondrocalcinosis, right ankle and foot
    M11.272 Other chondrocalcinosis, left ankle and foot
    M11.279 Other chondrocalcinosis, unspecified ankle and foot

M11.28 Other chondrocalcinosis, vertebrae
M11.29 Other chondrocalcinosis, multiple sites

✓5ᵗʰ M11.8 Other specified crystal arthropathies
M11.80 Other specified crystal arthropathies, unspecified site

✓6ᵗʰ M11.81 Other specified crystal arthropathies, shoulder
    M11.811 Other specified crystal arthropathies, right shoulder
    M11.812 Other specified crystal arthropathies, left shoulder
    M11.819 Other specified crystal arthropathies, unspecified shoulder

✓6ᵗʰ M11.82 Other specified crystal arthropathies, elbow
    M11.821 Other specified crystal arthropathies, right elbow
    M11.822 Other specified crystal arthropathies, left elbow
    M11.829 Other specified crystal arthropathies, unspecified elbow

✓6ᵗʰ M11.83 Other specified crystal arthropathies, wrist
    M11.831 Other specified crystal arthropathies, right wrist
    M11.832 Other specified crystal arthropathies, left wrist
    M11.839 Other specified crystal arthropathies, unspecified wrist

✓6ᵗʰ M11.84 Other specified crystal arthropathies, hand
    M11.841 Other specified crystal arthropathies, right hand
    M11.842 Other specified crystal arthropathies, left hand
    M11.849 Other specified crystal arthropathies, unspecified hand

✓6ᵗʰ M11.85 Other specified crystal arthropathies, hip
    M11.851 Other specified crystal arthropathies, right hip
    M11.852 Other specified crystal arthropathies, left hip
    M11.859 Other specified crystal arthropathies, unspecified hip

✓6ᵗʰ M11.86 Other specified crystal arthropathies, knee
    M11.861 Other specified crystal arthropathies, right knee
    M11.862 Other specified crystal arthropathies, left knee
    M11.869 Other specified crystal arthropathies, unspecified knee

✓6ᵗʰ M11.87 Other specified crystal arthropathies, ankle and foot
    M11.871 Other specified crystal arthropathies, right ankle and foot
    M11.872 Other specified crystal arthropathies, left ankle and foot
    M11.879 Other specified crystal arthropathies, unspecified ankle and foot

M11.88 Other specified crystal arthropathies, vertebrae
M11.89 Other specified crystal arthropathies, multiple sites

M11.9 Crystal arthropathy, unspecified

✓4ᵗʰ M12 Other and unspecified arthropathy
    EXCLUDES 1 arthrosis (M15-M19)
        cricoarytenoid arthropathy (J38.7)

✓5ᵗʰ M12.Ø Chronic postrheumatic arthropathy [Jaccoud]
M12.ØØ Chronic postrheumatic arthropathy [Jaccoud], unspecified site

✓6ᵗʰ M12.Ø1 Chronic postrheumatic arthropathy [Jaccoud], shoulder
    M12.Ø11 Chronic postrheumatic arthropathy [Jaccoud], right shoulder
    M12.Ø12 Chronic postrheumatic arthropathy [Jaccoud], left shoulder
    M12.Ø19 Chronic postrheumatic arthropathy [Jaccoud], unspecified shoulder

✓6ᵗʰ M12.Ø2 Chronic postrheumatic arthropathy [Jaccoud], elbow
    M12.Ø21 Chronic postrheumatic arthropathy [Jaccoud], right elbow
    M12.Ø22 Chronic postrheumatic arthropathy [Jaccoud], left elbow
    M12.Ø29 Chronic postrheumatic arthropathy [Jaccoud], unspecified elbow

✓6ᵗʰ M12.Ø3 Chronic postrheumatic arthropathy [Jaccoud], wrist
    M12.Ø31 Chronic postrheumatic arthropathy [Jaccoud], right wrist
    M12.Ø32 Chronic postrheumatic arthropathy [Jaccoud], left wrist
    M12.Ø39 Chronic postrheumatic arthropathy [Jaccoud], unspecified wrist

✓6ᵗʰ M12.Ø4 Chronic postrheumatic arthropathy [Jaccoud], hand
    M12.Ø41 Chronic postrheumatic arthropathy [Jaccoud], right hand
    M12.Ø42 Chronic postrheumatic arthropathy [Jaccoud], left hand
    M12.Ø49 Chronic postrheumatic arthropathy [Jaccoud], unspecified hand

✓6ᵗʰ M12.Ø5 Chronic postrheumatic arthropathy [Jaccoud], hip
    M12.Ø51 Chronic postrheumatic arthropathy [Jaccoud], right hip
    M12.Ø52 Chronic postrheumatic arthropathy [Jaccoud], left hip

EXCLUDES 1 Not coded here   EXCLUDES 2 Not included here   N Newborn Age: 0   P Pediatric Age: 0-17   M Maternity Age: 12-55   A Adult Age: 15-124

684   ICD-10-CM 2016

M12.059   **Chronic postrheumatic arthropathy [Jaccoud], unspecified hip**

✓6ᵗʰ   M12.06   Chronic postrheumatic arthropathy [Jaccoud], knee

M12.061   **Chronic postrheumatic arthropathy [Jaccoud], right knee**

M12.062   **Chronic postrheumatic arthropathy [Jaccoud], left knee**

M12.069   **Chronic postrheumatic arthropathy [Jaccoud], unspecified knee**

✓6ᵗʰ   M12.07   Chronic postrheumatic arthropathy [Jaccoud], ankle and foot

M12.071   **Chronic postrheumatic arthropathy [Jaccoud], right ankle and foot**

M12.072   **Chronic postrheumatic arthropathy [Jaccoud], left ankle and foot**

M12.079   **Chronic postrheumatic arthropathy [Jaccoud], unspecified ankle and foot**

M12.08   **Chronic postrheumatic arthropathy [Jaccoud], other specified site**

Chronic postrheumatic arthropathy [Jaccoud], vertebrae

M12.09   **Chronic postrheumatic arthropathy [Jaccoud], multiple sites**

✓5ᵗʰ   **M12.1   Kaschin-Beck disease**

Osteochondroarthrosis deformans endemica

M12.10   **Kaschin-Beck disease, unspecified site**

✓6ᵗʰ   M12.11   **Kaschin-Beck disease, shoulder**

M12.111   **Kaschin-Beck disease, right shoulder**

M12.112   **Kaschin-Beck disease, left shoulder**

M12.119   **Kaschin-Beck disease, unspecified shoulder**

✓6ᵗʰ   M12.12   **Kaschin-Beck disease, elbow**

M12.121   **Kaschin-Beck disease, right elbow**

M12.122   **Kaschin-Beck disease, left elbow**

M12.129   **Kaschin-Beck disease, unspecified elbow**

✓6ᵗʰ   M12.13   **Kaschin-Beck disease, wrist**

M12.131   **Kaschin-Beck disease, right wrist**

M12.132   **Kaschin-Beck disease, left wrist**

M12.139   **Kaschin-Beck disease, unspecified wrist**

✓6ᵗʰ   M12.14   **Kaschin-Beck disease, hand**

M12.141   **Kaschin-Beck disease, right hand**

M12.142   **Kaschin-Beck disease, left hand**

M12.149   **Kaschin-Beck disease, unspecified hand**

✓6ᵗʰ   M12.15   **Kaschin-Beck disease, hip**

M12.151   **Kaschin-Beck disease, right hip**

M12.152   **Kaschin-Beck disease, left hip**

M12.159   **Kaschin-Beck disease, unspecified hip**

✓6ᵗʰ   M12.16   **Kaschin-Beck disease, knee**

M12.161   **Kaschin-Beck disease, right knee**

M12.162   **Kaschin-Beck disease, left knee**

M12.169   **Kaschin-Beck disease, unspecified knee**

✓6ᵗʰ   M12.17   **Kaschin-Beck disease, ankle and foot**

M12.171   **Kaschin-Beck disease, right ankle and foot**

M12.172   **Kaschin-Beck disease, left ankle and foot**

M12.179   **Kaschin-Beck disease, unspecified ankle and foot**

M12.18   **Kaschin-Beck disease, vertebrae**

M12.19   **Kaschin-Beck disease, multiple sites**

✓5ᵗʰ   **M12.2   Villonodular synovitis (pigmented)**

M12.20   **Villonodular synovitis (pigmented), unspecified site**

✓6ᵗʰ   M12.21   Villonodular synovitis (pigmented), shoulder

M12.211   **Villonodular synovitis (pigmented), right shoulder**

M12.212   **Villonodular synovitis (pigmented), left shoulder**

M12.219   **Villonodular synovitis (pigmented), unspecified shoulder**

✓6ᵗʰ   M12.22   Villonodular synovitis (pigmented), elbow

M12.221   **Villonodular synovitis (pigmented), right elbow**

M12.222   **Villonodular synovitis (pigmented), left elbow**

M12.229   **Villonodular synovitis (pigmented), unspecified elbow**

✓6ᵗʰ   M12.23   Villonodular synovitis (pigmented), wrist

M12.231   **Villonodular synovitis (pigmented), right wrist**

M12.232   **Villonodular synovitis (pigmented), left wrist**

M12.239   **Villonodular synovitis (pigmented), unspecified wrist**

✓6ᵗʰ   M12.24   Villonodular synovitis (pigmented), hand

M12.241   **Villonodular synovitis (pigmented), right hand**

M12.242   **Villonodular synovitis (pigmented), left hand**

M12.249   **Villonodular synovitis (pigmented), unspecified hand**

✓6ᵗʰ   M12.25   Villonodular synovitis (pigmented), hip

M12.251   **Villonodular synovitis (pigmented), right hip**

M12.252   **Villonodular synovitis (pigmented), left hip**

M12.259   **Villonodular synovitis (pigmented), unspecified hip**

✓6ᵗʰ   M12.26   Villonodular synovitis (pigmented), knee

M12.261   **Villonodular synovitis (pigmented), right knee**

M12.262   **Villonodular synovitis (pigmented), left knee**

M12.269   **Villonodular synovitis (pigmented), unspecified knee**

✓6ᵗʰ   M12.27   Villonodular synovitis (pigmented), ankle and foot

M12.271   **Villonodular synovitis (pigmented), right ankle and foot**

M12.272   **Villonodular synovitis (pigmented), left ankle and foot**

M12.279   **Villonodular synovitis (pigmented), unspecified ankle and foot**

M12.28   **Villonodular synovitis (pigmented), other specified site**

Villonodular synovitis (pigmented), vertebrae

M12.29   **Villonodular synovitis (pigmented), multiple sites**

✓5ᵗʰ   **M12.3   Palindromic rheumatism**

M12.30   **Palindromic rheumatism, unspecified site**

✓6ᵗʰ   M12.31   Palindromic rheumatism, shoulder

M12.311   **Palindromic rheumatism, right shoulder**

M12.312   **Palindromic rheumatism, left shoulder**

M12.319   **Palindromic rheumatism, unspecified shoulder**

✓6ᵗʰ   M12.32   Palindromic rheumatism, elbow

M12.321   **Palindromic rheumatism, right elbow**

M12.322   **Palindromic rheumatism, left elbow**

M12.329   **Palindromic rheumatism, unspecified elbow**

✓6ᵗʰ   M12.33   Palindromic rheumatism, wrist

M12.331   **Palindromic rheumatism, right wrist**

M12.332   **Palindromic rheumatism, left wrist**

M12.339   **Palindromic rheumatism, unspecified wrist**

✓6ᵗʰ   M12.34   Palindromic rheumatism, hand

M12.341   **Palindromic rheumatism, right hand**

M12.342   **Palindromic rheumatism, left hand**

M12.349   **Palindromic rheumatism, unspecified hand**

✓6ᵗʰ   M12.35   Palindromic rheumatism, hip

M12.351   **Palindromic rheumatism, right hip**

M12.352   **Palindromic rheumatism, left hip**

M12.359   **Palindromic rheumatism, unspecified hip**

✓6ᵗʰ   M12.36   Palindromic rheumatism, knee

M12.361   **Palindromic rheumatism, right knee**

M12.362   **Palindromic rheumatism, left knee**

M12.369   **Palindromic rheumatism, unspecified knee**

✓6ᵗʰ   M12.37   Palindromic rheumatism, ankle and foot

M12.371   **Palindromic rheumatism, right ankle and foot**

M12.372   **Palindromic rheumatism, left ankle and foot**

☑ Additional Character Required   ✓x7ᵗʰ Placeholder Alert   Unspecified Dx   Other Specified Dx   Manifestation   ►◄ Revised Text   ● New Code   ▲ Revised Code Title

M12.379   **Palindromic rheumatism, unspecified ankle and foot**

M12.38   **Palindromic rheumatism, other specified site**
Palindromic rheumatism, vertebrae

M12.39   **Palindromic rheumatism,** multiple sites

✓5th M12.4   **Intermittent hydrarthrosis**

M12.40   **Intermittent hydrarthrosis, unspecified site**

✓6th M12.41   **Intermittent hydrarthrosis,** shoulder

M12.411   **Intermittent hydrarthrosis,** right shoulder
M12.412   **Intermittent hydrarthrosis,** left shoulder
M12.419   **Intermittent hydrarthrosis, unspecified shoulder**

✓6th M12.42   **Intermittent hydrarthrosis,** elbow

M12.421   **Intermittent hydrarthrosis,** right elbow
M12.422   **Intermittent hydrarthrosis,** left elbow
M12.429   **Intermittent hydrarthrosis, unspecified elbow**

✓6th M12.43   **Intermittent hydrarthrosis,** wrist

M12.431   **Intermittent hydrarthrosis,** right wrist
M12.432   **Intermittent hydrarthrosis,** left wrist
M12.439   **Intermittent hydrarthrosis, unspecified wrist**

✓6th M12.44   **Intermittent hydrarthrosis,** hand

M12.441   **Intermittent hydrarthrosis,** right hand
M12.442   **Intermittent hydrarthrosis,** left hand
M12.449   **Intermittent hydrarthrosis, unspecified hand**

✓6th M12.45   **Intermittent hydrarthrosis,** hip

M12.451   **Intermittent hydrarthrosis,** right hip
M12.452   **Intermittent hydrarthrosis,** left hip
M12.459   **Intermittent hydrarthrosis, unspecified hip**

✓6th M12.46   **Intermittent hydrarthrosis,** knee

M12.461   **Intermittent hydrarthrosis,** right knee
M12.462   **Intermittent hydrarthrosis,** left knee
M12.469   **Intermittent hydrarthrosis, unspecified knee**

✓6th M12.47   **Intermittent hydrarthrosis,** ankle and foot

M12.471   **Intermittent hydrarthrosis,** right ankle and foot
M12.472   **Intermittent hydrarthrosis,** left ankle and foot
M12.479   **Intermittent hydrarthrosis, unspecified ankle and foot**

M12.48   **Intermittent hydrarthrosis, other site**

M12.49   **Intermittent hydrarthrosis,** multiple sites

✓5th M12.5   **Traumatic arthropathy**

EXCLUDES 1   current injury–see Alphabetic Index
post-traumatic osteoarthritis NOS (M19.1-)
post-traumatic osteoarthritis of first carpometacarpal joint (M18.2-M18.3)
post-traumatic osteoarthritis of hip (M16.4-M16.5)
post-traumatic osteoarthritis of knee (M17.2-M17.3)
post-traumatic osteoarthritis of other single joints (M19.1-)

AHA: 2015, 1Q, 17

M12.50   **Traumatic arthropathy, unspecified site**

✓6th M12.51   **Traumatic arthropathy,** shoulder

M12.511   **Traumatic arthropathy,** right shoulder
M12.512   **Traumatic arthropathy,** left shoulder
M12.519   **Traumatic arthropathy, unspecified shoulder**

✓6th M12.52   **Traumatic arthropathy,** elbow

M12.521   **Traumatic arthropathy,** right elbow
M12.522   **Traumatic arthropathy,** left elbow
M12.529   **Traumatic arthropathy, unspecified elbow**

✓6th M12.53   **Traumatic arthropathy,** wrist

M12.531   **Traumatic arthropathy,** right wrist
M12.532   **Traumatic arthropathy,** left wrist
M12.539   **Traumatic arthropathy, unspecified wrist**

✓6th M12.54   **Traumatic arthropathy,** hand

M12.541   **Traumatic arthropathy,** right hand
M12.542   **Traumatic arthropathy,** left hand
M12.549   **Traumatic arthropathy, unspecified hand**

✓6th M12.55   **Traumatic arthropathy,** hip

M12.551   **Traumatic arthropathy,** right hip
M12.552   **Traumatic arthropathy,** left hip
M12.559   **Traumatic arthropathy, unspecified hip**

✓6th M12.56   **Traumatic arthropathy,** knee

M12.561   **Traumatic arthropathy,** right knee
M12.562   **Traumatic arthropathy,** left knee
M12.569   **Traumatic arthropathy, unspecified knee**

✓6th M12.57   **Traumatic arthropathy,** ankle and foot

M12.571   **Traumatic arthropathy,** right ankle and foot
M12.572   **Traumatic arthropathy,** left ankle and foot
M12.579   **Traumatic arthropathy, unspecified ankle and foot**

M12.58   **Traumatic arthropathy, other specified site**
Traumatic arthropathy, vertebrae

M12.59   **Traumatic arthropathy,** multiple sites

✓5th M12.8   **Other specific arthropathies, not elsewhere classified**
Transient arthropathy

M12.80   **Other specific arthropathies, not elsewhere classified, unspecified site**

✓6th M12.81   **Other specific arthropathies, not elsewhere classified,** shoulder

M12.811   **Other specific arthropathies, not elsewhere classified,** right shoulder
M12.812   **Other specific arthropathies, not elsewhere classified,** left shoulder
M12.819   **Other specific arthropathies, not elsewhere classified, unspecified shoulder**

✓6th M12.82   **Other specific arthropathies, not elsewhere classified,** elbow

M12.821   **Other specific arthropathies, not elsewhere classified,** right elbow
M12.822   **Other specific arthropathies, not elsewhere classified,** left elbow
M12.829   **Other specific arthropathies, not elsewhere classified, unspecified elbow**

✓6th M12.83   **Other specific arthropathies, not elsewhere classified,** wrist

M12.831   **Other specific arthropathies, not elsewhere classified,** right wrist
M12.832   **Other specific arthropathies, not elsewhere classified,** left wrist
M12.839   **Other specific arthropathies, not elsewhere classified, unspecified wrist**

✓6th M12.84   **Other specific arthropathies, not elsewhere classified,** hand

M12.841   **Other specific arthropathies, not elsewhere classified,** right hand
M12.842   **Other specific arthropathies, not elsewhere classified,** left hand
M12.849   **Other specific arthropathies, not elsewhere classified, unspecified hand**

✓6th M12.85   **Other specific arthropathies, not elsewhere classified,** hip

M12.851   **Other specific arthropathies, not elsewhere classified,** right hip
M12.852   **Other specific arthropathies, not elsewhere classified,** left hip
M12.859   **Other specific arthropathies, not elsewhere classified, unspecified hip**

✓6th M12.86   **Other specific arthropathies, not elsewhere classified,** knee

M12.861   **Other specific arthropathies, not elsewhere classified,** right knee
M12.862   **Other specific arthropathies, not elsewhere classified,** left knee
M12.869   **Other specific arthropathies, not elsewhere classified, unspecified knee**

✓6th M12.87   **Other specific arthropathies, not elsewhere classified,** ankle and foot

M12.871   **Other specific arthropathies, not elsewhere classified,** right ankle and foot
M12.872   **Other specific arthropathies, not elsewhere classified,** left ankle and foot

EXCLUDES 1 Not coded here   EXCLUDES 2 Not included here   N Newborn Age: 0   P Pediatric Age: 0-17   M Maternity Age: 12-55   A Adult Age: 15-124

686   ICD-10-CM 2016

M12.879 Other specific arthropathies, not elsewhere classified, unspecified ankle and foot

M12.88 Other specific arthropathies, not elsewhere classified, other specified site
Other specific arthropathies, not elsewhere classified, vertebrae

M12.89 Other specific arthropathies, not elsewhere classified, multiple sites

M12.9 Arthropathy, unspecified

√4ᵗʰ **M13 Other arthritis**
EXCLUDES 1   arthrosis (M15-M19)
osteoarthritis (M15-M19)

M13.0 Polyarthritis, unspecified

√5ᵗʰ M13.1 Monoarthritis, not elsewhere classified

M13.10 Monoarthritis, not elsewhere classified, unspecified site

√6ᵗʰ M13.11 Monoarthritis, not elsewhere classified, shoulder
M13.111 Monoarthritis, not elsewhere classified, right shoulder
M13.112 Monoarthritis, not elsewhere classified, left shoulder
M13.119 Monoarthritis, not elsewhere classified, unspecified shoulder

√6ᵗʰ M13.12 Monoarthritis, not elsewhere classified, elbow
M13.121 Monoarthritis, not elsewhere classified, right elbow
M13.122 Monoarthritis, not elsewhere classified, left elbow
M13.129 Monoarthritis, not elsewhere classified, unspecified elbow

√6ᵗʰ M13.13 Monoarthritis, not elsewhere classified, wrist
M13.131 Monoarthritis, not elsewhere classified, right wrist
M13.132 Monoarthritis, not elsewhere classified, left wrist
M13.139 Monoarthritis, not elsewhere classified, unspecified wrist

√6ᵗʰ M13.14 Monoarthritis, not elsewhere classified, hand
M13.141 Monoarthritis, not elsewhere classified, right hand
M13.142 Monoarthritis, not elsewhere classified, left hand
M13.149 Monoarthritis, not elsewhere classified, unspecified hand

√6ᵗʰ M13.15 Monoarthritis, not elsewhere classified, hip
M13.151 Monoarthritis, not elsewhere classified, right hip
M13.152 Monoarthritis, not elsewhere classified, left hip
M13.159 Monoarthritis, not elsewhere classified, unspecified hip

√6ᵗʰ M13.16 Monoarthritis, not elsewhere classified, knee
M13.161 Monoarthritis, not elsewhere classified, right knee
M13.162 Monoarthritis, not elsewhere classified, left knee
M13.169 Monoarthritis, not elsewhere classified, unspecified knee

√6ᵗʰ M13.17 Monoarthritis, not elsewhere classified, ankle and foot
M13.171 Monoarthritis, not elsewhere classified, right ankle and foot
M13.172 Monoarthritis, not elsewhere classified, left ankle and foot
M13.179 Monoarthritis, not elsewhere classified, unspecified ankle and foot

√5ᵗʰ M13.8 Other specified arthritis
Allergic arthritis
EXCLUDES 1   osteoarthritis (M15-M19)

M13.80 Other specified arthritis, unspecified site

√6ᵗʰ M13.81 Other specified arthritis, shoulder
M13.811 Other specified arthritis, right shoulder
M13.812 Other specified arthritis, left shoulder
M13.819 Other specified arthritis, unspecified shoulder

√6ᵗʰ M13.82 Other specified arthritis, elbow
M13.821 Other specified arthritis, right elbow
M13.822 Other specified arthritis, left elbow
M13.829 Other specified arthritis, unspecified elbow

√6ᵗʰ M13.83 Other specified arthritis, wrist
M13.831 Other specified arthritis, right wrist
M13.832 Other specified arthritis, left wrist
M13.839 Other specified arthritis, unspecified wrist

√6ᵗʰ M13.84 Other specified arthritis, hand
M13.841 Other specified arthritis, right hand
M13.842 Other specified arthritis, left hand
M13.849 Other specified arthritis, unspecified hand

√6ᵗʰ M13.85 Other specified arthritis, hip
M13.851 Other specified arthritis, right hip
M13.852 Other specified arthritis, left hip
M13.859 Other specified arthritis, unspecified hip

√6ᵗʰ M13.86 Other specified arthritis, knee
M13.861 Other specified arthritis, right knee
M13.862 Other specified arthritis, left knee
M13.869 Other specified arthritis, unspecified knee

√6ᵗʰ M13.87 Other specified arthritis, ankle and foot
M13.871 Other specified arthritis, right ankle and foot
M13.872 Other specified arthritis, left ankle and foot
M13.879 Other specified arthritis, unspecified ankle and foot

M13.88 Other specified arthritis, other site

M13.89 Other specified arthritis, multiple sites

√4ᵗʰ **M14 Arthropathies in other diseases classified elsewhere**
EXCLUDES 1   arthropathy in:
diabetes mellitus (E08-E13 with . 61-)
hematological disorders (M36.2-M36.3)
hypersensitivity reactions (M36.4)
neoplastic disease (M36.1)
neurosyphillis (A52.16)
sarcoidosis (D86.86)
enteropathic arthropathies (M07.-)
juvenile psoriatic arthropathy (L40.54)
lipoid dermatoarthritis (E78.81)

√5ᵗʰ M14.6 Charcôt's joint
Neuropathic arthropathy
EXCLUDES 1   Charcôt's joint in diabetes mellitus (E08-E13 with .610)
Charcôt's joint in tabes dorsalis (A52.16)

M14.60 Charcôt's joint, unspecified site

√6ᵗʰ M14.61 Charcôt's joint, shoulder
M14.611 Charcôt's joint, right shoulder
M14.612 Charcôt's joint, left shoulder
M14.619 Charcôt's joint, unspecified shoulder

√6ᵗʰ M14.62 Charcôt's joint, elbow
M14.621 Charcôt's joint, right elbow
M14.622 Charcôt's joint, left elbow
M14.629 Charcôt's joint, unspecified elbow

√6ᵗʰ M14.63 Charcôt's joint, wrist
M14.631 Charcôt's joint, right wrist
M14.632 Charcôt's joint, left wrist
M14.639 Charcôt's joint, unspecified wrist

√6ᵗʰ M14.64 Charcôt's joint, hand
M14.641 Charcôt's joint, right hand
M14.642 Charcôt's joint, left hand
M14.649 Charcôt's joint, unspecified hand

√6ᵗʰ M14.65 Charcôt's joint, hip
M14.651 Charcôt's joint, right hip
M14.652 Charcôt's joint, left hip
M14.659 Charcôt's joint, unspecified hip

√6ᵗʰ M14.66 Charcôt's joint, knee
M14.661 Charcôt's joint, right knee
M14.662 Charcôt's joint, left knee
M14.669 Charcôt's joint, unspecified knee

√6ᵗʰ M14.67 Charcôt's joint, ankle and foot
M14.671 Charcôt's joint, right ankle and foot
M14.672 Charcôt's joint, left ankle and foot

☑ Additional Character Required   √x7ᵗʰ Placeholder Alert   Unspecified Dx   Other Specified Dx   Manifestation   ►◄ Revised Text   ● New Code   ▲ Revised Code Title

M14.679   Charcôt's joint, unspecified ankle and foot

M14.68   Charcôt's joint, vertebrae

M14.69   Charcôt's joint, multiple sites

✓5ᵗʰ M14.8   Arthropathies in other specified diseases classified elsewhere

Code first underlying disease, such as:
amyloidosis (E85.-)
erythema multiforme (L51.-)
erythema nodosum (L52)
hemochromatosis (E83.11-)
hyperparathyroidism (E21.-)
hypothyroidism (E00-E03)
sickle-cell disorders (D57.-)
thyrotoxicosis [hyperthyroidism] (E05.-)
Whipple's disease (K90.81)

M14.80   *Arthropathies in other specified diseases classified elsewhere, unspecified site*

✓6ᵗʰ M14.81   **Arthropathies in other specified diseases classified elsewhere, shoulder**

M14.811   *Arthropathies in other specified diseases classified elsewhere, right shoulder*

M14.812   *Arthropathies in other specified diseases classified elsewhere, left shoulder*

M14.819   *Arthropathies in other specified diseases classified elsewhere, unspecified shoulder*

✓6ᵗʰ M14.82   **Arthropathies in other specified diseases classified elsewhere, elbow**

M14.821   *Arthropathies in other specified diseases classified elsewhere, right elbow*

M14.822   *Arthropathies in other specified diseases classified elsewhere, left elbow*

M14.829   *Arthropathies in other specified diseases classified elsewhere, unspecified elbow*

✓6ᵗʰ M14.83   **Arthropathies in other specified diseases classified elsewhere, wrist**

M14.831   *Arthropathies in other specified diseases classified elsewhere, right wrist*

M14.832   *Arthropathies in other specified diseases classified elsewhere, left wrist*

M14.839   *Arthropathies in other specified diseases classified elsewhere, unspecified wrist*

✓6ᵗʰ M14.84   **Arthropathies in other specified diseases classified elsewhere, hand**

M14.841   *Arthropathies in other specified diseases classified elsewhere, right hand*

M14.842   *Arthropathies in other specified diseases classified elsewhere, left hand*

M14.849   *Arthropathies in other specified diseases classified elsewhere, unspecified hand*

✓6ᵗʰ M14.85   **Arthropathies in other specified diseases classified elsewhere, hip**

M14.851   *Arthropathies in other specified diseases classified elsewhere, right hip*

M14.852   *Arthropathies in other specified diseases classified elsewhere, left hip*

M14.859   *Arthropathies in other specified diseases classified elsewhere, unspecified hip*

✓6ᵗʰ M14.86   **Arthropathies in other specified diseases classified elsewhere, knee**

M14.861   *Arthropathies in other specified diseases classified elsewhere, right knee*

M14.862   *Arthropathies in other specified diseases classified elsewhere, left knee*

M14.869   *Arthropathies in other specified diseases classified elsewhere, unspecified knee*

✓6ᵗʰ M14.87   **Arthropathies in other specified diseases classified elsewhere, ankle and foot**

M14.871   *Arthropathies in other specified diseases classified elsewhere, right ankle and foot*

M14.872   *Arthropathies in other specified diseases classified elsewhere, left ankle and foot*

M14.879   *Arthropathies in other specified diseases classified elsewhere, unspecified ankle and foot*

M14.88   *Arthropathies in other specified diseases classified elsewhere, vertebrae*

M14.89   *Arthropathies in other specified diseases classified elsewhere, multiple sites*

Osteoarthritis (M15-M19)

EXCLUDES 2   *osteoarthritis of spine (M47.-)*

✓4ᵗʰ M15   **Polyosteoarthritis**

INCLUDES   arthritis of multiple sites

EXCLUDES 1   *bilateral involvement of single joint (M16-M19)*

M15.0   **Primary generalized (osteo)arthritis**

M15.1   **Heberden's nodes (with arthropathy)**
Interphalangeal distal osteoarthritis

M15.2   **Bouchard's nodes (with arthropathy)**
Juxtaphalangeal distal osteoarthritis

M15.3   **Secondary multiple arthritis**
Post-traumatic polyosteoarthritis

M15.4   **Erosive (osteo)arthritis**

M15.8   **Other polyosteoarthritis**

M15.9   **Polyosteoarthritis, unspecified**
Generalized osteoarthritis NOS

✓4ᵗʰ M16   **Osteoarthritis of hip**

M16.0   **Bilateral primary osteoarthritis of hip**

✓5ᵗʰ M16.1   **Unilateral primary osteoarthritis of hip**
Primary osteoarthritis of hip NOS

M16.10   **Unilateral primary osteoarthritis, unspecified hip**

M16.11   **Unilateral primary osteoarthritis, right hip**

M16.12   **Unilateral primary osteoarthritis, left hip**

M16.2   **Bilateral osteoarthritis resulting from hip dysplasia**

✓5ᵗʰ M16.3   **Unilateral osteoarthritis resulting from hip dysplasia**
Dysplastic osteoarthritis of hip NOS

M16.30   **Unilateral osteoarthritis resulting from hip dysplasia, unspecified hip**

M16.31   **Unilateral osteoarthritis resulting from hip dysplasia, right hip**

M16.32   **Unilateral osteoarthritis resulting from hip dysplasia, left hip**

M16.4   **Bilateral post-traumatic osteoarthritis of hip**

✓5ᵗʰ M16.5   **Unilateral post-traumatic osteoarthritis of hip**
Post-traumatic osteoarthritis of hip NOS

M16.50   **Unilateral post-traumatic osteoarthritis, unspecified hip**

M16.51   **Unilateral post-traumatic osteoarthritis, right hip**

M16.52   **Unilateral post-traumatic osteoarthritis, left hip**

M16.6   **Other bilateral secondary osteoarthritis of hip**

M16.7   **Other unilateral secondary osteoarthritis of hip**
Secondary osteoarthritis of hip NOS

M16.9   **Osteoarthritis of hip, unspecified**

✓4ᵗʰ M17   **Osteoarthritis of knee**

M17.0   **Bilateral primary osteoarthritis of knee**

✓5ᵗʰ M17.1   **Unilateral primary osteoarthritis of knee**
Primary osteoarthritis of knee NOS

M17.10   **Unilateral primary osteoarthritis, unspecified knee**

M17.11   **Unilateral primary osteoarthritis, right knee**

M17.12   **Unilateral primary osteoarthritis, left knee**

M17.2   **Bilateral post-traumatic osteoarthritis of knee**

✓5ᵗʰ M17.3   **Unilateral post-traumatic osteoarthritis of knee**
Post-traumatic osteoarthritis of knee NOS

M17.30   **Unilateral post-traumatic osteoarthritis, unspecified knee**

M17.31   **Unilateral post-traumatic osteoarthritis, right knee**

M17.32   **Unilateral post-traumatic osteoarthritis, left knee**

M17.4   **Other bilateral secondary osteoarthritis of knee**

M17.5   **Other unilateral secondary osteoarthritis of knee**
Secondary osteoarthritis of knee NOS

M17.9   **Osteoarthritis of knee, unspecified**

✓4ᵗʰ M18   **Osteoarthritis of first carpometacarpal joint**

M18.0   **Bilateral primary osteoarthritis of first carpometacarpal joints**

✓5ᵗʰ M18.1   **Unilateral primary osteoarthritis of first carpometacarpal joint**
Primary osteoarthritis of first carpometacarpal joint NOS

M18.10   **Unilateral primary osteoarthritis of first carpometacarpal joint, unspecified hand**

M18.11   **Unilateral primary osteoarthritis of first carpometacarpal joint, right hand**

M18.12   **Unilateral primary osteoarthritis of first carpometacarpal joint, left hand**

EXCLUDES 1 Not coded here   EXCLUDES 2 Not included here   N Newborn Age: 0   P Pediatric Age: 0-17   M Maternity Age: 12-55   A Adult Age: 15-124

688   ICD-10-CM 2016

M18.2 Bilateral post-traumatic osteoarthritis of first carpometacarpal joints

✓5ᵗʰ M18.3 Unilateral post-traumatic osteoarthritis of first carpometacarpal joint
  Post-traumatic osteoarthritis of first carpometacarpal joint NOS

    M18.30 Unilateral post-traumatic osteoarthritis of first carpometacarpal joint, unspecified hand

    M18.31 Unilateral post-traumatic osteoarthritis of first carpometacarpal joint, right hand

    M18.32 Unilateral post-traumatic osteoarthritis of first carpometacarpal joint, left hand

M18.4 Other bilateral secondary osteoarthritis of first carpometacarpal joints

✓5ᵗʰ M18.5 Other unilateral secondary osteoarthritis of first carpometacarpal joint
  Secondary osteoarthritis of first carpometacarpal joint NOS

    M18.50 Other unilateral secondary osteoarthritis of first carpometacarpal joint, unspecified hand

    M18.51 Other unilateral secondary osteoarthritis of first carpometacarpal joint, right hand

    M18.52 Other unilateral secondary osteoarthritis of first carpometacarpal joint, left hand

M18.9 Osteoarthritis of first carpometacarpal joint, unspecified

✓4ᵗʰ M19 Other and unspecified osteoarthritis
    EXCLUDES 1   polyarthritis (M15.-)
    EXCLUDES 2   arthrosis of spine (M47.-)
              hallux rigidus (M20.2)
              osteoarthritis of spine (M47.-)

✓5ᵗʰ M19.0 Primary osteoarthritis of other joints

  ✓6ᵗʰ M19.01 Primary osteoarthritis, shoulder
    M19.011 Primary osteoarthritis, right shoulder
    M19.012 Primary osteoarthritis, left shoulder
    M19.019 Primary osteoarthritis, unspecified shoulder

  ✓6ᵗʰ M19.02 Primary osteoarthritis, elbow
    M19.021 Primary osteoarthritis, right elbow
    M19.022 Primary osteoarthritis, left elbow
    M19.029 Primary osteoarthritis, unspecified elbow

  ✓6ᵗʰ M19.03 Primary osteoarthritis, wrist
    M19.031 Primary osteoarthritis, right wrist
    M19.032 Primary osteoarthritis, left wrist
    M19.039 Primary osteoarthritis, unspecified wrist

  ✓6ᵗʰ M19.04 Primary osteoarthritis, hand
    EXCLUDES 2   primary osteoarthritis of first carpometacarpal joint (M18.0-, M18.1-)
    M19.041 Primary osteoarthritis, right hand
    M19.042 Primary osteoarthritis, left hand
    M19.049 Primary osteoarthritis, unspecified hand

  ✓6ᵗʰ M19.07 Primary osteoarthritis ankle and foot
    M19.071 Primary osteoarthritis, right ankle and foot
    M19.072 Primary osteoarthritis, left ankle and foot
    M19.079 Primary osteoarthritis, unspecified ankle and foot

✓5ᵗʰ M19.1 Post-traumatic osteoarthritis of other joints

  ✓6ᵗʰ M19.11 Post-traumatic osteoarthritis, shoulder
    M19.111 Post-traumatic osteoarthritis, right shoulder
    M19.112 Post-traumatic osteoarthritis, left shoulder
    M19.119 Post-traumatic osteoarthritis, unspecified shoulder

  ✓6ᵗʰ M19.12 Post-traumatic osteoarthritis, elbow
    M19.121 Post-traumatic osteoarthritis, right elbow
    M19.122 Post-traumatic osteoarthritis, left elbow
    M19.129 Post-traumatic osteoarthritis, unspecified elbow

  ✓6ᵗʰ M19.13 Post-traumatic osteoarthritis, wrist
    M19.131 Post-traumatic osteoarthritis, right wrist
    M19.132 Post-traumatic osteoarthritis, left wrist
    M19.139 Post-traumatic osteoarthritis, unspecified wrist

  ✓6ᵗʰ M19.14 Post-traumatic osteoarthritis, hand
    EXCLUDES 2   post-traumatic osteoarthritis of first carpometacarpal joint (M18.2-, M18.3-)
    M19.141 Post-traumatic osteoarthritis, right hand
    M19.142 Post-traumatic osteoarthritis, left hand
    M19.149 Post-traumatic osteoarthritis, unspecified hand

  ✓6ᵗʰ M19.17 Post-traumatic osteoarthritis, ankle and foot
    M19.171 Post-traumatic osteoarthritis, right ankle and foot
    M19.172 Post-traumatic osteoarthritis, left ankle and foot
    M19.179 Post-traumatic osteoarthritis, unspecified ankle and foot

✓5ᵗʰ M19.2 Secondary osteoarthritis of other joints

  ✓6ᵗʰ M19.21 Secondary osteoarthritis, shoulder
    M19.211 Secondary osteoarthritis, right shoulder
    M19.212 Secondary osteoarthritis, left shoulder
    M19.219 Secondary osteoarthritis, unspecified shoulder

  ✓6ᵗʰ M19.22 Secondary osteoarthritis, elbow
    M19.221 Secondary osteoarthritis, right elbow
    M19.222 Secondary osteoarthritis, left elbow
    M19.229 Secondary osteoarthritis, unspecified elbow

  ✓6ᵗʰ M19.23 Secondary osteoarthritis, wrist
    M19.231 Secondary osteoarthritis, right wrist
    M19.232 Secondary osteoarthritis, left wrist
    M19.239 Secondary osteoarthritis, unspecified wrist

  ✓6ᵗʰ M19.24 Secondary osteoarthritis, hand
    M19.241 Secondary osteoarthritis, right hand
    M19.242 Secondary osteoarthritis, left hand
    M19.249 Secondary osteoarthritis, unspecified hand

  ✓6ᵗʰ M19.27 Secondary osteoarthritis, ankle and foot
    M19.271 Secondary osteoarthritis, right ankle and foot
    M19.272 Secondary osteoarthritis, left ankle and foot
    M19.279 Secondary osteoarthritis, unspecified ankle and foot

✓5ᵗʰ M19.9 Osteoarthritis, unspecified site

    M19.90 Unspecified osteoarthritis, unspecified site
      Arthrosis NOSOsteoarthritis NOS
      Arthritis NOS

    M19.91 Primary osteoarthritis, unspecified site
      Primary osteoarthritis NOS

    M19.92 Post-traumatic osteoarthritis, unspecified site
      Post-traumatic osteoarthritis NOS

    M19.93 Secondary osteoarthritis, unspecified site
      Secondary osteoarthritis NOS

Other joint disorders (M20-M25)
EXCLUDES 2   joints of the spine (M40-M54)

✓4ᵗʰ M20 Acquired deformities of fingers and toes
    EXCLUDES 1   acquired absence of fingers and toes (Z89.-)
              congenital absence of fingers and toes (Q71.3-, Q72.3-)
              congenital deformities and malformations of fingers and toes (Q66-, Q68-Q70, Q74-)

✓5ᵗʰ M20.0 Deformity of finger(s)
    EXCLUDES 1   clubbing of fingers (R68.3)
              palmar fascial fibromatosis [Dupuytren] (M72.0)
              trigger finger (M65.3)

  ✓6ᵗʰ M20.00 Unspecified deformity of finger(s)
    M20.001 Unspecified deformity of right finger(s)
    M20.002 Unspecified deformity of left finger(s)
    M20.009 Unspecified deformity of unspecified finger(s)

  ✓6ᵗʰ M20.01 Mallet finger
    M20.011 Mallet finger of right finger(s)
    M20.012 Mallet finger of left finger(s)
    M20.019 Mallet finger of unspecified finger(s)

☑ Additional Character Required   ✓x7ᵗʰ Placeholder Alert   Unspecified Dx   Other Specified Dx   Manifestation   ▶◀ Revised Text   ● New Code   ▲ Revised Code Title

ICD-10-CM 2016   **689**

M18.2–M20.019

✓6ᵗʰ **M20.02** Boutonnière deformity
     M20.021 Boutonnière deformity of right finger(s)
     M20.022 Boutonnière deformity of left finger(s)
     M20.029 Boutonnière deformity of unspecified finger(s)

✓6ᵗʰ **M20.03** Swan-neck deformity
     M20.031 Swan-neck deformity of right finger(s)
     M20.032 Swan-neck deformity of left finger(s)
     M20.039 Swan-neck deformity of unspecified finger(s)

✓6ᵗʰ **M20.09** Other deformity of finger(s)
     M20.091 Other deformity of right finger(s)
     M20.092 Other deformity of left finger(s)
     M20.099 Other deformity of finger(s), unspecified finger(s)

✓6ᵗʰ **M20.1** Hallux valgus (acquired)
     Bunion
     M20.10 Hallux valgus (acquired), unspecified foot
     M20.11 Hallux valgus (acquired), right foot
     M20.12 Hallux valgus (acquired), left foot

✓5ᵗʰ **M20.2** Hallux rigidus
     M20.20 Hallux rigidus, unspecified foot
     M20.21 Hallux rigidus, right foot
     M20.22 Hallux rigidus, left foot

✓5ᵗʰ **M20.3** Hallux varus (acquired)
     M20.30 Hallux varus (acquired), unspecified foot
     M20.31 Hallux varus (acquired), right foot
     M20.32 Hallux varus (acquired), left foot

✓5ᵗʰ **M20.4** Other hammer toe(s) (acquired)
     M20.40 Other hammer toe(s) (acquired), unspecified foot
     M20.41 Other hammer toe(s) (acquired), right foot
     M20.42 Other hammer toe(s) (acquired), left foot

✓5ᵗʰ **M20.5** Other deformities of toe(s) (acquired)
   ✓6ᵗʰ **M20.5X** Other deformities of toe(s) (acquired)
     M20.5X1 Other deformities of toe(s) (acquired), right foot
     M20.5X2 Other deformities of toe(s) (acquired), left foot
     M20.5X9 Other deformities of toe(s) (acquired), unspecified foot

✓5ᵗʰ **M20.6** Acquired deformities of toe(s), unspecified
     M20.60 Acquired deformities of toe(s), unspecified, unspecified foot
     M20.61 Acquired deformities of toe(s), unspecified, right foot
     M20.62 Acquired deformities of toe(s), unspecified, left foot

✓4ᵗʰ **M21 Other acquired deformities of limbs**
   EXCLUDES 1 acquired absence of limb (Z89.-)
     congenital absence of limbs (Q71-Q73)
     congenital deformities and malformations of limbs (Q65-Q66, Q68-Q74)
   EXCLUDES 2 acquired deformities of fingers or toes (M20.-)
     coxa plana (M91.2)

✓5ᵗʰ **M21.0** Valgus deformity, not elsewhere classified
   EXCLUDES 1 metatarsus valgus (Q66.6)
     talipes calcaneovalgus (Q66.4)
     M21.00 Valgus deformity, not elsewhere classified, unspecified site

   ✓6ᵗʰ **M21.02** Valgus deformity, not elsewhere classified, elbow
     Cubitus valgus
     M21.021 Valgus deformity, not elsewhere classified, right elbow
     M21.022 Valgus deformity, not elsewhere classified, left elbow
     M21.029 Valgus deformity, not elsewhere classified, unspecified elbow

   ✓6ᵗʰ **M21.05** Valgus deformity, not elsewhere classified, hip
     M21.051 Valgus deformity, not elsewhere classified, right hip
     M21.052 Valgus deformity, not elsewhere classified, left hip
     M21.059 Valgus deformity, not elsewhere classified, unspecified hip

   ✓6ᵗʰ **M21.06** Valgus deformity, not elsewhere classified, knee
     Genu valgumKnock knee
     M21.061 Valgus deformity, not elsewhere classified, right knee
     M21.062 Valgus deformity, not elsewhere classified, left knee
     M21.069 Valgus deformity, not elsewhere classified, unspecified knee

   ✓6ᵗʰ **M21.07** Valgus deformity, not elsewhere classified, ankle
     M21.071 Valgus deformity, not elsewhere classified, right ankle
     M21.072 Valgus deformity, not elsewhere classified, left ankle
     M21.079 Valgus deformity, not elsewhere classified, unspecified ankle

✓5ᵗʰ **M21.1** Varus deformity, not elsewhere classified
   EXCLUDES 1 metatarsus varus (Q66.2)
     tibia vara (M92.5)
     M21.10 Varus deformity, not elsewhere classified, unspecified site

   ✓6ᵗʰ **M21.12** Varus deformity, not elsewhere classified, elbow
     Cubitus varus, elbow
     M21.121 Varus deformity, not elsewhere classified, right elbow
     M21.122 Varus deformity, not elsewhere classified, left elbow
     M21.129 Varus deformity, not elsewhere classified, unspecified elbow

   ✓6ᵗʰ **M21.15** Varus deformity, not elsewhere classified, hip
     M21.151 Varus deformity, not elsewhere classified, right hip
     M21.152 Varus deformity, not elsewhere classified, left hip
     M21.159 Varus deformity, not elsewhere classified, unspecified

   ✓6ᵗʰ **M21.16** Varus deformity, not elsewhere classified, knee
     Bow leg
     Genu varum
     M21.161 Varus deformity, not elsewhere classified, right knee
     M21.162 Varus deformity, not elsewhere classified, left knee
     M21.169 Varus deformity, not elsewhere classified, unspecified knee

   ✓6ᵗʰ **M21.17** Varus deformity, not elsewhere classified, ankle
     M21.171 Varus deformity, not elsewhere classified, right ankle
     M21.172 Varus deformity, not elsewhere classified, left ankle
     M21.179 Varus deformity, not elsewhere classified, unspecified ankle

✓5ᵗʰ **M21.2** Flexion deformity
     M21.20 Flexion deformity, unspecified site

   ✓6ᵗʰ **M21.21** Flexion deformity, shoulder
     M21.211 Flexion deformity, right shoulder
     M21.212 Flexion deformity, left shoulder
     M21.219 Flexion deformity, unspecified shoulder

   ✓6ᵗʰ **M21.22** Flexion deformity, elbow
     M21.221 Flexion deformity, right elbow
     M21.222 Flexion deformity, left elbow
     M21.229 Flexion deformity, unspecified elbow

   ✓6ᵗʰ **M21.23** Flexion deformity, wrist
     M21.231 Flexion deformity, right wrist
     M21.232 Flexion deformity, left wrist
     M21.239 Flexion deformity, unspecified wrist

   ✓6ᵗʰ **M21.24** Flexion deformity, finger joints
     M21.241 Flexion deformity, right finger joints
     M21.242 Flexion deformity, left finger joints
     M21.249 Flexion deformity, unspecified finger joints

   ✓6ᵗʰ **M21.25** Flexion deformity, hip
     M21.251 Flexion deformity, right hip
     M21.252 Flexion deformity, left hip
     M21.259 Flexion deformity, unspecified hip

EXCLUDES 1 Not coded here   **EXCLUDES 2** Not included here   N Newborn Age: 0   P Pediatric Age: 0-17   M Maternity Age: 12-55   A Adult Age: 15-124

690   ICD-10-CM 2016

✓6th **M21.26** Flexion deformity, knee
    M21.261 Flexion deformity, right knee
    M21.262 Flexion deformity, left knee
    M21.269 Flexion deformity, unspecified knee

✓6th **M21.27** Flexion deformity, ankle and toes
    M21.271 Flexion deformity, right ankle and toes
    M21.272 Flexion deformity, left ankle and toes
    M21.279 Flexion deformity, unspecified ankle and toes

✓5th **M21.3** Wrist or foot drop (acquired)

   ✓6th **M21.33** Wrist drop (acquired)
    M21.331 Wrist drop, right wrist
    M21.332 Wrist drop, left wrist
    M21.339 Wrist drop, unspecified wrist

   ✓6th **M21.37** Foot drop (acquired)
    M21.371 Foot drop, right foot
    M21.372 Foot drop, left foot
    M21.379 Foot drop, unspecified foot

✓5th **M21.4** Flat foot [pes planus] (acquired)
    EXCLUDES 1   congenital pes planus (Q66.5-)
    M21.40 Flat foot [pes planus] (acquired), unspecified foot
    M21.41 Flat foot [pes planus] (acquired), right foot
    M21.42 Flat foot [pes planus] (acquired), left foot

✓5th **M21.5** Acquired clawhand, clubhand, clawfoot and clubfoot
    EXCLUDES 1   clubfoot, not specified as acquired (Q66.89)

   ✓6th **M21.51** Acquired clawhand
    M21.511 Acquired clawhand, right hand
    M21.512 Acquired clawhand, left hand
    M21.519 Acquired clawhand, unspecified hand

   ✓6th **M21.52** Acquired clubhand
    M21.521 Acquired clubhand, right hand
    M21.522 Acquired clubhand, left hand
    M21.529 Acquired clubhand, unspecified hand

   ✓6th **M21.53** Acquired clawfoot
    M21.531 Acquired clawfoot, right foot
    M21.532 Acquired clawfoot, left foot
    M21.539 Acquired clawfoot, unspecified foot

   ✓6th **M21.54** Acquired clubfoot
    M21.541 Acquired clubfoot, right foot
    M21.542 Acquired clubfoot, left foot
    M21.549 Acquired clubfoot, unspecified foot

✓5th **M21.6** Other acquired deformities of foot
    EXCLUDES 2   deformities of toe (acquired) (M20.1-M20.6)

   ✓6th **M21.6X** Other acquired deformities of foot
    M21.6X1 Other acquired deformities of right foot
    M21.6X2 Other acquired deformities of left foot
    M21.6X9 Other acquired deformities of unspecified foot

✓5th **M21.7** Unequal limb length (acquired)
    NOTE   The site used should correspond to the shorter limb.
    M21.70 Unequal limb length (acquired), unspecified site

   ✓6th **M21.72** Unequal limb length (acquired), humerus
    M21.721 Unequal limb length (acquired), right humerus
    M21.722 Unequal limb length (acquired), left humerus
    M21.729 Unequal limb length (acquired), unspecified humerus

   ✓6th **M21.73** Unequal limb length (acquired), ulna and radius
    M21.731 Unequal limb length (acquired), right ulna
    M21.732 Unequal limb length (acquired), left ulna
    M21.733 Unequal limb length (acquired), right radius
    M21.734 Unequal limb length (acquired), left radius
    M21.739 Unequal limb length (acquired), unspecified ulna and radius

   ✓6th **M21.75** Unequal limb length (acquired), femur
    M21.751 Unequal limb length (acquired), right femur
    M21.752 Unequal limb length (acquired), left femur
    M21.759 Unequal limb length (acquired), unspecified femur

   ✓6th **M21.76** Unequal limb length (acquired), tibia and fibula
    M21.761 Unequal limb length (acquired), right tibia
    M21.762 Unequal limb length (acquired), left tibia
    M21.763 Unequal limb length (acquired), right fibula
    M21.764 Unequal limb length (acquired), left fibula
    M21.769 Unequal limb length (acquired), unspecified tibia and fibula

✓5th **M21.8** Other specified acquired deformities of limbs
    EXCLUDES 2   coxa plana (M91.2)
    M21.80 Other specified acquired deformities of unspecified limb

   ✓6th **M21.82** Other specified acquired deformities of upper arm
    M21.821 Other specified acquired deformities of right upper arm
    M21.822 Other specified acquired deformities of left upper arm
    M21.829 Other specified acquired deformities of unspecified upper arm

   ✓6th **M21.83** Other specified acquired deformities of forearm
    M21.831 Other specified acquired deformities of right forearm
    M21.832 Other specified acquired deformities of left forearm
    M21.839 Other specified acquired deformities of unspecified forearm

   ✓6th **M21.85** Other specified acquired deformities of thigh
    M21.851 Other specified acquired deformities of right thigh
    M21.852 Other specified acquired deformities of left thigh
    M21.859 Other specified acquired deformities of unspecified thigh

   ✓6th **M21.86** Other specified acquired deformities of lower leg
    M21.861 Other specified acquired deformities of right lower leg
    M21.862 Other specified acquired deformities of left lower leg
    M21.869 Other specified acquired deformities of unspecified lower leg

✓5th **M21.9** Unspecified acquired deformity of limb and hand
    M21.90 Unspecified acquired deformity of unspecified limb

   ✓6th **M21.92** Unspecified acquired deformity of upper arm
    M21.921 Unspecified acquired deformity of right upper arm
    M21.922 Unspecified acquired deformity of left upper arm
    M21.929 Unspecified acquired deformity of unspecified upper arm

   ✓6th **M21.93** Unspecified acquired deformity of forearm
    M21.931 Unspecified acquired deformity of right forearm
    M21.932 Unspecified acquired deformity of left forearm
    M21.939 Unspecified acquired deformity of unspecified forearm

   ✓6th **M21.94** Unspecified acquired deformity of hand
    M21.941 Unspecified acquired deformity of hand, right hand
    M21.942 Unspecified acquired deformity of hand, left hand
    M21.949 Unspecified acquired deformity of hand, unspecified hand

   ✓6th **M21.95** Unspecified acquired deformity of thigh
    M21.951 Unspecified acquired deformity of right thigh
    M21.952 Unspecified acquired deformity of left thigh
    M21.959 Unspecified acquired deformity of unspecified thigh

   ✓6th **M21.96** Unspecified acquired deformity of lower leg
    M21.961 Unspecified acquired deformity of right lower leg
    M21.962 Unspecified acquired deformity of left lower leg

☑ Additional Character Required   ✓x7th Placeholder Alert   Unspecified Dx   Other Specified Dx   Manifestation   ▶◀ Revised Text   ● New Code   ▲ Revised Code Title

M21.969 **Unspecified acquired deformity of unspecified lower leg**

✓4ᵗʰ **M22 Disorder of patella**
     EXCLUDES 1   traumatic dislocation of patella (S83.0-)

  ✓5ᵗʰ **M22.0 Recurrent dislocation of patella**
     M22.00 **Recurrent dislocation of patella, unspecified knee**
     M22.01 Recurrent dislocation of patella, right knee
     M22.02 Recurrent dislocation of patella, left knee

  ✓5ᵗʰ **M22.1 Recurrent subluxation of patella**
     Incomplete dislocation of patella
     M22.10 **Recurrent subluxation of patella, unspecified knee**
     M22.11 Recurrent subluxation of patella, right knee
     M22.12 Recurrent subluxation of patella, left knee

  ✓5ᵗʰ **M22.2 Patellofemoral disorders**
    ✓6ᵗʰ **M22.2X Patellofemoral disorders**
       M22.2X1 Patellofemoral disorders, right knee
       M22.2X2 Patellofemoral disorders, left knee
       M22.2X9 **Patellofemoral disorders, unspecified knee**

  ✓5ᵗʰ **M22.3 Other derangements of patella**
    ✓6ᵗʰ **M22.3X Other derangements of patella**
       M22.3X1 **Other derangements of patella, right knee**
       M22.3X2 **Other derangements of patella, left knee**
       M22.3X9 **Other derangements of patella, unspecified knee**

  ✓5ᵗʰ **M22.4 Chondromalacia patellae**
     M22.40 **Chondromalacia patellae, unspecified knee**
     M22.41 Chondromalacia patellae, right knee
     M22.42 Chondromalacia patellae, left knee

  ✓5ᵗʰ **M22.8 Other disorders of patella**
    ✓6ᵗʰ **M22.8X Other disorders of patella**
       M22.8X1 Other disorders of patella, right knee
       M22.8X2 Other disorders of patella, left knee
       M22.8X9 **Other disorders of patella, unspecified knee**

  ✓5ᵗʰ **M22.9 Unspecified disorder of patella**
     M22.90 **Unspecified disorder of patella, unspecified knee**
     M22.91 **Unspecified disorder of patella, right knee**
     M22.92 **Unspecified disorder of patella, left knee**

✓4ᵗʰ **M23 Internal derangement of knee**
     EXCLUDES 1   ankylosis (M24.66)
        current injury—see injury of knee and lower leg (S80-S89)
        deformity of knee (M21.-)
        osteochondritis dissecans (M93.2)
        recurrent dislocation or subluxation of joints (M24.4)
        recurrent dislocation or subluxation of patella (M22.0-M22.1)

  ✓5ᵗʰ **M23.0 Cystic meniscus**
    ✓6ᵗʰ **M23.00 Cystic meniscus, unspecified meniscus**
       Cystic meniscus, unspecified lateral meniscus
       Cystic meniscus, unspecified medial meniscus
       M23.000 Cystic meniscus, unspecified lateral meniscus, right knee
       M23.001 Cystic meniscus, unspecified lateral meniscus, left knee
       M23.002 **Cystic meniscus, unspecified lateral meniscus, unspecified knee**
       M23.003 Cystic meniscus, unspecified medial meniscus, right knee
       M23.004 Cystic meniscus, unspecified medial meniscus, left knee
       M23.005 **Cystic meniscus, unspecified medial meniscus, unspecified knee**
       M23.006 Cystic meniscus, unspecified meniscus, right knee
       M23.007 Cystic meniscus, unspecified meniscus, left knee
       M23.009 **Cystic meniscus, unspecified meniscus, unspecified knee**

    ✓6ᵗʰ **M23.01 Cystic meniscus, anterior horn of medial meniscus**
       M23.011 Cystic meniscus, anterior horn of medial meniscus, right knee
       M23.012 Cystic meniscus, anterior horn of medial meniscus, left knee

M23.019 **Cystic meniscus, anterior horn of medial meniscus, unspecified knee**

  ✓6ᵗʰ **M23.02 Cystic meniscus, posterior horn of medial meniscus**
     M23.021 Cystic meniscus, posterior horn of medial meniscus, right knee
     M23.022 Cystic meniscus, posterior horn of medial meniscus, left knee
     M23.029 **Cystic meniscus, posterior horn of medial meniscus, unspecified knee**

  ✓6ᵗʰ **M23.03 Cystic meniscus, other medial meniscus**
     M23.031 Cystic meniscus, other medial meniscus, right knee
     M23.032 Cystic meniscus, other medial meniscus, left knee
     M23.039 **Cystic meniscus, other medial meniscus, unspecified knee**

  ✓6ᵗʰ **M23.04 Cystic meniscus, anterior horn of lateral meniscus**
     M23.041 Cystic meniscus, anterior horn of lateral meniscus, right knee
     M23.042 Cystic meniscus, anterior horn of lateral meniscus, left knee
     M23.049 **Cystic meniscus, anterior horn of lateral meniscus, unspecified knee**

  ✓6ᵗʰ **M23.05 Cystic meniscus, posterior horn of lateral meniscus**
     M23.051 Cystic meniscus, posterior horn of lateral meniscus, right knee
     M23.052 Cystic meniscus, posterior horn of lateral meniscus, left knee
     M23.059 **Cystic meniscus, posterior horn of lateral meniscus, unspecified knee**

  ✓6ᵗʰ **M23.06 Cystic meniscus, other lateral meniscus**
     M23.061 Cystic meniscus, other lateral meniscus, right knee
     M23.062 Cystic meniscus, other lateral meniscus, left knee
     M23.069 **Cystic meniscus, other lateral meniscus, unspecified knee**

  ✓5ᵗʰ **M23.2 Derangement of meniscus due to old tear or injury**
     Old bucket-handle tear

    ✓6ᵗʰ **M23.20 Derangement of unspecified meniscus due to old tear or injury**
       Derangement of unspecified lateral meniscus due to old tear or injury
       Derangement of unspecified medial meniscus due to old tear or injury
       M23.200 Derangement of unspecified lateral meniscus due to old tear or injury, right knee
       M23.201 Derangement of unspecified lateral meniscus due to old tear or injury, left knee
       M23.202 **Derangement of unspecified lateral meniscus due to old tear or injury, unspecified knee**
       M23.203 Derangement of unspecified medial meniscus due to old tear or injury, right knee
       M23.204 Derangement of unspecified medial meniscus due to old tear or injury, left knee
       M23.205 **Derangement of unspecified medial meniscus due to old tear or injury, unspecified knee**
       M23.206 Derangement of unspecified meniscus due to old tear or injury, right knee
       M23.207 Derangement of unspecified meniscus due to old tear or injury, left knee
       M23.209 **Derangement of unspecified meniscus due to old tear or injury, unspecified knee**

    ✓6ᵗʰ **M23.21 Derangement of anterior horn of medial meniscus due to old tear or injury**
       M23.211 Derangement of anterior horn of medial meniscus due to old tear or injury, right knee
       M23.212 Derangement of anterior horn of medial meniscus due to old tear or injury, left knee

EXCLUDES 1 Not coded here   *EXCLUDES 2* Not included here   Ⓝ Newborn Age: 0   Ⓟ Pediatric Age: 0-17   Ⓜ Maternity Age: 12-55   Ⓐ Adult Age: 15-124

692   ICD-10-CM 2016

M23.219   Derangement of anterior horn of medial meniscus due to old tear or injury, unspecified knee

✓6th   **M23.22**   Derangement of posterior horn of medial meniscus due to old tear or injury

M23.221   Derangement of posterior horn of medial meniscus due to old tear or injury, right knee

M23.222   Derangement of posterior horn of medial meniscus due to old tear or injury, left knee

M23.229   Derangement of posterior horn of medial meniscus due to old tear or injury, unspecified knee

✓6th   **M23.23**   Derangement of other medial meniscus due to old tear or injury

M23.231   Derangement of other medial meniscus due to old tear or injury, right knee

M23.232   Derangement of other medial meniscus due to old tear or injury, left knee

M23.239   Derangement of other medial meniscus due to old tear or injury, unspecified knee

✓6th   **M23.24**   Derangement of anterior horn of lateral meniscus due to old tear or injury

M23.241   Derangement of anterior horn of lateral meniscus due to old tear or injury, right knee

M23.242   Derangement of anterior horn of lateral meniscus due to old tear or injury, left knee

M23.249   Derangement of anterior horn of lateral meniscus due to old tear or injury, unspecified knee

✓6th   **M23.25**   Derangement of posterior horn of lateral meniscus due to old tear or injury

M23.251   Derangement of posterior horn of lateral meniscus due to old tear or injury, right knee

M23.252   Derangement of posterior horn of lateral meniscus due to old tear or injury, left knee

M23.259   Derangement of posterior horn of lateral meniscus due to old tear or injury, unspecified knee

✓6th   **M23.26**   Derangement of other lateral meniscus due to old tear or injury

M23.261   Derangement of other lateral meniscus due to old tear or injury, right knee

M23.262   Derangement of other lateral meniscus due to old tear or injury, left knee

M23.269   Derangement of other lateral meniscus due to old tear or injury, unspecified knee

✓5th   **M23.3**   **Other meniscus derangements**
Degenerate meniscus
Detached meniscus
Retained meniscus

✓6th   **M23.30**   Other meniscus derangements, unspecified meniscus
Other meniscus derangements, unspecified lateral meniscus
Other meniscus derangements, unspecified medial meniscus

M23.300   Other meniscus derangements, unspecified lateral meniscus, right knee

M23.301   Other meniscus derangements, unspecified lateral meniscus, left knee

M23.302   Other meniscus derangements, unspecified lateral meniscus, unspecified knee

M23.303   Other meniscus derangements, unspecified medial meniscus, right knee

M23.304   Other meniscus derangements, unspecified medial meniscus, left knee

M23.305   Other meniscus derangements, unspecified medial meniscus, unspecified knee

M23.306   Other meniscus derangements, unspecified meniscus, right knee

M23.307   Other meniscus derangements, unspecified meniscus, left knee

M23.309   Other meniscus derangements, unspecified meniscus, unspecified knee

✓6th   **M23.31**   Other meniscus derangements, anterior horn of medial meniscus

M23.311   Other meniscus derangements, anterior horn of medial meniscus, right knee

M23.312   Other meniscus derangements, anterior horn of medial meniscus, left knee

M23.319   Other meniscus derangements, anterior horn of medial meniscus, unspecified knee

✓6th   **M23.32**   Other meniscus derangements, posterior horn of medial meniscus

M23.321   Other meniscus derangements, posterior horn of medial meniscus, right knee

M23.322   Other meniscus derangements, posterior horn of medial meniscus, left knee

M23.329   Other meniscus derangements, posterior horn of medial meniscus, unspecified knee

✓6th   **M23.33**   Other meniscus derangements, other medial meniscus

M23.331   Other meniscus derangements, other medial meniscus, right knee

M23.332   Other meniscus derangements, other medial meniscus, left knee

M23.339   Other meniscus derangements, other medial meniscus, unspecified knee

✓6th   **M23.34**   Other meniscus derangements, anterior horn of lateral meniscus

M23.341   Other meniscus derangements, anterior horn of lateral meniscus, right knee

M23.342   Other meniscus derangements, anterior horn of lateral meniscus, left knee

M23.349   Other meniscus derangements, anterior horn of lateral meniscus, unspecified knee

✓6th   **M23.35**   Other meniscus derangements, posterior horn of lateral meniscus

M23.351   Other meniscus derangements, posterior horn of lateral meniscus, right knee

M23.352   Other meniscus derangements, posterior horn of lateral meniscus, left knee

M23.359   Other meniscus derangements, posterior horn of lateral meniscus, unspecified knee

✓6th   **M23.36**   Other meniscus derangements, other lateral meniscus

M23.361   Other meniscus derangements, other lateral meniscus, right knee

M23.362   Other meniscus derangements, other lateral meniscus, left knee

M23.369   Other meniscus derangements, other lateral meniscus, unspecified knee

✓5th   **M23.4**   **Loose body in knee**

M23.40   Loose body in knee, unspecified knee

M23.41   Loose body in knee, right knee

M23.42   Loose body in knee, left knee

✓5th   **M23.5**   **Chronic instability of knee**

M23.50   Chronic instability of knee, unspecified knee

M23.51   Chronic instability of knee, right knee

M23.52   Chronic instability of knee, left knee

✓5th   **M23.6**   **Other spontaneous disruption of ligament(s) of knee**

✓6th   **M23.60**   Other spontaneous disruption of unspecified ligament of knee

M23.601   Other spontaneous disruption of unspecified ligament of right knee

M23.602   Other spontaneous disruption of unspecified ligament of left knee

M23.609   Other spontaneous disruption of unspecified ligament of unspecified knee

✓6th   **M23.61**   Other spontaneous disruption of anterior cruciate ligament of knee

M23.611   Other spontaneous disruption of anterior cruciate ligament of right knee

M23.612   Other spontaneous disruption of anterior cruciate ligament of left knee

M23.619   Other spontaneous disruption of anterior cruciate ligament of unspecified knee

---

✓ Additional Character Required   ✓x7th Placeholder Alert   Unspecified Dx   Other Specified Dx   Manifestation   ▶◀ Revised Text   ● New Code   ▲ Revised Code Title

✓6th **M23.62** Other spontaneous disruption of posterior cruciate ligament of knee

    M23.621 Other spontaneous disruption of posterior cruciate ligament of right knee

    M23.622 Other spontaneous disruption of posterior cruciate ligament of left knee

    M23.629 Other spontaneous disruption of posterior cruciate ligament of unspecified knee

✓6th **M23.63** Other spontaneous disruption of medial collateral ligament of knee

    M23.631 Other spontaneous disruption of medial collateral ligament of right knee

    M23.632 Other spontaneous disruption of medial collateral ligament of left knee

    M23.639 Other spontaneous disruption of medial collateral ligament of unspecified knee

✓6th **M23.64** Other spontaneous disruption of lateral collateral ligament of knee

    M23.641 Other spontaneous disruption of lateral collateral ligament of right knee

    M23.642 Other spontaneous disruption of lateral collateral ligament of left knee

    M23.649 Other spontaneous disruption of lateral collateral ligament of unspecified knee

✓6th **M23.67** Other spontaneous disruption of capsular ligament of knee

    M23.671 Other spontaneous disruption of capsular ligament of right knee

    M23.672 Other spontaneous disruption of capsular ligament of left knee

    M23.679 Other spontaneous disruption of capsular ligament of unspecified knee

✓5th **M23.8** Other internal derangements of knee

    Laxity of ligament of knee

    Snapping knee

✓6th **M23.8X** Other internal derangements of knee

    M23.8X1 Other internal derangements of right knee

    M23.8X2 Other internal derangements of left knee

    M23.8X9 Other internal derangements of unspecified knee

✓5th **M23.9** Unspecified internal derangement of knee

    M23.90 Unspecified internal derangement of unspecified knee

    M23.91 Unspecified internal derangement of right knee

    M23.92 Unspecified internal derangement of left knee

✓4th **M24** Other specific joint derangements

    EXCLUDES 1   current injury—see injury of joint by body region

    EXCLUDES 2   ganglion (M67.4)

       snapping knee (M23.8-)

       temporomandibular joint disorders (M26.6-)

✓5th **M24.0** Loose body in joint

    EXCLUDES 2   loose body in knee (M23.4)

    M24.00 Loose body in unspecified joint

✓6th **M24.01** Loose body in shoulder

    M24.011 Loose body in right shoulder

    M24.012 Loose body in left shoulder

    M24.019 Loose body in unspecified shoulder

✓6th **M24.02** Loose body in elbow

    M24.021 Loose body in right elbow

    M24.022 Loose body in left elbow

    M24.029 Loose body in unspecified elbow

✓6th **M24.03** Loose body in wrist

    M24.031 Loose body in right wrist

    M24.032 Loose body in left wrist

    M24.039 Loose body in unspecified wrist

✓6th **M24.04** Loose body in finger joints

    M24.041 Loose body in right finger joint(s)

    M24.042 Loose body in left finger joint(s)

    M24.049 Loose body in unspecified finger joint(s)

✓6th **M24.05** Loose body in hip

    M24.051 Loose body in right hip

    M24.052 Loose body in left hip

    M24.059 Loose body in unspecified hip

✓6th **M24.07** Loose body in ankle and toe joints

    M24.071 Loose body in right ankle

    M24.072 Loose body in left ankle

    M24.073 Loose body in unspecified ankle

    M24.074 Loose body in right toe joint(s)

    M24.075 Loose body in left toe joint(s)

    M24.076 Loose body in unspecified toe joints

    M24.08 Loose body, other site

✓5th **M24.1** Other articular cartilage disorders

    EXCLUDES 2   chondrocalcinosis (M11.1, M11.2-)

       internal derangement of knee (M23.-)

       metastatic calcification (E83.5)

       ochronosis (E70.2)

    M24.10 Other articular cartilage disorders, unspecified site

✓6th **M24.11** Other articular cartilage disorders, shoulder

    M24.111 Other articular cartilage disorders, right shoulder

    M24.112 Other articular cartilage disorders, left shoulder

    M24.119 Other articular cartilage disorders, unspecified shoulder

✓6th **M24.12** Other articular cartilage disorders, elbow

    M24.121 Other articular cartilage disorders, right elbow

    M24.122 Other articular cartilage disorders, left elbow

    M24.129 Other articular cartilage disorders, unspecified elbow

✓6th **M24.13** Other articular cartilage disorders, wrist

    M24.131 Other articular cartilage disorders, right wrist

    M24.132 Other articular cartilage disorders, left wrist

    M24.139 Other articular cartilage disorders, unspecified wrist

✓6th **M24.14** Other articular cartilage disorders, hand

    M24.141 Other articular cartilage disorders, right hand

    M24.142 Other articular cartilage disorders, left hand

    M24.149 Other articular cartilage disorders, unspecified hand

✓6th **M24.15** Other articular cartilage disorders, hip

    M24.151 Other articular cartilage disorders, right hip

    M24.152 Other articular cartilage disorders, left hip

    M24.159 Other articular cartilage disorders, unspecified hip

✓6th **M24.17** Other articular cartilage disorders, ankle and foot

    M24.171 Other articular cartilage disorders, right ankle

    M24.172 Other articular cartilage disorders, left ankle

    M24.173 Other articular cartilage disorders, unspecified ankle

    M24.174 Other articular cartilage disorders, right foot

    M24.175 Other articular cartilage disorders, left foot

    M24.176 Other articular cartilage disorders, unspecified foot

✓5th **M24.2** Disorder of ligament

    Instability secondary to old ligament injury

    Ligamentous laxity NOS

    EXCLUDES 1   familial ligamentous laxity (M35.7)

    EXCLUDES 2   internal derangement of knee (M23.5-M23.89)

    M24.20 Disorder of ligament, unspecified site

✓6th **M24.21** Disorder of ligament, shoulder

    M24.211 Disorder of ligament, right shoulder

    M24.212 Disorder of ligament, left shoulder

    M24.219 Disorder of ligament, unspecified shoulder

✓6th **M24.22** Disorder of ligament, elbow

    M24.221 Disorder of ligament, right elbow

    M24.222 Disorder of ligament, left elbow

    M24.229 Disorder of ligament, unspecified elbow

EXCLUDES 1 Not coded here   EXCLUDES 2 Not included here   N Newborn Age: 0   P Pediatric Age: 0-17   M Maternity Age: 12-55   A Adult Age: 15-124

694   ICD-10-CM 2016

√6ᵗʰ **M24.23 Disorder of ligament, wrist**
    M24.231 Disorder of ligament, right wrist
    M24.232 Disorder of ligament, left wrist
    M24.239 Disorder of ligament, unspecified wrist

√6ᵗʰ **M24.24 Disorder of ligament, hand**
    M24.241 Disorder of ligament, right hand
    M24.242 Disorder of ligament, left hand
    M24.249 Disorder of ligament, unspecified hand

√6ᵗʰ **M24.25 Disorder of ligament, hip**
    M24.251 Disorder of ligament, right hip
    M24.252 Disorder of ligament, left hip
    M24.259 Disorder of ligament, unspecified hip

√6ᵗʰ **M24.27 Disorder of ligament, ankle and foot**
    M24.271 Disorder of ligament, right ankle
    M24.272 Disorder of ligament, left ankle
    M24.273 Disorder of ligament, unspecified ankle
    M24.274 Disorder of ligament, right foot
    M24.275 Disorder of ligament, left foot
    M24.276 Disorder of ligament, unspecified foot

M24.28 Disorder of ligament, vertebrae

√5ᵗʰ **M24.3 Pathological dislocation of joint, not elsewhere classified**
   EXCLUDES 1 congenital dislocation or displacement of joint—see
           congenital malformations and deformations of
           the musculoskeletal system (Q65-Q79)
          current injury—see injury of joints and ligaments by
           body region
          recurrent dislocation of joint (M24.4-)

    M24.30 Pathological dislocation of unspecified joint, not
         elsewhere classified

√6ᵗʰ **M24.31 Pathological dislocation of shoulder, not elsewhere classified**
    M24.311 Pathological dislocation of right shoulder, not elsewhere classified
    M24.312 Pathological dislocation of left shoulder, not elsewhere classified
    M24.319 Pathological dislocation of unspecified shoulder, not elsewhere classified

√6ᵗʰ **M24.32 Pathological dislocation of elbow, not elsewhere classified**
    M24.321 Pathological dislocation of right elbow, not elsewhere classified
    M24.322 Pathological dislocation of left elbow, not elsewhere classified
    M24.329 Pathological dislocation of unspecified elbow, not elsewhere classified

√6ᵗʰ **M24.33 Pathological dislocation of wrist, not elsewhere classified**
    M24.331 Pathological dislocation of right wrist, not elsewhere classified
    M24.332 Pathological dislocation of left wrist, not elsewhere classified
    M24.339 Pathological dislocation of unspecified wrist, not elsewhere classified

√6ᵗʰ **M24.34 Pathological dislocation of hand, not elsewhere classified**
    M24.341 Pathological dislocation of right hand, not elsewhere classified
    M24.342 Pathological dislocation of left hand, not elsewhere classified
    M24.349 Pathological dislocation of unspecified hand, not elsewhere classified

√6ᵗʰ **M24.35 Pathological dislocation of hip, not elsewhere classified**
    M24.351 Pathological dislocation of right hip, not elsewhere classified
    M24.352 Pathological dislocation of left hip, not elsewhere classified
    M24.359 Pathological dislocation of unspecified hip, not elsewhere classified

√6ᵗʰ **M24.36 Pathological dislocation of knee, not elsewhere classified**
    M24.361 Pathological dislocation of right knee, not elsewhere classified
    M24.362 Pathological dislocation of left knee, not elsewhere classified

    M24.369 Pathological dislocation of unspecified knee, not elsewhere classified

√6ᵗʰ **M24.37 Pathological dislocation of ankle and foot, not elsewhere classified**
    M24.371 Pathological dislocation of right ankle, not elsewhere classified
    M24.372 Pathological dislocation of left ankle, not elsewhere classified
    M24.373 Pathological dislocation of unspecified ankle, not elsewhere classified
    M24.374 Pathological dislocation of right foot, not elsewhere classified
    M24.375 Pathological dislocation of left foot, not elsewhere classified
    M24.376 Pathological dislocation of unspecified foot, not elsewhere classified

√5ᵗʰ **M24.4 Recurrent dislocation of joint**
   Recurrent subluxation of joint
   EXCLUDES 2 recurrent dislocation of patella (M22.0-M22.1)
          recurrent vertebral dislocation (M43.3-, M43.4, M43.5-)

    M24.40 Recurrent dislocation, unspecified joint

√6ᵗʰ **M24.41 Recurrent dislocation, shoulder**
    M24.411 Recurrent dislocation, right shoulder
    M24.412 Recurrent dislocation, left shoulder
    M24.419 Recurrent dislocation, unspecified shoulder

√6ᵗʰ **M24.42 Recurrent dislocation, elbow**
    M24.421 Recurrent dislocation, right elbow
    M24.422 Recurrent dislocation, left elbow
    M24.429 Recurrent dislocation, unspecified elbow

√6ᵗʰ **M24.43 Recurrent dislocation, wrist**
    M24.431 Recurrent dislocation, right wrist
    M24.432 Recurrent dislocation, left wrist
    M24.439 Recurrent dislocation, unspecified wrist

√6ᵗʰ **M24.44 Recurrent dislocation, hand and finger(s)**
    M24.441 Recurrent dislocation, right hand
    M24.442 Recurrent dislocation, left hand
    M24.443 Recurrent dislocation, unspecified hand
    M24.444 Recurrent dislocation, right finger
    M24.445 Recurrent dislocation, left finger
    M24.446 Recurrent dislocation, unspecified finger

√6ᵗʰ **M24.45 Recurrent dislocation, hip**
    M24.451 Recurrent dislocation, right hip
    M24.452 Recurrent dislocation, left hip
    M24.459 Recurrent dislocation, unspecified hip

√6ᵗʰ **M24.46 Recurrent dislocation, knee**
    M24.461 Recurrent dislocation, right knee
    M24.462 Recurrent dislocation, left knee
    M24.469 Recurrent dislocation, unspecified knee

√6ᵗʰ **M24.47 Recurrent dislocation, ankle, foot and toes**
    M24.471 Recurrent dislocation, right ankle
    M24.472 Recurrent dislocation, left ankle
    M24.473 Recurrent dislocation, unspecified ankle
    M24.474 Recurrent dislocation, right foot
    M24.475 Recurrent dislocation, left foot
    M24.476 Recurrent dislocation, unspecified foot
    M24.477 Recurrent dislocation, right toe(s)
    M24.478 Recurrent dislocation, left toe(s)
    M24.479 Recurrent dislocation, unspecified toe(s)

√5ᵗʰ **M24.5 Contracture of joint**
   EXCLUDES 1 contracture of muscle without contracture of joint
           (M62.4-)
          contracture of tendon (sheath) without contracture of
           joint (M62.4-)
          Dupuytren's contracture (M72.0)
   EXCLUDES 2 acquired deformities of limbs (M20-M21)

    M24.50 Contracture, unspecified joint

√6ᵗʰ **M24.51 Contracture, shoulder**
    M24.511 Contracture, right shoulder
    M24.512 Contracture, left shoulder
    M24.519 Contracture, unspecified shoulder

√6ᵗʰ **M24.52 Contracture, elbow**
    M24.521 Contracture, right elbow
    M24.522 Contracture, left elbow

☑ Additional Character Required   ✓x7ᵗʰ Placeholder Alert   Unspecified Dx   Other Specified Dx   Manifestation   ▶◀ Revised Text   ● New Code   ▲ Revised Code Title

ICD-10-CM 2016   695

M24.529 **Contracture, unspecified elbow**

✓6ᵗʰ M24.53 Contracture, **wrist**

M24.531 **Contracture, right wrist**

M24.532 **Contracture, left wrist**

M24.539 **Contracture, unspecified wrist**

✓6ᵗʰ M24.54 Contracture, **hand**

M24.541 **Contracture, right hand**

M24.542 **Contracture, left hand**

M24.549 **Contracture, unspecified hand**

✓6ᵗʰ M24.55 Contracture, **hip**

M24.551 **Contracture, right hip**

M24.552 **Contracture, left hip**

M24.559 **Contracture, unspecified hip**

✓6ᵗʰ M24.56 Contracture, **knee**

M24.561 **Contracture, right knee**

M24.562 **Contracture, left knee**

M24.569 **Contracture, unspecified knee**

✓6ᵗʰ M24.57 Contracture, **ankle and foot**

M24.571 **Contracture, right ankle**

M24.572 **Contracture, left ankle**

M24.573 **Contracture, unspecified ankle**

M24.574 **Contracture, right foot**

M24.575 **Contracture, left foot**

M24.576 **Contracture, unspecified foot**

✓5ᵗʰ **M24.6 Ankylosis of joint**

EXCLUDES 1   *stiffness of joint without ankylosis (M25.6-)*

EXCLUDES 2   *spine (M43.2-)*

M24.60 **Ankylosis, unspecified joint**

✓6ᵗʰ M24.61 Ankylosis, **shoulder**

M24.611 **Ankylosis, right shoulder**

M24.612 **Ankylosis, left shoulder**

M24.619 **Ankylosis, unspecified shoulder**

✓6ᵗʰ M24.62 Ankylosis, **elbow**

M24.621 **Ankylosis, right elbow**

M24.622 **Ankylosis, left elbow**

M24.629 **Ankylosis, unspecified elbow**

✓6ᵗʰ M24.63 Ankylosis, **wrist**

M24.631 **Ankylosis, right wrist**

M24.632 **Ankylosis, left wrist**

M24.639 **Ankylosis, unspecified wrist**

✓6ᵗʰ M24.64 Ankylosis, **hand**

M24.641 **Ankylosis, right hand**

M24.642 **Ankylosis, left hand**

M24.649 **Ankylosis, unspecified hand**

✓6ᵗʰ M24.65 Ankylosis, **hip**

M24.651 **Ankylosis, right hip**

M24.652 **Ankylosis, left hip**

M24.659 **Ankylosis, unspecified hip**

✓6ᵗʰ M24.66 Ankylosis, **knee**

M24.661 **Ankylosis, right knee**

M24.662 **Ankylosis, left knee**

M24.669 **Ankylosis, unspecified knee**

✓6ᵗʰ M24.67 Ankylosis, **ankle and foot**

M24.671 **Ankylosis, right ankle**

M24.672 **Ankylosis, left ankle**

M24.673 **Ankylosis, unspecified ankle**

M24.674 **Ankylosis, right foot**

M24.675 **Ankylosis, left foot**

M24.676 **Ankylosis, unspecified foot**

M24.7 **Protrusio acetabuli**

✓5ᵗʰ M24.8 **Other specific joint derangements, not elsewhere classified**

EXCLUDES 2   *iliotibial band syndrome (M76.3)*

M24.80 **Other specific joint derangements of unspecified joint, not elsewhere classified**

✓6ᵗʰ M24.81 **Other specific joint derangements of shoulder, not elsewhere classified**

M24.811 **Other specific joint derangements of right shoulder, not elsewhere classified**

M24.812 **Other specific joint derangements of left shoulder, not elsewhere classified**

M24.819 **Other specific joint derangements of unspecified shoulder, not elsewhere classified**

✓6ᵗʰ M24.82 **Other specific joint derangements of elbow, not elsewhere classified**

M24.821 **Other specific joint derangements of right elbow, not elsewhere classified**

M24.822 **Other specific joint derangements of left elbow, not elsewhere classified**

M24.829 **Other specific joint derangements of unspecified elbow, not elsewhere classified**

✓6ᵗʰ M24.83 **Other specific joint derangements of wrist, not elsewhere classified**

M24.831 **Other specific joint derangements of right wrist, not elsewhere classified**

M24.832 **Other specific joint derangements of left wrist, not elsewhere classified**

M24.839 **Other specific joint derangements of unspecified wrist, not elsewhere classified**

✓6ᵗʰ M24.84 **Other specific joint derangements of hand, not elsewhere classified**

M24.841 **Other specific joint derangements of right hand, not elsewhere classified**

M24.842 **Other specific joint derangements of left hand, not elsewhere classified**

M24.849 **Other specific joint derangements of unspecified hand, not elsewhere classified**

✓6ᵗʰ M24.85 **Other specific joint derangements of hip, not elsewhere classified**

Irritable hip

M24.851 **Other specific joint derangements of right hip, not elsewhere classified**

M24.852 **Other specific joint derangements of left hip, not elsewhere classified**

M24.859 **Other specific joint derangements of unspecified hip, not elsewhere classified**

✓6ᵗʰ M24.87 **Other specific joint derangements of ankle and foot, not elsewhere classified**

M24.871 **Other specific joint derangements of right ankle, not elsewhere classified**

M24.872 **Other specific joint derangements of left ankle, not elsewhere classified**

M24.873 **Other specific joint derangements of unspecified ankle, not elsewhere classified**

M24.874 **Other specific joint derangements of right foot, not elsewhere classified**

M24.875 **Other specific joint derangements left foot, not elsewhere classified**

M24.876 **Other specific joint derangements of unspecified foot, not elsewhere classified**

M24.9 **Joint derangement, unspecified**

✓4ᵗʰ **M25 Other joint disorder, not elsewhere classified**

EXCLUDES 2   *abnormality of gait and mobility (R26.-)*
acquired deformities of limb (M20-M21)
calcification of bursa (M71.4-)
calcification of shoulder (joint) (M75.3)
calcification of tendon (M65.2-)
difficulty in walking (R26.2)
temporomandibular joint disorder (M26.6-)

✓5ᵗʰ **M25.0 Hemarthrosis**

EXCLUDES 1   *current injury—see injury of joint by body region*
hemophilic arthropathy (M36.2)

M25.00 **Hemarthrosis, unspecified joint**

✓6ᵗʰ M25.01 Hemarthrosis, **shoulder**

M25.011 **Hemarthrosis, right shoulder**

M25.012 **Hemarthrosis, left shoulder**

M25.019 **Hemarthrosis, unspecified shoulder**

✓6ᵗʰ M25.02 Hemarthrosis, **elbow**

M25.021 **Hemarthrosis, right elbow**

M25.022 **Hemarthrosis, left elbow**

M25.029 **Hemarthrosis, unspecified elbow**

✓6ᵗʰ M25.03 Hemarthrosis, **wrist**

M25.031 **Hemarthrosis, right wrist**

M25.032 **Hemarthrosis, left wrist**

M25.039 **Hemarthrosis, unspecified wrist**

EXCLUDES 1 Not coded here   *EXCLUDES 2* Not included here   **N** Newborn Age: 0   **P** Pediatric Age: 0-17   **M** Maternity Age: 12-55   **A** Adult Age: 15-124

696   ICD-10-CM 2016

✓6ᵗʰ **M25.04 Hemarthrosis,** hand
     M25.041 Hemarthrosis, right **hand**
     M25.042 Hemarthrosis, left **hand**
     M25.049 Hemarthrosis, unspecified hand

✓6ᵗʰ **M25.05 Hemarthrosis,** hip
     M25.051 Hemarthrosis, right **hip**
     M25.052 Hemarthrosis, left **hip**
     M25.059 Hemarthrosis, unspecified hip

✓6ᵗʰ **M25.06 Hemarthrosis,** knee
     M25.061 Hemarthrosis, right **knee**
     M25.062 Hemarthrosis, left **knee**
     M25.069 Hemarthrosis, unspecified knee

✓6ᵗʰ **M25.07 Hemarthrosis,** ankle and foot
     M25.071 Hemarthrosis, right **ankle**
     M25.072 Hemarthrosis, left **ankle**
     M25.073 Hemarthrosis, unspecified ankle
     M25.074 Hemarthrosis, right **foot**
     M25.075 Hemarthrosis, left **foot**
     M25.076 Hemarthrosis, unspecified foot

     M25.08 Hemarthrosis, other specified site
         Hemarthrosis, vertebrae

✓5ᵗʰ **M25.1 Fistula of joint**
     M25.10 Fistula, unspecified joint

✓6ᵗʰ **M25.11 Fistula,** shoulder
     M25.111 Fistula, right **shoulder**
     M25.112 Fistula, left **shoulder**
     M25.119 Fistula, unspecified shoulder

✓6ᵗʰ **M25.12 Fistula,** elbow
     M25.121 Fistula, right **elbow**
     M25.122 Fistula, left **elbow**
     M25.129 Fistula, unspecified elbow

✓6ᵗʰ **M25.13 Fistula,** wrist
     M25.131 Fistula, right **wrist**
     M25.132 Fistula, left **wrist**
     M25.139 Fistula, unspecified wrist

✓6ᵗʰ **M25.14 Fistula,** hand
     M25.141 Fistula, right **hand**
     M25.142 Fistula, left **hand**
     M25.149 Fistula, unspecified hand

✓6ᵗʰ **M25.15 Fistula,** hip
     M25.151 Fistula, right **hip**
     M25.152 Fistula, left **hip**
     M25.159 Fistula, unspecified hip

✓6ᵗʰ **M25.16 Fistula,** knee
     M25.161 Fistula, right **knee**
     M25.162 Fistula, left **knee**
     M25.169 Fistula, unspecified knee

✓6ᵗʰ **M25.17 Fistula,** ankle and foot
     M25.171 Fistula, right **ankle**
     M25.172 Fistula, left **ankle**
     M25.173 Fistula, unspecified ankle
     M25.174 Fistula, right **foot**
     M25.175 Fistula, left **foot**
     M25.176 Fistula, unspecified foot

     M25.18 Fistula, other specified site
         Fistula, vertebrae

✓5ᵗʰ **M25.2 Flail joint**
     M25.20 Flail joint, unspecified joint

✓6ᵗʰ **M25.21 Flail joint,** shoulder
     M25.211 Flail joint, right **shoulder**
     M25.212 Flail joint, left **shoulder**
     M25.219 Flail joint, unspecified shoulder

✓6ᵗʰ **M25.22 Flail joint,** elbow
     M25.221 Flail joint, right **elbow**
     M25.222 Flail joint, left **elbow**
     M25.229 Flail joint, unspecified elbow

✓6ᵗʰ **M25.23 Flail joint,** wrist
     M25.231 Flail joint, right **wrist**
     M25.232 Flail joint, left **wrist**
     M25.239 Flail joint, unspecified wrist

✓6ᵗʰ **M25.24 Flail joint,** hand
     M25.241 Flail joint, right **hand**
     M25.242 Flail joint, left **hand**
     M25.249 Flail joint, unspecified hand

✓6ᵗʰ **M25.25 Flail joint,** hip
     M25.251 Flail joint, right **hip**
     M25.252 Flail joint, left **hip**
     M25.259 Flail joint, unspecified hip

✓6ᵗʰ **M25.26 Flail joint,** knee
     M25.261 Flail joint, right **knee**
     M25.262 Flail joint, left **knee**
     M25.269 Flail joint, unspecified knee

✓6ᵗʰ **M25.27 Flail joint,** ankle and foot
     M25.271 Flail joint, right **ankle and foot**
     M25.272 Flail joint, left **ankle and foot**
     M25.279 Flail joint, unspecified ankle and foot

     M25.28 Flail joint, other site

✓5ᵗʰ **M25.3 Other instability of joint**
     EXCLUDES 1   *instability of joint secondary to old ligament injury (M24.2-)*
             instability of joint secondary to removal of joint prosthesis (M96.8-)
     EXCLUDES 2   *spinal instabilities (M53.2-)*

     M25.30 Other instability, unspecified joint

✓6ᵗʰ **M25.31 Other instability,** shoulder
     M25.311 Other instability, right **shoulder**
     M25.312 Other instability, left **shoulder**
     M25.319 Other instability, unspecified shoulder

✓6ᵗʰ **M25.32 Other instability,** elbow
     M25.321 Other instability, right **elbow**
     M25.322 Other instability, left **elbow**
     M25.329 Other instability, unspecified elbow

✓6ᵗʰ **M25.33 Other instability,** wrist
     M25.331 Other instability, right **wrist**
     M25.332 Other instability, left **wrist**
     M25.339 Other instability, unspecified wrist

✓6ᵗʰ **M25.34 Other instability,** hand
     M25.341 Other instability, right **hand**
     M25.342 Other instability, left **hand**
     M25.349 Other instability, unspecified hand

✓6ᵗʰ **M25.35 Other instability,** hip
     M25.351 Other instability, right **hip**
     M25.352 Other instability, left **hip**
     M25.359 Other instability, unspecified hip

✓6ᵗʰ **M25.36 Other instability,** knee
     M25.361 Other instability, right **knee**
     M25.362 Other instability, left **knee**
     M25.369 Other instability, unspecified knee

✓6ᵗʰ **M25.37 Other instability,** ankle and foot
     M25.371 Other instability, right **ankle**
     M25.372 Other instability, left **ankle**
     M25.373 Other instability, unspecified ankle
     M25.374 Other instability, right **foot**
     M25.375 Other instability, left **foot**
     M25.376 Other instability, unspecified foot

✓5ᵗʰ **M25.4 Effusion of joint**
     EXCLUDES 1   *hydrarthrosis in yaws (A66.6)*
             intermittent hydrarthrosis (M12.4-)
             other infective (teno)synovitis (M65.1-)

     M25.40 Effusion, unspecified joint

✓6ᵗʰ **M25.41 Effusion,** shoulder
     M25.411 Effusion, right **shoulder**
     M25.412 Effusion, left **shoulder**
     M25.419 Effusion, unspecified shoulder

✓6ᵗʰ **M25.42 Effusion,** elbow
     M25.421 Effusion, right **elbow**
     M25.422 Effusion, left **elbow**
     M25.429 Effusion, unspecified elbow

✓6ᵗʰ **M25.43 Effusion,** wrist
     M25.431 Effusion, right **wrist**
     M25.432 Effusion, left **wrist**
     M25.439 Effusion, unspecified wrist

✔ Additional Character Required   ✓x7ᵗʰ Placeholder Alert   <u>Unspecified Dx</u>   <u>Other Specified Dx</u>   Manifestation   ▶◀ Revised Text   ● New Code   ▲ Revised Code Title

√6ᵗʰ M25.44 Effusion, hand
- M25.441 Effusion, right hand
- M25.442 Effusion, left hand
- M25.449 Effusion, unspecified hand

√6ᵗʰ M25.45 Effusion, hip
- M25.451 Effusion, right hip
- M25.452 Effusion, left hip
- M25.459 Effusion, unspecified hip

√6ᵗʰ M25.46 Effusion, knee
- M25.461 Effusion, right knee
- M25.462 Effusion, left knee
- M25.469 Effusion, unspecified knee

√6ᵗʰ M25.47 Effusion, ankle and foot
- M25.471 Effusion, right ankle
- M25.472 Effusion, left ankle
- M25.473 Effusion, unspecified ankle
- M25.474 Effusion, right foot
- M25.475 Effusion, left foot
- M25.476 Effusion, unspecified foot

M25.48 Effusion, other site

√5ᵗʰ M25.5 Pain in joint
> EXCLUDES 2   pain in hand (M79.64-)
> pain in fingers (M79.64-)
> pain in foot (M79.67-)
> pain in limb (M79.6-)
> pain in toes (M79.67-)

M25.50 Pain in unspecified joint

√6ᵗʰ M25.51 Pain in shoulder
- M25.511 Pain in right shoulder
- M25.512 Pain in left shoulder
- M25.519 Pain in unspecified shoulder

√6ᵗʰ M25.52 Pain in elbow
- M25.521 Pain in right elbow
- M25.522 Pain in left elbow
- M25.529 Pain in unspecified elbow

√6ᵗʰ M25.53 Pain in wrist
- M25.531 Pain in right wrist
- M25.532 Pain in left wrist
- M25.539 Pain in unspecified wrist

√6ᵗʰ M25.55 Pain in hip
- M25.551 Pain in right hip
- M25.552 Pain in left hip
- M25.559 Pain in unspecified hip

√6ᵗʰ M25.56 Pain in knee
- M25.561 Pain in right knee
- M25.562 Pain in left knee
- M25.569 Pain in unspecified knee

√6ᵗʰ M25.57 Pain in ankle and joints of foot
- M25.571 Pain in right ankle and joints of right foot
- M25.572 Pain in left ankle and joints of left foot
- M25.579 Pain in unspecified ankle and joints of unspecified foot

√5ᵗʰ M25.6 Stiffness of joint, not elsewhere classified
> EXCLUDES 1   ankylosis of joint (M24.6-)
> contracture of joint (M24.5-)

M25.60 Stiffness of unspecified joint, not elsewhere classified

√6ᵗʰ M25.61 Stiffness of shoulder, not elsewhere classified
- M25.611 Stiffness of right shoulder, not elsewhere classified
- M25.612 Stiffness of left shoulder, not elsewhere classified
- M25.619 Stiffness of unspecified shoulder, not elsewhere classified

√6ᵗʰ M25.62 Stiffness of elbow, not elsewhere classified
- M25.621 Stiffness of right elbow, not elsewhere classified
- M25.622 Stiffness of left elbow, not elsewhere classified
- M25.629 Stiffness of unspecified elbow, not elsewhere classified

√6ᵗʰ M25.63 Stiffness of wrist, not elsewhere classified
- M25.631 Stiffness of right wrist, not elsewhere classified
- M25.632 Stiffness of left wrist, not elsewhere classified
- M25.639 Stiffness of unspecified wrist, not elsewhere classified

√6ᵗʰ M25.64 Stiffness of hand, not elsewhere classified
- M25.641 Stiffness of right hand, not elsewhere classified
- M25.642 Stiffness of left hand, not elsewhere classified
- M25.649 Stiffness of unspecified hand, not elsewhere classified

√6ᵗʰ M25.65 Stiffness of hip, not elsewhere classified
- M25.651 Stiffness of right hip, not elsewhere classified
- M25.652 Stiffness of left hip, not elsewhere classified
- M25.659 Stiffness of unspecified hip, not elsewhere classified

√6ᵗʰ M25.66 Stiffness of knee, not elsewhere classified
- M25.661 Stiffness of right knee, not elsewhere classified
- M25.662 Stiffness of left knee, not elsewhere classified
- M25.669 Stiffness of unspecified knee, not elsewhere classified

√6ᵗʰ M25.67 Stiffness of ankle and foot, not elsewhere classified
- M25.671 Stiffness of right ankle, not elsewhere classified
- M25.672 Stiffness of left ankle, not elsewhere classified
- M25.673 Stiffness of unspecified ankle, not elsewhere classified
- M25.674 Stiffness of right foot, not elsewhere classified
- M25.675 Stiffness of left foot, not elsewhere classified
- M25.676 Stiffness of unspecified foot, not elsewhere classified

√5ᵗʰ M25.7 Osteophyte

M25.70 Osteophyte, unspecified joint

√6ᵗʰ M25.71 Osteophyte, shoulder
- M25.711 Osteophyte, right shoulder
- M25.712 Osteophyte, left shoulder
- M25.719 Osteophyte, unspecified shoulder

√6ᵗʰ M25.72 Osteophyte, elbow
- M25.721 Osteophyte, right elbow
- M25.722 Osteophyte, left elbow
- M25.729 Osteophyte, unspecified elbow

√6ᵗʰ M25.73 Osteophyte, wrist
- M25.731 Osteophyte, right wrist
- M25.732 Osteophyte, left wrist
- M25.739 Osteophyte, unspecified wrist

√6ᵗʰ M25.74 Osteophyte, hand
- M25.741 Osteophyte, right hand
- M25.742 Osteophyte, left hand
- M25.749 Osteophyte, unspecified hand

√6ᵗʰ M25.75 Osteophyte, hip
- M25.751 Osteophyte, right hip
- M25.752 Osteophyte, left hip
- M25.759 Osteophyte, unspecified hip

√6ᵗʰ M25.76 Osteophyte, knee
- M25.761 Osteophyte, right knee
- M25.762 Osteophyte, left knee
- M25.769 Osteophyte, unspecified knee

√6ᵗʰ M25.77 Osteophyte, ankle and foot
- M25.771 Osteophyte, right ankle
- M25.772 Osteophyte, left ankle
- M25.773 Osteophyte, unspecified ankle
- M25.774 Osteophyte, right foot
- M25.775 Osteophyte, left foot
- M25.776 Osteophyte, unspecified foot

EXCLUDES 1 Not coded here   EXCLUDES 2 Not included here   N Newborn Age: 0   P Pediatric Age: 0-17   M Maternity Age: 12-55   A Adult Age: 15-124

698

ICD-10-CM 2016

M25.78 **Osteophyte,** vertebrae

☑5ᵗʰ M25.8 **Other specified joint disorders**

    M25.80 Other specified joint disorders, unspecified joint

    ☑6ᵗʰ M25.81 **Other specified joint disorders,** shoulder

       M25.811 **Other specified joint disorders,** right shoulder

       M25.812 **Other specified joint disorders,** left shoulder

       M25.819 **Other specified joint disorders, unspecified shoulder**

    ☑6ᵗʰ M25.82 **Other specified joint disorders,** elbow

       M25.821 **Other specified joint disorders,** right elbow

       M25.822 **Other specified joint disorders,** left elbow

       M25.829 **Other specified joint disorders, unspecified elbow**

    ☑6ᵗʰ M25.83 **Other specified joint disorders,** wrist

       M25.831 **Other specified joint disorders,** right wrist

       M25.832 **Other specified joint disorders,** left wrist

       M25.839 **Other specified joint disorders, unspecifiedwrist**

    ☑6ᵗʰ M25.84 **Other specified joint disorders,** hand

       M25.841 **Other specified joint disorders,** right hand

       M25.842 **Other specified joint disorders,** left hand

       M25.849 **Other specified joint disorders, unspecified hand**

    ☑6ᵗʰ M25.85 **Other specified joint disorders,** hip
       AHA: 2014, 4Q, 25

       M25.851 **Other specified joint disorders,** right hip

       M25.852 **Other specified joint disorders,** left hip

       M25.859 **Other specified joint disorders, unspecified hip**

    ☑6ᵗʰ M25.86 **Other specified joint disorders,** knee

       M25.861 **Other specified joint disorders,** right knee

       M25.862 **Other specified joint disorders,** left knee

       M25.869 **Other specified joint disorders, unspecified knee**

    ☑6ᵗʰ M25.87 **Other specified joint disorders,** ankle and foot

       M25.871 **Other specified joint disorders,** right ankle and foot

       M25.872 **Other specified joint disorders,** left ankle and foot

       M25.879 **Other specified joint disorders, unspecified ankle and foot**

    M25.9 **Joint disorder, unspecified**

Dentofacial anomalies [including malocclusion] and other disorders of jaw (M26-M27)

EXCLUDES 1   hemifacial atrophy or hypertrophy (Q67.4)
       unilateral condylar hyperplasia or hypoplasia (M27.8)

☑4ᵗʰ M26 **Dentofacial anomalies [including malocclusion]**

    ☑5ᵗʰ M26.0 **Major anomalies of jaw size**

       EXCLUDES 1   acromegaly (E22.0)
          Robin's syndrome (Q87.0)

       M26.00 **Unspecified anomaly of jaw size**

       M26.01 **Maxillary hyperplasia**

       M26.02 **Maxillary hypoplasia**
          AHA: 2014, 3Q, 23

       M26.03 **Mandibular hyperplasia**

       M26.04 **Mandibular hypoplasia**

       M26.05 **Macrogenia**

       M26.06 **Microgenia**

       M26.07 **Excessive tuberosity of jaw**
          Entire maxillary tuberosity

       M26.09 **Other specified anomalies of jaw size**

    ☑5ᵗʰ M26.1 **Anomalies of jaw-cranial base relationship**

       M26.10 **Unspecified anomaly of jaw-cranial base relationship**

       M26.11 **Maxillary asymmetry**

       M26.12 **Other jaw asymmetry**

       M26.19 **Other specified anomalies of jaw-cranial base relationship**

    ☑5ᵗʰ M26.2 **Anomalies of dental arch relationship**

       M26.20 **Unspecified anomaly of dental arch relationship**

    ☑6ᵗʰ M26.21 **Malocclusion, Angle's class**

       M26.211 **Malocclusion, Angle's** class I
          Neutro-occlusion

       M26.212 **Malocclusion, Angle's** class II
          Disto-occlusion Division I
          Disto-occlusion Division II

       M26.213 **Malocclusion, Angle's** class III
          Mesio-occlusion

       M26.219 **Malocclusion, Angle's class, unspecified**

    ☑6ᵗʰ M26.22 **Open occlusal relationship**

       M26.220 **Open** anterior **occlusal relationship**
          Anterior openbite

       M26.221 **Open** posterior **occlusal relationship**
          Posterior openbite

    M26.23 **Excessive horizontal overlap**
       Excessive horizontal overjet

    M26.24 **Reverse articulation**
       Crossbite (anterior) (posterior)

    M26.25 **Anomalies of interarch distance**

    M26.29 **Other anomalies of dental arch relationship**
       Midline deviation of dental arch
       Overbite (excessive) deep
       Overbite (excessive) horizontal
       Overbite (excessive) vertical
       Posterior lingual occlusion of mandibular teeth

    ☑5ᵗʰ M26.3 **Anomalies of tooth position of fully erupted tooth or teeth**
       EXCLUDES 2   embedded and impacted teeth (K01.-)

       M26.30 **Unspecified anomaly of tooth position of fully erupted tooth or teeth**
       Abnormal spacing of fully erupted tooth or teeth NOS
       Displacement of fully erupted tooth or teeth NOS
       Transposition of fully erupted tooth or teeth NOS

       M26.31 **Crowding of fully erupted teeth**

       M26.32 **Excessive spacing of fully erupted teeth**
       Diastema of fully erupted tooth or teeth NOS

       M26.33 **Horizontal displacement of fully erupted tooth or teeth**
       Tipped tooth or teeth
       Tipping of fully erupted tooth

       M26.34 **Vertical displacement of fully erupted tooth or teeth**
       Extruded tooth
       Infraeruption of tooth or teeth
       Supraeruption of tooth or teeth

       M26.35 **Rotation of fully erupted tooth or teeth**

       M26.36 **Insufficient interocclusal distance of fully erupted teeth (ridge)**
       Lack of adequate intermaxillary vertical dimension of fully erupted teeth

       M26.37 **Excessive interocclusal distance of fully erupted teeth**
       Excessive intermaxillary vertical dimension of fully erupted teeth
       Loss of occlusal vertical dimension of fully erupted teeth

       M26.39 **Other anomalies of tooth position of fully erupted tooth or teeth**

    M26.4 **Malocclusion, unspecified**

    ☑5ᵗʰ M26.5 **Dentofacial functional abnormalities**
       EXCLUDES 1   bruxism (F45.8)
          teeth-grinding NOS (F45.8)

       M26.50 **Dentofacial functional abnormalities, unspecified**

       M26.51 **Abnormal jaw closure**

       M26.52 **Limited mandibular range of motion**

       M26.53 **Deviation in opening and closing of the mandible**

       M26.54 **Insufficient anterior guidance**
       Insufficient anterior occlusal guidance

       M26.55 **Centric occlusion maximum intercuspation discrepancy**
       EXCLUDES 1   centric occlusion NOS (M26.59)

       M26.56 **Non-working side interference**
       Balancing side interference

       M26.57 **Lack of posterior occlusal support**

       M26.59 **Other dentofacial functional abnormalities**
       Centric occlusion (of teeth) NOS
       Malocclusion due to abnormal swallowing
       Malocclusion due to mouth breathing
       Malocclusion due to tongue, lip or finger habits

☑ Additional Character Required   ☑7ᵗʰ Placeholder Alert   Unspecified Dx   Other Specified Dx   Manifestation   ▶◀ Revised Text   ● New Code   ▲ Revised Code Title

ICD-10-CM 2016   **699**

✓5ᵗʰ **M26.6 Temporomandibular joint disorders**
> EXCLUDES 2   *current temporomandibular joint dislocation (S03.0)*
> *current temporomandibular joint sprain (S03.4)*

M26.60 Temporomandibular joint disorder, unspecified

M26.61 Adhesions and ankylosis of temporomandibular joint

M26.62 Arthralgia of temporomandibular joint

M26.63 Articular disc disorder of temporomandibular joint

M26.69 Other specified disorders of temporomandibular joint

✓5ᵗʰ **M26.7 Dental alveolar anomalies**

M26.70 Unspecified alveolar anomaly

M26.71 Alveolar maxillary hyperplasia

M26.72 Alveolar mandibular hyperplasia

M26.73 Alveolar maxillary hypoplasia

M26.74 Alveolar mandibular hypoplasia

M26.79 Other specified alveolar anomalies

✓5ᵗʰ **M26.8 Other dentofacial anomalies**

M26.81 Anterior soft tissue impingement
> Anterior soft tissue impingement on teeth

M26.82 Posterior soft tissue impingement
> Posterior soft tissue impingement on teeth

M26.89 Other dentofacial anomalies

M26.9 Dentofacial anomaly, unspecified

✓4ᵗʰ **M27 Other diseases of jaws**

M27.0 Developmental disorders of jaws
> Latent bone cyst of jaw   Torus mandibularis
> Stafne's cyst   Torus palatinus

M27.1 Giant cell granuloma, central
> Giant cell granuloma NOS
> EXCLUDES 1   *peripheral giant cell granuloma (K06.8)*

M27.2 Inflammatory conditions of jaws
> Osteitis of jaw(s)   Periostitis jaw(s)
> Osteomyelitis (neonatal) jaw(s)   Sequestrum of jaw bone
> Osteoradionecrosis jaw(s)
> Use additional code (W88-W90, X39.0) to identify radiation, if radiation-induced
> EXCLUDES 2   *osteonecrosis of jaw due to drug (M87.180)*

M27.3 Alveolitis of jaws
> Alveolar osteitis
> Dry socket

✓5ᵗʰ **M27.4 Other and unspecified cysts of jaw**
> EXCLUDES 1   *cysts of oral region (K09.-)*
> *latent bone cyst of jaw (M27.0)*
> *Stafne's cyst (M27.0)*

M27.40 Unspecified cyst of jaw
> Cyst of jaw NOS

M27.49 Other cysts of jaw
> Aneurysmal cyst of jaw
> Hemorrhagic cyst of jaw
> Traumatic cyst of jaw

✓5ᵗʰ **M27.5 Periradicular pathology associated with previous endodontic treatment**

M27.51 Perforation of root canal space due to endodontic treatment

M27.52 Endodontic overfill

M27.53 Endodontic underfill

M27.59 Other periradicular pathology associated with previous endodontic treatment

✓5ᵗʰ **M27.6 Endosseous dental implant failure**

M27.61 Osseointegration failure of dental implant
> Hemorrhagic complications of dental implant placement
> Iatrogenic osseointegration failure of dental implant
> Osseointegration failure of dental implant due to complications of systemic disease
> Osseointegration failure of dental implant due to poor bone quality
> Pre-integration failure of dental implant NOS
> Pre-osseointegration failure of dental implant

M27.62 Post-osseointegration biological failure of dental implant
> Failure of dental implant due to lack of attached gingiva
> Failure of dental implant due to occlusal trauma (caused by poor prosthetic design)
> Failure of dental implant due to parafunctional habits
> Failure of dental implant due to periodontal infection (peri-implantitis)
> Failure of dental implant due to poor oral hygiene
> Iatrogenic post-osseointegration failure of dental implant
> Post-osseointegration failure of dental implant due to complications of systemic disease

M27.63 Post-osseointegration mechanical failure of dental implant
> Failure of dental prosthesis causing loss of dental implant
> Fracture of dental implant
> EXCLUDES 2   *cracked tooth (K03.81)*
> *fractured dental restorative material with loss of material (K08.531)*
> *fractured dental restorative material without loss of material (K08.530)*
> *fractured tooth (S02.5)*

M27.69 Other endosseous dental implant failure
> Dental implant failure NOS

M27.8 Other specified diseases of jaws
> Cherubism   Unilateral condylar hyperplasia
> Exostosis   Unilateral condylar hypoplasia
> Fibrous dysplasia
> EXCLUDES 1   *jaw pain (R68.84)*

M27.9 Disease of jaws, unspecified

Systemic connective tissue disorders (M30-M36)

INCLUDES   autoimmune disease NOS
collagen (vascular) disease NOS
systemic autoimmune disease
systemic collagen (vascular) disease

EXCLUDES 1   *autoimmune disease, single organ or single cell-type—code to relevant condition category*

✓4ᵗʰ **M30 Polyarteritis nodosa and related conditions**
> EXCLUDES 1   *microscopic polyarteritis (M31.7)*

M30.0 Polyarteritis nodosa

M30.1 Polyarteritis with lung involvement [Churg-Strauss]
> Allergic granulomatous angiitis

M30.2 Juvenile polyarteritis

M30.3 Mucocutaneous lymph node syndrome [Kawasaki]

M30.8 Other conditions related to polyarteritis nodosa
> Polyangiitis overlap syndrome

✓4ᵗʰ **M31 Other necrotizing vasculopathies**

M31.0 Hypersensitivity angiitis
> Goodpasture's syndrome

M31.1 Thrombotic microangiopathy
> Thrombotic thrombocytopenic purpura

M31.2 Lethal midline granuloma

✓5ᵗʰ **M31.3 Wegener's granulomatosis**
> Necrotizing respiratory granulomatosis

M31.30 Wegener's granulomatosis without renal involvement
> Wegener's granulomatosis NOS

M31.31 Wegener's granulomatosis with renal involvement

M31.4 Aortic arch syndrome [Takayasu]

M31.5 Giant cell arteritis with polymyalgia rheumatica

M31.6 Other giant cell arteritis

M31.7 Microscopic polyangiitis
> Microscopic polyarteritis
> EXCLUDES 1   *polyarteritis nodosa (M30.0)*

M31.8 Other specified necrotizing vasculopathies
> Hypocomplementemic vasculitis
> Septic vasculitis

M31.9 Necrotizing vasculopathy, unspecified

✓4ᵗʰ **M32 Systemic lupus erythematosus (SLE)**
> EXCLUDES 1   *lupus erythematosus (discoid) (NOS) (L93.0)*

M32.0 Drug-induced systemic lupus erythematosus
> Use additional code for adverse effect, if applicable, to identify drug (T36-T50 with fifth or sixth character 5)

EXCLUDES 1 Not coded here   EXCLUDES 2 Not included here   N Newborn Age: 0   P Pediatric Age: 0-17   M Maternity Age: 12-55   A Adult Age: 15-124

✓5ᵗʰ **M32.1** Systemic lupus erythematosus with organ or system involvement

M32.10 Systemic lupus erythematosus, organ or system involvement unspecified

M32.11 Endocarditis in systemic lupus erythematosus
Libman-Sacks disease

M32.12 Pericarditis in systemic lupus erythematosus
Lupus pericarditis

M32.13 Lung involvement in systemic lupus erythematosus
Pleural effusion due to systemic lupus erythematosus

M32.14 Glomerular disease in systemic lupus erythematosus
Lupus renal disease NOS
AHA: 2013, 4Q, 125

M32.15 Tubulo-interstitial nephropathy in systemic lupus erythematosus

M32.19 Other organ or system involvement in systemic lupus erythematosus

M32.8 Other forms of systemic lupus erythematosus

M32.9 Systemic lupus erythematosus, unspecified
SLE NOS
Systemic lupus erythematosus NOS
Systemic lupus erythematosus without organ involvement

✓4ᵗʰ **M33** Dermatopolymyositis

✓5ᵗʰ **M33.0** Juvenile dermatopolymyositis

M33.00 Juvenile dermatopolymyositis, organ involvement unspecified

M33.01 Juvenile dermatopolymyositis with respiratory involvement

M33.02 Juvenile dermatopolymyositis with myopathy

M33.09 Juvenile dermatopolymyositis with other organ involvement

✓5ᵗʰ **M33.1** Other dermatopolymyositis

M33.10 Other dermatopolymyositis, organ involvement unspecified

M33.11 Other dermatopolymyositis with respiratory involvement

M33.12 Other dermatopolymyositis with myopathy

M33.19 Other dermatopolymyositis with other organ involvement

✓5ᵗʰ **M33.2** Polymyositis

M33.20 Polymyositis, organ involvement unspecified

M33.21 Polymyositis with respiratory involvement

M33.22 Polymyositis with myopathy

M33.29 Polymyositis with other organ involvement

✓5ᵗʰ **M33.9** Dermatopolymyositis, unspecified

M33.90 Dermatopolymyositis, unspecified, organ involvement unspecified

M33.91 Dermatopolymyositis, unspecified with respiratory involvement

M33.92 Dermatopolymyositis, unspecified with myopathy

M33.99 Dermatopolymyositis, unspecified with other organ involvement

✓4ᵗʰ **M34** Systemic sclerosis [scleroderma]
EXCLUDES 1   circumscribed scleroderma (L94.0)
neonatal scleroderma (P83.8)

M34.0 Progressive systemic sclerosis

M34.1 CR(E)ST syndrome
Combination of calcinosis, Raynaud's phenomenon, esophageal dysfunction, sclerodactyly, telangiectasia

M34.2 Systemic sclerosis induced by drug and chemical
Code first poisoning due to drug or toxin, if applicable (T36-T65 with fifth or sixth character 1-4 or 6)
Use additional code for adverse effect, if applicable, to identify drug (T36-T50 with fifth or sixth character 5)

✓5ᵗʰ **M34.8** Other forms of systemic sclerosis

M34.81 Systemic sclerosis with lung involvement

M34.82 Systemic sclerosis with myopathy

M34.83 Systemic sclerosis with polyneuropathy

M34.89 Other systemic sclerosis

M34.9 Systemic sclerosis, unspecified

✓4ᵗʰ **M35** Other systemic involvement of connective tissue
EXCLUDES 1   reactive perforating collagenosis (L87.1)

✓5ᵗʰ **M35.0** Sicca syndrome [Sjögren]

M35.00 Sicca syndrome, unspecified

M35.01 Sicca syndrome with keratoconjunctivitis

M35.02 Sicca syndrome with lung involvement

M35.03 Sicca syndrome with myopathy

M35.04 Sicca syndrome with tubulo-interstitial nephropathy
Renal tubular acidosis in sicca syndrome

M35.09 Sicca syndrome with other organ involvement

M35.1 Other overlap syndromes
Mixed connective tissue disease
EXCLUDES 1   polyangiitis overlap syndrome (M30.8)

M35.2 Behçet's disease

M35.3 Polymyalgia rheumatica
EXCLUDES 1   polymyalgia rheumatica with giant cell arteritis (M31.5)

M35.4 Diffuse (eosinophilic) fasciitis

M35.5 Multifocal fibrosclerosis

M35.6 Relapsing panniculitis [Weber-Christian]
EXCLUDES 1   lupus panniculitis (L93.2)
panniculitis NOS (M79.3-)

M35.7 Hypermobility syndrome
Familial ligamentous laxity
EXCLUDES 1   Ehlers-Danlos syndrome (Q79.6)
ligamentous laxity, NOS (M24.2-)

M35.8 Other specified systemic involvement of connective tissue

M35.9 Systemic involvement of connective tissue, unspecified
Autoimmune disease (systemic) NOS
Collagen (vascular) disease NOS

✓4ᵗʰ **M36** Systemic disorders of connective tissue in diseases classified elsewhere
EXCLUDES 2   arthropathies in diseases classified elsewhere (M14.-)

M36.0 Dermato(poly)myositis in neoplastic disease
Code first underlying neoplasm (C00-D49)

M36.1 Arthropathy in neoplastic disease
Code first underlying neoplasm, such as:
leukemia (C91-C95)
malignant histiocytosis (C96.A)
multiple myeloma (C90.0)

M36.2 Hemophilic arthropathy
Hemarthrosis in hemophilic arthropathy
Code first underlying disease, such as:
factor VIII deficiency (D66)
with vascular defect (D68.0)
factor IX deficiency (D67)
hemophilia (classical) (D66)
hemophilia B (D67)
hemophilia C (D68.1)

M36.3 Arthropathy in other blood disorders

M36.4 Arthropathy in hypersensitivity reactions classified elsewhere
Code first underlying disease, such as:
Henoch (-Schönlein) purpura (D69.0)
serum sickness (T80.6-)

M36.8 Systemic disorders of connective tissue in other diseases classified elsewhere
Code first underlying disease, such as:
alkaptonuria (E70.2)
hypogammaglobulinemia (D80.-)
ochronosis (E70.2)

DORSOPATHIES (M40-M54)

Deforming dorsopathies (M40-M43)

✓4ᵗʰ **M40** Kyphosis and lordosis
EXCLUDES 1   congenital kyphosis and lordosis (Q76.4)
kyphoscoliosis (M41.-)
postprocedural kyphosis and lordosis (M96.-)

✓5ᵗʰ **M40.0** Postural kyphosis
EXCLUDES 1   osteochondrosis of spine (M42.-)

M40.00 Postural kyphosis, site unspecified

M40.03 Postural kyphosis, cervicothoracic region

M40.04 Postural kyphosis, thoracic region

M40.05 Postural kyphosis, thoracolumbar region

✓5ᵗʰ **M40.1** Other secondary kyphosis

M40.10 Other secondary kyphosis, site unspecified

M40.12 Other secondary kyphosis, cervical region

M40.13 Other secondary kyphosis, cervicothoracic region

M40.14 Other secondary kyphosis, thoracic region

☑ Additional Character Required   ✓7ᵗʰ Placeholder Alert   Unspecified Dx   Other Specified Dx   Manifestation   ►◄ Revised Text   ● New Code   ▲ Revised Code Title

M40.15 Other secondary kyphosis, **thoracolumbar region**

✓5th **M40.2** Other and unspecified kyphosis

✓6th **M40.20** Unspecified **kyphosis**

M40.202 Unspecified kyphosis, **cervical region**

M40.203 Unspecified kyphosis, **cervicothoracic region**

M40.204 Unspecified kyphosis, **thoracic region**

M40.205 Unspecified kyphosis, **thoracolumbar region**

M40.209 Unspecified kyphosis, **site unspecified**

✓6th **M40.29** Other **kyphosis**

M40.292 Other kyphosis, **cervical region**

M40.293 Other kyphosis, **cervicothoracic region**

M40.294 Other kyphosis, **thoracic region**

M40.295 Other kyphosis, **thoracolumbar region**

M40.299 Other kyphosis, **site unspecified**

✓5th **M40.3** Flatback syndrome

M40.30 Flatback syndrome, **site unspecified**

M40.35 Flatback syndrome, **thoracolumbar region**

M40.36 Flatback syndrome, **lumbar region**

M40.37 Flatback syndrome, **lumbosacral region**

✓5th **M40.4** Postural lordosis

Acquired lordosis

M40.40 Postural lordosis, **site unspecified**

M40.45 Postural lordosis, **thoracolumbar region**

M40.46 Postural lordosis, **lumbar region**

M40.47 Postural lordosis, **lumbosacral region**

✓5th **M40.5** Lordosis, unspecified

M40.50 Lordosis, unspecified, **site unspecified**

M40.55 Lordosis, unspecified, **thoracolumbar region**

M40.56 Lordosis, unspecified, **lumbar region**

M40.57 Lordosis, unspecified, **lumbosacral region**

✓4th **M41 Scoliosis**

INCLUDES kyphoscoliosis

EXCLUDES 1 *congenital scoliosis due to bony malformation (Q76.3)*
congenital scoliosis NOS (Q67.5)
kyphoscoliotic heart disease (I27.1)
postprocedural scoliosis (M96.-)
postural congenital scoliosis (Q67.5)

✓5th **M41.0** Infantile idiopathic **scoliosis**

AHA: 2014, 4Q, 26

M41.00 Infantile idiopathic scoliosis, **site unspecified**

M41.02 Infantile idiopathic scoliosis, **cervical region**

M41.03 Infantile idiopathic scoliosis, **cervicothoracic region**

M41.04 Infantile idiopathic scoliosis, **thoracic region**

M41.05 Infantile idiopathic scoliosis, **thoracolumbar region**

M41.06 Infantile idiopathic scoliosis, **lumbar region**

M41.07 Infantile idiopathic scoliosis, **lumbosacral region**

M41.08 Infantile idiopathic scoliosis, **sacral and sacrococcygeal region**

✓5th **M41.1** Juvenile and adolescent idiopathic scoliosis

✓6th **M41.11** Juvenile idiopathic **scoliosis**

AHA: 2014, 4Q, 28

M41.112 Juvenile idiopathic scoliosis, **cervical region**

M41.113 Juvenile idiopathic scoliosis, **cervicothoracic region**

M41.114 Juvenile idiopathic scoliosis, **thoracic region**

M41.115 Juvenile idiopathic scoliosis, **thoracolumbar region**

M41.116 Juvenile idiopathic scoliosis, **lumbar region**

M41.117 Juvenile idiopathic scoliosis, **lumbosacral region**

M41.119 Juvenile idiopathic scoliosis, **site unspecified**

✓6th **M41.12** Adolescent **scoliosis**

M41.122 Adolescent idiopathic scoliosis, **cervical region**

M41.123 Adolescent idiopathic scoliosis, **cervicothoracic region**

M41.124 Adolescent idiopathic scoliosis, **thoracic region**

M41.125 Adolescent idiopathic scoliosis, **thoracolumbar region**

M41.126 Adolescent idiopathic scoliosis, **lumbar region**

M41.127 Adolescent idiopathic scoliosis, **lumbosacral region**

M41.129 Adolescent idiopathic scoliosis, **site unspecified**

✓5th **M41.2** Other idiopathic **scoliosis**

M41.20 Other idiopathic scoliosis, **site unspecified**

M41.22 Other idiopathic scoliosis, **cervical region**

M41.23 Other idiopathic scoliosis, **cervicothoracic region**

M41.24 Other idiopathic scoliosis, **thoracic region**

M41.25 Other idiopathic scoliosis, **thoracolumbar region**

M41.26 Other idiopathic scoliosis, **lumbar region**

M41.27 Other idiopathic scoliosis, **lumbosacral region**

✓5th **M41.3** Thoracogenic scoliosis

M41.30 Thoracogenic scoliosis, **site unspecified**

M41.34 Thoracogenic scoliosis, **thoracic region**

M41.35 Thoracogenic scoliosis, **thoracolumbar region**

✓5th **M41.4** Neuromuscular **scoliosis**

Scoliosis secondary to cerebral palsy, Friedreich's ataxia, poliomyelitis and other neuromuscular disorders

Code also underlying condition

AHA: 2014, 4Q, 27

M41.40 Neuromuscular scoliosis, **site unspecified**

M41.41 Neuromuscular scoliosis, **occipito-atlanto-axial region**

M41.42 Neuromuscular scoliosis, **cervical region**

M41.43 Neuromuscular scoliosis, **cervicothoracic region**

M41.44 Neuromuscular scoliosis, **thoracic region**

M41.45 Neuromuscular scoliosis, **thoracolumbar region**

M41.46 Neuromuscular scoliosis, **lumbar region**

M41.47 Neuromuscular scoliosis, **lumbosacral region**

✓5th **M41.5** Other secondary **scoliosis**

M41.50 Other secondary scoliosis, **site unspecified**

M41.52 Other secondary scoliosis, **cervical region**

M41.53 Other secondary scoliosis, **cervicothoracic region**

M41.54 Other secondary scoliosis, **thoracic region**

M41.55 Other secondary scoliosis, **thoracolumbar region**

M41.56 Other secondary scoliosis, **lumbar region**

M41.57 Other secondary scoliosis, **lumbosacral region**

✓5th **M41.8** Other forms of scoliosis

M41.80 Other forms of scoliosis, **site unspecified**

M41.82 Other forms of scoliosis, **cervical region**

M41.83 Other forms of scoliosis, **cervicothoracic region**

M41.84 Other forms of scoliosis, **thoracic region**

M41.85 Other forms of scoliosis, **thoracolumbar region**

M41.86 Other forms of scoliosis, **lumbar region**

M41.87 Other forms of scoliosis, **lumbosacral region**

M41.9 Scoliosis, unspecified

✓4th **M42 Spinal osteochondrosis**

✓5th **M42.0** Juvenile osteochondrosis of spine

Calvé's disease

Scheuermann's disease

EXCLUDES 1 *postural kyphosis (M40.0)*

M42.00 Juvenile osteochondrosis of spine, **site unspecified**

M42.01 Juvenile osteochondrosis of spine, **occipito-atlanto-axial region**

M42.02 Juvenile osteochondrosis of spine, **cervical region**

M42.03 Juvenile osteochondrosis of spine, **cervicothoracic region**

M42.04 Juvenile osteochondrosis of spine, **thoracic region**

M42.05 Juvenile osteochondrosis of spine, **thoracolumbar region**

M42.06 Juvenile osteochondrosis of spine, **lumbar region**

M42.07 Juvenile osteochondrosis of spine, **lumbosacral region**

M42.08 Juvenile osteochondrosis of spine, **sacral and sacrococcygeal region**

M42.09 Juvenile osteochondrosis of spine, **multiple sites in spine**

EXCLUDES 1 Not coded here   EXCLUDES 2 Not included here   N Newborn Age: 0   P Pediatric Age: 0-17   M Maternity Age: 12-55   A Adult Age: 15-124

√5ᵗʰ **M42.1** Adult **osteochondrosis of spine**

    M42.10 Adult osteochondrosis of spine, site unspecified   Ⓐ

    M42.11 Adult osteochondrosis of spine, occipito-atlanto-axial **region**   Ⓐ

    M42.12 Adult osteochondrosis of spine, cervical **region**   Ⓐ

    M42.13 Adult osteochondrosis of spine, cervicothoracic **region**   Ⓐ

    M42.14 Adult osteochondrosis of spine, thoracic **region**   Ⓐ

    M42.15 Adult osteochondrosis of spine, thoracolumbar **region**   Ⓐ

    M42.16 Adult osteochondrosis of spine, lumbar **region**   Ⓐ

    M42.17 Adult osteochondrosis of spine, lumbosacral **region**   Ⓐ

    M42.18 Adult osteochondrosis of spine, sacral and sacrococcygeal **region**   Ⓐ

    M42.19 Adult osteochondrosis of spine, multiple sites in spine   Ⓐ

   M42.9 Spinal osteochondrosis, unspecified

√4ᵗʰ **M43** Other **deforming dorsopathies**

    EXCLUDES 1   *congenital spondylolysis and spondylolisthesis (Q76.2)*
         hemivertebra (Q76.3-Q76.4)
         Klippel-Feil syndrome (Q76.1)
         lumbarization and sacralization (Q76.4)
         platyspondylisis (Q76.4)
         spina bifida occulta (Q76.0)
         spinal curvature in osteoporosis (M80.-)
         spinal curvature in Paget's disease of bone [osteitis deformans] (M88.-)

   √5ᵗʰ **M43.0** Spondylolysis

      EXCLUDES 1   *congenital spondylolysis (Q76.2)*
          spondylolisthesis (M43.1)

    M43.00 Spondylolysis, site unspecified

    M43.01 Spondylolysis, occipito-atlanto-axial **region**

    M43.02 Spondylolysis, cervical **region**

    M43.03 Spondylolysis, cervicothoracic **region**

    M43.04 Spondylolysis, thoracic **region**

    M43.05 Spondylolysis, thoracolumbar **region**

    M43.06 Spondylolysis, lumbar **region**

    M43.07 Spondylolysis, lumbosacral **region**

    M43.08 Spondylolysis, sacral and sacrococcygeal **region**

    M43.09 Spondylolysis, multiple sites in spine

   √5ᵗʰ **M43.1** Spondylolisthesis

      EXCLUDES 1   *acute traumatic of lumbosacral region (S33.1)*
          acute traumatic of sites other than lumbosacral— code to Fracture, vertebra, by region
          congenital spondylolisthesis (Q76.2)

    M43.10 Spondylolisthesis, site unspecified

    M43.11 Spondylolisthesis, occipito-atlanto-axial **region**

    M43.12 Spondylolisthesis, cervical **region**

    M43.13 Spondylolisthesis, cervicothoracic **region**

    M43.14 Spondylolisthesis, thoracic **region**

    M43.15 Spondylolisthesis, thoracolumbar **region**

    M43.16 Spondylolisthesis, lumbar **region**

    M43.17 Spondylolisthesis, lumbosacral **region**

    M43.18 Spondylolisthesis, sacral and sacrococcygeal **region**

    M43.19 Spondylolisthesis, multiple sites in spine

   √5ᵗʰ **M43.2** Fusion of spine

      Ankylosis of spinal joint

      EXCLUDES 1   *ankylosing spondylitis (M45.0-)*
          congenital fusion of spine (Q76.4)

      EXCLUDES 2   *arthrodesis status (Z98.1)*
          pseudoarthrosis after fusion or arthrodesis (M96.0)

    M43.20 Fusion of spine, site unspecified

    M43.21 Fusion of spine, occipito-atlanto-axial **region**

    M43.22 Fusion of spine, cervical **region**

    M43.23 Fusion of spine, cervicothoracic **region**

    M43.24 Fusion of spine, thoracic **region**

    M43.25 Fusion of spine, thoracolumbar **region**

    M43.26 Fusion of spine, lumbar **region**

    M43.27 Fusion of spine, lumbosacral **region**

    M43.28 Fusion of spine, sacral and sacrococcygeal **region**

   M43.3 Recurrent atlantoaxial dislocation with myelopathy

   M43.4 Other recurrent atlantoaxial dislocation

√5ᵗʰ **M43.5** Other **recurrent vertebral dislocation**

      EXCLUDES 1   *biomechanical lesions NEC (M99.-)*

   √6ᵗʰ **M43.5X** Other **recurrent vertebral dislocation**

    M43.5X2 Other recurrent vertebral dislocation, cervical **region**

    M43.5X3 Other recurrent vertebral dislocation, cervicothoracic **region**

    M43.5X4 Other recurrent vertebral dislocation, thoracic **region**

    M43.5X5 Other recurrent vertebral dislocation, thoracolumbar **region**

    M43.5X6 Other recurrent vertebral dislocation, lumbar **region**

    M43.5X7 Other recurrent vertebral dislocation, lumbosacral **region**

    M43.5X8 Other recurrent vertebral dislocation, sacral and sacrococcygeal **region**

    M43.5X9 Other recurrent vertebral dislocation, site unspecified

   M43.6 Torticollis

      EXCLUDES 1   *congenital (sternomastoid) torticollis (Q68.0)*
          current injury—see Injury, of spine, by body region
          ocular torticollis (R29.891)
          psychogenic torticollis (F45.8)
          spasmodic torticollis (G24.3)
          torticollis due to birth injury (P15.2)

   √5ᵗʰ **M43.8** Other **specified deforming dorsopathies**

      EXCLUDES 2   *kyphosis and lordosis (M40.-)*
          scoliosis (M41.-)

   √6ᵗʰ **M43.8X** Other **specified deforming dorsopathies**

    M43.8X1 Other specified deforming dorsopathies, occipito-atlanto-axial **region**

    M43.8X2 Other specified deforming dorsopathies, cervical **region**

    M43.8X3 Other specified deforming dorsopathies, cervicothoracic **region**

    M43.8X4 Other specified deforming dorsopathies, thoracic **region**

    M43.8X5 Other specified deforming dorsopathies, thoracolumbar **region**

    M43.8X6 Other specified deforming dorsopathies, lumbar **region**

    M43.8X7 Other specified deforming dorsopathies, lumbosacral **region**

    M43.8X8 Other specified deforming dorsopathies, sacral and sacrococcygeal **region**

    M43.8X9 Other specified deforming dorsopathies, site unspecified

   M43.9 Deforming dorsopathy, unspecified
      Curvature of spine NOS

Spondylopathies (M45-M49)

√4ᵗʰ **M45** Ankylosing **spondylitis**
      Rheumatoid arthritis of spine

      EXCLUDES 1   *arthropathy in Reiter's disease (M02.3-)*
          juvenile (ankylosing) spondylitis (M08.1)

      EXCLUDES 2   *Behçet's disease (M35.2)*

   M45.0 Ankylosing spondylitis of multiple sites in spine

   M45.1 Ankylosing spondylitis of occipito-atlanto-axial **region**

   M45.2 Ankylosing spondylitis of cervical **region**

   M45.3 Ankylosing spondylitis of cervicothoracic **region**

   M45.4 Ankylosing spondylitis of thoracic **region**

   M45.5 Ankylosing spondylitis of thoracolumbar **region**

   M45.6 Ankylosing spondylitis lumbar **region**

   M45.7 Ankylosing spondylitis of lumbosacral **region**

   M45.8 Ankylosing spondylitis sacral and sacrococcygeal **region**

   M45.9 Ankylosing spondylitis of unspecified sites in spine

√4ᵗʰ **M46** Other **inflammatory spondylopathies**

   √5ᵗʰ **M46.0** Spinal enthesopathy
      Disorder of ligamentous or muscular attachments of spine

    M46.00 Spinal enthesopathy, site unspecified

    M46.01 Spinal enthesopathy, occipito-atlanto-axial **region**

    M46.02 Spinal enthesopathy, cervical **region**

    M46.03 Spinal enthesopathy, cervicothoracic **region**

    M46.04 Spinal enthesopathy, thoracic **region**

☑ Additional Character Required   ✓ˣ⁷ᵗʰ Placeholder Alert   Unspecified Dx   Other Specified Dx   Manifestation   ►◄ Revised Text   ● New Code   ▲ Revised Code Title

Chapter 13. Diseases of the Musculoskeletal System and Connective Tissue

M46.05   **Spinal enthesopathy, thoracolumbar region**

M46.06   **Spinal enthesopathy, lumbar region**

M46.07   **Spinal enthesopathy, lumbosacral region**

M46.08   **Spinal enthesopathy, sacral and sacrococcygeal region**

M46.09   **Spinal enthesopathy, multiple sites in spine**

M46.1   Sacroiliitis, not elsewhere classified

✓5ᵗʰ   M46.2   Osteomyelitis of vertebra

M46.20   **Osteomyelitis of vertebra, site unspecified**

M46.21   **Osteomyelitis of vertebra, occipito-atlanto-axial region**

M46.22   **Osteomyelitis of vertebra, cervical region**

M46.23   **Osteomyelitis of vertebra, cervicothoracic region**

M46.24   **Osteomyelitis of vertebra, thoracic region**

M46.25   **Osteomyelitis of vertebra, thoracolumbar region**

M46.26   **Osteomyelitis of vertebra, lumbar region**

M46.27   **Osteomyelitis of vertebra, lumbosacral region**

M46.28   **Osteomyelitis of vertebra, sacral and sacrococcygeal region**

✓5ᵗʰ   M46.3   Infection of intervertebral disc (pyogenic)

Use additional code (B95-B97) to identify infectious agent

M46.30   **Infection of intervertebral disc (pyogenic), site unspecified**

M46.31   **Infection of intervertebral disc (pyogenic), occipito-atlanto-axial region**

M46.32   **Infection of intervertebral disc (pyogenic), cervical region**

M46.33   **Infection of intervertebral disc (pyogenic), cervicothoracic region**

M46.34   **Infection of intervertebral disc (pyogenic), thoracic region**

M46.35   **Infection of intervertebral disc (pyogenic), thoracolumbar region**

M46.36   **Infection of intervertebral disc (pyogenic), lumbar region**

M46.37   **Infection of intervertebral disc (pyogenic), lumbosacral region**

M46.38   **Infection of intervertebral disc (pyogenic), sacral and sacrococcygeal region**

M46.39   **Infection of intervertebral disc (pyogenic), multiple sites in spine**

✓5ᵗʰ   M46.4   Discitis, unspecified

M46.40   **Discitis, unspecified, site unspecified**   Ⓐ

M46.41   **Discitis, unspecified, occipito-atlanto-axial region**   Ⓐ

M46.42   **Discitis, unspecified, cervical region**   Ⓐ

M46.43   **Discitis, unspecified, cervicothoracic region**   Ⓐ

M46.44   **Discitis, unspecified, thoracic region**   Ⓐ

M46.45   **Discitis, unspecified, thoracolumbar region**   Ⓐ

M46.46   **Discitis, unspecified, lumbar region**   Ⓐ

M46.47   **Discitis, unspecified, lumbosacral region**   Ⓐ

M46.48   **Discitis, unspecified, sacral and sacrococcygeal region**   Ⓐ

M46.49   **Discitis, unspecified, multiple sites in spine**   Ⓐ

✓5ᵗʰ   M46.5   Other infective spondylopathies

M46.50   **Other infective spondylopathies, site unspecified**

M46.51   **Other infective spondylopathies, occipito-atlanto-axial region**

M46.52   **Other infective spondylopathies, cervical region**

M46.53   **Other infective spondylopathies, cervicothoracic region**

M46.54   **Other infective spondylopathies, thoracic region**

M46.55   **Other infective spondylopathies, thoracolumbar region**

M46.56   **Other infective spondylopathies, lumbar region**

M46.57   **Other infective spondylopathies, lumbosacral region**

M46.58   **Other infective spondylopathies, sacral and sacrococcygeal region**

M46.59   **Other infective spondylopathies, multiple sites in spine**

✓5ᵗʰ   M46.8   Other specified inflammatory spondylopathies

M46.80   **Other specified inflammatory spondylopathies, site unspecified**

M46.81   **Other specified inflammatory spondylopathies, occipito-atlanto-axial region**

M46.82   **Other specified inflammatory spondylopathies, cervical region**

M46.83   **Other specified inflammatory spondylopathies, cervicothoracic region**

M46.84   **Other specified inflammatory spondylopathies, thoracic region**

M46.85   **Other specified inflammatory spondylopathies, thoracolumbar region**

M46.86   **Other specified inflammatory spondylopathies, lumbar region**

M46.87   **Other specified inflammatory spondylopathies, lumbosacral region**

M46.88   **Other specified inflammatory spondylopathies, sacral and sacrococcygeal region**

M46.89   **Other specified inflammatory spondylopathies, multiple sites in spine**

✓5ᵗʰ   M46.9   Unspecified inflammatory spondylopathy

M46.90   **Unspecified inflammatory spondylopathy, site unspecified**

M46.91   **Unspecified inflammatory spondylopathy, occipito-atlanto-axial region**

M46.92   **Unspecified inflammatory spondylopathy, cervical region**

M46.93   **Unspecified inflammatory spondylopathy, cervicothoracic region**

M46.94   **Unspecified inflammatory spondylopathy, thoracic region**

M46.95   **Unspecified inflammatory spondylopathy, thoracolumbar region**

M46.96   **Unspecified inflammatory spondylopathy, lumbar region**

M46.97   **Unspecified inflammatory spondylopathy, lumbosacral region**

M46.98   **Unspecified inflammatory spondylopathy, sacral and sacrococcygeal region**

M46.99   **Unspecified inflammatory spondylopathy, multiple sites in spine**

✓4ᵗʰ   **M47   Spondylosis**

INCLUDES   arthrosis or osteoarthritis of spine
degeneration of facet joints

✓5ᵗʰ   M47.0   Anterior spinal and vertebral artery compression syndromes

✓6ᵗʰ   M47.01   Anterior spinal artery compression syndromes

M47.011   **Anterior spinal artery compression syndromes, occipito-atlanto-axial region**

M47.012   **Anterior spinal artery compression syndromes, cervical region**

M47.013   **Anterior spinal artery compression syndromes, cervicothoracic region**

M47.014   **Anterior spinal artery compression syndromes, thoracic region**

M47.015   **Anterior spinal artery compression syndromes, thoracolumbar region**

M47.016   **Anterior spinal artery compression syndromes, lumbar region**

M47.019   **Anterior spinal artery compression syndromes, site unspecified**

✓6ᵗʰ   M47.02   Vertebral artery compression syndromes

M47.021   **Vertebral artery compression syndromes, occipito-atlanto-axial region**

M47.022   **Vertebral artery compression syndromes, cervical region**

M47.029   **Vertebral artery compression syndromes, site unspecified**

✓5ᵗʰ   M47.1   Other spondylosis with myelopathy

Spondylogenic compression of spinal cord

EXCLUDES 1   *vertebral subluxation (M43.3-M43.5X9)*

M47.10   **Other spondylosis with myelopathy, site unspecified**

M47.11   **Other spondylosis with myelopathy, occipito-atlanto-axial region**

M47.12   **Other spondylosis with myelopathy, cervical region**

M47.13   **Other spondylosis with myelopathy, cervicothoracic region**

M47.14   **Other spondylosis with myelopathy, thoracic region**

EXCLUDES 1 Not coded here   EXCLUDES 2 Not included here   Ⓝ Newborn Age: 0   Ⓟ Pediatric Age: 0-17   Ⓜ Maternity Age: 12-55   Ⓐ Adult Age: 15-124

M47.15 Other spondylosis with myelopathy, thoracolumbar region

M47.16 Other spondylosis with myelopathy, lumbar region

✓5th **M47.2** Other spondylosis with radiculopathy

M47.20 Other spondylosis with radiculopathy, site unspecified

M47.21 Other spondylosis with radiculopathy, occipito-atlanto-axial region

M47.22 Other spondylosis with radiculopathy, cervical region

M47.23 Other spondylosis with radiculopathy, cervicothoracic region

M47.24 Other spondylosis with radiculopathy, thoracic region

M47.25 Other spondylosis with radiculopathy, thoracolumbar region

M47.26 Other spondylosis with radiculopathy, lumbar region

M47.27 Other spondylosis with radiculopathy, lumbosacral region

M47.28 Other spondylosis with radiculopathy, sacral and sacrococcygeal region

✓5th **M47.8** Other spondylosis

✓6th **M47.81** Spondylosis without myelopathy or radiculopathy

M47.811 Spondylosis without myelopathy or radiculopathy, occipito-atlanto-axial region

M47.812 Spondylosis without myelopathy or radiculopathy, cervical region

M47.813 Spondylosis without myelopathy or radiculopathy, cervicothoracic region

M47.814 Spondylosis without myelopathy or radiculopathy, thoracic region

M47.815 Spondylosis without myelopathy or radiculopathy, thoracolumbar region

M47.816 Spondylosis without myelopathy or radiculopathy, lumbar region

M47.817 Spondylosis without myelopathy or radiculopathy, lumbosacral region

M47.818 Spondylosis without myelopathy or radiculopathy, sacral and sacrococcygeal region

M47.819 Spondylosis without myelopathy or radiculopathy, site unspecified

✓6th **M47.89** Other spondylosis

M47.891 Other spondylosis, occipito-atlanto-axial region

M47.892 Other spondylosis, cervical region

M47.893 Other spondylosis, cervicothoracic region

M47.894 Other spondylosis, thoracic region

M47.895 Other spondylosis, thoracolumbar region

M47.896 Other spondylosis, lumbar region

M47.897 Other spondylosis, lumbosacral region

M47.898 Other spondylosis, sacral and sacrococcygeal region

M47.899 Other spondylosis, site unspecified

M47.9 Spondylosis, unspecified

✓4th **M48** Other spondylopathies

✓5th **M48.0** Spinal stenosis

Caudal stenosis

M48.00 Spinal stenosis, site unspecified Ⓐ

M48.01 Spinal stenosis, occipito-atlanto-axial region

M48.02 Spinal stenosis, cervical region

M48.03 Spinal stenosis, cervicothoracic region

M48.04 Spinal stenosis, thoracic region Ⓐ

M48.05 Spinal stenosis, thoracolumbar region Ⓐ

M48.06 Spinal stenosis, lumbar region Ⓐ

M48.07 Spinal stenosis, lumbosacral region Ⓐ

M48.08 Spinal stenosis, sacral and sacrococcygeal region Ⓐ

✓5th **M48.1** Ankylosing hyperostosis [Forestier]

Diffuse idiopathic skeletal hyperostosis [DISH]

M48.10 Ankylosing hyperostosis [Forestier], site unspecified

M48.11 Ankylosing hyperostosis [Forestier], occipito-atlanto-axial region

M48.12 Ankylosing hyperostosis [Forestier], cervical region

M48.13 Ankylosing hyperostosis [Forestier], cervicothoracic region

M48.14 Ankylosing hyperostosis [Forestier], thoracic region

M48.15 Ankylosing hyperostosis [Forestier], thoracolumbar region

M48.16 Ankylosing hyperostosis [Forestier], lumbar region

M48.17 Ankylosing hyperostosis [Forestier], lumbosacral region

M48.18 Ankylosing hyperostosis [Forestier], sacral and sacrococcygeal region

M48.19 Ankylosing hyperostosis [Forestier], multiple sites in spine

✓5th **M48.2** Kissing spine

M48.20 Kissing spine, site unspecified

M48.21 Kissing spine, occipito-atlanto-axial region

M48.22 Kissing spine, cervical region

M48.23 Kissing spine, cervicothoracic region

M48.24 Kissing spine, thoracic region

M48.25 Kissing spine, thoracolumbar region

M48.26 Kissing spine, lumbar region

M48.27 Kissing spine, lumbosacral region

✓5th **M48.3** Traumatic spondylopathy

M48.30 Traumatic spondylopathy, site unspecified

M48.31 Traumatic spondylopathy, occipito-atlanto-axial region

M48.32 Traumatic spondylopathy, cervical region

M48.33 Traumatic spondylopathy, cervicothoracic region

M48.34 Traumatic spondylopathy, thoracic region

M48.35 Traumatic spondylopathy, thoracolumbar region

M48.36 Traumatic spondylopathy, lumbar region

M48.37 Traumatic spondylopathy, lumbosacral region

M48.38 Traumatic spondylopathy, sacral and sacrococcygeal region

✓5th **M48.4** Fatigue fracture of vertebra

Stress fracture of vertebra

EXCLUDES 1 *pathological fracture NOS (M84.4-)*
pathological fracture of vertebra due to neoplasm (M84.58)
pathological fracture of vertebra due to other diagnosis (M84.68)
pathological fracture of vertebra due to osteoporosis (M80.-)
traumatic fracture of vertebrae (S12.0-S12.3-, S22.0-, S32.0-)

The appropriate 7th character is to be added to each code from subcategory M48.4.
A   initial encounter for fracture
D   subsequent encounter for fracture with routine healing
G   subsequent encounter for fracture with delayed healing
S   sequela of fracture

✓x7th **M48.40** Fatigue fracture of vertebra, site unspecified

✓x7th **M48.41** Fatigue fracture of vertebra, occipito-atlanto-axial region

✓x7th **M48.42** Fatigue fracture of vertebra, cervical region

✓x7th **M48.43** Fatigue fracture of vertebra, cervicothoracic region

✓x7th **M48.44** Fatigue fracture of vertebra, thoracic region

✓x7th **M48.45** Fatigue fracture of vertebra, thoracolumbar region

✓x7th **M48.46** Fatigue fracture of vertebra, lumbar region

✓x7th **M48.47** Fatigue fracture of vertebra, lumbosacral region

✓x7th **M48.48** Fatigue fracture of vertebra, sacral and sacrococcygeal region

---

✓ Additional Character Required   ✓x7th Placeholder Alert   Unspecified Dx   Other Specified Dx   Manifestation   ►◄ Revised Text   ● New Code   ▲ Revised Code Title

☑5th **M48.5 Collapsed vertebra, not elsewhere classified**
Collapsed vertebra NOS
Wedging of vertebra NOS
> **EXCLUDES 1** *current injury—see Injury of spine, by body region*
> *fatigue fracture of vertebra (M48.4)*
> *pathological fracture of vertebra due to neoplasm (M84.58)*
> *pathological fracture of vertebra due to other diagnosis (M84.68)*
> *pathological fracture of vertebra due to osteoporosis (M80.-)*
> *pathological fracture NOS (M84.4-)*
> *stress fracture of vertebra (M48.4-)*
> *traumatic fracture of vertebra (S12-, S22-, S32-)*

The appropriate 7th character is to be added to each code from subcategory M48.5.
A   initial encounter for fracture
D   subsequent encounter for fracture with routine healing
G   subsequent encounter for fracture with delayed healing
S   sequela of fracture

☑x7th **M48.50 Collapsed vertebra, not elsewhere classified, site unspecified**

☑x7th **M48.51 Collapsed vertebra, not elsewhere classified, occipito-atlanto-axial region**

☑x7th **M48.52 Collapsed vertebra, not elsewhere classified, cervical region**

☑x7th **M48.53 Collapsed vertebra, not elsewhere classified, cervicothoracic region**

☑x7th **M48.54 Collapsed vertebra, not elsewhere classified, thoracic region**

☑x7th **M48.55 Collapsed vertebra, not elsewhere classified, thoracolumbar region**

☑x7th **M48.56 Collapsed vertebra, not elsewhere classified, lumbar region**

☑x7th **M48.57 Collapsed vertebra, not elsewhere classified, lumbosacral region**

☑x7th **M48.58 Collapsed vertebra, not elsewhere classified, sacral and sacrococcygeal region**

☑5th **M48.8 Other specified spondylopathies**
Ossification of posterior longitudinal ligament

☑6th **M48.8X Other specified spondylopathies**

M48.8X1 Other specified spondylopathies, occipito-atlanto-axial region

M48.8X2 Other specified spondylopathies, cervical region

M48.8X3 Other specified spondylopathies, cervicothoracic region

M48.8X4 Other specified spondylopathies, thoracic region

M48.8X5 Other specified spondylopathies, thoracolumbar region

M48.8X6 Other specified spondylopathies, lumbar region

M48.8X7 Other specified spondylopathies, lumbosacral region

M48.8X8 Other specified spondylopathies, sacral and sacrococcygeal region

M48.8X9 Other specified spondylopathies, site unspecified

M48.9 Spondylopathy, unspecified

☑4th **M49 Spondylopathies in diseases classified elsewhere**
> **INCLUDES** curvature of spine in diseases classified elsewhere
> deformity of spine in diseases classified elsewhere
> kyphosis in diseases classified elsewhere
> scoliosis in diseases classified elsewhere
> spondylopathy in diseases classified elsewhere

Code first underlying disease, such as:
> *brucellosis (A23.-)*
> *Charcôt-Marie-Tooth disease (G60.0)*
> *enterobacterial infections (A01-A04)*
> *osteitis fibrosa cystica (E21.0)*
> **EXCLUDES 1** *curvature of spine in tuberculosis [Pott's] (A18.01)*
> *enteropathic arthropathies (M07.-)*
> *gonococcal spondylitis (A54.41)*
> *neuropathic [tabes dorsalis] spondylitis (A52.11)*
> *neuropathic spondylopathy in syringomyelia (G95.0)*
> *neuropathic spondylopathy in tabes dorsalis (A52.11)*
> *nonsyphilitic neuropathic spondylopathy NEC (G98.0)*
> *spondylitis in syphilis (acquired) (A52.77)*
> *tuberculous spondylitis (A18.01)*
> *typhoid fever spondylitis (A01.05)*

☑5th **M49.8 Spondylopathy in diseases classified elsewhere**

M49.80 *Spondylopathy in diseases classified elsewhere, site unspecified*

M49.81 *Spondylopathy in diseases classified elsewhere, occipito-atlanto-axial region*

M49.82 *Spondylopathy in diseases classified elsewhere, cervical region*

M49.83 *Spondylopathy in diseases classified elsewhere, cervicothoracic region*

M49.84 *Spondylopathy in diseases classified elsewhere, thoracic region*

M49.85 *Spondylopathy in diseases classified elsewhere, thoracolumbar region*

M49.86 *Spondylopathy in diseases classified elsewhere, lumbar region*

M49.87 *Spondylopathy in diseases classified elsewhere, lumbosacral region*

M49.88 *Spondylopathy in diseases classified elsewhere, sacral and sacrococcygeal region*

M49.89 *Spondylopathy in diseases classified elsewhere, multiple sites in spine*

Other dorsopathies (M50-M54)

> **EXCLUDES 1** *current injury—see injury of spine by body region*
> *discitis NOS (M46.4-)*

☑4th **M50 Cervical disc disorders**
> **NOTE** Code to the most superior level of disorder.
> **INCLUDES** cervicothoracic disc disorders with cervicalgia
> cervicothoracic disc disorders

☑5th **M50.0 Cervical disc disorder with myelopathy**

M50.00 Cervical disc disorder with myelopathy, unspecified cervical region 🅰

M50.01 Cervical disc disorder with myelopathy, high cervical region 🅰
C2-C3 disc disorder with myelopathy
C3-C4 disc disorder with myelopathy

M50.02 Cervical disc disorder with myelopathy, mid-cervical region 🅰
C4-C5 disc disorder with myelopathy
C5-C6 disc disorder with myelopathy
C6-C7 disc disorder with myelopathy

M50.03 Cervical disc disorder with myelopathy, cervicothoracic region 🅰
C7-T1 disc disorder with myelopathy

☑5th **M50.1 Cervical disc disorder with radiculopathy**
> **EXCLUDES 2** *brachial radiculitis NOS (M54.13)*

M50.10 Cervical disc disorder with radiculopathy, unspecified cervical region

M50.11 Cervical disc disorder with radiculopathy, high cervical region
C2-C3 disc disorder with radiculopathy
C3 radiculopathy due to disc disorder
C3-C4 disc disorder with radiculopathy
C4 radiculopathy due to disc disorder

M50.12 Cervical disc disorder with radiculopathy, mid-cervical region
C4-C5 disc disorder with radiculopathy
C5 radiculopathy due to disc disorder
C5-C6 disc disorder with radiculopathy
C6 radiculopathy due to disc disorder
C6-C7 disc disorder with radiculopathy
C7 radiculopathy due to disc disorder

M50.13 Cervical disc disorder with radiculopathy, cervicothoracic region
C7-T1 disc disorder with radiculopathy
C8 radiculopathy due to disc disorder

✓5th **M50.2 Other cervical disc displacement**

M50.20 Other cervical disc displacement, unspecified cervical region Ⓐ

M50.21 Other cervical disc displacement, high cervical region Ⓐ
Other C2-C3 cervical disc displacement
Other C3-C4 cervical disc displacement

M50.22 Other cervical disc displacement, mid-cervical region Ⓐ
Other C4-C5 cervical disc displacement
Other C5-C6 cervical disc displacement
Other C6-C7 cervical disc displacement

M50.23 Other cervical disc displacement, cervicothoracic region Ⓐ
Other C7-T1 cervical disc displacement

✓5th **M50.3 Other cervical disc degeneration**

M50.30 Other cervical disc degeneration, unspecified cervical region Ⓐ

M50.31 Other cervical disc degeneration, high cervical region Ⓐ
Other C2-C3 cervical disc degeneration
Other C3-C4 cervical disc degeneration

M50.32 Other cervical disc degeneration, mid-cervical region Ⓐ
Other C4-C5 cervical disc degeneration
Other C5-C6 cervical disc degeneration
Other C6-C7 cervical disc degeneration

M50.33 Other cervical disc degeneration, cervicothoracic region Ⓐ
Other C7-T1 cervical disc degeneration

✓5th **M50.8 Other cervical disc disorders**

M50.80 Other cervical disc disorders, unspecified cervical region Ⓐ

M50.81 Other cervical disc disorders, high cervical region Ⓐ
Other C2-C3 cervical disc disorders
Other C3-C4 cervical disc disorders

M50.82 Other cervical disc disorders, mid-cervical region Ⓐ
Other C4-C5 cervical disc disorders
Other C5-C6 cervical disc disorders
Other C6-C7 cervical disc disorders

M50.83 Other cervical disc disorders, cervicothoracic region Ⓐ
Other C7-T1 cervical disc disorders

✓5th **M50.9 Cervical disc disorder, unspecified**

M50.90 Cervical disc disorder, unspecified, unspecified cervical region Ⓐ

M50.91 Cervical disc disorder, unspecified, high cervical region Ⓐ
C2-C3 cervical disc disorder, unspecified
C3-C4 cervical disc disorder, unspecified

M50.92 Cervical disc disorder, unspecified, mid-cervical region Ⓐ
C4-C5 cervical disc disorder, unspecified
C5-C6 cervical disc disorder, unspecified
C6-C7 cervical disc disorder, unspecified

M50.93 Cervical disc disorder, unspecified, cervicothoracic region Ⓐ
C7-T1 cervical disc disorder, unspecified

✓4th **M51 Thoracic, thoracolumbar, and lumbosacral intervertebral disc disorders**
EXCLUDES 2   cervical and cervicothoracic disc disorders (M50.-)
sacral and sacrococcygeal disorders (M53.3)

✓5th **M51.0 Thoracic, thoracolumbar and lumbosacral intervertebral disc disorders with myelopathy**

M51.04 Intervertebral disc disorders with myelopathy, thoracic region Ⓐ

M51.05 Intervertebral disc disorders with myelopathy, thoracolumbar region Ⓐ

M51.06 Intervertebral disc disorders with myelopathy, lumbar region Ⓐ

✓5th **M51.1 Thoracic, thoracolumbar and lumbosacral intervertebral disc disorders with radiculopathy**
Sciatica due to intervertebral disc disorder
EXCLUDES 1   lumbar radiculitis NOS (M54.16)
sciatica NOS (M54.3)

M51.14 Intervertebral disc disorders with radiculopathy, thoracic region

M51.15 Intervertebral disc disorders with radiculopathy, thoracolumbar region

M51.16 Intervertebral disc disorders with radiculopathy, lumbar region

M51.17 Intervertebral disc disorders with radiculopathy, lumbosacral region

✓5th **M51.2 Other thoracic, thoracolumbar and lumbosacral intervertebral disc displacement**
Lumbago due to displacement of intervertebral disc

M51.24 Other intervertebral disc displacement, thoracic region Ⓐ

M51.25 Other intervertebral disc displacement, thoracolumbar region Ⓐ

M51.26 Other intervertebral disc displacement, lumbar region Ⓐ

M51.27 Other intervertebral disc displacement, lumbosacral region Ⓐ

✓5th **M51.3 Other thoracic, thoracolumbar and lumbosacral intervertebral disc degeneration**
AHA: 2013, 3Q, 22

M51.34 Other intervertebral disc degeneration, thoracic region Ⓐ

M51.35 Other intervertebral disc degeneration, thoracolumbar region Ⓐ

M51.36 Other intervertebral disc degeneration, lumbar region Ⓐ

M51.37 Other intervertebral disc degeneration, lumbosacral region Ⓐ

✓5th **M51.4 Schmorl's nodes**

M51.44 Schmorl's nodes, thoracic region Ⓐ

M51.45 Schmorl's nodes, thoracolumbar region Ⓐ

M51.46 Schmorl's nodes, lumbar region Ⓐ

M51.47 Schmorl's nodes, lumbosacral region Ⓐ

✓5th **M51.8 Other thoracic, thoracolumbar and lumbosacral intervertebral disc disorders**

M51.84 Other intervertebral disc disorders, thoracic region Ⓐ

M51.85 Other intervertebral disc disorders, thoracolumbar region Ⓐ

M51.86 Other intervertebral disc disorders, lumbar region Ⓐ

M51.87 Other intervertebral disc disorders, lumbosacral region Ⓐ

M51.9 Unspecified thoracic, thoracolumbar and lumbosacral intervertebral disc disorder Ⓐ

✓4th **M53 Other and unspecified dorsopathies, not elsewhere classified**

M53.0 Cervicocranial syndrome
Posterior cervical sympathetic syndrome

M53.1 Cervicobrachial syndrome
EXCLUDES 2   cervical disc disorder (M50.-)
thoracic outlet syndrome (G54.0)

✓5th **M53.2 Spinal instabilities**

✓6th **M53.2X Spinal instabilities**

M53.2X1 Spinal instabilities, occipito-atlanto-axial region

M53.2X2 Spinal instabilities, cervical region

M53.2X3 Spinal instabilities, cervicothoracic region

M53.2X4 Spinal instabilities, thoracic region

M53.2X5 Spinal instabilities, thoracolumbar region

M53.2X6 Spinal instabilities, lumbar region

M53.2X7 Spinal instabilities, lumbosacral region

M53.2X8 Spinal instabilities, sacral and sacrococcygeal region

M53.2X9 Spinal instabilities, site unspecified

✓ Additional Character Required   ✓x7th Placeholder Alert   Unspecified Dx   Other Specified Dx   Manifestation   ►◄ Revised Text   ● New Code   ▲ Revised Code Title

M53.3 Sacrococcygeal disorders, not elsewhere classified
Coccygodynia

✓5ᵗʰ **M53.8 Other specified dorsopathies**

M53.80 Other specified dorsopathies, site unspecified

M53.81 Other specified dorsopathies, occipito-atlanto-axial region

M53.82 Other specified dorsopathies, cervical region

M53.83 Other specified dorsopathies, cervicothoracic region

M53.84 Other specified dorsopathies, thoracic region

M53.85 Other specified dorsopathies, thoracolumbar region

M53.86 Other specified dorsopathies, lumbar region

M53.87 Other specified dorsopathies, lumbosacral region

M53.88 Other specified dorsopathies, sacral and sacrococcygeal region

M53.9 Dorsopathy, unspecified

✓4ᵗʰ **M54 Dorsalgia**

     EXCLUDES 1   psychogenic dorsalgia (F45.41)

✓5ᵗʰ **M54.0 Panniculitis affecting regions of neck and back**

     EXCLUDES 1   lupus panniculitis (L93.2)
                   panniculitis NOS (M79.3)
                   relapsing [Weber-Christian] panniculitis (M35.6)

M54.00 Panniculitis affecting regions of neck and back, site unspecified

M54.01 Panniculitis affecting regions of neck and back, occipito-atlanto-axial region

M54.02 Panniculitis affecting regions of neck and back, cervical region

M54.03 Panniculitis affecting regions of neck and back, cervicothoracic region

M54.04 Panniculitis affecting regions of neck and back, thoracic region

M54.05 Panniculitis affecting regions of neck and back, thoracolumbar region

M54.06 Panniculitis affecting regions of neck and back, lumbar region

M54.07 Panniculitis affecting regions of neck and back, lumbosacral region

M54.08 Panniculitis affecting regions of neck and back, sacral and sacrococcygeal region

M54.09 Panniculitis affecting regions, neck and back, multiple sites in spine

✓5ᵗʰ **M54.1 Radiculopathy**
Brachial neuritis or radiculitis NOS
Lumbar neuritis or radiculitis NOS
Lumbosacral neuritis or radiculitis NOS
Thoracic neuritis or radiculitis NOS
Radiculitis NOS

     EXCLUDES 1   neuralgia and neuritis NOS (M79.2)
                   radiculopathy with cervical disc disorder (M50.1)
                   radiculopathy with lumbar and other intervertebral disc disorder (M51.1-)
                   radiculopathy with spondylosis (M47.2-)

M54.10 Radiculopathy, site unspecified

M54.11 Radiculopathy, occipito-atlanto-axial region

M54.12 Radiculopathy, cervical region

M54.13 Radiculopathy, cervicothoracic region

M54.14 Radiculopathy, thoracic region

M54.15 Radiculopathy, thoracolumbar region

M54.16 Radiculopathy, lumbar region

M54.17 Radiculopathy, lumbosacral region

M54.18 Radiculopathy, sacral and sacrococcygeal region

M54.2 Cervicalgia

     EXCLUDES 1   cervicalgia due to intervertebral cervical disc disorder (M50.-)

✓5ᵗʰ **M54.3 Sciatica**

     EXCLUDES 1   lesion of sciatic nerve (G57.0)
                   sciatica due to intervertebral disc disorder (M51.1-)
                   sciatica with lumbago (M54.4-)

M54.30 Sciatica, unspecified side

M54.31 Sciatica, right side

M54.32 Sciatica, left side

✓5ᵗʰ **M54.4 Lumbago with sciatica**

     EXCLUDES 1   lumbago with sciatica due to intervertebral disc disorder (M51.1-)

M54.40 Lumbago with sciatica, unspecified side

M54.41 Lumbago with sciatica, right side

M54.42 Lumbago with sciatica, left side

M54.5 Low back pain
Loin pain
Lumbago NOS

     EXCLUDES 1   low back strain (S39.012)
                   lumbago due to intervertebral disc displacement (M51.2-)
                   lumbago with sciatica (M54.4-)

M54.6 Pain in thoracic spine

     EXCLUDES 1   pain in thoracic spine due to intervertebral disc disorder (M51.-)

✓5ᵗʰ **M54.8 Other dorsalgia**

     EXCLUDES 1   dorsalgia in thoracic region (M54.6)
                   low back pain (M54.5)

M54.81 Occipital neuralgia

M54.89 Other dorsalgia

M54.9 Dorsalgia, unspecified
Backache NOS   Back pain NOS

SOFT TISSUE DISORDERS (M60-M79)

Disorders of muscles (M60-M63)

     EXCLUDES 1   dermatopolymyositis (M33.-)
                   muscular dystrophies and myopathies (G71-G72)
                   myopathy in amyloidosis (E85.-)
                   myopathy in polyarteritis nodosa (M30.0)
                   myopathy in rheumatoid arthritis (M05.32)
                   myopathy in scleroderma (M34.-)
                   myopathy in Sjögren's syndrome (M35.03)
                   myopathy in systemic lupus erythematosus (M32.-)

✓4ᵗʰ **M60 Myositis**

     EXCLUDES 2   inclusion body myositis [IBM] (G72.41)

✓5ᵗʰ **M60.0 Infective myositis**
Tropical pyomyositis
Use additional code (B95-B97) to identify infectious agent

   ✓6ᵗʰ **M60.00 Infective myositis, unspecified site**

M60.000 Infective myositis, unspecified right arm
Infective myositis, right upper limb NOS

M60.001 Infective myositis, unspecified left arm
Infective myositis, left upper limb NOS

M60.002 Infective myositis, unspecified arm
Infective myositis, upper limb NOS

M60.003 Infective myositis, unspecified right leg
Infective myositis, right lower limb NOS

M60.004 Infective myositis, unspecified left leg
Infective myositis, left lower limb NOS

M60.005 Infective myositis, unspecified leg
Infective myositis, lower limb NOS

M60.009 Infective myositis, unspecified site

   ✓6ᵗʰ **M60.01 Infective myositis, shoulder**

M60.011 Infective myositis, right shoulder

M60.012 Infective myositis, left shoulder

M60.019 Infective myositis, unspecified shoulder

   ✓6ᵗʰ **M60.02 Infective myositis, upper arm**

M60.021 Infective myositis, right upper arm

M60.022 Infective myositis, left upper arm

M60.029 Infective myositis, unspecified upper arm

   ✓6ᵗʰ **M60.03 Infective myositis, forearm**

M60.031 Infective myositis, right forearm

M60.032 Infective myositis, left forearm

M60.039 Infective myositis, unspecified forearm

   ✓6ᵗʰ **M60.04 Infective myositis, hand and fingers**

M60.041 Infective myositis, right hand

M60.042 Infective myositis, left hand

M60.043 Infective myositis, unspecified hand

M60.044 Infective myositis, right finger(s)

M60.045 Infective myositis, left finger(s)

M60.046 Infective myositis, unspecified finger(s)

   ✓6ᵗʰ **M60.05 Infective myositis, thigh**

M60.051 Infective myositis, right thigh

M60.052 Infective myositis, left thigh

M60.059 Infective myositis, unspecified thigh

   ✓6ᵗʰ **M60.06 Infective myositis, lower leg**

M60.061 Infective myositis, right lower leg

EXCLUDES 1 Not coded here   *EXCLUDES 2* Not included here   N Newborn Age: 0   P Pediatric Age: 0-17   M Maternity Age: 12-55   A Adult Age: 15-124

708   ICD-10-CM 2016

　　　　M60.062　Infective myositis, left lower leg
　　　　M60.069　Infective myositis, unspecified lower leg
　　✓6ᵗʰ M60.07　Infective myositis, ankle, foot and toes
　　　　M60.070　Infective myositis, right ankle
　　　　M60.071　Infective myositis, left ankle
　　　　M60.072　Infective myositis, unspecified ankle
　　　　M60.073　Infective myositis, right foot
　　　　M60.074　Infective myositis, left foot
　　　　M60.075　Infective myositis, unspecified foot
　　　　M60.076　Infective myositis, right toe(s)
　　　　M60.077　Infective myositis, left toe(s)
　　　　M60.078　Infective myositis, unspecified toe(s)
　　M60.08　Infective myositis, other site
　　M60.09　Infective myositis, multiple sites
✓5ᵗʰ M60.1　Interstitial myositis
　　M60.10　Interstitial myositis of unspecified site
　　✓6ᵗʰ M60.11　Interstitial myositis, shoulder
　　　　M60.111　Interstitial myositis, right shoulder
　　　　M60.112　Interstitial myositis, left shoulder
　　　　M60.119　Interstitial myositis, unspecified shoulder
　　✓6ᵗʰ M60.12　Interstitial myositis, upper arm
　　　　M60.121　Interstitial myositis, right upper arm
　　　　M60.122　Interstitial myositis, left upper arm
　　　　M60.129　Interstitial myositis, unspecified upper arm
　　✓6ᵗʰ M60.13　Interstitial myositis, forearm
　　　　M60.131　Interstitial myositis, right forearm
　　　　M60.132　Interstitial myositis, left forearm
　　　　M60.139　Interstitial myositis, unspecified forearm
　　✓6ᵗʰ M60.14　Interstitial myositis, hand
　　　　M60.141　Interstitial myositis, right hand
　　　　M60.142　Interstitial myositis, left hand
　　　　M60.149　Interstitial myositis, unspecified hand
　　✓6ᵗʰ M60.15　Interstitial myositis, thigh
　　　　M60.151　Interstitial myositis, right thigh
　　　　M60.152　Interstitial myositis, left thigh
　　　　M60.159　Interstitial myositis, unspecified thigh
　　✓6ᵗʰ M60.16　Interstitial myositis, lower leg
　　　　M60.161　Interstitial myositis, right lower leg
　　　　M60.162　Interstitial myositis, left lower leg
　　　　M60.169　Interstitial myositis, unspecified lower leg
　　✓6ᵗʰ M60.17　Interstitial myositis, ankle and foot
　　　　M60.171　Interstitial myositis, right ankle and foot
　　　　M60.172　Interstitial myositis, left ankle and foot
　　　　M60.179　Interstitial myositis, unspecified ankle and foot
　　M60.18　Interstitial myositis, other site
　　M60.19　Interstitial myositis, multiple sites
✓5ᵗʰ M60.2　Foreign body granuloma of soft tissue, not elsewhere classified
　　　　Use additional code to identify the type of retained foreign body (Z18.-)
　　　　EXCLUDES 1　foreign body granuloma of skin and subcutaneous tissue (L92.3)
　　M60.20　Foreign body granuloma of soft tissue, not elsewhere classified, unspecified site
　　✓6ᵗʰ M60.21　Foreign body granuloma of soft tissue, not elsewhere classified, shoulder
　　　　M60.211　Foreign body granuloma of soft tissue, not elsewhere classified, right shoulder
　　　　M60.212　Foreign body granuloma of soft tissue, not elsewhere classified, left shoulder
　　　　M60.219　Foreign body granuloma of soft tissue, not elsewhere classified, unspecified shoulder
　　✓6ᵗʰ M60.22　Foreign body granuloma of soft tissue, not elsewhere classified, upper arm
　　　　M60.221　Foreign body granuloma of soft tissue, not elsewhere classified, right upper arm
　　　　M60.222　Foreign body granuloma of soft tissue, not elsewhere classified, left upper arm
　　　　M60.229　Foreign body granuloma of soft tissue, not elsewhere classified, unspecified upper arm

　　✓6ᵗʰ M60.23　Foreign body granuloma of soft tissue, not elsewhere classified, forearm
　　　　M60.231　Foreign body granuloma of soft tissue, not elsewhere classified, right forearm
　　　　M60.232　Foreign body granuloma of soft tissue, not elsewhere classified, left forearm
　　　　M60.239　Foreign body granuloma of soft tissue, not elsewhere classified, unspecified forearm
　　✓6ᵗʰ M60.24　Foreign body granuloma of soft tissue, not elsewhere classified, hand
　　　　M60.241　Foreign body granuloma of soft tissue, not elsewhere classified, right hand
　　　　M60.242　Foreign body granuloma of soft tissue, not elsewhere classified, left hand
　　　　M60.249　Foreign body granuloma of soft tissue, not elsewhere classified, unspecified hand
　　✓6ᵗʰ M60.25　Foreign body granuloma of soft tissue, not elsewhere classified, thigh
　　　　M60.251　Foreign body granuloma of soft tissue, not elsewhere classified, right thigh
　　　　M60.252　Foreign body granuloma of soft tissue, not elsewhere classified, left thigh
　　　　M60.259　Foreign body granuloma of soft tissue, not elsewhere classified, unspecified thigh
　　✓6ᵗʰ M60.26　Foreign body granuloma of soft tissue, not elsewhere classified, lower leg
　　　　M60.261　Foreign body granuloma of soft tissue, not elsewhere classified, right lower leg
　　　　M60.262　Foreign body granuloma of soft tissue, not elsewhere classified, left lower leg
　　　　M60.269　Foreign body granuloma of soft tissue, not elsewhere classified, unspecified lower leg
　　✓6ᵗʰ M60.27　Foreign body granuloma of soft tissue, not elsewhere classified, ankle and foot
　　　　M60.271　Foreign body granuloma of soft tissue, not elsewhere classified, right ankle and foot
　　　　M60.272　Foreign body granuloma of soft tissue, not elsewhere classified, left ankle and foot
　　　　M60.279　Foreign body granuloma of soft tissue, not elsewhere classified, unspecified ankle and foot
　　M60.28　Foreign body granuloma of soft tissue, not elsewhere classified, other site
✓5ᵗʰ M60.8　Other myositis
　　M60.80　Other myositis, unspecified site
　　✓6ᵗʰ M60.81　Other myositis shoulder
　　　　M60.811　Other myositis, right shoulder
　　　　M60.812　Other myositis, left shoulder
　　　　M60.819　Other myositis, unspecified shoulder
　　✓6ᵗʰ M60.82　Other myositis, upper arm
　　　　M60.821　Other myositis, right upper arm
　　　　M60.822　Other myositis, left upper arm
　　　　M60.829　Other myositis, unspecified upper arm
　　✓6ᵗʰ M60.83　Other myositis, forearm
　　　　M60.831　Other myositis, right forearm
　　　　M60.832　Other myositis, left forearm
　　　　M60.839　Other myositis, unspecified forearm
　　✓6ᵗʰ M60.84　Other myositis, hand
　　　　M60.841　Other myositis, right hand
　　　　M60.842　Other myositis, left hand
　　　　M60.849　Other myositis, unspecified hand
　　✓6ᵗʰ M60.85　Other myositis, thigh
　　　　M60.851　Other myositis, right thigh
　　　　M60.852　Other myositis, left thigh
　　　　M60.859　Other myositis, unspecified thigh
　　✓6ᵗʰ M60.86　Other myositis, lower leg
　　　　M60.861　Other myositis, right lower leg
　　　　M60.862　Other myositis, left lower leg
　　　　M60.869　Other myositis, unspecified lower leg
　　✓6ᵗʰ M60.87　Other myositis, ankle and foot
　　　　M60.871　Other myositis, right ankle and foot
　　　　M60.872　Other myositis, left ankle and foot
　　　　M60.879　Other myositis, unspecified ankle and foot
　　M60.88　Other myositis, other site
　　M60.89　Other myositis, multiple sites

✓ Additional Character Required　　ᵛˣ⁷ᵗʰ Placeholder Alert　　Unspecified Dx　　Other Specified Dx　　Manifestation　　▶◀ Revised Text　　● New Code　　▲ Revised Code Title

M60.9   **Myositis, unspecified**

√4th **M61**   **Calcification and ossification of muscle**

√5th   M61.0   Myositis ossificans traumatica

M61.00   **Myositis ossificans traumatica, unspecified site**

√6th   M61.01   Myositis ossificans traumatica, shoulder

M61.011   Myositis ossificans traumatica, right shoulder

M61.012   Myositis ossificans traumatica, left shoulder

M61.019   **Myositis ossificans traumatica, unspecified shoulder**

√6th   M61.02   Myositis ossificans traumatica, upper arm

M61.021   Myositis ossificans traumatica, right upper arm

M61.022   Myositis ossificans traumatica, left upper arm

M61.029   **Myositis ossificans traumatica, unspecified upper arm**

√6th   M61.03   Myositis ossificans traumatica, forearm

M61.031   Myositis ossificans traumatica, right forearm

M61.032   Myositis ossificans traumatica, left forearm

M61.039   **Myositis ossificans traumatica, unspecified forearm**

√6th   M61.04   Myositis ossificans traumatica, hand

M61.041   Myositis ossificans traumatica, right hand

M61.042   Myositis ossificans traumatica, left hand

M61.049   **Myositis ossificans traumatica, unspecified hand**

√6th   M61.05   Myositis ossificans traumatica, thigh

M61.051   Myositis ossificans traumatica, right thigh

M61.052   Myositis ossificans traumatica, left thigh

M61.059   **Myositis ossificans traumatica, unspecified thigh**

√6th   M61.06   Myositis ossificans traumatica, lower leg

M61.061   Myositis ossificans traumatica, right lower leg

M61.062   Myositis ossificans traumatica, left lower leg

M61.069   **Myositis ossificans traumatica, unspecified lower leg**

√6th   M61.07   Myositis ossificans traumatica, ankle and foot

M61.071   Myositis ossificans traumatica, right ankle and foot

M61.072   Myositis ossificans traumatica, left ankle and foot

M61.079   **Myositis ossificans traumatica, unspecified ankle and foot**

M61.08   **Myositis ossificans traumatica, other site**

M61.09   Myositis ossificans traumatica, multiple sites

√5th   M61.1   Myositis ossificans progressiva
Fibrodysplasia ossificans progressiva

M61.10   **Myositis ossificans progressiva, unspecified site**

√6th   M61.11   Myositis ossificans progressiva, shoulder

M61.111   Myositis ossificans progressiva, right shoulder

M61.112   Myositis ossificans progressiva, left shoulder

M61.119   **Myositis ossificans progressiva, unspecified shoulder**

√6th   M61.12   Myositis ossificans progressiva, upper arm

M61.121   Myositis ossificans progressiva, right upper arm

M61.122   Myositis ossificans progressiva, left upper arm

M61.129   **Myositis ossificans progressiva, unspecified arm**

√6th   M61.13   Myositis ossificans progressiva, forearm

M61.131   Myositis ossificans progressiva, right forearm

M61.132   Myositis ossificans progressiva, left forearm

M61.139   **Myositis ossificans progressiva, unspecified forearm**

√6th   M61.14   Myositis ossificans progressiva, hand and finger(s)

M61.141   Myositis ossificans progressiva, right hand

M61.142   Myositis ossificans progressiva, left hand

M61.143   **Myositis ossificans progressiva, unspecified hand**

M61.144   Myositis ossificans progressiva, right finger(s)

M61.145   Myositis ossificans progressiva, left finger(s)

M61.146   **Myositis ossificans progressiva, unspecified finger(s)**

√6th   M61.15   Myositis ossificans progressiva, thigh

M61.151   Myositis ossificans progressiva, right thigh

M61.152   Myositis ossificans progressiva, left thigh

M61.159   **Myositis ossificans progressiva, unspecified thigh**

√6th   M61.16   Myositis ossificans progressiva, lower leg

M61.161   Myositis ossificans progressiva, right lower leg

M61.162   Myositis ossificans progressiva, left lower leg

M61.169   **Myositis ossificans progressiva, unspecified lower leg**

√6th   M61.17   Myositis ossificans progressiva, ankle, foot and toe(s)

M61.171   Myositis ossificans progressiva, right ankle

M61.172   Myositis ossificans progressiva, left ankle

M61.173   **Myositis ossificans progressiva, unspecified ankle**

M61.174   Myositis ossificans progressiva, right foot

M61.175   Myositis ossificans progressiva, left foot

M61.176   **Myositis ossificans progressiva, unspecified foot**

M61.177   Myositis ossificans progressiva, right toe(s)

M61.178   Myositis ossificans progressiva, left toe(s)

M61.179   **Myositis ossificans progressiva, unspecified toe(s)**

M61.18   **Myositis ossificans progressiva, other site**

M61.19   Myositis ossificans progressiva, multiple sites

√5th   M61.2   Paralytic calcification and ossification of muscle
Myositis ossificans associated with quadriplegia or paraplegia

M61.20   **Paralytic calcification and ossification of muscle, unspecified site**

√6th   M61.21   Paralytic calcification and ossification of muscle, shoulder

M61.211   Paralytic calcification and ossification of muscle, right shoulder

M61.212   Paralytic calcification and ossification of muscle, left shoulder

M61.219   **Paralytic calcification and ossification of muscle, unspecified shoulder**

√6th   M61.22   Paralytic calcification and ossification of muscle, upper arm

M61.221   Paralytic calcification and ossification of muscle, right upper arm

M61.222   Paralytic calcification and ossification of muscle, left upper arm

M61.229   **Paralytic calcification and ossification of muscle, unspecified upper arm**

√6th   M61.23   Paralytic calcification and ossification of muscle, forearm

M61.231   Paralytic calcification and ossification of muscle, right forearm

M61.232   Paralytic calcification and ossification of muscle, left forearm

M61.239   **Paralytic calcification and ossification of muscle, unspecified forearm**

√6th   M61.24   Paralytic calcification and ossification of muscle, hand

M61.241   Paralytic calcification and ossification of muscle, right hand

M61.242   Paralytic calcification and ossification of muscle, left hand

---

EXCLUDES 1 Not coded here   EXCLUDES 2 Not included here   N Newborn Age: 0   P Pediatric Age: 0-17   M Maternity Age: 12-55   A Adult Age: 15-124

710   ICD-10-CM 2016

M61.249 **Paralytic calcification and ossification of muscle, unspecified hand**

✓6ᵗʰ M61.25 Paralytic calcification and ossification of muscle, thigh

    M61.251 Paralytic calcification and ossification of muscle, right thigh

    M61.252 Paralytic calcification and ossification of muscle, left thigh

    M61.259 **Paralytic calcification and ossification of muscle, unspecified thigh**

✓6ᵗʰ M61.26 Paralytic calcification and ossification of muscle, lower leg

    M61.261 Paralytic calcification and ossification of muscle, right lower leg

    M61.262 Paralytic calcification and ossification of muscle, left lower leg

    M61.269 **Paralytic calcification and ossification of muscle, unspecified lower leg**

✓6ᵗʰ M61.27 Paralytic calcification and ossification of muscle, ankle and foot

    M61.271 Paralytic calcification and ossification of muscle, right ankle and foot

    M61.272 Paralytic calcification and ossification of muscle, left ankle and foot

    M61.279 **Paralytic calcification and ossification of muscle, unspecified ankle and foot**

M61.28 **Paralytic calcification and ossification of muscle, other site**

M61.29 Paralytic calcification and ossification of muscle, multiple sites

✓5ᵗʰ M61.3 Calcification and ossification of muscles associated with burns

    Myositis ossificans associated with burns

M61.30 **Calcification and ossification of muscles associated with burns, unspecified site**

✓6ᵗʰ M61.31 Calcification and ossification of muscles associated with burns, shoulder

    M61.311 Calcification and ossification of muscles associated with burns, right shoulder

    M61.312 Calcification and ossification of muscles associated with burns, left shoulder

    M61.319 **Calcification and ossification of muscles associated with burns, unspecified shoulder**

✓6ᵗʰ M61.32 Calcification and ossification of muscles associated with burns, upper arm

    M61.321 Calcification and ossification of muscles associated with burns, right upper arm

    M61.322 Calcification and ossification of muscles associated with burns, left upper arm

    M61.329 **Calcification and ossification of muscles associated with burns, unspecified upper arm**

✓6ᵗʰ M61.33 Calcification and ossification of muscles associated with burns, forearm

    M61.331 Calcification and ossification of muscles associated with burns, right forearm

    M61.332 Calcification and ossification of muscles associated with burns, left forearm

    M61.339 **Calcification and ossification of muscles associated with burns, unspecified forearm**

✓6ᵗʰ M61.34 Calcification and ossification of muscles associated with burns, hand

    M61.341 Calcification and ossification of muscles associated with burns, right hand

    M61.342 Calcification and ossification of muscles associated with burns, left hand

    M61.349 **Calcification and ossification of muscles associated with burns, unspecified hand**

✓6ᵗʰ M61.35 Calcification and ossification of muscles associated with burns, thigh

    M61.351 Calcification and ossification of muscles associated with burns, right thigh

    M61.352 Calcification and ossification of muscles associated with burns, left thigh

    M61.359 **Calcification and ossification of muscles associated with burns, unspecified thigh**

✓6ᵗʰ M61.36 Calcification and ossification of muscles associated with burns, lower leg

    M61.361 Calcification and ossification of muscles associated with burns, right lower leg

    M61.362 Calcification and ossification of muscles associated with burns, left lower leg

    M61.369 **Calcification and ossification of muscles associated with burns, unspecified lower leg**

✓6ᵗʰ M61.37 Calcification and ossification of muscles associated with burns, ankle and foot

    M61.371 Calcification and ossification of muscles associated with burns, right ankle and foot

    M61.372 Calcification and ossification of muscles associated with burns, left ankle and foot

    M61.379 **Calcification and ossification of muscles associated with burns, unspecified ankle and foot**

M61.38 **Calcification and ossification of muscles associated with burns, other site**

M61.39 Calcification and ossification of muscles associated with burns, multiple sites

✓5ᵗʰ M61.4 Other calcification of muscle

    EXCLUDES 1   calcific tendinitis NOS (M65.2-)
                 calcific tendinitis of shoulder (M75.3)

M61.40 **Other calcification of muscle, unspecified site**

✓6ᵗʰ M61.41 Other calcification of muscle, shoulder

    M61.411 **Other calcification of muscle, right shoulder**

    M61.412 **Other calcification of muscle, left shoulder**

    M61.419 **Other calcification of muscle, unspecified shoulder**

✓6ᵗʰ M61.42 Other calcification of muscle, upper arm

    M61.421 **Other calcification of muscle, right upper arm**

    M61.422 **Other calcification of muscle, left upper arm**

    M61.429 **Other calcification of muscle, unspecified upper arm**

✓6ᵗʰ M61.43 Other calcification of muscle, forearm

    M61.431 **Other calcification of muscle, right forearm**

    M61.432 **Other calcification of muscle, left forearm**

    M61.439 **Other calcification of muscle, unspecified forearm**

✓6ᵗʰ M61.44 Other calcification of muscle, hand

    M61.441 **Other calcification of muscle, right hand**

    M61.442 **Other calcification of muscle, left hand**

    M61.449 **Other calcification of muscle, unspecified hand**

✓6ᵗʰ M61.45 Other calcification of muscle, thigh

    M61.451 **Other calcification of muscle, right thigh**

    M61.452 **Other calcification of muscle, left thigh**

    M61.459 **Other calcification of muscle, unspecified thigh**

✓6ᵗʰ M61.46 Other calcification of muscle, lower leg

    M61.461 **Other calcification of muscle, right lower leg**

    M61.462 **Other calcification of muscle, left lower leg**

    M61.469 **Other calcification of muscle, unspecified lower leg**

✓6ᵗʰ M61.47 Other calcification of muscle, ankle and foot

    M61.471 **Other calcification of muscle, right ankle and foot**

    M61.472 **Other calcification of muscle, left ankle and foot**

    M61.479 **Other calcification of muscle, unspecified ankle and foot**

M61.48 **Other calcification of muscle, other site**

M61.49 Other calcification of muscle, multiple sites

✓5ᵗʰ M61.5 Other ossification of muscle

M61.50 **Other ossification of muscle, unspecified site**

✓6ᵗʰ M61.51 Other ossification of muscle, shoulder

    M61.511 **Other ossification of muscle, right shoulder**

✓ Additional Character Required   ✓×7ᵗʰ Placeholder Alert   Unspecified Dx   Other Specified Dx   Manifestation   ►◄ Revised Text   ● New Code   ▲ Revised Code Title

ICD-10-CM 2016   **711**

M61.512 Other ossification of muscle, left shoulder
M61.519 Other ossification of muscle, unspecified shoulder

✓6ᵗʰ M61.52 Other ossification of muscle, upper arm
M61.521 Other ossification of muscle, right upper arm
M61.522 Other ossification of muscle, left upper arm
M61.529 Other ossification of muscle, unspecified upper arm

✓6ᵗʰ M61.53 Other ossification of muscle, forearm
M61.531 Other ossification of muscle, right forearm
M61.532 Other ossification of muscle, left forearm
M61.539 Other ossification of muscle, unspecified forearm

✓6ᵗʰ M61.54 Other ossification of muscle, hand
M61.541 Other ossification of muscle, right hand
M61.542 Other ossification of muscle, left hand
M61.549 Other ossification of muscle, unspecified hand

✓6ᵗʰ M61.55 Other ossification of muscle, thigh
M61.551 Other ossification of muscle, right thigh
M61.552 Other ossification of muscle, left thigh
M61.559 Other ossification of muscle, unspecified thigh

✓6ᵗʰ M61.56 Other ossification of muscle, lower leg
M61.561 Other ossification of muscle, right lower leg
M61.562 Other ossification of muscle, left lower leg
M61.569 Other ossification of muscle, unspecified lower leg

✓6ᵗʰ M61.57 Other ossification of muscle, ankle and foot
M61.571 Other ossification of muscle, right ankle and foot
M61.572 Other ossification of muscle, left ankle and foot
M61.579 Other ossification of muscle, unspecified ankle and foot

M61.58 Other ossification of muscle, other site
M61.59 Other ossification of muscle, multiple sites
M61.9 Calcification and ossification of muscle, unspecified

✓4ᵗʰ M62 Other disorders of muscle
EXCLUDES 1 alcoholic myopathy (G72.1)
cramp and spasm (R25.2)
drug-induced myopathy (G72.0)
myalgia (M79.1)
stiff-man syndrome (G25.82)
EXCLUDES 2 nontraumatic hematoma of muscle (M79.81)

✓5ᵗʰ M62.0 Separation of muscle (nontraumatic)
Diastasis of muscle
EXCLUDES 1 diastasis recti complicating pregnancy, labor and delivery (O71.8)
traumatic separation of muscle—see strain of muscle by body region

M62.00 Separation of muscle (nontraumatic), unspecified site

✓6ᵗʰ M62.01 Separation of muscle (nontraumatic), shoulder
M62.011 Separation of muscle (nontraumatic), right shoulder
M62.012 Separation of muscle (nontraumatic), left shoulder
M62.019 Separation of muscle (nontraumatic), unspecified shoulder

✓6ᵗʰ M62.02 Separation of muscle (nontraumatic), upper arm
M62.021 Separation of muscle (nontraumatic), right upper arm
M62.022 Separation of muscle (nontraumatic), left upper arm
M62.029 Separation of muscle (nontraumatic), unspecified upper arm

✓6ᵗʰ M62.03 Separation of muscle (nontraumatic), forearm
M62.031 Separation of muscle (nontraumatic), right forearm
M62.032 Separation of muscle (nontraumatic), left forearm

M62.039 Separation of muscle (nontraumatic), unspecified forearm

✓6ᵗʰ M62.04 Separation of muscle (nontraumatic), hand
M62.041 Separation of muscle (nontraumatic), right hand
M62.042 Separation of muscle (nontraumatic), left hand
M62.049 Separation of muscle (nontraumatic), unspecified hand

✓6ᵗʰ M62.05 Separation of muscle (nontraumatic), thigh
M62.051 Separation of muscle (nontraumatic), right thigh
M62.052 Separation of muscle (nontraumatic), left thigh
M62.059 Separation of muscle (nontraumatic), unspecified thigh

✓6ᵗʰ M62.06 Separation of muscle (nontraumatic), lower leg
M62.061 Separation of muscle (nontraumatic), right lower leg
M62.062 Separation of muscle (nontraumatic), left lower leg
M62.069 Separation of muscle (nontraumatic), unspecified lower leg

✓6ᵗʰ M62.07 Separation of muscle (nontraumatic), ankle and foot
M62.071 Separation of muscle (nontraumatic), right ankle and foot
M62.072 Separation of muscle (nontraumatic), left ankle and foot
M62.079 Separation of muscle (nontraumatic), unspecified ankle and foot

M62.08 Separation of muscle (nontraumatic), other site

✓5ᵗʰ M62.1 Other rupture of muscle (nontraumatic)
EXCLUDES 1 traumatic rupture of muscle—see strain of muscle by body region
EXCLUDES 2 rupture of tendon (M66.-)

M62.10 Other rupture of muscle (nontraumatic), unspecified site

✓6ᵗʰ M62.11 Other rupture of muscle (nontraumatic), shoulder
M62.111 Other rupture of muscle (nontraumatic), right shoulder
M62.112 Other rupture of muscle (nontraumatic), left shoulder
M62.119 Other rupture of muscle (nontraumatic), unspecified shoulder

✓6ᵗʰ M62.12 Other rupture of muscle (nontraumatic), upper arm
M62.121 Other rupture of muscle (nontraumatic), right upper arm
M62.122 Other rupture of muscle (nontraumatic), left upper arm
M62.129 Other rupture of muscle (nontraumatic), unspecified upper arm

✓6ᵗʰ M62.13 Other rupture of muscle (nontraumatic), forearm
M62.131 Other rupture of muscle (nontraumatic), right forearm
M62.132 Other rupture of muscle (nontraumatic), left forearm
M62.139 Other rupture of muscle (nontraumatic), unspecified forearm

✓6ᵗʰ M62.14 Other rupture of muscle (nontraumatic), hand
M62.141 Other rupture of muscle (nontraumatic), right hand
M62.142 Other rupture of muscle (nontraumatic), left hand
M62.149 Other rupture of muscle (nontraumatic), unspecified hand

✓6ᵗʰ M62.15 Other rupture of muscle (nontraumatic), thigh
M62.151 Other rupture of muscle (nontraumatic), right thigh
M62.152 Other rupture of muscle (nontraumatic), left thigh
M62.159 Other rupture of muscle (nontraumatic), unspecified thigh

✓6ᵗʰ M62.16 Other rupture of muscle (nontraumatic), lower leg
M62.161 Other rupture of muscle (nontraumatic), right lower leg
M62.162 Other rupture of muscle (nontraumatic), left lower leg

M62.169 **Other rupture of muscle (nontraumatic), unspecified lower leg**

✓6ᵗʰ M62.17 **Other rupture of muscle (nontraumatic),** ankle and foot

    M62.171 **Other rupture of muscle (nontraumatic), right ankle and foot**

    M62.172 **Other rupture of muscle (nontraumatic), left ankle and foot**

    M62.179 **Other rupture of muscle (nontraumatic), unspecified ankle and foot**

M62.18 **Other rupture of muscle (nontraumatic), other site**

✓5ᵗʰ M62.2 **Nontraumatic ischemic infarction of muscle**

    EXCLUDES 1 *compartment syndrome (traumatic) (T79.A-)*
       nontraumatic compartment syndrome (M79.A-)
       rhabdomyolysis (M62.82)
       traumatic ischemia of muscle (T79.6)
       Volkmann's ischemic contracture (T79.6)

M62.20 **Nontraumatic ischemic infarction of muscle, unspecified site**

✓6ᵗʰ M62.21 **Nontraumatic ischemic infarction of muscle, shoulder**

    M62.211 **Nontraumatic ischemic infarction of muscle, right shoulder**

    M62.212 **Nontraumatic ischemic infarction of muscle, left shoulder**

    M62.219 **Nontraumatic ischemic infarction of muscle, unspecified shoulder**

✓6ᵗʰ M62.22 **Nontraumatic ischemic infarction of muscle,** upper arm

    M62.221 **Nontraumatic ischemic infarction of muscle, right upper arm**

    M62.222 **Nontraumatic ischemic infarction of muscle, left upper arm**

    M62.229 **Nontraumatic ischemic infarction of muscle, unspecified upper arm**

✓6ᵗʰ M62.23 **Nontraumatic ischemic infarction of muscle,** forearm

    M62.231 **Nontraumatic ischemic infarction of muscle, right forearm**

    M62.232 **Nontraumatic ischemic infarction of muscle, left forearm**

    M62.239 **Nontraumatic ischemic infarction of muscle, unspecified forearm**

✓6ᵗʰ M62.24 **Nontraumatic ischemic infarction of muscle,** hand

    M62.241 **Nontraumatic ischemic infarction of muscle, right hand**

    M62.242 **Nontraumatic ischemic infarction of muscle, left hand**

    M62.249 **Nontraumatic ischemic infarction of muscle, unspecified hand**

✓6ᵗʰ M62.25 **Nontraumatic ischemic infarction of muscle,** thigh

    M62.251 **Nontraumatic ischemic infarction of muscle, right thigh**

    M62.252 **Nontraumatic ischemic infarction of muscle, left thigh**

    M62.259 **Nontraumatic ischemic infarction of muscle, unspecified thigh**

✓6ᵗʰ M62.26 **Nontraumatic ischemic infarction of muscle,** lower leg

    M62.261 **Nontraumatic ischemic infarction of muscle, right lower leg**

    M62.262 **Nontraumatic ischemic infarction of muscle, left lower leg**

    M62.269 **Nontraumatic ischemic infarction of muscle, unspecified lower leg**

✓6ᵗʰ M62.27 **Nontraumatic ischemic infarction of muscle,** ankle and foot

    M62.271 **Nontraumatic ischemic infarction of muscle, right ankle and foot**

    M62.272 **Nontraumatic ischemic infarction of muscle, left ankle and foot**

    M62.279 **Nontraumatic ischemic infarction of muscle, unspecified ankle and foot**

M62.28 **Nontraumatic ischemic infarction of muscle, other site**

M62.3 **Immobility syndrome (paraplegic)**

✓5ᵗʰ M62.4 **Contracture of muscle**

    Contracture of tendon (sheath)

    EXCLUDES 1 *contracture of joint (M24.5-)*

M62.40 **Contracture of muscle, unspecified site**

✓6ᵗʰ M62.41 **Contracture of muscle,** shoulder

    M62.411 **Contracture of muscle, right shoulder**

    M62.412 **Contracture of muscle, left shoulder**

    M62.419 **Contracture of muscle, unspecified shoulder**

✓6ᵗʰ M62.42 **Contracture of muscle,** upper arm

    M62.421 **Contracture of muscle, right upper arm**

    M62.422 **Contracture of muscle, left upper arm**

    M62.429 **Contracture of muscle, unspecified upper arm**

✓6ᵗʰ M62.43 **Contracture of muscle,** forearm

    M62.431 **Contracture of muscle, right forearm**

    M62.432 **Contracture of muscle, left forearm**

    M62.439 **Contracture of muscle, unspecified forearm**

✓6ᵗʰ M62.44 **Contracture of muscle,** hand

    M62.441 **Contracture of muscle, right hand**

    M62.442 **Contracture of muscle, left hand**

    M62.449 **Contracture of muscle, unspecified hand**

✓6ᵗʰ M62.45 **Contracture of muscle,** thigh

    M62.451 **Contracture of muscle, right thigh**

    M62.452 **Contracture of muscle, left thigh**

    M62.459 **Contracture of muscle, unspecified thigh**

✓6ᵗʰ M62.46 **Contracture of muscle,** lower leg

    M62.461 **Contracture of muscle, right lower leg**

    M62.462 **Contracture of muscle, left lower leg**

    M62.469 **Contracture of muscle, unspecified lower leg**

✓6ᵗʰ M62.47 **Contracture of muscle,** ankle and foot

    M62.471 **Contracture of muscle, right ankle and foot**

    M62.472 **Contracture of muscle, left ankle and foot**

    M62.479 **Contracture of muscle, unspecified ankle and foot**

M62.48 **Contracture of muscle, other site**

M62.49 **Contracture of muscle,** multiple sites

✓5ᵗʰ M62.5 **Muscle wasting and atrophy, not elsewhere classified**

    Disuse atrophy NEC

    EXCLUDES 1 *neuralgic amyotrophy (G54.5)*
       progressive muscular atrophy (G12.29)

    EXCLUDES 2 *pelvic muscle wasting (N81.84)*

M62.50 **Muscle wasting and atrophy, not elsewhere classified, unspecified site**

✓6ᵗʰ M62.51 **Muscle wasting and atrophy, not elsewhere classified,** shoulder

    M62.511 **Muscle wasting and atrophy, not elsewhere classified, right shoulder**

    M62.512 **Muscle wasting and atrophy, not elsewhere classified, left shoulder**

    M62.519 **Muscle wasting and atrophy, not elsewhere classified, unspecified shoulder**

✓6ᵗʰ M62.52 **Muscle wasting and atrophy, not elsewhere classified,** upper arm

    M62.521 **Muscle wasting and atrophy, not elsewhere classified, right upper arm**

    M62.522 **Muscle wasting and atrophy, not elsewhere classified, left upper arm**

    M62.529 **Muscle wasting and atrophy, not elsewhere classified, unspecified upper arm**

✓6ᵗʰ M62.53 **Muscle wasting and atrophy, not elsewhere classified,** forearm

    M62.531 **Muscle wasting and atrophy, not elsewhere classified, right forearm**

    M62.532 **Muscle wasting and atrophy, not elsewhere classified, left forearm**

    M62.539 **Muscle wasting and atrophy, not elsewhere classified, unspecified forearm**

☑ Additional Character Required   ᵛˣ7ᵗʰ Placeholder Alert   Unspecified Dx   Other Specified Dx   Manifestation   ▶◀ Revised Text   ● New Code   ▲ Revised Code Title

√6th **M62.54** **Muscle wasting and atrophy, not elsewhere classified, hand**

    M62.541 **Muscle wasting and atrophy, not elsewhere classified, right hand**

    M62.542 **Muscle wasting and atrophy, not elsewhere classified, left hand**

    M62.549 **Muscle wasting and atrophy, not elsewhere classified, unspecified hand**

√6th **M62.55** **Muscle wasting and atrophy, not elsewhere classified, thigh**

    M62.551 **Muscle wasting and atrophy, not elsewhere classified, right thigh**

    M62.552 **Muscle wasting and atrophy, not elsewhere classified, left thigh**

    M62.559 **Muscle wasting and atrophy, not elsewhere classified, unspecified thigh**

√6th **M62.56** **Muscle wasting and atrophy, not elsewhere classified, lower leg**

    M62.561 **Muscle wasting and atrophy, not elsewhere classified, right lower leg**

    M62.562 **Muscle wasting and atrophy, not elsewhere classified, left lower leg**

    M62.569 **Muscle wasting and atrophy, not elsewhere classified, unspecified lower leg**

√6th **M62.57** **Muscle wasting and atrophy, not elsewhere classified, ankle and foot**

    M62.571 **Muscle wasting and atrophy, not elsewhere classified, right ankle and foot**

    M62.572 **Muscle wasting and atrophy, not elsewhere classified, left ankle and foot**

    M62.579 **Muscle wasting and atrophy, not elsewhere classified, unspecified ankle and foot**

    M62.58 **Muscle wasting and atrophy, not elsewhere classified, other site**

    M62.59 **Muscle wasting and atrophy, not elsewhere classified, multiple sites**

√5th **M62.8** **Other specified disorders of muscle**

    EXCLUDES 2 *nontraumatic hematoma of muscle (M79.81)*

    M62.81 **Muscle weakness (generalized)**

    M62.82 **Rhabdomyolysis**

      EXCLUDES 1 *traumatic rhabdomyolysis (T79.6)*

√6th **M62.83** **Muscle spasm**

    M62.830 **Muscle spasm of back**

    M62.831 **Muscle spasm of calf**

      Charley-horse

    M62.838 **Other muscle spasm**

    M62.89 **Other specified disorders of muscle**

      Muscle (sheath) hernia

    M62.9 **Disorder of muscle, unspecified**

√4th **M63** **Disorders of muscle in diseases classified elsewhere**

    Code first underlying disease, such as:

      leprosy (A30.-)

      neoplasm (C49-, C79.89, D21-, D48.1)

      schistosomiasis (B65.-)

      trichinellosis (B75)

    EXCLUDES 1 *myopathy in cysticercosis (B69.81)*

      myopathy in endocrine diseases (G73.7)

      myopathy in metabolic diseases (G73.7)

      myopathy in sarcoidosis (D86.87)

      myopathy in secondary syphilis (A51.49)

      myopathy in syphilis (late) (A52.78)

      myopathy in toxoplasmosis (B58.82)

      myopathy in tuberculosis (A18.09)

√5th **M63.8** **Disorders of muscle in diseases classified elsewhere**

    M63.80 *Disorders of muscle in diseases classified elsewhere, unspecified site*

√6th **M63.81** **Disorders of muscle in diseases classified elsewhere, shoulder**

    M63.811 *Disorders of muscle in diseases classified elsewhere, right shoulder*

    M63.812 *Disorders of muscle in diseases classified elsewhere, left shoulder*

    M63.819 *Disorders of muscle in diseases classified elsewhere, unspecified shoulder*

√6th **M63.82** **Disorders of muscle in diseases classified elsewhere, upper arm**

    M63.821 *Disorders of muscle in diseases classified elsewhere, right upper arm*

    M63.822 *Disorders of muscle in diseases classified elsewhere, left upper arm*

    M63.829 *Disorders of muscle in diseases classified elsewhere, unspecified upper arm*

√6th **M63.83** **Disorders of muscle in diseases classified elsewhere, forearm**

    M63.831 *Disorders of muscle in diseases classified elsewhere, right forearm*

    M63.832 *Disorders of muscle in diseases classified elsewhere, left forearm*

    M63.839 *Disorders of muscle in diseases classified elsewhere, unspecified forearm*

√6th **M63.84** **Disorders of muscle in diseases classified elsewhere, hand**

    M63.841 *Disorders of muscle in diseases classified elsewhere, right hand*

    M63.842 *Disorders of muscle in diseases classified elsewhere, left hand*

    M63.849 *Disorders of muscle in diseases classified elsewhere, unspecified hand*

√6th **M63.85** **Disorders of muscle in diseases classified elsewhere, thigh**

    M63.851 *Disorders of muscle in diseases classified elsewhere, right thigh*

    M63.852 *Disorders of muscle in diseases classified elsewhere, left thigh*

    M63.859 *Disorders of muscle in diseases classified elsewhere, unspecified thigh*

√6th **M63.86** **Disorders of muscle in diseases classified elsewhere, lower leg**

    M63.861 *Disorders of muscle in diseases classified elsewhere, right lower leg*

    M63.862 *Disorders of muscle in diseases classified elsewhere, left lower leg*

    M63.869 *Disorders of muscle in diseases classified elsewhere, unspecified lower leg*

√6th **M63.87** **Disorders of muscle in diseases classified elsewhere, ankle and foot**

    M63.871 *Disorders of muscle in diseases classified elsewhere, right ankle and foot*

    M63.872 *Disorders of muscle in diseases classified elsewhere, left ankle and foot*

    M63.879 *Disorders of muscle in diseases classified elsewhere, unspecified ankle and foot*

    M63.88 *Disorders of muscle in diseases classified elsewhere, other site*

    M63.89 *Disorders of muscle in diseases classified elsewhere, multiple sites*

Disorders of synovium and tendon (M65-M67)

√4th **M65** **Synovitis and tenosynovitis**

    EXCLUDES 1 *chronic crepitant synovitis of hand and wrist (M70.0-)*

      current injury—see injury of ligament or tendon by body region

      soft tissue disorders related to use, overuse and pressure (M70.-)

√5th **M65.0** **Abscess of tendon sheath**

    Use additional code (B95-B96) to identify bacterial agent.

    M65.00 **Abscess of tendon sheath, unspecified site**

√6th **M65.01** **Abscess of tendon sheath, shoulder**

    M65.011 **Abscess of tendon sheath, right shoulder**

    M65.012 **Abscess of tendon sheath, left shoulder**

    M65.019 **Abscess of tendon sheath, unspecified shoulder**

√6th **M65.02** **Abscess of tendon sheath, upper arm**

    M65.021 **Abscess of tendon sheath, right upper arm**

    M65.022 **Abscess of tendon sheath, left upper arm**

    M65.029 **Abscess of tendon sheath, unspecified upper arm**

√6th **M65.03** **Abscess of tendon sheath, forearm**

    M65.031 **Abscess of tendon sheath, right forearm**

    M65.032 **Abscess of tendon sheath, left forearm**

    M65.039 **Abscess of tendon sheath, unspecified forearm**

EXCLUDES 1 Not coded here   *EXCLUDES 2* Not included here   N Newborn Age: 0   P Pediatric Age: 0-17   M Maternity Age: 12-55   A Adult Age: 15-124

714   ICD-10-CM 2016

☑6ᵗʰ **M65.04 Abscess of tendon sheath,** hand
 M65.041 Abscess of tendon sheath, right hand
 M65.042 Abscess of tendon sheath, left hand
 M65.049 Abscess of tendon sheath, unspecified hand

☑6ᵗʰ **M65.05 Abscess of tendon sheath,** thigh
 M65.051 Abscess of tendon sheath, right thigh
 M65.052 Abscess of tendon sheath, left thigh
 M65.059 Abscess of tendon sheath, unspecified thigh

☑6ᵗʰ **M65.06 Abscess of tendon sheath,** lower leg
 M65.061 Abscess of tendon sheath, right lower leg
 M65.062 Abscess of tendon sheath, left lower leg
 M65.069 Abscess of tendon sheath, unspecified lower leg

☑6ᵗʰ **M65.07 Abscess of tendon sheath,** ankle and foot
 M65.071 Abscess of tendon sheath, right ankle and foot
 M65.072 Abscess of tendon sheath, left ankle and foot
 M65.079 Abscess of tendon sheath, unspecified ankle and foot

 M65.08 Abscess of tendon sheath, other site

☑5ᵗʰ **M65.1 Other infective (teno)synovitis**
 M65.10 Other infective (teno)synovitis, unspecified site

☑6ᵗʰ **M65.11 Other infective (teno)synovitis,** shoulder
 M65.111 Other infective (teno)synovitis, right shoulder
 M65.112 Other infective (teno)synovitis, left shoulder
 M65.119 Other infective (teno)synovitis, unspecified shoulder

☑6ᵗʰ **M65.12 Other infective (teno)synovitis,** elbow
 M65.121 Other infective (teno)synovitis, right elbow
 M65.122 Other infective (teno)synovitis, left elbow
 M65.129 Other infective (teno)synovitis, unspecified elbow

☑6ᵗʰ **M65.13 Other infective (teno)synovitis,** wrist
 M65.131 Other infective (teno)synovitis, right wrist
 M65.132 Other infective (teno)synovitis, left wrist
 M65.139 Other infective (teno)synovitis, unspecified wrist

☑6ᵗʰ **M65.14 Other infective (teno)synovitis,** hand
 M65.141 Other infective (teno)synovitis, right hand
 M65.142 Other infective (teno)synovitis, left hand
 M65.149 Other infective (teno)synovitis, unspecified hand

☑6ᵗʰ **M65.15 Other infective (teno)synovitis,** hip
 M65.151 Other infective (teno)synovitis, right hip
 M65.152 Other infective (teno)synovitis, left hip
 M65.159 Other infective (teno)synovitis, unspecified hip

☑6ᵗʰ **M65.16 Other infective (teno)synovitis,** knee
 M65.161 Other infective (teno)synovitis, right knee
 M65.162 Other infective (teno)synovitis, left knee
 M65.169 Other infective (teno)synovitis, unspecified knee

☑6ᵗʰ **M65.17 Other infective (teno)synovitis,** ankle and foot
 M65.171 Other infective (teno)synovitis, right ankle and foot
 M65.172 Other infective (teno)synovitis, left ankle and foot
 M65.179 Other infective (teno)synovitis, unspecified ankle and foot

 M65.18 Other infective (teno)synovitis, other site
 M65.19 Other infective (teno)synovitis, multiple sites

☑5ᵗʰ **M65.2 Calcific tendinitis**
 EXCLUDES 1 tendinitis as classified in M75-M77
  calcified tendinitis of shoulder (M75.3)

 M65.20 Calcific tendinitis, unspecified site

☑6ᵗʰ **M65.22 Calcific tendinitis,** upper arm
 M65.221 Calcific tendinitis, right upper arm
 M65.222 Calcific tendinitis, left upper arm

 M65.229 Calcific tendinitis, unspecified upper arm

☑6ᵗʰ **M65.23 Calcific tendinitis,** forearm
 M65.231 Calcific tendinitis, right forearm
 M65.232 Calcific tendinitis, left forearm
 M65.239 Calcific tendinitis, unspecified forearm

☑6ᵗʰ **M65.24 Calcific tendinitis,** hand
 M65.241 Calcific tendinitis, right hand
 M65.242 Calcific tendinitis, left hand
 M65.249 Calcific tendinitis, unspecified hand

☑6ᵗʰ **M65.25 Calcific tendinitis,** thigh
 M65.251 Calcific tendinitis, right thigh
 M65.252 Calcific tendinitis, left thigh
 M65.259 Calcific tendinitis, unspecified thigh

☑6ᵗʰ **M65.26 Calcific tendinitis,** lower leg
 M65.261 Calcific tendinitis, right lower leg
 M65.262 Calcific tendinitis, left lower leg
 M65.269 Calcific tendinitis, unspecified lower leg

☑6ᵗʰ **M65.27 Calcific tendinitis,** ankle and foot
 M65.271 Calcific tendinitis, right ankle and foot
 M65.272 Calcific tendinitis, left ankle and foot
 M65.279 Calcific tendinitis, unspecified ankle and foot

 M65.28 Calcific tendinitis, other site
 M65.29 Calcific tendinitis, multiple sites

M65.3 Trigger finger
 Nodular tendinous disease
 M65.30 Trigger finger, unspecified finger

☑6ᵗʰ **M65.31 Trigger** thumb
 M65.311 Trigger thumb, right thumb
 M65.312 Trigger thumb, left thumb
 M65.319 Trigger thumb, unspecified thumb

☑6ᵗʰ **M65.32 Trigger finger,** index finger
 M65.321 Trigger finger, right index finger
 M65.322 Trigger finger, left index finger
 M65.329 Trigger finger, unspecified index finger

☑6ᵗʰ **M65.33 Trigger finger,** middle finger
 M65.331 Trigger finger, right middle finger
 M65.332 Trigger finger, left middle finger
 M65.339 Trigger finger, unspecified middle finger

☑6ᵗʰ **M65.34 Trigger finger,** ring finger
 M65.341 Trigger finger, right ring finger
 M65.342 Trigger finger, left ring finger
 M65.349 Trigger finger, unspecified ring finger

☑6ᵗʰ **M65.35 Trigger finger,** little finger
 M65.351 Trigger finger, right little finger
 M65.352 Trigger finger, left little finger
 M65.359 Trigger finger, unspecified little finger

M65.4 Radial styloid tenosynovitis [de Quervain]

☑5ᵗʰ **M65.8 Other synovitis and tenosynovitis**
 M65.80 Other synovitis and tenosynovitis, unspecified site

☑6ᵗʰ **M65.81 Other synovitis and tenosynovitis,** shoulder
 M65.811 Other synovitis and tenosynovitis, right shoulder
 M65.812 Other synovitis and tenosynovitis, left shoulder
 M65.819 Other synovitis and tenosynovitis, unspecified shoulder

☑6ᵗʰ **M65.82 Other synovitis and tenosynovitis,** upper arm
 M65.821 Other synovitis and tenosynovitis, right upper arm
 M65.822 Other synovitis and tenosynovitis, left upper arm
 M65.829 Other synovitis and tenosynovitis, unspecified upper arm

☑6ᵗʰ **M65.83 Other synovitis and tenosynovitis,** forearm
 M65.831 Other synovitis and tenosynovitis, right forearm
 M65.832 Other synovitis and tenosynovitis, left forearm
 M65.839 Other synovitis and tenosynovitis, unspecified forearm

---

☑ Additional Character Required   ☑×7ᵗʰ Placeholder Alert   Unspecified Dx   Other Specified Dx   Manifestation   ▶◀ Revised Text   ● New Code   ▲ Revised Code Title

✓6th **M65.84 Other synovitis and tenosynovitis, hand**
    M65.841 **Other synovitis and tenosynovitis, right hand**
    M65.842 **Other synovitis and tenosynovitis, left hand**
    M65.849 **Other synovitis and tenosynovitis, unspecified hand**

✓6th **M65.85 Other synovitis and tenosynovitis, thigh**
    M65.851 **Other synovitis and tenosynovitis, right thigh**
    M65.852 **Other synovitis and tenosynovitis, left thigh**
    M65.859 **Other synovitis and tenosynovitis, unspecified thigh**

✓6th **M65.86 Other synovitis and tenosynovitis, lower leg**
    M65.861 **Other synovitis and tenosynovitis, right lower leg**
    M65.862 **Other synovitis and tenosynovitis, left lower leg**
    M65.869 **Other synovitis and tenosynovitis, unspecified lower leg**

✓6th **M65.87 Other synovitis and tenosynovitis, ankle and foot**
    M65.871 **Other synovitis and tenosynovitis, right ankle and foot**
    M65.872 **Other synovitis and tenosynovitis, left ankle and foot**
    M65.879 **Other synovitis and tenosynovitis, unspecified ankle and foot**

M65.88 Other synovitis and tenosynovitis, other site
M65.89 Other synovitis and tenosynovitis, multiple sites

M65.9 Synovitis and tenosynovitis, unspecified

✓4th **M66 Spontaneous rupture of synovium and tendon**
    INCLUDES   rupture that occurs when a normal force is applied to tissues that are inferred to have less than normal strength
    EXCLUDES 2   rotator cuff syndrome (M75.1-)
         rupture where an abnormal force is applied to normal tissue—see injury of tendon by body region

M66.0 Rupture of popliteal cyst

✓5th **M66.1 Rupture of synovium**
    Rupture of synovial cyst
    EXCLUDES 2   rupture of popliteal cyst (M66.0)

    M66.10 Rupture of synovium, unspecified joint

✓6th **M66.11 Rupture of synovium, shoulder**
    M66.111 **Rupture of synovium, right shoulder**
    M66.112 **Rupture of synovium, left shoulder**
    M66.119 **Rupture of synovium, unspecified shoulder**

✓6th **M66.12 Rupture of synovium, elbow**
    M66.121 **Rupture of synovium, right elbow**
    M66.122 **Rupture of synovium, left elbow**
    M66.129 **Rupture of synovium, unspecified elbow**

✓6th **M66.13 Rupture of synovium, wrist**
    M66.131 **Rupture of synovium, right wrist**
    M66.132 **Rupture of synovium, left wrist**
    M66.139 **Rupture of synovium, unspecified wrist**

✓6th **M66.14 Rupture of synovium, hand and fingers**
    M66.141 **Rupture of synovium, right hand**
    M66.142 **Rupture of synovium, left hand**
    M66.143 **Rupture of synovium, unspecified hand**
    M66.144 **Rupture of synovium, right finger(s)**
    M66.145 **Rupture of synovium, left finger(s)**
    M66.146 **Rupture of synovium, unspecified finger(s)**

✓6th **M66.15 Rupture of synovium, hip**
    M66.151 **Rupture of synovium, right hip**
    M66.152 **Rupture of synovium, left hip**
    M66.159 **Rupture of synovium, unspecified hip**

✓6th **M66.17 Rupture of synovium, ankle, foot and toes**
    M66.171 **Rupture of synovium, right ankle**
    M66.172 **Rupture of synovium, left ankle**
    M66.173 **Rupture of synovium, unspecified ankle**
    M66.174 **Rupture of synovium, right foot**
    M66.175 **Rupture of synovium, left foot**

    M66.176 **Rupture of synovium, unspecified foot**
    M66.177 **Rupture of synovium, right toe(s)**
    M66.178 **Rupture of synovium, left toe(s)**
    M66.179 **Rupture of synovium, unspecified toe(s)**

    M66.18 Rupture of synovium, other site

✦ ✓5th **M66.2 Spontaneous rupture of extensor tendons**
    M66.20 Spontaneous rupture of extensor tendons, unspecified site

✓6th **M66.21 Spontaneous rupture of extensor tendons, shoulder**
    M66.211 **Spontaneous rupture of extensor tendons, right shoulder**
    M66.212 **Spontaneous rupture of extensor tendons, left shoulder**
    M66.219 **Spontaneous rupture of extensor tendons, unspecified shoulder**

✓6th **M66.22 Spontaneous rupture of extensor tendons, upper arm**
    M66.221 **Spontaneous rupture of extensor tendons, right upper arm**
    M66.222 **Spontaneous rupture of extensor tendons, left upper arm**
    M66.229 **Spontaneous rupture of extensor tendons, unspecified upper arm**

✓6th **M66.23 Spontaneous rupture of extensor tendons, forearm**
    M66.231 **Spontaneous rupture of extensor tendons, right forearm**
    M66.232 **Spontaneous rupture of extensor tendons, left forearm**
    M66.239 **Spontaneous rupture of extensor tendons, unspecified forearm**

✓6th **M66.24 Spontaneous rupture of extensor tendons, hand**
    M66.241 **Spontaneous rupture of extensor tendons, right hand**
    M66.242 **Spontaneous rupture of extensor tendons, left hand**
    M66.249 **Spontaneous rupture of extensor tendons, unspecified hand**

✓6th **M66.25 Spontaneous rupture of extensor tendons, thigh**
    M66.251 **Spontaneous rupture of extensor tendons, right thigh**
    M66.252 **Spontaneous rupture of extensor tendons, left thigh**
    M66.259 **Spontaneous rupture of extensor tendons, unspecified thigh**

✓6th **M66.26 Spontaneous rupture of extensor tendons, lower leg**
    M66.261 **Spontaneous rupture of extensor tendons, right lower leg**
    M66.262 **Spontaneous rupture of extensor tendons, left lower leg**
    M66.269 **Spontaneous rupture of extensor tendons, unspecified lower leg**

✓6th **M66.27 Spontaneous rupture of extensor tendons, ankle and foot**
    M66.271 **Spontaneous rupture of extensor tendons, right ankle and foot**
    M66.272 **Spontaneous rupture of extensor tendons, left ankle and foot**
    M66.279 **Spontaneous rupture of extensor tendons, unspecified ankle and foot**

    M66.28 Spontaneous rupture of extensor tendons, other site
    M66.29 Spontaneous rupture of extensor tendons, multiple sites

✦ ✓5th **M66.3 Spontaneous rupture of flexor tendons**
    M66.30 Spontaneous rupture of flexor tendons, unspecified site

✓6th **M66.31 Spontaneous rupture of flexor tendons, shoulder**
    M66.311 **Spontaneous rupture of flexor tendons, right shoulder**
    M66.312 **Spontaneous rupture of flexor tendons, left shoulder**
    M66.319 **Spontaneous rupture of flexor tendons, unspecified shoulder**

✓6th **M66.32 Spontaneous rupture of flexor tendons, upper arm**
    M66.321 **Spontaneous rupture of flexor tendons, right upper arm**

✦   Refer to the Muscle/Tendon Table at beginning of this chapter.

EXCLUDES 1 Not coded here   **EXCLUDES 2** Not included here   N Newborn Age: 0   P Pediatric Age: 0-17   M Maternity Age: 12-55   A Adult Age: 15-124

M66.322 Spontaneous rupture of flexor tendons, left **upper arm**

M66.329 Spontaneous rupture of flexor tendons, unspecified **upper arm**

√6ᵗʰ **M66.33** Spontaneous rupture of flexor tendons, **forearm**

    M66.331 Spontaneous rupture of flexor tendons, right **forearm**

    M66.332 Spontaneous rupture of flexor tendons, left **forearm**

    M66.339 Spontaneous rupture of flexor tendons, unspecified **forearm**

√6ᵗʰ **M66.34** Spontaneous rupture of flexor tendons, **hand**

    M66.341 Spontaneous rupture of flexor tendons, right **hand**

    M66.342 Spontaneous rupture of flexor tendons, left **hand**

    M66.349 Spontaneous rupture of flexor tendons, unspecified **hand**

√6ᵗʰ **M66.35** Spontaneous rupture of flexor tendons, **thigh**

    M66.351 Spontaneous rupture of flexor tendons, right **thigh**

    M66.352 Spontaneous rupture of flexor tendons, left **thigh**

    M66.359 Spontaneous rupture of flexor tendons, unspecified **thigh**

√6ᵗʰ **M66.36** Spontaneous rupture of flexor tendons, **lower leg**

    M66.361 Spontaneous rupture of flexor tendons, right **lower leg**

    M66.362 Spontaneous rupture of flexor tendons, left **lower leg**

    M66.369 Spontaneous rupture of flexor tendons, unspecified **lower leg**

√6ᵗʰ **M66.37** Spontaneous rupture of flexor tendons, **ankle and foot**

    M66.371 Spontaneous rupture of flexor tendons, right **ankle and foot**

    M66.372 Spontaneous rupture of flexor tendons, left **ankle and foot**

    M66.379 Spontaneous rupture of flexor tendons, unspecified **ankle and foot**

    M66.38 Spontaneous rupture of flexor tendons, other site

    M66.39 Spontaneous rupture of flexor tendons, **multiple** sites

✦ √5ᵗʰ **M66.8 Spontaneous rupture of other tendons**

    M66.80 Spontaneous rupture of other tendons, unspecified site

√6ᵗʰ **M66.81** Spontaneous rupture of other tendons, **shoulder**

    M66.811 Spontaneous rupture of other tendons, right **shoulder**

    M66.812 Spontaneous rupture of other tendons, left **shoulder**

    M66.819 Spontaneous rupture of other tendons, unspecified **shoulder**

√6ᵗʰ **M66.82** Spontaneous rupture of other tendons, **upper arm**

    M66.821 Spontaneous rupture of other tendons, right **upper arm**

    M66.822 Spontaneous rupture of other tendons, left **upper arm**

    M66.829 Spontaneous rupture of other tendons, unspecified **upper arm**

√6ᵗʰ **M66.83** Spontaneous rupture of other tendons, **forearm**

    M66.831 Spontaneous rupture of other tendons, right **forearm**

    M66.832 Spontaneous rupture of other tendons, left **forearm**

    M66.839 Spontaneous rupture of other tendons, unspecified **forearm**

√6ᵗʰ **M66.84** Spontaneous rupture of other tendons, **hand**

    M66.841 Spontaneous rupture of other tendons, right **hand**

    M66.842 Spontaneous rupture of other tendons, left **hand**

    M66.849 Spontaneous rupture of other tendons, unspecified **hand**

√6ᵗʰ **M66.85** Spontaneous rupture of other tendons, **thigh**

    M66.851 Spontaneous rupture of other tendons, right **thigh**

    M66.852 Spontaneous rupture of other tendons, left **thigh**

    M66.859 Spontaneous rupture of other tendons, unspecified **thigh**

√6ᵗʰ **M66.86** Spontaneous rupture of other tendons, **lower leg**

    M66.861 Spontaneous rupture of other tendons, right **lower leg**

    M66.862 Spontaneous rupture of other tendons, left **lower leg**

    M66.869 Spontaneous rupture of other tendons, unspecified **lower leg**

√6ᵗʰ **M66.87** Spontaneous rupture of other tendons, **ankle and foot**

    M66.871 Spontaneous rupture of other tendons, right **ankle and foot**

    M66.872 Spontaneous rupture of other tendons, left **ankle and foot**

    M66.879 Spontaneous rupture of other tendons, unspecified **ankle and foot**

    M66.88 Spontaneous rupture of other tendons, **other**

    M66.89 Spontaneous rupture of other tendons, **multiple** sites

  M66.9 Spontaneous rupture of unspecified tendon

    Rupture at musculotendinous junction, nontraumatic

√4ᵗʰ **M67 Other disorders of synovium and tendon**

    EXCLUDES 1   *palmar fascial fibromatosis [Dupuytren] (M72.0)*

          tendinitis NOS (M77.9-)

          xanthomatosis localized to tendons (E78.2)

√5ᵗʰ **M67.0 Short Achilles tendon (acquired)**

    M67.00 **Short Achilles tendon (acquired), unspecified ankle**

    M67.01 **Short Achilles tendon (acquired), right ankle**

    M67.02 **Short Achilles tendon (acquired), left ankle**

√5ᵗʰ **M67.2 Synovial hypertrophy, not elsewhere classified**

    EXCLUDES 1   *villonodular synovitis (pigmented) (M12.2-)*

    M67.20 Synovial hypertrophy, not elsewhere classified, unspecified site

√6ᵗʰ **M67.21** Synovial hypertrophy, not elsewhere classified, **shoulder**

    M67.211 Synovial hypertrophy, not elsewhere classified, right **shoulder**

    M67.212 Synovial hypertrophy, not elsewhere classified, left **shoulder**

    M67.219 Synovial hypertrophy, not elsewhere classified, unspecified **shoulder**

√6ᵗʰ **M67.22** Synovial hypertrophy, not elsewhere classified, **upper arm**

    M67.221 Synovial hypertrophy, not elsewhere classified, right **upper arm**

    M67.222 Synovial hypertrophy, not elsewhere classified, left **upper arm**

    M67.229 Synovial hypertrophy, not elsewhere classified, unspecified **upper arm**

√6ᵗʰ **M67.23** Synovial hypertrophy, not elsewhere classified, **forearm**

    M67.231 Synovial hypertrophy, not elsewhere classified, right **forearm**

    M67.232 Synovial hypertrophy, not elsewhere classified, left **forearm**

    M67.239 Synovial hypertrophy, not elsewhere classified, unspecified **forearm**

√6ᵗʰ **M67.24** Synovial hypertrophy, not elsewhere classified, **hand**

    M67.241 Synovial hypertrophy, not elsewhere classified, right **hand**

    M67.242 Synovial hypertrophy, not elsewhere classified, left **hand**

    M67.249 Synovial hypertrophy, not elsewhere classified, unspecified **hand**

√6ᵗʰ **M67.25** Synovial hypertrophy, not elsewhere classified, **thigh**

    M67.251 Synovial hypertrophy, not elsewhere classified, right **thigh**

✦ Refer to the Muscle/Tendon Table at beginning of this chapter.

☑ Additional Character Required   ✓ˣ⁷ᵗʰ Placeholder Alert   Unspecified Dx   Other Specified Dx   Manifestation   ▶◀ Revised Text   ● New Code   ▲ Revised Code Title

Chapter 13. Diseases of the Musculoskeletal System and Connective Tissue

M67.252–M67.843

         M67.252   Synovial hypertrophy, not elsewhere classified, left thigh

         M67.259   Synovial hypertrophy, not elsewhere classified, unspecified thigh

✓6th   M67.26   Synovial hypertrophy, not elsewhere classified, lower leg

         M67.261   Synovial hypertrophy, not elsewhere classified, right lower leg

         M67.262   Synovial hypertrophy, not elsewhere classified, left lower leg

         M67.269   Synovial hypertrophy, not elsewhere classified, unspecified lower leg

✓6th   M67.27   Synovial hypertrophy, not elsewhere classified, ankle and foot

         M67.271   Synovial hypertrophy, not elsewhere classified, right ankle and foot

         M67.272   Synovial hypertrophy, not elsewhere classified, left ankle and foot

         M67.279   Synovial hypertrophy, not elsewhere classified, unspecified ankle and foot

      M67.28   Synovial hypertrophy, not elsewhere classified, other site

      M67.29   Synovial hypertrophy, not elsewhere classified, multiple sites

✓5th   **M67.3   Transient synovitis**
Toxic synovitis
> *EXCLUDES 1*   palindromic rheumatism (M12.3-)

      M67.30   Transient synovitis, unspecified site

✓6th   M67.31   Transient synovitis, shoulder

         M67.311   Transient synovitis, right shoulder

         M67.312   Transient synovitis, left shoulder

         M67.319   Transient synovitis, unspecified shoulder

✓6th   M67.32   Transient synovitis, elbow

         M67.321   Transient synovitis, right elbow

         M67.322   Transient synovitis, left elbow

         M67.329   Transient synovitis, unspecified elbow

✓6th   M67.33   Transient synovitis, wrist

         M67.331   Transient synovitis, right wrist

         M67.332   Transient synovitis, left wrist

         M67.339   Transient synovitis, unspecified wrist

✓6th   M67.34   Transient synovitis, hand

         M67.341   Transient synovitis, right hand

         M67.342   Transient synovitis, left hand

         M67.349   Transient synovitis, unspecified hand

✓6th   M67.35   Transient synovitis, hip

         M67.351   Transient synovitis, right hip

         M67.352   Transient synovitis, left hip

         M67.359   Transient synovitis, unspecified hip

✓6th   M67.36   Transient synovitis, knee

         M67.361   Transient synovitis, right knee

         M67.362   Transient synovitis, left knee

         M67.369   Transient synovitis, unspecified knee

✓6th   M67.37   Transient synovitis, ankle and foot

         M67.371   Transient synovitis, right ankle and foot

         M67.372   Transient synovitis, left ankle and foot

         M67.379   Transient synovitis, unspecified ankle and foot

      M67.38   Transient synovitis, other site

      M67.39   Transient synovitis, multiple sites

✓5th   **M67.4   Ganglion**
Ganglion of joint or tendon (sheath)
> *EXCLUDES 1*   ganglion in yaws (A66.6)
> *EXCLUDES 2*   cyst of bursa (M71.2-M71.3)
>   cyst of synovium (M71.2-M71.3)

      M67.40   Ganglion, unspecified site

✓6th   M67.41   Ganglion, shoulder

         M67.411   Ganglion, right shoulder

         M67.412   Ganglion, left shoulder

         M67.419   Ganglion, unspecified shoulder

✓6th   M67.42   Ganglion, elbow

         M67.421   Ganglion, right elbow

         M67.422   Ganglion, left elbow

         M67.429   Ganglion, unspecified elbow

✓6th   M67.43   Ganglion, wrist

         M67.431   Ganglion, right wrist

         M67.432   Ganglion, left wrist

         M67.439   Ganglion, unspecified wrist

✓6th   M67.44   Ganglion, hand

         M67.441   Ganglion, right hand

         M67.442   Ganglion, left hand

         M67.449   Ganglion, unspecified hand

✓6th   M67.45   Ganglion, hip

         M67.451   Ganglion, right hip

         M67.452   Ganglion, left hip

         M67.459   Ganglion, unspecified hip

✓6th   M67.46   Ganglion, knee

         M67.461   Ganglion, right knee

         M67.462   Ganglion, left knee

         M67.469   Ganglion, unspecified knee

✓6th   M67.47   Ganglion, ankle and foot

         M67.471   Ganglion, right ankle and foot

         M67.472   Ganglion, left ankle and foot

         M67.479   Ganglion, unspecified ankle and foot

      M67.48   Ganglion, other site

      M67.49   Ganglion, multiple sites

✓5th   **M67.5   Plica syndrome**
Plica knee

      M67.50   Plica syndrome, unspecified knee

      M67.51   Plica syndrome, right knee

      M67.52   Plica syndrome, left knee

✓5th   **M67.8   Other specified disorders of synovium and tendon**

      M67.80   Other specified disorders of synovium and tendon, unspecified site

✓6th   M67.81   Other specified disorders of synovium and tendon, shoulder

         M67.811   Other specified disorders of synovium, right shoulder

         M67.812   Other specified disorders of synovium, left shoulder

         M67.813   Other specified disorders of tendon, right shoulder

         M67.814   Other specified disorders of tendon, left shoulder

         M67.819   Other specified disorders of synovium and tendon, unspecified shoulder

✓6th   M67.82   Other specified disorders of synovium and tendon, elbow

         M67.821   Other specified disorders of synovium, right elbow

         M67.822   Other specified disorders of synovium, left elbow

         M67.823   Other specified disorders of tendon, right elbow

         M67.824   Other specified disorders of tendon, left elbow

         M67.829   Other specified disorders of synovium and tendon, unspecified elbow

✓6th   M67.83   Other specified disorders of synovium and tendon, wrist

         M67.831   Other specified disorders of synovium, right wrist

         M67.832   Other specified disorders of synovium, left wrist

         M67.833   Other specified disorders of tendon, right wrist

         M67.834   Other specified disorders of tendon, left wrist

         M67.839   Other specified disorders of synovium and tendon, unspecified forearm

✓6th   M67.84   Other specified disorders of synovium and tendon, hand

         M67.841   Other specified disorders of synovium, right hand

         M67.842   Other specified disorders of synovium, left hand

         M67.843   Other specified disorders of tendon, right hand

EXCLUDES 1 Not coded here   *EXCLUDES 2* Not included here   N Newborn Age: 0   P Pediatric Age: 0-17   M Maternity Age: 12-55   A Adult Age: 15-124

718   ICD-10-CM 2016

M67.844   Other specified disorders of tendon, left hand

M67.849   Other specified disorders of synovium and tendon, unspecified hand

✓6ᵗʰ **M67.85 Other specified disorders of synovium and tendon, hip**

M67.851   Other specified disorders of synovium, right hip

M67.852   Other specified disorders of synovium, left hip

M67.853   Other specified disorders of tendon, right hip

M67.854   Other specified disorders of tendon, left hip

M67.859   Other specified disorders of synovium and tendon, unspecified hip

✓6ᵗʰ **M67.86 Other specified disorders of synovium and tendon, knee**

M67.861   Other specified disorders of synovium, right knee

M67.862   Other specified disorders of synovium, left knee

M67.863   Other specified disorders of tendon, right knee

M67.864   Other specified disorders of tendon, left knee

M67.869   Other specified disorders of synovium and tendon, unspecified knee

✓6ᵗʰ **M67.87 Other specified disorders of synovium and tendon, ankle and foot**

M67.871   Other specified disorders of synovium, right ankle and foot

M67.872   Other specified disorders of synovium, left ankle and foot

M67.873   Other specified disorders of tendon, right ankle and foot

M67.874   Other specified disorders of tendon, left ankle and foot

M67.879   Other specified disorders of synovium and tendon, unspecified ankle and foot

M67.88   Other specified disorders of synovium and tendon, other site

M67.89   Other specified disorders of synovium and tendon, multiple sites

✓5ᵗʰ **M67.9 Unspecified disorder of synovium and tendon**

M67.90   Unspecified disorder of synovium and tendon, unspecified site

✓6ᵗʰ **M67.91 Unspecified disorder of synovium and tendon, shoulder**

M67.911   Unspecified disorder of synovium and tendon, right shoulder

M67.912   Unspecified disorder of synovium and tendon, left shoulder

M67.919   Unspecified disorder of synovium and tendon, unspecified shoulder

✓6ᵗʰ **M67.92 Unspecified disorder of synovium and tendon, upper arm**

M67.921   Unspecified disorder of synovium and tendon, right upper arm

M67.922   Unspecified disorder of synovium and tendon, left upper arm

M67.929   Unspecified disorder of synovium and tendon, unspecified upper arm

✓6ᵗʰ **M67.93 Unspecified disorder of synovium and tendon, forearm**

M67.931   Unspecified disorder of synovium and tendon, right forearm

M67.932   Unspecified disorder of synovium and tendon, left forearm

M67.939   Unspecified disorder of synovium and tendon, unspecified forearm

✓6ᵗʰ **M67.94 Unspecified disorder of synovium and tendon, hand**

M67.941   Unspecified disorder of synovium and tendon, right hand

M67.942   Unspecified disorder of synovium and tendon, left hand

M67.949   Unspecified disorder of synovium and tendon, unspecified hand

✓6ᵗʰ **M67.95 Unspecified disorder of synovium and tendon, thigh**

M67.951   Unspecified disorder of synovium and tendon, right thigh

M67.952   Unspecified disorder of synovium and tendon, left thigh

M67.959   Unspecified disorder of synovium and tendon, unspecified thigh

✓6ᵗʰ **M67.96 Unspecified disorder of synovium and tendon, lower leg**

M67.961   Unspecified disorder of synovium and tendon, right lower leg

M67.962   Unspecified disorder of synovium and tendon, left lower leg

M67.969   Unspecified disorder of synovium and tendon, unspecified lower leg

✓6ᵗʰ **M67.97 Unspecified disorder of synovium and tendon, ankle and foot**

M67.971   Unspecified disorder of synovium and tendon, right ankle and foot

M67.972   Unspecified disorder of synovium and tendon, left ankle and foot

M67.979   Unspecified disorder of synovium and tendon, unspecified ankle and foot

M67.98   Unspecified disorder of synovium and tendon, other site

M67.99   Unspecified disorder of synovium and tendon, multiple sites

Other soft tissue disorders (M70-M79)

✓4ᵗʰ **M70 Soft tissue disorders related to use, overuse and pressure**

   INCLUDES   soft tissue disorders of occupational origin

   Use additional external cause code to identify activity causing disorder (Y93.-)

   EXCLUDES 1   *bursitis NOS (M71.9-)*

   EXCLUDES 2   *bursitis of shoulder (M75.5)*
         enthesopathies (M76-M77)
         pressure ulcer (pressure area) (L89.-)

✓5ᵗʰ **M70.0 Crepitant synovitis (acute) (chronic) of hand and wrist**

   ✓6ᵗʰ **M70.03 Crepitant synovitis (acute) (chronic), wrist**

M70.031   Crepitant synovitis (acute) (chronic), right wrist

M70.032   Crepitant synovitis (acute) (chronic), left wrist

M70.039   Crepitant synovitis (acute) (chronic), unspecified wrist

   ✓6ᵗʰ **M70.04 Crepitant synovitis (acute) (chronic), hand**

M70.041   Crepitant synovitis (acute) (chronic), right hand

M70.042   Crepitant synovitis (acute) (chronic), left hand

M70.049   Crepitant synovitis (acute) (chronic), unspecified hand

✓5ᵗʰ **M70.1 Bursitis of hand**

M70.10   Bursitis, unspecified hand

M70.11   Bursitis, right hand

M70.12   Bursitis, left hand

✓5ᵗʰ **M70.2 Olecranon bursitis**

M70.20   Olecranon bursitis, unspecified elbow

M70.21   Olecranon bursitis, right elbow

M70.22   Olecranon bursitis, left elbow

✓5ᵗʰ **M70.3 Other bursitis of elbow**

M70.30   Other bursitis of elbow, unspecified elbow

M70.31   Other bursitis of elbow, right elbow

M70.32   Other bursitis of elbow, left elbow

✓5ᵗʰ **M70.4 Prepatellar bursitis**

M70.40   Prepatellar bursitis, unspecified knee

M70.41   Prepatellar bursitis, right knee

M70.42   Prepatellar bursitis, left knee

✓5ᵗʰ **M70.5 Other bursitis of knee**

M70.50   Other bursitis of knee, unspecified knee

M70.51   Other bursitis of knee, right knee

M70.52   Other bursitis of knee, left knee

☑ Additional Character Required   ✓x7ᵗʰ Placeholder Alert   Unspecified Dx   Other Specified Dx   Manifestation   ▶◀ Revised Text   ● New Code   ▲ Revised Code Title

ICD-10-CM 2016   719

✓5ᵗʰ **M70.6** Trochanteric **bursitis**
Trochanteric tendinitis

    M70.60 **Trochanteric bursitis, unspecified hip**

    M70.61 **Trochanteric bursitis, right hip**

    M70.62 **Trochanteric bursitis, left hip**

✓5ᵗʰ **M70.7** Other bursitis of hip
Ischial bursitis

    M70.70 **Other bursitis of hip, unspecified hip**

    M70.71 **Other bursitis of hip, right hip**

    M70.72 **Other bursitis of hip, left hip**

✓5ᵗʰ **M70.8** Other soft tissue disorders related to use, overuse and pressure

    M70.80 **Other soft tissue disorders related to use, overuse and pressure of unspecified site**

✓6ᵗʰ   M70.81 **Other soft tissue disorders related to use, overuse and pressure of shoulder**

     M70.811 **Other soft tissue disorders related to use, overuse and pressure, right shoulder**

     M70.812 **Other soft tissue disorders related to use, overuse and pressure, left shoulder**

     M70.819 **Other soft tissue disorders related to use, overuse and pressure, unspecified shoulder**

✓6ᵗʰ   M70.82 **Other soft tissue disorders related to use, overuse and pressure of upper arm**

     M70.821 **Other soft tissue disorders related to use, overuse and pressure, right upper arm**

     M70.822 **Other soft tissue disorders related to use, overuse and pressure, left upper arm**

     M70.829 **Other soft tissue disorders related to use, overuse and pressure, unspecified upper arms**

✓6ᵗʰ   M70.83 **Other soft tissue disorders related to use, overuse and pressure of forearm**

     M70.831 **Other soft tissue disorders related to use, overuse and pressure, right forearm**

     M70.832 **Other soft tissue disorders related to use, overuse and pressure, left forearm**

     M70.839 **Other soft tissue disorders related to use, overuse and pressure, unspecified forearm**

✓6ᵗʰ   M70.84 **Other soft tissue disorders related to use, overuse and pressure of hand**

     M70.841 **Other soft tissue disorders related to use, overuse and pressure, right hand**

     M70.842 **Other soft tissue disorders related to use, overuse and pressure, left hand**

     M70.849 **Other soft tissue disorders related to use, overuse and pressure, unspecified hand**

✓6ᵗʰ   M70.85 **Other soft tissue disorders related to use, overuse and pressure of thigh**

     M70.851 **Other soft tissue disorders related to use, overuse and pressure, right thigh**

     M70.852 **Other soft tissue disorders related to use, overuse and pressure, left thigh**

     M70.859 **Other soft tissue disorders related to use, overuse and pressure, unspecified thigh**

✓6ᵗʰ   M70.86 **Other soft tissue disorders related to use, overuse and pressure lower leg**

     M70.861 **Other soft tissue disorders related to use, overuse and pressure, right lower leg**

     M70.862 **Other soft tissue disorders related to use, overuse and pressure, left lower leg**

     M70.869 **Other soft tissue disorders related to use, overuse and pressure, unspecified leg**

✓6ᵗʰ   M70.87 **Other soft tissue disorders related to use, overuse and pressure of ankle and foot**

     M70.871 **Other soft tissue disorders related to use, overuse and pressure, right ankle and foot**

     M70.872 **Other soft tissue disorders related to use, overuse and pressure, left ankle and foot**

     M70.879 **Other soft tissue disorders related to use, overuse and pressure, unspecified ankle and foot**

    M70.88 **Other soft tissue disorders related to use, overuse and pressure other site**

    M70.89 **Other soft tissue disorders related to use, overuse and pressure multiple sites**

✓5ᵗʰ **M70.9** Unspecified soft tissue disorder related to use, overuse and pressure

    M70.90 **Unspecified soft tissue disorder related to use, overuse and pressure of unspecified site**

✓6ᵗʰ   M70.91 **Unspecified soft tissue disorder related to use, overuse and pressure of shoulder**

     M70.911 **Unspecified soft tissue disorder related to use, overuse and pressure, right shoulder**

     M70.912 **Unspecified soft tissue disorder related to use, overuse and pressure, left shoulder**

     M70.919 **Unspecified soft tissue disorder related to use, overuse and pressure, unspecified shoulder**

✓6ᵗʰ   M70.92 **Unspecified soft tissue disorder related to use, overuse and pressure of upper arm**

     M70.921 **Unspecified soft tissue disorder related to use, overuse and pressure, right upper arm**

     M70.922 **Unspecified soft tissue disorder related to use, overuse and pressure, left upper arm**

     M70.929 **Unspecified soft tissue disorder related to use, overuse and pressure, unspecified upper arm**

✓6ᵗʰ   M70.93 **Unspecified soft tissue disorder related to use, overuse and pressure of forearm**

     M70.931 **Unspecified soft tissue disorder related to use, overuse and pressure, right forearm**

     M70.932 **Unspecified soft tissue disorder related to use, overuse and pressure, left forearm**

     M70.939 **Unspecified soft tissue disorder related to use, overuse and pressure, unspecified forearm**

✓6ᵗʰ   M70.94 **Unspecified soft tissue disorder related to use, overuse and pressure of hand**

     M70.941 **Unspecified soft tissue disorder related to use, overuse and pressure, right hand**

     M70.942 **Unspecified soft tissue disorder related to use, overuse and pressure, left hand**

     M70.949 **Unspecified soft tissue disorder related to use, overuse and pressure, unspecified hand**

✓6ᵗʰ   M70.95 **Unspecified soft tissue disorder related to use, overuse and pressure of thigh**

     M70.951 **Unspecified soft tissue disorder related to use, overuse and pressure, right thigh**

     M70.952 **Unspecified soft tissue disorder related to use, overuse and pressure, left thigh**

     M70.959 **Unspecified soft tissue disorder related to use, overuse and pressure, unspecified thigh**

✓6ᵗʰ   M70.96 **Unspecified soft tissue disorder related to use, overuse and pressure lower leg**

     M70.961 **Unspecified soft tissue disorder related to use, overuse and pressure, right lower leg**

     M70.962 **Unspecified soft tissue disorder related to use, overuse and pressure, left lower leg**

     M70.969 **Unspecified soft tissue disorder related to use, overuse and pressure, unspecified lower leg**

✓6ᵗʰ   M70.97 **Unspecified soft tissue disorder related to use, overuse and pressure of ankle and foot**

     M70.971 **Unspecified soft tissue disorder related to use, overuse and pressure, right ankle and foot**

     M70.972 **Unspecified soft tissue disorder related to use, overuse and pressure, left ankle and foot**

     M70.979 **Unspecified soft tissue disorder related to use, overuse and pressure, unspecified ankle and foot**

    M70.98 **Unspecified soft tissue disorder related to use, overuse and pressure other**

    M70.99 **Unspecified soft tissue disorder related to use, overuse and pressure multiple sites**

EXCLUDES 1 Not coded here   **EXCLUDES 2** Not included here   **N** Newborn Age: 0   **P** Pediatric Age: 0-17   **M** Maternity Age: 12-55   **A** Adult Age: 15-124

☑4ᵗʰ **M71 Other bursopathies**
> EXCLUDES 1   *bunion (M20.1)*
> *bursitis related to use, overuse or pressure (M70.-)*
> *enthesopathies (M76-M77)*

☑5ᵗʰ **M71.0 Abscess of bursa**
> Use additional code (B95.-, B96.-) to identify causative organism

    M71.00 Abscess of bursa, unspecified site

☑6ᵗʰ **M71.01 Abscess of bursa, shoulder**
      M71.011   Abscess of bursa, right shoulder
      M71.012   Abscess of bursa, left shoulder
      M71.019   Abscess of bursa, unspecified shoulder

☑6ᵗʰ **M71.02 Abscess of bursa, elbow**
      M71.021   Abscess of bursa, right elbow
      M71.022   Abscess of bursa, left elbow
      M71.029   Abscess of bursa, unspecified elbow

☑6ᵗʰ **M71.03 Abscess of bursa, wrist**
      M71.031   Abscess of bursa, right wrist
      M71.032   Abscess of bursa, left wrist
      M71.039   Abscess of bursa, unspecified wrist

☑6ᵗʰ **M71.04 Abscess of bursa, hand**
      M71.041   Abscess of bursa, right hand
      M71.042   Abscess of bursa, left hand
      M71.049   Abscess of bursa, unspecified hand

☑6ᵗʰ **M71.05 Abscess of bursa, hip**
      M71.051   Abscess of bursa, right hip
      M71.052   Abscess of bursa, left hip
      M71.059   Abscess of bursa, unspecified hip

☑6ᵗʰ **M71.06 Abscess of bursa, knee**
      M71.061   Abscess of bursa, right knee
      M71.062   Abscess of bursa, left knee
      M71.069   Abscess of bursa, unspecified knee

☑6ᵗʰ **M71.07 Abscess of bursa, ankle and foot**
      M71.071   Abscess of bursa, right ankle and foot
      M71.072   Abscess of bursa, left ankle and foot
      M71.079   Abscess of bursa, unspecified ankle and foot

    M71.08 Abscess of bursa, other site

    M71.09 Abscess of bursa, multiple sites

☑5ᵗʰ **M71.1 Other infective bursitis**
> Use additional code (B95.-, B96.-) to identify causative organism

    M71.10 Other infective bursitis, unspecified site

☑6ᵗʰ **M71.11 Other infective bursitis, shoulder**
      M71.111   Other infective bursitis, right shoulder
      M71.112   Other infective bursitis, left shoulder
      M71.119   Other infective bursitis, unspecified shoulder

☑6ᵗʰ **M71.12 Other infective bursitis, elbow**
      M71.121   Other infective bursitis, right elbow
      M71.122   Other infective bursitis, left elbow
      M71.129   Other infective bursitis, unspecified elbow

☑6ᵗʰ **M71.13 Other infective bursitis, wrist**
      M71.131   Other infective bursitis, right wrist
      M71.132   Other infective bursitis, left wrist
      M71.139   Other infective bursitis, unspecified wrist

☑6ᵗʰ **M71.14 Other infective bursitis, hand**
      M71.141   Other infective bursitis, right hand
      M71.142   Other infective bursitis, left hand
      M71.149   Other infective bursitis, unspecified hand

☑6ᵗʰ **M71.15 Other infective bursitis, hip**
      M71.151   Other infective bursitis, right hip
      M71.152   Other infective bursitis, left hip
      M71.159   Other infective bursitis, unspecified hip

☑6ᵗʰ **M71.16 Other infective bursitis, knee**
      M71.161   Other infective bursitis, right knee
      M71.162   Other infective bursitis, left knee
      M71.169   Other infective bursitis, unspecified knee

☑6ᵗʰ **M71.17 Other infective bursitis, ankle and foot**
      M71.171   Other infective bursitis, right ankle and foot
      M71.172   Other infective bursitis, left ankle and foot
      M71.179   Other infective bursitis, unspecified ankle and foot

    M71.18 Other infective bursitis, other site

    M71.19 Other infective bursitis, multiple sites

☑5ᵗʰ **M71.2 Synovial cyst of popliteal space [Baker]**
> EXCLUDES 1   *synovial cyst of popliteal space with rupture (M66.0)*

    M71.20 Synovial cyst of popliteal space [Baker], unspecified knee

    M71.21 Synovial cyst of popliteal space [Baker], right knee

    M71.22 Synovial cyst of popliteal space [Baker], left knee

☑5ᵗʰ **M71.3 Other bursal cyst**
> Synovial cyst NOS
> EXCLUDES 1   *synovial cyst with rupture (M66.1-)*

    M71.30 Other bursal cyst, unspecified site

☑6ᵗʰ **M71.31 Other bursal cyst, shoulder**
      M71.311   Other bursal cyst, right shoulder
      M71.312   Other bursal cyst, left shoulder
      M71.319   Other bursal cyst, unspecified shoulder

☑6ᵗʰ **M71.32 Other bursal cyst, elbow**
      M71.321   Other bursal cyst, right elbow
      M71.322   Other bursal cyst, left elbow
      M71.329   Other bursal cyst, unspecified elbow

☑6ᵗʰ **M71.33 Other bursal cyst, wrist**
      M71.331   Other bursal cyst, right wrist
      M71.332   Other bursal cyst, left wrist
      M71.339   Other bursal cyst, unspecified wrist

☑6ᵗʰ **M71.34 Other bursal cyst, hand**
      M71.341   Other bursal cyst, right hand
      M71.342   Other bursal cyst, left hand
      M71.349   Other bursal cyst, unspecified hand

☑6ᵗʰ **M71.35 Other bursal cyst, hip**
      M71.351   Other bursal cyst, right hip
      M71.352   Other bursal cyst, left hip
      M71.359   Other bursal cyst, unspecified hip

☑6ᵗʰ **M71.37 Other bursal cyst, ankle and foot**
      M71.371   Other bursal cyst, right ankle and foot
      M71.372   Other bursal cyst, left ankle and foot
      M71.379   Other bursal cyst, unspecified ankle and foot

    M71.38 Other bursal cyst, other site

    M71.39 Other bursal cyst, multiple sites

☑5ᵗʰ **M71.4 Calcium deposit in bursa**
> EXCLUDES 2   *calcium deposit in bursa of shoulder (M75.3)*

    M71.40 Calcium deposit in bursa, unspecified site

☑6ᵗʰ **M71.42 Calcium deposit in bursa, elbow**
      M71.421   Calcium deposit in bursa, right elbow
      M71.422   Calcium deposit in bursa, left elbow
      M71.429   Calcium deposit in bursa, unspecified elbow

☑6ᵗʰ **M71.43 Calcium deposit in bursa, wrist**
      M71.431   Calcium deposit in bursa, right wrist
      M71.432   Calcium deposit in bursa, left wrist
      M71.439   Calcium deposit in bursa, unspecified wrist

☑6ᵗʰ **M71.44 Calcium deposit in bursa, hand**
      M71.441   Calcium deposit in bursa, right hand
      M71.442   Calcium deposit in bursa, left hand
      M71.449   Calcium deposit in bursa, unspecified hand

☑6ᵗʰ **M71.45 Calcium deposit in bursa, hip**
      M71.451   Calcium deposit in bursa, right hip
      M71.452   Calcium deposit in bursa, left hip
      M71.459   Calcium deposit in bursa, unspecified hip

☑6ᵗʰ **M71.46 Calcium deposit in bursa, knee**
      M71.461   Calcium deposit in bursa, right knee
      M71.462   Calcium deposit in bursa, left knee
      M71.469   Calcium deposit in bursa, unspecified knee

☑6ᵗʰ **M71.47 Calcium deposit in bursa, ankle and foot**
      M71.471   Calcium deposit in bursa, right ankle and foot
      M71.472   Calcium deposit in bursa, left ankle and foot

---

☑ Additional Character Required   ☑x7ᵗʰ Placeholder Alert   Unspecified Dx   Other Specified Dx   Manifestation   ▶◀ Revised Text   ● New Code   ▲ Revised Code Title

M71.479 **Calcium deposit in bursa, unspecified ankle and foot**

M71.48 **Calcium deposit in bursa, other site**

M71.49 **Calcium deposit in bursa, multiple sites**

✓5th M71.5 **Other bursitis, not elsewhere classified**
> EXCLUDES 1 *bursitis NOS (M71.9-)*
> EXCLUDES 2 *bursitis of shoulder (M75.5)*
> *bursitis of tibial collateral [Pellegrini-Stieda] (M76.4)*

M71.50 **Other bursitis, not elsewhere classified, unspecified site**

✓6th M71.52 **Other bursitis, not elsewhere classified, elbow**

M71.521 **Other bursitis, not elsewhere classified, right elbow**

M71.522 **Other bursitis, not elsewhere classified, left elbow**

M71.529 **Other bursitis, not elsewhere classified, unspecified elbow**

✓6th M71.53 **Other bursitis, not elsewhere classified, wrist**

M71.531 **Other bursitis, not elsewhere classified, right wrist**

M71.532 **Other bursitis, not elsewhere classified, left wrist**

M71.539 **Other bursitis, not elsewhere classified, unspecified wrist**

✓6th M71.54 **Other bursitis, not elsewhere classified, hand**

M71.541 **Other bursitis, not elsewhere classified, right hand**

M71.542 **Other bursitis, not elsewhere classified, left hand**

M71.549 **Other bursitis, not elsewhere classified, unspecified hand**

✓6th M71.55 **Other bursitis, not elsewhere classified, hip**

M71.551 **Other bursitis, not elsewhere classified, right hip**

M71.552 **Other bursitis, not elsewhere classified, left hip**

M71.559 **Other bursitis, not elsewhere classified, unspecified hip**

✓6th M71.56 **Other bursitis, not elsewhere classified, knee**

M71.561 **Other bursitis, not elsewhere classified, right knee**

M71.562 **Other bursitis, not elsewhere classified, left knee**

M71.569 **Other bursitis, not elsewhere classified, unspecified knee**

✓6th M71.57 **Other bursitis, not elsewhere classified, ankle and foot**

M71.571 **Other bursitis, not elsewhere classified, right ankle and foot**

M71.572 **Other bursitis, not elsewhere classified, left ankle and foot**

M71.579 **Other bursitis, not elsewhere classified, unspecified ankle and foot**

M71.58 **Other bursitis, not elsewhere classified, other site**

✓5th M71.8 **Other specified bursopathies**

M71.80 **Other specified bursopathies, unspecified site**

✓6th M71.81 **Other specified bursopathies, shoulder**

M71.811 **Other specified bursopathies, right shoulder**

M71.812 **Other specified bursopathies, left shoulder**

M71.819 **Other specified bursopathies, unspecified shoulder**

✓6th M71.82 **Other specified bursopathies, elbow**

M71.821 **Other specified bursopathies, right elbow**

M71.822 **Other specified bursopathies, left elbow**

M71.829 **Other specified bursopathies, unspecified elbow**

✓6th M71.83 **Other specified bursopathies, wrist**

M71.831 **Other specified bursopathies, right wrist**

M71.832 **Other specified bursopathies, left wrist**

M71.839 **Other specified bursopathies, unspecified wrist**

✓6th M71.84 **Other specified bursopathies, hand**

M71.841 **Other specified bursopathies, right hand**

M71.842 **Other specified bursopathies, left hand**

M71.849 **Other specified bursopathies, unspecified hand**

✓6th M71.85 **Other specified bursopathies, hip**

M71.851 **Other specified bursopathies, right hip**

M71.852 **Other specified bursopathies, left hip**

M71.859 **Other specified bursopathies, unspecified hip**

✓6th M71.86 **Other specified bursopathies, knee**

M71.861 **Other specified bursopathies, right knee**

M71.862 **Other specified bursopathies, left knee**

M71.869 **Other specified bursopathies, unspecified knee**

✓6th M71.87 **Other specified bursopathies, ankle and foot**

M71.871 **Other specified bursopathies, right ankle and foot**

M71.872 **Other specified bursopathies, left ankle and foot**

M71.879 **Other specified bursopathies, unspecified ankle and foot**

M71.88 **Other specified bursopathies, other site**

M71.89 **Other specified bursopathies, multiple sites**

M71.9 **Bursopathy, unspecified**
Bursitis NOS

✓4th **M72 Fibroblastic disorders**
> EXCLUDES 2 *retroperitoneal fibromatosis (D48.3)*

M72.0 **Palmar fascial fibromatosis [Dupuytren]** Ⓐ

M72.1 **Knuckle pads**

M72.2 **Plantar fascial fibromatosis**
Plantar fasciitis

M72.4 **Pseudosarcomatous fibromatosis**
Nodular fasciitis

M72.6 **Necrotizing fasciitis**
Use additional code (B95.-, B96.-) to identify causative organism

M72.8 **Other fibroblastic disorders**
Abscess of fascia   Other infective fasciitis
Fasciitis NEC
Use additional code to (B95.-, B96.-) identify causative organism
> EXCLUDES 1 *diffuse (eosinophilic) fasciitis (M35.4)*
> *necrotizing fasciitis (M72.6)*
> *nodular fasciitis (M72.4)*
> *perirenal fasciitis NOS (N13.5)*
> *perirenal fasciitis with infection (N13.6)*
> *plantar fasciitis (M72.2)*

M72.9 **Fibroblastic disorder, unspecified**
Fasciitis NOS   Fibromatosis NOS

✓4th **M75 Shoulder lesions**
> EXCLUDES 2 *shoulder-hand syndrome (M89.0-)*

✓5th M75.0 **Adhesive capsulitis of shoulder**
Frozen shoulder
Periarthritis of shoulder

M75.00 **Adhesive capsulitis of unspecified shoulder**

M75.01 **Adhesive capsulitis of right shoulder**

M75.02 **Adhesive capsulitis of left shoulder**

✓5th M75.1 **Rotator cuff tear or rupture, not specified as traumatic**
Rotator cuff syndrome
Supraspinatus syndrome
Supraspinatus tear or rupture, not specified as traumatic
> EXCLUDES 1 *tear of rotator cuff, traumatic (S46.01-)*

✓6th M75.10 **Unspecified rotator cuff tear or rupture, not specified as traumatic**

M75.100 **Unspecified rotator cuff tear or rupture of unspecified shoulder, not specified as traumatic**

M75.101 **Unspecified rotator cuff tear or rupture of right shoulder, not specified as traumatic**

M75.102 **Unspecified rotator cuff tear or rupture of left shoulder, not specified as traumatic**

✓6th M75.11 **Incomplete rotator cuff tear or rupture not specified as traumatic**

M75.110 **Incomplete rotator cuff tear or rupture of unspecified shoulder, not specified as traumatic**

M75.111 **Incomplete rotator cuff tear or rupture of right shoulder, not specified as traumatic**

M75.112 **Incomplete rotator cuff tear or rupture of left shoulder, not specified as traumatic**

EXCLUDES 1 Not coded here   EXCLUDES 2 Not included here   Ⓝ Newborn Age: 0   Ⓟ Pediatric Age: 0-17   Ⓜ Maternity Age: 12-55   Ⓐ Adult Age: 15-124

722
ICD-10-CM 2016

✓6ᵗʰ **M75.12** Complete **rotator cuff tear or rupture not specified as traumatic**
    M75.120 **Complete rotator cuff tear or rupture of unspecified shoulder, not specified as traumatic**
    M75.121 **Complete rotator cuff tear or rupture of** right **shoulder, not specified as traumatic**
    M75.122 **Complete rotator cuff tear or rupture of** left **shoulder, not specified as traumatic**

✓5ᵗʰ **M75.2** Bicipital **tendinitis**
    M75.20 **Bicipital tendinitis, unspecified shoulder**
    M75.21 **Bicipital tendinitis,** right **shoulder**
    M75.22 **Bicipital tendinitis,** left **shoulder**

✓5ᵗʰ **M75.3** Calcific **tendinitis of shoulder**
    Calcified bursa of shoulder
    M75.30 **Calcific tendinitis of unspecified shoulder**
    M75.31 **Calcific tendinitis of** right **shoulder**
    M75.32 **Calcific tendinitis of** left **shoulder**

✓5ᵗʰ **M75.4** Impingement syndrome **of shoulder**
    M75.40 **Impingement syndrome of unspecified shoulder**
    M75.41 **Impingement syndrome of** right **shoulder**
    M75.42 **Impingement syndrome of** left **shoulder**

✓5ᵗʰ **M75.5** Bursitis **of shoulder**
    M75.50 **Bursitis of unspecified shoulder**
    M75.51 **Bursitis of** right **shoulder**
    M75.52 **Bursitis of** left **shoulder**

✓5ᵗʰ **M75.8** Other **shoulder lesions**
    M75.80 **Other shoulder lesions, unspecified shoulder**
    M75.81 **Other shoulder lesions,** right **shoulder**
    M75.82 **Other shoulder lesions,** left **shoulder**

✓5ᵗʰ **M75.9** Shoulder lesion, **unspecified**
    M75.90 **Shoulder lesion, unspecified, unspecified shoulder**
    M75.91 **Shoulder lesion, unspecified,** right **shoulder**
    M75.92 **Shoulder lesion, unspecified,** left **shoulder**

✓4ᵗʰ **M76** **Enthesopathies, lower limb, excluding foot**
    EXCLUDES 2 bursitis due to use, overuse and pressure (M70.-)
    enthesopathies of ankle and foot (M77.5-)

✓5ᵗʰ **M76.0** Gluteal **tendinitis**
    M76.00 **Gluteal tendinitis, unspecified hip**
    M76.01 **Gluteal tendinitis,** right **hip**
    M76.02 **Gluteal tendinitis,** left **hip**

✓5ᵗʰ **M76.1** Psoas **tendinitis**
    M76.10 **Psoas tendinitis, unspecified hip**
    M76.11 **Psoas tendinitis,** right **hip**
    M76.12 **Psoas tendinitis,** left **hip**

✓5ᵗʰ **M76.2** Iliac crest **spur**
    M76.20 **Iliac crest spur, unspecified hip**
    M76.21 **Iliac crest spur,** right **hip**
    M76.22 **Iliac crest spur,** left **hip**

✓5ᵗʰ **M76.3** Iliotibial band **syndrome**
    M76.30 **Iliotibial band syndrome, unspecified leg**
    M76.31 **Iliotibial band syndrome,** right **leg**
    M76.32 **Iliotibial band syndrome,** left **leg**

✓5ᵗʰ **M76.4** Tibial collateral **bursitis [Pellegrini-Stieda]**
    M76.40 **Tibial collateral bursitis [Pellegrini-Stieda], unspecified leg**
    M76.41 **Tibial collateral bursitis [Pellegrini-Stieda],** right **leg**
    M76.42 **Tibial collateral bursitis [Pellegrini-Stieda],** left **leg**

✓5ᵗʰ **M76.5** Patellar **tendinitis**
    M76.50 **Patellar tendinitis, unspecified knee**
    M76.51 **Patellar tendinitis,** right **knee**
    M76.52 **Patellar tendinitis,** left **knee**

✓5ᵗʰ **M76.6** Achilles **tendinitis**
    Achilles bursitis
    M76.60 **Achilles tendinitis, unspecified leg**
    M76.61 **Achilles tendinitis,** right **leg**
    M76.62 **Achilles tendinitis,** left **leg**

✓5ᵗʰ **M76.7** Peroneal **tendinitis**
    M76.70 **Peroneal tendinitis, unspecified leg**

    M76.71 **Peroneal tendinitis,** right **leg**
    M76.72 **Peroneal tendinitis,** left **leg**

✓5ᵗʰ **M76.8** Other **specified enthesopathies of lower limb, excluding foot**
    ✓6ᵗʰ **M76.81** Anterior tibial syndrome
      M76.811 **Anterior tibial syndrome,** right **leg**
      M76.812 **Anterior tibial syndrome,** left **leg**
      M76.819 **Anterior tibial syndrome, unspecified leg**
    ✓6ᵗʰ **M76.82** Posterior tibial tendinitis
      M76.821 **Posterior tibial tendinitis,** right **leg**
      M76.822 **Posterior tibial tendinitis,** left **leg**
      M76.829 **Posterior tibial tendinitis, unspecified leg**
    ✓6ᵗʰ **M76.89** Other specified enthesopathies of lower limb, excluding foot
      M76.891 **Other specified enthesopathies of** right **lower limb, excluding foot**
      M76.892 **Other specified enthesopathies of** left **lower limb, excluding foot**
      M76.899 **Other specified enthesopathies of unspecified lower limb, excluding foot**

    M76.9 **Unspecified enthesopathy, lower limb, excluding foot**

✓4ᵗʰ **M77** **Other enthesopathies**
    EXCLUDES 1 bursitis NOS (M71.9-)
    EXCLUDES 2 bursitis due to use, overuse and pressure (M70.-)
    osteophyte (M25.7)
    spinal enthesopathy (M46.0-)

✓5ᵗʰ **M77.0** Medial **epicondylitis**
    M77.00 **Medial epicondylitis, unspecified elbow**
    M77.01 **Medial epicondylitis,** right **elbow**
    M77.02 **Medial epicondylitis,** left **elbow**

✓5ᵗʰ **M77.1** Lateral **epicondylitis**
    Tennis elbow
    M77.10 **Lateral epicondylitis, unspecified elbow**
    M77.11 **Lateral epicondylitis,** right **elbow**
    M77.12 **Lateral epicondylitis,** left **elbow**

✓5ᵗʰ **M77.2** Periarthritis **of wrist**
    M77.20 **Periarthritis, unspecified wrist**
    M77.21 **Periarthritis,** right **wrist**
    M77.22 **Periarthritis,** left **wrist**

✓5ᵗʰ **M77.3** Calcaneal **spur**
    M77.30 **Calcaneal spur, unspecified foot**
    M77.31 **Calcaneal spur,** right **foot**
    M77.32 **Calcaneal spur,** left **foot**

✓5ᵗʰ **M77.4** Metatarsalgia
    EXCLUDES 1 Morton's metatarsalgia (G57.6)
    M77.40 **Metatarsalgia, unspecified foot**
    M77.41 **Metatarsalgia,** right **foot**
    M77.42 **Metatarsalgia,** left **foot**

✓5ᵗʰ **M77.5** Other **enthesopathy of foot**
    M77.50 **Other enthesopathy of unspecified foot**
    M77.51 **Other enthesopathy of** right **foot**
    M77.52 **Other enthesopathy of** left **foot**

    M77.8 **Other enthesopathies, not elsewhere classified**
    M77.9 **Enthesopathy, unspecified**
    Bone spur NOS   Periarthritis NOS
    Capsulitis NOS   Tendinitis NOS

✓4ᵗʰ **M79** **Other and unspecified soft tissue disorders, not elsewhere classified**
    EXCLUDES 1 psychogenic rheumatism (F45.8)
    soft tissue pain, psychogenic (F45.41)

    M79.0 **Rheumatism, unspecified**
    EXCLUDES 1 fibromyalgia (M79.7)
    palindromic rheumatism (M12.3-)

    M79.1 **Myalgia**
    Myofascial pain syndrome
    EXCLUDES 1 fibromyalgia (M79.7)
    myositis (M60.-)

    M79.2 **Neuralgia and neuritis, unspecified**
    EXCLUDES 1 brachial radiculitis NOS (M54.1)
    lumbosacral radiculitis NOS (M54.1)
    mononeuropathies (G56-G58)
    radiculitis NOS (M54.1)
    sciatica (M54.3-M54.4)

✔ Additional Character Required   ✔x7ᵗʰ Placeholder Alert   Unspecified Dx   Other Specified Dx   Manifestation   ►◄ Revised Text   ● New Code   ▲ Revised Code Title

ICD-10-CM 2016   723

M79.3 Panniculitis, unspecified
> EXCLUDES 1   lupus panniculitis (L93.2)
> neck and back panniculitis (M54.0-)
> relapsing [Weber-Christian] panniculitis (M35.6)

M79.4 Hypertrophy of (infrapatellar) fat pad

M79.5 Residual foreign body in soft tissue
> EXCLUDES 1   foreign body granuloma of skin and subcutaneous
> tissue (L92.3)
> foreign body granuloma of soft tissue (M60.2-)

√5th **M79.6 Pain in limb, hand, foot, fingers and toes**
> EXCLUDES 2   pain in joint (M25.5-)

  √6th **M79.60 Pain in limb, unspecified**
      M79.601 Pain in right arm
           Pain in right upper limb NOS
      M79.602 Pain in left arm
           Pain in left upper limb NOS
      M79.603 Pain in arm, unspecified
           Pain in upper limb NOS
      M79.604 Pain in right leg
           Pain in right lower limb NOS
      M79.605 Pain in left leg
           Pain in left lower limb NOS
      M79.606 Pain in leg, unspecified
           Pain in lower limb NOS
      M79.609 Pain in unspecified limb
           Pain in limb NOS

  √6th **M79.62 Pain in upper arm**
       Pain in axillary region
      M79.621 Pain in right upper arm
      M79.622 Pain in left upper arm
      M79.629 Pain in unspecified upper arm

  √6th **M79.63 Pain in forearm**
      M79.631 Pain in right forearm
      M79.632 Pain in left forearm
      M79.639 Pain in unspecified forearm

  √6th **M79.64 Pain in hand and fingers**
      M79.641 Pain in right hand
      M79.642 Pain in left hand
      M79.643 Pain in unspecified hand
      M79.644 Pain in right finger(s)
      M79.645 Pain in left finger(s)
      M79.646 Pain in unspecified finger(s)

  √6th **M79.65 Pain in thigh**
      M79.651 Pain in right thigh
      M79.652 Pain in left thigh
      M79.659 Pain in unspecified thigh

  √6th **M79.66 Pain in lower leg**
      M79.661 Pain in right lower leg
      M79.662 Pain in left lower leg
      M79.669 Pain in unspecified lower leg

  √6th **M79.67 Pain in foot and toes**
      M79.671 Pain in right foot
      M79.672 Pain in left foot
      M79.673 Pain in unspecified foot
      M79.674 Pain in right toe(s)
      M79.675 Pain in left toe(s)
      M79.676 Pain in unspecified toe(s)

M79.7 Fibromyalgia
     Fibromyositis   Myofibrositis
     Fibrositis

√5th **M79.A Nontraumatic compartment syndrome**
     Code first, if applicable, associated postprocedural complication
> EXCLUDES 1   compartment syndrome NOS (T79.A-)
> fibromyalgia (M79.7)
> nontraumatic ischemic infarction of muscle (M62.2-)
> traumatic compartment syndrome (T79.A-)

  √6th **M79.A1 Nontraumatic compartment syndrome of upper extremity**
       Nontraumatic compartment syndrome of shoulder, arm, forearm, wrist, hand, and fingers
      M79.A11 Nontraumatic compartment syndrome of right upper extremity
      M79.A12 Nontraumatic compartment syndrome of left upper extremity

      M79.A19 Nontraumatic compartment syndrome of unspecified upper extremity

  √6th **M79.A2 Nontraumatic compartment syndrome of lower extremity**
       Nontraumatic compartment syndrome of hip, buttock, thigh, leg, foot, and toes
      M79.A21 Nontraumatic compartment syndrome of right lower extremity
      M79.A22 Nontraumatic compartment syndrome of left lower extremity
      M79.A29 Nontraumatic compartment syndrome of unspecified lower extremity

  M79.A3 Nontraumatic compartment syndrome of abdomen

  M79.A9 Nontraumatic compartment syndrome of other sites

√5th **M79.8 Other specified soft tissue disorders**
  M79.81 Nontraumatic hematoma of soft tissue
       Nontraumatic hematoma of muscle
       Nontraumatic seroma of muscle and soft tissue

  M79.89 Other specified soft tissue disorders
       Polyalgia

M79.9 Soft tissue disorder, unspecified

OSTEOPATHIES AND CHONDROPATHIES (M80-M94)

Disorders of bone density and structure (M80-M85)

√4th **M80 Osteoporosis with current pathological fracture**
> INCLUDES   osteoporosis with current fragility fracture
> Use additional code to identify major osseous defect, if applicable (M89.7-)
> EXCLUDES 1   collapsed vertebra NOS (M48.5)
> pathological fracture NOS (M84.4)
> wedging of vertebra NOS (M48.5)
> EXCLUDES 2   personal history of (healed) osteoporosis fracture (Z87.310)

> The appropriate 7th character is to be added to each code from category M80.
> A   initial encounter for fracture
> D   subsequent encounter for fracture with routine healing
> G   subsequent encounter for fracture with delayed healing
> K   subsequent encounter for fracture with nonunion
> P   subsequent encounter for fracture with malunion
> S   sequela

√5th **M80.0 Age-related osteoporosis with current pathological fracture**
     Involutional osteoporosis with current pathological fracture
     Osteoporosis NOS with current pathological fracture
     Postmenopausal osteoporosis with current pathological fracture
     Senile osteoporosis with current pathological fracture

  √x7th **M80.00 Age-related osteoporosis with current pathological fracture, unspecified site**   A

  √6th **M80.01 Age-related osteoporosis with current pathological fracture, shoulder**
    √7th **M80.011 Age-related osteoporosis with current pathological fracture, right shoulder**   A
    √7th **M80.012 Age-related osteoporosis with current pathological fracture, left shoulder**   A
    √7th **M80.019 Age-related osteoporosis with current pathological fracture, unspecified shoulder**   A

  √6th **M80.02 Age-related osteoporosis with current pathological fracture, humerus**
    √7th **M80.021 Age-related osteoporosis with current pathological fracture, right humerus**   A
    √7th **M80.022 Age-related osteoporosis with current pathological fracture, left humerus**   A
    √7th **M80.029 Age-related osteoporosis with current pathological fracture, unspecified humerus**   A

  √6th **M80.03 Age-related osteoporosis with current pathological fracture, forearm**
     Age-related osteoporosis with current pathological fracture of wrist
    √7th **M80.031 Age-related osteoporosis with current pathological fracture, right forearm**   A
    √7th **M80.032 Age-related osteoporosis with current pathological fracture, left forearm**   A
    √7th **M80.039 Age-related osteoporosis with current pathological fracture, unspecified forearm**   A

EXCLUDES 1 Not coded here   EXCLUDES 2 Not included here   N Newborn Age: 0   P Pediatric Age: 0-17   M Maternity Age: 12-55   A Adult Age: 15-124

724   ICD-10-CM 2016

√6ᵗʰ **M80.04** Age-related osteoporosis with current pathological fracture, hand

 √7ᵗʰ **M80.041** Age-related osteoporosis with current pathological fracture, right hand △

 √7ᵗʰ **M80.042** Age-related osteoporosis with current pathological fracture, left hand △

 √7ᵗʰ **M80.049** Age-related osteoporosis with current pathological fracture, unspecified hand △

√6ᵗʰ **M80.05** Age-related osteoporosis with current pathological fracture, femur
 Age-related osteoporosis with current pathological fracture of hip

 √7ᵗʰ **M80.051** Age-related osteoporosis with current pathological fracture, right femur △

 √7ᵗʰ **M80.052** Age-related osteoporosis with current pathological fracture, left femur △

 √7ᵗʰ **M80.059** Age-related osteoporosis with current pathological fracture, unspecified femur △

√6ᵗʰ **M80.06** Age-related osteoporosis with current pathological fracture, lower leg

 √7ᵗʰ **M80.061** Age-related osteoporosis with current pathological fracture, right lower leg △

 √7ᵗʰ **M80.062** Age-related osteoporosis with current pathological fracture, left lower leg △

 √7ᵗʰ **M80.069** Age-related osteoporosis with current pathological fracture, unspecified lower leg △

√6ᵗʰ **M80.07** Age-related osteoporosis with current pathological fracture, ankle and foot

 √7ᵗʰ **M80.071** Age-related osteoporosis with current pathological fracture, right ankle and foot △

 √7ᵗʰ **M80.072** Age-related osteoporosis with current pathological fracture, left ankle and foot △

 √7ᵗʰ **M80.079** Age-related osteoporosis with current pathological fracture, unspecified ankle and foot △

√x7ᵗʰ **M80.08** Age-related osteoporosis with current pathological fracture, vertebra(e) △

√5ᵗʰ **M80.8** Other osteoporosis with current pathological fracture
 Drug-induced osteoporosis with current pathological fracture
 Idiopathic osteoporosis with current pathological fracture
 Osteoporosis of disuse with current pathological fracture
 Postoophorectomy osteoporosis with current pathological fracture
 Postsurgical malabsorption osteoporosis with current pathological fracture
 Post-traumatic osteoporosis with current pathological fracture
 Use additional code for adverse effect, if applicable, to identify drug (T36-T50 with fifth or sixth character 5)

√x7ᵗʰ **M80.80** Other osteoporosis with current pathological fracture, unspecified site

√6ᵗʰ **M80.81** Other osteoporosis with pathological fracture, shoulder

 √7ᵗʰ **M80.811** Other osteoporosis with current pathological fracture, right shoulder

 √7ᵗʰ **M80.812** Other osteoporosis with current pathological fracture, left shoulder

 √7ᵗʰ **M80.819** Other osteoporosis with current pathological fracture, unspecified shoulder

√6ᵗʰ **M80.82** Other osteoporosis with current pathological fracture, humerus

 √7ᵗʰ **M80.821** Other osteoporosis with current pathological fracture, right humerus

 √7ᵗʰ **M80.822** Other osteoporosis with current pathological fracture, left humerus

 √7ᵗʰ **M80.829** Other osteoporosis with current pathological fracture, unspecified humerus

√6ᵗʰ **M80.83** Other osteoporosis with current pathological fracture, forearm
 Other osteoporosis with current pathological fracture of wrist

 √7ᵗʰ **M80.831** Other osteoporosis with current pathological fracture, right forearm

 √7ᵗʰ **M80.832** Other osteoporosis with current pathological fracture, left forearm

 √7ᵗʰ **M80.839** Other osteoporosis with current pathological fracture, unspecified forearm

√6ᵗʰ **M80.84** Other osteoporosis with current pathological fracture, hand

 √7ᵗʰ **M80.841** Other osteoporosis with current pathological fracture, right hand

 √7ᵗʰ **M80.842** Other osteoporosis with current pathological fracture, left hand

 √7ᵗʰ **M80.849** Other osteoporosis with current pathological fracture, unspecified hand

√6ᵗʰ **M80.85** Other osteoporosis with current pathological fracture, femur
 Other osteoporosis with current pathological fracture of hip

 √7ᵗʰ **M80.851** Other osteoporosis with current pathological fracture, right femur

 √7ᵗʰ **M80.852** Other osteoporosis with current pathological fracture, left femur

 √7ᵗʰ **M80.859** Other osteoporosis with current pathological fracture, unspecified femur

√6ᵗʰ **M80.86** Other osteoporosis with current pathological fracture, lower leg

 √7ᵗʰ **M80.861** Other osteoporosis with current pathological fracture, right lower leg

 √7ᵗʰ **M80.862** Other osteoporosis with current pathological fracture, left lower leg

 √7ᵗʰ **M80.869** Other osteoporosis with current pathological fracture, unspecified lower leg

√6ᵗʰ **M80.87** Other osteoporosis with current pathological fracture, ankle and foot

 √7ᵗʰ **M80.871** Other osteoporosis with current pathological fracture, right ankle and foot

 √7ᵗʰ **M80.872** Other osteoporosis with current pathological fracture, left ankle and foot

 √7ᵗʰ **M80.879** Other osteoporosis with current pathological fracture, unspecified ankle and foot

√x7ᵗʰ **M80.88** Other osteoporosis with current pathological fracture, vertebra(e)

√4ᵗʰ **M81 Osteoporosis without current pathological fracture**
 Use additional code to identify:
  major osseous defect, if applicable (M89.7-)
  personal history of (healed) osteoporosis fracture, if applicable (Z87.310)
 EXCLUDES 1 osteoporosis with current pathological fracture (M80.-)
  Sudeck's atrophy (M89.0)

M81.0 Age-related osteoporosis without current pathological fracture △
 Involutional osteoporosis without current pathological fracture
 Osteoporosis NOS
 Postmenopausal osteoporosis without current pathological fracture
 Senile osteoporosis without current pathological fracture

M81.6 Localized osteoporosis [Lequesne]
 EXCLUDES 1 Sudeck's atrophy (M89.0)

M81.8 Other osteoporosis without current pathological fracture
 Drug-induced osteoporosis without current pathological fracture
 Idiopathic osteoporosis without current pathological fracture
 Osteoporosis of disuse without current pathological fracture
 Postoophorectomy osteoporosis without current pathological fracture
 Postsurgical malabsorption osteoporosis without current pathological fracture
 Post-traumatic osteoporosis without current pathological fracture
 Use additional code for adverse effect, if applicable, to identify drug (T36-T50 with fifth or sixth character 5)

√4ᵗʰ **M83 Adult osteomalacia**
 EXCLUDES 1 infantile and juvenile osteomalacia (E55.0)
  renal osteodystrophy (N25.0)
  rickets (active) (E55.0)
  rickets (active) sequelae (E64.3)
  vitamin D-resistant osteomalacia (E83.3)
  vitamin D-resistant rickets (active) (E83.3)

M83.0 Puerperal osteomalacia Ⓜ♀

M83.1 Senile osteomalacia △

☑ Additional Character Required   √x7ᵗʰ Placeholder Alert   Unspecified Dx   Other Specified Dx   Manifestation   ▶◀ Revised Text   ● New Code   ▲ Revised Code Title

M83.2 Adult osteomalacia **due to malabsorption**   🅰
    Postsurgical malabsorption osteomalacia in adults

M83.3 Adult osteomalacia **due to malnutrition**   🅰

M83.4 Aluminum bone disease

M83.5 Other **drug-induced** osteomalacia in adults   🅰
    Use additional code for adverse effect, if applicable, to identify drug (T36-T50 with fifth or sixth character 5)

M83.8 Other adult osteomalacia   🅰

M83.9 Adult osteomalacia, unspecified   🅰

✓4th **M84** **Disorder of continuity of bone**
    EXCLUDES 2 *traumatic fracture of bone-see fracture, by site*

  ✓5th **M84.3** **Stress fracture**
    Fatigue fracture   Stress fracture NOS
    March fracture   Stress reaction
    Use additional external cause code(s) to identify the cause of the stress fracture
    EXCLUDES 1 *pathological fracture NOS (M84.4-)*
        pathological fracture due to osteoporosis (M80.-)
        traumatic fracture (S12-, S22-, S32-, S42-, S52-, S62-, S72-, S82-, S92-)
    EXCLUDES 2 *personal history of (healed) stress (fatigue) fracture (Z87.312)*
        stress fracture of vertebra (M48.4-)

> The appropriate 7th character is to be added to each code from subcategory M84.3.
> A   initial encounter for fracture
> D   subsequent encounter for fracture with routine healing
> G   subsequent encounter for fracture with delayed healing
> K   subsequent encounter for fracture with nonunion
> P   subsequent encounter for fracture with malunion
> S   sequela

    ✓x7th **M84.30** **Stress fracture, unspecified site**

    ✓6th **M84.31** **Stress fracture, shoulder**
        ✓7th **M84.311** **Stress fracture, right shoulder**
        ✓7th **M84.312** **Stress fracture, left shoulder**
        ✓7th **M84.319** **Stress fracture, unspecified shoulder**

    ✓6th **M84.32** **Stress fracture, humerus**
        ✓7th **M84.321** **Stress fracture, right humerus**
        ✓7th **M84.322** **Stress fracture, left humerus**
        ✓7th **M84.329** **Stress fracture, unspecified humerus**

    ✓6th **M84.33** **Stress fracture, ulna and radius**
        ✓7th **M84.331** **Stress fracture, right ulna**
        ✓7th **M84.332** **Stress fracture, left ulna**
        ✓7th **M84.333** **Stress fracture, right radius**
        ✓7th **M84.334** **Stress fracture, left radius**
        ✓7th **M84.339** **Stress fracture, unspecified ulna and radius**

    ✓6th **M84.34** **Stress fracture, hand and fingers**
        ✓7th **M84.341** **Stress fracture, right hand**
        ✓7th **M84.342** **Stress fracture, left hand**
        ✓7th **M84.343** **Stress fracture, unspecified hand**
        ✓7th **M84.344** **Stress fracture, right finger(s)**
        ✓7th **M84.345** **Stress fracture, left finger(s)**
        ✓7th **M84.346** **Stress fracture, unspecified finger(s)**

    ✓6th **M84.35** **Stress fracture, pelvis and femur**
        Stress fracture, hip
        ✓7th **M84.350** **Stress fracture, pelvis**
        ✓7th **M84.351** **Stress fracture, right femur**
        ✓7th **M84.352** **Stress fracture, left femur**
        ✓7th **M84.353** **Stress fracture, unspecified femur**
        ✓7th **M84.359** **Stress fracture, hip, unspecified**

    ✓6th **M84.36** **Stress fracture, tibia and fibula**
        ✓7th **M84.361** **Stress fracture, right tibia**
        ✓7th **M84.362** **Stress fracture, left tibia**
        ✓7th **M84.363** **Stress fracture, right fibula**
        ✓7th **M84.364** **Stress fracture, left fibula**
        ✓7th **M84.369** **Stress fracture, unspecified tibia and fibula**

    ✓6th **M84.37** **Stress fracture, ankle, foot and toes**
        ✓7th **M84.371** **Stress fracture, right ankle**
        ✓7th **M84.372** **Stress fracture, left ankle**

        ✓7th **M84.373** **Stress fracture, unspecified ankle**
        ✓7th **M84.374** **Stress fracture, right foot**
        ✓7th **M84.375** **Stress fracture, left foot**
        ✓7th **M84.376** **Stress fracture, unspecified foot**
        ✓7th **M84.377** **Stress fracture, right toe(s)**
        ✓7th **M84.378** **Stress fracture, left toe(s)**
        ✓7th **M84.379** **Stress fracture, unspecified toe(s)**

    ✓x7th **M84.38** **Stress fracture, other site**
        EXCLUDES 2 *stress fracture of vertebra (M48.4-)*

  ✓5th **M84.4** **Pathological fracture, not elsewhere classified**
    Chronic fracture
    Pathological fracture NOS
    EXCLUDES 1 *collapsed vertebra NEC (M48.5)*
        pathological fracture in neoplastic disease (M84.5-)
        pathological fracture in osteoporosis (M80.-)
        pathological fracture in other disease (M84.6-)
        stress fracture (M84.3-)
        traumatic fracture (S12.-, S22.-, S32.-, S42.-, S52.-, S62.-, S72.-, S82.-, S92.-)
    EXCLUDES 2 *personal history of (healed) pathological fracture (Z87.311)*

> The appropriate 7th character is to be added to each code from subcategory M84.4.
> A   initial encounter for fracture
> D   subsequent encounter for fracture with routine healing
> G   subsequent encounter for fracture with delayed healing
> K   subsequent encounter for fracture with nonunion
> P   subsequent encounter for fracture with malunion
> S   sequela

    ✓x7th **M84.40** **Pathological fracture, unspecified site**

    ✓6th **M84.41** **Pathological fracture, shoulder**
        ✓7th **M84.411** **Pathological fracture, right shoulder**
        ✓7th **M84.412** **Pathological fracture, left shoulder**
        ✓7th **M84.419** **Pathological fracture, unspecified shoulder**

    ✓6th **M84.42** **Pathological fracture, humerus**
        ✓7th **M84.421** **Pathological fracture, right humerus**
        ✓7th **M84.422** **Pathological fracture, left humerus**
        ✓7th **M84.429** **Pathological fracture, unspecified humerus**

    ✓6th **M84.43** **Pathological fracture, ulna and radius**
        ✓7th **M84.431** **Pathological fracture, right ulna**
        ✓7th **M84.432** **Pathological fracture, left ulna**
        ✓7th **M84.433** **Pathological fracture, right radius**
        ✓7th **M84.434** **Pathological fracture, left radius**
        ✓7th **M84.439** **Pathological fracture, unspecified ulna and radius**

    ✓6th **M84.44** **Pathological fracture, hand and fingers**
        ✓7th **M84.441** **Pathological fracture, right hand**
        ✓7th **M84.442** **Pathological fracture, left hand**
        ✓7th **M84.443** **Pathological fracture, unspecified hand**
        ✓7th **M84.444** **Pathological fracture, right finger(s)**
        ✓7th **M84.445** **Pathological fracture, left finger(s)**
        ✓7th **M84.446** **Pathological fracture, unspecified finger(s)**

    ✓6th **M84.45** **Pathological fracture, femur and pelvis**
        ✓7th **M84.451** **Pathological fracture, right femur**
        ✓7th **M84.452** **Pathological fracture, left femur**
        ✓7th **M84.453** **Pathological fracture, unspecified femur**
        ✓7th **M84.454** **Pathological fracture, pelvis**
        ✓7th **M84.459** **Pathological fracture, hip, unspecified**

    ✓6th **M84.46** **Pathological fracture, tibia and fibula**
        ✓7th **M84.461** **Pathological fracture, right tibia**
        ✓7th **M84.462** **Pathological fracture, left tibia**
        ✓7th **M84.463** **Pathological fracture, right fibula**
        ✓7th **M84.464** **Pathological fracture, left fibula**
        ✓7th **M84.469** **Pathological fracture, unspecified tibia and fibula**

EXCLUDES 1 Not coded here   *EXCLUDES 2* Not included here   🅝 Newborn Age: 0   🅟 Pediatric Age: 0-17   🅜 Maternity Age: 12-55   🅐 Adult Age: 15-124

726   ICD-10-CM 2016

√6ᵗʰ **M84.47** Pathological fracture, ankle, foot and toes

     √7ᵗʰ **M84.471** Pathological fracture, right ankle

     √7ᵗʰ **M84.472** Pathological fracture, left ankle

     √7ᵗʰ **M84.473** Pathological fracture, unspecified ankle

     √7ᵗʰ **M84.474** Pathological fracture, right foot

     √7ᵗʰ **M84.475** Pathological fracture, left foot

     √7ᵗʰ **M84.476** Pathological fracture, unspecified foot

     √7ᵗʰ **M84.477** Pathological fracture, right toe(s)

     √7ᵗʰ **M84.478** Pathological fracture, left toe(s)

     √7ᵗʰ **M84.479** Pathological fracture, unspecified toe(s)

√x7ᵗʰ **M84.48** Pathological fracture, other site

√5ᵗʰ **M84.5** Pathological fracture in neoplastic disease

     Code also underlying neoplasm

> The appropriate 7th character is to be added to each code from subcategory M84.5.
> A   initial encounter for fracture
> D   subsequent encounter for fracture with routine healing
> G   subsequent encounter for fracture with delayed healing
> K   subsequent encounter for fracture with nonunion
> P   subsequent encounter for fracture with malunion
> S   sequela

√x7ᵗʰ **M84.50** Pathological fracture in neoplastic disease, unspecified site

√6ᵗʰ **M84.51** Pathological fracture in neoplastic disease, shoulder

     √7ᵗʰ **M84.511** Pathological fracture in neoplastic disease, right shoulder

     √7ᵗʰ **M84.512** Pathological fracture in neoplastic disease, left shoulder

     √7ᵗʰ **M84.519** Pathological fracture in neoplastic disease, unspecified shoulder

√6ᵗʰ **M84.52** Pathological fracture in neoplastic disease, humerus

     √7ᵗʰ **M84.521** Pathological fracture in neoplastic disease, right humerus

     √7ᵗʰ **M84.522** Pathological fracture in neoplastic disease, left humerus

     √7ᵗʰ **M84.529** Pathological fracture in neoplastic disease, unspecified humerus

√6ᵗʰ **M84.53** Pathological fracture in neoplastic disease, ulna and radius

     √7ᵗʰ **M84.531** Pathological fracture in neoplastic disease, right ulna

     √7ᵗʰ **M84.532** Pathological fracture in neoplastic disease, left ulna

     √7ᵗʰ **M84.533** Pathological fracture in neoplastic disease, right radius

     √7ᵗʰ **M84.534** Pathological fracture in neoplastic disease, left radius

     √7ᵗʰ **M84.539** Pathological fracture in neoplastic disease, unspecified ulna and radius

√6ᵗʰ **M84.54** Pathological fracture in neoplastic disease, hand

     √7ᵗʰ **M84.541** Pathological fracture in neoplastic disease, right hand

     √7ᵗʰ **M84.542** Pathological fracture in neoplastic disease, left hand

     √7ᵗʰ **M84.549** Pathological fracture in neoplastic disease, unspecified hand

√6ᵗʰ **M84.55** Pathological fracture in neoplastic disease, pelvis and femur

     √7ᵗʰ **M84.550** Pathological fracture in neoplastic disease, pelvis

     √7ᵗʰ **M84.551** Pathological fracture in neoplastic disease, right femur

     √7ᵗʰ **M84.552** Pathological fracture in neoplastic disease, left femur

     √7ᵗʰ **M84.553** Pathological fracture in neoplastic disease, unspecified femur

     √7ᵗʰ **M84.559** Pathological fracture in neoplastic disease, hip, unspecified

√6ᵗʰ **M84.56** Pathological fracture in neoplastic disease, tibia and fibula

     √7ᵗʰ **M84.561** Pathological fracture in neoplastic disease, right tibia

     √7ᵗʰ **M84.562** Pathological fracture in neoplastic disease, left tibia

     √7ᵗʰ **M84.563** Pathological fracture in neoplastic disease, right fibula

     √7ᵗʰ **M84.564** Pathological fracture in neoplastic disease, left fibula

     √7ᵗʰ **M84.569** Pathological fracture in neoplastic disease, unspecified tibia and fibula

√6ᵗʰ **M84.57** Pathological fracture in neoplastic disease, ankle and foot

     √7ᵗʰ **M84.571** Pathological fracture in neoplastic disease, right ankle

     √7ᵗʰ **M84.572** Pathological fracture in neoplastic disease, left ankle

     √7ᵗʰ **M84.573** Pathological fracture in neoplastic disease, unspecified ankle

     √7ᵗʰ **M84.574** Pathological fracture in neoplastic disease, right foot

     √7ᵗʰ **M84.575** Pathological fracture in neoplastic disease, left foot

     √7ᵗʰ **M84.576** Pathological fracture in neoplastic disease, unspecified foot

√x7ᵗʰ **M84.58** Pathological fracture in neoplastic disease, other specified site

     Pathological fracture in neoplastic disease, vertebrae

√5ᵗʰ **M84.6** Pathological fracture in other disease

     Code also underlying condition

     EXCLUDES 1   pathological fracture in osteoporosis (M80.-)

> The appropriate 7th character is to be added to each code from subcategory M84.6.
> A   initial encounter for fracture
> D   subsequent encounter for fracture with routine healing
> G   subsequent encounter for fracture with delayed healing
> K   subsequent encounter for fracture with nonunion
> P   subsequent encounter for fracture with malunion
> S   sequela

√x7ᵗʰ **M84.60** Pathological fracture in other disease, unspecified site

√6ᵗʰ **M84.61** Pathological fracture in other disease, shoulder

     √7ᵗʰ **M84.611** Pathological fracture in other disease, right shoulder

     √7ᵗʰ **M84.612** Pathological fracture in other disease, left shoulder

     √7ᵗʰ **M84.619** Pathological fracture in other disease, unspecified shoulder

√6ᵗʰ **M84.62** Pathological fracture in other disease, humerus

     √7ᵗʰ **M84.621** Pathological fracture in other disease, right humerus

     √7ᵗʰ **M84.622** Pathological fracture in other disease, left humerus

     √7ᵗʰ **M84.629** Pathological fracture in other disease, unspecified humerus

√6ᵗʰ **M84.63** Pathological fracture in other disease, ulna and radius

     √7ᵗʰ **M84.631** Pathological fracture in other disease, right ulna

     √7ᵗʰ **M84.632** Pathological fracture in other disease, left ulna

     √7ᵗʰ **M84.633** Pathological fracture in other disease, right radius

     √7ᵗʰ **M84.634** Pathological fracture in other disease, left radius

     √7ᵗʰ **M84.639** Pathological fracture in other disease, unspecified ulna and radius

√6ᵗʰ **M84.64** Pathological fracture in other disease, hand

     √7ᵗʰ **M84.641** Pathological fracture in other disease, right hand

     √7ᵗʰ **M84.642** Pathological fracture in other disease, left hand

     √7ᵗʰ **M84.649** Pathological fracture in other disease, unspecified hand

√6ᵗʰ **M84.65** Pathological fracture in other disease, pelvis and femur

     √7ᵗʰ **M84.650** Pathological fracture in other disease, pelvis

     √7ᵗʰ **M84.651** Pathological fracture in other disease, right femur

---

☑ Additional Character Required   √x7ᵗʰ Placeholder Alert   Unspecified Dx   Other Specified Dx   Manifestation   ▶◀ Revised Text   ● New Code   ▲ Revised Code Title

Chapter 13. Diseases of the Musculoskeletal System and Connective Tissue

✓7ᵗʰ **M84.652** Pathological fracture in other disease, left femur

✓7ᵗʰ **M84.653** Pathological fracture in other disease, unspecified femur

✓7ᵗʰ **M84.659** Pathological fracture in other disease, hip, unspecified

✓6ᵗʰ **M84.66** Pathological fracture in other disease, tibia and fibula

  ✓7ᵗʰ **M84.661** Pathological fracture in other disease, right tibia

  ✓7ᵗʰ **M84.662** Pathological fracture in other disease, left tibia

  ✓7ᵗʰ **M84.663** Pathological fracture in other disease, right fibula

  ✓7ᵗʰ **M84.664** Pathological fracture in other disease, left fibula

  ✓7ᵗʰ **M84.669** Pathological fracture in other disease, unspecified tibia and fibula

✓6ᵗʰ **M84.67** Pathological fracture in other disease, ankle and foot

  ✓7ᵗʰ **M84.671** Pathological fracture in other disease, right ankle

  ✓7ᵗʰ **M84.672** Pathological fracture in other disease, left ankle

  ✓7ᵗʰ **M84.673** Pathological fracture in other disease, unspecified ankle

  ✓7ᵗʰ **M84.674** Pathological fracture in other disease, right foot

  ✓7ᵗʰ **M84.675** Pathological fracture in other disease, left foot

  ✓7ᵗʰ **M84.676** Pathological fracture in other disease, unspecified foot

✓x7ᵗʰ **M84.68** Pathological fracture in other disease, other site

✓5ᵗʰ **M84.8** Other disorders of continuity of bone

  M84.80 Other disorders of continuity of bone, unspecified site

  ✓6ᵗʰ **M84.81** Other disorders of continuity of bone, shoulder

    M84.811 Other disorders of continuity of bone, right shoulder

    M84.812 Other disorders of continuity of bone, left shoulder

    M84.819 Other disorders of continuity of bone, unspecified shoulder

  ✓6ᵗʰ **M84.82** Other disorders of continuity of bone, humerus

    M84.821 Other disorders of continuity of bone, right humerus

    M84.822 Other disorders of continuity of bone, left humerus

    M84.829 Other disorders of continuity of bone, unspecified humerus

  ✓6ᵗʰ **M84.83** Other disorders of continuity of bone, ulna and radius

    M84.831 Other disorders of continuity of bone, right ulna

    M84.832 Other disorders of continuity of bone, left ulna

    M84.833 Other disorders of continuity of bone, right radius

    M84.834 Other disorders of continuity of bone, left radius

    M84.839 Other disorders of continuity of bone, unspecified ulna and radius

  ✓6ᵗʰ **M84.84** Other disorders of continuity of bone, hand

    M84.841 Other disorders of continuity of bone, right hand

    M84.842 Other disorders of continuity of bone, left hand

    M84.849 Other disorders of continuity of bone, unspecified hand

  ✓6ᵗʰ **M84.85** Other disorders of continuity of bone, pelvic region and thigh

    M84.851 Other disorders of continuity of bone, right pelvic region and thigh

    M84.852 Other disorders of continuity of bone, left pelvic region and thigh

    M84.859 Other disorders of continuity of bone, unspecified pelvic region and thigh

  ✓6ᵗʰ **M84.86** Other disorders of continuity of bone, tibia and fibula

    M84.861 Other disorders of continuity of bone, right tibia

    M84.862 Other disorders of continuity of bone, left tibia

    M84.863 Other disorders of continuity of bone, right fibula

    M84.864 Other disorders of continuity of bone, left fibula

    M84.869 Other disorders of continuity of bone, unspecified tibia and fibula

  ✓6ᵗʰ **M84.87** Other disorders of continuity of bone, ankle and foot

    M84.871 Other disorders of continuity of bone, right ankle and foot

    M84.872 Other disorders of continuity of bone, left ankle and foot

    M84.879 Other disorders of continuity of bone, unspecified ankle and foot

  M84.88 Other disorders of continuity of bone, other site

M84.9 Disorder of continuity of bone, unspecified

✓4ᵗʰ **M85** **Other disorders of bone density and structure**

  EXCLUDES 1   osteogenesis imperfecta (Q78.0)
        osteopetrosis (Q78.2)
        osteopoikilosis (Q78.8)
        polyostotic fibrous dysplasia (Q78.1)

✓5ᵗʰ **M85.0** Fibrous dysplasia (monostotic)

  EXCLUDES 2   fibrous dysplasia of jaw (M27.8)

  M85.00 Fibrous dysplasia (monostotic), unspecified site

  ✓6ᵗʰ **M85.01** Fibrous dysplasia (monostotic), shoulder

    M85.011 Fibrous dysplasia (monostotic), right shoulder

    M85.012 Fibrous dysplasia (monostotic), left shoulder

    M85.019 Fibrous dysplasia (monostotic), unspecified shoulder

  ✓6ᵗʰ **M85.02** Fibrous dysplasia (monostotic), upper arm

    M85.021 Fibrous dysplasia (monostotic), right upper arm

    M85.022 Fibrous dysplasia (monostotic), left upper arm

    M85.029 Fibrous dysplasia (monostotic), unspecified upper arm

  ✓6ᵗʰ **M85.03** Fibrous dysplasia (monostotic), forearm

    M85.031 Fibrous dysplasia (monostotic), right forearm

    M85.032 Fibrous dysplasia (monostotic), left forearm

    M85.039 Fibrous dysplasia (monostotic), unspecified forearm

  ✓6ᵗʰ **M85.04** Fibrous dysplasia (monostotic), hand

    M85.041 Fibrous dysplasia (monostotic), right hand

    M85.042 Fibrous dysplasia (monostotic), left hand

    M85.049 Fibrous dysplasia (monostotic), unspecified hand

  ✓6ᵗʰ **M85.05** Fibrous dysplasia (monostotic), thigh

    M85.051 Fibrous dysplasia (monostotic), right thigh

    M85.052 Fibrous dysplasia (monostotic), left thigh

    M85.059 Fibrous dysplasia (monostotic), unspecified thigh

  ✓6ᵗʰ **M85.06** Fibrous dysplasia (monostotic), lower leg

    M85.061 Fibrous dysplasia (monostotic), right lower leg

    M85.062 Fibrous dysplasia (monostotic), left lower leg

    M85.069 Fibrous dysplasia (monostotic), unspecified lower leg

  ✓6ᵗʰ **M85.07** Fibrous dysplasia (monostotic), ankle and foot

    M85.071 Fibrous dysplasia (monostotic), right ankle and foot

    M85.072 Fibrous dysplasia (monostotic), left ankle and foot

---

EXCLUDES 1 Not coded here   *EXCLUDES 2* Not included here   N Newborn Age: 0   P Pediatric Age: 0-17   M Maternity Age: 12-55   A Adult Age: 15-124

728   ICD-10-CM 2016

M85.Ø79   **Fibrous dysplasia (monostotic), unspecified ankle and foot**

M85.Ø8   **Fibrous dysplasia (monostotic), other site**

M85.Ø9   **Fibrous dysplasia (monostotic),** multiple sites

✓5ᵗʰ   **M85.1**   **Skeletal fluorosis**

    M85.1Ø   **Skeletal fluorosis, unspecified site**

    ✓6ᵗʰ   M85.11   **Skeletal fluorosis,** shoulder

       M85.111   **Skeletal fluorosis,** right **shoulder**

       M85.112   **Skeletal fluorosis,** left **shoulder**

       M85.119   **Skeletal fluorosis, unspecified shoulder**

    ✓6ᵗʰ   M85.12   **Skeletal fluorosis,** upper arm

       M85.121   **Skeletal fluorosis,** right **upper arm**

       M85.122   **Skeletal fluorosis,** left **upper arm**

       M85.129   **Skeletal fluorosis, unspecified upper arm**

    ✓6ᵗʰ   M85.13   **Skeletal fluorosis,** forearm

       M85.131   **Skeletal fluorosis,** right **forearm**

       M85.132   **Skeletal fluorosis,** left **forearm**

       M85.139   **Skeletal fluorosis, unspecified forearm**

    ✓6ᵗʰ   M85.14   **Skeletal fluorosis,** hand

       M85.141   **Skeletal fluorosis,** right **hand**

       M85.142   **Skeletal fluorosis,** left **hand**

       M85.149   **Skeletal fluorosis, unspecified hand**

    ✓6ᵗʰ   M85.15   **Skeletal fluorosis,** thigh

       M85.151   **Skeletal fluorosis,** right **thigh**

       M85.152   **Skeletal fluorosis,** left **thigh**

       M85.159   **Skeletal fluorosis, unspecified thigh**

    ✓6ᵗʰ   M85.16   **Skeletal fluorosis,** lower leg

       M85.161   **Skeletal fluorosis,** right **lower leg**

       M85.162   **Skeletal fluorosis,** left **lower leg**

       M85.169   **Skeletal fluorosis, unspecified lower leg**

    ✓6ᵗʰ   M85.17   **Skeletal fluorosis,** ankle and foot

       M85.171   **Skeletal fluorosis,** right **ankle and foot**

       M85.172   **Skeletal fluorosis,** left **ankle and foot**

       M85.179   **Skeletal fluorosis, unspecified ankle and foot**

    M85.18   **Skeletal fluorosis, other site**

    M85.19   **Skeletal fluorosis,** multiple sites

  M85.2   Hyperostosis of skull

✓5ᵗʰ   **M85.3**   Osteitis condensans

    M85.3Ø   **Osteitis condensans, unspecified site**

    ✓6ᵗʰ   M85.31   **Osteitis condensans,** shoulder

       M85.311   **Osteitis condensans,** right **shoulder**

       M85.312   **Osteitis condensans,** left **shoulder**

       M85.319   **Osteitis condensans, unspecified shoulder**

    ✓6ᵗʰ   M85.32   **Osteitis condensans,** upper arm

       M85.321   **Osteitis condensans,** right **upper arm**

       M85.322   **Osteitis condensans,** left **upper arm**

       M85.329   **Osteitis condensans, unspecified upper arm**

    ✓6ᵗʰ   M85.33   **Osteitis condensans,** forearm

       M85.331   **Osteitis condensans,** right **forearm**

       M85.332   **Osteitis condensans,** left **forearm**

       M85.339   **Osteitis condensans, unspecified forearm**

    ✓6ᵗʰ   M85.34   **Osteitis condensans,** hand

       M85.341   **Osteitis condensans,** right **hand**

       M85.342   **Osteitis condensans,** left **hand**

       M85.349   **Osteitis condensans, unspecified hand**

    ✓6ᵗʰ   M85.35   **Osteitis condensans,** thigh

       M85.351   **Osteitis condensans,** right **thigh**

       M85.352   **Osteitis condensans,** left **thigh**

       M85.359   **Osteitis condensans, unspecified thigh**

    ✓6ᵗʰ   M85.36   **Osteitis condensans,** lower leg

       M85.361   **Osteitis condensans,** right **lower leg**

       M85.362   **Osteitis condensans,** left **lower leg**

       M85.369   **Osteitis condensans, unspecified lower leg**

    ✓6ᵗʰ   M85.37   **Osteitis condensans,** ankle and foot

       M85.371   **Osteitis condensans,** right **ankle and foot**

       M85.372   **Osteitis condensans,** left **ankle and foot**

       M85.379   **Osteitis condensans, unspecified ankle and foot**

M85.38   **Osteitis condensans, other site**

M85.39   **Osteitis condensans,** multiple sites

✓5ᵗʰ   **M85.4**   Solitary **bone cyst**

    EXCLUDES 2   *solitary cyst of jaw (M27.4)*

    M85.4Ø   **Solitary bone cyst, unspecified site**

    ✓6ᵗʰ   M85.41   **Solitary bone cyst,** shoulder

       M85.411   **Solitary bone cyst,** right **shoulder**

       M85.412   **Solitary bone cyst,** left **shoulder**

       M85.419   **Solitary bone cyst, unspecified shoulder**

    ✓6ᵗʰ   M85.42   **Solitary bone cyst,** humerus

       M85.421   **Solitary bone cyst,** right **humerus**

       M85.422   **Solitary bone cyst,** left **humerus**

       M85.429   **Solitary bone cyst, unspecified humerus**

    ✓6ᵗʰ   M85.43   **Solitary bone cyst,** ulna and radius

       M85.431   **Solitary bone cyst,** right **ulna and radius**

       M85.432   **Solitary bone cyst,** left **ulna and radius**

       M85.439   **Solitary bone cyst, unspecified ulna and radius**

    ✓6ᵗʰ   M85.44   **Solitary bone cyst,** hand

       M85.441   **Solitary bone cyst,** right **hand**

       M85.442   **Solitary bone cyst,** left **hand**

       M85.449   **Solitary bone cyst, unspecified hand**

    ✓6ᵗʰ   M85.45   **Solitary bone cyst,** pelvis

       M85.451   **Solitary bone cyst,** right **pelvis**

       M85.452   **Solitary bone cyst,** left **pelvis**

       M85.459   **Solitary bone cyst, unspecified pelvis**

    ✓6ᵗʰ   M85.46   **Solitary bone cyst,** tibia and fibula

       M85.461   **Solitary bone cyst,** right **tibia and fibula**

       M85.462   **Solitary bone cyst,** left **tibia and fibula**

       M85.469   **Solitary bone cyst, unspecified tibia and fibula**

    ✓6ᵗʰ   M85.47   **Solitary bone cyst,** ankle and foot

       M85.471   **Solitary bone cyst,** right **ankle and foot**

       M85.472   **Solitary bone cyst,** left **ankle and foot**

       M85.479   **Solitary bone cyst, unspecified ankle and foot**

    M85.48   **Solitary bone cyst, other site**

✓5ᵗʰ   **M85.5**   Aneurysmal **bone cyst**

    EXCLUDES 2   *aneurysmal cyst of jaw (M27.4)*

    M85.5Ø   **Aneurysmal bone cyst, unspecified site**

    ✓6ᵗʰ   M85.51   **Aneurysmal bone cyst,** shoulder

       M85.511   **Aneurysmal bone cyst,** right **shoulder**

       M85.512   **Aneurysmal bone cyst,** left **shoulder**

       M85.519   **Aneurysmal bone cyst, unspecified shoulder**

    ✓6ᵗʰ   M85.52   **Aneurysmal bone cyst,** upper arm

       M85.521   **Aneurysmal bone cyst,** right **upper arm**

       M85.522   **Aneurysmal bone cyst,** left **upper arm**

       M85.529   **Aneurysmal bone cyst, unspecified upper arm**

    ✓6ᵗʰ   M85.53   **Aneurysmal bone cyst,** forearm

       M85.531   **Aneurysmal bone cyst,** right **forearm**

       M85.532   **Aneurysmal bone cyst,** left **forearm**

       M85.539   **Aneurysmal bone cyst, unspecified forearm**

    ✓6ᵗʰ   M85.54   **Aneurysmal bone cyst,** hand

       M85.541   **Aneurysmal bone cyst,** right **hand**

       M85.542   **Aneurysmal bone cyst,** left **hand**

       M85.549   **Aneurysmal bone cyst, unspecified hand**

    ✓6ᵗʰ   M85.55   **Aneurysmal bone cyst,** thigh

       M85.551   **Aneurysmal bone cyst,** right **thigh**

       M85.552   **Aneurysmal bone cyst,** left **thigh**

       M85.559   **Aneurysmal bone cyst, unspecified thigh**

    ✓6ᵗʰ   M85.56   **Aneurysmal bone cyst,** lower leg

       M85.561   **Aneurysmal bone cyst,** right **lower leg**

       M85.562   **Aneurysmal bone cyst,** left **lower leg**

       M85.569   **Aneurysmal bone cyst, unspecified lower leg**

    ✓6ᵗʰ   M85.57   **Aneurysmal bone cyst,** ankle and foot

       M85.571   **Aneurysmal bone cyst,** right **ankle and foot**

       M85.572   **Aneurysmal bone cyst,** left **ankle and foot**

☑ Additional Character Required   ✓7ᵗʰ Placeholder Alert   Unspecified Dx   Other Specified Dx   Manifestation   ►◄ Revised Text   ● New Code   ▲ Revised Code Title

M85.579 Aneurysmal bone cyst, unspecified ankle and foot

M85.58 Aneurysmal bone cyst, other site

M85.59 Aneurysmal bone cyst, multiple sites

✓5ᵗʰ **M85.6** Other cyst of bone
> **EXCLUDES 1** cyst of jaw NEC (M27.4)
> osteitis fibrosa cystica generalisata [von Recklinghausen's disease of bone] (E21.Ø)

M85.60 Other cyst of bone, unspecified site

✓6ᵗʰ **M85.61** Other cyst of bone, shoulder

M85.611 Other cyst of bone, right shoulder

M85.612 Other cyst of bone, left shoulder

M85.619 Other cyst of bone, unspecified shoulder

✓6ᵗʰ **M85.62** Other cyst of bone, upper arm

M85.621 Other cyst of bone, right upper arm

M85.622 Other cyst of bone, left upper arm

M85.629 Other cyst of bone, unspecified upper arm

✓6ᵗʰ **M85.63** Other cyst of bone, forearm

M85.631 Other cyst of bone, right forearm

M85.632 Other cyst of bone, left forearm

M85.639 Other cyst of bone, unspecified forearm

✓6ᵗʰ **M85.64** Other cyst of bone, hand

M85.641 Other cyst of bone, right hand

M85.642 Other cyst of bone, left hand

M85.649 Other cyst of bone, unspecified hand

✓6ᵗʰ **M85.65** Other cyst of bone, thigh

M85.651 Other cyst of bone, right thigh

M85.652 Other cyst of bone, left thigh

M85.659 Other cyst of bone, unspecified thigh

✓6ᵗʰ **M85.66** Other cyst of bone, lower leg

M85.661 Other cyst of bone, right lower leg

M85.662 Other cyst of bone, left lower leg

M85.669 Other cyst of bone, unspecified lower leg

✓6ᵗʰ **M85.67** Other cyst of bone, ankle and foot

M85.671 Other cyst of bone, right ankle and foot

M85.672 Other cyst of bone, left ankle and foot

M85.679 Other cyst of bone, unspecified ankle and foot

M85.68 Other cyst of bone, other site

M85.69 Other cyst of bone, multiple sites

✓5ᵗʰ **M85.8** Other specified disorders of bone density and structure
> Hyperostosis of bones, except skull
> Osteosclerosis, acquired
> **EXCLUDES 1** diffuse idiopathic skeletal hyperostosis [DISH] (M48.1)
> osteosclerosis congenita (Q77.4)
> osteosclerosis fragilitas (generalista) (Q78.2)
> osteosclerosis myelofibrosis (D75.81)

M85.80 Other specified disorders of bone density and structure, unspecified site

✓6ᵗʰ **M85.81** Other specified disorders of bone density and structure, shoulder

M85.811 Other specified disorders of bone density and structure, right shoulder

M85.812 Other specified disorders of bone density and structure, left shoulder

M85.819 Other specified disorders of bone density and structure, unspecified shoulder

✓6ᵗʰ **M85.82** Other specified disorders of bone density and structure, upper arm

M85.821 Other specified disorders of bone density and structure, right upper arm

M85.822 Other specified disorders of bone density and structure, left upper arm

M85.829 Other specified disorders of bone density and structure, unspecified upper arm

✓6ᵗʰ **M85.83** Other specified disorders of bone density and structure, forearm

M85.831 Other specified disorders of bone density and structure, right forearm

M85.832 Other specified disorders of bone density and structure, left forearm

M85.839 Other specified disorders of bone density and structure, unspecified forearm

✓6ᵗʰ **M85.84** Other specified disorders of bone density and structure, hand

M85.841 Other specified disorders of bone density and structure, right hand

M85.842 Other specified disorders of bone density and structure, left hand

M85.849 Other specified disorders of bone density and structure, unspecified hand

✓6ᵗʰ **M85.85** Other specified disorders of bone density and structure, thigh

M85.851 Other specified disorders of bone density and structure, right thigh

M85.852 Other specified disorders of bone density and structure, left thigh

M85.859 Other specified disorders of bone density and structure, unspecified thigh

✓6ᵗʰ **M85.86** Other specified disorders of bone density and structure, lower leg

M85.861 Other specified disorders of bone density and structure, right lower leg

M85.862 Other specified disorders of bone density and structure, left lower leg

M85.869 Other specified disorders of bone density and structure, unspecified lower leg

✓6ᵗʰ **M85.87** Other specified disorders of bone density and structure, ankle and foot

M85.871 Other specified disorders of bone density and structure, right ankle and foot

M85.872 Other specified disorders of bone density and structure, left ankle and foot

M85.879 Other specified disorders of bone density and structure, unspecified ankle and foot

M85.88 Other specified disorders of bone density and structure, other site

M85.89 Other specified disorders of bone density and structure, multiple sites

M85.9 Disorder of bone density and structure, unspecified

Other osteopathies (M86-M9Ø)
> **EXCLUDES 1** postprocedural osteopathies (M96.-)

✓4ᵗʰ **M86 Osteomyelitis**
> Use additional code (B95-B97) to identify infectious agent
> Use additional code to identify major osseous defect, if applicable (M89.7-)
> **EXCLUDES 1** osteomyelitis due to:
> echinococcus (B67.2)
> gonococcus (A54.43)
> salmonella (AØ2.24)
> **EXCLUDES 2** ostemyelitis of:
> orbit (HØ5.Ø-)
> petrous bone (H7Ø.2-)
> vertebra (M46.2-)

✓5ᵗʰ **M86.Ø** Acute hematogenous osteomyelitis

M86.ØØ Acute hematogenous osteomyelitis, unspecified site

✓6ᵗʰ **M86.Ø1** Acute hematogenous osteomyelitis, shoulder

M86.Ø11 Acute hematogenous osteomyelitis, right shoulder

M86.Ø12 Acute hematogenous osteomyelitis, left shoulder

M86.Ø19 Acute hematogenous osteomyelitis, unspecified shoulder

✓6ᵗʰ **M86.Ø2** Acute hematogenous osteomyelitis, humerus

M86.Ø21 Acute hematogenous osteomyelitis, right humerus

M86.Ø22 Acute hematogenous osteomyelitis, left humerus

M86.Ø29 Acute hematogenous osteomyelitis, unspecified humerus

✓6ᵗʰ **M86.Ø3** Acute hematogenous osteomyelitis, radius and ulna

M86.Ø31 Acute hematogenous osteomyelitis, right radius and ulna

M86.Ø32 Acute hematogenous osteomyelitis, left radius and ulna

M86.Ø39 Acute hematogenous osteomyelitis, unspecified radius and ulna

---

EXCLUDES 1 Not coded here   **EXCLUDES 2** Not included here   🔲 Newborn Age: 0   🅿 Pediatric Age: 0-17   🅼 Maternity Age: 12-55   🅰 Adult Age: 15-124

730
ICD-10-CM 2016

✓6th **M86.04 Acute hematogenous osteomyelitis,** hand
- M86.041 Acute hematogenous osteomyelitis, right hand
- M86.042 Acute hematogenous osteomyelitis, left hand
- M86.049 **Acute hematogenous osteomyelitis, unspecified hand**

✓6th **M86.05 Acute hematogenous osteomyelitis,** femur
- M86.051 Acute hematogenous osteomyelitis, right femur
- M86.052 Acute hematogenous osteomyelitis, left femur
- M86.059 **Acute hematogenous osteomyelitis, unspecified femur**

✓6th **M86.06 Acute hematogenous osteomyelitis,** tibia and fibula
- M86.061 Acute hematogenous osteomyelitis, right tibia and fibula
- M86.062 Acute hematogenous osteomyelitis, left tibia and fibula
- M86.069 **Acute hematogenous osteomyelitis, unspecified tibia and fibula**

✓6th **M86.07 Acute hematogenous osteomyelitis,** ankle and foot
- M86.071 Acute hematogenous osteomyelitis, right ankle and foot
- M86.072 Acute hematogenous osteomyelitis, left ankle and foot
- M86.079 **Acute hematogenous osteomyelitis, unspecified ankle and foot**

M86.08 Acute hematogenous osteomyelitis, other sites

M86.09 Acute hematogenous osteomyelitis, multiple sites

✓5th **M86.1** Other acute osteomyelitis
- **M86.10 Other acute osteomyelitis, unspecified site**

✓6th **M86.11 Other acute osteomyelitis,** shoulder
- M86.111 **Other acute osteomyelitis, right shoulder**
- M86.112 **Other acute osteomyelitis, left shoulder**
- M86.119 **Other acute osteomyelitis, unspecified shoulder**

✓6th **M86.12 Other acute osteomyelitis,** humerus
- M86.121 **Other acute osteomyelitis, right humerus**
- M86.122 **Other acute osteomyelitis, left humerus**
- M86.129 **Other acute osteomyelitis, unspecified humerus**

✓6th **M86.13 Other acute osteomyelitis,** radius and ulna
- M86.131 **Other acute osteomyelitis, right radius and ulna**
- M86.132 **Other acute osteomyelitis, left radius and ulna**
- M86.139 **Other acute osteomyelitis, unspecified radius and ulna**

✓6th **M86.14 Other acute osteomyelitis,** hand
- M86.141 **Other acute osteomyelitis, right hand**
- M86.142 **Other acute osteomyelitis, left hand**
- M86.149 **Other acute osteomyelitis, unspecified hand**

✓6th **M86.15 Other acute osteomyelitis,** femur
- M86.151 **Other acute osteomyelitis, right femur**
- M86.152 **Other acute osteomyelitis, left femur**
- M86.159 **Other acute osteomyelitis, unspecified femur**

✓6th **M86.16 Other acute osteomyelitis,** tibia and fibula
- M86.161 **Other acute osteomyelitis, right tibia and fibula**
- M86.162 **Other acute osteomyelitis, left tibia and fibula**
- M86.169 **Other acute osteomyelitis, unspecified tibia and fibula**

✓6th **M86.17 Other acute osteomyelitis,** ankle and foot
- M86.171 **Other acute osteomyelitis, right ankle and foot**
- M86.172 **Other acute osteomyelitis, left ankle and foot**
- M86.179 **Other acute osteomyelitis, unspecified ankle and foot**

M86.18 Other acute osteomyelitis, other site

M86.19 Other acute osteomyelitis, multiple sites

✓5th **M86.2** Subacute osteomyelitis
- **M86.20 Subacute osteomyelitis, unspecified site**

✓6th **M86.21 Subacute osteomyelitis,** shoulder
- M86.211 **Subacute osteomyelitis, right shoulder**
- M86.212 **Subacute osteomyelitis, left shoulder**
- M86.219 **Subacute osteomyelitis, unspecified shoulder**

✓6th **M86.22 Subacute osteomyelitis,** humerus
- M86.221 **Subacute osteomyelitis, right humerus**
- M86.222 **Subacute osteomyelitis, left humerus**
- M86.229 **Subacute osteomyelitis, unspecified humerus**

✓6th **M86.23 Subacute osteomyelitis,** radius and ulna
- M86.231 **Subacute osteomyelitis, right radius and ulna**
- M86.232 **Subacute osteomyelitis, left radius and ulna**
- M86.239 **Subacute osteomyelitis, unspecified radius and ulna**

✓6th **M86.24 Subacute osteomyelitis,** hand
- M86.241 **Subacute osteomyelitis, right hand**
- M86.242 **Subacute osteomyelitis, left hand**
- M86.249 **Subacute osteomyelitis, unspecified hand**

✓6th **M86.25 Subacute osteomyelitis,** femur
- M86.251 **Subacute osteomyelitis, right femur**
- M86.252 **Subacute osteomyelitis, left femur**
- M86.259 **Subacute osteomyelitis, unspecified femur**

✓6th **M86.26 Subacute osteomyelitis,** tibia and fibula
- M86.261 **Subacute osteomyelitis, right tibia and fibula**
- M86.262 **Subacute osteomyelitis, left tibia and fibula**
- M86.269 **Subacute osteomyelitis, unspecified tibia and fibula**

✓6th **M86.27 Subacute osteomyelitis,** ankle and foot
- M86.271 **Subacute osteomyelitis, right ankle and foot**
- M86.272 **Subacute osteomyelitis, left ankle and foot**
- M86.279 **Subacute osteomyelitis, unspecified ankle and foot**

M86.28 Subacute osteomyelitis, other site

M86.29 Subacute osteomyelitis, multiple sites

✓5th **M86.3** Chronic multifocal osteomyelitis
- **M86.30 Chronic multifocal osteomyelitis, unspecified site**

✓6th **M86.31 Chronic multifocal osteomyelitis,** shoulder
- M86.311 **Chronic multifocal osteomyelitis, right shoulder**
- M86.312 **Chronic multifocal osteomyelitis, left shoulder**
- M86.319 **Chronic multifocal osteomyelitis, unspecified shoulder**

✓6th **M86.32 Chronic multifocal osteomyelitis,** humerus
- M86.321 **Chronic multifocal osteomyelitis, right humerus**
- M86.322 **Chronic multifocal osteomyelitis, left humerus**
- M86.329 **Chronic multifocal osteomyelitis, unspecified humerus**

✓6th **M86.33 Chronic multifocal osteomyelitis,** radius and ulna
- M86.331 **Chronic multifocal osteomyelitis, right radius and ulna**
- M86.332 **Chronic multifocal osteomyelitis, left radius and ulna**
- M86.339 **Chronic multifocal osteomyelitis, unspecified radius and ulna**

✓6th **M86.34 Chronic multifocal osteomyelitis,** hand
- M86.341 **Chronic multifocal osteomyelitis, right hand**
- M86.342 **Chronic multifocal osteomyelitis, left hand**
- M86.349 **Chronic multifocal osteomyelitis, unspecified hand**

☑ Additional Character Required   ✓x7th Placeholder Alert   Unspecified Dx   Other Specified Dx   Manifestation   ▶◀ Revised Text   ● New Code   ▲ Revised Code Title

✓6ᵗʰ **M86.35** Chronic multifocal osteomyelitis, femur
     M86.351 Chronic multifocal osteomyelitis, right femur
     M86.352 Chronic multifocal osteomyelitis, left femur
     M86.359 Chronic multifocal osteomyelitis, unspecified femur

✓6ᵗʰ **M86.36** Chronic multifocal osteomyelitis, tibia and fibula
     M86.361 Chronic multifocal osteomyelitis, right tibia and fibula
     M86.362 Chronic multifocal osteomyelitis, left tibia and fibula
     M86.369 Chronic multifocal osteomyelitis, unspecified tibia and fibula

✓6ᵗʰ **M86.37** Chronic multifocal osteomyelitis, ankle and foot
     M86.371 Chronic multifocal osteomyelitis, right ankle and foot
     M86.372 Chronic multifocal osteomyelitis, left ankle and foot
     M86.379 Chronic multifocal osteomyelitis, unspecified ankle and foot

M86.38 Chronic multifocal osteomyelitis, other site
M86.39 Chronic multifocal osteomyelitis, multiple sites

✓5ᵗʰ **M86.4** Chronic osteomyelitis with draining sinus
     M86.40 Chronic osteomyelitis with draining sinus, unspecified site

✓6ᵗʰ **M86.41** Chronic osteomyelitis with draining sinus, shoulder
     M86.411 Chronic osteomyelitis with draining sinus, right shoulder
     M86.412 Chronic osteomyelitis with draining sinus, left shoulder
     M86.419 Chronic osteomyelitis with draining sinus, unspecified shoulder

✓6ᵗʰ **M86.42** Chronic osteomyelitis with draining sinus, humerus
     M86.421 Chronic osteomyelitis with draining sinus, right humerus
     M86.422 Chronic osteomyelitis with draining sinus, left humerus
     M86.429 Chronic osteomyelitis with draining sinus, unspecified humerus

✓6ᵗʰ **M86.43** Chronic osteomyelitis with draining sinus, radius and ulna
     M86.431 Chronic osteomyelitis with draining sinus, right radius and ulna
     M86.432 Chronic osteomyelitis with draining sinus, left radius and ulna
     M86.439 Chronic osteomyelitis with draining sinus, unspecified radius and ulna

✓6ᵗʰ **M86.44** Chronic osteomyelitis with draining sinus, hand
     M86.441 Chronic osteomyelitis with draining sinus, right hand
     M86.442 Chronic osteomyelitis with draining sinus, left hand
     M86.449 Chronic osteomyelitis with draining sinus, unspecified hand

✓6ᵗʰ **M86.45** Chronic osteomyelitis with draining sinus, femur
     M86.451 Chronic osteomyelitis with draining sinus, right femur
     M86.452 Chronic osteomyelitis with draining sinus, left femur
     M86.459 Chronic osteomyelitis with draining sinus, unspecified femur

✓6ᵗʰ **M86.46** Chronic osteomyelitis with draining sinus, tibia and fibula
     M86.461 Chronic osteomyelitis with draining sinus, right tibia and fibula
     M86.462 Chronic osteomyelitis with draining sinus, left tibia and fibula
     M86.469 Chronic osteomyelitis with draining sinus, unspecified tibia and fibula

✓6ᵗʰ **M86.47** Chronic osteomyelitis with draining sinus, ankle and foot
     M86.471 Chronic osteomyelitis with draining sinus, right ankle and foot
     M86.472 Chronic osteomyelitis with draining sinus, left ankle and foot

     M86.479 Chronic osteomyelitis with draining sinus, unspecified ankle and foot
M86.48 Chronic osteomyelitis with draining sinus, other site
M86.49 Chronic osteomyelitis with draining sinus, multiple sites

✓5ᵗʰ **M86.5** Other chronic hematogenous osteomyelitis
     M86.50 Other chronic hematogenous osteomyelitis, unspecified site

✓6ᵗʰ **M86.51** Other chronic hematogenous osteomyelitis, shoulder
     M86.511 Other chronic hematogenous osteomyelitis, right shoulder
     M86.512 Other chronic hematogenous osteomyelitis, left shoulder
     M86.519 Other chronic hematogenous osteomyelitis, unspecified shoulder

✓6ᵗʰ **M86.52** Other chronic hematogenous osteomyelitis, humerus
     M86.521 Other chronic hematogenous osteomyelitis, right humerus
     M86.522 Other chronic hematogenous osteomyelitis, left humerus
     M86.529 Other chronic hematogenous osteomyelitis, unspecified humerus

✓6ᵗʰ **M86.53** Other chronic hematogenous osteomyelitis, radius and ulna
     M86.531 Other chronic hematogenous osteomyelitis, right radius and ulna
     M86.532 Other chronic hematogenous osteomyelitis, left radius and ulna
     M86.539 Other chronic hematogenous osteomyelitis, unspecified radius and ulna

✓6ᵗʰ **M86.54** Other chronic hematogenous osteomyelitis, hand
     M86.541 Other chronic hematogenous osteomyelitis, right hand
     M86.542 Other chronic hematogenous osteomyelitis, left hand
     M86.549 Other chronic hematogenous osteomyelitis, unspecified hand

✓6ᵗʰ **M86.55** Other chronic hematogenous osteomyelitis, femur
     M86.551 Other chronic hematogenous osteomyelitis, right femur
     M86.552 Other chronic hematogenous osteomyelitis, left femur
     M86.559 Other chronic hematogenous osteomyelitis, unspecified femur

✓6ᵗʰ **M86.56** Other chronic hematogenous osteomyelitis, tibia and fibula
     M86.561 Other chronic hematogenous osteomyelitis, right tibia and fibula
     M86.562 Other chronic hematogenous osteomyelitis, left tibia and fibula
     M86.569 Other chronic hematogenous osteomyelitis, unspecified tibia and fibula

✓6ᵗʰ **M86.57** Other chronic hematogenous osteomyelitis, ankle and foot
     M86.571 Other chronic hematogenous osteomyelitis, right ankle and foot
     M86.572 Other chronic hematogenous osteomyelitis, left ankle and foot
     M86.579 Other chronic hematogenous osteomyelitis, unspecified ankle and foot

M86.58 Other chronic hematogenous osteomyelitis, other site
M86.59 Other chronic hematogenous osteomyelitis, multiple sites

✓5ᵗʰ **M86.6** Other chronic osteomyelitis
     M86.60 Other chronic osteomyelitis, unspecified site

✓6ᵗʰ **M86.61** Other chronic osteomyelitis, shoulder
     M86.611 Other chronic osteomyelitis, right shoulder
     M86.612 Other chronic osteomyelitis, left shoulder
     M86.619 Other chronic osteomyelitis, unspecified shoulder

✓6ᵗʰ **M86.62** Other chronic osteomyelitis, humerus
     M86.621 Other chronic osteomyelitis, right humerus

EXCLUDES 1 Not coded here   EXCLUDES 2 Not included here   N Newborn Age: 0   P Pediatric Age: 0-17   M Maternity Age: 12-55   A Adult Age: 15-124

732   ICD-10-CM 2016

     M86.622   **Other chronic osteomyelitis, left humerus**
     M86.629   **Other chronic osteomyelitis, unspecified humerus**

✓6ᵗʰ   **M86.63**   **Other chronic osteomyelitis, radius and ulna**
     M86.631   **Other chronic osteomyelitis, right radius and ulna**
     M86.632   **Other chronic osteomyelitis, left radius and ulna**
     M86.639   **Other chronic osteomyelitis, unspecified radius and ulna**

✓6ᵗʰ   **M86.64**   **Other chronic osteomyelitis, hand**
     M86.641   **Other chronic osteomyelitis, right hand**
     M86.642   **Other chronic osteomyelitis, left hand**
     M86.649   **Other chronic osteomyelitis, unspecified hand**

✓6ᵗʰ   **M86.65**   **Other chronic osteomyelitis, thigh**
     M86.651   **Other chronic osteomyelitis, right thigh**
     M86.652   **Other chronic osteomyelitis, left thigh**
     M86.659   **Other chronic osteomyelitis, unspecified thigh**

✓6ᵗʰ   **M86.66**   **Other chronic osteomyelitis, tibia and fibula**
     M86.661   **Other chronic osteomyelitis, right tibia and fibula**
     M86.662   **Other chronic osteomyelitis, left tibia and fibula**
     M86.669   **Other chronic osteomyelitis, unspecified tibia and fibula**

✓6ᵗʰ   **M86.67**   **Other chronic osteomyelitis, ankle and foot**
     M86.671   **Other chronic osteomyelitis, right ankle and foot**
     M86.672   **Other chronic osteomyelitis, left ankle and foot**
     M86.679   **Other chronic osteomyelitis, unspecified ankle and foot**

     M86.68   **Other chronic osteomyelitis, other site**
     M86.69   **Other chronic osteomyelitis, multiple sites**

✓5ᵗʰ   **M86.8**   **Other osteomyelitis**
     Brodie's abscess

     ✓6ᵗʰ   **M86.8X**   **Other osteomyelitis**
     M86.8X0   **Other osteomyelitis, multiple sites**
     M86.8X1   **Other osteomyelitis, shoulder**
     M86.8X2   **Other osteomyelitis, upper arm**
     M86.8X3   **Other osteomyelitis, forearm**
     M86.8X4   **Other osteomyelitis, hand**
     M86.8X5   **Other osteomyelitis, thigh**
     M86.8X6   **Other osteomyelitis, lower leg**
     M86.8X7   **Other osteomyelitis, ankle and foot**
     M86.8X8   **Other osteomyelitis, other site**
     M86.8X9   **Other osteomyelitis, unspecified sites**

     M86.9   **Osteomyelitis, unspecified**
     Infection of bone NOS   Periostitis without osteomyelitis

✓4ᵗʰ   **M87**   **Osteonecrosis**
     INCLUDES   avascular necrosis of bone
     Use additional code to identify major osseous defect, if applicable (M89.7-)
     EXCLUDES 1   juvenile osteonecrosis (M91-M92)
                   osteochondropathies (M90-M93)

✓5ᵗʰ   **M87.0**   **Idiopathic aseptic necrosis of bone**
     M87.00   **Idiopathic aseptic necrosis of unspecified bone**

     ✓6ᵗʰ   **M87.01**   **Idiopathic aseptic necrosis of shoulder**
     Idiopathic aseptic necrosis of clavicle and scapula
     M87.011   **Idiopathic aseptic necrosis of right shoulder**
     M87.012   **Idiopathic aseptic necrosis of left shoulder**
     M87.019   **Idiopathic aseptic necrosis of unspecified shoulder**

     ✓6ᵗʰ   **M87.02**   **Idiopathic aseptic necrosis of humerus**
     M87.021   **Idiopathic aseptic necrosis of right humerus**
     M87.022   **Idiopathic aseptic necrosis of left humerus**
     M87.029   **Idiopathic aseptic necrosis of unspecified humerus**

     ✓6ᵗʰ   **M87.03**   **Idiopathic aseptic necrosis of radius, ulna and carpus**
     M87.031   **Idiopathic aseptic necrosis of right radius**
     M87.032   **Idiopathic aseptic necrosis of left radius**

     M87.033   **Idiopathic aseptic necrosis of unspecified radius**
     M87.034   **Idiopathic aseptic necrosis of right ulna**
     M87.035   **Idiopathic aseptic necrosis of left ulna**
     M87.036   **Idiopathic aseptic necrosis of unspecified ulna**
     M87.037   **Idiopathic aseptic necrosis of right carpus**
     M87.038   **Idiopathic aseptic necrosis of left carpus**
     M87.039   **Idiopathic aseptic necrosis of unspecified carpus**

✓6ᵗʰ   **M87.04**   **Idiopathic aseptic necrosis of hand and fingers**
     Idiopathic aseptic necrosis of metacarpals and phalanges of hands
     M87.041   **Idiopathic aseptic necrosis of right hand**
     M87.042   **Idiopathic aseptic necrosis of left hand**
     M87.043   **Idiopathic aseptic necrosis of unspecified hand**
     M87.044   **Idiopathic aseptic necrosis of right finger(s)**
     M87.045   **Idiopathic aseptic necrosis of left finger(s)**
     M87.046   **Idiopathic aseptic necrosis of unspecified finger(s)**

✓6ᵗʰ   **M87.05**   **Idiopathic aseptic necrosis of pelvis and femur**
     M87.050   **Idiopathic aseptic necrosis of pelvis**
     M87.051   **Idiopathic aseptic necrosis of right femur**
     M87.052   **Idiopathic aseptic necrosis of left femur**
     M87.059   **Idiopathic aseptic necrosis of unspecified femur**
         Idiopathic aseptic necrosis of hip NOS

✓6ᵗʰ   **M87.06**   **Idiopathic aseptic necrosis of tibia and fibula**
     M87.061   **Idiopathic aseptic necrosis of right tibia**
     M87.062   **Idiopathic aseptic necrosis of left tibia**
     M87.063   **Idiopathic aseptic necrosis of unspecified tibia**
     M87.064   **Idiopathic aseptic necrosis of right fibula**
     M87.065   **Idiopathic aseptic necrosis of left fibula**
     M87.066   **Idiopathic aseptic necrosis of unspecified fibula**

✓6ᵗʰ   **M87.07**   **Idiopathic aseptic necrosis of ankle, foot and toes**
     Idiopathic aseptic necrosis of metatarsus, tarsus, and phalanges of toes
     M87.071   **Idiopathic aseptic necrosis of right ankle**
     M87.072   **Idiopathic aseptic necrosis of left ankle**
     M87.073   **Idiopathic aseptic necrosis of unspecified ankle**
     M87.074   **Idiopathic aseptic necrosis of right foot**
     M87.075   **Idiopathic aseptic necrosis of left foot**
     M87.076   **Idiopathic aseptic necrosis of unspecified foot**
     M87.077   **Idiopathic aseptic necrosis of right toe(s)**
     M87.078   **Idiopathic aseptic necrosis of left toe(s)**
     M87.079   **Idiopathic aseptic necrosis of unspecified toe(s)**

     M87.08   **Idiopathic aseptic necrosis of bone, other site**
     M87.09   **Idiopathic aseptic necrosis of bone, multiple sites**

✓5ᵗʰ   **M87.1**   **Osteonecrosis due to drugs**
     Use additional code for adverse effect, if applicable, to identify drug (T36-T50 with fifth or sixth character 5)
     M87.10   **Osteonecrosis due to drugs, unspecified bone**

     ✓6ᵗʰ   **M87.11**   **Osteonecrosis due to drugs, shoulder**
     M87.111   **Osteonecrosis due to drugs, right shoulder**
     M87.112   **Osteonecrosis due to drugs, left shoulder**
     M87.119   **Osteonecrosis due to drugs, unspecified shoulder**

     ✓6ᵗʰ   **M87.12**   **Osteonecrosis due to drugs, humerus**
     M87.121   **Osteonecrosis due to drugs, right humerus**
     M87.122   **Osteonecrosis due to drugs, left humerus**
     M87.129   **Osteonecrosis due to drugs, unspecified humerus**

     ✓6ᵗʰ   **M87.13**   **Osteonecrosis due to drugs of radius, ulna and carpus**
     M87.131   **Osteonecrosis due to drugs of right radius**
     M87.132   **Osteonecrosis due to drugs of left radius**
     M87.133   **Osteonecrosis due to drugs of unspecified radius**

✓ Additional Character Required   ✓x7ᵗʰ Placeholder Alert   Unspecified Dx   Other Specified Dx   Manifestation   ▶◀ Revised Text   ● New Code   ▲ Revised Code Title

ICD-10-CM 2016   733

M87.134 Osteonecrosis due to drugs of right ulna
M87.135 Osteonecrosis due to drugs of left ulna
M87.136 Osteonecrosis due to drugs of unspecified ulna
M87.137 Osteonecrosis due to drugs of right carpus
M87.138 Osteonecrosis due to drugs of left carpus
M87.139 Osteonecrosis due to drugs of unspecified carpus

✓6th M87.14 Osteonecrosis due to drugs, hand and fingers
M87.141 Osteonecrosis due to drugs, right hand
M87.142 Osteonecrosis due to drugs, left hand
M87.143 Osteonecrosis due to drugs, unspecified hand
M87.144 Osteonecrosis due to drugs, right finger(s)
M87.145 Osteonecrosis due to drugs, left finger(s)
M87.146 Osteonecrosis due to drugs, unspecified finger(s)

✓6th M87.15 Osteonecrosis due to drugs, pelvis and femur
M87.150 Osteonecrosis due to drugs, pelvis
M87.151 Osteonecrosis due to drugs, right femur
M87.152 Osteonecrosis due to drugs, left femur
M87.159 Osteonecrosis due to drugs, unspecified femur

✓6th M87.16 Osteonecrosis due to drugs, tibia and fibula
M87.161 Osteonecrosis due to drugs, right tibia
M87.162 Osteonecrosis due to drugs, left tibia
M87.163 Osteonecrosis due to drugs, unspecified tibia
M87.164 Osteonecrosis due to drugs, right fibula
M87.165 Osteonecrosis due to drugs, left fibula
M87.166 Osteonecrosis due to drugs, unspecified fibula

✓6th M87.17 Osteonecrosis due to drugs, ankle, foot and toes
M87.171 Osteonecrosis due to drugs, right ankle
M87.172 Osteonecrosis due to drugs, left ankle
M87.173 Osteonecrosis due to drugs, unspecified ankle
M87.174 Osteonecrosis due to drugs, right foot
M87.175 Osteonecrosis due to drugs, left foot
M87.176 Osteonecrosis due to drugs, unspecified foot
M87.177 Osteonecrosis due to drugs, right toe(s)
M87.178 Osteonecrosis due to drugs, left toe(s)
M87.179 Osteonecrosis due to drugs, unspecified toe(s)

✓6th M87.18 Osteonecrosis due to drugs, other site
M87.180 Osteonecrosis due to drugs, jaw
M87.188 Osteonecrosis due to drugs, other site
M87.19 Osteonecrosis due to drugs, multiple sites

✓5th M87.2 Osteonecrosis due to previous trauma
M87.20 Osteonecrosis due to previous trauma, unspecified bone

✓6th M87.21 Osteonecrosis due to previous trauma, shoulder
M87.211 Osteonecrosis due to previous trauma, right shoulder
M87.212 Osteonecrosis due to previous trauma, left shoulder
M87.219 Osteonecrosis due to previous trauma, unspecified shoulder

✓6th M87.22 Osteonecrosis due to previous trauma, humerus
M87.221 Osteonecrosis due to previous trauma, right humerus
M87.222 Osteonecrosis due to previous trauma, left humerus
M87.229 Osteonecrosis due to previous trauma, unspecified humerus

✓6th M87.23 Osteonecrosis due to previous trauma of radius, ulna and carpus
M87.231 Osteonecrosis due to previous trauma of right radius
M87.232 Osteonecrosis due to previous trauma of left radius
M87.233 Osteonecrosis due to previous trauma of unspecified radius

M87.234 Osteonecrosis due to previous trauma of right ulna
M87.235 Osteonecrosis due to previous trauma of left ulna
M87.236 Osteonecrosis due to previous trauma of unspecified ulna
M87.237 Osteonecrosis due to previous trauma of right carpus
M87.238 Osteonecrosis due to previous trauma of left carpus
M87.239 Osteonecrosis due to previous trauma of unspecified carpus

✓6th M87.24 Osteonecrosis due to previous trauma, hand and fingers
M87.241 Osteonecrosis due to previous trauma, right hand
M87.242 Osteonecrosis due to previous trauma, left hand
M87.243 Osteonecrosis due to previous trauma, unspecified hand
M87.244 Osteonecrosis due to previous trauma, right finger(s)
M87.245 Osteonecrosis due to previous trauma, left finger(s)
M87.246 Osteonecrosis due to previous trauma, unspecified finger(s)

✓6th M87.25 Osteonecrosis due to previous trauma, pelvis and femur
M87.250 Osteonecrosis due to previous trauma, pelvis
M87.251 Osteonecrosis due to previous trauma, right femur
M87.252 Osteonecrosis due to previous trauma, left femur
M87.256 Osteonecrosis due to previous trauma, unspecified femur

✓6th M87.26 Osteonecrosis due to previous trauma, tibia and fibula
M87.261 Osteonecrosis due to previous trauma, right tibia
M87.262 Osteonecrosis due to previous trauma, left tibia
M87.263 Osteonecrosis due to previous trauma, unspecified tibia
M87.264 Osteonecrosis due to previous trauma, right fibula
M87.265 Osteonecrosis due to previous trauma, left fibula
M87.266 Osteonecrosis due to previous trauma, unspecified fibula

✓6th M87.27 Osteonecrosis due to previous trauma, ankle, foot and toes
M87.271 Osteonecrosis due to previous trauma, right ankle
M87.272 Osteonecrosis due to previous trauma, left ankle
M87.273 Osteonecrosis due to previous trauma, unspecified ankle
M87.274 Osteonecrosis due to previous trauma, right foot
M87.275 Osteonecrosis due to previous trauma, left foot
M87.276 Osteonecrosis due to previous trauma, unspecified foot
M87.277 Osteonecrosis due to previous trauma, right toe(s)
M87.278 Osteonecrosis due to previous trauma, left toe(s)
M87.279 Osteonecrosis due to previous trauma, unspecified toe(s)

M87.28 Osteonecrosis due to previous trauma, other site
M87.29 Osteonecrosis due to previous trauma, multiple sites

✓5th M87.3 Other secondary osteonecrosis
M87.30 Other secondary osteonecrosis, unspecified bone

✓6th M87.31 Other secondary osteonecrosis, shoulder
M87.311 Other secondary osteonecrosis, right shoulder

EXCLUDES 1 Not coded here   EXCLUDES 2 Not included here   N Newborn Age: 0   P Pediatric Age: 0-17   M Maternity Age: 12-55   A Adult Age: 15-124

M87.312 Other secondary osteonecrosis, left shoulder

M87.319 Other secondary osteonecrosis, unspecified shoulder

✓6th M87.32 Other secondary osteonecrosis, humerus

M87.321 Other secondary osteonecrosis, right humerus

M87.322 Other secondary osteonecrosis, left humerus

M87.329 Other secondary osteonecrosis, unspecified humerus

✓6th M87.33 Other secondary osteonecrosis of radius, ulna and carpus

M87.331 Other secondary osteonecrosis of right radius

M87.332 Other secondary osteonecrosis of left radius

M87.333 Other secondary osteonecrosis of unspecified radius

M87.334 Other secondary osteonecrosis of right ulna

M87.335 Other secondary osteonecrosis of left ulna

M87.336 Other secondary osteonecrosis of unspecified ulna

M87.337 Other secondary osteonecrosis of right carpus

M87.338 Other secondary osteonecrosis of left carpus

M87.339 Other secondary osteonecrosis of unspecified carpus

✓6th M87.34 Other secondary osteonecrosis, hand and fingers

M87.341 Other secondary osteonecrosis, right hand

M87.342 Other secondary osteonecrosis, left hand

M87.343 Other secondary osteonecrosis, unspecified hand

M87.344 Other secondary osteonecrosis, right finger(s)

M87.345 Other secondary osteonecrosis, left finger(s)

M87.346 Other secondary osteonecrosis, unspecified finger(s)

✓6th M87.35 Other secondary osteonecrosis, pelvis and femur

M87.350 Other secondary osteonecrosis, pelvis

M87.351 Other secondary osteonecrosis, right femur

M87.352 Other secondary osteonecrosis, left femur

M87.353 Other secondary osteonecrosis, unspecified femur

✓6th M87.36 Other secondary osteonecrosis, tibia and fibula

M87.361 Other secondary osteonecrosis, right tibia

M87.362 Other secondary osteonecrosis, left tibia

M87.363 Other secondary osteonecrosis, unspecified tibia

M87.364 Other secondary osteonecrosis, right fibula

M87.365 Other secondary osteonecrosis, left fibula

M87.366 Other secondary osteonecrosis, unspecified fibula

✓6th M87.37 Other secondary osteonecrosis, ankle and foot

M87.371 Other secondary osteonecrosis, right ankle

M87.372 Other secondary osteonecrosis, left ankle

M87.373 Other secondary osteonecrosis, unspecified ankle

M87.374 Other secondary osteonecrosis, right foot

M87.375 Other secondary osteonecrosis, left foot

M87.376 Other secondary osteonecrosis, unspecified foot

M87.377 Other secondary osteonecrosis, right toe(s)

M87.378 Other secondary osteonecrosis, left toe(s)

M87.379 Other secondary osteonecrosis, unspecified toe(s)

M87.38 Other secondary osteonecrosis, other site

M87.39 Other secondary osteonecrosis, multiple sites

✓5th M87.8 Other osteonecrosis

M87.80 Other osteonecrosis, unspecified bone

✓6th M87.81 Other osteonecrosis, shoulder

M87.811 Other osteonecrosis, right shoulder

M87.812 Other osteonecrosis, left shoulder

M87.819 Other osteonecrosis, unspecified shoulder

✓6th M87.82 Other osteonecrosis, humerus

M87.821 Other osteonecrosis, right humerus

M87.822 Other osteonecrosis, left humerus

M87.829 Other osteonecrosis, unspecified humerus

✓6th M87.83 Other osteonecrosis of radius, ulna and carpus

M87.831 Other osteonecrosis of right radius

M87.832 Other osteonecrosis of left radius

M87.833 Other osteonecrosis of unspecified radius

M87.834 Other osteonecrosis of right ulna

M87.835 Other osteonecrosis of left ulna

M87.836 Other osteonecrosis of unspecified ulna

M87.837 Other osteonecrosis of right carpus

M87.838 Other osteonecrosis of left carpus

M87.839 Other osteonecrosis of unspecified carpus

✓6th M87.84 Other osteonecrosis, hand and fingers

M87.841 Other osteonecrosis, right hand

M87.842 Other osteonecrosis, left hand

M87.843 Other osteonecrosis, unspecified hand

M87.844 Other osteonecrosis, right finger(s)

M87.845 Other osteonecrosis, left finger(s)

M87.849 Other osteonecrosis, unspecified finger(s)

✓6th M87.85 Other osteonecrosis, pelvis and femur

M87.850 Other osteonecrosis, pelvis

M87.851 Other osteonecrosis, right femur

M87.852 Other osteonecrosis, left femur

M87.859 Other osteonecrosis, unspecified femur

✓6th M87.86 Other osteonecrosis, tibia and fibula

M87.861 Other osteonecrosis, right tibia

M87.862 Other osteonecrosis, left tibia

M87.863 Other osteonecrosis, unspecified tibia

M87.864 Other osteonecrosis, right fibula

M87.865 Other osteonecrosis, left fibula

M87.869 Other osteonecrosis, unspecified fibula

✓6th M87.87 Other osteonecrosis, ankle, foot and toes

M87.871 Other osteonecrosis, right ankle

M87.872 Other osteonecrosis, left ankle

M87.873 Other osteonecrosis, unspecified ankle

M87.874 Other osteonecrosis, right foot

M87.875 Other osteonecrosis, left foot

M87.876 Other osteonecrosis, unspecified foot

M87.877 Other osteonecrosis, right toe(s)

M87.878 Other osteonecrosis, left toe(s)

M87.879 Other osteonecrosis, unspecified toe(s)

M87.88 Other osteonecrosis, other site

M87.89 Other osteonecrosis, multiple sites

M87.9 Osteonecrosis, unspecified
Necrosis of bone NOS

✓4th **M88 Osteitis deformans [Paget's disease of bone]**
EXCLUDES 1 osteitis deformans in neoplastic disease (M90.6)

M88.0 Osteitis deformans of skull

M88.1 Osteitis deformans of vertebrae

✓5th M88.8 Osteitis deformans of other bones

✓6th M88.81 Osteitis deformans of shoulder

M88.811 Osteitis deformans of right shoulder

M88.812 Osteitis deformans of left shoulder

M88.819 Osteitis deformans of unspecified shoulder

✓6th M88.82 Osteitis deformans of upper arm

M88.821 Osteitis deformans of right upper arm

M88.822 Osteitis deformans of left upper arm

M88.829 Osteitis deformans of unspecified upper arm

✓6th M88.83 Osteitis deformans of forearm

M88.831 Osteitis deformans of right forearm

☑ Additional Character Required   ✓7th Placeholder Alert   Unspecified Dx   Other Specified Dx   Manifestation   ▶◀ Revised Text   ● New Code   ▲ Revised Code Title

M88.832   Osteitis deformans of left forearm
M88.839   **Osteitis deformans of unspecified forearm**

✓6ᵗʰ **M88.84**   Osteitis deformans of hand
    M88.841   Osteitis deformans of right hand
    M88.842   Osteitis deformans of left hand
    M88.849   **Osteitis deformans of unspecified hand**

✓6ᵗʰ **M88.85**   Osteitis deformans of thigh
    M88.851   Osteitis deformans of right thigh
    M88.852   Osteitis deformans of left thigh
    M88.859   **Osteitis deformans of unspecified thigh**

✓6ᵗʰ **M88.86**   Osteitis deformans of lower leg
    M88.861   Osteitis deformans of right lower leg
    M88.862   Osteitis deformans of left lower leg
    M88.869   **Osteitis deformans of unspecified lower leg**

✓6ᵗʰ **M88.87**   Osteitis deformans of ankle and foot
    M88.871   Osteitis deformans of right ankle and foot
    M88.872   Osteitis deformans of left ankle and foot
    M88.879   **Osteitis deformans of unspecified ankle and foot**

    M88.88   Osteitis deformans of other bones
       EXCLUDES 2   osteitis deformans of skull (M88.0)
                osteitis deformans of vertebrae (M88.1)

    M88.89   Osteitis deformans of multiple sites

   M88.9   **Osteitis deformans of unspecified bone**

✓4ᵗʰ **M89**   **Other disorders of bone**

✓5ᵗʰ **M89.0**   **Algoneurodystrophy**
    Shoulder-hand syndrome
    Sudeck's atrophy
     EXCLUDES 1   causalgia, lower limb (G57.7-)
              causalgia, upper limb (G56.4-)
              complex regional pain syndrome II, lower limb (G57.7-)
              complex regional pain syndrome II, upper limb (G56.4-)
              reflex sympathetic dystrophy (G90.5-)

    M89.00   **Algoneurodystrophy, unspecified site**

✓6ᵗʰ **M89.01**   Algoneurodystrophy, shoulder
    M89.011   Algoneurodystrophy, right shoulder
    M89.012   Algoneurodystrophy, left shoulder
    M89.019   **Algoneurodystrophy, unspecified shoulder**

✓6ᵗʰ **M89.02**   Algoneurodystrophy, upper arm
    M89.021   Algoneurodystrophy, right upper arm
    M89.022   Algoneurodystrophy, left upper arm
    M89.029   **Algoneurodystrophy, unspecified upper arm**

✓6ᵗʰ **M89.03**   Algoneurodystrophy, forearm
    M89.031   Algoneurodystrophy, right forearm
    M89.032   Algoneurodystrophy, left forearm
    M89.039   **Algoneurodystrophy, unspecified forearm**

✓6ᵗʰ **M89.04**   Algoneurodystrophy, hand
    M89.041   Algoneurodystrophy, right hand
    M89.042   Algoneurodystrophy, left hand
    M89.049   **Algoneurodystrophy, unspecified hand**

✓6ᵗʰ **M89.05**   Algoneurodystrophy, thigh
    M89.051   Algoneurodystrophy, right thigh
    M89.052   Algoneurodystrophy, left thigh
    M89.059   **Algoneurodystrophy, unspecified thigh**

✓6ᵗʰ **M89.06**   Algoneurodystrophy, lower leg
    M89.061   Algoneurodystrophy, right lower leg
    M89.062   Algoneurodystrophy, left lower leg
    M89.069   **Algoneurodystrophy, unspecified lower leg**

✓6ᵗʰ **M89.07**   Algoneurodystrophy, ankle and foot
    M89.071   Algoneurodystrophy, right ankle and foot
    M89.072   Algoneurodystrophy, left ankle and foot
    M89.079   **Algoneurodystrophy, unspecified ankle and foot**

    M89.08   **Algoneurodystrophy, other site**
    M89.09   Algoneurodystrophy, multiple sites

✓5ᵗʰ **M89.1**   **Physeal arrest**
    Arrest of growth plate   Growth plate arrest
    Epiphyseal arrest

✓6ᵗʰ **M89.12**   Physeal arrest, humerus
    M89.121   Complete physeal arrest, right proximal humerus
    M89.122   Complete physeal arrest, left proximal humerus
    M89.123   Partial physeal arrest, right proximal humerus
    M89.124   Partial physeal arrest, left proximal humerus
    M89.125   Complete physeal arrest, right distal humerus
    M89.126   Complete physeal arrest, left distal humerus
    M89.127   Partial physeal arrest, right distal humerus
    M89.128   Partial physeal arrest, left distal humerus
    M89.129   **Physeal arrest, humerus, unspecified**

✓6ᵗʰ **M89.13**   Physeal arrest, forearm
    M89.131   Complete physeal arrest, right distal radius
    M89.132   Complete physeal arrest, left distal radius
    M89.133   Partial physeal arrest, right distal radius
    M89.134   Partial physeal arrest, left distal radius
    M89.138   **Other physeal arrest of forearm**
    M89.139   **Physeal arrest, forearm, unspecified**

✓6ᵗʰ **M89.15**   Physeal arrest, femur
    M89.151   Complete physeal arrest, right proximal femur
    M89.152   Complete physeal arrest, left proximal femur
    M89.153   Partial physeal arrest, right proximal femur
    M89.154   Partial physeal arrest, left proximal femur
    M89.155   Complete physeal arrest, right distal femur
    M89.156   Complete physeal arrest, left distal femur
    M89.157   Partial physeal arrest, right distal femur
    M89.158   Partial physeal arrest, left distal femur
    M89.159   **Physeal arrest, femur, unspecified**

✓6ᵗʰ **M89.16**   Physeal arrest, lower leg
    M89.160   Complete physeal arrest, right proximal tibia
    M89.161   Complete physeal arrest, left proximal tibia
    M89.162   Partial physeal arrest, right proximal tibia
    M89.163   Partial physeal arrest, left proximal tibia
    M89.164   Complete physeal arrest, right distal tibia
    M89.165   Complete physeal arrest, left distal tibia
    M89.166   Partial physeal arrest, right distal tibia
    M89.167   Partial physeal arrest, left distal tibia
    M89.168   **Other physeal arrest of lower leg**
    M89.169   **Physeal arrest, lower leg, unspecified**

    M89.18   **Physeal arrest, other site**

✓5ᵗʰ **M89.2**   **Other disorders of bone development and growth**
    M89.20   **Other disorders of bone development and growth, unspecified site**

✓6ᵗʰ **M89.21**   Other disorders of bone development and growth, shoulder
    M89.211   **Other disorders of bone development and growth, right shoulder**
    M89.212   **Other disorders of bone development and growth, left shoulder**
    M89.219   **Other disorders of bone development and growth, unspecified shoulder**

✓6ᵗʰ **M89.22**   Other disorders of bone development and growth, humerus
    M89.221   **Other disorders of bone development and growth, right humerus**
    M89.222   **Other disorders of bone development and growth, left humerus**
    M89.229   **Other disorders of bone development and growth, unspecified humerus**

EXCLUDES 1 Not coded here   EXCLUDES 2 Not included here   N Newborn Age: 0   P Pediatric Age: 0-17   M Maternity Age: 12-55   A Adult Age: 15-124

736   ICD-10-CM 2016

✓6ᵗʰ **M89.23** **Other disorders of bone development and growth, ulna and radius**
     M89.231 Other disorders of bone development and growth, **right ulna**
     M89.232 Other disorders of bone development and growth, **left ulna**
     M89.233 Other disorders of bone development and growth, **right radius**
     M89.234 Other disorders of bone development and growth, **left radius**
     M89.239 Other disorders of bone development and growth, **unspecified ulna and radius**

✓6ᵗʰ **M89.24** **Other disorders of bone development and growth, hand**
     M89.241 Other disorders of bone development and growth, **right hand**
     M89.242 Other disorders of bone development and growth, **left hand**
     M89.249 Other disorders of bone development and growth, **unspecified hand**

✓6ᵗʰ **M89.25** **Other disorders of bone development and growth, femur**
     M89.251 Other disorders of bone development and growth, **right femur**
     M89.252 Other disorders of bone development and growth, **left femur**
     M89.259 Other disorders of bone development and growth, **unspecified femur**

✓6ᵗʰ **M89.26** **Other disorders of bone development and growth, tibia and fibula**
     M89.261 Other disorders of bone development and growth, **right tibia**
     M89.262 Other disorders of bone development and growth, **left tibia**
     M89.263 Other disorders of bone development and growth, **right fibula**
     M89.264 Other disorders of bone development and growth, **left fibula**
     M89.269 Other disorders of bone development and growth, **unspecified lower leg**

✓6ᵗʰ **M89.27** **Other disorders of bone development and growth, ankle and foot**
     M89.271 Other disorders of bone development and growth, **right ankle and foot**
     M89.272 Other disorders of bone development and growth, **left ankle and foot**
     M89.279 Other disorders of bone development and growth, **unspecified ankle and foot**

     M89.28 **Other disorders of bone development and growth, other site**

     M89.29 **Other disorders of bone development and growth, multiple sites**

✓5ᵗʰ **M89.3** **Hypertrophy of bone**
     M89.30 **Hypertrophy of bone, unspecified site**

✓6ᵗʰ **M89.31** **Hypertrophy of bone, shoulder**
     M89.311 Hypertrophy of bone, **right shoulder**
     M89.312 Hypertrophy of bone, **left shoulder**
     M89.319 Hypertrophy of bone, **unspecified shoulder**

✓6ᵗʰ **M89.32** **Hypertrophy of bone, humerus**
     M89.321 Hypertrophy of bone, **right humerus**
     M89.322 Hypertrophy of bone, **left humerus**
     M89.329 Hypertrophy of bone, **unspecified humerus**

✓6ᵗʰ **M89.33** **Hypertrophy of bone, ulna and radius**
     M89.331 Hypertrophy of bone, **right ulna**
     M89.332 Hypertrophy of bone, **left ulna**
     M89.333 Hypertrophy of bone, **right radius**
     M89.334 Hypertrophy of bone, **left radius**
     M89.339 Hypertrophy of bone, **unspecified ulna and radius**

✓6ᵗʰ **M89.34** **Hypertrophy of bone, hand**
     M89.341 Hypertrophy of bone, **right hand**
     M89.342 Hypertrophy of bone, **left hand**
     M89.349 Hypertrophy of bone, **unspecified hand**

✓6ᵗʰ **M89.35** **Hypertrophy of bone, femur**
     M89.351 Hypertrophy of bone, **right femur**
     M89.352 Hypertrophy of bone, **left femur**
     M89.359 Hypertrophy of bone, **unspecified femur**

✓6ᵗʰ **M89.36** **Hypertrophy of bone, tibia and fibula**
     M89.361 Hypertrophy of bone, **right tibia**
     M89.362 Hypertrophy of bone, **left tibia**
     M89.363 Hypertrophy of bone, **right fibula**
     M89.364 Hypertrophy of bone, **left fibula**
     M89.369 Hypertrophy of bone, **unspecified tibia and fibula**

✓6ᵗʰ **M89.37** **Hypertrophy of bone, ankle and foot**
     M89.371 Hypertrophy of bone, **right ankle and foot**
     M89.372 Hypertrophy of bone, **left ankle and foot**
     M89.379 Hypertrophy of bone, **unspecified ankle and foot**

     M89.38 **Hypertrophy of bone, other site**

     M89.39 **Hypertrophy of bone, multiple sites**

✓5ᵗʰ **M89.4** **Other hypertrophic osteoarthropathy**
     Marie-Bamberger disease   Pachydermoperiostosis

     M89.40 **Other hypertrophic osteoarthropathy, unspecified site**

✓6ᵗʰ **M89.41** **Other hypertrophic osteoarthropathy, shoulder**
     M89.411 Other hypertrophic osteoarthropathy, **right shoulder**
     M89.412 Other hypertrophic osteoarthropathy, **left shoulder**
     M89.419 Other hypertrophic osteoarthropathy, **unspecified shoulder**

✓6ᵗʰ **M89.42** **Other hypertrophic osteoarthropathy, upper arm**
     M89.421 Other hypertrophic osteoarthropathy, **right upper arm**
     M89.422 Other hypertrophic osteoarthropathy, **left upper arm**
     M89.429 Other hypertrophic osteoarthropathy, **unspecified upper arm**

✓6ᵗʰ **M89.43** **Other hypertrophic osteoarthropathy, forearm**
     M89.431 Other hypertrophic osteoarthropathy, **right forearm**
     M89.432 Other hypertrophic osteoarthropathy, **left forearm**
     M89.439 Other hypertrophic osteoarthropathy, **unspecified forearm**

✓6ᵗʰ **M89.44** **Other hypertrophic osteoarthropathy, hand**
     M89.441 Other hypertrophic osteoarthropathy, **right hand**
     M89.442 Other hypertrophic osteoarthropathy, **left hand**
     M89.449 Other hypertrophic osteoarthropathy, **unspecified hand**

✓6ᵗʰ **M89.45** **Other hypertrophic osteoarthropathy, thigh**
     M89.451 Other hypertrophic osteoarthropathy, **right thigh**
     M89.452 Other hypertrophic osteoarthropathy, **left thigh**
     M89.459 Other hypertrophic osteoarthropathy, **unspecified thigh**

✓6ᵗʰ **M89.46** **Other hypertrophic osteoarthropathy, lower leg**
     M89.461 Other hypertrophic osteoarthropathy, **right lower leg**
     M89.462 Other hypertrophic osteoarthropathy, **left lower leg**
     M89.469 Other hypertrophic osteoarthropathy, **unspecified lower leg**

✓6ᵗʰ **M89.47** **Other hypertrophic osteoarthropathy, ankle and foot**
     M89.471 Other hypertrophic osteoarthropathy, **right ankle and foot**
     M89.472 Other hypertrophic osteoarthropathy, **left ankle and foot**
     M89.479 Other hypertrophic osteoarthropathy, **unspecified ankle and foot**

     M89.48 **Other hypertrophic osteoarthropathy, other site**

     M89.49 **Other hypertrophic osteoarthropathy, multiple sites**

✓ Additional Character Required   ✓x7ᵗʰ Placeholder Alert   Unspecified Dx   Other Specified Dx   Manifestation   ►◄ Revised Text   ● New Code   ▲ Revised Code Title

✓5ᵗʰ M89.5 Osteolysis

Use additional code to identify major osseous defect, if applicable (M89.7-)

EXCLUDES 2   *periprosthetic osteolysis of internal prosthetic joint (T84.05-)*

    M89.50 Osteolysis, unspecified site

✓6ᵗʰ M89.51 Osteolysis, shoulder
- **M89.511 Osteolysis, right shoulder**
- **M89.512 Osteolysis, left shoulder**
- **M89.519 Osteolysis, unspecified shoulder**

✓6ᵗʰ M89.52 Osteolysis, upper arm
- **M89.521 Osteolysis, right upper arm**
- **M89.522 Osteolysis, left upper arm**
- **M89.529 Osteolysis, unspecified upper arm**

✓6ᵗʰ M89.53 Osteolysis, forearm
- **M89.531 Osteolysis, right forearm**
- **M89.532 Osteolysis, left forearm**
- **M89.539 Osteolysis, unspecified forearm**

✓6ᵗʰ M89.54 Osteolysis, hand
- **M89.541 Osteolysis, right hand**
- **M89.542 Osteolysis, left hand**
- **M89.549 Osteolysis, unspecified hand**

✓6ᵗʰ M89.55 Osteolysis, thigh
- **M89.551 Osteolysis, right thigh**
- **M89.552 Osteolysis, left thigh**
- **M89.559 Osteolysis, unspecified thigh**

✓6ᵗʰ M89.56 Osteolysis, lower leg
- **M89.561 Osteolysis, right lower leg**
- **M89.562 Osteolysis, left lower leg**
- **M89.569 Osteolysis, unspecified lower leg**

✓6ᵗʰ M89.57 Osteolysis, ankle and foot
- **M89.571 Osteolysis, right ankle and foot**
- **M89.572 Osteolysis, left ankle and foot**
- **M89.579 Osteolysis, unspecified ankle and foot**

    M89.58 Osteolysis, other site

    M89.59 Osteolysis, multiple sites

✓5ᵗʰ M89.6 Osteopathy after poliomyelitis

Use additional code (B91) to identify previous poliomyelitis

EXCLUDES 1   *postpolio syndrome (G14)*

    M89.60 Osteopathy after poliomyelitis, unspecified site

✓6ᵗʰ M89.61 Osteopathy after poliomyelitis, shoulder
- **M89.611 Osteopathy after poliomyelitis, right shoulder**
- **M89.612 Osteopathy after poliomyelitis, left shoulder**
- **M89.619 Osteopathy after poliomyelitis, unspecified shoulder**

✓6ᵗʰ M89.62 Osteopathy after poliomyelitis, upper arm
- **M89.621 Osteopathy after poliomyelitis, right upper arm**
- **M89.622 Osteopathy after poliomyelitis, left upper arm**
- **M89.629 Osteopathy after poliomyelitis, unspecified upper arm**

✓6ᵗʰ M89.63 Osteopathy after poliomyelitis, forearm
- **M89.631 Osteopathy after poliomyelitis, right forearm**
- **M89.632 Osteopathy after poliomyelitis, left forearm**
- **M89.639 Osteopathy after poliomyelitis, unspecified forearm**

✓6ᵗʰ M89.64 Osteopathy after poliomyelitis, hand
- **M89.641 Osteopathy after poliomyelitis, right hand**
- **M89.642 Osteopathy after poliomyelitis, left hand**
- **M89.649 Osteopathy after poliomyelitis, unspecified hand**

✓6ᵗʰ M89.65 Osteopathy after poliomyelitis, thigh
- **M89.651 Osteopathy after poliomyelitis, right thigh**
- **M89.652 Osteopathy after poliomyelitis, left thigh**
- **M89.659 Osteopathy after poliomyelitis, unspecified thigh**

✓6ᵗʰ M89.66 Osteopathy after poliomyelitis, lower leg
- **M89.661 Osteopathy after poliomyelitis, right lower leg**
- **M89.662 Osteopathy after poliomyelitis, left lower leg**
- **M89.669 Osteopathy after poliomyelitis, unspecified lower leg**

✓6ᵗʰ M89.67 Osteopathy after poliomyelitis, ankle and foot
- **M89.671 Osteopathy after poliomyelitis, right ankle and foot**
- **M89.672 Osteopathy after poliomyelitis, left ankle and foot**
- **M89.679 Osteopathy after poliomyelitis, unspecified ankle and foot**

    M89.68 Osteopathy after poliomyelitis, other site

    M89.69 Osteopathy after poliomyelitis, multiple sites

✓5ᵗʰ M89.7 Major osseous defect

Code first underlying disease, if known, such as:
aseptic necrosis of bone (M87.-)
malignant neoplasm of bone (C40.-)
osteolysis (M89.5)
osteomyelitis (M86.-)
osteonecrosis (M87.-)
osteoporosis (M80.-, M81.-)
periprosthetic osteolysis (T84.05-)

    M89.70 Major osseous defect, unspecified site

✓6ᵗʰ M89.71 Major osseous defect, shoulder region
Major osseous defect clavicle or scapula
- **M89.711 Major osseous defect, right shoulder region**
- **M89.712 Major osseous defect, left shoulder region**
- **M89.719 Major osseous defect, unspecified shoulder region**

✓6ᵗʰ M89.72 Major osseous defect, humerus
- **M89.721 Major osseous defect, right humerus**
- **M89.722 Major osseous defect, left humerus**
- **M89.729 Major osseous defect, unspecified humerus**

✓6ᵗʰ M89.73 Major osseous defect, forearm
Major osseous defect of radius and ulna
- **M89.731 Major osseous defect, right forearm**
- **M89.732 Major osseous defect, left forearm**
- **M89.739 Major osseous defect, unspecified forearm**

✓6ᵗʰ M89.74 Major osseous defect, hand
Major osseous defect of carpus, fingers, metacarpus
- **M89.741 Major osseous defect, right hand**
- **M89.742 Major osseous defect, left hand**
- **M89.749 Major osseous defect, unspecified hand**

✓6ᵗʰ M89.75 Major osseous defect, pelvic region and thigh
Major osseous defect of femur and pelvis
- **M89.751 Major osseous defect, right pelvic region and thigh**
- **M89.752 Major osseous defect, left pelvic region and thigh**
- **M89.759 Major osseous defect, unspecified pelvic region and thigh**

✓6ᵗʰ M89.76 Major osseous defect, lower leg
Major osseous defect of fibula and tibia
- **M89.761 Major osseous defect, right lower leg**
- **M89.762 Major osseous defect, left lower leg**
- **M89.769 Major osseous defect, unspecified lower leg**

✓6ᵗʰ M89.77 Major osseous defect, ankle and foot
Major osseous defect of metatarsus, tarsus, toes
- **M89.771 Major osseous defect, right ankle and foot**
- **M89.772 Major osseous defect, left ankle and foot**
- **M89.779 Major osseous defect, unspecified ankle and foot**

    M89.78 Major osseous defect, other site

    M89.79 Major osseous defect, multiple sites

✓5ᵗʰ M89.8 Other specified disorders of bone
Infantile cortical hyperostoses
Post-traumatic subperiosteal ossification

✓6ᵗʰ M89.8X Other specified disorders of bone
- **M89.8X0 Other specified disorders of bone, multiple sites**

EXCLUDES 1 Not coded here   EXCLUDES 2 Not included here   **N** Newborn Age: 0   **P** Pediatric Age: 0–17   **M** Maternity Age: 12–55   **A** Adult Age: 15–124

738   ICD-10-CM 2016

M89.8X1   **Other specified disorders of bone,** shoulder

M89.8X2   **Other specified disorders of bone,** upper arm

M89.8X3   **Other specified disorders of bone,** forearm

M89.8X4   **Other specified disorders of bone,** hand

M89.8X5   **Other specified disorders of bone,** thigh

M89.8X6   **Other specified disorders of bone,** lower leg

M89.8X7   **Other specified disorders of bone,** ankle and foot

M89.8X8   **Other specified disorders of bone, other site**

M89.8X9   **Other specified disorders of bone, unspecified site**

M89.9   Disorder of bone, unspecified

☑4ᵗʰ **M90   Osteopathies in diseases classified elsewhere**

     EXCLUDES 1   osteochondritis, osteomyelitis, and osteopathy (in):
       cryptococcosis (B45.3)
       diabetes mellitus (E08-E13 with .61-)
       gonococcal (A54.43)
       neurogenic syphilis (A52.11)
       renal osteodystrophy (N25.0)
       salmonellosis (A02.24)
       secondary syphilis (A51.46)
       syphilis (late) (A52.77)

☑5ᵗʰ **M90.5   Osteonecrosis in diseases classified elsewhere**

     Code first underlying disease, such as:
       caisson disease (T70.3)
       hemoglobinopathy (D50-D64)

M90.50   *Osteonecrosis in diseases classified elsewhere, unspecified site*

☑6ᵗʰ M90.51   **Osteonecrosis in diseases classified elsewhere,** shoulder

     M90.511   *Osteonecrosis in diseases classified elsewhere, right shoulder*

     M90.512   *Osteonecrosis in diseases classified elsewhere, left shoulder*

     M90.519   *Osteonecrosis in diseases classified elsewhere, unspecified shoulder*

☑6ᵗʰ M90.52   **Osteonecrosis in diseases classified elsewhere,** upper arm

     M90.521   *Osteonecrosis in diseases classified elsewhere, right upper arm*

     M90.522   *Osteonecrosis in diseases classified elsewhere, left upper arm*

     M90.529   *Osteonecrosis in diseases classified elsewhere, unspecified upper arm*

☑6ᵗʰ M90.53   **Osteonecrosis in diseases classified elsewhere,** forearm

     M90.531   *Osteonecrosis in diseases classified elsewhere, right forearm*

     M90.532   *Osteonecrosis in diseases classified elsewhere, left forearm*

     M90.539   *Osteonecrosis in diseases classified elsewhere, unspecified forearm*

☑6ᵗʰ M90.54   **Osteonecrosis in diseases classified elsewhere,** hand

     M90.541   *Osteonecrosis in diseases classified elsewhere, right hand*

     M90.542   *Osteonecrosis in diseases classified elsewhere, left hand*

     M90.549   *Osteonecrosis in diseases classified elsewhere, unspecified hand*

☑6ᵗʰ M90.55   **Osteonecrosis in diseases classified elsewhere,** thigh

     M90.551   *Osteonecrosis in diseases classified elsewhere, right thigh*

     M90.552   *Osteonecrosis in diseases classified elsewhere, left thigh*

     M90.559   *Osteonecrosis in diseases classified elsewhere, unspecified thigh*

☑6ᵗʰ M90.56   **Osteonecrosis in diseases classified elsewhere,** lower leg

     M90.561   *Osteonecrosis in diseases classified elsewhere, right lower leg*

     M90.562   *Osteonecrosis in diseases classified elsewhere, left lower leg*

     M90.569   *Osteonecrosis in diseases classified elsewhere, unspecified lower leg*

☑6ᵗʰ M90.57   **Osteonecrosis in diseases classified elsewhere,** ankle and foot

     M90.571   *Osteonecrosis in diseases classified elsewhere, right ankle and foot*

     M90.572   *Osteonecrosis in diseases classified elsewhere, left ankle and foot*

     M90.579   *Osteonecrosis in diseases classified elsewhere, unspecified ankle and foot*

M90.58   *Osteonecrosis in diseases classified elsewhere, other site*

M90.59   *Osteonecrosis in diseases classified elsewhere, multiple sites*

☑5ᵗʰ **M90.6   Osteitis deformans in neoplastic diseases**

     Osteitis deformans in malignant neoplasm of bone
     Code first the neoplasm (C40-, C41-)
     EXCLUDES 1   osteitis deformans [Paget's disease of bone] (M88.-)

M90.60   *Osteitis deformans in neoplastic diseases, unspecified site*

☑6ᵗʰ M90.61   **Osteitis deformans in neoplastic diseases,** shoulder

     M90.611   *Osteitis deformans in neoplastic diseases, right shoulder*

     M90.612   *Osteitis deformans in neoplastic diseases, left shoulder*

     M90.619   *Osteitis deformans in neoplastic diseases, unspecified shoulder*

☑6ᵗʰ M90.62   **Osteitis deformans in neoplastic diseases,** upper arm

     M90.621   *Osteitis deformans in neoplastic diseases, right upper arm*

     M90.622   *Osteitis deformans in neoplastic diseases, left upper arm*

     M90.629   *Osteitis deformans in neoplastic diseases, unspecified upper arm*

☑6ᵗʰ M90.63   **Osteitis deformans in neoplastic diseases,** forearm

     M90.631   *Osteitis deformans in neoplastic diseases, right forearm*

     M90.632   *Osteitis deformans in neoplastic diseases, left forearm*

     M90.639   *Osteitis deformans in neoplastic diseases, unspecified forearm*

☑6ᵗʰ M90.64   **Osteitis deformans in neoplastic diseases,** hand

     M90.641   *Osteitis deformans in neoplastic diseases, right hand*

     M90.642   *Osteitis deformans in neoplastic diseases, left hand*

     M90.649   *Osteitis deformans in neoplastic diseases, unspecified hand*

☑6ᵗʰ M90.65   **Osteitis deformans in neoplastic diseases,** thigh

     M90.651   *Osteitis deformans in neoplastic diseases, right thigh*

     M90.652   *Osteitis deformans in neoplastic diseases, left thigh*

     M90.659   *Osteitis deformans in neoplastic diseases, unspecified thigh*

☑6ᵗʰ M90.66   **Osteitis deformans in neoplastic diseases,** lower leg

     M90.661   *Osteitis deformans in neoplastic diseases, right lower leg*

     M90.662   *Osteitis deformans in neoplastic diseases, left lower leg*

     M90.669   *Osteitis deformans in neoplastic diseases, unspecified lower leg*

☑6ᵗʰ M90.67   **Osteitis deformans in neoplastic diseases,** ankle and foot

     M90.671   *Osteitis deformans in neoplastic diseases, right ankle and foot*

     M90.672   *Osteitis deformans in neoplastic diseases, left ankle and foot*

     M90.679   *Osteitis deformans in neoplastic diseases, unspecified ankle and foot*

M90.68   *Osteitis deformans in neoplastic diseases, other site*

M90.69   *Osteitis deformans in neoplastic diseases, multiple sites*

☑ Additional Character Required   ☑xₓ7ᵗʰ Placeholder Alert   Unspecified Dx   Other Specified Dx   Manifestation   ▶◀ Revised Text   ● New Code   ▲ Revised Code Title

✓5ᵗʰ **M90.8 Osteopathy in diseases classified elsewhere**
Code first underlying disease, such as:
    rickets (E55.0)
    vitamin-D-resistant rickets (E83.3)

    M90.80 *Osteopathy in diseases classified elsewhere, unspecified site*

✓6ᵗʰ **M90.81 Osteopathy in diseases classified elsewhere, shoulder**
    M90.811 *Osteopathy in diseases classified elsewhere, right shoulder*
    M90.812 *Osteopathy in diseases classified elsewhere, left shoulder*
    M90.819 *Osteopathy in diseases classified elsewhere, unspecified shoulder*

✓6ᵗʰ **M90.82 Osteopathy in diseases classified elsewhere, upper arm**
    M90.821 *Osteopathy in diseases classified elsewhere, right upper arm*
    M90.822 *Osteopathy in diseases classified elsewhere, left upper arm*
    M90.829 *Osteopathy in diseases classified elsewhere, unspecified upper arm*

✓6ᵗʰ **M90.83 Osteopathy in diseases classified elsewhere, forearm**
    M90.831 *Osteopathy in diseases classified elsewhere, right forearm*
    M90.832 *Osteopathy in diseases classified elsewhere, left forearm*
    M90.839 *Osteopathy in diseases classified elsewhere, unspecified forearm*

✓6ᵗʰ **M90.84 Osteopathy in diseases classified elsewhere, hand**
    M90.841 *Osteopathy in diseases classified elsewhere, right hand*
    M90.842 *Osteopathy in diseases classified elsewhere, left hand*
    M90.849 *Osteopathy in diseases classified elsewhere, unspecified hand*

✓6ᵗʰ **M90.85 Osteopathy in diseases classified elsewhere, thigh**
    M90.851 *Osteopathy in diseases classified elsewhere, right thigh*
    M90.852 *Osteopathy in diseases classified elsewhere, left thigh*
    M90.859 *Osteopathy in diseases classified elsewhere, unspecified thigh*

✓6ᵗʰ **M90.86 Osteopathy in diseases classified elsewhere, lower leg**
    M90.861 *Osteopathy in diseases classified elsewhere, right lower leg*
    M90.862 *Osteopathy in diseases classified elsewhere, left lower leg*
    M90.869 *Osteopathy in diseases classified elsewhere, unspecified lower leg*

✓6ᵗʰ **M90.87 Osteopathy in diseases classified elsewhere, ankle and foot**
    M90.871 *Osteopathy in diseases classified elsewhere, right ankle and foot*
    M90.872 *Osteopathy in diseases classified elsewhere, left ankle and foot*
    M90.879 *Osteopathy in diseases classified elsewhere, unspecified ankle and foot*

    M90.88 *Osteopathy in diseases classified elsewhere, other site*
    M90.89 *Osteopathy in diseases classified elsewhere, multiple sites*

Chondropathies (M91-M94)

EXCLUDES 1 *postprocedural chondropathies (M96.-)*

✓4ᵗʰ **M91 Juvenile osteochondrosis of hip and pelvis**
    EXCLUDES 1 *slipped upper femoral epiphysis (nontraumatic) (M93.0)*

M91.0 Juvenile osteochondrosis of pelvis
    Osteochondrosis (juvenile) of acetabulum
    Osteochondrosis (juvenile) of iliac crest [Buchanan]
    Osteochondrosis (juvenile) of ischiopubic synchondrosis [van Neck]
    Osteochondrosis (juvenile) of symphysis pubis [Pierson]

✓5ᵗʰ **M91.1 Juvenile osteochondrosis of head of femur [Legg-Calvé-Perthes]**
    M91.10 **Juvenile osteochondrosis of head of femur [Legg-Calvé-Perthes], unspecified leg**

    M91.11 **Juvenile osteochondrosis of head of femur [Legg-Calvé-Perthes], right leg**
    M91.12 **Juvenile osteochondrosis of head of femur [Legg-Calvé-Perthes], left leg**

✓5ᵗʰ **M91.2 Coxa plana**
    Hip deformity due to previous juvenile osteochondrosis
    M91.20 **Coxa plana, unspecified hip**
    M91.21 **Coxa plana, right hip**
    M91.22 **Coxa plana, left hip**

✓5ᵗʰ **M91.3 Pseudocoxalgia**
    M91.30 **Pseudocoxalgia, unspecified hip**
    M91.31 **Pseudocoxalgia, right hip**
    M91.32 **Pseudocoxalgia, left hip**

✓5ᵗʰ **M91.4 Coxa magna**
    M91.40 **Coxa magna, unspecified hip**
    M91.41 **Coxa magna, right hip**
    M91.42 **Coxa magna, left hip**

✓5ᵗʰ **M91.8 Other juvenile osteochondrosis of hip and pelvis**
    Juvenile osteochondrosis after reduction of congenital dislocation of hip
    M91.80 **Other juvenile osteochondrosis of hip and pelvis, unspecified leg**
    M91.81 **Other juvenile osteochondrosis of hip and pelvis, right leg**
    M91.82 **Other juvenile osteochondrosis of hip and pelvis, left leg**

✓5ᵗʰ **M91.9 Juvenile osteochondrosis of hip and pelvis, unspecified**
    M91.90 **Juvenile osteochondrosis of hip and pelvis, unspecified, unspecified leg**
    M91.91 **Juvenile osteochondrosis of hip and pelvis, unspecified, right leg**
    M91.92 **Juvenile osteochondrosis of hip and pelvis, unspecified, left leg**

✓4ᵗʰ **M92 Other juvenile osteochondrosis**

✓5ᵗʰ **M92.0 Juvenile osteochondrosis of humerus**
    Osteochondrosis (juvenile) of capitulum of humerus [Panner]
    Osteochondrosis (juvenile) of head of humerus [Haas]
    M92.00 **Juvenile osteochondrosis of humerus, unspecified arm**
    M92.01 **Juvenile osteochondrosis of humerus, right arm**
    M92.02 **Juvenile osteochondrosis of humerus, left arm**

✓5ᵗʰ **M92.1 Juvenile osteochondrosis of radius and ulna**
    Osteochondrosis (juvenile) of lower ulna [Burns]
    Osteochondrosis (juvenile) of radial head [Brailsford]
    M92.10 **Juvenile osteochondrosis of radius and ulna, unspecified arm**
    M92.11 **Juvenile osteochondrosis of radius and ulna, right arm**
    M92.12 **Juvenile osteochondrosis of radius and ulna, left arm**

✓5ᵗʰ **M92.2 Juvenile osteochondrosis, hand**
    ✓6ᵗʰ **M92.20** **Unspecified juvenile osteochondrosis, hand**
        M92.201 **Unspecified juvenile osteochondrosis, right hand**
        M92.202 **Unspecified juvenile osteochondrosis, left hand**
        M92.209 **Unspecified juvenile osteochondrosis, unspecified hand**

    ✓6ᵗʰ **M92.21** **Osteochondrosis (juvenile) of carpal lunate [Kienböck]**
        M92.211 **Osteochondrosis (juvenile) of carpal lunate [Kienböck], right hand**
        M92.212 **Osteochondrosis (juvenile) of carpal lunate [Kienböck], left hand**
        M92.219 **Osteochondrosis (juvenile) of carpal lunate [Kienböck], unspecified hand**

    ✓6ᵗʰ **M92.22** **Osteochondrosis (juvenile) of metacarpal heads [Mauclaire]**
        M92.221 **Osteochondrosis (juvenile) of metacarpal heads [Mauclaire], right hand**
        M92.222 **Osteochondrosis (juvenile) of metacarpal heads [Mauclaire], left hand**
        M92.229 **Osteochondrosis (juvenile) of metacarpal heads [Mauclaire], unspecified hand**

EXCLUDES 1 Not coded here   EXCLUDES 2 Not included here   N Newborn Age: 0   P Pediatric Age: 0-17   M Maternity Age: 12-55   A Adult Age: 15-124

☑6ᵗʰ **M92.29** Other juvenile osteochondrosis, hand

    M92.291 Other juvenile osteochondrosis, right hand

    M92.292 Other juvenile osteochondrosis, left hand

    M92.299 Other juvenile osteochondrosis, unspecified hand

☑5ᵗʰ **M92.3** Other juvenile osteochondrosis, upper limb

    M92.30 Other juvenile osteochondrosis, unspecified upper limb

    M92.31 Other juvenile osteochondrosis, right upper limb

    M92.32 Other juvenile osteochondrosis, left upper limb

☑5ᵗʰ **M92.4** Juvenile osteochondrosis of patella

    Osteochondrosis (juvenile) of primary patellar center [Köhler]

    Osteochondrosis (juvenile) of secondary patellar centre [Sinding Larsen]

    M92.40 Juvenile osteochondrosis of patella, unspecified knee

    M92.41 Juvenile osteochondrosis of patella, right knee

    M92.42 Juvenile osteochondrosis of patella, left knee

☑5ᵗʰ **M92.5** Juvenile osteochondrosis of tibia and fibula

    Osteochondrosis (juvenile) of proximal tibia [Blount]

    Osteochondrosis (juvenile) of tibial tubercle [Osgood-Schlatter]

    Tibia vara

    M92.50 Juvenile osteochondrosis of tibia and fibula, unspecified leg

    M92.51 Juvenile osteochondrosis of tibia and fibula, right leg

    M92.52 Juvenile osteochondrosis of tibia and fibula, left leg

☑5ᵗʰ **M92.6** Juvenile osteochondrosis of tarsus

    Osteochondrosis (juvenile) of calcaneum [Sever]

    Osteochondrosis (juvenile) of os tibiale externum [Haglund]

    Osteochondrosis (juvenile) of talus [Diaz]

    Osteochondrosis (juvenile) of tarsal navicular [Köhler]

    M92.60 Juvenile osteochondrosis of tarsus, unspecified ankle

    M92.61 Juvenile osteochondrosis of tarsus, right ankle

    M92.62 Juvenile osteochondrosis of tarsus, left ankle

☑5ᵗʰ **M92.7** Juvenile osteochondrosis of metatarsus

    Osteochondrosis (juvenile) of fifth metatarsus [Iselin]

    Osteochondrosis (juvenile) of second metatarsus [Freiberg]

    M92.70 Juvenile osteochondrosis of metatarsus, unspecified foot

    M92.71 Juvenile osteochondrosis of metatarsus, right foot

    M92.72 Juvenile osteochondrosis of metatarsus, left foot

M92.8 Other specified juvenile osteochondrosis

    Calcaneal apophysitis

M92.9 Juvenile osteochondrosis, unspecified

    Juvenile apophysitis NOS

    Juvenile epiphysitis NOS

    Juvenile osteochondritis NOS

    Juvenile osteochondrosis NOS

☑4ᵗʰ **M93 Other osteochondropathies**

    EXCLUDES 2   osteochondrosis of spine (M42.-)

☑5ᵗʰ **M93.0** Slipped upper femoral epiphysis (nontraumatic)

    Use additional code for associated chondrolysis (M94.3)

    ☑6ᵗʰ **M93.00** Unspecified slipped upper femoral epiphysis (nontraumatic)

      M93.001 Unspecified slipped upper femoral epiphysis (nontraumatic), right hip

      M93.002 Unspecified slipped upper femoral epiphysis (nontraumatic), left hip

      M93.003 Unspecified slipped upper femoral epiphysis (nontraumatic), unspecified hip

    ☑6ᵗʰ **M93.01** Acute slipped upper femoral epiphysis (nontraumatic)

      M93.011 Acute slipped upper femoral epiphysis (nontraumatic), right hip

      M93.012 Acute slipped upper femoral epiphysis (nontraumatic), left hip

      M93.013 Acute slipped upper femoral epiphysis (nontraumatic), unspecified hip

    ☑6ᵗʰ **M93.02** Chronic slipped upper femoral epiphysis (nontraumatic)

      M93.021 Chronic slipped upper femoral epiphysis (nontraumatic), right hip

      M93.022 Chronic slipped upper femoral epiphysis (nontraumatic), left hip

      M93.023 Chronic slipped upper femoral epiphysis (nontraumatic), unspecified hip

    ☑6ᵗʰ **M93.03** Acute on chronic slipped upper femoral epiphysis (nontraumatic)

      M93.031 Acute on chronic slipped upper femoral epiphysis (nontraumatic), right hip

      M93.032 Acute on chronic slipped upper femoral epiphysis (nontraumatic), left hip

      M93.033 Acute on chronic slipped upper femoral epiphysis (nontraumatic), unspecified hip

M93.1 Kienböck's disease of adults   A

    Adult osteochondrosis of carpal lunates

☑5ᵗʰ **M93.2** Osteochondritis dissecans

    M93.20 Osteochondritis dissecans of unspecified site

    ☑6ᵗʰ **M93.21** Osteochondritis dissecans of shoulder

      M93.211 Osteochondritis dissecans, right shoulder

      M93.212 Osteochondritis dissecans, left shoulder

      M93.219 Osteochondritis dissecans, unspecified shoulder

    ☑6ᵗʰ **M93.22** Osteochondritis dissecans of elbow

      M93.221 Osteochondritis dissecans, right elbow

      M93.222 Osteochondritis dissecans, left elbow

      M93.229 Osteochondritis dissecans, unspecified elbow

    ☑6ᵗʰ **M93.23** Osteochondritis dissecans of wrist

      M93.231 Osteochondritis dissecans, right wrist

      M93.232 Osteochondritis dissecans, left wrist

      M93.239 Osteochondritis dissecans, unspecified wrist

    ☑6ᵗʰ **M93.24** Osteochondritis dissecans of joints of hand

      M93.241 Osteochondritis dissecans, joints of right hand

      M93.242 Osteochondritis dissecans, joints of left hand

      M93.249 Osteochondritis dissecans, joints of unspecified hand

    ☑6ᵗʰ **M93.25** Osteochondritis dissecans of hip

      M93.251 Osteochondritis dissecans, right hip

      M93.252 Osteochondritis dissecans, left hip

      M93.259 Osteochondritis dissecans, unspecified hip

    ☑6ᵗʰ **M93.26** Osteochondritis dissecans knee

      M93.261 Osteochondritis dissecans, right knee

      M93.262 Osteochondritis dissecans, left knee

      M93.269 Osteochondritis dissecans, unspecified knee

    ☑6ᵗʰ **M93.27** Osteochondritis dissecans of ankle and joints of foot

      M93.271 Osteochondritis dissecans, right ankle and joints of right foot

      M93.272 Osteochondritis dissecans, left ankle and joints of left foot

      M93.279 Osteochondritis dissecans, unspecified ankle and joints of foot

    M93.28 Osteochondritis dissecans other site

    M93.29 Osteochondritis dissecans multiple sites

☑5ᵗʰ **M93.8** Other specified osteochondropathies

    M93.80 Other specified osteochondropathies of unspecified site

    ☑6ᵗʰ **M93.81** Other specified osteochondropathies of shoulder

      M93.811 Other specified osteochondropathies, right shoulder

      M93.812 Other specified osteochondropathies, left shoulder

      M93.819 Other specified osteochondropathies, unspecified shoulder

    ☑6ᵗʰ **M93.82** Other specified osteochondropathies of upper arm

      M93.821 Other specified osteochondropathies, right upper arm

      M93.822 Other specified osteochondropathies, left upper arm

      M93.829 Other specified osteochondropathies, unspecified upper arm

☑ Additional Character Required   ✓×7ᵗʰ Placeholder Alert   Unspecified Dx   Other Specified Dx   Manifestation   ▶◀ Revised Text   ● New Code   ▲ Revised Code Title

ICD-10-CM 2016   **741**

✓6th **M93.83 Other specified osteochondropathies of** forearm

    M93.831 Other specified osteochondropathies, right forearm

    M93.832 Other specified osteochondropathies, left forearm

    M93.839 Other specified osteochondropathies, unspecified forearm

✓6th **M93.84 Other specified osteochondropathies of** hand

    M93.841 Other specified osteochondropathies, right hand

    M93.842 Other specified osteochondropathies, left hand

    M93.849 Other specified osteochondropathies, unspecified hand

✓6th **M93.85 Other specified osteochondropathies of** thigh

    M93.851 Other specified osteochondropathies, right thigh

    M93.852 Other specified osteochondropathies, left thigh

    M93.859 Other specified osteochondropathies, unspecified thigh

✓6th **M93.86 Other specified osteochondropathies** lower leg

    M93.861 Other specified osteochondropathies, right lower leg

    M93.862 Other specified osteochondropathies, left lower leg

    M93.869 Other specified osteochondropathies, unspecified lower leg

✓6th **M93.87 Other specified osteochondropathies of** ankle and foot

    M93.871 Other specified osteochondropathies, right ankle and foot

    M93.872 Other specified osteochondropathies, left ankle and foot

    M93.879 Other specified osteochondropathies, unspecified ankle and foot

M93.88 Other specified osteochondropathies other site

M93.89 Other specified osteochondropathies multiple sites

✓5th **M93.9 Osteochondropathy, unspecified**

    Apophysitis NOS   Osteochondritis NOS
    Epiphysitis NOS   Osteochondrosis NOS

    M93.90 Osteochondropathy, unspecified of unspecified site

✓6th **M93.91 Osteochondropathy, unspecified of** shoulder

    M93.911 Osteochondropathy, unspecified, right shoulder

    M93.912 Osteochondropathy, unspecified, left shoulder

    M93.919 Osteochondropathy, unspecified, unspecified shoulder

✓6th **M93.92 Osteochondropathy, unspecified of** upper arm

    M93.921 Osteochondropathy, unspecified, right upper arm

    M93.922 Osteochondropathy, unspecified, left upper arm

    M93.929 Osteochondropathy, unspecified, unspecified upper arm

✓6th **M93.93 Osteochondropathy, unspecified of** forearm

    M93.931 Osteochondropathy, unspecified, right forearm

    M93.932 Osteochondropathy, unspecified, left forearm

    M93.939 Osteochondropathy, unspecified, unspecified forearm

✓6th **M93.94 Osteochondropathy, unspecified of** hand

    M93.941 Osteochondropathy, unspecified, right hand

    M93.942 Osteochondropathy, unspecified, left hand

    M93.949 Osteochondropathy, unspecified, unspecified hand

✓6th **M93.95 Osteochondropathy, unspecified of** thigh

    M93.951 Osteochondropathy, unspecified, right thigh

    M93.952 Osteochondropathy, unspecified, left thigh

    M93.959 Osteochondropathy, unspecified, unspecified thigh

✓6th **M93.96 Osteochondropathy, unspecified** lower leg

    M93.961 Osteochondropathy, unspecified, right lower leg

    M93.962 Osteochondropathy, unspecified, left lower leg

    M93.969 Osteochondropathy, unspecified, unspecified lower leg

✓6th **M93.97 Osteochondropathy, unspecified of** ankle and foot

    M93.971 Osteochondropathy, unspecified, right ankle and foot

    M93.972 Osteochondropathy, unspecified, left ankle and foot

    M93.979 Osteochondropathy, unspecified, unspecified ankle and foot

M93.98 Osteochondropathy, unspecified other site

M93.99 Osteochondropathy, unspecified multiple sites

✓4th **M94 Other disorders of cartilage**

    M94.0 Chondrocostal junction syndrome [Tietze]

        Costochondritis

    M94.1 Relapsing polychondritis

✓5th **M94.2 Chondromalacia**

    EXCLUDES 1 *chondromalacia patellae (M22.4)*

    M94.20 Chondromalacia, unspecified site

✓6th **M94.21 Chondromalacia,** shoulder

    M94.211 Chondromalacia, right shoulder

    M94.212 Chondromalacia, left shoulder

    M94.219 Chondromalacia, unspecified shoulder

✓6th **M94.22 Chondromalacia,** elbow

    M94.221 Chondromalacia, right elbow

    M94.222 Chondromalacia, left elbow

    M94.229 Chondromalacia, unspecified elbow

✓6th **M94.23 Chondromalacia,** wrist

    M94.231 Chondromalacia, right wrist

    M94.232 Chondromalacia, left wrist

    M94.239 Chondromalacia, unspecified wrist

✓6th **M94.24 Chondromalacia,** joints of hand

    M94.241 Chondromalacia, joints of right hand

    M94.242 Chondromalacia, joints of left hand

    M94.249 Chondromalacia, joints of unspecified hand

✓6th **M94.25 Chondromalacia,** hip

    M94.251 Chondromalacia, right hip

    M94.252 Chondromalacia, left hip

    M94.259 Chondromalacia, unspecified hip

✓6th **M94.26 Chondromalacia,** knee

    M94.261 Chondromalacia, right knee

    M94.262 Chondromalacia, left knee

    M94.269 Chondromalacia, unspecified knee

✓6th **M94.27 Chondromalacia,** ankle and joints of foot

    M94.271 Chondromalacia, right ankle and joints of right foot

    M94.272 Chondromalacia, left ankle and joints of left foot

    M94.279 Chondromalacia, unspecified ankle and joints of foot

M94.28 Chondromalacia, other site

M94.29 Chondromalacia, multiple sites

✓5th **M94.3 Chondrolysis**

    Code first any associated slipped upper femoral epiphysis (nontraumatic) (M93.0-)

✓6th **M94.35 Chondrolysis, hip**

    M94.351 Chondrolysis, right hip

    M94.352 Chondrolysis, left hip

    M94.359 Chondrolysis, unspecified hip

✓5th **M94.8 Other specified disorders of cartilage**

✓6th **M94.8X Other specified disorders of cartilage**

    M94.8X0 Other specified disorders of cartilage, multiple sites

    M94.8X1 Other specified disorders of cartilage, shoulder

    M94.8X2 Other specified disorders of cartilage, upper arm

EXCLUDES 1 Not coded here   EXCLUDES 2 Not included here   N Newborn Age: 0   P Pediatric Age: 0-17   M Maternity Age: 12-55   A Adult Age: 15-124

742   ICD-10-CM 2016

M94.8X3   **Other specified disorders of cartilage, forearm**

M94.8X4   **Other specified disorders of cartilage, hand**

M94.8X5   **Other specified disorders of cartilage, thigh**

M94.8X6   **Other specified disorders of cartilage, lower leg**

M94.8X7   **Other specified disorders of cartilage, ankle and foot**

M94.8X8   **Other specified disorders of cartilage, other site**

M94.8X9   **Other specified disorders of cartilage, unspecified sites**

M94.9   **Disorder of cartilage, unspecified**

Other disorders of the musculoskeletal system and connective tissue (M95)

✓4ᵗʰ M95   Other acquired deformities of musculoskeletal system and connective tissue

    EXCLUDES 2   *acquired absence of limbs and organs (Z89-Z90)*
                   acquired deformities of limbs (M20-M21)
                   congenital malformations and deformations of the musculoskeletal system (Q65-Q79)
                   deforming dorsopathies (M40-M43)
                   dentofacial anomalies [including malocclusion] (M26.-)
                   postprocedural musculoskeletal disorders (M96.-)

M95.0   **Acquired deformity of nose**
      EXCLUDES 2   *deviated nasal septum (J34.2)*

✓5ᵗʰ M95.1   **Cauliflower ear**
      EXCLUDES 2   *other acquired deformities of ear (H61.1)*

    M95.10   **Cauliflower ear, unspecified ear**

    M95.11   **Cauliflower ear, right ear**

    M95.12   **Cauliflower ear, left ear**

M95.2   **Other acquired deformity of head**

M95.3   **Acquired deformity of neck**

M95.4   **Acquired deformity of chest and rib**
      AHA: 2014, 4Q, 26-27

M95.5   **Acquired deformity of pelvis**
      EXCLUDES 1   *maternal care for known or suspected disproportion (O33.-)*

M95.8   **Other specified acquired deformities of musculoskeletal system**

M95.9   **Acquired deformity of musculoskeletal system, unspecified**

Intraoperative and postprocedural complications and disorders of musculoskeletal system, not elsewhere classified (M96)

✓4ᵗʰ M96   Intraoperative and postprocedural complications and disorders of musculoskeletal system, not elsewhere classified

    EXCLUDES 2   *arthropathy following intestinal bypass (M02.0-)*
                   complications of internal orthopedic prosthetic devices, implants and grafts (T84.-)
                   disorders associated with osteoporosis (M80)
                   presence of functional implants and other devices (Z96-Z97)

M96.0   **Pseudarthrosis after fusion or arthrodesis**

M96.1   **Postlaminectomy syndrome, not elsewhere classified**   ▲

M96.2   **Postradiation kyphosis**

M96.3   **Postlaminectomy kyphosis**

M96.4   **Postsurgical lordosis**

M96.5   **Postradiation scoliosis**

✓5ᵗʰ M96.6   **Fracture of bone following insertion of orthopedic implant, joint prosthesis, or bone plate**
      Intraoperative fracture of bone during insertion of orthopedic implant, joint prosthesis, or bone plate
      EXCLUDES 2   *complication of internal orthopedic devices, implants or grafts (T84.-)*

   ✓6ᵗʰ M96.62   **Fracture of humerus following insertion of orthopedic implant, joint prosthesis, or bone plate**

      M96.621   **Fracture of humerus following insertion of orthopedic implant, joint prosthesis, or bone plate, right arm**

      M96.622   **Fracture of humerus following insertion of orthopedic implant, joint prosthesis, or bone plate, left arm**

      M96.629   **Fracture of humerus following insertion of orthopedic implant, joint prosthesis, or bone plate, unspecified arm**

✓6ᵗʰ M96.63   **Fracture of radius or ulna following insertion of orthopedic implant, joint prosthesis, or bone plate**

      M96.631   **Fracture of radius or ulna following insertion of orthopedic implant, joint prosthesis, or bone plate, right arm**

      M96.632   **Fracture of radius or ulna following insertion of orthopedic implant, joint prosthesis, or bone plate, left arm**

      M96.639   **Fracture of radius or ulna following insertion of orthopedic implant, joint prosthesis, or bone plate, unspecified arm**

M96.65   **Fracture of pelvis following insertion of orthopedic implant, joint prosthesis, or bone plate**

✓6ᵗʰ M96.66   **Fracture of femur following insertion of orthopedic implant, joint prosthesis, or bone plate**

      M96.661   **Fracture of femur following insertion of orthopedic implant, joint prosthesis, or bone plate, right leg**

      M96.662   **Fracture of femur following insertion of orthopedic implant, joint prosthesis, or bone plate, left leg**

      M96.669   **Fracture of femur following insertion of orthopedic implant, joint prosthesis, or bone plate, unspecified leg**

✓6ᵗʰ M96.67   **Fracture of tibia or fibula following insertion of orthopedic implant, joint prosthesis, or bone plate**

      M96.671   **Fracture of tibia or fibula following insertion of orthopedic implant, joint prosthesis, or bone plate, right leg**

      M96.672   **Fracture of tibia or fibula following insertion of orthopedic implant, joint prosthesis, or bone plate, left leg**

      M96.679   **Fracture of tibia or fibula following insertion of orthopedic implant, joint prosthesis, or bone plate, unspecified leg**

M96.69   **Fracture of other bone following insertion of orthopedic implant, joint prosthesis, or bone plate**

✓5ᵗʰ M96.8   **Other intraoperative and postprocedural complications and disorders of musculoskeletal system, not elsewhere classified**

   ✓6ᵗʰ M96.81   **Intraoperative hemorrhage and hematoma of a musculoskeletal structure complicating a procedure**
      EXCLUDES 1   *intraoperative hemorrhage and hematoma of a musculoskeletal structure due to accidental puncture and laceration during a procedure (M96.82-)*

      M96.810   **Intraoperative hemorrhage and hematoma of a musculoskeletal structure complicating a musculoskeletal system procedure**

      M96.811   **Intraoperative hemorrhage and hematoma of a musculoskeletal structure complicating other procedure**

   ✓6ᵗʰ M96.82   **Accidental puncture and laceration of a musculoskeletal structure during a procedure**

      M96.820   **Accidental puncture and laceration of a musculoskeletal structure during a musculoskeletal system procedure**

      M96.821   **Accidental puncture and laceration of a musculoskeletal structure during other procedure**

   ✓6ᵗʰ M96.83   **Postprocedural hemorrhage and hematoma of a musculoskeletal structure following a procedure**

      M96.830   **Postprocedural hemorrhage and hematoma of a musculoskeletal structure following a musculoskeletal system procedure**

      M96.831   **Postprocedural hemorrhage and hematoma of a musculoskeletal structure following other procedure**

M96.89   **Other intraoperative and postprocedural complications and disorders of the musculoskeletal system**
      Instability of joint secondary to removal of joint prosthesis
      Use additional code, if applicable, to further specify disorder

---

✓ Additional Character Required   ✓·1ᵗʰ Placeholder Alert   Unspecified Dx   Other Specified Dx   Manifestation   ►◄ Revised Text   ● New Code   ▲ Revised Code Title

ICD-10-CM 2016   **743**

Biomechanical lesions, not elsewhere classified (M99)

✓4ᵗʰ M99 Biomechanical lesions, not elsewhere classified

> **NOTE** This category should not be used if the condition can be classified elsewhere.

✓5ᵗʰ M99.0 Segmental and somatic dysfunction
- M99.00 Segmental and somatic dysfunction of head region
- M99.01 Segmental and somatic dysfunction of cervical region
- M99.02 Segmental and somatic dysfunction of thoracic region
- M99.03 Segmental and somatic dysfunction of lumbar region
- M99.04 Segmental and somatic dysfunction of sacral region
- M99.05 Segmental and somatic dysfunction of pelvic region
- M99.06 Segmental and somatic dysfunction of lower extremity
- M99.07 Segmental and somatic dysfunction of upper extremity
- M99.08 Segmental and somatic dysfunction of rib cage
- M99.09 Segmental and somatic dysfunction of abdomen and other regions

✓5ᵗʰ M99.1 Subluxation complex (vertebral)
- M99.10 Subluxation complex (vertebral) of head region
- M99.11 Subluxation complex (vertebral) of cervical region
- M99.12 Subluxation complex (vertebral) of thoracic region
- M99.13 Subluxation complex (vertebral) of lumbar region
- M99.14 Subluxation complex (vertebral) of sacral region
- M99.15 Subluxation complex (vertebral) of pelvic region
- M99.16 Subluxation complex (vertebral) of lower extremity
- M99.17 Subluxation complex (vertebral) of upper extremity
- M99.18 Subluxation complex (vertebral) of rib cage
- M99.19 Subluxation complex (vertebral) of abdomen and other regions

✓5ᵗʰ M99.2 Subluxation stenosis of neural canal
- M99.20 Subluxation stenosis of neural canal of head region
- M99.21 Subluxation stenosis of neural canal of cervical region
- M99.22 Subluxation stenosis of neural canal of thoracic region Ⓐ
- M99.23 Subluxation stenosis of neural canal of lumbar region Ⓐ
- M99.24 Subluxation stenosis of neural canal of sacral region Ⓐ
- M99.25 Subluxation stenosis of neural canal of pelvic region Ⓐ
- M99.26 Subluxation stenosis of neural canal of lower extremity Ⓐ
- M99.27 Subluxation stenosis of neural canal of upper extremity Ⓐ
- M99.28 Subluxation stenosis of neural canal of rib cage Ⓐ
- M99.29 Subluxation stenosis of neural canal of abdomen and other regions Ⓐ

✓5ᵗʰ M99.3 Osseous stenosis of neural canal
- M99.30 Osseous stenosis of neural canal of head region
- M99.31 Osseous stenosis of neural canal of cervical region
- M99.32 Osseous stenosis of neural canal of thoracic region Ⓐ
- M99.33 Osseous stenosis of neural canal of lumbar region Ⓐ
- M99.34 Osseous stenosis of neural canal of sacral region Ⓐ
- M99.35 Osseous stenosis of neural canal of pelvic region Ⓐ
- M99.36 Osseous stenosis of neural canal of lower extremity Ⓐ
- M99.37 Osseous stenosis of neural canal of upper extremity Ⓐ
- M99.38 Osseous stenosis of neural canal of rib cage Ⓐ
- M99.39 Osseous stenosis of neural canal of abdomen and other regions Ⓐ

✓5ᵗʰ M99.4 Connective tissue stenosis of neural canal
- M99.40 Connective tissue stenosis of neural canal of head region

- M99.41 Connective tissue stenosis of neural canal of cervical region
- M99.42 Connective tissue stenosis of neural canal of thoracic region Ⓐ
- M99.43 Connective tissue stenosis of neural canal of lumbar region Ⓐ
- M99.44 Connective tissue stenosis of neural canal of sacral region Ⓐ
- M99.45 Connective tissue stenosis of neural canal of pelvic region Ⓐ
- M99.46 Connective tissue stenosis of neural canal of lower extremity Ⓐ
- M99.47 Connective tissue stenosis of neural canal of upper extremity Ⓐ
- M99.48 Connective tissue stenosis of neural canal of rib cage Ⓐ
- M99.49 Connective tissue stenosis of neural canal of abdomen and other regions Ⓐ

✓5ᵗʰ M99.5 Intervertebral disc stenosis of neural canal
- M99.50 Intervertebral disc stenosis of neural canal of head region
- M99.51 Intervertebral disc stenosis of neural canal of cervical region
- M99.52 Intervertebral disc stenosis of neural canal of thoracic region Ⓐ
- M99.53 Intervertebral disc stenosis of neural canal of lumbar region Ⓐ
- M99.54 Intervertebral disc stenosis of neural canal of sacral region Ⓐ
- M99.55 Intervertebral disc stenosis of neural canal of pelvic region Ⓐ
- M99.56 Intervertebral disc stenosis of neural canal of lower extremity Ⓐ
- M99.57 Intervertebral disc stenosis of neural canal of upper extremity Ⓐ
- M99.58 Intervertebral disc stenosis of neural canal of rib cage Ⓐ
- M99.59 Intervertebral disc stenosis of neural canal of abdomen and other regions Ⓐ

✓5ᵗʰ M99.6 Osseous and subluxation stenosis of intervertebral foramina
- M99.60 Osseous and subluxation stenosis of intervertebral foramina of head region
- M99.61 Osseous and subluxation stenosis of intervertebral foramina of cervical region
- M99.62 Osseous and subluxation stenosis of intervertebral foramina of thoracic region Ⓐ
- M99.63 Osseous and subluxation stenosis of intervertebral foramina of lumbar region Ⓐ
- M99.64 Osseous and subluxation stenosis of intervertebral foramina of sacral region Ⓐ
- M99.65 Osseous and subluxation stenosis of intervertebral foramina of pelvic region Ⓐ
- M99.66 Osseous and subluxation stenosis of intervertebral foramina of lower extremity Ⓐ
- M99.67 Osseous and subluxation stenosis of intervertebral foramina of upper extremity Ⓐ
- M99.68 Osseous and subluxation stenosis of intervertebral foramina of rib cage Ⓐ
- M99.69 Osseous and subluxation stenosis of intervertebral foramina of abdomen and other regions Ⓐ

✓5ᵗʰ M99.7 Connective tissue and disc stenosis of intervertebral foramina
- M99.70 Connective tissue and disc stenosis of intervertebral foramina of head region
- M99.71 Connective tissue and disc stenosis of intervertebral foramina of cervical region
- M99.72 Connective tissue and disc stenosis of intervertebral foramina of thoracic region Ⓐ
- M99.73 Connective tissue and disc stenosis of intervertebral foramina of lumbar region Ⓐ
- M99.74 Connective tissue and disc stenosis of intervertebral foramina of sacral region Ⓐ
- M99.75 Connective tissue and disc stenosis of intervertebral foramina of pelvic region Ⓐ
- M99.76 Connective tissue and disc stenosis of intervertebral foramina of lower extremity Ⓐ

EXCLUDES 1 Not coded here   *EXCLUDES 2* Not included here   Ⓝ Newborn Age: 0   Ⓟ Pediatric Age: 0-17   Ⓜ Maternity Age: 12-55   Ⓐ Adult Age: 15-124

744   ICD-10-CM 2016

M99.77   **Connective tissue and disc stenosis of**   🄰
      intervertebral foramina of upper extremity

M99.78   **Connective tissue and disc stenosis of**   🄰
      intervertebral foramina of rib cage

M99.79   **Connective tissue and disc stenosis of**   🄰
      intervertebral foramina of abdomen and other
      regions

☑5ᵗʰ   **M99.8**   Other **biomechanical lesions**

M99.80   **Other biomechanical lesions of** head **region**

M99.81   **Other biomechanical lesions of** cervical **region**

M99.82   **Other biomechanical lesions of** thoracic **region**

M99.83   **Other biomechanical lesions of** lumbar **region**

M99.84   **Other biomechanical lesions of** sacral **region**

M99.85   **Other biomechanical lesions of** pelvic **region**

M99.86   **Other biomechanical lesions of** lower extremity

M99.87   **Other biomechanical lesions of** upper extremity

M99.88   **Other biomechanical lesions of** rib cage

M99.89   **Other biomechanical lesions of** abdomen and other
      regions

M99.9   **Biomechanical lesion, unspecified**

☑ Additional Character Required   ☑ˣ⁷ᵗʰ Placeholder Alert   Unspecified Dx   Other Specified Dx   Manifestation   ▶◀ Revised Text   ● New Code   ▲ Revised Code Title

Chapter 14. Diseases of Genitourinary System (NØØ–N99)

Chapter Specific Guidelines with Coding Examples

The chapter specific guidelines from the ICD-10-CM Official Guidelines for Coding and Reporting have been provided below. Along with these guidelines are coding examples, contained in the shaded boxes, that have been developed to help illustrate the coding and/or sequencing guidance found in these guidelines.

a. Chronic kidney disease

1) Stages of chronic kidney disease (CKD)

The ICD-10-CM classifies CKD based on severity. The severity of CKD is designated by stages 1-5. Stage 2, code N18.2, equates to mild CKD; stage 3, code N18.3, equates to moderate CKD; and stage 4, code N18.4, equates to severe CKD. Code N18.6, End stage renal disease (ESRD), is assigned when the provider has documented end-stage-renal disease (ESRD).

If both a stage of CKD and ESRD are documented, assign code N18.6 only.

> Stage 5 chronic kidney disease with ESRD requiring chronic dialysis
>
> **N18.6**   **End stage renal disease**
>
> **Z99.2**   **Dependence on renal dialysis**
>
> *Explanation:* The diagnostic statement indicates the patient has chronic kidney disease, documented both as stage 5 and as ESRD requiring chronic dialysis. Code N18.6 End stage renal disease (ESRD), is assigned when the provider has documented end-stage-renal disease (ESRD). If both a stage of CKD and ESRD are documented, assign code N18.6 only.

2) Chronic kidney disease and kidney transplant status

Patients who have undergone kidney transplant may still have some form of chronic kidney disease (CKD) because the kidney transplant may not fully restore kidney function. Therefore, the presence of CKD alone does not constitute a transplant complication. Assign the appropriate N18 code for the patient's stage of CKD and code Z94.Ø, Kidney transplant status. If a transplant complication such as failure or rejection or other transplant complication is documented, see section I.C.19.g for information on coding complications of a kidney transplant. If the documentation is unclear as to whether the patient has a complication of the transplant, query the provider.

> Patient with residual chronic kidney disease stage 1 after kidney transplant
>
> **N18.1**   **Chronic kidney disease, stage 1**
>
> **Z94.Ø**   **Kidney transplant status**
>
> *Explanation:* Patients who have undergone kidney transplant may still have some form of chronic kidney disease (CKD) because the kidney transplant may not fully restore kidney function. The presence of CKD alone does not constitute a transplant complication. Assign the appropriate N18 code for the patient's stage of CKD and code Z94.Ø Kidney transplant status.

3) Chronic kidney disease with other conditions

Patients with CKD may also suffer from other serious conditions, most commonly diabetes mellitus and hypertension. The sequencing of the CKD code in relationship to codes for other contributing conditions is based on the conventions in the Tabular List.

See I.C.9. Hypertensive chronic kidney disease.

See I.C.19. Chronic kidney disease and kidney transplant complications.

> Type 1 diabetic chronic kidney disease, stage 2
>
> **E1Ø.22**   **Type 1 diabetes mellitus with diabetic chronic kidney disease**
>
> **N18.2**   **Chronic kidney disease, stage 2 (mild)**
>
> *Explanation:* Patients with CKD may also suffer from other serious conditions such as diabetes mellitus. The sequencing of the CKD code in relationship to codes for other contributing conditions is based on the conventions in the Tabular List. Diabetic CKD code E1Ø.22 includes an instructional note to "Use additional code to identify stage of chronic kidney disease (N18.1–N18.6)," thus providing sequencing direction.

Chapter 14. Diseases of the Genitourinary System (N00-N99)

> EXCLUDES 2   *certain conditions originating in the perinatal period (P04-P96)*
> *certain infectious and parasitic diseases (A00-B99)*
> *complications of pregnancy, childbirth and the puerperium (O00-O9A)*
> *congenital malformations, deformations and chromosomal abnormalities (Q00-Q99)*
> *endocrine, nutritional and metabolic diseases (E00-E88)*
> *injury, poisoning and certain other consequences of external causes (S00-T88)*
> *neoplasms (C00-D49)*
> *symptoms, signs and abnormal clinical and laboratory findings, not elsewhere classified (R00-R94)*

This chapter contains the following blocks:

N00-N08	Glomerular diseases
N10-N16	Renal tubulo-interstitial diseases
N17-N19	Acute kidney failure and chronic kidney disease
N20-N23	Urolithiasis
N25-N29	Other disorders of kidney and ureter
N30-N39	Other diseases of the urinary system
N40-N53	Diseases of male genital organs
N60-N65	Disorders of breast
N70-N77	Inflammatory diseases of female pelvic organs
N80-N98	Noninflammatory disorders of female genital tract
N99	Intraoperative and postprocedural complications and disorders of genitourinary system, not elsewhere classified

Glomerular diseases (N00-N08)

Code also any associated kidney failure (N17-N19).

> EXCLUDES 1   *hypertensive chronic kidney disease (I12.-)*

✓4ᵗʰ N00   Acute nephritic syndrome
> INCLUDES   acute glomerular disease
> acute glomerulonephritis
> acute nephritis
>
> EXCLUDES 1   *acute tubulo-interstitial nephritis (N10)*
> *nephritic syndrome NOS (N05.-)*

N00.0   Acute nephritic syndrome with minor glomerular abnormality
> Acute nephritic syndrome with minimal change lesion

N00.1   Acute nephritic syndrome with focal and segmental glomerular lesions
> Acute nephritic syndrome with focal and segmental hyalinosis
> Acute nephritic syndrome with focal and segmental sclerosis
> Acute nephritic syndrome with focal glomerulonephritis

N00.2   Acute nephritic syndrome with diffuse membranous glomerulonephritis

N00.3   Acute nephritic syndrome with diffuse mesangial proliferative glomerulonephritis

N00.4   Acute nephritic syndrome with diffuse endocapillary proliferative glomerulonephritis

N00.5   Acute nephritic syndrome with diffuse mesangiocapillary glomerulonephritis
> Acute nephritic syndrome with membranoproliferative glomerulonephritis, types 1 and 3, or NOS

N00.6   Acute nephritic syndrome with dense deposit disease
> Acute nephritic syndrome with membranoproliferative glomerulonephritis, type 2

N00.7   Acute nephritic syndrome with diffuse crescentic glomerulonephritis
> Acute nephritic syndrome with extracapillary glomerulonephritis

N00.8   Acute nephritic syndrome with other morphologic changes
> Acute nephritic syndrome with proliferative glomerulonephritis NOS

N00.9   Acute nephritic syndrome with unspecified morphologic changes

✓4ᵗʰ N01   Rapidly progressive nephritic syndrome
> INCLUDES   rapidly progressive glomerular disease
> rapidly progressive glomerulonephritis
> rapidly progressive nephritis
>
> EXCLUDES 1   *nephritic syndrome NOS (N05.-)*

N01.0   Rapidly progressive nephritic syndrome with minor glomerular abnormality
> Rapidly progressive nephritic syndrome with minimal change lesion

N01.1   Rapidly progressive nephritic syndrome with focal and segmental glomerular lesions
> Rapidly progressive nephritic syndrome with focal and segmental hyalinosis
> Rapidly progressive nephritic syndrome with focal and segmental sclerosis
> Rapidly progressive nephritic syndrome with focal glomerulonephritis

N01.2   Rapidly progressive nephritic syndrome with diffuse membranous glomerulonephritis

N01.3   Rapidly progressive nephritic syndrome with diffuse mesangial proliferative glomerulonephritis

N01.4   Rapidly progressive nephritic syndrome with diffuse endocapillary proliferative glomerulonephritis

N01.5   Rapidly progressive nephritic syndrome with diffuse mesangiocapillary glomerulonephritis
> Rapidly progressive nephritic syndrome with membranoproliferative glomerulonephritis, types 1 and 3, or NOS

N01.6   Rapidly progressive nephritic syndrome with dense deposit disease
> Rapidly progressive nephritic syndrome with membranoproliferative glomerulonephritis, type 2

N01.7   Rapidly progressive nephritic syndrome with diffuse crescentic glomerulonephritis
> Rapidly progressive nephritic syndrome with extracapillary glomerulonephritis

N01.8   Rapidly progressive nephritic syndrome with other morphologic changes
> Rapidly progressive nephritic syndrome with proliferative glomerulonephritis NOS

N01.9   Rapidly progressive nephritic syndrome with unspecified morphologic changes

✓4ᵗʰ N02   Recurrent and persistent hematuria
> EXCLUDES 1   *acute cystitis with hematuria (N30.01)*
> *hematuria NOS (R31.9)*
> *hematuria not associated with specified morphologic lesions (R31.-)*

N02.0   Recurrent and persistent hematuria with minor glomerular abnormality
> Recurrent and persistent hematuria with minimal change lesion

N02.1   Recurrent and persistent hematuria with focal and segmental glomerular lesions
> Recurrent and persistent hematuria with focal and segmental hyalinosis
> Recurrent and persistent hematuria with focal and segmental sclerosis
> Recurrent and persistent hematuria with focal glomerulonephritis

N02.2   Recurrent and persistent hematuria with diffuse membranous glomerulonephritis

N02.3   Recurrent and persistent hematuria with diffuse mesangial proliferative glomerulonephritis

N02.4   Recurrent and persistent hematuria with diffuse endocapillary proliferative glomerulonephritis

N02.5   Recurrent and persistent hematuria with diffuse mesangiocapillary glomerulonephritis
> Recurrent and persistent hematuria with membranoproliferative glomerulonephritis, types 1 and 3, or NOS

N02.6   Recurrent and persistent hematuria with dense deposit disease
> Recurrent and persistent hematuria with membranoproliferative glomerulonephritis, type 2

N02.7   Recurrent and persistent hematuria with diffuse crescentic glomerulonephritis
> Recurrent and persistent hematuria with extracapillary glomerulonephritis

N02.8   Recurrent and persistent hematuria with other morphologic changes
> Recurrent and persistent hematuria with proliferative glomerulonephritis NOS

N02.9   Recurrent and persistent hematuria with unspecified morphologic changes

☑ Additional Character Required   ✓x7ᵗʰ Placeholder Alert   Unspecified Dx   Other Specified Dx   Manifestation   ►◄ Revised Text   ● New Code   ▲ Revised Code Title

ICD-10-CM 2016   **747**

☑4ᵗʰ N03   **Chronic nephritic syndrome**

     INCLUDES   chronic glomerular disease
                chronic glomerulonephritis
                chronic nephritis

     EXCLUDES 1   *chronic tubulo-interstitial nephritis (N11.-)*
                diffuse sclerosing glomerulonephritis (N05.8-)
                nephritic syndrome NOS (N05.-)

N03.0   **Chronic nephritic syndrome with minor glomerular abnormality**
     Chronic nephritic syndrome with minimal change lesion

N03.1   **Chronic nephritic syndrome with focal and segmental glomerular lesions**
     Chronic nephritic syndrome with focal and segmental hyalinosis
     Chronic nephritic syndrome with focal and segmental sclerosis
     Chronic nephritic syndrome with focal glomerulonephritis

N03.2   **Chronic nephritic syndrome with diffuse membranous glomerulonephritis**

N03.3   **Chronic nephritic syndrome with diffuse mesangial proliferative glomerulonephritis**

N03.4   **Chronic nephritic syndrome with diffuse endocapillary proliferative glomerulonephritis**

N03.5   **Chronic nephritic syndrome with diffuse mesangiocapillary glomerulonephritis**
     Chronic nephritic syndrome with membranoproliferative glomerulonephritis, types 1 and 3, or NOS

N03.6   **Chronic nephritic syndrome with dense deposit disease**
     Chronic nephritic syndrome with membranoproliferative glomerulonephritis, type 2

N03.7   **Chronic nephritic syndrome with diffuse crescentic glomerulonephritis**
     Chronic nephritic syndrome with extracapillary glomerulonephritis

N03.8   **Chronic nephritic syndrome with other morphologic changes**
     Chronic nephritic syndrome with proliferative glomerulonephritis NOS

N03.9   **Chronic nephritic syndrome with unspecified morphologic changes**

☑4ᵗʰ N04   **Nephrotic syndrome**

     INCLUDES   congenital nephrotic syndrome
                lipoid nephrosis

N04.0   **Nephrotic syndrome with minor glomerular abnormality**
     Nephrotic syndrome with minimal change lesion

N04.1   **Nephrotic syndrome with focal and segmental glomerular lesions**
     Nephrotic syndrome with focal and segmental hyalinosis
     Nephrotic syndrome with focal and segmental sclerosis
     Nephrotic syndrome with focal glomerulonephritis

N04.2   **Nephrotic syndrome with diffuse membranous glomerulonephritis**

N04.3   **Nephrotic syndrome with diffuse mesangial proliferative glomerulonephritis**

N04.4   **Nephrotic syndrome with diffuse endocapillary proliferative glomerulonephritis**

N04.5   **Nephrotic syndrome with diffuse mesangiocapillary glomerulonephritis**
     Nephrotic syndrome with membranoproliferative glomerulonephritis, types 1 and 3, or NOS

N04.6   **Nephrotic syndrome with dense deposit disease**
     Nephrotic syndrome with membranoproliferative glomerulonephritis, type 2

N04.7   **Nephrotic syndrome with diffuse crescentic glomerulonephritis**
     Nephrotic syndrome with extracapillary glomerulonephritis

N04.8   **Nephrotic syndrome with other morphologic changes**
     Nephrotic syndrome with proliferative glomerulonephritis NOS

N04.9   **Nephrotic syndrome with unspecified morphologic changes**

☑4ᵗʰ N05   **Unspecified nephritic syndrome**

     INCLUDES   glomerular disease NOS
                glomerulonephritis NOS
                nephritis NOS
                nephropathy NOS and renal disease NOS with morphological lesion specified in .0-.8

     EXCLUDES 1   *nephropathy NOS with no stated morphological lesion (N28.9)*
                renal disease NOS with no stated morphological lesion (N28.9)
                tubulo-interstitial nephritis NOS (N12)

N05.0   **Unspecified nephritic syndrome with minor glomerular abnormality**
     Unspecified nephritic syndrome with minimal change lesion

N05.1   **Unspecified nephritic syndrome with focal and segmental glomerular lesions**
     Unspecified nephritic syndrome with focal and segmental hyalinosis
     Unspecified nephritic syndrome with focal and segmental sclerosis
     Unspecified nephritic syndrome with focal glomerulonephritis

N05.2   **Unspecified nephritic syndrome with diffuse membranous glomerulonephritis**

N05.3   **Unspecified nephritic syndrome with diffuse mesangial proliferative glomerulonephritis**

N05.4   **Unspecified nephritic syndrome with diffuse endocapillary proliferative glomerulonephritis**

N05.5   **Unspecified nephritic syndrome with diffuse mesangiocapillary glomerulonephritis**
     Unspecified nephritic syndrome with membranoproliferative glomerulonephritis, types 1 and 3, or NOS

N05.6   **Unspecified nephritic syndrome with dense deposit disease**
     Unspecified nephritic syndrome with membranoproliferative glomerulonephritis, type 2

N05.7   **Unspecified nephritic syndrome with diffuse crescentic glomerulonephritis**
     Unspecified nephritic syndrome with extracapillary glomerulonephritis

N05.8   **Unspecified nephritic syndrome with other morphologic changes**
     Unspecified nephritic syndrome with proliferative glomerulonephritis NOS

N05.9   **Unspecified nephritic syndrome with unspecified morphologic changes**

☑4ᵗʰ N06   **Isolated proteinuria with specified morphological lesion**

     EXCLUDES 1   *proteinuria not associated with specific morphologic lesions (R80.0)*

N06.0   **Isolated proteinuria with minor glomerular abnormality**
     Isolated proteinuria with minimal change lesion

N06.1   **Isolated proteinuria with focal and segmental glomerular lesions**
     Isolated proteinuria with focal and segmental hyalinosis
     Isolated proteinuria with focal and segmental sclerosis
     Isolated proteinuria with focal glomerulonephritis

N06.2   **Isolated proteinuria with diffuse membranous glomerulonephritis**

N06.3   **Isolated proteinuria with diffuse mesangial proliferative glomerulonephritis**

N06.4   **Isolated proteinuria with diffuse endocapillary proliferative glomerulonephritis**

N06.5   **Isolated proteinuria with diffuse mesangiocapillary glomerulonephritis**
     Isolated proteinuria with membranoproliferative glomerulonephritis, types 1 and 3, or NOS

N06.6   **Isolated proteinuria with dense deposit disease**
     Isolated proteinuria with membranoproliferative glomerulonephritis, type 2

N06.7   **Isolated proteinuria with diffuse crescentic glomerulonephritis**
     Isolated proteinuria with extracapillary glomerulonephritis

N06.8   **Isolated proteinuria with other morphologic lesion**
     Isolated proteinuria with proliferative glomerulonephritis NOS

N06.9   **Isolated proteinuria with unspecified morphologic lesion**

☑4ᵗʰ N07   **Hereditary nephropathy, not elsewhere classified**

     EXCLUDES 2   *Alport's syndrome (Q87.81-)*
                hereditary amyloid nephropathy (E85.-)
                nail patella syndrome (Q87.2)
                non-neuropathic heredofamilial amyloidosis (E85.-)

N07.0   **Hereditary nephropathy, not elsewhere classified with minor glomerular abnormality**
     Hereditary nephropathy, not elsewhere classified with minimal change lesion

N07.1   **Hereditary nephropathy, not elsewhere classified with focal and segmental glomerular lesions**
     Hereditary nephropathy, not elsewhere classified with focal and segmental hyalinosis
     Hereditary nephropathy, not elsewhere classified with focal and segmental sclerosis
     Hereditary nephropathy, not elsewhere classified with focal glomerulonephritis

N07.2   **Hereditary nephropathy, not elsewhere classified with diffuse membranous glomerulonephritis**

N07.3   **Hereditary nephropathy, not elsewhere classified with diffuse mesangial proliferative glomerulonephritis**

EXCLUDES 1 Not coded here   **EXCLUDES 2** Not included here   **N** Newborn Age: 0   **P** Pediatric Age: 0-17   **M** Maternity Age: 12-55   **A** Adult Age: 15-124

748   ICD-10-CM 2016

NØ7.4 Hereditary nephropathy, not elsewhere classified with diffuse endocapillary proliferative glomerulonephritis

NØ7.5 Hereditary nephropathy, not elsewhere classified with diffuse mesangiocapillary glomerulonephritis
Hereditary nephropathy, not elsewhere classified with membranoproliferative glomerulonephritis, types 1 and 3, or NOS

NØ7.6 Hereditary nephropathy, not elsewhere classified with dense deposit disease
Hereditary nephropathy, not elsewhere classified with membranoproliferative glomerulonephritis, type 2

NØ7.7 Hereditary nephropathy, not elsewhere classified with diffuse crescentic glomerulonephritis
Hereditary nephropathy, not elsewhere classified with extracapillary glomerulonephritis

NØ7.8 Hereditary nephropathy, not elsewhere classified with other morphologic lesions
Hereditary nephropathy, not elsewhere classified with proliferative glomerulonephritis NOS

NØ7.9 Hereditary nephropathy, not elsewhere classified with unspecified morphologic lesions

NØ8 Glomerular disorders in diseases classified elsewhere
Glomerulonephritis
Nephritis
Nephropathy
Code first underlying disease, such as:
amyloidosis (E85.-)
congenital syphilis (A5Ø.5)
cryoglobulinemia (D89.1)
disseminated intravascular coagulation (D65)
gout (M1A.-, M1Ø.-)
microscopic polyangiitis (M31.7)
multiple myeloma (C9Ø.Ø-)
sepsis (A4Ø.Ø-A41.9)
sickle-cell disease (D57.Ø-D57.8)
EXCLUDES 1   *glomerulonephritis, nephritis and nephropathy (in):*
antiglomerular basement membrane disease (M31.Ø)
diabetes (EØ8-E13 with .21)
gonococcal (A54.21)
Goodpasture's syndrome (M31.Ø)
hemolytic-uremic syndrome (D59.3)
lupus (M32.14)
mumps (B26.83)
syphilis (A52.75)
systemic lupus erythematosus (M32.14)
Wegener's granulomatosis (M31.31)
pyelonephritis in diseases classified elsewhere (N16)
renal tubulo-interstitial disorders classified elsewhere (N16)

Renal tubulo-interstitial diseases (N1Ø-N16)

INCLUDES   pyelonephritis
EXCLUDES 1   *pyeloureteritis cystica (N28.85)*

N1Ø Acute tubulo-interstitial nephritis
Acute infectious interstitial nephritis
Acute pyelitis
Acute pyelonephritis
Hemoglobin nephrosis
Myoglobin nephrosis
Use additional code (B95-B97), to identify infectious agent

☑4ᵗʰ N11 Chronic tubulo-interstitial nephritis
INCLUDES   chronic infectious interstitial nephritis
chronic pyelitis
chronic pyelonephritis
Use additional code (B95-B97), to identify infectious agent

N11.Ø Nonobstructive reflux-associated chronic pyelonephritis
Pyelonephritis (chronic) associated with (vesicoureteral) reflux
EXCLUDES 1   *vesicoureteral reflux NOS (N13.7Ø)*

N11.1 Chronic obstructive pyelonephritis
Pyelonephritis (chronic) associated with anomaly of pelviureteric junction
Pyelonephritis (chronic) associated with anomaly of pyeloureteric junction
Pyelonephritis (chronic) associated with crossing of vessel
Pyelonephritis (chronic) associated with kinking of ureter
Pyelonephritis (chronic) associated with obstruction of ureter
Pyelonephritis (chronic) associated with stricture of pelviureteric junction
Pyelonephritis (chronic) associated with stricture of ureter
EXCLUDES 1   *calculous pyelonephritis (N2Ø.9)*
obstructive uropathy (N13.-)

N11.8 Other chronic tubulo-interstitial nephritis
Nonobstructive chronic pyelonephritis NOS

N11.9 Chronic tubulo-interstitial nephritis, unspecified
Chronic interstitial nephritis NOS
Chronic pyelitis NOS
Chronic pyelonephritis NOS

N12 Tubulo-interstitial nephritis, not specified as acute or chronic
Interstitial nephritis NOS
Pyelitis NOS
Pyelonephritis NOS
EXCLUDES 1   *calculous pyelonephritis (N2Ø.9)*

☑4ᵗʰ N13 Obstructive and reflux uropathy
EXCLUDES 2   *calculus of kidney and ureter without hydronephrosis (N2Ø.-)*
congenital obstructive defects of renal pelvis and ureter (Q62.Ø-Q62.3)
hydronephrosis with ureteropelvic junction obstruction (Q62.1)
obstructive pyelonephritis (N11.1)

N13.1 Hydronephrosis with ureteral stricture, not elsewhere classified
EXCLUDES 1   *hydronephrosis with ureteral stricture with infection (N13.6)*

N13.2 Hydronephrosis with renal and ureteral calculous obstruction
EXCLUDES 1   *hydronephrosis with renal and ureteral calculous obstruction with infection (N13.6)*

☑5ᵗʰ N13.3 Other and unspecified hydronephrosis
EXCLUDES 1   *hydronephrosis with infection (N13.6)*

    N13.3Ø Unspecified hydronephrosis

    N13.39 Other hydronephrosis

N13.4 Hydroureter
EXCLUDES 1   *congenital hydroureter (Q62.3-)*
hydroureter with infection (N13.6)
vesicoureteral-reflux with hydroureter (N13.73-)

N13.5 Crossing vessel and stricture of ureter without hydronephrosis
Kinking and stricture of ureter without hydronephrosis
EXCLUDES 1   *crossing vessel and stricture of ureter without hydronephrosis with infection (N13.6)*

N13.6 Pyonephrosis
Conditions in N13.1-N13.5 with infection
Obstructive uropathy with infection
Use additional code (B95-B97), to identify infectious agent

☑5ᵗʰ N13.7 Vesicoureteral-reflux
EXCLUDES 1   *reflux-associated pyelonephritis (N11.Ø)*

    N13.7Ø Vesicoureteral-reflux, unspecified
    Vesicoureteral-reflux NOS

    N13.71 Vesicoureteral-reflux without reflux nephropathy

    ☑6ᵗʰ N13.72 Vesicoureteral-reflux with reflux nephropathy without hydroureter

        N13.721 Vesicoureteral-reflux with reflux nephropathy without hydroureter, unilateral

        N13.722 Vesicoureteral-reflux with reflux nephropathy without hydroureter, bilateral

        N13.729 Vesicoureteral-reflux with reflux nephropathy without hydroureter, unspecified

    ☑6ᵗʰ N13.73 Vesicoureteral-reflux with reflux nephropathy with hydroureter

        N13.731 Vesicoureteral-reflux with reflux nephropathy with hydroureter, unilateral

        N13.732 Vesicoureteral-reflux with reflux nephropathy with hydroureter, bilateral

        N13.739 Vesicoureteral-reflux with reflux nephropathy with hydroureter, unspecified

N13.8 Other obstructive and reflux uropathy
Urinary tract obstruction due to specified cause
Code first, if applicable, any causal condition, such as: enlarged prostate (N4Ø.1)

N13.9 Obstructive and reflux uropathy, unspecified
Urinary tract obstruction NOS

☑4ᵗʰ N14 Drug- and heavy-metal-induced tubulo-interstitial and tubular conditions
Code first poisoning due to drug or toxin, if applicable (T36-T65 with fifth or sixth character 1-4 or 6)
Use additional code for adverse effect, if applicable, to identify drug (T36-T5Ø with fifth or sixth character 5)

N14.0 Analgesic nephropathy

☑ Additional Character Required   ☑ₓ7ᵗʰ Placeholder Alert   Unspecified Dx   Other Specified Dx   Manifestation   ►◄ Revised Text   ● New Code   ▲ Revised Code Title

ICD-10-CM 2016   749

N14.1 Nephropathy induced by other drugs, medicants and biological substances

N14.2 Nephropathy induced by unspecified drug, medicant or biological substance

N14.3 Nephropathy induced by heavy metals

N14.4 Toxic nephropathy, not elsewhere classified

✓4ᵗʰ **N15 Other renal tubulo-interstitial diseases**

N15.0 Balkan nephropathy
Balkan endemic nephropathy

N15.1 Renal and perinephric abscess

N15.8 Other specified renal tubulo-interstitial diseases

N15.9 Renal tubulo-interstitial disease, unspecified
Infection of kidney NOS
EXCLUDES 1 *urinary tract infection NOS (N39.0)*

N16 *Renal tubulo-interstitial disorders in diseases classified elsewhere*
Pyelonephritis
Tubulo-interstitial nephritis
Code first underlying disease, such as:
brucellosis (A23.0-A23.9)
cryoglobulinemia (D89.1)
glycogen storage disease (E74.0)
leukemia (C91-C95)
lymphoma (C81.0-C85.9, C96.0-C96.9)
multiple myeloma (C90.0-)
sepsis (A40.0-A41.9)
Wilson's disease (E83.0)
EXCLUDES 1 *diphtheritic pyelonephritis and tubulo-interstitial nephritis (A36.84)*
pyelonephritis and tubulo-interstitial nephritis in candidiasis (B37.49)
pyelonephritis and tubulo-interstitial nephritis in cystinosis (E72.04)
pyelonephritis and tubulo-interstitial nephritis in salmonella infection (A02.25)
pyelonephritis and tubulo-interstitial nephritis in sarcoidosis (D86.84)
pyelonephritis and tubulo-interstitial nephritis in sicca syndrome [Sjogren's] (M35.04)
pyelonephritis and tubulo-interstitial nephritis in systemic lupus erythematosus (M32.15)
pyelonephritis and tubulo-interstitial nephritis in toxoplasmosis (B58.83)
renal tubular degeneration in diabetes (E08-E13 with .29)
syphilitic pyelonephritis and tubulo-interstitial nephritis (A52.75)

Acute kidney failure and chronic kidney disease (N17-N19)

EXCLUDES 2 *congenital renal failure (P96.0)*
drug- and heavy-metal-induced tubulo-interstitial and tubular conditions (N14.-)
extrarenal uremia (R39.2)
hemolytic-uremic syndrome (D59.3)
hepatorenal syndrome (K76.7)
postpartum hepatorenal syndrome (O90.4)
posttraumatic renal failure (T79.5)
prerenal uremia (R39.2)
renal failure complicating abortion or ectopic or molar pregnancy (O00-O07, O08.4)
renal failure following labor and delivery (O90.4)
renal failure postprocedural (N99.0)

✓4ᵗʰ **N17 Acute kidney failure**
Code also associated underlying condition
EXCLUDES 1 *posttraumatic renal failure (T79.5)*
AHA: 2013, 4Q, 124

N17.0 Acute kidney failure with tubular necrosis
Acute tubular necrosis
Renal tubular necrosis
Tubular necrosis NOS

N17.1 Acute kidney failure with acute cortical necrosis
Acute cortical necrosis
Cortical necrosis NOS
Renal cortical necrosis

N17.2 Acute kidney failure with medullary necrosis
Medullary [papillary] necrosis NOS
Acute medullary [papillary] necrosis
Renal medullary [papillary] necrosis

N17.8 Other acute kidney failure

N17.9 Acute kidney failure, unspecified
Acute kidney injury (nontraumatic)
EXCLUDES 2 *traumatic kidney injury (S37.0-)*

✓4ᵗʰ **N18 Chronic kidney disease (CKD)**
Code first any associated:
diabetic chronic kidney disease (E08.22, E09.22, E10.22, E11.22, E13.22)
hypertensive chronic kidney disease (I12-, I13-)
Use additional code to identify kidney transplant status, if applicable, (Z94.0)
AHA: 2013, 1Q, 24

N18.1 Chronic kidney disease, stage 1

N18.2 Chronic kidney disease, stage 2 (mild)

N18.3 Chronic kidney disease, stage 3 (moderate)

N18.4 Chronic kidney disease, stage 4 (severe)

N18.5 Chronic kidney disease, stage 5
EXCLUDES 1 *chronic kidney disease, stage 5 requiring chronic dialysis (N18.6)*

N18.6 End stage renal disease
Chronic kidney disease requiring chronic dialysis
Use additional code to identify dialysis status (Z99.2)
AHA: 2013, 4Q, 124-125

N18.9 Chronic kidney disease, unspecified
Chronic renal disease
Chronic renal failure NOS
Chronic renal insufficiency
Chronic uremia

N19 Unspecified kidney failure
Uremia NOS
EXCLUDES 1 *acute kidney failure (N17.-)*
chronic kidney disease (N18.-)
chronic uremia (N18.9)
extrarenal uremia (R39.2)
prerenal uremia (R39.2)
renal insufficiency (acute) (N28.9)
uremia of newborn (P96.0)

Urolithiasis (N20-N23)

✓4ᵗʰ **N20 Calculus of kidney and ureter**
Calculous pyelonephritis
EXCLUDES 1 *nephrocalcinosis (E83.5)*
that with hydronephrosis (N13.2)

N20.0 Calculus of kidney
Nephrolithiasis NOS
Renal calculus
Renal stone
Staghorn calculus
Stone in kidney

N20.1 Calculus of ureter
Ureteric stone

N20.2 Calculus of kidney with calculus of ureter

N20.9 Urinary calculus, unspecified

✓4ᵗʰ **N21 Calculus of lower urinary tract**
Calculus of lower urinary tract with cystitis and urethritis

N21.0 Calculus in bladder
Calculus in diverticulum of bladder
Urinary bladder stone
EXCLUDES 2 *staghorn calculus (N20.0)*

N21.1 Calculus in urethra
EXCLUDES 2 *calculus of prostate (N42.0)*

N21.8 Other lower urinary tract calculus

N21.9 Calculus of lower urinary tract, unspecified
EXCLUDES 1 *calculus of urinary tract NOS (N20.9)*

N22 *Calculus of urinary tract in diseases classified elsewhere*
Code first underlying disease, such as:
gout (M1A.-, M10.-)
schistosomiasis (B65.0-B65.9)

N23 Unspecified renal colic

EXCLUDES 1 Not coded here   EXCLUDES 2 Not included here   N Newborn Age: 0   P Pediatric Age: 0-17   M Maternity Age: 12-55   A Adult Age: 15-124

750

ICD-10-CM 2016

Chapter 14. Diseases of Genitourinary System

N14.1–N23

Other disorders of kidney and ureter (N25-N29)

EXCLUDES 2   *disorders of kidney and ureter with urolithiasis (N20-N23)*

☑4ᵗʰ **N25 Disorders resulting from impaired renal tubular function**
    EXCLUDES 1   *metabolic disorders classifiable to E70-E88*

    N25.0 Renal osteodystrophy
        Azotemic osteodystrophy
        Phosphate-losing tubular disorders
        Renal rickets
        Renal short stature

    N25.1 Nephrogenic diabetes insipidus
        EXCLUDES 1   *diabetes insipidus NOS (E23.2)*

    ☑5ᵗʰ **N25.8 Other disorders resulting from impaired renal tubular function**

        N25.81 Secondary hyperparathyroidism of renal origin
            EXCLUDES 1   *secondary hyperparathyroidism, non-renal (E21.1)*

        N25.89 Other disorders resulting from impaired renal tubular function
            Hypokalemic nephropathy
            Lightwood-Albright syndrome
            Renal tubular acidosis NOS

    N25.9 Disorder resulting from impaired renal tubular function, unspecified

☑4ᵗʰ **N26 Unspecified contracted kidney**
    EXCLUDES 1   *contracted kidney due to hypertension (I12.-)*
                diffuse sclerosing glomerulonephritis (N05.8-)
                hypertensive nephrosclerosis (arteriolar) (arteriosclerotic) (I12.-)
                small kidney of unknown cause (N27.-)

    N26.1 Atrophy of kidney (terminal)

    N26.2 Page kidney

    N26.9 Renal sclerosis, unspecified

☑4ᵗʰ **N27 Small kidney of unknown cause**
    INCLUDES   oligonephronia

    N27.0 Small kidney, unilateral

    N27.1 Small kidney, bilateral

    N27.9 Small kidney, unspecified

☑4ᵗʰ **N28 Other disorders of kidney and ureter, not elsewhere classified**

    N28.0 Ischemia and infarction of kidney
        Renal artery embolism   Renal artery thrombosis
        Renal artery obstruction   Renal infarct
        Renal artery occlusion
        EXCLUDES 1   *atherosclerosis of renal artery (extrarenal part) (I70.1)*
                  congenital stenosis of renal artery (Q27.1)
                  Goldblatt's kidney (I70.1)

    N28.1 Cyst of kidney, acquired
        Cyst (multiple)(solitary) of kidney, acquired
        EXCLUDES 1   *cystic kidney disease (congenital) (Q61.-)*

    ☑5ᵗʰ **N28.8 Other specified disorders of kidney and ureter**
        EXCLUDES 1   *hydroureter (N13.4)*
                  ureteric stricture with hydronephrosis (N13.1)
                  ureteric stricture without hydronephrosis (N13.5)

        N28.81 Hypertrophy of kidney

        N28.82 Megaloureter

        N28.83 Nephroptosis

        N28.84 Pyelitis cystica

        N28.85 Pyeloureteritis cystica

        N28.86 Ureteritis cystica

        N28.89 Other specified disorders of kidney and ureter

    N28.9 Disorder of kidney and ureter, unspecified
        Nephropathy NOS
        Renal disease (acute) NOS
        Renal insufficiency (acute)
        EXCLUDES 1   *chronic renal insufficiency (N18.9)*
                  unspecified nephritic syndrome (N05.-)

N29 Other disorders of kidney and ureter in diseases classified elsewhere
    Code first underlying disease, such as:
        amyloidosis (E85.-)
        nephrocalcinosis (E83.5)
        schistosomiasis (B65.0-B65.9)
    EXCLUDES 1   *disorders of kidney and ureter in:*
            cystinosis (E72.0)
            gonorrhea (A54.21)
            syphilis (A52.75)
            tuberculosis (A18.11)

Other diseases of the urinary system (N30-N39)

EXCLUDES 1   *urinary infection (complicating):*
        abortion or ectopic or molar pregnancy (-O07, O08.8)
        pregnancy, childbirth and the puerperium (O23-, O75.3, O86.2-)

☑4ᵗʰ **N30 Cystitis**
    Use additional code to identify infectious agent (B95-B97)
    EXCLUDES 1   *prostatocystitis (N41.3)*

    ☑5ᵗʰ **N30.0 Acute cystitis**
        EXCLUDES 1   *irradiation cystitis (N30.4-)*
                  trigonitis (N30.3-)

        N30.00 Acute cystitis without hematuria

        N30.01 Acute cystitis with hematuria

    ☑5ᵗʰ **N30.1 Interstitial cystitis (chronic)**

        N30.10 Interstitial cystitis (chronic) without hematuria

        N30.11 Interstitial cystitis (chronic) with hematuria

    ☑5ᵗʰ **N30.2 Other chronic cystitis**

        N30.20 Other chronic cystitis without hematuria

        N30.21 Other chronic cystitis with hematuria

    ☑5ᵗʰ **N30.3 Trigonitis**
        Urethrotrigonitis

        N30.30 Trigonitis without hematuria

        N30.31 Trigonitis with hematuria

    ☑5ᵗʰ **N30.4 Irradiation cystitis**

        N30.40 Irradiation cystitis without hematuria

        N30.41 Irradiation cystitis with hematuria

    ☑5ᵗʰ **N30.8 Other cystitis**
        Abscess of bladder

        N30.80 Other cystitis without hematuria

        N30.81 Other cystitis with hematuria

    ☑5ᵗʰ **N30.9 Cystitis, unspecified**

        N30.90 Cystitis, unspecified without hematuria

        N30.91 Cystitis, unspecified with hematuria

☑4ᵗʰ **N31 Neuromuscular dysfunction of bladder, not elsewhere classified**
    Use additional code to identify any associated urinary incontinence (N39.3-N39.4-)
    EXCLUDES 1   *cord bladder NOS (G95.89)*
                  neurogenic bladder due to cauda equina syndrome (G83.4)
                  neuromuscular dysfunction due to spinal cord lesion (G95.89)

    N31.0 Uninhibited neuropathic bladder, not elsewhere classified

    N31.1 Reflex neuropathic bladder, not elsewhere classified

    N31.2 Flaccid neuropathic bladder, not elsewhere classified
        Atonic (motor) (sensory) neuropathic bladder
        Autonomous neuropathic bladder
        Nonreflex neuropathic bladder

    N31.8 Other neuromuscular dysfunction of bladder

    N31.9 Neuromuscular dysfunction of bladder, unspecified
        Neurogenic bladder dysfunction NOS

☑4ᵗʰ **N32 Other disorders of bladder**
    EXCLUDES 2   *calculus of bladder (N21.0)*
                  cystocele (N81.1-)
                  hernia or prolapse of bladder, female (N81.1-)

    N32.0 Bladder-neck obstruction
        Bladder-neck stenosis (acquired)
        EXCLUDES 1   *congenital bladder-neck obstruction (Q64.3-)*

    N32.1 Vesicointestinal fistula
        Vesicorectal fistula

    N32.2 Vesical fistula, not elsewhere classified
        EXCLUDES 1   *fistula between bladder and female genital tract (N82.0-N82.1)*

    N32.3 Diverticulum of bladder
        EXCLUDES 1   *congenital diverticulum of bladder (Q64.6)*
                  diverticulitis of bladder (N30.8-)

    ☑5ᵗʰ **N32.8 Other specified disorders of bladder**

        N32.81 Overactive bladder
            Detrusor muscle hyperactivity
            EXCLUDES 1   *frequent urination due to specified bladder condition—code to condition*

        N32.89 Other specified disorders of bladder
            Bladder hemorrhage
            Bladder hypertrophy
            Calcified bladder
            Contracted bladder

    N32.9 Bladder disorder, unspecified

☑ Additional Character Required   ✓x7ᵗʰ Placeholder Alert   Unspecified Dx   Other Specified Dx   Manifestation   ►◄ Revised Text   ● New Code   ▲ Revised Code Title

N33   **Bladder disorders in diseases classified elsewhere**
Code first underlying disease, such as:
   schistosomiasis (B65.0-B65.9)
   EXCLUDES 1   *bladder disorder in syphilis (A52.76)*
       bladder disorder in tuberculosis (A18.12)
       candidal cystitis (B37.41)
       chlamydial cystitis (A56.01)
       cystitis in gonorrhea (A54.01)
       cystitis in neurogenic bladder (N31.-)
       diphtheritic cystitis (A36.85)
       neurogenic bladder (N31.-)
       syphilitic cystitis (A52.76)
       trichomonal cystitis (A59.03)

✓4th **N34**   **Urethritis and urethral syndrome**
Use additional code (B95-B97), to identify infectious agent
   EXCLUDES 2   *Reiter's disease (M02.3-)*
       urethritis in diseases with a predominantly sexual mode of
        transmission (A50-A64)
       urethrotrigonitis (N30.3-)

  N34.0   **Urethral abscess**
    Abscess (of) Cowper's gland
    Abscess (of) Littrés gland
    Abscess (of) urethral (gland)
    Periurethral abscess
      EXCLUDES 1   *urethral caruncle (N36.2)*

  N34.1   **Nonspecific urethritis**
    Nongonococcal urethritis
    Nonvenereal urethritis

  N34.2   **Other urethritis**
    Meatitis, urethral
    Postmenopausal urethritis
    Ulcer of urethra (meatus)
    Urethritis NOS

  N34.3   **Urethral syndrome, unspecified**

✓4th **N35**   **Urethral stricture**
   EXCLUDES 1   *congenital urethral stricture (Q64.3-)*
       postprocedural urethral stricture (N99.1-)

 ✓5th **N35.0**   **Post-traumatic urethral stricture**
    Urethral stricture due to injury
      EXCLUDES 1   *postprocedural urethral stricture (N99.1-)*

   ✓6th **N35.01**   **Post-traumatic urethral stricture, male**
     N35.010   **Post-traumatic urethral stricture, male, meatal**   ♂
     N35.011   **Post-traumatic bulbous urethral stricture**
     N35.012   **Post-traumatic membranous urethral stricture**
     N35.013   **Post-traumatic anterior urethral stricture**
     N35.014   **Post-traumatic urethral stricture, male, unspecified**   ♂

   ✓6th **N35.02**   **Post-traumatic urethral stricture, female**
     N35.021   **Urethral stricture due to childbirth**   ♀
     N35.028   **Other post-traumatic urethral stricture, female**   ♀

 ✓5th **N35.1**   **Postinfective urethral stricture, not elsewhere classified**
      EXCLUDES 1   *urethral stricture associated with schistosomiasis (B65-, N29)*
        gonococcal urethral stricture (A54.01)
        syphilitic urethral stricture (A52.76)

   ✓6th **N35.11**   **Postinfective urethral stricture, not elsewhere classified, male**
     N35.111   **Postinfective urethral stricture, not elsewhere classified, male, meatal**   ♂
     N35.112   **Postinfective bulbous urethral stricture, not elsewhere classified**
     N35.113   **Postinfective membranous urethral stricture, not elsewhere classified**
     N35.114   **Postinfective anterior urethral stricture, not elsewhere classified**
     N35.119   **Postinfective urethral stricture, not elsewhere classified, male, unspecified**   ♂

    N35.12   **Postinfective urethral stricture, not elsewhere classified, female**   ♀

  N35.8   **Other urethral stricture**
      EXCLUDES 1   *postprocedural urethral stricture (N99.1-)*

  N35.9   **Urethral stricture, unspecified**

✓4th **N36**   **Other disorders of urethra**

  N36.0   **Urethral fistula**
    Urethroperineal fistula
    Urethrorectal fistula
    Urinary fistula NOS
      EXCLUDES 1   *urethroscrotal fistula (N50.8)*
        urethrovaginal fistula (N82.1)
        urethrovesicovaginal fistula (N82.1)

  N36.1   **Urethral diverticulum**

  N36.2   **Urethral caruncle**

 ✓5th **N36.4**   **Urethral functional and muscular disorders**
    Use additional code to identify associated urinary stress incontinence (N39.3)

    N36.41   **Hypermobility of urethra**
    N36.42   **Intrinsic sphincter deficiency (ISD)**
    N36.43   **Combined hypermobility of urethra and intrinsic sphincter deficiency**
    N36.44   **Muscular disorders of urethra**
      Bladder sphincter dyssynergy

  N36.5   **Urethral false passage**

  N36.8   **Other specified disorders of urethra**

  N36.9   **Urethral disorder, unspecified**

N37   **Urethral disorders in diseases classified elsewhere**
Code first underlying disease
   EXCLUDES 1   *urethritis (in):*
       candidal infection (B37.41)
       chlamydial (A56.01)
       gonorrhea (A54.01)
       syphilis (A52.76)
       trichomonal infection (A59.03)
       tuberculosis (A18.13)

✓4th **N39**   **Other disorders of urinary system**
   EXCLUDES 2   *hematuria NOS (R31.-)*
       recurrent or persistent hematuria (N02.-)
       recurrent or persistent hematuria with specified morphological lesion (N02.-)
       proteinuria NOS (R80.-)

  N39.0   **Urinary tract infection, site not specified**
    Use additional code (B95-B97), to identify infectious agent
      EXCLUDES 1   *candidiasis of urinary tract (B37.4-)*
        neonatal urinary tract infection (P39.3)
        urinary tract infection of specified site, such as:
         cystitis (N30.-)
         urethritis (N34.-)
    AHA: 2012, 4Q, 94

  N39.3   **Stress incontinence (female) (male)**
    Code also any associated overactive bladder (N32.81)
      EXCLUDES 1   *mixed incontinence (N39.46)*

 ✓5th **N39.4**   **Other specified urinary incontinence**
    Code also any associated overactive bladder (N32.81)
      EXCLUDES 1   *enuresis NOS (R32)*
        functional urinary incontinence (R39.81)
        urinary incontinence associated with cognitive impairment (R39.81)
        urinary incontinence NOS (R32)
        urinary incontinence of nonorganic origin (F98.0)

    N39.41   **Urge incontinence**
      EXCLUDES 1   *mixed incontinence (N39.46)*
    N39.42   **Incontinence without sensory awareness**
    N39.43   **Post-void dribbling**
    N39.44   **Nocturnal enuresis**
    N39.45   **Continuous leakage**
    N39.46   **Mixed incontinence**
      Urge and stress incontinence

   ✓6th **N39.49**   **Other specified urinary incontinence**
     N39.490   **Overflow incontinence**
     N39.498   **Other specified urinary incontinence**
       Reflex incontinence
       Total incontinence

  N39.8   **Other specified disorders of urinary system**

  N39.9   **Disorder of urinary system, unspecified**

EXCLUDES 1 Not coded here   EXCLUDES 2 Not included here   N Newborn Age: 0   P Pediatric Age: 0-17   M Maternity Age: 12-55   A Adult Age: 15-124

752   ICD-10-CM 2016

Diseases of male genital organs (N40-N53)

☑️4ᵗʰ N40 Enlarged prostate
Adenofibromatous hypertrophy of prostate
Benign hypertrophy of the prostate
Benign prostatic hyperplasia
Benign prostatic hypertrophy
BPH
Nodular prostate
Polyp of prostate
     EXCLUDES 1   benign neoplasms of prostate (adenoma, benign)
                       (fibroadenoma) (fibroma) (myoma) (D29.1)
     EXCLUDES 2   malignant neoplasm of prostate (C61)

N40.0 Enlarged prostate without lower urinary tract symptoms A♂
Enlarged prostate NOS
Enlarged prostate without LUTS

N40.1 Enlarged prostate with lower urinary tract symptoms A♂
Enlarged prostate with LUTS
Use additional code for associated symptoms, when specified:
    incomplete bladder emptying (R39.14)
    nocturia (R35.1)
    straining on urination (R39.16)
    urinary frequency (R35.0)
    urinary hesitancy (R39.11)
    urinary incontinence (N39.4-)
    urinary obstruction (N13.8)
    urinary retention (R33.8)
    urinary urgency (R39.15)
    weak urinary stream (R39.12)

N40.2 Nodular prostate without lower urinary tract symptoms A♂
Nodular prostate without LUTS

N40.3 Nodular prostate with lower urinary tract symptoms A♂
Use additional code for associated symptoms, when specified:
    incomplete bladder emptying (R39.14)
    nocturia (R35.1)
    straining on urination (R39.16)
    urinary frequency (R35.0)
    urinary hesitancy (R39.11)
    urinary incontinence (N39.4-)
    urinary obstruction (N13.8)
    urinary retention (R33.8)
    urinary urgency (R39.15)
    weak urinary stream (R39.12)

☑️4ᵗʰ N41 Inflammatory diseases of prostate
Use additional code (B95-B97), to identify infectious agent

N41.0 Acute prostatitis A♂
N41.1 Chronic prostatitis A♂
N41.2 Abscess of prostate A♂
N41.3 Prostatocystitis A♂
N41.4 Granulomatous prostatitis A♂
N41.8 Other inflammatory diseases of prostate A♂
N41.9 Inflammatory disease of prostate, unspecified A♂
Prostatitis NOS

☑️4ᵗʰ N42 Other and unspecified disorders of prostate

N42.0 Calculus of prostate A♂
Prostatic stone

N42.1 Congestion and hemorrhage of prostate A♂
     EXCLUDES 1   enlarged prostate (N40.-)
                 hematuria (R31.-)
                 hyperplasia of prostate (N40.-)
                 inflammatory diseases of prostate (N41.-)

N42.3 Dysplasia of prostate ♂
Prostatic intraepithelial neoplasia I (PIN I)
Prostatic intraepithelial neoplasia II (PIN II)
     EXCLUDES 1   prostatic intraepithelial neoplasia III (PIN III) (D07.5)

☑️5ᵗʰ N42.8 Other specified disorders of prostate
    N42.81 Prostatodynia syndrome A♂
      Painful prostate syndrome
    N42.82 Prostatosis syndrome A♂
    N42.83 Cyst of prostate A♂
    N42.89 Other specified disorders of prostate A♂
N42.9 Disorder of prostate, unspecified A♂

☑️4ᵗʰ N43 Hydrocele and spermatocele
     INCLUDES   hydrocele of spermatic cord, testis or tunica vaginalis
     EXCLUDES 1   congenital hydrocele (P83.5)

N43.0 Encysted hydrocele ♂
N43.1 Infected hydrocele ♂
Use additional code (B95-B97), to identify infectious agent

N43.2 Other hydrocele ♂
N43.3 Hydrocele, unspecified ♂
☑️5ᵗʰ N43.4 Spermatocele of epididymis
     Spermatic cyst
    N43.40 Spermatocele of epididymis, unspecified ♂
    N43.41 Spermatocele of epididymis, single ♂
    N43.42 Spermatocele of epididymis, multiple ♂

☑️4ᵗʰ N44 Noninflammatory disorders of testis
☑️5ᵗʰ N44.0 Torsion of testis
    N44.00 Torsion of testis, unspecified ♂
    N44.01 Extravaginal torsion of spermatic cord ♂
    N44.02 Intravaginal torsion of spermatic cord ♂
      Torsion of spermatic cord NOS
    N44.03 Torsion of appendix testis ♂
    N44.04 Torsion of appendix epididymis ♂
N44.1 Cyst of tunica albuginea testis ♂
N44.2 Benign cyst of testis ♂
N44.8 Other noninflammatory disorders of the testis ♂

☑️4ᵗʰ N45 Orchitis and epididymitis
Use additional code (B95-B97), to identify infectious agent

N45.1 Epididymitis ♂
N45.2 Orchitis ♂
N45.3 Epididymo-orchitis ♂
N45.4 Abscess of epididymis or testis ♂

☑️4ᵗʰ N46 Male infertility
     EXCLUDES 1   vasectomy status (Z98.52)

☑️5ᵗʰ N46.0 Azoospermia
Absolute male infertility
Male infertility due to germinal (cell) aplasia
Male infertility due to spermatogenic arrest (complete)
    N46.01 Organic azoospermia A♂
      Azoospermia NOS
    ☑️6ᵗʰ N46.02 Azoospermia due to extratesticular causes
      Code also associated cause
      N46.021 Azoospermia due to drug therapy A♂
      N46.022 Azoospermia due to infection A♂
      N46.023 Azoospermia due to obstruction of A♂
         efferent ducts
      N46.024 Azoospermia due to radiation A♂
      N46.025 Azoospermia due to systemic disease A♂
      N46.029 Azoospermia due to other A♂
         extratesticular causes

☑️5ᵗʰ N46.1 Oligospermia
Male infertility due to germinal cell desquamation
Male infertility due to hypospermatogenesis
Male infertility due to incomplete spermatogenic arrest
    N46.11 Organic oligospermia A♂
      Oligospermia NOS
    ☑️6ᵗʰ N46.12 Oligospermia due to extratesticular causes
      Code also associated cause
      N46.121 Oligospermia due to drug therapy A♂
      N46.122 Oligospermia due to infection A♂
      N46.123 Oligospermia due to obstruction of A♂
         efferent ducts
      N46.124 Oligospermia due to radiation A♂
      N46.125 Oligospermia due to systemic disease A♂
      N46.129 Oligospermia due to other A♂
         extratesticular causes
N46.8 Other male infertility A♂
N46.9 Male infertility, unspecified A♂

☑️4ᵗʰ N47 Disorders of prepuce
N47.0 Adherent prepuce, newborn N♂
N47.1 Phimosis ♂
N47.2 Paraphimosis ♂
N47.3 Deficient foreskin ♂
N47.4 Benign cyst of prepuce ♂
N47.5 Adhesions of prepuce and glans penis ♂
N47.6 Balanoposthitis ♂
    Use additional code (B95-B97), to identify infectious agent
     EXCLUDES 1   balanitis (N48.1)
N47.7 Other inflammatory diseases of prepuce ♂
    Use additional code (B95-B97), to identify infectious agent

---

☑️ Additional Character Required   ✓x7ᵗʰ Placeholder Alert   Unspecified Dx   Other Specified Dx   Manifestation   ▶◀ Revised Text   ● New Code   ▲ Revised Code Title

N47.8　Other disorders of prepuce ♂

✓4th N48　Other disorders of penis

N48.0　Leukoplakia of penis ♂
Balanitis xerotica obliterans
Kraurosis of penis
Lichen sclerosus of external male genital organs
EXCLUDES 1　*carcinoma in situ of penis (D07.4)*

N48.1　Balanitis ♂
Use additional code (B95-B97), to identify infectious agent
EXCLUDES 1　*amebic balanitis (A06.8)*
balanitis xerotica obliterans (N48.0)
candidal balanitis (B37.42)
gonococcal balanitis (A54.23)
herpesviral [herpes simplex] balanitis (A60.01)

✓5th N48.2　Other inflammatory disorders of penis
Use additional code (B95-B97), to identify infectious agent
EXCLUDES 1　*balanitis (N48.1)*
balanitis xerotica obliterans (N48.0)
balanoposthitis (N47.6)

N48.21　Abscess of corpus cavernosum and penis ♂
N48.22　Cellulitis of corpus cavernosum and penis ♂
N48.29　Other inflammatory disorders of penis ♂

✓5th N48.3　Priapism
Painful erection
Code first underlying cause

N48.30　Priapism, unspecified ♂
N48.31　Priapism due to trauma ♂
N48.32　*Priapism due to disease classified elsewhere* ♂
N48.33　Priapism, drug-induced ♂
N48.39　Other priapism ♂

N48.5　Ulcer of penis ♂

N48.6　Induration penis plastica A♂
Peyronie's disease
Plastic induration of penis

✓5th N48.8　Other specified disorders of penis

N48.81　Thrombosis of superficial vein of penis ♂
N48.82　Acquired torsion of penis ♂
Acquired torsion of penis NOS
EXCLUDES 1　*congenital torsion of penis (Q55.63)*
N48.83　Acquired buried penis ♂
EXCLUDES 1　*congenital hidden penis (Q55.64)*
N48.89　Other specified disorders of penis ♂

N48.9　Disorder of penis, unspecified ♂

✓4th N49　Inflammatory disorders of male genital organs, not elsewhere classified
Use additional code (B95-B97), to identify infectious agent
EXCLUDES 1　*inflammation of penis (N48.1, N48.2-)*
orchitis and epididymitis (N45.-)

N49.0　Inflammatory disorders of seminal vesicle ♂
Vesiculitis NOS

N49.1　Inflammatory disorders of spermatic cord, tunica vaginalis and vas deferens ♂
Vasitis

N49.2　Inflammatory disorders of scrotum ♂

N49.3　Fournier gangrene ♂

N49.8　Inflammatory disorders of other specified male genital organs ♂
Inflammation of multiple sites in male genital organs

N49.9　Inflammatory disorder of unspecified male genital organ ♂
Abscess of unspecified male genital organ
Boil of unspecified male genital organ
Carbuncle of unspecified male genital organ
Cellulitis of unspecified male genital organ

✓4th N50　Other and unspecified disorders of male genital organs
EXCLUDES 2　*torsion of testis (N44.0-)*

N50.0　Atrophy of testis ♂

N50.1　Vascular disorders of male genital organs ♂
Hematocele, NOS, of male genital organs
Hemorrhage of male genital organs
Thrombosis of male genital organs

N50.3　Cyst of epididymis ♂

N50.8　Other specified disorders of male genital organs ♂
Atrophy of scrotum, seminal vesicle, spermatic cord, tunica vaginalis and vas deferens
Chylocele, tunica vaginalis (nonfilarial) NOS
Edema of scrotum, seminal vesicle, spermatic cord, testis, tunica vaginalis and vas deferens
Hypertrophy of scrotum, seminal vesicle, spermatic cord, testis, tunica vaginalis and vas deferens
Stricture of spermatic cord, tunica vaginalis, and vas deferens
Ulcer of scrotum, seminal vesicle, spermatic cord, testis, tunica vaginalis and vas deferens
Urethroscrotal fistula

N50.9　Disorder of male genital organs, unspecified ♂

N51　*Disorders of male genital organs in diseases classified elsewhere* ♂
Code first underlying disease, such as:
filariasis (B74.0-B74.9)
EXCLUDES 1　*amebic balanitis (A06.8)*
candidal balanitis (B37.42)
gonococcal balanitis (A54.23)
gonococcal prostatitis (A54.22)
herpesviral [herpes simplex] balanitis (A60.01)
trichomonal prostatitis (A59.02)
tuberculous prostatitis (A18.14)

✓4th N52　Male erectile dysfunction
EXCLUDES 1　*psychogenic impotence (F52.21)*

✓5th N52.0　Vasculogenic erectile dysfunction

N52.01　Erectile dysfunction due to arterial insufficiency A♂
N52.02　Corporo-venous occlusive erectile dysfunction A♂
N52.03　Combined arterial insufficiency and corporo-venous occlusive erectile dysfunction A♂

N52.1　*Erectile dysfunction due to diseases classified elsewhere* A♂
Code first underlying disease

N52.2　Drug-induced erectile dysfunction A♂

✓5th N52.3　Post-surgical erectile dysfunction

N52.31　Erectile dysfunction following radical prostatectomy A♂
N52.32　Erectile dysfunction following radical cystectomy A♂
N52.33　Erectile dysfunction following urethral surgery A♂
N52.34　Erectile dysfunction following simple prostatectomy A♂
N52.39　Other post-surgical erectile dysfunction A♂

N52.8　Other male erectile dysfunction A♂

N52.9　Male erectile dysfunction, unspecified A♂
Impotence NOS

✓4th N53　Other male sexual dysfunction
EXCLUDES 1　*psychogenic sexual dysfunction (F52.-)*

✓5th N53.1　Ejaculatory dysfunction
EXCLUDES 1　*premature ejaculation (F52.4)*

N53.11　Retarded ejaculation A♂
N53.12　Painful ejaculation ♂
N53.13　Anejaculatory orgasm A♂
N53.14　Retrograde ejaculation A♂
N53.19　Other ejaculatory dysfunction A♂
Ejaculatory dysfunction NOS

N53.8　Other male sexual dysfunction ♂

N53.9　Unspecified male sexual dysfunction ♂

Disorders of breast (N60-N65)

EXCLUDES 1　*disorders of breast associated with childbirth (O91-O92)*

✓4th N60　Benign mammary dysplasia
INCLUDES　fibrocystic mastopathy

✓5th N60.0　Solitary cyst of breast
Cyst of breast

N60.01　Solitary cyst of right breast
N60.02　Solitary cyst of left breast
N60.09　Solitary cyst of unspecified breast

✓5th N60.1　Diffuse cystic mastopathy
Cystic breast
Fibrocystic disease of breast
EXCLUDES 1　*diffuse cystic mastopathy with epithelial proliferation (N60.3-)*

N60.11　Diffuse cystic mastopathy of right breast A
N60.12　Diffuse cystic mastopathy of left breast A

EXCLUDES 1 Not coded here　　EXCLUDES 2 Not included here　　N Newborn Age: 0　　P Pediatric Age: 0-17　　M Maternity Age: 12-55　　A Adult Age: 15-124

N60.19 **Diffuse cystic mastopathy of unspecified breast** 🅰

✓5ᵗʰ N60.2 **Fibroadenosis of breast**
Adenofibrosis of breast
EXCLUDES 2   *fibroadenoma of breast (D24.-)*

  N60.21 **Fibroadenosis of right breast**
  N60.22 **Fibroadenosis of left breast**
  N60.29 **Fibroadenosis of unspecified breast**

✓5ᵗʰ N60.3 **Fibrosclerosis of breast**
Cystic mastopathy with epithelial proliferation

  N60.31 **Fibrosclerosis of right breast**
  N60.32 **Fibrosclerosis of left breast**
  N60.39 **Fibrosclerosis of unspecified breast**

✓5ᵗʰ N60.4 **Mammary duct ectasia**

  N60.41 **Mammary duct ectasia of right breast**
  N60.42 **Mammary duct ectasia of left breast**
  N60.49 **Mammary duct ectasia of unspecified breast**

✓5ᵗʰ N60.8 **Other benign mammary dysplasias**

  N60.81 **Other benign mammary dysplasias of right breast**
  N60.82 **Other benign mammary dysplasias of left breast**
  N60.89 **Other benign mammary dysplasias of unspecified breast**

✓5ᵗʰ N60.9 **Unspecified benign mammary dysplasia**

  N60.91 **Unspecified benign mammary dysplasia of right breast**
  N60.92 **Unspecified benign mammary dysplasia of left breast**
  N60.99 **Unspecified benign mammary dysplasia of unspecified breast**

N61 **Inflammatory disorders of breast**
Abscess (acute) (chronic) (nonpuerperal) of areola
Abscess (acute) (chronic) (nonpuerperal) of breast
Carbuncle of breast
Infective mastitis (acute) (subacute) (nonpuerperal)
Mastitis (acute) (subacute) (nonpuerperal) NOS
EXCLUDES 1   *inflammatory carcinoma of breast (C50.9)*
      inflammatory disorder of breast associated with childbirth (O91.-)
      neonatal infective mastitis (P39.0)
      thrombophlebitis of breast [Mondor's disease] (I80.8)

N62 **Hypertrophy of breast**
Gynecomastia
Hypertrophy of breast NOS
Massive pubertal hypertrophy of breast
EXCLUDES 1   *breast engorgement of newborn (P83.4)*
      disproportion of reconstructed breast (N65.1)

N63 **Unspecified lump in breast**
Nodule(s) NOS in breast

✓4ᵗʰ N64 **Other disorders of breast**
EXCLUDES 2   *mechanical complication of breast prosthesis and implant (T85.4-)*

N64.0 **Fissure and fistula of nipple**

N64.1 **Fat necrosis of breast**
Fat necrosis (segmental) of breast
Code first breast necrosis due to breast graft (T85.89)

N64.2 **Atrophy of breast**

N64.3 **Galactorrhea not associated with childbirth**

N64.4 **Mastodynia**

✓5ᵗʰ N64.5 **Other signs and symptoms in breast**
EXCLUDES 2   *abnormal findings on diagnostic imaging of breast (R92.-)*

  N64.51 **Induration of breast**
  N64.52 **Nipple discharge**
      EXCLUDES 1   *abnormal findings in nipple discharge (R89.-)*
  N64.53 **Retraction of nipple**
  N64.59 **Other signs and symptoms in breast**

✓5ᵗʰ N64.8 **Other specified disorders of breast**

  N64.81 **Ptosis of breast** 🅰
      EXCLUDES 1   *ptosis of native breast in relation to reconstructed breast (N65.1)*
  N64.82 **Hypoplasia of breast** 🅰
      Micromastia
      EXCLUDES 1   *congenital absence of breast (Q83.0)*
      hypoplasia of native breast in relation to reconstructed breast (N65.1)

  N64.89 **Other specified disorders of breast**
      Galactocele
      Subinvolution of breast (postlactational)

N64.9 **Disorder of breast, unspecified**

✓4ᵗʰ N65 **Deformity and disproportion of reconstructed breast**

N65.0 **Deformity of reconstructed breast** 🅰
Contour irregularity in reconstructed breast
Excess tissue in reconstructed breast
Misshapen reconstructed breast

N65.1 **Disproportion of reconstructed breast** 🅰
Breast asymmetry between native breast and reconstructed breast
Disproportion between native breast and reconstructed breast

Inflammatory diseases of female pelvic organs (N70-N77)

EXCLUDES 1   *inflammatory diseases of female pelvic organs complicating:*
      abortion or ectopic or molar pregnancy (O00-O07, O08.0)
      pregnancy, childbirth and the puerperium (O23-, O75.3, O85, O86-)

✓4ᵗʰ N70 **Salpingitis and oophoritis**
INCLUDES   abscess (of) fallopian tube
      abscess (of) ovary
      pyosalpinx
      salpingo-oophoritis
      tubo-ovarian abscess
      tubo-ovarian inflammatory disease
Use additional code (B95-B97), to identify infectious agent
EXCLUDES 1   *gonococcal infection (A54.24)*
      tuberculous infection (A18.17)

✓5ᵗʰ N70.0 **Acute salpingitis and oophoritis**

  N70.01 **Acute salpingitis** ♀
  N70.02 **Acute oophoritis** ♀
  N70.03 **Acute salpingitis and oophoritis** ♀

✓5ᵗʰ N70.1 **Chronic salpingitis and oophoritis**
Hydrosalpinx

  N70.11 **Chronic salpingitis** ♀
  N70.12 **Chronic oophoritis** ♀
  N70.13 **Chronic salpingitis and oophoritis** ♀

✓5ᵗʰ N70.9 **Salpingitis and oophoritis, unspecified**

  N70.91 **Salpingitis, unspecified** ♀
  N70.92 **Oophoritis, unspecified** ♀
  N70.93 **Salpingitis and oophoritis, unspecified** ♀

✓4ᵗʰ N71 **Inflammatory disease of uterus, except cervix**
Endo (myo) metritis   Pyometra
Metritis   Uterine abscess
Myometritis
Use additional code (B95-B97), to identify infectious agent
EXCLUDES 1   *hyperplastic endometritis (N85.0-)*
      infection of uterus following delivery (O85, O86.-)

N71.0 **Acute inflammatory disease of uterus** ♀
N71.1 **Chronic inflammatory disease of uterus** ♀
N71.9 **Inflammatory disease of uterus, unspecified** ♀

N72 **Inflammatory disease of cervix uteri** ♀
Cervicitis (with or without erosion or ectropion)
Endocervicitis (with or without erosion or ectropion)
Exocervicitis (with or without erosion or ectropion)
Use additional code (B95-B97), to identify infectious agent
EXCLUDES 1   *erosion and ectropion of cervix without cervicitis (N86)*

✓4ᵗʰ N73 **Other female pelvic inflammatory diseases**
Use additional code (B95-B97), to identify infectious agent

N73.0 **Acute parametritis and pelvic cellulitis** ♀
Abscess of broad ligament
Abscess of parametrium
Pelvic cellulitis, female

N73.1 **Chronic parametritis and pelvic cellulitis** ♀
Any condition in N73.0 specified as chronic
EXCLUDES 1   *tuberculous parametritis and pelvic cellultis (A18.17)*

N73.2 **Unspecified parametritis and pelvic cellulitis** ♀
Any condition in N73.0 unspecified whether acute or chronic

N73.3 **Female acute pelvic peritonitis** ♀
N73.4 **Female chronic pelvic peritonitis** ♀
EXCLUDES 1   *tuberculous pelvic (female) peritonitis (A18.17)*

N73.5 **Female pelvic peritonitis, unspecified** ♀
N73.6 **Female pelvic peritoneal adhesions (postinfective)** ♀
EXCLUDES 2   *postprocedural pelvic peritoneal adhesions (N99.4)*
AHA: 2014, 1Q, 6

✓ Additional Character Required   ✓ˣ⁷ᵗʰ Placeholder Alert   Unspecified Dx   Other Specified Dx   Manifestation   ►◄ Revised Text   ● New Code   ▲ Revised Code Title

Chapter 14. Diseases of Genitourinary System

N73.8   **Other specified female pelvic inflammatory diseases** ♀

N73.9   **Female pelvic inflammatory disease, unspecified** ♀
Female pelvic infection or inflammation NOS

N74   *Female pelvic inflammatory disorders in diseases classified elsewhere* ♀
Code first underlying disease
EXCLUDES 1   chlamydial cervicitis (A56.02)
chlamydial pelvic inflammatory disease (A56.11)
gonococcal cervicitis (A54.03)
gonococcal pelvic inflammatory disease (A54.24)
herpesviral [herpes simplex] cervicitis (A60.03)
herpesviral [herpes simplex] pelvic inflammatory disease (A60.09)
syphilitic cervicitis (A52.76)
syphilitic pelvic inflammatory disease (A52.76)
trichomonal cervicitis (A59.09)
tuberculous cervicitis (A18.16)
tuberculous pelvic inflammatory disease (A18.17)

✓4th **N75**   **Diseases of Bartholin's gland**

N75.0   **Cyst** of Bartholin's gland ♀

N75.1   **Abscess** of Bartholin's gland ♀

N75.8   **Other diseases of Bartholin's gland** ♀
Bartholinitis

N75.9   **Disease of Bartholin's gland, unspecified** ♀

✓4th **N76**   **Other inflammation of vagina and vulva**
Use additional code (B95-B97), to identify infectious agent
EXCLUDES 2   senile (atrophic) vaginitis (N95.2)
vulvar vestibulitis (N94.810)

N76.0   **Acute vaginitis** ♀
Acute vulvovaginitis
Vaginitis NOS
Vulvovaginitis NOS

N76.1   **Subacute and chronic vaginitis** ♀
Chronic vulvovaginitis
Subacute vulvovaginitis

N76.2   **Acute vulvitis** ♀
Vulvitis NOS

N76.3   **Subacute and chronic vulvitis** ♀

N76.4   **Abscess of vulva** ♀
Furuncle of vulva

N76.5   **Ulceration of vagina** ♀

N76.6   **Ulceration of vulva** ♀

✓5th **N76.8**   **Other specified inflammation of vagina and vulva**

N76.81   **Mucositis (ulcerative) of vagina and vulva** ♀
Code also type of associated therapy, such as:
antineoplastic and immunosuppressive drugs (T45.1X-)
radiological procedure and radiotherapy (Y84.2)
EXCLUDES 2   gastrointestinal mucositis (ulcerative) (K92.81)
nasal mucositis (ulcerative) (J34.81)
oral mucositis (ulcerative) (K12.3-)

N76.89   **Other specified inflammation of vagina and vulva** ♀

✓4th **N77**   **Vulvovaginal ulceration and inflammation in diseases classified elsewhere**

N77.0   *Ulceration of vulva in diseases classified elsewhere* ♀
Code first underlying disease, such as:
Behçet's disease (M35.2)
EXCLUDES 1   ulceration of vulva in gonococcal infection (A54.02)
ulceration of vulva in herpesviral [herpes simplex] infection (A60.04)
ulceration of vulva in syphilis (A51.0)
ulceration of vulva in tuberculosis (A18.18)

N77.1   *Vaginitis, vulvitis and vulvovaginitis in diseases classified elsewhere* ♀
Code first underlying disease, such as:
pinworm (B80)
EXCLUDES 1   candidal vulvovaginitis (B37.3)
chlamydial vulvovaginitis (A56.02)
gonococcal vulvovaginitis (A54.02)
herpesviral [herpes simplex] vulvovaginitis (A60.04)
trichomonal vulvovaginitis (A59.01)
tuberculous vulvovaginitis (A18.18)
vulvovaginitis in early syphilis (A51.0)
vulvovaginitis in late syphilis (A52.76)

Noninflammatory disorders of female genital tract (N80-N98)

✓4th **N80**   **Endometriosis**

N80.0   **Endometriosis of** uterus ♀
Adenomyosis
EXCLUDES 1   stromal endometriosis (D39.0)

N80.1   **Endometriosis of** ovary ♀

N80.2   **Endometriosis of** fallopian tube ♀

N80.3   **Endometriosis of** pelvic peritoneum ♀

N80.4   **Endometriosis of** rectovaginal septum and vagina ♀

N80.5   **Endometriosis of** intestine ♀

N80.6   **Endometriosis in** cutaneous scar ♀

N80.8   **Other endometriosis** ♀

N80.9   **Endometriosis, unspecified** ♀

✓4th **N81**   **Female genital prolapse**
EXCLUDES 1   genital prolapse complicating pregnancy, labor or delivery (O34.5-)
prolapse and hernia of ovary and fallopian tube (N83.4)
prolapse of vaginal vault after hysterectomy (N99.3)

N81.0   **Urethrocele** ♀
EXCLUDES 1   urethrocele with cystocele (N81.1-)
urethrocele with prolapse of uterus (N81.2-N81.4)

✓5th **N81.1**   **Cystocele**
Cystocele with urethrocele
Cystourethrocele
EXCLUDES 1   cystocele with prolapse of uterus (N81.2-N81.4)

N81.10   **Cystocele, unspecified** ♀
Prolapse of (anterior) vaginal wall NOS

N81.11   **Cystocele,** midline ♀

N81.12   **Cystocele,** lateral ♀
Paravaginal cystocele

N81.2   **Incomplete** uterovaginal prolapse ♀
First degree uterine prolapse
Prolapse of cervix NOS
Second degree uterine prolapse
EXCLUDES 1   cervical stump prolaspe (N81.85)

N81.3   **Complete** uterovaginal prolapse ♀
Procidentia (uteri) NOS
Third degree uterine prolapse

N81.4   **Uterovaginal prolapse, unspecified** ♀
Prolapse of uterus NOS

N81.5   **Vaginal enterocele** ♀
EXCLUDES 1   enterocele with prolapse of uterus (N81.2-N81.4)

N81.6   **Rectocele** ♀
Prolapse of posterior vaginal wall
Use additional code for any associated fecal incontinence, if applicable (R15.-)
EXCLUDES 2   perineocele (N81.81)
rectal prolapse (K62.3)
rectocele with prolapse of uterus (N81.2-N81.4)

✓5th **N81.8**   **Other female genital prolapse**

N81.81   **Perineocele** ♀

N81.82   **Incompetence or weakening of** pubocervical tissue ♀

N81.83   **Incompetence or weakening of** rectovaginal tissue ♀

N81.84   **Pelvic muscle wasting** ♀
Disuse atrophy of pelvic muscles and anal sphincter

N81.85   **Cervical stump prolapse** ♀

N81.89   **Other female genital prolapse** ♀
Deficient perineum
Old laceration of muscles of pelvic floor

N81.9   **Female genital prolapse, unspecified** ♀

✓4th **N82**   **Fistulae involving female genital tract**
EXCLUDES 1   vesicointestinal fistulae (N32.1)

N82.0   **Vesicovaginal** fistula ♀

N82.1   **Other female urinary-genital tract fistulae** ♀
Cervicovesical fistula
Ureterovaginal fistula
Urethrovaginal fistula
Uteroureteric fistula
Uterovesical fistula

N82.2   **Fistula of vagina to** small intestine ♀

N82.3   **Fistula of vagina to** large intestine ♀
Rectovaginal fistula

EXCLUDES 1 Not coded here   **EXCLUDES 2** Not included here   N Newborn Age: 0   P Pediatric Age: 0-17   M Maternity Age: 12-55   A Adult Age: 15-124

756   ICD-10-CM 2016

N82.4　**Other female intestinal-genital tract fistulae**　♀
Intestinouterine fistula

N82.5　**Female genital tract-skin fistulae**　♀
Uterus to abdominal wall fistula
Vaginoperineal fistula

N82.8　**Other female genital tract fistulae**　♀

N82.9　**Female genital tract fistula, unspecified**　♀

✓4ᵗʰ　N83　**Noninflammatory disorders of ovary, fallopian tube and broad ligament**
EXCLUDES 2　*hydrosalpinx (N70.1-)*

N83.0　**Follicular cyst of ovary**　♀
Cyst of graafian follicle
Hemorrhagic follicular cyst (of ovary)

N83.1　**Corpus luteum cyst**　♀
Hemorrhagic corpus luteum cyst

✓5ᵗʰ　N83.2　**Other and unspecified ovarian cysts**
EXCLUDES 1　*developmental ovarian cyst (Q50.1)*
neoplastic ovarian cyst (D27.-)
polycystic ovarian syndrome (E28.2)
Stein-Leventhal syndrome (E28.2)

N83.20　**Unspecified ovarian cysts**　♀

N83.29　**Other ovarian cysts**　♀
Retention cyst of ovary
Simple cyst of ovary

✓5ᵗʰ　N83.3　**Acquired atrophy of ovary and fallopian tube**
N83.31　**Acquired atrophy of ovary**　♀
N83.32　**Acquired atrophy of fallopian tube**　♀
N83.33　**Acquired atrophy of ovary and fallopian tube**　♀

N83.4　**Prolapse and hernia of ovary and fallopian tube**　♀

✓5ᵗʰ　N83.5　**Torsion of ovary, ovarian pedicle and fallopian tube**
Torsion of accessory tube
N83.51　**Torsion of ovary and ovarian pedicle**　♀
N83.52　**Torsion of fallopian tube**　♀
Torsion of hydatid of Morgagni
N83.53　**Torsion of ovary, ovarian pedicle and fallopian tube**　♀

N83.6　**Hematosalpinx**　♀
EXCLUDES 1　*hematosalpinx (with) (in):*
hematocolpos (N89.7)
hematometra (N85.7)
tubal pregnancy (O00.1)

N83.7　**Hematoma of broad ligament**　♀

N83.8　**Other noninflammatory disorders of ovary, fallopian tube and broad ligament**　♀
Broad ligament laceration syndrome [Allen-Masters]

N83.9　**Noninflammatory disorder of ovary, fallopian tube and broad ligament, unspecified**　♀

✓4ᵗʰ　N84　**Polyp of female genital tract**
EXCLUDES 1　*adenomatous polyp (D28.-)*
placental polyp (O90.89)

N84.0　**Polyp of corpus uteri**　♀
Polyp of endometrium
Polyp of uterus NOS
EXCLUDES 1　*polypoid endometrial hyperplasia (N85.0-)*

N84.1　**Polyp of cervix uteri**　♀
Mucous polyp of cervix

N84.2　**Polyp of vagina**　♀

N84.3　**Polyp of vulva**　♀
Polyp of labia

N84.8　**Polyp of other parts of female genital tract**　♀

N84.9　**Polyp of female genital tract, unspecified**　♀

✓4ᵗʰ　N85　**Other noninflammatory disorders of uterus, except cervix**
EXCLUDES 1　*endometriosis (N80.-)*
inflammatory diseases of uterus (N71.-)
noninflammatory disorders of cervix, except malposition (N86-N88)
polyp of corpus uteri (N84.0)
uterine prolapse (N81.-)

✓5ᵗʰ　N85.0　**Endometrial hyperplasia**
N85.00　**Endometrial hyperplasia, unspecified**　♀
Hyperplasia (adenomatous) (cystic) (glandular) of endometrium
Hyperplastic endometritis

N85.01　**Benign endometrial hyperplasia**　♀
Endometrial hyperplasia (complex) (simple) without atypia

N85.02　**Endometrial intraepithelial neoplasia [EIN]**　♀
Endometrial hyperplasia with atypia
EXCLUDES 1　*malignant neoplasm of endometrium (with endometrial intraepithelial neoplasia [EIN]) (C54.1)*

N85.2　**Hypertrophy of uterus**　♀
Bulky or enlarged uterus
EXCLUDES 1　*puerperal hypertrophy of uterus (O90.89)*

N85.3　**Subinvolution of uterus**　♀
EXCLUDES 1　*puerperal subinvolution of uterus (O90.89)*

N85.4　**Malposition of uterus**　♀
Anteversion of uterus　　　Retroversion of uterus
Retroflexion of uterus
EXCLUDES 1　*malposition of uterus complicating pregnancy, labor or delivery (O34.5-, O65.5)*

N85.5　**Inversion of uterus**　♀
EXCLUDES 1　*current obstetric trauma (O71.2)*
postpartum inversion of uterus (O71.2)

N85.6　**Intrauterine synechiae**　♀

N85.7　**Hematometra**　♀
Hematosalpinx with hematometra
EXCLUDES 1　*hematometra with hematocolpos (N89.7)*

N85.8　**Other specified noninflammatory disorders of uterus**　♀
Atrophy of uterus, acquired
Fibrosis of uterus NOS

N85.9　**Noninflammatory disorder of uterus, unspecified**　♀
Disorder of uterus NOS

N86　**Erosion and ectropion of cervix uteri**　♀
Decubitus (trophic) ulcer of cervix
Eversion of cervix
EXCLUDES 1　*erosion and ectropion of cervix with cervicitis (N72)*

✓4ᵗʰ　N87　**Dysplasia of cervix uteri**
EXCLUDES 1　*abnormal results from cervical cytologic examination without histologic confirmation (R87.61-)*
carcinoma in situ of cervix uteri (D06.-)
cervical intraepithelial neoplasia III [CIN III] (D06.-)
HGSIL of cervix (R87.613)
severe dysplasia of cervix uteri (D06.-)

N87.0　**Mild cervical dysplasia**　♀
Cervical intraepithelial neoplasia I [CIN I]

N87.1　**Moderate cervical dysplasia**　♀
Cervical intraepithelial neoplasia II [CIN II]

N87.9　**Dysplasia of cervix uteri, unspecified**　♀
Anaplasia of cervix　　　Cervical dysplasia NOS
Cervical atypism

✓4ᵗʰ　N88　**Other noninflammatory disorders of cervix uteri**
EXCLUDES 2　*inflammatory disease of cervix (N72)*
polyp of cervix (N84.1)

N88.0　**Leukoplakia of cervix uteri**　♀

N88.1　**Old laceration of cervix uteri**　♀
Adhesions of cervix
EXCLUDES 1　*current obstetric trauma (O71.3)*

N88.2　**Stricture and stenosis of cervix uteri**　♀
EXCLUDES 1　*stricture and stenosis of cervix uteri complicating labor (O65.5)*

N88.3　**Incompetence of cervix uteri**　♀
Investigation and management of (suspected) cervical incompetence in a nonpregnant woman
EXCLUDES 1　*cervical incompetence complicating pregnancy (O34.3-)*

N88.4　**Hypertrophic elongation of cervix uteri**　♀

N88.8　**Other specified noninflammatory disorders of cervix uteri**　♀
EXCLUDES 1　*current obstetric trauma (O71.3)*

N88.9　**Noninflammatory disorder of cervix uteri, unspecified**　♀

✓4ᵗʰ　N89　**Other noninflammatory disorders of vagina**
EXCLUDES 1　*abnormal results from vaginal cytologic examination without histologic confirmation (R87.62-)*
carcinoma in situ of vagina (D07.2)
HGSIL of vagina (R87.623)
inflammation of vagina (N76.-)
senile (atrophic) vaginitis (N95.2)
severe dysplasia of vagina (D07.2)
trichomonal leukorrhea (A59.00)
vaginal intraepithelial neoplasia [VAIN], grade III (D07.2)

N89.0　**Mild vaginal dysplasia**　♀
Vaginal intraepithelial neoplasia [VAIN], grade I

✓　Additional Character Required　　✓ᴺ⁷ᵗʰ Placeholder Alert　　Unspecified Dx　　Other Specified Dx　　Manifestation　　▶◀ Revised Text　　● New Code　　▲ Revised Code Title

N89.1 Moderate **vaginal dysplasia**   ♀
  Vaginal intraepithelial neoplasia [VAIN], grade II

N89.3 **Dysplasia of vagina, unspecified**   ♀

N89.4 **Leukoplakia of vagina**   ♀

N89.5 **Stricture and atresia of vagina**   ♀
  Vaginal adhesions
  Vaginal stenosis
  EXCLUDES 1 *congenital atresia or stricture (Q52.4)*
        postprocedural adhesions of vagina (N99.2)

N89.6 **Tight hymenal ring**   ♀
  Rigid hymen
  Tight introitus
  EXCLUDES 1 *imperforate hymen (Q52.3)*

N89.7 **Hematocolpos**   ♀
  Hematocolpos with hematometra or hematosalpinx

N89.8 **Other specified noninflammatory disorders of vagina**   ♀
  Leukorrhea NOS
  Old vaginal laceration
  Pessary ulcer of vagina
  EXCLUDES 1 *current obstetric trauma (O70-, O71.4, O71.7-O71.8)*
        old laceration involving muscles of pelvic floor (N81.8)

N89.9 **Noninflammatory disorder of vagina, unspecified**   ♀

√4ᵗʰ N90 **Other noninflammatory disorders of vulva and perineum**
  EXCLUDES 1 *anogenital (venereal) warts (A63.0)*
        carcinoma in situ of vulva (D07.1)
        condyloma acuminatum (A63.0)
        current obstetric trauma (O70-, O71.7-O71.8)
        inflammation of vulva (N76.-)
        severe dysplasia of vulva (D07.1)
        vulvar intraepithelial neoplasm III [VIN III] (D07.1)

N90.0 Mild **vulvar dysplasia**   ♀
  Vulvar intraepithelial neoplasia [VIN], grade I

N90.1 Moderate **vulvar dysplasia**   ♀
  Vulvar intraepithelial neoplasia [VIN], grade II

N90.3 **Dysplasia of vulva, unspecified**   ♀

N90.4 **Leukoplakia of vulva**   ♀
  Dystrophy of vulva
  Kraurosis of vulva
  Lichen sclerosus of external female genital organs

N90.5 **Atrophy of vulva**   ♀
  Stenosis of vulva

N90.6 **Hypertrophy of vulva**   ♀
  Hypertrophy of labia

N90.7 **Vulvar cyst**   ♀

√5ᵗʰ N90.8 **Other specified noninflammatory disorders of vulva and perineum**

  √6ᵗʰ N90.81 **Female genital mutilation status**
    Female genital cutting status

    N90.810 **Female genital mutilation status, unspecified**   ♀
      Female genital cutting status, unspecified
      Female genital mutilation status NOS

    N90.811 **Female genital mutilation** Type I **status** ♀
      Clitorectomy status
      Female genital cutting Type I status

    N90.812 **Female genital mutilation** Type II **status** ♀
      Clitorectomy with excision of labia minora status
      Female genital cutting Type II status

    N90.813 **Female genital mutilation** Type III **status** ♀
      Female genital cutting Type III status
      Infibulation status

    N90.818 **Other female genital mutilation status**   ♀
      Female genital cutting Type IV status
      Female genital mutilation Type IV status
      Other female genital cutting status

  N90.89 **Other specified noninflammatory disorders of vulva and perineum**   ♀
    Adhesions of vulva   Hypertrophy of clitoris

N90.9 **Noninflammatory disorder of vulva and perineum, unspecified**   ♀

√4ᵗʰ N91 **Absent, scanty and rare menstruation**
  EXCLUDES 1 *ovarian dysfunction (E28.-)*

N91.0 **Primary amenorrhea**   ♀

N91.1 **Secondary amenorrhea**   ♀

N91.2 **Amenorrhea, unspecified**   ♀

N91.3 **Primary oligomenorrhea**   ♀

N91.4 **Secondary oligomenorrhea**   ♀

N91.5 **Oligomenorrhea, unspecified**   ♀
  Hypomenorrhea NOS

√4ᵗʰ N92 **Excessive, frequent and irregular menstruation**
  EXCLUDES 1 *postmenopausal bleeding (N95.0)*
        precocious puberty (menstruation) (E30.1)

N92.0 **Excessive and frequent menstruation** with regular cycle   ♀
  Heavy periods NOS
  Menorrhagia NOS
  Polymenorrhea

N92.1 **Excessive and frequent menstruation** with irregular cycle   ♀
  Irregular intermenstrual bleeding
  Irregular, shortened intervals between menstrual bleeding
  Menometrorrhagia
  Metrorrhagia

N92.2 **Excessive menstruation at puberty**   ℙ♀
  Excessive bleeding associated with onset of menstrual periods
  Pubertal menorrhagia
  Puberty bleeding

N92.3 **Ovulation bleeding**   ♀
  Regular intermenstrual bleeding

N92.4 **Excessive bleeding in the premenopausal period**   ♀
  Climacteric menorrhagia or metrorrhagia
  Menopausal menorrhagia or metrorrhagia
  Preclimacteric menorrhagia or metrorrhagia
  Premenopausal menorrhagia or metrorrhagia

N92.5 **Other specified irregular menstruation**   ♀

N92.6 **Irregular menstruation, unspecified**   ♀
  Irregular bleeding NOS
  Irregular periods NOS
  EXCLUDES 1 *irregular menstruation with:*
        lengthened intervals or scanty bleeding (N91.3-N91.5)
        shortened intervals or excessive bleeding (N92.1)

√4ᵗʰ N93 **Other abnormal uterine and vaginal bleeding**
  EXCLUDES 1 *neonatal vaginal hemorrhage (P54.6)*
        precocious puberty (menstruation) (E30.1)
        pseudomenses (P54.6)

N93.0 **Postcoital and contact bleeding**   ♀

N93.8 **Other specified abnormal uterine and vaginal bleeding**   ♀
  Dysfunctional or functional uterine or vaginal bleeding NOS

N93.9 **Abnormal uterine and vaginal bleeding, unspecified**   ♀

√4ᵗʰ N94 **Pain and other conditions associated with female genital organs and menstrual cycle**

N94.0 **Mittelschmerz**   ♀

N94.1 **Dyspareunia**   ♀
  EXCLUDES 1 *psychogenic dyspareunia (F52.6)*

N94.2 **Vaginismus**   ♀
  EXCLUDES 1 *psychogenic vaginismus (F52.5)*

N94.3 **Premenstrual tension syndrome**   ♀
  Premenstrual dysphoric disorder
  Code also associated menstrual migraine (G43.82-, G43.83-)

N94.4 **Primary dysmenorrhea**   ♀

N94.5 **Secondary dysmenorrhea**   ♀

N94.6 **Dysmenorrhea, unspecified**   ♀
  EXCLUDES 1 *psychogenic dysmenorrhea (F45.8)*

√5ᵗʰ N94.8 **Other specified conditions associated with female genital organs and menstrual cycle**

  √6ᵗʰ N94.81 **Vulvodynia**

    N94.810 **Vulvar vestibulitis**   ♀

    N94.818 **Other vulvodynia**   ♀

    N94.819 **Vulvodynia, unspecified**   ♀
      Vulvodynia NOS

  N94.89 **Other specified conditions associated with female genital organs and menstrual cycle**   ♀

N94.9 **Unspecified condition associated with female genital organs and menstrual cycle**   ♀

√4ᵗʰ N95 **Menopausal and other perimenopausal disorders**
  Menopausal and other perimenopausal disorders due to naturally occurring (age-related) menopause and perimenopause
  EXCLUDES 1 *excessive bleeding in the premenopausal period (N92.4)*
        menopausal and perimenopausal disorders due to artificial or premature menopause (E89.4-, E28.31-)
        premature menopause (E28.31-)
  EXCLUDES 2 *postmenopausal osteoporosis (M81.0-)*
        postmenopausal osteoporosis with current pathological fracture (M80.0-)
        postmenopausal urethritis (N34.2)

N95.0 **Postmenopausal bleeding**   ♀

EXCLUDES 1 Not coded here   *EXCLUDES 2* Not included here   ℕ Newborn Age: 0   ℙ Pediatric Age: 0-17   Ⓜ Maternity Age: 12-55   Ⓐ Adult Age: 15-124

N95.1 Menopausal and female climacteric states ♀
Symptoms such as flushing, sleeplessness, headache, lack of concentration, associated with natural (age-related) menopause
Use additional code for associated symptoms
EXCLUDES 1   asymptomatic menopausal state (Z78.0)
symptoms associated with artificial menopause (E89.41)
symptoms associated with premature menopause (E28.310)

N95.2 Postmenopausal atrophic vaginitis ♀
Senile (atrophic) vaginitis

N95.8 Other specified menopausal and perimenopausal disorders ♀

N95.9 Unspecified menopausal and perimenopausal disorder ♀

N96 Recurrent pregnancy loss ♀
Investigation or care in a nonpregnant woman with history of recurrent pregnancy loss
EXCLUDES 1   recurrent pregnancy loss with current pregnancy (O26.2-)

✓4ᵗʰ N97 Female infertility
INCLUDES   inability to achieve a pregnancy
sterility, female NOS
EXCLUDES 1   female infertility associated with:
hypopituitarism (E23.0)
Stein-Leventhal syndrome (E28.2)
EXCLUDES 2   incompetence of cervix uteri (N88.3)

N97.0 Female infertility associated with anovulation ♀

N97.1 Female infertility of tubal origin ♀
Female infertility associated with congenital anomaly of tube
Female infertility due to tubal block
Female infertility due to tubal occlusion
Female infertility due to tubal stenosis

N97.2 Female infertility of uterine origin ♀
Female infertility associated with congenital anomaly of uterus
Female infertility due to nonimplantation of ovum

N97.8 Female infertility of other origin ♀

N97.9 Female infertility, unspecified ♀

✓4ᵗʰ N98 Complications associated with artificial fertilization

N98.0 Infection associated with artificial insemination ♀

N98.1 Hyperstimulation of ovaries ♀
Hyperstimulation of ovaries NOS
Hyperstimulation of ovaries associated with induced ovulation

N98.2 Complications of attempted introduction of fertilized ovum following in vitro fertilization ♀

N98.3 Complications of attempted introduction of embryo in embryo transfer ♀

N98.8 Other complications associated with artificial fertilization ♀

N98.9 Complication associated with artificial fertilization, unspecified ♀

Intraoperative and postprocedural complications and disorders of genitourinary system, not elsewhere classified (N99)

✓4ᵗʰ N99 Intraoperative and postprocedural complications and disorders of genitourinary system, not elsewhere classified
EXCLUDES 2   irradiation cystitis (N30.4-)
postoophorectomy osteoporosis with current pathological fracture (M80.8-)
postoophorectomy osteoporosis without current pathological fracture (M81.8)

N99.0 Postprocedural (acute) (chronic) kidney failure
Use additional code to type of kidney disease

✓5ᵗʰ N99.1 Postprocedural urethral stricture
Postcatheterization urethral stricture

✓6ᵗʰ N99.11 Postprocedural urethral stricture, male
N99.110 Postprocedural urethral stricture, male, meatal ♂
N99.111 Postprocedural bulbous urethral stricture
N99.112 Postprocedural membranous urethral stricture
N99.113 Postprocedural anterior urethral stricture
N99.114 Postprocedural urethral stricture, male unspecified ♂

N99.12 Postprocedural urethral stricture, female ♀

N99.2 Postprocedural adhesions of vagina ♀

N99.3 Prolapse of vaginal vault after hysterectomy ♀

N99.4 Postprocedural pelvic peritoneal adhesions
EXCLUDES 2   pelvic peritoneal adhesions NOS (N73.6)
postinfective pelvic peritoneal adhesions (N73.6)

✓5ᵗʰ N99.5 Complications of stoma of urinary tract
EXCLUDES 2   mechanical complication of urinary (indwelling) catheter (T83.0-)

✓6ᵗʰ N99.51 Complication of cystostomy
N99.510 Cystostomy hemorrhage
N99.511 Cystostomy infection
N99.512 Cystostomy malfunction
N99.518 Other cystostomy complication

✓6ᵗʰ N99.52 Complication of other external stoma of urinary tract
N99.520 Hemorrhage of other external stoma of urinary tract
N99.521 Infection of other external stoma of urinary tract
N99.522 Malfunction of other external stoma of urinary tract
N99.528 Other complication of other external stoma of urinary tract

✓6ᵗʰ N99.53 Complication of other stoma of urinary tract
N99.530 Hemorrhage of other stoma of urinary tract
N99.531 Infection of other stoma of urinary tract
N99.532 Malfunction of other stoma of urinary tract
N99.538 Other complication of other stoma of urinary tract

✓5ᵗʰ N99.6 Intraoperative hemorrhage and hematoma of a genitourinary system organ or structure complicating a procedure
EXCLUDES 1   intraoperative hemorrhage and hematoma of a genitourinary system organ or structure due to accidental puncture or laceration during a procedure (N99.7-)

N99.61 Intraoperative hemorrhage and hematoma of a genitourinary system organ or structure complicating a genitourinary system procedure

N99.62 Intraoperative hemorrhage and hematoma of a genitourinary system organ or structure complicating other procedure

✓5ᵗʰ N99.7 Accidental puncture and laceration of a genitourinary system organ or structure during a procedure

N99.71 Accidental puncture and laceration of a genitourinary system organ or structure during a genitourinary system procedure

N99.72 Accidental puncture and laceration of a genitourinary system organ or structure during other procedure

✓5ᵗʰ N99.8 Other intraoperative and postprocedural complications and disorders of genitourinary system

N99.81 Other intraoperative complications of genitourinary system

✓6ᵗʰ N99.82 Postprocedural hemorrhage and hematoma of a genitourinary system organ or structure following a procedure
N99.820 Postprocedural hemorrhage and hematoma of a genitourinary system organ or structure following a genitourinary system procedure
N99.821 Postprocedural hemorrhage and hematoma of a genitourinary system organ or structure following other procedure

N99.83 Residual ovary syndrome ♀

N99.89 Other postprocedural complications and disorders of genitourinary system

---

☑ Additional Character Required   *✓x7ᵗʰ* Placeholder Alert   Unspecified Dx   Other Specified Dx   Manifestation   ▶◀ Revised Text   ● New Code   ▲ Revised Code Title

Chapter 15. Pregnancy, Childbirth, and the Puerperium (O00–O9A)

Chapter Specific Guidelines with Coding Examples

The chapter specific guidelines from the ICD-10-CM Official Guidelines for Coding and Reporting have been provided below. Along with these guidelines are coding examples, contained in the shaded boxes, that have been developed to help illustrate the coding and/or sequencing guidance found in these guidelines.

a. General rules for obstetric cases

1) Codes from chapter 15 and sequencing priority

Obstetric cases require codes from chapter 15, codes in the range O00-O9A, Pregnancy, Childbirth, and the Puerperium. Chapter 15 codes have sequencing priority over codes from other chapters. Additional codes from other chapters may be used in conjunction with chapter 15 codes to further specify conditions. Should the provider document that the pregnancy is incidental to the encounter, then code Z33.1, Pregnant state, incidental, should be used in place of any chapter 15 codes. It is the provider's responsibility to state that the condition being treated is not affecting the pregnancy.

> Bladder abscess in pregnant patient at 25 weeks' gestation
>
> **O23.12**   **Infections of bladder in pregnancy, second trimester**
>
> **N30.80**   **Other cystitis without hematuria**
>
> **Z3A.25**   **25 weeks gestation of pregnancy**
>
> *Explanation:* The documentation does not indicate that the pregnancy is incidental or in any way unaffected by the bladder abscess; therefore, an obstetrics code should be sequenced first. An additional code was provided to identify the specific bladder condition as this information is not called out specifically in the obstetrics code.

2) Chapter 15 codes used only on the maternal record

Chapter 15 codes are to be used only on the maternal record, <u>never</u> on the record of the newborn.

3) Final character for trimester

The majority of codes in Chapter 15 have a final character indicating the trimester of pregnancy. The timeframes for the trimesters are indicated at the beginning of the chapter. If trimester is not a component of a code, it is because the condition always occurs in a specific trimester, or the concept of trimester of pregnancy is not applicable. Certain codes have characters for only certain trimesters because the condition does not occur in all trimesters, but it may occur in more than just one.

Assignment of the final character for trimester should be based on the provider's documentation of the trimester (or number of weeks) for the current admission/encounter. This applies to the assignment of trimester for pre-existing conditions as well as those that develop during or are due to the pregnancy. The provider's documentation of the number of weeks may be used to assign the appropriate code identifying the trimester.

Whenever delivery occurs during the current admission, and there is an "in childbirth" option for the obstetric complication being coded, the "in childbirth" code should be assigned.

> Pregnant patient at 21 weeks' gestation admitted with excessive vomiting
>
> **O21.2**   **Late vomiting of pregnancy**
>
> **Z3A.21**   **21 weeks gestation of pregnancy**
>
> *Explanation:* Category O21 classifies vomiting in pregnancy. Although code selection is based on whether the vomiting is before or after 20 completed weeks, these codes are not further classified by trimester. If vomiting only in the second trimester was documented, the provider should be queried for the specific week of gestation, as this will affect code selection.

4) Selection of trimester for inpatient admissions that encompass more than one trimester

In instances when a patient is admitted to a hospital for complications of pregnancy during one trimester and remains in the hospital into a subsequent trimester, the trimester character for the antepartum complication code should be assigned on the basis of the trimester when the complication developed, not the trimester of the discharge. If the condition developed prior to the current admission/encounter or represents a pre-existing condition, the trimester character for the trimester at the time of the admission/encounter should be assigned.

> Patient admitted at 27 6/7 weeks' gestation for hemorrhaging from placenta previa; three days after admission at 28 1/7 weeks' gestation, she developed gestational hypertension
>
> **O44.12**   **Placenta previa with hemorrhage, second trimester**
>
> **O13.3**   **Gestational [pregnancy-induced] hypertension without significant proteinuria, third trimester**
>
> **Z3A.27**   **27 weeks gestation of pregnancy**
>
> *Explanation:* The patient presented with hemorrhaging from placenta previa while still in her 27th week, which falls within the second trimester. The gestational hypertension did not occur until three days after admission, putting the patient in her 28th week of pregnancy or what is considered to be the third trimester. The weeks of gestation captured by a code from category Z3A should represent only the gestational weeks upon admission.

5) Unspecified trimester

Each category that includes codes for trimester has a code for "unspecified trimester." The "unspecified trimester" code should rarely be used, such as when the documentation in the record is insufficient to determine the trimester and it is not possible to obtain clarification.

6) 7th character for fetus identification

Where applicable, a 7th character is to be assigned for certain categories (O31, O32, O33.3 - O33.6, O35, O36, O40, O41, O60.1, O60.2, O64, and O69) to identify the fetus for which the complication code applies.

Assign 7th character "0":

- For single gestations
- When the documentation in the record is insufficient to determine the fetus affected and it is not possible to obtain clarification.
- When it is not possible to clinically determine which fetus is affected.

> Maternal patient with twin gestations is seen after ultrasound identifies fetus B to be in breech presentation
>
> **O32.1XX2**   **Maternal care for breech presentation, fetus 2**
>
> *Explanation:* The documentation indicates that although there are two fetuses, only one fetus is determined to be in breech presentation. Whether fetus 2 or fetus B is used, the coder can assign the seventh character of 2 to identify the second fetus as the one in breech.

b. Selection of OB principal or first-listed diagnosis

1) Routine outpatient prenatal visits

For routine outpatient prenatal visits when no complications are present, a code from category Z34, Encounter for supervision of normal pregnancy, should be used as the first-listed diagnosis. These codes should not be used in conjunction with chapter 15 codes.

2) Prenatal outpatient visits for high-risk patients

For routine prenatal outpatient visits for patients with high-risk pregnancies, a code from category O09, Supervision of high-risk pregnancy, should be used as the first-listed diagnosis. Secondary chapter 15 codes may be used in conjunction with these codes if appropriate.

3) Episodes when no delivery occurs

In episodes when no delivery occurs, the principal diagnosis should correspond to the principal complication of the pregnancy which necessitated the encounter. Should more than one complication exist, all of which are treated or monitored, any of the complications codes may be sequenced first.

4) When a delivery occurs

When a delivery occurs, the principal diagnosis should correspond to the main circumstances or complication of the delivery. In cases of cesarean delivery, the selection of the principal diagnosis should be the condition established after study that was responsible for the patient's admission. If the patient was admitted with a condition that resulted in the performance of a cesarean procedure, that condition should be selected as the principal diagnosis. If the reason for the admission/encounter was unrelated to the condition resulting in the cesarean delivery, the condition related to the reason for the admission/encounter should be selected as the principal diagnosis.

Maternal patient with diet-controlled gestational diabetes was admitted at 38 weeks' gestation in obstructed labor due to footling presentation; cesarean performed for the malpresentation

O64.8XX0	**Obstructed labor due to other malposition and malpresentation, fetus not applicable or unspecified**
O24.420	**Gestational diabetes mellitus in childbirth, diet controlled**
Z3A.38	**38 weeks gestation of pregnancy**
Z37.0	**Single live birth**

Explanation: The obstructed labor necessitated the cesarean procedure.

At 39 weeks' gestation, a maternal patient presents with hemorrhage with coagulation defect; the next day the patient goes into labor and eventually delivers via cesarean section due to arrested active phase of labor

O46.003	**Antepartum hemorrhage with coagulation defect, unspecified, third trimester**
O62.1	**Secondary uterine inertia**
Z3A.39	**39 weeks gestation of pregnancy**
Z37.0	**Single live birth**

Explanation: The patient was admitted because of the antepartum hemorrhage with coagulation defect. The arrested active phase, although the reason for the cesarean delivery, did not develop until later into the stay.

5) Outcome of delivery

A code from category Z37, Outcome of delivery, should be included on every maternal record when a delivery has occurred. These codes are not to be used on subsequent records or on the newborn record.

c. Pre-existing conditions versus conditions due to the pregnancy

Certain categories in Chapter 15 distinguish between conditions of the mother that existed prior to pregnancy (pre-existing) and those that are a direct result of pregnancy. When assigning codes from Chapter 15, it is important to assess if a condition was pre-existing prior to pregnancy or developed during or due to the pregnancy in order to assign the correct code.

Categories that do not distinguish between pre-existing and pregnancy-related conditions may be used for either. It is acceptable to use codes specifically for the puerperium with codes complicating pregnancy and childbirth if a condition arises postpartum during the delivery encounter.

d. Pre-existing hypertension in pregnancy

Category O10, Pre-existing hypertension complicating pregnancy, childbirth and the puerperium, includes codes for hypertensive heart and hypertensive chronic kidney disease. When assigning one of the O10 codes that includes hypertensive heart disease or hypertensive chronic kidney disease, it is necessary to add a secondary code from the appropriate hypertension category to specify the type of heart failure or chronic kidney disease.

See Section I.C.9. Hypertension.

e. Fetal conditions affecting the management of the mother

1) Codes from categories O35 and O36

Codes from categories O35, Maternal care for known or suspected fetal abnormality and damage, and O36, Maternal care for other fetal problems, are assigned only when the fetal condition is actually responsible for modifying the management of the mother, i.e., by requiring diagnostic studies, additional observation, special care, or termination of pregnancy. The fact that the fetal condition exists does not justify assigning a code from this series to the mother's record.

A patient is seen for spotting 15 weeks into her pregnancy; the doctors also suspect fetal hydrocephalus

O26.852	**Spotting complicating pregnancy**
Z3A.15	**15 weeks gestation of pregnancy**

Explanation: Whether the fetal hydrocephalus was suspected or confirmed, an additional code is not warranted for this condition as the documentation does not indicate that this fetal condition is in any way altering the management of the mother or complicating her pregnancy.

2) In utero surgery

In cases when surgery is performed on the fetus, a diagnosis code from category O35, Maternal care for known or suspected fetal abnormality and damage, should be assigned identifying the fetal condition. Assign the appropriate procedure code for the procedure performed.

No code from Chapter 16, the perinatal codes, should be used on the mother's record to identify fetal conditions. Surgery performed in utero on a fetus is still to be coded as an obstetric encounter.

f. HIV infection in pregnancy, childbirth and the puerperium

During pregnancy, childbirth or the puerperium, a patient admitted because of an HIV-related illness should receive a principal diagnosis from subcategory O98.7-, Human immunodeficiency [HIV] disease complicating pregnancy, childbirth and the puerperium, followed by the code(s) for the HIV-related illness(es).

Patients with asymptomatic HIV infection status admitted during pregnancy, childbirth, or the puerperium should receive codes of O98.7- and Z21, Asymptomatic human immunodeficiency virus [HIV] infection status.

A previously asymptomatic HIV patient who is 13 weeks pregnant is admitted with oral thrush

O98.711	**Human immunodeficiency virus [HIV] disease complicating pregnancy, first trimester**
B20	**Human immunodeficiency virus [HIV] disease**
B37.0	**Candidal stomatitis**
Z3A.13	**13 weeks gestation of pregnancy**

Explanation: Because oral thrush is an HIV-related condition, this patient is now considered to have HIV disease. An obstetrics code indicating that HIV is complicating the pregnancy is coded first, followed by B20 for HIV disease as well as a code for the oral thrush.

g. Diabetes mellitus in pregnancy

Diabetes mellitus is a significant complicating factor in pregnancy. Pregnant women who are diabetic should be assigned a code from category O24, Diabetes mellitus in pregnancy, childbirth, and the puerperium, first, followed by the appropriate diabetes code(s) (E08-E13) from Chapter 4.

h. Long term use of insulin

Code Z79.4, Long-term (current) use of insulin, should also be assigned if the diabetes mellitus is being treated with insulin.

i. Gestational (pregnancy induced) diabetes

Gestational (pregnancy induced) diabetes can occur during the second and third trimester of pregnancy in women who were not diabetic prior to pregnancy. Gestational diabetes can cause complications in the pregnancy similar to those of pre-existing diabetes mellitus. It also puts the woman at greater risk of developing diabetes after the pregnancy. Codes for gestational diabetes are in subcategory O24.4, Gestational diabetes mellitus. No other code from category O24, Diabetes mellitus in pregnancy, childbirth, and the puerperium, should be used with a code from O24.4.

The codes under subcategory O24.4 include diet controlled and insulin controlled. If a patient with gestational diabetes is treated with both diet and insulin, only the code for insulin-controlled is required.

Code Z79.4, Long-term (current) use of insulin, should not be assigned with codes from subcategory O24.4.

An abnormal glucose tolerance in pregnancy is assigned a code from subcategory O99.81, Abnormal glucose complicating pregnancy, childbirth, and the puerperium.

j. Sepsis and septic shock complicating abortion, pregnancy, childbirth and the puerperium

When assigning a chapter 15 code for sepsis complicating abortion, pregnancy, childbirth, and the puerperium, a code for the specific type of infection should be assigned as an additional diagnosis. If severe sepsis is present, a code from subcategory R65.2, Severe sepsis, and code(s) for associated organ dysfunction(s) should also be assigned as additional diagnoses.

Patient is seen several days after a miscarriage with sepsis; cultures return MSSA

O03.87	**Sepsis following complete or unspecified spontaneous abortion**
B95.61	**Methicillin susceptible Staphylococcus aureus infection as the cause of diseases classified elsewhere**

Explanation: The type of infection that caused this patient to become septic was methicillin susceptible *Staphylococcus aureus* (MSSA), which as a secondary code helps capture all aspects related to this patient's septic condition.

k. Puerperal sepsis

Code O85, Puerperal sepsis, should be assigned with a secondary code to identify the causal organism (e.g., for a bacterial infection, assign a code from category B95-B96, Bacterial infections in conditions classified elsewhere). A code from category A40, Streptococcal sepsis, or A41, Other sepsis, should not be used for puerperal sepsis. If applicable, use additional codes to identify severe sepsis (R65.2-) and any associated acute organ dysfunction.

l. Alcohol and tobacco use during pregnancy, childbirth and the puerperium

1) Alcohol use during pregnancy, childbirth and the puerperium

Codes under subcategory O99.31, Alcohol use complicating pregnancy, childbirth, and the puerperium, should be assigned for any pregnancy case when a mother uses alcohol during the pregnancy or postpartum. A secondary code from category F10, Alcohol related disorders, should also be assigned to identify manifestations of the alcohol use.

2) Tobacco use during pregnancy, childbirth and the puerperium

Codes under subcategory O99.33, Smoking (tobacco) complicating pregnancy, childbirth, and the puerperium, should be assigned for any pregnancy case when a mother uses any type of tobacco product during the pregnancy or postpartum. A secondary code from category F17, Nicotine dependence, should also be assigned to identify the type of nicotine dependence.

m. Poisoning, toxic effects, adverse effects and underdosing in a pregnant patient

A code from subcategory O9A.2, Injury, poisoning and certain other consequences of external causes complicating pregnancy, childbirth, and the puerperium, should be sequenced first, followed by the appropriate injury, poisoning, toxic effect, adverse effect or underdosing code, and then the additional code(s) that specifies the condition caused by the poisoning, toxic effect, adverse effect or underdosing.

See Section I.C.19. Adverse effects, poisoning, underdosing and toxic effects.

Patient admitted with accidental carbon monoxide poisoning from a gas heating implement; the patient is 18 weeks' pregnant

O9A.212	**Injury, poisoning and certain other consequences of external causes complicating pregnancy, second trimester**
T58.11XA	**Toxic effect of carbon monoxide from utility gas, accidental (unintentional), initial encounter**
Z3A.18	**18 weeks gestation of pregnancy**

Explanation: Although the carbon monoxide poisoning is the reason the patient was admitted, a code from the obstetrics chapter must be sequenced first. Chapter 15 codes have sequencing priority over codes from other chapters.

n. Normal delivery, code O80

1) Encounter for full term uncomplicated delivery

Code O80 should be assigned when a woman is admitted for a full-term normal delivery and delivers a single, healthy infant without any complications antepartum, during the delivery, or postpartum during the delivery episode. Code O80 is always a principal diagnosis. It is not to be used if any other code from chapter 15 is needed to describe a current complication of the antenatal, delivery, or perinatal period. Additional codes from other chapters may be used with code O80 if they are not related to or are in any way complicating the pregnancy.

2) Uncomplicated delivery with resolved antepartum complication

Code O80 may be used if the patient had a complication at some point during the pregnancy, but the complication is not present at the time of the admission for delivery.

Patient presents in labor at 39 weeks' gestation and delivers a healthy newborn; patient had abnormal glucose levels in her first trimester, which have since resolved

O80	**Encounter for full-term uncomplicated delivery**
Z37.0	**Single live birth**

Explanation: The abnormal glucose levels during the first trimester cannot be coded if they are not affecting the patient's current trimester. Without additional complications associated with the pregnancy, fetus, or mother, code O80 is appropriate.

3) Outcome of delivery for O80

Z37.0, Single live birth, is the only outcome of delivery code appropriate for use with O80.

o. The peripartum and postpartum periods

1) Peripartum and postpartum periods

The postpartum period begins immediately after delivery and continues for six weeks following delivery. The peripartum period is defined as the last month of pregnancy to five months postpartum.

2) Peripartum and postpartum complication

A postpartum complication is any complication occurring within the six-week period.

3) Pregnancy-related complications after 6 week period

Chapter 15 codes may also be used to describe pregnancy-related complications after the peripartum or postpartum period if the provider documents that a condition is pregnancy related.

Patient admitted for varicose veins. She had a baby boy three months ago; the varicose veins started to appear one month ago. The doctor attributes the patient's pregnancy as the cause of the varicose veins, which continue to be painful and bother the patient. She is seeking surgical relief.

O87.4	**Varicose veins of the lower extremity in the puerperium**

Explanation: Although the varicose veins occurred several months after the delivery of the newborn, the doctor attributed the varicose veins to pregnancy and therefore a code from chapter 15 is appropriate.

4) Admission for routine postpartum care following delivery outside hospital

When the mother delivers outside the hospital prior to admission and is admitted for routine postpartum care and no complications are noted, code Z39.0, Encounter for care and examination of mother immediately after delivery, should be assigned as the principal diagnosis.

5) Pregnancy associated cardiomyopathy

Pregnancy associated cardiomyopathy, code O90.3, is unique in that it may be diagnosed in the third trimester of pregnancy but may continue to progress months after delivery. For this reason, it is referred to as peripartum cardiomyopathy. Code O90.3 is only for use when the cardiomyopathy develops as a result of pregnancy in a woman who did not have pre-existing heart disease.

p. Code O94, Sequelae of complication of pregnancy, childbirth, and the puerperium

1) Code O94

Code O94, Sequelae of complication of pregnancy, childbirth, and the puerperium, is for use in those cases when an initial complication of a pregnancy develops a sequelae requiring care or treatment at a future date.

2) After the initial postpartum period

This code may be used at any time after the initial postpartum period.

3) Sequencing of code O94

This code, like all sequela codes, is to be sequenced following the code describing the sequelae of the complication.

q. Termination of pregnancy and spontaneous abortions

1) Abortion with liveborn fetus

When an attempted termination of pregnancy results in a liveborn fetus, assign code Z33.2, Encounter for elective termination of pregnancy and a code from category Z37, Outcome of Delivery.

2) Retained products of conception following an abortion

Subsequent encounters for retained products of conception following a spontaneous abortion or elective termination of pregnancy are assigned the appropriate code from category O03, Spontaneous abortion, or codes O07.4, Failed attempted termination of pregnancy without complication and Z33.2, Encounter for elective termination of pregnancy. This advice is appropriate even when the patient was discharged previously with a discharge diagnosis of complete abortion.

> Patient was seen two days ago for complete spontaneous abortion but returns today for urinary tract infection (UTI) with ultrasound showing retained products of conception
>
> **O03.38   Urinary tract infection following incomplete spontaneous abortion**
>
> *Explanation:* Although the diagnosis from the patient's previous stay indicated that the patient had a complete abortion, it is now determined that there were actually retained products of conception (POC). An abortion with retained POC is considered incomplete and in this case resulted in the patient developing a UTI.

3) Complications leading to abortion

Codes from Chapter 15 may be used as additional codes to identify any documented complications of the pregnancy in conjunction with codes in categories in O07 and O08.

r. Abuse in a pregnant patient

For suspected or confirmed cases of abuse of a pregnant patient, a code(s) from subcategories O9A.3, Physical abuse complicating pregnancy, childbirth, and the puerperium, O9A.4, Sexual abuse complicating pregnancy, childbirth, and the puerperium, and O9A.5, Psychological abuse complicating pregnancy, childbirth, and the puerperium, should be sequenced first, followed by the appropriate codes (if applicable) to identify any associated current injury due to physical abuse, sexual abuse, and the perpetrator of abuse.

See Section I.C.19. Adult and child abuse, neglect and other maltreatment.

Chapter 15. Pregnancy, Childbirth and the Puerperium (O00-O9A)

NOTE CODES FROM THIS CHAPTER ARE FOR USE ONLY ON MATERNAL RECORDS, NEVER ON NEWBORN RECORDS.

Codes from this chapter are for use for conditions related to or aggravated by the pregnancy, childbirth, or by the puerperium (maternal causes or obstetric causes).

NOTE Trimesters are counted from the first day of the last menstrual period. They are defined as follows:

1st trimester- less than 14 weeks 0 days
2nd trimester- 14 weeks 0 days to less than 28 weeks 0 days
3rd trimester- 28 weeks 0 days until delivery.

Use additional code from category Z3A, Weeks of gestation, to identify the specific week of the pregnancy

EXCLUDES1 supervision of normal pregnancy (Z34.-)
EXCLUDES2 mental and behavioral disorders associated with the puerperium (F53)
obstetrical tetanus (A34)
postpartum necrosis of pituitary gland (E23.0)
puerperal osteomalacia (M83.0)

AHA: 2014, 3Q, 17

This chapter contains the following blocks:

O00-O08	Pregnancy with abortive outcome
O09	Supervision of high risk pregnancy
O10-O16	Edema, proteinuria and hypertensive disorders in pregnancy, childbirth and the puerperium
O20-O29	Other maternal disorders predominantly related to pregnancy
O30-O48	Maternal care related to the fetus and amniotic cavity and possible delivery problems
O60-O77	Complications of labor and delivery
O80, O82	Encounter for delivery
O85-O92	Complications predominantly related to the puerperium
O94-O9A	Other obstetric conditions, not elsewhere classified

Pregnancy with abortive outcome (O00-O08)

EXCLUDES1 continuing pregnancy in multiple gestation after abortion of one fetus or more (O31.1-, O31.3-)

✓4ᵗʰ **O00 Ectopic pregnancy**
INCLUDES ruptured ectopic pregnancy
Use additional code from category O08 to identify any associated complication
AHA: 2014, 3Q, 17

O00.0 Abdominal pregnancy Ⓜ♀
EXCLUDES1 maternal care for viable fetus in abdominal pregnancy (O36.7-)

O00.1 Tubal pregnancy Ⓜ♀
Fallopian pregnancy
Rupture of (fallopian) tube due to pregnancy
Tubal abortion

O00.2 Ovarian pregnancy Ⓜ♀

O00.8 Other ectopic pregnancy Ⓜ♀
Cervical pregnancy
Cornual pregnancy
Intraligamentous pregnancy
Mural pregnancy

O00.9 Ectopic pregnancy, unspecified Ⓜ♀

✓4ᵗʰ **O01 Hydatidiform mole**
Use additional code from category O08 to identify any associated complication
EXCLUDES1 chorioadenoma (destruens) (D39.2)
malignant hydatidiform mole (D39.2)
AHA: 2014, 3Q, 17

O01.0 Classical hydatidiform mole Ⓜ♀
Complete hydatidiform mole

O01.1 Incomplete and partial hydatidiform mole Ⓜ♀

O01.9 Hydatidiform mole, unspecified Ⓜ♀
Trophoblastic disease NOS
Vesicular mole NOS

✓4ᵗʰ **O02 Other abnormal products of conception**
Use additional code from category O08 to identify any associated complication
EXCLUDES1 papyraceous fetus (O31.0-)
AHA: 2014, 3Q, 17

O02.0 Blighted ovum and nonhydatidiform mole Ⓜ♀
Carneous mole
Fleshy mole
Intrauterine mole NOS
Molar pregnancy NEC
Pathological ovum

O02.1 Missed abortion Ⓜ♀
Early fetal death, before completion of 20 weeks of gestation, with retention of dead fetus
EXCLUDES1 failed induced abortion (O07.-)
fetal death (intrauterine) (late) (O36.4)
missed abortion with blighted ovum (O02.0)
missed abortion with hydatidiform mole (O01.-)
missed abortion with nonhydatidiform (O02.0)
missed abortion with other abnormal products of conception (O02.8-)
missed delivery (O36.4)
stillbirth (P95)

✓5ᵗʰ **O02.8 Other specified abnormal products of conception**
EXCLUDES1 abnormal products of conception with blighted ovum (O02.0)
abnormal products of conception with hydatidiform mole (O01.-)
abnormal products of conception with nonhydatidiform mole (O02.0)

O02.81 Inappropriate change in quantitative human chorionic gonadotropin (hCG) in early pregnancy Ⓜ♀
Biochemical pregnancy
Chemical pregnancy
Inappropriate level of quantitative human chorionic gonadotropin (hCG) for gestational age in early pregnancy

O02.89 Other abnormal products of conception Ⓜ♀

O02.9 Abnormal product of conception, unspecified Ⓜ♀

✓4ᵗʰ **O03 Spontaneous abortion**
NOTE Incomplete abortion includes retained products of conception following spontaneous abortion
INCLUDES miscarriage

O03.0 Genital tract and pelvic infection following incomplete spontaneous abortion Ⓜ♀
Endometritis following incomplete spontaneous abortion
Oophoritis following incomplete spontaneous abortion
Parametritis following incomplete spontaneous abortion
Pelvic peritonitis following incomplete spontaneous abortion
Salpingitis following incomplete spontaneous abortion
Salpingo-oophoritis following incomplete spontaneous abortion
EXCLUDES1 sepsis following incomplete spontaneous abortion (O03.37)
urinary tract infection following incomplete spontaneous abortion (O03.38)

O03.1 Delayed or excessive hemorrhage following incomplete spontaneous abortion Ⓜ♀
Afibrinogenemia following incomplete spontaneous abortion
Defibrination syndrome following incomplete spontaneous abortion
Hemolysis following incomplete spontaneous abortion
Intravascular coagulation following incomplete spontaneous abortion

O03.2 Embolism following incomplete spontaneous abortion Ⓜ♀
Air embolism following incomplete spontaneous abortion
Amniotic fluid embolism following incomplete spontaneous abortion
Blood-clot embolism following incomplete spontaneous abortion
Embolism NOS following incomplete spontaneous abortion
Fat embolism following incomplete spontaneous abortion
Pulmonary embolism following incomplete spontaneous abortion
Pyemic embolism following incomplete spontaneous abortion
Septic or septicopyemic embolism following incomplete spontaneous abortion
Soap embolism following incomplete spontaneous abortion

✓5ᵗʰ **O03.3 Other and unspecified complications following incomplete spontaneous abortion**

O03.30 Unspecified complication following incomplete spontaneous abortion Ⓜ♀

O03.31 Shock following incomplete spontaneous abortion Ⓜ♀
Circulatory collapse following incomplete spontaneous abortion
Shock (postprocedural) following incomplete spontaneous abortion
EXCLUDES1 shock due to infection following incomplete spontaneous abortion (O03.37)

EXCLUDES1 Not coded here   **EXCLUDES2** Not included here   Ⓝ Newborn Age: 0   Ⓟ Pediatric Age: 0-17   Ⓜ Maternity Age: 12-55   Ⓐ Adult Age: 15-124

O03.32   Renal failure **following incomplete spontaneous**   Ⅿ♀ **abortion**
> Kidney failure (acute) following incomplete spontaneous abortion
> Oliguria following incomplete spontaneous abortion
> Renal shutdown following incomplete spontaneous abortion
> Renal tubular necrosis following incomplete spontaneous abortion
> Uremia following incomplete spontaneous abortion

O03.33   Metabolic disorder **following incomplete**   Ⅿ♀ **spontaneous abortion**

O03.34   Damage to pelvic organs **following incomplete**   Ⅿ♀ **spontaneous abortion**
> Laceration, perforation, tear or chemical damage of bladder following incomplete spontaneous abortion
> Laceration, perforation, tear or chemical damage of bowel following incomplete spontaneous abortion
> Laceration, perforation, tear or chemical damage of broad ligament following incomplete spontaneous abortion
> Laceration, perforation, tear or chemical damage of cervix following incomplete spontaneous abortion
> Laceration, perforation, tear or chemical damage of periurethral tissue following incomplete spontaneous abortion
> Laceration, perforation, tear or chemical damage of uterus following incomplete spontaneous abortion
> Laceration, perforation, tear or chemical damage of vagina following incomplete spontaneous abortion

O03.35   Other venous complications following incomplete spontaneous abortion   Ⅿ♀

O03.36   Cardiac arrest **following incomplete**   Ⅿ♀ **spontaneousabortion**

O03.37   Sepsis **following incomplete spontaneous**   Ⅿ♀ **abortion**
> Use additional code to identify infectious agent (B95-B97)
> Use additional code to identify severe sepsis, if applicable (R65.2-)
> **EXCLUDES 1** *septic or septicopyemic embolism following incomplete spontaneous abortion (O03.2)*

O03.38   Urinary tract infection **following incomplete**   Ⅿ♀ **spontaneous abortion**
> Cystitis following incomplete spontaneous abortion

O03.39   Incomplete spontaneous abortion with other complications   Ⅿ♀

O03.4   Incomplete **spontaneous abortion** without complication   Ⅿ♀

O03.5   Genital tract and pelvic infection **following** complete or   Ⅿ♀ unspecified **spontaneous abortion**
> Endometritis following complete or unspecified spontaneous abortion
> Oophoritis following complete or unspecified spontaneous abortion
> Parametritis following complete or unspecified spontaneous abortion
> Pelvic peritonitis following complete or unspecified spontaneous abortion
> Salpingitis following complete or unspecified spontaneous abortion
> Salpingo-oophoritis following complete or unspecified spontaneous abortion
> **EXCLUDES 1** *sepsis following complete or unspecified spontaneous abortion (O03.87)*
> *urinary tract infection following complete or unspecified spontaneous abortion (O03.88)*

O03.6   Delayed or excessive hemorrhage **following complete or**   Ⅿ♀ unspecified **spontaneous abortion**
> Afibrinogenemia following complete or unspecified spontaneous abortion
> Defibrination syndrome following complete or unspecified spontaneous abortion
> Hemolysis following complete or unspecified spontaneous abortion
> Intravascular coagulation following complete or unspecified spontaneous abortion

O03.7   Embolism **following** complete or unspecified   Ⅿ♀ **spontaneous abortion**
> Air embolism following complete or unspecified spontaneous abortion
> Amniotic fluid embolism following complete or unspecified spontaneous abortion
> Blood-clot embolism following complete or unspecified spontaneous abortion
> Embolism NOS following complete or unspecified spontaneous abortion
> Fat embolism following complete or unspecified spontaneous abortion
> Pulmonary embolism following complete or unspecified spontaneous abortion
> Pyemic embolism following complete or unspecified spontaneous abortion
> Septic or septicopyemic embolism following complete or unspecified spontaneous abortion
> Soap embolism following complete or unspecified spontaneous abortion

✓5ᵗʰ **O03.8**   Other **and unspecified** complications **following** complete or unspecified **spontaneous abortion**

O03.80   Unspecified complication following complete or   Ⅿ♀ unspecified spontaneous abortion

O03.81   Shock **following complete or unspecified**   Ⅿ♀ **spontaneous abortion**
> Circulatory collapse following complete or unspecified spontaneous abortion
> Shock (postprocedural) following complete or unspecified spontaneous abortion
> **EXCLUDES 1** *shock due to infection following complete or unspecified spontaneous abortion (O03.87)*

O03.82   Renal failure **following complete or unspecified**   Ⅿ♀ **spontaneous abortion**
> Kidney failure (acute) following complete or unspecified spontaneous abortion
> Oliguria following complete or unspecified spontaneous abortion
> Renal shutdown following complete or unspecified spontaneous abortion
> Renal tubular necrosis following complete or unspecified spontaneous abortion
> Uremia following complete or unspecified spontaneous abortion

O03.83   Metabolic **disorder following complete or**   Ⅿ♀ **unspecified spontaneous abortion**

O03.84   Damage to pelvic organs **following complete or**   Ⅿ♀ **unspecified spontaneous abortion**
> Laceration, perforation, tear or chemical damage of bladder following complete or unspecified spontaneous abortion
> Laceration, perforation, tear or chemical damage of bowel following complete or unspecified spontaneous abortion
> Laceration, perforation, tear or chemical damage of broad ligament following complete or unspecified spontaneous abortion
> Laceration, perforation, tear or chemical damage of cervix following complete or unspecified spontaneous abortion
> Laceration, perforation, tear or chemical damage of periurethral tissue following complete or unspecified spontaneous abortion
> Laceration, perforation, tear or chemical damage of uterus following complete or unspecified spontaneous abortion
> Laceration, perforation, tear or chemical damage of vagina following complete or unspecified spontaneous abortion

O03.85   Other venous complications following complete   Ⅿ♀ or unspecified spontaneous abortion

O03.86   Cardiac arrest **following complete or unspecified**   Ⅿ♀ **spontaneous abortion**

O03.87   Sepsis **following complete or unspecified**   Ⅿ♀ **spontaneous abortion**
> Use additional code to identify infectious agent (B95-B97)
> Use additional code to identify severe sepsis, if applicable (R65.2-)
> **EXCLUDES 1** *septic or septicopyemic embolism following complete or unspecified spontaneous abortion (O03.7)*

✅ Additional Character Required   **ᵛˣᵗ** Placeholder Alert   Unspecified Dx   Other Specified Dx   Manifestation   ▶◀ Revised Text   ● New Code   ▲ Revised Code Title

O03.88   **Urinary tract infection following complete or**   Ⓜ♀
     unspecified spontaneous abortion
       Cystitis following complete or unspecified
         spontaneous abortion

O03.89   **Complete or unspecified spontaneous abortion**   Ⓜ♀
     with other complications

O03.9   **Complete or unspecified spontaneous abortion** without   Ⓜ♀
  complication
     Miscarriage NOS
     Spontaneous abortion NOS

✓4ᵗʰ **O04**   **Complications following (induced) termination of pregnancy**
    INCLUDES   complications following (induced) termination of pregnancy
    EXCLUDES 1   *encounter for elective termination of pregnancy, uncomplicated*
        (Z33.2)
       failed attempted termination of pregnancy (O07.-)

O04.5   **Genital tract and pelvic infection following (induced)**   Ⓜ♀
  termination of pregnancy
     Endometritis following (induced) termination of pregnancy
     Oophoritis following (induced) termination of pregnancy
     Parametritis following (induced) termination of pregnancy
     Pelvic peritonitis following (induced) termination of pregnancy
     Salpingitis following (induced) termination of pregnancy
     Salpingo-oophoritis following (induced) termination of
       pregnancy
      EXCLUDES 1   *sepsis following (induced) termination of pregnancy*
         (O04.87)
        urinary tract infection following (induced) termination
         of pregnancy (O04.88)

O04.6   **Delayed or excessive hemorrhage following (induced)**   Ⓜ♀
  termination of pregnancy
     Afibrinogenemia following (induced) termination of pregnancy
     Defibrination syndrome following (induced) termination of
       pregnancy
     Hemolysis following (induced) termination of pregnancy
     Intravascular coagulation following (induced) termination of
       pregnancy

O04.7   **Embolism following (induced) termination of pregnancy**   Ⓜ♀
     Air embolism following (induced) termination of pregnancy
     Amniotic fluid embolism following (induced) termination of
       pregnancy
     Blood-clot embolism following (induced) termination of
       pregnancy
     Embolism NOS following (induced) termination of pregnancy
     Fat embolism following (induced) termination of pregnancy
     Pulmonary embolism following (induced) termination of
       pregnancy
     Pyemic embolism following (induced) termination of pregnancy
     Septic or septicopyemic embolism following (induced)
       termination of pregnancy
     Soap embolism following (induced) termination of pregnancy

✓5ᵗʰ **O04.8**   **(Induced) termination of pregnancy with** other **and**
  unspecified complications

O04.80   **(Induced) termination of pregnancy with**   Ⓜ♀
     unspecified complications

O04.81   **Shock following (induced) termination of**   Ⓜ♀
     pregnancy
       Circulatory collapse following (induced) termination of
         pregnancy
       Shock (postprocedural) following (induced)
         termination of pregnancy
      EXCLUDES 1   *shock due to infection following (induced)*
         termination of pregnancy (O04.87)

O04.82   **Renal failure following (induced) termination**   Ⓜ♀
     of pregnancy
       Kidney failure (acute) following (induced) termination
         of pregnancy
       Oliguria following (induced) termination of pregnancy
       Renal shutdown following (induced) termination of
         pregnancy
       Renal tubular necrosis following (induced) termination
         of pregnancy
       Uremia following (induced) termination of pregnancy

O04.83   **Metabolic disorder following (induced)**   Ⓜ♀
     termination of pregnancy

O04.84   **Damage to pelvic organs following (induced)**   Ⓜ♀
  termination of pregnancy
     Laceration, perforation, tear or chemical damage of
       bladder following (induced) termination of
       pregnancy
     Laceration, perforation, tear or chemical damage of
       bowel following (induced) termination of
       pregnancy
     Laceration, perforation, tear or chemical damage of
       broad ligament following (induced) termination
       of pregnancy
     Laceration, perforation, tear or chemical damage of
       cervix following (induced) termination of
       pregnancy
     Laceration, perforation, tear or chemical damage of
       periurethral tissue following (induced)
       termination of pregnancy
     Laceration, perforation, tear or chemical damage of
       uterus following (induced) termination of
       pregnancy
     Laceration, perforation, tear or chemical damage of
       vagina following (induced) termination of
       pregnancy

O04.85   **Other** venous **complications following (induced)**   Ⓜ♀
     termination of pregnancy

O04.86   **Cardiac arrest following (induced) termination**   Ⓜ♀
     of pregnancy

O04.87   **Sepsis following (induced) termination of**   Ⓜ♀
     pregnancy
       Use additional code to identify infectious agent
         (B95-B97)
       Use additional code to identify severe sepsis, if
         applicable (R65.2-)
      EXCLUDES 1   *septic or septicopyemic embolism following*
         (induced) termination of pregnancy
         (O04.7)

O04.88   **Urinary tract infection following (induced)**   Ⓜ♀
     termination of pregnancy
       Cystitis following (induced) termination of pregnancy

O04.89   **(Induced) termination of pregnancy with other**   Ⓜ♀
     complications

✓4ᵗʰ **O07**   **Failed attempted termination of pregnancy**
    INCLUDES   failure of attempted induction of termination of pregnancy
        incomplete elective abortion
    EXCLUDES 1   *incomplete spontaneous abortion (O03.0-)*

O07.0   **Genital tract and pelvic infection following failed**   Ⓜ♀
  attempted termination of pregnancy
     Endometritis following failed attempted termination of
       pregnancy
     Oophoritis following failed attempted termination of pregnancy
     Parametritis following failed attempted termination of
       pregnancy
     Pelvic peritonitis following failed attempted termination of
       pregnancy
     Salpingitis following failed attempted termination of pregnancy
     Salpingo-oophoritis following failed attempted termination of
       pregnancy
      EXCLUDES 1   *sepsis following failed attempted termination of*
         pregnancy (O07.37)
        urinary tract infection following failed attempted
         termination of pregnancy (O07.38)

O07.1   **Delayed or excessive hemorrhage following failed**   Ⓜ♀
  attempted termination of pregnancy
     Afibrinogenemia following failed attempted termination of
       pregnancy
     Defibrination syndrome following failed attempted termination
       of pregnancy
     Hemolysis following failed attempted termination of pregnancy
     Intravascular coagulation following failed attempted
       termination of pregnancy

EXCLUDES 1 Not coded here   EXCLUDES 2 Not included here   Ⓝ Newborn Age: 0   Ⓟ Pediatric Age: 0-17   Ⓜ Maternity Age: 12-55   Ⓐ Adult Age: 15-124

766   ICD-10-CM 2016

O07.2 **Embolism** following failed attempted termination of pregnancy   Ⓜ♀

    Air embolism following failed attempted termination of pregnancy
    Amniotic fluid embolism following failed attempted termination of pregnancy
    Blood-clot embolism following failed attempted termination of pregnancy
    Embolism NOS following failed attempted termination of pregnancy
    Fat embolism following failed attempted termination of pregnancy
    Pulmonary embolism following failed attempted termination of pregnancy
    Pyemic embolism following failed attempted termination of pregnancy
    Septic or septicopyemic embolism following failed attempted termination of pregnancy
    Soap embolism following failed attempted termination of pregnancy

✓5ᵗʰ **O07.3** **Failed attempted termination of pregnancy with** other **and** unspecified **complications**

  O07.30 **Failed attempted termination of pregnancy with unspecified complications**   Ⓜ♀

  O07.31 **Shock** following failed attempted termination of pregnancy   Ⓜ♀
      Circulatory collapse following failed attempted termination of pregnancy
      Shock (postprocedural) following failed attempted termination of pregnancy
      EXCLUDES 1 *shock due to infection following failed attempted termination of pregnancy (O07.37)*

  O07.32 **Renal failure** following failed attempted termination of pregnancy   Ⓜ♀
      Kidney failure (acute) following failed attempted termination of pregnancy
      Oliguria following failed attempted termination of pregnancy
      Renal shutdown following failed attempted termination of pregnancy
      Renal tubular necrosis following failed attempted termination of pregnancy
      Uremia following failed attempted termination of pregnancy

  O07.33 **Metabolic disorder** following failed attempted termination of pregnancy   Ⓜ♀

  O07.34 **Damage to pelvic organs** following failed attempted termination of pregnancy   Ⓜ♀
      Laceration, perforation, tear or chemical damage of bladder following failed attempted termination of pregnancy
      Laceration, perforation, tear or chemical damage of bowel following failed attempted termination of pregnancy
      Laceration, perforation, tear or chemical damage of broad ligament following failed attempted termination of pregnancy
      Laceration, perforation, tear or chemical damage of cervix following failed attempted termination of pregnancy
      Laceration, perforation, tear or chemical damage of periurethral tissue following failed attempted termination of pregnancy
      Laceration, perforation, tear or chemical damage of uterus following failed attempted termination of pregnancy
      Laceration, perforation, tear or chemical damage of vagina following failed attempted termination of pregnancy

  O07.35 **Other** venous **complications following failed attempted termination of pregnancy**   Ⓜ♀

  O07.36 **Cardiac arrest** following failed attempted termination of pregnancy   Ⓜ♀

  O07.37 **Sepsis** following failed attempted termination of pregnancy   Ⓜ♀
      Use additional code to identify infectious agent (B95-B97)
      Use additional code to identify severe sepsis, if applicable (R65.2-)
      EXCLUDES 1 *septic or septicopyemic embolism following failed attempted termination of pregnancy (O07.2)*

  O07.38 **Urinary tract infection** following failed attempted termination of pregnancy   Ⓜ♀
      Cystitis following failed attempted termination of pregnancy

  O07.39 **Failed attempted termination of pregnancy with other complications**   Ⓜ♀

O07.4 **Failed attempted termination of pregnancy** without complication   Ⓜ♀

✓4ᵗʰ **O08** **Complications following ectopic and molar** **pregnancy**
    This category is for use with categories O00-O02 to identify any associated complications

O08.0 **Genital tract and pelvic infection** following ectopic and molar pregnancy   Ⓜ♀
    Endometritis following ectopic and molar pregnancy
    Oophoritis following ectopic and molar pregnancy
    Parametritis following ectopic and molar pregnancy
    Pelvic peritonitis following ectopic and molar pregnancy
    Salpingitis following ectopic and molar pregnancy
    Salpingo-oophoritis following ectopic and molar pregnancy
    EXCLUDES 1 *sepsis following ectopic and molar pregnancy (O08.82)*
      urinary tract infection (O08.83)

O08.1 **Delayed or excessive hemorrhage** following ectopic and molar pregnancy   Ⓜ♀
    Afibrinogenemia following ectopic and molar pregnancy
    Defibrination syndrome following ectopic and molar pregnancy
    Hemolysis following ectopic and molar pregnancy
    Intravascular coagulation following ectopic and molar pregnancy
    EXCLUDES 1 *delayed or excessive hemorrhage due to incomplete abortion (O03.1)*

O08.2 **Embolism** following ectopic and molar pregnancy   Ⓜ♀
    Air embolism following ectopic and molar pregnancy
    Amniotic fluid embolism following ectopic and molar pregnancy
    Blood-clot embolism following ectopic and molar pregnancy
    Embolism NOS following ectopic and molar pregnancy
    Fat embolism following ectopic and molar pregnancy
    Pulmonary embolism following ectopic and molar pregnancy
    Pyemic embolism following ectopic and molar pregnancy
    Septic or septicopyemic embolism following ectopic and molar pregnancy
    Soap embolism following ectopic and molar pregnancy

O08.3 **Shock** following ectopic and molar pregnancy   Ⓜ♀
    Circulatory collapse following ectopic and molar pregnancy
    Shock (postprocedural) following ectopic and molar pregnancy
    EXCLUDES 1 *shock due to infection following ectopic and molar pregnancy (O08.82)*

O08.4 **Renal failure** following ectopic and molar pregnancy   Ⓜ♀
    Kidney failure (acute) following ectopic and molar pregnancy
    Oliguria following ectopic and molar pregnancy
    Renal shutdown following ectopic and molar pregnancy
    Renal tubular necrosis following ectopic and molar pregnancy
    Uremia following ectopic and molar pregnancy

O08.5 **Metabolic disorders** following an ectopic and molar pregnancy   Ⓜ♀

O08.6 **Damage to pelvic organs and tissues** following an ectopic and molar pregnancy   Ⓜ♀
    Laceration, perforation, tear or chemical damage of bladder following an ectopic and molar pregnancy
    Laceration, perforation, tear or chemical damage of bowel following an ectopic and molar pregnancy
    Laceration, perforation, tear or chemical damage of broad ligament following an ectopic and molar pregnancy
    Laceration, perforation, tear or chemical damage of cervix following an ectopic and molar pregnancy
    Laceration, perforation, tear or chemical damage of periurethral tissue following an ectopic and molar pregnancy
    Laceration, perforation, tear or chemical damage of uterus following an ectopic and molar pregnancy
    Laceration, perforation, tear or chemical damage of vagina following an ectopic and molar pregnancy

O08.7 **Other** venous **complications following an ectopic and molar pregnancy**   Ⓜ♀

☑ Additional Character Required   ✓ˣ⁷ᵗʰ Placeholder Alert   Unspecified Dx   Other Specified Dx   Manifestation   ▶◀ Revised Text   ● New Code   ▲ Revised Code Title

ICD-10-CM 2016   **767**

✓5ᵗʰ O08.8　Other complications following an ectopic and molar pregnancy

　　O08.81　Cardiac arrest following an ectopic and molar pregnancy Ⓜ♀

　　O08.82　Sepsis following ectopic and molar pregnancy Ⓜ♀
　　　　Use additional code to identify infectious agent (B95-B97)
　　　　Use additional code to identify severe sepsis, if applicable (R65.2-)
　　　　EXCLUDES 1 *septic or septicopyemic embolism following ectopic and molar pregnancy (O08.2)*

　　O08.83　Urinary tract infection following an ectopic and molar pregnancy Ⓜ♀
　　　　Cystitis following an ectopic and molar pregnancy

　　O08.89　Other complications following an ectopic and molar pregnancy Ⓜ♀

O08.9　Unspecified complication following an ectopic and molar pregnancy Ⓜ♀

Supervision of high risk pregnancy (O09)

✓4ᵗʰ O09　Supervision of high risk pregnancy

　✓5ᵗʰ O09.0　Supervision of pregnancy with history of infertility

　　O09.00　Supervision of pregnancy with history of infertility, unspecified trimester Ⓜ♀

　　O09.01　Supervision of pregnancy with history of infertility, first trimester Ⓜ♀

　　O09.02　Supervision of pregnancy with history of infertility, second trimester Ⓜ♀

　　O09.03　Supervision of pregnancy with history of infertility, third trimester Ⓜ♀

　✓5ᵗʰ O09.1　Supervision of pregnancy with history of ectopic or molar pregnancy

　　O09.10　Supervision of pregnancy with history of ectopic or molar pregnancy, unspecified trimester Ⓜ♀

　　O09.11　Supervision of pregnancy with history of ectopic or molar pregnancy, first trimester Ⓜ♀

　　O09.12　Supervision of pregnancy with history of ectopic or molar pregnancy, second trimester Ⓜ♀

　　O09.13　Supervision of pregnancy with history of ectopic or molar pregnancy, third trimester Ⓜ♀

　✓5ᵗʰ O09.2　Supervision of pregnancy with other poor reproductive or obstetric history
　　　EXCLUDES 2 *pregnancy care for patient with history of recurrent pregnancy loss (O26.2-)*

　　✓6ᵗʰ O09.21　Supervision of pregnancy with history of pre-term labor

　　　O09.211　Supervision of pregnancy with history of pre-term labor, first trimester Ⓜ♀

　　　O09.212　Supervision of pregnancy with history of pre-term labor, second trimester Ⓜ♀

　　　O09.213　Supervision of pregnancy with history of pre-term labor, third trimester Ⓜ♀

　　　O09.219　Supervision of pregnancy with history of pre-term labor, unspecified trimester Ⓜ♀

　　✓6ᵗʰ O09.29　Supervision of pregnancy with other poor reproductive or obstetric history
　　　　Supervision of pregnancy with history of neonatal death
　　　　Supervision of pregnancy with history of stillbirth

　　　O09.291　Supervision of pregnancy with other poor reproductive or obstetric history, first trimester Ⓜ♀

　　　O09.292　Supervision of pregnancy with other poor reproductive or obstetric history, second trimester Ⓜ♀

　　　O09.293　Supervision of pregnancy with other poor reproductive or obstetric history, third trimester Ⓜ♀

　　　O09.299　Supervision of pregnancy with other poor reproductive or obstetric history, unspecified trimester Ⓜ♀

　✓5ᵗʰ O09.3　Supervision of pregnancy with insufficient antenatal care
　　　Supervision of concealed pregnancy
　　　Supervision of hidden pregnancy

　　O09.30　Supervision of pregnancy with insufficient antenatal care, unspecified trimester Ⓜ♀

　　O09.31　Supervision of pregnancy with insufficient antenatal care, first trimester Ⓜ♀

　　O09.32　Supervision of pregnancy with insufficient antenatal care, second trimester Ⓜ♀

　　O09.33　Supervision of pregnancy with insufficient antenatal care, third trimester Ⓜ♀

　✓5ᵗʰ O09.4　Supervision of pregnancy with grand multiparity

　　O09.40　Supervision of pregnancy with grand multiparity, unspecified trimester Ⓜ♀

　　O09.41　Supervision of pregnancy with grand multiparity, first trimester Ⓜ♀

　　O09.42　Supervision of pregnancy with grand multiparity, second trimester Ⓜ♀

　　O09.43　Supervision of pregnancy with grand multiparity, third trimester Ⓜ♀

　✓5ᵗʰ O09.5　Supervision of elderly primigravida and multigravida
　　　Pregnancy for a female 35 years and older at expected date of delivery

　　✓6ᵗʰ O09.51　Supervision of elderly primigravida

　　　O09.511　Supervision of elderly primigravida, first trimester Ⓜ♀

　　　O09.512　Supervision of elderly primigravida, second trimester Ⓜ♀

　　　O09.513　Supervision of elderly primigravida, third trimester Ⓜ♀

　　　O09.519　Supervision of elderly primigravida, unspecified trimester Ⓜ♀

　　✓6ᵗʰ O09.52　Supervision of elderly multigravida

　　　O09.521　Supervision of elderly multigravida, first trimester Ⓜ♀

　　　O09.522　Supervision of elderly multigravida, second trimester Ⓜ♀

　　　O09.523　Supervision of elderly multigravida, third trimester Ⓜ♀

　　　O09.529　Supervision of elderly multigravida, unspecified trimester Ⓜ♀

　✓5ᵗʰ O09.6　Supervision of young primigravida and multigravida
　　　Supervision of pregnancy for a female less than 16 years old at expected date of delivery

　　✓6ᵗʰ O09.61　Supervision of young primigravida

　　　O09.611　Supervision of young primigravida, first trimester Ⓜ♀

　　　O09.612　Supervision of young primigravida, second trimester Ⓜ♀

　　　O09.613　Supervision of young primigravida, third trimester Ⓜ♀

　　　O09.619　Supervision of young primigravida, unspecified trimester Ⓜ♀

　　✓6ᵗʰ O09.62　Supervision of young multigravida

　　　O09.621　Supervision of young multigravida, first trimester Ⓜ♀

　　　O09.622　Supervision of young multigravida, second trimester Ⓜ♀

　　　O09.623　Supervision of young multigravida, third trimester Ⓜ♀

　　　O09.629　Supervision of young multigravida, unspecified trimester Ⓜ♀

　✓5ᵗʰ O09.7　Supervision of high risk pregnancy due to social problems

　　O09.70　Supervision of high risk pregnancy due to social problems, unspecified trimester Ⓜ♀

　　O09.71　Supervision of high risk pregnancy due to social problems, first trimester Ⓜ♀

　　O09.72　Supervision of high risk pregnancy due to social problems, second trimester Ⓜ♀

　　O09.73　Supervision of high risk pregnancy due to social problems, third trimester Ⓜ♀

　✓5ᵗʰ O09.8　Supervision of other high risk pregnancies

　　✓6ᵗʰ O09.81　Supervision of pregnancy resulting from assisted reproductive technology
　　　　Supervision of pregnancy resulting from in-vitro fertilization

　　　O09.811　Supervision of pregnancy resulting from assisted reproductive technology, first trimester Ⓜ♀

　　　O09.812　Supervision of pregnancy resulting from assisted reproductive technology, second trimester Ⓜ♀

EXCLUDES 1 Not coded here　　　**EXCLUDES 2** Not included here　　　Ⓝ Newborn Age: 0　　Ⓟ Pediatric Age: 0-17　　Ⓜ Maternity Age: 12-55　　Ⓐ Adult Age: 15-124

768　　ICD-10-CM 2016

O09.813   Supervision of pregnancy resulting from assisted reproductive technology, third trimester   Ⓜ♀

O09.819   **Supervision of pregnancy resulting from assisted reproductive technology, unspecified trimester**   Ⓜ♀

✓6ᵗʰ **O09.82**   Supervision of pregnancy with history of in utero procedure during previous pregnancy

     O09.821   Supervision of pregnancy with history of in utero procedure during previous pregnancy, first trimester   Ⓜ♀

     O09.822   Supervision of pregnancy with history of in utero procedure during previous pregnancy, second trimester   Ⓜ♀

     O09.823   Supervision of pregnancy with history of in utero procedure during previous pregnancy, third trimester   Ⓜ♀

     O09.829   **Supervision of pregnancy with history of in utero procedure during previous pregnancy, unspecified trimester**   Ⓜ♀

         EXCLUDES 1   *supervision of pregnancy affected by in utero procedure during current pregnancy (O35.7)*

✓6ᵗʰ **O09.89**   Supervision of other high risk pregnancies

     O09.891   **Supervision of other high risk pregnancies, first trimester**   Ⓜ♀

     O09.892   **Supervision of other high risk pregnancies, second trimester**   Ⓜ♀

     O09.893   **Supervision of other high risk pregnancies, third trimester**   Ⓜ♀

     O09.899   **Supervision of other high risk pregnancies, unspecified trimester**   Ⓜ♀

✓5ᵗʰ **O09.9**   Supervision of high risk pregnancy, unspecified

     O09.90   **Supervision of high risk pregnancy, unspecified, unspecified trimester**   Ⓜ♀

     O09.91   **Supervision of high risk pregnancy, unspecified, first trimester**   Ⓜ♀

     O09.92   **Supervision of high risk pregnancy, unspecified, second trimester**   Ⓜ♀

     O09.93   **Supervision of high risk pregnancy, unspecified, third trimester**   Ⓜ♀

Edema, proteinuria and hypertensive disorders in pregnancy, childbirth and the puerperium (O10-O16)

✓4ᵗʰ **O10**   Pre-existing hypertension complicating pregnancy, childbirth and the puerperium

     Pre-existing hypertension with pre-existing proteinuria complicating pregnancy, childbirth and the puerperium

     EXCLUDES 2   *pre-existing hypertension with superimposed pre-eclampsia complicating pregnancy, childbirth and the puerperium (O11.-)*

✓5ᵗʰ **O10.0**   Pre-existing essential hypertension complicating pregnancy, childbirth and the puerperium

     Any condition in I10 specified as a reason for obstetric care during pregnancy, childbirth or the puerperium

✓6ᵗʰ **O10.01**   Pre-existing essential hypertension complicating pregnancy

     O10.011   **Pre-existing essential hypertension complicating pregnancy, first trimester**   Ⓜ♀

     O10.012   **Pre-existing essential hypertension complicating pregnancy, second trimester**   Ⓜ♀

     O10.013   **Pre-existing essential hypertension complicating pregnancy, third trimester**   Ⓜ♀

     O10.019   **Pre-existing essential hypertension complicating pregnancy, unspecified trimester**   Ⓜ♀

   O10.02   **Pre-existing essential hypertension complicating childbirth**   Ⓜ♀

   O10.03   **Pre-existing essential hypertension complicating the puerperium**   Ⓜ♀

✓5ᵗʰ **O10.1**   Pre-existing hypertensive heart disease complicating pregnancy, childbirth and the puerperium

     Any condition in I11 specified as a reason for obstetric care during pregnancy, childbirth or the puerperium

     Use additional code from I11 to identify the type of hypertensive heart disease

✓6ᵗʰ **O10.11**   Pre-existing hypertensive heart disease complicating pregnancy

     O10.111   **Pre-existing hypertensive heart disease complicating pregnancy, first trimester**   Ⓜ♀

     O10.112   **Pre-existing hypertensive heart disease complicating pregnancy, second trimester**   Ⓜ♀

     O10.113   **Pre-existing hypertensive heart disease complicating pregnancy, third trimester**   Ⓜ♀

     O10.119   **Pre-existing hypertensive heart disease complicating pregnancy, unspecified trimester**   Ⓜ♀

   O10.12   **Pre-existing hypertensive heart disease complicating childbirth**   Ⓜ♀

   O10.13   **Pre-existing hypertensive heart disease complicating the puerperium**   Ⓜ♀

✓5ᵗʰ **O10.2**   Pre-existing hypertensive chronic kidney disease complicating pregnancy, childbirth and the puerperium

     Any condition in I12 specified as a reason for obstetric care during pregnancy, childbirth or the puerperium

     Use additional code from I12 to identify the type of hypertensive chronic kidney disease

✓6ᵗʰ **O10.21**   Pre-existing hypertensive chronic kidney disease complicating pregnancy

     O10.211   **Pre-existing hypertensive chronic kidney disease complicating pregnancy, first trimester**   Ⓜ♀

     O10.212   **Pre-existing hypertensive chronic kidney disease complicating pregnancy, second trimester**   Ⓜ♀

     O10.213   **Pre-existing hypertensive chronic kidney disease complicating pregnancy, third trimester**   Ⓜ♀

     O10.219   **Pre-existing hypertensive chronic kidney disease complicating pregnancy, unspecified trimester**   Ⓜ♀

   O10.22   **Pre-existing hypertensive chronic kidney disease complicating childbirth**   Ⓜ♀

   O10.23   **Pre-existing hypertensive chronic kidney disease complicating the puerperium**   Ⓜ♀

✓5ᵗʰ **O10.3**   Pre-existing hypertensive heart and chronic kidney disease complicating pregnancy, childbirth and the puerperium

     Any condition in I13 specified as a reason for obstetric care during pregnancy, childbirth or the puerperium

     Use additional code from I13 to identify the type of hypertensive heart and chronic kidney disease

✓6ᵗʰ **O10.31**   Pre-existing hypertensive heart and chronic kidney disease complicating pregnancy

     O10.311   **Pre-existing hypertensive heart and chronic kidney disease complicating pregnancy, first trimester**   Ⓜ♀

     O10.312   **Pre-existing hypertensive heart and chronic kidney disease complicating pregnancy, second trimester**   Ⓜ♀

     O10.313   **Pre-existing hypertensive heart and chronic kidney disease complicating pregnancy, third trimester**   Ⓜ♀

     O10.319   **Pre-existing hypertensive heart and chronic kidney disease complicating pregnancy, unspecified trimester**   Ⓜ♀

   O10.32   **Pre-existing hypertensive heart and chronic kidney disease complicating childbirth**   Ⓜ♀

   O10.33   **Pre-existing hypertensive heart and chronic kidney disease complicating the puerperium**   Ⓜ♀

☑ Additional Character Required   ✓ˣ7ᵗʰ Placeholder Alert   Unspecified Dx   Other Specified Dx   Manifestation   ►◄ Revised Text   ● New Code   ▲ Revised Code Title

ICD-10-CM 2016   769

Chapter 15. Pregnancy, Childbirth, and the Puerperium

✓5ᵗʰ **O10.4 Pre-existing** secondary **hypertension complicating pregnancy, childbirth and the puerperium**
Any condition in I15 specified as a reason for obstetric care during pregnancy, childbirth or the puerperium
Use additional code from I15 to identify the type of secondary hypertension

    ✓6ᵗʰ **O10.41 Pre-existing secondary hypertension complicating** pregnancy

        O10.411 Pre-existing secondary hypertension complicating pregnancy, first trimester Ⓜ♀

        O10.412 Pre-existing secondary hypertension complicating pregnancy, second trimester Ⓜ♀

        O10.413 Pre-existing secondary hypertension complicating pregnancy, third trimester Ⓜ♀

        O10.419 Pre-existing secondary hypertension complicating pregnancy, unspecified trimester Ⓜ♀

    O10.42 Pre-existing secondary hypertension complicating childbirth Ⓜ♀

    O10.43 Pre-existing secondary hypertension complicating the puerperium Ⓜ♀

✓5ᵗʰ **O10.9 Unspecified** pre-existing hypertension complicating **pregnancy, childbirth and the puerperium**

    ✓6ᵗʰ **O10.91 Unspecified pre-existing hypertension complicating** pregnancy

        O10.911 Unspecified pre-existing hypertension complicating pregnancy, first trimester Ⓜ♀

        O10.912 Unspecified pre-existing hypertension complicating pregnancy, second trimester Ⓜ♀

        O10.913 Unspecified pre-existing hypertension complicating pregnancy, third trimester Ⓜ♀

        O10.919 Unspecified pre-existing hypertension complicating pregnancy, unspecified trimester Ⓜ♀

    O10.92 Unspecified pre-existing hypertension complicating childbirth Ⓜ♀

    O10.93 Unspecified pre-existing hypertension complicating the puerperium Ⓜ♀

✓4ᵗʰ **O11 Pre-existing hypertension with pre-eclampsia**
Conditions in O10 complicated by pre-eclampsia
Pre-eclampsia superimposed pre-existing hypertension
Use additional code from O10 to identify the type of hypertension

    O11.1 Pre-existing hypertension with pre-eclampsia, first trimester Ⓜ♀

    O11.2 Pre-existing hypertension with pre-eclampsia, second trimester Ⓜ♀

    O11.3 Pre-existing hypertension with pre-eclampsia, third trimester Ⓜ♀

    O11.9 Pre-existing hypertension with pre-eclampsia, unspecified trimester Ⓜ♀

✓4ᵗʰ **O12 Gestational [pregnancy-induced] edema and proteinuria without hypertension**

    ✓5ᵗʰ **O12.0 Gestational** edema

        O12.00 Gestational edema, unspecified trimester Ⓜ♀

        O12.01 Gestational edema, first trimester Ⓜ♀

        O12.02 Gestational edema, second trimester Ⓜ♀

        O12.03 Gestational edema, third trimester Ⓜ♀

    ✓5ᵗʰ **O12.1 Gestational** proteinuria

        O12.10 Gestational proteinuria, unspecified trimester Ⓜ♀

        O12.11 Gestational proteinuria, first trimester Ⓜ♀

        O12.12 Gestational proteinuria, second trimester Ⓜ♀

        O12.13 Gestational proteinuria, third trimester Ⓜ♀

    ✓5ᵗʰ **O12.2 Gestational** edema with proteinuria

        O12.20 Gestational edema with proteinuria, unspecified trimester Ⓜ♀

        O12.21 Gestational edema with proteinuria, first trimester Ⓜ♀

        O12.22 Gestational edema with proteinuria, second trimester Ⓜ♀

        O12.23 Gestational edema with proteinuria, third trimester Ⓜ♀

✓4ᵗʰ **O13 Gestational [pregnancy-induced] hypertension without significant proteinuria**
INCLUDES gestational hypertension NOS

    O13.1 Gestational [pregnancy-induced] hypertension without significant proteinuria, first trimester Ⓜ♀

    O13.2 Gestational [pregnancy-induced] hypertension without significant proteinuria, second trimester Ⓜ♀

    O13.3 Gestational [pregnancy-induced] hypertension without significant proteinuria, third trimester Ⓜ♀

    O13.9 Gestational [pregnancy-induced] hypertension without significant proteinuria, unspecified trimester Ⓜ♀

✓4ᵗʰ **O14 Pre-eclampsia**
EXCLUDES 1 pre-existing hypertension with pre-eclampsia (O11)

    ✓5ᵗʰ **O14.0 Mild to moderate pre-eclampsia**

        O14.00 Mild to moderate pre-eclampsia, unspecified trimester Ⓜ♀

        O14.02 Mild to moderate pre-eclampsia, second trimester Ⓜ♀

        O14.03 Mild to moderate pre-eclampsia, third trimester Ⓜ♀

    ✓5ᵗʰ **O14.1 Severe pre-eclampsia**
        EXCLUDES 1 HELLP syndrome (O14.2-)

        O14.10 Severe pre-eclampsia, unspecified trimester Ⓜ♀

        O14.12 Severe pre-eclampsia, second trimester Ⓜ♀

        O14.13 Severe pre-eclampsia, third trimester Ⓜ♀

    ✓5ᵗʰ **O14.2 HELLP syndrome**
Severe pre-eclampsia with hemolysis, elevated liver enzymes and low platelet count (HELLP)

        O14.20 HELLP syndrome (HELLP), unspecified trimester Ⓜ♀

        O14.22 HELLP syndrome (HELLP), second trimester Ⓜ♀

        O14.23 HELLP syndrome (HELLP), third trimester Ⓜ♀

    ✓5ᵗʰ **O14.9 Unspecified pre-eclampsia**

        O14.90 Unspecified pre-eclampsia, unspecified trimester Ⓜ♀

        O14.92 Unspecified pre-eclampsia, second trimester Ⓜ♀

        O14.93 Unspecified pre-eclampsia, third trimester Ⓜ♀

✓4ᵗʰ **O15 Eclampsia**
INCLUDES convulsions following conditions in O10-O14 and O16

    ✓5ᵗʰ **O15.0 Eclampsia in** pregnancy

        O15.00 Eclampsia in pregnancy, unspecified trimester Ⓜ♀

        O15.02 Eclampsia in pregnancy, second trimester Ⓜ♀

        O15.03 Eclampsia in pregnancy, third trimester Ⓜ♀

    O15.1 Eclampsia in labor Ⓜ♀

    O15.2 Eclampsia in the puerperium Ⓜ♀

    O15.9 Eclampsia, unspecified as to time period Ⓜ♀
    Eclampsia NOS

✓4ᵗʰ **O16 Unspecified maternal hypertension**

    O16.1 Unspecified maternal hypertension, first trimester Ⓜ♀

    O16.2 Unspecified maternal hypertension, second trimester Ⓜ♀

    O16.3 Unspecified maternal hypertension, third trimester Ⓜ♀

    O16.9 Unspecified maternal hypertension, unspecified trimester Ⓜ♀

Other maternal disorders predominantly related to pregnancy (O20-O29)

EXCLUDES 2 maternal care related to the fetus and amniotic cavity and possible delivery problems (O30-O48)
maternal diseases classifiable elsewhere but complicating pregnancy, labor and delivery, and the puerperium (O98-O99)

✓4ᵗʰ **O20 Hemorrhage in early pregnancy**
Hemorrhage before completion of 20 weeks gestation
EXCLUDES 1 pregnancy with abortive outcome (O00-O08)

    O20.0 Threatened abortion Ⓜ♀
    Hemorrhage specified as due to threatened abortion

    O20.8 Other hemorrhage in early pregnancy Ⓜ♀

    O20.9 Hemorrhage in early pregnancy, unspecified Ⓜ♀

✓4ᵗʰ **O21 Excessive vomiting in pregnancy**

    O21.0 Mild hyperemesis gravidarum Ⓜ♀
    Hyperemesis gravidarum, mild or unspecified, starting before the end of the 20th week of gestation

---

EXCLUDES 1 Not coded here   EXCLUDES 2 Not included here   Ⓝ Newborn Age: 0   Ⓟ Pediatric Age: 0-17   Ⓜ Maternity Age: 12-55   Ⓐ Adult Age: 15-124

O21.1 **Hyperemesis gravidarum with** metabolic disturbance   Ⓜ♀
     Hyperemesis gravidarum, starting before the end of the 20th week of gestation, with metabolic disturbance such as carbohydrate depletion
     Hyperemesis gravidarum, starting before the end of the 20th week of gestation, with metabolic disturbance such as dehydration
     Hyperemesis gravidarum, starting before the end of the 20th week of gestation, with metabolic disturbance such as electrolyte imbalance

O21.2 Late **vomiting of pregnancy**   Ⓜ♀
     Excessive vomiting starting after 20 completed weeks of gestation

O21.8 **Other vomiting complicating pregnancy**   Ⓜ♀
     Vomiting due to diseases classified elsewhere, complicating pregnancy
     Use additional code, to identify cause

O21.9 **Vomiting of pregnancy, unspecified**   Ⓜ♀

✔4ᵗʰ **O22** **Venous complications and hemorrhoids in pregnancy**
     EXCLUDES 1   venous complications of:
       abortion NOS (O03.9)
       ectopic or molar pregnancy (O08.7)
       failed attempted abortion (O07.35)
       induced abortion (O04.85)
       spontaneous abortion (O03.89)
     EXCLUDES 2   obstetric pulmonary embolism (O88.-)
       venous complications and hemorrhoids of childbirth and the puerperium (O87.-)

✔5ᵗʰ **O22.0** Varicose veins of lower extremity **in pregnancy**
     Varicose veins NOS in pregnancy

     O22.00 **Varicose veins of lower extremity in pregnancy, unspecified trimester**   Ⓜ♀

     O22.01 **Varicose veins of lower extremity in pregnancy,** Ⓜ♀ **first trimester**

     O22.02 **Varicose veins of lower extremity in pregnancy,** Ⓜ♀ **second trimester**

     O22.03 **Varicose veins of lower extremity in pregnancy,** Ⓜ♀ **third trimester**

✔5ᵗʰ **O22.1** Genital varices **in pregnancy**
     Perineal varices in pregnancy
     Vaginal varices in pregnancy
     Vulval varices in pregnancy

     O22.10 **Genital varices in pregnancy, unspecified** Ⓜ♀ **trimester**

     O22.11 **Genital varices in pregnancy,** first trimester   Ⓜ♀

     O22.12 **Genital varices in pregnancy,** second trimester   Ⓜ♀

     O22.13 **Genital varices in pregnancy,** third trimester   Ⓜ♀

✔5ᵗʰ **O22.2** Superficial thrombophlebitis **in pregnancy**
     Phlebitis in pregnancy NOS
     Thrombophlebitis of legs in pregnancy
     Thrombosis in pregnancy NOS
     Use additional code to identify the superficial thrombophlebitis (I80.0-)

     O22.20 **Superficial thrombophlebitis in pregnancy,** Ⓜ♀ **unspecified trimester**

     O22.21 **Superficial thrombophlebitis in pregnancy,** Ⓜ♀ **first trimester**

     O22.22 **Superficial thrombophlebitis in pregnancy,** Ⓜ♀ **second trimester**

     O22.23 **Superficial thrombophlebitis in pregnancy,** Ⓜ♀ **third trimester**

✔5ᵗʰ **O22.3** Deep phlebothrombosis **in pregnancy**
     Deep vein thrombosis, antepartum
     Use additional code to identify the deep vein thrombosis (I82.4-, I82.5-, I82.62-. I82.72-)
     Use additional code, if applicable, for associated long-term (current) use of anticoagulants (Z79.01)

     O22.30 **Deep phlebothrombosis in pregnancy,** Ⓜ♀ **unspecified trimester**

     O22.31 **Deep phlebothrombosis in pregnancy,** Ⓜ♀ **first trimester**

     O22.32 **Deep phlebothrombosis in pregnancy,** Ⓜ♀ **second trimester**

     O22.33 **Deep phlebothrombosis in pregnancy,** Ⓜ♀ **third trimester**

✔5ᵗʰ **O22.4** Hemorrhoids **in pregnancy**

     O22.40 **Hemorrhoids in pregnancy, unspecified** Ⓜ♀ **trimester**

     O22.41 **Hemorrhoids in pregnancy,** first trimester   Ⓜ♀

     O22.42 **Hemorrhoids in pregnancy,** second trimester   Ⓜ♀

     O22.43 **Hemorrhoids in pregnancy,** third trimester   Ⓜ♀

✔5ᵗʰ **O22.5** Cerebral venous thrombosis **in pregnancy**
     Cerebrovenous sinus thrombosis in pregnancy

     O22.50 **Cerebral venous thrombosis in pregnancy,** Ⓜ♀ **unspecified trimester**

     O22.51 **Cerebral venous thrombosis in pregnancy,** Ⓜ♀ **first trimester**

     O22.52 **Cerebral venous thrombosis in pregnancy,** Ⓜ♀ **second trimester**

     O22.53 **Cerebral venous thrombosis in pregnancy,** Ⓜ♀ **third trimester**

✔5ᵗʰ **O22.8** Other venous complications **in pregnancy**

     ✔6ᵗʰ **O22.8X** Other **venous complications in pregnancy**

       O22.8X1 **Other venous complications in** Ⓜ♀ **pregnancy,** first trimester

       O22.8X2 **Other venous complications in** Ⓜ♀ **pregnancy,** second trimester

       O22.8X3 **Other venous complications in** Ⓜ♀ **pregnancy,** third trimester

       O22.8X9 **Other venous complications in** Ⓜ♀ **pregnancy, unspecified trimester**

✔5ᵗʰ **O22.9** Venous complication **in pregnancy,** unspecified
     Gestational phlebitis NOS
     Gestational phlebopathy NOS
     Gestational thrombosis NOS

     O22.90 **Venous complication in pregnancy, unspecified,** Ⓜ♀ **unspecified trimester**

     O22.91 **Venous complication in pregnancy, unspecified,** Ⓜ♀ **first trimester**

     O22.92 **Venous complication in pregnancy, unspecified,** Ⓜ♀ **second trimester**

     O22.93 **Venous complication in pregnancy, unspecified,** Ⓜ♀ **third trimester**

✔4ᵗʰ **O23** **Infections of genitourinary tract in pregnancy**
     Use additional code to identify organism (B95.-, B96.-)
     EXCLUDES 2   gonococcal infections complicating pregnancy, childbirth and the puerperium (O98.2)
       infections with a predominantly sexual mode of transmission NOS complicating pregnancy, childbirth and the puerperium (O98.3)
       syphilis complicating pregnancy, childbirth and the puerperium (O98.1)
       tuberculosis of genitourinary system complicating pregnancy, childbirth and the puerperium (O98.0)
       venereal disease NOS complicating pregnancy, childbirth and the puerperium (O98.3)

✔5ᵗʰ **O23.0** **Infections of** kidney **in pregnancy**
     Pyelonephritis in pregnancy

     O23.00 **Infections of kidney in pregnancy, unspecified** Ⓜ♀ **trimester**

     O23.01 **Infections of kidney in pregnancy,** first trimester Ⓜ♀

     O23.02 **Infections of kidney in pregnancy,** second Ⓜ♀ **trimester**

     O23.03 **Infections of kidney in pregnancy,** third Ⓜ♀ **trimester**

✔5ᵗʰ **O23.1** **Infections of** bladder **in pregnancy**

     O23.10 **Infections of bladder in pregnancy,** Ⓜ♀ **unspecified trimester**

     O23.11 **Infections of bladder in pregnancy,** Ⓜ♀ **first trimester**

     O23.12 **Infections of bladder in pregnancy,** Ⓜ♀ **second trimester**

     O23.13 **Infections of bladder in pregnancy,** Ⓜ♀ **third trimester**

✔5ᵗʰ **O23.2** **Infections of** urethra **in pregnancy**

     O23.20 **Infections of urethra in pregnancy,** Ⓜ♀ **unspecified trimester**

     O23.21 **Infections of urethra in pregnancy,** Ⓜ♀ **first trimester**

     O23.22 **Infections of urethra in pregnancy,** Ⓜ♀ **second trimester**

✔ Additional Character Required   ▪ₓ7ᵗʰ Placeholder Alert   Unspecified Dx   Other Specified Dx   Manifestation   ▶◀ Revised Text   ● New Code   ▲ Revised Code Title

O23.23   Infections of urethra in pregnancy, third trimester   Ⓜ♀

✓5ᵗʰ **O23.3**   Infections of other parts of urinary tract in pregnancy

    O23.30   Infections of other parts of urinary tract in pregnancy, unspecified trimester   Ⓜ♀

    O23.31   Infections of other parts of urinary tract in pregnancy, first trimester   Ⓜ♀

    O23.32   Infections of other parts of urinary tract in pregnancy, second trimester   Ⓜ♀

    O23.33   Infections of other parts of urinary tract in pregnancy, third trimester   Ⓜ♀

✓5ᵗʰ **O23.4**   Unspecified infection of urinary tract in pregnancy

    O23.40   Unspecified infection of urinary tract in pregnancy, unspecified trimester   Ⓜ♀

    O23.41   Unspecified infection of urinary tract in pregnancy, first trimester   Ⓜ♀

    O23.42   Unspecified infection of urinary tract in pregnancy, second trimester   Ⓜ♀

    O23.43   Unspecified infection of urinary tract in pregnancy, third trimester   Ⓜ♀

✓5ᵗʰ **O23.5**   Infections of the genital tract in pregnancy

  ✓6ᵗʰ **O23.51**   Infection of cervix in pregnancy

    O23.511   Infections of cervix in pregnancy, first trimester   Ⓜ♀

    O23.512   Infections of cervix in pregnancy, second trimester   Ⓜ♀

    O23.513   Infections of cervix in pregnancy, third trimester   Ⓜ♀

    O23.519   Infections of cervix in pregnancy, unspecified trimester   Ⓜ♀

  ✓6ᵗʰ **O23.52**   Salpingo-oophoritis in pregnancy
    Oophoritis in pregnancy
    Salpingitis in pregnancy

    O23.521   Salpingo-oophoritis in pregnancy, first trimester   Ⓜ♀

    O23.522   Salpingo-oophoritis in pregnancy, second trimester   Ⓜ♀

    O23.523   Salpingo-oophoritis in pregnancy, third trimester   Ⓜ♀

    O23.529   Salpingo-oophoritis in pregnancy, unspecified trimester   Ⓜ♀

  ✓6ᵗʰ **O23.59**   Infection of other part of genital tract in pregnancy

    O23.591   Infection of other part of genital tract in pregnancy, first trimester   Ⓜ♀

    O23.592   Infection of other part of genital tract in pregnancy, second trimester   Ⓜ♀

    O23.593   Infection of other part of genital tract in pregnancy, third trimester   Ⓜ♀

    O23.599   Infection of other part of genital tract in pregnancy, unspecified trimester   Ⓜ♀

✓5ᵗʰ **O23.9**   Unspecified genitourinary tract infection in pregnancy
    Genitourinary tract infection in pregnancy NOS

    O23.90   Unspecified genitourinary tract infection in pregnancy, unspecified trimester   Ⓜ♀

    O23.91   Unspecified genitourinary tract infection in pregnancy, first trimester   Ⓜ♀

    O23.92   Unspecified genitourinary tract infection in pregnancy, second trimester   Ⓜ♀

    O23.93   Unspecified genitourinary tract infection in pregnancy, third trimester   Ⓜ♀

✓4ᵗʰ **O24**   Diabetes mellitus in pregnancy, childbirth, and the puerperium

  ✓5ᵗʰ **O24.0**   Pre-existing diabetes mellitus, type 1, in pregnancy, childbirth and the puerperium
    Juvenile onset diabetes mellitus, in pregnancy, childbirth and the puerperium
    Ketosis-prone diabetes mellitus in pregnancy, childbirth and the puerperium
    Use additional code from category E10 to further identify any manifestations

   ✓6ᵗʰ **O24.01**   Pre-existing diabetes mellitus, type 1, in pregnancy

    O24.011   Pre-existing diabetes mellitus, type 1, in pregnancy, first trimester   Ⓜ♀

    O24.012   Pre-existing diabetes mellitus, type 1, in pregnancy, second trimester   Ⓜ♀

    O24.013   Pre-existing diabetes mellitus, type 1, in pregnancy, third trimester   Ⓜ♀

    O24.019   Pre-existing diabetes mellitus, type 1, in pregnancy, unspecified trimester   Ⓜ♀

   O24.02   Pre-existing diabetes mellitus, type 1, in childbirth   Ⓜ♀

   O24.03   Pre-existing diabetes mellitus, type 1, in the puerperium   Ⓜ♀

  ✓5ᵗʰ **O24.1**   Pre-existing diabetes mellitus, type 2, in pregnancy, childbirth and the puerperium
    Insulin-resistant diabetes mellitus in pregnancy, childbirth and the puerperium
    Use additional code (for):
      from category E11 to further identify any manifestations
      long-term (current) use of insulin (Z79.4)

   ✓6ᵗʰ **O24.11**   Pre-existing diabetes mellitus, type 2, in pregnancy

    O24.111   Pre-existing diabetes mellitus, type 2, in pregnancy, first trimester   Ⓜ♀

    O24.112   Pre-existing diabetes mellitus, type 2, in pregnancy, second trimester   Ⓜ♀

    O24.113   Pre-existing diabetes mellitus, type 2, in pregnancy, third trimester   Ⓜ♀

    O24.119   Pre-existing diabetes mellitus, type 2, in pregnancy, unspecified trimester   Ⓜ♀

   O24.12   Pre-existing diabetes mellitus, type 2, in childbirth   Ⓜ♀

   O24.13   Pre-existing diabetes mellitus, type 2, in the puerperium   Ⓜ♀

  ✓5ᵗʰ **O24.3**   Unspecified pre-existing diabetes mellitus in pregnancy, childbirth and the puerperium
    Use additional code (for):
      from category E11 to further identify any manifestation
      long-term (current) use of insulin (Z79.4)

   ✓6ᵗʰ **O24.31**   Unspecified pre-existing diabetes mellitus in pregnancy

    O24.311   Unspecified pre-existing diabetes mellitus in pregnancy, first trimester   Ⓜ♀

    O24.312   Unspecified pre-existing diabetes mellitus in pregnancy, second trimester   Ⓜ♀

    O24.313   Unspecified pre-existing diabetes mellitus in pregnancy, third trimester   Ⓜ♀

    O24.319   Unspecified pre-existing diabetes mellitus in pregnancy, unspecified trimester   Ⓜ♀

   O24.32   Unspecified pre-existing diabetes mellitus in childbirth   Ⓜ♀

   O24.33   Unspecified pre-existing diabetes mellitus in the puerperium   Ⓜ♀

  ✓5ᵗʰ **O24.4**   Gestational diabetes mellitus
    Diabetes mellitus arising in pregnancy
    Gestational diabetes mellitus NOS

   ✓6ᵗʰ **O24.41**   Gestational diabetes mellitus in pregnancy

    O24.410   Gestational diabetes mellitus in pregnancy, diet controlled   Ⓜ♀

    O24.414   Gestational diabetes mellitus in pregnancy, insulin controlled   Ⓜ♀

    O24.419   Gestational diabetes mellitus in pregnancy, unspecified control   Ⓜ♀

   ✓6ᵗʰ **O24.42**   Gestational diabetes mellitus in childbirth

    O24.420   Gestational diabetes mellitus in childbirth, diet controlled   Ⓜ♀

    O24.424   Gestational diabetes mellitus in childbirth, insulin controlled   Ⓜ♀

    O24.429   Gestational diabetes mellitus in childbirth, unspecified control   Ⓜ♀

   ✓6ᵗʰ **O24.43**   Gestational diabetes mellitus in the puerperium

    O24.430   Gestational diabetes mellitus in the puerperium, diet controlled   Ⓜ♀

    O24.434   Gestational diabetes mellitus in the puerperium, insulin controlled   Ⓜ♀

    O24.439   Gestational diabetes mellitus in the puerperium, unspecified control   Ⓜ♀

EXCLUDES 1 Not coded here   **EXCLUDES 2** Not included here   Ⓝ Newborn Age: 0   Ⓟ Pediatric Age: 0-17   Ⓜ Maternity Age: 12-55   Ⓐ Adult Age: 15-124

772   ICD-10-CM 2016

✓5th **O24.8** Other pre-existing diabetes mellitus in pregnancy, childbirth, and the puerperium
　　Use additional code (for):
　　　from categories E08, E09 and E13 to further identify any manifestation
　　　long-term (current) use of insulin (Z79.4)

✓6th **O24.81** Other pre-existing diabetes mellitus in pregnancy
　　O24.811 Other pre-existing diabetes mellitus in pregnancy, first trimester   M♀
　　O24.812 Other pre-existing diabetes mellitus in pregnancy, second trimester   M♀
　　O24.813 Other pre-existing diabetes mellitus in pregnancy, third trimester   M♀
　　O24.819 Other pre-existing diabetes mellitus in pregnancy, unspecified trimester   M♀

O24.82 Other pre-existing diabetes mellitus in childbirth   M♀

O24.83 Other pre-existing diabetes mellitus in the puerperium   M♀

✓5th **O24.9** Unspecified diabetes mellitus in pregnancy, childbirth and the puerperium
　　Use additional code for long-term (current) use of insulin (Z79.4)

✓6th **O24.91** Unspecified diabetes mellitus in pregnancy
　　O24.911 Unspecified diabetes mellitus in pregnancy, first trimester   M♀
　　O24.912 Unspecified diabetes mellitus in pregnancy, second trimester   M♀
　　O24.913 Unspecified diabetes mellitus in pregnancy, third trimester   M♀
　　O24.919 Unspecified diabetes mellitus in pregnancy, unspecified trimester   M♀

O24.92 Unspecified diabetes mellitus in childbirth   M♀

O24.93 Unspecified diabetes mellitus in the puerperium   M♀

✓4th **O25** Malnutrition in pregnancy, childbirth and the puerperium

✓5th **O25.1** Malnutrition in pregnancy
　O25.10 Malnutrition in pregnancy, unspecified trimester   M♀
　O25.11 Malnutrition in pregnancy, first trimester   M♀
　O25.12 Malnutrition in pregnancy, second trimester   M♀
　O25.13 Malnutrition in pregnancy, third trimester   M♀

O25.2 Malnutrition in childbirth   M♀

O25.3 Malnutrition in the puerperium   M♀

✓4th **O26** Maternal care for other conditions predominantly related to pregnancy

✓5th **O26.0** Excessive weight gain in pregnancy
　EXCLUDES 2　gestational edema (O12.0, O12.2)
　O26.00 Excessive weight gain in pregnancy, unspecified trimester   M♀
　O26.01 Excessive weight gain in pregnancy, first trimester   M♀
　O26.02 Excessive weight gain in pregnancy, second trimester   M♀
　O26.03 Excessive weight gain in pregnancy, third trimester   M♀

✓5th **O26.1** Low weight gain in pregnancy
　O26.10 Low weight gain in pregnancy, unspecified trimester   M♀
　O26.11 Low weight gain in pregnancy, first trimester   M♀
　O26.12 Low weight gain in pregnancy, second trimester   M♀
　O26.13 Low weight gain in pregnancy, third trimester   M♀

✓5th **O26.2** Pregnancy care for patient with recurrent pregnancy loss
　O26.20 Pregnancy care for patient with recurrent pregnancy loss, unspecified trimester   M♀
　O26.21 Pregnancy care for patient with recurrent pregnancy loss, first trimester   M♀
　O26.22 Pregnancy care for patient with recurrent pregnancy loss, second trimester   M♀
　O26.23 Pregnancy care for patient with recurrent pregnancy loss, third trimester   M♀

✓5th **O26.3** Retained intrauterine contraceptive device in pregnancy
　O26.30 Retained intrauterine contraceptive device in pregnancy, unspecified trimester   M♀
　O26.31 Retained intrauterine contraceptive device in pregnancy, first trimester   M♀

O26.32 Retained intrauterine contraceptive device in pregnancy, second trimester   M♀

O26.33 Retained intrauterine contraceptive device in pregnancy, third trimester   M♀

✓5th **O26.4** Herpes gestationis
　O26.40 Herpes gestationis, unspecified trimester   M♀
　O26.41 Herpes gestationis, first trimester   M♀
　O26.42 Herpes gestationis, second trimester   M♀
　O26.43 Herpes gestationis, third trimester   M♀

✓5th **O26.5** Maternal hypotension syndrome
　　Supine hypotensive syndrome
　O26.50 Maternal hypotension syndrome, unspecified trimester   M♀
　O26.51 Maternal hypotension syndrome, first trimester   M♀
　O26.52 Maternal hypotension syndrome, second trimester   M♀
　O26.53 Maternal hypotension syndrome, third trimester   M♀

✓5th **O26.6** Liver and biliary tract disorders in pregnancy, childbirth and the puerperium
　　Use additional code to identify the specific disorder
　　EXCLUDES 2　hepatorenal syndrome following labor and delivery (O90.4)

✓6th **O26.61** Liver and biliary tract disorders in pregnancy
　　O26.611 Liver and biliary tract disorders in pregnancy, first trimester   M♀
　　O26.612 Liver and biliary tract disorders in pregnancy, second trimester   M♀
　　O26.613 Liver and biliary tract disorders in pregnancy, third trimester   M♀
　　O26.619 Liver and biliary tract disorders in pregnancy, unspecified trimester   M♀

O26.62 Liver and biliary tract disorders in childbirth   M♀

O26.63 Liver and biliary tract disorders in the puerperium   M♀

✓5th **O26.7** Subluxation of symphysis (pubis) in pregnancy, childbirth and the puerperium
　　EXCLUDES 1　traumatic separation of symphysis (pubis) during childbirth (O71.6)

✓6th **O26.71** Subluxation of symphysis (pubis) in pregnancy
　　O26.711 Subluxation of symphysis (pubis) in pregnancy, first trimester   M♀
　　O26.712 Subluxation of symphysis (pubis) in pregnancy, second trimester   M♀
　　O26.713 Subluxation of symphysis (pubis) in pregnancy, third trimester   M♀
　　O26.719 Subluxation of symphysis (pubis) in pregnancy, unspecified trimester   M♀

O26.72 Subluxation of symphysis (pubis) in childbirth   M♀

O26.73 Subluxation of symphysis (pubis) in the puerperium   M♀

✓5th **O26.8** Other specified pregnancy related conditions

✓6th **O26.81** Pregnancy related exhaustion and fatigue
　　O26.811 Pregnancy related exhaustion and fatigue, first trimester   M♀
　　O26.812 Pregnancy related exhaustion and fatigue, second trimester   M♀
　　O26.813 Pregnancy related exhaustion and fatigue, third trimester   M♀
　　O26.819 Pregnancy related exhaustion and fatigue, unspecified trimester   M♀

✓6th **O26.82** Pregnancy related peripheral neuritis
　　O26.821 Pregnancy related peripheral neuritis, first trimester   M♀
　　O26.822 Pregnancy related peripheral neuritis, second trimester   M♀
　　O26.823 Pregnancy related peripheral neuritis, third trimester   M♀
　　O26.829 Pregnancy related peripheral neuritis, unspecified trimester   M♀

✓6th **O26.83** Pregnancy related renal disease
　　Use additional code to identify the specific disorder
　　O26.831 Pregnancy related renal disease, first trimester   M♀
　　O26.832 Pregnancy related renal disease, second trimester   M♀

✓ Additional Character Required   ✓x7th Placeholder Alert   Unspecified Dx   Other Specified Dx   Manifestation   ▶◀ Revised Text   ● New Code   ▲ Revised Code Title

O26.833 Pregnancy related renal disease, third trimester Ⓜ♀

O26.839 Pregnancy related renal disease, unspecified trimester Ⓜ♀

√6ᵗʰ **O26.84** Uterine size-date discrepancy complicating pregnancy
> EXCLUDES 1 encounter for suspected problem with fetal growth ruled out (Z03.74)

O26.841 Uterine size-date discrepancy, first trimester Ⓜ♀

O26.842 Uterine size-date discrepancy, second trimester Ⓜ♀

O26.843 Uterine size-date discrepancy, third trimester Ⓜ♀

O26.849 Uterine size-date discrepancy, unspecified trimester Ⓜ♀

√6ᵗʰ **O26.85** Spotting complicating pregnancy

O26.851 Spotting complicating pregnancy, first trimester Ⓜ♀

O26.852 Spotting complicating pregnancy, second trimester Ⓜ♀

O26.853 Spotting complicating pregnancy, third trimester Ⓜ♀

O26.859 Spotting complicating pregnancy, unspecified trimester Ⓜ♀

O26.86 Pruritic urticarial papules and plaques of pregnancy (PUPPP) Ⓜ♀
> Polymorphic eruption of pregnancy

√6ᵗʰ **O26.87** Cervical shortening
> EXCLUDES 1 encounter for suspected cervical shortening ruled out (Z03.75)

O26.872 Cervical shortening, second trimester Ⓜ♀

O26.873 Cervical shortening, third trimester Ⓜ♀

O26.879 Cervical shortening, unspecified trimester Ⓜ♀

√6ᵗʰ **O26.89** Other specified pregnancy related conditions

O26.891 Other specified pregnancy related conditions, first trimester Ⓜ♀

O26.892 Other specified pregnancy related conditions, second trimester Ⓜ♀

O26.893 Other specified pregnancy related conditions, third trimester Ⓜ♀

O26.899 Other specified pregnancy related conditions, unspecified trimester Ⓜ♀

√5ᵗʰ **O26.9** Pregnancy related conditions, unspecified

O26.90 Pregnancy related conditions, unspecified, unspecified trimester Ⓜ♀

O26.91 Pregnancy related conditions, unspecified, first trimester Ⓜ♀

O26.92 Pregnancy related conditions, unspecified, second trimester Ⓜ♀

O26.93 Pregnancy related conditions, unspecified, third trimester Ⓜ♀

√4ᵗʰ **O28** Abnormal findings on antenatal screening of mother
> EXCLUDES 1 diagnostic findings classified elsewhere—see Alphabetical Index

O28.0 Abnormal hematological finding on antenatal screening of mother Ⓜ♀

O28.1 Abnormal biochemical finding on antenatal screening of mother Ⓜ♀

O28.2 Abnormal cytological finding on antenatal screening of mother Ⓜ♀

O28.3 Abnormal ultrasonic finding on antenatal screening of mother Ⓜ♀

O28.4 Abnormal radiological finding on antenatal screening of mother Ⓜ♀

O28.5 Abnormal chromosomal and genetic finding on antenatal screening of mother Ⓜ♀

O28.8 Other abnormal findings on antenatal screening of mother Ⓜ♀

O28.9 Unspecified abnormal findings on antenatal screening of mother Ⓜ♀

√4ᵗʰ **O29** Complications of anesthesia during pregnancy
> INCLUDES maternal complications arising from the administration of a general, regional or local anesthetic, analgesic or other sedation during pregnancy

Use additional code, if necessary, to identify the complication
> EXCLUDES 2 complications of anesthesia during labor and delivery (O74.-)
> complications of anesthesia during the puerperium (O89.-)

√5ᵗʰ **O29.0** Pulmonary complications of anesthesia during pregnancy

√6ᵗʰ **O29.01** Aspiration pneumonitis due to anesthesia during pregnancy
> Inhalation of stomach contents or secretions NOS due to anesthesia during pregnancy
> Mendelson's syndrome due to anesthesia during pregnancy

O29.011 Aspiration pneumonitis due to anesthesia during pregnancy, first trimester Ⓜ♀

O29.012 Aspiration pneumonitis due to anesthesia during pregnancy, second trimester Ⓜ♀

O29.013 Aspiration pneumonitis due to anesthesia during pregnancy, third trimester Ⓜ♀

O29.019 Aspiration pneumonitis due to anesthesia during pregnancy, unspecified trimester Ⓜ♀

√6ᵗʰ **O29.02** Pressure collapse of lung due to anesthesia during pregnancy

O29.021 Pressure collapse of lung due to anesthesia during pregnancy, first trimester Ⓜ♀

O29.022 Pressure collapse of lung due to anesthesia during pregnancy, second trimester Ⓜ♀

O29.023 Pressure collapse of lung due to anesthesia during pregnancy, third trimester Ⓜ♀

O29.029 Pressure collapse of lung due to anesthesia during pregnancy, unspecified trimester Ⓜ♀

√6ᵗʰ **O29.09** Other pulmonary complications of anesthesia during pregnancy

O29.091 Other pulmonary complications of anesthesia during pregnancy, first trimester Ⓜ♀

O29.092 Other pulmonary complications of anesthesia during pregnancy, second trimester Ⓜ♀

O29.093 Other pulmonary complications of anesthesia during pregnancy, third trimester Ⓜ♀

O29.099 Other pulmonary complications of anesthesia during pregnancy, unspecified trimester Ⓜ♀

√5ᵗʰ **O29.1** Cardiac complications of anesthesia during pregnancy

√6ᵗʰ **O29.11** Cardiac arrest due to anesthesia during pregnancy

O29.111 Cardiac arrest due to anesthesia during pregnancy, first trimester Ⓜ♀

O29.112 Cardiac arrest due to anesthesia during pregnancy, second trimester Ⓜ♀

O29.113 Cardiac arrest due to anesthesia during pregnancy, third trimester Ⓜ♀

O29.119 Cardiac arrest due to anesthesia during pregnancy, unspecified trimester Ⓜ♀

√6ᵗʰ **O29.12** Cardiac failure due to anesthesia during pregnancy

O29.121 Cardiac failure due to anesthesia during pregnancy, first trimester Ⓜ♀

O29.122 Cardiac failure due to anesthesia during pregnancy, second trimester Ⓜ♀

O29.123 Cardiac failure due to anesthesia during pregnancy, third trimester Ⓜ♀

O29.129 Cardiac failure due to anesthesia during pregnancy, unspecified trimester Ⓜ♀

√6ᵗʰ **O29.19** Other cardiac complications of anesthesia during pregnancy

O29.191 Other cardiac complications of anesthesia during pregnancy, first trimester Ⓜ♀

EXCLUDES 1 Not coded here   EXCLUDES 2 Not included here   Ⓝ Newborn Age: 0   Ⓟ Pediatric Age: 0-17   Ⓜ Maternity Age: 12-55   Ⓐ Adult Age: 15-124

774   ICD-10-CM 2016

O29.192 Other cardiac complications of anesthesia during pregnancy, second trimester Ⓜ♀

O29.193 Other cardiac complications of anesthesia during pregnancy, third trimester Ⓜ♀

O29.199 Other cardiac complications of anesthesia during pregnancy, unspecified trimester Ⓜ♀

✓5ᵗʰ **O29.2** Central nervous system complications of anesthesia during pregnancy

  ✓6ᵗʰ **O29.21** Cerebral anoxia due to anesthesia during pregnancy

    O29.211 Cerebral anoxia due to anesthesia during pregnancy, first trimester Ⓜ♀

    O29.212 Cerebral anoxia due to anesthesia during pregnancy, second trimester Ⓜ♀

    O29.213 Cerebral anoxia due to anesthesia during pregnancy, third trimester Ⓜ♀

    O29.219 Cerebral anoxia due to anesthesia during pregnancy, unspecified trimester Ⓜ♀

  ✓6ᵗʰ **O29.29** Other central nervous system complications of anesthesia during pregnancy

    O29.291 Other central nervous system complications of anesthesia during pregnancy, first trimester Ⓜ♀

    O29.292 Other central nervous system complications of anesthesia during pregnancy, second trimester Ⓜ♀

    O29.293 Other central nervous system complications of anesthesia during pregnancy, third trimester Ⓜ♀

    O29.299 Other central nervous system complications of anesthesia during pregnancy, unspecified trimester Ⓜ♀

✓5ᵗʰ **O29.3** Toxic reaction to local anesthesia during pregnancy

  ✓6ᵗʰ **O29.3X** Toxic reaction to local anesthesia during pregnancy

    O29.3X1 Toxic reaction to local anesthesia during pregnancy, first trimester Ⓜ♀

    O29.3X2 Toxic reaction to local anesthesia during pregnancy, second trimester Ⓜ♀

    O29.3X3 Toxic reaction to local anesthesia during pregnancy, third trimester Ⓜ♀

    O29.3X9 Toxic reaction to local anesthesia during pregnancy, unspecified trimester Ⓜ♀

✓5ᵗʰ **O29.4** Spinal and epidural anesthesia induced headache during pregnancy

  O29.40 Spinal and epidural anesthesia induced headache during pregnancy, unspecified trimester Ⓜ♀

  O29.41 Spinal and epidural anesthesia induced headache during pregnancy, first trimester Ⓜ♀

  O29.42 Spinal and epidural anesthesia induced headache during pregnancy, second trimester Ⓜ♀

  O29.43 Spinal and epidural anesthesia induced headache during pregnancy, third trimester Ⓜ♀

✓5ᵗʰ **O29.5** Other complications of spinal and epidural anesthesia during pregnancy

  ✓6ᵗʰ **O29.5X** Other complications of spinal and epidural anesthesia during pregnancy

    O29.5X1 Other complications of spinal and epidural anesthesia during pregnancy, first trimester Ⓜ♀

    O29.5X2 Other complications of spinal and epidural anesthesia during pregnancy, second trimester Ⓜ♀

    O29.5X3 Other complications of spinal and epidural anesthesia during pregnancy, third trimester Ⓜ♀

    O29.5X9 Other complications of spinal and epidural anesthesia during pregnancy, unspecified trimester Ⓜ♀

✓5ᵗʰ **O29.6** Failed or difficult intubation for anesthesia during pregnancy

  O29.60 Failed or difficult intubation for anesthesia during pregnancy, unspecified trimester Ⓜ♀

  O29.61 Failed or difficult intubation for anesthesia during pregnancy, first trimester Ⓜ♀

  O29.62 Failed or difficult intubation for anesthesia during pregnancy, second trimester Ⓜ♀

O29.63 Failed or difficult intubation for anesthesia during pregnancy, third trimester Ⓜ♀

✓5ᵗʰ **O29.8** Other complications of anesthesia during pregnancy

  ✓6ᵗʰ **O29.8X** Other complications of anesthesia during pregnancy

    O29.8X1 Other complications of anesthesia during pregnancy, first trimester Ⓜ♀

    O29.8X2 Other complications of anesthesia during pregnancy, second trimester Ⓜ♀

    O29.8X3 Other complications of anesthesia during pregnancy, third trimester Ⓜ♀

    O29.8X9 Other complications of anesthesia during pregnancy, unspecified trimester Ⓜ♀

✓5ᵗʰ **O29.9** Unspecified complication of anesthesia during pregnancy

  O29.90 Unspecified complication of anesthesia during pregnancy, unspecified trimester Ⓜ♀

  O29.91 Unspecified complication of anesthesia during pregnancy, first trimester Ⓜ♀

  O29.92 Unspecified complication of anesthesia during pregnancy, second trimester Ⓜ♀

  O29.93 Unspecified complication of anesthesia during pregnancy, third trimester Ⓜ♀

Maternal care related to the fetus and amniotic cavity and possible delivery problems (O30-O48)

✓4ᵗʰ **O30** Multiple gestation

Code also any complications specific to multiple gestation

  ✓5ᵗʰ **O30.0** Twin pregnancy

    ✓6ᵗʰ **O30.00** Twin pregnancy, unspecified number of placenta and unspecified number of amniotic sacs

      O30.001 Twin pregnancy, unspecified number of placenta and unspecified number of amniotic sacs, first trimester Ⓜ♀

      O30.002 Twin pregnancy, unspecified number of placenta and unspecified number of amniotic sacs, second trimester Ⓜ♀

      O30.003 Twin pregnancy, unspecified number of placenta and unspecified number of amniotic sacs, third trimester Ⓜ♀

      O30.009 Twin pregnancy, unspecified number of placenta and unspecified number of amniotic sacs, unspecified trimester Ⓜ♀

    ✓6ᵗʰ **O30.01** Twin pregnancy, monochorionic/monoamniotic
Twin pregnancy, one placenta, one amniotic sac
EXCLUDES 1 conjoined twins (O30.02-)

      O30.011 Twin pregnancy, monochorionic/monoamniotic, first trimester Ⓜ♀

      O30.012 Twin pregnancy, monochorionic/monoamniotic, second trimester Ⓜ♀

      O30.013 Twin pregnancy, monochorionic/monoamniotic, third trimester Ⓜ♀

      O30.019 Twin pregnancy, monochorionic/monoamniotic, unspecified trimester Ⓜ♀

    ✓6ᵗʰ **O30.02** Conjoined twin pregnancy

      O30.021 Conjoined twin pregnancy, first trimester Ⓜ♀

      O30.022 Conjoined twin pregnancy, second trimester Ⓜ♀

      O30.023 Conjoined twin pregnancy, third trimester Ⓜ♀

      O30.029 Conjoined twin pregnancy, unspecified trimester Ⓜ♀

    ✓6ᵗʰ **O30.03** Twin pregnancy, monochorionic/diamniotic
Twin pregnancy, one placenta, two amniotic sacs

      O30.031 Twin pregnancy, monochorionic/diamniotic, first trimester Ⓜ♀

      O30.032 Twin pregnancy, monochorionic/diamniotic, second trimester Ⓜ♀

      O30.033 Twin pregnancy, monochorionic/diamniotic, third trimester Ⓜ♀

      O30.039 Twin pregnancy, monochorionic/diamniotic, unspecified trimester Ⓜ♀

    ✓6ᵗʰ **O30.04** Twin pregnancy, dichorionic/diamniotic
Twin pregnancy, two placentae, two amniotic sacs

      O30.041 Twin pregnancy, dichorionic/diamniotic, first trimester Ⓜ♀

      O30.042 Twin pregnancy, dichorionic/diamniotic, second trimester Ⓜ♀

☑ Additional Character Required   ᵛˣ⁷ᵗʰ Placeholder Alert   Unspecified Dx   Other Specified Dx   Manifestation   ▶◀ Revised Text   ● New Code   ▲ Revised Code Title

ICD-10-CM 2016   775

Chapter 15. Pregnancy, Childbirth, and the Puerperium

O30.043 Twin pregnancy, dichorionic/diamniotic, third trimester Ⓜ♀

O30.049 Twin pregnancy, dichorionic/diamniotic, unspecified trimester Ⓜ♀

✓6ᵗʰ O30.09 Twin pregnancy, unable to determine number of placenta and number of amniotic sacs

O30.091 Twin pregnancy, unable to determine number of placenta and number of amniotic sacs, first trimester Ⓜ♀

O30.092 Twin pregnancy, unable to determine number of placenta and number of amniotic sacs, second trimester Ⓜ♀

O30.093 Twin pregnancy, unable to determine number of placenta and number of amniotic sacs, third trimester Ⓜ♀

O30.099 Twin pregnancy, unable to determine number of placenta and number of amniotic sacs, unspecified trimester Ⓜ♀

✓5ᵗʰ O30.1 Triplet pregnancy

✓6ᵗʰ O30.10 Triplet pregnancy, unspecified number of placenta and unspecified number of amniotic sacs

O30.101 Triplet pregnancy, unspecified number of placenta and unspecified number of amniotic sacs, first trimester Ⓜ♀

O30.102 Triplet pregnancy, unspecified number of placenta and unspecified number of amniotic sacs, second trimester Ⓜ♀

O30.103 Triplet pregnancy, unspecified number of placenta and unspecified number of amniotic sacs, third trimester Ⓜ♀

O30.109 Triplet pregnancy, unspecified number of placenta and unspecified number of amniotic sacs, unspecified trimester Ⓜ♀

✓6ᵗʰ O30.11 Triplet pregnancy with two or more monochorionic fetuses

O30.111 Triplet pregnancy with two or more monochorionic fetuses, first trimester Ⓜ♀

O30.112 Triplet pregnancy with two or more monochorionic fetuses, second trimester Ⓜ♀

O30.113 Triplet pregnancy with two or more monochorionic fetuses, third trimester Ⓜ♀

O30.119 Triplet pregnancy with two or more monochorionic fetuses, unspecified trimester Ⓜ♀

✓6ᵗʰ O30.12 Triplet pregnancy with two or more monoamniotic fetuses

O30.121 Triplet pregnancy with two or more monoamniotic fetuses, first trimester Ⓜ♀

O30.122 Triplet pregnancy with two or more monoamniotic fetuses, second trimester Ⓜ♀

O30.123 Triplet pregnancy with two or more monoamniotic fetuses, third trimester Ⓜ♀

O30.129 Triplet pregnancy with two or more monoamniotic fetuses, unspecified trimester Ⓜ♀

✓6ᵗʰ O30.19 Triplet pregnancy, unable to determine number of placenta and number of amniotic sacs

O30.191 Triplet pregnancy, unable to determine number of placenta and number of amniotic sacs, first trimester Ⓜ♀

O30.192 Triplet pregnancy, unable to determine number of placenta and number of amniotic sacs, second trimester Ⓜ♀

O30.193 Triplet pregnancy, unable to determine number of placenta and number of amniotic sacs, third trimester Ⓜ♀

O30.199 Triplet pregnancy, unable to determine number of placenta and number of amniotic sacs, unspecified trimester Ⓜ♀

✓6ᵗʰ O30.2 Quadruplet pregnancy

✓6ᵗʰ O30.20 Quadruplet pregnancy, unspecified number of placenta and unspecified number of amniotic sacs

O30.201 Quadruplet pregnancy, unspecified number of placenta and unspecified number of amniotic sacs, first trimester Ⓜ♀

O30.202 Quadruplet pregnancy, unspecified number of placenta and unspecified number of amniotic sacs, second trimester Ⓜ♀

O30.203 Quadruplet pregnancy, unspecified number of placenta and unspecified number of amniotic sacs, third trimester Ⓜ♀

O30.209 Quadruplet pregnancy, unspecified number of placenta and unspecified number of amniotic sacs, unspecified trimester Ⓜ♀

✓6ᵗʰ O30.21 Quadruplet pregnancy with two or more monochorionic fetuses

O30.211 Quadruplet pregnancy with two or more monochorionic fetuses, first trimester Ⓜ♀

O30.212 Quadruplet pregnancy with two or more monochorionic fetuses, second trimester Ⓜ♀

O30.213 Quadruplet pregnancy with two or more monochorionic fetuses, third trimester Ⓜ♀

O30.219 Quadruplet pregnancy with two or more monochorionic fetuses, unspecified trimester Ⓜ♀

✓6ᵗʰ O30.22 Quadruplet pregnancy with two or more monoamniotic fetuses

O30.221 Quadruplet pregnancy with two or more monoamniotic fetuses, first trimester Ⓜ♀

O30.222 Quadruplet pregnancy with two or more monoamniotic fetuses, second trimester Ⓜ♀

O30.223 Quadruplet pregnancy with two or more monoamniotic fetuses, third trimester Ⓜ♀

O30.229 Quadruplet pregnancy with two or more monoamniotic fetuses, unspecified trimester Ⓜ♀

✓6ᵗʰ O30.29 Quadruplet pregnancy, unable to determine number of placenta and number of amniotic sacs

O30.291 Quadruplet pregnancy, unable to determine number of placenta and number of amniotic sacs, first trimester Ⓜ♀

O30.292 Quadruplet pregnancy, unable to determine number of placenta and number of amniotic sacs, second trimester Ⓜ♀

O30.293 Quadruplet pregnancy, unable to determine number of placenta and number of amniotic sacs, third trimester Ⓜ♀

O30.299 Quadruplet pregnancy, unable to determine number of placenta and number of amniotic sacs, unspecified Ⓜ♀

✓5ᵗʰ O30.8 Other specified multiple gestation
Multiple gestation pregnancy greater than quadruplets

✓6ᵗʰ O30.80 Other specified multiple gestation, unspecified number of placenta and unspecified number of amniotic sacs

O30.801 Other specified multiple gestation, unspecified number of placenta and unspecified number of amniotic sacs, first trimester Ⓜ♀

O30.802 Other specified multiple gestation, unspecified number of placenta and unspecified number of amniotic sacs, second trimester Ⓜ♀

EXCLUDES 1 Not coded here   EXCLUDES 2 Not included here   Ⓝ Newborn Age: 0   Ⓟ Pediatric Age: 0-17   Ⓜ Maternity Age: 12-55   Ⓐ Adult Age: 15-124

776   ICD-10-CM 2016

O30.803   **Other specified multiple gestation, unspecified number of placenta and unspecified number of amniotic sacs, third trimester**   Ⓜ♀

O30.809   **Other specified multiple gestation, unspecified number of placenta and unspecified number of amniotic sacs, unspecified trimester**   Ⓜ♀

✓6ᵗʰ **O30.81**   **Other specified multiple gestation with two or more monochorionic fetuses**

O30.811   **Other specified multiple gestation with two or more monochorionic fetuses, first trimester**   Ⓜ♀

O30.812   **Other specified multiple gestation with two or more monochorionic fetuses, second trimester**   Ⓜ♀

O30.813   **Other specified multiple gestation with two or more monochorionic fetuses, third trimester**   Ⓜ♀

O30.819   **Other specified multiple gestation with two or more monochorionic fetuses, unspecified trimester**   Ⓜ♀

✓6ᵗʰ **O30.82**   **Other specified multiple gestation with two or more monoamniotic fetuses**

O30.821   **Other specified multiple gestation with two or more monoamniotic fetuses, first trimester**   Ⓜ♀

O30.822   **Other specified multiple gestation with two or more monoamniotic fetuses, second trimester**   Ⓜ♀

O30.823   **Other specified multiple gestation with two or more monoamniotic fetuses, third trimester**   Ⓜ♀

O30.829   **Other specified multiple gestation with two or more monoamniotic fetuses, unspecified trimester**   Ⓜ♀

✓6ᵗʰ **O30.89**   **Other specified multiple gestation, unable to determine number of placenta and number of amniotic sacs**

O30.891   **Other specified multiple gestation, unable to determine number of placenta and number of amniotic sacs, first trimester**   Ⓜ♀

O30.892   **Other specified multiple gestation, unable to determine number of placenta and number of amniotic sacs, second trimester**   Ⓜ♀

O30.893   **Other specified multiple gestation, unable to determine number of placenta and number of amniotic sacs, third trimester**   Ⓜ♀

O30.899   **Other specified multiple gestation, unable to determine number of placenta and number of amniotic sacs, unspecified trimester**   Ⓜ♀

✓5ᵗʰ **O30.9**   **Multiple gestation, unspecified**
Multiple pregnancy NOS

O30.90   **Multiple gestation, unspecified, unspecified trimester**   Ⓜ♀

O30.91   **Multiple gestation, unspecified, first trimester**   Ⓜ♀

O30.92   **Multiple gestation, unspecified, second trimester**   Ⓜ♀

O30.93   **Multiple gestation, unspecified, third trimester**   Ⓜ♀

✓4ᵗʰ **O31**   **Complications specific to multiple gestation**
EXCLUDES 2   *delayed delivery of second twin, triplet, etc. (O63.2)*
malpresentation of one fetus or more (O32.9)
placental transfusion syndromes (O43.0-)
AHA: 2012, 4Q, 107

One of the following 7th characters is to be assigned to each code under category O31. 7th character 0 is for single gestations and multiple gestations where the fetus is unspecified. 7th characters 1 through 9 are for cases of multiple gestations to identify the fetus for which the code applies. The appropriate code from category O30, Multiple gestation, must also be assigned when assigning a code from category O31 that has a 7th character of 1 through 9.

0	not applicable or unspecified	4	fetus 4
1	fetus 1	5	fetus 5
2	fetus 2	9	other fetus
3	fetus 3		

✓5ᵗʰ **O31.0**   **Papyraceous fetus**
Fetus compressus

✓x7ᵗʰ   **O31.00**   **Papyraceous fetus, unspecified trimester**   Ⓜ♀

✓x7ᵗʰ   **O31.01**   **Papyraceous fetus, first trimester**   Ⓜ♀

✓x7ᵗʰ   **O31.02**   **Papyraceous fetus, second trimester**   Ⓜ♀

✓x7ᵗʰ   **O31.03**   **Papyraceous fetus, third trimester**   Ⓜ♀

✓5ᵗʰ **O31.1**   **Continuing pregnancy after spontaneous abortion of one fetus or more**

✓x7ᵗʰ   **O31.10**   **Continuing pregnancy after spontaneous abortion of one fetus or more, unspecified trimester**   Ⓜ♀

✓x7ᵗʰ   **O31.11**   **Continuing pregnancy after spontaneous abortion of one fetus or more, first trimester**   Ⓜ♀

✓x7ᵗʰ   **O31.12**   **Continuing pregnancy after spontaneous abortion of one fetus or more, second trimester**   Ⓜ♀

✓x7ᵗʰ   **O31.13**   **Continuing pregnancy after spontaneous abortion of one fetus or more, third trimester**   Ⓜ♀

✓5ᵗʰ **O31.2**   **Continuing pregnancy after intrauterine death of one fetus or more**

✓x7ᵗʰ   **O31.20**   **Continuing pregnancy after intrauterine death of one fetus or more, unspecified trimester**   Ⓜ♀

✓x7ᵗʰ   **O31.21**   **Continuing pregnancy after intrauterine death of one fetus or more, first trimester**   Ⓜ♀

✓x7ᵗʰ   **O31.22**   **Continuing pregnancy after intrauterine death of one fetus or more, second trimester**   Ⓜ♀

✓x7ᵗʰ   **O31.23**   **Continuing pregnancy after intrauterine death of one fetus or more, third trimester**   Ⓜ♀

✓5ᵗʰ **O31.3**   **Continuing pregnancy after elective fetal reduction of one fetus or more**
Continuing pregnancy after selective termination of one fetus or more

✓x7ᵗʰ   **O31.30**   **Continuing pregnancy after elective fetal reduction of one fetus or more, unspecified trimester**   Ⓜ♀

✓x7ᵗʰ   **O31.31**   **Continuing pregnancy after elective fetal reduction of one fetus or more, first trimester**   Ⓜ♀

✓x7ᵗʰ   **O31.32**   **Continuing pregnancy after elective fetal reduction of one fetus or more, second trimester**   Ⓜ♀

✓x7ᵗʰ   **O31.33**   **Continuing pregnancy after elective fetal reduction of one fetus or more, third trimester**   Ⓜ♀

✓5ᵗʰ **O31.8**   **Other complications specific to multiple gestation**

✓6ᵗʰ **O31.8X**   **Other complications specific to multiple gestation**

✓7ᵗʰ   **O31.8X1**   **Other complications specific to multiple gestation, first trimester**   Ⓜ♀

✓7ᵗʰ   **O31.8X2**   **Other complications specific to multiple gestation, second trimester**   Ⓜ♀

✓7ᵗʰ   **O31.8X3**   **Other complications specific to multiple gestation, third trimester**   Ⓜ♀

✓7ᵗʰ   **O31.8X9**   **Other complications specific to multiple gestation, unspecified trimester**   Ⓜ♀

☑ Additional Character Required   ✓x7ᵗʰ Placeholder Alert   Unspecified Dx   Other Specified Dx   Manifestation   ▶◀ Revised Text   ● New Code   ▲ Revised Code Title

ICD-10-CM 2016   777

✓4th **O32 Maternal care for malpresentation of fetus**

INCLUDES the listed conditions as a reason for observation, hospitalization or other obstetric care of the mother, or for cesarean delivery before onset of labor

EXCLUDES 1 *malpresentation of fetus with obstructed labor (O64.-)*

AHA: 2012, 4Q, 107

One of the following 7th characters is to be assigned to each code under category O32. 7th character 0 is for single gestations and multiple gestations where the fetus is unspecified. 7th characters 1 through 9 are for cases of multiple gestations to identify the fetus for which the code applies. The appropriate code from category O30, Multiple gestation, must also be assigned when assigning a code from category O32 that has a 7th character of 1 through 9.

0	not applicable or unspecified	4	fetus 4
1	fetus 1	5	fetus 5
2	fetus 2	9	other fetus
3	fetus 3		

✓x7th **O32.0 Maternal care for unstable lie** Ⓜ♀

✓x7th **O32.1 Maternal care for breech presentation** Ⓜ♀
     Maternal care for buttocks presentation
     Maternal care for complete breech
     Maternal care for frank breech
     EXCLUDES 1 *footling presentation (O32.8)*
          incomplete breech (O32.8)

✓x7th **O32.2 Maternal care for transverse and oblique lie** Ⓜ♀
     Maternal care for oblique presentation
     Maternal care for transverse presentation

✓x7th **O32.3 Maternal care for face, brow and chin presentation** Ⓜ♀

✓x7th **O32.4 Maternal care for high head at term** Ⓜ♀
     Maternal care for failure of head to enter pelvic brim

✓x7th **O32.6 Maternal care for compound presentation** Ⓜ♀

✓x7th **O32.8 Maternal care for other malpresentation of fetus** Ⓜ♀
     Maternal care for footling presentation
     Maternal care for incomplete breech

✓x7th **O32.9 Maternal care for malpresentation of fetus, unspecified** Ⓜ♀

✓4th **O33 Maternal care for disproportion**

INCLUDES the listed conditions as a reason for observation, hospitalization or other obstetric care of the mother, or for cesarean delivery before onset of labor

EXCLUDES 1 *disproportion with obstructed labor (O65-O66)*

O33.0 Maternal care for disproportion due to deformity of maternal pelvic bones Ⓜ♀
     Maternal care for disproportion due to pelvic deformity causing disproportion NOS

O33.1 Maternal care for disproportion due to generally contracted pelvis Ⓜ♀
     Maternal care for disproportion due to contracted pelvis NOS causing disproportion

O33.2 Maternal care for disproportion due to inlet contraction of pelvis Ⓜ♀
     Maternal care for disproportion due to inlet contraction (pelvis) causing disproportion

✓x7th **O33.3 Maternal care for disproportion due to outlet contraction of pelvis** Ⓜ♀
     Maternal care for disproportion due to mid-cavity contraction (pelvis)
     Maternal care for disproportion due to outlet contraction (pelvis)

One of the following 7th characters is to be assigned to code O33.3. 7th character 0 is for single gestations and multiple gestations where the fetus is unspecified. 7th characters 1 through 9 are for cases of multiple gestations to identify the fetus for which the code applies. The appropriate code from category O30, Multiple gestation, must also be assigned when assigning code O33.3 with a 7th character of 1 through 9.

0	not applicable or unspecified	4	fetus 4
1	fetus 1	5	fetus 5
2	fetus 2	9	other fetus
3	fetus 3		

✓x7th **O33.4 Maternal care for disproportion of mixed maternal and fetal origin** Ⓜ♀

One of the following 7th characters is to be assigned to code O33.4. 7th character 0 is for single gestations and multiple gestations where the fetus is unspecified. 7th characters 1 through 9 are for cases of multiple gestations to identify the fetus for which the code applies. The appropriate code from category O30, Multiple gestation, must also be assigned when assigning code O33.4 with a 7th character of 1 through 9.

0	not applicable or unspecified	4	fetus 4
1	fetus 1	5	fetus 5
2	fetus 2	9	other fetus
3	fetus 3		

✓x7th **O33.5 Maternal care for disproportion due to unusually large fetus** Ⓜ♀
     Maternal care for disproportion due to disproportion of fetal origin with normally formed fetus
     Maternal care for disproportion due to fetal disproportion NOS

One of the following 7th characters is to be assigned to code O33.5. 7th character 0 is for single gestations and multiple gestations where the fetus is unspecified. 7th characters 1 through 9 are for cases of multiple gestations to identify the fetus for which the code applies. The appropriate code from category O30, Multiple gestation, must also be assigned when assigning code O33.5 with a 7th character of 1 through 9.

0	not applicable or unspecified	4	fetus 4
1	fetus 1	5	fetus 5
2	fetus 2	9	other fetus
3	fetus 3		

✓x7th **O33.6 Maternal care for disproportion due to hydrocephalic fetus** Ⓜ♀

One of the following 7th characters is to be assigned to code O33.6. 7th character 0 is for single gestations and multiple gestations where the fetus is unspecified. 7th characters 1 through 9 are for cases of multiple gestations to identify the fetus for which the code applies. The appropriate code from category O30, Multiple gestation, must also be assigned when assigning code O33.6 with a 7th character of 1 through 9.

0	not applicable or unspecified	4	fetus 4
1	fetus 1	5	fetus 5
2	fetus 2	9	other fetus
3	fetus 3		

O33.7 Maternal care for disproportion due to other fetal deformities Ⓜ♀
     Maternal care for disproportion due to fetal ascites
     Maternal care for disproportion due to fetal hydrops
     Maternal care for disproportion due to fetal meningomyelocele
     Maternal care for disproportion due to fetal sacral teratoma
     Maternal care for disproportion due to fetal tumor
     EXCLUDES 1 *obstructed labor due to other fetal deformities (O66.3)*

O33.8 Maternal care for disproportion of other origin Ⓜ♀

O33.9 Maternal care for disproportion, unspecified Ⓜ♀
     Maternal care for disproportion due to cephalopelvic disproportion NOS
     Maternal care for disproportion due to fetopelvic disproportion NOS

✓4th **O34 Maternal care for abnormality of pelvic organs**

INCLUDES the listed conditions as a reason for hospitalization or other obstetric care of the mother, or for cesarean delivery before onset of labor

     Code first any associated obstructed labor (O65.5)
     Use additional code for specific condition

✓5th **O34.0 Maternal care for congenital malformation of uterus**

     O34.00 Maternal care for unspecified congenital malformation of uterus, unspecified trimester Ⓜ♀

     O34.01 Maternal care for unspecified congenital malformation of uterus, first trimester Ⓜ♀

     O34.02 Maternal care for unspecified congenital malformation of uterus, second trimester Ⓜ♀

     O34.03 Maternal care for unspecified congenital malformation of uterus, third trimester Ⓜ♀

✓5th **O34.1 Maternal care for benign tumor of corpus uteri**
     EXCLUDES 2 *maternal care for benign tumor of cervix (O34.4-)*
          maternal care for malignant neoplasm of uterus (O9A.1-)

     O34.10 Maternal care for benign tumor of corpus uteri, unspecified trimester Ⓜ♀

     O34.11 Maternal care for benign tumor of corpus uteri, first trimester Ⓜ♀

EXCLUDES 1 Not coded here   **EXCLUDES 2** Not included here   N Newborn Age: 0   P Pediatric Age: 0-17   Ⓜ Maternity Age: 12-55   A Adult Age: 15-124

O34.12   **Maternal care for benign tumor of corpus uteri, second trimester**   Ⓜ♀

O34.13   **Maternal care for benign tumor of corpus uteri, third trimester**   Ⓜ♀

✓5ᵗʰ   **O34.2   Maternal care due to uterine scar from previous surgery**

O34.21   **Maternal care for scar from previous cesarean delivery**   Ⓜ♀

O34.29   **Maternal care due to uterine scar from other previous surgery**   Ⓜ♀

✓5ᵗʰ   **O34.3   Maternal care for cervical incompetence**
     Maternal care for cerclage with or without cervical incompetence
     Maternal care for Shirodkar suture with or without cervical incompetence

O34.30   **Maternal care for cervical incompetence, unspecified trimester**   Ⓜ♀

O34.31   **Maternal care for cervical incompetence, first trimester**   Ⓜ♀

O34.32   **Maternal care for cervical incompetence, second trimester**   Ⓜ♀

O34.33   **Maternal care for cervical incompetence, third trimester**   Ⓜ♀

✓5ᵗʰ   **O34.4   Maternal care for other abnormalities of cervix**

O34.40   **Maternal care for other abnormalities of cervix, unspecified trimester**   Ⓜ♀

O34.41   **Maternal care for other abnormalities of cervix, first trimester**   Ⓜ♀

O34.42   **Maternal care for other abnormalities of cervix, second trimester**   Ⓜ♀

O34.43   **Maternal care for other abnormalities of cervix, third trimester**   Ⓜ♀

✓5ᵗʰ   **O34.5   Maternal care for other abnormalities of gravid uterus**

✓6ᵗʰ   **O34.51   Maternal care for incarceration of gravid uterus**

O34.511   **Maternal care for incarceration of gravid uterus, first trimester**   Ⓜ♀

O34.512   **Maternal care for incarceration of gravid uterus, second trimester**   Ⓜ♀

O34.513   **Maternal care for incarceration of gravid uterus, third trimester**   Ⓜ♀

O34.519   **Maternal care for incarceration of gravid uterus, unspecified trimester**   Ⓜ♀

✓6ᵗʰ   **O34.52   Maternal care for prolapse of gravid uterus**

O34.521   **Maternal care for prolapse of gravid uterus, first trimester**   Ⓜ♀

O34.522   **Maternal care for prolapse of gravid uterus, second trimester**   Ⓜ♀

O34.523   **Maternal care for prolapse of gravid uterus, third trimester**   Ⓜ♀

O34.529   **Maternal care for prolapse of gravid uterus, unspecified trimester**   Ⓜ♀

✓6ᵗʰ   **O34.53   Maternal care for retroversion of gravid uterus**

O34.531   **Maternal care for retroversion of gravid uterus, first trimester**   Ⓜ♀

O34.532   **Maternal care for retroversion of gravid uterus, second trimester**   Ⓜ♀

O34.533   **Maternal care for retroversion of gravid uterus, third trimester**   Ⓜ♀

O34.539   **Maternal care for retroversion of gravid uterus, unspecified trimester**   Ⓜ♀

✓6ᵗʰ   **O34.59   Maternal care for other abnormalities of gravid uterus**

O34.591   **Maternal care for other abnormalities of gravid uterus, first trimester**   Ⓜ♀

O34.592   **Maternal care for other abnormalities of gravid uterus, second trimester**   Ⓜ♀

O34.593   **Maternal care for other abnormalities of gravid uterus, third trimester**   Ⓜ♀

O34.599   **Maternal care for other abnormalities of gravid uterus, unspecified trimester**   Ⓜ♀

✓5ᵗʰ   **O34.6   Maternal care for abnormality of vagina**
     EXCLUDES 2   *maternal care for vaginal varices in pregnancy (O22.1-)*

O34.60   **Maternal care for abnormality of vagina, unspecified trimester**   Ⓜ♀

O34.61   **Maternal care for abnormality of vagina, first trimester**   Ⓜ♀

O34.62   **Maternal care for abnormality of vagina, second trimester**   Ⓜ♀

O34.63   **Maternal care for abnormality of vagina, third trimester**   Ⓜ♀

✓5ᵗʰ   **O34.7   Maternal care for abnormality of vulva and perineum**
     EXCLUDES 2   *maternal care for perineal and vulval varices in pregnancy (O22.1-)*

O34.70   **Maternal care for abnormality of vulva and perineum, unspecified trimester**   Ⓜ♀

O34.71   **Maternal care for abnormality of vulva and perineum, first trimester**   Ⓜ♀

O34.72   **Maternal care for abnormality of vulva and perineum, second trimester**   Ⓜ♀

O34.73   **Maternal care for abnormality of vulva and perineum, third trimester**   Ⓜ♀

✓5ᵗʰ   **O34.8   Maternal care for other abnormalities of pelvic organs**

O34.80   **Maternal care for other abnormalities of pelvic organs, unspecified trimester**   Ⓜ♀

O34.81   **Maternal care for other abnormalities of pelvic organs, first trimester**   Ⓜ♀

O34.82   **Maternal care for other abnormalities of pelvic organs, second trimester**   Ⓜ♀

O34.83   **Maternal care for other abnormalities of pelvic organs, third trimester**   Ⓜ♀

✓5ᵗʰ   **O34.9   Maternal care for abnormality of pelvic organ, unspecified**

O34.90   **Maternal care for abnormality of pelvic organ, unspecified, unspecified trimester**   Ⓜ♀

O34.91   **Maternal care for abnormality of pelvic organ, unspecified, first trimester**   Ⓜ♀

O34.92   **Maternal care for abnormality of pelvic organ, unspecified, second trimester**   Ⓜ♀

O34.93   **Maternal care for abnormality of pelvic organ, unspecified, third trimester**   Ⓜ♀

✓4ᵗʰ   **O35   Maternal care for known or suspected fetal abnormality and damage**
     INCLUDES   the listed conditions in the fetus as a reason for hospitalization or other obstetric care to the mother, or for termination of pregnancy
     Code also any associated maternal condition
     EXCLUDES 1   *encounter for suspected maternal and fetal conditions ruled out (Z03.7-)*

One of the following 7th characters is to be assigned to each code under category O35. 7th character 0 is for single gestations and multiple gestations where the fetus is unspecified. 7th characters 1 through 9 are for cases of multiple gestations to identify the fetus for which the code applies. The appropriate code from category O30, Multiple gestation, must also be assigned when assigning a code from category O35 that has a 7th character of 1 through 9.

0	not applicable or unspecified	4	fetus 4
1	fetus 1	5	fetus 5
2	fetus 2	9	other fetus
3	fetus 3		

✓x7ᵗʰ   **O35.0   Maternal care for (suspected) central nervous system malformation in fetus**   Ⓜ♀
     Maternal care for fetal anencephaly
     Maternal care for fetal hydrocephalus
     Maternal care for fetal spina bifida
     EXCLUDES 2   *chromosomal abnormality in fetus (O35.1)*

✓x7ᵗʰ   **O35.1   Maternal care for (suspected) chromosomal abnormality in fetus**   Ⓜ♀

✓x7ᵗʰ   **O35.2   Maternal care for (suspected) hereditary disease in fetus**   Ⓜ♀
     EXCLUDES 2   *chromosomal abnormality in fetus (O35.1)*

✓x7ᵗʰ   **O35.3   Maternal care for (suspected) damage to fetus from viral disease in mother**   Ⓜ♀
     Maternal care for damage to fetus from maternal cytomegalovirus infection
     Maternal care for damage to fetus from maternal rubella

✓x7ᵗʰ   **O35.4   Maternal care for (suspected) damage to fetus from alcohol**   Ⓜ♀

✓x7ᵗʰ   **O35.5   Maternal care for (suspected) damage to fetus by drugs**   Ⓜ♀
     Maternal care for damage to fetus from drug addiction

✓x7ᵗʰ   **O35.6   Maternal care for (suspected) damage to fetus by radiation**   Ⓜ♀

✓ Additional Character Required   ✓x7ᵗʰ Placeholder Alert   Unspecified Dx   Other Specified Dx   Manifestation   ▶◀ Revised Text   ● New Code   ▲ Revised Code Title

ICD-10-CM 2016   **779**

Chapter 15. Pregnancy, Childbirth, and the Puerperium

035.7–036.73

√x7ᵗʰ **O35.7** **Maternal care for (suspected) damage to fetus by other medical procedures**   Ⓜ♀
     Maternal care for damage to fetus by amniocentesis
     Maternal care for damage to fetus by biopsy procedures
     Maternal care for damage to fetus by hematological investigation
     Maternal care for damage to fetus by intrauterine contraceptive device
     Maternal care for damage to fetus by intrauterine surgery

√x7ᵗʰ **O35.8** **Maternal care for other (suspected) fetal abnormality and damage**   Ⓜ♀
     Maternal care for damage to fetus from maternal listeriosis
     Maternal care for damage to fetus from maternal toxoplasmosis

√x7ᵗʰ **O35.9** **Maternal care for (suspected) fetal abnormality and damage, unspecified**   Ⓜ♀

√4ᵗʰ **O36** **Maternal care for other fetal problems**
     INCLUDES   the listed conditions in the fetus as a reason for hospitalization or other obstetric care of the mother, or for termination of pregnancy
     EXCLUDES 1   *encounter for suspected maternal and fetal conditions ruled out (Z03.7-)*
         placental transfusion syndromes (O43.0-)
     EXCLUDES 2   *labor and delivery complicated by fetal stress (O77.-)*

> One of the following 7th characters is to be assigned to each code under category O36. 7th character 0 is for single gestations and multiple gestations where the fetus is unspecified. 7th characters 1 through 9 are for cases of multiple gestations to identify the fetus for which the code applies. The appropriate code from category O30, Multiple gestation, must also be assigned when assigning a code from category O36 that has a 7th character of 1 through 9.
> | | | | |
> |---|---|---|---|
> | 0 | not applicable or unspecified | 4 | fetus 4 |
> | 1 | fetus 1 | 5 | fetus 5 |
> | 2 | fetus 2 | 9 | other fetus |
> | 3 | fetus 3 | | |

√5ᵗʰ **O36.0** **Maternal care for rhesus isoimmunization**
     Maternal care for Rh incompatibility (with hydrops fetalis)

   √6ᵗʰ **O36.01** **Maternal care for anti-D [Rh] antibodies**
       AHA: 2014, 4Q, 17

     √7ᵗʰ **O36.011** **Maternal care for anti-D [Rh] antibodies, first trimester**   Ⓜ♀

     √7ᵗʰ **O36.012** **Maternal care for anti-D [Rh] antibodies, second trimester**   Ⓜ♀

     √7ᵗʰ **O36.013** **Maternal care for anti-D [Rh] antibodies, third trimester**   Ⓜ♀

     √7ᵗʰ **O36.019** **Maternal care for anti-D [Rh] antibodies, unspecified trimester**   Ⓜ♀

   √6ᵗʰ **O36.09** **Maternal care for other rhesus isoimmunization**

     √7ᵗʰ **O36.091** **Maternal care for other rhesus isoimmunization, first trimester**   Ⓜ♀

     √7ᵗʰ **O36.092** **Maternal care for other rhesus isoimmunization, second trimester**   Ⓜ♀

     √7ᵗʰ **O36.093** **Maternal care for other rhesus isoimmunization, third trimester**   Ⓜ♀

     √7ᵗʰ **O36.099** **Maternal care for other rhesus isoimmunization, unspecified trimester**   Ⓜ♀

√5ᵗʰ **O36.1** **Maternal care for other isoimmunization**
     Maternal care for ABO isoimmunization

   √6ᵗʰ **O36.11** **Maternal care for Anti-A sensitization**
     Maternal care for isoimmunization NOS (with hydrops fetalis)

     √7ᵗʰ **O36.111** **Maternal care for Anti-A sensitization, first trimester**   Ⓜ♀

     √7ᵗʰ **O36.112** **Maternal care for Anti-A sensitization, second trimester**   Ⓜ♀

     √7ᵗʰ **O36.113** **Maternal care for Anti-A sensitization, third trimester**   Ⓜ♀

     √7ᵗʰ **O36.119** **Maternal care for Anti-A sensitization, unspecified trimester**   Ⓜ♀

   √6ᵗʰ **O36.19** **Maternal care for other isoimmunization**
     Maternal care for Anti-B sensitization

     √7ᵗʰ **O36.191** **Maternal care for other isoimmunization, first trimester**   Ⓜ♀

     √7ᵗʰ **O36.192** **Maternal care for other isoimmunization, second trimester**   Ⓜ♀

     √7ᵗʰ **O36.193** **Maternal care for other isoimmunization, third trimester**   ♀

     √7ᵗʰ **O36.199** **Maternal care for other isoimmunization, unspecified trimester**   Ⓜ♀

√5ᵗʰ **O36.2** **Maternal care for hydrops fetalis**
     Maternal care for hydrops fetalis NOS
     Maternal care for hydrops fetalis not associated with isoimmunization
     EXCLUDES 1   *hydrops fetalis associated with ABO isoimmunization (O36.1-)*
         hydrops fetalis associated with rhesus isoimmunization (O36.0-)

   √x7ᵗʰ **O36.20** **Maternal care for hydrops fetalis, unspecified trimester**   Ⓜ♀

   √x7ᵗʰ **O36.21** **Maternal care for hydrops fetalis, first trimester**   Ⓜ♀

   √x7ᵗʰ **O36.22** **Maternal care for hydrops fetalis, second trimester**   Ⓜ♀

   √x7ᵗʰ **O36.23** **Maternal care for hydrops fetalis, third trimester**   Ⓜ♀

√x7ᵗʰ **O36.4** **Maternal care for intrauterine death**   Ⓜ♀
     Maternal care for intrauterine fetal death NOS
     Maternal care for intrauterine fetal death after completion of 20 weeks of gestation
     Maternal care for late fetal death
     Maternal care for missed delivery
     EXCLUDES 1   *missed abortion (O02.1)*
         stillbirth (P95)

√5ᵗʰ **O36.5** **Maternal care for known or suspected poor fetal growth**

   √6ᵗʰ **O36.51** **Maternal care for known or suspected placental insufficiency**

     √7ᵗʰ **O36.511** **Maternal care for known or suspected placental insufficiency, first trimester**   Ⓜ♀

     √7ᵗʰ **O36.512** **Maternal care for known or suspected placental insufficiency, second trimester**   Ⓜ♀

     √7ᵗʰ **O36.513** **Maternal care for known or suspected placental insufficiency, third trimester**   Ⓜ♀

     √7ᵗʰ **O36.519** **Maternal care for known or suspected placental insufficiency, unspecified trimester**   Ⓜ♀

   √6ᵗʰ **O36.59** **Maternal care for other known or suspected poor fetal growth**
     Maternal care for known or suspected light-for-dates NOS
     Maternal care for known or suspected small-for-dates NOS

     √7ᵗʰ **O36.591** **Maternal care for other known or suspected poor fetal growth, first trimester**   Ⓜ♀

     √7ᵗʰ **O36.592** **Maternal care for other known or suspected poor fetal growth, second trimester**   Ⓜ♀

     √7ᵗʰ **O36.593** **Maternal care for other known or suspected poor fetal growth, third trimester**   Ⓜ♀

     √7ᵗʰ **O36.599** **Maternal care for other known or suspected poor fetal growth, unspecified trimester**   Ⓜ♀

√5ᵗʰ **O36.6** **Maternal care for excessive fetal growth**
     Maternal care for known or suspected large-for-dates

   √x7ᵗʰ **O36.60** **Maternal care for excessive fetal growth, unspecified trimester**   Ⓜ♀

   √x7ᵗʰ **O36.61** **Maternal care for excessive fetal growth, first trimester**   Ⓜ♀

   √x7ᵗʰ **O36.62** **Maternal care for excessive fetal growth, second trimester**   Ⓜ♀

   √x7ᵗʰ **O36.63** **Maternal care for excessive fetal growth, third trimester**   Ⓜ♀

√5ᵗʰ **O36.7** **Maternal care for viable fetus in abdominal pregnancy**

   √x7ᵗʰ **O36.70** **Maternal care for viable fetus in abdominal pregnancy, unspecified trimester**   Ⓜ♀

   √x7ᵗʰ **O36.71** **Maternal care for viable fetus in abdominal pregnancy, first trimester**   Ⓜ♀

   √x7ᵗʰ **O36.72** **Maternal care for viable fetus in abdominal pregnancy, second trimester**   Ⓜ♀

   √x7ᵗʰ **O36.73** **Maternal care for viable fetus in abdominal pregnancy, third trimester**   Ⓜ♀

EXCLUDES 1 Not coded here   **EXCLUDES 2** Not included here   Ⓝ Newborn Age: 0   Ⓟ Pediatric Age: 0-17   Ⓜ Maternity Age: 12-55   Ⓐ Adult Age: 15-124

780   **ICD-10-CM 2016**

✓5ᵗʰ **O36.8 Maternal care for other specified fetal problems**

   ✓x7ᵗʰ **O36.80 Pregnancy with inconclusive fetal viability** Ⓜ♀
       Encounter to determine fetal viability of pregnancy

   ✓6ᵗʰ **O36.81 Decreased fetal movements**

      ✓7ᵗʰ **O36.812 Decreased fetal movements, second** Ⓜ♀
         trimester

      ✓7ᵗʰ **O36.813 Decreased fetal movements, third** Ⓜ♀
         trimester

      ✓7ᵗʰ **O36.819 Decreased fetal movements,** Ⓜ♀
         unspecified trimester

   ✓6ᵗʰ **O36.82 Fetal anemia and thrombocytopenia**

      ✓7ᵗʰ **O36.821 Fetal anemia and thrombocytopenia,** Ⓜ♀
         first trimester

      ✓7ᵗʰ **O36.822 Fetal anemia and thrombocytopenia,** Ⓜ♀
         second trimester

      ✓7ᵗʰ **O36.823 Fetal anemia and thrombocytopenia,** Ⓜ♀
         third trimester

      ✓7ᵗʰ **O36.829 Fetal anemia and thrombocytopenia,** Ⓜ♀
         unspecified trimester

   ✓6ᵗʰ **O36.89 Maternal care for other specified fetal problems**

      ✓7ᵗʰ **O36.891 Maternal care for other specified fetal** Ⓜ♀
         problems, first trimester

      ✓7ᵗʰ **O36.892 Maternal care for other specified fetal** Ⓜ♀
         problems, second trimester

      ✓7ᵗʰ **O36.893 Maternal care for other specified fetal** Ⓜ♀
         problems, third trimester

      ✓7ᵗʰ **O36.899 Maternal care for other specified fetal** Ⓜ♀
         problems, unspecified trimester

✓5ᵗʰ **O36.9 Maternal care for fetal problem, unspecified**

   ✓x7ᵗʰ **O36.90 Maternal care for fetal problem, unspecified,** Ⓜ♀
       unspecified trimester

   ✓x7ᵗʰ **O36.91 Maternal care for fetal problem, unspecified,** Ⓜ♀
       first trimester

   ✓x7ᵗʰ **O36.92 Maternal care for fetal problem, unspecified,** Ⓜ♀
       second trimester

   ✓x7ᵗʰ **O36.93 Maternal care for fetal problem, unspecified,** Ⓜ♀
       third trimester

✓4ᵗʰ **O40 Polyhydramnios**
   Hydramnios
   EXCLUDES 1 encounter for suspected maternal and fetal conditions ruled out
      (Z03.7-)

> One of the following 7th characters is to be assigned to each code under category O40. 7th character 0 is for single gestations and multiple gestations where the fetus is unspecified. 7th characters 1 through 9 are for cases of multiple gestations to identify the fetus for which the code applies. The appropriate code from category O30, Multiple gestation, must also be assigned when assigning a code from category O40 that has a 7th character of 1 through 9.
>
> 0   not applicable or unspecified   4   fetus 4
> 1   fetus 1   5   fetus 5
> 2   fetus 2   9   other fetus
> 3   fetus 3

  ✓x7ᵗʰ **O40.1 Polyhydramnios, first trimester** Ⓜ♀
  ✓x7ᵗʰ **O40.2 Polyhydramnios, second trimester** Ⓜ♀
  ✓x7ᵗʰ **O40.3 Polyhydramnios, third trimester** Ⓜ♀
  ✓x7ᵗʰ **O40.9 Polyhydramnios, unspecified trimester** Ⓜ♀

✓4ᵗʰ **O41 Other disorders of amniotic fluid and membranes**
   EXCLUDES 1 encounter for suspected maternal and fetal conditions ruled out
      (Z03.7-)

> One of the following 7th characters is to be assigned to each code under category O41. 7th character 0 is for single gestations and multiple gestations where the fetus is unspecified. 7th characters 1 through 9 are for cases of multiple gestations to identify the fetus for which the code applies. The appropriate code from category O30, Multiple gestation, must also be assigned when assigning a code from category O41 that has a 7th character of 1 through 9.
>
> 0   not applicable or unspecified   4   fetus 4
> 1   fetus 1   5   fetus 5
> 2   fetus 2   9   other fetus
> 3   fetus 3

  ✓5ᵗʰ **O41.0 Oligohydramnios**
     Oligohydramnios without rupture of membranes

    ✓x7ᵗʰ **O41.00 Oligohydramnios, unspecified trimester** Ⓜ♀
    ✓x7ᵗʰ **O41.01 Oligohydramnios, first trimester** Ⓜ♀

    ✓x7ᵗʰ **O41.02 Oligohydramnios, second trimester** Ⓜ♀
    ✓x7ᵗʰ **O41.03 Oligohydramnios, third trimester** Ⓜ♀

  ✓5ᵗʰ **O41.1 Infection of amniotic sac and membranes**

    ✓6ᵗʰ **O41.10 Infection of amniotic sac and membranes,**
       unspecified

      ✓7ᵗʰ **O41.101 Infection of amniotic sac and** Ⓜ♀
         membranes, unspecified, first
         trimester

      ✓7ᵗʰ **O41.102 Infection of amniotic sac and** Ⓜ♀
         membranes, unspecified, second
         trimester

      ✓7ᵗʰ **O41.103 Infection of amniotic sac and** Ⓜ♀
         membranes, unspecified, third
         trimester

      ✓7ᵗʰ **O41.109 Infection of amniotic sac and** Ⓜ♀
         membranes, unspecified, unspecified
         trimester

    ✓6ᵗʰ **O41.12 Chorioamnionitis**

      ✓7ᵗʰ **O41.121 Chorioamnionitis, first trimester** Ⓜ♀
      ✓7ᵗʰ **O41.122 Chorioamnionitis, second trimester** Ⓜ♀
      ✓7ᵗʰ **O41.123 Chorioamnionitis, third trimester** Ⓜ♀
      ✓7ᵗʰ **O41.129 Chorioamnionitis, unspecified** Ⓜ♀
         trimester

    ✓6ᵗʰ **O41.14 Placentitis**

      ✓7ᵗʰ **O41.141 Placentitis, first trimester** Ⓜ♀
      ✓7ᵗʰ **O41.142 Placentitis, second trimester** Ⓜ♀
      ✓7ᵗʰ **O41.143 Placentitis, third trimester** Ⓜ♀
      ✓7ᵗʰ **O41.149 Placentitis, unspecified trimester** Ⓜ♀

  ✓5ᵗʰ **O41.8 Other specified disorders of amniotic fluid and membranes**

    ✓6ᵗʰ **O41.8X Other specified disorders of amniotic fluid and**
       membranes

      ✓7ᵗʰ **O41.8X1 Other specified disorders of amniotic** Ⓜ♀
         fluid and membranes, first trimester

      ✓7ᵗʰ **O41.8X2 Other specified disorders of amniotic** Ⓜ♀
         fluid and membranes, second trimester

      ✓7ᵗʰ **O41.8X3 Other specified disorders of amniotic** Ⓜ♀
         fluid and membranes, third trimester

      ✓7ᵗʰ **O41.8X9 Other specified disorders of amniotic** Ⓜ♀
         fluid and membranes, unspecified
         trimester

  ✓5ᵗʰ **O41.9 Disorder of amniotic fluid and membranes, unspecified**

    ✓x7ᵗʰ **O41.90 Disorder of amniotic fluid and membranes,** Ⓜ♀
       unspecified, unspecified trimester

    ✓x7ᵗʰ **O41.91 Disorder of amniotic fluid and membranes,** Ⓜ♀
       unspecified, first trimester

    ✓x7ᵗʰ **O41.92 Disorder of amniotic fluid and membranes,** Ⓜ♀
       unspecified, second trimester

    ✓x7ᵗʰ **O41.93 Disorder of amniotic fluid and membranes,** Ⓜ♀
       unspecified, third trimester

✓4ᵗʰ **O42 Premature rupture of membranes**

  ✓5ᵗʰ **O42.0 Premature rupture of membranes, onset of labor within 24 hours of rupture**

     O42.00 Premature rupture of membranes, onset of Ⓜ♀
       labor within 24 hours of rupture, unspecified
       weeks of gestation

    ✓6ᵗʰ **O42.01 Preterm premature rupture of membranes,**
       onset of labor within 24 hours of rupture
       Premature rupture of membranes before 37
         completed weeks of gestation

       O42.011 Preterm premature rupture of Ⓜ♀
         membranes, onset of labor within 24
         hours of rupture, first trimester

       O42.012 Preterm premature rupture of Ⓜ♀
         membranes, onset of labor within 24
         hours of rupture, second trimester

       O42.013 Preterm premature rupture of Ⓜ♀
         membranes, onset of labor within 24
         hours of rupture, third trimester

       O42.019 Preterm premature rupture of Ⓜ♀
         membranes, onset of labor within 24
         hours of rupture, unspecified trimester

     O42.02 Full-term premature rupture of membranes, Ⓜ♀
       onset of labor within 24 hours of rupture
       Premature rupture of membranes after 37 completed
        weeks of gestation

✓ Additional Character Required   ✓x7ᵗʰ Placeholder Alert   Unspecified Dx   Other Specified Dx   Manifestation   ▶◀ Revised Text   ● New Code   ▲ Revised Code Title

√5ᵗʰ **O42.1** **Premature rupture of membranes, onset of labor more than 24 hours following rupture**

    O42.10 Premature rupture of membranes, onset of labor more than 24 hours following rupture, unspecified weeks of gestation   Ⓜ♀

    √6ᵗʰ **O42.11** **Preterm premature rupture of membranes, onset of labor more than 24 hours following rupture**
      Premature rupture of membranes before 37 completed weeks of gestation

      O42.111 Preterm premature rupture of membranes, onset of labor more than 24 hours following rupture, first trimester   Ⓜ♀

      O42.112 Preterm premature rupture of membranes, onset of labor more than 24 hours following rupture, second trimester   Ⓜ♀

      O42.113 Preterm premature rupture of membranes, onset of labor more than 24 hours following rupture, third trimester   Ⓜ♀

      O42.119 Preterm premature rupture of membranes, onset of labor more than 24 hours following rupture, unspecified trimester   Ⓜ♀

    O42.12 Full-term premature rupture of membranes, onset of labor more than 24 hours following rupture   Ⓜ♀
      Premature rupture of membranes after 37 completed weeks of gestation

√5ᵗʰ **O42.9** **Premature rupture of membranes, unspecified as to length of time between rupture and onset of labor**

    O42.90 Premature rupture of membranes, unspecified as to length of time between rupture and onset of labor, unspecified weeks of gestation   Ⓜ♀

    √6ᵗʰ **O42.91** **Preterm premature rupture of membranes, unspecified as to length of time between rupture and onset of labor**
      Premature rupture of membranes before 37 completed weeks of gestation

      O42.911 Preterm premature rupture of membranes, unspecified as to length of time between rupture and onset of labor, first trimester   Ⓜ♀

      O42.912 Preterm premature rupture of membranes, unspecified as to length of time between rupture and onset of labor, second trimester   Ⓜ♀

      O42.913 Preterm premature rupture of membranes, unspecified as to length of time between rupture and onset of labor, third trimester   Ⓜ♀

      O42.919 Preterm premature rupture of membranes, unspecified as to length of time between rupture and onset of labor, unspecified trimester   Ⓜ♀

    O42.92 Full-term premature rupture of membranes, unspecified as to length of time between rupture and onset of labor   Ⓜ♀
      Premature rupture of membranes after 37 completed weeks of gestation

√4ᵗʰ **O43** **Placental disorders**

    EXCLUDES 2   *maternal care for poor fetal growth due to placental insufficiency (O36.5-)*
       placenta previa (O44.-)
       placental polyp (O90.89)
       placentitis (O41.14-)
       premature separation of placenta [abruptio placentae] (O45.-)

√5ᵗʰ **O43.0** **Placental transfusion syndromes**

    √6ᵗʰ **O43.01** **Fetomaternal placental transfusion syndrome**
      Maternofetal placental transfusion syndrome

      O43.011 Fetomaternal placental transfusion syndrome, first trimester   Ⓜ♀

      O43.012 Fetomaternal placental transfusion syndrome, second trimester   Ⓜ♀

      O43.013 Fetomaternal placental transfusion syndrome, third trimester   Ⓜ♀

      O43.019 Fetomaternal placental transfusion syndrome, unspecified trimester   Ⓜ♀

    √6ᵗʰ **O43.02** **Fetus-to-fetus placental transfusion syndrome**

      O43.021 Fetus-to-fetus placental transfusion syndrome, first trimester   Ⓜ♀

      O43.022 Fetus-to-fetus placental transfusion syndrome, second trimester   Ⓜ♀

      O43.023 Fetus-to-fetus placental transfusion syndrome, third trimester   Ⓜ♀

      O43.029 Fetus-to-fetus placental transfusion syndrome, unspecified trimester   Ⓜ♀

√5ᵗʰ **O43.1** **Malformation of placenta**

    √6ᵗʰ **O43.10** **Malformation of placenta, unspecified**
      Abnormal placenta NOS

      O43.101 Malformation of placenta, unspecified, first trimester   Ⓜ♀

      O43.102 Malformation of placenta, unspecified, second trimester   Ⓜ♀

      O43.103 Malformation of placenta, unspecified, third trimester   Ⓜ♀

      O43.109 Malformation of placenta, unspecified, unspecified trimester   Ⓜ♀

    √6ᵗʰ **O43.11** **Circumvallate placenta**

      O43.111 Circumvallate placenta, first trimester   Ⓜ♀

      O43.112 Circumvallate placenta, second trimester   Ⓜ♀

      O43.113 Circumvallate placenta, third trimester   Ⓜ♀

      O43.119 Circumvallate placenta, unspecified trimester   Ⓜ♀

    √6ᵗʰ **O43.12** **Velamentous insertion of umbilical cord**

      O43.121 Velamentous insertion of umbilical cord, first trimester   Ⓜ♀

      O43.122 Velamentous insertion of umbilical cord, second trimester   Ⓜ♀

      O43.123 Velamentous insertion of umbilical cord, third trimester   Ⓜ♀

      O43.129 Velamentous insertion of umbilical cord, unspecified trimester   Ⓜ♀

    √6ᵗʰ **O43.19** **Other malformation of placenta**

      O43.191 Other malformation of placenta, first trimester   Ⓜ♀

      O43.192 Other malformation of placenta, second trimester   Ⓜ♀

      O43.193 Other malformation of placenta, third trimester   Ⓜ♀

      O43.199 Other malformation of placenta, unspecified trimester   Ⓜ♀

√5ᵗʰ **O43.2** **Morbidly adherent placenta**
    Code also associated third stage postpartum hemorrhage, if applicable (O72.0)
     EXCLUDES 1   *retained placenta (O73.-)*

    √6ᵗʰ **O43.21** **Placenta accreta**

      O43.211 Placenta accreta, first trimester   Ⓜ♀
      O43.212 Placenta accreta, second trimester   Ⓜ♀
      O43.213 Placenta accreta, third trimester   Ⓜ♀
      O43.219 Placenta accreta, unspecified trimester   Ⓜ♀

    √6ᵗʰ **O43.22** **Placenta increta**

      O43.221 Placenta increta, first trimester   Ⓜ♀
      O43.222 Placenta increta, second trimester   Ⓜ♀
      O43.223 Placenta increta, third trimester   Ⓜ♀
      O43.229 Placenta increta, unspecified trimester   Ⓜ♀

    √6ᵗʰ **O43.23** **Placenta percreta**

      O43.231 Placenta percreta, first trimester   Ⓜ♀
      O43.232 Placenta percreta, second trimester   Ⓜ♀
      O43.233 Placenta percreta, third trimester   Ⓜ♀
      O43.239 Placenta percreta, unspecified trimester   Ⓜ♀

√5ᵗʰ **O43.8** **Other placental disorders**

    √6ᵗʰ **O43.81** **Placental infarction**

      O43.811 Placental infarction, first trimester   Ⓜ♀
      O43.812 Placental infarction, second trimester   Ⓜ♀
      O43.813 Placental infarction, third trimester   Ⓜ♀
      O43.819 Placental infarction, unspecified trimester   Ⓜ♀

EXCLUDES 1 Not coded here   *EXCLUDES 2* Not included here   Ⓝ Newborn Age: 0   Ⓟ Pediatric Age: 0-17   Ⓜ Maternity Age: 12-55   Ⓐ Adult Age: 15-124

✓6ᵗʰ **O43.89 Other placental disorders**
     Placental dysfunction

     O43.891 Other placental disorders, first trimester Ⓜ♀
     O43.892 Other placental disorders, second trimester Ⓜ♀
     O43.893 Other placental disorders, third trimester Ⓜ♀
     O43.899 Other placental disorders, unspecified trimester Ⓜ♀

✓5ᵗʰ **O43.9 Unspecified placental disorder**

     O43.90 Unspecified placental disorder, unspecified trimester Ⓜ♀
     O43.91 Unspecified placental disorder, first trimester Ⓜ♀
     O43.92 Unspecified placental disorder, second trimester Ⓜ♀
     O43.93 Unspecified placental disorder, third trimester Ⓜ♀

✓4ᵗʰ **O44 Placenta previa**

✓5ᵗʰ **O44.0 Placenta previa specified as without hemorrhage**
     Low implantation of placenta specified as without hemorrhage

     O44.00 Placenta previa specified as without hemorrhage, unspecified trimester Ⓜ♀
     O44.01 Placenta previa specified as without hemorrhage, first trimester Ⓜ♀
     O44.02 Placenta previa specified as without hemorrhage, second trimester Ⓜ♀
     O44.03 Placenta previa specified as without hemorrhage, third trimester Ⓜ♀

✓5ᵗʰ **O44.1 Placenta previa with hemorrhage**
     Low implantation of placenta, NOS or with hemorrhage
     Marginal placenta previa, NOS or with hemorrhage
     Partial placenta previa, NOS or with hemorrhage
     Total placenta previa, NOS or with hemorrhage
     EXCLUDES 1   *labor and delivery complicated by hemorrhage from vasa previa (O69.4)*

     O44.10 Placenta previa with hemorrhage, unspecified trimester Ⓜ♀
     O44.11 Placenta previa with hemorrhage, first trimester Ⓜ♀
     O44.12 Placenta previa with hemorrhage, second trimester Ⓜ♀
     O44.13 Placenta previa with hemorrhage, third trimester Ⓜ♀

✓4ᵗʰ **O45 Premature separation of placenta [abruptio placentae]**

✓5ᵗʰ **O45.0 Premature separation of placenta with coagulation defect**

✓6ᵗʰ **O45.00 Premature separation of placenta with coagulation defect, unspecified**

     O45.001 Premature separation of placenta with coagulation defect, unspecified, first trimester Ⓜ♀
     O45.002 Premature separation of placenta with coagulation defect, unspecified, second trimester Ⓜ♀
     O45.003 Premature separation of placenta with coagulation defect, unspecified, third trimester Ⓜ♀
     O45.009 Premature separation of placenta with coagulation defect, unspecified, unspecified trimester Ⓜ♀

✓6ᵗʰ **O45.01 Premature separation of placenta with afibrinogenemia**
     Premature separation of placenta with hypofibrinogenemia

     O45.011 Premature separation of placenta with afibrinogenemia, first trimester Ⓜ♀
     O45.012 Premature separation of placenta with afibrinogenemia, second trimester Ⓜ♀
     O45.013 Premature separation of placenta with afibrinogenemia, third trimester Ⓜ♀
     O45.019 Premature separation of placenta with afibrinogenemia, unspecified trimester Ⓜ♀

✓6ᵗʰ **O45.02 Premature separation of placenta with disseminated intravascular coagulation**

     O45.021 Premature separation of placenta with disseminated intravascular coagulation, first trimester Ⓜ♀

     O45.022 Premature separation of placenta with disseminated intravascular coagulation, second trimester Ⓜ♀
     O45.023 Premature separation of placenta with disseminated intravascular coagulation, third trimester Ⓜ♀
     O45.029 Premature separation of placenta with disseminated intravascular coagulation, unspecified trimester Ⓜ♀

✓6ᵗʰ **O45.09 Premature separation of placenta with other coagulation defect**

     O45.091 Premature separation of placenta with other coagulation defect, first trimester Ⓜ♀
     O45.092 Premature separation of placenta with other coagulation defect, second trimester Ⓜ♀
     O45.093 Premature separation of placenta with other coagulation defect, third trimester Ⓜ♀
     O45.099 Premature separation of placenta with other coagulation defect, unspecified trimester Ⓜ♀

✓5ᵗʰ **O45.8 Other premature separation of placenta**

✓6ᵗʰ **O45.8X Other premature separation of placenta**

     O45.8X1 Other premature separation of placenta, first trimester Ⓜ♀
     O45.8X2 Other premature separation of placenta, second trimester Ⓜ♀
     O45.8X3 Other premature separation of placenta, third trimester Ⓜ♀
     O45.8X9 Other premature separation of placenta, unspecified trimester Ⓜ♀

✓5ᵗʰ **O45.9 Premature separation of placenta, unspecified**
     Abruptio placentae NOS

     O45.90 Premature separation of placenta, unspecified, unspecified trimester Ⓜ♀
     O45.91 Premature separation of placenta, unspecified, first trimester Ⓜ♀
     O45.92 Premature separation of placenta, unspecified, second trimester Ⓜ♀
     O45.93 Premature separation of placenta, unspecified, third trimester Ⓜ♀

✓4ᵗʰ **O46 Antepartum hemorrhage, not elsewhere classified**
     EXCLUDES 1   *hemorrhage in early pregnancy (O20.-)*
     intrapartum hemorrhage NEC (O67.-)
     placenta previa (O44.-)
     premature separation of placenta [abruptio placentae] (O45.-)

✓5ᵗʰ **O46.0 Antepartum hemorrhage with coagulation defect**

✓6ᵗʰ **O46.00 Antepartum hemorrhage with coagulation defect, unspecified**

     O46.001 Antepartum hemorrhage with coagulation defect, unspecified, first trimester Ⓜ♀
     O46.002 Antepartum hemorrhage with coagulation defect, unspecified, second trimester Ⓜ♀
     O46.003 Antepartum hemorrhage with coagulation defect, unspecified, third trimester Ⓜ♀
     O46.009 Antepartum hemorrhage with coagulation defect, unspecified, unspecified trimester Ⓜ♀

✓6ᵗʰ **O46.01 Antepartum hemorrhage with afibrinogenemia**
     Antepartum hemorrhage with hypofibrinogenemia

     O46.011 Antepartum hemorrhage with afibrinogenemia, first trimester Ⓜ♀
     O46.012 Antepartum hemorrhage with afibrinogenemia, second trimester Ⓜ♀
     O46.013 Antepartum hemorrhage with afibrinogenemia, third trimester Ⓜ♀
     O46.019 Antepartum hemorrhage with afibrinogenemia, unspecified trimester Ⓜ♀

✓6ᵗʰ **O46.02 Antepartum hemorrhage with disseminated intravascular coagulation**

     O46.021 Antepartum hemorrhage with disseminated intravascular coagulation, first trimester Ⓜ♀

✓ Additional Character Required   ✓7ᵗʰ Placeholder Alert   Unspecified Dx   Other Specified Dx   Manifestation   ►◄ Revised Text   ● New Code   ▲ Revised Code Title

     O46.022 **Antepartum hemorrhage with disseminated intravascular coagulation, second trimester** Ⓜ♀

     O46.023 **Antepartum hemorrhage with disseminated intravascular coagulation, third trimester** Ⓜ♀

     O46.029 **Antepartum hemorrhage with disseminated intravascular coagulation, unspecified trimester** Ⓜ♀

   ✓6ᵗʰ **O46.09** **Antepartum hemorrhage with** other **coagulation defect**

     O46.091 **Antepartum hemorrhage with other coagulation defect,** first trimester Ⓜ♀

     O46.092 **Antepartum hemorrhage with other coagulation defect,** second trimester Ⓜ♀

     O46.093 **Antepartum hemorrhage with other coagulation defect,** third trimester Ⓜ♀

     O46.099 **Antepartum hemorrhage with other coagulation defect, unspecified trimester** Ⓜ♀

✓5ᵗʰ **O46.8** **Other** antepartum hemorrhage

   ✓6ᵗʰ **O46.8X** **Other** antepartum hemorrhage

     O46.8X1 **Other antepartum hemorrhage,** first trimester Ⓜ♀

     O46.8X2 **Other antepartum hemorrhage,** second trimester Ⓜ♀

     O46.8X3 **Other antepartum hemorrhage,** third trimester Ⓜ♀

     O46.8X9 **Other antepartum hemorrhage, unspecified trimester** Ⓜ♀

✓5ᵗʰ **O46.9** **Antepartum hemorrhage,** unspecified

     O46.90 **Antepartum hemorrhage, unspecified, unspecified trimester** Ⓜ♀

     O46.91 **Antepartum hemorrhage, unspecified,** first trimester Ⓜ♀

     O46.92 **Antepartum hemorrhage, unspecified,** second trimester Ⓜ♀

     O46.93 **Antepartum hemorrhage, unspecified,** third trimester Ⓜ♀

✓4ᵗʰ **O47** **False labor**
Braxton Hicks contractions
Threatened labor
EXCLUDES 1   preterm labor (O60.-)

✓5ᵗʰ **O47.0** **False labor** before 37 completed weeks of gestation

     O47.00 **False labor before 37 completed weeks of gestation, unspecified trimester** Ⓜ♀

     O47.02 **False labor before 37 completed weeks of gestation,** second trimester Ⓜ♀

     O47.03 **False labor before 37 completed weeks of gestation,** third trimester Ⓜ♀

   O47.1 **False labor** at or after 37 completed weeks of gestation Ⓜ♀

   O47.9 **False labor, unspecified** Ⓜ♀

✓4ᵗʰ **O48** **Late pregnancy**

   O48.0 **Post-term pregnancy** ♀
Pregnancy over 40 completed weeks to 42 completed weeks gestation

   O48.1 **Prolonged pregnancy** Ⓜ♀
Pregnancy which has advanced beyond 42 completed weeks gestation

Complications of labor and delivery (O60-O77)

✓4ᵗʰ **O60** **Preterm labor**
INCLUDES   onset (spontaneous) of labor before 37 completed weeks of gestation
EXCLUDES 1   false labor (O47.0-)
     threatened labor NOS (O47.0-)

✓5ᵗʰ **O60.0** **Preterm labor** without delivery

     O60.00 **Preterm labor without delivery, unspecified trimester** Ⓜ♀

     O60.02 **Preterm labor without delivery,** second trimester Ⓜ♀

     O60.03 **Preterm labor without delivery,** third trimester Ⓜ♀

✓5ᵗʰ **O60.1** **Preterm labor** with preterm delivery

One of the following 7th characters is to be assigned to each code under subcategory O60.1. 7th character 0 is for single gestations and multiple gestations where the fetus is unspecified. 7th characters 1 through 9 are for cases of multiple gestations to identify the fetus for which the code applies. The appropriate code from category O30, Multiple gestation, must also be assigned when assigning a code from subcategory O60.1 that has a 7th character of 1 through 9.
0   not applicable or unspecified   4   fetus 4
1   fetus 1   5   fetus 5
2   fetus 2   9   other fetus
3   fetus 3

   ✓x7ᵗʰ **O60.10** **Preterm labor with preterm delivery, unspecified trimester** Ⓜ♀
Preterm labor with delivery NOS

   ✓x7ᵗʰ **O60.12** **Preterm labor second trimester with preterm delivery** second trimester Ⓜ♀

   ✓x7ᵗʰ **O60.13** **Preterm labor second trimester with preterm delivery** third trimester Ⓜ♀

   ✓x7ᵗʰ **O60.14** **Preterm labor third trimester with preterm delivery** third trimester Ⓜ♀

✓5ᵗʰ **O60.2** **Term delivery with preterm labor**

One of the following 7th characters is to be assigned to each code under subcategory O60.2. 7th character 0 is for single gestations and multiple gestations where the fetus is unspecified. 7th characters 1 through 9 are for cases of multiple gestations to identify the fetus for which the code applies. The appropriate code from category O30, Multiple gestation, must also be assigned when assigning a code from subcategory O60.2 that has a 7th character of 1 through 9.
0   not applicable or unspecified   4   fetus 4
1   fetus 1   5   fetus 5
2   fetus 2   9   other fetus
3   fetus 3

   ✓x7ᵗʰ **O60.20** **Term delivery with preterm labor, unspecified trimester** Ⓜ♀

   ✓x7ᵗʰ **O60.22** **Term delivery with preterm labor,** second trimester Ⓜ♀

   ✓x7ᵗʰ **O60.23** **Term delivery with preterm labor,** third trimester Ⓜ♀

✓4ᵗʰ **O61** **Failed induction of labor**

   O61.0 **Failed** medical **induction of labor** Ⓜ♀
Failed induction (of labor) by oxytocin
Failed induction (of labor) by prostaglandins

   O61.1 **Failed** instrumental **induction of labor** Ⓜ♀
Failed mechanical induction (of labor)
Failed surgical induction (of labor)

   O61.8 **Other failed induction of labor** Ⓜ♀

   O61.9 **Failed induction of labor, unspecified** Ⓜ♀

✓4ᵗʰ **O62** **Abnormalities of forces of labor**

   O62.0 **Primary inadequate contractions** Ⓜ♀
Failure of cervical dilatation
Primary hypotonic uterine dysfunction
Uterine inertia during latent phase of labor

   O62.1 **Secondary uterine inertia** Ⓜ♀
Arrested active phase of labor
Secondary hypotonic uterine dysfunction

   O62.2 **Other uterine inertia** Ⓜ♀
Atony of uterus without hemorrhage
Atony of uterus NOS
Desultory labor
Hypotonic uterine dysfunction NOS
Irregular labor
Poor contractions
Slow slope active phase of labor
Uterine inertia NOS
EXCLUDES 1   atony of uterus with hemorrhage (postpartum) (O72.1)
     postpartum atony of uterus without hemorrhage (O75.89)

   O62.3 **Precipitate labor** Ⓜ♀

O62.4 Hypertonic, incoordinate, and prolonged uterine contractions   Ⓜ♀
Cervical spasm
Contraction ring dystocia
Dyscoordinate labor
Hour-glass contraction of uterus
Hypertonic uterine dysfunction
Incoordinate uterine action
Tetanic contractions
Uterine dystocia NOS
Uterine spasm
EXCLUDES 1   *dystocia (fetal) (maternal) NOS (O66.9)*

O62.8 Other abnormalities of forces of labor   Ⓜ♀

O62.9 Abnormality of forces of labor, unspecified   Ⓜ♀

✓4ᵗʰ **O63 Long labor**

O63.0 Prolonged first stage (of labor)   Ⓜ♀

O63.1 Prolonged second stage (of labor)   Ⓜ♀

O63.2 Delayed delivery of second twin, triplet, etc.   Ⓜ♀

O63.9 Long labor, unspecified   Ⓜ♀
Prolonged labor NOS

✓4ᵗʰ **O64 Obstructed labor due to malposition and malpresentation of fetus**

One of the following 7th characters is to be assigned to each code under category O64. 7th character 0 is for single gestations and multiple gestations where the fetus is unspecified. 7th characters 1 through 9 are for cases of multiple gestations to identify the fetus for which the code applies. The appropriate code from category O30, Multiple gestation, must also be assigned when assigning a code from category O64 that has a 7th character of 1 through 9.
0	not applicable or unspecified	4	fetus 4
1	fetus 1	5	fetus 5
2	fetus 2	9	other fetus
3	fetus 3		

✓x7ᵗʰ **O64.0 Obstructed labor due to incomplete rotation of fetal head**   Ⓜ♀
Deep transverse arrest
Obstructed labor due to persistent occipitoiliac (position)
Obstructed labor due to persistent occipitoposterior (position)
Obstructed labor due to persistent occipitosacral (position)
Obstructed labor due to persistent occipitotransverse (position)

✓x7ᵗʰ **O64.1 Obstructed labor due to breech presentation**   Ⓜ♀
Obstructed labor due to buttocks presentation
Obstructed labor due to complete breech presentation
Obstructed labor due to frank breech presentation

✓x7ᵗʰ **O64.2 Obstructed labor due to face presentation**   Ⓜ♀
Obstructed labor due to chin presentation

✓x7ᵗʰ **O64.3 Obstructed labor due to brow presentation**   Ⓜ♀

✓x7ᵗʰ **O64.4 Obstructed labor due to shoulder presentation**   Ⓜ♀
Prolapsed arm
EXCLUDES 1   *impacted shoulders (O66.0)*
shoulder dystocia (O66.0)

✓x7ᵗʰ **O64.5 Obstructed labor due to compound presentation**   Ⓜ♀

✓x7ᵗʰ **O64.8 Obstructed labor due to other malposition and malpresentation**   Ⓜ♀
Obstructed labor due to footling presentation
Obstructed labor due to incomplete breech presentation

✓x7ᵗʰ **O64.9 Obstructed labor due to malposition and malpresentation, unspecified**   Ⓜ♀

✓4ᵗʰ **O65 Obstructed labor due to maternal pelvic abnormality**

O65.0 Obstructed labor due to deformed pelvis   Ⓜ♀

O65.1 Obstructed labor due to generally contracted pelvis   Ⓜ♀

O65.2 Obstructed labor due to pelvic inlet contraction   Ⓜ♀

O65.3 Obstructed labor due to pelvic outlet and mid-cavity contraction   Ⓜ♀

O65.4 Obstructed labor due to fetopelvic disproportion, unspecified   Ⓜ♀
EXCLUDES 1   *dystocia due to abnormality of fetus (O66.2-O66.3)*

O65.5 Obstructed labor due to abnormality of maternal pelvic organs   Ⓜ♀
Obstructed labor due to conditions listed in O34-
Use additional code to identify abnormality of pelvic organs (O34.-)

O65.8 Obstructed labor due to other maternal pelvic abnormalities   Ⓜ♀

O65.9 Obstructed labor due to maternal pelvic abnormality, unspecified   Ⓜ♀

✓4ᵗʰ **O66 Other obstructed labor**

O66.0 Obstructed labor due to shoulder dystocia   Ⓜ♀
Impacted shoulders

O66.1 Obstructed labor due to locked twins   Ⓜ♀

O66.2 Obstructed labor due to unusually large fetus   Ⓜ♀

O66.3 Obstructed labor due to other abnormalities of fetus   Ⓜ♀
Dystocia due to fetal ascites
Dystocia due to fetal hydrops
Dystocia due to fetal meningomyelocele
Dystocia due to fetal sacral teratoma
Dystocia due to fetal tumor
Dystocia due to hydrocephalic fetus
Use additional code to identify cause of obstruction

✓5ᵗʰ **O66.4 Failed trial of labor**

O66.40 Failed trial of labor, unspecified   Ⓜ♀

O66.41 Failed attempted vaginal birth after previous cesarean delivery   Ⓜ♀
Code first rupture of uterus, if applicable (O71.0-, O71.1)

O66.5 Attempted application of vacuum extractor and forceps   Ⓜ♀
Attempted application of vacuum or forceps, with subsequent delivery by forceps or cesarean delivery

O66.6 Obstructed labor due to other multiple fetuses   Ⓜ♀

O66.8 Other specified obstructed labor   Ⓜ♀
Use additional code to identify cause of obstruction

O66.9 Obstructed labor, unspecified   Ⓜ♀
Dystocia NOS
Fetal dystocia NOS
Maternal dystocia NOS

✓4ᵗʰ **O67 Labor and delivery complicated by intrapartum hemorrhage, not elsewhere classified**
EXCLUDES 1   *antepartum hemorrhage NEC (O46.-)*
placenta previa (O44.-)
premature separation of placenta [abruptio placentae] (O45.-)
EXCLUDES 1   *postpartum hemorrhage (O72.-)*

O67.0 Intrapartum hemorrhage with coagulation defect   Ⓜ♀
Intrapartum hemorrhage (excessive) associated with afibrinogenemia
Intrapartum hemorrhage (excessive) associated with disseminated intravascular coagulation
Intrapartum hemorrhage (excessive) associated with hyperfibrinolysis
Intrapartum hemorrhage (excessive) associated with hypofibrinogenemia

O67.8 Other intrapartum hemorrhage   Ⓜ♀
Excessive intrapartum hemorrhage

O67.9 Intrapartum hemorrhage, unspecified   Ⓜ♀

O68 Labor and delivery complicated by abnormality of fetal acid-base balance   Ⓜ♀
Fetal acidemia complicating labor and delivery
Fetal acidosis complicating labor and delivery
Fetal alkalosis complicating labor and delivery
Fetal metabolic acidemia complicating labor and delivery
EXCLUDES 1   *fetal stress NOS (O77.9)*
labor and delivery complicated by electrocardiographic evidence of fetal stress (O77.8)
labor and delivery complicated by ultrasonic evidence of fetal stress (O77.8)
EXCLUDES 2   *abnormality in fetal heart rate or rhythm (O76)*
labor and delivery complicated by meconium in amniotic fluid (O77.0)

✓4ᵗʰ **O69 Labor and delivery complicated by umbilical cord complications**

One of the following 7th characters is to be assigned to each code under category O69. 7th character 0 is for single gestations and multiple gestations where the fetus is unspecified. 7th characters 1 through 9 are for cases of multiple gestations to identify the fetus for which the code applies. The appropriate code from category O30, Multiple gestation, must also be assigned when assigning a code from category O69 that has a 7th character of 1 through 9.
0	not applicable or unspecified	4	fetus 4
1	fetus 1	5	fetus 5
2	fetus 2	9	other fetus
3	fetus 3		

✓x7ᵗʰ **O69.0 Labor and delivery complicated by prolapse of cord**   Ⓜ♀

✓x7ᵗʰ **O69.1 Labor and delivery complicated by cord around neck, with compression**   Ⓜ♀
EXCLUDES 1   *labor and delivery complicated by cord around neck, without compression (O69.81)*

✓ Additional Character Required   ✓x7ᵗʰ Placeholder Alert   Unspecified Dx   Other Specified Dx   Manifestation   ▶◀ Revised Text   ● New Code   ▲ Revised Code Title

√x7ᵗʰ O69.2 Labor and delivery complicated by other cord entanglement, with compression Ⓜ♀
    Labor and delivery complicated by compression of cord NOS
    Labor and delivery complicated by entanglement of cords of twins in monoamniotic sac
    Labor and delivery complicated by knot in cord
    EXCLUDES 1   *labor and delivery complicated by other cord entanglement, without compression (O69.82)*

√x7ᵗʰ O69.3 Labor and delivery complicated by short cord Ⓜ♀

√x7ᵗʰ O69.4 Labor and delivery complicated by vasa previa Ⓜ♀
    Labor and delivery complicated by hemorrhage from vasa previa

√x7ᵗʰ O69.5 Labor and delivery complicated by vascular lesion of cord Ⓜ♀
    Labor and delivery complicated by cord bruising
    Labor and delivery complicated by cord hematoma
    Labor and delivery complicated by thrombosis of umbilical vessels

√5ᵗʰ O69.8 Labor and delivery complicated by other cord complications

    √x7ᵗʰ O69.81 Labor and delivery complicated by cord around neck, without compression Ⓜ♀

    √x7ᵗʰ O69.82 Labor and delivery complicated by other cord entanglement, without compression Ⓜ♀

    √x7ᵗʰ O69.89 Labor and delivery complicated by other cord complications Ⓜ♀

√x7ᵗʰ O69.9 Labor and delivery complicated by cord complication, unspecified Ⓜ♀

√4ᵗʰ O70 Perineal laceration during delivery
    Episiotomy extended by laceration
    EXCLUDES 1   *obstetric high vaginal laceration alone (O71.4)*

    O70.0 First degree perineal laceration during delivery Ⓜ♀
      Perineal laceration, rupture or tear involving fourchette during delivery
      Perineal laceration, rupture or tear involving labia during delivery
      Perineal laceration, rupture or tear involving skin during delivery
      Perineal laceration, rupture or tear involving vagina during delivery
      Perineal laceration, rupture or tear involving vulva during delivery
      Slight perineal laceration, rupture or tear during delivery

    O70.1 Second degree perineal laceration during delivery Ⓜ♀
      Perineal laceration, rupture or tear during delivery as in O70.0, also involving pelvic floor
      Perineal laceration, rupture or tear during delivery as in O70.0, also involving perineal muscles
      Perineal laceration, rupture or tear during delivery as in O70.0, also involving vaginal muscles
      EXCLUDES 1   *perineal laceration involving anal sphincter (O70.2)*

    O70.2 Third degree perineal laceration during delivery Ⓜ♀
      Perineal laceration, rupture or tear during delivery as in O70.1, also involving anal sphincter
      Perineal laceration, rupture or tear during delivery as in O70.1, also involving rectovaginal septum
      Perineal laceration, rupture or tear during delivery as in O70.1, also involving sphincter NOS
      EXCLUDES 1   *anal sphincter tear during delivery without third degree perineal laceration (O70.4)*
          perineal laceration involving anal or rectal mucosa (O70.3)

    O70.3 Fourth degree perineal laceration during delivery Ⓜ♀
      Perineal laceration, rupture or tear during delivery as in O70.2, also involving anal mucosa
      Perineal laceration, rupture or tear during delivery as in O70.2, also involving rectal mucosa

    O70.4 Anal sphincter tear complicating delivery, not associated with third degree laceration Ⓜ♀
      EXCLUDES 1   *anal sphincter tear with third degree perineal laceration (O70.2)*

    O70.9 Perineal laceration during delivery, unspecified Ⓜ♀

√4ᵗʰ O71 Other obstetric trauma
    Obstetric damage from instruments

    √5ᵗʰ O71.0 Rupture of uterus (spontaneous) before onset of labor
      EXCLUDES 1   *disruption of (current) cesarean delivery wound (O90.0)*
          laceration of (uterus), NEC (O71.81)

      O71.00 Rupture of uterus before onset of labor, unspecified trimester Ⓜ♀

      O71.02 Rupture of uterus before onset of labor, second trimester Ⓜ♀

O71.03 Rupture of uterus before onset of labor, third trimester Ⓜ♀

O71.1 Rupture of uterus during labor Ⓜ♀
    Rupture of uterus not stated as occurring before onset of labor
    EXCLUDES 1   *disruption of cesarean delivery wound (O90.0)*
        laceration of uterus, NEC (O71.81)

O71.2 Postpartum inversion of uterus Ⓜ♀

O71.3 Obstetric laceration of cervix Ⓜ♀
    Annular detachment of cervix

O71.4 Obstetric high vaginal laceration alone Ⓜ♀
    Laceration of vaginal wall without perineal laceration
    EXCLUDES 1   *obstetric high vaginal laceration with perineal laceration (O70.-)*

O71.5 Other obstetric injury to pelvic organs Ⓜ♀
    Obstetric injury to bladder
    Obstetric injury to urethra
    EXCLUDES 2   *obstetric periurethral trauma (O71.82)*
    AHA: 2014, 4Q, 18

O71.6 Obstetric damage to pelvic joints and ligaments Ⓜ♀
    Obstetric avulsion of inner symphyseal cartilage
    Obstetric damage to coccyx
    Obstetric traumatic separation of symphysis (pubis)

O71.7 Obstetric hematoma of pelvis Ⓜ♀
    Obstetric hematoma of perineum
    Obstetric hematoma of vagina
    Obstetric hematoma of vulva

√5ᵗʰ O71.8 Other specified obstetric trauma

    O71.81 Laceration of uterus, not elsewhere classified Ⓜ♀

    O71.82 Other specified trauma to perineum and vulva Ⓜ♀
      Obstetric periurethral trauma
      AHA: 2014, 4Q, 18

    O71.89 Other specified obstetric trauma Ⓜ♀

O71.9 Obstetric trauma, unspecified Ⓜ♀

√4ᵗʰ O72 Postpartum hemorrhage
    INCLUDES   hemorrhage after delivery of fetus or infant

    O72.0 Third-stage hemorrhage Ⓜ♀
      Hemorrhage associated with retained, trapped or adherent placenta
      Retained placenta NOS
      Code also type of adherent placenta (O43.2-)

    O72.1 Other immediate postpartum hemorrhage Ⓜ♀
      Hemorrhage following delivery of placenta
      Postpartum hemorrhage (atonic) NOS
      Uterine atony with hemorrhage
      EXCLUDES 1   *uterine atony NOS (O62.2)*
          uterine atony without hemorrhage (O62.2)
          postpartum atony of uterus without hemorrhage (O75.89)

    O72.2 Delayed and secondary postpartum hemorrhage Ⓜ♀
      Hemorrhage associated with retained portions of placenta or membranes after the first 24 hours following delivery of placenta
      Retained products of conception NOS, following delivery

    O72.3 Postpartum coagulation defects Ⓜ♀
      Postpartum afibrinogenemia
      Postpartum fibrinolysis

√4ᵗʰ O73 Retained placenta and membranes, without hemorrhage
    EXCLUDES 1   *placenta accreta (O43.21-)*
        placenta increta (O43.22-)
        placenta percreta (O43.23-)

    O73.0 Retained placenta without hemorrhage Ⓜ♀
      Adherent placenta, without hemorrhage
      Trapped placenta without hemorrhage

    O73.1 Retained portions of placenta and membranes, without hemorrhage Ⓜ♀
      Retained products of conception following delivery, without hemorrhage

√4ᵗʰ O74 Complications of anesthesia during labor and delivery
    INCLUDES   maternal complications arising from the administration of a general, regional or local anesthetic, analgesic or other sedation during labor and delivery
    Use additional code, if applicable, to identify specific complication

    O74.0 Aspiration pneumonitis due to anesthesia during labor and delivery Ⓜ♀
      Inhalation of stomach contents or secretions NOS due to anesthesia during labor and delivery
      Mendelson's syndrome due to anesthesia during labor and delivery

---

EXCLUDES 1 Not coded here   *EXCLUDES 2* Not included here   Ⓝ Newborn Age: 0   Ⓟ Pediatric Age: 0-17   Ⓜ Maternity Age: 12-55   Ⓐ Adult Age: 15-124

O74.1 Other pulmonary complications of anesthesia during labor and delivery   Ⓜ♀

O74.2 Cardiac complications of anesthesia during labor and delivery   Ⓜ♀

O74.3 Central nervous system complications of anesthesia during labor and delivery   Ⓜ♀

O74.4 Toxic reaction to local anesthesia during labor and delivery   Ⓜ♀

O74.5 Spinal and epidural anesthesia-induced headache during labor and delivery   Ⓜ♀

O74.6 Other complications of spinal and epidural anesthesia during labor and delivery   Ⓜ♀

O74.7 Failed or difficult intubation for anesthesia during labor and delivery   Ⓜ♀

O74.8 Other complications of anesthesia during labor and delivery   Ⓜ♀

O74.9 Complication of anesthesia during labor and delivery, unspecified   Ⓜ♀

✓4ᵗʰ **O75** Other complications of labor and delivery, not elsewhere classified

> EXCLUDES 2   puerperal (postpartum) infection (O86.-)
> puerperal (postpartum) sepsis (O85)

O75.0 Maternal distress during labor and delivery   Ⓜ♀

O75.1 Shock during or following labor and delivery   Ⓜ♀
Obstetric shock following labor and delivery

O75.2 Pyrexia during labor, not elsewhere classified   Ⓜ♀

O75.3 Other infection during labor   Ⓜ♀
Sepsis during labor
Use additional code (B95-B97), to identify infectious agent

O75.4 Other complications of obstetric surgery and procedures   Ⓜ♀
Cardiac arrest following obstetric surgery or procedures
Cardiac failure following obstetric surgery or procedures
Cerebral anoxia following obstetric surgery or procedures
Pulmonary edema following obstetric surgery or procedures
Use additional code to identify specific complication

> EXCLUDES 2   complications of anesthesia during labor and delivery (O74.-)
> disruption of obstetrical (surgical) wound (O90.0-O90.1)
> hematoma of obstetrical (surgical) wound (O90.2)
> infection of obstetrical (surgical) wound (O86.0)

O75.5 Delayed delivery after artificial rupture of membranes   Ⓜ♀

✓5ᵗʰ **O75.8** Other specified complications of labor and delivery

O75.81 Maternal exhaustion complicating labor and delivery   Ⓜ♀

O75.82 Onset (spontaneous) of labor after 37 completed weeks of gestation but before 39 completed weeks gestation, with delivery by (planned) cesarean section   Ⓜ♀
Delivery by (planned) cesarean section occurring after 37 completed weeks of gestation but before 39 completed weeks gestation due to (spontaneous) onset of labor
Code first to specify reason for planned cesarean section such as:
  cephalopelvic disproportion (normally formed fetus) (O33.9)
  previous cesarean delivery (O34.21)

O75.89 Other specified complications of labor and delivery   Ⓜ♀

O75.9 Complication of labor and delivery, unspecified   Ⓜ♀

O76 Abnormality in fetal heart rate and rhythm complicating labor and delivery   Ⓜ♀
Depressed fetal heart rate tones complicating labor and delivery
Fetal bradycardia complicating labor and delivery
Fetal heart rate abnormal variability complicating labor and delivery
Fetal heart rate decelerations complicating labor and delivery
Fetal heart rate irregularity complicating labor and delivery
Fetal tachycardia complicating labor and delivery
Non-reassuring fetal heart rate or rhythm complicating labor and delivery

> EXCLUDES 1   fetal stress NOS (O77.9)
> labor and delivery complicated by electrocardiographic evidence of fetal stress (O77.8)
> labor and delivery complicated by ultrasonic evidence of fetal stress (O77.8)

> EXCLUDES 2   fetal metabolic acidemia (O68)
> other fetal stress (O77.0-O77.1)

AHA: 2013, 4Q, 118

✓4ᵗʰ **O77** Other fetal stress complicating labor and delivery

O77.0 Labor and delivery complicated by meconium in amniotic fluid   Ⓜ♀
AHA: 2013, 4Q, 117-118

O77.1 Fetal stress in labor or delivery due to drug administration   Ⓜ♀

O77.8 Labor and delivery complicated by other evidence of fetal stress   Ⓜ♀
Labor and delivery complicated by electrocardiographic evidence of fetal stress
Labor and delivery complicated by ultrasonic evidence of fetal stress

> EXCLUDES 1   abnormality in fetal heart rate or rhythm (O76)
> abnormality of fetal acid-base balance (O68)
> fetal metabolic acidemia (O68)

O77.9 Labor and delivery complicated by fetal stress, unspecified   Ⓜ♀

> EXCLUDES 1   abnormality in fetal heart rate or rhythm (O76)
> abnormality of fetal acid-base balance (O68)
> fetal metabolic acidemia (O68)

Encounter for delivery (O80, O82)

O80 Encounter for full-term uncomplicated delivery   Ⓜ♀

> NOTE   Delivery requiring minimal or no assistance, with or without episiotomy, without fetal manipulation [e.g., rotation version] or instrumentation [forceps] of a spontaneous, cephalic, vaginal, full-term, single, live-born infant. This code is for use as a single diagnosis code and is not to be used with any other code from chapter 15.

Use additional code to indicate outcome of delivery (Z37.0)
AHA: 2014, 2Q, 9

O82 Encounter for cesarean delivery without indication   Ⓜ♀
Use additional code to indicate outcome of delivery (Z37.0)

Complications predominantly related to the puerperium (O85-O92)

> EXCLUDES 2   mental and behavioral disorders associated with the puerperium (F53)
> obstetrical tetanus (A34)
> puerperal osteomalacia (M83.0)

O85 Puerperal sepsis   Ⓜ♀
Postpartum sepsis
Puerperal peritonitis
Puerperal pyemia
Use additional code (B95-B97), to identify infectious agent
Use additional code (R65.2-) to identify severe sepsis, if applicable

> EXCLUDES 1   fever of unknown origin following delivery (O86.4)
> genital tract infection following delivery (O86.1-)
> obstetric pyemic and septic embolism (O88.3-)
> puerperal septic thrombophlebitis (O86.81)
> urinary tract infection following delivery (O86.2-)

> EXCLUDES 2   sepsis during labor (O75.3)

✓4ᵗʰ **O86** Other puerperal infections
Use additional code (B95-B97), to identify infectious agent

> EXCLUDES 2   infection during labor (O75.3)
> obstetrical tetanus (A34)

O86.0 Infection of obstetric surgical wound   Ⓜ♀
Infected cesarean delivery wound following delivery
Infected perineal repair following delivery

✓5ᵗʰ **O86.1** Other infection of genital tract following delivery

O86.11 Cervicitis following delivery   Ⓜ♀
O86.12 Endometritis following delivery   Ⓜ♀
O86.13 Vaginitis following delivery   Ⓜ♀
O86.19 Other infection of genital tract following delivery   Ⓜ♀

✓5ᵗʰ **O86.2** Urinary tract infection following delivery

O86.20 Urinary tract infection following delivery, unspecified   Ⓜ♀
Puerperal urinary tract infection NOS
O86.21 Infection of kidney following delivery   Ⓜ♀
O86.22 Infection of bladder following delivery   Ⓜ♀
Infection of urethra following delivery
O86.29 Other urinary tract infection following delivery   Ⓜ♀

O86.4 Pyrexia of unknown origin following delivery   Ⓜ♀
Puerperal infection NOS following delivery
Puerperal pyrexia NOS following delivery

> EXCLUDES 2   pyrexia during labor (O75.2)

☑ Additional Character Required   ✓ᵡᵀ Placeholder Alert   Unspecified Dx   Other Specified Dx   Manifestation   ▶◀ Revised Text   ● New Code   ▲ Revised Code Title

✓5ᵗʰ **O86.8** **Other specified puerperal infections**

     O86.81 **Puerperal** septic thrombophlebitis   Ⓜ♀

     O86.89 **Other specified puerperal infections**   Ⓜ♀

✓4ᵗʰ **O87** **Venous complications and hemorrhoids in the puerperium**
Venous complications in labor, delivery and the puerperium
   EXCLUDES 2   *obstetric embolism (O88.-)*
       puerperal septic thrombophlebitis (O86.81)
       venous complications in pregnancy (O22.-)

   O87.0 **Superficial thrombophlebitis in the puerperium**   Ⓜ♀
Puerperal phlebitis NOS
Puerperal thrombosis NOS

   O87.1 **Deep phlebothrombosis in the puerperium**   Ⓜ♀
Deep vein thrombosis, postpartum
Pelvic thrombophlebitis, postpartum
Use additional code to identify the deep vein thrombosis (I82.4-, I82.5-, I82.62-. I82.72-)
Use additional code, if applicable, for associated long-term (current) use of anticoagulants (Z79.01)

   O87.2 **Hemorrhoids in the puerperium**   Ⓜ♀

   O87.3 **Cerebral venous thrombosis in the puerperium**   Ⓜ♀
Cerebrovenous sinus thrombosis in the puerperium

   O87.4 **Varicose veins of lower extremity in the puerperium**   Ⓜ♀

   O87.8 **Other venous complications in the puerperium**   Ⓜ♀
Genital varices in the puerperium

   O87.9 **Venous complication in the puerperium, unspecified**   Ⓜ♀
Puerperal phlebopathy NOS

✓4ᵗʰ **O88** **Obstetric embolism**
   EXCLUDES 1   *embolism complicating abortion NOS (O03.2)*
       embolism complicating ectopic or molar pregnancy (O08.2)
       embolism complicating failed attempted abortion (O07.2)
       embolism complicating induced abortion (O04.7)
       embolism complicating spontaneous abortion (O03.2, O03.7)

   ✓5ᵗʰ **O88.0** **Obstetric** air embolism

     ✓6ᵗʰ **O88.01** **Obstetric air embolism in** pregnancy

       O88.011 **Air embolism in pregnancy, first trimester**   Ⓜ♀

       O88.012 **Air embolism in pregnancy, second trimester**   Ⓜ♀

       O88.013 **Air embolism in pregnancy, third trimester**   Ⓜ♀

       O88.019 **Air embolism in pregnancy, unspecified trimester**   Ⓜ♀

     O88.02 **Air embolism in** childbirth   Ⓜ♀

     O88.03 **Air embolism in the** puerperium   Ⓜ♀

   ✓5ᵗʰ **O88.1** **Amniotic fluid** embolism
Anaphylactoid syndrome in pregnancy

     ✓6ᵗʰ **O88.11** **Amniotic fluid embolism in** pregnancy

       O88.111 **Amniotic fluid embolism in pregnancy, first trimester**   Ⓜ♀

       O88.112 **Amniotic fluid embolism in pregnancy, second trimester**   Ⓜ♀

       O88.113 **Amniotic fluid embolism in pregnancy, third trimester**   Ⓜ♀

       O88.119 **Amniotic fluid embolism in pregnancy, unspecified trimester**   Ⓜ♀

     O88.12 **Amniotic fluid embolism in** childbirth   Ⓜ♀

     O88.13 **Amniotic fluid embolism in the** puerperium   Ⓜ♀

   ✓5ᵗʰ **O88.2** **Obstetric** thromboembolism

     ✓6ᵗʰ **O88.21** **Thromboembolism in** pregnancy
Obstetric (pulmonary) embolism NOS

       O88.211 **Thromboembolism in pregnancy, first trimester**   Ⓜ♀

       O88.212 **Thromboembolism in pregnancy, second trimester**   Ⓜ♀

       O88.213 **Thromboembolism in pregnancy, third trimester**   Ⓜ♀

       O88.219 **Thromboembolism in pregnancy, unspecified trimester**   Ⓜ♀

     O88.22 **Thromboembolism in** childbirth   Ⓜ♀

     O88.23 **Thromboembolism in the** puerperium   Ⓜ♀
Puerperal (pulmonary) embolism NOS

   ✓5ᵗʰ **O88.3** **Obstetric pyemic and septic embolism**

     ✓6ᵗʰ **O88.31** **Pyemic and septic embolism in** pregnancy

       O88.311 **Pyemic and septic embolism in pregnancy, first trimester**   Ⓜ♀

       O88.312 **Pyemic and septic embolism in pregnancy, second trimester**   Ⓜ♀

       O88.313 **Pyemic and septic embolism in pregnancy, third trimester**   Ⓜ♀

       O88.319 **Pyemic and septic embolism in pregnancy, unspecified trimester**   Ⓜ♀

     O88.32 **Pyemic and septic embolism in childbirth**   Ⓜ♀

     O88.33 **Pyemic and septic embolism in the puerperium**   Ⓜ♀

   ✓5ᵗʰ **O88.8** **Other obstetric embolism**
Obstetric fat embolism

     ✓6ᵗʰ **O88.81** **Other embolism in pregnancy**

       O88.811 **Other embolism in pregnancy, first trimester**   Ⓜ♀

       O88.812 **Other embolism in pregnancy, second trimester**   Ⓜ♀

       O88.813 **Other embolism in pregnancy, third trimester**   Ⓜ♀

       O88.819 **Other embolism in pregnancy, unspecified trimester**   Ⓜ♀

     O88.82 **Other embolism in childbirth**   Ⓜ♀

     O88.83 **Other embolism in the puerperium**   Ⓜ♀

✓4ᵗʰ **O89** **Complications of anesthesia during the puerperium**
   INCLUDES   maternal complications arising from the administration of a general, regional or local anesthetic, analgesic or other sedation during the puerperium
Use additional code, if applicable, to identify specific complication

   ✓5ᵗʰ **O89.0** **Pulmonary complications of anesthesia during the puerperium**

     O89.01 **Aspiration pneumonitis due to anesthesia during the puerperium**   Ⓜ♀
Inhalation of stomach contents or secretions NOS due to anesthesia during the puerperium
Mendelson's syndrome due to anesthesia during the puerperium

     O89.09 **Other pulmonary complications of anesthesia during the puerperium**   Ⓜ♀

   O89.1 **Cardiac complications of anesthesia during the puerperium**   Ⓜ♀

   O89.2 **Central nervous system complications of anesthesia during the puerperium**   Ⓜ♀

   O89.3 **Toxic reaction to local anesthesia during the puerperium**   Ⓜ♀

   O89.4 **Spinal and epidural anesthesia-induced headache during the puerperium**   Ⓜ♀

   O89.5 **Other complications of spinal and epidural anesthesia during the puerperium**   Ⓜ♀

   O89.6 **Failed or difficult intubation for anesthesia during the puerperium**   Ⓜ♀

   O89.8 **Other complications of anesthesia during the puerperium**   Ⓜ♀

   O89.9 **Complication of anesthesia during the puerperium, unspecified**   Ⓜ♀

✓4ᵗʰ **O90** **Complications of the puerperium, not elsewhere classified**

   O90.0 **Disruption of cesarean delivery wound**   Ⓜ♀
Dehiscence of cesarean delivery wound
     EXCLUDES 1   *rupture of uterus (spontaneous) before onset of labor (O71.0-)*
       rupture of uterus during labor (O71.1)

   O90.1 **Disruption of perineal obstetric wound**   Ⓜ♀
Disruption of wound of episiotomy
Disruption of wound of perineal laceration
Secondary perineal tear

   O90.2 **Hematoma of obstetric wound**   Ⓜ♀

   O90.3 **Peripartum cardiomyopathy**   Ⓜ♀
Conditions in I42- arising during pregnancy and the puerperium
     EXCLUDES 1   *pre-existing heart disease complicating pregnancy and the puerperium (O99.4-)*

   O90.4 **Postpartum acute kidney failure**   Ⓜ♀
Hepatorenal syndrome following labor and delivery

   O90.5 **Postpartum thyroiditis**   Ⓜ♀

   O90.6 **Postpartum mood disturbance**   Ⓜ♀
Postpartum blues
Postpartum dysphoria
Postpartum sadness
     EXCLUDES 1   *postpartum depression (F53)*
       puerperal psychosis (F53)

EXCLUDES 1 Not coded here   EXCLUDES 2 Not included here   Ⓝ Newborn Age: 0   Ⓟ Pediatric Age: 0–17   Ⓜ Maternity Age: 12–55   Ⓐ Adult Age: 15–124

788   ICD-10-CM 2016

✓5ᵗʰ O90.8   **Other complications of the puerperium, not elsewhere classified**

     O90.81   **Anemia of the puerperium**   Ⓜ♀
         Postpartum anemia NOS
         EXCLUDES 1   *pre-existing anemia complicating the puerperium (O99.03)*

     O90.89   **Other complications of the puerperium, not elsewhere classified**   Ⓜ♀
         Placental polyp

     O90.9   **Complication of the puerperium, unspecified**   Ⓜ♀

✓4ᵗʰ O91   **Infections of breast associated with pregnancy, the puerperium and lactation**
     Use additional code to identify infection

✓5ᵗʰ O91.0   **Infection of nipple associated with pregnancy, the puerperium and lactation**

     ✓6ᵗʰ O91.01   **Infection of nipple associated with pregnancy**
         Gestational abscess of nipple

         O91.011   **Infection of nipple associated with pregnancy, first trimester**   Ⓜ♀

         O91.012   **Infection of nipple associated with pregnancy, second trimester**   Ⓜ♀

         O91.013   **Infection of nipple associated with pregnancy, third trimester**   Ⓜ♀

         O91.019   **Infection of nipple associated with pregnancy, unspecified trimester**   Ⓜ♀

     O91.02   **Infection of nipple associated with the puerperium**   Ⓜ♀
         Puerperal abscess of nipple

     O91.03   **Infection of nipple associated with lactation**   Ⓜ♀
         Abscess of nipple associated with lactation

✓5ᵗʰ O91.1   **Abscess of breast associated with pregnancy, the puerperium and lactation**

     ✓6ᵗʰ O91.11   **Abscess of breast associated with pregnancy**
         Gestational mammary abscess
         Gestational purulent mastitis
         Gestational subareolar abscess

         O91.111   **Abscess of breast associated with pregnancy, first trimester**   Ⓜ♀

         O91.112   **Abscess of breast associated with pregnancy, second trimester**   Ⓜ♀

         O91.113   **Abscess of breast associated with pregnancy, third trimester**   Ⓜ♀

         O91.119   **Abscess of breast associated with pregnancy, unspecified trimester**   Ⓜ♀

     O91.12   **Abscess of breast associated with the puerperium**   Ⓜ♀
         Puerperal mammary abscess
         Puerperal purulent mastitis
         Puerperal subareolar abscess

     O91.13   **Abscess of breast associated with lactation**   Ⓜ♀
         Mammary abscess associated with lactation
         Purulent mastitis associated with lactation
         Subareolar abscess associated with lactation

✓5ᵗʰ O91.2   **Nonpurulent mastitis associated with pregnancy, the puerperium and lactation**

     ✓6ᵗʰ O91.21   **Nonpurulent mastitis associated with pregnancy**
         Gestational interstitial mastitis
         Gestational lymphangitis of breast
         Gestational mastitis NOS
         Gestational parenchymatous mastitis

         O91.211   **Nonpurulent mastitis associated with pregnancy, first trimester**   Ⓜ♀

         O91.212   **Nonpurulent mastitis associated with pregnancy, second trimester**   Ⓜ♀

         O91.213   **Nonpurulent mastitis associated with pregnancy, third trimester**   Ⓜ♀

         O91.219   **Nonpurulent mastitis associated with pregnancy, unspecified trimester**   Ⓜ♀

     O91.22   **Nonpurulent mastitis associated with the puerperium**   Ⓜ♀
         Puerperal interstitial mastitis
         Puerperal lymphangitis of breast
         Puerperal mastitis NOS
         Puerperal parenchymatous mastitis

     O91.23   **Nonpurulent mastitis associated with lactation**   Ⓜ♀
         Interstitial mastitis associated with lactation
         Lymphangitis of breast associated with lactation
         Mastitis NOS associated with lactation
         Parenchymatous mastitis associated with lactation

✓4ᵗʰ O92   **Other disorders of breast and disorders of lactation associated with pregnancy and the puerperium**

✓5ᵗʰ O92.0   **Retracted nipple associated with pregnancy, the puerperium, and lactation**

     ✓6ᵗʰ O92.01   **Retracted nipple associated with pregnancy**

         O92.011   **Retracted nipple associated with pregnancy, first trimester**   Ⓜ♀

         O92.012   **Retracted nipple associated with pregnancy, second trimester**   Ⓜ♀

         O92.013   **Retracted nipple associated with pregnancy, third trimester**   Ⓜ♀

         O92.019   **Retracted nipple associated with pregnancy, unspecified trimester**   Ⓜ♀

     O92.02   **Retracted nipple associated with the puerperium**   Ⓜ♀

     O92.03   **Retracted nipple associated with lactation**   Ⓜ♀

✓5ᵗʰ O92.1   **Cracked nipple associated with pregnancy, the puerperium, and lactation**
     Fissure of nipple, gestational or puerperal

     ✓6ᵗʰ O92.11   **Cracked nipple associated with pregnancy**

         O92.111   **Cracked nipple associated with pregnancy, first trimester**   Ⓜ♀

         O92.112   **Cracked nipple associated with pregnancy, second trimester**   Ⓜ♀

         O92.113   **Cracked nipple associated with pregnancy, third trimester**   Ⓜ♀

         O92.119   **Cracked nipple associated with pregnancy, unspecified trimester**   Ⓜ♀

     O92.12   **Cracked nipple associated with the puerperium**   Ⓜ♀

     O92.13   **Cracked nipple associated with lactation**   Ⓜ♀

✓5ᵗʰ O92.2   **Other and unspecified disorders of breast associated with pregnancy and the puerperium**

     O92.20   **Unspecified disorder of breast associated with pregnancy and the puerperium**   Ⓜ♀

     O92.29   **Other disorders of breast associated with pregnancy and the puerperium**   Ⓜ♀

     O92.3   **Agalactia**   Ⓜ♀
         Primary agalactia
         EXCLUDES 1   *elective agalactia (O92.5)*
                 secondary agalactia (O92.5)
                 therapeutic agalactia (O92.5)

     O92.4   **Hypogalactia**   Ⓜ♀

     O92.5   **Suppressed lactation**   Ⓜ♀
         Elective agalactia
         Secondary agalactia
         Therapeutic agalactia
         EXCLUDES 1   *primary agalactia (O92.3)*

     O92.6   **Galactorrhea**   Ⓜ♀

✓5ᵗʰ O92.7   **Other and unspecified disorders of lactation**

     O92.70   **Unspecified disorders of lactation**   Ⓜ♀

     O92.79   **Other disorders of lactation**   Ⓜ♀
         Puerperal galactocele

Other obstetric conditions, not elsewhere classified (O94-O9A)

O94   **Sequelae of complication of pregnancy, childbirth, and the puerperium**   Ⓜ♀

     NOTE   This category is to be used to indicate conditions in O00-O77.-, O85-O94 and O98-O9A.- as the cause of late effects. The sequelae include conditions specified as such, or as late effects, which may occur at any time after the puerperium.

     Code first condition resulting from (sequela) of complication of pregnancy, childbirth, and the puerperium

---

☑ Additional Character Required   ✓x7ᵗʰ Placeholder Alert   Unspecified Dx   Other Specified Dx   Manifestation   ▶◀ Revised Text   ● New Code   ▲ Revised Code Title

Chapter 15. Pregnancy, Childbirth, and the Puerperium

O98–O98.73

✓4th **O98 Maternal infectious and parasitic diseases classifiable elsewhere but complicating pregnancy, childbirth and the puerperium**

INCLUDES the listed conditions when complicating the pregnant state, when aggravated by the pregnancy, or as a reason for obstetric care

Use additional code (Chapter 1), to identify specific infectious or parasitic disease

EXCLUDES 2 herpes gestationis (O26.4-)
infectious carrier state (O99.82-, O99.83-)
obstetrical tetanus (A34)
puerperal infection (O86.-)
puerperal sepsis (O85)
when the reason for maternal care is that the disease is known or suspected to have affected the fetus (O35-O36)

✓5th **O98.0 Tuberculosis complicating pregnancy, childbirth and the puerperium**

Conditions in A15-A19

✓6th **O98.01 Tuberculosis complicating pregnancy**

O98.011 Tuberculosis complicating pregnancy, first trimester Ⓜ♀

O98.012 Tuberculosis complicating pregnancy, second trimester Ⓜ♀

O98.013 Tuberculosis complicating pregnancy, third trimester Ⓜ♀

O98.019 Tuberculosis complicating pregnancy, unspecified trimester Ⓜ♀

O98.02 Tuberculosis complicating childbirth Ⓜ♀

O98.03 Tuberculosis complicating the puerperium Ⓜ♀

✓5th **O98.1 Syphilis complicating pregnancy, childbirth and the puerperium**

Conditions in A50-A53

✓6th **O98.11 Syphilis complicating pregnancy**

O98.111 Syphilis complicating pregnancy, first trimester Ⓜ♀

O98.112 Syphilis complicating pregnancy, second trimester Ⓜ♀

O98.113 Syphilis complicating pregnancy, third trimester Ⓜ♀

O98.119 Syphilis complicating pregnancy, unspecified trimester Ⓜ♀

O98.12 Syphilis complicating childbirth Ⓜ♀

O98.13 Syphilis complicating the puerperium Ⓜ♀

✓5th **O98.2 Gonorrhea complicating pregnancy, childbirth and the puerperium**

Conditions in A54-

✓6th **O98.21 Gonorrhea complicating pregnancy**

O98.211 Gonorrhea complicating pregnancy, first trimester Ⓜ♀

O98.212 Gonorrhea complicating pregnancy, second trimester Ⓜ♀

O98.213 Gonorrhea complicating pregnancy, third trimester Ⓜ♀

O98.219 Gonorrhea complicating pregnancy, unspecified trimester Ⓜ♀

O98.22 Gonorrhea complicating childbirth Ⓜ♀

O98.23 Gonorrhea complicating the puerperium Ⓜ♀

✓5th **O98.3 Other infections with a predominantly sexual mode of transmission complicating pregnancy, childbirth and the puerperium**

Conditions in A55-A64

✓6th **O98.31 Other infections with a predominantly sexual mode of transmission complicating pregnancy**

O98.311 Other infections with a predominantly sexual mode of transmission complicating pregnancy, first trimester Ⓜ♀

O98.312 Other infections with a predominantly sexual mode of transmission complicating pregnancy, second trimester Ⓜ♀

O98.313 Other infections with a predominantly sexual mode of transmission complicating pregnancy, third trimester Ⓜ♀

O98.319 Other infections with a predominantly sexual mode of transmission complicating pregnancy, unspecified trimester Ⓜ♀

O98.32 Other infections with a predominantly sexual mode of transmission complicating childbirth Ⓜ♀

O98.33 Other infections with a predominantly sexual mode of transmission complicating the puerperium Ⓜ♀

✓5th **O98.4 Viral hepatitis complicating pregnancy, childbirth and the puerperium**

Conditions in B15-B19

✓6th **O98.41 Viral hepatitis complicating pregnancy**

O98.411 Viral hepatitis complicating pregnancy, first trimester Ⓜ♀

O98.412 Viral hepatitis complicating pregnancy, second trimester Ⓜ♀

O98.413 Viral hepatitis complicating pregnancy, third trimester Ⓜ♀

O98.419 Viral hepatitis complicating pregnancy, unspecified trimester Ⓜ♀

O98.42 Viral hepatitis complicating childbirth Ⓜ♀

O98.43 Viral hepatitis complicating the puerperium Ⓜ♀

✓5th **O98.5 Other viral diseases complicating pregnancy, childbirth and the puerperium**

Conditions in A80-B09, B25-B34, R87.81-, R87.82-

EXCLUDES 1 human immunodeficiency virus [HIV] disease complicating pregnancy, childbirth and the puerperium (O98.7-)

✓6th **O98.51 Other viral diseases complicating pregnancy**

O98.511 Other viral diseases complicating pregnancy, first trimester Ⓜ♀

O98.512 Other viral diseases complicating pregnancy, second trimester Ⓜ♀

O98.513 Other viral diseases complicating pregnancy, third trimester Ⓜ♀

O98.519 Other viral diseases complicating pregnancy, unspecified trimester Ⓜ♀

O98.52 Other viral diseases complicating childbirth Ⓜ♀

O98.53 Other viral diseases complicating the puerperium Ⓜ♀

✓5th **O98.6 Protozoal diseases complicating pregnancy, childbirth and the puerperium**

Conditions in B50-B64

✓6th **O98.61 Protozoal diseases complicating pregnancy**

O98.611 Protozoal diseases complicating pregnancy, first trimester Ⓜ♀

O98.612 Protozoal diseases complicating pregnancy, second trimester Ⓜ♀

O98.613 Protozoal diseases complicating pregnancy, third trimester Ⓜ♀

O98.619 Protozoal diseases complicating pregnancy, unspecified trimester Ⓜ♀

O98.62 Protozoal diseases complicating childbirth Ⓜ♀

O98.63 Protozoal diseases complicating the puerperium Ⓜ♀

✓5th **O98.7 Human immunodeficiency virus [HIV] disease complicating pregnancy, childbirth and the puerperium**

Use additional code to identify the type of HIV disease:
acquired immune deficiency syndrome (AIDS) (B20)
asymptomatic HIV status (Z21)
HIV positive NOS (Z21)
symptomatic HIV disease (B20)

✓6th **O98.71 Human immunodeficiency virus [HIV] disease complicating pregnancy**

O98.711 Human immunodeficiency virus [HIV] disease complicating pregnancy, first trimester Ⓜ♀

O98.712 Human immunodeficiency virus [HIV] disease complicating pregnancy, second trimester Ⓜ♀

O98.713 Human immunodeficiency virus [HIV] disease complicating pregnancy, third trimester Ⓜ♀

O98.719 Human immunodeficiency virus [HIV] disease complicating pregnancy, unspecified trimester Ⓜ♀

O98.72 Human immunodeficiency virus [HIV] disease complicating childbirth Ⓜ♀

O98.73 Human immunodeficiency virus [HIV] disease complicating the puerperium Ⓜ♀

EXCLUDES 1 Not coded here   EXCLUDES 2 Not included here   Ⓝ Newborn Age: 0   Ⓟ Pediatric Age: 0-17   Ⓜ Maternity Age: 12-55   Ⓐ Adult Age: 15-124

790   ICD-10-CM 2016

✓5ᵗʰ **O98.8** Other maternal infectious and parasitic diseases complicating pregnancy, childbirth and the puerperium

   ✓6ᵗʰ **O98.81** Other maternal infectious and parasitic diseases complicating pregnancy

      O98.811 Other maternal infectious and parasitic diseases complicating pregnancy, first trimester   Ⓜ♀

      O98.812 Other maternal infectious and parasitic diseases complicating pregnancy, second trimester   Ⓜ♀

      O98.813 Other maternal infectious and parasitic diseases complicating pregnancy, third trimester   Ⓜ♀

      O98.819 Other maternal infectious and parasitic diseases complicating pregnancy, unspecified trimester   Ⓜ♀

   O98.82 Other maternal infectious and parasitic diseases complicating childbirth   Ⓜ♀

   O98.83 Other maternal infectious and parasitic diseases complicating the puerperium   Ⓜ♀

✓5ᵗʰ **O98.9** Unspecified maternal infectious and parasitic disease complicating pregnancy, childbirth and the puerperium

   ✓6ᵗʰ **O98.91** Unspecified maternal infectious and parasitic disease complicating pregnancy

      O98.911 Unspecified maternal infectious and parasitic disease complicating pregnancy, first trimester   Ⓜ♀

      O98.912 Unspecified maternal infectious and parasitic disease complicating pregnancy, second trimester   Ⓜ♀

      O98.913 Unspecified maternal infectious and parasitic disease complicating pregnancy, third trimester   Ⓜ♀

      O98.919 Unspecified maternal infectious and parasitic disease complicating pregnancy, unspecified trimester   Ⓜ♀

   O98.92 Unspecified maternal infectious and parasitic disease complicating childbirth   Ⓜ♀

   O98.93 Unspecified maternal infectious and parasitic disease complicating the puerperium   Ⓜ♀

✓4ᵗʰ **O99** Other maternal diseases classifiable elsewhere but complicating pregnancy, childbirth and the puerperium

   INCLUDES conditions which complicate the pregnant state, are aggravated by the pregnancy or are a main reason for obstetric care

   Use additional code to identify specific condition

   EXCLUDES 2 *when the reason for maternal care is that the condition is known or suspected to have affected the fetus (O35-O36)*

  ✓5ᵗʰ **O99.0** Anemia complicating pregnancy, childbirth and the puerperium

    Conditions in D50-D64

    EXCLUDES 1 *anemia arising in the puerperium (O90.81)*
       postpartum anemia NOS (O90.81)

   ✓6ᵗʰ **O99.01** Anemia complicating pregnancy

      O99.011 Anemia complicating pregnancy, first trimester   Ⓜ♀

      O99.012 Anemia complicating pregnancy, second trimester   Ⓜ♀

      O99.013 Anemia complicating pregnancy, third trimester   Ⓜ♀

      O99.019 Anemia complicating pregnancy, unspecified trimester   Ⓜ♀

   O99.02 Anemia complicating childbirth   Ⓜ♀

   O99.03 Anemia complicating the puerperium   Ⓜ♀

    EXCLUDES 1 *postpartum anemia not pre-existing prior to delivery (O90.81)*

✓5ᵗʰ **O99.1** Other diseases of the blood and blood-forming organs and certain disorders involving the immune mechanism complicating pregnancy, childbirth and the puerperium

   Conditions in D65-D89

   EXCLUDES 2 *hemorrhage with coagulation defects (O45.-, O46.0-, O67.0, O72.3)*

  ✓6ᵗʰ **O99.11** Other diseases of the blood and blood-forming organs and certain disorders involving the immune mechanism complicating pregnancy

      O99.111 Other diseases of the blood and blood-forming organs and certain disorders involving the immune mechanism complicating pregnancy, first trimester   Ⓜ♀

      O99.112 Other diseases of the blood and blood-forming organs and certain disorders involving the immune mechanism complicating pregnancy, second trimester   Ⓜ♀

      O99.113 Other diseases of the blood and blood-forming organs and certain disorders involving the immune mechanism complicating pregnancy, third trimester   Ⓜ♀

      O99.119 Other diseases of the blood and blood-forming organs and certain disorders involving the immune mechanism complicating pregnancy, unspecified trimester   Ⓜ♀

   O99.12 Other diseases of the blood and blood-forming organs and certain disorders involving the immune mechanism complicating childbirth   Ⓜ♀

   O99.13 Other diseases of the blood and blood-forming organs and certain disorders involving the immune mechanism complicating the puerperium   Ⓜ♀

✓5ᵗʰ **O99.2** Endocrine, nutritional and metabolic diseases complicating pregnancy, childbirth and the puerperium

   Conditions in E00-E88

   EXCLUDES 2 *diabetes mellitus (O24.-)*
       malnutrition (O25.-)
       postpartum thyroiditis (O90.5)

  ✓6ᵗʰ **O99.21** Obesity complicating pregnancy, childbirth, and the puerperium

    Use additional code to identify the type of obesity (E66.-)

      O99.210 Obesity complicating pregnancy, unspecified trimester   Ⓜ♀

      O99.211 Obesity complicating pregnancy, first trimester   Ⓜ♀

      O99.212 Obesity complicating pregnancy, second trimester   Ⓜ♀

      O99.213 Obesity complicating pregnancy, third trimester   Ⓜ♀

      O99.214 Obesity complicating childbirth   Ⓜ♀

      O99.215 Obesity complicating the puerperium   Ⓜ♀

  ✓6ᵗʰ **O99.28** Other endocrine, nutritional and metabolic diseases complicating pregnancy, childbirth and the puerperium

      O99.280 Endocrine, nutritional and metabolic diseases complicating pregnancy, unspecified trimester   Ⓜ♀

      O99.281 Endocrine, nutritional and metabolic diseases complicating pregnancy, first trimester   Ⓜ♀

      O99.282 Endocrine, nutritional and metabolic diseases complicating pregnancy, second trimester   Ⓜ♀

      O99.283 Endocrine, nutritional and metabolic diseases complicating pregnancy, third trimester   Ⓜ♀

      O99.284 Endocrine, nutritional and metabolic diseases complicating childbirth   Ⓜ♀

      O99.285 Endocrine, nutritional and metabolic diseases complicating the puerperium   Ⓜ♀

☑ Additional Character Required   ✓x7ᵗʰ Placeholder Alert   Unspecified Dx   Other Specified Dx   Manifestation   ▶◀ Revised Text   ● New Code   ▲ Revised Code Title

ICD-10-CM 2016   791

Chapter 15. Pregnancy, Childbirth, and the Puerperium

O99.3–O99.63

✓5ᵗʰ **O99.3** Mental disorders and diseases of the nervous system complicating pregnancy, childbirth and the puerperium

  ✓6ᵗʰ **O99.31** Alcohol use complicating pregnancy, childbirth, and the puerperium
       Use additional code(s) from F10 to identify manifestations of the alcohol use

       O99.310 Alcohol use complicating pregnancy, unspecified trimester   Ⓜ♀
       O99.311 Alcohol use complicating pregnancy, first trimester   Ⓜ♀
       O99.312 Alcohol use complicating pregnancy, second trimester   Ⓜ♀
       O99.313 Alcohol use complicating pregnancy, third trimester   Ⓜ♀
       O99.314 Alcohol use complicating childbirth   Ⓜ♀
       O99.315 Alcohol use complicating the puerperium   Ⓜ♀

  ✓6ᵗʰ **O99.32** Drug use complicating pregnancy, childbirth, and the puerperium
       Use additional code(s) from F11-F16 and F18-F19 to identify manifestations of the drug use

       O99.320 Drug use complicating pregnancy, unspecified trimester   Ⓜ♀
       O99.321 Drug use complicating pregnancy, first trimester   Ⓜ♀
       O99.322 Drug use complicating pregnancy, second trimester   Ⓜ♀
       O99.323 Drug use complicating pregnancy, third trimester   Ⓜ♀
       O99.324 Drug use complicating childbirth   Ⓜ♀
       O99.325 Drug use complicating the puerperium   Ⓜ♀

  ✓6ᵗʰ **O99.33** Smoking (tobacco) complicating pregnancy, childbirth, and the puerperium
       Use additional code from F17 to identify type of tobacco

       O99.330 Smoking (tobacco) complicating pregnancy, unspecified trimester   Ⓜ♀
       O99.331 Smoking (tobacco) complicating pregnancy, first trimester   Ⓜ♀
       O99.332 Smoking (tobacco) complicating pregnancy, second trimester   Ⓜ♀
       O99.333 Smoking (tobacco) complicating pregnancy, third trimester   Ⓜ♀
       O99.334 Smoking (tobacco) complicating childbirth   Ⓜ♀
       O99.335 Smoking (tobacco) complicating the puerperium   Ⓜ♀

  ✓6ᵗʰ **O99.34** Other mental disorders complicating pregnancy, childbirth, and the puerperium
       Conditions in F01-F09 and F20-F99
       EXCLUDES 2   postpartum mood disturbance (O90.6)
               postnatal psychosis (F53)
               puerperal psychosis (F53)

       O99.340 Other mental disorders complicating pregnancy, unspecified trimester   Ⓜ♀
       O99.341 Other mental disorders complicating pregnancy, first trimester   Ⓜ♀
       O99.342 Other mental disorders complicating pregnancy, second trimester   Ⓜ♀
       O99.343 Other mental disorders complicating pregnancy, third trimester   Ⓜ♀
       O99.344 Other mental disorders complicating childbirth   Ⓜ♀
       O99.345 Other mental disorders complicating the puerperium   Ⓜ♀

  ✓6ᵗʰ **O99.35** Diseases of the nervous system complicating pregnancy, childbirth, and the puerperium
       Conditions in G00-G99
       EXCLUDES 2   pregnancy related peripheral neuritis (O26.8-)

       O99.350 Diseases of the nervous system complicating pregnancy, unspecified trimester   Ⓜ♀
       O99.351 Diseases of the nervous system complicating pregnancy, first trimester   Ⓜ♀
       O99.352 Diseases of the nervous system complicating pregnancy, second trimester   Ⓜ♀

       O99.353 Diseases of the nervous system complicating pregnancy, third trimester   Ⓜ♀
       O99.354 Diseases of the nervous system complicating childbirth   Ⓜ♀
       O99.355 Diseases of the nervous system complicating the puerperium   Ⓜ♀

✓5ᵗʰ **O99.4** Diseases of the circulatory system complicating pregnancy, childbirth and the puerperium
     Conditions in I00-I99
     EXCLUDES 1   peripartum cardiomyopathy (O90.3)
     EXCLUDES 2   hypertensive disorders (O10-O16)
              obstetric embolism (O88.-)
              venous complications and cerebrovenous sinus thrombosis in labor, childbirth and the puerperium (O87.-)
              venous complications and cerebrovenous sinus thrombosis in pregnancy (O22.-)

  ✓6ᵗʰ **O99.41** Diseases of the circulatory system complicating pregnancy

       O99.411 Diseases of the circulatory system complicating pregnancy, first trimester   Ⓜ♀
       O99.412 Diseases of the circulatory system complicating pregnancy, second trimester   Ⓜ♀
       O99.413 Diseases of the circulatory system complicating pregnancy, third trimester   Ⓜ♀
       O99.419 Diseases of the circulatory system complicating pregnancy, unspecified trimester   Ⓜ♀

  O99.42 Diseases of the circulatory system complicating childbirth   Ⓜ♀

  O99.43 Diseases of the circulatory system complicating the puerperium   Ⓜ♀

✓5ᵗʰ **O99.5** Diseases of the respiratory system complicating pregnancy, childbirth and the puerperium
     Conditions in J00-J99

  ✓6ᵗʰ **O99.51** Diseases of the respiratory system complicating pregnancy

       O99.511 Diseases of the respiratory system complicating pregnancy, first trimester   Ⓜ♀
       O99.512 Diseases of the respiratory system complicating pregnancy, second trimester   Ⓜ♀
       O99.513 Diseases of the respiratory system complicating pregnancy, third trimester   Ⓜ♀
       O99.519 Diseases of the respiratory system complicating pregnancy, unspecified trimester   Ⓜ♀

  O99.52 Diseases of the respiratory system complicating childbirth   Ⓜ♀

  O99.53 Diseases of the respiratory system complicating the puerperium   Ⓜ♀

✓5ᵗʰ **O99.6** Diseases of the digestive system complicating pregnancy, childbirth and the puerperium
     Conditions in K00-K93
     EXCLUDES 2   liver and biliary tract disorders in pregnancy, childbirth and the puerperium (O26.6-)

  ✓6ᵗʰ **O99.61** Diseases of the digestive system complicating pregnancy

       O99.611 Diseases of the digestive system complicating pregnancy, first trimester   Ⓜ♀
       O99.612 Diseases of the digestive system complicating pregnancy, second trimester   Ⓜ♀
       O99.613 Diseases of the digestive system complicating pregnancy, third trimester   Ⓜ♀
       O99.619 Diseases of the digestive system complicating pregnancy, unspecified trimester   Ⓜ♀

  O99.62 Diseases of the digestive system complicating childbirth   Ⓜ♀

  O99.63 Diseases of the digestive system complicating the puerperium   Ⓜ♀

EXCLUDES 1 Not coded here   EXCLUDES 2 Not included here   Ⓝ Newborn Age: 0   Ⓟ Pediatric Age: 0-17   Ⓜ Maternity Age: 12-55   Ⓐ Adult Age: 15-124

792   ICD-10-CM 2016

✓5ᵗʰ O99.7 Diseases of the skin and subcutaneous **tissue complicating pregnancy, childbirth and the puerperium**
     Conditions in L00-L99
     EXCLUDES 2   *herpes gestationis (O26.4)*
          pruritic urticarial papules and plaques of pregnancy (PUPPP) (O26.86)

    ✓6ᵗʰ O99.71 Diseases of the skin and subcutaneous tissue complicating pregnancy
       O99.711 Diseases of the skin and subcutaneous tissue complicating pregnancy, first trimester   Ⓜ♀
       O99.712 Diseases of the skin and subcutaneous tissue complicating pregnancy, second trimester   Ⓜ♀
       O99.713 Diseases of the skin and subcutaneous tissue complicating pregnancy, third trimester   Ⓜ♀
       O99.719 Diseases of the skin and subcutaneous tissue complicating pregnancy, unspecified trimester   Ⓜ♀

    O99.72 Diseases of the skin and subcutaneous tissue complicating childbirth   Ⓜ♀
    O99.73 Diseases of the skin and subcutaneous tissue complicating the puerperium   Ⓜ♀

✓5ᵗʰ O99.8 Other specified diseases and conditions complicating pregnancy, childbirth and the puerperium
     Conditions in D00-D48, H00-H95, M00-N99, and Q00-Q99
     Use additional code to identify condition
     EXCLUDES 2   *genitourinary infections in pregnancy (O23.-)*
          infection of genitourinary tract following delivery (O86.1-O86.3)
          malignant neoplasm complicating pregnancy, childbirth and the puerperium (O9A.1-)
          maternal care for known or suspected abnormality of maternal pelvic organs (O34.-)
          postpartum acute kidney failure (O90.4)
          traumatic injuries in pregnancy (O9A.2)

    ✓6ᵗʰ O99.81 Abnormal glucose complicating pregnancy, childbirth and the puerperium
       EXCLUDES 1   *gestational diabetes (O24.4-)*
       O99.810 Abnormal glucose complicating pregnancy   Ⓜ♀
       O99.814 Abnormal glucose complicating childbirth   Ⓜ♀
       O99.815 Abnormal glucose complicating the puerperium   Ⓜ♀

    ✓6ᵗʰ O99.82 Streptococcus B carrier state complicating pregnancy, childbirth and the puerperium
       O99.820 Streptococcus B carrier state complicating pregnancy   Ⓜ♀
       O99.824 Streptococcus B carrier state complicating childbirth   Ⓜ♀
       O99.825 Streptococcus B carrier state complicating the puerperium   Ⓜ♀

    ✓6ᵗʰ O99.83 Other infection carrier state complicating pregnancy, childbirth and the puerperium
       Use additional code to identify the carrier state (Z22.-)
       O99.830 Other infection carrier state complicating pregnancy   Ⓜ♀
       O99.834 Other infection carrier state complicating childbirth   Ⓜ♀
       O99.835 Other infection carrier state complicating the puerperium   Ⓜ♀

    ✓6ᵗʰ O99.84 Bariatric surgery status complicating pregnancy, childbirth and the puerperium
       Gastric banding status complicating pregnancy, childbirth and the puerperium
       Gastric bypass status for obesity complicating pregnancy, childbirth and the puerperium
       Obesity surgery status complicating pregnancy, childbirth and the puerperium
       O99.840 Bariatric surgery status complicating pregnancy, unspecified trimester   Ⓜ♀
       O99.841 Bariatric surgery status complicating pregnancy, first trimester   Ⓜ♀
       O99.842 Bariatric surgery status complicating pregnancy, second trimester   Ⓜ♀
       O99.843 Bariatric surgery status complicating pregnancy, third trimester   Ⓜ♀

       O99.844 Bariatric surgery status complicating childbirth   Ⓜ♀
       O99.845 Bariatric surgery status complicating the puerperium   Ⓜ♀
    O99.89 Other specified diseases and conditions complicating pregnancy, childbirth and the puerperium   Ⓜ♀

✓4ᵗʰ O9A Maternal malignant neoplasms, traumatic injuries and abuse classifiable elsewhere but complicating pregnancy, childbirth and the puerperium

    ✓5ᵗʰ O9A.1 Malignant neoplasm complicating pregnancy, childbirth and the puerperium
       Conditions in C00-C96
       Use additional code to identify neoplasm
       EXCLUDES 2   *maternal care for benign tumor of corpus uteri (O34.1-)*
          maternal care for benign tumor of cervix (O34.4-)

     ✓6ᵗʰ O9A.11 Malignant neoplasm complicating pregnancy
         O9A.111 Malignant neoplasm complicating pregnancy, first trimester   Ⓜ♀
         O9A.112 Malignant neoplasm complicating pregnancy, second trimester   Ⓜ♀
         O9A.113 Malignant neoplasm complicating pregnancy, third trimester   Ⓜ♀
         O9A.119 Malignant neoplasm complicating pregnancy, unspecified trimester   Ⓜ♀

     O9A.12 Malignant neoplasm complicating childbirth   Ⓜ♀
     O9A.13 Malignant neoplasm complicating the puerperium   Ⓜ♀

    ✓5ᵗʰ O9A.2 Injury, poisoning and certain other consequences of external causes complicating pregnancy, childbirth and the puerperium
       Conditions in S00-T88, except T74 and T76
       Use additional code(s) to identify the injury or poisoning
       EXCLUDES 2   *physical, sexual and psychological abuse complicating pregnancy, childbirth and the puerperium (O9A.3-, O9A.4-, O9A.5-)*

     ✓6ᵗʰ O9A.21 Injury, poisoning and certain other consequences of external causes complicating pregnancy
         O9A.211 Injury, poisoning and certain other consequences of external causes complicating pregnancy, first trimester   Ⓜ♀
         O9A.212 Injury, poisoning and certain other consequences of external causes complicating pregnancy, second trimester   Ⓜ♀
         O9A.213 Injury, poisoning and certain other consequences of external causes complicating pregnancy, third trimester   Ⓜ♀
         O9A.219 Injury, poisoning and certain other consequences of external causes complicating pregnancy, unspecified trimester   Ⓜ♀

     O9A.22 Injury, poisoning and certain other consequences of external causes complicating childbirth   Ⓜ♀
     O9A.23 Injury, poisoning and certain other consequencesof external causes complicating the puerperium   Ⓜ♀

    ✓5ᵗʰ O9A.3 Physical abuse complicating pregnancy, childbirth and the puerperium
       Conditions in T74.11 or T76.11
       Use additional code (if applicable):
         to identify any associated current injury due to physical abuse
         to identify the perpetrator of abuse (Y07.-)
       EXCLUDES 2   *sexual abuse complicating pregnancy, childbirth and the puerperium (O9A.4)*

     ✓6ᵗʰ O9A.31 Physical abuse complicating pregnancy
         O9A.311 Physical abuse complicating pregnancy, first trimester   Ⓜ♀
         O9A.312 Physical abuse complicating pregnancy,second trimester   Ⓜ♀
         O9A.313 Physical abuse complicating pregnancy, third trimester   Ⓜ♀
         O9A.319 Physical abuse complicating pregnancy,unspecified trimester   Ⓜ♀

     O9A.32 Physical abuse complicating childbirth   Ⓜ♀
     O9A.33 Physical abuse complicating the puerperium   Ⓜ♀

☑ Additional Character Required   ✓×7ᵗʰ Placeholder Alert   Unspecified Dx   Other Specified Dx   Manifestation   ▶◀ Revised Text   ● New Code   ▲ Revised Code Title

Chapter 15. Pregnancy, Childbirth, and the Puerperium *(side margin)*

√5ᵗʰ **O9A.4 Sexual abuse complicating pregnancy, childbirth and the puerperium**
Conditions in T74.21 or T76.21
Use additional code (if applicable):
   to identify any associated current injury due to sexual abuse
   to identify the perpetrator of abuse (YØ7.-)

√6ᵗʰ **O9A.41 Sexual abuse complicating pregnancy**

    O9A.411 Sexual abuse complicating pregnancy, Ⓜ♀
            first trimester

    O9A.412 Sexual abuse complicating pregnancy, Ⓜ♀
            second trimester

    O9A.413 Sexual abuse complicating pregnancy, Ⓜ♀
            third trimester

    O9A.419 Sexual abuse complicating   Ⓜ♀
            pregnancy, unspecified trimester

 O9A.42 Sexual abuse complicating childbirth   Ⓜ♀

 O9A.43 Sexual abuse complicating the puerperium   Ⓜ♀

√5ᵗʰ **O9A.5 Psychological abuse complicating pregnancy, childbirth and the puerperium**
Conditions in T74.31 or T76.31
Use additional code to identify the perpetrator of abuse (YØ7.-)

√6ᵗʰ **O9A.51 Psychological abuse complicating pregnancy**

    O9A.511 Psychological abuse complicating Ⓜ♀
            pregnancy, first trimester

    O9A.512 Psychological abuse complicating Ⓜ♀
            pregnancy, second trimester

    O9A.513 Psychological abuse complicating Ⓜ♀
            pregnancy, third trimester

    O9A.519 Psychological abuse complicating Ⓜ♀
            pregnancy, unspecified trimester

 O9A.52 Psychological abuse complicating childbirth Ⓜ♀

 O9A.53 Psychological abuse complicating the   Ⓜ♀
     puerperium

EXCLUDES 1 Not coded here   EXCLUDES 2 Not included here   Ⓝ Newborn Age: 0   Ⓟ Pediatric Age: 0-17   Ⓜ Maternity Age: 12-55   Ⓐ Adult Age: 15-124

794   ICD-10-CM 2016

Chapter 16.Certain Conditions Originating in the Perinatal Period (P00–P96)

Chapter Specific Guidelines with Coding Examples

The chapter specific guidelines from the ICD-10-CM Official Guidelines for Coding and Reporting have been provided below. Along with these guidelines are coding examples, contained in the shaded boxes, that have been developed to help illustrate the coding and/or sequencing guidance found in these guidelines.

For coding and reporting purposes the perinatal period is defined as before birth through the 28th day following birth. The following guidelines are provided for reporting purposes

a. General Perinatal Rules

1) Use of chapter 16 codes

Codes in this chapter are never for use on the maternal record. Codes from Chapter 15, the obstetric chapter, are never permitted on the newborn record. Chapter 16 codes may be used throughout the life of the patient if the condition is still present.

2) Principal diagnosis for birth record

When coding the birth episode in a newborn record, assign a code from category Z38, Liveborn infants according to place of birth and type of delivery, as the principal diagnosis. A code from category Z38 is assigned only once, to a newborn at the time of birth. If a newborn is transferred to another institution, a code from category Z38 should not be used at the receiving hospital.

A code from category Z38 is used only on the newborn record, not on the mother's record.

> Newborn delivered via vaginal delivery in Rural Hospital A, experienced meconium aspiration resulting in pneumonia. Rural hospital A is not equipped to handle the extensive respiratory therapy this baby needs and transfers the patient to Metropolis Hospital B, where the pneumonia resolves and the newborn is eventually discharged.
>
> *Rural hospital A*
>
> **Z38.00**   **Single liveborn infant, delivered vaginally**
>
> **P24.01**   **Meconium aspiration with respiratory symptoms**
>
> *Metropolis hospital B*
>
> **P24.01**   **Meconium aspiration with respiratory symptoms**
>
> *Explanation:* A code from category Z38 is a one-time use only code. The hospital that actually delivered the newborn, in this case Rural Hospital A, can append a code from category Z38 but for the delivery admission only. Once the patient is transferred or discharged, the Z38 category no longer applies for that patient.
>
> The reason for the transfer to Metropolis hospital B was for the respiratory symptoms (pneumonia) the newborn was exhibiting secondary to aspirating meconium.

3) Use of codes from other chapters with codes from chapter 16

Codes from other chapters may be used with codes from chapter 16 if the codes from the other chapters provide more specific detail. Codes for signs and symptoms may be assigned when a definitive diagnosis has not been established. If the reason for the encounter is a perinatal condition, the code from chapter 16 should be sequenced first.

4) Use of chapter 16 codes after the perinatal period

Should a condition originate in the perinatal period, and continue throughout the life of the patient, the perinatal code should continue to be used regardless of the patient's age.

> A 7-year-old patient with history of birth injury that resulted in Erb's palsy is seen for subscapularis release
>
> **P14.0**   **Erb's paralysis due to birth injury**
>
> *Explanation:* Although in this instance Erb's palsy is specifically related to a birth injury, it has not resolved and continues to be a health concern. A perinatal code is appropriate even though this patient is beyond the perinatal period.

5) Birth process or community acquired conditions

If a newborn has a condition that may be either due to the birth process or community acquired and the documentation does not indicate which it is, the default is due to the birth process and the code from Chapter 16 should be used. If the condition is community-acquired, a code from Chapter 16 should not be assigned.

6) Code all clinically significant conditions

All clinically significant conditions noted on routine newborn examination should be coded. A condition is clinically significant if it requires:

clinical evaluation; or

therapeutic treatment; or

diagnostic procedures; or

extended length of hospital stay; or

increased nursing care and/or monitoring; or

has implications for future health care needs

Note: The perinatal guidelines listed above are the same as the general coding guidelines for "additional diagnoses", except for the final point regarding implications for future health care needs. Codes should be assigned for conditions that have been specified by the provider as having implications for future health care needs.

b. Observation and evaluation of newborns for suspected conditions not found

Reserved for future expansion

c. Coding additional perinatal diagnoses

1) Assigning codes for conditions that require treatment

Assign codes for conditions that require treatment or further investigation, prolong the length of stay, or require resource utilization.

2) Codes for conditions specified as having implications for future health care needs

Assign codes for conditions that have been specified by the provider as having implications for future health care needs.

Note: This guideline should not be used for adult patients.

> An abnormal noise was heard in the left hip of a post-term newborn during a physical examination. The pediatrician would like to follow the patient after discharge as a hip click can be an early sign of hip dysplasia. The newborn was delivered via cesarean at 41 weeks.
>
> **Z38.01**   **Single liveborn infant, delivered by cesarean**
>
> **P08.21**   **Post-term newborn**
>
> **R29.4**   **Clicking hip**
>
> *Explanation:* The abnormal hip noise or click is appended as a secondary diagnosis not only because it is an abnormal finding upon examination, but also due to its potential to be part of a bigger health issue. The hip dysplasia has not yet been diagnosed and does not warrant a code at this time.

d. Prematurity and fetal growth retardation

Providers utilize different criteria in determining prematurity. A code for prematurity should not be assigned unless it is documented. Assignment of codes in categories P05, Disorders of newborn related to slow fetal growth and fetal malnutrition, and P07, Disorders of newborn related to short gestation and low birth weight, not elsewhere classified, should be based on the recorded birth weight and estimated gestational age. Codes from category P05 should not be assigned with codes from category P07.

When both birth weight and gestational age are available, two codes from category P07 should be assigned, with the code for birth weight sequenced before the code for gestational age.

e. Low birth weight and immaturity status

Codes from category P07, Disorders of newborn related to short gestation and low birth weight, not elsewhere classified, are for use for a child or adult who was premature or had a low birth weight as a newborn and this is affecting the patient's current health status.

See Section I.C.21. Factors influencing health status and contact with health services, Status.

A 35-year-old patient, who weighed 659 grams at birth, is seen for heart disease documented as being a consequence of the low birth weight

I51.9   **Heart disease, unspecified**

P07.02   **Extremely low birth weight newborn, 500–749 grams**

Explanation: A code from subcategories P07.0- and P07.1- is appropriate, regardless of the age of the patient, as long as the documentation provides a clear link between the patient's current illness and the low birth weight.

f. Bacterial Sepsis of Newborn

Category P36, Bacterial sepsis of newborn, includes congenital sepsis. If a perinate is documented as having sepsis without documentation of congenital or community acquired, the default is congenital and a code from category P36 should be assigned. If the P36 code includes the causal organism, an additional code from category B95, Streptococcus, Staphylococcus, and Enterococcus as the cause of diseases classified elsewhere, or B96, Other bacterial agents as the cause of diseases classified elsewhere, should not be assigned. If the P36 code does not include the causal organism, assign an additional code from category B96. If applicable,

use additional codes to identify severe sepsis (R65.2-) and any associated acute organ dysfunction.

A full-term infant develops severe sepsis 24 hours after discharge from the hospital and is readmitted; cultures identified *E. coli* as the infective agent

P36.4   **Sepsis of newborn due to Escherichia coli**

R65.20   **Severe sepsis without septic shock**

Explanation: Even though this newborn was discharged and could have acquired *E. coli* from his/her external environment, due to the lack of documentation specifying specifically how this pathogen was acquired, the default is to code the *E. coli* sepsis as congenital. A code from chapter 1, "Certain Infectious and Parasitic Diseases," is not required because the perinatal sepsis code identifies both the sepsis and the bacteria causing the sepsis.

g. Stillbirth

Code P95, Stillbirth, is only for use in institutions that maintain separate records for stillbirths. No other code should be used with P95. Code P95 should not be used on the mother's record.

Chapter 16. Certain Conditions Originating in the Perinatal Period (P00-P96)

NOTE   Codes from this chapter are for use on newborn records only, never on maternal records.

INCLUDES   conditions that have their origin in the fetal or perinatal period (before birth through the first 28 days after birth) even if morbidity occurs later

EXCLUDES 2   congenital malformations, deformations and chromosomal abnormalities (Q00-Q99)
endocrine, nutritional and metabolic diseases (E00-E88)
injury, poisoning and certain other consequences of external causes (S00-T88)
neoplasms (C00-D49)
tetanus neonatorum (A33)

This chapter contains the following blocks:

P00-P04	Newborn affected by maternal factors and by complications of pregnancy, labor, and delivery
P05-P08	Disorders of newborn related to length of gestation and fetal growth
P09	Abnormal findings on neonatal screening
P10-P15	Birth trauma
P19-P29	Respiratory and cardiovascular disorders specific to the perinatal period
P35-P39	Infections specific to the perinatal period
P50-P61	Hemorrhagic and hematological disorders of newborn
P70-P74	Transitory endocrine and metabolic disorders specific to newborn
P76-P78	Digestive system disorders of newborn
P80-P83	Conditions involving the integument and temperature regulation of newborn
P84	Other problems with newborn
P90-P96	Other disorders originating in the perinatal period

Newborn affected by maternal factors and by complications of pregnancy, labor, and delivery (P00-P04)

NOTE   These codes are for use when the listed maternal conditions are specified as the cause of confirmed morbidity or potential morbidity which have their origin in the perinatal period (before birth through the first 28 days after birth). Codes from these categories are also for use for newborns who are suspected of having an abnormal condition resulting from exposure from the mother or the birth process, but without signs or symptoms, and, which after examination and observation, is found not to exist. These codes may be used even if treatment is begun for a suspected condition that is ruled out.

✓4ᵗʰ P00 Newborn (suspected to be) affected by maternal conditions that may be unrelated to present pregnancy

Code first any current condition in newborn

EXCLUDES 2   newborn (suspected to be) affected by maternal complications of pregnancy (P01.-)
newborn affected by maternal endocrine and metabolic disorders (P70-P74)
newborn affected by noxious substances transmitted via placenta or breast milk (P04.-)

P00.0 Newborn (suspected to be) affected by maternal hypertensive disorders   N
Newborn (suspected to be) affected by maternal conditions classifiable to O10-O11, O13-O16

P00.1 Newborn (suspected to be) affected by maternal renal and urinary tract diseases   N
Newborn (suspected to be) affected by maternal conditions classifiable to N00-N39

P00.2 Newborn (suspected to be) affected by maternal infectious and parasitic diseases   N
Newborn (suspected to be) affected by maternal infectious disease classifiable to A00-B99, J09 and J10

EXCLUDES 1   infections specific to the perinatal period (P35-P39)
maternal genital tract or other localized infections (P00.8)

P00.3 Newborn (suspected to be) affected by other maternal circulatory and respiratory diseases   N
Newborn (suspected to be) affected by maternal conditions classifiable to I00-I99, J00-J99, Q20-Q34 and not included in P00.0, P00.2

P00.4 Newborn (suspected to be) affected by maternal nutritional disorders   N
Newborn (suspected to be) affected by maternal disorders classifiable to E40-E64
Maternal malnutrition NOS

P00.5 Newborn (suspected to be) affected by maternal injury   N
Newborn (suspected to be) affected by maternal conditions classifiable to O9A.2-

P00.6 Newborn (suspected to be) affected by surgical procedure on mother   N
Newborn (suspected to be) affected by amniocentesis

EXCLUDES 1   Cesarean delivery for present delivery (P03.4)
damage to placenta from amniocentesis, Cesarean delivery or surgical induction (P02.1)
previous surgery to uterus or pelvic organs (P03.89)

EXCLUDES 2   newborn affected by complication of (fetal) intrauterine procedure (P96.5)

P00.7 Newborn (suspected to be) affected by other medical procedures on mother, not elsewhere classified   N
Newborn (suspected to be) affected by radiation to mother

EXCLUDES 1   damage to placenta from amniocentesis, cesarean delivery or surgical induction (P02.1)
newborn affected by other complications of labor and delivery (P03.-)

✓5ᵗʰ P00.8 Newborn (suspected to be) affected by other maternal conditions

P00.81 Newborn (suspected to be) affected by periodontal disease in mother   N

P00.89 Newborn (suspected to be) affected by other maternal conditions   N
Newborn (suspected to be) affected by conditions classifiable to T80-T88
Newborn (suspected to be) affected by maternal genital tract or other localized infections
Newborn (suspected to be) affected by maternal systemic lupus erythematosus

P00.9 Newborn (suspected to be) affected by unspecified maternal condition   N

✓4ᵗʰ P01 Newborn (suspected to be) affected by maternal complications of pregnancy

Code first any current condition in newborn

P01.0 Newborn (suspected to be) affected by incompetent cervix   N

P01.1 Newborn (suspected to be) affected by premature rupture of membranes   N

P01.2 Newborn (suspected to be) affected by oligohydramnios   N

EXCLUDES 1   oligohydramnios due to premature rupture of membranes (P01.1)

P01.3 Newborn (suspected to be) affected by polyhydramnios   N
Newborn (suspected to be) affected by hydramnios

P01.4 Newborn (suspected to be) affected by ectopic pregnancy   N
Newborn (suspected to be) affected by abdominal pregnancy

P01.5 Newborn (suspected to be) affected by multiple pregnancy   N
Newborn (suspected to be) affected by triplet (pregnancy)
Newborn (suspected to be) affected by twin (pregnancy)

P01.6 Newborn (suspected to be) affected by maternal death   N

P01.7 Newborn (suspected to be) affected by malpresentation before labor   N
Newborn (suspected to be) affected by breech presentation before labor
Newborn (suspected to be) affected by external version before labor
Newborn (suspected to be) affected by face presentation before labor
Newborn (suspected to be) affected by transverse lie before labor
Newborn (suspected to be) affected by unstable lie before labor

P01.8 Newborn (suspected to be) affected by other maternal complications of pregnancy   N

P01.9 Newborn (suspected to be) affected by maternal complication of pregnancy, unspecified   N

✓4ᵗʰ P02 Newborn (suspected to be) affected by complications of placenta, cord and membranes

Code first any current condition in newborn

P02.0 Newborn (suspected to be) affected by placenta previa   N

P02.1 Newborn (suspected to be) affected by other forms of placental separation and hemorrhage   N
Newborn (suspected to be) affected by abruptio placenta
Newborn (suspected to be) affected by accidental hemorrhage
Newborn (suspected to be) affected by antepartum hemorrhage
Newborn (suspected to be) affected by damage to placenta from amniocentesis, cesarean delivery or surgical induction
Newborn (suspected to be) affected by maternal blood loss
Newborn (suspected to be) affected by premature separation of placenta

---

☑ Additional Character Required   ✗x7ᵗʰ Placeholder Alert   Unspecified Dx   Other Specified Dx   Manifestation   ▶◀ Revised Text   ● New Code   ▲ Revised Code Title

Chapter 16. Certain Conditions Originating in the Perinatal Period

✓5ᵗʰ **P02.2** **Newborn (suspected to be) affected by other and unspecified morphological and functional abnormalities of placenta**

    P02.20 **Newborn (suspected to be) affected by unspecified morphological and functional abnormalities of placenta** Ⓝ

    P02.29 **Newborn (suspected to be) affected by other morphological and functional abnormalities of placenta** Ⓝ

        Newborn (suspected to be) affected by placental dysfunction

        Newborn (suspected to be) affected by placental infarction

        Newborn (suspected to be) affected by placental insufficiency

P02.3 **Newborn (suspected to be) affected by placental transfusion syndromes** Ⓝ

    Newborn (suspected to be) affected by placental and cord abnormalities resulting in twin-to-twin or other transplacental transfusion

P02.4 **Newborn (suspected to be) affected by prolapsed cord** Ⓝ

P02.5 **Newborn (suspected to be) affected by other compression of umbilical cord** Ⓝ

    Newborn (suspected to be) affected by umbilical cord (tightly) around neck

    Newborn (suspected to be) affected by entanglement of umbilical cord

    Newborn (suspected to be) affected by knot in umbilical cord

✓5ᵗʰ **P02.6** **Newborn (suspected to be) affected by other and unspecified conditions of umbilical cord**

    P02.60 **Newborn (suspected to be) affected by unspecified conditions of umbilical cord** Ⓝ

    P02.69 **Newborn (suspected to be) affected by other conditions of umbilical cord** Ⓝ

        Newborn (suspected to be) affected by short umbilical cord

        Newborn (suspected to be) affected by vasa previa

        EXCLUDES 1   *newborn affected by single umbilical artery (Q27.0)*

P02.7 **Newborn (suspected to be) affected by chorioamnionitis** Ⓝ

    Newborn (suspected to be) affected by amnionitis

    Newborn (suspected to be) affected by membranitis

    Newborn (suspected to be) affected by placentitis

P02.8 **Newborn (suspected to be) affected by other abnormalities of membranes** Ⓝ

P02.9 **Newborn (suspected to be) affected by abnormality of membranes, unspecified** Ⓝ

✓4ᵗʰ **P03** **Newborn (suspected to be) affected by other complications of labor and delivery**

    Code first any current condition in newborn

P03.0 **Newborn (suspected to be) affected by breech delivery and extraction** Ⓝ

P03.1 **Newborn (suspected to be) affected by other malpresentation, malposition and disproportion during labor and delivery** Ⓝ

    Newborn (suspected to be) affected by contracted pelvis

    Newborn (suspected to be) affected by conditions classifiable to O64-O66

    Newborn (suspected to be) affected by persistent occipitoposterior

    Newborn (suspected to be) affected by transverse lie

P03.2 **Newborn (suspected to be) affected by forceps delivery** Ⓝ

P03.3 **Newborn (suspected to be) affected by delivery by vacuum extractor [ventouse]** Ⓝ

P03.4 **Newborn (suspected to be) affected by Cesarean delivery** Ⓝ

P03.5 **Newborn (suspected to be) affected by precipitate delivery** Ⓝ

    Newborn (suspected to be) affected by rapid second stage

P03.6 **Newborn (suspected to be) affected by abnormal uterine contractions** Ⓝ

    Newborn (suspected to be) affected by conditions classifiable to O62-, except O62.3

    Newborn (suspected to be) affected by hypertonic labor

    Newborn (suspected to be) affected by uterine inertia

✓5ᵗʰ **P03.8** **Newborn (suspected to be) affected by other specified complications of labor and delivery**

    ✓6ᵗʰ **P03.81** **Newborn (suspected to be) affected by abnormality in fetal (intrauterine) heart rate or rhythm**

        EXCLUDES 1   *neonatal cardiac dysrhythmia (P29.1-)*

        P03.810 **Newborn (suspected to be) affected by abnormality in fetal (intrauterine) heart rate or rhythm before the onset of labor** Ⓝ

        P03.811 **Newborn (suspected to be) affected by abnormality in fetal (intrauterine) heart rate or rhythm during labor** Ⓝ

        P03.819 **Newborn (suspected to be) affected by abnormality in fetal (intrauterine) heart rate or rhythm, unspecified as to time of onset** Ⓝ

    P03.82 **Meconium passage during delivery**

        EXCLUDES 1   *meconium aspiration (P24.00, P24.01)*

        meconium staining (P96.83)

    P03.89 **Newborn (suspected to be) affected by other specified complications of labor and delivery**

        Newborn (suspected to be) affected by abnormality of maternal soft tissues

        Newborn (suspected to be) affected by conditions classifiable to O60-O75 and by procedures used in labor and delivery not included in P02- and P03.0-P03.6

        Newborn (suspected to be) affected by induction of labor

P03.9 **Newborn (suspected to be) affected by complication of labor and delivery, unspecified** Ⓝ

✓4ᵗʰ **P04** **Newborn (suspected to be) affected by noxious substances transmitted via placenta or breast milk**

    INCLUDES   nonteratogenic effects of substances transmitted via placenta

    EXCLUDES 2   *congenital malformations (Q00-Q99)*

        neonatal jaundice from excessive hemolysis due to drugs or toxins transmitted from mother (P58.4)

        newborn in contact with and (suspected) exposures hazardous to health not transmitted via placenta or breast milk (Z77.-)

P04.0 **Newborn (suspected to be) affected by maternal anesthesia and analgesia in pregnancy, labor and delivery** Ⓝ

    Newborn (suspected to be) affected by reactions and intoxications from maternal opiates and tranquilizers administered during labor and delivery

P04.1 **Newborn (suspected to be) affected by other maternal medication** Ⓝ

    Newborn (suspected to be) affected by cancer chemotherapy

    Newborn (suspected to be) affected by cytotoxic drugs

    EXCLUDES 1   *dysmorphism due to warfarin (Q86.2)*

        fetal hydantoin syndrome (Q86.1)

        maternal use of drugs of addiction (P04.4-)

P04.2 **Newborn (suspected to be) affected by maternal use of tobacco** Ⓝ

    Newborn (suspected to be) affected by exposure in utero to tobacco smoke

    EXCLUDES 2   *newborn exposure to environmental tobacco smoke (P96.81)*

P04.3 **Newborn (suspected to be) affected by maternal use of alcohol** Ⓝ

    EXCLUDES 1   *fetal alcohol syndrome (Q86.0)*

✓5ᵗʰ **P04.4** **Newborn (suspected to be) affected by maternal use of drugs of addiction**

    P04.41 **Newborn (suspected to be) affected by maternal use of cocaine** Ⓝ

        "Crack baby"

    P04.49 **Newborn (suspected to be) affected by maternal use of other drugs of addiction** Ⓝ

        EXCLUDES 2   *newborn (suspected to be) affected by maternal anesthesia and analgesia (P04.0)*

        withdrawal symptoms from maternal use of drugs of addiction (P96.1)

P04.5 **Newborn (suspected to be) affected by maternal use of nutritional chemical substances** Ⓝ

P04.6 **Newborn (suspected to be) affected by maternal exposure to environmental chemical substances** Ⓝ

P04.8 **Newborn (suspected to be) affected by other maternal noxious substances** Ⓝ

P04.9 **Newborn (suspected to be) affected by maternal noxious substance, unspecified** Ⓝ

EXCLUDES 1 Not coded here   *EXCLUDES 2* Not included here   Ⓝ Newborn Age: 0   Ⓟ Pediatric Age: 0-17   Ⓜ Maternity Age: 12-55   Ⓐ Adult Age: 15-124

798   ICD-10-CM 2016

Disorders of newborn related to length of gestation and fetal growth (P05-P08)

✓4ᵗʰ **P05**   **Disorders of newborn related to slow fetal growth and fetal malnutrition**

    ✓5ᵗʰ **P05.0**   **Newborn light for gestational age**
       Newborn light-for-dates

       P05.00   **Newborn light for gestational age, unspecified weight**   N

       P05.01   **Newborn light for gestational age, less than 500 grams**   N

       P05.02   **Newborn light for gestational age, 500-749 grams**   N

       P05.03   **Newborn light for gestational age, 750-999 grams**   N

       P05.04   **Newborn light for gestational age, 1000-1249 grams**   N

       P05.05   **Newborn light for gestational age, 1250-1499 grams**   N

       P05.06   **Newborn light for gestational age, 1500-1749 grams**   N

       P05.07   **Newborn light for gestational age, 1750-1999 grams**   N

       P05.08   **Newborn light for gestational age, 2000-2499 grams**   N

    ✓5ᵗʰ **P05.1**   **Newborn small for gestational age**
       Newborn small-and-light-for-dates
       Newborn small-for-dates

       P05.10   **Newborn small for gestational age, unspecified weight**   N

       P05.11   **Newborn small for gestational age, less than 500 grams**   N

       P05.12   **Newborn small for gestational age, 500-749 grams**   N

       P05.13   **Newborn small for gestational age, 750-999 grams**   N

       P05.14   **Newborn small for gestational age, 1000-1249 grams**   N

       P05.15   **Newborn small for gestational age, 1250-1499 grams**   N

       P05.16   **Newborn small for gestational age, 1500-1749 grams**   N

       P05.17   **Newborn small for gestational age, 1750-1999 grams**   N

       P05.18   **Newborn small for gestational age, 2000-2499 grams**   N

    P05.2   **Newborn affected by fetal (intrauterine) malnutrition not light or small for gestational age**   N
       Infant, not light or small for gestational age, showing signs of fetal malnutrition, such as dry, peeling skin and loss of subcutaneous tissue
       EXCLUDES 1   *newborn affected by fetal malnutrition with light for gestational age (P05.0-)*
          newborn affected by fetal malnutrition with small for gestational age (P05.1-)

    P05.9   **Newborn affected by slow intrauterine growth, unspecified**   N
       Newborn affected by fetal growth retardation NOS

✓4ᵗʰ **P07**   **Disorders of newborn related to short gestation and low birth weight, not elsewhere classified**
       NOTE   When both birth weight and gestational age of the newborn are available, both should be coded with birth weight sequenced before gestational age
       INCLUDES   The listed conditions, without further specification, as the cause of morbidity or additional care, in newborn
       EXCLUDES 1   *low birth weight due to slow fetal growth and fetal malnutrition (P05.-)*

    ✓5ᵗʰ **P07.0**   **Extremely low birth weight newborn**
       Newborn birth weight 999 g. or less

       P07.00   **Extremely low birth weight newborn, unspecified weight**   N

       P07.01   **Extremely low birth weight newborn, less than 500 grams**   N

       P07.02   **Extremely low birth weight newborn, 500-749 grams**   N

       P07.03   **Extremely low birth weight newborn, 750-999 grams**   N

    ✓5ᵗʰ **P07.1**   **Other low birth weight newborn**
       Newborn birth weight 1000-2499 g.

       P07.10   **Other low birth weight newborn, unspecified weight**   N

       P07.14   **Other low birth weight newborn, 1000-1249 grams**   N

       P07.15   **Other low birth weight newborn, 1250-1499 grams**   N

       P07.16   **Other low birth weight newborn, 1500-1749 grams**   N

       P07.17   **Other low birth weight newborn, 1750-1999 grams**   N

       P07.18   **Other low birth weight newborn, 2000-2499 grams**   N

    ✓5ᵗʰ **P07.2**   **Extreme immaturity of newborn**
       Less than 28 completed weeks (less than 196 completed days) of gestation.

       P07.20   **Extreme immaturity of newborn, unspecified weeks of gestation**   N
          Gestational age less than 28 completed weeks NOS

       P07.21   **Extreme immaturity of newborn, gestational age less than 23 completed weeks**   N
          Extreme immaturity of newborn, gestational age less than 23 weeks, 0 days

       P07.22   **Extreme immaturity of newborn, gestational age 23 completed weeks**   N
          Extreme immaturity of newborn, gestational age 23 weeks, 0 days through 23 weeks, 6 days

       P07.23   **Extreme immaturity of newborn, gestational age 24 completed weeks**   N
          Extreme immaturity of newborn, gestational age 24 weeks, 0 days through 24 weeks, 6 days

       P07.24   **Extreme immaturity of newborn, gestational age 25 completed weeks**   N
          Extreme immaturity of newborn, gestational age 25 weeks, 0 days through 25 weeks, 6 days

       P07.25   **Extreme immaturity of newborn, gestational age 26 completed weeks**   N
          Extreme immaturity of newborn, gestational age 26 weeks, 0 days through 26 weeks, 6 days

       P07.26   **Extreme immaturity of newborn, gestational age 27 completed weeks**   N
          Extreme immaturity of newborn, gestational age 27 weeks, 0 days through 27 weeks, 6 days

    ✓5ᵗʰ **P07.3**   **Preterm [premature] newborn [other]**
       28 completed weeks or more but less than 37 completed weeks (196 completed days but less than 259 completed days) of gestation
       Prematurity NOS

       P07.30   **Preterm newborn, unspecified weeks of gestation**   N

       P07.31   **Preterm newborn, gestational age 28 completed weeks**   N
          Preterm newborn, gestational age 28 weeks, 0 days through 28 weeks, 6 days

       P07.32   **Preterm newborn, gestational age 29 completed weeks**   N
          Preterm newborn, gestational age 29 weeks, 0 days through 29 weeks, 6 days

       P07.33   **Preterm newborn, gestational age 30 completed weeks**   N
          Preterm newborn, gestational age 30 weeks, 0 days through 30 weeks, 6 days

       P07.34   **Preterm newborn, gestational age 31 completed weeks**   N
          Preterm newborn, gestational age 31 weeks, 0 days through 31 weeks, 6 days

       P07.35   **Preterm newborn, gestational age 32 completed weeks**   N
          Preterm newborn, gestational age 32 weeks, 0 days through 32 weeks, 6 days

       P07.36   **Preterm newborn, gestational age 33 completed weeks**   N
          Preterm newborn, gestational age 33 weeks, 0 days through 33 weeks, 6 days

       P07.37   **Preterm newborn, gestational age 34 completed weeks**   N
          Preterm newborn, gestational age 34 weeks, 0 days through 34 weeks, 6 days

---

✓ Additional Character Required   ✓x7ᵗʰ Placeholder Alert   Unspecified Dx   Other Specified Dx   Manifestation   ►◄ Revised Text   ● New Code   ▲ Revised Code Title

P07.38   **Preterm newborn, gestational age 35 completed weeks**   N
> Preterm newborn, gestational age 35 weeks, Ø days through 35 weeks, 6 days

P07.39   **Preterm newborn, gestational age 36 completed weeks**   N
> Preterm newborn, gestational age 36 weeks, Ø days through 36 weeks, 6 days

✓4ᵗʰ **P08**   **Disorders of newborn related to long gestation and high birth weight**
> NOTE   When both birth weight and gestational age of the newborn are available, priority of assignment should be given to birth weight
>
> INCLUDES   the listed conditions, without further specification, as causes of morbidity or additional care, in newborn

P08.0   **Exceptionally large newborn baby**   N
> Usually implies a birth weight of 4500 g. or more
>
> EXCLUDES 1   *syndrome of infant of diabetic mother (P70.1)*
> *syndrome of infant of mother with gestational diabetes (P70.0)*

P08.1   **Other heavy for gestational age newborn**   N
> Other newborn heavy- or large-for-dates regardless of period of gestation
> Usually implies a birth weight of 4000 g. to 4499 g.
>
> EXCLUDES 1   *newborn with a birth weight of 4500 or more (P08.0)*
> *syndrome of infant of diabetic mother (P70.1)*
> *syndrome of infant of mother with gestational diabetes (P70.0).*

✓5ᵗʰ **P08.2**   **Late newborn, not heavy for gestational age**
> AHA: 2014, 1Q, 14

P08.21   **Post-term newborn**   N
> Newborn with gestation period over 40 completed weeks to 42 completed weeks

P08.22   **Prolonged gestation of newborn**   N
> Newborn with gestation period over 42 completed weeks (294 days or more), not heavy- or large-for-dates.
> Postmaturity NOS

Abnormal findings on neonatal screening (P09)

P09   **Abnormal findings on neonatal screening**   N
> Use additional code to identify signs, symptoms and conditions associated with the screening
>
> EXCLUDES 2   *nonspecific serologic evidence of human immunodeficiency virus [HIV] (R75)*

Birth trauma (P10-P15)

✓4ᵗʰ **P10**   **Intracranial laceration and hemorrhage due to birth injury**
> EXCLUDES 1   *intracranial hemorrhage of newborn NOS (P52.9)*
> *intracranial hemorrhage of newborn due to anoxia or hypoxia (P52.-)*
> *nontraumatic intracranial hemorrhage of newborn (P52.-)*

P10.0   **Subdural hemorrhage due to birth injury**   N
> Subdural hematoma (localized) due to birth injury
>
> EXCLUDES 1   *subdural hemorrhage accompanying tentorial tear (P10.4)*

P10.1   **Cerebral hemorrhage due to birth injury**   N

P10.2   **Intraventricular hemorrhage due to birth injury**   N

P10.3   **Subarachnoid hemorrhage due to birth injury**   N

P10.4   **Tentorial tear due to birth injury**   N

P10.8   **Other intracranial lacerations and hemorrhages due to birth injury**   N

P10.9   **Unspecified intracranial laceration and hemorrhage due to birth injury**   N

✓4ᵗʰ **P11**   **Other birth injuries to central nervous system**

P11.0   **Cerebral edema due to birth injury**   N

P11.1   **Other specified brain damage due to birth injury**   N

P11.2   **Unspecified brain damage due to birth injury**   N

P11.3   **Birth injury to facial nerve**   N
> Facial palsy due to birth injury

P11.4   **Birth injury to other cranial nerves**   N

P11.5   **Birth injury to spine and spinal cord**   N
> Fracture of spine due to birth injury

P11.9   **Birth injury to central nervous system, unspecified**   N

✓4ᵗʰ **P12**   **Birth injury to scalp**

P12.0   **Cephalhematoma due to birth injury**   N

P12.1   **Chignon (from vacuum extraction) due to birth injury**   N

P12.2   **Epicranial subaponeurotic hemorrhage due to birth injury**   N
> Subgaleal hemorrhage

P12.3   **Bruising of scalp due to birth injury**   N

P12.4   **Injury of scalp of newborn due to monitoring equipment**   N
> Sampling incision of scalp of newborn
> Scalp clip (electrode) injury of newborn

✓5ᵗʰ **P12.8**   **Other birth injuries to scalp**

P12.81   **Caput succedaneum**   N

P12.89   **Other birth injuries to scalp**   N

P12.9   **Birth injury to scalp, unspecified**   N

✓4ᵗʰ **P13**   **Birth injury to skeleton**
> EXCLUDES 2   *birth injury to spine (P11.5)*

P13.0   **Fracture of skull due to birth injury**   N

P13.1   **Other birth injuries to skull**   N
> EXCLUDES 1   *cephalhematoma (P12.0)*

P13.2   **Birth injury to femur**   N

P13.3   **Birth injury to other long bones**   N

P13.4   **Fracture of clavicle due to birth injury**   N

P13.8   **Birth injuries to other parts of skeleton**   N

P13.9   **Birth injury to skeleton, unspecified**   N

✓4ᵗʰ **P14**   **Birth injury to peripheral nervous system**

P14.0   **Erb's paralysis due to birth injury**   N

P14.1   **Klumpke's paralysis due to birth injury**   N

P14.2   **Phrenic nerve paralysis due to birth injury**   N

P14.3   **Other brachial plexus birth injuries**   N

P14.8   **Birth injuries to other parts of peripheral nervous system**   N

P14.9   **Birth injury to peripheral nervous system, unspecified**   N

✓4ᵗʰ **P15**   **Other birth injuries**

P15.0   **Birth injury to liver**   N
> Rupture of liver due to birth injury

P15.1   **Birth injury to spleen**   N
> Rupture of spleen due to birth injury

P15.2   **Sternomastoid injury due to birth injury**   N

P15.3   **Birth injury to eye**   N
> Subconjunctival hemorrhage due to birth injury
> Traumatic glaucoma due to birth injury

P15.4   **Birth injury to face**   N
> Facial congestion due to birth injury

P15.5   **Birth injury to external genitalia**   N

P15.6   **Subcutaneous fat necrosis due to birth injury**   N

P15.8   **Other specified birth injuries**   N

P15.9   **Birth injury, unspecified**   N

Respiratory and cardiovascular disorders specific to the perinatal period (P19-P29)

✓4ᵗʰ **P19**   **Metabolic acidemia in newborn**
> Metabolic acidemia in newborn

P19.0   **Metabolic acidemia in newborn first noted before onset of labor**   N

P19.1   **Metabolic acidemia in newborn first noted during labor**   N

P19.2   **Metabolic acidemia noted at birth**   N

P19.9   **Metabolic acidemia, unspecified**   N

✓4ᵗʰ **P22**   **Respiratory distress of newborn**
> EXCLUDES 1   *respiratory arrest of newborn (P28.81)*
> *respiratory failure of newborn NOS (P28.5)*

P22.0   **Respiratory distress syndrome of newborn**   N
> Cardiorespiratory distress syndrome of newborn
> Hyaline membrane disease
> Idiopathic respiratory distress syndrome [IRDS or RDS] of newborn
> Pulmonary hypoperfusion syndrome
> Respiratory distress syndrome, type I

P22.1   **Transient tachypnea of newborn**   N
> Idiopathic tachypnea of newborn
> Respiratory distress syndrome, type II
> Wet lung syndrome

P22.8   **Other respiratory distress of newborn**   N

P22.9   **Respiratory distress of newborn, unspecified**   N

EXCLUDES 1 Not coded here   EXCLUDES 2 Not included here   N Newborn Age: 0   P Pediatric Age: 0-17   M Maternity Age: 12-55   A Adult Age: 15-124

800   ICD-10-CM 2016

√4ᵗʰ **P23 Congenital pneumonia**
     INCLUDES   infective pneumonia acquired in utero or during birth
     EXCLUDES 1   *neonatal pneumonia resulting from aspiration (P24.-)*

     P23.0 Congenital pneumonia due to viral agent   N
         Use additional code (B97) to identify organism
         EXCLUDES 1   *congenital rubella pneumonitis (P35.0)*

     P23.1 Congenital pneumonia due to Chlamydia   N
     P23.2 Congenital pneumonia due to staphylococcus   N
     P23.3 Congenital pneumonia due to streptococcus, group B   N
     P23.4 Congenital pneumonia due to Escherichia coli   N
     P23.5 Congenital pneumonia due to Pseudomonas   N
     P23.6 Congenital pneumonia due to other bacterial agents   N
         Congenital pneumonia due to Hemophilus influenzae
         Congenital pneumonia due to Klebsiella pneumoniae
         Congenital pneumonia due to Mycoplasma
         Congenital pneumonia due to Streptococcus, except group B
         Use additional code (B95-B96) to identify organism

     P23.8 Congenital pneumonia due to other organisms   N
     P23.9 Congenital pneumonia, unspecified   N

√4ᵗʰ **P24 Neonatal aspiration**
     INCLUDES   aspiration in utero and during delivery

   √5ᵗʰ **P24.0 Meconium aspiration**
     EXCLUDES 1   *meconium passage (without aspiration) during delivery*
         (P03.82)
         meconium staining (P96.83)

       P24.00 Meconium aspiration without respiratory   N
         symptoms
         Meconium aspiration NOS

       P24.01 Meconium aspiration with respiratory symptoms   N
         Meconium aspiration pneumonia
         Meconium aspiration pneumonitis
         Meconium aspiration syndrome NOS
         Use additional code to identify any secondary
         pulmonary hypertension, if applicable (I27.2)

   √5ᵗʰ **P24.1 Neonatal aspiration of (clear) amniotic fluid and mucus**
     Neonatal aspiration of liquor (amnii)

       P24.10 Neonatal aspiration of (clear) amniotic fluid and   N
         mucus without respiratory symptoms
         Neonatal aspiration of amniotic fluid and mucus NOS

       P24.11 Neonatal aspiration of (clear) amniotic fluid and   N
         mucus with respiratory symptoms
         Neonatal aspiration of amniotic fluid and mucus with
         pneumonia
         Neonatal aspiration of amniotic fluid and mucus with
         pneumonitis
         Use additional code to identify any secondary
         pulmonary hypertension, if applicable (I27.2)

   √5ᵗʰ **P24.2 Neonatal aspiration of blood**

       P24.20 Neonatal aspiration of blood without respiratory   N
         symptoms
         Neonatal aspiration of blood NOS

       P24.21 Neonatal aspiration of blood with respiratory   N
         symptoms
         Neonatal aspiration of blood with pneumonia
         Neonatal aspiration of blood with pneumonitis
         Use additional code to identify any secondary
         pulmonary hypertension, if applicable (I27.2)

   √5ᵗʰ **P24.3 Neonatal aspiration of milk and regurgitated food**
     Neonatal aspiration of stomach contents

       P24.30 Neonatal aspiration of milk and regurgitated   N
         food without respiratory symptoms
         Neonatal aspiration of milk and regurgitated food NOS

       P24.31 Neonatal aspiration of milk and regurgitated   N
         food with respiratory symptoms
         Neonatal aspiration of milk and regurgitated food with
         pneumonia
         Neonatal aspiration of milk and regurgitated food with
         pneumonitis
         Use additional code to identify any secondary
         pulmonary hypertension, if applicable (I27.2)

   √5ᵗʰ **P24.8 Other neonatal aspiration**

       P24.80 Other neonatal aspiration without respiratory   N
         symptoms
         Neonatal aspiration NEC

       P24.81 Other neonatal aspiration with respiratory   N
         symptoms
         Neonatal aspiration pneumonia NEC
         Neonatal aspiration with pneumonitis NEC
         Neonatal aspiration with pneumonia NOS
         Neonatal aspiration with pneumonitis NOS
         Use additional code to identify any secondary
         pulmonary hypertension, if applicable (I27.2)

     P24.9 Neonatal aspiration, unspecified   N

√4ᵗʰ **P25 Interstitial emphysema and related conditions originating in the perinatal period**

     P25.0 Interstitial emphysema originating in the perinatal period   N
     P25.1 Pneumothorax originating in the perinatal period   N
     P25.2 Pneumomediastinum originating in the perinatal period   N
     P25.3 Pneumopericardium originating in the perinatal period   N
     P25.8 Other conditions related to interstitial emphysema   N
         originating in the perinatal period

√4ᵗʰ **P26 Pulmonary hemorrhage originating in the perinatal period**
     EXCLUDES 1   *acute idiopathic hemorrhage in infants over 28 days old*
         (R04.81)

     P26.0 Tracheobronchial hemorrhage originating in the   N
         perinatal period
     P26.1 Massive pulmonary hemorrhage originating in the   N
         perinatal period
     P26.8 Other pulmonary hemorrhages originating in the   N
         perinatal period
     P26.9 Unspecified pulmonary hemorrhage originating   N
         in the perinatal period

√4ᵗʰ **P27 Chronic respiratory disease originating in the perinatal period**
     EXCLUDES 1   *respiratory distress of newborn (P22.0-P22.9)*

     P27.0 Wilson-Mikity syndrome
         Pulmonary dysmaturity
     P27.1 Bronchopulmonary dysplasia originating in the perinatal
         period
     P27.8 Other chronic respiratory diseases originating in the perinatal
         period
         Congenital pulmonary fibrosis
         Ventilator lung in newborn
     P27.9 Unspecified chronic respiratory disease originating in the
         perinatal period

√4ᵗʰ **P28 Other respiratory conditions originating in the perinatal period**
     EXCLUDES 1   *congenital malformations of the respiratory system (Q30-Q34)*

     P28.0 Primary atelectasis of newborn   N
         Primary failure to expand terminal respiratory units
         Pulmonary hypoplasia associated with short gestation
         Pulmonary immaturity NOS

   √5ᵗʰ **P28.1 Other and unspecified atelectasis of newborn**

       P28.10 Unspecified atelectasis of newborn   N
         Atelectasis of newborn NOS

       P28.11 Resorption atelectasis without respiratory   N
         distress syndrome
         EXCLUDES 1   *resorption atelectasis with respiratory*
            distress syndrome (P22.0)

       P28.19 Other atelectasis of newborn   N
         Partial atelectasis of newborn
         Secondary atelectasis of newborn

     P28.2 Cyanotic attacks of newborn   N
         EXCLUDES 1   *apnea of newborn (P28.3-P28.4)*

     P28.3 Primary sleep apnea of newborn   N
         Central sleep apnea of newborn
         Obstructive sleep apnea of newborn
         Sleep apnea of newborn NOS

     P28.4 Other apnea of newborn   N
         Apnea of prematurity
         Obstructive apnea of newborn
         EXCLUDES 1   *obstructive sleep apnea of newborn (P28.3)*

     P28.5 Respiratory failure of newborn   N
         EXCLUDES 1   *respiratory arrest of newborn (P28.81)*
            respiratory distress of newborn (P22.0-)

   √5ᵗʰ **P28.8 Other specified respiratory conditions of newborn**

       P28.81 Respiratory arrest of newborn   N
       P28.89 Other specified respiratory conditions of   N
         newborn
         Congenital laryngeal stridor
         Sniffles in newborn
         Snuffles in newborn
         EXCLUDES 1   *early congenital syphilitic rhinitis (A50.05)*

☑ Additional Character Required   ✓ˣ⁷ Placeholder Alert   Unspecified Dx   Other Specified Dx   Manifestation   ▶◀ Revised Text   ● New Code   ▲ Revised Code Title

P28.9   **Respiratory condition of newborn, unspecified**   N
Respiratory depression in newborn

✓4ᵗʰ **P29** **Cardiovascular disorders originating in the perinatal period**
EXCLUDES 1   congenital malformations of the circulatory system (Q20-Q28)

P29.0   **Neonatal cardiac failure**   N

✓5ᵗʰ **P29.1**   **Neonatal cardiac dysrhythmia**

    P29.11   **Neonatal** tachycardia   N

    P29.12   **Neonatal** bradycardia   N

P29.2   **Neonatal hypertension**   N

P29.3   **Persistent fetal circulation**   N
Delayed closure of ductus arteriosus
(Persistent) pulmonary hypertension of newborn

P29.4   **Transient myocardial ischemia in newborn**   N

✓5ᵗʰ **P29.8**   **Other cardiovascular disorders originating in the perinatal period**

    P29.81   **Cardiac arrest of newborn**   N

    P29.89   **Other cardiovascular disorders originating in the perinatal period**   N
AHA: 2014, 4Q, 23

P29.9   **Cardiovascular disorder originating in the perinatal period, unspecified**   N

Infections specific to the perinatal period (P35-P39)

Infections acquired in utero, during birth via the umbilicus, or during the first 28 days after birth
EXCLUDES 2   asymptomatic human immunodeficiency virus [HIV] infection status (Z21)
congenital gonococcal infection (A54.-)
congenital pneumonia (P23.-)
congenital syphilis (A50.-)
human immunodeficiency virus [HIV] disease (B20)
infant botulism (A48.51)
infectious diseases not specific to the perinatal period (A00-B99, J09, J10-)
intestinal infectious disease (A00-A09)
laboratory evidence of human immunodeficiency virus [HIV] (R75)
tetanus neonatorum (A33)

✓4ᵗʰ **P35** **Congenital viral diseases**
INCLUDES   infections acquired in utero or during birth

P35.0   **Congenital** rubella **syndrome**   N
Congenital rubella pneumonitis

P35.1   **Congenital** cytomegalovirus **infection**   N

P35.2   **Congenital** herpesviral [herpes simplex] **infection**   N

P35.3   **Congenital** viral hepatitis   N

P35.8   **Other congenital viral diseases**   N
Congenital varicella [chickenpox]

P35.9   **Congenital viral disease, unspecified**   N

✓4ᵗʰ **P36** **Bacterial sepsis of newborn**
INCLUDES   congenital sepsis
Use additional code(s), if applicable, to identify severe sepsis (R65.2-) and associated acute organ dysfunction(s)

P36.0   **Sepsis of newborn due to** streptococcus, group B   N

✓5ᵗʰ **P36.1**   **Sepsis of newborn due to other and unspecified streptococci**

    P36.10   **Sepsis of newborn due to unspecified streptococci**   N

    P36.19   **Sepsis of newborn due to other streptococci**   N

P36.2   **Sepsis of newborn due to** Staphylococcus aureus   N

✓5ᵗʰ **P36.3**   **Sepsis of newborn due to other and unspecified staphylococci**

    P36.30   **Sepsis of newborn due to unspecified staphylococci**   N

    P36.39   **Sepsis of newborn due to other staphylococci**   N

P36.4   **Sepsis of newborn due to** Escherichia coli   N

P36.5   **Sepsis of newborn due to** anaerobes   N

P36.8   **Other** bacterial sepsis **of newborn**   N
Use additional code from category B96 to identify organism

P36.9   **Bacterial sepsis of newborn, unspecified**   N

✓4ᵗʰ **P37** **Other congenital infectious and parasitic diseases**
EXCLUDES 2   congenital syphilis (A50.-)
infectious neonatal diarrhea (A00-A09)
necrotizing enterocolitis in newborn (P77.-)
noninfectious neonatal diarrhea (P78.3)
ophthalmia neonatorum due to gonococcus (A54.31)
tetanus neonatorum (A33)

P37.0   **Congenital** tuberculosis   N

P37.1   **Congenital** toxoplasmosis   N
Hydrocephalus due to congenital toxoplasmosis

P37.2   **Neonatal (disseminated)** listeriosis   N

P37.3   **Congenital** falciparum malaria   N

P37.4   **Other congenital** malaria   N

P37.5   **Neonatal** candidiasis   N

P37.8   **Other specified congenital infectious and parasitic diseases**   N

P37.9   **Congenital infectious or parasitic disease, unspecified**   N

✓4ᵗʰ **P38** **Omphalitis of newborn**
EXCLUDES 1   omphalitis not of newborn (L08.82)
tetanus omphalitis (A33)
umbilical hemorrhage of newborn (P51.-)

P38.1   **Omphalitis** with mild hemorrhage   N

P38.9   **Omphalitis** without hemorrhage   N
Omphalitis of newborn NOS

✓4ᵗʰ **P39** **Other infections specific to the perinatal period**
Use additional code to identify organism or specific infection

P39.0   **Neonatal infective** mastitis   N
EXCLUDES 1   breast engorgement of newborn (P83.4)
noninfective mastitis of newborn (P83.4)

P39.1   **Neonatal** conjunctivitis and dacryocystitis   N
Neonatal chlamydial conjunctivitis
Ophthalmia neonatorum NOS
EXCLUDES 1   gonococcal conjunctivitis (A54.31)

P39.2   **Intra-amniotic** infection affecting newborn, not elsewhere classified   N

P39.3   **Neonatal** urinary tract **infection**   N

P39.4   **Neonatal** skin infection   N
Neonatal pyoderma
EXCLUDES 1   pemphigus neonatorum (L00)
staphylococcal scalded skin syndrome (L00)

P39.8   **Other specified infections specific to the perinatal period**   N

P39.9   **Infection specific to the perinatal period, unspecified**   N

Hemorrhagic and hematological disorders of newborn (P50-P61)

EXCLUDES 1   congenital stenosis and stricture of bile ducts (Q44.3)
Crigler-Najjar syndrome (E80.5)
Dubin-Johnson syndrome (E80.6)
Gilbert syndrome (E80.4)
hereditary hemolytic anemias (D55-D58)

✓4ᵗʰ **P50** **Newborn affected by intrauterine (fetal)** blood loss
EXCLUDES 1   congenital anemia from intrauterine (fetal) blood loss (P61.3)

P50.0   **Newborn affected by intrauterine (fetal) blood loss from** vasa previa   N

P50.1   **Newborn affected by intrauterine (fetal) blood loss from** ruptured cord   N

P50.2   **Newborn affected by intrauterine (fetal) blood loss from** placenta   N

P50.3   **Newborn affected by hemorrhage into** co-twin   N

P50.4   **Newborn affected by hemorrhage into** maternal circulation   N

P50.5   **Newborn affected by intrauterine (fetal) blood loss from** cut end of co-twin's cord   N

P50.8   **Newborn affected by other intrauterine (fetal) blood loss**   N

P50.9   **Newborn affected by intrauterine (fetal) blood loss, unspecified**   N
Newborn affected by fetal hemorrhage NOS

✓4ᵗʰ **P51** **Umbilical** hemorrhage **of newborn**
EXCLUDES 1   omphalitis with mild hemorrhage (P38.1)
umbilical hemorrhage from cut end of co-twins cord (P50.5)

P51.0   **Massive** umbilical hemorrhage of newborn   N

P51.8   **Other umbilical hemorrhages of newborn**   N
Slipped umbilical ligature NOS

P51.9   **Umbilical hemorrhage of newborn, unspecified**   N

EXCLUDES 1 Not coded here   *EXCLUDES 2* Not included here   N Newborn Age: 0   P Pediatric Age: 0-17   M Maternity Age: 12-55   A Adult Age: 15-124

✓4th **P52 Intracranial nontraumatic hemorrhage of newborn**
Intracranial hemorrhage due to anoxia or hypoxia
    EXCLUDES 1   *intracranial hemorrhage due to birth injury (P10.-)*
               intracranial hemorrhage due to other injury (S06.-)

   P52.0 Intraventricular (nontraumatic) hemorrhage, grade 1, of newborn   N
         Subependymal hemorrhage (without intraventricular extension)
         Bleeding into germinal matrix

   P52.1 Intraventricular (nontraumatic) hemorrhage, grade 2, of newborn   N
         Subependymal hemorrhage with intraventricular extension
         Bleeding into ventricle

   ✓5th **P52.2 Intraventricular (nontraumatic) hemorrhage, grade 3 and grade 4, of newborn**

       P52.21 Intraventricular (nontraumatic) hemorrhage, grade 3, of newborn   N
              Subependymal hemorrhage with intraventricular extension with enlargement of ventricle

       P52.22 Intraventricular (nontraumatic) hemorrhage, grade 4, of newborn   N
              Bleeding into cerebral cortex
              Subependymal hemorrhage with intracerebral extension

   P52.3 Unspecified intraventricular (nontraumatic) hemorrhage of newborn   N

   P52.4 Intracerebral (nontraumatic) hemorrhage of newborn   N

   P52.5 Subarachnoid (nontraumatic) hemorrhage of newborn   N

   P52.6 Cerebellar (nontraumatic) and posterior fossa hemorrhage of newborn   N

   P52.8 Other intracranial (nontraumatic) hemorrhages of newborn   N

   P52.9 Intracranial (nontraumatic) hemorrhage of newborn, unspecified   N

P53 Hemorrhagic disease of newborn   N
   Vitamin K deficiency of newborn

✓4th **P54 Other neonatal hemorrhages**
    EXCLUDES 1   *newborn affected by (intrauterine) blood loss (P50.-)*
               pulmonary hemorrhage originating in the perinatal period (P26.-)

   P54.0 Neonatal hematemesis   N
     EXCLUDES 1   *neonatal hematemesis due to swallowed maternal blood (P78.2)*

   P54.1 Neonatal melena   N
     EXCLUDES 1   *neonatal melena due to swallowed maternal blood (P78.2)*

   P54.2 Neonatal rectal hemorrhage   N

   P54.3 Other neonatal gastrointestinal hemorrhage   N

   P54.4 Neonatal adrenal hemorrhage   N

   P54.5 Neonatal cutaneous hemorrhage   N
         Neonatal bruising
         Neonatal ecchymoses
         Neonatal petechiae
         Neonatal superficial hematomata
     EXCLUDES 2   *bruising of scalp due to birth injury (P12.3)*
               cephalhematoma due to birth injury (P12.0)

   P54.6 Neonatal vaginal hemorrhage   N ♀
         Neonatal pseudomenses

   P54.8 Other specified neonatal hemorrhages   N
   P54.9 Neonatal hemorrhage, unspecified   N

✓4th **P55 Hemolytic disease of newborn**
   P55.0 Rh isoimmunization of newborn   N
   P55.1 ABO isoimmunization of newborn   N
   P55.8 Other hemolytic diseases of newborn   N
   P55.9 Hemolytic disease of newborn, unspecified   N

✓4th **P56 Hydrops fetalis due to hemolytic disease**
    EXCLUDES 1   *hydrops fetalis NOS (P83.2)*
   P56.0 Hydrops fetalis due to isoimmunization   N
   ✓5th **P56.9 Hydrops fetalis due to other and unspecified hemolytic disease**
       P56.90 Hydrops fetalis due to unspecified hemolytic disease   N
       P56.99 Hydrops fetalis due to other hemolytic disease   N

✓4th **P57 Kernicterus**
   P57.0 Kernicterus due to isoimmunization   N
   P57.8 Other specified kernicterus   N
     EXCLUDES 1   *Crigler-Najjar syndrome (E80.5)*
   P57.9 Kernicterus, unspecified   N

✓4th **P58 Neonatal jaundice due to other excessive hemolysis**
    EXCLUDES 1   *jaundice due to isoimmunization (P55-P57)*
   P58.0 Neonatal jaundice due to bruising   N
   P58.1 Neonatal jaundice due to bleeding   N
   P58.2 Neonatal jaundice due to infection   N
   P58.3 Neonatal jaundice due to polycythemia   N
   ✓5th **P58.4 Neonatal jaundice due to drugs or toxins transmitted from mother or given to newborn**
         Code first poisoning due to drug or toxin, if applicable (T36-T65 with fifth or sixth character 1-4 or 6)
         Use additional code for adverse effect, if applicable, to identify drug (T36-T50 with fifth or sixth character 5)
       P58.41 Neonatal jaundice due to drugs or toxins transmitted from mother   N
       P58.42 Neonatal jaundice due to drugs or toxins given to newborn   N
   P58.5 Neonatal jaundice due to swallowed maternal blood   N
   P58.8 Neonatal jaundice due to other specified excessive hemolysis   N
   P58.9 Neonatal jaundice due to excessive hemolysis, unspecified   N

✓4th **P59 Neonatal jaundice from other and unspecified causes**
    EXCLUDES 1   *jaundice due to inborn errors of metabolism (E70-E88)*
               kernicterus (P57.-)
   P59.0 Neonatal jaundice associated with preterm delivery   N
         Hyperbilirubinemia of prematurity
         Jaundice due to delayed conjugation associated with preterm delivery
   P59.1 Inspissated bile syndrome   N
   ✓5th **P59.2 Neonatal jaundice from other and unspecified hepatocellular damage**
     EXCLUDES 1   *congenital viral hepatitis (P35.3)*
       P59.20 Neonatal jaundice from unspecified hepatocellular damage   N
       P59.29 Neonatal jaundice from other hepatocellular damage   N
           Neonatal giant cell hepatitis
           Neonatal (idiopathic) hepatitis
   P59.3 Neonatal jaundice from breast milk inhibitor   N
   P59.8 Neonatal jaundice from other specified causes   N
   P59.9 Neonatal jaundice, unspecified   N
         Neonatal physiological jaundice (intense)(prolonged) NOS

P60 Disseminated intravascular coagulation of newborn   N
   Defibrination syndrome of newborn

✓4th **P61 Other perinatal hematological disorders**
    EXCLUDES 1   *transient hypogammaglobulinemia of infancy (D80.7)*
   P61.0 Transient neonatal thrombocytopenia   N
         Neonatal thrombocytopenia due to exchange transfusion
         Neonatal thrombocytopenia due to idiopathic maternal thrombocytopenia
         Neonatal thrombocytopenia due to isoimmunization
   P61.1 Polycythemia neonatorum   N
   P61.2 Anemia of prematurity   N
   P61.3 Congenital anemia from fetal blood loss   N
   P61.4 Other congenital anemias, not elsewhere classified   N
         Congenital anemia NOS
   P61.5 Transient neonatal neutropenia   N
     EXCLUDES 1   *congenital neutropenia (nontransient) (D70.0)*
   P61.6 Other transient neonatal disorders of coagulation   N
   P61.8 Other specified perinatal hematological disorders   N
   P61.9 Perinatal hematological disorder, unspecified   N

☑ Additional Character Required   ✓x7th Placeholder Alert   Unspecified Dx   Other Specified Dx   Manifestation   ▶◀ Revised Text   ● New Code   ▲ Revised Code Title

Chapter 16. Certain Conditions Originating in the Perinatal Period

P70–P83.30

Transitory endocrine and metabolic disorders specific to newborn (P70-P74)

INCLUDES transitory endocrine and metabolic disturbances caused by the infant's response to maternal endocrine and metabolic factors, or its adjustment to extrauterine environment

✓4ᵗʰ **P70 Transitory disorders of carbohydrate metabolism specific to newborn**

P70.0 Syndrome of infant of mother with gestational diabetes N
Newborn (with hypoglycemia) affected by maternal gestational diabetes
EXCLUDES 1 newborn (with hypoglycemia) affected by maternal (pre-existing) diabetes mellitus (P70.1)
syndrome of infant of a diabetic mother (P70.1)

P70.1 Syndrome of infant of a diabetic mother N
Newborn (with hypoglycemia) affected by maternal (pre-existing) diabetes mellitus
EXCLUDES 1 newborn (with hypoglycemia) affected by maternal gestational diabetes (P70.0)
syndrome of infant of mother with gestational diabetes (P70.0)

P70.2 Neonatal diabetes mellitus N

P70.3 Iatrogenic neonatal hypoglycemia N

P70.4 Other neonatal hypoglycemia N
Transitory neonatal hypoglycemia

P70.8 Other transitory disorders of carbohydrate metabolism of newborn N

P70.9 Transitory disorder of carbohydrate metabolism of newborn, unspecified N

✓4ᵗʰ **P71 Transitory neonatal disorders of calcium and magnesium metabolism**

P71.0 Cow's milk hypocalcemia in newborn N

P71.1 Other neonatal hypocalcemia N
EXCLUDES 1 neonatal hypoparathyroidism (P71.4)

P71.2 Neonatal hypomagnesemia N

P71.3 Neonatal tetany without calcium or magnesium deficiency N
Neonatal tetany NOS

P71.4 Transitory neonatal hypoparathyroidism N

P71.8 Other transitory neonatal disorders of calcium and magnesium metabolism N

P71.9 Transitory neonatal disorder of calcium and magnesium metabolism, unspecified N

✓4ᵗʰ **P72 Other transitory neonatal endocrine disorders**
EXCLUDES 1 congenital hypothyroidism with or without goiter (E03.0-E03.1)
dyshormogenetic goiter (E07.1)
Pendred's syndrome (E07.1)

P72.0 Neonatal goiter, not elsewhere classified N
Transitory congenital goiter with normal functioning

P72.1 Transitory neonatal hyperthyroidism N
Neonatal thyrotoxicosis

P72.2 Other transitory neonatal disorders of thyroid function, not elsewhere classified N
Transitory neonatal hypothyroidism

P72.8 Other specified transitory neonatal endocrine disorders N

P72.9 Transitory neonatal endocrine disorder, unspecified N

✓4ᵗʰ **P74 Other transitory neonatal electrolyte and metabolic disturbances**

P74.0 Late metabolic acidosis of newborn N
EXCLUDES 1 (fetal) metabolic acidosis of newborn (P19)

P74.1 Dehydration of newborn N

P74.2 Disturbances of sodium balance of newborn N

P74.3 Disturbances of potassium balance of newborn N

P74.4 Other transitory electrolyte disturbances of newborn N

P74.5 Transitory tyrosinemia of newborn N

P74.6 Transitory hyperammonemia of newborn N

P74.8 Other transitory metabolic disturbances of newborn N
Amino-acid metabolic disorders described as transitory

P74.9 Transitory metabolic disturbance of newborn, unspecified N

Digestive system disorders of newborn (P76-P78)

✓4ᵗʰ **P76 Other intestinal obstruction of newborn**

P76.0 Meconium plug syndrome N
Meconium ileus NOS
EXCLUDES 1 meconium ileus in cystic fibrosis (E84.11)

P76.1 Transitory ileus of newborn N
EXCLUDES 1 Hirschsprung's disease (Q43.1)

P76.2 Intestinal obstruction due to inspissated milk N

P76.8 Other specified intestinal obstruction of newborn N
EXCLUDES 1 intestinal obstruction classifiable to K56-

P76.9 Intestinal obstruction of newborn, unspecified N

✓4ᵗʰ **P77 Necrotizing enterocolitis of newborn**

P77.1 Stage 1 necrotizing enterocolitis in newborn N
Necrotizing enterocolitis without pneumatosis, without perforation

P77.2 Stage 2 necrotizing enterocolitis in newborn N
Necrotizing enterocolitis with pneumatosis, without perforation

P77.3 Stage 3 necrotizing enterocolitis in newborn N
Necrotizing enterocolitis with perforation
Necrotizing enterocolitis with pneumatosis and perforation

P77.9 Necrotizing enterocolitis in newborn, unspecified N
Necrotizing enterocolitis in newborn, NOS

✓4ᵗʰ **P78 Other perinatal digestive system disorders**
EXCLUDES 1 cystic fibrosis (E84.0-E84.9)
neonatal gastrointestinal hemorrhages (P54.0-P54.3)

P78.0 Perinatal intestinal perforation N
Meconium peritonitis

P78.1 Other neonatal peritonitis N
Neonatal peritonitis NOS

P78.2 Neonatal hematemesis and melena due to swallowed maternal blood N

P78.3 Noninfective neonatal diarrhea N
Neonatal diarrhea NOS

✓5ᵗʰ **P78.8 Other specified perinatal digestive system disorders**
P78.81 Congenital cirrhosis (of liver) N
P78.82 Peptic ulcer of newborn N
P78.83 Newborn esophageal reflux N
Neonatal esophageal reflux
P78.89 Other specified perinatal digestive system disorders N

P78.9 Perinatal digestive system disorder, unspecified N

Conditions involving the integument and temperature regulation of newborn (P80-P83)

✓4ᵗʰ **P80 Hypothermia of newborn**

P80.0 Cold injury syndrome N
Severe and usually chronic hypothermia associated with a pink flushed appearance, edema and neurological and biochemical abnormalities.
EXCLUDES 1 mild hypothermia of newborn (P80.8)

P80.8 Other hypothermia of newborn N
Mild hypothermia of newborn

P80.9 Hypothermia of newborn, unspecified N

✓4ᵗʰ **P81 Other disturbances of temperature regulation of newborn**

P81.0 Environmental hyperthermia of newborn N

P81.8 Other specified disturbances of temperature regulation of newborn N

P81.9 Disturbance of temperature regulation of newborn, unspecified N
Fever of newborn NOS

✓4ᵗʰ **P83 Other conditions of integument specific to newborn**
EXCLUDES 1 congenital malformations of skin and integument (Q80-Q84)
hydrops fetalis due to hemolytic disease (P56.-)
neonatal skin infection (P39.4)
staphylococcal scalded skin syndrome (L00)
EXCLUDES 2 cradle cap (L21.0)
diaper [napkin] dermatitis (L22)

P83.0 Sclerema neonatorum N

P83.1 Neonatal erythema toxicum N

P83.2 Hydrops fetalis not due to hemolytic disease N
Hydrops fetalis NOS

✓5ᵗʰ **P83.3 Other and unspecified edema specific to newborn**
P83.30 Unspecified edema specific to newborn N

EXCLUDES 1 Not coded here   **EXCLUDES 2** Not included here   N Newborn Age: 0   P Pediatric Age: 0-17   M Maternity Age: 12-55   A Adult Age: 15-124

804   ICD-10-CM 2016

    P83.39   Other edema specific to newborn   N

P83.4   **Breast engorgement of newborn**   N
     Noninfective mastitis of newborn

P83.5   **Congenital hydrocele**   ♂

P83.6   **Umbilical polyp of newborn**

P83.8   **Other specified conditions of integument specific to newborn**   N
     Bronze baby syndrome
     Neonatal scleroderma
     Urticaria neonatorum

P83.9   **Condition of the integument specific to newborn, unspecified**   N

Other problems with newborn (P84)

P84   **Other problems with newborn**   N
     Acidemia of newborn
     Acidosis of newborn
     Anoxia of newborn NOS
     Asphyxia of newborn NOS
     Hypercapnia of newborn
     Hypoxemia of newborn
     Hypoxia of newborn NOS
     Mixed metabolic and respiratory acidosis of newborn
     EXCLUDES 1   *intracranial hemorrhage due to anoxia or hypoxia (P52.-)*
         hypoxic ischemic encephalopathy [HIE] (P91.6-)
         late metabolic acidosis of newborn (P74.0)

Other disorders originating in the perinatal period (P90-P96)

P90   **Convulsions of newborn**   N
     EXCLUDES 1   *benign myoclonic epilepsy in infancy (G40.3-)*
         benign neonatal convulsions (familial) (G40.3-)

✓4th **P91**   **Other disturbances of cerebral status of newborn**

    P91.0   **Neonatal cerebral ischemia**   N

    P91.1   **Acquired periventricular cysts of newborn**   N

    P91.2   **Neonatal cerebral leukomalacia**   N
         Periventricular leukomalacia

    P91.3   **Neonatal cerebral irritability**   N

    P91.4   **Neonatal cerebral depression**   N

    P91.5   **Neonatal coma**   N

    ✓5th **P91.6**   **Hypoxic ischemic encephalopathy [HIE]**

        P91.60   **Hypoxic ischemic encephalopathy [HIE], unspecified**   N

        P91.61   **Mild hypoxic ischemic encephalopathy [HIE]**   N

        P91.62   **Moderate hypoxic ischemic encephalopathy [HIE]**   N

        P91.63   **Severe hypoxic ischemic encephalopathy [HIE]**   N

    P91.8   **Other specified disturbances of cerebral status of newborn**   N

    P91.9   **Disturbance of cerebral status of newborn, unspecified**   N

✓4th **P92**   **Feeding problems of newborn**
     EXCLUDES 1   *feeding problems in child over 28 days old (R63.3)*

    ✓5th **P92.0**   **Vomiting of newborn**
         EXCLUDES 1   *vomiting of child over 28 days old (R11.-)*

        P92.01   **Bilious vomiting of newborn**   N
             EXCLUDES 1   *bilious vomiting in child over 28 days old (R11.14)*

        P92.09   **Other vomiting of newborn**   N
             EXCLUDES 1   *regurgitation of food in newborn (P92.1)*

    P92.1   **Regurgitation and rumination of newborn**   N

    P92.2   **Slow feeding of newborn**   N

    P92.3   **Underfeeding of newborn**   N

    P92.4   **Overfeeding of newborn**   N

    P92.5   **Neonatal difficulty in feeding at breast**   N

    P92.6   **Failure to thrive in newborn**   N
         EXCLUDES 1   *failure to thrive in child over 28 days old (R62.51)*

    P92.8   **Other feeding problems of newborn**   N

    P92.9   **Feeding problem of newborn, unspecified**   N

✓4th **P93**   **Reactions and intoxications due to drugs administered to newborn**
     INCLUDES   reactions and intoxications due to drugs administered to fetus affecting newborn
     EXCLUDES 1   *jaundice due to drugs or toxins transmitted from mother or given to newborn (P58.4-)*
         reactions and intoxications from maternal opiates, tranquilizers and other medication (P04.0-P04.1, P04.4)
         withdrawal symptoms from maternal use of drugs of addiction (P96.1)
         withdrawal symptoms from therapeutic use of drugs in newborn (P96.2)

    P93.0   **Grey baby syndrome**   N
         Grey syndrome from chloramphenicol administration in newborn

    P93.8   **Other reactions and intoxications due to drugs administered to newborn**   N
         Use additional code for adverse effect, if applicable, to identify drug (T36-T50 with fifth or sixth character 5)

✓4th **P94**   **Disorders of muscle tone of newborn**

    P94.0   **Transient neonatal myasthenia gravis**   N
         EXCLUDES 1   *myasthenia gravis (G70.0)*

    P94.1   **Congenital hypertonia**   N

    P94.2   **Congenital hypotonia**   N
         Floppy baby syndrome, unspecified

    P94.8   **Other disorders of muscle tone of newborn**   N

    P94.9   **Disorder of muscle tone of newborn, unspecified**   N

P95   **Stillbirth**   N
     Deadborn fetus NOS
     Fetal death of unspecified cause
     Stillbirth NOS
     EXCLUDES 1   *maternal care for intrauterine death (O36.4)*
         missed abortion (O02.1)
         outcome of delivery, stillbirth (Z37.1, Z37.3, Z37.4, Z37.7)

✓4th **P96**   **Other conditions originating in the perinatal period**

    P96.0   **Congenital renal failure**   N
         Uremia of newborn

    P96.1   **Neonatal withdrawal symptoms from maternal use of drugs of addiction**   N
         Drug withdrawal syndrome in infant of dependent mother
         Neonatal abstinence syndrome
         EXCLUDES 1   *reactions and intoxications from maternal opiates and tranquilizers administered during labor and delivery (P04.0)*

    P96.2   **Withdrawal symptoms from therapeutic use of drugs in newborn**   N

    P96.3   **Wide cranial sutures of newborn**   N
         Neonatal craniotabes

    P96.5   **Complication to newborn due to (fetal) intrauterine procedure**   N
         EXCLUDES 2   *newborn (suspected to be) affected by amniocentesis (P00.6)*

    ✓5th **P96.8**   **Other specified conditions originating in the perinatal period**

        P96.81   **Exposure to (parental) (environmental) tobacco smoke in the perinatal period**
             EXCLUDES 2   *newborn affected by in utero exposure to tobacco (P04.2)*
                  exposure to environmental tobacco smoke after the perinatal period (Z77.22)

        P96.82   **Delayed separation of umbilical cord**   N

        P96.83   **Meconium staining**   N
             EXCLUDES 1   *meconium aspiration (P24.00, P24.01)*
                  meconium passage during delivery (P03.82)

        P96.89   **Other specified conditions originating in the perinatal period**   N
             Use additional code to specify condition

    P96.9   **Condition originating in the perinatal period, unspecified**   N
         Congenital debility NOS

✓ Additional Character Required   ✓x7th Placeholder Alert   Unspecified Dx   Other Specified Dx   Manifestation   ►◄ Revised Text   ● New Code   ▲ Revised Code Title

Chapter 17. Congenital Malformations, Deformations, and Chromosomal Abnormalities (Q00–Q99)

Chapter Specific Guidelines with Coding Examples

The chapter specific guidelines from the ICD-10-CM Official Guidelines for Coding and Reporting have been provided below. Along with these guidelines are coding examples, contained in the shaded boxes, that have been developed to help illustrate the coding and/or sequencing guidance found in these guidelines.

Assign an appropriate code(s) from categories Q00–Q99, Congenital malformations, deformations, and chromosomal abnormalities when a malformation/deformation or chromosomal abnormality is documented. A malformation/deformation/or chromosomal abnormality may be the principal/first-listed diagnosis on a record or a secondary diagnosis.

When a malformation/deformation/or chromosomal abnormality does not have a unique code assignment, assign additional code(s) for any manifestations that may be present.

When the code assignment specifically identifies the malformation/deformation/or chromosomal abnormality, manifestations that are an inherent component of the anomaly should not be coded separately. Additional codes should be assigned for manifestations that are not an inherent component.

8-day-old infant with tetralogy of Fallot and pulmonary stenosis

Q21.3   **Tetralogy of Fallot**

Explanation: Pulmonary stenosis is inherent in the disease process of tetralogy of Fallot. When the code assignment specifically identifies the malformation/deformation/or chromosomal abnormality, manifestations that are inherent components of the anomaly should not be coded separately.

7-month-old infant with Down syndrome and common atrioventricular canal

Q90.9   **Down syndrome, unspecified**

Q21.2   **Atrioventricular septal defect**

Explanation: While a common atrioventricular canal is often associated with patients with Down syndrome, this manifestation is not an inherent component and may be reported separately. When the code assignment specifically identifies the anomaly, manifestations that are inherent components of the condition should not be coded separately. Additional codes should be assigned for manifestations that are not inherent components.

Codes from Chapter 17 may be used throughout the life of the patient. If a congenital malformation or deformity has been corrected, a personal history code should be used to identify the history of the malformation or deformity. Although present at birth, malformation/deformation/or chromosomal abnormality may not be identified until later in life. Whenever the condition is diagnosed by the physician, it is appropriate to assign a code from codes Q00-Q99. For the birth admission, the appropriate code from category Z38, Liveborn infants, according to place of birth and type of delivery, should be sequenced as the principal diagnosis, followed by any congenital anomaly codes, Q00- Q99.

Three-year-old with history of corrected ventricular septal defect

Z87.74   **Personal history of (corrected) congenital malformations of heart and circulatory system**

Explanation: If a congenital malformation or deformity has been corrected, a personal history code should be used to identify the history of the malformation or deformity.

Forty-year-old man with headaches diagnosed with congenital arteriovenous malformation by brain scan

Q28.2   **Arteriovenous malformation of cerebral vessels**

Explanation: Although present at birth, malformations may not be identified until later in life. Whenever the condition is diagnosed by the physician, it is appropriate to assign a code from the range Q00–Q99.

Newborn with anencephaly delivered vaginally in hospital

Z38.00   **Single liveborn infant, delivered vaginally**

Q00.0   **Anencephaly**

Explanation: For the birth admission, the appropriate code from category Z38 Liveborn infants, according to place of birth and type of delivery, should be sequenced as the principal diagnosis, followed by any congenital anomaly codes, Q00–Q99.

Chapter 17. Congenital Malformations, Deformations and Chromosomal Abnormalities(Q00-Q99)

NOTE Codes from this chapter are not for use on maternal or fetal records.

EXCLUDES 2 inborn errors of metabolism (E70-E88)

This chapter contains the following blocks:

Q00-Q07	Congenital malformations of the nervous system
Q10-Q18	Congenital malformations of eye, ear, face and neck
Q20-Q28	Congenital malformations of the circulatory system
Q30-Q34	Congenital malformations of the respiratory system
Q35-Q37	Cleft lip and cleft palate
Q38-Q45	Other congenital malformations of the digestive system
Q50-Q56	Congenital malformations of genital organs
Q60-Q64	Congenital malformations of the urinary system
Q65-Q79	Congenital malformations and deformations of the musculoskeletal system
Q80-Q89	Other congenital malformations
Q90-Q99	Chromosomal abnormalities, not elsewhere classified

Congenital malformations of the nervous system (Q00-Q07)

☑4ᵗʰ **Q00   Anencephaly and similar malformations**

Q00.0   Anencephaly
Acephaly
Acrania
Amyelencephaly
Hemianencephaly
Hemicephaly

Q00.1   Craniorachischisis

Q00.2   Iniencephaly

☑4ᵗʰ **Q01   Encephalocele**
INCLUDES   Arnold-Chiari syndrome, type III
encephalocystocele
encephalomyelocele
hydroencephalocele
hydromeningocele, cranial
meningocele, cerebral
meningoencephalocele
EXCLUDES 1   Meckel-Gruber syndrome (Q61.9)

Q01.0   Frontal encephalocele

Q01.1   Nasofrontal encephalocele

Q01.2   Occipital encephalocele

Q01.8   Encephalocele of other sites

Q01.9   Encephalocele, unspecified

Q02   Microcephaly
INCLUDES   hydromicrocephaly
micrencephalon
EXCLUDES 1   Meckel-Gruber syndrome (Q61.9)

☑4ᵗʰ **Q03   Congenital hydrocephalus**
INCLUDES   hydrocephalus in newborn
EXCLUDES 1   Arnold-Chiari syndrome, type II (Q07.0-)
acquired hydrocephalus (G91.-)
hydrocephalus due to congenital toxoplasmosis (P37.1)
hydrocephalus with spina bifida (Q05.0-Q05.4)

Q03.0   Malformations of aqueduct of Sylvius
Anomaly of aqueduct of Sylvius
Obstruction of aqueduct of Sylvius, congenital
Stenosis of aqueduct of Sylvius

Q03.1   Atresia of foramina of Magendie and Luschka
Dandy-Walker syndrome

Q03.8   Other congenital hydrocephalus

Q03.9   Congenital hydrocephalus, unspecified

☑4ᵗʰ **Q04   Other congenital malformations of brain**
EXCLUDES 1   cyclopia (Q87.0)
macrocephaly (Q75.3)

Q04.0   Congenital malformations of corpus callosum
Agenesis of corpus callosum

Q04.1   Arhinencephaly

Q04.2   Holoprosencephaly

Q04.3   Other reduction deformities of brain
Absence of part of brain
Agenesis of part of brain
Agyria
Aplasia of part of brain
Hydranencephaly
Hypoplasia of part of brain
Lissencephaly
Microgyria
Pachygyria
EXCLUDES 1   congenital malformations of corpus callosum (Q04.0)

Q04.4   Septo-optic dysplasia of brain

Q04.5   Megalencephaly

Q04.6   Congenital cerebral cysts
Porencephaly
Schizencephaly
EXCLUDES 1   acquired porencephalic cyst (G93.0)

Q04.8   Other specified congenital malformations of brain
Arnold-Chiari syndrome, type IV
Macrogyria

Q04.9   Congenital malformation of brain, unspecified
Congenital anomaly NOS of brain
Congenital deformity NOS of brain
Congenital disease or lesion NOS of brain
Multiple anomalies NOS of brain, congenital

☑4ᵗʰ **Q05   Spina bifida**
Hydromeningocele (spinal)
Meningocele (spinal)
Meningomyelocele
Myelocele
Myelomeningocele
Rachischisis
Spina bifida (aperta)(cystica)
Syringomyelocele
Use additional code for any associated paraplegia (paraparesis) (G82.2-)
EXCLUDES 1   Arnold-Chiari syndrome, type II (Q07.0-)
spina bifida occulta (Q76.0)

Q05.0   Cervical spina bifida with hydrocephalus

Q05.1   Thoracic spina bifida with hydrocephalus
Dorsal spina bifida with hydrocephalus
Thoracolumbar spina bifida with hydrocephalus

Q05.2   Lumbar spina bifida with hydrocephalus
Lumbosacral spina bifida with hydrocephalus

Q05.3   Sacral spina bifida with hydrocephalus

Q05.4   Unspecified spina bifida with hydrocephalus

Q05.5   Cervical spina bifida without hydrocephalus

Q05.6   Thoracic spina bifida without hydrocephalus
Dorsal spina bifida NOS
Thoracolumbar spina bifida NOS

Q05.7   Lumbar spina bifida without hydrocephalus
Lumbosacral spina bifida NOS

Q05.8   Sacral spina bifida without hydrocephalus

Q05.9   Spina bifida, unspecified

☑4ᵗʰ **Q06   Other congenital malformations of spinal cord**

Q06.0   Amyelia

Q06.1   Hypoplasia and dysplasia of spinal cord
Atelomyelia
Myelatelia
Myelodysplasia of spinal cord

Q06.2   Diastematomyelia

Q06.3   Other congenital cauda equina malformations

Q06.4   Hydromyelia
Hydrorachis

Q06.8   Other specified congenital malformations of spinal cord

Q06.9   Congenital malformation of spinal cord, unspecified
Congenital anomaly NOS of spinal cord
Congenital deformity NOS of spinal cord
Congenital disease or lesion NOS of spinal cord

☑4ᵗʰ **Q07   Other congenital malformations of nervous system**
EXCLUDES 2   congenital central alveolar hypoventilation syndrome (G47.35)
familial dysautonomia [Riley-Day] (G90.1)
neurofibromatosis (nonmalignant) (Q85.0-)

☑5ᵗʰ **Q07.0   Arnold-Chiari syndrome**
Arnold-Chiari syndrome, type II
EXCLUDES 1   Arnold-Chiari syndrome, type III (Q01.-)
Arnold-Chiari syndrome, type IV (Q04.8)

Q07.00   Arnold-Chiari syndrome without spina bifida or hydrocephalus

---

☑ Additional Character Required   ☑ᵡ7ᵗʰ Placeholder Alert   Unspecified Dx   Other Specified Dx   Manifestation   ►◄ Revised Text   ● New Code   ▲ Revised Code Title

Q07.01 Arnold-Chiari syndrome with spina bifida

Q07.02 Arnold-Chiari syndrome with hydrocephalus

Q07.03 Arnold-Chiari syndrome with spina bifida and hydrocephalus

Q07.8 Other specified congenital malformations of nervous system
Agenesis of nerve
Displacement of brachial plexus
Jaw-winking syndrome
Marcus Gunn's syndrome

Q07.9 Congenital malformation of nervous system, unspecified
Congenital anomaly NOS of nervous system
Congenital deformity NOS of nervous system
Congenital disease or lesion NOS of nervous system

Congenital malformations of eye, ear, face and neck (Q10-Q18)

EXCLUDES 2 cleft lip and cleft palate (Q35-Q37)
congenital malformation of cervical spine (Q05.0, Q05.5, Q67.5, Q76.0-Q76.4)
congenital malformation of larynx (Q31.-)
congenital malformation of lip NEC (Q38.0)
congenital malformation of nose (Q30.-)
congenital malformation of parathyroid gland (Q89.2)
congenital malformation of thyroid gland (Q89.2)

✓4ᵗʰ **Q10 Congenital malformations of** eyelid, lacrimal apparatus and orbit
EXCLUDES 1 cryptophthalmos NOS (Q11.2)
cryptophthalmos syndrome (Q87.0)

Q10.0 Congenital ptosis

Q10.1 Congenital ectropion

Q10.2 Congenital entropion

Q10.3 Other congenital malformations of eyelid
Ablepharon
Blepharophimosis, congenital
Coloboma of eyelid
Congenital absence or agenesis of cilia
Congenital absence or agenesis of eyelid
Congenital accessory eyelid
Congenital accessory eye muscle
Congenital malformation of eyelid NOS

Q10.4 Absence and agenesis of lacrimal apparatus
Congenital absence of punctum lacrimale

Q10.5 Congenital stenosis and stricture of lacrimal duct

Q10.6 Other congenital malformations of lacrimal apparatus
Congenital malformation of lacrimal apparatus NOS

Q10.7 Congenital malformation of orbit

✓4ᵗʰ **Q11 Anophthalmos, microphthalmos and macrophthalmos**

Q11.0 Cystic eyeball

Q11.1 Other anophthalmos
Anophthalmos NOS
Agenesis of eye
Aplasia of eye

Q11.2 Microphthalmos
Cryptophthalmos NOS
Dysplasia of eye
Hypoplasia of eye
Rudimentary eye
EXCLUDES 1 cryptophthalmos syndrome (Q87.0)

Q11.3 Macrophthalmos
EXCLUDES 1 macrophthalmos in congenital glaucoma (Q15.0)

✓4ᵗʰ **Q12 Congenital lens malformations**

Q12.0 Congenital cataract

Q12.1 Congenital displaced lens

Q12.2 Coloboma of lens

Q12.3 Congenital aphakia

Q12.4 Spherophakia

Q12.8 Other congenital lens malformations
Microphakia

Q12.9 Congenital lens malformation, unspecified

✓4ᵗʰ **Q13 Congenital malformations of** anterior segment of eye

Q13.0 Coloboma of iris
Coloboma NOS

Q13.1 Absence of iris
Aniridia
Use additional code for associated glaucoma (H42)

Q13.2 Other congenital malformations of iris
Anisocoria, congenital
Atresia of pupil
Congenital malformation of iris NOS
Corectopia

Q13.3 Congenital corneal opacity

Q13.4 Other congenital corneal malformations
Congenital malformation of cornea NOS
Microcornea
Peter's anomaly

Q13.5 Blue sclera

✓5ᵗʰ **Q13.8 Other congenital malformations of anterior segment of eye**

Q13.81 Rieger's anomaly
Use additional code for associated glaucoma (H42)

Q13.89 Other congenital malformations of anterior segment of eye

Q13.9 Congenital malformation of anterior segment of eye, unspecified

✓4ᵗʰ **Q14 Congenital malformations of** posterior segment of eye
EXCLUDES 2 optic nerve hypoplasia (H47.03-)

Q14.0 Congenital malformation of vitreous humor
Congenital vitreous opacity

Q14.1 Congenital malformation of retina
Congenital retinal aneurysm

Q14.2 Congenital malformation of optic disc
Coloboma of optic disc

Q14.3 Congenital malformation of choroid

Q14.8 Other congenital malformations of posterior segment of eye
Coloboma of the fundus

Q14.9 Congenital malformation of posterior segment of eye, unspecified

✓4ᵗʰ **Q15 Other congenital malformations of** eye
EXCLUDES 1 congenital nystagmus (H55.01)
ocular albinism (E70.31-)
optic nerve hypoplasia (H47.03-)
retinitis pigmentosa (H35.52)

Q15.0 Congenital glaucoma
Axenfeld's anomaly
Buphthalmos
Glaucoma of childhood
Glaucoma of newborn
Hydrophthalmos
Keratoglobus, congenital, with glaucoma
Macrocornea with glaucoma
Macrophthalmos in congenital glaucoma
Megalocornea with glaucoma

Q15.8 Other specified congenital malformations of eye

Q15.9 Congenital malformation of eye, unspecified
Congenital anomaly of eye
Congenital deformity of eye

✓4ᵗʰ **Q16 Congenital malformations of** ear causing impairment of hearing
EXCLUDES 1 congenital deafness (H90.-)

Q16.0 Congenital absence of (ear) auricle

Q16.1 Congenital absence, atresia and stricture of auditory canal (external)
Congenital atresia or stricture of osseous meatus

Q16.2 Absence of eustachian tube

Q16.3 Congenital malformation of ear ossicles
Congenital fusion of ear ossicles

Q16.4 Other congenital malformations of middle ear
Congenital malformation of middle ear NOS

Q16.5 Congenital malformation of inner ear
Congenital anomaly of membranous labyrinth
Congenital anomaly of organ of Corti

Q16.9 Congenital malformation of ear causing impairment of hearing, unspecified
Congenital absence of ear NOS

✓4ᵗʰ **Q17 Other congenital malformations of** ear
EXCLUDES 1 congenital malformations of ear with impairment of hearing (Q16.0- Q16.9)
preauricular sinus (Q18.1)

Q17.0 Accessory auricle
Accessory tragus
Polyotia
Preauricular appendage or tag
Supernumerary ear
Supernumerary lobule

Q17.1 Macrotia

EXCLUDES 1 Not coded here   EXCLUDES 2 Not included here   🄽 Newborn Age: 0   🄿 Pediatric Age: 0-17   🄼 Maternity Age: 12-55   🄰 Adult Age: 15-124

Q17.2   **Microtia**

Q17.3   **Other misshapen ear**
Pointed ear

Q17.4   **Misplaced ear**
Low-set ears
EXCLUDES 1   *cervical auricle (Q18.2)*

Q17.5   **Prominent ear**
Bat ear

Q17.8   **Other specified congenital malformations of ear**
Congenital absence of lobe of ear

Q17.9   **Congenital malformation of ear, unspecified**
Congenital anomaly of ear NOS

✓4th **Q18**   **Other congenital malformations of face and neck**
EXCLUDES 1   *cleft lip and cleft palate (Q35-Q37)*
conditions classified to Q67.0-Q67.4
congenital malformations of skull and face bones (Q75.-)
cyclopia (Q87.0)
dentofacial anomalies [including malocclusion] (M26.-)
malformation syndromes affecting facial appearance (Q87.0)
persistent thyroglossal duct (Q89.2)

Q18.0   **Sinus, fistula and cyst of branchial cleft**
Branchial vestige

Q18.1   **Preauricular sinus and cyst**
Fistula of auricle, congenital
Cervicoaural fistula

Q18.2   **Other branchial cleft malformations**
Branchial cleft malformation NOS
Cervical auricle
Otocephaly

Q18.3   **Webbing of neck**
Pterygium colli

Q18.4   **Macrostomia**

Q18.5   **Microstomia**

Q18.6   **Macrocheilia**
Hypertrophy of lip, congenital

Q18.7   **Microcheilia**

Q18.8   **Other specified congenital malformations of face and neck**
Medial cyst of face and neck
Medial fistula of face and neck
Medial sinus of face and neck

Q18.9   **Congenital malformation of face and neck, unspecified**
Congenital anomaly NOS of face and neck

Congenital malformations of the circulatory system (Q20-Q28)

✓4th **Q20**   **Congenital malformations of cardiac chambers and connections**
EXCLUDES 1   *dextrocardia with situs inversus (Q89.3)*
mirror-image atrial arrangement with situs inversus (Q89.3)

Q20.0   **Common arterial trunk**
Persistent truncus arteriosus
EXCLUDES 1   *aortic septal defect (Q21.4)*

Q20.1   **Double outlet right ventricle**
Taussig-Bing syndrome

Q20.2   **Double outlet left ventricle**

Q20.3   **Discordant ventriculoarterial connection**
Dextrotransposition of aorta
Transposition of great vessels (complete)

Q20.4   **Double inlet ventricle**
Common ventricle
Cor triloculare biatriatum
Single ventricle

Q20.5   **Discordant atrioventricular connection**
Corrected transposition
Levotransposition
Ventricular inversion

Q20.6   **Isomerism of atrial appendages**
Isomerism of atrial appendages with asplenia or polysplenia

Q20.8   **Other congenital malformations of cardiac chambers and connections**
Cor binoculare

Q20.9   **Congenital malformation of cardiac chambers and connections, unspecified**

✓4th **Q21**   **Congenital malformations of cardiac septa**
EXCLUDES 1   *acquired cardiac septal defect (I51.0)*

Q21.0   **Ventricular septal defect**
Roger's disease

Q21.1   **Atrial septal defect**
Coronary sinus defect
Patent or persistent foramen ovale
Patent or persistent ostium secundum defect (type II)
Patent or persistent sinus venosus defect

Q21.2   **Atrioventricular septal defect**
Common atrioventricular canal
Endocardial cushion defect
Ostium primum atrial septal defect (type I)

Q21.3   **Tetralogy of Fallot**
Ventricular septal defect with pulmonary stenosis or atresia, dextroposition of aorta and hypertrophy of right ventricle.
AHA: 2014, 3Q, 16

Q21.4   **Aortopulmonary septal defect**
Aortic septal defect
Aortopulmonary window

Q21.8   **Other congenital malformations of cardiac septa**
Eisenmenger's defect
Pentalogy of Fallot
EXCLUDES 1   *Eisenmenger's complex (I27.8)*
Eisenmenger's syndrome (I27.8)

Q21.9   **Congenital malformation of cardiac septum, unspecified**
Septal (heart) defect NOS

✓4th **Q22**   **Congenital malformations of pulmonary and tricuspid valves**

Q22.0   **Pulmonary valve atresia**

Q22.1   **Congenital pulmonary valve stenosis**

Q22.2   **Congenital pulmonary valve insufficiency**
Congenital pulmonary valve regurgitation

Q22.3   **Other congenital malformations of pulmonary valve**
Congenital malformation of pulmonary valve NOS
Supernumerary cusps of pulmonary valve

Q22.4   **Congenital tricuspid stenosis**
Congenital tricuspid atresia

Q22.5   **Ebstein's anomaly**

Q22.6   **Hypoplastic right heart syndrome**

Q22.8   **Other congenital malformations of tricuspid valve**

Q22.9   **Congenital malformation of tricuspid valve, unspecified**

✓4th **Q23**   **Congenital malformations of aortic and mitral valves**

Q23.0   **Congenital stenosis of aortic valve**
Congenital aortic atresia
Congenital aortic stenosis NOS
EXCLUDES 1   *congenital stenosis of aortic valve in hypoplastic left heart syndrome (Q23.4)*
congenital subaortic stenosis (Q24.4)
supravalvular aortic stenosis (congenital) (Q25.3)

Q23.1   **Congenital insufficiency of aortic valve**
Bicuspid aortic valve
Congenital aortic insufficiency

Q23.2   **Congenital mitral stenosis**
Congenital mitral atresia

Q23.3   **Congenital mitral insufficiency**

Q23.4   **Hypoplastic left heart syndrome**

Q23.8   **Other congenital malformations of aortic and mitral valves**

Q23.9   **Congenital malformation of aortic and mitral valves, unspecified**

✓4th **Q24**   **Other congenital malformations of heart**
EXCLUDES 1   *endocardial fibroelastosis (I42.4)*

Q24.0   **Dextrocardia**
EXCLUDES 1   *dextrocardia with situs inversus (Q89.3)*
isomerism of atrial appendages (with asplenia or polysplenia) (Q20.6)
mirror-image atrial arrangement with situs inversus (Q89.3)

Q24.1   **Levocardia**

Q24.2   **Cor triatriatum**

Q24.3   **Pulmonary infundibular stenosis**
Subvalvular pulmonic stenosis

Q24.4   **Congenital subaortic stenosis**

Q24.5   **Malformation of coronary vessels**
Congenital coronary (artery) aneurysm

Q24.6   **Congenital heart block**

Q24.8   **Other specified congenital malformations of heart**
Congenital diverticulum of left ventricle
Congenital malformation of myocardium
Congenital malformation of pericardium
Malposition of heart
Uhl's disease

✓ Additional Character Required   ✓7th Placeholder Alert   Unspecified Dx   Other Specified Dx   Manifestation   ▶◀ Revised Text   ● New Code   ▲ Revised Code Title

Q24.9 Congenital malformation of heart, unspecified
Congenital anomaly of heart
Congenital disease of heart

✓4ᵗʰ **Q25 Congenital malformations of great arteries**

Q25.0 Patent ductus arteriosus
Patent ductus Botallo
Persistent ductus arteriosus

Q25.1 Coarctation of aorta
Coarctation of aorta (preductal) (postductal)

Q25.2 Atresia of aorta

Q25.3 Supravalvular aortic stenosis
EXCLUDES 1 *congenital aortic stenosis NOS (Q23.0)*
congenital stenosis of aortic valve (Q23.0)

Q25.4 Other congenital malformations of aorta
Absence of aorta
Aneurysm of sinus of Valsalva (ruptured)
Aplasia of aorta
Congenital aneurysm of aorta
Congenital malformations of aorta
Congenital dilatation of aorta
Double aortic arch [vascular ring of aorta]
Hypoplasia of aorta
Persistent convolutions of aortic arch
Persistent right aortic arch
EXCLUDES 1 *hypoplasia of aorta in hypoplastic left heart syndrome (Q23.4)*

Q25.5 Atresia of pulmonary artery

Q25.6 Stenosis of pulmonary artery
Supravalvular pulmonary stenosis

✓5ᵗʰ **Q25.7 Other congenital malformations of pulmonary artery**

Q25.71 Coarctation of pulmonary artery

Q25.72 Congenital pulmonary arteriovenous malformation
Congenital pulmonary arteriovenous aneurysm

Q25.79 Other congenital malformations of pulmonary artery
Aberrant pulmonary artery
Agenesis of pulmonary artery
Congenital aneurysm of pulmonary artery
Congenital anomaly of pulmonary artery
Hypoplasia of pulmonary artery

Q25.8 Other congenital malformations of other great arteries

Q25.9 Congenital malformation of great arteries, unspecified

✓4ᵗʰ **Q26 Congenital malformations of great veins**

Q26.0 Congenital stenosis of vena cava
Congenital stenosis of vena cava (inferior)(superior)

Q26.1 Persistent left superior vena cava

Q26.2 Total anomalous pulmonary venous connection
Total anomalous pulmonary venous return [TAPVR], subdiaphragmatic
Total anomalous pulmonary venous return [TAPVR], supradiaphragmatic

Q26.3 Partial anomalous pulmonary venous connection
Partial anomalous pulmonary venous return

Q26.4 Anomalous pulmonary venous connection, unspecified

Q26.5 Anomalous portal venous connection

Q26.6 Portal vein-hepatic artery fistula

Q26.8 Other congenital malformations of great veins
Absence of vena cava (inferior) (superior)
Azygos continuation of inferior vena cava
Persistent left posterior cardinal vein
Scimitar syndrome

Q26.9 Congenital malformation of great vein, unspecified
Congenital anomaly of vena cava (inferior) (superior) NOS

✓4ᵗʰ **Q27 Other congenital malformations of peripheral vascular system**
EXCLUDES 2 *anomalies of cerebral and precerebral vessels (Q28.0-Q28.3)*
anomalies of coronary vessels (Q24.5)
anomalies of pulmonary artery (Q25.5-Q25.7)
congenital retinal aneurysm (Q14.1)
hemangioma and lymphangioma (D18.-)

Q27.0 Congenital absence and hypoplasia of umbilical artery
Single umbilical artery

Q27.1 Congenital renal artery stenosis

Q27.2 Other congenital malformations of renal artery
Congenital malformation of renal artery NOS
Multiple renal arteries

✓5ᵗʰ **Q27.3 Arteriovenous malformation (peripheral)**
Arteriovenous aneurysm
EXCLUDES 1 *acquired arteriovenous aneurysm (I77.0)*
EXCLUDES 2 *arteriovenous malformation of cerebral vessels (Q28.2)*
arteriovenous malformation of precerebral vessels (Q28.0)

Q27.30 Arteriovenous malformation, site unspecified

Q27.31 Arteriovenous malformation of vessel of upper limb

Q27.32 Arteriovenous malformation of vessel of lower limb

Q27.33 Arteriovenous malformation of digestive system vessel

Q27.34 Arteriovenous malformation of renal vessel

Q27.39 Arteriovenous malformation, other site

Q27.4 Congenital phlebectasia

Q27.8 Other specified congenital malformations of peripheral vascular system
Absence of peripheral vascular system
Atresia of peripheral vascular system
Congenital aneurysm (peripheral)
Congenital stricture, artery
Congenital varix
EXCLUDES 1 *arteriovenous malformation (Q27.3-)*

Q27.9 Congenital malformation of peripheral vascular system, unspecified
Anomaly of artery or vein NOS

✓4ᵗʰ **Q28 Other congenital malformations of circulatory system**
EXCLUDES 1 *congenital aneurysm NOS (Q27.8)*
congenital coronary aneurysm (Q24.5)
ruptured cerebral arteriovenous malformation (I60.8)
ruptured malformation of precerebral vessels (I72.0)
EXCLUDES 2 *congenital peripheral aneurysm (Q27.8)*
congenital pulmonary aneurysm (Q25.79)
congenital retinal aneurysm (Q14.1)

Q28.0 Arteriovenous malformation of precerebral vessels
Congenital arteriovenous precerebral aneurysm (nonruptured)

Q28.1 Other malformations of precerebral vessels
Congenital malformation of precerebral vessels NOS
Congenital precerebral aneurysm (nonruptured)

Q28.2 Arteriovenous malformation of cerebral vessels
Arteriovenous malformation of brain NOS
Congenital arteriovenous cerebral aneurysm (nonruptured)

Q28.3 Other malformations of cerebral vessels
Congenital cerebral aneurysm (nonruptured)
Congenital malformation of cerebral vessels NOS
Developmental venous anomaly

Q28.8 Other specified congenital malformations of circulatory system
Congenital aneurysm, specified site NEC
Spinal vessel anomaly

Q28.9 Congenital malformation of circulatory system, unspecified

Congenital malformations of the respiratory system (Q30-Q34)

✓4ᵗʰ **Q30 Congenital malformations of nose**
EXCLUDES 1 *congenital deviation of nasal septum (Q67.4)*

Q30.0 Choanal atresia
Atresia of nares (anterior) (posterior)
Congenital stenosis of nares (anterior) (posterior)

Q30.1 Agenesis and underdevelopment of nose
Congenital absent of nose

Q30.2 Fissured, notched and cleft nose

Q30.3 Congenital perforated nasal septum

Q30.8 Other congenital malformations of nose
Accessory nose
Congenital anomaly of nasal sinus wall

Q30.9 Congenital malformation of nose, unspecified

✓4ᵗʰ **Q31 Congenital malformations of larynx**
EXCLUDES 1 *congenital laryngeal stridor NOS (P28.89)*

Q31.0 Web of larynx
Glottic web of larynx
Subglottic web of larynx
Web of larynx NOS

Q31.1 Congenital subglottic stenosis

Q31.2 Laryngeal hypoplasia

Q31.3 Laryngocele

Q31.5 Congenital laryngomalacia

EXCLUDES 1 Not coded here   EXCLUDES 2 Not included here   N Newborn Age: 0   P Pediatric Age: 0-17   M Maternity Age: 12-55   A Adult Age: 15-124

ICD-10-CM 2016

Q31.8 Other congenital malformations of larynx
Absence of larynx
Agenesis of larynx
Atresia of larynx
Congenital cleft thyroid cartilage
Congenital fissure of epiglottis
Congenital stenosis of larynx NEC
Posterior cleft of cricoid cartilage

Q31.9 Congenital malformation of larynx, unspecified

✓4ᵗʰ **Q32 Congenital malformations of trachea and bronchus**
     EXCLUDES 1   congenital bronchiectasis (Q33.4)

Q32.0 Congenital tracheomalacia

Q32.1 Other congenital malformations of trachea
Atresia of trachea
Congenital anomaly of tracheal cartilage
Congenital dilatation of trachea
Congenital malformation of trachea
Congenital stenosis of trachea
Congenital tracheocele

Q32.2 Congenital bronchomalacia

Q32.3 Congenital stenosis of bronchus

Q32.4 Other congenital malformations of bronchus
Absence of bronchus
Agenesis of bronchus
Atresia of bronchus
Congenital diverticulum of bronchus
Congenital malformation of bronchus NOS

✓4ᵗʰ **Q33 Congenital malformations of lung**

Q33.0 Congenital cystic lung
Congenital cystic lung disease
Congenital honeycomb lung
Congenital polycystic lung disease
     EXCLUDES 1   cystic fibrosis (E84.0)
            cystic lung disease, acquired or unspecified (J98.4)

Q33.1 Accessory lobe of lung
Azygos lobe (fissured), lung

Q33.2 Sequestration of lung

Q33.3 Agenesis of lung
Congenital absence of lung (lobe)

Q33.4 Congenital bronchiectasis

Q33.5 Ectopic tissue in lung

Q33.6 Congenital hypoplasia and dysplasia of lung
     EXCLUDES 1   pulmonary hypoplasia associated with short gestation
            (P28.0)

Q33.8 Other congenital malformations of lung

Q33.9 Congenital malformation of lung, unspecified

✓4ᵗʰ **Q34 Other congenital malformations of respiratory system**
     EXCLUDES 2   congenital central alveolar hypoventilation syndrome (G47.35)

Q34.0 Anomaly of pleura

Q34.1 Congenital cyst of mediastinum

Q34.8 Other specified congenital malformations of respiratory system
Atresia of nasopharynx

Q34.9 Congenital malformation of respiratory system, unspecified
Congenital absence of respiratory system
Congenital anomaly of respiratory system NOS

Cleft lip and cleft palate (Q35-Q37)

Use additional code to identify associated malformation of the nose (Q30.2)
EXCLUDES 1   Robin's syndrome (Q87.0)

✓4ᵗʰ **Q35 Cleft palate**
     INCLUDES   fissure of palate
            palatoschisis
     EXCLUDES 1   cleft palate with cleft lip (Q37.-)

Q35.1 Cleft hard palate

Q35.3 Cleft soft palate

Q35.5 Cleft hard palate with cleft soft palate

Q35.7 Cleft uvula

Q35.9 Cleft palate, unspecified
Cleft palate NOS

✓4ᵗʰ **Q36 Cleft lip**
Cheiloschisis
Congenital fissure of lip
Harelip
Labium leporinum
     EXCLUDES 1   cleft lip with cleft palate (Q37.-)

Q36.0 Cleft lip, bilateral

Q36.1 Cleft lip, median

Q36.9 Cleft lip, unilateral
Cleft lip NOS

✓4ᵗʰ **Q37 Cleft palate with cleft lip**
Cheilopalatoschisis

Q37.0 Cleft hard palate with bilateral cleft lip

Q37.1 Cleft hard palate with unilateral cleft lip
Cleft hard palate with cleft lip NOS

Q37.2 Cleft soft palate with bilateral cleft lip

Q37.3 Cleft soft palate with unilateral cleft lip
Cleft soft palate with cleft lip NOS

Q37.4 Cleft hard and soft palate with bilateral cleft lip

Q37.5 Cleft hard and soft palate with unilateral cleft lip
Cleft hard and soft palate with cleft lip NOS

Q37.8 Unspecified cleft palate with bilateral cleft lip

Q37.9 Unspecified cleft palate with unilateral cleft lip
Cleft palate with cleft lip NOS

Other congenital malformations of the digestive system (Q38-Q45)

✓4ᵗʰ **Q38 Other congenital malformations of tongue, mouth and pharynx**
     EXCLUDES 1   dentofacial anomalies (M26.-)
            macrostomia (Q18.4)
            microstomia (Q18.5)

Q38.0 Congenital malformations of lips, not elsewhere classified
Congenital fistula of lip
Congenital malformation of lip NOS
Van der Woude's syndrome
     EXCLUDES 1   cleft lip (Q36.-)
            cleft lip with cleft palate (Q37.-)
            macrocheilia (Q18.6)
            microcheilia (Q18.7)

Q38.1 Ankyloglossia
Tongue tie

Q38.2 Macroglossia
Congenital hypertrophy of tongue

Q38.3 Other congenital malformations of tongue
Aglossia
Bifid tongue
Congenital adhesion of tongue
Congenital fissure of tongue
Congenital malformation of tongue NOS
Double tongue
Hypoglossia
Hypoplasia of tongue
Microglossia

Q38.4 Congenital malformations of salivary glands and ducts
Atresia of salivary glands and ducts
Congenital absence of salivary glands and ducts
Congenital accessory salivary glands and ducts
Congenital fistula of salivary gland

Q38.5 Congenital malformations of palate, not elsewhere classified
Congenital absence of uvula
Congenital malformation of palate NOS
Congenital high arched palate
     EXCLUDES 1   cleft palate (Q35.-)
            cleft palate with cleft lip (Q37.-)

Q38.6 Other congenital malformations of mouth
Congenital malformation of mouth NOS

Q38.7 Congenital pharyngeal pouch
Congenital diverticulum of pharynx
     EXCLUDES 1   pharyngeal pouch syndrome (D82.1)

Q38.8 Other congenital malformations of pharynx
Congenital malformation of pharynx NOS
Imperforate pharynx

✓4ᵗʰ **Q39 Congenital malformations of esophagus**

Q39.0 Atresia of esophagus without fistula
Atresia of esophagus NOS

Q39.1 Atresia of esophagus with tracheo-esophageal fistula
Atresia of esophagus with broncho-esophageal fistula

✓ Additional Character Required   ✓7ᵗʰ Placeholder Alert   Unspecified Dx   Other Specified Dx   Manifestation   ▶◀ Revised Text   ● New Code   ▲ Revised Code Title

Q39.2 Congenital tracheo-esophageal fistula without atresia
Congenital tracheo-esophageal fistula NOS

Q39.3 Congenital stenosis and stricture of esophagus

Q39.4 Esophageal web

Q39.5 Congenital dilatation of esophagus
Congenital cardiospasm

Q39.6 Congenital diverticulum of esophagus
Congenital esophageal pouch

Q39.8 Other congenital malformations of esophagus
Congenital absence of esophagus
Congenital displacement of esophagus
Congenital duplication of esophagus

Q39.9 Congenital malformation of esophagus, unspecified

✓4ᵗʰ **Q40 Other congenital malformations of upper alimentary tract**

Q40.0 Congenital hypertrophic pyloric stenosis
Congenital or infantile constriction
Congenital or infantile hypertrophy
Congenital or infantile spasm
Congenital or infantile stenosis
Congenital or infantile stricture

Q40.1 Congenital hiatus hernia
Congenital displacement of cardia through esophageal hiatus
EXCLUDES 1 *congenital diaphragmatic hernia (Q79.0)*

Q40.2 Other specified congenital malformations of stomach
Congenital displacement of stomach
Congenital diverticulum of stomach
Congenital hourglass stomach
Congenital duplication of stomach
Megalogastria
Microgastria

Q40.3 Congenital malformation of stomach, unspecified

Q40.8 Other specified congenital malformations of upper alimentary tract

Q40.9 Congenital malformation of upper alimentary tract, unspecified
Congenital anomaly of upper alimentary tract
Congenital deformity of upper alimentary tract

✓4ᵗʰ **Q41 Congenital absence, atresia and stenosis of small intestine**
Congenital obstruction, occlusion or stricture of small intestine or intestine NOS
EXCLUDES 1 *cystic fibrosis with intestinal manifestation (E84.11)*
meconium ileus NOS (without cystic fibrosis) (P76.0)

Q41.0 Congenital absence, atresia and stenosis of duodenum

Q41.1 Congenital absence, atresia and stenosis of jejunum
Apple peel syndrome
Imperforate jejunum

Q41.2 Congenital absence, atresia and stenosis of ileum

Q41.8 Congenital absence, atresia and stenosis of other specified parts of small intestine

Q41.9 Congenital absence, atresia and stenosis of small intestine, part unspecified
Congenital absence, atresia and stenosis of intestine NOS

✓4ᵗʰ **Q42 Congenital absence, atresia and stenosis of large intestine**
Congenital obstruction, occlusion and stricture of large intestine

Q42.0 Congenital absence, atresia and stenosis of rectum with fistula

Q42.1 Congenital absence, atresia and stenosis of rectum without fistula

Q42.2 Congenital absence, atresia and stenosis of anus with fistula

Q42.3 Congenital absence, atresia and stenosis of anus without fistula
Imperforate anus

Q42.8 Congenital absence, atresia and stenosis of other parts of large intestine

Q42.9 Congenital absence, atresia and stenosis of large intestine, part unspecified

✓4ᵗʰ **Q43 Other congenital malformations of intestine**

Q43.0 Meckel's diverticulum (displaced) (hypertrophic)
Persistent omphalomesenteric duct
Persistent vitelline duct

Q43.1 Hirschsprung's disease
Aganglionosis
Congenital (aganglionic) megacolon

Q43.2 Other congenital functional disorders of colon
Congenital dilatation of colon

Q43.3 Congenital malformations of intestinal fixation
Congenital omental, anomalous adhesions [bands]
Congenital peritoneal adhesions [bands]
Incomplete rotation of cecum and colon
Insufficient rotation of cecum and colon
Jackson's membrane
Malrotation of colon
Rotation failure of cecum and colon
Universal mesentery

Q43.4 Duplication of intestine

Q43.5 Ectopic anus

Q43.6 Congenital fistula of rectum and anus
EXCLUDES 1 *congenital fistula of anus with absence, atresia and stenosis (Q42.2)*
congenital fistula of rectum with absence, atresia and stenosis (Q42.0)
congenital rectovaginal fistula (Q52.2)
congenital urethrorectal fistula (Q64.73)
pilonidal fistula or sinus (L05.-)

Q43.7 Persistent cloaca
Cloaca NOS

Q43.8 Other specified congenital malformations of intestine
Congenital blind loop syndrome
Congenital diverticulitis, colon
Congenital diverticulum, intestine
Dolichocolon
Megaloappendix
Megaloduodenum
Microcolon
Transposition of appendix
Transposition of colon
Transposition of intestine
AHA: 2013, 2Q, 31

Q43.9 Congenital malformation of intestine, unspecified

✓4ᵗʰ **Q44 Congenital malformations of gallbladder, bile ducts and liver**

Q44.0 Agenesis, aplasia and hypoplasia of gallbladder
Congenital absence of gallbladder

Q44.1 Other congenital malformations of gallbladder
Congenital malformation of gallbladder NOS
Intrahepatic gallbladder

Q44.2 Atresia of bile ducts

Q44.3 Congenital stenosis and stricture of bile ducts

Q44.4 Choledochal cyst

Q44.5 Other congenital malformations of bile ducts
Accessory hepatic duct
Biliary duct duplication
Congenital malformation of bile duct NOS
Cystic duct duplication

Q44.6 Cystic disease of liver
Fibrocystic disease of liver

Q44.7 Other congenital malformations of liver
Accessory liver
Alagille's syndrome
Congenital absence of liver
Congenital hepatomegaly
Congenital malformation of liver NOS

✓4ᵗʰ **Q45 Other congenital malformations of digestive system**
EXCLUDES 2 *congenital diaphragmatic hernia (Q79.0)*
congenital hiatus hernia (Q40.1)

Q45.0 Agenesis, aplasia and hypoplasia of pancreas
Congenital absence of pancreas

Q45.1 Annular pancreas

Q45.2 Congenital pancreatic cyst

Q45.3 Other congenital malformations of pancreas and pancreatic duct
Accessory pancreas
Congenital malformation of pancreas or pancreatic duct NOS
EXCLUDES 1 *congenital diabetes mellitus (E10.-)*
cystic fibrosis (E84.0-E84.9)
fibrocystic disease of pancreas (E84.-)
neonatal diabetes mellitus (P70.2)

Q45.8 Other specified congenital malformations of digestive system
Absence (complete) (partial) of alimentary tract NOS
Duplication of digestive system
Malposition, congenital of digestive system

Q45.9 Congenital malformation of digestive system, unspecified
Congenital anomaly of digestive system
Congenital deformity of digestive system

EXCLUDES 1 Not coded here   EXCLUDES 2 Not included here   Ⓝ Newborn Age: 0   Ⓟ Pediatric Age: 0-17   Ⓜ Maternity Age: 12-55   Ⓐ Adult Age: 15-124

Congenital malformations of genital organs (Q50-Q56)

EXCLUDES 1   androgen insensitivity syndrome (E34.5-)
syndromes associated with anomalies in the number and form of chromosomes (Q90-Q99)

✓4ᵗʰ **Q50 Congenital malformations of** ovaries, fallopian tubes and broad ligaments

✓5ᵗʰ **Q50.0 Congenital absence of** ovary
     EXCLUDES 1   Turner's syndrome (Q96.-)

   Q50.01 Congenital absence of ovary, unilateral   ♀
   Q50.02 Congenital absence of ovary, bilateral   ♀

Q50.1 Developmental ovarian cyst   ♀
Q50.2 Congenital torsion **of ovary**   ♀

✓5ᵗʰ **Q50.3 Other** congenital malformations of ovary

   Q50.31 Accessory ovary   ♀
   Q50.32 Ovarian streak   ♀
     46, XX with streak gonads
   Q50.39 Other congenital malformation of ovary   ♀
     Congenital malformation of ovary NOS

Q50.4 Embryonic cyst of fallopian tube   ♀
   Fimbrial cyst

Q50.5 Embryonic cyst of broad ligament   ♀
   Epoophoron cyst
   Parovarian cyst

Q50.6 Other congenital malformations of fallopian tube and broad ligament   ♀
   Absence of fallopian tube and broad ligament
   Accessory fallopian tube and broad ligament
   Atresia of fallopian tube and broad ligament
   Congenital malformation of fallopian tube or broad ligament NOS

✓4ᵗʰ **Q51 Congenital malformations of** uterus and cervix

Q51.0 Agenesis and aplasia of uterus   ♀
   Congenital absence of uterus

✓5ᵗʰ **Q51.1 Doubling of uterus with doubling of cervix and vagina**

   Q51.10 Doubling of uterus with doubling of cervix and vagina without obstruction   ♀
     Doubling of uterus with doubling of cervix and vagina NOS
   Q51.11 Doubling of uterus with doubling of cervix and vagina with obstruction   ♀

Q51.2 Other doubling **of uterus**   ♀
   Doubling of uterus NOS
   Septate uterus, complete or partial

Q51.3 Bicornate uterus   ♀
   Bicornate uterus, complete or partial

Q51.4 Unicornate uterus   ♀
   Unicornate uterus with or without a separate uterine horn
   Uterus with only one functioning horn

Q51.5 Agenesis and aplasia of cervix   ♀
   Congenital absence of cervix

Q51.6 Embryonic cyst **of cervix**   ♀
Q51.7 Congenital fistulae **between uterus and digestive and urinary tracts**   ♀

✓5ᵗʰ **Q51.8 Other** congenital malformations of uterus and cervix

   ✓6ᵗʰ **Q51.81 Other congenital malformations of** uterus
     Q51.810 Arcuate uterus   ♀
       Arcuatus uterus
     Q51.811 Hypoplasia of uterus   ♀
     Q51.818 Other congenital malformations of uterus   ♀
       Müllerian anomaly of uterus NEC
   ✓6ᵗʰ **Q51.82 Other congenital malformations of** cervix
     Q51.820 Cervical duplication   ♀
     Q51.821 Hypoplasia of cervix   ♀
     Q51.828 Other congenital malformations of cervix   ♀

Q51.9 Congenital malformation of uterus and cervix, unspecified   ♀

✓4ᵗʰ **Q52 Other congenital malformations of** female genitalia

Q52.0 Congenital absence **of** vagina   ♀
   Vaginal agenesis, total or partial

✓5ᵗʰ **Q52.1 Doubling of vagina**
   EXCLUDES 1   doubling of vagina with doubling of uterus and cervix (Q51.1-)

   Q52.10 Doubling of vagina, unspecified   ♀
     Septate vagina NOS

   Q52.11 Transverse vaginal septum   ♀
   Q52.12 Longitudinal vaginal septum   ♀
     Longitudinal vaginal septum with or without obstruction

Q52.2 Congenital rectovaginal fistula   ♀
   EXCLUDES 1   cloaca (Q43.7)

Q52.3 Imperforate hymen   ♀
Q52.4 Other congenital malformations of vagina   ♀
   Canal of Nuck cyst, congenital
   Congenital malformation of vagina NOS
   Embryonic vaginal cyst
   Gartner's duct cyst

Q52.5 Fusion of labia   ♀
Q52.6 Congenital malformation of clitoris   ♀

✓5ᵗʰ **Q52.7 Other and unspecified congenital malformations of vulva**

   Q52.70 Unspecified congenital malformations of vulva   ♀
     Congenital malformation of vulva NOS
   Q52.71 Congenital absence **of vulva**   ♀
   Q52.79 Other congenital malformations of vulva   ♀
     Congenital cyst of vulva

Q52.8 Other specified congenital malformations of female genitalia   ♀
Q52.9 Congenital malformation of female genitalia, unspecified   ♀

✓4ᵗʰ **Q53 Undescended and ectopic** testicle

✓5ᵗʰ **Q53.0 Ectopic** testis

   Q53.00 Ectopic testis, unspecified   ♂
   Q53.01 Ectopic testis, unilateral   ♂
   Q53.02 Ectopic testes, bilateral   ♂

✓5ᵗʰ **Q53.1 Undescended** testicle, unilateral

   Q53.10 Unspecified undescended testicle, unilateral   ♂
   Q53.11 Abdominal testis, unilateral   ♂
   Q53.12 Ectopic perineal testis, unilateral   ♂

✓5ᵗʰ **Q53.2 Undescended** testicle, bilateral

   Q53.20 Undescended testicle, unspecified, bilateral   ♂
   Q53.21 Abdominal testis, bilateral   ♂
   Q53.22 Ectopic perineal testis, bilateral   ♂

Q53.9 Undescended testicle, unspecified   ♂
   Cryptorchism NOS

✓4ᵗʰ **Q54 Hypospadias**
   EXCLUDES 1   epispadias (Q64.0)

Q54.0 Hypospadias, balanic   ♂
   Hypospadias, coronal
   Hypospadias, glandular

Q54.1 Hypospadias, penile   ♂
Q54.2 Hypospadias, penoscrotal   ♂
Q54.3 Hypospadias, perineal   ♂
Q54.4 Congenital chordee   ♂
   Chordee without hypospadias

Q54.8 Other hypospadias   ♂
   Hypospadias with intersex state

Q54.9 Hypospadias, unspecified   ♂

✓4ᵗʰ **Q55 Other congenital malformations of** male genital organs
   EXCLUDES 1   congenital hydrocele (P83.5)
     hypospadias (Q54.-)

Q55.0 Absence and aplasia of testis   ♂
   Monorchism

Q55.1 Hypoplasia of testis and scrotum   ♂
   Fusion of testes

✓5ᵗʰ **Q55.2 Other and unspecified congenital malformations of** testis and scrotum

   Q55.20 Unspecified congenital malformations of testis and scrotum   ♂
     Congenital malformation of testis or scrotum NOS
   Q55.21 Polyorchism   ♂
   Q55.22 Retractile testis   ♂
   Q55.23 Scrotal transposition   ♂
   Q55.29 Other congenital malformations of testis and scrotum   ♂

Q55.3 Atresia of vas deferens   ♂
   Code first any associated cystic fibrosis (E84.-)

☑ Additional Character Required   ✓7ᵗʰ Placeholder Alert   Unspecified Dx   Other Specified Dx   Manifestation   ►◄ Revised Text   ● New Code   ▲ Revised Code Title

Q55.4 **Other congenital malformations of vas deferens, epididymis, seminal vesicles and prostate** ♂
Absence or aplasia of prostate
Absence or aplasia of spermatic cord
Congenital malformation of vas deferens, epididymis, seminal vesicles or prostate NOS

Q55.5 **Congenital absence and aplasia of penis** ♂

✓5ᵗʰ **Q55.6** **Other congenital malformations of penis**

     Q55.61 **Curvature of penis (lateral)** ♂

     Q55.62 **Hypoplasia of penis** ♂
         Micropenis

     Q55.63 **Congenital torsion of penis** ♂
         EXCLUDES 1   acquired torsion of penis (N48.82)

     Q55.64 **Hidden penis** ♂
         Buried penis
         Concealed penis
         EXCLUDES 1   acquired buried penis (N48.83)

     Q55.69 **Other congenital malformation of penis** ♂
         Congenital malformation of penis NOS

Q55.7 **Congenital vasocutaneous fistula** ♂

Q55.8 **Other specified congenital malformations of male genital organs** ♂

Q55.9 **Congenital malformation of male genital organ, unspecified** ♂
Congenital anomaly of male genital organ
Congenital deformity of male genital organ

✓4ᵗʰ **Q56** **Indeterminate sex and pseudohermaphroditism**
     EXCLUDES 1   46, XX true hermaphrodite (Q99.1)
         androgen insensitivity syndrome (E34.5-)
         chimera 46, XX/46, XY true hermaphrodite (Q99.0)
         female pseudohermaphroditism with adrenocortical disorder (E25.-)
         pseudohermaphroditism with specified chromosomal anomaly (Q96-Q99)
         pure gonadal dysgenesis (Q99.1)

Q56.0 **Hermaphroditism, not elsewhere classified**
Ovotestis

Q56.1 **Male pseudohermaphroditism, not elsewhere classified** ♂
46, XY with streak gonads
Male pseudohermaphroditism NOS

Q56.2 **Female pseudohermaphroditism, not elsewhere classified** ♀
Female pseudohermaphroditism NOS

Q56.3 **Pseudohermaphroditism, unspecified**

Q56.4 **Indeterminate sex, unspecified**
Ambiguous genitalia

Congenital malformations of the urinary system (Q60-Q64)

✓4ᵗʰ **Q60** **Renal agenesis and other reduction defects of kidney**
Congenital absence of kidney
Congenital atrophy of kidney
Infantile atrophy of kidney

Q60.0 **Renal agenesis, unilateral**

Q60.1 **Renal agenesis, bilateral**

Q60.2 **Renal agenesis, unspecified**

Q60.3 **Renal hypoplasia, unilateral**

Q60.4 **Renal hypoplasia, bilateral**

Q60.5 **Renal hypoplasia, unspecified**

Q60.6 **Potter's syndrome**

✓4ᵗʰ **Q61** **Cystic kidney disease**
     EXCLUDES 1   acquired cyst of kidney (N28.1)
         Potter's syndrome (Q60.6)

✓5ᵗʰ **Q61.0** **Congenital renal cyst**

     Q61.00 **Congenital renal cyst, unspecified**
         Cyst of kidney NOS (congenital)

     Q61.01 **Congenital single renal cyst**

     Q61.02 **Congenital multiple renal cysts**

✓5ᵗʰ **Q61.1** **Polycystic kidney, infantile type**
     Polycystic kidney, autosomal recessive

     Q61.11 **Cystic dilatation of collecting ducts**

     Q61.19 **Other polycystic kidney, infantile type**

Q61.2 **Polycystic kidney, adult type**
Polycystic kidney, autosomal dominant

Q61.3 **Polycystic kidney, unspecified**

Q61.4 **Renal dysplasia**
Multicystic dysplastic kidney
Multicystic kidney (development)
Multicystic kidney disease
Multicystic renal dysplasia
     EXCLUDES 1   polycystic kidney disease (Q61.11-Q61.3)

Q61.5 **Medullary cystic kidney**
Nephronopthisis
Sponge kidney NOS

Q61.8 **Other cystic kidney diseases**
Fibrocystic kidney
Fibrocystic renal degeneration or disease

Q61.9 **Cystic kidney disease, unspecified**
Meckel-Gruber syndrome

✓4ᵗʰ **Q62** **Congenital obstructive defects of renal pelvis and congenital malformations of ureter**

Q62.0 **Congenital hydronephrosis**

✓5ᵗʰ **Q62.1** **Congenital occlusion of ureter**
     Atresia and stenosis of ureter

     Q62.10 **Congenital occlusion of ureter, unspecified**

     Q62.11 **Congenital occlusion of ureteropelvic junction**

     Q62.12 **Congenital occlusion of ureterovesical orifice**

Q62.2 **Congenital megaureter**
Congenital dilatation of ureter

✓5ᵗʰ **Q62.3** **Other obstructive defects of renal pelvis and ureter**

     Q62.31 **Congenital ureterocele, orthotopic**

     Q62.32 **Cecoureterocele**
         Ectopic ureterocele

     Q62.39 **Other obstructive defects of renal pelvis and ureter**
         Ureteropelvic junction obstruction NOS

Q62.4 **Agenesis of ureter**
Congenital absence ureter

Q62.5 **Duplication of ureter**
Accessory ureter
Double ureter

✓5ᵗʰ **Q62.6** **Malposition of ureter**

     Q62.60 **Malposition of ureter, unspecified**

     Q62.61 **Deviation of ureter**

     Q62.62 **Displacement of ureter**

     Q62.63 **Anomalous implantation of ureter**
         Ectopia of ureter
         Ectopic ureter

     Q62.69 **Other malposition of ureter**

Q62.7 **Congenital vesico-uretero-renal reflux**

Q62.8 **Other congenital malformations of ureter**
Anomaly of ureter NOS

✓4ᵗʰ **Q63** **Other congenital malformations of kidney**
     EXCLUDES 1   congenital nephrotic syndrome (N04.-)

Q63.0 **Accessory kidney**

Q63.1 **Lobulated, fused and horseshoe kidney**

Q63.2 **Ectopic kidney**
Congenital displaced kidney
Malrotation of kidney

Q63.3 **Hyperplastic and giant kidney**
Compensatory hypertrophy of kidney

Q63.8 **Other specified congenital malformations of kidney**
Congenital renal calculi

Q63.9 **Congenital malformation of kidney, unspecified**

✓4ᵗʰ **Q64** **Other congenital malformations of urinary system**

Q64.0 **Epispadias** ♂
     EXCLUDES 1   hypospadias (Q54.-)

✓5ᵗʰ **Q64.1** **Exstrophy of urinary bladder**

     Q64.10 **Exstrophy of urinary bladder, unspecified**
         Ectopia vesicae

     Q64.11 **Supravesical fissure of urinary bladder**

     Q64.12 **Cloacal extrophy of urinary bladder**

     Q64.19 **Other exstrophy of urinary bladder**
         Extroversion of bladder

Q64.2 **Congenital posterior urethral valves**

✓5ᵗʰ **Q64.3** **Other atresia and stenosis of urethra and bladder neck**

     Q64.31 **Congenital bladder neck obstruction**
         Congenital obstruction of vesicourethral orifice

     Q64.32 **Congenital stricture of urethra**

     Q64.33 **Congenital stricture of urinary meatus**

EXCLUDES 1 Not coded here   *EXCLUDES 2* Not included here   N Newborn Age: 0   P Pediatric Age: 0-17   M Maternity Age: 12-55   A Adult Age: 15-124

Q64.39   **Other atresia and stenosis of urethra and bladder neck**
Atresia and stenosis of urethra and bladder neck NOS

Q64.4   **Malformation of urachus**
Cyst of urachus
Patent urachus
Prolapse of urachus

Q64.5   **Congenital absence of bladder and urethra**

Q64.6   **Congenital diverticulum of bladder**

☑5ᵗʰ **Q64.7**   **Other and unspecified congenital malformations of bladder and urethra**
EXCLUDES 1   *congenital prolapse of bladder (mucosa) (Q79.4)*

    Q64.70   **Unspecified congenital malformation of bladder and urethra**
      Malformation of bladder or urethra NOS

    Q64.71   **Congenital prolapse of urethra**

    Q64.72   **Congenital prolapse of urinary meatus**

    Q64.73   **Congenital urethrorectal fistula**

    Q64.74   **Double urethra**

    Q64.75   **Double urinary meatus**

    Q64.79   **Other congenital malformations of bladder and urethra**

Q64.8   **Other specified congenital malformations of urinary system**

Q64.9   **Congenital malformation of urinary system, unspecified**
Congenital anomaly NOS of urinary system
Congenital deformity NOS of urinary system

Congenital malformations and deformations of the musculoskeletal system (Q65-Q79)

☑4ᵗʰ **Q65**   **Congenital deformities of hip**
EXCLUDES 1   *clicking hip (R29.4)*

☑5ᵗʰ **Q65.0**   **Congenital dislocation of hip, unilateral**

    Q65.00   **Congenital dislocation of unspecified hip, unilateral**

    Q65.01   **Congenital dislocation of right hip, unilateral**

    Q65.02   **Congenital dislocation of left hip, unilateral**

Q65.1   **Congenital dislocation of hip, bilateral**

Q65.2   **Congenital dislocation of hip, unspecified**

☑5ᵗʰ **Q65.3**   **Congenital partial dislocation of hip, unilateral**

    Q65.30   **Congenital partial dislocation of unspecified hip, unilateral**

    Q65.31   **Congenital partial dislocation of right hip, unilateral**

    Q65.32   **Congenital partial dislocation of left hip, unilateral**

Q65.4   **Congenital partial dislocation of hip, bilateral**

Q65.5   **Congenital partial dislocation of hip, unspecified**

Q65.6   **Congenital unstable hip**
Congenital dislocatable hip

☑5ᵗʰ **Q65.8**   **Other congenital deformities of hip**

    Q65.81   **Congenital coxa valga**

    Q65.82   **Congenital coxa vara**

    Q65.89   **Other specified congenital deformities of hip**
      Anteversion of femoral neck
      Congenital acetabular dysplasia

Q65.9   **Congenital deformity of hip, unspecified**

☑4ᵗʰ **Q66**   **Congenital deformities of feet**
EXCLUDES 1   *reduction defects of feet (Q72.-)*
      valgus deformities (acquired) (M21.0-)
      varus deformities (acquired) (M21.1-)

Q66.0   **Congenital talipes equinovarus**

Q66.1   **Congenital talipes calcaneovarus**

Q66.2   **Congenital metatarsus (primus) varus**

Q66.3   **Other congenital varus deformities of feet**
Hallux varus, congenital

Q66.4   **Congenital talipes calcaneovalgus**

☑5ᵗʰ **Q66.5**   **Congenital pes planus**
Congenital flat foot
Congenital rigid flat foot
Congenital spastic (everted) flat foot
EXCLUDES 1   *pes planus, acquired (M21.4)*

    Q66.50   **Congenital pes planus, unspecified foot**

    Q66.51   **Congenital pes planus, right foot**

    Q66.52   **Congenital pes planus, left foot**

Q66.6   **Other congenital valgus deformities of feet**
Congenital metatarsus valgus

Q66.7   **Congenital pes cavus**

☑5ᵗʰ **Q66.8**   Other congenital deformities of feet

    Q66.80   **Congenital vertical talus deformity, unspecified foot**

    Q66.81   **Congenital vertical talus deformity, right foot**

    Q66.82   **Congenital vertical talus deformity, left foot**

    Q66.89   **Other specified congenital deformities of feet**
      Congenital asymmetric talipes
      Congenital clubfoot NOS
      Congenital talipes NOS
      Congenital tarsal coalition
      Hammer toe, congenital

Q66.9   **Congenital deformity of feet, unspecified**

☑4ᵗʰ **Q67**   Other congenital musculoskeletal deformities of **head, face, spine and chest**
EXCLUDES 1   *congenital malformation syndromes classified to Q87-Potter's syndrome (Q60.6)*

Q67.0   **Congenital facial asymmetry**

Q67.1   **Congenital compression facies**

Q67.2   Dolichocephaly

Q67.3   Plagiocephaly

Q67.4   **Other congenital deformities of skull, face and jaw**
Congenital depressions in skull
Congenital hemifacial atrophy or hypertrophy
Deviation of nasal septum, congenital
Squashed or bent nose, congenital
EXCLUDES 1   *dentofacial anomalies [including malocclusion] (M26.-)*
      syphilitic saddle nose (A50.5)

Q67.5   **Congenital deformity of spine**
Congenital postural scoliosis
Congenital scoliosis NOS
EXCLUDES 1   *infantile idiopathic scoliosis (M41.0)*
      scoliosis due to congenital bony malformation (Q76.3)
AHA: 2014, 4Q, 26

Q67.6   Pectus excavatum
Congenital funnel chest

Q67.7   Pectus carinatum
Congenital pigeon chest

Q67.8   **Other congenital deformities of chest**
Congenital deformity of chest wall NOS

☑4ᵗʰ **Q68**   Other **congenital musculoskeletal deformities**
EXCLUDES 1   *reduction defects of limb(s) (Q71-Q73)*
EXCLUDES 2   *congenital myotonic chondrodystrophy (G71.13)*

Q68.0   **Congenital deformity of sternocleidomastoid muscle**
Congenital contracture of sternocleidomastoid (muscle)
Congenital (sternomastoid) torticollis
Sternomastoid tumor (congenital)

Q68.1   **Congenital deformity of finger(s) and hand**
Congenital clubfinger
Spade-like hand (congenital)

Q68.2   **Congenital deformity of knee**
Congenital dislocation of knee
Congenital genu recurvatum

Q68.3   **Congenital bowing of femur**
EXCLUDES 1   *anteversion of femur (neck) (Q65.89)*

Q68.4   **Congenital bowing of tibia and fibula**

Q68.5   **Congenital bowing of long bones of leg, unspecified**

Q68.6   Discoid meniscus

Q68.8   **Other specified congenital musculoskeletal deformities**
Congenital deformity of clavicle
Congenital deformity of elbow
Congenital deformity of forearm
Congenital deformity of scapula
Congenital deformity of wrist
Congenital dislocation of elbow
Congenital dislocation of shoulder
Congenital dislocation of wrist

☑4ᵗʰ **Q69**   Polydactyly

Q69.0   **Accessory finger(s)**

Q69.1   **Accessory thumb(s)**

Q69.2   **Accessory toe(s)**
Accessory hallux

Q69.9   **Polydactyly, unspecified**
Supernumerary digit(s) NOS

☑4ᵗʰ **Q70**   Syndactyly

☑5ᵗʰ **Q70.0**   Fused fingers
Complex syndactyly of fingers with synostosis

    Q70.00   **Fused fingers, unspecified hand**

☑ Additional Character Required   ☑xᵗʰ Placeholder Alert   Unspecified Dx   Other Specified Dx   Manifestation   ▶◀ Revised Text   ● New Code   ▲ Revised Code Title

Q70.01 **Fused fingers, right hand**
Q70.02 **Fused fingers, left hand**
Q70.03 **Fused fingers, bilateral**

✓5th **Q70.1** Webbed fingers
Simple syndactyly of fingers without synostosis
Q70.10 **Webbed fingers, unspecified hand**
Q70.11 **Webbed fingers, right hand**
Q70.12 **Webbed fingers, left hand**
Q70.13 **Webbed fingers, bilateral**

✓5th **Q70.2** Fused toes
Complex syndactyly of toes with synostosis
Q70.20 **Fused toes, unspecified foot**
Q70.21 **Fused toes, right foot**
Q70.22 **Fused toes, left foot**
Q70.23 **Fused toes, bilateral**

✓5th **Q70.3** Webbed toes
Simple syndactyly of toes without synostosis
Q70.30 **Webbed toes, unspecified foot**
Q70.31 **Webbed toes, right foot**
Q70.32 **Webbed toes, left foot**
Q70.33 **Webbed toes, bilateral**

Q70.4 Polysyndactyly, unspecified
EXCLUDES 1 specified syndactyly of hand and feet—code to specified conditions (Q70.0-Q70.3-)

Q70.9 Syndactyly, unspecified
Symphalangy NOS

✓4th **Q71 Reduction defects of upper limb**

✓5th **Q71.0** Congenital complete absence of upper limb
Q71.00 **Congenital complete absence of unspecified upper limb**
Q71.01 **Congenital complete absence of right upper limb**
Q71.02 **Congenital complete absence of left upper limb**
Q71.03 **Congenital complete absence of upper limb, bilateral**

✓5th **Q71.1** Congenital absence of upper arm and forearm with hand present
Q71.10 **Congenital absence of unspecified upper arm and forearm with hand present**
Q71.11 **Congenital absence of right upper arm and forearm with hand present**
Q71.12 **Congenital absence of left upper arm and forearm with hand present**
Q71.13 **Congenital absence of upper arm and forearm with hand present, bilateral**

✓5th **Q71.2** Congenital absence of both forearm and hand
Q71.20 **Congenital absence of both forearm and hand, unspecified upper limb**
Q71.21 **Congenital absence of both forearm and hand, right upper limb**
Q71.22 **Congenital absence of both forearm and hand, left upper limb**
Q71.23 **Congenital absence of both forearm and hand, bilateral**

✓5th **Q71.3** Congenital absence of hand and finger
Q71.30 **Congenital absence of unspecified hand and finger**
Q71.31 **Congenital absence of right hand and finger**
Q71.32 **Congenital absence of left hand and finger**
Q71.33 **Congenital absence of hand and finger, bilateral**

✓5th **Q71.4** Longitudinal reduction defect of radius
Clubhand (congenital)
Radial clubhand
Q71.40 **Longitudinal reduction defect of unspecified radius**
Q71.41 **Longitudinal reduction defect of right radius**
Q71.42 **Longitudinal reduction defect of left radius**
Q71.43 **Longitudinal reduction defect of radius, bilateral**

✓5th **Q71.5** Longitudinal reduction defect of ulna
Q71.50 **Longitudinal reduction defect of unspecified ulna**
Q71.51 **Longitudinal reduction defect of right ulna**
Q71.52 **Longitudinal reduction defect of left ulna**
Q71.53 **Longitudinal reduction defect of ulna, bilateral**

✓5th **Q71.6** Lobster-claw hand
Q71.60 **Lobster-claw hand, unspecified hand**

Q71.61 **Lobster-claw right hand**
Q71.62 **Lobster-claw left hand**
Q71.63 **Lobster-claw hand, bilateral**

✓5th **Q71.8** Other reduction defects of upper limb
✓6th **Q71.81** Congenital shortening of upper limb
Q71.811 **Congenital shortening of right upper limb**
Q71.812 **Congenital shortening of left upper limb**
Q71.813 **Congenital shortening of upper limb, bilateral**
Q71.819 **Congenital shortening of unspecified upper limb**

✓6th **Q71.89** Other reduction defects of upper limb
Q71.891 **Other reduction defects of right upper limb**
Q71.892 **Other reduction defects of left upper limb**
Q71.893 **Other reduction defects of upper limb, bilateral**
Q71.899 **Other reduction defects of unspecified upper limb**

✓5th **Q71.9** Unspecified reduction defect of upper limb
Q71.90 **Unspecified reduction defect of unspecified upper limb**
Q71.91 **Unspecified reduction defect of right upper limb**
Q71.92 **Unspecified reduction defect of left upper limb**
Q71.93 **Unspecified reduction defect of upper limb, bilateral**

✓4th **Q72 Reduction defects of lower limb**

✓5th **Q72.0** Congenital complete absence of lower limb
Q72.00 **Congenital complete absence of unspecified lower limb**
Q72.01 **Congenital complete absence of right lower limb**
Q72.02 **Congenital complete absence of left lower limb**
Q72.03 **Congenital complete absence of lower limb, bilateral**

✓5th **Q72.1** Congenital absence of thigh and lower leg with foot present
Q72.10 **Congenital absence of unspecified thigh and lower leg with foot present**
Q72.11 **Congenital absence of right thigh and lower leg with foot present**
Q72.12 **Congenital absence of left thigh and lower leg with foot present**
Q72.13 **Congenital absence of thigh and lower leg with foot present, bilateral**

✓5th **Q72.2** Congenital absence of both lower leg and foot
Q72.20 **Congenital absence of both lower leg and foot, unspecified lower limb**
Q72.21 **Congenital absence of both lower leg and foot, right lower limb**
Q72.22 **Congenital absence of both lower leg and foot, left lower limb**
Q72.23 **Congenital absence of both lower leg and foot, bilateral**

✓5th **Q72.3** Congenital absence of foot and toe(s)
Q72.30 **Congenital absence of unspecified foot and toe(s)**
Q72.31 **Congenital absence of right foot and toe(s)**
Q72.32 **Congenital absence of left foot and toe(s)**
Q72.33 **Congenital absence of foot and toe(s), bilateral**

✓5th **Q72.4** Longitudinal reduction defect of femur
Proximal femoral focal deficiency
Q72.40 **Longitudinal reduction defect of unspecified femur**
Q72.41 **Longitudinal reduction defect of right femur**
Q72.42 **Longitudinal reduction defect of left femur**
Q72.43 **Longitudinal reduction defect of femur, bilateral**

✓5th **Q72.5** Longitudinal reduction defect of tibia
Q72.50 **Longitudinal reduction defect of unspecified tibia**
Q72.51 **Longitudinal reduction defect of right tibia**
Q72.52 **Longitudinal reduction defect of left tibia**
Q72.53 **Longitudinal reduction defect of tibia, bilateral**

✓5th **Q72.6** Longitudinal reduction defect of fibula
Q72.60 **Longitudinal reduction defect of unspecified fibula**
Q72.61 **Longitudinal reduction defect of right fibula**
Q72.62 **Longitudinal reduction defect of left fibula**
Q72.63 **Longitudinal reduction defect of fibula, bilateral**

EXCLUDES 1 Not coded here   EXCLUDES 2 Not included here   N Newborn Age: 0   P Pediatric Age: 0-17   M Maternity Age: 12-55   A Adult Age: 15-124

816   ICD-10-CM 2016

☑5ᵗʰ **Q72.7** Split foot
- **Q72.70** Split foot, unspecified lower limb
- **Q72.71** Split foot, right lower limb
- **Q72.72** Split foot, left lower limb
- **Q72.73** Split foot, bilateral

☑5ᵗʰ **Q72.8** Other reduction defects of lower limb
- ☑6ᵗʰ **Q72.81** Congenital shortening of lower limb
  - **Q72.811** Congenital shortening of right lower limb
  - **Q72.812** Congenital shortening of left lower limb
  - **Q72.813** Congenital shortening of lower limb, bilateral
  - **Q72.819** Congenital shortening of unspecified lower limb
- ☑6ᵗʰ **Q72.89** Other reduction defects of lower limb
  - **Q72.891** Other reduction defects of right lower limb
  - **Q72.892** Other reduction defects of left lower limb
  - **Q72.893** Other reduction defects of lower limb, bilateral
  - **Q72.899** Other reduction defects of unspecified lower limb

☑5ᵗʰ **Q72.9** Unspecified reduction defect of lower limb
- **Q72.90** Unspecified reduction defect of unspecified lower limb
- **Q72.91** Unspecified reduction defect of right lower limb
- **Q72.92** Unspecified reduction defect of left lower limb
- **Q72.93** Unspecified reduction defect of lower limb, bilateral

☑4ᵗʰ **Q73** Reduction defects of unspecified limb
- **Q73.0** Congenital absence of unspecified limb(s)
  - Amelia NOS
- **Q73.1** Phocomelia, unspecified limb(s)
  - Phocomelia NOS
- **Q73.8** Other reduction defects of unspecified limb(s)
  - Longitudinal reduction deformity of unspecified limb(s)
  - Ectromelia of limb NOS
  - Hemimelia of limb NOS
  - Reduction defect of limb NOS

☑4ᵗʰ **Q74** Other congenital malformations of limb(s)
- EXCLUDES 1   polydactyly (Q69.-)
  - reduction defect of limb (Q71-Q73)
  - syndactyly (Q70.-)
- **Q74.0** Other congenital malformations of upper limb(s), including shoulder girdle
  - Accessory carpal bones
  - Cleidocranial dysostosis
  - Congenital pseudarthrosis of clavicle
  - Macrodactylia (fingers)
  - Madelung's deformity
  - Radioulnar synostosis
  - Sprengel's deformity
  - Triphalangeal thumb
- **Q74.1** Congenital malformation of knee
  - Congenital absence of patella
  - Congenital dislocation of patella
  - Congenital genu valgum
  - Congenital genu varum
  - Rudimentary patella
  - EXCLUDES 1   congenital dislocation of knee (Q68.2)
    - congenital genu recurvatum (Q68.2)
    - nail patella syndrome (Q87.2)
- **Q74.2** Other congenital malformations of lower limb(s), including pelvic girdle
  - Congenital fusion of sacroiliac joint
  - Congenital malformation of ankle joint
  - Congenital malformation of sacroiliac joint
  - EXCLUDES 1   anteversion of femur (neck) (Q65.89)
- **Q74.3** Arthrogryposis multiplex congenita
- **Q74.8** Other specified congenital malformations of limb(s)
- **Q74.9** Unspecified congenital malformation of limb(s)
  - Congenital anomaly of limb(s) NOS

☑4ᵗʰ **Q75** Other congenital malformations of skull and face bones
- EXCLUDES 1   congenital malformation of face NOS (Q18.-)
  - congenital malformation syndromes classified to Q87.-
  - dentofacial anomalies [including malocclusion] (M26.-)
  - musculoskeletal deformities of head and face (Q67.0-Q67.4)
  - skull defects associated with congenital anomalies of brain such as:
    - anencephaly (Q00.0)
    - encephalocele (Q01.-)
    - hydrocephalus (Q03.-)
    - microcephaly (Q02)
- **Q75.0** Craniosynostosis
  - Acrocephaly
  - Imperfect fusion of skull
  - Oxycephaly
  - Trigonocephaly
- **Q75.1** Craniofacial dysostosis
  - Crouzon's disease
- **Q75.2** Hypertelorism
- **Q75.3** Macrocephaly
- **Q75.4** Mandibulofacial dysostosis
  - Franceschetti syndrome
  - Treacher Collins syndrome
- **Q75.5** Oculomandibular dysostosis
- **Q75.8** Other specified congenital malformations of skull and face bones
  - Absence of skull bone, congenital
  - Congenital deformity of forehead
  - Platybasia
- **Q75.9** Congenital malformation of skull and face bones, unspecified
  - Congenital anomaly of face bones NOS
  - Congenital anomaly of skull NOS

☑4ᵗʰ **Q76** Congenital malformations of spine and bony thorax
- EXCLUDES 1   congenital musculoskeletal deformities of spine and chest (Q67.5-Q67.8)
- **Q76.0** Spina bifida occulta
  - EXCLUDES 1   meningocele (spinal) (Q05.-)
    - spina bifida (aperta) (cystica) (Q05.-)
- **Q76.1** Klippel-Feil syndrome
  - Cervical fusion syndrome
- **Q76.2** Congenital spondylolisthesis
  - Congenital spondylolysis
  - EXCLUDES 1   spondylolisthesis (acquired) (M43.1-)
    - spondylolysis (acquired) (M43.0-)
- **Q76.3** Congenital scoliosis due to congenital bony malformation
  - Hemivertebra fusion or failure of segmentation with scoliosis
- ☑5ᵗʰ **Q76.4** Other congenital malformations of spine, not associated with scoliosis
  - ☑6ᵗʰ **Q76.41** Congenital kyphosis
    - **Q76.411** Congenital kyphosis, occipito-atlanto-axial region
    - **Q76.412** Congenital kyphosis, cervical region
    - **Q76.413** Congenital kyphosis, cervicothoracic region
    - **Q76.414** Congenital kyphosis, thoracic region
    - **Q76.415** Congenital kyphosis, thoracolumbar region
    - **Q76.419** Congenital kyphosis, unspecified region
  - ☑6ᵗʰ **Q76.42** Congenital lordosis
    - **Q76.425** Congenital lordosis, thoracolumbar region
    - **Q76.426** Congenital lordosis, lumbar region
    - **Q76.427** Congenital lordosis, lumbosacral region
    - **Q76.428** Congenital lordosis, sacral and sacrococcygeal region
    - **Q76.429** Congenital lordosis, unspecified region
  - **Q76.49** Other congenital malformations of spine, not associated with scoliosis
    - Congenital absence of vertebra NOS
    - Congenital fusion of spine NOS
    - Congenital malformation of lumbosacral (joint) (region) NOS
    - Congenital malformation of spine NOS
    - Hemivertebra NOS
    - Malformation of spine NOS
    - Platyspondylisis NOS
    - Supernumerary vertebra NOS
- **Q76.5** Cervical rib
  - Supernumerary rib in cervical region

☑ Additional Character Required   ☑x7ᵗʰ Placeholder Alert   Unspecified Dx   Other Specified Dx   Manifestation   ▶◀ Revised Text   ● New Code   ▲ Revised Code Title

CD-10-CM 2016   817

Q76.6 **Other congenital malformations of ribs**
Accessory rib
Congenital absence of rib
Congenital fusion of ribs
Congenital malformation of ribs NOS
EXCLUDES 1 short rib syndrome (Q77.2)

Q76.7 **Congenital malformation of sternum**
Congenital absence of sternum
Sternum bifidum

Q76.8 **Other congenital malformations of bony thorax**

Q76.9 **Congenital malformation of bony thorax, unspecified**

✓4ᵗʰ **Q77** **Osteochondrodysplasia with defects of growth of tubular bones and spine**
EXCLUDES 1 mucopolysaccharidosis (E76.0-E76.3)
EXCLUDES 2 congenital myotonic chondrodystrophy (G71.13)

Q77.0 **Achondrogenesis**
Hypochondrogenesis

Q77.1 **Thanatophoric short stature**

Q77.2 **Short rib syndrome**
Asphyxiating thoracic dysplasia [Jeune]

Q77.3 **Chondrodysplasia punctata**
EXCLUDES 1 Rhizomelic chondrodysplasia punctata (E71.43)

Q77.4 **Achondroplasia**
Hypochondroplasia
Osteosclerosis congenita

Q77.5 **Diastrophic dysplasia**

Q77.6 **Chondroectodermal dysplasia**
Ellis-van Creveld syndrome

Q77.7 **Spondyloepiphyseal dysplasia**

Q77.8 **Other osteochondrodysplasia with defects of growth of tubular bones and spine**

Q77.9 **Osteochondrodysplasia with defects of growth of tubular bones and spine, unspecified**

✓4ᵗʰ **Q78** **Other osteochondrodysplasias**
EXCLUDES 2 congenital myotonic chondrodystrophy (G71.13)

Q78.0 **Osteogenesis imperfecta**
Fragilitas ossium
Osteopsathyrosis

Q78.1 **Polyostotic fibrous dysplasia**
Albright(-McCune)(-Sternberg) syndrome

Q78.2 **Osteopetrosis**
Albers-Schönberg syndrome
Osteosclerosis NOS

Q78.3 **Progressive diaphyseal dysplasia**
Camurati-Engelmann syndrome

Q78.4 **Enchondromatosis**
Maffucci's syndrome
Ollier's disease

Q78.5 **Metaphyseal dysplasia**
Pyle's syndrome

Q78.6 **Multiple congenital exostoses**
Diaphyseal aclasis

Q78.8 **Other specified osteochondrodysplasias**
Osteopoikilosis

Q78.9 **Osteochondrodysplasia, unspecified**
Chondrodystrophy NOS
Osteodystrophy NOS

✓4ᵗʰ **Q79** **Congenital malformations of musculoskeletal system, not elsewhere classified**
EXCLUDES 2 congenital (sternomastoid) torticollis (Q68.0)

Q79.0 **Congenital diaphragmatic hernia**
EXCLUDES 1 congenital hiatus hernia (Q40.1)

Q79.1 **Other congenital malformations of diaphragm**
Absence of diaphragm
Congenital malformation of diaphragm NOS
Eventration of diaphragm

Q79.2 **Exomphalos**
Omphalocele
EXCLUDES 1 umbilical hernia (K42.-)

Q79.3 **Gastroschisis**

Q79.4 **Prune belly syndrome**
Congenital prolapse of bladder mucosa
Eagle-Barrett syndrome

✓5ᵗʰ **Q79.5** **Other congenital malformations of abdominal wall**
EXCLUDES 1 umbilical hernia (K42.-)

Q79.51 **Congenital hernia of bladder**

Q79.59 **Other congenital malformations of abdominal wall**

Q79.6 **Ehlers-Danlos syndrome**

Q79.8 **Other congenital malformations of musculoskeletal system**
Absence of muscle
Absence of tendon
Accessory muscle
Amyotrophia congenita
Congenital constricting bands
Congenital shortening of tendon
Poland syndrome

Q79.9 **Congenital malformation of musculoskeletal system, unspecified**
Congenital anomaly of musculoskeletal system NOS
Congenital deformity of musculoskeletal system NOS

Other congenital malformations (Q80-Q89)

✓4ᵗʰ **Q80** **Congenital ichthyosis**
EXCLUDES 1 Refsum's disease (G60.1)

Q80.0 **Ichthyosis vulgaris**

Q80.1 **X-linked ichthyosis**

Q80.2 **Lamellar ichthyosis**
Collodion baby

Q80.3 **Congenital bullous ichthyosiform erythroderma**

Q80.4 **Harlequin fetus**

Q80.8 **Other congenital ichthyosis**

Q80.9 **Congenital ichthyosis, unspecified**

✓4ᵗʰ **Q81** **Epidermolysis bullosa**

Q81.0 **Epidermolysis bullosa simplex**
EXCLUDES 1 Cockayne's syndrome (Q87.1)

Q81.1 **Epidermolysis bullosa letalis**
Herlitz' syndrome

Q81.2 **Epidermolysis bullosa dystrophica**

Q81.8 **Other epidermolysis bullosa**

Q81.9 **Epidermolysis bullosa, unspecified**

✓4ᵗʰ **Q82** **Other congenital malformations of skin**
EXCLUDES 1 acrodermatitis enteropathica (E83.2)
congenital erythropoietic porphyria (E80.0)
pilonidal cyst or sinus (L05.-)
Sturge-Weber (-Dimitri) syndrome (Q85.8)

Q82.0 **Hereditary lymphedema**

Q82.1 **Xeroderma pigmentosum**

Q82.2 **Mastocytosis**
Urticaria pigmentosa
EXCLUDES 1 malignant mastocytosis (C96.2)

Q82.3 **Incontinentia pigmenti**

Q82.4 **Ectodermal dysplasia (anhidrotic)**
EXCLUDES 1 Ellis-van Creveld syndrome (Q77.6)

Q82.5 **Congenital non-neoplastic nevus**
Birthmark NOS   Strawberry Nevus
Flammeus Nevus   Vascular Nevus NOS
Portwine Nevus   Verrucous Nevus
Sanguineous Nevus
EXCLUDES 2 araneus nevus (I78.1)
café au lait spots (L81.3)
lentigo (L81.4)
melanocytic nevus (D22.-)
nevus NOS (D22.-)
pigmented nevus (D22.-)
spider nevus (I78.1)
stellar nevus (I78.1)

Q82.8 **Other specified congenital malformations of skin**
Abnormal palmar creases
Accessory skin tags
Benign familial pemphigus [Hailey-Hailey]
Congenital poikiloderma
Cutis laxa (hyperelastica)
Dermatoglyphic anomalies
Inherited keratosis palmaris et plantaris
Keratosis follicularis [Darier-White]
EXCLUDES 1 Ehlers-Danlos syndrome (Q79.6)

Q82.9 **Congenital malformation of skin, unspecified**

✓4ᵗʰ **Q83** **Congenital malformations of breast**
EXCLUDES 2 absence of pectoral muscle (Q79.8)
hypoplasia of breast (N64.82)
micromastia (N64.82)

Q83.0 **Congenital absence of breast with absent nipple**

EXCLUDES 1 Not coded here   *EXCLUDES 2* Not included here   N Newborn Age: 0   P Pediatric Age: 0-17   M Maternity Age: 12-55   A Adult Age: 15-124

Q83.1   Accessory breast
Supernumerary breast

Q83.2   Absent nipple

Q83.3   Accessory nipple
Supernumerary nipple

Q83.8   Other congenital malformations of breast

Q83.9   Congenital malformation of breast, unspecified

✔4ᵗʰ **Q84**   **Other congenital malformations of integument**

Q84.0   Congenital alopecia
Congenital atrichosis

Q84.1   Congenital morphological disturbances of hair, not
elsewhere classified
Beaded hair   Pili annulati
Monilethrix
EXCLUDES 1   *Menkes' kinky hair syndrome (E83.0)*

Q84.2   Other congenital malformations of hair
Congenital hypertrichosis
Congenital malformation of hair NOS
Persistent lanugo

Q84.3   Anonychia
EXCLUDES 1   *nail patella syndrome (Q87.2)*

Q84.4   Congenital leukonychia

Q84.5   Enlarged and hypertrophic nails
Congenital onychauxis   Pachyonychia

Q84.6   Other congenital malformations of nails
Congenital clubnail
Congenital koilonychia
Congenital malformation of nail NOS

Q84.8   Other specified congenital malformations of integument
Aplasia cutis congenita

Q84.9   Congenital malformation of integument, unspecified
Congenital anomaly of integument NOS
Congenital deformity of integument NOS

✔4ᵗʰ **Q85**   **Phakomatoses, not elsewhere classified**
EXCLUDES 1   *ataxia telangiectasia [Louis-Bar] (G11.3)*
familial dysautonomia [Riley-Day] (G90.1)

✔5ᵗʰ **Q85.0**   Neurofibromatosis (nonmalignant)

Q85.00   **Neurofibromatosis, unspecified**

Q85.01   **Neurofibromatosis, type 1**
Von Recklinghausen disease

Q85.02   **Neurofibromatosis, type 2**
Acoustic neurofibromatosis

Q85.03   **Schwannomatosis**

Q85.09   **Other neurofibromatosis**

Q85.1   Tuberous sclerosis
Bourneville's disease
Epiloia

Q85.8   Other phakomatoses, not elsewhere classified
Peutz-Jeghers Syndrome
Sturge-Weber(-Dimitri) syndrome
von Hippel-Lindau syndrome
EXCLUDES 1   *Meckel-Gruber syndrome (Q61.9)*

Q85.9   Phakomatosis, unspecified
Hamartosis NOS

✔4ᵗʰ **Q86**   **Congenital malformation syndromes due to known exogenous
causes, not elsewhere classified**
EXCLUDES 2   *iodine-deficiency-related hypothyroidism (E00-E02)*
*nonteratogenic effects of substances transmitted via placenta
or breast milk (P04.-)*

Q86.0   Fetal alcohol syndrome (dysmorphic)

Q86.1   Fetal hydantoin syndrome   N
Meadow's syndrome

Q86.2   Dysmorphism due to warfarin

Q86.8   Other congenital malformation syndromes due to known
exogenous causes

✔4ᵗʰ **Q87**   **Other specified congenital malformation syndromes affecting
multiple systems**
Use additional code(s) to identify all associated manifestations

Q87.0   Congenital malformation syndromes predominantly
affecting facial appearance
Acrocephalopolysyndactyly   Robin syndrome
Acrocephalosyndactyly [Apert]   Whistling face
Cryptophthalmos syndrome
Cyclopia
Goldenhar syndrome
Moebius syndrome
Oro-facial-digital syndrome

Q87.1   Congenital malformation syndromes predominantly
associated with short stature
Aarskog syndrome   Robinow-Silverman-Smith
Cockayne syndrome   syndrome
De Lange syndrome   Russell-Silver syndrome
Dubowitz syndrome   Seckel syndrome
Noonan syndrome
Prader-Willi syndrome
EXCLUDES 1   *Ellis-van Creveld syndrome (Q77.6)*
Smith-Lemli-Opitz syndrome (E78.72)

Q87.2   Congenital malformation syndromes predominantly
involving limbs
Holt-Oram syndrome
Klippel-Trenaunay-Weber syndrome
Nail patella syndrome
Rubinstein-Taybi syndrome
Sirenomelia syndrome
Thrombocytopenia with absent radius [TAR] syndrome
VATER syndrome

Q87.3   Congenital malformation syndromes involving early
overgrowth
Beckwith-Wiedemann syndrome   Weaver syndrome
Sotos syndrome

✔5ᵗʰ **Q87.4**   Marfan's syndrome

Q87.40   **Marfan's syndrome, unspecified**

✔6ᵗʰ **Q87.41**   **Marfan's syndrome with cardiovascular
manifestations**

Q87.410   **Marfan's syndrome with aortic dilation**

Q87.418   **Marfan's syndrome with other
cardiovascular manifestations**

Q87.42   **Marfan's syndrome with ocular manifestations**

Q87.43   **Marfan's syndrome with skeletal manifestation**

Q87.5   Other congenital malformation syndromes with other
skeletal changes

✔5ᵗʰ **Q87.8**   Other specified congenital malformation syndromes, not
elsewhere classified
EXCLUDES 1   *Zellweger syndrome (E71.510)*

Q87.81   Alport syndrome
Use additional code to identify stage of chronic kidney
disease (N18.1-N18.6)

Q87.89   Other specified congenital malformation
syndromes, not elsewhere classified
Laurence-Moon (-Bardet)-Biedl syndrome

✔4ᵗʰ **Q89**   **Other congenital malformations, not elsewhere classified**

✔5ᵗʰ **Q89.0**   Congenital absence and malformations of spleen
EXCLUDES 1   *isomerism of atrial appendages (with asplenia or
polysplenia) (Q20.6)*

Q89.01   Asplenia (congenital)

Q89.09   Congenital malformations of spleen
Congenital splenomegaly

Q89.1   Congenital malformations of adrenal gland
EXCLUDES 1   *adrenogenital disorders (E25.-)*
congenital adrenal hyperplasia (E25.0)

Q89.2   Congenital malformations of other endocrine glands
Congenital malformation of parathyroid or thyroid gland
Persistent thyroglossal duct
Thyroglossal cyst
EXCLUDES 1   *congenital goiter (E03.0)*
congenital hypothyroidism (E03.1)

Q89.3   Situs inversus
Dextrocardia with situs inversus
Mirror-image atrial arrangement with situs inversus
Situs inversus or transversus abdominalis
Situs inversus or transversus thoracis
Transposition of abdominal viscera
Transposition of thoracic viscera
EXCLUDES 1   *dextrocardia NOS (Q24.0)*

Q89.4   Conjoined twins
Craniopagus   Pygopagus
Dicephaly   Thoracopagus

Q89.7   Multiple congenital malformations, not elsewhere classified
Multiple congenital anomalies NOS
Multiple congenital deformities NOS
EXCLUDES 1   *congenital malformation syndromes affecting multiple
systems (Q87.-)*

Q89.8   Other specified congenital malformations
Use additional code(s) to identify all associated manifestations

Q89.9   Congenital malformation, unspecified
Congenital anomaly NOS   Congenital deformity NOS

✔ Additional Character Required   ✔x7ᵗʰ Placeholder Alert   Unspecified Dx   Other Specified Dx   Manifestation   ►◄ Revised Text   ● New Code   ▲ Revised Code Title

Chapter 17. Congenital Malformations, Deformations, and Chromosomal Abnormalities

Q90–Q99.9

Chromosomal abnormalities, not elsewhere classified (Q90-Q99)

EXCLUDES 2   *mitochondrial metabolic disorders (E88.4-)*

✓4ᵗʰ **Q90 Down syndrome**
    Use additional code(s) to identify any associated physical conditions and degree of intellectual disabilities (F70-F79)

Q90.0 Trisomy 21, nonmosaicism (meiotic nondisjunction)

Q90.1 Trisomy 21, mosaicism (mitotic nondisjunction)

Q90.2 Trisomy 21, translocation

Q90.9 Down syndrome, unspecified
    Trisomy 21 NOS

✓4ᵗʰ **Q91 Trisomy 18 and Trisomy 13**

Q91.0 Trisomy 18, nonmosaicism (meiotic nondisjunction)

Q91.1 Trisomy 18, mosaicism (mitotic nondisjunction)

Q91.2 Trisomy 18, translocation

Q91.3 Trisomy 18, unspecified

Q91.4 Trisomy 13, nonmosaicism (meiotic nondisjunction)

Q91.5 Trisomy 13, mosaicism (mitotic nondisjunction)

Q91.6 Trisomy 13, translocation

Q91.7 Trisomy 13, unspecified

✓4ᵗʰ **Q92 Other trisomies and partial trisomies of the autosomes, not elsewhere classified**
    INCLUDES   unbalanced translocations and insertions
    EXCLUDES 1   *trisomies of chromosomes 13, 18, 21 (Q90-Q91)*

Q92.0 Whole chromosome trisomy, nonmosaicism (meiotic nondisjunction)

Q92.1 Whole chromosome trisomy, mosaicism (mitotic nondisjunction)

Q92.2 Partial trisomy
    Less than whole arm duplicated
    Whole arm or more duplicated
    EXCLUDES 1   *partial trisomy due to unbalanced translocation (Q92.5)*

Q92.5 Duplications with other complex rearrangements
    Partial trisomy due to unbalanced translocations
    Code also any associated deletions due to unbalanced translocations, inversions and insertions (Q93.7)

✓5ᵗʰ **Q92.6 Marker chromosomes**
    Trisomies due to dicentrics
    Trisomies due to extra rings
    Trisomies due to isochromosomes
    Individual with marker heterochromatin

    Q92.61 Marker chromosomes in normal individual

    Q92.62 Marker chromosomes in abnormal individual

Q92.7 Triploidy and polyploidy

Q92.8 Other specified trisomies and partial trisomies of autosomes
    Duplications identified by fluorescence in situ hybridization (FISH)
    Duplications identified by in situ hybridization (ISH)
    Duplications seen only at prometaphase

Q92.9 Trisomy and partial trisomy of autosomes, unspecified

✓4ᵗʰ **Q93 Monosomies and deletions from the autosomes, not elsewhere classified**

Q93.0 Whole chromosome monosomy, nonmosaicism (meiotic nondisjunction)

Q93.1 Whole chromosome monosomy, mosaicism (mitotic nondisjunction)

Q93.2 Chromosome replaced with ring, dicentric or isochromosome

Q93.3 Deletion of short arm of chromosome 4
    Wolff-Hirschorn syndrome

Q93.4 Deletion of short arm of chromosome 5
    Cri-du-chat syndrome

Q93.5 Other deletions of part of a chromosome
    Angelman syndrome

Q93.7 Deletions with other complex rearrangements
    Deletions due to unbalanced translocations, inversions and insertions
    Code also any associated duplications due to unbalanced translocations, inversions and insertions (Q92.5)

✓5ᵗʰ **Q93.8 Other deletions from the autosomes**

    Q93.81 Velo-cardio-facial syndrome
        Deletion 22q11.2

    Q93.88 Other microdeletions
        Miller-Dieker syndrome
        Smith-Magenis syndrome

    Q93.89 Other deletions from the autosomes
        Deletions identified by fluorescence in situ hybridization (FISH)
        Deletions identified by in situ hybridization (ISH)
        Deletions seen only at prometaphase

Q93.9 Deletion from autosomes, unspecified

✓4ᵗʰ **Q95 Balanced rearrangements and structural markers, not elsewhere classified**
    INCLUDES   Robertsonian and balanced reciprocal translocations and insertions

Q95.0 Balanced translocation and insertion in normal individual

Q95.1 Chromosome inversion in normal individual

Q95.2 Balanced autosomal rearrangement in abnormal individual

Q95.3 Balanced sex/autosomal rearrangement in abnormal individual

Q95.5 Individual with autosomal fragile site

Q95.8 Other balanced rearrangements and structural markers

Q95.9 Balanced rearrangement and structural marker, unspecified

✓4ᵗʰ **Q96 Turner's syndrome**
    EXCLUDES 1   *Noonan syndrome (Q87.1)*

Q96.0 Karyotype 45, X   ♀

Q96.1 Karyotype 46, X iso (Xq)   ♀
    Karyotype 46, isochromosome Xq

Q96.2 Karyotype 46, X with abnormal sex chromosome, except iso (Xq)   ♀
    Karyotype 46, X with abnormal sex chromosome, except isochromosome Xq

Q96.3 Mosaicism, 45, X/46, XX or XY   ♀

Q96.4 Mosaicism, 45, X/other cell line(s) with abnormal sex chromosome   ♀

Q96.8 Other variants of Turner's syndrome   ♀

Q96.9 Turner's syndrome, unspecified   ♀

✓4ᵗʰ **Q97 Other sex chromosome abnormalities, female phenotype, not elsewhere classified**
    EXCLUDES 1   *Turner's syndrome (Q96.-)*

Q97.0 Karyotype 47, XXX   ♀

Q97.1 Female with more than three X chromosomes   ♀

Q97.2 Mosaicism, lines with various numbers of X chromosomes   ♀

Q97.3 Female with 46, XY karyotype   ♀

Q97.8 Other specified sex chromosome abnormalities, female phenotype   ♀

Q97.9 Sex chromosome abnormality, female phenotype, unspecified   ♀

✓4ᵗʰ **Q98 Other sex chromosome abnormalities, male phenotype, not elsewhere classified**

Q98.0 Klinefelter syndrome karyotype 47, XXY   ♂

Q98.1 Klinefelter syndrome, male with more than two X chromosomes   ♂

Q98.3 Other male with 46, XX karyotype   ♂

Q98.4 Klinefelter syndrome, unspecified   ♂

Q98.5 Karyotype 47, XYY   ♂

Q98.6 Male with structurally abnormal sex chromosome   ♂

Q98.7 Male with sex chromosome mosaicism   ♂

Q98.8 Other specified sex chromosome abnormalities, male phenotype   ♂

Q98.9 Sex chromosome abnormality, male phenotype, unspecified   ♂

✓4ᵗʰ **Q99 Other chromosome abnormalities, not elsewhere classified**

Q99.0 Chimera 46, XX/46, XY
    Chimera 46, XX/46, XY true hermaphrodite

Q99.1 46, XX true hermaphrodite
    46, XX with streak gonads   Pure gonadal dysgenesis
    46, XY with streak gonads

Q99.2 Fragile X chromosome
    Fragile X syndrome

Q99.8 Other specified chromosome abnormalities

Q99.9 Chromosomal abnormality, unspecified

EXCLUDES 1 Not coded here   EXCLUDES 2 Not included here   N Newborn Age: 0   P Pediatric Age: 0-17   M Maternity Age: 12-55   A Adult Age: 15-124

Chapter 18. Symptoms, Signs, and Abnormal Clinical and Laboratory Findings, Not Elsewhere Classified (R00–R99)

Chapter Specific Guidelines with Coding Examples

The chapter specific guidelines from the ICD-10-CM Official Guidelines for Coding and Reporting have been provided below. Along with these guidelines are coding examples, contained in the shaded boxes, that have been developed to help illustrate the coding and/or sequencing guidance found in these guidelines.

Chapter 18 includes symptoms, signs, abnormal results of clinical or other investigative procedures, and ill-defined conditions regarding which no diagnosis classifiable elsewhere is recorded. Signs and symptoms that point to a specific diagnosis have been assigned to a category in other chapters of the classification.

a. Use of symptom codes

Codes that describe symptoms and signs are acceptable for reporting purposes when a related definitive diagnosis has not been established (confirmed) by the provider.

> Chest pain of unknown origin
>
> **R07.9   Chest pain, unspecified**
>
> *Explanation:* Codes that describe symptoms such as chest pain are acceptable for reporting purposes when the provider has not established (confirmed) a related definitive diagnosis.

b. Use of a symptom code with a definitive diagnosis code

Codes for signs and symptoms may be reported in addition to a related definitive diagnosis when the sign or symptom is not routinely associated with that diagnosis, such as the various signs and symptoms associated with complex syndromes. The definitive diagnosis code should be sequenced before the symptom code.

Signs or symptoms that are associated routinely with a disease process should not be assigned as additional codes, unless otherwise instructed by the classification.

> Pneumonia with hemoptysis
>
> **J18.9   Pneumonia, unspecified organism**
>
> **R04.2   Hemoptysis**
>
> *Explanation:* Codes for signs and symptoms may be reported in addition to a related definitive diagnosis when the sign or symptom is not routinely associated with that diagnosis.

> Abdominal pain due to acute appendicitis
>
> **K35.80   Unspecified acute appendicitis**
>
> *Explanation:* Codes for signs or symptoms routinely associated with a disease process should not be assigned unless the classification instructs otherwise.

c. Combination codes that include symptoms

ICD-10-CM contains a number of combination codes that identify both the definitive diagnosis and common symptoms of that diagnosis. When using one of these combination codes, an additional code should not be assigned for the symptom.

> Acute gastritis with hemorrhage
>
> **K29.01   Acute gastritis with bleeding**
>
> *Explanation:* When a combination code identifies both the definitive diagnosis and the symptom, an additional code should not be assigned for the symptom.

d. Repeated falls

Code R29.6, Repeated falls, is for use for encounters when a patient has recently fallen and the reason for the fall is being investigated.

Code Z91.81, History of falling, is for use when a patient has fallen in the past and is at risk for future falls. When appropriate, both codes R29.6 and Z91.81 may be assigned together.

e. Coma scale

The coma scale codes (R40.2-) can be used in conjunction with traumatic brain injury codes, acute cerebrovascular disease or sequelae of cerebrovascular disease codes. These codes are primarily for use by trauma registries, but they may be used in any setting where this information is collected. The coma scale codes should be sequenced after the diagnosis code(s).

These codes, one from each subcategory, are needed to complete the scale. The 7th character indicates when the scale was recorded. The 7th character should match for all three codes.

At a minimum, report the initial score documented on presentation at your facility. This may be a score from the emergency medicine technician (EMT) or in the emergency department. If desired, a facility may choose to capture multiple coma scale scores.

Assign code R40.24, Glasgow coma scale, total score, when only the total score is documented in the medical record and not the individual score(s).

> 23-year-old man found down after unknown injury with skull fracture and with concussion and loss of consciousness of unknown duration. EMS evaluated the patient in the field and reported the individual Glasgow coma scores:
>
> Eye opening response—3: eyes open to speech
>
> Verbal response—4: confused but coherent speech
>
> Motor response—6: obeys commands fully
>
> **S02.0XXA   Fracture of vault of skull, initial encounter for closed fracture**
>
> **S06.0X9A   Concussion with loss of consciousness of unspecified duration, initial encounter**
>
> **R40.2131   Coma scale, eyes open, to sound, in the field [EMT or ambulance]**
>
> **R40.2241   Coma scale, best verbal response, confused conversation, in the field [EMT or ambulance]**
>
> **R40.2361   Coma scale, best motor response, obeys commands, in the field [EMT or ambulance]**
>
> *Explanation:* When individual scores for the Glasgow coma scale are documented, one code from each category is needed to complete the scale. The seventh character indicates when the scale was recorded and should match for all three codes. Assign code R40.24 Glasgow coma scale, total score, when only the total and not the individual score(s) is documented in the medical record.

f. Functional quadriplegia

Functional quadriplegia (code R53.2) is the lack of ability to use one's limbs or to ambulate due to extreme debility. It is not associated with neurologic deficit or injury, and code R53.2 should not be used for cases of neurologic quadriplegia. It should only be assigned if functional quadriplegia is specifically documented in the medical record.

g. SIRS due to non-infectious process

The systemic inflammatory response syndrome (SIRS) can develop as a result of certain non-infectious disease processes, such as trauma, malignant neoplasm, or pancreatitis. When SIRS is documented with a noninfectious condition, and no subsequent infection is documented, the code for the underlying condition, such as an injury, should be assigned, followed by code R65.10, Systemic inflammatory response syndrome (SIRS) of non-infectious origin without acute organ dysfunction, or code R65.11, Systemic inflammatory response syndrome (SIRS) of non-infectious origin with acute organ dysfunction. If an associated acute organ dysfunction is documented, the appropriate code(s) for the specific type of organ dysfunction(s) should be assigned in addition to code R65.11. If acute organ dysfunction is documented, but it cannot be determined if the acute organ dysfunction is associated with SIRS or due to another condition (e.g., directly due to the trauma), the provider should be queried.

Systemic inflammatory response syndrome (SIRS) due to acute gallstone pancreatitis

K85.1   **Biliary acute pancreatitis**

R65.10   **Systemic inflammatory response syndrome (SIRS) of noninfectious origin without acute organ dysfunction**

Explanation: When SIRS is documented with a noninfectious condition without subsequent infection documented, the code for the underlying condition such as pancreatitis should be assigned followed by the appropriate code for SIRS of noninfectious origin, either with or without associated organ dysfunction.

h. Death NOS

Code R99, Ill-defined and unknown cause of mortality, is only for use in the very limited circumstance when a patient who has already died is brought into an emergency department or other healthcare facility and is pronounced dead upon arrival. It does not represent the discharge disposition of death.

Chapter 18. Symptoms, Signs and Abnormal Clinical and Laboratory Findings, Not Elsewhere Classified (R00-R99)

NOTE This chapter includes symptoms, signs, abnormal results of clinical or other investigative procedures, and ill-defined conditions regarding which no diagnosis classifiable elsewhere is recorded.

Signs and symptoms that point rather definitely to a given diagnosis have been assigned to a category in other chapters of the classification. In general, categories in this chapter include the less well-defined conditions and symptoms that, without the necessary study of the case to establish a final diagnosis, point perhaps equally to two or more diseases or to two or more systems of the body. Practically all categories in the chapter could be designated "not otherwise specified", "unknown etiology" or "transient". The Alphabetical Index should be consulted to determine which symptoms and signs are to be allocated here and which to other chapters. The residual subcategories, numbered .8, are generally provided for other relevant symptoms that cannot be allocated elsewhere in the classification.

The conditions and signs or symptoms included in categories R00-R94 consist of:

(a)   cases for which no more specific diagnosis can be made even after all the facts bearing on the case have been investigated;

(b)   signs or symptoms existing at the time of initial encounter that proved to be transient and whose causes could not be determined;

(c)   provisional diagnosis in a patient who failed to return for further investigation or care;

(d)   cases referred elsewhere for investigation or treatment before the diagnosis was made;

(e)   cases in which a more precise diagnosis was not available for any other reason;

(f)   certain symptoms, for which supplementary information is provided, that represent important problems in medical care in their own right.

EXCLUDES 2 *abnormal findings on antenatal screening of mother (O28.-)*
certain conditions originating in the perinatal period (P04-P96)
signs and symptoms classified in the body system chapters
signs and symptoms of breast (N63, N64.5)

This chapter contains the following blocks:

R00-R09	Symptoms and signs involving the circulatory and respiratory systems
R10-R19	Symptoms and signs involving the digestive system and abdomen
R20-R23	Symptoms and signs involving the skin and subcutaneous tissue
R25-R29	Symptoms and signs involving the nervous and musculoskeletal systems
R30-R39	Symptoms and signs involving the genitourinary system
R40-R46	Symptoms and signs involving cognition, perception, emotional state and behavior
R47-R49	Symptoms and signs involving speech and voice
R50-R69	General symptoms and signs
R70-R79	Abnormal findings on examination of blood, without diagnosis
R80-R82	Abnormal findings on examination of urine, without diagnosis
R83-R89	Abnormal findings on examination of other body fluids, substances and tissues, without diagnosis
R90-R94	Abnormal findings on diagnostic imaging and in function studies, without diagnosis
R97	Abnormal tumor markers
R99	Ill-defined and unknown cause of mortality

Symptoms and signs involving the circulatory and respiratory systems (R00-R09)

4th R00 Abnormalities of heart beat
EXCLUDES 1 *abnormalities originating in the perinatal period (P29.1-)*
specified arrhythmias (I47-I49)

R00.0 Tachycardia, unspecified
Rapid heart beat
Sinoauricular tachycardia NOS
Sinus [sinusal] tachycardia NOS
EXCLUDES 1 *neonatal tachycardia (P29.11)*
paroxysmal tachycardia (I47.-)

R00.1 Bradycardia, unspecified
Sinoatrial bradycardia
Sinus bradycardia
Slow heart beat
Vagal bradycardia
Use additional code for adverse effect, if applicable, to identify drug (T36-T50 with fifth or sixth character 5)
EXCLUDES 1 *neonatal bradycardia (P29.12)*

R00.2 Palpitations
Awareness of heart beat

R00.8 Other abnormalities of heart beat

R00.9 Unspecified abnormalities of heart beat

✓4th R01 Cardiac murmurs and other cardiac sounds
EXCLUDES 1 *cardiac murmurs and sounds originating in the perinatal period (P29.8)*

R01.0 Benign and innocent cardiac murmurs
Functional cardiac murmur

R01.1 Cardiac murmur, unspecified
Cardiac bruit NOS
Heart murmur NOS

R01.2 Other cardiac sounds
Cardiac dullness, increased or decreased
Precordial friction

✓4th R03 Abnormal blood-pressure reading, *without diagnosis*

R03.0 Elevated blood-pressure reading, without diagnosis of hypertension
NOTE This category is to be used to record an episode of elevated blood pressure in a patient in whom no formal diagnosis of hypertension has been made, or as an isolated incidental finding.

R03.1 Nonspecific low blood-pressure reading
EXCLUDES 1 *hypotension (I95.-)*
maternal hypotension syndrome (O26.5-)
neurogenic orthostatic hypotension (G90.3)

✓4th R04 Hemorrhage from respiratory passages

R04.0 Epistaxis
Hemorrhage from nose
Nosebleed

R04.1 Hemorrhage from throat
EXCLUDES 2 *hemoptysis (R04.2)*

R04.2 Hemoptysis
Blood-stained sputum
Cough with hemorrhage
AHA: 2013, 4Q, 118

✓5th R04.8 Hemorrhage from other sites in respiratory passages

R04.81 Acute idiopathic pulmonary hemorrhage in infants   **P**
AIPHI
Acute idiopathic hemorrhage in infants over 28 days old
EXCLUDES 1 *perinatal pulmonary hemorrhage (P26.-)*
von Willebrand's disease (D68.0)

R04.89 Hemorrhage from other sites in respiratory passages
Pulmonary hemorrhage NOS

R04.9 Hemorrhage from respiratory passages, unspecified

R05 Cough
EXCLUDES 1 *cough with hemorrhage (R04.2)*
smoker's cough (J41.0)

✓4th R06 Abnormalities of breathing
EXCLUDES 1 *acute respiratory distress syndrome (J80)*
respiratory arrest (R09.2)
respiratory arrest of newborn (P28.81)
respiratory distress syndrome of newborn (P22.-)
respiratory failure (J96.-)
respiratory failure of newborn (P28.5)

✓5th R06.0 Dyspnea
EXCLUDES 1 *tachypnea NOS (R06.82)*
transient tachypnea of newborn (P22.1)

R06.00 Dyspnea, unspecified

R06.01 Orthopnea

R06.02 Shortness of breath

R06.09 Other forms of dyspnea

R06.1 Stridor
EXCLUDES 1 *congenital laryngeal stridor (P28.89)*
laryngismus (stridulus) (J38.5)

R06.2 Wheezing
EXCLUDES 1 *asthma (J45.-)*

R06.3 Periodic breathing
Cheyne-Stokes breathing

R06.4 Hyperventilation
EXCLUDES 1 *psychogenic hyperventilation (F45.8)*

R06.5 Mouth breathing
EXCLUDES 2 *dry mouth NOS (R68.2)*

☑ Additional Character Required   ☑x7th Placeholder Alert   Unspecified Dx   Other Specified Dx   Manifestation   ▶◀ Revised Text   ● New Code   ▲ Revised Code Title

R06.6 Hiccough
> *EXCLUDES 1*   *psychogenic hiccough (F45.8)*

R06.7 Sneezing

✓5th **R06.8 Other abnormalities of breathing**

    R06.81 Apnea, not elsewhere classified
        Apnea NOS
> *EXCLUDES 1*   *apnea (of) newborn (P28.4)*
>   *sleep apnea (G47.3-)*
>   *sleep apnea of newborn (primary) (P28.3)*

    R06.82 Tachypnea, not elsewhere classified
        Tachypnea NOS
> *EXCLUDES 1*   *transitory tachypnea of newborn (P22.1)*

    R06.83 Snoring

    R06.89 Other abnormalities of breathing
        Breath-holding (spells)
        Sighing

R06.9 Unspecified abnormalities of breathing

✓4th **R07 Pain in throat and chest**
> *EXCLUDES 1*   *epidemic myalgia (B33.0)*
> *EXCLUDES 2*   *jaw pain (R68.84)*
>   *pain in breast (N64.4)*

    R07.0 Pain in throat
> *EXCLUDES 1*   *chronic sore throat (J31.2)*
>   *sore throat (acute) NOS (J02.9)*
> *EXCLUDES 2*   *dysphagia (R13.1-)*
>   *pain in neck (M54.2)*

    R07.1 Chest pain on breathing
        Painful respiration

    R07.2 Precordial pain

✓5th   **R07.8 Other chest pain**

    R07.81 Pleurodynia
        Pleurodynia NOS
> *EXCLUDES 1*   *epidemic pleurodynia (B33.0)*

    R07.82 Intercostal pain

    R07.89 Other chest pain
        Anterior chest-wall pain NOS

    R07.9 Chest pain, unspecified

✓4th **R09 Other symptoms and signs involving the circulatory and respiratory system**
> *EXCLUDES 1*   *acute respiratory distress syndrome (J80)*
>   *respiratory arrest of newborn (P28.81)*
>   *respiratory distress syndrome of newborn (P22.0)*
>   *respiratory failure (J96.-)*
>   *respiratory failure of newborn (P28.5)*

✓5th   **R09.0 Asphyxia and hypoxemia**
> *EXCLUDES 1*   *asphyxia due to carbon monoxide (T58.-)*
>   *asphyxia due to foreign body in respiratory tract (T17.-)*
>   *birth (intrauterine) asphyxia (P84)*
>   *hypercapnia (R06.4)*
>   *hyperventilation (R06.4)*
>   *traumatic asphyxia (T71.-)*

    R09.01 Asphyxia

    R09.02 Hypoxemia

    R09.1 Pleurisy
> *EXCLUDES 1*   *pleurisy with effusion (J90)*

    R09.2 Respiratory arrest
        Cardiorespiratory failure
> *EXCLUDES 1*   *cardiac arrest (I46.-)*
>   *respiratory arrest of newborn (P28.81)*
>   *respiratory distress of newborn (P22.0)*
>   *respiratory failure (J96.-)*
>   *respiratory failure of newborn (P28.5)*
>   *respiratory insufficiency (R06.89)*
>   *respiratory insufficiency of newborn (P28.5)*

    R09.3 Abnormal sputum
        Abnormal amount of sputum
        Abnormal color of sputum
        Abnormal odor of sputum
        Excessive sputum
> *EXCLUDES 1*   *blood-stained sputum (R04.2)*

✓5th   **R09.8 Other specified symptoms and signs involving the circulatory and respiratory systems**

    R09.81 Nasal congestion

    R09.82 Postnasal drip

    R09.89 Other specified symptoms and signs involving the circulatory and respiratory systems
        Abnormal chest percussion
        Bruit (arterial)
        Chest tympany
        Choking sensation
        Feeling of foreign body in throat
        Friction sounds in chest
        Rales
        Weak pulse
> *EXCLUDES 2*   *foreign body in throat (T17.2-)*
>   *wheezing (R06.2)*

Symptoms and signs involving the digestive system and abdomen (R10-R19)

> *EXCLUDES 1*   *congenital or infantile pylorospasm (Q40.0)*
>   *gastrointestinal hemorrhage (K92.0-K92.2)*
>   *intestinal obstruction (K56.-)*
>   *newborn gastrointestinal hemorrhage (P54.0-P54.3)*
>   *newborn intestinal obstruction (P76.-)*
>   *pylorospasm (K31.3)*
>   *signs and symptoms involving the urinary system (R30-R39)*
>   *symptoms referable to female genital organs (N94.-)*
>   *symptoms referable to male genital organs male (N48-N50)*

✓4th **R10 Abdominal and pelvic pain**
> *EXCLUDES 1*   *renal colic (N23)*
> *EXCLUDES 2*   *dorsalgia (M54.-)*
>   *flatulence and related conditions (R14.-)*

    R10.0 Acute abdomen
        Severe abdominal pain (generalized) (with abdominal rigidity)
> *EXCLUDES 1*   *abdominal rigidity NOS (R19.3)*
>   *generalized abdominal pain NOS (R10.84)*
>   *localized abdominal pain (R10.1-R10.3-)*

✓5th   **R10.1 Pain localized to upper abdomen**

    R10.10 Upper abdominal pain, unspecified

    R10.11 Right upper quadrant pain

    R10.12 Left upper quadrant pain

    R10.13 Epigastric pain
        Dyspepsia
> *EXCLUDES 1*   *functional dyspepsia (K30)*

    R10.2 Pelvic and perineal pain
> *EXCLUDES 1*   *vulvodynia (N94.81)*

✓5th   **R10.3 Pain localized to other parts of lower abdomen**

    R10.30 Lower abdominal pain, unspecified

    R10.31 Right lower quadrant pain

    R10.32 Left lower quadrant pain

    R10.33 Periumbilical pain

✓5th   **R10.8 Other abdominal pain**

✓6th   **R10.81 Abdominal tenderness**
        Abdominal tenderness NOS

    R10.811 Right upper quadrant abdominal tenderness

    R10.812 Left upper quadrant abdominal tenderness

    R10.813 Right lower quadrant abdominal tenderness

    R10.814 Left lower quadrant abdominal tenderness

    R10.815 Periumbilic abdominal tenderness

    R10.816 Epigastric abdominal tenderness

    R10.817 Generalized abdominal tenderness

    R10.819 Abdominal tenderness, unspecified site

✓6th   **R10.82 Rebound abdominal tenderness**

    R10.821 Right upper quadrant rebound abdominal tenderness

    R10.822 Left upper quadrant rebound abdominal tenderness

    R10.823 Right lower quadrant rebound abdominal tenderness

    R10.824 Left lower quadrant rebound abdominal tenderness

    R10.825 Periumbilic rebound abdominal tenderness

    R10.826 Epigastric rebound abdominal tenderness

    R10.827 Generalized rebound abdominal tenderness

    R10.829 Rebound abdominal tenderness, unspecified site

EXCLUDES 1 Not coded here   *EXCLUDES 2* Not included here   N Newborn Age: 0   P Pediatric Age: 0-17   M Maternity Age: 12-55   A Adult Age: 15-124

824   ICD-10-CM 2016

R10.83 **Colic** P
    Colic NOS
    Infantile colic
    EXCLUDES 1   *colic in adult and child over 12 months old*
        (R10.84)

R10.84 **Generalized abdominal pain**
    EXCLUDES 1   *generalized abdominal pain associated with*
        acute abdomen (R10.0)

R10.9 **Unspecified abdominal pain**

√4th **R11** **Nausea and vomiting**
    EXCLUDES 1   *cyclical vomiting associated with migraine (G43.A-)*
        excessive vomiting in pregnancy (O21.-)
        hematemesis (K92.0)
        neonatal hematemesis (P54.0)
        newborn vomiting (P92.0-)
        psychogenic vomiting (F50.8)
        vomiting associated with bulimia nervosa (F50.2)
        vomiting following gastrointestinal surgery (K91.0)

R11.0 **Nausea**
    Nausea NOS
    Nausea without vomiting

√5th **R11.1** **Vomiting**
    R11.10 **Vomiting, unspecified**
        Vomiting NOS
    R11.11 **Vomiting without nausea**
    R11.12 **Projectile vomiting**
    R11.13 **Vomiting of fecal matter**
    R11.14 **Bilious vomiting**
        Bilious emesis

R11.2 **Nausea with vomiting, unspecified**
    Persistent nausea with vomiting NOS

R12 **Heartburn**
    EXCLUDES 1   *dyspepsia NOS (R10.13)*
        functional dyspepsia (K30)

√4th **R13** **Aphagia and dysphagia**
    R13.0 **Aphagia**
        Inability to swallow
        EXCLUDES 1   *psychogenic aphagia (F50.9)*

√5th **R13.1** **Dysphagia**
    Code first, if applicable, dysphagia following cerebrovascular
        disease (I69. with final characters -91)
    EXCLUDES 1   *psychogenic dysphagia (F45.8)*
    R13.10 **Dysphagia, unspecified**
        Difficulty in swallowing NOS
    R13.11 **Dysphagia, oral phase**
    R13.12 **Dysphagia, oropharyngeal phase**
    R13.13 **Dysphagia, pharyngeal phase**
    R13.14 **Dysphagia, pharyngoesophageal phase**
    R13.19 **Other dysphagia**
        Cervical dysphagia
        Neurogenic dysphagia

√4th **R14** **Flatulence and related conditions**
    EXCLUDES 1   *psychogenic aerophagy (F45.8)*
    R14.0 **Abdominal distension (gaseous)**
        Bloating
        Tympanites (abdominal) (intestinal)
    R14.1 **Gas pain**
    R14.2 **Eructation**
    R14.3 **Flatulence**

√4th **R15** **Fecal incontinence**
    Encopresis NOS
    EXCLUDES 1   *fecal incontinence of nonorganic origin (F98.1)*
    R15.0 **Incomplete defecation**
        EXCLUDES 1   *constipation (K59.0-)*
           fecal impaction (K56.41)
    R15.1 **Fecal smearing**
        Fecal soiling
    R15.2 **Fecal urgency**
    R15.9 **Full incontinence of feces**
        Fecal incontinence NOS

√4th **R16** **Hepatomegaly and splenomegaly, not elsewhere classified**
    R16.0 **Hepatomegaly, not elsewhere classified**
        Hepatomegaly NOS
    R16.1 **Splenomegaly, not elsewhere classified**
        Splenomegaly NOS

R16.2 **Hepatomegaly with splenomegaly, not elsewhere classified**
    Hepatosplenomegaly NOS

R17 **Unspecified jaundice**
    EXCLUDES 1   *neonatal jaundice (P55, P57-P59)*

√4th **R18** **Ascites**
    INCLUDES   fluid in peritoneal cavity
    EXCLUDES 1   *ascites in alcoholic cirrhosis (K70.31)*
        ascites in alcoholic hepatitis (K70.11)
        ascites in toxic liver disease with chronic active hepatitis
           (K71.51)

R18.0 **Malignant ascites**
    Code first malignancy, such as:
        malignant neoplasm of ovary (C56.-)
        secondary malignant neoplasm of retroperitoneum and
           peritoneum (C78.6)

R18.8 **Other ascites**
    Ascites NOS
    Peritoneal effusion (chronic)

√4th **R19** **Other symptoms and signs involving the digestive system and abdomen**
    EXCLUDES 1   *acute abdomen (R10.0)*

√5th **R19.0** **Intra-abdominal and pelvic swelling, mass and lump**
    EXCLUDES 1   *abdominal distension (gaseous) (R14.-)*
        ascites (R18.-)
    R19.00 **Intra-abdominal and pelvic swelling, mass and lump, unspecified site**
    R19.01 **Right upper quadrant abdominal swelling, mass and lump**
    R19.02 **Left upper quadrant abdominal swelling, mass and lump**
    R19.03 **Right lower quadrant abdominal swelling, mass and lump**
    R19.04 **Left lower quadrant abdominal swelling, mass and lump**
    R19.05 **Periumbilic swelling, mass or lump**
        Diffuse or generalized umbilical swelling or mass
    R19.06 **Epigastric swelling, mass or lump**
    R19.07 **Generalized intra-abdominal and pelvic swelling, mass and lump**
        Diffuse or generalized intra-abdominal swelling or
           mass NOS
        Diffuse or generalized pelvic swelling or mass NOS
    R19.09 **Other intra-abdominal and pelvic swelling, mass and lump**

√5th **R19.1** **Abnormal bowel sounds**
    R19.11 **Absent bowel sounds**
    R19.12 **Hyperactive bowel sounds**
    R19.15 **Other abnormal bowel sounds**
        Abnormal bowel sounds NOS

R19.2 **Visible peristalsis**
    Hyperperistalsis

√5th **R19.3** **Abdominal rigidity**
    EXCLUDES 1   *abdominal rigidity with severe abdominal pain (R10.0)*
    R19.30 **Abdominal rigidity, unspecified site**
    R19.31 **Right upper quadrant abdominal rigidity**
    R19.32 **Left upper quadrant abdominal rigidity**
    R19.33 **Right lower quadrant abdominal rigidity**
    R19.34 **Left lower quadrant abdominal rigidity**
    R19.35 **Periumbilic abdominal rigidity**
    R19.36 **Epigastric abdominal rigidity**
    R19.37 **Generalized abdominal rigidity**

R19.4 **Change in bowel habit**
    EXCLUDES 1   *constipation (K59.0-)*
        functional diarrhea (K59.1)

R19.5 **Other fecal abnormalities**
    Abnormal stool color
    Bulky stools
    Mucus in stools
    Occult blood in feces
    Occult blood in stools
    EXCLUDES 1   *melena (K92.1)*
        neonatal melena (P54.1)

R19.6 **Halitosis**

☑ Additional Character Required   x̄ T̄ Placeholder Alert   Unspecified Dx   Other Specified Dx   Manifestation   ►◄ Revised Text   ● New Code   ▲ Revised Code Title

R19.7 Diarrhea, unspecified
Diarrhea NOS
EXCLUDES 1 functional diarrhea (K59.1)
neonatal diarrhea (P78.3)
psychogenic diarrhea (F45.8)

R19.8 Other specified symptoms and signs involving the digestive system and abdomen

Symptoms and signs involving the skin and subcutaneous tissue (R20-R23)

EXCLUDES 2 symptoms relating to breast (N64.4-N64.5)

✓4ᵗʰ **R20 Disturbances of skin sensation**
EXCLUDES 1 dissociative anesthesia and sensory loss (F44.6)
psychogenic disturbances (F45.8)

R20.0 Anesthesia of skin

R20.1 Hypoesthesia of skin

R20.2 Paresthesia of skin
Formication
Pins and needles
Tingling skin
EXCLUDES 1 acroparesthesia (I73.8)

R20.3 Hyperesthesia

R20.8 Other disturbances of skin sensation

R20.9 Unspecified disturbances of skin sensation

R21 Rash and other nonspecific skin eruption
Rash NOS
EXCLUDES 1 specified type of rash—code to condition
vesicular eruption (R23.8)

✓4ᵗʰ **R22 Localized swelling, mass and lump of skin and subcutaneous tissue**
Subcutaneous nodules (localized)(superficial)
EXCLUDES 1 abnormal findings on diagnostic imaging (R90-R93)
edema (R60.-)
enlarged lymph nodes (R59.-)
localized adiposity (E65)
swelling of joint (M25.4-)

R22.0 Localized swelling, mass and lump, head

R22.1 Localized swelling, mass and lump, neck

R22.2 Localized swelling, mass and lump, trunk
EXCLUDES 1 intra-abdominal or pelvic mass and lump (R19.0-)
intra-abdominal or pelvic swelling (R19.0-)
EXCLUDES 2 breast mass and lump (N63)

✓5ᵗʰ **R22.3 Localized swelling, mass and lump, upper limb**
R22.30 Localized swelling, mass and lump, unspecified upper limb
R22.31 Localized swelling, mass and lump, right upper limb
R22.32 Localized swelling, mass and lump, left upper limb
R22.33 Localized swelling, mass and lump, upper limb, bilateral

✓5ᵗʰ **R22.4 Localized swelling, mass and lump, lower limb**
R22.40 Localized swelling, mass and lump, unspecified lower limb
R22.41 Localized swelling, mass and lump, right lower limb
R22.42 Localized swelling, mass and lump, left lower limb
R22.43 Localized swelling, mass and lump, lower limb, bilateral

R22.9 Localized swelling, mass and lump, unspecified

✓4ᵗʰ **R23 Other skin changes**
R23.0 Cyanosis
EXCLUDES 1 acrocyanosis (I73.8)
cyanotic attacks of newborn (P28.2)

R23.1 Pallor
Clammy skin

R23.2 Flushing
Excessive blushing
Code first, if applicable, menopausal and female climacteric states (N95.1)

R23.3 Spontaneous ecchymoses
Petechiae
EXCLUDES 1 ecchymoses of newborn (P54.5)
purpura (D69.-)

R23.4 Changes in skin texture
Desquamation of skin
Induration of skin
Scaling of skin
EXCLUDES 1 epidermal thickening NOS (L85.9)

R23.8 Other skin changes

R23.9 Unspecified skin changes

Symptoms and signs involving the nervous and musculoskeletal systems (R25-R29)

✓4ᵗʰ **R25 Abnormal involuntary movements**
EXCLUDES 1 specific movement disorders (G20-G26)
stereotyped movement disorders (F98.4)
tic disorders (F95.-)

R25.0 Abnormal head movements

R25.1 Tremor, unspecified
EXCLUDES 1 chorea NOS (G25.5)
essential tremor (G25.0)
hysterical tremor (F44.4)
intention tremor (G25.2)

R25.2 Cramp and spasm
EXCLUDES 2 carpopedal spasm (R29.0)
charley-horse (M62.831)
infantile spasms (G40.4-)
muscle spasm of back (M62.830)
muscle spasm of calf (M62.831)

R25.3 Fasciculation
Twitching NOS

R25.8 Other abnormal involuntary movements

R25.9 Unspecified abnormal involuntary movements

✓4ᵗʰ **R26 Abnormalities of gait and mobility**
EXCLUDES 1 ataxia NOS (R27.0)
hereditary ataxia (G11.-)
locomotor (syphilitic) ataxia (A52.11)
immobility syndrome (paraplegic) (M62.3)

R26.0 Ataxic gait
Staggering gait

R26.1 Paralytic gait
Spastic gait

R26.2 Difficulty in walking, not elsewhere classified
EXCLUDES 1 falling (R29.6)
unsteadiness on feet (R26.81)

✓5ᵗʰ **R26.8 Other abnormalities of gait and mobility**
R26.81 Unsteadiness on feet
R26.89 Other abnormalities of gait and mobility

R26.9 Unspecified abnormalities of gait and mobility

✓4ᵗʰ **R27 Other lack of coordination**
EXCLUDES 1 ataxic gait (R26.0)
hereditary ataxia (G11.-)
vertigo NOS (R42)

R27.0 Ataxia, unspecified
EXCLUDES 1 ataxia following cerebrovascular disease (I69. with final characters -93)

R27.8 Other lack of coordination

R27.9 Unspecified lack of coordination

✓4ᵗʰ **R29 Other symptoms and signs involving the nervous and musculoskeletal systems**
R29.0 Tetany
Carpopedal spasm
EXCLUDES 1 hysterical tetany (F44.5)
neonatal tetany (P71.3)
parathyroid tetany (E20.9)
post-thyroidectomy tetany (E89.2)

R29.1 Meningismus

R29.2 Abnormal reflex
EXCLUDES 2 abnormal pupillary reflex (H57.0)
hyperactive gag reflex (J39.2)
vasovagal reaction or syncope (R55)

R29.3 Abnormal posture

R29.4 Clicking hip
EXCLUDES 1 congenital deformities of hip (Q65.-)

R29.5 Transient paralysis
Code first any associated spinal cord injury (S14.0, S14.1-, S24.0, S24.1-, S34.0-, S34.1-)
EXCLUDES 1 transient ischemic attack (G45.9)

R29.6 Repeated falls
Falling
Tendency to fall
EXCLUDES 2 at risk for falling (Z91.81)
history of falling (Z91.81)

EXCLUDES 1 Not coded here   *EXCLUDES 2* Not included here   **N** Newborn Age: 0   **P** Pediatric Age: 0-17   **M** Maternity Age: 12-55   **A** Adult Age: 15-124

✓5th R29.8 Other symptoms and signs involving the nervous and musculoskeletal systems

   ✓6th R29.81 Other symptoms and signs involving the nervous system

      R29.810 Facial weakness
         Facial droop
         EXCLUDES 1 *Bell's palsy (G51.0)*
               facial weakness following cere-brovascular disease (I69. with final characters -92)

      R29.818 Other symptoms and signs involving the nervous system

   ✓6th R29.89 Other symptoms and signs involving the musculoskeletal system
      EXCLUDES 2 *pain in limb (M79.6-)*

      R29.890 Loss of height
         EXCLUDES 1 *osteoporosis (M80-M81)*

      R29.891 Ocular torticollis
         EXCLUDES 1 *congenital (sternomastoid) torticollis Q68.0*
               psychogenic torticollis (F45.8)
               spasmodic torticollis (G24.3)
               torticollis due to birth injury (P15.8)
               torticollis NOS M43.6

      R29.898 Other symptoms and signs involving the musculoskeletal system

✓5th R29.9 Unspecified symptoms and signs involving the nervous and musculoskeletal systems

   R29.90 Unspecified symptoms and signs involving the nervous system

   R29.91 Unspecified symptoms and signs involving the musculoskeletal system

Symptoms and signs involving the genitourinary system (R30-R39)

✓4th R30 Pain associated with micturition
   EXCLUDES 1 *psychogenic pain associated with micturition (F45.8)*

   R30.0 Dysuria
      Strangury

   R30.1 Vesical tenesmus

   R30.9 Painful micturition, unspecified
      Painful urination NOS

✓4th R31 Hematuria
   EXCLUDES 1 *hematuria included with underlying conditions, such as:*
         acute cystitis with hematuria (N30.01)
         recurrent and persistent hematuria in glomerular diseases (N02.-)

   R31.0 Gross hematuria

   R31.1 Benign essential microscopic hematuria

   R31.2 Other microscopic hematuria

   R31.9 Hematuria, unspecified

R32 Unspecified urinary incontinence
   Enuresis NOS
   EXCLUDES 1 *functional urinary incontinence (R39.81)*
         nonorganic enuresis (F98.0)
         stress incontinence and other specified urinary incontinence (N39.3-N39.4-)
         urinary incontinence associated with cognitive impairment (R39.81)

✓4th R33 Retention of urine
   EXCLUDES 1 *psychogenic retention of urine (F45.8)*

   R33.0 Drug induced retention of urine
      Use additional code for adverse effect, if applicable, to identify drug (T36-T50 with fifth or sixth character 5)

   R33.8 Other retention of urine
      Code first, if applicable, any causal condition, such as:
         enlarged prostate (N40.1)

   R33.9 Retention of urine, unspecified

R34 Anuria and oliguria
   EXCLUDES 1 *anuria and oliguria complicating abortion or ectopic or molar pregnancy (O00-O07, O08.4)*
         anuria and oliguria complicating pregnancy (O26.83-)
         anuria and oliguria complicating the puerperium (O90.4)

✓4th R35 Polyuria
   Code first, if applicable, any causal condition, such as:
      enlarged prostate (N40.1)
      EXCLUDES 1 *psychogenic polyuria (F45.8)*

   R35.0 Frequency of micturition

   R35.1 Nocturia

   R35.8 Other polyuria
      Polyuria NOS

✓4th R36 Urethral discharge

   R36.0 Urethral discharge without blood

   R36.1 Hematospermia   ♂

   R36.9 Urethral discharge, unspecified
      Penile discharge NOS
      Urethrorrhea

R37 Sexual dysfunction, unspecified

✓4th R39 Other and unspecified symptoms and signs involving the genitourinary system

   R39.0 Extravasation of urine

   ✓5th R39.1 Other difficulties with micturition
      Code first, if applicable, any causal condition, such as:
         enlarged prostate (N40.1)

      R39.11 Hesitancy of micturition

      R39.12 Poor urinary stream
         Weak urinary steam

      R39.13 Splitting of urinary stream

      R39.14 Feeling of incomplete bladder emptying

      R39.15 Urgency of urination
         EXCLUDES 1 *urge incontinence (N39.41, N39.46)*

      R39.16 Straining to void

      R39.19 Other difficulties with micturition

   R39.2 Extrarenal uremia
      Prerenal uremia
      EXCLUDES 1 *uremia NOS (N19)*

   ✓5th R39.8 Other symptoms and signs involving the genitourinary system

      R39.81 Functional urinary incontinence
         Urinary incontinence due to cognitive impairment, or severe physical disability or immobility
         EXCLUDES 1 *stress incontinence and other specified urinary incontinence (N39.3-N39.4-)*
               urinary incontinence NOS (R32)

      R39.89 Other symptoms and signs involving the genitourinary system

   R39.9 Unspecified symptoms and signs involving the genitourinary system

Symptoms and signs involving cognition, perception, emotional state and behavior (R40-R46)

EXCLUDES 1 *symptoms and signs constituting part of a pattern of mental disorder (F01-F99)*

✓4th R40 Somnolence, stupor and coma
   EXCLUDES 1 *neonatal coma (P91.5)*
         somnolence, stupor and coma in diabetes (E08-E13)
         somnolence, stupor and coma in hepatic failure (K72.-)
         somnolence, stupor and coma in hypoglycemia (nondiabetic) (E15)

   R40.0 Somnolence
      Drowsiness
      EXCLUDES 1 *coma (R40.2-)*

   R40.1 Stupor
      Catatonic stupor
      Semicoma
      EXCLUDES 1 *catatonic schizophrenia (F20.2)*
               coma (R40.2-)
               depressive stupor (F31-F33)
               dissociative stupor (F44.2)
               manic stupor (F30.2)

☑ Additional Character Required   ✗7th Placeholder Alert   Unspecified Dx   Other Specified Dx   Manifestation   ▶◀ Revised Text   ● New Code   ▲ Revised Code Title

Chapter 18. Symptoms, Signs, and Abnormal Clinical and Laboratory Findings, Not Elsewhere Classified

✓5th **R40.2** **Coma**
Code first any associated:
  fracture of skull (S02.-)
  intracranial injury (S06.-)
> **NOTE** One code from subcategories R40.21-R40.23 is required to complete the coma scale
AHA: 2014, 1Q, 19

    R40.20 **Unspecified coma**
      Coma NOS
      Unconsciousness NOS

    ✓6th **R40.21** **Coma scale, eyes open**

> The following appropriate 7th character is to be added to subcategory R40.21-.
> 0   unspecified time
> 1   in the field [EMT or ambulance]
> 2   at arrival to emergency department
> 3   at hospital admission
> 4   24 hours or more after hospital admission

      ✓7th **R40.211** **Coma scale, eyes open, never**
      ✓7th **R40.212** **Coma scale, eyes open, to pain**
      ✓7th **R40.213** **Coma scale, eyes open, to sound**
      ✓7th **R40.214** **Coma scale, eyes open, spontaneous**

    ✓6th **R40.22** **Coma scale, best verbal response**

> The following appropriate 7th character is to be added to subcategory R40.22-.
> 0   unspecified time
> 1   in the field [EMT or ambulance]
> 2   at arrival to emergency department
> 3   at hospital admission
> 4   24 hours or more after hospital admission

      ✓7th **R40.221** **Coma scale, best verbal response, none**
      ✓7th **R40.222** **Coma scale, best verbal response, incomprehensible words**
      ✓7th **R40.223** **Coma scale, best verbal response, inappropriate words**
      ✓7th **R40.224** **Coma scale, best verbal response, confused conversation**
      ✓7th **R40.225** **Coma scale, best verbal response, oriented**

    ✓6th **R40.23** **Coma scale, best motor response**

> The following appropriate 7th character is to be added to subcategory R40.23-.
> 0   unspecified time
> 1   in the field [EMT or ambulance]
> 2   at arrival to emergency department
> 3   at hospital admission
> 4   24 hours or more after hospital admission

      ✓7th **R40.231** **Coma scale, best motor response, none**
      ✓7th **R40.232** **Coma scale, best motor response, extension**
      ✓7th **R40.233** **Coma scale, best motor response, abnormal**
      ✓7th **R40.234** **Coma scale, best motor response, flexion withdrawal**
      ✓7th **R40.235** **Coma scale, best motor response, localizes pain**
      ✓7th **R40.236** **Coma scale, best motor response, obeys commands**

    ✓6th **R40.24** **Glasgow coma scale, total score**
      Use codes R40.21- through R40.23- only when the individual score(s) are documented
      R40.241 **Glasgow coma scale score 13-15**
      R40.242 **Glasgow coma scale score 9-12**
      R40.243 **Glasgow coma scale score 3-8**
      R40.244 **Other coma, without documented Glasgow coma scale score, or with partial score reported**

R40.3 **Persistent vegetative state**
R40.4 **Transient alteration of awareness**

✓4th **R41** **Other symptoms and signs involving cognitive functions and awareness**
> **EXCLUDES 1** dissociative [conversion] disorders (F44.-)
> mild cognitive impairment, so stated (G31.84)

    R41.0 **Disorientation, unspecified**
      Confusion NOS
      Delirium NOS

    R41.1 **Anterograde amnesia**
    R41.2 **Retrograde amnesia**
    R41.3 **Other amnesia**
      Amnesia NOS
      Memory loss NOS
> **EXCLUDES 1** amnestic disorder due to known physiologic condition (F04)
> amnestic syndrome due to psychoactive substance use (F10-F19 with 5th character .6)
> mild memory disturbance due to known physiological condition (F06.8)
> transient global amnesia (G45.4)

    R41.4 **Neurologic neglect syndrome**
      Asomatognosia
      Hemi-akinesia
      Hemi-inattention
      Hemispatial neglect
      Left-sided neglect
      Sensory neglect
      Visuospatial neglect
> **EXCLUDES 1** visuospatial deficit (R41.842)

    ✓5th **R41.8** **Other symptoms and signs involving cognitive functions and awareness**
      R41.81 **Age-related cognitive decline** 🅐
        Senility NOS

      R41.82 **Altered mental status, unspecified**
        Change in mental status NOS
> **EXCLUDES 1** altered level of consciousness (R40.-)
> altered mental status due to known condition—code to condition
> delirium NOS (R41.0)
        AHA: 2012, 4Q, 97

      R41.83 **Borderline intellectual functioning**
        IQ level 71 to 84
> **EXCLUDES 1** intellectual disabilities (F70-F79)

      ✓6th **R41.84** **Other specified cognitive deficit**
        R41.840 **Attention and concentration deficit**
> **EXCLUDES 1** attention-deficit hyperactivity disorders (F90.-)
        R41.841 **Cognitive communication deficit**
        R41.842 **Visuospatial deficit**
        R41.843 **Psychomotor deficit**
        R41.844 **Frontal lobe and executive function deficit**

      R41.89 **Other symptoms and signs involving cognitive functions and awareness**
        Anosognosia

    R41.9 **Unspecified symptoms and signs involving cognitive functions and awareness**

R42 **Dizziness and giddiness**
    Light-headedness
    Vertigo NOS
> **EXCLUDES 1** vertiginous syndromes (H81.-)
> vertigo from infrasound (T75.23)

✓4th **R43** **Disturbances of smell and taste**
    R43.0 **Anosmia**
    R43.1 **Parosmia**
    R43.2 **Parageusia**
    R43.8 **Other disturbances of smell and taste**
      Mixed disturbance of smell and taste
    R43.9 **Unspecified disturbances of smell and taste**

EXCLUDES 1 Not coded here   **EXCLUDES 2** Not included here   **N** Newborn Age: 0   **P** Pediatric Age: 0-17   **M** Maternity Age: 12-55   **A** Adult Age: 15-124

828   ICD-10-CM 2016

4ᵗʰ R44 Other symptoms and signs involving general sensations and perceptions

EXCLUDES 1   *alcoholic hallucinations (F1.5)*
    hallucinations in drug psychosis (F11–F19 with .5)
    hallucinations in mood disorders with psychotic symptoms (F30.2, F31.5, F32.3, F33.3)
    hallucinations in schizophrenia, schizotypal and delusional disorders (F20–F29)

EXCLUDES 2   *disturbances of skin sensation (R20.-)*

R44.0 Auditory hallucinations

R44.1 Visual hallucinations

R44.2 Other hallucinations

R44.3 Hallucinations, unspecified

R44.8 Other symptoms and signs involving general sensations and perceptions

R44.9 Unspecified symptoms and signs involving general sensations and perceptions

4ᵗʰ R45 Symptoms and signs involving emotional state

R45.0 Nervousness
    Nervous tension

R45.1 Restlessness and agitation

R45.2 Unhappiness

R45.3 Demoralization and apathy
EXCLUDES 1   *anhedonia (R45.84)*

R45.4 Irritability and anger

R45.5 Hostility

R45.6 Violent behavior

R45.7 State of emotional shock and stress, unspecified

✓5ᵗʰ R45.8 Other symptoms and signs involving emotional state

    R45.81 Low self-esteem

    R45.82 Worries

    R45.83 Excessive crying of child, adolescent or adult
    EXCLUDES 1   *excessive crying of infant (baby) R68.11*

    R45.84 Anhedonia

    ✓6ᵗʰ R45.85 Homicidal and suicidal ideations
    EXCLUDES 1   *suicide attempt (T14.91)*

        R45.850 Homicidal ideations

        R45.851 Suicidal ideations

    R45.86 Emotional lability

    R45.87 Impulsiveness

    R45.89 Other symptoms and signs involving emotional state

4ᵗʰ R46 Symptoms and signs involving appearance and behavior

EXCLUDES 1   *appearance and behavior in schizophrenia, schizotypal and delusional disorders (F20-F29)*
    mental and behavioral disorders (F01-F99)

R46.0 Very low level of personal hygiene

R46.1 Bizarre personal appearance

R46.2 Strange and inexplicable behavior

R46.3 Overactivity

R46.4 Slowness and poor responsiveness
EXCLUDES 1   *stupor (R40.1)*

R46.5 Suspiciousness and marked evasiveness

R46.6 Undue concern and preoccupation with stressful events

R46.7 Verbosity and circumstantial detail obscuring reason for contact

✓5ᵗʰ R46.8 Other symptoms and signs involving appearance and behavior

    R46.81 Obsessive-compulsive behavior
    EXCLUDES 1   *obsessive-compulsive disorder (F42)*

    R46.89 Other symptoms and signs involving appearance and behavior

Symptoms and signs involving speech and voice (R47-R49)

✓4ᵗʰ R47 Speech disturbances, not elsewhere classified

EXCLUDES 1   *autism (F84.0)*
    cluttering (F80.81)
    specific developmental disorders of speech and language (F80.-)
    stuttering (F80.81)

✓5ᵗʰ R47.0 Dysphasia and aphasia

    R47.01 Aphasia
    EXCLUDES 1   *aphasia following cerebrovascular disease (I69. with final characters -20)*
        progressive isolated aphasia (G31.01)

    R47.02 Dysphasia
    EXCLUDES 1   *dysphasia following cerebrovascular disease (I69. with final characters -21)*

R47.1 Dysarthria and anarthria
EXCLUDES 1   *dysarthria following cerebrovascular disease (I69. with final characters -22)*

✓5ᵗʰ R47.8 Other speech disturbances
EXCLUDES 1   *dysarthria following cerebrovascular disease (I69. with final characters -28)*

    R47.81 Slurred speech

    R47.82 Fluency disorder in conditions classified elsewhere
    Stuttering in conditions classified elsewhere
    Code first underlying disease or condition, such as:
    Parkinson's disease (G20)
    EXCLUDES 1   *adult onset fluency disorder (F98.5)*
        childhood onset fluency disorder (F80.81)
        fluency disorder (stuttering) following cerebrovascular disease (I69. with final characters-23)

    R47.89 Other speech disturbances

R47.9 Unspecified speech disturbances

✓4ᵗʰ R48 Dyslexia and other symbolic dysfunctions, not elsewhere classified

EXCLUDES 1   *specific developmental disorders of scholastic skills (F81.-)*

R48.0 Dyslexia and alexia

R48.1 Agnosia
    Astereognosia (astereognosis)
    Autotopagnosia
    EXCLUDES 1   *visual object agnosia (R48.3)*

R48.2 Apraxia
EXCLUDES 1   *apraxia following cerebrovascular disease (I69. with final characters -90)*

R48.3 Visual agnosia
    Prosopagnosia
    Simultanagnosia (asimultagnosia)

R48.8 Other symbolic dysfunctions
    Acalculia
    Agraphia

R48.9 Unspecified symbolic dysfunctions

✓4ᵗʰ R49 Voice and resonance disorders

EXCLUDES 1   *psychogenic voice and resonance disorders (F44.4)*

R49.0 Dysphonia
    Hoarseness

R49.1 Aphonia
    Loss of voice

✓5ᵗʰ R49.2 Hypernasality and hyponasality

    R49.21 Hypernasality

    R49.22 Hyponasality

R49.8 Other voice and resonance disorders

R49.9 Unspecified voice and resonance disorder
    Change in voice NOS
    Resonance disorder NOS

Chapter 18. Symptoms, Signs, and Abnormal Clinical and Laboratory Findings, Not Elsewhere Classified

R44–R49.9

☑ Additional Character Required   ✓×7ᵗʰ Placeholder Alert   Unspecified Dx   Other Specified Dx   Manifestation   ▶◀ Revised Text   ● New Code   ▲ Revised Code Title

General symptoms and signs (R50-R69)

✓4ᵗʰ R50　Fever of other and unknown origin
> EXCLUDES 1　chills without fever (R68.83)
> febrile convulsions (R56.0-)
> fever of unknown origin during labor (O75.2)
> fever of unknown origin in newborn (P81.9)
> hypothermia due to illness (R68.0)
> malignant hyperthermia due to anesthesia (T88.3)
> puerperal pyrexia NOS (O86.4)

R50.2　Drug induced fever
> Use additional code for adverse effect, if applicable, to identify drug (T36-T50 with fifth or sixth character 5)
> EXCLUDES 1　postvaccination (postimmunization) fever (R50.83)

✓5ᵗʰ R50.8　Other specified fever

R50.81　Fever presenting with conditions classified elsewhere
> Code first underlying condition when associated fever is present, such as with:
> leukemia (C91-C95)
> neutropenia (D70.-)
> sickle-cell disease (D57.-)
> AHA: 2014, 4Q, 22

R50.82　Postprocedural fever
> EXCLUDES 1　postprocedural infection (T81.4)
> posttransfusion fever (R50.84)
> postvaccination (postimmunization) fever (R50.83)

R50.83　Postvaccination fever
> Postimmunization fever

R50.84　Febrile nonhemolytic transfusion reaction
> FNHTR
> Posttransfusion fever

R50.9　Fever, unspecified
> Fever NOS
> Fever of unknown origin [FUO]
> Fever with chills
> Fever with rigors
> Hyperpyrexia NOS
> Persistent fever
> Pyrexia NOS

R51　Headache
> Facial pain NOS
> EXCLUDES 1　atypical face pain (G50.1)
> migraine and other headache syndromes (G43-G44)
> trigeminal neuralgia (G50.0)

R52　Pain, unspecified
> Acute pain NOS
> Generalized pain NOS
> Pain NOS
> EXCLUDES 1　acute and chronic pain, not elsewhere classified (G89.-)
> localized pain, unspecified type—code to pain by site, such as:
> abdomen pain (R10.-)
> back pain (M54.9)
> breast pain (N64.4)
> chest pain (R07.1-R07.9)
> ear pain (H92.0-)
> eye pain (H57.1)
> headache (R51)
> joint pain (M25.5-)
> limb pain (M79.6-)
> lumbar region pain (M54.5)
> pelvic and perineal pain (R10.2)
> renal colic (N23)
> shoulder pain (M25.51-)
> spine pain (M54.-)
> throat pain (R07.0)
> tongue pain (K14.6)
> tooth pain (K08.8)
> pain disorders exclusively related to psychological factors (F45.41)

✓4ᵗʰ R53　Malaise and fatigue

R53.0　Neoplastic (malignant) related fatigue
> Code first associated neoplasm

R53.1　Weakness
> Asthenia NOS
> EXCLUDES 1　age-related weakness (R54)
> muscle weakness (M62.8-)
> senile asthenia (R54)
> AHA: 2015, 1Q, 25

R53.2　Functional quadriplegia
> Complete immobility due to severe physical disability or frailty
> EXCLUDES 1　frailty NOS (R54)
> hysterical paralysis (F44.4)
> immobility syndrome (M62.3)
> neurologic quadriplegia (G82.5-)
> quadriplegia (G82.50)

✓5ᵗʰ R53.8　Other malaise and fatigue
> EXCLUDES 1　combat exhaustion and fatigue (F43.0)
> congenital debility (P96.9)
> exhaustion and fatigue due to depressive episode (F32.-)
> exhaustion and fatigue due to excessive exertion (T73.3)
> exhaustion and fatigue due to exposure (T73.2)
> exhaustion and fatigue due to heat (T67.-)
> exhaustion and fatigue due to pregnancy (O26.8-)
> exhaustion and fatigue due to recurrent depressive episode (F33)
> exhaustion and fatigue due to senile debility (R54)

R53.81　Other malaise
> Chronic debility
> Debility NOS
> General physical deterioration
> Malaise NOS
> Nervous debility
> EXCLUDES 1　age-related physical debility (R54)

R53.82　Chronic fatigue, unspecified
> Chronic fatigue syndrome NOS
> EXCLUDES 1　postviral fatigue syndrome (G93.3)

R53.83　Other fatigue
> Fatigue NOS
> Lack of energy
> Lethargy
> Tiredness

R54　Age-related physical debility
> Frailty
> Old age
> Senescence
> Senile asthenia
> Senile debility
> EXCLUDES 1　age-related cognitive decline (R41.81)
> senile psychosis (F03)
> senility NOS (R41.81)

R55　Syncope and collapse
> Blackout
> Fainting
> Vasovagal attack
> EXCLUDES 1　cardiogenic shock (R57.0)
> carotid sinus syncope (G90.01)
> heat syncope (T67.1)
> neurocirculatory asthenia (F45.8)
> neurogenic orthostatic hypotension (G90.3)
> orthostatic hypotension (I95.1)
> postprocedural shock (T81.1-)
> psychogenic syncope (F48.8)
> shock NOS (R57.9)
> shock complicating or following abortion or ectopic or molar pregnancy (O00-O07, O08.3)
> shock complicating or following labor and delivery (O75.1)
> Stokes-Adams attack (I45.9)
> unconsciousness NOS (R40.2-)

✓4ᵗʰ R56　Convulsions, not elsewhere classified
> EXCLUDES 1　dissociative convulsions and seizures (F44.5)
> epileptic convulsions and seizures (G40.-)
> newborn convulsions and seizures (P90)

✓5ᵗʰ R56.0　Febrile convulsions

R56.00　Simple febrile convulsions
> Febrile convulsion NOS
> Febrile seizure NOS

R56.01　Complex febrile convulsions
> Atypical febrile seizure
> Complex febrile seizure
> Complicated febrile seizure
> EXCLUDES 1　status epilepticus (G40.901)

R56.1　Post traumatic seizures
> EXCLUDES 1　post traumatic epilepsy (G40.-)

EXCLUDES 1 Not coded here　　　EXCLUDES 2 Not included here　　　N Newborn Age: 0　　　P Pediatric Age: 0-17　　　M Maternity Age: 12-55　　　A Adult Age: 15-124

830　　　ICD-10-CM 2016

R56.9 Unspecified convulsions
Convulsion disorder
Fit NOS
Recurrent convulsions
Seizure(s) (convulsive) NOS

✓4ᵗʰ **R57 Shock, not elsewhere classified**
EXCLUDES 1 *anaphylactic shock NOS (T78.2)*
anaphylactic reaction or shock due to adverse food reaction (T78.0-)
anaphylactic shock due to adverse effect of correct drug or medicament properly administered (T88.6)
anaphylactic shock due to serum (T80.5-)
anesthetic shock (T88.3)
electric shock (T75.4)
obstetric shock (O75.1)
postprocedural shock (T81.1-)
psychic shock (F43.0)
septic shock (R65.21)
shock complicating or following ectopic or molar pregnancy (O00-O07, O08.3)
shock due to lightning (T75.01)
traumatic shock (T79.4)
toxic shock syndrome (A48.3)

R57.0 Cardiogenic shock

R57.1 Hypovolemic shock

R57.8 Other shock

R57.9 Shock, unspecified
Failure of peripheral circulation NOS

R58 Hemorrhage, not elsewhere classified
Hemorrhage NOS
EXCLUDES 1 *hemorrhage included with underlying conditions, such as:*
acute duodenal ulcer with hemorrhage (K26.0)
acute gastritis with bleeding (K29.01)
ulcerative enterocolitis with rectal bleeding (K51.01)

✓4ᵗʰ **R59 Enlarged lymph nodes**
INCLUDES swollen glands
EXCLUDES 1 *acute lymphadenitis (L04.-)*
chronic lymphadenitis (I88.1)
lymphadenitis NOS (I88.9)
mesenteric (acute) (chronic) lymphadenitis (I88.0)

R59.0 Localized enlarged lymph nodes

R59.1 Generalized enlarged lymph nodes
Lymphadenopathy NOS

R59.9 Enlarged lymph nodes, unspecified

✓4ᵗʰ **R60 Edema, not elsewhere classified**
EXCLUDES 1 *angioneurotic edema (T78.3)*
ascites (R18.-)
cerebral edema (G93.6)
cerebral edema due to birth injury (P11.0)
edema of larynx (J38.4)
edema of nasopharynx (J39.2)
edema of pharynx (J39.2)
gestational edema (O12.0-)
hereditary edema (Q82.0)
hydrops fetalis NOS (P83.2)
hydrothorax (J94.8)
nutritional edema (E40-E46)
hydrops fetalis NOS (P83.2)
newborn edema (P83.3)
pulmonary edema (J81.-)

R60.0 Localized edema

R60.1 Generalized edema

R60.9 Edema, unspecified
Fluid retention NOS

R61 Generalized hyperhidrosis
Excessive sweating
Night sweats
Secondary hyperhidrosis
Code first, if applicable, menopausal and female climacteric states (N95.1)
EXCLUDES 1 *focal (primary) (secondary) hyperhidrosis (L74.5-)*
Frey's syndrome (L74.52)
localized (primary) (secondary) hyperhidrosis (L74.5-)

✓4ᵗʰ **R62 Lack of expected normal physiological development in childhood and adults**
EXCLUDES 1 *delayed puberty (E30.0)*
gonadal dysgenesis (Q99.1)
hypopituitarism (E23.0)

R62.0 Delayed milestone in childhood   ℗
Delayed attainment of expected physiological developmental stage
Late talker
Late walker

✓5ᵗʰ **R62.5 Other and unspecified lack of expected normal physiological development in childhood**
EXCLUDES 1 *HIV disease resulting in failure to thrive (B20)*
physical retardation due to malnutrition (E45)

R62.50 Unspecified lack of expected normal physiological development in childhood   ℗
Infantilism NOS

R62.51 Failure to thrive (child)   ℗
Failure to gain weight
EXCLUDES 1 *failure to thrive in child under 28 days old (P92.6)*

R62.52 Short stature (child)   ℗
Lack of growth
Physical retardation
Short stature NOS
EXCLUDES 1 *short stature due to endocrine disorder (E34.3)*

R62.59 Other lack of expected normal physiological development in childhood   ℗

R62.7 Adult failure to thrive   Ⓐ

✓4ᵗʰ **R63 Symptoms and signs concerning food and fluid intake**
EXCLUDES 1 *bulimia NOS (F50.2)*
eating disorders of nonorganic origin (F50.-)
malnutrition (E40-E46)

R63.0 Anorexia
Loss of appetite
EXCLUDES 1 *anorexia nervosa (F50.0-)*
loss of appetite of nonorganic origin (F50.8)

R63.1 Polydipsia
Excessive thirst

R63.2 Polyphagia
Excessive eating
Hyperalimentation NOS

R63.3 Feeding difficulties
Feeding problem (elderly) (infant) NOS
EXCLUDES 1 *feeding problems of newborn (P92.-)*
infant feeding disorder of nonorganic origin (F98.2-)

R63.4 Abnormal weight loss

R63.5 Abnormal weight gain
EXCLUDES 1 *excessive weight gain in pregnancy (O26.0-)*
obesity (E66.-)

R63.6 Underweight
Use additional code to identify body mass index (BMI), if known (Z68.-)
EXCLUDES 1 *abnormal weight loss (R63.4)*
anorexia nervosa (F50.0-)
malnutrition (E40-E46)

R63.8 Other symptoms and signs concerning food and fluid intake

R64 Cachexia
Wasting syndrome
Code first underlying condition, if known
EXCLUDES 1 *abnormal weight loss (R63.4)*
nutritional marasmus (E41)

✓4ᵗʰ **R65 Symptoms and signs specifically associated with systemic inflammation and infection**

✓5ᵗʰ **R65.1 Systemic inflammatory response syndrome [SIRS] of non-infectious origin**
Code first underlying condition, such as:
heatstroke (T67.0)
injury and trauma (S00-T88)
EXCLUDES 1 *sepsis—code to infection*
severe sepsis (R65.2)

R65.10 Systemic inflammatory response syndrome [SIRS] of non-infectious origin without acute organ dysfunction
Systemic inflammatory response syndrome (SIRS) NOS

✅ Additional Character Required   ✓x7ᵗʰ Placeholder Alert   Unspecified Dx   Other Specified Dx   Manifestation   ▶◀ Revised Text   ● New Code   ▲ Revised Code Title

R65.11 **Systemic inflammatory response syndrome [SIRS] of non-infectious origin** with acute organ dysfunction
Use additional code to identify specific acute organ dysfunction, such as:
acute kidney failure (N17.-)
acute respiratory failure (J96.0-)
critical illness myopathy (G72.81)
critical illness polyneuropathy (G62.81)
disseminated intravascular coagulopathy [DIC] (D65)
encephalopathy (metabolic) (septic) (G93.41)
hepatic failure (K72.0-)

✓5th **R65.2** **Severe sepsis**
Infection with associated acute organ dysfunction
Sepsis with acute organ dysfunction
Sepsis with multiple organ dysfunction
Systemic inflammatory response syndrome due to infectious process with acute organ dysfunction
Code first underlying infection, such as:
infection following a procedure (T81.4)
infections following infusion, transfusion and therapeutic injection (T80.2-)
puerperal sepsis (O85)
sepsis following complete or unspecified spontaneous abortion (O03.87)
sepsis following ectopic and molar pregnancy (O08.82)
sepsis following incomplete spontaneous abortion (O03.37)
sepsis following (induced) termination of pregnancy (O04.87)
sepsis NOS (A41.9)
Use additional code to identify specific acute organ dysfunction, such as:
acute kidney failure (N17.-)
acute respiratory failure (J96.0-)
critical illness myopathy (G72.81)
critical illness polyneuropathy (G62.81)
disseminated intravascular coagulopathy [DIC] (D65)
encephalopathy (metabolic) (septic) (G93.41)
hepatic failure (K72.0-)

R65.20 **Severe sepsis** without septic shock
Severe sepsis NOS
AHA: 2013, 4Q, 119

R65.21 **Severe sepsis** with septic shock

✓4th **R68** **Other general symptoms and signs**

R68.0 **Hypothermia, not associated with low environmental temperature**
EXCLUDES1   hypothermia due to anesthesia (T88.51)
hypothermia due to low environmental temperature (T68)
hypothermia NOS (accidental) (T68)
newborn hypothermia (P80.-)

✓5th **R68.1** **Nonspecific symptoms peculiar to infancy**
EXCLUDES1   colic, infantile (R10.83)
neonatal cerebral irritability (P91.3)
teething syndrome (K00.7)

R68.11 **Excessive crying of infant (baby)**   P
EXCLUDES1   excessive crying of child, adolescent, or adult (R45.83)

R68.12 **Fussy infant (baby)**   P
Irritable infant

R68.13 **Apparent life threatening event in infant [ALTE]**   P
Apparent life threatening event in newborn
Code first confirmed diagnosis, if known
Use additional code(s) for associated signs and symptoms if no confirmed diagnosis established, or if signs and symptoms are not associated routinely with confirmed diagnosis, or provide additional information for cause of ALTE

R68.19 **Other nonspecific symptoms peculiar to infancy**   P

R68.2 **Dry mouth, unspecified**
EXCLUDES1   dry mouth due to dehydration (E86.0)
dry mouth due to sicca syndrome [Sjögren] (M35.0-)
salivary gland hyposecretion (K11.7)

R68.3 **Clubbing of fingers**
Clubbing of nails
EXCLUDES1   congenital clubfinger (Q68.1)

✓5th **R68.8** **Other general symptoms and signs**

R68.81 **Early satiety**

R68.82 **Decreased libido**   A
Decreased sexual desire

R68.83 **Chills (without fever)**
Chills NOS
EXCLUDES1   chills with fever (R50.9)

R68.84 **Jaw pain**
Mandibular pain
Maxilla pain
EXCLUDES1   temporomandibular joint arthralgia (M26.62)

R68.89 **Other general symptoms and signs**

R69 **Illness, unspecified**
Unknown and unspecified cases of morbidity

Abnormal findings on examination of blood, without diagnosis (R70-R79)

EXCLUDES1   abnormalities (of)(on):
abnormal findings on antenatal screening of mother (O28.-)
coagulation hemorrhagic disorders (D65-D68)
lipids (E78.-)
platelets and thrombocytes (D69.-)
white blood cells classified elsewhere (D70-D72)
diagnostic abnormal findings classified elsewhere—see Alphabetical Index
hemorrhagic and hematological disorders of newborn (P50-P61)

✓4th **R70** **Elevated erythrocyte sedimentation rate and abnormality of plasma viscosity**

R70.0 **Elevated erythrocyte sedimentation rate**

R70.1 **Abnormal plasma viscosity**

✓4th **R71** **Abnormality of red blood cells**
EXCLUDES1   anemias (D50-D64)
anemia of premature infant (P61.2)
benign (familial) polycythemia (D75.0)
congenital anemias (P61.2-P61.4)
newborn anemia due to isoimmunization (P55.-)
polycythemia neonatorum (P61.1)
polycythemia NOS (D75.1)
polycythemia vera (D45)
secondary polycythemia (D75.1)

R71.0 **Precipitous drop in hematocrit**
Drop (precipitous) in hemoglobin
Drop in hematocrit

R71.8 **Other abnormality of red blood cells**
Abnormal red-cell morphology NOS
Abnormal red-cell volume NOS
Anisocytosis
Poikilocytosis

✓4th **R73** **Elevated blood glucose level**
EXCLUDES1   diabetes mellitus (E08-E13)
diabetes mellitus in pregnancy, childbirth and the puerperium (O24.-)
neonatal disorders (P70.0-P70.2)
postsurgical hypoinsulinemia (E89.1)

✓5th **R73.0** **Abnormal glucose**
EXCLUDES1   abnormal glucose in pregnancy (O99.81-)
diabetes mellitus (E08-E13)
dysmetabolic syndrome X (E88.81)
gestational diabetes (O24.4-)
glycosuria (R81)
hypoglycemia (E16.2)

R73.01 **Impaired fasting glucose**
Elevated fasting glucose

R73.02 **Impaired glucose tolerance (oral)**
Elevated glucose tolerance

R73.09 **Other abnormal glucose**
Abnormal glucose NOS
Abnormal non-fasting glucose tolerance
Latent diabetes
Prediabetes

R73.9 **Hyperglycemia, unspecified**

✓4th **R74** **Abnormal serum enzyme levels**

R74.0 **Nonspecific elevation of levels of transaminase and lactic acid dehydrogenase [LDH]**

R74.8 **Abnormal levels of other serum enzymes**
Abnormal level of acid phosphatase
Abnormal level of alkaline phosphatase
Abnormal level of amylase
Abnormal level of lipase [triacylglycerol lipase]

R74.9 **Abnormal serum enzyme level, unspecified**

EXCLUDES1 Not coded here   EXCLUDES2 Not included here   N Newborn Age: 0   P Pediatric Age: 0-17   M Maternity Age: 12-55   A Adult Age: 15-124

832   ICD-10-CM 2016

R75 Inconclusive laboratory evidence of human immunodeficiency virus [HIV]

Nonconclusive HIV-test finding in infants

EXCLUDES 1   *asymptomatic human immunodeficiency virus [HIV] infection status (Z21)*

human immunodeficiency virus [HIV] disease (B20)

✓4th R76 Other abnormal immunological findings in serum

R76.0 Raised antibody titer

EXCLUDES 1   *isoimmunization in pregnancy (O36.0–O36.1)*

isoimmunization affecting newborn (P55.-)

✓5th R76.1 Nonspecific reaction to test for tuberculosis

R76.11 Nonspecific reaction to tuberculin skin test without active tuberculosis

Abnormal result of Mantoux test

PPD positive

Tuberculin (skin test) positive

Tuberculin (skin test) reactor

EXCLUDES 1   *nonspecific reaction to cell mediated immunity measurement of gamma interferon antigen response without active tuberculosis (R76.12)*

R76.12 Nonspecific reaction to cell mediated immunity measurement of gamma interferon antigen response without active tuberculosis

Nonspecific reaction to QuantiFERON-TB test (QFT) without active tuberculosis

EXCLUDES 1   *nonspecific reaction to tuberculin skin test without active tuberculosis (R76.11)*

positive tuberculin skin test (R76.11)

R76.8 Other specified abnormal immunological findings in serum

Raised level of immunoglobulins NOS

R76.9 Abnormal immunological finding in serum, unspecified

✓4th R77 Other abnormalities of plasma proteins

EXCLUDES 1   *disorders of plasma-protein metabolism (E88.0)*

R77.0 Abnormality of albumin

R77.1 Abnormality of globulin

Hyperglobulinemia NOS

R77.2 Abnormality of alphafetoprotein

R77.8 Other specified abnormalities of plasma proteins

R77.9 Abnormality of plasma protein, unspecified

✓4th R78 Findings of drugs and other substances, not normally found in blood

Use additional code to identify any retained foreign body, if applicable (Z18.-)

EXCLUDES 1   *mental or behavioral disorders due to psychoactive substance use (F10-F19)*

R78.0 Finding of alcohol **in blood**

Use additional external cause code (Y90.-), for detail regarding alcohol level

R78.1 Finding of opiate **drug in blood**

R78.2 Finding of cocaine **in blood**

R78.3 Finding of hallucinogen **in blood**

R78.4 Finding of other drugs of addictive potential **in blood**

R78.5 Finding of other psychotropic **drug in blood**

R78.6 Finding of steroid **agent in blood**

✓5th R78.7 Finding of abnormal level of heavy metals **in blood**

R78.71 Abnormal lead **level in blood**

EXCLUDES 1   *lead poisoning (T56.0-)*

R78.79 Finding of abnormal level of heavy metals **in blood**

✓5th R78.8 Finding of other specified substances, not normally found in blood

R78.81 Bacteremia

EXCLUDES 1   *sepsis—code to specified infection (A00-B99)*

R78.89 Finding of other specified substances, not normally found in blood

Finding of abnormal level of lithium in blood

R78.9 Finding of unspecified substance, not normally found in blood

✓4th R79 Other abnormal findings of blood chemistry

Use additional code to identify any retained foreign body, if applicable (Z18.-)

EXCLUDES 1   *abnormality of fluid, electrolyte or acid-base balance (E86-E87)*

asymptomatic hyperuricemia (E79.0)

hyperglycemia NOS (R73.9)

hypoglycemia NOS (E16.2)

neonatal hypoglycemia (P70.3-P70.4)

specific findings indicating disorder of amino-acid metabolism (E70-E72)

specific findings indicating disorder of carbohydrate metabolism (E73-E74)

specific findings indicating disorder of lipid metabolism (E75.-)

R79.0 Abnormal level of blood mineral

Abnormal blood level of cobalt

Abnormal blood level of copper

Abnormal blood level of iron

Abnormal blood level of magnesium

Abnormal blood level of mineral NEC

Abnormal blood level of zinc

EXCLUDES 1   *abnormal level of lithium (R78.89)*

disorders of mineral metabolism (E83.-)

neonatal hypomagnesemia (P71.2)

nutritional mineral deficiency (E58-E61)

R79.1 Abnormal coagulation profile

Abnormal or prolonged bleeding time

Abnormal or prolonged coagulation time

Abnormal or prolonged partial thromboplastin time [PTT]

Abnormal or prolonged prothrombin time [PT]

EXCLUDES 1   *coagulation defects (D68.-)*

✓5th R79.8 Other specified abnormal findings of blood chemistry

R79.81 Abnormal blood-gas **level**

R79.82 Elevated C-reactive protein [CRP]

R79.89 Other specified abnormal findings of blood chemistry

R79.9 Abnormal finding of blood chemistry, unspecified

Abnormal findings on examination of urine, without diagnosis (R80-R82)

EXCLUDES 1   *abnormal findings on antenatal screening of mother (O28.-)*

diagnostic abnormal findings classified elsewhere—see Alphabetical Index

specific findings indicating disorder of amino-acid metabolism (E70-E72)

specific findings indicating disorder of carbohydrate metabolism (E73-E74)

✓4th R80 Proteinuria

EXCLUDES 1   *gestational proteinuria (O12.1-)*

R80.0 Isolated proteinuria

Idiopathic proteinuria

EXCLUDES 1   *isolated proteinuria with specific morphological lesion (N06.-)*

R80.1 Persistent proteinuria, unspecified

R80.2 Orthostatic proteinuria, unspecified

Postural proteinuria

R80.3 Bence Jones proteinuria

R80.8 Other proteinuria

R80.9 Proteinuria, unspecified

Albuminuria NOS

R81 Glycosuria

EXCLUDES 1   *renal glycosuria (E74.8)*

✓4th R82 Other and unspecified abnormal findings in urine

Chromoabnormalities in urine

Use additional code to identify any retained foreign body, if applicable (Z18.-)

EXCLUDES 2   *hematuria (R31.-)*

R82.0 Chyluria

EXCLUDES 1   *filarial chyluria (B74.-)*

R82.1 Myoglobinuria

R82.2 Biliuria

R82.3 Hemoglobinuria

EXCLUDES 1   *hemoglobinuria due to hemolysis from external causes NEC (D59.6)*

hemoglobinuria due to paroxysmal nocturnal [Marchiafava-Micheli] (D59.5)

R82.4 Acetonuria

Ketonuria

☑ Additional Character Required   ✓x7th Placeholder Alert   Unspecified Dx   Other Specified Dx   Manifestation   ▶◀ Revised Text   ● New Code   ▲ Revised Code Title

R82.5 Elevated urine levels of drugs, medicaments and biological substances
Elevated urine levels of catecholamines
Elevated urine levels of indoleacetic acid
Elevated urine levels of 17-ketosteroids
Elevated urine levels of steroids

R82.6 Abnormal urine levels of substances chiefly nonmedicinal as to source
Abnormal urine level of heavy metals

R82.7 Abnormal findings on microbiological examination of urine
Positive culture findings of urine
EXCLUDES 1 colonization status (Z22.-)

R82.8 Abnormal findings on cytological and histological examination of urine

✓5ᵗʰ **R82.9 Other and unspecified abnormal findings in urine**

R82.90 Unspecified abnormal findings in urine

R82.91 Other chromoabnormalities of urine
Chromoconversion (dipstick)
Idiopathic dipstick converts positive for blood with no cellular forms in sediment
EXCLUDES 1 hemoglobinuria (R82.3)
myoglobinuria (R82.1)

R82.99 Other abnormal findings in urine
Cells and casts in urine
Crystalluria
Melanuria

Abnormal findings on examination of other body fluids, substances and tissues, without diagnosis (R83-R89)

EXCLUDES 1 abnormal findings on antenatal screening of mother (O28.-)
diagnostic abnormal findings classified elsewhere—see Alphabetical Index
EXCLUDES 2 abnormal findings on examination of blood, without diagnosis (R70-R79)
abnormal findings on examination of urine, without diagnosis (R80-R82)
abnormal tumor markers (R97.-)

✓4ᵗʰ **R83 Abnormal findings in cerebrospinal fluid**

R83.0 Abnormal level of enzymes in cerebrospinal fluid

R83.1 Abnormal level of hormones in cerebrospinal fluid

R83.2 Abnormal level of other drugs, medicaments and biological substances in cerebrospinal fluid

R83.3 Abnormal level of substances chiefly nonmedicinal as to source in cerebrospinal fluid

R83.4 Abnormal immunological findings in cerebrospinal fluid

R83.5 Abnormal microbiological findings in cerebrospinal fluid
Positive culture findings in cerebrospinal fluid
EXCLUDES 1 colonization status (Z22.-)

R83.6 Abnormal cytological findings in cerebrospinal fluid

R83.8 Other abnormal findings in cerebrospinal fluid
Abnormal chromosomal findings in cerebrospinal fluid

R83.9 Unspecified abnormal finding in cerebrospinal fluid

✓4ᵗʰ **R84 Abnormal findings in specimens from respiratory organs and thorax**
Abnormal findings in bronchial washings
Abnormal findings in nasal secretions
Abnormal findings in pleural fluid
Abnormal findings in sputum
Abnormal findings in throat scrapings
EXCLUDES 1 blood-stained sputum (R04.2)

R84.0 Abnormal level of enzymes in specimens from respiratory organs and thorax

R84.1 Abnormal level of hormones in specimens from respiratory organs and thorax

R84.2 Abnormal level of other drugs, medicaments and biological substances in specimens from respiratory organs and thorax

R84.3 Abnormal level of substances chiefly nonmedicinal as to source in specimens from respiratory organs and thorax

R84.4 Abnormal immunological findings in specimens from respiratory organs and thorax

R84.5 Abnormal microbiological findings in specimens from respiratory organs and thorax
Positive culture findings in specimens from respiratory organs and thorax
EXCLUDES 1 colonization status (Z22.-)

R84.6 Abnormal cytological findings in specimens from respiratory organs and thorax

R84.7 Abnormal histological findings in specimens from respiratory organs and thorax

R84.8 Other abnormal findings in specimens from respiratory organs and thorax
Abnormal chromosomal findings in specimens from respiratory organs and thorax

R84.9 Unspecified abnormal finding in specimens from respiratory organs and thorax

✓4ᵗʰ **R85 Abnormal findings in specimens from digestive organs and abdominal cavity**
INCLUDES abnormal findings in peritoneal fluid
abnormal findings in saliva
EXCLUDES 1 cloudy peritoneal dialysis effluent (R88.0)
fecal abnormalities (R19.5)

R85.0 Abnormal level of enzymes in specimens from digestive organs and abdominal cavity

R85.1 Abnormal level of hormones in specimens from digestive organs and abdominal cavity

R85.2 Abnormal level of other drugs, medicaments and biological substances in specimens from digestive organs and abdominal cavity

R85.3 Abnormal level of substances chiefly nonmedicinal as to source in specimens from digestive organs and abdominal cavity

R85.4 Abnormal immunological findings in specimens from digestive organs and abdominal cavity

R85.5 Abnormal microbiological findings in specimens from digestive organs and abdominal cavity
Positive culture findings in specimens from digestive organs and abdominal cavity
EXCLUDES 1 colonization status (Z22.-)

✓5ᵗʰ **R85.6 Abnormal cytological findings in specimens from digestive organs and abdominal cavity**

✓6ᵗʰ **R85.61 Abnormal cytologic smear of anus**
EXCLUDES 1 abnormal cytological findings in specimens from other digestive organs and abdominal cavity (R85.69)
anal intraepithelial neoplasia I [AIN I] (K62.82)
anal intraepithelial neoplasia II [AIN II] (K62.82)
anal intraepithelial neoplasia III [AIN III] (D01.3)
carcinoma in situ of anus (histologically confirmed) (D01.3)
dysplasia (mild) (moderate) of anus (histologically confirmed) (K62.82)
severe dysplasia of anus (histologically confirmed) (D01.3)
EXCLUDES 2 anal high risk human papillomavirus (HPV) DNA test positive (R85.81)
anal low risk human papillomavirus (HPV) DNA test positive (R85.82)

R85.610 Atypical squamous cells of undetermined significance on cytologic smear of anus [ASC-US]

R85.611 Atypical squamous cells cannot exclude high grade squamous intraepithelial lesion on cytologic smear of anus [ASC-H]

R85.612 Low grade squamous intraepithelial lesion on cytologic smear of anus [LGSIL]

R85.613 High grade squamous intraepithelial lesion on cytologic smear of anus [HGSIL]

R85.614 Cytologic evidence of malignancy on smear of anus

R85.615 Unsatisfactory cytologic smear of anus
Inadequate sample of cytologic smear of anus

R85.616 Satisfactory anal smear but lacking transformation zone

R85.618 Other abnormal cytological findings on specimens from anus

R85.619 Unspecified abnormal cytological findings in specimens from anus
Abnormal anal cytology NOS
Atypical glandular cells of anus NOS

R85.69 Abnormal cytological findings in specimens from other digestive organs and abdominal cavity

R85.7 Abnormal histological findings in specimens from digestive organs and abdominal cavity

---

EXCLUDES 1 Not coded here   *EXCLUDES 2* Not included here   ℕ Newborn Age: 0   ℙ Pediatric Age: 0-17   Ⓜ Maternity Age: 12-55   Ⓐ Adult Age: 15-124

834
ICD-10-CM 2016

☑5ᵗʰ **R85.8** Other abnormal findings in specimens from digestive organs and abdominal cavity

    R85.81 Anal high risk human papillomavirus [HPV] DNA test positive

       EXCLUDES 1   anogenital warts due to human papillomavirus (HPV) (A63.0)
            condyloma acuminatum (A63.0)

    R85.82 Anal low risk human papillomavirus [HPV] DNA test positive

       Use additional code for associated human papillomavirus (B97.7)

    R85.89 Other abnormal findings in specimens from digestive organs and abdominal cavity

       Abnormal chromosomal findings in specimens from digestive organs and abdominal cavity

R85.9 Unspecified abnormal finding in specimens from digestive organs and abdominal cavity

☑4ᵗʰ **R86** Abnormal findings in specimens from male genital organs

    INCLUDES   abnormal findings in prostatic secretions
            abnormal findings in semen, seminal fluid
            abnormal spermatozoa

    EXCLUDES 1   azoospermia (N46.0-)
            oligospermia (N46.1-)

R86.0 Abnormal level of enzymes in specimens from male genital organs   ♂

R86.1 Abnormal level of hormones in specimens from male genital organs   ♂

R86.2 Abnormal level of other drugs, medicaments and biological substances in specimens from male genital organs   ♂

R86.3 Abnormal level of substances chiefly nonmedicinal as to source in specimens from male genital organs   ♂

R86.4 Abnormal immunological findings in specimens from male genital organs   ♂

R86.5 Abnormal microbiological findings in specimens from male genital organs   ♂

    Positive culture findings in specimens from male genital organs

    EXCLUDES 1   colonization status (Z22.-)

R86.6 Abnormal cytological findings in specimens from male genital organs   ♂

R86.7 Abnormal histological findings in specimens from male genital organs   ♂

R86.8 Other abnormal findings in specimens from male genital organs   ♂

    Abnormal chromosomal findings in specimens from male genital organs

R86.9 Unspecified abnormal finding in specimens from male genital organs   ♂

☑4ᵗʰ **R87** Abnormal findings in specimens from female genital organs

    Abnormal findings in secretion and smears from cervix uteri
    Abnormal findings in secretion and smears from vagina
    Abnormal findings in secretion and smears from vulva

R87.0 Abnormal level of enzymes in specimens from female genital organs   ♀

R87.1 Abnormal level of hormones in specimens from female genital organs   ♀

R87.2 Abnormal level of other drugs, medicaments and biological substances in specimens from female genital organs   ♀

R87.3 Abnormal level of substances chiefly nonmedicinal as to source in specimens from female genital organs   ♀

R87.4 Abnormal immunological findings in specimens from female genital organs   ♀

R87.5 Abnormal microbiological findings in specimens from female genital organs   ♀

    Positive culture findings in specimens from female genital organs

    EXCLUDES 1   colonization status (Z22.-)

☑5ᵗʰ **R87.6** Abnormal cytological findings in specimens from female genital organs

    ☑6ᵗʰ **R87.61** Abnormal cytological findings in specimens from cervix uteri

       EXCLUDES 1   abnormal cytological findings in specimens from other female genital organs (R87.69)
            abnormal cytological findings in specimens from vagina (R87.62-)
            carcinoma in situ of cervix uteri (histologically confirmed) (D06.-)
            cervical intraepithelial neoplasia I [CIN I] (N87.0)
            cervical intraepithelial neoplasia II [CIN II] (N87.1)
            cervical intraepithelial neoplasia III [CIN III] (D06.-)
            dysplasia (mild) (moderate) of cervix uteri (histologically confirmed) (N87.-)
            severe dysplasia of cervix uteri (histologically confirmed) (D06.-)

       EXCLUDES 2   cervical high risk human papillomavirus (HPV) DNA test positive (R87.810)
            cervical low risk human papillomavirus (HPV) DNA test positive (R87.820)

    R87.610 Atypical squamous cells of undetermined significance on cytologic smear of cervix [ASC-US]   ♀

    R87.611 Atypical squamous cells cannot exclude high grade squamous intraepithelial lesion on cytologic smear of cervix [ASC-H]   ♀

    R87.612 Low grade squamous intraepithelial lesion on cytologic smear of cervix [LGSIL]   ♀

    R87.613 High grade squamous intraepithelial lesion on cytologic smear of cervix [HGSIL]   ♀

    R87.614 Cytologic evidence of malignancy on smear of cervix   ♀

    R87.615 Unsatisfactory cytologic smear of cervix   ♀

       Inadequate sample of cytologic smear of cervix

    R87.616 Satisfactory cervical smear but lacking transformation zone   ♀

    R87.618 Other abnormal cytological findings on specimens from cervix uteri   ♀

    R87.619 Unspecified abnormal cytological findings in specimens from cervix uteri   ♀

       Abnormal cervical cytology NOS
       Abnormal Papanicolaou smear of cervix NOS
       Abnormal thin preparation smear of cervix NOS
       Atypical endocervical cells of cervix NOS
       Atypical endometrial cells of cervix NOS
       Atypical glandular cells of cervix NOS

☑ Additional Character Required   ☑7ᵗʰ Placeholder Alert   Unspecified Dx   Other Specified Dx   Manifestation   ►◄ Revised Text   ● New Code   ▲ Revised Code Title

Chapter 18. Symptoms, Signs, and Abnormal Clinical and Laboratory Findings, Not Elsewhere Classified

✓6ᵗʰ **R87.62** **Abnormal cytological findings in specimens from vagina**

Use additional code to identify acquired absence of uterus and cervix, if applicable (Z90.71-)

EXCLUDES 1   *abnormal cytological findings in specimens from cervix uteri (R87.61-)*

abnormal cytological findings in specimens from other female genital organs (R87.69)

carcinoma in situ of vagina (histologically confirmed) (D07.2)

dysplasia (mild) (moderate) of vagina (histologically confirmed) (N89.-)

severe dysplasia of vagina (histologically confirmed) (D07.2)

vaginal intraepithelial neoplasia I [VAIN I] (N89.0)

vaginal intraepithelial neoplasia II [VAIN II] (N09.1)

vaginal intraepithelial neoplasia III [VAIN III] (D07.2)

EXCLUDES 2   *vaginal high risk human papillomavirus (HPV) DNA test positive (R87.811)*

vaginal low risk human papillomavirus (HPV) DNA test positive (R87.821)

R87.620 **Atypical squamous cells of undetermined significance on cytologic smear of vagina [ASC-US]** ♀

R87.621 **Atypical squamous cells cannot exclude high grade squamous intraepithelial lesion on cytologic smear of vagina [ASC-H]** ♀

R87.622 **Low grade squamous intraepithelial lesion on cytologic smear of vagina [LGSIL]** ♀

R87.623 **High grade squamous intraepithelial lesion on cytologic smear of vagina [HGSIL]** ♀

R87.624 **Cytologic evidence of malignancy on smear of vagina** ♀

R87.625 **Unsatisfactory cytologic smear of vagina** ♀

Inadequate sample of cytologic smear of vagina

R87.628 **Other abnormal cytological findings on specimens from vagina** ♀

R87.629 **Unspecified abnormal cytological findings in specimens from vagina** ♀

Abnormal Papanicolaou smear of vagina NOS

Abnormal thin preparation smear of vagina NOS

Abnormal vaginal cytology NOS

Atypical endocervical cells of vagina NOS

Atypical endometrial cells of vagina NOS

Atypical glandular cells of vagina NOS

R87.69 **Abnormal cytological findings in specimens from other female genital organs** ♀

Abnormal cytological findings in specimens from female genital organs NOS

EXCLUDES 1   *dysplasia of vulva (histologically confirmed) (N90.0-N90.3)*

R87.7 **Abnormal histological findings in specimens from female genital organs** ♀

EXCLUDES 1   *carcinoma in situ (histologically confirmed) of female genital organs (D06-D07.3)*

cervical intraepithelial neoplasia I [CIN I] (N87.0)

cervical intraepithelial neoplasia II [CIN II] (N87.1)

cervical intraepithelial neoplasia III [CIN III] (D06.-)

dysplasia (mild) (moderate) of cervix uteri (histologically confirmed) (N87.-)

dysplasia (mild) (moderate) of vagina (histologically confirmed) (N89.-)

severe dysplasia of cervix uteri (histologically confirmed) (D06.-)

severe dysplasia of vagina (histologically confirmed) (D07.2)

vaginal intraepithelial neoplasia I [VAIN I] (N89.0)

vaginal intraepithelial neoplasia II [VAIN II] (N89.1)

vaginal intraepithelial neoplasia III [VAIN III] (D07.2)

✓5ᵗʰ **R87.8** **Other abnormal findings in specimens from female genital organs**

✓6ᵗʰ **R87.81** **High risk human papillomavirus [HPV] DNA test positive from female genital organs**

EXCLUDES 1   *anogenital warts due to human papillomavirus (HPV) (A63.0)*

condyloma acuminatum (A63.0)

R87.810 **Cervical high risk human papillomavirus [HPV] DNA test positive** ♀

R87.811 **Vaginal high risk human papillomavirus [HPV] DNA test positive** ♀

✓6ᵗʰ **R87.82** **Low risk human papillomavirus [HPV] DNA test positive from female genital organs**

Use additional code for associated human papillomavirus (B97.7)

R87.820 **Cervical low risk human papillomavirus [HPV] DNA test positive** ♀

R87.821 **Vaginal low risk human papillomavirus [HPV] DNA test positive** ♀

R87.89 **Other abnormal findings in specimens from female genital organs** ♀

Abnormal chromosomal findings in specimens from female genital organs

R87.9 **Unspecified abnormal finding in specimens from female genital organs** ♀

✓4ᵗʰ **R88** **Abnormal findings in other body fluids and substances**

R88.0 **Cloudy (hemodialysis) (peritoneal) dialysis effluent**

R88.8 **Abnormal findings in other body fluids and substances**

✓4ᵗʰ **R89** **Abnormal findings in specimens from other organs, systems and tissues**

INCLUDES   abnormal findings in nipple discharge

abnormal findings in synovial fluid

abnormal findings in wound secretions

R89.0 **Abnormal level of enzymes in specimens from other organs, systems and tissues**

R89.1 **Abnormal level of hormones in specimens from other organs, systems and tissues**

R89.2 **Abnormal level of other drugs, medicaments and biological substances in specimens from other organs, systems and tissues**

R89.3 **Abnormal level of substances chiefly nonmedicinal as to source in specimens from other organs, systems and tissues**

R89.4 **Abnormal immunological findings in specimens from other organs, systems and tissues**

R89.5 **Abnormal microbiological findings in specimens from other organs, systems and tissues**

Positive culture findings in specimens from other organs, systems and tissues

EXCLUDES 1   *colonization status (Z22.-)*

R89.6 **Abnormal cytological findings in specimens from other organs, systems and tissues**

R89.7 **Abnormal histological findings in specimens from other organs, systems and tissues**

R89.8 **Other abnormal findings in specimens from other organs, systems and tissues**

Abnormal chromosomal findings in specimens from other organs, systems and tissues

R89.9 **Unspecified abnormal finding in specimens from other organs, systems and tissues**

EXCLUDES 1 Not coded here   EXCLUDES 2 Not included here   N Newborn Age: 0   P Pediatric Age: 0-17   M Maternity Age: 12-55   A Adult Age: 15-124

836

ICD-10-CM 2016

R87.62–R89.9

Abnormal findings on diagnostic imaging and in function studies, without diagnosis (R90-R94)

INCLUDES	nonspecific abnormal findings on diagnostic imaging by computerized axial tomography [CAT scan]
	nonspecific abnormal findings on diagnostic imaging by magnetic resonance imaging [MRI][NMR]
	nonspecific abnormal findings on diagnostic imaging by positron emission tomography [PET scan]
	nonspecific abnormal findings on diagnostic imaging by thermography
	nonspecific abnormal findings on diagnostic imaging by ultrasound [echogram]
	nonspecific abnormal findings on diagnostic imaging by X-ray examination

EXCLUDES 1   abnormal findings on antenatal screening of mother (O28.-)
          diagnostic abnormal findings classified elsewhere—see Alphabetical Index

✓4th R90   Abnormal findings on diagnostic imaging of central nervous system

R90.0   Intracranial space-occupying lesion found on diagnostic imaging of central nervous system

✓5th R90.8   Other abnormal findings on diagnostic imaging of central nervous system

     R90.81   Abnormal echoencephalogram

     R90.82   White matter disease, unspecified

     R90.89   Other abnormal findings on diagnostic imaging of central nervous system
            Other cerebrovascular abnormality found on diagnostic imaging of central nervous system

✓4th R91   Abnormal findings on diagnostic imaging of lung

R91.1   Solitary pulmonary nodule
      Coin lesion lung
      Solitary pulmonary nodule, subsegmental branch of the bronchial tree

R91.8   Other nonspecific abnormal finding of lung field
      Lung mass NOS found on diagnostic imaging of lung
      Pulmonary infiltrate NOS
      Shadow, lung

✓4th R92   Abnormal and inconclusive findings on diagnostic imaging of breast

R92.0   Mammographic microcalcification found on diagnostic imaging of breast
     EXCLUDES 2   mammographic calcification (calculus) found on diagnostic imaging of breast (R92.1)

R92.1   Mammographic calcification found on diagnostic imaging of breast
      Mammographic calculus found on diagnostic imaging of breast

R92.2   Inconclusive mammogram
      Dense breasts NOS
      Inconclusive mammogram NEC
      Inconclusive mammography due to dense breasts
      Inconclusive mammography NEC
      AHA: 2015, 1Q, 24

R92.8   Other abnormal and inconclusive findings on diagnostic imaging of breast

✓4th R93   Abnormal findings on diagnostic imaging of other body structures

R93.0   Abnormal findings on diagnostic imaging of skull and head, not elsewhere classified
     EXCLUDES 1   intracranial space-occupying lesion found on diagnostic imaging (R90.0)

R93.1   Abnormal findings on diagnostic imaging of heart and coronary circulation
      Abnormal echocardiogram NOS
      Abnormal heart shadow

R93.2   Abnormal findings on diagnostic imaging of liver and biliary tract
      Nonvisualization of gallbladder

R93.3   Abnormal findings on diagnostic imaging of other parts of digestive tract

R93.4   Abnormal findings on diagnostic imaging of urinary organs
      Filling defect of bladder found on diagnostic imaging
      Filling defect of kidney found on diagnostic imaging
      Filling defect of ureter found on diagnostic imaging
     EXCLUDES 1   hypertrophy of kidney (N28.81)

R93.5   Abnormal findings on diagnostic imaging of other abdominal regions, including retroperitoneum

R93.6   Abnormal findings on diagnostic imaging of limbs
     EXCLUDES 2   abnormal finding in skin and subcutaneous tissue (R93.8)

R93.7   Abnormal findings on diagnostic imaging of other parts of musculoskeletal system
     EXCLUDES 2   abnormal findings on diagnostic imaging of skull (R93.0)

R93.8   Abnormal findings on diagnostic imaging of other specified body structures
      Abnormal finding by radioisotope localization of placenta
      Abnormal radiological finding in skin and subcutaneous tissue
      Mediastinal shift

R93.9   Diagnostic imaging inconclusive due to excess body fat of patient

✓4th R94   Abnormal results of function studies

INCLUDES	abnormal results of radionuclide [radioisotope] uptake studies
	abnormal results of scintigraphy

✓5th R94.0   Abnormal results of function studies of central nervous system

     R94.01   Abnormal electroencephalogram [EEG]

     R94.02   Abnormal brain scan

     R94.09   Abnormal results of other function studies of central nervous system

✓5th R94.1   Abnormal results of function studies of peripheral nervous system and special senses

     ✓6th R94.11   Abnormal results of function studies of eye

         R94.110   Abnormal electro-oculogram [EOG]

         R94.111   Abnormal electroretinogram [ERG]
             Abnormal retinal function study

         R94.112   Abnormal visually evoked potential [VEP]

         R94.113   Abnormal oculomotor study

         R94.118   Abnormal results of other function studies of eye

     ✓6th R94.12   Abnormal results of function studies of ear and other special senses

         R94.120   Abnormal auditory function study

         R94.121   Abnormal vestibular function study

         R94.128   Abnormal results of other function studies of ear and other special senses

     ✓6th R94.13   Abnormal results of function studies of peripheral nervous system

         R94.130   Abnormal response to nerve stimulation, unspecified

         R94.131   Abnormal electromyogram [EMG]
            EXCLUDES 1   electromyogram of eye (R94.113)

         R94.138   Abnormal results of other function studies of peripheral nervous system

R94.2   Abnormal results of pulmonary function studies
      Reduced ventilatory capacity
      Reduced vital capacity

✓5th R94.3   Abnormal results of cardiovascular function studies

     R94.30   Abnormal result of cardiovascular function study, unspecified

     R94.31   Abnormal electrocardiogram [ECG] [EKG]
         EXCLUDES 1   long QT syndrome (I45.81)

     R94.39   Abnormal result of other cardiovascular function study
         Abnormal electrophysiological intracardiac studies
         Abnormal phonocardiogram
         Abnormal vectorcardiogram

R94.4   Abnormal results of kidney function studies
      Abnormal renal function test

R94.5   Abnormal results of liver function studies

R94.6   Abnormal results of thyroid function studies

R94.7   Abnormal results of other endocrine function studies
     EXCLUDES 2   abnormal glucose (R73.0-)

R94.8   Abnormal results of function studies of other organs and systems
      Abnormal basal metabolic rate [BMR]
      Abnormal bladder function test
      Abnormal splenic function test

✓ Additional Character Required   ✓7th Placeholder Alert   Unspecified Dx   Other Specified Dx   Manifestation   ►◄ Revised Text   ● New Code   ▲ Revised Code Title

Abnormal tumor markers (R97)

R97 **Abnormal tumor markers**
    Elevated tumor associated antigens [TAA]
    Elevated tumor specific antigens [TSA]

    R97.0 **Elevated carcinoembryonic antigen [CEA]**

    R97.1 **Elevated cancer antigen 125 [CA 125]**   ♀

    R97.2 **Elevated prostate specific antigen [PSA]**   🅐 ♂

    R97.8 **Other abnormal tumor markers**

Ill-defined and unknown cause of mortality (R99)

R99 **Ill-defined and unknown cause of mortality**
    Death (unexplained) NOS
    Unspecified cause of mortality

EXCLUDES 1 Not coded here   EXCLUDES 2 Not included here   N Newborn Age: 0   P Pediatric Age: 0-17   M Maternity Age: 12-55   A Adult Age: 15-124

838

ICD-10-CM 2016

Chapter 19. Injury, Poisoning, and Certain Other Consequences of External Causes (S00–T88)

Chapter Specific Guidelines with Coding Examples

The chapter specific guidelines from the ICD-10-CM Official Guidelines for Coding and Reporting have been provided below. Along with these guidelines are coding examples, contained in the shaded boxes, that have been developed to help illustrate the coding and/or sequencing guidance found in these guidelines.

a. Application of 7th Characters in Chapter 19

Most categories in chapter 19 have a 7th character requirement for each applicable code. Most categories in this chapter have three 7th character values (with the exception of fractures): A, initial encounter, D, subsequent encounter and S, sequela. Categories for traumatic fractures have additional 7th character values. While the patient may be seen by a new or different provider over the course of treatment for an injury, assignment of the 7th character is based on whether the patient is undergoing active treatment and not whether the provider is seeing the patient for the first time.

For complication codes, active treatment refers to treatment for the condition described by the code, even though it may be related to an earlier precipitating problem. For example, code T84.50XA, Infection and inflammatory reaction due to unspecified internal joint prosthesis, initial encounter, is used when active treatment is provided for the infection, even though the condition relates to the prosthetic device, implant or graft that was placed at a previous encounter.

7th character "A", initial encounter is used while the patient is receiving active treatment for the condition. Examples of active treatment are: surgical treatment, emergency department encounter, and evaluation and continuing treatment by the same or a different physician.

> Patient admitted after fall from a skateboard onto the sidewalk, x-rays identify a nondisplaced fracture to the distal pole of the right scaphoid bone. The patient is placed in a cast.
>
> **S62.014A**   **Nondisplaced fracture of distal pole of navicular [scaphoid] bone of right wrist, initial encounter for closed fracture**
>
> **V00.131A**   **Fall from skateboard, initial encounter**
>
> **Y92.480**   **Sidewalk as the place of occurrence of the external cause**
>
> **Y93.51**   **Activity, roller skating (inline) and skateboarding**
>
> **Y99.8**   **Other external cause status**
>
> *Explanation:* This fracture would be coded with a seventh character A for initial encounter because the patient received x-rays to identify the site of the fracture and treatment was rendered; this would be considered active treatment.

7th character "D" subsequent encounter is used for encounters after the patient has received active treatment of the condition and is receiving routine care for the condition during the healing or recovery phase. Examples of subsequent care are: cast change or removal, an x-ray to check healing status of fracture, removal of external or internal fixation device, medication adjustment, other aftercare and follow up visits following treatment of the injury or condition.

> Patient admitted after fall from a skateboard onto the sidewalk resulted in casting of the right arm. X-rays are taken to evaluate how well the nondisplaced fracture to the distal pole of the right scaphoid bone is healing. The physician feels the fracture is healing appropriately; no adjustments to the cast are made.
>
> **S62.014D**   **Nondisplaced fracture of distal pole of navicular [scaphoid] bone of right wrist, subsequent encounter for fracture with routine healing**
>
> **V00.131D**   **Fall from skateboard, subsequent encounter**
>
> *Explanation:* This fracture would be coded with a seventh character D for subsequent encounter, whether the same physician who provided the initial cast application or a different physician is now seeing the patient. Although the patient received x-rays, the intent of the x-rays was to assess how the fracture was healing. There was no active treatment rendered and the visit is therefore considered a subsequent encounter.

The aftercare Z codes should not be used for aftercare for conditions such as injuries or poisonings, where 7th characters are provided to identify subsequent care. For example, for aftercare of an injury, assign the acute injury code with the 7th character "D" (subsequent encounter).

7th character "S", sequela, is for use for complications or conditions that arise as a direct result of a condition, such as scar formation after a burn. The scars are sequelae of the burn. When using 7th character "S", it is necessary to use both the injury code that precipitated the sequela and the code for the sequela itself. The "S" is added only to the injury code, not the sequela code. The 7th character "S" identifies the injury responsible for the sequela. The specific type of sequela (e.g. scar) is sequenced first, followed by the injury code.

See Section I.B.10 Sequelae, (Late Effects)

> Patient with a history of a nondisplaced fracture to the distal pole of the right scaphoid bone due to a fall from a skateboard is admitted for evaluation of arthritis to the right wrist that has developed as a consequence of the traumatic fracture.
>
> **M12.531**   **Traumatic arthropathy, right wrist**
>
> **S62.014S**   **Nondisplaced fracture of distal pole of navicular [scaphoid] bone of right wrist, sequela**
>
> **V00.131S**   **Fall from skateboard, sequela**
>
> *Explanation:* The code identifying the specific sequela condition (traumatic arthritis) should be coded first followed by the injury that instigated the development of the sequela (fracture). The scaphoid fracture injury code is given a 7th character S for sequela to represent its role as the inciting injury. The fracture has healed and is not being managed or treated on this admit and therefore is not applicable as a first listed or principal diagnosis. However, it is directly related to the development of the arthritis and should be appended as a secondary code to signify this cause and effect relationship.

b. Coding of injuries

When coding injuries, assign separate codes for each injury unless a combination code is provided, in which case the combination code is assigned. Code T07, Unspecified multiple injuries should not be assigned in the inpatient setting unless information for a more specific code is not available. Traumatic injury codes (S00-T14.9) are not to be used for normal, healing surgical wounds or to identify complications of surgical wounds.

> 11-year-old girl fell from her horse, resulting in a laceration to her right forearm with several large pieces of wooden fragments embedded in the wound as well as abrasions to her right ear; in addition, her right shoulder was dislocated
>
> **S43.004A**   **Unspecified dislocation of right shoulder joint, initial encounter**
>
> **S51.821A**   **Laceration with foreign body of right forearm, initial encounter**
>
> **S00.411A**   **Abrasion of right ear, initial encounter**
>
> **V80.010A**   **Animal-rider injured by fall from or being thrown from horse in noncollision accident, initial encounter**
>
> **Y93.52**   **Activity, horseback riding**
>
> *Explanation:* Each separate injury should be reported. The patient's injury to the forearm is reported with one combination code that captures both the laceration and the foreign body.

The code for the most serious injury, as determined by the provider and the focus of treatment, is sequenced first.

1) Superficial injuries

Superficial injuries such as abrasions or contusions are not coded when associated with more severe injuries of the same site.

2) Primary injury with damage to nerves/blood vessels

When a primary injury results in minor damage to peripheral nerves or blood vessels, the primary injury is sequenced first with additional code(s) for injuries to nerves and spinal cord (such as category S04), and/or injury to blood vessels (such as category S15). When the primary injury is to the blood vessels or nerves, that injury should be sequenced first.

Chapter 19. Injury, Poisoning, and Certain Other Consequences of External Causes

c. Coding of traumatic fractures

The principles of multiple coding of injuries should be followed in coding fractures. Fractures of specified sites are coded individually by site in accordance with both the provisions within categories S02, S12, S22, S32, S42, S49, S52, S59, S62, S72, S79, S82, S89, S92 and the level of detail furnished by medical record content.

A fracture not indicated as open or closed should be coded to closed. A fracture not indicated whether displaced or not displaced should be coded to displaced.

More specific guidelines are as follows:

1) Initial vs. Subsequent Encounter for Fractures

Traumatic fractures are coded using the appropriate 7th character for initial encounter (A, B, C) while the patient is receiving active treatment for the fracture. Examples of active treatment are: surgical treatment, emergency department encounter, and evaluation and continuing (ongoing) treatment by the same or different physician. The appropriate 7th character for initial encounter should also be assigned for a patient who delayed seeking treatment for the fracture or nonunion.

Fractures are coded using the appropriate 7th character for subsequent care for encounters after the patient has completed active treatment of the fracture and is receiving routine care for the fracture during the healing or recovery phase. Examples of fracture aftercare are: cast change or removal, an x-ray to check healing status of fracture, removal of external or internal fixation device, medication adjustment, and follow-up visits following fracture treatment.

Care for complications of surgical treatment for fracture repairs during the healing or recovery phase should be coded with the appropriate complication codes.

Care of complications of fractures, such as malunion and nonunion, should be reported with the appropriate 7th character for subsequent care with nonunion (K, M, N,) or subsequent care with malunion (P, Q, R).

Malunion/nonunion: The appropriate 7th character for initial encounter should also be assigned for a patient who delayed seeking treatment for the fracture or nonunion.

Female patient fell during a hiking excursion almost six months ago and until recently did not feel she needed to seek medical attention for her left ankle pain; x-rays show nonunion of lateral malleolus and surgery has been scheduled

S82.862A	**Displaced Maisonneuve's fracture of left leg, initial encounter for closed fracture**
W01.0XXA	**Fall on same level from slipping, tripping and stumbling without subsequent striking against object, initial encounter**
Y92.821	**Forest as place of occurrence of the external cause**
Y93.01	**Activity, walking, marching and hiking**
Y99.8	**Other external cause status**

Explanation: A seventh character of A is used for the lateral malleolus nonunion fracture to signify that the fracture is receiving active treatment. The delayed care for the fracture has resulted in a nonunion, but capturing the nonunion in the seventh character is trumped by the provision of active care.

A code from category M80, not a traumatic fracture code, should be used for any patient with known osteoporosis who suffers a fracture, even if the patient had a minor fall or trauma, if that fall or trauma would not usually break a normal, healthy bone.

See Section I.C.13. Osteoporosis.

The aftercare Z codes should not be used for aftercare for traumatic fractures. For aftercare of a traumatic fracture, assign the acute fracture code with the appropriate 7th character.

2) Multiple fractures sequencing

Multiple fractures are sequenced in accordance with the severity of the fracture.

d. Coding of burns and corrosions

The ICD-10-CM makes a distinction between burns and corrosions. The burn codes are for thermal burns, except sunburns, that come from a heat source, such as a fire or hot appliance. The burn codes are also for burns resulting from electricity and radiation. Corrosions are burns due to chemicals. The guidelines are the same for burns and corrosions.

Current burns (T20-T25) are classified by depth, extent and by agent (X code). Burns are classified by depth as first degree (erythema), second

---

degree (blistering), and third degree (full-thickness involvement). Burns of the eye and internal organs (T26-T28) are classified by site, but not by degree.

1) Sequencing of burn and related condition codes

Sequence first the code that reflects the highest degree of burn when more than one burn is present.

a. When the reason for the admission or encounter is for treatment of external multiple burns, sequence first the code that reflects the burn of the highest degree.

b. When a patient has both internal and external burns, the circumstances of admission govern the selection of the principal diagnosis or first-listed diagnosis.

c. When a patient is admitted for burn injuries and other related conditions such as smoke inhalation and/or respiratory failure the circumstances of admission govern the selection of the principal or first-listed diagnosis.

Patient admitted with minor first-degree burns to multiple sites of her right and left hands as well as severe smoke inhalation. While she was sleeping at home, a candle on her dresser lit the bedroom curtains on fire.

T59.811A	**Toxic effect of smoke, accidental (unintentional), initial encounter**
J70.5	**Respiratory conditions due to smoke inhalation**
T23.191A	**Burn of first degree of multiple sites of right wrist and hand, initial encounter**
T23.192A	**Burn of first degree of multiple sites of left wrist and hand, initial encounter**
X08.8XXA	**Exposure to other specified smoke, fire and flames, initial encounter**
Y92.003	**Bedroom of unspecified non-institutional (private) residence as the place of occurrence of the external cause**
Y93.84	**Activity, sleeping**

Explanation: Based on the documentation, the inhalation injury is more severe than the first-degree burns and is sequenced first. The burns to the hands are appended as secondary diagnoses.

---

2) Burns of the same local site

Classify burns of the same local site (three-character category level, T20-T28) but of different degrees to the subcategory identifying the highest degree recorded in the diagnosis.

10-year-old male patient is admitted for third-degree burns of his right palm and second-degree burns of multiple right fingers; right thumb not affected

T23.351A	**Burn of third degree of right palm, initial encounter**

Explanation: Although there is a code for second-degree burns of multiple fingers, not including the thumb (T23.131-), this code falls in the same three-digit category that the third-degree burn of the right palm falls under, category T23. Only the subcategory identifying the highest degree is captured when different burn degrees are classified to a single category.

Patient is admitted with third-degree burns of the scalp as well as second-degree burns to the back of the right hand

T20.35XA	**Burn of third degree of scalp [any part], initial encounter**
T23.261A	**Burn of second degree of back of right hand, initial encounter**

Explanation: Since burns to the hand and scalp are classified to two different three-digit categories, both burns may be reported as they represent distinct sites.

---

3) Non-healing burns

Non-healing burns are coded as acute burns.

Necrosis of burned skin should be coded as a non-healed burn.

4) Infected burn

For any documented infected burn site, use an additional code for the infection.

5) Assign separate codes for each burn site

When coding burns, assign separate codes for each burn site. Category T30, Burn and corrosion, body region unspecified is extremely vague and should rarely be used.

6) Burns and Corrosions Classified According to Extent of Body Surface Involved

Assign codes from category T31, Burns classified according to extent of body surface involved, or T32, Corrosions classified according to extent of body surface involved, when the site of the burn is not specified or when there is a need for additional data. It is advisable to use category T31 as additional coding when needed to provide data for evaluating burn mortality, such as that needed by burn units. It is also advisable to use category T31 as an additional code for reporting purposes when there is mention of a third-degree burn involving 20 percent or more of the body surface.

Categories T31 and T32 are based on the classic "rule of nines" in estimating body surface involved: head and neck are assigned nine percent, each arm nine percent, each leg 18 percent, the anterior trunk 18 percent, posterior trunk 18 percent, and genitalia one percent. Providers may change these percentage assignments where necessary to accommodate infants and children who have proportionately larger heads than adults, and patients who have large buttocks, thighs, or abdomen that involve burns.

> Patient seen for dressing change after he accidentally spilled acetic acid on himself two days ago. The second-degree burns to his right thigh, covering about 3 percent of his body surface, are healing appropriately.
>
> | **T54.2X1D** | **Toxic effect of corrosive acids and acid-like substances, accidental (unintentional), subsequent encounter** |
> |---|---|
> | **T24.611D** | **Corrosion of second degree of right thigh, subsequent encounter** |
> | **T32.0** | **Corrosions involving less than 10% of body surface** |
>
> *Explanation:* Code T32.0 provides additional information as to how much of the patient's body was affected by the corrosive substance.

7) Encounters for treatment of sequela of burns

Encounters for the treatment of the late effects of burns or corrosions (i.e., scars or joint contractures) should be coded with a burn or corrosion code with the 7th character "S" for sequela.

8) Sequelae with a late effect code and current burn

When appropriate, both a code for a current burn or corrosion with 7th character "A" or "D" and a burn or corrosion code with 7th character "S" may be assigned on the same record (when both a current burn and sequelae of an old burn exist). Burns and corrosions do not heal at the same rate and a current healing wound may still exist with sequela of a healed burn or corrosion.

See Section I.B.10 Sequela (Late Effects)

> Female patient seen for second-degree burn to the left ear; she also has significant scarring on her left elbow from a third-degree burn from childhood
>
> | **T20.212A** | **Burn of second degree of left ear [any part, except ear drum], initial encounter** |
> |---|---|
> | **L90.5** | **Scar conditions and fibrosis of skin** |
> | **T22.322S** | **Burn of third degree of left elbow, sequela** |
>
> *Explanation:* The patient is being seen for management of a current second-degree burn, which is reflected in the code by appending the seventh character of A, indicating active treatment or management of this burn. The elbow scarring is a sequela of a previous third-degree burn. The sequela condition precedes the original burn injury, which is appended with a seventh character of S.

9) Use of an external cause code with burns and corrosions

An external cause code should be used with burns and corrosions to identify the source and intent of the burn, as well as the place where it occurred.

e. Adverse effects, poisoning, underdosing and toxic effects

Codes in categories T36-T65 are combination codes that include the substance that was taken as well as the intent. No additional external cause code is required for poisonings, toxic effects, adverse effects and underdosing codes.

1) Do not code directly from the Table of Drugs

Do not code directly from the Table of Drugs and Chemicals. Always refer back to the Tabular List.

2) Use as many codes as necessary to describe

Use as many codes as necessary to describe completely all drugs, medicinal or biological substances.

3) If the same code would describe the causative agent

If the same code would describe the causative agent for more than one adverse reaction, poisoning, toxic effect or underdosing, assign the code only once.

4) If two or more drugs, medicinal or biological substances

If two or more drugs, medicinal or biological substances are reported, code each individually unless a combination code is listed in the Table of Drugs and Chemicals.

5) The occurrence of drug toxicity is classified in ICD-10-CM as follows:

(a) Adverse effect

When coding an adverse effect of a drug that has been correctly prescribed and properly administered, assign the appropriate code for the nature of the adverse effect followed by the appropriate code for the adverse effect of the drug (T36-T50). The code for the drug should have a 5th or 6th character "5" (for example T36.0X5-) Examples of the nature of an adverse effect are tachycardia, delirium, gastrointestinal hemorrhaging, vomiting, hypokalemia, hepatitis, renal failure, or respiratory failure.

> Patient seen for stomach pain and jaundice, indicated by physician as possible side-effects of Inderal, recently started for hypertension. Inderal was discontinued and the patient switched to Atenolol instead.
>
> | **R10.9** | **Unspecified abdominal pain** |
> |---|---|
> | **R17** | **Unspecified jaundice** |
> | **T44.7X5A** | **Adverse effect of beta-adrenoreceptor antagonists, initial encounter** |
> | **I10** | **Essential (primary) hypertension** |
>
> *Explanation:* The side-effects caused by the drug are listed first, followed by the code for the adverse effect of the drug to capture the specific drug that was used.

(b) Poisoning

When coding a poisoning or reaction to the improper use of a medication (e.g., overdose, wrong substance given or taken in error, wrong route of administration), first assign the appropriate code from categories T36-T50. The poisoning codes have an associated intent as their 5th or 6th character (accidental, intentional self-harm, assault and undetermined. Use additional code(s) for all manifestations of poisonings.

If there is also a diagnosis of abuse or dependence of the substance, the abuse or dependence is assigned as an additional code.

Examples of poisoning include:

(i) Error was made in drug prescription

Errors made in drug prescription or in the administration of the drug by provider, nurse, patient, or other person.

(ii) Overdose of a drug intentionally taken

If an overdose of a drug was intentionally taken or administered and resulted in drug toxicity, it would be coded as a poisoning.

(iii) Nonprescribed drug taken with correctly prescribed and properly administered drug

If a nonprescribed drug or medicinal agent was taken in combination with a correctly prescribed and properly administered drug, any drug toxicity or other reaction resulting from the interaction of the two drugs would be classified as a poisoning.

(iv) Interaction of drug(s) and alcohol

When a reaction results from the interaction of a drug(s) and alcohol, this would be classified as poisoning.

See Section I.C.4. if poisoning is the result of insulin pump malfunctions.

(c) Underdosing

Underdosing refers to taking less of a medication than is prescribed by a provider or a manufacturer's instruction. For underdosing, assign the code from categories T36-T50 (fifth or sixth character "6").

Codes for underdosing should never be assigned as principal or first-listed codes. If a patient has a relapse or exacerbation of the medical condition for which the drug is prescribed because of the reduction in dose, then the medical condition itself should be coded.

Noncompliance (Z91.12-, Z91.13-) or complication of care (Y63.6-Y63.9) codes are to be used with an underdosing code to indicate intent, if known.

> Patient admitted for atrial fibrillation with history of chronic atrial fibrillation for which she is prescribed amiodarone. Financial concerns have left the patient unable to pay for her prescriptions and she has been skipping her amiodarone dose every other day to offset the cost.
>
> | I48.2 | **Chronic atrial fibrillation** |
> |---|---|
> | **T46.2X6A** | **Underdosing of other antidysrhythmic drugs, initial encounter** |
> | **Z91.120** | **Patient's intentional underdosing of medication regimen due to financial hardship** |
>
> *Explanation:* By skipping her amiodarone pill every other day, the patient's atrial fibrillation returned. The condition for which the drug was being taken is reported first, followed by an underdosing code to show that the patient was not adhering to her prescription regiment. The Z code helps elaborate on the patient's social and/or economic circumstances that led to the patient taking less then what she was prescribed.

(d) Toxic effects

When a harmful substance is ingested or comes in contact with a person, this is classified as a toxic effect. The toxic effect codes are in categories T51-T65.

Toxic effect codes have an associated intent: accidental, intentional self-harm, assault and undetermined.

f. Adult and child abuse, neglect and other maltreatment

Sequence first the appropriate code from categories T74.- (Adult and child abuse, neglect and other maltreatment, confirmed) or T76.- (Adult and child abuse, neglect and other maltreatment, suspected) for abuse, neglect and other maltreatment, followed by any accompanying mental health or injury code(s).

If the documentation in the medical record states abuse or neglect it is coded as confirmed (T74.-). It is coded as suspected if it is documented as suspected (T76.-).

For cases of confirmed abuse or neglect an external cause code from the assault section (X92-Y08) should be added to identify the cause of any physical injuries. A perpetrator code (Y07) should be added when the perpetrator of the abuse is known. For suspected cases of abuse or neglect, do not report external cause or perpetrator code.

If a suspected case of abuse, neglect or mistreatment is ruled out during an encounter code Z04.71, Encounter for examination and observation following alleged physical adult abuse, ruled out, or code Z04.72, Encounter for examination and observation following alleged child physical abuse, ruled out, should be used, not a code from T76.

If a suspected case of alleged rape or sexual abuse is ruled out during an encounter code Z04.41, Encounter for examination and observation following alleged physical adult abuse, ruled out, or code Z04.42, Encounter for examination and observation following alleged rape or sexual abuse, ruled out, should be used, not a code from T76.

See Section I.C.15. Abuse in a pregnant patient.

g. Complications of care

1) General guidelines for complications of care

(a) Documentation of complications of care

See Section I.B.16. for information on documentation of complications of care.

2) Pain due to medical devices

Pain associated with devices, implants or grafts left in a surgical site (for example painful hip prosthesis) is assigned to the appropriate code(s) found in Chapter 19, Injury, poisoning, and certain other consequences of external causes. Specific codes for pain due to medical devices are found in the T code section of the ICD-10-CM. Use additional code(s) from category G89 to identify acute or chronic pain due to presence of the device, implant or graft (G89.18 or G89.28).

> Chronic left breast pain secondary to breast implant
>
> | **T85.84XA** | **Pain due to internal prosthetic devices, implants and grafts, not elsewhere classified, initial encounter** |
> |---|---|
> | N64.4 | **Mastodynia** |
> | G89.28 | **Other chronic postprocedural pain** |
>
> *Explanation:* As the pain is a complication related to the breast implant, the complication code is sequenced first. The T code does not describe the site or type of pain, so additional codes may be appended to indicate that the patient is experiencing chronic pain in the breast.

3) Transplant complications

(a) Transplant complications other than kidney

Codes under category T86, Complications of transplanted organs and tissues, are for use for both complications and rejection of transplanted organs. A transplant complication code is only assigned if the complication affects the function of the transplanted organ. Two codes are required to fully describe a transplant complication: the appropriate code from category T86 and a secondary code that identifies the complication.

Pre-existing conditions or conditions that develop after the transplant are not coded as complications unless they affect the function of the transplanted organs.

See I.C.21. for transplant organ removal status

See I.C.2. for malignant neoplasm associated with transplanted organ

(b) Kidney transplant complications

Patients who have undergone kidney transplant may still have some form of chronic kidney disease (CKD) because the kidney transplant may not fully restore kidney function. Code T86.1- should be assigned for documented complications of a kidney transplant, such as transplant failure or rejection or other transplant complication. Code T86.1- should not be assigned for post kidney transplant patients who have chronic kidney (CKD) unless a transplant complication such as transplant failure or rejection is documented. If the documentation is unclear as to whether the patient has a complication of the transplant, query the provider.

Conditions that affect the function of the transplanted kidney, other than CKD, should be assigned a code from subcategory T86.1, Complications of transplanted organ, Kidney, and a secondary code that identifies the complication.

For patients with CKD following a kidney transplant, but who do not have a complication such as failure or rejection, *see section I.C.14. Chronic kidney disease and kidney transplant status.*

> Patient seen for chronic kidney disease stage 2; history of successful kidney transplant with no complications identified
>
> | **N18.2** | **Chronic kidney disease, stage 2 (mild)** |
> |---|---|
> | **Z94.0** | **Kidney transplant status** |
>
> *Explanation:* This patient's stage 2 CKD is not indicated as being due to the transplanted kidney but instead is just the residual disease the patient had prior to the transplant.

4) Complication codes that include the external cause

As with certain other T codes, some of the complications of care codes have the external cause included in the code. The code includes the nature of the complication as well as the type of procedure that caused the complication. No external cause code indicating the type of procedure is necessary for these codes.

5) Complications of care codes within the body system chapters

Intraoperative and postprocedural complication codes are found within the body system chapters with codes specific to the organs and structures of that body system. These codes should be sequenced first, followed by a code(s) for the specific complication, if applicable.

> During a spinal fusion procedure, the surgeon inadvertently punctured the dura. The midline durotomy was repaired, and the fusion procedure was completed.
>
> | **G97.41** | **Accidental puncture or laceration of dura during a procedure** |
> |---|---|
>
> *Explanation:* The accidental durotomy is not coded to an injury code in chapter 19 but instead is categorized to the nervous system chapter.

Muscle/Tendon Table

CD-10-CM categorizes certain muscles and tendons in the upper and lower extremities by their action (e.g., extension, flexion), their anatomical location (e.g., posterior, anterior), and/or whether they are intrinsic or extrinsic to a certain anatomical area. The Muscle/Tendon Table is provided at the beginning of chapters 13 and 19 as a resource to help users when code selection depends on one or more of these characteristics. The categories and/or subcategories that relate to this table are identified by the icon ✦. Please note that this table is not all-inclusive, and proper code assignment should be based on the provider's documentation.

Body Region	Muscle	Extensor Tendon	Flexor Tendon	Other Tendon
Shoulder				
	Deltoid	Posterior deltoid	Anterior deltoid	
	Rotator cuff			
	Infraspinatus			Infraspinatus
	Subscapularis			Subscapularis
	Supraspinatus			Supraspinatus
	Teres minor			Teres minor
	Teres major	Teres major		
Upper arm				
	Anterior muscles			
	Biceps brachii — long head		Biceps brachii — long head	
	Biceps brachii — short head		Biceps brachii — short head	
	Brachialis		Brachialis	
	Coracobrachialis		Coracobrachialis	
	Posterior muscles			
	Triceps brachii	Triceps brachii		
Forearm				
	Anterior muscles			
	Flexors			
	Deep			
	Flexor digitorum profundus		Flexor digitorum profundus	
	Flexor pollicis longus		Flexor pollicis longus	
	Intermediate			
	Flexor digitorum superficialis		Flexor digitorum superficialis	
	Superficial			
	Flexor carpi radialis		Flexor carpi radialis	
	Flexor carpi ulnaris		Flexor carpi ulnaris	
	Palmaris longus		Palmaris longus	
	Pronators			
	Pronator quadratus			Pronator quadratus
	Pronator teres			Pronator teres
	Posterior muscles			
	Extensors			
	Deep			
	Abductor pollicis longus			Abductor pollicis longus
	Extensor indicis	Extensor indicis		
	Extensor pollicis brevis	Extensor pollicis brevis		
	Extensor pollicis longus	Extensor pollicis longus		
	Superficial			
	Brachioradialis			Brachioradialis
	Extensor carpi radialis brevis	Extensor carpi radialis brevis		
	Extensor carpi radialis longus	Extensor carpi radialis longus		
	Extensor carpi ulnaris	Extensor carpi ulnaris		
	Extensor digiti minimi	Extensor digiti minimi		
	Extensor digitorum	Extensor digitorum		
	Anconeus	Anconeus		
	Supinator			Supinator

Chapter 19. Injury, Poisoning, and Certain Other Consequences of External Causes

Body Region	Muscle	Extensor Tendon	Flexor Tendon	Other Tendon
Hand				
Extrinsic — attach to a site in the forearm as well as a site in the hand with action related to hand movement at the wrist				
	Extensor carpi radialis brevis	Extensor carpi radialis brevis		
	Extensor carpi radialis longus	Extensor carpie radialis longus		
	Extensor carpi ulnaris	Extensor carpi ulnaris		
	Flexor carpi radialis		Flexor carpi radialis	
	Flexor carpi ulnaris		Flexor carpi ulnaris	
	Flexor digitorum superficialis		Flexor digitorum superficialis	
	Palmaris longus		Palmaris longus	
Extrinsic — attach to a site in the forearm as well as a site in the hand with action in the hand related to finger movement				
	Adductor pollicis longus			Adductor pollicis longus
	Extensor digiti minimi	Extensor digiti minimi		
	Extensor digitorum	Extensor digitorum		
	Extensor indicis	Extensor indicis		
	Flexor digitorum profundus		Flexor digitorum profundus	
	Flexor digitorum superficialis		Flexor digitorum superficialis	
Extrinsic — attach to a site in the forearm as well as a site in the hand with action in the hand related to thumb movement				
	Extensor pollicis brevis	Extensor pollicis brevis		
	Extensor pollicis longus	Extensor pollicis longus		
	Flexor pollicis longus		Flexor pollicis longus	
Intrinsic — found within the hand only				
	Adductor pollicis			Adductor pollicis
	Dorsal interossei	Dorsal interossei	Dorsal interossei	
	Lumbricals	Lumbricals	Lumbricals	
	Palmaris brevis			Palmaris brevis
	Palmar interossei	Palmar interossei	Palmar interossei	
	Hypothenar muscles			
	Abductor digiti minimi			Abductor digiti minimi
	Flexor digiti minimi brevis		Flexor digiti minimi brevis	
	Oppenens digiti minimi		Oppenens digiti minimi	
	Thenar muscles			
	Abductor pollicis brevis			Abductor pollicis brevis
	Flexor pollicis brevis		Flexor pollicis brevis	
	Oppenens pollicis		Oppenens pollicis	
Thigh				
	Anterior muscles			
	Iliopsoas		Iliopsoas	
	Pectineus		Pectineus	
	Quadriceps	Quadriceps		
	Rectus femoris	Rectus femoris — Extends knee	Rectus femoris — Flexes hip	
	Vastus intermedius	Vastus intermedius		
	Vastus lateralis	Vastus lateralis		
	Vastus medialis	Vastus medialis		
	Sartorius		Sartorius	
	Medial muscles			
	Adductor brevis			Adductor brevis
	Adductor longus			Adductor longus
	Adductor magnus			Adductor magnus
	Gracilis			Gracilis
	Obturator externus			Obturator externus
	Posterior muscles			
	Hamstring	Hamstring — Extends hip	Hamstring — Flexes knee	
	Biceps femoris	Biceps femoris	Biceps femoris	
	Semimembranosus	Semimembranosus	Semimembranosus	
	Semitendinosus	Semitendinosus	Semitendinosus	

Body Region	Muscle	Extensor Tendon	Flexor Tendon	Other Tendon
Lower leg				
	Anterior muscles			
	Extensor digitorum longus	Extensor digitorum longus		
	Extensor hallucis longus	Extensor hallucis longus		
	Fibularis (peroneus) tertius	Fibularis (peroneus) tertius		
	Tibialis anterior	Tibialis anterior		Tibialis anterior
	Lateral muscles			
	Fibularis (peroneus) brevis		Fibularis (peroneus) brevis	
	Fibularis (peroneus) longus		Fibularis (peroneus) longus	
	Posterior muscles			
	Deep			
	Flexor digitorum longus		Flexor digitorum longus	
	Flexor hallucis longus		Flexor hallucis longus	
	Popliteus		Popliteus	
	Tibialis posterior		Tibialis posterior	
	Superficial			
	Gastrocnemius		Gastrocnemius	
	Plantaris		Plantaris	
	Soleus		Soleus	
				Calcaneal (Achilles)
Ankle/Foot				
Extrinsic — attach to a site in the lower leg as well as a site in the foot with action related to foot movement at the ankle				
	Plantaris		Plantaris	
	Soleus		Soleus	
	Tibialis anterior	Tibialis anterior		
	Tibialis posterior		Tibialis posterior	
Extrinsic — attach to a site in the lower leg as well as a site in the foot with action in the foot related to toe movement				
	Extensor digitorum longus	Extensor digitorum longus		
	Extensor hallicus longus	Extensor hallicus longus		
	Flexor digitorum longus		Flexor digitorum longus	
	Flexor hallucis longus		Flexor hallucis longus	
Intrinsic — found within the ankle/foot only				
	Dorsal muscles			
	Extensor digitorum brevis	Extensor digitorum brevis		
	Extensor hallucis brevis	Extensor hallucis brevis		
	Plantar muscles			
	Abductor digiti minimi		Abductor digiti minimi	
	Abductor hallucis		Abductor hallucis	
	Dorsal interossei	Dorsal interossei	Dorsal interossei	
	Flexor digiti minimi brevis		Flexor digiti minimi brevis	
	Flexor digitorum brevis		Flexor digitorum brevis	
	Flexor hallucis brevis		Flexor hallucis brevis	
	Lumbricals	Lumbricals	Lumbricals	
	Quadratus plantae		Quadratus plantae	
	Plantar interossei	Plantar interossei	Plantar interossei	

Chapter 19. Injury, Poisoning and Certain Other Consequences of External Causes (S00-T88)

NOTE   Use secondary code(s) from Chapter 20, External causes of morbidity, to indicate cause of injury. Codes within the T section that include the external cause do not require an additional external cause code.

Use additional code to identify any retained foreign body, if applicable (Z18.-)

EXCLUDES 1   birth trauma (P10-P15)
     obstetric trauma (O70-O71)

NOTE   The chapter uses the S-section for coding different types of injuries related to single body regions and the T-section to cover injuries to unspecified body regions as well as poisoning and certain other consequences of external causes.

AHA: 2015, 1Q, 3-21

This chapter contains the following blocks:

S00-S09	Injuries to the head
S10-S19	Injuries to the neck
S20-S29	Injuries to the thorax
S30-S39	Injuries to the abdomen, lower back, lumbar spine, pelvis and external genitals
S40-S49	Injuries to the shoulder and upper arm
S50-S59	Injuries to the elbow and forearm
S60-S69	Injuries to the wrist, hand and fingers
S70-S79	Injuries to the hip and thigh
S80-S89	Injuries to the knee and lower leg
S90-S99	Injuries to the ankle and foot
T07	Injuries involving multiple body regions
T14	Injury of unspecified body region
T15-T19	Effects of foreign body entering through natural orifice
T20-T25	Burns and corrosions of external body surface, specified by site
T26-T28	Burns and corrosions confined to eye and internal organs
T30-T32	Burns and corrosions of multiple and unspecified body regions
T33-T34	Frostbite
T36-T50	Poisoning by, adverse effect of and underdosing of drugs, medicaments and biological substances
T51-T65	Toxic effects of substances chiefly nonmedicinal as to source
T66-T78	Other and unspecified effects of external causes
T79	Certain early complications of trauma
T80-T88	Complications of surgical and medical care, not elsewhere classified

Injuries to the head (S00-S09)

INCLUDES   injuries of ear
     injuries of eye
     injuries of face [any part]
     injuries of gum
     injuries of jaw
     injuries of oral cavity
     injuries of palate
     injuries of periocular area
     injuries of scalp
     injuries of temporomandibular joint area
     injuries of tongue
     injuries of tooth

Code also for any associated infection

EXCLUDES 2   burns and corrosions (T20-T32)
     effects of foreign body in ear (T16)
     effects of foreign body in larynx (T17.3)
     effects of foreign body in mouth NOS (T18.0)
     effects of foreign body in nose (T17.0-T17.1)
     effects of foreign body in pharynx (T17.2)
     effects of foreign body on external eye (T15.-)
     frostbite (T33-T34)
     insect bite or sting, venomous (T63.4)

√4ᵗʰ S00   **Superficial injury of head**

     EXCLUDES 1   diffuse cerebral contusion (S06.2-)
         focal cerebral contusion (S06.3-)
         injury of eye and orbit (S05.-)
         open wound of head (S01.-)

> The appropriate 7th character is to be added to each code from category S00.
> A   initial encounter
> D   subsequent encounter
> S   sequela

   √5ᵗʰ S00.0   **Superficial injury of scalp**

     √x7ᵗʰ S00.00   **Unspecified superficial injury of scalp**

     √x7ᵗʰ S00.01   **Abrasion of scalp**

     √x7ᵗʰ S00.02   **Blister (nonthermal) of scalp**

     √x7ᵗʰ S00.03   **Contusion of scalp**
           Bruise of scalp
           Hematoma of scalp

     √x7ᵗʰ S00.04   **External constriction of part of scalp**

     √x7ᵗʰ S00.05   **Superficial foreign body of scalp**
           Splinter in the scalp

     √x7ᵗʰ S00.06   **Insect bite (nonvenomous) of scalp**

     √x7ᵗʰ S00.07   **Other superficial bite of scalp**
         EXCLUDES 1   open bite of scalp (S01.05)

   √5ᵗʰ S00.1   **Contusion of eyelid and periocular area**
       Black eye
     EXCLUDES 2   contusion of eyeball and orbital tissues (S05.1)

     √x7ᵗʰ S00.10   **Contusion of unspecified eyelid and periocular area**

     √x7ᵗʰ S00.11   **Contusion of right eyelid and periocular area**

     √x7ᵗʰ S00.12   **Contusion of left eyelid and periocular area**

   √5ᵗʰ S00.2   **Other and unspecified superficial injuries of eyelid and periocular area**
     EXCLUDES 2   superficial injury of conjunctiva and cornea (S05.0-)

     √6ᵗʰ S00.20   **Unspecified superficial injury of eyelid and periocular area**

       √7ᵗʰ S00.201   **Unspecified superficial injury of right eyelid and periocular area**

       √7ᵗʰ S00.202   **Unspecified superficial injury of left eyelid and periocular area**

       √7ᵗʰ S00.209   **Unspecified superficial injury of unspecified eyelid and periocular area**

     √6ᵗʰ S00.21   **Abrasion of eyelid and periocular area**

       √7ᵗʰ S00.211   **Abrasion of right eyelid and periocular area**

       √7ᵗʰ S00.212   **Abrasion of left eyelid and periocular area**

       √7ᵗʰ S00.219   **Abrasion of unspecified eyelid and periocular area**

     √6ᵗʰ S00.22   **Blister (nonthermal) of eyelid and periocular area**

       √7ᵗʰ S00.221   **Blister (nonthermal) of right eyelid and periocular area**

       √7ᵗʰ S00.222   **Blister (nonthermal) of left eyelid and periocular area**

       √7ᵗʰ S00.229   **Blister (nonthermal) of unspecified eyelid and periocular area**

     √6ᵗʰ S00.24   **External constriction of eyelid and periocular area**

       √7ᵗʰ S00.241   **External constriction of right eyelid and periocular area**

       √7ᵗʰ S00.242   **External constriction of left eyelid and periocular area**

       √7ᵗʰ S00.249   **External constriction of unspecified eyelid and periocular area**

     √6ᵗʰ S00.25   **Superficial foreign body of eyelid and periocular area**
         Splinter of eyelid and periocular area
         EXCLUDES 2   retained foreign body in eyelid (H02.81-)

       √7ᵗʰ S00.251   **Superficial foreign body of right eyelid and periocular area**

       √7ᵗʰ S00.252   **Superficial foreign body of left eyelid and periocular area**

       √7ᵗʰ S00.259   **Superficial foreign body of unspecified eyelid and periocular area**

     √6ᵗʰ S00.26   **Insect bite (nonvenomous) of eyelid and periocular area**

       √7ᵗʰ S00.261   **Insect bite (nonvenomous) of right eyelid and periocular area**

       √7ᵗʰ S00.262   **Insect bite (nonvenomous) of left eyelid and periocular area**

       √7ᵗʰ S00.269   **Insect bite (nonvenomous) of unspecified eyelid and periocular area**

     √6ᵗʰ S00.27   **Other superficial bite of eyelid and periocular area**
       EXCLUDES 1   open bite of eyelid and periocular area (S01.15)

       √7ᵗʰ S00.271   **Other superficial bite of right eyelid and periocular area**

       √7ᵗʰ S00.272   **Other superficial bite of left eyelid and periocular area**

       √7ᵗʰ S00.279   **Other superficial bite of unspecified eyelid and periocular area**

EXCLUDES 1 Not coded here   **EXCLUDES 2** Not included here   N Newborn Age: 0   P Pediatric Age: 0-17   M Maternity Age: 12-55   A Adult Age: 15-124

846   ICD-10-CM 2016

√5ᵗʰ **S00.3**   Superficial injury of nose

  √x7ᵗʰ **S00.30**   **Unspecified superficial injury of nose**

  √x7ᵗʰ **S00.31**   Abrasion of nose

  √x7ᵗʰ **S00.32**   Blister (nonthermal) of nose

  √x7ᵗʰ **S00.33**   Contusion of nose
       Bruise of nose
       Hematoma of nose

  √x7ᵗʰ **S00.34**   External constriction of nose

  √x7ᵗʰ **S00.35**   Superficial foreign body of nose
       Splinter in the nose

  √x7ᵗʰ **S00.36**   Insect bite (nonvenomous) of nose

  √x7ᵗʰ **S00.37**   Other superficial bite of nose
       EXCLUDES 1   *open bite of nose (S01.25)*

√5ᵗʰ **S00.4**   Superficial injury of ear

  √6ᵗʰ **S00.40**   Unspecified superficial injury of ear

    √7ᵗʰ **S00.401**   Unspecified superficial injury of right ear

    √7ᵗʰ **S00.402**   Unspecified superficial injury of left ear

    √7ᵗʰ **S00.409**   Unspecified superficial injury of unspecified ear

  √6ᵗʰ **S00.41**   Abrasion of ear

    √7ᵗʰ **S00.411**   Abrasion of right ear

    √7ᵗʰ **S00.412**   Abrasion of left ear

    √7ᵗʰ **S00.419**   Abrasion of unspecified ear

  √6ᵗʰ **S00.42**   Blister (nonthermal) of ear

    √7ᵗʰ **S00.421**   Blister (nonthermal) of right ear

    √7ᵗʰ **S00.422**   Blister (nonthermal) of left ear

    √7ᵗʰ **S00.429**   Blister (nonthermal) of unspecified ear

  √6ᵗʰ **S00.43**   Contusion of ear
       Bruise of ear
       Hematoma of ear

    √7ᵗʰ **S00.431**   Contusion of right ear

    √7ᵗʰ **S00.432**   Contusion of left ear

    √7ᵗʰ **S00.439**   Contusion of unspecified ear

  √6ᵗʰ **S00.44**   External constriction of ear

    √7ᵗʰ **S00.441**   External constriction of right ear

    √7ᵗʰ **S00.442**   External constriction of left ear

    √7ᵗʰ **S00.449**   External constriction of unspecified ear

  √6ᵗʰ **S00.45**   Superficial foreign body of ear
       Splinter in the ear

    √7ᵗʰ **S00.451**   Superficial foreign body of right ear

    √7ᵗʰ **S00.452**   Superficial foreign body of left ear

    √7ᵗʰ **S00.459**   Superficial foreign body of unspecified ear

  √6ᵗʰ **S00.46**   Insect bite (nonvenomous) of ear

    √7ᵗʰ **S00.461**   Insect bite (nonvenomous) of right ear

    √7ᵗʰ **S00.462**   Insect bite (nonvenomous) of left ear

    √7ᵗʰ **S00.469**   Insect bite (nonvenomous) of unspecified ear

  √6ᵗʰ **S00.47**   Other superficial bite of ear
       EXCLUDES 1   *open bite of ear (S01.35)*

    √7ᵗʰ **S00.471**   Other superficial bite of right ear

    √7ᵗʰ **S00.472**   Other superficial bite of left ear

    √7ᵗʰ **S00.479**   Other superficial bite of unspecified ear

√5ᵗʰ **S00.5**   Superficial injury of lip and oral cavity

  √6ᵗʰ **S00.50**   Unspecified superficial injury of lip and oral cavity

    √7ᵗʰ **S00.501**   Unspecified superficial injury of lip

    √7ᵗʰ **S00.502**   Unspecified superficial injury of oral cavity

  √6ᵗʰ **S00.51**   Abrasion of lip and oral cavity

    √7ᵗʰ **S00.511**   Abrasion of lip

    √7ᵗʰ **S00.512**   Abrasion of oral cavity

  √6ᵗʰ **S00.52**   Blister (nonthermal) of lip and oral cavity

    √7ᵗʰ **S00.521**   Blister (nonthermal) of lip

    √7ᵗʰ **S00.522**   Blister (nonthermal) of oral cavity

  √6ᵗʰ **S00.53**   Contusion of lip and oral cavity

    √7ᵗʰ **S00.531**   Contusion of lip
       Bruise of lip
       Hematoma of oral cavity

    √7ᵗʰ **S00.532**   Contusion of oral cavity
       Bruise of lip
       Hematoma of oral cavity

  √6ᵗʰ **S00.54**   External constriction of lip and oral cavity

    √7ᵗʰ **S00.541**   External constriction of lip

    √7ᵗʰ **S00.542**   External constriction of oral cavity

  √6ᵗʰ **S00.55**   Superficial foreign body of lip and oral cavity

    √7ᵗʰ **S00.551**   Superficial foreign body of lip
       Splinter of lip and oral cavity

    √7ᵗʰ **S00.552**   Superficial foreign body of oral cavity
       Splinter of lip and oral cavity

  √6ᵗʰ **S00.56**   Insect bite (nonvenomous) of lip and oral cavity

    √7ᵗʰ **S00.561**   Insect bite (nonvenomous) of lip

    √7ᵗʰ **S00.562**   Insect bite (nonvenomous) of oral cavity

  √6ᵗʰ **S00.57**   Other superficial bite of lip and oral cavity

    √7ᵗʰ **S00.571**   Other superficial bite of lip
       EXCLUDES 1   *open bite of lip (S01.551)*

    √7ᵗʰ **S00.572**   Other superficial bite of oral cavity
       EXCLUDES 1   *open bite of oral cavity (S01.552)*

√5ᵗʰ **S00.8**   Superficial injury of other parts of head

  √x7ᵗʰ **S00.80**   **Unspecified superficial injury of other part of head**

  √x7ᵗʰ **S00.81**   Abrasion of other part of head

  √x7ᵗʰ **S00.82**   Blister (nonthermal) of other part of head

  √x7ᵗʰ **S00.83**   Contusion of other part of head
       Bruise of other part of head
       Hematoma of other part of head

  √x7ᵗʰ **S00.84**   External constriction of other part of head

  √x7ᵗʰ **S00.85**   Superficial foreign body of other part of head
       Splinter in other part of head

  √x7ᵗʰ **S00.86**   Insect bite (nonvenomous) of other part of head

  √x7ᵗʰ **S00.87**   Other superficial bite of other part of head
       EXCLUDES 1   *open bite of other part of head (S01.85)*

√5ᵗʰ **S00.9**   Superficial injury of unspecified part of head

  √x7ᵗʰ **S00.90**   **Unspecified superficial injury of unspecified part of head**

  √x7ᵗʰ **S00.91**   Abrasion of unspecified part of head

  √x7ᵗʰ **S00.92**   Blister (nonthermal) of unspecified part of head

  √x7ᵗʰ **S00.93**   Contusion of unspecified part of head
       Bruise of head
       Hematoma of head

  √x7ᵗʰ **S00.94**   External constriction of unspecified part of head

  √x7ᵗʰ **S00.95**   Superficial foreign body of unspecified part of head
       Splinter of head

  √x7ᵗʰ **S00.96**   Insect bite (nonvenomous) of unspecified part of head

  √x7ᵗʰ **S00.97**   Other superficial bite of unspecified part of head
       EXCLUDES 1   *open bite of head (S01.95)*

√4ᵗʰ **S01**   **Open wound of head**
     Code also any associated:
       injury of cranial nerve (S04.-)
       injury of muscle and tendon of head (S09.1-)
       intracranial injury (S06.-)
       wound infection
     EXCLUDES 1   *open skull fracture (S02- with 7th character B)*
     EXCLUDES 2   *injury of eye and orbit (S05.-)*
                  traumatic amputation of part of head (S08.-)

> The appropriate 7th character is to be added to each code from category S01.
> A   initial encounter
> D   subsequent encounter
> S   sequela

√5ᵗʰ **S01.0**   Open wound of scalp
     EXCLUDES 1   *avulsion of scalp (S08.0)*

  √x7ᵗʰ **S01.00**   **Unspecified open wound of scalp**

  √x7ᵗʰ **S01.01**   Laceration without foreign body of scalp

  √x7ᵗʰ **S01.02**   Laceration with foreign body of scalp

  √x7ᵗʰ **S01.03**   Puncture wound without foreign body of scalp

  √x7ᵗʰ **S01.04**   Puncture wound with foreign body of scalp

  √x7ᵗʰ **S01.05**   Open bite of scalp
       Bite of scalp NOS
       EXCLUDES 1   *superficial bite of scalp (S00.06, S00.07-)*

☑ Additional Character Required   √x7ᵗʰ Placeholder Alert   Unspecified Dx   Other Specified Dx   Manifestation   ▶◀ Revised Text   ● New Code   ▲ Revised Code Title

√5ᵗʰ S01.1   Open wound of eyelid and periocular area
Open wound of eyelid and periocular area with or without involvement of lacrimal passages

√6ᵗʰ S01.10   Unspecified open wound of eyelid and periocular area

√7ᵗʰ S01.101   Unspecified open wound of right eyelid and periocular area

√7ᵗʰ S01.102   Unspecified open wound of left eyelid and periocular area

√7ᵗʰ S01.109   Unspecified open wound of unspecified eyelid and periocular area

√6ᵗʰ S01.11   Laceration without foreign body of eyelid and periocular area

√7ᵗʰ S01.111   Laceration without foreign body of right eyelid and periocular area

√7ᵗʰ S01.112   Laceration without foreign body of left eyelid and periocular area

√7ᵗʰ S01.119   Laceration without foreign body of unspecified eyelid and periocular area

√6ᵗʰ S01.12   Laceration with foreign body of eyelid and periocular area

√7ᵗʰ S01.121   Laceration with foreign body of right eyelid and periocular area

√7ᵗʰ S01.122   Laceration with foreign body of left eyelid and periocular area

√7ᵗʰ S01.129   Laceration with foreign body of unspecified eyelid and periocular area

√6ᵗʰ S01.13   Puncture wound without foreign body of eyelid and periocular area

√7ᵗʰ S01.131   Puncture wound without foreign body of right eyelid and periocular area

√7ᵗʰ S01.132   Puncture wound without foreign body of left eyelid and periocular area

√7ᵗʰ S01.139   Puncture wound without foreign body of unspecified eyelid and periocular area

√6ᵗʰ S01.14   Puncture wound with foreign body of eyelid and periocular area

√7ᵗʰ S01.141   Puncture wound with foreign body of right eyelid and periocular area

√7ᵗʰ S01.142   Puncture wound with foreign body of left eyelid and periocular area

√7ᵗʰ S01.149   Puncture wound with foreign body of unspecified eyelid and periocular area

√6ᵗʰ S01.15   Open bite of eyelid and periocular area
Bite of eyelid and periocular area NOS
> **EXCLUDES 1** superficial bite of eyelid and periocular area (S00.26, S00.27)

√7ᵗʰ S01.151   Open bite of right eyelid and periocular area

√7ᵗʰ S01.152   Open bite of left eyelid and periocular area

√7ᵗʰ S01.159   Open bite of unspecified eyelid and periocular area

√5ᵗʰ S01.2   Open wound of nose

√x7ᵗʰ S01.20   Unspecified open wound of nose

√x7ᵗʰ S01.21   Laceration without foreign body of nose

√x7ᵗʰ S01.22   Laceration with foreign body of nose

√x7ᵗʰ S01.23   Puncture wound without foreign body of nose

√x7ᵗʰ S01.24   Puncture wound with foreign body of nose

√x7ᵗʰ S01.25   Open bite of nose
Bite of nose NOS
> **EXCLUDES 1** superficial bite of nose (S00.36, S00.37)

√5ᵗʰ S01.3   Open wound of ear

√6ᵗʰ S01.30   Unspecified open wound of ear

√7ᵗʰ S01.301   Unspecified open wound of right ear

√7ᵗʰ S01.302   Unspecified open wound of left ear

√7ᵗʰ S01.309   Unspecified open wound of unspecified ear

√6ᵗʰ S01.31   Laceration without foreign body of ear

√7ᵗʰ S01.311   Laceration without foreign body of right ear

√7ᵗʰ S01.312   Laceration without foreign body of left ear

√7ᵗʰ S01.319   Laceration without foreign body of unspecified ear

√6ᵗʰ S01.32   Laceration with foreign body of ear

√7ᵗʰ S01.321   Laceration with foreign body of right ear

√7ᵗʰ S01.322   Laceration with foreign body of left ear

√7ᵗʰ S01.329   Laceration with foreign body of unspecified ear

√6ᵗʰ S01.33   Puncture wound without foreign body of ear

√7ᵗʰ S01.331   Puncture wound without foreign body of right ear

√7ᵗʰ S01.332   Puncture wound without foreign body of left ear

√7ᵗʰ S01.339   Puncture wound without foreign body of unspecified ear

√6ᵗʰ S01.34   Puncture wound with foreign body of ear

√7ᵗʰ S01.341   Puncture wound with foreign body of right ear

√7ᵗʰ S01.342   Puncture wound with foreign body of left ear

√7ᵗʰ S01.349   Puncture wound with foreign body of unspecified ear

√6ᵗʰ S01.35   Open bite of ear
Bite of ear NOS
> **EXCLUDES 1** superficial bite of ear (S00.46, S00.47)

√7ᵗʰ S01.351   Open bite of right ear

√7ᵗʰ S01.352   Open bite of left ear

√7ᵗʰ S01.359   Open bite of unspecified ear

√5ᵗʰ S01.4   Open wound of cheek and temporomandibular area

√6ᵗʰ S01.40   Unspecified open wound of cheek and temporomandibular area

√7ᵗʰ S01.401   Unspecified open wound of right cheek and temporomandibular area

√7ᵗʰ S01.402   Unspecified open wound of left cheek and temporomandibular area

√7ᵗʰ S01.409   Unspecified open wound of unspecified cheek and temporomandibular area

√6ᵗʰ S01.41   Laceration without foreign body of cheek and temporomandibular area

√7ᵗʰ S01.411   Laceration without foreign body of right cheek and temporomandibular area

√7ᵗʰ S01.412   Laceration without foreign body of left cheek and temporomandibular area

√7ᵗʰ S01.419   Laceration without foreign body of unspecified cheek and temporomandibular area

√6ᵗʰ S01.42   Laceration with foreign body of cheek and temporomandibular area

√7ᵗʰ S01.421   Laceration with foreign body of right cheek and temporomandibular area

√7ᵗʰ S01.422   Laceration with foreign body of left cheek and temporomandibular area

√7ᵗʰ S01.429   Laceration with foreign body of unspecified cheek and temporomandibular area

√6ᵗʰ S01.43   Puncture wound without foreign body of cheek and temporomandibular area

√7ᵗʰ S01.431   Puncture wound without foreign body of right cheek and temporomandibular area

√7ᵗʰ S01.432   Puncture wound without foreign body of left cheek and temporomandibular area

√7ᵗʰ S01.439   Puncture wound without foreign body of unspecified cheek and temporomandibular area

√6ᵗʰ S01.44   Puncture wound with foreign body of cheek and temporomandibular area

√7ᵗʰ S01.441   Puncture wound with foreign body of right cheek and temporomandibular area

√7ᵗʰ S01.442   Puncture wound with foreign body of left cheek and temporomandibular area

√7ᵗʰ S01.449   Puncture wound with foreign body of unspecified cheek and temporomandibular area

EXCLUDES 1 Not coded here   **EXCLUDES 2** Not included here   **N** Newborn Age: 0   **P** Pediatric Age: 0-17   **M** Maternity Age: 12-55   **A** Adult Age: 15-124

848   ICD-10-CM 2016

✓6ᵗʰ S01.45　Open bite of cheek and temporomandibular area
　　　Bite of cheek and temporomandibular area NOS
　　　*EXCLUDES 2　superficial bite of cheek and
　　　　　　temporomandibular area (S00.86,
　　　　　　S00.87)*

　　**✓7ᵗʰ S01.451　Open bite of right cheek and
　　　　　temporomandibular area**

　　**✓7ᵗʰ S01.452　Open bite of left cheek and
　　　　　temporomandibular area**

　　**✓7ᵗʰ S01.459　Open bite of unspecified cheek and
　　　　　temporomandibular area**

✓5ᵗʰ S01.5　Open wound of lip and oral cavity
　　*EXCLUDES 2　tooth dislocation (S03.2)
　　　　　tooth fracture (S02.5)*

　✓6ᵗʰ S01.50　Unspecified open wound of lip and oral cavity
　　✓7ᵗʰ S01.501　Unspecified open wound of lip
　　✓7ᵗʰ S01.502　Unspecified open wound of oral cavity

　**✓6ᵗʰ S01.51　Laceration of lip and oral cavity without foreign
　　　body**
　　✓7ᵗʰ S01.511　Laceration without foreign body of lip
　　**✓7ᵗʰ S01.512　Laceration without foreign body of oral
　　　　　cavity**

　✓6ᵗʰ S01.52　Laceration of lip and oral cavity with foreign body
　　✓7ᵗʰ S01.521　Laceration with foreign body of lip
　　✓7ᵗʰ S01.522　Laceration with foreign body of oral cavity

　**✓6ᵗʰ S01.53　Puncture wound of lip and oral cavity without
　　　foreign body**
　　**✓7ᵗʰ S01.531　Puncture wound without foreign body of
　　　　　lip**
　　**✓7ᵗʰ S01.532　Puncture wound without foreign body of
　　　　　oral cavity**

　**✓6ᵗʰ S01.54　Puncture wound of lip and oral cavity with foreign
　　　body**
　　✓7ᵗʰ S01.541　Puncture wound with foreign body of lip
　　**✓7ᵗʰ S01.542　Puncture wound with foreign body of oral
　　　　　cavity**

　✓6ᵗʰ S01.55　Open bite of lip and oral cavity
　　✓7ᵗʰ S01.551　Open bite of lip
　　　　　Bite of lip NOS
　　　　　EXCLUDES 1　superficial bite of lip (S00.571)

　　✓7ᵗʰ S01.552　Open bite of oral cavity
　　　　　Bite of oral cavity NOS
　　　　　*EXCLUDES 1　superficial bite of oral cavity
　　　　　　　(S00.572)*

✓5ᵗʰ S01.8　Open wound of other parts of head
　✓x7ᵗʰ S01.80　Unspecified open wound of other part of head
　**✓x7ᵗʰ S01.81　Laceration without foreign body of other part of
　　　head**
　✓x7ᵗʰ S01.82　Laceration with foreign body of other part of head
　**✓x7ᵗʰ S01.83　Puncture wound without foreign body of other part
　　　of head**
　**✓x7ᵗʰ S01.84　Puncture wound with foreign body of other part of
　　　head**
　✓x7ᵗʰ S01.85　Open bite of other part of head
　　　　Bite of other part of head NOS
　　　　EXCLUDES 1　superficial bite of other part of head (S00.85)

✓5ᵗʰ S01.9　Open wound of unspecified part of head
　✓x7ᵗʰ S01.90　Unspecified open wound of unspecified part of head
　**✓x7ᵗʰ S01.91　Laceration without foreign body of unspecified part
　　　of head**
　**✓x7ᵗʰ S01.92　Laceration with foreign body of unspecified part of
　　　head**
　**✓x7ᵗʰ S01.93　Puncture wound without foreign body of
　　　unspecified part of head**
　**✓x7ᵗʰ S01.94　Puncture wound with foreign body of unspecified
　　　part of head**
　✓x7ᵗʰ S01.95　Open bite of unspecified part of head
　　　　Bite of head NOS
　　　　EXCLUDES 1　superficial bite of head NOS (S00.97)

✓4ᵗʰ S02　Fracture of skull and facial bones
　　NOTE　A fracture not indicated as open or closed should be coded to
　　　closed.
　　Code also any associated intracranial injury (S06.-).

　┌───┐
　│ The appropriate 7th character is to be added to each code from
　│ category S02.
　│ A　initial encounter for closed fracture
　│ B　initial encounter for open fracture
　│ D　subsequent encounter for fracture with routine healing
　│ G　subsequent encounter for fracture with delayed healing
　│ K　subsequent encounter for fracture with nonunion
　│ S　sequela
　└───┘

✓x7ᵗʰ S02.0　Fracture of vault of skull
　　　Fracture of frontal bone
　　　Fracture of parietal bone

✓5ᵗʰ S02.1　Fracture of base of skull
　　EXCLUDES 1　orbit NOS (S02.8)
　　EXCLUDES 2　orbital floor (S02.3-)

　✓x7ᵗʰ S02.10　Unspecified fracture of base of skull

　✓6ᵗʰ S02.11　Fracture of occiput
　　✓7ᵗʰ S02.110　Type I occipital condyle fracture
　　✓7ᵗʰ S02.111　Type II occipital condyle fracture
　　✓7ᵗʰ S02.112　Type III occipital condyle fracture
　　✓7ᵗʰ S02.113　Unspecified occipital condyle fracture
　　✓7ᵗʰ S02.118　Other fracture of occiput
　　✓7ᵗʰ S02.119　Unspecified fracture of occiput

　✓x7ᵗʰ S02.19　Other fracture of base of skull
　　　　Fracture of anterior fossa of base of skull
　　　　Fracture of ethmoid sinus
　　　　Fracture of frontal sinus
　　　　Fracture of middle fossa of base of skull
　　　　Fracture of orbital roof
　　　　Fracture of posterior fossa of base of skull
　　　　Fracture of sphenoid
　　　　Fracture of temporal bone

✓x7ᵗʰ S02.2　Fracture of nasal bones

✓x7ᵗʰ S02.3　Fracture of orbital floor
　　EXCLUDES 1　orbit NOS (S02.8)
　　EXCLUDES 2　orbital roof (S02.1-)

✓5ᵗʰ S02.4　Fracture of malar, maxillary and zygoma bones
　　　Fracture of superior maxilla
　　　Fracture of upper jaw (bone)
　　　Fracture of zygomatic process of temporal bone

　**✓6ᵗʰ S02.40　Fracture of malar, maxillary and zygoma bones,
　　　unspecified**
　　✓7ᵗʰ S02.400　Malar fracture unspecified
　　✓7ᵗʰ S02.401　Maxillary fracture, unspecified
　　✓7ᵗʰ S02.402　Zygomatic fracture, unspecified

　✓6ᵗʰ S02.41　LeFort fracture
　　✓7ᵗʰ S02.411　LeFort I fracture
　　✓7ᵗʰ S02.412　LeFort II fracture
　　✓7ᵗʰ S02.413　LeFort III fracture

　✓x7ᵗʰ S02.42　Fracture of alveolus of maxilla

✓x7ᵗʰ S02.5　Fracture of tooth (traumatic)
　　　Broken tooth
　　　EXCLUDES 1　cracked tooth (nontraumatic) (K03.81)

✓5ᵗʰ S02.6　Fracture of mandible
　　　Fracture of lower jaw (bone)

　✓6ᵗʰ S02.60　Fracture of mandible, unspecified
　　**✓7ᵗʰ S02.600　Fracture of unspecified part of body of
　　　　　mandible**
　　✓7ᵗʰ S02.609　Fracture of mandible, unspecified

　✓x7ᵗʰ S02.61　Fracture of condylar process of mandible
　✓x7ᵗʰ S02.62　Fracture of subcondylar process of mandible
　✓x7ᵗʰ S02.63　Fracture of coronoid process of mandible
　✓x7ᵗʰ S02.64　Fracture of ramus of mandible
　✓x7ᵗʰ S02.65　Fracture of angle of mandible
　✓x7ᵗʰ S02.66　Fracture of symphysis of mandible
　✓x7ᵗʰ S02.67　Fracture of alveolus of mandible
　✓x7ᵗʰ S02.69　Fracture of mandible of other specified site

✓ Additional Character Required　✓x7ᵗʰ Placeholder Alert　　Unspecified Dx　　Other Specified Dx　　Manifestation　　▶◀ Revised Text　　● New Code　　▲ Revised Code Title

ICD-10-CM 2016　　　　　　　　　　　　　　　　　　　　　　　　　849

√x7ᵗʰ **S02.8** **Fractures of other specified skull and facial bones**
Fracture of orbit NOS
Fracture of palate
EXCLUDES 1 *fracture of orbital floor (S02.3-)*
fracture of orbital roof (S02.1-)

√5ᵗʰ **S02.9** **Fracture of unspecified skull and facial bones**

√x7ᵗʰ **S02.91** **Unspecified fracture of skull**

√x7ᵗʰ **S02.92** **Unspecified fracture of facial bones**

√4ᵗʰ **S03** **Dislocation and sprain of joints and ligaments of head**
INCLUDES avulsion of joint (capsule) or ligament of head
laceration of cartilage, joint (capsule) or ligament of head
sprain of cartilage, joint (capsule) or ligament of head
traumatic hemarthrosis of joint or ligament of head
traumatic rupture of joint or ligament of head
traumatic subluxation of joint or ligament of head
traumatic tear of joint or ligament of head
Code also any associated open wound
EXCLUDES 2 *strain of muscle or tendon of head (S09.1)*

The appropriate 7th character is to be added to each code from category S03.
A   initial encounter
D   subsequent encounter
S   sequela

√x7ᵗʰ **S03.0** **Dislocation of jaw**
Dislocation of jaw (cartilage) (meniscus)
Dislocation of mandible
Dislocation of temporomandibular (joint)

√x7ᵗʰ **S03.1** **Dislocation of septal cartilage of nose**

√x7ᵗʰ **S03.2** **Dislocation of tooth**

√x7ᵗʰ **S03.4** **Sprain of jaw**
Sprain of temporomandibular (joint) (ligament)

√x7ᵗʰ **S03.8** **Sprain of joints and ligaments of other parts of head**

√x7ᵗʰ **S03.9** **Sprain of joints and ligaments of unspecified parts of head**

√4ᵗʰ **S04** **Injury of cranial nerve**
The selection of side should be based on the side of the body being affected
Codes first any associated intracranial injury (S06.-)
Code also any associated:
open wound of head (S01.-)
skull fracture (S02.-)

The appropriate 7th character is to be added to each code from category S04.
A   initial encounter
D   subsequent encounter
S   sequela

√5ᵗʰ **S04.0** **Injury of optic nerve and pathways**
Use additional code to identify any visual field defect or blindness (H53.4-, H54)

√6ᵗʰ **S04.01** **Injury of optic nerve**
Injury of 2nd cranial nerve

√7ᵗʰ **S04.011** **Injury of optic nerve, right eye**

√7ᵗʰ **S04.012** **Injury of optic nerve, left eye**

√7ᵗʰ **S04.019** **Injury of optic nerve, unspecified eye**
Injury of optic nerve NOS

√x7ᵗʰ **S04.02** **Injury of optic chiasm**

√6ᵗʰ **S04.03** **Injury of optic tract and pathways**
Injury of optic radiation

√7ᵗʰ **S04.031** **Injury of optic tract and pathways, right eye**

√7ᵗʰ **S04.032** **Injury of optic tract and pathways, left eye**

√7ᵗʰ **S04.039** **Injury of optic tract and pathways, unspecified eye**
Injury of optic tract and pathways NOS

√6ᵗʰ **S04.04** **Injury of visual cortex**

√7ᵗʰ **S04.041** **Injury of visual cortex, right eye**

√7ᵗʰ **S04.042** **Injury of visual cortex, left eye**

√7ᵗʰ **S04.049** **Injury of visual cortex, unspecified eye**
Injury of visual cortex NOS

√5ᵗʰ **S04.1** **Injury of oculomotor nerve**
Injury of 3rd cranial nerve

√x7ᵗʰ **S04.10** **Injury of oculomotor nerve, unspecified side**

√x7ᵗʰ **S04.11** **Injury of oculomotor nerve, right side**

√x7ᵗʰ **S04.12** **Injury of oculomotor nerve, left side**

√5ᵗʰ **S04.2** **Injury of trochlear nerve**
Injury of 4th cranial nerve

√x7ᵗʰ **S04.20** **Injury of trochlear nerve, unspecified side**

√x7ᵗʰ **S04.21** **Injury of trochlear nerve, right side**

√x7ᵗʰ **S04.22** **Injury of trochlear nerve, left side**

√5ᵗʰ **S04.3** **Injury of trigeminal nerve**
Injury of 5th cranial nerve

√x7ᵗʰ **S04.30** **Injury of trigeminal nerve, unspecified side**

√x7ᵗʰ **S04.31** **Injury of trigeminal nerve, right side**

√x7ᵗʰ **S04.32** **Injury of trigeminal nerve, left side**

√5ᵗʰ **S04.4** **Injury of abducent nerve**
Injury of 6th cranial nerve

√x7ᵗʰ **S04.40** **Injury of abducent nerve, unspecified side**

√x7ᵗʰ **S04.41** **Injury of abducent nerve, right side**

√x7ᵗʰ **S04.42** **Injury of abducent nerve, left side**

√5ᵗʰ **S04.5** **Injury of facial nerve**
Injury of 7th cranial nerve

√x7ᵗʰ **S04.50** **Injury of facial nerve, unspecified side**

√x7ᵗʰ **S04.51** **Injury of facial nerve, right side**

√x7ᵗʰ **S04.52** **Injury of facial nerve, left side**

√5ᵗʰ **S04.6** **Injury of acoustic nerve**
Injury of auditory nerve
Injury of 8th cranial nerve

√x7ᵗʰ **S04.60** **Injury of acoustic nerve, unspecified side**

√x7ᵗʰ **S04.61** **Injury of acoustic nerve, right side**

√x7ᵗʰ **S04.62** **Injury of acoustic nerve, left side**

√5ᵗʰ **S04.7** **Injury of accessory nerve**
Injury of 11th cranial nerve

√x7ᵗʰ **S04.70** **Injury of accessory nerve, unspecified side**

√x7ᵗʰ **S04.71** **Injury of accessory nerve, right side**

√x7ᵗʰ **S04.72** **Injury of accessory nerve, left side**

√5ᵗʰ **S04.8** **Injury of other cranial nerves**

√6ᵗʰ **S04.81** **Injury of olfactory [1st] nerve**

√7ᵗʰ **S04.811** **Injury of olfactory [1st] nerve, right side**

√7ᵗʰ **S04.812** **Injury of olfactory [1st] nerve, left side**

√7ᵗʰ **S04.819** **Injury of olfactory [1st] nerve, unspecified side**

√6ᵗʰ **S04.89** **Injury of other cranial nerves**
Injury of vagus [10th] nerve

√7ᵗʰ **S04.891** **Injury of other cranial nerves, right side**

√7ᵗʰ **S04.892** **Injury of other cranial nerves, left side**

√7ᵗʰ **S04.899** **Injury of other cranial nerves, unspecified side**

√x7ᵗʰ **S04.9** **Injury of unspecified cranial nerve**

√4ᵗʰ **S05** **Injury of eye and orbit**
Open wound of eye and orbit
EXCLUDES 2 *2nd cranial [optic] nerve injury (S04.0-)*
3rd cranial [oculomotor] nerve injury (S04.1-)
open wound of eyelid and periocular area (S01.1-)
orbital bone fracture (S02.1-, S02.3-, S02.8-)
superficial injury of eyelid (S00.1-S00.2)

The appropriate 7th character is to be added to each code from category S05.
A   initial encounter
D   subsequent encounter
S   sequela

√5ᵗʰ **S05.0** **Injury of conjunctiva and corneal abrasion without foreign body**
EXCLUDES 1 *foreign body in conjunctival sac (T15.1)*
foreign body in cornea (T15.0)

√x7ᵗʰ **S05.00** **Injury of conjunctiva and corneal abrasion without foreign body, unspecified eye**

√x7ᵗʰ **S05.01** **Injury of conjunctiva and corneal abrasion without foreign body, right eye**

√x7ᵗʰ **S05.02** **Injury of conjunctiva and corneal abrasion without foreign body, left eye**

EXCLUDES 1 Not coded here   *EXCLUDES 2* Not included here   Ⓝ Newborn Age: 0   Ⓟ Pediatric Age: 0-17   Ⓜ Maternity Age: 12-55   Ⓐ Adult Age: 15-124

850

ICD-10-CM 2016

✓5ᵗʰ **S05.1** **Contusion** of eyeball and orbital tissues
    Traumatic hyphema
    EXCLUDES 2   *black eye NOS (S00.1)*
                  contusion of eyelid and periocular area (S00.1)

    ✓x7ᵗʰ **S05.10** **Contusion** of eyeball and orbital tissues, **unspecified eye**

    ✓x7ᵗʰ **S05.11** **Contusion** of eyeball and orbital tissues, **right eye**

    ✓x7ᵗʰ **S05.12** **Contusion** of eyeball and orbital tissues, **left eye**

✓5ᵗʰ **S05.2** **Ocular laceration and rupture** with prolapse or loss of intraocular tissue

    ✓x7ᵗʰ **S05.20** **Ocular laceration and rupture** with prolapse or loss of intraocular tissue, **unspecified eye**

    ✓x7ᵗʰ **S05.21** **Ocular laceration and rupture** with prolapse or loss of intraocular tissue, **right eye**

    ✓x7ᵗʰ **S05.22** **Ocular laceration and rupture** with prolapse or loss of intraocular tissue, **left eye**

✓5ᵗʰ **S05.3** **Ocular laceration** without prolapse or loss of intraocular tissue
    Laceration of eye NOS

    ✓x7ᵗʰ **S05.30** **Ocular laceration** without prolapse or loss of intraocular tissue, **unspecified eye**

    ✓x7ᵗʰ **S05.31** **Ocular laceration** without prolapse or loss of intraocular tissue, **right eye**

    ✓x7ᵗʰ **S05.32** **Ocular laceration** without prolapse or loss of intraocular tissue, **left eye**

✓5ᵗʰ **S05.4** **Penetrating wound** of orbit with or without foreign body
    EXCLUDES 2   *retained (old) foreign body following penetrating wound in orbit (H05.5-)*

    ✓x7ᵗʰ **S05.40** **Penetrating wound** of orbit with or without foreign body, **unspecified eye**

    ✓x7ᵗʰ **S05.41** **Penetrating wound** of orbit with or without foreign body, **right eye**

    ✓x7ᵗʰ **S05.42** **Penetrating wound** of orbit with or without foreign body, **left eye**

✓5ᵗʰ **S05.5** **Penetrating wound** with foreign body of eyeball
    EXCLUDES 2   *retained (old) intraocular foreign body (H44.6-, H44.7)*

    ✓x7ᵗʰ **S05.50** **Penetrating wound** with foreign body of **unspecified eyeball**

    ✓x7ᵗʰ **S05.51** **Penetrating wound** with foreign body of **right eyeball**

    ✓x7ᵗʰ **S05.52** **Penetrating wound** with foreign body of **left** eyeball

✓5ᵗʰ **S05.6** **Penetrating wound** without foreign body of eyeball
    Ocular penetration NOS

    ✓x7ᵗʰ **S05.60** **Penetrating wound** without foreign body of **unspecified eyeball**

    ✓x7ᵗʰ **S05.61** **Penetrating wound** without foreign body of **right eyeball**

    ✓x7ᵗʰ **S05.62** **Penetrating wound** without foreign body of **left eyeball**

✓5ᵗʰ **S05.7** **Avulsion of eye**
    Traumatic enucleation

    ✓x7ᵗʰ **S05.70** **Avulsion of unspecified eye**

    ✓x7ᵗʰ **S05.71** **Avulsion of right eye**

    ✓x7ᵗʰ **S05.72** **Avulsion of left eye**

✓5ᵗʰ **S05.8** **Other injuries** of eye and orbit
    Lacrimal duct injury

    ✓6ᵗʰ **S05.8X** **Other** injuries of eye and orbit

       ✓7ᵗʰ **S05.8X1** **Other injuries of right eye and orbit**

       ✓7ᵗʰ **S05.8X2** **Other injuries of left eye and orbit**

       ✓7ᵗʰ **S05.8X9** **Other injuries of unspecified eye and orbit**

✓5ᵗʰ **S05.9** **Unspecified** injury of eye and orbit
    Injury of eye NOS

    ✓x7ᵗʰ **S05.90** **Unspecified injury of unspecified eye and orbit**

    ✓x7ᵗʰ **S05.91** **Unspecified injury of right eye and orbit**

    ✓x7ᵗʰ **S05.92** **Unspecified injury of left eye and orbit**

✓4ᵗʰ **S06** **Intracranial injury**
    Traumatic brain injury
    Code also any associated:
       open wound of head (S01.-)
       skull fracture (S02.-)
    EXCLUDES 1   *head injury NOS (S09.90)*

    The appropriate 7th character is to be added to each code from category S06.
    A   initial encounter
    D   subsequent encounter
    S   sequela

    ✓5ᵗʰ **S06.0** **Concussion**
       Commotio cerebri
       EXCLUDES 1   *concussion with other intracranial injuries classified in category S06—code to specified intracranial injury*

       ✓6ᵗʰ **S06.0X** **Concussion**

          ✓7ᵗʰ **S06.0X0** **Concussion without loss of consciousness**

          ✓7ᵗʰ **S06.0X1** **Concussion with loss of consciousness of 30 minutes or less**

          ✓7ᵗʰ **S06.0X2** **Concussion with loss of consciousness of 31 minutes to 59 minutes**

          ✓7ᵗʰ **S06.0X3** **Concussion with loss of consciousness of 1 hour to 5 hours 59 minutes**

          ✓7ᵗʰ **S06.0X4** **Concussion with loss of consciousness of 6 hours to 24 hours**

          ✓7ᵗʰ **S06.0X5** **Concussion with loss of consciousness greater than 24 hours with return to pre-existing conscious level**

          ✓7ᵗʰ **S06.0X6** **Concussion with loss of consciousness greater than 24 hours without return to pre-existing conscious level with patient surviving**

          ✓7ᵗʰ **S06.0X7** **Concussion with loss of consciousness of any duration with death due to brain injury prior to regaining consciousness**

          ✓7ᵗʰ **S06.0X8** **Concussion with loss of consciousness of any duration with death due to other cause prior to regaining consciousness**

          ✓7ᵗʰ **S06.0X9** **Concussion with loss of consciousness of unspecified duration**
             Concussion NOS

    ✓5ᵗʰ **S06.1** **Traumatic cerebral edema**
       Diffuse traumatic cerebral edema
       Focal traumatic cerebral edema

       ✓6ᵗʰ **S06.1X** **Traumatic cerebral edema**

          ✓7ᵗʰ **S06.1X0** **Traumatic cerebral edema without loss of consciousness**

          ✓7ᵗʰ **S06.1X1** **Traumatic cerebral edema with loss of consciousness of 30 minutes or less**

          ✓7ᵗʰ **S06.1X2** **Traumatic cerebral edema with loss of consciousness of 31 minutes to 59 minutes**

          ✓7ᵗʰ **S06.1X3** **Traumatic cerebral edema with loss of consciousness of 1 hour to 5 hours 59 minutes**

          ✓7ᵗʰ **S06.1X4** **Traumatic cerebral edema with loss of consciousness of 6 hours to 24 hours**

          ✓7ᵗʰ **S06.1X5** **Traumatic cerebral edema with loss of consciousness greater than 24 hours with return to pre-existing conscious level**

          ✓7ᵗʰ **S06.1X6** **Traumatic cerebral edema with loss of consciousness greater than 24 hours without return to pre-existing conscious level with patient surviving**

          ✓7ᵗʰ **S06.1X7** **Traumatic cerebral edema with loss of consciousness of any duration with death due to brain injury prior to regaining consciousness**

          ✓7ᵗʰ **S06.1X8** **Traumatic cerebral edema with loss of consciousness of any duration with death due to other cause prior to regaining consciousness**

          ✓7ᵗʰ **S06.1X9** **Traumatic cerebral edema with loss of consciousness of unspecified duration**
             Traumatic cerebral edema NOS

✓ Additional Character Required   ✓x7ᵗʰ Placeholder Alert   Unspecified Dx   Other Specified Dx   Manifestation   ▶◀ Revised Text   ● New Code   ▲ Revised Code Title

√5ᵗʰ **S06.2 Diffuse traumatic brain injury**
Diffuse axonal brain injury
EXCLUDES 1   traumatic diffuse cerebral edema (S06.1X-)

√6ᵗʰ **S06.2X**   Diffuse traumatic brain injury

√7ᵗʰ **S06.2X0**   **Diffuse traumatic brain injury** without loss of consciousness

√7ᵗʰ **S06.2X1**   **Diffuse traumatic brain injury with loss of consciousness of** 30 minutes or less

√7ᵗʰ **S06.2X2**   **Diffuse traumatic brain injury with loss of consciousness of** 31 minutes to 59 minutes

√7ᵗʰ **S06.2X3**   **Diffuse traumatic brain injury with loss of consciousness of** 1 hour to 5 hours 59 minutes

√7ᵗʰ **S06.2X4**   **Diffuse traumatic brain injury with loss of consciousness of** 6 hours to 24 hours

√7ᵗʰ **S06.2X5**   **Diffuse traumatic brain injury with loss of consciousness** greater than 24 hours with return to pre-existing conscious levels

√7ᵗʰ **S06.2X6**   **Diffuse traumatic brain injury with loss of consciousness** greater than 24 hours without return to pre-existing conscious level with patient surviving

√7ᵗʰ **S06.2X7**   **Diffuse traumatic brain injury with loss of consciousness of** any duration with death due to brain injury prior to regaining consciousness

√7ᵗʰ **S06.2X8**   **Diffuse traumatic brain injury with loss of consciousness of** any duration with death due to **other** cause prior to regaining consciousness

√7ᵗʰ **S06.2X9**   **Diffuse traumatic brain injury with loss of consciousness of unspecified duration**
Diffuse traumatic brain injury NOS

√5ᵗʰ **S06.3 Focal traumatic brain injury**
EXCLUDES 1   any condition classifiable to S06.4-S06.6 focal cerebral edema (S06.1)

√6ᵗʰ **S06.30**   Unspecified **focal traumatic brain injury**

√7ᵗʰ **S06.300**   **Unspecified focal traumatic brain injury** without loss of consciousness

√7ᵗʰ **S06.301**   **Unspecified focal traumatic brain injury with loss of consciousness of** 30 minutes or less

√7ᵗʰ **S06.302**   **Unspecified focal traumatic brain injury with loss of consciousness of** 31 minutes to 59 minutes

√7ᵗʰ **S06.303**   **Unspecified focal traumatic brain injury with loss of consciousness of** 1 hour to 5 hours 59 minutes

√7ᵗʰ **S06.304**   **Unspecified focal traumatic brain injury with loss of consciousness of** 6 hours to 24 hours

√7ᵗʰ **S06.305**   **Unspecified focal traumatic brain injury with loss of consciousness** greater than 24 hours with return to pre-existing conscious level

√7ᵗʰ **S06.306**   **Unspecified focal traumatic brain injury with loss of consciousness** greater than 24 hours without return to pre-existing conscious level with patient surviving

√7ᵗʰ **S06.307**   **Unspecified focal traumatic brain injury with loss of consciousness of** any duration with death due to brain injury prior to regaining consciousness

√7ᵗʰ **S06.308**   **Unspecified focal traumatic brain injury with loss of consciousness of** any duration with death due to **other** cause prior to regaining consciousness

√7ᵗʰ **S06.309**   **Unspecified focal traumatic brain injury with loss of consciousness of unspecified duration**
Unspecified focal traumatic brain injury NOS

√6ᵗʰ **S06.31**   Contusion and laceration of right cerebrum

√7ᵗʰ **S06.310**   **Contusion and laceration of right cerebrum** without loss of consciousness

√7ᵗʰ **S06.311**   **Contusion and laceration of right cerebrum with loss of consciousness of** 3 minutes or less

√7ᵗʰ **S06.312**   **Contusion and laceration of right cerebrum with loss of consciousness of** 3 minutes to 59 minutes

√7ᵗʰ **S06.313**   **Contusion and laceration of right cerebrum with loss of consciousness of** 1 hour to 5 hours 59 minutes

√7ᵗʰ **S06.314**   **Contusion and laceration of right cerebrum with loss of consciousness of** 6 hours to 24 hours

√7ᵗʰ **S06.315**   **Contusion and laceration of right cerebrum with loss of consciousness** greater than 24 hours with return to pre-existing conscious level

√7ᵗʰ **S06.316**   **Contusion and laceration of right cerebrum with loss of consciousness** greater than 24 hours without return to pre-existing conscious level with patient surviving

√7ᵗʰ **S06.317**   **Contusion and laceration of right cerebrum with loss of consciousness of** any duration with death due to brain injury prior to regaining consciousness

√7ᵗʰ **S06.318**   **Contusion and laceration of right cerebrum with loss of consciousness of** any duration with death due to **other** cause prior to regaining consciousness

√7ᵗʰ **S06.319**   **Contusion and laceration of right cerebrum with loss of consciousness of unspecified duration**
Contusion and laceration of right cerebrum NOS

√6ᵗʰ **S06.32**   Contusion and laceration of left cerebrum

√7ᵗʰ **S06.320**   **Contusion and laceration of left cerebrum** without loss of consciousness

√7ᵗʰ **S06.321**   **Contusion and laceration of left cerebrum with loss of consciousness of** 30 minutes or less

√7ᵗʰ **S06.322**   **Contusion and laceration of left cerebrum with loss of consciousness of** 31 minutes to 59 minutes

√7ᵗʰ **S06.323**   **Contusion and laceration of left cerebrum with loss of consciousness of** 1 hour to 5 hours 59 minutes

√7ᵗʰ **S06.324**   **Contusion and laceration of left cerebrum with loss of consciousness of** 6 hours to 24 hours

√7ᵗʰ **S06.325**   **Contusion and laceration of left cerebrum with loss of consciousness** greater than 24 hours with return to pre-existing conscious level

√7ᵗʰ **S06.326**   **Contusion and laceration of left cerebrum with loss of consciousness** greater than 24 hours without return to pre-existing conscious level with patient surviving

√7ᵗʰ **S06.327**   **Contusion and laceration of left cerebrum with loss of consciousness of** any duration with death due to brain injury prior to regaining consciousness

√7ᵗʰ **S06.328**   **Contusion and laceration of left cerebrum with loss of consciousness of** any duration with death due to **other** cause prior to regaining consciousness

√7ᵗʰ **S06.329**   **Contusion and laceration of left cerebrum with loss of consciousness of unspecified duration**
Contusion and laceration of left cerebrum NOS

√6ᵗʰ **S06.33**   Contusion and laceration of cerebrum, unspecified

√7ᵗʰ **S06.330**   **Contusion and laceration of cerebrum, unspecified, without loss of consciousness**

√7ᵗʰ **S06.331**   **Contusion and laceration of cerebrum, unspecified, with loss of consciousness of** 30 minutes or less

√7ᵗʰ **S06.332**   **Contusion and laceration of cerebrum, unspecified, with loss of consciousness of** 31 minutes to 59 minutes

---

EXCLUDES 1 Not coded here   *EXCLUDES 2* Not included here   **N** Newborn Age: 0   **P** Pediatric Age: 0-17   **M** Maternity Age: 12-55   **A** Adult Age: 15-124

852   ICD-10-CM 2016

✓7th **S06.333** **Contusion and laceration of cerebrum, unspecified, with loss of consciousness of** 1 hour to 5 hours 59 minutes

✓7th **S06.334** **Contusion and laceration of cerebrum, unspecified, with loss of consciousness of** 6 hours to 24 hours

✓7th **S06.335** **Contusion and laceration of cerebrum, unspecified, with loss of consciousness** greater than 24 hours with return to pre-existing conscious level

✓7th **S06.336** **Contusion and laceration of cerebrum, unspecified, with loss of consciousness** greater than 24 hours without return to pre-existing conscious level with patient surviving

✓7th **S06.337** **Contusion and laceration of cerebrum, unspecified, with loss of consciousness of** any duration with death due to brain injury prior to regaining consciousness

✓7th **S06.338** **Contusion and laceration of cerebrum, unspecified, with loss of consciousness of** any duration with death due to other cause prior to regaining consciousness

✓7th **S06.339** **Contusion and laceration of cerebrum, unspecified, with loss of consciousness of unspecified duration**
Contusion and laceration of cerebrum NOS

✓6th **S06.34** **Traumatic hemorrhage of** right cerebrum
Traumatic intracerebral hemorrhage and hematoma of right cerebrum

✓7th **S06.340** **Traumatic hemorrhage of right cerebrum** without loss of consciousness

✓7th **S06.341** **Traumatic hemorrhage of right cerebrum with loss of consciousness of** 30 minutes or less

✓7th **S06.342** **Traumatic hemorrhage of right cerebrum with loss of consciousness of** 31 minutes to 59 minutes

✓7th **S06.343** **Traumatic hemorrhage of right cerebrum with loss of consciousness of** 1 hours to 5 hours 59 minutes

✓7th **S06.344** **Traumatic hemorrhage of right cerebrum with loss of consciousness of** 6 hours to 24 hours

✓7th **S06.345** **Traumatic hemorrhage of right cerebrum with loss of consciousness** greater than 24 hours with return to pre-existing conscious level

✓7th **S06.346** **Traumatic hemorrhage of right cerebrum with loss of consciousness** greater than 24 hours without return to pre-existing conscious level with patient surviving

✓7th **S06.347** **Traumatic hemorrhage of right cerebrum with loss of consciousness of** any duration with death due to brain injury prior to regaining consciousness

✓7th **S06.348** **Traumatic hemorrhage of right cerebrum with loss of consciousness of** any duration with death due to other cause prior to regaining consciousness

✓7th **S06.349** **Traumatic hemorrhage of right cerebrum with loss of consciousness of unspecified duration**
Traumatic hemorrhage of right cerebrum NOS

✓6th **S06.35** **Traumatic hemorrhage of** left cerebrum
Traumatic intracerebral hemorrhage and hematoma of left cerebrum

✓7th **S06.350** **Traumatic hemorrhage of left cerebrum** without loss of consciousness

✓7th **S06.351** **Traumatic hemorrhage of left cerebrum with loss of consciousness of** 30 minutes or less

✓7th **S06.352** **Traumatic hemorrhage of left cerebrum with loss of consciousness of** 31 minutes to 59 minutes

✓7th **S06.353** **Traumatic hemorrhage of left cerebrum with loss of consciousness of** 1 hours to 5 hours 59 minutes

✓7th **S06.354** **Traumatic hemorrhage of left cerebrum with loss of consciousness of** 6 hours to 24 hours

✓7th **S06.355** **Traumatic hemorrhage of left cerebrum with loss of consciousness** greater than 24 hours with return to pre-existing conscious level

✓7th **S06.356** **Traumatic hemorrhage of left cerebrum with loss of consciousness** greater than 24 hours without return to pre-existing conscious level with patient surviving

✓7th **S06.357** **Traumatic hemorrhage of left cerebrum with loss of consciousness of** any duration with death due to brain injury prior to regaining consciousness

✓7th **S06.358** **Traumatic hemorrhage of left cerebrum with loss of consciousness of** any duration with death due to other cause prior to regaining consciousness

✓7th **S06.359** **Traumatic hemorrhage of left cerebrum with loss of consciousness of unspecified duration**
Traumatic hemorrhage of left cerebrum NOS

✓6th **S06.36** **Traumatic hemorrhage of** cerebrum, unspecified
Traumatic intracerebral hemorrhage and hematoma, unspecified

✓7th **S06.360** **Traumatic hemorrhage of cerebrum, unspecified,** without loss of consciousness

✓7th **S06.361** **Traumatic hemorrhage of cerebrum, unspecified, with loss of consciousness of** 30 minutes or less

✓7th **S06.362** **Traumatic hemorrhage of cerebrum, unspecified, with loss of consciousness of** 31 minutes to 59 minutes

✓7th **S06.363** **Traumatic hemorrhage of cerebrum, unspecified, with loss of consciousness of** 1 hours to 5 hours 59 minutes

✓7th **S06.364** **Traumatic hemorrhage of cerebrum, unspecified, with loss of consciousness of** 6 hours to 24 hours

✓7th **S06.365** **Traumatic hemorrhage of cerebrum, unspecified, with loss of consciousness** greater than 24 hours with return to pre-existing conscious level

✓7th **S06.366** **Traumatic hemorrhage of cerebrum, unspecified, with loss of consciousness** greater than 24 hours without return to pre-existing conscious level with patient surviving

✓7th **S06.367** **Traumatic hemorrhage of cerebrum, unspecified, with loss of consciousness of** any duration with death due to brain injury prior to regaining consciousness

✓7th **S06.368** **Traumatic hemorrhage of cerebrum, unspecified, with loss of consciousness of** any duration with death due to other cause prior to regaining consciousness

✓7th **S06.369** **Traumatic hemorrhage of cerebrum, unspecified, with loss of consciousness of unspecified duration**
Traumatic hemorrhage of cerebrum NOS

✓6th **S06.37** **Contusion, laceration, and hemorrhage of** cerebellum

✓7th **S06.370** **Contusion, laceration, and hemorrhage of cerebellum** without loss of consciousness

✓7th **S06.371** **Contusion, laceration, and hemorrhage of cerebellum with loss of consciousness of** 30 minutes or less

✓7th **S06.372** **Contusion, laceration, and hemorrhage of cerebellum with loss of consciousness of** 31 minutes to 59 minutes

✓7th **S06.373** **Contusion, laceration, and hemorrhage of cerebellum with loss of consciousness of** 1 hour to 5 hours 59 minutes

✓7th **S06.374** **Contusion, laceration, and hemorrhage of cerebellum with loss of consciousness of** 6 hours to 24 hours

---

☑ Additional Character Required   ✓7th Placeholder Alert   Unspecified Dx   Other Specified Dx   Manifestation   ►◄ Revised Text   ● New Code   ▲ Revised Code Title

√7th **S06.375** **Contusion, laceration, and hemorrhage of cerebellum with loss of consciousness greater than 24 hours with return to pre-existing conscious level**

√7th **S06.376** **Contusion, laceration, and hemorrhage of cerebellum with loss of consciousness greater than 24 hours without return to pre-existing conscious level with patient surviving**

√7th **S06.377** **Contusion, laceration, and hemorrhage of cerebellum with loss of consciousness of any duration with death due to brain injury prior to regaining consciousness**

√7th **S06.378** **Contusion, laceration, and hemorrhage of cerebellum with loss of consciousness of any duration with death due to other cause prior to regaining consciousness**

√7th **S06.379** **Contusion, laceration, and hemorrhage of cerebellum with loss of consciousness of unspecified duration**
Contusion, laceration, and hemorrhage of cerebellum NOS

√6th **S06.38** **Contusion, laceration, and hemorrhage of brainstem**

√7th **S06.380** **Contusion, laceration, and hemorrhage of brainstem without loss of consciousness**

√7th **S06.381** **Contusion, laceration, and hemorrhage of brainstem with loss of consciousness of 30 minutes or less**

√7th **S06.382** **Contusion, laceration, and hemorrhage of brainstem with loss of consciousness of 31 minutes to 59 minutes**

√7th **S06.383** **Contusion, laceration, and hemorrhage of brainstem with loss of consciousness of 1 hour to 5 hours 59 minutes**

√7th **S06.384** **Contusion, laceration, and hemorrhage of brainstem with loss of consciousness of 6 hours to 24 hours**

√7th **S06.385** **Contusion, laceration, and hemorrhage of brainstem with loss of consciousness greater than 24 hours with return to pre-existing conscious level**

√7th **S06.386** **Contusion, laceration, and hemorrhage of brainstem with loss of consciousness greater than 24 hours without return to pre-existing conscious level with patient surviving**

√7th **S06.387** **Contusion, laceration, and hemorrhage of brainstem with loss of consciousness of any duration with death due to brain injury prior to regaining consciousness**

√7th **S06.388** **Contusion, laceration, and hemorrhage of brainstem with loss of consciousness of any duration with death due to other cause prior to regaining consciousness**

√7th **S06.389** **Contusion, laceration, and hemorrhage of brainstem with loss of consciousness of unspecified duration**
Contusion, laceration, and hemorrhage of brainstem NOS

√5th **S06.4** **Epidural hemorrhage**
Extradural hemorrhage NOS
Extradural hemorrhage (traumatic)

√6th **S06.4X** **Epidural hemorrhage**

√7th **S06.4X0** **Epidural hemorrhage without loss of consciousness**

√7th **S06.4X1** **Epidural hemorrhage with loss of consciousness of 30 minutes or less**

√7th **S06.4X2** **Epidural hemorrhage with loss of consciousness of 31 minutes to 59 minutes**

√7th **S06.4X3** **Epidural hemorrhage with loss of consciousness of 1 hour to 5 hours 59 minutes**

√7th **S06.4X4** **Epidural hemorrhage with loss of consciousness of 6 hours to 24 hours**

√7th **S06.4X5** **Epidural hemorrhage with loss of consciousness greater than 24 hours with return to pre-existing conscious level**

√7th **S06.4X6** **Epidural hemorrhage with loss of consciousness greater than 24 hours without return to pre-existing conscious level with patient surviving**

√7th **S06.4X7** **Epidural hemorrhage with loss of consciousness of any duration with death due to brain injury prior to regaining consciousness**

√7th **S06.4X8** **Epidural hemorrhage with loss of consciousness of any duration with death due to other causes prior to regaining consciousness**

√7th **S06.4X9** **Epidural hemorrhage with loss of consciousness of unspecified duration**
Epidural hemorrhage NOS

√5th **S06.5** **Traumatic subdural hemorrhage**

√6th **S06.5X** **Traumatic subdural hemorrhage**

√7th **S06.5X0** **Traumatic subdural hemorrhage without loss of consciousness**

√7th **S06.5X1** **Traumatic subdural hemorrhage with loss of consciousness of 30 minutes or less**

√7th **S06.5X2** **Traumatic subdural hemorrhage with loss of consciousness of 31 minutes to 59 minutes**

√7th **S06.5X3** **Traumatic subdural hemorrhage with loss of consciousness of 1 hour to 5 hours 59 minutes**

√7th **S06.5X4** **Traumatic subdural hemorrhage with loss of consciousness of 6 hours to 24 hours**

√7th **S06.5X5** **Traumatic subdural hemorrhage with loss of consciousness greater than 24 hours with return to pre-existing conscious level**

√7th **S06.5X6** **Traumatic subdural hemorrhage with loss of consciousness greater than 24 hours without return to pre-existing conscious level with patient surviving**

√7th **S06.5X7** **Traumatic subdural hemorrhage with loss of consciousness of any duration with death due to brain injury before regaining consciousness**

√7th **S06.5X8** **Traumatic subdural hemorrhage with loss of consciousness of any duration with death due to other cause before regaining consciousness**

√7th **S06.5X9** **Traumatic subdural hemorrhage with loss of consciousness of unspecified duration**
Traumatic subdural hemorrhage NOS

√5th **S06.6** **Traumatic subarachnoid hemorrhage**

√6th **S06.6X** **Traumatic subarachnoid hemorrhage**

√7th **S06.6X0** **Traumatic subarachnoid hemorrhage without loss of consciousness**

√7th **S06.6X1** **Traumatic subarachnoid hemorrhage with loss of consciousness of 30 minutes or less**

√7th **S06.6X2** **Traumatic subarachnoid hemorrhage with loss of consciousness of 31 minutes to 59 minutes**

√7th **S06.6X3** **Traumatic subarachnoid hemorrhage with loss of consciousness of 1 hour to 5 hours 59 minutes**

√7th **S06.6X4** **Traumatic subarachnoid hemorrhage with loss of consciousness of 6 hours to 24 hours**

√7th **S06.6X5** **Traumatic subarachnoid hemorrhage with loss of consciousness greater than 24 hours with return to pre-existing conscious level**

√7th **S06.6X6** **Traumatic subarachnoid hemorrhage with loss of consciousness greater than 24 hours without return to pre-existing conscious level with patient surviving**

√7th **S06.6X7** **Traumatic subarachnoid hemorrhage with loss of consciousness of any duration with death due to brain injury prior to regaining consciousness**

√7th **S06.6X8** **Traumatic subarachnoid hemorrhage with loss of consciousness of any duration with death due to other cause prior to regaining consciousness**

EXCLUDES 1 Not coded here   EXCLUDES 2 Not included here   N Newborn Age: 0   P Pediatric Age: 0-17   M Maternity Age: 12-55   A Adult Age: 15-124

854

ICD-10-CM 2016

✓7ᵗʰ **S06.6X9 Traumatic subarachnoid hemorrhage with loss of consciousness of unspecified duration**
Traumatic subarachnoid hemorrhage NOS

✓5ᵗʰ **S06.8 Other specified intracranial injuries**

✓6ᵗʰ **S06.81 Injury of right internal carotid artery, intracranial portion, not elsewhere classified**

✓7ᵗʰ **S06.810 Injury of right internal carotid artery, intracranial portion, not elsewhere classified without loss of consciousness**

✓7ᵗʰ **S06.811 Injury of right internal carotid artery, intracranial portion, not elsewhere classified with loss of consciousness of 30 minutes or less**

✓7ᵗʰ **S06.812 Injury of right internal carotid artery, intracranial portion, not elsewhere classified with loss of consciousness of 31 minutes to 59 minutes**

✓7ᵗʰ **S06.813 Injury of right internal carotid artery, intracranial portion, not elsewhere classified with loss of consciousness of 1 hour to 5 hours 59 minutes**

✓7ᵗʰ **S06.814 Injury of right internal carotid artery, intracranial portion, not elsewhere classified with loss of consciousness of 6 hours to 24 hours**

✓7ᵗʰ **S06.815 Injury of right internal carotid artery, intracranial portion, not elsewhere classified with loss of consciousness greater than 24 hours with return to pre-existing conscious level**

✓7ᵗʰ **S06.816 Injury of right internal carotid artery, intracranial portion, not elsewhere classified with loss of consciousness greater than 24 hours without return to pre-existing conscious level with patient surviving**

✓7ᵗʰ **S06.817 Injury of right internal carotid artery, intracranial portion, not elsewhere classified with loss of consciousness of any duration with death due to brain injury prior to regaining consciousness**

✓7ᵗʰ **S06.818 Injury of right internal carotid artery, intracranial portion, not elsewhere classified with loss of consciousness of any duration with death due to other cause prior to regaining consciousness**

✓7ᵗʰ **S06.819 Injury of right internal carotid artery, intracranial portion, not elsewhere classified with loss of consciousness of unspecified duration**
Injury of right internal carotid artery, intracranial portion, not elsewhere classified NOS

✓6ᵗʰ **S06.82 Injury of left internal carotid artery, intracranial portion, not elsewhere classified**

✓7ᵗʰ **S06.820 Injury of left internal carotid artery, intracranial portion, not elsewhere classified without loss of consciousness**

✓7ᵗʰ **S06.821 Injury of left internal carotid artery, intracranial portion, not elsewhere classified with loss of consciousness of 30 minutes or less**

✓7ᵗʰ **S06.822 Injury of left internal carotid artery, intracranial portion, not elsewhere classified with loss of consciousness of 31 minutes to 59 minutes**

✓7ᵗʰ **S06.823 Injury of left internal carotid artery, intracranial portion, not elsewhere classified with loss of consciousness of 1 hour to 5 hours 59 minutes**

✓7ᵗʰ **S06.824 Injury of left internal carotid artery, intracranial portion, not elsewhere classified with loss of consciousness of 6 hours to 24 hours**

✓7ᵗʰ **S06.825 Injury of left internal carotid artery, intracranial portion, not elsewhere classified with loss of consciousness greater than 24 hours with return to pre-existing conscious level**

✓7ᵗʰ **S06.826 Injury of left internal carotid artery, intracranial portion, not elsewhere classified with loss of consciousness greater than 24 hours without return to pre-existing conscious level with patient surviving**

✓7ᵗʰ **S06.827 Injury of left internal carotid artery, intracranial portion, not elsewhere classified with loss of consciousness of any duration with death due to brain injury prior to regaining consciousness**

✓7ᵗʰ **S06.828 Injury of left internal carotid artery, intracranial portion, not elsewhere classified with loss of consciousness of any duration with death due to other cause prior to regaining consciousness**

✓7ᵗʰ **S06.829 Injury of left internal carotid artery, intracranial portion, not elsewhere classified with loss of consciousness of unspecified duration**
Injury of left internal carotid artery, intracranial portion, not elsewhere classified NOS

✓6ᵗʰ **S06.89 Other specified intracranial injury**

✓7ᵗʰ **S06.890 Other specified intracranial injury without loss of consciousness**

✓7ᵗʰ **S06.891 Other specified intracranial injury with loss of consciousness of 30 minutes or less**

✓7ᵗʰ **S06.892 Other specified intracranial injury with loss of consciousness of 31 minutes to 59 minutes**

✓7ᵗʰ **S06.893 Other specified intracranial injury with loss of consciousness of 1 hour to 5 hours 59 minutes**

✓7ᵗʰ **S06.894 Other specified intracranial injury with loss of consciousness of 6 hours to 24 hours**

✓7ᵗʰ **S06.895 Other specified intracranial injury with loss of consciousness greater than 24 hours with return to pre-existing conscious level**

✓7ᵗʰ **S06.896 Other specified intracranial injury with loss of consciousness greater than 24 hours without return to pre-existing conscious level with patient surviving**

✓7ᵗʰ **S06.897 Other specified intracranial injury with loss of consciousness of any duration with death due to brain injury prior to regaining consciousness**

✓7ᵗʰ **S06.898 Other specified intracranial injury with loss of consciousness of any duration with death due to other cause prior to regaining consciousness**

✓7ᵗʰ **S06.899 Other specified intracranial injury with loss of consciousness of unspecified duration**

✓5ᵗʰ **S06.9 Unspecified intracranial injury**
Brain injury NOS
Head injury NOS with loss of consciousness
EXCLUDES 1   head injury NOS (S09.90)

✓6ᵗʰ **S06.9X Unspecified intracranial injury**

✓7ᵗʰ **S06.9X0 Unspecified intracranial injury without loss of consciousness**

✓7ᵗʰ **S06.9X1 Unspecified intracranial injury with loss of consciousness of 30 minutes or less**

✓7ᵗʰ **S06.9X2 Unspecified intracranial injury with loss of consciousness of 31 minutes to 59 minutes**

✓7ᵗʰ **S06.9X3 Unspecified intracranial injury with loss of consciousness of 1 hour to 5 hours 59 minutes**

✓7ᵗʰ **S06.9X4 Unspecified intracranial injury with loss of consciousness of 6 hours to 24 hours**

✓7ᵗʰ **S06.9X5 Unspecified intracranial injury with loss of consciousness greater than 24 hours with return to pre-existing conscious level**

✓7ᵗʰ **S06.9X6 Unspecified intracranial injury with loss of consciousness greater than 24 hours without return to pre-existing conscious level with patient surviving**

✓ Additional Character Required   ✓ˣ7ᵗʰ Placeholder Alert   Unspecified Dx   Other Specified Dx   Manifestation   ▶◀ Revised Text   ● New Code   ▲ Revised Code Title

√7ᵗʰ **S06.9X7** **Unspecified intracranial injury with loss of consciousness of** any duration with death due to brain injury prior to regaining consciousness

√7ᵗʰ **S06.9X8** **Unspecified intracranial injury with loss of consciousness of** any duration with death due to **other** cause prior to regaining consciousness

√7ᵗʰ **S06.9X9** **Unspecified intracranial injury with loss of consciousness of unspecified duration**

√4ᵗʰ **S07** **Crushing injury of head**
Use additional code for all associated injuries, such as:
intracranial injuries (S06.-)
skull fractures (S02.-)

The appropriate 7th character is to be added to each code from category S07.
A   initial encounter
D   subsequent encounter
S   sequela

√x7ᵗʰ **S07.0** **Crushing injury of** face

√x7ᵗʰ **S07.1** **Crushing injury of** skull

√x7ᵗʰ **S07.8** **Crushing injury of other parts of head**

√x7ᵗʰ **S07.9** **Crushing injury of head, part unspecified**

√4ᵗʰ **S08** **Avulsion and traumatic amputation of part of head**
NOTE   An amputation not identified as partial or complete should be coded to complete

The appropriate 7th character is to be added to each code from category S08.
A   initial encounter
D   subsequent encounter
S   sequela

√x7ᵗʰ **S08.0** **Avulsion of** scalp

√5ᵗʰ **S08.1** **Traumatic amputation of** ear

     √6ᵗʰ **S08.11** **Complete traumatic amputation of ear**

         √7ᵗʰ **S08.111** **Complete traumatic amputation of** right ear

         √7ᵗʰ **S08.112** **Complete traumatic amputation of** left ear

         √7ᵗʰ **S08.119** **Complete traumatic amputation of unspecified ear**

     √6ᵗʰ **S08.12** **Partial traumatic amputation of ear**

         √7ᵗʰ **S08.121** **Partial traumatic amputation of** right ear

         √7ᵗʰ **S08.122** **Partial traumatic amputation of** left ear

         √7ᵗʰ **S08.129** **Partial traumatic amputation of unspecified ear**

√5ᵗʰ **S08.8** **Traumatic amputation of** other parts of head

     √6ᵗʰ **S08.81** **Traumatic amputation of** nose

         √7ᵗʰ **S08.811** **Complete** traumatic amputation of nose

         √7ᵗʰ **S08.812** **Partial** traumatic amputation of nose

     √x7ᵗʰ **S08.89** **Traumatic amputation of other parts of head**

√4ᵗʰ **S09** **Other and unspecified injuries of head**

The appropriate 7th character is to be added to each code from category S09.
A   initial encounter
D   subsequent encounter
S   sequela

√x7ᵗʰ **S09.0** **Injury of** blood vessels **of head, not elsewhere classified**
EXCLUDES 1   injury of cerebral blood vessels (S06.-)
injury of precerebral blood vessels (S15.-)

√5ᵗʰ **S09.1** **Injury of** muscle and tendon **of head**
Code also any associated open wound (S01.-)
EXCLUDES 2   sprain to joints and ligament of head (S03.9)

     √x7ᵗʰ **S09.10** **Unspecified injury of muscle and tendon of head**
Injury of muscle and tendon of head NOS

     √x7ᵗʰ **S09.11** **Strain of muscle and tendon of head**

     √x7ᵗʰ **S09.12** **Laceration of muscle and tendon of head**

     √x7ᵗʰ **S09.19** **Other specified injury of muscle and tendon of head**

√5ᵗʰ **S09.2** **Traumatic rupture of** ear drum
EXCLUDES 1   traumatic rupture of ear drum due to blast injury (S09.31-)

     √x7ᵗʰ **S09.20** **Traumatic rupture of unspecified ear drum**

     √x7ᵗʰ **S09.21** **Traumatic rupture of** right **ear drum**

     √x7ᵗʰ **S09.22** **Traumatic rupture of** left **ear drum**

√5ᵗʰ **S09.3** **Other specified and unspecified injury of middle and inner ear**
EXCLUDES 1   injury to ear NOS (S09.91-)
EXCLUDES 2   injury to external ear (S00.4-, S01.3-, S08.1-)

     √6ᵗʰ **S09.30** **Unspecified injury of** middle and inner ear

         √7ᵗʰ **S09.301** **Unspecified injury of** right **middle and inner ear**

         √7ᵗʰ **S09.302** **Unspecified injury of** left **middle and inner ear**

         √7ᵗʰ **S09.309** **Unspecified injury of unspecified middle and inner ear**

     √6ᵗʰ **S09.31** **Primary** blast injury **of ear**
Blast injury of ear NOS

         √7ᵗʰ **S09.311** **Primary blast injury of** right **ear**

         √7ᵗʰ **S09.312** **Primary blast injury of** left **ear**

         √7ᵗʰ **S09.313** **Primary blast injury of ear, bilateral**

         √7ᵗʰ **S09.319** **Primary blast injury of unspecified ear**

     √6ᵗʰ **S09.39** **Other** specified injury of middle and inner ear
Secondary blast injury to ear

         √7ᵗʰ **S09.391** **Other specified injury of** right **middle and inner ear**

         √7ᵗʰ **S09.392** **Other specified injury of** left **middle and inner ear**

         √7ᵗʰ **S09.399** **Other specified injury of unspecified middle and inner ear**

√x7ᵗʰ **S09.8** **Other specified injuries of head**

√5ᵗʰ **S09.9** **Unspecified injury of face and head**

     √x7ᵗʰ **S09.90** **Unspecified injury of** head
Head injury NOS
EXCLUDES 1   brain injury NOS (S06.9-)
head injury NOS with loss of consciousness (S06.9-)
intracranial injury NOS (S06.9-)

     √x7ᵗʰ **S09.91** **Unspecified injury of** ear
Injury of ear NOS

     √x7ᵗʰ **S09.92** **Unspecified injury of** nose
Injury of nose NOS

     √x7ᵗʰ **S09.93** **Unspecified injury of** face
Injury of face NOS

Injuries to the neck (S10-S19)

INCLUDES   injuries of nape
injuries of supraclavicular region
injuries of throat
EXCLUDES 2   burns and corrosions (T20-T32)
effects of foreign body in esophagus (T18.1)
effects of foreign body in larynx (T17.3)
effects of foreign body in pharynx (T17.2)
effects of foreign body in trachea (T17.4)
frostbite (T33-T34)
insect bite or sting, venomous (T63.4)

√4ᵗʰ **S10** **Superficial injury of neck**

The appropriate 7th character is to be added to each code from category S10.
A   initial encounter
D   subsequent encounter
S   sequela

√x7ᵗʰ **S10.0** **Contusion of throat**
Contusion of cervical esophagus
Contusion of larynx
Contusion of pharynx
Contusion of trachea

√5ᵗʰ **S10.1** **Other and unspecified superficial injuries of throat**

     √x7ᵗʰ **S10.10** **Unspecified superficial injuries of throat**

     √x7ᵗʰ **S10.11** **Abrasion of throat**

     √x7ᵗʰ **S10.12** **Blister (nonthermal) of throat**

     √x7ᵗʰ **S10.14** **External constriction of part of throat**

     √x7ᵗʰ **S10.15** **Superficial** foreign body **of throat**
Splinter in the throat

     √x7ᵗʰ **S10.16** **Insect bite (nonvenomous) of throat**

     √x7ᵗʰ **S10.17** **Other superficial** bite **of throat**
EXCLUDES 1   open bite of throat (S11.85)

EXCLUDES 1 Not coded here   *EXCLUDES 2* Not included here   N Newborn Age: 0   P Pediatric Age: 0-17   M Maternity Age: 12-55   A Adult Age: 15-124

856   ICD-10-CM 2016

√5ᵗʰ **S10.8 Superficial injury of other specified parts of neck**

√x7ᵗʰ **S10.80 Unspecified superficial injury of other specified part of neck**

√x7ᵗʰ **S10.81 Abrasion of other specified part of neck**

√x7ᵗʰ **S10.82 Blister (nonthermal) of other specified part of neck**

√x7ᵗʰ **S10.83 Contusion of other specified part of neck**

√x7ᵗʰ **S10.84 External constriction of other specified part of neck**

√x7ᵗʰ **S10.85 Superficial foreign body of other specified part of neck**
Splinter in other specified part of neck

√x7ᵗʰ **S10.86 Insect bite of other specified part of neck**

√x7ᵗʰ **S10.87 Other superficial bite of other specified part of neck**
EXCLUDES 1   open bite of other specified parts of neck (S11.85)

√5ᵗʰ **S10.9 Superficial injury of unspecified part of neck**

√x7ᵗʰ **S10.90 Unspecified superficial injury of unspecified part of neck**

√x7ᵗʰ **S10.91 Abrasion of unspecified part of neck**

√x7ᵗʰ **S10.92 Blister (nonthermal) of unspecified part of neck**

√x7ᵗʰ **S10.93 Contusion of unspecified part of neck**

√x7ᵗʰ **S10.94 External constriction of unspecified part of neck**

√x7ᵗʰ **S10.95 Superficial foreign body of unspecified part of neck**

√x7ᵗʰ **S10.96 Insect bite of unspecified part of neck**

√x7ᵗʰ **S10.97 Other superficial bite of unspecified part of neck**

4ᵗʰ **S11 Open wound of neck**
Code also any associated:
spinal cord injury (S14.0, S14.1-)
wound infection
EXCLUDES 2   open fracture of vertebra (S12- with 7th character B)

The appropriate 7th character is to be added to each code from category S11.
A   initial encounter
D   subsequent encounter
S   sequela

√5ᵗʰ **S11.0 Open wound of larynx and trachea**

√6ᵗʰ **S11.01 Open wound of larynx**
EXCLUDES 2   open wound of vocal cord (S11.03)

√7ᵗʰ **S11.011 Laceration without foreign body of larynx**

√7ᵗʰ **S11.012 Laceration with foreign body of larynx**

√7ᵗʰ **S11.013 Puncture wound without foreign body of larynx**

√7ᵗʰ **S11.014 Puncture wound with foreign body of larynx**

√7ᵗʰ **S11.015 Open bite of larynx**
Bite of larynx NOS

√7ᵗʰ **S11.019 Unspecified open wound of larynx**

√6ᵗʰ **S11.02 Open wound of trachea**
Open wound of cervical trachea
Open wound of trachea NOS
EXCLUDES 2   open wound of thoracic trachea (S27.5-)

√7ᵗʰ **S11.021 Laceration without foreign body of trachea**

√7ᵗʰ **S11.022 Laceration with foreign body of trachea**

√7ᵗʰ **S11.023 Puncture wound without foreign body of trachea**

√7ᵗʰ **S11.024 Puncture wound with foreign body of trachea**

√7ᵗʰ **S11.025 Open bite of trachea**
Bite of trachea NOS

√7ᵗʰ **S11.029 Unspecified open wound of trachea**

√6ᵗʰ **S11.03 Open wound of vocal cord**

√7ᵗʰ **S11.031 Laceration without foreign body of vocal cord**

√7ᵗʰ **S11.032 Laceration with foreign body of vocal cord**

√7ᵗʰ **S11.033 Puncture wound without foreign body of vocal cord**

√7ᵗʰ **S11.034 Puncture wound with foreign body of vocal cord**

√7ᵗʰ **S11.035 Open bite of vocal cord**
Bite of vocal cord NOS

√7ᵗʰ **S11.039 Unspecified open wound of vocal cord**

√5ᵗʰ **S11.1 Open wound of thyroid gland**

√x7ᵗʰ **S11.10 Unspecified open wound of thyroid gland**

√x7ᵗʰ **S11.11 Laceration without foreign body of thyroid gland**

√x7ᵗʰ **S11.12 Laceration with foreign body of thyroid gland**

√x7ᵗʰ **S11.13 Puncture wound without foreign body of thyroid gland**

√x7ᵗʰ **S11.14 Puncture wound with foreign body of thyroid gland**

√x7ᵗʰ **S11.15 Open bite of thyroid gland**
Bite of thyroid gland NOS

√5ᵗʰ **S11.2 Open wound of pharynx and cervical esophagus**
EXCLUDES 1   open wound of esophagus NOS (S27.8-)

√x7ᵗʰ **S11.20 Unspecified open wound of pharynx and cervical esophagus**

√x7ᵗʰ **S11.21 Laceration without foreign body of pharynx and cervical esophagus**

√x7ᵗʰ **S11.22 Laceration with foreign body of pharynx and cervical esophagus**

√x7ᵗʰ **S11.23 Puncture wound without foreign body of pharynx and cervical esophagus**

√x7ᵗʰ **S11.24 Puncture wound with foreign body of pharynx and cervical esophagus**

√x7ᵗʰ **S11.25 Open bite of pharynx and cervical esophagus**
Bite of pharynx and cervical esophagus NOS

√5ᵗʰ **S11.8 Open wound of other specified parts of neck**

√x7ᵗʰ **S11.80 Unspecified open wound of other specified part of neck**

√x7ᵗʰ **S11.81 Laceration without foreign body of other specified part of neck**

√x7ᵗʰ **S11.82 Laceration with foreign body of other specified part of neck**

√x7ᵗʰ **S11.83 Puncture wound without foreign body of other specified part of neck**

√x7ᵗʰ **S11.84 Puncture wound with foreign body of other specified part of neck**

√x7ᵗʰ **S11.85 Open bite of other specified part of neck**
Bite of other specified part of neck NOS
EXCLUDES 1   superficial bite of other specified part of neck (S10.87)

√x7ᵗʰ **S11.89 Other open wound of other specified part of neck**

√5ᵗʰ **S11.9 Open wound of unspecified part of neck**

√x7ᵗʰ **S11.90 Unspecified open wound of unspecified part of neck**

√x7ᵗʰ **S11.91 Laceration without foreign body of unspecified part of neck**

√x7ᵗʰ **S11.92 Laceration with foreign body of unspecified part of neck**

√x7ᵗʰ **S11.93 Puncture wound without foreign body of unspecified part of neck**

√x7ᵗʰ **S11.94 Puncture wound with foreign body of unspecified part of neck**

√x7ᵗʰ **S11.95 Open bite of unspecified part of neck**
Bite of neck NOS
EXCLUDES 1   superficial bite of neck (S10.97)

✓ Additional Character Required   √x7ᵗʰ Placeholder Alert   Unspecified Dx   Other Specified Dx   Manifestation   ▶◀ Revised Text   ● New Code   ▲ Revised Code Title

√4th **S12 Fracture of cervical vertebra and other parts of neck**

> NOTE   A fracture not indicated as nondisplaced or displaced should be coded to displaced.
> A fracture not indicated as open or closed should be coded to closed.

> INCLUDES   fracture of cervical neural arch
> fracture of cervical spine
> fracture of cervical spinous process
> fracture of cervical transverse process
> fracture of cervical vertebral arch
> fracture of neck

Code first any associated cervical spinal cord injury (S14.0, S14.1-)

> The appropriate 7th character is to be added to all codes from subcategories S12.0-S12.6.
> A   initial encounter for closed fracture
> B   initial encounter for open fracture
> D   subsequent encounter for fracture with routine healing
> G   subsequent encounter for fracture with delayed healing
> K   subsequent encounter for fracture with nonunion
> S   sequela

√5th **S12.0 Fracture of first cervical vertebra**
Atlas

     √6th **S12.00 Unspecified fracture of first cervical vertebra**

         √7th **S12.000 Unspecified displaced fracture of first cervical vertebra**

         √7th **S12.001 Unspecified nondisplaced fracture of first cervical vertebra**

     √x7th **S12.01 Stable burst fracture of first cervical vertebra**

     √x7th **S12.02 Unstable burst fracture of first cervical vertebra**

     √6th **S12.03 Posterior arch fracture of first cervical vertebra**

         √7th **S12.030 Displaced posterior arch fracture of first cervical vertebra**

         √7th **S12.031 Nondisplaced posterior arch fracture of first cervical vertebra**

     √6th **S12.04 Lateral mass fracture of first cervical vertebra**

         √7th **S12.040 Displaced lateral mass fracture of first cervical vertebra**

         √7th **S12.041 Nondisplaced lateral mass fracture of first cervical vertebra**

     √6th **S12.09 Other fracture of first cervical vertebra**

         √7th **S12.090 Other displaced fracture of first cervical vertebra**

         √7th **S12.091 Other nondisplaced fracture of first cervical vertebra**

√5th **S12.1 Fracture of second cervical vertebra**
Axis

     √6th **S12.10 Unspecified fracture of second cervical vertebra**

         √7th **S12.100 Unspecified displaced fracture of second cervical vertebra**

         √7th **S12.101 Unspecified nondisplaced fracture of second cervical vertebra**

     √6th **S12.11 Type II dens fracture**

         √7th **S12.110 Anterior displaced Type II dens fracture**

         √7th **S12.111 Posterior displaced Type II dens fracture**

         √7th **S12.112 Nondisplaced Type II dens fracture**

     √6th **S12.12 Other dens fracture**

         √7th **S12.120 Other displaced dens fracture**

         √7th **S12.121 Other nondisplaced dens fracture**

     √6th **S12.13 Unspecified traumatic spondylolisthesis of second cervical vertebra**

         √7th **S12.130 Unspecified traumatic displaced spondylolisthesis of second cervical vertebra**

         √7th **S12.131 Unspecified traumatic nondisplaced spondylolisthesis of second cervical vertebra**

     √x7th **S12.14 Type III traumatic spondylolisthesis of second cervical vertebra**

     √6th **S12.15 Other traumatic spondylolisthesis of second cervical vertebra**

         √7th **S12.150 Other traumatic displaced spondylolisthesis of second cervical vertebra**

         √7th **S12.151 Other traumatic nondisplaced spondylolisthesis of second cervical vertebra**

     √6th **S12.19 Other fracture of second cervical vertebra**

         √7th **S12.190 Other displaced fracture of second cervic vertebra**

         √7th **S12.191 Other nondisplaced fracture of second cervical vertebra**

√5th **S12.2 Fracture of third cervical vertebra**

     √6th **S12.20 Unspecified fracture of third cervical vertebra**

         √7th **S12.200 Unspecified displaced fracture of third cervical vertebra**

         √7th **S12.201 Unspecified nondisplaced fracture of third cervical vertebra**

     √6th **S12.23 Unspecified traumatic spondylolisthesis of third cervical vertebra**

         √7th **S12.230 Unspecified traumatic displaced spondylolisthesis of third cervical vertebra**

         √7th **S12.231 Unspecified traumatic nondisplaced spondylolisthesis of third cervical vertebra**

     √x7th **S12.24 Type III traumatic spondylolisthesis of third cervical vertebra**

     √6th **S12.25 Other traumatic spondylolisthesis of third cervical vertebra**

         √7th **S12.250 Other traumatic displaced spondylolisthesis of third cervical vertebra**

         √7th **S12.251 Other traumatic nondisplaced spondylolisthesis of third cervical vertebra**

     √6th **S12.29 Other fracture of third cervical vertebra**

         √7th **S12.290 Other displaced fracture of third cervical vertebra**

         √7th **S12.291 Other nondisplaced fracture of third cervical vertebra**

√5th **S12.3 Fracture of fourth cervical vertebra**

     √6th **S12.30 Unspecified fracture of fourth cervical vertebra**

         √7th **S12.300 Unspecified displaced fracture of fourth cervical vertebra**

         √7th **S12.301 Unspecified nondisplaced fracture of fourth cervical vertebra**

     √6th **S12.33 Unspecified traumatic spondylolisthesis of fourth cervical vertebra**

         √7th **S12.330 Unspecified traumatic displaced spondylolisthesis of fourth cervical vertebra**

         √7th **S12.331 Unspecified traumatic nondisplaced spondylolisthesis of fourth cervical vertebra**

     √x7th **S12.34 Type III traumatic spondylolisthesis of fourth cervical vertebra**

     √6th **S12.35 Other traumatic spondylolisthesis of fourth cervical vertebra**

         √7th **S12.350 Other traumatic displaced spondylolisthesis of fourth cervical vertebra**

         √7th **S12.351 Other traumatic nondisplaced spondylolisthesis of fourth cervical vertebra**

     √6th **S12.39 Other fracture of fourth cervical vertebra**

         √7th **S12.390 Other displaced fracture of fourth cervical vertebra**

         √7th **S12.391 Other nondisplaced fracture of fourth cervical vertebra**

√5th **S12.4 Fracture of fifth cervical vertebra**

     √6th **S12.40 Unspecified fracture of fifth cervical vertebra**

         √7th **S12.400 Unspecified displaced fracture of fifth cervical vertebra**

         √7th **S12.401 Unspecified nondisplaced fracture of fifth cervical vertebra**

EXCLUDES1 Not coded here   EXCLUDES2 Not included here   N Newborn Age: 0   P Pediatric Age: 0-17   M Maternity Age: 12-55   A Adult Age: 15-124

858   ICD-10-CM 2016

✓6ᵗʰ **S12.43** Unspecified **traumatic** spondylolisthesis of fifth cervical vertebra

　✓7ᵗʰ **S12.430** Unspecified traumatic displaced spondylolisthesis of fifth cervical vertebra

　✓7ᵗʰ **S12.431** Unspecified traumatic nondisplaced spondylolisthesis of fifth cervical vertebra

✓x7ᵗʰ **S12.44** Type III **traumatic** spondylolisthesis of fifth cervical vertebra

✓6ᵗʰ **S12.45** Other **traumatic** spondylolisthesis of fifth cervical vertebra

　✓7ᵗʰ **S12.450** Other traumatic displaced spondylolisthesis of fifth cervical vertebra

　✓7ᵗʰ **S12.451** Other traumatic nondisplaced spondylolisthesis of fifth cervical vertebra

✓6ᵗʰ **S12.49** Other fracture of fifth cervical vertebra

　✓7ᵗʰ **S12.490** Other displaced fracture of fifth cervical vertebra

　✓7ᵗʰ **S12.491** Other nondisplaced fracture of fifth cervical vertebra

✓5ᵗʰ **S12.5** Fracture of sixth cervical vertebra

　✓6ᵗʰ **S12.50** Unspecified fracture of sixth cervical vertebra

　　✓7ᵗʰ **S12.500** Unspecified displaced fracture of sixth cervical vertebra

　　✓7ᵗʰ **S12.501** Unspecified nondisplaced fracture of sixth cervical vertebra

　✓6ᵗʰ **S12.53** Unspecified **traumatic** spondylolisthesis of sixth cervical vertebra

　　✓7ᵗʰ **S12.530** Unspecified traumatic displaced spondylolisthesis of sixth cervical vertebra

　　✓7ᵗʰ **S12.531** Unspecified traumatic nondisplaced spondylolisthesis of sixth cervical vertebra

　✓x7ᵗʰ **S12.54** Type III **traumatic** spondylolisthesis of sixth cervical vertebra

　✓6ᵗʰ **S12.55** Other **traumatic** spondylolisthesis of sixth cervical vertebra

　　✓7ᵗʰ **S12.550** Other traumatic displaced spondylolisthesis of sixth cervical vertebra

　　✓7ᵗʰ **S12.551** Other traumatic nondisplaced spondylolisthesis of sixth cervical vertebra

　✓6ᵗʰ **S12.59** Other fracture of sixth cervical vertebra

　　✓7ᵗʰ **S12.590** Other displaced fracture of sixth cervical vertebra

　　✓7ᵗʰ **S12.591** Other nondisplaced fracture of sixth cervical vertebra

✓5ᵗʰ **S12.6** Fracture of seventh cervical vertebra

　✓6ᵗʰ **S12.60** Unspecified fracture of seventh cervical vertebra

　　✓7ᵗʰ **S12.600** Unspecified displaced fracture of seventh cervical vertebra

　　✓7ᵗʰ **S12.601** Unspecified nondisplaced fracture of seventh cervical vertebra

　✓6ᵗʰ **S12.63** Unspecified **traumatic** spondylolisthesis of seventh cervical vertebra

　　✓7ᵗʰ **S12.630** Unspecified traumatic displaced spondylolisthesis of seventh cervical vertebra

　　✓7ᵗʰ **S12.631** Unspecified traumatic nondisplaced spondylolisthesis of seventh cervical vertebra

　✓x7ᵗʰ **S12.64** Type III **traumatic** spondylolisthesis of seventh cervical vertebra

　✓6ᵗʰ **S12.65** Other **traumatic** spondylolisthesis of seventh cervical vertebra

　　✓7ᵗʰ **S12.650** Other traumatic displaced spondylolisthesis of seventh cervical vertebra

　　✓7ᵗʰ **S12.651** Other traumatic nondisplaced spondylolisthesis of seventh cervical vertebra

　✓6ᵗʰ **S12.69** Other fracture of seventh cervical vertebra

　　✓7ᵗʰ **S12.690** Other displaced fracture of seventh cervical vertebra

✓7ᵗʰ **S12.691** Other nondisplaced fracture of seventh cervical vertebra

✓x7ᵗʰ **S12.8** **Fracture of other parts of neck**
Hyoid bone　　　　　　Thyroid cartilage
Larynx　　　　　　　　Trachea

The appropriate 7th character is to be added to code S12.8.
A　initial encounter
D　subsequent encounter
S　sequela

✓x7ᵗʰ **S12.9** **Fracture of neck, unspecified**
Fracture of cervical spine NOS
Fracture of cervical vertebra NOS
Fracture of neck NOS

The appropriate 7th character is to be added to code S12.9.
A　initial encounter
D　subsequent encounter
S　sequela

✓4ᵗʰ **S13** **Dislocation and sprain of joints and ligaments at neck level**
　INCLUDES　avulsion of joint or ligament at neck level
　　　　　　laceration of cartilage, joint or ligament at neck level
　　　　　　sprain of cartilage, joint or ligament at neck level
　　　　　　traumatic hemarthrosis of joint or ligament at neck level
　　　　　　traumatic rupture of joint or ligament at neck level
　　　　　　traumatic subluxation of joint or ligament at neck level
　　　　　　traumatic tear of joint or ligament at neck level
Code also any associated open wound
　EXCLUDES 2　strain of muscle or tendon at neck level (S16.1)

The appropriate 7th character is to be added to each code from category S13.
A　initial encounter
D　subsequent encounter
S　sequela

✓x7ᵗʰ **S13.0** **Traumatic rupture of cervical intervertebral disc**
　EXCLUDES 1　rupture or displacement (nontraumatic) of cervical intervertebral disc NOS (M50.-)

✓5ᵗʰ **S13.1** **Subluxation and dislocation of cervical vertebrae**
Code also any associated:
　open wound of neck (S11.-)
　spinal cord injury (S14.1-)
　EXCLUDES 2　fracture of cervical vertebrae (S12.0--S12.3-)

　✓6ᵗʰ **S13.10** Subluxation and dislocation of unspecified cervical vertebrae

　　✓7ᵗʰ **S13.100** Subluxation of unspecified cervical vertebrae

　　✓7ᵗʰ **S13.101** Dislocation of unspecified cervical vertebrae

　✓6ᵗʰ **S13.11** Subluxation and dislocation of C0/C1 cervical vertebrae
　　　Subluxation and dislocation of atlantooccipital joint
　　　Subluxation and dislocation of atloidooccipital joint
　　　Subluxation and dislocation of occipitoatloid joint

　　✓7ᵗʰ **S13.110** Subluxation of C0/C1 cervical vertebrae

　　✓7ᵗʰ **S13.111** Dislocation of C0/C1 cervical vertebrae

　✓6ᵗʰ **S13.12** Subluxation and dislocation of C1/C2 cervical vertebrae
　　　Subluxation and dislocation of atlantoaxial joint

　　✓7ᵗʰ **S13.120** Subluxation of C1/C2 cervical vertebrae

　　✓7ᵗʰ **S13.121** Dislocation of C1/C2 cervical vertebrae

　✓6ᵗʰ **S13.13** Subluxation and dislocation of C2/C3 cervical vertebrae

　　✓7ᵗʰ **S13.130** Subluxation of C2/C3 cervical vertebrae

　　✓7ᵗʰ **S13.131** Dislocation of C2/C3 cervical vertebrae

　✓6ᵗʰ **S13.14** Subluxation and dislocation of C3/C4 cervical vertebrae

　　✓7ᵗʰ **S13.140** Subluxation of C3/C4 cervical vertebrae

　　✓7ᵗʰ **S13.141** Dislocation of C3/C4 cervical vertebrae

　✓6ᵗʰ **S13.15** Subluxation and dislocation of C4/C5 cervical vertebrae

　　✓7ᵗʰ **S13.150** Subluxation of C4/C5 cervical vertebrae

　　✓7ᵗʰ **S13.151** Dislocation of C4/C5 cervical vertebrae

　✓6ᵗʰ **S13.16** Subluxation and dislocation of C5/C6 cervical vertebrae

　　✓7ᵗʰ **S13.160** Subluxation of C5/C6 cervical vertebrae

　　✓7ᵗʰ **S13.161** Dislocation of C5/C6 cervical vertebrae

☑ Additional Character Required　　✓x7ᵗʰ Placeholder Alert　　Unspecified Dx　　Other Specified Dx　　Manifestation　　▶◀ Revised Text　　● New Code　　▲ Revised Code Title

√6ᵗʰ S13.17   **Subluxation and dislocation of C6/C7 cervical vertebrae**

     √7ᵗʰ S13.170   Subluxation of C6/C7 cervical vertebrae

     √7ᵗʰ S13.171   Dislocation of C6/C7 cervical vertebrae

√6ᵗʰ S13.18   **Subluxation and dislocation of C7/T1 cervical vertebrae**

     √7ᵗʰ S13.180   Subluxation of C7/T1 cervical vertebrae

     √7ᵗʰ S13.181   Dislocation of C7/T1 cervical vertebrae

√5ᵗʰ S13.2   Dislocation of other and unspecified parts of neck

     √x7ᵗʰ S13.20   **Dislocation of unspecified parts of neck**

     √x7ᵗʰ S13.29   **Dislocation of other parts of neck**

√x7ᵗʰ S13.4   Sprain of ligaments of cervical spine

     Sprain of anterior longitudinal (ligament), cervical
     Sprain of atlanto-axial (joints)
     Sprain of atlanto-occipital (joints)
     Whiplash injury of cervical spine

√x7ᵗʰ S13.5   Sprain of thyroid region

     Sprain of cricoarytenoid (joint) (ligament)
     Sprain of cricothyroid (joint) (ligament)
     Sprain of thyroid cartilage

√x7ᵗʰ S13.8   **Sprain of joints and ligaments of other parts of neck**

√x7ᵗʰ S13.9   **Sprain of joints and ligaments of unspecified parts of neck**

√4ᵗʰ S14   **Injury of nerves and spinal cord at neck level**

> **NOTE**   Code to highest level of cervical cord injury.

Code also any associated:
     fracture of cervical vertebra (S12.0- -S12.6-)
     open wound of neck (S11.-)
     transient paralysis (R29.5)

> The appropriate 7th character is to be added to each code from category S14.
> A   initial encounter
> D   subsequent encounter
> S   sequela

√x7ᵗʰ S14.0   **Concussion and edema of cervical spinal cord**

√5ᵗʰ S14.1   Other and unspecified injuries of cervical spinal cord

     √6ᵗʰ S14.10   Unspecified injury of cervical spinal cord

         √7ᵗʰ S14.101   **Unspecified injury at C1 level of cervical spinal cord**

         √7ᵗʰ S14.102   **Unspecified injury at C2 level of cervical spinal cord**

         √7ᵗʰ S14.103   **Unspecified injury at C3 level of cervical spinal cord**

         √7ᵗʰ S14.104   **Unspecified injury at C4 level of cervical spinal cord**

         √7ᵗʰ S14.105   **Unspecified injury at C5 level of cervical spinal cord**

         √7ᵗʰ S14.106   **Unspecified injury at C6 level of cervical spinal cord**

         √7ᵗʰ S14.107   **Unspecified injury at C7 level of cervical spinal cord**

         √7ᵗʰ S14.108   **Unspecified injury at C8 level of cervical spinal cord**

         √7ᵗʰ S14.109   **Unspecified injury at unspecified level of cervical spinal cord**

            Injury of cervical spinal cord NOS

     √6ᵗʰ S14.11   Complete lesion of cervical spinal cord

         √7ᵗʰ S14.111   **Complete lesion at C1 level of cervical spinal cord**

         √7ᵗʰ S14.112   **Complete lesion at C2 level of cervical spinal cord**

         √7ᵗʰ S14.113   **Complete lesion at C3 level of cervical spinal cord**

         √7ᵗʰ S14.114   **Complete lesion at C4 level of cervical spinal cord**

         √7ᵗʰ S14.115   **Complete lesion at C5 level of cervical spinal cord**

         √7ᵗʰ S14.116   **Complete lesion at C6 level of cervical spinal cord**

         √7ᵗʰ S14.117   **Complete lesion at C7 level of cervical spinal cord**

         √7ᵗʰ S14.118   **Complete lesion at C8 level of cervical spinal cord**

         √7ᵗʰ S14.119   **Complete lesion at unspecified level of cervical spinal cord**

√6ᵗʰ S14.12   Central cord syndrome of cervical spinal cord

     √7ᵗʰ S14.121   **Central cord syndrome at C1 level of cervical spinal cord**

     √7ᵗʰ S14.122   **Central cord syndrome at C2 level of cervical spinal cord**

     √7ᵗʰ S14.123   **Central cord syndrome at C3 level of cervical spinal cord**

     √7ᵗʰ S14.124   **Central cord syndrome at C4 level of cervical spinal cord**

     √7ᵗʰ S14.125   **Central cord syndrome at C5 level of cervical spinal cord**

     √7ᵗʰ S14.126   **Central cord syndrome at C6 level of cervical spinal cord**

     √7ᵗʰ S14.127   **Central cord syndrome at C7 level of cervical spinal cord**

     √7ᵗʰ S14.128   **Central cord syndrome at C8 level of cervical spinal cord**

     √7ᵗʰ S14.129   **Central cord syndrome at unspecified level of cervical spinal cord**

√6ᵗʰ S14.13   Anterior cord syndrome of cervical spinal cord

     √7ᵗʰ S14.131   **Anterior cord syndrome at C1 level of cervical spinal cord**

     √7ᵗʰ S14.132   **Anterior cord syndrome at C2 level of cervical spinal cord**

     √7ᵗʰ S14.133   **Anterior cord syndrome at C3 level of cervical spinal cord**

     √7ᵗʰ S14.134   **Anterior cord syndrome at C4 level of cervical spinal cord**

     √7ᵗʰ S14.135   **Anterior cord syndrome at C5 level of cervical spinal cord**

     √7ᵗʰ S14.136   **Anterior cord syndrome at C6 level of cervical spinal cord**

     √7ᵗʰ S14.137   **Anterior cord syndrome at C7 level of cervical spinal cord**

     √7ᵗʰ S14.138   **Anterior cord syndrome at C8 level of cervical spinal cord**

     √7ᵗʰ S14.139   **Anterior cord syndrome at unspecified level of cervical spinal cord**

√6ᵗʰ S14.14   Brown-Séquard syndrome of cervical spinal cord

     √7ᵗʰ S14.141   **Brown-Séquard syndrome at C1 level of cervical spinal cord**

     √7ᵗʰ S14.142   **Brown-Séquard syndrome at C2 level of cervical spinal cord**

     √7ᵗʰ S14.143   **Brown-Séquard syndrome at C3 level of cervical spinal cord**

     √7ᵗʰ S14.144   **Brown-Séquard syndrome at C4 level of cervical spinal cord**

     √7ᵗʰ S14.145   **Brown-Séquard syndrome at C5 level of cervical spinal cord**

     √7ᵗʰ S14.146   **Brown-Séquard syndrome at C6 level of cervical spinal cord**

     √7ᵗʰ S14.147   **Brown-Séquard syndrome at C7 level of cervical spinal cord**

     √7ᵗʰ S14.148   **Brown-Séquard syndrome at C8 level of cervical spinal cord**

     √7ᵗʰ S14.149   **Brown-Séquard syndrome at unspecified level of cervical spinal cord**

√6ᵗʰ S14.15   Other incomplete lesions of cervical spinal cord

     Incomplete lesion of cervical spinal cord NOS
     Posterior cord syndrome of cervical spinal cord

     √7ᵗʰ S14.151   **Other incomplete lesion at C1 level of cervical spinal cord**

     √7ᵗʰ S14.152   **Other incomplete lesion at C2 level of cervical spinal cord**

     √7ᵗʰ S14.153   **Other incomplete lesion at C3 level of cervical spinal cord**

     √7ᵗʰ S14.154   **Other incomplete lesion at C4 level of cervical spinal cord**

     √7ᵗʰ S14.155   **Other incomplete lesion at C5 level of cervical spinal cord**

     √7ᵗʰ S14.156   **Other incomplete lesion at C6 level of cervical spinal cord**

     √7ᵗʰ S14.157   **Other incomplete lesion at C7 level of cervical spinal cord**

EXCLUDES 1 Not coded here   **EXCLUDES 2** Not included here   **N** Newborn Age: 0   **P** Pediatric Age: 0-17   **M** Maternity Age: 12-55   **A** Adult Age: 15-124

860   ICD-10-CM 201

☑7ᵗʰ **S14.158** Other incomplete lesion at C8 level of cervical spinal cord

☑7ᵗʰ **S14.159** Other incomplete lesion at unspecified level of cervical spinal cord

✓x7ᵗʰ **S14.2** Injury of nerve root of cervical spine

✓x7ᵗʰ **S14.3** Injury of brachial plexus

✓x7ᵗʰ **S14.4** Injury of peripheral nerves of neck

✓x7ᵗʰ **S14.5** Injury of cervical sympathetic nerves

✓x7ᵗʰ **S14.8** Injury of other specified nerves of neck

✓x7ᵗʰ **S14.9** Injury of unspecified nerves of neck

◰ S15 **Injury of blood vessels at neck level**
Code also any associated open wound (S11.-)

> The appropriate 7th character is to be added to each code from category S15.
> A   initial encounter
> D   subsequent encounter
> S   sequela

✓5ᵗʰ **S15.0** **Injury of carotid artery of neck**
Injury of carotid artery (common) (external) (internal, extracranial portion)
Injury of carotid artery NOS
EXCLUDES 1   injury of internal carotid artery, intracranial portion (S06.8)

✓6ᵗʰ **S15.00** Unspecified injury of carotid artery

☑7ᵗʰ **S15.001** Unspecified injury of right carotid artery

☑7ᵗʰ **S15.002** Unspecified injury of left carotid artery

☑7ᵗʰ **S15.009** Unspecified injury of unspecified carotid artery

✓6ᵗʰ **S15.01** Minor laceration of carotid artery
Incomplete transection of carotid artery
Laceration of carotid artery NOS
Superficial laceration of carotid artery

☑7ᵗʰ **S15.011** Minor laceration of right carotid artery

☑7ᵗʰ **S15.012** Minor laceration of left carotid artery

☑7ᵗʰ **S15.019** Minor laceration of unspecified carotid artery

✓6ᵗʰ **S15.02** Major laceration of carotid artery
Complete transection of carotid artery
Traumatic rupture of carotid artery

☑7ᵗʰ **S15.021** Major laceration of right carotid artery

☑7ᵗʰ **S15.022** Major laceration of left carotid artery

☑7ᵗʰ **S15.029** Major laceration of unspecified carotid artery

✓6ᵗʰ **S15.09** Other specified injury of carotid artery

☑7ᵗʰ **S15.091** Other specified injury of right carotid artery

☑7ᵗʰ **S15.092** Other specified injury of left carotid artery

☑7ᵗʰ **S15.099** Other specified injury of unspecified carotid artery

✓5ᵗʰ **S15.1** **Injury of vertebral artery**

✓6ᵗʰ **S15.10** Unspecified injury of vertebral artery

☑7ᵗʰ **S15.101** Unspecified injury of right vertebral artery

☑7ᵗʰ **S15.102** Unspecified injury of left vertebral artery

☑7ᵗʰ **S15.109** Unspecified injury of unspecified vertebral artery

✓6ᵗʰ **S15.11** Minor laceration of vertebral artery
Incomplete transection of vertebral artery
Laceration of vertebral artery NOS
Superficial laceration of vertebral artery

☑7ᵗʰ **S15.111** Minor laceration of right vertebral artery

☑7ᵗʰ **S15.112** Minor laceration of left vertebral artery

☑7ᵗʰ **S15.119** Minor laceration of unspecified vertebral artery

✓6ᵗʰ **S15.12** Major laceration of vertebral artery
Complete transection of vertebral artery
Traumatic rupture of vertebral artery

☑7ᵗʰ **S15.121** Major laceration of right vertebral artery

☑7ᵗʰ **S15.122** Major laceration of left vertebral artery

☑7ᵗʰ **S15.129** Major laceration of unspecified vertebral artery

☑7ᵗʰ **S15.19** Other specified injury of vertebral artery

☑7ᵗʰ **S15.191** Other specified injury of right vertebral artery

☑7ᵗʰ **S15.192** Other specified injury of left vertebral artery

☑7ᵗʰ **S15.199** Other specified injury of unspecified vertebral artery

✓5ᵗʰ **S15.2** **Injury of external jugular vein**

✓6ᵗʰ **S15.20** Unspecified injury of external jugular vein

☑7ᵗʰ **S15.201** Unspecified injury of right external jugular vein

☑7ᵗʰ **S15.202** Unspecified injury of left external jugular vein

☑7ᵗʰ **S15.209** Unspecified injury of unspecified external jugular vein

✓6ᵗʰ **S15.21** Minor laceration of external jugular vein
Incomplete transection of external jugular vein
Laceration of external jugular vein NOS
Superficial laceration of external jugular vein

☑7ᵗʰ **S15.211** Minor laceration of right external jugular vein

☑7ᵗʰ **S15.212** Minor laceration of left external jugular vein

☑7ᵗʰ **S15.219** Minor laceration of unspecified external jugular vein

✓6ᵗʰ **S15.22** Major laceration of external jugular vein
Complete transection of external jugular vein
Traumatic rupture of external jugular vein

☑7ᵗʰ **S15.221** Major laceration of right external jugular vein

☑7ᵗʰ **S15.222** Major laceration of left external jugular vein

☑7ᵗʰ **S15.229** Major laceration of unspecified external jugular vein

✓6ᵗʰ **S15.29** Other specified injury of external jugular vein

☑7ᵗʰ **S15.291** Other specified injury of right external jugular vein

☑7ᵗʰ **S15.292** Other specified injury of left external jugular vein

☑7ᵗʰ **S15.299** Other specified injury of unspecified external jugular vein

✓5ᵗʰ **S15.3** **Injury of internal jugular vein**

✓6ᵗʰ **S15.30** Unspecified injury of internal jugular vein

☑7ᵗʰ **S15.301** Unspecified injury of right internal jugular vein

☑7ᵗʰ **S15.302** Unspecified injury of left internal jugular vein

☑7ᵗʰ **S15.309** Unspecified injury of unspecified internal jugular vein

✓6ᵗʰ **S15.31** Minor laceration of internal jugular vein
Incomplete transection of internal jugular vein
Laceration of internal jugular vein NOS
Superficial laceration of internal jugular vein

☑7ᵗʰ **S15.311** Minor laceration of right internal jugular vein

☑7ᵗʰ **S15.312** Minor laceration of left internal jugular vein

☑7ᵗʰ **S15.319** Minor laceration of unspecified internal jugular vein

✓6ᵗʰ **S15.32** Major laceration of internal jugular vein
Complete transection of internal jugular vein
Traumatic rupture of internal jugular vein

☑7ᵗʰ **S15.321** Major laceration of right internal jugular vein

☑7ᵗʰ **S15.322** Major laceration of left internal jugular vein

☑7ᵗʰ **S15.329** Major laceration of unspecified internal jugular vein

✓6ᵗʰ **S15.39** Other specified injury of internal jugular vein

☑7ᵗʰ **S15.391** Other specified injury of right internal jugular vein

☑7ᵗʰ **S15.392** Other specified injury of left internal jugular vein

☑7ᵗʰ **S15.399** Other specified injury of unspecified internal jugular vein

---

☑ Additional Character Required   ✓x7ᵗʰ Placeholder Alert   Unspecified Dx   Other Specified Dx   Manifestation   ▶◀ Revised Text   ● New Code   ▲ Revised Code Title

√x7ᵗʰ **S15.8 Injury of other specified blood vessels at neck level**

√x7ᵗʰ **S15.9 Injury of unspecified blood vessel at neck level**

√4ᵗʰ **S16 Injury of muscle, fascia and tendon at neck level**
Code also any associated open wound (S11.-)
EXCLUDES 2 *sprain of joint or ligament at neck level (S13.9)*

The appropriate 7th character is to be added to each code from category S16.
A   initial encounter
D   subsequent encounter
S   sequela

√x7ᵗʰ **S16.1 Strain of muscle, fascia and tendon at neck level**

√x7ᵗʰ **S16.2 Laceration of muscle, fascia and tendon at neck level**

√x7ᵗʰ **S16.8 Other specified injury of muscle, fascia and tendon at neck level**

√x7ᵗʰ **S16.9 Unspecified injury of muscle, fascia and tendon at neck level**

√4ᵗʰ **S17 Crushing injury of neck**
Use additional code for all associated injuries, such as:
injury of blood vessels (S15.-)
open wound of neck (S11.-)
spinal cord injury (S14.0, S14.1-)
vertebral fracture (S12.0- -S12.3-)

The appropriate 7th character is to be added to each code from category S17.
A   initial encounter
D   subsequent encounter
S   sequela

√x7ᵗʰ **S17.0 Crushing injury of larynx and trachea**

√x7ᵗʰ **S17.8 Crushing injury of other specified parts of neck**

√x7ᵗʰ **S17.9 Crushing injury of neck, part unspecified**

√4ᵗʰ **S19 Other specified and unspecified injuries of neck**

The appropriate 7th character is to be added to each code from category S19.
A   initial encounter
D   subsequent encounter
S   sequela

√5ᵗʰ **S19.8 Other specified injuries of neck**

√x7ᵗʰ **S19.80 Other specified injuries of unspecified part of neck**

√x7ᵗʰ **S19.81 Other specified injuries of larynx**

√x7ᵗʰ **S19.82 Other specified injuries of cervical trachea**
EXCLUDES 2 *other specified injury of thoracic trachea (S27.5-)*

√x7ᵗʰ **S19.83 Other specified injuries of vocal cord**

√x7ᵗʰ **S19.84 Other specified injuries of thyroid gland**

√x7ᵗʰ **S19.85 Other specified injuries of pharynx and cervical esophagus**

√x7ᵗʰ **S19.89 Other specified injuries of other specified part of neck**

√x7ᵗʰ **S19.9 Unspecified injury of neck**

Injuries to the thorax (S20-S29)

INCLUDES   injuries of breast
injuries of chest (wall)
injuries of interscapular area
EXCLUDES 2 *burns and corrosions (T20-T32)*
effects of foreign body in bronchus (T17.5)
effects of foreign body in esophagus (T18.1)
effects of foreign body in lung (T17.8)
effects of foreign body in trachea (T17.4)
frostbite (T33-T34)
injuries of axilla
injuries of clavicle
injuries of scapular region
injuries of shoulder
insect bite or sting, venomous (T63.4)

√4ᵗʰ **S20 Superficial injury of thorax**

The appropriate 7th character is to be added to each code from category S20.
A   initial encounter
D   subsequent encounter
S   sequela

√5ᵗʰ **S20.0 Contusion of breast**

√x7ᵗʰ **S20.00 Contusion of breast, unspecified breast**

√x7ᵗʰ **S20.01 Contusion of right breast**

√x7ᵗʰ **S20.02 Contusion of left breast**

√5ᵗʰ **S20.1 Other and unspecified superficial injuries of breast**

√6ᵗʰ **S20.10 Unspecified superficial injuries of breast**

√7ᵗʰ **S20.101 Unspecified superficial injuries of breast, right breast**

√7ᵗʰ **S20.102 Unspecified superficial injuries of breast, left breast**

√7ᵗʰ **S20.109 Unspecified superficial injuries of breast, unspecified breast**

√6ᵗʰ **S20.11 Abrasion of breast**

√7ᵗʰ **S20.111 Abrasion of breast, right breast**

√7ᵗʰ **S20.112 Abrasion of breast, left breast**

√7ᵗʰ **S20.119 Abrasion of breast, unspecified breast**

√6ᵗʰ **S20.12 Blister (nonthermal) of breast**

√7ᵗʰ **S20.121 Blister (nonthermal) of breast, right breast**

√7ᵗʰ **S20.122 Blister (nonthermal) of breast, left breast**

√7ᵗʰ **S20.129 Blister (nonthermal) of breast, unspecified breast**

√6ᵗʰ **S20.14 External constriction of part of breast**

√7ᵗʰ **S20.141 External constriction of part of breast, right breast**

√7ᵗʰ **S20.142 External constriction of part of breast, left breast**

√7ᵗʰ **S20.149 External constriction of part of breast, unspecified breast**

√6ᵗʰ **S20.15 Superficial foreign body of breast**
Splinter in the breast

√7ᵗʰ **S20.151 Superficial foreign body of breast, right breast**

√7ᵗʰ **S20.152 Superficial foreign body of breast, left breast**

√7ᵗʰ **S20.159 Superficial foreign body of breast, unspecified breast**

√6ᵗʰ **S20.16 Insect bite (nonvenomous) of breast**

√7ᵗʰ **S20.161 Insect bite (nonvenomous) of breast, right breast**

√7ᵗʰ **S20.162 Insect bite (nonvenomous) of breast, left breast**

√7ᵗʰ **S20.169 Insect bite (nonvenomous) of breast, unspecified breast**

√6ᵗʰ **S20.17 Other superficial bite of breast**
EXCLUDES 1 *open bite of breast (S21.05-)*

√7ᵗʰ **S20.171 Other superficial bite of breast, right breast**

√7ᵗʰ **S20.172 Other superficial bite of breast, left breast**

√7ᵗʰ **S20.179 Other superficial bite of breast, unspecified breast**

√5ᵗʰ **S20.2 Contusion of thorax**

√x7ᵗʰ **S20.20 Contusion of thorax, unspecified**

√6ᵗʰ **S20.21 Contusion of front wall of thorax**

√7ᵗʰ **S20.211 Contusion of right front wall of thorax**

√7ᵗʰ **S20.212 Contusion of left front wall of thorax**

√7ᵗʰ **S20.219 Contusion of unspecified front wall of thorax**

√6ᵗʰ **S20.22 Contusion of back wall of thorax**

√7ᵗʰ **S20.221 Contusion of right back wall of thorax**

√7ᵗʰ **S20.222 Contusion of left back wall of thorax**

√7ᵗʰ **S20.229 Contusion of unspecified back wall of thorax**

√5ᵗʰ **S20.3 Other and unspecified superficial injuries of front wall of thorax**

√6ᵗʰ **S20.30 Unspecified superficial injuries of front wall of thorax**

√7ᵗʰ **S20.301 Unspecified superficial injuries of right front wall of thorax**

√7ᵗʰ **S20.302 Unspecified superficial injuries of left front wall of thorax**

√7ᵗʰ **S20.309 Unspecified superficial injuries of unspecified front wall of thorax**

√6ᵗʰ **S20.31 Abrasion of front wall of thorax**

√7ᵗʰ **S20.311 Abrasion of right front wall of thorax**

EXCLUDES 1 Not coded here   EXCLUDES 2 Not included here   N Newborn Age: 0   P Pediatric Age: 0-17   M Maternity Age: 12-55   A Adult Age: 15-124

862   ICD-10-CM 201

✓7th **S20.312** Abrasion of left front wall of thorax

✓7th **S20.319** Abrasion of unspecified front wall of thorax

✓6th **S20.32** Blister (nonthermal) of front wall of thorax

✓7th **S20.321** Blister (nonthermal) of right front wall of thorax

✓7th **S20.322** Blister (nonthermal) of left front wall of thorax

✓7th **S20.329** Blister (nonthermal) of unspecified front wall of thorax

✓6th **S20.34** External constriction of front wall of thorax

✓7th **S20.341** External constriction of right front wall of thorax

✓7th **S20.342** External constriction of left front wall of thorax

✓7th **S20.349** External constriction of unspecified front wall of thorax

✓6th **S20.35** Superficial foreign body of front wall of thorax
Splinter in front wall of thorax

✓7th **S20.351** Superficial foreign body of right front wall of thorax

✓7th **S20.352** Superficial foreign body of left front wall of thorax

✓7th **S20.359** Superficial foreign body of unspecified front wall of thorax

✓6th **S20.36** Insect bite (nonvenomous) of front wall of thorax

✓7th **S20.361** Insect bite (nonvenomous) of right front wall of thorax

✓7th **S20.362** Insect bite (nonvenomous) of left front wall of thorax

✓7th **S20.369** Insect bite (nonvenomous) of unspecified front wall of thorax

✓6th **S20.37** Other superficial bite of front wall of thorax
EXCLUDES 1   open bite of front wall of thorax (S21.14)

✓7th **S20.371** Other superficial bite of right front wall of thorax

✓7th **S20.372** Other superficial bite of left front wall of thorax

✓7th **S20.379** Other superficial bite of unspecified front wall of thorax

✓5th **S20.4** Other and unspecified superficial injuries of back wall of thorax

✓6th **S20.40** Unspecified superficial injuries of back wall of thorax

✓7th **S20.401** Unspecified superficial injuries of right back wall of thorax

✓7th **S20.402** Unspecified superficial injuries of left back wall of thorax

✓7th **S20.409** Unspecified superficial injuries of unspecified back wall of thorax

✓6th **S20.41** Abrasion of back wall of thorax

✓7th **S20.411** Abrasion of right back wall of thorax

✓7th **S20.412** Abrasion of left back wall of thorax

✓7th **S20.419** Abrasion of unspecified back wall of thorax

✓6th **S20.42** Blister (nonthermal) of back wall of thorax

✓7th **S20.421** Blister (nonthermal) of right back wall of thorax

✓7th **S20.422** Blister (nonthermal) of left back wall of thorax

✓7th **S20.429** Blister (nonthermal) of unspecified back wall of thorax

✓6th **S20.44** External constriction of back wall of thorax

✓7th **S20.441** External constriction of right back wall of thorax

✓7th **S20.442** External constriction of left back wall of thorax

✓7th **S20.449** External constriction of unspecified back wall of thorax

✓6th **S20.45** Superficial foreign body of back wall of thorax
Splinter of back wall of thorax

✓7th **S20.451** Superficial foreign body of right back wall of thorax

✓7th **S20.452** Superficial foreign body of left back wall of thorax

✓7th **S20.459** Superficial foreign body of unspecified back wall of thorax

✓6th **S20.46** Insect bite (nonvenomous) of back wall of thorax

✓7th **S20.461** Insect bite (nonvenomous) of right back wall of thorax

✓7th **S20.462** Insect bite (nonvenomous) of left back wall of thorax

✓7th **S20.469** Insect bite (nonvenomous) of unspecified back wall of thorax

✓6th **S20.47** Other superficial bite of back wall of thorax
EXCLUDES 1   open bite of back wall of thorax (S21.24)

✓7th **S20.471** Other superficial bite of right back wall of thorax

✓7th **S20.472** Other superficial bite of left back wall of thorax

✓7th **S20.479** Other superficial bite of unspecified back wall of thorax

✓5th **S20.9** Superficial injury of unspecified parts of thorax
EXCLUDES 1   contusion of thorax NOS (S20.20)

✓x7th **S20.90** Unspecified superficial injury of unspecified parts of thorax
Superficial injury of thoracic wall NOS

✓x7th **S20.91** Abrasion of unspecified parts of thorax

✓x7th **S20.92** Blister (nonthermal) of unspecified parts of thorax

✓x7th **S20.94** External constriction of unspecified parts of thorax

✓x7th **S20.95** Superficial foreign body of unspecified parts of thorax
Splinter in thorax NOS

✓x7th **S20.96** Insect bite (nonvenomous) of unspecified parts of thorax

✓x7th **S20.97** Other superficial bite of unspecified parts of thorax
EXCLUDES 1   open bite of thorax NOS (S21.95)

✓4th **S21** **Open wound of thorax**
Code also any associated injury, such as:
injury of heart (S26.-)
injury of intrathoracic organs (S27.-)
rib fracture (S22.3-, S22.4-)
spinal cord injury (S24.0-, S24.1-)
traumatic hemopneumothorax (S27.3)
traumatic hemothorax (S27.1)
traumatic pneumothorax (S27.0)
wound infection
EXCLUDES 1   traumatic amputation (partial) of thorax (S28.1)

The appropriate 7th character is to be added to each code from category S21.
A   initial encounter
D   subsequent encounter
S   sequela

✓5th **S21.0** Open wound of breast

✓6th **S21.00** Unspecified open wound of breast

✓7th **S21.001** Unspecified open wound of right breast

✓7th **S21.002** Unspecified open wound of left breast

✓7th **S21.009** Unspecified open wound of unspecified breast

✓6th **S21.01** Laceration without foreign body of breast

✓7th **S21.011** Laceration without foreign body of right breast

✓7th **S21.012** Laceration without foreign body of left breast

✓7th **S21.019** Laceration without foreign body of unspecified breast

✓6th **S21.02** Laceration with foreign body of breast

✓7th **S21.021** Laceration with foreign body of right breast

✓7th **S21.022** Laceration with foreign body of left breast

✓7th **S21.029** Laceration with foreign body of unspecified breast

✓6th **S21.03** Puncture wound without foreign body of breast

✓7th **S21.031** Puncture wound without foreign body of right breast

✓7th **S21.032** Puncture wound without foreign body of left breast

---

✓ Additional Character Required   ✓x7th Placeholder Alert   Unspecified Dx   Other Specified Dx   Manifestation   ▶◀ Revised Text   ● New Code   ▲ Revised Code Title

✓7ᵗʰ **S21.039 Puncture wound without foreign body of unspecified breast**

✓6ᵗʰ **S21.04** Puncture wound with foreign body of breast

✓7ᵗʰ **S21.041 Puncture wound with foreign body of right breast**

✓7ᵗʰ **S21.042 Puncture wound with foreign body of left breast**

✓7ᵗʰ **S21.049 Puncture wound with foreign body of unspecified breast**

✓6ᵗʰ **S21.05** Open bite of breast
Bite of breast NOS
EXCLUDES 1 superficial bite of breast (S20.17)

✓7ᵗʰ **S21.051 Open bite of right breast**

✓7ᵗʰ **S21.052 Open bite of left breast**

✓7ᵗʰ **S21.059 Open bite of unspecified breast**

✓6ᵗʰ **S21.1** Open wound of front wall of thorax without penetration into thoracic cavity
Open wound of chest without penetration into thoracic cavity

✓6ᵗʰ **S21.10** Unspecified open wound of front wall of thorax without penetration into thoracic cavity

✓7ᵗʰ **S21.101 Unspecified open wound of right front wall of thorax without penetration into thoracic cavity**

✓7ᵗʰ **S21.102 Unspecified open wound of left front wall of thorax without penetration into thoracic cavity**

✓7ᵗʰ **S21.109 Unspecified open wound of unspecified front wall of thorax without penetration into thoracic cavity**

✓6ᵗʰ **S21.11** Laceration without foreign body of front wall of thorax without penetration into thoracic cavity

✓7ᵗʰ **S21.111 Laceration without foreign body of right front wall of thorax without penetration into thoracic cavity**

✓7ᵗʰ **S21.112 Laceration without foreign body of left front wall of thorax without penetration into thoracic cavity**

✓7ᵗʰ **S21.119 Laceration without foreign body of unspecified front wall of thorax without penetration into thoracic cavity**

✓6ᵗʰ **S21.12** Laceration with foreign body of front wall of thorax without penetration into thoracic cavity

✓7ᵗʰ **S21.121 Laceration with foreign body of right front wall of thorax without penetration into thoracic cavity**

✓7ᵗʰ **S21.122 Laceration with foreign body of left front wall of thorax without penetration into thoracic cavity**

✓7ᵗʰ **S21.129 Laceration with foreign body of unspecified front wall of thorax without penetration into thoracic cavity**

✓6ᵗʰ **S21.13** Puncture wound without foreign body of front wall of thorax without penetration into thoracic cavity

✓7ᵗʰ **S21.131 Puncture wound without foreign body of right front wall of thorax without penetration into thoracic cavity**

✓7ᵗʰ **S21.132 Puncture wound without foreign body of left front wall of thorax without penetration into thoracic cavity**

✓7ᵗʰ **S21.139 Puncture wound without foreign body of unspecified front wall of thorax without penetration into thoracic cavity**

✓6ᵗʰ **S21.14** Puncture wound with foreign body of front wall of thorax without penetration into thoracic cavity

✓7ᵗʰ **S21.141 Puncture wound with foreign body of right front wall of thorax without penetration into thoracic cavity**

✓7ᵗʰ **S21.142 Puncture wound with foreign body of left front wall of thorax without penetration into thoracic cavity**

✓7ᵗʰ **S21.149 Puncture wound with foreign body of unspecified front wall of thorax without penetration into thoracic cavity**

✓6ᵗʰ **S21.15** Open bite of front wall of thorax without penetration into thoracic cavity
Bite of front wall of thorax NOS
EXCLUDES 1 superficial bite of front wall of thorax (S20.3

✓7ᵗʰ **S21.151 Open bite of right front wall of thorax without penetration into thoracic cavity**

✓7ᵗʰ **S21.152 Open bite of left front wall of thorax without penetration into thoracic cavity**

✓7ᵗʰ **S21.159 Open bite of unspecified front wall of thorax without penetration into thoracic cavity**

✓5ᵗʰ **S21.2** Open wound of back wall of thorax without penetration into thoracic cavity

✓6ᵗʰ **S21.20** Unspecified open wound of back wall of thorax without penetration into thoracic cavity

✓7ᵗʰ **S21.201 Unspecified open wound of right back wall of thorax without penetration into thoracic cavity**

✓7ᵗʰ **S21.202 Unspecified open wound of left back wall of thorax without penetration into thoracic cavity**

✓7ᵗʰ **S21.209 Unspecified open wound of unspecified back wall of thorax without penetration into thoracic cavity**

✓6ᵗʰ **S21.21** Laceration without foreign body of back wall of thorax without penetration into thoracic cavity

✓7ᵗʰ **S21.211 Laceration without foreign body of right back wall of thorax without penetration into thoracic cavity**

✓7ᵗʰ **S21.212 Laceration without foreign body of left back wall of thorax without penetration into thoracic cavity**

✓7ᵗʰ **S21.219 Laceration without foreign body of unspecified back wall of thorax without penetration into thoracic cavity**

✓6ᵗʰ **S21.22** Laceration with foreign body of back wall of thorax without penetration into thoracic cavity

✓7ᵗʰ **S21.221 Laceration with foreign body of right back wall of thorax without penetration into thoracic cavity**

✓7ᵗʰ **S21.222 Laceration with foreign body of left back wall of thorax without penetration into thoracic cavity**

✓7ᵗʰ **S21.229 Laceration with foreign body of unspecified back wall of thorax without penetration into thoracic cavity**

✓6ᵗʰ **S21.23** Puncture wound without foreign body of back wall of thorax without penetration into thoracic cavity

✓7ᵗʰ **S21.231 Puncture wound without foreign body of right back wall of thorax without penetration into thoracic cavity**

✓7ᵗʰ **S21.232 Puncture wound without foreign body of left back wall of thorax without penetration into thoracic cavity**

✓7ᵗʰ **S21.239 Puncture wound without foreign body of unspecified back wall of thorax without penetration into thoracic cavity**

✓6ᵗʰ **S21.24** Puncture wound with foreign body of back wall of thorax without penetration into thoracic cavity

✓7ᵗʰ **S21.241 Puncture wound with foreign body of right back wall of thorax without penetration into thoracic cavity**

✓7ᵗʰ **S21.242 Puncture wound with foreign body of left back wall of thorax without penetration into thoracic cavity**

✓7ᵗʰ **S21.249 Puncture wound with foreign body of unspecified back wall of thorax without penetration into thoracic cavity**

✓6ᵗʰ **S21.25** Open bite of back wall of thorax without penetration into thoracic cavity
Bite of back wall of thorax NOS
EXCLUDES 1 superficial bite of back wall of thorax (S20.47

✓7ᵗʰ **S21.251 Open bite of right back wall of thorax without penetration into thoracic cavity**

✓7ᵗʰ **S21.252 Open bite of left back wall of thorax without penetration into thoracic cavity**

EXCLUDES 1 Not coded here   *EXCLUDES 2* Not included here   N Newborn Age: 0   P Pediatric Age: 0-17   M Maternity Age: 12-55   A Adult Age: 15-124

864

ICD-10-CM 201

√7ᵗʰ **S21.259** **Open bite of unspecified back wall of thorax without penetration into thoracic cavity**

√5ᵗʰ **S21.3** **Open wound of** front wall of thorax with penetration **into thoracic cavity**
    Open wound of chest with penetration into thoracic cavity

  √6ᵗʰ **S21.30** Unspecified **open wound of front wall of thorax with penetration into thoracic cavity**

    √7ᵗʰ **S21.301** **Unspecified open wound of** right **front wall of thorax with penetration into thoracic cavity**

    √7ᵗʰ **S21.302** **Unspecified open wound of** left **front wall of thorax with penetration into thoracic cavity**

    √7ᵗʰ **S21.309** **Unspecified open wound of unspecified front wall of thorax with penetration into thoracic cavity**

  √6ᵗʰ **S21.31** Laceration without foreign body **of front wall of thorax with penetration into thoracic cavity**

    √7ᵗʰ **S21.311** **Laceration without foreign body of** right **front wall of thorax with penetration into thoracic cavity**

    √7ᵗʰ **S21.312** **Laceration without foreign body of** left **front wall of thorax with penetration into thoracic cavity**

    √7ᵗʰ **S21.319** **Laceration without foreign body of unspecified front wall of thorax with penetration into thoracic cavity**

  √6ᵗʰ **S21.32** Laceration with foreign body **of front wall of thorax with penetration into thoracic cavity**

    √7ᵗʰ **S21.321** **Laceration with foreign body of** right **front wall of thorax with penetration into thoracic cavity**

    √7ᵗʰ **S21.322** **Laceration with foreign body of** left **front wall of thorax with penetration into thoracic cavity**

    √7ᵗʰ **S21.329** **Laceration with foreign body of unspecified front wall of thorax with penetration into thoracic cavity**

  √6ᵗʰ **S21.33** Puncture wound without foreign body **of front wall of thorax with penetration into thoracic cavity**

    √7ᵗʰ **S21.331** **Puncture wound without foreign body of** right **front wall of thorax with penetration into thoracic cavity**

    √7ᵗʰ **S21.332** **Puncture wound without foreign body of** left **front wall of thorax with penetration into thoracic cavity**

    √7ᵗʰ **S21.339** **Puncture wound without foreign body of unspecified front wall of thorax with penetration into thoracic cavity**

  √6ᵗʰ **S21.34** Puncture wound with foreign body **of front wall of thorax with penetration into thoracic cavity**

    √7ᵗʰ **S21.341** **Puncture wound with foreign body of** right **front wall of thorax with penetration into thoracic cavity**

    √7ᵗʰ **S21.342** **Puncture wound with foreign body of** left **front wall of thorax with penetration into thoracic cavity**

    √7ᵗʰ **S21.349** **Puncture wound with foreign body of unspecified front wall of thorax with penetration into thoracic cavity**

  √6ᵗʰ **S21.35** Open bite **of front wall of thorax with penetration into thoracic cavity**
    EXCLUDES 1   *superficial bite of front wall of thorax (S20.37)*

    √7ᵗʰ **S21.351** **Open bite of** right **front wall of thorax with penetration into thoracic cavity**

    √7ᵗʰ **S21.352** **Open bite of** left **front wall of thorax with penetration into thoracic cavity**

    √7ᵗʰ **S21.359** **Open bite of unspecified front wall of thorax with penetration into thoracic cavity**

√5ᵗʰ **S21.4** **Open wound of** back wall of thorax with penetration **into thoracic cavity**

  √6ᵗʰ **S21.40** Unspecified **open wound of back wall of thorax with penetration into thoracic cavity**

    √7ᵗʰ **S21.401** **Unspecified open wound of** right **back wall of thorax with penetration into thoracic cavity**

    √7ᵗʰ **S21.402** **Unspecified open wound of** left **back wall of thorax with penetration into thoracic cavity**

    √7ᵗʰ **S21.409** **Unspecified open wound of unspecified back wall of thorax with penetration into thoracic cavity**

  √6ᵗʰ **S21.41** Laceration without foreign body **of back wall of thorax with penetration into thoracic cavity**

    √7ᵗʰ **S21.411** **Laceration without foreign body of** right **back wall of thorax with penetration into thoracic cavity**

    √7ᵗʰ **S21.412** **Laceration without foreign body of** left **back wall of thorax with penetration into thoracic cavity**

    √7ᵗʰ **S21.419** **Laceration without foreign body of unspecified back wall of thorax with penetration into thoracic cavity**

  √6ᵗʰ **S21.42** Laceration with foreign body **of back wall of thorax with penetration into thoracic cavity**

    √7ᵗʰ **S21.421** **Laceration with foreign body of** right **back wall of thorax with penetration into thoracic cavity**

    √7ᵗʰ **S21.422** **Laceration with foreign body of** left **back wall of thorax with penetration into thoracic cavity**

    √7ᵗʰ **S21.429** **Laceration with foreign body of unspecified back wall of thorax with penetration into thoracic cavity**

  √6ᵗʰ **S21.43** Puncture wound without foreign body **of back wall of thorax with penetration into thoracic cavity**

    √7ᵗʰ **S21.431** **Puncture wound without foreign body of** right **back wall of thorax with penetration into thoracic cavity**

    √7ᵗʰ **S21.432** **Puncture wound without foreign body of** left **back wall of thorax with penetration into thoracic cavity**

    √7ᵗʰ **S21.439** **Puncture wound without foreign body of unspecified back wall of thorax with penetration into thoracic cavity**

  √6ᵗʰ **S21.44** Puncture wound with foreign body **of back wall of thorax with penetration into thoracic cavity**

    √7ᵗʰ **S21.441** **Puncture wound with foreign body of** right **back wall of thorax with penetration into thoracic cavity**

    √7ᵗʰ **S21.442** **Puncture wound with foreign body of** left **back wall of thorax with penetration into thoracic cavity**

    √7ᵗʰ **S21.449** **Puncture wound with foreign body of unspecified back wall of thorax with penetration into thoracic cavity**

  √6ᵗʰ **S21.45** Open bite **of back wall of thorax with penetration into thoracic cavity**
    Bite of back wall of thorax NOS
    EXCLUDES 1   *superficial bite of back wall of thorax (S20.47)*

    √7ᵗʰ **S21.451** **Open bite of** right **back wall of thorax with penetration into thoracic cavity**

    √7ᵗʰ **S21.452** **Open bite of** left **back wall of thorax with penetration into thoracic cavity**

    √7ᵗʰ **S21.459** **Open bite of unspecified back wall of thorax with penetration into thoracic cavity**

√5ᵗʰ **S21.9** **Open wound of unspecified part of thorax**
    Open wound of thoracic wall NOS

  √x7ᵗʰ **S21.90** **Unspecified open wound of unspecified part of thorax**

  √x7ᵗʰ **S21.91** Laceration without foreign body **of unspecified part of thorax**

  √x7ᵗʰ **S21.92** Laceration with foreign body **of unspecified part of thorax**

  √x7ᵗʰ **S21.93** Puncture wound without foreign body **of unspecified part of thorax**

  √x7ᵗʰ **S21.94** Puncture wound with foreign body **of unspecified part of thorax**

  √x7ᵗʰ **S21.95** Open bite **of unspecified part of thorax**
    EXCLUDES 1   *superficial bite of thorax (S20.97)*

◀ Additional Character Required   √x7ᵗʰ Placeholder Alert   Unspecified Dx   Other Specified Dx   Manifestation   ▶◀ Revised Text   ● New Code   ▲ Revised Code Title

D-10-CM 2016   865

✓4ᵗʰ S22   Fracture of rib(s), sternum and thoracic spine

> **NOTE**   A fracture not indicated as nondisplaced or displaced should be coded to displaced.
> A fracture not indicated as open or closed should be coded to closed.
>
> **INCLUDES**   fracture of thoracic neural arch
> fracture of thoracic spinous process
> fracture of thoracic transverse process
> fracture of thoracic vertebra
> fracture of thoracic vertebral arch
>
> Code first any associated:
>   injury of intrathoracic organ (S27.-)
>   spinal cord injury (S24.Ø-, S24.1-)
> **EXCLUDES 1**   *transection of thorax (S28.1)*
> **EXCLUDES 2**   *fracture of clavicle (S42.Ø-)*
>   *fracture of scapula (S42.1-)*

> The appropriate 7th character is to be added to each code from category S22.
> A   initial encounter for closed fracture
> B   initial encounter for open fracture
> D   subsequent encounter for fracture with routine healing
> G   subsequent encounter for fracture with delayed healing
> K   subsequent encounter for fracture with nonunion
> S   sequela

✓5ᵗʰ S22.Ø   Fracture of thoracic vertebra

  ✓6ᵗʰ S22.ØØ   Fracture of unspecified thoracic vertebra

    ✓7ᵗʰ S22.ØØØ   Wedge compression fracture of unspecified thoracic vertebra

    ✓7ᵗʰ S22.ØØ1   Stable burst fracture of unspecified thoracic vertebra

    ✓7ᵗʰ S22.ØØ2   Unstable burst fracture of unspecified thoracic vertebra

    ✓7ᵗʰ S22.ØØ8   Other fracture of unspecified thoracic vertebra

    ✓7ᵗʰ S22.ØØ9   Unspecified fracture of unspecified thoracic vertebra

  ✓6ᵗʰ S22.Ø1   Fracture of first thoracic vertebra

    ✓7ᵗʰ S22.Ø1Ø   Wedge compression fracture of first thoracic vertebra

    ✓7ᵗʰ S22.Ø11   Stable burst fracture of first thoracic vertebra

    ✓7ᵗʰ S22.Ø12   Unstable burst fracture of first thoracic vertebra

    ✓7ᵗʰ S22.Ø18   Other fracture of first thoracic vertebra

    ✓7ᵗʰ S22.Ø19   Unspecified fracture of first thoracic vertebra

  ✓6ᵗʰ S22.Ø2   Fracture of second thoracic vertebra

    ✓7ᵗʰ S22.Ø2Ø   Wedge compression fracture of second thoracic vertebra

    ✓7ᵗʰ S22.Ø21   Stable burst fracture of second thoracic vertebra

    ✓7ᵗʰ S22.Ø22   Unstable burst fracture of second thoracic vertebra

    ✓7ᵗʰ S22.Ø28   Other fracture of second thoracic vertebra

    ✓7ᵗʰ S22.Ø29   Unspecified fracture of second thoracic vertebra

  ✓6ᵗʰ S22.Ø3   Fracture of third thoracic vertebra

    ✓7ᵗʰ S22.Ø3Ø   Wedge compression fracture of third thoracic vertebra

    ✓7ᵗʰ S22.Ø31   Stable burst fracture of third thoracic vertebra

    ✓7ᵗʰ S22.Ø32   Unstable burst fracture of third thoracic vertebra

    ✓7ᵗʰ S22.Ø38   Other fracture of third thoracic vertebra

    ✓7ᵗʰ S22.Ø39   Unspecified fracture of third thoracic vertebra

  ✓6ᵗʰ S22.Ø4   Fracture of fourth thoracic vertebra

    ✓7ᵗʰ S22.Ø4Ø   Wedge compression fracture of fourth thoracic vertebra

    ✓7ᵗʰ S22.Ø41   Stable burst fracture of fourth thoracic vertebra

    ✓7ᵗʰ S22.Ø42   Unstable burst fracture of fourth thoracic vertebra

    ✓7ᵗʰ S22.Ø48   Other fracture of fourth thoracic vertebra

    ✓7ᵗʰ S22.Ø49   Unspecified fracture of fourth thoracic vertebra

  ✓6ᵗʰ S22.Ø5   Fracture of T5-T6 vertebra

    ✓7ᵗʰ S22.Ø5Ø   Wedge compression fracture of T5-T6 vertebra

    ✓7ᵗʰ S22.Ø51   Stable burst fracture of T5-T6 vertebra

    ✓7ᵗʰ S22.Ø52   Unstable burst fracture of T5-T6 vertebra

    ✓7ᵗʰ S22.Ø58   Other fracture of T5-T6 vertebra

    ✓7ᵗʰ S22.Ø59   Unspecified fracture of T5-T6 vertebra

  ✓6ᵗʰ S22.Ø6   Fracture of T7-T8 vertebra

    ✓7ᵗʰ S22.Ø6Ø   Wedge compression fracture of T7-T8 vertebra

    ✓7ᵗʰ S22.Ø61   Stable burst fracture of T7-T8 vertebra

    ✓7ᵗʰ S22.Ø62   Unstable burst fracture of T7-T8 vertebra

    ✓7ᵗʰ S22.Ø68   Other fracture of T7-T8 thoracic vertebra

    ✓7ᵗʰ S22.Ø69   Unspecified fracture of T7-T8 vertebra

  ✓6ᵗʰ S22.Ø7   Fracture of T9-T1Ø vertebra

    ✓7ᵗʰ S22.Ø7Ø   Wedge compression fracture of T9-T1Ø vertebra

    ✓7ᵗʰ S22.Ø71   Stable burst fracture of T9-T1Ø vertebra

    ✓7ᵗʰ S22.Ø72   Unstable burst fracture of T9-T1Ø vertebra

    ✓7ᵗʰ S22.Ø78   Other fracture of T9-T1Ø vertebra

    ✓7ᵗʰ S22.Ø79   Unspecified fracture of T9-T1Ø vertebra

  ✓6ᵗʰ S22.Ø8   Fracture of T11-T12 vertebra

    ✓7ᵗʰ S22.Ø8Ø   Wedge compression fracture of T11-T12 vertebra

    ✓7ᵗʰ S22.Ø81   Stable burst fracture of T11-T12 vertebra

    ✓7ᵗʰ S22.Ø82   Unstable burst fracture of T11-T12 vertebra

    ✓7ᵗʰ S22.Ø88   Other fracture of T11-T12 vertebra

    ✓7ᵗʰ S22.Ø89   Unspecified fracture of T11-T12 vertebra

✓5ᵗʰ S22.2   Fracture of sternum

  ✓x7ᵗʰ S22.2Ø   Unspecified fracture of sternum

  ✓x7ᵗʰ S22.21   Fracture of manubrium

  ✓x7ᵗʰ S22.22   Fracture of body of sternum

  ✓x7ᵗʰ S22.23   Sternal manubrial dissociation

  ✓x7ᵗʰ S22.24   Fracture of xiphoid process

✓5ᵗʰ S22.3   Fracture of one rib

  ✓x7ᵗʰ S22.31   Fracture of one rib, right side

  ✓x7ᵗʰ S22.32   Fracture of one rib, left side

  ✓x7ᵗʰ S22.39   Fracture of one rib, unspecified side

✓5ᵗʰ S22.4   Multiple fractures of ribs

> Fractures of two or more ribs
> **EXCLUDES 1**   *flail chest (S22.5-)*

  ✓x7ᵗʰ S22.41   Multiple fractures of ribs, right side

  ✓x7ᵗʰ S22.42   Multiple fractures of ribs, left side

  ✓x7ᵗʰ S22.43   Multiple fractures of ribs, bilateral

  ✓x7ᵗʰ S22.49   Multiple fractures of ribs, unspecified side

✓x7ᵗʰ S22.5   Flail chest

✓x7ᵗʰ S22.9   Fracture of bony thorax, part unspecified

✓4ᵗʰ S23   Dislocation and sprain of joints and ligaments of thorax

> **INCLUDES**   avulsion of joint or ligament of thorax
> laceration of cartilage, joint or ligament of thorax
> sprain of cartilage, joint or ligament of thorax
> traumatic hemarthrosis of joint or ligament of thorax
> traumatic rupture of joint or ligament of thorax
> traumatic subluxation of joint or ligament of thorax
> traumatic tear of joint or ligament of thorax
>
> Code also any associated open wound
> **EXCLUDES 2**   *dislocation, sprain of sternoclavicular joint (S43.2, S43.6)*
>   *strain of muscle or tendon of thorax (S29.Ø1-)*

> The appropriate 7th character is to be added to each code from category S23.
> A   initial encounter
> D   subsequent encounter
> S   sequela

✓x7ᵗʰ S23.Ø   Traumatic rupture of thoracic intervertebral disc

> **EXCLUDES 1**   *rupture or displacement (nontraumatic) of thoracic intervertebral disc NOS (M51- with fifth character 4)*

EXCLUDES 1 Not coded here   **EXCLUDES 2** Not included here   **N** Newborn Age: 0   **P** Pediatric Age: 0-17   **M** Maternity Age: 12-55   **A** Adult Age: 15-12

866   ICD-10-CM 2Ø

√5ᵗʰ **S23.1** **Subluxation and dislocation of thoracic vertebra**
Code also any associated
open wound of thorax (S21.-)
spinal cord injury (S24.0-, S24.1-)
EXCLUDES 2 *fracture of thoracic vertebrae (S22.0-)*

√6ᵗʰ **S23.10** **Subluxation and dislocation of unspecified thoracic vertebra**

√7ᵗʰ **S23.100** Subluxation of unspecified thoracic vertebra

√7ᵗʰ **S23.101** Dislocation of unspecified thoracic vertebra

√6ᵗʰ **S23.11** **Subluxation and dislocation of T1/T2 thoracic vertebra**

√7ᵗʰ **S23.110** Subluxation of T1/T2 thoracic vertebra

√7ᵗʰ **S23.111** Dislocation of T1/T2 thoracic vertebra

√6ᵗʰ **S23.12** **Subluxation and dislocation of T2/T3-T3/T4 thoracic vertebra**

√7ᵗʰ **S23.120** Subluxation of T2/T3 thoracic vertebra

√7ᵗʰ **S23.121** Dislocation of T2/T3 thoracic vertebra

√7ᵗʰ **S23.122** Subluxation of T3/T4 thoracic vertebra

√7ᵗʰ **S23.123** Dislocation of T3/T4 thoracic vertebra

√6ᵗʰ **S23.13** **Subluxation and dislocation of T4/T5-T5/T6 thoracic vertebra**

√7ᵗʰ **S23.130** Subluxation of T4/T5 thoracic vertebra

√7ᵗʰ **S23.131** Dislocation of T4/T5 thoracic vertebra

√7ᵗʰ **S23.132** Subluxation of T5/T6 thoracic vertebra

√7ᵗʰ **S23.133** Dislocation of T5/T6 thoracic vertebra

√6ᵗʰ **S23.14** **Subluxation and dislocation of T6/T7-T7/T8 thoracic vertebra**

√7ᵗʰ **S23.140** Subluxation of T6/T7 thoracic vertebra

√7ᵗʰ **S23.141** Dislocation of T6/T7 thoracic vertebra

√7ᵗʰ **S23.142** Subluxation of T7/T8 thoracic vertebra

√7ᵗʰ **S23.143** Dislocation of T7/T8 thoracic vertebra

√6ᵗʰ **S23.15** **Subluxation and dislocation of T8/T9-T9/T10 thoracic vertebra**

√7ᵗʰ **S23.150** Subluxation of T8/T9 thoracic vertebra

√7ᵗʰ **S23.151** Dislocation of T8/T9 thoracic vertebra

√7ᵗʰ **S23.152** Subluxation of T9/T10 thoracic vertebra

√7ᵗʰ **S23.153** Dislocation of T9/T10 thoracic vertebra

√6ᵗʰ **S23.16** **Subluxation and dislocation of T10/T11-T11/T12 thoracic vertebra**

√7ᵗʰ **S23.160** Subluxation of T10/T11 thoracic vertebra

√7ᵗʰ **S23.161** Dislocation of T10/T11 thoracic vertebra

√7ᵗʰ **S23.162** Subluxation of T11/T12 thoracic vertebra

√7ᵗʰ **S23.163** Dislocation of T11/T12 thoracic vertebra

√6ᵗʰ **S23.17** **Subluxation and dislocation of T12/L1 thoracic vertebra**

√7ᵗʰ **S23.170** Subluxation of T12/L1 thoracic vertebra

√7ᵗʰ **S23.171** Dislocation of T12/L1 thoracic vertebra

√5ᵗʰ **S23.2** **Dislocation of other and unspecified parts of thorax**

√×7ᵗʰ **S23.20** Dislocation of unspecified part of thorax

√×7ᵗʰ **S23.29** Dislocation of other parts of thorax

√×7ᵗʰ **S23.3** **Sprain of ligaments of thoracic spine**

√5ᵗʰ **S23.4** **Sprain of ribs and sternum**

√×7ᵗʰ **S23.41** Sprain of ribs

√6ᵗʰ **S23.42** Sprain of sternum

√7ᵗʰ **S23.420** Sprain of sternoclavicular (joint) (ligament)

√7ᵗʰ **S23.421** Sprain of chondrosternal joint

√7ᵗʰ **S23.428** Other sprain of sternum

√7ᵗʰ **S23.429** Unspecified sprain of sternum

√×7ᵗʰ **S23.8** **Sprain of other specified parts of thorax**

√×7ᵗʰ **S23.9** **Sprain of unspecified parts of thorax**

√4ᵗʰ **S24** **Injury of nerves and spinal cord at thorax level**
NOTE Code to highest level of thoracic spinal cord injury.
Injuries to the spinal cord (S24.0 and S24.1) refer to the cord level and not bone level injury, and can affect nerve roots at and below the level given.
Code also any associated:
fracture of thoracic vertebra (S22.0-)
open wound of thorax (S21.-)
transient paralysis (R29.5)
EXCLUDES 2 *injury of brachial plexus (S14.3)*

The appropriate 7th character is to be added to each code from category S24.
A   initial encounter
D   subsequent encounter
S   sequela

√×7ᵗʰ **S24.0** **Concussion and edema of thoracic spinal cord**

√5ᵗʰ **S24.1** **Other and unspecified injuries of thoracic spinal cord**

√6ᵗʰ **S24.10** Unspecified injury of thoracic spinal cord

√7ᵗʰ **S24.101** Unspecified injury at T1 level of thoracic spinal cord

√7ᵗʰ **S24.102** Unspecified injury at T2-T6 level of thoracic spinal cord

√7ᵗʰ **S24.103** Unspecified injury at T7-T10 level of thoracic spinal cord

√7ᵗʰ **S24.104** Unspecified injury at T11-T12 level of thoracic spinal cord

√7ᵗʰ **S24.109** Unspecified injury at unspecified level of thoracic spinal cord
Injury of thoracic spinal cord NOS

√6ᵗʰ **S24.11** Complete lesion of thoracic spinal cord

√7ᵗʰ **S24.111** Complete lesion at T1 level of thoracic spinal cord

√7ᵗʰ **S24.112** Complete lesion at T2-T6 level of thoracic spinal cord

√7ᵗʰ **S24.113** Complete lesion at T7-T10 level of thoracic spinal cord

√7ᵗʰ **S24.114** Complete lesion at T11-T12 level of thoracic spinal cord

√7ᵗʰ **S24.119** Complete lesion at unspecified level of thoracic spinal cord

√6ᵗʰ **S24.13** Anterior cord syndrome of thoracic spinal cord

√7ᵗʰ **S24.131** Anterior cord syndrome at T1 level of thoracic spinal cord

√7ᵗʰ **S24.132** Anterior cord syndrome at T2-T6 level of thoracic spinal cord

√7ᵗʰ **S24.133** Anterior cord syndrome at T7-T10 level of thoracic spinal cord

√7ᵗʰ **S24.134** Anterior cord syndrome at T11-T12 level of thoracic spinal cord

√7ᵗʰ **S24.139** Anterior cord syndrome at unspecified level of thoracic spinal cord

√6ᵗʰ **S24.14** Brown-Séquard syndrome of thoracic spinal cord

√7ᵗʰ **S24.141** Brown-Séquard syndrome at T1 level of thoracic spinal cord

√7ᵗʰ **S24.142** Brown-Séquard syndrome at T2-T6 level of thoracic spinal cord

√7ᵗʰ **S24.143** Brown-Séquard syndrome at T7-T10 level of thoracic spinal cord

√7ᵗʰ **S24.144** Brown-Séquard syndrome at T11-T12 level of thoracic spinal cord

√7ᵗʰ **S24.149** Brown-Séquard syndrome at unspecified level of thoracic spinal cord

√6ᵗʰ **S24.15** Other incomplete lesions of thoracic spinal cord
Incomplete lesion of thoracic spinal cord NOS
Posterior cord syndrome of thoracic spinal cord

√7ᵗʰ **S24.151** Other incomplete lesion at T1 level of thoracic spinal cord

√7ᵗʰ **S24.152** Other incomplete lesion at T2-T6 level of thoracic spinal cord

√7ᵗʰ **S24.153** Other incomplete lesion at T7-T10 level of thoracic spinal cord

√7ᵗʰ **S24.154** Other incomplete lesion at T11-T12 level of thoracic spinal cord

√7ᵗʰ **S24.159** Other incomplete lesion at unspecified level of thoracic spinal cord

Additional Character Required   √×7ᵗʰ Placeholder Alert   Unspecified Dx   Other Specified Dx   Manifestation   ►◄ Revised Text   ● New Code   ▲ Revised Code Title

D-10-CM 2016   867

√x7ᵗʰ **S24.2** Injury of nerve root of thoracic spine

√x7ᵗʰ **S24.3** Injury of peripheral nerves of thorax

√x7ᵗʰ **S24.4** Injury of thoracic sympathetic nervous system
　　　Injury of cardiac plexus
　　　Injury of esophageal plexus
　　　Injury of pulmonary plexus
　　　Injury of stellate ganglion
　　　Injury of thoracic sympathetic ganglion

√x7ᵗʰ **S24.8** Injury of other specified nerves of thorax

√x7ᵗʰ **S24.9** Injury of unspecified nerve of thorax

√4ᵗʰ **S25** **Injury of blood vessels of thorax**
　　　Code also any associated open wound (S21.-)

> The appropriate 7th character is to be added to each code from category S25.
> A　initial encounter
> D　subsequent encounter
> S　sequela

√5ᵗʰ **S25.0** Injury of thoracic aorta
　　　Injury of aorta NOS

　√x7ᵗʰ **S25.00** **Unspecified injury of thoracic aorta**

　√x7ᵗʰ **S25.01** **Minor laceration of thoracic aorta**
　　　Incomplete transection of thoracic aorta
　　　Laceration of thoracic aorta NOS
　　　Superficial laceration of thoracic aorta

　√x7ᵗʰ **S25.02** **Major laceration of thoracic aorta**
　　　Complete transection of thoracic aorta
　　　Traumatic rupture of thoracic aorta

　√x7ᵗʰ **S25.09** **Other specified injury of thoracic aorta**

√5ᵗʰ **S25.1** Injury of innominate or subclavian artery

　√6ᵗʰ **S25.10** Unspecified injury of innominate or subclavian artery

　　√7ᵗʰ **S25.101** **Unspecified injury of right innominate or subclavian artery**

　　√7ᵗʰ **S25.102** **Unspecified injury of left innominate or subclavian artery**

　　√7ᵗʰ **S25.109** **Unspecified injury of unspecified innominate or subclavian artery**

　√6ᵗʰ **S25.11** Minor laceration of innominate or subclavian artery
　　　Incomplete transection of innominate or subclavian artery
　　　Laceration of innominate or subclavian artery NOS
　　　Superficial laceration of innominate or subclavian artery

　　√7ᵗʰ **S25.111** **Minor laceration of right innominate or subclavian artery**

　　√7ᵗʰ **S25.112** **Minor laceration of left innominate or subclavian artery**

　　√7ᵗʰ **S25.119** **Minor laceration of unspecified innominate or subclavian artery**

　√6ᵗʰ **S25.12** Major laceration of innominate or subclavian artery
　　　Complete transection of innominate or subclavian artery
　　　Traumatic rupture of innominate or subclavian artery

　　√7ᵗʰ **S25.121** **Major laceration of right innominate or subclavian artery**

　　√7ᵗʰ **S25.122** **Major laceration of left innominate or subclavian artery**

　　√7ᵗʰ **S25.129** **Major laceration of unspecified innominate or subclavian artery**

　√6ᵗʰ **S25.19** Other specified injury of innominate or subclavian artery

　　√7ᵗʰ **S25.191** **Other specified injury of right innominate or subclavian artery**

　　√7ᵗʰ **S25.192** **Other specified injury of left innominate or subclavian artery**

　　√7ᵗʰ **S25.199** **Other specified injury of unspecified innominate or subclavian artery**

√5ᵗʰ **S25.2** Injury of superior vena cava
　　　Injury of vena cava NOS

　√x7ᵗʰ **S25.20** **Unspecified injury of superior vena cava**

　√x7ᵗʰ **S25.21** **Minor laceration of superior vena cava**
　　　Incomplete transection of superior vena cava
　　　Laceration of superior vena cava NOS
　　　Superficial laceration of superior vena cava

　√x7ᵗʰ **S25.22** **Major laceration of superior vena cava**
　　　Complete transection of superior vena cava
　　　Traumatic rupture of superior vena cava

　√x7ᵗʰ **S25.29** **Other specified injury of superior vena cava**

√5ᵗʰ **S25.3** Injury of innominate or subclavian vein

　√6ᵗʰ **S25.30** Unspecified injury of innominate or subclavian ve

　　√7ᵗʰ **S25.301** **Unspecified injury of right innominate subclavian vein**

　　√7ᵗʰ **S25.302** **Unspecified injury of left innominate or subclavian vein**

　　√7ᵗʰ **S25.309** **Unspecified injury of unspecified innominate or subclavian vein**

　√6ᵗʰ **S25.31** Minor laceration of innominate or subclavian vein
　　　Incomplete transection of innominate or subclavian vein
　　　Laceration of innominate or subclavian vein NOS
　　　Superficial laceration of innominate or subclavian v

　　√7ᵗʰ **S25.311** **Minor laceration of right innominate or subclavian vein**

　　√7ᵗʰ **S25.312** **Minor laceration of left innominate or subclavian vein**

　　√7ᵗʰ **S25.319** **Minor laceration of unspecified innominate or subclavian vein**

　√6ᵗʰ **S25.32** Major laceration of innominate or subclavian vein
　　　Complete transection of innominate or subclavian vein
　　　Traumatic rupture of innominate or subclavian vein

　　√7ᵗʰ **S25.321** **Major laceration of right innominate or subclavian vein**

　　√7ᵗʰ **S25.322** **Major laceration of left innominate or subclavian vein**

　　√7ᵗʰ **S25.329** **Major laceration of unspecified innominate or subclavian vein**

　√6ᵗʰ **S25.39** Other specified injury of innominate or subclavian vein

　　√7ᵗʰ **S25.391** **Other specified injury of right innomina or subclavian vein**

　　√7ᵗʰ **S25.392** **Other specified injury of left innominate or subclavian vein**

　　√7ᵗʰ **S25.399** **Other specified injury of unspecified innominate or subclavian vein**

√5ᵗʰ **S25.4** Injury of pulmonary blood vessels

　√6ᵗʰ **S25.40** Unspecified injury of pulmonary blood vessels

　　√7ᵗʰ **S25.401** **Unspecified injury of right pulmonary blood vessels**

　　√7ᵗʰ **S25.402** **Unspecified injury of left pulmonary blo vessels**

　　√7ᵗʰ **S25.409** **Unspecified injury of unspecified pulmonary blood vessels**

　√6ᵗʰ **S25.41** Minor laceration of pulmonary blood vessels
　　　Incomplete transection of pulmonary blood vessels
　　　Laceration of pulmonary blood vessels NOS
　　　Superficial laceration of pulmonary blood vessels

　　√7ᵗʰ **S25.411** **Minor laceration of right pulmonary blo vessels**

　　√7ᵗʰ **S25.412** **Minor laceration of left pulmonary bloo vessels**

　　√7ᵗʰ **S25.419** **Minor laceration of unspecified pulmonary blood vessels**

　√6ᵗʰ **S25.42** Major laceration of pulmonary blood vessels
　　　Complete transection of pulmonary blood vessels
　　　Traumatic rupture of pulmonary blood vessels

　　√7ᵗʰ **S25.421** **Major laceration of right pulmonary bloo vessels**

　　√7ᵗʰ **S25.422** **Major laceration of left pulmonary bloo vessels**

　　√7ᵗʰ **S25.429** **Major laceration of unspecified pulmonary blood vessels**

　√6ᵗʰ **S25.49** Other specified injury of pulmonary blood vessels

　　√7ᵗʰ **S25.491** **Other specified injury of right pulmonar blood vessels**

　　√7ᵗʰ **S25.492** **Other specified injury of left pulmonary blood vessels**

　　√7ᵗʰ **S25.499** **Other specified injury of unspecified pulmonary blood vessels**

EXCLUDES 1 Not coded here　　**EXCLUDES 2** Not included here　　Ⓝ Newborn Age: 0　　Ⓟ Pediatric Age: 0-17　　Ⓜ Maternity Age: 12-55　　Ⓐ Adult Age: 15-1

S25.5   Injury of intercostal blood vessels

  S25.50   Unspecified injury of intercostal blood vessels

    S25.501   Unspecified injury of intercostal blood vessels, right side

    S25.502   Unspecified injury of intercostal blood vessels, left side

    S25.509   Unspecified injury of intercostal blood vessels, unspecified side

  S25.51   Laceration of intercostal blood vessels

    S25.511   Laceration of intercostal blood vessels, right side

    S25.512   Laceration of intercostal blood vessels, left side

    S25.519   Laceration of intercostal blood vessels, unspecified side

  S25.59   Other specified injury of intercostal blood vessels

    S25.591   Other specified injury of intercostal blood vessels, right side

    S25.592   Other specified injury of intercostal blood vessels, left side

    S25.599   Other specified injury of intercostal blood vessels, unspecified side

S25.8   Injury of other blood vessels of thorax

    Injury of azygos vein   Injury of mammary artery or vein

  S25.80   Unspecified injury of other blood vessels of thorax

    S25.801   Unspecified injury of other blood vessels of thorax, right side

    S25.802   Unspecified injury of other blood vessels of thorax, left side

    S25.809   Unspecified injury of other blood vessels of thorax, unspecified side

  S25.81   Laceration of other blood vessels of thorax

    S25.811   Laceration of other blood vessels of thorax, right side

    S25.812   Laceration of other blood vessels of thorax, left side

    S25.819   Laceration of other blood vessels of thorax, unspecified side

  S25.89   Other specified injury of other blood vessels of thorax

    S25.891   Other specified injury of other blood vessels of thorax, right side

    S25.892   Other specified injury of other blood vessels of thorax, left side

    S25.899   Other specified injury of other blood vessels of thorax, unspecified side

S25.9   Injury of unspecified blood vessel of thorax

  S25.90   Unspecified injury of unspecified blood vessel of thorax

  S25.91   Laceration of unspecified blood vessel of thorax

  S25.99   Other specified injury of unspecified blood vessel of thorax

S26   Injury of heart

    Code also any associated:
      open wound of thorax (S21.-)
      traumatic hemopneumothorax (S27.2)
      traumatic hemothorax (S27.1)
      traumatic pneumothorax (S27.0)

    The appropriate 7th character is to be added to each code from category S26.
    A   initial encounter
    D   subsequent encounter
    S   sequela

  S26.0   Injury of heart with hemopericardium

    S26.00   Unspecified injury of heart with hemopericardium

    S26.01   Contusion of heart with hemopericardium

    S26.02   Laceration of heart with hemopericardium

      S26.020   Mild laceration of heart with hemopericardium
        Laceration of heart without penetration of heart chamber

      S26.021   Moderate laceration of heart with hemopericardium
        Laceration of heart with penetration of heart chamber

      S26.022   Major laceration of heart with hemopericardium
        Laceration of heart with penetration of multiple heart chambers

    S26.09   Other injury of heart with hemopericardium

  S26.1   Injury of heart without hemopericardium

    S26.10   Unspecified injury of heart without hemopericardium

    S26.11   Contusion of heart without hemopericardium

    S26.12   Laceration of heart without hemopericardium

    S26.19   Other injury of heart without hemopericardium

  S26.9   Injury of heart, unspecified with or without hemopericardium

    S26.90   Unspecified injury of heart, unspecified with or without hemopericardium

    S26.91   Contusion of heart, unspecified with or without hemopericardium

    S26.92   Laceration of heart, unspecified with or without hemopericardium
      Laceration of heart NOS

    S26.99   Other injury of heart, unspecified with or without hemopericardium

S27   Injury of other and unspecified intrathoracic organs

    Code also any associated open wound of thorax (S21.-)
    EXCLUDES 2   injury of cervical esophagus (S10-S19)
              injury of trachea (cervical) (S10-S19)

    The appropriate 7th character is to be added to each code from category S27.
    A   initial encounter
    D   subsequent encounter
    S   sequela

  S27.0   Traumatic pneumothorax
    EXCLUDES 1   spontaneous pneumothorax (J93.-)

  S27.1   Traumatic hemothorax

  S27.2   Traumatic hemopneumothorax

  S27.3   Other and unspecified injuries of lung

    S27.30   Unspecified injury of lung

      S27.301   Unspecified injury of lung, unilateral

      S27.302   Unspecified injury of lung, bilateral

      S27.309   Unspecified injury of lung, unspecified

    S27.31   Primary blast injury of lung
      Blast injury of lung NOS

      S27.311   Primary blast injury of lung, unilateral

      S27.312   Primary blast injury of lung, bilateral

      S27.319   Primary blast injury of lung, unspecified

    S27.32   Contusion of lung

      S27.321   Contusion of lung, unilateral

      S27.322   Contusion of lung, bilateral

      S27.329   Contusion of lung, unspecified

    S27.33   Laceration of lung

      S27.331   Laceration of lung, unilateral

      S27.332   Laceration of lung, bilateral

      S27.339   Laceration of lung, unspecified

    S27.39   Other injuries of lung
      Secondary blast injury of lung

      S27.391   Other injuries of lung, unilateral

      S27.392   Other injuries of lung, bilateral

      S27.399   Other injuries of lung, unspecified

  S27.4   Injury of bronchus

    S27.40   Unspecified injury of bronchus

      S27.401   Unspecified injury of bronchus, unilateral

      S27.402   Unspecified injury of bronchus, bilateral

      S27.409   Unspecified injury of bronchus, unspecified

    S27.41   Primary blast injury of bronchus
      Blast injury of bronchus NOS

      S27.411   Primary blast injury of bronchus, unilateral

◀ Additional Character Required   ✓x7ᵗʰ Placeholder Alert   Unspecified Dx   Other Specified Dx   Manifestation   ▶◀ Revised Text   ● New Code   ▲ Revised Code Title

D-10-CM 2016   869

√7ᵗʰ **S27.412** **Primary blast injury of bronchus,** bilateral

√7ᵗʰ **S27.419** **Primary blast injury of bronchus,**
unspecified

√6ᵗʰ **S27.42** Contusion of bronchus

√7ᵗʰ **S27.421** **Contusion of bronchus,** unilateral

√7ᵗʰ **S27.422** **Contusion of bronchus,** bilateral

√7ᵗʰ **S27.429** **Contusion of bronchus, unspecified**

√6ᵗʰ **S27.43** Laceration of bronchus

√7ᵗʰ **S27.431** **Laceration of bronchus,** unilateral

√7ᵗʰ **S27.432** **Laceration of bronchus,** bilateral

√7ᵗʰ **S27.439** **Laceration of bronchus, unspecified**

√6ᵗʰ **S27.49** Other injury of bronchus
Secondary blast injury of bronchus

√7ᵗʰ **S27.491** **Other injury of bronchus,** unilateral

√7ᵗʰ **S27.492** **Other injury of bronchus,** bilateral

√7ᵗʰ **S27.499** **Other injury of bronchus, unspecified**

√5ᵗʰ **S27.5** Injury of thoracic trachea

√x7ᵗʰ **S27.50** **Unspecified injury of thoracic trachea**

√x7ᵗʰ **S27.51** **Primary blast injury of thoracic trachea**
Blast injury of thoracic trachea NOS

√x7ᵗʰ **S27.52** **Contusion of thoracic trachea**

√x7ᵗʰ **S27.53** **Laceration of thoracic trachea**

√x7ᵗʰ **S27.59** **Other injury of thoracic trachea**
Secondary blast injury of thoracic trachea

√5ᵗʰ **S27.6** Injury of pleura

√x7ᵗʰ **S27.60** **Unspecified injury of pleura**

√x7ᵗʰ **S27.63** **Laceration of pleura**

√x7ᵗʰ **S27.69** **Other injury of pleura**

√5ᵗʰ **S27.8** Injury of other specified intrathoracic organs

√6ᵗʰ **S27.80** Injury of diaphragm

√7ᵗʰ **S27.802** **Contusion of diaphragm**

√7ᵗʰ **S27.803** **Laceration of diaphragm**

√7ᵗʰ **S27.808** **Other injury of diaphragm**

√7ᵗʰ **S27.809** **Unspecified injury of diaphragm**

√6ᵗʰ **S27.81** Injury of esophagus (thoracic part)

√7ᵗʰ **S27.812** **Contusion of esophagus (thoracic part)**

√7ᵗʰ **S27.813** **Laceration of esophagus (thoracic part)**

√7ᵗʰ **S27.818** **Other injury of esophagus (thoracic part)**

√7ᵗʰ **S27.819** **Unspecified injury of esophagus (thoracic part)**

√6ᵗʰ **S27.89** Injury of other specified intrathoracic organs
Injury of lymphatic thoracic duct
Injury of thymus gland

√7ᵗʰ **S27.892** **Contusion of other specified intrathoracic organs**

√7ᵗʰ **S27.893** **Laceration of other specified intrathoracic organs**

√7ᵗʰ **S27.898** **Other injury of other specified intrathoracic organs**

√7ᵗʰ **S27.899** **Unspecified injury of other specified intrathoracic organs**

√x7ᵗʰ **S27.9** Injury of unspecified intrathoracic organ

√4ᵗʰ **S28** **Crushing injury of thorax, and traumatic amputation of part of thorax**

The appropriate 7th character is to be added to each code from category S28.
A   initial encounter
D   subsequent encounter
S   sequela

√x7ᵗʰ **S28.0** **Crushed chest**
Use additional code for all associated injuries
EXCLUDES 1   flail chest (S22.5)

√x7ᵗʰ **S28.1** **Traumatic amputation (partial) of** part of thorax, except breast

√5ᵗʰ **S28.2** **Traumatic amputation of** breast

√6ᵗʰ **S28.21** Complete traumatic amputation of breast
Traumatic amputation of breast NOS

√7ᵗʰ **S28.211** **Complete traumatic amputation of** right breast

√7ᵗʰ **S28.212** **Complete traumatic amputation of** left breast

√7ᵗʰ **S28.219** **Complete traumatic amputation of unspecified breast**

√6ᵗʰ **S28.22** Partial traumatic amputation of breast

√7ᵗʰ **S28.221** **Partial traumatic amputation of** right breast

√7ᵗʰ **S28.222** **Partial traumatic amputation of** left breast

√7ᵗʰ **S28.229** **Partial traumatic amputation of unspecified breast**

√4ᵗʰ **S29** **Other and unspecified injuries of thorax**
Code also any associated open wound (S21.-)

The appropriate 7th character is to be added to each code from category S29.
A   initial encounter
D   subsequent encounter
S   sequela

√5ᵗʰ **S29.0** Injury of muscle and tendon at thorax level

√6ᵗʰ **S29.00** Unspecified injury of muscle and tendon of thorax

√7ᵗʰ **S29.001** **Unspecified injury of muscle and tendon of** front **wall of thorax**

√7ᵗʰ **S29.002** **Unspecified injury of muscle and tendon of** back **wall of thorax**

√7ᵗʰ **S29.009** **Unspecified injury of muscle and tendon of unspecified wall of thorax**

√6ᵗʰ **S29.01** Strain of muscle and tendon of thorax

√7ᵗʰ **S29.011** **Strain of muscle and tendon of** front wall **of thorax**

√7ᵗʰ **S29.012** **Strain of muscle and tendon of** back wall **of thorax**

√7ᵗʰ **S29.019** **Strain of muscle and tendon of unspecified wall of thorax**

√6ᵗʰ **S29.02** Laceration of muscle and tendon of thorax

√7ᵗʰ **S29.021** **Laceration of muscle and tendon of** front **wall of thorax**

√7ᵗʰ **S29.022** **Laceration of muscle and tendon of** back **wall of thorax**

√7ᵗʰ **S29.029** **Laceration of muscle and tendon of unspecified wall of thorax**

√6ᵗʰ **S29.09** Other injury of muscle and tendon of thorax

√7ᵗʰ **S29.091** **Other injury of muscle and tendon of** front **wall of thorax**

√7ᵗʰ **S29.092** **Other injury of muscle and tendon of** back **wall of thorax**

√7ᵗʰ **S29.099** **Other injury of muscle and tendon of unspecified wall of thorax**

√x7ᵗʰ **S29.8** **Other specified injuries of thorax**

√x7ᵗʰ **S29.9** **Unspecified injury of thorax**

Injuries to the abdomen, lower back, lumbar spine, pelvis and external genitals (S30-S39)

INCLUDES   injuries to the abdominal wall
injuries to the anus
injuries to the buttock
injuries to the external genitalia
injuries to the flank
injuries to the groin
EXCLUDES 2   burns and corrosions (T20-T32)
effects of foreign body in anus and rectum (T18.5)
effects of foreign body in genitourinary tract (T19.-)
effects of foreign body in stomach, small intestine and colon (T18.2-T18.4)
frostbite (T33-T34)
insect bite or sting, venomous (T63.4)

√4ᵗʰ **S30** **Superficial injury of abdomen, lower back, pelvis and external genitals**
EXCLUDES 2   superficial injury of hip (S70.-)

The appropriate 7th character is to be added to each code from category S30.
A   initial encounter
D   subsequent encounter
S   sequela

√x7ᵗʰ **S30.0** **Contusion of lower back and pelvis**
Contusion of buttock

EXCLUDES 1 Not coded here   *EXCLUDES 2* Not included here   N Newborn Age: 0   P Pediatric Age: 0-17   M Maternity Age: 12-55   A Adult Age: 15-12

870

ICD-10-CM 201

✓x7ᵗʰ S30.1　Contusion of abdominal wall
　　　Contusion of flank　　　　Contusion of groin

✓5ᵗʰ S30.2　Contusion of external genital organs
　　✓6ᵗʰ S30.20　Contusion of unspecified external genital organ
　　　　✓7ᵗʰ S30.201　Contusion of unspecified external genital organ, male ♂
　　　　✓7ᵗʰ S30.202　Contusion of unspecified external genital organ, female ♀
　　✓x7ᵗʰ S30.21　Contusion of penis ♂
　　✓x7ᵗʰ S30.22　Contusion of scrotum and testes ♂
　　✓x7ᵗʰ S30.23　Contusion of vagina and vulva ♀

✓x7ᵗʰ S30.3　Contusion of anus

✓5ᵗʰ S30.8　Other superficial injuries of abdomen, lower back, pelvis and external genitals
　　✓6ᵗʰ S30.81　Abrasion of abdomen, lower back, pelvis and external genitals
　　　　✓7ᵗʰ S30.810　Abrasion of lower back and pelvis
　　　　✓7ᵗʰ S30.811　Abrasion of abdominal wall
　　　　✓7ᵗʰ S30.812　Abrasion of penis ♂
　　　　✓7ᵗʰ S30.813　Abrasion of scrotum and testes ♂
　　　　✓7ᵗʰ S30.814　Abrasion of vagina and vulva ♀
　　　　✓7ᵗʰ S30.815　Abrasion of unspecified external genital organs, male ♂
　　　　✓7ᵗʰ S30.816　Abrasion of unspecified external genital organs, female ♀
　　　　✓7ᵗʰ S30.817　Abrasion of anus
　　✓6ᵗʰ S30.82　Blister (nonthermal) of abdomen, lower back, pelvis and external genitals
　　　　✓7ᵗʰ S30.820　Blister (nonthermal) of lower back and pelvis
　　　　✓7ᵗʰ S30.821　Blister (nonthermal) of abdominal wall
　　　　✓7ᵗʰ S30.822　Blister (nonthermal) of penis ♂
　　　　✓7ᵗʰ S30.823　Blister (nonthermal) of scrotum and testes ♂
　　　　✓7ᵗʰ S30.824　Blister (nonthermal) of vagina and vulva ♀
　　　　✓7ᵗʰ S30.825　Blister (nonthermal) of unspecified external genital organs, male ♂
　　　　✓7ᵗʰ S30.826　Blister (nonthermal) of unspecified external genital organs, female ♀
　　　　✓7ᵗʰ S30.827　Blister (nonthermal) of anus
　　✓6ᵗʰ S30.84　External constriction of abdomen, lower back, pelvis and external genitals
　　　　✓7ᵗʰ S30.840　External constriction of lower back and pelvis
　　　　✓7ᵗʰ S30.841　External constriction of abdominal wall
　　　　✓7ᵗʰ S30.842　External constriction of penis ♂
　　　　　　Hair tourniquet syndrome of penis
　　　　　　Use additional cause code to identify the constricting item (W49.0-)
　　　　✓7ᵗʰ S30.843　External constriction of scrotum and testes ♂
　　　　✓7ᵗʰ S30.844　External constriction of vagina and vulva ♀
　　　　✓7ᵗʰ S30.845　External constriction of unspecified external genital organs, male ♂
　　　　✓7ᵗʰ S30.846　External constriction of unspecified external genital organs, female ♀
　　✓6ᵗʰ S30.85　Superficial foreign body of abdomen, lower back, pelvis and external genitals
　　　　　Splinter in the abdomen, lower back, pelvis and external genitals
　　　　✓7ᵗʰ S30.850　Superficial foreign body of lower back and pelvis
　　　　✓7ᵗʰ S30.851　Superficial foreign body of abdominal wall
　　　　✓7ᵗʰ S30.852　Superficial foreign body of penis ♂
　　　　✓7ᵗʰ S30.853　Superficial foreign body of scrotum and testes ♂
　　　　✓7ᵗʰ S30.854　Superficial foreign body of vagina and vulva ♀
　　　　✓7ᵗʰ S30.855　Superficial foreign body of unspecified external genital organs, male ♂

✓7ᵗʰ S30.856　Superficial foreign body of unspecified external genital organs, female ♀
✓7ᵗʰ S30.857　Superficial foreign body of anus
✓6ᵗʰ S30.86　Insect bite (nonvenomous) of abdomen, lower back, pelvis and external genitals
　　✓7ᵗʰ S30.860　Insect bite (nonvenomous) of lower back and pelvis
　　✓7ᵗʰ S30.861　Insect bite (nonvenomous) of abdominal wall
　　✓7ᵗʰ S30.862　Insect bite (nonvenomous) of penis ♂
　　✓7ᵗʰ S30.863　Insect bite (nonvenomous) of scrotum and testes ♂
　　✓7ᵗʰ S30.864　Insect bite (nonvenomous) of vagina and vulva ♀
　　✓7ᵗʰ S30.865　Insect bite (nonvenomous) of unspecified external genital organs, male ♂
　　✓7ᵗʰ S30.866　Insect bite (nonvenomous) of unspecified external genital organs, female ♀
　　✓7ᵗʰ S30.867　Insect bite (nonvenomous) of anus
✓6ᵗʰ S30.87　Other superficial bite of abdomen, lower back, pelvis and external genitals
　　EXCLUDES 1　open bite of abdomen, lower back, pelvis and external genitals (S31.05, S31.15, S31.25, S31.35, S31.45, S31.55)
　　✓7ᵗʰ S30.870　Other superficial bite of lower back and pelvis
　　✓7ᵗʰ S30.871　Other superficial bite of abdominal wall
　　✓7ᵗʰ S30.872　Other superficial bite of penis ♂
　　✓7ᵗʰ S30.873　Other superficial bite of scrotum and testes ♂
　　✓7ᵗʰ S30.874　Other superficial bite of vagina and vulva ♀
　　✓7ᵗʰ S30.875　Other superficial bite of unspecified external genital organs, male ♂
　　✓7ᵗʰ S30.876　Other superficial bite of unspecified external genital organs, female ♀
　　✓7ᵗʰ S30.877　Other superficial bite of anus

✓5ᵗʰ S30.9　Unspecified superficial injury of abdomen, lower back, pelvis and external genitals
　　✓x7ᵗʰ S30.91　Unspecified superficial injury of lower back and pelvis
　　✓x7ᵗʰ S30.92　Unspecified superficial injury of abdominal wall
　　✓x7ᵗʰ S30.93　Unspecified superficial injury of penis ♂
　　✓x7ᵗʰ S30.94　Unspecified superficial injury of scrotum and testes ♂
　　✓x7ᵗʰ S30.95　Unspecified superficial injury of vagina and vulva ♀
　　✓x7ᵗʰ S30.96　Unspecified superficial injury of unspecified external genital organs, male ♂
　　✓x7ᵗʰ S30.97　Unspecified superficial injury of unspecified external genital organs, female ♀
　　✓x7ᵗʰ S30.98　Unspecified superficial injury of anus

✓4ᵗʰ S31　Open wound of abdomen, lower back, pelvis and external genitals
　　Code also any associated:
　　　spinal cord injury (S24.0, S24.1-, S34.0-, S34.1-)
　　　wound infection
　　EXCLUDES 1　traumatic amputation of part of abdomen, lower back and pelvis (S38.2-, S38.3)
　　EXCLUDES 2　open wound of hip (S71.00-S71.02)
　　　　　　　open fracture of pelvis (S32.1--S32.9 with 7th character B)

　　The appropriate 7th character is to be added to each code from category S31.
　　A　initial encounter
　　D　subsequent encounter
　　S　sequela

✓5ᵗʰ S31.0　Open wound of lower back and pelvis
　　✓6ᵗʰ S31.00　Unspecified open wound of lower back and pelvis
　　　　✓7ᵗʰ S31.000　Unspecified open wound of lower back and pelvis without penetration into retroperitoneum
　　　　　　Unspecified open wound of lower back and pelvis NOS

✓7ᵗʰ **S31.001** **Unspecified open wound of lower back and pelvis** with penetration into retroperitoneum

✓6ᵗʰ **S31.01** Laceration without foreign body **of lower back and pelvis**

✓7ᵗʰ **S31.010** **Laceration without foreign body of lower back and pelvis** without penetration into retroperitoneum
Laceration without foreign body of lower back and pelvis NOS

✓7ᵗʰ **S31.011** **Laceration without foreign body of lower back and pelvis** with penetration into retroperitoneum

✓6ᵗʰ **S31.02** Laceration with foreign body **of lower back and pelvis**

✓7ᵗʰ **S31.020** **Laceration with foreign body of lower back and pelvis** without penetration into retroperitoneum
Laceration with foreign body of lower back and pelvis NOS

✓7ᵗʰ **S31.021** **Laceration with foreign body of lower back and pelvis** with penetration into retroperitoneum

✓6ᵗʰ **S31.03** Puncture wound without foreign body **of lower back and pelvis**

✓7ᵗʰ **S31.030** **Puncture wound without foreign body of lower back and pelvis** without penetration into retroperitoneum
Puncture wound without foreign body of lower back and pelvis NOS

✓7ᵗʰ **S31.031** **Puncture wound without foreign body of lower back and pelvis** with penetration into retroperitoneum

✓6ᵗʰ **S31.04** Puncture wound with foreign body **of lower back and pelvis**

✓7ᵗʰ **S31.040** **Puncture wound with foreign body of lower back and pelvis** without penetration into retroperitoneum
Puncture wound with foreign body of lower back and pelvis NOS

✓7ᵗʰ **S31.041** **Puncture wound with foreign body of lower back and pelvis** with penetration into retroperitoneum

✓6ᵗʰ **S31.05** Open bite **of lower back and pelvis**
Bite of lower back and pelvis NOS
EXCLUDES 1 *superficial bite of lower back and pelvis (S30.860, S30.870)*

✓7ᵗʰ **S31.050** **Open bite of lower back and pelvis** without penetration into retroperitoneum
Open bite of lower back and pelvis NOS

✓7ᵗʰ **S31.051** **Open bite of lower back and pelvis** with penetration into retroperitoneum

✓5ᵗʰ **S31.1** Open wound of abdominal wall without penetration into peritoneal cavity
Open wound of abdominal wall NOS
EXCLUDES 2 *open wound of abdominal wall with penetration into peritoneal cavity (S31.6-)*

✓6ᵗʰ **S31.10** Unspecified open wound of abdominal wall without penetration into peritoneal cavity

✓7ᵗʰ **S31.100** **Unspecified open wound of abdominal wall,** right upper quadrant **without penetration into peritoneal cavity**

✓7ᵗʰ **S31.101** **Unspecified open wound of abdominal wall,** left upper quadrant **without penetration into peritoneal cavity**

✓7ᵗʰ **S31.102** **Unspecified open wound of abdominal wall,** epigastric region **without penetration into peritoneal cavity**

✓7ᵗʰ **S31.103** **Unspecified open wound of abdominal wall,** right lower quadrant **without penetration into peritoneal cavity**

✓7ᵗʰ **S31.104** **Unspecified open wound of abdominal wall,** left lower quadrant **without penetration into peritoneal cavity**

✓7ᵗʰ **S31.105** **Unspecified open wound of abdominal wall,** periumbilic region **without penetration into peritoneal cavity**

✓7ᵗʰ **S31.109** **Unspecified open wound of abdominal wall, unspecified quadrant without penetration into peritoneal cavity**
Unspecified open wound of abdominal w NOS

✓6ᵗʰ **S31.11** Laceration without foreign body **of abdominal wa** without penetration into peritoneal cavity

✓7ᵗʰ **S31.110** **Laceration without foreign body of abdominal wall,** right upper quadrant **without penetration into peritoneal cav**

✓7ᵗʰ **S31.111** **Laceration without foreign body of abdominal wall,** left upper quadrant **without penetration into peritoneal cav**

✓7ᵗʰ **S31.112** **Laceration without foreign body of abdominal wall,** epigastric region **witho penetration into peritoneal cavity**

✓7ᵗʰ **S31.113** **Laceration without foreign body of abdominal wall,** right lower quadrant **without penetration into peritoneal cav**

✓7ᵗʰ **S31.114** **Laceration without foreign body of abdominal wall,** left lower quadrant **without penetration into peritoneal cav**

✓7ᵗʰ **S31.115** **Laceration without foreign body of abdominal wall,** periumbilic region **without penetration into peritoneal cav**

✓7ᵗʰ **S31.119** **Laceration without foreign body of abdominal wall, unspecified quadrant without penetration into peritoneal cav**

✓6ᵗʰ **S31.12** Laceration with foreign body **of abdominal wall** without penetration into peritoneal cavity

✓7ᵗʰ **S31.120** **Laceration of abdominal wall with forei body,** right upper quadrant **without penetration into peritoneal cavity**

✓7ᵗʰ **S31.121** **Laceration of abdominal wall with forei body,** left upper quadrant **without penetration into peritoneal cavity**

✓7ᵗʰ **S31.122** **Laceration of abdominal wall with forei body,** epigastric region **without penetration into peritoneal cavity**

✓7ᵗʰ **S31.123** **Laceration of abdominal wall with forei body,** right lower quadrant **without penetration into peritoneal cavity**

✓7ᵗʰ **S31.124** **Laceration of abdominal wall with forei body,** left lower quadrant **without penetration into peritoneal cavity**

✓7ᵗʰ **S31.125** **Laceration of abdominal wall with forei body,** periumbilic region **without penetration into peritoneal cavity**

✓7ᵗʰ **S31.129** **Laceration of abdominal wall with forei body, unspecified quadrant without penetration into peritoneal cavity**

✓6ᵗʰ **S31.13** Puncture wound **of abdominal wall without foreig body without penetration into peritoneal cavity**

✓7ᵗʰ **S31.130** **Puncture wound of abdominal wall without foreign body,** right upper quadrant **without penetration into peritoneal cavity**

✓7ᵗʰ **S31.131** **Puncture wound of abdominal wall without foreign body,** left upper quadra **without penetration into peritoneal cav**

✓7ᵗʰ **S31.132** **Puncture wound of abdominal wall without foreign body,** epigastric region **without penetration into peritoneal cav**

✓7ᵗʰ **S31.133** **Puncture wound of abdominal wall without foreign body,** right lower quadrant **without penetration into peritoneal cavity**

✓7ᵗʰ **S31.134** **Puncture wound of abdominal wall without foreign body,** left lower quadra **without penetration into peritoneal cav**

✓7ᵗʰ **S31.135** **Puncture wound of abdominal wall without foreign body,** periumbilic regio **without penetration into peritoneal cav**

✓7ᵗʰ **S31.139** **Puncture wound of abdominal wall without foreign body, unspecified quadrant without penetration into peritoneal cavity**

√6ᵗʰ **S31.14** Puncture wound of abdominal wall with foreign body without penetration into peritoneal cavity

    √7ᵗʰ **S31.140** Puncture wound of abdominal wall with foreign body, right upper quadrant without penetration into peritoneal cavity

    √7ᵗʰ **S31.141** Puncture wound of abdominal wall with foreign body, left upper quadrant without penetration into peritoneal cavity

    √7ᵗʰ **S31.142** Puncture wound of abdominal wall with foreign body, epigastric region without penetration into peritoneal cavity

    √7ᵗʰ **S31.143** Puncture wound of abdominal wall with foreign body, right lower quadrant without penetration into peritoneal cavity

    √7ᵗʰ **S31.144** Puncture wound of abdominal wall with foreign body, left lower quadrant without penetration into peritoneal cavity

    √7ᵗʰ **S31.145** Puncture wound of abdominal wall with foreign body, periumbilic region without penetration into peritoneal cavity

    √7ᵗʰ **S31.149** Puncture wound of abdominal wall with foreign body, unspecified quadrant without penetration into peritoneal cavity

√6ᵗʰ **S31.15** Open bite of abdominal wall without penetration into peritoneal cavity
    Bite of abdominal wall NOS
    EXCLUDES 1   superficial bite of abdominal wall (S30.871)

    √7ᵗʰ **S31.150** Open bite of abdominal wall, right upper quadrant without penetration into peritoneal cavity

    √7ᵗʰ **S31.151** Open bite of abdominal wall, left upper quadrant without penetration into peritoneal cavity

    √7ᵗʰ **S31.152** Open bite of abdominal wall, epigastric region without penetration into peritoneal cavity

    √7ᵗʰ **S31.153** Open bite of abdominal wall, right lower quadrant without penetration into peritoneal cavity

    √7ᵗʰ **S31.154** Open bite of abdominal wall, left lower quadrant without penetration into peritoneal cavity

    √7ᵗʰ **S31.155** Open bite of abdominal wall, periumbilic region without penetration into peritoneal cavity

    √7ᵗʰ **S31.159** Open bite of abdominal wall, unspecified quadrant without penetration into peritoneal cavity

√5ᵗʰ **S31.2** Open wound of penis

   √x7ᵗʰ **S31.20** Unspecified open wound of penis   ♂

   √x7ᵗʰ **S31.21** Laceration without foreign body of penis   ♂

   √x7ᵗʰ **S31.22** Laceration with foreign body of penis   ♂

   √x7ᵗʰ **S31.23** Puncture wound without foreign body of penis   ♂

   √x7ᵗʰ **S31.24** Puncture wound with foreign body of penis   ♂

   √x7ᵗʰ **S31.25** Open bite of penis   ♂
    Bite of penis NOS
    EXCLUDES 1   superficial bite of penis (S30.862, S30.872)

√5ᵗʰ **S31.3** Open wound of scrotum and testes

   √x7ᵗʰ **S31.30** Unspecified open wound of scrotum and testes   ♂

   √x7ᵗʰ **S31.31** Laceration without foreign body of scrotum and testes   ♂

   √x7ᵗʰ **S31.32** Laceration with foreign body of scrotum and testes   ♂

   √x7ᵗʰ **S31.33** Puncture wound without foreign body of scrotum and testes   ♂

   √x7ᵗʰ **S31.34** Puncture wound with foreign body of scrotum and testes   ♂

   √x7ᵗʰ **S31.35** Open bite of scrotum and testes   ♂
    Bite of scrotum and testes NOS
    EXCLUDES 1   superficial bite of scrotum and testes (S30.863, S30.873)

√5ᵗʰ **S31.4** Open wound of vagina and vulva
    EXCLUDES 1   injury to vagina and vulva during delivery (O70-, O71.4)

   √x7ᵗʰ **S31.40** Unspecified open wound of vagina and vulva   ♀

   √x7ᵗʰ **S31.41** Laceration without foreign body of vagina and vulva   ♀

   √x7ᵗʰ **S31.42** Laceration with foreign body of vagina and vulva   ♀

   √x7ᵗʰ **S31.43** Puncture wound without foreign body of vagina and vulva   ♀

   √x7ᵗʰ **S31.44** Puncture wound with foreign body of vagina and vulva   ♀

   √x7ᵗʰ **S31.45** Open bite of vagina and vulva   ♀
    Bite of vagina and vulva NOS
    EXCLUDES 1   superficial bite of vagina and vulva (S30.864, S30.874)

√5ᵗʰ **S31.5** Open wound of unspecified external genital organs
    EXCLUDES 1   traumatic amputation of external genital organs (S38.21, S38.22)

   √6ᵗʰ **S31.50** Unspecified open wound of unspecified external genital organs

    √7ᵗʰ **S31.501** Unspecified open wound of unspecified external genital organs, male   ♂

    √7ᵗʰ **S31.502** Unspecified open wound of unspecified external genital organs, female   ♀

   √6ᵗʰ **S31.51** Laceration without foreign body of unspecified external genital organs

    √7ᵗʰ **S31.511** Laceration without foreign body of unspecified external genital organs, male   ♂

    √7ᵗʰ **S31.512** Laceration without foreign body of unspecified external genital organs, female   ♀

   √6ᵗʰ **S31.52** Laceration with foreign body of unspecified external genital organs

    √7ᵗʰ **S31.521** Laceration with foreign body of unspecified external genital organs, male   ♂

    √7ᵗʰ **S31.522** Laceration with foreign body of unspecified external genital organs, female   ♀

   √6ᵗʰ **S31.53** Puncture wound without foreign body of unspecified external genital organs

    √7ᵗʰ **S31.531** Puncture wound without foreign body of unspecified external genital organs, male   ♂

    √7ᵗʰ **S31.532** Puncture wound without foreign body of unspecified external genital organs, female   ♀

   √6ᵗʰ **S31.54** Puncture wound with foreign body of unspecified external genital organs

    √7ᵗʰ **S31.541** Puncture wound with foreign body of unspecified external genital organs, male   ♂

    √7ᵗʰ **S31.542** Puncture wound with foreign body of unspecified external genital organs, female   ♀

   √6ᵗʰ **S31.55** Open bite of unspecified external genital organs
    Bite of unspecified external genital organs NOS
    EXCLUDES 1   superficial bite of unspecified external genital organs (S30.865, S30.866, S30.875, S30.876)

    √7ᵗʰ **S31.551** Open bite of unspecified external genital organs, male   ♂

    √7ᵗʰ **S31.552** Open bite of unspecified external genital organs, female   ♀

√5ᵗʰ **S31.6** Open wound of abdominal wall with penetration into peritoneal cavity

   √6ᵗʰ **S31.60** Unspecified open wound of abdominal wall with penetration into peritoneal cavity

    √7ᵗʰ **S31.600** Unspecified open wound of abdominal wall, right upper quadrant with penetration into peritoneal cavity

    √7ᵗʰ **S31.601** Unspecified open wound of abdominal wall, left upper quadrant with penetration into peritoneal cavity

    √7ᵗʰ **S31.602** Unspecified open wound of abdominal wall, epigastric region with penetration into peritoneal cavity

    √7ᵗʰ **S31.603** Unspecified open wound of abdominal wall, right lower quadrant with penetration into peritoneal cavity

◀ Additional Character Required   √x7ᵗʰ Placeholder Alert   Unspecified Dx   Other Specified Dx   Manifestation   ▶◀ Revised Text   ● New Code   ▲ Revised Code Title

D-10-CM 2016   873

√7ᵗʰ **S31.604** **Unspecified open wound of abdominal wall, left lower quadrant with penetration into peritoneal cavity**

√7ᵗʰ **S31.605** **Unspecified open wound of abdominal wall, periumbilic region with penetration into peritoneal cavity**

√7ᵗʰ **S31.609** **Unspecified open wound of abdominal wall, unspecified quadrant with penetration into peritoneal cavity**

√6ᵗʰ **S31.61** Laceration without foreign body of abdominal wall with penetration into peritoneal cavity

√7ᵗʰ **S31.610** **Laceration without foreign body of abdominal wall, right upper quadrant with penetration into peritoneal cavity**

√7ᵗʰ **S31.611** **Laceration without foreign body of abdominal wall, left lower quadrant with penetration into peritoneal cavity**

√7ᵗʰ **S31.612** **Laceration without foreign body of abdominal wall, epigastric region with penetration into peritoneal cavity**

√7ᵗʰ **S31.613** **Laceration without foreign body of abdominal wall, right lower quadrant with penetration into peritoneal cavity**

√7ᵗʰ **S31.614** **Laceration without foreign body of abdominal wall, left lower quadrant with penetration into peritoneal cavity**

√7ᵗʰ **S31.615** **Laceration without foreign body of abdominal wall, periumbilic region with penetration into peritoneal cavity**

√7ᵗʰ **S31.619** **Laceration without foreign body of abdominal wall, unspecified quadrant with penetration into peritoneal cavity**

√6ᵗʰ **S31.62** Laceration with foreign body of abdominal wall with penetration into peritoneal cavity

√7ᵗʰ **S31.620** **Laceration with foreign body of abdominal wall, right upper quadrant with penetration into peritoneal cavity**

√7ᵗʰ **S31.621** **Laceration with foreign body of abdominal wall, left upper quadrant with penetration into peritoneal cavity**

√7ᵗʰ **S31.622** **Laceration with foreign body of abdominal wall, epigastric region with penetration into peritoneal cavity**

√7ᵗʰ **S31.623** **Laceration with foreign body of abdominal wall, right lower quadrant with penetration into peritoneal cavity**

√7ᵗʰ **S31.624** **Laceration with foreign body of abdominal wall, left lower quadrant with penetration into peritoneal cavity**

√7ᵗʰ **S31.625** **Laceration with foreign body of abdominal wall, periumbilic region with penetration into peritoneal cavity**

√7ᵗʰ **S31.629** **Laceration with foreign body of abdominal wall, unspecified quadrant with penetration into peritoneal cavity**

√6ᵗʰ **S31.63** Puncture wound without foreign body of abdominal wall with penetration into peritoneal cavity

√7ᵗʰ **S31.630** **Puncture wound without foreign body of abdominal wall, right upper quadrant with penetration into peritoneal cavity**

√7ᵗʰ **S31.631** **Puncture wound without foreign body of abdominal wall, left upper quadrant with penetration into peritoneal cavity**

√7ᵗʰ **S31.632** **Puncture wound without foreign body of abdominal wall, epigastric region with penetration into peritoneal cavity**

√7ᵗʰ **S31.633** **Puncture wound without foreign body of abdominal wall, right lower quadrant with penetration into peritoneal cavity**

√7ᵗʰ **S31.634** **Puncture wound without foreign body of abdominal wall, left lower quadrant with penetration into peritoneal cavity**

√7ᵗʰ **S31.635** **Puncture wound without foreign body of abdominal wall, periumbilic region with penetration into peritoneal cavity**

√7ᵗʰ **S31.639** **Puncture wound without foreign body of abdominal wall, unspecified quadrant with penetration into peritoneal cavity**

√6ᵗʰ **S31.64** Puncture wound with foreign body of abdominal wall with penetration into peritoneal cavity

√7ᵗʰ **S31.640** **Puncture wound with foreign body of abdominal wall, right upper quadrant with penetration into peritoneal cavity**

√7ᵗʰ **S31.641** **Puncture wound with foreign body of abdominal wall, left upper quadrant with penetration into peritoneal cavity**

√7ᵗʰ **S31.642** **Puncture wound with foreign body of abdominal wall, epigastric region with penetration into peritoneal cavity**

√7ᵗʰ **S31.643** **Puncture wound with foreign body of abdominal wall, right lower quadrant with penetration into peritoneal cavity**

√7ᵗʰ **S31.644** **Puncture wound with foreign body of abdominal wall, left lower quadrant with penetration into peritoneal cavity**

√7ᵗʰ **S31.645** **Puncture wound with foreign body of abdominal wall, periumbilic region with penetration into peritoneal cavity**

√7ᵗʰ **S31.649** **Puncture wound with foreign body of abdominal wall, unspecified quadrant with penetration into peritoneal cavity**

√6ᵗʰ **S31.65** Open bite of abdominal wall with penetration into peritoneal cavity

    EXCLUDES 1 superficial bite of abdominal wall (S30.861, S30.871)

√7ᵗʰ **S31.650** **Open bite of abdominal wall, right upper quadrant with penetration into peritoneal cavity**

√7ᵗʰ **S31.651** **Open bite of abdominal wall, left upper quadrant with penetration into peritoneal cavity**

√7ᵗʰ **S31.652** **Open bite of abdominal wall, epigastric region with penetration into peritoneal cavity**

√7ᵗʰ **S31.653** **Open bite of abdominal wall, right lower quadrant with penetration into peritoneal cavity**

√7ᵗʰ **S31.654** **Open bite of abdominal wall, left lower quadrant with penetration into peritoneal cavity**

√7ᵗʰ **S31.655** **Open bite of abdominal wall, periumbilic region with penetration into peritoneal cavity**

√7ᵗʰ **S31.659** **Open bite of abdominal wall, unspecified quadrant with penetration into peritoneal cavity**

√5ᵗʰ **S31.8** Open wound of other parts of abdomen, lower back and pelvis

√6ᵗʰ **S31.80** Open wound of unspecified buttock

√7ᵗʰ **S31.801** Laceration without foreign body of unspecified buttock

√7ᵗʰ **S31.802** Laceration with foreign body of unspecified buttock

√7ᵗʰ **S31.803** Puncture wound without foreign body of unspecified buttock

√7ᵗʰ **S31.804** Puncture wound with foreign body of unspecified buttock

√7ᵗʰ **S31.805** Open bite of unspecified buttock
    Bite of buttock NOS
    EXCLUDES 1 superficial bite of buttock (S30.870)

√7ᵗʰ **S31.809** Unspecified open wound of unspecified buttock

√6ᵗʰ **S31.81** Open wound of right buttock

√7ᵗʰ **S31.811** Laceration without foreign body of right buttock

√7ᵗʰ **S31.812** Laceration with foreign body of right buttock

√7ᵗʰ **S31.813** Puncture wound without foreign body of right buttock

√7ᵗʰ **S31.814** Puncture wound with foreign body of right buttock

√7ᵗʰ **S31.815** Open bite of right buttock
    Bite of right buttock NOS
    EXCLUDES 1 superficial bite of buttock (S30.870)

EXCLUDES 1 Not coded here   **EXCLUDES 2** Not included here   N Newborn Age: 0   P Pediatric Age: 0-17   M Maternity Age: 12-55   A Adult Age: 15-12

874

ICD-10-CM 201

√7ᵗʰ **S31.819** Unspecified open wound of right buttock

√6ᵗʰ **S31.82** Open wound of left buttock

　√7ᵗʰ **S31.821** Laceration without foreign body of left buttock

　√7ᵗʰ **S31.822** Laceration with foreign body of left buttock

　√7ᵗʰ **S31.823** Puncture wound without foreign body of left buttock

　√7ᵗʰ **S31.824** Puncture wound with foreign body of left buttock

　√7ᵗʰ **S31.825** Open bite of left buttock
　　　Bite of left buttock NOS
　　　EXCLUDES 1 *superficial bite of buttock (S30.870)*

　√7ᵗʰ **S31.829** Unspecified open wound of left buttock

√6ᵗʰ **S31.83** Open wound of anus

　√7ᵗʰ **S31.831** Laceration without foreign body of anus

　√7ᵗʰ **S31.832** Laceration with foreign body of anus

　√7ᵗʰ **S31.833** Puncture wound without foreign body of anus

　√7ᵗʰ **S31.834** Puncture wound with foreign body of anus

　√7ᵗʰ **S31.835** Open bite of anus
　　　Bite of anus NOS
　　　EXCLUDES 1 *superficial bite of anus (S30.877)*

　√7ᵗʰ **S31.839** Unspecified open wound of anus

√4ᵗʰ **S32** **Fracture of lumbar spine and pelvis**

　NOTE　A fracture not indicated as displaced or nondisplaced should be coded to displaced.
　　　A fracture not indicated as opened or closed should be coded to closed.

　INCLUDES　fracture of lumbosacral neural arch
　　　fracture of lumbosacral spinous process
　　　fracture of lumbosacral transverse process
　　　fracture of lumbosacral vertebra
　　　fracture of lumbosacral vertebral arch

Code first any associated spinal cord and spinal nerve injury (S34.-)
　EXCLUDES 1 *transection of abdomen (S38.3)*
　EXCLUDES 2 *fracture of hip NOS (S72.0-)*
AHA: 2012, 4Q, 93

The appropriate 7th character is to be added to each code from category S32.
A　initial encounter for closed fracture
B　initial encounter for open fracture
D　subsequent encounter for fracture with routine healing
G　subsequent encounter for fracture with delayed healing
K　subsequent encounter for fracture with nonunion
S　sequela

√5ᵗʰ **S32.0** Fracture of lumbar vertebra
　　　Fracture of lumbar spine NOS

√6ᵗʰ **S32.00** Fracture of unspecified lumbar vertebra

　√7ᵗʰ **S32.000** Wedge compression fracture of unspecified lumbar vertebra

　√7ᵗʰ **S32.001** Stable burst fracture of unspecified lumbar vertebra

　√7ᵗʰ **S32.002** Unstable burst fracture of unspecified lumbar vertebra

　√7ᵗʰ **S32.008** Other fracture of unspecified lumbar vertebra

　√7ᵗʰ **S32.009** Unspecified fracture of unspecified lumbar vertebra

√6ᵗʰ **S32.01** Fracture of first lumbar vertebra

　√7ᵗʰ **S32.010** Wedge compression fracture of first lumbar vertebra

　√7ᵗʰ **S32.011** Stable burst fracture of first lumbar vertebra

　√7ᵗʰ **S32.012** Unstable burst fracture of first lumbar vertebra

　√7ᵗʰ **S32.018** Other fracture of first lumbar vertebra

　√7ᵗʰ **S32.019** Unspecified fracture of first lumbar vertebra

√6ᵗʰ **S32.02** Fracture of second lumbar vertebra

　√7ᵗʰ **S32.020** Wedge compression fracture of second lumbar vertebra

　√7ᵗʰ **S32.021** Stable burst fracture of second lumbar vertebra

　√7ᵗʰ **S32.022** Unstable burst fracture of second lumbar vertebra

　√7ᵗʰ **S32.028** Other fracture of second lumbar vertebra

　√7ᵗʰ **S32.029** Unspecified fracture of second lumbar vertebra

√6ᵗʰ **S32.03** Fracture of third lumbar vertebra

　√7ᵗʰ **S32.030** Wedge compression fracture of third lumbar vertebra

　√7ᵗʰ **S32.031** Stable burst fracture of third lumbar vertebra

　√7ᵗʰ **S32.032** Unstable burst fracture of third lumbar vertebra

　√7ᵗʰ **S32.038** Other fracture of third lumbar vertebra

　√7ᵗʰ **S32.039** Unspecified fracture of third lumbar vertebra

√6ᵗʰ **S32.04** Fracture of fourth lumbar vertebra

　√7ᵗʰ **S32.040** Wedge compression fracture of fourth lumbar vertebra

　√7ᵗʰ **S32.041** Stable burst fracture of fourth lumbar vertebra

　√7ᵗʰ **S32.042** Unstable burst fracture of fourth lumbar vertebra

　√7ᵗʰ **S32.048** Other fracture of fourth lumbar vertebra

　√7ᵗʰ **S32.049** Unspecified fracture of fourth lumbar vertebra

√6ᵗʰ **S32.05** Fracture of fifth lumbar vertebra

　√7ᵗʰ **S32.050** Wedge compression fracture of fifth lumbar vertebra

　√7ᵗʰ **S32.051** Stable burst fracture of fifth lumbar vertebra

　√7ᵗʰ **S32.052** Unstable burst fracture of fifth lumbar vertebra

　√7ᵗʰ **S32.058** Other fracture of fifth lumbar vertebra

　√7ᵗʰ **S32.059** Unspecified fracture of fifth lumbar vertebra

√5ᵗʰ **S32.1** Fracture of sacrum
　NOTE　For vertical fractures, code to most medial fracture extension.
　　　Use two codes if both a vertical and transverse fracture are present.
　　Code also any associated fracture of pelvic ring (S32.8-)

√x7ᵗʰ **S32.10** Unspecified fracture of sacrum

√6ᵗʰ **S32.11** Zone I fracture of sacrum
　　　Vertical sacral ala fracture of sacrum

　√7ᵗʰ **S32.110** Nondisplaced Zone I fracture of sacrum

　√7ᵗʰ **S32.111** Minimally displaced Zone I fracture of sacrum

　√7ᵗʰ **S32.112** Severely displaced Zone I fracture of sacrum

　√7ᵗʰ **S32.119** Unspecified Zone I fracture of sacrum

√6ᵗʰ **S32.12** Zone II fracture of sacrum
　　　Vertical foraminal region fracture of sacrum

　√7ᵗʰ **S32.120** Nondisplaced Zone II fracture of sacrum

　√7ᵗʰ **S32.121** Minimally displaced Zone II fracture of sacrum

　√7ᵗʰ **S32.122** Severely displaced Zone II fracture of sacrum

　√7ᵗʰ **S32.129** Unspecified Zone II fracture of sacrum

√6ᵗʰ **S32.13** Zone III fracture of sacrum
　　　Vertical fracture into spinal canal region of sacrum

　√7ᵗʰ **S32.130** Nondisplaced Zone III fracture of sacrum

　√7ᵗʰ **S32.131** Minimally displaced Zone III fracture of sacrum

　√7ᵗʰ **S32.132** Severely displaced Zone III fracture of sacrum

　√7ᵗʰ **S32.139** Unspecified Zone III fracture of sacrum

√x7ᵗʰ **S32.14** Type 1 fracture of sacrum
　　　Transverse flexion fracture of sacrum without displacement

√x7ᵗʰ **S32.15** Type 2 fracture of sacrum
　　　Transverse flexion fracture of sacrum with posterior displacement

■ Additional Character Required　√x7ᵗʰ Placeholder Alert　Unspecified Dx　Other Specified Dx　Manifestation　▶◀ Revised Text　● New Code　▲ Revised Code Title

-10-CM 2016　　　　875

√x7th **S32.16** Type 3 **fracture of sacrum**
Transverse extension fracture of sacrum with anterior displacement

√x7th **S32.17** Type 4 **fracture of sacrum**
Transverse segmental comminution of upper sacrum

√x7th **S32.19** **Other fracture of sacrum**

√x7th **S32.2** Fracture of coccyx

√5th **S32.3** Fracture of ilium

EXCLUDES 1 *fracture of ilium with associated disruption of pelvic ring (S32.8-)*

√6th **S32.30** Unspecified **fracture of ilium**

√7th **S32.301** **Unspecified fracture of right ilium**

√7th **S32.302** **Unspecified fracture of left ilium**

√7th **S32.309** **Unspecified fracture of unspecified ilium**

√6th **S32.31** Avulsion **fracture of ilium**

√7th **S32.311** Displaced **avulsion fracture of right** ilium

√7th **S32.312** Displaced **avulsion fracture of left** ilium

√7th **S32.313** Displaced **avulsion fracture of unspecified ilium**

√7th **S32.314** Nondisplaced **avulsion fracture of right** ilium

√7th **S32.315** Nondisplaced **avulsion fracture of left** ilium

√7th **S32.316** Nondisplaced **avulsion fracture of unspecified ilium**

√6th **S32.39** Other **fracture of ilium**

√7th **S32.391** **Other fracture of right ilium**

√7th **S32.392** **Other fracture of left ilium**

√7th **S32.399** **Other fracture of unspecified ilium**

√5th **S32.4** Fracture of acetabulum
Code also any associated fracture of pelvic ring (S32.8-)

√6th **S32.40** Unspecified **fracture of acetabulum**

√7th **S32.401** **Unspecified fracture of right acetabulum**

√7th **S32.402** **Unspecified fracture of left acetabulum**

√7th **S32.409** **Unspecified fracture of unspecified acetabulum**

√6th **S32.41** Fracture of anterior wall **of acetabulum**

√7th **S32.411** Displaced **fracture of anterior wall of right acetabulum**

√7th **S32.412** Displaced **fracture of anterior wall of left acetabulum**

√7th **S32.413** Displaced **fracture of anterior wall of unspecified acetabulum**

√7th **S32.414** Nondisplaced **fracture of anterior wall of right acetabulum**

√7th **S32.415** Nondisplaced **fracture of anterior wall of left acetabulum**

√7th **S32.416** Nondisplaced **fracture of anterior wall of unspecified acetabulum**

√6th **S32.42** Fracture of posterior wall **of acetabulum**

√7th **S32.421** Displaced **fracture of posterior wall of right acetabulum**

√7th **S32.422** Displaced **fracture of posterior wall of left acetabulum**

√7th **S32.423** Displaced **fracture of posterior wall of unspecified acetabulum**

√7th **S32.424** Nondisplaced **fracture of posterior wall of right acetabulum**

√7th **S32.425** Nondisplaced **fracture of posterior wall of left acetabulum**

√7th **S32.426** Nondisplaced **fracture of posterior wall of unspecified acetabulum**

√6th **S32.43** Fracture of anterior column [iliopubic] **of acetabulum**

√7th **S32.431** Displaced **fracture of anterior column [iliopubic] of right acetabulum**

√7th **S32.432** Displaced **fracture of anterior column [iliopubic] of left acetabulum**

√7th **S32.433** Displaced **fracture of anterior column [iliopubic] of unspecified acetabulum**

√7th **S32.434** Nondisplaced **fracture of anterior column [iliopubic] of right acetabulum**

√7th **S32.435** Nondisplaced **fracture of anterior colum [iliopubic] of left acetabulum**

√7th **S32.436** Nondisplaced **fracture of anterior colum [iliopubic] of unspecified acetabulum**

√6th **S32.44** Fracture of posterior column [ilioischial] of acetabulum

√7th **S32.441** Displaced **fracture of posterior column [ilioischial] of right acetabulum**

√7th **S32.442** Displaced **fracture of posterior column [ilioischial] of left acetabulum**

√7th **S32.443** Displaced **fracture of posterior column [ilioischial] of unspecified acetabulum**

√7th **S32.444** Nondisplaced **fracture of posterior colum [ilioischial] of right acetabulum**

√7th **S32.445** Nondisplaced **fracture of posterior colum [ilioischial] of left acetabulum**

√7th **S32.446** Nondisplaced **fracture of posterior colum [ilioischial] of unspecified acetabulum**

√6th **S32.45** Transverse **fracture of acetabulum**

√7th **S32.451** Displaced **transverse fracture of right acetabulum**

√7th **S32.452** Displaced **transverse fracture of left acetabulum**

√7th **S32.453** Displaced **transverse fracture of unspecified acetabulum**

√7th **S32.454** Nondisplaced **transverse fracture of right acetabulum**

√7th **S32.455** Nondisplaced **transverse fracture of left acetabulum**

√7th **S32.456** Nondisplaced **transverse fracture of unspecified acetabulum**

√6th **S32.46** Associated transverse-posterior **fracture of acetabulum**

√7th **S32.461** Displaced **associated transverse-posterior fracture of right acetabulum**

√7th **S32.462** Displaced **associated transverse-posterior fracture of left acetabulum**

√7th **S32.463** Displaced **associated transverse-posterior fracture of unspecified acetabulum**

√7th **S32.464** Nondisplaced **associated transverse-posterior fracture of right acetabulum**

√7th **S32.465** Nondisplaced **associated transverse-posterior fracture of left acetabulum**

√7th **S32.466** Nondisplaced **associated transverse-posterior fracture of unspecified acetabulum**

√6th **S32.47** Fracture of medial wall **of acetabulum**

√7th **S32.471** Displaced **fracture of medial wall of right acetabulum**

√7th **S32.472** Displaced **fracture of medial wall of left acetabulum**

√7th **S32.473** Displaced **fracture of medial wall of unspecified acetabulum**

√7th **S32.474** Nondisplaced **fracture of medial wall of right acetabulum**

√7th **S32.475** Nondisplaced **fracture of medial wall of left acetabulum**

√7th **S32.476** Nondisplaced **fracture of medial wall of unspecified acetabulum**

√6th **S32.48** Dome fracture **of acetabulum**

√7th **S32.481** Displaced **dome fracture of right acetabulum**

√7th **S32.482** Displaced **dome fracture of left acetabulum**

√7th **S32.483** Displaced **dome fracture of unspecified acetabulum**

√7th **S32.484** Nondisplaced **dome fracture of right acetabulum**

√7th **S32.485** Nondisplaced **dome fracture of left acetabulum**

√7th **S32.486** Nondisplaced **dome fracture of unspecified acetabulum**

EXCLUDES 1 Not coded here   EXCLUDES 2 Not included here   N Newborn Age: 0   P Pediatric Age: 0-17   M Maternity Age: 12-55   A Adult Age: 15-12

876   ICD-10-CM 201

✓6ᵗʰ **S32.49** Other specified fracture of acetabulum

　　✓7ᵗʰ **S32.491** Other specified fracture of right acetabulum

　　✓7ᵗʰ **S32.492** Other specified fracture of left acetabulum

　　✓7ᵗʰ **S32.499** Other specified fracture of unspecified acetabulum

✓5ᵗʰ **S32.5** Fracture of pubis

　　EXCLUDES 1　*fracture of pubis with associated disruption of pelvic ring (S32.8-)*

　✓6ᵗʰ **S32.50** Unspecified fracture of pubis

　　✓7ᵗʰ **S32.501** Unspecified fracture of right pubis

　　✓7ᵗʰ **S32.502** Unspecified fracture of left pubis

　　✓7ᵗʰ **S32.509** Unspecified fracture of unspecified pubis

　✓6ᵗʰ **S32.51** Fracture of superior rim of pubis

　　✓7ᵗʰ **S32.511** Fracture of superior rim of right pubis

　　✓7ᵗʰ **S32.512** Fracture of superior rim of left pubis

　　✓7ᵗʰ **S32.519** Fracture of superior rim of unspecified pubis

　✓6ᵗʰ **S32.59** Other specified fracture of pubis

　　✓7ᵗʰ **S32.591** Other specified fracture of right pubis

　　✓7ᵗʰ **S32.592** Other specified fracture of left pubis

　　✓7ᵗʰ **S32.599** Other specified fracture of unspecified pubis

✓5ᵗʰ **S32.6** Fracture of ischium

　　EXCLUDES 1　*fracture of ischium with associated disruption of pelvic ring (S32.8-)*

　✓6ᵗʰ **S32.60** Unspecified fracture of ischium

　　✓7ᵗʰ **S32.601** Unspecified fracture of right ischium

　　✓7ᵗʰ **S32.602** Unspecified fracture of left ischium

　　✓7ᵗʰ **S32.609** Unspecified fracture of unspecified ischium

　✓6ᵗʰ **S32.61** Avulsion fracture of ischium

　　✓7ᵗʰ **S32.611** Displaced avulsion fracture of right ischium

　　✓7ᵗʰ **S32.612** Displaced avulsion fracture of left ischium

　　✓7ᵗʰ **S32.613** Displaced avulsion fracture of unspecified ischium

　　✓7ᵗʰ **S32.614** Nondisplaced avulsion fracture of right ischium

　　✓7ᵗʰ **S32.615** Nondisplaced avulsion fracture of left ischium

　　✓7ᵗʰ **S32.616** Nondisplaced avulsion fracture of unspecified ischium

　✓6ᵗʰ **S32.69** Other specified fracture of ischium

　　✓7ᵗʰ **S32.691** Other specified fracture of right ischium

　　✓7ᵗʰ **S32.692** Other specified fracture of left ischium

　　✓7ᵗʰ **S32.699** Other specified fracture of unspecified ischium

✓5ᵗʰ **S32.8** Fracture of other parts of pelvis

　　Code also any associated:
　　　fracture of acetabulum (S32.4-)
　　　sacral fracture (S32.1-)

　✓6ᵗʰ **S32.81** Multiple fractures of pelvis with disruption of pelvic ring

　　　Multiple pelvic fractures with disruption of pelvic circle

　　✓7ᵗʰ **S32.810** Multiple fractures of pelvis with stable disruption of pelvic ring

　　✓7ᵗʰ **S32.811** Multiple fractures of pelvis with unstable disruption of pelvic ring

　✓x7ᵗʰ **S32.82** Multiple fractures of pelvis without disruption of pelvic ring

　　　Multiple pelvic fractures without disruption of pelvic circle

　✓x7ᵗʰ **S32.89** Fracture of other parts of pelvis

✓x7ᵗʰ **S32.9** Fracture of unspecified parts of lumbosacral spine and pelvis

　　Fracture of lumbosacral spine NOS
　　Fracture of pelvis NOS
　　AHA: 2012, 4Q, 93

✓4ᵗʰ **S33** Dislocation and sprain of joints and ligaments of lumbar spine and pelvis

　　INCLUDES　avulsion of joint or ligament of lumbar spine and pelvis
　　　laceration of cartilage, joint or ligament of lumbar spine and pelvis
　　　sprain of cartilage, joint or ligament of lumbar spine and pelvis
　　　traumatic hemarthrosis of joint or ligament of lumbar spine and pelvis
　　　traumatic rupture of joint or ligament of lumbar spine and pelvis
　　　traumatic subluxation of joint or ligament of lumbar spine and pelvis
　　　traumatic tear of joint or ligament of lumbar spine and pelvis

　　Code also any associated open wound

　　EXCLUDES 1　*nontraumatic rupture or displacement of lumbar intervertebral disc NOS (M51.-)*
　　　obstetric damage to pelvic joints and ligaments (O71.6)

　　EXCLUDES 2　*dislocation and sprain of joints and ligaments of hip (S73.-)*
　　　strain of muscle of lower back and pelvis (S39.01-)

　　The appropriate 7th character is to be added to each code from category S33.
　　A　initial encounter
　　D　subsequent encounter
　　S　sequela

　✓x7ᵗʰ **S33.0** Traumatic rupture of lumbar intervertebral disc

　　　EXCLUDES 1　*rupture or displacement (nontraumatic) of lumbar intervertebral disc NOS (M51- with fifth character 6)*

　✓5ᵗʰ **S33.1** Subluxation and dislocation of lumbar vertebra

　　　Code also any associated:
　　　　open wound of abdomen, lower back and pelvis (S31)
　　　　spinal cord injury (S24.0, S24.1-, S34.0-, S34.1-)
　　　EXCLUDES 2　*fracture of lumbar vertebrae (S32.0-)*

　　✓6ᵗʰ **S33.10** Subluxation and dislocation of unspecified lumbar vertebra

　　　✓7ᵗʰ **S33.100** Subluxation of unspecified lumbar vertebra

　　　✓7ᵗʰ **S33.101** Dislocation of unspecified lumbar vertebra

　　✓6ᵗʰ **S33.11** Subluxation and dislocation of L1/L2 lumbar vertebra

　　　✓7ᵗʰ **S33.110** Subluxation of L1/L2 lumbar vertebra

　　　✓7ᵗʰ **S33.111** Dislocation of L1/L2 lumbar vertebra

　　✓6ᵗʰ **S33.12** Subluxation and dislocation of L2/L3 lumbar vertebra

　　　✓7ᵗʰ **S33.120** Subluxation of L2/L3 lumbar vertebra

　　　✓7ᵗʰ **S33.121** Dislocation of L2/L3 lumbar vertebra

　　✓6ᵗʰ **S33.13** Subluxation and dislocation of L3/L4 lumbar vertebra

　　　✓7ᵗʰ **S33.130** Subluxation of L3/L4 lumbar vertebra

　　　✓7ᵗʰ **S33.131** Dislocation of L3/L4 lumbar vertebra

　　✓6ᵗʰ **S33.14** Subluxation and dislocation of L4/L5 lumbar vertebra

　　　✓7ᵗʰ **S33.140** Subluxation of L4/L5 lumbar vertebra

　　　✓7ᵗʰ **S33.141** Dislocation of L4/L5 lumbar vertebra

　✓x7ᵗʰ **S33.2** Dislocation of sacroiliac and sacrococcygeal joint

　✓5ᵗʰ **S33.3** Dislocation of other and unspecified parts of lumbar spine and pelvis

　　✓x7ᵗʰ **S33.30** Dislocation of unspecified parts of lumbar spine and pelvis

　　✓x7ᵗʰ **S33.39** Dislocation of other parts of lumbar spine and pelvis

　✓x7ᵗʰ **S33.4** Traumatic rupture of symphysis pubis

　✓x7ᵗʰ **S33.5** Sprain of ligaments of lumbar spine

　✓x7ᵗʰ **S33.6** Sprain of sacroiliac joint

　✓x7ᵗʰ **S33.8** Sprain of other parts of lumbar spine and pelvis

　✓x7ᵗʰ **S33.9** Sprain of unspecified parts of lumbar spine and pelvis

Additional Character Required　　✓x7ᵗʰ Placeholder Alert　　Unspecified Dx　　Other Specified Dx　　Manifestation　　►◄ Revised Text　　● New Code　　▲ Revised Code Title

✓4ᵗʰ S34 Injury of lumbar and sacral spinal cord and nerves at abdomen, lower back and pelvis level

> **NOTE** Code to highest level of lumbar cord injury.
> Injuries to the spinal cord (S34.0 and S34.1) refer to the cord level and not bone level injury, and can affect nerve roots at and below the level given.

Code also any associated:
    fracture of vertebra (S22.0-, S32.0-)
    open wound of abdomen, lower back and pelvis (S31.-)
    transient paralysis (R29.5)

The appropriate 7th character is to be added to each code from category S34.
A   initial encounter
D   subsequent encounter
S   sequela

✓5ᵗʰ S34.0 Concussion and edema of lumbar and sacral spinal cord

  ✓x7ᵗʰ S34.01 Concussion and edema of lumbar spinal cord

  ✓x7ᵗʰ S34.02 Concussion and edema of sacral spinal cord
    Concussion and edema of conus medullaris

✓5ᵗʰ S34.1 Other and unspecified injury of lumbar and sacral spinal cord

  ✓6ᵗʰ S34.10 Unspecified injury to lumbar spinal cord

    ✓7ᵗʰ S34.101 Unspecified injury to L1 level of lumbar spinal cord

    ✓7ᵗʰ S34.102 Unspecified injury to L2 level of lumbar spinal cord

    ✓7ᵗʰ S34.103 Unspecified injury to L3 level of lumbar spinal cord

    ✓7ᵗʰ S34.104 Unspecified injury to L4 level of lumbar spinal cord

    ✓7ᵗʰ S34.105 Unspecified injury to L5 level of lumbar spinal cord

    ✓7ᵗʰ S34.109 Unspecified injury to unspecified level of lumbar spinal cord

  ✓6ᵗʰ S34.11 Complete lesion of lumbar spinal cord

    ✓7ᵗʰ S34.111 Complete lesion of L1 level of lumbar spinal cord

    ✓7ᵗʰ S34.112 Complete lesion of L2 level of lumbar spinal cord

    ✓7ᵗʰ S34.113 Complete lesion of L3 level of lumbar spinal cord

    ✓7ᵗʰ S34.114 Complete lesion of L4 level of lumbar spinal cord

    ✓7ᵗʰ S34.115 Complete lesion of L5 level of lumbar spinal cord

    ✓7ᵗʰ S34.119 Complete lesion of unspecified level of lumbar spinal cord

  ✓6ᵗʰ S34.12 Incomplete lesion of lumbar spinal cord

    ✓7ᵗʰ S34.121 Incomplete lesion of L1 level of lumbar spinal cord

    ✓7ᵗʰ S34.122 Incomplete lesion of L2 level of lumbar spinal cord

    ✓7ᵗʰ S34.123 Incomplete lesion of L3 level of lumbar spinal cord

    ✓7ᵗʰ S34.124 Incomplete lesion of L4 level of lumbar spinal cord

    ✓7ᵗʰ S34.125 Incomplete lesion of L5 level of lumbar spinal cord

    ✓7ᵗʰ S34.129 Incomplete lesion of unspecified level of lumbar spinal cord

  ✓6ᵗʰ S34.13 Other and unspecified injury to sacral spinal cord
    Other injury to conus medullaris

    ✓7ᵗʰ S34.131 Complete lesion of sacral spinal cord
      Complete lesion of conus medullaris

    ✓7ᵗʰ S34.132 Incomplete lesion of sacral spinal cord
      Incomplete lesion of conus medullaris

    ✓7ᵗʰ S34.139 Unspecified injury to sacral spinal cord
      Unspecified injury of conus medullaris

✓5ᵗʰ S34.2 Injury of nerve root of lumbar and sacral spine

  ✓x7ᵗʰ S34.21 Injury of nerve root of lumbar spine

  ✓x7ᵗʰ S34.22 Injury of nerve root of sacral spine

✓x7ᵗʰ S34.3 Injury of cauda equina

✓x7ᵗʰ S34.4 Injury of lumbosacral plexus

✓x7ᵗʰ S34.5 Injury of lumbar, sacral and pelvic sympathetic nerves
    Injury of celiac ganglion or plexus
    Injury of hypogastric plexus
    Injury of mesenteric plexus (inferior) (superior)
    Injury of splanchnic nerve

✓x7ᵗʰ S34.6 Injury of peripheral nerve(s) at abdomen, lower back and pelvis level

✓x7ᵗʰ S34.8 Injury of other nerves at abdomen, lower back and pelvis level

✓x7ᵗʰ S34.9 Injury of unspecified nerves at abdomen, lower back and pelvis level

✓4ᵗʰ S35 Injury of blood vessels at abdomen, lower back and pelvis level
Code also any associated open wound (S31.-)

The appropriate 7th character is to be added to each code from category S35.
A   initial encounter
D   subsequent encounter
S   sequela

✓5ᵗʰ S35.0 Injury of abdominal aorta
  EXCLUDES 1 injury of aorta NOS (S25.0)

  ✓x7ᵗʰ S35.00 Unspecified injury of abdominal aorta

  ✓x7ᵗʰ S35.01 Minor laceration of abdominal aorta
    Incomplete transection of abdominal aorta
    Laceration of abdominal aorta NOS
    Superficial laceration of abdominal aorta

  ✓x7ᵗʰ S35.02 Major laceration of abdominal aorta
    Complete transection of abdominal aorta
    Traumatic rupture of abdominal aorta

  ✓x7ᵗʰ S35.09 Other injury of abdominal aorta

✓5ᵗʰ S35.1 Injury of inferior vena cava
    Injury of hepatic vein
  EXCLUDES 1 injury of vena cava NOS (S25.2)

  ✓x7ᵗʰ S35.10 Unspecified injury of inferior vena cava

  ✓x7ᵗʰ S35.11 Minor laceration of inferior vena cava
    Incomplete transection of inferior vena cava
    Laceration of inferior vena cava NOS
    Superficial laceration of inferior vena cava

  ✓x7ᵗʰ S35.12 Major laceration of inferior vena cava
    Complete transection of inferior vena cava
    Traumatic rupture of inferior vena cava

  ✓x7ᵗʰ S35.19 Other injury of inferior vena cava

✓5ᵗʰ S35.2 Injury of celiac or mesenteric artery and branches

  ✓6ᵗʰ S35.21 Injury of celiac artery

    ✓7ᵗʰ S35.211 Minor laceration of celiac artery
      Incomplete transection of celiac artery
      Laceration of celiac artery NOS
      Superficial laceration of celiac artery

    ✓7ᵗʰ S35.212 Major laceration of celiac artery
      Complete transection of celiac artery
      Traumatic rupture of celiac artery

    ✓7ᵗʰ S35.218 Other injury of celiac artery

    ✓7ᵗʰ S35.219 Unspecified injury of celiac artery

  ✓6ᵗʰ S35.22 Injury of superior mesenteric artery

    ✓7ᵗʰ S35.221 Minor laceration of superior mesenteric artery
      Incomplete transection of superior mesenteric artery
      Laceration of superior mesenteric artery NOS
      Superficial laceration of superior mesenteric artery

    ✓7ᵗʰ S35.222 Major laceration of superior mesenteric artery
      Complete transection of superior mesenteric artery
      Traumatic rupture of superior mesenteric artery

    ✓7ᵗʰ S35.228 Other injury of superior mesenteric artery

    ✓7ᵗʰ S35.229 Unspecified injury of superior mesenteric artery

EXCLUDES 1 Not coded here   **EXCLUDES 2** Not included here   **N** Newborn Age: 0   **P** Pediatric Age: 0-17   **M** Maternity Age: 12-55   **A** Adult Age: 15-12

878   ICD-10-CM 20

√6th **S35.23** **Injury of** inferior mesenteric artery

    √7th **S35.231** **Minor laceration of inferior mesenteric artery**
        Incomplete transection of inferior mesenteric artery
        Laceration of inferior mesenteric artery NOS
        Superficial laceration of inferior mesenteric artery

    √7th **S35.232** **Major laceration of inferior mesenteric artery**
        Complete transection of inferior mesenteric artery
        Traumatic rupture of inferior mesenteric artery

    √7th **S35.238** **Other injury of inferior mesenteric artery**

    √7th **S35.239** **Unspecified injury of inferior mesenteric artery**

√6th **S35.29** **Injury of** branches of celiac and mesenteric artery
    Injury of gastric artery
    Injury of gastroduodenal artery
    Injury of hepatic artery
    Injury of splenic artery

    √7th **S35.291** **Minor laceration of branches of celiac and mesenteric artery**
        Incomplete transection of branches of celiac and mesenteric artery
        Laceration of branches of celiac and mesenteric artery NOS
        Superficial laceration of branches of celiac and mesenteric artery

    √7th **S35.292** **Major laceration of branches of celiac and mesenteric artery**
        Complete transection of branches of celiac and mesenteric artery
        Traumatic rupture of branches of celiac and mesenteric artery

    √7th **S35.298** **Other injury of branches of celiac and mesenteric artery**

    √7th **S35.299** **Unspecified injury of branches of celiac and mesenteric artery**

√5th **S35.3** **Injury of portal or splenic vein and branches**

√6th **S35.31** **Injury of** portal vein

    √7th **S35.311** **Laceration of portal vein**

    √7th **S35.318** **Other specified injury of portal vein**

    √7th **S35.319** **Unspecified injury of portal vein**

√6th **S35.32** **Injury of** splenic vein

    √7th **S35.321** **Laceration of splenic vein**

    √7th **S35.328** **Other specified injury of splenic vein**

    √7th **S35.329** **Unspecified injury of splenic vein**

√6th **S35.33** **Injury of** superior mesenteric vein

    √7th **S35.331** **Laceration of superior mesenteric vein**

    √7th **S35.338** **Other specified injury of superior mesenteric vein**

    √7th **S35.339** **Unspecified injury of superior mesenteric vein**

√6th **S35.34** **Injury of** inferior mesenteric vein

    √7th **S35.341** **Laceration of inferior mesenteric vein**

    √7th **S35.348** **Other specified injury of inferior mesenteric vein**

    √7th **S35.349** **Unspecified injury of inferior mesenteric vein**

√5th **S35.4** **Injury of** renal blood vessels

√6th **S35.40** **Unspecified injury of renal blood vessel**

    √7th **S35.401** **Unspecified injury of** right **renal** artery

    √7th **S35.402** **Unspecified injury of** left **renal** artery

    √7th **S35.403** **Unspecified injury of unspecified renal artery**

    √7th **S35.404** **Unspecified injury of** right **renal** vein

    √7th **S35.405** **Unspecified injury of** left **renal** vein

    √7th **S35.406** **Unspecified injury of unspecified renal vein**

√6th **S35.41** **Laceration of renal blood vessel**

    √7th **S35.411** **Laceration of** right **renal** artery

    √7th **S35.412** **Laceration of** left **renal** artery

    √7th **S35.413** **Laceration of unspecified renal artery**

    √7th **S35.414** **Laceration of** right **renal** vein

    √7th **S35.415** **Laceration of** left **renal** vein

    √7th **S35.416** **Laceration of unspecified renal vein**

√6th **S35.49** **Other specified injury of renal blood vessel**

    √7th **S35.491** **Other specified injury of** right **renal** artery

    √7th **S35.492** **Other specified injury of** left **renal** artery

    √7th **S35.493** **Other specified injury of unspecified renal artery**

    √7th **S35.494** **Other specified injury of** right **renal** vein

    √7th **S35.495** **Other specified injury of** left **renal** vein

    √7th **S35.496** **Other specified injury of unspecified renal vein**

√5th **S35.5** **Injury of** iliac blood vessels

    √x7th **S35.50** **Injury of unspecified iliac blood vessel(s)**

√6th **S35.51** **Injury of** iliac artery or vein
    Injury of hypogastric artery or vein

    √7th **S35.511** **Injury of** right **iliac** artery

    √7th **S35.512** **Injury of** left **iliac** artery

    √7th **S35.513** **Injury of unspecified iliac artery**

    √7th **S35.514** **Injury of** right **iliac** vein

    √7th **S35.515** **Injury of** left **iliac** vein

    √7th **S35.516** **Injury of unspecified iliac vein**

√6th **S35.53** **Injury of** uterine artery or vein

    √7th **S35.531** **Injury of** right **uterine** artery   ♀

    √7th **S35.532** **Injury of** left **uterine** artery   ♀

    √7th **S35.533** **Injury of unspecified uterine artery**   ♀

    √7th **S35.534** **Injury of** right **uterine** vein   ♀

    √7th **S35.535** **Injury of** left **uterine** vein   ♀

    √7th **S35.536** **Injury of unspecified uterine vein**   ♀

    √x7th **S35.59** **Injury of other iliac blood vessels**

√5th **S35.8** **Injury of other blood vessels at abdomen, lower back and pelvis level**
    Injury of ovarian artery or vein

√6th **S35.8X** **Injury of** other **blood vessels at abdomen, lower back and pelvis level**

    √7th **S35.8X1** **Laceration of other blood vessels at abdomen, lower back and pelvis level**

    √7th **S35.8X8** **Other specified injury of other blood vessels at abdomen, lower back and pelvis level**

    √7th **S35.8X9** **Unspecified injury of other blood vessels at abdomen, lower back and pelvis level**

√5th **S35.9** **Injury of** unspecified **blood vessel at abdomen, lower back and pelvis level**

    √x7th **S35.90** **Unspecified injury of unspecified blood vessel at abdomen, lower back and pelvis level**

    √x7th **S35.91** **Laceration of unspecified blood vessel at abdomen, lower back and pelvis level**

    √x7th **S35.99** **Other specified injury of unspecified blood vessel at abdomen, lower back and pelvis level**

√4th **S36** **Injury of intra-abdominal organs**
    Code also any associated open wound (S31.-)

> The appropriate 7th character is to be added to each code from category S36.
> A   initial encounter
> D   subsequent encounter
> S   sequela

√5th **S36.0** **Injury of** spleen

    √x7th **S36.00** **Unspecified injury of spleen**

√6th **S36.02** **Contusion of spleen**

    √7th **S36.020** **Minor contusion of spleen**
        Contusion of spleen less than 2 cm

    √7th **S36.021** **Major contusion of spleen**
        Contusion of spleen greater than 2 cm

    √7th **S36.029** **Unspecified contusion of spleen**

√6th **S36.03** **Laceration of spleen**

    √7th **S36.030** **Superficial (capsular) laceration of spleen**
        Laceration of spleen less than 1cm
        Minor laceration of spleen

☑ Additional Character Required   √x7th Placeholder Alert   Unspecified Dx   Other Specified Dx   Manifestation   ►◄ Revised Text   ● New Code   ▲ Revised Code Title

CD-10-CM 2016   879

Chapter 19. Injury, Poisoning, and Certain Other Consequences of External Causes

S36.031–S36.519

- √7ᵗʰ **S36.031** Moderate **laceration of spleen**
  Laceration of spleen 1 to 3 cm
- √7ᵗʰ **S36.032** Major **laceration of spleen**
  Avulsion of spleen
  Laceration of spleen greater than 3 cm
  Massive laceration of spleen
  Multiple moderate lacerations of spleen
  Stellate laceration of spleen
- √7ᵗʰ **S36.039** Unspecified laceration of spleen
- √x7ᵗʰ **S36.09** Other injury of spleen

√5ᵗʰ **S36.1 Injury of liver and gallbladder and bile duct**
- √6ᵗʰ **S36.11** Injury of liver
  - √7ᵗʰ **S36.112** Contusion of liver
  - √7ᵗʰ **S36.113** Laceration of liver, unspecified degree
  - √7ᵗʰ **S36.114** Minor laceration of liver
    Laceration involving capsule only, or, without significant involvement of hepatic parenchyma [i.e., less than 1cm deep]
  - √7ᵗʰ **S36.115** Moderate laceration of liver
    Laceration involving parenchyma but without major disruption of parenchyma [i.e., less than 10 cm long and less than 3 cm deep]
  - √7ᵗʰ **S36.116** Major laceration of liver
    Laceration with significant disruption of hepatic parenchyma [i.e., greater than 10 cm long and 3 cm deep]
    Multiple moderate lacerations, with or without hematoma
    Stellate laceration of liver
  - √7ᵗʰ **S36.118** Other injury of liver
  - √7ᵗʰ **S36.119** Unspecified injury of liver
- √6ᵗʰ **S36.12** Injury of gallbladder
  - √7ᵗʰ **S36.122** Contusion of gallbladder
  - √7ᵗʰ **S36.123** Laceration of gallbladder
  - √7ᵗʰ **S36.128** Other injury of gallbladder
  - √7ᵗʰ **S36.129** Unspecified injury of gallbladder
- √x7ᵗʰ **S36.13** Injury of bile duct

√5ᵗʰ **S36.2 Injury of pancreas**
- √6ᵗʰ **S36.20** Unspecified injury of pancreas
  - √7ᵗʰ **S36.200** Unspecified injury of head of pancreas
  - √7ᵗʰ **S36.201** Unspecified injury of body of pancreas
  - √7ᵗʰ **S36.202** Unspecified injury of tail of pancreas
  - √7ᵗʰ **S36.209** Unspecified injury of unspecified part of pancreas
- √6ᵗʰ **S36.22** Contusion of pancreas
  - √7ᵗʰ **S36.220** Contusion of head of pancreas
  - √7ᵗʰ **S36.221** Contusion of body of pancreas
  - √7ᵗʰ **S36.222** Contusion of tail of pancreas
  - √7ᵗʰ **S36.229** Contusion of unspecified part of pancreas
- √6ᵗʰ **S36.23** Laceration of pancreas, unspecified degree
  - √7ᵗʰ **S36.230** Laceration of head of pancreas, unspecified degree
  - √7ᵗʰ **S36.231** Laceration of body of pancreas, unspecified degree
  - √7ᵗʰ **S36.232** Laceration of tail of pancreas, unspecified degree
  - √7ᵗʰ **S36.239** Laceration of unspecified part of pancreas, unspecified degree
- √6ᵗʰ **S36.24** Minor laceration of pancreas
  - √7ᵗʰ **S36.240** Minor laceration of head of pancreas
  - √7ᵗʰ **S36.241** Minor laceration of body of pancreas
  - √7ᵗʰ **S36.242** Minor laceration of tail of pancreas
  - √7ᵗʰ **S36.249** Minor laceration of unspecified part of pancreas
- √6ᵗʰ **S36.25** Moderate laceration of pancreas
  - √7ᵗʰ **S36.250** Moderate laceration of head of pancreas
  - √7ᵗʰ **S36.251** Moderate laceration of body of pancreas
  - √7ᵗʰ **S36.252** Moderate laceration of tail of pancreas
  - √7ᵗʰ **S36.259** Moderate laceration of unspecified part of pancreas

- √6ᵗʰ **S36.26** Major laceration of pancreas
  - √7ᵗʰ **S36.260** Major laceration of head of pancreas
  - √7ᵗʰ **S36.261** Major laceration of body of pancreas
  - √7ᵗʰ **S36.262** Major laceration of tail of pancreas
  - √7ᵗʰ **S36.269** Major laceration of unspecified part of pancreas
- √6ᵗʰ **S36.29** Other injury of pancreas
  - √7ᵗʰ **S36.290** Other injury of head of pancreas
  - √7ᵗʰ **S36.291** Other injury of body of pancreas
  - √7ᵗʰ **S36.292** Other injury of tail of pancreas
  - √7ᵗʰ **S36.299** Other injury of unspecified part of pancreas

√5ᵗʰ **S36.3 Injury of stomach**
- √x7ᵗʰ **S36.30** Unspecified injury of stomach
- √x7ᵗʰ **S36.32** Contusion of stomach
- √x7ᵗʰ **S36.33** Laceration of stomach
- √x7ᵗʰ **S36.39** Other injury of stomach

√5ᵗʰ **S36.4 Injury of small intestine**
- √6ᵗʰ **S36.40** Unspecified injury of small intestine
  - √7ᵗʰ **S36.400** Unspecified injury of duodenum
  - √7ᵗʰ **S36.408** Unspecified injury of other part of small intestine
  - √7ᵗʰ **S36.409** Unspecified injury of unspecified part of small intestine
- √6ᵗʰ **S36.41** Primary blast injury of small intestine
  Blast injury of small intestine NOS
  - √7ᵗʰ **S36.410** Primary blast injury of duodenum
  - √7ᵗʰ **S36.418** Primary blast injury of other part of small intestine
  - √7ᵗʰ **S36.419** Primary blast injury of unspecified part of small intestine
- √6ᵗʰ **S36.42** Contusion of small intestine
  - √7ᵗʰ **S36.420** Contusion of duodenum
  - √7ᵗʰ **S36.428** Contusion of other part of small intestine
  - √7ᵗʰ **S36.429** Contusion of unspecified part of small intestine
- √6ᵗʰ **S36.43** Laceration of small intestine
  - √7ᵗʰ **S36.430** Laceration of duodenum
  - √7ᵗʰ **S36.438** Laceration of other part of small intestine
  - √7ᵗʰ **S36.439** Laceration of unspecified part of small intestine
- √6ᵗʰ **S36.49** Other injury of small intestine
  - √7ᵗʰ **S36.490** Other injury of duodenum
  - √7ᵗʰ **S36.498** Other injury of other part of small intestine
  - √7ᵗʰ **S36.499** Other injury of unspecified part of small intestine

√5ᵗʰ **S36.5 Injury of colon**
  EXCLUDES 2 injury of rectum (S36.6-)
- √6ᵗʰ **S36.50** Unspecified injury of colon
  - √7ᵗʰ **S36.500** Unspecified injury of ascending [right] colon
  - √7ᵗʰ **S36.501** Unspecified injury of transverse colon
  - √7ᵗʰ **S36.502** Unspecified injury of descending [left] colon
  - √7ᵗʰ **S36.503** Unspecified injury of sigmoid colon
  - √7ᵗʰ **S36.508** Unspecified injury of other part of colon
  - √7ᵗʰ **S36.509** Unspecified injury of unspecified part of colon
- √6ᵗʰ **S36.51** Primary blast injury of colon
  Blast injury of colon NOS
  - √7ᵗʰ **S36.510** Primary blast injury of ascending [right] colon
  - √7ᵗʰ **S36.511** Primary blast injury of transverse colon
  - √7ᵗʰ **S36.512** Primary blast injury of descending [left] colon
  - √7ᵗʰ **S36.513** Primary blast injury of sigmoid colon
  - √7ᵗʰ **S36.518** Primary blast injury of other part of colon
  - √7ᵗʰ **S36.519** Primary blast injury of unspecified part of colon

EXCLUDES 1 Not coded here   EXCLUDES 2 Not included here   N Newborn Age: 0   P Pediatric Age: 0-17   M Maternity Age: 12-55   A Adult Age: 15-124

880

ICD-10-CM 2016

☑6ᵗʰ **S36.52** Contusion of colon
- ☑7ᵗʰ **S36.520** Contusion of ascending [right] colon
- ☑7ᵗʰ **S36.521** Contusion of transverse colon
- ☑7ᵗʰ **S36.522** Contusion of descending [left] colon
- ☑7ᵗʰ **S36.523** Contusion of sigmoid colon
- ☑7ᵗʰ **S36.528** Contusion of other part of colon
- ☑7ᵗʰ **S36.529** Contusion of unspecified part of colon

☑6ᵗʰ **S36.53** Laceration of colon
- ☑7ᵗʰ **S36.530** Laceration of ascending [right] colon
- ☑7ᵗʰ **S36.531** Laceration of transverse colon
- ☑7ᵗʰ **S36.532** Laceration of descending [left] colon
- ☑7ᵗʰ **S36.533** Laceration of sigmoid colon
- ☑7ᵗʰ **S36.538** Laceration of other part of colon
- ☑7ᵗʰ **S36.539** Laceration of unspecified part of colon

☑6ᵗʰ **S36.59** Other injury of colon
    Secondary blast injury of colon
- ☑7ᵗʰ **S36.590** Other injury of ascending [right] colon
- ☑7ᵗʰ **S36.591** Other injury of transverse colon
- ☑7ᵗʰ **S36.592** Other injury of descending [left] colon
- ☑7ᵗʰ **S36.593** Other injury of sigmoid colon
- ☑7ᵗʰ **S36.598** Other injury of other part of colon
- ☑7ᵗʰ **S36.599** Other injury of unspecified part of colon

☑5ᵗʰ **S36.6 Injury of rectum**
- ☑x7ᵗʰ **S36.60** Unspecified injury of rectum
- ☑x7ᵗʰ **S36.61** Primary blast injury of rectum
    Blast injury of rectum NOS
- ☑x7ᵗʰ **S36.62** Contusion of rectum
- ☑x7ᵗʰ **S36.63** Laceration of rectum
- ☑x7ᵗʰ **S36.69** Other injury of rectum
    Secondary blast injury of rectum

☑5ᵗʰ **S36.8 Injury of other intra-abdominal organs**
- ☑x7ᵗʰ **S36.81** Injury of peritoneum
- ☑6ᵗʰ **S36.89** Injury of other intra-abdominal organs
    Injury of retroperitoneum
  - ☑7ᵗʰ **S36.892** Contusion of other intra-abdominal organs
  - ☑7ᵗʰ **S36.893** Laceration of other intra-abdominal organs
  - ☑7ᵗʰ **S36.898** Other injury of other intra-abdominal organs
  - ☑7ᵗʰ **S36.899** Unspecified injury of other intra-abdominal organs

☑5ᵗʰ **S36.9 Injury of unspecified intra-abdominal organ**
- ☑x7ᵗʰ **S36.90** Unspecified injury of unspecified intra-abdominal organ
- ☑x7ᵗʰ **S36.92** Contusion of unspecified intra-abdominal organ
- ☑x7ᵗʰ **S36.93** Laceration of unspecified intra-abdominal organ
- ☑x7ᵗʰ **S36.99** Other injury of unspecified intra-abdominal organ

4ᵗʰ **S37 Injury of urinary and pelvic organs**
    Code also any associated open wound (S31.-)
    EXCLUDES 1   obstetric trauma to pelvic organs (O71.-)
    EXCLUDES 2   injury of peritoneum (S36.81)
                 injury of retroperitoneum (S36.89-)

    The appropriate 7th character is to be added to each code from category S37.
    A   initial encounter
    D   subsequent encounter
    S   sequela

☑5ᵗʰ **S37.0 Injury of kidney**
    EXCLUDES 2   acute kidney injury (nontraumatic) (N17.9)
- ☑6ᵗʰ **S37.00** Unspecified injury of kidney
  - ☑7ᵗʰ **S37.001** Unspecified injury of right kidney
  - ☑7ᵗʰ **S37.002** Unspecified injury of left kidney
  - ☑7ᵗʰ **S37.009** Unspecified injury of unspecified kidney
- ☑6ᵗʰ **S37.01** Minor contusion of kidney
    Contusion of kidney less than 2 cm
    Contusion of kidney NOS
  - ☑7ᵗʰ **S37.011** Minor contusion of right kidney
  - ☑7ᵗʰ **S37.012** Minor contusion of left kidney
  - ☑7ᵗʰ **S37.019** Minor contusion of unspecified kidney

☑6ᵗʰ **S37.02** Major contusion of kidney
    Contusion of kidney greater than 2 cm
- ☑7ᵗʰ **S37.021** Major contusion of right kidney
- ☑7ᵗʰ **S37.022** Major contusion of left kidney
- ☑7ᵗʰ **S37.029** Major contusion of unspecified kidney

☑6ᵗʰ **S37.03** Laceration of kidney, unspecified degree
- ☑7ᵗʰ **S37.031** Laceration of right kidney, unspecified degree
- ☑7ᵗʰ **S37.032** Laceration of left kidney, unspecified degree
- ☑7ᵗʰ **S37.039** Laceration of unspecified kidney, unspecified degree

☑6ᵗʰ **S37.04** Minor laceration of kidney
    Laceration of kidney less than 1 cm
- ☑7ᵗʰ **S37.041** Minor laceration of right kidney
- ☑7ᵗʰ **S37.042** Minor laceration of left kidney
- ☑7ᵗʰ **S37.049** Minor laceration of unspecified kidney

☑6ᵗʰ **S37.05** Moderate laceration of kidney
    Laceration of kidney 1 to 3 cm
- ☑7ᵗʰ **S37.051** Moderate laceration of right kidney
- ☑7ᵗʰ **S37.052** Moderate laceration of left kidney
- ☑7ᵗʰ **S37.059** Moderate laceration of unspecified kidney

☑6ᵗʰ **S37.06** Major laceration of kidney
    Avulsion of kidney
    Laceration of kidney greater than 3 cm
    Massive laceration of kidney
    Multiple moderate lacerations of kidney
    Stellate laceration of kidney
- ☑7ᵗʰ **S37.061** Major laceration of right kidney
- ☑7ᵗʰ **S37.062** Major laceration of left kidney
- ☑7ᵗʰ **S37.069** Major laceration of unspecified kidney

☑6ᵗʰ **S37.09** Other injury of kidney
- ☑7ᵗʰ **S37.091** Other injury of right kidney
- ☑7ᵗʰ **S37.092** Other injury of left kidney
- ☑7ᵗʰ **S37.099** Other injury of unspecified kidney

☑5ᵗʰ **S37.1 Injury of ureter**
- ☑x7ᵗʰ **S37.10** Unspecified injury of ureter
- ☑x7ᵗʰ **S37.12** Contusion of ureter
- ☑x7ᵗʰ **S37.13** Laceration of ureter
- ☑x7ᵗʰ **S37.19** Other injury of ureter

☑5ᵗʰ **S37.2 Injury of bladder**
- ☑x7ᵗʰ **S37.20** Unspecified injury of bladder
- ☑x7ᵗʰ **S37.22** Contusion of bladder
- ☑x7ᵗʰ **S37.23** Laceration of bladder
- ☑x7ᵗʰ **S37.29** Other injury of bladder

☑5ᵗʰ **S37.3 Injury of urethra**
- ☑x7ᵗʰ **S37.30** Unspecified injury of urethra
- ☑x7ᵗʰ **S37.32** Contusion of urethra
- ☑x7ᵗʰ **S37.33** Laceration of urethra
- ☑x7ᵗʰ **S37.39** Other injury of urethra

☑5ᵗʰ **S37.4 Injury of ovary**
- ☑6ᵗʰ **S37.40** Unspecified injury of ovary
  - ☑7ᵗʰ **S37.401** Unspecified injury of ovary, unilateral   ♀
  - ☑7ᵗʰ **S37.402** Unspecified injury of ovary, bilateral   ♀
  - ☑7ᵗʰ **S37.409** Unspecified injury of ovary, unspecified ♀
- ☑6ᵗʰ **S37.42** Contusion of ovary
  - ☑7ᵗʰ **S37.421** Contusion of ovary, unilateral   ♀
  - ☑7ᵗʰ **S37.422** Contusion of ovary, bilateral   ♀
  - ☑7ᵗʰ **S37.429** Contusion of ovary, unspecified   ♀
- ☑6ᵗʰ **S37.43** Laceration of ovary
  - ☑7ᵗʰ **S37.431** Laceration of ovary, unilateral   ♀
  - ☑7ᵗʰ **S37.432** Laceration of ovary, bilateral   ♀
  - ☑7ᵗʰ **S37.439** Laceration of ovary, unspecified   ♀
- ☑6ᵗʰ **S37.49** Other injury of ovary
  - ☑7ᵗʰ **S37.491** Other injury of ovary, unilateral   ♀
  - ☑7ᵗʰ **S37.492** Other injury of ovary, bilateral   ♀
  - ☑7ᵗʰ **S37.499** Other injury of ovary, unspecified
    ♀

◀ Additional Character Required   ☑x7ᵗʰ Placeholder Alert   Unspecified Dx   Other Specified Dx   Manifestation   ▶◀ Revised Text   ● New Code   ▲ Revised Code Title

✓5ᵗʰ S37.5 Injury of fallopian tube

S37.50 Unspecified injury of fallopian tube

✓7ᵗʰ **S37.501 Unspecified injury of fallopian tube, unilateral** ♀

✓7ᵗʰ **S37.502 Unspecified injury of fallopian tube, bilateral** ♀

✓7ᵗʰ **S37.509 Unspecified injury of fallopian tube, unspecified** ♀

✓6ᵗʰ **S37.51 Primary blast injury of fallopian tube**
Blast injury of fallopian tube NOS

✓7ᵗʰ **S37.511 Primary blast injury of fallopian tube, unilateral** ♀

✓7ᵗʰ **S37.512 Primary blast injury of fallopian tube, bilateral** ♀

✓7ᵗʰ **S37.519 Primary blast injury of fallopian tube, unspecified** ♀

✓6ᵗʰ **S37.52 Contusion of fallopian tube**

✓7ᵗʰ **S37.521 Contusion of fallopian tube, unilateral** ♀

✓7ᵗʰ **S37.522 Contusion of fallopian tube, bilateral** ♀

✓7ᵗʰ **S37.529 Contusion of fallopian tube, unspecified** ♀

✓6ᵗʰ **S37.53 Laceration of fallopian tube**

✓7ᵗʰ **S37.531 Laceration of fallopian tube, unilateral** ♀

✓7ᵗʰ **S37.532 Laceration of fallopian tube, bilateral** ♀

✓7ᵗʰ **S37.539 Laceration of fallopian tube, unspecified** ♀

✓6ᵗʰ **S37.59 Other injury of fallopian tube**
Secondary blast injury of fallopian tube

✓7ᵗʰ **S37.591 Other injury of fallopian tube, unilateral** ♀

✓7ᵗʰ **S37.592 Other injury of fallopian tube, bilateral** ♀

✓7ᵗʰ **S37.599 Other injury of fallopian tube, unspecified** ♀

✓5ᵗʰ S37.6 Injury of uterus

EXCLUDES 1   injury to gravid uterus (O9A.2-)
injury to uterus during delivery (O71.-)

✓x7ᵗʰ **S37.60 Unspecified injury of uterus** ♀

✓x7ᵗʰ **S37.62 Contusion of uterus** ♀

✓x7ᵗʰ **S37.63 Laceration of uterus** ♀

✓x7ᵗʰ **S37.69 Other injury of uterus** ♀

✓5ᵗʰ S37.8 Injury of other urinary and pelvic organs

✓6ᵗʰ **S37.81 Injury of adrenal gland**

✓7ᵗʰ **S37.812 Contusion of adrenal gland**

✓7ᵗʰ **S37.813 Laceration of adrenal gland**

✓7ᵗʰ **S37.818 Other injury of adrenal gland**

✓7ᵗʰ **S37.819 Unspecified injury of adrenal gland**

✓6ᵗʰ **S37.82 Injury of prostate**

✓7ᵗʰ **S37.822 Contusion of prostate** ♂

✓7ᵗʰ **S37.823 Laceration of prostate** ♂

✓7ᵗʰ **S37.828 Other injury of prostate** ♂

✓7ᵗʰ **S37.829 Unspecified injury of prostate** ♂

✓6ᵗʰ **S37.89 Injury of other urinary and pelvic organ**

✓7ᵗʰ **S37.892 Contusion of other urinary and pelvic organ**

✓7ᵗʰ **S37.893 Laceration of other urinary and pelvic organ**

✓7ᵗʰ **S37.898 Other injury of other urinary and pelvic organ**

✓7ᵗʰ **S37.899 Unspecified injury of other urinary and pelvic organ**

✓5ᵗʰ S37.9 Injury of unspecified urinary and pelvic organ

✓x7ᵗʰ **S37.90 Unspecified injury of unspecified urinary and pelvic organ**

✓x7ᵗʰ **S37.92 Contusion of unspecified urinary and pelvic organ**

✓x7ᵗʰ **S37.93 Laceration of unspecified urinary and pelvic organ**

✓x7ᵗʰ **S37.99 Other injury of unspecified urinary and pelvic organ**

✓4ᵗʰ S38 Crushing injury and traumatic amputation of abdomen, lower back, pelvis and external genitals

NOTE   An amputation not identified as partial or complete shoulc be coded to complete.

The appropriate 7th character is to be added to each code from category S38.
A   initial encounter
D   subsequent encounter
S   sequela

✓5ᵗʰ S38.0 Crushing injury of external genital organs
Use additional code for any associated injuries

✓6ᵗʰ **S38.00 Crushing injury of unspecified external genital organs**

✓7ᵗʰ **S38.001 Crushing injury of unspecified external genital organs, male**

✓7ᵗʰ **S38.002 Crushing injury of unspecified external genital organs, female**

✓x7ᵗʰ **S38.01 Crushing injury of penis**

✓x7ᵗʰ **S38.02 Crushing injury of scrotum and testis**

✓x7ᵗʰ **S38.03 Crushing injury of vulva**

✓x7ᵗʰ **S38.1 Crushing injury of abdomen, lower back, and pelvis**
Use additional code for all associated injuries, such as:
fracture of thoracic or lumbar spine and pelvis (S22.0-, S32-)
injury to intra-abdominal organs (S36.-)
injury to urinary and pelvic organs (S37.-)
open wound of abdominal wall (S31.-)
spinal cord injury (S34.0, S34.1-)

EXCLUDES 2   crushing injury of external genital organs (S38.0-)

✓5ᵗʰ S38.2 Traumatic amputation of external genital organs

✓6ᵗʰ **S38.21 Traumatic amputation of female external genital organs**
Traumatic amputation of clitoris
Traumatic amputation of labium (majus) (minus)
Traumatic amputation of vulva

✓7ᵗʰ **S38.211 Complete traumatic amputation of female external genital organs**

✓7ᵗʰ **S38.212 Partial traumatic amputation of female external genital organs**

✓6ᵗʰ **S38.22 Traumatic amputation of penis**

✓7ᵗʰ **S38.221 Complete traumatic amputation of penis**

✓7ᵗʰ **S38.222 Partial traumatic amputation of penis**

✓6ᵗʰ **S38.23 Traumatic amputation of scrotum and testis**

✓7ᵗʰ **S38.231 Complete traumatic amputation of scrotum and testis**

✓7ᵗʰ **S38.232 Partial traumatic amputation of scrotum and testis**

✓x7ᵗʰ **S38.3 Transection (partial) of abdomen**

✓4ᵗʰ S39 Other and unspecified injuries of abdomen, lower back, pelvis and external genitals
Code also any associated open wound (S31.-)

EXCLUDES 2   sprain of joints and ligaments of lumbar spine and pelvis (S33.)

The appropriate 7th character is to be added to each code from category S39.
A   initial encounter
D   subsequent encounter
S   sequela

✓5ᵗʰ S39.0 Injury of muscle, fascia and tendon of abdomen, lower back and pelvis

✓6ᵗʰ **S39.00 Unspecified injury of muscle, fascia and tendon of abdomen, lower back and pelvis**

✓7ᵗʰ **S39.001 Unspecified injury of muscle, fascia and tendon of abdomen**

✓7ᵗʰ **S39.002 Unspecified injury of muscle, fascia and tendon of lower back**

✓7ᵗʰ **S39.003 Unspecified injury of muscle, fascia and tendon of pelvis**

✓6ᵗʰ **S39.01 Strain of muscle, fascia and tendon of abdomen, lower back and pelvis**

✓7ᵗʰ **S39.011 Strain of muscle, fascia and tendon of abdomen**

✓7ᵗʰ **S39.012 Strain of muscle, fascia and tendon of lower back**

EXCLUDES 1 Not coded here   EXCLUDES 2 Not included here   N Newborn Age: 0   P Pediatric Age: 0-17   M Maternity Age: 12-55   A Adult Age: 15-12

882

ICD-10-CM 20⬤

✓7ᵗʰ **S39.013** **Strain of muscle, fascia and tendon of pelvis**

✓6ᵗʰ **S39.02** Laceration **of muscle, fascia and tendon of abdomen, lower back and pelvis**

  ✓7ᵗʰ **S39.021** **Laceration of muscle, fascia and tendon of** abdomen

  ✓7ᵗʰ **S39.022** **Laceration of muscle, fascia and tendon of** lower back

  ✓7ᵗʰ **S39.023** **Laceration of muscle, fascia and tendon of** pelvis

✓6ᵗʰ **S39.09** Other **injury of muscle, fascia and tendon of abdomen, lower back and pelvis**

  ✓7ᵗʰ **S39.091** **Other injury of muscle, fascia and tendon of** abdomen

  ✓7ᵗʰ **S39.092** **Other injury of muscle, fascia and tendon of** lower back

  ✓7ᵗʰ **S39.093** **Other injury of muscle, fascia and tendon of** pelvis

✓5ᵗʰ **S39.8** Other **specified injuries of abdomen, lower back, pelvis and external genitals**

  ✓x7ᵗʰ **S39.81** **Other specified injuries of** abdomen

  ✓x7ᵗʰ **S39.82** **Other specified injuries of** lower back

  ✓x7ᵗʰ **S39.83** **Other specified injuries of** pelvis

  ✓6ᵗʰ **S39.84** **Other specified injuries of** external genitals

    ✓7ᵗʰ **S39.840** **Fracture of** corpus cavernosum penis   ♂

    ✓7ᵗʰ **S39.848** **Other specified injuries of external genitals**

✓5ᵗʰ **S39.9** Unspecified **injury of abdomen, lower back, pelvis and external genitals**

  ✓x7ᵗʰ **S39.91** **Unspecified injury of** abdomen

  ✓x7ᵗʰ **S39.92** **Unspecified injury of** lower back

  ✓x7ᵗʰ **S39.93** **Unspecified injury of** pelvis

  ✓x7ᵗʰ **S39.94** **Unspecified injury of** external genitals

Injuries to the shoulder and upper arm (S40-S49)

INCLUDES   injuries of axilla
         injuries of scapular region
EXCLUDES 2   burns and corrosions (T20-T32)
         frostbite (T33-T34)
         injuries of elbow (S50-S59)
         insect bite or sting, venomous (T63.4)

1ˢᵗ **S40** **Superficial injury of shoulder and upper arm**

The appropriate 7th character is to be added to each code from category S40.
A   initial encounter
D   subsequent encounter
S   sequela

✓5ᵗʰ **S40.0** Contusion **of shoulder and upper arm**

  ✓6ᵗʰ **S40.01** **Contusion of** shoulder

    ✓7ᵗʰ **S40.011** **Contusion of** right **shoulder**

    ✓7ᵗʰ **S40.012** **Contusion of** left **shoulder**

    ✓7ᵗʰ **S40.019** **Contusion of unspecified shoulder**

  ✓6ᵗʰ **S40.02** **Contusion of** upper arm

    ✓7ᵗʰ **S40.021** **Contusion of** right **upper arm**

    ✓7ᵗʰ **S40.022** **Contusion of** left **upper arm**

    ✓7ᵗʰ **S40.029** **Contusion of unspecified upper arm**

✓5ᵗʰ **S40.2** Other **superficial injuries of shoulder**

  ✓6ᵗʰ **S40.21** Abrasion **of shoulder**

    ✓7ᵗʰ **S40.211** **Abrasion of** right **shoulder**

    ✓7ᵗʰ **S40.212** **Abrasion of** left **shoulder**

    ✓7ᵗʰ **S40.219** **Abrasion of unspecified shoulder**

  ✓6ᵗʰ **S40.22** Blister (nonthermal) **of shoulder**

    ✓7ᵗʰ **S40.221** **Blister (nonthermal) of** right **shoulder**

    ✓7ᵗʰ **S40.222** **Blister (nonthermal) of** left **shoulder**

    ✓7ᵗʰ **S40.229** **Blister (nonthermal) of unspecified shoulder**

  ✓6ᵗʰ **S40.24** External constriction **of shoulder**

    ✓7ᵗʰ **S40.241** **External constriction of** right **shoulder**

    ✓7ᵗʰ **S40.242** **External constriction of** left **shoulder**

    ✓7ᵗʰ **S40.249** **External constriction of unspecified shoulder**

✓6ᵗʰ **S40.25** **Superficial** foreign body **of shoulder**
     Splinter in the shoulder

  ✓7ᵗʰ **S40.251** **Superficial foreign body of** right **shoulder**

  ✓7ᵗʰ **S40.252** **Superficial foreign body of** left **shoulder**

  ✓7ᵗʰ **S40.259** **Superficial foreign body of unspecified shoulder**

✓6ᵗʰ **S40.26** Insect bite (nonvenomous) **of shoulder**

  ✓7ᵗʰ **S40.261** **Insect bite (nonvenomous) of** right **shoulder**

  ✓7ᵗʰ **S40.262** **Insect bite (nonvenomous) of** left **shoulder**

  ✓7ᵗʰ **S40.269** **Insect bite (nonvenomous) of unspecified shoulder**

✓6ᵗʰ **S40.27** Other **superficial** bite **of shoulder**
     EXCLUDES 1   open bite of shoulder (S41.05)

  ✓7ᵗʰ **S40.271** **Other superficial bite of** right **shoulder**

  ✓7ᵗʰ **S40.272** **Other superficial bite of** left **shoulder**

  ✓7ᵗʰ **S40.279** **Other superficial bite of unspecified shoulder**

✓5ᵗʰ **S40.8** Other **superficial injuries of upper arm**

  ✓6ᵗʰ **S40.81** Abrasion **of upper arm**

    ✓7ᵗʰ **S40.811** **Abrasion of** right **upper arm**

    ✓7ᵗʰ **S40.812** **Abrasion of** left **upper arm**

    ✓7ᵗʰ **S40.819** **Abrasion of unspecified upper arm**

  ✓6ᵗʰ **S40.82** Blister (nonthermal) **of upper arm**

    ✓7ᵗʰ **S40.821** **Blister (nonthermal) of** right **upper arm**

    ✓7ᵗʰ **S40.822** **Blister (nonthermal) of** left **upper arm**

    ✓7ᵗʰ **S40.829** **Blister (nonthermal) of unspecified upper arm**

  ✓6ᵗʰ **S40.84** External constriction **of upper arm**

    ✓7ᵗʰ **S40.841** **External constriction of** right **upper arm**

    ✓7ᵗʰ **S40.842** **External constriction of** left **upper arm**

    ✓7ᵗʰ **S40.849** **External constriction of unspecified upper arm**

  ✓6ᵗʰ **S40.85** **Superficial** foreign body **of upper arm**
       Splinter in the upper arm

    ✓7ᵗʰ **S40.851** **Superficial foreign body of** right **upper arm**

    ✓7ᵗʰ **S40.852** **Superficial foreign body of** left **upper arm**

    ✓7ᵗʰ **S40.859** **Superficial foreign body of unspecified upper arm**

  ✓6ᵗʰ **S40.86** Insect bite (nonvenomous) **of upper arm**

    ✓7ᵗʰ **S40.861** **Insect bite (nonvenomous) of** right **upper arm**

    ✓7ᵗʰ **S40.862** **Insect bite (nonvenomous) of** left **upper arm**

    ✓7ᵗʰ **S40.869** **Insect bite (nonvenomous) of unspecified upper arm**

  ✓6ᵗʰ **S40.87** Other **superficial** bite **of upper arm**
       EXCLUDES 1   open bite of upper arm (S41.14)
       EXCLUDES 2   other superficial bite of shoulder (S40.27-)

    ✓7ᵗʰ **S40.871** **Other superficial bite of** right **upper arm**

    ✓7ᵗʰ **S40.872** **Other superficial bite of** left **upper arm**

    ✓7ᵗʰ **S40.879** **Other superficial bite of unspecified upper arm**

✓5ᵗʰ **S40.9** Unspecified **superficial injury of shoulder and upper arm**

  ✓6ᵗʰ **S40.91** **Unspecified superficial injury of** shoulder

    ✓7ᵗʰ **S40.911** **Unspecified superficial injury of** right **shoulder**

    ✓7ᵗʰ **S40.912** **Unspecified superficial injury of** left **shoulder**

    ✓7ᵗʰ **S40.919** **Unspecified superficial injury of unspecified shoulder**

  ✓6ᵗʰ **S40.92** **Unspecified superficial injury of** upper arm

    ✓7ᵗʰ **S40.921** **Unspecified superficial injury of** right **upper arm**

    ✓7ᵗʰ **S40.922** **Unspecified superficial injury of** left **upper arm**

    ✓7ᵗʰ **S40.929** **Unspecified superficial injury of unspecified upper arm**

✓ Additional Character Required   ✓x7ᵗʰ Placeholder Alert   Unspecified Dx   Other Specified Dx   Manifestation   ►◄ Revised Text   ● New Code   ▲ Revised Code Title

Chapter 19. Injury, Poisoning, and Certain Other Consequences of External Causes

S41–S42.026

√4ᵗʰ **S41 Open wound of shoulder and upper arm**

Code also any associated wound infection

EXCLUDES 1 traumatic amputation of shoulder and upper arm (S48.-)

EXCLUDES 2 open fracture of shoulder and upper arm (S42.- with 7th character B or C)

The appropriate 7th character is to be added to each code from category S41.

A   initial encounter
D   subsequent encounter
S   sequela

√5ᵗʰ **S41.0 Open wound of shoulder**

√6ᵗʰ **S41.00 Unspecified open wound of shoulder**

√7ᵗʰ **S41.001 Unspecified open wound of right shoulder**

√7ᵗʰ **S41.002 Unspecified open wound of left shoulder**

√7ᵗʰ **S41.009 Unspecified open wound of unspecified shoulder**

√6ᵗʰ **S41.01 Laceration without foreign body of shoulder**

√7ᵗʰ **S41.011 Laceration without foreign body of right shoulder**

√7ᵗʰ **S41.012 Laceration without foreign body of left shoulder**

√7ᵗʰ **S41.019 Laceration without foreign body of unspecified shoulder**

√6ᵗʰ **S41.02 Laceration with foreign body of shoulder**

√7ᵗʰ **S41.021 Laceration with foreign body of right shoulder**

√7ᵗʰ **S41.022 Laceration with foreign body of left shoulder**

√7ᵗʰ **S41.029 Laceration with foreign body of unspecified shoulder**

√6ᵗʰ **S41.03 Puncture wound without foreign body of shoulder**

√7ᵗʰ **S41.031 Puncture wound without foreign body of right shoulder**

√7ᵗʰ **S41.032 Puncture wound without foreign body of left shoulder**

√7ᵗʰ **S41.039 Puncture wound without foreign body of unspecified shoulder**

√6ᵗʰ **S41.04 Puncture wound with foreign body of shoulder**

√7ᵗʰ **S41.041 Puncture wound with foreign body of right shoulder**

√7ᵗʰ **S41.042 Puncture wound with foreign body of left shoulder**

√7ᵗʰ **S41.049 Puncture wound with foreign body of unspecified shoulder**

√6ᵗʰ **S41.05 Open bite of shoulder**

Bite of shoulder NOS

EXCLUDES 1 superficial bite of shoulder (S40.27)

√7ᵗʰ **S41.051 Open bite of right shoulder**

√7ᵗʰ **S41.052 Open bite of left shoulder**

√7ᵗʰ **S41.059 Open bite of unspecified shoulder**

√5ᵗʰ **S41.1 Open wound of upper arm**

√6ᵗʰ **S41.10 Unspecified open wound of upper arm**

√7ᵗʰ **S41.101 Unspecified open wound of right upper arm**

√7ᵗʰ **S41.102 Unspecified open wound of left upper arm**

√7ᵗʰ **S41.109 Unspecified open wound of unspecified upper arm**

√6ᵗʰ **S41.11 Laceration without foreign body of upper arm**

√7ᵗʰ **S41.111 Laceration without foreign body of right upper arm**

√7ᵗʰ **S41.112 Laceration without foreign body of left upper arm**

√7ᵗʰ **S41.119 Laceration without foreign body of unspecified upper arm**

√6ᵗʰ **S41.12 Laceration with foreign body of upper arm**

√7ᵗʰ **S41.121 Laceration with foreign body of right upper arm**

√7ᵗʰ **S41.122 Laceration with foreign body of left upper arm**

√7ᵗʰ **S41.129 Laceration with foreign body of unspecified upper arm**

√6ᵗʰ **S41.13 Puncture wound without foreign body of upper ar**

√7ᵗʰ **S41.131 Puncture wound without foreign body o right upper arm**

√7ᵗʰ **S41.132 Puncture wound without foreign body o left upper arm**

√7ᵗʰ **S41.139 Puncture wound without foreign body o unspecified upper arm**

√6ᵗʰ **S41.14 Puncture wound with foreign body of upper arm**

√7ᵗʰ **S41.141 Puncture wound with foreign body of right upper arm**

√7ᵗʰ **S41.142 Puncture wound with foreign body of le upper arm**

√7ᵗʰ **S41.149 Puncture wound with foreign body of unspecified upper arm**

√6ᵗʰ **S41.15 Open bite of upper arm**

Bite of upper arm NOS

EXCLUDES 1 superficial bite of upper arm (S40.87)

√7ᵗʰ **S41.151 Open bite of right upper arm**

√7ᵗʰ **S41.152 Open bite of left upper arm**

√7ᵗʰ **S41.159 Open bite of unspecified upper arm**

√4ᵗʰ **S42 Fracture of shoulder and upper arm**

NOTE A fracture not indicated as displaced or nondisplaced shoul be coded to displaced.

A fracture not indicated as open or closed should be coded to closed.

EXCLUDES 1 traumatic amputation of shoulder and upper arm (S48.-)

The appropriate 7th character is to be added to all codes from category S42 [unless otherwise indicated].

A   initial encounter for closed fracture
B   initial encounter for open fracture
D   subsequent encounter for fracture with routine healing
G   subsequent encounter for fracture with delayed healing
K   subsequent encounter for fracture with nonunion
P   subsequent encounter for fracture with malunion
S   sequela

√5ᵗʰ **S42.0 Fracture of clavicle**

√6ᵗʰ **S42.00 Fracture of unspecified part of clavicle**

√7ᵗʰ **S42.001 Fracture of unspecified part of right clavicle**

√7ᵗʰ **S42.002 Fracture of unspecified part of left clavic**

√7ᵗʰ **S42.009 Fracture of unspecified part of unspecifie clavicle**

AHA: 2012, 4Q, 93

√6ᵗʰ **S42.01 Fracture of sternal end of clavicle**

√7ᵗʰ **S42.011 Anterior displaced fracture of sternal end of right clavicle**

√7ᵗʰ **S42.012 Anterior displaced fracture of sternal end of left clavicle**

√7ᵗʰ **S42.013 Anterior displaced fracture of sternal end of unspecified clavicle**

Displaced fracture of sternal end of clavicl NOS

√7ᵗʰ **S42.014 Posterior displaced fracture of sternal en of right clavicle**

√7ᵗʰ **S42.015 Posterior displaced fracture of sternal end of left clavicle**

√7ᵗʰ **S42.016 Posterior displaced fracture of sternal en of unspecified clavicle**

√7ᵗʰ **S42.017 Nondisplaced fracture of sternal end of right clavicle**

√7ᵗʰ **S42.018 Nondisplaced fracture of sternal end of left clavicle**

√7ᵗʰ **S42.019 Nondisplaced fracture of sternal end of unspecified clavicle**

√6ᵗʰ **S42.02 Fracture of shaft of clavicle**

√7ᵗʰ **S42.021 Displaced fracture of shaft of right clavic**

√7ᵗʰ **S42.022 Displaced fracture of shaft of left clavicle**

√7ᵗʰ **S42.023 Displaced fracture of shaft of unspecified clavicle**

√7ᵗʰ **S42.024 Nondisplaced fracture of shaft of right clavicle**

√7ᵗʰ **S42.025 Nondisplaced fracture of shaft of left clavicle**

√7ᵗʰ **S42.026 Nondisplaced fracture of shaft of unspecified clavicle**

EXCLUDES 1 Not coded here   *EXCLUDES 2* Not included here   N Newborn Age: 0   P Pediatric Age: 0-17   M Maternity Age: 12-55   A Adult Age: 15-12

884   ICD-10-CM 201

√6ᵗʰ **S42.03** **Fracture of** lateral end **of clavicle**
Fracture of acromial end of clavicle

√7ᵗʰ **S42.031** Displaced **fracture of lateral end of** right **clavicle**

√7ᵗʰ **S42.032** Displaced **fracture of lateral end of** left **clavicle**

√7ᵗʰ **S42.033** Displaced **fracture of lateral end of unspecified clavicle**

√7ᵗʰ **S42.034** Nondisplaced **fracture of lateral end of** right **clavicle**

√7ᵗʰ **S42.035** Nondisplaced **fracture of lateral end of** left **clavicle**

√7ᵗʰ **S42.036** Nondisplaced **fracture of lateral end of unspecified clavicle**

√5ᵗʰ **S42.1** **Fracture of** scapula

√6ᵗʰ **S42.10** **Fracture of** unspecified **part of scapula**

√7ᵗʰ **S42.101** **Fracture of unspecified part of scapula,** right **shoulder**

√7ᵗʰ **S42.102** **Fracture of unspecified part of scapula,** left **shoulder**

√7ᵗʰ **S42.109** **Fracture of unspecified part of scapula, unspecified shoulder**

√6ᵗʰ **S42.11** **Fracture of** body **of scapula**

√7ᵗʰ **S42.111** Displaced **fracture of body of scapula,** right **shoulder**

√7ᵗʰ **S42.112** Displaced **fracture of body of scapula,** left **shoulder**

√7ᵗʰ **S42.113** Displaced **fracture of body of scapula, unspecified shoulder**

√7ᵗʰ **S42.114** Nondisplaced **fracture of body of scapula,** right **shoulder**

√7ᵗʰ **S42.115** Nondisplaced **fracture of body of scapula,** left **shoulder**

√7ᵗʰ **S42.116** Nondisplaced **fracture of body of scapula, unspecified shoulder**

√6ᵗʰ **S42.12** **Fracture of** acromial process

√7ᵗʰ **S42.121** Displaced **fracture of acromial process,** right **shoulder**

√7ᵗʰ **S42.122** Displaced **fracture of acromial process,** left **shoulder**

√7ᵗʰ **S42.123** Displaced **fracture of acromial process, unspecified shoulder**

√7ᵗʰ **S42.124** Nondisplaced **fracture of acromial process, right shoulder**

√7ᵗʰ **S42.125** Nondisplaced **fracture of acromial process, left shoulder**

√7ᵗʰ **S42.126** Nondisplaced **fracture of acromial process, unspecified shoulder**

√6ᵗʰ **S42.13** **Fracture of** coracoid process

√7ᵗʰ **S42.131** Displaced **fracture of coracoid process,** right **shoulder**

√7ᵗʰ **S42.132** Displaced **fracture of coracoid process,** left **shoulder**

√7ᵗʰ **S42.133** Displaced **fracture of coracoid process, unspecified shoulder**

√7ᵗʰ **S42.134** Nondisplaced **fracture of coracoid process, right shoulder**

√7ᵗʰ **S42.135** Nondisplaced **fracture of coracoid process, left shoulder**

√7ᵗʰ **S42.136** Nondisplaced **fracture of coracoid process, unspecified shoulder**

√6ᵗʰ **S42.14** **Fracture of** glenoid cavity **of scapula**

√7ᵗʰ **S42.141** Displaced **fracture of glenoid cavity of scapula, right shoulder**

√7ᵗʰ **S42.142** Displaced **fracture of glenoid cavity of scapula, left shoulder**

√7ᵗʰ **S42.143** Displaced **fracture of glenoid cavity of scapula, unspecified shoulder**

√7ᵗʰ **S42.144** Nondisplaced **fracture of glenoid cavity of scapula, right shoulder**

√7ᵗʰ **S42.145** Nondisplaced **fracture of glenoid cavity of scapula, left shoulder**

√7ᵗʰ **S42.146** Nondisplaced **fracture of glenoid cavity of scapula, unspecified shoulder**

√6ᵗʰ **S42.15** **Fracture of** neck **of scapula**

√7ᵗʰ **S42.151** Displaced **fracture of neck of scapula,** right **shoulder**

√7ᵗʰ **S42.152** Displaced **fracture of neck of scapula,** left **shoulder**

√7ᵗʰ **S42.153** Displaced **fracture of neck of scapula, unspecified shoulder**

√7ᵗʰ **S42.154** Nondisplaced **fracture of neck of scapula,** right **shoulder**

√7ᵗʰ **S42.155** Nondisplaced **fracture of neck of scapula,** left **shoulder**

√7ᵗʰ **S42.156** Nondisplaced **fracture of neck of scapula, unspecified shoulder**

√6ᵗʰ **S42.19** **Fracture of** other **part of scapula**

√7ᵗʰ **S42.191** **Fracture of other part of scapula,** right **shoulder**

√7ᵗʰ **S42.192** **Fracture of other part of scapula,** left **shoulder**

√7ᵗʰ **S42.199** **Fracture of other part of scapula, unspecified shoulder**

√5ᵗʰ **S42.2** **Fracture of** upper end of humerus
Fracture of proximal end of humerus

EXCLUDES 2 *fracture of shaft of humerus (S42.3-)*
physeal fracture of upper end of humerus (S49.0-)

√6ᵗʰ **S42.20** Unspecified **fracture of upper end of humerus**

√7ᵗʰ **S42.201** **Unspecified fracture of upper end of** right **humerus**

√7ᵗʰ **S42.202** **Unspecified fracture of upper end of** left **humerus**

√7ᵗʰ **S42.209** **Unspecified fracture of upper end of unspecified humerus**

√6ᵗʰ **S42.21** Unspecified **fracture of** surgical neck **of humerus**
Fracture of neck of humerus NOS

√7ᵗʰ **S42.211** **Unspecified** displaced **fracture of surgical neck of** right **humerus**

√7ᵗʰ **S42.212** **Unspecified** displaced **fracture of surgical neck of** left **humerus**

√7ᵗʰ **S42.213** **Unspecified** displaced **fracture of surgical neck of unspecified humerus**

√7ᵗʰ **S42.214** **Unspecified** nondisplaced **fracture of surgical neck of** right **humerus**

√7ᵗʰ **S42.215** **Unspecified** nondisplaced **fracture of surgical neck of** left **humerus**

√7ᵗʰ **S42.216** **Unspecified** nondisplaced **fracture of surgical neck of unspecified humerus**

√6ᵗʰ **S42.22** 2-part **fracture of** surgical neck **of humerus**

√7ᵗʰ **S42.221** **2-part** displaced **fracture of surgical neck of** right **humerus**

√7ᵗʰ **S42.222** **2-part** displaced **fracture of surgical neck of** left **humerus**

√7ᵗʰ **S42.223** **2-part** displaced **fracture of surgical neck of unspecified humerus**

√7ᵗʰ **S42.224** **2-part** nondisplaced **fracture of surgical neck of** right **humerus**

√7ᵗʰ **S42.225** **2-part** nondisplaced **fracture of surgical neck of** left **humerus**

√7ᵗʰ **S42.226** **2-part** nondisplaced **fracture of surgical neck of unspecified humerus**

√6ᵗʰ **S42.23** 3-part **fracture of** surgical neck **of humerus**

√7ᵗʰ **S42.231** **3-part fracture of surgical neck of** right **humerus**

√7ᵗʰ **S42.232** **3-part fracture of surgical neck of** left **humerus**

√7ᵗʰ **S42.239** **3-part fracture of surgical neck of unspecified humerus**

√6ᵗʰ **S42.24** 4-part **fracture of** surgical neck **of humerus**

√7ᵗʰ **S42.241** **4-part fracture of surgical neck of** right **humerus**

√7ᵗʰ **S42.242** **4-part fracture of surgical neck of** left **humerus**

√7ᵗʰ **S42.249** **4-part fracture of surgical neck of unspecified humerus**

☑ Additional Character Required   √x7ᵗʰ Placeholder Alert   Unspecified Dx   Other Specified Dx   Manifestation   ▶◀ Revised Text   ● New Code   ▲ Revised Code Title

CD-10-CM 2016   885

✓6ᵗʰ S42.25 Fracture of greater tuberosity of humerus

✓7ᵗʰ S42.251 Displaced fracture of greater tuberosity of right humerus

✓7ᵗʰ S42.252 Displaced fracture of greater tuberosity of left humerus

✓7ᵗʰ S42.253 Displaced fracture of greater tuberosity of unspecified humerus

✓7ᵗʰ S42.254 Nondisplaced fracture of greater tuberosity of right humerus

✓7ᵗʰ S42.255 Nondisplaced fracture of greater tuberosity of left humerus

✓7ᵗʰ S42.256 Nondisplaced fracture of greater tuberosity of unspecified humerus

✓6ᵗʰ S42.26 Fracture of lesser tuberosity of humerus

✓7ᵗʰ S42.261 Displaced fracture of lesser tuberosity of right humerus

✓7ᵗʰ S42.262 Displaced fracture of lesser tuberosity of left humerus

✓7ᵗʰ S42.263 Displaced fracture of lesser tuberosity of unspecified humerus

✓7ᵗʰ S42.264 Nondisplaced fracture of lesser tuberosity of right humerus

✓7ᵗʰ S42.265 Nondisplaced fracture of lesser tuberosity of left humerus

✓7ᵗʰ S42.266 Nondisplaced fracture of lesser tuberosity of unspecified humerus

✓6ᵗʰ S42.27 Torus fracture of upper end of humerus

> The appropriate 7th character is to be added to all codes in subcategory S42.27.
> A   initial encounter for closed fracture
> D   subsequent encounter for fracture with routine healing
> G   subsequent encounter for fracture with delayed healing
> K   subsequent encounter for fracture with nonunion
> P   subsequent encounter for fracture with malunion
> S   sequela

✓7ᵗʰ S42.271 Torus fracture of upper end of right humerus

✓7ᵗʰ S42.272 Torus fracture of upper end of left humerus

✓7ᵗʰ S42.279 Torus fracture of upper end of unspecified humerus

✓6ᵗʰ S42.29 Other fracture of upper end of humerus
Fracture of anatomical neck of humerus
Fracture of articular head of humerus

✓7ᵗʰ S42.291 Other displaced fracture of upper end of right humerus

✓7ᵗʰ S42.292 Other displaced fracture of upper end of left humerus

✓7ᵗʰ S42.293 Other displaced fracture of upper end of unspecified humerus

✓7ᵗʰ S42.294 Other nondisplaced fracture of upper end of right humerus

✓7ᵗʰ S42.295 Other nondisplaced fracture of upper end of left humerus

✓7ᵗʰ S42.296 Other nondisplaced fracture of upper end of unspecified humerus

✓5ᵗʰ S42.3 Fracture of shaft of humerus
Fracture of humerus NOS
Fracture of upper arm NOS
> EXCLUDES 2   physeal fractures of upper end of humerus (S49.Ø-)
> physeal fractures of lower end of humerus (S49.1-)

✓6ᵗʰ S42.3Ø Unspecified fracture of shaft of humerus

✓7ᵗʰ S42.3Ø1 Unspecified fracture of shaft of humerus, right arm

✓7ᵗʰ S42.3Ø2 Unspecified fracture of shaft of humerus, left arm

✓7ᵗʰ S42.3Ø9 Unspecified fracture of shaft of humerus, unspecified arm

✓6ᵗʰ S42.31 Greenstick fracture of shaft of humerus

> The appropriate 7th character is to be added to all codes in subcategory S42.31.
> A   initial encounter for closed fracture
> D   subsequent encounter for fracture with routin healing
> G   subsequent encounter for fracture with delaye healing
> K   subsequent encounter for fracture with nonunion
> P   subsequent encounter for fracture with malunion
> S   sequela

✓7ᵗʰ S42.311 Greenstick fracture of shaft of humerus, right arm

✓7ᵗʰ S42.312 Greenstick fracture of shaft of humerus, left arm

✓7ᵗʰ S42.319 Greenstick fracture of shaft of humerus, unspecified arm

✓6ᵗʰ S42.32 Transverse fracture of shaft of humerus

✓7ᵗʰ S42.321 Displaced transverse fracture of shaft of humerus, right arm

✓7ᵗʰ S42.322 Displaced transverse fracture of shaft of humerus, left arm

✓7ᵗʰ S42.323 Displaced transverse fracture of shaft of humerus, unspecified arm

✓7ᵗʰ S42.324 Nondisplaced transverse fracture of shaft of humerus, right arm

✓7ᵗʰ S42.325 Nondisplaced transverse fracture of shaft of humerus, left arm

✓7ᵗʰ S42.326 Nondisplaced transverse fracture of shaft of humerus, unspecified arm

✓6ᵗʰ S42.33 Oblique fracture of shaft of humerus

✓7ᵗʰ S42.331 Displaced oblique fracture of shaft of humerus, right arm

✓7ᵗʰ S42.332 Displaced oblique fracture of shaft of humerus, left arm

✓7ᵗʰ S42.333 Displaced oblique fracture of shaft of humerus, unspecified arm

✓7ᵗʰ S42.334 Nondisplaced oblique fracture of shaft of humerus, right arm

✓7ᵗʰ S42.335 Nondisplaced oblique fracture of shaft of humerus, left arm

✓7ᵗʰ S42.336 Nondisplaced oblique fracture of shaft of humerus, unspecified arm

✓6ᵗʰ S42.34 Spiral fracture of shaft of humerus

✓7ᵗʰ S42.341 Displaced spiral fracture of shaft of humerus, right arm

✓7ᵗʰ S42.342 Displaced spiral fracture of shaft of humerus, left arm

✓7ᵗʰ S42.343 Displaced spiral fracture of shaft of humerus, unspecified arm

✓7ᵗʰ S42.344 Nondisplaced spiral fracture of shaft of humerus, right arm

✓7ᵗʰ S42.345 Nondisplaced spiral fracture of shaft of humerus, left arm

✓7ᵗʰ S42.346 Nondisplaced spiral fracture of shaft of humerus, unspecified arm

✓6ᵗʰ S42.35 Comminuted fracture of shaft of humerus

✓7ᵗʰ S42.351 Displaced comminuted fracture of shaft of humerus, right arm

✓7ᵗʰ S42.352 Displaced comminuted fracture of shaft of humerus, left arm

✓7ᵗʰ S42.353 Displaced comminuted fracture of shaft of humerus, unspecified arm

✓7ᵗʰ S42.354 Nondisplaced comminuted fracture of shaft of humerus, right arm

✓7ᵗʰ S42.355 Nondisplaced comminuted fracture of shaft of humerus, left arm

✓7ᵗʰ S42.356 Nondisplaced comminuted fracture of shaft of humerus, unspecified arm

✓6ᵗʰ S42.36 Segmental fracture of shaft of humerus

✓7ᵗʰ S42.361 Displaced segmental fracture of shaft of humerus, right arm

---

EXCLUDES 1 Not coded here   EXCLUDES 2 Not included here   N Newborn Age: 0   P Pediatric Age: 0-17   M Maternity Age: 12-55   A Adult Age: 15-124

886   ICD-10-CM 201

☑7ᵗʰ **S42.362** Displaced segmental fracture of shaft of humerus, left arm

☑7ᵗʰ **S42.363** Displaced segmental fracture of shaft of humerus, unspecified arm

☑7ᵗʰ **S42.364** Nondisplaced segmental fracture of shaft of humerus, right arm

☑7ᵗʰ **S42.365** Nondisplaced segmental fracture of shaft of humerus, left arm

☑7ᵗʰ **S42.366** Nondisplaced segmental fracture of shaft of humerus, unspecified arm

☑6ᵗʰ **S42.39** Other fracture of shaft of humerus

☑7ᵗʰ **S42.391** Other fracture of shaft of right humerus

☑7ᵗʰ **S42.392** Other fracture of shaft of left humerus

☑7ᵗʰ **S42.399** Other fracture of shaft of unspecified humerus

☑5ᵗʰ **S42.4** Fracture of lower end of humerus
Fracture of distal end of humerus

    EXCLUDES 2   *fracture of shaft of humerus (S42.3-)*
        physeal fracture of lower end of humerus (S49.1-)

☑6ᵗʰ **S42.40** Unspecified fracture of lower end of humerus
Fracture of elbow NOS

☑7ᵗʰ **S42.401** Unspecified fracture of lower end of right humerus

☑7ᵗʰ **S42.402** Unspecified fracture of lower end of left humerus

☑7ᵗʰ **S42.409** Unspecified fracture of lower end of unspecified humerus

☑6ᵗʰ **S42.41** Simple supracondylar fracture without intercondylar fracture of humerus

☑7ᵗʰ **S42.411** Displaced simple supracondylar fracture without intercondylar fracture of right humerus

☑7ᵗʰ **S42.412** Displaced simple supracondylar fracture without intercondylar fracture of left humerus

☑7ᵗʰ **S42.413** Displaced simple supracondylar fracture without intercondylar fracture of unspecified humerus

☑7ᵗʰ **S42.414** Nondisplaced simple supracondylar fracture without intercondylar fracture of right humerus

☑7ᵗʰ **S42.415** Nondisplaced simple supracondylar fracture without intercondylar fracture of left humerus

☑7ᵗʰ **S42.416** Nondisplaced simple supracondylar fracture without intercondylar fracture of unspecified humerus

☑6ᵗʰ **S42.42** Comminuted supracondylar fracture without intercondylar fracture of humerus

☑7ᵗʰ **S42.421** Displaced comminuted supracondylar fracture without intercondylar fracture of right humerus

☑7ᵗʰ **S42.422** Displaced comminuted supracondylar fracture without intercondylar fracture of left humerus

☑7ᵗʰ **S42.423** Displaced comminuted supracondylar fracture without intercondylar fracture of unspecified humerus

☑7ᵗʰ **S42.424** Nondisplaced comminuted supracondylar fracture without intercondylar fracture of right humerus

☑7ᵗʰ **S42.425** Nondisplaced comminuted supracondylar fracture without intercondylar fracture of left humerus

☑7ᵗʰ **S42.426** Nondisplaced comminuted supracondylar fracture without intercondylar fracture of unspecified humerus

☑6ᵗʰ **S42.43** Fracture (avulsion) of lateral epicondyle of humerus

☑7ᵗʰ **S42.431** Displaced fracture (avulsion) of lateral epicondyle of right humerus

☑7ᵗʰ **S42.432** Displaced fracture (avulsion) of lateral epicondyle of left humerus

☑7ᵗʰ **S42.433** Displaced fracture (avulsion) of lateral epicondyle of unspecified humerus

☑7ᵗʰ **S42.434** Nondisplaced fracture (avulsion) of lateral epicondyle of right humerus

☑7ᵗʰ **S42.435** Nondisplaced fracture (avulsion) of lateral epicondyle of left humerus

☑7ᵗʰ **S42.436** Nondisplaced fracture (avulsion) of lateral epicondyle of unspecified humerus

☑6ᵗʰ **S42.44** Fracture (avulsion) of medial epicondyle of humerus

S42.441 Displaced fracture (avulsion) of medial epicondyle of right humerus

☑7ᵗʰ **S42.442** Displaced fracture (avulsion) of medial epicondyle of left humerus

☑7ᵗʰ **S42.443** Displaced fracture (avulsion) of medial epicondyle of unspecified humerus

☑7ᵗʰ **S42.444** Nondisplaced fracture (avulsion) of medial epicondyle of right humerus

☑7ᵗʰ **S42.445** Nondisplaced fracture (avulsion) of medial epicondyle of left humerus

☑7ᵗʰ **S42.446** Nondisplaced fracture (avulsion) of medial epicondyle of unspecified humerus

☑7ᵗʰ **S42.447** Incarcerated fracture (avulsion) of medial epicondyle of right humerus

☑7ᵗʰ **S42.448** Incarcerated fracture (avulsion) of medial epicondyle of left humerus

☑7ᵗʰ **S42.449** Incarcerated fracture (avulsion) of medial epicondyle of unspecified humerus

☑6ᵗʰ **S42.45** Fracture of lateral condyle of humerus
Fracture of capitellum of humerus

☑7ᵗʰ **S42.451** Displaced fracture of lateral condyle of right humerus

☑7ᵗʰ **S42.452** Displaced fracture of lateral condyle of left humerus

☑7ᵗʰ **S42.453** Displaced fracture of lateral condyle of unspecified humerus

☑7ᵗʰ **S42.454** Nondisplaced fracture of lateral condyle of right humerus

☑7ᵗʰ **S42.455** Nondisplaced fracture of lateral condyle of left humerus

☑7ᵗʰ **S42.456** Nondisplaced fracture of lateral condyle of unspecified humerus

☑6ᵗʰ **S42.46** Fracture of medial condyle of humerus
Trochlea fracture of humerus

☑7ᵗʰ **S42.461** Displaced fracture of medial condyle of right humerus

☑7ᵗʰ **S42.462** Displaced fracture of medial condyle of left humerus

☑7ᵗʰ **S42.463** Displaced fracture of medial condyle of unspecified humerus

☑7ᵗʰ **S42.464** Nondisplaced fracture of medial condyle of right humerus

☑7ᵗʰ **S42.465** Nondisplaced fracture of medial condyle of left humerus

☑7ᵗʰ **S42.466** Nondisplaced fracture of medial condyle of unspecified humerus

☑6ᵗʰ **S42.47** Transcondylar fracture of humerus

☑7ᵗʰ **S42.471** Displaced transcondylar fracture of right humerus

☑7ᵗʰ **S42.472** Displaced transcondylar fracture of left humerus

☑7ᵗʰ **S42.473** Displaced transcondylar fracture of unspecified humerus

☑7ᵗʰ **S42.474** Nondisplaced transcondylar fracture of right humerus

☑7ᵗʰ **S42.475** Nondisplaced transcondylar fracture of left humerus

☑7ᵗʰ **S42.476** Nondisplaced transcondylar fracture of unspecified humerus

◢ Additional Character Required   ☑7ᵗʰ Placeholder Alert   Unspecified Dx   Other Specified Dx   Manifestation   ▶◀ Revised Text   ● New Code   ▲ Revised Code Title

D-10-CM 2016   887

√6ᵗʰ **S42.48**   **Torus fracture of lower end of humerus**

> The appropriate 7th character is to be added to all codes in subcategory S42.48.
> A   initial encounter for closed fracture
> D   subsequent encounter for fracture with routine healing
> G   subsequent encounter for fracture with delayed healing
> K   subsequent encounter for fracture with nonunion
> P   subsequent encounter for fracture with malunion
> S   sequela

     √7ᵗʰ **S42.481**   **Torus fracture of lower end of** right humerus

     √7ᵗʰ **S42.482**   **Torus fracture of lower end of** left humerus

     √7ᵗʰ **S42.489**   **Torus fracture of lower end of unspecified humerus**

√6ᵗʰ **S42.49**   Other **fracture of lower end of humerus**

     √7ᵗʰ **S42.491**   **Other** displaced **fracture of lower end of** right **humerus**

     √7ᵗʰ **S42.492**   **Other** displaced **fracture of lower end of** left **humerus**

     √7ᵗʰ **S42.493**   **Other** displaced **fracture of lower end of unspecified humerus**

     √7ᵗʰ **S42.494**   **Other** nondisplaced **fracture of lower end of** right **humerus**

     √7ᵗʰ **S42.495**   **Other** nondisplaced **fracture of lower end of** left **humerus**

     √7ᵗʰ **S42.496**   **Other** nondisplaced **fracture of lower end of unspecified humerus**

√5ᵗʰ **S42.9**   **Fracture of** shoulder girdle, part unspecified
     Fracture of shoulder NOS

     √x7ᵗʰ **S42.90**   **Fracture of unspecified shoulder girdle, part unspecified**

     √x7ᵗʰ **S42.91**   **Fracture of** right **shoulder girdle, part unspecified**

     √x7ᵗʰ **S42.92**   **Fracture of** left **shoulder girdle, part unspecified**

√4ᵗʰ **S43**   **Dislocation and sprain of joints and ligaments of shoulder girdle**

> INCLUDES   avulsion of joint or ligament of shoulder girdle
> laceration of cartilage, joint or ligament of shoulder girdle
> sprain of cartilage, joint or ligament of shoulder girdle
> traumatic hemarthrosis of joint or ligament of shoulder girdle
> traumatic rupture of joint or ligament of shoulder girdle
> traumatic subluxation of joint or ligament of shoulder girdle
> traumatic tear of joint or ligament of shoulder girdle

   Code also any associated open wound
   EXCLUDES 2   *strain of muscle, fascia and tendon of shoulder and upper arm (S46.-)*

> The appropriate 7th character is to be added to each code from category S43.
> A   initial encounter
> D   subsequent encounter
> S   sequela

√5ᵗʰ **S43.0**   **Subluxation and dislocation of** shoulder joint
     Dislocation of glenohumeral joint
     Subluxation of glenohumeral joint

     √6ᵗʰ **S43.00**   **Unspecified subluxation and dislocation of shoulder joint**
       Dislocation of humerus NOS
       Subluxation of humerus NOS

       √7ᵗʰ **S43.001**   **Unspecified** subluxation of right **shoulder joint**

       √7ᵗʰ **S43.002**   **Unspecified** subluxation of left **shoulder joint**

       √7ᵗʰ **S43.003**   **Unspecified** subluxation of unspecified **shoulder joint**

       √7ᵗʰ **S43.004**   **Unspecified** dislocation of right **shoulder joint**

       √7ᵗʰ **S43.005**   **Unspecified** dislocation of left **shoulder joint**

       √7ᵗʰ **S43.006**   **Unspecified** dislocation of unspecified **shoulder joint**

     √6ᵗʰ **S43.01**   Anterior **subluxation and dislocation of humerus**

       √7ᵗʰ **S43.011**   **Anterior** subluxation of right **humerus**

       √7ᵗʰ **S43.012**   **Anterior** subluxation of left **humerus**

       √7ᵗʰ **S43.013**   **Anterior** subluxation of unspecified **humerus**

       √7ᵗʰ **S43.014**   **Anterior** dislocation of right **humerus**

       √7ᵗʰ **S43.015**   **Anterior** dislocation of left **humerus**

       √7ᵗʰ **S43.016**   **Anterior** dislocation of unspecified **humerus**

     √6ᵗʰ **S43.02**   Posterior **subluxation and dislocation of humerus**

       √7ᵗʰ **S43.021**   **Posterior** subluxation of right **humerus**

       √7ᵗʰ **S43.022**   **Posterior** subluxation of left **humerus**

       √7ᵗʰ **S43.023**   **Posterior** subluxation of unspecified **humerus**

       √7ᵗʰ **S43.024**   **Posterior** dislocation of right **humerus**

       √7ᵗʰ **S43.025**   **Posterior** dislocation of left **humerus**

       √7ᵗʰ **S43.026**   **Posterior** dislocation of unspecified **humerus**

     √6ᵗʰ **S43.03**   Inferior **subluxation and dislocation of humerus**

       √7ᵗʰ **S43.031**   **Inferior** subluxation of right **humerus**

       √7ᵗʰ **S43.032**   **Inferior** subluxation of left **humerus**

       √7ᵗʰ **S43.033**   **Inferior** subluxation of unspecified **humerus**

       √7ᵗʰ **S43.034**   **Inferior** dislocation of right **humerus**

       √7ᵗʰ **S43.035**   **Inferior** dislocation of left **humerus**

       √7ᵗʰ **S43.036**   **Inferior** dislocation of unspecified **humerus**

     √6ᵗʰ **S43.08**   Other **subluxation and dislocation of shoulder join**

       √7ᵗʰ **S43.081**   **Other** subluxation of right **shoulder join**

       √7ᵗʰ **S43.082**   **Other** subluxation of left **shoulder joint**

       √7ᵗʰ **S43.083**   **Other** subluxation of unspecified **should joint**

       √7ᵗʰ **S43.084**   **Other** dislocation of right **shoulder joint**

       √7ᵗʰ **S43.085**   **Other** dislocation of left **shoulder joint**

       √7ᵗʰ **S43.086**   **Other** dislocation of unspecified **shoulde joint**

√5ᵗʰ **S43.1**   **Subluxation and dislocation of** acromioclavicular joint

     √6ᵗʰ **S43.10**   Unspecified **dislocation of acromioclavicular joint**

       √7ᵗʰ **S43.101**   **Unspecified dislocation of** right **acromioclavicular joint**

       √7ᵗʰ **S43.102**   **Unspecified dislocation of** left **acromioclavicular joint**

       √7ᵗʰ **S43.109**   **Unspecified dislocation of unspecified acromioclavicular joint**

     √6ᵗʰ **S43.11**   Subluxation **of acromioclavicular joint**

       √7ᵗʰ **S43.111**   **Subluxation of** right **acromioclavicular joint**

       √7ᵗʰ **S43.112**   **Subluxation of** left **acromioclavicular joi**

       √7ᵗʰ **S43.119**   **Subluxation of unspecified acromioclavicular joint**

     √6ᵗʰ **S43.12**   Dislocation **of acromioclavicular joint,** 100%-200% displacement

       √7ᵗʰ **S43.121**   **Dislocation of** right **acromioclavicular joint, 100%-200% displacement**

       √7ᵗʰ **S43.122**   **Dislocation of** left **acromioclavicular join 100%-200% displacement**

       √7ᵗʰ **S43.129**   **Dislocation of unspecified acromioclavicular joint, 100%-200% displacement**

     √6ᵗʰ **S43.13**   Dislocation **of acromioclavicular joint,** greater than 200% displacement

       √7ᵗʰ **S43.131**   **Dislocation of** right **acromioclavicular joint, greater than 200% displacement**

       √7ᵗʰ **S43.132**   **Dislocation of** left **acromioclavicular join greater than 200% displacement**

       √7ᵗʰ **S43.139**   **Dislocation of unspecified acromioclavicular joint, greater than 200% displacement**

     √6ᵗʰ **S43.14**   Inferior **dislocation of acromioclavicular joint**

       √7ᵗʰ **S43.141**   **Inferior dislocation of** right **acromioclavicular joint**

       √7ᵗʰ **S43.142**   **Inferior dislocation of** left **acromioclavicular joint**

       √7ᵗʰ **S43.149**   **Inferior dislocation of unspecified acromioclavicular joint**

EXCLUDES 1 Not coded here   EXCLUDES 2 Not included here   N Newborn Age: 0   P Pediatric Age: 0-17   M Maternity Age: 12-55   A Adult Age: 15-12

888

ICD-10-CM 20

✓6th **S43.15** Posterior dislocation of **acromioclavicular joint**

   ✓7th **S43.151** Posterior dislocation of right acromioclavicular joint

   ✓7th **S43.152** Posterior dislocation of left acromioclavicular joint

   ✓7th **S43.159** Posterior dislocation of unspecified acromioclavicular joint

✓5th **S43.2** Subluxation and dislocation of sternoclavicular joint

  ✓6th **S43.20** Unspecified subluxation and dislocation of sternoclavicular joint

   ✓7th **S43.201** Unspecified subluxation of right sternoclavicular joint

   ✓7th **S43.202** Unspecified subluxation of left sternoclavicular joint

   ✓7th **S43.203** Unspecified subluxation of unspecified sternoclavicular joint

   ✓7th **S43.204** Unspecified dislocation of right sternoclavicular joint

   ✓7th **S43.205** Unspecified dislocation of left sternoclavicular joint

   ✓7th **S43.206** Unspecified dislocation of unspecified sternoclavicular joint

  ✓6th **S43.21** Anterior subluxation and dislocation of sternoclavicular joint

   ✓7th **S43.211** Anterior subluxation of right sternoclavicular joint

   ✓7th **S43.212** Anterior subluxation of left sternoclavicular joint

   ✓7th **S43.213** Anterior subluxation of unspecified sternoclavicular joint

   ✓7th **S43.214** Anterior dislocation of right sternoclavicular joint

   ✓7th **S43.215** Anterior dislocation of left sternoclavicular joint

   ✓7th **S43.216** Anterior dislocation of unspecified sternoclavicular joint

  ✓6th **S43.22** Posterior subluxation and dislocation of sternoclavicular joint

   ✓7th **S43.221** Posterior subluxation of right sternoclavicular joint

   ✓7th **S43.222** Posterior subluxation of left sternoclavicular joint

   ✓7th **S43.223** Posterior subluxation of unspecified sternoclavicular joint

   ✓7th **S43.224** Posterior dislocation of right sternoclavicular joint

   ✓7th **S43.225** Posterior dislocation of left sternoclavicular joint

   ✓7th **S43.226** Posterior dislocation of unspecified sternoclavicular joint

✓5th **S43.3** Subluxation and dislocation of other and unspecified parts of shoulder girdle

  ✓6th **S43.30** Subluxation and dislocation of unspecified parts of shoulder girdle
      Dislocation of shoulder girdle NOS
      Subluxation of shoulder girdle NOS

   ✓7th **S43.301** Subluxation of unspecified parts of right shoulder girdle

   ✓7th **S43.302** Subluxation of unspecified parts of left shoulder girdle

   ✓7th **S43.303** Subluxation of unspecified parts of unspecified shoulder girdle

   ✓7th **S43.304** Dislocation of unspecified parts of right shoulder girdle

   ✓7th **S43.305** Dislocation of unspecified parts of left shoulder girdle

   ✓7th **S43.306** Dislocation of unspecified parts of unspecified shoulder girdle

  ✓6th **S43.31** Subluxation and dislocation of scapula

   ✓7th **S43.311** Subluxation of right scapula

   ✓7th **S43.312** Subluxation of left scapula

   ✓7th **S43.313** Subluxation of unspecified scapula

   ✓7th **S43.314** Dislocation of right scapula

   ✓7th **S43.315** Dislocation of left scapula

   ✓7th **S43.316** Dislocation of unspecified scapula

  ✓6th **S43.39** Subluxation and dislocation of other parts of shoulder girdle

   ✓7th **S43.391** Subluxation of other parts of right shoulder girdle

   ✓7th **S43.392** Subluxation of other parts of left shoulder girdle

   ✓7th **S43.393** Subluxation of other parts of unspecified shoulder girdle

   ✓7th **S43.394** Dislocation of other parts of right shoulder girdle

   ✓7th **S43.395** Dislocation of other parts of left shoulder girdle

   ✓7th **S43.396** Dislocation of other parts of unspecified shoulder girdle

✓5th **S43.4** Sprain of shoulder joint

  ✓6th **S43.40** Unspecified sprain of shoulder joint

   ✓7th **S43.401** Unspecified sprain of right shoulder joint

   ✓7th **S43.402** Unspecified sprain of left shoulder joint

   ✓7th **S43.409** Unspecified sprain of unspecified shoulder joint

  ✓6th **S43.41** Sprain of coracohumeral (ligament)

   ✓7th **S43.411** Sprain of right coracohumeral (ligament)

   ✓7th **S43.412** Sprain of left coracohumeral (ligament)

   ✓7th **S43.419** Sprain of unspecified coracohumeral (ligament)

  ✓6th **S43.42** Sprain of rotator cuff capsule

      EXCLUDES 1 rotator cuff syndrome (complete) (incomplete), not specified as traumatic (M75.1-)
      EXCLUDES 2 injury of tendon of rotator cuff (S46.0-)

   ✓7th **S43.421** Sprain of right rotator cuff capsule

   ✓7th **S43.422** Sprain of left rotator cuff capsule

   ✓7th **S43.429** Sprain of unspecified rotator cuff capsule

  ✓6th **S43.43** Superior glenoid labrum lesion
      SLAP lesion

   ✓7th **S43.431** Superior glenoid labrum lesion of right shoulder

   ✓7th **S43.432** Superior glenoid labrum lesion of left shoulder

   ✓7th **S43.439** Superior glenoid labrum lesion of unspecified shoulder

  ✓6th **S43.49** Other sprain of shoulder joint

   ✓7th **S43.491** Other sprain of right shoulder joint

   ✓7th **S43.492** Other sprain of left shoulder joint

   ✓7th **S43.499** Other sprain of unspecified shoulder joint

✓5th **S43.5** Sprain of acromioclavicular joint
      Sprain of acromioclavicular ligament

  ✓x7th **S43.50** Sprain of unspecified acromioclavicular joint

  ✓x7th **S43.51** Sprain of right acromioclavicular joint

  ✓x7th **S43.52** Sprain of left acromioclavicular joint

✓5th **S43.6** Sprain of sternoclavicular joint

  ✓x7th **S43.60** Sprain of unspecified sternoclavicular joint

  ✓x7th **S43.61** Sprain of right sternoclavicular joint

  ✓x7th **S43.62** Sprain of left sternoclavicular joint

✓5th **S43.8** Sprain of other specified parts of shoulder girdle

  ✓x7th **S43.80** Sprain of other specified parts of unspecified shoulder girdle

  ✓x7th **S43.81** Sprain of other specified parts of right shoulder girdle

  ✓x7th **S43.82** Sprain of other specified parts of left shoulder girdle

✓5th **S43.9** Sprain of unspecified parts of shoulder girdle

  ✓x7th **S43.90** Sprain of unspecified parts of unspecified shoulder girdle
      Sprain of shoulder girdle NOS

  ✓x7th **S43.91** Sprain of unspecified parts of right shoulder girdle

  ✓x7th **S43.92** Sprain of unspecified parts of left shoulder girdle

---

✓ Additional Character Required   ✓x7th Placeholder Alert   Unspecified Dx   Other Specified Dx   Manifestation   ►◄ Revised Text   ● New Code   ▲ Revised Code Title

√4ᵗʰ **S44 Injury of nerves at shoulder and upper arm level**
Code also any associated open wound (S41.-)
EXCLUDES 2 injury of brachial plexus (S14.3-)

The appropriate 7th character is to be added to each code from category S44.
A   initial encounter
D   subsequent encounter
S   sequela

√5ᵗʰ **S44.0 Injury of ulnar nerve at upper arm level**
EXCLUDES 1 ulnar nerve NOS (S54.0)

√x7ᵗʰ **S44.00 Injury of ulnar nerve at upper arm level, unspecified arm**

√x7ᵗʰ **S44.01 Injury of ulnar nerve at upper arm level, right arm**

√x7ᵗʰ **S44.02 Injury of ulnar nerve at upper arm level, left arm**

√5ᵗʰ **S44.1 Injury of median nerve at upper arm level**
EXCLUDES 1 median nerve NOS (S54.1)

√x7ᵗʰ **S44.10 Injury of median nerve at upper arm level, unspecified arm**

√x7ᵗʰ **S44.11 Injury of median nerve at upper arm level, right arm**

√x7ᵗʰ **S44.12 Injury of median nerve at upper arm level, left arm**

√5ᵗʰ **S44.2 Injury of radial nerve at upper arm level**
EXCLUDES 1 radial nerve NOS (S54.2)

√x7ᵗʰ **S44.20 Injury of radial nerve at upper arm level, unspecified arm**

√x7ᵗʰ **S44.21 Injury of radial nerve at upper arm level, right arm**

√x7ᵗʰ **S44.22 Injury of radial nerve at upper arm level, left arm**

√5ᵗʰ **S44.3 Injury of axillary nerve**

√x7ᵗʰ **S44.30 Injury of axillary nerve, unspecified arm**

√x7ᵗʰ **S44.31 Injury of axillary nerve, right arm**

√x7ᵗʰ **S44.32 Injury of axillary nerve, left arm**

√5ᵗʰ **S44.4 Injury of musculocutaneous nerve**

√x7ᵗʰ **S44.40 Injury of musculocutaneous nerve, unspecified arm**

√x7ᵗʰ **S44.41 Injury of musculocutaneous nerve, right arm**

√x7ᵗʰ **S44.42 Injury of musculocutaneous nerve, left arm**

√5ᵗʰ **S44.5 Injury of cutaneous sensory nerve at shoulder and upper arm level**

√x7ᵗʰ **S44.50 Injury of cutaneous sensory nerve at shoulder and upper arm level, unspecified arm**

√x7ᵗʰ **S44.51 Injury of cutaneous sensory nerve at shoulder and upper arm level, right arm**

√x7ᵗʰ **S44.52 Injury of cutaneous sensory nerve at shoulder and upper arm level, left arm**

√5ᵗʰ **S44.8 Injury of other nerves at shoulder and upper arm level**

√6ᵗʰ **S44.8X Injury of other nerves at shoulder and upper arm level**

√7ᵗʰ **S44.8X1 Injury of other nerves at shoulder and upper arm level, right arm**

√7ᵗʰ **S44.8X2 Injury of other nerves at shoulder and upper arm level, left arm**

√7ᵗʰ **S44.8X9 Injury of other nerves at shoulder and upper arm level, unspecified arm**

√5ᵗʰ **S44.9 Injury of unspecified nerve at shoulder and upper arm level**

√x7ᵗʰ **S44.90 Injury of unspecified nerve at shoulder and upper arm level, unspecified arm**

√x7ᵗʰ **S44.91 Injury of unspecified nerve at shoulder and upper arm level, right arm**

√x7ᵗʰ **S44.92 Injury of unspecified nerve at shoulder and upper arm level, left arm**

√4ᵗʰ **S45 Injury of blood vessels at shoulder and upper arm level**
Code also any associated open wound (S41.-)
EXCLUDES 2 injury of subclavian artery (S25.1)
injury of subclavian vein (S25.3)

The appropriate 7th character is to be added to each code from category S45.
A   initial encounter
D   subsequent encounter
S   sequela

√5ᵗʰ **S45.0 Injury of axillary artery**

√6ᵗʰ **S45.00 Unspecified injury of axillary artery**

√7ᵗʰ **S45.001 Unspecified injury of axillary artery, right side**

√7ᵗʰ **S45.002 Unspecified injury of axillary artery, left side**

√7ᵗʰ **S45.009 Unspecified injury of axillary artery, unspecified side**

√6ᵗʰ **S45.01 Laceration of axillary artery**

√7ᵗʰ **S45.011 Laceration of axillary artery, right side**

√7ᵗʰ **S45.012 Laceration of axillary artery, left side**

√7ᵗʰ **S45.019 Laceration of axillary artery, unspecified side**

√6ᵗʰ **S45.09 Other specified injury of axillary artery**

√7ᵗʰ **S45.091 Other specified injury of axillary artery, right side**

√7ᵗʰ **S45.092 Other specified injury of axillary artery, left side**

√7ᵗʰ **S45.099 Other specified injury of axillary artery, unspecified side**

√5ᵗʰ **S45.1 Injury of brachial artery**

√6ᵗʰ **S45.10 Unspecified injury of brachial artery**

√7ᵗʰ **S45.101 Unspecified injury of brachial artery, right side**

√7ᵗʰ **S45.102 Unspecified injury of brachial artery, left side**

√7ᵗʰ **S45.109 Unspecified injury of brachial artery, unspecified side**

√6ᵗʰ **S45.11 Laceration of brachial artery**

√7ᵗʰ **S45.111 Laceration of brachial artery, right side**

√7ᵗʰ **S45.112 Laceration of brachial artery, left side**

√7ᵗʰ **S45.119 Laceration of brachial artery, unspecified side**

√6ᵗʰ **S45.19 Other specified injury of brachial artery**

√7ᵗʰ **S45.191 Other specified injury of brachial artery, right side**

√7ᵗʰ **S45.192 Other specified injury of brachial artery, left side**

√7ᵗʰ **S45.199 Other specified injury of brachial artery, unspecified side**

√5ᵗʰ **S45.2 Injury of axillary or brachial vein**

√6ᵗʰ **S45.20 Unspecified injury of axillary or brachial vein**

√7ᵗʰ **S45.201 Unspecified injury of axillary or brachial vein, right side**

√7ᵗʰ **S45.202 Unspecified injury of axillary or brachial vein, left side**

√7ᵗʰ **S45.209 Unspecified injury of axillary or brachial vein, unspecified side**

√6ᵗʰ **S45.21 Laceration of axillary or brachial vein**

√7ᵗʰ **S45.211 Laceration of axillary or brachial vein, right side**

√7ᵗʰ **S45.212 Laceration of axillary or brachial vein, left side**

√7ᵗʰ **S45.219 Laceration of axillary or brachial vein, unspecified side**

√6ᵗʰ **S45.29 Other specified injury of axillary or brachial vein**

√7ᵗʰ **S45.291 Other specified injury of axillary or brachial vein, right side**

√7ᵗʰ **S45.292 Other specified injury of axillary or brachial vein, left side**

√7ᵗʰ **S45.299 Other specified injury of axillary or brachial vein, unspecified side**

√5ᵗʰ **S45.3 Injury of superficial vein at shoulder and upper arm level**

√6ᵗʰ **S45.30 Unspecified injury of superficial vein at shoulder and upper arm level**

√7ᵗʰ **S45.301 Unspecified injury of superficial vein at shoulder and upper arm level, right arm**

√7ᵗʰ **S45.302 Unspecified injury of superficial vein at shoulder and upper arm level, left arm**

√7ᵗʰ **S45.309 Unspecified injury of superficial vein at shoulder and upper arm level, unspecified arm**

√6ᵗʰ **S45.31 Laceration of superficial vein at shoulder and upper arm level**

√7ᵗʰ **S45.311 Laceration of superficial vein at shoulder and upper arm level, right arm**

✓7ᵗʰ **S45.312** Laceration of superficial vein at shoulder and upper arm level, left arm

✓7ᵗʰ **S45.319** Laceration of superficial vein at shoulder and upper arm level, unspecified arm

✓6ᵗʰ **S45.39** Other specified injury of superficial vein at shoulder and upper arm level

✓7ᵗʰ **S45.391** Other specified injury of superficial vein at shoulder and upper arm level, right arm

✓7ᵗʰ **S45.392** Other specified injury of superficial vein at shoulder and upper arm level, left arm

✓7ᵗʰ **S45.399** Other specified injury of superficial vein at shoulder and upper arm level, unspecified arm

✓5ᵗʰ **S45.8** Injury of other specified blood vessels at shoulder and upper arm level

✓6ᵗʰ **S45.80** Unspecified injury of other specified blood vessels at shoulder and upper arm level

✓7ᵗʰ **S45.801** Unspecified injury of other specified blood vessels at shoulder and upper arm level, right arm

✓7ᵗʰ **S45.802** Unspecified injury of other specified blood vessels at shoulder and upper arm level, left arm

✓7ᵗʰ **S45.809** Unspecified injury of other specified blood vessels at shoulder and upper arm level, unspecified arm

✓6ᵗʰ **S45.81** Laceration of other specified blood vessels at shoulder and upper arm level

✓7ᵗʰ **S45.811** Laceration of other specified blood vessels at shoulder and upper arm level, right arm

✓7ᵗʰ **S45.812** Laceration of other specified blood vessels at shoulder and upper arm level, left arm

✓7ᵗʰ **S45.819** Laceration of other specified blood vessels at shoulder and upper arm level, unspecified arm

✓6ᵗʰ **S45.89** Other specified injury of other specified blood vessels at shoulder and upper arm level

✓7ᵗʰ **S45.891** Other specified injury of other specified blood vessels at shoulder and upper arm level, right arm

✓7ᵗʰ **S45.892** Other specified injury of other specified blood vessels at shoulder and upper arm level, left arm

✓7ᵗʰ **S45.899** Other specified injury of other specified blood vessels at shoulder and upper arm level, unspecified arm

✓5ᵗʰ **S45.9** Injury of unspecified blood vessel at shoulder and upper arm level

✓6ᵗʰ **S45.90** Unspecified injury of unspecified blood vessel at shoulder and upper arm level

✓7ᵗʰ **S45.901** Unspecified injury of unspecified blood vessel at shoulder and upper arm level, right arm

✓7ᵗʰ **S45.902** Unspecified injury of unspecified blood vessel at shoulder and upper arm level, left arm

✓7ᵗʰ **S45.909** Unspecified injury of unspecified blood vessel at shoulder and upper arm level, unspecified arm

✓6ᵗʰ **S45.91** Laceration of unspecified blood vessel at shoulder and upper arm level

✓7ᵗʰ **S45.911** Laceration of unspecified blood vessel at shoulder and upper arm level, right arm

✓7ᵗʰ **S45.912** Laceration of unspecified blood vessel at shoulder and upper arm level, left arm

✓7ᵗʰ **S45.919** Laceration of unspecified blood vessel at shoulder and upper arm level, unspecified arm

✓6ᵗʰ **S45.99** Other specified injury of unspecified blood vessel at shoulder and upper arm level

✓7ᵗʰ **S45.991** Other specified injury of unspecified blood vessel at shoulder and upper arm level, right arm

✓7ᵗʰ **S45.992** Other specified injury of unspecified blood vessel at shoulder and upper arm level, left arm

---

✓7ᵗʰ **S45.999** Other specified injury of unspecified blood vessel at shoulder and upper arm level, unspecified arm

✦ ✓4ᵗʰ **S46 Injury of muscle, fascia and tendon at shoulder and upper arm level**

Code also any associated open wound (S41.-)

EXCLUDES 2   injury of muscle, fascia and tendon at elbow (S56.-)
sprain of joints and ligaments of shoulder girdle (S43.9)

The appropriate 7th character is to be added to each code from category S46.
A   initial encounter
D   subsequent encounter
S   sequela

✓5ᵗʰ **S46.0** Injury of muscle(s) and tendon(s) of the rotator cuff of shoulder

✓6ᵗʰ **S46.00** Unspecified injury of muscle(s) and tendon(s) of the rotator cuff of shoulder

✓7ᵗʰ **S46.001** Unspecified injury of muscle(s) and tendon(s) of the rotator cuff of right shoulder

✓7ᵗʰ **S46.002** Unspecified injury of muscle(s) and tendon(s) of the rotator cuff of left shoulder

✓7ᵗʰ **S46.009** Unspecified injury of muscle(s) and tendon(s) of the rotator cuff of unspecified shoulder

✓6ᵗʰ **S46.01** Strain of muscle(s) and tendon(s) of the rotator cuff of shoulder

✓7ᵗʰ **S46.011** Strain of muscle(s) and tendon(s) of the rotator cuff of right shoulder

✓7ᵗʰ **S46.012** Strain of muscle(s) and tendon(s) of the rotator cuff of left shoulder

✓7ᵗʰ **S46.019** Strain of muscle(s) and tendon(s) of the rotator cuff of unspecified shoulder

✓6ᵗʰ **S46.02** Laceration of muscle(s) and tendon(s) of the rotator cuff of shoulder

✓7ᵗʰ **S46.021** Laceration of muscle(s) and tendon(s) of the rotator cuff of right shoulder

✓7ᵗʰ **S46.022** Laceration of muscle(s) and tendon(s) of the rotator cuff of left shoulder

✓7ᵗʰ **S46.029** Laceration of muscle(s) and tendon(s) of the rotator cuff of unspecified shoulder

✓6ᵗʰ **S46.09** Other injury of muscle(s) and tendon(s) of the rotator cuff of shoulder

✓7ᵗʰ **S46.091** Other injury of muscle(s) and tendon(s) of the rotator cuff of right shoulder

✓7ᵗʰ **S46.092** Other injury of muscle(s) and tendon(s) of the rotator cuff of left shoulder

✓7ᵗʰ **S46.099** Other injury of muscle(s) and tendon(s) of the rotator cuff of unspecified shoulder

✓5ᵗʰ **S46.1** Injury of muscle, fascia and tendon of long head of biceps

✓6ᵗʰ **S46.10** Unspecified injury of muscle, fascia and tendon of long head of biceps

✓7ᵗʰ **S46.101** Unspecified injury of muscle, fascia and tendon of long head of biceps, right arm

✓7ᵗʰ **S46.102** Unspecified injury of muscle, fascia and tendon of long head of biceps, left arm

✓7ᵗʰ **S46.109** Unspecified injury of muscle, fascia and tendon of long head of biceps, unspecified arm

✓6ᵗʰ **S46.11** Strain of muscle, fascia and tendon of long head of biceps

✓7ᵗʰ **S46.111** Strain of muscle, fascia and tendon of long head of biceps, right arm

✓7ᵗʰ **S46.112** Strain of muscle, fascia and tendon of long head of biceps, left arm

✓7ᵗʰ **S46.119** Strain of muscle, fascia and tendon of long head of biceps, unspecified arm

✓6ᵗʰ **S46.12** Laceration of muscle, fascia and tendon of long head of biceps

✓7ᵗʰ **S46.121** Laceration of muscle, fascia and tendon of long head of biceps, right arm

✓7ᵗʰ **S46.122** Laceration of muscle, fascia and tendon of long head of biceps, left arm

---

✦ Refer to the Muscle/Tendon Table at the beginning of this chapter.

☑ Additional Character Required   ✓7ᵗʰ Placeholder Alert   Unspecified Dx   Other Specified Dx   Manifestation   ▶◀ Revised Text   ● New Code   ▲ Revised Code Title

☑7ᵗʰ **S46.129** Laceration of muscle, fascia and tendon of long head of biceps, unspecified arm

☑6ᵗʰ **S46.19** Other injury of muscle, fascia and tendon of long head of biceps

    ☑7ᵗʰ **S46.191** Other injury of muscle, fascia and tendon of long head of biceps, **right** arm

    ☑7ᵗʰ **S46.192** Other injury of muscle, fascia and tendon of long head of biceps, **left** arm

    ☑7ᵗʰ **S46.199** Other injury of muscle, fascia and tendon of long head of biceps, **unspecified** arm

☑5ᵗʰ **S46.2** Injury of muscle, fascia and tendon of other parts of biceps

    ☑6ᵗʰ **S46.20** Unspecified injury of muscle, fascia and tendon of other parts of biceps

       ☑7ᵗʰ **S46.201** Unspecified injury of muscle, fascia and tendon of other parts of biceps, **right** arm

       ☑7ᵗʰ **S46.202** Unspecified injury of muscle, fascia and tendon of other parts of biceps, **left** arm

       ☑7ᵗʰ **S46.209** Unspecified injury of muscle, fascia and tendon of other parts of biceps, **unspecified** arm

    ☑6ᵗʰ **S46.21** Strain of muscle, fascia and tendon of other parts of biceps

       ☑7ᵗʰ **S46.211** Strain of muscle, fascia and tendon of other parts of biceps, **right** arm

       ☑7ᵗʰ **S46.212** Strain of muscle, fascia and tendon of other parts of biceps, **left** arm

       ☑7ᵗʰ **S46.219** Strain of muscle, fascia and tendon of other parts of biceps, **unspecified** arm

    ☑6ᵗʰ **S46.22** Laceration of muscle, fascia and tendon of other parts of biceps

       ☑7ᵗʰ **S46.221** Laceration of muscle, fascia and tendon of other parts of biceps, **right** arm

       ☑7ᵗʰ **S46.222** Laceration of muscle, fascia and tendon of other parts of biceps, **left** arm

       ☑7ᵗʰ **S46.229** Laceration of muscle, fascia and tendon of other parts of biceps, **unspecified** arm

    ☑6ᵗʰ **S46.29** Other injury of muscle, fascia and tendon of other parts of biceps

       ☑7ᵗʰ **S46.291** Other injury of muscle, fascia and tendon of other parts of biceps, **right** arm

       ☑7ᵗʰ **S46.292** Other injury of muscle, fascia and tendon of other parts of biceps, **left** arm

       ☑7ᵗʰ **S46.299** Other injury of muscle, fascia and tendon of other parts of biceps, **unspecified** arm

☑5ᵗʰ **S46.3** Injury of muscle, fascia and tendon of triceps

    ☑6ᵗʰ **S46.30** Unspecified injury of muscle, fascia and tendon of triceps

       ☑7ᵗʰ **S46.301** Unspecified injury of muscle, fascia and tendon of triceps, **right** arm

       ☑7ᵗʰ **S46.302** Unspecified injury of muscle, fascia and tendon of triceps, **left** arm

       ☑7ᵗʰ **S46.309** Unspecified injury of muscle, fascia and tendon of triceps, **unspecified** arm

    ☑6ᵗʰ **S46.31** Strain of muscle, fascia and tendon of triceps

       ☑7ᵗʰ **S46.311** Strain of muscle, fascia and tendon of triceps, **right** arm

       ☑7ᵗʰ **S46.312** Strain of muscle, fascia and tendon of triceps, **left** arm

       ☑7ᵗʰ **S46.319** Strain of muscle, fascia and tendon of triceps, **unspecified** arm

    ☑6ᵗʰ **S46.32** Laceration of muscle, fascia and tendon of triceps

       ☑7ᵗʰ **S46.321** Laceration of muscle, fascia and tendon of triceps, **right** arm

       ☑7ᵗʰ **S46.322** Laceration of muscle, fascia and tendon of triceps, **left** arm

       ☑7ᵗʰ **S46.329** Laceration of muscle, fascia and tendon of triceps, **unspecified** arm

    ☑6ᵗʰ **S46.39** Other injury of muscle, fascia and tendon of triceps

       ☑7ᵗʰ **S46.391** Other injury of muscle, fascia and tendon of triceps, **right** arm

       ☑7ᵗʰ **S46.392** Other injury of muscle, fascia and tendon of triceps, **left** arm

       ☑7ᵗʰ **S46.399** Other injury of muscle, fascia and tendon of triceps, **unspecified** arm

☑5ᵗʰ **S46.8** Injury of other muscles, fascia and tendons at shoulder and upper arm level

    ☑6ᵗʰ **S46.80** Unspecified injury of other muscles, fascia and tendons at shoulder and upper arm level

       ☑7ᵗʰ **S46.801** Unspecified injury of other muscles, fascia and tendons at shoulder and upper arm level, **right** arm

       ☑7ᵗʰ **S46.802** Unspecified injury of other muscles, fascia and tendons at shoulder and upper arm level, **left** arm

       ☑7ᵗʰ **S46.809** Unspecified injury of other muscles, fascia and tendons at shoulder and upper arm level, **unspecified arm**

    ☑6ᵗʰ **S46.81** Strain of other muscles, fascia and tendons at shoulder and upper arm level

       ☑7ᵗʰ **S46.811** Strain of other muscles, fascia and tendons at shoulder and upper arm level, **right arm**

       ☑7ᵗʰ **S46.812** Strain of other muscles, fascia and tendons at shoulder and upper arm level, **left** arm

       ☑7ᵗʰ **S46.819** Strain of other muscles, fascia and tendons at shoulder and upper arm level, **unspecified** arm

    ☑6ᵗʰ **S46.82** Laceration of other muscles, fascia and tendons at shoulder and upper arm level

       ☑7ᵗʰ **S46.821** Laceration of other muscles, fascia and tendons at shoulder and upper arm level, **right arm**

       ☑7ᵗʰ **S46.822** Laceration of other muscles, fascia and tendons at shoulder and upper arm level, **left** arm

       ☑7ᵗʰ **S46.829** Laceration of other muscles, fascia and tendons at shoulder and upper arm level, **unspecified arm**

    ☑6ᵗʰ **S46.89** Other injury of other muscles, fascia and tendons at shoulder and upper arm level

       ☑7ᵗʰ **S46.891** Other injury of other muscles, fascia and tendons at shoulder and upper arm level, **right arm**

       ☑7ᵗʰ **S46.892** Other injury of other muscles, fascia and tendons at shoulder and upper arm level, **left** arm

       ☑7ᵗʰ **S46.899** Other injury of other muscles, fascia and tendons at shoulder and upper arm level, **unspecified arm**

☑5ᵗʰ **S46.9** Injury of unspecified muscle, fascia and tendon at shoulder and upper arm level

    ☑6ᵗʰ **S46.90** Unspecified injury of unspecified muscle, fascia and tendon at shoulder and upper arm level

       ☑7ᵗʰ **S46.901** Unspecified injury of unspecified muscle, fascia and tendon at shoulder and upper arm level, **right** arm

       ☑7ᵗʰ **S46.902** Unspecified injury of unspecified muscle, fascia and tendon at shoulder and upper arm level, **left** arm

       ☑7ᵗʰ **S46.909** Unspecified injury of unspecified muscle, fascia and tendon at shoulder and upper arm level, **unspecified** arm

    ☑6ᵗʰ **S46.91** Strain of unspecified muscle, fascia and tendon at shoulder and upper arm level

       ☑7ᵗʰ **S46.911** Strain of unspecified muscle, fascia and tendon at shoulder and upper arm level, **right** arm

       ☑7ᵗʰ **S46.912** Strain of unspecified muscle, fascia and tendon at shoulder and upper arm level, **left** arm

       ☑7ᵗʰ **S46.919** Strain of unspecified muscle, fascia and tendon at shoulder and upper arm level, **unspecified** arm

    ☑6ᵗʰ **S46.92** Laceration of unspecified muscle, fascia and tendon at shoulder and upper arm level

       ☑7ᵗʰ **S46.921** Laceration of unspecified muscle, fascia and tendon at shoulder and upper arm level, **right** arm

       ☑7ᵗʰ **S46.922** Laceration of unspecified muscle, fascia and tendon at shoulder and upper arm level, **left** arm

---

EXCLUDES 1 Not coded here   **EXCLUDES 2** Not included here   **N** Newborn Age: 0   **P** Pediatric Age: 0-17   **M** Maternity Age: 12-55   **A** Adult Age: 15-124

892

ICD-10-CM 2016

√7ᵗʰ **S46.929**   **Laceration of unspecified muscle, fascia and tendon at shoulder and upper arm level, unspecified arm**

√6ᵗʰ **S46.99**   Other **injury of unspecified muscle, fascia and tendon at shoulder and upper arm level**

√7ᵗʰ **S46.991**   **Other injury of unspecified muscle, fascia and tendon at shoulder and upper arm level,** right **arm**

√7ᵗʰ **S46.992**   **Other injury of unspecified muscle, fascia and tendon at shoulder and upper arm level,** left **arm**

√7ᵗʰ **S46.999**   **Other injury of unspecified muscle, fascia and tendon at shoulder and upper arm level, unspecified arm**

√4ᵗʰ **S47**   **Crushing injury of shoulder and upper arm**

Use additional code for all associated injuries

EXCLUDES 2   *crushing injury of elbow (S57.0-)*

The appropriate 7th character is to be added to each code from category S47.
A   initial encounter
D   subsequent encounter
S   sequela

√x7ᵗʰ **S47.1**   **Crushing injury of** right **shoulder and upper arm**

√x7ᵗʰ **S47.2**   **Crushing injury of** left **shoulder and upper arm**

√x7ᵗʰ **S47.9**   **Crushing injury of shoulder and upper arm, unspecified arm**

√4ᵗʰ **S48**   **Traumatic amputation of shoulder and upper arm**

NOTE   An amputation not identified as partial or complete should be coded to complete.

EXCLUDES 1   *traumatic amputation at elbow level (S58.0)*

The appropriate 7th character is to be added to each code from category S48.
A   initial encounter
D   subsequent encounter
S   sequela

√5ᵗʰ **S48.0**   **Traumatic amputation at** shoulder joint

√6ᵗʰ **S48.01**   Complete **traumatic amputation at shoulder joint**

√7ᵗʰ **S48.011**   **Complete traumatic amputation at** right **shoulder joint**

√7ᵗʰ **S48.012**   **Complete traumatic amputation at** left **shoulder joint**

√7ᵗʰ **S48.019**   **Complete traumatic amputation at unspecified shoulder joint**

√6ᵗʰ **S48.02**   Partial **traumatic amputation at shoulder joint**

√7ᵗʰ **S48.021**   **Partial traumatic amputation at** right **shoulder joint**

√7ᵗʰ **S48.022**   **Partial traumatic amputation at** left **shoulder joint**

√7ᵗʰ **S48.029**   **Partial traumatic amputation at unspecified shoulder joint**

√5ᵗʰ **S48.1**   **Traumatic amputation at** level between shoulder and elbow

√6ᵗʰ **S48.11**   Complete **traumatic amputation at level between shoulder and elbow**

√7ᵗʰ **S48.111**   **Complete traumatic amputation at level between** right **shoulder and elbow**

√7ᵗʰ **S48.112**   **Complete traumatic amputation at level between** left **shoulder and elbow**

√7ᵗʰ **S48.119**   **Complete traumatic amputation at level between unspecified shoulder and elbow**

√6ᵗʰ **S48.12**   Partial **traumatic amputation at level between shoulder and elbow**

√7ᵗʰ **S48.121**   **Partial traumatic amputation at level between** right **shoulder and elbow**

√7ᵗʰ **S48.122**   **Partial traumatic amputation at level between** left **shoulder and elbow**

√7ᵗʰ **S48.129**   **Partial traumatic amputation at level between unspecified shoulder and elbow**

√5ᵗʰ **S48.9**   **Traumatic amputation of shoulder and upper arm,** level unspecified

√6ᵗʰ **S48.91**   Complete **traumatic amputation of shoulder and upper arm, level unspecified**

√7ᵗʰ **S48.911**   **Complete traumatic amputation of** right **shoulder and upper arm, level unspecified**

√7ᵗʰ **S48.912**   **Complete traumatic amputation of** left **shoulder and upper arm, level unspecified**

√7ᵗʰ **S48.919**   **Complete traumatic amputation of unspecified shoulder and upper arm, level unspecified**

√6ᵗʰ **S48.92**   Partial **traumatic amputation of shoulder and upper arm, level unspecified**

√7ᵗʰ **S48.921**   **Partial traumatic amputation of** right **shoulder and upper arm, level unspecified**

√7ᵗʰ **S48.922**   **Partial traumatic amputation of** left **shoulder and upper arm, level unspecified**

√7ᵗʰ **S48.929**   **Partial traumatic amputation of unspecified shoulder and upper arm, level unspecified**

√4ᵗʰ **S49**   **Other and unspecified injuries of shoulder and upper arm**

The appropriate 7th character is to be added to each code from subcategories S49.0 and S49.1.
A   initial encounter for closed fracture
D   subsequent encounter for fracture with routine healing
G   subsequent encounter for fracture with delayed healing
K   subsequent encounter for fracture with nonunion
P   subsequent encounter for fracture with malunion
S   sequela

√5ᵗʰ **S49.0**   Physeal **fracture of** upper end of humerus

√6ᵗʰ **S49.00**   Unspecified **physeal fracture of upper end of humerus**

√7ᵗʰ **S49.001**   **Unspecified physeal fracture of upper end of humerus,** right **arm**

√7ᵗʰ **S49.002**   **Unspecified physeal fracture of upper end of humerus,** left **arm**

√7ᵗʰ **S49.009**   **Unspecified physeal fracture of upper end of humerus, unspecified arm**

√6ᵗʰ **S49.01**   **Salter-Harris Type I physeal fracture of upper end of humerus**

√7ᵗʰ **S49.011**   **Salter-Harris Type I physeal fracture of upper end of humerus,** right **arm**

√7ᵗʰ **S49.012**   **Salter-Harris Type I physeal fracture of upper end of humerus,** left **arm**

√7ᵗʰ **S49.019**   **Salter-Harris Type I physeal fracture of upper end of humerus, unspecified arm**

√6ᵗʰ **S49.02**   **Salter-Harris Type II physeal fracture of upper end of humerus**

√7ᵗʰ **S49.021**   **Salter-Harris Type II physeal fracture of upper end of humerus,** right **arm**

√7ᵗʰ **S49.022**   **Salter-Harris Type II physeal fracture of upper end of humerus,** left **arm**

√7ᵗʰ **S49.029**   **Salter-Harris Type II physeal fracture of upper end of humerus, unspecified arm**

√6ᵗʰ **S49.03**   **Salter-Harris Type III physeal fracture of upper end of humerus**

√7ᵗʰ **S49.031**   **Salter Harris Type III physeal fracture of upper end of humerus,** right **arm**

√7ᵗʰ **S49.032**   **Salter-Harris Type III physeal fracture of upper end of humerus,** left **arm**

√7ᵗʰ **S49.039**   **Salter-Harris Type III physeal fracture of upper end of humerus, unspecified arm**

√6ᵗʰ **S49.04**   **Salter-Harris Type IV physeal fracture of upper end of humerus**

√7ᵗʰ **S49.041**   **Salter-Harris Type IV physeal fracture of upper end of humerus,** right **arm**

√7ᵗʰ **S49.042**   **Salter-Harris Type IV physeal fracture of upper end of humerus,** left **arm**

√7ᵗʰ **S49.049**   **Salter-Harris Type IV physeal fracture of upper end of humerus, unspecified arm**

√6ᵗʰ **S49.09**   Other **physeal fracture of upper end of humerus**

√7ᵗʰ **S49.091**   **Other physeal fracture of upper end of humerus,** right **arm**

√7ᵗʰ **S49.092**   **Other physeal fracture of upper end of humerus,** left **arm**

√7ᵗʰ **S49.099**   **Other physeal fracture of upper end of humerus, unspecified arm**

√5ᵗʰ **S49.1**   Physeal **fracture of** lower end of humerus

√6ᵗʰ **S49.10**   Unspecified **physeal fracture of lower end of humerus**

√7ᵗʰ **S49.101**   **Unspecified physeal fracture of lower end of humerus,** right **arm**

☑ Additional Character Required   √x7ᵗʰ Placeholder Alert   Unspecified Dx   Other Specified Dx   Manifestation   ▶◀ Revised Text   ● New Code   ▲ Revised Code Title

ICD-10-CM 2016   **893**

S46.929–S49.101

√7ᵗʰ **S49.102** Unspecified physeal fracture of lower end of humerus, **left** arm

√7ᵗʰ **S49.109** Unspecified physeal fracture of lower end of humerus, **unspecified** arm

√6ᵗʰ **S49.11** Salter-Harris Type I physeal fracture of lower end of humerus

     √7ᵗʰ **S49.111** Salter-Harris Type I physeal fracture of lower end of humerus, **right** arm

     √7ᵗʰ **S49.112** Salter-Harris Type I physeal fracture of lower end of humerus, **left** arm

     √7ᵗʰ **S49.119** Salter-Harris Type I physeal fracture of lower end of humerus, **unspecified** arm

√6ᵗʰ **S49.12** Salter-Harris Type II physeal fracture of lower end of humerus

     √7ᵗʰ **S49.121** Salter-Harris Type II physeal fracture of lower end of humerus, **right** arm

     √7ᵗʰ **S49.122** Salter-Harris Type II physeal fracture of lower end of humerus, **left** arm

     √7ᵗʰ **S49.129** Salter-Harris Type II physeal fracture of lower end of humerus, **unspecified** arm

√6ᵗʰ **S49.13** Salter Harris Type III physeal fracture of lower end of humerus

     √7ᵗʰ **S49.131** Salter Harris Type III physeal fracture of lower end of humerus, **right** arm

     √7ᵗʰ **S49.132** Salter Harris Type III physeal fracture of lower end of humerus, **left** arm

     √7ᵗʰ **S49.139** Salter Harris Type III physeal fracture of lower end of humerus, **unspecified** arm

√6ᵗʰ **S49.14** Salter-Harris Type IV physeal fracture of lower end of humerus

     √7ᵗʰ **S49.141** Salter-Harris Type IV physeal fracture of lower end of humerus, **right** arm

     √7ᵗʰ **S49.142** Salter-Harris Type IV physeal fracture of lower end of humerus, **left** arm

     √7ᵗʰ **S49.149** Salter-Harris Type IV physeal fracture of lower end of humerus, **unspecified** arm

√6ᵗʰ **S49.19** Other physeal fracture of lower end of humerus

     √7ᵗʰ **S49.191** Other physeal fracture of lower end of humerus, **right** arm

     √7ᵗʰ **S49.192** Other physeal fracture of lower end of humerus, **left** arm

     √7ᵗʰ **S49.199** Other physeal fracture of lower end of humerus, **unspecified** arm

√5ᵗʰ **S49.8** Other specified injuries of shoulder and upper arm

The appropriate 7th character is to be added to each code in subcategory S49.8.
A   initial encounter
D   subsequent encounter
S   sequela

√x7ᵗʰ **S49.80** Other specified injuries of shoulder and upper arm, **unspecified** arm

√x7ᵗʰ **S49.81** Other specified injuries of **right** shoulder and upper arm

√x7ᵗʰ **S49.82** Other specified injuries of **left** shoulder and upper arm

√5ᵗʰ **S49.9** Unspecified injury of shoulder and upper arm

The appropriate 7th character is to be added to each code in subcategory S49.9.
A   initial encounter
D   subsequent encounter
S   sequela

√x7ᵗʰ **S49.90** Unspecified injury of shoulder and upper arm, **unspecified** arm

√x7ᵗʰ **S49.91** Unspecified injury of **right** shoulder and upper arm

√x7ᵗʰ **S49.92** Unspecified injury of **left** shoulder and upper arm

Injuries to the elbow and forearm (S50-S59)

EXCLUDES 2   burns and corrosions (T20-T32)
     frostbite (T33-T34)
     injuries of wrist and hand (S60-S69)
     insect bite or sting, venomous (T63.4)

√4ᵗʰ **S50** Superficial injury of elbow and forearm

EXCLUDES 2   superficial injury of wrist and hand (S60.-)

The appropriate 7th character is to be added to each code from category S50.
A   initial encounter
D   subsequent encounter
S   sequela

√5ᵗʰ **S50.0** Contusion of elbow

     √x7ᵗʰ **S50.00** Contusion of unspecified elbow

     √x7ᵗʰ **S50.01** Contusion of right elbow

     √x7ᵗʰ **S50.02** Contusion of left elbow

√5ᵗʰ **S50.1** Contusion of forearm

     √x7ᵗʰ **S50.10** Contusion of unspecified forearm

     √x7ᵗʰ **S50.11** Contusion of right forearm

     √x7ᵗʰ **S50.12** Contusion of left forearm

√5ᵗʰ **S50.3** Other superficial injuries of elbow

     √6ᵗʰ **S50.31** Abrasion of elbow

         √7ᵗʰ **S50.311** Abrasion of right elbow

         √7ᵗʰ **S50.312** Abrasion of left elbow

         √7ᵗʰ **S50.319** Abrasion of unspecified elbow

     √6ᵗʰ **S50.32** Blister (nonthermal) of elbow

         √7ᵗʰ **S50.321** Blister (nonthermal) of right elbow

         √7ᵗʰ **S50.322** Blister (nonthermal) of left elbow

         √7ᵗʰ **S50.329** Blister (nonthermal) of unspecified elbow

     √6ᵗʰ **S50.34** External constriction of elbow

         √7ᵗʰ **S50.341** External constriction of right elbow

         √7ᵗʰ **S50.342** External constriction of left elbow

         √7ᵗʰ **S50.349** External constriction of unspecified elbow

     √6ᵗʰ **S50.35** Superficial foreign body of elbow
         Splinter in the elbow

         √7ᵗʰ **S50.351** Superficial foreign body of right elbow

         √7ᵗʰ **S50.352** Superficial foreign body of left elbow

         √7ᵗʰ **S50.359** Superficial foreign body of unspecified elbow

     √6ᵗʰ **S50.36** Insect bite (nonvenomous) of elbow

         √7ᵗʰ **S50.361** Insect bite (nonvenomous) of right elbow

         √7ᵗʰ **S50.362** Insect bite (nonvenomous) of left elbow

         √7ᵗʰ **S50.369** Insect bite (nonvenomous) of unspecified elbow

     √6ᵗʰ **S50.37** Other superficial bite of elbow

         EXCLUDES 1   open bite of elbow (S51.05)

         √7ᵗʰ **S50.371** Other superficial bite of right elbow

         √7ᵗʰ **S50.372** Other superficial bite of left elbow

         √7ᵗʰ **S50.379** Other superficial bite of unspecified elbow

√5ᵗʰ **S50.8** Other superficial injuries of forearm

     √6ᵗʰ **S50.81** Abrasion of forearm

         √7ᵗʰ **S50.811** Abrasion of right forearm

         √7ᵗʰ **S50.812** Abrasion of left forearm

         √7ᵗʰ **S50.819** Abrasion of unspecified forearm

     √6ᵗʰ **S50.82** Blister (nonthermal) of forearm

         √7ᵗʰ **S50.821** Blister (nonthermal) of right forearm

         √7ᵗʰ **S50.822** Blister (nonthermal) of left forearm

         √7ᵗʰ **S50.829** Blister (nonthermal) of unspecified forearm

     √6ᵗʰ **S50.84** External constriction of forearm

         √7ᵗʰ **S50.841** External constriction of right forearm

         √7ᵗʰ **S50.842** External constriction of left forearm

         √7ᵗʰ **S50.849** External constriction of unspecified forearm

     √6ᵗʰ **S50.85** Superficial foreign body of forearm
         Splinter in the forearm

         √7ᵗʰ **S50.851** Superficial foreign body of right forearm

         √7ᵗʰ **S50.852** Superficial foreign body of left forearm

EXCLUDES 1 Not coded here   *EXCLUDES 2* Not included here   Ⓝ Newborn Age: 0   Ⓟ Pediatric Age: 0-17   Ⓜ Maternity Age: 12-55   Ⓐ Adult Age: 15-124

894   ICD-10-CM 2016

√7th **S50.859** Superficial foreign body of unspecified forearm

√6th **S50.86** Insect bite (nonvenomous) of forearm

√7th **S50.861** Insect bite (nonvenomous) of right forearm

√7th **S50.862** Insect bite (nonvenomous) of left forearm

√7th **S50.869** Insect bite (nonvenomous) of unspecified forearm

√6th **S50.87** Other superficial bite of forearm
  EXCLUDES 1 open bite of forearm (S51.85)

√7th **S50.871** Other superficial bite of right forearm

√7th **S50.872** Other superficial bite of left forearm

√7th **S50.879** Other superficial bite of unspecified forearm

√5th **S50.9** Unspecified superficial injury of elbow and forearm

√6th **S50.90** Unspecified superficial injury of elbow

√7th **S50.901** Unspecified superficial injury of right elbow

√7th **S50.902** Unspecified superficial injury of left elbow

√7th **S50.909** Unspecified superficial injury of unspecified elbow

√6th **S50.91** Unspecified superficial injury of forearm

√7th **S50.911** Unspecified superficial injury of right forearm

√7th **S50.912** Unspecified superficial injury of left forearm

√7th **S50.919** Unspecified superficial injury of unspecified forearm

√4th **S51** Open wound of elbow and forearm
  Code also any associated wound infection
  EXCLUDES 1 open fracture of elbow and forearm (S52- with open fracture 7th character)
    traumatic amputation of elbow and forearm (S58.-)
  EXCLUDES 2 open wound of wrist and hand (S61.-)

  The appropriate 7th character is to be added to each code from category S51.
  A   initial encounter
  D   subsequent encounter
  S   sequela

√5th **S51.0** Open wound of elbow

√6th **S51.00** Unspecified open wound of elbow

√7th **S51.001** Unspecified open wound of right elbow
  AHA: 2012, 4Q, 108

√7th **S51.002** Unspecified open wound of left elbow

√7th **S51.009** Unspecified open wound of unspecified elbow
  Open wound of elbow NOS

√6th **S51.01** Laceration without foreign body of elbow

√7th **S51.011** Laceration without foreign body of right elbow

√7th **S51.012** Laceration without foreign body of left elbow

√7th **S51.019** Laceration without foreign body of unspecified elbow

√6th **S51.02** Laceration with foreign body of elbow

√7th **S51.021** Laceration with foreign body of right elbow

√7th **S51.022** Laceration with foreign body of left elbow

√7th **S51.029** Laceration with foreign body of unspecified elbow

√6th **S51.03** Puncture wound without foreign body of elbow

√7th **S51.031** Puncture wound without foreign body of right elbow

√7th **S51.032** Puncture wound without foreign body of left elbow

√7th **S51.039** Puncture wound without foreign body of unspecified elbow

√6th **S51.04** Puncture wound with foreign body of elbow

√7th **S51.041** Puncture wound with foreign body of right elbow

√7th **S51.042** Puncture wound with foreign body of left elbow

√7th **S51.049** Puncture wound with foreign body of unspecified elbow

√6th **S51.05** Open bite of elbow
  Bite of elbow NOS
  EXCLUDES 1 superficial bite of elbow (S50.36, S50.37)

√7th **S51.051** Open bite, right elbow

√7th **S51.052** Open bite, left elbow

√7th **S51.059** Open bite, unspecified elbow

√5th **S51.8** Open wound of forearm
  EXCLUDES 2 open wound of elbow (S51.0-)

√6th **S51.80** Unspecified open wound of forearm

√7th **S51.801** Unspecified open wound of right forearm

√7th **S51.802** Unspecified open wound of left forearm

√7th **S51.809** Unspecified open wound of unspecified forearm
  Open wound of forearm NOS

√6th **S51.81** Laceration without foreign body of forearm

√7th **S51.811** Laceration without foreign body of right forearm

√7th **S51.812** Laceration without foreign body of left forearm

√7th **S51.819** Laceration without foreign body of unspecified forearm

√6th **S51.82** Laceration with foreign body of forearm

√7th **S51.821** Laceration with foreign body of right forearm

√7th **S51.822** Laceration with foreign body of left forearm

√7th **S51.829** Laceration with foreign body of unspecified forearm

√6th **S51.83** Puncture wound without foreign body of forearm

√7th **S51.831** Puncture wound without foreign body of right forearm

√7th **S51.832** Puncture wound without foreign body of left forearm

√7th **S51.839** Puncture wound without foreign body of unspecified forearm

√6th **S51.84** Puncture wound with foreign body of forearm

√7th **S51.841** Puncture wound with foreign body of right forearm

√7th **S51.842** Puncture wound with foreign body of left forearm

√7th **S51.849** Puncture wound with foreign body of unspecified forearm

√6th **S51.85** Open bite of forearm
  Bite of forearm NOS
  EXCLUDES 1 superficial bite of forearm (S50.86, S50.87)

√7th **S51.851** Open bite of right forearm

√7th **S51.852** Open bite of left forearm

√7th **S51.859** Open bite of unspecified forearm

√4ᵗʰ S52 Fracture of forearm

> **NOTE** A fracture not indicated as displaced or nondisplaced should be coded to displaced.
> A fracture not indicated as open or closed should be coded to closed.
> The open fracture designations are based on the Gustilo open fracture classification.

EXCLUDES 1 traumatic amputation of forearm (S58.-)
EXCLUDES 2 fracture at wrist and hand level (S62.-)

The appropriate 7th character is to be added to all codes from category S52 [unless otherwise indicated].
A   initial encounter for closed fracture
B   initial encounter for open fracture type I or II
      initial encounter for open fracture NOS
C   initial encounter for open fracture type IIIA, IIIB, or IIIC
D   subsequent encounter for closed fracture with routine healing
E   subsequent encounter for open fracture type I or II with routine healing
F   subsequent encounter for open fracture type IIIA, IIIB, or IIIC with routine healing
G   subsequent encounter for closed fracture with delayed healing
H   subsequent encounter for open fracture type I or II with delayed healing
J   subsequent encounter for open fracture type IIIA, IIIB, or IIIC with delayed healing
K   subsequent encounter for closed fracture with nonunion
M   subsequent encounter for open fracture type I or II with nonunion
N   subsequent encounter for open fracture type IIIA, IIIB, or IIIC with nonunion
P   subsequent encounter for closed fracture with malunion
Q   subsequent encounter for open fracture type I or II with malunion
R   subsequent encounter for open fracture type IIIA, IIIB, or IIIC with malunion
S   sequela

√5ᵗʰ S52.0 Fracture of upper end of ulna
Fracture of proximal end of ulna
EXCLUDES 2 fracture of elbow NOS (S42.40-)
      fractures of shaft of ulna (S52.2-)

√6ᵗʰ S52.00 Unspecified fracture of upper end of ulna
√7ᵗʰ S52.001 Unspecified fracture of upper end of right ulna
√7ᵗʰ S52.002 Unspecified fracture of upper end of left ulna
√7ᵗʰ S52.009 Unspecified fracture of upper end of unspecified ulna

√6ᵗʰ S52.01 Torus fracture of upper end of ulna

The appropriate 7th character is to be added to all codes in subcategory S52.01.
A   initial encounter for closed fracture
D   subsequent encounter for fracture with routine healing
G   subsequent encounter for fracture with delayed healing
K   subsequent encounter for fracture with nonunion
P   subsequent encounter for fracture with malunion
S   sequela

√7ᵗʰ S52.011 Torus fracture of upper end of right ulna
√7ᵗʰ S52.012 Torus fracture of upper end of left ulna
√7ᵗʰ S52.019 Torus fracture of upper end of unspecified ulna

√6ᵗʰ S52.02 Fracture of olecranon process without intraarticular extension of ulna
√7ᵗʰ S52.021 Displaced fracture of olecranon process without intraarticular extension of right ulna
√7ᵗʰ S52.022 Displaced fracture of olecranon process without intraarticular extension of left ulna
√7ᵗʰ S52.023 Displaced fracture of olecranon process without intraarticular extension of unspecified ulna
√7ᵗʰ S52.024 Nondisplaced fracture of olecranon process without intraarticular extension of right ulna

√7ᵗʰ S52.025 Nondisplaced fracture of olecranon process without intraarticular extension of left ulna
√7ᵗʰ S52.026 Nondisplaced fracture of olecranon process without intraarticular extension of unspecified ulna

√6ᵗʰ S52.03 Fracture of olecranon process with intraarticular extension of ulna
√7ᵗʰ S52.031 Displaced fracture of olecranon process with intraarticular extension of right ulna
√7ᵗʰ S52.032 Displaced fracture of olecranon process with intraarticular extension of left ulna
√7ᵗʰ S52.033 Displaced fracture of olecranon process with intraarticular extension of unspecified ulna
√7ᵗʰ S52.034 Nondisplaced fracture of olecranon process with intraarticular extension of right ulna
√7ᵗʰ S52.035 Nondisplaced fracture of olecranon process with intraarticular extension of left ulna
√7ᵗʰ S52.036 Nondisplaced fracture of olecranon process with intraarticular extension of unspecified ulna

√6ᵗʰ S52.04 Fracture of coronoid process of ulna
√7ᵗʰ S52.041 Displaced fracture of coronoid process of right ulna
√7ᵗʰ S52.042 Displaced fracture of coronoid process of left ulna
√7ᵗʰ S52.043 Displaced fracture of coronoid process of unspecified ulna
√7ᵗʰ S52.044 Nondisplaced fracture of coronoid process of right ulna
√7ᵗʰ S52.045 Nondisplaced fracture of coronoid process of left ulna
√7ᵗʰ S52.046 Nondisplaced fracture of coronoid process of unspecified ulna

√6ᵗʰ S52.09 Other fracture of upper end of ulna
√7ᵗʰ S52.091 Other fracture of upper end of right ulna
√7ᵗʰ S52.092 Other fracture of upper end of left ulna
√7ᵗʰ S52.099 Other fracture of upper end of unspecified ulna

√5ᵗʰ S52.1 Fracture of upper end of radius
Fracture of proximal end of radius
EXCLUDES 2 physeal fractures of upper end of radius (S59.2-)
      fracture of shaft of radius (S52.3-)

√6ᵗʰ S52.10 Unspecified fracture of upper end of radius
√7ᵗʰ S52.101 Unspecified fracture of upper end of right radius
√7ᵗʰ S52.102 Unspecified fracture of upper end of left radius
√7ᵗʰ S52.109 Unspecified fracture of upper end of unspecified radius

√6ᵗʰ S52.11 Torus fracture of upper end of radius

The appropriate 7th character is to be added to all codes in subcategory S52.11.
A   initial encounter for closed fracture
D   subsequent encounter for fracture with routine healing
G   subsequent encounter for fracture with delayed healing
K   subsequent encounter for fracture with nonunion
P   subsequent encounter for fracture with malunion
S   sequela

√7ᵗʰ S52.111 Torus fracture of upper end of right radius
√7ᵗʰ S52.112 Torus fracture of upper end of left radius
√7ᵗʰ S52.119 Torus fracture of upper end of unspecified radius

√6ᵗʰ S52.12 Fracture of head of radius
√7ᵗʰ S52.121 Displaced fracture of head of right radius
√7ᵗʰ S52.122 Displaced fracture of head of left radius
√7ᵗʰ S52.123 Displaced fracture of head of unspecified radius

EXCLUDES 1 Not coded here   **EXCLUDES 2** Not included here   **N** Newborn Age: 0   **P** Pediatric Age: 0-17   **M** Maternity Age: 12-55   **A** Adult Age: 15-124

896   ICD-10-CM 2016

√7th **S52.124** Nondisplaced **fracture of head of** right **radius**

√7th **S52.125** Nondisplaced **fracture of head of** left **radius**

√7th **S52.126** Nondisplaced **fracture of head of unspecified radius**

√6th **S52.13** Fracture of **neck of radius**

    √7th **S52.131** Displaced **fracture of neck of** right **radius**

    √7th **S52.132** Displaced **fracture of neck of** left **radius**

    √7th **S52.133** Displaced **fracture of neck of unspecified radius**

    √7th **S52.134** Nondisplaced **fracture of neck of** right **radius**

    √7th **S52.135** Nondisplaced **fracture of neck of** left **radius**

    √7th **S52.136** Nondisplaced **fracture of neck of unspecified radius**

√6th **S52.18** Other **fracture of upper end of radius**

    √7th **S52.181** Other fracture of upper end of right radius

    √7th **S52.182** Other fracture of upper end of left radius

    √7th **S52.189** Other fracture of upper end of unspecified radius

√5th **S52.2** Fracture of **shaft of ulna**

    √6th **S52.20** Unspecified **fracture of shaft of ulna**
       Fracture of ulna NOS

       √7th **S52.201** Unspecified fracture of shaft of right ulna

       √7th **S52.202** Unspecified fracture of shaft of left ulna

       √7th **S52.209** Unspecified fracture of shaft of unspecified ulna

    √6th **S52.21** Greenstick **fracture of shaft of ulna**

The appropriate 7th character is to be added to all codes in subcategory S52.21.
A   initial encounter for closed fracture
D   subsequent encounter for fracture with routine healing
G   subsequent encounter for fracture with delayed healing
K   subsequent encounter for fracture with nonunion
P   subsequent encounter for fracture with malunion
S   sequela

       √7th **S52.211** Greenstick fracture of shaft of right ulna

       √7th **S52.212** Greenstick fracture of shaft of left ulna

       √7th **S52.219** Greenstick fracture of shaft of unspecified ulna

    √6th **S52.22** Transverse **fracture of shaft of ulna**

       √7th **S52.221** Displaced **transverse fracture of shaft of** right **ulna**

       √7th **S52.222** Displaced **transverse fracture of shaft of** left **ulna**

       √7th **S52.223** Displaced **transverse fracture of shaft of unspecified ulna**

       √7th **S52.224** Nondisplaced **transverse fracture of shaft of** right **ulna**

       √7th **S52.225** Nondisplaced **transverse fracture of shaft of** left **ulna**

       √7th **S52.226** Nondisplaced **transverse fracture of shaft of unspecified ulna**

    √6th **S52.23** Oblique **fracture of shaft of ulna**

       √7th **S52.231** Displaced **oblique fracture of shaft of** right **ulna**

       √7th **S52.232** Displaced **oblique fracture of shaft of** left **ulna**

       √7th **S52.233** Displaced **oblique fracture of shaft of unspecified ulna**

       √7th **S52.234** Nondisplaced **oblique fracture of shaft of** right **ulna**

       √7th **S52.235** Nondisplaced **oblique fracture of shaft of** left **ulna**

       √7th **S52.236** Nondisplaced **oblique fracture of shaft of unspecified ulna**

    √6th **S52.24** Spiral **fracture of shaft of ulna**

√7th **S52.241** Displaced **spiral fracture of shaft of ulna,** right **arm**

√7th **S52.242** Displaced **spiral fracture of shaft of ulna,** left **arm**

√7th **S52.243** Displaced **spiral fracture of shaft of ulna, unspecified arm**

√7th **S52.244** Nondisplaced **spiral fracture of shaft of ulna,** right **arm**

√7th **S52.245** Nondisplaced **spiral fracture of shaft of ulna,** left **arm**

√7th **S52.246** Nondisplaced **spiral fracture of shaft of ulna, unspecified arm**

√6th **S52.25** Comminuted **fracture of shaft of ulna**

    √7th **S52.251** Displaced **comminuted fracture of shaft of ulna,** right **arm**

    √7th **S52.252** Displaced **comminuted fracture of shaft of ulna,** left **arm**

    √7th **S52.253** Displaced **comminuted fracture of shaft of ulna, unspecified arm**

    √7th **S52.254** Nondisplaced **comminuted fracture of shaft of ulna,** right **arm**

    √7th **S52.255** Nondisplaced **comminuted fracture of shaft of ulna,** left **arm**

    √7th **S52.256** Nondisplaced **comminuted fracture of shaft of ulna, unspecified arm**

√6th **S52.26** Segmental **fracture of shaft of ulna**

    √7th **S52.261** Displaced **segmental fracture of shaft of ulna,** right **arm**

    √7th **S52.262** Displaced **segmental fracture of shaft of ulna,** left **arm**

    √7th **S52.263** Displaced **segmental fracture of shaft of ulna, unspecified arm**

    √7th **S52.264** Nondisplaced **segmental fracture of shaft of ulna,** right **arm**

    √7th **S52.265** Nondisplaced **segmental fracture of shaft of ulna,** left **arm**

    √7th **S52.266** Nondisplaced **segmental fracture of shaft of ulna, unspecified arm**

√6th **S52.27** Monteggia's **fracture of ulna**
       Fracture of upper shaft of ulna with dislocation of radial head

    √7th **S52.271** Monteggia's **fracture of** right **ulna**

    √7th **S52.272** Monteggia's **fracture of** left **ulna**

    √7th **S52.279** Monteggia's **fracture of unspecified ulna**

√6th **S52.28** Bent bone **of ulna**

    √7th **S52.281** Bent bone **of** right **ulna**

    √7th **S52.282** Bent bone **of** left **ulna**

    √7th **S52.283** Bent bone **of unspecified ulna**

√6th **S52.29** Other **fracture of shaft of ulna**

    √7th **S52.291** Other fracture of shaft of right ulna

    √7th **S52.292** Other fracture of shaft of left ulna

    √7th **S52.299** Other fracture of shaft of unspecified ulna

√5th **S52.3** Fracture of **shaft of radius**

    √6th **S52.30** Unspecified **fracture of shaft of radius**

       √7th **S52.301** Unspecified fracture of shaft of right radius

       √7th **S52.302** Unspecified fracture of shaft of left radius

       √7th **S52.309** Unspecified fracture of shaft of unspecified radius

    √6th **S52.31** Greenstick **fracture of shaft of radius**

The appropriate 7th character is to be added to all codes in subcategory S52.31.
A   initial encounter for closed fracture
D   subsequent encounter for fracture with routine healing
G   subsequent encounter for fracture with delayed healing
K   subsequent encounter for fracture with nonunion
P   subsequent encounter for fracture with malunion
S   sequela

       √7th **S52.311** Greenstick fracture of shaft of radius, right arm

✔ Additional Character Required   √x7th Placeholder Alert   Unspecified Dx   Other Specified Dx   Manifestation   ▶◀ Revised Text   ● New Code   ▲ Revised Code Title

ICD-10-CM 2016   897

√7ᵗʰ **S52.312** Greenstick fracture of shaft of radius, left arm

√7ᵗʰ **S52.319** **Greenstick fracture of shaft of radius, unspecified arm**

√6ᵗʰ **S52.32** Transverse fracture of shaft of radius

√7ᵗʰ **S52.321** Displaced **transverse** fracture of shaft of right radius

√7ᵗʰ **S52.322** Displaced **transverse** fracture of shaft of left radius

√7ᵗʰ **S52.323** **Displaced transverse fracture of shaft of unspecified radius**

√7ᵗʰ **S52.324** Nondisplaced **transverse** fracture of shaft of right radius

√7ᵗʰ **S52.325** Nondisplaced **transverse** fracture of shaft of left radius

√7ᵗʰ **S52.326** **Nondisplaced transverse fracture of shaft of unspecified radius**

√6ᵗʰ **S52.33** Oblique fracture of shaft of radius

√7ᵗʰ **S52.331** Displaced **oblique** fracture of shaft of right radius

√7ᵗʰ **S52.332** Displaced **oblique** fracture of shaft of left radius

√7ᵗʰ **S52.333** **Displaced oblique fracture of shaft of unspecified radius**

√7ᵗʰ **S52.334** Nondisplaced **oblique** fracture of shaft of right radius

√7ᵗʰ **S52.335** Nondisplaced **oblique** fracture of shaft of left radius

√7ᵗʰ **S52.336** **Nondisplaced oblique fracture of shaft of unspecified radius**

√6ᵗʰ **S52.34** Spiral fracture of shaft of radius

√7ᵗʰ **S52.341** Displaced **spiral** fracture of shaft of radius, right arm

√7ᵗʰ **S52.342** Displaced **spiral** fracture of shaft of radius, left arm

√7ᵗʰ **S52.343** **Displaced spiral fracture of shaft of radius, unspecified arm**

√7ᵗʰ **S52.344** Nondisplaced **spiral** fracture of shaft of radius, right arm

√7ᵗʰ **S52.345** Nondisplaced **spiral** fracture of shaft of radius, left arm

√7ᵗʰ **S52.346** **Nondisplaced spiral fracture of shaft of radius, unspecified arm**

√6ᵗʰ **S52.35** Comminuted fracture of shaft of radius

√7ᵗʰ **S52.351** Displaced **comminuted** fracture of shaft of radius, right arm

√7ᵗʰ **S52.352** Displaced **comminuted** fracture of shaft of radius, left arm

√7ᵗʰ **S52.353** **Displaced comminuted fracture of shaft of radius, unspecified arm**

√7ᵗʰ **S52.354** Nondisplaced **comminuted** fracture of shaft of radius, right arm

√7ᵗʰ **S52.355** Nondisplaced **comminuted** fracture of shaft of radius, left arm

√7ᵗʰ **S52.356** **Nondisplaced comminuted fracture of shaft of radius, unspecified arm**

√6ᵗʰ **S52.36** Segmental fracture of shaft of radius

√7ᵗʰ **S52.361** Displaced **segmental** fracture of shaft of radius, right arm

√7ᵗʰ **S52.362** Displaced **segmental** fracture of shaft of radius, left arm

√7ᵗʰ **S52.363** **Displaced segmental fracture of shaft of radius, unspecified arm**

√7ᵗʰ **S52.364** Nondisplaced **segmental** fracture of shaft of radius, right arm

√7ᵗʰ **S52.365** Nondisplaced **segmental** fracture of shaft of radius, left arm

√7ᵗʰ **S52.366** **Nondisplaced segmental fracture of shaft of radius, unspecified arm**

√6ᵗʰ **S52.37** Galeazzi's fracture
Fracture of lower shaft of radius with radioulnar joint dislocation

√7ᵗʰ **S52.371** **Galeazzi's fracture of** right **radius**

√7ᵗʰ **S52.372** **Galeazzi's fracture of** left **radius**

√7ᵗʰ **S52.379** **Galeazzi's fracture of unspecified radius**

√6ᵗʰ **S52.38** Bent bone of radius

√7ᵗʰ **S52.381** Bent bone of right radius

√7ᵗʰ **S52.382** Bent bone of left radius

√7ᵗʰ **S52.389** Bent bone of unspecified radius

√6ᵗʰ **S52.39** Other fracture of shaft of radius

√7ᵗʰ **S52.391** Other fracture of shaft of radius, right arm

√7ᵗʰ **S52.392** Other fracture of shaft of radius, left arm

√7ᵗʰ **S52.399** Other fracture of shaft of radius, unspecified arm

√5ᵗʰ **S52.5** Fracture of lower end of radius
Fracture of distal end of radius
EXCLUDES 2 *physeal fractures of lower end of radius (S59.2-)*

√6ᵗʰ **S52.50** Unspecified fracture of the lower end of radius

√7ᵗʰ **S52.501** **Unspecified** fracture of the lower end of right radius

√7ᵗʰ **S52.502** **Unspecified** fracture of the lower end of left radius

√7ᵗʰ **S52.509** **Unspecified fracture of the lower end of unspecified radius**

√6ᵗʰ **S52.51** Fracture of radial styloid process

√7ᵗʰ **S52.511** Displaced fracture of right radial styloid process

√7ᵗʰ **S52.512** Displaced fracture of left radial styloid process

√7ᵗʰ **S52.513** **Displaced fracture of unspecified radial styloid process**

√7ᵗʰ **S52.514** Nondisplaced fracture of right radial styloid process

√7ᵗʰ **S52.515** Nondisplaced fracture of left radial styloid process

√7ᵗʰ **S52.516** **Nondisplaced fracture of unspecified radial styloid process**

√6ᵗʰ **S52.52** Torus fracture of lower end of radius

> The appropriate 7th character is to be added to all codes in subcategory S52.52.
> A   initial encounter for closed fracture
> D   subsequent encounter for fracture with routine healing
> G   subsequent encounter for fracture with delayed healing
> K   subsequent encounter for fracture with nonunion
> P   subsequent encounter for fracture with malunion
> S   sequela

√7ᵗʰ **S52.521** Torus fracture of lower end of right radius

√7ᵗʰ **S52.522** Torus fracture of lower end of left radius

√7ᵗʰ **S52.529** **Torus fracture of lower end of unspecified radius**

√6ᵗʰ **S52.53** Colles' fracture

√7ᵗʰ **S52.531** **Colles' fracture of** right **radius**

√7ᵗʰ **S52.532** **Colles' fracture of** left **radius**

√7ᵗʰ **S52.539** **Colles' fracture of unspecified radius**

√6ᵗʰ **S52.54** Smith's fracture

√7ᵗʰ **S52.541** **Smith's fracture of** right **radius**

√7ᵗʰ **S52.542** **Smith's fracture of** left **radius**

√7ᵗʰ **S52.549** **Smith's fracture of unspecified radius**

√6ᵗʰ **S52.55** Other extraarticular fracture of lower end of radius

√7ᵗʰ **S52.551** **Other extraarticular fracture of lower end of** right **radius**

√7ᵗʰ **S52.552** **Other extraarticular fracture of lower end of** left **radius**

√7ᵗʰ **S52.559** **Other extraarticular fracture of lower end of unspecified radius**

√6ᵗʰ **S52.56** Barton's fracture

√7ᵗʰ **S52.561** Barton's fracture of right radius

√7ᵗʰ **S52.562** Barton's fracture of left radius

√7ᵗʰ **S52.569** **Barton's fracture of unspecified radius**

√6ᵗʰ **S52.57** Other intraarticular fracture of lower end of radius

√7ᵗʰ **S52.571** **Other intraarticular fracture of lower end of** right **radius**

EXCLUDES 1 Not coded here   *EXCLUDES 2* Not included here   N Newborn Age: 0   P Pediatric Age: 0-17   M Maternity Age: 12-55   A Adult Age: 15-124

√7ᵗʰ **S52.572** **Other intraarticular fracture of lower end of left radius**

√7ᵗʰ **S52.579** **Other intraarticular fracture of lower end of unspecified radius**

√6ᵗʰ **S52.59** Other fractures of lower end of radius

√7ᵗʰ **S52.591** **Other fractures of lower end of right radius**

√7ᵗʰ **S52.592** **Other fractures of lower end of left radius**

√7ᵗʰ **S52.599** **Other fractures of lower end of unspecified radius**

√5ᵗʰ **S52.6** Fracture of lower end of ulna

√6ᵗʰ **S52.60** Unspecified fracture of lower end of ulna

√7ᵗʰ **S52.601** **Unspecified fracture of lower end of right ulna**

√7ᵗʰ **S52.602** **Unspecified fracture of lower end of left ulna**

√7ᵗʰ **S52.609** **Unspecified fracture of lower end of unspecified ulna**

√6ᵗʰ **S52.61** Fracture of ulna styloid process

√7ᵗʰ **S52.611** **Displaced fracture of right ulna styloid process**

√7ᵗʰ **S52.612** **Displaced fracture of left ulna styloid process**

√7ᵗʰ **S52.613** **Displaced fracture of unspecified ulna styloid process**

√7ᵗʰ **S52.614** **Nondisplaced fracture of right ulna styloid process**

√7ᵗʰ **S52.615** **Nondisplaced fracture of left ulna styloid process**

√7ᵗʰ **S52.616** **Nondisplaced fracture of unspecified ulna styloid process**

√6ᵗʰ **S52.62** Torus fracture of lower end of ulna

> The appropriate 7th character is to be added to all codes in subcategory S52.62.
> A   initial encounter for closed fracture
> D   subsequent encounter for fracture with routine healing
> G   subsequent encounter for fracture with delayed healing
> K   subsequent encounter for fracture with nonunion
> P   subsequent encounter for fracture with malunion
> S   sequela

√7ᵗʰ **S52.621** **Torus fracture of lower end of right ulna**

√7ᵗʰ **S52.622** **Torus fracture of lower end of left ulna**

√7ᵗʰ **S52.629** **Torus fracture of lower end of unspecified ulna**

√6ᵗʰ **S52.69** Other fracture of lower end of ulna

√7ᵗʰ **S52.691** **Other fracture of lower end of right ulna**

√7ᵗʰ **S52.692** **Other fracture of lower end of left ulna**

√7ᵗʰ **S52.699** **Other fracture of lower end of unspecified ulna**

√5ᵗʰ **S52.9** Unspecified fracture of forearm

√x7ᵗʰ **S52.90** Unspecified fracture of unspecified forearm

√x7ᵗʰ **S52.91** Unspecified fracture of right forearm

√x7ᵗʰ **S52.92** Unspecified fracture of left forearm

√4ᵗʰ **S53** **Dislocation and sprain of joints and ligaments of elbow**

INCLUDES   avulsion of joint or ligament of elbow
laceration of cartilage, joint or ligament of elbow
sprain of cartilage, joint or ligament of elbow
traumatic hemarthrosis of joint or ligament of elbow
traumatic rupture of joint or ligament of elbow
traumatic subluxation of joint or ligament of elbow
traumatic tear of joint or ligament of elbow

Code also any associated open wound

EXCLUDES 2   strain of muscle, fascia and tendon at forearm level (S56.-)

> The appropriate 7th character is to be added to each code from category S53.
> A   initial encounter
> D   subsequent encounter
> S   sequela

√5ᵗʰ **S53.0** Subluxation and dislocation of radial head
Dislocation of radiohumeral joint
Subluxation of radiohumeral joint
EXCLUDES 1   Monteggia's fracture-dislocation (S52.27-)

√6ᵗʰ **S53.00** Unspecified subluxation and dislocation of radial head

√7ᵗʰ **S53.001** **Unspecified subluxation of right radial head**

√7ᵗʰ **S53.002** **Unspecified subluxation of left radial head**

√7ᵗʰ **S53.003** **Unspecified subluxation of unspecified radial head**

√7ᵗʰ **S53.004** **Unspecified dislocation of right radial head**

√7ᵗʰ **S53.005** **Unspecified dislocation of left radial head**

√7ᵗʰ **S53.006** **Unspecified dislocation of unspecified radial head**

√6ᵗʰ **S53.01** Anterior subluxation and dislocation of radial head
Anteriomedial subluxation and dislocation of radial head

√7ᵗʰ **S53.011** **Anterior subluxation of right radial head**

√7ᵗʰ **S53.012** **Anterior subluxation of left radial head**

√7ᵗʰ **S53.013** **Anterior subluxation of unspecified radial head**

√7ᵗʰ **S53.014** **Anterior dislocation of right radial head**

√7ᵗʰ **S53.015** **Anterior dislocation of left radial head**

√7ᵗʰ **S53.016** **Anterior dislocation of unspecified radial head**

√6ᵗʰ **S53.02** Posterior subluxation and dislocation of radial head
Posteriolateral subluxation and dislocation of radial head

√7ᵗʰ **S53.021** **Posterior subluxation of right radial head**

√7ᵗʰ **S53.022** **Posterior subluxation of left radial head**

√7ᵗʰ **S53.023** **Posterior subluxation of unspecified radial head**

√7ᵗʰ **S53.024** **Posterior dislocation of right radial head**

√7ᵗʰ **S53.025** **Posterior dislocation of left radial head**

√7ᵗʰ **S53.026** **Posterior dislocation of unspecified radial head**

√6ᵗʰ **S53.03** Nursemaid's elbow

√7ᵗʰ **S53.031** **Nursemaid's elbow, right elbow**

√7ᵗʰ **S53.032** **Nursemaid's elbow, left elbow**

√7ᵗʰ **S53.033** **Nursemaid's elbow, unspecified elbow**

√6ᵗʰ **S53.09** Other subluxation and dislocation of radial head

√7ᵗʰ **S53.091** **Other subluxation of right radial head**

√7ᵗʰ **S53.092** **Other subluxation of left radial head**

√7ᵗʰ **S53.093** **Other subluxation of unspecified radial head**

√7ᵗʰ **S53.094** **Other dislocation of right radial head**

√7ᵗʰ **S53.095** **Other dislocation of left radial head**

√7ᵗʰ **S53.096** **Other dislocation of unspecified radial head**

√5ᵗʰ **S53.1** Subluxation and dislocation of ulnohumeral joint
Subluxation and dislocation of elbow NOS
EXCLUDES 1   dislocation of radial head alone (S53.0-)

√6ᵗʰ **S53.10** Unspecified subluxation and dislocation of ulnohumeral joint

√7ᵗʰ **S53.101** **Unspecified subluxation of right ulnohumeral joint**

√7ᵗʰ **S53.102** **Unspecified subluxation of left ulnohumeral joint**

√7ᵗʰ **S53.103** **Unspecified subluxation of unspecified ulnohumeral joint**

√7ᵗʰ **S53.104** **Unspecified dislocation of right ulnohumeral joint**

√7ᵗʰ **S53.105** **Unspecified dislocation of left ulnohumeral joint**

√7ᵗʰ **S53.106** **Unspecified dislocation of unspecified ulnohumeral joint**

√6ᵗʰ **S53.11** Anterior subluxation and dislocation of ulnohumeral joint

√7ᵗʰ **S53.111** **Anterior subluxation of right ulnohumeral joint**

☑ Additional Character Required   √x7ᵗʰ Placeholder Alert   Unspecified Dx   Other Specified Dx   Manifestation   ►◄ Revised Text   ● New Code   ▲ Revised Code Title

✓7ᵗʰ **S53.112 Anterior** subluxation of **left** ulnohumeral joint

✓7ᵗʰ **S53.113 Anterior** subluxation of **unspecified** ulnohumeral joint

✓7ᵗʰ **S53.114 Anterior** dislocation of **right** ulnohumeral joint
AHA: 2012, 4Q, 108

✓7ᵗʰ **S53.115 Anterior** dislocation of **left** ulnohumeral joint

✓7ᵗʰ **S53.116 Anterior** dislocation of **unspecified** ulnohumeral joint

✓6ᵗʰ **S53.12 Posterior** subluxation and dislocation of ulnohumeral joint

✓7ᵗʰ **S53.121 Posterior** subluxation of **right** ulnohumeral joint

✓7ᵗʰ **S53.122 Posterior** subluxation of **left** ulnohumeral joint

✓7ᵗʰ **S53.123 Posterior** subluxation of **unspecified** ulnohumeral joint

✓7ᵗʰ **S53.124 Posterior** dislocation of **right** ulnohumeral joint

✓7ᵗʰ **S53.125 Posterior** dislocation of **left** ulnohumeral joint

✓7ᵗʰ **S53.126 Posterior** dislocation of **unspecified** ulnohumeral joint

✓6ᵗʰ **S53.13 Medial** subluxation and dislocation of ulnohumeral joint

✓7ᵗʰ **S53.131 Medial** subluxation of **right** ulnohumeral joint

✓7ᵗʰ **S53.132 Medial** subluxation of **left** ulnohumeral joint

✓7ᵗʰ **S53.133 Medial** subluxation of **unspecified** ulnohumeral joint

✓7ᵗʰ **S53.134 Medial** dislocation of **right** ulnohumeral joint

✓7ᵗʰ **S53.135 Medial** dislocation of **left** ulnohumeral joint

✓7ᵗʰ **S53.136 Medial** dislocation of **unspecified** ulnohumeral joint

✓6ᵗʰ **S53.14 Lateral** subluxation and dislocation of ulnohumeral joint

✓7ᵗʰ **S53.141 Lateral** subluxation of **right** ulnohumeral joint

✓7ᵗʰ **S53.142 Lateral** subluxation of **left** ulnohumeral joint

✓7ᵗʰ **S53.143 Lateral** subluxation of **unspecified** ulnohumeral joint

✓7ᵗʰ **S53.144 Lateral** dislocation of **right** ulnohumeral joint

✓7ᵗʰ **S53.145 Lateral** dislocation of **left** ulnohumeral joint

✓7ᵗʰ **S53.146 Lateral** dislocation of **unspecified** ulnohumeral joint

✓6ᵗʰ **S53.19 Other** subluxation and dislocation of ulnohumeral joint

✓7ᵗʰ **S53.191 Other** subluxation of **right** ulnohumeral joint

✓7ᵗʰ **S53.192 Other** subluxation of **left** ulnohumeral joint

✓7ᵗʰ **S53.193 Other** subluxation of **unspecified** ulnohumeral joint

✓7ᵗʰ **S53.194 Other** dislocation of **right** ulnohumeral joint

✓7ᵗʰ **S53.195 Other** dislocation of **left** ulnohumeral joint

✓7ᵗʰ **S53.196 Other** dislocation of **unspecified** ulnohumeral joint

✓5ᵗʰ **S53.2 Traumatic rupture of** radial collateral ligament
EXCLUDES 1 sprain of radial collateral ligament NOS (S53.43-)

✓x7ᵗʰ **S53.20 Traumatic rupture of unspecified radial collateral ligament**

✓x7ᵗʰ **S53.21 Traumatic rupture of** right radial collateral ligament

✓x7ᵗʰ **S53.22 Traumatic rupture of** left radial collateral ligament

✓5ᵗʰ **S53.3 Traumatic rupture of** ulnar collateral ligament
EXCLUDES 1 sprain of ulnar collateral ligament (S53.44-)

✓x7ᵗʰ **S53.30 Traumatic rupture of unspecified ulnar collateral ligament**

✓x7ᵗʰ **S53.31 Traumatic rupture of** right ulnar collateral ligament

✓x7ᵗʰ **S53.32 Traumatic rupture of** left ulnar collateral ligament

✓5ᵗʰ **S53.4 Sprain of** elbow
EXCLUDES 2 traumatic rupture of radial collateral ligament (S53.2-)
traumatic rupture of ulnar collateral ligament (S53.3-)

✓6ᵗʰ **S53.40 Unspecified sprain of** elbow

✓7ᵗʰ **S53.401 Unspecified sprain of** right **elbow**

✓7ᵗʰ **S53.402 Unspecified sprain of** left **elbow**

✓7ᵗʰ **S53.409 Unspecified sprain of unspecified elbow**
Sprain of elbow NOS

✓6ᵗʰ **S53.41 Radiohumeral (joint) sprain**

✓7ᵗʰ **S53.411 Radiohumeral (joint) sprain of** right **elbow**

✓7ᵗʰ **S53.412 Radiohumeral (joint) sprain of** left **elbow**

✓7ᵗʰ **S53.419 Radiohumeral (joint) sprain of unspecified elbow**

✓6ᵗʰ **S53.42 Ulnohumeral (joint) sprain**

✓7ᵗʰ **S53.421 Ulnohumeral (joint) sprain of** right **elbow**

✓7ᵗʰ **S53.422 Ulnohumeral (joint) sprain of** left **elbow**

✓7ᵗʰ **S53.429 Ulnohumeral (joint) sprain of unspecified elbow**

✓6ᵗʰ **S53.43 Radial collateral ligament sprain**

✓7ᵗʰ **S53.431 Radial collateral ligament sprain of** right **elbow**

✓7ᵗʰ **S53.432 Radial collateral ligament sprain of** left **elbow**

✓7ᵗʰ **S53.439 Radial collateral ligament sprain of unspecified elbow**

✓6ᵗʰ **S53.44 Ulnar collateral ligament sprain**

✓7ᵗʰ **S53.441 Ulnar collateral ligament sprain of** right **elbow**

✓7ᵗʰ **S53.442 Ulnar collateral ligament sprain of** left **elbow**

✓7ᵗʰ **S53.449 Ulnar collateral ligament sprain of unspecified elbow**

✓6ᵗʰ **S53.49 Other sprain of** elbow

✓7ᵗʰ **S53.491 Other sprain of** right **elbow**

✓7ᵗʰ **S53.492 Other sprain of** left **elbow**

✓7ᵗʰ **S53.499 Other sprain of unspecified elbow**

✓4ᵗʰ **S54 Injury of nerves at forearm level**
Code also any associated open wound (S51.-)
EXCLUDES 2 injury of nerves at wrist and hand level (S64.-)

The appropriate 7th character is to be added to each code from category S54.
A   initial encounter
D   subsequent encounter
S   sequela

✓5ᵗʰ **S54.0 Injury of** ulnar **nerve at forearm level**
Injury of ulnar nerve NOS

✓x7ᵗʰ **S54.00 Injury of ulnar nerve at forearm level, unspecified arm**

✓x7ᵗʰ **S54.01 Injury of ulnar nerve at forearm level,** right **arm**

✓x7ᵗʰ **S54.02 Injury of ulnar nerve at forearm level,** left **arm**

✓5ᵗʰ **S54.1 Injury of** median **nerve at forearm level**
Injury of median nerve NOS

✓x7ᵗʰ **S54.10 Injury of median nerve at forearm level, unspecified arm**

✓x7ᵗʰ **S54.11 Injury of median nerve at forearm level,** right **arm**

✓x7ᵗʰ **S54.12 Injury of median nerve at forearm level,** left **arm**

✓5ᵗʰ **S54.2 Injury of** radial **nerve at forearm level**
Injury of radial nerve NOS

✓x7ᵗʰ **S54.20 Injury of radial nerve at forearm level, unspecified arm**

✓x7ᵗʰ **S54.21 Injury of radial nerve at forearm level,** right **arm**

✓x7ᵗʰ **S54.22 Injury of radial nerve at forearm level,** left **arm**

✓5ᵗʰ **S54.3 Injury of** cutaneous sensory **nerve at forearm level**

✓x7ᵗʰ **S54.30 Injury of cutaneous sensory nerve at forearm level, unspecified arm**

EXCLUDES 1 Not coded here   *EXCLUDES 2* Not included here   Ⓝ Newborn Age: 0   Ⓟ Pediatric Age: 0-17   Ⓜ Maternity Age: 12-55   Ⓐ Adult Age: 15-124

900   ICD-10-CM 2016

✓x7ᵗʰ **S54.31** Injury of cutaneous sensory nerve at forearm level, right **arm**

✓x7ᵗʰ **S54.32** Injury of cutaneous sensory nerve at forearm level, left **arm**

✓5ᵗʰ **S54.8** Injury of other nerves at forearm level

    ✓6ᵗʰ **S54.8X** Unspecified injury of other nerves at forearm level

       ✓7ᵗʰ **S54.8X1** Unspecified injury of other nerves at forearm level, right **arm**

       ✓7ᵗʰ **S54.8X2** Unspecified injury of other nerves at forearm level, left **arm**

       ✓7ᵗʰ **S54.8X9** Unspecified injury of other nerves at forearm level, unspecified **arm**

✓5ᵗʰ **S54.9** Injury of unspecified nerve at forearm level

    ✓x7ᵗʰ **S54.90** Injury of unspecified nerve at forearm level, unspecified **arm**

    ✓x7ᵗʰ **S54.91** Injury of unspecified nerve at forearm level, right **arm**

    ✓x7ᵗʰ **S54.92** Injury of unspecified nerve at forearm level, left **arm**

✓4ᵗʰ **S55** Injury of blood vessels at forearm level

    Code also any associated open wound (S51.-)

    EXCLUDES 2   injury of blood vessels at wrist and hand level (S65.-)
               injury of brachial vessels (S45.1-S45.2)

    The appropriate 7th character is to be added to each code from category S55.
    A   initial encounter
    D   subsequent encounter
    S   sequela

✓5ᵗʰ **S55.0** Injury of ulnar artery at forearm level

    ✓6ᵗʰ **S55.00** Unspecified injury of ulnar artery at forearm level

       ✓7ᵗʰ **S55.001** Unspecified injury of ulnar artery at forearm level, right **arm**

       ✓7ᵗʰ **S55.002** Unspecified injury of ulnar artery at forearm level, left **arm**

       ✓7ᵗʰ **S55.009** Unspecified injury of ulnar artery at forearm level, unspecified **arm**

    ✓6ᵗʰ **S55.01** Laceration of ulnar artery at forearm level

       ✓7ᵗʰ **S55.011** Laceration of ulnar artery at forearm level, right **arm**

       ✓7ᵗʰ **S55.012** Laceration of ulnar artery at forearm level, left **arm**

       ✓7ᵗʰ **S55.019** Laceration of ulnar artery at forearm level, unspecified **arm**

    ✓6ᵗʰ **S55.09** Other specified injury of ulnar artery at forearm level

       ✓7ᵗʰ **S55.091** Other specified injury of ulnar artery at forearm level, right **arm**

       ✓7ᵗʰ **S55.092** Other specified injury of ulnar artery at forearm level, left **arm**

       ✓7ᵗʰ **S55.099** Other specified injury of ulnar artery at forearm level, unspecified **arm**

✓5ᵗʰ **S55.1** Injury of radial artery at forearm level

    ✓6ᵗʰ **S55.10** Unspecified injury of radial artery at forearm level

       ✓7ᵗʰ **S55.101** Unspecified injury of radial artery at forearm level, right **arm**

       ✓7ᵗʰ **S55.102** Unspecified injury of radial artery at forearm level, left **arm**

       ✓7ᵗʰ **S55.109** Unspecified injury of radial artery at forearm level, unspecified **arm**

    ✓6ᵗʰ **S55.11** Laceration of radial artery at forearm level

       ✓7ᵗʰ **S55.111** Laceration of radial artery at forearm level, right **arm**

       ✓7ᵗʰ **S55.112** Laceration of radial artery at forearm level, left **arm**

       ✓7ᵗʰ **S55.119** Laceration of radial artery at forearm level, unspecified **arm**

    ✓6ᵗʰ **S55.19** Other specified injury of radial artery at forearm level

       ✓7ᵗʰ **S55.191** Other specified injury of radial artery at forearm level, right **arm**

       ✓7ᵗʰ **S55.192** Other specified injury of radial artery at forearm level, left **arm**

       ✓7ᵗʰ **S55.199** Other specified injury of radial artery at forearm level, unspecified **arm**

✓5ᵗʰ **S55.2** Injury of vein at forearm level

    ✓6ᵗʰ **S55.20** Unspecified injury of vein at forearm level

       ✓7ᵗʰ **S55.201** Unspecified injury of vein at forearm level, right **arm**

       ✓7ᵗʰ **S55.202** Unspecified injury of vein at forearm level, left **arm**

       ✓7ᵗʰ **S55.209** Unspecified injury of vein at forearm level, unspecified **arm**

    ✓6ᵗʰ **S55.21** Laceration of vein at forearm level

       ✓7ᵗʰ **S55.211** Laceration of vein at forearm level, right **arm**

       ✓7ᵗʰ **S55.212** Laceration of vein at forearm level, left **arm**

       ✓7ᵗʰ **S55.219** Laceration of vein at forearm level, unspecified **arm**

    ✓6ᵗʰ **S55.29** Other specified injury of vein at forearm level

       ✓7ᵗʰ **S55.291** Other specified injury of vein at forearm level, right **arm**

       ✓7ᵗʰ **S55.292** Other specified injury of vein at forearm level, left **arm**

       ✓7ᵗʰ **S55.299** Other specified injury of vein at forearm level, unspecified **arm**

✓5ᵗʰ **S55.8** Injury of other blood vessels at forearm level

    ✓6ᵗʰ **S55.80** Unspecified injury of other blood vessels at forearm level

       ✓7ᵗʰ **S55.801** Unspecified injury of other blood vessels at forearm level, right **arm**

       ✓7ᵗʰ **S55.802** Unspecified injury of other blood vessels at forearm level, left **arm**

       ✓7ᵗʰ **S55.809** Unspecified injury of other blood vessels at forearm level, unspecified **arm**

    ✓6ᵗʰ **S55.81** Laceration of other blood vessels at forearm level

       ✓7ᵗʰ **S55.811** Laceration of other blood vessels at forearm level, right **arm**

       ✓7ᵗʰ **S55.812** Laceration of other blood vessels at forearm level, left **arm**

       ✓7ᵗʰ **S55.819** Laceration of other blood vessels at forearm level, unspecified **arm**

    ✓6ᵗʰ **S55.89** Other specified injury of other blood vessels at forearm level

       ✓7ᵗʰ **S55.891** Other specified injury of other blood vessels at forearm level, right **arm**

       ✓7ᵗʰ **S55.892** Other specified injury of other blood vessels at forearm level, left **arm**

       ✓7ᵗʰ **S55.899** Other specified injury of other blood vessels at forearm level, unspecified **arm**

✓5ᵗʰ **S55.9** Injury of unspecified blood vessel at forearm level

    ✓6ᵗʰ **S55.90** Unspecified injury of unspecified blood vessel at forearm level

       ✓7ᵗʰ **S55.901** Unspecified injury of unspecified blood vessel at forearm level, right **arm**

       ✓7ᵗʰ **S55.902** Unspecified injury of unspecified blood vessel at forearm level, left **arm**

       ✓7ᵗʰ **S55.909** Unspecified injury of unspecified blood vessel at forearm level, unspecified **arm**

    ✓6ᵗʰ **S55.91** Laceration of unspecified blood vessel at forearm level

       ✓7ᵗʰ **S55.911** Laceration of unspecified blood vessel at forearm level, right **arm**

       ✓7ᵗʰ **S55.912** Laceration of unspecified blood vessel at forearm level, left **arm**

       ✓7ᵗʰ **S55.919** Laceration of unspecified blood vessel at forearm level, unspecified **arm**

    ✓6ᵗʰ **S55.99** Other specified injury of unspecified blood vessel at forearm level

       ✓7ᵗʰ **S55.991** Other specified injury of unspecified blood vessel at forearm level, right **arm**

       ✓7ᵗʰ **S55.992** Other specified injury of unspecified blood vessel at forearm level, left **arm**

       ✓7ᵗʰ **S55.999** Other specified injury of unspecified blood vessel at forearm level, unspecified **arm**

✓ Additional Character Required   ✓x7ᵗʰ Placeholder Alert   Unspecified Dx   Other Specified Dx   Manifestation   ►◄ Revised Text   ● New Code   ▲ Revised Code Title

✓4ᵗʰ S56 Injury of muscle, fascia and tendon at forearm level

Code also any associated open wound (S51.-)

EXCLUDES 2   injury of muscle, fascia and tendon at or below wrist (S66.-)
sprain of joints and ligaments of elbow (S53.4-)

> The appropriate 7th character is to be added to each code from category S56.
> A   initial encounter
> D   subsequent encounter
> S   sequela

✓5ᵗʰ S56.0 Injury of flexor muscle, fascia and tendon of thumb at forearm level

   ✓6ᵗʰ S56.00 Unspecified injury of flexor muscle, fascia and tendon of thumb at forearm level

     ✓7ᵗʰ **S56.001 Unspecified injury of flexor muscle, fascia and tendon of right thumb at forearm level**

     ✓7ᵗʰ **S56.002 Unspecified injury of flexor muscle, fascia and tendon of left thumb at forearm level**

     ✓7ᵗʰ **S56.009 Unspecified injury of flexor muscle, fascia and tendon of unspecified thumb at forearm level**

   ✓6ᵗʰ S56.01 Strain of flexor muscle, fascia and tendon of thumb at forearm level

     ✓7ᵗʰ **S56.011 Strain of flexor muscle, fascia and tendon of right thumb at forearm level**

     ✓7ᵗʰ **S56.012 Strain of flexor muscle, fascia and tendon of left thumb at forearm level**

     ✓7ᵗʰ **S56.019 Strain of flexor muscle, fascia and tendon of unspecified thumb at forearm level**

   ✓6ᵗʰ S56.02 Laceration of flexor muscle, fascia and tendon of thumb at forearm level

     ✓7ᵗʰ **S56.021 Laceration of flexor muscle, fascia and tendon of right thumb at forearm level**

     ✓7ᵗʰ **S56.022 Laceration of flexor muscle, fascia and tendon of left thumb at forearm level**

     ✓7ᵗʰ **S56.029 Laceration of flexor muscle, fascia and tendon of unspecified thumb at forearm level**

   ✓6ᵗʰ S56.09 Other injury of flexor muscle, fascia and tendon of thumb at forearm level

     ✓7ᵗʰ **S56.091 Other injury of flexor muscle, fascia and tendon of right thumb at forearm level**

     ✓7ᵗʰ **S56.092 Other injury of flexor muscle, fascia and tendon of left thumb at forearm level**

     ✓7ᵗʰ **S56.099 Other injury of flexor muscle, fascia and tendon of unspecified thumb at forearm level**

✓5ᵗʰ S56.1 Injury of flexor muscle, fascia and tendon of other and unspecified finger at forearm level

   ✓6ᵗʰ S56.10 Unspecified injury of flexor muscle, fascia and tendon of other and unspecified finger at forearm level

     ✓7ᵗʰ **S56.101 Unspecified injury of flexor muscle, fascia and tendon of right index finger at forearm level**

     ✓7ᵗʰ **S56.102 Unspecified injury of flexor muscle, fascia and tendon of left index finger at forearm level**

     ✓7ᵗʰ **S56.103 Unspecified injury of flexor muscle, fascia and tendon of right middle finger at forearm level**

     ✓7ᵗʰ **S56.104 Unspecified injury of flexor muscle, fascia and tendon of left middle finger at forearm level**

     ✓7ᵗʰ **S56.105 Unspecified injury of flexor muscle, fascia and tendon of right ring finger at forearm level**

     ✓7ᵗʰ **S56.106 Unspecified injury of flexor muscle, fascia and tendon of left ring finger at forearm level**

     ✓7ᵗʰ **S56.107 Unspecified injury of flexor muscle, fascia and tendon of right little finger at forearm level**

     ✓7ᵗʰ **S56.108 Unspecified injury of flexor muscle, fascia and tendon of left little finger at forearm level**

     ✓7ᵗʰ **S56.109 Unspecified injury of flexor muscle, fascia and tendon of unspecified finger at forearm level**

   ✓6ᵗʰ S56.11 Strain of flexor muscle, fascia and tendon of other and unspecified finger at forearm level

     ✓7ᵗʰ **S56.111 Strain of flexor muscle, fascia and tendon of right index finger at forearm level**

     ✓7ᵗʰ **S56.112 Strain of flexor muscle, fascia and tendon of left index finger at forearm level**

     ✓7ᵗʰ **S56.113 Strain of flexor muscle, fascia and tendon of right middle finger at forearm level**

     ✓7ᵗʰ **S56.114 Strain of flexor muscle, fascia and tendon of left middle finger at forearm level**

     ✓7ᵗʰ **S56.115 Strain of flexor muscle, fascia and tendon of right ring finger at forearm level**

     ✓7ᵗʰ **S56.116 Strain of flexor muscle, fascia and tendon of left ring finger at forearm level**

     ✓7ᵗʰ **S56.117 Strain of flexor muscle, fascia and tendon of right little finger at forearm level**

     ✓7ᵗʰ **S56.118 Strain of flexor muscle, fascia and tendon of left little finger at forearm level**

     ✓7ᵗʰ **S56.119 Strain of flexor muscle, fascia and tendon of finger of unspecified finger at forearm level**

   ✓6ᵗʰ S56.12 Laceration of flexor muscle, fascia and tendon of other and unspecified finger at forearm level

     ✓7ᵗʰ **S56.121 Laceration of flexor muscle, fascia and tendon of right index finger at forearm level**

     ✓7ᵗʰ **S56.122 Laceration of flexor muscle, fascia and tendon of left index finger at forearm level**

     ✓7ᵗʰ **S56.123 Laceration of flexor muscle, fascia and tendon of right middle finger at forearm level**

     ✓7ᵗʰ **S56.124 Laceration of flexor muscle, fascia and tendon of left middle finger at forearm level**

     ✓7ᵗʰ **S56.125 Laceration of flexor muscle, fascia and tendon of right ring finger at forearm level**

     ✓7ᵗʰ **S56.126 Laceration of flexor muscle, fascia and tendon of left ring finger at forearm level**

     ✓7ᵗʰ **S56.127 Laceration of flexor muscle, fascia and tendon of right little finger at forearm level**

     ✓7ᵗʰ **S56.128 Laceration of flexor muscle, fascia and tendon of left little finger at forearm level**

     ✓7ᵗʰ **S56.129 Laceration of flexor muscle, fascia and tendon of unspecified finger at forearm level**

   ✓6ᵗʰ S56.19 Other injury of flexor muscle, fascia and tendon of other and unspecified finger at forearm level

     ✓7ᵗʰ **S56.191 Other injury of flexor muscle, fascia and tendon of right index finger at forearm level**

     ✓7ᵗʰ **S56.192 Other injury of flexor muscle, fascia and tendon of left index finger at forearm level**

     ✓7ᵗʰ **S56.193 Other injury of flexor muscle, fascia and tendon of right middle finger at forearm level**

     ✓7ᵗʰ **S56.194 Other injury of flexor muscle, fascia and tendon of left middle finger at forearm level**

     ✓7ᵗʰ **S56.195 Other injury of flexor muscle, fascia and tendon of right ring finger at forearm level**

     ✓7ᵗʰ **S56.196 Other injury of flexor muscle, fascia and tendon of left ring finger at forearm level**

     ✓7ᵗʰ **S56.197 Other injury of flexor muscle, fascia and tendon of right little finger at forearm level**

     ✓7ᵗʰ **S56.198 Other injury of flexor muscle, fascia and tendon of left little finger at forearm level**

     ✓7ᵗʰ **S56.199 Other injury of flexor muscle, fascia and tendon of unspecified finger at forearm level**

✦ Refer to the Muscle/Tendon Table at the beginning of this chapter.

EXCLUDES 1 Not coded here   *EXCLUDES 2* Not included here   Ⓝ Newborn Age: 0   Ⓟ Pediatric Age: 0-17   Ⓜ Maternity Age: 12-55   Ⓐ Adult Age: 15-124

902

ICD-10-CM 2016

✓5ᵗʰ **S56.2** Injury of other flexor muscle, fascia and tendon at forearm level

  ✓6ᵗʰ **S56.20** Unspecified injury of other flexor muscle, fascia and tendon at forearm level

    ✓7ᵗʰ **S56.201** Unspecified injury of other flexor muscle, fascia and tendon at forearm level, right arm

    ✓7ᵗʰ **S56.202** Unspecified injury of other flexor muscle, fascia and tendon at forearm level, left arm

    ✓7ᵗʰ **S56.209** Unspecified injury of other flexor muscle, fascia and tendon at forearm level, unspecified arm

  ✓6ᵗʰ **S56.21** Strain of other flexor muscle, fascia and tendon at forearm level

    ✓7ᵗʰ **S56.211** Strain of other flexor muscle, fascia and tendon at forearm level, right arm

    ✓7ᵗʰ **S56.212** Strain of other flexor muscle, fascia and tendon at forearm level, left arm

    ✓7ᵗʰ **S56.219** Strain of other flexor muscle, fascia and tendon at forearm level, unspecified arm

  ✓6ᵗʰ **S56.22** Laceration of other flexor muscle, fascia and tendon at forearm level

    ✓7ᵗʰ **S56.221** Laceration of other flexor muscle, fascia and tendon at forearm level, right arm

    ✓7ᵗʰ **S56.222** Laceration of other flexor muscle, fascia and tendon at forearm level, left arm

    ✓7ᵗʰ **S56.229** Laceration of other flexor muscle, fascia and tendon at forearm level, unspecified arm

  ✓6ᵗʰ **S56.29** Other injury of other flexor muscle, fascia and tendon at forearm level

    ✓7ᵗʰ **S56.291** Other injury of other flexor muscle, fascia and tendon at forearm level, right arm

    ✓7ᵗʰ **S56.292** Other injury of other flexor muscle, fascia and tendon at forearm level, left arm

    ✓7ᵗʰ **S56.299** Other injury of other flexor muscle, fascia and tendon at forearm level, unspecified arm

✓5ᵗʰ **S56.3** Injury of extensor or abductor muscles, fascia and tendons of thumb at forearm level

  ✓6ᵗʰ **S56.30** Unspecified injury of extensor or abductor muscles, fascia and tendons of thumb at forearm level

    ✓7ᵗʰ **S56.301** Unspecified injury of extensor or abductor muscles, fascia and tendons of right thumb at forearm level

    ✓7ᵗʰ **S56.302** Unspecified injury of extensor or abductor muscles, fascia and tendons of left thumb at forearm level

    ✓7ᵗʰ **S56.309** Unspecified injury of extensor or abductor muscles, fascia and tendons of unspecified thumb at forearm level

  ✓6ᵗʰ **S56.31** Strain of extensor or abductor muscles, fascia and tendons of thumb at forearm level

    ✓7ᵗʰ **S56.311** Strain of extensor or abductor muscles, fascia and tendons of right thumb at forearm level

    ✓7ᵗʰ **S56.312** Strain of extensor or abductor muscles, fascia and tendons of left thumb at forearm level

    ✓7ᵗʰ **S56.319** Strain of extensor or abductor muscles, fascia and tendons of unspecified thumb at forearm level

  ✓6ᵗʰ **S56.32** Laceration of extensor or abductor muscles, fascia and tendons of thumb at forearm level

    ✓7ᵗʰ **S56.321** Laceration of extensor or abductor muscles, fascia and tendons of right thumb at forearm level

    ✓7ᵗʰ **S56.322** Laceration of extensor or abductor muscles, fascia and tendons of left thumb at forearm level

    ✓7ᵗʰ **S56.329** Laceration of extensor or abductor muscles, fascia and tendons of unspecified thumb at forearm level

  ✓6ᵗʰ **S56.39** Other injury of extensor or abductor muscles, fascia and tendons of thumb at forearm level

    ✓7ᵗʰ **S56.391** Other injury of extensor or abductor muscles, fascia and tendons of right thumb at forearm level

    ✓7ᵗʰ **S56.392** Other injury of extensor or abductor muscles, fascia and tendons of left thumb at forearm level

    ✓7ᵗʰ **S56.399** Other injury of extensor or abductor muscles, fascia and tendons of unspecified thumb at forearm level

✓5ᵗʰ **S56.4** Injury of extensor muscle, fascia and tendon of other and unspecified finger at forearm level

  ✓6ᵗʰ **S56.40** Unspecified injury of extensor muscle, fascia and tendon of other and unspecified finger at forearm level

    ✓7ᵗʰ **S56.401** Unspecified injury of extensor muscle, fascia and tendon of right index finger at forearm level

    ✓7ᵗʰ **S56.402** Unspecified injury of extensor muscle, fascia and tendon of left index finger at forearm level

    ✓7ᵗʰ **S56.403** Unspecified injury of extensor muscle, fascia and tendon of right middle finger at forearm level

    ✓7ᵗʰ **S56.404** Unspecified injury of extensor muscle, fascia and tendon of left middle finger at forearm level

    ✓7ᵗʰ **S56.405** Unspecified injury of extensor muscle, fascia and tendon of right ring finger at forearm level

    ✓7ᵗʰ **S56.406** Unspecified injury of extensor muscle, fascia and tendon of left ring finger at forearm level

    ✓7ᵗʰ **S56.407** Unspecified injury of extensor muscle, fascia and tendon of right little finger at forearm level

    ✓7ᵗʰ **S56.408** Unspecified injury of extensor muscle, fascia and tendon of left little finger at forearm level

    ✓7ᵗʰ **S56.409** Unspecified injury of extensor muscle, fascia and tendon of unspecified finger at forearm level

  ✓6ᵗʰ **S56.41** Strain of extensor muscle, fascia and tendon of other and unspecified finger at forearm level

    ✓7ᵗʰ **S56.411** Strain of extensor muscle, fascia and tendon of right index finger at forearm level

    ✓7ᵗʰ **S56.412** Strain of extensor muscle, fascia and tendon of left index finger at forearm level

    ✓7ᵗʰ **S56.413** Strain of extensor muscle, fascia and tendon of right middle finger at forearm level

    ✓7ᵗʰ **S56.414** Strain of extensor muscle, fascia and tendon of left middle finger at forearm level

    ✓7ᵗʰ **S56.415** Strain of extensor muscle, fascia and tendon of right ring finger at forearm level

    ✓7ᵗʰ **S56.416** Strain of extensor muscle, fascia and tendon of left ring finger at forearm level

    ✓7ᵗʰ **S56.417** Strain of extensor muscle, fascia and tendon of right little finger at forearm level

    ✓7ᵗʰ **S56.418** Strain of extensor muscle, fascia and tendon of left little finger at forearm level

    ✓7ᵗʰ **S56.419** Strain of extensor muscle, fascia and tendon of finger, unspecified finger at forearm level

  ✓6ᵗʰ **S56.42** Laceration of extensor muscle, fascia and tendon of other and unspecified finger at forearm level

    ✓7ᵗʰ **S56.421** Laceration of extensor muscle, fascia and tendon of right index finger at forearm level

    ✓7ᵗʰ **S56.422** Laceration of extensor muscle, fascia and tendon of left index finger at forearm level

    ✓7ᵗʰ **S56.423** Laceration of extensor muscle, fascia and tendon of right middle finger at forearm level

☑ Additional Character Required   ᵥₓ7 Placeholder Alert   Unspecified Dx   Other Specified Dx   Manifestation   ▶◀ Revised Text   ● New Code   ▲ Revised Code Title

ICD-10-CM 2016   903

✓7ᵗʰ **S56.424** Laceration of extensor muscle, fascia and tendon of left middle finger at forearm level

✓7ᵗʰ **S56.425** Laceration of extensor muscle, fascia and tendon of right ring finger at forearm level

✓7ᵗʰ **S56.426** Laceration of extensor muscle, fascia and tendon of left ring finger at forearm level

✓7ᵗʰ **S56.427** Laceration of extensor muscle, fascia and tendon of right little finger at forearm level

✓7ᵗʰ **S56.428** Laceration of extensor muscle, fascia and tendon of left little finger at forearm level

✓7ᵗʰ **S56.429** Laceration of extensor muscle, fascia and tendon of unspecified finger at forearm level

✓6ᵗʰ **S56.49** Other injury of extensor muscle, fascia and tendon of other and unspecified finger at forearm level

✓7ᵗʰ **S56.491** Other injury of extensor muscle, fascia and tendon of right index finger at forearm level

✓7ᵗʰ **S56.492** Other injury of extensor muscle, fascia and tendon of left index finger at forearm level

✓7ᵗʰ **S56.493** Other injury of extensor muscle, fascia and tendon of right middle finger at forearm level

✓7ᵗʰ **S56.494** Other injury of extensor muscle, fascia and tendon of left middle finger at forearm level

✓7ᵗʰ **S56.495** Other injury of extensor muscle, fascia and tendon of right ring finger at forearm level

✓7ᵗʰ **S56.496** Other injury of extensor muscle, fascia and tendon of left ring finger at forearm level

✓7ᵗʰ **S56.497** Other injury of extensor muscle, fascia and tendon of right little finger at forearm level

✓7ᵗʰ **S56.498** Other injury of extensor muscle, fascia and tendon of left little finger at forearm level

✓7ᵗʰ **S56.499** Other injury of extensor muscle, fascia and tendon of unspecified finger at forearm level

✓5ᵗʰ **S56.5** Injury of other extensor muscle, fascia and tendon at forearm level

✓6ᵗʰ **S56.50** Unspecified injury of other extensor muscle, fascia and tendon at forearm level

✓7ᵗʰ **S56.501** Unspecified injury of other extensor muscle, fascia and tendon at forearm level, right arm

✓7ᵗʰ **S56.502** Unspecified injury of other extensor muscle, fascia and tendon at forearm level, left arm

✓7ᵗʰ **S56.509** Unspecified injury of other extensor muscle, fascia and tendon at forearm level, unspecified arm

✓6ᵗʰ **S56.51** Strain of other extensor muscle, fascia and tendon at forearm level

✓7ᵗʰ **S56.511** Strain of other extensor muscle, fascia and tendon at forearm level, right arm

✓7ᵗʰ **S56.512** Strain of other extensor muscle, fascia and tendon at forearm level, left arm

✓7ᵗʰ **S56.519** Strain of other extensor muscle, fascia and tendon at forearm level, unspecified arm

✓6ᵗʰ **S56.52** Laceration of other extensor muscle, fascia and tendon at forearm level

✓7ᵗʰ **S56.521** Laceration of other extensor muscle, fascia and tendon at forearm level, right arm

✓7ᵗʰ **S56.522** Laceration of other extensor muscle, fascia and tendon at forearm level, left arm

✓7ᵗʰ **S56.529** Laceration of other extensor muscle, fascia and tendon at forearm level, unspecified arm

✓6ᵗʰ **S56.59** Other injury of other extensor muscle, fascia and tendon at forearm level

✓7ᵗʰ **S56.591** Other injury of other extensor muscle, fascia and tendon at forearm level, right arm

✓7ᵗʰ **S56.592** Other injury of other extensor muscle, fascia and tendon at forearm level, left arm

✓7ᵗʰ **S56.599** Other injury of other extensor muscle, fascia and tendon at forearm level, unspecified arm

✓5ᵗʰ **S56.8** Injury of other muscles, fascia and tendons at forearm level

✓6ᵗʰ **S56.80** Unspecified injury of other muscles, fascia and tendons at forearm level

✓7ᵗʰ **S56.801** Unspecified injury of other muscles, fascia and tendons at forearm level, right arm

✓7ᵗʰ **S56.802** Unspecified injury of other muscles, fascia and tendons at forearm level, left arm

✓7ᵗʰ **S56.809** Unspecified injury of other muscles, fascia and tendons at forearm level, unspecified arm

✓6ᵗʰ **S56.81** Strain of other muscles, fascia and tendons at forearm level

✓7ᵗʰ **S56.811** Strain of other muscles, fascia and tendons at forearm level, right arm

✓7ᵗʰ **S56.812** Strain of other muscles, fascia and tendons at forearm level, left arm

✓7ᵗʰ **S56.819** Strain of other muscles, fascia and tendons at forearm level, unspecified arm

✓6ᵗʰ **S56.82** Laceration of other muscles, fascia and tendons at forearm level

✓7ᵗʰ **S56.821** Laceration of other muscles, fascia and tendons at forearm level, right arm

✓7ᵗʰ **S56.822** Laceration of other muscles, fascia and tendons at forearm level, left arm

✓7ᵗʰ **S56.829** Laceration of other muscles, fascia and tendons at forearm level, unspecified arm

✓6ᵗʰ **S56.89** Other injury of other muscles, fascia and tendons at forearm level

✓7ᵗʰ **S56.891** Other injury of other muscles, fascia and tendons at forearm level, right arm

✓7ᵗʰ **S56.892** Other injury of other muscles, fascia and tendons at forearm level, left arm

✓7ᵗʰ **S56.899** Other injury of other muscles, fascia and tendons at forearm level, unspecified arm

✓5ᵗʰ **S56.9** Injury of unspecified muscles, fascia and tendons at forearm level

✓6ᵗʰ **S56.90** Unspecified injury of unspecified muscles, fascia and tendons at forearm level

✓7ᵗʰ **S56.901** Unspecified injury of unspecified muscles, fascia and tendons at forearm level, right arm

✓7ᵗʰ **S56.902** Unspecified injury of unspecified muscles, fascia and tendons at forearm level, left arm

✓7ᵗʰ **S56.909** Unspecified injury of unspecified muscles, fascia and tendons at forearm level, unspecified arm

✓6ᵗʰ **S56.91** Strain of unspecified muscles, fascia and tendons at forearm level

✓7ᵗʰ **S56.911** Strain of unspecified muscles, fascia and tendons at forearm level, right arm

✓7ᵗʰ **S56.912** Strain of unspecified muscles, fascia and tendons at forearm level, left arm

✓7ᵗʰ **S56.919** Strain of unspecified muscles, fascia and tendons at forearm level, unspecified arm

✓6ᵗʰ **S56.92** Laceration of unspecified muscles, fascia and tendons at forearm level

✓7ᵗʰ **S56.921** Laceration of unspecified muscles, fascia and tendons at forearm level, right arm

✓7ᵗʰ **S56.922** Laceration of unspecified muscles, fascia and tendons at forearm level, left arm

✓7ᵗʰ **S56.929** Laceration of unspecified muscles, fascia and tendons at forearm level, unspecified arm

✓6ᵗʰ **S56.99** Other injury of unspecified muscles, fascia and tendons at forearm level

✓7ᵗʰ **S56.991** Other injury of unspecified muscles, fascia and tendons at forearm level, right arm

✓7ᵗʰ **S56.992** Other injury of unspecified muscles, fascia and tendons at forearm level, left arm

---

EXCLUDES 1 Not coded here   EXCLUDES 2 Not included here   N Newborn Age: 0   P Pediatric Age: 0-17   M Maternity Age: 12-55   A Adult Age: 15-124

☑7ᵗʰ **S56.999** Other injury of unspecified muscles, fascia and tendons at forearm level, unspecified arm

☑4ᵗʰ **S57** **Crushing injury of elbow and forearm**
Use additional code(s) for all associated injuries
EXCLUDES 2 *crushing injury of wrist and hand (S67.-)*

> The appropriate 7th character is to be added to each code from category S57.
> A   initial encounter
> D   subsequent encounter
> S   sequela

☑5ᵗʰ **S57.0** **Crushing injury of elbow**
  ☑x7ᵗʰ **S57.00** Crushing injury of unspecified elbow
  ☑x7ᵗʰ **S57.01** Crushing injury of right elbow
  ☑x7ᵗʰ **S57.02** Crushing injury of left elbow

☑5ᵗʰ **S57.8** **Crushing injury of forearm**
  ☑x7ᵗʰ **S57.80** Crushing injury of unspecified forearm
  ☑x7ᵗʰ **S57.81** Crushing injury of right forearm
  ☑x7ᵗʰ **S57.82** Crushing injury of left forearm

☑4ᵗʰ **S58** **Traumatic amputation of elbow and forearm**
  NOTE   An amputation not identified as partial or complete should be coded to complete.
  EXCLUDES 1 *traumatic amputation of wrist and hand (S68.-)*

> The appropriate 7th character is to be added to each code from category S58.
> A   initial encounter
> D   subsequent encounter
> S   sequela

☑5ᵗʰ **S58.0** **Traumatic amputation at elbow level**
  ☑6ᵗʰ **S58.01** Complete traumatic amputation at elbow level
    ☑7ᵗʰ **S58.011** Complete traumatic amputation at elbow level, right arm
    ☑7ᵗʰ **S58.012** Complete traumatic amputation at elbow level, left arm
    ☑7ᵗʰ **S58.019** Complete traumatic amputation at elbow level, unspecified arm
  ☑6ᵗʰ **S58.02** Partial traumatic amputation at elbow level
    ☑7ᵗʰ **S58.021** Partial traumatic amputation at elbow level, right arm
    ☑7ᵗʰ **S58.022** Partial traumatic amputation at elbow level, left arm
    ☑7ᵗʰ **S58.029** Partial traumatic amputation at elbow level, unspecified arm

☑5ᵗʰ **S58.1** **Traumatic amputation at level between elbow and wrist**
  ☑6ᵗʰ **S58.11** Complete traumatic amputation at level between elbow and wrist
    ☑7ᵗʰ **S58.111** Complete traumatic amputation at level between elbow and wrist, right arm
    ☑7ᵗʰ **S58.112** Complete traumatic amputation at level between elbow and wrist, left arm
    ☑7ᵗʰ **S58.119** Complete traumatic amputation at level between elbow and wrist, unspecified arm
  ☑6ᵗʰ **S58.12** Partial traumatic amputation at level between elbow and wrist
    ☑7ᵗʰ **S58.121** Partial traumatic amputation at level between elbow and wrist, right arm
    ☑7ᵗʰ **S58.122** Partial traumatic amputation at level between elbow and wrist, left arm
    ☑7ᵗʰ **S58.129** Partial traumatic amputation at level between elbow and wrist, unspecified arm

☑5ᵗʰ **S58.9** **Traumatic amputation of forearm, level unspecified**
  EXCLUDES 1 *traumatic amputation of wrist (S68.-)*
  ☑6ᵗʰ **S58.91** Complete traumatic amputation of forearm, level unspecified
    ☑7ᵗʰ **S58.911** Complete traumatic amputation of right forearm, level unspecified
    ☑7ᵗʰ **S58.912** Complete traumatic amputation of left forearm, level unspecified
    ☑7ᵗʰ **S58.919** Complete traumatic amputation of unspecified forearm, level unspecified

  ☑6ᵗʰ **S58.92** Partial traumatic amputation of forearm, level unspecified
    ☑7ᵗʰ **S58.921** Partial traumatic amputation of right forearm, level unspecified
    ☑7ᵗʰ **S58.922** Partial traumatic amputation of left forearm, level unspecified
    ☑7ᵗʰ **S58.929** Partial traumatic amputation of unspecified forearm, level unspecified

☑4ᵗʰ **S59** **Other and unspecified injuries of elbow and forearm**
  EXCLUDES 2 *other and unspecified injuries of wrist and hand (S69.-)*

> The appropriate 7th character is to be added to each code from subcategories S59.0, S59.1, and S59.2.
> A   initial encounter for closed fracture
> D   subsequent encounter for fracture with routine healing
> G   subsequent encounter for fracture with delayed healing
> K   subsequent encounter for fracture with nonunion
> P   subsequent encounter for fracture with malunion
> S   sequela

☑5ᵗʰ **S59.0** **Physeal fracture of lower end of ulna**
  ☑6ᵗʰ **S59.00** Unspecified physeal fracture of lower end of ulna
    ☑7ᵗʰ **S59.001** Unspecified physeal fracture of lower end of ulna, right arm
    ☑7ᵗʰ **S59.002** Unspecified physeal fracture of lower end of ulna, left arm
    ☑7ᵗʰ **S59.009** Unspecified physeal fracture of lower end of ulna, unspecified arm
  ☑6ᵗʰ **S59.01** Salter-Harris Type I physeal fracture of lower end of ulna
    ☑7ᵗʰ **S59.011** Salter-Harris Type I physeal fracture of lower end of ulna, right arm
    ☑7ᵗʰ **S59.012** Salter-Harris Type I physeal fracture of lower end of ulna, left arm
    ☑7ᵗʰ **S59.019** Salter-Harris Type I physeal fracture of lower end of ulna, unspecified arm
  ☑6ᵗʰ **S59.02** Salter-Harris Type II physeal fracture of lower end of ulna
    ☑7ᵗʰ **S59.021** Salter-Harris Type II physeal fracture of lower end of ulna, right arm
    ☑7ᵗʰ **S59.022** Salter-Harris Type II physeal fracture of lower end of ulna, left arm
    ☑7ᵗʰ **S59.029** Salter-Harris Type II physeal fracture of lower end of ulna, unspecified arm
  ☑6ᵗʰ **S59.03** Salter-Harris Type III physeal fracture of lower end of ulna
    ☑7ᵗʰ **S59.031** Salter-Harris Type III physeal fracture of lower end of ulna, right arm
    ☑7ᵗʰ **S59.032** Salter-Harris Type III physeal fracture of lower end of ulna, left arm
    ☑7ᵗʰ **S59.039** Salter-Harris Type III physeal fracture of lower end of ulna, unspecified arm
  ☑6ᵗʰ **S59.04** Salter-Harris Type IV physeal fracture of lower end of ulna
    ☑7ᵗʰ **S59.041** Salter-Harris Type IV physeal fracture of lower end of ulna, right arm
    ☑7ᵗʰ **S59.042** Salter-Harris Type IV physeal fracture of lower end of ulna, left arm
    ☑7ᵗʰ **S59.049** Salter-Harris Type IV physeal fracture of lower end of ulna, unspecified arm
  ☑6ᵗʰ **S59.09** Other physeal fracture of lower end of ulna
    ☑7ᵗʰ **S59.091** Other physeal fracture of lower end of ulna, right arm
    ☑7ᵗʰ **S59.092** Other physeal fracture of lower end of ulna, left arm
    ☑7ᵗʰ **S59.099** Other physeal fracture of lower end of ulna, unspecified arm

☑5ᵗʰ **S59.1** **Physeal fracture of upper end of radius**
  ☑6ᵗʰ **S59.10** Unspecified physeal fracture of upper end of radius
    ☑7ᵗʰ **S59.101** Unspecified physeal fracture of upper end of radius, right arm
    ☑7ᵗʰ **S59.102** Unspecified physeal fracture of upper end of radius, left arm
    ☑7ᵗʰ **S59.109** Unspecified physeal fracture of upper end of radius, unspecified arm

√6th **S59.11** Salter-Harris Type I physeal fracture of upper end of radius

- √7th **S59.111** Salter-Harris Type I physeal fracture of upper end of radius, right arm
- √7th **S59.112** Salter-Harris Type I physeal fracture of upper end of radius, left arm
- √7th **S59.119** Salter-Harris Type I physeal fracture of upper end of radius, unspecified arm

√6th **S59.12** Salter-Harris Type II physeal fracture of upper end of radius

- √7th **S59.121** Salter-Harris Type II physeal fracture of upper end of radius, right arm
- √7th **S59.122** Salter-Harris Type II physeal fracture of upper end of radius, left arm
- √7th **S59.129** Salter-Harris Type II physeal fracture of upper end of radius, unspecified arm

√6th **S59.13** Salter-Harris Type III physeal fracture of upper end of radius

- √7th **S59.131** Salter-Harris Type III physeal fracture of upper end of radius, right arm
- √7th **S59.132** Salter-Harris Type III physeal fracture of upper end of radius, left arm
- √7th **S59.139** Salter-Harris Type III physeal fracture of upper end of radius, unspecified arm

√6th **S59.14** Salter-Harris Type IV physeal fracture of upper end of radius

- √7th **S59.141** Salter-Harris Type IV physeal fracture of upper end of radius, right arm
- √7th **S59.142** Salter-Harris Type IV physeal fracture of upper end of radius, left arm
- √7th **S59.149** Salter-Harris Type IV physeal fracture of upper end of radius, unspecified arm

√6th **S59.19** Other physeal fracture of upper end of radius

- √7th **S59.191** Other physeal fracture of upper end of radius, right arm
- √7th **S59.192** Other physeal fracture of upper end of radius, left arm
- √7th **S59.199** Other physeal fracture of upper end of radius, unspecified arm

√5th **S59.2** Physeal fracture of lower end of radius

√6th **S59.20** Unspecified physeal fracture of lower end of radius

- √7th **S59.201** Unspecified physeal fracture of lower end of radius, right arm
- √7th **S59.202** Unspecified physeal fracture of lower end of radius, left arm
- √7th **S59.209** Unspecified physeal fracture of lower end of radius, unspecified arm

√6th **S59.21** Salter-Harris Type I physeal fracture of lower end of radius

- √7th **S59.211** Salter-Harris Type I physeal fracture of lower end of radius, right arm
- √7th **S59.212** Salter-Harris Type I physeal fracture of lower end of radius, left arm
- √7th **S59.219** Salter-Harris Type I physeal fracture of lower end of radius, unspecified arm

√6th **S59.22** Salter-Harris Type II physeal fracture of lower end of radius

- √7th **S59.221** Salter-Harris Type II physeal fracture of lower end of radius, right arm
- √7th **S59.222** Salter-Harris Type II physeal fracture of lower end of radius, left arm
- √7th **S59.229** Salter-Harris Type II physeal fracture of lower end of radius, unspecified arm

√6th **S59.23** Salter-Harris Type III physeal fracture of lower end of radius

- √7th **S59.231** Salter-Harris Type III physeal fracture of lower end of radius, right arm
- √7th **S59.232** Salter-Harris Type III physeal fracture of lower end of radius, left arm
- √7th **S59.239** Salter-Harris Type III physeal fracture of lower end of radius, unspecified arm

√6th **S59.24** Salter-Harris Type IV physeal fracture of lower end of radius

- √7th **S59.241** Salter-Harris Type IV physeal fracture of lower end of radius, right arm

- √7th **S59.242** Salter-Harris Type IV physeal fracture of lower end of radius, left arm
- √7th **S59.249** Salter-Harris Type IV physeal fracture of lower end of radius, unspecified arm

√6th **S59.29** Other physeal fracture of lower end of radius

- √7th **S59.291** Other physeal fracture of lower end of radius, right arm
- √7th **S59.292** Other physeal fracture of lower end of radius, left arm
- √7th **S59.299** Other physeal fracture of lower end of radius, unspecified arm

√5th **S59.8** Other specified injuries of elbow and forearm

The appropriate 7th character is to be added to each code in subcategory S59.8.
A　initial encounter
D　subsequent encounter
S　sequela

√6th **S59.80** Other specified injuries of elbow

- √7th **S59.801** Other specified injuries of right elbow
- √7th **S59.802** Other specified injuries of left elbow
- √7th **S59.809** Other specified injuries of unspecified elbow

√6th **S59.81** Other specified injuries of forearm

- √7th **S59.811** Other specified injuries right forearm
- √7th **S59.812** Other specified injuries left forearm
- √7th **S59.819** Other specified injuries unspecified forearm

√5th **S59.9** Unspecified injury of elbow and forearm

The appropriate 7th character is to be added to each code in subcategory S59.9.
A　initial encounter
D　subsequent encounter
S　sequela

√6th **S59.90** Unspecified injury of elbow

- √7th **S59.901** Unspecified injury of right elbow
- √7th **S59.902** Unspecified injury of left elbow
- √7th **S59.909** Unspecified injury of unspecified elbow

√6th **S59.91** Unspecified injury of forearm

- √7th **S59.911** Unspecified injury of right forearm
- √7th **S59.912** Unspecified injury of left forearm
- √7th **S59.919** Unspecified injury of unspecified forearm

Injuries to the wrist, hand and fingers (S60-S69)

EXCLUDES 2　burns and corrosions (T20-T32)
frostbite (T33-T34)
insect bite or sting, venomous (T63.4)

√4th **S60** Superficial injury of wrist, hand and fingers

The appropriate 7th character is to be added to each code from category S60.
A　initial encounter
D　subsequent encounter
S　sequela

√5th **S60.0** Contusion of finger without damage to nail

EXCLUDES 1　contusion involving nail (matrix) (S60.1)

√x7th **S60.00** Contusion of unspecified finger without damage to nail

Contusion of finger(s) NOS

√6th **S60.01** Contusion of thumb without damage to nail

- √7th **S60.011** Contusion of right thumb without damage to nail
- √7th **S60.012** Contusion of left thumb without damage to nail
- √7th **S60.019** Contusion of unspecified thumb without damage to nail

√6th **S60.02** Contusion of index finger without damage to nail

- √7th **S60.021** Contusion of right index finger without damage to nail
- √7th **S60.022** Contusion of left index finger without damage to nail
- √7th **S60.029** Contusion of unspecified index finger without damage to nail

✓6ᵗʰ	**S60.03**	**Contusion of** middle finger **without damage to nail**
✓7ᵗʰ	**S60.031**	**Contusion of** right **middle finger without damage to nail**
✓7ᵗʰ	**S60.032**	**Contusion of** left **middle finger without damage to nail**
✓7ᵗʰ	**S60.039**	**Contusion of unspecified middle finger without damage to nail**
✓6ᵗʰ	**S60.04**	**Contusion of** ring finger **without damage to nail**
✓7ᵗʰ	**S60.041**	**Contusion of** right **ring finger without damage to nail**
✓7ᵗʰ	**S60.042**	**Contusion of** left **ring finger without damage to nail**
✓7ᵗʰ	**S60.049**	**Contusion of unspecified ring finger without damage to nail**
✓6ᵗʰ	**S60.05**	**Contusion of** little finger **without damage to nail**
✓7ᵗʰ	**S60.051**	**Contusion of** right **little finger without damage to nail**
✓7ᵗʰ	**S60.052**	**Contusion of** left **little finger without damage to nail**
✓7ᵗʰ	**S60.059**	**Contusion of unspecified little finger without damage to nail**

✓5ᵗʰ S60.1 Contusion of finger with damage to nail

✓ₓ7ᵗʰ	**S60.10**	**Contusion of unspecified finger with damage to nail**
✓6ᵗʰ	**S60.11**	**Contusion of** thumb with damage to nail
✓7ᵗʰ	**S60.111**	**Contusion of** right **thumb with damage to nail**
✓7ᵗʰ	**S60.112**	**Contusion of** left **thumb with damage to nail**
✓7ᵗʰ	**S60.119**	**Contusion of unspecified thumb with damage to nail**
✓6ᵗʰ	**S60.12**	**Contusion of** index finger with damage to nail
✓7ᵗʰ	**S60.121**	**Contusion of** right **index finger with damage to nail**
✓7ᵗʰ	**S60.122**	**Contusion of** left **index finger with damage to nail**
✓7ᵗʰ	**S60.129**	**Contusion of unspecified index finger with damage to nail**
✓6ᵗʰ	**S60.13**	**Contusion of** middle finger with damage to nail
✓7ᵗʰ	**S60.131**	**Contusion of** right **middle finger with damage to nail**
✓7ᵗʰ	**S60.132**	**Contusion of** left **middle finger with damage to nail**
✓7ᵗʰ	**S60.139**	**Contusion of unspecified middle finger with damage to nail**
✓6ᵗʰ	**S60.14**	**Contusion of** ring finger with damage to nail
✓7ᵗʰ	**S60.141**	**Contusion of** right **ring finger with damage to nail**
✓7ᵗʰ	**S60.142**	**Contusion of** left **ring finger with damage to nail**
✓7ᵗʰ	**S60.149**	**Contusion of unspecified ring finger with damage to nail**
✓6ᵗʰ	**S60.15**	**Contusion of** little finger with damage to nail
✓7ᵗʰ	**S60.151**	**Contusion of** right **little finger with damage to nail**
✓7ᵗʰ	**S60.152**	**Contusion of** left **little finger with damage to nail**
✓7ᵗʰ	**S60.159**	**Contusion of unspecified little finger with damage to nail**

✓5ᵗʰ S60.2 Contusion of wrist and hand

     EXCLUDES 2 *contusion of fingers (S60.0-, S60.1-)*

✓6ᵗʰ	**S60.21**	**Contusion of** wrist
✓7ᵗʰ	**S60.211**	**Contusion of** right **wrist**
✓7ᵗʰ	**S60.212**	**Contusion of** left **wrist**
✓7ᵗʰ	**S60.219**	**Contusion of unspecified wrist**
✓6ᵗʰ	**S60.22**	**Contusion of** hand
✓7ᵗʰ	**S60.221**	**Contusion of** right **hand**
✓7ᵗʰ	**S60.222**	**Contusion of** left **hand**
✓7ᵗʰ	**S60.229**	**Contusion of unspecified hand**

✓5ᵗʰ S60.3 Other superficial injuries of thumb

✓6ᵗʰ	**S60.31**	**Abrasion of** thumb
✓7ᵗʰ	**S60.311**	**Abrasion of** right **thumb**
✓7ᵗʰ	**S60.312**	**Abrasion of** left **thumb**

✓7ᵗʰ	**S60.319**	**Abrasion of unspecified thumb**
✓6ᵗʰ	**S60.32**	**Blister (nonthermal) of** thumb
✓7ᵗʰ	**S60.321**	**Blister (nonthermal) of** right **thumb**
✓7ᵗʰ	**S60.322**	**Blister (nonthermal) of** left **thumb**
✓7ᵗʰ	**S60.329**	**Blister (nonthermal) of unspecified thumb**
✓6ᵗʰ	**S60.34**	**External constriction of** thumb

     Hair tourniquet syndrome of thumb
     Use additional cause code to identify the constricting item (W49.0-)

✓7ᵗʰ	**S60.341**	**External constriction of** right **thumb**
✓7ᵗʰ	**S60.342**	**External constriction of** left **thumb**
✓7ᵗʰ	**S60.349**	**External constriction of unspecified thumb**
✓6ᵗʰ	**S60.35**	**Superficial** foreign body **of thumb**

     Splinter in the thumb

✓7ᵗʰ	**S60.351**	**Superficial foreign body of** right **thumb**
✓7ᵗʰ	**S60.352**	**Superficial foreign body of** left **thumb**
✓7ᵗʰ	**S60.359**	**Superficial foreign body of unspecified thumb**
✓6ᵗʰ	**S60.36**	**Insect bite (nonvenomous) of** thumb
✓7ᵗʰ	**S60.361**	**Insect bite (nonvenomous) of** right **thumb**
✓7ᵗʰ	**S60.362**	**Insect bite (nonvenomous) of** left **thumb**
✓7ᵗʰ	**S60.369**	**Insect bite (nonvenomous) of unspecified thumb**
✓6ᵗʰ	**S60.37**	**Other superficial** bite **of thumb**

     EXCLUDES 1 *open bite of thumb (S61.05-, S61.15-)*

✓7ᵗʰ	**S60.371**	**Other superficial bite of** right **thumb**
✓7ᵗʰ	**S60.372**	**Other superficial bite of** left **thumb**
✓7ᵗʰ	**S60.379**	**Other superficial bite of unspecified thumb**
✓6ᵗʰ	**S60.39**	**Other superficial injuries of** thumb
✓7ᵗʰ	**S60.391**	**Other superficial injuries of** right **thumb**
✓7ᵗʰ	**S60.392**	**Other superficial injuries of** left **thumb**
✓7ᵗʰ	**S60.399**	**Other superficial injuries of unspecified thumb**

✓5ᵗʰ S60.4 Other superficial injuries of other fingers

✓6ᵗʰ	**S60.41**	**Abrasion of** fingers
✓7ᵗʰ	**S60.410**	**Abrasion of** right index **finger**
✓7ᵗʰ	**S60.411**	**Abrasion of** left index **finger**
✓7ᵗʰ	**S60.412**	**Abrasion of** right middle **finger**
✓7ᵗʰ	**S60.413**	**Abrasion of** left middle **finger**
✓7ᵗʰ	**S60.414**	**Abrasion of** right ring **finger**
✓7ᵗʰ	**S60.415**	**Abrasion of** left ring **finger**
✓7ᵗʰ	**S60.416**	**Abrasion of** right little **finger**
✓7ᵗʰ	**S60.417**	**Abrasion of** left little **finger**
✓7ᵗʰ	**S60.418**	**Abrasion of other finger**

     Abrasion of specified finger with unspecified laterality

✓7ᵗʰ	**S60.419**	**Abrasion of unspecified finger**
✓6ᵗʰ	**S60.42**	**Blister (nonthermal) of** fingers
✓7ᵗʰ	**S60.420**	**Blister (nonthermal) of** right index **finger**
✓7ᵗʰ	**S60.421**	**Blister (nonthermal) of** left index **finger**
✓7ᵗʰ	**S60.422**	**Blister (nonthermal) of** right middle **finger**
✓7ᵗʰ	**S60.423**	**Blister (nonthermal) of** left middle **finger**
✓7ᵗʰ	**S60.424**	**Blister (nonthermal) of** right ring **finger**
✓7ᵗʰ	**S60.425**	**Blister (nonthermal) of** left ring **finger**
✓7ᵗʰ	**S60.426**	**Blister (nonthermal) of** right little **finger**
✓7ᵗʰ	**S60.427**	**Blister (nonthermal) of** left little **finger**
✓7ᵗʰ	**S60.428**	**Blister (nonthermal) of other finger**

     Blister (nonthermal) of specified finger with unspecified laterality

✓7ᵗʰ	**S60.429**	**Blister (nonthermal) of unspecified finger**
✓6ᵗʰ	**S60.44**	**External constriction of** fingers

     Hair tourniquet syndrome of finger
     Use additional cause code to identify the constricting item (W49.0-)

✓7ᵗʰ	**S60.440**	**External constriction of** right index **finger**
✓7ᵗʰ	**S60.441**	**External constriction of** left index **finger**
✓7ᵗʰ	**S60.442**	**External constriction of** right middle **finger**
✓7ᵗʰ	**S60.443**	**External constriction of** left middle **finger**

✓ Additional Character Required   ✓ₓ7ᵗʰ Placeholder Alert   Unspecified Dx   Other Specified Dx   Manifestation   ►◄ Revised Text   ● New Code   ▲ Revised Code Title

ICD-10-CM 2016   907

✓7ᵗʰ **S60.444** External constriction of right ring finger

✓7ᵗʰ **S60.445** External constriction of left ring finger

✓7ᵗʰ **S60.446** External constriction of right little finger

✓7ᵗʰ **S60.447** External constriction of left little finger

✓7ᵗʰ **S60.448** **External constriction of other finger**
External constriction of specified finger with unspecified laterality

✓7ᵗʰ **S60.449** **External constriction of unspecified finger**

✓6ᵗʰ **S60.45** **Superficial foreign body of fingers**
Splinter in the finger(s)

✓7ᵗʰ **S60.450** **Superficial foreign body of right index finger**

✓7ᵗʰ **S60.451** **Superficial foreign body of left index finger**

✓7ᵗʰ **S60.452** **Superficial foreign body of right middle finger**

✓7ᵗʰ **S60.453** **Superficial foreign body of left middle finger**

✓7ᵗʰ **S60.454** **Superficial foreign body of right ring finger**

✓7ᵗʰ **S60.455** **Superficial foreign body of left ring finger**

✓7ᵗʰ **S60.456** **Superficial foreign body of right little finger**

✓7ᵗʰ **S60.457** **Superficial foreign body of left little finger**

✓7ᵗʰ **S60.458** **Superficial foreign body of other finger**
Superficial foreign body of specified finger with unspecified laterality

✓7ᵗʰ **S60.459** **Superficial foreign body of unspecified finger**

✓6ᵗʰ **S60.46** **Insect bite (nonvenomous) of fingers**

✓7ᵗʰ **S60.460** **Insect bite (nonvenomous) of right index finger**

✓7ᵗʰ **S60.461** **Insect bite (nonvenomous) of left index finger**

✓7ᵗʰ **S60.462** **Insect bite (nonvenomous) of right middle finger**

✓7ᵗʰ **S60.463** **Insect bite (nonvenomous) of left middle finger**

✓7ᵗʰ **S60.464** **Insect bite (nonvenomous) of right ring finger**

✓7ᵗʰ **S60.465** **Insect bite (nonvenomous) of left ring finger**

✓7ᵗʰ **S60.466** **Insect bite (nonvenomous) of right little finger**

✓7ᵗʰ **S60.467** **Insect bite (nonvenomous) of left little finger**

✓7ᵗʰ **S60.468** **Insect bite (nonvenomous) of other finger**
Insect bite (nonvenomous) of specified finger with unspecified laterality

✓7ᵗʰ **S60.469** **Insect bite (nonvenomous) of unspecified finger**

✓6ᵗʰ **S60.47** **Other superficial bite of fingers**
EXCLUDES 1 open bite of fingers (S61.25-, S61.35-)

✓7ᵗʰ **S60.470** **Other superficial bite of right index finger**

✓7ᵗʰ **S60.471** **Other superficial bite of left index finger**

✓7ᵗʰ **S60.472** **Other superficial bite of right middle finger**

✓7ᵗʰ **S60.473** **Other superficial bite of left middle finger**

✓7ᵗʰ **S60.474** **Other superficial bite of right ring finger**

✓7ᵗʰ **S60.475** **Other superficial bite of left ring finger**

✓7ᵗʰ **S60.476** **Other superficial bite of right little finger**

✓7ᵗʰ **S60.477** **Other superficial bite of left little finger**

✓7ᵗʰ **S60.478** **Other superficial bite of other finger**
Other superficial bite of specified finger with unspecified laterality

✓7ᵗʰ **S60.479** **Other superficial bite of unspecified finger**

✓5ᵗʰ **S60.5** **Other superficial injuries of hand**
EXCLUDES 2 superficial injuries of fingers (S60.3-, S60.4-)

✓6ᵗʰ **S60.51** **Abrasion of hand**

✓7ᵗʰ **S60.511** Abrasion of right hand

✓7ᵗʰ **S60.512** Abrasion of left hand

✓7ᵗʰ **S60.519** **Abrasion of unspecified hand**

✓6ᵗʰ **S60.52** Blister (nonthermal) of hand

✓7ᵗʰ **S60.521** Blister (nonthermal) of right hand

✓7ᵗʰ **S60.522** Blister (nonthermal) of left hand

✓7ᵗʰ **S60.529** Blister (nonthermal) of unspecified hand

✓6ᵗʰ **S60.54** External constriction of hand

✓7ᵗʰ **S60.541** External constriction of right hand

✓7ᵗʰ **S60.542** External constriction of left hand

✓7ᵗʰ **S60.549** External constriction of unspecified hand

✓6ᵗʰ **S60.55** Superficial foreign body of hand
Splinter in the hand

✓7ᵗʰ **S60.551** Superficial foreign body of right hand

✓7ᵗʰ **S60.552** Superficial foreign body of left hand

✓7ᵗʰ **S60.559** **Superficial foreign body of unspecified hand**

✓6ᵗʰ **S60.56** Insect bite (nonvenomous) of hand

✓7ᵗʰ **S60.561** Insect bite (nonvenomous) of right hand

✓7ᵗʰ **S60.562** Insect bite (nonvenomous) of left hand

✓7ᵗʰ **S60.569** Insect bite (nonvenomous) of unspecified hand

✓6ᵗʰ **S60.57** Other superficial bite of hand
EXCLUDES 1 open bite of hand (S61.45-)

✓7ᵗʰ **S60.571** **Other superficial bite of hand of right hand**

✓7ᵗʰ **S60.572** **Other superficial bite of hand of left hand**

✓7ᵗʰ **S60.579** **Other superficial bite of hand of unspecified hand**

✓5ᵗʰ **S60.8** **Other superficial injuries of wrist**

✓6ᵗʰ **S60.81** **Abrasion of wrist**

✓7ᵗʰ **S60.811** Abrasion of right wrist

✓7ᵗʰ **S60.812** Abrasion of left wrist

✓7ᵗʰ **S60.819** Abrasion of unspecified wrist

✓6ᵗʰ **S60.82** Blister (nonthermal) of wrist

✓7ᵗʰ **S60.821** Blister (nonthermal) of right wrist

✓7ᵗʰ **S60.822** Blister (nonthermal) of left wrist

✓7ᵗʰ **S60.829** **Blister (nonthermal) of unspecified wrist**

✓6ᵗʰ **S60.84** External constriction of wrist

✓7ᵗʰ **S60.841** External constriction of right wrist

✓7ᵗʰ **S60.842** External constriction of left wrist

✓7ᵗʰ **S60.849** External constriction of unspecified wrist

✓6ᵗʰ **S60.85** Superficial foreign body of wrist
Splinter in the wrist

✓7ᵗʰ **S60.851** Superficial foreign body of right wrist

✓7ᵗʰ **S60.852** Superficial foreign body of left wrist

✓7ᵗʰ **S60.859** **Superficial foreign body of unspecified wrist**

✓6ᵗʰ **S60.86** Insect bite (nonvenomous) of wrist

✓7ᵗʰ **S60.861** Insect bite (nonvenomous) of right wrist

✓7ᵗʰ **S60.862** Insect bite (nonvenomous) of left wrist

✓7ᵗʰ **S60.869** **Insect bite (nonvenomous) of unspecified wrist**

✓6ᵗʰ **S60.87** Other superficial bite of wrist
EXCLUDES 1 open bite of wrist (S61.55)

✓7ᵗʰ **S60.871** **Other superficial bite of right wrist**

✓7ᵗʰ **S60.872** **Other superficial bite of left wrist**

✓7ᵗʰ **S60.879** **Other superficial bite of unspecified wrist**

✓5ᵗʰ **S60.9** **Unspecified superficial injury of wrist, hand and fingers**

✓6ᵗʰ **S60.91** **Unspecified superficial injury of wrist**

✓7ᵗʰ **S60.911** **Unspecified superficial injury of right wrist**

✓7ᵗʰ **S60.912** **Unspecified superficial injury of left wrist**

✓7ᵗʰ **S60.919** **Unspecified superficial injury of unspecified wrist**

✓6ᵗʰ **S60.92** **Unspecified superficial injury of hand**

✓7ᵗʰ **S60.921** **Unspecified superficial injury of right hand**

✓7ᵗʰ **S60.922** **Unspecified superficial injury of left hand**

✓7ᵗʰ **S60.929** **Unspecified superficial injury of unspecified hand**

EXCLUDES 1 Not coded here   *EXCLUDES 2* Not included here   Ⓝ Newborn Age: 0   Ⓟ Pediatric Age: 0-17   Ⓜ Maternity Age: 12-55   Ⓐ Adult Age: 15-124

908   ICD-10-CM 2016

✓6ᵗʰ **S60.93** **Unspecified superficial injury of** thumb

    ✓7ᵗʰ **S60.931** **Unspecified superficial injury of** right **thumb**

    ✓7ᵗʰ **S60.932** **Unspecified superficial injury of** left **thumb**

    ✓7ᵗʰ **S60.939** **Unspecified superficial injury of unspecified thumb**

✓6ᵗʰ **S60.94** **Unspecified superficial injury of other** fingers

    ✓7ᵗʰ **S60.940** **Unspecified superficial injury of** right index **finger**

    ✓7ᵗʰ **S60.941** **Unspecified superficial injury of** left index **finger**

    ✓7ᵗʰ **S60.942** **Unspecified superficial injury of** right middle **finger**

    ✓7ᵗʰ **S60.943** **Unspecified superficial injury of** left middle **finger**

    ✓7ᵗʰ **S60.944** **Unspecified superficial injury of** right ring **finger**

    ✓7ᵗʰ **S60.945** **Unspecified superficial injury of** left ring **finger**

    ✓7ᵗʰ **S60.946** **Unspecified superficial injury of** right little **finger**

    ✓7ᵗʰ **S60.947** **Unspecified superficial injury of** left little **finger**

    ✓7ᵗʰ **S60.948** **Unspecified superficial injury of other finger**
         Unspecified superficial injury of specified finger with unspecified laterality

    ✓7ᵗʰ **S60.949** **Unspecified superficial injury of unspecified finger**

✓4ᵗʰ **S61** **Open wound of wrist, hand and fingers**
     Code also any associated wound infection
     EXCLUDES 1   open fracture of wrist, hand and finger (S62- with 7th character B)
          traumatic amputation of wrist and hand (S68.-)

> The appropriate 7th character is to be added to each code from category S61.
> A   initial encounter
> D   subsequent encounter
> S   sequela

✓5ᵗʰ **S61.0** **Open wound of** thumb without damage to nail
     EXCLUDES 1   open wound of thumb with damage to nail (S61.1-)

    ✓6ᵗʰ **S61.00** Unspecified **open wound of thumb without damage to nail**

        ✓7ᵗʰ **S61.001** **Unspecified open wound of** right **thumb without damage to nail**

        ✓7ᵗʰ **S61.002** **Unspecified open wound of** left **thumb without damage to nail**

        ✓7ᵗʰ **S61.009** **Unspecified open wound of unspecified thumb without damage to nail**

    ✓6ᵗʰ **S61.01** Laceration without foreign body **of thumb without damage to nail**

        ✓7ᵗʰ **S61.011** **Laceration without foreign body of** right **thumb without damage to nail**

        ✓7ᵗʰ **S61.012** **Laceration without foreign body of** left **thumb without damage to nail**

        ✓7ᵗʰ **S61.019** **Laceration without foreign body of unspecified thumb without damage to nail**

    ✓6ᵗʰ **S61.02** Laceration with foreign body **of thumb without damage to nail**

        ✓7ᵗʰ **S61.021** **Laceration with foreign body of** right **thumb without damage to nail**

        ✓7ᵗʰ **S61.022** **Laceration with foreign body of** left **thumb without damage to nail**

        ✓7ᵗʰ **S61.029** **Laceration with foreign body of unspecified thumb without damage to nail**

    ✓6ᵗʰ **S61.03** Puncture wound without foreign body **of thumb without damage to nail**

        ✓7ᵗʰ **S61.031** **Puncture wound without foreign body of** right **thumb without damage to nail**

        ✓7ᵗʰ **S61.032** **Puncture wound without foreign body of** left **thumb without damage to nail**

        ✓7ᵗʰ **S61.039** **Puncture wound without foreign body of unspecified thumb without damage to nail**

✓6ᵗʰ **S61.04** Puncture wound with foreign body **of thumb without damage to nail**

    ✓7ᵗʰ **S61.041** **Puncture wound with foreign body of** right **thumb without damage to nail**

    ✓7ᵗʰ **S61.042** **Puncture wound with foreign body of** left **thumb without damage to nail**

    ✓7ᵗʰ **S61.049** **Puncture wound with foreign body of unspecified thumb without damage to nail**

✓6ᵗʰ **S61.05** Open bite **of thumb without damage to nail**
     Bite of thumb NOS
     EXCLUDES 1   superficial bite of thumb (S60.36-, S60.37-)

    ✓7ᵗʰ **S61.051** **Open bite of** right **thumb without damage to nail**

    ✓7ᵗʰ **S61.052** **Open bite of** left **thumb without damage to nail**

    ✓7ᵗʰ **S61.059** **Open bite of unspecified thumb without damage to nail**

✓5ᵗʰ **S61.1** **Open wound of** thumb with damage to nail

    ✓6ᵗʰ **S61.10** Unspecified **open wound of thumb with damage to nail**

        ✓7ᵗʰ **S61.101** **Unspecified open wound of** right **thumb with damage to nail**

        ✓7ᵗʰ **S61.102** **Unspecified open wound of** left **thumb with damage to nail**

        ✓7ᵗʰ **S61.109** **Unspecified open wound of unspecified thumb with damage to nail**

    ✓6ᵗʰ **S61.11** Laceration without foreign body **of thumb with damage to nail**

        ✓7ᵗʰ **S61.111** **Laceration without foreign body of** right **thumb with damage to nail**

        ✓7ᵗʰ **S61.112** **Laceration without foreign body of** left **thumb with damage to nail**

        ✓7ᵗʰ **S61.119** **Laceration without foreign body of unspecified thumb with damage to nail**

    ✓6ᵗʰ **S61.12** Laceration with foreign body **of thumb with damage to nail**

        ✓7ᵗʰ **S61.121** **Laceration with foreign body of** right **thumb with damage to nail**

        ✓7ᵗʰ **S61.122** **Laceration with foreign body of** left **thumb with damage to nail**

        ✓7ᵗʰ **S61.129** **Laceration with foreign body of unspecified thumb with damage to nail**

    ✓6ᵗʰ **S61.13** Puncture wound without foreign body **of thumb with damage to nail**

        ✓7ᵗʰ **S61.131** **Puncture wound without foreign body of** right **thumb with damage to nail**

        ✓7ᵗʰ **S61.132** **Puncture wound without foreign body of** left **thumb with damage to nail**

        ✓7ᵗʰ **S61.139** **Puncture wound without foreign body of unspecified thumb with damage to nail**

    ✓6ᵗʰ **S61.14** Puncture wound with foreign body **of thumb with damage to nail**

        ✓7ᵗʰ **S61.141** **Puncture wound with foreign body of** right **thumb with damage to nail**

        ✓7ᵗʰ **S61.142** **Puncture wound with foreign body of** left **thumb with damage to nail**

        ✓7ᵗʰ **S61.149** **Puncture wound with foreign body of unspecified thumb with damage to nail**

    ✓6ᵗʰ **S61.15** Open bite **of thumb** with damage to nail
         Bite of thumb with damage to nail NOS
         EXCLUDES 1   superficial bite of thumb (S60.36-, S60.37-)

        ✓7ᵗʰ **S61.151** **Open bite of** right **thumb with damage to nail**

        ✓7ᵗʰ **S61.152** **Open bite of** left **thumb with damage to nail**

        ✓7ᵗʰ **S61.159** **Open bite of unspecified thumb with damage to nail**

✅ Additional Character Required   ✓x7ᵗʰ Placeholder Alert   Unspecified Dx   Other Specified Dx   Manifestation   ▶◀ Revised Text   ● New Code   ▲ Revised Code Title

Chapter 19. Injury, Poisoning, and Certain Other Consequences of External Causes

✓5ᵗʰ **S61.2 Open wound of** other finger without damage to nail
> *EXCLUDES 1*   open wound of finger involving nail (matrix) (S61.3-)
> *EXCLUDES 2*   open wound of thumb without damage to nail (S61.0-)

✓6ᵗʰ **S61.20** Unspecified **open wound of other finger without damage to nail**

✓7ᵗʰ **S61.200** Unspecified open wound of right index finger without damage to nail

✓7ᵗʰ **S61.201** Unspecified open wound of left index finger without damage to nail

✓7ᵗʰ **S61.202** Unspecified open wound of right middle finger without damage to nail

✓7ᵗʰ **S61.203** Unspecified open wound of left middle finger without damage to nail

✓7ᵗʰ **S61.204** Unspecified open wound of right ring finger without damage to nail

✓7ᵗʰ **S61.205** Unspecified open wound of left ring finger without damage to nail

✓7ᵗʰ **S61.206** Unspecified open wound of right little finger without damage to nail

✓7ᵗʰ **S61.207** Unspecified open wound of left little finger without damage to nail

✓7ᵗʰ **S61.208** Unspecified open wound of other finger without damage to nail
> Unspecified open wound of specified finger with unspecified laterality without damage to nail

✓7ᵗʰ **S61.209** Unspecified open wound of unspecified finger without damage to nail

✓6ᵗʰ **S61.21** Laceration without foreign body of finger without damage to nail

✓7ᵗʰ **S61.210** Laceration without foreign body of right index finger without damage to nail

✓7ᵗʰ **S61.211** Laceration without foreign body of left index finger without damage to nail

✓7ᵗʰ **S61.212** Laceration without foreign body of right middle finger without damage to nail

✓7ᵗʰ **S61.213** Laceration without foreign body of left middle finger without damage to nail

✓7ᵗʰ **S61.214** Laceration without foreign body of right ring finger without damage to nail

✓7ᵗʰ **S61.215** Laceration without foreign body of left ring finger without damage to nail

✓7ᵗʰ **S61.216** Laceration without foreign body of right little finger without damage to nail

✓7ᵗʰ **S61.217** Laceration without foreign body of left little finger without damage to nail

✓7ᵗʰ **S61.218** Laceration without foreign body of other finger without damage to nail
> Laceration without foreign body of specified finger with unspecified laterality without damage to nail

✓7ᵗʰ **S61.219** Laceration without foreign body of unspecified finger without damage to nail

✓6ᵗʰ **S61.22** Laceration with foreign body of finger without damage to nail

✓7ᵗʰ **S61.220** Laceration with foreign body of right index finger without damage to nail

✓7ᵗʰ **S61.221** Laceration with foreign body of left index finger without damage to nail

✓7ᵗʰ **S61.222** Laceration with foreign body of right middle finger without damage to nail

✓7ᵗʰ **S61.223** Laceration with foreign body of left middle finger without damage to nail

✓7ᵗʰ **S61.224** Laceration with foreign body of right ring finger without damage to nail

✓7ᵗʰ **S61.225** Laceration with foreign body of left ring finger without damage to nail

✓7ᵗʰ **S61.226** Laceration with foreign body of right little finger without damage to nail

✓7ᵗʰ **S61.227** Laceration with foreign body of left little finger without damage to nail

✓7ᵗʰ **S61.228** Laceration with foreign body of other finger without damage to nail
> Laceration with foreign body of specified finger with unspecified laterality without damage to nail

✓7ᵗʰ **S61.229** Laceration with foreign body of unspecified finger without damage to nail

✓6ᵗʰ **S61.23** Puncture wound without foreign body of finger without damage to nail

✓7ᵗʰ **S61.230** Puncture wound without foreign body of right index finger without damage to nail

✓7ᵗʰ **S61.231** Puncture wound without foreign body of left index finger without damage to nail

✓7ᵗʰ **S61.232** Puncture wound without foreign body of right middle finger without damage to nail

✓7ᵗʰ **S61.233** Puncture wound without foreign body of left middle finger without damage to nail

✓7ᵗʰ **S61.234** Puncture wound without foreign body of right ring finger without damage to nail

✓7ᵗʰ **S61.235** Puncture wound without foreign body of left ring finger without damage to nail

✓7ᵗʰ **S61.236** Puncture wound without foreign body of right little finger without damage to nail

✓7ᵗʰ **S61.237** Puncture wound without foreign body of left little finger without damage to nail

✓7ᵗʰ **S61.238** Puncture wound without foreign body of other finger without damage to nail
> Puncture wound without foreign body of specified finger with unspecified laterality without damage to nail

✓7ᵗʰ **S61.239** Puncture wound without foreign body of unspecified finger without damage to nail

✓6ᵗʰ **S61.24** Puncture wound with foreign body of finger without damage to nail

✓7ᵗʰ **S61.240** Puncture wound with foreign body of right index finger without damage to nail

✓7ᵗʰ **S61.241** Puncture wound with foreign body of left index finger without damage to nail

✓7ᵗʰ **S61.242** Puncture wound with foreign body of right middle finger without damage to nail

✓7ᵗʰ **S61.243** Puncture wound with foreign body of left middle finger without damage to nail

✓7ᵗʰ **S61.244** Puncture wound with foreign body of right ring finger without damage to nail

✓7ᵗʰ **S61.245** Puncture wound with foreign body of left ring finger without damage to nail

✓7ᵗʰ **S61.246** Puncture wound with foreign body of right little finger without damage to nail

✓7ᵗʰ **S61.247** Puncture wound with foreign body of left little finger without damage to nail

✓7ᵗʰ **S61.248** Puncture wound with foreign body of other finger without damage to nail
> Puncture wound with foreign body of specified finger with unspecified laterality without damage to nail

✓7ᵗʰ **S61.249** Puncture wound with foreign body of unspecified finger without damage to nail

✓6ᵗʰ **S61.25** Open bite of finger without damage to nail
> Bite of finger without damage to nail NOS
> *EXCLUDES 1*   superficial bite of finger (S60.46-, S60.47-)

✓7ᵗʰ **S61.250** Open bite of right index finger without damage to nail

✓7ᵗʰ **S61.251** Open bite of left index finger without damage to nail

✓7ᵗʰ **S61.252** Open bite of right middle finger without damage to nail

✓7ᵗʰ **S61.253** Open bite of left middle finger without damage to nail

✓7ᵗʰ **S61.254** Open bite of right ring finger without damage to nail

✓7ᵗʰ **S61.255** Open bite of left ring finger without damage to nail

✓7ᵗʰ **S61.256** Open bite of right little finger without damage to nail

✓7ᵗʰ **S61.257** Open bite of left little finger without damage to nail

---

EXCLUDES 1 Not coded here   *EXCLUDES 2* Not included here   N Newborn Age: 0   P Pediatric Age: 0-17   M Maternity Age: 12-55   A Adult Age: 15-124

910   ICD-10-CM 2016

☑7ᵗʰ **S61.258 Open bite of other finger without damage to nail**
Open bite of specified finger with unspecified laterality without damage to nail

☑7ᵗʰ **S61.259 Open bite of unspecified finger without damage to nail**

☑5ᵗʰ **S61.3 Open wound of** other finger with damage to nail

☑6ᵗʰ **S61.30 Unspecified open wound of finger with damage to nail**

☑7ᵗʰ **S61.300 Unspecified open wound of** right index finger with damage to nail

☑7ᵗʰ **S61.301 Unspecified open wound of** left index finger with damage to nail

☑7ᵗʰ **S61.302 Unspecified open wound of** right middle finger with damage to nail

☑7ᵗʰ **S61.303 Unspecified open wound of** left middle finger with damage to nail

☑7ᵗʰ **S61.304 Unspecified open wound of** right ring finger with damage to nail

☑7ᵗʰ **S61.305 Unspecified open wound of** left ring **finger with damage to nail**

☑7ᵗʰ **S61.306 Unspecified open wound of** right little finger with damage to nail

☑7ᵗʰ **S61.307 Unspecified open wound of** left little finger with damage to nail

☑7ᵗʰ **S61.308 Unspecified open wound of other finger with damage to nail**
Unspecified open wound of specified finger with unspecified laterality with damage to nail

☑7ᵗʰ **S61.309 Unspecified open wound of unspecified finger with damage to nail**

☑6ᵗʰ **S61.31 Laceration without foreign body of finger with damage to nail**

☑7ᵗʰ **S61.310 Laceration without foreign body of** right index finger with damage to nail

☑7ᵗʰ **S61.311 Laceration without foreign body of** left index finger with damage to nail

☑7ᵗʰ **S61.312 Laceration without foreign body of** right middle finger with damage to nail

☑7ᵗʰ **S61.313 Laceration without foreign body of** left middle finger with damage to nail

☑7ᵗʰ **S61.314 Laceration without foreign body of** right ring finger with damage to nail

☑7ᵗʰ **S61.315 Laceration without foreign body of** left ring finger with damage to nail

☑7ᵗʰ **S61.316 Laceration without foreign body of** right little finger with damage to nail

☑7ᵗʰ **S61.317 Laceration without foreign body of** left little finger with damage to nail

☑7ᵗʰ **S61.318 Laceration without foreign body of other finger with damage to nail**
Laceration without foreign body of specified finger with unspecified laterality with damage to nail

☑7ᵗʰ **S61.319 Laceration without foreign body of unspecified finger with damage to nail**

☑6ᵗʰ **S61.32 Laceration with foreign body of finger with damage to nail**

☑7ᵗʰ **S61.320 Laceration with foreign body of** right index finger with damage to nail

☑7ᵗʰ **S61.321 Laceration with foreign body of** left index finger with damage to nail

☑7ᵗʰ **S61.322 Laceration with foreign body of** right middle finger with damage to nail

☑7ᵗʰ **S61.323 Laceration with foreign body of** left middle finger with damage to nail

☑7ᵗʰ **S61.324 Laceration with foreign body of** right ring finger with damage to nail

☑7ᵗʰ **S61.325 Laceration with foreign body of** left ring finger with damage to nail

☑7ᵗʰ **S61.326 Laceration with foreign body of** right little finger with damage to nail

☑7ᵗʰ **S61.327 Laceration with foreign body of** left little finger with damage to nail

☑7ᵗʰ **S61.328 Laceration with foreign body of other finger with damage to nail**
Laceration with foreign body of specified finger with unspecified laterality with damage to nail

☑7ᵗʰ **S61.329 Laceration with foreign body of unspecified finger with damage to nail**

☑6ᵗʰ **S61.33 Puncture wound without foreign body of finger with damage to nail**

☑7ᵗʰ **S61.330 Puncture wound without foreign body of** right index finger with damage to nail

☑7ᵗʰ **S61.331 Puncture wound without foreign body of** left index finger with damage to nail

☑7ᵗʰ **S61.332 Puncture wound without foreign body of** right middle finger with damage to nail

☑7ᵗʰ **S61.333 Puncture wound without foreign body of** left middle finger with damage to nail

☑7ᵗʰ **S61.334 Puncture wound without foreign body of** right ring finger with damage to nail

☑7ᵗʰ **S61.335 Puncture wound without foreign body of** left ring finger with damage to nail

☑7ᵗʰ **S61.336 Puncture wound without foreign body of** right little finger with damage to nail

☑7ᵗʰ **S61.337 Puncture wound without foreign body of** left little finger with damage to nail

☑7ᵗʰ **S61.338 Puncture wound without foreign body of other finger with damage to nail**
Puncture wound without foreign body of specified finger with unspecified laterality with damage to nail

☑7ᵗʰ **S61.339 Puncture wound without foreign body of unspecified finger with damage to nail**

☑6ᵗʰ **S61.34 Puncture wound with foreign body of finger with damage to nail**

☑7ᵗʰ **S61.340 Puncture wound with foreign body of** right index finger with damage to nail

☑7ᵗʰ **S61.341 Puncture wound with foreign body of** left index finger with damage to nail

☑7ᵗʰ **S61.342 Puncture wound with foreign body of** right middle finger with damage to nail

☑7ᵗʰ **S61.343 Puncture wound with foreign body of** left middle finger with damage to nail

☑7ᵗʰ **S61.344 Puncture wound with foreign body of** right ring finger with damage to nail

☑7ᵗʰ **S61.345 Puncture wound with foreign body of** left ring finger with damage to nail

☑7ᵗʰ **S61.346 Puncture wound with foreign body of** right little finger with damage to nail

☑7ᵗʰ **S61.347 Puncture wound with foreign body of** left little finger with damage to nail

☑7ᵗʰ **S61.348 Puncture wound with foreign body of other finger with damage to nail**
Puncture wound with foreign body of specified finger with unspecified laterality with damage to nail

☑7ᵗʰ **S61.349 Puncture wound with foreign body of unspecified finger with damage to nail**

☑6ᵗʰ **S61.35 Open bite** of finger with damage to nail
Bite of finger with damage to nail NOS
EXCLUDES 1 *superficial bite of finger (S60.46-, S60.47-)*

☑7ᵗʰ **S61.350 Open bite of** right index finger with damage to nail

☑7ᵗʰ **S61.351 Open bite of** left index finger with damage to nail

☑7ᵗʰ **S61.352 Open bite of** right middle finger with damage to nail

☑7ᵗʰ **S61.353 Open bite of** left middle finger with damage to nail

☑7ᵗʰ **S61.354 Open bite of** right ring finger with damage to nail

☑7ᵗʰ **S61.355 Open bite of** left ring finger with damage to nail

☑7ᵗʰ **S61.356 Open bite of** right little finger with damage to nail

☑7ᵗʰ **S61.357 Open bite of** left little finger with damage to nail

☑ Additional Character Required   ☑7ᵗʰ Placeholder Alert   Unspecified Dx   Other Specified Dx   Manifestation   ►◄ Revised Text   ● New Code   ▲ Revised Code Title

ICD-10-CM 2016   911

    ✓7ᵗʰ **S61.358** **Open bite of other finger with damage to nail**

        Open bite of specified finger with unspecified laterality with damage to nail

    ✓7ᵗʰ **S61.359** **Open bite of unspecified finger with damage to nail**

✓5ᵗʰ **S61.4** **Open wound of hand**

   ✓6ᵗʰ **S61.40** **Unspecified open wound of hand**

    ✓7ᵗʰ **S61.401** **Unspecified open wound of right hand**

    ✓7ᵗʰ **S61.402** **Unspecified open wound of left hand**

    ✓7ᵗʰ **S61.409** **Unspecified open wound of unspecified hand**

   ✓6ᵗʰ **S61.41** **Laceration without foreign body of hand**

    ✓7ᵗʰ **S61.411** **Laceration without foreign body of right hand**

    ✓7ᵗʰ **S61.412** **Laceration without foreign body of left hand**

    ✓7ᵗʰ **S61.419** **Laceration without foreign body of unspecified hand**

   ✓6ᵗʰ **S61.42** **Laceration with foreign body of hand**

    ✓7ᵗʰ **S61.421** **Laceration with foreign body of right hand**

    ✓7ᵗʰ **S61.422** **Laceration with foreign body of left hand**

    ✓7ᵗʰ **S61.429** **Laceration with foreign body of unspecified hand**

   ✓6ᵗʰ **S61.43** **Puncture wound without foreign body of hand**

    ✓7ᵗʰ **S61.431** **Puncture wound without foreign body of right hand**

    ✓7ᵗʰ **S61.432** **Puncture wound without foreign body of left hand**

    ✓7ᵗʰ **S61.439** **Puncture wound without foreign body of unspecified hand**

   ✓6ᵗʰ **S61.44** **Puncture wound with foreign body of hand**

    ✓7ᵗʰ **S61.441** **Puncture wound with foreign body of right hand**

    ✓7ᵗʰ **S61.442** **Puncture wound with foreign body of left hand**

    ✓7ᵗʰ **S61.449** **Puncture wound with foreign body of unspecified hand**

   ✓6ᵗʰ **S61.45** **Open bite of hand**

      Bite of hand NOS

      EXCLUDES 1   superficial bite of hand (S60.56-, S60.57-)

    ✓7ᵗʰ **S61.451** **Open bite of right hand**

    ✓7ᵗʰ **S61.452** **Open bite of left hand**

    ✓7ᵗʰ **S61.459** **Open bite of unspecified hand**

✓5ᵗʰ **S61.5** **Open wound of wrist**

   ✓6ᵗʰ **S61.50** **Unspecified open wound of wrist**

    ✓7ᵗʰ **S61.501** **Unspecified open wound of right wrist**

    ✓7ᵗʰ **S61.502** **Unspecified open wound of left wrist**

    ✓7ᵗʰ **S61.509** **Unspecified open wound of unspecified wrist**

   ✓6ᵗʰ **S61.51** **Laceration without foreign body of wrist**

    ✓7ᵗʰ **S61.511** **Laceration without foreign body of right wrist**

    ✓7ᵗʰ **S61.512** **Laceration without foreign body of left wrist**

    ✓7ᵗʰ **S61.519** **Laceration without foreign body of unspecified wrist**

   ✓6ᵗʰ **S61.52** **Laceration with foreign body of wrist**

    ✓7ᵗʰ **S61.521** **Laceration with foreign body of right wrist**

    ✓7ᵗʰ **S61.522** **Laceration with foreign body of left wrist**

    ✓7ᵗʰ **S61.529** **Laceration with foreign body of unspecified wrist**

   ✓6ᵗʰ **S61.53** **Puncture wound without foreign body of wrist**

    ✓7ᵗʰ **S61.531** **Puncture wound without foreign body of right wrist**

    ✓7ᵗʰ **S61.532** **Puncture wound without foreign body of left wrist**

    ✓7ᵗʰ **S61.539** **Puncture wound without foreign body of unspecified wrist**

   ✓6ᵗʰ **S61.54** **Puncture wound with foreign body of wrist**

    ✓7ᵗʰ **S61.541** **Puncture wound with foreign body of right wrist**

    ✓7ᵗʰ **S61.542** **Puncture wound with foreign body of left wrist**

    ✓7ᵗʰ **S61.549** **Puncture wound with foreign body of unspecified wrist**

   ✓6ᵗʰ **S61.55** **Open bite of wrist**

      Bite of wrist NOS

      EXCLUDES 1   superficial bite of wrist (S60.86-, S60.87-)

    ✓7ᵗʰ **S61.551** **Open bite of right wrist**

    ✓7ᵗʰ **S61.552** **Open bite of left wrist**

    ✓7ᵗʰ **S61.559** **Open bite of unspecified wrist**

✓4ᵗʰ **S62** **Fracture at wrist and hand level**

  NOTE   A fracture not indicated as displaced or nondisplaced should be coded to displaced.

      A fracture not indicated as open or closed should be coded to closed.

  EXCLUDES 1   traumatic amputation of wrist and hand (S68.-)

  EXCLUDES 2   fracture of distal parts of ulna and radius (S52.-)

The appropriate 7th character is to be added to each code from category S62.

A   initial encounter for closed fracture
B   initial encounter for open fracture
D   subsequent encounter for fracture with routine healing
G   subsequent encounter for fracture with delayed healing
K   subsequent encounter for fracture with nonunion
P   subsequent encounter for fracture with malunion
S   sequela

✓5ᵗʰ **S62.0** **Fracture of navicular [scaphoid] bone of wrist**

   ✓6ᵗʰ **S62.00** **Unspecified fracture of navicular [scaphoid] bone of wrist**

    ✓7ᵗʰ **S62.001** **Unspecified fracture of navicular [scaphoid] bone of right wrist**

    ✓7ᵗʰ **S62.002** **Unspecified fracture of navicular [scaphoid] bone of left wrist**

      AHA: 2012, 4Q, 106

    ✓7ᵗʰ **S62.009** **Unspecified fracture of navicular [scaphoid] bone of unspecified wrist**

   ✓6ᵗʰ **S62.01** **Fracture of distal pole of navicular [scaphoid] bone of wrist**

      Fracture of volar tuberosity of navicular [scaphoid] bone of wrist

    ✓7ᵗʰ **S62.011** **Displaced fracture of distal pole of navicular [scaphoid] bone of right wrist**

    ✓7ᵗʰ **S62.012** **Displaced fracture of distal pole of navicular [scaphoid] bone of left wrist**

    ✓7ᵗʰ **S62.013** **Displaced fracture of distal pole of navicular [scaphoid] bone of unspecified wrist**

    ✓7ᵗʰ **S62.014** **Nondisplaced fracture of distal pole of navicular [scaphoid] bone of right wrist**

    ✓7ᵗʰ **S62.015** **Nondisplaced fracture of distal pole of navicular [scaphoid] bone of left wrist**

    ✓7ᵗʰ **S62.016** **Nondisplaced fracture of distal pole of navicular [scaphoid] bone of unspecified wrist**

   ✓6ᵗʰ **S62.02** **Fracture of middle third of navicular [scaphoid] bone of wrist**

    ✓7ᵗʰ **S62.021** **Displaced fracture of middle third of navicular [scaphoid] bone of right wrist**

    ✓7ᵗʰ **S62.022** **Displaced fracture of middle third of navicular [scaphoid] bone of left wrist**

    ✓7ᵗʰ **S62.023** **Displaced fracture of middle third of navicular [scaphoid] bone of unspecified wrist**

    ✓7ᵗʰ **S62.024** **Nondisplaced fracture of middle third of navicular [scaphoid] bone of right wrist**

    ✓7ᵗʰ **S62.025** **Nondisplaced fracture of middle third of navicular [scaphoid] bone of left wrist**

    ✓7ᵗʰ **S62.026** **Nondisplaced fracture of middle third of navicular [scaphoid] bone of unspecified wrist**

   ✓6ᵗʰ **S62.03** **Fracture of proximal third of navicular [scaphoid] bone of wrist**

    ✓7ᵗʰ **S62.031** **Displaced fracture of proximal third of navicular [scaphoid] bone of right wrist**

    ✓7ᵗʰ **S62.032** **Displaced fracture of proximal third of navicular [scaphoid] bone of left wrist**

EXCLUDES 1 Not coded here   *EXCLUDES 2* Not included here   N Newborn Age: 0   P Pediatric Age: 0-17   M Maternity Age: 12-55   A Adult Age: 15-124

912   ICD-10-CM 2016

√7ᵗʰ **S62.033** Displaced **fracture of proximal third of navicular [scaphoid] bone of unspecified wrist**

√7ᵗʰ **S62.034** Nondisplaced **fracture of proximal third of navicular [scaphoid] bone of right wrist**

√7ᵗʰ **S62.035** Nondisplaced **fracture of proximal third of navicular [scaphoid] bone of left wrist**

√7ᵗʰ **S62.036** Nondisplaced **fracture of proximal third of navicular [scaphoid] bone of unspecified wrist**

√5ᵗʰ **S62.1** **Fracture of other and unspecified carpal bone(s)**

     EXCLUDES 2   fracture of scaphoid of wrist (S62.0-)

√6ᵗʰ **S62.10** **Fracture of unspecified carpal bone**
     Fracture of wrist NOS

√7ᵗʰ **S62.101** **Fracture of unspecified carpal bone, right wrist**

√7ᵗʰ **S62.102** **Fracture of unspecified carpal bone, left wrist**
     AHA: 2012, 4Q, 95

√7ᵗʰ **S62.109** **Fracture of unspecified carpal bone, unspecified wrist**

√6ᵗʰ **S62.11** **Fracture of triquetrum [cuneiform] bone of wrist**

√7ᵗʰ **S62.111** Displaced **fracture of triquetrum [cuneiform] bone, right wrist**

√7ᵗʰ **S62.112** Displaced **fracture of triquetrum [cuneiform] bone, left wrist**

√7ᵗʰ **S62.113** Displaced **fracture of triquetrum [cuneiform] bone, unspecified wrist**

√7ᵗʰ **S62.114** Nondisplaced **fracture of triquetrum [cuneiform] bone, right wrist**

√7ᵗʰ **S62.115** Nondisplaced **fracture of triquetrum [cuneiform] bone, left wrist**

√7ᵗʰ **S62.116** Nondisplaced **fracture of triquetrum [cuneiform] bone, unspecified wrist**

√6ᵗʰ **S62.12** **Fracture of lunate [semilunar]**

√7ᵗʰ **S62.121** Displaced **fracture of lunate [semilunar], right wrist**

√7ᵗʰ **S62.122** Displaced **fracture of lunate [semilunar], left wrist**

√7ᵗʰ **S62.123** Displaced **fracture of lunate [semilunar], unspecified wrist**

√7ᵗʰ **S62.124** Nondisplaced **fracture of lunate [semilunar], right wrist**

√7ᵗʰ **S62.125** Nondisplaced **fracture of lunate [semilunar], left wrist**

√7ᵗʰ **S62.126** Nondisplaced **fracture of lunate [semilunar], unspecified wrist**

√6ᵗʰ **S62.13** **Fracture of capitate [os magnum] bone**

√7ᵗʰ **S62.131** Displaced **fracture of capitate [os magnum] bone, right wrist**

√7ᵗʰ **S62.132** Displaced **fracture of capitate [os magnum] bone, left wrist**

√7ᵗʰ **S62.133** Displaced **fracture of capitate [os magnum] bone, unspecified wrist**

√7ᵗʰ **S62.134** Nondisplaced **fracture of capitate [os magnum] bone, right wrist**

√7ᵗʰ **S62.135** Nondisplaced **fracture of capitate [os magnum] bone, left wrist**

√7ᵗʰ **S62.136** Nondisplaced **fracture of capitate [os magnum] bone, unspecified wrist**

√6ᵗʰ **S62.14** **Fracture of body of hamate [unciform] bone**
     Fracture of hamate [unciform] bone NOS

√7ᵗʰ **S62.141** Displaced **fracture of body of hamate [unciform] bone, right wrist**

√7ᵗʰ **S62.142** Displaced **fracture of body of hamate [unciform] bone, left wrist**

√7ᵗʰ **S62.143** Displaced **fracture of body of hamate [unciform] bone, unspecified wrist**

√7ᵗʰ **S62.144** Nondisplaced **fracture of body of hamate [unciform] bone, right wrist**

√7ᵗʰ **S62.145** Nondisplaced **fracture of body of hamate [unciform] bone, left wrist**

√7ᵗʰ **S62.146** Nondisplaced **fracture of body of hamate [unciform] bone, unspecified wrist**

√6ᵗʰ **S62.15** **Fracture of hook process of hamate [unciform] bone**
     Fracture of unciform process of hamate [unciform] bone

√7ᵗʰ **S62.151** Displaced **fracture of hook process of hamate [unciform] bone, right wrist**

√7ᵗʰ **S62.152** Displaced **fracture of hook process of hamate [unciform] bone, left wrist**

√7ᵗʰ **S62.153** Displaced **fracture of hook process of hamate [unciform] bone, unspecified wrist**

√7ᵗʰ **S62.154** Nondisplaced **fracture of hook process of hamate [unciform] bone, right wrist**

√7ᵗʰ **S62.155** Nondisplaced **fracture of hook process of hamate [unciform] bone, left wrist**

√7ᵗʰ **S62.156** Nondisplaced **fracture of hook process of hamate [unciform] bone, unspecified wrist**

√6ᵗʰ **S62.16** **Fracture of pisiform**

√7ᵗʰ **S62.161** Displaced **fracture of pisiform, right wrist**

√7ᵗʰ **S62.162** Displaced **fracture of pisiform, left wrist**

√7ᵗʰ **S62.163** Displaced **fracture of pisiform, unspecified wrist**

√7ᵗʰ **S62.164** Nondisplaced **fracture of pisiform, right wrist**

√7ᵗʰ **S62.165** Nondisplaced **fracture of pisiform, left wrist**

√7ᵗʰ **S62.166** Nondisplaced **fracture of pisiform, unspecified wrist**

√6ᵗʰ **S62.17** **Fracture of trapezium [larger multangular]**

√7ᵗʰ **S62.171** Displaced **fracture of trapezium [larger multangular], right wrist**

√7ᵗʰ **S62.172** Displaced **fracture of trapezium [larger multangular], left wrist**

√7ᵗʰ **S62.173** Displaced **fracture of trapezium [larger multangular], unspecified wrist**

√7ᵗʰ **S62.174** Nondisplaced **fracture of trapezium [larger multangular], right wrist**

√7ᵗʰ **S62.175** Nondisplaced **fracture of trapezium [larger multangular], left wrist**

√7ᵗʰ **S62.176** Nondisplaced **fracture of trapezium [larger multangular], unspecified wrist**

√6ᵗʰ **S62.18** **Fracture of trapezoid [smaller multangular]**

√7ᵗʰ **S62.181** Displaced **fracture of trapezoid [smaller multangular], right wrist**

√7ᵗʰ **S62.182** Displaced **fracture of trapezoid [smaller multangular], left wrist**

√7ᵗʰ **S62.183** Displaced **fracture of trapezoid [smaller multangular], unspecified wrist**

√7ᵗʰ **S62.184** Nondisplaced **fracture of trapezoid [smaller multangular], right wrist**

√7ᵗʰ **S62.185** Nondisplaced **fracture of trapezoid [smaller multangular], left wrist**

√7ᵗʰ **S62.186** Nondisplaced **fracture of trapezoid [smaller multangular], unspecified wrist**

√5ᵗʰ **S62.2** **Fracture of first metacarpal bone**

√6ᵗʰ **S62.20** Unspecified **fracture of first metacarpal bone**

√7ᵗʰ **S62.201** **Unspecified fracture of first metacarpal bone, right hand**

√7ᵗʰ **S62.202** **Unspecified fracture of first metacarpal bone, left hand**

√7ᵗʰ **S62.209** **Unspecified fracture of first metacarpal bone, unspecified hand**

√6ᵗʰ **S62.21** Bennett's **fracture**

√7ᵗʰ **S62.211** **Bennett's fracture, right hand**

√7ᵗʰ **S62.212** **Bennett's fracture, left hand**

√7ᵗʰ **S62.213** **Bennett's fracture, unspecified hand**

√6ᵗʰ **S62.22** Rolando's **fracture**

√7ᵗʰ **S62.221** Displaced **Rolando's fracture, right hand**

√7ᵗʰ **S62.222** Displaced **Rolando's fracture, left hand**

√7ᵗʰ **S62.223** Displaced **Rolando's fracture, unspecified hand**

√7ᵗʰ **S62.224** Nondisplaced **Rolando's fracture, right hand**

√7ᵗʰ **S62.225** Nondisplaced **Rolando's fracture, left hand**

☑ Additional Character Required   √7ₓ7ᵗʰ Placeholder Alert   Unspecified Dx   Other Specified Dx   Manifestation   ▶◀ Revised Text   ● New Code   ▲ Revised Code Title

ICD-10-CM 2016   913

✓7th **S62.226** Nondisplaced Rolando's fracture, unspecified hand

✓6th **S62.23** Other fracture of base of first metacarpal bone

✓7th **S62.231** Other displaced fracture of base of first metacarpal bone, right hand

✓7th **S62.232** Other displaced fracture of base of first metacarpal bone, left hand

✓7th **S62.233** Other displaced fracture of base of first metacarpal bone, unspecified hand

✓7th **S62.234** Other nondisplaced fracture of base of first metacarpal bone, right hand

✓7th **S62.235** Other nondisplaced fracture of base of first metacarpal bone, left hand

✓7th **S62.236** Other nondisplaced fracture of base of first metacarpal bone, unspecified hand

✓6th **S62.24** Fracture of shaft of first metacarpal bone

✓7th **S62.241** Displaced fracture of shaft of first metacarpal bone, right hand

✓7th **S62.242** Displaced fracture of shaft of first metacarpal bone, left hand

✓7th **S62.243** Displaced fracture of shaft of first metacarpal bone, unspecified hand

✓7th **S62.244** Nondisplaced fracture of shaft of first metacarpal bone, right hand

✓7th **S62.245** Nondisplaced fracture of shaft of first metacarpal bone, left hand

✓7th **S62.246** Nondisplaced fracture of shaft of first metacarpal bone, unspecified hand

✓6th **S62.25** Fracture of neck of first metacarpal bone

✓7th **S62.251** Displaced fracture of neck of first metacarpal bone, right hand

✓7th **S62.252** Displaced fracture of neck of first metacarpal bone, left hand

✓7th **S62.253** Displaced fracture of neck of first metacarpal bone, unspecified hand

✓7th **S62.254** Nondisplaced fracture of neck of first metacarpal bone, right hand

✓7th **S62.255** Nondisplaced fracture of neck of first metacarpal bone, left hand

✓7th **S62.256** Nondisplaced fracture of neck of first metacarpal bone, unspecified hand

✓6th **S62.29** Other fracture of first metacarpal bone

✓7th **S62.291** Other fracture of first metacarpal bone, right hand

✓7th **S62.292** Other fracture of first metacarpal bone, left hand

✓7th **S62.299** Other fracture of first metacarpal bone, unspecified hand

✓5th **S62.3** Fracture of other and unspecified metacarpal bone

   EXCLUDES 2   fracture of first metacarpal bone (S62.2-)

✓6th **S62.30** Unspecified fracture of other metacarpal bone

✓7th **S62.300** Unspecified fracture of second metacarpal bone, right hand

✓7th **S62.301** Unspecified fracture of second metacarpal bone, left hand

✓7th **S62.302** Unspecified fracture of third metacarpal bone, right hand

✓7th **S62.303** Unspecified fracture of third metacarpal bone, left hand

✓7th **S62.304** Unspecified fracture of fourth metacarpal bone, right hand

✓7th **S62.305** Unspecified fracture of fourth metacarpal bone, left hand

✓7th **S62.306** Unspecified fracture of fifth metacarpal bone, right hand

✓7th **S62.307** Unspecified fracture of fifth metacarpal bone, left hand

✓7th **S62.308** Unspecified fracture of other metacarpal bone

    Unspecified fracture of specified metacarpal bone with unspecified laterality

✓7th **S62.309** Unspecified fracture of unspecified metacarpal bone

✓6th **S62.31** Displaced fracture of base of other metacarpal bone

✓7th **S62.310** Displaced fracture of base of second metacarpal bone, right hand

✓7th **S62.311** Displaced fracture of base of second metacarpal bone, left hand

✓7th **S62.312** Displaced fracture of base of third metacarpal bone, right hand

✓7th **S62.313** Displaced fracture of base of third metacarpal bone, left hand

✓7th **S62.314** Displaced fracture of base of fourth metacarpal bone, right hand

✓7th **S62.315** Displaced fracture of base of fourth metacarpal bone, left hand

✓7th **S62.316** Displaced fracture of base of fifth metacarpal bone, right hand

✓7th **S62.317** Displaced fracture of base of fifth metacarpal bone, left hand

✓7th **S62.318** Displaced fracture of base of other metacarpal bone

    Displaced fracture of base of specified metacarpal bone with unspecified laterality

✓7th **S62.319** Displaced fracture of base of unspecified metacarpal bone

✓6th **S62.32** Displaced fracture of shaft of other metacarpal bone

✓7th **S62.320** Displaced fracture of shaft of second metacarpal bone, right hand

✓7th **S62.321** Displaced fracture of shaft of second metacarpal bone, left hand

✓7th **S62.322** Displaced fracture of shaft of third metacarpal bone, right hand

✓7th **S62.323** Displaced fracture of shaft of third metacarpal bone, left hand

✓7th **S62.324** Displaced fracture of shaft of fourth metacarpal bone, right hand

✓7th **S62.325** Displaced fracture of shaft of fourth metacarpal bone, left hand

✓7th **S62.326** Displaced fracture of shaft of fifth metacarpal bone, right hand

✓7th **S62.327** Displaced fracture of shaft of fifth metacarpal bone, left hand

✓7th **S62.328** Displaced fracture of shaft of other metacarpal bone

    Displaced fracture of shaft of specified metacarpal bone with unspecified laterality

✓7th **S62.329** Displaced fracture of shaft of unspecified metacarpal bone

✓6th **S62.33** Displaced fracture of neck of other metacarpal bone

✓7th **S62.330** Displaced fracture of neck of second metacarpal bone, right hand

✓7th **S62.331** Displaced fracture of neck of second metacarpal bone, left hand

✓7th **S62.332** Displaced fracture of neck of third metacarpal bone, right hand

✓7th **S62.333** Displaced fracture of neck of third metacarpal bone, left hand

✓7th **S62.334** Displaced fracture of neck of fourth metacarpal bone, right hand

✓7th **S62.335** Displaced fracture of neck of fourth metacarpal bone, left hand

✓7th **S62.336** Displaced fracture of neck of fifth metacarpal bone, right hand

✓7th **S62.337** Displaced fracture of neck of fifth metacarpal bone, left hand

✓7th **S62.338** Displaced fracture of neck of other metacarpal bone

    Displaced fracture of neck of specified metacarpal bone with unspecified laterality

✓7th **S62.339** Displaced fracture of neck of unspecified metacarpal bone

EXCLUDES 1 Not coded here   **EXCLUDES 2** Not included here   **N** Newborn Age: 0   **P** Pediatric Age: 0-17   **M** Maternity Age: 12-55   **A** Adult Age: 15-124

914   ICD-10-CM 2016

✓6ᵗʰ **S62.34** Nondisplaced fracture of base of other metacarpal bone

- ✓7ᵗʰ **S62.340** Nondisplaced fracture of base of second metacarpal bone, right hand
- ✓7ᵗʰ **S62.341** Nondisplaced fracture of base of second metacarpal bone, left hand
- ✓7ᵗʰ **S62.342** Nondisplaced fracture of base of third metacarpal bone, right hand
- ✓7ᵗʰ **S62.343** Nondisplaced fracture of base of third metacarpal bone, left hand
- ✓7ᵗʰ **S62.344** Nondisplaced fracture of base of fourth metacarpal bone, right hand
- ✓7ᵗʰ **S62.345** Nondisplaced fracture of base of fourth metacarpal bone, left hand
- ✓7ᵗʰ **S62.346** Nondisplaced fracture of base of fifth metacarpal bone, right hand
- ✓7ᵗʰ **S62.347** Nondisplaced fracture of base of fifth metacarpal bone, left hand
- ✓7ᵗʰ **S62.348** Nondisplaced fracture of base of other metacarpal bone
  - Nondisplaced fracture of base of specified metacarpal bone with unspecified laterality
- ✓7ᵗʰ **S62.349** Nondisplaced fracture of base of unspecified metacarpal bone

✓6ᵗʰ **S62.35** Nondisplaced fracture of shaft of other metacarpal bone

- ✓7ᵗʰ **S62.350** Nondisplaced fracture of shaft of second metacarpal bone, right hand
- ✓7ᵗʰ **S62.351** Nondisplaced fracture of shaft of second metacarpal bone, left hand
- ✓7ᵗʰ **S62.352** Nondisplaced fracture of shaft of third metacarpal bone, right hand
- ✓7ᵗʰ **S62.353** Nondisplaced fracture of shaft of third metacarpal bone, left hand
- ✓7ᵗʰ **S62.354** Nondisplaced fracture of shaft of fourth metacarpal bone, right hand
- ✓7ᵗʰ **S62.355** Nondisplaced fracture of shaft of fourth metacarpal bone, left hand
- ✓7ᵗʰ **S62.356** Nondisplaced fracture of shaft of fifth metacarpal bone, right hand
- ✓7ᵗʰ **S62.357** Nondisplaced fracture of shaft of fifth metacarpal bone, left hand
- ✓7ᵗʰ **S62.358** Nondisplaced fracture of shaft of other metacarpal bone
  - Nondisplaced fracture of shaft of specified metacarpal bone with unspecified laterality
- ✓7ᵗʰ **S62.359** Nondisplaced fracture of shaft of unspecified metacarpal bone

✓6ᵗʰ **S62.36** Nondisplaced fracture of neck of other metacarpal bone

- ✓7ᵗʰ **S62.360** Nondisplaced fracture of neck of second metacarpal bone, right hand
- ✓7ᵗʰ **S62.361** Nondisplaced fracture of neck of second metacarpal bone, left hand
- ✓7ᵗʰ **S62.362** Nondisplaced fracture of neck of third metacarpal bone, right hand
- ✓7ᵗʰ **S62.363** Nondisplaced fracture of neck of third metacarpal bone, left hand
- ✓7ᵗʰ **S62.364** Nondisplaced fracture of neck of fourth metacarpal bone, right hand
- ✓7ᵗʰ **S62.365** Nondisplaced fracture of neck of fourth metacarpal bone, left hand
- ✓7ᵗʰ **S62.366** Nondisplaced fracture of neck of fifth metacarpal bone, right hand
- ✓7ᵗʰ **S62.367** Nondisplaced fracture of neck of fifth metacarpal bone, left hand
- ✓7ᵗʰ **S62.368** Nondisplaced fracture of neck of other metacarpal bone
  - Nondisplaced fracture of neck of specified metacarpal bone with unspecified laterality
- ✓7ᵗʰ **S62.369** Nondisplaced fracture of neck of unspecified metacarpal bone

✓6ᵗʰ **S62.39** Other fracture of other metacarpal bone

- ✓7ᵗʰ **S62.390** Other fracture of second metacarpal bone, right hand
- ✓7ᵗʰ **S62.391** Other fracture of second metacarpal bone, left hand
- ✓7ᵗʰ **S62.392** Other fracture of third metacarpal bone, right hand
- ✓7ᵗʰ **S62.393** Other fracture of third metacarpal bone, left hand
- ✓7ᵗʰ **S62.394** Other fracture of fourth metacarpal bone, right hand
- ✓7ᵗʰ **S62.395** Other fracture of fourth metacarpal bone, left hand
- ✓7ᵗʰ **S62.396** Other fracture of fifth metacarpal bone, right hand
- ✓7ᵗʰ **S62.397** Other fracture of fifth metacarpal bone, left hand
- ✓7ᵗʰ **S62.398** Other fracture of other metacarpal bone
  - Other fracture of specified metacarpal bone with unspecified laterality
- ✓7ᵗʰ **S62.399** Other fracture of unspecified metacarpal bone

✓5ᵗʰ **S62.5** Fracture of thumb

✓6ᵗʰ **S62.50** Fracture of unspecified phalanx of thumb

- ✓7ᵗʰ **S62.501** Fracture of unspecified phalanx of right thumb
- ✓7ᵗʰ **S62.502** Fracture of unspecified phalanx of left thumb
- ✓7ᵗʰ **S62.509** Fracture of unspecified phalanx of unspecified thumb

✓6ᵗʰ **S62.51** Fracture of proximal phalanx of thumb

- ✓7ᵗʰ **S62.511** Displaced fracture of proximal phalanx of right thumb
- ✓7ᵗʰ **S62.512** Displaced fracture of proximal phalanx of left thumb
- ✓7ᵗʰ **S62.513** Displaced fracture of proximal phalanx of unspecified thumb
- ✓7ᵗʰ **S62.514** Nondisplaced fracture of proximal phalanx of right thumb
- ✓7ᵗʰ **S62.515** Nondisplaced fracture of proximal phalanx of left thumb
- ✓7ᵗʰ **S62.516** Nondisplaced fracture of proximal phalanx of unspecified thumb

✓6ᵗʰ **S62.52** Fracture of distal phalanx of thumb

- ✓7ᵗʰ **S62.521** Displaced fracture of distal phalanx of right thumb
- ✓7ᵗʰ **S62.522** Displaced fracture of distal phalanx of left thumb
- ✓7ᵗʰ **S62.523** Displaced fracture of distal phalanx of unspecified thumb
- ✓7ᵗʰ **S62.524** Nondisplaced fracture of distal phalanx of right thumb
- ✓7ᵗʰ **S62.525** Nondisplaced fracture of distal phalanx of left thumb
- ✓7ᵗʰ **S62.526** Nondisplaced fracture of distal phalanx of unspecified thumb

✓5ᵗʰ **S62.6** Fracture of other and unspecified finger(s)

     EXCLUDES 2   fracture of thumb (S62.5-)

✓6ᵗʰ **S62.60** Fracture of unspecified phalanx of finger

- ✓7ᵗʰ **S62.600** Fracture of unspecified phalanx of right index finger
- ✓7ᵗʰ **S62.601** Fracture of unspecified phalanx of left index finger
- ✓7ᵗʰ **S62.602** Fracture of unspecified phalanx of right middle finger
- ✓7ᵗʰ **S62.603** Fracture of unspecified phalanx of left middle finger
- ✓7ᵗʰ **S62.604** Fracture of unspecified phalanx of right ring finger
- ✓7ᵗʰ **S62.605** Fracture of unspecified phalanx of left ring finger
- ✓7ᵗʰ **S62.606** Fracture of unspecified phalanx of right little finger
- ✓7ᵗʰ **S62.607** Fracture of unspecified phalanx of left little finger

---

☑ Additional Character Required   ✓ˣ7ᵗʰ Placeholder Alert   Unspecified Dx   Other Specified Dx   Manifestation   ▶◀ Revised Text   ● New Code   ▲ Revised Code Title

√7ᵗʰ **S62.6Ø8 Fracture of unspecified phalanx of other finger**
Fracture of unspecified phalanx of specified finger with unspecified laterality

√7ᵗʰ **S62.6Ø9 Fracture of unspecified phalanx of unspecified finger**

√6ᵗʰ **S62.61** Displaced **fracture of proximal phalanx** of finger

√7ᵗʰ **S62.61Ø Displaced fracture of proximal phalanx of right index finger**

√7ᵗʰ **S62.611 Displaced fracture of proximal phalanx of left index finger**

√7ᵗʰ **S62.612 Displaced fracture of proximal phalanx of right middle finger**

√7ᵗʰ **S62.613 Displaced fracture of proximal phalanx of left middle finger**

√7ᵗʰ **S62.614 Displaced fracture of proximal phalanx of right ring finger**

√7ᵗʰ **S62.615 Displaced fracture of proximal phalanx of left ring finger**

√7ᵗʰ **S62.616 Displaced fracture of proximal phalanx of right little finger**

√7ᵗʰ **S62.617 Displaced fracture of proximal phalanx of left little finger**

√7ᵗʰ **S62.618 Displaced fracture of proximal phalanx of other finger**
Displaced fracture of proximal phalanx of specified finger with unspecified laterality

√7ᵗʰ **S62.619 Displaced fracture of proximal phalanx of unspecified finger**

√6ᵗʰ **S62.62** Displaced **fracture of medial phalanx** of finger

√7ᵗʰ **S62.62Ø Displaced fracture of medial phalanx of right index finger**

√7ᵗʰ **S62.621 Displaced fracture of medial phalanx of left index finger**

√7ᵗʰ **S62.622 Displaced fracture of medial phalanx of right middle finger**

√7ᵗʰ **S62.623 Displaced fracture of medial phalanx of left middle finger**

√7ᵗʰ **S62.624 Displaced fracture of medial phalanx of right ring finger**

√7ᵗʰ **S62.625 Displaced fracture of medial phalanx of left ring finger**

√7ᵗʰ **S62.626 Displaced fracture of medial phalanx of right little finger**

√7ᵗʰ **S62.627 Displaced fracture of medial phalanx of left little finger**

√7ᵗʰ **S62.628 Displaced fracture of medial phalanx of other finger**
Displaced fracture of medial phalanx of specified finger with unspecified laterality

√7ᵗʰ **S62.629 Displaced fracture of medial phalanx of unspecified finger**

√6ᵗʰ **S62.63** Displaced **fracture of distal phalanx** of finger

√7ᵗʰ **S62.63Ø Displaced fracture of distal phalanx of right index finger**

√7ᵗʰ **S62.631 Displaced fracture of distal phalanx of left index finger**

√7ᵗʰ **S62.632 Displaced fracture of distal phalanx of right middle finger**

√7ᵗʰ **S62.633 Displaced fracture of distal phalanx of left middle finger**

√7ᵗʰ **S62.634 Displaced fracture of distal phalanx of right ring finger**

√7ᵗʰ **S62.635 Displaced fracture of distal phalanx of left ring finger**

√7ᵗʰ **S62.636 Displaced fracture of distal phalanx of right little finger**

√7ᵗʰ **S62.637 Displaced fracture of distal phalanx of left little finger**

√7ᵗʰ **S62.638 Displaced fracture of distal phalanx of other finger**
Displaced fracture of distal phalanx of specified finger with unspecified laterality

√7ᵗʰ **S62.639 Displaced fracture of distal phalanx of unspecified finger**

√6ᵗʰ **S62.64** Nondisplaced **fracture of proximal phalanx** of finger

√7ᵗʰ **S62.64Ø Nondisplaced fracture of proximal phalanx of right index finger**

√7ᵗʰ **S62.641 Nondisplaced fracture of proximal phalanx of left index finger**

√7ᵗʰ **S62.642 Nondisplaced fracture of proximal phalanx of right middle finger**

√7ᵗʰ **S62.643 Nondisplaced fracture of proximal phalanx of left middle finger**

√7ᵗʰ **S62.644 Nondisplaced fracture of proximal phalanx of right ring finger**

√7ᵗʰ **S62.645 Nondisplaced fracture of proximal phalanx of left ring finger**

√7ᵗʰ **S62.646 Nondisplaced fracture of proximal phalanx of right little finger**

√7ᵗʰ **S62.647 Nondisplaced fracture of proximal phalanx of left little finger**

√7ᵗʰ **S62.648 Nondisplaced fracture of proximal phalanx of other finger**
Nondisplaced fracture of proximal phalanx of specified finger with unspecified laterality

√7ᵗʰ **S62.649 Nondisplaced fracture of proximal phalanx of unspecified finger**

√6ᵗʰ **S62.65** Nondisplaced **fracture of medial phalanx** of finger

√7ᵗʰ **S62.65Ø Nondisplaced fracture of medial phalanx of right index finger**

√7ᵗʰ **S62.651 Nondisplaced fracture of medial phalanx of left index finger**

√7ᵗʰ **S62.652 Nondisplaced fracture of medial phalanx of right middle finger**

√7ᵗʰ **S62.653 Nondisplaced fracture of medial phalanx of left middle finger**

√7ᵗʰ **S62.654 Nondisplaced fracture of medial phalanx of right ring finger**

√7ᵗʰ **S62.655 Nondisplaced fracture of medial phalanx of left ring finger**

√7ᵗʰ **S62.656 Nondisplaced fracture of medial phalanx of right little finger**

√7ᵗʰ **S62.657 Nondisplaced fracture of medial phalanx of left little finger**

√7ᵗʰ **S62.658 Nondisplaced fracture of medial phalanx of other finger**
Nondisplaced fracture of medial phalanx of specified finger with unspecified laterality

√7ᵗʰ **S62.659 Nondisplaced fracture of medial phalanx of unspecified finger**

√6ᵗʰ **S62.66** Nondisplaced **fracture of distal phalanx** of finger

√7ᵗʰ **S62.66Ø Nondisplaced fracture of distal phalanx of right index finger**

√7ᵗʰ **S62.661 Nondisplaced fracture of distal phalanx of left index finger**

√7ᵗʰ **S62.662 Nondisplaced fracture of distal phalanx of right middle finger**

√7ᵗʰ **S62.663 Nondisplaced fracture of distal phalanx of left middle finger**

√7ᵗʰ **S62.664 Nondisplaced fracture of distal phalanx of right ring finger**

√7ᵗʰ **S62.665 Nondisplaced fracture of distal phalanx of left ring finger**

√7ᵗʰ **S62.666 Nondisplaced fracture of distal phalanx of right little finger**

√7ᵗʰ **S62.667 Nondisplaced fracture of distal phalanx of left little finger**

√7ᵗʰ **S62.668 Nondisplaced fracture of distal phalanx of other finger**
Nondisplaced fracture of distal phalanx of specified finger with unspecified laterality

√7ᵗʰ **S62.669 Nondisplaced fracture of distal phalanx of unspecified finger**

EXCLUDES 1 Not coded here   **EXCLUDES 2** Not included here   **N** Newborn Age: 0   **P** Pediatric Age: 0-17   **M** Maternity Age: 12-55   **A** Adult Age: 15-124

916

ICD-10-CM 2016

☑5th **S62.9** Unspecified fracture of wrist and hand

√x7th **S62.90** Unspecified fracture of unspecified wrist and hand

√x7th **S62.91** Unspecified fracture of right wrist and hand

√x7th **S62.92** Unspecified fracture of left wrist and hand

☑4th **S63** **Dislocation and sprain of joints and ligaments at wrist and hand level**

INCLUDES avulsion of joint or ligament at wrist and hand level

laceration of cartilage, joint or ligament at wrist and hand level

sprain of cartilage, joint or ligament at wrist and hand level

traumatic hemarthrosis of joint or ligament at wrist and hand level

traumatic rupture of joint or ligament at wrist and hand level

traumatic subluxation of joint or ligament at wrist and hand level

traumatic tear of joint or ligament at wrist and hand level

Code also any associated open wound

EXCLUDES 2 *strain of muscle, fascia and tendon of wrist and hand (S66.-)*

The appropriate 7th character is to be added to each code from category S63.
A   initial encounter
D   subsequent encounter
S   sequela

☑5th **S63.0** **Subluxation and dislocation of** wrist and hand joints

√6th **S63.00** **Unspecified subluxation and dislocation of wrist and hand**

Dislocation of carpal bone NOS
Dislocation of distal end of radius NOS
Subluxation of carpal bone NOS
Subluxation of distal end of radius NOS

√7th **S63.001** **Unspecified** subluxation **of** right **wrist and hand**

√7th **S63.002** **Unspecified** subluxation **of** left **wrist and hand**

√7th **S63.003** **Unspecified** subluxation **of unspecified wrist and hand**

√7th **S63.004** **Unspecified** dislocation **of** right **wrist and hand**

√7th **S63.005** **Unspecified** dislocation **of** left **wrist and hand**

√7th **S63.006** **Unspecified** dislocation **of unspecified wrist and hand**

√6th **S63.01** **Subluxation and dislocation of** distal radioulnar joint

√7th **S63.011** Subluxation **of distal radioulnar joint of** right **wrist**

√7th **S63.012** Subluxation **of distal radioulnar joint of** left **wrist**

√7th **S63.013** Subluxation **of distal radioulnar joint of unspecified wrist**

√7th **S63.014** Dislocation **of distal radioulnar joint of** right **wrist**

√7th **S63.015** Dislocation **of distal radioulnar joint of** left **wrist**

√7th **S63.016** Dislocation **of distal radioulnar joint of unspecified wrist**

√6th **S63.02** **Subluxation and dislocation of** radiocarpal **joint**

√7th **S63.021** Subluxation **of radiocarpal joint of** right **wrist**

√7th **S63.022** Subluxation **of radiocarpal joint of** left **wrist**

√7th **S63.023** Subluxation **of radiocarpal joint of unspecified wrist**

√7th **S63.024** Dislocation **of radiocarpal joint of** right **wrist**

√7th **S63.025** Dislocation **of radiocarpal joint of** left **wrist**

√7th **S63.026** Dislocation **of radiocarpal joint of unspecified wrist**

√6th **S63.03** **Subluxation and dislocation of** midcarpal **joint**

√7th **S63.031** Subluxation **of midcarpal joint of** right **wrist**

√7th **S63.032** Subluxation **of midcarpal joint of** left **wrist**

√7th **S63.033** Subluxation **of midcarpal joint of unspecified wrist**

√7th **S63.034** Dislocation **of midcarpal joint of** right **wrist**

√7th **S63.035** Dislocation **of midcarpal joint of** left **wrist**

√7th **S63.036** Dislocation **of midcarpal joint of unspecified wrist**

√6th **S63.04** **Subluxation and dislocation of** carpometacarpal **joint of** thumb

EXCLUDES 2 *interphalangeal subluxation and dislocation of thumb (S63.1-)*

√7th **S63.041** Subluxation **of carpometacarpal joint of** right **thumb**

√7th **S63.042** Subluxation **of carpometacarpal joint of** left **thumb**

√7th **S63.043** Subluxation **of carpometacarpal joint of unspecified thumb**

√7th **S63.044** Dislocation **of carpometacarpal joint of** right **thumb**

√7th **S63.045** Dislocation **of carpometacarpal joint of** left **thumb**

√7th **S63.046** Dislocation **of carpometacarpal joint of unspecified thumb**

√6th **S63.05** **Subluxation and dislocation of** other carpometacarpal **joint**

EXCLUDES 2 *subluxation and dislocation of carpometacarpal joint of thumb (S63.04-)*

√7th **S63.051** Subluxation **of other carpometacarpal joint of** right **hand**

√7th **S63.052** Subluxation **of other carpometacarpal joint of** left **hand**

√7th **S63.053** Subluxation **of other carpometacarpal joint of unspecified hand**

√7th **S63.054** Dislocation **of other carpometacarpal joint of** right **hand**

√7th **S63.055** Dislocation **of other carpometacarpal joint of** left **hand**

√7th **S63.056** Dislocation **of other carpometacarpal joint of unspecified hand**

√6th **S63.06** **Subluxation and dislocation of** metacarpal (bone), proximal end

√7th **S63.061** Subluxation **of metacarpal (bone), proximal end of** right **hand**

√7th **S63.062** Subluxation **of metacarpal (bone), proximal end of** left **hand**

√7th **S63.063** Subluxation **of metacarpal (bone), proximal end of unspecified hand**

√7th **S63.064** Dislocation **of metacarpal (bone), proximal end of** right **hand**

√7th **S63.065** Dislocation **of metacarpal (bone), proximal end of** left **hand**

√7th **S63.066** Dislocation **of metacarpal (bone), proximal end of unspecified hand**

√6th **S63.07** **Subluxation and dislocation of** distal end of ulna

√7th **S63.071** Subluxation **of distal end of** right **ulna**

√7th **S63.072** Subluxation **of distal end of** left **ulna**

√7th **S63.073** Subluxation **of distal end of unspecified ulna**

√7th **S63.074** Dislocation **of distal end of** right **ulna**

√7th **S63.075** Dislocation **of distal end of** left **ulna**

√7th **S63.076** Dislocation **of distal end of unspecified ulna**

√6th **S63.09** **Other subluxation and dislocation of** wrist and hand

√7th **S63.091** **Other** subluxation **of** right **wrist and hand**

√7th **S63.092** **Other** subluxation **of** left **wrist and hand**

√7th **S63.093** **Other** subluxation **of unspecified wrist and hand**

√7th **S63.094** **Other** dislocation **of** right **wrist and hand**

√7th **S63.095** **Other** dislocation **of** left **wrist and hand**

√7th **S63.096** **Other** dislocation **of unspecified wrist and hand**

☑5th **S63.1** **Subluxation and dislocation of** thumb

√6th **S63.10** **Unspecified subluxation and dislocation of thumb**

√7th **S63.101** **Unspecified** subluxation **of** right **thumb**

√7th **S63.102** **Unspecified** subluxation **of** left **thumb**

☑ Additional Character Required   √x7th Placeholder Alert   Unspecified Dx   Other Specified Dx   Manifestation   ▶◀ Revised Text   ● New Code   ▲ Revised Code Title

√7ᵗʰ **S63.103** Unspecified subluxation of unspecified thumb

√7ᵗʰ **S63.104** Unspecified dislocation of right thumb

√7ᵗʰ **S63.105** Unspecified dislocation of left thumb

√7ᵗʰ **S63.106** Unspecified dislocation of unspecified thumb

√6ᵗʰ **S63.11** Subluxation and dislocation of metacarpophalangeal joint of thumb

√7ᵗʰ **S63.111** Subluxation of metacarpophalangeal joint of right thumb

√7ᵗʰ **S63.112** Subluxation of metacarpophalangeal joint of left thumb

√7ᵗʰ **S63.113** Subluxation of metacarpophalangeal joint of unspecified thumb

√7ᵗʰ **S63.114** Dislocation of metacarpophalangeal joint of right thumb

√7ᵗʰ **S63.115** Dislocation of metacarpophalangeal joint of left thumb

√7ᵗʰ **S63.116** Dislocation of metacarpophalangeal joint of unspecified thumb

√6ᵗʰ **S63.12** Subluxation and dislocation of unspecified interphalangeal joint of thumb

√7ᵗʰ **S63.121** Subluxation of unspecified interphalangeal joint of right thumb

√7ᵗʰ **S63.122** Subluxation of unspecified interphalangeal joint of left thumb

√7ᵗʰ **S63.123** Subluxation of unspecified interphalangeal joint of unspecified thumb

√7ᵗʰ **S63.124** Dislocation of unspecified interphalangeal joint of right thumb

√7ᵗʰ **S63.125** Dislocation of unspecified interphalangeal joint of left thumb

√7ᵗʰ **S63.126** Dislocation of unspecified interphalangeal joint of unspecified thumb

√6ᵗʰ **S63.13** Subluxation and dislocation of proximal interphalangeal joint of thumb

√7ᵗʰ **S63.131** Subluxation of proximal interphalangeal joint of right thumb

√7ᵗʰ **S63.132** Subluxation of proximal interphalangeal joint of left thumb

√7ᵗʰ **S63.133** Subluxation of proximal interphalangeal joint of unspecified thumb

√7ᵗʰ **S63.134** Dislocation of proximal interphalangeal joint of right thumb

√7ᵗʰ **S63.135** Dislocation of proximal interphalangeal joint of left thumb

√7ᵗʰ **S63.136** Dislocation of proximal interphalangeal joint of unspecified thumb

√6ᵗʰ **S63.14** Subluxation and dislocation of distal interphalangeal joint of thumb

√7ᵗʰ **S63.141** Subluxation of distal interphalangeal joint of right thumb

√7ᵗʰ **S63.142** Subluxation of distal interphalangeal joint of left thumb

√7ᵗʰ **S63.143** Subluxation of distal interphalangeal joint of unspecified thumb

√7ᵗʰ **S63.144** Dislocation of distal interphalangeal joint of right thumb

√7ᵗʰ **S63.145** Dislocation of distal interphalangeal joint of left thumb

√7ᵗʰ **S63.146** Dislocation of distal interphalangeal joint of unspecified thumb

√5ᵗʰ **S63.2** Subluxation and dislocation of other finger(s)

EXCLUDES 2 subluxation and dislocation of thumb (S63.1-)

√6ᵗʰ **S63.20** Unspecified subluxation of other finger

√7ᵗʰ **S63.200** Unspecified subluxation of right index finger

√7ᵗʰ **S63.201** Unspecified subluxation of left index finger

√7ᵗʰ **S63.202** Unspecified subluxation of right middle finger

√7ᵗʰ **S63.203** Unspecified subluxation of left middle finger

√7ᵗʰ **S63.204** Unspecified subluxation of right ring finger

√7ᵗʰ **S63.205** Unspecified subluxation of left ring finger

√7ᵗʰ **S63.206** Unspecified subluxation of right little finger

√7ᵗʰ **S63.207** Unspecified subluxation of left little finger

√7ᵗʰ **S63.208** Unspecified subluxation of other finger
Unspecified subluxation of specified finger with unspecified laterality

√7ᵗʰ **S63.209** Unspecified subluxation of unspecified finger

√6ᵗʰ **S63.21** Subluxation of metacarpophalangeal joint of finger

√7ᵗʰ **S63.210** Subluxation of metacarpophalangeal joint of right index finger

√7ᵗʰ **S63.211** Subluxation of metacarpophalangeal joint of left index finger

√7ᵗʰ **S63.212** Subluxation of metacarpophalangeal joint of right middle finger

√7ᵗʰ **S63.213** Subluxation of metacarpophalangeal joint of left middle finger

√7ᵗʰ **S63.214** Subluxation of metacarpophalangeal joint of right ring finger

√7ᵗʰ **S63.215** Subluxation of metacarpophalangeal joint of left ring finger

√7ᵗʰ **S63.216** Subluxation of metacarpophalangeal joint of right little finger

√7ᵗʰ **S63.217** Subluxation of metacarpophalangeal joint of left little finger

√7ᵗʰ **S63.218** Subluxation of metacarpophalangeal joint of other finger
Subluxation of metacarpophalangeal joint of specified finger with unspecified laterality

√7ᵗʰ **S63.219** Subluxation of metacarpophalangeal joint of unspecified finger

√6ᵗʰ **S63.22** Subluxation of unspecified interphalangeal joint of finger

√7ᵗʰ **S63.220** Subluxation of unspecified interphalangeal joint of right index finger

√7ᵗʰ **S63.221** Subluxation of unspecified interphalangeal joint of left index finger

√7ᵗʰ **S63.222** Subluxation of unspecified interphalangeal joint of right middle finger

√7ᵗʰ **S63.223** Subluxation of unspecified interphalangeal joint of left middle finger

√7ᵗʰ **S63.224** Subluxation of unspecified interphalangeal joint of right ring finger

√7ᵗʰ **S63.225** Subluxation of unspecified interphalangeal joint of left ring finger

√7ᵗʰ **S63.226** Subluxation of unspecified interphalangeal joint of right little finger

√7ᵗʰ **S63.227** Subluxation of unspecified interphalangeal joint of left little finger

√7ᵗʰ **S63.228** Subluxation of unspecified interphalangeal joint of other finger
Subluxation of unspecified interphalangeal joint of specified finger with unspecified laterality

√7ᵗʰ **S63.229** Subluxation of unspecified interphalangeal joint of unspecified finger

√6ᵗʰ **S63.23** Subluxation of proximal interphalangeal joint of finger

√7ᵗʰ **S63.230** Subluxation of proximal interphalangeal joint of right index finger

√7ᵗʰ **S63.231** Subluxation of proximal interphalangeal joint of left index finger

√7ᵗʰ **S63.232** Subluxation of proximal interphalangeal joint of right middle finger

√7ᵗʰ **S63.233** Subluxation of proximal interphalangeal joint of left middle finger

√7ᵗʰ **S63.234** Subluxation of proximal interphalangeal joint of right ring finger

√7ᵗʰ **S63.235** Subluxation of proximal interphalangeal joint of left ring finger

EXCLUDES 1 Not coded here   *EXCLUDES 2* Not included here   N Newborn Age: 0   P Pediatric Age: 0-17   M Maternity Age: 12-55   A Adult Age: 15-124

918

ICD-10-CM 2016

√7ᵗʰ **S63.236** **Subluxation of proximal interphalangeal joint of** right little **finger**

√7ᵗʰ **S63.237** **Subluxation of proximal interphalangeal joint of** left little **finger**

√7ᵗʰ **S63.238** **Subluxation of proximal interphalangeal joint of other finger**
Subluxation of proximal interphalangeal joint of specified finger with unspecified laterality

√7ᵗʰ **S63.239** **Subluxation of proximal interphalangeal joint of unspecified finger**

√6ᵗʰ **S63.24** **Subluxation of** distal interphalangeal **joint of finger**

√7ᵗʰ **S63.240** **Subluxation of distal interphalangeal joint of** right index **finger**

√7ᵗʰ **S63.241** **Subluxation of distal interphalangeal joint of** left index **finger**

√7ᵗʰ **S63.242** **Subluxation of distal interphalangeal joint of** right middle **finger**

√7ᵗʰ **S63.243** **Subluxation of distal interphalangeal joint of** left middle **finger**

√7ᵗʰ **S63.244** **Subluxation of distal interphalangeal joint of** right ring **finger**

√7ᵗʰ **S63.245** **Subluxation of distal interphalangeal joint of** left ring **finger**

√7ᵗʰ **S63.246** **Subluxation of distal interphalangeal joint of** right little **finger**

√7ᵗʰ **S63.247** **Subluxation of distal interphalangeal joint of** left little **finger**

√7ᵗʰ **S63.248** **Subluxation of distal interphalangeal joint of other finger**
Subluxation of distal interphalangeal joint of specified finger with unspecified laterality

√7ᵗʰ **S63.249** **Subluxation of distal interphalangeal joint of unspecified finger**

√6ᵗʰ **S63.25** **Unspecified dislocation of** other **finger**

√7ᵗʰ **S63.250** **Unspecified dislocation of** right index **finger**

√7ᵗʰ **S63.251** **Unspecified dislocation of** left index **finger**

√7ᵗʰ **S63.252** **Unspecified dislocation of** right middle **finger**

√7ᵗʰ **S63.253** **Unspecified dislocation of** left middle **finger**

√7ᵗʰ **S63.254** **Unspecified dislocation of** right ring **finger**

√7ᵗʰ **S63.255** **Unspecified dislocation of** left ring **finger**

√7ᵗʰ **S63.256** **Unspecified dislocation of** right little **finger**

√7ᵗʰ **S63.257** **Unspecified dislocation of** left little **finger**

√7ᵗʰ **S63.258** **Unspecified dislocation of other finger**
Unspecified dislocation of specified finger with unspecified laterality

√7ᵗʰ **S63.259** **Unspecified dislocation of unspecified finger**
Unspecified dislocation of specified finger with unspecified laterality

√6ᵗʰ **S63.26** **Dislocation of** metacarpophalangeal joint **of finger**

√7ᵗʰ **S63.260** **Dislocation of metacarpophalangeal joint of** right index **finger**

√7ᵗʰ **S63.261** **Dislocation of metacarpophalangeal joint of** left index **finger**

√7ᵗʰ **S63.262** **Dislocation of metacarpophalangeal joint of** right middle **finger**

√7ᵗʰ **S63.263** **Dislocation of metacarpophalangeal joint of** left middle **finger**

√7ᵗʰ **S63.264** **Dislocation of metacarpophalangeal joint of** right ring **finger**

√7ᵗʰ **S63.265** **Dislocation of metacarpophalangeal joint of** left ring **finger**

√7ᵗʰ **S63.266** **Dislocation of metacarpophalangeal joint of** right little **finger**

√7ᵗʰ **S63.267** **Dislocation of metacarpophalangeal joint of** left little **finger**

√7ᵗʰ **S63.268** **Dislocation of metacarpophalangeal joint of other finger**
Dislocation of metacarpophalangeal joint of specified finger with unspecified laterality

√7ᵗʰ **S63.269** **Dislocation of metacarpophalangeal joint of unspecified finger**

√6ᵗʰ **S63.27** **Dislocation of unspecified** interphalangeal joint **of finger**

√7ᵗʰ **S63.270** **Dislocation of unspecified interphalangeal joint of** right index **finger**

√7ᵗʰ **S63.271** **Dislocation of unspecified interphalangeal joint of** left index **finger**

√7ᵗʰ **S63.272** **Dislocation of unspecified interphalangeal joint of** right middle **finger**

√7ᵗʰ **S63.273** **Dislocation of unspecified interphalangeal joint of** left middle **finger**

√7ᵗʰ **S63.274** **Dislocation of unspecified interphalangeal joint of** right ring **finger**

√7ᵗʰ **S63.275** **Dislocation of unspecified interphalangeal joint of** left ring **finger**

√7ᵗʰ **S63.276** **Dislocation of unspecified interphalangeal joint of** right little **finger**

√7ᵗʰ **S63.277** **Dislocation of unspecified interphalangeal joint of** left little **finger**

√7ᵗʰ **S63.278** **Dislocation of unspecified interphalangeal joint of other finger**
Dislocation of unspecified interphalangeal joint of specified finger with unspecified laterality

√7ᵗʰ **S63.279** **Dislocation of unspecified interphalangeal joint of unspecified finger**
Dislocation of unspecified interphalangeal joint of specified finger without specified laterality

√6ᵗʰ **S63.28** **Dislocation of** proximal interphalangeal joint **of finger**

√7ᵗʰ **S63.280** **Dislocation of proximal interphalangeal joint of** right index **finger**

√7ᵗʰ **S63.281** **Dislocation of proximal interphalangeal joint of** left index **finger**

√7ᵗʰ **S63.282** **Dislocation of proximal interphalangeal joint of** right middle **finger**

√7ᵗʰ **S63.283** **Dislocation of proximal interphalangeal joint of** left middle **finger**

√7ᵗʰ **S63.284** **Dislocation of proximal interphalangeal joint of** right ring **finger**

√7ᵗʰ **S63.285** **Dislocation of proximal interphalangeal joint of** left ring **finger**

√7ᵗʰ **S63.286** **Dislocation of proximal interphalangeal joint of** right little **finger**

√7ᵗʰ **S63.287** **Dislocation of proximal interphalangeal joint of** left little **finger**

√7ᵗʰ **S63.288** **Dislocation of proximal interphalangeal joint of other finger**
Dislocation of proximal interphalangeal joint of specified finger with unspecified laterality

√7ᵗʰ **S63.289** **Dislocation of proximal interphalangeal joint of unspecified finger**

√6ᵗʰ **S63.29** **Dislocation of** distal interphalangeal joint **of finger**

√7ᵗʰ **S63.290** **Dislocation of distal interphalangeal joint of** right index **finger**

√7ᵗʰ **S63.291** **Dislocation of distal interphalangeal joint of** left index **finger**

√7ᵗʰ **S63.292** **Dislocation of distal interphalangeal joint of** right middle **finger**

√7ᵗʰ **S63.293** **Dislocation of distal interphalangeal joint of** left middle **finger**

√7ᵗʰ **S63.294** **Dislocation of distal interphalangeal joint of** right ring **finger**

√7ᵗʰ **S63.295** **Dislocation of distal interphalangeal joint of** left ring **finger**

√7ᵗʰ **S63.296** **Dislocation of distal interphalangeal joint of** right little **finger**

Chapter 19. Injury, Poisoning, and Certain Other Consequences of External Causes

S63.297 Dislocation of distal interphalangeal joint of left little finger

S63.298 Dislocation of distal interphalangeal joint of other finger
Dislocation of distal interphalangeal joint of specified finger with unspecified laterality

S63.299 Dislocation of distal interphalangeal joint of unspecified finger

S63.3 Traumatic rupture of ligament of wrist

  S63.30 Traumatic rupture of unspecified ligament of wrist

    S63.301 Traumatic rupture of unspecified ligament of right wrist

    S63.302 Traumatic rupture of unspecified ligament of left wrist

    S63.309 Traumatic rupture of unspecified ligament of unspecified wrist

  S63.31 Traumatic rupture of collateral ligament of wrist

    S63.311 Traumatic rupture of collateral ligament of right wrist

    S63.312 Traumatic rupture of collateral ligament of left wrist

    S63.319 Traumatic rupture of collateral ligament of unspecified wrist

  S63.32 Traumatic rupture of radiocarpal ligament

    S63.321 Traumatic rupture of right radiocarpal ligament

    S63.322 Traumatic rupture of left radiocarpal ligament

    S63.329 Traumatic rupture of unspecified radiocarpal ligament

  S63.33 Traumatic rupture of ulnocarpal (palmar) ligament

    S63.331 Traumatic rupture of right ulnocarpal (palmar) ligament

    S63.332 Traumatic rupture of left ulnocarpal (palmar) ligament

    S63.339 Traumatic rupture of unspecified ulnocarpal (palmar) ligament

  S63.39 Traumatic rupture of other ligament of wrist

    S63.391 Traumatic rupture of other ligament of right wrist

    S63.392 Traumatic rupture of other ligament of left wrist

    S63.399 Traumatic rupture of other ligament of unspecified wrist

S63.4 Traumatic rupture of ligament of finger at metacarpophalangeal and interphalangeal joint(s)

  S63.40 Traumatic rupture of unspecified ligament of finger at metacarpophalangeal and interphalangeal joint

    S63.400 Traumatic rupture of unspecified ligament of right index finger at metacarpophalangeal and interphalangeal joint

    S63.401 Traumatic rupture of unspecified ligament of left index finger at metacarpophalangeal and interphalangeal joint

    S63.402 Traumatic rupture of unspecified ligament of right middle finger at metacarpophalangeal and interphalangeal joint

    S63.403 Traumatic rupture of unspecified ligament of left middle finger at metacarpophalangeal and interphalangeal joint

    S63.404 Traumatic rupture of unspecified ligament of right ring finger at metacarpophalangeal and interphalangeal joint

    S63.405 Traumatic rupture of unspecified ligament of left ring finger at metacarpophalangeal and interphalangeal joint

    S63.406 Traumatic rupture of unspecified ligament of right little finger at metacarpophalangeal and interphalangeal joint

    S63.407 Traumatic rupture of unspecified ligament of left little finger at metacarpophalangeal and interphalangeal joint

    S63.408 Traumatic rupture of unspecified ligament of other finger at metacarpophalangeal and interphalangeal joint
Traumatic rupture of unspecified ligament of specified finger with unspecified laterality at metacarpophalangeal and interphalangeal joint

    S63.409 Traumatic rupture of unspecified ligament of unspecified finger at metacarpophalangeal and interphalangeal joint

  S63.41 Traumatic rupture of collateral ligament of finger at metacarpophalangeal and interphalangeal joint

    S63.410 Traumatic rupture of collateral ligament of right index finger at metacarpophalangeal and interphalangeal joint

    S63.411 Traumatic rupture of collateral ligament of left index finger at metacarpophalangeal and interphalangeal joint

    S63.412 Traumatic rupture of collateral ligament of right middle finger at metacarpophalangeal and interphalangeal joint

    S63.413 Traumatic rupture of collateral ligament of left middle finger at metacarpophalangeal and interphalangeal joint

    S63.414 Traumatic rupture of collateral ligament of right ring finger at metacarpophalangeal and interphalangeal joint

    S63.415 Traumatic rupture of collateral ligament of left ring finger at metacarpophalangeal and interphalangeal joint

    S63.416 Traumatic rupture of collateral ligament of right little finger at metacarpophalangeal and interphalangeal joint

    S63.417 Traumatic rupture of collateral ligament of left little finger at metacarpophalangeal and interphalangeal joint

    S63.418 Traumatic rupture of collateral ligament of other finger at metacarpophalangeal and interphalangeal joint
Traumatic rupture of collateral ligament of specified finger with unspecified laterality at metacarpophalangeal and interphalangeal joint

    S63.419 Traumatic rupture of collateral ligament of unspecified finger at metacarpophalangeal and interphalangeal joint

  S63.42 Traumatic rupture of palmar ligament of finger at metacarpophalangeal and interphalangeal joint

    S63.420 Traumatic rupture of palmar ligament of right index finger at metacarpophalangeal and interphalangeal joint

    S63.421 Traumatic rupture of palmar ligament of left index finger at metacarpophalangeal and interphalangeal joint

    S63.422 Traumatic rupture of palmar ligament of right middle finger at metacarpophalangeal and interphalangeal joint

    S63.423 Traumatic rupture of palmar ligament of left middle finger at metacarpophalangeal and interphalangeal joint

    S63.424 Traumatic rupture of palmar ligament of right ring finger at metacarpophalangeal and interphalangeal joint

    S63.425 Traumatic rupture of palmar ligament of left ring finger at metacarpophalangeal and interphalangeal joint

    S63.426 Traumatic rupture of palmar ligament of right little finger at metacarpophalangeal and interphalangeal joint

    S63.427 Traumatic rupture of palmar ligament of left little finger at metacarpophalangeal and interphalangeal joint

    S63.428 Traumatic rupture of palmar ligament of other finger at metacarpophalangeal and interphalangeal joint
Traumatic rupture of palmar ligament of specified finger with unspecified laterality at metacarpophalangeal and interphalangeal joint

EXCLUDES 1 Not coded here   EXCLUDES 2 Not included here   N Newborn Age: 0   P Pediatric Age: 0-17   M Maternity Age: 12-55   A Adult Age: 15-124

920   ICD-10-CM 2016

√7ᵗʰ **S63.429** Traumatic rupture of palmar ligament of unspecified finger at metacarpophalangeal and interphalangeal joint

√6ᵗʰ **S63.43** Traumatic rupture of volar plate of finger at metacarpophalangeal and interphalangeal joint

√7ᵗʰ **S63.430** Traumatic rupture of volar plate of right index finger at metacarpophalangeal and interphalangeal joint

√7ᵗʰ **S63.431** Traumatic rupture of volar plate of left index finger at metacarpophalangeal and interphalangeal joint

√7ᵗʰ **S63.432** Traumatic rupture of volar plate of right middle finger at metacarpophalangeal and interphalangeal joint

√7ᵗʰ **S63.433** Traumatic rupture of volar plate of left middle finger at metacarpophalangeal and interphalangeal joint

√7ᵗʰ **S63.434** Traumatic rupture of volar plate of right ring finger at metacarpophalangeal and interphalangeal joint

√7ᵗʰ **S63.435** Traumatic rupture of volar plate of left ring finger at metacarpophalangeal and interphalangeal joint

√7ᵗʰ **S63.436** Traumatic rupture of volar plate of right little finger at metacarpophalangeal and interphalangeal joint

√7ᵗʰ **S63.437** Traumatic rupture of volar plate of left little finger at metacarpophalangeal and interphalangeal joint

√7ᵗʰ **S63.438** Traumatic rupture of volar plate of other finger at metacarpophalangeal and interphalangeal joint

Traumatic rupture of volar plate of specified finger with unspecified laterality at metacarpophalangeal and interphalangeal joint

√7ᵗʰ **S63.439** Traumatic rupture of volar plate of unspecified finger at metacarpophalangeal and interphalangeal joint

√6ᵗʰ **S63.49** Traumatic rupture of other ligament of finger at metacarpophalangeal and interphalangeal joint

√7ᵗʰ **S63.490** Traumatic rupture of other ligament of right index finger at metacarpophalangeal and interphalangeal joint

√7ᵗʰ **S63.491** Traumatic rupture of other ligament of left index finger at metacarpophalangeal and interphalangeal joint

√7ᵗʰ **S63.492** Traumatic rupture of other ligament of right middle finger at metacarpophalangeal and interphalangeal joint

√7ᵗʰ **S63.493** Traumatic rupture of other ligament of left middle finger at metacarpophalangeal and interphalangeal joint

√7ᵗʰ **S63.494** Traumatic rupture of other ligament of right ring finger at metacarpophalangeal and interphalangeal joint

√7ᵗʰ **S63.495** Traumatic rupture of other ligament of left ring finger at metacarpophalangeal and interphalangeal joint

√7ᵗʰ **S63.496** Traumatic rupture of other ligament of right little finger at metacarpophalangeal and interphalangeal joint

√7ᵗʰ **S63.497** Traumatic rupture of other ligament of left little finger at metacarpophalangeal and interphalangeal joint

√7ᵗʰ **S63.498** Traumatic rupture of other ligament of other finger at metacarpophalangeal and interphalangeal joint

Traumatic rupture of ligament of specified finger with unspecified laterality at metacarpophalangeal and interphalangeal joint

√7ᵗʰ **S63.499** Traumatic rupture of other ligament of unspecified finger at metacarpophalangeal and interphalangeal joint

√5ᵗʰ **S63.5** Other and unspecified sprain of wrist

√6ᵗʰ **S63.50** Unspecified sprain of wrist

√7ᵗʰ **S63.501** Unspecified sprain of right wrist

√7ᵗʰ **S63.502** Unspecified sprain of left wrist

√7ᵗʰ **S63.509** Unspecified sprain of unspecified wrist

√6ᵗʰ **S63.51** Sprain of carpal (joint)

√7ᵗʰ **S63.511** Sprain of carpal joint of right wrist

√7ᵗʰ **S63.512** Sprain of carpal joint of left wrist

√7ᵗʰ **S63.519** Sprain of carpal joint of unspecified wrist

√6ᵗʰ **S63.52** Sprain of radiocarpal joint

EXCLUDES 1   *traumatic rupture of radiocarpal ligament (S63.32-)*

√7ᵗʰ **S63.521** Sprain of radiocarpal joint of right wrist

√7ᵗʰ **S63.522** Sprain of radiocarpal joint of left wrist

√7ᵗʰ **S63.529** Sprain of radiocarpal joint of unspecified wrist

√6ᵗʰ **S63.59** Other specified sprain of wrist

√7ᵗʰ **S63.591** Other specified sprain of right wrist

√7ᵗʰ **S63.592** Other specified sprain of left wrist

√7ᵗʰ **S63.599** Other specified sprain of unspecified wrist

√5ᵗʰ **S63.6** Other and unspecified sprain of finger(s)

EXCLUDES 1   *traumatic rupture of ligament of finger at metacarpophalangeal and interphalangeal joint(s) (S63.4-)*

√6ᵗʰ **S63.60** Unspecified sprain of thumb

√7ᵗʰ **S63.601** Unspecified sprain of right thumb

√7ᵗʰ **S63.602** Unspecified sprain of left thumb

√7ᵗʰ **S63.609** Unspecified sprain of unspecified thumb

√6ᵗʰ **S63.61** Unspecified sprain of other and unspecified finger(s)

√7ᵗʰ **S63.610** Unspecified sprain of right index finger

√7ᵗʰ **S63.611** Unspecified sprain of left index finger

√7ᵗʰ **S63.612** Unspecified sprain of right middle finger

√7ᵗʰ **S63.613** Unspecified sprain of left middle finger

√7ᵗʰ **S63.614** Unspecified sprain of right ring finger

√7ᵗʰ **S63.615** Unspecified sprain of left ring finger

√7ᵗʰ **S63.616** Unspecified sprain of right little finger

√7ᵗʰ **S63.617** Unspecified sprain of left little finger

√7ᵗʰ **S63.618** Unspecified sprain of other finger

Unspecified sprain of specified finger with unspecified laterality

√7ᵗʰ **S63.619** Unspecified sprain of unspecified finger

√6ᵗʰ **S63.62** Sprain of interphalangeal joint of thumb

√7ᵗʰ **S63.621** Sprain of interphalangeal joint of right thumb

√7ᵗʰ **S63.622** Sprain of interphalangeal joint of left thumb

√7ᵗʰ **S63.629** Sprain of interphalangeal joint of unspecified thumb

√6ᵗʰ **S63.63** Sprain of interphalangeal joint of other and unspecified finger(s)

√7ᵗʰ **S63.630** Sprain of interphalangeal joint of right index finger

√7ᵗʰ **S63.631** Sprain of interphalangeal joint of left index finger

√7ᵗʰ **S63.632** Sprain of interphalangeal joint of right middle finger

√7ᵗʰ **S63.633** Sprain of interphalangeal joint of left middle finger

√7ᵗʰ **S63.634** Sprain of interphalangeal joint of right ring finger

√7ᵗʰ **S63.635** Sprain of interphalangeal joint of left ring finger

√7ᵗʰ **S63.636** Sprain of interphalangeal joint of right little finger

√7ᵗʰ **S63.637** Sprain of interphalangeal joint of left little finger

√7ᵗʰ **S63.638** Sprain of interphalangeal joint of other finger

√7ᵗʰ **S63.639** Sprain of interphalangeal joint of unspecified finger

√6ᵗʰ **S63.64** Sprain of metacarpophalangeal joint of thumb

√7ᵗʰ **S63.641** Sprain of metacarpophalangeal joint of right thumb

√7ᵗʰ **S63.642** Sprain of metacarpophalangeal joint of left thumb

---

☑ Additional Character Required   √ₓ7ᵗʰ Placeholder Alert   Unspecified Dx   Other Specified Dx   Manifestation   ▶◀ Revised Text   ● New Code   ▲ Revised Code Title

√7ᵗʰ **S63.649** **Sprain of metacarpophalangeal joint of unspecified thumb**

√6ᵗʰ **S63.65** Sprain of metacarpophalangeal joint of other and unspecified finger(s)

√7ᵗʰ **S63.650** **Sprain of metacarpophalangeal joint of right index finger**

√7ᵗʰ **S63.651** **Sprain of metacarpophalangeal joint of left index finger**

√7ᵗʰ **S63.652** **Sprain of metacarpophalangeal joint of right middle finger**

√7ᵗʰ **S63.653** **Sprain of metacarpophalangeal joint of left middle finger**

√7ᵗʰ **S63.654** **Sprain of metacarpophalangeal joint of right ring finger**

√7ᵗʰ **S63.655** **Sprain of metacarpophalangeal joint of left ring finger**

√7ᵗʰ **S63.656** **Sprain of metacarpophalangeal joint of right little finger**

√7ᵗʰ **S63.657** **Sprain of metacarpophalangeal joint of left little finger**

√7ᵗʰ **S63.658** **Sprain of metacarpophalangeal joint of other finger**
Sprain of metacarpophalangeal joint of specified finger with unspecified laterality

√7ᵗʰ **S63.659** **Sprain of metacarpophalangeal joint of unspecified finger**

√6ᵗʰ **S63.68** **Other sprain of thumb**

√7ᵗʰ **S63.681** **Other sprain of right thumb**

√7ᵗʰ **S63.682** **Other sprain of left thumb**

√7ᵗʰ **S63.689** **Other sprain of unspecified thumb**

√6ᵗʰ **S63.69** **Other sprain of other and unspecified finger(s)**

√7ᵗʰ **S63.690** **Other sprain of right index finger**

√7ᵗʰ **S63.691** **Other sprain of left index finger**

√7ᵗʰ **S63.692** **Other sprain of right middle finger**

√7ᵗʰ **S63.693** **Other sprain of left middle finger**

√7ᵗʰ **S63.694** **Other sprain of right ring finger**

√7ᵗʰ **S63.695** **Other sprain of left ring finger**

√7ᵗʰ **S63.696** **Other sprain of right little finger**

√7ᵗʰ **S63.697** **Other sprain of left little finger**

√7ᵗʰ **S63.698** **Other sprain of other finger**
Other sprain of specified finger with unspecified laterality

√7ᵗʰ **S63.699** **Other sprain of unspecified finger**

√5ᵗʰ **S63.8** Sprain of other part of wrist and hand

√6ᵗʰ **S63.8X** Sprain of other part of wrist and hand

√7ᵗʰ **S63.8X1** **Sprain of other part of right wrist and hand**

√7ᵗʰ **S63.8X2** **Sprain of other part of left wrist and hand**

√7ᵗʰ **S63.8X9** **Sprain of other part of unspecified wrist and hand**

√5ᵗʰ **S63.9** Sprain of unspecified part of wrist and hand

√x7ᵗʰ **S63.90** **Sprain of unspecified part of unspecified wrist and hand**

√x7ᵗʰ **S63.91** **Sprain of unspecified part of right wrist and hand**

√x7ᵗʰ **S63.92** **Sprain of unspecified part of left wrist and hand**

√4ᵗʰ **S64** **Injury of nerves at wrist and hand level**
Code also any associated open wound (S61.-)

The appropriate 7th character is to be added to each code from category S64.
A   initial encounter
D   subsequent encounter
S   sequela

√5ᵗʰ **S64.0** Injury of ulnar nerve at wrist and hand level

√x7ᵗʰ **S64.00** **Injury of ulnar nerve at wrist and hand level of unspecified arm**

√x7ᵗʰ **S64.01** **Injury of ulnar nerve at wrist and hand level of right arm**

√x7ᵗʰ **S64.02** **Injury of ulnar nerve at wrist and hand level of left arm**

√5ᵗʰ **S64.1** Injury of median nerve at wrist and hand level

√x7ᵗʰ **S64.10** **Injury of median nerve at wrist and hand level of unspecified arm**

√x7ᵗʰ **S64.11** **Injury of median nerve at wrist and hand level of right arm**

√x7ᵗʰ **S64.12** **Injury of median nerve at wrist and hand level of left arm**

√5ᵗʰ **S64.2** Injury of radial nerve at wrist and hand level

√x7ᵗʰ **S64.20** **Injury of radial nerve at wrist and hand level of unspecified arm**

√x7ᵗʰ **S64.21** **Injury of radial nerve at wrist and hand level of right arm**

√x7ᵗʰ **S64.22** **Injury of radial nerve at wrist and hand level of left arm**

√5ᵗʰ **S64.3** Injury of digital nerve of thumb

√x7ᵗʰ **S64.30** **Injury of digital nerve of unspecified thumb**

√x7ᵗʰ **S64.31** Injury of digital nerve of right thumb

√x7ᵗʰ **S64.32** **Injury of digital nerve of left thumb**

√5ᵗʰ **S64.4** Injury of digital nerve of other and unspecified finger

√x7ᵗʰ **S64.40** **Injury of digital nerve of unspecified finger**

√6ᵗʰ **S64.49** **Injury of digital nerve of other finger**

√7ᵗʰ **S64.490** **Injury of digital nerve of right index finger**

√7ᵗʰ **S64.491** **Injury of digital nerve of left index finger**

√7ᵗʰ **S64.492** **Injury of digital nerve of right middle finger**

√7ᵗʰ **S64.493** **Injury of digital nerve of left middle finger**

√7ᵗʰ **S64.494** **Injury of digital nerve of right ring finger**

√7ᵗʰ **S64.495** **Injury of digital nerve of left ring finger**

√7ᵗʰ **S64.496** **Injury of digital nerve of right little finger**

√7ᵗʰ **S64.497** **Injury of digital nerve of left little finger**

√7ᵗʰ **S64.498** **Injury of digital nerve of other finger**
Injury of digital nerve of specified finger with unspecified laterality

√5ᵗʰ **S64.8** Injury of other nerves at wrist and hand level

√6ᵗʰ **S64.8X** Injury of other nerves at wrist and hand level

√7ᵗʰ **S64.8X1** **Injury of other nerves at wrist and hand level of right arm**

√7ᵗʰ **S64.8X2** **Injury of other nerves at wrist and hand level of left arm**

√7ᵗʰ **S64.8X9** **Injury of other nerves at wrist and hand level of unspecified arm**

√5ᵗʰ **S64.9** Injury of unspecified nerve at wrist and hand level

√x7ᵗʰ **S64.90** **Injury of unspecified nerve at wrist and hand level of unspecified arm**

√x7ᵗʰ **S64.91** **Injury of unspecified nerve at wrist and hand level of right arm**

√x7ᵗʰ **S64.92** **Injury of unspecified nerve at wrist and hand level of left arm**

√4ᵗʰ **S65** **Injury of blood vessels at wrist and hand level**
Code also any associated open wound (S61.-)

The appropriate 7th character is to be added to each code from category S65.
A   initial encounter
D   subsequent encounter
S   sequela

√5ᵗʰ **S65.0** Injury of ulnar artery at wrist and hand level

√6ᵗʰ **S65.00** **Unspecified injury of ulnar artery at wrist and hand level**

√7ᵗʰ **S65.001** **Unspecified injury of ulnar artery at wrist and hand level of right arm**

√7ᵗʰ **S65.002** **Unspecified injury of ulnar artery at wrist and hand level of left arm**

√7ᵗʰ **S65.009** **Unspecified injury of ulnar artery at wrist and hand level of unspecified arm**

√6ᵗʰ **S65.01** Laceration of ulnar artery at wrist and hand level

√7ᵗʰ **S65.011** **Laceration of ulnar artery at wrist and hand level of right arm**

√7ᵗʰ **S65.012** **Laceration of ulnar artery at wrist and hand level of left arm**

√7ᵗʰ **S65.019** **Laceration of ulnar artery at wrist and hand level of unspecified arm**

EXCLUDES 1 Not coded here   *EXCLUDES 2* Not included here   N Newborn Age: 0   P Pediatric Age: 0-17   M Maternity Age: 12-55   A Adult Age: 15-124

922   ICD-10-CM 2016

✓6th **S65.09** Other specified injury of ulnar artery at wrist and hand level

  ✓7th **S65.091** Other specified injury of ulnar artery at wrist and hand level of right arm

  ✓7th **S65.092** Other specified injury of ulnar artery at wrist and hand level of left arm

  ✓7th **S65.099** Other specified injury of ulnar artery at wrist and hand level of unspecified arm

✓5th **S65.1** Injury of radial artery at wrist and hand level

 ✓6th **S65.10** Unspecified injury of radial artery at wrist and hand level

  ✓7th **S65.101** Unspecified injury of radial artery at wrist and hand level of right arm

  ✓7th **S65.102** Unspecified injury of radial artery at wrist and hand level of left arm

  ✓7th **S65.109** Unspecified injury of radial artery at wrist and hand level of unspecified arm

 ✓6th **S65.11** Laceration of radial artery at wrist and hand level

  ✓7th **S65.111** Laceration of radial artery at wrist and hand level of right arm

  ✓7th **S65.112** Laceration of radial artery at wrist and hand level of left arm

  ✓7th **S65.119** Laceration of radial artery at wrist and hand level of unspecified arm

 ✓6th **S65.19** Other specified injury of radial artery at wrist and hand level

  ✓7th **S65.191** Other specified injury of radial artery at wrist and hand level of right arm

  ✓7th **S65.192** Other specified injury of radial artery at wrist and hand level of left arm

  ✓7th **S65.199** Other specified injury of radial artery at wrist and hand level of unspecified arm

✓5th **S65.2** Injury of superficial palmar arch

 ✓6th **S65.20** Unspecified injury of superficial palmar arch

  ✓7th **S65.201** Unspecified injury of superficial palmar arch of right hand

  ✓7th **S65.202** Unspecified injury of superficial palmar arch of left hand

  ✓7th **S65.209** Unspecified injury of superficial palmar arch of unspecified hand

 ✓6th **S65.21** Laceration of superficial palmar arch

  ✓7th **S65.211** Laceration of superficial palmar arch of right hand

  ✓7th **S65.212** Laceration of superficial palmar arch of left hand

  ✓7th **S65.219** Laceration of superficial palmar arch of unspecified hand

 ✓6th **S65.29** Other specified injury of superficial palmar arch

  ✓7th **S65.291** Other specified injury of superficial palmar arch of right hand

  ✓7th **S65.292** Other specified injury of superficial palmar arch of left hand

  ✓7th **S65.299** Other specified injury of superficial palmar arch of unspecified hand

✓5th **S65.3** Injury of deep palmar arch

 ✓6th **S65.30** Unspecified injury of deep palmar arch

  ✓7th **S65.301** Unspecified injury of deep palmar arch of right hand

  ✓7th **S65.302** Unspecified injury of deep palmar arch of left hand

  ✓7th **S65.309** Unspecified injury of deep palmar arch of unspecified hand

 ✓6th **S65.31** Laceration of deep palmar arch

  ✓7th **S65.311** Laceration of deep palmar arch of right hand

  ✓7th **S65.312** Laceration of deep palmar arch of left hand

  ✓7th **S65.319** Laceration of deep palmar arch of unspecified hand

 ✓6th **S65.39** Other specified injury of deep palmar arch

  ✓7th **S65.391** Other specified injury of deep palmar arch of right hand

  ✓7th **S65.392** Other specified injury of deep palmar arch of left hand

  ✓7th **S65.399** Other specified injury of deep palmar arch of unspecified hand

✓5th **S65.4** Injury of blood vessel of thumb

 ✓6th **S65.40** Unspecified injury of blood vessel of thumb

  ✓7th **S65.401** Unspecified injury of blood vessel of right thumb

  ✓7th **S65.402** Unspecified injury of blood vessel of left thumb

  ✓7th **S65.409** Unspecified injury of blood vessel of unspecified thumb

 ✓6th **S65.41** Laceration of blood vessel of thumb

  ✓7th **S65.411** Laceration of blood vessel of right thumb

  ✓7th **S65.412** Laceration of blood vessel of left thumb

  ✓7th **S65.419** Laceration of blood vessel of unspecified thumb

 ✓6th **S65.49** Other specified injury of blood vessel of thumb

  ✓7th **S65.491** Other specified injury of blood vessel of right thumb

  ✓7th **S65.492** Other specified injury of blood vessel of left thumb

  ✓7th **S65.499** Other specified injury of blood vessel of unspecified thumb

✓5th **S65.5** Injury of blood vessel of other and unspecified finger

 ✓6th **S65.50** Unspecified injury of blood vessel of other and unspecified finger

  ✓7th **S65.500** Unspecified injury of blood vessel of right index finger

  ✓7th **S65.501** Unspecified injury of blood vessel of left index finger

  ✓7th **S65.502** Unspecified injury of blood vessel of right middle finger

  ✓7th **S65.503** Unspecified injury of blood vessel of left middle finger

  ✓7th **S65.504** Unspecified injury of blood vessel of right ring finger

  ✓7th **S65.505** Unspecified injury of blood vessel of left ring finger

  ✓7th **S65.506** Unspecified injury of blood vessel of right little finger

  ✓7th **S65.507** Unspecified injury of blood vessel of left little finger

  ✓7th **S65.508** Unspecified injury of blood vessel of other finger
Unspecified injury of blood vessel of specified finger with unspecified laterality

  ✓7th **S65.509** Unspecified injury of blood vessel of unspecified finger

 ✓6th **S65.51** Laceration of blood vessel of other and unspecified finger

  ✓7th **S65.510** Laceration of blood vessel of right index finger

  ✓7th **S65.511** Laceration of blood vessel of left index finger

  ✓7th **S65.512** Laceration of blood vessel of right middle finger

  ✓7th **S65.513** Laceration of blood vessel of left middle finger

  ✓7th **S65.514** Laceration of blood vessel of right ring finger

  ✓7th **S65.515** Laceration of blood vessel of left ring finger

  ✓7th **S65.516** Laceration of blood vessel of right little finger

  ✓7th **S65.517** Laceration of blood vessel of left little finger

  ✓7th **S65.518** Laceration of blood vessel of other finger
Laceration of blood vessel of specified finger with unspecified laterality

  ✓7th **S65.519** Laceration of blood vessel of unspecified finger

---

☑ Additional Character Required   ✓x7th Placeholder Alert   Unspecified Dx   Other Specified Dx   Manifestation   ▶◀ Revised Text   ● New Code   ▲ Revised Code Title

√6ᵗʰ **S65.59** Other specified injury of blood vessel of other and unspecified finger

   √7ᵗʰ **S65.590** Other specified injury of blood vessel of right index finger

   √7ᵗʰ **S65.591** Other specified injury of blood vessel of left index finger

   √7ᵗʰ **S65.592** Other specified injury of blood vessel of right middle finger

   √7ᵗʰ **S65.593** Other specified injury of blood vessel of left middle finger

   √7ᵗʰ **S65.594** Other specified injury of blood vessel of right ring finger

   √7ᵗʰ **S65.595** Other specified injury of blood vessel of left ring finger

   √7ᵗʰ **S65.596** Other specified injury of blood vessel of right little finger

   √7ᵗʰ **S65.597** Other specified injury of blood vessel of left little finger

   √7ᵗʰ **S65.598** Other specified injury of blood vessel of other finger

          Other specified injury of blood vessel of specified finger with unspecified laterality

   √7ᵗʰ **S65.599** Other specified injury of blood vessel of unspecified finger

√5ᵗʰ **S65.8** Injury of other blood vessels at wrist and hand level

  √6ᵗʰ **S65.80** Unspecified injury of other blood vessels at wrist and hand level

   √7ᵗʰ **S65.801** Unspecified injury of other blood vessels at wrist and hand level of right arm

   √7ᵗʰ **S65.802** Unspecified injury of other blood vessels at wrist and hand level of left arm

   √7ᵗʰ **S65.809** Unspecified injury of other blood vessels at wrist and hand level of unspecified arm

  √6ᵗʰ **S65.81** Laceration of other blood vessels at wrist and hand level

   √7ᵗʰ **S65.811** Laceration of other blood vessels at wrist and hand level of right arm

   √7ᵗʰ **S65.812** Laceration of other blood vessels at wrist and hand level of left arm

   √7ᵗʰ **S65.819** Laceration of other blood vessels at wrist and hand level of unspecified arm

  √6ᵗʰ **S65.89** Other specified injury of other blood vessels at wrist and hand level

   √7ᵗʰ **S65.891** Other specified injury of other blood vessels at wrist and hand level of right arm

   √7ᵗʰ **S65.892** Other specified injury of other blood vessels at wrist and hand level of left arm

   √7ᵗʰ **S65.899** Other specified injury of other blood vessels at wrist and hand level of unspecified arm

√5ᵗʰ **S65.9** Injury of unspecified blood vessel at wrist and hand level

  √6ᵗʰ **S65.90** Unspecified injury of unspecified blood vessel at wrist and hand level

   √7ᵗʰ **S65.901** Unspecified injury of unspecified blood vessel at wrist and hand level of right arm

   √7ᵗʰ **S65.902** Unspecified injury of unspecified blood vessel at wrist and hand level of left arm

   √7ᵗʰ **S65.909** Unspecified injury of unspecified blood vessel at wrist and hand level of unspecified arm

  √6ᵗʰ **S65.91** Laceration of unspecified blood vessel at wrist and hand level

   √7ᵗʰ **S65.911** Laceration of unspecified blood vessel at wrist and hand level of right arm

   √7ᵗʰ **S65.912** Laceration of unspecified blood vessel at wrist and hand level of left arm

   √7ᵗʰ **S65.919** Laceration of unspecified blood vessel at wrist and hand level of unspecified arm

  √6ᵗʰ **S65.99** Other specified injury of unspecified blood vessel at wrist and hand level

   √7ᵗʰ **S65.991** Other specified injury of unspecified blood vessel at wrist and hand of right arm

   √7ᵗʰ **S65.992** Other specified injury of unspecified blood vessel at wrist and hand of left arm

   √7ᵗʰ **S65.999** Other specified injury of unspecified blood vessel at wrist and hand of unspecified arm

◆ √4ᵗʰ **S66 Injury of muscle, fascia and tendon at wrist and hand level**

    Code also any associated open wound (S61.-)

    EXCLUDES 2   sprain of joints and ligaments of wrist and hand (S63.-)

    The appropriate 7th character is to be added to each code from category S66.
    A   initial encounter
    D   subsequent encounter
    S   sequela

√5ᵗʰ **S66.0** Injury of long flexor muscle, fascia and tendon of thumb at wrist and hand level

  √6ᵗʰ **S66.00** Unspecified injury of long flexor muscle, fascia and tendon of thumb at wrist and hand level

   √7ᵗʰ **S66.001** Unspecified injury of long flexor muscle, fascia and tendon of right thumb at wrist and hand level

   √7ᵗʰ **S66.002** Unspecified injury of long flexor muscle, fascia and tendon of left thumb at wrist and hand level

   √7ᵗʰ **S66.009** Unspecified injury of long flexor muscle, fascia and tendon of unspecified thumb at wrist and hand level

  √6ᵗʰ **S66.01** Strain of long flexor muscle, fascia and tendon of thumb at wrist and hand level

   √7ᵗʰ **S66.011** Strain of long flexor muscle, fascia and tendon of right thumb at wrist and hand level

   √7ᵗʰ **S66.012** Strain of long flexor muscle, fascia and tendon of left thumb at wrist and hand level

   √7ᵗʰ **S66.019** Strain of long flexor muscle, fascia and tendon of unspecified thumb at wrist and hand level

  √6ᵗʰ **S66.02** Laceration of long flexor muscle, fascia and tendon of thumb at wrist and hand level

   √7ᵗʰ **S66.021** Laceration of long flexor muscle, fascia and tendon of right thumb at wrist and hand level

   √7ᵗʰ **S66.022** Laceration of long flexor muscle, fascia and tendon of left thumb at wrist and hand level

   √7ᵗʰ **S66.029** Laceration of long flexor muscle, fascia and tendon of unspecified thumb at wrist and hand level

  √6ᵗʰ **S66.09** Other specified injury of long flexor muscle, fascia and tendon of thumb at wrist and hand level

   √7ᵗʰ **S66.091** Other specified injury of long flexor muscle, fascia and tendon of right thumb at wrist and hand level

   √7ᵗʰ **S66.092** Other specified injury of long flexor muscle, fascia and tendon of left thumb at wrist and hand level

   √7ᵗʰ **S66.099** Other specified injury of long flexor muscle, fascia and tendon of unspecified thumb at wrist and hand level

√5ᵗʰ **S66.1** Injury of flexor muscle, fascia and tendon of other and unspecified finger at wrist and hand level

    EXCLUDES 2   Injury of long flexor muscle, fascia and tendon of thumb at wrist and hand level (S66.0-)

  √6ᵗʰ **S66.10** Unspecified injury of flexor muscle, fascia and tendon of other and unspecified finger at wrist and hand level

   √7ᵗʰ **S66.100** Unspecified injury of flexor muscle, fascia and tendon of right index finger at wrist and hand level

   √7ᵗʰ **S66.101** Unspecified injury of flexor muscle, fascia and tendon of left index finger at wrist and hand level

   √7ᵗʰ **S66.102** Unspecified injury of flexor muscle, fascia and tendon of right middle finger at wrist and hand level

   √7ᵗʰ **S66.103** Unspecified injury of flexor muscle, fascia and tendon of left middle finger at wrist and hand level

◆ Refer to the Muscle/Tendon Table at beginning of this chapter.

EXCLUDES 1 Not coded here   *EXCLUDES 2* Not included here   N Newborn Age: 0   P Pediatric Age: 0-17   M Maternity Age: 12-55   A Adult Age: 15-124

924   ICD-10-CM 2016

√7ᵗʰ **S66.104** **Unspecified injury of flexor muscle, fascia and tendon of right ring finger at wrist and hand level**

√7ᵗʰ **S66.105** **Unspecified injury of flexor muscle, fascia and tendon of left ring finger at wrist and hand level**

√7ᵗʰ **S66.106** **Unspecified injury of flexor muscle, fascia and tendon of right little finger at wrist and hand level**

√7ᵗʰ **S66.107** **Unspecified injury of flexor muscle, fascia and tendon of left little finger at wrist and hand level**

√7ᵗʰ **S66.108** **Unspecified injury of flexor muscle, fascia and tendon of other finger at wrist and hand level**
Unspecified injury of flexor muscle, fascia and tendon of specified finger with unspecified laterality at wrist and hand level

√7ᵗʰ **S66.109** **Unspecified injury of flexor muscle, fascia and tendon of unspecified finger at wrist and hand level**

√6ᵗʰ **S66.11** Strain of flexor muscle, fascia and tendon of other and unspecified finger at wrist and hand level

√7ᵗʰ **S66.110** **Strain of flexor muscle, fascia and tendon of right index finger at wrist and hand level**

√7ᵗʰ **S66.111** **Strain of flexor muscle, fascia and tendon of left index finger at wrist and hand level**

√7ᵗʰ **S66.112** **Strain of flexor muscle, fascia and tendon of right middle finger at wrist and hand level**

√7ᵗʰ **S66.113** **Strain of flexor muscle, fascia and tendon of left middle finger at wrist and hand level**

√7ᵗʰ **S66.114** **Strain of flexor muscle, fascia and tendon of right ring finger at wrist and hand level**

√7ᵗʰ **S66.115** **Strain of flexor muscle, fascia and tendon of left ring finger at wrist and hand level**

√7ᵗʰ **S66.116** **Strain of flexor muscle, fascia and tendon of right little finger at wrist and hand level**

√7ᵗʰ **S66.117** **Strain of flexor muscle, fascia and tendon of left little finger at wrist and hand level**

√7ᵗʰ **S66.118** **Strain of flexor muscle, fascia and tendon of other finger at wrist and hand level**
Strain of flexor muscle, fascia and tendon of specified finger with unspecified laterality at wrist and hand level

√7ᵗʰ **S66.119** **Strain of flexor muscle, fascia and tendon of unspecified finger at wrist and hand level**

√6ᵗʰ **S66.12** Laceration of flexor muscle, fascia and tendon of other and unspecified finger at wrist and hand level

√7ᵗʰ **S66.120** **Laceration of flexor muscle, fascia and tendon of right index finger at wrist and hand level**

√7ᵗʰ **S66.121** **Laceration of flexor muscle, fascia and tendon of left index finger at wrist and hand level**

√7ᵗʰ **S66.122** **Laceration of flexor muscle, fascia and tendon of right middle finger at wrist and hand level**

√7ᵗʰ **S66.123** **Laceration of flexor muscle, fascia and tendon of left middle finger at wrist and hand level**

√7ᵗʰ **S66.124** **Laceration of flexor muscle, fascia and tendon of right ring finger at wrist and hand level**

√7ᵗʰ **S66.125** **Laceration of flexor muscle, fascia and tendon of left ring finger at wrist and hand level**

√7ᵗʰ **S66.126** **Laceration of flexor muscle, fascia and tendon of right little finger at wrist and hand level**

√7ᵗʰ **S66.127** **Laceration of flexor muscle, fascia and tendon of left little finger at wrist and hand level**

√7ᵗʰ **S66.128** **Laceration of flexor muscle, fascia and tendon of other finger at wrist and hand level**
Laceration of flexor muscle, fascia and tendon of specified finger with unspecified laterality at wrist and hand level

√7ᵗʰ **S66.129** **Laceration of flexor muscle, fascia and tendon of unspecified finger at wrist and hand level**

√6ᵗʰ **S66.19** Other injury of flexor muscle, fascia and tendon of other and unspecified finger at wrist and hand level

√7ᵗʰ **S66.190** **Other injury of flexor muscle, fascia and tendon of right index finger at wrist and hand level**

√7ᵗʰ **S66.191** **Other injury of flexor muscle, fascia and tendon of left index finger at wrist and hand level**

√7ᵗʰ **S66.192** **Other injury of flexor muscle, fascia and tendon of right middle finger at wrist and hand level**

√7ᵗʰ **S66.193** **Other injury of flexor muscle, fascia and tendon of left middle finger at wrist and hand level**

√7ᵗʰ **S66.194** **Other injury of flexor muscle, fascia and tendon of right ring finger at wrist and hand level**

√7ᵗʰ **S66.195** **Other injury of flexor muscle, fascia and tendon of left ring finger at wrist and hand level**

√7ᵗʰ **S66.196** **Other injury of flexor muscle, fascia and tendon of right little finger at wrist and hand level**

√7ᵗʰ **S66.197** **Other injury of flexor muscle, fascia and tendon of left little finger at wrist and hand level**

√7ᵗʰ **S66.198** **Other injury of flexor muscle, fascia and tendon of other finger at wrist and hand level**
Other injury of flexor muscle, fascia and tendon of specified finger with unspecified laterality at wrist and hand level

√7ᵗʰ **S66.199** **Other injury of flexor muscle, fascia and tendon of unspecified finger at wrist and hand level**

√5ᵗʰ **S66.2** Injury of extensor muscle, fascia and tendon of thumb at wrist and hand level

√6ᵗʰ **S66.20** Unspecified injury of extensor muscle, fascia and tendon of thumb at wrist and hand level

√7ᵗʰ **S66.201** **Unspecified injury of extensor muscle, fascia and tendon of right thumb at wrist and hand level**

√7ᵗʰ **S66.202** **Unspecified injury of extensor muscle, fascia and tendon of left thumb at wrist and hand level**

√7ᵗʰ **S66.209** **Unspecified injury of extensor muscle, fascia and tendon of unspecified thumb at wrist and hand level**

√6ᵗʰ **S66.21** Strain of extensor muscle, fascia and tendon of thumb at wrist and hand level

√7ᵗʰ **S66.211** **Strain of extensor muscle, fascia and tendon of right thumb at wrist and hand level**

√7ᵗʰ **S66.212** **Strain of extensor muscle, fascia and tendon of left thumb at wrist and hand level**

√7ᵗʰ **S66.219** **Strain of extensor muscle, fascia and tendon of unspecified thumb at wrist and hand level**

√6ᵗʰ **S66.22** Laceration of extensor muscle, fascia and tendon of thumb at wrist and hand level

√7ᵗʰ **S66.221** **Laceration of extensor muscle, fascia and tendon of right thumb at wrist and hand level**

√7ᵗʰ **S66.222** **Laceration of extensor muscle, fascia and tendon of left thumb at wrist and hand level**

☑ Additional Character Required   ✓x7ᵗʰ Placeholder Alert   Unspecified Dx   Other Specified Dx   Manifestation   ▶◀ Revised Text   ● New Code   ▲ Revised Code Title

ICD-10-CM 2016   925

✓7ᵗʰ S66.229 Laceration of extensor muscle, fascia and tendon of unspecified thumb at wrist and hand level

✓6ᵗʰ S66.29 Other specified injury of extensor muscle, fascia and tendon of thumb at wrist and hand level

✓7ᵗʰ S66.291 Other specified injury of extensor muscle, fascia and tendon of right thumb at wrist and hand level

✓7ᵗʰ S66.292 Other specified injury of extensor muscle, fascia and tendon of left thumb at wrist and hand level

✓7ᵗʰ S66.299 Other specified injury of extensor muscle, fascia and tendon of unspecified thumb at wrist and hand level

✓5ᵗʰ S66.3 Injury of extensor muscle, fascia and tendon of other and unspecified finger at wrist and hand level

> *EXCLUDES 2*   Injury of extensor muscle, fascia and tendon of thumb at wrist and hand level (S66.2-)

✓6ᵗʰ S66.30 Unspecified injury of extensor muscle, fascia and tendon of other and unspecified finger at wrist and hand level

✓7ᵗʰ S66.300 Unspecified injury of extensor muscle, fascia and tendon of right index finger at wrist and hand level

✓7ᵗʰ S66.301 Unspecified injury of extensor muscle, fascia and tendon of left index finger at wrist and hand level

✓7ᵗʰ S66.302 Unspecified injury of extensor muscle, fascia and tendon of right middle finger at wrist and hand level

✓7ᵗʰ S66.303 Unspecified injury of extensor muscle, fascia and tendon of left middle finger at wrist and hand level

✓7ᵗʰ S66.304 Unspecified injury of extensor muscle, fascia and tendon of right ring finger at wrist and hand level

✓7ᵗʰ S66.305 Unspecified injury of extensor muscle, fascia and tendon of left ring finger at wrist and hand level

✓7ᵗʰ S66.306 Unspecified injury of extensor muscle, fascia and tendon of right little finger at wrist and hand level

✓7ᵗʰ S66.307 Unspecified injury of extensor muscle, fascia and tendon of left little finger at wrist and hand level

✓7ᵗʰ S66.308 Unspecified injury of extensor muscle, fascia and tendon of other finger at wrist and hand level

> Unspecified injury of extensor muscle, fascia and tendon of specified finger with unspecified laterality at wrist and hand level

✓7ᵗʰ S66.309 Unspecified injury of extensor muscle, fascia and tendon of unspecified finger at wrist and hand level

✓6ᵗʰ S66.31 Strain of extensor muscle, fascia and tendon of other and unspecified finger at wrist and hand level

✓7ᵗʰ S66.310 Strain of extensor muscle, fascia and tendon of right index finger at wrist and hand level

✓7ᵗʰ S66.311 Strain of extensor muscle, fascia and tendon of left index finger at wrist and hand level

✓7ᵗʰ S66.312 Strain of extensor muscle, fascia and tendon of right middle finger at wrist and hand level

✓7ᵗʰ S66.313 Strain of extensor muscle, fascia and tendon of left middle finger at wrist and hand level

✓7ᵗʰ S66.314 Strain of extensor muscle, fascia and tendon of right ring finger at wrist and hand level

✓7ᵗʰ S66.315 Strain of extensor muscle, fascia and tendon of left ring finger at wrist and hand level

✓7ᵗʰ S66.316 Strain of extensor muscle, fascia and tendon of right little finger at wrist and hand level

✓7ᵗʰ S66.317 Strain of extensor muscle, fascia and tendon of left little finger at wrist and hand level

✓7ᵗʰ S66.318 Strain of extensor muscle, fascia and tendon of other finger at wrist and hand level

> Strain of extensor muscle, fascia and tendon of specified finger with unspecified laterality at wrist and hand level

✓7ᵗʰ S66.319 Strain of extensor muscle, fascia and tendon of unspecified finger at wrist and hand level

✓6ᵗʰ S66.32 Laceration of extensor muscle, fascia and tendon of other and unspecified finger at wrist and hand level

✓7ᵗʰ S66.320 Laceration of extensor muscle, fascia and tendon of right index finger at wrist and hand level

✓7ᵗʰ S66.321 Laceration of extensor muscle, fascia and tendon of left index finger at wrist and hand level

✓7ᵗʰ S66.322 Laceration of extensor muscle, fascia and tendon of right middle finger at wrist and hand level

✓7ᵗʰ S66.323 Laceration of extensor muscle, fascia and tendon of left middle finger at wrist and hand level

✓7ᵗʰ S66.324 Laceration of extensor muscle, fascia and tendon of right ring finger at wrist and hand level

✓7ᵗʰ S66.325 Laceration of extensor muscle, fascia and tendon of left ring finger at wrist and hand level

✓7ᵗʰ S66.326 Laceration of extensor muscle, fascia and tendon of right little finger at wrist and hand level

✓7ᵗʰ S66.327 Laceration of extensor muscle, fascia and tendon of left little finger at wrist and hand level

✓7ᵗʰ S66.328 Laceration of extensor muscle, fascia and tendon of other finger at wrist and hand level

> Laceration of extensor muscle, fascia and tendon of specified finger with unspecified laterality at wrist and hand level

✓7ᵗʰ S66.329 Laceration of extensor muscle, fascia and tendon of unspecified finger at wrist and hand level

✓6ᵗʰ S66.39 Other injury of extensor muscle, fascia and tendon of other and unspecified finger at wrist and hand level

✓7ᵗʰ S66.390 Other injury of extensor muscle, fascia and tendon of right index finger at wrist and hand level

✓7ᵗʰ S66.391 Other injury of extensor muscle, fascia and tendon of left index finger at wrist and hand level

✓7ᵗʰ S66.392 Other injury of extensor muscle, fascia and tendon of right middle finger at wrist and hand level

✓7ᵗʰ S66.393 Other injury of extensor muscle, fascia and tendon of left middle finger at wrist and hand level

✓7ᵗʰ S66.394 Other injury of extensor muscle, fascia and tendon of right ring finger at wrist and hand level

✓7ᵗʰ S66.395 Other injury of extensor muscle, fascia and tendon of left ring finger at wrist and hand level

✓7ᵗʰ S66.396 Other injury of extensor muscle, fascia and tendon of right little finger at wrist and hand level

✓7ᵗʰ S66.397 Other injury of extensor muscle, fascia and tendon of left little finger at wrist and hand level

EXCLUDES 1 Not coded here   *EXCLUDES 2* Not included here   **N** Newborn Age: 0   **P** Pediatric Age: 0-17   **M** Maternity Age: 12-55   **A** Adult Age: 15-124

926

ICD-10-CM 2016

✓7ᵗʰ **S66.398** **Other injury of extensor muscle, fascia and tendon of other finger at wrist and hand level**

Other injury of extensor muscle, fascia and tendon of specified finger with unspecified laterality at wrist and hand level

✓7ᵗʰ **S66.399** **Other injury of extensor muscle, fascia and tendon of unspecified finger at wrist and hand level**

✓5ᵗʰ **S66.4** **Injury of** intrinsic muscle, fascia and tendon of **thumb at wrist and hand level**

✓6ᵗʰ **S66.40** **Unspecified injury of intrinsic muscle, fascia and tendon of thumb at wrist and hand level**

✓7ᵗʰ **S66.401** **Unspecified injury of intrinsic muscle, fascia and tendon of right thumb at wrist and hand level**

✓7ᵗʰ **S66.402** **Unspecified injury of intrinsic muscle, fascia and tendon of left thumb at wrist and hand level**

✓7ᵗʰ **S66.409** **Unspecified injury of intrinsic muscle, fascia and tendon of unspecified thumb at wrist and hand level**

✓6ᵗʰ **S66.41** **Strain of intrinsic muscle, fascia and tendon of thumb at wrist and hand level**

✓7ᵗʰ **S66.411** **Strain of intrinsic muscle, fascia and tendon of right thumb at wrist and hand level**

✓7ᵗʰ **S66.412** **Strain of intrinsic muscle, fascia and tendon of left thumb at wrist and hand level**

✓7ᵗʰ **S66.419** **Strain of intrinsic muscle, fascia and tendon of unspecified thumb at wrist and hand level**

✓6ᵗʰ **S66.42** **Laceration of intrinsic muscle, fascia and tendon of thumb at wrist and hand level**

✓7ᵗʰ **S66.421** **Laceration of intrinsic muscle, fascia and tendon of right thumb at wrist and hand level**

✓7ᵗʰ **S66.422** **Laceration of intrinsic muscle, fascia and tendon of left thumb at wrist and hand level**

✓7ᵗʰ **S66.429** **Laceration of intrinsic muscle, fascia and tendon of unspecified thumb at wrist and hand level**

✓6ᵗʰ **S66.49** **Other specified injury of intrinsic muscle, fascia and tendon of thumb at wrist and hand level**

✓7ᵗʰ **S66.491** **Other specified injury of intrinsic muscle, fascia and tendon of right thumb at wrist and hand level**

✓7ᵗʰ **S66.492** **Other specified injury of intrinsic muscle, fascia and tendon of left thumb at wrist and hand level**

✓7ᵗʰ **S66.499** **Other specified injury of intrinsic muscle, fascia and tendon of unspecified thumb at wrist and hand level**

✓5ᵗʰ **S66.5** **Injury of** intrinsic muscle, fascia and tendon of other and **unspecified finger at wrist and hand level**

> **EXCLUDES 2**   *injury of intrinsic muscle, fascia and tendon of thumb at wrist and hand level (S66.4-)*

✓6ᵗʰ **S66.50** **Unspecified injury of intrinsic muscle, fascia and tendon of other and unspecified finger at wrist and hand level**

✓7ᵗʰ **S66.500** **Unspecified injury of intrinsic muscle, fascia and tendon of right index finger at wrist and hand level**

✓7ᵗʰ **S66.501** **Unspecified injury of intrinsic muscle, fascia and tendon of left index finger at wrist and hand level**

✓7ᵗʰ **S66.502** **Unspecified injury of intrinsic muscle, fascia and tendon of right middle finger at wrist and hand level**

✓7ᵗʰ **S66.503** **Unspecified injury of intrinsic muscle, fascia and tendon of left middle finger at wrist and hand level**

✓7ᵗʰ **S66.504** **Unspecified injury of intrinsic muscle, fascia and tendon of right ring finger at wrist and hand level**

✓7ᵗʰ **S66.505** **Unspecified injury of intrinsic muscle, fascia and tendon of left ring finger at wrist and hand level**

✓7ᵗʰ **S66.506** **Unspecified injury of intrinsic muscle, fascia and tendon of right little finger at wrist and hand level**

✓7ᵗʰ **S66.507** **Unspecified injury of intrinsic muscle, fascia and tendon of left little finger at wrist and hand level**

✓7ᵗʰ **S66.508** **Unspecified injury of intrinsic muscle, fascia and tendon of other finger at wrist and hand level**

Unspecified injury of intrinsic muscle, fascia and tendon of specified finger with unspecified laterality at wrist and hand level

✓7ᵗʰ **S66.509** **Unspecified injury of intrinsic muscle, fascia and tendon of unspecified finger at wrist and hand level**

✓6ᵗʰ **S66.51** **Strain of intrinsic muscle, fascia and tendon of** other **and unspecified finger at wrist and hand level**

✓7ᵗʰ **S66.510** **Strain of intrinsic muscle, fascia and tendon of right index finger at wrist and hand level**

✓7ᵗʰ **S66.511** **Strain of intrinsic muscle, fascia and tendon of left index finger at wrist and hand level**

✓7ᵗʰ **S66.512** **Strain of intrinsic muscle, fascia and tendon of right middle finger at wrist and hand level**

✓7ᵗʰ **S66.513** **Strain of intrinsic muscle, fascia and tendon of left middle finger at wrist and hand level**

✓7ᵗʰ **S66.514** **Strain of intrinsic muscle, fascia and tendon of right ring finger at wrist and hand level**

✓7ᵗʰ **S66.515** **Strain of intrinsic muscle, fascia and tendon of left ring finger at wrist and hand level**

✓7ᵗʰ **S66.516** **Strain of intrinsic muscle, fascia and tendon of right little finger at wrist and hand level**

✓7ᵗʰ **S66.517** **Strain of intrinsic muscle, fascia and tendon of left little finger at wrist and hand level**

✓7ᵗʰ **S66.518** **Strain of intrinsic muscle, fascia and tendon of other finger at wrist and hand level**

Strain of intrinsic muscle, fascia and tendon of specified finger with unspecified laterality at wrist and hand level

✓7ᵗʰ **S66.519** **Strain of intrinsic muscle, fascia and tendon of unspecified finger at wrist and hand level**

✓6ᵗʰ **S66.52** **Laceration of intrinsic muscle, fascia and tendon of other and unspecified finger at wrist and hand level**

✓7ᵗʰ **S66.520** **Laceration of intrinsic muscle, fascia and tendon of right index finger at wrist and hand level**

✓7ᵗʰ **S66.521** **Laceration of intrinsic muscle, fascia and tendon of left index finger at wrist and hand level**

✓7ᵗʰ **S66.522** **Laceration of intrinsic muscle, fascia and tendon of right middle finger at wrist and hand level**

✓7ᵗʰ **S66.523** **Laceration of intrinsic muscle, fascia and tendon of left middle finger at wrist and hand level**

✓7ᵗʰ **S66.524** **Laceration of intrinsic muscle, fascia and tendon of right ring finger at wrist and hand level**

✓7ᵗʰ **S66.525** **Laceration of intrinsic muscle, fascia and tendon of left ring finger at wrist and hand level**

✓7ᵗʰ **S66.526** **Laceration of intrinsic muscle, fascia and tendon of right little finger at wrist and hand level**

✓7ᵗʰ **S66.527** **Laceration of intrinsic muscle, fascia and tendon of left little finger at wrist and hand level**

✓ Additional Character Required   ✓x7ᵗʰ Placeholder Alert   Unspecified Dx   Other Specified Dx   Manifestation   ▶◀ Revised Text   ● New Code   ▲ Revised Code Title

✓7th **S66.528** **Laceration of intrinsic muscle, fascia and tendon of other finger at wrist and hand level**

Laceration of intrinsic muscle, fascia and tendon of specified finger with unspecified laterality at wrist and hand level

✓7th **S66.529** **Laceration of intrinsic muscle, fascia and tendon of unspecified finger at wrist and hand level**

✓6th **S66.59** Other **injury of intrinsic muscle, fascia and tendon of other and unspecified finger at wrist and hand level**

✓7th **S66.590** **Other injury of intrinsic muscle, fascia and tendon of** right index **finger at wrist and hand level**

✓7th **S66.591** **Other injury of intrinsic muscle, fascia and tendon of** left index **finger at wrist and hand level**

✓7th **S66.592** **Other injury of intrinsic muscle, fascia and tendon of** right middle **finger at wrist and hand level**

✓7th **S66.593** **Other injury of intrinsic muscle, fascia and tendon of** left middle **finger at wrist and hand level**

✓7th **S66.594** **Other injury of intrinsic muscle, fascia and tendon of** right ring **finger at wrist and hand level**

✓7th **S66.595** **Other injury of intrinsic muscle, fascia and tendon of** left ring **finger at wrist and hand level**

✓7th **S66.596** **Other injury of intrinsic muscle, fascia and tendon of** right little **finger at wrist and hand level**

✓7th **S66.597** **Other injury of intrinsic muscle, fascia and tendon of** left little **finger at wrist and hand level**

✓7th **S66.598** **Other injury of intrinsic muscle, fascia and tendon of other finger at wrist and hand level**

Other injury of intrinsic muscle, fascia and tendon of specified finger with unspecified laterality at wrist and hand level

✓7th **S66.599** **Other injury of intrinsic muscle, fascia and tendon of unspecified finger at wrist and hand level**

✓5th **S66.8** **Injury of** other specified muscles, **fascia and tendons at wrist and hand level**

✓6th **S66.80** Unspecified **injury of other specified muscles, fascia and tendons at wrist and hand level**

✓7th **S66.801** **Unspecified injury of other specified muscles, fascia and tendons at wrist and hand level,** right **hand**

✓7th **S66.802** **Unspecified injury of other specified muscles, fascia and tendons at wrist and hand level,** left **hand**

✓7th **S66.809** **Unspecified injury of other specified muscles, fascia and tendons at wrist and hand level, unspecified hand**

✓6th **S66.81** Strain **of other specified muscles, fascia and tendons at wrist and hand level**

✓7th **S66.811** **Strain of other specified muscles, fascia and tendons at wrist and hand level,** right **hand**

✓7th **S66.812** **Strain of other specified muscles, fascia and tendons at wrist and hand level,** left **hand**

✓7th **S66.819** **Strain of other specified muscles, fascia and tendons at wrist and hand level, unspecified hand**

✓6th **S66.82** Laceration **of other specified muscles, fascia and tendons at wrist and hand level**

✓7th **S66.821** **Laceration of other specified muscles, fascia and tendons at wrist and hand level,** right **hand**

✓7th **S66.822** **Laceration of other specified muscles, fascia and tendons at wrist and hand level,** left **hand**

✓7th **S66.829** **Laceration of other specified muscles, fascia and tendons at wrist and hand level, unspecified hand**

✓6th **S66.89** Other **injury of other specified muscles, fascia and tendons at wrist and hand level**

✓7th **S66.891** **Other injury of other specified muscles, fascia and tendons at wrist and hand level,** right **hand**

✓7th **S66.892** **Other injury of other specified muscles, fascia and tendons at wrist and hand level,** left **hand**

✓7th **S66.899** **Other injury of other specified muscles, fascia and tendons at wrist and hand level, unspecified hand**

✓5th **S66.9** **Injury of** unspecified muscle, **fascia and tendon at wrist and hand level**

✓6th **S66.90** Unspecified **injury of unspecified muscle, fascia and tendon at wrist and hand level**

✓7th **S66.901** **Unspecified injury of unspecified muscle, fascia and tendon at wrist and hand level,** right **hand**

✓7th **S66.902** **Unspecified injury of unspecified muscle, fascia and tendon at wrist and hand level,** left **hand**

✓7th **S66.909** **Unspecified injury of unspecified muscle, fascia and tendon at wrist and hand level, unspecified hand**

✓6th **S66.91** Strain **of unspecified muscle, fascia and tendon at wrist and hand level**

✓7th **S66.911** **Strain of unspecified muscle, fascia and tendon at wrist and hand level,** right **hand**

✓7th **S66.912** **Strain of unspecified muscle, fascia and tendon at wrist and hand level,** left **hand**

✓7th **S66.919** **Strain of unspecified muscle, fascia and tendon at wrist and hand level, unspecified hand**

✓6th **S66.92** Laceration **of unspecified muscle, fascia and tendon at wrist and hand level**

✓7th **S66.921** **Laceration of unspecified muscle, fascia and tendon at wrist and hand level,** right **hand**

✓7th **S66.922** **Laceration of unspecified muscle, fascia and tendon at wrist and hand level,** left **hand**

✓7th **S66.929** **Laceration of unspecified muscle, fascia and tendon at wrist and hand level, unspecified hand**

✓6th **S66.99** Other **injury of unspecified muscle, fascia and tendon at wrist and hand level**

✓7th **S66.991** **Other injury of unspecified muscle, fascia and tendon at wrist and hand level,** right **hand**

✓7th **S66.992** **Other injury of unspecified muscle, fascia and tendon at wrist and hand level,** left **hand**

✓7th **S66.999** **Other injury of unspecified muscle, fascia and tendon at wrist and hand level, unspecified hand**

EXCLUDES 1 Not coded here   *EXCLUDES 2* Not included here   N Newborn Age: 0   P Pediatric Age: 0-17   M Maternity Age: 12-55   A Adult Age: 15-124

928   ICD-10-CM 2016

✓4ᵗʰ **S67 Crushing injury of wrist, hand and fingers**
Use additional code for all associated injuries, such as:
    fracture of wrist and hand (S62.-)
    open wound of wrist and hand (S61.-)

The appropriate 7th character is to be added to each code from category S67.
  A   initial encounter
  D   subsequent encounter
  S   sequela

✓5ᵗʰ **S67.0 Crushing injury of thumb**
  ✓x7ᵗʰ **S67.00 Crushing injury of unspecified thumb**
  ✓x7ᵗʰ **S67.01 Crushing injury of right thumb**
  ✓x7ᵗʰ **S67.02 Crushing injury of left thumb**

✓5ᵗʰ **S67.1 Crushing injury of other and unspecified finger(s)**
    EXCLUDES 2   *crushing injury of thumb (S67.0-)*
  ✓x7ᵗʰ **S67.10 Crushing injury of unspecified finger(s)**
  ✓6ᵗʰ **S67.19 Crushing injury of other finger(s)**
    ✓7ᵗʰ **S67.190 Crushing injury of right index finger**
    ✓7ᵗʰ **S67.191 Crushing injury of left index finger**
    ✓7ᵗʰ **S67.192 Crushing injury of right middle finger**
    ✓7ᵗʰ **S67.193 Crushing injury of left middle finger**
    ✓7ᵗʰ **S67.194 Crushing injury of right ring finger**
    ✓7ᵗʰ **S67.195 Crushing injury of left ring finger**
    ✓7ᵗʰ **S67.196 Crushing injury of right little finger**
    ✓7ᵗʰ **S67.197 Crushing injury of left little finger**
    ✓7ᵗʰ **S67.198 Crushing injury of other finger**
        Crushing injury of specified finger with unspecified laterality

✓5ᵗʰ **S67.2 Crushing injury of hand**
    EXCLUDES 2   *crushing injury of fingers (S67.1-)*
              crushing injury of thumb (S67.0-)
  ✓x7ᵗʰ **S67.20 Crushing injury of unspecified hand**
  ✓x7ᵗʰ **S67.21 Crushing injury of right hand**
  ✓x7ᵗʰ **S67.22 Crushing injury of left hand**

✓5ᵗʰ **S67.3 Crushing injury of wrist**
  ✓x7ᵗʰ **S67.30 Crushing injury of unspecified wrist**
  ✓x7ᵗʰ **S67.31 Crushing injury of right wrist**
  ✓x7ᵗʰ **S67.32 Crushing injury of left wrist**

✓5ᵗʰ **S67.4 Crushing injury of wrist and hand**
    EXCLUDES 1   *crushing injury of hand alone (S67.2-)*
              crushing injury of wrist alone (S67.3-)
    EXCLUDES 2   *crushing injury of fingers (S67.1-)*
              crushing injury of thumb (S67.0-)
  ✓x7ᵗʰ **S67.40 Crushing injury of unspecified wrist and hand**
  ✓x7ᵗʰ **S67.41 Crushing injury of right wrist and hand**
  ✓x7ᵗʰ **S67.42 Crushing injury of left wrist and hand**

✓5ᵗʰ **S67.9 Crushing injury of unspecified part(s) of wrist, hand and fingers**
  ✓x7ᵗʰ **S67.90 Crushing injury of unspecified part(s) of unspecified wrist, hand and fingers**
  ✓x7ᵗʰ **S67.91 Crushing injury of unspecified part(s) of right wrist, hand and fingers**
  ✓x7ᵗʰ **S67.92 Crushing injury of unspecified part(s) of left wrist, hand and fingers**

✓4ᵗʰ **S68 Traumatic amputation of wrist, hand and fingers**
    NOTE   An amputation not identified as partial or complete should be coded to complete.

The appropriate 7th character is to be added to each code from category S68.
  A   initial encounter
  D   subsequent encounter
  S   sequela

✓5ᵗʰ **S68.0 Traumatic metacarpophalangeal amputation of thumb**
    Traumatic amputation of thumb NOS
  ✓6ᵗʰ **S68.01 Complete traumatic metacarpophalangeal amputation of thumb**
    ✓7ᵗʰ **S68.011 Complete traumatic metacarpophalangeal amputation of right thumb**
    ✓7ᵗʰ **S68.012 Complete traumatic metacarpophalangeal amputation of left thumb**

    ✓7ᵗʰ **S68.019 Complete traumatic metacarpophalangeal amputation of unspecified thumb**
  ✓6ᵗʰ **S68.02 Partial traumatic metacarpophalangeal amputation of thumb**
    ✓7ᵗʰ **S68.021 Partial traumatic metacarpophalangeal amputation of right thumb**
    ✓7ᵗʰ **S68.022 Partial traumatic metacarpophalangeal amputation of left thumb**
    ✓7ᵗʰ **S68.029 Partial traumatic metacarpophalangeal amputation of unspecified thumb**

✓5ᵗʰ **S68.1 Traumatic metacarpophalangeal amputation of other and unspecified finger**
    Traumatic amputation of finger NOS
    EXCLUDES 2   *traumatic metacarpophalangeal amputation of thumb (S68.0-)*
  ✓6ᵗʰ **S68.11 Complete traumatic metacarpophalangeal amputation of other and unspecified finger**
    ✓7ᵗʰ **S68.110 Complete traumatic metacarpophalangeal amputation of right index finger**
    ✓7ᵗʰ **S68.111 Complete traumatic metacarpophalangeal amputation of left index finger**
    ✓7ᵗʰ **S68.112 Complete traumatic metacarpophalangeal amputation of right middle finger**
    ✓7ᵗʰ **S68.113 Complete traumatic metacarpophalangeal amputation of left middle finger**
    ✓7ᵗʰ **S68.114 Complete traumatic metacarpophalangeal amputation of right ring finger**
    ✓7ᵗʰ **S68.115 Complete traumatic metacarpophalangeal amputation of left ring finger**
    ✓7ᵗʰ **S68.116 Complete traumatic metacarpophalangeal amputation of right little finger**
    ✓7ᵗʰ **S68.117 Complete traumatic metacarpophalangeal amputation of left little finger**
    ✓7ᵗʰ **S68.118 Complete traumatic metacarpophalangeal amputation of other finger**
        Complete traumatic metacarpophalangeal amputation of specified finger with unspecified laterality
    ✓7ᵗʰ **S68.119 Complete traumatic metacarpophalangeal amputation of unspecified finger**

  ✓6ᵗʰ **S68.12 Partial traumatic metacarpophalangeal amputation of other and unspecified finger**
    ✓7ᵗʰ **S68.120 Partial traumatic metacarpophalangeal amputation of right index finger**
    ✓7ᵗʰ **S68.121 Partial traumatic metacarpophalangeal amputation of left index finger**
    ✓7ᵗʰ **S68.122 Partial traumatic metacarpophalangeal amputation of right middle finger**
    ✓7ᵗʰ **S68.123 Partial traumatic metacarpophalangeal amputation of left middle finger**
    ✓7ᵗʰ **S68.124 Partial traumatic metacarpophalangeal amputation of right ring finger**
    ✓7ᵗʰ **S68.125 Partial traumatic metacarpophalangeal amputation of left ring finger**
    ✓7ᵗʰ **S68.126 Partial traumatic metacarpophalangeal amputation of right little finger**
    ✓7ᵗʰ **S68.127 Partial traumatic metacarpophalangeal amputation of left little finger**
    ✓7ᵗʰ **S68.128 Partial traumatic metacarpophalangeal amputation of other finger**
        Partial traumatic metacarpophalangeal amputation of specified finger with unspecified laterality
    ✓7ᵗʰ **S68.129 Partial traumatic metacarpophalangeal amputation of unspecified finger**

☑ Additional Character Required   ✓x7ᵗʰ Placeholder Alert   Unspecified Dx   Other Specified Dx   Manifestation   ▶◀ Revised Text   ● New Code   ▲ Revised Code Title

√5ᵗʰ **S68.4** **Traumatic amputation of** hand at wrist level
Traumatic amputation of hand NOS
Traumatic amputation of wrist

  √6ᵗʰ **S68.41** **Complete traumatic amputation of hand at wrist level**

    √7ᵗʰ **S68.411** **Complete traumatic amputation of** right **hand at wrist level**

    √7ᵗʰ **S68.412** **Complete traumatic amputation of** left **hand at wrist level**

    √7ᵗʰ **S68.419** **Complete traumatic amputation of unspecified hand at wrist level**

  √6ᵗʰ **S68.42** **Partial traumatic amputation of hand at wrist level**

    √7ᵗʰ **S68.421** **Partial traumatic amputation of** right **hand at wrist level**

    √7ᵗʰ **S68.422** **Partial traumatic amputation of** left **hand at wrist level**

    √7ᵗʰ **S68.429** **Partial traumatic amputation of unspecified hand at wrist level**

√5ᵗʰ **S68.5** **Traumatic** transphalangeal **amputation of** thumb
Traumatic interphalangeal joint amputation of thumb

  √6ᵗʰ **S68.51** **Complete traumatic transphalangeal amputation of thumb**

    √7ᵗʰ **S68.511** **Complete traumatic transphalangeal amputation of** right **thumb**

    √7ᵗʰ **S68.512** **Complete traumatic transphalangeal amputation of** left **thumb**

    √7ᵗʰ **S68.519** **Complete traumatic transphalangeal amputation of unspecified thumb**

  √6ᵗʰ **S68.52** **Partial traumatic transphalangeal amputation of thumb**

    √7ᵗʰ **S68.521** **Partial traumatic transphalangeal amputation of** right **thumb**

    √7ᵗʰ **S68.522** **Partial traumatic transphalangeal amputation of** left **thumb**

    √7ᵗʰ **S68.529** **Partial traumatic transphalangeal amputation of unspecified thumb**

√5ᵗʰ **S68.6** **Traumatic** transphalangeal **amputation of** other and unspecified finger

  √6ᵗʰ **S68.61** **Complete traumatic transphalangeal amputation of other and unspecified finger(s)**

    √7ᵗʰ **S68.610** **Complete traumatic transphalangeal amputation of** right index **finger**

    √7ᵗʰ **S68.611** **Complete traumatic transphalangeal amputation of** left index **finger**

    √7ᵗʰ **S68.612** **Complete traumatic transphalangeal amputation of** right middle **finger**

    √7ᵗʰ **S68.613** **Complete traumatic transphalangeal amputation of** left middle **finger**

    √7ᵗʰ **S68.614** **Complete traumatic transphalangeal amputation of** right ring **finger**

    √7ᵗʰ **S68.615** **Complete traumatic transphalangeal amputation of** left ring **finger**

    √7ᵗʰ **S68.616** **Complete traumatic transphalangeal amputation of** right little **finger**

    √7ᵗʰ **S68.617** **Complete traumatic transphalangeal amputation of** left little **finger**

    √7ᵗʰ **S68.618** **Complete traumatic transphalangeal amputation of other finger**
Complete traumatic transphalangeal amputation of specified finger with unspecified laterality

    √7ᵗʰ **S68.619** **Complete traumatic transphalangeal amputation of unspecified finger**

  √6ᵗʰ **S68.62** **Partial traumatic transphalangeal amputation of other and unspecified finger**

    √7ᵗʰ **S68.620** **Partial traumatic transphalangeal amputation of** right index **finger**

    √7ᵗʰ **S68.621** **Partial traumatic transphalangeal amputation of** left index **finger**

    √7ᵗʰ **S68.622** **Partial traumatic transphalangeal amputation of** right middle **finger**

    √7ᵗʰ **S68.623** **Partial traumatic transphalangeal amputation of** left middle **finger**

    √7ᵗʰ **S68.624** **Partial traumatic transphalangeal amputation of** right ring **finger**

    √7ᵗʰ **S68.625** **Partial traumatic transphalangeal amputation of** left ring **finger**

    √7ᵗʰ **S68.626** **Partial traumatic transphalangeal amputation of** right little **finger**

    √7ᵗʰ **S68.627** **Partial traumatic transphalangeal amputation of** left little **finger**

    √7ᵗʰ **S68.628** **Partial traumatic transphalangeal amputation of other finger**
Partial traumatic transphalangeal amputation of specified finger with unspecified laterality

    √7ᵗʰ **S68.629** **Partial traumatic transphalangeal amputation of unspecified finger**

√5ᵗʰ **S68.7** **Traumatic** transmetacarpal **amputation of** hand

  √6ᵗʰ **S68.71** **Complete traumatic transmetacarpal amputation of hand**

    √7ᵗʰ **S68.711** **Complete traumatic transmetacarpal amputation of** right **hand**

    √7ᵗʰ **S68.712** **Complete traumatic transmetacarpal amputation of** left **hand**

    √7ᵗʰ **S68.719** **Complete traumatic transmetacarpal amputation of unspecified hand**

  √6ᵗʰ **S68.72** **Partial traumatic transmetacarpal amputation of hand**

    √7ᵗʰ **S68.721** **Partial traumatic transmetacarpal amputation of** right **hand**

    √7ᵗʰ **S68.722** **Partial traumatic transmetacarpal amputation of** left **hand**

    √7ᵗʰ **S68.729** **Partial traumatic transmetacarpal amputation of unspecified hand**

√4ᵗʰ **S69** **Other and unspecified injuries of wrist, hand and finger(s)**

> The appropriate 7th character is to be added to each code from category S69.
> A   initial encounter
> D   subsequent encounter
> S   sequela

  √5ᵗʰ **S69.8** **Other specified injuries of wrist, hand and finger(s)**

    √x7ᵗʰ **S69.80** **Other specified injuries of unspecified wrist, hand and finger(s)**

    √x7ᵗʰ **S69.81** **Other specified injuries of** right **wrist, hand and finger(s)**

    √x7ᵗʰ **S69.82** **Other specified injuries of** left **wrist, hand and finger(s)**

  √5ᵗʰ **S69.9** **Unspecified injury of wrist, hand and finger(s)**

    √x7ᵗʰ **S69.90** **Unspecified injury of unspecified wrist, hand and finger(s)**

    √x7ᵗʰ **S69.91** **Unspecified injury of** right **wrist, hand and finger(s)**

    √x7ᵗʰ **S69.92** **Unspecified injury of** left **wrist, hand and finger(s)**

Injuries to the hip and thigh (S70-S79)

EXCLUDES 2 *burns and corrosions (T20-T32)*
frostbite (T33-T34)
snake bite (T63.0-)
venomous insect bite or sting (T63.4-)

√4ᵗʰ **S70** **Superficial injury of hip and thigh**

> The appropriate 7th character is to be added to each code from category S70.
> A   initial encounter
> D   subsequent encounter
> S   sequela

  √5ᵗʰ **S70.0** **Contusion of** hip

    √x7ᵗʰ **S70.00** **Contusion of unspecified hip**

    √x7ᵗʰ **S70.01** **Contusion of** right **hip**

    √x7ᵗʰ **S70.02** **Contusion of** left **hip**

  √5ᵗʰ **S70.1** **Contusion of** thigh

    √x7ᵗʰ **S70.10** **Contusion of unspecified thigh**

    √x7ᵗʰ **S70.11** **Contusion of** right **thigh**

    √x7ᵗʰ **S70.12** **Contusion of** left **thigh**

  √5ᵗʰ **S70.2** **Other superficial injuries of** hip

    √6ᵗʰ **S70.21** **Abrasion of hip**

      √7ᵗʰ **S70.211** **Abrasion,** right **hip**

      √7ᵗʰ **S70.212** **Abrasion,** left **hip**

EXCLUDES 1 Not coded here   *EXCLUDES 2* Not included here   N Newborn Age: 0   P Pediatric Age: 0-17   M Maternity Age: 12-55   A Adult Age: 15-124

930   ICD-10-CM 2016

√7ᵗʰ **S70.219** **Abrasion, unspecified hip**

√6ᵗʰ **S70.22** Blister (nonthermal) of hip

√7ᵗʰ **S70.221** Blister (nonthermal), right hip

√7ᵗʰ **S70.222** Blister (nonthermal), left hip

√7ᵗʰ **S70.229** **Blister (nonthermal), unspecified hip**

√6ᵗʰ **S70.24** External constriction of hip

√7ᵗʰ **S70.241** External constriction, right hip

√7ᵗʰ **S70.242** External constriction, left hip

√7ᵗʰ **S70.249** **External constriction, unspecified hip**

√6ᵗʰ **S70.25** Superficial foreign body of hip
Splinter in the hip

√7ᵗʰ **S70.251** Superficial foreign body, right hip

√7ᵗʰ **S70.252** Superficial foreign body, left hip

√7ᵗʰ **S70.259** **Superficial foreign body, unspecified hip**

√6ᵗʰ **S70.26** Insect bite (nonvenomous) of hip

√7ᵗʰ **S70.261** Insect bite (nonvenomous), right hip

√7ᵗʰ **S70.262** Insect bite (nonvenomous), left hip

√7ᵗʰ **S70.269** **Insect bite (nonvenomous), unspecified hip**

√6ᵗʰ **S70.27** Other superficial bite of hip
EXCLUDES 1 *open bite of hip (S71.05-)*

√7ᵗʰ **S70.271** Other superficial bite of hip, right hip

√7ᵗʰ **S70.272** Other superficial bite of hip, left hip

√7ᵗʰ **S70.279** **Other superficial bite of hip, unspecified hip**

√5ᵗʰ **S70.3** Other superficial injuries of thigh

√6ᵗʰ **S70.31** Abrasion of thigh

√7ᵗʰ **S70.311** Abrasion, right thigh

√7ᵗʰ **S70.312** Abrasion, left thigh

√7ᵗʰ **S70.319** Abrasion, unspecified thigh

√6ᵗʰ **S70.32** Blister (nonthermal) of thigh

√7ᵗʰ **S70.321** Blister (nonthermal), right thigh

√7ᵗʰ **S70.322** Blister (nonthermal), left thigh

√7ᵗʰ **S70.329** **Blister (nonthermal), unspecified thigh**

√6ᵗʰ **S70.34** External constriction of thigh

√7ᵗʰ **S70.341** External constriction, right thigh

√7ᵗʰ **S70.342** External constriction, left thigh

√7ᵗʰ **S70.349** **External constriction, unspecified thigh**

√6ᵗʰ **S70.35** Superficial foreign body of thigh
Splinter in the thigh

√7ᵗʰ **S70.351** Superficial foreign body, right thigh

√7ᵗʰ **S70.352** Superficial foreign body, left thigh

√7ᵗʰ **S70.359** **Superficial foreign body, unspecified thigh**

√6ᵗʰ **S70.36** Insect bite (nonvenomous) of thigh

√7ᵗʰ **S70.361** Insect bite (nonvenomous), right thigh

√7ᵗʰ **S70.362** Insect bite (nonvenomous), left thigh

√7ᵗʰ **S70.369** **Insect bite (nonvenomous), unspecified thigh**

√6ᵗʰ **S70.37** Other superficial bite of thigh
EXCLUDES 1 *open bite of thigh (S71.15)*

√7ᵗʰ **S70.371** **Other superficial bite of right thigh**

√7ᵗʰ **S70.372** **Other superficial bite of left thigh**

√7ᵗʰ **S70.379** **Other superficial bite of unspecified thigh**

√5ᵗʰ **S70.9** Unspecified superficial injury of hip and thigh

√6ᵗʰ **S70.91** Unspecified superficial injury of hip

√7ᵗʰ **S70.911** Unspecified superficial injury of right hip

√7ᵗʰ **S70.912** Unspecified superficial injury of left hip

√7ᵗʰ **S70.919** Unspecified superficial injury of unspecified hip

√6ᵗʰ **S70.92** Unspecified superficial injury of thigh

√7ᵗʰ **S70.921** Unspecified superficial injury of right thigh

√7ᵗʰ **S70.922** Unspecified superficial injury of left thigh

√7ᵗʰ **S70.929** Unspecified superficial injury of unspecified thigh

√4ᵗʰ **S71** Open wound of hip and thigh
Code also any associated wound infection
EXCLUDES 1 *open fracture of hip and thigh (S72.-)*
traumatic amputation of hip and thigh (S78.-)
EXCLUDES 2 *bite of venomous animal (T63.-)*
open wound of ankle, foot and toes (S91.-)
open wound of knee and lower leg (S81.-)

The appropriate 7th character is to be added to each code
from category S71.
A   initial encounter
D   subsequent encounter
S   sequela

√5ᵗʰ **S71.0** Open wound of hip

√6ᵗʰ **S71.00** Unspecified open wound of hip

√7ᵗʰ **S71.001** Unspecified open wound, right hip

√7ᵗʰ **S71.002** Unspecified open wound, left hip

√7ᵗʰ **S71.009** Unspecified open wound, unspecified hip

√6ᵗʰ **S71.01** Laceration without foreign body of hip

√7ᵗʰ **S71.011** Laceration without foreign body, right hip

√7ᵗʰ **S71.012** Laceration without foreign body, left hip

√7ᵗʰ **S71.019** **Laceration without foreign body, unspecified hip**

√6ᵗʰ **S71.02** Laceration with foreign body of hip

√7ᵗʰ **S71.021** Laceration with foreign body, right hip

√7ᵗʰ **S71.022** Laceration with foreign body, left hip

√7ᵗʰ **S71.029** **Laceration with foreign body, unspecified hip**

√6ᵗʰ **S71.03** Puncture wound without foreign body of hip

√7ᵗʰ **S71.031** Puncture wound without foreign body, right hip

√7ᵗʰ **S71.032** Puncture wound without foreign body, left hip

√7ᵗʰ **S71.039** **Puncture wound without foreign body, unspecified hip**

√6ᵗʰ **S71.04** Puncture wound with foreign body of hip

√7ᵗʰ **S71.041** Puncture wound with foreign body, right hip

√7ᵗʰ **S71.042** Puncture wound with foreign body, left hip

√7ᵗʰ **S71.049** **Puncture wound with foreign body, unspecified hip**

√6ᵗʰ **S71.05** Open bite of hip
Bite of hip NOS
EXCLUDES 1 *superficial bite of hip (S70.26, S70.27)*

√7ᵗʰ **S71.051** Open bite, right hip

√7ᵗʰ **S71.052** Open bite, left hip

√7ᵗʰ **S71.059** **Open bite, unspecified hip**

√5ᵗʰ **S71.1** Open wound of thigh

√6ᵗʰ **S71.10** Unspecified open wound of thigh

√7ᵗʰ **S71.101** Unspecified open wound, right thigh

√7ᵗʰ **S71.102** Unspecified open wound, left thigh

√7ᵗʰ **S71.109** **Unspecified open wound, unspecified thigh**

√6ᵗʰ **S71.11** Laceration without foreign body of thigh

√7ᵗʰ **S71.111** Laceration without foreign body, right thigh

√7ᵗʰ **S71.112** Laceration without foreign body, left thigh

√7ᵗʰ **S71.119** **Laceration without foreign body, unspecified thigh**

√6ᵗʰ **S71.12** Laceration with foreign body of thigh

√7ᵗʰ **S71.121** Laceration with foreign body, right thigh

√7ᵗʰ **S71.122** Laceration with foreign body, left thigh

√7ᵗʰ **S71.129** **Laceration with foreign body, unspecified thigh**

√6ᵗʰ **S71.13** Puncture wound without foreign body of thigh

√7ᵗʰ **S71.131** Puncture wound without foreign body, right thigh

√7ᵗʰ **S71.132** Puncture wound without foreign body, left thigh

√7ᵗʰ **S71.139** **Puncture wound without foreign body, unspecified thigh**

☑ Additional Character Required   √x7ᵗʰ Placeholder Alert   Unspecified Dx   Other Specified Dx   Manifestation   ►◄ Revised Text   ● New Code   ▲ Revised Code Title

ICD-10-CM 2016   **931**

Chapter 19. Injury, Poisoning, and Certain Other Consequences of External Causes

S70.219–S71.139

√6ᵗʰ S71.14 Puncture wound with foreign body of thigh

    √7ᵗʰ **S71.141 Puncture wound with foreign body, right thigh**

    √7ᵗʰ **S71.142 Puncture wound with foreign body, left thigh**

    √7ᵗʰ **S71.149 Puncture wound with foreign body, unspecified thigh**

√6ᵗʰ S71.15 Open bite of thigh
    Bite of thigh NOS
    EXCLUDES 1   *superficial bite of thigh (S70.37-)*

    √7ᵗʰ **S71.151 Open bite, right thigh**

    √7ᵗʰ **S71.152 Open bite, left thigh**

    √7ᵗʰ **S71.159 Open bite, unspecified thigh**

√4ᵗʰ S72   Fracture of femur
    NOTE   A fracture not indicated as displaced or nondisplaced should be coded to displaced.
        The open fracture designations are based on the Gustilo open fracture classification.
        A fracture not indicated as open or closed should be coded to closed.
    EXCLUDES 1 *traumatic amputation of hip and thigh (S78.-)*
    EXCLUDES 2 *fracture of foot (S92.-)*
             fracture of lower leg and ankle (S82.-)
             periprosthetic fracture of prosthetic implant of hip (T84.040, T84.041)
    AHA: 2015, 1Q, 17; 2013, 4Q, 128

> The appropriate 7th character is to be added to all codes from category S72 [unless otherwise indicated].
> A   initial encounter for closed fracture
> B   initial encounter for open fracture type I or II
>   initial encounter for open fracture NOS
> C   initial encounter for open fracture type IIIA, IIIB, or IIIC
> D   subsequent encounter for closed fracture with routine healing
> E   subsequent encounter for open fracture type I or II with routine healing
> F   subsequent encounter for open fracture type IIIA, IIIB, or IIIC with routine healing
> G   subsequent encounter for closed fracture with delayed healing
> H   subsequent encounter for open fracture type I or II with delayed healing
> J   subsequent encounter for open fracture type IIIA, IIIB, or IIIC with delayed healing
> K   subsequent encounter for closed fracture with nonunion
> M   subsequent encounter for open fracture type I or II with nonunion
> N   subsequent encounter for open fracture type IIIA, IIIB, or IIIC with nonunion
> P   subsequent encounter for closed fracture with malunion
> Q   subsequent encounter for open fracture type I or II with malunion
> R   subsequent encounter for open fracture type IIIA, IIIB, or IIIC with malunion
> S   sequela

√5ᵗʰ S72.0   Fracture of head and neck of femur
    EXCLUDES 2 *physeal fracture of upper end of femur (S79.0-)*

√6ᵗʰ S72.00 Fracture of unspecified part of neck of femur
    Fracture of hip NOSFracture of neck of femur NOS

    √7ᵗʰ **S72.001 Fracture of unspecified part of neck of right femur**

    √7ᵗʰ **S72.002 Fracture of unspecified part of neck of left femur**

    √7ᵗʰ **S72.009 Fracture of unspecified part of neck of unspecified femur**

√6ᵗʰ S72.01 Unspecified intracapsular fracture of femur
    Subcapital fracture of femur

    √7ᵗʰ **S72.011 Unspecified intracapsular fracture of right femur**

    √7ᵗʰ **S72.012 Unspecified intracapsular fracture of left femur**

    √7ᵗʰ **S72.019 Unspecified intracapsular fracture of unspecified femur**

√6ᵗʰ S72.02 Fracture of epiphysis (separation) (upper) of femur
    Transepiphyseal fracture of femur
    EXCLUDES 1 *capital femoral epiphyseal fracture (pediatric) of femur (S79.01-)*
           Salter-Harris Type I physeal fracture of upper end of femur (S79.01-)

    √7ᵗʰ **S72.021 Displaced fracture of epiphysis (separation) (upper) of right femur**

    √7ᵗʰ **S72.022 Displaced fracture of epiphysis (separation) (upper) of left femur**

    √7ᵗʰ **S72.023 Displaced fracture of epiphysis (separation) (upper) of unspecified femur**

    √7ᵗʰ **S72.024 Nondisplaced fracture of epiphysis (separation) (upper) of right femur**

    √7ᵗʰ **S72.025 Nondisplaced fracture of epiphysis (separation) (upper) of left femur**

    √7ᵗʰ **S72.026 Nondisplaced fracture of epiphysis (separation) (upper) of unspecified femur**

√6ᵗʰ S72.03 Midcervical fracture of femur
    Transcervical fracture of femur NOS

    √7ᵗʰ **S72.031 Displaced midcervical fracture of right femur**

    √7ᵗʰ **S72.032 Displaced midcervical fracture of left femur**

    √7ᵗʰ **S72.033 Displaced midcervical fracture of unspecified femur**

    √7ᵗʰ **S72.034 Nondisplaced midcervical fracture of right femur**

    √7ᵗʰ **S72.035 Nondisplaced midcervical fracture of left femur**

    √7ᵗʰ **S72.036 Nondisplaced midcervical fracture of unspecified femur**

√6ᵗʰ S72.04 Fracture of base of neck of femur
    Cervicotrochanteric fracture of femur

    √7ᵗʰ **S72.041 Displaced fracture of base of neck of right femur**

    √7ᵗʰ **S72.042 Displaced fracture of base of neck of left femur**

    √7ᵗʰ **S72.043 Displaced fracture of base of neck of unspecified femur**

    √7ᵗʰ **S72.044 Nondisplaced fracture of base of neck of right femur**

    √7ᵗʰ **S72.045 Nondisplaced fracture of base of neck of left femur**

    √7ᵗʰ **S72.046 Nondisplaced fracture of base of neck of unspecified femur**

√6ᵗʰ S72.05 Unspecified fracture of head of femur
    Fracture of head of femur NOS

    √7ᵗʰ **S72.051 Unspecified fracture of head of right femur**

    √7ᵗʰ **S72.052 Unspecified fracture of head of left femur**

    √7ᵗʰ **S72.059 Unspecified fracture of head of unspecified femur**

√6ᵗʰ S72.06 Articular fracture of head of femur

    √7ᵗʰ **S72.061 Displaced articular fracture of head of right femur**

    √7ᵗʰ **S72.062 Displaced articular fracture of head of left femur**

    √7ᵗʰ **S72.063 Displaced articular fracture of head of unspecified femur**

    √7ᵗʰ **S72.064 Nondisplaced articular fracture of head of right femur**

    √7ᵗʰ **S72.065 Nondisplaced articular fracture of head of left femur**

    √7ᵗʰ **S72.066 Nondisplaced articular fracture of head of unspecified femur**

√6ᵗʰ S72.09 Other fracture of head and neck of femur

    √7ᵗʰ **S72.091 Other fracture of head and neck of right femur**

    √7ᵗʰ **S72.092 Other fracture of head and neck of left femur**

    √7ᵗʰ **S72.099 Other fracture of head and neck of unspecified femur**

EXCLUDES 1 Not coded here   EXCLUDES 2 Not included here   N Newborn Age: 0   P Pediatric Age: 0-17   M Maternity Age: 12-55   A Adult Age: 15-124

✓5th S72.1   Pertrochanteric **fracture**

   ✓6th S72.10   Unspecified trochanteric **fracture of femur**
       Fracture of trochanter NOS

     ✓7th S72.101   **Unspecified trochanteric fracture of** right **femur**

     ✓7th S72.102   **Unspecified trochanteric fracture of** left **femur**

     ✓7th S72.109   **Unspecified trochanteric fracture of unspecified femur**

   ✓6th S72.11   **Fracture of** greater trochanter **of femur**

     ✓7th S72.111   **Displaced fracture of greater trochanter of** right **femur**

     ✓7th S72.112   **Displaced fracture of greater trochanter of** left **femur**

     ✓7th S72.113   Displaced **fracture of greater trochanter of unspecified femur**

     ✓7th S72.114   **Nondisplaced fracture of greater trochanter of** right **femur**

     ✓7th S72.115   **Nondisplaced fracture of greater trochanter of** left **femur**

     ✓7th S72.116   Nondisplaced **fracture of greater trochanter of unspecified femur**

   ✓6th S72.12   **Fracture of** lesser trochanter **of femur**

     ✓7th S72.121   **Displaced fracture of lesser trochanter of** right **femur**

     ✓7th S72.122   **Displaced fracture of lesser trochanter of** left **femur**

     ✓7th S72.123   Displaced **fracture of lesser trochanter of unspecified femur**

     ✓7th S72.124   **Nondisplaced fracture of lesser trochanter of** right **femur**

     ✓7th S72.125   **Nondisplaced fracture of lesser trochanter of** left **femur**

     ✓7th S72.126   Nondisplaced **fracture of lesser trochanter of unspecified femur**

   ✓6th S72.13   Apophyseal **fracture of femur**
     EXCLUDES 1   *chronic (nontraumatic) slipped upper femoral epiphysis (M93.0-)*

     ✓7th S72.131   **Displaced apophyseal fracture of** right **femur**

     ✓7th S72.132   **Displaced apophyseal fracture of** left **femur**

     ✓7th S72.133   Displaced **apophyseal fracture of unspecified femur**

     ✓7th S72.134   **Nondisplaced apophyseal fracture of** right **femur**

     ✓7th S72.135   **Nondisplaced apophyseal fracture of** left **femur**

     ✓7th S72.136   Nondisplaced **apophyseal fracture of unspecified femur**

   ✓6th S72.14   Intertrochanteric **fracture of femur**

     ✓7th S72.141   **Displaced intertrochanteric fracture of** right **femur**

     ✓7th S72.142   **Displaced intertrochanteric fracture of** left **femur**

     ✓7th S72.143   Displaced **intertrochanteric fracture of unspecified femur**

     ✓7th S72.144   **Nondisplaced intertrochanteric fracture of** right **femur**

     ✓7th S72.145   **Nondisplaced intertrochanteric fracture of** left **femur**

     ✓7th S72.146   Nondisplaced **intertrochanteric fracture of unspecified femur**

✓5th S72.2   Subtrochanteric **fracture of femur**

   ✓x7th S72.21   Displaced **subtrochanteric fracture of** right **femur**

   ✓x7th S72.22   Displaced **subtrochanteric fracture of** left **femur**

   ✓x7th S72.23   Displaced **subtrochanteric fracture of unspecified femur**

   ✓x7th S72.24   Nondisplaced **subtrochanteric fracture of** right **femur**

   ✓x7th S72.25   Nondisplaced **subtrochanteric fracture of** left **femur**

   ✓x7th S72.26   Nondisplaced **subtrochanteric fracture of unspecified femur**

✓5th S72.3   Fracture of shaft **of femur**

   ✓6th S72.30   Unspecified **fracture of shaft of femur**

     ✓7th S72.301   **Unspecified fracture of shaft of** right **femur**

     ✓7th S72.302   **Unspecified fracture of shaft of** left **femur**

     ✓7th S72.309   **Unspecified fracture of shaft of unspecified femur**

   ✓6th S72.32   Transverse **fracture of shaft of femur**

     ✓7th S72.321   **Displaced transverse fracture of shaft of** right **femur**

     ✓7th S72.322   **Displaced transverse fracture of shaft of** left **femur**

     ✓7th S72.323   Displaced **transverse fracture of shaft of unspecified femur**

     ✓7th S72.324   **Nondisplaced transverse fracture of shaft of** right **femur**

     ✓7th S72.325   **Nondisplaced transverse fracture of shaft of** left **femur**

     ✓7th S72.326   Nondisplaced **transverse fracture of shaft of unspecified femur**

   ✓6th S72.33   Oblique **fracture of shaft of femur**

     ✓7th S72.331   **Displaced oblique fracture of shaft of** right **femur**

     ✓7th S72.332   **Displaced oblique fracture of shaft of** left **femur**

     ✓7th S72.333   Displaced **oblique fracture of shaft of unspecified femur**

     ✓7th S72.334   **Nondisplaced oblique fracture of shaft of** right **femur**

     ✓7th S72.335   **Nondisplaced oblique fracture of shaft of** left **femur**

     ✓7th S72.336   Nondisplaced **oblique fracture of shaft of unspecified femur**

   ✓6th S72.34   Spiral **fracture of shaft of femur**

     ✓7th S72.341   **Displaced spiral fracture of shaft of** right **femur**

     ✓7th S72.342   **Displaced spiral fracture of shaft of** left **femur**

     ✓7th S72.343   Displaced **spiral fracture of shaft of unspecified femur**

     ✓7th S72.344   **Nondisplaced spiral fracture of shaft of** right **femur**

     ✓7th S72.345   **Nondisplaced spiral fracture of shaft of** left **femur**

     ✓7th S72.346   Nondisplaced **spiral fracture of shaft of unspecified femur**

   ✓6th S72.35   Comminuted **fracture of shaft of femur**

     ✓7th S72.351   **Displaced comminuted fracture of shaft of** right **femur**

     ✓7th S72.352   **Displaced comminuted fracture of shaft of** left **femur**

     ✓7th S72.353   Displaced **comminuted fracture of shaft of unspecified femur**

     ✓7th S72.354   **Nondisplaced comminuted fracture of shaft of** right **femur**

     ✓7th S72.355   **Nondisplaced comminuted fracture of shaft of** left **femur**

     ✓7th S72.356   Nondisplaced **comminuted fracture of shaft of unspecified femur**

   ✓6th S72.36   Segmental **fracture of shaft of femur**

     ✓7th S72.361   **Displaced segmental fracture of shaft of** right **femur**

     ✓7th S72.362   **Displaced segmental fracture of shaft of** left **femur**

     ✓7th S72.363   Displaced **segmental fracture of shaft of unspecified femur**

     ✓7th S72.364   **Nondisplaced segmental fracture of shaft of** right **femur**

     ✓7th S72.365   **Nondisplaced segmental fracture of shaft of** left **femur**

     ✓7th S72.366   Nondisplaced **segmental fracture of shaft of unspecified femur**

✔ Additional Character Required   ✔x7th Placeholder Alert   Unspecified Dx   Other Specified Dx   Manifestation   ▶◀ Revised Text   ● New Code   ▲ Revised Code Title

√6ᵗʰ **S72.39** Other fracture of shaft of femur

√7ᵗʰ **S72.391** **Other fracture of shaft of right femur**

√7ᵗʰ **S72.392** **Other fracture of shaft of left femur**

√7ᵗʰ **S72.399** **Other fracture of shaft of unspecified femur**

√5ᵗʰ **S72.4** Fracture of lower end of femur

Fracture of distal end of femur

EXCLUDES 2 *fracture of shaft of femur (S72.3-)*
physeal fracture of lower end of femur (S79.1-)

√6ᵗʰ **S72.40** Unspecified fracture of lower end of femur

√7ᵗʰ **S72.401** **Unspecified fracture of lower end of right femur**

√7ᵗʰ **S72.402** **Unspecified fracture of lower end of left femur**

√7ᵗʰ **S72.409** **Unspecified fracture of lower end of unspecified femur**

√6ᵗʰ **S72.41** Unspecified condyle fracture of lower end of femur

Condyle fracture of femur NOS

√7ᵗʰ **S72.411** **Displaced unspecified condyle fracture of lower end of right femur**

√7ᵗʰ **S72.412** **Displaced unspecified condyle fracture of lower end of left femur**

√7ᵗʰ **S72.413** **Displaced unspecified condyle fracture of lower end of unspecified femur**

√7ᵗʰ **S72.414** **Nondisplaced unspecified condyle fracture of lower end of right femur**

√7ᵗʰ **S72.415** **Nondisplaced unspecified condyle fracture of lower end of left femur**

√7ᵗʰ **S72.416** **Nondisplaced unspecified condyle fracture of lower end of unspecified femur**

√6ᵗʰ **S72.42** Fracture of lateral condyle of femur

√7ᵗʰ **S72.421** **Displaced fracture of lateral condyle of right femur**

√7ᵗʰ **S72.422** **Displaced fracture of lateral condyle of left femur**

√7ᵗʰ **S72.423** **Displaced fracture of lateral condyle of unspecified femur**

√7ᵗʰ **S72.424** **Nondisplaced fracture of lateral condyle of right femur**

√7ᵗʰ **S72.425** **Nondisplaced fracture of lateral condyle of left femur**

√7ᵗʰ **S72.426** **Nondisplaced fracture of lateral condyle of unspecified femur**

√6ᵗʰ **S72.43** Fracture of medial condyle of femur

√7ᵗʰ **S72.431** **Displaced fracture of medial condyle of right femur**

√7ᵗʰ **S72.432** **Displaced fracture of medial condyle of left femur**

√7ᵗʰ **S72.433** **Displaced fracture of medial condyle of unspecified femur**

√7ᵗʰ **S72.434** **Nondisplaced fracture of medial condyle of right femur**

√7ᵗʰ **S72.435** **Nondisplaced fracture of medial condyle of left femur**

√7ᵗʰ **S72.436** **Nondisplaced fracture of medial condyle of unspecified femur**

√6ᵗʰ **S72.44** Fracture of lower epiphysis (separation) of femur

EXCLUDES 1 *Salter-Harris Type I physeal fracture of lower end of femur (S79.11-)*

√7ᵗʰ **S72.441** **Displaced fracture of lower epiphysis (separation) of right femur**

√7ᵗʰ **S72.442** **Displaced fracture of lower epiphysis (separation) of left femur**

√7ᵗʰ **S72.443** **Displaced fracture of lower epiphysis (separation) of unspecified femur**

√7ᵗʰ **S72.444** **Nondisplaced fracture of lower epiphysis (separation) of right femur**

√7ᵗʰ **S72.445** **Nondisplaced fracture of lower epiphysis (separation) of left femur**

√7ᵗʰ **S72.446** **Nondisplaced fracture of lower epiphysis (separation) of unspecified femur**

√6ᵗʰ **S72.45** Supracondylar fracture without intracondylar extension of lower end of femur

Supracondylar fracture of lower end of femur NOS

EXCLUDES 1 *supracondylar fracture with intracondylar extension of lower end of femur (S72.46-)*

√7ᵗʰ **S72.451** **Displaced supracondylar fracture without intracondylar extension of lower end of right femur**

√7ᵗʰ **S72.452** **Displaced supracondylar fracture without intracondylar extension of lower end of left femur**

√7ᵗʰ **S72.453** **Displaced supracondylar fracture without intracondylar extension of lower end of unspecified femur**

√7ᵗʰ **S72.454** **Nondisplaced supracondylar fracture without intracondylar extension of lower end of right femur**

√7ᵗʰ **S72.455** **Nondisplaced supracondylar fracture without intracondylar extension of lower end of left femur**

√7ᵗʰ **S72.456** **Nondisplaced supracondylar fracture without intracondylar extension of lower end of unspecified femur**

√6ᵗʰ **S72.46** Supracondylar fracture with intracondylar extension of lower end of femur

EXCLUDES 1 *supracondylar fracture without intracondylar extension of lower end of femur (S72.45-)*

√7ᵗʰ **S72.461** **Displaced supracondylar fracture with intracondylar extension of lower end of right femur**

√7ᵗʰ **S72.462** **Displaced supracondylar fracture with intracondylar extension of lower end of left femur**

√7ᵗʰ **S72.463** **Displaced supracondylar fracture with intracondylar extension of lower end of unspecified femur**

√7ᵗʰ **S72.464** **Nondisplaced supracondylar fracture with intracondylar extension of lower end of right femur**

√7ᵗʰ **S72.465** **Nondisplaced supracondylar fracture with intracondylar extension of lower end of left femur**

√7ᵗʰ **S72.466** **Nondisplaced supracondylar fracture with intracondylar extension of lower end of unspecified femur**

√6ᵗʰ **S72.47** Torus fracture of lower end of femur

The appropriate 7th character is to be added to all codes in subcategory S72.47.
A   initial encounter for closed fracture
D   subsequent encounter for fracture with routine healing
G   subsequent encounter for fracture with delayed healing
K   subsequent encounter for fracture with nonunion
P   subsequent encounter for fracture with malunion
S   sequela

√7ᵗʰ **S72.471** Torus fracture of lower end of right femur

√7ᵗʰ **S72.472** Torus fracture of lower end of left femur

√7ᵗʰ **S72.479** Torus fracture of lower end of unspecified femur

√6ᵗʰ **S72.49** Other fracture of lower end of femur

√7ᵗʰ **S72.491** Other fracture of lower end of right femur

√7ᵗʰ **S72.492** Other fracture of lower end of left femur

√7ᵗʰ **S72.499** Other fracture of lower end of unspecified femur

√5ᵗʰ **S72.8** Other fracture of femur

√6ᵗʰ **S72.8X** Other fracture of femur

√7ᵗʰ **S72.8X1** Other fracture of right femur

√7ᵗʰ **S72.8X2** Other fracture of left femur

√7ᵗʰ **S72.8X9** Other fracture of unspecified femur

EXCLUDES 1 Not coded here   EXCLUDES 2 Not included here   N Newborn Age: 0   P Pediatric Age: 0-17   M Maternity Age: 12-55   A Adult Age: 15-124

934   ICD-10-CM 2016

✓5ᵗʰ **S72.9   Unspecified fracture of femur**
Fracture of thigh NOS
Fracture of upper leg NOS
EXCLUDES 1   *fracture of hip NOS (S72.00-, S72.01-)*

✓x7ᵗʰ **S72.90   Unspecified fracture of unspecified femur**
AHA: 2012, 4Q, 93

✓x7ᵗʰ **S72.91   Unspecified fracture of right femur**

✓x7ᵗʰ **S72.92   Unspecified fracture of left femur**

✓4ᵗʰ **S73   Dislocation and sprain of joint and ligaments of hip**
INCLUDES   avulsion of joint or ligament of hip
laceration of cartilage, joint or ligament of hip
sprain of cartilage, joint or ligament of hip
traumatic hemarthrosis of joint or ligament of hip
traumatic rupture of joint or ligament of hip
traumatic subluxation of joint or ligament of hip
traumatic tear of joint or ligament of hip
Code also any associated open wound
EXCLUDES 2   *strain of muscle, fascia and tendon of hip and thigh (S76.-)*

The appropriate 7th character is to be added to each code from category S73.
A   initial encounter
D   subsequent encounter
S   sequela

✓5ᵗʰ **S73.0   Subluxation and dislocation of hip**
EXCLUDES 2   *dislocation and subluxation of hip prosthesis (T84.020, T84.021)*

✓6ᵗʰ **S73.00   Unspecified subluxation and dislocation of hip**
Dislocation of hip NOS
Subluxation of hip NOS

✓7ᵗʰ **S73.001   Unspecified subluxation of right hip**

✓7ᵗʰ **S73.002   Unspecified subluxation of left hip**

✓7ᵗʰ **S73.003   Unspecified subluxation of unspecified hip**

✓7ᵗʰ **S73.004   Unspecified dislocation of right hip**

✓7ᵗʰ **S73.005   Unspecified dislocation of left hip**

✓7ᵗʰ **S73.006   Unspecified dislocation of unspecified hip**

✓6ᵗʰ **S73.01   Posterior subluxation and dislocation of hip**

✓7ᵗʰ **S73.011   Posterior subluxation of right hip**

✓7ᵗʰ **S73.012   Posterior subluxation of left hip**

✓7ᵗʰ **S73.013   Posterior subluxation of unspecified hip**

✓7ᵗʰ **S73.014   Posterior dislocation of right hip**

✓7ᵗʰ **S73.015   Posterior dislocation of left hip**

✓7ᵗʰ **S73.016   Posterior dislocation of unspecified hip**

✓6ᵗʰ **S73.02   Obturator subluxation and dislocation of hip**

✓7ᵗʰ **S73.021   Obturator subluxation of right hip**

✓7ᵗʰ **S73.022   Obturator subluxation of left hip**

✓7ᵗʰ **S73.023   Obturator subluxation of unspecified hip**

✓7ᵗʰ **S73.024   Obturator dislocation of right hip**

✓7ᵗʰ **S73.025   Obturator dislocation of left hip**

✓7ᵗʰ **S73.026   Obturator dislocation of unspecified hip**

✓6ᵗʰ **S73.03   Other anterior dislocation of hip**

✓7ᵗʰ **S73.031   Other anterior subluxation of right hip**

✓7ᵗʰ **S73.032   Other anterior subluxation of left hip**

✓7ᵗʰ **S73.033   Other anterior subluxation of unspecified hip**

✓7ᵗʰ **S73.034   Other anterior dislocation of right hip**

✓7ᵗʰ **S73.035   Other anterior dislocation of left hip**

✓7ᵗʰ **S73.036   Other anterior dislocation of unspecified hip**

✓6ᵗʰ **S73.04   Central dislocation of hip**

✓7ᵗʰ **S73.041   Central subluxation of right hip**

✓7ᵗʰ **S73.042   Central subluxation of left hip**

✓7ᵗʰ **S73.043   Central subluxation of unspecified hip**

✓7ᵗʰ **S73.044   Central dislocation of right hip**

✓7ᵗʰ **S73.045   Central dislocation of left hip**

✓7ᵗʰ **S73.046   Central dislocation of unspecified hip**

✓5ᵗʰ **S73.1   Sprain of hip**
AHA: 2014, 4Q, 25

✓6ᵗʰ **S73.10   Unspecified sprain of hip**

✓7ᵗʰ **S73.101   Unspecified sprain of right hip**

✓7ᵗʰ **S73.102   Unspecified sprain of left hip**

✓7ᵗʰ **S73.109   Unspecified sprain of unspecified hip**

✓6ᵗʰ **S73.11   Iliofemoral ligament sprain of hip**

✓7ᵗʰ **S73.111   Iliofemoral ligament sprain of right hip**

✓7ᵗʰ **S73.112   Iliofemoral ligament sprain of left hip**

✓7ᵗʰ **S73.119   Iliofemoral ligament sprain of unspecified hip**

✓6ᵗʰ **S73.12   Ischiocapsular (ligament) sprain of hip**

✓7ᵗʰ **S73.121   Ischiocapsular ligament sprain of right hip**

✓7ᵗʰ **S73.122   Ischiocapsular ligament sprain of left hip**

✓7ᵗʰ **S73.129   Ischiocapsular ligament sprain of unspecified hip**

✓6ᵗʰ **S73.19   Other sprain of hip**

✓7ᵗʰ **S73.191   Other sprain of right hip**

✓7ᵗʰ **S73.192   Other sprain of left hip**

✓7ᵗʰ **S73.199   Other sprain of unspecified hip**

✓4ᵗʰ **S74   Injury of nerves at hip and thigh level**
Code also any associated open wound (S71.-)
EXCLUDES 2   *injury of nerves at ankle and foot level (S94.-)*
injury of nerves at lower leg level (S84.-)

The appropriate 7th character is to be added to each code from category S74.
A   initial encounter
D   subsequent encounter
S   sequela

✓5ᵗʰ **S74.0   Injury of sciatic nerve at hip and thigh level**

✓x7ᵗʰ **S74.00   Injury of sciatic nerve at hip and thigh level, unspecified leg**

✓x7ᵗʰ **S74.01   Injury of sciatic nerve at hip and thigh level, right leg**

✓x7ᵗʰ **S74.02   Injury of sciatic nerve at hip and thigh level, left leg**

✓5ᵗʰ **S74.1   Injury of femoral nerve at hip and thigh level**

✓x7ᵗʰ **S74.10   Injury of femoral nerve at hip and thigh level, unspecified leg**

✓x7ᵗʰ **S74.11   Injury of femoral nerve at hip and thigh level, right leg**

✓x7ᵗʰ **S74.12   Injury of femoral nerve at hip and thigh level, left leg**

✓5ᵗʰ **S74.2   Injury of cutaneous sensory nerve at hip and thigh level**

✓x7ᵗʰ **S74.20   Injury of cutaneous sensory nerve at hip and thigh level, unspecified leg**

✓x7ᵗʰ **S74.21   Injury of cutaneous sensory nerve at hip and high level, right leg**

✓x7ᵗʰ **S74.22   Injury of cutaneous sensory nerve at hip and thigh level, left leg**

✓5ᵗʰ **S74.8   Injury of other nerves at hip and thigh level**

✓6ᵗʰ **S74.8X   Injury of other nerves at hip and thigh level**

✓7ᵗʰ **S74.8X1   Injury of other nerves at hip and thigh level, right leg**

✓7ᵗʰ **S74.8X2   Injury of other nerves at hip and thigh level, left leg**

✓7ᵗʰ **S74.8X9   Injury of other nerves at hip and thigh level, unspecified leg**

✓5ᵗʰ **S74.9   Injury of unspecified nerve at hip and thigh level**

✓x7ᵗʰ **S74.90   Injury of unspecified nerve at hip and thigh level, unspecified leg**

✓x7ᵗʰ **S74.91   Injury of unspecified nerve at hip and thigh level, right leg**

✓x7ᵗʰ **S74.92   Injury of unspecified nerve at hip and thigh level, left leg**

√4ᵗʰ S75 Injury of blood vessels at hip and thigh level

Code also any associated open wound (S71.-)

EXCLUDES 2   injury of blood vessels at lower leg level (S85.-)
injury of popliteal artery (S85.0)

The appropriate 7th character is to be added to each code from category S75.
A   initial encounter
D   subsequent encounter
S   sequela

√5ᵗʰ S75.0 Injury of femoral artery

    √6ᵗʰ S75.00 Unspecified injury of femoral artery

        √7ᵗʰ S75.001 Unspecified injury of femoral artery, right leg

        √7ᵗʰ S75.002 Unspecified injury of femoral artery, left leg

        √7ᵗʰ S75.009 Unspecified injury of femoral artery, unspecified leg

    √6ᵗʰ S75.01 Minor laceration of femoral artery
Incomplete transection of femoral artery
Laceration of femoral artery NOS
Superficial laceration of femoral artery

        √7ᵗʰ S75.011 Minor laceration of femoral artery, right leg

        √7ᵗʰ S75.012 Minor laceration of femoral artery, left leg

        √7ᵗʰ S75.019 Minor laceration of femoral artery, unspecified leg

    √6ᵗʰ S75.02 Major laceration of femoral artery
Complete transection of femoral artery
Traumatic rupture of femoral artery

        √7ᵗʰ S75.021 Major laceration of femoral artery, right leg

        √7ᵗʰ S75.022 Major laceration of femoral artery, left leg

        √7ᵗʰ S75.029 Major laceration of femoral artery, unspecified leg

    √6ᵗʰ S75.09 Other specified injury of femoral artery

        √7ᵗʰ S75.091 Other specified injury of femoral artery, right leg

        √7ᵗʰ S75.092 Other specified injury of femoral artery, left leg

        √7ᵗʰ S75.099 Other specified injury of femoral artery, unspecified leg

√5ᵗʰ S75.1 Injury of femoral vein at hip and thigh level

    √6ᵗʰ S75.10 Unspecified injury of femoral vein at hip and thigh level

        √7ᵗʰ S75.101 Unspecified injury of femoral vein at hip and thigh level, right leg

        √7ᵗʰ S75.102 Unspecified injury of femoral vein at hip and thigh level, left leg

        √7ᵗʰ S75.109 Unspecified injury of femoral vein at hip and thigh level, unspecified leg

    √6ᵗʰ S75.11 Minor laceration of femoral vein at hip and thigh level
Incomplete transection of femoral vein at hip and thigh level
Laceration of femoral vein at hip and thigh level NOS
Superficial laceration of femoral vein at hip and thigh level

        √7ᵗʰ S75.111 Minor laceration of femoral vein at hip and thigh level, right leg

        √7ᵗʰ S75.112 Minor laceration of femoral vein at hip and thigh level, left leg

        √7ᵗʰ S75.119 Minor laceration of femoral vein at hip and thigh level, unspecified leg

    √6ᵗʰ S75.12 Major laceration of femoral vein at hip and thigh level
Complete transection of femoral vein at hip and thigh level
Traumatic rupture of femoral vein at hip and thigh level

        √7ᵗʰ S75.121 Major laceration of femoral vein at hip and thigh level, right leg

        √7ᵗʰ S75.122 Major laceration of femoral vein at hip and thigh level, left leg

        √7ᵗʰ S75.129 Major laceration of femoral vein at hip and thigh level, unspecified leg

    √6ᵗʰ S75.19 Other specified injury of femoral vein at hip and thigh level

        √7ᵗʰ S75.191 Other specified injury of femoral vein at hip and thigh level, right leg

        √7ᵗʰ S75.192 Other specified injury of femoral vein at hip and thigh level, left leg

        √7ᵗʰ S75.199 Other specified injury of femoral vein at hip and thigh level, unspecified leg

√5ᵗʰ S75.2 Injury of greater saphenous vein at hip and thigh level

EXCLUDES 1   greater saphenous vein NOS (S85.3)

    √6ᵗʰ S75.20 Unspecified injury of greater saphenous vein at hip and thigh level

        √7ᵗʰ S75.201 Unspecified injury of greater saphenous vein at hip and thigh level, right leg

        √7ᵗʰ S75.202 Unspecified injury of greater saphenous vein at hip and thigh level, left leg

        √7ᵗʰ S75.209 Unspecified injury of greater saphenous vein at hip and thigh level, unspecified leg

    √6ᵗʰ S75.21 Minor laceration of greater saphenous vein at hip and thigh level
Incomplete transection of greater saphenous vein at hip and thigh level
Laceration of greater saphenous vein at hip and thigh level NOS
Superficial laceration of greater saphenous vein at hip and thigh level

        √7ᵗʰ S75.211 Minor laceration of greater saphenous vein at hip and thigh level, right leg

        √7ᵗʰ S75.212 Minor laceration of greater saphenous vein at hip and thigh level, left leg

        √7ᵗʰ S75.219 Minor laceration of greater saphenous vein at hip and thigh level, unspecified leg

    √6ᵗʰ S75.22 Major laceration of greater saphenous vein at hip and thigh level
Complete transection of greater saphenous vein at hip and thigh level
Traumatic rupture of greater saphenous vein at hip and thigh level

        √7ᵗʰ S75.221 Major laceration of greater saphenous vein at hip and thigh level, right leg

        √7ᵗʰ S75.222 Major laceration of greater saphenous vein at hip and thigh level, left leg

        √7ᵗʰ S75.229 Major laceration of greater saphenous vein at hip and thigh level, unspecified leg

    √6ᵗʰ S75.29 Other specified injury of greater saphenous vein at hip and thigh level

        √7ᵗʰ S75.291 Other specified injury of greater saphenous vein at hip and thigh level, right leg

        √7ᵗʰ S75.292 Other specified injury of greater saphenous vein at hip and thigh level, left leg

        √7ᵗʰ S75.299 Other specified injury of greater saphenous vein at hip and thigh level, unspecified leg

√5ᵗʰ S75.8 Injury of other blood vessels at hip and thigh level

    √6ᵗʰ S75.80 Unspecified injury of other blood vessels at hip and thigh level

        √7ᵗʰ S75.801 Unspecified injury of other blood vessels at hip and thigh level, right leg

        √7ᵗʰ S75.802 Unspecified injury of other blood vessels at hip and thigh level, left leg

        √7ᵗʰ S75.809 Unspecified injury of other blood vessels at hip and thigh level, unspecified leg

    √6ᵗʰ S75.81 Laceration of other blood vessels at hip and thigh level

        √7ᵗʰ S75.811 Laceration of other blood vessels at hip and thigh level, right leg

        √7ᵗʰ S75.812 Laceration of other blood vessels at hip and thigh level, left leg

        √7ᵗʰ S75.819 Laceration of other blood vessels at hip and thigh level, unspecified leg

    √6ᵗʰ S75.89 Other specified injury of other blood vessels at hip and thigh level

        √7ᵗʰ S75.891 Other specified injury of other blood vessels at hip and thigh level, right leg

---

EXCLUDES 1 Not coded here   *EXCLUDES 2* Not included here   N Newborn Age: 0   P Pediatric Age: 0-17   M Maternity Age: 12-55   A Adult Age: 15-124

936   ICD-10-CM 2016

✓7ᵗʰ	**S75.892**	**Other specified injury of other blood vessels at hip and thigh level, left leg**
✓7ᵗʰ	**S75.899**	**Other specified injury of other blood vessels at hip and thigh level, unspecified leg**

✓5ᵗʰ **S75.9 Injury of unspecified blood vessel at hip and thigh level**

✓6ᵗʰ **S75.90 Unspecified injury of unspecified blood vessel at hip and thigh level**

✓7ᵗʰ	**S75.901**	**Unspecified injury of unspecified blood vessel at hip and thigh level, right leg**
✓7ᵗʰ	**S75.902**	**Unspecified injury of unspecified blood vessel at hip and thigh level, left leg**
✓7ᵗʰ	**S75.909**	**Unspecified injury of unspecified blood vessel at hip and thigh level, unspecified leg**

✓6ᵗʰ **S75.91 Laceration of unspecified blood vessel at hip and thigh level**

✓7ᵗʰ	**S75.911**	**Laceration of unspecified blood vessel at hip and thigh level, right leg**
✓7ᵗʰ	**S75.912**	**Laceration of unspecified blood vessel at hip and thigh level, left leg**
✓7ᵗʰ	**S75.919**	**Laceration of unspecified blood vessel at hip and thigh level, unspecified leg**

✓6ᵗʰ **S75.99 Other specified injury of unspecified blood vessel at hip and thigh level**

✓7ᵗʰ	**S75.991**	**Other specified injury of unspecified blood vessel at hip and thigh level, right leg**
✓7ᵗʰ	**S75.992**	**Other specified injury of unspecified blood vessel at hip and thigh level, left leg**
✓7ᵗʰ	**S75.999**	**Other specified injury of unspecified blood vessel at hip and thigh level, unspecified leg**

✦ ✓4ᵗʰ **S76 Injury of muscle, fascia and tendon at hip and thigh level**

Code also any associated open wound (S71.-)

EXCLUDES 2 *injury of muscle, fascia and tendon at lower leg level (S86)*
sprain of joint and ligament of hip (S73.1)

> The appropriate 7th character is to be added to each code from category S76.
> A   initial encounter
> D   subsequent encounter
> S   sequela

✓5ᵗʰ **S76.0 Injury of muscle, fascia and tendon of hip**

✓6ᵗʰ **S76.00 Unspecified injury of muscle, fascia and tendon of hip**

✓7ᵗʰ	**S76.001**	**Unspecified injury of muscle, fascia and tendon of right hip**
✓7ᵗʰ	**S76.002**	**Unspecified injury of muscle, fascia and tendon of left hip**
✓7ᵗʰ	**S76.009**	**Unspecified injury of muscle, fascia and tendon of unspecified hip**

✓6ᵗʰ **S76.01 Strain of muscle, fascia and tendon of hip**

✓7ᵗʰ	**S76.011**	**Strain of muscle, fascia and tendon of right hip**
✓7ᵗʰ	**S76.012**	**Strain of muscle, fascia and tendon of left hip**
✓7ᵗʰ	**S76.019**	**Strain of muscle, fascia and tendon of unspecified hip**

✓6ᵗʰ **S76.02 Laceration of muscle, fascia and tendon of hip**

✓7ᵗʰ	**S76.021**	**Laceration of muscle, fascia and tendon of right hip**
✓7ᵗʰ	**S76.022**	**Laceration of muscle, fascia and tendon of left hip**
✓7ᵗʰ	**S76.029**	**Laceration of muscle, fascia and tendon of unspecified hip**

✓6ᵗʰ **S76.09 Other specified injury of muscle, fascia and tendon of hip**

✓7ᵗʰ	**S76.091**	**Other specified injury of muscle, fascia and tendon of right hip**
✓7ᵗʰ	**S76.092**	**Other specified injury of muscle, fascia and tendon of left hip**
✓7ᵗʰ	**S76.099**	**Other specified injury of muscle, fascia and tendon of unspecified hip**

✓5ᵗʰ **S76.1 Injury of quadriceps muscle, fascia and tendon**

Injury of patellar ligament (tendon)

✓6ᵗʰ **S76.10 Unspecified injury of quadriceps muscle, fascia and tendon**

✓7ᵗʰ	**S76.101**	**Unspecified injury of right quadriceps muscle, fascia and tendon**
✓7ᵗʰ	**S76.102**	**Unspecified injury of left quadriceps muscle, fascia and tendon**
✓7ᵗʰ	**S76.109**	**Unspecified injury of unspecified quadriceps muscle, fascia and tendon**

✓6ᵗʰ **S76.11 Strain of quadriceps muscle, fascia and tendon**

✓7ᵗʰ	**S76.111**	**Strain of right quadriceps muscle, fascia and tendon**
✓7ᵗʰ	**S76.112**	**Strain of left quadriceps muscle, fascia and tendon**
✓7ᵗʰ	**S76.119**	**Strain of unspecified quadriceps muscle, fascia and tendon**

✓6ᵗʰ **S76.12 Laceration of quadriceps muscle, fascia and tendon**

✓7ᵗʰ	**S76.121**	**Laceration of right quadriceps muscle, fascia and tendon**
✓7ᵗʰ	**S76.122**	**Laceration of left quadriceps muscle, fascia and tendon**
✓7ᵗʰ	**S76.129**	**Laceration of unspecified quadriceps muscle, fascia and tendon**

✓6ᵗʰ **S76.19 Other specified injury of quadriceps muscle, fascia and tendon**

✓7ᵗʰ	**S76.191**	**Other specified injury of right quadriceps muscle, fascia and tendon**
✓7ᵗʰ	**S76.192**	**Other specified injury of left quadriceps muscle, fascia and tendon**
✓7ᵗʰ	**S76.199**	**Other specified injury of unspecified quadriceps muscle, fascia and tendon**

✓5ᵗʰ **S76.2 Injury of adductor muscle, fascia and tendon of thigh**

✓6ᵗʰ **S76.20 Unspecified injury of adductor muscle, fascia and tendon of thigh**

✓7ᵗʰ	**S76.201**	**Unspecified injury of adductor muscle, fascia and tendon of right thigh**
✓7ᵗʰ	**S76.202**	**Unspecified injury of adductor muscle, fascia and tendon of left thigh**
✓7ᵗʰ	**S76.209**	**Unspecified injury of adductor muscle, fascia and tendon of unspecified thigh**

✓6ᵗʰ **S76.21 Strain of adductor muscle, fascia and tendon of thigh**

✓7ᵗʰ	**S76.211**	**Strain of adductor muscle, fascia and tendon of right thigh**
✓7ᵗʰ	**S76.212**	**Strain of adductor muscle, fascia and tendon of left thigh**
✓7ᵗʰ	**S76.219**	**Strain of adductor muscle, fascia and tendon of unspecified thigh**

✓6ᵗʰ **S76.22 Laceration of adductor muscle, fascia and tendon of thigh**

✓7ᵗʰ	**S76.221**	**Laceration of adductor muscle, fascia and tendon of right thigh**
✓7ᵗʰ	**S76.222**	**Laceration of adductor muscle, fascia and tendon of left thigh**
✓7ᵗʰ	**S76.229**	**Laceration of adductor muscle, fascia and tendon of unspecified thigh**

✓6ᵗʰ **S76.29 Other injury of adductor muscle, fascia and tendon of thigh**

✓7ᵗʰ	**S76.291**	**Other injury of adductor muscle, fascia and tendon of right thigh**
✓7ᵗʰ	**S76.292**	**Other injury of adductor muscle, fascia and tendon of left thigh**
✓7ᵗʰ	**S76.299**	**Other injury of adductor muscle, fascia and tendon of unspecified thigh**

✓5ᵗʰ **S76.3 Injury of muscle, fascia and tendon of the posterior muscle group at thigh level**

✓6ᵗʰ **S76.30 Unspecified injury of muscle, fascia and tendon of the posterior muscle group at thigh level**

✓7ᵗʰ	**S76.301**	**Unspecified injury of muscle, fascia and tendon of the posterior muscle group at thigh level, right thigh**

✦ Refer to the Muscle/Tendon Table at beginning of this chapter.

☑ Additional Character Required   ✓x7ᵗʰ Placeholder Alert   Unspecified Dx   Other Specified Dx   Manifestation   ►◄ Revised Text   ● New Code   ▲ Revised Code Title

√7th **S76.302** Unspecified injury of muscle, fascia and tendon of the posterior muscle group at thigh level, **left thigh**

√7th **S76.309** Unspecified injury of muscle, fascia and tendon of the posterior muscle group at thigh level, **unspecified thigh**

√6th **S76.31** Strain of muscle, fascia and tendon of the posterior muscle group at thigh level

√7th **S76.311** Strain of muscle, fascia and tendon of the posterior muscle group at thigh level, **right thigh**

√7th **S76.312** Strain of muscle, fascia and tendon of the posterior muscle group at thigh level, **left thigh**

√7th **S76.319** Strain of muscle, fascia and tendon of the posterior muscle group at thigh level, **unspecified thigh**

√6th **S76.32** Laceration of muscle, fascia and tendon of the posterior muscle group at thigh level

√7th **S76.321** Laceration of muscle, fascia and tendon of the posterior muscle group at thigh level, **right thigh**

√7th **S76.322** Laceration of muscle, fascia and tendon of the posterior muscle group at thigh level, **left thigh**

√7th **S76.329** Laceration of muscle, fascia and tendon of the posterior muscle group at thigh level, **unspecified thigh**

√6th **S76.39** Other specified injury of muscle, fascia and tendon of the posterior muscle group at thigh level

√7th **S76.391** Other specified injury of muscle, fascia and tendon of the posterior muscle group at thigh level, **right thigh**

√7th **S76.392** Other specified injury of muscle, fascia and tendon of the posterior muscle group at thigh level, **left thigh**

√7th **S76.399** Other specified injury of muscle, fascia and tendon of the posterior muscle group at thigh level, **unspecified thigh**

√5th **S76.8** Injury of other specified muscles, fascia and tendons at thigh level

√6th **S76.80** Unspecified injury of other specified muscles, fascia and tendons at thigh level

√7th **S76.801** Unspecified injury of other specified muscles, fascia and tendons at thigh level, **right thigh**

√7th **S76.802** Unspecified injury of other specified muscles, fascia and tendons at thigh level, **left thigh**

√7th **S76.809** Unspecified injury of other specified muscles, fascia and tendons at thigh level, **unspecified thigh**

√6th **S76.81** Strain of other specified muscles, fascia and tendons at thigh level

√7th **S76.811** Strain of other specified muscles, fascia and tendons at thigh level, **right thigh**

√7th **S76.812** Strain of other specified muscles, fascia and tendons at thigh level, **left thigh**

√7th **S76.819** Strain of other specified muscles, fascia and tendons at thigh level, **unspecified thigh**

√6th **S76.82** Laceration of other specified muscles, fascia and tendons at thigh level

√7th **S76.821** Laceration of other specified muscles, fascia and tendons at thigh level, **right thigh**

√7th **S76.822** Laceration of other specified muscles, fascia and tendons at thigh level, **left thigh**

√7th **S76.829** Laceration of other specified muscles, fascia and tendons at thigh level, **unspecified thigh**

√6th **S76.89** Other injury of other specified muscles, fascia and tendons at thigh level

√7th **S76.891** Other injury of other specified muscles, fascia and tendons at thigh level, **right thigh**

√7th **S76.892** Other injury of other specified muscles, fascia and tendons at thigh level, **left thigh**

√7th **S76.899** Other injury of other specified muscles, fascia and tendons at thigh level, **unspecified thigh**

√5th **S76.9** Injury of **unspecified** muscles, fascia and tendons at thigh level

√6th **S76.90** Unspecified injury of unspecified muscles, fascia and tendons at thigh level

√7th **S76.901** Unspecified injury of unspecified muscles, fascia and tendons at thigh level, **right thigh**

√7th **S76.902** Unspecified injury of unspecified muscles, fascia and tendons at thigh level, **left thigh**

√7th **S76.909** Unspecified injury of unspecified muscles, fascia and tendons at thigh level, **unspecified thigh**

√6th **S76.91** Strain of unspecified muscles, fascia and tendons at thigh level

√7th **S76.911** Strain of unspecified muscles, fascia and tendons at thigh level, **right thigh**

√7th **S76.912** Strain of unspecified muscles, fascia and tendons at thigh level, **left thigh**

√7th **S76.919** Strain of unspecified muscles, fascia and tendons at thigh level, **unspecified thigh**

√6th **S76.92** Laceration of unspecified muscles, fascia and tendons at thigh level

√7th **S76.921** Laceration of unspecified muscles, fascia and tendons at thigh level, **right thigh**

√7th **S76.922** Laceration of unspecified muscles, fascia and tendons at thigh level, **left thigh**

√7th **S76.929** Laceration of unspecified muscles, fascia and tendons at thigh level, **unspecified thigh**

√6th **S76.99** Other specified injury of unspecified muscles, fascia and tendons at thigh level

√7th **S76.991** Other specified injury of unspecified muscles, fascia and tendons at thigh level, **right thigh**

√7th **S76.992** Other specified injury of unspecified muscles, fascia and tendons at thigh level, **left thigh**

√7th **S76.999** Other specified injury of unspecified muscles, fascia and tendons at thigh level, **unspecified thigh**

√4th **S77** **Crushing injury of hip and thigh**

Use additional code(s) for all associated injuries

EXCLUDES 2   *crushing injury of ankle and foot (S97.-)*
             crushing injury of lower leg (S87.-)

The appropriate 7th character is to be added to each code from category S77.
A   initial encounter
D   subsequent encounter
S   sequela

√5th **S77.0** **Crushing injury of** hip

√x7th **S77.00** **Crushing injury of** unspecified hip

√x7th **S77.01** **Crushing injury of** right hip

√x7th **S77.02** **Crushing injury of** left hip

√5th **S77.1** **Crushing injury of** thigh

√x7th **S77.10** **Crushing injury of** unspecified thigh

√x7th **S77.11** **Crushing injury of** right thigh

√x7th **S77.12** **Crushing injury of** left thigh

√5th **S77.2** **Crushing injury of** hip with thigh

√x7th **S77.20** **Crushing injury of** unspecified hip with thigh

√x7th **S77.21** **Crushing injury of** right hip with thigh

√x7th **S77.22** **Crushing injury of** left hip with thigh

EXCLUDES 1 Not coded here   EXCLUDES 2 Not included here   N Newborn Age: 0   P Pediatric Age: 0-17   M Maternity Age: 12-55   A Adult Age: 15-124

☑4ᵗʰ **S78** **Traumatic amputation of hip and thigh**

> **NOTE** An amputation not identified as partial or complete should be coded to complete.
>
> **EXCLUDES 1** *traumatic amputation of knee (S88.0-)*

> The appropriate 7th character is to be added to each code from category S78.
> A   initial encounter
> D   subsequent encounter
> S   sequela

☑5ᵗʰ **S78.0** **Traumatic amputation at hip joint**

     ☑6ᵗʰ **S78.01** **Complete** traumatic amputation at hip joint

         ☑7ᵗʰ **S78.011** **Complete traumatic amputation at** right **hip joint**

         ☑7ᵗʰ **S78.012** **Complete traumatic amputation at** left **hip joint**

         ☑7ᵗʰ **S78.019** **Complete traumatic amputation at unspecified hip joint**

     ☑6ᵗʰ **S78.02** **Partial** traumatic amputation at hip joint

         ☑7ᵗʰ **S78.021** **Partial traumatic amputation at** right **hip joint**

         ☑7ᵗʰ **S78.022** **Partial traumatic amputation at** left **hip joint**

         ☑7ᵗʰ **S78.029** **Partial traumatic amputation at unspecified hip joint**

☑5ᵗʰ **S78.1** **Traumatic amputation at level between hip and knee**

> **EXCLUDES 1** *traumatic amputation of knee (S88.0-)*

     ☑6ᵗʰ **S78.11** **Complete** traumatic amputation at level between hip and knee

         ☑7ᵗʰ **S78.111** **Complete traumatic amputation at level between** right **hip and knee**

         ☑7ᵗʰ **S78.112** **Complete traumatic amputation at level between** left **hip and knee**

         ☑7ᵗʰ **S78.119** **Complete traumatic amputation at level between unspecified hip and knee**

     ☑6ᵗʰ **S78.12** **Partial** traumatic amputation at level between hip and knee

         ☑7ᵗʰ **S78.121** **Partial traumatic amputation at level between** right **hip and knee**

         ☑7ᵗʰ **S78.122** **Partial traumatic amputation at level between** left **hip and knee**

         ☑7ᵗʰ **S78.129** **Partial traumatic amputation at level between unspecified hip and knee**

☑5ᵗʰ **S78.9** **Traumatic amputation of hip and thigh, level unspecified**

     ☑6ᵗʰ **S78.91** **Complete** traumatic amputation of hip and thigh, level unspecified

         ☑7ᵗʰ **S78.911** **Complete traumatic amputation of** right **hip and thigh, level unspecified**

         ☑7ᵗʰ **S78.912** **Complete traumatic amputation of** left **hip and thigh, level unspecified**

         ☑7ᵗʰ **S78.919** **Complete traumatic amputation of unspecified hip and thigh, level unspecified**

     ☑6ᵗʰ **S78.92** **Partial** traumatic amputation of hip and thigh, level unspecified

         ☑7ᵗʰ **S78.921** **Partial traumatic amputation of** right **hip and thigh, level unspecified**

         ☑7ᵗʰ **S78.922** **Partial traumatic amputation of** left **hip and thigh, level unspecified**

         ☑7ᵗʰ **S78.929** **Partial traumatic amputation of unspecified hip and thigh, level unspecified**

☑4ᵗʰ **S79** **Other and unspecified injuries of hip and thigh**

☑5ᵗʰ **S79.0** **Physeal fracture of upper end of femur**

> **NOTE** A fracture not indicated as open or closed should be coded to closed.
>
> **EXCLUDES 1** *apophyseal fracture of upper end of femur (S72.13-)*
> *nontraumatic slipped upper femoral epiphysis (M93.0-)*

> The appropriate 7th character is to be added to each code from subcategory S79.0.
> A   initial encounter for closed fracture
> D   subsequent encounter for fracture with routine healing
> G   subsequent encounter for fracture with delayed healing
> K   subsequent encounter for fracture with nonunion
> P   subsequent encounter for fracture with malunion
> S   sequela

     ☑6ᵗʰ **S79.00** **Unspecified** physeal fracture of upper end of femur

         ☑7ᵗʰ **S79.001** **Unspecified physeal fracture of upper end of** right **femur**

         ☑7ᵗʰ **S79.002** **Unspecified physeal fracture of upper end of** left **femur**

         ☑7ᵗʰ **S79.009** **Unspecified physeal fracture of upper end of unspecified femur**

     ☑6ᵗʰ **S79.01** **Salter-Harris Type I** physeal fracture of upper end of femur

         Acute on chronic slipped capital femoral epiphysis (traumatic)
         Acute slipped capital femoral epiphysis (traumatic)
         Capital femoral epiphyseal fracture

> **EXCLUDES 1** *chronic slipped upper femoral epiphysis (nontraumatic) (M93.02-)*

         ☑7ᵗʰ **S79.011** **Salter-Harris Type I physeal fracture of upper end of** right **femur**

         ☑7ᵗʰ **S79.012** **Salter-Harris Type I physeal fracture of upper end of** left **femur**

         ☑7ᵗʰ **S79.019** **Salter-Harris Type I physeal fracture of upper end of unspecified femur**

     ☑6ᵗʰ **S79.09** **Other** physeal fracture of upper end of femur

         ☑7ᵗʰ **S79.091** **Other physeal fracture of upper end of** right **femur**

         ☑7ᵗʰ **S79.092** **Other physeal fracture of upper end of** left **femur**

         ☑7ᵗʰ **S79.099** **Other physeal fracture of upper end of unspecified femur**

☑5ᵗʰ **S79.1** **Physeal fracture of lower end of femur**

> **NOTE** A fracture not indicated as open or closed should be coded to closed.

> The appropriate 7th character is to be added to each code from subcategory S79.1.
> A   initial encounter for closed fracture
> D   subsequent encounter for fracture with routine healing
> G   subsequent encounter for fracture with delayed healing
> K   subsequent encounter for fracture with nonunion
> P   subsequent encounter for fracture with malunion
> S   sequela

     ☑6ᵗʰ **S79.10** **Unspecified** physeal fracture of lower end of femur

         ☑7ᵗʰ **S79.101** **Unspecified physeal fracture of lower end of** right **femur**

         ☑7ᵗʰ **S79.102** **Unspecified physeal fracture of lower end of** left **femur**

         ☑7ᵗʰ **S79.109** **Unspecified physeal fracture of lower end of unspecified femur**

     ☑6ᵗʰ **S79.11** **Salter-Harris Type I** physeal fracture of lower end of femur

         ☑7ᵗʰ **S79.111** **Salter-Harris Type I physeal fracture of lower end of** right **femur**

         ☑7ᵗʰ **S79.112** **Salter-Harris Type I physeal fracture of lower end of** left **femur**

         ☑7ᵗʰ **S79.119** **Salter-Harris Type I physeal fracture of lower end of unspecified femur**

     ☑6ᵗʰ **S79.12** **Salter-Harris Type II** physeal fracture of lower end of femur

         ☑7ᵗʰ **S79.121** **Salter-Harris Type II physeal fracture of lower end of** right **femur**

         ☑7ᵗʰ **S79.122** **Salter-Harris Type II physeal fracture of lower end of** left **femur**

         ☑7ᵗʰ **S79.129** **Salter-Harris Type II physeal fracture of lower end of unspecified femur**

☑ Additional Character Required   ☑x7ᵗʰ Placeholder Alert   Unspecified Dx   Other Specified Dx   Manifestation   ▶◀ Revised Text   ● New Code   ▲ Revised Code Title

√6ᵗʰ **S79.13** **Salter-Harris Type III physeal fracture of lower end of femur**
- √7ᵗʰ **S79.131** **Salter-Harris Type III physeal fracture of lower end of right femur**
- √7ᵗʰ **S79.132** **Salter-Harris Type III physeal fracture of lower end of left femur**
- √7ᵗʰ **S79.139** **Salter-Harris Type III physeal fracture of lower end of unspecified femur**

√6ᵗʰ **S79.14** **Salter-Harris Type IV physeal fracture of lower end of femur**
- √7ᵗʰ **S79.141** **Salter-Harris Type IV physeal fracture of lower end of right femur**
- √7ᵗʰ **S79.142** **Salter-Harris Type IV physeal fracture of lower end of left femur**
- √7ᵗʰ **S79.149** **Salter-Harris Type IV physeal fracture of lower end of unspecified femur**

√6ᵗʰ **S79.19** **Other physeal fracture of lower end of femur**
- √7ᵗʰ **S79.191** **Other physeal fracture of lower end of right femur**
- √7ᵗʰ **S79.192** **Other physeal fracture of lower end of left femur**
- √7ᵗʰ **S79.199** **Other physeal fracture of lower end of unspecified femur**

√5ᵗʰ **S79.8** **Other specified injuries of hip and thigh**

> The appropriate 7th character is to be added to each code in subcategory S79.8.
> A   initial encounter
> D   subsequent encounter
> S   sequela

√6ᵗʰ **S79.81** **Other specified injuries of hip**
- √7ᵗʰ **S79.811** **Other specified injuries of right hip**
- √7ᵗʰ **S79.812** **Other specified injuries of left hip**
- √7ᵗʰ **S79.819** **Other specified injuries of unspecified hip**

√6ᵗʰ **S79.82** **Other specified injuries of thigh**
- √7ᵗʰ **S79.821** **Other specified injuries of right thigh**
- √7ᵗʰ **S79.822** **Other specified injuries of left thigh**
- √7ᵗʰ **S79.829** **Other specified injuries of unspecified thigh**

√5ᵗʰ **S79.9** **Unspecified injury of hip and thigh**

> The appropriate 7th character is to be added to each code in subcategory S79.9.
> A   initial encounter
> D   subsequent encounter
> S   sequela

√6ᵗʰ **S79.91** **Unspecified injury of hip**
- √7ᵗʰ **S79.911** **Unspecified injury of right hip**
- √7ᵗʰ **S79.912** **Unspecified injury of left hip**
- √7ᵗʰ **S79.919** **Unspecified injury of unspecified hip**

√6ᵗʰ **S79.92** **Unspecified injury of thigh**
- √7ᵗʰ **S79.921** **Unspecified injury of right thigh**
- √7ᵗʰ **S79.922** **Unspecified injury of left thigh**
- √7ᵗʰ **S79.929** **Unspecified injury of unspecified thigh**

Injuries to the knee and lower leg (S80-S89)

EXCLUDES 2   burns and corrosions (T20-T32)
frostbite (T33-T34)
injuries of ankle and foot, except fracture of ankle and malleolus (S90-S99)
insect bite or sting, venomous (T63.4)

√4ᵗʰ **S80** **Superficial injury of knee and lower leg**
EXCLUDES 2   superficial injury of ankle and foot (S90.-)

> The appropriate 7th character is to be added to each code from category S80.
> A   initial encounter
> D   subsequent encounter
> S   sequela

√5ᵗʰ **S80.0** **Contusion of knee**
- √×7ᵗʰ **S80.00** **Contusion of unspecified knee**
- √×7ᵗʰ **S80.01** **Contusion of right knee**
- √×7ᵗʰ **S80.02** **Contusion of left knee**

√5ᵗʰ **S80.1** **Contusion of lower leg**
- √×7ᵗʰ **S80.10** **Contusion of unspecified lower leg**

√×7ᵗʰ **S80.11** **Contusion of right lower leg**
√×7ᵗʰ **S80.12** **Contusion of left lower leg**

√5ᵗʰ **S80.2** **Other superficial injuries of knee**
√6ᵗʰ **S80.21** **Abrasion of knee**
- √7ᵗʰ **S80.211** **Abrasion, right knee**
- √7ᵗʰ **S80.212** **Abrasion, left knee**
- √7ᵗʰ **S80.219** **Abrasion, unspecified knee**

√6ᵗʰ **S80.22** **Blister (nonthermal) of knee**
- √7ᵗʰ **S80.221** **Blister (nonthermal), right knee**
- √7ᵗʰ **S80.222** **Blister (nonthermal), left knee**
- √7ᵗʰ **S80.229** **Blister (nonthermal), unspecified knee**

√6ᵗʰ **S80.24** **External constriction of knee**
- √7ᵗʰ **S80.241** **External constriction, right knee**
- √7ᵗʰ **S80.242** **External constriction, left knee**
- √7ᵗʰ **S80.249** **External constriction, unspecified knee**

√6ᵗʰ **S80.25** **Superficial foreign body of knee**
Splinter in the knee
- √7ᵗʰ **S80.251** **Superficial foreign body, right knee**
- √7ᵗʰ **S80.252** **Superficial foreign body, left knee**
- √7ᵗʰ **S80.259** **Superficial foreign body, unspecified knee**

√6ᵗʰ **S80.26** **Insect bite (nonvenomous) of knee**
- √7ᵗʰ **S80.261** **Insect bite (nonvenomous), right knee**
- √7ᵗʰ **S80.262** **Insect bite (nonvenomous), left knee**
- √7ᵗʰ **S80.269** **Insect bite (nonvenomous), unspecified knee**

√6ᵗʰ **S80.27** **Other superficial bite of knee**
EXCLUDES 1   open bite of knee (S81.05-)
- √7ᵗʰ **S80.271** **Other superficial bite of right knee**
- √7ᵗʰ **S80.272** **Other superficial bite of left knee**
- √7ᵗʰ **S80.279** **Other superficial bite of unspecified knee**

√5ᵗʰ **S80.8** **Other superficial injuries of lower leg**
√6ᵗʰ **S80.81** **Abrasion of lower leg**
- √7ᵗʰ **S80.811** **Abrasion, right lower leg**
- √7ᵗʰ **S80.812** **Abrasion, left lower leg**
- √7ᵗʰ **S80.819** **Abrasion, unspecified lower leg**

√6ᵗʰ **S80.82** **Blister (nonthermal) of lower leg**
- √7ᵗʰ **S80.821** **Blister (nonthermal), right lower leg**
- √7ᵗʰ **S80.822** **Blister (nonthermal), left lower leg**
- √7ᵗʰ **S80.829** **Blister (nonthermal), unspecified lower leg**

√6ᵗʰ **S80.84** **External constriction of lower leg**
- √7ᵗʰ **S80.841** **External constriction, right lower leg**
- √7ᵗʰ **S80.842** **External constriction, left lower leg**
- √7ᵗʰ **S80.849** **External constriction, unspecified lower leg**

√6ᵗʰ **S80.85** **Superficial foreign body of lower leg**
Splinter in the lower leg
- √7ᵗʰ **S80.851** **Superficial foreign body, right lower leg**
- √7ᵗʰ **S80.852** **Superficial foreign body, left lower leg**
- √7ᵗʰ **S80.859** **Superficial foreign body, unspecified lower leg**

√6ᵗʰ **S80.86** **Insect bite (nonvenomous) of lower leg**
- √7ᵗʰ **S80.861** **Insect bite (nonvenomous), right lower leg**
- √7ᵗʰ **S80.862** **Insect bite (nonvenomous), left lower leg**
- √7ᵗʰ **S80.869** **Insect bite (nonvenomous), unspecified lower leg**

√6ᵗʰ **S80.87** **Other superficial bite of lower leg**
EXCLUDES 1   open bite of lower leg (S81.85-)
- √7ᵗʰ **S80.871** **Other superficial bite, right lower leg**
- √7ᵗʰ **S80.872** **Other superficial bite, left lower leg**
- √7ᵗʰ **S80.879** **Other superficial bite, unspecified lower leg**

√5ᵗʰ **S80.9** **Unspecified superficial injury of knee and lower leg**
√6ᵗʰ **S80.91** **Unspecified superficial injury of knee**
- √7ᵗʰ **S80.911** **Unspecified superficial injury of right knee**
- √7ᵗʰ **S80.912** **Unspecified superficial injury of left knee**
- √7ᵗʰ **S80.919** **Unspecified superficial injury of unspecified knee**

EXCLUDES 1 Not coded here   EXCLUDES 2 Not included here   N Newborn Age: 0   P Pediatric Age: 0-17   M Maternity Age: 12-55   A Adult Age: 15-124

940

ICD-10-CM 2016

✓6ᵗʰ **S80.92** Unspecified superficial injury of lower leg

     ✓7ᵗʰ **S80.921** **Unspecified superficial injury of right lower leg**

     ✓7ᵗʰ **S80.922** **Unspecified superficial injury of left lower leg**

     ✓7ᵗʰ **S80.929** **Unspecified superficial injury of unspecified lower leg**

✓4ᵗʰ **S81** **Open wound of knee and lower leg**

     Code also any associated wound infection

     EXCLUDES 1   *open fracture of knee and lower leg (S82.-)*

                  traumatic amputation of lower leg (S88.-)

     EXCLUDES 2   *open wound of ankle and foot (S91.-)*

     The appropriate 7th character is to be added to each code from category S81.
     A   initial encounter
     D   subsequent encounter
     S   sequela

   ✓5ᵗʰ **S81.0** **Open wound of knee**

     ✓6ᵗʰ **S81.00** Unspecified open wound of knee

       ✓7ᵗʰ **S81.001** **Unspecified open wound, right knee**

       ✓7ᵗʰ **S81.002** **Unspecified open wound, left knee**

       ✓7ᵗʰ **S81.009** **Unspecified open wound, unspecified knee**

     ✓6ᵗʰ **S81.01** Laceration without foreign body of knee

       ✓7ᵗʰ **S81.011** **Laceration without foreign body, right knee**

       ✓7ᵗʰ **S81.012** **Laceration without foreign body, left knee**

       ✓7ᵗʰ **S81.019** **Laceration without foreign body, unspecified knee**

     ✓6ᵗʰ **S81.02** Laceration with foreign body of knee

       ✓7ᵗʰ **S81.021** **Laceration with foreign body, right knee**

       ✓7ᵗʰ **S81.022** **Laceration with foreign body, left knee**

       ✓7ᵗʰ **S81.029** **Laceration with foreign body, unspecified knee**

     ✓6ᵗʰ **S81.03** Puncture wound without foreign body of knee

       ✓7ᵗʰ **S81.031** **Puncture wound without foreign body, right knee**

       ✓7ᵗʰ **S81.032** **Puncture wound without foreign body, left knee**

       ✓7ᵗʰ **S81.039** **Puncture wound without foreign body, unspecified knee**

     ✓6ᵗʰ **S81.04** Puncture wound with foreign body of knee

       ✓7ᵗʰ **S81.041** **Puncture wound with foreign body, right knee**

       ✓7ᵗʰ **S81.042** **Puncture wound with foreign body, left knee**

       ✓7ᵗʰ **S81.049** **Puncture wound with foreign body, unspecified knee**

     ✓6ᵗʰ **S81.05** Open bite of knee

        Bite of knee NOS

          EXCLUDES 1   *superficial bite of knee (S80.27-)*

       ✓7ᵗʰ **S81.051** **Open bite, right knee**

       ✓7ᵗʰ **S81.052** **Open bite, left knee**

       ✓7ᵗʰ **S81.059** **Open bite, unspecified knee**

   ✓5ᵗʰ **S81.8** **Open wound of lower leg**

     ✓6ᵗʰ **S81.80** Unspecified open wound of lower leg

       ✓7ᵗʰ **S81.801** **Unspecified open wound, right lower leg**

       ✓7ᵗʰ **S81.802** **Unspecified open wound, left lower leg**

       ✓7ᵗʰ **S81.809** **Unspecified open wound, unspecified lower leg**

     ✓6ᵗʰ **S81.81** Laceration without foreign body of lower leg

       ✓7ᵗʰ **S81.811** **Laceration without foreign body, right lower leg**

       ✓7ᵗʰ **S81.812** **Laceration without foreign body, left lower leg**

       ✓7ᵗʰ **S81.819** **Laceration without foreign body, unspecified lower leg**

     ✓6ᵗʰ **S81.82** Laceration with foreign body of lower leg

       ✓7ᵗʰ **S81.821** **Laceration with foreign body, right lower leg**

       ✓7ᵗʰ **S81.822** **Laceration with foreign body, left lower leg**

       ✓7ᵗʰ **S81.829** **Laceration with foreign body, unspecified lower leg**

     ✓6ᵗʰ **S81.83** Puncture wound without foreign body of lower leg

       ✓7ᵗʰ **S81.831** **Puncture wound without foreign body, right lower leg**

       ✓7ᵗʰ **S81.832** **Puncture wound without foreign body, left lower leg**

       ✓7ᵗʰ **S81.839** **Puncture wound without foreign body, unspecified lower leg**

     ✓6ᵗʰ **S81.84** Puncture wound with foreign body of lower leg

       ✓7ᵗʰ **S81.841** **Puncture wound with foreign body, right lower leg**

       ✓7ᵗʰ **S81.842** **Puncture wound with foreign body, left lower leg**

       ✓7ᵗʰ **S81.849** **Puncture wound with foreign body, unspecified lower leg**

     ✓6ᵗʰ **S81.85** Open bite of lower leg

        Bite of lower leg NOS

          EXCLUDES 1   *superficial bite of lower leg (S80.86-, S80.87-)*

       ✓7ᵗʰ **S81.851** **Open bite, right lower leg**

       ✓7ᵗʰ **S81.852** **Open bite, left lower leg**

       ✓7ᵗʰ **S81.859** **Open bite, unspecified lower leg**

✓4ᵗʰ **S82** **Fracture of lower leg, including ankle**

     NOTE   A fracture not indicated as displaced or nondisplaced should be coded to displaced.

             A fracture not designated as open or closed should be coded to closed.

             The open fracture designations are based on the Gustilo open fracture classification.

     INCLUDES   fracture of malleolus

     EXCLUDES 1   *traumatic amputation of lower leg (S88.-)*

     EXCLUDES 2   *fracture of foot, except ankle (S92.-)*

                     periprosthetic fracture of prosthetic implant of knee (T84.042, T84.043)

     The appropriate 7th character is to be added to all codes from category S82 [unless otherwise indicated].
     A   initial encounter for closed fracture
     B   initial encounter for open fracture type I or II
           initial encounter for open fracture NOS
     C   initial encounter for open fracture type IIIA, IIIB, or IIIC
     D   subsequent encounter for closed fracture with routine healing
     E   subsequent encounter for open fracture type I or II with routine healing
     F   subsequent encounter for open fracture type IIIA, IIIB, or IIIC with routine healing
     G   subsequent encounter for closed fracture with delayed healing
     H   subsequent encounter for open fracture type I or II with delayed healing
     J   subsequent encounter for open fracture type IIIA, IIIB or IIIC with delayed healing
     K   subsequent encounter for closed fracture with nonunion
     M   subsequent encounter for open fracture type I or II with nonunion
     N   subsequent encounter for open fracture type IIIA, IIIB or IIIC with nonunion
     P   subsequent encounter for closed fracture with malunion
     Q   subsequent encounter for open fracture type I or II with malunion
     R   subsequent encounter for open fracture type IIIA, IIIB or IIIC with malunion
     S   sequela

   ✓5ᵗʰ **S82.0** **Fracture of patella**

       Knee cap

     ✓6ᵗʰ **S82.00** Unspecified fracture of patella

       ✓7ᵗʰ **S82.001** **Unspecified fracture of right patella**

       ✓7ᵗʰ **S82.002** **Unspecified fracture of left patella**

       ✓7ᵗʰ **S82.009** **Unspecified fracture of unspecified patella**

     ✓6ᵗʰ **S82.01** Osteochondral fracture of patella

       ✓7ᵗʰ **S82.011** **Displaced osteochondral fracture of right patella**

       ✓7ᵗʰ **S82.012** **Displaced osteochondral fracture of left patella**

✓ Additional Character Required   ✓x7ᵗʰ Placeholder Alert   Unspecified Dx   Other Specified Dx   Manifestation   ►◄ Revised Text   ● New Code   ▲ Revised Code Title

√7ᵗʰ **S82.013** Displaced **osteochondral fracture of unspecified patella**

√7ᵗʰ **S82.014** Nondisplaced **osteochondral fracture of right patella**

√7ᵗʰ **S82.015** Nondisplaced **osteochondral fracture of left patella**

√7ᵗʰ **S82.016** Nondisplaced **osteochondral fracture of unspecified patella**

√6ᵗʰ **S82.02** Longitudinal **fracture of patella**

√7ᵗʰ **S82.021** Displaced **longitudinal fracture of right patella**

√7ᵗʰ **S82.022** Displaced **longitudinal fracture of left patella**

√7ᵗʰ **S82.023** Displaced **longitudinal fracture of unspecified patella**

√7ᵗʰ **S82.024** Nondisplaced **longitudinal fracture of right patella**

√7ᵗʰ **S82.025** Nondisplaced **longitudinal fracture of left patella**

√7ᵗʰ **S82.026** Nondisplaced **longitudinal fracture of unspecified patella**

√6ᵗʰ **S82.03** Transverse **fracture of patella**

√7ᵗʰ **S82.031** Displaced **transverse fracture of right patella**

√7ᵗʰ **S82.032** Displaced **transverse fracture of left patella**

√7ᵗʰ **S82.033** Displaced **transverse fracture of unspecified patella**

√7ᵗʰ **S82.034** Nondisplaced **transverse fracture of right patella**

√7ᵗʰ **S82.035** Nondisplaced **transverse fracture of left patella**

√7ᵗʰ **S82.036** Nondisplaced **transverse fracture of unspecified patella**

√6ᵗʰ **S82.04** Comminuted **fracture of patella**

√7ᵗʰ **S82.041** Displaced **comminuted fracture of right patella**

√7ᵗʰ **S82.042** Displaced **comminuted fracture of left patella**

√7ᵗʰ **S82.043** Displaced **comminuted fracture of unspecified patella**

√7ᵗʰ **S82.044** Nondisplaced **comminuted fracture of right patella**

√7ᵗʰ **S82.045** Nondisplaced **comminuted fracture of left patella**

√7ᵗʰ **S82.046** Nondisplaced **comminuted fracture of unspecified patella**

√6ᵗʰ **S82.09** Other **fracture of patella**

√7ᵗʰ **S82.091** Other fracture of right **patella**

√7ᵗʰ **S82.092** Other fracture of left **patella**

√7ᵗʰ **S82.099** Other fracture of unspecified **patella**

√5ᵗʰ **S82.1** Fracture of **upper end of tibia**
Fracture of proximal end of tibia
> EXCLUDES 2   *fracture of shaft of tibia (S82.2-)*
> *physeal fracture of upper end of tibia (S89.0-)*

√6ᵗʰ **S82.10** Unspecified **fracture of upper end of tibia**

√7ᵗʰ **S82.101** Unspecified fracture of upper end of right **tibia**

√7ᵗʰ **S82.102** Unspecified fracture of upper end of left **tibia**

√7ᵗʰ **S82.109** Unspecified fracture of upper end of **unspecified tibia**

√6ᵗʰ **S82.11** Fracture of **tibial spine**

√7ᵗʰ **S82.111** Displaced fracture of right **tibial spine**

√7ᵗʰ **S82.112** Displaced fracture of left **tibial spine**

√7ᵗʰ **S82.113** Displaced **fracture of unspecified tibial spine**

√7ᵗʰ **S82.114** Nondisplaced fracture of right **tibial spine**

√7ᵗʰ **S82.115** Nondisplaced fracture of left **tibial spine**

√7ᵗʰ **S82.116** Nondisplaced **fracture of unspecified tibial spine**

√6ᵗʰ **S82.12** Fracture of lateral condyle **of tibia**

√7ᵗʰ **S82.121** Displaced **fracture of lateral condyle of right tibia**

√7ᵗʰ **S82.122** Displaced **fracture of lateral condyle of left tibia**

√7ᵗʰ **S82.123** Displaced **fracture of lateral condyle of unspecified tibia**

√7ᵗʰ **S82.124** Nondisplaced **fracture of lateral condyle of right tibia**

√7ᵗʰ **S82.125** Nondisplaced **fracture of lateral condyle of left tibia**

√7ᵗʰ **S82.126** Nondisplaced **fracture of lateral condyle of unspecified tibia**

√6ᵗʰ **S82.13** Fracture of medial condyle **of tibia**

√7ᵗʰ **S82.131** Displaced **fracture of medial condyle of right tibia**

√7ᵗʰ **S82.132** Displaced **fracture of medial condyle of left tibia**

√7ᵗʰ **S82.133** Displaced **fracture of medial condyle of unspecified tibia**

√7ᵗʰ **S82.134** Nondisplaced **fracture of medial condyle of right tibia**

√7ᵗʰ **S82.135** Nondisplaced **fracture of medial condyle of left tibia**

√7ᵗʰ **S82.136** Nondisplaced **fracture of medial condyle of unspecified tibia**

√6ᵗʰ **S82.14** Bicondylar **fracture of tibia**
Fracture of tibial plateau NOS

√7ᵗʰ **S82.141** Displaced **bicondylar fracture of right tibia**

√7ᵗʰ **S82.142** Displaced **bicondylar fracture of left tibia**

√7ᵗʰ **S82.143** Displaced **bicondylar fracture of unspecified tibia**

√7ᵗʰ **S82.144** Nondisplaced **bicondylar fracture of right tibia**

√7ᵗʰ **S82.145** Nondisplaced **bicondylar fracture of left tibia**

√7ᵗʰ **S82.146** Nondisplaced **bicondylar fracture of unspecified tibia**

√6ᵗʰ **S82.15** Fracture of **tibial tuberosity**

√7ᵗʰ **S82.151** Displaced fracture of right **tibial tuberosity**

√7ᵗʰ **S82.152** Displaced fracture of left **tibial tuberosity**

√7ᵗʰ **S82.153** Displaced **fracture of unspecified tibial tuberosity**

√7ᵗʰ **S82.154** Nondisplaced fracture of right **tibial tuberosity**

√7ᵗʰ **S82.155** Nondisplaced fracture of left **tibial tuberosity**

√7ᵗʰ **S82.156** Nondisplaced **fracture of unspecified tibial tuberosity**

√6ᵗʰ **S82.16** Torus **fracture of upper end of tibia**

> The appropriate 7th character is to be added to all codes in subcategory S82.16.
> A   initial encounter for closed fracture
> D   subsequent encounter for fracture with routine healing
> G   subsequent encounter for fracture with delayed healing
> K   subsequent encounter for fracture with nonunion
> P   subsequent encounter for fracture with malunion
> S   sequela

√7ᵗʰ **S82.161** Torus fracture of upper end of right **tibia**

√7ᵗʰ **S82.162** Torus fracture of upper end of left **tibia**

√7ᵗʰ **S82.169** Torus fracture of upper end of unspecified **tibia**

√6ᵗʰ **S82.19** Other **fracture of upper end of tibia**

√7ᵗʰ **S82.191** Other fracture of upper end of right **tibia**

√7ᵗʰ **S82.192** Other fracture of upper end of left **tibia**

√7ᵗʰ **S82.199** Other fracture of upper end of unspecified **tibia**

✓5ᵗʰ **S82.2** **Fracture of** shaft of tibia

  ✓6ᵗʰ **S82.20** **Unspecified** fracture of shaft of tibia
        Fracture of tibia NOS

    ✓7ᵗʰ **S82.201** **Unspecified** fracture of shaft of right tibia

    ✓7ᵗʰ **S82.202** **Unspecified** fracture of shaft of left tibia

    ✓7ᵗʰ **S82.209** **Unspecified** fracture of shaft of unspecified tibia

  ✓6ᵗʰ **S82.22** **Transverse** fracture of shaft of tibia

    ✓7ᵗʰ **S82.221** **Displaced** transverse fracture of shaft of right tibia

    ✓7ᵗʰ **S82.222** **Displaced** transverse fracture of shaft of left tibia

    ✓7ᵗʰ **S82.223** **Displaced** transverse fracture of shaft of unspecified tibia

    ✓7ᵗʰ **S82.224** **Nondisplaced** transverse fracture of shaft of right tibia

    ✓7ᵗʰ **S82.225** **Nondisplaced** transverse fracture of shaft of left tibia

    ✓7ᵗʰ **S82.226** **Nondisplaced** transverse fracture of shaft of unspecified tibia

  ✓6ᵗʰ **S82.23** **Oblique** fracture of shaft of tibia

    ✓7ᵗʰ **S82.231** **Displaced** oblique fracture of shaft of right tibia

    ✓7ᵗʰ **S82.232** **Displaced** oblique fracture of shaft of left tibia

    ✓7ᵗʰ **S82.233** **Displaced** oblique fracture of shaft of unspecified tibia

    ✓7ᵗʰ **S82.234** **Nondisplaced** oblique fracture of shaft of right tibia

    ✓7ᵗʰ **S82.235** **Nondisplaced** oblique fracture of shaft of left tibia

    ✓7ᵗʰ **S82.236** **Nondisplaced** oblique fracture of shaft of unspecified tibia

  ✓6ᵗʰ **S82.24** **Spiral** fracture of shaft of tibia
        Toddler fracture

    ✓7ᵗʰ **S82.241** **Displaced** spiral fracture of shaft of right tibia

    ✓7ᵗʰ **S82.242** **Displaced** spiral fracture of shaft of left tibia

    ✓7ᵗʰ **S82.243** **Displaced** spiral fracture of shaft of unspecified tibia

    ✓7ᵗʰ **S82.244** **Nondisplaced** spiral fracture of shaft of right tibia

    ✓7ᵗʰ **S82.245** **Nondisplaced** spiral fracture of shaft of left tibia

    ✓7ᵗʰ **S82.246** **Nondisplaced** spiral fracture of shaft of unspecified tibia

  ✓6ᵗʰ **S82.25** **Comminuted** fracture of shaft of tibia

    ✓7ᵗʰ **S82.251** **Displaced** comminuted fracture of shaft of right tibia

    ✓7ᵗʰ **S82.252** **Displaced** comminuted fracture of shaft of left tibia

    ✓7ᵗʰ **S82.253** **Displaced** comminuted fracture of shaft of unspecified tibia

    ✓7ᵗʰ **S82.254** **Nondisplaced** comminuted fracture of shaft of right tibia

    ✓7ᵗʰ **S82.255** **Nondisplaced** comminuted fracture of shaft of left tibia

    ✓7ᵗʰ **S82.256** **Nondisplaced** comminuted fracture of shaft of unspecified tibia

  ✓6ᵗʰ **S82.26** **Segmental** fracture of shaft of tibia

    ✓7ᵗʰ **S82.261** **Displaced** segmental fracture of shaft of right tibia

    ✓7ᵗʰ **S82.262** **Displaced** segmental fracture of shaft of left tibia

    ✓7ᵗʰ **S82.263** **Displaced** segmental fracture of shaft of unspecified tibia

    ✓7ᵗʰ **S82.264** **Nondisplaced** segmental fracture of shaft of right tibia

    ✓7ᵗʰ **S82.265** **Nondisplaced** segmental fracture of shaft of left tibia

    ✓7ᵗʰ **S82.266** **Nondisplaced** segmental fracture of shaft of unspecified tibia

  ✓6ᵗʰ **S82.29** **Other** fracture of shaft of tibia

    ✓7ᵗʰ **S82.291** **Other fracture of shaft of right tibia**

    ✓7ᵗʰ **S82.292** **Other fracture of shaft of left tibia**

    ✓7ᵗʰ **S82.299** **Other fracture of shaft of unspecified tibia**

✓5ᵗʰ **S82.3** **Fracture of** lower end of tibia

  EXCLUDES 1 *bimalleolar fracture of lower leg (S82.84-)*
               fracture of medial malleolus alone (S82.5-)
               Maisonneuve's fracture (S82.86-)
               pilon fracture of distal tibia (S82.87-)
               trimalleolar fractures of lower leg (S82.85-)

  ✓6ᵗʰ **S82.30** **Unspecified** fracture of lower end of tibia

    ✓7ᵗʰ **S82.301** **Unspecified fracture of lower end of right tibia**

    ✓7ᵗʰ **S82.302** **Unspecified fracture of lower end of left tibia**

    ✓7ᵗʰ **S82.309** **Unspecified fracture of lower end of unspecified tibia**

  ✓6ᵗʰ **S82.31** **Torus** fracture of lower end of tibia

> The appropriate 7th character is to be added to all codes in subcategory S82.31.
> A   initial encounter for closed fracture
> D   subsequent encounter for fracture with routine healing
> G   subsequent encounter for fracture with delayed healing
> K   subsequent encounter for fracture with nonunion
> P   subsequent encounter for fracture with malunion
> S   sequela

    ✓7ᵗʰ **S82.311** Torus fracture of lower end of right tibia

    ✓7ᵗʰ **S82.312** Torus fracture of lower end of left tibia

    ✓7ᵗʰ **S82.319** **Torus fracture of lower end of unspecified tibia**

  ✓6ᵗʰ **S82.39** **Other** fracture of lower end of tibia
        AHA: 2015, 1Q, 25

    ✓7ᵗʰ **S82.391** **Other fracture of lower end of right tibia**

    ✓7ᵗʰ **S82.392** **Other fracture of lower end of left tibia**

    ✓7ᵗʰ **S82.399** **Other fracture of lower end of unspecified tibia**

✓5ᵗʰ **S82.4** **Fracture of** shaft of fibula

  EXCLUDES 2 *fracture of lateral malleolus alone (S82.6-)*

  ✓6ᵗʰ **S82.40** **Unspecified** fracture of shaft of fibula

    ✓7ᵗʰ **S82.401** **Unspecified fracture of shaft of right fibula**

    ✓7ᵗʰ **S82.402** **Unspecified fracture of shaft of left fibula**

    ✓7ᵗʰ **S82.409** **Unspecified fracture of shaft of unspecified fibula**

  ✓6ᵗʰ **S82.42** **Transverse** fracture of shaft of fibula

    ✓7ᵗʰ **S82.421** **Displaced** transverse fracture of shaft of right fibula

    ✓7ᵗʰ **S82.422** **Displaced** transverse fracture of shaft of left fibula

    ✓7ᵗʰ **S82.423** **Displaced transverse fracture of shaft of unspecified fibula**

    ✓7ᵗʰ **S82.424** **Nondisplaced** transverse fracture of shaft of right fibula

    ✓7ᵗʰ **S82.425** **Nondisplaced** transverse fracture of shaft of left fibula

    ✓7ᵗʰ **S82.426** **Nondisplaced transverse fracture of shaft of unspecified fibula**

  ✓6ᵗʰ **S82.43** **Oblique** fracture of shaft of fibula

    ✓7ᵗʰ **S82.431** **Displaced** oblique fracture of shaft of right fibula

    ✓7ᵗʰ **S82.432** **Displaced** oblique fracture of shaft of left fibula

    ✓7ᵗʰ **S82.433** **Displaced oblique fracture of shaft of unspecified fibula**

    ✓7ᵗʰ **S82.434** **Nondisplaced** oblique fracture of shaft of right fibula

    ✓7ᵗʰ **S82.435** **Nondisplaced** oblique fracture of shaft of left fibula

    ✓7ᵗʰ **S82.436** **Nondisplaced oblique fracture of shaft of unspecified fibula**

✓ Additional Character Required   ✓x7ᵗʰ Placeholder Alert   Unspecified Dx   Other Specified Dx   Manifestation   ▶◀ Revised Text   ● New Code   ▲ Revised Code Title

ICD-10-CM 2016   **943**

√6ᵗʰ **S82.44** Spiral fracture of shaft of fibula

√7ᵗʰ **S82.441** Displaced spiral fracture of shaft of right fibula

√7ᵗʰ **S82.442** Displaced spiral fracture of shaft of left fibula

√7ᵗʰ **S82.443** Displaced spiral fracture of shaft of unspecified fibula

√7ᵗʰ **S82.444** Nondisplaced spiral fracture of shaft of right fibula

√7ᵗʰ **S82.445** Nondisplaced spiral fracture of shaft of left fibula

√7ᵗʰ **S82.446** Nondisplaced spiral fracture of shaft of unspecified fibula

√6ᵗʰ **S82.45** Comminuted fracture of shaft of fibula

√7ᵗʰ **S82.451** Displaced comminuted fracture of shaft of right fibula

√7ᵗʰ **S82.452** Displaced comminuted fracture of shaft of left fibula

√7ᵗʰ **S82.453** Displaced comminuted fracture of shaft of unspecified fibula

√7ᵗʰ **S82.454** Nondisplaced comminuted fracture of shaft of right fibula

√7ᵗʰ **S82.455** Nondisplaced comminuted fracture of shaft of left fibula

√7ᵗʰ **S82.456** Nondisplaced comminuted fracture of shaft of unspecified fibula

√6ᵗʰ **S82.46** Segmental fracture of shaft of fibula

√7ᵗʰ **S82.461** Displaced segmental fracture of shaft of right fibula

√7ᵗʰ **S82.462** Displaced segmental fracture of shaft of left fibula

√7ᵗʰ **S82.463** Displaced segmental fracture of shaft of unspecified fibula

√7ᵗʰ **S82.464** Nondisplaced segmental fracture of shaft of right fibula

√7ᵗʰ **S82.465** Nondisplaced segmental fracture of shaft of left fibula

√7ᵗʰ **S82.466** Nondisplaced segmental fracture of shaft of unspecified fibula

√6ᵗʰ **S82.49** Other fracture of shaft of fibula

√7ᵗʰ **S82.491** Other fracture of shaft of right fibula

√7ᵗʰ **S82.492** Other fracture of shaft of left fibula

√7ᵗʰ **S82.499** Other fracture of shaft of unspecified fibula

√5ᵗʰ **S82.5** Fracture of medial malleolus

EXCLUDES 1 pilon fracture of distal tibia (S82.87-)
Salter-Harris type III of lower end of tibia (S89.13-)
Salter-Harris type IV of lower end of tibia (S89.14-)

√x 7ᵗʰ **S82.51** Displaced fracture of medial malleolus of right tibia

√x 7ᵗʰ **S82.52** Displaced fracture of medial malleolus of left tibia

√x 7ᵗʰ **S82.53** Displaced fracture of medial malleolus of unspecified tibia

√x 7ᵗʰ **S82.54** Nondisplaced fracture of medial malleolus of right tibia

√x 7ᵗʰ **S82.55** Nondisplaced fracture of medial malleolus of left tibia

√x 7ᵗʰ **S82.56** Nondisplaced fracture of medial malleolus of unspecified tibia

√5ᵗʰ **S82.6** Fracture of lateral malleolus

EXCLUDES 1 pilon fracture of distal tibia (S82.87-)

√x 7ᵗʰ **S82.61** Displaced fracture of lateral malleolus of right fibula

√x 7ᵗʰ **S82.62** Displaced fracture of lateral malleolus of left fibula

√x 7ᵗʰ **S82.63** Displaced fracture of lateral malleolus of unspecified fibula

√x 7ᵗʰ **S82.64** Nondisplaced fracture of lateral malleolus of right fibula

√x 7ᵗʰ **S82.65** Nondisplaced fracture of lateral malleolus of left fibula

√x 7ᵗʰ **S82.66** Nondisplaced fracture of lateral malleolus of unspecified fibula

√5ᵗʰ **S82.8** Other fractures of lower leg

√6ᵗʰ **S82.81** Torus fracture of upper end of fibula

> The appropriate 7th character is to be added to all codes in subcategory S82.81.
> A   initial encounter for closed fracture
> D   subsequent encounter for fracture with routine healing
> G   subsequent encounter for fracture with delayed healing
> K   subsequent encounter for fracture with nonunion
> P   subsequent encounter for fracture with malunion
> S   sequela

√7ᵗʰ **S82.811** Torus fracture of upper end of right fibula

√7ᵗʰ **S82.812** Torus fracture of upper end of left fibula

√7ᵗʰ **S82.819** Torus fracture of upper end of unspecified fibula

√6ᵗʰ **S82.82** Torus fracture of lower end of fibula

> The appropriate 7th character is to be added to all codes in subcategory S82.82.
> A   initial encounter for closed fracture
> D   subsequent encounter for fracture with routine healing
> G   subsequent encounter for fracture with delayed healing
> K   subsequent encounter for fracture with nonunion
> P   subsequent encounter for fracture with malunion
> S   sequela

√7ᵗʰ **S82.821** Torus fracture of lower end of right fibula

√7ᵗʰ **S82.822** Torus fracture of lower end of left fibula

√7ᵗʰ **S82.829** Torus fracture of lower end of unspecified fibula

√6ᵗʰ **S82.83** Other fracture of upper and lower end of fibula
AHA: 2015, 1Q, 25

√7ᵗʰ **S82.831** Other fracture of upper and lower end of right fibula

√7ᵗʰ **S82.832** Other fracture of upper and lower end of left fibula

√7ᵗʰ **S82.839** Other fracture of upper and lower end of unspecified fibula

√6ᵗʰ **S82.84** Bimalleolar fracture of lower leg

√7ᵗʰ **S82.841** Displaced bimalleolar fracture of right lower leg

√7ᵗʰ **S82.842** Displaced bimalleolar fracture of left lower leg

√7ᵗʰ **S82.843** Displaced bimalleolar fracture of unspecified lower leg

√7ᵗʰ **S82.844** Nondisplaced bimalleolar fracture of right lower leg

√7ᵗʰ **S82.845** Nondisplaced bimalleolar fracture of left lower leg

√7ᵗʰ **S82.846** Nondisplaced bimalleolar fracture of unspecified lower leg

√6ᵗʰ **S82.85** Trimalleolar fracture of lower leg

√7ᵗʰ **S82.851** Displaced trimalleolar fracture of right lower leg

√7ᵗʰ **S82.852** Displaced trimalleolar fracture of left lower leg

√7ᵗʰ **S82.853** Displaced trimalleolar fracture of unspecified lower leg

√7ᵗʰ **S82.854** Nondisplaced trimalleolar fracture of right lower leg

√7ᵗʰ **S82.855** Nondisplaced trimalleolar fracture of left lower leg

√7ᵗʰ **S82.856** Nondisplaced trimalleolar fracture of unspecified lower leg

√6ᵗʰ **S82.86** Maisonneuve's fracture

√7ᵗʰ **S82.861** Displaced Maisonneuve's fracture of right leg

√7ᵗʰ **S82.862** Displaced Maisonneuve's fracture of left leg

---

EXCLUDES 1 Not coded here   **EXCLUDES 2** Not included here   N Newborn Age: 0   P Pediatric Age: 0-17   M Maternity Age: 12-55   A Adult Age: 15-124

√7ᵗʰ **S82.863** Displaced Maisonneuve's fracture of unspecified leg

√7ᵗʰ **S82.864** Nondisplaced Maisonneuve's fracture of right leg

√7ᵗʰ **S82.865** Nondisplaced Maisonneuve's fracture of left leg

√7ᵗʰ **S82.866** Nondisplaced Maisonneuve's fracture of unspecified leg

√6ᵗʰ **S82.87** Pilon fracture of tibia

√7ᵗʰ **S82.871** Displaced pilon fracture of right tibia

√7ᵗʰ **S82.872** Displaced pilon fracture of left tibia

√7ᵗʰ **S82.873** Displaced pilon fracture of unspecified tibia

√7ᵗʰ **S82.874** Nondisplaced pilon fracture of right tibia

√7ᵗʰ **S82.875** Nondisplaced pilon fracture of left tibia

√7ᵗʰ **S82.876** Nondisplaced pilon fracture of unspecified tibia

√6ᵗʰ **S82.89** Other fractures of lower leg
　　　　　Fracture of ankle NOS

√7ᵗʰ **S82.891** Other fracture of right lower leg

√7ᵗʰ **S82.892** Other fracture of left lower leg

√7ᵗʰ **S82.899** Other fracture of unspecified lower leg

√5ᵗʰ **S82.9** Unspecified fracture of lower leg

√×7ᵗʰ **S82.90** Unspecified fracture of unspecified lower leg

√×7ᵗʰ **S82.91** Unspecified fracture of right lower leg

√×7ᵗʰ **S82.92** Unspecified fracture of left lower leg

√4ᵗʰ **S83** Dislocation and sprain of joints and ligaments of knee
　　INCLUDES　avulsion of joint or ligament of knee
　　　　　　laceration of cartilage, joint or ligament of knee
　　　　　　sprain of cartilage, joint or ligament of knee
　　　　　　traumatic hemarthrosis of joint or ligament of knee
　　　　　　traumatic rupture of joint or ligament of knee
　　　　　　traumatic subluxation of joint or ligament of knee
　　　　　　traumatic tear of joint or ligament of knee
　　Code also any associated open wound
　　EXCLUDES 1　derangement of patella (M22.0-M22.3)
　　　　　　injury of patellar ligament (tendon) (S76.1-)
　　　　　　internal derangement of knee (M23.-)
　　　　　　old dislocation of knee (M24.36)
　　　　　　pathological dislocation of knee (M24.36)
　　　　　　recurrent dislocation of knee (M22.0)
　　EXCLUDES 2　strain of muscle, fascia and tendon of lower leg (S86.-)

The appropriate 7th character is to be added to each code from category S83.
A　initial encounter
D　subsequent encounter
S　sequela

√5ᵗʰ **S83.0** Subluxation and dislocation of patella

√6ᵗʰ **S83.00** Unspecified subluxation and dislocation of patella

√7ᵗʰ **S83.001** Unspecified subluxation of right patella

√7ᵗʰ **S83.002** Unspecified subluxation of left patella

√7ᵗʰ **S83.003** Unspecified subluxation of unspecified patella

√7ᵗʰ **S83.004** Unspecified dislocation of right patella

√7ᵗʰ **S83.005** Unspecified dislocation of left patella

√7ᵗʰ **S83.006** Unspecified dislocation of unspecified patella

√6ᵗʰ **S83.01** Lateral subluxation and dislocation of patella

√7ᵗʰ **S83.011** Lateral subluxation of right patella

√7ᵗʰ **S83.012** Lateral subluxation of left patella

√7ᵗʰ **S83.013** Lateral subluxation of unspecified patella

√7ᵗʰ **S83.014** Lateral dislocation of right patella

√7ᵗʰ **S83.015** Lateral dislocation of left patella

√7ᵗʰ **S83.016** Lateral dislocation of unspecified patella

√6ᵗʰ **S83.09** Other subluxation and dislocation of patella

√7ᵗʰ **S83.091** Other subluxation of right patella

√7ᵗʰ **S83.092** Other subluxation of left patella

√7ᵗʰ **S83.093** Other subluxation of unspecified patella

√7ᵗʰ **S83.094** Other dislocation of right patella

√7ᵗʰ **S83.095** Other dislocation of left patella

√7ᵗʰ **S83.096** Other dislocation of unspecified patella

√5ᵗʰ **S83.1** Subluxation and dislocation of knee
　　EXCLUDES 2　instability of knee prosthesis (T84.022, T84.023)

√6ᵗʰ **S83.10** Unspecified subluxation and dislocation of knee

√7ᵗʰ **S83.101** Unspecified subluxation of right knee

√7ᵗʰ **S83.102** Unspecified subluxation of left knee

√7ᵗʰ **S83.103** Unspecified subluxation of unspecified knee

√7ᵗʰ **S83.104** Unspecified dislocation of right knee

√7ᵗʰ **S83.105** Unspecified dislocation of left knee

√7ᵗʰ **S83.106** Unspecified dislocation of unspecified knee

√6ᵗʰ **S83.11** Anterior subluxation and dislocation of proximal end of tibia
　　　　　Posterior subluxation and dislocation of distal end of femur

√7ᵗʰ **S83.111** Anterior subluxation of proximal end of tibia, right knee

√7ᵗʰ **S83.112** Anterior subluxation of proximal end of tibia, left knee

√7ᵗʰ **S83.113** Anterior subluxation of proximal end of tibia, unspecified knee

√7ᵗʰ **S83.114** Anterior dislocation of proximal end of tibia, right knee

√7ᵗʰ **S83.115** Anterior dislocation of proximal end of tibia, left knee

√7ᵗʰ **S83.116** Anterior dislocation of proximal end of tibia, unspecified knee

√6ᵗʰ **S83.12** Posterior subluxation and dislocation of proximal end of tibia
　　　　　Anterior dislocation of distal end of femur

√7ᵗʰ **S83.121** Posterior subluxation of proximal end of tibia, right knee

√7ᵗʰ **S83.122** Posterior subluxation of proximal end of tibia, left knee

√7ᵗʰ **S83.123** Posterior subluxation of proximal end of tibia, unspecified knee

√7ᵗʰ **S83.124** Posterior dislocation of proximal end of tibia, right knee

√7ᵗʰ **S83.125** Posterior dislocation of proximal end of tibia, left knee

√7ᵗʰ **S83.126** Posterior dislocation of proximal end of tibia, unspecified knee

√6ᵗʰ **S83.13** Medial subluxation and dislocation of proximal end of tibia

√7ᵗʰ **S83.131** Medial subluxation of proximal end of tibia, right knee

√7ᵗʰ **S83.132** Medial subluxation of proximal end of tibia, left knee

√7ᵗʰ **S83.133** Medial subluxation of proximal end of tibia, unspecified knee

√7ᵗʰ **S83.134** Medial dislocation of proximal end of tibia, right knee

√7ᵗʰ **S83.135** Medial dislocation of proximal end of tibia, left knee

√7ᵗʰ **S83.136** Medial dislocation of proximal end of tibia, unspecified knee

√6ᵗʰ **S83.14** Lateral subluxation and dislocation of proximal end of tibia

√7ᵗʰ **S83.141** Lateral subluxation of proximal end of tibia, right knee

√7ᵗʰ **S83.142** Lateral subluxation of proximal end of tibia, left knee

√7ᵗʰ **S83.143** Lateral subluxation of proximal end of tibia, unspecified knee

√7ᵗʰ **S83.144** Lateral dislocation of proximal end of tibia, right knee

√7ᵗʰ **S83.145** Lateral dislocation of proximal end of tibia, left knee

√7ᵗʰ **S83.146** Lateral dislocation of proximal end of tibia, unspecified knee

√6ᵗʰ **S83.19** Other subluxation and dislocation of knee

√7ᵗʰ **S83.191** Other subluxation of right knee

√7ᵗʰ **S83.192** Other subluxation of left knee

√7ᵗʰ **S83.193** Other subluxation of unspecified knee

☑ Additional Character Required　√×7ᵗʰ Placeholder Alert　Unspecified Dx　Other Specified Dx　Manifestation　▶◀ Revised Text　● New Code　▲ Revised Code Title

ICD-10-CM 2016　　　　　　　　　　　　　　　　　　　　　　　　　　　　　　**945**

√7ᵗʰ **S83.194** **Other dislocation of right knee**

√7ᵗʰ **S83.195** **Other dislocation of left knee**

√7ᵗʰ **S83.196** **Other dislocation of unspecified knee**

√5ᵗʰ **S83.2** Tear of meniscus, current injury

> *EXCLUDES 1* old bucket-handle tear (M23.2)

√6ᵗʰ **S83.20** **Tear of unspecified meniscus, current injury**
Tear of meniscus of knee NOS

√7ᵗʰ **S83.200** **Bucket-handle tear of unspecified meniscus, current injury, right knee**

√7ᵗʰ **S83.201** **Bucket-handle tear of unspecified meniscus, current injury, left knee**

√7ᵗʰ **S83.202** **Bucket-handle tear of unspecified meniscus, current injury, unspecified knee**

√7ᵗʰ **S83.203** **Other tear of unspecified meniscus, current injury, right knee**

√7ᵗʰ **S83.204** **Other tear of unspecified meniscus, current injury, left knee**

√7ᵗʰ **S83.205** **Other tear of unspecified meniscus, current injury, unspecified knee**

√7ᵗʰ **S83.206** **Unspecified tear of unspecified meniscus, current injury, right knee**

√7ᵗʰ **S83.207** **Unspecified tear of unspecified meniscus, current injury, left knee**

√7ᵗʰ **S83.209** **Unspecified tear of unspecified meniscus, current injury, unspecified knee**

√6ᵗʰ **S83.21** **Bucket-handle tear of medial meniscus, current injury**

√7ᵗʰ **S83.211** **Bucket-handle tear of medial meniscus, current injury, right knee**

√7ᵗʰ **S83.212** **Bucket-handle tear of medial meniscus, current injury, left knee**

√7ᵗʰ **S83.219** **Bucket-handle tear of medial meniscus, current injury, unspecified knee**

√6ᵗʰ **S83.22** **Peripheral tear of medial meniscus, current injury**

√7ᵗʰ **S83.221** **Peripheral tear of medial meniscus, current injury, right knee**

√7ᵗʰ **S83.222** **Peripheral tear of medial meniscus, current injury, left knee**

√7ᵗʰ **S83.229** **Peripheral tear of medial meniscus, current injury, unspecified knee**

√6ᵗʰ **S83.23** **Complex tear of medial meniscus, current injury**

√7ᵗʰ **S83.231** **Complex tear of medial meniscus, current injury, right knee**

√7ᵗʰ **S83.232** **Complex tear of medial meniscus, current injury, left knee**

√7ᵗʰ **S83.239** **Complex tear of medial meniscus, current injury, unspecified knee**

√6ᵗʰ **S83.24** **Other tear of medial meniscus, current injury**

√7ᵗʰ **S83.241** **Other tear of medial meniscus, current injury, right knee**

√7ᵗʰ **S83.242** **Other tear of medial meniscus, current injury, left knee**

√7ᵗʰ **S83.249** **Other tear of medial meniscus, current injury, unspecified knee**

√6ᵗʰ **S83.25** **Bucket-handle tear of lateral meniscus, current injury**

√7ᵗʰ **S83.251** **Bucket-handle tear of lateral meniscus, current injury, right knee**

√7ᵗʰ **S83.252** **Bucket-handle tear of lateral meniscus, current injury, left knee**

√7ᵗʰ **S83.259** **Bucket-handle tear of lateral meniscus, current injury, unspecified knee**

√6ᵗʰ **S83.26** **Peripheral tear of lateral meniscus, current injury**

√7ᵗʰ **S83.261** **Peripheral tear of lateral meniscus, current injury, right knee**

√7ᵗʰ **S83.262** **Peripheral tear of lateral meniscus, current injury, left knee**

√7ᵗʰ **S83.269** **Peripheral tear of lateral meniscus, current injury, unspecified knee**

√6ᵗʰ **S83.27** **Complex tear of lateral meniscus, current injury**

√7ᵗʰ **S83.271** **Complex tear of lateral meniscus, current injury, right knee**

√7ᵗʰ **S83.272** **Complex tear of lateral meniscus, current injury, left knee**

√7ᵗʰ **S83.279** **Complex tear of lateral meniscus, current injury, unspecified knee**

√6ᵗʰ **S83.28** **Other tear of lateral meniscus, current injury**

√7ᵗʰ **S83.281** **Other tear of lateral meniscus, current injury, right knee**

√7ᵗʰ **S83.282** **Other tear of lateral meniscus, current injury, left knee**

√7ᵗʰ **S83.289** **Other tear of lateral meniscus, current injury, unspecified knee**

√5ᵗʰ **S83.3** Tear of articular cartilage of knee, current

√x7ᵗʰ **S83.30** **Tear of articular cartilage of unspecified knee, current**

√x7ᵗʰ **S83.31** **Tear of articular cartilage of right knee, current**

√x7ᵗʰ **S83.32** **Tear of articular cartilage of left knee, current**

√5ᵗʰ **S83.4** Sprain of collateral ligament of knee

√6ᵗʰ **S83.40** **Sprain of unspecified collateral ligament of knee**

√7ᵗʰ **S83.401** **Sprain of unspecified collateral ligament of right knee**

√7ᵗʰ **S83.402** **Sprain of unspecified collateral ligament of left knee**

√7ᵗʰ **S83.409** **Sprain of unspecified collateral ligament of unspecified knee**

√6ᵗʰ **S83.41** **Sprain of medial collateral ligament of knee**
Sprain of tibial collateral ligament

√7ᵗʰ **S83.411** **Sprain of medial collateral ligament of right knee**

√7ᵗʰ **S83.412** **Sprain of medial collateral ligament of left knee**

√7ᵗʰ **S83.419** **Sprain of medial collateral ligament of unspecified knee**

√6ᵗʰ **S83.42** **Sprain of lateral collateral ligament of knee**
Sprain of fibular collateral ligament

√7ᵗʰ **S83.421** **Sprain of lateral collateral ligament of right knee**

√7ᵗʰ **S83.422** **Sprain of lateral collateral ligament of left knee**

√7ᵗʰ **S83.429** **Sprain of lateral collateral ligament of unspecified knee**

√5ᵗʰ **S83.5** Sprain of cruciate ligament of knee

√6ᵗʰ **S83.50** **Sprain of unspecified cruciate ligament of knee**

√7ᵗʰ **S83.501** **Sprain of unspecified cruciate ligament of right knee**

√7ᵗʰ **S83.502** **Sprain of unspecified cruciate ligament of left knee**

√7ᵗʰ **S83.509** **Sprain of unspecified cruciate ligament of unspecified knee**

√6ᵗʰ **S83.51** **Sprain of anterior cruciate ligament of knee**

√7ᵗʰ **S83.511** **Sprain of anterior cruciate ligament of right knee**

√7ᵗʰ **S83.512** **Sprain of anterior cruciate ligament of left knee**

√7ᵗʰ **S83.519** **Sprain of anterior cruciate ligament of unspecified knee**

√6ᵗʰ **S83.52** **Sprain of posterior cruciate ligament of knee**

√7ᵗʰ **S83.521** **Sprain of posterior cruciate ligament of right knee**

√7ᵗʰ **S83.522** **Sprain of posterior cruciate ligament of left knee**

√7ᵗʰ **S83.529** **Sprain of posterior cruciate ligament of unspecified knee**

√5ᵗʰ **S83.6** Sprain of the superior tibiofibular joint and ligament

√x7ᵗʰ **S83.60** **Sprain of the superior tibiofibular joint and ligament, unspecified knee**

√x7ᵗʰ **S83.61** **Sprain of the superior tibiofibular joint and ligament, right knee**

√x7ᵗʰ **S83.62** **Sprain of the superior tibiofibular joint and ligament, left knee**

√5ᵗʰ **S83.8** Sprain of other specified parts of knee

√6ᵗʰ **S83.8X** **Sprain of other specified parts of knee**

√7ᵗʰ **S83.8X1** **Sprain of other specified parts of right knee**

√7ᵗʰ **S83.8X2** **Sprain of other specified parts of left knee**

EXCLUDES 1 Not coded here   *EXCLUDES 2* Not included here   N Newborn Age: 0   P Pediatric Age: 0-17   M Maternity Age: 12-55   A Adult Age: 15-124

946   ICD-10-CM 2016

☑7ᵗʰ **S83.8X9**   **Sprain of other specified parts of unspecified knee**

☑5ᵗʰ **S83.9**   **Sprain of** unspecified **site of knee**

   ☑x7ᵗʰ **S83.90**   **Sprain of unspecified site of unspecified knee**

   ☑x7ᵗʰ **S83.91**   **Sprain of unspecified site of right knee**

   ☑x7ᵗʰ **S83.92**   **Sprain of unspecified site of left knee**

☑4ᵗʰ **S84**   **Injury of nerves at lower leg level**

   Code also any associated open wound (S81.-)

   EXCLUDES 2   *injury of nerves at ankle and foot level (S94.-)*

   The appropriate 7th character is to be added to each code from category S84.
   A   initial encounter
   D   subsequent encounter
   S   sequela

   ☑5ᵗʰ **S84.0**   **Injury of** tibial nerve **at lower leg level**

     ☑x7ᵗʰ **S84.00**   **Injury of tibial nerve at lower leg level, unspecified leg**

     ☑x7ᵗʰ **S84.01**   **Injury of tibial nerve at lower leg level, right leg**

     ☑x7ᵗʰ **S84.02**   **Injury of tibial nerve at lower leg level, left leg**

   ☑5ᵗʰ **S84.1**   **Injury of** peroneal nerve **at lower leg level**

     ☑x7ᵗʰ **S84.10**   **Injury of peroneal nerve at lower leg level, unspecified leg**

     ☑x7ᵗʰ **S84.11**   **Injury of peroneal nerve at lower leg level, right leg**

     ☑x7ᵗʰ **S84.12**   **Injury of peroneal nerve at lower leg level, left leg**

   ☑5ᵗʰ **S84.2**   **Injury of** cutaneous sensory nerve **at lower leg level**

     ☑x7ᵗʰ **S84.20**   **Injury of cutaneous sensory nerve at lower leg level, unspecified leg**

     ☑x7ᵗʰ **S84.21**   **Injury of cutaneous sensory nerve at lower leg level, right leg**

     ☑x7ᵗʰ **S84.22**   **Injury of cutaneous sensory nerve at lower leg level, left leg**

   ☑5ᵗʰ **S84.8**   **Injury of** other nerves **at lower leg level**

     ☑6ᵗʰ **S84.80**   **Injury of other nerves at lower leg level**

       ☑7ᵗʰ **S84.801**   **Injury of other nerves at lower leg level, right leg**

       ☑7ᵗʰ **S84.802**   **Injury of other nerves at lower leg level, left leg**

       ☑7ᵗʰ **S84.809**   **Injury of other nerves at lower leg level, unspecified leg**

   ☑5ᵗʰ **S84.9**   **Injury of** unspecified nerve **at lower leg level**

     ☑x7ᵗʰ **S84.90**   **Injury of unspecified nerve at lower leg level, unspecified leg**

     ☑x7ᵗʰ **S84.91**   **Injury of unspecified nerve at lower leg level, right leg**

     ☑x7ᵗʰ **S84.92**   **Injury of unspecified nerve at lower leg level, left leg**

☑4ᵗʰ **S85**   **Injury of blood vessels at lower leg level**

   Code also any associated open wound (S81.-)

   EXCLUDES 2   *injury of blood vessels at ankle and foot level (S95.-)*

   The appropriate 7th character is to be added to each code from category S85.
   A   initial encounter
   D   subsequent encounter
   S   sequela

   ☑5ᵗʰ **S85.0**   **Injury of** popliteal artery

     ☑6ᵗʰ **S85.00**   **Unspecified injury of popliteal artery**

       ☑7ᵗʰ **S85.001**   **Unspecified injury of popliteal artery, right leg**

       ☑7ᵗʰ **S85.002**   **Unspecified injury of popliteal artery, left leg**

       ☑7ᵗʰ **S85.009**   **Unspecified injury of popliteal artery, unspecified leg**

     ☑6ᵗʰ **S85.01**   **Laceration of popliteal artery**

       ☑7ᵗʰ **S85.011**   **Laceration of popliteal artery, right leg**

       ☑7ᵗʰ **S85.012**   **Laceration of popliteal artery, left leg**

       ☑7ᵗʰ **S85.019**   **Laceration of popliteal artery, unspecified leg**

     ☑6ᵗʰ **S85.09**   **Other** specified injury of popliteal artery

       ☑7ᵗʰ **S85.091**   **Other specified injury of popliteal artery, right leg**

       ☑7ᵗʰ **S85.092**   **Other specified injury of popliteal artery, left leg**

       ☑7ᵗʰ **S85.099**   **Other specified injury of popliteal artery, unspecified leg**

   ☑5ᵗʰ **S85.1**   **Injury of** tibial artery

     ☑6ᵗʰ **S85.10**   **Unspecified injury of unspecified tibial artery**
       Injury of tibial artery NOS

       ☑7ᵗʰ **S85.101**   **Unspecified injury of unspecified tibial artery, right leg**

       ☑7ᵗʰ **S85.102**   **Unspecified injury of unspecified tibial artery, left leg**

       ☑7ᵗʰ **S85.109**   **Unspecified injury of unspecified tibial artery, unspecified leg**

     ☑6ᵗʰ **S85.11**   **Laceration of** unspecified **tibial artery**

       ☑7ᵗʰ **S85.111**   **Laceration of unspecified tibial artery, right leg**

       ☑7ᵗʰ **S85.112**   **Laceration of unspecified tibial artery, left leg**

       ☑7ᵗʰ **S85.119**   **Laceration of unspecified tibial artery, unspecified leg**

     ☑6ᵗʰ **S85.12**   **Other** specified injury of unspecified **tibial artery**

       ☑7ᵗʰ **S85.121**   **Other specified injury of unspecified tibial artery, right leg**

       ☑7ᵗʰ **S85.122**   **Other specified injury of unspecified tibial artery, left leg**

       ☑7ᵗʰ **S85.129**   **Other specified injury of unspecified tibial artery, unspecified leg**

     ☑6ᵗʰ **S85.13**   **Unspecified** injury of anterior **tibial artery**

       ☑7ᵗʰ **S85.131**   **Unspecified injury of anterior tibial artery, right leg**

       ☑7ᵗʰ **S85.132**   **Unspecified injury of anterior tibial artery, left leg**

       ☑7ᵗʰ **S85.139**   **Unspecified injury of anterior tibial artery, unspecified leg**

     ☑6ᵗʰ **S85.14**   **Laceration** of anterior **tibial artery**

       ☑7ᵗʰ **S85.141**   **Laceration of anterior tibial artery, right leg**

       ☑7ᵗʰ **S85.142**   **Laceration of anterior tibial artery, left leg**

       ☑7ᵗʰ **S85.149**   **Laceration of anterior tibial artery, unspecified leg**

     ☑6ᵗʰ **S85.15**   **Other** specified injury of anterior **tibial artery**

       ☑7ᵗʰ **S85.151**   **Other specified injury of anterior tibial artery, right leg**

       ☑7ᵗʰ **S85.152**   **Other specified injury of anterior tibial artery, left leg**

       ☑7ᵗʰ **S85.159**   **Other specified injury of anterior tibial artery, unspecified leg**

     ☑6ᵗʰ **S85.16**   **Unspecified** injury of posterior **tibial artery**

       ☑7ᵗʰ **S85.161**   **Unspecified injury of posterior tibial artery, right leg**

       ☑7ᵗʰ **S85.162**   **Unspecified injury of posterior tibial artery, left leg**

       ☑7ᵗʰ **S85.169**   **Unspecified injury of posterior tibial artery, unspecified leg**

     ☑6ᵗʰ **S85.17**   **Laceration of** posterior **tibial artery**

       ☑7ᵗʰ **S85.171**   **Laceration of posterior tibial artery, right leg**

       ☑7ᵗʰ **S85.172**   **Laceration of posterior tibial artery, left leg**

       ☑7ᵗʰ **S85.179**   **Laceration of posterior tibial artery, unspecified leg**

     ☑6ᵗʰ **S85.18**   **Other** specified injury of posterior **tibial artery**

       ☑7ᵗʰ **S85.181**   **Other specified injury of posterior tibial artery, right leg**

       ☑7ᵗʰ **S85.182**   **Other specified injury of posterior tibial artery, left leg**

       ☑7ᵗʰ **S85.189**   **Other specified injury of posterior tibial artery, unspecified leg**

   ☑5ᵗʰ **S85.2**   **Injury of** peroneal **artery**

     ☑6ᵗʰ **S85.20**   **Unspecified** injury of peroneal **artery**

       ☑7ᵗʰ **S85.201**   **Unspecified injury of peroneal artery, right leg**

       ☑7ᵗʰ **S85.202**   **Unspecified injury of peroneal artery, left leg**

       ☑7ᵗʰ **S85.209**   **Unspecified injury of peroneal artery, unspecified leg**

☑ Additional Character Required   ☑x7ᵗʰ Placeholder Alert   Unspecified Dx   Other Specified Dx   Manifestation   ▶◀ Revised Text   ● New Code   ▲ Revised Code Title

ICD-10-CM 2016   **947**

√6ᵗʰ **S85.21** Laceration of peroneal artery
- √7ᵗʰ **S85.211** Laceration of peroneal artery, right leg
- √7ᵗʰ **S85.212** Laceration of peroneal artery, left leg
- √7ᵗʰ **S85.219** Laceration of peroneal artery, unspecified leg

√6ᵗʰ **S85.29** Other specified injury of peroneal artery
- √7ᵗʰ **S85.291** Other specified injury of peroneal artery, right leg
- √7ᵗʰ **S85.292** Other specified injury of peroneal artery, left leg
- √7ᵗʰ **S85.299** Other specified injury of peroneal artery, unspecified leg

√5ᵗʰ **S85.3** Injury of greater saphenous vein at lower leg level
Injury of greater saphenous vein NOS
Injury of saphenous vein NOS

√6ᵗʰ **S85.30** Unspecified injury of greater saphenous vein at lower leg level
- √7ᵗʰ **S85.301** Unspecified injury of greater saphenous vein at lower leg level, right leg
- √7ᵗʰ **S85.302** Unspecified injury of greater saphenous vein at lower leg level, left leg
- √7ᵗʰ **S85.309** Unspecified injury of greater saphenous vein at lower leg level, unspecified leg

√6ᵗʰ **S85.31** Laceration of greater saphenous vein at lower leg level
- √7ᵗʰ **S85.311** Laceration of greater saphenous vein at lower leg level, right leg
- √7ᵗʰ **S85.312** Laceration of greater saphenous vein at lower leg level, left leg
- √7ᵗʰ **S85.319** Laceration of greater saphenous vein at lower leg level, unspecified leg

√6ᵗʰ **S85.39** Other specified injury of greater saphenous vein at lower leg level
- √7ᵗʰ **S85.391** Other specified injury of greater saphenous vein at lower leg level, right leg
- √7ᵗʰ **S85.392** Other specified injury of greater saphenous vein at lower leg level, left leg
- √7ᵗʰ **S85.399** Other specified injury of greater saphenous vein at lower leg level, unspecified leg

√5ᵗʰ **S85.4** Injury of lesser saphenous vein at lower leg level

√6ᵗʰ **S85.40** Unspecified injury of lesser saphenous vein at lower leg level
- √7ᵗʰ **S85.401** Unspecified injury of lesser saphenous vein at lower leg level, right leg
- √7ᵗʰ **S85.402** Unspecified injury of lesser saphenous vein at lower leg level, left leg
- √7ᵗʰ **S85.409** Unspecified injury of lesser saphenous vein at lower leg level, unspecified leg

√6ᵗʰ **S85.41** Laceration of lesser saphenous vein at lower leg level
- √7ᵗʰ **S85.411** Laceration of lesser saphenous vein at lower leg level, right leg
- √7ᵗʰ **S85.412** Laceration of lesser saphenous vein at lower leg level, left leg
- √7ᵗʰ **S85.419** Laceration of lesser saphenous vein at lower leg level, unspecified leg

√6ᵗʰ **S85.49** Other specified injury of lesser saphenous vein at lower leg level
- √7ᵗʰ **S85.491** Other specified injury of lesser saphenous vein at lower leg level, right leg
- √7ᵗʰ **S85.492** Other specified injury of lesser saphenous vein at lower leg level, left leg
- √7ᵗʰ **S85.499** Other specified injury of lesser saphenous vein at lower leg level, unspecified leg

√5ᵗʰ **S85.5** Injury of popliteal vein

√6ᵗʰ **S85.50** Unspecified injury of popliteal vein
- √7ᵗʰ **S85.501** Unspecified injury of popliteal vein, right leg
- √7ᵗʰ **S85.502** Unspecified injury of popliteal vein, left leg
- √7ᵗʰ **S85.509** Unspecified injury of popliteal vein, unspecified leg

√6ᵗʰ **S85.51** Laceration of popliteal vein
- √7ᵗʰ **S85.511** Laceration of popliteal vein, right leg
- √7ᵗʰ **S85.512** Laceration of popliteal vein, left leg
- √7ᵗʰ **S85.519** Laceration of popliteal vein, unspecified leg

√6ᵗʰ **S85.59** Other specified injury of popliteal vein
- √7ᵗʰ **S85.591** Other specified injury of popliteal vein, right leg
- √7ᵗʰ **S85.592** Other specified injury of popliteal vein, left leg
- √7ᵗʰ **S85.599** Other specified injury of popliteal vein, unspecified leg

√5ᵗʰ **S85.8** Injury of other blood vessels at lower leg level

√6ᵗʰ **S85.80** Unspecified injury of other blood vessels at lower leg level
- √7ᵗʰ **S85.801** Unspecified injury of other blood vessels at lower leg level, right leg
- √7ᵗʰ **S85.802** Unspecified injury of other blood vessels at lower leg level, left leg
- √7ᵗʰ **S85.809** Unspecified injury of other blood vessels at lower leg level, unspecified leg

√6ᵗʰ **S85.81** Laceration of other blood vessels at lower leg level
- √7ᵗʰ **S85.811** Laceration of other blood vessels at lower leg level, right leg
- √7ᵗʰ **S85.812** Laceration of other blood vessels at lower leg level, left leg
- √7ᵗʰ **S85.819** Laceration of other blood vessels at lower leg level, unspecified leg

√6ᵗʰ **S85.89** Other specified injury of other blood vessels at lower leg level
- √7ᵗʰ **S85.891** Other specified injury of other blood vessels at lower leg level, right leg
- √7ᵗʰ **S85.892** Other specified injury of other blood vessels at lower leg level, left leg
- √7ᵗʰ **S85.899** Other specified injury of other blood vessels at lower leg level, unspecified leg

√5ᵗʰ **S85.9** Injury of unspecified blood vessel at lower leg level

√6ᵗʰ **S85.90** Unspecified injury of unspecified blood vessel at lower leg level
- √7ᵗʰ **S85.901** Unspecified injury of unspecified blood vessel at lower leg level, right leg
- √7ᵗʰ **S85.902** Unspecified injury of unspecified blood vessel at lower leg level, left leg
- √7ᵗʰ **S85.909** Unspecified injury of unspecified blood vessel at lower leg level, unspecified leg

√6ᵗʰ **S85.91** Laceration of unspecified blood vessel at lower leg level
- √7ᵗʰ **S85.911** Laceration of unspecified blood vessel at lower leg level, right leg
- √7ᵗʰ **S85.912** Laceration of unspecified blood vessel at lower leg level, left leg
- √7ᵗʰ **S85.919** Laceration of unspecified blood vessel at lower leg level, unspecified leg

√6ᵗʰ **S85.99** Other specified injury of unspecified blood vessel at lower leg level
- √7ᵗʰ **S85.991** Other specified injury of unspecified blood vessel at lower leg level, right leg
- √7ᵗʰ **S85.992** Other specified injury of unspecified blood vessel at lower leg level, left leg
- √7ᵗʰ **S85.999** Other specified injury of unspecified blood vessel at lower leg level, unspecified leg

EXCLUDES 1 Not coded here   **EXCLUDES 2** Not included here   N Newborn Age: 0   P Pediatric Age: 0-17   M Maternity Age: 12-55   A Adult Age: 15-124

948

ICD-10-CM 2016

✦ ✓4ᵗʰ S86 Injury of muscle, fascia and tendon at lower leg level

Code also any associated open wound (S81.-)

EXCLUDES 2   injury of muscle, fascia and tendon at ankle (S96.-)
injury of patellar ligament (tendon) (S76.1-)
sprain of joints and ligaments of knee (S83.-)

The appropriate 7th character is to be added to each code from category S86.
A   initial encounter
D   subsequent encounter
S   sequela

✓5ᵗʰ **S86.0**   **Injury of** Achilles tendon

   ✓6ᵗʰ **S86.00**   **Unspecified injury of Achilles tendon**

     ✓7ᵗʰ **S86.001**   **Unspecified injury of** right **Achilles tendon**

     ✓7ᵗʰ **S86.002**   **Unspecified injury of** left **Achilles tendon**

     ✓7ᵗʰ **S86.009**   **Unspecified injury of unspecified Achilles tendon**

   ✓6ᵗʰ **S86.01**   **Strain of Achilles tendon**

     ✓7ᵗʰ **S86.011**   **Strain of** right **Achilles tendon**

     ✓7ᵗʰ **S86.012**   **Strain of** left **Achilles tendon**

     ✓7ᵗʰ **S86.019**   **Strain of unspecified Achilles tendon**

   ✓6ᵗʰ **S86.02**   **Laceration of Achilles tendon**

     ✓7ᵗʰ **S86.021**   **Laceration of** right **Achilles tendon**

     ✓7ᵗʰ **S86.022**   **Laceration of** left **Achilles tendon**

     ✓7ᵗʰ **S86.029**   **Laceration of unspecified Achilles tendon**

   ✓6ᵗʰ **S86.09**   **Other** specified injury of Achilles tendon

     ✓7ᵗʰ **S86.091**   **Other specified injury of** right **Achilles tendon**

     ✓7ᵗʰ **S86.092**   **Other specified injury of** left **Achilles tendon**

     ✓7ᵗʰ **S86.099**   **Other specified injury of unspecified Achilles tendon**

✓5ᵗʰ **S86.1**   **Injury of other muscle(s) and tendon(s) of** posterior muscle group **at lower leg level**

   ✓6ᵗʰ **S86.10**   **Unspecified** injury of other muscle(s) and tendon(s) of posterior muscle group at lower leg level

     ✓7ᵗʰ **S86.101**   **Unspecified injury of other muscle(s) and tendon(s) of posterior muscle group at lower leg level,** right **leg**

     ✓7ᵗʰ **S86.102**   **Unspecified injury of other muscle(s) and tendon(s) of posterior muscle group at lower leg level,** left **leg**

     ✓7ᵗʰ **S86.109**   **Unspecified injury of other muscle(s) and tendon(s) of posterior muscle group at lower leg level, unspecified leg**

   ✓6ᵗʰ **S86.11**   **Strain** of other muscle(s) and tendon(s) of posterior muscle group at lower leg level

     ✓7ᵗʰ **S86.111**   **Strain of other muscle(s) and tendon(s) of posterior muscle group at lower leg level,** right **leg**

     ✓7ᵗʰ **S86.112**   **Strain of other muscle(s) and tendon(s) of posterior muscle group at lower leg level,** left **leg**

     ✓7ᵗʰ **S86.119**   **Strain of other muscle(s) and tendon(s) of posterior muscle group at lower leg level, unspecified leg**

   ✓6ᵗʰ **S86.12**   **Laceration** of other muscle(s) and tendon(s) of posterior muscle group at lower leg level

     ✓7ᵗʰ **S86.121**   **Laceration of other muscle(s) and tendon(s) of posterior muscle group at lower leg level,** right **leg**

     ✓7ᵗʰ **S86.122**   **Laceration of other muscle(s) and tendon(s) of posterior muscle group at lower leg level,** left **leg**

     ✓7ᵗʰ **S86.129**   **Laceration of other muscle(s) and tendon(s) of posterior muscle group at lower leg level, unspecified leg**

   ✓6ᵗʰ **S86.19**   **Other** injury of other muscle(s) and tendon(s) of posterior muscle group at lower leg level

     ✓7ᵗʰ **S86.191**   **Other injury of other muscle(s) and tendon(s) of posterior muscle group at lower leg level,** right **leg**

     ✓7ᵗʰ **S86.192**   **Other injury of other muscle(s) and tendon(s) of posterior muscle group at lower leg level,** left **leg**

     ✓7ᵗʰ **S86.199**   **Other injury of other muscle(s) and tendon(s) of posterior muscle group at lower leg level, unspecified leg**

✓5ᵗʰ **S86.2**   **Injury of muscle(s) and tendon(s) of** anterior muscle group **at lower leg level**

   ✓6ᵗʰ **S86.20**   **Unspecified** injury of muscle(s) and tendon(s) of anterior muscle group at lower leg level

     ✓7ᵗʰ **S86.201**   **Unspecified injury of muscle(s) and tendon(s) of anterior muscle group at lower leg level,** right **leg**

     ✓7ᵗʰ **S86.202**   **Unspecified injury of muscle(s) and tendon(s) of anterior muscle group at lower leg level,** left **leg**

     ✓7ᵗʰ **S86.209**   **Unspecified injury of muscle(s) and tendon(s) of anterior muscle group at lower leg level, unspecified leg**

   ✓6ᵗʰ **S86.21**   **Strain of muscle(s) and tendon(s) of anterior muscle group at lower leg level**

     ✓7ᵗʰ **S86.211**   **Strain of muscle(s) and tendon(s) of anterior muscle group at lower leg level,** right **leg**

     ✓7ᵗʰ **S86.212**   **Strain of muscle(s) and tendon(s) of anterior muscle group at lower leg level,** left **leg**

     ✓7ᵗʰ **S86.219**   **Strain of muscle(s) and tendon(s) of anterior muscle group at lower leg level, unspecified leg**

   ✓6ᵗʰ **S86.22**   **Laceration** of muscle(s) and tendon(s) of anterior muscle group at lower leg level

     ✓7ᵗʰ **S86.221**   **Laceration of muscle(s) and tendon(s) of anterior muscle group at lower leg level,** right **leg**

     ✓7ᵗʰ **S86.222**   **Laceration of muscle(s) and tendon(s) of anterior muscle group at lower leg level,** left **leg**

     ✓7ᵗʰ **S86.229**   **Laceration of muscle(s) and tendon(s) of anterior muscle group at lower leg level, unspecified leg**

   ✓6ᵗʰ **S86.29**   **Other** injury of muscle(s) and tendon(s) of anterior muscle group at lower leg level

     ✓7ᵗʰ **S86.291**   **Other injury of muscle(s) and tendon(s) of anterior muscle group at lower leg level,** right **leg**

     ✓7ᵗʰ **S86.292**   **Other injury of muscle(s) and tendon(s) of anterior muscle group at lower leg level,** left **leg**

     ✓7ᵗʰ **S86.299**   **Other injury of muscle(s) and tendon(s) of anterior muscle group at lower leg level, unspecified leg**

✓5ᵗʰ **S86.3**   **Injury of muscle(s) and tendon(s) of** peroneal muscle group **at lower leg level**

   ✓6ᵗʰ **S86.30**   **Unspecified** injury of muscle(s) and tendon(s) of peroneal muscle group at lower leg level

     ✓7ᵗʰ **S86.301**   **Unspecified injury of muscle(s) and tendon(s) of peroneal muscle group at lower leg level,** right **leg**

     ✓7ᵗʰ **S86.302**   **Unspecified injury of muscle(s) and tendon(s) of peroneal muscle group at lower leg level,** left **leg**

     ✓7ᵗʰ **S86.309**   **Unspecified injury of muscle(s) and tendon(s) of peroneal muscle group at lower leg level, unspecified leg**

   ✓6ᵗʰ **S86.31**   **Strain of muscle(s) and tendon(s) of peroneal muscle group at lower leg level**

     ✓7ᵗʰ **S86.311**   **Strain of muscle(s) and tendon(s) of peroneal muscle group at lower leg level,** right **leg**

     ✓7ᵗʰ **S86.312**   **Strain of muscle(s) and tendon(s) of peroneal muscle group at lower leg level,** left **leg**

     ✓7ᵗʰ **S86.319**   **Strain of muscle(s) and tendon(s) of peroneal muscle group at lower leg level, unspecified leg**

✦   Refer to the Muscle/Tendon Table at beginning of this chapter.

☑ Additional Character Required   ✓x7ᵗʰ Placeholder Alert   Unspecified Dx   Other Specified Dx   Manifestation   ▶◀ Revised Text   ● New Code   ▲ Revised Code Title

√6ᵗʰ **S86.32** Laceration of muscle(s) and tendon(s) of peroneal muscle group at lower leg level

     √7ᵗʰ **S86.321** Laceration of muscle(s) and tendon(s) of peroneal muscle group at lower leg level, right leg

     √7ᵗʰ **S86.322** Laceration of muscle(s) and tendon(s) of peroneal muscle group at lower leg level, left leg

     √7ᵗʰ **S86.329** Laceration of muscle(s) and tendon(s) of peroneal muscle group at lower leg level, unspecified leg

√6ᵗʰ **S86.39** Other injury of muscle(s) and tendon(s) of peroneal muscle group at lower leg level

     √7ᵗʰ **S86.391** Other injury of muscle(s) and tendon(s) of peroneal muscle group at lower leg level, right leg

     √7ᵗʰ **S86.392** Other injury of muscle(s) and tendon(s) of peroneal muscle group at lower leg level, left leg

     √7ᵗʰ **S86.399** Other injury of muscle(s) and tendon(s) of peroneal muscle group at lower leg level, unspecified leg

√5ᵗʰ **S86.8** Injury of other muscles and tendons at lower leg level

√6ᵗʰ **S86.80** Unspecified injury of other muscles and tendons at lower leg level

     √7ᵗʰ **S86.801** Unspecified injury of other muscle(s) and tendon(s) at lower leg level, right leg

     √7ᵗʰ **S86.802** Unspecified injury of other muscle(s) and tendon(s) at lower leg level, left leg

     √7ᵗʰ **S86.809** Unspecified injury of other muscle(s) and tendon(s) at lower leg level, unspecified leg

√6ᵗʰ **S86.81** Strain of other muscles and tendons at lower leg level

     √7ᵗʰ **S86.811** Strain of other muscle(s) and tendon(s) at lower leg level, right leg

     √7ᵗʰ **S86.812** Strain of other muscle(s) and tendon(s) at lower leg level, left leg

     √7ᵗʰ **S86.819** Strain of other muscle(s) and tendon(s) at lower leg level, unspecified leg

√6ᵗʰ **S86.82** Laceration of other muscles and tendons at lower leg level

     √7ᵗʰ **S86.821** Laceration of other muscle(s) and tendon(s) at lower leg level, right leg

     √7ᵗʰ **S86.822** Laceration of other muscle(s) and tendon(s) at lower leg level, left leg

     √7ᵗʰ **S86.829** Laceration of other muscle(s) and tendon(s) at lower leg level, unspecified leg

√6ᵗʰ **S86.89** Other injury of other muscles and tendons at lower leg level

     √7ᵗʰ **S86.891** Other injury of other muscle(s) and tendon(s) at lower leg level, right leg

     √7ᵗʰ **S86.892** Other injury of other muscle(s) and tendon(s) at lower leg level, left leg

     √7ᵗʰ **S86.899** Other injury of other muscle(s) and tendon(s) at lower leg level, unspecified leg

√5ᵗʰ **S86.9** Injury of unspecified muscle and tendon at lower leg level

√6ᵗʰ **S86.90** Unspecified injury of unspecified muscle and tendon at lower leg level

     √7ᵗʰ **S86.901** Unspecified injury of unspecified muscle(s) and tendon(s) at lower leg level, right leg

     √7ᵗʰ **S86.902** Unspecified injury of unspecified muscle(s) and tendon(s) at lower leg level, left leg

     √7ᵗʰ **S86.909** Unspecified injury of unspecified muscle(s) and tendon(s) at lower leg level, unspecified leg

√6ᵗʰ **S86.91** Strain of unspecified muscle and tendon at lower leg level

     √7ᵗʰ **S86.911** Strain of unspecified muscle(s) and tendon(s) at lower leg level, right leg

     √7ᵗʰ **S86.912** Strain of unspecified muscle(s) and tendon(s) at lower leg level, left leg

     √7ᵗʰ **S86.919** Strain of unspecified muscle(s) and tendon(s) at lower leg level, unspecified leg

√6ᵗʰ **S86.92** Laceration of unspecified muscle and tendon at lower leg level

     √7ᵗʰ **S86.921** Laceration of unspecified muscle(s) and tendon(s) at lower leg level, right leg

     √7ᵗʰ **S86.922** Laceration of unspecified muscle(s) and tendon(s) at lower leg level, left leg

     √7ᵗʰ **S86.929** Laceration of unspecified muscle(s) and tendon(s) at lower leg level, unspecified leg

√6ᵗʰ **S86.99** Other injury of unspecified muscle and tendon at lower leg level

     √7ᵗʰ **S86.991** Other injury of unspecified muscle(s) and tendon(s) at lower leg level, right leg

     √7ᵗʰ **S86.992** Other injury of unspecified muscle(s) and tendon(s) at lower leg level, left leg

     √7ᵗʰ **S86.999** Other injury of unspecified muscle(s) and tendon(s) at lower leg level, unspecified leg

√4ᵗʰ **S87 Crushing injury of lower leg**

Use additional code(s) for all associated injuries

EXCLUDES 2   crushing injury of ankle and foot (S97.-)

> The appropriate 7th character is to be added to each code from category S87.
> A   initial encounter
> D   subsequent encounter
> S   sequela

√5ᵗʰ **S87.0** Crushing injury of knee

     √x7ᵗʰ **S87.00** Crushing injury of unspecified knee

     √x7ᵗʰ **S87.01** Crushing injury of right knee

     √x7ᵗʰ **S87.02** Crushing injury of left knee

√5ᵗʰ **S87.8** Crushing injury of lower leg

     √x7ᵗʰ **S87.80** Crushing injury of unspecified lower leg

     √x7ᵗʰ **S87.81** Crushing injury of right lower leg

     √x7ᵗʰ **S87.82** Crushing injury of left lower leg

√4ᵗʰ **S88 Traumatic amputation of lower leg**

NOTE   An amputation not identified as partial or complete should be coded to complete.

EXCLUDES 1   traumatic amputation of ankle and foot (S98.-)

> The appropriate 7th character is to be added to each code from category S88.
> A   initial encounter
> D   subsequent encounter
> S   sequela

√5ᵗʰ **S88.0** Traumatic amputation at knee level

√6ᵗʰ **S88.01** Complete traumatic amputation at knee level

     √7ᵗʰ **S88.011** Complete traumatic amputation at knee level, right lower leg

     √7ᵗʰ **S88.012** Complete traumatic amputation at knee level, left lower leg

     √7ᵗʰ **S88.019** Complete traumatic amputation at knee level, unspecified lower leg

√6ᵗʰ **S88.02** Partial traumatic amputation at knee level

     √7ᵗʰ **S88.021** Partial traumatic amputation at knee level, right lower leg

     √7ᵗʰ **S88.022** Partial traumatic amputation at knee level, left lower leg

     √7ᵗʰ **S88.029** Partial traumatic amputation at knee level, unspecified lower leg

√5ᵗʰ **S88.1** Traumatic amputation at level between knee and ankle

√6ᵗʰ **S88.11** Complete traumatic amputation at level between knee and ankle

     √7ᵗʰ **S88.111** Complete traumatic amputation at level between knee and ankle, right lower leg

     √7ᵗʰ **S88.112** Complete traumatic amputation at level between knee and ankle, left lower leg

     √7ᵗʰ **S88.119** Complete traumatic amputation at level between knee and ankle, unspecified lower leg

---

EXCLUDES 1 Not coded here   *EXCLUDES 2* Not included here   **N** Newborn Age: 0   **P** Pediatric Age: 0-17   **M** Maternity Age: 12-55   **A** Adult Age: 15-124

☑6ᵗʰ **S88.12** Partial **traumatic amputation at level between knee and ankle**

    ☑7ᵗʰ **S88.121** Partial **traumatic amputation at level between knee and ankle, right lower leg**

    ☑7ᵗʰ **S88.122** Partial **traumatic amputation at level between knee and ankle, left lower leg**

    ☑7ᵗʰ **S88.129** Partial **traumatic amputation at level between knee and ankle, unspecified lower leg**

☑5ᵗʰ **S88.9** Traumatic amputation of lower leg, **level unspecified**

  ☑6ᵗʰ **S88.91** Complete **traumatic amputation of lower leg, level unspecified**

    ☑7ᵗʰ **S88.911** Complete **traumatic amputation of right lower leg, level unspecified**

    ☑7ᵗʰ **S88.912** Complete **traumatic amputation of left lower leg, level unspecified**

    ☑7ᵗʰ **S88.919** Complete **traumatic amputation of unspecified lower leg, level unspecified**

  ☑6ᵗʰ **S88.92** Partial **traumatic amputation of lower leg, level unspecified**

    ☑7ᵗʰ **S88.921** Partial **traumatic amputation of right lower leg, level unspecified**

    ☑7ᵗʰ **S88.922** Partial **traumatic amputation of left lower leg, level unspecified**

    ☑7ᵗʰ **S88.929** Partial **traumatic amputation of unspecified lower leg, level unspecified**

☑4ᵗʰ **S89** **Other and unspecified injuries of lower leg**

    NOTE   A fracture not indicated as open or closed should be coded to closed.

    EXCLUDES 2   *other and unspecified injuries of ankle and foot (S99.-)*

> The appropriate 7th character is to be added to each code from subcategories S89.0, S89.1, S89.2, and S89.3.
> A   initial encounter for closed fracture
> D   subsequent encounter for fracture with routine healing
> G   subsequent encounter for fracture with delayed healing
> K   subsequent encounter for fracture with nonunion
> P   subsequent encounter for fracture with malunion
> S   sequela

☑5ᵗʰ **S89.0** Physeal **fracture of upper end of tibia**

  ☑6ᵗʰ **S89.00** Unspecified **physeal fracture of upper end of tibia**

    ☑7ᵗʰ **S89.001** Unspecified **physeal fracture of upper end of right tibia**

    ☑7ᵗʰ **S89.002** Unspecified **physeal fracture of upper end of left tibia**

    ☑7ᵗʰ **S89.009** Unspecified **physeal fracture of upper end of unspecified tibia**

  ☑6ᵗʰ **S89.01** Salter-Harris Type I **physeal fracture of upper end of tibia**

    ☑7ᵗʰ **S89.011** Salter-Harris Type I **physeal fracture of upper end of right tibia**

    ☑7ᵗʰ **S89.012** Salter-Harris Type I **physeal fracture of upper end of left tibia**

    ☑7ᵗʰ **S89.019** Salter-Harris Type I **physeal fracture of upper end of unspecified tibia**

  ☑6ᵗʰ **S89.02** Salter-Harris Type II **physeal fracture of upper end of tibia**

    ☑7ᵗʰ **S89.021** Salter-Harris Type II **physeal fracture of upper end of right tibia**

    ☑7ᵗʰ **S89.022** Salter-Harris Type II **physeal fracture of upper end of left tibia**

    ☑7ᵗʰ **S89.029** Salter-Harris Type II **physeal fracture of upper end of unspecified tibia**

  ☑6ᵗʰ **S89.03** Salter-Harris Type III **physeal fracture of upper end of tibia**

    ☑7ᵗʰ **S89.031** Salter-Harris Type III **physeal fracture of upper end of right tibia**

    ☑7ᵗʰ **S89.032** Salter-Harris Type III **physeal fracture of upper end of left tibia**

    ☑7ᵗʰ **S89.039** Salter-Harris Type III **physeal fracture of upper end of unspecified tibia**

  ☑6ᵗʰ **S89.04** Salter-Harris Type IV **physeal fracture of upper end of tibia**

    ☑7ᵗʰ **S89.041** Salter-Harris Type IV **physeal fracture of upper end of right tibia**

    ☑7ᵗʰ **S89.042** Salter-Harris Type IV **physeal fracture of upper end of left tibia**

    ☑7ᵗʰ **S89.049** Salter-Harris Type IV **physeal fracture of upper end of unspecified tibia**

  ☑6ᵗʰ **S89.09** Other physeal **fracture of upper end of tibia**

    ☑7ᵗʰ **S89.091** Other physeal **fracture of upper end of right tibia**

    ☑7ᵗʰ **S89.092** Other physeal **fracture of upper end of left tibia**

    ☑7ᵗʰ **S89.099** Other physeal **fracture of upper end of unspecified tibia**

☑5ᵗʰ **S89.1** Physeal fracture of **lower end of tibia**

  ☑6ᵗʰ **S89.10** Unspecified **physeal fracture of lower end of tibia**

    ☑7ᵗʰ **S89.101** Unspecified **physeal fracture of lower end of right tibia**

    ☑7ᵗʰ **S89.102** Unspecified **physeal fracture of lower end of left tibia**

    ☑7ᵗʰ **S89.109** Unspecified **physeal fracture of lower end of unspecified tibia**

  ☑6ᵗʰ **S89.11** Salter-Harris Type I **physeal fracture of ower end of tibia**

    ☑7ᵗʰ **S89.111** Salter-Harris Type I **physeal fracture of lower end of right tibia**

    ☑7ᵗʰ **S89.112** Salter-Harris Type I **physeal fracture of lower end of left tibia**

    ☑7ᵗʰ **S89.119** Salter-Harris Type I **physeal fracture of lower end of unspecified tibia**

  ☑6ᵗʰ **S89.12** Salter-Harris Type II **physeal fracture of lower end of tibia**

    ☑7ᵗʰ **S89.121** Salter-Harris Type II **physeal fracture of lower end of right tibia**

    ☑7ᵗʰ **S89.122** Salter-Harris Type II **physeal fracture of lower end of left tibia**

    ☑7ᵗʰ **S89.129** Salter-Harris Type II **physeal fracture of lower end of unspecified tibia**

  ☑6ᵗʰ **S89.13** Salter-Harris Type III **physeal fracture of lower end of tibia**

    EXCLUDES 1 *fracture of medial malleolus (adult) (S82.5-)*

    ☑7ᵗʰ **S89.131** Salter-Harris Type III **physeal fracture of lower end of right tibia**

    ☑7ᵗʰ **S89.132** Salter-Harris Type III **physeal fracture of lower end of left tibia**

    ☑7ᵗʰ **S89.139** Salter-Harris Type III **physeal fracture of lower end of unspecified tibia**

  ☑6ᵗʰ **S89.14** Salter-Harris Type IV **physeal fracture of lower end of tibia**

    EXCLUDES 1 *fracture of medial malleolus (adult) (S82.5-)*

    ☑7ᵗʰ **S89.141** Salter-Harris Type IV **physeal fracture of lower end of right tibia**

    ☑7ᵗʰ **S89.142** Salter-Harris Type IV **physeal fracture of lower end of left tibia**

    ☑7ᵗʰ **S89.149** Salter-Harris Type IV **physeal fracture of lower end of unspecified tibia**

  ☑6ᵗʰ **S89.19** Other **physeal fracture of lower end of tibia**

    ☑7ᵗʰ **S89.191** Other **physeal fracture of lower end of right tibia**

    ☑7ᵗʰ **S89.192** Other **physeal fracture of lower end of left tibia**

    ☑7ᵗʰ **S89.199** Other **physeal fracture of lower end of unspecified tibia**

☑5ᵗʰ **S89.2** Physeal fracture of **upper end of fibula**

  ☑6ᵗʰ **S89.20** Unspecified **physeal fracture of upper end of fibula**

    ☑7ᵗʰ **S89.201** Unspecified **physeal fracture of upper end of right fibula**

    ☑7ᵗʰ **S89.202** Unspecified **physeal fracture of upper end of left fibula**

    ☑7ᵗʰ **S89.209** Unspecified **physeal fracture of upper end of unspecified fibula**

  ☑6ᵗʰ **S89.21** Salter-Harris Type I **physeal fracture of upper end of fibula**

    ☑7ᵗʰ **S89.211** Salter-Harris Type I **physeal fracture of upper end of right fibula**

    ☑7ᵗʰ **S89.212** Salter-Harris Type I **physeal fracture of upper end of left fibula**

☑ Additional Character Required   ᵛˣ7ᵗʰ Placeholder Alert   Unspecified Dx   Other Specified Dx   Manifestation   ▶◀ Revised Text   ● New Code   ▲ Revised Code Title

√7ᵗʰ **S89.219** **Salter-Harris Type I physeal fracture of upper end of unspecified fibula**

√6ᵗʰ **S89.22** Salter-Harris Type II physeal fracture of upper end of fibula

√7ᵗʰ **S89.221** **Salter-Harris Type II physeal fracture of upper end of right fibula**

√7ᵗʰ **S89.222** **Salter-Harris Type II physeal fracture of upper end of left fibula**

√7ᵗʰ **S89.229** **Salter-Harris Type II physeal fracture of upper end of unspecified fibula**

√6ᵗʰ **S89.29** Other physeal fracture of upper end of fibula

√7ᵗʰ **S89.291** **Other physeal fracture of upper end of right fibula**

√7ᵗʰ **S89.292** **Other physeal fracture of upper end of left fibula**

√7ᵗʰ **S89.299** **Other physeal fracture of upper end of unspecified fibula**

√5ᵗʰ **S89.3** Physeal fracture of lower end of fibula

√6ᵗʰ **S89.30** Unspecified physeal fracture of lower end of fibula

√7ᵗʰ **S89.301** **Unspecified physeal fracture of lower end of right fibula**

√7ᵗʰ **S89.302** **Unspecified physeal fracture of lower end of left fibula**

√7ᵗʰ **S89.309** **Unspecified physeal fracture of lower end of unspecified fibula**

√6ᵗʰ **S89.31** Salter-Harris Type I physeal fracture of lower end of fibula

√7ᵗʰ **S89.311** **Salter-Harris Type I physeal fracture of lower end of right fibula**

√7ᵗʰ **S89.312** **Salter-Harris Type I physeal fracture of lower end of left fibula**

√7ᵗʰ **S89.319** **Salter-Harris Type I physeal fracture of lower end of unspecified fibula**

√6ᵗʰ **S89.32** Salter-Harris Type II physeal fracture of lower end of fibula

√7ᵗʰ **S89.321** **Salter-Harris Type II physeal fracture of lower end of right fibula**

√7ᵗʰ **S89.322** **Salter-Harris Type II physeal fracture of lower end of left fibula**

√7ᵗʰ **S89.329** **Salter-Harris Type II physeal fracture of lower end of unspecified fibula**

√6ᵗʰ **S89.39** Other physeal fracture of lower end of fibula

√7ᵗʰ **S89.391** **Other physeal fracture of lower end of right fibula**

√7ᵗʰ **S89.392** **Other physeal fracture of lower end of left fibula**

√7ᵗʰ **S89.399** **Other physeal fracture of lower end of unspecified fibula**

√5ᵗʰ **S89.8** Other specified injuries of lower leg

The appropriate 7th character is to be added to each code in subcategory S89.8.
A   initial encounter
D   subsequent encounter
S   sequela

√x7ᵗʰ **S89.80** **Other specified injuries of unspecified lower leg**

√x7ᵗʰ **S89.81** **Other specified injuries of right lower leg**

√x7ᵗʰ **S89.82** **Other specified injuries of left lower leg**

√5ᵗʰ **S89.9** Unspecified injury of lower leg

The appropriate 7th character is to be added to each code in subcategory S89.9.
A   initial encounter
D   subsequent encounter
S   sequela

√x7ᵗʰ **S89.90** **Unspecified injury of unspecified lower leg**

√x7ᵗʰ **S89.91** **Unspecified injury of right lower leg**

√x7ᵗʰ **S89.92** **Unspecified injury of left lower leg**

Injuries to the ankle and foot (S90-S99)

EXCLUDES 2 *burns and corrosions (T20-T32)*
fracture of ankle and malleolus (S82.-)
frostbite (T33-T34)
insect bite or sting, venomous (T63.4)

√4ᵗʰ **S90** **Superficial injury of ankle, foot and toes**

The appropriate 7th character is to be added to each code from category S90.
A   initial encounter
D   subsequent encounter
S   sequela

√5ᵗʰ **S90.0** Contusion of ankle

√x7ᵗʰ **S90.00** **Contusion of unspecified ankle**

√x7ᵗʰ **S90.01** **Contusion of right ankle**

√x7ᵗʰ **S90.02** **Contusion of left ankle**

√5ᵗʰ **S90.1** Contusion of toe without damage to nail

√6ᵗʰ **S90.11** Contusion of great toe without damage to nail

√7ᵗʰ **S90.111** **Contusion of right great toe without damage to nail**

√7ᵗʰ **S90.112** **Contusion of left great toe without damage to nail**

√7ᵗʰ **S90.119** **Contusion of unspecified great toe without damage to nail**

√6ᵗʰ **S90.12** Contusion of lesser toe without damage to nail

√7ᵗʰ **S90.121** **Contusion of right lesser toe(s) without damage to nail**

√7ᵗʰ **S90.122** **Contusion of left lesser toe(s) without damage to nail**

√7ᵗʰ **S90.129** **Contusion of unspecified lesser toe(s) without damage to nail**
Contusion of toe NOS

√5ᵗʰ **S90.2** Contusion of toe with damage to nail

√6ᵗʰ **S90.21** Contusion of great toe with damage to nail

√7ᵗʰ **S90.211** **Contusion of right great toe with damage to nail**

√7ᵗʰ **S90.212** **Contusion of left great toe with damage to nail**

√7ᵗʰ **S90.219** **Contusion of unspecified great toe with damage to nail**

√6ᵗʰ **S90.22** Contusion of lesser toe with damage to nail

√7ᵗʰ **S90.221** **Contusion of right lesser toe(s) with damage to nail**

√7ᵗʰ **S90.222** **Contusion of left lesser toe(s) with damage to nail**

√7ᵗʰ **S90.229** **Contusion of unspecified lesser toe(s) with damage to nail**

√5ᵗʰ **S90.3** Contusion of foot
EXCLUDES 2 *contusion of toes (S90.1-, S90.2-)*

√x7ᵗʰ **S90.30** **Contusion of unspecified foot**
Contusion of foot NOS

√x7ᵗʰ **S90.31** **Contusion of right foot**

√x7ᵗʰ **S90.32** **Contusion of left foot**

√5ᵗʰ **S90.4** Other superficial injuries of toe

√6ᵗʰ **S90.41** Abrasion of toe

√7ᵗʰ **S90.411** **Abrasion, right great toe**

√7ᵗʰ **S90.412** **Abrasion, left great toe**

√7ᵗʰ **S90.413** **Abrasion, unspecified great toe**

√7ᵗʰ **S90.414** **Abrasion, right lesser toe(s)**

√7ᵗʰ **S90.415** **Abrasion, left lesser toe(s)**

√7ᵗʰ **S90.416** **Abrasion, unspecified lesser toe(s)**

√6ᵗʰ **S90.42** Blister (nonthermal) of toe

√7ᵗʰ **S90.421** **Blister (nonthermal), right great toe**

√7ᵗʰ **S90.422** **Blister (nonthermal), left great toe**

√7ᵗʰ **S90.423** **Blister (nonthermal), unspecified great toe**

√7ᵗʰ **S90.424** **Blister (nonthermal), right lesser toe(s)**

√7ᵗʰ **S90.425** **Blister (nonthermal), left lesser toe(s)**

√7ᵗʰ **S90.426** **Blister (nonthermal), unspecified lesser toe(s)**

EXCLUDES 1 Not coded here   EXCLUDES 2 Not included here   N Newborn Age: 0   P Pediatric Age: 0-17   M Maternity Age: 12-55   A Adult Age: 15-124

952

ICD-10-CM 2016

✓6ᵗʰ **S90.44 External constriction of toe**
    Hair tourniquet syndrome of toe
- ✓7ᵗʰ **S90.441 External constriction, right great toe**
- ✓7ᵗʰ **S90.442 External constriction, left great toe**
- ✓7ᵗʰ **S90.443 External constriction, unspecified great toe**
- ✓7ᵗʰ **S90.444 External constriction, right lesser toe(s)**
- ✓7ᵗʰ **S90.445 External constriction, left lesser toe(s)**
- ✓7ᵗʰ **S90.446 External constriction, unspecified lesser toe(s)**

✓6ᵗʰ **S90.45 Superficial foreign body of toe**
    Splinter in the toe
- ✓7ᵗʰ **S90.451 Superficial foreign body, right great toe**
- ✓7ᵗʰ **S90.452 Superficial foreign body, left great toe**
- ✓7ᵗʰ **S90.453 Superficial foreign body, unspecified great toe**
- ✓7ᵗʰ **S90.454 Superficial foreign body, right lesser toe(s)**
- ✓7ᵗʰ **S90.455 Superficial foreign body, left lesser toe(s)**
- ✓7ᵗʰ **S90.456 Superficial foreign body, unspecified lesser toe(s)**

✓6ᵗʰ **S90.46 Insect bite (nonvenomous) of toe**
- ✓7ᵗʰ **S90.461 Insect bite (nonvenomous), right great toe**
- ✓7ᵗʰ **S90.462 Insect bite (nonvenomous), left great toe**
- ✓7ᵗʰ **S90.463 Insect bite (nonvenomous), unspecified great toe**
- ✓7ᵗʰ **S90.464 Insect bite (nonvenomous), right lesser toe(s)**
- ✓7ᵗʰ **S90.465 Insect bite (nonvenomous), left lesser toe(s)**
- ✓7ᵗʰ **S90.466 Insect bite (nonvenomous), unspecified lesser toe(s)**

✓6ᵗʰ **S90.47 Other superficial bite of toe**
    EXCLUDES 1 *open bite of toe (S91.15-, S91.25-)*
- ✓7ᵗʰ **S90.471 Other superficial bite of right great toe**
- ✓7ᵗʰ **S90.472 Other superficial bite of left great toe**
- ✓7ᵗʰ **S90.473 Other superficial bite of unspecified great toe**
- ✓7ᵗʰ **S90.474 Other superficial bite of right lesser toe(s)**
- ✓7ᵗʰ **S90.475 Other superficial bite of left lesser toe(s)**
- ✓7ᵗʰ **S90.476 Other superficial bite of unspecified lesser toe(s)**

✓5ᵗʰ **S90.5 Other superficial injuries of ankle**

✓6ᵗʰ **S90.51 Abrasion of ankle**
- ✓7ᵗʰ **S90.511 Abrasion, right ankle**
- ✓7ᵗʰ **S90.512 Abrasion, left ankle**
- ✓7ᵗʰ **S90.519 Abrasion, unspecified ankle**

✓6ᵗʰ **S90.52 Blister (nonthermal) of ankle**
- ✓7ᵗʰ **S90.521 Blister (nonthermal), right ankle**
- ✓7ᵗʰ **S90.522 Blister (nonthermal), left ankle**
- ✓7ᵗʰ **S90.529 Blister (nonthermal), unspecified ankle**

✓6ᵗʰ **S90.54 External constriction of ankle**
- ✓7ᵗʰ **S90.541 External constriction, right ankle**
- ✓7ᵗʰ **S90.542 External constriction, left ankle**
- ✓7ᵗʰ **S90.549 External constriction, unspecified ankle**

✓6ᵗʰ **S90.55 Superficial foreign body of ankle**
    Splinter in the ankle
- ✓7ᵗʰ **S90.551 Superficial foreign body, right ankle**
- ✓7ᵗʰ **S90.552 Superficial foreign body, left ankle**
- ✓7ᵗʰ **S90.559 Superficial foreign body, unspecified ankle**

✓6ᵗʰ **S90.56 Insect bite (nonvenomous) of ankle**
- ✓7ᵗʰ **S90.561 Insect bite (nonvenomous), right ankle**
- ✓7ᵗʰ **S90.562 Insect bite (nonvenomous), left ankle**
- ✓7ᵗʰ **S90.569 Insect bite (nonvenomous), unspecified ankle**

✓6ᵗʰ **S90.57 Other superficial bite of ankle**
    EXCLUDES 1 *open bite of ankle (S91.05-)*
- ✓7ᵗʰ **S90.571 Other superficial bite of ankle, right ankle**
- ✓7ᵗʰ **S90.572 Other superficial bite of ankle, left ankle**
- ✓7ᵗʰ **S90.579 Other superficial bite of ankle, unspecified ankle**

✓5ᵗʰ **S90.8 Other superficial injuries of foot**

✓6ᵗʰ **S90.81 Abrasion of foot**
- ✓7ᵗʰ **S90.811 Abrasion, right foot**
- ✓7ᵗʰ **S90.812 Abrasion, left foot**
- ✓7ᵗʰ **S90.819 Abrasion, unspecified foot**

✓6ᵗʰ **S90.82 Blister (nonthermal) of foot**
- ✓7ᵗʰ **S90.821 Blister (nonthermal), right foot**
- ✓7ᵗʰ **S90.822 Blister (nonthermal), left foot**
- ✓7ᵗʰ **S90.829 Blister (nonthermal), unspecified foot**

✓6ᵗʰ **S90.84 External constriction of foot**
- ✓7ᵗʰ **S90.841 External constriction, right foot**
- ✓7ᵗʰ **S90.842 External constriction, left foot**
- ✓7ᵗʰ **S90.849 External constriction, unspecified foot**

✓6ᵗʰ **S90.85 Superficial foreign body of foot**
    Splinter in the foot
- ✓7ᵗʰ **S90.851 Superficial foreign body, right foot**
- ✓7ᵗʰ **S90.852 Superficial foreign body, left foot**
- ✓7ᵗʰ **S90.859 Superficial foreign body, unspecified foot**

✓6ᵗʰ **S90.86 Insect bite (nonvenomous) of foot**
- ✓7ᵗʰ **S90.861 Insect bite (nonvenomous), right foot**
- ✓7ᵗʰ **S90.862 Insect bite (nonvenomous), left foot**
- ✓7ᵗʰ **S90.869 Insect bite (nonvenomous), unspecified foot**

✓6ᵗʰ **S90.87 Other superficial bite of foot**
    EXCLUDES 1 *open bite of foot (S91.35-)*
- ✓7ᵗʰ **S90.871 Other superficial bite of right foot**
- ✓7ᵗʰ **S90.872 Other superficial bite of left foot**
- ✓7ᵗʰ **S90.879 Other superficial bite of unspecified foot**

✓5ᵗʰ **S90.9 Unspecified superficial injury of ankle, foot and toe**

✓6ᵗʰ **S90.91 Unspecified superficial injury of ankle**
- ✓7ᵗʰ **S90.911 Unspecified superficial injury of right ankle**
- ✓7ᵗʰ **S90.912 Unspecified superficial injury of left ankle**
- ✓7ᵗʰ **S90.919 Unspecified superficial injury of unspecified ankle**

✓6ᵗʰ **S90.92 Unspecified superficial injury of foot**
- ✓7ᵗʰ **S90.921 Unspecified superficial injury of right foot**
- ✓7ᵗʰ **S90.922 Unspecified superficial injury of left foot**
- ✓7ᵗʰ **S90.929 Unspecified superficial injury of unspecified foot**

✓6ᵗʰ **S90.93 Unspecified superficial injury of toes**
- ✓7ᵗʰ **S90.931 Unspecified superficial injury of right great toe**
- ✓7ᵗʰ **S90.932 Unspecified superficial injury of left great toe**
- ✓7ᵗʰ **S90.933 Unspecified superficial injury of unspecified great toe**
- ✓7ᵗʰ **S90.934 Unspecified superficial injury of right lesser toe(s)**
- ✓7ᵗʰ **S90.935 Unspecified superficial injury of left lesser toe(s)**
- ✓7ᵗʰ **S90.936 Unspecified superficial injury of unspecified lesser toe(s)**

☑ Additional Character Required   ✓ₓ7ᵗʰ Placeholder Alert   Unspecified Dx   Other Specified Dx   Manifestation   ►◄ Revised Text   ● New Code   ▲ Revised Code Title

✓4ᵗʰ S91　Open wound of ankle, foot and toes
Code also any associated wound infection
EXCLUDES 1　open fracture of ankle, foot and toes (S92-with 7th character B)
traumatic amputation of ankle and foot (S98.-)

The appropriate 7th character is to be added to each code from category S91.
A　　initial encounter
D　　subsequent encounter
S　　sequela

✓5ᵗʰ S91.0　Open wound of ankle
✓6ᵗʰ S91.00　Unspecified open wound of ankle
　✓7ᵗʰ S91.001　Unspecified open wound, right ankle
　✓7ᵗʰ S91.002　Unspecified open wound, left ankle
　✓7ᵗʰ S91.009　Unspecified open wound, unspecified ankle

✓6ᵗʰ S91.01　Laceration without foreign body of ankle
　✓7ᵗʰ S91.011　Laceration without foreign body, right ankle
　✓7ᵗʰ S91.012　Laceration without foreign body, left ankle
　✓7ᵗʰ S91.019　Laceration without foreign body, unspecified ankle

✓6ᵗʰ S91.02　Laceration with foreign body of ankle
　✓7ᵗʰ S91.021　Laceration with foreign body, right ankle
　✓7ᵗʰ S91.022　Laceration with foreign body, left ankle
　✓7ᵗʰ S91.029　Laceration with foreign body, unspecified ankle

✓6ᵗʰ S91.03　Puncture wound without foreign body of ankle
　✓7ᵗʰ S91.031　Puncture wound without foreign body, right ankle
　✓7ᵗʰ S91.032　Puncture wound without foreign body, left ankle
　✓7ᵗʰ S91.039　Puncture wound without foreign body, unspecified ankle

✓6ᵗʰ S91.04　Puncture wound with foreign body of ankle
　✓7ᵗʰ S91.041　Puncture wound with foreign body, right ankle
　✓7ᵗʰ S91.042　Puncture wound with foreign body, left ankle
　✓7ᵗʰ S91.049　Puncture wound with foreign body, unspecified ankle

✓6ᵗʰ S91.05　Open bite of ankle
EXCLUDES 1　superficial bite of ankle (S90.56-, S90.57-)
　✓7ᵗʰ S91.051　Open bite, right ankle
　✓7ᵗʰ S91.052　Open bite, left ankle
　✓7ᵗʰ S91.059　Open bite, unspecified ankle

✓5ᵗʰ S91.1　Open wound of toe without damage to nail
✓6ᵗʰ S91.10　Unspecified open wound of toe without damage to nail
　✓7ᵗʰ S91.101　Unspecified open wound of right great toe without damage to nail
　✓7ᵗʰ S91.102　Unspecified open wound of left great toe without damage to nail
　✓7ᵗʰ S91.103　Unspecified open wound of unspecified great toe without damage to nail
　✓7ᵗʰ S91.104　Unspecified open wound of right lesser toe(s) without damage to nail
　✓7ᵗʰ S91.105　Unspecified open wound of left lesser toe(s) without damage to nail
　✓7ᵗʰ S91.106　Unspecified open wound of unspecified lesser toe(s) without damage to nail
　✓7ᵗʰ S91.109　Unspecified open wound of unspecified toe(s) without damage to nail

✓6ᵗʰ S91.11　Laceration without foreign body of toe without damage to nail
　✓7ᵗʰ S91.111　Laceration without foreign body of right great toe without damage to nail
　✓7ᵗʰ S91.112　Laceration without foreign body of left great toe without damage to nail
　✓7ᵗʰ S91.113　Laceration without foreign body of unspecified great toe without damage to nail
　✓7ᵗʰ S91.114　Laceration without foreign body of right lesser toe(s) without damage to nail
　✓7ᵗʰ S91.115　Laceration without foreign body of left lesser toe(s) without damage to nail
　✓7ᵗʰ S91.116　Laceration without foreign body of unspecified lesser toe(s) without damage to nail
　✓7ᵗʰ S91.119　Laceration without foreign body of unspecified toe without damage to nail

✓6ᵗʰ S91.12　Laceration with foreign body of toe without damage to nail
　✓7ᵗʰ S91.121　Laceration with foreign body of right great toe without damage to nail
　✓7ᵗʰ S91.122　Laceration with foreign body of left great toe without damage to nail
　✓7ᵗʰ S91.123　Laceration with foreign body of unspecified great toe without damage to nail
　✓7ᵗʰ S91.124　Laceration with foreign body of right lesser toe(s) without damage to nail
　✓7ᵗʰ S91.125　Laceration with foreign body of left lesser toe(s) without damage to nail
　✓7ᵗʰ S91.126　Laceration with foreign body of unspecified lesser toe(s) without damage to nail
　✓7ᵗʰ S91.129　Laceration with foreign body of unspecified toe(s) without damage to nail

✓6ᵗʰ S91.13　Puncture wound without foreign body of toe without damage to nail
　✓7ᵗʰ S91.131　Puncture wound without foreign body of right great toe without damage to nail
　✓7ᵗʰ S91.132　Puncture wound without foreign body of left great toe without damage to nail
　✓7ᵗʰ S91.133　Puncture wound without foreign body of unspecified great toe without damage to nail
　✓7ᵗʰ S91.134　Puncture wound without foreign body of right lesser toe(s) without damage to nail
　✓7ᵗʰ S91.135　Puncture wound without foreign body of left lesser toe(s) without damage to nail
　✓7ᵗʰ S91.136　Puncture wound without foreign body of unspecified lesser toe(s) without damage to nail
　✓7ᵗʰ S91.139　Puncture wound without foreign body of unspecified toe(s) without damage to nail

✓6ᵗʰ S91.14　Puncture wound with foreign body of toe without damage to nail
　✓7ᵗʰ S91.141　Puncture wound with foreign body of right great toe without damage to nail
　✓7ᵗʰ S91.142　Puncture wound with foreign body of left great toe without damage to nail
　✓7ᵗʰ S91.143　Puncture wound with foreign body of unspecified great toe without damage to nail
　✓7ᵗʰ S91.144　Puncture wound with foreign body of right lesser toe(s) without damage to nail
　✓7ᵗʰ S91.145　Puncture wound with foreign body of left lesser toe(s) without damage to nail
　✓7ᵗʰ S91.146　Puncture wound with foreign body of unspecified lesser toe(s) without damage to nail
　✓7ᵗʰ S91.149　Puncture wound with foreign body of unspecified toe(s) without damage to nail

✓6ᵗʰ S91.15　Open bite of toe without damage to nail
Bite of toe NOS
EXCLUDES 1　superficial bite of toe (S90.46-, S90.47-)
　✓7ᵗʰ S91.151　Open bite of right great toe without damage to nail
　✓7ᵗʰ S91.152　Open bite of left great toe without damage to nail
　✓7ᵗʰ S91.153　Open bite of unspecified great toe without damage to nail
　✓7ᵗʰ S91.154　Open bite of right lesser toe(s) without damage to nail
　✓7ᵗʰ S91.155　Open bite of left lesser toe(s) without damage to nail

✓7ᵗʰ **S91.156** **Open bite of unspecified lesser toe(s) without damage to nail**

✓7ᵗʰ **S91.159** **Open bite of unspecified toe(s) without damage to nail**

✓5ᵗʰ **S91.2** Open wound of toe with damage to nail

✓6ᵗʰ **S91.20** Unspecified open wound of toe with damage to nail

✓7ᵗʰ **S91.201** **Unspecified open wound of right great toe with damage to nail**

✓7ᵗʰ **S91.202** **Unspecified open wound of left great toe with damage to nail**

✓7ᵗʰ **S91.203** **Unspecified open wound of unspecified great toe with damage to nail**

✓7ᵗʰ **S91.204** **Unspecified open wound of right lesser toe(s) with damage to nail**

✓7ᵗʰ **S91.205** **Unspecified open wound of left lesser toe(s) with damage to nail**

✓7ᵗʰ **S91.206** **Unspecified open wound of unspecified lesser toe(s) with damage to nail**

✓7ᵗʰ **S91.209** **Unspecified open wound of unspecified toe(s) with damage to nail**

✓6ᵗʰ **S91.21** Laceration without foreign body of toe with damage to nail

✓7ᵗʰ **S91.211** **Laceration without foreign body of right great toe with damage to nail**

✓7ᵗʰ **S91.212** **Laceration without foreign body of left great toe with damage to nail**

✓7ᵗʰ **S91.213** **Laceration without foreign body of unspecified great toe with damage to nail**

✓7ᵗʰ **S91.214** **Laceration without foreign body of right lesser toe(s) with damage to nail**

✓7ᵗʰ **S91.215** **Laceration without foreign body of left lesser toe(s) with damage to nail**

✓7ᵗʰ **S91.216** **Laceration without foreign body of unspecified lesser toe(s) with damage to nail**

✓7ᵗʰ **S91.219** **Laceration without foreign body of unspecified toe(s) with damage to nail**

✓6ᵗʰ **S91.22** Laceration with foreign body of toe with damage to nail

✓7ᵗʰ **S91.221** **Laceration with foreign body of right great toe with damage to nail**

✓7ᵗʰ **S91.222** **Laceration with foreign body of left great toe with damage to nail**

✓7ᵗʰ **S91.223** **Laceration with foreign body of unspecified great toe with damage to nail**

✓7ᵗʰ **S91.224** **Laceration with foreign body of right lesser toe(s) with damage to nail**

✓7ᵗʰ **S91.225** **Laceration with foreign body of left lesser toe(s) with damage to nail**

✓7ᵗʰ **S91.226** **Laceration with foreign body of unspecified lesser toe(s) with damage to nail**

✓7ᵗʰ **S91.229** **Laceration with foreign body of unspecified toe(s) with damage to nail**

✓6ᵗʰ **S91.23** Puncture wound without foreign body of toe with damage to nail

✓7ᵗʰ **S91.231** **Puncture wound without foreign body of right great toe with damage to nail**

✓7ᵗʰ **S91.232** **Puncture wound without foreign body of left great toe with damage to nail**

✓7ᵗʰ **S91.233** **Puncture wound without foreign body of unspecified great toe with damage to nail**

✓7ᵗʰ **S91.234** **Puncture wound without foreign body of right lesser toe(s) with damage to nail**

✓7ᵗʰ **S91.235** **Puncture wound without foreign body of left lesser toe(s) with damage to nail**

✓7ᵗʰ **S91.236** **Puncture wound without foreign body of unspecified lesser toe(s) with damage to nail**

✓7ᵗʰ **S91.239** **Puncture wound without foreign body of unspecified toe(s) with damage to nail**

✓6ᵗʰ **S91.24** Puncture wound with foreign body of toe with damage to nail

✓7ᵗʰ **S91.241** **Puncture wound with foreign body of right great toe with damage to nail**

✓7ᵗʰ **S91.242** **Puncture wound with foreign body of left great toe with damage to nail**

✓7ᵗʰ **S91.243** **Puncture wound with foreign body of unspecified great toe with damage to nail**

✓7ᵗʰ **S91.244** **Puncture wound with foreign body of right lesser toe(s) with damage to nail**

✓7ᵗʰ **S91.245** **Puncture wound with foreign body of left lesser toe(s) with damage to nail**

✓7ᵗʰ **S91.246** **Puncture wound with foreign body of unspecified lesser toe(s) with damage to nail**

✓7ᵗʰ **S91.249** **Puncture wound with foreign body of unspecified toe(s) with damage to nail**

✓6ᵗʰ **S91.25** Open bite of toe with damage to nail
Bite of toe with damage to nail NOS
EXCLUDES 1 *superficial bite of toe (S90.46-, S90.47-)*

✓7ᵗʰ **S91.251** **Open bite of right great toe with damage to nail**

✓7ᵗʰ **S91.252** **Open bite of left great toe with damage to nail**

✓7ᵗʰ **S91.253** **Open bite of unspecified great toe with damage to nail**

✓7ᵗʰ **S91.254** **Open bite of right lesser toe(s) with damage to nail**

✓7ᵗʰ **S91.255** **Open bite of left lesser toe(s) with damage to nail**

✓7ᵗʰ **S91.256** **Open bite of unspecified lesser toe(s) with damage to nail**

✓7ᵗʰ **S91.259** **Open bite of unspecified toe(s) with damage to nail**

✓5ᵗʰ **S91.3** Open wound of foot

✓6ᵗʰ **S91.30** Unspecified open wound of foot

✓7ᵗʰ **S91.301** **Unspecified open wound, right foot**

✓7ᵗʰ **S91.302** **Unspecified open wound, left foot**

✓7ᵗʰ **S91.309** **Unspecified open wound, unspecified foot**

✓6ᵗʰ **S91.31** Laceration without foreign body of foot

✓7ᵗʰ **S91.311** **Laceration without foreign body, right foot**

✓7ᵗʰ **S91.312** **Laceration without foreign body, left foot**

✓7ᵗʰ **S91.319** **Laceration without foreign body, unspecified foot**

✓6ᵗʰ **S91.32** Laceration with foreign body of foot

✓7ᵗʰ **S91.321** **Laceration with foreign body, right foot**

✓7ᵗʰ **S91.322** **Laceration with foreign body, left foot**

✓7ᵗʰ **S91.329** **Laceration with foreign body, unspecified foot**

✓6ᵗʰ **S91.33** Puncture wound without foreign body of foot

✓7ᵗʰ **S91.331** **Puncture wound without foreign body, right foot**

✓7ᵗʰ **S91.332** **Puncture wound without foreign body, left foot**

✓7ᵗʰ **S91.339** **Puncture wound without foreign body, unspecified foot**

✓6ᵗʰ **S91.34** Puncture wound with foreign body of foot

✓7ᵗʰ **S91.341** **Puncture wound with foreign body, right foot**

✓7ᵗʰ **S91.342** **Puncture wound with foreign body, left foot**

✓7ᵗʰ **S91.349** **Puncture wound with foreign body, unspecified foot**

✓6ᵗʰ **S91.35** Open bite of foot
EXCLUDES 1 *superficial bite of foot (S90.86-, S90.87-)*

✓7ᵗʰ **S91.351** **Open bite, right foot**

✓7ᵗʰ **S91.352** **Open bite, left foot**

✓7ᵗʰ **S91.359** **Open bite, unspecified foot**

✓ Additional Character Required   ✓x7ᵗʰ Placeholder Alert   Unspecified Dx   Other Specified Dx   Manifestation   ▶◀ Revised Text   ● New Code   ▲ Revised Code Title

✓4ᵗʰ **S92   Fracture of foot and toe, except ankle**

> **NOTE**   A fracture not indicated as displaced or nondisplaced should be coded to displaced.
> A fracture not indicated as open or closed should be coded to closed.
>
> *EXCLUDES 1*   traumatic amputation of ankle and foot (S98.-)
> *EXCLUDES 2*   fracture of ankle (S82.-)
>   fracture of malleolus (S82.-)

> The appropriate 7th character is to be added to each code from category S92.
> A   initial encounter for closed fracture
> B   initial encounter for open fracture
> D   subsequent encounter for fracture with routine healing
> G   subsequent encounter for fracture with delayed healing
> K   subsequent encounter for fracture with nonunion
> P   subsequent encounter for fracture with malunion
> S   sequela

✓5ᵗʰ **S92.0   Fracture of calcaneus**
     Heel bone
     Os calcis

   ✓6ᵗʰ **S92.00   Unspecified fracture of calcaneus**
     ✓7ᵗʰ **S92.001   Unspecified fracture of right calcaneus**
     ✓7ᵗʰ **S92.002   Unspecified fracture of left calcaneus**
     ✓7ᵗʰ **S92.009   Unspecified fracture of unspecified calcaneus**

   ✓6ᵗʰ **S92.01   Fracture of body of calcaneus**
     ✓7ᵗʰ **S92.011   Displaced fracture of body of right calcaneus**
     ✓7ᵗʰ **S92.012   Displaced fracture of body of left calcaneus**
     ✓7ᵗʰ **S92.013   Displaced fracture of body of unspecified calcaneus**
     ✓7ᵗʰ **S92.014   Nondisplaced fracture of body of right calcaneus**
     ✓7ᵗʰ **S92.015   Nondisplaced fracture of body of left calcaneus**
     ✓7ᵗʰ **S92.016   Nondisplaced fracture of body of unspecified calcaneus**

   ✓6ᵗʰ **S92.02   Fracture of anterior process of calcaneus**
     ✓7ᵗʰ **S92.021   Displaced fracture of anterior process of right calcaneus**
     ✓7ᵗʰ **S92.022   Displaced fracture of anterior process of left calcaneus**
     ✓7ᵗʰ **S92.023   Displaced fracture of anterior process of unspecified calcaneus**
     ✓7ᵗʰ **S92.024   Nondisplaced fracture of anterior process of right calcaneus**
     ✓7ᵗʰ **S92.025   Nondisplaced fracture of anterior process of left calcaneus**
     ✓7ᵗʰ **S92.026   Nondisplaced fracture of anterior process of unspecified calcaneus**

   ✓6ᵗʰ **S92.03   Avulsion fracture of tuberosity of calcaneus**
     ✓7ᵗʰ **S92.031   Displaced avulsion fracture of tuberosity of right calcaneus**
     ✓7ᵗʰ **S92.032   Displaced avulsion fracture of tuberosity of left calcaneus**
     ✓7ᵗʰ **S92.033   Displaced avulsion fracture of tuberosity of unspecified calcaneus**
     ✓7ᵗʰ **S92.034   Nondisplaced avulsion fracture of tuberosity of right calcaneus**
     ✓7ᵗʰ **S92.035   Nondisplaced avulsion fracture of tuberosity of left calcaneus**
     ✓7ᵗʰ **S92.036   Nondisplaced avulsion fracture of tuberosity of unspecified calcaneus**

   ✓6ᵗʰ **S92.04   Other fracture of tuberosity of calcaneus**
     ✓7ᵗʰ **S92.041   Displaced other fracture of tuberosity of right calcaneus**
     ✓7ᵗʰ **S92.042   Displaced other fracture of tuberosity of left calcaneus**
     ✓7ᵗʰ **S92.043   Displaced other fracture of tuberosity of unspecified calcaneus**
     ✓7ᵗʰ **S92.044   Nondisplaced other fracture of tuberosity of right calcaneus**
     ✓7ᵗʰ **S92.045   Nondisplaced other fracture of tuberosity of left calcaneus**
     ✓7ᵗʰ **S92.046   Nondisplaced other fracture of tuberosity of unspecified calcaneus**

   ✓6ᵗʰ **S92.05   Other extraarticular fracture of calcaneus**
     ✓7ᵗʰ **S92.051   Displaced other extraarticular fracture of right calcaneus**
     ✓7ᵗʰ **S92.052   Displaced other extraarticular fracture of left calcaneus**
     ✓7ᵗʰ **S92.053   Displaced other extraarticular fracture of unspecified calcaneus**
     ✓7ᵗʰ **S92.054   Nondisplaced other extraarticular fracture of right calcaneus**
     ✓7ᵗʰ **S92.055   Nondisplaced other extraarticular fracture of left calcaneus**
     ✓7ᵗʰ **S92.056   Nondisplaced other extraarticular fracture of unspecified calcaneus**

   ✓6ᵗʰ **S92.06   Intraarticular fracture of calcaneus**
     ✓7ᵗʰ **S92.061   Displaced intraarticular fracture of right calcaneus**
     ✓7ᵗʰ **S92.062   Displaced intraarticular fracture of left calcaneus**
     ✓7ᵗʰ **S92.063   Displaced intraarticular fracture of unspecified calcaneus**
     ✓7ᵗʰ **S92.064   Nondisplaced intraarticular fracture of right calcaneus**
     ✓7ᵗʰ **S92.065   Nondisplaced intraarticular fracture of left calcaneus**
     ✓7ᵗʰ **S92.066   Nondisplaced intraarticular fracture of unspecified calcaneus**

✓5ᵗʰ **S92.1   Fracture of talus**
     Astragalus

   ✓6ᵗʰ **S92.10   Unspecified fracture of talus**
     ✓7ᵗʰ **S92.101   Unspecified fracture of right talus**
     ✓7ᵗʰ **S92.102   Unspecified fracture of left talus**
     ✓7ᵗʰ **S92.109   Unspecified fracture of unspecified talus**

   ✓6ᵗʰ **S92.11   Fracture of neck of talus**
     ✓7ᵗʰ **S92.111   Displaced fracture of neck of right talus**
     ✓7ᵗʰ **S92.112   Displaced fracture of neck of left talus**
     ✓7ᵗʰ **S92.113   Displaced fracture of neck of unspecified talus**
     ✓7ᵗʰ **S92.114   Nondisplaced fracture of neck of right talus**
     ✓7ᵗʰ **S92.115   Nondisplaced fracture of neck of left talus**
     ✓7ᵗʰ **S92.116   Nondisplaced fracture of neck of unspecified talus**

   ✓6ᵗʰ **S92.12   Fracture of body of talus**
     ✓7ᵗʰ **S92.121   Displaced fracture of body of right talus**
     ✓7ᵗʰ **S92.122   Displaced fracture of body of left talus**
     ✓7ᵗʰ **S92.123   Displaced fracture of body of unspecified talus**
     ✓7ᵗʰ **S92.124   Nondisplaced fracture of body of right talus**
     ✓7ᵗʰ **S92.125   Nondisplaced fracture of body of left talus**
     ✓7ᵗʰ **S92.126   Nondisplaced fracture of body of unspecified talus**

   ✓6ᵗʰ **S92.13   Fracture of posterior process of talus**
     ✓7ᵗʰ **S92.131   Displaced fracture of posterior process of right talus**
     ✓7ᵗʰ **S92.132   Displaced fracture of posterior process of left talus**
     ✓7ᵗʰ **S92.133   Displaced fracture of posterior process of unspecified talus**
     ✓7ᵗʰ **S92.134   Nondisplaced fracture of posterior process of right talus**
     ✓7ᵗʰ **S92.135   Nondisplaced fracture of posterior process of left talus**
     ✓7ᵗʰ **S92.136   Nondisplaced fracture of posterior process of unspecified talus**

   ✓6ᵗʰ **S92.14   Dome fracture of talus**
     EXCLUDES 1   osteochondritis dissecans (M93.2)
     ✓7ᵗʰ **S92.141   Displaced dome fracture of right talus**
     ✓7ᵗʰ **S92.142   Displaced dome fracture of left talus**
     ✓7ᵗʰ **S92.143   Displaced dome fracture of unspecified talus**

EXCLUDES 1 Not coded here   *EXCLUDES 2* Not included here   N Newborn Age: 0   P Pediatric Age: 0-17   M Maternity Age: 12-55   A Adult Age: 15-124

956   ICD-10-CM 2016

√7th **S92.144** Nondisplaced **dome fracture of** right **talus**

√7th **S92.145** Nondisplaced **dome fracture of** left **talus**

√7th **S92.146** Nondisplaced **dome fracture of unspecified talus**

√6th **S92.15** Avulsion **fracture (chip fracture) of talus**

√7th **S92.151** Displaced **avulsion fracture (chip fracture) of** right **talus**

√7th **S92.152** Displaced **avulsion fracture (chip fracture) of** left **talus**

√7th **S92.153** Displaced **avulsion fracture (chip fracture) of unspecified talus**

√7th **S92.154** Nondisplaced **avulsion fracture (chip fracture) of** right **talus**

√7th **S92.155** Nondisplaced **avulsion fracture (chip fracture) of** left **talus**

√7th **S92.156** Nondisplaced **avulsion fracture (chip fracture) of unspecified talus**

√6th **S92.19** Other **fracture of talus**

√7th **S92.191** Other **fracture of** right **talus**

√7th **S92.192** Other **fracture of** left **talus**

√7th **S92.199** Other **fracture of unspecified talus**

√5th **S92.2** Fracture of other and unspecified tarsal bone(s)

√6th **S92.20** Fracture of **unspecified tarsal bone(s)**

√7th **S92.201** Fracture of unspecified tarsal bone(s) of **right foot**

√7th **S92.202** Fracture of unspecified tarsal bone(s) of **left foot**

√7th **S92.209** Fracture of unspecified tarsal bone(s) of **unspecified foot**

√6th **S92.21** Fracture of **cuboid bone**

√7th **S92.211** Displaced **fracture of cuboid bone of** right **foot**

√7th **S92.212** Displaced **fracture of cuboid bone of** left **foot**

√7th **S92.213** Displaced **fracture of cuboid bone of unspecified foot**

√7th **S92.214** Nondisplaced **fracture of cuboid bone of** right **foot**

√7th **S92.215** Nondisplaced **fracture of cuboid bone of** left **foot**

√7th **S92.216** Nondisplaced **fracture of cuboid bone of unspecified foot**

√6th **S92.22** Fracture of **lateral cuneiform**

√7th **S92.221** Displaced **fracture of lateral cuneiform of** right **foot**

√7th **S92.222** Displaced **fracture of lateral cuneiform of** left **foot**

√7th **S92.223** Displaced **fracture of lateral cuneiform of unspecified foot**

√7th **S92.224** Nondisplaced **fracture of lateral cuneiform of** right **foot**

√7th **S92.225** Nondisplaced **fracture of lateral cuneiform of** left **foot**

√7th **S92.226** Nondisplaced **fracture of lateral cuneiform of unspecified foot**

√6th **S92.23** Fracture of **intermediate cuneiform**

√7th **S92.231** Displaced **fracture of intermediate cuneiform of** right **foot**

√7th **S92.232** Displaced **fracture of intermediate cuneiform of** left **foot**

√7th **S92.233** Displaced **fracture of intermediate cuneiform of unspecified foot**

√7th **S92.234** Nondisplaced **fracture of intermediate cuneiform of** right **foot**

√7th **S92.235** Nondisplaced **fracture of intermediate cuneiform of** left **foot**

√7th **S92.236** Nondisplaced **fracture of intermediate cuneiform of unspecified foot**

√6th **S92.24** Fracture of **medial cuneiform**

√7th **S92.241** Displaced **fracture of medial cuneiform of** right **foot**

√7th **S92.242** Displaced **fracture of medial cuneiform of** left **foot**

√7th **S92.243** Displaced **fracture of medial cuneiform of unspecified foot**

√7th **S92.244** Nondisplaced **fracture of medial cuneiform of** right **foot**

√7th **S92.245** Nondisplaced **fracture of medial cuneiform of** left **foot**

√7th **S92.246** Nondisplaced **fracture of medial cuneiform of unspecified foot**

√6th **S92.25** Fracture of **navicular [scaphoid] of foot**

√7th **S92.251** Displaced **fracture of navicular [scaphoid] of** right **foot**

√7th **S92.252** Displaced **fracture of navicular [scaphoid] of** left **foot**

√7th **S92.253** Displaced **fracture of navicular [scaphoid] of unspecified foot**

√7th **S92.254** Nondisplaced **fracture of navicular [scaphoid] of** right **foot**

√7th **S92.255** Nondisplaced **fracture of navicular [scaphoid] of** left **foot**

√7th **S92.256** Nondisplaced **fracture of navicular [scaphoid] of unspecified foot**

√5th **S92.3** Fracture of metatarsal bone(s)

√6th **S92.30** Fracture of **unspecified metatarsal bone(s)**

√7th **S92.301** Fracture of unspecified metatarsal **bone(s),** right **foot**

√7th **S92.302** Fracture of unspecified metatarsal **bone(s),** left **foot**

√7th **S92.309** Fracture of unspecified metatarsal **bone(s), unspecified foot**

√6th **S92.31** Fracture of **first metatarsal bone**

√7th **S92.311** Displaced **fracture of first metatarsal bone,** right **foot**

√7th **S92.312** Displaced **fracture of first metatarsal bone,** left **foot**

√7th **S92.313** Displaced **fracture of first metatarsal bone, unspecified foot**

√7th **S92.314** Nondisplaced **fracture of first metatarsal bone,** right **foot**

√7th **S92.315** Nondisplaced **fracture of first metatarsal bone,** left **foot**

√7th **S92.316** Nondisplaced **fracture of first metatarsal bone, unspecified foot**

√6th **S92.32** Fracture of **second metatarsal bone**

√7th **S92.321** Displaced **fracture of second metatarsal bone,** right **foot**

√7th **S92.322** Displaced **fracture of second metatarsal bone,** left **foot**

√7th **S92.323** Displaced **fracture of second metatarsal bone, unspecified foot**

√7th **S92.324** Nondisplaced **fracture of second metatarsal bone,** right **foot**

√7th **S92.325** Nondisplaced **fracture of second metatarsal bone,** left **foot**

√7th **S92.326** Nondisplaced **fracture of second metatarsal bone, unspecified foot**

√6th **S92.33** Fracture of **third metatarsal bone**

√7th **S92.331** Displaced **fracture of third metatarsal bone,** right **foot**

√7th **S92.332** Displaced **fracture of third metatarsal bone,** left **foot**

√7th **S92.333** Displaced **fracture of third metatarsal bone, unspecified foot**

√7th **S92.334** Nondisplaced **fracture of third metatarsal bone,** right **foot**

√7th **S92.335** Nondisplaced **fracture of third metatarsal bone,** left **foot**

√7th **S92.336** Nondisplaced **fracture of third metatarsal bone, unspecified foot**

√6th **S92.34** Fracture of **fourth metatarsal bone**

√7th **S92.341** Displaced **fracture of fourth metatarsal bone,** right **foot**

√7th **S92.342** Displaced **fracture of fourth metatarsal bone,** left **foot**

√7th **S92.343** Displaced **fracture of fourth metatarsal bone, unspecified foot**

☑ Additional Character Required　√x7th Placeholder Alert　Unspecified Dx　Other Specified Dx　Manifestation　▶◀ Revised Text　● New Code　▲ Revised Code Title

☑7ᵗʰ **S92.344** Nondisplaced fracture of fourth metatarsal bone, right foot

☑7ᵗʰ **S92.345** Nondisplaced fracture of fourth metatarsal bone, left foot

☑7ᵗʰ **S92.346** Nondisplaced fracture of fourth metatarsal bone, unspecified foot

☑6ᵗʰ **S92.35** Fracture of fifth metatarsal bone

☑7ᵗʰ **S92.351** Displaced fracture of fifth metatarsal bone, right foot

☑7ᵗʰ **S92.352** Displaced fracture of fifth metatarsal bone, left foot

☑7ᵗʰ **S92.353** Displaced fracture of fifth metatarsal bone, unspecified foot

☑7ᵗʰ **S92.354** Nondisplaced fracture of fifth metatarsal bone, right foot

☑7ᵗʰ **S92.355** Nondisplaced fracture of fifth metatarsal bone, left foot

☑7ᵗʰ **S92.356** Nondisplaced fracture of fifth metatarsal bone, unspecified foot

☑5ᵗʰ **S92.4** Fracture of great toe

☑6ᵗʰ **S92.40** Unspecified fracture of great toe

☑7ᵗʰ **S92.401** Displaced unspecified fracture of right great toe

☑7ᵗʰ **S92.402** Displaced unspecified fracture of left great toe

☑7ᵗʰ **S92.403** Displaced unspecified fracture of unspecified great toe

☑7ᵗʰ **S92.404** Nondisplaced unspecified fracture of right great toe

☑7ᵗʰ **S92.405** Nondisplaced unspecified fracture of left great toe

☑7ᵗʰ **S92.406** Nondisplaced unspecified fracture of unspecified great toe

☑6ᵗʰ **S92.41** Fracture of proximal phalanx of great toe

☑7ᵗʰ **S92.411** Displaced fracture of proximal phalanx of right great toe

☑7ᵗʰ **S92.412** Displaced fracture of proximal phalanx of left great toe

☑7ᵗʰ **S92.413** Displaced fracture of proximal phalanx of unspecified great toe

☑7ᵗʰ **S92.414** Nondisplaced fracture of proximal phalanx of right great toe

☑7ᵗʰ **S92.415** Nondisplaced fracture of proximal phalanx of left great toe

☑7ᵗʰ **S92.416** Nondisplaced fracture of proximal phalanx of unspecified great toe

☑6ᵗʰ **S92.42** Fracture of distal phalanx of great toe

☑7ᵗʰ **S92.421** Displaced fracture of distal phalanx of right great toe

☑7ᵗʰ **S92.422** Displaced fracture of distal phalanx of left great toe

☑7ᵗʰ **S92.423** Displaced fracture of distal phalanx of unspecified great toe

☑7ᵗʰ **S92.424** Nondisplaced fracture of distal phalanx of right great toe

☑7ᵗʰ **S92.425** Nondisplaced fracture of distal phalanx of left great toe

☑7ᵗʰ **S92.426** Nondisplaced fracture of distal phalanx of unspecified great toe

☑6ᵗʰ **S92.49** Other fracture of great toe

☑7ᵗʰ **S92.491** Other fracture of right great toe

☑7ᵗʰ **S92.492** Other fracture of left great toe

☑7ᵗʰ **S92.499** Other fracture of unspecified great toe

☑5ᵗʰ **S92.5** Fracture of lesser toe(s)

☑6ᵗʰ **S92.50** Unspecified fracture of lesser toe(s)

☑7ᵗʰ **S92.501** Displaced unspecified fracture of right lesser toe(s)

☑7ᵗʰ **S92.502** Displaced unspecified fracture of left lesser toe(s)

☑7ᵗʰ **S92.503** Displaced unspecified fracture of unspecified lesser toe(s)

☑7ᵗʰ **S92.504** Nondisplaced unspecified fracture of right lesser toe(s)

☑7ᵗʰ **S92.505** Nondisplaced unspecified fracture of left lesser toe(s)

☑7ᵗʰ **S92.506** Nondisplaced unspecified fracture of unspecified lesser toe(s)

☑6ᵗʰ **S92.51** Fracture of proximal phalanx of lesser toe(s)

☑7ᵗʰ **S92.511** Displaced fracture of proximal phalanx of right lesser toe(s)

☑7ᵗʰ **S92.512** Displaced fracture of proximal phalanx of left lesser toe(s)

☑7ᵗʰ **S92.513** Displaced fracture of proximal phalanx of unspecified lesser toe(s)

☑7ᵗʰ **S92.514** Nondisplaced fracture of proximal phalanx of right lesser toe(s)

☑7ᵗʰ **S92.515** Nondisplaced fracture of proximal phalanx of left lesser toe(s)

☑7ᵗʰ **S92.516** Nondisplaced fracture of proximal phalanx of unspecified lesser toe(s)

☑6ᵗʰ **S92.52** Fracture of medial phalanx of lesser toe(s)

☑7ᵗʰ **S92.521** Displaced fracture of medial phalanx of right lesser toe(s)

☑7ᵗʰ **S92.522** Displaced fracture of medial phalanx of left lesser toe(s)

☑7ᵗʰ **S92.523** Displaced fracture of medial phalanx of unspecified lesser toe(s)

☑7ᵗʰ **S92.524** Nondisplaced fracture of medial phalanx of right lesser toe(s)

☑7ᵗʰ **S92.525** Nondisplaced fracture of medial phalanx of left lesser toe(s)

☑7ᵗʰ **S92.526** Nondisplaced fracture of medial phalanx of unspecified lesser toe(s)

☑6ᵗʰ **S92.53** Fracture of distal phalanx of lesser toe(s)

☑7ᵗʰ **S92.531** Displaced fracture of distal phalanx of right lesser toe(s)

☑7ᵗʰ **S92.532** Displaced fracture of distal phalanx of left lesser toe(s)

☑7ᵗʰ **S92.533** Displaced fracture of distal phalanx of unspecified lesser toe(s)

☑7ᵗʰ **S92.534** Nondisplaced fracture of distal phalanx of right lesser toe(s)

☑7ᵗʰ **S92.535** Nondisplaced fracture of distal phalanx of left lesser toe(s)

☑7ᵗʰ **S92.536** Nondisplaced fracture of distal phalanx of unspecified lesser toe(s)

☑6ᵗʰ **S92.59** Other fracture of lesser toe(s)

☑7ᵗʰ **S92.591** Other fracture of right lesser toe(s)

☑7ᵗʰ **S92.592** Other fracture of left lesser toe(s)

☑7ᵗʰ **S92.599** Other fracture of unspecified lesser toe(s)

☑5ᵗʰ **S92.9** Unspecified fracture of foot and toe

☑6ᵗʰ **S92.90** Unspecified fracture of foot

☑7ᵗʰ **S92.901** Unspecified fracture of right foot

☑7ᵗʰ **S92.902** Unspecified fracture of left foot

☑7ᵗʰ **S92.909** Unspecified fracture of unspecified foot

☑6ᵗʰ **S92.91** Unspecified fracture of toe

☑7ᵗʰ **S92.911** Unspecified fracture of right toe(s)

☑7ᵗʰ **S92.912** Unspecified fracture of left toe(s)

☑7ᵗʰ **S92.919** Unspecified fracture of unspecified toe(s)

EXCLUDES 1 Not coded here   *EXCLUDES 2* Not included here   Ⓝ Newborn Age: 0   Ⓟ Pediatric Age: 0-17   Ⓜ Maternity Age: 12-55   Ⓐ Adult Age: 15-124

958   ICD-10-CM 2016

✓4ᵗʰ S93 Dislocation and sprain of joints and ligaments at ankle, foot and toe level

INCLUDES   avulsion of joint or ligament of ankle, foot and toe
laceration of cartilage, joint or ligament of ankle, foot and toe
sprain of cartilage, joint or ligament of ankle, foot and toe
traumatic hemarthrosis of joint or ligament of ankle, foot and toe
traumatic rupture of joint or ligament of ankle, foot and toe
traumatic subluxation of joint or ligament of ankle, foot and toe
traumatic tear of joint or ligament of ankle, foot and toe

Code also any associated open wound

EXCLUDES 2   *strain of muscle and tendon of ankle and foot (S96.-)*

> The appropriate 7th character is to be added to each code from category S93.
> A   initial encounter
> D   subsequent encounter
> S   sequela

✓5ᵗʰ S93.0 Subluxation and dislocation of ankle joint
Subluxation and dislocation of astragalus
Subluxation and dislocation of fibula, lower end
Subluxation and dislocation of talus
Subluxation and dislocation of tibia, lower end

✓x7ᵗʰ   **S93.01**   Subluxation of right ankle joint
✓x7ᵗʰ   **S93.02**   Subluxation of left ankle joint
✓x7ᵗʰ   **S93.03**   Subluxation of unspecified ankle joint
✓x7ᵗʰ   **S93.04**   Dislocation of right ankle joint
✓x7ᵗʰ   **S93.05**   Dislocation of left ankle joint
✓x7ᵗʰ   **S93.06**   Dislocation of unspecified ankle joint

✓5ᵗʰ S93.1 Subluxation and dislocation of toe

✓6ᵗʰ   **S93.10**   Unspecified subluxation and dislocation of toe
Dislocation of toe NOS
Subluxation of toe NOS

✓7ᵗʰ   **S93.101**   Unspecified subluxation of right toe(s)
✓7ᵗʰ   **S93.102**   Unspecified subluxation of left toe(s)
✓7ᵗʰ   **S93.103**   Unspecified subluxation of unspecified toe(s)
✓7ᵗʰ   **S93.104**   Unspecified dislocation of right toe(s)
✓7ᵗʰ   **S93.105**   Unspecified dislocation of left toe(s)
✓7ᵗʰ   **S93.106**   Unspecified dislocation of unspecified toe(s)

✓6ᵗʰ   **S93.11**   Dislocation of interphalangeal joint

✓7ᵗʰ   **S93.111**   Dislocation of interphalangeal joint of right great toe
✓7ᵗʰ   **S93.112**   Dislocation of interphalangeal joint of left great toe
✓7ᵗʰ   **S93.113**   Dislocation of interphalangeal joint of unspecified great toe
✓7ᵗʰ   **S93.114**   Dislocation of interphalangeal joint of right lesser toe(s)
✓7ᵗʰ   **S93.115**   Dislocation of interphalangeal joint of left lesser toe(s)
✓7ᵗʰ   **S93.116**   Dislocation of interphalangeal joint of unspecified lesser toe(s)
✓7ᵗʰ   **S93.119**   Dislocation of interphalangeal joint of unspecified toe(s)

✓6ᵗʰ   **S93.12**   Dislocation of metatarsophalangeal joint

✓7ᵗʰ   **S93.121**   Dislocation of metatarsophalangeal joint of right great toe
✓7ᵗʰ   **S93.122**   Dislocation of metatarsophalangeal joint of left great toe
✓7ᵗʰ   **S93.123**   Dislocation of metatarsophalangeal joint of unspecified great toe
✓7ᵗʰ   **S93.124**   Dislocation of metatarsophalangeal joint of right lesser toe(s)
✓7ᵗʰ   **S93.125**   Dislocation of metatarsophalangeal joint of left lesser toe(s)
✓7ᵗʰ   **S93.126**   Dislocation of metatarsophalangeal joint of unspecified lesser toe(s)
✓7ᵗʰ   **S93.129**   Dislocation of metatarsophalangeal joint of unspecified toe(s)

✓6ᵗʰ   **S93.13**   Subluxation of interphalangeal joint

✓7ᵗʰ   **S93.131**   Subluxation of interphalangeal joint of right great toe
✓7ᵗʰ   **S93.132**   Subluxation of interphalangeal joint of left great toe
✓7ᵗʰ   **S93.133**   Subluxation of interphalangeal joint of unspecified great toe
✓7ᵗʰ   **S93.134**   Subluxation of interphalangeal joint of right lesser toe(s)
✓7ᵗʰ   **S93.135**   Subluxation of interphalangeal joint of left lesser toe(s)
✓7ᵗʰ   **S93.136**   Subluxation of interphalangeal joint of unspecified lesser toe(s)
✓7ᵗʰ   **S93.139**   Subluxation of interphalangeal joint of unspecified toe(s)

✓6ᵗʰ   **S93.14**   Subluxation of metatarsophalangeal joint

✓7ᵗʰ   **S93.141**   Subluxation of metatarsophalangeal joint of right great toe
✓7ᵗʰ   **S93.142**   Subluxation of metatarsophalangeal joint of left great toe
✓7ᵗʰ   **S93.143**   Subluxation of metatarsophalangeal joint of unspecified great toe
✓7ᵗʰ   **S93.144**   Subluxation of metatarsophalangeal joint of right lesser toe(s)
✓7ᵗʰ   **S93.145**   Subluxation of metatarsophalangeal joint of left lesser toe(s)
✓7ᵗʰ   **S93.146**   Subluxation of metatarsophalangeal joint of unspecified lesser toe(s)
✓7ᵗʰ   **S93.149**   Subluxation of metatarsophalangeal joint of unspecified toe(s)

✓5ᵗʰ S93.3 Subluxation and dislocation of foot

EXCLUDES 2   *dislocation of toe (S93.1-)*

✓6ᵗʰ   **S93.30**   Unspecified subluxation and dislocation of foot
Dislocation of foot NOS
Subluxation of foot NOS

✓7ᵗʰ   **S93.301**   Unspecified subluxation of right foot
✓7ᵗʰ   **S93.302**   Unspecified subluxation of left foot
✓7ᵗʰ   **S93.303**   Unspecified subluxation of unspecified foot
✓7ᵗʰ   **S93.304**   Unspecified dislocation of right foot
✓7ᵗʰ   **S93.305**   Unspecified dislocation of left foot
✓7ᵗʰ   **S93.306**   Unspecified dislocation of unspecified foot

✓6ᵗʰ   **S93.31**   Subluxation and dislocation of tarsal joint

✓7ᵗʰ   **S93.311**   Subluxation of tarsal joint of right foot
✓7ᵗʰ   **S93.312**   Subluxation of tarsal joint of left foot
✓7ᵗʰ   **S93.313**   Subluxation of tarsal joint of unspecified foot
✓7ᵗʰ   **S93.314**   Dislocation of tarsal joint of right foot
✓7ᵗʰ   **S93.315**   Dislocation of tarsal joint of left foot
✓7ᵗʰ   **S93.316**   Dislocation of tarsal joint of unspecified foot

✓6ᵗʰ   **S93.32**   Subluxation and dislocation of tarsometatarsal joint

✓7ᵗʰ   **S93.321**   Subluxation of tarsometatarsal joint of right foot
✓7ᵗʰ   **S93.322**   Subluxation of tarsometatarsal joint of left foot
✓7ᵗʰ   **S93.323**   Subluxation of tarsometatarsal joint of unspecified foot
✓7ᵗʰ   **S93.324**   Dislocation of tarsometatarsal joint of right foot
✓7ᵗʰ   **S93.325**   Dislocation of tarsometatarsal joint of left foot
✓7ᵗʰ   **S93.326**   Dislocation of tarsometatarsal joint of unspecified foot

✓6ᵗʰ   **S93.33**   Other subluxation and dislocation of foot

✓7ᵗʰ   **S93.331**   Other subluxation of right foot
✓7ᵗʰ   **S93.332**   Other subluxation of left foot
✓7ᵗʰ   **S93.333**   Other subluxation of unspecified foot
✓7ᵗʰ   **S93.334**   Other dislocation of right foot
✓7ᵗʰ   **S93.335**   Other dislocation of left foot
✓7ᵗʰ   **S93.336**   Other dislocation of unspecified foot

✓ Additional Character Required   ✓x7ᵗʰ Placeholder Alert   Unspecified Dx   Other Specified Dx   Manifestation   ►◄ Revised Text   ● New Code   ▲ Revised Code Title

✓5th **S93.4** **Sprain of** ankle
    EXCLUDES 2 *injury of Achilles tendon (S86.0-)*

  ✓6th **S93.40** **Sprain of** unspecified **ligament of ankle**
      Sprain of ankle NOS
      Sprained ankle NOS

    ✓7th **S93.401** **Sprain of unspecified ligament of** right **ankle**

    ✓7th **S93.402** **Sprain of unspecified ligament of** left **ankle**

    ✓7th **S93.409** **Sprain of unspecified ligament of unspecified ankle**

  ✓6th **S93.41** **Sprain of** calcaneofibular **ligament**

    ✓7th **S93.411** **Sprain of calcaneofibular ligament of** right **ankle**

    ✓7th **S93.412** **Sprain of calcaneofibular ligament of** left **ankle**

    ✓7th **S93.419** **Sprain of calcaneofibular ligament of unspecified ankle**

  ✓6th **S93.42** **Sprain of** deltoid **ligament**

    ✓7th **S93.421** **Sprain of deltoid ligament of** right **ankle**

    ✓7th **S93.422** **Sprain of deltoid ligament of** left **ankle**

    ✓7th **S93.429** **Sprain of deltoid ligament of unspecified ankle**

  ✓6th **S93.43** **Sprain of** tibiofibular **ligament**

    ✓7th **S93.431** **Sprain of tibiofibular ligament of** right **ankle**

    ✓7th **S93.432** **Sprain of tibiofibular ligament of** left **ankle**

    ✓7th **S93.439** **Sprain of tibiofibular ligament of unspecified ankle**

  ✓6th **S93.49** **Sprain of** other **ligament of ankle**
      Sprain of internal collateral ligament
      Sprain of talofibular ligament

    ✓7th **S93.491** **Sprain of other ligament of** right **ankle**

    ✓7th **S93.492** **Sprain of other ligament of** left **ankle**

    ✓7th **S93.499** **Sprain of other ligament of unspecified ankle**

✓5th **S93.5** **Sprain of** toe

  ✓6th **S93.50** **Unspecified sprain of toe**

    ✓7th **S93.501** **Unspecified sprain of** right great **toe**

    ✓7th **S93.502** **Unspecified sprain of** left great **toe**

    ✓7th **S93.503** **Unspecified sprain of unspecified great toe**

    ✓7th **S93.504** **Unspecified sprain of** right lesser **toe(s)**

    ✓7th **S93.505** **Unspecified sprain of** left lesser **toe(s)**

    ✓7th **S93.506** **Unspecified sprain of unspecified lesser toe(s)**

    ✓7th **S93.509** **Unspecified sprain of unspecified toe(s)**

  ✓6th **S93.51** **Sprain of** interphalangeal joint **of toe**

    ✓7th **S93.511** **Sprain of interphalangeal joint of** right great **toe**

    ✓7th **S93.512** **Sprain of interphalangeal joint of** left great **toe**

    ✓7th **S93.513** **Sprain of interphalangeal joint of unspecified great toe**

    ✓7th **S93.514** **Sprain of interphalangeal joint of** right lesser **toe(s)**

    ✓7th **S93.515** **Sprain of interphalangeal joint of** left lesser **toe(s)**

    ✓7th **S93.516** **Sprain of interphalangeal joint of unspecified lesser toe(s)**

    ✓7th **S93.519** **Sprain of interphalangeal joint of unspecified toe(s)**

  ✓6th **S93.52** **Sprain of** metatarsophalangeal joint **of toe**

    ✓7th **S93.521** **Sprain of metatarsophalangeal joint of** right great **toe**

    ✓7th **S93.522** **Sprain of metatarsophalangeal joint of** left great **toe**

    ✓7th **S93.523** **Sprain of metatarsophalangeal joint of unspecified great toe**

    ✓7th **S93.524** **Sprain of metatarsophalangeal joint of** right lesser **toe(s)**

    ✓7th **S93.525** **Sprain of metatarsophalangeal joint of** left lesser **toe(s)**

    ✓7th **S93.526** **Sprain of metatarsophalangeal joint of unspecified lesser toe(s)**

    ✓7th **S93.529** **Sprain of metatarsophalangeal joint of unspecified toe(s)**

✓5th **S93.6** **Sprain of** foot
    EXCLUDES 2 *sprain of metatarsophalangeal joint of toe (S93.52-)*
            sprain of toe (S93.5-)

  ✓6th **S93.60** **Unspecified sprain of foot**

    ✓7th **S93.601** **Unspecified sprain of** right **foot**

    ✓7th **S93.602** **Unspecified sprain of** left **foot**

    ✓7th **S93.609** **Unspecified sprain of unspecified foot**

  ✓6th **S93.61** **Sprain of** tarsal ligament **of foot**

    ✓7th **S93.611** **Sprain of tarsal ligament of** right **foot**

    ✓7th **S93.612** **Sprain of tarsal ligament of** left **foot**

    ✓7th **S93.619** **Sprain of tarsal ligament of unspecified foot**

  ✓6th **S93.62** **Sprain of** tarsometatarsal ligament **of foot**

    ✓7th **S93.621** **Sprain of tarsometatarsal ligament of** right **foot**

    ✓7th **S93.622** **Sprain of tarsometatarsal ligament of** left **foot**

    ✓7th **S93.629** **Sprain of tarsometatarsal ligament of unspecified foot**

  ✓6th **S93.69** **Other sprain of foot**

    ✓7th **S93.691** **Other sprain of** right **foot**

    ✓7th **S93.692** **Other sprain of** left **foot**

    ✓7th **S93.699** **Other sprain of unspecified foot**

✓4th **S94** **Injury of nerves at ankle and foot level**
    Code also any associated open wound (S91.-)

    The appropriate 7th character is to be added to each code from category S94.
    A   initial encounter
    D   subsequent encounter
    S   sequela

  ✓5th **S94.0** **Injury of** lateral plantar **nerve**

    ✓x7th **S94.00** **Injury of lateral plantar nerve, unspecified leg**

    ✓x7th **S94.01** **Injury of lateral plantar nerve,** right **leg**

    ✓x7th **S94.02** **Injury of lateral plantar nerve,** left **leg**

  ✓5th **S94.1** **Injury of** medial plantar **nerve**

    ✓x7th **S94.10** **Injury of medial plantar nerve, unspecified leg**

    ✓x7th **S94.11** **Injury of medial plantar nerve,** right **leg**

    ✓x7th **S94.12** **Injury of medial plantar nerve,** left **leg**

  ✓5th **S94.2** **Injury of** deep peroneal **nerve at ankle and foot level**
      Injury of terminal, lateral branch of deep peroneal nerve

    ✓x7th **S94.20** **Injury of deep peroneal nerve at ankle and foot level, unspecified leg**

    ✓x7th **S94.21** **Injury of deep peroneal nerve at ankle and foot level,** right **leg**

    ✓x7th **S94.22** **Injury of deep peroneal nerve at ankle and foot level,** left **leg**

  ✓5th **S94.3** **Injury of** cutaneous sensory **nerve at ankle and foot level**

    ✓x7th **S94.30** **Injury of cutaneous sensory nerve at ankle and foot level, unspecified leg**

    ✓x7th **S94.31** **Injury of cutaneous sensory nerve at ankle and foot level,** right **leg**

    ✓x7th **S94.32** **Injury of cutaneous sensory nerve at ankle and foot level,** left **leg**

  ✓5th **S94.8** **Injury of** other **nerves at ankle and foot level**

    ✓6th **S94.8X** **Injury of other nerves at ankle and foot level**

      ✓7th **S94.8X1** **Injury of other nerves at ankle and foot level,** right **leg**

      ✓7th **S94.8X2** **Injury of other nerves at ankle and foot level,** left **leg**

      ✓7th **S94.8X9** **Injury of other nerves at ankle and foot level, unspecified leg**

  ✓5th **S94.9** **Injury of** unspecified **nerve at ankle and foot level**

    ✓x7th **S94.90** **Injury of unspecified nerve at ankle and foot level, unspecified leg**

✓x7ᵗʰ **S94.91** Injury of unspecified nerve at ankle and foot level, right leg

✓x7ᵗʰ **S94.92** Injury of unspecified nerve at ankle and foot level, left leg

✓4ᵗʰ **S95** **Injury of blood vessels at ankle and foot level**
   Code also any associated open wound (S91.-)
   EXCLUDES 2 *injury of posterior tibial artery and vein (S85.1-, S85.8-)*

   The appropriate 7th character is to be added to each code from category S95.
   A   initial encounter
   D   subsequent encounter
   S   sequela

✓5ᵗʰ **S95.0** **Injury of dorsal artery of foot**
   ✓6ᵗʰ **S95.00** Unspecified injury of dorsal artery of foot
      ✓7ᵗʰ **S95.001** Unspecified injury of dorsal artery of right foot
      ✓7ᵗʰ **S95.002** Unspecified injury of dorsal artery of left foot
      ✓7ᵗʰ **S95.009** Unspecified injury of dorsal artery of unspecified foot
   ✓6ᵗʰ **S95.01** Laceration of dorsal artery of foot
      ✓7ᵗʰ **S95.011** Laceration of dorsal artery of right foot
      ✓7ᵗʰ **S95.012** Laceration of dorsal artery of left foot
      ✓7ᵗʰ **S95.019** Laceration of dorsal artery of unspecified foot
   ✓6ᵗʰ **S95.09** Other specified injury of dorsal artery of foot
      ✓7ᵗʰ **S95.091** Other specified injury of dorsal artery of right foot
      ✓7ᵗʰ **S95.092** Other specified injury of dorsal artery of left foot
      ✓7ᵗʰ **S95.099** Other specified injury of dorsal artery of unspecified foot

✓5ᵗʰ **S95.1** **Injury of plantar artery of foot**
   ✓6ᵗʰ **S95.10** Unspecified injury of plantar artery of foot
      ✓7ᵗʰ **S95.101** Unspecified injury of plantar artery of right foot
      ✓7ᵗʰ **S95.102** Unspecified injury of plantar artery of left foot
      ✓7ᵗʰ **S95.109** Unspecified injury of plantar artery of unspecified foot
   ✓6ᵗʰ **S95.11** Laceration of plantar artery of foot
      ✓7ᵗʰ **S95.111** Laceration of plantar artery of right foot
      ✓7ᵗʰ **S95.112** Laceration of plantar artery of left foot
      ✓7ᵗʰ **S95.119** Laceration of plantar artery of unspecified foot
   ✓6ᵗʰ **S95.19** Other specified injury of plantar artery of foot
      ✓7ᵗʰ **S95.191** Other specified injury of plantar artery of right foot
      ✓7ᵗʰ **S95.192** Other specified injury of plantar artery of left foot
      ✓7ᵗʰ **S95.199** Other specified injury of plantar artery of unspecified foot

✓5ᵗʰ **S95.2** **Injury of dorsal vein of foot**
   ✓6ᵗʰ **S95.20** Unspecified injury of dorsal vein of foot
      ✓7ᵗʰ **S95.201** Unspecified injury of dorsal vein of right foot
      ✓7ᵗʰ **S95.202** Unspecified injury of dorsal vein of left foot
      ✓7ᵗʰ **S95.209** Unspecified injury of dorsal vein of unspecified foot
   ✓6ᵗʰ **S95.21** Laceration of dorsal vein of foot
      ✓7ᵗʰ **S95.211** Laceration of dorsal vein of right foot
      ✓7ᵗʰ **S95.212** Laceration of dorsal vein of left foot
      ✓7ᵗʰ **S95.219** Laceration of dorsal vein of unspecified foot
   ✓6ᵗʰ **S95.29** Other specified injury of dorsal vein of foot
      ✓7ᵗʰ **S95.291** Other specified injury of dorsal vein of right foot
      ✓7ᵗʰ **S95.292** Other specified injury of dorsal vein of left foot

      ✓7ᵗʰ **S95.299** Other specified injury of dorsal vein of unspecified foot

✓5ᵗʰ **S95.8** **Injury of other blood vessels at ankle and foot level**
   ✓6ᵗʰ **S95.80** Unspecified injury of other blood vessels at ankle and foot level
      ✓7ᵗʰ **S95.801** Unspecified injury of other blood vessels at ankle and foot level, right leg
      ✓7ᵗʰ **S95.802** Unspecified injury of other blood vessels at ankle and foot level, left leg
      ✓7ᵗʰ **S95.809** Unspecified injury of other blood vessels at ankle and foot level, unspecified leg
   ✓6ᵗʰ **S95.81** Laceration of other blood vessels at ankle and foot level
      ✓7ᵗʰ **S95.811** Laceration of other blood vessels at ankle and foot level, right leg
      ✓7ᵗʰ **S95.812** Laceration of other blood vessels at ankle and foot level, left leg
      ✓7ᵗʰ **S95.819** Laceration of other blood vessels at ankle and foot level, unspecified leg
   ✓6ᵗʰ **S95.89** Other specified injury of other blood vessels at ankle and foot level
      ✓7ᵗʰ **S95.891** Other specified injury of other blood vessels at ankle and foot level, right leg
      ✓7ᵗʰ **S95.892** Other specified injury of other blood vessels at ankle and foot level, left leg
      ✓7ᵗʰ **S95.899** Other specified injury of other blood vessels at ankle and foot level, unspecified leg

✓5ᵗʰ **S95.9** **Injury of unspecified blood vessel at ankle and foot level**
   ✓6ᵗʰ **S95.90** Unspecified injury of unspecified blood vessel at ankle and foot level
      ✓7ᵗʰ **S95.901** Unspecified injury of unspecified blood vessel at ankle and foot level, right leg
      ✓7ᵗʰ **S95.902** Unspecified injury of unspecified blood vessel at ankle and foot level, left leg
      ✓7ᵗʰ **S95.909** Unspecified injury of unspecified blood vessel at ankle and foot level, unspecified leg
   ✓6ᵗʰ **S95.91** Laceration of unspecified blood vessel at ankle and foot level
      ✓7ᵗʰ **S95.911** Laceration of unspecified blood vessel at ankle and foot level, right leg
      ✓7ᵗʰ **S95.912** Laceration of unspecified blood vessel at ankle and foot level, left leg
      ✓7ᵗʰ **S95.919** Laceration of unspecified blood vessel at ankle and foot level, unspecified leg
   ✓6ᵗʰ **S95.99** Other specified injury of unspecified blood vessel at ankle and foot level
      ✓7ᵗʰ **S95.991** Other specified injury of unspecified blood vessel at ankle and foot level, right leg
      ✓7ᵗʰ **S95.992** Other specified injury of unspecified blood vessel at ankle and foot level, left leg
      ✓7ᵗʰ **S95.999** Other specified injury of unspecified blood vessel at ankle and foot level, unspecified leg

✦ ✓4ᵗʰ **S96 Injury of muscle and tendon at ankle and foot level**
   Code also any associated open wound (S91.-)
   EXCLUDES 2 *injury of Achilles tendon (S86.0-)*
                sprain of joints and ligaments of ankle and foot (S93.-)

   The appropriate 7th character is to be added to each code from category S96.
   A   initial encounter
   D   subsequent encounter
   S   sequela

✓5ᵗʰ **S96.0** **Injury of muscle and tendon of long flexor muscle of toe at ankle and foot level**
   ✓6ᵗʰ **S96.00** Unspecified injury of muscle and tendon of long flexor muscle of toe at ankle and foot level
      ✓7ᵗʰ **S96.001** Unspecified injury of muscle and tendon of long flexor muscle of toe at ankle and foot level, right foot

---

✦ Refer to the Muscle/Tendon Table at beginning of this chapter.

✓ Additional Character Required   ✓x7ᵗʰ Placeholder Alert   Unspecified Dx   Other Specified Dx   Manifestation   ▶◀ Revised Text   ● New Code   ▲ Revised Code Title

☑7ᵗʰ S96.002 Unspecified injury of muscle and tendon of long flexor muscle of toe at ankle and foot level, **left** foot

☑7ᵗʰ S96.009 Unspecified injury of muscle and tendon of long flexor muscle of toe at ankle and foot level, unspecified foot

☑6ᵗʰ S96.01 Strain of muscle and tendon of long flexor muscle of toe at ankle and foot level

  ☑7ᵗʰ S96.011 Strain of muscle and tendon of long flexor muscle of toe at ankle and foot level, **right** foot

  ☑7ᵗʰ S96.012 Strain of muscle and tendon of long flexor muscle of toe at ankle and foot level, **left** foot

  ☑7ᵗʰ S96.019 Strain of muscle and tendon of long flexor muscle of toe at ankle and foot level, unspecified foot

☑6ᵗʰ S96.02 Laceration of muscle and tendon of long flexor muscle of toe at ankle and foot level

  ☑7ᵗʰ S96.021 Laceration of muscle and tendon of long flexor muscle of toe at ankle and foot level, **right** foot

  ☑7ᵗʰ S96.022 Laceration of muscle and tendon of long flexor muscle of toe at ankle and foot level, **left** foot

  ☑7ᵗʰ S96.029 Laceration of muscle and tendon of long flexor muscle of toe at ankle and foot level, unspecified foot

☑6ᵗʰ S96.09 Other injury of muscle and tendon of long flexor muscle of toe at ankle and foot level

  ☑7ᵗʰ S96.091 Other injury of muscle and tendon of long flexor muscle of toe at ankle and foot level, **right** foot

  ☑7ᵗʰ S96.092 Other injury of muscle and tendon of long flexor muscle of toe at ankle and foot level, **left** foot

  ☑7ᵗʰ S96.099 Other injury of muscle and tendon of long flexor muscle of toe at ankle and foot level, unspecified foot

☑5ᵗʰ S96.1 Injury of muscle and tendon of long extensor muscle of toe at ankle and foot level

☑6ᵗʰ S96.10 Unspecified injury of muscle and tendon of long extensor muscle of toe at ankle and foot level

  ☑7ᵗʰ S96.101 Unspecified injury of muscle and tendon of long extensor muscle of toe at ankle and foot level, **right** foot

  ☑7ᵗʰ S96.102 Unspecified injury of muscle and tendon of long extensor muscle of toe at ankle and foot level, **left** foot

  ☑7ᵗʰ S96.109 Unspecified injury of muscle and tendon of long extensor muscle of toe at ankle and foot level, unspecified foot

☑6ᵗʰ S96.11 Strain of muscle and tendon of long extensor muscle of toe at ankle and foot level

  ☑7ᵗʰ S96.111 Strain of muscle and tendon of long extensor muscle of toe at ankle and foot level, **right** foot

  ☑7ᵗʰ S96.112 Strain of muscle and tendon of long extensor muscle of toe at ankle and foot level, **left** foot

  ☑7ᵗʰ S96.119 Strain of muscle and tendon of long extensor muscle of toe at ankle and foot level, unspecified foot

☑6ᵗʰ S96.12 Laceration of muscle and tendon of long extensor muscle of toe at ankle and foot level

  ☑7ᵗʰ S96.121 Laceration of muscle and tendon of long extensor muscle of toe at ankle and foot level, **right** foot

  ☑7ᵗʰ S96.122 Laceration of muscle and tendon of long extensor muscle of toe at ankle and foot level, **left** foot

  ☑7ᵗʰ S96.129 Laceration of muscle and tendon of long extensor muscle of toe at ankle and foot level, unspecified foot

☑6ᵗʰ S96.19 Other specified injury of muscle and tendon of long extensor muscle of toe at ankle and foot level

  ☑7ᵗʰ S96.191 Other specified injury of muscle and tendon of long extensor muscle of toe at ankle and foot level, **right** foot

  ☑7ᵗʰ S96.192 Other specified injury of muscle and tendon of long extensor muscle of toe at ankle and foot level, **left** foot

  ☑7ᵗʰ S96.199 Other specified injury of muscle and tendon of long extensor muscle of toe at ankle and foot level, unspecified foot

☑5ᵗʰ S96.2 Injury of intrinsic muscle and tendon at ankle and foot level

☑6ᵗʰ S96.20 Unspecified injury of intrinsic muscle and tendon at ankle and foot level

  ☑7ᵗʰ S96.201 Unspecified injury of intrinsic muscle and tendon at ankle and foot level, **right** foot

  ☑7ᵗʰ S96.202 Unspecified injury of intrinsic muscle and tendon at ankle and foot level, **left** foot

  ☑7ᵗʰ S96.209 Unspecified injury of intrinsic muscle and tendon at ankle and foot level, unspecified foot

☑6ᵗʰ S96.21 Strain of intrinsic muscle and tendon at ankle and foot level

  ☑7ᵗʰ S96.211 Strain of intrinsic muscle and tendon at ankle and foot level, **right** foot

  ☑7ᵗʰ S96.212 Strain of intrinsic muscle and tendon at ankle and foot level, **left** foot

  ☑7ᵗʰ S96.219 Strain of intrinsic muscle and tendon at ankle and foot level, unspecified foot

☑6ᵗʰ S96.22 Laceration of intrinsic muscle and tendon at ankle and foot level

  ☑7ᵗʰ S96.221 Laceration of intrinsic muscle and tendon at ankle and foot level, **right** foot

  ☑7ᵗʰ S96.222 Laceration of intrinsic muscle and tendon at ankle and foot level, **left** foot

  ☑7ᵗʰ S96.229 Laceration of intrinsic muscle and tendon at ankle and foot level, unspecified foot

☑6ᵗʰ S96.29 Other specified injury of intrinsic muscle and tendon at ankle and foot level

  ☑7ᵗʰ S96.291 Other specified injury of intrinsic muscle and tendon at ankle and foot level, **right** foot

  ☑7ᵗʰ S96.292 Other specified injury of intrinsic muscle and tendon at ankle and foot level, **left** foot

  ☑7ᵗʰ S96.299 Other specified injury of intrinsic muscle and tendon at ankle and foot level, unspecified foot

☑5ᵗʰ S96.8 Injury of other specified muscles and tendons at ankle and foot level

☑6ᵗʰ S96.80 Unspecified injury of other specified muscles and tendons at ankle and foot level

  ☑7ᵗʰ S96.801 Unspecified injury of other specified muscles and tendons at ankle and foot level, **right** foot

  ☑7ᵗʰ S96.802 Unspecified injury of other specified muscles and tendons at ankle and foot level, **left** foot

  ☑7ᵗʰ S96.809 Unspecified injury of other specified muscles and tendons at ankle and foot level, unspecified foot

☑6ᵗʰ S96.81 Strain of other specified muscles and tendons at ankle and foot level

  ☑7ᵗʰ S96.811 Strain of other specified muscles and tendons at ankle and foot level, **right** foot

  ☑7ᵗʰ S96.812 Strain of other specified muscles and tendons at ankle and foot level, **left** foot

  ☑7ᵗʰ S96.819 Strain of other specified muscles and tendons at ankle and foot level, unspecified foot

☑6ᵗʰ S96.82 Laceration of other specified muscles and tendons at ankle and foot level

  ☑7ᵗʰ S96.821 Laceration of other specified muscles and tendons at ankle and foot level, **right** foot

  ☑7ᵗʰ S96.822 Laceration of other specified muscles and tendons at ankle and foot level, **left** foot

EXCLUDES 1 Not coded here   *EXCLUDES 2* Not included here   N Newborn Age: 0   P Pediatric Age: 0-17   M Maternity Age: 12-55   A Adult Age: 15-124

962   ICD-10-CM 2016

✓7ᵗʰ **S96.829** Laceration of other specified muscles and tendons at ankle and foot level, unspecified foot

✓6ᵗʰ **S96.89** Other specified injury of other specified muscles and tendons at ankle and foot level

  ✓7ᵗʰ **S96.891** Other specified injury of other specified muscles and tendons at ankle and foot level, right foot

  ✓7ᵗʰ **S96.892** Other specified injury of other specified muscles and tendons at ankle and foot level, left foot

  ✓7ᵗʰ **S96.899** Other specified injury of other specified muscles and tendons at ankle and foot level, unspecified foot

✓5ᵗʰ **S96.9** Injury of unspecified muscle and tendon at ankle and foot level

✓6ᵗʰ **S96.90** Unspecified injury of unspecified muscle and tendon at ankle and foot level

  ✓7ᵗʰ **S96.901** Unspecified injury of unspecified muscle and tendon at ankle and foot level, right foot

  ✓7ᵗʰ **S96.902** Unspecified injury of unspecified muscle and tendon at ankle and foot level, left foot

  ✓7ᵗʰ **S96.909** Unspecified injury of unspecified muscle and tendon at ankle and foot level, unspecified foot

✓6ᵗʰ **S96.91** Strain of unspecified muscle and tendon at ankle and foot level

  ✓7ᵗʰ **S96.911** Strain of unspecified muscle and tendon at ankle and foot level, right foot

  ✓7ᵗʰ **S96.912** Strain of unspecified muscle and tendon at ankle and foot level, left foot

  ✓7ᵗʰ **S96.919** Strain of unspecified muscle and tendon at ankle and foot level, unspecified foot

✓6ᵗʰ **S96.92** Laceration of unspecified muscle and tendon at ankle and foot level

  ✓7ᵗʰ **S96.921** Laceration of unspecified muscle and tendon at ankle and foot level, right foot

  ✓7ᵗʰ **S96.922** Laceration of unspecified muscle and tendon at ankle and foot level, left foot

  ✓7ᵗʰ **S96.929** Laceration of unspecified muscle and tendon at ankle and foot level, unspecified foot

✓6ᵗʰ **S96.99** Other specified injury of unspecified muscle and tendon at ankle and foot level

  ✓7ᵗʰ **S96.991** Other specified injury of unspecified muscle and tendon at ankle and foot level, right foot

  ✓7ᵗʰ **S96.992** Other specified injury of unspecified muscle and tendon at ankle and foot level, left foot

  ✓7ᵗʰ **S96.999** Other specified injury of unspecified muscle and tendon at ankle and foot level, unspecified foot

✓4ᵗʰ **S97** Crushing injury of ankle and foot

Use additional code(s) for all associated injuries

> The appropriate 7th character is to be added to each code from category S97.
> A   initial encounter
> D   subsequent encounter
> S   sequela

✓5ᵗʰ **S97.0** Crushing injury of ankle

✓x7ᵗʰ **S97.00** Crushing injury of unspecified ankle

✓x7ᵗʰ **S97.01** Crushing injury of right ankle

✓x7ᵗʰ **S97.02** Crushing injury of left ankle

✓5ᵗʰ **S97.1** Crushing injury of toe

✓6ᵗʰ **S97.10** Crushing injury of unspecified toe(s)

  ✓7ᵗʰ **S97.101** Crushing injury of unspecified right toe(s)

  ✓7ᵗʰ **S97.102** Crushing injury of unspecified left toe(s)

  ✓7ᵗʰ **S97.109** Crushing injury of unspecified toe(s)
       Crushing injury of toe NOS

✓6ᵗʰ **S97.11** Crushing injury of great toe

  ✓7ᵗʰ **S97.111** Crushing injury of right great toe

  ✓7ᵗʰ **S97.112** Crushing injury of left great toe

  ✓7ᵗʰ **S97.119** Crushing injury of unspecified great toe

✓6ᵗʰ **S97.12** Crushing injury of lesser toe(s)

  ✓7ᵗʰ **S97.121** Crushing injury of right lesser toe(s)

  ✓7ᵗʰ **S97.122** Crushing injury of left lesser toe(s)

  ✓7ᵗʰ **S97.129** Crushing injury of unspecified lesser toe(s)

✓5ᵗʰ **S97.8** Crushing injury of foot

✓x7ᵗʰ **S97.80** Crushing injury of unspecified foot
       Crushing injury of foot NOS

✓x7ᵗʰ **S97.81** Crushing injury of right foot

✓x7ᵗʰ **S97.82** Crushing injury of left foot

✓4ᵗʰ **S98** Traumatic amputation of ankle and foot

An amputation not identified as partial or complete should be coded to complete

> The appropriate 7th character is to be added to each code from category S98.
> A   initial encounter
> D   subsequent encounter
> S   sequela

✓5ᵗʰ **S98.0** Traumatic amputation of foot at ankle level

✓6ᵗʰ **S98.01** Complete traumatic amputation of foot at ankle level

  ✓7ᵗʰ **S98.011** Complete traumatic amputation of right foot at ankle level

  ✓7ᵗʰ **S98.012** Complete traumatic amputation of left foot at ankle level

  ✓7ᵗʰ **S98.019** Complete traumatic amputation of unspecified foot at ankle level

✓6ᵗʰ **S98.02** Partial traumatic amputation of foot at ankle level

  ✓7ᵗʰ **S98.021** Partial traumatic amputation of right foot at ankle level

  ✓7ᵗʰ **S98.022** Partial traumatic amputation of left foot at ankle level

  ✓7ᵗʰ **S98.029** Partial traumatic amputation of unspecified foot at ankle level

✓5ᵗʰ **S98.1** Traumatic amputation of one toe

✓6ᵗʰ **S98.11** Complete traumatic amputation of great toe

  ✓7ᵗʰ **S98.111** Complete traumatic amputation of right great toe

  ✓7ᵗʰ **S98.112** Complete traumatic amputation of left great toe

  ✓7ᵗʰ **S98.119** Complete traumatic amputation of unspecified great toe

✓6ᵗʰ **S98.12** Partial traumatic amputation of great toe

  ✓7ᵗʰ **S98.121** Partial traumatic amputation of right great toe

  ✓7ᵗʰ **S98.122** Partial traumatic amputation of left great toe

  ✓7ᵗʰ **S98.129** Partial traumatic amputation of unspecified great toe

✓6ᵗʰ **S98.13** Complete traumatic amputation of one lesser toe
       Traumatic amputation of toe NOS

  ✓7ᵗʰ **S98.131** Complete traumatic amputation of one right lesser toe

  ✓7ᵗʰ **S98.132** Complete traumatic amputation of one left lesser toe

  ✓7ᵗʰ **S98.139** Complete traumatic amputation of one unspecified lesser toe

✓6ᵗʰ **S98.14** Partial traumatic amputation of one lesser toe

  ✓7ᵗʰ **S98.141** Partial traumatic amputation of one right lesser toe

  ✓7ᵗʰ **S98.142** Partial traumatic amputation of one left lesser toe

  ✓7ᵗʰ **S98.149** Partial traumatic amputation of one unspecified lesser toe

✓5ᵗʰ **S98.2** Traumatic amputation of two or more lesser toes

✓6ᵗʰ **S98.21** Complete traumatic amputation of two or more lesser toes

  ✓7ᵗʰ **S98.211** Complete traumatic amputation of two or more right lesser toes

  ✓7ᵗʰ **S98.212** Complete traumatic amputation of two or more left lesser toes

  ✓7ᵗʰ **S98.219** Complete traumatic amputation of two or more unspecified lesser toes

---

☑ Additional Character Required   ✓x7ᵗʰ Placeholder Alert   Unspecified Dx   Other Specified Dx   Manifestation   ▶◀ Revised Text   ● New Code   ▲ Revised Code Title

ICD-10-CM 2016   963

✓6ᵗʰ **S98.22**   **Partial** traumatic amputation of two or more lesser toes

   ✓7ᵗʰ **S98.221**   **Partial traumatic amputation of two or more right lesser toes**

   ✓7ᵗʰ **S98.222**   **Partial traumatic amputation of two or more left lesser toes**

   ✓7ᵗʰ **S98.229**   **Partial traumatic amputation of two or more unspecified lesser toes**

✓5ᵗʰ **S98.3**   **Traumatic amputation of** midfoot

  ✓6ᵗʰ **S98.31**   **Complete** traumatic amputation of midfoot

   ✓7ᵗʰ **S98.311**   **Complete traumatic amputation of right midfoot**

   ✓7ᵗʰ **S98.312**   **Complete traumatic amputation of left midfoot**

   ✓7ᵗʰ **S98.319**   **Complete traumatic amputation of unspecified midfoot**

  ✓6ᵗʰ **S98.32**   **Partial traumatic amputation of midfoot**

   ✓7ᵗʰ **S98.321**   **Partial traumatic amputation of right midfoot**

   ✓7ᵗʰ **S98.322**   **Partial traumatic amputation of left midfoot**

   ✓7ᵗʰ **S98.329**   **Partial traumatic amputation of unspecified midfoot**

✓5ᵗʰ **S98.9**   **Traumatic amputation of** foot, level unspecified

  ✓6ᵗʰ **S98.91**   **Complete** traumatic amputation of foot, level unspecified

   ✓7ᵗʰ **S98.911**   **Complete traumatic amputation of right foot, level unspecified**

   ✓7ᵗʰ **S98.912**   **Complete traumatic amputation of left foot, level unspecified**

   ✓7ᵗʰ **S98.919**   **Complete traumatic amputation of unspecified foot, level unspecified**

  ✓6ᵗʰ **S98.92**   **Partial** traumatic amputation of foot, level unspecified

   ✓7ᵗʰ **S98.921**   **Partial traumatic amputation of right foot, level unspecified**

   ✓7ᵗʰ **S98.922**   **Partial traumatic amputation of left foot, level unspecified**

   ✓7ᵗʰ **S98.929**   **Partial traumatic amputation of unspecified foot, level unspecified**

✓4ᵗʰ **S99**   **Other and unspecified injuries of ankle and foot**

> The appropriate 7th character is to be added to each code from category S99.
> A   initial encounter
> D   subsequent encounter
> S   sequela

  ✓5ᵗʰ **S99.8**   **Other** specified injuries of ankle and foot

   ✓6ᵗʰ **S99.81**   **Other specified injuries of** ankle

    ✓7ᵗʰ **S99.811**   **Other specified injuries of right ankle**

    ✓7ᵗʰ **S99.812**   **Other specified injuries of left ankle**

    ✓7ᵗʰ **S99.819**   **Other specified injuries of unspecified ankle**

   ✓6ᵗʰ **S99.82**   **Other specified injuries of** foot

    ✓7ᵗʰ **S99.821**   **Other specified injuries of right foot**

    ✓7ᵗʰ **S99.822**   **Other specified injuries of left foot**

    ✓7ᵗʰ **S99.829**   **Other specified injuries of unspecified foot**

  ✓5ᵗʰ **S99.9**   **Unspecified** injury of ankle and foot

   ✓6ᵗʰ **S99.91**   **Unspecified injury of** ankle

    ✓7ᵗʰ **S99.911**   **Unspecified injury of right ankle**

    ✓7ᵗʰ **S99.912**   **Unspecified injury of left ankle**

    ✓7ᵗʰ **S99.919**   **Unspecified injury of unspecified ankle**

   ✓6ᵗʰ **S99.92**   **Unspecified injury of** foot

    ✓7ᵗʰ **S99.921**   **Unspecified injury of right foot**

    ✓7ᵗʰ **S99.922**   **Unspecified injury of left foot**

    ✓7ᵗʰ **S99.929**   **Unspecified injury of unspecified foot**

Injury, Poisoning And Certain Other Consequences Of External Causes (T07-T88)

Injuries involving multiple body regions (T07)

EXCLUDES 1   *burns and corrosions (T20-T32)*
frostbite (T33-T34)
insect bite or sting, venomous (T63.4)
sunburn (L55.-)

T07   **Unspecified multiple injuries**
   EXCLUDES 1   *injury NOS (T14)*

Injury of unspecified body region (T14)

✓4ᵗʰ **T14**   **Injury of unspecified body region**
   EXCLUDES 1   *multiple unspecified injuries (T07)*

  T14.8   **Other injury of unspecified body region**
   Abrasion NOS
   Contusion NOS
   Crush injury NOS
   Fracture NOS
   Skin injury NOS
   Vascular injury NOS

  ✓5ᵗʰ **T14.9**   **Unspecified injury**

   T14.90   **Injury, unspecified**
    Injury NOS

   T14.91   **Suicide attempt**
    Attempted suicide NOS

Effects of foreign body entering through natural orifice (T15-T19)

EXCLUDES 2   *foreign body accidentally left in operation wound (T81.5-)*
foreign body in penetrating wound—See open wound by body region
residual foreign body in soft tissue (M79.5)
splinter, without open wound—See superficial injury by body region

✓4ᵗʰ **T15**   **Foreign body on external eye**
   EXCLUDES 2   *foreign body in penetrating wound of orbit and eye ball (S05.4-, S05.5-)*
    open wound of eyelid and periocular area (S01.1-)
    retained foreign body in eyelid (H02.8-)
    retained (old) foreign body in penetrating wound of orbit and eye ball (H05.5-, H44.6-, H44.7-)
    superficial foreign body of eyelid and periocular area (S00.25-)

> The appropriate 7th character is to be added to each code from category T15.
> A   initial encounter
> D   subsequent encounter
> S   sequela

  ✓5ᵗʰ **T15.0**   **Foreign body in** cornea

   ✓x7ᵗʰ **T15.00**   **Foreign body in cornea, unspecified eye**

   ✓x7ᵗʰ **T15.01**   **Foreign body in cornea, right eye**

   ✓x7ᵗʰ **T15.02**   **Foreign body in cornea, left eye**

  ✓5ᵗʰ **T15.1**   **Foreign body in** conjunctival sac

   ✓x7ᵗʰ **T15.10**   **Foreign body in conjunctival sac, unspecified eye**

   ✓x7ᵗʰ **T15.11**   **Foreign body in conjunctival sac, right eye**

   ✓x7ᵗʰ **T15.12**   **Foreign body in conjunctival sac, left eye**

  ✓5ᵗʰ **T15.8**   **Foreign body in other and** multiple parts **of external eye**
   Foreign body in lacrimal punctum

   ✓x7ᵗʰ **T15.80**   **Foreign body in other and multiple parts of external eye, unspecified eye**

   ✓x7ᵗʰ **T15.81**   **Foreign body in other and multiple parts of external eye, right eye**

   ✓x7ᵗʰ **T15.82**   **Foreign body in other and multiple parts of external eye, left eye**

  ✓5ᵗʰ **T15.9**   **Foreign body on external eye,** part unspecified

   ✓x7ᵗʰ **T15.90**   **Foreign body on external eye, part unspecified, unspecified eye**

   ✓x7ᵗʰ **T15.91**   **Foreign body on external eye, part unspecified, right eye**

   ✓x7ᵗʰ **T15.92**   **Foreign body on external eye, part unspecified, left eye**

EXCLUDES 1 Not coded here   *EXCLUDES 2* Not included here   N Newborn Age: 0   P Pediatric Age: 0-17   M Maternity Age: 12-55   A Adult Age: 15-124

964   ICD-10-CM 2016

✓4ᵗʰ **T16**   **Foreign body in ear**
Foreign body in auditory canal

> The appropriate 7th character is to be added to each code from category T16.
> A   initial encounter
> D   subsequent encounter
> S   sequela

✓x7ᵗʰ   **T16.1**   **Foreign body in right ear**

✓x7ᵗʰ   **T16.2**   **Foreign body in left ear**

✓x7ᵗʰ   **T16.9**   **Foreign body in ear, unspecified ear**

✓4ᵗʰ **T17**   **Foreign body in respiratory tract**

> The appropriate 7th character is to be added to each code from category T17.
> A   initial encounter
> D   subsequent encounter
> S   sequela

✓x7ᵗʰ   **T17.0**   **Foreign body in nasal sinus**

✓x7ᵗʰ   **T17.1**   **Foreign body in nostril**
Foreign body in nose NOS

✓5ᵗʰ   **T17.2**   **Foreign body in pharynx**
Foreign body in nasopharynx
Foreign body in throat NOS

    ✓6ᵗʰ   **T17.20**   **Unspecified foreign body in pharynx**

       ✓7ᵗʰ   **T17.200**   **Unspecified foreign body in pharynx causing asphyxiation**

       ✓7ᵗʰ   **T17.208**   **Unspecified foreign body in pharynx causing other injury**

    ✓6ᵗʰ   **T17.21**   **Gastric contents in pharynx**
Aspiration of gastric contents into pharynx
Vomitus in pharynx

       ✓7ᵗʰ   **T17.210**   **Gastric contents in pharynx causing asphyxiation**

       ✓7ᵗʰ   **T17.218**   **Gastric contents in pharynx causing other injury**

    ✓6ᵗʰ   **T17.22**   **Food in pharynx**
Bones in pharynx
Seeds in pharynx

       ✓7ᵗʰ   **T17.220**   **Food in pharynx causing asphyxiation**

       ✓7ᵗʰ   **T17.228**   **Food in pharynx causing other injury**

    ✓6ᵗʰ   **T17.29**   **Other foreign object in pharynx**

       ✓7ᵗʰ   **T17.290**   **Other foreign object in pharynx causing asphyxiation**

       ✓7ᵗʰ   **T17.298**   **Other foreign object in pharynx causing other injury**

✓5ᵗʰ   **T17.3**   **Foreign body in larynx**

    ✓6ᵗʰ   **T17.30**   **Unspecified foreign body in larynx**

       ✓7ᵗʰ   **T17.300**   **Unspecified foreign body in larynx causing asphyxiation**

       ✓7ᵗʰ   **T17.308**   **Unspecified foreign body in larynx causing other injury**

    ✓6ᵗʰ   **T17.31**   **Gastric contents in larynx**
Aspiration of gastric contents into larynx
Vomitus in larynx

       ✓7ᵗʰ   **T17.310**   **Gastric contents in larynx causing asphyxiation**

       ✓7ᵗʰ   **T17.318**   **Gastric contents in larynx causing other injury**

    ✓6ᵗʰ   **T17.32**   **Food in larynx**
Bones in larynx
Seeds in larynx

       ✓7ᵗʰ   **T17.320**   **Food in larynx causing asphyxiation**

       ✓7ᵗʰ   **T17.328**   **Food in larynx causing other injury**

    ✓6ᵗʰ   **T17.39**   **Other foreign object in larynx**

       ✓7ᵗʰ   **T17.390**   **Other foreign object in larynx causing asphyxiation**

       ✓7ᵗʰ   **T17.398**   **Other foreign object in larynx causing other injury**

✓5ᵗʰ   **T17.4**   **Foreign body in trachea**

    ✓6ᵗʰ   **T17.40**   **Unspecified foreign body in trachea**

       ✓7ᵗʰ   **T17.400**   **Unspecified foreign body in trachea causing asphyxiation**

       ✓7ᵗʰ   **T17.408**   **Unspecified foreign body in trachea causing other injury**

    ✓6ᵗʰ   **T17.41**   **Gastric contents in trachea**
Aspiration of gastric contents into trachea
Vomitus in trachea

       ✓7ᵗʰ   **T17.410**   **Gastric contents in trachea causing asphyxiation**

       ✓7ᵗʰ   **T17.418**   **Gastric contents in trachea causing other injury**

    ✓6ᵗʰ   **T17.42**   **Food in trachea**
Bones in trachea
Seeds in trachea

       ✓7ᵗʰ   **T17.420**   **Food in trachea causing asphyxiation**

       ✓7ᵗʰ   **T17.428**   **Food in trachea causing other injury**

    ✓6ᵗʰ   **T17.49**   **Other foreign object in trachea**

       ✓7ᵗʰ   **T17.490**   **Other foreign object in trachea causing asphyxiation**

       ✓7ᵗʰ   **T17.498**   **Other foreign object in trachea causing other injury**

✓5ᵗʰ   **T17.5**   **Foreign body in bronchus**

    ✓6ᵗʰ   **T17.50**   **Unspecified foreign body in bronchus**

       ✓7ᵗʰ   **T17.500**   **Unspecified foreign body in bronchus causing asphyxiation**

       ✓7ᵗʰ   **T17.508**   **Unspecified foreign body in bronchus causing other injury**

    ✓6ᵗʰ   **T17.51**   **Gastric contents in bronchus**
Aspiration of gastric contents into bronchus
Vomitus in bronchus

       ✓7ᵗʰ   **T17.510**   **Gastric contents in bronchus causing asphyxiation**

       ✓7ᵗʰ   **T17.518**   **Gastric contents in bronchus causing other injury**

    ✓6ᵗʰ   **T17.52**   **Food in bronchus**
Bones in bronchusSeeds in bronchus

       ✓7ᵗʰ   **T17.520**   **Food in bronchus causing asphyxiation**

       ✓7ᵗʰ   **T17.528**   **Food in bronchus causing other injury**

    ✓6ᵗʰ   **T17.59**   **Other foreign object in bronchus**

       ✓7ᵗʰ   **T17.590**   **Other foreign object in bronchus causing asphyxiation**

       ✓7ᵗʰ   **T17.598**   **Other foreign object in bronchus causing other injury**

✓5ᵗʰ   **T17.8**   **Foreign body in other parts of respiratory tract**
Foreign body in bronchioles
Foreign body in lung

    ✓6ᵗʰ   **T17.80**   **Unspecified foreign body in other parts of respiratory tract**

       ✓7ᵗʰ   **T17.800**   **Unspecified foreign body in other parts of respiratory tract causing asphyxiation**

       ✓7ᵗʰ   **T17.808**   **Unspecified foreign body in other parts of respiratory tract causing other injury**

    ✓6ᵗʰ   **T17.81**   **Gastric contents in other parts of respiratory tract**
Aspiration of gastric contents into other parts of respiratory tract
Vomitus in other parts of respiratory tract

       ✓7ᵗʰ   **T17.810**   **Gastric contents in other parts of respiratory tract causing asphyxiation**

       ✓7ᵗʰ   **T17.818**   **Gastric contents in other parts of respiratory tract causing other injury**

    ✓6ᵗʰ   **T17.82**   **Food in other parts of respiratory tract**
Bones in other parts of respiratory tract
Seeds in other parts of respiratory tract

       ✓7ᵗʰ   **T17.820**   **Food in other parts of respiratory tract causing asphyxiation**

       ✓7ᵗʰ   **T17.828**   **Food in other parts of respiratory tract causing other injury**

    ✓6ᵗʰ   **T17.89**   **Other foreign object in other parts of respiratory tract**

       ✓7ᵗʰ   **T17.890**   **Other foreign object in other parts of respiratory tract causing asphyxiation**

       ✓7ᵗʰ   **T17.898**   **Other foreign object in other parts of respiratory tract causing other injury**

☑ Additional Character Required   ✓x7ᵗʰ Placeholder Alert   Unspecified Dx   Other Specified Dx   Manifestation   ▶◀ Revised Text   ● New Code   ▲ Revised Code Title

Chapter 19. Injury, Poisoning, and Certain Other Consequences of External Causes

T17.9–T20.05

√5ᵗʰ **T17.9　Foreign body in respiratory tract**, part unspecified
- √6ᵗʰ **T17.90　Unspecified foreign body in respiratory tract, part unspecified**
  - √7ᵗʰ **T17.900　Unspecified foreign body in respiratory tract, part unspecified** causing asphyxiation
  - √7ᵗʰ **T17.908　Unspecified foreign body in respiratory tract, part unspecified** causing other injury
- √6ᵗʰ **T17.91　Gastric contents in respiratory tract, part unspecified**
  Aspiration of gastric contents into respiratory tract, part unspecified
  Vomitus in trachea respiratory tract, part unspecified
  - √7ᵗʰ **T17.910　Gastric contents in respiratory tract, part unspecified** causing asphyxiation
  - √7ᵗʰ **T17.918　Gastric contents in respiratory tract, part unspecified** causing other injury
- √6ᵗʰ **T17.92　Food in respiratory tract, part unspecified**
  Bones in respiratory tract, part unspecified
  Seeds in respiratory tract, part unspecified
  - √7ᵗʰ **T17.920　Food in respiratory tract, part unspecified** causing asphyxiation
  - √7ᵗʰ **T17.928　Food in respiratory tract, part unspecified** causing other injury
- √6ᵗʰ **T17.99　Other foreign object in respiratory tract, part unspecified**
  - √7ᵗʰ **T17.990　Other foreign object in respiratory tract, part unspecified in** causing asphyxiation
  - √7ᵗʰ **T17.998　Other foreign object in respiratory tract, part unspecified** causing other injury

√4ᵗʰ **T18　Foreign body in alimentary tract**
> EXCLUDES 2　foreign body in pharynx (T17.2-)

The appropriate 7th character is to be added to each code from category T18.
A　initial encounter
D　subsequent encounter
S　sequela

√x7ᵗʰ **T18.0　Foreign body in mouth**
√5ᵗʰ **T18.1　Foreign body in esophagus**
> EXCLUDES 2　foreign body in respiratory tract (T17.-)

- √6ᵗʰ **T18.10　Unspecified foreign body in esophagus**
  - √7ᵗʰ **T18.100　Unspecified foreign body in esophagus causing compression of trachea**
    Unspecified foreign body in esophagus causing obstruction of respiration
  - √7ᵗʰ **T18.108　Unspecified foreign body in esophagus causing other injury**
- √6ᵗʰ **T18.11　Gastric contents in esophagus**
  Vomitus in esophagus
  - √7ᵗʰ **T18.110　Gastric contents in esophagus causing compression of trachea**
    Gastric contents in esophagus causing obstruction of respiration
  - √7ᵗʰ **T18.118　Gastric contents in esophagus causing other injury**
- √6ᵗʰ **T18.12　Food in esophagus**
  Bones in esophagus
  Seeds in esophagus
  - √7ᵗʰ **T18.120　Food in esophagus causing compression of trachea**
    Food in esophagus causing obstruction of respiration
  - √7ᵗʰ **T18.128　Food in esophagus causing other injury**
- √6ᵗʰ **T18.19　Other foreign object in esophagus**
  AHA: 2015, 1Q, 23
  - √7ᵗʰ **T18.190　Other foreign object in esophagus causing compression of trachea**
    Other foreign body in esophagus causing obstruction of respiration
  - √7ᵗʰ **T18.198　Other foreign object in esophagus causing other injury**

√x7ᵗʰ **T18.2　Foreign body in stomach**
√x7ᵗʰ **T18.3　Foreign body in small intestine**
√x7ᵗʰ **T18.4　Foreign body in colon**

√x7ᵗʰ **T18.5　Foreign body in anus and rectum**
　Foreign body in rectosigmoid (junction)
√x7ᵗʰ **T18.8　Foreign body in other parts of alimentary tract**
√x7ᵗʰ **T18.9　Foreign body of alimentary tract, part unspecified**
　Foreign body in digestive system NOS
　Swallowed foreign body NOS

√4ᵗʰ **T19　Foreign body in genitourinary tract**
> EXCLUDES 2　complications due to implanted mesh (T83.7-)
> mechanical complications of contraceptive device (intrauterine) (vaginal) (T83.3-)
> presence of contraceptive device (intrauterine) (vaginal) (Z97.5)

The appropriate 7th character is to be added to each code from category T19.
A　initial encounter
D　subsequent encounter
S　sequela

√x7ᵗʰ **T19.0　Foreign body in urethra**
√x7ᵗʰ **T19.1　Foreign body in bladder**
√x7ᵗʰ **T19.2　Foreign body in vulva and vagina**　♀
√x7ᵗʰ **T19.3　Foreign body in uterus**　♀
√x7ᵗʰ **T19.4　Foreign body in penis**　♂
√x7ᵗʰ **T19.8　Foreign body in other parts of genitourinary tract**
√x7ᵗʰ **T19.9　Foreign body in genitourinary tract, part unspecified**

Burns and corrosions (T20-T32)

> INCLUDES　burns (thermal) from electrical heating appliances
> burns (thermal) from electricity
> burns (thermal) from flame
> burns (thermal) from friction
> burns (thermal) from hot air and hot gases
> burns (thermal) from hot objects
> burns (thermal) from lightning
> burns (thermal) from radiation
> chemical burn [corrosion] (external) (internal)
> scalds
> EXCLUDES 2　erythema [dermatitis] ab igne (L59.0)
> radiation-related disorders of the skin and subcutaneous tissue (L55-L59)
> sunburn (L55.-)

Burns and corrosions of external body surface, specified by site (T20-T25)

> INCLUDES　burns and corrosions of first degree [erythema]
> burns and corrosions of second degree [blisters] [epidermal loss]
> burns and corrosions of third degree [deep necrosis of underlying tissue] [full-thickness skin loss]

Use additional code from category T31 or T32 to identify the extent of body surface involved

√4ᵗʰ **T20　Burn and corrosion of head, face, and neck**
> EXCLUDES 2　burn and corrosion of ear drum (T28.41, T28.91)
> burn and corrosion of eye and adnexa (T26.-)
> burn and corrosion of mouth and pharynx (T28.0)
> AHA: 2015, 1Q, 18-19

The appropriate 7th character is to be added to each code from category T20.
A　initial encounter
D　subsequent encounter
S　sequela

√5ᵗʰ **T20.0　Burn of unspecified degree of head, face, and neck**
　Use additional external cause code to identify the source, place and intent of the burn (X00-X19, X75-X77, X96-X98, Y92)
- √x7ᵗʰ **T20.00　Burn of unspecified degree of head, face, and neck, unspecified site**
- √6ᵗʰ **T20.01　Burn of unspecified degree of ear [any part, except ear drum]**
  > EXCLUDES 2　burn of ear drum (T28.41-)
  - √7ᵗʰ **T20.011　Burn of unspecified degree of right ear [any part, except ear drum]**
  - √7ᵗʰ **T20.012　Burn of unspecified degree of left ear [any part, except ear drum]**
  - √7ᵗʰ **T20.019　Burn of unspecified degree of unspecified ear [any part, except ear drum]**
- √x7ᵗʰ **T20.02　Burn of unspecified degree of lip(s)**
- √x7ᵗʰ **T20.03　Burn of unspecified degree of chin**
- √x7ᵗʰ **T20.04　Burn of unspecified degree of nose (septum)**
- √x7ᵗʰ **T20.05　Burn of unspecified degree of scalp [any part]**

✓x7ᵗʰ **T20.06** **Burn of unspecified degree of** forehead and cheek

✓x7ᵗʰ **T20.07** **Burn of unspecified degree of** neck

✓x7ᵗʰ **T20.09** **Burn of unspecified degree of** multiple sites **of head, face, and neck**

✓5ᵗʰ **T20.1** **Burn of** first degree **of head, face, and neck**
Use additional external cause code to identify the source, place and intent of the burn (X00-X19, X75-X77, X96-X98, Y92)

✓x7ᵗʰ **T20.10** **Burn of first degree of head, face, and neck, unspecified site**

✓6ᵗʰ **T20.11** **Burn of first degree of** ear [any part, except ear drum]
EXCLUDES 2   *burn of ear drum (T28.41-)*

✓7ᵗʰ **T20.111** **Burn of first degree of** right **ear [any part, except ear drum]**

✓7ᵗʰ **T20.112** **Burn of first degree of** left **ear [any part, except ear drum]**

✓7ᵗʰ **T20.119** **Burn of first degree of unspecified ear [any part, except ear drum]**

✓x7ᵗʰ **T20.12** **Burn of first degree of** lip(s)

✓x7ᵗʰ **T20.13** **Burn of first degree of** chin

✓x7ᵗʰ **T20.14** **Burn of first degree of** nose (septum)

✓x7ᵗʰ **T20.15** **Burn of first degree of** scalp [any part]

✓x7ᵗʰ **T20.16** **Burn of first degree of** forehead and cheek

✓x7ᵗʰ **T20.17** **Burn of first degree of** neck

✓x7ᵗʰ **T20.19** **Burn of first degree of** multiple sites **of head, face, and neck**

✓5ᵗʰ **T20.2** **Burn of** second degree **of head, face, and neck**
Use additional external cause code to identify the source, place and intent of the burn (X00-X19, X75-X77, X96-X98, Y92)

✓x7ᵗʰ **T20.20** **Burn of second degree of head, face, and neck, unspecified site**

✓6ᵗʰ **T20.21** **Burn of second degree of** ear [any part, except ear drum]
EXCLUDES 2   *burn of ear drum (T28.41-)*

✓7ᵗʰ **T20.211** **Burn of second degree of** right **ear [any part, except ear drum]**

✓7ᵗʰ **T20.212** **Burn of second degree of** left **ear [any part, except ear drum]**

✓7ᵗʰ **T20.219** **Burn of second degree of unspecified ear [any part, except ear drum]**

✓x7ᵗʰ **T20.22** **Burn of second degree of** lip(s)

✓x7ᵗʰ **T20.23** **Burn of second degree of** chin

✓x7ᵗʰ **T20.24** **Burn of second degree of** nose (septum)

✓x7ᵗʰ **T20.25** **Burn of second degree of** scalp [any part]

✓x7ᵗʰ **T20.26** **Burn of second degree of** forehead and cheek

✓x7ᵗʰ **T20.27** **Burn of second degree of** neck

✓x7ᵗʰ **T20.29** **Burn of second degree of** multiple sites **of head, face, and neck**

✓5ᵗʰ **T20.3** **Burn of** third degree **of head, face, and neck**
Use additional external cause code to identify the source, place and intent of the burn (X00-X19, X75-X77, X96-X98, Y92)

✓x7ᵗʰ **T20.30** **Burn of third degree of head, face, and neck, unspecified site**

✓6ᵗʰ **T20.31** **Burn of third degree of** ear [any part, except ear drum]
EXCLUDES 2   *burn of ear drum (T28.41-)*
AHA: 2015, 1Q, 18

✓7ᵗʰ **T20.311** **Burn of third degree of** right **ear [any part, except ear drum]**

✓7ᵗʰ **T20.312** **Burn of third degree of** left **ear [any part, except ear drum]**

✓7ᵗʰ **T20.319** **Burn of third degree of unspecified ear [any part, except ear drum]**

✓x7ᵗʰ **T20.32** **Burn of third degree of** lip(s)

✓x7ᵗʰ **T20.33** **Burn of third degree of** chin

✓x7ᵗʰ **T20.34** **Burn of third degree of** nose (septum)

✓x7ᵗʰ **T20.35** **Burn of third degree of** scalp [any part]

✓x7ᵗʰ **T20.36** **Burn of third degree of** forehead and cheek

✓x7ᵗʰ **T20.37** **Burn of third degree of** neck

✓x7ᵗʰ **T20.39** **Burn of third degree of** multiple sites **of head, face, and neck**

✓5ᵗʰ **T20.4** **Corrosion of** unspecified degree **of head, face, and neck**
Code first (T51-T65) to identify chemical and intent
Use additional external cause code to identify place (Y92)

✓x7ᵗʰ **T20.40** **Corrosion of unspecified degree of head, face, and neck, unspecified site**

✓6ᵗʰ **T20.41** **Corrosion of unspecified degree of** ear [any part, except ear drum]
EXCLUDES 2   *corrosion of ear drum (T28.91-)*

✓7ᵗʰ **T20.411** **Corrosion of unspecified degree of** right **ear [any part, except ear drum]**

✓7ᵗʰ **T20.412** **Corrosion of unspecified degree of** left **ear [any part, except ear drum]**

✓7ᵗʰ **T20.419** **Corrosion of unspecified degree of unspecified ear [any part, except ear drum]**

✓x7ᵗʰ **T20.42** **Corrosion of unspecified degree of** lip(s)

✓x7ᵗʰ **T20.43** **Corrosion of unspecified degree of** chin

✓x7ᵗʰ **T20.44** **Corrosion of unspecified degree of** nose (septum)

✓x7ᵗʰ **T20.45** **Corrosion of unspecified degree of** scalp [any part]

✓x7ᵗʰ **T20.46** **Corrosion of unspecified degree of** forehead and cheek

✓x7ᵗʰ **T20.47** **Corrosion of unspecified degree of** neck

✓x7ᵗʰ **T20.49** **Corrosion of unspecified degree of** multiple sites **of head, face, and neck**

✓5ᵗʰ **T20.5** **Corrosion of** first degree **of head, face, and neck**
Code first (T51-T65) to identify chemical and intent
Use additional external cause code to identify place (Y92)

✓x7ᵗʰ **T20.50** **Corrosion of first degree of head, face, and neck, unspecified site**

✓6ᵗʰ **T20.51** **Corrosion of first degree of** ear [any part, except ear drum]
EXCLUDES 2   *corrosion of ear drum (T28.91-)*

✓7ᵗʰ **T20.511** **Corrosion of first degree of** right **ear [any part, except ear drum]**

✓7ᵗʰ **T20.512** **Corrosion of first degree of** left **ear [any part, except ear drum]**

✓7ᵗʰ **T20.519** **Corrosion of first degree of unspecified ear [any part, except ear drum]**

✓x7ᵗʰ **T20.52** **Corrosion of first degree of** lip(s)

✓x7ᵗʰ **T20.53** **Corrosion of first degree of** chin

✓x7ᵗʰ **T20.54** **Corrosion of first degree of** nose (septum)

✓x7ᵗʰ **T20.55** **Corrosion of first degree of** scalp [any part]

✓x7ᵗʰ **T20.56** **Corrosion of first degree of** forehead and cheek

✓x7ᵗʰ **T20.57** **Corrosion of first degree of** neck

✓x7ᵗʰ **T20.59** **Corrosion of first degree of** multiple sites **of head, face, and neck**

✓5ᵗʰ **T20.6** **Corrosion of** second degree **of head, face, and neck**
Code first (T51-T65) to identify chemical and intent
Use additional external cause code to identify place (Y92)

✓x7ᵗʰ **T20.60** **Corrosion of second degree of head, face, and neck, unspecified site**

✓6ᵗʰ **T20.61** **Corrosion of second degree of** ear [any part, except ear drum]
EXCLUDES 2   *corrosion of ear drum (T28.91-)*

✓7ᵗʰ **T20.611** **Corrosion of second degree of** right **ear [any part, except ear drum]**

✓7ᵗʰ **T20.612** **Corrosion of second degree of** left **ear [any part, except ear drum]**

✓7ᵗʰ **T20.619** **Corrosion of second degree of unspecified ear [any part, except ear drum]**

✓x7ᵗʰ **T20.62** **Corrosion of second degree of** lip(s)

✓x7ᵗʰ **T20.63** **Corrosion of second degree of** chin

✓x7ᵗʰ **T20.64** **Corrosion of second degree of** nose (septum)

✓x7ᵗʰ **T20.65** **Corrosion of second degree of** scalp [any part]

✓x7ᵗʰ **T20.66** **Corrosion of second degree of** forehead and cheek

✓x7ᵗʰ **T20.67** **Corrosion of second degree of** neck

✓x7ᵗʰ **T20.69** **Corrosion of second degree of** multiple sites **of head, face, and neck**

✓ Additional Character Required   ✓x7ᵗʰ Placeholder Alert   Unspecified Dx   Other Specified Dx   Manifestation   ▶◀ Revised Text   ● New Code   ▲ Revised Code Title

Chapter 19. Injury, Poisoning, and Certain Other Consequences of External Causes (side margin)

T20.7–T21.45 (side margin)

✓5ᵗʰ **T20.7 Corrosion of** third degree **of head, face, and neck**
Code first (T51-T65) to identify chemical and intent
Use additional external cause code to identify place (Y92)

✓ₓ7ᵗʰ **T20.70 Corrosion of third degree of head, face, and neck, unspecified site**

✓6ᵗʰ **T20.71 Corrosion of third degree of** ear [any part, except ear drum]
EXCLUDES 2 *corrosion of ear drum (T28.91-)*

✓7ᵗʰ **T20.711 Corrosion of third degree of** right **ear [any part, except ear drum]**

✓7ᵗʰ **T20.712 Corrosion of third degree of** left **ear [any part, except ear drum]**

✓7ᵗʰ **T20.719 Corrosion of third degree of unspecified ear [any part, except ear drum]**

✓ₓ7ᵗʰ **T20.72 Corrosion of third degree of** lip(s)

✓ₓ7ᵗʰ **T20.73 Corrosion of third degree of** chin

✓ₓ7ᵗʰ **T20.74 Corrosion of third degree of** nose (septum)

✓ₓ7ᵗʰ **T20.75 Corrosion of third degree of** scalp [any part]

✓ₓ7ᵗʰ **T20.76 Corrosion of third degree of** forehead and cheek

✓ₓ7ᵗʰ **T20.77 Corrosion of third degree of** neck

✓ₓ7ᵗʰ **T20.79 Corrosion of third degree of** multiple sites **of head, face, and neck**

✓4ᵗʰ **T21 Burn and corrosion of trunk**
Burns and corrosion of hip region
EXCLUDES 2 *burns and corrosion of axilla (T22.- with fifth character 4)*
burns and corrosion of scapular region (T22.- with fifth character 6)
burns and corrosion of shoulder (T22.- with fifth character 5)

The appropriate 7th character is to be added to each code from category T21.
A   initial encounter
D   subsequent encounter
S   sequela

✓5ᵗʰ **T21.0 Burn of** unspecified degree **of trunk**
Use additional external cause code to identify the source, place and intent of the burn (X00-X19, X75-X77, X96-X98, Y92)

✓ₓ7ᵗʰ **T21.00 Burn of unspecified degree of trunk, unspecified site**

✓ₓ7ᵗʰ **T21.01 Burn of unspecified degree of** chest wall
Burn of of unspecified degree of breast

✓ₓ7ᵗʰ **T21.02 Burn of unspecified degree of** abdominal wall
Burn of unspecified degree of flank
Burn of unspecified degree of groin

✓ₓ7ᵗʰ **T21.03 Burn of unspecified degree of** upper back
Burn of unspecified degree of interscapular region

✓ₓ7ᵗʰ **T21.04 Burn of unspecified degree of** lower back

✓ₓ7ᵗʰ **T21.05 Burn of unspecified degree of** buttock
Burn of unspecified degree of anus

✓ₓ7ᵗʰ **T21.06 Burn of unspecified degree of** male genital region ♂
Burn of unspecified degree of penis
Burn of unspecified degree of scrotum
Burn of unspecified degree of testis

✓ₓ7ᵗʰ **T21.07 Burn of unspecified degree of** female genital region ♀
Burn of unspecified degree of labium (majus) (minus)
Burn of unspecified degree of perineum
Burn of unspecified degree of vulva
EXCLUDES 2 *burn of vagina (T28.3)*

✓ₓ7ᵗʰ **T21.09 Burn of unspecified degree of other site of trunk**

✓5ᵗʰ **T21.1 Burn of** first degree **of trunk**
Use additional external cause code to identify the source, place and intent of the burn (X00-X19, X75-X77, X96-X98, Y92)

✓ₓ7ᵗʰ **T21.10 Burn of first degree of trunk, unspecified site**

✓ₓ7ᵗʰ **T21.11 Burn of first degree of** chest wall
Burn of first degree of breast

✓ₓ7ᵗʰ **T21.12 Burn of first degree of** abdominal wall
Burn of first degree of flank
Burn of first degree of groin

✓ₓ7ᵗʰ **T21.13 Burn of first degree of** upper back
Burn of first degree of interscapular region

✓ₓ7ᵗʰ **T21.14 Burn of first degree of** lower back

✓ₓ7ᵗʰ **T21.15 Burn of first degree of** buttock
Burn of first degree of anus

✓ₓ7ᵗʰ **T21.16 Burn of first degree of** male genital region ♂
Burn of first degree of penis
Burn of first degree of scrotum
Burn of first degree of testis

✓ₓ7ᵗʰ **T21.17 Burn of first degree of** female genital region ♀
Burn of first degree of labium (majus) (minus)
Burn of first degree of perineum
Burn of first degree of vulva
EXCLUDES 2 *burn of vagina (T28.3)*

✓ₓ7ᵗʰ **T21.19 Burn of first degree of other site of trunk**

✓5ᵗʰ **T21.2 Burn of** second degree **of trunk**
Use additional external cause code to identify the source, place and intent of the burn (X00-X19, X75-X77, X96-X98, Y92)

✓ₓ7ᵗʰ **T21.20 Burn of second degree of trunk, unspecified site**

✓ₓ7ᵗʰ **T21.21 Burn of second degree of** chest wall
Burn of second degree of breast

✓ₓ7ᵗʰ **T21.22 Burn of second degree of** abdominal wall
Burn of second degree of flank
Burn of second degree of groin

✓ₓ7ᵗʰ **T21.23 Burn of second degree of** upper back
Burn of second degree of interscapular region

✓ₓ7ᵗʰ **T21.24 Burn of second degree of** lower back

✓ₓ7ᵗʰ **T21.25 Burn of second degree of** buttock
Burn of second degree of anus

✓ₓ7ᵗʰ **T21.26 Burn of second degree of** male genital region ♂
Burn of second degree of penis
Burn of second degree of scrotum
Burn of second degree of testis

✓ₓ7ᵗʰ **T21.27 Burn of second degree of** female genital region ♀
Burn of second degree of labium (majus) (minus)
Burn of second degree of perineum
Burn of second degree of vulva
EXCLUDES 2 *burn of vagina (T28.3)*

✓ₓ7ᵗʰ **T21.29 Burn of second degree of other site of trunk**

✓5ᵗʰ **T21.3 Burn of** third degree **of trunk**
Use additional external cause code to identify the source, place and intent of the burn (X00-X19, X75-X77, X96-X98, Y92)

✓ₓ7ᵗʰ **T21.30 Burn of third degree of trunk, unspecified site**

✓ₓ7ᵗʰ **T21.31 Burn of third degree of** chest wall
Burn of third degree of breast

✓ₓ7ᵗʰ **T21.32 Burn of third degree of** abdominal wall
Burn of third degree of flank
Burn of third degree of groin

✓ₓ7ᵗʰ **T21.33 Burn of third degree of** upper back
Burn of third degree of interscapular region

✓ₓ7ᵗʰ **T21.34 Burn of third degree of** lower back

✓ₓ7ᵗʰ **T21.35 Burn of third degree of** buttock
Burn of third degree of anus

✓ₓ7ᵗʰ **T21.36 Burn of third degree of** male genital region ♂
Burn of third degree of penis
Burn of third degree of scrotum
Burn of third degree of testis

✓ₓ7ᵗʰ **T21.37 Burn of third degree of** female genital region ♀
Burn of third degree of labium (majus) (minus)
Burn of third degree of perineum
Burn of third degree of vulva
EXCLUDES 2 *burn of vagina (T28.3)*

✓ₓ7ᵗʰ **T21.39 Burn of third degree of other site of trunk**

✓5ᵗʰ **T21.4 Corrosion of** unspecified degree **of trunk**
Code first (T51-T65) to identify chemical and intent
Use additional external cause code to identify place (Y92)

✓ₓ7ᵗʰ **T21.40 Corrosion of unspecified degree of trunk, unspecified site**

✓ₓ7ᵗʰ **T21.41 Corrosion of unspecified degree of** chest wall
Corrosion of unspecified degree of breast

✓ₓ7ᵗʰ **T21.42 Corrosion of unspecified degree of** abdominal wall
Corrosion of unspecified degree of flank
Corrosion of unspecified degree of groin

✓ₓ7ᵗʰ **T21.43 Corrosion of unspecified degree of** upper back
Corrosion of unspecified degree of interscapular region

✓ₓ7ᵗʰ **T21.44 Corrosion of unspecified degree of** lower back

✓ₓ7ᵗʰ **T21.45 Corrosion of unspecified degree of** buttock
Corrosion of unspecified degree of anus

EXCLUDES 1 Not coded here   EXCLUDES 2 Not included here   N Newborn Age: 0   P Pediatric Age: 0-17   M Maternity Age: 12-55   A Adult Age: 15-124

968   **ICD-10-CM 2016**

✓x7ᵗʰ **T21.46** **Corrosion of unspecified degree of** male genital ♂
region
Corrosion of unspecified degree of penis
Corrosion of unspecified degree of scrotum
Corrosion of unspecified degree of testis

✓x7ᵗʰ **T21.47** **Corrosion of unspecified degree of** female genital ♀
region
Corrosion of unspecified degree of labium (majus)
(minus)
Corrosion of unspecified degree of perineum
Corrosion of unspecified degree of vulva
EXCLUDES 2   *corrosion of vagina (T28.8)*

✓x7ᵗʰ **T21.49** **Corrosion of unspecified degree of other site of**
trunk

✓5ᵗʰ **T21.5** **Corrosion of** first degree **of trunk**
Code first (T51-T65) to identify chemical and intent
Use additional external cause code to identify place (Y92)

✓x7ᵗʰ **T21.50** **Corrosion of first degree of trunk, unspecified site**

✓x7ᵗʰ **T21.51** **Corrosion of first degree of** chest wall
Corrosion of first degree of breast

✓x7ᵗʰ **T21.52** **Corrosion of first degree of** abdominal wall
Corrosion of first degree of flank
Corrosion of first degree of groin

✓x7ᵗʰ **T21.53** **Corrosion of first degree of** upper back
Corrosion of first degree of interscapular region

✓x7ᵗʰ **T21.54** **Corrosion of first degree of** lower back

✓x7ᵗʰ **T21.55** **Corrosion of first degree of** buttock
Corrosion of first degree of anus

✓x7ᵗʰ **T21.56** **Corrosion of first degree of** male genital region ♂
Corrosion of first degree of penis
Corrosion of first degree of scrotum
Corrosion of first degree of testis

✓x7ᵗʰ **T21.57** **Corrosion of first degree of** female genital region ♀
Corrosion of first degree of labium (majus) (minus)
Corrosion of first degree of perineum
Corrosion of first degree of vulva
EXCLUDES 2   *corrosion of vagina (T28.8)*

✓x7ᵗʰ **T21.59** **Corrosion of first degree of other site of trunk**

✓5ᵗʰ **T21.6** **Corrosion of** second degree **of trunk**
Code first (T51-T65) to identify chemical and intent
Use additional external cause code to identify place (Y92)

✓x7ᵗʰ **T21.60** **Corrosion of second degree of trunk, unspecified site**

✓x7ᵗʰ **T21.61** **Corrosion of second degree of** chest wall
Corrosion of second degree of breast

✓x7ᵗʰ **T21.62** **Corrosion of second degree of** abdominal wall
Corrosion of second degree of flank
Corrosion of second degree of groin

✓x7ᵗʰ **T21.63** **Corrosion of second degree of** upper back
Corrosion of second degree of interscapular region

✓x7ᵗʰ **T21.64** **Corrosion of second degree of** lower back

✓x7ᵗʰ **T21.65** **Corrosion of second degree of** buttock
Corrosion of second degree of anus

✓x7ᵗʰ **T21.66** **Corrosion of second degree of** male genital region ♂
Corrosion of second degree of penis
Corrosion of second degree of scrotum
Corrosion of second degree of testis

✓x7ᵗʰ **T21.67** **Corrosion of second degree of** female genital ♀
region
Corrosion of second degree of labium (majus) (minus)
Corrosion of second degree of perineum
Corrosion of second degree of vulva
EXCLUDES 2   *corrosion of vagina (T28.8)*

✓x7ᵗʰ **T21.69** **Corrosion of second degree of other site of trunk**

✓5ᵗʰ **T21.7** **Corrosion of** third degree **of trunk**
Code first (T51-T65) to identify chemical and intent
Use additional external cause code to identify place (Y92)

✓x7ᵗʰ **T21.70** **Corrosion of third degree of trunk, unspecified site**

✓x7ᵗʰ **T21.71** **Corrosion of third degree of** chest wall
Corrosion of third degree of breast

✓x7ᵗʰ **T21.72** **Corrosion of third degree of** abdominal wall
Corrosion of third degree of flank
Corrosion of third degree of groin

✓x7ᵗʰ **T21.73** **Corrosion of third degree of** upper back
Corrosion of third degree of interscapular region

✓x7ᵗʰ **T21.74** **Corrosion of third degree of** lower back

✓x7ᵗʰ **T21.75** **Corrosion of third degree of** buttock
Corrosion of third degree of anus

✓x7ᵗʰ **T21.76** **Corrosion of third degree of** male genital region ♂
Corrosion of third degree of penis
Corrosion of third degree of scrotum
Corrosion of third degree of testis

✓x7ᵗʰ **T21.77** **Corrosion of third degree of** female genital region ♀
Corrosion of third degree of labium (majus) (minus)
Corrosion of third degree of perineum
Corrosion of third degree of vulva
EXCLUDES 2   *corrosion of vagina (T28.8)*

✓x7ᵗʰ **T21.79** **Corrosion of third degree of other site of trunk**

✓4ᵗʰ **T22** **Burn and corrosion of shoulder and upper limb, except wrist and**
hand
EXCLUDES 2   *burn and corrosion of interscapular region (T21.-)*
burn and corrosion of wrist and hand (T23.-)

> The appropriate 7th character is to be added to each code from
> category T22.
> A   initial encounter
> D   subsequent encounter
> S   sequela

✓5ᵗʰ **T22.0** **Burn of** unspecified degree **of shoulder and upper limb,**
except wrist and hand
Use additional external cause code to identify the source, place
and intent of the burn (X00-X19, X75-X77, X96-X98, Y92)

✓x7ᵗʰ **T22.00** **Burn of unspecified degree of shoulder and upper**
limb, except wrist and hand, unspecified site

✓6ᵗʰ **T22.01** **Burn of unspecified degree of** forearm

✓7ᵗʰ **T22.011** **Burn of unspecified degree of** right
forearm

✓7ᵗʰ **T22.012** **Burn of unspecified degree of** left forearm

✓7ᵗʰ **T22.019** **Burn of unspecified degree of** unspecified
forearm

✓6ᵗʰ **T22.02** **Burn of unspecified degree of** elbow

✓7ᵗʰ **T22.021** **Burn of unspecified degree of** right elbow

✓7ᵗʰ **T22.022** **Burn of unspecified degree of** left elbow

✓7ᵗʰ **T22.029** **Burn of unspecified degree of** unspecified
elbow

✓6ᵗʰ **T22.03** **Burn of unspecified degree of** upper arm

✓7ᵗʰ **T22.031** **Burn of unspecified degree of** right upper
arm

✓7ᵗʰ **T22.032** **Burn of unspecified degree of** left upper
arm

✓7ᵗʰ **T22.039** **Burn of unspecified degree of** unspecified
upper arm

✓6ᵗʰ **T22.04** **Burn of unspecified degree of** axilla

✓7ᵗʰ **T22.041** **Burn of unspecified degree of** right axilla

✓7ᵗʰ **T22.042** **Burn of unspecified degree of** left axilla

✓7ᵗʰ **T22.049** **Burn of unspecified degree of** unspecified
axilla

✓6ᵗʰ **T22.05** **Burn of unspecified degree of** shoulder

✓7ᵗʰ **T22.051** **Burn of unspecified degree of** right
shoulder

✓7ᵗʰ **T22.052** **Burn of unspecified degree of** left
shoulder

✓7ᵗʰ **T22.059** **Burn of unspecified degree of** unspecified
shoulder

✓6ᵗʰ **T22.06** **Burn of unspecified degree of** scapular region

✓7ᵗʰ **T22.061** **Burn of unspecified degree of** right
scapular region

✓7ᵗʰ **T22.062** **Burn of unspecified degree of** left scapular
region

✓7ᵗʰ **T22.069** **Burn of unspecified degree of** unspecified
scapular region

✓6ᵗʰ **T22.09** **Burn of unspecified degree of** multiple sites of
shoulder and upper limb, except wrist and hand

✓7ᵗʰ **T22.091** **Burn of unspecified degree of multiple**
sites of right shoulder and upper limb,
except wrist and hand

✓7ᵗʰ **T22.092** **Burn of unspecified degree of multiple**
sites of left shoulder and upper limb,
except wrist and hand

✓ Additional Character Required   ✓x7ᵗʰ Placeholder Alert   Unspecified Dx   Other Specified Dx   Manifestation   ▶◀ Revised Text   ● New Code   ▲ Revised Code Title

√7th **T22.099** **Burn of unspecified degree of multiple sites of unspecified shoulder and upper limb, except wrist and hand**

√5th **T22.1** **Burn of** first degree **of shoulder and upper limb, except wrist and hand**
> Use additional external cause code to identify the source, place and intent of the burn (X00-X19, X75-X77, X96-X98, Y92)

√x7th **T22.10** **Burn of first degree of shoulder and upper limb, except wrist and hand,** unspecified site

√6th **T22.11** **Burn of first degree of** forearm
- √7th **T22.111** Burn of first degree of right forearm
- √7th **T22.112** Burn of first degree of left forearm
- √7th **T22.119** **Burn of first degree of unspecified forearm**

√6th **T22.12** **Burn of first degree of** elbow
- √7th **T22.121** Burn of first degree of right elbow
- √7th **T22.122** Burn of first degree of left elbow
- √7th **T22.129** **Burn of first degree of unspecified elbow**

√6th **T22.13** **Burn of first degree of** upper arm
- √7th **T22.131** Burn of first degree of right upper arm
- √7th **T22.132** Burn of first degree of left upper arm
- √7th **T22.139** **Burn of first degree of unspecified upper arm**

√6th **T22.14** **Burn of first degree of** axilla
- √7th **T22.141** Burn of first degree of right axilla
- √7th **T22.142** Burn of first degree of left axilla
- √7th **T22.149** **Burn of first degree of unspecified axilla**

√6th **T22.15** **Burn of first degree of** shoulder
- √7th **T22.151** Burn of first degree of right shoulder
- √7th **T22.152** Burn of first degree of left shoulder
- √7th **T22.159** **Burn of first degree of unspecified shoulder**

√6th **T22.16** **Burn of first degree of** scapular region
- √7th **T22.161** **Burn of first degree of** right scapular region
- √7th **T22.162** Burn of first degree of left scapular region
- √7th **T22.169** **Burn of first degree of unspecified scapular region**

√6th **T22.19** **Burn of first degree of** multiple sites **of shoulder and upper limb, except wrist and hand**
- √7th **T22.191** Burn of first degree of multiple sites of right shoulder and upper limb, except wrist and hand
- √7th **T22.192** Burn of first degree of multiple sites of left shoulder and upper limb, except wrist and hand
- √7th **T22.199** **Burn of first degree of multiple sites of unspecified shoulder and upper limb, except wrist and hand**

√5th **T22.2** **Burn of** second degree **of shoulder and upper limb, except wrist and hand**
> Use additional external cause code to identify the source, place and intent of the burn (X00-X19, X75-X77, X96-X98, Y92)

√x7th **T22.20** **Burn of second degree of shoulder and upper limb, except wrist and hand, unspecified site**

√6th **T22.21** **Burn of second degree of** forearm
- √7th **T22.211** Burn of second degree of right forearm
- √7th **T22.212** Burn of second degree of left forearm
- √7th **T22.219** **Burn of second degree of unspecified forearm**

√6th **T22.22** **Burn of second degree of** elbow
- √7th **T22.221** Burn of second degree of right elbow
- √7th **T22.222** Burn of second degree of left elbow
- √7th **T22.229** **Burn of second degree of unspecified elbow**

√6th **T22.23** **Burn of second degree of** upper arm
- √7th **T22.231** Burn of second degree of right upper arm
- √7th **T22.232** Burn of second degree of left upper arm
- √7th **T22.239** **Burn of second degree of unspecified upper arm**

√6th **T22.24** **Burn of second degree of** axilla
- √7th **T22.241** Burn of second degree of right axilla
- √7th **T22.242** Burn of second degree of left axilla
- √7th **T22.249** **Burn of second degree of unspecified axilla**

√6th **T22.25** **Burn of second degree of** shoulder
- √7th **T22.251** Burn of second degree of right shoulder
- √7th **T22.252** Burn of second degree of left shoulder
- √7th **T22.259** **Burn of second degree of unspecified shoulder**

√6th **T22.26** **Burn of second degree of** scapular region
- √7th **T22.261** **Burn of second degree of** right scapular region
- √7th **T22.262** Burn of second degree of left scapular region
- √7th **T22.269** **Burn of second degree of unspecified scapular region**

√6th **T22.29** **Burn of second degree of** multiple sites **of shoulder and upper limb, except wrist and hand**
- √7th **T22.291** Burn of second degree of multiple sites of right shoulder and upper limb, except wrist and hand
- √7th **T22.292** Burn of second degree of multiple sites of left shoulder and upper limb, except wrist and hand
- √7th **T22.299** **Burn of second degree of multiple sites of unspecified shoulder and upper limb, except wrist and hand**

√5th **T22.3** **Burn of** third degree **of shoulder and upper limb, except wrist and hand**
> Use additional external cause code to identify the source, place and intent of the burn (X00-X19, X75-X77, X96-X98, Y92)

√x7th **T22.30** **Burn of third degree of shoulder and upper limb, except wrist and hand, unspecified site**

√6th **T22.31** **Burn of third degree of** forearm
- √7th **T22.311** Burn of third degree of right forearm
- √7th **T22.312** Burn of third degree of left forearm
- √7th **T22.319** **Burn of third degree of unspecified forearm**

√6th **T22.32** **Burn of third degree of** elbow
- √7th **T22.321** Burn of third degree of right elbow
- √7th **T22.322** Burn of third degree of left elbow
- √7th **T22.329** **Burn of third degree of unspecified elbow**

√6th **T22.33** **Burn of third degree of** upper arm
- √7th **T22.331** Burn of third degree of right upper arm
- √7th **T22.332** Burn of third degree of left upper arm
- √7th **T22.339** **Burn of third degree of unspecified upper arm**

√6th **T22.34** **Burn of third degree of** axilla
- √7th **T22.341** Burn of third degree of right axilla
- √7th **T22.342** Burn of third degree of left axilla
- √7th **T22.349** **Burn of third degree of unspecified axilla**

√6th **T22.35** **Burn of third degree of** shoulder
- √7th **T22.351** Burn of third degree of right shoulder
- √7th **T22.352** Burn of third degree of left shoulder
- √7th **T22.359** **Burn of third degree of unspecified shoulder**

√6th **T22.36** **Burn of third degree of** scapular region
- √7th **T22.361** **Burn of third degree of** right scapular region
- √7th **T22.362** Burn of third degree of left scapular region
- √7th **T22.369** **Burn of third degree of unspecified scapular region**

√6th **T22.39** **Burn of third degree of** multiple sites **of shoulder and upper limb, except wrist and hand**
- √7th **T22.391** Burn of third degree of multiple sites of right shoulder and upper limb, except wrist and hand
- √7th **T22.392** Burn of third degree of multiple sites of left shoulder and upper limb, except wrist and hand

EXCLUDES 1 Not coded here | EXCLUDES 2 Not included here | N Newborn Age: 0 | P Pediatric Age: 0-17 | M Maternity Age: 12-55 | A Adult Age: 15-124

970

ICD-10-CM 2016

✓7ᵗʰ **T22.399** **Burn of third degree of multiple sites of unspecified shoulder and upper limb, except wrist and hand**

✓5ᵗʰ **T22.4** **Corrosion of** unspecified degree **of shoulder and upper limb, except wrist and hand**
 Code first (T51-T65) to identify chemical and intent
 Use additional external cause code to identify place (Y92)

 ✓x7ᵗʰ **T22.40** **Corrosion of unspecified degree of shoulder and upper limb, except wrist and hand, unspecified site**

 ✓6ᵗʰ **T22.41** **Corrosion of unspecified degree of** forearm
  ✓7ᵗʰ **T22.411** **Corrosion of unspecified degree of** right **forearm**
  ✓7ᵗʰ **T22.412** **Corrosion of unspecified degree of** left **forearm**
  ✓7ᵗʰ **T22.419** **Corrosion of unspecified degree of unspecified forearm**

 ✓6ᵗʰ **T22.42** **Corrosion of unspecified degree of** elbow
  ✓7ᵗʰ **T22.421** **Corrosion of unspecified degree of** right **elbow**
  ✓7ᵗʰ **T22.422** **Corrosion of unspecified degree of** left **elbow**
  ✓7ᵗʰ **T22.429** **Corrosion of unspecified degree of unspecified elbow**

 ✓6ᵗʰ **T22.43** **Corrosion of unspecified degree of** upper arm
  ✓7ᵗʰ **T22.431** **Corrosion of unspecified degree of** right **upper arm**
  ✓7ᵗʰ **T22.432** **Corrosion of unspecified degree of** left **upper arm**
  ✓7ᵗʰ **T22.439** **Corrosion of unspecified degree of unspecified upper arm**

 ✓6ᵗʰ **T22.44** **Corrosion of unspecified degree of** axilla
  ✓7ᵗʰ **T22.441** **Corrosion of unspecified degree of** right **axilla**
  ✓7ᵗʰ **T22.442** **Corrosion of unspecified degree of** left **axilla**
  ✓7ᵗʰ **T22.449** **Corrosion of unspecified degree of unspecified axilla**

 ✓6ᵗʰ **T22.45** **Corrosion of unspecified degree of** shoulder
  ✓7ᵗʰ **T22.451** **Corrosion of unspecified degree of** right **shoulder**
  ✓7ᵗʰ **T22.452** **Corrosion of unspecified degree of** left **shoulder**
  ✓7ᵗʰ **T22.459** **Corrosion of unspecified degree of unspecified shoulder**

 ✓6ᵗʰ **T22.46** **Corrosion of unspecified degree of** scapular region
  ✓7ᵗʰ **T22.461** **Corrosion of unspecified degree of** right **scapular region**
  ✓7ᵗʰ **T22.462** **Corrosion of unspecified degree of** left **scapular region**
  ✓7ᵗʰ **T22.469** **Corrosion of unspecified degree of unspecified scapular region**

 ✓6ᵗʰ **T22.49** **Corrosion of unspecified degree of** multiple sites **of shoulder and upper limb, except wrist and hand**
  ✓7ᵗʰ **T22.491** **Corrosion of unspecified degree of multiple sites of** right **shoulder and upper limb, except wrist and hand**
  ✓7ᵗʰ **T22.492** **Corrosion of unspecified degree of multiple sites of** left **shoulder and upper limb, except wrist and hand**
  ✓7ᵗʰ **T22.499** **Corrosion of unspecified degree of multiple sites of unspecified shoulder and upper limb, except wrist and hand**

✓5ᵗʰ **T22.5** **Corrosion of** first degree **of shoulder and upper limb, except wrist and hand**
 Code first (T51-T65) to identify chemical and intent
 Use additional external cause code to identify place (Y92)

 ✓x7ᵗʰ **T22.50** **Corrosion of first degree of shoulder and upper limb, except wrist and hand unspecified site**

 ✓6ᵗʰ **T22.51** **Corrosion of first degree of** forearm
  ✓7ᵗʰ **T22.511** **Corrosion of first degree of** right **forearm**
  ✓7ᵗʰ **T22.512** **Corrosion of first degree of** left **forearm**
  ✓7ᵗʰ **T22.519** **Corrosion of first degree of unspecified forearm**

 ✓6ᵗʰ **T22.52** **Corrosion of first degree of** elbow
  ✓7ᵗʰ **T22.521** **Corrosion of first degree of** right **elbow**
  ✓7ᵗʰ **T22.522** **Corrosion of first degree of** left **elbow**
  ✓7ᵗʰ **T22.529** **Corrosion of first degree of unspecified elbow**

 ✓6ᵗʰ **T22.53** **Corrosion of first degree of** upper arm
  ✓7ᵗʰ **T22.531** **Corrosion of first degree of** right **upper arm**
  ✓7ᵗʰ **T22.532** **Corrosion of first degree of** left **upper arm**
  ✓7ᵗʰ **T22.539** **Corrosion of first degree of unspecified upper arm**

 ✓6ᵗʰ **T22.54** **Corrosion of first degree of** axilla
  ✓7ᵗʰ **T22.541** **Corrosion of first degree of** right **axilla**
  ✓7ᵗʰ **T22.542** **Corrosion of first degree of** left **axilla**
  ✓7ᵗʰ **T22.549** **Corrosion of first degree of unspecified axilla**

 ✓6ᵗʰ **T22.55** **Corrosion of first degree of** shoulder
  ✓7ᵗʰ **T22.551** **Corrosion of first degree of** right **shoulder**
  ✓7ᵗʰ **T22.552** **Corrosion of first degree of** left **shoulder**
  ✓7ᵗʰ **T22.559** **Corrosion of first degree of unspecified shoulder**

 ✓6ᵗʰ **T22.56** **Corrosion of first degree of** scapular region
  ✓7ᵗʰ **T22.561** **Corrosion of first degree of** right **scapular region**
  ✓7ᵗʰ **T22.562** **Corrosion of first degree of** left **scapular region**
  ✓7ᵗʰ **T22.569** **Corrosion of first degree of unspecified scapular region**

 ✓6ᵗʰ **T22.59** **Corrosion of first degree of** multiple sites **of shoulder and upper limb, except wrist and hand**
  ✓7ᵗʰ **T22.591** **Corrosion of first degree of multiple sites of** right **shoulder and upper limb, except wrist and hand**
  ✓7ᵗʰ **T22.592** **Corrosion of first degree of multiple sites of** left **shoulder and upper limb, except wrist and hand**
  ✓7ᵗʰ **T22.599** **Corrosion of first degree of multiple sites of unspecified shoulder and upper limb, except wrist and hand**

✓5ᵗʰ **T22.6** **Corrosion of** second degree **of shoulder and upper limb, except wrist and hand**
 Code first (T51-T65) to identify chemical and intent
 Use additional external cause code to identify place (Y92)

 ✓x7ᵗʰ **T22.60** **Corrosion of second degree of shoulder and upper limb, except wrist and hand, unspecified site**

 ✓6ᵗʰ **T22.61** **Corrosion of second degree of** forearm
  ✓7ᵗʰ **T22.611** **Corrosion of second degree of** right **forearm**
  ✓7ᵗʰ **T22.612** **Corrosion of second degree of** left **forearm**
  ✓7ᵗʰ **T22.619** **Corrosion of second degree of unspecified forearm**

 ✓6ᵗʰ **T22.62** **Corrosion of second degree of** elbow
  ✓7ᵗʰ **T22.621** **Corrosion of second degree of** right **elbow**
  ✓7ᵗʰ **T22.622** **Corrosion of second degree of** left **elbow**
  ✓7ᵗʰ **T22.629** **Corrosion of second degree of unspecified elbow**

 ✓6ᵗʰ **T22.63** **Corrosion of second degree of** upper arm
  ✓7ᵗʰ **T22.631** **Corrosion of second degree of** right **upper arm**
  ✓7ᵗʰ **T22.632** **Corrosion of second degree of** left **upper arm**
  ✓7ᵗʰ **T22.639** **Corrosion of second degree of unspecified upper arm**

 ✓6ᵗʰ **T22.64** **Corrosion of second degree of** axilla
  ✓7ᵗʰ **T22.641** **Corrosion of second degree of** right **axilla**
  ✓7ᵗʰ **T22.642** **Corrosion of second degree of** left **axilla**
  ✓7ᵗʰ **T22.649** **Corrosion of second degree of unspecified axilla**

 ✓6ᵗʰ **T22.65** **Corrosion of second degree of** shoulder
  ✓7ᵗʰ **T22.651** **Corrosion of second degree of** right **shoulder**
  ✓7ᵗʰ **T22.652** **Corrosion of second degree of** left **shoulder**

✓ Additional Character Required ✓x7ᵗʰ Placeholder Alert Unspecified Dx Other Specified Dx Manifestation ►◄ Revised Text ● New Code ▲ Revised Code Title

✓7ᵗʰ T22.659 Corrosion of second degree of unspecified shoulder

✓6ᵗʰ T22.66 Corrosion of second degree of scapular region

     ✓7ᵗʰ T22.661 Corrosion of second degree of right scapular region

     ✓7ᵗʰ T22.662 Corrosion of second degree of left scapular region

     ✓7ᵗʰ T22.669 Corrosion of second degree of unspecified scapular region

✓6ᵗʰ T22.69 Corrosion of second degree of multiple sites of shoulder and upper limb, except wrist and hand

     ✓7ᵗʰ T22.691 Corrosion of second degree of multiple sites of right shoulder and upper limb, except wrist and hand

     ✓7ᵗʰ T22.692 Corrosion of second degree of multiple sites of left shoulder and upper limb, except wrist and hand

     ✓7ᵗʰ T22.699 Corrosion of second degree of multiple sites of unspecified shoulder and upper limb, except wrist and hand

✓5ᵗʰ T22.7 Corrosion of third degree of shoulder and upper limb, except wrist and hand

> Code first (T51-T65) to identify chemical and intent
> Use additional external cause code to identify place (Y92)

✓x7ᵗʰ T22.70 Corrosion of third degree of shoulder and upper limb, except wrist and hand, unspecified site

✓6ᵗʰ T22.71 Corrosion of third degree of forearm

     ✓7ᵗʰ T22.711 Corrosion of third degree of right forearm

     ✓7ᵗʰ T22.712 Corrosion of third degree of left forearm

     ✓7ᵗʰ T22.719 Corrosion of third degree of unspecified forearm

✓6ᵗʰ T22.72 Corrosion of third degree of elbow

     ✓7ᵗʰ T22.721 Corrosion of third degree of right elbow

     ✓7ᵗʰ T22.722 Corrosion of third degree of left elbow

     ✓7ᵗʰ T22.729 Corrosion of third degree of unspecified elbow

✓6ᵗʰ T22.73 Corrosion of third degree of upper arm

     ✓7ᵗʰ T22.731 Corrosion of third degree of right upper arm

     ✓7ᵗʰ T22.732 Corrosion of third degree of left upper arm

     ✓7ᵗʰ T22.739 Corrosion of third degree of unspecified upper arm

✓6ᵗʰ T22.74 Corrosion of third degree of axilla

     ✓7ᵗʰ T22.741 Corrosion of third degree of right axilla

     ✓7ᵗʰ T22.742 Corrosion of third degree of left axilla

     ✓7ᵗʰ T22.749 Corrosion of third degree of unspecified axilla

✓6ᵗʰ T22.75 Corrosion of third degree of shoulder

     ✓7ᵗʰ T22.751 Corrosion of third degree of right shoulder

     ✓7ᵗʰ T22.752 Corrosion of third degree of left shoulder

     ✓7ᵗʰ T22.759 Corrosion of third degree of unspecified shoulder

✓6ᵗʰ T22.76 Corrosion of third degree of scapular region

     ✓7ᵗʰ T22.761 Corrosion of third degree of right scapular region

     ✓7ᵗʰ T22.762 Corrosion of third degree of left scapular region

     ✓7ᵗʰ T22.769 Corrosion of third degree of unspecified scapular region

✓6ᵗʰ T22.79 Corrosion of third degree of multiple sites of shoulder and upper limb, except wrist and hand

     ✓7ᵗʰ T22.791 Corrosion of third degree of multiple sites of right shoulder and upper limb, except wrist and hand

     ✓7ᵗʰ T22.792 Corrosion of third degree of multiple sites of left shoulder and upper limb, except wrist and hand

     ✓7ᵗʰ T22.799 Corrosion of third degree of multiple sites of unspecified shoulder and upper limb, except wrist and hand

✓4ᵗʰ T23 Burn and corrosion of wrist and hand

AHA: 2015, 1Q, 19

> The appropriate 7th character is to be added to each code from category T23.
> A   initial encounter
> D   subsequent encounter
> S   sequela

✓5ᵗʰ T23.0 Burn of unspecified degree of wrist and hand

> Use additional external cause code to identify the source, place and intent of the burn (X00-X19, X75-X77, X96-X98, Y92)

✓6ᵗʰ T23.00 Burn of unspecified degree of hand, unspecified site

     ✓7ᵗʰ T23.001 Burn of unspecified degree of right hand, unspecified site

     ✓7ᵗʰ T23.002 Burn of unspecified degree of left hand, unspecified site

     ✓7ᵗʰ T23.009 Burn of unspecified degree of unspecified hand, unspecified site

✓6ᵗʰ T23.01 Burn of unspecified degree of thumb (nail)

     ✓7ᵗʰ T23.011 Burn of unspecified degree of right thumb (nail)

     ✓7ᵗʰ T23.012 Burn of unspecified degree of left thumb (nail)

     ✓7ᵗʰ T23.019 Burn of unspecified degree of unspecified thumb (nail)

✓6ᵗʰ T23.02 Burn of unspecified degree of single finger (nail) except thumb

     ✓7ᵗʰ T23.021 Burn of unspecified degree of single right finger (nail) except thumb

     ✓7ᵗʰ T23.022 Burn of unspecified degree of single left finger (nail) except thumb

     ✓7ᵗʰ T23.029 Burn of unspecified degree of unspecified single finger (nail) except thumb

✓6ᵗʰ T23.03 Burn of unspecified degree of multiple fingers (nail), not including thumb

     ✓7ᵗʰ T23.031 Burn of unspecified degree of multiple right fingers (nail), not including thumb

     ✓7ᵗʰ T23.032 Burn of unspecified degree of multiple left fingers (nail), not including thumb

     ✓7ᵗʰ T23.039 Burn of unspecified degree of unspecified multiple fingers (nail), not including thumb

✓6ᵗʰ T23.04 Burn of unspecified degree of multiple fingers (nail), including thumb

     ✓7ᵗʰ T23.041 Burn of unspecified degree of multiple right fingers (nail), including thumb

     ✓7ᵗʰ T23.042 Burn of unspecified degree of multiple left fingers (nail), including thumb

     ✓7ᵗʰ T23.049 Burn of unspecified degree of unspecified multiple fingers (nail), including thumb

✓6ᵗʰ T23.05 Burn of unspecified degree of palm

     ✓7ᵗʰ T23.051 Burn of unspecified degree of right palm

     ✓7ᵗʰ T23.052 Burn of unspecified degree of left palm

     ✓7ᵗʰ T23.059 Burn of unspecified degree of unspecified palm

✓6ᵗʰ T23.06 Burn of unspecified degree of back of hand

     ✓7ᵗʰ T23.061 Burn of unspecified degree of back of right hand

     ✓7ᵗʰ T23.062 Burn of unspecified degree of back of left hand

     ✓7ᵗʰ T23.069 Burn of unspecified degree of back of unspecified hand

✓6ᵗʰ T23.07 Burn of unspecified degree of wrist

     ✓7ᵗʰ T23.071 Burn of unspecified degree of right wrist

     ✓7ᵗʰ T23.072 Burn of unspecified degree of left wrist

     ✓7ᵗʰ T23.079 Burn of unspecified degree of unspecified wrist

✓6ᵗʰ T23.09 Burn of unspecified degree of multiple sites of wrist and hand

     ✓7ᵗʰ T23.091 Burn of unspecified degree of multiple sites of right wrist and hand

     ✓7ᵗʰ T23.092 Burn of unspecified degree of multiple sites of left wrist and hand

     ✓7ᵗʰ T23.099 Burn of unspecified degree of multiple sites of unspecified wrist and hand

EXCLUDES 1 Not coded here   **EXCLUDES 2** Not included here   **N** Newborn Age: 0   **P** Pediatric Age: 0-17   **M** Maternity Age: 12-55   **A** Adult Age: 15-124

972   ICD-10-CM 2016

✓5ᵗʰ **T23.1**   **Burn of** first degree **of wrist and hand**
Use additional external cause code to identify the source, place and intent of the burn (X00-X19, X75-X77, X96-X98, Y92)

✓6ᵗʰ   **T23.10**   **Burn of first degree of hand,** unspecified site

    ✓7ᵗʰ   **T23.101**   **Burn of first degree of** right **hand, unspecified site**

    ✓7ᵗʰ   **T23.102**   **Burn of first degree of** left **hand, unspecified site**

    ✓7ᵗʰ   **T23.109**   **Burn of first degree of unspecified hand, unspecified site**

✓6ᵗʰ   **T23.11**   **Burn of first degree of** thumb (nail)

    ✓7ᵗʰ   **T23.111**   **Burn of first degree of** right **thumb (nail)**

    ✓7ᵗʰ   **T23.112**   **Burn of first degree of** left **thumb (nail)**

    ✓7ᵗʰ   **T23.119**   **Burn of first degree of unspecified thumb (nail)**

✓6ᵗʰ   **T23.12**   **Burn of first degree of** single finger (nail) except **thumb**

    ✓7ᵗʰ   **T23.121**   **Burn of first degree of single** right **finger (nail) except thumb**

    ✓7ᵗʰ   **T23.122**   **Burn of first degree of single** left **finger (nail) except thumb**

    ✓7ᵗʰ   **T23.129**   **Burn of first degree of unspecified single finger (nail) except thumb**

✓6ᵗʰ   **T23.13**   **Burn of first degree of** multiple fingers (nail), not including thumb

    ✓7ᵗʰ   **T23.131**   **Burn of first degree of multiple** right **fingers (nail), not including thumb**

    ✓7ᵗʰ   **T23.132**   **Burn of first degree of multiple** left **fingers (nail), not including thumb**

    ✓7ᵗʰ   **T23.139**   **Burn of first degree of unspecified multiple fingers (nail), not including thumb**

✓6ᵗʰ   **T23.14**   **Burn of first degree of** multiple fingers (nail), including thumb

    ✓7ᵗʰ   **T23.141**   **Burn of first degree of multiple** right **fingers (nail), including thumb**

    ✓7ᵗʰ   **T23.142**   **Burn of first degree of multiple** left **fingers (nail), including thumb**

    ✓7ᵗʰ   **T23.149**   **Burn of first degree of unspecified multiple fingers (nail), including thumb**

✓6ᵗʰ   **T23.15**   **Burn of first degree of** palm

    ✓7ᵗʰ   **T23.151**   **Burn of first degree of** right **palm**

    ✓7ᵗʰ   **T23.152**   **Burn of first degree of** left **palm**

    ✓7ᵗʰ   **T23.159**   **Burn of first degree of unspecified palm**

✓6ᵗʰ   **T23.16**   **Burn of first degree of** back of hand

    ✓7ᵗʰ   **T23.161**   **Burn of first degree of back of** right **hand**

    ✓7ᵗʰ   **T23.162**   **Burn of first degree of back of** left **hand**

    ✓7ᵗʰ   **T23.169**   **Burn of first degree of back of unspecified hand**

✓6ᵗʰ   **T23.17**   **Burn of first degree of** wrist

    ✓7ᵗʰ   **T23.171**   **Burn of first degree of** right **wrist**

    ✓7ᵗʰ   **T23.172**   **Burn of first degree of** left **wrist**

    ✓7ᵗʰ   **T23.179**   **Burn of first degree of unspecified wrist**

✓6ᵗʰ   **T23.19**   **Burn of first degree of** multiple sites **of wrist and hand**

    ✓7ᵗʰ   **T23.191**   **Burn of first degree of multiple sites of** right **wrist and hand**

    ✓7ᵗʰ   **T23.192**   **Burn of first degree of multiple sites of** left **wrist and hand**

    ✓7ᵗʰ   **T23.199**   **Burn of first degree of multiple sites of unspecified wrist and hand**

✓5ᵗʰ **T23.2**   **Burn of** second degree **of wrist and hand**
Use additional external cause code to identify the source, place and intent of the burn (X00-X19, X75-X77, X96-X98, Y92)

✓6ᵗʰ   **T23.20**   **Burn of second degree of hand,** unspecified site

    ✓7ᵗʰ   **T23.201**   **Burn of second degree of** right **hand, unspecified site**

    ✓7ᵗʰ   **T23.202**   **Burn of second degree of** left **hand, unspecified site**

    ✓7ᵗʰ   **T23.209**   **Burn of second degree of unspecified hand, unspecified site**

✓6ᵗʰ   **T23.21**   **Burn of second degree of** thumb (nail)

    ✓7ᵗʰ   **T23.211**   **Burn of second degree of** right **thumb (nail)**

    ✓7ᵗʰ   **T23.212**   **Burn of second degree of** left **thumb (nail)**

    ✓7ᵗʰ   **T23.219**   **Burn of second degree of unspecified thumb (nail)**

✓6ᵗʰ   **T23.22**   **Burn of second degree of** single finger (nail) except **thumb**

    ✓7ᵗʰ   **T23.221**   **Burn of second degree of single** right **finger (nail) except thumb**

    ✓7ᵗʰ   **T23.222**   **Burn of second degree of single** left **finger (nail) except thumb**

    ✓7ᵗʰ   **T23.229**   **Burn of second degree of unspecified single finger (nail) except thumb**

✓6ᵗʰ   **T23.23**   **Burn of second degree of** multiple fingers (nail), not including thumb

    ✓7ᵗʰ   **T23.231**   **Burn of second degree of multiple** right **fingers (nail), not including thumb**

    ✓7ᵗʰ   **T23.232**   **Burn of second degree of multiple** left **fingers (nail), not including thumb**

    ✓7ᵗʰ   **T23.239**   **Burn of second degree of unspecified multiple fingers (nail), not including thumb**

✓6ᵗʰ   **T23.24**   **Burn of second degree of** multiple fingers (nail), including thumb

    ✓7ᵗʰ   **T23.241**   **Burn of second degree of multiple** right **fingers (nail), including thumb**

    ✓7ᵗʰ   **T23.242**   **Burn of second degree of multiple** left **fingers (nail), including thumb**

    ✓7ᵗʰ   **T23.249**   **Burn of second degree of unspecified multiple fingers (nail), including thumb**

✓6ᵗʰ   **T23.25**   **Burn of second degree of** palm

    ✓7ᵗʰ   **T23.251**   **Burn of second degree of** right **palm**

    ✓7ᵗʰ   **T23.252**   **Burn of second degree of** left **palm**

    ✓7ᵗʰ   **T23.259**   **Burn of second degree of unspecified palm**

✓6ᵗʰ   **T23.26**   **Burn of second degree of** back of hand

    ✓7ᵗʰ   **T23.261**   **Burn of second degree of back of** right **hand**

    ✓7ᵗʰ   **T23.262**   **Burn of second degree of back of** left **hand**

    ✓7ᵗʰ   **T23.269**   **Burn of second degree of back of unspecified hand**

✓6ᵗʰ   **T23.27**   **Burn of second degree of** wrist

    ✓7ᵗʰ   **T23.271**   **Burn of second degree of** right **wrist**

    ✓7ᵗʰ   **T23.272**   **Burn of second degree of** left **wrist**

    ✓7ᵗʰ   **T23.279**   **Burn of second degree of unspecified wrist**

✓6ᵗʰ   **T23.29**   **Burn of second degree of** multiple sites **of wrist and hand**

    ✓7ᵗʰ   **T23.291**   **Burn of second degree of multiple sites of** right **wrist and hand**

    ✓7ᵗʰ   **T23.292**   **Burn of second degree of multiple sites of** left **wrist and hand**

    ✓7ᵗʰ   **T23.299**   **Burn of second degree of multiple sites of unspecified wrist and hand**

✓5ᵗʰ **T23.3**   **Burn of** third degree **of wrist and hand**
Use additional external cause code to identify the source, place and intent of the burn (X00-X19, X75-X77, X96-X98, Y92)

✓6ᵗʰ   **T23.30**   **Burn of third degree of hand,** unspecified site

    ✓7ᵗʰ   **T23.301**   **Burn of third degree of** right **hand, unspecified site**

    ✓7ᵗʰ   **T23.302**   **Burn of third degree of** left **hand, unspecified site**

    ✓7ᵗʰ   **T23.309**   **Burn of third degree of unspecified hand, unspecified site**

✓6ᵗʰ   **T23.31**   **Burn of third degree of** thumb (nail)

    ✓7ᵗʰ   **T23.311**   **Burn of third degree of** right **thumb (nail)**

    ✓7ᵗʰ   **T23.312**   **Burn of third degree of** left **thumb (nail)**

    ✓7ᵗʰ   **T23.319**   **Burn of third degree of unspecified thumb (nail)**

✓6ᵗʰ   **T23.32**   **Burn of third degree of** single finger (nail) except **thumb**

    ✓7ᵗʰ   **T23.321**   **Burn of third degree of single** right **finger (nail) except thumb**

☑ Additional Character Required   ✓xʗᵗʰ Placeholder Alert   Unspecified Dx   Other Specified Dx   Manifestation   ►◄ Revised Text   ● New Code   ▲ Revised Code Title

ICD-10-CM 2016   973

✓7th **T23.322** Burn of third degree of single left finger (nail) except thumb

✓7th **T23.329** Burn of third degree of unspecified single finger (nail) except thumb

✓6th **T23.33** Burn of third degree of multiple fingers (nail), not including thumb

    ✓7th **T23.331** Burn of third degree of multiple right fingers (nail), not including thumb

    ✓7th **T23.332** Burn of third degree of multiple left fingers (nail), not including thumb

    ✓7th **T23.339** Burn of third degree of unspecified multiple fingers (nail), not including thumb

✓6th **T23.34** Burn of third degree of multiple fingers (nail), including thumb

    ✓7th **T23.341** Burn of third degree of multiple right fingers (nail), including thumb

    ✓7th **T23.342** Burn of third degree of multiple left fingers (nail), including thumb

    ✓7th **T23.349** Burn of third degree of unspecified multiple fingers (nail), including thumb

✓6th **T23.35** Burn of third degree of palm

    ✓7th **T23.351** Burn of third degree of right palm

    ✓7th **T23.352** Burn of third degree of left palm

    ✓7th **T23.359** Burn of third degree of unspecified palm

✓6th **T23.36** Burn of third degree of back of hand

    ✓7th **T23.361** Burn of third degree of back of right hand

    ✓7th **T23.362** Burn of third degree of back of left hand

    ✓7th **T23.369** Burn of third degree of back of unspecified hand

✓6th **T23.37** Burn of third degree of wrist

    ✓7th **T23.371** Burn of third degree of right wrist

    ✓7th **T23.372** Burn of third degree of left wrist

    ✓7th **T23.379** Burn of third degree of unspecified wrist

✓6th **T23.39** Burn of third degree of multiple sites of wrist and hand

    ✓7th **T23.391** Burn of third degree of multiple sites of right wrist and hand

    ✓7th **T23.392** Burn of third degree of multiple sites of left wrist and hand

    ✓7th **T23.399** Burn of third degree of multiple sites of unspecified wrist and hand

✓5th **T23.4** Corrosion of unspecified degree of wrist and hand

    Code first (T51-T65) to identify chemical and intent
    Use additional external cause code to identify place (Y92)

✓6th **T23.40** Corrosion of unspecified degree of hand, unspecified site

    ✓7th **T23.401** Corrosion of unspecified degree of right hand, unspecified site

    ✓7th **T23.402** Corrosion of unspecified degree of left hand, unspecified site

    ✓7th **T23.409** Corrosion of unspecified degree of unspecified hand, unspecified site

✓6th **T23.41** Corrosion of unspecified degree of thumb (nail)

    ✓7th **T23.411** Corrosion of unspecified degree of right thumb (nail)

    ✓7th **T23.412** Corrosion of unspecified degree of left thumb (nail)

    ✓7th **T23.419** Corrosion of unspecified degree of unspecified thumb (nail)

✓6th **T23.42** Corrosion of unspecified degree of single finger (nail) except thumb

    ✓7th **T23.421** Corrosion of unspecified degree of single right finger (nail) except thumb

    ✓7th **T23.422** Corrosion of unspecified degree of single left finger (nail) except thumb

    ✓7th **T23.429** Corrosion of unspecified degree of unspecified single finger (nail) except thumb

✓6th **T23.43** Corrosion of unspecified degree of multiple fingers (nail), not including thumb

    ✓7th **T23.431** Corrosion of unspecified degree of multiple right fingers (nail), not including thumb

✓7th **T23.432** Corrosion of unspecified degree of multiple left fingers (nail), not including thumb

✓7th **T23.439** Corrosion of unspecified degree of unspecified multiple fingers (nail), not including thumb

✓6th **T23.44** Corrosion of unspecified degree of multiple fingers (nail), including thumb

    ✓7th **T23.441** Corrosion of unspecified degree of multiple right fingers (nail), including thumb

    ✓7th **T23.442** Corrosion of unspecified degree of multiple left fingers (nail), including thumb

    ✓7th **T23.449** Corrosion of unspecified degree of unspecified multiple fingers (nail), including thumb

✓6th **T23.45** Corrosion of unspecified degree of palm

    ✓7th **T23.451** Corrosion of unspecified degree of right palm

    ✓7th **T23.452** Corrosion of unspecified degree of left palm

    ✓7th **T23.459** Corrosion of unspecified degree of unspecified palm

✓6th **T23.46** Corrosion of unspecified degree of back of hand

    ✓7th **T23.461** Corrosion of unspecified degree of back of right hand

    ✓7th **T23.462** Corrosion of unspecified degree of back of left hand

    ✓7th **T23.469** Corrosion of unspecified degree of back of unspecified hand

✓6th **T23.47** Corrosion of unspecified degree of wrist

    ✓7th **T23.471** Corrosion of unspecified degree of right wrist

    ✓7th **T23.472** Corrosion of unspecified degree of left wrist

    ✓7th **T23.479** Corrosion of unspecified degree of unspecified wrist

✓6th **T23.49** Corrosion of unspecified degree of multiple sites of wrist and hand

    ✓7th **T23.491** Corrosion of unspecified degree of multiple sites of right wrist and hand

    ✓7th **T23.492** Corrosion of unspecified degree of multiple sites of left wrist and hand

    ✓7th **T23.499** Corrosion of unspecified degree of multiple sites of unspecified wrist and hand

✓5th **T23.5** Corrosion of first degree of wrist and hand

    Code first (T51-T65) to identify chemical and intent
    Use additional external cause code to identify place (Y92)

✓6th **T23.50** Corrosion of first degree of hand, unspecified site

    ✓7th **T23.501** Corrosion of first degree of right hand, unspecified site

    ✓7th **T23.502** Corrosion of first degree of left hand, unspecified site

    ✓7th **T23.509** Corrosion of first degree of unspecified hand, unspecified site

✓6th **T23.51** Corrosion of first degree of thumb (nail)

    ✓7th **T23.511** Corrosion of first degree of right thumb (nail)

    ✓7th **T23.512** Corrosion of first degree of left thumb (nail)

    ✓7th **T23.519** Corrosion of first degree of unspecified thumb (nail)

✓6th **T23.52** Corrosion of first degree of single finger (nail) except thumb

    ✓7th **T23.521** Corrosion of first degree of single right finger (nail) except thumb

    ✓7th **T23.522** Corrosion of first degree of single left finger (nail) except thumb

    ✓7th **T23.529** Corrosion of first degree of unspecified single finger (nail) except thumb

EXCLUDES 1 Not coded here   EXCLUDES 2 Not included here   N Newborn Age: 0   P Pediatric Age: 0-17   M Maternity Age: 12-55   A Adult Age: 15-124

974

ICD-10-CM 2016

√6ᵗʰ **T23.53** Corrosion of first degree of multiple fingers (nail), not including thumb
  √7ᵗʰ **T23.531** Corrosion of first degree of multiple right fingers (nail), not including thumb
  √7ᵗʰ **T23.532** Corrosion of first degree of multiple left fingers (nail), not including thumb
  √7ᵗʰ **T23.539** Corrosion of first degree of unspecified multiple fingers (nail), not including thumb

√6ᵗʰ **T23.54** Corrosion of first degree of multiple fingers (nail), including thumb
  √7ᵗʰ **T23.541** Corrosion of first degree of multiple right fingers (nail), including thumb
  √7ᵗʰ **T23.542** Corrosion of first degree of multiple left fingers (nail), including thumb
  √7ᵗʰ **T23.549** Corrosion of first degree of unspecified multiple fingers (nail), including thumb

√6ᵗʰ **T23.55** Corrosion of first degree of palm
  √7ᵗʰ **T23.551** Corrosion of first degree of right palm
  √7ᵗʰ **T23.552** Corrosion of first degree of left palm
  √7ᵗʰ **T23.559** Corrosion of first degree of unspecified palm

√6ᵗʰ **T23.56** Corrosion of first degree of back of hand
  √7ᵗʰ **T23.561** Corrosion of first degree of back of right hand
  √7ᵗʰ **T23.562** Corrosion of first degree of back of left hand
  √7ᵗʰ **T23.569** Corrosion of first degree of back of unspecified hand

√6ᵗʰ **T23.57** Corrosion of first degree of wrist
  √7ᵗʰ **T23.571** Corrosion of first degree of right wrist
  √7ᵗʰ **T23.572** Corrosion of first degree of left wrist
  √7ᵗʰ **T23.579** Corrosion of first degree of unspecified wrist

√6ᵗʰ **T23.59** Corrosion of first degree of multiple sites of wrist and hand
  √7ᵗʰ **T23.591** Corrosion of first degree of multiple sites of right wrist and hand
  √7ᵗʰ **T23.592** Corrosion of first degree of multiple sites of left wrist and hand
  √7ᵗʰ **T23.599** Corrosion of first degree of multiple sites of unspecified wrist and hand

√5ᵗʰ **T23.6** Corrosion of second degree of wrist and hand
  Code first (T51-T65) to identify chemical and intent
  Use additional external cause code to identify place (Y92)

√6ᵗʰ **T23.60** Corrosion of second degree of hand, unspecified site
  √7ᵗʰ **T23.601** Corrosion of second degree of right hand, unspecified site
  √7ᵗʰ **T23.602** Corrosion of second degree of left hand, unspecified site
  √7ᵗʰ **T23.609** Corrosion of second degree of unspecified hand, unspecified site

√6ᵗʰ **T23.61** Corrosion of second degree of thumb (nail)
  √7ᵗʰ **T23.611** Corrosion of second degree of right thumb (nail)
  √7ᵗʰ **T23.612** Corrosion of second degree of left thumb (nail)
  √7ᵗʰ **T23.619** Corrosion of second degree of unspecified thumb (nail)

√6ᵗʰ **T23.62** Corrosion of second degree of single finger (nail) except thumb
  √7ᵗʰ **T23.621** Corrosion of second degree of single right finger (nail) except thumb
  √7ᵗʰ **T23.622** Corrosion of second degree of single left finger (nail) except thumb
  √7ᵗʰ **T23.629** Corrosion of second degree of unspecified single finger (nail) except thumb

√6ᵗʰ **T23.63** Corrosion of second degree of multiple fingers (nail), not including thumb
  √7ᵗʰ **T23.631** Corrosion of second degree of multiple right fingers (nail), not including thumb
  √7ᵗʰ **T23.632** Corrosion of second degree of multiple left fingers (nail), not including thumb

  √7ᵗʰ **T23.639** Corrosion of second degree of unspecified multiple fingers (nail), not including thumb

√6ᵗʰ **T23.64** Corrosion of second degree of multiple fingers (nail), including thumb
  √7ᵗʰ **T23.641** Corrosion of second degree of multiple right fingers (nail), including thumb
  √7ᵗʰ **T23.642** Corrosion of second degree of multiple left fingers (nail), including thumb
  √7ᵗʰ **T23.649** Corrosion of second degree of unspecified multiple fingers (nail), including thumb

√6ᵗʰ **T23.65** Corrosion of second degree of palm
  √7ᵗʰ **T23.651** Corrosion of second degree of right palm
  √7ᵗʰ **T23.652** Corrosion of second degree of left palm
  √7ᵗʰ **T23.659** Corrosion of second degree of unspecified palm

√6ᵗʰ **T23.66** Corrosion of second degree of back of hand
  √7ᵗʰ **T23.661** Corrosion of second degree back of right hand
  √7ᵗʰ **T23.662** Corrosion of second degree back of left hand
  √7ᵗʰ **T23.669** Corrosion of second degree back of unspecified hand

√6ᵗʰ **T23.67** Corrosion of second degree of wrist
  √7ᵗʰ **T23.671** Corrosion of second degree of right wrist
  √7ᵗʰ **T23.672** Corrosion of second degree of left wrist
  √7ᵗʰ **T23.679** Corrosion of second degree of unspecified wrist

√6ᵗʰ **T23.69** Corrosion of second degree of multiple sites of wrist and hand
  √7ᵗʰ **T23.691** Corrosion of second degree of multiple sites of right wrist and hand
  √7ᵗʰ **T23.692** Corrosion of second degree of multiple sites of left wrist and hand
  √7ᵗʰ **T23.699** Corrosion of second degree of multiple sites of unspecified wrist and hand

√5ᵗʰ **T23.7** Corrosion of third degree of wrist and hand
  Code first (T51-T65) to identify chemical and intent
  Use additional external cause code to identify place (Y92)

√6ᵗʰ **T23.70** Corrosion of third degree of hand, unspecified site
  √7ᵗʰ **T23.701** Corrosion of third degree of right hand, unspecified site
  √7ᵗʰ **T23.702** Corrosion of third degree of left hand, unspecified site
  √7ᵗʰ **T23.709** Corrosion of third degree of unspecified hand, unspecified site

√6ᵗʰ **T23.71** Corrosion of third degree of thumb (nail)
  √7ᵗʰ **T23.711** Corrosion of third degree of right thumb (nail)
  √7ᵗʰ **T23.712** Corrosion of third degree of left thumb (nail)
  √7ᵗʰ **T23.719** Corrosion of third degree of unspecified thumb (nail)

√6ᵗʰ **T23.72** Corrosion of third degree of single finger (nail) except thumb
  √7ᵗʰ **T23.721** Corrosion of third degree of single right finger (nail) except thumb
  √7ᵗʰ **T23.722** Corrosion of third degree of single left finger (nail) except thumb
  √7ᵗʰ **T23.729** Corrosion of third degree of unspecified single finger (nail) except thumb

√6ᵗʰ **T23.73** Corrosion of third degree of multiple fingers (nail), not including thumb
  √7ᵗʰ **T23.731** Corrosion of third degree of multiple right fingers (nail), not including thumb
  √7ᵗʰ **T23.732** Corrosion of third degree of multiple left fingers (nail), not including thumb
  √7ᵗʰ **T23.739** Corrosion of third degree of unspecified multiple fingers (nail), not including thumb

☑ Additional Character Required √x7ᵗʰ Placeholder Alert Unspecified Dx Other Specified Dx Manifestation ►◄ Revised Text ● New Code ▲ Revised Code Title

ICD-10-CM 2016 975

✓6ᵗʰ **T23.74** Corrosion of third degree of multiple fingers (nail), including thumb

   ✓7ᵗʰ **T23.741** Corrosion of third degree of multiple right fingers (nail), including thumb

   ✓7ᵗʰ **T23.742** Corrosion of third degree of multiple left fingers (nail), including thumb

   ✓7ᵗʰ **T23.749** Corrosion of third degree of unspecified multiple fingers (nail), including thumb

✓6ᵗʰ **T23.75** Corrosion of third degree of palm

   ✓7ᵗʰ **T23.751** Corrosion of third degree of right palm

   ✓7ᵗʰ **T23.752** Corrosion of third degree of left palm

   ✓7ᵗʰ **T23.759** Corrosion of third degree of unspecified palm

✓6ᵗʰ **T23.76** Corrosion of third degree of back of hand

   ✓7ᵗʰ **T23.761** Corrosion of third degree of back of right hand

   ✓7ᵗʰ **T23.762** Corrosion of third degree of back of left hand

   ✓7ᵗʰ **T23.769** Corrosion of third degree back of unspecified hand

✓6ᵗʰ **T23.77** Corrosion of third degree of wrist

   ✓7ᵗʰ **T23.771** Corrosion of third degree of right wrist

   ✓7ᵗʰ **T23.772** Corrosion of third degree of left wrist

   ✓7ᵗʰ **T23.779** Corrosion of third degree of unspecified wrist

✓6ᵗʰ **T23.79** Corrosion of third degree of multiple sites of wrist and hand

   ✓7ᵗʰ **T23.791** Corrosion of third degree of multiple sites of right wrist and hand

   ✓7ᵗʰ **T23.792** Corrosion of third degree of multiple sites of left wrist and hand

   ✓7ᵗʰ **T23.799** Corrosion of third degree of multiple sites of unspecified wrist and hand

✓4ᵗʰ **T24** Burn and corrosion of lower limb, except ankle and foot

   EXCLUDES 2   burn and corrosion of ankle and foot (T25.-)
                    burn and corrosion of hip region (T21.-)

   The appropriate 7th character is to be added to each code from category T24.
   A   initial encounter
   D   subsequent encounter
   S   sequela

✓5ᵗʰ **T24.0** Burn of unspecified degree of lower limb, except ankle and foot

   Use additional external cause code to identify the source, place and intent of the burn (X00-X19, X75-X77, X96-X98, Y92)

   ✓6ᵗʰ **T24.00** Burn of unspecified degree of unspecified site of lower limb, except ankle and foot

      ✓7ᵗʰ **T24.001** Burn of unspecified degree of unspecified site of right lower limb, except ankle and foot

      ✓7ᵗʰ **T24.002** Burn of unspecified degree of unspecified site of left lower limb, except ankle and foot

      ✓7ᵗʰ **T24.009** Burn of unspecified degree of unspecified site of unspecified lower limb, except ankle and foot

   ✓6ᵗʰ **T24.01** Burn of unspecified degree of thigh

      ✓7ᵗʰ **T24.011** Burn of unspecified degree of right thigh

      ✓7ᵗʰ **T24.012** Burn of unspecified degree of left thigh

      ✓7ᵗʰ **T24.019** Burn of unspecified degree of unspecified thigh

   ✓6ᵗʰ **T24.02** Burn of unspecified degree of knee

      ✓7ᵗʰ **T24.021** Burn of unspecified degree of right knee

      ✓7ᵗʰ **T24.022** Burn of unspecified degree of left knee

      ✓7ᵗʰ **T24.029** Burn of unspecified degree of unspecified knee

   ✓6ᵗʰ **T24.03** Burn of unspecified degree of lower leg

      ✓7ᵗʰ **T24.031** Burn of unspecified degree of right lower leg

      ✓7ᵗʰ **T24.032** Burn of unspecified degree of left lower leg

      ✓7ᵗʰ **T24.039** Burn of unspecified degree of unspecified lower leg

✓6ᵗʰ **T24.09** Burn of unspecified degree of multiple sites of lower limb, except ankle and foot

   ✓7ᵗʰ **T24.091** Burn of unspecified degree of multiple sites of right lower limb, except ankle and foot

   ✓7ᵗʰ **T24.092** Burn of unspecified degree of multiple sites of left lower limb, except ankle and foot

   ✓7ᵗʰ **T24.099** Burn of unspecified degree of multiple sites of unspecified lower limb, except ankle and foot

✓5ᵗʰ **T24.1** Burn of first degree of lower limb, except ankle and foot

   Use additional external cause code to identify the source, place and intent of the burn (X00-X19, X75-X77, X96-X98, Y92)

   ✓6ᵗʰ **T24.10** Burn of first degree of unspecified site of lower limb, except ankle and foot

      ✓7ᵗʰ **T24.101** Burn of first degree of unspecified site of right lower limb, except ankle and foot

      ✓7ᵗʰ **T24.102** Burn of first degree of unspecified site of left lower limb, except ankle and foot

      ✓7ᵗʰ **T24.109** Burn of first degree of unspecified site of unspecified lower limb, except ankle and foot

   ✓6ᵗʰ **T24.11** Burn of first degree of thigh

      ✓7ᵗʰ **T24.111** Burn of first degree of right thigh

      ✓7ᵗʰ **T24.112** Burn of first degree of left thigh

      ✓7ᵗʰ **T24.119** Burn of first degree of unspecified thigh

   ✓6ᵗʰ **T24.12** Burn of first degree of knee

      ✓7ᵗʰ **T24.121** Burn of first degree of right knee

      ✓7ᵗʰ **T24.122** Burn of first degree of left knee

      ✓7ᵗʰ **T24.129** Burn of first degree of unspecified knee

   ✓6ᵗʰ **T24.13** Burn of first degree of lower leg

      ✓7ᵗʰ **T24.131** Burn of first degree of right lower leg

      ✓7ᵗʰ **T24.132** Burn of first degree of left lower leg

      ✓7ᵗʰ **T24.139** Burn of first degree of unspecified lower leg

   ✓6ᵗʰ **T24.19** Burn of first degree of multiple sites of lower limb, except ankle and foot

      ✓7ᵗʰ **T24.191** Burn of first degree of multiple sites of right lower limb, except ankle and foot

      ✓7ᵗʰ **T24.192** Burn of first degree of multiple sites of left lower limb, except ankle and foot

      ✓7ᵗʰ **T24.199** Burn of first degree of multiple sites of unspecified lower limb, except ankle and foot

✓5ᵗʰ **T24.2** Burn of second degree of lower limb, except ankle and foot

   Use additional external cause code to identify the source, place and intent of the burn (X00-X19, X75-X77, X96-X98, Y92)

   ✓6ᵗʰ **T24.20** Burn of second degree of unspecified site of lower limb, except ankle and foot

      ✓7ᵗʰ **T24.201** Burn of second degree of unspecified site of right lower limb, except ankle and foot

      ✓7ᵗʰ **T24.202** Burn of second degree of unspecified site of left lower limb, except ankle and foot

      ✓7ᵗʰ **T24.209** Burn of second degree of unspecified site of unspecified lower limb, except ankle and foot

   ✓6ᵗʰ **T24.21** Burn of second degree of thigh

      ✓7ᵗʰ **T24.211** Burn of second degree of right thigh

      ✓7ᵗʰ **T24.212** Burn of second degree of left thigh

      ✓7ᵗʰ **T24.219** Burn of second degree of unspecified thigh

   ✓6ᵗʰ **T24.22** Burn of second degree of knee

      ✓7ᵗʰ **T24.221** Burn of second degree of right knee

      ✓7ᵗʰ **T24.222** Burn of second degree of left knee

      ✓7ᵗʰ **T24.229** Burn of second degree of unspecified knee

   ✓6ᵗʰ **T24.23** Burn of second degree of lower leg

      ✓7ᵗʰ **T24.231** Burn of second degree of right lower leg

      ✓7ᵗʰ **T24.232** Burn of second degree of left lower leg

      ✓7ᵗʰ **T24.239** Burn of second degree of unspecified lower leg

EXCLUDES 1 Not coded here   EXCLUDES 2 Not included here   N Newborn Age: 0   P Pediatric Age: 0-17   M Maternity Age: 12-55   A Adult Age: 15-124

976   ICD-10-CM 2016

✓6ᵗʰ **T24.29 Burn of second degree of multiple sites of lower limb, except ankle and foot**

   ✓7ᵗʰ **T24.291** Burn of second degree of multiple sites of right lower limb, except ankle and foot

   ✓7ᵗʰ **T24.292** Burn of second degree of multiple sites of left lower limb, except ankle and foot

   ✓7ᵗʰ **T24.299** Burn of second degree of multiple sites of unspecified lower limb, except ankle and foot

✓5ᵗʰ **T24.3 Burn of third degree of lower limb, except ankle and foot**

Use additional external cause code to identify the source, place and intent of the burn (X00-X19, X75-X77, X96-X98, Y92)

✓6ᵗʰ **T24.30 Burn of third degree of unspecified site of lower limb, except ankle and foot**

   ✓7ᵗʰ **T24.301** Burn of third degree of unspecified site of right lower limb, except ankle and foot

   ✓7ᵗʰ **T24.302** Burn of third degree of unspecified site of left lower limb, except ankle and foot

   ✓7ᵗʰ **T24.309** Burn of third degree of unspecified site of unspecified lower limb, except ankle and foot

✓6ᵗʰ **T24.31 Burn of third degree of thigh**

   ✓7ᵗʰ **T24.311** Burn of third degree of right thigh

   ✓7ᵗʰ **T24.312** Burn of third degree of left thigh

   ✓7ᵗʰ **T24.319** Burn of third degree of unspecified thigh

✓6ᵗʰ **T24.32 Burn of third degree of knee**

   ✓7ᵗʰ **T24.321** Burn of third degree of right knee

   ✓7ᵗʰ **T24.322** Burn of third degree of left knee

   ✓7ᵗʰ **T24.329** Burn of third degree of unspecified knee

✓6ᵗʰ **T24.33 Burn of third degree of lower leg**

   ✓7ᵗʰ **T24.331** Burn of third degree of right lower leg

   ✓7ᵗʰ **T24.332** Burn of third degree of left lower leg

   ✓7ᵗʰ **T24.339** Burn of third degree of unspecified lower leg

✓6ᵗʰ **T24.39 Burn of third degree of multiple sites of lower limb, except ankle and foot**

   ✓7ᵗʰ **T24.391** Burn of third degree of multiple sites of right lower limb, except ankle and foot

   ✓7ᵗʰ **T24.392** Burn of third degree of multiple sites of left lower limb, except ankle and foot

   ✓7ᵗʰ **T24.399** Burn of third degree of multiple sites of unspecified lower limb, except ankle and foot

✓5ᵗʰ **T24.4 Corrosion of unspecified degree of lower limb, except ankle and foot**

Code first (T51-T65) to identify chemical and intent
Use additional external cause code to identify place (Y92)

✓6ᵗʰ **T24.40 Corrosion of unspecified degree of unspecified site of lower limb, except ankle and foot**

   ✓7ᵗʰ **T24.401** Corrosion of unspecified degree of unspecified site of right lower limb, except ankle and foot

   ✓7ᵗʰ **T24.402** Corrosion of unspecified degree of unspecified site of left lower limb, except ankle and foot

   ✓7ᵗʰ **T24.409** Corrosion of unspecified degree of unspecified site of unspecified lower limb, except ankle and foot

✓6ᵗʰ **T24.41 Corrosion of unspecified degree of thigh**

   ✓7ᵗʰ **T24.411** Corrosion of unspecified degree of right thigh

   ✓7ᵗʰ **T24.412** Corrosion of unspecified degree of left thigh

   ✓7ᵗʰ **T24.419** Corrosion of unspecified degree of unspecified thigh

✓6ᵗʰ **T24.42 Corrosion of unspecified degree of knee**

   ✓7ᵗʰ **T24.421** Corrosion of unspecified degree of right knee

   ✓7ᵗʰ **T24.422** Corrosion of unspecified degree of left knee

   ✓7ᵗʰ **T24.429** Corrosion of unspecified degree of unspecified knee

✓6ᵗʰ **T24.43 Corrosion of unspecified degree of lower leg**

   ✓7ᵗʰ **T24.431** Corrosion of unspecified degree of right lower leg

   ✓7ᵗʰ **T24.432** Corrosion of unspecified degree of left lower leg

   ✓7ᵗʰ **T24.439** Corrosion of unspecified degree of unspecified lower leg

✓6ᵗʰ **T24.49 Corrosion of unspecified degree of multiple sites of lower limb, except ankle and foot**

   ✓7ᵗʰ **T24.491** Corrosion of unspecified degree of multiple sites of right lower limb, except ankle and foot

   ✓7ᵗʰ **T24.492** Corrosion of unspecified degree of multiple sites of left lower limb, except ankle and foot

   ✓7ᵗʰ **T24.499** Corrosion of unspecified degree of multiple sites of unspecified lower limb, except ankle and foot

✓5ᵗʰ **T24.5 Corrosion of first degree of lower limb, except ankle and foot**

Code first (T51-T65) to identify chemical and intent
Use additional external cause code to identify place (Y92)

✓6ᵗʰ **T24.50 Corrosion of first degree of unspecified site of lower limb, except ankle and foot**

   ✓7ᵗʰ **T24.501** Corrosion of first degree of unspecified site of right lower limb, except ankle and foot

   ✓7ᵗʰ **T24.502** Corrosion of first degree of unspecified site of left lower limb, except ankle and foot

   ✓7ᵗʰ **T24.509** Corrosion of first degree of unspecified site of unspecified lower limb, except ankle and foot

✓6ᵗʰ **T24.51 Corrosion of first degree of thigh**

   ✓7ᵗʰ **T24.511** Corrosion of first degree of right thigh

   ✓7ᵗʰ **T24.512** Corrosion of first degree of left thigh

   ✓7ᵗʰ **T24.519** Corrosion of first degree of unspecified thigh

✓6ᵗʰ **T24.52 Corrosion of first degree of knee**

   ✓7ᵗʰ **T24.521** Corrosion of first degree of right knee

   ✓7ᵗʰ **T24.522** Corrosion of first degree of left knee

   ✓7ᵗʰ **T24.529** Corrosion of first degree of unspecified knee

✓6ᵗʰ **T24.53 Corrosion of first degree of lower leg**

   ✓7ᵗʰ **T24.531** Corrosion of first degree of right lower leg

   ✓7ᵗʰ **T24.532** Corrosion of first degree of left lower leg

   ✓7ᵗʰ **T24.539** Corrosion of first degree of unspecified lower leg

✓6ᵗʰ **T24.59 Corrosion of first degree of multiple sites of lower limb, except ankle and foot**

   ✓7ᵗʰ **T24.591** Corrosion of first degree of multiple sites of right lower limb, except ankle and foot

   ✓7ᵗʰ **T24.592** Corrosion of first degree of multiple sites of left lower limb, except ankle and foot

   ✓7ᵗʰ **T24.599** Corrosion of first degree of multiple sites of unspecified lower limb, except ankle and foot

✓5ᵗʰ **T24.6 Corrosion of second degree of lower limb, except ankle and foot**

Code first (T51-T65) to identify chemical and intent
Use additional external cause code to identify place (Y92)

✓6ᵗʰ **T24.60 Corrosion of second degree of unspecified site of lower limb, except ankle and foot**

   ✓7ᵗʰ **T24.601** Corrosion of second degree of unspecified site of right lower limb, except ankle and foot

   ✓7ᵗʰ **T24.602** Corrosion of second degree of unspecified site of left lower limb, except ankle and foot

   ✓7ᵗʰ **T24.609** Corrosion of second degree of unspecified site of unspecified lower limb, except ankle and foot

✓6ᵗʰ **T24.61 Corrosion of second degree of thigh**

   ✓7ᵗʰ **T24.611** Corrosion of second degree of right thigh

   ✓7ᵗʰ **T24.612** Corrosion of second degree of left thigh

✓ Additional Character Required   ✓7ᵗʰ Placeholder Alert   Unspecified Dx   Other Specified Dx   Manifestation   ▶◀ Revised Text   ● New Code   ▲ Revised Code Title

ICD-10-CM 2016   977

✓7ᵗʰ **T24.619** Corrosion of second degree of unspecified thigh

✓6ᵗʰ **T24.62** Corrosion of second degree of knee

　✓7ᵗʰ **T24.621** Corrosion of second degree of right knee

　✓7ᵗʰ **T24.622** Corrosion of second degree of left knee

　✓7ᵗʰ **T24.629** Corrosion of second degree of unspecified knee

✓6ᵗʰ **T24.63** Corrosion of second degree of lower leg

　✓7ᵗʰ **T24.631** Corrosion of second degree of right lower leg

　✓7ᵗʰ **T24.632** Corrosion of second degree of left lower leg

　✓7ᵗʰ **T24.639** Corrosion of second degree of unspecified lower leg

✓6ᵗʰ **T24.69** Corrosion of second degree of multiple sites of lower limb, except ankle and foot

　✓7ᵗʰ **T24.691** Corrosion of second degree of multiple sites of right lower limb, except ankle and foot

　✓7ᵗʰ **T24.692** Corrosion of second degree of multiple sites of left lower limb, except ankle and foot

　✓7ᵗʰ **T24.699** Corrosion of second degree of multiple sites of unspecified lower limb, except ankle and foot

✓5ᵗʰ **T24.7** Corrosion of third degree of lower limb, except ankle and foot

Code first (T51-T65) to identify chemical and intent
Use additional external cause code to identify place (Y92)

✓6ᵗʰ **T24.70** Corrosion of third degree of unspecified site of lower limb, except ankle and foot

　✓7ᵗʰ **T24.701** Corrosion of third degree of unspecified site of right lower limb, except ankle and foot

　✓7ᵗʰ **T24.702** Corrosion of third degree of unspecified site of left lower limb, except ankle and foot

　✓7ᵗʰ **T24.709** Corrosion of third degree of unspecified site of unspecified lower limb, except ankle and foot

✓6ᵗʰ **T24.71** Corrosion of third degree of thigh

　✓7ᵗʰ **T24.711** Corrosion of third degree of right thigh

　✓7ᵗʰ **T24.712** Corrosion of third degree of left thigh

　✓7ᵗʰ **T24.719** Corrosion of third degree of unspecified thigh

✓6ᵗʰ **T24.72** Corrosion of third degree of knee

　✓7ᵗʰ **T24.721** Corrosion of third degree of right knee

　✓7ᵗʰ **T24.722** Corrosion of third degree of left knee

　✓7ᵗʰ **T24.729** Corrosion of third degree of unspecified knee

✓6ᵗʰ **T24.73** Corrosion of third degree of lower leg

　✓7ᵗʰ **T24.731** Corrosion of third degree of right lower leg

　✓7ᵗʰ **T24.732** Corrosion of third degree of left lower leg

　✓7ᵗʰ **T24.739** Corrosion of third degree of unspecified lower leg

✓6ᵗʰ **T24.79** Corrosion of third degree of multiple sites of lower limb, except ankle and foot

　✓7ᵗʰ **T24.791** Corrosion of third degree of multiple sites of right lower limb, except ankle and foot

　✓7ᵗʰ **T24.792** Corrosion of third degree of multiple sites of left lower limb, except ankle and foot

　✓7ᵗʰ **T24.799** Corrosion of third degree of multiple sites of unspecified lower limb, except ankle and foot

✓4ᵗʰ **T25** Burn and corrosion of ankle and foot

The appropriate 7th character is to be added to each code from category T25.
A　initial encounter
D　subsequent encounter
S　sequela

✓5ᵗʰ **T25.0** Burn of unspecified degree of ankle and foot

Use additional external cause code to identify the source, place and intent of the burn (X00-X19, X75-X77, X96-X98, Y92)

✓6ᵗʰ **T25.01** Burn of unspecified degree of ankle

　✓7ᵗʰ **T25.011** Burn of unspecified degree of right ankle

　✓7ᵗʰ **T25.012** Burn of unspecified degree of left ankle

　✓7ᵗʰ **T25.019** Burn of unspecified degree of unspecified ankle

✓6ᵗʰ **T25.02** Burn of unspecified degree of foot

EXCLUDES 2 burn of unspecified degree of toe(s) (nail) (T25.03-)

　✓7ᵗʰ **T25.021** Burn of unspecified degree of right foot

　✓7ᵗʰ **T25.022** Burn of unspecified degree of left foot

　✓7ᵗʰ **T25.029** Burn of unspecified degree of unspecified foot

✓6ᵗʰ **T25.03** Burn of unspecified degree of toe(s) (nail)

　✓7ᵗʰ **T25.031** Burn of unspecified degree of right toe(s) (nail)

　✓7ᵗʰ **T25.032** Burn of unspecified degree of left toe(s) (nail)

　✓7ᵗʰ **T25.039** Burn of unspecified degree of unspecified toe(s) (nail)

✓6ᵗʰ **T25.09** Burn of unspecified degree of multiple sites of ankle and foot

　✓7ᵗʰ **T25.091** Burn of unspecified degree of multiple sites of right ankle and foot

　✓7ᵗʰ **T25.092** Burn of unspecified degree of multiple sites of left ankle and foot

　✓7ᵗʰ **T25.099** Burn of unspecified degree of multiple sites of unspecified ankle and foot

✓5ᵗʰ **T25.1** Burn of first degree of ankle and foot

Use additional external cause code to identify the source, place and intent of the burn (X00-X19, X75-X77, X96-X98, Y92)

✓6ᵗʰ **T25.11** Burn of first degree of ankle

　✓7ᵗʰ **T25.111** Burn of first degree of right ankle

　✓7ᵗʰ **T25.112** Burn of first degree of left ankle

　✓7ᵗʰ **T25.119** Burn of first degree of unspecified ankle

✓6ᵗʰ **T25.12** Burn of first degree of foot

EXCLUDES 2 burn of first degree of toe(s) (nail) (T25.13-)

　✓7ᵗʰ **T25.121** Burn of first degree of right foot

　✓7ᵗʰ **T25.122** Burn of first degree of left foot

　✓7ᵗʰ **T25.129** Burn of first degree of unspecified foot

✓6ᵗʰ **T25.13** Burn of first degree of toe(s) (nail)

　✓7ᵗʰ **T25.131** Burn of first degree of right toe(s) (nail)

　✓7ᵗʰ **T25.132** Burn of first degree of left toe(s) (nail)

　✓7ᵗʰ **T25.139** Burn of first degree of unspecified toe(s) (nail)

✓6ᵗʰ **T25.19** Burn of first degree of multiple sites of ankle and foot

　✓7ᵗʰ **T25.191** Burn of first degree of multiple sites of right ankle and foot

　✓7ᵗʰ **T25.192** Burn of first degree of multiple sites of left ankle and foot

　✓7ᵗʰ **T25.199** Burn of first degree of multiple sites of unspecified ankle and foot

✓5ᵗʰ **T25.2** Burn of second degree of ankle and foot

Use additional external cause code to identify the source, place and intent of the burn (X00-X19, X75-X77, X96-X98, Y92)

✓6ᵗʰ **T25.21** Burn of second degree of ankle

　✓7ᵗʰ **T25.211** Burn of second degree of right ankle

　✓7ᵗʰ **T25.212** Burn of second degree of left ankle

　✓7ᵗʰ **T25.219** Burn of second degree of unspecified ankle

EXCLUDES 1 Not coded here　　*EXCLUDES 2* Not included here　　**N** Newborn Age: 0　　**P** Pediatric Age: 0-17　　**M** Maternity Age: 12-55　　**A** Adult Age: 15-124

978　　ICD-10-CM 2016

√6ᵗʰ **T25.22** Burn of second degree of **foot**
> EXCLUDES 2 *burn of second degree of toe(s) (nail) (T25.23-)*

    √7ᵗʰ **T25.221** Burn of second degree of **right** foot
    √7ᵗʰ **T25.222** Burn of second degree of **left** foot
    √7ᵗʰ **T25.229** Burn of second degree of **unspecified foot**

√6ᵗʰ **T25.23** Burn of second degree of **toe(s) (nail)**
    √7ᵗʰ **T25.231** Burn of second degree of **right** toe(s) (nail)
    √7ᵗʰ **T25.232** Burn of second degree of **left** toe(s) (nail)
    √7ᵗʰ **T25.239** Burn of second degree of **unspecified toe(s) (nail)**

√6ᵗʰ **T25.29** Burn of second degree of **multiple sites** of ankle and foot
    √7ᵗʰ **T25.291** Burn of second degree of multiple sites of **right** ankle and foot
    √7ᵗʰ **T25.292** Burn of second degree of multiple sites of **left** ankle and foot
    √7ᵗʰ **T25.299** Burn of second degree of multiple sites of **unspecified ankle and foot**

√5ᵗʰ **T25.3** Burn of **third degree** of ankle and foot
> Use additional external cause code to identify the source, place and intent of the burn (X00-X19, X75-X77, X96-X98, Y92)

√6ᵗʰ **T25.31** Burn of third degree of **ankle**
    √7ᵗʰ **T25.311** Burn of third degree of **right** ankle
    √7ᵗʰ **T25.312** Burn of third degree of **left** ankle
    √7ᵗʰ **T25.319** Burn of third degree of **unspecified ankle**

√6ᵗʰ **T25.32** Burn of third degree of **foot**
> EXCLUDES 2 *burn of third degree of toe(s) (nail) (T25.33)*

    √7ᵗʰ **T25.321** Burn of third degree of **right** foot
    √7ᵗʰ **T25.322** Burn of third degree of **left** foot
    √7ᵗʰ **T25.329** Burn of third degree of **unspecified foot**

√6ᵗʰ **T25.33** Burn of third degree of **toe(s) (nail)**
    √7ᵗʰ **T25.331** Burn of third degree of **right** toe(s) (nail)
    √7ᵗʰ **T25.332** Burn of third degree of **left** toe(s) (nail)
    √7ᵗʰ **T25.339** Burn of third degree of **unspecified toe(s) (nail)**

√6ᵗʰ **T25.39** Burn of third degree of **multiple sites** of ankle and foot
    √7ᵗʰ **T25.391** Burn of third degree of multiple sites of **right** ankle and foot
    √7ᵗʰ **T25.392** Burn of third degree of multiple sites of **left** ankle and foot
    √7ᵗʰ **T25.399** Burn of third degree of multiple sites of **unspecified ankle and foot**

√5ᵗʰ **T25.4** Corrosion of **unspecified degree** of ankle and foot
> Code first (T51-T65) to identify chemical and intent
> Use additional external cause code to identify place (Y92)

√6ᵗʰ **T25.41** Corrosion of unspecified degree of **ankle**
    √7ᵗʰ **T25.411** Corrosion of unspecified degree of **right ankle**
    √7ᵗʰ **T25.412** Corrosion of unspecified degree of **left ankle**
    √7ᵗʰ **T25.419** Corrosion of unspecified degree of **unspecified ankle**

√6ᵗʰ **T25.42** Corrosion of unspecified degree of **foot**
> EXCLUDES 2 *corrosion of unspecified degree of toe(s) (nail) (T25.43-)*

    √7ᵗʰ **T25.421** Corrosion of unspecified degree of **right foot**
    √7ᵗʰ **T25.422** Corrosion of unspecified degree of **left foot**
    √7ᵗʰ **T25.429** Corrosion of unspecified degree of **unspecified foot**

√6ᵗʰ **T25.43** Corrosion of unspecified degree of **toe(s) (nail)**
    √7ᵗʰ **T25.431** Corrosion of unspecified degree of **right toe(s) (nail)**
    √7ᵗʰ **T25.432** Corrosion of unspecified degree of **left toe(s) (nail)**
    √7ᵗʰ **T25.439** Corrosion of unspecified degree of **unspecified toe(s) (nail)**

√6ᵗʰ **T25.49** Corrosion of unspecified degree of **multiple sites** of ankle and foot
    √7ᵗʰ **T25.491** Corrosion of unspecified degree of multiple sites of **right ankle and foot**
    √7ᵗʰ **T25.492** Corrosion of unspecified degree of multiple sites of **left ankle and foot**
    √7ᵗʰ **T25.499** Corrosion of unspecified degree of multiple sites of **unspecified ankle and foot**

√5ᵗʰ **T25.5** Corrosion of **first degree** of ankle and foot
> Code first (T51-T65) to identify chemical and intent
> Use additional external cause code to identify place (Y92)

√6ᵗʰ **T25.51** Corrosion of first degree of **ankle**
    √7ᵗʰ **T25.511** Corrosion of first degree of **right** ankle
    √7ᵗʰ **T25.512** Corrosion of first degree of **left** ankle
    √7ᵗʰ **T25.519** Corrosion of first degree of **unspecified ankle**

√6ᵗʰ **T25.52** Corrosion of first degree of **foot**
> EXCLUDES 2 *corrosion of first degree of toe(s) (nail) (T25.53-)*

    √7ᵗʰ **T25.521** Corrosion of first degree of **right** foot
    √7ᵗʰ **T25.522** Corrosion of first degree of **left** foot
    √7ᵗʰ **T25.529** Corrosion of first degree of **unspecified foot**

√6ᵗʰ **T25.53** Corrosion of first degree of **toe(s) (nail)**
    √7ᵗʰ **T25.531** Corrosion of first degree of **right** toe(s) (nail)
    √7ᵗʰ **T25.532** Corrosion of first degree of **left** toe(s) (nail)
    √7ᵗʰ **T25.539** Corrosion of first degree of **unspecified toe(s) (nail)**

√6ᵗʰ **T25.59** Corrosion of first degree of **multiple sites** of ankle and foot
    √7ᵗʰ **T25.591** Corrosion of first degree of multiple sites of **right** ankle and foot
    √7ᵗʰ **T25.592** Corrosion of first degree of multiple sites of **left** ankle and foot
    √7ᵗʰ **T25.599** Corrosion of first degree of multiple sites of **unspecified ankle and foot**

√5ᵗʰ **T25.6** Corrosion of **second degree** of ankle and foot
> Code first (T51-T65) to identify chemical and intent
> Use additional external cause code to identify place (Y92)

√6ᵗʰ **T25.61** Corrosion of second degree of **ankle**
    √7ᵗʰ **T25.611** Corrosion of second degree of **right** ankle
    √7ᵗʰ **T25.612** Corrosion of second degree of **left** ankle
    √7ᵗʰ **T25.619** Corrosion of second degree of **unspecified ankle**

√6ᵗʰ **T25.62** Corrosion of second degree of **foot**
> EXCLUDES 2 *corrosion of second degree of toe(s) (nail) (T25.63-)*

    √7ᵗʰ **T25.621** Corrosion of second degree of **right** foot
    √7ᵗʰ **T25.622** Corrosion of second degree of **left** foot
    √7ᵗʰ **T25.629** Corrosion of second degree of **unspecified foot**

√6ᵗʰ **T25.63** Corrosion of second degree of **toe(s) (nail)**
    √7ᵗʰ **T25.631** Corrosion of second degree of **right** toe(s) (nail)
    √7ᵗʰ **T25.632** Corrosion of second degree of **left** toe(s) (nail)
    √7ᵗʰ **T25.639** Corrosion of second degree of **unspecified toe(s) (nail)**

√6ᵗʰ **T25.69** Corrosion of second degree of **multiple sites** of ankle and foot
    √7ᵗʰ **T25.691** Corrosion of second degree of **right** ankle and foot
    √7ᵗʰ **T25.692** Corrosion of second degree of **left** ankle and foot
    √7ᵗʰ **T25.699** Corrosion of second degree of **unspecified ankle and foot**

√5ᵗʰ **T25.7** Corrosion of **third degree** of ankle and foot
> Code first (T51-T65) to identify chemical and intent
> Use additional external cause code to identify place (Y92)

√6ᵗʰ **T25.71** Corrosion of third degree of **ankle**
    √7ᵗʰ **T25.711** Corrosion of third degree of **right** ankle

---

☑ Additional Character Required   ✔x7ᵗʰ Placeholder Alert   Unspecified Dx   Other Specified Dx   Manifestation   ▶◀ Revised Text   ● New Code   ▲ Revised Code Title

Chapter 19. Injury, Poisoning, and Certain Other Consequences of External Causes
T25.712–T28.3

- ✓7th **T25.712** Corrosion of third degree of left ankle
- ✓7th **T25.719** **Corrosion of third degree of unspecified ankle**
- ✓6th **T25.72** Corrosion of third degree of foot
  - EXCLUDES 2 *corrosion of third degree of toe(s) (nail) (T25.73-)*
  - ✓7th **T25.721** **Corrosion of third degree of right foot**
  - ✓7th **T25.722** **Corrosion of third degree of left foot**
  - ✓7th **T25.729** **Corrosion of third degree of unspecified foot**
- ✓6th **T25.73** Corrosion of third degree of toe(s) (nail)
  - ✓7th **T25.731** **Corrosion of third degree of right toe(s) (nail)**
  - ✓7th **T25.732** **Corrosion of third degree of left toe(s) (nail)**
  - ✓7th **T25.739** **Corrosion of third degree of unspecified toe(s) (nail)**
- ✓6th **T25.79** Corrosion of third degree of multiple sites of ankle and foot
  - ✓7th **T25.791** **Corrosion of third degree of multiple sites of right ankle and foot**
  - ✓7th **T25.792** **Corrosion of third degree of multiple sites of left ankle and foot**
  - ✓7th **T25.799** **Corrosion of third degree of multiple sites of unspecified ankle and foot**

Burns and corrosions confined to eye and internal organs (T26-T28)

✓4th **T26** **Burn and corrosion confined to eye and adnexa**

> The appropriate 7th character is to be added to each code from category T26.
> A   initial encounter
> D   subsequent encounter
> S   sequela

- ✓5th **T26.0** **Burn of eyelid and periocular area**
  - Use additional external cause code to identify the source, place and intent of the burn (X00-X19, X75-X77, X96-X98, Y92)
  - ✓x7th **T26.00** **Burn of unspecified eyelid and periocular area**
  - ✓x7th **T26.01** **Burn of right eyelid and periocular area**
  - ✓x7th **T26.02** **Burn of left eyelid and periocular area**
- ✓5th **T26.1** **Burn of cornea and conjunctival sac**
  - Use additional external cause code to identify the source, place and intent of the burn (X00-X19, X75-X77, X96-X98, Y92)
  - ✓x7th **T26.10** **Burn of cornea and conjunctival sac, unspecified eye**
  - ✓x7th **T26.11** **Burn of cornea and conjunctival sac, right eye**
  - ✓x7th **T26.12** **Burn of cornea and conjunctival sac, left eye**
- ✓5th **T26.2** **Burn with resulting rupture and destruction of eyeball**
  - Use additional external cause code to identify the source, place and intent of the burn (X00-X19, X75-X77, X96-X98, Y92)
  - ✓x7th **T26.20** **Burn with resulting rupture and destruction of unspecified eyeball**
  - ✓x7th **T26.21** **Burn with resulting rupture and destruction of right eyeball**
  - ✓x7th **T26.22** **Burn with resulting rupture and destruction of left eyeball**
- ✓5th **T26.3** **Burns of other specified parts of eye and adnexa**
  - Use additional external cause code to identify the source, place and intent of the burn (X00-X19, X75-X77, X96-X98, Y92)
  - ✓x7th **T26.30** **Burns of other specified parts of unspecified eye and adnexa**
  - ✓x7th **T26.31** **Burns of other specified parts of right eye and adnexa**
  - ✓x7th **T26.32** **Burns of other specified parts of left eye and adnexa**
- ✓5th **T26.4** **Burn of eye and adnexa, part unspecified**
  - Use additional external cause code to identify the source, place and intent of the burn (X00-X19, X75-X77, X96-X98, Y92)
  - ✓x7th **T26.40** **Burn of unspecified eye and adnexa, part unspecified**
  - ✓x7th **T26.41** **Burn of right eye and adnexa, part unspecified**
  - ✓x7th **T26.42** **Burn of left eye and adnexa, part unspecified**

- ✓5th **T26.5** **Corrosion of eyelid and periocular area**
  - Code first (T51-T65) to identify chemical and intent
  - Use additional external cause code to identify place (Y92)
  - ✓x7th **T26.50** **Corrosion of unspecified eyelid and periocular area**
  - ✓x7th **T26.51** **Corrosion of right eyelid and periocular area**
  - ✓x7th **T26.52** **Corrosion of left eyelid and periocular area**
- ✓5th **T26.6** **Corrosion of cornea and conjunctival sac**
  - Code first (T51-T65) to identify chemical and intent
  - Use additional external cause code to identify place (Y92)
  - ✓x7th **T26.60** **Corrosion of cornea and conjunctival sac, unspecified eye**
  - ✓x7th **T26.61** **Corrosion of cornea and conjunctival sac, right eye**
  - ✓x7th **T26.62** **Corrosion of cornea and conjunctival sac, left eye**
- ✓5th **T26.7** **Corrosion with resulting rupture and destruction of eyeball**
  - Code first (T51-T65) to identify chemical and intent
  - Use additional external cause code to identify place (Y92)
  - ✓x7th **T26.70** **Corrosion with resulting rupture and destruction of unspecified eyeball**
  - ✓x7th **T26.71** **Corrosion with resulting rupture and destruction of right eyeball**
  - ✓x7th **T26.72** **Corrosion with resulting rupture and destruction of left eyeball**
- ✓5th **T26.8** **Corrosions of other specified parts of eye and adnexa**
  - Code first (T51-T65) to identify chemical and intent
  - Use additional external cause code to identify place (Y92)
  - ✓x7th **T26.80** **Corrosions of other specified parts of unspecified eye and adnexa**
  - ✓x7th **T26.81** **Corrosions of other specified parts of right eye and adnexa**
  - ✓x7th **T26.82** **Corrosions of other specified parts of left eye and adnexa**
- ✓5th **T26.9** **Corrosion of eye and adnexa, part unspecified**
  - Code first (T51-T65) to identify chemical and intent
  - Use additional external cause code to identify place (Y92)
  - ✓x7th **T26.90** **Corrosion of unspecified eye and adnexa, part unspecified**
  - ✓x7th **T26.91** **Corrosion of right eye and adnexa, part unspecified**
  - ✓x7th **T26.92** **Corrosion of left eye and adnexa, part unspecified**

✓4th **T27** **Burn and corrosion of respiratory tract**
> Use additional external cause code to identify the source and intent of the burn (X00-X19, X75-X77, X96-X98)
> Use additional external cause code to identify place (Y92)

> The appropriate 7th character is to be added to each code from category T27.
> A   initial encounter
> D   subsequent encounter
> S   sequela

- ✓x7th **T27.0** **Burn of larynx and trachea**
- ✓x7th **T27.1** **Burn involving larynx and trachea with lung**
- ✓x7th **T27.2** **Burn of other parts of respiratory tract**
  - Burn of thoracic cavity
- ✓x7th **T27.3** **Burn of respiratory tract, part unspecified**
  - Code first (T51-T65) to identify chemical and intent for codes T27.4-T27.7
- ✓x7th **T27.4** **Corrosion of larynx and trachea**
- ✓x7th **T27.5** **Corrosion involving larynx and trachea with lung**
- ✓x7th **T27.6** **Corrosion of other parts of respiratory tract**
- ✓x7th **T27.7** **Corrosion of respiratory tract, part unspecified**

✓4th **T28** **Burn and corrosion of other internal organs**
> Use additional external cause code to identify the source and intent of the burn (X00- X19, X75-X77, X96-X98)
> Use additional external cause code to identify place (Y92)

> The appropriate 7th character is to be added to each code from category T28.
> A   initial encounter
> D   subsequent encounter
> S   sequela

- ✓x7th **T28.0** **Burn of mouth and pharynx**
- ✓x7th **T28.1** **Burn of esophagus**
- ✓x7th **T28.2** **Burn of other parts of alimentary tract**
- ✓x7th **T28.3** **Burn of internal genitourinary organs**

EXCLUDES 1 Not coded here   EXCLUDES 2 Not included here   N Newborn Age: 0   P Pediatric Age: 0-17   M Maternity Age: 12-55   A Adult Age: 15-124

980   ICD-10-CM 2016

✓5th **T28.4** **Burns of other and unspecified internal organs**
- ✓x7th **T28.40** **Burn of unspecified internal organ**
- ✓6th **T28.41** **Burn of** ear drum
  - ✓7th **T28.411** **Burn of right ear drum**
  - ✓7th **T28.412** **Burn of left ear drum**
  - ✓7th **T28.419** **Burn of unspecified ear drum**
- ✓x7th **T28.49** **Burn of other internal organ**
  Code first (T51-T65) to identify chemical and intent for T28.5-T28.9-

✓x7th **T28.5** **Corrosion of** mouth and pharynx

✓x7th **T28.6** **Corrosion of** esophagus

✓x7th **T28.7** **Corrosion of other parts of** alimentary tract

✓x7th **T28.8** **Corrosion of internal** genitourinary organs

✓5th **T28.9** **Corrosions of other and unspecified internal organs**
- ✓x7th **T28.90** **Corrosions of unspecified internal organs**
- ✓6th **T28.91** **Corrosions of** ear drum
  - ✓7th **T28.911** **Corrosions of right ear drum**
  - ✓7th **T28.912** **Corrosions of left ear drum**
  - ✓7th **T28.919** **Corrosions of unspecified ear drum**
- ✓x7th **T28.99** **Corrosions of other internal organs**

Burns and corrosions of multiple and unspecified body regions (T30-T32)

✓4th **T30** **Burn and corrosion, body region unspecified**
- **T30.0** **Burn of unspecified body region, unspecified degree**
  NOTE This code is not for inpatient use. Code to specified site and degree of burns.
  Burn NOS
  Multiple burns NOS
- **T30.4** **Corrosion of unspecified body region, unspecified degree**
  NOTE This code is not for inpatient use. Code to specified site and degree of corrosion.
  Corrosion NOS
  Multiple corrosion NOS

✓4th **T31** **Burns classified according to extent of body surface involved**
  NOTE This category is to be used as the primary code only when the site of the burn is unspecified. It should be used as a supplementary code with categories T20-T25 when the site is specified.
- **T31.0** **Burns involving** less than 10% of body surface
- ✓5th **T31.1** **Burns involving** 10-19% **of body surface**
  - **T31.10** **Burns involving 10-19% of body surface with** 0% to 9% third degree **burns**
    Burns involving 10-19% of body surface NOS
  - **T31.11** **Burns involving 10-19% of body surface with** 10-19% third degree **burns**
- ✓5th **T31.2** **Burns involving** 20-29% **of body surface**
  - **T31.20** **Burns involving 20-29% of body surface with** 0% to 9% third degree **burns**
    Burns involving 20-29% of body surface NOS
  - **T31.21** **Burns involving 20-29% of body surface with** 10-19% third degree **burns**
  - **T31.22** **Burns involving 20-29% of body surface with** 20-29% third degree **burns**
- ✓5th **T31.3** **Burns involving** 30-39% **of body surface**
  - **T31.30** **Burns involving 30-39% of body surface with** 0% to 9% third degree **burns**
    Burns involving 30-39% of body surface NOS
  - **T31.31** **Burns involving 30-39% of body surface with** 10-19% third degree **burns**
  - **T31.32** **Burns involving 30-39% of body surface with** 20-29% third degree **burns**
  - **T31.33** **Burns involving 30-39% of body surface with** 30-39% third degree **burns**
- ✓5th **T31.4** **Burns involving** 40-49% **of body surface**
  - **T31.40** **Burns involving 40-49% of body surface with** 0% to 9% third degree **burns**
    Burns involving 40-49% of body surface NOS
  - **T31.41** **Burns involving 40-49% of body surface with** 10-19% third degree **burns**
  - **T31.42** **Burns involving 40-49% of body surface with** 20-29% third degree **burns**
  - **T31.43** **Burns involving 40-49% of body surface with** 30-39% third degree **burns**
  - **T31.44** **Burns involving 40-49% of body surface with** 40-49% third degree **burns**
- ✓5th **T31.5** **Burns involving** 50-59% **of body surface**
  - **T31.50** **Burns involving 50-59% of body surface with** 0% to 9% third degree **burns**
    Burns involving 50-59% of body surface NOS
  - **T31.51** **Burns involving 50-59% of body surface with** 10-19% third degree **burns**
  - **T31.52** **Burns involving 50-59% of body surface with** 20-29% third degree **burns**
  - **T31.53** **Burns involving 50-59% of body surface with** 30-39% third degree **burns**
  - **T31.54** **Burns involving 50-59% of body surface with** 40-49% third degree **burns**
  - **T31.55** **Burns involving 50-59% of body surface with** 50-59% third degree **burns**
- ✓5th **T31.6** **Burns involving** 60-69% **of body surface**
  - **T31.60** **Burns involving 60-69% of body surface with** 0% to 9% third degree **burns**
    Burns involving 60-69% of body surface NOS
  - **T31.61** **Burns involving 60-69% of body surface with** 10-19% third degree **burns**
  - **T31.62** **Burns involving 60-69% of body surface with** 20-29% third degree **burns**
  - **T31.63** **Burns involving 60-69% of body surface with** 30-39% third degree **burns**
  - **T31.64** **Burns involving 60-69% of body surface with** 40-49% third degree **burns**
  - **T31.65** **Burns involving 60-69% of body surface with** 50-59% third degree **burns**
  - **T31.66** **Burns involving 60-69% of body surface with** 60-69% third degree **burns**
- ✓5th **T31.7** **Burns involving** 70-79% **of body surface**
  - **T31.70** **Burns involving 70-79% of body surface with** 0% to 9% third degree **burns**
    Burns involving 70-79% of body surface NOS
  - **T31.71** **Burns involving 70-79% of body surface with** 10-19% third degree **burns**
  - **T31.72** **Burns involving 70-79% of body surface with** 20-29% third degree **burns**
  - **T31.73** **Burns involving 70-79% of body surface with** 30-39% third degree **burns**
  - **T31.74** **Burns involving 70-79% of body surface with** 40-49% third degree **burns**
  - **T31.75** **Burns involving 70-79% of body surface with** 50-59% third degree **burns**
  - **T31.76** **Burns involving 70-79% of body surface with** 60-69% third degree **burns**
  - **T31.77** **Burns involving 70-79% of body surface with** 70-79% third degree **burns**
- ✓5th **T31.8** **Burns involving** 80-89% **of body surface**
  - **T31.80** **Burns involving 80-89% of body surface with** 0% to 9% third degree **burns**
    Burns involving 80-89% of body surface NOS
  - **T31.81** **Burns involving 80-89% of body surface with** 10-19% third degree **burns**
  - **T31.82** **Burns involving 80-89% of body surface with** 20-29% third degree **burns**
  - **T31.83** **Burns involving 80-89% of body surface with** 30-39% third degree **burns**
  - **T31.84** **Burns involving 80-89% of body surface with** 40-49% third degree **burns**
  - **T31.85** **Burns involving 80-89% of body surface with** 50-59% third degree **burns**
  - **T31.86** **Burns involving 80-89% of body surface with** 60-69% third degree **burns**
  - **T31.87** **Burns involving 80-89% of body surface with** 70-79% third degree **burns**
  - **T31.88** **Burns involving 80-89% of body surface with** 80-89% third degree **burns**
- ✓5th **T31.9** **Burns involving** 90% or more **of body surface**
  - **T31.90** **Burns involving 90% or more of body surface with** 0% to 9% third degree **burns**
    Burns involving 90% or more of body surface NOS

☑ Additional Character Required   ✓x7th Placeholder Alert   Unspecified Dx   Other Specified Dx   Manifestation   ►◄ Revised Text   ● New Code   ▲ Revised Code Title

T31.91 Burns involving 90% or more of body surface with 10-19% third degree **burns**

T31.92 Burns involving 90% or more of body surface with 20-29% third degree **burns**

T31.93 Burns involving 90% or more of body surface with 30-39% third degree **burns**

T31.94 Burns involving 90% or more of body surface with 40-49% third degree **burns**

T31.95 Burns involving 90% or more of body surface with 50-59% third degree **burns**

T31.96 Burns involving 90% or more of body surface with 60-69% third degree **burns**

T31.97 Burns involving 90% or more of body surface with 70-79% third degree **burns**

T31.98 Burns involving 90% or more of body surface with 80-89% third degree **burns**

T31.99 Burns involving 90% or more of body surface with 90% or more third degree **burns**

√4ᵗʰ **T32** Corrosions **classified** according to extent of body surface involved

> **NOTE** This category is to be used as the primary code only when the site of the corrosion is unspecified. It may be used as a supplementary code with categories T20-T25 when the site is specified.

T32.0 Corrosions involving less than 10% of body surface

√5ᵗʰ **T32.1** Corrosions involving 10-19% of body surface

T32.10 Corrosions involving 10-19% of body surface with 0% to 9% third degree **corrosion**
Corrosions involving 10-19% of body surface NOS

T32.11 Corrosions involving 10-19% of body surface with 10-19% third degree **corrosion**

√5ᵗʰ **T32.2** Corrosions involving 20-29% of body surface

T32.20 Corrosions involving 20-29% of body surface with 0% to 9% third degree **corrosion**

T32.21 Corrosions involving 20-29% of body surface with 10-19% third degree **corrosion**

T32.22 Corrosions involving 20-29% of body surface with 20-29% third degree **corrosion**

√5ᵗʰ **T32.3** Corrosions involving 30-39% of body surface

T32.30 Corrosions involving 30-39% of body surface with 0% to 9% third degree **corrosion**

T32.31 Corrosions involving 30-39% of body surface with 10-19% third degree **corrosion**

T32.32 Corrosions involving 30-39% of body surface with 20-29% third degree **corrosion**

T32.33 Corrosions involving 30-39% of body surface with 30-39% third degree **corrosion**

√5ᵗʰ **T32.4** Corrosions involving 40-49% of body surface

T32.40 Corrosions involving 40-49% of body surface with 0% to 9% third degree **corrosion**

T32.41 Corrosions involving 40-49% of body surface with 10-19% third degree **corrosion**

T32.42 Corrosions involving 40-49% of body surface with 20-29% third degree **corrosion**

T32.43 Corrosions involving 40-49% of body surface with 30-39% third degree **corrosion**

T32.44 Corrosions involving 40-49% of body surface with 40-49% third degree **corrosion**

√5ᵗʰ **T32.5** Corrosions involving 50-59% of body surface

T32.50 Corrosions involving 50-59% of body surface with 0% to 9% third degree **corrosion**

T32.51 Corrosions involving 50-59% of body surface with 10-19% third degree **corrosion**

T32.52 Corrosions involving 50-59% of body surface with 20-29% third degree **corrosion**

T32.53 Corrosions involving 50-59% of body surface with 30-39% third degree **corrosion**

T32.54 Corrosions involving 50-59% of body surface with 40-49% third degree **corrosion**

T32.55 Corrosions involving 50-59% of body surface with 50-59% third degree **corrosion**

√5ᵗʰ **T32.6** Corrosions involving 60-69% of body surface

T32.60 Corrosions involving 60-69% of body surface with 0% to 9% third degree **corrosion**

T32.61 Corrosions involving 60-69% of body surface with 10-19% third degree **corrosion**

T32.62 Corrosions involving 60-69% of body surface with 20-29% third degree **corrosion**

T32.63 Corrosions involving 60-69% of body surface with 30-39% third degree **corrosion**

T32.64 Corrosions involving 60-69% of body surface with 40-49% third degree **corrosion**

T32.65 Corrosions involving 60-69% of body surface with 50-59% third degree **corrosion**

T32.66 Corrosions involving 60-69% of body surface with 60-69% third degree **corrosion**

√5ᵗʰ **T32.7** Corrosions involving 70-79% of body surface

T32.70 Corrosions involving 70-79% of body surface with 0% to 9% third degree **corrosion**

T32.71 Corrosions involving 70-79% of body surface with 10-19% third degree **corrosion**

T32.72 Corrosions involving 70-79% of body surface with 20-29% third degree **corrosion**

T32.73 Corrosions involving 70-79% of body surface with 30-39% third degree **corrosion**

T32.74 Corrosions involving 70-79% of body surface with 40-49% third degree **corrosion**

T32.75 Corrosions involving 70-79% of body surface with 50-59% third degree **corrosion**

T32.76 Corrosions involving 70-79% of body surface with 60-69% third degree **corrosion**

T32.77 Corrosions involving 70-79% of body surface with 70-79% third degree **corrosion**

√5ᵗʰ **T32.8** Corrosions involving 80-89% of body surface

T32.80 Corrosions involving 80-89% of body surface with 0% to 9% third degree **corrosion**

T32.81 Corrosions involving 80-89% of body surface with 10-19% third degree **corrosion**

T32.82 Corrosions involving 80-89% of body surface with 20-29% third degree **corrosion**

T32.83 Corrosions involving 80-89% of body surface with 30-39% third degree **corrosion**

T32.84 Corrosions involving 80-89% of body surface with 40-49% third degree **corrosion**

T32.85 Corrosions involving 80-89% of body surface with 50-59% third degree **corrosion**

T32.86 Corrosions involving 80-89% of body surface with 60-69% third degree **corrosion**

T32.87 Corrosions involving 80-89% of body surface with 70-79% third degree **corrosion**

T32.88 Corrosions involving 80-89% of body surface with 80-89% third degree **corrosion**

√5ᵗʰ **T32.9** Corrosions involving 90% or more of body surface

T32.90 Corrosions involving 90% or more of body surface with 0% to 9% third degree **corrosion**

T32.91 Corrosions involving 90% or more of body surface with 10-19% third degree **corrosion**

T32.92 Corrosions involving 90% or more of body surface with 20-29% third degree **corrosion**

T32.93 Corrosions involving 90% or more of body surface with 30-39% third degree **corrosion**

T32.94 Corrosions involving 90% or more of body surface with 40-49% third degree **corrosion**

T32.95 Corrosions involving 90% or more of body surface with 50-59% third degree **corrosion**

T32.96 Corrosions involving 90% or more of body surface with 60-69% third degree **corrosion**

T32.97 Corrosions involving 90% or more of body surface with 70-79% third degree **corrosion**

T32.98 Corrosions involving 90% or more of body surface with 80-89% third degree **corrosion**

T32.99 Corrosions involving 90% or more of body surface with 90% or more third degree **corrosion**

EXCLUDES 1 Not coded here   EXCLUDES 2 Not included here   N Newborn Age: 0   P Pediatric Age: 0-17   M Maternity Age: 12-55   A Adult Age: 15-124

982   ICD-10-CM 2016

Frostbite (T33-T34)

EXCLUDES 2   hypothermia and other effects of reduced temperature (T68, T69-)

✓4ᵗʰ **T33**   **Superficial frostbite**

    INCLUDES   frostbite with partial thickness skin loss

> The appropriate 7th character is to be added to each code from category T33.
> A   initial encounter
> D   subsequent encounter
> S   sequela

✓5ᵗʰ   **T33.0**   Superficial frostbite of head

    ✓6ᵗʰ   **T33.01**   **Superficial frostbite of** ear

      ✓7ᵗʰ   **T33.011**   **Superficial frostbite of** right **ear**

      ✓7ᵗʰ   **T33.012**   **Superficial frostbite of** left **ear**

      ✓7ᵗʰ   **T33.019**   **Superficial frostbite of unspecified ear**

    ✓x7ᵗʰ   **T33.02**   **Superficial frostbite of** nose

    ✓x7ᵗʰ   **T33.09**   **Superficial frostbite of other** part of head

✓x7ᵗʰ   **T33.1**   Superficial frostbite of neck

✓x7ᵗʰ   **T33.2**   Superficial frostbite of thorax

✓x7ᵗʰ   **T33.3**   Superficial frostbite of abdominal wall, lower back and pelvis

✓5ᵗʰ   **T33.4**   Superficial frostbite of arm

    EXCLUDES 2   superficial frostbite of wrist and hand (T33.5-)

    ✓x7ᵗʰ   **T33.40**   **Superficial frostbite of unspecified arm**

    ✓x7ᵗʰ   **T33.41**   **Superficial frostbite of** right **arm**

    ✓x7ᵗʰ   **T33.42**   **Superficial frostbite of** left **arm**

✓5ᵗʰ   **T33.5**   Superficial frostbite of wrist, hand, and fingers

    ✓6ᵗʰ   **T33.51**   **Superficial frostbite of** wrist

      ✓7ᵗʰ   **T33.511**   **Superficial frostbite of** right **wrist**

      ✓7ᵗʰ   **T33.512**   **Superficial frostbite of** left **wrist**

      ✓7ᵗʰ   **T33.519**   **Superficial frostbite of unspecified wrist**

    ✓6ᵗʰ   **T33.52**   **Superficial frostbite of** hand

      EXCLUDES 2   superficial frostbite of fingers (T33.53-)

      ✓7ᵗʰ   **T33.521**   **Superficial frostbite of** right **hand**

      ✓7ᵗʰ   **T33.522**   **Superficial frostbite of** left **hand**

      ✓7ᵗʰ   **T33.529**   **Superficial frostbite of unspecified hand**

    ✓6ᵗʰ   **T33.53**   **Superficial frostbite of** finger(s)

      ✓7ᵗʰ   **T33.531**   **Superficial frostbite of** right **finger(s)**

      ✓7ᵗʰ   **T33.532**   **Superficial frostbite of** left **finger(s)**

      ✓7ᵗʰ   **T33.539**   **Superficial frostbite of unspecified finger(s)**

✓5ᵗʰ   **T33.6**   Superficial frostbite of hip and thigh

    ✓x7ᵗʰ   **T33.60**   **Superficial frostbite of unspecified hip and thigh**

    ✓x7ᵗʰ   **T33.61**   **Superficial frostbite of** right **hip and thigh**

    ✓x7ᵗʰ   **T33.62**   **Superficial frostbite of** left **hip and thigh**

✓5ᵗʰ   **T33.7**   Superficial frostbite of knee and lower leg

    EXCLUDES 2   superficial frostbite of ankle and foot (T33.8-)

    ✓x7ᵗʰ   **T33.70**   **Superficial frostbite of unspecified knee and lower leg**

    ✓x7ᵗʰ   **T33.71**   **Superficial frostbite of** right **knee and lower leg**

    ✓x7ᵗʰ   **T33.72**   **Superficial frostbite of** left **knee and lower leg**

✓5ᵗʰ   **T33.8**   Superficial frostbite of ankle, foot, and toe(s)

    ✓6ᵗʰ   **T33.81**   **Superficial frostbite of** ankle

      ✓7ᵗʰ   **T33.811**   **Superficial frostbite of** right **ankle**

      ✓7ᵗʰ   **T33.812**   **Superficial frostbite of** left **ankle**

      ✓7ᵗʰ   **T33.819**   **Superficial frostbite of unspecified ankle**

    ✓6ᵗʰ   **T33.82**   **Superficial frostbite of** foot

      ✓7ᵗʰ   **T33.821**   **Superficial frostbite of** right **foot**

      ✓7ᵗʰ   **T33.822**   **Superficial frostbite of** left **foot**

      ✓7ᵗʰ   **T33.829**   **Superficial frostbite of unspecified foot**

    ✓6ᵗʰ   **T33.83**   **Superficial frostbite of** toe(s)

      ✓7ᵗʰ   **T33.831**   **Superficial frostbite of** right **toe(s)**

      ✓7ᵗʰ   **T33.832**   **Superficial frostbite of** left **toe(s)**

      ✓7ᵗʰ   **T33.839**   **Superficial frostbite of unspecified toe(s)**

✓5ᵗʰ   **T33.9**   Superficial frostbite of other and unspecified sites

    ✓x7ᵗʰ   **T33.90**   **Superficial frostbite of unspecified sites**
> Superficial frostbite NOS

    ✓x7ᵗʰ   **T33.99**   **Superficial frostbite of other sites**
> Superficial frostbite of leg NOS
> Superficial frostbite of trunk NOS

✓4ᵗʰ **T34**   **Frostbite with tissue necrosis**

> The appropriate 7th character is to be added to each code from category T34.
> A   initial encounter
> D   subsequent encounter
> S   sequela

✓5ᵗʰ   **T34.0**   Frostbite with tissue necrosis of head

    ✓6ᵗʰ   **T34.01**   **Frostbite with tissue necrosis of** ear

      ✓7ᵗʰ   **T34.011**   **Frostbite with tissue necrosis of** right **ear**

      ✓7ᵗʰ   **T34.012**   **Frostbite with tissue necrosis of** left **ear**

      ✓7ᵗʰ   **T34.019**   **Frostbite with tissue necrosis of unspecified ear**

    ✓x7ᵗʰ   **T34.02**   **Frostbite with tissue necrosis of** nose

    ✓x7ᵗʰ   **T34.09**   **Frostbite with tissue necrosis of other part of head**

✓x7ᵗʰ   **T34.1**   Frostbite with tissue necrosis of neck

✓x7ᵗʰ   **T34.2**   Frostbite with tissue necrosis of thorax

✓x7ᵗʰ   **T34.3**   Frostbite with tissue necrosis of abdominal wall, lower back and pelvis

✓5ᵗʰ   **T34.4**   Frostbite with tissue necrosis of arm

    EXCLUDES 2   frostbite with tissue necrosis of wrist and hand (T34.5-)

    ✓x7ᵗʰ   **T34.40**   **Frostbite with tissue necrosis of unspecified arm**

    ✓x7ᵗʰ   **T34.41**   **Frostbite with tissue necrosis of** right **arm**

    ✓x7ᵗʰ   **T34.42**   **Frostbite with tissue necrosis of** left **arm**

✓5ᵗʰ   **T34.5**   Frostbite with tissue necrosis of wrist, hand, and finger(s)

    ✓6ᵗʰ   **T34.51**   **Frostbite with tissue necrosis of** wrist

      ✓7ᵗʰ   **T34.511**   **Frostbite with tissue necrosis of** right **wrist**

      ✓7ᵗʰ   **T34.512**   **Frostbite with tissue necrosis of** left **wrist**

      ✓7ᵗʰ   **T34.519**   **Frostbite with tissue necrosis of unspecified wrist**

    ✓6ᵗʰ   **T34.52**   **Frostbite with tissue necrosis of** hand

      EXCLUDES 2   frostbite with tissue necrosis of finger(s) (T34.53-)

      ✓7ᵗʰ   **T34.521**   **Frostbite with tissue necrosis of** right **hand**

      ✓7ᵗʰ   **T34.522**   **Frostbite with tissue necrosis of** left **hand**

      ✓7ᵗʰ   **T34.529**   **Frostbite with tissue necrosis of unspecified hand**

    ✓6ᵗʰ   **T34.53**   **Frostbite with tissue necrosis of** finger(s)

      ✓7ᵗʰ   **T34.531**   **Frostbite with tissue necrosis of** right **finger(s)**

      ✓7ᵗʰ   **T34.532**   **Frostbite with tissue necrosis of** left **finger(s)**

      ✓7ᵗʰ   **T34.539**   **Frostbite with tissue necrosis of unspecified finger(s)**

✓5ᵗʰ   **T34.6**   Frostbite with tissue necrosis of hip and thigh

    ✓x7ᵗʰ   **T34.60**   **Frostbite with tissue necrosis of unspecified hip and thigh**

    ✓x7ᵗʰ   **T34.61**   **Frostbite with tissue necrosis of** right **hip and thigh**

    ✓x7ᵗʰ   **T34.62**   **Frostbite with tissue necrosis of** left **hip and thigh**

✓5ᵗʰ   **T34.7**   Frostbite with tissue necrosis of knee and lower leg

    EXCLUDES 2   frostbite with tissue necrosis of ankle and foot (T34.8-)

    ✓x7ᵗʰ   **T34.70**   **Frostbite with tissue necrosis of unspecified knee and lower leg**

    ✓x7ᵗʰ   **T34.71**   **Frostbite with tissue necrosis of** right **knee and lower leg**

    ✓x7ᵗʰ   **T34.72**   **Frostbite with tissue necrosis of** left **knee and lower leg**

✓5ᵗʰ   **T34.8**   Frostbite with tissue necrosis of ankle, foot, and toe(s)

    ✓6ᵗʰ   **T34.81**   **Frostbite with tissue necrosis of** ankle

      ✓7ᵗʰ   **T34.811**   **Frostbite with tissue necrosis of** right **ankle**

      ✓7ᵗʰ   **T34.812**   **Frostbite with tissue necrosis of** left **ankle**

      ✓7ᵗʰ   **T34.819**   **Frostbite with tissue necrosis of unspecified ankle**

    ✓6ᵗʰ   **T34.82**   **Frostbite with tissue necrosis of** foot

      ✓7ᵗʰ   **T34.821**   **Frostbite with tissue necrosis of** right **foot**

      ✓7ᵗʰ   **T34.822**   **Frostbite with tissue necrosis of** left **foot**

      ✓7ᵗʰ   **T34.829**   **Frostbite with tissue necrosis of unspecified foot**

☑ Additional Character Required   ✓x7ᵗʰ Placeholder Alert   Unspecified Dx   Other Specified Dx   Manifestation   ▶◀ Revised Text   ● New Code   ▲ Revised Code Title

✓6ᵗʰ **T34.83**   **Frostbite with tissue necrosis of** toe(s)

    ✓7ᵗʰ **T34.831**   **Frostbite with tissue necrosis of** right toe(s)

    ✓7ᵗʰ **T34.832**   **Frostbite with tissue necrosis of** left toe(s)

    ✓7ᵗʰ **T34.839**   **Frostbite with tissue necrosis of unspecified toe(s)**

✓5ᵗʰ **T34.9**   **Frostbite with tissue necrosis of other and unspecified sites**

    ✓x7ᵗʰ **T34.90**   **Frostbite with tissue necrosis of unspecified sites**
       Frostbite with tissue necrosis NOS

    ✓x7ᵗʰ **T34.99**   **Frostbite with tissue necrosis of other sites**
       Frostbite with tissue necrosis of leg NOS
       Frostbite with tissue necrosis of trunk NOS

Poisoning by, adverse effects of and underdosing of drugs, medicaments and biological substances (T36-T50)

INCLUDES   adverse effect of correct substance properly administered
    poisoning by overdose of substance
    poisoning by wrong substance given or taken in error
    underdosing by (inadvertently) (deliberately) taking less substance than prescribed or instructed

Code first, for adverse effects, the nature of the adverse effect, such as:
    adverse effect NOS (T88.7)
    aspirin gastritis (K29.-)
    blood disorders (D56-D76)
    contact dermatitis (L23-L25)
    dermatitis due to substances taken internally (L27.-)
    nephropathy (N14.0-N14.2)

NOTE   The drug giving rise to the adverse effect should be identified by use of codes from categories T36-T50 with fifth or sixth character 5.

Use additional code(s) to specify:
    manifestations of poisoning
    underdosing or failure in dosage during medical and surgical care (Y63.6, Y63.8-Y63.9)
    underdosing of medication regimen (Z91.12-, Z91.13-)

EXCLUDES 1   *toxic reaction to local anesthesia in pregnancy (O29.3-)*
EXCLUDES 2   *abuse and dependence of psychoactive substances (F10-F19)*
    abuse of non-dependence-producing substances (F55.-)
    drug reaction and poisoning affecting newborn (P00-P96)
    pathological drug intoxication (inebriation) (F10-F19)

✓4ᵗʰ **T36**   **Poisoning by, adverse effect of and underdosing of systemic antibiotics**

    EXCLUDES 1   *antineoplastic antibiotics (T45.1-)*
       locally applied antibiotic NEC (T49.0)
       topically used antibiotic for ear, nose and throat (T49.6)
       topically used antibiotic for eye (T49.5)

    The appropriate 7th character is to be added to each code from category T36.
    A   initial encounter
    D   subsequent encounter
    S   sequela

✓5ᵗʰ **T36.0**   **Poisoning by, adverse effect of and underdosing of penicillins**

    ✓6ᵗʰ **T36.0X**   **Poisoning by, adverse effect of and underdosing of penicillins**

       ✓7ᵗʰ **T36.0X1**   **Poisoning by penicillins,** accidental (unintentional)
          Poisoning by penicillins NOS

       ✓7ᵗʰ **T36.0X2**   **Poisoning by penicillins,** intentional self-harm

       ✓7ᵗʰ **T36.0X3**   **Poisoning by penicillins,** assault

       ✓7ᵗʰ **T36.0X4**   **Poisoning by penicillins,** undetermined

       ✓7ᵗʰ **T36.0X5**   **Adverse effect of penicillins**

       ✓7ᵗʰ **T36.0X6**   **Underdosing of penicillins**

✓5ᵗʰ **T36.1**   **Poisoning by, adverse effect of and underdosing of cephalosporins and other beta-lactam antibiotics**

    ✓6ᵗʰ **T36.1X**   **Poisoning by, adverse effect of and underdosing of cephalosporins and other beta-lactam antibiotics**

       ✓7ᵗʰ **T36.1X1**   **Poisoning by cephalosporins and other beta-lactam antibiotics,** accidental (unintentional)
          Poisoning by cephalosporins and other beta-lactam antibiotics NOS

       ✓7ᵗʰ **T36.1X2**   **Poisoning by cephalosporins and other beta-lactam antibiotics,** intentional self-harm

       ✓7ᵗʰ **T36.1X3**   **Poisoning by cephalosporins and other beta-lactam antibiotics,** assault

       ✓7ᵗʰ **T36.1X4**   **Poisoning by cephalosporins and other beta-lactam antibiotics,** undetermined

       ✓7ᵗʰ **T36.1X5**   **Adverse effect of cephalosporins and other beta-lactam antibiotics**

       ✓7ᵗʰ **T36.1X6**   **Underdosing of cephalosporins and other beta-lactam antibiotics**

✓5ᵗʰ **T36.2**   **Poisoning by, adverse effect of and underdosing of chloramphenicol group**

    ✓6ᵗʰ **T36.2X**   **Poisoning by, adverse effect of and underdosing of chloramphenicol group**

       ✓7ᵗʰ **T36.2X1**   **Poisoning by chloramphenicol group,** accidental (unintentional)
          Poisoning by chloramphenicol group NOS

       ✓7ᵗʰ **T36.2X2**   **Poisoning by chloramphenicol group,** intentional self-harm

       ✓7ᵗʰ **T36.2X3**   **Poisoning by chloramphenicol group,** assault

       ✓7ᵗʰ **T36.2X4**   **Poisoning by chloramphenicol group,** undetermined

       ✓7ᵗʰ **T36.2X5**   **Adverse effect of chloramphenicol group**

       ✓7ᵗʰ **T36.2X6**   **Underdosing of chloramphenicol group**

✓5ᵗʰ **T36.3**   **Poisoning by, adverse effect of and underdosing of macrolides**

    ✓6ᵗʰ **T36.3X**   **Poisoning by, adverse effect of and underdosing of macrolides**

       ✓7ᵗʰ **T36.3X1**   **Poisoning by macrolides,** accidental (unintentional)
          Poisoning by macrolides NOS

       ✓7ᵗʰ **T36.3X2**   **Poisoning by macrolides,** intentional self-harm

       ✓7ᵗʰ **T36.3X3**   **Poisoning by macrolides,** assault

       ✓7ᵗʰ **T36.3X4**   **Poisoning by macrolides,** undetermined

       ✓7ᵗʰ **T36.3X5**   **Adverse effect of macrolides**

       ✓7ᵗʰ **T36.3X6**   **Underdosing of macrolides**

✓5ᵗʰ **T36.4**   **Poisoning by, adverse effect of and underdosing of tetracyclines**

    ✓6ᵗʰ **T36.4X**   **Poisoning by, adverse effect of and underdosing of tetracyclines**

       ✓7ᵗʰ **T36.4X1**   **Poisoning by tetracyclines,** accidental (unintentional)
          Poisoning by tetracyclines NOS

       ✓7ᵗʰ **T36.4X2**   **Poisoning by tetracyclines,** intentional self-harm

       ✓7ᵗʰ **T36.4X3**   **Poisoning by tetracyclines,** assault

       ✓7ᵗʰ **T36.4X4**   **Poisoning by tetracyclines,** undetermined

       ✓7ᵗʰ **T36.4X5**   **Adverse effect of tetracyclines**

       ✓7ᵗʰ **T36.4X6**   **Underdosing of tetracyclines**

✓5ᵗʰ **T36.5**   **Poisoning by, adverse effect of and underdosing of aminoglycosides**
      Poisoning by, adverse effect of and underdosing of streptomycin

    ✓6ᵗʰ **T36.5X**   **Poisoning by, adverse effect of and underdosing of aminoglycosides**

       ✓7ᵗʰ **T36.5X1**   **Poisoning by aminoglycosides,** accidental (unintentional)
          Poisoning by aminoglycosides NOS

       ✓7ᵗʰ **T36.5X2**   **Poisoning by aminoglycosides,** intentional self-harm

       ✓7ᵗʰ **T36.5X3**   **Poisoning by aminoglycosides,** assault

       ✓7ᵗʰ **T36.5X4**   **Poisoning by aminoglycosides,** undetermined

       ✓7ᵗʰ **T36.5X5**   **Adverse effect of aminoglycosides**

       ✓7ᵗʰ **T36.5X6**   **Underdosing of aminoglycosides**

✓5ᵗʰ **T36.6**   **Poisoning by, adverse effect of and underdosing of rifampicins**

    ✓6ᵗʰ **T36.6X**   **Poisoning by, adverse effect of and underdosing of rifampicins**

       ✓7ᵗʰ **T36.6X1**   **Poisoning by rifampicins,** accidental (unintentional)
          Poisoning by rifampicins NOS

       ✓7ᵗʰ **T36.6X2**   **Poisoning by rifampicins,** intentional self-harm

       ✓7ᵗʰ **T36.6X3**   **Poisoning by rifampicins,** assault

       ✓7ᵗʰ **T36.6X4**   **Poisoning by rifampicins,** undetermined

---

EXCLUDES 1 Not coded here   **EXCLUDES 2** Not included here   **N** Newborn Age: 0   **P** Pediatric Age: 0-17   **M** Maternity Age: 12-55   **A** Adult Age: 15-124

984   ICD-10-CM 2016

✓7ᵗʰ **T36.6X5** Adverse effect of rifampicins

✓7ᵗʰ **T36.6X6** Underdosing of rifampicins

✓5ᵗʰ **T36.7** Poisoning by, adverse effect of and underdosing of antifungal antibiotics, systemically used

  ✓6ᵗʰ **T36.7X** Poisoning by, adverse effect of and underdosing of antifungal antibiotics, systemically used

    ✓7ᵗʰ **T36.7X1** Poisoning by antifungal antibiotics, systemically used, accidental (unintentional)
Poisoning by antifungal antibiotics, systemically used NOS

    ✓7ᵗʰ **T36.7X2** Poisoning by antifungal antibiotics, systemically used, intentional self-harm

    ✓7ᵗʰ **T36.7X3** Poisoning by antifungal antibiotics, systemically used, assault

    ✓7ᵗʰ **T36.7X4** Poisoning by antifungal antibiotics, systemically used, undetermined

    ✓7ᵗʰ **T36.7X5** Adverse effect of antifungal antibiotics, systemically used

    ✓7ᵗʰ **T36.7X6** Underdosing of antifungal antibiotics, systemically used

✓5ᵗʰ **T36.8** Poisoning by, adverse effect of and underdosing of other systemic antibiotics

  ✓6ᵗʰ **T36.8X** Poisoning by, adverse effect of and underdosing of other systemic antibiotics

    ✓7ᵗʰ **T36.8X1** Poisoning by other systemic antibiotics, accidental (unintentional)
Poisoning by other systemic antibiotics NOS

    ✓7ᵗʰ **T36.8X2** Poisoning by other systemic antibiotics, intentional self-harm

    ✓7ᵗʰ **T36.8X3** Poisoning by other systemic antibiotics, assault

    ✓7ᵗʰ **T36.8X4** Poisoning by other systemic antibiotics, undetermined

    ✓7ᵗʰ **T36.8X5** Adverse effect of other systemic antibiotics

    ✓7ᵗʰ **T36.8X6** Underdosing of other systemic antibiotics

✓5ᵗʰ **T36.9** Poisoning by, adverse effect of and underdosing of unspecified systemic antibiotic

  ✓×7ᵗʰ **T36.91** Poisoning by unspecified systemic antibiotic, accidental (unintentional)
Poisoning by systemic antibiotic NOS

  ✓×7ᵗʰ **T36.92** Poisoning by unspecified systemic antibiotic, intentional self-harm

  ✓×7ᵗʰ **T36.93** Poisoning by unspecified systemic antibiotic, assault

  ✓×7ᵗʰ **T36.94** Poisoning by unspecified systemic antibiotic, undetermined

  ✓×7ᵗʰ **T36.95** Adverse effect of unspecified systemic antibiotic

  ✓×7ᵗʰ **T36.96** Underdosing of unspecified systemic antibiotic

✓4ᵗʰ **T37** Poisoning by, adverse effect of and underdosing of other systemic anti-infectives and antiparasitics

EXCLUDES 1 *anti-infectives topically used for ear, nose and throat (T49.6-)*
anti-infectives topically used for eye (T49.5-)
locally applied anti-infectives NEC (T49.0-)

The appropriate 7th character is to be added to each code from category T37.
A   initial encounter
D   subsequent encounter
S   sequela

✓5ᵗʰ **T37.0** Poisoning by, adverse effect of and underdosing of sulfonamides

  ✓6ᵗʰ **T37.0X** Poisoning by, adverse effect of and underdosing of sulfonamides

    ✓7ᵗʰ **T37.0X1** Poisoning by sulfonamides, accidental (unintentional)
Poisoning by sulfonamides NOS

    ✓7ᵗʰ **T37.0X2** Poisoning by sulfonamides, intentional self-harm

    ✓7ᵗʰ **T37.0X3** Poisoning by sulfonamides, assault

    ✓7ᵗʰ **T37.0X4** Poisoning by sulfonamides, undetermined

    ✓7ᵗʰ **T37.0X5** Adverse effect of sulfonamides

    ✓7ᵗʰ **T37.0X6** Underdosing of sulfonamides

✓5ᵗʰ **T37.1** Poisoning by, adverse effect of and underdosing of antimycobacterial drugs

EXCLUDES 1 *rifampicins (T36.6-)*
streptomycin (T36.5-)

  ✓6ᵗʰ **T37.1X** Poisoning by, adverse effect of and underdosing of antimycobacterial drugs

    ✓7ᵗʰ **T37.1X1** Poisoning by antimycobacterial drugs, accidental (unintentional)
Poisoning by antimycobacterial drugs NOS

    ✓7ᵗʰ **T37.1X2** Poisoning by antimycobacterial drugs, intentional self-harm

    ✓7ᵗʰ **T37.1X3** Poisoning by antimycobacterial drugs, assault

    ✓7ᵗʰ **T37.1X4** Poisoning by antimycobacterial drugs, undetermined

    ✓7ᵗʰ **T37.1X5** Adverse effect of antimycobacterial drugs

    ✓7ᵗʰ **T37.1X6** Underdosing of antimycobacterial drugs

✓5ᵗʰ **T37.2** Poisoning by, adverse effect of and underdosing of antimalarials and drugs acting on other blood protozoa

EXCLUDES 1 *hydroxyquinoline derivatives (T37.8-)*

  ✓6ᵗʰ **T37.2X** Poisoning by, adverse effect of and underdosing of antimalarials and drugs acting on other blood protozoa

    ✓7ᵗʰ **T37.2X1** Poisoning by antimalarials and drugs acting on other blood protozoa, accidental (unintentional)
Poisoning by antimalarials and drugs acting on other blood protozoa NOS

    ✓7ᵗʰ **T37.2X2** Poisoning by antimalarials and drugs acting on other blood protozoa, intentional self-harm

    ✓7ᵗʰ **T37.2X3** Poisoning by antimalarials and drugs acting on other blood protozoa, assault

    ✓7ᵗʰ **T37.2X4** Poisoning by antimalarials and drugs acting on other blood protozoa, undetermined

    ✓7ᵗʰ **T37.2X5** Adverse effect of antimalarials and drugs acting on other blood protozoa

    ✓7ᵗʰ **T37.2X6** Underdosing of antimalarials and drugs acting on other blood protozoa

✓5ᵗʰ **T37.3** Poisoning by, adverse effect of and underdosing of other antiprotozoal drugs

  ✓6ᵗʰ **T37.3X** Poisoning by, adverse effect of and underdosing of other antiprotozoal drugs

    ✓7ᵗʰ **T37.3X1** Poisoning by other antiprotozoal drugs, accidental (unintentional)
Poisoning by other antiprotozoal drugs NOS

    ✓7ᵗʰ **T37.3X2** Poisoning by other antiprotozoal drugs, intentional self-harm

    ✓7ᵗʰ **T37.3X3** Poisoning by other antiprotozoal drugs, assault

    ✓7ᵗʰ **T37.3X4** Poisoning by other antiprotozoal drugs, undetermined

    ✓7ᵗʰ **T37.3X5** Adverse effect of other antiprotozoal drugs

    ✓7ᵗʰ **T37.3X6** Underdosing of other antiprotozoal drugs

✓5ᵗʰ **T37.4** Poisoning by, adverse effect of and underdosing of anthelminthics

  ✓6ᵗʰ **T37.4X** Poisoning by, adverse effect of and underdosing of anthelminthics

    ✓7ᵗʰ **T37.4X1** Poisoning by anthelminthics, accidental (unintentional)
Poisoning by anthelminthics NOS

    ✓7ᵗʰ **T37.4X2** Poisoning by anthelminthics, intentional self-harm

    ✓7ᵗʰ **T37.4X3** Poisoning by anthelminthics, assault

    ✓7ᵗʰ **T37.4X4** Poisoning by anthelminthics, undetermined

    ✓7ᵗʰ **T37.4X5** Adverse effect of anthelminthics

    ✓7ᵗʰ **T37.4X6** Underdosing of anthelminthics

✓ Additional Character Required   ✓×7ᵗʰ Placeholder Alert   Unspecified Dx   Other Specified Dx   Manifestation   ▶◀ Revised Text   ● New Code   ▲ Revised Code Title

Chapter 19. Injury, Poisoning, and Certain Other Consequences of External Causes

✓5ᵗʰ **T37.5 Poisoning by, adverse effect of and underdosing of antiviral drugs**

> EXCLUDES1   amantadine (T42.8-)
> cytarabine (T45.1-)

✓6ᵗʰ **T37.5X Poisoning by, adverse effect of and underdosing of antiviral drugs**

> ✓7ᵗʰ **T37.5X1 Poisoning by antiviral drugs, accidental (unintentional)**
> Poisoning by antiviral drugs NOS

> ✓7ᵗʰ **T37.5X2 Poisoning by antiviral drugs, intentional self-harm**

> ✓7ᵗʰ **T37.5X3 Poisoning by antiviral drugs, assault**

> ✓7ᵗʰ **T37.5X4 Poisoning by antiviral drugs, undetermined**

> ✓7ᵗʰ **T37.5X5 Adverse effect of antiviral drugs**

> ✓7ᵗʰ **T37.5X6 Underdosing of antiviral drugs**

✓5ᵗʰ **T37.8 Poisoning by, adverse effect of and underdosing of other specified systemic anti-infectives and antiparasitics**
Poisoning by, adverse effect of and underdosing of hydroxyquinoline derivatives

> EXCLUDES1   antimalarial drugs (T37.2-)

✓6ᵗʰ **T37.8X Poisoning by, adverse effect of and underdosing of other specified systemic anti-infectives and antiparasitics**

> ✓7ᵗʰ **T37.8X1 Poisoning by other specified systemic anti-infectives and antiparasitics, accidental (unintentional)**
> Poisoning by other specified systemic anti-infectives and antiparasitics NOS

> ✓7ᵗʰ **T37.8X2 Poisoning by other specified systemic anti-infectives and antiparasitics, intentional self-harm**

> ✓7ᵗʰ **T37.8X3 Poisoning by other specified systemic anti-infectives and antiparasitics, assault**

> ✓7ᵗʰ **T37.8X4 Poisoning by other specified systemic anti-infectives and antiparasitics, undetermined**

> ✓7ᵗʰ **T37.8X5 Adverse effect of other specified systemic anti-infectives and antiparasitics**

> ✓7ᵗʰ **T37.8X6 Underdosing of other specified systemic anti-infectives and antiparasitics**

✓5ᵗʰ **T37.9 Poisoning by, adverse effect of and underdosing of unspecified systemic anti-infective and antiparasitics**

> ✓x7ᵗʰ **T37.91 Poisoning by unspecified systemic anti-infective and antiparasitics, accidental (unintentional)**
> Poisoning by, adverse effect of and underdosing of systemic anti-infective and antiparasitics NOS

> ✓x7ᵗʰ **T37.92 Poisoning by unspecified systemic anti-infective and antiparasitics, intentional self-harm**

> ✓x7ᵗʰ **T37.93 Poisoning by unspecified systemic anti-infective and antiparasitics, assault**

> ✓x7ᵗʰ **T37.94 Poisoning by unspecified systemic anti-infective and antiparasitics, undetermined**

> ✓x7ᵗʰ **T37.95 Adverse effect of unspecified systemic anti-infective and antiparasitic**

> ✓x7ᵗʰ **T37.96 Underdosing of unspecified systemic anti-infectives and antiparasitics**

✓4ᵗʰ **T38 Poisoning by, adverse effect of and underdosing of hormones and their synthetic substitutes and antagonists, not elsewhere classified**

> EXCLUDES1   mineralocorticoids and their antagonists (T50.0-)
> oxytocic hormones (T48.0-)
> parathyroid hormones and derivatives (T50.9-)

> The appropriate 7th character is to be added to each code from category T38.
> A   initial encounter
> D   subsequent encounter
> S   sequela

✓5ᵗʰ **T38.0 Poisoning by, adverse effect of and underdosing of glucocorticoids and synthetic analogues**

> EXCLUDES1   glucocorticoids, topically used (T49.-)

✓6ᵗʰ **T38.0X Poisoning by, adverse effect of and underdosing of glucocorticoids and synthetic analogues**

> ✓7ᵗʰ **T38.0X1 Poisoning by glucocorticoids and synthetic analogues, accidental (unintentional)**
> Poisoning by glucocorticoids and synthetic analogues NOS

> ✓7ᵗʰ **T38.0X2 Poisoning by glucocorticoids and synthetic analogues, intentional self-harm**

> ✓7ᵗʰ **T38.0X3 Poisoning by glucocorticoids and synthetic analogues, assault**

> ✓7ᵗʰ **T38.0X4 Poisoning by glucocorticoids and synthetic analogues, undetermined**

> ✓7ᵗʰ **T38.0X5 Adverse effect of glucocorticoids and synthetic analogues**

> ✓7ᵗʰ **T38.0X6 Underdosing of glucocorticoids and synthetic analogues**

✓5ᵗʰ **T38.1 Poisoning by, adverse effect of and underdosing of thyroid hormones and substitutes**

✓6ᵗʰ **T38.1X Poisoning by, adverse effect of and underdosing of thyroid hormones and substitutes**

> ✓7ᵗʰ **T38.1X1 Poisoning by thyroid hormones and substitutes, accidental (unintentional)**
> Poisoning by thyroid hormones and substitutes NOS

> ✓7ᵗʰ **T38.1X2 Poisoning by thyroid hormones and substitutes, intentional self-harm**

> ✓7ᵗʰ **T38.1X3 Poisoning by thyroid hormones and substitutes, assault**

> ✓7ᵗʰ **T38.1X4 Poisoning by thyroid hormones and substitutes, undetermined**

> ✓7ᵗʰ **T38.1X5 Adverse effect of thyroid hormones and substitutes**

> ✓7ᵗʰ **T38.1X6 Underdosing of thyroid hormones and substitutes**

✓5ᵗʰ **T38.2 Poisoning by, adverse effect of and underdosing of antithyroid drugs**

✓6ᵗʰ **T38.2X Poisoning by, adverse effect of and underdosing of antithyroid drugs**

> ✓7ᵗʰ **T38.2X1 Poisoning by antithyroid drugs, accidental (unintentional)**
> Poisoning by antithyroid drugs NOS

> ✓7ᵗʰ **T38.2X2 Poisoning by antithyroid drugs, intentional self-harm**

> ✓7ᵗʰ **T38.2X3 Poisoning by antithyroid drugs, assault**

> ✓7ᵗʰ **T38.2X4 Poisoning by antithyroid drugs, undetermined**

> ✓7ᵗʰ **T38.2X5 Adverse effect of antithyroid drugs**

> ✓7ᵗʰ **T38.2X6 Underdosing of antithyroid drugs**

✓5ᵗʰ **T38.3 Poisoning by, adverse effect of and underdosing of insulin and oral hypoglycemic [antidiabetic] drugs**

✓6ᵗʰ **T38.3X Poisoning by, adverse effect of and underdosing of insulin and oral hypoglycemic [antidiabetic] drugs**

> ✓7ᵗʰ **T38.3X1 Poisoning by insulin and oral hypoglycemic [antidiabetic] drugs, accidental (unintentional)**
> Poisoning by insulin and oral hypoglycemic [antidiabetic] drugs NOS

> ✓7ᵗʰ **T38.3X2 Poisoning by insulin and oral hypoglycemic [antidiabetic] drugs, intentional self-harm**

EXCLUDES1 Not coded here   EXCLUDES2 Not included here   N Newborn Age: 0   P Pediatric Age: 0-17   M Maternity Age: 12-55   A Adult Age: 15-124

986   ICD-10-CM 2016

☑7ᵗʰ **T38.3X3** **Poisoning by insulin and oral hypoglycemic [antidiabetic] drugs,** assault

☑7ᵗʰ **T38.3X4** **Poisoning by insulin and oral hypoglycemic [antidiabetic] drugs,** undetermined

☑7ᵗʰ **T38.3X5** Adverse effect **of insulin and oral hypoglycemic [antidiabetic] drugs**

☑7ᵗʰ **T38.3X6** Underdosing **of insulin and oral hypoglycemic [antidiabetic] drugs**

☑5ᵗʰ **T38.4** **Poisoning by, adverse effect of and underdosing of oral contraceptives**
Poisoning by, adverse effect of and underdosing of multiple- and single-ingredient oral contraceptive preparations

☑6ᵗʰ **T38.4X** **Poisoning by, adverse effect of and underdosing of** oral contraceptives

☑7ᵗʰ **T38.4X1** **Poisoning by oral contraceptives,** accidental (unintentional)
Poisoning by oral contraceptives NOS

☑7ᵗʰ **T38.4X2** **Poisoning by oral contraceptives,** intentional self-harm

☑7ᵗʰ **T38.4X3** **Poisoning by oral contraceptives,** assault

☑7ᵗʰ **T38.4X4** **Poisoning by oral contraceptives,** undetermined

☑7ᵗʰ **T38.4X5** Adverse effect **of oral contraceptives**

☑7ᵗʰ **T38.4X6** Underdosing **of oral contraceptives**

☑5ᵗʰ **T38.5** **Poisoning by, adverse effect of and underdosing of other estrogens and progestogens**
Poisoning by, adverse effect of and underdosing of estrogens and progestogens mixtures and substitutes

☑6ᵗʰ **T38.5X** **Poisoning by, adverse effect of and underdosing of other** estrogens and progestogens

☑7ᵗʰ **T38.5X1** **Poisoning by other estrogens and progestogens,** accidental (unintentional)
Poisoning by other estrogens and progestogens NOS

☑7ᵗʰ **T38.5X2** **Poisoning by other estrogens and progestogens,** intentional self-harm

☑7ᵗʰ **T38.5X3** **Poisoning by other estrogens and progestogens,** assault

☑7ᵗʰ **T38.5X4** **Poisoning by other estrogens and progestogens,** undetermined

☑7ᵗʰ **T38.5X5** Adverse effect **of other estrogens and progestogens**

☑7ᵗʰ **T38.5X6** Underdosing **of other estrogens and progestogens**

☑5ᵗʰ **T38.6** **Poisoning by, adverse effect of and underdosing of antigonadotrophins, antiestrogens, antiandrogens, not elsewhere classified**
Poisoning by, adverse effect of and underdosing of tamoxifen

☑6ᵗʰ **T38.6X** **Poisoning by, adverse effect of and underdosing of** antigonadotrophins, antiestrogens, antiandrogens, not elsewhere classified

☑7ᵗʰ **T38.6X1** **Poisoning by antigonadotrophins, antiestrogens, antiandrogens, not elsewhere classified,** accidental (unintentional)
Poisoning by antigonadotrophins, antiestrogens, antiandrogens, not elsewhere classified NOS

☑7ᵗʰ **T38.6X2** **Poisoning by antigonadotrophins, antiestrogens, antiandrogens, not elsewhere classified,** intentional self-harm

☑7ᵗʰ **T38.6X3** **Poisoning by antigonadotrophins, antiestrogens, antiandrogens, not elsewhere classified,** assault

☑7ᵗʰ **T38.6X4** **Poisoning by antigonadotrophins, antiestrogens, antiandrogens, not elsewhere classified,** undetermined

☑7ᵗʰ **T38.6X5** Adverse effect **of antigonadotrophins, antiestrogens, antiandrogens, not elsewhere classified**

☑7ᵗʰ **T38.6X6** Underdosing **of antigonadotrophins, antiestrogens, antiandrogens, not elsewhere classified**

☑5ᵗʰ **T38.7** **Poisoning by, adverse effect of and underdosing of androgens and anabolic congeners**

☑6ᵗʰ **T38.7X** **Poisoning by, adverse effect of and underdosing of** androgens and anabolic congeners

☑7ᵗʰ **T38.7X1** **Poisoning by androgens and anabolic congeners,** accidental (unintentional)
Poisoning by androgens and anabolic congeners NOS

☑7ᵗʰ **T38.7X2** **Poisoning by androgens and anabolic congeners,** intentional self-harm

☑7ᵗʰ **T38.7X3** **Poisoning by androgens and anabolic congeners,** assault

☑7ᵗʰ **T38.7X4** **Poisoning by androgens and anabolic congeners,** undetermined

☑7ᵗʰ **T38.7X5** Adverse effect **of androgens and anabolic congeners**

☑7ᵗʰ **T38.7X6** Underdosing **of androgens and anabolic congeners**

☑5ᵗʰ **T38.8** **Poisoning by, adverse effect of and underdosing of other and unspecified hormones and synthetic substitutes**

☑6ᵗʰ **T38.80** **Poisoning by, adverse effect of and underdosing of** unspecified hormones and synthetic substitutes

☑7ᵗʰ **T38.801** **Poisoning by unspecified hormones and synthetic substitutes,** accidental (unintentional)
Poisoning by unspecified hormones and synthetic substitutes NOS

☑7ᵗʰ **T38.802** **Poisoning by unspecified hormones and synthetic substitutes,** intentional self-harm

☑7ᵗʰ **T38.803** **Poisoning by unspecified hormones and synthetic substitutes,** assault

☑7ᵗʰ **T38.804** **Poisoning by unspecified hormones and synthetic substitutes,** undetermined

☑7ᵗʰ **T38.805** Adverse effect **of unspecified hormones and synthetic substitutes**

☑7ᵗʰ **T38.806** Underdosing **of unspecified hormones and synthetic substitutes**

☑6ᵗʰ **T38.81** **Poisoning by, adverse effect of and underdosing of** anterior pituitary [adenohypophyseal] hormones

☑7ᵗʰ **T38.811** **Poisoning by anterior pituitary [adenohypophyseal] hormones,** accidental (unintentional)
Poisoning by anterior pituitary [adenohypophyseal] hormones NOS

☑7ᵗʰ **T38.812** **Poisoning by anterior pituitary [adenohypophyseal] hormones,** intentional self-harm

☑7ᵗʰ **T38.813** **Poisoning by anterior pituitary [adenohypophyseal] hormones,** assault

☑7ᵗʰ **T38.814** **Poisoning by anterior pituitary [adenohypophyseal] hormones,** undetermined

☑7ᵗʰ **T38.815** Adverse effect **of anterior pituitary [adenohypophyseal] hormones**

☑7ᵗʰ **T38.816** Underdosing **of anterior pituitary [adenohypophyseal] hormones**

☑6ᵗʰ **T38.89** **Poisoning by, adverse effect of and underdosing of** other hormones and synthetic substitutes

☑7ᵗʰ **T38.891** **Poisoning by other hormones and synthetic substitutes,** accidental (unintentional)
Poisoning by other hormones and synthetic substitutes NOS

☑7ᵗʰ **T38.892** **Poisoning by other hormones and synthetic substitutes,** intentional self-harm

☑7ᵗʰ **T38.893** **Poisoning by other hormones and synthetic substitutes,** assault

☑7ᵗʰ **T38.894** **Poisoning by other hormones and synthetic substitutes,** undetermined

☑7ᵗʰ **T38.895** Adverse effect **of other hormones and synthetic substitutes**

☑7ᵗʰ **T38.896** Underdosing **of other hormones and synthetic substitutes**

☑ Additional Character Required   ☑ᵡ7ᵡ Placeholder Alert   Unspecified Dx   Other Specified Dx   Manifestation   ▶◀ Revised Text   ● New Code   ▲ Revised Code Title

√5th **T38.9** Poisoning by, adverse effect of and underdosing of other and unspecified hormone antagonists

√6th **T38.90** Poisoning by, adverse effect of and underdosing of unspecified hormone antagonists

√7th **T38.901** Poisoning by unspecified hormone antagonists, accidental (unintentional)
Poisoning by unspecified hormone antagonists NOS

√7th **T38.902** Poisoning by unspecified hormone antagonists, intentional self-harm

√7th **T38.903** Poisoning by unspecified hormone antagonists, assault

√7th **T38.904** Poisoning by unspecified hormone antagonists, undetermined

√7th **T38.905** Adverse effect of unspecified hormone antagonists

√7th **T38.906** Underdosing of unspecified hormone antagonists

√6th **T38.99** Poisoning by, adverse effect of and underdosing of other hormone antagonists

√7th **T38.991** Poisoning by other hormone antagonists, accidental (unintentional)
Poisoning by other hormone antagonists NOS

√7th **T38.992** Poisoning by other hormone antagonists, intentional self-harm

√7th **T38.993** Poisoning by other hormone antagonists, assault

√7th **T38.994** Poisoning by other hormone antagonists, undetermined

√7th **T38.995** Adverse effect of other hormone antagonists

√7th **T38.996** Underdosing of other hormone antagonists

√4th **T39** Poisoning by, adverse effect of and underdosing of nonopioid analgesics, antipyretics and antirheumatics

The appropriate 7th character is to be added to each code from category T39.
A   initial encounter
D   subsequent encounter
S   sequela

√5th **T39.0** Poisoning by, adverse effect of and underdosing of salicylates

√6th **T39.01** Poisoning by, adverse effect of and underdosing of aspirin
Poisoning by, adverse effect of and underdosing of acetylsalicylic acid

√7th **T39.011** Poisoning by aspirin, accidental (unintentional)

√7th **T39.012** Poisoning by aspirin, intentional self-harm

√7th **T39.013** Poisoning by aspirin, assault

√7th **T39.014** Poisoning by aspirin, undetermined

√7th **T39.015** Adverse effect of aspirin

√7th **T39.016** Underdosing of aspirin

√6th **T39.09** Poisoning by, adverse effect of and underdosing of other salicylates

√7th **T39.091** Poisoning by salicylates, accidental (unintentional)
Poisoning by salicylates NOS

√7th **T39.092** Poisoning by salicylates, intentional self-harm

√7th **T39.093** Poisoning by salicylates, assault

√7th **T39.094** Poisoning by salicylates, undetermined

√7th **T39.095** Adverse effect of salicylates

√7th **T39.096** Underdosing of salicylates

√5th **T39.1** Poisoning by, adverse effect of and underdosing of 4-Aminophenol derivatives

√6th **T39.1X** Poisoning by, adverse effect of and underdosing of 4-Aminophenol derivatives

√7th **T39.1X1** Poisoning by 4-Aminophenol derivatives, accidental (unintentional)
Poisoning by 4-Aminophenol derivatives NOS

√7th **T39.1X2** Poisoning by 4-Aminophenol derivatives, intentional self-harm

√7th **T39.1X3** Poisoning by 4-Aminophenol derivatives, assault

√7th **T39.1X4** Poisoning by 4-Aminophenol derivatives, undetermined

√7th **T39.1X5** Adverse effect of 4-Aminophenol derivatives

√7th **T39.1X6** Underdosing of 4-Aminophenol derivatives

√5th **T39.2** Poisoning by, adverse effect of and underdosing of pyrazolone derivatives

√6th **T39.2X** Poisoning by, adverse effect of and underdosing of pyrazolone derivatives

√7th **T39.2X1** Poisoning by pyrazolone derivatives, accidental (unintentional)
Poisoning by pyrazolone derivatives NOS

√7th **T39.2X2** Poisoning by pyrazolone derivatives, intentional self-harm

√7th **T39.2X3** Poisoning by pyrazolone derivatives, assault

√7th **T39.2X4** Poisoning by pyrazolone derivatives, undetermined

√7th **T39.2X5** Adverse effect of pyrazolone derivatives

√7th **T39.2X6** Underdosing of pyrazolone derivatives

√5th **T39.3** Poisoning by, adverse effect of and underdosing of other nonsteroidal anti-inflammatory drugs [NSAID]

√6th **T39.31** Poisoning by, adverse effect of and underdosing of propionic acid derivatives
Poisoning by, adverse effect of and underdosing of fenoprofen
Poisoning by, adverse effect of and underdosing of flurbiprofen
Poisoning by, adverse effect of and underdosing of ibuprofen
Poisoning by, adverse effect of and underdosing of ketoprofen
Poisoning by, adverse effect of and underdosing of naproxen
Poisoning by, adverse effect of and underdosing of oxaprozin

√7th **T39.311** Poisoning by propionic acid derivatives, accidental (unintentional)

√7th **T39.312** Poisoning by propionic acid derivatives, intentional self-harm

√7th **T39.313** Poisoning by propionic acid derivatives, assault

√7th **T39.314** Poisoning by propionic acid derivatives, undetermined

√7th **T39.315** Adverse effect of propionic acid derivatives

√7th **T39.316** Underdosing of propionic acid derivatives

√6th **T39.39** Poisoning by, adverse effect of and underdosing of other nonsteroidal anti-inflammatory drugs [NSAID]

√7th **T39.391** Poisoning by other nonsteroidal anti-inflammatory drugs [NSAID], accidental (unintentional)
Poisoning by other nonsteroidal anti-inflammatory drugs NOS

√7th **T39.392** Poisoning by other nonsteroidal anti-inflammatory drugs [NSAID], intentional self-harm

√7th **T39.393** Poisoning by other nonsteroidal anti-inflammatory drugs [NSAID], assault

√7th **T39.394** Poisoning by other nonsteroidal anti-inflammatory drugs [NSAID], undetermined

√7th **T39.395** Adverse effect of other nonsteroidal anti-inflammatory drugs [NSAID]

√7th **T39.396** Underdosing of other nonsteroidal anti-inflammatory drugs [NSAID]

EXCLUDES 1 Not coded here   EXCLUDES 2 Not included here   N Newborn Age: 0   P Pediatric Age: 0-17   M Maternity Age: 12-55   A Adult Age: 15-124

988
ICD-10-CM 2016

☑5ʰ T39.4 Poisoning by, adverse effect of and underdosing of antirheumatics, not elsewhere classified

> EXCLUDES 1   poisoning by, adverse effect of and underdosing of glucocorticoids (T38.0-)
> poisoning by, adverse effect of and underdosing of salicylates (T39.0-)

> **☑6ʰ T39.4X Poisoning by, adverse effect of and underdosing of antirheumatics, not elsewhere classified**

>> ☑7ʰ **T39.4X1** Poisoning by antirheumatics, not elsewhere classified, accidental (unintentional)
>>> Poisoning by antirheumatics, not elsewhere classified NOS

>> ☑7ʰ **T39.4X2** Poisoning by antirheumatics, not elsewhere classified, intentional self-harm

>> ☑7ʰ **T39.4X3** Poisoning by antirheumatics, not elsewhere classified, assault

>> ☑7ʰ **T39.4X4** Poisoning by antirheumatics, not elsewhere classified, undetermined

>> ☑7ʰ **T39.4X5** Adverse effect of antirheumatics, not elsewhere classified

>> ☑7ʰ **T39.4X6** Underdosing of antirheumatics, not elsewhere classified

☑5ʰ T39.8 Poisoning by, adverse effect of and underdosing of other nonopioid analgesics and antipyretics, not elsewhere classified

> **☑6ʰ T39.8X Poisoning by, adverse effect of and underdosing of other nonopioid analgesics and antipyretics, not elsewhere classified**

>> ☑7ʰ **T39.8X1** Poisoning by other nonopioid analgesics and antipyretics, not elsewhere classified, accidental (unintentional)
>>> Poisoning by other nonopioid analgesics and antipyretics, not elsewhere classified NOS

>> ☑7ʰ **T39.8X2** Poisoning by other nonopioid analgesics and antipyretics, not elsewhere classified, intentional self-harm

>> ☑7ʰ **T39.8X3** Poisoning by other nonopioid analgesics and antipyretics, not elsewhere classified, assault

>> ☑7ʰ **T39.8X4** Poisoning by other nonopioid analgesics and antipyretics, not elsewhere classified, undetermined

>> ☑7ʰ **T39.8X5** Adverse effect of other nonopioid analgesics and antipyretics, not elsewhere classified

>> ☑7ʰ **T39.8X6** Underdosing of other nonopioid analgesics and antipyretics, not elsewhere classified

☑5ʰ T39.9 Poisoning by, adverse effect of and underdosing of unspecified nonopioid analgesic, antipyretic and antirheumatic

> ☑x7ʰ **T39.91** Poisoning by unspecified nonopioid analgesic, antipyretic and antirheumatic, accidental (unintentional)
>> Poisoning by nonopioid analgesic, antipyretic and antirheumatic NOS

> ☑x7ʰ **T39.92** Poisoning by unspecified nonopioid analgesic, antipyretic and antirheumatic, intentional self-harm

> ☑x7ʰ **T39.93** Poisoning by unspecified nonopioid analgesic, antipyretic and antirheumatic, assault

> ☑x7ʰ **T39.94** Poisoning by unspecified nonopioid analgesic, antipyretic and antirheumatic, undetermined

> ☑x7ʰ **T39.95** Adverse effect of unspecified nonopioid analgesic, antipyretic and antirheumatic

> ☑x7ʰ **T39.96** Underdosing of unspecified nonopioid analgesic, antipyretic and antirheumatic

☑4ʰ T40 Poisoning by, adverse effect of and underdosing of narcotics and psychodysleptics [hallucinogens]

> EXCLUDES 2   drug dependence and related mental and behavioral disorders due to psychoactive substance use (F10-F19-)

> The appropriate 7th character is to be added to each code from category T40.
> A   initial encounter
> D   subsequent encounter
> S   sequela

☑5ʰ T40.0 Poisoning by, adverse effect of and underdosing of opium

> **☑6ʰ T40.0X Poisoning by, adverse effect of and underdosing of opium**

>> ☑7ʰ **T40.0X1** Poisoning by opium, accidental (unintentional)
>>> Poisoning by opium NOS

>> ☑7ʰ **T40.0X2** Poisoning by opium, intentional self-harm

>> ☑7ʰ **T40.0X3** Poisoning by opium, assault

>> ☑7ʰ **T40.0X4** Poisoning by opium, undetermined

>> ☑7ʰ **T40.0X5** Adverse effect of opium

>> ☑7ʰ **T40.0X6** Underdosing of opium

☑5ʰ T40.1 Poisoning by and adverse effect of heroin

> **☑6ʰ T40.1X Poisoning by and adverse effect of heroin**

>> ☑7ʰ **T40.1X1** Poisoning by heroin, accidental (unintentional)
>>> Poisoning by heroin NOS

>> ☑7ʰ **T40.1X2** Poisoning by heroin, intentional self-harm

>> ☑7ʰ **T40.1X3** Poisoning by heroin, assault

>> ☑7ʰ **T40.1X4** Poisoning by heroin, undetermined

☑5ʰ T40.2 Poisoning by, adverse effect of and underdosing of other opioids

> **☑6ʰ T40.2X Poisoning by, adverse effect of and underdosing of other opioids**

>> ☑7ʰ **T40.2X1** Poisoning by other opioids, accidental (unintentional)
>>> Poisoning by other opioids NOS

>> ☑7ʰ **T40.2X2** Poisoning by other opioids, intentional self-harm

>> ☑7ʰ **T40.2X3** Poisoning by other opioids, assault

>> ☑7ʰ **T40.2X4** Poisoning by other opioids, undetermined

>> ☑7ʰ **T40.2X5** Adverse effect of other opioids

>> ☑7ʰ **T40.2X6** Underdosing of other opioids

☑5ʰ T40.3 Poisoning by, adverse effect of and underdosing of methadone

> **☑6ʰ T40.3X Poisoning by, adverse effect of and underdosing of methadone**

>> ☑7ʰ **T40.3X1** Poisoning by methadone, accidental (unintentional)
>>> Poisoning by methadone NOS

>> ☑7ʰ **T40.3X2** Poisoning by methadone, intentional self-harm

>> ☑7ʰ **T40.3X3** Poisoning by methadone, assault

>> ☑7ʰ **T40.3X4** Poisoning by methadone, undetermined

>> ☑7ʰ **T40.3X5** Adverse effect of methadone

>> ☑7ʰ **T40.3X6** Underdosing of methadone

☑5ʰ T40.4 Poisoning by, adverse effect of and underdosing of other synthetic narcotics

> **☑6ʰ T40.4X Poisoning by, adverse effect of and underdosing of other synthetic narcotics**

>> ☑7ʰ **T40.4X1** Poisoning by other synthetic narcotics, accidental (unintentional)
>>> Poisoning by other synthetic narcotics NOS

>> ☑7ʰ **T40.4X2** Poisoning by other synthetic narcotics, intentional self-harm

>> ☑7ʰ **T40.4X3** Poisoning by other synthetic narcotics, assault

>> ☑7ʰ **T40.4X4** Poisoning by other synthetic narcotics, undetermined

>> ☑7ʰ **T40.4X5** Adverse effect of other synthetic narcotics

>> ☑7ʰ **T40.4X6** Underdosing of other synthetic narcotics

☑ Additional Character Required   ☑x7ʰ Placeholder Alert   Unspecified Dx   Other Specified Dx   Manifestation   ▶◀ Revised Text   ● New Code   ▲ Revised Code Title

ICD-10-CM 2016   989

√5ᵗʰ **T40.5** Poisoning by, adverse effect of and underdosing of cocaine

    √6ᵗʰ **T40.5X** Poisoning by, adverse effect of and underdosing of cocaine

        √7ᵗʰ **T40.5X1** Poisoning by cocaine, accidental (unintentional)
             Poisoning by cocaine NOS

        √7ᵗʰ **T40.5X2** Poisoning by cocaine, intentional self-harm

        √7ᵗʰ **T40.5X3** Poisoning by cocaine, assault

        √7ᵗʰ **T40.5X4** Poisoning by cocaine, undetermined

        √7ᵗʰ **T40.5X5** Adverse effect of cocaine

        √7ᵗʰ **T40.5X6** Underdosing of cocaine

√5ᵗʰ **T40.6** Poisoning by, adverse effect of and underdosing of other and unspecified narcotics

    √6ᵗʰ **T40.60** Poisoning by, adverse effect of and underdosing of unspecified narcotics

        √7ᵗʰ **T40.601** Poisoning by unspecified narcotics, accidental (unintentional)
             Poisoning by narcotics NOS

        √7ᵗʰ **T40.602** Poisoning by unspecified narcotics, intentional self-harm

        √7ᵗʰ **T40.603** Poisoning by unspecified narcotics, assault

        √7ᵗʰ **T40.604** Poisoning by unspecified narcotics, undetermined

        √7ᵗʰ **T40.605** Adverse effect of unspecified narcotics

        √7ᵗʰ **T40.606** Underdosing of unspecified narcotics

    √6ᵗʰ **T40.69** Poisoning by, adverse effect of and underdosing of other narcotics

        √7ᵗʰ **T40.691** Poisoning by other narcotics, accidental (unintentional)
             Poisoning by other narcotics NOS

        √7ᵗʰ **T40.692** Poisoning by other narcotics, intentional self-harm

        √7ᵗʰ **T40.693** Poisoning by other narcotics, assault

        √7ᵗʰ **T40.694** Poisoning by other narcotics, undetermined

        √7ᵗʰ **T40.695** Adverse effect of other narcotics

        √7ᵗʰ **T40.696** Underdosing of other narcotics

√5ᵗʰ **T40.7** Poisoning by, adverse effect of and underdosing of cannabis (derivatives)

    √6ᵗʰ **T40.7X** Poisoning by, adverse effect of and underdosing of cannabis (derivatives)

        √7ᵗʰ **T40.7X1** Poisoning by cannabis (derivatives), accidental (unintentional)
             Poisoning by cannabis NOS

        √7ᵗʰ **T40.7X2** Poisoning by cannabis (derivatives), intentional self-harm

        √7ᵗʰ **T40.7X3** Poisoning by cannabis (derivatives), assault

        √7ᵗʰ **T40.7X4** Poisoning by cannabis (derivatives), undetermined

        √7ᵗʰ **T40.7X5** Adverse effect of cannabis (derivatives)

        √7ᵗʰ **T40.7X6** Underdosing of cannabis (derivatives)

√5ᵗʰ **T40.8** Poisoning by and adverse effect of lysergide [LSD]

    √6ᵗʰ **T40.8X** Poisoning by and adverse effect of lysergide [LSD]

        √7ᵗʰ **T40.8X1** Poisoning by lysergide [LSD], accidental (unintentional)
             Poisoning by lysergide [LSD]NOS

        √7ᵗʰ **T40.8X2** Poisoning by lysergide [LSD], intentional self-harm

        √7ᵗʰ **T40.8X3** Poisoning by lysergide [LSD], assault

        √7ᵗʰ **T40.8X4** Poisoning by lysergide [LSD], undetermined

√5ᵗʰ **T40.9** Poisoning by, adverse effect of and underdosing of other and unspecified psychodysleptics [hallucinogens]

    √6ᵗʰ **T40.90** Poisoning by, adverse effect of and underdosing of unspecified psychodysleptics [hallucinogens]

        √7ᵗʰ **T40.901** Poisoning by unspecified psychodysleptics [hallucinogens], accidental (unintentional)

        √7ᵗʰ **T40.902** Poisoning by unspecified psychodysleptics [hallucinogens], intentional self-harm

        √7ᵗʰ **T40.903** Poisoning by unspecified psychodysleptics [hallucinogens], assault

        √7ᵗʰ **T40.904** Poisoning by unspecified psychodysleptics [hallucinogens], undetermined

        √7ᵗʰ **T40.905** Adverse effect of unspecified psychodysleptics [hallucinogens]

        √7ᵗʰ **T40.906** Underdosing of unspecified psychodysleptics

    √6ᵗʰ **T40.99** Poisoning by, adverse effect of and underdosing of other psychodysleptics [hallucinogens]

        √7ᵗʰ **T40.991** Poisoning by other psychodysleptics [hallucinogens], accidental (unintentional)
             Poisoning by other psychodysleptics [hallucinogens] NOS

        √7ᵗʰ **T40.992** Poisoning by other psychodysleptics [hallucinogens], intentional self-harm

        √7ᵗʰ **T40.993** Poisoning by other psychodysleptics [hallucinogens], assault

        √7ᵗʰ **T40.994** Poisoning by other psychodysleptics [hallucinogens], undetermined

        √7ᵗʰ **T40.995** Adverse effect of other psychodysleptics [hallucinogens]

        √7ᵗʰ **T40.996** Underdosing of other psychodysleptics

√4ᵗʰ **T41** Poisoning by, adverse effect of and underdosing of anesthetics and therapeutic gases

    EXCLUDES 1   benzodiazepines (T42.4-)
               cocaine (T40.5-)
               complications of anesthesia during labor and delivery (O74.-)
               complications of anesthesia during pregnancy (O29.-)
               complications of anesthesia during the puerperium (O89.-)
               opioids (T40.0-T40.2-)

    The appropriate 7th character is to be added to each code from category T41.
    A   initial encounter
    D   subsequent encounter
    S   sequela

√5ᵗʰ **T41.0** Poisoning by, adverse effect of and underdosing of inhaled anesthetics

    EXCLUDES 1   oxygen (T41.5-)

    √6ᵗʰ **T41.0X** Poisoning by, adverse effect of and underdosing of inhaled anesthetics

        √7ᵗʰ **T41.0X1** Poisoning by inhaled anesthetics, accidental (unintentional)
             Poisoning by inhaled anesthetics NOS

        √7ᵗʰ **T41.0X2** Poisoning by inhaled anesthetics, intentional self-harm

        √7ᵗʰ **T41.0X3** Poisoning by inhaled anesthetics, assault

        √7ᵗʰ **T41.0X4** Poisoning by inhaled anesthetics, undetermined

        √7ᵗʰ **T41.0X5** Adverse effect of inhaled anesthetics

        √7ᵗʰ **T41.0X6** Underdosing of inhaled anesthetics

√5ᵗʰ **T41.1** Poisoning by, adverse effect of and underdosing of intravenous anesthetics
         Poisoning by, adverse effect of and underdosing of thiobarbiturates

    √6ᵗʰ **T41.1X** Poisoning by, adverse effect of and underdosing of intravenous anesthetics

        √7ᵗʰ **T41.1X1** Poisoning by intravenous anesthetics, accidental (unintentional)
             Poisoning by intravenous anesthetics NOS

        √7ᵗʰ **T41.1X2** Poisoning by intravenous anesthetics, intentional self-harm

        √7ᵗʰ **T41.1X3** Poisoning by intravenous anesthetics, assault

        √7ᵗʰ **T41.1X4** Poisoning by intravenous anesthetics, undetermined

        √7ᵗʰ **T41.1X5** Adverse effect of intravenous anesthetics

        √7ᵗʰ **T41.1X6** Underdosing of intravenous anesthetics

EXCLUDES 1 Not coded here   **EXCLUDES 2** Not included here   N Newborn Age: 0   P Pediatric Age: 0-17   M Maternity Age: 12-55   A Adult Age: 15-124

990   ICD-10-CM 2016

☑5ᵗʰ **T41.2** **Poisoning by, adverse effect of and underdosing of other and unspecified general anesthetics**

  ☑6ᵗʰ **T41.20** **Poisoning by, adverse effect of and underdosing of unspecified general anesthetics**

    ☑7ᵗʰ **T41.201** **Poisoning by unspecified general anesthetics, accidental (unintentional)**
       Poisoning by general anesthetics NOS

    ☑7ᵗʰ **T41.202** **Poisoning by unspecified general anesthetics, intentional self-harm**

    ☑7ᵗʰ **T41.203** **Poisoning by unspecified general anesthetics, assault**

    ☑7ᵗʰ **T41.204** **Poisoning by unspecified general anesthetics, undetermined**

    ☑7ᵗʰ **T41.205** **Adverse effect of unspecified general anesthetics**

    ☑7ᵗʰ **T41.206** **Underdosing of unspecified general anesthetics**

  ☑6ᵗʰ **T41.29** **Poisoning by, adverse effect of and underdosing of other general anesthetics**

    ☑7ᵗʰ **T41.291** **Poisoning by other general anesthetics, accidental (unintentional)**
       Poisoning by other general anesthetics NOS

    ☑7ᵗʰ **T41.292** **Poisoning by other general anesthetics, intentional self-harm**

    ☑7ᵗʰ **T41.293** **Poisoning by other general anesthetics, assault**

    ☑7ᵗʰ **T41.294** **Poisoning by other general anesthetics, undetermined**

    ☑7ᵗʰ **T41.295** **Adverse effect of other general anesthetics**

    ☑7ᵗʰ **T41.296** **Underdosing of other general anesthetics**

☑5ᵗʰ **T41.3** **Poisoning by, adverse effect of and underdosing of local anesthetics**
  Cocaine (topical)
  EXCLUDES 2   poisoning by cocaine used as a central nervous system stimulant (T40.5X1-T40.5X4)

  ☑6ᵗʰ **T41.3X** **Poisoning by, adverse effect of and underdosing of local anesthetics**

    ☑7ᵗʰ **T41.3X1** **Poisoning by local anesthetics, accidental (unintentional)**
       Poisoning by local anesthetics NOS

    ☑7ᵗʰ **T41.3X2** **Poisoning by local anesthetics, intentional self-harm**

    ☑7ᵗʰ **T41.3X3** **Poisoning by local anesthetics, assault**

    ☑7ᵗʰ **T41.3X4** **Poisoning by local anesthetics, undetermined**

    ☑7ᵗʰ **T41.3X5** **Adverse effect of local anesthetics**

    ☑7ᵗʰ **T41.3X6** **Underdosing of local anesthetics**

☑5ᵗʰ **T41.4** **Poisoning by, adverse effect of and underdosing of unspecified anesthetic**

  ☑x7ᵗʰ **T41.41** **Poisoning by unspecified anesthetic, accidental (unintentional)**
    Poisoning by anesthetic NOS

  ☑x7ᵗʰ **T41.42** **Poisoning by unspecified anesthetic, intentional self-harm**

  ☑x7ᵗʰ **T41.43** **Poisoning by unspecified anesthetic, assault**

  ☑x7ᵗʰ **T41.44** **Poisoning by unspecified anesthetic, undetermined**

  ☑x7ᵗʰ **T41.45** **Adverse effect of unspecified anesthetic**

  ☑x7ᵗʰ **T41.46** **Underdosing of unspecified anesthetics**

☑5ᵗʰ **T41.5** **Poisoning by, adverse effect of and underdosing of therapeutic gases**

  ☑6ᵗʰ **T41.5X** **Poisoning by, adverse effect of and underdosing of therapeutic gases**

    ☑7ᵗʰ **T41.5X1** **Poisoning by therapeutic gases, accidental (unintentional)**
       Poisoning by therapeutic gases NOS

    ☑7ᵗʰ **T41.5X2** **Poisoning by therapeutic gases, intentional self-harm**

    ☑7ᵗʰ **T41.5X3** **Poisoning by therapeutic gases, assault**

    ☑7ᵗʰ **T41.5X4** **Poisoning by therapeutic gases, undetermined**

    ☑7ᵗʰ **T41.5X5** **Adverse effect of therapeutic gases**

    ☑7ᵗʰ **T41.5X6** **Underdosing of therapeutic gases**

☑4ᵗʰ **T42** **Poisoning by, adverse effect of and underdosing of antiepileptic, sedative- hypnotic and antiparkinsonism drugs**
  EXCLUDES 2   drug dependence and related mental and behavioral disorders due to psychoactive substance use (F10.--F19.-)

  The appropriate 7th character is to be added to each code from category T42.
  A   initial encounter
  D   subsequent encounter
  S   sequela

☑5ᵗʰ **T42.0** **Poisoning by, adverse effect of and underdosing of hydantoin derivatives**

  ☑6ᵗʰ **T42.0X** **Poisoning by, adverse effect of and underdosing of hydantoin derivatives**

    ☑7ᵗʰ **T42.0X1** **Poisoning by hydantoin derivatives, accidental (unintentional)**
       Poisoning by hydantoin derivatives NOS

    ☑7ᵗʰ **T42.0X2** **Poisoning by hydantoin derivatives, intentional self-harm**

    ☑7ᵗʰ **T42.0X3** **Poisoning by hydantoin derivatives, assault**

    ☑7ᵗʰ **T42.0X4** **Poisoning by hydantoin derivatives, undetermined**

    ☑7ᵗʰ **T42.0X5** **Adverse effect of hydantoin derivatives**

    ☑7ᵗʰ **T42.0X6** **Underdosing of hydantoin derivatives**

☑5ᵗʰ **T42.1** **Poisoning by, adverse effect of and underdosing of iminostilbenes**
  Poisoning by, adverse effect of and underdosing of carbamazepine

  ☑6ᵗʰ **T42.1X** **Poisoning by, adverse effect of and underdosing of iminostilbenes**

    ☑7ᵗʰ **T42.1X1** **Poisoning by iminostilbenes, accidental (unintentional)**
       Poisoning by iminostilbenes NOS

    ☑7ᵗʰ **T42.1X2** **Poisoning by iminostilbenes, intentional self-harm**

    ☑7ᵗʰ **T42.1X3** **Poisoning by iminostilbenes, assault**

    ☑7ᵗʰ **T42.1X4** **Poisoning by iminostilbenes, undetermined**

    ☑7ᵗʰ **T42.1X5** **Adverse effect of iminostilbenes**

    ☑7ᵗʰ **T42.1X6** **Underdosing of iminostilbenes**

☑5ᵗʰ **T42.2** **Poisoning by, adverse effect of and underdosing of succinimides and oxazolidinediones**

  ☑6ᵗʰ **T42.2X** **Poisoning by, adverse effect of and underdosing of succinimides and oxazolidinediones**

    ☑7ᵗʰ **T42.2X1** **Poisoning by succinimides and oxazolidinediones, accidental (unintentional)**
       Poisoning by succinimides and oxazolidinediones NOS

    ☑7ᵗʰ **T42.2X2** **Poisoning by succinimides and oxazolidinediones, intentional self-harm**

    ☑7ᵗʰ **T42.2X3** **Poisoning by succinimides and oxazolidinediones, assault**

    ☑7ᵗʰ **T42.2X4** **Poisoning by succinimides and oxazolidinediones, undetermined**

    ☑7ᵗʰ **T42.2X5** **Adverse effect of succinimides and oxazolidinediones**

    ☑7ᵗʰ **T42.2X6** **Underdosing of succinimides and oxazolidinediones**

☑5ᵗʰ **T42.3** **Poisoning by, adverse effect of and underdosing of barbiturates**
  EXCLUDES 1   poisoning by, adverse effect of and underdosing of thiobarbiturates (T41.1-)

  ☑6ᵗʰ **T42.3X** **Poisoning by, adverse effect of and underdosing of barbiturates**

    ☑7ᵗʰ **T42.3X1** **Poisoning by barbiturates, accidental (unintentional)**
       Poisoning by barbiturates NOS

    ☑7ᵗʰ **T42.3X2** **Poisoning by barbiturates, intentional self-harm**

    ☑7ᵗʰ **T42.3X3** **Poisoning by barbiturates, assault**

    ☑7ᵗʰ **T42.3X4** **Poisoning by barbiturates, undetermined**

    ☑7ᵗʰ **T42.3X5** **Adverse effect of barbiturates**

    ☑7ᵗʰ **T42.3X6** **Underdosing of barbiturates**

☑ Additional Character Required   ☑x7ᵗʰ Placeholder Alert   Unspecified Dx   Other Specified Dx   Manifestation   ▶◀ Revised Text   ● New Code   ▲ Revised Code Title

✓5ᵗʰ T42.4 Poisoning by, adverse effect of and underdosing of benzodiazepines

    ✓6ᵗʰ T42.4X Poisoning by, adverse effect of and underdosing of benzodiazepines

        ✓7ᵗʰ T42.4X1 Poisoning by benzodiazepines, accidental (unintentional)
            Poisoning by benzodiazepines NOS

        ✓7ᵗʰ T42.4X2 Poisoning by benzodiazepines, intentional self-harm

        ✓7ᵗʰ T42.4X3 Poisoning by benzodiazepines, assault

        ✓7ᵗʰ T42.4X4 Poisoning by benzodiazepines, undetermined

        ✓7ᵗʰ T42.4X5 Adverse effect of benzodiazepines

        ✓7ᵗʰ T42.4X6 Underdosing of benzodiazepines

✓5ᵗʰ T42.5 Poisoning by, adverse effect of and underdosing of mixed antiepileptics

    ✓6ᵗʰ T42.5X Poisoning by, adverse effect of and underdosing of antiepileptics

        ✓7ᵗʰ T42.5X1 Poisoning by mixed antiepileptics, accidental (unintentional)
            Poisoning by mixed antiepileptics NOS

        ✓7ᵗʰ T42.5X2 Poisoning by mixed antiepileptics, intentional self-harm

        ✓7ᵗʰ T42.5X3 Poisoning by mixed antiepileptics, assault

        ✓7ᵗʰ T42.5X4 Poisoning by mixed antiepileptics, undetermined

        ✓7ᵗʰ T42.5X5 Adverse effect of mixed antiepileptics

        ✓7ᵗʰ T42.5X6 Underdosing of mixed antiepileptics

✓5ᵗʰ T42.6 Poisoning by, adverse effect of and underdosing of other antiepileptic and sedative-hypnotic drugs
    Poisoning by, adverse effect of and underdosing of methaqualone
    Poisoning by, adverse effect of and underdosing of valproic acid
    EXCLUDES 1   poisoning by, adverse effect of and underdosing of carbamazepine (T42.1-)

    ✓6ᵗʰ T42.6X Poisoning by, adverse effect of and underdosing of other antiepileptic and sedative-hypnotic drugs

        ✓7ᵗʰ T42.6X1 Poisoning by other antiepileptic and sedative-hypnotic drugs, accidental (unintentional)
            Poisoning by other antiepileptic and sedative-hypnotic drugs NOS

        ✓7ᵗʰ T42.6X2 Poisoning by other antiepileptic and sedative-hypnotic drugs, intentional self-harm

        ✓7ᵗʰ T42.6X3 Poisoning by other antiepileptic and sedative-hypnotic drugs, assault

        ✓7ᵗʰ T42.6X4 Poisoning by other antiepileptic and sedative-hypnotic drugs, undetermined

        ✓7ᵗʰ T42.6X5 Adverse effect of other antiepileptic and sedative-hypnotic drugs

        ✓7ᵗʰ T42.6X6 Underdosing of other antiepileptic and sedative-hypnotic drugs

✓5ᵗʰ T42.7 Poisoning by, adverse effect of and underdosing of unspecified antiepileptic and sedative-hypnotic drugs

    ✓x7ᵗʰ T42.71 Poisoning by unspecified antiepileptic and sedative-hypnotic drugs, accidental (unintentional)
        Poisoning by antiepileptic and sedative-hypnotic drugs NOS

    ✓x7ᵗʰ T42.72 Poisoning by unspecified antiepileptic and sedative-hypnotic drugs, intentional self-harm

    ✓x7ᵗʰ T42.73 Poisoning by unspecified antiepileptic and sedative-hypnotic drugs, assault

    ✓x7ᵗʰ T42.74 Poisoning by unspecified antiepileptic and sedative-hypnotic drugs, undetermined

    ✓x7ᵗʰ T42.75 Adverse effect of unspecified antiepileptic and sedative-hypnotic drugs

    ✓x7ᵗʰ T42.76 Underdosing of unspecified antiepileptic and sedative-hypnotic drugs

✓5ᵗʰ T42.8 Poisoning by, adverse effect of and underdosing of antiparkinsonism drugs and other central muscle-tone depressants
    Poisoning by, adverse effect of and underdosing of amantadine

    ✓6ᵗʰ T42.8X Poisoning by, adverse effect of and underdosing of antiparkinsonism drugs and other central muscle-tone depressants

        ✓7ᵗʰ T42.8X1 Poisoning by antiparkinsonism drugs and other central muscle-tone depressants, accidental (unintentional)
            Poisoning by antiparkinsonism drugs and other central muscle-tone depressants NOS

        ✓7ᵗʰ T42.8X2 Poisoning by antiparkinsonism drugs and other central muscle-tone depressants, intentional self-harm

        ✓7ᵗʰ T42.8X3 Poisoning by antiparkinsonism drugs and other central muscle-tone depressants, assault

        ✓7ᵗʰ T42.8X4 Poisoning by antiparkinsonism drugs and other central muscle-tone depressants, undetermined

        ✓7ᵗʰ T42.8X5 Adverse effect of antiparkinsonism drugs and other central muscle-tone depressants

        ✓7ᵗʰ T42.8X6 Underdosing of antiparkinsonism drugs and other central muscle-tone depressants

✓4ᵗʰ T43 Poisoning by, adverse effect of and underdosing of psychotropic drugs, not elsewhere classified
    EXCLUDES 1   appetite depressants (T50.5-)
             barbiturates (T42.3-)
             benzodiazepines (T42.4-)
             methaqualone (T42.6-)
             psychodysleptics [hallucinogens] (T40.7-T40.9-)
    EXCLUDES 2   drug dependence and related mental and behavioral disorders due to psychoactive substance use (F10.- -F19.-)

    The appropriate 7th character is to be added to each code from category T43.
    A   initial encounter
    D   subsequent encounter
    S   sequela

    ✓5ᵗʰ T43.0 Poisoning by, adverse effect of and underdosing of tricyclic and tetracyclic antidepressants

        ✓6ᵗʰ T43.01 Poisoning by, adverse effect of and underdosing of tricyclic antidepressants

            ✓7ᵗʰ T43.011 Poisoning by tricyclic antidepressants, accidental (unintentional)
                Poisoning by tricyclic antidepressants NOS

            ✓7ᵗʰ T43.012 Poisoning by tricyclic antidepressants, intentional self-harm

            ✓7ᵗʰ T43.013 Poisoning by tricyclic antidepressants, assault

            ✓7ᵗʰ T43.014 Poisoning by tricyclic antidepressants, undetermined

            ✓7ᵗʰ T43.015 Adverse effect of tricyclic antidepressants

            ✓7ᵗʰ T43.016 Underdosing of tricyclic antidepressants

        ✓6ᵗʰ T43.02 Poisoning by, adverse effect of and underdosing of tetracyclic antidepressants

            ✓7ᵗʰ T43.021 Poisoning by tetracyclic antidepressants, accidental (unintentional)
                Poisoning by tetracyclic antidepressants NOS

            ✓7ᵗʰ T43.022 Poisoning by tetracyclic antidepressants, intentional self-harm

            ✓7ᵗʰ T43.023 Poisoning by tetracyclic antidepressants, assault

            ✓7ᵗʰ T43.024 Poisoning by tetracyclic antidepressants, undetermined

            ✓7ᵗʰ T43.025 Adverse effect of tetracyclic antidepressants

            ✓7ᵗʰ T43.026 Underdosing of tetracyclic antidepressants

EXCLUDES 1 Not coded here   *EXCLUDES 2* Not included here   N Newborn Age: 0   P Pediatric Age: 0-17   M Maternity Age: 12-55   A Adult Age: 15-124

992   ICD-10-CM 2016

✓5ᵗʰ **T43.1** **Poisoning by, adverse effect of and underdosing of monoamine-oxidase-inhibitor antidepressants**

✓6ᵗʰ **T43.1X** **Poisoning by, adverse effect of and underdosing of** monoamine-oxidase-inhibitor antidepressants

✓7ᵗʰ **T43.1X1** **Poisoning by monoamine-oxidase-inhibitor antidepressants,** accidental **(unintentional)**
Poisoning by monoamine-oxidase-inhibitor antidepressants NOS

✓7ᵗʰ **T43.1X2** **Poisoning by monoamine-oxidase-inhibitor antidepressants,** intentional self-harm

✓7ᵗʰ **T43.1X3** **Poisoning by monoamine-oxidase-inhibitor antidepressants,** assault

✓7ᵗʰ **T43.1X4** **Poisoning by monoamine-oxidase-inhibitor antidepressants,** undetermined

✓7ᵗʰ **T43.1X5** Adverse effect **of monoamine-oxidase-inhibitor antidepressants**

✓7ᵗʰ **T43.1X6** Underdosing **of monoamine-oxidase-inhibitor antidepressants**

✓5ᵗʰ **T43.2** **Poisoning by, adverse effect of and underdosing of other and unspecified antidepressants**

✓6ᵗʰ **T43.20** **Poisoning by, adverse effect of and underdosing of** unspecified antidepressants

✓7ᵗʰ **T43.201** **Poisoning by unspecified antidepressants,** accidental **(unintentional)**
Poisoning by antidepressants NOS

✓7ᵗʰ **T43.202** **Poisoning by unspecified antidepressants,** intentional self-harm

✓7ᵗʰ **T43.203** **Poisoning by unspecified antidepressants,** assault

✓7ᵗʰ **T43.204** **Poisoning by unspecified antidepressants,** undetermined

✓7ᵗʰ **T43.205** Adverse effect **of unspecified antidepressants**

✓7ᵗʰ **T43.206** Underdosing **of unspecified antidepressants**

✓6ᵗʰ **T43.21** **Poisoning by, adverse effect of and underdosing of** selective serotonin and norepinephrine reuptake inhibitors
Poisoning by, adverse effect of and underdosing of SSNRI antidepressants

✓7ᵗʰ **T43.211** **Poisoning by selective serotonin and norepinephrine reuptake inhibitors,** accidental **(unintentional)**

✓7ᵗʰ **T43.212** **Poisoning by selective serotonin and norepinephrine reuptake inhibitors,** intentional self-harm

✓7ᵗʰ **T43.213** **Poisoning by selective serotonin and norepinephrine reuptake inhibitors,** assault

✓7ᵗʰ **T43.214** **Poisoning by selective serotonin and norepinephrine reuptake inhibitors,** undetermined

✓7ᵗʰ **T43.215** Adverse effect **of selective serotonin and norepinephrine reuptake inhibitors**

✓7ᵗʰ **T43.216** Underdosing **of selective serotonin and norepinephrine reuptake inhibitors**

✓6ᵗʰ **T43.22** **Poisoning by, adverse effect of and underdosing of** selective serotonin reuptake inhibitors
Poisoning by, adverse effect of and underdosing of SSRI antidepressants

✓7ᵗʰ **T43.221** **Poisoning by selective serotonin reuptake inhibitors,** accidental **(unintentional)**

✓7ᵗʰ **T43.222** **Poisoning by selective serotonin reuptake inhibitors,** intentional self-harm

✓7ᵗʰ **T43.223** **Poisoning by selective serotonin reuptake inhibitors,** assault

✓7ᵗʰ **T43.224** **Poisoning by selective serotonin reuptake inhibitors,** undetermined

✓7ᵗʰ **T43.225** Adverse effect **of selective serotonin reuptake inhibitors**

✓7ᵗʰ **T43.226** Underdosing **of selective serotonin reuptake inhibitors**

✓6ᵗʰ **T43.29** **Poisoning by, adverse effect of and underdosing of** other antidepressants

✓7ᵗʰ **T43.291** Poisoning by other antidepressants, accidental **(unintentional)**
Poisoning by other antidepressants NOS

✓7ᵗʰ **T43.292** Poisoning by other antidepressants, intentional self-harm

✓7ᵗʰ **T43.293** Poisoning by other antidepressants, assault

✓7ᵗʰ **T43.294** Poisoning by other antidepressants, undetermined

✓7ᵗʰ **T43.295** Adverse effect **of other antidepressants**

✓7ᵗʰ **T43.296** Underdosing of other antidepressants

✓5ᵗʰ **T43.3** **Poisoning by, adverse effect of and underdosing of phenothiazine antipsychotics and neuroleptics**

✓6ᵗʰ **T43.3X** **Poisoning by, adverse effect of and underdosing of** phenothiazine antipsychotics and neuroleptics

✓7ᵗʰ **T43.3X1** **Poisoning by phenothiazine antipsychotics and neuroleptics,** accidental **(unintentional)**
Poisoning by phenothiazine antipsychotics and neuroleptics NOS

✓7ᵗʰ **T43.3X2** **Poisoning by phenothiazine antipsychotics and neuroleptics,** intentional self-harm

✓7ᵗʰ **T43.3X3** **Poisoning by phenothiazine antipsychotics and neuroleptics,** assault

✓7ᵗʰ **T43.3X4** **Poisoning by phenothiazine antipsychotics and neuroleptics,** undetermined

✓7ᵗʰ **T43.3X5** Adverse effect **of phenothiazine antipsychotics and neuroleptics**

✓7ᵗʰ **T43.3X6** Underdosing **of phenothiazine antipsychotics and neuroleptics**

✓5ᵗʰ **T43.4** **Poisoning by, adverse effect of and underdosing of butyrophenone and thiothixene neuroleptics**

✓6ᵗʰ **T43.4X** **Poisoning by, adverse effect of and underdosing of** butyrophenone and thiothixene neuroleptics

✓7ᵗʰ **T43.4X1** **Poisoning by butyrophenone and thiothixene neuroleptics,** accidental **(unintentional)**
Poisoning by butyrophenone and thiothixene neuroleptics NOS

✓7ᵗʰ **T43.4X2** **Poisoning by butyrophenone and thiothixene neuroleptics,** intentional self-harm

✓7ᵗʰ **T43.4X3** **Poisoning by butyrophenone and thiothixene neuroleptics,** assault

✓7ᵗʰ **T43.4X4** **Poisoning by butyrophenone and thiothixene neuroleptics,** undetermined

✓7ᵗʰ **T43.4X5** Adverse effect **of butyrophenone and thiothixene neuroleptics**

✓7ᵗʰ **T43.4X6** Underdosing **of butyrophenone and thiothixene neuroleptics**

✓5ᵗʰ **T43.5** **Poisoning by, adverse effect of and underdosing of other and unspecified antipsychotics and neuroleptics**
EXCLUDES 1 *poisoning by, adverse effect of and underdosing of rauwolfia (T46.5-)*

✓6ᵗʰ **T43.50** **Poisoning by, adverse effect of and underdosing of** unspecified antipsychotics and neuroleptics

✓7ᵗʰ **T43.501** Poisoning by unspecified antipsychotics and neuroleptics, accidental **(unintentional)**
Poisoning by antipsychotics and neuroleptics NOS

✓7ᵗʰ **T43.502** Poisoning by unspecified antipsychotics and neuroleptics, intentional self-harm

✓7ᵗʰ **T43.503** Poisoning by unspecified antipsychotics and neuroleptics, assault

✓7ᵗʰ **T43.504** Poisoning by unspecified antipsychotics and neuroleptics, undetermined

✓7ᵗʰ **T43.505** Adverse effect **of unspecified antipsychotics and neuroleptics**

✓7ᵗʰ **T43.506** Underdosing **of unspecified antipsychotics and neuroleptics**

☑ Additional Character Required   ✓ₓ7ᵗʰ Placeholder Alert   Unspecified Dx   Other Specified Dx   Manifestation   ▶◀ Revised Text   ● New Code   ▲ Revised Code Title

√6ᵗʰ **T43.59** **Poisoning by, adverse effect of and underdosing of other antipsychotics and neuroleptics**

     √7ᵗʰ **T43.591** **Poisoning by other antipsychotics and neuroleptics, accidental (unintentional)**
         Poisoning by other antipsychotics and neuroleptics NOS

     √7ᵗʰ **T43.592** **Poisoning by other antipsychotics and neuroleptics, intentional self-harm**

     √7ᵗʰ **T43.593** **Poisoning by other antipsychotics and neuroleptics, assault**

     √7ᵗʰ **T43.594** **Poisoning by other antipsychotics and neuroleptics, undetermined**

     √7ᵗʰ **T43.595** **Adverse effect of other antipsychotics and neuroleptics**

     √7ᵗʰ **T43.596** **Underdosing of other antipsychotics and neuroleptics**

√5ᵗʰ **T43.6** **Poisoning by, adverse effect of and underdosing of psychostimulants**

     EXCLUDES 1   *poisoning by, adverse effect of and underdosing of cocaine (T40.5-)*

     √6ᵗʰ **T43.60** **Poisoning by, adverse effect of and underdosing of unspecified psychostimulant**

         √7ᵗʰ **T43.601** **Poisoning by unspecified psychostimulants, accidental (unintentional)**
             Poisoning by psychostimulants NOS

         √7ᵗʰ **T43.602** **Poisoning by unspecified psychostimulants, intentional self-harm**

         √7ᵗʰ **T43.603** **Poisoning by unspecified psychostimulants, assault**

         √7ᵗʰ **T43.604** **Poisoning by unspecified psychostimulants, undetermined**

         √7ᵗʰ **T43.605** **Adverse effect of unspecified psychostimulants**

         √7ᵗʰ **T43.606** **Underdosing of unspecified psychostimulants**

     √6ᵗʰ **T43.61** **Poisoning by, adverse effect of and underdosing of caffeine**

         √7ᵗʰ **T43.611** **Poisoning by caffeine, accidental (unintentional)**
             Poisoning by caffeine NOS

         √7ᵗʰ **T43.612** **Poisoning by caffeine, intentional self-harm**

         √7ᵗʰ **T43.613** **Poisoning by caffeine, assault**

         √7ᵗʰ **T43.614** **Poisoning by caffeine, undetermined**

         √7ᵗʰ **T43.615** **Adverse effect of caffeine**

         √7ᵗʰ **T43.616** **Underdosing of caffeine**

     √6ᵗʰ **T43.62** **Poisoning by, adverse effect of and underdosing of amphetamines**
         Poisoning by, adverse effect of and underdosing of methamphetamines

         √7ᵗʰ **T43.621** **Poisoning by amphetamines, accidental (unintentional)**
             Poisoning by amphetamines NOS

         √7ᵗʰ **T43.622** **Poisoning by amphetamines, intentional self-harm**

         √7ᵗʰ **T43.623** **Poisoning by amphetamines, assault**

         √7ᵗʰ **T43.624** **Poisoning by amphetamines, undetermined**

         √7ᵗʰ **T43.625** **Adverse effect of amphetamines**

         √7ᵗʰ **T43.626** **Underdosing of amphetamines**

     √6ᵗʰ **T43.63** **Poisoning by, adverse effect of and underdosing of methylphenidate**

         √7ᵗʰ **T43.631** **Poisoning by methylphenidate, accidental (unintentional)**
             Poisoning by methylphenidate NOS

         √7ᵗʰ **T43.632** **Poisoning by methylphenidate, intentional self-harm**

         √7ᵗʰ **T43.633** **Poisoning by methylphenidate, assault**

         √7ᵗʰ **T43.634** **Poisoning by methylphenidate, undetermined**

         √7ᵗʰ **T43.635** **Adverse effect of methylphenidate**

         √7ᵗʰ **T43.636** **Underdosing of methylphenidate**

√6ᵗʰ **T43.69** **Poisoning by, adverse effect of and underdosing of other psychostimulants**

     √7ᵗʰ **T43.691** **Poisoning by other psychostimulants, accidental (unintentional)**
         Poisoning by other psychostimulants NOS

     √7ᵗʰ **T43.692** **Poisoning by other psychostimulants, intentional self-harm**

     √7ᵗʰ **T43.693** **Poisoning by other psychostimulants, assault**

     √7ᵗʰ **T43.694** **Poisoning by other psychostimulants, undetermined**

     √7ᵗʰ **T43.695** **Adverse effect of other psychostimulants**

     √7ᵗʰ **T43.696** **Underdosing of other psychostimulants**

√5ᵗʰ **T43.8** **Poisoning by, adverse effect of and underdosing of other psychotropic drugs**

     √6ᵗʰ **T43.8X** **Poisoning by, adverse effect of and underdosing of other psychotropic drugs**

         √7ᵗʰ **T43.8X1** **Poisoning by other psychotropic drugs, accidental (unintentional)**
             Poisoning by other psychotropic drugs NOS

         √7ᵗʰ **T43.8X2** **Poisoning by other psychotropic drugs, intentional self-harm**

         √7ᵗʰ **T43.8X3** **Poisoning by other psychotropic drugs, assault**

         √7ᵗʰ **T43.8X4** **Poisoning by other psychotropic drugs, undetermined**

         √7ᵗʰ **T43.8X5** **Adverse effect of other psychotropic drugs**

         √7ᵗʰ **T43.8X6** **Underdosing of other psychotropic drugs**

√5ᵗʰ **T43.9** **Poisoning by, adverse effect of and underdosing of unspecified psychotropic drug**

     √x7ᵗʰ **T43.91** **Poisoning by unspecified psychotropic drug, accidental (unintentional)**
         Poisoning by psychotropic drug NOS

     √x7ᵗʰ **T43.92** **Poisoning by unspecified psychotropic drug, intentional self-harm**

     √x7ᵗʰ **T43.93** **Poisoning by unspecified psychotropic drug, assault**

     √x7ᵗʰ **T43.94** **Poisoning by unspecified psychotropic drug, undetermined**

     √x7ᵗʰ **T43.95** **Adverse effect of unspecified psychotropic drug**

     √x7ᵗʰ **T43.96** **Underdosing of unspecified psychotropic drug**

√4ᵗʰ **T44** **Poisoning by, adverse effect of and underdosing of drugs primarily affecting the autonomic nervous system**

> The appropriate 7th character is to be added to each code from category T44.
> A   initial encounter
> D   subsequent encounter
> S   sequela

√5ᵗʰ **T44.0** **Poisoning by, adverse effect of and underdosing of anticholinesterase agents**

     √6ᵗʰ **T44.0X** **Poisoning by, adverse effect of and underdosing of anticholinesterase agents**

         √7ᵗʰ **T44.0X1** **Poisoning by anticholinesterase agents, accidental (unintentional)**
             Poisoning by anticholinesterase agents NOS

         √7ᵗʰ **T44.0X2** **Poisoning by anticholinesterase agents, intentional self-harm**

         √7ᵗʰ **T44.0X3** **Poisoning by anticholinesterase agents, assault**

         √7ᵗʰ **T44.0X4** **Poisoning by anticholinesterase agents, undetermined**

         √7ᵗʰ **T44.0X5** **Adverse effect of anticholinesterase agents**

         √7ᵗʰ **T44.0X6** **Underdosing of anticholinesterase agents**

√5ᵗʰ **T44.1** **Poisoning by, adverse effect of and underdosing of other parasympathomimetics [cholinergics]**

     √6ᵗʰ **T44.1X** **Poisoning by, adverse effect of and underdosing of other parasympathomimetics [cholinergics]**

         √7ᵗʰ **T44.1X1** **Poisoning by other parasympathomimetics [cholinergics], accidental (unintentional)**
         Poisoning by other parasympathomimetics [cholinergics] NOS

         √7ᵗʰ **T44.1X2** **Poisoning by other parasympathomimetics [cholinergics], intentional self-harm**

EXCLUDES 1 Not coded here   **EXCLUDES 2** Not included here   N Newborn Age: 0   P Pediatric Age: 0-17   M Maternity Age: 12-55   A Adult Age: 15-124

994   ICD-10-CM 2016

✓7th **T44.1X3** Poisoning by other parasympathomimetics [cholinergics], assault

✓7th **T44.1X4** Poisoning by other parasympathomimetics [cholinergics], undetermined

✓7th **T44.1X5** Adverse effect of other parasympathomimetics [cholinergics]

✓7th **T44.1X6** Underdosing of other parasympathomimetics

✓5th **T44.2** Poisoning by, adverse effect of and underdosing of ganglionic blocking drugs

✓6th **T44.2X** Poisoning by, adverse effect of and underdosing of ganglionic blocking drugs

✓7th **T44.2X1** Poisoning by ganglionic blocking drugs, accidental (unintentional)
Poisoning by ganglionic blocking drugs NOS

✓7th **T44.2X2** Poisoning by ganglionic blocking drugs, intentional self-harm

✓7th **T44.2X3** Poisoning by ganglionic blocking drugs, assault

✓7th **T44.2X4** Poisoning by ganglionic blocking drugs, undetermined

✓7th **T44.2X5** Adverse effect of ganglionic blocking drugs

✓7th **T44.2X6** Underdosing of ganglionic blocking drugs

✓5th **T44.3** Poisoning by, adverse effect of and underdosing of other parasympatholytics [anticholinergics and antimuscarinics] and spasmolytics
Poisoning by, adverse effect of and underdosing of papaverine

✓6th **T44.3X** Poisoning by, adverse effect of and underdosing of other parasympatholytics [anticholinergics and antimuscarinics] and spasmolytics

✓7th **T44.3X1** Poisoning by other parasympatholytics [anticholinergics and antimuscarinics] and spasmolytics, accidental (unintentional)
Poisoning by other parasympatholytics [anticholinergics and antimuscarinics] and spasmolytics NOS

✓7th **T44.3X2** Poisoning by other parasympatholytics [anticholinergics and antimuscarinics] and spasmolytics, intentional self-harm

✓7th **T44.3X3** Poisoning by other parasympatholytics [anticholinergics and antimuscarinics] and spasmolytics, assault

✓7th **T44.3X4** Poisoning by other parasympatholytics [anticholinergics and antimuscarinics] and spasmolytics, undetermined

✓7th **T44.3X5** Adverse effect of other parasympatholytics [anticholinergics and antimuscarinics] and spasmolytics

✓7th **T44.3X6** Underdosing of other parasympatholytics [anticholinergics and antimuscarinics] and spasmolytics

✓5th **T44.4** Poisoning by, adverse effect of and underdosing of predominantly alpha-adrenoreceptor agonists
Poisoning by, adverse effect of and underdosing of metaraminol

✓6th **T44.4X** Poisoning by, adverse effect of and underdosing of predominantly alpha-adrenoreceptor agonists

✓7th **T44.4X1** Poisoning by predominantly alpha-adrenoreceptor agonists, accidental (unintentional)
Poisoning by predominantly alpha-adrenoreceptor agonists NOS

✓7th **T44.4X2** Poisoning by predominantly alpha-adrenoreceptor agonists, intentional self-harm

✓7th **T44.4X3** Poisoning by predominantly alpha-adrenoreceptor agonists, assault

✓7th **T44.4X4** Poisoning by predominantly alpha-adrenoreceptor agonists, undetermined

✓7th **T44.4X5** Adverse effect of predominantly alpha-adrenoreceptor agonists

✓7th **T44.4X6** Underdosing of predominantly alpha-adrenoreceptor agonists

✓5th **T44.5** Poisoning by, adverse effect of and underdosing of predominantly beta-adrenoreceptor agonists
EXCLUDES 1   poisoning by, adverse effect of and underdosing of beta-adrenoreceptor agonists used in asthma therapy (T48.6-)

✓6th **T44.5X** Poisoning by, adverse effect of and underdosing of predominantly beta-adrenoreceptor agonists

✓7th **T44.5X1** Poisoning by predominantly beta-adrenoreceptor agonists, accidental (unintentional)
Poisoning by predominantly beta-adrenoreceptor agonists NOS

✓7th **T44.5X2** Poisoning by predominantly beta-adrenoreceptor agonists, intentional self-harm

✓7th **T44.5X3** Poisoning by predominantly beta-adrenoreceptor agonists, assault

✓7th **T44.5X4** Poisoning by predominantly beta-adrenoreceptor agonists, undetermined

✓7th **T44.5X5** Adverse effect of predominantly beta-adrenoreceptor agonists

✓7th **T44.5X6** Underdosing of predominantly beta-adrenoreceptor agonists

✓5th **T44.6** Poisoning by, adverse effect of and underdosing of alpha-adrenoreceptor antagonists
EXCLUDES 1   poisoning by, adverse effect of and underdosing of ergot alkaloids (T48.0)

✓6th **T44.6X** Poisoning by, adverse effect of and underdosing of alpha-adrenoreceptor antagonists

✓7th **T44.6X1** Poisoning by alpha-adrenoreceptor antagonists, accidental (unintentional)
Poisoning by alpha-adrenoreceptor antagonists NOS

✓7th **T44.6X2** Poisoning by alpha-adrenoreceptor antagonists, intentional self-harm

✓7th **T44.6X3** Poisoning by alpha-adrenoreceptor antagonists, assault

✓7th **T44.6X4** Poisoning by alpha-adrenoreceptor antagonists, undetermined

✓7th **T44.6X5** Adverse effect of alpha-adrenoreceptor antagonists

✓7th **T44.6X6** Underdosing of alpha-adrenoreceptor antagonists

✓5th **T44.7** Poisoning by, adverse effect of and underdosing of beta-adrenoreceptor antagonists

✓6th **T44.7X** Poisoning by, adverse effect of and underdosing of beta-adrenoreceptor antagonists

✓7th **T44.7X1** Poisoning by beta-adrenoreceptor antagonists, accidental (unintentional)
Poisoning by beta-adrenoreceptor antagonists NOS

✓7th **T44.7X2** Poisoning by beta-adrenoreceptor antagonists, intentional self-harm

✓7th **T44.7X3** Poisoning by beta-adrenoreceptor antagonists, assault

✓7th **T44.7X4** Poisoning by beta-adrenoreceptor antagonists, undetermined

✓7th **T44.7X5** Adverse effect of beta-adrenoreceptor antagonists

✓7th **T44.7X6** Underdosing of beta-adrenoreceptor antagonists

✓5th **T44.8** Poisoning by, adverse effect of and underdosing of centrally-acting and adrenergic-neuron- blocking agents
EXCLUDES 1   poisoning by, adverse effect of and underdosing of clonidine (T46.5)
poisoning by, adverse effect of and underdosing of guanethidine (T46.5)

✓6th **T44.8X** Poisoning by, adverse effect of and underdosing of centrally-acting and adrenergic-neuron-blocking agents

✓7th **T44.8X1** Poisoning by centrally-acting and adrenergic-neuron-blocking agents, accidental (unintentional)
Poisoning by centrally-acting and adrenergic-neuron-blocking agents NOS

☑ Additional Character Required   ✓x7th Placeholder Alert   Unspecified Dx   Other Specified Dx   Manifestation   ▶◀ Revised Text   ● New Code   ▲ Revised Code Title

Chapter 19. Injury, Poisoning, and Certain Other Consequences of External Causes

T44.8X2 Poisoning by centrally-acting and adrenergic-neuron-blocking agents, **intentional self-harm**

T44.8X3 Poisoning by centrally-acting and adrenergic-neuron-blocking agents, **assault**

T44.8X4 Poisoning by centrally-acting and adrenergic-neuron-blocking agents, **undetermined**

T44.8X5 Adverse effect of centrally-acting and adrenergic-neuron-blocking agents

T44.8X6 Underdosing of centrally-acting and adrenergic-neuron-blocking agents

T44.9 Poisoning by, adverse effect of and underdosing of other and unspecified drugs primarily affecting the autonomic nervous system
Poisoning by, adverse effect of and underdosing of drug stimulating both alpha and beta-adrenoreceptors

T44.90 Poisoning by, adverse effect of and underdosing of unspecified drugs primarily affecting the autonomic nervous system

T44.901 Poisoning by unspecified drugs primarily affecting the autonomic nervous system, **accidental (unintentional)**
Poisoning by unspecified drugs primarily affecting the autonomic nervous system NOS

T44.902 Poisoning by unspecified drugs primarily affecting the autonomic nervous system, **intentional self-harm**

T44.903 Poisoning by unspecified drugs primarily affecting the autonomic nervous system, **assault**

T44.904 Poisoning by unspecified drugs primarily affecting the autonomic nervous system, **undetermined**

T44.905 Adverse effect of unspecified drugs primarily affecting the autonomic nervous system

T44.906 Underdosing of unspecified drugs primarily affecting the autonomic nervous system

T44.99 Poisoning by, adverse effect of and underdosing of other drugs primarily affecting the autonomic nervous system

T44.991 Poisoning by other drug primarily affecting the autonomic nervous system, **accidental (unintentional)**
Poisoning by other drugs primarily affecting the autonomic nervous system NOS

T44.992 Poisoning by other drug primarily affecting the autonomic nervous system, **intentional self-harm**

T44.993 Poisoning by other drug primarily affecting the autonomic nervous system, **assault**

T44.994 Poisoning by other drug primarily affecting the autonomic nervous system, **undetermined**

T44.995 Adverse effect of other drug primarily affecting the autonomic nervous system

T44.996 Underdosing of other drug primarily affecting the autonomic nervous system

T45 Poisoning by, adverse effect of and underdosing of primarily systemic and hematological agents, not elsewhere classified

The appropriate 7th character is to be added to each code from category T45.
A   initial encounter
D   subsequent encounter
S   sequela

T45.0 Poisoning by, adverse effect of and underdosing of antiallergic and antiemetic drugs
EXCLUDES 1 poisoning by, adverse effect of and underdosing of phenothiazine-based neuroleptics (T43.3)

T45.0X Poisoning by, adverse effect of and underdosing of antiallergic and antiemetic drugs

T45.0X1 Poisoning by antiallergic and antiemetic drugs, **accidental (unintentional)**
Poisoning by antiallergic and antiemetic drugs NOS

T45.0X2 Poisoning by antiallergic and antiemetic drugs, **intentional self-harm**

T45.0X3 Poisoning by antiallergic and antiemetic drugs, **assault**

T45.0X4 Poisoning by antiallergic and antiemetic drugs, **undetermined**

T45.0X5 Adverse effect of antiallergic and antiemetic drugs

T45.0X6 Underdosing of antiallergic and antiemetic drugs

T45.1 Poisoning by, adverse effect of and underdosing of antineoplastic and immunosuppressive drugs
EXCLUDES 1 poisoning by, adverse effect of and underdosing of tamoxifen (T38.6)
AHA: 2014, 4Q, 22

T45.1X Poisoning by, adverse effect of and underdosing of antineoplastic and immunosuppressive drugs

T45.1X1 Poisoning by antineoplastic and immunosuppressive drugs, **accidental (unintentional)**
Poisoning by antineoplastic and immunosuppressive drugs NOS

T45.1X2 Poisoning by antineoplastic and immunosuppressive drugs, **intentional self-harm**

T45.1X3 Poisoning by antineoplastic and immunosuppressive drugs, **assault**

T45.1X4 Poisoning by antineoplastic and immunosuppressive drugs, **undetermined**

T45.1X5 Adverse effect of antineoplastic and immunosuppressive drugs

T45.1X6 Underdosing of antineoplastic and immunosuppressive drugs

T45.2 Poisoning by, adverse effect of and underdosing of vitamins
EXCLUDES 2 poisoning by, adverse effect of and underdosing of iron (T45.4)
poisoning by, adverse effect of and underdosing of nicotinic acid (derivatives) (T46.7)
poisoning by, adverse effect of and underdosing of vitamin K (T45.7)

T45.2X Poisoning by, adverse effect of and underdosing of vitamins

T45.2X1 Poisoning by vitamins, **accidental (unintentional)**
Poisoning by vitamins NOS

T45.2X2 Poisoning by vitamins, **intentional self-harm**

T45.2X3 Poisoning by vitamins, **assault**

T45.2X4 Poisoning by vitamins, **undetermined**

T45.2X5 Adverse effect of vitamins

T45.2X6 Underdosing of vitamins
EXCLUDES 1 vitamin deficiencies (E50-E56)

T45.3 Poisoning by, adverse effect of and underdosing of enzymes

T45.3X Poisoning by, adverse effect of and underdosing of enzymes

T45.3X1 Poisoning by enzymes, **accidental (unintentional)**
Poisoning by enzymes NOS

T45.3X2 Poisoning by enzymes, **intentional self-harm**

EXCLUDES 1 Not coded here   **EXCLUDES 2** Not included here   **N** Newborn Age: 0   **P** Pediatric Age: 0-17   **M** Maternity Age: 12-55   **A** Adult Age: 15-124

996   ICD-10-CM 2016

☑7ᵗʰ **T45.3X3**   **Poisoning by enzymes,** assault

☑7ᵗʰ **T45.3X4**   **Poisoning by enzymes,** undetermined

☑7ᵗʰ **T45.3X5**   Adverse effect **of enzymes**

☑7ᵗʰ **T45.3X6**   Underdosing **of enzymes**

☑5ᵗʰ **T45.4**   **Poisoning by, adverse effect of and underdosing of iron and its compounds**

    ☑6ᵗʰ **T45.4X**   **Poisoning by, adverse effect of and underdosing of iron and its compounds**

       T45.4X1   **Poisoning by iron and its compounds,** accidental **(unintentional)**
             Poisoning by iron and its compounds NOS

       ☑7ᵗʰ **T45.4X2**   **Poisoning by iron and its compounds,** intentional self-harm

       ☑7ᵗʰ **T45.4X3**   **Poisoning by iron and its compounds,** assault

       ☑7ᵗʰ **T45.4X4**   **Poisoning by iron and its compounds,** undetermined

       ☑7ᵗʰ **T45.4X5**   Adverse effect **of iron and its compounds**

       ☑7ᵗʰ **T45.4X6**   Underdosing **of iron and its compounds**
           EXCLUDES 1   iron deficiency (E61.1)

☑5ᵗʰ **T45.5**   **Poisoning by, adverse effect of and underdosing of anticoagulants and antithrombotic drugs**

    ☑6ᵗʰ **T45.51**   **Poisoning by, adverse effect of and underdosing of anticoagulants**

       ☑7ᵗʰ **T45.511**   **Poisoning by anticoagulants,** accidental **(unintentional)**
             Poisoning by anticoagulants NOS

       ☑7ᵗʰ **T45.512**   **Poisoning by anticoagulants,** intentional self-harm

       ☑7ᵗʰ **T45.513**   **Poisoning by anticoagulants,** assault

       ☑7ᵗʰ **T45.514**   **Poisoning by anticoagulants,** undetermined

       ☑7ᵗʰ **T45.515**   Adverse effect **of anticoagulants**
             AHA: 2013, 2Q, 34

       ☑7ᵗʰ **T45.516**   Underdosing **of anticoagulants**

    ☑6ᵗʰ **T45.52**   **Poisoning by, adverse effect of and underdosing of antithrombotic drugs**
        Poisoning by, adverse effect of and underdosing of antiplatelet drugs
        EXCLUDES 2   poisoning by, adverse effect of and underdosing of aspirin (T39.Ø1-)
                poisoning by, adverse effect of and underdosing of acetylsalicylic acid (T39.Ø1-)

       ☑7ᵗʰ **T45.521**   **Poisoning by antithrombotic drugs,** accidental **(unintentional)**
             Poisoning by antithrombotic drug NOS

       ☑7ᵗʰ **T45.522**   **Poisoning by antithrombotic drugs,** intentional self-harm

       ☑7ᵗʰ **T45.523**   **Poisoning by antithrombotic drugs,** assault

       ☑7ᵗʰ **T45.524**   **Poisoning by antithrombotic drugs,** undetermined

       ☑7ᵗʰ **T45.525**   Adverse effect **of antithrombotic drugs**

       ☑7ᵗʰ **T45.526**   Underdosing **of antithrombotic drugs**

☑5ᵗʰ **T45.6**   **Poisoning by, adverse effect of and underdosing of fibrinolysis-affecting drugs**

    ☑6ᵗʰ **T45.6Ø**   **Poisoning by, adverse effect of and underdosing of unspecified fibrinolysis-affecting drugs**

       ☑7ᵗʰ **T45.6Ø1**   **Poisoning by unspecified fibrinolysis-affecting drugs,** accidental **(unintentional)**
             Poisoning by fibrinolysis-affecting drug NOS

       ☑7ᵗʰ **T45.6Ø2**   **Poisoning by unspecified fibrinolysis-affecting drugs,** intentional self-harm

       ☑7ᵗʰ **T45.6Ø3**   **Poisoning by unspecified fibrinolysis-affecting drugs,** assault

       ☑7ᵗʰ **T45.6Ø4**   **Poisoning by unspecified fibrinolysis-affecting drugs,** undetermined

       ☑7ᵗʰ **T45.6Ø5**   Adverse effect **of unspecified fibrinolysis-affecting drugs**

       ☑7ᵗʰ **T45.6Ø6**   Underdosing **of unspecified fibrinolysis-affecting drugs**

☑6ᵗʰ **T45.61**   **Poisoning by, adverse effect of and underdosing of thrombolytic drugs**

       ☑7ᵗʰ **T45.611**   **Poisoning by thrombolytic drug,** accidental **(unintentional)**
             Poisoning by thrombolytic drug NOS

       ☑7ᵗʰ **T45.612**   **Poisoning by thrombolytic drug,** intentional self-harm

       ☑7ᵗʰ **T45.613**   **Poisoning by thrombolytic drug,** assault

       ☑7ᵗʰ **T45.614**   **Poisoning by thrombolytic drug,** undetermined

       ☑7ᵗʰ **T45.615**   Adverse effect **of thrombolytic drugs**

       ☑7ᵗʰ **T45.616**   Underdosing **of thrombolytic drugs**

☑6ᵗʰ **T45.62**   **Poisoning by, adverse effect of and underdosing of hemostatic drugs**

       ☑7ᵗʰ **T45.621**   **Poisoning by hemostatic drug,** accidental **(unintentional)**
             Poisoning by hemostatic drug NOS

       ☑7ᵗʰ **T45.622**   **Poisoning by hemostatic drug,** intentional self-harm

       ☑7ᵗʰ **T45.623**   **Poisoning by hemostatic drug,** assault

       ☑7ᵗʰ **T45.624**   **Poisoning by hemostatic drug,** undetermined

       ☑7ᵗʰ **T45.625**   Adverse effect **of hemostatic drug**

       ☑7ᵗʰ **T45.626**   Underdosing **of hemostatic drugs**

☑6ᵗʰ **T45.69**   **Poisoning by, adverse effect of and underdosing of other fibrinolysis-affecting drugs**

       ☑7ᵗʰ **T45.691**   **Poisoning by other fibrinolysis-affecting drugs,** accidental **(unintentional)**
             Poisoning by other fibrinolysis-affecting drug NOS

       ☑7ᵗʰ **T45.692**   **Poisoning by other fibrinolysis-affecting drugs,** intentional self-harm

       ☑7ᵗʰ **T45.693**   **Poisoning by other fibrinolysis-affecting drugs,** assault

       ☑7ᵗʰ **T45.694**   **Poisoning by other fibrinolysis-affecting drugs,** undetermined

       ☑7ᵗʰ **T45.695**   Adverse effect **of other fibrinolysis-affecting drugs**

       ☑7ᵗʰ **T45.696**   Underdosing **of other fibrinolysis-affecting drugs**

☑5ᵗʰ **T45.7**   **Poisoning by, adverse effect of and underdosing of anticoagulant antagonists, vitamin K and other coagulants**

    ☑6ᵗʰ **T45.7X**   **Poisoning by, adverse effect of and underdosing of anticoagulant antagonists, vitamin K and other coagulants**

       ☑7ᵗʰ **T45.7X1**   **Poisoning by anticoagulant antagonists, vitamin K and other coagulants,** accidental **(unintentional)**
             Poisoning by anticoagulant antagonists, vitamin K and other coagulants NOS

       ☑7ᵗʰ **T45.7X2**   **Poisoning by anticoagulant antagonists, vitamin K and other coagulants,** intentional self-harm

       ☑7ᵗʰ **T45.7X3**   **Poisoning by anticoagulant antagonists, vitamin K and other coagulants,** assault

       ☑7ᵗʰ **T45.7X4**   **Poisoning by anticoagulant antagonists, vitamin K and other coagulants,** undetermined

       ☑7ᵗʰ **T45.7X5**   Adverse effect **of anticoagulant antagonists, vitamin K and other coagulants**

       ☑7ᵗʰ **T45.7X6**   Underdosing **of anticoagulant antagonist, vitamin K and other coagulants**
             EXCLUDES 1   vitamin K deficiency (E56.1)

☑ Additional Character Required   ☑ₓ7ᵗʰ Placeholder Alert   Unspecified Dx   Other Specified Dx   Manifestation   ▶◀ Revised Text   ● New Code   ▲ Revised Code Title

✓5th **T45.8** **Poisoning by, adverse effect of and underdosing of** other **primarily systemic and hematological agents**

Poisoning by, adverse effect of and underdosing of liver preparations and other antianemic agents

Poisoning by, adverse effect of and underdosing of natural blood and blood products

Poisoning by, adverse effect of and underdosing of plasma substitute

EXCLUDES 2   poisoning by, adverse effect of and underdosing of immunoglobulin (T50.Z1)

poisoning by, adverse effect of and underdosing of iron (T45.4)

transfusion reactions (T80.-)

✓6th **T45.8X** **Poisoning by, adverse effect of and underdosing of** other **primarily systemic and hematological agents**

✓7th **T45.8X1** **Poisoning by other primarily systemic and hematological agents,** accidental **(unintentional)**

Poisoning by other primarily systemic and hematological agents NOS

✓7th **T45.8X2** **Poisoning by other primarily systemic and hematological agents,** intentional self-harm

✓7th **T45.8X3** **Poisoning by other primarily systemic and hematological agents,** assault

✓7th **T45.8X4** **Poisoning by other primarily systemic and hematological agents,** undetermined

✓7th **T45.8X5** Adverse effect **of other primarily systemic and hematological agents**

✓7th **T45.8X6** Underdosing **of other primarily systemic and hematological agents**

✓5th **T45.9** **Poisoning by, adverse effect of and underdosing of** unspecified **primarily systemic and hematological agent**

✓x 7th **T45.91** **Poisoning by unspecified primarily systemic and hematological agent,** accidental **(unintentional)**

Poisoning by primarily systemic and hematological agent NOS

✓x 7th **T45.92** **Poisoning by unspecified primarily systemic and hematological agent,** intentional self-harm

✓x 7th **T45.93** **Poisoning by unspecified primarily systemic and hematological agent,** assault

✓x 7th **T45.94** **Poisoning by unspecified primarily systemic and hematological agent,** undetermined

✓x 7th **T45.95** Adverse effect **of unspecified primarily systemic and hematological agent**

✓x 7th **T45.96** Underdosing **of unspecified primarily systemic and hematological agent**

✓4th **T46** **Poisoning by, adverse effect of and underdosing of agents primarily affecting the cardiovascular system**

EXCLUDES 1   poisoning by, adverse effect of and underdosing of metaraminol (T44.4)

The appropriate 7th character is to be added to each code from category T46.

A   initial encounter
D   subsequent encounter
S   sequela

✓5th **T46.0** **Poisoning by, adverse effect of and underdosing of cardiac-stimulant glycosides and drugs of similar action**

✓6th **T46.0X** **Poisoning by, adverse effect of and underdosing of** cardiac-stimulant glycosides **and drugs of similar action**

✓7th **T46.0X1** **Poisoning by cardiac-stimulant glycosides and drugs of similar action,** accidental **(unintentional)**

Poisoning by cardiac-stimulant glycosides and drugs of similar action NOS

✓7th **T46.0X2** **Poisoning by cardiac-stimulant glycosides and drugs of similar action,** intentional self-harm

✓7th **T46.0X3** **Poisoning by cardiac-stimulant glycosides and drugs of similar action,** assault

✓7th **T46.0X4** **Poisoning by cardiac-stimulant glycosides and drugs of similar action,** undetermined

✓7th **T46.0X5** Adverse effect **of cardiac-stimulant glycosides and drugs of similar action**

✓7th **T46.0X6** Underdosing **of cardiac-stimulant glycosides and drugs of similar action**

✓5th **T46.1** **Poisoning by, adverse effect of and underdosing of calcium-channel blockers**

✓6th **T46.1X** **Poisoning by, adverse effect of and underdosing of** calcium-channel blockers

✓7th **T46.1X1** **Poisoning by calcium-channel blockers,** accidental **(unintentional)**

Poisoning by calcium-channel blockers NOS

✓7th **T46.1X2** **Poisoning by calcium-channel blockers,** intentional self-harm

✓7th **T46.1X3** **Poisoning by calcium-channel blockers,** assault

✓7th **T46.1X4** **Poisoning by calcium-channel blockers,** undetermined

✓7th **T46.1X5** Adverse effect **of calcium-channel blockers**

✓7th **T46.1X6** Underdosing **of calcium-channel blockers**

✓5th **T46.2** **Poisoning by, adverse effect of and underdosing of other antidysrhythmic drugs, not elsewhere classified**

EXCLUDES 1   poisoning by, adverse effect of and underdosing of beta-adrenoreceptor antagonists (T44.7-)

✓6th **T46.2X** **Poisoning by, adverse effect of and underdosing of** other antidysrhythmic **drugs**

✓7th **T46.2X1** **Poisoning by other antidysrhythmic drugs,** accidental **(unintentional)**

Poisoning by other antidysrhythmic drugs NOS

✓7th **T46.2X2** **Poisoning by other antidysrhythmic drugs,** intentional self-harm

✓7th **T46.2X3** **Poisoning by other antidysrhythmic drugs,** assault

✓7th **T46.2X4** **Poisoning by other antidysrhythmic drugs,** undetermined

✓7th **T46.2X5** Adverse effect **of other antidysrhythmic drugs**

✓7th **T46.2X6** Underdosing **of other antidysrhythmic drugs**

✓5th **T46.3** **Poisoning by, adverse effect of and underdosing of coronary vasodilators**

Poisoning by, adverse effect of and underdosing of dipyridamole

EXCLUDES 1   poisoning by, adverse effect of and underdosing of calcium-channel blockers (T46.1)

✓6th **T46.3X** **Poisoning by, adverse effect of and underdosing of** coronary vasodilators

✓7th **T46.3X1** **Poisoning by coronary vasodilators,** accidental **(unintentional)**

Poisoning by coronary vasodilators NOS

✓7th **T46.3X2** **Poisoning by coronary vasodilators,** intentional self-harm

✓7th **T46.3X3** **Poisoning by coronary vasodilators,** assault

✓7th **T46.3X4** **Poisoning by coronary vasodilators,** undetermined

✓7th **T46.3X5** Adverse effect **of coronary vasodilators**

✓7th **T46.3X6** Underdosing **of coronary vasodilators**

✓5th **T46.4** **Poisoning by, adverse effect of and underdosing of angiotensin-converting-enzyme inhibitors**

✓6th **T46.4X** **Poisoning by, adverse effect of and underdosing of** angiotensin-converting-enzyme inhibitors

✓7th **T46.4X1** **Poisoning by angiotensin-converting-enzyme inhibitors,** accidental **(unintentional)**

Poisoning by angiotensin-converting-enzyme inhibitors NOS

✓7th **T46.4X2** **Poisoning by angiotensin-converting-enzyme inhibitors,** intentional self-harm

✓7th **T46.4X3** **Poisoning by angiotensin-converting-enzyme inhibitors,** assault

✓7th **T46.4X4** **Poisoning by angiotensin-converting-enzyme inhibitors,** undetermined

✓7th **T46.4X5** Adverse effect **of angiotensin-converting-enzyme inhibitors**

✓7th **T46.4X6** Underdosing **of angiotensin-converting-enzyme inhibitors**

EXCLUDES 1 Not coded here   EXCLUDES 2 Not included here   N Newborn Age: 0   P Pediatric Age: 0-17   M Maternity Age: 12-55   A Adult Age: 15-124

998   ICD-10-CM 2016

✓5ᵗʰ T46.5 Poisoning by, adverse effect of and underdosing of other antihypertensive drugs

> EXCLUDES 2   *poisoning by, adverse effect of and underdosing of beta-adrenoreceptor antagonists (T44.7)*
> *poisoning by, adverse effect of and underdosing of calcium-channel blockers (T46.1)*
> *poisoning by, adverse effect of and underdosing of diuretics (T50.0-T50.2)*

✓6ᵗʰ T46.5X Poisoning, adverse effect of and underdosing of other antihypertensive drugs

    ✓7ᵗʰ **T46.5X1 Poisoning by other antihypertensive drugs, accidental (unintentional)**
       Poisoning by other antihypertensive drugs NOS

    ✓7ᵗʰ **T46.5X2 Poisoning by other antihypertensive drugs, intentional self-harm**

    ✓7ᵗʰ **T46.5X3 Poisoning by other antihypertensive drugs, assault**

    ✓7ᵗʰ **T46.5X4 Poisoning by other antihypertensive drugs, undetermined**

    ✓7ᵗʰ **T46.5X5 Adverse effect of other antihypertensive drugs**

    ✓7ᵗʰ **T46.5X6 Underdosing of other antihypertensive drugs**

✓5ᵗʰ T46.6 Poisoning by, adverse effect of and underdosing of antihyperlipidemic and antiarteriosclerotic drugs

✓6ᵗʰ T46.6X Poisoning by, adverse effect of and underdosing of antihyperlipidemic and antiarteriosclerotic drugs

    ✓7ᵗʰ **T46.6X1 Poisoning by antihyperlipidemic and antiarteriosclerotic drugs, accidental (unintentional)**
       Poisoning by antihyperlipidemic and antiarteriosclerotic drugs NOS

    ✓7ᵗʰ **T46.6X2 Poisoning by antihyperlipidemic and antiarteriosclerotic drugs, intentional self-harm**

    ✓7ᵗʰ **T46.6X3 Poisoning by antihyperlipidemic and antiarteriosclerotic drugs, assault**

    ✓7ᵗʰ **T46.6X4 Poisoning by antihyperlipidemic and antiarteriosclerotic drugs, undetermined**

    ✓7ᵗʰ **T46.6X5 Adverse effect of antihyperlipidemic and antiarteriosclerotic drugs**

    ✓7ᵗʰ **T46.6X6 Underdosing of antihyperlipidemic and antiarteriosclerotic drugs**

✓5ᵗʰ T46.7 Poisoning by, adverse effect of and underdosing of peripheral vasodilators
    Poisoning by, adverse effect of and underdosing of nicotinic acid (derivatives)

> EXCLUDES 1   *poisoning by, adverse effect of and underdosing of papaverine (T44.3)*

✓6ᵗʰ T46.7X Poisoning by, adverse effect of and underdosing of peripheral vasodilators

    ✓7ᵗʰ **T46.7X1 Poisoning by peripheral vasodilators, accidental (unintentional)**
       Poisoning by peripheral vasodilators NOS

    ✓7ᵗʰ **T46.7X2 Poisoning by peripheral vasodilators, intentional self-harm**

    ✓7ᵗʰ **T46.7X3 Poisoning by peripheral vasodilators, assault**

    ✓7ᵗʰ **T46.7X4 Poisoning by peripheral vasodilators, undetermined**

    ✓7ᵗʰ **T46.7X5 Adverse effect of peripheral vasodilators**

    ✓7ᵗʰ **T46.7X6 Underdosing of peripheral vasodilators**

✓5ᵗʰ T46.8 Poisoning by, adverse effect of and underdosing of antivaricose drugs, including sclerosing agents

✓6ᵗʰ T46.8X Poisoning by, adverse effect of and underdosing of antivaricose drugs, including sclerosing agents

    ✓7ᵗʰ **T46.8X1 Poisoning by antivaricose drugs, including sclerosing agents, accidental (unintentional)**
       Poisoning by antivaricose drugs, including sclerosing agents NOS

    ✓7ᵗʰ **T46.8X2 Poisoning by antivaricose drugs, including sclerosing agents, intentional self-harm**

    ✓7ᵗʰ **T46.8X3 Poisoning by antivaricose drugs, including sclerosing agents, assault**

    ✓7ᵗʰ **T46.8X4 Poisoning by antivaricose drugs, including sclerosing agents, undetermined**

    ✓7ᵗʰ **T46.8X5 Adverse effect of antivaricose drugs, including sclerosing agents**

    ✓7ᵗʰ **T46.8X6 Underdosing of antivaricose drugs, including sclerosing agents**

✓5ᵗʰ T46.9 Poisoning by, adverse effect of and underdosing of other and unspecified agents primarily affecting the cardiovascular system

✓6ᵗʰ T46.90 Poisoning by, adverse effect of and underdosing of unspecified agents primarily affecting the cardiovascular system

    ✓7ᵗʰ **T46.901 Poisoning by unspecified agents primarily affecting the cardiovascular system, accidental (unintentional)**

    ✓7ᵗʰ **T46.902 Poisoning by unspecified agents primarily affecting the cardiovascular system, intentional self-harm**

    ✓7ᵗʰ **T46.903 Poisoning by unspecified agents primarily affecting the cardiovascular system, assault**

    ✓7ᵗʰ **T46.904 Poisoning by unspecified agents primarily affecting the cardiovascular system, undetermined**

    ✓7ᵗʰ **T46.905 Adverse effect of unspecified agents primarily affecting the cardiovascular system**

    ✓7ᵗʰ **T46.906 Underdosing of unspecified agents primarily affecting the cardiovascular system**

✓6ᵗʰ T46.99 Poisoning by, adverse effect of and underdosing of other agents primarily affecting the cardiovascular system

    ✓7ᵗʰ **T46.991 Poisoning by other agents primarily affecting the cardiovascular system, accidental (unintentional)**

    ✓7ᵗʰ **T46.992 Poisoning by other agents primarily affecting the cardiovascular system, intentional self-harm**

    ✓7ᵗʰ **T46.993 Poisoning by other agents primarily affecting the cardiovascular system, assault**

    ✓7ᵗʰ **T46.994 Poisoning by other agents primarily affecting the cardiovascular system, undetermined**

    ✓7ᵗʰ **T46.995 Adverse effect of other agents primarily affecting the cardiovascular system**

    ✓7ᵗʰ **T46.996 Underdosing of other agents primarily affecting the cardiovascular system**

✓4ᵗʰ T47 Poisoning by, adverse effect of and underdosing of agents primarily affecting the gastrointestinal system

> The appropriate 7th character is to be added to each code from category T47.
> A   initial encounter
> D   subsequent encounter
> S   sequela

✓5ᵗʰ T47.0 Poisoning by, adverse effect of and underdosing of histamine H2-receptor blockers

✓6ᵗʰ T47.0X Poisoning by, adverse effect of and underdosing of histamine H2-receptor blockers

    ✓7ᵗʰ **T47.0X1 Poisoning by histamine H2-receptor blockers, accidental (unintentional)**
       Poisoning by histamine H2-receptor blockers NOS

    ✓7ᵗʰ **T47.0X2 Poisoning by histamine H2-receptor blockers, intentional self-harm**

    ✓7ᵗʰ **T47.0X3 Poisoning by histamine H2-receptor blockers, assault**

    ✓7ᵗʰ **T47.0X4 Poisoning by histamine H2-receptor blockers, undetermined**

    ✓7ᵗʰ **T47.0X5 Adverse effect of histamine H2-receptor blockers**

    ✓7ᵗʰ **T47.0X6 Underdosing of histamine H2-receptor blockers**

✓ Additional Character Required   ✓x7ᵗʰ Placeholder Alert   Unspecified Dx   Other Specified Dx   Manifestation   ►◄ Revised Text   ● New Code   ▲ Revised Code Title

☑5th **T47.1** **Poisoning by, adverse effect of and underdosing of other antacids and anti-gastric-secretion drugs**

     ☑6th **T47.1X** **Poisoning by, adverse effect of and underdosing of** other antacids and anti-gastric-secretion **drugs**

         ☑7th **T47.1X1** **Poisoning by other antacids and anti-gastric-secretion drugs,** accidental **(unintentional)**
                 Poisoning by other antacids and anti-gastric-secretion drugs NOS

         ☑7th **T47.1X2** **Poisoning by other antacids and anti-gastric-secretion drugs,** intentional self-harm

         ☑7th **T47.1X3** **Poisoning by other antacids and anti-gastric-secretion drugs,** assault

         ☑7th **T47.1X4** **Poisoning by other antacids and anti-gastric-secretion drugs, undetermined**

         ☑7th **T47.1X5** Adverse effect **of other antacids and anti-gastric-secretion drugs**

         ☑7th **T47.1X6** Underdosing **of other antacids and anti-gastric-secretion drugs**

☑5th **T47.2** **Poisoning by, adverse effect of and underdosing of stimulant laxatives**

     ☑6th **T47.2X** **Poisoning by, adverse effect of and underdosing of** stimulant laxatives

         ☑7th **T47.2X1** **Poisoning by stimulant laxatives,** accidental **(unintentional)**
                 Poisoning by stimulant laxatives NOS

         ☑7th **T47.2X2** **Poisoning by stimulant laxatives,** intentional self-harm

         ☑7th **T47.2X3** **Poisoning by stimulant laxatives,** assault

         ☑7th **T47.2X4** **Poisoning by stimulant laxatives, undetermined**

         ☑7th **T47.2X5** Adverse effect **of stimulant laxatives**

         ☑7th **T47.2X6** Underdosing **of stimulant laxatives**

☑5th **T47.3** **Poisoning by, adverse effect of and underdosing of saline and osmotic laxatives**

     ☑6th **T47.3X** **Poisoning by and adverse effect of** saline and osmotic laxatives

         ☑7th **T47.3X1** **Poisoning by saline and osmotic laxatives,** accidental **(unintentional)**
                 Poisoning by saline and osmotic laxatives NOS

         ☑7th **T47.3X2** **Poisoning by saline and osmotic laxatives,** intentional self-harm

         ☑7th **T47.3X3** **Poisoning by saline and osmotic laxatives, assault**

         ☑7th **T47.3X4** **Poisoning by saline and osmotic laxatives, undetermined**

         ☑7th **T47.3X5** Adverse effect **of saline and osmotic laxatives**

         ☑7th **T47.3X6** Underdosing **of saline and osmotic laxatives**

☑5th **T47.4** **Poisoning by, adverse effect of and underdosing of other laxatives**

     ☑6th **T47.4X** **Poisoning by, adverse effect of and underdosing of** other laxatives

         ☑7th **T47.4X1** **Poisoning by other laxatives,** accidental **(unintentional)**
                 Poisoning by other laxatives NOS

         ☑7th **T47.4X2** **Poisoning by other laxatives,** intentional self-harm

         ☑7th **T47.4X3** **Poisoning by other laxatives,** assault

         ☑7th **T47.4X4** **Poisoning by other laxatives, undetermined**

         ☑7th **T47.4X5** Adverse effect **of other laxatives**

         ☑7th **T47.4X6** Underdosing **of other laxatives**

☑5th **T47.5** **Poisoning by, adverse effect of and underdosing of digestants**

     ☑6th **T47.5X** **Poisoning by, adverse effect of and underdosing of** digestants

         ☑7th **T47.5X1** **Poisoning by digestants,** accidental **(unintentional)**
                 Poisoning by digestants NOS

         ☑7th **T47.5X2** **Poisoning by digestants,** intentional self-harm

         ☑7th **T47.5X3** **Poisoning by digestants,** assault

         ☑7th **T47.5X4** **Poisoning by digestants,** undetermined

         ☑7th **T47.5X5** Adverse effect **of digestants**

         ☑7th **T47.5X6** Underdosing **of digestants**

☑5th **T47.6** **Poisoning by, adverse effect of and underdosing of antidiarrheal drugs**

     EXCLUDES 2   *poisoning by, adverse effect of and underdosing of systemic antibiotics and other anti-infectives (T36-T37)*

     ☑6th **T47.6X** **Poisoning by, adverse effect of and underdosing of** antidiarrheal **drugs**

         ☑7th **T47.6X1** **Poisoning by antidiarrheal drugs,** accidental **(unintentional)**
                 Poisoning by antidiarrheal drugs NOS

         ☑7th **T47.6X2** **Poisoning by antidiarrheal drugs,** intentional self-harm

         ☑7th **T47.6X3** **Poisoning by antidiarrheal drugs,** assault

         ☑7th **T47.6X4** **Poisoning by antidiarrheal drugs, undetermined**

         ☑7th **T47.6X5** Adverse effect **of antidiarrheal drugs**

         ☑7th **T47.6X6** Underdosing **of antidiarrheal drugs**

☑5th **T47.7** **Poisoning by, adverse effect of and underdosing of emetics**

     ☑6th **T47.7X** **Poisoning by, adverse effect of and underdosing of** emetics

         ☑7th **T47.7X1** **Poisoning by emetics,** accidental **(unintentional)**
                 Poisoning by emetics NOS

         ☑7th **T47.7X2** **Poisoning by emetics,** intentional self-harm

         ☑7th **T47.7X3** **Poisoning by emetics,** assault

         ☑7th **T47.7X4** **Poisoning by emetics,** undetermined

         ☑7th **T47.7X5** Adverse effect **of emetics**

         ☑7th **T47.7X6** Underdosing **of emetics**

☑5th **T47.8** **Poisoning by, adverse effect of and underdosing of other** agents primarily affecting gastrointestinal system

     ☑6th **T47.8X** **Poisoning by, adverse effect of and underdosing of** other **agents primarily affecting gastrointestinal system**

         ☑7th **T47.8X1** **Poisoning by other agents primarily affecting gastrointestinal system, accidental (unintentional)**
                 Poisoning by other agents primarily affecting gastrointestinal system NOS

         ☑7th **T47.8X2** **Poisoning by other agents primarily affecting gastrointestinal system, intentional self-harm**

         ☑7th **T47.8X3** **Poisoning by other agents primarily affecting gastrointestinal system, assault**

         ☑7th **T47.8X4** **Poisoning by other agents primarily affecting gastrointestinal system, undetermined**

         ☑7th **T47.8X5** Adverse effect **of other agents primarily affecting gastrointestinal system**

         ☑7th **T47.8X6** Underdosing **of other agents primarily affecting gastrointestinal system**

☑5th **T47.9** **Poisoning by, adverse effect of and underdosing of** unspecified **agents primarily affecting the gastrointestinal system**

     ☑x7th **T47.91** **Poisoning by unspecified agents primarily affecting the gastrointestinal system,** accidental **(unintentional)**
         Poisoning by agents primarily affecting the gastrointestinal system NOS

     ☑x7th **T47.92** **Poisoning by unspecified agents primarily affecting the gastrointestinal system,** intentional self-harm

     ☑x7th **T47.93** **Poisoning by unspecified agents primarily affecting the gastrointestinal system,** assault

     ☑x7th **T47.94** **Poisoning by unspecified agents primarily affecting the gastrointestinal system,** undetermined

     ☑x7th **T47.95** Adverse effect **of unspecified agents primarily affecting the gastrointestinal system**

     ☑x7th **T47.96** Underdosing **of unspecified agents primarily affecting the gastrointestinal system**

EXCLUDES 1 Not coded here   *EXCLUDES 2* Not included here   N Newborn Age: 0   P Pediatric Age: 0-17   M Maternity Age: 12-55   A Adult Age: 15-124

1000   ICD-10-CM 2016

☑4ᵗʰ **T48**   **Poisoning by, adverse effect of and underdosing of agents primarily acting on smooth and skeletal muscles and the respiratory system**

> The appropriate 7th character is to be added to each code from category T48.
> A   initial encounter
> D   subsequent encounter
> S   sequela

☑5ᵗʰ **T48.0**   **Poisoning by, adverse effect of and underdosing of oxytocic drugs**

     EXCLUDES 1   poisoning by, adverse effect of and underdosing of estrogens, progestogens and antagonists (T38.4-T38.6)

   ☑6ᵗʰ **T48.0X**   **Poisoning by, adverse effect of and underdosing of oxytocic drugs**

     ☑7ᵗʰ **T48.0X1**   **Poisoning by oxytocic drugs, accidental (unintentional)**
         Poisoning by oxytocic drugs NOS

     ☑7ᵗʰ **T48.0X2**   **Poisoning by oxytocic drugs, intentional self-harm**

     ☑7ᵗʰ **T48.0X3**   **Poisoning by oxytocic drugs, assault**

     ☑7ᵗʰ **T48.0X4**   **Poisoning by oxytocic drugs, undetermined**

     ☑7ᵗʰ **T48.0X5**   **Adverse effect of oxytocic drugs**

     ☑7ᵗʰ **T48.0X6**   **Underdosing of oxytocic drugs**

☑5ᵗʰ **T48.1**   **Poisoning by, adverse effect of and underdosing of skeletal muscle relaxants [neuromuscular blocking agents]**

   ☑6ᵗʰ **T48.1X**   **Poisoning by, adverse effect of and underdosing of skeletal muscle relaxants [neuromuscular blocking agents]**

     ☑7ᵗʰ **T48.1X1**   **Poisoning by skeletal muscle relaxants [neuromuscular blocking agents], accidental (unintentional)**
         Poisoning by skeletal muscle relaxants [neuromuscular blocking agents] NOS

     ☑7ᵗʰ **T48.1X2**   **Poisoning by skeletal muscle relaxants [neuromuscular blocking agents], intentional self-harm**

     ☑7ᵗʰ **T48.1X3**   **Poisoning by skeletal muscle relaxants [neuromuscular blocking agents], assault**

     ☑7ᵗʰ **T48.1X4**   **Poisoning by skeletal muscle relaxants [neuromuscular blocking agents], undetermined**

     ☑7ᵗʰ **T48.1X5**   **Adverse effect of skeletal muscle relaxants [neuromuscular blocking agents]**

     ☑7ᵗʰ **T48.1X6**   **Underdosing of skeletal muscle relaxants [neuromuscular blocking agents]**

☑5ᵗʰ **T48.2**   **Poisoning by, adverse effect of and underdosing of other and unspecified drugs acting on muscles**

   ☑6ᵗʰ **T48.20**   **Poisoning by, adverse effect of and underdosing of unspecified drugs acting on muscles**

     ☑7ᵗʰ **T48.201**   **Poisoning by unspecified drugs acting on muscles, accidental (unintentional)**
         Poisoning by unspecified drugs acting on muscles NOS

     ☑7ᵗʰ **T48.202**   **Poisoning by unspecified drugs acting on muscles, intentional self-harm**

     ☑7ᵗʰ **T48.203**   **Poisoning by unspecified drugs acting on muscles, assault**

     ☑7ᵗʰ **T48.204**   **Poisoning by unspecified drugs acting on muscles, undetermined**

     ☑7ᵗʰ **T48.205**   **Adverse effect of unspecified drugs acting on muscles**

     ☑7ᵗʰ **T48.206**   **Underdosing of unspecified drugs acting on muscles**

   ☑6ᵗʰ **T48.29**   **Poisoning by, adverse effect of and underdosing of other drugs acting on muscles**

     ☑7ᵗʰ **T48.291**   **Poisoning by other drugs acting on muscles, accidental (unintentional)**
         Poisoning by other drugs acting on muscles NOS

     ☑7ᵗʰ **T48.292**   **Poisoning by other drugs acting on muscles, intentional self-harm**

     ☑7ᵗʰ **T48.293**   **Poisoning by other drugs acting on muscles, assault**

     ☑7ᵗʰ **T48.294**   **Poisoning by other drugs acting on muscles, undetermined**

     ☑7ᵗʰ **T48.295**   **Adverse effect of other drugs acting on muscles**

     ☑7ᵗʰ **T48.296**   **Underdosing of other drugs acting on muscles**

☑5ᵗʰ **T48.3**   **Poisoning by, adverse effect of and underdosing of antitussives**

   ☑6ᵗʰ **T48.3X**   **Poisoning by, adverse effect of and underdosing of antitussives**

     ☑7ᵗʰ **T48.3X1**   **Poisoning by antitussives, accidental (unintentional)**
         Poisoning by antitussives NOS

     ☑7ᵗʰ **T48.3X2**   **Poisoning by antitussives, intentional self-harm**

     ☑7ᵗʰ **T48.3X3**   **Poisoning by antitussives, assault**

     ☑7ᵗʰ **T48.3X4**   **Poisoning by antitussives, undetermined**

     ☑7ᵗʰ **T48.3X5**   **Adverse effect of antitussives**

     ☑7ᵗʰ **T48.3X6**   **Underdosing of antitussives**

☑5ᵗʰ **T48.4**   **Poisoning by, adverse effect of and underdosing of expectorants**

   ☑6ᵗʰ **T48.4X**   **Poisoning by, adverse effect of and underdosing of expectorants**

     ☑7ᵗʰ **T48.4X1**   **Poisoning by expectorants, accidental (unintentional)**
         Poisoning by expectorants NOS

     ☑7ᵗʰ **T48.4X2**   **Poisoning by expectorants, intentional self-harm**

     ☑7ᵗʰ **T48.4X3**   **Poisoning by expectorants, assault**

     ☑7ᵗʰ **T48.4X4**   **Poisoning by expectorants, undetermined**

     ☑7ᵗʰ **T48.4X5**   **Adverse effect of expectorants**

     ☑7ᵗʰ **T48.4X6**   **Underdosing of expectorants**

☑5ᵗʰ **T48.5**   **Poisoning by, adverse effect of and underdosing of other anti-common-cold drugs**

     Poisoning by, adverse effect of and underdosing of decongestants

     EXCLUDES 2   poisoning by, adverse effect of and underdosing of antipyretics, NEC (T39.9-)
         poisoning by, adverse effect of and underdosing of non-steroidal antiinflammatory drugs (T39.3-)
         poisoning by, adverse effect of and underdosing of salicylates (T39.0-)

   ☑6ᵗʰ **T48.5X**   **Poisoning by, adverse effect of and underdosing of other anti-common-cold drugs**

     ☑7ᵗʰ **T48.5X1**   **Poisoning by other anti-common-cold drugs, accidental (unintentional)**
         Poisoning by other anti-common-cold drugs NOS

     ☑7ᵗʰ **T48.5X2**   **Poisoning by other anti-common-cold drugs, intentional self-harm**

     ☑7ᵗʰ **T48.5X3**   **Poisoning by other anti-common-cold drugs, assault**

     ☑7ᵗʰ **T48.5X4**   **Poisoning by other anti-common-cold drugs, undetermined**

     ☑7ᵗʰ **T48.5X5**   **Adverse effect of other anti-common-cold drugs**

     ☑7ᵗʰ **T48.5X6**   **Underdosing of other anti-common-cold drugs**

☑5ᵗʰ **T48.6**   **Poisoning by, adverse effect of and underdosing of antiasthmatics, not elsewhere classified**

     Poisoning by, adverse effect of and underdosing of beta-adrenoreceptor agonists used in asthma therapy

     EXCLUDES 1   poisoning by, adverse effect of and underdosing of anterior pituitary [adenohypophyseal] hormones (T38.8)
         poisoning by, adverse effect of and underdosing of beta-adrenoreceptor agonists not used in asthma therapy (T44.5)

   ☑6ᵗʰ **T48.6X**   **Poisoning by, adverse effect of and underdosing of antiasthmatics**

     ☑7ᵗʰ **T48.6X1**   **Poisoning by antiasthmatics, accidental (unintentional)**
         Poisoning by antiasthmatics NOS

     ☑7ᵗʰ **T48.6X2**   **Poisoning by antiasthmatics, intentional self-harm**

     ☑7ᵗʰ **T48.6X3**   **Poisoning by antiasthmatics, assault**

     ☑7ᵗʰ **T48.6X4**   **Poisoning by antiasthmatics, undetermined**

     ☑7ᵗʰ **T48.6X5**   **Adverse effect of antiasthmatics**

☑ Additional Character Required   ☑7ᵗʰ Placeholder Alert   Unspecified Dx   Other Specified Dx   Manifestation   ►◄ Revised Text   ● New Code   ▲ Revised Code Title

Chapter 19. Injury, Poisoning, and Certain Other Consequences of External Causes

T48.6X6–T49.4X6

✓7ᵗʰ **T48.6X6**   Underdosing of antiasthmatics

✓5ᵗʰ **T48.9**   **Poisoning by, adverse effect of and underdosing of other and unspecified** agents primarily acting on the respiratory system

✓6ᵗʰ **T48.90**   **Poisoning by, adverse effect of and underdosing of unspecified** agents primarily acting on the respiratory system

✓7ᵗʰ **T48.901**   **Poisoning by unspecified agents primarily acting on the respiratory system, accidental (unintentional)**

✓7ᵗʰ **T48.902**   **Poisoning by unspecified agents primarily acting on the respiratory system, intentional self-harm**

✓7ᵗʰ **T48.903**   **Poisoning by unspecified agents primarily acting on the respiratory system, assault**

✓7ᵗʰ **T48.904**   **Poisoning by unspecified agents primarily acting on the respiratory system, undetermined**

✓7ᵗʰ **T48.905**   Adverse effect of unspecified agents primarily acting on the respiratory system

✓7ᵗʰ **T48.906**   Underdosing of unspecified agents primarily acting on the respiratory system

✓6ᵗʰ **T48.99**   **Poisoning by, adverse effect of and underdosing of other** agents primarily acting on the respiratory system

✓7ᵗʰ **T48.991**   **Poisoning by other agents primarily acting on the respiratory system, accidental (unintentional)**

✓7ᵗʰ **T48.992**   **Poisoning by other agents primarily acting on the respiratory system, intentional self-harm**

✓7ᵗʰ **T48.993**   **Poisoning by other agents primarily acting on the respiratory system, assault**

✓7ᵗʰ **T48.994**   **Poisoning by other agents primarily acting on the respiratory system, undetermined**

✓7ᵗʰ **T48.995**   Adverse effect of other agents primarily acting on the respiratory system

✓7ᵗʰ **T48.996**   Underdosing of other agents primarily acting on the respiratory system

✓4ᵗʰ **T49**   **Poisoning by, adverse effect of and underdosing of topical agents primarily affecting skin and mucous membrane and by ophthalmological, otorhinolaryngological and dental drugs**
Poisoning by, adverse effect of and underdosing of glucocorticoids, topically used

The appropriate 7th character is to be added to each code from category T49.
A   initial encounter
D   subsequent encounter
S   sequela

✓5ᵗʰ **T49.0**   **Poisoning by, adverse effect of and underdosing of local antifungal, anti-infective and anti-inflammatory drugs**

✓6ᵗʰ **T49.0X**   **Poisoning by, adverse effect of and underdosing of local antifungal, anti-infective and anti-inflammatory drugs**

✓7ᵗʰ **T49.0X1**   **Poisoning by local antifungal, anti-infective and anti-inflammatory drugs, accidental (unintentional)**
Poisoning by local antifungal, anti-infective and anti-inflammatory drugs NOS

✓7ᵗʰ **T49.0X2**   **Poisoning by local antifungal, anti-infective and anti-inflammatory drugs, intentional self-harm**

✓7ᵗʰ **T49.0X3**   **Poisoning by local antifungal, anti-infective and anti-inflammatory drugs, assault**

✓7ᵗʰ **T49.0X4**   **Poisoning by local antifungal, anti-infective and anti-inflammatory drugs, undetermined**

✓7ᵗʰ **T49.0X5**   Adverse effect of local antifungal, anti-infective and anti-inflammatory drugs

✓7ᵗʰ **T49.0X6**   Underdosing of local antifungal, anti-infective and anti-inflammatory drugs

✓5ᵗʰ **T49.1**   **Poisoning by, adverse effect of and underdosing of antipruritics**

✓6ᵗʰ **T49.1X**   **Poisoning by, adverse effect of and underdosing of antipruritics**

✓7ᵗʰ **T49.1X1**   **Poisoning by antipruritics, accidental (unintentional)**
Poisoning by antipruritics NOS

✓7ᵗʰ **T49.1X2**   **Poisoning by antipruritics, intentional self-harm**

✓7ᵗʰ **T49.1X3**   **Poisoning by antipruritics, assault**

✓7ᵗʰ **T49.1X4**   **Poisoning by antipruritics, undetermined**

✓7ᵗʰ **T49.1X5**   Adverse effect of antipruritics

✓7ᵗʰ **T49.1X6**   Underdosing of antipruritics

✓5ᵗʰ **T49.2**   **Poisoning by, adverse effect of and underdosing of local astringents and local detergents**

✓6ᵗʰ **T49.2X**   **Poisoning by, adverse effect of and underdosing of local astringents and local detergents**

✓7ᵗʰ **T49.2X1**   **Poisoning by local astringents and local detergents, accidental (unintentional)**
Poisoning by local astringents and local detergents NOS

✓7ᵗʰ **T49.2X2**   **Poisoning by local astringents and local detergents, intentional self-harm**

✓7ᵗʰ **T49.2X3**   **Poisoning by local astringents and local detergents, assault**

✓7ᵗʰ **T49.2X4**   **Poisoning by local astringents and local detergents, undetermined**

✓7ᵗʰ **T49.2X5**   Adverse effect of local astringents and local detergents

✓7ᵗʰ **T49.2X6**   Underdosing of local astringents and local detergents

✓5ᵗʰ **T49.3**   **Poisoning by, adverse effect of and underdosing of emollients, demulcents and protectants**

✓6ᵗʰ **T49.3X**   **Poisoning by, adverse effect of and underdosing of emollients, demulcents and protectants**

✓7ᵗʰ **T49.3X1**   **Poisoning by emollients, demulcents and protectants, accidental (unintentional)**
Poisoning by emollients, demulcents and protectants NOS

✓7ᵗʰ **T49.3X2**   **Poisoning by emollients, demulcents and protectants, intentional self-harm**

✓7ᵗʰ **T49.3X3**   **Poisoning by emollients, demulcents and protectants, assault**

✓7ᵗʰ **T49.3X4**   **Poisoning by emollients, demulcents and protectants, undetermined**

✓7ᵗʰ **T49.3X5**   Adverse effect of emollients, demulcents and protectants

✓7ᵗʰ **T49.3X6**   Underdosing of emollients, demulcents and protectants

✓5ᵗʰ **T49.4**   **Poisoning by, adverse effect of and underdosing of keratolytics, keratoplastics, and other hair treatment drugs and preparations**

✓6ᵗʰ **T49.4X**   **Poisoning by, adverse effect of and underdosing of keratolytics, keratoplastics, and other hair treatment drugs and preparations**

✓7ᵗʰ **T49.4X1**   **Poisoning by keratolytics, keratoplastics, and other hair treatment drugs and preparations, accidental (unintentional)**
Poisoning by keratolytics, keratoplastics, and other hair treatment drugs and preparations NOS

✓7ᵗʰ **T49.4X2**   **Poisoning by keratolytics, keratoplastics, and other hair treatment drugs and preparations, intentional self-harm**

✓7ᵗʰ **T49.4X3**   **Poisoning by keratolytics, keratoplastics, and other hair treatment drugs and preparations, assault**

✓7ᵗʰ **T49.4X4**   **Poisoning by keratolytics, keratoplastics, and other hair treatment drugs and preparations, undetermined**

✓7ᵗʰ **T49.4X5**   Adverse effect of keratolytics, keratoplastics, and other hair treatment drugs and preparations

✓7ᵗʰ **T49.4X6**   Underdosing of keratolytics, keratoplastics, and other hair treatment drugs and preparations

EXCLUDES 1 Not coded here   **EXCLUDES 2** Not included here   **N** Newborn Age: 0   **P** Pediatric Age: 0-17   **M** Maternity Age: 12-55   **A** Adult Age: 15-124

1002   ICD-10-CM 2016

✓5th **T49.5** **Poisoning by, adverse effect of and underdosing of ophthalmological drugs and preparations**

✓6th **T49.5X** **Poisoning by, adverse effect of and underdosing of** ophthalmological **drugs and preparations**

✓7th **T49.5X1** **Poisoning by ophthalmological drugs and preparations, accidental (unintentional)**
Poisoning by ophthalmological drugs and preparations NOS

✓7th **T49.5X2** **Poisoning by ophthalmological drugs and preparations, intentional self-harm**

✓7th **T49.5X3** **Poisoning by ophthalmological drugs and preparations, assault**

✓7th **T49.5X4** **Poisoning by ophthalmological drugs and preparations, undetermined**

✓7th **T49.5X5** **Adverse effect of ophthalmological drugs and preparations**

✓7th **T49.5X6** **Underdosing of ophthalmological drugs and preparations**

✓5th **T49.6** **Poisoning by, adverse effect of and underdosing of otorhinolaryngological drugs and preparations**

✓6th **T49.6X** **Poisoning by, adverse effect of and underdosing of** otorhinolaryngological **drugs and preparations**

✓7th **T49.6X1** **Poisoning by otorhinolaryngological drugs and preparations, accidental (unintentional)**
Poisoning by otorhinolaryngological drugs and preparations NOS

✓7th **T49.6X2** **Poisoning by otorhinolaryngological drugs and preparations, intentional self-harm**

✓7th **T49.6X3** **Poisoning by otorhinolaryngological drugs and preparations, assault**

✓7th **T49.6X4** **Poisoning by otorhinolaryngological drugs and preparations, undetermined**

✓7th **T49.6X5** **Adverse effect of otorhinolaryngological drugs and preparations**

✓7th **T49.6X6** **Underdosing of otorhinolaryngological drugs and preparations**

✓5th **T49.7** **Poisoning by, adverse effect of and underdosing of dental drugs, topically applied**

✓6th **T49.7X** **Poisoning by, adverse effect of and underdosing of** dental **drugs, topically applied**

✓7th **T49.7X1** **Poisoning by dental drugs, topically applied, accidental (unintentional)**
Poisoning by dental drugs, topically applied NOS

✓7th **T49.7X2** **Poisoning by dental drugs, topically applied, intentional self-harm**

✓7th **T49.7X3** **Poisoning by dental drugs, topically applied, assault**

✓7th **T49.7X4** **Poisoning by dental drugs, topically applied, undetermined**

✓7th **T49.7X5** **Adverse effect of dental drugs, topically applied**

✓7th **T49.7X6** **Underdosing of dental drugs, topically applied**

✓5th **T49.8** **Poisoning by, adverse effect of and underdosing of other topical agents**
Poisoning by, adverse effect of and underdosing of spermicides

✓6th **T49.8X** **Poisoning by, adverse effect of and underdosing of** other **topical agents**

✓7th **T49.8X1** **Poisoning by other topical agents, accidental (unintentional)**
Poisoning by other topical agents NOS

✓7th **T49.8X2** **Poisoning by other topical agents, intentional self-harm**

✓7th **T49.8X3** **Poisoning by other topical agents, assault**

✓7th **T49.8X4** **Poisoning by other topical agents, undetermined**

✓7th **T49.8X5** **Adverse effect of other topical agents**

✓7th **T49.8X6** **Underdosing of other topical agents**

✓5th **T49.9** **Poisoning by, adverse effect of and underdosing of** unspecified **topical agent**

✓x7th **T49.91** **Poisoning by unspecified topical agent, accidental (unintentional)**

✓x7th **T49.92** **Poisoning by unspecified topical agent, intentional self-harm**

✓x7th **T49.93** **Poisoning by unspecified topical agent, assault**

✓x7th **T49.94** **Poisoning by unspecified topical agent, undetermined**

✓x7th **T49.95** **Adverse effect of unspecified topical agent**

✓x7th **T49.96** **Underdosing of unspecified topical agent**

✓4th **T50** **Poisoning by, adverse effect of and underdosing of diuretics and other and unspecified drugs, medicaments and biological substances**

> The appropriate 7th character is to be added to each code from category T50.
> A   initial encounter
> D   subsequent encounter
> S   sequela

✓5th **T50.0** **Poisoning by, adverse effect of and underdosing of mineralocorticoids and their antagonists**

✓6th **T50.0X** **Poisoning by, adverse effect of and underdosing of** mineralocorticoids **and their antagonists**

✓7th **T50.0X1** **Poisoning by mineralocorticoids and their antagonists, accidental (unintentional)**
Poisoning by mineralocorticoids and their antagonists NOS

✓7th **T50.0X2** **Poisoning by mineralocorticoids and their antagonists, intentional self-harm**

✓7th **T50.0X3** **Poisoning by mineralocorticoids and their antagonists, assault**

✓7th **T50.0X4** **Poisoning by mineralocorticoids and their antagonists, undetermined**

✓7th **T50.0X5** **Adverse effect of mineralocorticoids and their antagonists**

✓7th **T50.0X6** **Underdosing of mineralocorticoids and their antagonists**

✓5th **T50.1** **Poisoning by, adverse effect of and underdosing of loop [high-ceiling] diuretics**

✓6th **T50.1X** **Poisoning by, adverse effect of and underdosing of** loop [high-ceiling] diuretics

✓7th **T50.1X1** **Poisoning by loop [high-ceiling] diuretics, accidental (unintentional)**
Poisoning by loop [high-ceiling] diuretics NOS

✓7th **T50.1X2** **Poisoning by loop [high-ceiling] diuretics, intentional self-harm**

✓7th **T50.1X3** **Poisoning by loop [high-ceiling] diuretics, assault**

✓7th **T50.1X4** **Poisoning by loop [high-ceiling] diuretics, undetermined**

✓7th **T50.1X5** **Adverse effect of loop [high-ceiling] diuretics**

✓7th **T50.1X6** **Underdosing of loop [high-ceiling] diuretics**

✓5th **T50.2** **Poisoning by, adverse effect of and underdosing of carbonic-anhydrase inhibitors, benzothiadiazides and other diuretics**
Poisoning by, adverse effect of and underdosing of acetazolamide

✓6th **T50.2X** **Poisoning by, adverse effect of and underdosing of** carbonic-anhydrase inhibitors, benzothiadiazides and other diuretics

✓7th **T50.2X1** **Poisoning by carbonic-anhydrase inhibitors, benzothiadiazides and other diuretics, accidental (unintentional)**
Poisoning by carbonic-anhydrase inhibitors, benzothiadiazides and other diuretics NOS

✓7th **T50.2X2** **Poisoning by carbonic-anhydrase inhibitors, benzothiadiazides and other diuretics, intentional self-harm**

✓7th **T50.2X3** **Poisoning by carbonic-anhydrase inhibitors, benzothiadiazides and other diuretics, assault**

✓7th **T50.2X4** **Poisoning by carbonic-anhydrase inhibitors, benzothiadiazides and other diuretics, undetermined**

✓7th **T50.2X5** **Adverse effect of carbonic-anhydrase inhibitors, benzothiadiazides and other diuretics**

✓ Additional Character Required   ✓x7th Placeholder Alert   Unspecified Dx   Other Specified Dx   Manifestation   ►◄ Revised Text   ● New Code   ▲ Revised Code Title

✓7ᵗʰ **T50.2X6** Underdosing of carbonic-anhydrase inhibitors, benzothiadiazides and other diuretics

✓5ᵗʰ **T50.3** Poisoning by, adverse effect of and underdosing of electrolytic, caloric and water-balance agents
Poisoning by, adverse effect of and underdosing of oral rehydration salts

✓6ᵗʰ **T50.3X** Poisoning by, adverse effect of and underdosing of electrolytic, caloric and water-balance agents

✓7ᵗʰ **T50.3X1** Poisoning by electrolytic, caloric and water-balance agents, accidental (unintentional)
Poisoning by electrolytic, caloric and water-balance agents NOS

✓7ᵗʰ **T50.3X2** Poisoning by electrolytic, caloric and water-balance agents, intentional self-harm

✓7ᵗʰ **T50.3X3** Poisoning by electrolytic, caloric and water-balance agents, assault

✓7ᵗʰ **T50.3X4** Poisoning by electrolytic, caloric and water-balance agents, undetermined

✓7ᵗʰ **T50.3X5** Adverse effect of electrolytic, caloric and water-balance agents

✓7ᵗʰ **T50.3X6** Underdosing of electrolytic, caloric and water-balance agents

✓5ᵗʰ **T50.4** Poisoning by, adverse effect of and underdosing of drugs affecting uric acid metabolism

✓6ᵗʰ **T50.4X** Poisoning by, adverse effect of and underdosing of drugs affecting uric acid metabolism

✓7ᵗʰ **T50.4X1** Poisoning by drugs affecting uric acid metabolism, accidental (unintentional)
Poisoning by drugs affecting uric acid metabolism NOS

✓7ᵗʰ **T50.4X2** Poisoning by drugs affecting uric acid metabolism, intentional self-harm

✓7ᵗʰ **T50.4X3** Poisoning by drugs affecting uric acid metabolism, assault

✓7ᵗʰ **T50.4X4** Poisoning by drugs affecting uric acid metabolism, undetermined

✓7ᵗʰ **T50.4X5** Adverse effect of drugs affecting uric acid metabolism

✓7ᵗʰ **T50.4X6** Underdosing of drugs affecting uric acid metabolism

✓5ᵗʰ **T50.5** Poisoning by, adverse effect of and underdosing of appetite depressants

✓6ᵗʰ **T50.5X** Poisoning by, adverse effect of and underdosing of appetite depressants

✓7ᵗʰ **T50.5X1** Poisoning by appetite depressants, accidental (unintentional)
Poisoning by appetite depressants NOS

✓7ᵗʰ **T50.5X2** Poisoning by appetite depressants, intentional self-harm

✓7ᵗʰ **T50.5X3** Poisoning by appetite depressants, assault

✓7ᵗʰ **T50.5X4** Poisoning by appetite depressants, undetermined

✓7ᵗʰ **T50.5X5** Adverse effect of appetite depressants

✓7ᵗʰ **T50.5X6** Underdosing of appetite depressants

✓5ᵗʰ **T50.6** Poisoning by, adverse effect of and underdosing of antidotes and chelating agents
Poisoning by, adverse effect of and underdosing of alcohol deterrents

✓6ᵗʰ **T50.6X** Poisoning by, adverse effect of and underdosing of antidotes and chelating agents

✓7ᵗʰ **T50.6X1** Poisoning by antidotes and chelating agents, accidental (unintentional)
Poisoning by antidotes and chelating agents NOS

✓7ᵗʰ **T50.6X2** Poisoning by antidotes and chelating agents, intentional self-harm

✓7ᵗʰ **T50.6X3** Poisoning by antidotes and chelating agents, assault

✓7ᵗʰ **T50.6X4** Poisoning by antidotes and chelating agents, undetermined

✓7ᵗʰ **T50.6X5** Adverse effect of antidotes and chelating agents

✓7ᵗʰ **T50.6X6** Underdosing of antidotes and chelating agents

✓5ᵗʰ **T50.7** Poisoning by, adverse effect of and underdosing of analeptics and opioid receptor antagonists

✓6ᵗʰ **T50.7X** Poisoning by, adverse effect of and underdosing of analeptics and opioid receptor antagonists

✓7ᵗʰ **T50.7X1** Poisoning by analeptics and opioid receptor antagonists, accidental (unintentional)
Poisoning by analeptics and opioid receptor antagonists NOS

✓7ᵗʰ **T50.7X2** Poisoning by analeptics and opioid receptor antagonists, intentional self-harm

✓7ᵗʰ **T50.7X3** Poisoning by analeptics and opioid receptor antagonists, assault

✓7ᵗʰ **T50.7X4** Poisoning by analeptics and opioid receptor antagonists, undetermined

✓7ᵗʰ **T50.7X5** Adverse effect of analeptics and opioid receptor antagonists

✓7ᵗʰ **T50.7X6** Underdosing of analeptics and opioid receptor antagonists

✓5ᵗʰ **T50.8** Poisoning by, adverse effect of and underdosing of diagnostic agents

✓6ᵗʰ **T50.8X** Poisoning by, adverse effect of and underdosing of diagnostic agents

✓7ᵗʰ **T50.8X1** Poisoning by diagnostic agents, accidental (unintentional)
Poisoning by diagnostic agents NOS

✓7ᵗʰ **T50.8X2** Poisoning by diagnostic agents, intentional self-harm

✓7ᵗʰ **T50.8X3** Poisoning by diagnostic agents, assault

✓7ᵗʰ **T50.8X4** Poisoning by diagnostic agents, undetermined

✓7ᵗʰ **T50.8X5** Adverse effect of diagnostic agents

✓7ᵗʰ **T50.8X6** Underdosing of diagnostic agents

✓5ᵗʰ **T50.A** Poisoning by, adverse effect of and underdosing of bacterial vaccines

✓6ᵗʰ **T50.A1** Poisoning by, adverse effect of and underdosing of pertussis vaccine, including combinations with a pertussis component

✓7ᵗʰ **T50.A11** Poisoning by pertussis vaccine, including combinations with a pertussis component, accidental (unintentional)

✓7ᵗʰ **T50.A12** Poisoning by pertussis vaccine, including combinations with a pertussis component, intentional self-harm

✓7ᵗʰ **T50.A13** Poisoning by pertussis vaccine, including combinations with a pertussis component, assault

✓7ᵗʰ **T50.A14** Poisoning by pertussis vaccine, including combinations with a pertussis component, undetermined

✓7ᵗʰ **T50.A15** Adverse effect of pertussis vaccine, including combinations with a pertussis component

✓7ᵗʰ **T50.A16** Underdosing of pertussis vaccine, including combinations with a pertussis component

✓6ᵗʰ **T50.A2** Poisoning by, adverse effect of and underdosing of mixed bacterial vaccines without a pertussis component

✓7ᵗʰ **T50.A21** Poisoning by mixed bacterial vaccines without a pertussis component, accidental (unintentional)

✓7ᵗʰ **T50.A22** Poisoning by mixed bacterial vaccines without a pertussis component, intentional self-harm

✓7ᵗʰ **T50.A23** Poisoning by mixed bacterial vaccines without a pertussis component, assault

✓7ᵗʰ **T50.A24** Poisoning by mixed bacterial vaccines without a pertussis component, undetermined

✓7ᵗʰ **T50.A25** Adverse effect of mixed bacterial vaccines without a pertussis component

✓7ᵗʰ **T50.A26** Underdosing of mixed bacterial vaccines without a pertussis component

EXCLUDES 1 Not coded here　　**EXCLUDES 2** Not included here　　Ⓝ Newborn Age: 0　　Ⓟ Pediatric Age: 0-17　　Ⓜ Maternity Age: 12-55　　Ⓐ Adult Age: 15-124

1004　　ICD-10-CM 2016

✓6th **T50.A9** Poisoning by, adverse effect of and underdosing of other bacterial vaccines

  ✓7th **T50.A91** **Poisoning by other bacterial vaccines, accidental (unintentional)**

  ✓7th **T50.A92** **Poisoning by other bacterial vaccines, intentional self-harm**

  ✓7th **T50.A93** **Poisoning by other bacterial vaccines, assault**

  ✓7th **T50.A94** **Poisoning by other bacterial vaccines, undetermined**

  ✓7th **T50.A95** Adverse effect of other bacterial vaccines

  ✓7th **T50.A96** Underdosing of other bacterial vaccines

✓5th **T50.B** Poisoning by, adverse effect of and underdosing of viral vaccines

  ✓6th **T50.B1** Poisoning by, adverse effect of and underdosing of smallpox vaccines

    ✓7th **T50.B11** **Poisoning by smallpox vaccines, accidental (unintentional)**

    ✓7th **T50.B12** **Poisoning by smallpox vaccines, intentional self-harm**

    ✓7th **T50.B13** **Poisoning by smallpox vaccines, assault**

    ✓7th **T50.B14** **Poisoning by smallpox vaccines, undetermined**

    ✓7th **T50.B15** Adverse effect of smallpox vaccines

    ✓7th **T50.B16** Underdosing of smallpox vaccines

  ✓6th **T50.B9** Poisoning by, adverse effect of and underdosing of other viral vaccines

    ✓7th **T50.B91** **Poisoning by other viral vaccines, accidental (unintentional)**

    ✓7th **T50.B92** **Poisoning by other viral vaccines, intentional self-harm**

    ✓7th **T50.B93** **Poisoning by other viral vaccines, assault**

    ✓7th **T50.B94** **Poisoning by other viral vaccines, undetermined**

    ✓7th **T50.B95** Adverse effect of other viral vaccines

    ✓7th **T50.B96** Underdosing of other viral vaccines

✓5th **T50.Z** Poisoning by, adverse effect of and underdosing of other vaccines and biological substances

  ✓6th **T50.Z1** Poisoning by, adverse effect of and underdosing of immunoglobulin

    ✓7th **T50.Z11** **Poisoning by immunoglobulin, accidental (unintentional)**

    ✓7th **T50.Z12** **Poisoning by immunoglobulin, intentional self-harm**

    ✓7th **T50.Z13** **Poisoning by immunoglobulin, assault**

    ✓7th **T50.Z14** **Poisoning by immunoglobulin, undetermined**

    ✓7th **T50.Z15** Adverse effect of immunoglobulin

    ✓7th **T50.Z16** Underdosing of immunoglobulin

  ✓6th **T50.Z9** Poisoning by, adverse effect of and underdosing of other vaccines and biological substances

    ✓7th **T50.Z91** **Poisoning by other vaccines and biological substances, accidental (unintentional)**

    ✓7th **T50.Z92** **Poisoning by other vaccines and biological substances, intentional self-harm**

    ✓7th **T50.Z93** **Poisoning by other vaccines and biological substances, assault**

    ✓7th **T50.Z94** **Poisoning by other vaccines and biological substances, undetermined**

    ✓7th **T50.Z95** Adverse effect of other vaccines and biological substances

    ✓7th **T50.Z96** Underdosing of other vaccines and biological substances

✓5th **T50.9** Poisoning by, adverse effect of and underdosing of other and unspecified drugs, medicaments and biological substances
AHA: 2015, 1Q, 21

  ✓6th **T50.90** Poisoning by, adverse effect of and underdosing of unspecified drugs, medicaments and biological substances

    ✓7th **T50.901** **Poisoning by unspecified drugs, medicaments and biological substances, accidental (unintentional)**

    ✓7th **T50.902** **Poisoning by unspecified drugs, medicaments and biological substances, intentional self-harm**

    ✓7th **T50.903** **Poisoning by unspecified drugs, medicaments and biological substances, assault**

    ✓7th **T50.904** **Poisoning by unspecified drugs, medicaments and biological substances, undetermined**

    ✓7th **T50.905** Adverse effect of unspecified drugs, medicaments and biological substances

    ✓7th **T50.906** Underdosing of unspecified drugs, medicaments and biological substances

  ✓6th **T50.99** Poisoning by, adverse effect of and underdosing of other drugs, medicaments and biological substances

    ✓7th **T50.991** **Poisoning by other drugs, medicaments and biological substances, accidental (unintentional)**

    ✓7th **T50.992** **Poisoning by other drugs, medicaments and biological substances, intentional self-harm**

    ✓7th **T50.993** **Poisoning by other drugs, medicaments and biological substances, assault**

    ✓7th **T50.994** **Poisoning by other drugs, medicaments and biological substances, undetermined**

    ✓7th **T50.995** Adverse effect of other drugs, medicaments and biological substances

    ✓7th **T50.996** Underdosing of other drugs, medicaments and biological substances

Toxic effects of substances chiefly nonmedicinal as to source (T51-T65)

  NOTE   When no intent is indicated code to accidental. Undetermined intent is only for use when there is specific documentation in the record that the intent of the toxic effect cannot be determined.

Use additional code(s) for all associated manifestations of toxic effect, such as:
personal history of foreign body fully removed (Z87.821)
respiratory conditions due to external agents (J60-J70)
to identify any retained foreign body, if applicable (Z18.-)

EXCLUDES 1   contact with and (suspected) exposure to toxic substances (Z77.-)

✓4th **T51** **Toxic effect of alcohol**

> The appropriate 7th character is to be added to each code from category T51.
> A   initial encounter
> D   subsequent encounter
> S   sequela

✓5th **T51.0** **Toxic effect of ethanol**
Toxic effect of ethyl alcohol

  EXCLUDES 2   acute alcohol intoxication or 'hangover' effects (F10.129, F10.229, F10.929)
drunkenness (F10.129, F10.229, F10.929)
pathological alcohol intoxication (F10.129, F10.229, F10.929)

  ✓6th **T51.0X** Toxic effect of ethanol

    ✓7th **T51.0X1** **Toxic effect of ethanol, accidental (unintentional)**
Toxic effect of ethanol NOS

    ✓7th **T51.0X2** **Toxic effect of ethanol, intentional self-harm**

    ✓7th **T51.0X3** **Toxic effect of ethanol, assault**

    ✓7th **T51.0X4** **Toxic effect of ethanol, undetermined**

✓5th **T51.1** **Toxic effect of methanol**
Toxic effect of methyl alcohol

  ✓6th **T51.1X** Toxic effect of methanol

    ✓7th **T51.1X1** **Toxic effect of methanol, accidental (unintentional)**
Toxic effect of methanol NOS

    ✓7th **T51.1X2** **Toxic effect of methanol, intentional self-harm**

    ✓7th **T51.1X3** **Toxic effect of methanol, assault**

    ✓7th **T51.1X4** **Toxic effect of methanol, undetermined**

✓5th **T51.2** **Toxic effect of 2-Propanol**
Toxic effect of isopropyl alcohol

  ✓6th **T51.2X** Toxic effect of 2-Propanol

    ✓7th **T51.2X1** **Toxic effect of 2-Propanol, accidental (unintentional)**
Toxic effect of 2-Propanol NOS

    ✓7th **T51.2X2** **Toxic effect of 2-Propanol, intentional self-harm**

☑ Additional Character Required   ☑x7th Placeholder Alert   Unspecified Dx   Other Specified Dx   Manifestation   ►◄ Revised Text   ● New Code   ▲ Revised Code Title

✓7ᵗʰ **T51.2X3** **Toxic effect of 2-Propanol,** assault

✓7ᵗʰ **T51.2X4** **Toxic effect of 2-Propanol,** undetermined

✓5ᵗʰ **T51.3** **Toxic effect of fusel oil**
Toxic effect of amyl alcohol
Toxic effect of butyl [1-butanol] alcohol
Toxic effect of propyl [1-propanol] alcohol

    ✓6ᵗʰ **T51.3X** **Toxic effect of** fusel oil

      ✓7ᵗʰ **T51.3X1** **Toxic effect of fusel oil,** accidental **(unintentional)**
Toxic effect of fusel oil NOS

      ✓7ᵗʰ **T51.3X2** **Toxic effect of fusel oil,** intentional self-harm

      ✓7ᵗʰ **T51.3X3** **Toxic effect of fusel oil,** assault

      ✓7ᵗʰ **T51.3X4** **Toxic effect of fusel oil,** undetermined

✓5ᵗʰ **T51.8** **Toxic effect of other alcohols**

    ✓6ᵗʰ **T51.8X** **Toxic effect of** other alcohols

      ✓7ᵗʰ **T51.8X1** **Toxic effect of other alcohols,** accidental **(unintentional)**
Toxic effect of other alcohols NOS

      ✓7ᵗʰ **T51.8X2** **Toxic effect of other alcohols,** intentional self-harm

      ✓7ᵗʰ **T51.8X3** **Toxic effect of other alcohols,** assault

      ✓7ᵗʰ **T51.8X4** **Toxic effect of other alcohols,** undetermined

✓5ᵗʰ **T51.9** **Toxic effect of** unspecified **alcohol**

    ✓×7ᵗʰ **T51.91** **Toxic effect of unspecified alcohol,** accidental **(unintentional)**

    ✓×7ᵗʰ **T51.92** **Toxic effect of unspecified alcohol,** intentional self-harm

    ✓×7ᵗʰ **T51.93** **Toxic effect of unspecified alcohol,** assault

    ✓×7ᵗʰ **T51.94** **Toxic effect of unspecified alcohol,** undetermined

✓4ᵗʰ **T52** **Toxic effect of organic solvents**

    EXCLUDES 1   halogen derivatives of aliphatic and aromatic hydrocarbons (T53.-)

> The appropriate 7th character is to be added to each code from category T52.
> A   initial encounter
> D   subsequent encounter
> S   sequela

✓5ᵗʰ **T52.0** **Toxic effects of petroleum products**
Toxic effects of ether petroleum
Toxic effects of gasoline [petrol]
Toxic effects of kerosene [paraffin oil]
Toxic effects of naphtha petroleum
Toxic effects of paraffin wax
Toxic effects of spirit petroleum

    ✓6ᵗʰ **T52.0X** **Toxic effects of** petroleum products

      ✓7ᵗʰ **T52.0X1** **Toxic effect of petroleum products,** accidental **(unintentional)**
Toxic effects of petroleum products NOS

      ✓7ᵗʰ **T52.0X2** **Toxic effect of petroleum products,** intentional self-harm

      ✓7ᵗʰ **T52.0X3** **Toxic effect of petroleum products,** assault

      ✓7ᵗʰ **T52.0X4** **Toxic effect of petroleum products,** undetermined

✓5ᵗʰ **T52.1** **Toxic effects of benzene**

    EXCLUDES 1   homologues of benzene (T52.2)
nitroderivatives and aminoderivatives of benzene and its homologues (T65.3)

    ✓6ᵗʰ **T52.1X** **Toxic effects of** benzene

      ✓7ᵗʰ **T52.1X1** **Toxic effect of benzene,** accidental **(unintentional)**
Toxic effects of benzene NOS

      ✓7ᵗʰ **T52.1X2** **Toxic effect of benzene,** intentional self-harm

      ✓7ᵗʰ **T52.1X3** **Toxic effect of benzene,** assault

      ✓7ᵗʰ **T52.1X4** **Toxic effect of benzene,** undetermined

✓5ᵗʰ **T52.2** **Toxic effects of homologues of benzene**
Toxic effects of toluene [methylbenzene]
Toxic effects of xylene [dimethylbenzene]

    ✓6ᵗʰ **T52.2X** **Toxic effects of** homologues of benzene

      ✓7ᵗʰ **T52.2X1** **Toxic effect of homologues of benzene,** accidental **(unintentional)**
Toxic effects of homologues of benzene NOS

      ✓7ᵗʰ **T52.2X2** **Toxic effect of homologues of benzene,** intentional self-harm

      ✓7ᵗʰ **T52.2X3** **Toxic effect of homologues of benzene,** assault

      ✓7ᵗʰ **T52.2X4** **Toxic effect of homologues of benzene,** undetermined

✓5ᵗʰ **T52.3** **Toxic effects of glycols**

    ✓6ᵗʰ **T52.3X** **Toxic effects of** glycols

      ✓7ᵗʰ **T52.3X1** **Toxic effect of glycols,** accidental **(unintentional)**
Toxic effects of glycols NOS

      ✓7ᵗʰ **T52.3X2** **Toxic effect of glycols,** intentional self-harm

      ✓7ᵗʰ **T52.3X3** **Toxic effect of glycols,** assault

      ✓7ᵗʰ **T52.3X4** **Toxic effect of glycols,** undetermined

✓5ᵗʰ **T52.4** **Toxic effects of ketones**

    ✓6ᵗʰ **T52.4X** **Toxic effects of** ketones

      ✓7ᵗʰ **T52.4X1** **Toxic effect of ketones,** accidental **(unintentional)**
Toxic effects of ketones NOS

      ✓7ᵗʰ **T52.4X2** **Toxic effect of ketones,** intentional self-harm

      ✓7ᵗʰ **T52.4X3** **Toxic effect of ketones,** assault

      ✓7ᵗʰ **T52.4X4** **Toxic effect of ketones,** undetermined

✓5ᵗʰ **T52.8** **Toxic effects of other organic solvents**

    ✓6ᵗʰ **T52.8X** **Toxic effects of** other organic solvents

      ✓7ᵗʰ **T52.8X1** **Toxic effect of other organic solvents,** accidental **(unintentional)**
Toxic effects of other organic solvents NOS

      ✓7ᵗʰ **T52.8X2** **Toxic effect of other organic solvents,** intentional self-harm

      ✓7ᵗʰ **T52.8X3** **Toxic effect of other organic solvents,** assault

      ✓7ᵗʰ **T52.8X4** **Toxic effect of other organic solvents,** undetermined

✓5ᵗʰ **T52.9** **Toxic effects of** unspecified **organic solvent**

    ✓×7ᵗʰ **T52.91** **Toxic effect of unspecified organic solvent,** accidental **(unintentional)**

    ✓×7ᵗʰ **T52.92** **Toxic effect of unspecified organic solvent,** intentional self-harm

    ✓×7ᵗʰ **T52.93** **Toxic effect of unspecified organic solvent,** assault

    ✓×7ᵗʰ **T52.94** **Toxic effect of unspecified organic solvent,** undetermined

✓4ᵗʰ **T53** **Toxic effect of halogen derivatives of aliphatic and aromatic hydrocarbons**

> The appropriate 7th character is to be added to each code from category T53.
> A   initial encounter
> D   subsequent encounter
> S   sequela

✓5ᵗʰ **T53.0** **Toxic effects of carbon tetrachloride**
Toxic effects of tetrachloromethane

    ✓6ᵗʰ **T53.0X** **Toxic effects of** carbon tetrachloride

      ✓7ᵗʰ **T53.0X1** **Toxic effect of carbon tetrachloride,** accidental **(unintentional)**
Toxic effects of carbon tetrachloride NOS

      ✓7ᵗʰ **T53.0X2** **Toxic effect of carbon tetrachloride,** intentional self-harm

      ✓7ᵗʰ **T53.0X3** **Toxic effect of carbon tetrachloride,** assault

      ✓7ᵗʰ **T53.0X4** **Toxic effect of carbon tetrachloride,** undetermined

---

EXCLUDES 1 Not coded here   *EXCLUDES 2* Not included here   Ⓝ Newborn Age: 0   Ⓟ Pediatric Age: 0-17   Ⓜ Maternity Age: 12-55   Ⓐ Adult Age: 15-124

1006   ICD-10-CM 2016

☑5ᵗʰ **T53.1 Toxic effects of chloroform**
Toxic effects of trichloromethane

  ☑6ᵗʰ **T53.1X Toxic effects of** chloroform

    ☑7ᵗʰ **T53.1X1 Toxic effect of chloroform,** accidental (unintentional)
Toxic effects of chloroform NOS

    ☑7ᵗʰ **T53.1X2 Toxic effect of chloroform,** intentional self-harm

    ☑7ᵗʰ **T53.1X3 Toxic effect of chloroform,** assault

    ☑7ᵗʰ **T53.1X4 Toxic effect of chloroform,** undetermined

☑5ᵗʰ **T53.2 Toxic effects of trichloroethylene**
Toxic effects of trichloroethene

  ☑6ᵗʰ **T53.2X Toxic effects of** trichloroethylene

    ☑7ᵗʰ **T53.2X1 Toxic effect of trichloroethylene,** accidental (unintentional)
Toxic effects of trichloroethylene NOS

    ☑7ᵗʰ **T53.2X2 Toxic effect of trichloroethylene,** intentional self-harm

    ☑7ᵗʰ **T53.2X3 Toxic effect of trichloroethylene,** assault

    ☑7ᵗʰ **T53.2X4 Toxic effect of trichloroethylene,** undetermined

☑5ᵗʰ **T53.3 Toxic effects of tetrachloroethylene**
Toxic effects of perchloroethylene
Toxic effect of tetrachloroethene

  ☑6ᵗʰ **T53.3X Toxic effects of** tetrachloroethylene

    ☑7ᵗʰ **T53.3X1 Toxic effect of tetrachloroethylene,** accidental (unintentional)
Toxic effects of tetrachloroethylene NOS

    ☑7ᵗʰ **T53.3X2 Toxic effect of tetrachloroethylene,** intentional self-harm

    ☑7ᵗʰ **T53.3X3 Toxic effect of tetrachloroethylene,** assault

    ☑7ᵗʰ **T53.3X4 Toxic effect of tetrachloroethylene,** undetermined

☑5ᵗʰ **T53.4 Toxic effects of dichloromethane**
Toxic effects of methylene chloride

  ☑6ᵗʰ **T53.4X Toxic effects of** dichloromethane

    ☑7ᵗʰ **T53.4X1 Toxic effect of dichloromethane,** accidental (unintentional)
Toxic effects of dichloromethane NOS

    ☑7ᵗʰ **T53.4X2 Toxic effect of dichloromethane,** intentional self-harm

    ☑7ᵗʰ **T53.4X3 Toxic effect of dichloromethane,** assault

    ☑7ᵗʰ **T53.4X4 Toxic effect of dichloromethane,** undetermined

☑5ᵗʰ **T53.5 Toxic effects of chlorofluorocarbons**

  ☑6ᵗʰ **T53.5X Toxic effects of** chlorofluorocarbons

    ☑7ᵗʰ **T53.5X1 Toxic effect of chlorofluorocarbons,** accidental (unintentional)
Toxic effects of chlorofluorocarbons NOS

    ☑7ᵗʰ **T53.5X2 Toxic effect of chlorofluorocarbons,** intentional self-harm

    ☑7ᵗʰ **T53.5X3 Toxic effect of chlorofluorocarbons,** assault

    ☑7ᵗʰ **T53.5X4 Toxic effect of chlorofluorocarbons,** undetermined

☑5ᵗʰ **T53.6 Toxic effects of other halogen derivatives of aliphatic hydrocarbons**

  ☑6ᵗʰ **T53.6X Toxic effects of other** halogen derivatives of aliphatic hydrocarbons

    ☑7ᵗʰ **T53.6X1 Toxic effect of other halogen derivatives of aliphatic hydrocarbons,** accidental (unintentional)
Toxic effects of other halogen derivatives of aliphatic hydrocarbons NOS

    ☑7ᵗʰ **T53.6X2 Toxic effect of other halogen derivatives of aliphatic hydrocarbons,** intentional self-harm

    ☑7ᵗʰ **T53.6X3 Toxic effect of other halogen derivatives of aliphatic hydrocarbons,** assault

    ☑7ᵗʰ **T53.6X4 Toxic effect of other halogen derivatives of aliphatic hydrocarbons,** undetermined

☑5ᵗʰ **T53.7 Toxic effects of other halogen derivatives of aromatic hydrocarbons**

  ☑6ᵗʰ **T53.7X Toxic effects of other** halogen derivatives of aromatic hydrocarbons

    ☑7ᵗʰ **T53.7X1 Toxic effect of other halogen derivatives of aromatic hydrocarbons,** accidental (unintentional)
Toxic effects of other halogen derivatives of aromatic hydrocarbons NOS

    ☑7ᵗʰ **T53.7X2 Toxic effect of other halogen derivatives of aromatic hydrocarbons,** intentional self-harm

    ☑7ᵗʰ **T53.7X3 Toxic effect of other halogen derivatives of aromatic hydrocarbons,** assault

    ☑7ᵗʰ **T53.7X4 Toxic effect of other halogen derivatives of aromatic hydrocarbons,** undetermined

☑5ᵗʰ **T53.9 Toxic effects of** unspecified halogen derivatives of aliphatic and aromatic hydrocarbons

  ☑x7ᵗʰ **T53.91 Toxic effect of unspecified halogen derivatives of aliphatic and aromatic hydrocarbons,** accidental (unintentional)

  ☑x7ᵗʰ **T53.92 Toxic effect of unspecified halogen derivatives of aliphatic and aromatic hydrocarbons,** intentional self-harm

  ☑x7ᵗʰ **T53.93 Toxic effect of unspecified halogen derivatives of aliphatic and aromatic hydrocarbons,** assault

  ☑x7ᵗʰ **T53.94 Toxic effect of unspecified halogen derivatives of aliphatic and aromatic hydrocarbons,** undetermined

☑4ᵗʰ **T54 Toxic effect of corrosive substances**

> The appropriate 7th character is to be added to each code from category T54.
> A   initial encounter
> D   subsequent encounter
> S   sequela

☑5ᵗʰ **T54.0 Toxic effects of phenol and phenol homologues**

  ☑6ᵗʰ **T54.0X Toxic effects of** phenol and phenol homologues

    ☑7ᵗʰ **T54.0X1 Toxic effect of phenol and phenol homologues,** accidental (unintentional)
Toxic effects of phenol and phenol homologues NOS

    ☑7ᵗʰ **T54.0X2 Toxic effect of phenol and phenol homologues,** intentional self-harm

    ☑7ᵗʰ **T54.0X3 Toxic effect of phenol and phenol homologues,** assault

    ☑7ᵗʰ **T54.0X4 Toxic effect of phenol and phenol homologues,** undetermined

☑5ᵗʰ **T54.1 Toxic effects of other corrosive organic compounds**

  ☑6ᵗʰ **T54.1X Toxic effects of** other corrosive organic compounds

    ☑7ᵗʰ **T54.1X1 Toxic effect of other corrosive organic compounds,** accidental (unintentional)
Toxic effects of other corrosive organic compounds NOS

    ☑7ᵗʰ **T54.1X2 Toxic effect of other corrosive organic compounds,** intentional self-harm

    ☑7ᵗʰ **T54.1X3 Toxic effect of other corrosive organic compounds,** assault

    ☑7ᵗʰ **T54.1X4 Toxic effect of other corrosive organic compounds,** undetermined

☑5ᵗʰ **T54.2 Toxic effects of corrosive acids and acid-like substances**
Toxic effects of hydrochloric acid
Toxic effects of sulfuric acid

  ☑6ᵗʰ **T54.2X Toxic effects of corrosive** acids and acid-like substances

    ☑7ᵗʰ **T54.2X1 Toxic effect of corrosive acids and acid-like substances,** accidental (unintentional)
Toxic effects of corrosive acids and acid-like substances NOS

    ☑7ᵗʰ **T54.2X2 Toxic effect of corrosive acids and acid-like substances,** intentional self-harm

    ☑7ᵗʰ **T54.2X3 Toxic effect of corrosive acids and acid-like substances,** assault

    ☑7ᵗʰ **T54.2X4 Toxic effect of corrosive acids and acid-like substances,** undetermined

---

☑ Additional Character Required   ☑x7ᵗʰ Placeholder Alert   Unspecified Dx   Other Specified Dx   Manifestation   ▶◀ Revised Text   ● New Code   ▲ Revised Code Title

✓5th **T54.3 Toxic effects of corrosive alkalis and alkali-like substances**
     Toxic effects of potassium hydroxide
     Toxic effects of sodium hydroxide

   ✓6th **T54.3X Toxic effects of corrosive** alkalis and alkali-like substances

     ✓7th **T54.3X1 Toxic effect of corrosive alkalis and alkali-like substances, accidental (unintentional)**
       Toxic effects of corrosive alkalis and alkali-like substances NOS

     ✓7th **T54.3X2 Toxic effect of corrosive alkalis and alkali-like substances, intentional self-harm**

     ✓7th **T54.3X3 Toxic effect of corrosive alkalis and alkali-like substances, assault**

     ✓7th **T54.3X4 Toxic effect of corrosive alkalis and alkali-like substances, undetermined**

✓5th **T54.9 Toxic effects of** unspecified **corrosive substance**

   ✓x7th **T54.91 Toxic effect of unspecified corrosive substance, accidental (unintentional)**

   ✓x7th **T54.92 Toxic effect of unspecified corrosive substance, intentional self-harm**

   ✓x7th **T54.93 Toxic effect of unspecified corrosive substance, assault**

   ✓x7th **T54.94 Toxic effect of unspecified corrosive substance, undetermined**

✓4th **T55 Toxic effect of soaps and detergents**

> The appropriate 7th character is to be added to each code from category T55.
> A   initial encounter
> D   subsequent encounter
> S   sequela

✓5th **T55.0 Toxic effect of soaps**

   ✓6th **T55.0X Toxic effect of** soaps

     ✓7th **T55.0X1 Toxic effect of soaps, accidental (unintentional)**
       Toxic effect of soaps NOS

     ✓7th **T55.0X2 Toxic effect of soaps, intentional self-harm**

     ✓7th **T55.0X3 Toxic effect of soaps, assault**

     ✓7th **T55.0X4 Toxic effect of soaps, undetermined**

✓5th **T55.1 Toxic effect of detergents**

   ✓6th **T55.1X Toxic effect of** detergents

     ✓7th **T55.1X1 Toxic effect of detergents, accidental (unintentional)**
       Toxic effect of detergents NOS

     ✓7th **T55.1X2 Toxic effect of detergents, intentional self-harm**

     ✓7th **T55.1X3 Toxic effect of detergents, assault**

     ✓7th **T55.1X4 Toxic effect of detergents, undetermined**

✓4th **T56 Toxic effect of metals**
   INCLUDES toxic effects of fumes and vapors of metals
       toxic effects of metals from all sources, except medicinal substances

   Use additional code to identify any retained metal foreign body, if applicable (Z18.0-, T18.1-)
   EXCLUDES 1 *arsenic and its compounds (T57.0)*
       manganese and its compounds (T57.2)

> The appropriate 7th character is to be added to each code from category T56.
> A   initial encounter
> D   subsequent encounter
> S   sequela

✓5th **T56.0 Toxic effects of lead and its compounds**

   ✓6th **T56.0X Toxic effects of** lead **and its compounds**

     ✓7th **T56.0X1 Toxic effect of lead and its compounds, accidental (unintentional)**
       Toxic effects of lead and its compounds NOS

     ✓7th **T56.0X2 Toxic effect of lead and its compounds, intentional self-harm**

     ✓7th **T56.0X3 Toxic effect of lead and its compounds, assault**

     ✓7th **T56.0X4 Toxic effect of lead and its compounds, undetermined**

✓5th **T56.1 Toxic effects of mercury and its compounds**

   ✓6th **T56.1X Toxic effects of** mercury **and its compounds**

     ✓7th **T56.1X1 Toxic effect of mercury and its compounds, accidental (unintentional)**
       Toxic effects of mercury and its compounds NOS

     ✓7th **T56.1X2 Toxic effect of mercury and its compounds, intentional self-harm**

     ✓7th **T56.1X3 Toxic effect of mercury and its compounds, assault**

     ✓7th **T56.1X4 Toxic effect of mercury and its compounds, undetermined**

✓5th **T56.2 Toxic effects of chromium and its compounds**

   ✓6th **T56.2X Toxic effects of** chromium **and its compounds**

     ✓7th **T56.2X1 Toxic effect of chromium and its compounds, accidental (unintentional)**
       Toxic effects of chromium and its compounds NOS

     ✓7th **T56.2X2 Toxic effect of chromium and its compounds, intentional self-harm**

     ✓7th **T56.2X3 Toxic effect of chromium and its compounds, assault**

     ✓7th **T56.2X4 Toxic effect of chromium and its compounds, undetermined**

✓5th **T56.3 Toxic effects of** cadmium **and its compounds**

   ✓6th **T56.3X Toxic effects of cadmium and its compounds**

     ✓7th **T56.3X1 Toxic effect of cadmium and its compounds, accidental (unintentional)**
       Toxic effects of cadmium and its compounds NOS

     ✓7th **T56.3X2 Toxic effect of cadmium and its compounds, intentional self-harm**

     ✓7th **T56.3X3 Toxic effect of cadmium and its compounds, assault**

     ✓7th **T56.3X4 Toxic effect of cadmium and its compounds, undetermined**

✓5th **T56.4 Toxic effects of copper and its compounds**

   ✓6th **T56.4X Toxic effects of** copper **and its compounds**

     ✓7th **T56.4X1 Toxic effect of copper and its compounds, accidental (unintentional)**
       Toxic effects of copper and its compounds NOS

     ✓7th **T56.4X2 Toxic effect of copper and its compounds, intentional self-harm**

     ✓7th **T56.4X3 Toxic effect of copper and its compounds, assault**

     ✓7th **T56.4X4 Toxic effect of copper and its compounds, undetermined**

✓5th **T56.5 Toxic effects of zinc and its compounds**

   ✓6th **T56.5X Toxic effects of** zinc **and its compounds**

     ✓7th **T56.5X1 Toxic effect of zinc and its compounds, accidental (unintentional)**
       Toxic effects of zinc and its compounds NOS

     ✓7th **T56.5X2 Toxic effect of zinc and its compounds, intentional self-harm**

     ✓7th **T56.5X3 Toxic effect of zinc and its compounds, assault**

     ✓7th **T56.5X4 Toxic effect of zinc and its compounds, undetermined**

✓5th **T56.6 Toxic effects of tin and its compounds**

   ✓6th **T56.6X Toxic effects of** tin **and its compounds**

     ✓7th **T56.6X1 Toxic effect of tin and its compounds, accidental (unintentional)**
       Toxic effects of tin and its compounds NOS

     ✓7th **T56.6X2 Toxic effect of tin and its compounds, intentional self-harm**

     ✓7th **T56.6X3 Toxic effect of tin and its compounds, assault**

     ✓7th **T56.6X4 Toxic effect of tin and its compounds, undetermined**

√5ᵗʰ **T56.7** **Toxic effects of beryllium and its compounds**

  √6ᵗʰ **T56.7X** **Toxic effects of beryllium and its compounds**

    √7ᵗʰ **T56.7X1** **Toxic effect of beryllium and its compounds,** accidental (unintentional)
        Toxic effects of beryllium and its compounds NOS

    √7ᵗʰ **T56.7X2** **Toxic effect of beryllium and its compounds,** intentional self-harm

    √7ᵗʰ **T56.7X3** **Toxic effect of beryllium and its compounds,** assault

    √7ᵗʰ **T56.7X4** **Toxic effect of beryllium and its compounds,** undetermined

√5ᵗʰ **T56.8** **Toxic effects of other metals**

  √6ᵗʰ **T56.81** **Toxic effect of thallium**

    √7ᵗʰ **T56.811** **Toxic effect of thallium,** accidental (unintentional)
        Toxic effect of thallium NOS

    √7ᵗʰ **T56.812** **Toxic effect of thallium,** intentional self-harm

    √7ᵗʰ **T56.813** **Toxic effect of thallium,** assault

    √7ᵗʰ **T56.814** **Toxic effect of thallium,** undetermined

  √6ᵗʰ **T56.89** **Toxic effects of other metals**

    √7ᵗʰ **T56.891** **Toxic effect of other metals,** accidental (unintentional)
        Toxic effects of other metals NOS

    √7ᵗʰ **T56.892** **Toxic effect of other metals,** intentional self-harm

    √7ᵗʰ **T56.893** **Toxic effect of other metals,** assault

    √7ᵗʰ **T56.894** **Toxic effect of other metals,** undetermined

√5ᵗʰ **T56.9** **Toxic effects of unspecified metal**

  √x7ᵗʰ **T56.91** **Toxic effect of unspecified metal,** accidental (unintentional)

  √x7ᵗʰ **T56.92** **Toxic effect of unspecified metal,** intentional self-harm

  √x7ᵗʰ **T56.93** **Toxic effect of unspecified metal,** assault

  √x7ᵗʰ **T56.94** **Toxic effect of unspecified metal,** undetermined

√4ᵗʰ **T57** **Toxic effect of other inorganic substances**

> The appropriate 7th character is to be added to each code from category T57.
> A   initial encounter
> D   subsequent encounter
> S   sequela

√5ᵗʰ **T57.0** **Toxic effect of arsenic and its compounds**

  √6ᵗʰ **T57.0X** **Toxic effect of arsenic and its compounds**

    √7ᵗʰ **T57.0X1** **Toxic effect of arsenic and its compounds,** accidental (unintentional)
        Toxic effect of arsenic and its compounds NOS

    √7ᵗʰ **T57.0X2** **Toxic effect of arsenic and its compounds,** intentional self-harm

    √7ᵗʰ **T57.0X3** **Toxic effect of arsenic and its compounds,** assault

    √7ᵗʰ **T57.0X4** **Toxic effect of arsenic and its compounds,** undetermined

√5ᵗʰ **T57.1** **Toxic effect of phosphorus and its compounds**
    EXCLUDES 1 organophosphate insecticides (T60.0)

  √6ᵗʰ **T57.1X** **Toxic effect of phosphorus and its compounds**

    √7ᵗʰ **T57.1X1** **Toxic effect of phosphorus and its compounds,** accidental (unintentional)
        Toxic effect of phosphorus and its compounds NOS

    √7ᵗʰ **T57.1X2** **Toxic effect of phosphorus and its compounds,** intentional self-harm

    √7ᵗʰ **T57.1X3** **Toxic effect of phosphorus and its compounds,** assault

    √7ᵗʰ **T57.1X4** **Toxic effect of phosphorus and its compounds,** undetermined

√5ᵗʰ **T57.2** **Toxic effect of manganese and its compounds**

  √6ᵗʰ **T57.2X** **Toxic effect of manganese and its compounds**

    √7ᵗʰ **T57.2X1** **Toxic effect of manganese and its compounds,** accidental (unintentional)
        Toxic effect of manganese and its compounds NOS

    √7ᵗʰ **T57.2X2** **Toxic effect of manganese and its compounds,** intentional self-harm

    √7ᵗʰ **T57.2X3** **Toxic effect of manganese and its compounds,** assault

    √7ᵗʰ **T57.2X4** **Toxic effect of manganese and its compounds,** undetermined

√5ᵗʰ **T57.3** **Toxic effect of hydrogen cyanide**

  √6ᵗʰ **T57.3X** **Toxic effect of hydrogen cyanide**

    √7ᵗʰ **T57.3X1** **Toxic effect of hydrogen cyanide,** accidental (unintentional)
        Toxic effect of hydrogen cyanide NOS

    √7ᵗʰ **T57.3X2** **Toxic effect of hydrogen cyanide,** intentional self-harm

    √7ᵗʰ **T57.3X3** **Toxic effect of hydrogen cyanide,** assault

    √7ᵗʰ **T57.3X4** **Toxic effect of hydrogen cyanide,** undetermined

√5ᵗʰ **T57.8** **Toxic effect of other specified inorganic substances**

  √6ᵗʰ **T57.8X** **Toxic effect of other specified inorganic substances**

    √7ᵗʰ **T57.8X1** **Toxic effect of other specified inorganic substances,** accidental (unintentional)
        Toxic effect of other specified inorganic substances NOS

    √7ᵗʰ **T57.8X2** **Toxic effect of other specified inorganic substances,** intentional self-harm

    √7ᵗʰ **T57.8X3** **Toxic effect of other specified inorganic substances,** assault

    √7ᵗʰ **T57.8X4** **Toxic effect of other specified inorganic substances,** undetermined

√5ᵗʰ **T57.9** **Toxic effect of unspecified inorganic substance**

  √x7ᵗʰ **T57.91** **Toxic effect of unspecified inorganic substance,** accidental (unintentional)

  √x7ᵗʰ **T57.92** **Toxic effect of unspecified inorganic substance,** intentional self-harm

  √x7ᵗʰ **T57.93** **Toxic effect of unspecified inorganic substance,** assault

  √x7ᵗʰ **T57.94** **Toxic effect of unspecified inorganic substance,** undetermined

√4ᵗʰ **T58** **Toxic effect of carbon monoxide**
  INCLUDES asphyxiation from carbon monoxide
         toxic effect of carbon monoxide from all sources

> The appropriate 7th character is to be added to each code from category T58.
> A   initial encounter
> D   subsequent encounter
> S   sequela

√5ᵗʰ **T58.0** **Toxic effect of carbon monoxide from motor vehicle exhaust**
    Toxic effect of exhaust gas from gas engine
    Toxic effect of exhaust gas from motor pump

  √x7ᵗʰ **T58.01** **Toxic effect of carbon monoxide from motor vehicle exhaust,** accidental (unintentional)

  √x7ᵗʰ **T58.02** **Toxic effect of carbon monoxide from motor vehicle exhaust,** intentional self-harm

  √x7ᵗʰ **T58.03** **Toxic effect of carbon monoxide from motor vehicle exhaust,** assault

  √x7ᵗʰ **T58.04** **Toxic effect of carbon monoxide from motor vehicle exhaust,** undetermined

√5ᵗʰ **T58.1** **Toxic effect of carbon monoxide from utility gas**
    Toxic effect of acetylene
    Toxic effect of gas NOS used for lighting, heating, cooking
    Toxic effect of water gas

  √x7ᵗʰ **T58.11** **Toxic effect of carbon monoxide from utility gas,** accidental (unintentional)

  √x7ᵗʰ **T58.12** **Toxic effect of carbon monoxide from utility gas,** intentional self-harm

  √x7ᵗʰ **T58.13** **Toxic effect of carbon monoxide from utility gas,** assault

  √x7ᵗʰ **T58.14** **Toxic effect of carbon monoxide from utility gas,** undetermined

---

☑ Additional Character Required   √x7ᵗʰ Placeholder Alert   Unspecified Dx   Other Specified Dx   Manifestation   ►◄ Revised Text   ● New Code   ▲ Revised Code Title

✓5ᵗʰ **T58.2** **Toxic effect of carbon monoxide** from incomplete combustion of other domestic fuels
     Toxic effect of carbon monoxide from incomplete combustion of coal, coke, kerosene, wood

   ✓6ᵗʰ **T58.2X** **Toxic effect of carbon monoxide from incomplete combustion of other domestic fuels**

      ✓7ᵗʰ **T58.2X1** **Toxic effect of carbon monoxide from incomplete combustion of other domestic fuels, accidental (unintentional)**

      ✓7ᵗʰ **T58.2X2** **Toxic effect of carbon monoxide from incomplete combustion of other domestic fuels, intentional self-harm**

      ✓7ᵗʰ **T58.2X3** **Toxic effect of carbon monoxide from incomplete combustion of other domestic fuels, assault**

      ✓7ᵗʰ **T58.2X4** **Toxic effect of carbon monoxide from incomplete combustion of other domestic fuels, undetermined**

✓5ᵗʰ **T58.8** **Toxic effect of carbon monoxide** from other source
     Toxic effect of carbon monoxide from blast furnace gas
     Toxic effect of carbon monoxide from fuels in industrial use
     Toxic effect of carbon monoxide from kiln vapor

   ✓6ᵗʰ **T58.8X** **Toxic effect of carbon monoxide from other source**

      ✓7ᵗʰ **T58.8X1** **Toxic effect of carbon monoxide from other source, accidental (unintentional)**

      ✓7ᵗʰ **T58.8X2** **Toxic effect of carbon monoxide from other source, intentional self-harm**

      ✓7ᵗʰ **T58.8X3** **Toxic effect of carbon monoxide from other source, assault**

      ✓7ᵗʰ **T58.8X4** **Toxic effect of carbon monoxide from other source, undetermined**

✓5ᵗʰ **T58.9** **Toxic effect of carbon monoxide** from unspecified source

   ✓x 7ᵗʰ **T58.91** **Toxic effect of carbon monoxide from unspecified source, accidental (unintentional)**

   ✓x 7ᵗʰ **T58.92** **Toxic effect of carbon monoxide from unspecified source, intentional self-harm**

   ✓x 7ᵗʰ **T58.93** **Toxic effect of carbon monoxide from unspecified source, assault**

   ✓x 7ᵗʰ **T58.94** **Toxic effect of carbon monoxide from unspecified source, undetermined**

✓4ᵗʰ **T59** **Toxic effect of other gases, fumes and vapors**
   INCLUDES aerosol propellants
   EXCLUDES 1 *chlorofluorocarbons (T53.5)*

> The appropriate 7th character is to be added to each code from category T59.
> A   initial encounter
> D   subsequent encounter
> S   sequela

✓5ᵗʰ **T59.0** **Toxic effect of nitrogen oxides**

   ✓6ᵗʰ **T59.0X** **Toxic effect of nitrogen oxides**

      ✓7ᵗʰ **T59.0X1** **Toxic effect of nitrogen oxides, accidental (unintentional)**
            Toxic effect of nitrogen oxides NOS

      ✓7ᵗʰ **T59.0X2** **Toxic effect of nitrogen oxides, intentional self-harm**

      ✓7ᵗʰ **T59.0X3** **Toxic effect of nitrogen oxides, assault**

      ✓7ᵗʰ **T59.0X4** **Toxic effect of nitrogen oxides, undetermined**

✓5ᵗʰ **T59.1** **Toxic effect of sulfur dioxide**

   ✓6ᵗʰ **T59.1X** **Toxic effect of sulfur dioxide**

      ✓7ᵗʰ **T59.1X1** **Toxic effect of sulfur dioxide, accidental (unintentional)**
            Toxic effect of sulfur dioxide NOS

      ✓7ᵗʰ **T59.1X2** **Toxic effect of sulfur dioxide, intentional self-harm**

      ✓7ᵗʰ **T59.1X3** **Toxic effect of sulfur dioxide, assault**

      ✓7ᵗʰ **T59.1X4** **Toxic effect of sulfur dioxide, undetermined**

✓5ᵗʰ **T59.2** **Toxic effect of formaldehyde**

   ✓6ᵗʰ **T59.2X** **Toxic effect of formaldehyde**

      ✓7ᵗʰ **T59.2X1** **Toxic effect of formaldehyde, accidental (unintentional)**
            Toxic effect of formaldehyde NOS

      ✓7ᵗʰ **T59.2X2** **Toxic effect of formaldehyde, intentional self-harm**

      ✓7ᵗʰ **T59.2X3** **Toxic effect of formaldehyde, assault**

      ✓7ᵗʰ **T59.2X4** **Toxic effect of formaldehyde, undetermined**

✓5ᵗʰ **T59.3** **Toxic effect of lacrimogenic gas**
     Toxic effect of tear gas

   ✓6ᵗʰ **T59.3X** **Toxic effect of lacrimogenic gas**

      ✓7ᵗʰ **T59.3X1** **Toxic effect of lacrimogenic gas, accidental (unintentional)**
            Toxic effect of lacrimogenic gas NOS

      ✓7ᵗʰ **T59.3X2** **Toxic effect of lacrimogenic gas, intentional self-harm**

      ✓7ᵗʰ **T59.3X3** **Toxic effect of lacrimogenic gas, assault**

      ✓7ᵗʰ **T59.3X4** **Toxic effect of lacrimogenic gas, undetermined**

✓5ᵗʰ **T59.4** **Toxic effect of chlorine gas**

   ✓6ᵗʰ **T59.4X** **Toxic effect of chlorine gas**

      ✓7ᵗʰ **T59.4X1** **Toxic effect of chlorine gas, accidental (unintentional)**
            Toxic effect of chlorine gas NOS

      ✓7ᵗʰ **T59.4X2** **Toxic effect of chlorine gas, intentional self-harm**

      ✓7ᵗʰ **T59.4X3** **Toxic effect of chlorine gas, assault**

      ✓7ᵗʰ **T59.4X4** **Toxic effect of chlorine gas, undetermined**

✓5ᵗʰ **T59.5** **Toxic effect of fluorine gas and hydrogen fluoride**

   ✓6ᵗʰ **T59.5X** **Toxic effect of fluorine gas and hydrogen fluoride**

      ✓7ᵗʰ **T59.5X1** **Toxic effect of fluorine gas and hydrogen fluoride, accidental (unintentional)**
            Toxic effect of fluorine gas and hydrogen fluoride NOS

      ✓7ᵗʰ **T59.5X2** **Toxic effect of fluorine gas and hydrogen fluoride, intentional self-harm**

      ✓7ᵗʰ **T59.5X3** **Toxic effect of fluorine gas and hydrogen fluoride, assault**

      ✓7ᵗʰ **T59.5X4** **Toxic effect of fluorine gas and hydrogen fluoride, undetermined**

✓5ᵗʰ **T59.6** **Toxic effect of hydrogen sulfide**

   ✓6ᵗʰ **T59.6X** **Toxic effect of hydrogen sulfide**

      ✓7ᵗʰ **T59.6X1** **Toxic effect of hydrogen sulfide, accidental (unintentional)**
            Toxic effect of hydrogen sulfide NOS

      ✓7ᵗʰ **T59.6X2** **Toxic effect of hydrogen sulfide, intentional self-harm**

      ✓7ᵗʰ **T59.6X3** **Toxic effect of hydrogen sulfide, assault**

      ✓7ᵗʰ **T59.6X4** **Toxic effect of hydrogen sulfide, undetermined**

✓5ᵗʰ **T59.7** **Toxic effect of carbon dioxide**

   ✓6ᵗʰ **T59.7X** **Toxic effect of carbon dioxide**

      ✓7ᵗʰ **T59.7X1** **Toxic effect of carbon dioxide, accidental (unintentional)**
            Toxic effect of carbon dioxide NOS

      ✓7ᵗʰ **T59.7X2** **Toxic effect of carbon dioxide, intentional self-harm**

      ✓7ᵗʰ **T59.7X3** **Toxic effect of carbon dioxide, assault**

      ✓7ᵗʰ **T59.7X4** **Toxic effect of carbon dioxide, undetermined**

✓5ᵗʰ **T59.8** **Toxic effect of other specified gases, fumes and vapors**

   ✓6ᵗʰ **T59.81** **Toxic effect of smoke**
       Smoke inhalation
       EXCLUDES 2 *toxic effect of cigarette (tobacco) smoke (T65.22-)*

      ✓7ᵗʰ **T59.811** **Toxic effect of smoke, accidental (unintentional)**
            Toxic effect of smoke NOS
            AHA: 2013, 4Q, 121

      ✓7ᵗʰ **T59.812** **Toxic effect of smoke, intentional self-harm**

      ✓7ᵗʰ **T59.813** **Toxic effect of smoke, assault**

      ✓7ᵗʰ **T59.814** **Toxic effect of smoke, undetermined**

   ✓6ᵗʰ **T59.89** **Toxic effect of other specified gases, fumes and vapors**

      ✓7ᵗʰ **T59.891** **Toxic effect of other specified gases, fumes and vapors, accidental (unintentional)**

EXCLUDES 1 Not coded here   **EXCLUDES 2** Not included here   **N** Newborn Age: 0   **P** Pediatric Age: 0-17   **M** Maternity Age: 12-55   **A** Adult Age: 15-124

1010   ICD-10-CM 2016

√7ᵗʰ **T59.892** **Toxic effect of other specified gases, fumes and vapors, intentional self-harm**

√7ᵗʰ **T59.893** **Toxic effect of other specified gases, fumes and vapors, assault**

√7ᵗʰ **T59.894** **Toxic effect of other specified gases, fumes and vapors, undetermined**

√5ᵗʰ **T59.9** **Toxic effect of unspecified gases, fumes and vapors**

√x7ᵗʰ **T59.91** **Toxic effect of unspecified gases, fumes and vapors, accidental (unintentional)**

√x7ᵗʰ **T59.92** **Toxic effect of unspecified gases, fumes and vapors, intentional self-harm**

√x7ᵗʰ **T59.93** **Toxic effect of unspecified gases, fumes and vapors, assault**

√x7ᵗʰ **T59.94** **Toxic effect of unspecified gases, fumes and vapors, undetermined**

√4ᵗʰ **T60** **Toxic effect of pesticides**

INCLUDES   toxic effect of wood preservatives

The appropriate 7th character is to be added to each code from category T60.
A   initial encounter
D   subsequent encounter
S   sequela

√5ᵗʰ **T60.0** **Toxic effect of organophosphate and carbamate insecticides**

√6ᵗʰ **T60.0X** **Toxic effect of organophosphate and carbamate insecticides**

√7ᵗʰ **T60.0X1** **Toxic effect of organophosphate and carbamate insecticides, accidental (unintentional)**
Toxic effect of organophosphate and carbamate insecticides NOS

√7ᵗʰ **T60.0X2** **Toxic effect of organophosphate and carbamate insecticides, intentional self-harm**

√7ᵗʰ **T60.0X3** **Toxic effect of organophosphate and carbamate insecticides, assault**

√7ᵗʰ **T60.0X4** **Toxic effect of organophosphate and carbamate insecticides, undetermined**

√5ᵗʰ **T60.1** **Toxic effect of halogenated insecticides**

EXCLUDES 1   chlorinated hydrocarbon (T53.-)

√6ᵗʰ **T60.1X** **Toxic effect of halogenated insecticides**

√7ᵗʰ **T60.1X1** **Toxic effect of halogenated insecticides, accidental (unintentional)**
Toxic effect of halogenated insecticides NOS

√7ᵗʰ **T60.1X2** **Toxic effect of halogenated insecticides, intentional self-harm**

√7ᵗʰ **T60.1X3** **Toxic effect of halogenated insecticides, assault**

√7ᵗʰ **T60.1X4** **Toxic effect of halogenated insecticides, undetermined**

√5ᵗʰ **T60.2** **Toxic effect of other insecticides**

√6ᵗʰ **T60.2X** **Toxic effect of other insecticides**

√7ᵗʰ **T60.2X1** **Toxic effect of other insecticides, accidental (unintentional)**
Toxic effect of other insecticides NOS

√7ᵗʰ **T60.2X2** **Toxic effect of other insecticides, intentional self-harm**

√7ᵗʰ **T60.2X3** **Toxic effect of other insecticides, assault**

√7ᵗʰ **T60.2X4** **Toxic effect of other insecticides, undetermined**

√5ᵗʰ **T60.3** **Toxic effect of herbicides and fungicides**

√6ᵗʰ **T60.3X** **Toxic effect of herbicides and fungicides**

√7ᵗʰ **T60.3X1** **Toxic effect of herbicides and fungicides, accidental (unintentional)**
Toxic effect of herbicides and fungicides NOS

√7ᵗʰ **T60.3X2** **Toxic effect of herbicides and fungicides, intentional self-harm**

√7ᵗʰ **T60.3X3** **Toxic effect of herbicides and fungicides, assault**

√7ᵗʰ **T60.3X4** **Toxic effect of herbicides and fungicides, undetermined**

√5ᵗʰ **T60.4** **Toxic effect of rodenticides**

EXCLUDES 1   strychnine and its salts (T65.1)
thallium (T56.81-)

√6ᵗʰ **T60.4X** **Toxic effect of rodenticides**

√7ᵗʰ **T60.4X1** **Toxic effect of rodenticides, accidental (unintentional)**
Toxic effect of rodenticides NOS

√7ᵗʰ **T60.4X2** **Toxic effect of rodenticides, intentional self-harm**

√7ᵗʰ **T60.4X3** **Toxic effect of rodenticides, assault**

√7ᵗʰ **T60.4X4** **Toxic effect of rodenticides, undetermined**

√5ᵗʰ **T60.8** **Toxic effect of other pesticides**

√6ᵗʰ **T60.8X** **Toxic effect of other pesticides**

√7ᵗʰ **T60.8X1** **Toxic effect of other pesticides, accidental (unintentional)**
Toxic effect of other pesticides NOS

√7ᵗʰ **T60.8X2** **Toxic effect of other pesticides, intentional self-harm**

√7ᵗʰ **T60.8X3** **Toxic effect of other pesticides, assault**

√7ᵗʰ **T60.8X4** **Toxic effect of other pesticides, undetermined**

√5ᵗʰ **T60.9** **Toxic effect of unspecified pesticide**

√x7ᵗʰ **T60.91** **Toxic effect of unspecified pesticide, accidental (unintentional)**

√x7ᵗʰ **T60.92** **Toxic effect of unspecified pesticide, intentional self-harm**

√x7ᵗʰ **T60.93** **Toxic effect of unspecified pesticide, assault**

√x7ᵗʰ **T60.94** **Toxic effect of unspecified pesticide, undetermined**

√4ᵗʰ **T61** **Toxic effect of noxious substances eaten as seafood**

EXCLUDES 1   allergic reaction to food, such as:
anaphylactic reaction or shock due to adverse food reaction (T78.0-)
dermatitis (L23.6, L25.4, L27.2)
gastroenteritis (noninfective) (K52.2)
bacterial foodborne intoxications (A05.-)
toxic effect of aflatoxin and other mycotoxins (T64)
toxic effect of cyanides (T65.0-)
toxic effect of harmful algae bloom (T65.82-)
toxic effect of hydrogen cyanide (T57.3-)
toxic effect of mercury (T56.1-)
toxic effect of red tide (T65.82-)

The appropriate 7th character is to be added to each code from category T61.
A   initial encounter
D   subsequent encounter
S   sequela

√5ᵗʰ **T61.0** **Ciguatera fish poisoning**

√x7ᵗʰ **T61.01** **Ciguatera fish poisoning, accidental (unintentional)**

√x7ᵗʰ **T61.02** **Ciguatera fish poisoning, intentional self-harm**

√x7ᵗʰ **T61.03** **Ciguatera fish poisoning, assault**

√x7ᵗʰ **T61.04** **Ciguatera fish poisoning, undetermined**

√5ᵗʰ **T61.1** **Scombroid fish poisoning**
Histamine-like syndrome

√x7ᵗʰ **T61.11** **Scombroid fish poisoning, accidental (unintentional)**

√x7ᵗʰ **T61.12** **Scombroid fish poisoning, intentional self-harm**

√x7ᵗʰ **T61.13** **Scombroid fish poisoning, assault**

√x7ᵗʰ **T61.14** **Scombroid fish poisoning, undetermined**

√5ᵗʰ **T61.7** **Other fish and shellfish poisoning**

√6ᵗʰ **T61.77** **Other fish poisoning**

√7ᵗʰ **T61.771** **Other fish poisoning, accidental (unintentional)**

√7ᵗʰ **T61.772** **Other fish poisoning, intentional self-harm**

√7ᵗʰ **T61.773** **Other fish poisoning, assault**

√7ᵗʰ **T61.774** **Other fish poisoning, undetermined**

√6ᵗʰ **T61.78** **Other shellfish poisoning**

√7ᵗʰ **T61.781** **Other shellfish poisoning, accidental (unintentional)**

√7ᵗʰ **T61.782** **Other shellfish poisoning, intentional self-harm**

√7ᵗʰ **T61.783** **Other shellfish poisoning, assault**

√7ᵗʰ **T61.784** **Other shellfish poisoning, undetermined**

✔ Additional Character Required   √x7ᵗʰ Placeholder Alert   Unspecified Dx   Other Specified Dx   Manifestation   ►◄ Revised Text   ● New Code   ▲ Revised Code Title

✓5ᵗʰ **T61.8** **Toxic effect of other seafood**

    ✓6ᵗʰ **T61.8X** **Toxic effect of** other seafood

       ✓7ᵗʰ **T61.8X1** **Toxic effect of other seafood, accidental (unintentional)**

       ✓7ᵗʰ **T61.8X2** **Toxic effect of other seafood, intentional self-harm**

       ✓7ᵗʰ **T61.8X3** **Toxic effect of other seafood, assault**

       ✓7ᵗʰ **T61.8X4** **Toxic effect of other seafood, undetermined**

✓5ᵗʰ **T61.9** **Toxic effect of** unspecified **seafood**

    ✓x7ᵗʰ **T61.91** **Toxic effect of unspecified seafood, accidental (unintentional)**

    ✓x7ᵗʰ **T61.92** **Toxic effect of unspecified seafood, intentional self-harm**

    ✓x7ᵗʰ **T61.93** **Toxic effect of unspecified seafood, assault**

    ✓x7ᵗʰ **T61.94** **Toxic effect of unspecified seafood, undetermined**

✓4ᵗʰ **T62** **Toxic effect of other noxious substances eaten as food**

    EXCLUDES 1   *allergic reaction to food, such as:*
       anaphylactic shock (reaction) due to adverse food reaction (T78.0-)
       dermatitis (L23.6, L25.4, L27.2)
       gastroenteritis (noninfective) (K52.2)
       bacterial food borne intoxications (A05.-)
       toxic effect of aflatoxin and other mycotoxins (T64)
       toxic effect of cyanides (T65.0-)
       toxic effect of hydrogen cyanide (T57.3-)
       toxic effect of mercury (T56.1-)

    The appropriate 7th character is to be added to each code from category T62.
    A   initial encounter
    D   subsequent encounter
    S   sequela

✓5ᵗʰ **T62.0** **Toxic effect of ingested mushrooms**

    ✓6ᵗʰ **T62.0X** **Toxic effect of** ingested mushrooms

       ✓7ᵗʰ **T62.0X1** **Toxic effect of ingested mushrooms, accidental (unintentional)**
          Toxic effect of ingested mushrooms NOS

       ✓7ᵗʰ **T62.0X2** **Toxic effect of ingested mushrooms, intentional self-harm**

       ✓7ᵗʰ **T62.0X3** **Toxic effect of ingested mushrooms, assault**

       ✓7ᵗʰ **T62.0X4** **Toxic effect of ingested mushrooms, undetermined**

✓5ᵗʰ **T62.1** **Toxic effect of ingested berries**

    ✓6ᵗʰ **T62.1X** **Toxic effect of** ingested berries

       ✓7ᵗʰ **T62.1X1** **Toxic effect of ingested berries, accidental (unintentional)**
          Toxic effect of ingested berries NOS

       ✓7ᵗʰ **T62.1X2** **Toxic effect of ingested berries, intentional self-harm**

       ✓7ᵗʰ **T62.1X3** **Toxic effect of ingested berries, assault**

       ✓7ᵗʰ **T62.1X4** **Toxic effect of ingested berries, undetermined**

✓5ᵗʰ **T62.2** **Toxic effect of other ingested (parts of) plant(s)**

    ✓6ᵗʰ **T62.2X** **Toxic effect of** other ingested (parts of) plant(s)

       ✓7ᵗʰ **T62.2X1** **Toxic effect of other ingested (parts of) plant(s), accidental (unintentional)**
          Toxic effect of other ingested (parts of) plant(s) NOS

       ✓7ᵗʰ **T62.2X2** **Toxic effect of other ingested (parts of) plant(s), intentional self-harm**

       ✓7ᵗʰ **T62.2X3** **Toxic effect of other ingested (parts of) plant(s), assault**

       ✓7ᵗʰ **T62.2X4** **Toxic effect of other ingested (parts of) plant(s), undetermined**

✓5ᵗʰ **T62.8** **Toxic effect of other specified** noxious substances eaten as food

    ✓6ᵗʰ **T62.8X** **Toxic effect of** other specified noxious substances eaten as food

       ✓7ᵗʰ **T62.8X1** **Toxic effect of other specified noxious substances eaten as food, accidental (unintentional)**
          Toxic effect of other specified noxious substances eaten as food NOS

       ✓7ᵗʰ **T62.8X2** **Toxic effect of other specified noxious substances eaten as food, intentional self-harm**

       ✓7ᵗʰ **T62.8X3** **Toxic effect of other specified noxious substances eaten as food, assault**

       ✓7ᵗʰ **T62.8X4** **Toxic effect of other specified noxious substances eaten as food, undetermined**

✓5ᵗʰ **T62.9** **Toxic effect of** unspecified **noxious substance eaten as food**

    ✓x7ᵗʰ **T62.91** **Toxic effect of unspecified noxious substance eaten as food, accidental (unintentional)**
       Toxic effect of unspecified noxious substance eaten as food NOS

    ✓x7ᵗʰ **T62.92** **Toxic effect of unspecified noxious substance eaten as food, intentional self-harm**

    ✓x7ᵗʰ **T62.93** **Toxic effect of unspecified noxious substance eaten as food, assault**

    ✓x7ᵗʰ **T62.94** **Toxic effect of unspecified noxious substance eaten as food, undetermined**

✓4ᵗʰ **T63** **Toxic effect of contact with venomous animals and plants**

    INCLUDES   bite or touch of venomous animal
       pricked or stuck by thorn or leaf

    EXCLUDES 2   *ingestion of toxic animal or plant (T61.-, T62.-)*

    The appropriate 7th character is to be added to each code from category T63.
    A   initial encounter
    D   subsequent encounter
    S   sequela

✓5ᵗʰ **T63.0** **Toxic effect of** snake venom

    ✓6ᵗʰ **T63.00** **Toxic effect of** unspecified **snake venom**

       ✓7ᵗʰ **T63.001** **Toxic effect of unspecified snake venom, accidental (unintentional)**
          Toxic effect of unspecified snake venom NOS

       ✓7ᵗʰ **T63.002** **Toxic effect of unspecified snake venom, intentional self-harm**

       ✓7ᵗʰ **T63.003** **Toxic effect of unspecified snake venom, assault**

       ✓7ᵗʰ **T63.004** **Toxic effect of unspecified snake venom, undetermined**

    ✓6ᵗʰ **T63.01** **Toxic effect of** rattlesnake **venom**

       ✓7ᵗʰ **T63.011** **Toxic effect of rattlesnake venom, accidental (unintentional)**
          Toxic effect of rattlesnake venom NOS

       ✓7ᵗʰ **T63.012** **Toxic effect of rattlesnake venom, intentional self-harm**

       ✓7ᵗʰ **T63.013** **Toxic effect of rattlesnake venom, assault**

       ✓7ᵗʰ **T63.014** **Toxic effect of rattlesnake venom, undetermined**

    ✓6ᵗʰ **T63.02** **Toxic effect of** coral snake **venom**

       ✓7ᵗʰ **T63.021** **Toxic effect of coral snake venom, accidental (unintentional)**
          Toxic effect of coral snake venom NOS

       ✓7ᵗʰ **T63.022** **Toxic effect of coral snake venom, intentional self-harm**

       ✓7ᵗʰ **T63.023** **Toxic effect of coral snake venom, assault**

       ✓7ᵗʰ **T63.024** **Toxic effect of coral snake venom, undetermined**

    ✓6ᵗʰ **T63.03** **Toxic effect of** taipan **venom**

       ✓7ᵗʰ **T63.031** **Toxic effect of taipan venom, accidental (unintentional)**
          Toxic effect of taipan venom NOS

       ✓7ᵗʰ **T63.032** **Toxic effect of taipan venom, intentional self-harm**

       ✓7ᵗʰ **T63.033** **Toxic effect of taipan venom, assault**

       ✓7ᵗʰ **T63.034** **Toxic effect of taipan venom, undetermined**

    ✓6ᵗʰ **T63.04** **Toxic effect of** cobra **venom**

       ✓7ᵗʰ **T63.041** **Toxic effect of cobra venom, accidental (unintentional)**
          Toxic effect of cobra venom NOS

       ✓7ᵗʰ **T63.042** **Toxic effect of cobra venom, intentional self-harm**

       ✓7ᵗʰ **T63.043** **Toxic effect of cobra venom, assault**

EXCLUDES 1 Not coded here   EXCLUDES 2 Not included here   N Newborn Age: 0   P Pediatric Age: 0-17   M Maternity Age: 12-55   A Adult Age: 15-124

☑7ᵗʰ **T63.044 Toxic effect of cobra venom,** undetermined

☑6ᵗʰ **T63.06 Toxic effect of venom of** other North and South American snake

    ☑7ᵗʰ **T63.061 Toxic effect of venom of other North and South American snake,** accidental (unintentional)
        Toxic effect of venom of other North and South American snake NOS

    ☑7ᵗʰ **T63.062 Toxic effect of venom of other North and South American snake,** intentional self-harm

    ☑7ᵗʰ **T63.063 Toxic effect of venom of other North and South American snake,** assault

    ☑7ᵗʰ **T63.064 Toxic effect of venom of other North and South American snake,** undetermined

☑6ᵗʰ **T63.07 Toxic effect of venom of** other Australian snake

    ☑7ᵗʰ **T63.071 Toxic effect of venom of other Australian snake,** accidental (unintentional)
        Toxic effect of venom of other Australian snake NOS

    ☑7ᵗʰ **T63.072 Toxic effect of venom of other Australian snake,** intentional self-harm

    ☑7ᵗʰ **T63.073 Toxic effect of venom of other Australian snake,** assault

    ☑7ᵗʰ **T63.074 Toxic effect of venom of other Australian snake,** undetermined

☑6ᵗʰ **T63.08 Toxic effect of venom of** other African and Asian snake

    ☑7ᵗʰ **T63.081 Toxic effect of venom of other African and Asian snake,** accidental (unintentional)
        Toxic effect of venom of other African and Asian snake NOS

    ☑7ᵗʰ **T63.082 Toxic effect of venom of other African and Asian snake,** intentional self-harm

    ☑7ᵗʰ **T63.083 Toxic effect of venom of other African and Asian snake,** assault

    ☑7ᵗʰ **T63.084 Toxic effect of venom of other African and Asian snake,** undetermined

☑6ᵗʰ **T63.09 Toxic effect of venom of** other snake

    ☑7ᵗʰ **T63.091 Toxic effect of venom of other snake,** accidental (unintentional)
        Toxic effect of venom of other snake NOS

    ☑7ᵗʰ **T63.092 Toxic effect of venom of other snake,** intentional self-harm

    ☑7ᵗʰ **T63.093 Toxic effect of venom of other snake,** assault

    ☑7ᵗʰ **T63.094 Toxic effect of venom of other snake,** undetermined

☑5ᵗʰ **T63.1 Toxic effect of venom of** other reptiles

☑6ᵗʰ **T63.11 Toxic effect of venom of** gila monster

    ☑7ᵗʰ **T63.111 Toxic effect of venom of gila monster,** accidental (unintentional)
        Toxic effect of venom of gila monster NOS

    ☑7ᵗʰ **T63.112 Toxic effect of venom of gila monster,** intentional self-harm

    ☑7ᵗʰ **T63.113 Toxic effect of venom of gila monster,** assault

    ☑7ᵗʰ **T63.114 Toxic effect of venom of gila monster,** undetermined

☑6ᵗʰ **T63.12 Toxic effect of venom of** other venomous lizard

    ☑7ᵗʰ **T63.121 Toxic effect of venom of other venomous lizard,** accidental (unintentional)
        Toxic effect of venom of other venomous lizard NOS

    ☑7ᵗʰ **T63.122 Toxic effect of venom of other venomous lizard,** intentional self-harm

    ☑7ᵗʰ **T63.123 Toxic effect of venom of other venomous lizard,** assault

    ☑7ᵗʰ **T63.124 Toxic effect of venom of other venomous lizard,** undetermined

☑6ᵗʰ **T63.19 Toxic effect of venom of** other reptiles

    ☑7ᵗʰ **T63.191 Toxic effect of venom of other reptiles,** accidental (unintentional)
        Toxic effect of venom of other reptiles NOS

    ☑7ᵗʰ **T63.192 Toxic effect of venom of other reptiles,** intentional self-harm

    ☑7ᵗʰ **T63.193 Toxic effect of venom of other reptiles,** assault

    ☑7ᵗʰ **T63.194 Toxic effect of venom of other reptiles,** undetermined

☑5ᵗʰ **T63.2 Toxic effect of venom of** scorpion

☑6ᵗʰ **T63.2X Toxic effect of venom of scorpion**

    ☑7ᵗʰ **T63.2X1 Toxic effect of venom of scorpion,** accidental (unintentional)
        Toxic effect of venom of scorpion NOS

    ☑7ᵗʰ **T63.2X2 Toxic effect of venom of scorpion,** intentional self-harm

    ☑7ᵗʰ **T63.2X3 Toxic effect of venom of scorpion,** assault

    ☑7ᵗʰ **T63.2X4 Toxic effect of venom of scorpion,** undetermined

☑5ᵗʰ **T63.3 Toxic effect of venom of** spider

☑6ᵗʰ **T63.30 Toxic effect of** unspecified spider venom

    ☑7ᵗʰ **T63.301 Toxic effect of unspecified spider venom,** accidental (unintentional)

    ☑7ᵗʰ **T63.302 Toxic effect of unspecified spider venom,** intentional self-harm

    ☑7ᵗʰ **T63.303 Toxic effect of unspecified spider venom,** assault

    ☑7ᵗʰ **T63.304 Toxic effect of unspecified spider venom,** undetermined

☑6ᵗʰ **T63.31 Toxic effect of venom of** black widow spider

    ☑7ᵗʰ **T63.311 Toxic effect of venom of black widow spider,** accidental (unintentional)

    ☑7ᵗʰ **T63.312 Toxic effect of venom of black widow spider,** intentional self-harm

    ☑7ᵗʰ **T63.313 Toxic effect of venom of black widow spider,** assault

    ☑7ᵗʰ **T63.314 Toxic effect of venom of black widow spider,** undetermined

☑6ᵗʰ **T63.32 Toxic effect of venom of** tarantula

    ☑7ᵗʰ **T63.321 Toxic effect of venom of tarantula,** accidental (unintentional)

    ☑7ᵗʰ **T63.322 Toxic effect of venom of tarantula,** intentional self-harm

    ☑7ᵗʰ **T63.323 Toxic effect of venom of tarantula,** assault

    ☑7ᵗʰ **T63.324 Toxic effect of venom of tarantula,** undetermined

☑6ᵗʰ **T63.33 Toxic effect of venom of** brown recluse spider

    ☑7ᵗʰ **T63.331 Toxic effect of venom of brown recluse spider,** accidental (unintentional)

    ☑7ᵗʰ **T63.332 Toxic effect of venom of brown recluse spider,** intentional self-harm

    ☑7ᵗʰ **T63.333 Toxic effect of venom of brown recluse spider,** assault

    ☑7ᵗʰ **T63.334 Toxic effect of venom of brown recluse spider,** undetermined

☑6ᵗʰ **T63.39 Toxic effect of venom of** other spider

    ☑7ᵗʰ **T63.391 Toxic effect of venom of other spider,** accidental (unintentional)

    ☑7ᵗʰ **T63.392 Toxic effect of venom of other spider,** intentional self-harm

    ☑7ᵗʰ **T63.393 Toxic effect of venom of other spider,** assault

    ☑7ᵗʰ **T63.394 Toxic effect of venom of other spider,** undetermined

☑5ᵗʰ **T63.4 Toxic effect of venom of** other arthropods

☑6ᵗʰ **T63.41 Toxic effect of venom of** centipedes and venomous millipedes

    ☑7ᵗʰ **T63.411 Toxic effect of venom of centipedes and venomous millipedes,** accidental (unintentional)

    ☑7ᵗʰ **T63.412 Toxic effect of venom of centipedes and venomous millipedes,** intentional self-harm

    ☑7ᵗʰ **T63.413 Toxic effect of venom of centipedes and venomous millipedes,** assault

    ☑7ᵗʰ **T63.414 Toxic effect of venom of centipedes and venomous millipedes,** undetermined

---

☑ Additional Character Required   ☒x7ᵗʰ Placeholder Alert   Unspecified Dx   Other Specified Dx   Manifestation   ►◄ Revised Text   ● New Code   ▲ Revised Code Title

√6ᵗʰ **T63.42** **Toxic effect of venom of** ants

   √7ᵗʰ **T63.421** **Toxic effect of venom of ants,** accidental **(unintentional)**

   √7ᵗʰ **T63.422** **Toxic effect of venom of ants,** intentional self-harm

   √7ᵗʰ **T63.423** **Toxic effect of venom of ants,** assault

   √7ᵗʰ **T63.424** **Toxic effect of venom of ants,** undetermined

√6ᵗʰ **T63.43** **Toxic effect of venom of** caterpillars

   √7ᵗʰ **T63.431** **Toxic effect of venom of caterpillars,** accidental **(unintentional)**

   √7ᵗʰ **T63.432** **Toxic effect of venom of caterpillars,** intentional self-harm

   √7ᵗʰ **T63.433** **Toxic effect of venom of caterpillars,** assault

   √7ᵗʰ **T63.434** **Toxic effect of venom of caterpillars,** undetermined

√6ᵗʰ **T63.44** **Toxic effect of venom of** bees

   √7ᵗʰ **T63.441** **Toxic effect of venom of bees,** accidental **(unintentional)**

   √7ᵗʰ **T63.442** **Toxic effect of venom of bees,** intentional self-harm

   √7ᵗʰ **T63.443** **Toxic effect of venom of bees,** assault

   √7ᵗʰ **T63.444** **Toxic effect of venom of bees,** undetermined

√6ᵗʰ **T63.45** **Toxic effect of venom of** hornets

   √7ᵗʰ **T63.451** **Toxic effect of venom of hornets,** accidental **(unintentional)**

   √7ᵗʰ **T63.452** **Toxic effect of venom of hornets,** intentional self-harm

   √7ᵗʰ **T63.453** **Toxic effect of venom of hornets,** assault

   √7ᵗʰ **T63.454** **Toxic effect of venom of hornets,** undetermined

√6ᵗʰ **T63.46** **Toxic effect of venom of** wasps
          Toxic effect of yellow jacket

   √7ᵗʰ **T63.461** **Toxic effect of venom of wasps,** accidental **(unintentional)**

   √7ᵗʰ **T63.462** **Toxic effect of venom of wasps,** intentional self-harm

   √7ᵗʰ **T63.463** **Toxic effect of venom of wasps,** assault

   √7ᵗʰ **T63.464** **Toxic effect of venom of wasps,** undetermined

√6ᵗʰ **T63.48** **Toxic effect of venom of** other arthropod

   √7ᵗʰ **T63.481** **Toxic effect of venom of other arthropod,** accidental **(unintentional)**

   √7ᵗʰ **T63.482** **Toxic effect of venom of other arthropod,** intentional self-harm

   √7ᵗʰ **T63.483** **Toxic effect of venom of other arthropod,** assault

   √7ᵗʰ **T63.484** **Toxic effect of venom of other arthropod,** undetermined

√5ᵗʰ **T63.5** **Toxic effect of contact with** venomous fish
   EXCLUDES 2   *poisoning by ingestion of fish (T61.-)*

√6ᵗʰ **T63.51** **Toxic effect of contact with** stingray

   √7ᵗʰ **T63.511** **Toxic effect of contact with stingray,** accidental **(unintentional)**

   √7ᵗʰ **T63.512** **Toxic effect of contact with stingray,** intentional self-harm

   √7ᵗʰ **T63.513** **Toxic effect of contact with stingray,** assault

   √7ᵗʰ **T63.514** **Toxic effect of contact with stingray,** undetermined

√6ᵗʰ **T63.59** **Toxic effect of contact with** other venomous fish

   √7ᵗʰ **T63.591** **Toxic effect of contact with other venomous fish,** accidental **(unintentional)**

   √7ᵗʰ **T63.592** **Toxic effect of contact with other venomous fish,** intentional self-harm

   √7ᵗʰ **T63.593** **Toxic effect of contact with other venomous fish,** assault

   √7ᵗʰ **T63.594** **Toxic effect of contact with other venomous fish,** undetermined

√5ᵗʰ **T63.6** **Toxic effect of contact with other** venomous marine animals
   EXCLUDES 1   *sea-snake venom (T63.09)*
   EXCLUDES 2   *poisoning by ingestion of shellfish (T61.78-)*

√6ᵗʰ **T63.61** **Toxic effect of contact with** Portugese Man-o-war
          Toxic effect of contact with bluebottle

   √7ᵗʰ **T63.611** **Toxic effect of contact with Portugese Man-o-war,** accidental **(unintentional)**

   √7ᵗʰ **T63.612** **Toxic effect of contact with Portugese Man-o-war,** intentional self-harm

   √7ᵗʰ **T63.613** **Toxic effect of contact with Portugese Man-o-war,** assault

   √7ᵗʰ **T63.614** **Toxic effect of contact with Portugese Man-o-war,** undetermined

√6ᵗʰ **T63.62** **Toxic effect of contact with** other jellyfish

   √7ᵗʰ **T63.621** **Toxic effect of contact with other jellyfish,** accidental **(unintentional)**

   √7ᵗʰ **T63.622** **Toxic effect of contact with other jellyfish,** intentional self-harm

   √7ᵗʰ **T63.623** **Toxic effect of contact with other jellyfish,** assault

   √7ᵗʰ **T63.624** **Toxic effect of contact with other jellyfish,** undetermined

√6ᵗʰ **T63.63** **Toxic effect of contact with** sea anemone

   √7ᵗʰ **T63.631** **Toxic effect of contact with sea anemone,** accidental **(unintentional)**

   √7ᵗʰ **T63.632** **Toxic effect of contact with sea anemone,** intentional self-harm

   √7ᵗʰ **T63.633** **Toxic effect of contact with sea anemone,** assault

   √7ᵗʰ **T63.634** **Toxic effect of contact with sea anemone,** undetermined

√6ᵗʰ **T63.69** **Toxic effect of contact with** other venomous marine animals

   √7ᵗʰ **T63.691** **Toxic effect of contact with other venomous marine animals,** accidental **(unintentional)**

   √7ᵗʰ **T63.692** **Toxic effect of contact with other venomous marine animals,** intentional self-harm

   √7ᵗʰ **T63.693** **Toxic effect of contact with other venomous marine animals,** assault

   √7ᵗʰ **T63.694** **Toxic effect of contact with other venomous marine animals,** undetermined

√5ᵗʰ **T63.7** **Toxic effect of contact with** venomous plant

√6ᵗʰ **T63.71** **Toxic effect of contact with venomous** marine plant

   √7ᵗʰ **T63.711** **Toxic effect of contact with venomous marine plant,** accidental **(unintentional)**

   √7ᵗʰ **T63.712** **Toxic effect of contact with venomous marine plant,** intentional self-harm

   √7ᵗʰ **T63.713** **Toxic effect of contact with venomous marine plant,** assault

   √7ᵗʰ **T63.714** **Toxic effect of contact with venomous marine plant,** undetermined

√6ᵗʰ **T63.79** **Toxic effect of contact with** other venomous plant

   √7ᵗʰ **T63.791** **Toxic effect of contact with other venomous plant,** accidental **(unintentional)**

   √7ᵗʰ **T63.792** **Toxic effect of contact with other venomous plant,** intentional self-harm

   √7ᵗʰ **T63.793** **Toxic effect of contact with other venomous plant,** assault

   √7ᵗʰ **T63.794** **Toxic effect of contact with other venomous plant,** undetermined

√5ᵗʰ **T63.8** **Toxic effect of contact with** other venomous animals

√6ᵗʰ **T63.81** **Toxic effect of contact with venomous** frog
   EXCLUDES 1   *contact with nonvenomous frog (W62.0)*

   √7ᵗʰ **T63.811** **Toxic effect of contact with venomous frog,** accidental **(unintentional)**

   √7ᵗʰ **T63.812** **Toxic effect of contact with venomous frog,** intentional self-harm

   √7ᵗʰ **T63.813** **Toxic effect of contact with venomous frog,** assault

   √7ᵗʰ **T63.814** **Toxic effect of contact with venomous frog,** undetermined

EXCLUDES 1 Not coded here   *EXCLUDES 2* Not included here   N Newborn Age: 0   P Pediatric Age: 0-17   M Maternity Age: 12-55   A Adult Age: 15-124

1014   ICD-10-CM 2016

✓6th T63.82 Toxic effect of contact with venomous toad
    EXCLUDES 1   contact with nonvenomous toad (W62.1)

    ✓7th T63.821 Toxic effect of contact with venomous toad, accidental (unintentional)

    ✓7th T63.822 Toxic effect of contact with venomous toad, intentional self-harm

    ✓7th T63.823 Toxic effect of contact with venomous toad, assault

    ✓7th T63.824 Toxic effect of contact with venomous toad, undetermined

✓6th T63.83 Toxic effect of contact with other venomous amphibian
    EXCLUDES 1   contact with nonvenomous amphibian (W62.9)

    ✓7th T63.831 Toxic effect of contact with other venomous amphibian, accidental (unintentional)

    ✓7th T63.832 Toxic effect of contact with other venomous amphibian, intentional self-harm

    ✓7th T63.833 Toxic effect of contact with other venomous amphibian, assault

    ✓7th T63.834 Toxic effect of contact with other venomous amphibian, undetermined

✓6th T63.89 Toxic effect of contact with other venomous animals

    ✓7th T63.891 Toxic effect of contact with other venomous animals, accidental (unintentional)

    ✓7th T63.892 Toxic effect of contact with other venomous animals, intentional self-harm

    ✓7th T63.893 Toxic effect of contact with other venomous animals, assault

    ✓7th T63.894 Toxic effect of contact with other venomous animals, undetermined

✓5th T63.9 Toxic effect of contact with unspecified venomous animal

    ✓x7th T63.91 Toxic effect of contact with unspecified venomous animal, accidental (unintentional)

    ✓x7th T63.92 Toxic effect of contact with unspecified venomous animal, intentional self-harm

    ✓x7th T63.93 Toxic effect of contact with unspecified venomous animal, assault

    ✓x7th T63.94 Toxic effect of contact with unspecified venomous animal, undetermined

✓4th T64 Toxic effect of aflatoxin and other mycotoxin food contaminants

> The appropriate 7th character is to be added to each code from category T64.
> A   initial encounter
> D   subsequent encounter
> S   sequela

✓5th T64.0 Toxic effect of aflatoxin

    ✓x7th T64.01 Toxic effect of aflatoxin, accidental (unintentional)

    ✓x7th T64.02 Toxic effect of aflatoxin, intentional self-harm

    ✓x7th T64.03 Toxic effect of aflatoxin, assault

    ✓x7th T64.04 Toxic effect of aflatoxin, undetermined

✓5th T64.8 Toxic effect of other mycotoxin food contaminants

    ✓x7th T64.81 Toxic effect of other mycotoxin food contaminants, accidental (unintentional)

    ✓x7th T64.82 Toxic effect of other mycotoxin food contaminants, intentional self-harm

    ✓x7th T64.83 Toxic effect of other mycotoxin food contaminants, assault

    ✓x7th T64.84 Toxic effect of other mycotoxin food contaminants, undetermined

✓4th T65 Toxic effect of other and unspecified substances

> The appropriate 7th character is to be added to each code from category T65.
> A   initial encounter
> D   subsequent encounter
> S   sequela

✓5th T65.0 Toxic effect of cyanides
    EXCLUDES 1   hydrogen cyanide (T57.3-)

    ✓6th T65.0X Toxic effect of cyanides

      ✓7th T65.0X1 Toxic effect of cyanides, accidental (unintentional)
        Toxic effect of cyanides NOS

      ✓7th T65.0X2 Toxic effect of cyanides, intentional self-harm

      ✓7th T65.0X3 Toxic effect of cyanides, assault

      ✓7th T65.0X4 Toxic effect of cyanides, undetermined

✓5th T65.1 Toxic effect of strychnine and its salts

    ✓6th T65.1X Toxic effect of strychnine and its salts

      ✓7th T65.1X1 Toxic effect of strychnine and its salts, accidental (unintentional)
        Toxic effect of strychnine and its salts NOS

      ✓7th T65.1X2 Toxic effect of strychnine and its salts, intentional self-harm

      ✓7th T65.1X3 Toxic effect of strychnine and its salts, assault

      ✓7th T65.1X4 Toxic effect of strychnine and its salts, undetermined

✓5th T65.2 Toxic effect of tobacco and nicotine
    EXCLUDES 2   nicotine dependence (F17.-)

    ✓6th T65.21 Toxic effect of chewing tobacco

      ✓7th T65.211 Toxic effect of chewing tobacco, accidental (unintentional)
        Toxic effect of chewing tobacco NOS

      ✓7th T65.212 Toxic effect of chewing tobacco, intentional self-harm

      ✓7th T65.213 Toxic effect of chewing tobacco, assault

      ✓7th T65.214 Toxic effect of chewing tobacco, undetermined

    ✓6th T65.22 Toxic effect of tobacco cigarettes
      Toxic effect of tobacco smoke
      Use additional code for exposure to second hand tobacco smoke (Z57.31, Z77.22)

      ✓7th T65.221 Toxic effect of tobacco cigarettes, accidental (unintentional)
        Toxic effect of tobacco cigarettes NOS

      ✓7th T65.222 Toxic effect of tobacco cigarettes, intentional self-harm

      ✓7th T65.223 Toxic effect of tobacco cigarettes, assault

      ✓7th T65.224 Toxic effect of tobacco cigarettes, undetermined

    ✓6th T65.29 Toxic effect of other tobacco and nicotine

      ✓7th T65.291 Toxic effect of other tobacco and nicotine, accidental (unintentional)
        Toxic effect of other tobacco and nicotine NOS

      ✓7th T65.292 Toxic effect of other tobacco and nicotine, intentional self-harm

      ✓7th T65.293 Toxic effect of other tobacco and nicotine, assault

      ✓7th T65.294 Toxic effect of other tobacco and nicotine, undetermined

✓5th T65.3 Toxic effect of nitroderivatives and aminoderivatives of benzene and its homologues
    Toxic effect of anilin [benzenamine]
    Toxic effect of nitrobenzene
    Toxic effect of trinitrotoluene

    ✓6th T65.3X Toxic effect of nitroderivatives and aminoderivatives of benzene and its homologues

      ✓7th T65.3X1 Toxic effect of nitroderivatives and aminoderivatives of benzene and its homologues, accidental (unintentional)
        Toxic effect of nitroderivatives and aminoderivatives of benzene and its homologues NOS

✓ Additional Character Required   ✓x7th Placeholder Alert   Unspecified Dx   Other Specified Dx   Manifestation   ►◄ Revised Text   ● New Code   ▲ Revised Code Title

ICD-10-CM 2016   1015

✓7ᵗʰ **T65.3X2 Toxic effect of nitroderivatives and aminoderivatives of benzene and its homologues, intentional self-harm**

✓7ᵗʰ **T65.3X3 Toxic effect of nitroderivatives and aminoderivatives of benzene and its homologues, assault**

✓7ᵗʰ **T65.3X4 Toxic effect of nitroderivatives and aminoderivatives of benzene and its homologues, undetermined**

✓5ᵗʰ **T65.4 Toxic effect of carbon disulfide**

✓6ᵗʰ **T65.4X Toxic effect of carbon disulfide**

✓7ᵗʰ **T65.4X1 Toxic effect of carbon disulfide, accidental (unintentional)**
Toxic effect of carbon disulfide NOS

✓7ᵗʰ **T65.4X2 Toxic effect of carbon disulfide, intentional self-harm**

✓7ᵗʰ **T65.4X3 Toxic effect of carbon disulfide, assault**

✓7ᵗʰ **T65.4X4 Toxic effect of carbon disulfide, undetermined**

✓5ᵗʰ **T65.5 Toxic effect of nitroglycerin and other nitric acids and esters**
Toxic effect of 1,2,3-Propanetriol trinitrate

✓6ᵗʰ **T65.5X Toxic effect of nitroglycerin and other nitric acids and esters**

✓7ᵗʰ **T65.5X1 Toxic effect of nitroglycerin and other nitric acids and esters, accidental (unintentional)**
Toxic effect of nitroglycerin and other nitric acids and esters NOS

✓7ᵗʰ **T65.5X2 Toxic effect of nitroglycerin and other nitric acids and esters, intentional self-harm**

✓7ᵗʰ **T65.5X3 Toxic effect of nitroglycerin and other nitric acids and esters, assault**

✓7ᵗʰ **T65.5X4 Toxic effect of nitroglycerin and other nitric acids and esters, undetermined**

✓5ᵗʰ **T65.6 Toxic effect of paints and dyes, not elsewhere classified**

✓6ᵗʰ **T65.6X Toxic effect of paints and dyes, not elsewhere classified**

✓7ᵗʰ **T65.6X1 Toxic effect of paints and dyes, not elsewhere classified, accidental (unintentional)**
Toxic effect of paints and dyes NOS

✓7ᵗʰ **T65.6X2 Toxic effect of paints and dyes, not elsewhere classified, intentional self-harm**

✓7ᵗʰ **T65.6X3 Toxic effect of paints and dyes, not elsewhere classified, assault**

✓7ᵗʰ **T65.6X4 Toxic effect of paints and dyes, not elsewhere classified, undetermined**

✓5ᵗʰ **T65.8 Toxic effect of other specified substances**

✓6ᵗʰ **T65.81 Toxic effect of latex**

✓7ᵗʰ **T65.811 Toxic effect of latex, accidental (unintentional)**
Toxic effect of latex NOS

✓7ᵗʰ **T65.812 Toxic effect of latex, intentional self-harm**

✓7ᵗʰ **T65.813 Toxic effect of latex, assault**

✓7ᵗʰ **T65.814 Toxic effect of latex, undetermined**

✓6ᵗʰ **T65.82 Toxic effect of harmful algae and algae toxins**
Toxic effect of (harmful) algae bloom NOS
Toxic effect of blue-green algae bloom
Toxic effect of brown tide
Toxic effect of cyanobacteria bloom
Toxic effect of Florida red tide
Toxic effect of pfiesteria piscicida
Toxic effect of red tide

✓7ᵗʰ **T65.821 Toxic effect of harmful algae and algae toxins, accidental (unintentional)**
Toxic effect of harmful algae and algae toxins NOS

✓7ᵗʰ **T65.822 Toxic effect of harmful algae and algae toxins, intentional self-harm**

✓7ᵗʰ **T65.823 Toxic effect of harmful algae and algae toxins, assault**

✓7ᵗʰ **T65.824 Toxic effect of harmful algae and algae toxins, undetermined**

✓6ᵗʰ **T65.83 Toxic effect of fiberglass**

✓7ᵗʰ **T65.831 Toxic effect of fiberglass, accidental (unintentional)**
Toxic effect of fiberglass NOS

✓7ᵗʰ **T65.832 Toxic effect of fiberglass, intentional self-harm**

✓7ᵗʰ **T65.833 Toxic effect of fiberglass, assault**

✓7ᵗʰ **T65.834 Toxic effect of fiberglass, undetermined**

✓6ᵗʰ **T65.89 Toxic effect of other specified substances**

✓7ᵗʰ **T65.891 Toxic effect of other specified substances, accidental (unintentional)**
Toxic effect of other specified substances NOS

✓7ᵗʰ **T65.892 Toxic effect of other specified substances, intentional self-harm**

✓7ᵗʰ **T65.893 Toxic effect of other specified substances, assault**

✓7ᵗʰ **T65.894 Toxic effect of other specified substances, undetermined**

✓5ᵗʰ **T65.9 Toxic effect of unspecified substance**

✓x7ᵗʰ **T65.91 Toxic effect of unspecified substance, accidental (unintentional)**
Poisoning NOS

✓x7ᵗʰ **T65.92 Toxic effect of unspecified substance, intentional self-harm**

✓x7ᵗʰ **T65.93 Toxic effect of unspecified substance, assault**

✓x7ᵗʰ **T65.94 Toxic effect of unspecified substance, undetermined**

Other and unspecified effects of external causes (T66-T78)

✓x7ᵗʰ **T66 Radiation sickness, unspecified**

EXCLUDES 1 *specified adverse effects of radiation, such as:*
burns (T20-T31)
leukemia (C91-C95)
radiation gastroenteritis and colitis (K52.0)
radiation pneumonitis (J70.0)
radiation related disorders of the skin and subcutaneous tissue (L55-L59)
radiation sunburn (L55.-)

The appropriate 7th character is to be added to code T66.
A   initial encounter
D   subsequent encounter
S   sequela

✓4ᵗʰ **T67 Effects of heat and light**

EXCLUDES 1 *erythema [dermatitis] ab igne (L59.0)*
malignant hyperpyrexia due to anesthesia (T88.3)
radiation-related disorders of the skin and subcutaneous tissue (L55-L59)

EXCLUDES 2 *burns (T20-T31)*
sunburn (L55.-)
sweat disorder due to heat (L74-L75)

The appropriate 7th character is to be added to each code from category T67.
A   initial encounter
D   subsequent encounter
S   sequela

✓x7ᵗʰ **T67.0 Heatstroke and sunstroke**
Heat apoplexy   Siriasis
Heat pyrexia   Thermoplegia
Use additional code(s) to identify any associated complications of heatstroke, such as:
coma and stupor (R40.-)
systemic inflammatory response syndrome (R65.1-)

✓x7ᵗʰ **T67.1 Heat syncope**
Heat collapse

✓x7ᵗʰ **T67.2 Heat cramp**

✓x7ᵗʰ **T67.3 Heat exhaustion, anhydrotic**
Heat prostration due to water depletion
EXCLUDES 1 *heat exhaustion due to salt depletion (T67.4)*

✓x7ᵗʰ **T67.4 Heat exhaustion due to salt depletion**
Heat prostration due to salt (and water) depletion

✓x7ᵗʰ **T67.5 Heat exhaustion, unspecified**
Heat prostration NOS

✓x7ᵗʰ **T67.6 Heat fatigue, transient**

✓x7ᵗʰ **T67.7 Heat edema**

✓x7ᵗʰ **T67.8 Other effects of heat and light**

√x 7ᵗʰ **T67.9** **Effect of heat and light, unspecified**

√x 7ᵗʰ **T68** **Hypothermia**
Accidental hypothermia   Hypothermia NOS
Use additional code to identify source of exposure:
    exposure to excessive cold of man-made origin (W93)
    exposure to excessive cold of natural origin (X31)
    EXCLUDES 1 *hypothermia following anesthesia (T88.51)*
        hypothermia not associated with low environmental
            temperature (R68.0)
        hypothermia of newborn (P80.-)
    EXCLUDES 2 *frostbite (T33-T34)*

The appropriate 7th character is to be added to code T68.
A   initial encounter
D   subsequent encounter
S   sequela

√4ᵗʰ **T69** **Other effects of reduced temperature**
Use additional code to identify source of exposure:
    exposure to excessive cold of man-made origin (W93)
    exposure to excessive cold of natural origin (X31)
    EXCLUDES 2 *frostbite (T33-T34)*

The appropriate 7th character is to be added to each code from
category T69.
A   initial encounter
D   subsequent encounter
S   sequela

√5ᵗʰ **T69.0** **Immersion hand and foot**
    √6ᵗʰ **T69.01** **Immersion hand**
        √7ᵗʰ **T69.011** **Immersion hand, right hand**
        √7ᵗʰ **T69.012** **Immersion hand, left hand**
        √7ᵗʰ **T69.019** **Immersion hand, unspecified hand**
    √6ᵗʰ **T69.02** **Immersion foot**
        Trench foot
        √7ᵗʰ **T69.021** **Immersion foot, right foot**
        √7ᵗʰ **T69.022** **Immersion foot, left foot**
        √7ᵗʰ **T69.029** **Immersion foot, unspecified foot**
√x 7ᵗʰ **T69.1** **Chilblains**
√x 7ᵗʰ **T69.8** **Other specified effects of reduced temperature**
√x 7ᵗʰ **T69.9** **Effect of reduced temperature, unspecified**

√4ᵗʰ **T70** **Effects of air pressure and water pressure**

The appropriate 7th character is to be added to each code from
category T70.
A   initial encounter
D   subsequent encounter
S   sequela

√x 7ᵗʰ **T70.0** **Otitic barotrauma**
Aero-otitis media
Effects of change in ambient atmospheric pressure or water
    pressure on ears

√x 7ᵗʰ **T70.1** **Sinus barotrauma**
Aerosinusitis
Effects of change in ambient atmospheric pressure on sinuses

√5ᵗʰ **T70.2** **Other and unspecified effects of high altitude**
    EXCLUDES 2 *polycythemia due to high altitude (D75.1)*
    √x 7ᵗʰ **T70.20** **Unspecified effects of high altitude**
    √x 7ᵗʰ **T70.29** **Other effects of high altitude**
        Alpine sickness
        Anoxia due to high altitude
        Barotrauma NOS
        Hypobaropathy
        Mountain sickness

√x 7ᵗʰ **T70.3** **Caisson disease [decompression sickness]**
Compressed-air disease
Diver's palsy or paralysis

√x 7ᵗʰ **T70.4** **Effects of high-pressure fluids**
Hydraulic jet injection (industrial)
Pneumatic jet injection (industrial)
Traumatic jet injection (industrial)

√x 7ᵗʰ **T70.8** **Other effects of air pressure and water pressure**
√x 7ᵗʰ **T70.9** **Effect of air pressure and water pressure, unspecified**

√4ᵗʰ **T71** **Asphyxiation**
Mechanical suffocation
Traumatic suffocation
    EXCLUDES 1 *acute respiratory distress (syndrome) (J80)*
        anoxia due to high altitude (T70.2)
        asphyxia NOS (R09.01)
        asphyxia from carbon monoxide (T58.-)
        asphyxia from inhalation of food or foreign body (T17.-)
        asphyxia from other gases, fumes and vapors (T59.-)
        respiratory distress (syndrome) in newborn (P22.-)

The appropriate 7th character is to be added to each code from
category T71.
A   initial encounter
D   subsequent encounter
S   sequela

√5ᵗʰ **T71.1** **Asphyxiation due to mechanical threat to breathing**
Suffocation due to mechanical threat to breathing
    √6ᵗʰ **T71.11** **Asphyxiation due to smothering under pillow**
        √7ᵗʰ **T71.111** **Asphyxiation due to smothering under
            pillow, accidental**
            Asphyxiation due to smothering under
                pillow NOS
        √7ᵗʰ **T71.112** **Asphyxiation due to smothering under
            pillow, intentional self-harm**
        √7ᵗʰ **T71.113** **Asphyxiation due to smothering under
            pillow, assault**
        √7ᵗʰ **T71.114** **Asphyxiation due to smothering under
            pillow, undetermined**
    √6ᵗʰ **T71.12** **Asphyxiation due to plastic bag**
        √7ᵗʰ **T71.121** **Asphyxiation due to plastic bag,
            accidental**
            Asphyxiation due to plastic bag NOS
        √7ᵗʰ **T71.122** **Asphyxiation due to plastic bag,
            intentional self-harm**
        √7ᵗʰ **T71.123** **Asphyxiation due to plastic bag, assault**
        √7ᵗʰ **T71.124** **Asphyxiation due to plastic bag,
            undetermined**
    √6ᵗʰ **T71.13** **Asphyxiation due to being trapped in bed linens**
        √7ᵗʰ **T71.131** **Asphyxiation due to being trapped in bed
            linens, accidental**
            Asphyxiation due to being trapped in bed
                linens NOS
        √7ᵗʰ **T71.132** **Asphyxiation due to being trapped in bed
            linens, intentional self-harm**
        √7ᵗʰ **T71.133** **Asphyxiation due to being trapped in bed
            linens, assault**
        √7ᵗʰ **T71.134** **Asphyxiation due to being trapped in bed
            linens, undetermined**
    √6ᵗʰ **T71.14** **Asphyxiation due to smothering under another
        person's body (in bed)**
        √7ᵗʰ **T71.141** **Asphyxiation due to smothering under
            another person's body (in bed), accidental**
            Asphyxiation due to smothering under
                another person's body (in bed) NOS
        √7ᵗʰ **T71.143** **Asphyxiation due to smothering under
            another person's body (in bed), assault**
        √7ᵗʰ **T71.144** **Asphyxiation due to smothering under
            another person's body (in bed),
            undetermined**
    √6ᵗʰ **T71.15** **Asphyxiation due to smothering in furniture**
        √7ᵗʰ **T71.151** **Asphyxiation due to smothering in
            furniture, accidental**
            Asphyxiation due to smothering in
                furniture NOS
        √7ᵗʰ **T71.152** **Asphyxiation due to smothering in
            furniture, intentional self-harm**
        √7ᵗʰ **T71.153** **Asphyxiation due to smothering in
            furniture, assault**
        √7ᵗʰ **T71.154** **Asphyxiation due to smothering in
            furniture, undetermined**

✓ Additional Character Required   √x 7ᵗʰ Placeholder Alert   Unspecified Dx   Other Specified Dx   Manifestation   ▶◀ Revised Text   ● New Code   ▲ Revised Code Title

Chapter 19. Injury, Poisoning, and Certain Other Consequences of External Causes

√6ᵗʰ **T71.16** **Asphyxiation due to** hanging
Hanging by window shade cord
Use additional code for any associated injuries, such as:
    crushing injury of neck (S17.-)
    fracture of cervical vertebrae (S12.Ø-S12.2-)
    open wound of neck (S11.-)

    √7ᵗʰ **T71.161** **Asphyxiation due to hanging,** accidental
Asphyxiation due to hanging NOS
Hanging NOS

    √7ᵗʰ **T71.162** **Asphyxiation due to hanging,** intentional self-harm

    √7ᵗʰ **T71.163** **Asphyxiation due to hanging,** assault

    √7ᵗʰ **T71.164** **Asphyxiation due to hanging,** undetermined

√6ᵗʰ **T71.19** **Asphyxiation due to mechanical threat to breathing due to other causes**

    √7ᵗʰ **T71.191** **Asphyxiation due to mechanical threat to breathing due to other causes,** accidental
Asphyxiation due to other causes NOS

    √7ᵗʰ **T71.192** **Asphyxiation due to mechanical threat to breathing due to other causes,** intentional self-harm

    √7ᵗʰ **T71.193** **Asphyxiation due to mechanical threat to breathing due to other causes,** assault

    √7ᵗʰ **T71.194** **Asphyxiation due to mechanical threat to breathing due to other causes,** undetermined

√5ᵗʰ **T71.2** **Asphyxiation due to** systemic oxygen deficiency due to low oxygen content in ambient air
Suffocation due to systemic oxygen deficiency due to low oxygen content in ambient air

    √x7ᵗʰ **T71.2Ø** **Asphyxiation due to systemic oxygen deficiency due to low oxygen content in ambient air due to unspecified cause**

    √x7ᵗʰ **T71.21** **Asphyxiation due to** cave-in or falling earth
Use additional code for any associated cataclysm (X34-X38)

√6ᵗʰ **T71.22** **Asphyxiation due to** being trapped in a car trunk

    √7ᵗʰ **T71.221** **Asphyxiation due to being trapped in a car trunk,** accidental

    √7ᵗʰ **T71.222** **Asphyxiation due to being trapped in a car trunk,** intentional self-harm

    √7ᵗʰ **T71.223** **Asphyxiation due to being trapped in a car trunk,** assault

    √7ᵗʰ **T71.224** **Asphyxiation due to being trapped in a car trunk,** undetermined

√6ᵗʰ **T71.23** **Asphyxiation due to being** trapped in a **(discarded) refrigerator**

    √7ᵗʰ **T71.231** **Asphyxiation due to being trapped in a (discarded) refrigerator,** accidental

    √7ᵗʰ **T71.232** **Asphyxiation due to being trapped in a (discarded) refrigerator,** intentional self-harm

    √7ᵗʰ **T71.233** **Asphyxiation due to being trapped in a (discarded) refrigerator,** assault

    √7ᵗʰ **T71.234** **Asphyxiation due to being trapped in a (discarded) refrigerator,** undetermined

    √x7ᵗʰ **T71.29** **Asphyxiation due to being trapped in other low oxygen environment**

√x7ᵗʰ **T71.9** **Asphyxiation due to unspecified cause**
Suffocation (by strangulation) due to unspecified cause
Suffocation NOS
Systemic oxygen deficiency due to low oxygen content in ambient air due to unspecified cause
Systemic oxygen deficiency due to mechanical threat to breathing due to unspecified cause
Traumatic asphyxia NOS

√4ᵗʰ **T73** **Effects of other deprivation**

The appropriate 7th character is to be added to each code from category T73.
A   initial encounter
D   subsequent encounter
S   sequela

√x7ᵗʰ **T73.Ø** **Starvation**
Deprivation of food

√x7ᵗʰ **T73.1** **Deprivation of water**

√x7ᵗʰ **T73.2** **Exhaustion due to exposure**

√x7ᵗʰ **T73.3** **Exhaustion due to excessive exertion**
Exhaustion due to overexertion

√x7ᵗʰ **T73.8** **Other effects of deprivation**

√x7ᵗʰ **T73.9** **Effect of deprivation, unspecified**

√4ᵗʰ **T74** **Adult and child abuse, neglect and other maltreatment, confirmed**
Use additional code, if applicable, to identify any associated current injury
Use additional external cause code to identify perpetrator, if known (YØ7.-)
EXCLUDES 1   abuse and maltreatment in pregnancy (O9A.3-, O9A.4-, O9A.5-)
        adult and child maltreatment, suspected (T76.-)

The appropriate 7th character is to be added to each code from category T74.
A   initial encounter
D   subsequent encounter
S   sequela

√5ᵗʰ **T74.Ø** **Neglect or abandonment, confirmed**

    √x7ᵗʰ **T74.Ø1** **Adult neglect or abandonment, confirmed** Ⓐ

    √x7ᵗʰ **T74.Ø2** **Child neglect or abandonment, confirmed** Ⓟ

√5ᵗʰ **T74.1** **Physical abuse, confirmed**
EXCLUDES 2   sexual abuse (T74.2-)

    √x7ᵗʰ **T74.11** **Adult physical abuse, confirmed** Ⓐ

    √x7ᵗʰ **T74.12** **Child physical abuse, confirmed** Ⓟ
        EXCLUDES 2   shaken infant syndrome (T74.4)

√5ᵗʰ **T74.2** **Sexual abuse, confirmed**
Rape, confirmed
Sexual assault, confirmed

    √x7ᵗʰ **T74.21** **Adult sexual abuse, confirmed** Ⓐ

    √x7ᵗʰ **T74.22** **Child sexual abuse, confirmed** Ⓟ

√5ᵗʰ **T74.3** **Psychological abuse, confirmed**

    √x7ᵗʰ **T74.31** **Adult psychological abuse, confirmed** Ⓐ

    √x7ᵗʰ **T74.32** **Child psychological abuse, confirmed** Ⓟ

√x7ᵗʰ **T74.4** **Shaken infant syndrome** Ⓟ

√5ᵗʰ **T74.9** **Unspecified maltreatment, confirmed**

    √x7ᵗʰ **T74.91** **Unspecified** adult **maltreatment, confirmed** Ⓐ

    √x7ᵗʰ **T74.92** **Unspecified** child **maltreatment, confirmed** Ⓟ

√4ᵗʰ **T75** **Other and unspecified effects of other external causes**
EXCLUDES 1   adverse effects NEC (T78.-)
EXCLUDES 2   burns (electric) (T2Ø-T31)

The appropriate 7th character is to be added to each code from category T75.
A   initial encounter
D   subsequent encounter
S   sequela

√5ᵗʰ **T75.Ø** **Effects of lightning**
Struck by lightning

    √x7ᵗʰ **T75.ØØ** **Unspecified effects of lightning**
Struck by lightning NOS

    √x7ᵗʰ **T75.Ø1** **Shock due to being struck by lightning**

    √x7ᵗʰ **T75.Ø9** **Other effects of lightning**
Use additional code for other effects of lightning

√x7ᵗʰ **T75.1** **Unspecified effects of drowning and nonfatal submersion**
Immersion
EXCLUDES 1   specified effects of drowning—code to effects

√5ᵗʰ **T75.2** **Effects of vibration**

    √x7ᵗʰ **T75.2Ø** **Unspecified effects of vibration**

    √x7ᵗʰ **T75.21** **Pneumatic hammer syndrome**

    √x7ᵗʰ **T75.22** **Traumatic vasospastic syndrome**

    √x7ᵗʰ **T75.23** **Vertigo from infrasound**
EXCLUDES 1   vertigo NOS (R42)

    √x7ᵗʰ **T75.29** **Other effects of vibration**

√x7ᵗʰ **T75.3** **Motion sickness**
Airsickness
Seasickness
Travel sickness
Use additional external cause code to identify vehicle or type of motion (Y92.81-, Y93.5-)

EXCLUDES 1 Not coded here   *EXCLUDES 2* Not included here   Ⓝ Newborn Age: 0   Ⓟ Pediatric Age: 0-17   Ⓜ Maternity Age: 12-55   Ⓐ Adult Age: 15-124

1018   ICD-10-CM 2016

✓x7ᵗʰ **T75.4 Electrocution**
　　　Shock from electric current
　　　Shock from electroshock gun (taser)

✓5ᵗʰ **T75.8 Other specified effects of external causes**

　　✓x7ᵗʰ **T75.81 Effects of abnormal gravitation [G] forces**

　　✓x7ᵗʰ **T75.82 Effects of weightlessness**

　　✓x7ᵗʰ **T75.89 Other specified effects of external causes**

✓4ᵗʰ **T76 Adult and child abuse, neglect and other maltreatment, suspected**
　　　Use additional code, if applicable, to identify any associated current injury
　　　EXCLUDES 1　*adult and child maltreatment, confirmed (T74.-)*
　　　　　suspected abuse and maltreatment in pregnancy (O9A.3-, O9A.4-, O9A.5-)
　　　　　suspected adult physical abuse, ruled out (Z04.71)
　　　　　suspected adult sexual abuse, ruled out (Z04.41)
　　　　　suspected child physical abuse, ruled out (Z04.72)
　　　　　suspected child sexual abuse, ruled out (Z04.42)

　　The appropriate 7th character is to be added to each code from category T76.
　　A　initial encounter
　　D　subsequent encounter
　　S　sequela

✓5ᵗʰ **T76.0 Neglect or abandonment, suspected**

　　✓x7ᵗʰ **T76.01 Adult neglect or abandonment, suspected**　Ⓐ

　　✓x7ᵗʰ **T76.02 Child neglect or abandonment, suspected**　Ⓟ

✓5ᵗʰ **T76.1 Physical abuse, suspected**

　　✓x7ᵗʰ **T76.11 Adult physical abuse, suspected**　Ⓐ

　　✓x7ᵗʰ **T76.12 Child physical abuse, suspected**　Ⓟ

✓5ᵗʰ **T76.2 Sexual abuse, suspected**
　　　Rape, suspected
　　　Sexual abuse, suspected
　　　EXCLUDES 1　*alleged abuse, ruled out (Z04.7)*

　　✓x7ᵗʰ **T76.21 Adult sexual abuse, suspected**　Ⓐ

　　✓x7ᵗʰ **T76.22 Child sexual abuse, suspected**　Ⓟ

✓5ᵗʰ **T76.3 Psychological abuse, suspected**

　　✓x7ᵗʰ **T76.31 Adult psychological abuse, suspected**　Ⓐ

　　✓x7ᵗʰ **T76.32 Child psychological abuse, suspected**　Ⓟ

✓5ᵗʰ **T76.9 Unspecified maltreatment, suspected**

　　✓x7ᵗʰ **T76.91 Unspecified adult maltreatment, suspected**　Ⓐ

　　✓x7ᵗʰ **T76.92 Unspecified child maltreatment, suspected**　Ⓟ

✓4ᵗʰ **T78 Adverse effects, not elsewhere classified**
　　　EXCLUDES 2　*complications of surgical and medical care NEC (T80-T88)*

　　The appropriate 7th character is to be added to each code from category T78.
　　A　initial encounter
　　D　subsequent encounter
　　S　sequela

✓5ᵗʰ **T78.0 Anaphylactic reaction due to food**
　　　Anaphylactic reaction due to adverse food reaction
　　　Anaphylactic shock or reaction due to nonpoisonous foods
　　　Anaphylactoid reaction due to food

　　✓x7ᵗʰ **T78.00 Anaphylactic reaction due to unspecified food**

　　✓x7ᵗʰ **T78.01 Anaphylactic reaction due to peanuts**

　　✓x7ᵗʰ **T78.02 Anaphylactic reaction due to shellfish (crustaceans)**

　　✓x7ᵗʰ **T78.03 Anaphylactic reaction due to other fish**

　　✓x7ᵗʰ **T78.04 Anaphylactic reaction due to fruits and vegetables**

　　✓x7ᵗʰ **T78.05 Anaphylactic reaction due to tree nuts and seeds**
　　　　　EXCLUDES 1　*anaphylactic reaction due to peanuts (T78.01)*

　　✓x7ᵗʰ **T78.06 Anaphylactic reaction due to food additives**

　　✓x7ᵗʰ **T78.07 Anaphylactic reaction due to milk and dairy products**

　　✓x7ᵗʰ **T78.08 Anaphylactic reaction due to eggs**

　　✓x7ᵗʰ **T78.09 Anaphylactic reaction due to other food products**

✓x7ᵗʰ **T78.1 Other adverse food reactions, not elsewhere classified**
　　　Use additional code to identify the type of reaction
　　　EXCLUDES 1　*anaphylactic reaction or shock due to adverse food reaction (T78.0-)*
　　　　　anaphylactic reaction due to food (T78.0-)
　　　　　bacterial food borne intoxications (A05.-)
　　　EXCLUDES 2　*allergic and dietetic gastroenteritis and colitis (K52.2)*
　　　　　allergic rhinitis due to food (J30.5)
　　　　　dermatitis due to food in contact with skin (L23.6, L24.6, L25.4)
　　　　　dermatitis due to ingested food (L27.2)

✓x7ᵗʰ **T78.2 Anaphylactic shock, unspecified**
　　　Allergic shock
　　　Anaphylactic reaction
　　　Anaphylaxis
　　　EXCLUDES 1　*anaphylactic reaction or shock due to adverse effect of correct medicinal substance properly administered (T88.6)*
　　　　　anaphylactic reaction or shock due to adverse food reaction (T78.0-)
　　　　　anaphylactic reaction or shock due to serum (T80.5-)

✓x7ᵗʰ **T78.3 Angioneurotic edema**
　　　Allergic angioedema
　　　Giant urticaria
　　　Quincke's edema
　　　EXCLUDES 1　*serum urticaria (T80.6-)*
　　　　　urticaria (L50.-)

✓5ᵗʰ **T78.4 Other and unspecified allergy**
　　　EXCLUDES 1　*specified types of allergic reaction such as:*
　　　　　allergic diarrhea (K52.2)
　　　　　allergic gastroenteritis and colitis (K52.2)
　　　　　dermatitis (L23-L25, L27-)
　　　　　hay fever (J30.1)

　　✓x7ᵗʰ **T78.40 Allergy, unspecified**
　　　　　Allergic reaction NOS
　　　　　Hypersensitivity NOS

　　✓x7ᵗʰ **T78.41 Arthus phenomenon**
　　　　　Arthus reaction

　　✓x7ᵗʰ **T78.49 Other allergy**

✓x7ᵗʰ **T78.8 Other adverse effects, not elsewhere classified**

Certain early complications of trauma (T79)

✓4ᵗʰ **T79 Certain early complications of trauma, not elsewhere classified**
　　　EXCLUDES 2　*acute respiratory distress syndrome (J80)*
　　　　　complications occurring during or following medical procedures (T80-T88)
　　　　　complications of surgical and medical care NEC (T80-T88)
　　　　　newborn respiratory distress syndrome (P22.0)

　　The appropriate 7th character is to be added to each code from category T79.
　　A　initial encounter
　　D　subsequent encounter
　　S　sequela

　　✓x7ᵗʰ **T79.0 Air embolism (traumatic)**
　　　　　EXCLUDES 1　*air embolism complicating abortion or ectopic or molar pregnancy (O00-O07, O08.2)*
　　　　　　air embolism complicating pregnancy, childbirth and the puerperium (O88.0)
　　　　　　air embolism following infusion, transfusion, and therapeutic injection (T80.0)
　　　　　　air embolism following procedure NEC (T81.7-)

　　✓x7ᵗʰ **T79.1 Fat embolism (traumatic)**
　　　　　EXCLUDES 1　*fat embolism complicating:*
　　　　　　abortion or ectopic or molar pregnancy (O00-O07, O08.2)
　　　　　　pregnancy, childbirth and the puerperium (O88.8)

　　✓x7ᵗʰ **T79.2 Traumatic secondary and recurrent hemorrhage and seroma**

☑ Additional Character Required　✓x7ᵗʰ Placeholder Alert　Unspecified Dx　Other Specified Dx　Manifestation　▶◀ Revised Text　● New Code　▲ Revised Code Title

ICD-10-CM 2016　　　　　　　　　　　　　　　　　　　　　　　　　　　　　　　　　　　　　**1019**

√x7ᵗʰ **T79.4 Traumatic shock**

Shock (immediate) (delayed) following injury

> EXCLUDES 1   anaphylactic shock due to adverse food reaction (T78.0-)
> anaphylactic shock due to correct medicinal substance properly administered (T88.6)
> anaphylactic shock due to serum (T80.5-)
> anaphylactic shock NOS (T78.2)
> anesthetic shock (T88.2)
> electric shock (T75.4)
> nontraumatic shock NEC (R57.-)
> obstetric shock (O75.1)
> postprocedural shock (T81.1-)
> septic shock (R65.21)
> shock complicating abortion or ectopic or molar pregnancy (O00-O07, O08.3)
> shock due to lightning (T75.01)
> shock NOS (R57.9)

√x7ᵗʰ **T79.5 Traumatic anuria**

Crush syndrome
Renal failure following crushing

√x7ᵗʰ **T79.6 Traumatic ischemia of muscle**

Traumatic rhabdomyolysis
Volkmann's ischemic contracture

> EXCLUDES 2   anterior tibial syndrome (M76.8)
> compartment syndrome (traumatic) (T79.A-)
> nontraumatic ischemia of muscle (M62.2-)

√x7ᵗʰ **T79.7 Traumatic subcutaneous emphysema**

> EXCLUDES 1   emphysema NOS (J43)
> emphysema (subcutaneous) resulting from a procedure (T81.82)

√5ᵗʰ **T79.A Traumatic compartment syndrome**

> EXCLUDES 1   fibromyalgia (M79.7)
> nontraumatic compartment syndrome (M79.A-)
> traumatic ischemic infarction of muscle (T79.6)

√x7ᵗʰ **T79.A0 Compartment syndrome, unspecified**

Compartment syndrome NOS

√6ᵗʰ **T79.A1 Traumatic compartment syndrome of upper extremity**

Traumatic compartment syndrome of shoulder, arm, forearm, wrist, hand, and fingers

√7ᵗʰ **T79.A11 Traumatic compartment syndrome of right upper extremity**

√7ᵗʰ **T79.A12 Traumatic compartment syndrome of left upper extremity**

√7ᵗʰ **T79.A19 Traumatic compartment syndrome of unspecified upper extremity**

√6ᵗʰ **T79.A2 Traumatic compartment syndrome of lower extremity**

Traumatic compartment syndrome of hip, buttock, thigh, leg, foot, and toes

√7ᵗʰ **T79.A21 Traumatic compartment syndrome of right lower extremity**

√7ᵗʰ **T79.A22 Traumatic compartment syndrome of left lower extremity**

√7ᵗʰ **T79.A29 Traumatic compartment syndrome of unspecified lower extremity**

√x7ᵗʰ **T79.A3 Traumatic compartment syndrome of abdomen**

√x7ᵗʰ **T79.A9 Traumatic compartment syndrome of other sites**

√x7ᵗʰ **T79.8 Other early complications of trauma**

√x7ᵗʰ **T79.9 Unspecified early complication of trauma**

Complications of surgical and medical care, not elsewhere classified (T80-T88)

Use additional code for adverse effect, if applicable, to identify drug (T36-T50 with fifth or sixth character 5)

Use additional code(s) to identify the specified condition resulting from the complication

Use additional code to identify devices involved and details of circumstances (Y62-Y82)

> EXCLUDES 2   any encounters with medical care for postprocedural conditions in which no complications are present, such as:
> artificial opening status (Z93.-)
> closure of external stoma (Z43.-)
> fitting and adjustment of external prosthetic device (Z44.-)
> burns and corrosions from local applications and irradiation (T20-T32)
> complications of surgical procedures during pregnancy, childbirth and the puerperium (O00-O9A)
> mechanical complication of respirator [ventilator] (J95.850)
> poisoning and toxic effects of drugs and chemicals (T36-T65 with fifth or sixth character 1-4 or 6)
> postprocedural fever (R50.82)
> specified complications classified elsewhere, such as:
> cerebrospinal fluid leak from spinal puncture (G97.0)
> colostomy malfunction (K94.0-)
> disorders of fluid and electrolyte imbalance (E86-E87)
> functional disturbances following cardiac surgery (I97.0-I97.1)
> intraoperative and postprocedural complications of specified body systems (D78.-, E36.-, E89.-, G97.3-, G97.4, H59.3-, H59.-, H95.2-, H95.3, I97.4-, I97.5, J95.6-, J95.7, K91.6-, L76.-, M96.-, N99.-)
> ostomy complications (J95.0-, K94.-, N99.5-)
> postgastric surgery syndromes (K91.1)
> postlaminectomy syndrome NEC (M96.1)
> postmastectomy lymphedema syndrome (I97.2)
> postsurgical blind-loop syndrome (K91.2)
> ventilator associated pneumonia (J95.851)

AHA: 2015, 1Q, 15

√4ᵗʰ **T80 Complications following infusion, transfusion and therapeutic injection**

> INCLUDES   complications following perfusion
> EXCLUDES 2   bone marrow transplant rejection (T86.01)
> febrile nonhemolytic transfusion reaction (R50.84)
> fluid overload due to transfusion (E87.71)
> posttransfusion purpura (D69.51)
> transfusion associated circulatory overload (TACO) (E87.71)
> transfusion (red blood cell) associated hemochromatosis (E83.111)
> transfusion related acute lung injury (TRALI) (J95.84)

> The appropriate 7th character is to be added to each code from category T80.
> A   initial encounter
> D   subsequent encounter
> S   sequela

√x7ᵗʰ **T80.0 Air embolism following infusion, transfusion and therapeutic injection**

√x7ᵗʰ **T80.1 Vascular complications following infusion, transfusion and therapeutic injection**

Use additional code to identify the vascular complication

> EXCLUDES 2   extravasation of vesicant agent (T80.81-)
> infiltration of vesicant agent (T80.81-)
> postprocedural vascular complications (T81.7-)
> vascular complications specified as due to prosthetic devices, implants and grafts (T82.8-, T83.8, T84.8-, T85.8)

EXCLUDES 1   Not coded here   EXCLUDES 2   Not included here   N Newborn Age: 0   P Pediatric Age: 0-17   M Maternity Age: 12-55   A Adult Age: 15-124

1020

ICD-10-CM 2016

✓5th **T80.2** **Infections following infusion, transfusion and therapeutic injection**

Use additional code to identify the specific infection, such as: sepsis (A41.9)

Use additional code (R65.2-) to identify severe sepsis, if applicable

EXCLUDES 2   *infections specified as due to prosthetic devices, implants and grafts (T82.6-T82.7, T83.5-T83.6, T84.5-T84.7, T85.7)*
postprocedural infections (T81.4)

✓6th **T80.21** **Infection due to central venous catheter**

✓7th **T80.211** **Bloodstream infection due to central venous catheter**

Catheter-related bloodstream infection (CRBSI) NOS

Central line-associated bloodstream infection (CLABSI)

Bloodstream infection due to Hickman catheter

Bloodstream infection due to peripherally inserted central catheter (PICC)

Bloodstream infection due to portacath (port-a-cath)

Bloodstream infection due to triple lumen catheter

Bloodstream infection due to umbilical venous catheter

✓7th **T80.212** **Local infection due to central venous catheter**

Exit or insertion site infection

Local infection due to Hickman catheter

Local infection due to peripherally inserted central catheter (PICC)

Local infection due to portacath (port-a-cath)

Local infection due to triple lumen catheter

Local infection due to umbilical venous catheter

Port or reservoir infection

Tunnel infection

✓7th **T80.218** **Other infection due to central venous catheter**

Other central line-associated infection

Other infection due to Hickman catheter

Other infection due to peripherally inserted central catheter (PICC)

Other infection due to portacath (port-a-cath)

Other infection due to triple lumen catheter

Other infection due to umbilical venous catheter

✓7th **T80.219** **Unspecified infection due to central venous catheter**

Central line-associated infection NOS

Unspecified infection due to Hickman catheter

Unspecified infection due to peripherally inserted central catheter (PICC)

Unspecified infection due to portacath (port-a-cath)

Unspecified infection due to triple lumen catheter

Unspecified infection due to umbilical venous catheter

✓x7th **T80.22** **Acute infection following transfusion, infusion, or injection of blood and blood products**

✓x7th **T80.29** **Infection following other infusion, transfusion and therapeutic injection**

✓5th **T80.3** **ABO incompatibility reaction due to transfusion of blood or blood products**

EXCLUDES 1   *minor blood group antigens reactions (Duffy) (E) (K(ell)) (Kidd) (Lewis) (M) (N) (P) (S) (T80.A)*

✓x7th **T80.30** **ABO incompatibility reaction due to transfusion of blood or blood products, unspecified**

ABO incompatibility blood transfusion NOS

Reaction to ABO incompatibility from transfusion NOS

✓6th **T80.31** **ABO incompatibility with hemolytic transfusion reaction**

✓7th **T80.310** **ABO incompatibility with acute hemolytic transfusion reaction**

ABO incompatibility with hemolytic transfusion reaction less than 24 hours after transfusion

Acute hemolytic transfusion reaction (AHTR) due to ABO incompatibility

✓7th **T80.311** **ABO incompatibility with delayed hemolytic transfusion reaction**

ABO incompatibility with hemolytic transfusion reaction 24 hours or more after transfusion

Delayed hemolytic transfusion reaction (DHTR) due to ABO incompatibility

✓7th **T80.319** **ABO incompatibility with hemolytic transfusion reaction, unspecified**

ABO incompatibility with hemolytic transfusion reaction at unspecified time after transfusion

Hemolytic transfusion reaction (HTR) due to ABO incompatibility NOS

✓x7th **T80.39** **Other ABO incompatibility reaction due to transfusion of blood or blood products**

Delayed serologic transfusion reaction (DSTR) from ABO incompatibility

Other ABO incompatible blood transfusion

Other reaction to ABO incompatible blood transfusion

✓x7th **T80.4** **Rh incompatibility reaction due to transfusion of blood or blood products**

Reaction due to incompatibility of Rh antigens (C) (c) (D) (E) (e)

✓x7th **T80.40** **Rh incompatibility reaction due to transfusion of blood or blood products, unspecified**

Reaction due to Rh factor in transfusion NOS

Rh incompatible blood transfusion NOS

✓6th **T80.41** **Rh incompatibility with hemolytic transfusion reaction**

✓7th **T80.410** **Rh incompatibility with acute hemolytic transfusion reaction**

Acute hemolytic transfusion reaction (AHTR) due to Rh incompatibility

Rh incompatibility with hemolytic transfusion reaction less than 24 hours after transfusion

✓7th **T80.411** **Rh incompatibility with delayed hemolytic transfusion reaction**

Delayed hemolytic transfusion reaction (DHTR) due to Rh incompatibility

Rh incompatibility with hemolytic transfusion reaction 24 hours or more after transfusion

✓7th **T80.419** **Rh incompatibility with hemolytic transfusion reaction, unspecified**

Hemolytic transfusion reaction (HTR) due to Rh incompatibility NOS

Rh incompatibility with hemolytic transfusion reaction at unspecified time after transfusion

✓x7th **T80.49** **Other Rh incompatibility reaction due to transfusion of blood or blood products**

Delayed serologic transfusion reaction (DSTR) from Rh incompatibility

Other reaction to Rh incompatible blood transfusion

✓5th **T80.A** **Non-ABO incompatibility reaction due to transfusion of blood or blood products**

Reaction due to incompatibility of minor antigens (Duffy) (Kell) (Kidd) (Lewis) (M) (N) (P) (S)

✓x7th **T80.A0** **Non-ABO incompatibility reaction due to transfusion of blood or blood products, unspecified**

Non-ABO antigen incompatibility reaction from transfusion NOS

✓6th **T80.A1** **Non-ABO incompatibility with hemolytic transfusion reaction**

✓7th **T80.A10** **Non-ABO incompatibility with acute hemolytic transfusion reaction**

Acute hemolytic transfusion reaction (AHTR) due to non-ABO incompatibility

Non-ABO incompatibility with hemolytic transfusion reaction less than 24 hours after transfusion

---

✔ Additional Character Required   ✓x7th Placeholder Alert   Unspecified Dx   Other Specified Dx   Manifestation   ▶◀ Revised Text   ● New Code   ▲ Revised Code Title

✓7ᵗʰ **T80.A11** **Non-ABO incompatibility with** delayed hemolytic transfusion reaction
Delayed hemolytic transfusion reaction (DHTR) due to non-ABO incompatibility
Non-ABO incompatibility with hemolytic transfusion reaction 24 or more hours after transfusion

✓7ᵗʰ **T80.A19** **Non-ABO incompatibility with hemolytic transfusion reaction, unspecified**
Hemolytic transfusion reaction (HTR) due to non-ABO incompatibility NOS
Non-ABO incompatibility with hemolytic transfusion reaction at unspecified time after transfusion

✓x7ᵗʰ **T80.A9** **Other non-ABO incompatibility reaction due to transfusion of blood or blood products**
Delayed serologic transfusion reaction (DSTR) from non-ABO incompatibility
Other reaction to non-ABO incompatible blood transfusion

✓5ᵗʰ **T80.5** **Anaphylactic reaction due to serum**
Allergic shock due to serum
Anaphylactic shock due to serum
Anaphylactoid reaction due to serum
Anaphylaxis due to serum
EXCLUDES 1   *ABO incompatibility reaction due to transfusion of blood or blood products (T80.3-)*
allergic reaction or shock NOS (T78.2)
anaphylactic reaction or shock NOS (T78.2)
anaphylactic reaction or shock due to adverse effect of correct medicinal substance properly administered (T88.6)
other serum reaction (T80.6-)

✓x7ᵗʰ **T80.51** **Anaphylactic reaction due to** administration of blood and blood products

✓x7ᵗʰ **T80.52** **Anaphylactic reaction due to** vaccination

✓x7ᵗʰ **T80.59** **Anaphylactic reaction due to other serum**

✓5ᵗʰ **T80.6** **Other serum reactions**
Intoxication by serum
Protein sickness
Serum rash
Serum sickness
Serum urticaria
EXCLUDES 2   *serum hepatitis (B16.-)*

✓x7ᵗʰ **T80.61** **Other serum reaction** due to administration of blood and blood products

✓x7ᵗʰ **T80.62** **Other serum reaction** due to vaccination

✓x7ᵗʰ **T80.69** **Other serum reaction due to other** serum

✓5ᵗʰ **T80.8** **Other complications following infusion, transfusion and therapeutic injection**

✓6ᵗʰ **T80.81** **Extravasation of vesicant agent**
Infiltration of vesicant agent

✓7ᵗʰ **T80.810** **Extravasation of vesicant antineoplastic chemotherapy**
Infiltration of vesicant antineoplastic chemotherapy

✓7ᵗʰ **T80.818** **Extravasation of other vesicant agent**
Infiltration of other vesicant agent

✓x7ᵗʰ **T80.89** **Other complications following infusion, transfusion and therapeutic injection**
Delayed serologic transfusion reaction (DSTR), unspecified incompatibility
Use additional code to identify graft-versus-host reaction, if applicable, (D89.81-)

✓5ᵗʰ **T80.9** **Unspecified complication following infusion, transfusion and therapeutic injection**

✓x7ᵗʰ **T80.90** **Unspecified complication** following infusion and therapeutic injection

✓6ᵗʰ **T80.91** **Hemolytic transfusion reaction, unspecified incompatibility**
EXCLUDES 1   *ABO incompatibility with hemolytic transfusion reaction (T80.31-)*
Non-ABO incompatibility with hemolytic transfusion reaction (T80.A1-)
Rh incompatibility with hemolytic transfusion reaction (T80.41-)

✓7ᵗʰ **T80.910** **Acute hemolytic transfusion reaction, unspecified incompatibility**

✓7ᵗʰ **T80.911** **Delayed hemolytic transfusion reaction, unspecified incompatibility**

✓7ᵗʰ **T80.919** **Hemolytic transfusion reaction, unspecified incompatibility, unspecified as acute or delayed**
Hemolytic transfusion reaction NOS

✓x7ᵗʰ **T80.92** **Unspecified transfusion reaction**
Transfusion reaction NOS

✓4ᵗʰ **T81** **Complications of procedures, not elsewhere classified**
Use additional code for adverse effect, if applicable, to identify drug (T36-T50 with fifth or sixth character 5)
EXCLUDES 2   *complications following immunization (T88.0-T88.1)*
complications following infusion, transfusion and therapeutic injection (T80.-)
complications of transplanted organs and tissue (T86.-)
specified complications classified elsewhere, such as:
complication of prosthetic devices, implants and grafts (T02-T05)
dermatitis due to drugs and medicaments (L23.3, L24.4, L25.1, L27.0-L27.1)
endosseous dental implant failure (M27.6-)
floppy iris syndrome (IFIS) (intraoperative) (H21.81)
intraoperative and postprocedural complications of specific body system (D78.-, E36.-, E89.-, G97.3-, G97.4, H59.3-, H59.-, H95.2-, H95.3, I97.4-, I97.5, J95, K91.-, L76.-, M96.-, N99.-)
ostomy complications (J95.0-, K94.-, N99.5-)
plateau iris syndrome (post-iridectomy) (postprocedural) (H21.82)
poisoning and toxic effects of drugs and chemicals (T36-T65 with fifth or sixth character 1-4 or 6)

The appropriate 7th character is to be added to each code from category T81.
A   initial encounter
D   subsequent encounter
S   sequela

✓5ᵗʰ **T81.1** **Postprocedural shock**
Shock during or resulting from a procedure, not elsewhere classified
EXCLUDES 1   *anaphylactic shock due to correct substance properly administered (T88.6)*
anaphylactic shock due to serum (T80.5-)
anaphylactic shock NOS (T78.2)
anesthetic shock (T88.2)
electric shock (T75.4)
obstetric shock (O75.1)
septic shock (R65.21)
shock following abortion or ectopic or molar pregnancy (O00-O07, O08.3)
traumatic shock (T79.4)

✓x7ᵗʰ **T81.10** **Postprocedural shock unspecified**
Collapse NOS during or resulting from a procedure, not elsewhere classified
Postprocedural failure of peripheral circulation
Postprocedural shock NOS

✓x7ᵗʰ **T81.11** **Postprocedural cardiogenic shock**

✓x7ᵗʰ **T81.12** **Postprocedural septic shock**
Postprocedural endotoxic shock during or resulting from a procedure, not elsewhere classified
Postprocedural gram-negative shock during or resulting from a procedure, not elsewhere classified
Code first underlying infection
Use additional code, to identify any associated acute organ dysfunction, if applicable

✓x7ᵗʰ **T81.19** **Other postprocedural shock**
Postprocedural hypovolemic shock

✓5ᵗʰ **T81.3** **Disruption of wound, not elsewhere classified**
Disruption of any suture materials or other closure methods
EXCLUDES 1   *breakdown (mechanical) of permanent sutures (T85.612)*
displacement of permanent sutures (T85.622)
disruption of cesarean delivery wound (O90.0)
disruption of perineal obstetric wound (O90.1)
mechanical complication of permanent sutures NEC (T85.692)
AHA: 2014, 1Q, 23

✓x7ᵗʰ **T81.30** **Disruption of wound, unspecified**
Disruption of wound NOS

✓x7ᵗʰ **T81.31** **Disruption of** external operation (surgical) wound, **not elsewhere classified**
Dehiscence of operation wound NOS
Disruption of operation wound NOS
Disruption or dehiscence of closure of cornea
Disruption or dehiscence of closure of mucosa
Disruption or dehiscence of closure of skin and subcutaneous tissue
Full-thickness skin disruption or dehiscence
Superficial disruption or dehiscence of operation wound
> EXCLUDES 1 dehiscence of amputation stump (T87.81)

✓x7ᵗʰ **T81.32** **Disruption of** internal operation (surgical) wound, **not elsewhere classified**
Deep disruption or dehiscence of operation wound NOS
Disruption or dehiscence of closure of internal organ or other internal tissue
Disruption or dehiscence of closure of muscle or muscle flap
Disruption or dehiscence of closure of ribs or rib cage
Disruption or dehiscence of closure of skull or craniotomy
Disruption or dehiscence of closure of sternum or sternotomy
Disruption or dehiscence of closure of tendon or ligament
Disruption or dehiscence of closure of superficial or muscular fascia

✓x7ᵗʰ **T81.33** **Disruption of** traumatic injury **wound** repair
Disruption or dehiscence of closure of traumatic laceration (external) (internal)

✓x7ᵗʰ **T81.4** **Infection following a procedure**
Intra-abdominal abscess following a procedure
Postprocedural infection, not elsewhere classified
Sepsis following a procedure
Stitch abscess following a procedure
Subphrenic abscess following a procedure
Wound abscess following a procedure
Use additional code to identify infection
Use additional code (R65.2-) to identify severe sepsis, if applicable
> EXCLUDES 1 obstetric surgical wound infection (O86.0)
> postprocedural fever NOS (R50.82)
> postprocedural retroperitoneal abscess (K68.11)
> EXCLUDES 2 bleb associated endophthalmitis (H59.4-)
> infection due to infusion, transfusion and therapeutic injection (T80.2-)
> infection due to prosthetic devices, implants and grafts (T82.6-T82.7, T83.5-T83.6, T84.5-T84.7, T85.7)

AHA: 2014, 1Q, 23

✓5ᵗʰ **T81.5** **Complications of** foreign body accidentally left in body following procedure
AHA: 2014, 4Q, 24

✓6ᵗʰ **T81.50** **Unspecified** complication of foreign body accidentally left in body following procedure

✓7ᵗʰ **T81.500** **Unspecified complication of foreign body accidentally left in body following** surgical operation

✓7ᵗʰ **T81.501** **Unspecified complication of foreign body accidentally left in body following** infusion or transfusion

✓7ᵗʰ **T81.502** **Unspecified complication of foreign body accidentally left in body following** kidney dialysis

✓7ᵗʰ **T81.503** **Unspecified complication of foreign body accidentally left in body following** injection or immunization

✓7ᵗʰ **T81.504** **Unspecified complication of foreign body accidentally left in body following** endoscopic examination

✓7ᵗʰ **T81.505** **Unspecified complication of foreign body accidentally left in body following** heart catheterization

✓7ᵗʰ **T81.506** **Unspecified complication of foreign body accidentally left in body following** aspiration, puncture or other catheterization

✓7ᵗʰ **T81.507** **Unspecified complication of foreign body accidentally left in body following** removal of catheter or packing

✓7ᵗʰ **T81.508** **Unspecified complication of foreign body accidentally left in body following other procedure**

✓7ᵗʰ **T81.509** **Unspecified complication of foreign body accidentally left in body following unspecified procedure**

✓6ᵗʰ **T81.51** **Adhesions** due to foreign body accidentally left in body following procedure

✓7ᵗʰ **T81.510** **Adhesions due to foreign body accidentally left in body following** surgical operation

✓7ᵗʰ **T81.511** **Adhesions due to foreign body accidentally left in body following** infusion or transfusion

✓7ᵗʰ **T81.512** **Adhesions due to foreign body accidentally left in body following** kidney dialysis

✓7ᵗʰ **T81.513** **Adhesions due to foreign body accidentally left in body following** injection or immunization

✓7ᵗʰ **T81.514** **Adhesions due to foreign body accidentally left in body following** endoscopic examination

✓7ᵗʰ **T81.515** **Adhesions due to foreign body accidentally left in body following** heart catheterization

✓7ᵗʰ **T81.516** **Adhesions due to foreign body accidentally left in body following** aspiration, puncture or other catheterization

✓7ᵗʰ **T81.517** **Adhesions due to foreign body accidentally left in body following** removal of catheter or packing

✓7ᵗʰ **T81.518** **Adhesions due to foreign body accidentally left in body following other procedure**

✓7ᵗʰ **T81.519** **Adhesions due to foreign body accidentally left in body following unspecified procedure**

✓6ᵗʰ **T81.52** **Obstruction** due to foreign body accidentally left in body following procedure

✓7ᵗʰ **T81.520** **Obstruction due to foreign body accidentally left in body following** surgical operation

✓7ᵗʰ **T81.521** **Obstruction due to foreign body accidentally left in body following** infusion or transfusion

✓7ᵗʰ **T81.522** **Obstruction due to foreign body accidentally left in body following** kidney dialysis

✓7ᵗʰ **T81.523** **Obstruction due to foreign body accidentally left in body following** injection or immunization

✓7ᵗʰ **T81.524** **Obstruction due to foreign body accidentally left in body following** endoscopic examination

✓7ᵗʰ **T81.525** **Obstruction due to foreign body accidentally left in body following** heart catheterization

✓7ᵗʰ **T81.526** **Obstruction due to foreign body accidentally left in body following** aspiration, puncture or other catheterization

✓7ᵗʰ **T81.527** **Obstruction due to foreign body accidentally left in body following** removal of catheter or packing

✓7ᵗʰ **T81.528** **Obstruction due to foreign body accidentally left in body following other procedure**

✓7ᵗʰ **T81.529** **Obstruction due to foreign body accidentally left in body following unspecified procedure**

✓6ᵗʰ **T81.53** **Perforation** due to foreign body accidentally left in body following procedure

✓7ᵗʰ **T81.530** **Perforation due to foreign body accidentally left in body following** surgical operation

---

✓ Additional Character Required   ✓x7ᵗʰ Placeholder Alert   Unspecified Dx   Other Specified Dx   Manifestation   ►◄ Revised Text   ● New Code   ▲ Revised Code Title

T81.531 Perforation due to foreign body accidentally left in body following **infusion or transfusion**

T81.532 Perforation due to foreign body accidentally left in body following **kidney dialysis**

T81.533 Perforation due to foreign body accidentally left in body following **injection or immunization**

T81.534 Perforation due to foreign body accidentally left in body following **endoscopic examination**

T81.535 Perforation due to foreign body accidentally left in body following **heart catheterization**

T81.536 Perforation due to foreign body accidentally left in body following **aspiration, puncture or other catheterization**

T81.537 Perforation due to foreign body accidentally left in body following **removal of catheter or packing**

T81.538 Perforation due to foreign body accidentally left in body following **other procedure**

T81.539 Perforation due to foreign body accidentally left in body following **unspecified procedure**

T81.59 Other complications of foreign body accidentally left in body following procedure

> EXCLUDES 2   obstruction or perforation due to prosthetic devices and implants intentionally left in body (T82.0-T82.5, T83.0-T83.4, T83.7, T84.0-T84.4, T85.0-T85.6)

T81.590 Other complications of foreign body accidentally left in body following **surgical operation**

T81.591 Other complications of foreign body accidentally left in body following **infusion or transfusion**

T81.592 Other complications of foreign body accidentally left in body following **kidney dialysis**

T81.593 Other complications of foreign body accidentally left in body following **injection or immunization**

T81.594 Other complications of foreign body accidentally left in body following **endoscopic examination**

T81.595 Other complications of foreign body accidentally left in body following **heart catheterization**

T81.596 Other complications of foreign body accidentally left in body following **aspiration, puncture or other catheterization**

T81.597 Other complications of foreign body accidentally left in body following **removal of catheter or packing**

T81.598 Other complications of foreign body accidentally left in body following **other procedure**

T81.599 Other complications of foreign body accidentally left in body following **unspecified procedure**

T81.6 Acute reaction to foreign substance accidentally left during a procedure

> EXCLUDES 2   complications of foreign body accidentally left in body cavity or operation wound following procedure (T81.5-)

T81.60 Unspecified acute reaction to foreign substance accidentally left during a procedure

T81.61 Aseptic peritonitis due to foreign substance accidentally left during a procedure
Chemical peritonitis

T81.69 Other acute reaction to foreign substance accidentally left during a procedure

T81.7 Vascular complications following a procedure, not elsewhere classified
Air embolism following procedure NEC
Phlebitis or thrombophlebitis resulting from a procedure

> EXCLUDES 1   embolism complicating abortion or ectopic or molar pregnancy (O00-O07, O08.2)
> embolism complicating pregnancy, childbirth and the puerperium (O88.-)
> traumatic embolism (T79.0)

> EXCLUDES 2   embolism due to prosthetic devices, implants and grafts (T82.8-, T83.8, T84.8-, T85.8)
> embolism following infusion, transfusion and therapeutic injection (T80.0)

T81.71 Complication of artery following a procedure, not elsewhere classified

T81.710 Complication of **mesenteric** artery following a procedure, not elsewhere classified

T81.711 Complication of **renal** artery following a procedure, not elsewhere classified

T81.718 Complication of **other artery** following a procedure, not elsewhere classified

T81.719 Complication of **unspecified artery** following a procedure, not elsewhere classified

T81.72 Complication of **vein** following a procedure, not elsewhere classified

T81.8 Other complications of procedures, not elsewhere classified

> EXCLUDES 2   hypothermia following anesthesia (T88.51)
> malignant hyperpyrexia due to anesthesia (T88.3)

T81.81 Complication of inhalation therapy

T81.82 Emphysema (subcutaneous) resulting from a procedure

T81.83 Persistent postprocedural fistula

T81.89 Other complications of procedures, not elsewhere classified
Use additional code to specify complication, such as: postprocedural delirium (F05)
AHA: 2014, 1Q, 23

T81.9 Unspecified complication of procedure

T82 Complications of cardiac and vascular prosthetic devices, implants and grafts

> EXCLUDES 2   failure and rejection of transplanted organs and tissue (T86.-)

> The appropriate 7th character is to be added to each code from category T82.
> A   initial encounter
> D   subsequent encounter
> S   sequela

T82.0 Mechanical complication of **heart valve prosthesis**
Mechanical complication of artificial heart valve

> EXCLUDES 1   mechanical complication of biological heart valve graft (T82.22-)

T82.01 Breakdown (mechanical) of heart valve prosthesis

T82.02 Displacement of heart valve prosthesis
Malposition of heart valve prosthesis

T82.03 Leakage of heart valve prosthesis

T82.09 Other mechanical complication of heart valve prosthesis
Obstruction (mechanical) of heart valve prosthesis
Perforation of heart valve prosthesis
Protrusion of heart valve prosthesis

T82.1 Mechanical complication of **cardiac electronic device**

T82.11 Breakdown (mechanical) of cardiac electronic device

T82.110 Breakdown (mechanical) of cardiac **electrode**

T82.111 Breakdown (mechanical) of cardiac **pulse generator (battery)**

T82.118 Breakdown (mechanical) of other cardiac **electronic device**

T82.119 Breakdown (mechanical) of unspecified cardiac electronic device

T82.12 Displacement of cardiac electronic device
Malposition of cardiac electronic device

T82.120 Displacement of **cardiac electrode**

T82.121 Displacement of cardiac **pulse generator (battery)**

EXCLUDES 1 Not coded here   EXCLUDES 2 Not included here   N Newborn Age: 0   P Pediatric Age: 0-17   M Maternity Age: 12-55   A Adult Age: 15-124

1024   ICD-10-CM 2016

✓7ᵗʰ **T82.128** Displacement of other cardiac electronic device

✓7ᵗʰ **T82.129** Displacement of unspecified cardiac electronic device

✓6ᵗʰ **T82.19** Other mechanical complication of cardiac electronic device
> Leakage of cardiac electronic device
> Obstruction of cardiac electronic device
> Perforation of cardiac electronic device
> Protrusion of cardiac electronic device

✓7ᵗʰ **T82.190** Other mechanical complication of cardiac electrode

✓7ᵗʰ **T82.191** Other mechanical complication of cardiac pulse generator (battery)

✓7ᵗʰ **T82.198** Other mechanical complication of other cardiac electronic device

✓7ᵗʰ **T82.199** Other mechanical complication of unspecified cardiac device

✓5ᵗʰ **T82.2** Mechanical complication of coronary artery bypass graft and biological heart valve graft
> EXCLUDES 1   mechanical complication of artificial heart valve prosthesis (T82.0-)

✓6ᵗʰ **T82.21** Mechanical complication of coronary artery bypass graft

✓7ᵗʰ **T82.211** Breakdown (mechanical) of coronary artery bypass graft

✓7ᵗʰ **T82.212** Displacement of coronary artery bypass graft
> Malposition of coronary artery bypass graft

✓7ᵗʰ **T82.213** Leakage of coronary artery bypass graft

✓7ᵗʰ **T82.218** Other mechanical complication of coronary artery bypass graft
> Obstruction, mechanical of coronary artery bypass graft
> Perforation of coronary artery bypass graft
> Protrusion of coronary artery bypass graft

✓6ᵗʰ **T82.22** Mechanical complication of biological heart valve graft

✓7ᵗʰ **T82.221** Breakdown (mechanical) of biological heart valve graft

✓7ᵗʰ **T82.222** Displacement of biological heart valve graft
> Malposition of biological heart valve graft

✓7ᵗʰ **T82.223** Leakage of biological heart valve graft

✓7ᵗʰ **T82.228** Other mechanical complication of biological heart valve graft
> Obstruction of biological heart valve graft
> Perforation of biological heart valve graft
> Protrusion of biological heart valve graft

✓5ᵗʰ **T82.3** Mechanical complication of other vascular grafts

✓6ᵗʰ **T82.31** Breakdown (mechanical) of other vascular grafts

✓7ᵗʰ **T82.310** Breakdown (mechanical) of aortic (bifurcation) graft (replacement)

✓7ᵗʰ **T82.311** Breakdown (mechanical) of carotid arterial graft (bypass)

✓7ᵗʰ **T82.312** Breakdown (mechanical) of femoral arterial graft (bypass)

✓7ᵗʰ **T82.318** Breakdown (mechanical) of other vascular grafts

✓7ᵗʰ **T82.319** Breakdown (mechanical) of unspecified vascular grafts

✓6ᵗʰ **T82.32** Displacement of other vascular grafts
> Malposition of other vascular grafts

✓7ᵗʰ **T82.320** Displacement of aortic (bifurcation) graft (replacement)

✓7ᵗʰ **T82.321** Displacement of carotid arterial graft (bypass)

✓7ᵗʰ **T82.322** Displacement of femoral arterial graft (bypass)

✓7ᵗʰ **T82.328** Displacement of other vascular grafts

✓7ᵗʰ **T82.329** Displacement of unspecified vascular grafts

✓6ᵗʰ **T82.33** Leakage of other vascular grafts

✓7ᵗʰ **T82.330** Leakage of aortic (bifurcation) graft (replacement)

✓7ᵗʰ **T82.331** Leakage of carotid arterial graft (bypass)

✓7ᵗʰ **T82.332** Leakage of femoral arterial graft (bypass)

✓7ᵗʰ **T82.338** Leakage of other vascular grafts

✓7ᵗʰ **T82.339** Leakage of unspecified vascular graft

✓6ᵗʰ **T82.39** Other mechanical complication of other vascular grafts
> Obstruction (mechanical) of other vascular grafts
> Perforation of other vascular grafts
> Protrusion of other vascular grafts

✓7ᵗʰ **T82.390** Other mechanical complication of aortic (bifurcation) graft (replacement)

✓7ᵗʰ **T82.391** Other mechanical complication of carotid arterial graft (bypass)

✓7ᵗʰ **T82.392** Other mechanical complication of femoral arterial graft (bypass)

✓7ᵗʰ **T82.398** Other mechanical complication of other vascular grafts

✓7ᵗʰ **T82.399** Other mechanical complication of unspecified vascular grafts

✓5ᵗʰ **T82.4** Mechanical complication of vascular dialysis catheter
> Mechanical complication of hemodialysis catheter
> EXCLUDES 1   mechanical complication of intraperitoneal dialysis catheter (T85.62)

✓x7ᵗʰ **T82.41** Breakdown (mechanical) of vascular dialysis catheter

✓x7ᵗʰ **T82.42** Displacement of vascular dialysis catheter
> Malposition of vascular dialysis catheter

✓x7ᵗʰ **T82.43** Leakage of vascular dialysis catheter

✓x7ᵗʰ **T82.49** Other complication of vascular dialysis catheter
> Obstruction (mechanical) of vascular dialysis catheter
> Perforation of vascular dialysis catheter
> Protrusion of vascular dialysis catheter

✓5ᵗʰ **T82.5** Mechanical complication of other cardiac and vascular devices and implants
> EXCLUDES 2   mechanical complication of epidural and subdural infusion catheter (T85.61)

✓6ᵗʰ **T82.51** Breakdown (mechanical) of other cardiac and vascular devices and implants

✓7ᵗʰ **T82.510** Breakdown (mechanical) of surgically created arteriovenous fistula

✓7ᵗʰ **T82.511** Breakdown (mechanical) of surgically created arteriovenous shunt

✓7ᵗʰ **T82.512** Breakdown (mechanical) of artificial heart

✓7ᵗʰ **T82.513** Breakdown (mechanical) of balloon (counterpulsation) device

✓7ᵗʰ **T82.514** Breakdown (mechanical) of infusion catheter

✓7ᵗʰ **T82.515** Breakdown (mechanical) of umbrella device

✓7ᵗʰ **T82.518** Breakdown (mechanical) of other cardiac and vascular devices and implants

✓7ᵗʰ **T82.519** Breakdown (mechanical) of unspecified cardiac and vascular devices and implants

✓6ᵗʰ **T82.52** Displacement of other cardiac and vascular devices and implants
> Malposition of other cardiac and vascular devices and implants

✓7ᵗʰ **T82.520** Displacement of surgically created arteriovenous fistula

✓7ᵗʰ **T82.521** Displacement of surgically created arteriovenous shunt

✓7ᵗʰ **T82.522** Displacement of artificial heart

✓7ᵗʰ **T82.523** Displacement of balloon (counterpulsation) device

✓7ᵗʰ **T82.524** Displacement of infusion catheter

✓7ᵗʰ **T82.525** Displacement of umbrella device

✓7ᵗʰ **T82.528** Displacement of other cardiac and vascular devices and implants

✓7ᵗʰ **T82.529** Displacement of unspecified cardiac and vascular devices and implants

✓6ᵗʰ **T82.53** Leakage of other cardiac and vascular devices and implants

✓7ᵗʰ **T82.530** Leakage of surgically created arteriovenous fistula

✓7ᵗʰ **T82.531** Leakage of surgically created arteriovenous shunt

✓ Additional Character Required   ✓x7ᵗʰ Placeholder Alert   Unspecified Dx   Other Specified Dx   Manifestation   ►◄ Revised Text   ● New Code   ▲ Revised Code Title

ICD-10-CM 2016   1025

Chapter 19. Injury, Poisoning, and Certain Other Consequences of External Causes

✓7ᵗʰ **T82.532 Leakage of** artificial heart

✓7ᵗʰ **T82.533 Leakage of** balloon (counterpulsation) device

✓7ᵗʰ **T82.534 Leakage of** infusion catheter

✓7ᵗʰ **T82.535 Leakage of** umbrella device

✓7ᵗʰ **T82.538 Leakage of other cardiac and vascular devices and implants**

✓7ᵗʰ **T82.539 Leakage of unspecified cardiac and vascular devices and implants**

✓6ᵗʰ **T82.59 Other** mechanical complication of other cardiac and vascular devices and implants

Obstruction (mechanical) of other cardiac and vascular devices and implants
Perforation of other cardiac and vascular devices and implants
Protrusion of other cardiac and vascular devices and implants

✓7ᵗʰ **T82.590 Other mechanical complication of surgically created arteriovenous fistula**

✓7ᵗʰ **T82.591 Other mechanical complication of surgically created arteriovenous shunt**

✓7ᵗʰ **T82.592 Other mechanical complication of** artificial heart

✓7ᵗʰ **T82.593 Other mechanical complication of** balloon (counterpulsation) device

✓7ᵗʰ **T82.594 Other mechanical complication of** infusion catheter

✓7ᵗʰ **T82.595 Other mechanical complication of** umbrella device

✓7ᵗʰ **T82.598 Other mechanical complication of other cardiac and vascular devices and implants**

✓7ᵗʰ **T82.599 Other mechanical complication of unspecified cardiac and vascular devices and implants**

✓x7ᵗʰ **T82.6 Infection and inflammatory reaction due to** cardiac valve prosthesis

Use additional code to identify infection

✓x7ᵗʰ **T82.7 Infection and inflammatory reaction due to** other cardiac and vascular devices, implants and grafts

Use additional code to identify infection

✓5ᵗʰ **T82.8 Other specified complications** of cardiac and vascular prosthetic devices, implants and grafts

✓6ᵗʰ **T82.81 Embolism** of cardiac and vascular prosthetic devices, implants and grafts

✓7ᵗʰ **T82.817 Embolism of** cardiac prosthetic devices, implants and grafts

✓7ᵗʰ **T82.818 Embolism of** vascular prosthetic devices, implants and grafts

✓6ᵗʰ **T82.82 Fibrosis** of cardiac and vascular prosthetic devices, implants and grafts

✓7ᵗʰ **T82.827 Fibrosis of** cardiac prosthetic devices, implants and grafts

✓7ᵗʰ **T82.828 Fibrosis of** vascular prosthetic devices, implants and grafts

✓6ᵗʰ **T82.83 Hemorrhage** of cardiac and vascular prosthetic devices, implants and grafts

✓7ᵗʰ **T82.837 Hemorrhage of** cardiac prosthetic devices, implants and grafts

✓7ᵗʰ **T82.838 Hemorrhage of** vascular prosthetic devices, implants and grafts

✓6ᵗʰ **T82.84 Pain** from cardiac and vascular prosthetic devices, implants and grafts

✓7ᵗʰ **T82.847 Pain from** cardiac prosthetic devices, implants and grafts

✓7ᵗʰ **T82.848 Pain from** vascular prosthetic devices, implants and grafts

✓6ᵗʰ **T82.85 Stenosis** of cardiac and vascular prosthetic devices, implants and grafts

✓7ᵗʰ **T82.857 Stenosis of** cardiac prosthetic devices, implants and grafts

✓7ᵗʰ **T82.858 Stenosis of** vascular prosthetic devices, implants and grafts

✓6ᵗʰ **T82.86 Thrombosis** of cardiac and vascular prosthetic devices, implants and grafts

✓7ᵗʰ **T82.867 Thrombosis of** cardiac prosthetic devices, implants and grafts

✓7ᵗʰ **T82.868 Thrombosis of** vascular prosthetic devices, implants and grafts

✓6ᵗʰ **T82.89 Other** specified complication of cardiac and vascular prosthetic devices, implants and grafts

✓7ᵗʰ **T82.897 Other specified complication of** cardiac prosthetic devices, implants and grafts

✓7ᵗʰ **T82.898 Other specified complication of** vascular prosthetic devices, implants and grafts

✓x7ᵗʰ **T82.9 Unspecified complication of cardiac and vascular prosthetic device, implant and graft**

✓4ᵗʰ **T83 Complications of genitourinary prosthetic devices, implants and grafts**

EXCLUDES 2 failure and rejection of transplanted organs and tissue (T86.-)

The appropriate 7th character is to be added to each code from category T83.
A   initial encounter
D   subsequent encounter
S   sequela

✓5ᵗʰ **T83.0 Mechanical complication of** urinary (indwelling) catheter

EXCLUDES 2 complications of stoma of urinary tract (N99.5-)

✓6ᵗʰ **T83.01 Breakdown** (mechanical) of urinary (indwelling) catheter

✓7ᵗʰ **T83.010 Breakdown (mechanical) of** cystostomy catheter

✓7ᵗʰ **T83.018 Breakdown (mechanical) of other indwelling** urethral **catheter**

✓6ᵗʰ **T83.02 Displacement** of urinary (indwelling) catheter

Malposition of urinary (indwelling) catheter

✓7ᵗʰ **T83.020 Displacement of** cystostomy **catheter**

✓7ᵗʰ **T83.028 Displacement of other indwelling** urethral **catheter**

✓6ᵗʰ **T83.03 Leakage** of urinary (indwelling) catheter

✓7ᵗʰ **T83.030 Leakage of** cystostomy **catheter**

✓7ᵗʰ **T83.038 Leakage of other indwelling** urethral **catheter**

✓6ᵗʰ **T83.09 Other** mechanical complication of urinary (indwelling) catheter

Obstruction (mechanical) of urinary (indwelling) catheter
Perforation of urinary (indwelling) catheter
Protrusion of urinary (indwelling) catheter

✓7ᵗʰ **T83.090 Other mechanical complication of** cystostomy **catheter**

✓7ᵗʰ **T83.098 Other mechanical complication of other indwelling** urethral **catheter**

✓5ᵗʰ **T83.1 Mechanical complication of** other urinary devices and implants

✓6ᵗʰ **T83.11 Breakdown** (mechanical) of other urinary devices and implants

✓7ᵗʰ **T83.110 Breakdown (mechanical) of urinary** electronic stimulator device

✓7ᵗʰ **T83.111 Breakdown (mechanical) of urinary** sphincter implant

✓7ᵗʰ **T83.112 Breakdown (mechanical) of urinary** stent

✓7ᵗʰ **T83.118 Breakdown (mechanical) of other urinary devices and implants**

✓6ᵗʰ **T83.12 Displacement** of other urinary devices and implants

Malposition of other urinary devices and implants

✓7ᵗʰ **T83.120 Displacement of urinary** electronic stimulator device

✓7ᵗʰ **T83.121 Displacement of urinary** sphincter implant

✓7ᵗʰ **T83.122 Displacement of urinary** stent

✓7ᵗʰ **T83.128 Displacement of other urinary devices and implants**

✓6ᵗʰ **T83.19 Other** mechanical complication of other urinary devices and implants

Leakage of other urinary devices and implants
Obstruction (mechanical) of other urinary devices and implants
Perforation of other urinary devices and implants
Protrusion of other urinary devices and implants

✓7ᵗʰ **T83.190 Other mechanical complication of urinary** electronic stimulator device

EXCLUDES 1 Not coded here   EXCLUDES 2 Not included here   N Newborn Age: 0   P Pediatric Age: 0-17   M Maternity Age: 12-55   A Adult Age: 15-124

1026

ICD-10-CM 2016

√7ᵗʰ **T83.191** **Other mechanical complication of urinary sphincter implant**

√7ᵗʰ **T83.192** **Other mechanical complication of urinary stent**

√7ᵗʰ **T83.198** **Other mechanical complication of other urinary devices and implants**

√5ᵗʰ **T83.2** Mechanical complication of graft of urinary organ

√x7ᵗʰ **T83.21** Breakdown (mechanical) of graft of urinary organ

√x7ᵗʰ **T83.22** Displacement of graft of urinary organ
Malposition of graft of urinary organ

√x7ᵗʰ **T83.23** Leakage of graft of urinary organ

√x7ᵗʰ **T83.29** **Other mechanical complication of graft of urinary organ**
Obstruction (mechanical) of graft of urinary organ
Perforation of graft of urinary organ
Protrusion of graft of urinary organ

√5ᵗʰ **T83.3** Mechanical complication of intrauterine contraceptive device

¹ √x7ᵗʰ **T83.31** Breakdown (mechanical) of intrauterine contraceptive device   Ⓜ♀

¹ √x7ᵗʰ **T83.32** Displacement of intrauterine contraceptive device   Ⓜ♀
Malposition of intrauterine contraceptive device

¹ √x7ᵗʰ **T83.39** **Other mechanical complication of intrauterine contraceptive device**   Ⓜ♀
Leakage of intrauterine contraceptive device
Obstruction (mechanical) of intrauterine contraceptive device
Perforation of intrauterine contraceptive device
Protrusion of intrauterine contraceptive device

√5ᵗʰ **T83.4** Mechanical complication of other prosthetic devices, implants and grafts of genital tract

√6ᵗʰ **T83.41** Breakdown (mechanical) of other prosthetic devices, implants and grafts of genital tract

√7ᵗʰ **T83.410** **Breakdown (mechanical) of penile (implanted) prosthesis**   ♂

√7ᵗʰ **T83.418** **Breakdown (mechanical) of other prosthetic devices, implants and grafts of genital tract**

√6ᵗʰ **T83.42** Displacement of other prosthetic devices, implants and grafts of genital tract
Malposition of other prosthetic devices, implants and grafts of genital tract

√7ᵗʰ **T83.420** **Displacement of penile (implanted) prosthesis**   ♂

√7ᵗʰ **T83.428** **Displacement of other prosthetic devices, implants and grafts of genital tract**

√6ᵗʰ **T83.49** Other mechanical complication of other prosthetic devices, implants and grafts of genital tract
Leakage of other prosthetic devices, implants and grafts of genital tract
Obstruction, mechanical of other prosthetic devices, implants and grafts of genital tract
Perforation of other prosthetic devices, implants and grafts of genital tract
Protrusion of other prosthetic devices, implants and grafts of genital tract

√7ᵗʰ **T83.490** **Other mechanical complication of penile (implanted) prosthesis**   ♂

√7ᵗʰ **T83.498** **Other mechanical complication of other prosthetic devices, implants and grafts of genital tract**

√5ᵗʰ **T83.5** Infection and inflammatory reaction due to prosthetic device, implant and graft in urinary system
Use additional code to identify infection

√x7ᵗʰ **T83.51** Infection and inflammatory reaction due to indwelling urinary catheter
EXCLUDES 2 complications of stoma of urinary tract (N99.5-)

√x7ᵗʰ **T83.59** Infection and inflammatory reaction due to prosthetic device, implant and graft in urinary system

√x7ᵗʰ **T83.6** Infection and inflammatory reaction due to prosthetic device, implant and graft in genital tract
Use additional code to identify infection

√5ᵗʰ **T83.7** Complications due to implanted mesh and other prosthetic materials

√6ᵗʰ **T83.71** Erosion of implanted mesh and other prosthetic materials to surrounding organ or tissue

√7ᵗʰ **T83.711** Erosion of implanted vaginal mesh and other prosthetic materials to surrounding organ or tissue   ♀
Erosion of implanted vaginal mesh and other prosthetic materials into pelvic floor muscles

√7ᵗʰ **T83.718** **Erosion of other implanted mesh and other prosthetic materials to surrounding organ or tissue**

√6ᵗʰ **T83.72** Exposure of implanted mesh and other prosthetic materials into surrounding organ or tissue

√7ᵗʰ **T83.721** Exposure of implanted vaginal mesh and other prosthetic materials into vagina   ♀
Exposure of implanted vaginal mesh and other prosthetic materials through vaginal wall

√7ᵗʰ **T83.728** **Exposure of other implanted mesh and other prosthetic materials to surrounding organ or tissue**

√5ᵗʰ **T83.8** Other specified complications of genitourinary prosthetic devices, implants and grafts

√x7ᵗʰ **T83.81** Embolism of genitourinary prosthetic devices, implants and grafts

√x7ᵗʰ **T83.82** Fibrosis of genitourinary prosthetic devices, implants and grafts

√x7ᵗʰ **T83.83** Hemorrhage of genitourinary prosthetic devices, implants and grafts

√x7ᵗʰ **T83.84** Pain from genitourinary prosthetic devices, implants and grafts

√x7ᵗʰ **T83.85** Stenosis of genitourinary prosthetic devices, implants and grafts

√x7ᵗʰ **T83.86** Thrombosis of genitourinary prosthetic devices, implants and grafts

√x7ᵗʰ **T83.89** **Other specified complication of genitourinary prosthetic devices, implants and grafts**

√x7ᵗʰ **T83.9** **Unspecified complication of genitourinary prosthetic device, implant and graft**

√4ᵗʰ **T84** **Complications of internal orthopedic prosthetic devices, implants and grafts**
EXCLUDES 2 failure and rejection of transplanted organs and tissues (T86.-)
fracture of bone following insertion of orthopedic implant, joint prosthesis or bone plate (M96.6)

The appropriate 7th character is to be added to each code from category T84.
A   initial encounter
D   subsequent encounter
S   sequela

√5ᵗʰ **T84.0** **Mechanical complication of internal joint prosthesis**

√6ᵗʰ **T84.01** Broken internal joint prosthesis
Breakage (fracture) of prosthetic joint
Broken prosthetic joint implant
EXCLUDES 1 periprosthetic joint implant fracture (T84.04)

√7ᵗʰ **T84.010** Broken internal right hip prosthesis

√7ᵗʰ **T84.011** Broken internal left hip prosthesis

√7ᵗʰ **T84.012** Broken internal right knee prosthesis

√7ᵗʰ **T84.013** Broken internal left knee prosthesis

√7ᵗʰ **T84.018** **Broken internal joint prosthesis, other site**
Use additional code to identify the joint (Z96.6-)

√7ᵗʰ **T84.019** **Broken internal joint prosthesis, unspecified site**

√6ᵗʰ **T84.02** Dislocation of internal joint prosthesis
Instability of internal joint prosthesis
Subluxation of internal joint prosthesis

√7ᵗʰ **T84.020** Dislocation of internal right hip prosthesis

√7ᵗʰ **T84.021** Dislocation of internal left hip prosthesis

√7ᵗʰ **T84.022** Instability of internal right knee prosthesis

√7ᵗʰ **T84.023** Instability of internal left knee prosthesis

---

¹ Maternity diagnosis only when code is reported using 7th character A for initial encounter.

☑ Additional Character Required   √x7ᵗʰ Placeholder Alert   Unspecified Dx   Other Specified Dx   Manifestation   ►◄ Revised Text   ● New Code   ▲ Revised Code Title

ICD-10-CM 2016   **1027**

√7ᵗʰ **T84.028 Dislocation of other internal joint prosthesis**
Use additional code to identify the joint (Z96.6-)

√7ᵗʰ **T84.029 Dislocation of unspecified internal joint prosthesis**

√6ᵗʰ **T84.03 Mechanical loosening of internal prosthetic joint**
Aseptic loosening of prosthetic joint

√7ᵗʰ **T84.030 Mechanical loosening of internal right hip prosthetic joint**

√7ᵗʰ **T84.031 Mechanical loosening of internal left hip prosthetic joint**

√7ᵗʰ **T84.032 Mechanical loosening of internal right knee prosthetic joint**

√7ᵗʰ **T84.033 Mechanical loosening of internal left knee prosthetic joint**

√7ᵗʰ **T84.038 Mechanical loosening of other internal prosthetic joint**
Use additional code to identify the joint (Z96.6-)

√7ᵗʰ **T84.039 Mechanical loosening of unspecified internal prosthetic joint**

√6ᵗʰ **T84.04 Periprosthetic fracture around internal prosthetic joint**
EXCLUDES 2   breakage (fracture) of prosthetic joint (T84.01)

√7ᵗʰ **T84.040 Periprosthetic fracture around internal prosthetic right hip joint**

√7ᵗʰ **T84.041 Periprosthetic fracture around internal prosthetic left hip joint**

√7ᵗʰ **T84.042 Periprosthetic fracture around internal prosthetic right knee joint**

√7ᵗʰ **T84.043 Periprosthetic fracture around internal prosthetic left knee joint**

√7ᵗʰ **T84.048 Periprosthetic fracture around other internal prosthetic joint**
Use additional code to identify the joint (Z96.6-)

√7ᵗʰ **T84.049 Periprosthetic fracture around unspecified internal prosthetic joint**

√6ᵗʰ **T84.05 Periprosthetic osteolysis of internal prosthetic joint**
Use additional code to identify major osseous defect, if applicable (M89.7-)

√7ᵗʰ **T84.050 Periprosthetic osteolysis of internal prosthetic right hip joint**

√7ᵗʰ **T84.051 Periprosthetic osteolysis of internal prosthetic left hip joint**

√7ᵗʰ **T84.052 Periprosthetic osteolysis of internal prosthetic right knee joint**

√7ᵗʰ **T84.053 Periprosthetic osteolysis of internal prosthetic left knee joint**

√7ᵗʰ **T84.058 Periprosthetic osteolysis of other internal prosthetic joint**
Use additional code to identify the joint (Z96.6-)

√7ᵗʰ **T84.059 Periprosthetic osteolysis of unspecified internal prosthetic joint**

√6ᵗʰ **T84.06 Wear of articular bearing surface of internal prosthetic joint**

√7ᵗʰ **T84.060 Wear of articular bearing surface of internal prosthetic right hip joint**

√7ᵗʰ **T84.061 Wear of articular bearing surface of internal prosthetic left hip joint**

√7ᵗʰ **T84.062 Wear of articular bearing surface of internal prosthetic right knee joint**

√7ᵗʰ **T84.063 Wear of articular bearing surface of internal prosthetic left knee joint**

√7ᵗʰ **T84.068 Wear of articular bearing surface of other internal prosthetic joint**
Use additional code to identify the joint (Z96.6-)

√7ᵗʰ **T84.069 Wear of articular bearing surface of unspecified internal prosthetic joint**

√6ᵗʰ **T84.09 Other mechanical complication of internal joint prosthesis**
Prosthetic joint implant failure NOS

√7ᵗʰ **T84.090 Other mechanical complication of internal right hip prosthesis**

√7ᵗʰ **T84.091 Other mechanical complication of internal left hip prosthesis**

√7ᵗʰ **T84.092 Other mechanical complication of internal right knee prosthesis**

√7ᵗʰ **T84.093 Other mechanical complication of internal left knee prosthesis**

√7ᵗʰ **T84.098 Other mechanical complication of other internal joint prosthesis**
Use additional code to identify the joint (Z96.6-)

√7ᵗʰ **T84.099 Other mechanical complication of unspecified internal joint prosthesis**

√5ᵗʰ **T84.1 Mechanical complication of internal fixation device of bones of limb**
EXCLUDES 2   mechanical complication of internal fixation device of bones of feet (T84.2-)
mechanical complication of internal fixation device of bones of fingers (T84.2-)
mechanical complication of internal fixation device of bones of hands (T84.2-)
mechanical complication of internal fixation device of bones of toes (T84.2-)

√6ᵗʰ **T84.11 Breakdown (mechanical) of internal fixation device of bones of limb**

√7ᵗʰ **T84.110 Breakdown (mechanical) of internal fixation device of right humerus**

√7ᵗʰ **T84.111 Breakdown (mechanical) of internal fixation device of left humerus**

√7ᵗʰ **T84.112 Breakdown (mechanical) of internal fixation device of bone of right forearm**

√7ᵗʰ **T84.113 Breakdown (mechanical) of internal fixation device of bone of left forearm**

√7ᵗʰ **T84.114 Breakdown (mechanical) of internal fixation device of right femur**

√7ᵗʰ **T84.115 Breakdown (mechanical) of internal fixation device of left femur**

√7ᵗʰ **T84.116 Breakdown (mechanical) of internal fixation device of bone of right lower leg**

√7ᵗʰ **T84.117 Breakdown (mechanical) of internal fixation device of bone of left lower leg**

√7ᵗʰ **T84.119 Breakdown (mechanical) of internal fixation device of unspecified bone of limb**

√6ᵗʰ **T84.12 Displacement of internal fixation device of bones of limb**
Malposition of internal fixation device of bones of limb

√7ᵗʰ **T84.120 Displacement of internal fixation device of right humerus**

√7ᵗʰ **T84.121 Displacement of internal fixation device of left humerus**

√7ᵗʰ **T84.122 Displacement of internal fixation device of bone of right forearm**

√7ᵗʰ **T84.123 Displacement of internal fixation device of bone of left forearm**

√7ᵗʰ **T84.124 Displacement of internal fixation device of right femur**

√7ᵗʰ **T84.125 Displacement of internal fixation device of left femur**

√7ᵗʰ **T84.126 Displacement of internal fixation device of bone of right lower leg**

√7ᵗʰ **T84.127 Displacement of internal fixation device of bone of left lower leg**

√7ᵗʰ **T84.129 Displacement of internal fixation device of unspecified bone of limb**

√6ᵗʰ **T84.19 Other mechanical complication of internal fixation device of bones of limb**
Obstruction (mechanical) of internal fixation device of bones of limb
Perforation of internal fixation device of bones of limb
Protrusion of internal fixation device of bones of limb

√7ᵗʰ **T84.190 Other mechanical complication of internal fixation device of right humerus**

√7ᵗʰ **T84.191 Other mechanical complication of internal fixation device of left humerus**

✓7ᵗʰ T84.192 Other mechanical complication of internal fixation device of bone of right forearm

✓7ᵗʰ T84.193 Other mechanical complication of internal fixation device of bone of left forearm

✓7ᵗʰ T84.194 Other mechanical complication of internal fixation device of right femur

✓7ᵗʰ T84.195 Other mechanical complication of internal fixation device of left femur

✓7ᵗʰ T84.196 Other mechanical complication of internal fixation device of bone of right lower leg

✓7ᵗʰ T84.197 Other mechanical complication of internal fixation device of bone of left lower leg

✓7ᵗʰ T84.199 Other mechanical complication of internal fixation device of unspecified bone of limb

✓5ᵗʰ T84.2 Mechanical complication of internal fixation device of other bones

✓6ᵗʰ T84.21 Breakdown (mechanical) of internal fixation device of other bones

✓7ᵗʰ T84.210 Breakdown (mechanical) of internal fixation device of bones of hand and fingers

✓7ᵗʰ T84.213 Breakdown (mechanical) of internal fixation device of bones of foot and toes

✓7ᵗʰ T84.216 Breakdown (mechanical) of internal fixation device of vertebrae

✓7ᵗʰ T84.218 Breakdown (mechanical) of internal fixation device of other bones

✓6ᵗʰ T84.22 Displacement of internal fixation device of other bones
Malposition of internal fixation device of other bones

✓7ᵗʰ T84.220 Displacement of internal fixation device of bones of hand and fingers

✓7ᵗʰ T84.223 Displacement of internal fixation device of bones of foot and toes

✓7ᵗʰ T84.226 Displacement of internal fixation device of vertebrae

✓7ᵗʰ T84.228 Displacement of internal fixation device of other bones

✓6ᵗʰ T84.29 Other mechanical complication of internal fixation device of other bones
Obstruction (mechanical) of internal fixation device of other bones
Perforation of internal fixation device of other bones
Protrusion of internal fixation device of other bones

✓7ᵗʰ T84.290 Other mechanical complication of internal fixation device of bones of hand and fingers

✓7ᵗʰ T84.293 Other mechanical complication of internal fixation device of bones of foot and toes

✓7ᵗʰ T84.296 Other mechanical complication of internal fixation device of vertebrae

✓7ᵗʰ T84.298 Other mechanical complication of internal fixation device of other bones

✓5ᵗʰ T84.3 Mechanical complication of other bone devices, implants and grafts
EXCLUDES 2 other complications of bone graft (T86.83-)

✓6ᵗʰ T84.31 Breakdown (mechanical) of other bone devices, implants and grafts

✓7ᵗʰ T84.310 Breakdown (mechanical) of electronic bone stimulator

✓7ᵗʰ T84.318 Breakdown (mechanical) of other bone devices, implants and grafts

✓6ᵗʰ T84.32 Displacement of other bone devices, implants and grafts
Malposition of other bone devices, implants and grafts

✓7ᵗʰ T84.320 Displacement of electronic bone stimulator

✓7ᵗʰ T84.328 Displacement of other bone devices, implants and grafts
AHA: 2014, 4Q, 28

✓6ᵗʰ T84.39 Other mechanical complication of other bone devices, implants and grafts
Obstruction (mechanical) of other bone devices, implants and grafts
Perforation of other bone devices, implants and grafts
Protrusion of other bone devices, implants and grafts

✓7ᵗʰ T84.390 Other mechanical complication of electronic bone stimulator

✓7ᵗʰ T84.398 Other mechanical complication of other bone devices, implants and grafts

✓5ᵗʰ T84.4 Mechanical complication of other internal orthopedic devices, implants and grafts

✓6ᵗʰ T84.41 Breakdown (mechanical) of other internal orthopedic devices, implants and grafts

✓7ᵗʰ T84.410 Breakdown (mechanical) of muscle and tendon graft

✓7ᵗʰ T84.418 Breakdown (mechanical) of other internal orthopedic devices, implants and grafts

✓6ᵗʰ T84.42 Displacement of other internal orthopedic devices, implants and grafts
Malposition of other internal orthopedic devices, implants and grafts

✓7ᵗʰ T84.420 Displacement of muscle and tendon graft

✓7ᵗʰ T84.428 Displacement of other internal orthopedic devices, implants and grafts

✓6ᵗʰ T84.49 Other mechanical complication of other internal orthopedic devices, implants and grafts
Mechanical complication of other internal orthopedic devices, implants and grafts NOS
Obstruction (mechanical) of other internal orthopedic devices, implants and grafts
Perforation of other internal orthopedic devices, implants and grafts
Protrusion of other internal orthopedic devices, implants and grafts

✓7ᵗʰ T84.490 Other mechanical complication of muscle and tendon graft

✓7ᵗʰ T84.498 Other mechanical complication of other internal orthopedic devices, implants and grafts

✓5ᵗʰ T84.5 Infection and inflammatory reaction due to internal joint prosthesis
Use additional code to identify infection
AHA: 2015, 1Q, 16

✓x7ᵗʰ T84.50 Infection and inflammatory reaction due to unspecified internal joint prosthesis

✓x7ᵗʰ T84.51 Infection and inflammatory reaction due to internal right hip prosthesis

✓x7ᵗʰ T84.52 Infection and inflammatory reaction due to internal left hip prosthesis

✓x7ᵗʰ T84.53 Infection and inflammatory reaction due to internal right knee prosthesis

✓x7ᵗʰ T84.54 Infection and inflammatory reaction due to internal left knee prosthesis

✓x7ᵗʰ T84.59 Infection and inflammatory reaction due to other internal joint prosthesis

✓5ᵗʰ T84.6 Infection and inflammatory reaction due to internal fixation device
Use additional code to identify infection

✓x7ᵗʰ T84.60 Infection and inflammatory reaction due to internal fixation device of unspecified site

✓6ᵗʰ T84.61 Infection and inflammatory reaction due to internal fixation device of arm

✓7ᵗʰ T84.610 Infection and inflammatory reaction due to internal fixation device of right humerus

✓7ᵗʰ T84.611 Infection and inflammatory reaction due to internal fixation device of left humerus

✓7ᵗʰ T84.612 Infection and inflammatory reaction due to internal fixation device of right radius

✓7ᵗʰ T84.613 Infection and inflammatory reaction due to internal fixation device of left radius

✓7ᵗʰ T84.614 Infection and inflammatory reaction due to internal fixation device of right ulna

✓7ᵗʰ T84.615 Infection and inflammatory reaction due to internal fixation device of left ulna

---

✓ Additional Character Required   ✓x7ᵗʰ Placeholder Alert   Unspecified Dx   Other Specified Dx   Manifestation   ▶◀ Revised Text   ● New Code   ▲ Revised Code Title

Chapter 19. Injury, Poisoning, and Certain Other Consequences of External Causes *(left margin)*

☑7ᵗʰ **T84.619** Infection and inflammatory reaction due to internal fixation device of unspecified bone of arm

☑6ᵗʰ **T84.62** Infection and inflammatory reaction due to internal fixation device of leg

☑7ᵗʰ **T84.620** Infection and inflammatory reaction due to internal fixation device of right femur

☑7ᵗʰ **T84.621** Infection and inflammatory reaction due to internal fixation device of left femur

☑7ᵗʰ **T84.622** Infection and inflammatory reaction due to internal fixation device of right tibia

☑7ᵗʰ **T84.623** Infection and inflammatory reaction due to internal fixation device of left tibia

☑7ᵗʰ **T84.624** Infection and inflammatory reaction due to internal fixation device of right fibula

☑7ᵗʰ **T84.625** Infection and inflammatory reaction due to internal fixation device of left fibula

☑7ᵗʰ **T84.629** Infection and inflammatory reaction due to internal fixation device of unspecified bone of leg

☑x7ᵗʰ **T84.63** Infection and inflammatory reaction due to internal fixation device of spine

☑x7ᵗʰ **T84.69** Infection and inflammatory reaction due to internal fixation device of other site

☑x7ᵗʰ **T84.7** Infection and inflammatory reaction due to other internal orthopedic prosthetic devices, implants and grafts
Use additional code to identify infection

☑5ᵗʰ **T84.8** Other specified complications of internal orthopedic prosthetic devices, implants and grafts

☑x7ᵗʰ **T84.81** Embolism due to internal orthopedic prosthetic devices, implants and grafts

☑x7ᵗʰ **T84.82** Fibrosis due to internal orthopedic prosthetic devices, implants and grafts

☑x7ᵗʰ **T84.83** Hemorrhage due to internal orthopedic prosthetic devices, implants and grafts

☑x7ᵗʰ **T84.84** Pain due to internal orthopedic prosthetic devices, implants and grafts

☑x7ᵗʰ **T84.85** Stenosis due to internal orthopedic prosthetic devices, implants and grafts

☑x7ᵗʰ **T84.86** Thrombosis due to internal orthopedic prosthetic devices, implants and grafts

☑x7ᵗʰ **T84.89** Other specified complication of internal orthopedic prosthetic devices, implants and grafts

☑x7ᵗʰ **T84.9** Unspecified complication of internal orthopedic prosthetic device, implant and graft

☑4ᵗʰ **T85** Complications of other internal prosthetic devices, implants and grafts
EXCLUDES 2 failure and rejection of transplanted organs and tissue (T86.-)

The appropriate 7th character is to be added to each code from category T85.
A   initial encounter
D   subsequent encounter
S   sequela

☑5ᵗʰ **T85.0** Mechanical complication of ventricular intracranial (communicating) shunt

☑x7ᵗʰ **T85.01** Breakdown (mechanical) of ventricular intracranial (communicating) shunt

☑x7ᵗʰ **T85.02** Displacement of ventricular intracranial (communicating) shunt
Malposition of ventricular intracranial (communicating) shunt

☑x7ᵗʰ **T85.03** Leakage of ventricular intracranial (communicating) shunt

☑x7ᵗʰ **T85.09** Other mechanical complication of ventricular intracranial (communicating) shunt
Obstruction (mechanical) of ventricular intracranial (communicating) shunt
Perforation of ventricular intracranial (communicating) shunt
Protrusion of ventricular intracranial (communicating) shunt

☑5ᵗʰ **T85.1** Mechanical complication of implanted electronic stimulator of nervous system

☑6ᵗʰ **T85.11** Breakdown (mechanical) of implanted electronic stimulator of nervous system

☑7ᵗʰ **T85.110** Breakdown (mechanical) of implanted electronic neurostimulator (electrode) of brain

☑7ᵗʰ **T85.111** Breakdown (mechanical) of implanted electronic neurostimulator (electrode) of peripheral nerve

☑7ᵗʰ **T85.112** Breakdown (mechanical) of implanted electronic neurostimulator (electrode) of spinal cord

☑7ᵗʰ **T85.118** Breakdown (mechanical) of other implanted electronic stimulator of nervous system

☑6ᵗʰ **T85.12** Displacement of implanted electronic stimulator of nervous system
Malposition of implanted electronic stimulator of nervous system

☑7ᵗʰ **T85.120** Displacement of implanted electronic neurostimulator (electrode) of brain

☑7ᵗʰ **T85.121** Displacement of implanted electronic neurostimulator (electrode) of peripheral nerve

☑7ᵗʰ **T85.122** Displacement of implanted electronic neurostimulator (electrode) of spinal cord

☑7ᵗʰ **T85.128** Displacement of other implanted electronic stimulator of nervous system

☑6ᵗʰ **T85.19** Other mechanical complication of implanted electronic stimulator of nervous system
Leakage of implanted electronic stimulator of nervous system
Obstruction (mechanical) of implanted electronic stimulator of nervous system
Perforation of implanted electronic stimulator of nervous system
Protrusion of implanted electronic stimulator of nervous system

☑7ᵗʰ **T85.190** Other mechanical complication of implanted electronic neurostimulator (electrode) of brain

☑7ᵗʰ **T85.191** Other mechanical complication of implanted electronic neurostimulator (electrode) of peripheral nerve

☑7ᵗʰ **T85.192** Other mechanical complication of implanted electronic neurostimulator (electrode) of spinal cord

☑7ᵗʰ **T85.199** Other mechanical complication of other implanted electronic stimulator of nervous system

☑5ᵗʰ **T85.2** Mechanical complication of intraocular lens

☑x7ᵗʰ **T85.21** Breakdown (mechanical) of intraocular lens

☑x7ᵗʰ **T85.22** Displacement of intraocular lens
Malposition of intraocular lens

☑x7ᵗʰ **T85.29** Other mechanical complication of intraocular lens
Obstruction (mechanical) of intraocular lens
Perforation of intraocular lens
Protrusion of intraocular lens

☑5ᵗʰ **T85.3** Mechanical complication of other ocular prosthetic devices, implants and grafts
EXCLUDES 2 other complications of corneal graft (T86.84-)

☑6ᵗʰ **T85.31** Breakdown (mechanical) of other ocular prosthetic devices, implants and grafts

☑7ᵗʰ **T85.310** Breakdown (mechanical) of prosthetic orbit of right eye

☑7ᵗʰ **T85.311** Breakdown (mechanical) of prosthetic orbit of left eye

☑7ᵗʰ **T85.318** Breakdown (mechanical) of other ocular prosthetic devices, implants and grafts

☑6ᵗʰ **T85.32** Displacement of other ocular prosthetic devices, implants and grafts
Malposition of other ocular prosthetic devices, implants and grafts

☑7ᵗʰ **T85.320** Displacement of prosthetic orbit of right eye

☑7ᵗʰ **T85.321** Displacement of prosthetic orbit of left eye

EXCLUDES 1 Not coded here   *EXCLUDES 2* Not included here   N Newborn Age: 0   P Pediatric Age: 0-17   M Maternity Age: 12-55   A Adult Age: 15-124

1030   ICD-10-CM 2016

☑7ᵗʰ **T85.328** **Displacement of other ocular prosthetic devices, implants and grafts**

☑6ᵗʰ **T85.39** **Other** mechanical complication of other ocular prosthetic devices, implants and grafts
Obstruction (mechanical) of other ocular prosthetic devices, implants and grafts
Perforation of other ocular prosthetic devices, implants and grafts
Protrusion of other ocular prosthetic devices, implants and grafts

☑7ᵗʰ **T85.390** **Other mechanical complication of prosthetic orbit of** right eye

☑7ᵗʰ **T85.391** **Other mechanical complication of prosthetic orbit of** left eye

☑7ᵗʰ **T85.398** **Other mechanical complication of other ocular prosthetic devices, implants and grafts**

☑5ᵗʰ **T85.4** **Mechanical complication of** breast prosthesis and implant

✓x 7ᵗʰ **T85.41** **Breakdown (mechanical) of breast prosthesis and implant**

✓x 7ᵗʰ **T85.42** **Displacement of breast prosthesis and implant**
Malposition of breast prosthesis and implant

✓x 7ᵗʰ **T85.43** **Leakage of breast prosthesis and implant**

✓x 7ᵗʰ **T85.44** **Capsular contracture of breast implant**

✓x 7ᵗʰ **T85.49** **Other mechanical complication of breast prosthesis and implant**
Obstruction (mechanical) of breast prosthesis and implant
Perforation of breast prosthesis and implant
Protrusion of breast prosthesis and Implant

☑5ᵗʰ **T85.5** **Mechanical complication of** gastrointestinal prosthetic devices, implants and grafts

☑6ᵗʰ **T85.51** **Breakdown (mechanical) of gastrointestinal prosthetic devices, implants and grafts**

☑7ᵗʰ **T85.510** **Breakdown (mechanical) of** bile duct prosthesis

☑7ᵗʰ **T85.511** **Breakdown (mechanical) of** esophageal anti-reflux **device**

☑7ᵗʰ **T85.518** **Breakdown (mechanical) of other gastrointestinal prosthetic devices, implants and grafts**

☑6ᵗʰ **T85.52** **Displacement of gastrointestinal prosthetic devices, implants and grafts**
Malposition of gastrointestinal prosthetic devices, implants and grafts

☑7ᵗʰ **T85.520** **Displacement of** bile duct **prosthesis**

☑7ᵗʰ **T85.521** **Displacement of** esophageal anti-reflux **device**

☑7ᵗʰ **T85.528** **Displacement of other gastrointestinal prosthetic devices, implants and grafts**

☑6ᵗʰ **T85.59** **Other** mechanical complication of gastrointestinal prosthetic devices, implants and grafts
Obstruction, mechanical of gastrointestinal prosthetic devices, implants and grafts
Perforation of gastrointestinal prosthetic devices, implants and grafts
Protrusion of gastrointestinal prosthetic devices, implants and grafts

☑7ᵗʰ **T85.590** **Other mechanical complication of** bile duct **prosthesis**

☑7ᵗʰ **T85.591** **Other mechanical complication of** esophageal anti-reflux **device**

☑7ᵗʰ **T85.598** **Other mechanical complication of other gastrointestinal prosthetic devices, implants and grafts**

☑5ᵗʰ **T85.6** **Mechanical complication of** other specified internal and external prosthetic devices, implants and grafts

☑6ᵗʰ **T85.61** **Breakdown (mechanical) of other specified internal prosthetic devices, implants and grafts**

☑7ᵗʰ **T85.610** **Breakdown (mechanical) of** epidural and subdural infusion catheter

☑7ᵗʰ **T85.611** **Breakdown (mechanical) of** intraperitoneal dialysis catheter
EXCLUDES 1 *mechanical complication of vascular dialysis catheter (T82.4-)*

☑7ᵗʰ **T85.612** **Breakdown (mechanical) of** permanent sutures
EXCLUDES 1 *mechanical complication of permanent (wire) suture used in bone repair (T84.1-T84.2)*

☑7ᵗʰ **T85.613** **Breakdown (mechanical) of** artificial skin graft and decellularized allodermis
Failure of artificial skin graft and decellularized allodermis
Non-adherence of artificial skin graft and decellularized allodermis
Poor incorporation of artificial skin graft and decellularized allodermis
Shearing of artificial skin graft and decellularized allodermis

☑7ᵗʰ **T85.614** **Breakdown (mechanical) of** insulin pump

☑7ᵗʰ **T85.618** **Breakdown (mechanical) of other specified internal prosthetic devices, implants and grafts**

☑6ᵗʰ **T85.62** **Displacement of other specified internal prosthetic devices, implants and grafts**
Malposition of other specified internal prosthetic devices, implants and grafts

☑7ᵗʰ **T85.620** **Displacement of** epidural and subdural infusion catheter

☑7ᵗʰ **T85.621** **Displacement of** intraperitoneal dialysis catheter
EXCLUDES 1 *mechanical complication of vascular dialysis catheter (T82.4-)*

☑7ᵗʰ **T85.622** **Displacement of** permanent sutures
EXCLUDES 1 *mechanical complication of permanent (wire) suture used in bone repair (T84.1-T84.2)*

☑7ᵗʰ **T85.623** **Displacement of** artificial skin graft and decellularized allodermis
Dislodgement of artificial skin graft and decellularized allodermis
Displacement of artificial skin graft and decellularized allodermis

☑7ᵗʰ **T85.624** **Displacement of** insulin pump

☑7ᵗʰ **T85.628** **Displacement of other specified internal prosthetic devices, implants and grafts**

☑6ᵗʰ **T85.63** **Leakage of** other specified internal prosthetic devices, implants and grafts

☑7ᵗʰ **T85.630** **Leakage of** epidural and subdural infusion catheter

☑7ᵗʰ **T85.631** **Leakage of** intraperitoneal dialysis catheter
EXCLUDES 1 *mechanical complication of vascular dialysis catheter (T82.4)*

☑7ᵗʰ **T85.633** **Leakage of** insulin pump

☑7ᵗʰ **T85.638** **Leakage of other specified internal prosthetic devices, implants and grafts**

☑6ᵗʰ **T85.69** **Other** mechanical complication of other specified internal prosthetic devices, implants and grafts
Obstruction, mechanical of other specified internal prosthetic devices, implants and grafts
Perforation of other specified internal prosthetic devices, implants and grafts
Protrusion of other specified internal prosthetic devices, implants and grafts

☑7ᵗʰ **T85.690** **Other mechanical complication of** epidural and subdural infusion catheter

☑7ᵗʰ **T85.691** **Other mechanical complication of** intraperitoneal dialysis catheter
EXCLUDES 1 *mechanical complication of vascular dialysis catheter (T82.4)*

☑7ᵗʰ **T85.692** **Other mechanical complication of** permanent sutures
EXCLUDES 1 *mechanical complication of permanent (wire) suture used in bone repair (T84.1-T84.2)*

☑7ᵗʰ **T85.693** **Other mechanical complication of** artificial skin graft and decellularized allodermis

---

☑ Additional Character Required   ✓x 7ᵗʰ Placeholder Alert   Unspecified Dx   Other Specified Dx   Manifestation   ▶◀ Revised Text   ● New Code   ▲ Revised Code Title

✓7ᵗʰ **T85.694** **Other mechanical complication of** insulin pump

✓7ᵗʰ **T85.698** **Other mechanical complication of other specified internal prosthetic devices, implants and grafts**
　　　　Mechanical complication of nonabsorbable surgical material NOS

✓5ᵗʰ **T85.7** **Infection and inflammatory reaction due to other internal prosthetic devices, implants and grafts**
　　Use additional code to identify infection

✓x7ᵗʰ **T85.71** **Infection and inflammatory reaction due to peritoneal dialysis catheter**

✓x7ᵗʰ **T85.72** **Infection and inflammatory reaction due to** insulin pump

✓x7ᵗʰ **T85.79** **Infection and inflammatory reaction due to other internal prosthetic devices, implants and grafts**

✓6ᵗʰ **T85.8** **Other specified complications of internal prosthetic devices, implants and grafts, not elsewhere classified**

✓x7ᵗʰ **T85.81** **Embolism due to internal prosthetic devices, implants and grafts, not elsewhere classified**

✓x7ᵗʰ **T85.82** **Fibrosis due to internal prosthetic devices, implants and grafts, not elsewhere classified**

✓x7ᵗʰ **T85.83** **Hemorrhage due to internal prosthetic devices, implants and grafts, not elsewhere classified**

✓x7ᵗʰ **T85.84** **Pain due to internal prosthetic devices, implants and grafts, not elsewhere classified**

✓x7ᵗʰ **T85.85** **Stenosis due to internal prosthetic devices, implants and grafts, not elsewhere classified**

✓x7ᵗʰ **T85.86** **Thrombosis due to internal prosthetic devices, implants and grafts, not elsewhere classified**

✓x7ᵗʰ **T85.89** **Other specified complication of internal prosthetic devices, implants and grafts, not elsewhere classified**

✓x7ᵗʰ **T85.9** **Unspecified complication of internal prosthetic device, implant and graft**
　　Complication of internal prosthetic device, implant and graft NOS

✓4ᵗʰ **T86** **Complications of transplanted organs and tissue**
　　Use additional code to identify other transplant complications, such as:
　　graft-versus-host disease (D89.81-)
　　malignancy associated with organ transplant (C80.2)
　　post-transplant lymphoproliferative disorders (PTLD) (D47.Z1)

✓5ᵗʰ **T86.0** **Complications of** bone marrow **transplant**

T86.00 **Unspecified complication of bone marrow transplant**

T86.01 **Bone marrow transplant** rejection

T86.02 **Bone marrow transplant** failure

T86.03 **Bone marrow transplant** infection

T86.09 **Other complications of bone marrow transplant**

✓5ᵗʰ **T86.1** **Complications of** kidney **transplant**

T86.10 **Unspecified complication of kidney transplant**

T86.11 **Kidney transplant** rejection

T86.12 **Kidney transplant** failure
　　AHA: 2013, 1Q, 24

T86.13 **Kidney transplant** infection
　　Use additional code to specify infection

T86.19 **Other complication of kidney transplant**

✓5ᵗʰ **T86.2** **Complications of** heart **transplant**
　　EXCLUDES 1　complication of:
　　　artificial heart device (T82.5)
　　　heart-lung transplant (T86.3)

T86.20 **Unspecified complication of heart transplant**

T86.21 **Heart transplant** rejection

T86.22 **Heart transplant** failure

T86.23 **Heart transplant** infection
　　Use additional code to specify infection

✓6ᵗʰ **T86.29** **Other complications of heart transplant**

T86.290 **Cardiac allograft vasculopathy**
　　EXCLUDES 1　atherosclerosis of coronary arteries (I25.75-, I25.76-, I25.81-)

T86.298 **Other complications of heart transplant**

✓5ᵗʰ **T86.3** **Complications of** heart-lung **transplant**

T86.30 **Unspecified complication of heart-lung transplant**

T86.31 **Heart-lung transplant** rejection

T86.32 **Heart-lung transplant** failure

T86.33 **Heart-lung transplant** infection
　　Use additional code to specify infection

T86.39 **Other complications of heart-lung transplant**

✓5ᵗʰ **T86.4** **Complications of** liver **transplant**

T86.40 **Unspecified complication of liver transplant**

T86.41 **Liver transplant** rejection

T86.42 **Liver transplant** failure

T86.43 **Liver transplant** infection
　　Use additional code to identify infection, such as:
　　cytomegalovirus (CMV) infection (B25.-)

T86.49 **Other complications of liver transplant**

T86.5 **Complications of** stem cell **transplant**
　　Complications from stem cells from peripheral blood
　　Complications from stem cells from umbilical cord

✓5ᵗʰ **T86.8** **Complications of** other **transplanted organs and tissues**

✓6ᵗʰ **T86.81** **Complications of** lung **transplant**
　　EXCLUDES 1　complication of heart-lung transplant (T86.3-)

T86.810 **Lung transplant** rejection

T86.811 **Lung transplant** failure

T86.812 **Lung transplant** infection
　　Use additional code to specify infection

T86.818 **Other complications of lung transplant**

T86.819 **Unspecified complication of lung transplant**

✓6ᵗʰ **T86.82** **Complications of** skin graft (allograft) (autograft)
　　EXCLUDES 2　complication of artificial skin graft (T85.693)

T86.820 **Skin graft (allograft)** rejection

T86.821 **Skin graft (allograft) (autograft)** failure

T86.822 **Skin graft (allograft) (autograft)** infection
　　Use additional code to specify infection

T86.828 **Other complications of skin graft (allograft) (autograft)**

T86.829 **Unspecified complication of skin graft (allograft) (autograft)**

✓6ᵗʰ **T86.83** **Complications of** bone graft
　　EXCLUDES 2　mechanical complications of bone graft (T84.3-)

T86.830 **Bone graft** rejection

T86.831 **Bone graft** failure

T86.832 **Bone graft** infection
　　Use additional code to specify infection

T86.838 **Other complications of bone graft**

T86.839 **Unspecified complication of bone graft**

✓6ᵗʰ **T86.84** **Complications of** corneal **transplant**
　　EXCLUDES 2　mechanical complications of corneal graft (T85.3-)

T86.840 **Corneal transplant** rejection

T86.841 **Corneal transplant** failure

T86.842 **Corneal transplant** infection
　　Use additional code to specify infection

T86.848 **Other complications of corneal transplant**

T86.849 **Unspecified complication of corneal transplant**

✓6ᵗʰ **T86.85** **Complication of** intestine **transplant**

T86.850 **Intestine transplant** rejection

T86.851 **Intestine transplant** failure

T86.852 **Intestine transplant** infection
　　Use additional code to specify infection

T86.858 **Other complications of intestine transplant**

T86.859 **Unspecified complication of intestine transplant**

✓6ᵗʰ **T86.89** **Complications of** other **transplanted tissue**
　　Transplant failure or rejection of pancreas

T86.890 **Other transplanted tissue** rejection

T86.891 **Other transplanted tissue** failure

T86.892 **Other transplanted tissue** infection
　　Use additional code to specify infection

EXCLUDES 1　Not coded here　　　EXCLUDES 2　Not included here　　　N Newborn Age: 0　　　P Pediatric Age: 0-17　　　M Maternity Age: 12-55　　　A Adult Age: 15-124

1032　　　ICD-10-CM 2016

T86.898 **Other complications of other transplanted tissue**

T86.899 **Unspecified complication of other transplanted tissue**

✓5ᵗʰ **T86.9 Complication of** unspecified transplanted organ and tissue

T86.90 **Unspecified complication of unspecified transplanted organ and tissue**

T86.91 **Unspecified transplanted organ and tissue** rejection

T86.92 **Unspecified transplanted organ and tissue** failure

T86.93 **Unspecified transplanted organ and tissue** infection
Use additional code to specify infection

T86.99 **Other complications of unspecified transplanted organ and tissue**

✓4ᵗʰ **T87 Complications peculiar to reattachment and amputation**

✓5ᵗʰ **T87.0 Complications of reattached (part of)** upper extremity

✓6ᵗʰ **T87.0X Complications of reattached (part of) upper extremity**

T87.0X1 **Complications of reattached (part of)** right upper extremity

T87.0X2 **Complications of reattached (part of)** left upper extremity

T87.0X9 **Complications of reattached (part of) unspecified upper extremity**

✓5ᵗʰ **T87.1 Complications of reattached (part of)** lower extremity

✓6ᵗʰ **T87.1X Complications of reattached (part of) lower extremity**

T87.1X1 **Complications of reattached (part of)** right lower extremity

T87.1X2 **Complications of reattached (part of)** left lower extremity

T87.1X9 **Complications of reattached (part of) unspecified lower extremity**

T87.2 **Complications of other reattached body part**

✓5ᵗʰ **T87.3 Neuroma of amputation stump**

T87.30 **Neuroma of amputation stump, unspecified extremity**

T87.31 **Neuroma of amputation stump,** right upper extremity

T87.32 **Neuroma of amputation stump,** left upper extremity

T87.33 **Neuroma of amputation stump,** right lower extremity

T87.34 **Neuroma of amputation stump,** left lower extremity

✓5ᵗʰ **T87.4 Infection** of amputation stump

T87.40 **Infection of amputation stump, unspecified extremity**

T87.41 **Infection of amputation stump,** right upper extremity

T87.42 **Infection of amputation stump,** left upper extremity

T87.43 **Infection of amputation stump,** right lower extremity

T87.44 **Infection of amputation stump,** left lower extremity

✓5ᵗʰ **T87.5 Necrosis of amputation stump**

T87.50 **Necrosis of amputation stump, unspecified extremity**

T87.51 **Necrosis of amputation stump,** right upper extremity

T87.52 **Necrosis of amputation stump,** left upper extremity

T87.53 **Necrosis of amputation stump,** right lower extremity

T87.54 **Necrosis of amputation stump,** left lower extremity

✓5ᵗʰ **T87.8 Other complications of amputation stump**

T87.81 **Dehiscence** of amputation stump

T87.89 **Other complications of amputation stump**
Amputation stump contracture
Amputation stump contracture of next proximal joint
Amputation stump flexion
Amputation stump edema
Amputation stump hematoma
EXCLUDES 2 *phantom limb syndrome (G54.6-G54.7)*

T87.9 **Unspecified complications of amputation stump**

✓4ᵗʰ **T88 Other complications of surgical and medical care, not elsewhere classified**

EXCLUDES 2 *complication following infusion, transfusion and therapeutic injection (T80.-)*
complication following procedure NEC (T81.-)
complications of anesthesia in labor and delivery (O74.-)
complications of anesthesia in pregnancy (O29.-)
complications of anesthesia in puerperium (O89.-)
complications of devices, implants and grafts (T82-T85)
complications of obstetric surgery and procedure (O75.4)
dermatitis due to drugs and medicaments (L23.3, L24.4, L25.1, L27.0-L27.1)
poisoning and toxic effects of drugs and chemicals (T36-T65 with fifth or sixth character 1-4 or 6)
specified complications classified elsewhere

The appropriate 7th character is to be added to each code from category T88.
A   initial encounter
D   subsequent encounter
S   sequela

✓x7ᵗʰ **T88.0 Infection following immunization**
Sepsis following immunization

✓x7ᵗʰ **T88.1 Other complications following immunization, not elsewhere classified**
Generalized vaccinia
Rash following immunization
EXCLUDES 1 *vaccinia not from vaccine (B08.011)*
EXCLUDES 2 *anaphylactic shock due to serum (T80.5-)*
other serum reactions (T80.6-)
postimmunization arthropathy (M02.2)
postimmunization encephalitis (G04.02)
postimmunization fever (R50.83)

✓x7ᵗʰ **T88.2 Shock due to anesthesia**
Use additional code for adverse effect, if applicable, to identify drug (T41.- with fifth or sixth character 5)
EXCLUDES 1 *complications of anesthesia (in):*
labor and delivery (O74.-)
postprocedural shock NOS (T81.1-)
pregnancy (O29.-)
puerperium (O89.-)

✓x7ᵗʰ **T88.3 Malignant hyperthermia due to anesthesia**
Use additional code for adverse effect, if applicable, to identify drug (T41.- with fifth or sixth character 5)

✓x7ᵗʰ **T88.4 Failed or difficult intubation**

✓5ᵗʰ **T88.5 Other complications of anesthesia**
Use additional code for adverse effect, if applicable, to identify drug (T41.- with fifth or sixth character 5)

✓x7ᵗʰ **T88.51 Hypothermia following anesthesia**

✓x7ᵗʰ **T88.52 Failed moderate sedation during procedure**
Failed conscious sedation during procedure
EXCLUDES 2 *personal history of failed moderate sedation (Z92.83)*

✓x7ᵗʰ **T88.59 Other complications of anesthesia**

✓x7ᵗʰ **T88.6 Anaphylactic reaction due to adverse effect of correct drug or medicament properly administered**
Anaphylactic shock due to adverse effect of correct drug or medicament properly administered
Anaphylactoid reaction NOS
Use additional code for adverse effect, if applicable, to identify drug (T36-T50 with fifth or sixth character 5)
EXCLUDES 1 *anaphylactic reaction due to serum (T80.5-)*
anaphylactic shock or reaction due to adverse food reaction (T78.0-)

☑ Additional Character Required   ✓x7ᵗʰ Placeholder Alert   Unspecified Dx   Other Specified Dx   Manifestation   ▶◀ Revised Text   ● New Code   ▲ Revised Code Title

ICD-10-CM 2016   1033

√x 7ᵗʰ **T88.7** **Unspecified adverse effect of drug or medicament**
Drug hypersensitivity NOS
Drug reaction NOS
Use additional code for adverse effect, if applicable, to identify
drug (T36-T50 with fifth or sixth character 5)
EXCLUDES 1 specified adverse effects of drugs and medicaments
(A00-R94 and T80-T88.6, T88.8)

√x 7ᵗʰ **T88.8** **Other specified complications of surgical and medical care,
not elsewhere classified**
Use additional code to identify the complication

√x 7ᵗʰ **T88.9** **Complication of surgical and medical care, unspecified**

EXCLUDES 1 Not coded here   EXCLUDES 2 Not included here   N Newborn Age: 0   P Pediatric Age: 0-17   M Maternity Age: 12-55   A Adult Age: 15-124

Chapter 20. External Causes of Morbidity (V00–Y99)

Chapter Specific Guidelines with Coding Examples

The chapter specific guidelines from the ICD-10-CM Official Guidelines for Coding and Reporting have been provided below. Along with these guidelines are coding examples, contained in the shaded boxes, that have been developed to help illustrate the coding and/or sequencing guidance found in these guidelines.

The external causes of morbidity codes should never be sequenced as the first-listed or principal diagnosis.

External cause codes are intended to provide data for injury research and evaluation of injury prevention strategies. These codes capture how the injury or health condition happened (cause), the intent (unintentional or accidental; or intentional, such as suicide or assault), the place where the event occurred, the activity of the patient at the time of the event, and the person's status (e.g., civilian, military).

There is no national requirement for mandatory ICD-10-CM external cause code reporting. Unless a provider is subject to a state-based external cause code reporting mandate or these codes are required by a particular payer, reporting of ICD-10-CM codes in Chapter 20, External Causes of Morbidity, is not required. In the absence of a mandatory reporting requirement, providers are encouraged to voluntarily report external cause codes, as they provide valuable data for injury research and evaluation of injury prevention strategies.

a. General external cause coding guidelines

1) Used with any code in the range of A00.0–T88.9, Z00–Z99

An external cause code may be used with any code in the range of A00.0–T88.9, Z00–Z99, classification that is a health condition due to an external cause. Though they are most applicable to injuries, they are also valid for use with such things as infections or diseases due to an external source, and other health conditions, such as a heart attack that occurs during strenuous physical activity.

Actinic reticuloid due to tanning bed use

L57.1	**Actinic reticuloid**
W89.1XXA	**Exposure to tanning bed, initial encounter**

Explanation: An external cause code may be used with any code in the range of A00.0–T88.9, Z00–Z99, classifications that describe health conditions due to an external cause. Code W89.1 Exposure to tanning bed requires a seventh character of A to report this initial encounter, with a placeholder X for the fifth and sixth characters.

---

2) External cause code used for length of treatment

Assign the external cause code, with the appropriate 7th character (initial encounter, subsequent encounter or sequela) for each encounter for which the injury or condition is being treated.

Most categories in chapter 20 have a 7th character requirement for each applicable code. Most categories in this chapter have three 7th character values: A, initial encounter, D, subsequent encounter and S, sequela. While the patient may be seen by a new or different provider over the course of treatment for an injury or condition, assignment of the 7th character for external cause should match the 7th character of the code assigned for the associated injury or condition for the encounter.

3) Use the full range of external cause codes

Use the full range of external cause codes to completely describe the cause, the intent, the place of occurrence, and if applicable, the activity of the patient at the time of the event, and the patient's status, for all injuries, and other health conditions due to an external cause.

4) Assign as many external cause codes as necessary

Assign as many external cause codes as necessary to fully explain each cause. If only one external code can be recorded, assign the code most related to the principal diagnosis.

5) The selection of the appropriate external cause code

The selection of the appropriate external cause code is guided by the Alphabetic Index of External Causes and by Inclusion and Exclusion notes in the Tabular List.

6) External cause code can never be a principal diagnosis

An external cause code can never be a principal (first-listed) diagnosis.

7) Combination external cause codes

Certain of the external cause codes are combination codes that identify sequential events that result in an injury, such as a fall which results in striking against an object. The injury may be due to either event or both.

The combination external cause code used should correspond to the sequence of events regardless of which caused the most serious injury.

Toddler tripped and fell while walking and struck his head on an end table, sustaining a scalp contusion

S00.03XA	**Contusion of scalp, initial encounter**
W01.190A	**Fall on same level from slipping, tripping and stumbling with subsequent striking against furniture, initial encounter**

Explanation: Combination external cause codes identify sequential events that result in an injury, such as a fall resulting in striking against an object. The injury may be due to either or both events.

---

8) No external cause code needed in certain circumstances

No external cause code from Chapter 20 is needed if the external cause and intent are included in a code from another chapter (e.g. T36.0X1-Poisoning by penicillins, accidental (unintentional)).

b. Place of occurrence guideline

Codes from category Y92, Place of occurrence of the external cause, are secondary codes for use after other external cause codes to identify the location of the patient at the time of injury or other condition.

Generally, a place of occurrence code is assigned only once, at the initial encounter for treatment. However, in the rare instance that a new injury occurs during hospitalization, an additional place of occurrence code may be assigned. No 7th characters are used for Y92.

Do not use place of occurrence code Y92.9 if the place is not stated or is not applicable.

A farmer was working in his barn and sustained a foot contusion when the horse stepped on his left foot

S90.32XA	**Contusion of left foot, initial encounter**
W55.19XA	**Other contact with horse, initial encounter**
Y92.71	**Barn as the place of occurrence of the external cause**

Explanation: A place-of-occurrence code from category Y92 is assigned at the initial encounter to identify the location of the patient at the time the injury occurred.

---

c. Activity code

Assign a code from category Y93, Activity code, to describe the activity of the patient at the time the injury or other health condition occurred.

An activity code is used only once, at the initial encounter for treatment. Only one code from Y93 should be recorded on a medical record.

The activity codes are not applicable to poisonings, adverse effects, misadventures or sequela.

Do not assign Y93.9, Unspecified activity, if the activity is not stated.

A code from category Y93 is appropriate for use with external cause and intent codes if identifying the activity provides additional information about the event.

Ranch hand who was grooming a horse sustained a foot contusion when the horse stepped on his left foot

S90.32XA	**Contusion of left foot, initial encounter**
W55.19XA	**Other contact with horse, initial encounter**
Y93.K3	**Activity, grooming and shearing an animal**

Explanation: One activity code from category Y93 is assigned at the initial encounter only to describe the activity of the patient at the time the injury occurred.

---

d. Place of occurrence, activity, and status codes used with other external cause code

When applicable, place of occurrence, activity, and external cause status codes are sequenced after the main external cause code(s). Regardless of the number of external cause codes assigned, there should be only one place of occurrence code, one activity code, and one external cause status code assigned to an encounter.

e. If the reporting format limits the number of external cause codes

If the reporting format limits the number of external cause codes that can be used in reporting clinical data, report the code for the cause/intent most related to the principal diagnosis. If the format permits, capture of additional external cause codes, the cause/intent, including medical misadventures, of the additional events should be reported rather than the codes for place, activity, or external status.

f. Multiple external cause coding guidelines

More than one external cause code is required to fully describe the external cause of an illness or injury. The assignment of external cause codes should be sequenced in the following priority:

If two or more events cause separate injuries, an external cause code should be assigned for each cause. The first-listed external cause code will be selected in the following order:

External codes for child and adult abuse take priority over all other external cause codes.

See Section I.C.19., Child and Adult abuse guidelines.

External cause codes for terrorism events take priority over all other external cause codes except child and adult abuse.

External cause codes for cataclysmic events take priority over all other external cause codes except child and adult abuse and terrorism.

External cause codes for transport accidents take priority over all other external cause codes except cataclysmic events, child and adult abuse and terrorism.

Activity and external cause status codes are assigned following all causal (intent) external cause codes.

The first-listed external cause code should correspond to the cause of the most serious diagnosis due to an assault, accident, or self-harm, following the order of hierarchy listed above..

> 30-year-old man accidentally discharged his hunting rifle, sustaining an open gunshot wound to the right thigh, which caused him to fall down the stairs, resulting in closed displaced comminuted fracture of his left radial shaft
>
> | | |
> |---|---|
> | **S71.101A** | **Unspecified open wound, right thigh, initial encounter** |
> | **W33.02XA** | **Accidental discharge of hunting rifle, initial encounter** |
> | **S52.352A** | **Displaced comminuted fracture of shaft of radius, left arm, initial encounter for closed fracture** |
> | **W10.9XXA** | **Fall (on) (from) unspecified stairs and steps, initial encounter** |
>
> *Explanation:* If two or more events cause separate injuries, an external cause code should be assigned for each cause.

g. Child and adult abuse guideline

Adult and child abuse, neglect and maltreatment are classified as assault. Any of the assault codes may be used to indicate the external cause of any injury resulting from the confirmed abuse.

For confirmed cases of abuse, neglect and maltreatment, when the perpetrator is known, a code from Y07, Perpetrator of maltreatment and neglect, should accompany any other assault codes.

See Section I.C.19. Adult and child abuse, neglect and other maltreatment

h. Unknown or Undetermined Intent Guideline

If the intent (accident, self-harm, assault) of the cause of an injury or other condition is unknown or unspecified, code the intent as accidental intent. All transport accident categories assume accidental intent.

1) Use of undetermined intent

External cause codes for events of undetermined intent are only for use if the documentation in the record specifies that the intent cannot be determined.

i. Sequelae (late effects) of external cause guidelines

1) Sequelae external cause codes

Sequela are reported using the external cause code with the 7th character "S" for sequela. These codes should be used with any report of a late effect or sequela resulting from a previous injury.

See Section I.B.10 Sequela (Late Effects)

2) Sequela external cause code with a related current injury

A sequela external cause code should never be used with a related current nature of injury code.

3) Use of sequela external cause codes for subsequent visits

Use a late effect external cause code for subsequent visits when a late effect of the initial injury is being treated. Do not use a late effect external cause code for subsequent visits for follow-up care (e.g., to assess healing,

to receive rehabilitative therapy) of the injury when no late effect of the injury has been documented.

j. Terrorism guidelines

1) Cause of injury identified by the Federal Government (FBI) as terrorism

When the cause of an injury is identified by the Federal Government (FBI) as terrorism, the first-listed external cause code should be a code from category Y38, Terrorism. The definition of terrorism employed by the FBI is found at the inclusion note at the beginning of category Y38. Use additional code for place of occurrence (Y92.-). More than one Y38 code may be assigned if the injury is the result of more than one mechanism of terrorism.

2) Cause of an injury is suspected to be the result of terrorism

When the cause of an injury is suspected to be the result of terrorism a code from category Y38 should not be assigned. Suspected cases should be classified as assault.

3) Code Y38.9, Terrorism, secondary effects

Assign code Y38.9, Terrorism, secondary effects, for conditions occurring subsequent to the terrorist event. This code should not be assigned for conditions that are due to the initial terrorist act.

It is acceptable to assign code Y38.9 with another code from Y38 if there is an injury due to the initial terrorist event and an injury that is a subsequent result of the terrorist event.

k. External cause status

A code from category Y99, External cause status, should be assigned whenever any other external cause code is assigned for an encounter, including an Activity code, except for the events noted below. Assign a code from category Y99, External cause status, to indicate the work status of the person at the time the event occurred. The status code indicates whether the event occurred during military activity, whether a non-military person was at work, whether an individual including a student or volunteer was involved in a non-work activity at the time of the causal event.

A code from Y99, External cause status, should be assigned, when applicable, with other external cause codes, such as transport accidents and falls. The external cause status codes are not applicable to poisonings, adverse effects, misadventures or late effects.

Do not assign a code from category Y99 if no other external cause codes (cause, activity) are applicable for the encounter.

An external cause status code is used only once, at the initial encounter for treatment. Only one code from Y99 should be recorded on a medical record.

Do not assign code Y99.9, Unspecified external cause status, if the status is not stated.

Chapter 20. External Causes of Morbidity (V00-Y99)

NOTE　This chapter permits the classification of environmental events and circumstances as the cause of injury, and other adverse effects. Where a code from this section is applicable, it is intended that it shall be used secondary to a code from another chapter of the Classification indicating the nature of the condition. Most often, the condition will be classifiable to Chapter 19, Injury, poisoning and certain other consequences of external causes (S00-T88). Other conditions that may be stated to be due to external causes are classified in Chapters I to XVIII. For these conditions, codes from Chapter 20 should be used to provide additional information as to the cause of the condition.

This chapter contains the following blocks:

V00-X58	Accidents
V00-V99	Transport accidents
V00-V09	Pedestrian injured in transport accident
V10-V19	Pedal cycle rider injured in transport accident
V20-V29	Motorcycle rider injured in transport accident
V30-V39	Occupant of three-wheeled motor vehicle injured in transport accident
V40-V49	Car occupant injured in transport accident
V50-V59	Occupant of pick-up truck or van injured in transport accident
V60-V69	Occupant of heavy transport vehicle injured in transport accident
V70-V79	Bus occupant injured in transport accident
V80-V89	Other land transport accidents
V90-V94	Water transport accidents
V95-V97	Air and space transport accidents
V98-V99	Other and unspecified transport accidents
W00-X58	Other external causes of accidental injury
W00-W19	Slipping, tripping, stumbling and falls
W20-W49	Exposure to inanimate mechanical forces
W50-W64	Exposure to animate mechanical forces
W65-W74	Accidental non-transport drowning and submersion
W85-W99	Exposure to electric current, radiation and extreme ambient air temperature and pressure
X00-X08	Exposure to smoke, fire and flames
X10-X19	Contact with heat and hot substances
X30-X39	Exposure to forces of nature
X52-X58	Accidental exposure to other specified factors
X71-X83	Intentional self-harm
X92-Y08	Assault
Y21-Y33	Event of undetermined intent
Y35-Y38	Legal intervention, operations of war, military operations, and terrorism
Y62-Y84	Complications of medical and surgical care
Y62-Y69	Misadventures to patients during surgical and medical care
Y70-Y82	Medical devices associated with adverse incidents in diagnostic and therapeutic use
Y83-Y84	Surgical and other medical procedures as the cause of abnormal reaction of the patient, or of later complication, without mention of misadventure at the time of the procedure
Y90-Y99	Supplementary factors related to causes of morbidity classified elsewhere

Accidents (V00-X58)

Transport accidents (V00-V99)

NOTE　This section is structured in 12 groups. Those relating to land transport accidents (V01-V89) reflect the victim's mode of transport and are subdivided to identify the victim's 'counterpart' or the type of event. The vehicle of which the injured person is an occupant is identified in the first two characters since it is seen as the most important factor to identify for prevention purposes. A transport accident is one in which the vehicle involved must be moving or running or in use for transport purposes at the time of the accident.

Use additional code to identify:
  airbag injury (W22.1)
  type of street or road (Y92.4-)
  use of cellular telephone and other electronic equipment at the time of the transport accident (Y93.C-)

EXCLUDES1　*agricultural vehicles in stationary use or maintenance (W31.-)*
assault by crashing of motor vehicle (Y03.-)
automobile or motor cycle in stationary use or maintenance—code to type of accident
crashing of motor vehicle, undetermined intent (Y32)
intentional self-harm by crashing of motor vehicle (X82)

EXCLUDES2　*transport accidents due to cataclysm (X34-X38)*

NOTE　Definitions of transport vehicles:
  (a) A transport accident is any accident involving a device designed primarily for, or used at the time primarily for, conveying persons or good from one place to another.

  (b) A public highway [trafficway] or street is the entire width between property lines (or other boundary lines) of land open to the public as a matter of right or custom for purposes of moving persons or property from one place to another. A roadway is that part of the public highway designed, improved and customarily used for vehicular traffic.

  (c) A traffic accident is any vehicle accident occurring on the public highway [i.e. originating on, terminating on, or involving a vehicle partially on the highway]. A vehicle accident is assumed to have occurred on the public highway unless another place is specified, except in the case of accidents involving only off-road motor vehicles, which are classified as nontraffic accidents unless the contrary is stated.

  (d) A nontraffic accident is any vehicle accident that occurs entirely in any place other than a public highway.

  (e) A pedestrian is any person involved in an accident who was not at the time of the accident riding in or on a motor vehicle, railway train, streetcar or animal-drawn or other vehicle, or on a pedal cycle or animal. This includes, a person changing a tire or working on a parked car. It also includes the use of a pedestrian conveyance such as a baby carriage, ice-skates, roller skates, a skateboard, nonmotorized or motorized wheelchair, motorized mobility scooter, or nonmotorized scooter.

  (f) A driver is an occupant of a transport vehicle who is operating or intending to operate it.

  (g) A passenger is any occupant of a transport vehicle other than the driver, except a person traveling on the outside of the vehicle.

  (h) A person on the outside of a vehicle is any person being transported by a vehicle but not occupying the space normally reserved for the driver or passengers, or the space intended for the transport of property. This includes the body, bumper, fender, roof, running board or step of a vehicle.

  (i) A pedal cycle is any land transport vehicle operated solely by nonmotorized pedals including a bicycle or tricycle.

  (j) A pedal cyclist is any person riding a pedal cycle or in a sidecar or trailer attached to a pedal cycle.

  (k) A motorcycle is a two-wheeled motor vehicle with one or two riding saddles and sometimes with a third wheel for the support of a sidecar. The sidecar is considered part of the motorcycle.

  (l) A motorcycle rider is any person riding a motorcycle or in a sidecar or trailer attached to the motorcycle.

  (m) A three-wheeled motor vehicle is a motorized tricycle designed primarily for on-road use. This includes a motor-driven tricycle, a motorized rickshaw, or a three-wheeled motor car.

  (n) A car [automobile] is a four-wheeled motor vehicle designed primarily for carrying up to 7 persons. A trailer being towed by the car is considered part of the car.

  (o) A pick-up truck or van is a four or six-wheeled motor vehicle designed for carrying passengers as well as property or cargo weighing less than the local limit for classification as a heavy goods vehicle, and not requiring a special driver's license. This includes a minivan and a sport-utility vehicle (SUV).

  (p) A heavy transport vehicle is a motor vehicle designed primarily for carrying property, meeting local criteria for classification as a heavy goods vehicle in terms of weight and requiring a special driver's license.

  (q) A bus (coach) is a motor vehicle designed or adapted primarily for carrying more than 10 passengers, and requiring a special driver's license.

  (r) A railway train or railway vehicle is any device, with or without freight or passenger cars couple to it, designed for traffic on a railway track. This includes subterranean (subways) or elevated trains.

  (s) A streetcar, is a device designed and used primarily for transporting passengers within a municipality, running on rails, usually subject to normal traffic control signals, and operated principally on a right-of-way that forms part of the roadway. This includes a tram or trolley that runs on rails. A trailer being towed by a streetcar is considered part of the streetcar.

  (t) A special vehicle mainly used on industrial premises is a motor vehicle designed primarily for use within the buildings and premises of industrial or commercial establishments. This includes battery-powered trucks, forklifts, coal-cars in a coal mine, logging cars and trucks used in mines or quarries.

  (u) A special vehicle mainly used in agriculture is a motor vehicle designed specifically for use in farming and agriculture (horticulture), to work the land, tend and harvest crops and transport materials on the farm. This includes harvesters, farm machinery and tractor and trailers.

(v) A special construction vehicle is a motor vehicle designed specifically for use on construction and demolition sites. This includes bulldozers, diggers, earth levellers, dump trucks, backhoes, front-end loaders, pavers, and mechanical shovels.

(w) A special all-terrain vehicle is a motor vehicle of special design to enable it to negotiate over rough or soft terrain, snow or sand. This includes snow mobiles, All-terrain vehicles (ATV), and dune buggies. It does not include passenger vehicle designated as Sport Utility Vehicles. (SUV)

(x) A watercraft is any device designed for transporting passengers or goods on water. This includes motor or sailboats, ships, and hovercraft.

(y) An aircraft is any device for transporting passengers or goods in the air. This includes hot-air balloons, gliders, helicopters and airplanes.

(z) A military vehicle is any motorized vehicle operating on a public roadway owned by the military and being operated by a member of the military.

Pedestrian injured in transport accident (V00-V09)

INCLUDES person changing tire on transport vehicle
person examining engine of vehicle broken down in (on side of) road

EXCLUDES 1 fall due to non-transport collision with other person (W03)
pedestrian on foot falling (slipping) on ice and snow (W00.-)
struck or bumped by another person (W51)

✓4ᵗʰ **V00 Pedestrian conveyance accident**

Use additional place of occurrence and activity external cause codes, if known (Y92-, Y93-)

EXCLUDES 1 collision with another person without fall (W51)
fall due to person on foot colliding with another person on foot (W03)
fall from non-moving wheelchair, nonmotorized scooter and motorized mobility scooter without collision (W05.-)
pedestrian (conveyance) collision with other land transport vehicle (V01-V09)
pedestrian on foot falling (slipping) on ice and snow (W00.-)

The appropriate 7th character is to be added to each code from category V00.
A   initial encounter
D   subsequent encounter
S   sequela

✓5ᵗʰ **V00.0 Pedestrian on foot injured in collision with pedestrian conveyance**

✓x7ᵗʰ **V00.01 Pedestrian on foot injured in collision with roller-skater**

✓x7ᵗʰ **V00.02 Pedestrian on foot injured in collision with skateboarder**

✓x7ᵗʰ **V00.09 Pedestrian on foot injured in collision with other pedestrian conveyance**

✓5ᵗʰ **V00.1 Rolling-type pedestrian conveyance accident**

EXCLUDES 1 accident with babystroller (V00.82-)
accident with motorized mobility scooter (V00.83-)
accident with wheelchair (powered) (V00.81-)

✓6ᵗʰ **V00.11 In-line roller-skate accident**

✓7ᵗʰ **V00.111 Fall from in-line roller-skates**

✓7ᵗʰ **V00.112 In-line roller-skater colliding with stationary object**

✓7ᵗʰ **V00.118 Other in-line roller-skate accident**
EXCLUDES 1 roller-skater collision with other land transport vehicle (V01-V09 with 5th character 1)

✓6ᵗʰ **V00.12 Non-in-line roller-skate accident**

✓7ᵗʰ **V00.121 Fall from non-in-line roller-skates**

✓7ᵗʰ **V00.122 Non-in-line roller-skater colliding with stationary object**

✓7ᵗʰ **V00.128 Other non-in-line roller-skating accident**
EXCLUDES 1 roller-skater collision with other land transport vehicle (V01-V09 with 5th character 1)

✓6ᵗʰ **V00.13 Skateboard accident**

✓7ᵗʰ **V00.131 Fall from skateboard**

✓7ᵗʰ **V00.132 Skateboarder colliding with stationary object**

✓7ᵗʰ **V00.138 Other skateboard accident**
EXCLUDES 1 skateboarder collision with other land transport vehicle (V01-V09 with 5th character 2)

✓6ᵗʰ **V00.14 Scooter (nonmotorized) accident**
EXCLUDES 1 motorscooter accident (V20-V29)

✓7ᵗʰ **V00.141 Fall from scooter (nonmotorized)**

✓7ᵗʰ **V00.142 Scooter (nonmotorized) colliding with stationary object**

✓7ᵗʰ **V00.148 Other scooter (nonmotorized) accident**
EXCLUDES 1 scooter (nonmotorized) collision with other land transport vehicle (V01-V09 with fifth character 9)

✓6ᵗʰ **V00.15 Heelies accident**
Rolling shoe
Wheeled shoe
Wheelies accident

✓7ᵗʰ **V00.151 Fall from heelies**

✓7ᵗʰ **V00.152 Heelies colliding with stationary object**

✓7ᵗʰ **V00.158 Other heelies accident**

✓6ᵗʰ **V00.18 Accident on other rolling-type pedestrian conveyance**

✓7ᵗʰ **V00.181 Fall from other rolling-type pedestrian conveyance**

✓7ᵗʰ **V00.182 Pedestrian on other rolling-type pedestrian conveyance colliding with stationary object**

✓7ᵗʰ **V00.188 Other accident on other rolling-type pedestrian conveyance**

✓5ᵗʰ **V00.2 Gliding-type pedestrian conveyance accident**

✓6ᵗʰ **V00.21 Ice-skates accident**

✓7ᵗʰ **V00.211 Fall from ice-skates**

✓7ᵗʰ **V00.212 Ice-skater colliding with stationary object**

✓7ᵗʰ **V00.218 Other ice-skates accident**
EXCLUDES 1 ice-skater collision with other land transport vehicle (V01-V09 with 5th digit 9)

✓6ᵗʰ **V00.22 Sled accident**

✓7ᵗʰ **V00.221 Fall from sled**

✓7ᵗʰ **V00.222 Sledder colliding with stationary object**

✓7ᵗʰ **V00.228 Other sled accident**
EXCLUDES 1 sled collision with other land transport vehicle (V01-V09 with 5th digit 9)

✓6ᵗʰ **V00.28 Other gliding-type pedestrian conveyance accident**

✓7ᵗʰ **V00.281 Fall from other gliding-type pedestrian conveyance**

✓7ᵗʰ **V00.282 Pedestrian on other gliding-type pedestrian conveyance colliding with stationary object**

✓7ᵗʰ **V00.288 Other accident on other gliding-type pedestrian conveyance**
EXCLUDES 1 gliding-type pedestrian conveyance collision with other land transport vehicle (V01-V09 with 5th digit 9)

✓5ᵗʰ **V00.3 Flat-bottomed pedestrian conveyance accident**

✓6ᵗʰ **V00.31 Snowboard accident**

✓7ᵗʰ **V00.311 Fall from snowboard**

✓7ᵗʰ **V00.312 Snowboarder colliding with stationary object**

✓7ᵗʰ **V00.318 Other snowboard accident**
EXCLUDES 1 snowboarder collision with other land transport vehicle (V01-V09 with 5th digit 9)

✓6ᵗʰ **V00.32 Snow-ski accident**

✓7ᵗʰ **V00.321 Fall from snow-skis**

✓7ᵗʰ **V00.322 Snow-skier colliding with stationary object**

✓7ᵗʰ **V00.328 Other snow-ski accident**
EXCLUDES 1 snow-skier collision with other land transport vehicle (V01-V09 with 5th digit 9)

✓6ᵗʰ **V00.38** Other flat-bottomed **pedestrian conveyance accident**

    ✓7ᵗʰ **V00.381** **Fall from other flat-bottomed pedestrian conveyance**

    ✓7ᵗʰ **V00.382** **Pedestrian on other flat-bottomed pedestrian conveyance** colliding with stationary object

    ✓7ᵗʰ **V00.388** **Other accident on other flat-bottomed pedestrian conveyance**

✓5ᵗʰ **V00.8** **Accident on other pedestrian conveyance**

    ✓6ᵗʰ **V00.81** **Accident with** wheelchair (powered)

       ✓7ᵗʰ **V00.811** **Fall from moving wheelchair (powered)**
          EXCLUDES 1   *fall from non-moving wheelchair (W05.0)*

       ✓7ᵗʰ **V00.812** **Wheelchair (powered)** colliding with stationary object

       ✓7ᵗʰ **V00.818** **Other accident with wheelchair (powered)**

    ✓6ᵗʰ **V00.82** **Accident with** babystroller

       ✓7ᵗʰ **V00.821** **Fall from babystroller**

       ✓7ᵗʰ **V00.822** **Babystroller** colliding with stationary object

       ✓7ᵗʰ **V00.828** **Other accident with babystroller**

    ✓6ᵗʰ **V00.83** **Accident with** motorized mobility scooter

       V00.831 **Fall from motorized mobility scooter**
          EXCLUDES 1   *fall from non-moving motorized mobility scooter (W05.2)*

       V00.832 **Motorized mobility scooter** colliding with stationary object

       V00.838 **Other accident with motorized mobility scooter**

    ✓6ᵗʰ **V00.89** **Accident on** other **pedestrian** conveyance

       ✓7ᵗʰ **V00.891** **Fall from other pedestrian conveyance**

       ✓7ᵗʰ **V00.892** **Pedestrian on other pedestrian conveyance** colliding with stationary object

       ✓7ᵗʰ **V00.898** **Other accident on other pedestrian conveyance**
          EXCLUDES 1   *other pedestrian (conveyance) collision with other land transport vehicle (V01-V09 with 5th digit 9)*

✓4ᵗʰ **V01** **Pedestrian injured in collision with pedal cycle**

The appropriate 7th character is to be added to each code from category V01.
A   initial encounter
D   subsequent encounter
S   sequela

✓5ᵗʰ **V01.0** **Pedestrian injured in collision with pedal cycle in** nontraffic accident

    ✓x7ᵗʰ **V01.00** **Pedestrian** on foot **injured in collision with pedal cycle in nontraffic accident**
       Pedestrian NOS injured in collision with pedal cycle in nontraffic accident

    ✓x7ᵗʰ **V01.01** **Pedestrian** on roller-skates **injured in collision with pedal cycle in nontraffic accident**

    ✓x7ᵗʰ **V01.02** **Pedestrian** on skateboard **injured in collision with pedal cycle in nontraffic accident**

    ✓x7ᵗʰ **V01.09** **Pedestrian with other** conveyance **injured in collision with pedal cycle in nontraffic accident**
       Pedestrian with babystroller injured in collision with pedal cycle in nontraffic accident
       Pedestrian on ice-skates injured in collision with pedal cycle in nontraffic accident
       Pedestrian on nonmotorized scooter injured in collision with pedal cycle in nontraffic accident
       Pedestrian on sled injured in collision with pedal cycle in nontraffic accident
       Pedestrian on snowboard injured in collision with pedal cycle in nontraffic accident
       Pedestrian on snow-skis injured in collision with pedal cycle in nontraffic accident
       Pedestrian in wheelchair (powered) injured in collision with pedal cycle in nontraffic accident
       Pedestrian in motorized mobility scooter injured in collision with pedal cycle in nontraffic accident

✓5ᵗʰ **V01.1** **Pedestrian injured in collision with pedal cycle in** traffic accident

    ✓x7ᵗʰ **V01.10** **Pedestrian** on foot **injured in collision with pedal cycle in traffic accident**
       Pedestrian NOS injured in collision with pedal cycle in traffic accident

    ✓x7ᵗʰ **V01.11** **Pedestrian** on roller-skates **injured in collision with pedal cycle in traffic accident**

    ✓x7ᵗʰ **V01.12** **Pedestrian** on skateboard **injured in collision with pedal cycle in traffic accident**

    ✓x7ᵗʰ **V01.19** **Pedestrian with other** conveyance **injured in collision with pedal cycle in traffic accident**
       Pedestrian with babystroller injured in collision with pedal cycle in traffic accident
       Pedestrian on ice-skates injured in collision with pedal cycle in traffic accident
       Pedestrian on nonmotorized scooter injured in collision with pedal cycle in traffic accident
       Pedestrian on sled injured in collision with pedal cycle in traffic accident
       Pedestrian on snowboard injured in collision with pedal cycle in traffic accident
       Pedestrian on snow-skis injured in collision with pedal cycle in traffic accident
       Pedestrian in wheelchair (powered) injured in collision with pedal cycle in traffic accident
       Pedestrian in motorized mobility scooter injured in collision with pedal cycle in traffic accident

✓5ᵗʰ **V01.9** **Pedestrian injured in collision with pedal cycle,** unspecified whether traffic or nontraffic accident

    ✓x7ᵗʰ **V01.90** **Pedestrian** on foot **injured in collision with pedal cycle, unspecified whether traffic or nontraffic accident**
       Pedestrian NOS injured in collision with pedal cycle, unspecified whether traffic or nontraffic accident

    ✓x7ᵗʰ **V01.91** **Pedestrian** on roller-skates **injured in collision with pedal cycle, unspecified whether traffic or nontraffic accident**

    ✓x7ᵗʰ **V01.92** **Pedestrian** on skateboard **injured in collision with pedal cycle, unspecified whether traffic or nontraffic accident**

    ✓x7ᵗʰ **V01.99** **Pedestrian with other** conveyance **injured in collision with pedal cycle, unspecified whether traffic or nontraffic accident**
       Pedestrian with babystroller injured in collision with pedal cycle, unspecified whether traffic or nontraffic accident
       Pedestrian on ice-skates injured in collision with pedal cycle unspecified, whether traffic or nontraffic accident
       Pedestrian on nonmotorized scooter injured in collision with pedal cycle, unspecified whether traffic or nontraffic accident
       Pedestrian on sled injured in collision with pedal cycle unspecified, whether traffic or nontraffic accident
       Pedestrian on snowboard injured in collision with pedal cycle, unspecified whether traffic or nontraffic accident
       Pedestrian on snow-skis injured in collision with pedal cycle, unspecified whether traffic or nontraffic accident
       Pedestrian in wheelchair (powered) injured in collision with pedal cycle, unspecified whether traffic or nontraffic accident
       Pedestrian in motorized mobility scooter injured in collision with pedal cycle, unspecified whether traffic or nontraffic accident

✓4ᵗʰ **V02** **Pedestrian injured in collision with two- or three-wheeled motor vehicle**

The appropriate 7th character is to be added to each code from category V02.
A   initial encounter
D   subsequent encounter
S   sequela

✓5ᵗʰ **V02.0** **Pedestrian injured in collision with two- or three-wheeled motor vehicle in** nontraffic accident

    ✓x7ᵗʰ **V02.00** **Pedestrian** on foot **injured in collision with two- or three-wheeled motor vehicle in nontraffic accident**
       Pedestrian NOS injured in collision with two- or three-wheeled motor vehicle in nontraffic accident

✓ Additional Character Required   ✓x7ᵗʰ Placeholder Alert   Unspecified Dx   Other Specified Dx   Manifestation   ▶◀ Revised Text   ● New Code   ▲ Revised Code Title

ICD-10-CM 2016   1039

√x7th **V02.01** **Pedestrian** on roller-skates **injured in collision with two- or three-wheeled motor vehicle in nontraffic accident**

√x7th **V02.02** **Pedestrian** on skateboard **injured in collision with two- or three-wheeled motor vehicle in nontraffic accident**

√x7th **V02.09** **Pedestrian with other** conveyance **injured in collision with two- or three-wheeled motor vehicle in nontraffic accident**

Pedestrian with babystroller injured in collision with two- or three-wheeled motor vehicle in nontraffic accident

Pedestrian on ice-skates injured in collision with two- or three-wheeled motor vehicle in nontraffic accident

Pedestrian on nonmotorized scooter injured in collision with two- or three-wheeled motor vehicle in nontraffic accident

Pedestrian on sled injured in collision with two- or three-wheeled motor vehicle in nontraffic accident

Pedestrian on snowboard injured in collision with two- or three-wheeled motor vehicle in nontraffic accident

Pedestrian on snow-skis injured in collision with two- or three-wheeled motor vehicle in nontraffic accident

Pedestrian in wheelchair (powered) injured in collision with two- or three-wheeled motor vehicle in nontraffic accident

Pedestrian in motorized mobility scooter injured in collision with two- or three-wheeled motor vehicle in nontraffic accident

√5th **V02.1** **Pedestrian injured in collision with two- or three-wheeled motor vehicle in** traffic accident

√x7th **V02.10** **Pedestrian** on foot **injured in collision with two- or three-wheeled motor vehicle in traffic accident**

Pedestrian NOS injured in collision with two- or three-wheeled motor vehicle in traffic accident

√x7th **V02.11** **Pedestrian** on roller-skates **injured in collision with two- or three-wheeled motor vehicle in traffic accident**

√x7th **V02.12** **Pedestrian** on skateboard **injured in collision with two- or three-wheeled motor vehicle in traffic accident**

√x7th **V02.19** **Pedestrian with other** conveyance **injured in collision with two- or three-wheeled motor vehicle in traffic accident**

Pedestrian with babystroller injured in collision with two- or three-wheeled motor vehicle in traffic accident

Pedestrian on ice-skates injured in collision with two- or three-wheeled motor vehicle in traffic accident

Pedestrian on nonmotorized scooter injured in collision with two- or three-wheeled motor vehicle in traffic accident

Pedestrian on sled injured in collision with two- or three-wheeled motor vehicle in traffic accident

Pedestrian on snowboard injured in collision with two- or three-wheeled motor vehicle in traffic accident

Pedestrian on snow-skis injured in collision with two- or three-wheeled motor vehicle in traffic accident

Pedestrian in wheelchair (powered) injured in collision with two- or three-wheeled motor vehicle in traffic accident

Pedestrian in motorized mobility scooter injured in collision with two- or three-wheeled motor vehicle in traffic accident

√5th **V02.9** **Pedestrian injured in collision with two- or three-wheeled motor vehicle,** unspecified whether traffic or nontraffic accident

√x7th **V02.90** **Pedestrian** on foot **injured in collision with two- or three-wheeled motor vehicle, unspecified whether traffic or nontraffic accident**

Pedestrian NOS injured in collision with two- or three-wheeled motor vehicle, unspecified whether traffic or nontraffic accident

√x7th **V02.91** **Pedestrian** on roller-skates **injured in collision with two- or three-wheeled motor vehicle, unspecified whether traffic or nontraffic accident**

√x7th **V02.92** **Pedestrian** on skateboard **injured in collision with two- or three-wheeled motor vehicle, unspecified whether traffic or nontraffic accident**

√x7th **V02.99** **Pedestrian with other** conveyance **injured in collision with two- or three-wheeled motor vehicle, unspecified whether traffic or nontraffic accident**

Pedestrian with babystroller injured in collision with two- or three-wheeled motor vehicle, unspecified whether traffic or nontraffic accident

Pedestrian on ice-skates injured in collision with two- or three-wheeled motor vehicle, unspecified whether traffic or nontraffic accident

Pedestrian on nonmotorized scooter injured in collision with two- or three-wheeled motor vehicle, unspecified whether traffic or nontraffic accident

Pedestrian on sled injured in collision with two- or three-wheeled motor vehicle, unspecified whether traffic or nontraffic accident

Pedestrian on snowboard injured in collision with two- or three-wheeled motor vehicle, unspecified whether traffic or nontraffic accident

Pedestrian on snow-skis injured in collision with two- or three-wheeled motor vehicle, unspecified whether traffic or nontraffic accident

Pedestrian in wheelchair (powered) injured in collision with two- or three-wheeled motor vehicle, unspecified whether traffic or nontraffic accident

Pedestrian in motorized mobility scooter injured in collision with two- or three-wheeled motor vehicle, unspecified whether traffic or nontraffic accident

√4th **V03** **Pedestrian injured in collision with car, pick-up truck or van**

The appropriate 7th character is to be added to each code from category V03.
A   initial encounter
D   subsequent encounter
S   sequela

√5th **V03.0** **Pedestrian injured in collision with car, pick-up truck or van in** nontraffic accident

√x7th **V03.00** **Pedestrian** on foot **injured in collision with car, pick-up truck or van in nontraffic accident**

Pedestrian NOS injured in collision with car, pick-up truck or van in nontraffic accident

√x7th **V03.01** **Pedestrian** on roller-skates **injured in collision with car, pick-up truck or van in nontraffic accident**

√x7th **V03.02** **Pedestrian** on skateboard **injured in collision with car, pick-up truck or van in nontraffic accident**

√x7th **V03.09** **Pedestrian with other** conveyance **injured in collision with car, pick-up truck or van in nontraffic accident**

Pedestrian with babystroller injured in collision with car, pick-up truck or van in nontraffic accident

Pedestrian on ice-skates injured in collision with car, pick-up truck or van in nontraffic accident

Pedestrian on nonmotorized scooter injured in collision with car, pick-up truck or van in nontraffic accident

Pedestrian on sled injured in collision with car, pick-up truck or van in nontraffic accident

Pedestrian on snowboard injured in collision with car, pick-up truck or van in nontraffic accident

Pedestrian on snow-skis injured in collision with car, pick-up truck or van in nontraffic accident

Pedestrian in wheelchair (powered) injured in collision with car, pick-up truck or van in nontraffic accident

Pedestrian in motorized mobility scooter injured in collision with car, pick-up truck or van in nontraffic accident

√5th **V03.1** **Pedestrian injured in collision with car, pick-up truck or van in** traffic accident

√x7th **V03.10** **Pedestrian** on foot **injured in collision with car, pick-up truck or van in traffic accident**

Pedestrian NOS injured in collision with car, pick-up truck or van in traffic accident

√x7th **V03.11** **Pedestrian** on roller-skates **injured in collision with car, pick-up truck or van in traffic accident**

√x7th **V03.12** **Pedestrian** on skateboard **injured in collision with car, pick-up truck or van in traffic accident**

EXCLUDES 1 Not coded here   EXCLUDES 2 Not included here   N Newborn Age: 0   P Pediatric Age: 0-17   M Maternity Age: 12-55   A Adult Age: 15-124

☑x7ᵗʰ **V03.19 Pedestrian with other conveyance injured in collision with car, pick-up truck or van in traffic accident**

Pedestrian with babystroller injured in collision with car, pick-up truck or van in traffic accident

Pedestrian on ice-skates injured in collision with car, pick-up truck or van in traffic accident

Pedestrian on nonmotorized scooter injured in collision with car, pick-up truck or van in traffic accident

Pedestrian on sled injured in collision with car, pick-up truck or van in traffic accident

Pedestrian on snowboard injured in collision with car, pick-up truck or van in traffic accident

Pedestrian on snow-skis injured in collision with car, pick-up truck or van in traffic accident

Pedestrian in wheelchair (powered) injured in collision with car, pick-up truck or van in traffic accident

Pedestrian in motorized mobility scooter injured in collision with car, pick-up truck or van in traffic accident

☑5ᵗʰ **V03.9 Pedestrian injured in collision with car, pick-up truck or van, unspecified whether traffic or nontraffic accident**

☑x7ᵗʰ **V03.90 Pedestrian on foot injured in collision with car, pick-up truck or van, unspecified whether traffic or nontraffic accident**

Pedestrian NOS injured in collision with car, pick-up truck or van, unspecified whether traffic or nontraffic accident

☑x7ᵗʰ **V03.91 Pedestrian on roller-skates injured in collision with car, pick-up truck or van, unspecified whether traffic or nontraffic accident**

☑x7ᵗʰ **V03.92 Pedestrian on skateboard injured in collision with car, pick-up truck or van, unspecified whether traffic or nontraffic accident**

☑x7ᵗʰ **V03.99 Pedestrian with other conveyance injured in collision with car, pick-up truck or van, unspecified whether traffic or nontraffic accident**

Pedestrian with babystroller injured in collision with car, pick-up truck or van, unspecified whether traffic or nontraffic accident

Pedestrian on ice-skates injured in collision with car, pick-up truck or van, unspecified whether traffic or nontraffic accident

Pedestrian on nonmotorized scooter injured in collision with car, pick-up truck or van, unspecified whether traffic or nontraffic accident

Pedestrian on sled injured in collision with car, pick-up truck or van in nontraffic accident

Pedestrian on snowboard injured in collision with car, pick-up truck or van, unspecified whether traffic or nontraffic accident

Pedestrian on snow-skis injured in collision with car, pick-up truck or van, unspecified whether traffic or nontraffic accident

Pedestrian in wheelchair (powered) injured in collision with car, pick-up truck or van, unspecified whether traffic or nontraffic accident

Pedestrian in motorized mobility scooter injured in collision with car, pick-up truck or van, unspecified whether traffic or nontraffic accident

☑4ᵗʰ **V04 Pedestrian injured in collision with heavy transport vehicle or bus**

EXCLUDES 1   *pedestrian injured in collision with military vehicle (V09.01, V09.21)*

The appropriate 7th character is to be added to each code from category V04.
A   initial encounter
D   subsequent encounter
S   sequela

☑5ᵗʰ **V04.0 Pedestrian injured in collision with heavy transport vehicle or bus in nontraffic accident**

☑x7ᵗʰ **V04.00 Pedestrian on foot injured in collision with heavy transport vehicle or bus in nontraffic accident**

Pedestrian NOS injured in collision with heavy transport vehicle or bus in nontraffic accident

☑x7ᵗʰ **V04.01 Pedestrian on roller-skates injured in collision with heavy transport vehicle or bus in nontraffic accident**

☑x7ᵗʰ **V04.02 Pedestrian on skateboard injured in collision with heavy transport vehicle or bus in nontraffic accident**

☑x7ᵗʰ **V04.09 Pedestrian with other conveyance injured in collision with heavy transport vehicle or bus in nontraffic accident**

Pedestrian with babystroller injured in collision with heavy transport vehicle or bus in nontraffic accident

Pedestrian on ice-skates injured in collision with heavy transport vehicle or bus in nontraffic accident

Pedestrian on nonmotorized scooter injured in collision with heavy transport vehicle or bus in nontraffic accident

Pedestrian on sled injured in collision with heavy transport vehicle or bus in nontraffic accident

Pedestrian on snowboard injured in collision with heavy transport vehicle or bus in nontraffic accident

Pedestrian on snow-skis injured in collision with heavy transport vehicle or bus in nontraffic accident

Pedestrian in wheelchair (powered) injured in collision with heavy transport vehicle or bus in nontraffic accident

Pedestrian in motorized mobility scooter injured in collision with heavy transport vehicle or bus in nontraffic accident

☑5ᵗʰ **V04.1 Pedestrian injured in collision with heavy transport vehicle or bus in traffic accident**

☑x7ᵗʰ **V04.10 Pedestrian on foot injured in collision with heavy transport vehicle or bus in traffic accident**

Pedestrian NOS injured in collision with heavy transport vehicle or bus in traffic accident

☑x7ᵗʰ **V04.11 Pedestrian on roller-skates injured in collision with heavy transport vehicle or bus in traffic accident**

☑x7ᵗʰ **V04.12 Pedestrian on skateboard injured in collision with heavy transport vehicle or bus in traffic accident**

☑x7ᵗʰ **V04.19 Pedestrian with other conveyance injured in collision with heavy transport vehicle or bus in traffic accident**

Pedestrian with babystroller injured in collision with heavy transport vehicle or bus in traffic accident

Pedestrian on ice-skates injured in collision with heavy transport vehicle or bus in traffic accident

Pedestrian on nonmotorized scooter injured in collision with heavy transport vehicle or bus in traffic accident

Pedestrian on sled injured in collision with heavy transport vehicle or bus in traffic accident

Pedestrian on snowboard injured in collision with heavy transport vehicle or bus in traffic accident

Pedestrian on snow-skis injured in collision with heavy transport vehicle or bus in traffic accident

Pedestrian in wheelchair (powered) injured in collision with heavy transport vehicle or bus in traffic accident

Pedestrian in motorized mobility scooter injured in collision with heavy transport vehicle or bus in traffic accident

☑5ᵗʰ **V04.9 Pedestrian injured in collision with heavy transport vehicle or bus, unspecified whether traffic or nontraffic accident**

☑x7ᵗʰ **V04.90 Pedestrian on foot injured in collision with heavy transport vehicle or bus, unspecified whether traffic or nontraffic accident**

Pedestrian NOS injured in collision with heavy transport vehicle or bus, unspecified whether traffic or nontraffic accident

☑x7ᵗʰ **V04.91 Pedestrian on roller-skates injured in collision with heavy transport vehicle or bus, unspecified whether traffic or nontraffic accident**

☑x7ᵗʰ **V04.92 Pedestrian on skateboard injured in collision with heavy transport vehicle or bus, unspecified whether traffic or nontraffic accident**

☑ Additional Character Required   ☑x7ᵗʰ Placeholder Alert   Unspecified Dx   Other Specified Dx   Manifestation   ▶◀ Revised Text   ● New Code   ▲ Revised Code Title

√x7th **V04.99** **Pedestrian with other conveyance injured in collision with heavy transport vehicle or bus, unspecified whether traffic or nontraffic accident**

Pedestrian with babystroller injured in collision with heavy transport vehicle or bus, unspecified whether traffic or nontraffic accident

Pedestrian on ice-skates injured in collision with heavy transport vehicle or bus, unspecified whether traffic or nontraffic accident

Pedestrian on nonmotorized scooter injured in collision with heavy transport vehicle or bus, unspecified whether traffic or nontraffic accident

Pedestrian on sled injured in collision with heavy transport vehicle or bus, unspecified whether traffic or nontraffic accident

Pedestrian on snowboard injured in collision with heavy transport vehicle or bus, unspecified whether traffic or nontraffic accident

Pedestrian on snow-skis injured in collision with heavy transport vehicle or bus, unspecified whether traffic or nontraffic accident

Pedestrian in wheelchair (powered) injured in collision with heavy transport vehicle or bus, unspecified whether traffic or nontraffic accident

Pedestrian in motorized mobility scooter injured in collision with heavy transport vehicle or bus, unspecified whether traffic or nontraffic accident

√4th **V05** **Pedestrian injured in collision with railway train or railway vehicle**

The appropriate 7th character is to be added to each code from category V05.
A   initial encounter
D   subsequent encounter
S   sequela

√5th **V05.0** **Pedestrian injured in collision with railway train or railway vehicle in nontraffic accident**

√x7th **V05.00** **Pedestrian on foot injured in collision with railway train or railway vehicle in nontraffic accident**

Pedestrian NOS injured in collision with railway train or railway vehicle in nontraffic accident

√x7th **V05.01** **Pedestrian on roller-skates injured in collision with railway train or railway vehicle in nontraffic accident**

√x7th **V05.02** **Pedestrian on skateboard injured in collision with railway train or railway vehicle in nontraffic accident**

√x7th **V05.09** **Pedestrian with other conveyance injured in collision with railway train or railway vehicle in nontraffic accident**

Pedestrian with babystroller injured in collision with railway train or railway vehicle in nontraffic accident

Pedestrian on ice-skates injured in collision with railway train or railway vehicle in nontraffic accident

Pedestrian on nonmotorized scooter injured in collision with railway train or railway vehicle in nontraffic accident

Pedestrian on sled injured in collision with railway train or railway vehicle in nontraffic accident

Pedestrian on snowboard injured in collision with railway train or railway vehicle in nontraffic accident

Pedestrian on snow-skis injured in collision with railway train or railway vehicle in nontraffic accident

Pedestrian in wheelchair (powered) injured in collision with railway train or railway vehicle in nontraffic accident

Pedestrian in motorized mobility scooter injured in collision with railway train or railway vehicle in nontraffic accident

√5th **V05.1** **Pedestrian injured in collision with railway train or railway vehicle in traffic accident**

√x7th **V05.10** **Pedestrian on foot injured in collision with railway train or railway vehicle in traffic accident**

Pedestrian NOS injured in collision with railway train or railway vehicle in traffic accident

√x7th **V05.11** **Pedestrian on roller-skates injured in collision with railway train or railway vehicle in traffic accident**

√x7th **V05.12** **Pedestrian on skateboard injured in collision with railway train or railway vehicle in traffic accident**

√x7th **V05.19** **Pedestrian with other conveyance injured in collision with railway train or railway vehicle in traffic accident**

Pedestrian with babystroller injured in collision with railway train or railway vehicle in traffic accident

Pedestrian on ice-skates injured in collision with railway train or railway vehicle in traffic accident

Pedestrian on nonmotorized scooter injured in collision with railway train or railway vehicle in traffic accident

Pedestrian on sled injured in collision with railway train or railway vehicle in traffic accident

Pedestrian on snowboard injured in collision with railway train or railway vehicle in traffic accident

Pedestrian on snow-skis injured in collision with railway train or railway vehicle in traffic accident

Pedestrian in wheelchair (powered) injured in collision with railway train or railway vehicle in traffic accident

Pedestrian in motorized mobility scooter injured in collision with railway train or railway vehicle in traffic accident

√5th **V05.9** **Pedestrian injured in collision with railway train or railway vehicle, unspecified whether traffic or nontraffic accident**

√x7th **V05.90** **Pedestrian on foot injured in collision with railway train or railway vehicle, unspecified whether traffic or nontraffic accident**

Pedestrian NOS injured in collision with railway train or railway vehicle, unspecified whether traffic or nontraffic accident

√x7th **V05.91** **Pedestrian on roller-skates injured in collision with railway train or railway vehicle, unspecified whether traffic or nontraffic accident**

√x7th **V05.92** **Pedestrian on skateboard injured in collision with railway train or railway vehicle, unspecified whether traffic or nontraffic accident**

√x7th **V05.99** **Pedestrian with other conveyance injured in collision with railway train or railway vehicle, unspecified whether traffic or nontraffic accident**

Pedestrian with babystroller injured in collision with railway train or railway vehicle, unspecified whether traffic or nontraffic

Pedestrian on ice-skates injured in collision with railway train or railway vehicle, unspecified whether traffic or nontraffic

Pedestrian on nonmotorized scooter injured in collision with railway train or railway vehicle, unspecified whether traffic or nontraffic

Pedestrian on sled injured in collision with railway train or railway vehicle, unspecified whether traffic or nontraffic

Pedestrian on snowboard injured in collision with railway train or railway vehicle, unspecified whether traffic or nontraffic

Pedestrian on snow-skis injured in collision with railway train or railway vehicle, unspecified whether traffic or nontraffic

Pedestrian in wheelchair (powered) injured in collision with railway train or railway vehicle, unspecified whether traffic or nontraffic

Pedestrian in motorized mobility scooter injured in collision with railway train or railway vehicle, unspecified whether traffic or nontraffic

√4th **V06** **Pedestrian injured in collision with other nonmotor vehicle**

INCLUDES   collision with animal-drawn vehicle, animal being ridden, nonpowered streetcar

EXCLUDES 1   pedestrian injured in collision with pedestrian conveyance (V00.0-)

The appropriate 7th character is to be added to each code from category V06.
A   initial encounter
D   subsequent encounter
S   sequela

√5th **V06.0** **Pedestrian injured in collision with other nonmotor vehicle in nontraffic accident**

√x7th **V06.00** **Pedestrian on foot injured in collision with other nonmotor vehicle in nontraffic accident**

Pedestrian NOS injured in collision with other nonmotor vehicle in nontraffic accident

√x7th **V06.01** **Pedestrian on roller-skates injured in collision with other nonmotor vehicle in nontraffic accident**

EXCLUDES 1 Not coded here   EXCLUDES 2 Not included here   N Newborn Age: 0   P Pediatric Age: 0-17   M Maternity Age: 12-55   A Adult Age: 15-124

1042   ICD-10-CM 2016

√x 7ᵗʰ **V06.02** **Pedestrian** on skateboard **injured in collision with other nonmotor vehicle in nontraffic accident**

√x 7ᵗʰ **V06.09** **Pedestrian with other** conveyance **injured in collision with other nonmotor vehicle in nontraffic accident**

    Pedestrian with babystroller injured in collision with other nonmotor vehicle in nontraffic accident

    Pedestrian on ice-skates injured in collision with other nonmotor vehicle in nontraffic accident

    Pedestrian on nonmotorized scooter injured in collision with other nonmotor vehicle in nontraffic accident

    Pedestrian on sled injured in collision with other nonmotor vehicle in nontraffic accident

    Pedestrian on snowboard injured in collision with other nonmotor vehicle in nontraffic accident

    Pedestrian on snow-skis injured in collision with other nonmotor vehicle in nontraffic accident

    Pedestrian in wheelchair (powered) injured in collision with other nonmotor vehicle in nontraffic accident

    Pedestrian in motorized mobility scooter injured in collision with other nonmotor vehicle in nontraffic accident

√5ᵗʰ **V06.1** **Pedestrian injured in collision with other nonmotor vehicle** in traffic accident

√x 7ᵗʰ **V06.10** **Pedestrian** on foot **injured in collision with other nonmotor vehicle in traffic accident**

    Pedestrian NOS injured in collision with other nonmotor vehicle in traffic accident

√x 7ᵗʰ **V06.11** **Pedestrian** on roller-skates **injured in collision with other nonmotor vehicle in traffic accident**

√x 7ᵗʰ **V06.12** **Pedestrian** on skateboard **injured in collision with other nonmotor vehicle in traffic accident**

√x 7ᵗʰ **V06.19** **Pedestrian with other** conveyance **injured in collision with other nonmotor vehicle in traffic accident**

    Pedestrian with babystroller injured in collision with other nonmotor vehicle in nontraffic accident

    Pedestrian on ice-skates injured in collision with other nonmotor vehicle in traffic accident

    Pedestrian on nonmotorized scooter injured in collision with other nonmotor vehicle in traffic accident

    Pedestrian on sled injured in collision with other nonmotor vehicle in traffic accident

    Pedestrian on snowboard injured in collision with other nonmotor vehicle in traffic accident

    Pedestrian on snow-skis injured in collision with other nonmotor vehicle in traffic accident

    Pedestrian in wheelchair (powered) injured in collision with other nonmotor vehicle in traffic accident

    Pedestrian in motorized mobility scooter injured in collision with other nonmotor vehicle in traffic accident

√5ᵗʰ **V06.9** **Pedestrian injured in collision with other nonmotor vehicle, unspecified whether traffic or nontraffic accident**

√x 7ᵗʰ **V06.90** **Pedestrian** on foot **injured in collision with other nonmotor vehicle, unspecified whether traffic or nontraffic accident**

    Pedestrian NOS injured in collision with other nonmotor vehicle, unspecified whether traffic or nontraffic accident

√x 7ᵗʰ **V06.91** **Pedestrian** on roller-skates **injured in collision with other nonmotor vehicle, unspecified whether traffic or nontraffic accident**

√x 7ᵗʰ **V06.92** **Pedestrian** on skateboard **injured in collision with other nonmotor vehicle, unspecified whether traffic or nontraffic accident**

√x 7ᵗʰ **V06.99** **Pedestrian with other** conveyance **injured in collision with other nonmotor vehicle, unspecified whether traffic or nontraffic accident**

    Pedestrian with babystroller injured in collision with other nonmotor vehicle, unspecified whether traffic or nontraffic accident

    Pedestrian on ice-skates injured in collision with other nonmotor vehicle, unspecified whether traffic or nontraffic accident

    Pedestrian on nonmotorized scooter injured in collision with other nonmotor vehicle, unspecified whether traffic or nontraffic accident

    Pedestrian on sled injured in collision with other nonmotor vehicle, unspecified whether traffic or nontraffic accident

    Pedestrian on snowboard injured in collision with other nonmotor vehicle, unspecified whether traffic or nontraffic accident

    Pedestrian on snow-skis injured in collision with other nonmotor vehicle, unspecified whether traffic or nontraffic accident

    Pedestrian in wheelchair (powered) injured in collision with other nonmotor vehicle, unspecified whether traffic or nontraffic accident

    Pedestrian in motorized mobility scooter injured in collision with other nonmotor vehicle, unspecified whether traffic or nontraffic accident

√4ᵗʰ **V09** **Pedestrian injured in other and unspecified transport accidents**

The appropriate 7th character is to be added to each code from category V09.
A   initial encounter
D   subsequent encounter
S   sequela

√5ᵗʰ **V09.0** **Pedestrian injured in** nontraffic **accident involving** other **and unspecified motor vehicles**

√x 7ᵗʰ **V09.00** **Pedestrian injured in nontraffic accident involving unspecified motor vehicles**

√x 7ᵗʰ **V09.01** **Pedestrian injured in nontraffic accident involving** military **vehicle**

√x 7ᵗʰ **V09.09** **Pedestrian injured in nontraffic accident involving other motor vehicles**

    Pedestrian injured in nontraffic accident by special vehicle

√x 7ᵗʰ **V09.1** **Pedestrian injured in unspecified** nontraffic **accident**

√5ᵗʰ **V09.2** **Pedestrian injured in** traffic accident **involving other and unspecified motor vehicles**

√x 7ᵗʰ **V09.20** **Pedestrian injured in traffic accident involving unspecified motor vehicles**

√x 7ᵗʰ **V09.21** **Pedestrian injured in traffic accident involving** military **vehicle**

√x 7ᵗʰ **V09.29** **Pedestrian injured in traffic accident involving other motor vehicles**

√x 7ᵗʰ **V09.3** **Pedestrian injured in unspecified** traffic **accident**

√x 7ᵗʰ **V09.9** **Pedestrian injured in unspecified** transport **accident**

Pedal cycle rider injured in transport accident (V10–V19)

INCLUDES   any non-motorized vehicle, excluding an animal-drawn vehicle, or a sidecar or trailer attached to the pedal cycle

EXCLUDES 2   rupture of pedal cycle tire (W37.0)

√4ᵗʰ **V10** **Pedal cycle rider injured in collision with pedestrian or animal**

EXCLUDES 1   pedal cycle rider collision with animal-drawn vehicle or animal being ridden (V16.-)

The appropriate 7th character is to be added to each code from category V10.
A   initial encounter
D   subsequent encounter
S   sequela

√x 7ᵗʰ **V10.0** **Pedal cycle** driver **injured in collision with pedestrian or animal** in nontraffic accident

√x 7ᵗʰ **V10.1** **Pedal cycle** passenger **injured in collision with pedestrian or animal** in nontraffic accident

√x 7ᵗʰ **V10.2** **Unspecified pedal cyclist injured in collision with pedestrian or animal** in nontraffic accident

√x 7ᵗʰ **V10.3** Person boarding or alighting **a pedal cycle injured in collision with pedestrian or animal**

√x 7ᵗʰ **V10.4** **Pedal cycle** driver **injured in collision with pedestrian or animal** in traffic accident

---

☑ Additional Character Required   √x 7ᵗʰ Placeholder Alert   Unspecified Dx   Other Specified Dx   Manifestation   ▶◀ Revised Text   ● New Code   ▲ Revised Code Title

ICD-10-CM 2016   1043

Chapter 20. External Causes of Morbidity

V10.5–V16.9

√x7ᵗʰ **V10.5** **Pedal cycle** passenger **injured in collision with pedestrian or animal** in traffic accident

√x7ᵗʰ **V10.9** **Unspecified pedal cyclist injured in collision with pedestrian or animal** in traffic accident

✓4ᵗʰ **V11 Pedal cycle rider injured in collision with other pedal cycle**

> The appropriate 7th character is to be added to each code from category V11.
> A   initial encounter
> D   subsequent encounter
> S   sequela

√x7ᵗʰ **V11.0** **Pedal cycle** driver **injured in collision with other pedal cycle** in nontraffic accident

√x7ᵗʰ **V11.1** **Pedal cycle** passenger **injured in collision with other pedal cycle** in nontraffic accident

√x7ᵗʰ **V11.2** **Unspecified pedal cyclist injured in collision with other pedal cycle** in nontraffic accident

√x7ᵗʰ **V11.3** **Person boarding or alighting a pedal cycle injured in collision with other pedal cycle**

√x7ᵗʰ **V11.4** **Pedal cycle** driver **injured in collision with other pedal cycle** in traffic accident

√x7ᵗʰ **V11.5** **Pedal cycle** passenger **injured in collision with other pedal cycle** in traffic accident

√x7ᵗʰ **V11.9** **Unspecified pedal cyclist injured in collision with other pedal cycle** in traffic accident

✓4ᵗʰ **V12 Pedal cycle rider injured in collision with two- or three-wheeled motor vehicle**

> The appropriate 7th character is to be added to each code from category V12.
> A   initial encounter
> D   subsequent encounter
> S   sequela

√x7ᵗʰ **V12.0** **Pedal cycle** driver **injured in collision with two- or three-wheeled motor vehicle** in nontraffic accident

√x7ᵗʰ **V12.1** **Pedal cycle** passenger **injured in collision with two- or three-wheeled motor vehicle** in nontraffic accident

√x7ᵗʰ **V12.2** **Unspecified pedal cyclist injured in collision with two- or three-wheeled motor vehicle** in nontraffic accident

√x7ᵗʰ **V12.3** **Person boarding or alighting a pedal cycle injured in collision with two- or three-wheeled motor vehicle**

√x7ᵗʰ **V12.4** **Pedal cycle** driver **injured in collision with two- or three-wheeled motor vehicle** in traffic accident

√x7ᵗʰ **V12.5** **Pedal cycle** passenger **injured in collision with two- or three-wheeled motor vehicle** in traffic accident

√x7ᵗʰ **V12.9** **Unspecified pedal cyclist injured in collision with two- or three-wheeled motor vehicle** in traffic accident

✓4ᵗʰ **V13 Pedal cycle rider injured in collision with car, pick-up truck or van**

> The appropriate 7th character is to be added to each code from category V13.
> A   initial encounter
> D   subsequent encounter
> S   sequela

√x7ᵗʰ **V13.0** **Pedal cycle** driver **injured in collision with car, pick-up truck or van** in nontraffic accident

√x7ᵗʰ **V13.1** **Pedal cycle** passenger **injured in collision with car, pick-up truck or van** in nontraffic accident

√x7ᵗʰ **V13.2** **Unspecified pedal cyclist injured in collision with car, pick-up truck or van** in nontraffic accident

√x7ᵗʰ **V13.3** **Person boarding or alighting a pedal cycle injured in collision with car, pick-up truck or van**

√x7ᵗʰ **V13.4** **Pedal cycle** driver **injured in collision with car, pick-up truck or van** in traffic accident

√x7ᵗʰ **V13.5** **Pedal cycle** passenger **injured in collision with car, pick-up truck or van** in traffic accident

√x7ᵗʰ **V13.9** **Unspecified pedal cyclist injured in collision with car, pick-up truck or van** in traffic accident

✓4ᵗʰ **V14 Pedal cycle rider injured in collision with heavy transport vehicle or bus**

> EXCLUDES 1   pedal cycle rider injured in collision with military vehicle (V19.81)

> The appropriate 7th character is to be added to each code from category V14.
> A   initial encounter
> D   subsequent encounter
> S   sequela

√x7ᵗʰ **V14.0** **Pedal cycle** driver **injured in collision with heavy transport vehicle or bus** in nontraffic accident

√x7ᵗʰ **V14.1** **Pedal cycle** passenger **injured in collision with heavy transport vehicle or bus** in nontraffic accident

√x7ᵗʰ **V14.2** **Unspecified pedal cyclist injured in collision with heavy transport vehicle or bus** in nontraffic accident

√x7ᵗʰ **V14.3** **Person boarding or alighting a pedal cycle injured in collision with heavy transport vehicle or bus**

√x7ᵗʰ **V14.4** **Pedal cycle** driver **injured in collision with heavy transport vehicle or bus** in traffic accident

√x7ᵗʰ **V14.5** **Pedal cycle** passenger **injured in collision with heavy transport vehicle or bus** in traffic accident

√x7ᵗʰ **V14.9** **Unspecified pedal cyclist injured in collision with heavy transport vehicle or bus** in traffic accident

✓4ᵗʰ **V15 Pedal cycle rider injured in collision with railway train or railway vehicle**

> The appropriate 7th character is to be added to each code from category V15.
> A   initial encounter
> D   subsequent encounter
> S   sequela

√x7ᵗʰ **V15.0** **Pedal cycle** driver **injured in collision with railway train or railway vehicle** in nontraffic accident

√x7ᵗʰ **V15.1** **Pedal cycle** passenger **injured in collision with railway train or railway vehicle** in nontraffic accident

√x7ᵗʰ **V15.2** **Unspecified pedal cyclist injured in collision with railway train or railway vehicle** in nontraffic accident

√x7ᵗʰ **V15.3** **Person boarding or alighting a pedal cycle injured in collision with railway train or railway vehicle**

√x7ᵗʰ **V15.4** **Pedal cycle** driver **injured in collision with railway train or railway vehicle** in traffic accident

√x7ᵗʰ **V15.5** **Pedal cycle** passenger **injured in collision with railway train or railway vehicle** in traffic accident

√x7ᵗʰ **V15.9** **Unspecified pedal cyclist injured in collision with railway train or railway vehicle** in traffic accident

✓4ᵗʰ **V16 Pedal cycle rider injured in collision with other nonmotor vehicle**

> INCLUDES   collision with animal-drawn vehicle, animal being ridden, streetcar

> The appropriate 7th character is to be added to each code from category V16.
> A   initial encounter
> D   subsequent encounter
> S   sequela

√x7ᵗʰ **V16.0** **Pedal cycle** driver **injured in collision with other nonmotor vehicle** in nontraffic accident

√x7ᵗʰ **V16.1** **Pedal cycle** passenger **injured in collision with other nonmotor vehicle** in nontraffic accident

√x7ᵗʰ **V16.2** **Unspecified pedal cyclist injured in collision with other nonmotor vehicle** in nontraffic accident

√x7ᵗʰ **V16.3** **Person boarding or alighting a pedal cycle injured in collision with other nonmotor vehicle** in nontraffic accident

√x7ᵗʰ **V16.4** **Pedal cycle** driver **injured in collision with other nonmotor vehicle** in traffic accident

√x7ᵗʰ **V16.5** **Pedal cycle** passenger **injured in collision with other nonmotor vehicle** in traffic accident

√x7ᵗʰ **V16.9** **Unspecified pedal cyclist injured in collision with other nonmotor vehicle** in traffic accident

EXCLUDES 1 Not coded here   EXCLUDES 2 Not included here   N Newborn Age: 0   P Pediatric Age: 0-17   M Maternity Age: 12-55   A Adult Age: 15-124

1044   ICD-10-CM 2016

✓4th **V17 Pedal cycle rider injured in collision with fixed or stationary object**

> The appropriate 7th character is to be added to each code from category V17.
> A   initial encounter
> D   subsequent encounter
> S   sequela

✓x7th **V17.0 Pedal cycle driver injured in collision with fixed or stationary object in nontraffic accident**

✓x7th **V17.1 Pedal cycle passenger injured in collision with fixed or stationary object in nontraffic accident**

✓x7th **V17.2 Unspecified pedal cyclist injured in collision with fixed or stationary object in nontraffic accident**

✓x7th **V17.3 Person boarding or alighting a pedal cycle injured in collision with fixed or stationary object**

✓x7th **V17.4 Pedal cycle driver injured in collision with fixed or stationary object in traffic accident**

✓x7th **V17.5 Pedal cycle passenger injured in collision with fixed or stationary object in traffic accident**

✓x7th **V17.9 Unspecified pedal cyclist injured in collision with fixed or stationary object in traffic accident**

✓4th **V18 Pedal cycle rider injured in noncollision transport accident**

> INCLUDES   fall or thrown from pedal cycle (without antecedent collision)
> overturning pedal cycle NOS
> overturning pedal cycle without collision

> The appropriate 7th character is to be added to each code from category V18.
> A   initial encounter
> D   subsequent encounter
> S   sequela

✓x7th **V18.0 Pedal cycle driver injured in noncollision transport accident in nontraffic accident**

✓x7th **V18.1 Pedal cycle passenger injured in noncollision transport accident in nontraffic accident**

✓x7th **V18.2 Unspecified pedal cyclist injured in noncollision transport accident in nontraffic accident**

✓x7th **V18.3 Person boarding or alighting a pedal cycle injured in noncollision transport accident**

✓x7th **V18.4 Pedal cycle driver injured in noncollision transport accident in traffic accident**

✓x7th **V18.5 Pedal cycle passenger injured in noncollision transport accident in traffic accident**

✓x7th **V18.9 Unspecified pedal cyclist injured in noncollision transport accident in traffic accident**

✓4th **V19 Pedal cycle rider injured in other and unspecified transport accidents**

> The appropriate 7th character is to be added to each code from category V19.
> A   initial encounter
> D   subsequent encounter
> S   sequela

✓5th **V19.0 Pedal cycle driver injured in collision with other and unspecified motor vehicles in nontraffic accident**

   ✓x7th **V19.00 Pedal cycle driver injured in collision with unspecified motor vehicles in nontraffic accident**

   ✓x7th **V19.09 Pedal cycle driver injured in collision with other motor vehicles in nontraffic accident**

✓5th **V19.1 Pedal cycle passenger injured in collision with other and unspecified motor vehicles in nontraffic accident**

   ✓x7th **V19.10 Pedal cycle passenger injured in collision with unspecified motor vehicles in nontraffic accident**

   ✓x7th **V19.19 Pedal cycle passenger injured in collision with other motor vehicles in nontraffic accident**

✓5th **V19.2 Unspecified pedal cyclist injured in collision with other and unspecified motor vehicles in nontraffic accident**

   ✓x7th **V19.20 Unspecified pedal cyclist injured in collision with unspecified motor vehicles in nontraffic accident**
> Pedal cycle collision NOS, nontraffic

   ✓x7th **V19.29 Unspecified pedal cyclist injured in collision with other motor vehicles in nontraffic accident**

✓x7th **V19.3 Pedal cyclist (driver) (passenger) injured in unspecified nontraffic accident**
> Pedal cycle accident NOS, nontraffic
> Pedal cyclist injured in nontraffic accident NOS

✓5th **V19.4 Pedal cycle driver injured in collision with other and unspecified motor vehicles in traffic accident**

   ✓x7th **V19.40 Pedal cycle driver injured in collision with unspecified motor vehicles in traffic accident**

   ✓x7th **V19.49 Pedal cycle driver injured in collision with other motor vehicles in traffic accident**

✓5th **V19.5 Pedal cycle passenger injured in collision with other and unspecified motor vehicles in traffic accident**

   ✓x7th **V19.50 Pedal cycle passenger injured in collision with unspecified motor vehicles in traffic accident**

   ✓x7th **V19.59 Pedal cycle passenger injured in collision with other motor vehicles in traffic accident**

✓5th **V19.6 Unspecified pedal cyclist injured in collision with other and unspecified motor vehicles in traffic accident**

   ✓x7th **V19.60 Unspecified pedal cyclist injured in collision with unspecified motor vehicles in traffic accident**
> Pedal cycle collision NOS (traffic)

   ✓x7th **V19.69 Unspecified pedal cyclist injured in collision with other motor vehicles in traffic accident**

✓5th **V19.8 Pedal cyclist (driver) (passenger) injured in other specified transport accidents**

   ✓x7th **V19.81 Pedal cyclist (driver) (passenger) injured in transport accident with military vehicle**

   ✓x7th **V19.88 Pedal cyclist (driver) (passenger) injured in other specified transport accidents**

✓x7th **V19.9 Pedal cyclist (driver) (passenger) injured in unspecified traffic accident**
> Pedal cycle accident NOS

Motorcycle rider injured in transport accident (V20-V29)

> INCLUDES   moped
> motorcycle with sidecar
> motorized bicycle
> motor scooter
> EXCLUDES 1   three-wheeled motor vehicle (V30-V39)

✓4th **V20 Motorcycle rider injured in collision with pedestrian or animal**
> EXCLUDES 1   motorcycle rider collision with animal-drawn vehicle or animal being ridden (V26.-)

> The appropriate 7th character is to be added to each code from category V20.
> A   initial encounter
> D   subsequent encounter
> S   sequela

✓x7th **V20.0 Motorcycle driver injured in collision with pedestrian or animal in nontraffic accident**

✓x7th **V20.1 Motorcycle passenger injured in collision with pedestrian or animal in nontraffic accident**

✓x7th **V20.2 Unspecified motorcycle rider injured in collision with pedestrian or animal in nontraffic accident**

✓x7th **V20.3 Person boarding or alighting a motorcycle injured in collision with pedestrian or animal**

✓x7th **V20.4 Motorcycle driver injured in collision with pedestrian or animal in traffic accident**

✓x7th **V20.5 Motorcycle passenger injured in collision with pedestrian or animal in traffic accident**

✓x7th **V20.9 Unspecified motorcycle rider injured in collision with pedestrian or animal in traffic accident**

✓4th **V21 Motorcycle rider injured in collision with pedal cycle**

> The appropriate 7th character is to be added to each code from category V21.
> A   initial encounter
> D   subsequent encounter
> S   sequela

✓x7th **V21.0 Motorcycle driver injured in collision with pedal cycle in nontraffic accident**

✓x7th **V21.1 Motorcycle passenger injured in collision with pedal cycle in nontraffic accident**

✓x7th **V21.2 Unspecified motorcycle rider injured in collision with pedal cycle in nontraffic accident**

✓x7th **V21.3 Person boarding or alighting a motorcycle injured in collision with pedal cycle**

✓ Additional Character Required   ✓x7th Placeholder Alert   Unspecified Dx   Other Specified Dx   Manifestation   ►◄ Revised Text   ● New Code   ▲ Revised Code Title

√x7th **V21.4 Motorcycle driver injured in collision with pedal cycle in traffic accident**

√x7th **V21.5 Motorcycle passenger injured in collision with pedal cycle in traffic accident**

√x7th **V21.9 Unspecified motorcycle rider injured in collision with pedal cycle in traffic accident**

√4th **V22 Motorcycle rider injured in collision with two- or three-wheeled motor vehicle**

The appropriate 7th character is to be added to each code from category V22.
A   initial encounter
D   subsequent encounter
S   sequela

√x7th **V22.0 Motorcycle driver injured in collision with two- or three-wheeled motor vehicle in nontraffic accident**

√x7th **V22.1 Motorcycle passenger injured in collision with two- or three-wheeled motor vehicle in nontraffic accident**

√x7th **V22.2 Unspecified motorcycle rider injured in collision with two- or three-wheeled motor vehicle in nontraffic accident**

√x7th **V22.3 Person boarding or alighting a motorcycle injured in collision with two- or three-wheeled motor vehicle**

√x7th **V22.4 Motorcycle driver injured in collision with two- or three-wheeled motor vehicle in traffic accident**

√x7th **V22.5 Motorcycle passenger injured in collision with two- or three-wheeled motor vehicle in traffic accident**

√x7th **V22.9 Unspecified motorcycle rider injured in collision with two- or three-wheeled motor vehicle in traffic accident**

√4th **V23 Motorcycle rider injured in collision with car, pick-up truck or van**

The appropriate 7th character is to be added to each code from category V23.
A   initial encounter
D   subsequent encounter
S   sequela

√x7th **V23.0 Motorcycle driver injured in collision with car, pick-up truck or van in nontraffic accident**

√x7th **V23.1 Motorcycle passenger injured in collision with car, pick-up truck or van in nontraffic accident**

√x7th **V23.2 Unspecified motorcycle rider injured in collision with car, pick-up truck or van in nontraffic accident**

√x7th **V23.3 Person boarding or alighting a motorcycle injured in collision with car, pick-up truck or van**

√x7th **V23.4 Motorcycle driver injured in collision with car, pick-up truck or van in traffic accident**

√x7th **V23.5 Motorcycle passenger injured in collision with car, pick-up truck or van in traffic accident**

√x7th **V23.9 Unspecified motorcycle rider injured in collision with car, pick-up truck or van in traffic accident**

√4th **V24 Motorcycle rider injured in collision with heavy transport vehicle or bus**

EXCLUDES 1   motorcycle rider injured in collision with military vehicle (V29.81)

The appropriate 7th character is to be added to each code from category V24.
A   initial encounter
D   subsequent encounter
S   sequela

√x7th **V24.0 Motorcycle driver injured in collision with heavy transport vehicle or bus in nontraffic accident**

√x7th **V24.1 Motorcycle passenger injured in collision with heavy transport vehicle or bus in nontraffic accident**

√x7th **V24.2 Unspecified motorcycle rider injured in collision with heavy transport vehicle or bus in nontraffic accident**

√x7th **V24.3 Person boarding or alighting a motorcycle injured in collision with heavy transport vehicle or bus**

√x7th **V24.4 Motorcycle driver injured in collision with heavy transport vehicle or bus in traffic accident**

√x7th **V24.5 Motorcycle passenger injured in collision with heavy transport vehicle or bus in traffic accident**

√x7th **V24.9 Unspecified motorcycle rider injured in collision with heavy transport vehicle or bus in traffic accident**

√4th **V25 Motorcycle rider injured in collision with railway train or railway vehicle**

The appropriate 7th character is to be added to each code from category V25.
A   initial encounter
D   subsequent encounter
S   sequela

√x7th **V25.0 Motorcycle driver injured in collision with railway train or railway vehicle in nontraffic accident**

√x7th **V25.1 Motorcycle passenger injured in collision with railway train or railway vehicle in nontraffic accident**

√x7th **V25.2 Unspecified motorcycle rider injured in collision with railway train or railway vehicle in nontraffic accident**

√x7th **V25.3 Person boarding or alighting a motorcycle injured in collision with railway train or railway vehicle**

√x7th **V25.4 Motorcycle driver injured in collision with railway train or railway vehicle in traffic accident**

√x7th **V25.5 Motorcycle passenger injured in collision with railway train or railway vehicle in traffic accident**

√x7th **V25.9 Unspecified motorcycle rider injured in collision with railway train or railway vehicle in traffic accident**

√4th **V26 Motorcycle rider injured in collision with other nonmotor vehicle**

INCLUDES   collision with animal-drawn vehicle, animal being ridden, streetcar

The appropriate 7th character is to be added to each code from category V26.
A   initial encounter
D   subsequent encounter
S   sequela

√x7th **V26.0 Motorcycle driver injured in collision with other nonmotor vehicle in nontraffic accident**

√x7th **V26.1 Motorcycle passenger injured in collision with other nonmotor vehicle in nontraffic accident**

√x7th **V26.2 Unspecified motorcycle rider injured in collision with other nonmotor vehicle in nontraffic accident**

√x7th **V26.3 Person boarding or alighting a motorcycle injured in collision with other nonmotor vehicle**

√x7th **V26.4 Motorcycle driver injured in collision with other nonmotor vehicle in traffic accident**

√x7th **V26.5 Motorcycle passenger injured in collision with other nonmotor vehicle in traffic accident**

√x7th **V26.9 Unspecified motorcycle rider injured in collision with other nonmotor vehicle in traffic accident**

√4th **V27 Motorcycle rider injured in collision with fixed or stationary object**

The appropriate 7th character is to be added to each code from category V27.
A   initial encounter
D   subsequent encounter
S   sequela

√x7th **V27.0 Motorcycle driver injured in collision with fixed or stationary object in nontraffic accident**

√x7th **V27.1 Motorcycle passenger injured in collision with fixed or stationary object in nontraffic accident**

√x7th **V27.2 Unspecified motorcycle rider injured in collision with fixed or stationary object in nontraffic accident**

√x7th **V27.3 Person boarding or alighting a motorcycle injured in collision with fixed or stationary object**

√x7th **V27.4 Motorcycle driver injured in collision with fixed or stationary object in traffic accident**

√x7th **V27.5 Motorcycle passenger injured in collision with fixed or stationary object in traffic accident**

√x7th **V27.9 Unspecified motorcycle rider injured in collision with fixed or stationary object in traffic accident**

✓4th V28 Motorcycle rider injured in noncollision transport accident

INCLUDES   fall or thrown from motorcycle (without antecedent collision)
overturning motorcycle NOS
overturning motorcycle without collision

The appropriate 7th character is to be added to each code from category V28.
A   initial encounter
D   subsequent encounter
S   sequela

✓x7th **V28.0**   **Motorcycle driver injured in noncollision transport accident in nontraffic accident**

✓x7th **V28.1**   **Motorcycle passenger injured in noncollision transport accident in nontraffic accident**

✓x7th **V28.2**   **Unspecified motorcycle rider injured in noncollision transport accident in nontraffic accident**

✓x7th **V28.3**   **Person boarding or alighting a motorcycle injured in noncollision transport accident**

✓x7th **V28.4**   **Motorcycle driver injured in noncollision transport accident in traffic accident**

✓x7th **V28.5**   **Motorcycle passenger injured in noncollision transport accident in traffic accident**

✓x7th **V28.9**   **Unspecified motorcycle rider injured in noncollision transport accident in traffic accident**

✓4th V29 Motorcycle rider injured in other and unspecified transport accidents

The appropriate 7th character is to be added to each code from category V29.
A   initial encounter
D   subsequent encounter
S   sequela

✓5th **V29.0**   **Motorcycle driver injured in collision with other and unspecified motor vehicles in nontraffic accident**

    ✓x7th **V29.00**   **Motorcycle driver injured in collision with unspecified motor vehicles in nontraffic accident**

    ✓x7th **V29.09**   **Motorcycle driver injured in collision with other motor vehicles in nontraffic accident**

✓5th **V29.1**   **Motorcycle passenger injured in collision with other and unspecified motor vehicles in nontraffic accident**

    ✓x7th **V29.10**   **Motorcycle passenger injured in collision with unspecified motor vehicles in nontraffic accident**

    ✓x7th **V29.19**   **Motorcycle passenger injured in collision with other motor vehicles in nontraffic accident**

✓5th **V29.2**   **Unspecified motorcycle rider injured in collision with other and unspecified motor vehicles in nontraffic accident**

    ✓x7th **V29.20**   **Unspecified motorcycle rider injured in collision with unspecified motor vehicles in nontraffic accident**
        Motorcycle collision NOS, nontraffic

    ✓x7th **V29.29**   **Unspecified motorcycle rider injured in collision with other motor vehicles in nontraffic accident**

✓x7th **V29.3**   **Motorcycle rider (driver) (passenger) injured in unspecified nontraffic accident**
      Motorcycle accident NOS, nontraffic
      Motorcycle rider injured in nontraffic accident NOS

✓5th **V29.4**   **Motorcycle driver injured in collision with other and unspecified motor vehicles in traffic accident**

    ✓x7th **V29.40**   **Motorcycle driver injured in collision with unspecified motor vehicles in traffic accident**

    ✓x7th **V29.49**   **Motorcycle driver injured in collision with other motor vehicles in traffic accident**

✓5th **V29.5**   **Motorcycle passenger injured in collision with other and unspecified motor vehicles in traffic accident**

    ✓x7th **V29.50**   **Motorcycle passenger injured in collision with unspecified motor vehicles in traffic accident**

    ✓x7th **V29.59**   **Motorcycle passenger injured in collision with other motor vehicles in traffic accident**

✓5th **V29.6**   **Unspecified motorcycle rider injured in collision with other and unspecified motor vehicles in traffic accident**

    ✓x7th **V29.60**   **Unspecified motorcycle rider injured in collision with unspecified motor vehicles in traffic accident**
        Motorcycle collision NOS (traffic)

    ✓x7th **V29.69**   **Unspecified motorcycle rider injured in collision with other motor vehicles in traffic accident**

    ✓5th **V29.8**   **Motorcycle rider (driver) (passenger) injured in other specified transport accidents**

      ✓x7th **V29.81**   **Motorcycle rider (driver) (passenger) injured in transport accident with military vehicle**

      ✓x7th **V29.88**   **Motorcycle rider (driver) (passenger) injured in other specified transport accidents**

✓x7th **V29.9**   **Motorcycle rider (driver) (passenger) injured in unspecified traffic accident**
      Motorcycle accident NOS

Occupant of three-wheeled motor vehicle injured in transport accident (V30-V39)

INCLUDES   motorized tricycle
motorized rickshaw
three-wheeled motor car
EXCLUDES 1   all-terrain vehicles (V86.-)
motorcycle with sidecar (V20-V29)
vehicle designed primarily for off-road use (V86.-)

✓4th V30 Occupant of three-wheeled motor vehicle injured in collision with pedestrian or animal

EXCLUDES 1   three-wheeled motor vehicle collision with animal-drawn vehicle or animal being ridden (V36.-)

The appropriate 7th character is to be added to each code from category V30.
A   initial encounter
D   subsequent encounter
S   sequela

✓x7th **V30.0**   **Driver of three-wheeled motor vehicle injured in collision with pedestrian or animal in nontraffic accident**

✓x7th **V30.1**   **Passenger in three-wheeled motor vehicle injured in collision with pedestrian or animal in nontraffic accident**

✓x7th **V30.2**   **Person on outside of three-wheeled motor vehicle injured in collision with pedestrian or animal in nontraffic accident**

✓x7th **V30.3**   **Unspecified occupant of three-wheeled motor vehicle injured in collision with pedestrian or animal in nontraffic accident**

✓x7th **V30.4**   **Person boarding or alighting a three-wheeled motor vehicle injured in collision with pedestrian or animal**

✓x7th **V30.5**   **Driver of three-wheeled motor vehicle injured in collision with pedestrian or animal in traffic accident**

✓x7th **V30.6**   **Passenger in three-wheeled motor vehicle injured in collision with pedestrian or animal in traffic accident**

✓x7th **V30.7**   **Person on outside of three-wheeled motor vehicle injured in collision with pedestrian or animal in traffic accident**

✓x7th **V30.9**   **Unspecified occupant of three-wheeled motor vehicle injured in collision with pedestrian or animal in traffic accident**

✓4th V31 Occupant of three-wheeled motor vehicle injured in collision with pedal cycle

The appropriate 7th character is to be added to each code from category V31.
A   initial encounter
D   subsequent encounter
S   sequela

✓x7th **V31.0**   **Driver of three-wheeled motor vehicle injured in collision with pedal cycle in nontraffic accident**

✓x7th **V31.1**   **Passenger in three-wheeled motor vehicle injured in collision with pedal cycle in nontraffic accident**

✓x7th **V31.2**   **Person on outside of three-wheeled motor vehicle injured in collision with pedal cycle in nontraffic accident**

✓x7th **V31.3**   **Unspecified occupant of three-wheeled motor vehicle injured in collision with pedal cycle in nontraffic accident**

✓x7th **V31.4**   **Person boarding or alighting a three-wheeled motor vehicle injured in collision with pedal cycle**

✓x7th **V31.5**   **Driver of three-wheeled motor vehicle injured in collision with pedal cycle in traffic accident**

✓x7th **V31.6**   **Passenger in three-wheeled motor vehicle injured in collision with pedal cycle in traffic accident**

✓x7th **V31.7**   **Person on outside of three-wheeled motor vehicle injured in collision with pedal cycle in traffic accident**

✓x7th **V31.9**   **Unspecified occupant of three-wheeled motor vehicle injured in collision with pedal cycle in traffic accident**

✓ Additional Character Required   ✓x7th Placeholder Alert   Unspecified Dx   Other Specified Dx   Manifestation   ▶◀ Revised Text   ● New Code   ▲ Revised Code Title

✓4ᵗʰ **V32 Occupant of three-wheeled motor vehicle injured in collision with two- or three-wheeled motor vehicle**

> The appropriate 7th character is to be added to each code from category V32.
> A   initial encounter
> D   subsequent encounter
> S   sequela

✓x7ᵗʰ **V32.0 Driver** of three-wheeled motor vehicle injured in collision with two- or three-wheeled motor vehicle **in nontraffic accident**

✓x7ᵗʰ **V32.1 Passenger** in three-wheeled motor vehicle injured in collision with two- or three-wheeled motor vehicle **in nontraffic accident**

✓x7ᵗʰ **V32.2 Person on outside** of three-wheeled motor vehicle injured in collision with two- or three-wheeled motor vehicle **in nontraffic accident**

✓x7ᵗʰ **V32.3 Unspecified occupant** of three-wheeled motor vehicle injured in collision with two- or three-wheeled motor vehicle **in nontraffic accident**

✓x7ᵗʰ **V32.4 Person boarding or alighting** a three-wheeled motor vehicle injured in collision with two- or three-wheeled motor vehicle

✓x7ᵗʰ **V32.5 Driver** of three-wheeled motor vehicle injured in collision with two- or three-wheeled motor vehicle **in traffic accident**

✓x7ᵗʰ **V32.6 Passenger** in three-wheeled motor vehicle injured in collision with two- or three-wheeled motor vehicle **in traffic accident**

✓x7ᵗʰ **V32.7 Person on outside** of three-wheeled motor vehicle injured in collision with two- or three-wheeled motor vehicle **in traffic accident**

✓x7ᵗʰ **V32.9 Unspecified occupant** of three-wheeled motor vehicle injured in collision with two- or three-wheeled motor vehicle **in traffic accident**

✓4ᵗʰ **V33 Occupant of three-wheeled motor vehicle injured in collision with car, pick-up truck or van**

> The appropriate 7th character is to be added to each code from category V33.
> A   initial encounter
> D   subsequent encounter
> S   sequela

✓x7ᵗʰ **V33.0 Driver** of three-wheeled motor vehicle injured in collision with car, pick-up truck or van **in nontraffic accident**

✓x7ᵗʰ **V33.1 Passenger** in three-wheeled motor vehicle injured in collision with car, pick-up truck or van **in nontraffic accident**

✓x7ᵗʰ **V33.2 Person on outside** of three-wheeled motor vehicle injured in collision with car, pick-up truck or van **in nontraffic accident**

✓x7ᵗʰ **V33.3 Unspecified occupant** of three-wheeled motor vehicle injured in collision with car, pick-up truck or van **in nontraffic accident**

✓x7ᵗʰ **V33.4 Person** boarding or alighting a three-wheeled motor vehicle injured in collision with car, pick-up truck or van

✓x7ᵗʰ **V33.5 Driver** of three-wheeled motor vehicle injured in collision with car, pick-up truck or van **in traffic accident**

✓x7ᵗʰ **V33.6 Passenger** in three-wheeled motor vehicle injured in collision with car, pick-up truck or van **in traffic accident**

✓x7ᵗʰ **V33.7 Person on outside** of three-wheeled motor vehicle injured in collision with car, pick-up truck or van **in traffic accident**

✓x7ᵗʰ **V33.9 Unspecified occupant** of three-wheeled motor vehicle injured in collision with car, pick-up truck or van **in traffic accident**

✓4ᵗʰ **V34 Occupant of three-wheeled motor vehicle injured in collision with heavy transport vehicle or bus**

> **EXCLUDES 1** *occupant of three-wheeled motor vehicle injured in collision with military vehicle (V39.81)*

> The appropriate 7th character is to be added to each code from category V34.
> A   initial encounter
> D   subsequent encounter
> S   sequela

✓x7ᵗʰ **V34.0 Driver** of three-wheeled motor vehicle injured in collision with heavy transport vehicle or bus **in nontraffic accident**

✓x7ᵗʰ **V34.1 Passenger** in three-wheeled motor vehicle injured in collision with heavy transport vehicle or bus **in nontraffic accident**

✓x7ᵗʰ **V34.2 Person on outside** of three-wheeled motor vehicle injured in collision with heavy transport vehicle or bus **in nontraffic accident**

✓x7ᵗʰ **V34.3 Unspecified occupant** of three-wheeled motor vehicle injured in collision with heavy transport vehicle or bus **in nontraffic accident**

✓x7ᵗʰ **V34.4 Person boarding or alighting** a three-wheeled motor vehicle injured in collision with heavy transport vehicle or bus

✓x7ᵗʰ **V34.5 Driver** of three-wheeled motor vehicle injured in collision with heavy transport vehicle or bus **in traffic accident**

✓x7ᵗʰ **V34.6 Passenger** in three-wheeled motor vehicle injured in collision with heavy transport vehicle or bus **in traffic accident**

✓x7ᵗʰ **V34.7 Person on outside** of three-wheeled motor vehicle injured in collision with heavy transport vehicle or bus **in traffic accident**

✓x7ᵗʰ **V34.9 Unspecified occupant** of three-wheeled motor vehicle injured in collision with heavy transport vehicle or bus **in traffic accident**

✓4ᵗʰ **V35 Occupant of three-wheeled motor vehicle injured in collision with railway train or railway vehicle**

> The appropriate 7th character is to be added to each code from category V35.
> A   initial encounter
> D   subsequent encounter
> S   sequela

✓x7ᵗʰ **V35.0 Driver** of three-wheeled motor vehicle injured in collision with railway train or railway vehicle **in nontraffic accident**

✓x7ᵗʰ **V35.1 Passenger** in three-wheeled motor vehicle injured in collision with railway train or railway vehicle **in nontraffic accident**

✓x7ᵗʰ **V35.2 Person on outside** of three-wheeled motor vehicle injured in collision with railway train or railway vehicle **in nontraffic accident**

✓x7ᵗʰ **V35.3 Unspecified occupant** of three-wheeled motor vehicle injured in collision with railway train or railway vehicle **in nontraffic accident**

✓x7ᵗʰ **V35.4 Person boarding or alighting** a three-wheeled motor vehicle injured in collision with railway train or railway vehicle

✓x7ᵗʰ **V35.5 Driver** of three-wheeled motor vehicle injured in collision with railway train or railway vehicle **in traffic accident**

✓x7ᵗʰ **V35.6 Passenger** in three-wheeled motor vehicle injured in collision with railway train or railway vehicle **in traffic accident**

✓x7ᵗʰ **V35.7 Person on outside** of three-wheeled motor vehicle injured in collision with railway train or railway vehicle **in traffic accident**

✓x7ᵗʰ **V35.9 Unspecified occupant** of three-wheeled motor vehicle injured in collision with railway train or railway vehicle **in traffic accident**

✓4ᵗʰ **V36 Occupant of three-wheeled motor vehicle injured in collision with other nonmotor vehicle**
> **INCLUDES** collision with animal-drawn vehicle, animal being ridden, streetcar

> The appropriate 7th character is to be added to each code from category V36.
> A   initial encounter
> D   subsequent encounter
> S   sequela

✓x7ᵗʰ **V36.0 Driver** of three-wheeled motor vehicle injured in collision with other nonmotor vehicle **in nontraffic accident**

✓x7ᵗʰ **V36.1 Passenger** in three-wheeled motor vehicle injured in collision with other nonmotor vehicle **in nontraffic accident**

✓x7ᵗʰ **V36.2 Person on outside** of three-wheeled motor vehicle injured in collision with other nonmotor vehicle **in nontraffic accident**

✓x7ᵗʰ **V36.3 Unspecified occupant** of three-wheeled motor vehicle injured in collision with other nonmotor vehicle **in nontraffic accident**

✓x7ᵗʰ **V36.4 Person boarding or alighting** a three-wheeled motor vehicle injured in collision with other nonmotor vehicle

✓x7ᵗʰ **V36.5 Driver** of three-wheeled motor vehicle injured in collision with other nonmotor vehicle **in traffic accident**

✓x7ᵗʰ **V36.6 Passenger** in three-wheeled motor vehicle injured in collision with other nonmotor vehicle **in traffic accident**

✓x7ᵗʰ **V36.7 Person on outside** of three-wheeled motor vehicle injured in collision with other nonmotor vehicle **in traffic accident**

✓x7ᵗʰ **V36.9 Unspecified occupant** of three-wheeled motor vehicle injured in collision with other nonmotor vehicle **in traffic accident**

EXCLUDES 1 Not coded here   **EXCLUDES 2** Not included here   **N** Newborn Age: 0   **P** Pediatric Age: 0-17   **M** Maternity Age: 12-55   **A** Adult Age: 15-124

1048   ICD-10-CM 2016

✓4th **V37 Occupant of three-wheeled motor vehicle injured in collision with fixed or stationary object**

The appropriate 7th character is to be added to each code from category V37.
A   initial encounter
D   subsequent encounter
S   sequela

✓x7th **V37.0** Driver of three-wheeled motor vehicle injured in collision with fixed or stationary object in nontraffic accident

✓x7th **V37.1** Passenger in three-wheeled motor vehicle injured in collision with fixed or stationary object in nontraffic accident

✓x7th **V37.2** Person on outside of three-wheeled motor vehicle injured in collision with fixed or stationary object in nontraffic accident

✓x7th **V37.3** Unspecified occupant of three-wheeled motor vehicle injured in collision with fixed or stationary object in nontraffic accident

✓x7th **V37.4** Person boarding or alighting a three-wheeled motor vehicle injured in collision with fixed or stationary object

✓x7th **V37.5** Driver of three-wheeled motor vehicle injured in collision with fixed or stationary object in traffic accident

✓x7th **V37.6** Passenger in three-wheeled motor vehicle injured in collision with fixed or stationary object in traffic accident

✓x7th **V37.7** Person on outside of three-wheeled motor vehicle injured in collision with fixed or stationary object in traffic accident

✓x7th **V37.9** Unspecified occupant of three-wheeled motor vehicle injured in collision with fixed or stationary object in traffic accident

✓4th **V38 Occupant of three-wheeled motor vehicle injured in noncollision transport accident**

INCLUDES   fall or thrown from three-wheeled motor vehicle
overturning of three-wheeled motor vehicle NOS
overturning of three-wheeled motor vehicle without collision

The appropriate 7th character is to be added to each code from category V38.
A   initial encounter
D   subsequent encounter
S   sequela

✓x7th **V38.0** Driver of three-wheeled motor vehicle injured in noncollision transport accident in nontraffic accident

✓x7th **V38.1** Passenger in three-wheeled motor vehicle injured in noncollision transport accident in nontraffic accident

✓x7th **V38.2** Person on outside of three-wheeled motor vehicle injured in noncollision transport accident in nontraffic accident

✓x7th **V38.3** Unspecified occupant of three-wheeled motor vehicle injured in noncollision transport accident in nontraffic accident

✓x7th **V38.4** Person boarding or alighting a three-wheeled motor vehicle injured in noncollision transport accident

✓x7th **V38.5** Driver of three-wheeled motor vehicle injured in noncollision transport accident in traffic accident

✓x7th **V38.6** Passenger in three-wheeled motor vehicle injured in noncollision transport accident in traffic accident

✓x7th **V38.7** Person on outside of three-wheeled motor vehicle injured in noncollision transport accident in traffic accident

✓x7th **V38.9** Unspecified occupant of three-wheeled motor vehicle injured in noncollision transport accident in traffic accident

✓4th **V39 Occupant of three-wheeled motor vehicle injured in other and unspecified transport accidents**

The appropriate 7th character is to be added to each code from category V39.
A   initial encounter
D   subsequent encounter
S   sequela

✓5th **V39.0** Driver of three-wheeled motor vehicle injured in collision with other and unspecified motor vehicles in nontraffic accident

✓x7th **V39.00** Driver of three-wheeled motor vehicle injured in collision with unspecified motor vehicles in nontraffic accident

✓x7th **V39.09** Driver of three-wheeled motor vehicle injured in collision with other motor vehicles in nontraffic accident

✓5th **V39.1** Passenger in three-wheeled motor vehicle injured in collision with other and unspecified motor vehicles in nontraffic accident

✓x7th **V39.10** Passenger in three-wheeled motor vehicle injured in collision with unspecified motor vehicles in nontraffic accident

✓x7th **V39.19** Passenger in three-wheeled motor vehicle injured in collision with other motor vehicles in nontraffic accident

✓5th **V39.2** Unspecified occupant of three-wheeled motor vehicle injured in collision with other and unspecified motor vehicles in nontraffic accident

✓x7th **V39.20** Unspecified occupant of three-wheeled motor vehicle injured in collision with unspecified motor vehicles in nontraffic accident
Collision NOS involving three-wheeled motor vehicle, nontraffic

✓x7th **V39.29** Unspecified occupant of three-wheeled motor vehicle injured in collision with other motor vehicles in nontraffic accident

✓x7th **V39.3** Occupant (driver) (passenger) of three-wheeled motor vehicle injured in unspecified nontraffic accident
Accident NOS involving three-wheeled motor vehicle, nontraffic
Occupant of three-wheeled motor vehicle injured in nontraffic accident NOS

✓5th **V39.4** Driver of three-wheeled motor vehicle injured in collision with other and unspecified motor vehicles in traffic accident

✓x7th **V39.40** Driver of three-wheeled motor vehicle injured in collision with unspecified motor vehicles in traffic accident

✓x7th **V39.49** Driver of three-wheeled motor vehicle injured in collision with other motor vehicles in traffic accident

✓5th **V39.5** Passenger in three-wheeled motor vehicle injured in collision with other and unspecified motor vehicles in traffic accident

✓x7th **V39.50** Passenger in three-wheeled motor vehicle injured in collision with unspecified motor vehicles in traffic accident

✓x7th **V39.59** Passenger in three-wheeled motor vehicle injured in collision with other motor vehicles in traffic accident

✓5th **V39.6** Unspecified occupant of three-wheeled motor vehicle injured in collision with other and unspecified motor vehicles in traffic accident

✓x7th **V39.60** Unspecified occupant of three-wheeled motor vehicle injured in collision with unspecified motor vehicles in traffic accident
Collision NOS involving three-wheeled motor vehicle (traffic)

✓x7th **V39.69** Unspecified occupant of three-wheeled motor vehicle injured in collision with other motor vehicles in traffic accident

✓5th **V39.8** Occupant (driver) (passenger) of three-wheeled motor vehicle injured in other specified transport accidents

✓x7th **V39.81** Occupant (driver) (passenger) of three-wheeled motor vehicle injured in transport accident with military vehicle

✓x7th **V39.89** Occupant (driver) (passenger) of three-wheeled motor vehicle injured in other specified transport accidents

✓x7th **V39.9** Occupant (driver) (passenger) of three-wheeled motor vehicle injured in unspecified traffic accident
Accident NOS involving three-wheeled motor vehicle

☑ Additional Character Required   ✓x7th Placeholder Alert   Unspecified Dx   Other Specified Dx   Manifestation   ▶◀ Revised Text   ● New Code   ▲ Revised Code Title

Car occupant injured in transport accident (V40-V49)

INCLUDES   a four-wheeled motor vehicle designed primarily for carrying passengers
automobile (pulling a trailer or camper)

EXCLUDES 1   bus (V50-V59)
minibus (V50-V59)
minivan (V50-V59)
motorcoach (V70-V79)
pick-up truck (V50-V59)
sport utility vehicle (SUV) (V50-V59)

✓4ᵗʰ V40   **Car occupant injured in collision with pedestrian or animal**

> **EXCLUDES 1**   car collision with animal-drawn vehicle or animal being ridden (V46.-)

> The appropriate 7th character is to be added to each code from category V40.
> A   initial encounter
> D   subsequent encounter
> S   sequela

✓x7ᵗʰ V40.0   **Car driver** injured in collision with pedestrian or animal in nontraffic accident

✓x7ᵗʰ V40.1   **Car passenger** injured in collision with pedestrian or animal in nontraffic accident

✓x7ᵗʰ V40.2   **Person on outside** of car injured in collision with pedestrian or animal in nontraffic accident

✓x7ᵗʰ V40.3   **Unspecified car occupant** injured in collision with pedestrian or animal in nontraffic accident

✓x7ᵗʰ V40.4   **Person boarding or alighting** a car injured in collision with pedestrian or animal

✓x7ᵗʰ V40.5   **Car driver** injured in collision with pedestrian or animal in traffic accident

✓x7ᵗʰ V40.6   **Car passenger** injured in collision with pedestrian or animal in traffic accident

✓x7ᵗʰ V40.7   **Person on outside** of car injured in collision with pedestrian or animal in traffic accident

✓x7ᵗʰ V40.9   **Unspecified car occupant** injured in collision with pedestrian or animal in traffic accident

✓4ᵗʰ V41   **Car occupant injured in collision with pedal cycle**

> The appropriate 7th character is to be added to each code from category V41.
> A   initial encounter
> D   subsequent encounter
> S   sequela

✓x7ᵗʰ V41.0   **Car driver** injured in collision with pedal cycle in nontraffic accident

✓x7ᵗʰ V41.1   **Car passenger** injured in collision with pedal cycle in nontraffic accident

✓x7ᵗʰ V41.2   **Person on outside** of car injured in collision with pedal cycle in nontraffic accident

✓x7ᵗʰ V41.3   **Unspecified car occupant** injured in collision with pedal cycle in nontraffic accident

✓x7ᵗʰ V41.4   **Person boarding or alighting** a car injured in collision with pedal cycle

✓x7ᵗʰ V41.5   **Car driver** injured in collision with pedal cycle in traffic accident

✓x7ᵗʰ V41.6   **Car passenger** injured in collision with pedal cycle in traffic accident

✓x7ᵗʰ V41.7   **Person on outside** of car injured in collision with pedal cycle in traffic accident

✓x7ᵗʰ V41.9   **Unspecified car occupant** injured in collision with pedal cycle in traffic accident

✓4ᵗʰ V42   **Car occupant injured in collision with two- or three-wheeled motor vehicle**

> The appropriate 7th character is to be added to each code from category V42.
> A   initial encounter
> D   subsequent encounter
> S   sequela

✓x7ᵗʰ V42.0   **Car driver** injured in collision with two- or three-wheeled motor vehicle in nontraffic accident

✓x7ᵗʰ V42.1   **Car passenger** injured in collision with two- or three-wheeled motor vehicle in nontraffic accident

✓x7ᵗʰ V42.2   **Person on outside** of car injured in collision with two- or three-wheeled motor vehicle in nontraffic accident

✓x7ᵗʰ V42.3   **Unspecified car occupant** injured in collision with two- or three-wheeled motor vehicle in nontraffic accident

✓x7ᵗʰ V42.4   **Person boarding or alighting** a car injured in collision with two- or three-wheeled motor vehicle

✓x7ᵗʰ V42.5   **Car driver** injured in collision with two- or three-wheeled motor vehicle in traffic accident

✓x7ᵗʰ V42.6   **Car passenger** injured in collision with two- or three-wheeled motor vehicle in traffic accident

✓x7ᵗʰ V42.7   **Person on outside** of car injured in collision with two- or three-wheeled motor vehicle in traffic accident

✓x7ᵗʰ V42.9   **Unspecified car occupant** injured in collision with two- or three-wheeled motor vehicle in traffic accident

✓4ᵗʰ V43   **Car occupant injured in collision with car, pick-up truck or van**

> The appropriate 7th character is to be added to each code from category V43.
> A   initial encounter
> D   subsequent encounter
> S   sequela

✓5ᵗʰ V43.0   **Car driver** injured in collision with car, pick-up truck or van in nontraffic accident

    ✓x7ᵗʰ V43.01   **Car driver** injured in collision with sport utility vehicle in nontraffic accident

    ✓x7ᵗʰ V43.02   **Car driver** injured in collision with other type car in nontraffic accident

    ✓x7ᵗʰ V43.03   **Car driver** injured in collision with pick-up truck in nontraffic accident

    ✓x7ᵗʰ V43.04   **Car driver** injured in collision with van in nontraffic accident

✓5ᵗʰ V43.1   **Car passenger** injured in collision with car, pick-up truck or van in nontraffic accident

    ✓x7ᵗʰ V43.11   **Car passenger** injured in collision with sport utility vehicle in nontraffic accident

    ✓x7ᵗʰ V43.12   **Car passenger** injured in collision with other type car in nontraffic accident

    ✓x7ᵗʰ V43.13   **Car passenger** injured in collision with pick-up in nontraffic accident

    ✓x7ᵗʰ V43.14   **Car passenger** injured in collision with van in nontraffic accident

✓5ᵗʰ V43.2   **Person on outside** of car injured in collision with car, pick-up truck or van in nontraffic accident

    ✓x7ᵗʰ V43.21   **Person on outside** of car injured in collision with sport utility vehicle in nontraffic accident

    ✓x7ᵗʰ V43.22   **Person on outside** of car injured in collision with other type car in nontraffic accident

    ✓x7ᵗʰ V43.23   **Person on outside** of car injured in collision with pick-up truck in nontraffic accident

    ✓x7ᵗʰ V43.24   **Person on outside** of car injured in collision with van in nontraffic accident

✓5ᵗʰ V43.3   **Unspecified car occupant** injured in collision with car, pick-up truck or van in nontraffic accident

    ✓x7ᵗʰ V43.31   **Unspecified car occupant** injured in collision with sport utility vehicle in nontraffic accident

    ✓x7ᵗʰ V43.32   **Unspecified car occupant** injured in collision with other type car in nontraffic accident

    ✓x7ᵗʰ V43.33   **Unspecified car occupant** injured in collision with pick-up truck in nontraffic accident

    ✓x7ᵗʰ V43.34   **Unspecified car occupant** injured in collision with van in nontraffic accident

✓5ᵗʰ V43.4   **Person boarding or alighting** a car injured in collision with car, pick-up truck or van

    ✓x7ᵗʰ V43.41   **Person boarding or alighting** a car injured in collision with sport utility vehicle

    ✓x7ᵗʰ V43.42   **Person boarding or alighting** a car injured in collision with other type car

    ✓x7ᵗʰ V43.43   **Person boarding or alighting** a car injured in collision with pick-up truck

    ✓x7ᵗʰ V43.44   **Person boarding or alighting** a car injured in collision with van

✓5ᵗʰ V43.5   **Car driver** injured in collision with car, pick-up truck or van in traffic accident

    ✓x7ᵗʰ V43.51   **Car driver** injured in collision with sport utility vehicle in traffic accident

---

EXCLUDES 1 Not coded here   **EXCLUDES 2** Not included here   **N** Newborn Age: 0   **P** Pediatric Age: 0-17   **M** Maternity Age: 12-55   **A** Adult Age: 15-124

1050   ICD-10-CM 2016

Chapter 20. External Causes of Morbidity

✓x7ᵗʰ **V43.52** Car driver injured in collision with other type car in traffic accident

✓x7ᵗʰ **V43.53** Car driver injured in collision with pick-up truck in traffic accident

✓x7ᵗʰ **V43.54** Car driver injured in collision with van in traffic accident

✓5ᵗʰ **V43.6** Car passenger injured in collision with car, pick-up truck or van in traffic accident

✓x7ᵗʰ **V43.61** Car passenger injured in collision with sport utility vehicle in traffic accident

✓x7ᵗʰ **V43.62** Car passenger injured in collision with other type car in traffic accident

✓x7ᵗʰ **V43.63** Car passenger injured in collision with pick-up truck in traffic accident

✓x7ᵗʰ **V43.64** Car passenger injured in collision with van in traffic accident

✓5ᵗʰ **V43.7** Person on outside of car injured in collision with car, pick-up truck or van in traffic accident

✓x7ᵗʰ **V43.71** Person on outside of car injured in collision with sport utility vehicle in traffic accident

✓x7ᵗʰ **V43.72** Person on outside of car injured in collision with other type car in traffic accident

✓x7ᵗʰ **V43.73** Person on outside of car injured in collision with pick-up truck in traffic accident

✓x7ᵗʰ **V43.74** Person on outside of car injured in collision with van in traffic accident

✓5ᵗʰ **V43.9** Unspecified car occupant injured in collision with car, pick-up truck or van in traffic accident

✓x7ᵗʰ **V43.91** Unspecified car occupant injured in collision with sport utility vehicle in traffic accident

✓x7ᵗʰ **V43.92** Unspecified car occupant injured in collision with other type car in traffic accident

✓x7ᵗʰ **V43.93** Unspecified car occupant injured in collision with pick-up truck in traffic accident

✓x7ᵗʰ **V43.94** Unspecified car occupant injured in collision with van in traffic accident

✓4ᵗʰ **V44** Car occupant injured in collision with heavy transport vehicle or bus

> EXCLUDES 1   car occupant injured in collision with military vehicle (V49.81)

> The appropriate 7th character is to be added to each code from category V44.
> A   initial encounter
> D   subsequent encounter
> S   sequela

✓x7ᵗʰ **V44.0** Car driver injured in collision with heavy transport vehicle or bus in nontraffic accident

✓x7ᵗʰ **V44.1** Car passenger injured in collision with heavy transport vehicle or bus in nontraffic accident

✓x7ᵗʰ **V44.2** Person on outside of car injured in collision with heavy transport vehicle or bus in nontraffic accident

✓x7ᵗʰ **V44.3** Unspecified car occupant injured in collision with heavy transport vehicle or bus in nontraffic accident

✓x7ᵗʰ **V44.4** Person boarding or alighting a car injured in collision with heavy transport vehicle or bus

✓x7ᵗʰ **V44.5** Car driver injured in collision with heavy transport vehicle or bus in traffic accident

✓x7ᵗʰ **V44.6** Car passenger injured in collision with heavy transport vehicle or bus in traffic accident

✓x7ᵗʰ **V44.7** Person on outside of car injured in collision with heavy transport vehicle or bus in traffic accident

✓x7ᵗʰ **V44.9** Unspecified car occupant injured in collision with heavy transport vehicle or bus in traffic accident

✓4ᵗʰ **V45** Car occupant injured in collision with railway train or railway vehicle

> The appropriate 7th character is to be added to each code from category V45.
> A   initial encounter
> D   subsequent encounter
> S   sequela

✓x7ᵗʰ **V45.0** Car driver injured in collision with railway train or railway vehicle in nontraffic accident

✓x7ᵗʰ **V45.1** Car passenger injured in collision with railway train or railway vehicle in nontraffic accident

✓x7ᵗʰ **V45.2** Person on outside of car injured in collision with railway train or railway vehicle in nontraffic accident

✓x7ᵗʰ **V45.3** Unspecified car occupant injured in collision with railway train or railway vehicle in nontraffic accident

✓x7ᵗʰ **V45.4** Person boarding or alighting a car injured in collision with railway train or railway vehicle

✓x7ᵗʰ **V45.5** Car driver injured in collision with railway train or railway vehicle in traffic accident

✓x7ᵗʰ **V45.6** Car passenger injured in collision with railway train or railway vehicle in traffic accident

✓x7ᵗʰ **V45.7** Person on outside of car injured in collision with railway train or railway vehicle in traffic accident

✓x7ᵗʰ **V45.9** Unspecified car occupant injured in collision with railway train or railway vehicle in traffic accident

✓4ᵗʰ **V46** Car occupant injured in collision with other nonmotor vehicle

> INCLUDES   collision with animal-drawn vehicle, animal being ridden, streetcar

> The appropriate 7th character is to be added to each code from category V46.
> A   initial encounter
> D   subsequent encounter
> S   sequela

✓x7ᵗʰ **V46.0** Car driver injured in collision with other nonmotor vehicle in nontraffic accident

✓x7ᵗʰ **V46.1** Car passenger injured in collision with other nonmotor vehicle in nontraffic accident

✓x7ᵗʰ **V46.2** Person on outside of car injured in collision with other nonmotor vehicle in nontraffic accident

✓x7ᵗʰ **V46.3** Unspecified car occupant injured in collision with other nonmotor vehicle in nontraffic accident

✓x7ᵗʰ **V46.4** Person boarding or alighting a car injured in collision with other nonmotor vehicle

✓x7ᵗʰ **V46.5** Car driver injured in collision with other nonmotor vehicle in traffic accident

✓x7ᵗʰ **V46.6** Car passenger injured in collision with other nonmotor vehicle in traffic accident

✓x7ᵗʰ **V46.7** Person on outside of car injured in collision with other nonmotor vehicle in traffic accident

✓x7ᵗʰ **V46.9** Unspecified car occupant injured in collision with other nonmotor vehicle in traffic accident

✓4ᵗʰ **V47** Car occupant injured in collision with fixed or stationary object

> The appropriate 7th character is to be added to each code from category V47.
> A   initial encounter
> D   subsequent encounter
> S   sequela

✓5ᵗʰ **V47.0** Car driver injured in collision with fixed or stationary object in nontraffic accident

✓x7ᵗʰ **V47.01** Driver of sport utility vehicle injured in collision with fixed or stationary object in nontraffic accident

✓x7ᵗʰ **V47.02** Driver of other type car injured in collision with fixed or stationary object in nontraffic accident

✓5ᵗʰ **V47.1** Car passenger injured in collision with fixed or stationary object in nontraffic accident

✓x7ᵗʰ **V47.11** Passenger of sport utility vehicle injured in collision with fixed or stationary object in nontraffic accident

✓x7ᵗʰ **V47.12** Passenger of other type car injured in collision with fixed or stationary object in nontraffic accident

✓x7ᵗʰ **V47.2** Person on outside of car injured in collision with fixed or stationary object in nontraffic accident

✓5ᵗʰ **V47.3** Unspecified car occupant injured in collision with fixed or stationary object in nontraffic accident

✓x7ᵗʰ **V47.31** Unspecified occupant of sport utility vehicle injured in collision with fixed or stationary object in nontraffic accident

✓x7ᵗʰ **V47.32** Unspecified occupant of other type car injured in collision with fixed or stationary object in nontraffic accident

✓x7ᵗʰ **V47.4** Person boarding or alighting a car injured in collision with fixed or stationary object

✓5ᵗʰ **V47.5** Car driver injured in collision with fixed or stationary object in traffic accident

✓x7ᵗʰ **V47.51** Driver of sport utility vehicle injured in collision with fixed or stationary object in traffic accident

---

✓ Additional Character Required   ✓x7ᵗʰ Placeholder Alert   Unspecified Dx   Other Specified Dx   Manifestation   ▶◀ Revised Text   ● New Code   ▲ Revised Code Title

Chapter 20. External Causes of Morbidity

√x7ᵗʰ **V47.52** Driver of other type car injured in collision with fixed or stationary object in traffic accident

√5ᵗʰ **V47.6** Car passenger injured in collision with fixed or stationary object in traffic accident

    √x7ᵗʰ **V47.61** Passenger of sport utility vehicle injured in collision with fixed or stationary object in traffic accident

    √x7ᵗʰ **V47.62** Passenger of other type car injured in collision with fixed or stationary object in traffic accident

√x7ᵗʰ **V47.7** Person on outside of car injured in collision with fixed or stationary object in traffic accident

√5ᵗʰ **V47.9** Unspecified car occupant injured in collision with fixed or stationary object in traffic accident

    √x7ᵗʰ **V47.91** Unspecified occupant of sport utility vehicle injured in collision with fixed or stationary object in traffic accident

    √x7ᵗʰ **V47.92** Unspecified occupant of other type car injured in collision with fixed or stationary object in traffic accident

√4ᵗʰ **V48** Car occupant injured in noncollision transport accident

    INCLUDES   overturning car NOS
                   overturning car without collision

    The appropriate 7th character is to be added to each code from category V48.
    A   initial encounter
    D   subsequent encounter
    S   sequela

√x7ᵗʰ **V48.0** Car driver injured in noncollision transport accident in nontraffic accident

√x7ᵗʰ **V48.1** Car passenger injured in noncollision transport accident in nontraffic accident

√x7ᵗʰ **V48.2** Person on outside of car injured in noncollision transport accident in nontraffic accident

√x7ᵗʰ **V48.3** Unspecified car occupant injured in noncollision transport accident in nontraffic accident

√x7ᵗʰ **V48.4** Person boarding or alighting a car injured in noncollision transport accident

√x7ᵗʰ **V48.5** Car driver injured in noncollision transport accident in traffic accident

√x7ᵗʰ **V48.6** Car passenger injured in noncollision transport accident in traffic accident

√x7ᵗʰ **V48.7** Person on outside of car injured in noncollision transport accident in traffic accident

√x7ᵗʰ **V48.9** Unspecified car occupant injured in noncollision transport accident in traffic accident

√4ᵗʰ **V49** Car occupant injured in other and unspecified transport accidents

    The appropriate 7th character is to be added to each code from category V49.
    A   initial encounter
    D   subsequent encounter
    S   sequela

√5ᵗʰ **V49.0** Driver injured in collision with other and unspecified motor vehicles in nontraffic accident

    √x7ᵗʰ **V49.00** Driver injured in collision with unspecified motor vehicles in nontraffic accident

    √x7ᵗʰ **V49.09** Driver injured in collision with other motor vehicles in nontraffic accident

√5ᵗʰ **V49.1** Passenger injured in collision with other and unspecified motor vehicles in nontraffic accident

    √x7ᵗʰ **V49.10** Passenger injured in collision with unspecified motor vehicles in nontraffic accident

    √x7ᵗʰ **V49.19** Passenger injured in collision with other motor vehicles in nontraffic accident

√5ᵗʰ **V49.2** Unspecified car occupant injured in collision with other and unspecified motor vehicles in nontraffic accident

    √x7ᵗʰ **V49.20** Unspecified car occupant injured in collision with unspecified motor vehicles in nontraffic accident
          Car collision NOS, nontraffic

    √x7ᵗʰ **V49.29** Unspecified car occupant injured in collision with other motor vehicles in nontraffic accident

√x7ᵗʰ **V49.3** Car occupant (driver) (passenger) injured in unspecified nontraffic accident
    Car accident NOS, nontraffic
    Car occupant injured in nontraffic accident NOS

√5ᵗʰ **V49.4** Driver injured in collision with other and unspecified motor vehicles in traffic accident

    √x7ᵗʰ **V49.40** Driver injured in collision with unspecified motor vehicles in traffic accident

    √x7ᵗʰ **V49.49** Driver injured in collision with other motor vehicles in traffic accident

√5ᵗʰ **V49.5** Passenger injured in collision with other and unspecified motor vehicles in traffic accident

    √x7ᵗʰ **V49.50** Passenger injured in collision with unspecified motor vehicles in traffic accident

    √x7ᵗʰ **V49.59** Passenger injured in collision with other motor vehicles in traffic accident

√5ᵗʰ **V49.6** Unspecified car occupant injured in collision with other and unspecified motor vehicles in traffic accident

    √x7ᵗʰ **V49.60** Unspecified car occupant injured in collision with unspecified motor vehicles in traffic accident
          Car collision NOS (traffic)

    √x7ᵗʰ **V49.69** Unspecified car occupant injured in collision with other motor vehicles in traffic accident

√5ᵗʰ **V49.8** Car occupant (driver) (passenger) injured in other specified transport accidents

    √x7ᵗʰ **V49.81** Car occupant (driver) (passenger) injured in transport accident with military vehicle

    √x7ᵗʰ **V49.88** Car occupant (driver) (passenger) injured in other specified transport accidents

√x7ᵗʰ **V49.9** Car occupant (driver) (passenger) injured in unspecified traffic accident
    Car accident NOS

Occupant of pick-up truck or van injured in transport accident (V50-V59)

    INCLUDES   a four or six wheel motor vehicle designed primarily for carrying passengers and property but weighing less than the local limit for classification as a heavy goods vehicle
                   minibus
                   minivan
                   sport utility vehicle (SUV)
                   truck
                   van
    EXCLUDES 1   heavy transport vehicle (V60-V69)

√4ᵗʰ **V50** Occupant of pick-up truck or van injured in collision with pedestrian or animal
    EXCLUDES 1   pick-up truck or van collision with animal-drawn vehicle or animal being ridden (V56.-)

    The appropriate 7th character is to be added to each code from category V50.
    A   initial encounter
    D   subsequent encounter
    S   sequela

√x7ᵗʰ **V50.0** Driver of pick-up truck or van injured in collision with pedestrian or animal in nontraffic accident

√x7ᵗʰ **V50.1** Passenger in pick-up truck or van injured in collision with pedestrian or animal in nontraffic accident

√x7ᵗʰ **V50.2** Person on outside of pick-up truck or van injured in collision with pedestrian or animal in nontraffic accident

√x7ᵗʰ **V50.3** Unspecified occupant of pick-up truck or van injured in collision with pedestrian or animal in nontraffic accident

√x7ᵗʰ **V50.4** Person boarding or alighting a pick-up truck or van injured in collision with pedestrian or animal

√x7ᵗʰ **V50.5** Driver of pick-up truck or van injured in collision with pedestrian or animal in traffic accident

√x7ᵗʰ **V50.6** Passenger in pick-up truck or van injured in collision with pedestrian or animal in traffic accident

√x7ᵗʰ **V50.7** Person on outside of pick-up truck or van injured in collision with pedestrian or animal in traffic accident

√x7ᵗʰ **V50.9** Unspecified occupant of pick-up truck or van injured in collision with pedestrian or animal in traffic accident

EXCLUDES 1 Not coded here   EXCLUDES 2 Not included here   N Newborn Age: 0   P Pediatric Age: 0-17   M Maternity Age: 12-55   A Adult Age: 15-124

1052   ICD-10-CM 2016

✓4th V51 Occupant of pick-up truck or van injured in collision with pedal cycle

> The appropriate 7th character is to be added to each code from category V51.
> A   initial encounter
> D   subsequent encounter
> S   sequela

✓x7th **V51.0** Driver of pick-up truck or van injured in collision with pedal cycle in nontraffic accident

✓x7th **V51.1** Passenger in pick-up truck or van injured in collision with pedal cycle in nontraffic accident

✓x7th **V51.2** Person on outside of pick-up truck or van injured in collision with pedal cycle in nontraffic accident

✓x7th **V51.3** Unspecified occupant of pick-up truck or van injured in collision with pedal cycle in nontraffic accident

✓x7th **V51.4** Person boarding or alighting a pick-up truck or van injured in collision with pedal cycle

✓x7th **V51.5** Driver of pick-up truck or van injured in collision with pedal cycle in traffic accident

✓x7th **V51.6** Passenger in pick-up truck or van injured in collision with pedal cycle in traffic accident

✓x7th **V51.7** Person on outside of pick-up truck or van injured in collision with pedal cycle in traffic accident

✓x7th **V51.9** Unspecified occupant of pick-up truck or van injured in collision with pedal cycle in traffic accident

✓4th V52 Occupant of pick-up truck or van injured in collision with two- or three-wheeled motor vehicle

> The appropriate 7th character is to be added to each code from category V52.
> A   initial encounter
> D   subsequent encounter
> S   sequela

✓x7th **V52.0** Driver of pick-up truck or van injured in collision with two- or three-wheeled motor vehicle in nontraffic accident

✓x7th **V52.1** Passenger in pick-up truck or van injured in collision with two- or three-wheeled motor vehicle in nontraffic accident

✓x7th **V52.2** Person on outside of pick-up truck or van injured in collision with two- or three-wheeled motor vehicle in nontraffic accident

✓x7th **V52.3** Unspecified occupant of pick-up truck or van injured in collision with two- or three-wheeled motor vehicle in nontraffic accident

✓x7th **V52.4** Person boarding or alighting a pick-up truck or van injured in collision with two- or three-wheeled motor vehicle

✓x7th **V52.5** Driver of pick-up truck or van injured in collision with two- or three-wheeled motor vehicle in traffic accident

✓x7th **V52.6** Passenger in pick-up truck or van injured in collision with two- or three-wheeled motor vehicle in traffic accident

✓x7th **V52.7** Person on outside of pick-up truck or van injured in collision with two- or three-wheeled motor vehicle in traffic accident

✓x7th **V52.9** Unspecified occupant of pick-up truck or van injured in collision with two- or three-wheeled motor vehicle in traffic accident

✓4th V53 Occupant of pick-up truck or van injured in collision with car, pick-up truck or van

> The appropriate 7th character is to be added to each code from category V53.
> A   initial encounter
> D   subsequent encounter
> S   sequela

✓x7th **V53.0** Driver of pick-up truck or van injured in collision with car, pick-up truck or van in nontraffic accident

✓x7th **V53.1** Passenger in pick-up truck or van injured in collision with car, pick-up truck or van in nontraffic accident

✓x7th **V53.2** Person on outside of pick-up truck or van injured in collision with car, pick-up truck or van in nontraffic accident

✓x7th **V53.3** Unspecified occupant of pick-up truck or van injured in collision with car, pick-up truck or van in nontraffic accident

✓x7th **V53.4** Person boarding or alighting a pick-up truck or van injured in collision with car, pick-up truck or van

✓x7th **V53.5** Driver of pick-up truck or van injured in collision with car, pick-up truck or van in traffic accident

✓x7th **V53.6** Passenger in pick-up truck or van injured in collision with car, pick-up truck or van in traffic accident

✓x7th **V53.7** Person on outside of pick-up truck or van injured in collision with car, pick-up truck or van in traffic accident

✓x7th **V53.9** Unspecified occupant of pick-up truck or van injured in collision with car, pick-up truck or van in traffic accident

✓4th V54 Occupant of pick-up truck or van injured in collision with heavy transport vehicle or bus

> **EXCLUDES 1**   occupant of pick-up truck or van injured in collision with military vehicle (V59.81)

> The appropriate 7th character is to be added to each code from category V54.
> A   initial encounter
> D   subsequent encounter
> S   sequela

✓x7th **V54.0** Driver of pick-up truck or van injured in collision with heavy transport vehicle or bus in nontraffic accident

✓x7th **V54.1** Passenger in pick-up truck or van injured in collision with heavy transport vehicle or bus in nontraffic accident

✓x7th **V54.2** Person on outside of pick-up truck or van injured in collision with heavy transport vehicle or bus in nontraffic accident

✓x7th **V54.3** Unspecified occupant of pick-up truck or van injured in collision with heavy transport vehicle or bus in nontraffic accident

✓x7th **V54.4** Person boarding or alighting a pick-up truck or van injured in collision with heavy transport vehicle or bus

✓x7th **V54.5** Driver of pick-up truck or van injured in collision with heavy transport vehicle or bus in traffic accident

✓x7th **V54.6** Passenger in pick-up truck or van injured in collision with heavy transport vehicle or bus in traffic accident

✓x7th **V54.7** Person on outside of pick-up truck or van injured in collision with heavy transport vehicle or bus in traffic accident

✓x7th **V54.9** Unspecified occupant of pick-up truck or van injured in collision with heavy transport vehicle or bus in traffic accident

✓4th V55 Occupant of pick-up truck or van injured in collision with railway train or railway vehicle

> The appropriate 7th character is to be added to each code from category V55.
> A   initial encounter
> D   subsequent encounter
> S   sequela

✓x7th **V55.0** Driver of pick-up truck or van injured in collision with railway train or railway vehicle in nontraffic accident

✓x7th **V55.1** Passenger in pick-up truck or van injured in collision with railway train or railway vehicle in nontraffic accident

✓x7th **V55.2** Person on outside of pick-up truck or van injured in collision with railway train or railway vehicle in nontraffic accident

✓x7th **V55.3** Unspecified occupant of pick-up truck or van injured in collision with railway train or railway vehicle in nontraffic accident

✓x7th **V55.4** Person boarding or alighting a pick-up truck or van injured in collision with railway train or railway vehicle

✓x7th **V55.5** Driver of pick-up truck or van injured in collision with railway train or railway vehicle in traffic accident

✓x7th **V55.6** Passenger in pick-up truck or van injured in collision with railway train or railway vehicle in traffic accident

✓x7th **V55.7** Person on outside of pick-up truck or van injured in collision with railway train or railway vehicle in traffic accident

✓x7th **V55.9** Unspecified occupant of pick-up truck or van injured in collision with railway train or railway vehicle in traffic accident

✓4th V56 Occupant of pick-up truck or van injured in collision with other nonmotor vehicle

> **INCLUDES**   collision with animal-drawn vehicle, animal being ridden, streetcar

> The appropriate 7th character is to be added to each code from category V56.
> A   initial encounter
> D   subsequent encounter
> S   sequela

✓x7th **V56.0** Driver of pick-up truck or van injured in collision with other nonmotor vehicle in nontraffic accident

✓x7th **V56.1** Passenger in pick-up truck or van injured in collision with other nonmotor vehicle in nontraffic accident

---

✓ Additional Character Required   ✓x7th Placeholder Alert   Unspecified Dx   Other Specified Dx   Manifestation   ▶◀ Revised Text   ● New Code   ▲ Revised Code Title

✓x7ᵗʰ **V56.2** Person on outside of pick-up truck or van injured in collision with other nonmotor vehicle in nontraffic accident

✓x7ᵗʰ **V56.3** Unspecified occupant of pick-up truck or van injured in collision with other nonmotor vehicle in nontraffic accident

✓x7ᵗʰ **V56.4** Person boarding or alighting a pick-up truck or van injured in collision with other nonmotor vehicle

✓x7ᵗʰ **V56.5** Driver of pick-up truck or van injured in collision with other nonmotor vehicle in traffic accident

✓x7ᵗʰ **V56.6** Passenger in pick-up truck or van injured in collision with other nonmotor vehicle in traffic accident

✓x7ᵗʰ **V56.7** Person on outside of pick-up truck or van injured in collision with other nonmotor vehicle in traffic accident

✓x7ᵗʰ **V56.9** Unspecified occupant of pick-up truck or van injured in collision with other nonmotor vehicle in traffic accident

✓4ᵗʰ **V57 Occupant of pick-up truck or van injured in collision with fixed or stationary object**

> The appropriate 7th character is to be added to each code from category V57.
> A   initial encounter
> D   subsequent encounter
> S   sequela

✓x7ᵗʰ **V57.0** Driver of pick-up truck or van injured in collision with fixed or stationary object in nontraffic accident

✓x7ᵗʰ **V57.1** Passenger in pick-up truck or van injured in collision with fixed or stationary object in nontraffic accident

✓x7ᵗʰ **V57.2** Person on outside of pick-up truck or van injured in collision with fixed or stationary object in nontraffic accident

✓x7ᵗʰ **V57.3** Unspecified occupant of pick-up truck or van injured in collision with fixed or stationary object in nontraffic accident

✓x7ᵗʰ **V57.4** Person boarding or alighting a pick-up truck or van injured in collision with fixed or stationary object

✓x7ᵗʰ **V57.5** Driver of pick-up truck or van injured in collision with fixed or stationary object in traffic accident

✓x7ᵗʰ **V57.6** Passenger in pick-up truck or van injured in collision with fixed or stationary object in traffic accident

✓x7ᵗʰ **V57.7** Person on outside of pick-up truck or van injured in collision with fixed or stationary object in traffic accident

✓x7ᵗʰ **V57.9** Unspecified occupant of pick-up truck or van injured in collision with fixed or stationary object in traffic accident

✓4ᵗʰ **V58 Occupant of pick-up truck or van injured in noncollision transport accident**

> INCLUDES   overturning pick-up truck or van NOS
>   overturning pick-up truck or van without collision

> The appropriate 7th character is to be added to each code from category V58.
> A   initial encounter
> D   subsequent encounter
> S   sequela

✓x7ᵗʰ **V58.0** Driver of pick-up truck or van injured in noncollision transport accident in nontraffic accident

✓x7ᵗʰ **V58.1** Passenger in pick-up truck or van injured in noncollision transport accident in nontraffic accident

✓x7ᵗʰ **V58.2** Person on outside of pick-up truck or van injured in noncollision transport accident in nontraffic accident

✓x7ᵗʰ **V58.3** Unspecified occupant of pick-up truck or van injured in noncollision transport accident in nontraffic accident

✓x7ᵗʰ **V58.4** Person boarding or alighting a pick-up truck or van injured in noncollision transport accident

✓x7ᵗʰ **V58.5** Driver of pick-up truck or van injured in noncollision transport accident in traffic accident

✓x7ᵗʰ **V58.6** Passenger in pick-up truck or van injured in noncollision transport accident in traffic accident

✓x7ᵗʰ **V58.7** Person on outside of pick-up truck or van injured in noncollision transport accident in traffic accident

✓x7ᵗʰ **V58.9** Unspecified occupant of pick-up truck or van injured in noncollision transport accident in traffic accident

✓4ᵗʰ **V59 Occupant of pick-up truck or van injured in other and unspecified transport accidents**

> The appropriate 7th character is to be added to each code from category V59.
> A   initial encounter
> D   subsequent encounter
> S   sequela

✓5ᵗʰ **V59.0** Driver of pick-up truck or van injured in collision with other and unspecified motor vehicles in nontraffic accident

✓x7ᵗʰ **V59.00** Driver of pick-up truck or van injured in collision with unspecified motor vehicles in nontraffic accident

✓x7ᵗʰ **V59.09** Driver of pick-up truck or van injured in collision with other motor vehicles in nontraffic accident

✓5ᵗʰ **V59.1** Passenger in pick-up truck or van injured in collision with other and unspecified motor vehicles in nontraffic accident

✓x7ᵗʰ **V59.10** Passenger in pick-up truck or van injured in collision with unspecified motor vehicles in nontraffic accident

✓x7ᵗʰ **V59.19** Passenger in pick-up truck or van injured in collision with other motor vehicles in nontraffic accident

✓5ᵗʰ **V59.2** Unspecified occupant of pick-up truck or van injured in collision with other and unspecified motor vehicles in nontraffic accident

✓x7ᵗʰ **V59.20** Unspecified occupant of pick-up truck or van injured in collision with unspecified motor vehicles in nontraffic accident
> Collision NOS involving pick-up truck or van, nontraffic

✓x7ᵗʰ **V59.29** Unspecified occupant of pick-up truck or van injured in collision with other motor vehicles in nontraffic accident

✓x7ᵗʰ **V59.3** Occupant (driver) (passenger) of pick-up truck or van injured in unspecified nontraffic accident
> Accident NOS involving pick-up truck or van, nontraffic
> Occupant of pick-up truck or van injured in nontraffic accident NOS

✓5ᵗʰ **V59.4** Driver of pick-up truck or van injured in collision with other and unspecified motor vehicles in traffic accident

✓x7ᵗʰ **V59.40** Driver of pick-up truck or van injured in collision with unspecified motor vehicles in traffic accident

✓x7ᵗʰ **V59.49** Driver of pick-up truck or van injured in collision with other motor vehicles in traffic accident

✓5ᵗʰ **V59.5** Passenger in pick-up truck or van injured in collision with other and unspecified motor vehicles in traffic accident

✓x7ᵗʰ **V59.50** Passenger in pick-up truck or van injured in collision with unspecified motor vehicles in traffic accident

✓x7ᵗʰ **V59.59** Passenger in pick-up truck or van injured in collision with other motor vehicles in traffic accident

✓5ᵗʰ **V59.6** Unspecified occupant of pick-up truck or van injured in collision with other and unspecified motor vehicles in traffic accident

✓x7ᵗʰ **V59.60** Unspecified occupant of pick-up truck or van injured in collision with unspecified motor vehicles in traffic accident
> Collision NOS involving pick-up truck or van (traffic)

✓x7ᵗʰ **V59.69** Unspecified occupant of pick-up truck or van injured in collision with other motor vehicles in traffic accident

✓5ᵗʰ **V59.8** Occupant (driver) (passenger) of pick-up truck or van injured in other specified transport accidents

✓x7ᵗʰ **V59.81** Occupant (driver) (passenger) of pick-up truck or van injured in transport accident with military vehicle

✓x7ᵗʰ **V59.88** Occupant (driver) (passenger) of pick-up truck or van injured in other specified transport accidents

✓x7ᵗʰ **V59.9** Occupant (driver) (passenger) of pick-up truck or van injured in unspecified traffic accident
> Accident NOS involving pick-up truck or van

EXCLUDES 1 Not coded here   EXCLUDES 2 Not included here   N Newborn Age: 0   P Pediatric Age: 0-17   M Maternity Age: 12-55   A Adult Age: 15-124

1054   ICD-10-CM 2016

Occupant of heavy transport vehicle injured in transport accident (V60-V69)

> **INCLUDES**   18 wheeler
> armored car
> panel truck
>
> **EXCLUDES 1**   bus
> motorcoach

✓4ᵗʰ V60   **Occupant of heavy transport vehicle injured in collision with pedestrian or animal**

> **EXCLUDES 1**   *heavy transport vehicle collision with animal-drawn vehicle or animal being ridden (V66.-)*

> The appropriate 7th character is to be added to each code from category V60.
> A   initial encounter
> D   subsequent encounter
> S   sequela

✓x7ᵗʰ V60.0   Driver of heavy transport vehicle injured in collision with pedestrian or animal in nontraffic accident

✓x7ᵗʰ V60.1   Passenger in heavy transport vehicle injured in collision with pedestrian or animal in nontraffic accident

✓x7ᵗʰ V60.2   Person on outside of heavy transport vehicle injured in collision with pedestrian or animal in nontraffic accident

✓x7ᵗʰ V60.3   Unspecified occupant of heavy transport vehicle injured in collision with pedestrian or animal in nontraffic accident

✓x7ᵗʰ V60.4   Person boarding or alighting a heavy transport vehicle injured in collision with pedestrian or animal

✓x7ᵗʰ V60.5   Driver of heavy transport vehicle injured in collision with pedestrian or animal in traffic accident

✓x7ᵗʰ V60.6   Passenger in heavy transport vehicle injured in collision with pedestrian or animal in traffic accident

✓x7ᵗʰ V60.7   Person on outside of heavy transport vehicle injured in collision with pedestrian or animal in traffic accident

✓x7ᵗʰ V60.9   Unspecified occupant of heavy transport vehicle injured in collision with pedestrian or animal in traffic accident

✓4ᵗʰ V61   **Occupant of heavy transport vehicle injured in collision with pedal cycle**

> The appropriate 7th character is to be added to each code from category V61.
> A   initial encounter
> D   subsequent encounter
> S   sequela

✓x7ᵗʰ V61.0   Driver of heavy transport vehicle injured in collision with pedal cycle in nontraffic accident

✓x7ᵗʰ V61.1   Passenger in heavy transport vehicle injured in collision with pedal cycle in nontraffic accident

✓x7ᵗʰ V61.2   Person on outside of heavy transport vehicle injured in collision with pedal cycle in nontraffic accident

✓x7ᵗʰ V61.3   Unspecified occupant of heavy transport vehicle injured in collision with pedal cycle in nontraffic accident

✓x7ᵗʰ V61.4   Person boarding or alighting a heavy transport vehicle injured in collision with pedal cycle while boarding or alighting

✓x7ᵗʰ V61.5   Driver of heavy transport vehicle injured in collision with pedal cycle in traffic accident

✓x7ᵗʰ V61.6   Passenger in heavy transport vehicle injured in collision with pedal cycle in traffic accident

✓x7ᵗʰ V61.7   Person on outside of heavy transport vehicle injured in collision with pedal cycle in traffic accident

✓x7ᵗʰ V61.9   Unspecified occupant of heavy transport vehicle injured in collision with pedal cycle in traffic accident

✓4ᵗʰ V62   **Occupant of heavy transport vehicle injured in collision with two- or three-wheeled motor vehicle**

> The appropriate 7th character is to be added to each code from category V62.
> A   initial encounter
> D   subsequent encounter
> S   sequela

✓x7ᵗʰ V62.0   Driver of heavy transport vehicle injured in collision with two- or three-wheeled motor vehicle in nontraffic accident

✓x7ᵗʰ V62.1   Passenger in heavy transport vehicle injured in collision with two- or three-wheeled motor vehicle in nontraffic accident

✓x7ᵗʰ V62.2   Person on outside of heavy transport vehicle injured in collision with two- or three-wheeled motor vehicle in nontraffic accident

✓x7ᵗʰ V62.3   Unspecified occupant of heavy transport vehicle injured in collision with two- or three-wheeled motor vehicle in nontraffic accident

✓x7ᵗʰ V62.4   Person boarding or alighting a heavy transport vehicle injured in collision with two- or three-wheeled motor vehicle

✓x7ᵗʰ V62.5   Driver of heavy transport vehicle injured in collision with two- or three-wheeled motor vehicle in traffic accident

✓x7ᵗʰ V62.6   Passenger in heavy transport vehicle injured in collision with two- or three-wheeled motor vehicle in traffic accident

✓x7ᵗʰ V62.7   Person on outside of heavy transport vehicle injured in collision with two- or three-wheeled motor vehicle in traffic accident

✓x7ᵗʰ V62.9   Unspecified occupant of heavy transport vehicle injured in collision with two- or three-wheeled motor vehicle in traffic accident

✓4ᵗʰ V63   **Occupant of heavy transport vehicle injured in collision with car, pick-up truck or van**

> The appropriate 7th character is to be added to each code from category V63.
> A   initial encounter
> D   subsequent encounter
> S   sequela

✓x7ᵗʰ V63.0   Driver of heavy transport vehicle injured in collision with car, pick-up truck or van in nontraffic accident

✓x7ᵗʰ V63.1   Passenger in heavy transport vehicle injured in collision with car, pick-up truck or van in nontraffic accident

✓x7ᵗʰ V63.2   Person on outside of heavy transport vehicle injured in collision with car, pick-up truck or van in nontraffic accident

✓x7ᵗʰ V63.3   Unspecified occupant of heavy transport vehicle injured in collision with car, pick-up truck or van in nontraffic accident

✓x7ᵗʰ V63.4   Person boarding or alighting a heavy transport vehicle injured in collision with car, pick-up truck or van

✓x7ᵗʰ V63.5   Driver of heavy transport vehicle injured in collision with car, pick-up truck or van in traffic accident

✓x7ᵗʰ V63.6   Passenger in heavy transport vehicle injured in collision with car, pick-up truck or van in traffic accident

✓x7ᵗʰ V63.7   Person on outside of heavy transport vehicle injured in collision with car, pick-up truck or van in traffic accident

✓x7ᵗʰ V63.9   Unspecified occupant of heavy transport vehicle injured in collision with car, pick-up truck or van in traffic accident

✓4ᵗʰ V64   **Occupant of heavy transport vehicle injured in collision with heavy transport vehicle or bus**

> **EXCLUDES 1**   *occupant of heavy transport vehicle injured in collision with military vehicle (V69.81)*

> The appropriate 7th character is to be added to each code from category V64.
> A   initial encounter
> D   subsequent encounter
> S   sequela

✓x7ᵗʰ V64.0   Driver of heavy transport vehicle injured in collision with heavy transport vehicle or bus in nontraffic accident

✓x7ᵗʰ V64.1   Passenger in heavy transport vehicle injured in collision with heavy transport vehicle or bus in nontraffic accident

✓x7ᵗʰ V64.2   Person on outside of heavy transport vehicle injured in collision with heavy transport vehicle or bus in nontraffic accident

✓x7ᵗʰ V64.3   Unspecified occupant of heavy transport vehicle injured in collision with heavy transport vehicle or bus in nontraffic accident

✓x7ᵗʰ V64.4   Person boarding or alighting a heavy transport vehicle injured in collision with heavy transport vehicle or bus while boarding or alighting

✓x7ᵗʰ V64.5   Driver of heavy transport vehicle injured in collision with heavy transport vehicle or bus in traffic accident

✓x7ᵗʰ V64.6   Passenger in heavy transport vehicle injured in collision with heavy transport vehicle or bus in traffic accident

✓x7ᵗʰ V64.7   Person on outside of heavy transport vehicle injured in collision with heavy transport vehicle or bus in traffic accident

✓x7ᵗʰ V64.9   Unspecified occupant of heavy transport vehicle injured in collision with heavy transport vehicle or bus in traffic accident

---

✔ Additional Character Required   ✓x7ᵗʰ Placeholder Alert   Unspecified Dx   Other Specified Dx   Manifestation   ▶◀ Revised Text   ● New Code   ▲ Revised Code Title

✓4ᵗʰ V65 Occupant of heavy transport vehicle injured in collision with railway train or railway vehicle

The appropriate 7th character is to be added to each code from category V65.
A   initial encounter
D   subsequent encounter
S   sequela

✓x7ᵗʰ **V65.0** Driver of heavy transport vehicle injured in collision with railway train or railway vehicle in nontraffic accident

✓x7ᵗʰ **V65.1** Passenger in heavy transport vehicle injured in collision with railway train or railway vehicle in nontraffic accident

✓x7ᵗʰ **V65.2** Person on outside of heavy transport vehicle injured in collision with railway train or railway vehicle in nontraffic accident

✓x7ᵗʰ **V65.3** Unspecified occupant of heavy transport vehicle injured in collision with railway train or railway vehicle in nontraffic accident

✓x7ᵗʰ **V65.4** Person boarding or alighting a heavy transport vehicle injured in collision with railway train or railway vehicle

✓x7ᵗʰ **V65.5** Driver of heavy transport vehicle injured in collision with railway train or railway vehicle in traffic accident

✓x7ᵗʰ **V65.6** Passenger in heavy transport vehicle injured in collision with railway train or railway vehicle in traffic accident

✓x7ᵗʰ **V65.7** Person on outside of heavy transport vehicle injured in collision with railway train or railway vehicle in traffic accident

✓x7ᵗʰ **V65.9** Unspecified occupant of heavy transport vehicle injured in collision with railway train or railway vehicle in traffic accident

✓4ᵗʰ V66 Occupant of heavy transport vehicle injured in collision with other nonmotor vehicle

INCLUDES   collision with animal-drawn vehicle, animal being ridden, streetcar

The appropriate 7th character is to be added to each code from category V66.
A   initial encounter
D   subsequent encounter
S   sequela

✓x7ᵗʰ **V66.0** Driver of heavy transport vehicle injured in collision with other nonmotor vehicle in nontraffic accident

✓x7ᵗʰ **V66.1** Passenger in heavy transport vehicle injured in collision with other nonmotor vehicle in nontraffic accident

✓x7ᵗʰ **V66.2** Person on outside of heavy transport vehicle injured in collision with other nonmotor vehicle in nontraffic accident

✓x7ᵗʰ **V66.3** Unspecified occupant of heavy transport vehicle injured in collision with other nonmotor vehicle in nontraffic accident

✓x7ᵗʰ **V66.4** Person boarding or alighting a heavy transport vehicle injured in collision with other nonmotor vehicle

✓x7ᵗʰ **V66.5** Driver of heavy transport vehicle injured in collision with other nonmotor vehicle in traffic accident

✓x7ᵗʰ **V66.6** Passenger in heavy transport vehicle injured in collision with other nonmotor vehicle in traffic accident

✓x7ᵗʰ **V66.7** Person on outside of heavy transport vehicle injured in collision with other nonmotor vehicle in traffic accident

✓x7ᵗʰ **V66.9** Unspecified occupant of heavy transport vehicle injured in collision with other nonmotor vehicle in traffic accident

✓4ᵗʰ V67 Occupant of heavy transport vehicle injured in collision with fixed or stationary object

The appropriate 7th character is to be added to each code from category V67.
A   initial encounter
D   subsequent encounter
S   sequela

✓x7ᵗʰ **V67.0** Driver of heavy transport vehicle injured in collision with fixed or stationary object in nontraffic accident

✓x7ᵗʰ **V67.1** Passenger in heavy transport vehicle injured in collision with fixed or stationary object in nontraffic accident

✓x7ᵗʰ **V67.2** Person on outside of heavy transport vehicle injured in collision with fixed or stationary object in nontraffic accident

✓x7ᵗʰ **V67.3** Unspecified occupant of heavy transport vehicle injured in collision with fixed or stationary object in nontraffic accident

✓x7ᵗʰ **V67.4** Person boarding or alighting a heavy transport vehicle injured in collision with fixed or stationary object

✓x7ᵗʰ **V67.5** Driver of heavy transport vehicle injured in collision with fixed or stationary object in traffic accident

✓x7ᵗʰ **V67.6** Passenger in heavy transport vehicle injured in collision with fixed or stationary object in traffic accident

✓x7ᵗʰ **V67.7** Person on outside of heavy transport vehicle injured in collision with fixed or stationary object in traffic accident

✓x7ᵗʰ **V67.9** Unspecified occupant of heavy transport vehicle injured in collision with fixed or stationary object in traffic accident

✓4ᵗʰ V68 Occupant of heavy transport vehicle injured in noncollision transport accident

INCLUDES   overturning heavy transport vehicle NOS
overturning heavy transport vehicle without collision

The appropriate 7th character is to be added to each code from category V68.
A   initial encounter
D   subsequent encounter
S   sequela

✓x7ᵗʰ **V68.0** Driver of heavy transport vehicle injured in noncollision transport accident in nontraffic accident

✓x7ᵗʰ **V68.1** Passenger in heavy transport vehicle injured in noncollision transport accident in nontraffic accident

✓x7ᵗʰ **V68.2** Person on outside of heavy transport vehicle injured in noncollision transport accident in nontraffic accident

✓x7ᵗʰ **V68.3** Unspecified occupant of heavy transport vehicle injured in noncollision transport accident in nontraffic accident

✓x7ᵗʰ **V68.4** Person boarding or alighting a heavy transport vehicle injured in noncollision transport accident

✓x7ᵗʰ **V68.5** Driver of heavy transport vehicle injured in noncollision transport accident in traffic accident

✓x7ᵗʰ **V68.6** Passenger in heavy transport vehicle injured in noncollision transport accident in traffic accident

✓x7ᵗʰ **V68.7** Person on outside of heavy transport vehicle injured in noncollision transport accident in traffic accident

✓x7ᵗʰ **V68.9** Unspecified occupant of heavy transport vehicle injured in noncollision transport accident in traffic accident

✓4ᵗʰ V69 Occupant of heavy transport vehicle injured in other and unspecified transport accidents

The appropriate 7th character is to be added to each code from category V69.
A   initial encounter
D   subsequent encounter
S   sequela

✓5ᵗʰ **V69.0** Driver of heavy transport vehicle injured in collision with other and unspecified motor vehicles in nontraffic accident

   ✓x7ᵗʰ **V69.00** Driver of heavy transport vehicle injured in collision with unspecified motor vehicles in nontraffic accident

   ✓x7ᵗʰ **V69.09** Driver of heavy transport vehicle injured in collision with other motor vehicles in nontraffic accident

✓5ᵗʰ **V69.1** Passenger in heavy transport vehicle injured in collision with other and unspecified motor vehicles in nontraffic accident

   ✓x7ᵗʰ **V69.10** Passenger in heavy transport vehicle injured in collision with unspecified motor vehicles in nontraffic accident

   ✓x7ᵗʰ **V69.19** Passenger in heavy transport vehicle injured in collision with other motor vehicles in nontraffic accident

✓5ᵗʰ **V69.2** Unspecified occupant of heavy transport vehicle injured in collision with other and unspecified motor vehicles in nontraffic accident

   ✓x7ᵗʰ **V69.20** Unspecified occupant of heavy transport vehicle injured in collision with unspecified motor vehicles in nontraffic accident
     Collision NOS involving heavy transport vehicle, nontraffic

   ✓x7ᵗʰ **V69.29** Unspecified occupant of heavy transport vehicle injured in collision with other motor vehicles in nontraffic accident

✓x7ᵗʰ **V69.3** Occupant (driver) (passenger) of heavy transport vehicle injured in unspecified nontraffic accident
   Accident NOS involving heavy transport vehicle, nontraffic
   Occupant of heavy transport vehicle injured in nontraffic accident NOS

EXCLUDES 1 Not coded here   EXCLUDES 2 Not included here   N Newborn Age: 0   P Pediatric Age: 0-17   M Maternity Age: 12-55   A Adult Age: 15-124

1056   ICD-10-CM 2016

√5ᵗʰ **V69.4** Driver of heavy transport vehicle injured in collision with other and unspecified motor vehicles in traffic accident

   √x7ᵗʰ **V69.40** Driver of heavy transport vehicle injured in collision with unspecified motor vehicles in traffic accident

   √x7ᵗʰ **V69.49** Driver of heavy transport vehicle injured in collision with other motor vehicles in traffic accident

√5ᵗʰ **V69.5** Passenger in heavy transport vehicle injured in collision with other and unspecified motor vehicles in traffic accident

   √x7ᵗʰ **V69.50** Passenger in heavy transport vehicle injured in collision with unspecified motor vehicles in traffic accident

   √x7ᵗʰ **V69.59** Passenger in heavy transport vehicle injured in collision with other motor vehicles in traffic accident

√5ᵗʰ **V69.6** Unspecified occupant of heavy transport vehicle injured in collision with other and unspecified motor vehicles in traffic accident

   √x7ᵗʰ **V69.60** Unspecified occupant of heavy transport vehicle injured in collision with unspecified motor vehicles in traffic accident

      Collision NOS involving heavy transport vehicle (traffic)

   √x7ᵗʰ **V69.69** Unspecified occupant of heavy transport vehicle injured in collision with other motor vehicles in traffic accident

√5ᵗʰ **V69.8** Occupant (driver) (passenger) of heavy transport vehicle injured in other specified transport accidents

   √x7ᵗʰ **V69.81** Occupant (driver) (passenger) of heavy transport vehicle injured in transport accidents with military vehicle

   √x7ᵗʰ **V69.88** Occupant (driver) (passenger) of heavy transport vehicle injured in other specified transport accidents

√x7ᵗʰ **V69.9** Occupant (driver) (passenger) of heavy transport vehicle injured in unspecified traffic accident

     Accident NOS involving heavy transport vehicle

Bus occupant injured in transport accident (V70-V79)

INCLUDES   motorcoach
EXCLUDES1   minibus (V50-V59)

√4ᵗʰ **V70** Bus occupant injured in collision with pedestrian or animal

  EXCLUDES1   bus collision with animal-drawn vehicle or animal being ridden (V76.-)

The appropriate 7th character is to be added to each code from category V70.
A   initial encounter
D   subsequent encounter
S   sequela

√x7ᵗʰ **V70.0** Driver of bus injured in collision with pedestrian or animal in nontraffic accident

√x7ᵗʰ **V70.1** Passenger on bus injured in collision with pedestrian or animal in nontraffic accident

√x7ᵗʰ **V70.2** Person on outside of bus injured in collision with pedestrian or animal in nontraffic accident

√x7ᵗʰ **V70.3** Unspecified occupant of bus injured in collision with pedestrian or animal in nontraffic accident

√x7ᵗʰ **V70.4** Person boarding or alighting from bus injured in collision with pedestrian or animal

√x7ᵗʰ **V70.5** Driver of bus injured in collision with pedestrian or animal in traffic accident

√x7ᵗʰ **V70.6** Passenger on bus injured in collision with pedestrian or animal in traffic accident

√x7ᵗʰ **V70.7** Person on outside of bus injured in collision with pedestrian or animal in traffic accident

√x7ᵗʰ **V70.9** Unspecified occupant of bus injured in collision with pedestrian or animal in traffic accident

√4ᵗʰ **V71** Bus occupant injured in collision with pedal cycle

The appropriate 7th character is to be added to each code from category V71.
A   initial encounter
D   subsequent encounter
S   sequela

√x7ᵗʰ **V71.0** Driver of bus injured in collision with pedal cycle in nontraffic accident

√x7ᵗʰ **V71.1** Passenger on bus injured in collision with pedal cycle in nontraffic accident

√x7ᵗʰ **V71.2** Person on outside of bus injured in collision with pedal cycle in nontraffic accident

√x7ᵗʰ **V71.3** Unspecified occupant of bus injured in collision with pedal cycle in nontraffic accident

√x7ᵗʰ **V71.4** Person boarding or alighting from bus injured in collision with pedal cycle

√x7ᵗʰ **V71.5** Driver of bus injured in collision with pedal cycle in traffic accident

√x7ᵗʰ **V71.6** Passenger on bus injured in collision with pedal cycle in traffic accident

√x7ᵗʰ **V71.7** Person on outside of bus injured in collision with pedal cycle in traffic accident

√x7ᵗʰ **V71.9** Unspecified occupant of bus injured in collision with pedal cycle in traffic accident

√4ᵗʰ **V72** Bus occupant injured in collision with two- or three-wheeled motor vehicle

The appropriate 7th character is to be added to each code from category V72.
A   initial encounter
D   subsequent encounter
S   sequela

√x7ᵗʰ **V72.0** Driver of bus injured in collision with two- or three-wheeled motor vehicle in nontraffic accident

√x7ᵗʰ **V72.1** Passenger on bus injured in collision with two- or three-wheeled motor vehicle in nontraffic accident

√x7ᵗʰ **V72.2** Person on outside of bus injured in collision with two- or three-wheeled motor vehicle in nontraffic accident

√x7ᵗʰ **V72.3** Unspecified occupant of bus injured in collision with two- or three-wheeled motor vehicle in nontraffic accident

√x7ᵗʰ **V72.4** Person boarding or alighting from bus injured in collision with two- or three-wheeled motor vehicle

√x7ᵗʰ **V72.5** Driver of bus injured in collision with two- or three-wheeled motor vehicle in traffic accident

√x7ᵗʰ **V72.6** Passenger on bus injured in collision with two- or three-wheeled motor vehicle in traffic accident

√x7ᵗʰ **V72.7** Person on outside of bus injured in collision with two- or three-wheeled motor vehicle in traffic accident

√x7ᵗʰ **V72.9** Unspecified occupant of bus injured in collision with two- or three-wheeled motor vehicle in traffic accident

√4ᵗʰ **V73** Bus occupant injured in collision with car, pick-up truck or van

The appropriate 7th character is to be added to each code from category V73.
A   initial encounter
D   subsequent encounter
S   sequela

√x7ᵗʰ **V73.0** Driver of bus injured in collision with car, pick-up truck or van in nontraffic accident

√x7ᵗʰ **V73.1** Passenger on bus injured in collision with car, pick-up truck or van in nontraffic accident

√x7ᵗʰ **V73.2** Person on outside of bus injured in collision with car, pick-up truck or van in nontraffic accident

√x7ᵗʰ **V73.3** Unspecified occupant of bus injured in collision with car, pick-up truck or van in nontraffic accident

√x7ᵗʰ **V73.4** Person boarding or alighting from bus injured in collision with car, pick-up truck or van

√x7ᵗʰ **V73.5** Driver of bus injured in collision with car, pick-up truck or van in traffic accident

√x7ᵗʰ **V73.6** Passenger on bus injured in collision with car, pick-up truck or van in traffic accident

√x7ᵗʰ **V73.7** Person on outside of bus injured in collision with car, pick-up truck or van in traffic accident

√x7ᵗʰ **V73.9** Unspecified occupant of bus injured in collision with car, pick-up truck or van in traffic accident

√4ᵗʰ **V74** Bus occupant injured in collision with heavy transport vehicle or bus

  EXCLUDES1   bus occupant injured in collision with military vehicle (V79.81)

The appropriate 7th character is to be added to each code from category V74.
A   initial encounter
D   subsequent encounter
S   sequela

√x7ᵗʰ **V74.0** Driver of bus injured in collision with heavy transport vehicle or bus in nontraffic accident

---

✓ Additional Character Required   √x7ᵗʰ Placeholder Alert   Unspecified Dx   Other Specified Dx   Manifestation   ▶◀ Revised Text   ● New Code   ▲ Revised Code Title

Chapter 2Ø. External Causes of Morbidity

V74.1–V79.19

√x7ᵗʰ **V74.1** Passenger on bus injured in collision with heavy transport vehicle or bus in nontraffic accident

√x7ᵗʰ **V74.2** Person on outside of bus injured in collision with heavy transport vehicle or bus in nontraffic accident

√x7ᵗʰ **V74.3** Unspecified occupant of bus injured in collision with heavy transport vehicle or bus in nontraffic accident

√x7ᵗʰ **V74.4** Person boarding or alighting from bus injured in collision with heavy transport vehicle or bus

√x7ᵗʰ **V74.5** Driver of bus injured in collision with heavy transport vehicle or bus in traffic accident

√x7ᵗʰ **V74.6** Passenger on bus injured in collision with heavy transport vehicle or bus in traffic accident

√x7ᵗʰ **V74.7** Person on outside of bus injured in collision with heavy transport vehicle or bus in traffic accident

√x7ᵗʰ **V74.9** Unspecified occupant of bus injured in collision with heavy transport vehicle or bus in traffic accident

✓4ᵗʰ **V75** Bus occupant injured in collision with railway train or railway vehicle

The appropriate 7th character is to be added to each code from category V75.
A   initial encounter
D   subsequent encounter
S   sequela

√x7ᵗʰ **V75.Ø** Driver of bus injured in collision with railway train or railway vehicle in nontraffic accident

√x7ᵗʰ **V75.1** Passenger on bus injured in collision with railway train or railway vehicle in nontraffic accident

√x7ᵗʰ **V75.2** Person on outside of bus injured in collision with railway train or railway vehicle in nontraffic accident

√x7ᵗʰ **V75.3** Unspecified occupant of bus injured in collision with railway train or railway vehicle in nontraffic accident

√x7ᵗʰ **V75.4** Person boarding or alighting from bus injured in collision with railway train or railway vehicle

√x7ᵗʰ **V75.5** Driver of bus injured in collision with railway train or railway vehicle in traffic accident

√x7ᵗʰ **V75.6** Passenger on bus injured in collision with railway train or railway vehicle in traffic accident

√x7ᵗʰ **V75.7** Person on outside of bus injured in collision with railway train or railway vehicle in traffic accident

√x7ᵗʰ **V75.9** Unspecified occupant of bus injured in collision with railway train or railway vehicle in traffic accident

✓4ᵗʰ **V76** Bus occupant injured in collision with other nonmotor vehicle

INCLUDES   collision with animal-drawn vehicle, animal being ridden, streetcar

The appropriate 7th character is to be added to each code from category V76.
A   initial encounter
D   subsequent encounter
S   sequela

√x7ᵗʰ **V76.Ø** Driver of bus injured in collision with other nonmotor vehicle in nontraffic accident

√x7ᵗʰ **V76.1** Passenger on bus injured in collision with other nonmotor vehicle in nontraffic accident

√x7ᵗʰ **V76.2** Person on outside of bus injured in collision with other nonmotor vehicle in nontraffic accident

√x7ᵗʰ **V76.3** Unspecified occupant of bus injured in collision with other nonmotor vehicle in nontraffic accident

√x7ᵗʰ **V76.4** Person boarding or alighting from bus injured in collision with other nonmotor vehicle

√x7ᵗʰ **V76.5** Driver of bus injured in collision with other nonmotor vehicle in traffic accident

√x7ᵗʰ **V76.6** Passenger on bus injured in collision with other nonmotor vehicle in traffic accident

√x7ᵗʰ **V76.7** Person on outside of bus injured in collision with other nonmotor vehicle in traffic accident

√x7ᵗʰ **V76.9** Unspecified occupant of bus injured in collision with other nonmotor vehicle in traffic accident

✓4ᵗʰ **V77** Bus occupant injured in collision with fixed or stationary object

The appropriate 7th character is to be added to each code from category V77.
A   initial encounter
D   subsequent encounter
S   sequela

√x7ᵗʰ **V77.Ø** Driver of bus injured in collision with fixed or stationary object in nontraffic accident

√x7ᵗʰ **V77.1** Passenger on bus injured in collision with fixed or stationary object in nontraffic accident

√x7ᵗʰ **V77.2** Person on outside of bus injured in collision with fixed or stationary object in nontraffic accident

√x7ᵗʰ **V77.3** Unspecified occupant of bus injured in collision with fixed or stationary object in nontraffic accident

√x7ᵗʰ **V77.4** Person boarding or alighting from bus injured in collision with fixed or stationary object

√x7ᵗʰ **V77.5** Driver of bus injured in collision with fixed or stationary object in traffic accident

√x7ᵗʰ **V77.6** Passenger on bus injured in collision with fixed or stationary object in traffic accident

√x7ᵗʰ **V77.7** Person on outside of bus injured in collision with fixed or stationary object in traffic accident

√x7ᵗʰ **V77.9** Unspecified occupant of bus injured in collision with fixed or stationary object in traffic accident

✓4ᵗʰ **V78** Bus occupant injured in noncollision transport accident

INCLUDES   overturning bus NOS
       overturning bus without collision

The appropriate 7th character is to be added to each code from category V78.
A   initial encounter
D   subsequent encounter
S   sequela

√x7ᵗʰ **V78.Ø** Driver of bus injured in noncollision transport accident in nontraffic accident

√x7ᵗʰ **V78.1** Passenger on bus injured in noncollision transport accident in nontraffic accident

√x7ᵗʰ **V78.2** Person on outside of bus injured in noncollision transport accident in nontraffic accident

√x7ᵗʰ **V78.3** Unspecified occupant of bus injured in noncollision transport accident in nontraffic accident

√x7ᵗʰ **V78.4** Person boarding or alighting from bus injured in noncollision transport accident

√x7ᵗʰ **V78.5** Driver of bus injured in noncollision transport accident in traffic accident

√x7ᵗʰ **V78.6** Passenger on bus injured in noncollision transport accident in traffic accident

√x7ᵗʰ **V78.7** Person on outside of bus injured in noncollision transport accident in traffic accident

√x7ᵗʰ **V78.9** Unspecified occupant of bus injured in noncollision transport accident in traffic accident

✓4ᵗʰ **V79** Bus occupant injured in other and unspecified transport accidents

The appropriate 7th character is to be added to each code from category V79.
A   initial encounter
D   subsequent encounter
S   sequela

✓5ᵗʰ **V79.Ø** Driver of bus injured in collision with other and unspecified motor vehicles in nontraffic accident

√x7ᵗʰ   **V79.ØØ** Driver of bus injured in collision with unspecified motor vehicles in nontraffic accident

√x7ᵗʰ   **V79.Ø9** Driver of bus injured in collision with other motor vehicles in nontraffic accident

✓5ᵗʰ **V79.1** Passenger on bus injured in collision with other and unspecified motor vehicles in nontraffic accident

√x7ᵗʰ   **V79.1Ø** Passenger on bus injured in collision with unspecified motor vehicles in nontraffic accident

√x7ᵗʰ   **V79.19** Passenger on bus injured in collision with other motor vehicles in nontraffic accident

EXCLUDES 1 Not coded here   EXCLUDES 2 Not included here   Ⓝ Newborn Age: 0   Ⓟ Pediatric Age: 0-17   Ⓜ Maternity Age: 12-55   Ⓐ Adult Age: 15-12

1058   ICD-10-CM 201

✓5ᵗʰ **V79.2** Unspecified bus occupant injured in collision with other and unspecified motor vehicles in nontraffic accident

  ✓x7ᵗʰ **V79.20** Unspecified bus occupant injured in collision with unspecified motor vehicles in nontraffic accident
       Bus collision NOS, nontraffic

  ✓x7ᵗʰ **V79.29** Unspecified bus occupant injured in collision with other motor vehicles in nontraffic accident

✓x7ᵗʰ **V79.3** Bus occupant (driver) (passenger) injured in unspecified nontraffic accident
       Bus accident NOS, nontraffic
       Bus occupant injured in nontraffic accident NOS

✓5ᵗʰ **V79.4** Driver of bus injured in collision with other and unspecified motor vehicles in traffic accident

  ✓x7ᵗʰ **V79.40** Driver of bus injured in collision with unspecified motor vehicles in traffic accident

  ✓x7ᵗʰ **V79.49** Driver of bus injured in collision with other motor vehicles in traffic accident

✓5ᵗʰ **V79.5** Passenger on bus injured in collision with other and unspecified motor vehicles in traffic accident

  ✓x7ᵗʰ **V79.50** Passenger on bus injured in collision with unspecified motor vehicles in traffic accident

  ✓x7ᵗʰ **V79.59** Passenger on bus injured in collision with other motor vehicles in traffic accident

✓5ᵗʰ **V79.6** Unspecified bus occupant injured in collision with other and unspecified motor vehicles in traffic accident

  ✓x7ᵗʰ **V79.60** Unspecified bus occupant injured in collision with unspecified motor vehicles in traffic accident
       Bus collision NOS (traffic)

  ✓x7ᵗʰ **V79.69** Unspecified bus occupant injured in collision with other motor vehicles in traffic accident

✓5ᵗʰ **V79.8** Bus occupant (driver) (passenger) injured in other specified transport accidents

  ✓x7ᵗʰ **V79.81** Bus occupant (driver) (passenger) injured in transport accidents with military vehicle

  ✓x7ᵗʰ **V79.88** Bus occupant (driver) (passenger) injured in other specified transport accidents

✓x7ᵗʰ **V79.9** Bus occupant (driver) (passenger) injured in unspecified traffic accident
       Bus accident NOS

Other land transport accidents (V80-V89)

4ᵗʰ **V80** Animal-rider or occupant of animal-drawn vehicle injured in transport accident

> The appropriate 7th character is to be added to each code from category V80.
> A   initial encounter
> D   subsequent encounter
> S   sequela

✓5ᵗʰ **V80.0** Animal-rider or occupant of animal drawn vehicle injured by fall from or being thrown from animal or animal-drawn vehicle in noncollision accident

  ✓6ᵗʰ **V80.01** Animal-rider injured by fall from or being thrown from animal in noncollision accident

    ✓7ᵗʰ **V80.010** Animal-rider injured by fall from or being thrown from horse in noncollision accident

    ✓7ᵗʰ **V80.018** Animal-rider injured by fall from or being thrown from other animal in noncollision accident

  ✓x7ᵗʰ **V80.02** Occupant of animal-drawn vehicle injured by fall from or being thrown from animal-drawn vehicle in noncollision accident
       Overturning animal-drawn vehicle NOS
       Overturning animal-drawn vehicle without collision

✓5ᵗʰ **V80.1** Animal-rider or occupant of animal-drawn vehicle injured in collision with pedestrian or animal

  EXCLUDES 1 *animal-rider or animal-drawn vehicle collision with animal-drawn vehicle or animal being ridden (V80.7)*

  ✓x7ᵗʰ **V80.11** Animal-rider injured in collision with pedestrian or animal

  ✓x7ᵗʰ **V80.12** Occupant of animal-drawn vehicle injured in collision with pedestrian or animal

✓5ᵗʰ **V80.2** Animal-rider or occupant of animal-drawn vehicle injured in collision with pedal cycle

  ✓x7ᵗʰ **V80.21** Animal-rider injured in collision with pedal cycle

  ✓x7ᵗʰ **V80.22** Occupant of animal-drawn vehicle injured in collision with pedal cycle

✓5ᵗʰ **V80.3** Animal-rider or occupant of animal-drawn vehicle injured in collision with two- or three-wheeled motor vehicle

  ✓x7ᵗʰ **V80.31** Animal-rider injured in collision with two- or three-wheeled motor vehicle

  ✓x7ᵗʰ **V80.32** Occupant of animal-drawn vehicle injured in collision with two- or three-wheeled motor vehicle

✓5ᵗʰ **V80.4** Animal-rider or occupant of animal-drawn vehicle injured in collision with car, pick-up truck, van, heavy transport vehicle or bus

  EXCLUDES 1 *animal-rider injured in collision with military vehicle (V80.910)*
        occupant of animal-drawn vehicle injured in collision with military vehicle (V80.920)

  ✓x7ᵗʰ **V80.41** Animal-rider injured in collision with car, pick-up truck, van, heavy transport vehicle or bus

  ✓x7ᵗʰ **V80.42** Occupant of animal-drawn vehicle injured in collision with car, pick-up truck, van, heavy transport vehicle or bus

✓5ᵗʰ **V80.5** Animal-rider or occupant of animal-drawn vehicle injured in collision with other specified motor vehicle

  ✓x7ᵗʰ **V80.51** Animal-rider injured in collision with other specified motor vehicle

  ✓x7ᵗʰ **V80.52** Occupant of animal-drawn vehicle injured in collision with other specified motor vehicle

✓5ᵗʰ **V80.6** Animal-rider or occupant of animal-drawn vehicle injured in collision with railway train or railway vehicle

  ✓x7ᵗʰ **V80.61** Animal-rider injured in collision with railway train or railway vehicle

  ✓x7ᵗʰ **V80.62** Occupant of animal-drawn vehicle injured in collision with railway train or railway vehicle

✓5ᵗʰ **V80.7** Animal-rider or occupant of animal-drawn vehicle injured in collision with other nonmotor vehicles

  ✓6ᵗʰ **V80.71** Animal-rider or occupant of animal-drawn vehicle injured in collision with animal being ridden

    ✓7ᵗʰ **V80.710** Animal-rider injured in collision with other animal being ridden

    ✓7ᵗʰ **V80.711** Occupant of animal-drawn vehicle injured in collision with animal being ridden

  ✓6ᵗʰ **V80.72** Animal-rider or occupant of animal-drawn vehicle injured in collision with other animal-drawn vehicle

    ✓7ᵗʰ **V80.720** Animal-rider injured in collision with animal-drawn vehicle

    ✓7ᵗʰ **V80.721** Occupant of animal-drawn vehicle injured in collision with other animal-drawn vehicle

  ✓6ᵗʰ **V80.73** Animal-rider or occupant of animal-drawn vehicle injured in collision with streetcar

    ✓7ᵗʰ **V80.730** Animal-rider injured in collision with streetcar

    ✓7ᵗʰ **V80.731** Occupant of animal-drawn vehicle injured in collision with streetcar

  ✓6ᵗʰ **V80.79** Animal-rider or occupant of animal-drawn vehicle injured in collision with other nonmotor vehicles

    ✓7ᵗʰ **V80.790** Animal-rider injured in collision with other nonmotor vehicles

    ✓7ᵗʰ **V80.791** Occupant of animal-drawn vehicle injured in collision with other nonmotor vehicles

✓5ᵗʰ **V80.8** Animal-rider or occupant of animal-drawn vehicle injured in collision with fixed or stationary object

  ✓x7ᵗʰ **V80.81** Animal-rider injured in collision with fixed or stationary object

  ✓x7ᵗʰ **V80.82** Occupant of animal-drawn vehicle injured in collision with fixed or stationary object

✓5ᵗʰ **V80.9** Animal-rider or occupant of animal-drawn vehicle injured in other and unspecified transport accidents

  ✓6ᵗʰ **V80.91** Animal-rider injured in other and unspecified transport accidents

    ✓7ᵗʰ **V80.910** Animal-rider injured in transport accident with military vehicle

    ✓7ᵗʰ **V80.918** Animal-rider injured in other transport accident

---

✓ Additional Character Required   ✓x7ᵗʰ Placeholder Alert   Unspecified Dx   Other Specified Dx   Manifestation   ▶◀ Revised Text   ● New Code   ▲ Revised Code Title

✓7ᵗʰ **V80.919** **Animal-rider injured in unspecified transport accident**
Animal rider accident NOS

✓6ᵗʰ **V80.92** **Occupant of animal-drawn vehicle injured in other and unspecified transport accidents**

✓7ᵗʰ **V80.920** **Occupant of animal-drawn vehicle injured in transport accident with military vehicle**

✓7ᵗʰ **V80.928** **Occupant of animal-drawn vehicle injured in other transport accident**

✓7ᵗʰ **V80.929** **Occupant of animal-drawn vehicle injured in unspecified transport accident**
Animal-drawn vehicle accident NOS

✓4ᵗʰ **V81** **Occupant of railway train or railway vehicle injured in transport accident**

INCLUDES   derailment of railway train or railway vehicle
person on outside of train

EXCLUDES 1   *streetcar (V82.-)*

The appropriate 7th character is to be added to each code from category V81.
A   initial encounter
D   subsequent encounter
S   sequela

✓x7ᵗʰ **V81.0** **Occupant of railway train or railway vehicle injured in collision with motor vehicle in nontraffic accident**
EXCLUDES 1   *occupant of railway train or railway vehicle injured due to collision with military vehicle (V81.83)*

✓x7ᵗʰ **V81.1** **Occupant of railway train or railway vehicle injured in collision with motor vehicle in traffic accident**
EXCLUDES 1   *occupant of railway train or railway vehicle injured due to collision with military vehicle (V81.83)*

✓x7ᵗʰ **V81.2** **Occupant of railway train or railway vehicle injured in collision with or hit by rolling stock**

✓x7ᵗʰ **V81.3** **Occupant of railway train or railway vehicle injured in collision with other object**
Railway collision NOS

✓x7ᵗʰ **V81.4** **Person injured while boarding or alighting from railway train or railway vehicle**

✓x7ᵗʰ **V81.5** **Occupant of railway train or railway vehicle injured by fall in railway train or railway vehicle**

✓x7ᵗʰ **V81.6** **Occupant of railway train or railway vehicle injured by fall from railway train or railway vehicle**

✓x7ᵗʰ **V81.7** **Occupant of railway train or railway vehicle injured in derailment without antecedent collision**

✓5ᵗʰ **V81.8** **Occupant of railway train or railway vehicle injured in other specified railway accidents**

✓x7ᵗʰ **V81.81** **Occupant of railway train or railway vehicle injured due to explosion or fire on train**

✓x7ᵗʰ **V81.82** **Occupant of railway train or railway vehicle injured due to object falling onto train**
Occupant of railway train or railway vehicle injured due to falling earth onto train
Occupant of railway train or railway vehicle injured due to falling rocks onto train
Occupant of railway train or railway vehicle injured due to falling snow onto train
Occupant of railway train or railway vehicle injured due to falling trees onto train

✓x7ᵗʰ **V81.83** **Occupant of railway train or railway vehicle injured due to collision with military vehicle**

✓x7ᵗʰ **V81.89** **Occupant of railway train or railway vehicle injured due to other specified railway accident**

✓x7ᵗʰ **V81.9** **Occupant of railway train or railway vehicle injured in unspecified railway accident**
Railway accident NOS

✓4ᵗʰ **V82** **Occupant of powered streetcar injured in transport accident**
INCLUDES   interurban electric car
person on outside of streetcar
tram (car)
trolley (car)

EXCLUDES 1   *bus (V70-V79)*
motorcoach (V70-V79)
nonpowered streetcar (V76.-)
train (V81.-)

The appropriate 7th character is to be added to each code from category V82.
A   initial encounter
D   subsequent encounter
S   sequela

✓x7ᵗʰ **V82.0** **Occupant of streetcar injured in collision with motor vehicle in nontraffic accident**

✓x7ᵗʰ **V82.1** **Occupant of streetcar injured in collision with motor vehicle in traffic accident**

✓x7ᵗʰ **V82.2** **Occupant of streetcar injured in collision with or hit by rolling stock**

✓x7ᵗʰ **V82.3** **Occupant of streetcar injured in collision with other object**
EXCLUDES 1   *collision with animal-drawn vehicle or animal being ridden (V82.8)*

✓x7ᵗʰ **V82.4** **Person injured while boarding or alighting from streetcar**

✓x7ᵗʰ **V82.5** **Occupant of streetcar injured by fall in streetcar**
EXCLUDES 1   *fall in streetcar:*
while boarding or alighting (V82.4)
with antecedent collision (V82.0-V82.3)

✓x7ᵗʰ **V82.6** **Occupant of streetcar injured by fall from streetcar**
EXCLUDES 1   *fall from streetcar:*
while boarding or alighting (V82.4)
with antecedent collision (V82.0-V82.3)

✓x7ᵗʰ **V82.7** **Occupant of streetcar injured in derailment without antecedent collision**
EXCLUDES 1   *occupant of streetcar injured in derailment with antecedent collision (V82.0-V82.3)*

✓x7ᵗʰ **V82.8** **Occupant of streetcar injured in other specified transport accidents**
Streetcar collision with military vehicle
Streetcar collision with train or nonmotor vehicles

✓x7ᵗʰ **V82.9** **Occupant of streetcar injured in unspecified traffic accident**
Streetcar accident NOS

✓4ᵗʰ **V83** **Occupant of special vehicle mainly used on industrial premises injured in transport accident**
INCLUDES   battery-powered airport passenger vehicle
battery-powered truck (baggage) (mail)
coal-car in mine
forklift (truck)
logging car
self-propelled industrial truck
station baggage truck (powered)
tram, truck, or tub (powered) in mine or quarry

EXCLUDES 1   *special construction vehicles (V85.-)*
special industrial vehicle in stationary use or maintenance (W31.-)

The appropriate 7th character is to be added to each code from category V83.
A   initial encounter
D   subsequent encounter
S   sequela

✓x7ᵗʰ **V83.0** **Driver of special industrial vehicle injured in traffic accident**

✓x7ᵗʰ **V83.1** **Passenger of special industrial vehicle injured in traffic accident**

✓x7ᵗʰ **V83.2** **Person on outside of special industrial vehicle injured in traffic accident**

✓x7ᵗʰ **V83.3** **Unspecified occupant of special industrial vehicle injured in traffic accident**

✓x7ᵗʰ **V83.4** **Person injured while boarding or alighting from special industrial vehicle**

✓x7ᵗʰ **V83.5** **Driver of special industrial vehicle injured in nontraffic accident**

✓x7ᵗʰ **V83.6** **Passenger of special industrial vehicle injured in nontraffic accident**

✓x7ᵗʰ **V83.7** **Person on outside of special industrial vehicle injured in nontraffic accident**

EXCLUDES 1 Not coded here   EXCLUDES 2 Not included here   N Newborn Age: 0   P Pediatric Age: 0-17   M Maternity Age: 12-55   A Adult Age: 15-12-

1060   ICD-10-CM 201◼

✓x7th **V83.9** **Unspecified occupant of special industrial vehicle injured in nontraffic accident**
Special-industrial-vehicle accident NOS

✓4th **V84** **Occupant of special vehicle mainly used in agriculture injured in transport accident**
INCLUDES self-propelled farm machinery
tractor (and trailer)
EXCLUDES 1 *animal-powered farm machinery accident (W30.8-)*
contact with combine harvester (W30.0)
special agricultural vehicle in stationary use or maintenance (W30.-)

The appropriate 7th character is to be added to each code from category V84.
A　initial encounter
D　subsequent encounter
S　sequela

✓x7th **V84.0** **Driver** of special agricultural vehicle injured in traffic accident

✓x7th **V84.1** **Passenger** of special agricultural vehicle injured in traffic accident

✓x7th **V84.2** **Person on outside** of special agricultural vehicle injured in traffic accident

✓x7th **V84.3** **Unspecified occupant of special agricultural vehicle injured in traffic accident**

✓x7th **V84.4** **Person injured while** boarding or alighting **from special agricultural vehicle**

✓x7th **V84.5** **Driver** of special agricultural vehicle injured in nontraffic accident

✓x7th **V84.6** **Passenger** of special agricultural vehicle injured in nontraffic accident

✓x7th **V84.7** **Person on outside** of special agricultural vehicle injured in nontraffic accident

✓x7th **V84.9** **Unspecified occupant of special agricultural vehicle injured in nontraffic accident**
Special-agricultural vehicle accident NOS

✓4th **V85** **Occupant of special construction vehicle injured in transport accident**
INCLUDES bulldozer
digger
dump truck
earth-leveller
mechanical shovel
road-roller
EXCLUDES 1 *special industrial vehicle (V83.-)*
special construction vehicle in stationary use or maintenance (W31.-)

The appropriate 7th character is to be added to each code from category V85.
A　initial encounter
D　subsequent encounter
S　sequela

✓x7th **V85.0** **Driver** of special construction vehicle injured in traffic accident

✓x7th **V85.1** **Passenger** of special construction vehicle injured in traffic accident

✓x7th **V85.2** **Person on outside** of special construction vehicle injured in traffic accident

✓x7th **V85.3** **Unspecified occupant of special construction vehicle injured in traffic accident**

✓x7th **V85.4** **Person injured while** boarding or alighting **from special construction vehicle**

✓x7th **V85.5** **Driver** of special construction vehicle injured in nontraffic accident

✓x7th **V85.6** **Passenger** of special construction vehicle injured in nontraffic accident

✓x7th **V85.7** **Person on outside** of special construction vehicle injured in nontraffic accident

✓x7th **V85.9** **Unspecified occupant of special construction vehicle injured in nontraffic accident**
Special-construction-vehicle accident NOS

✓4th **V86** **Occupant of special all-terrain or other off-road motor vehicle, injured in transport accident**
EXCLUDES 1 *special all-terrain vehicle in stationary use or maintenance (W31.-)*
sport-utility vehicle (V50-V59)
three-wheeled motor vehicle designed for on-road use (V30-V39)

The appropriate 7th character is to be added to each code from category V86.
A　initial encounter
D　subsequent encounter
S　sequela

✓5th **V86.0** **Driver** of special all-terrain or other off-road motor vehicle injured in traffic accident

✓x7th **V86.01** **Driver of** ambulance **or** fire engine **injured in traffic accident**

✓x7th **V86.02** **Driver of** snowmobile **injured in traffic accident**

✓x7th **V86.03** **Driver of** dune buggy **injured in traffic accident**

✓x7th **V86.04** **Driver of** military vehicle **injured in traffic accident**

✓x7th **V86.09** **Driver of other special all-terrain or other off-road motor vehicle injured in traffic accident**
Driver of dirt bike injured in traffic accident
Driver of go cart injured in traffic accident
Driver of golf cart injured in traffic accident

✓5th **V86.1** **Passenger** of special all-terrain or other off-road motor vehicle injured in traffic accident

✓x7th **V86.11** **Passenger of** ambulance **or** fire engine **injured in traffic accident**

✓x7th **V86.12** **Passenger of** snowmobile **injured in traffic accident**

✓x7th **V86.13** **Passenger of** dune buggy **injured in traffic accident**

✓x7th **V86.14** **Passenger of** military vehicle **injured in traffic accident**

✓x7th **V86.19** **Passenger of other special all-terrain or other off-road motor vehicle injured in traffic accident**
Passenger of dirt bike injured in traffic accident
Passenger of go cart injured in traffic accident
Passenger of golf cart injured in traffic accident

✓5th **V86.2** **Person on outside** of special all-terrain or other off-road motor vehicle injured in traffic accident

✓x7th **V86.21** **Person on outside of** ambulance **or** fire engine **injured in traffic accident**

✓x7th **V86.22** **Person on outside of** snowmobile **injured in traffic accident**

✓x7th **V86.23** **Person on outside of** dune buggy **injured in traffic accident**

✓x7th **V86.24** **Person on outside of** military vehicle **injured in traffic accident**

✓x7th **V86.29** **Person on outside of other special all-terrain or other off-road motor vehicle injured in traffic accident**
Person on outside of dirt bike injured in traffic accident
Person on outside of go cart in traffic accident
Person on outside of golf cart injured in traffic accident

✓5th **V86.3** **Unspecified occupant** of special all-terrain or other off-road motor vehicle injured in traffic accident

✓x7th **V86.31** **Unspecified occupant of** ambulance **or** fire engine **injured in traffic accident**

✓x7th **V86.32** **Unspecified occupant of** snowmobile **injured in traffic accident**

✓x7th **V86.33** **Unspecified occupant of** dune buggy **injured in traffic accident**

✓x7th **V86.34** **Unspecified occupant of** military vehicle **injured in traffic accident**

✓x7th **V86.39** **Unspecified occupant of other special all-terrain or other off-road motor vehicle injured in traffic accident**
Unspecified occupant of dirt bike injured in traffic accident
Unspecified occupant of go cart injured in traffic accident
Unspecified occupant of golf cart injured in traffic accident

✓5th **V86.4** **Person injured while** boarding or alighting **from special all-terrain or other off-road motor vehicle**

✓x7th **V86.41** **Person injured while boarding or alighting from** ambulance **or** fire engine

---

✓ Additional Character Required　　✓x7th Placeholder Alert　　Unspecified Dx　　Other Specified Dx　　Manifestation　　▶◀ Revised Text　　● New Code　　▲ Revised Code Title

√x7ᵗʰ **V86.42** **Person injured while boarding or alighting from snowmobile**

√x7ᵗʰ **V86.43** **Person injured while boarding or alighting from dune buggy**

√x7ᵗʰ **V86.44** **Person injured while boarding or alighting from military vehicle**

√x7ᵗʰ **V86.49** **Person injured while boarding or alighting from other special all-terrain or other off-road motor vehicle**

Person injured while boarding or alighting from dirt bike

Person injured while boarding or alighting from go cart

Person injured while boarding or alighting from golf cart

√5ᵗʰ **V86.5** **Driver of special all-terrain or other off-road vehicle injured in nontraffic accident**

√x7ᵗʰ **V86.51** **Driver of ambulance or fire engine injured in nontraffic accident**

√x7ᵗʰ **V86.52** **Driver of snowmobile injured in nontraffic accident**

√x7ᵗʰ **V86.53** **Driver of dune buggy injured in nontraffic accident**

√x7ᵗʰ **V86.54** **Driver of military vehicle injured in nontraffic accident**

√x7ᵗʰ **V86.59** **Driver of other special all-terrain or other off-road motor vehicle injured in nontraffic accident**

Driver of dirt bike injured in nontraffic accident

Driver of go cart injured in nontraffic accident

Driver of golf cart injured in nontraffic accident

√5ᵗʰ **V86.6** **Passenger of special all-terrain or other off-road motor vehicle injured in nontraffic accident**

√x7ᵗʰ **V86.61** **Passenger of ambulance or fire engine injured in nontraffic accident**

√x7ᵗʰ **V86.62** **Passenger of snowmobile injured in nontraffic accident**

√x7ᵗʰ **V86.63** **Passenger of dune buggy injured in nontraffic accident**

√x7ᵗʰ **V86.64** **Passenger of military vehicle injured in nontraffic accident**

√x7ᵗʰ **V86.69** **Passenger of other special all-terrain or other off-road motor vehicle injured in nontraffic accident**

Passenger of dirt bike injured in nontraffic accident

Passenger of go cart injured in nontraffic accident

Passenger of golf cart injured in nontraffic accident

√5ᵗʰ **V86.7** **Person on outside of special all-terrain or other off-road motor vehicle injured in nontraffic accident**

√x7ᵗʰ **V86.71** **Person on outside of ambulance or fire engine injured in nontraffic accident**

√x7ᵗʰ **V86.72** **Person on outside of snowmobile injured in nontraffic accident**

√x7ᵗʰ **V86.73** **Person on outside of dune buggy injured in nontraffic accident**

√x7ᵗʰ **V86.74** **Person on outside of military vehicle injured in nontraffic accident**

√x7ᵗʰ **V86.79** **Person on outside of other special all-terrain or other off-road motor vehicles injured in nontraffic accident**

Person on outside of dirt bike injured in nontraffic accident

Person on outside of go cart injured in nontraffic accident

Person on outside of golf cart injured in nontraffic accident

√5ᵗʰ **V86.9** **Unspecified occupant of special all-terrain or other off-road motor vehicle injured in nontraffic accident**

√x7ᵗʰ **V86.91** **Unspecified occupant of ambulance or fire engine injured in nontraffic accident**

√x7ᵗʰ **V86.92** **Unspecified occupant of snowmobile injured in nontraffic accident**

√x7ᵗʰ **V86.93** **Unspecified occupant of dune buggy injured in nontraffic accident**

√x7ᵗʰ **V86.94** **Unspecified occupant of military vehicle injured in nontraffic accident**

√x7ᵗʰ **V86.99** **Unspecified occupant of other special all-terrain or other off-road motor vehicle injured in nontraffic accident**

All-terrain motor-vehicle accident NOS

Off-road motor-vehicle accident NOS

Other motor-vehicle accident NOS

Unspecified occupant of dirt bike injured in nontraffic accident

Unspecified occupant of go cart injured in nontraffic accident

Unspecified occupant of golf cart injured in nontraffic accident

√4ᵗʰ **V87** **Traffic accident of specified type but victim's mode of transport unknown**

EXCLUDES 1   collision involving:

pedal cycle (V10-V19)

pedestrian (V01-V09)

The appropriate 7th character is to be added to each code from category V87.

A   initial encounter

D   subsequent encounter

S   sequela

√x7ᵗʰ **V87.0** **Person injured in collision between car and two- or three-wheeled powered vehicle (traffic)**

√x7ᵗʰ **V87.1** **Person injured in collision between other motor vehicle and two- or three-wheeled motor vehicle (traffic)**

√x7ᵗʰ **V87.2** **Person injured in collision between car and pick-up truck or van (traffic)**

√x7ᵗʰ **V87.3** **Person injured in collision between car and bus (traffic)**

√x7ᵗʰ **V87.4** **Person injured in collision between car and heavy transport vehicle (traffic)**

√x7ᵗʰ **V87.5** **Person injured in collision between heavy transport vehicle and bus (traffic)**

√x7ᵗʰ **V87.6** **Person injured in collision between railway train or railway vehicle and car (traffic)**

√x7ᵗʰ **V87.7** **Person injured in collision between other specified motor vehicles (traffic)**

√x7ᵗʰ **V87.8** **Person injured in other specified noncollision transport accidents involving motor vehicle (traffic)**

√x7ᵗʰ **V87.9** **Person injured in other specified (collision)(noncollision) transport accidents involving nonmotor vehicle (traffic)**

√4ᵗʰ **V88** **Nontraffic accident of specified type but victim's mode of transport unknown**

EXCLUDES 1   collision involving:

pedal cycle (V10-V19)

pedestrian (V01-V09)

The appropriate 7th character is to be added to each code from category V88.

A   initial encounter

D   subsequent encounter

S   sequela

√x7ᵗʰ **V88.0** **Person injured in collision between car and two- or three-wheeled motor vehicle, nontraffic**

√x7ᵗʰ **V88.1** **Person injured in collision between other motor vehicle and two- or three-wheeled motor vehicle, nontraffic**

√x7ᵗʰ **V88.2** **Person injured in collision between car and pick-up truck or van, nontraffic**

√x7ᵗʰ **V88.3** **Person injured in collision between car and bus, nontraffic**

√x7ᵗʰ **V88.4** **Person injured in collision between car and heavy transport vehicle, nontraffic**

√x7ᵗʰ **V88.5** **Person injured in collision between heavy transport vehicle and bus, nontraffic**

√x7ᵗʰ **V88.6** **Person injured in collision between railway train or railway vehicle and car, nontraffic**

√x7ᵗʰ **V88.7** **Person injured in collision between other specified motor vehicle, nontraffic**

√x7ᵗʰ **V88.8** **Person injured in other specified noncollision transport accidents involving motor vehicle, nontraffic**

√x7ᵗʰ **V88.9** **Person injured in other specified (collision)(noncollision) transport accidents involving nonmotor vehicle, nontraffic**

EXCLUDES 1 Not coded here   EXCLUDES 2 Not included here   N Newborn Age: 0   P Pediatric Age: 0-17   M Maternity Age: 12-55   A Adult Age: 15-124

1062   ICD-10-CM 201

◢ V89 Motor- or nonmotor-vehicle accident, type of vehicle unspecified

The appropriate 7th character is to be added to each code from category V89.
A   initial encounter
D   subsequent encounter
S   sequela

✓x7ᵗʰ V89.0 Person injured in unspecified motor-vehicle accident, nontraffic
Motor-vehicle accident NOS, nontraffic

✓x7ᵗʰ V89.1 Person injured in unspecified nonmotor-vehicle accident, nontraffic
Nonmotor-vehicle accident NOS (nontraffic)

✓x7ᵗʰ V89.2 Person injured in unspecified motor-vehicle accident, traffic
Motor-vehicle accident [MVA] NOS
Road (traffic) accident [RTA] NOS

✓x7ᵗʰ V89.3 Person injured in unspecified nonmotor-vehicle accident, traffic
Nonmotor-vehicle traffic accident NOS

✓x7ᵗʰ V89.9 Person injured in unspecified vehicle accident
Collision NOS

Water transport accidents (V90-V94)

◢ V90 Drowning and submersion due to accident to watercraft

EXCLUDES 1   civilian water transport accident involving military watercraft (V94.81-)
fall into water not from watercraft (W16.-)
military watercraft accident in military or war operations (Y36.0-, Y37.0-)
water-transport-related drowning or submersion without accident to watercraft (V92.-)

The appropriate 7th character is to be added to each code from category V90.
A   initial encounter
D   subsequent encounter
S   sequela

✓5ᵗʰ V90.0 Drowning and submersion due to watercraft overturning

✓x7ᵗʰ V90.00 Drowning and submersion due to merchant ship overturning

✓x7ᵗʰ V90.01 Drowning and submersion due to passenger ship overturning
Drowning and submersion due to Ferry-boat overturning
Drowning and submersion due to Liner overturning

✓x7ᵗʰ V90.02 Drowning and submersion due to fishing boat overturning

✓x7ᵗʰ V90.03 Drowning and submersion due to other powered watercraft overturning
Drowning and submersion due to Hovercraft (on open water) overturning
Drowning and submersion due to Jet ski overturning

✓x7ᵗʰ V90.04 Drowning and submersion due to sailboat overturning

✓x7ᵗʰ V90.05 Drowning and submersion due to canoe or kayak overturning

✓x7ᵗʰ V90.06 Drowning and submersion due to (nonpowered) inflatable craft overturning

✓x7ᵗʰ V90.08 Drowning and submersion due to other unpowered watercraft overturning
Drowning and submersion due to windsurfer overturning

✓x7ᵗʰ V90.09 Drowning and submersion due to unspecified watercraft overturning
Drowning and submersion due to boat NOS overturning
Drowning and submersion due to ship NOS overturning
Drowning and submersion due to watercraft NOS overturning

✓5ᵗʰ V90.1 Drowning and submersion due to watercraft sinking

✓x7ᵗʰ V90.10 Drowning and submersion due to merchant ship sinking

✓x7ᵗʰ V90.11 Drowning and submersion due to passenger ship sinking
Drowning and submersion due to Ferry-boat sinking
Drowning and submersion due to Liner sinking

✓x7ᵗʰ V90.12 Drowning and submersion due to fishing boat sinking

✓x7ᵗʰ V90.13 Drowning and submersion due to other powered watercraft sinking
Drowning and submersion due to Hovercraft (on open water) sinking
Drowning and submersion due to Jet ski sinking

✓x7ᵗʰ V90.14 Drowning and submersion due to sailboat sinking

✓x7ᵗʰ V90.15 Drowning and submersion due to canoe or kayak sinking

✓x7ᵗʰ V90.16 Drowning and submersion due to (nonpowered) inflatable craft sinking

✓x7ᵗʰ V90.18 Drowning and submersion due to other unpowered watercraft sinking

✓x7ᵗʰ V90.19 Drowning and submersion due to unspecified watercraft sinking
Drowning and submersion due to boat NOS sinking
Drowning and submersion due to ship NOS sinking
Drowning and submersion due to watercraft NOS sinking

✓5ᵗʰ V90.2 Drowning and submersion due to falling or jumping from burning watercraft

✓x7ᵗʰ V90.20 Drowning and submersion due to falling or jumping from burning merchant ship

✓x7ᵗʰ V90.21 Drowning and submersion due to falling or jumping from burning passenger ship
Drowning and submersion due to falling or jumping from burning Ferry-boat
Drowning and submersion due to falling or jumping from burning Liner

✓x7ᵗʰ V90.22 Drowning and submersion due to falling or jumping from burning fishing boat

✓x7ᵗʰ V90.23 Drowning and submersion due to falling or jumping from other burning powered watercraft
Drowning and submersion due to falling and jumping from burning Hovercraft (on open water)
Drowning and submersion due to falling and jumping from burning Jet ski

✓x7ᵗʰ V90.24 Drowning and submersion due to falling or jumping from burning sailboat

✓x7ᵗʰ V90.25 Drowning and submersion due to falling or jumping from burning canoe or kayak

✓x7ᵗʰ V90.26 Drowning and submersion due to falling or jumping from burning (nonpowered) inflatable craft

✓x7ᵗʰ V90.27 Drowning and submersion due to falling or jumping from burning water-skis

✓x7ᵗʰ V90.28 Drowning and submersion due to falling or jumping from other burning unpowered watercraft
Drowning and submersion due to falling and jumping from burning surf-board
Drowning and submersion due to falling and jumping from burning windsurfer

✓x7ᵗʰ V90.29 Drowning and submersion due to falling or jumping from unspecified burning watercraft
Drowning and submersion due to falling or jumping from burning boat NOS
Drowning and submersion due to falling or jumping from burning ship NOS
Drowning and submersion due to falling or jumping from burning watercraft NOS

✓5ᵗʰ V90.3 Drowning and submersion due to falling or jumping from crushed watercraft

✓x7ᵗʰ V90.30 Drowning and submersion due to falling or jumping from crushed merchant ship

✓x7ᵗʰ V90.31 Drowning and submersion due to falling or jumping from crushed passenger ship
Drowning and submersion due to falling and jumping from crushed Ferry boat
Drowning and submersion due to falling and jumping from crushed Liner

✓x7ᵗʰ V90.32 Drowning and submersion due to falling or jumping from crushed fishing boat

✓x7ᵗʰ V90.33 Drowning and submersion due to falling or jumping from other crushed powered watercraft
Drowning and submersion due to falling and jumping from crushed Hovercraft
Drowning and submersion due to falling and jumping from crushed Jet ski

✓x7ᵗʰ V90.34 Drowning and submersion due to falling or jumping from crushed sailboat

■ Additional Character Required   ✓x7ᵗʰ Placeholder Alert   Unspecified Dx   Other Specified Dx   Manifestation   ►◄ Revised Text   ● New Code   ▲ Revised Code Title

D-10-CM 2016   1063

☑7ᵗʰ **V90.35** **Drowning and submersion due to falling or jumping from crushed canoe or kayak**

☑7ᵗʰ **V90.36** **Drowning and submersion due to falling or jumping from crushed (nonpowered) inflatable craft**

☑7ᵗʰ **V90.37** **Drowning and submersion due to falling or jumping from crushed water-skis**

☑7ᵗʰ **V90.38** **Drowning and submersion due to falling or jumping from other crushed unpowered watercraft**
Drowning and submersion due to falling and jumping from crushed surf-board
Drowning and submersion due to falling and jumping from crushed windsurfer

☑7ᵗʰ **V90.39** **Drowning and submersion due to falling or jumping from crushed unspecified watercraft**
Drowning and submersion due to falling and jumping from crushed boat NOS
Drowning and submersion due to falling and jumping from crushed ship NOS
Drowning and submersion due to falling and jumping from crushed watercraft NOS

☑5ᵗʰ **V90.8** **Drowning and submersion due to other accident to watercraft**

☑7ᵗʰ **V90.80** **Drowning and submersion due to other accident to merchant ship**

☑7ᵗʰ **V90.81** **Drowning and submersion due to other accident to passenger ship**
Drowning and submersion due to other accident to Ferry-boat
Drowning and submersion due to other accident to Liner

☑7ᵗʰ **V90.82** **Drowning and submersion due to other accident to fishing boat**

☑7ᵗʰ **V90.83** **Drowning and submersion due to other accident to other powered watercraft**
Drowning and submersion due to other accident to Hovercraft (on open water)
Drowning and submersion due to other accident to Jet ski

☑7ᵗʰ **V90.84** **Drowning and submersion due to other accident to sailboat**

☑7ᵗʰ **V90.85** **Drowning and submersion due to other accident to canoe or kayak**

☑7ᵗʰ **V90.86** **Drowning and submersion due to other accident to (nonpowered) inflatable craft**

☑7ᵗʰ **V90.87** **Drowning and submersion due to other accident to water-skis**

☑7ᵗʰ **V90.88** **Drowning and submersion due to other accident to other unpowered watercraft**
Drowning and submersion due to other accident to surf-board
Drowning and submersion due to other accident to windsurfer

☑7ᵗʰ **V90.89** **Drowning and submersion due to other accident to unspecified watercraft**
Drowning and submersion due to other accident to boat NOS
Drowning and submersion due to other accident to ship NOS
Drowning and submersion due to other accident to watercraft NOS

☑4ᵗʰ **V91** **Other injury due to accident to watercraft**
INCLUDES   any injury except drowning and submersion as a result of an accident to watercraft
EXCLUDES 1   civilian water transport accident involving military watercraft (V94.81-)
military watercraft accident in military or war operations (Y36, Y37.-)
EXCLUDES 2   drowning and submersion due to accident to watercraft (V90.-)

The appropriate 7th character is to be added to each code from category V91.
A   initial encounter
D   subsequent encounter
S   sequela

☑5ᵗʰ **V91.0** **Burn due to watercraft on fire**
EXCLUDES 1   burn from localized fire or explosion on board ship without accident to watercraft (V93.-)

☑7ᵗʰ **V91.00** **Burn due to merchant ship on fire**

☑7ᵗʰ **V91.01** **Burn due to passenger ship on fire**
Burn due to Ferry-boat on fire
Burn due to Liner on fire

☑7ᵗʰ **V91.02** **Burn due to fishing boat on fire**

☑7ᵗʰ **V91.03** **Burn due to other powered watercraft on fire**
Burn due to Hovercraft (on open water) on fire
Burn due to Jet ski on fire

☑7ᵗʰ **V91.04** **Burn due to sailboat on fire**

☑7ᵗʰ **V91.05** **Burn due to canoe or kayak on fire**

☑7ᵗʰ **V91.06** **Burn due to (nonpowered) inflatable craft on fire**

☑7ᵗʰ **V91.07** **Burn due to water-skis on fire**

☑7ᵗʰ **V91.08** **Burn due to other unpowered watercraft on fire**

☑7ᵗʰ **V91.09** **Burn due to unspecified watercraft on fire**
Burn due to boat NOS on fire
Burn due to ship NOS on fire
Burn due to watercraft NOS on fire

☑5ᵗʰ **V91.1** **Crushed between watercraft and other watercraft or other object due to collision**
Crushed by lifeboat after abandoning ship in a collision
NOTE   Select the specified type of watercraft that the victim was on at the time of the collision

☑7ᵗʰ **V91.10** **Crushed between merchant ship and other watercraft or other object due to collision**

☑7ᵗʰ **V91.11** **Crushed between passenger ship and other watercraft or other object due to collision**
Crushed between Ferry-boat and other watercraft or other object due to collision
Crushed between Liner and other watercraft or other object due to collision

☑7ᵗʰ **V91.12** **Crushed between fishing boat and other watercraft or other object due to collision**

☑7ᵗʰ **V91.13** **Crushed between other powered watercraft and other watercraft or other object due to collision**
Crushed between Hovercraft (on open water) and other watercraft or other object due to collision
Crushed between Jet ski and other watercraft or other object due to collision

☑7ᵗʰ **V91.14** **Crushed between sailboat and other watercraft or other object due to collision**

☑7ᵗʰ **V91.15** **Crushed between canoe or kayak and other watercraft or other object due to collision**

☑7ᵗʰ **V91.16** **Crushed between (nonpowered) inflatable craft and other watercraft or other object due to collision**

☑7ᵗʰ **V91.18** **Crushed between other unpowered watercraft and other watercraft or other object due to collision**
Crushed between surfboard and other watercraft or other object due to collision
Crushed between windsurfer and other watercraft or other object due to collision

☑7ᵗʰ **V91.19** **Crushed between unspecified watercraft and other watercraft or other object due to collision**
Crushed between boat NOS and other watercraft or other object due to collision
Crushed between ship NOS and other watercraft or other object due to collision
Crushed between watercraft NOS and other watercraft or other object due to collision

☑5ᵗʰ **V91.2** **Fall due to collision between watercraft and other watercraft or other object**
Fall while remaining on watercraft after collision
NOTE   Select the specified type of watercraft that the victim was on at the time of the collision.
EXCLUDES 1   crushed between watercraft and other watercraft and other object due to collision (V91.1-)
drowning and submersion due to falling from crushed watercraft (V90.3-)

☑7ᵗʰ **V91.20** **Fall due to collision between merchant ship and other watercraft or other object**

☑7ᵗʰ **V91.21** **Fall due to collision between passenger ship and other watercraft or other object**
Fall due to collision between Ferry-boat and other watercraft or other object
Fall due to collision between Liner and other watercraft or other object

☑7ᵗʰ **V91.22** **Fall due to collision between fishing boat and other watercraft or other object**

EXCLUDES 1 Not coded here   EXCLUDES 2 Not included here   N Newborn Age: 0   P Pediatric Age: 0-17   M Maternity Age: 12-55   A Adult Age: 15-12

1064
ICD-10-CM 201

√x 7ᵗʰ **V91.23** **Fall due to collision between other** powered **watercraft and other watercraft or other object**
> Fall due to collision between Hovercraft (on open water) and other watercraft or other object
> Fall due to collision between Jet ski and other watercraft or other object

√x 7ᵗʰ **V91.24** **Fall due to collision between** sailboat **and other watercraft or other object**

√x 7ᵗʰ **V91.25** **Fall due to collision between** canoe or kayak **and other watercraft or other object**

√x 7ᵗʰ **V91.26** **Fall due to collision between (nonpowered)** inflatable craft **and other watercraft or other object**

√x 7ᵗʰ **V91.29** **Fall due to collision between unspecified watercraft and other watercraft or other object**
> Fall due to collision between boat NOS and other watercraft or other object
> Fall due to collision between ship NOS and other watercraft or other object
> Fall due to collision between watercraft NOS and other watercraft or other object

√ 5ᵗʰ **V91.3** **Hit or struck by falling object due to accident to watercraft**
> Hit or struck by falling object (part of damaged watercraft or other object) after falling or jumping from damaged watercraft
>
> *EXCLUDES 2*   *drowning or submersion due to fall or jumping from damaged watercraft (V90.2-, V90.3-)*

√x 7ᵗʰ **V91.30** **Hit or struck by falling object due to accident to** merchant ship

√x 7ᵗʰ **V91.31** **Hit or struck by falling object due to accident to** passenger ship
> Hit or struck by falling object due to accident to Ferry-boat
> Hit or struck by falling object due to accident to Liner

√x 7ᵗʰ **V91.32** **Hit or struck by falling object due to accident to** fishing boat

√x 7ᵗʰ **V91.33** **Hit or struck by falling object due to accident to other** powered **watercraft**
> Hit or struck by falling object due to accident to Hovercraft (on open water)
> Hit or struck by falling object due to accident to Jet ski

√x 7ᵗʰ **V91.34** **Hit or struck by falling object due to accident to** sailboat

√x 7ᵗʰ **V91.35** **Hit or struck by falling object due to accident to** canoe or kayak

√x 7ᵗʰ **V91.36** **Hit or struck by falling object due to accident to (nonpowered)** inflatable craft

√x 7ᵗʰ **V91.37** **Hit or struck by falling object due to accident to** water-skis
> Hit by water-skis after jumping off of waterskis

√x 7ᵗʰ **V91.38** **Hit or struck by falling object due to accident to other** unpowered **watercraft**
> Hit or struck by surf-board after falling off damaged surf-board
> Hit or struck by object after falling off damaged windsurfer

√x 7ᵗʰ **V91.39** **Hit or struck by falling object due to accident to unspecified watercraft**
> Hit or struck by falling object due to accident to boat NOS
> Hit or struck by falling object due to accident to ship NOS
> Hit or struck by falling object due to accident to watercraft NOS

√ 5ᵗʰ **V91.8** **Other injury due to other accident to watercraft**

√x 7ᵗʰ **V91.80** **Other injury due to other accident to** merchant ship

√x 7ᵗʰ **V91.81** **Other injury due to other accident to** passenger ship
> Other injury due to other accident to Ferry-boat
> Other injury due to other accident to Liner

√x 7ᵗʰ **V91.82** **Other injury due to other accident to** fishing boat

√x 7ᵗʰ **V91.83** **Other injury due to other accident to other** powered **watercraft**
> Other injury due to other accident to Hovercraft (on open water)
> Other injury due to other accident to Jet ski

√x 7ᵗʰ **V91.84** **Other injury due to other accident to** sailboat

√x 7ᵗʰ **V91.85** **Other injury due to other accident to** canoe or kayak

√x 7ᵗʰ **V91.86** **Other injury due to other accident to (nonpowered)** inflatable craft

√x 7ᵗʰ **V91.87** **Other injury due to other accident to** water-skis

√x 7ᵗʰ **V91.88** **Other injury due to other accident to other** unpowered **watercraft**
> Other injury due to other accident to surf-board
> Other injury due to other accident to windsurfer

√x 7ᵗʰ **V91.89** **Other injury due to other accident to unspecified watercraft**
> Other injury due to other accident to boat NOS
> Other injury due to other accident to ship NOS
> Other injury due to other accident to watercraft NOS

√ 4ᵗʰ **V92** **Drowning and submersion due to accident on board watercraft, without accident to watercraft**
> *EXCLUDES 1*   *civilian water transport accident involving military watercraft (V94.81-)*
> *drowning or submersion due to accident to watercraft (V90-V91)*
> *drowning or submersion of diver who voluntarily jumps from boat not involved in an accident (W16.711, W16.721)*
> *fall into water without watercraft (W16.-)*
> *military watercraft accident in military or war operations (Y36, Y37)*

> The appropriate 7th character is to be added to each code from category V92.
> A   initial encounter
> D   subsequent encounter
> S   sequela

√ 5ᵗʰ **V92.0** **Drowning and submersion due to** fall off **watercraft**
> Drowning and submersion due to fall from gangplank of watercraft
> Drowning and submersion due to fall overboard watercraft
>
> *EXCLUDES 2*   *hitting head on object or bottom of body of water due to fall from watercraft (V94.0-)*

√x 7ᵗʰ **V92.00** **Drowning and submersion due to fall off** merchant ship

√x 7ᵗʰ **V92.01** **Drowning and submersion due to fall off** passenger ship
> Drowning and submersion due to fall off Ferry-boat
> Drowning and submersion due to fall off Liner

√x 7ᵗʰ **V92.02** **Drowning and submersion due to fall off** fishing boat

√x 7ᵗʰ **V92.03** **Drowning and submersion due to fall off other** powered **watercraft**
> Drowning and submersion due to fall off Hovercraft (on open water)
> Drowning and submersion due to fall off Jet ski

√x 7ᵗʰ **V92.04** **Drowning and submersion due to fall off** sailboat

√x 7ᵗʰ **V92.05** **Drowning and submersion due to fall off** canoe or kayak

√x 7ᵗʰ **V92.06** **Drowning and submersion due to fall off (nonpowered)** inflatable craft

√x 7ᵗʰ **V92.07** **Drowning and submersion due to fall off** water-skis
> *EXCLUDES 1*   *drowning and submersion due to falling off burning water-skis (V90.27)*
> *drowning and submersion due to falling off crushed water-skis (V90.37)*
> *hit by boat while water-skiing NOS (V94.X)*

√x 7ᵗʰ **V92.08** **Drowning and submersion due to fall off other** unpowered **watercraft**
> Drowning and submersion due to fall off surf-board
> Drowning and submersion due to fall off windsurfer
>
> *EXCLUDES 1*   *drowning and submersion due to fall off burning unpowered watercraft (V90.28)*
> *drowning and submersion due to fall off crushed unpowered watercraft (V90.38)*
> *drowning and submersion due to fall off damaged unpowered watercraft (V90.88)*
> *drowning and submersion due to rider of nonpowered watercraft being hit by other watercraft (V94.-)*
> *other injury due to rider of nonpowered watercraft being hit by other watercraft (V94.-)*

√x 7ᵗʰ **V92.09** **Drowning and submersion due to fall off unspecified watercraft**
> Drowning and submersion due to fall off boat NOS
> Drowning and submersion due to fall off ship
> Drowning and submersion due to fall off watercraft NOS

Additional Character Required   🔲x 7ᵗʰ Placeholder Alert   Unspecified Dx   Other Specified Dx   Manifestation   ▶◀ Revised Text   ● New Code   ▲ Revised Code Title

✓5ᵗʰ **V92.1 Drowning and submersion due to being thrown overboard by motion of watercraft**
> EXCLUDES 1 *drowning and submersion due to fall off surf-board (V92.08)*
> *drowning and submersion due to fall off water-skis (V92.07)*
> *drowning and submersion due to fall off windsurfer (V92.08)*

✓x7ᵗʰ **V92.10 Drowning and submersion due to being thrown overboard by motion of merchant ship**

✓x7ᵗʰ **V92.11 Drowning and submersion due to being thrown overboard by motion of passenger ship**
> Drowning and submersion due to being thrown overboard by motion of Ferry-boat
> Drowning and submersion due to being thrown overboard by motion of Liner

✓x7ᵗʰ **V92.12 Drowning and submersion due to being thrown overboard by motion of fishing boat**

✓x7ᵗʰ **V92.13 Drowning and submersion due to being thrown overboard by motion of other powered watercraft**
> Drowning and submersion due to being thrown overboard by motion of Hovercraft

✓x7ᵗʰ **V92.14 Drowning and submersion due to being thrown overboard by motion of sailboat**

✓x7ᵗʰ **V92.15 Drowning and submersion due to being thrown overboard by motion of canoe or kayak**

✓x7ᵗʰ **V92.16 Drowning and submersion due to being thrown overboard by motion of (nonpowered) inflatable craft**

✓x7ᵗʰ **V92.19 Drowning and submersion due to being thrown overboard by motion of unspecified watercraft**
> Drowning and submersion due to being thrown overboard by motion of boat NOS
> Drowning and submersion due to being thrown overboard by motion of ship NOS
> Drowning and submersion due to being thrown overboard by motion of watercraft NOS

✓5ᵗʰ **V92.2 Drowning and submersion due to being washed overboard from watercraft**
> Code first any associated cataclysm (X37.0-)

✓x7ᵗʰ **V92.20 Drowning and submersion due to being washed overboard from merchant ship**

✓x7ᵗʰ **V92.21 Drowning and submersion due to being washed overboard from passenger ship**
> Drowning and submersion due to being washed overboard from Ferry-boat
> Drowning and submersion due to being washed overboard from Liner

✓x7ᵗʰ **V92.22 Drowning and submersion due to being washed overboard from fishing boat**

✓x7ᵗʰ **V92.23 Drowning and submersion due to being washed overboard from other powered watercraft**
> Drowning and submersion due to being washed overboard from Hovercraft (on open water)
> Drowning and submersion due to being washed overboard from Jet ski

✓x7ᵗʰ **V92.24 Drowning and submersion due to being washed overboard from sailboat**

✓x7ᵗʰ **V92.25 Drowning and submersion due to being washed overboard from canoe or kayak**

✓x7ᵗʰ **V92.26 Drowning and submersion due to being washed overboard from (nonpowered) inflatable craft**

✓x7ᵗʰ **V92.27 Drowning and submersion due to being washed overboard from water-skis**
> EXCLUDES 1 *drowning and submersion due to fall off water-skis (V92.07)*

✓x7ᵗʰ **V92.28 Drowning and submersion due to being washed overboard from other unpowered watercraft**
> Drowning and submersion due to being washed overboard from surf-board
> Drowning and submersion due to being washed overboard from windsurfer

✓x7ᵗʰ **V92.29 Drowning and submersion due to being washed overboard from unspecified watercraft**
> Drowning and submersion due to being washed overboard from boat NOS
> Drowning and submersion due to being washed overboard from ship NOS
> Drowning and submersion due to being washed overboard from watercraft NOS

✓4ᵗʰ **V93 Other injury due to accident on board watercraft, without accident to watercraft**
> EXCLUDES 1 *civilian water transport accident involving military watercraft (V94.81-)*
> *other injury due to accident to watercraft (V91.-)*
> *military watercraft accident in military or war operations (Y36, Y37.-)*
> EXCLUDES 2 *drowning and submersion due to accident on board watercraft without accident to watercraft (V92.-)*

> The appropriate 7th character is to be added to each code from category V93.
> A   initial encounter
> D   subsequent encounter
> S   sequela

✓5ᵗʰ **V93.0 Burn due to localized fire on board watercraft**
> EXCLUDES 1 *burn due to watercraft on fire (V91.0-)*

✓x7ᵗʰ **V93.00 Burn due to localized fire on board merchant vessel**

✓x7ᵗʰ **V93.01 Burn due to localized fire on board passenger vessel**
> Burn due to localized fire on board Ferry-boat
> Burn due to localized fire on board Liner

✓x7ᵗʰ **V93.02 Burn due to localized fire on board fishing boat**

✓x7ᵗʰ **V93.03 Burn due to localized fire on board other powered watercraft**
> Burn due to localized fire on board Hovercraft
> Burn due to localized fire on board Jet ski

✓x7ᵗʰ **V93.04 Burn due to localized fire on board sailboat**

✓x7ᵗʰ **V93.09 Burn due to localized fire on board unspecified watercraft**
> Burn due to localized fire on board boat NOS
> Burn due to localized fire on board ship NOS
> Burn due to localized fire on board watercraft NOS

✓5ᵗʰ **V93.1 Other burn on board watercraft**
> Burn due to source other than fire on board watercraft
> EXCLUDES 1 *burn due to watercraft on fire (V91.0-)*

✓x7ᵗʰ **V93.10 Other burn on board merchant vessel**

✓x7ᵗʰ **V93.11 Other burn on board passenger vessel**
> Other burn on board Ferry-boat
> Other burn on board Liner

✓x7ᵗʰ **V93.12 Other burn on board fishing boat**

✓x7ᵗʰ **V93.13 Other burn on board other powered watercraft**
> Other burn on board Hovercraft
> Other burn on board Jet ski

✓x7ᵗʰ **V93.14 Other burn on board sailboat**

✓x7ᵗʰ **V93.19 Other burn on board unspecified watercraft**
> Other burn on board boat NOS
> Other burn on board ship NOS
> Other burn on board watercraft NOS

✓5ᵗʰ **V93.2 Heat exposure on board watercraft**
> EXCLUDES 1 *exposure to man-made heat not aboard watercraft (W92)*
> *exposure to natural heat while on board watercraft (X30)*
> *exposure to sunlight while on board watercraft (X32)*
> EXCLUDES 2 *burn due to fire on board watercraft (V93.0-)*

✓x7ᵗʰ **V93.20 Heat exposure on board merchant ship**

✓x7ᵗʰ **V93.21 Heat exposure on board passenger ship**
> Heat exposure on board Ferry-boat
> Heat exposure on board Liner

✓x7ᵗʰ **V93.22 Heat exposure on board fishing boat**

✓x7ᵗʰ **V93.23 Heat exposure on board other powered watercraft**
> Heat exposure on board hovercraft

✓x7ᵗʰ **V93.24 Heat exposure on board sailboat**

✓x7ᵗʰ **V93.29 Heat exposure on board unspecified watercraft**
> Heat exposure on board boat NOS
> Heat exposure on board ship NOS
> Heat exposure on board watercraft NOS

✓5ᵗʰ **V93.3 Fall on board watercraft**
> EXCLUDES 1 *fall due to collision of watercraft (V91.2-)*

✓x7ᵗʰ **V93.30 Fall on board merchant ship**

✓x7ᵗʰ **V93.31 Fall on board passenger ship**
> Fall on board Ferry-boat
> Fall on board Liner

✓x7ᵗʰ **V93.32 Fall on board fishing boat**

EXCLUDES 1 Not coded here   EXCLUDES 2 Not included here   N Newborn Age: 0   P Pediatric Age: 0-17   M Maternity Age: 12-55   A Adult Age: 15-1

√x7ᵗʰ **V93.33 Fall on board other powered watercraft**
Fall on board Hovercraft (on open water)
Fall on board Jet ski

√x7ᵗʰ **V93.34 Fall on board sailboat**

√x7ᵗʰ **V93.35 Fall on board canoe or kayak**

√x7ᵗʰ **V93.36 Fall on board (nonpowered) inflatable craft**

√x7ᵗʰ **V93.38 Fall on board other unpowered watercraft**

√x7ᵗʰ **V93.39 Fall on board unspecified watercraft**
Fall on board boat NOS
Fall on board ship NOS
Fall on board watercraft NOS

√5ᵗʰ **V93.4 Struck by falling object on board watercraft**
Hit by falling object on board watercraft
> **EXCLUDES 1** struck by falling object due to accident to watercraft (V91.3)

√x7ᵗʰ **V93.40 Struck by falling object on merchant ship**

√x7ᵗʰ **V93.41 Struck by falling object on passenger ship**
Struck by falling object on Ferry-boat
Struck by falling object on Liner

√x7ᵗʰ **V93.42 Struck by falling object on fishing boat**

√x7ᵗʰ **V93.43 Struck by falling object on other powered watercraft**
Struck by falling object on Hovercraft

√x7ᵗʰ **V93.44 Struck by falling object on sailboat**

√x7ᵗʰ **V93.48 Struck by falling object on other unpowered watercraft**

√x7ᵗʰ **V93.49 Struck by falling object on unspecified watercraft**

√5ᵗʰ **V93.5 Explosion on board watercraft**
Boiler explosion on steamship
> **EXCLUDES 2** fire on board watercraft (V93.0-)

√x7ᵗʰ **V93.50 Explosion on board merchant ship**

√x7ᵗʰ **V93.51 Explosion on board passenger ship**
Explosion on board Ferry-boat
Explosion on board Liner

√x7ᵗʰ **V93.52 Explosion on board fishing boat**

√x7ᵗʰ **V93.53 Explosion on board other powered watercraft**
Explosion on board Hovercraft
Explosion on board Jet ski

√x7ᵗʰ **V93.54 Explosion on board sailboat**

√x7ᵗʰ **V93.59 Explosion on board unspecified watercraft**
Explosion on board boat NOS
Explosion on board ship NOS
Explosion on board watercraft NOS

√5ᵗʰ **V93.6 Machinery accident on board watercraft**
> **EXCLUDES 1** machinery explosion on board watercraft (V93.4-)
> machinery fire on board watercraft (V93.0-)

√x7ᵗʰ **V93.60 Machinery accident on board merchant ship**

√x7ᵗʰ **V93.61 Machinery accident on board passenger ship**
Machinery accident on board Ferry-boat
Machinery accident on board Liner

√x7ᵗʰ **V93.62 Machinery accident on board fishing boat**

√x7ᵗʰ **V93.63 Machinery accident on board other powered watercraft**
Machinery accident on board Hovercraft

√x7ᵗʰ **V93.64 Machinery accident on board sailboat**

√x7ᵗʰ **V93.69 Machinery accident on board unspecified watercraft**
Machinery accident on board boat NOS
Machinery accident on board ship NOS
Machinery accident on board watercraft NOS

√5ᵗʰ **V93.8 Other injury due to other accident on board watercraft**
Accidental poisoning by gases or fumes on watercraft

√x7ᵗʰ **V93.80 Other injury due to other accident on board merchant ship**

√x7ᵗʰ **V93.81 Other injury due to other accident on board passenger ship**
Other injury due to other accident on board Ferry-boat
Other injury due to other accident on board Liner

√x7ᵗʰ **V93.82 Other injury due to other accident on board fishing boat**

√x7ᵗʰ **V93.83 Other injury due to other accident on board other powered watercraft**
Other injury due to other accident on board Hovercraft
Other injury due to other accident on board Jet ski

√x7ᵗʰ **V93.84 Other injury due to other accident on board sailboat**

√x7ᵗʰ **V93.85 Other injury due to other accident on board canoe or kayak**

√x7ᵗʰ **V93.86 Other injury due to other accident on board (nonpowered) inflatable craft**

√x7ᵗʰ **V93.87 Other injury due to other accident on board water-skis**
Hit or struck by object while waterskiing

√x7ᵗʰ **V93.88 Other injury due to other accident on board other unpowered watercraft**
Hit or struck by object while surfing
Hit or struck by object while on board windsurfer

√x7ᵗʰ **V93.89 Other injury due to other accident on board unspecified watercraft**
Other injury due to other accident on board boat NOS
Other injury due to other accident on board ship NOS
Other injury due to other accident on board watercraft NOS

√4ᵗʰ **V94 Other and unspecified water transport accidents**
> **EXCLUDES 1** military watercraft accidents in military or war operations (Y36, Y37)

> The appropriate 7th character is to be added to each code from category V94.
> A   initial encounter
> D   subsequent encounter
> S   sequela

√x7ᵗʰ **V94.0 Hitting object or bottom of body of water due to fall from watercraft**
> **EXCLUDES 2** drowning and submersion due to fall from watercraft (V92.0-)

√5ᵗʰ **V94.1 Bather struck by watercraft**
Swimmer hit by watercraft

√x7ᵗʰ **V94.11 Bather struck by powered watercraft**

√x7ᵗʰ **V94.12 Bather struck by nonpowered watercraft**

√5ᵗʰ **V94.2 Rider of nonpowered watercraft struck by other watercraft**

√x7ᵗʰ **V94.21 Rider of nonpowered watercraft struck by other nonpowered watercraft**
Canoer hit by other nonpowered watercraft
Surfer hit by other nonpowered watercraft
Windsurfer hit by other nonpowered watercraft

√x7ᵗʰ **V94.22 Rider of nonpowered watercraft struck by powered watercraft**
Canoer hit by motorboat
Surfer hit by motorboat
Windsurfer hit by motorboat

√5ᵗʰ **V94.3 Injury to rider of (inflatable) watercraft being pulled behind other watercraft**

√x7ᵗʰ **V94.31 Injury to rider of (inflatable) recreational watercraft being pulled behind other watercraft**
Injury to rider of inner-tube pulled behind motor boat

√x7ᵗʰ **V94.32 Injury to rider of non-recreational watercraft being pulled behind other watercraft**
Injury to occupant of dingy being pulled behind boat or ship
Injury to occupant of life-raft being pulled behind boat or ship

√x7ᵗʰ **V94.4 Injury to barefoot water-skier**
Injury to person being pulled behind boat or ship

√5ᵗʰ **V94.8 Other water transport accident**

√6ᵗʰ **V94.81 Water transport accident involving military watercraft**

√7ᵗʰ **V94.810 Civilian watercraft involved in water transport accident with military watercraft**
Passenger on civilian watercraft injured due to accident with military watercraft

√7ᵗʰ **V94.811 Civilian in water injured by military watercraft**

√7ᵗʰ **V94.818 Other water transport accident involving military watercraft**

√x7ᵗʰ **V94.89 Other water transport accident**

√x7ᵗʰ **V94.9 Unspecified water transport accident**
Water transport accident NOS

Additional Character Required   √x7ᵗʰ Placeholder Alert   Unspecified Dx   Other Specified Dx   Manifestation   ▶◀ Revised Text   ● New Code   ▲ Revised Code Title

Chapter 20. External Causes of Morbidity

Air and space transport accidents (V95-V97)

EXCLUDES 1 military aircraft accidents in military or war operations (Y36, Y37)

✓4th V95 Accident to powered aircraft causing injury to occupant

> The appropriate 7th character is to be added to each code from category V95.
> A   initial encounter
> D   subsequent encounter
> S   sequela

✓5th V95.0 Helicopter accident injuring occupant

  ✓7th V95.00 Unspecified helicopter accident injuring occupant

  ✓7th V95.01 Helicopter crash injuring occupant

  ✓7th V95.02 Forced landing of helicopter injuring occupant

  ✓7th V95.03 Helicopter collision injuring occupant
> Helicopter collision with any object, fixed, movable or moving

  ✓7th V95.04 Helicopter fire injuring occupant

  ✓7th V95.05 Helicopter explosion injuring occupant

  ✓7th V95.09 Other helicopter accident injuring occupant

✓5th V95.1 Ultralight, microlight or powered-glider accident injuring occupant

  ✓7th V95.10 Unspecified ultralight, microlight or powered-glider accident injuring occupant

  ✓7th V95.11 Ultralight, microlight or powered-glider crash injuring occupant

  ✓7th V95.12 Forced landing of ultralight, microlight or powered-glider injuring occupant

  ✓7th V95.13 Ultralight, microlight or powered-glider collision injuring occupant
> Ultralight, microlight or powered-glider collision with any object, fixed, movable or moving

  ✓7th V95.14 Ultralight, microlight or powered-glider fire injuring occupant

  ✓7th V95.15 Ultralight, microlight or powered-glider explosion injuring occupant

  ✓7th V95.19 Other ultralight, microlight or powered-glider accident injuring occupant

✓5th V95.2 Other private fixed-wing aircraft accident injuring occupant

  ✓7th V95.20 Unspecified accident to other private fixed-wing aircraft, injuring occupant

  ✓7th V95.21 Other private fixed-wing aircraft crash injuring occupant

  ✓7th V95.22 Forced landing of other private fixed-wing aircraft injuring occupant

  ✓7th V95.23 Other private fixed-wing aircraft collision injuring occupant
> Other private fixed-wing aircraft collision with any object, fixed, movable or moving

  ✓7th V95.24 Other private fixed-wing aircraft fire injuring occupant

  ✓7th V95.25 Other private fixed-wing aircraft explosion injuring occupant

  ✓7th V95.29 Other accident to other private fixed-wing aircraft injuring occupant

✓5th V95.3 Commercial fixed-wing aircraft accident injuring occupant

  ✓7th V95.30 Unspecified accident to commercial fixed-wing aircraft injuring occupant

  ✓7th V95.31 Commercial fixed-wing aircraft crash injuring occupant

  ✓7th V95.32 Forced landing of commercial fixed-wing aircraft injuring occupant

  ✓7th V95.33 Commercial fixed-wing aircraft collision injuring occupant
> Commercial fixed-wing aircraft collision with any object, fixed, movable or moving

  ✓7th V95.34 Commercial fixed-wing aircraft fire injuring occupant

  ✓7th V95.35 Commercial fixed-wing aircraft explosion injuring occupant

  ✓7th V95.39 Other accident to commercial fixed-wing aircraft injuring occupant

✓5th V95.4 Spacecraft accident injuring occupant

  ✓7th V95.40 Unspecified spacecraft accident injuring occupant

  ✓x7th V95.41 Spacecraft crash injuring occupant

  ✓x7th V95.42 Forced landing of spacecraft injuring occupant

  ✓x7th V95.43 Spacecraft collision injuring occupant
> Spacecraft collision with any object, fixed, moveable or moving

  ✓x7th V95.44 Spacecraft fire injuring occupant

  ✓x7th V95.45 Spacecraft explosion injuring occupant

  ✓x7th V95.49 Other spacecraft accident injuring occupant

✓x7th V95.8 Other powered aircraft accidents injuring occupant

✓x7th V95.9 Unspecified aircraft accident injuring occupant
> Aircraft accident NOS
> Air transport accident NOS

✓4th V96 Accident to nonpowered aircraft causing injury to occupant

> The appropriate 7th character is to be added to each code from category V96.
> A   initial encounter
> D   subsequent encounter
> S   sequela

✓5th V96.0 Balloon accident injuring occupant

  ✓x7th V96.00 Unspecified balloon accident injuring occupant

  ✓x7th V96.01 Balloon crash injuring occupant

  ✓x7th V96.02 Forced landing of balloon injuring occupant

  ✓x7th V96.03 Balloon collision injuring occupant
> Balloon collision with any object, fixed, moveable or moving

  ✓x7th V96.04 Balloon fire injuring occupant

  ✓x7th V96.05 Balloon explosion injuring occupant

  ✓x7th V96.09 Other balloon accident injuring occupant

✓5th V96.1 Hang-glider accident injuring occupant

  ✓x7th V96.10 Unspecified hang-glider accident injuring occupant

  ✓x7th V96.11 Hang-glider crash injuring occupant

  ✓x7th V96.12 Forced landing of hang-glider injuring occupant

  ✓x7th V96.13 Hang-glider collision injuring occupant
> Hang-glider collision with any object, fixed, moveable or moving

  ✓x7th V96.14 Hang-glider fire injuring occupant

  ✓x7th V96.15 Hang-glider explosion injuring occupant

  ✓x7th V96.19 Other hang-glider accident injuring occupant

✓5th V96.2 Glider (nonpowered) accident injuring occupant

  ✓x7th V96.20 Unspecified glider (nonpowered) accident injuring occupant

  ✓x7th V96.21 Glider (nonpowered) crash injuring occupant

  ✓x7th V96.22 Forced landing of glider (nonpowered) injuring occupant

  ✓x7th V96.23 Glider (nonpowered) collision injuring occupant
> Glider (nonpowered) collision with any object, fixed, moveable or moving

  ✓x7th V96.24 Glider (nonpowered) fire injuring occupant

  ✓x7th V96.25 Glider (nonpowered) explosion injuring occupant

  ✓x7th V96.29 Other glider (nonpowered) accident injuring occupant

✓x7th V96.8 Other nonpowered-aircraft accidents injuring occupant
> Kite carrying a person accident injuring occupant

✓x7th V96.9 Unspecified nonpowered-aircraft accident injuring occupant
> Nonpowered-aircraft accident NOS

✓4th V97 Other specified air transport accidents

> The appropriate 7th character is to be added to each code from category V97.
> A   initial encounter
> D   subsequent encounter
> S   sequela

✓x7th V97.0 Occupant of aircraft injured in other specified air transport accidents
> Fall in, on or from aircraft in air transport accident
> *EXCLUDES 1* accident while boarding or alighting aircraft (V97.1)

✓x7th V97.1 Person injured while boarding or alighting from aircraft

✓5th V97.2 Parachutist accident

  ✓x7th V97.21 Parachutist entangled in object
> Parachutist landing in tree

  ✓x7th V97.22 Parachutist injured on landing

EXCLUDES 1 Not coded here   *EXCLUDES 2* Not included here   N Newborn Age: 0   P Pediatric Age: 0-17   M Maternity Age: 12-55   A Adult Age: 15-12

1068   ICD-10-CM 20

   ✓7ᵗʰ **V97.29**   **Other parachutist accident**

✓5ᵗʰ **V97.3**   **Person on ground injured in air transport accident**

   ✓6ᵗʰ **V97.31**   **Hit by object falling from aircraft**
                Hit by crashing aircraft
                Injured by aircraft hitting house
                Injured by aircraft hitting car

   ✓x7ᵗʰ **V97.32**   **Injured by rotating propeller**

   ✓x7ᵗʰ **V97.33**   **Sucked into jet engine**

   ✓x7ᵗʰ **V97.39**   **Other injury to person on ground due to air transport accident**

✓5ᵗʰ **V97.8**   **Other air transport accidents, not elsewhere classified**
      EXCLUDES 1   *aircraft accident NOS (V95.9)*
                   exposure to changes in air pressure during ascent or descent (W94.-)

   ✓6ᵗʰ **V97.81**   **Air transport accident involving military aircraft**

      ✓7ᵗʰ **V97.810**   **Civilian aircraft involved in air transport accident with military aircraft**
                      Passenger in civilian aircraft injured due to accident with military aircraft

      ✓7ᵗʰ **V97.811**   **Civilian injured by military aircraft**

      ✓7ᵗʰ **V97.818**   **Other air transport accident involving military aircraft**

   ✓x7ᵗʰ **V97.89**   **Other air transport accidents, not elsewhere classified**
                Injury from machinery on aircraft

Other and unspecified transport accidents (V98-V99)

   EXCLUDES 1   *vehicle accident, type of vehicle unspecified (V89.-)*

4ᵗʰ **V98**   **Other specified transport accidents**

    The appropriate 7th character is to be added to each code from category V98.
    A   initial encounter
    D   subsequent encounter
    S   sequela

  ✓x7ᵗʰ **V98.0**   **Accident to, on or involving cable-car, not on rails**
              Caught or dragged by cable-car, not on rails
              Fall or jump from cable-car, not on rails
              Object thrown from or in cable-car, not on rails

  ✓x7ᵗʰ **V98.1**   **Accident to, on or involving land-yacht**

  ✓x7ᵗʰ **V98.2**   **Accident to, on or involving ice yacht**

  ✓x7ᵗʰ **V98.3**   **Accident to, on or involving ski lift**
              Accident to, on or involving ski chair-lift
              Accident to, on or involving ski-lift with gondola

  ✓x7ᵗʰ **V98.8**   **Other specified transport accidents**

x7ᵗʰ **V99**   **Unspecified transport accident**

    The appropriate 7th character is to be added to code V99.
    A   initial encounter
    D   subsequent encounter
    S   sequela

OTHER EXTERNAL CAUSES OF ACCIDENTAL INJURY (W00-X58)

Slipping, tripping, stumbling and falls (W00-W19)

   EXCLUDES 1   *assault involving a fall (Y01-Y02)*
                   fall from animal (V80.-)
                   fall (in) (from) machinery (in operation) (W28-W31)
                   fall (in) (from) transport vehicle (V01-V99)
                   intentional self-harm involving a fall (X80-X81)
   EXCLUDES 2   *at risk for fall (history of fall) (Z91.81)*
                   fall (in) (from) burning building (X00.-)
                   fall into fire (X00-X04, X08-X09)

4ᵗʰ **W00**   **Fall due to ice and snow**
      INCLUDES   pedestrian on foot falling (slipping) on ice and snow
      EXCLUDES 1   *fall on (from) ice and snow involving pedestrian conveyance (V00.-)*
                   fall from stairs and steps not due to ice and snow (W10.-)

    The appropriate 7th character is to be added to each code from category W00.
    A   initial encounter
    D   subsequent encounter
    S   sequela

  ✓x7ᵗʰ **W00.0**   **Fall on same level due to ice and snow**

  ✓x7ᵗʰ **W00.1**   **Fall from stairs and steps due to ice and snow**

  ✓x7ᵗʰ **W00.2**   **Other fall from one level to another due to ice and snow**

  ✓x7ᵗʰ **W00.9**   **Unspecified fall due to ice and snow**

✓4ᵗʰ **W01**   **Fall on same level from slipping, tripping and stumbling**
      INCLUDES   fall on moving sidewalk
      EXCLUDES 1   *fall due to bumping (striking) against object (W18.0-)*
                   fall in shower or bathtub (W18.2-)
                   fall on same level NOS (W18.30)
                   fall on same level from slipping, tripping and stumbling due to ice or snow (W00.0)
                   fall off or from toilet (W18.1-)
                   slipping, tripping and stumbling NOS (W18.40)
                   slipping, tripping and stumbling without falling (W18.4-)

    The appropriate 7th character is to be added to each code from category W01.
    A   initial encounter
    D   subsequent encounter
    S   sequela

  ✓x7ᵗʰ **W01.0**   **Fall on same level from slipping, tripping and stumbling without subsequent striking against object**
              Falling over animal

  ✓5ᵗʰ **W01.1**   **Fall on same level from slipping, tripping and stumbling with subsequent striking against object**

    ✓x7ᵗʰ **W01.10**   **Fall on same level from slipping, tripping and stumbling with subsequent striking against unspecified object**

    ✓6ᵗʰ **W01.11**   **Fall on same level from slipping, tripping and stumbling with subsequent striking against sharp object**

      ✓7ᵗʰ **W01.110**   **Fall on same level from slipping, tripping and stumbling with subsequent striking against sharp glass**

      ✓7ᵗʰ **W01.111**   **Fall on same level from slipping, tripping and stumbling with subsequent striking against power tool or machine**

      ✓7ᵗʰ **W01.118**   **Fall on same level from slipping, tripping and stumbling with subsequent striking against other sharp object**

      ✓7ᵗʰ **W01.119**   **Fall on same level from slipping, tripping and stumbling with subsequent striking against unspecified sharp object**

    ✓6ᵗʰ **W01.19**   **Fall on same level from slipping, tripping and stumbling with subsequent striking against other object**

      ✓7ᵗʰ **W01.190**   **Fall on same level from slipping, tripping and stumbling with subsequent striking against furniture**

      ✓7ᵗʰ **W01.198**   **Fall on same level from slipping, tripping and stumbling with subsequent striking against other object**

  ✓x7ᵗʰ **W03**   **Other fall on same level due to collision with another person**
         Fall due to non-transport collision with other person
      EXCLUDES 1   *collision with another person without fall (W51)*
                   crushed or pushed by a crowd or human stampede (W52)
                   fall involving pedestrian conveyance (V00-V09)
                   fall due to ice or snow (W00)
                   fall on same level NOS (W18.30)
     AHA: 2012, 4Q, 108

    The appropriate 7th character is to be added to code W03.
    A   initial encounter
    D   subsequent encounter
    S   sequela

  ✓x7ᵗʰ **W04**   **Fall while being carried or supported by other persons**
         Accidentally dropped while being carried

    The appropriate 7th character is to be added to code W04.
    A   initial encounter
    D   subsequent encounter
    S   sequela

✓ Additional Character Required   x7ᵗʰ Placeholder Alert   Unspecified Dx   Other Specified Dx   Manifestation   ▶◀ Revised Text   ● New Code   ▲ Revised Code Title

✓4th **W05 Fall from non-moving wheelchair, nonmotorized scooter and motorized mobility scooter**

> EXCLUDES 1   *fall from moving wheelchair (powered) (V00.811)*
> *fall from moving motorized mobility scooter (V00.831)*
> *fall from nonmotorized scooter (V00.141)*

> The appropriate 7th character is to be added to each code from category W05.
> A   initial encounter
> D   subsequent encounter
> S   sequela

✓x7th **W05.0 Fall from non-moving wheelchair**

✓x7th **W05.1 Fall from non-moving nonmotorized scooter**

✓x7th **W05.2 Fall from non-moving motorized mobility scooter**

✓x7th **W06 Fall from bed**

> The appropriate 7th character is to be added to code W06.
> A   initial encounter
> D   subsequent encounter
> S   sequela

✓x7th **W07 Fall from chair**

> The appropriate 7th character is to be added to code W07.
> A   initial encounter
> D   subsequent encounter
> S   sequela

✓x7th **W08 Fall from other furniture**

> The appropriate 7th character is to be added to code W08.
> A   initial encounter
> D   subsequent encounter
> S   sequela

✓4th **W09 Fall on and from playground equipment**

> EXCLUDES 1   *fall involving recreational machinery (W31)*

> The appropriate 7th character is to be added to each code from category W09.
> A   initial encounter
> D   subsequent encounter
> S   sequela

✓x7th **W09.0 Fall on or from playground slide**

✓x7th **W09.1 Fall from playground swing**

✓x7th **W09.2 Fall on or from jungle gym**

✓x7th **W09.8 Fall on or from other playground equipment**

✓4th **W10 Fall on and from stairs and steps**

> EXCLUDES 1   *Fall from stairs and steps due to ice and snow (W00.1)*

> The appropriate 7th character is to be added to each code from category W10.
> A   initial encounter
> D   subsequent encounter
> S   sequela

✓x7th **W10.0 Fall (on)(from) escalator**

✓x7th **W10.1 Fall (on)(from) sidewalk curb**

✓x7th **W10.2 Fall (on)(from) incline**
> Fall (on) (from) ramp

✓x7th **W10.8 Fall (on) (from) other stairs and steps**

✓x7th **W10.9 Fall (on) (from) unspecified stairs and steps**

✓x7th **W11 Fall on and from ladder**

> The appropriate 7th character is to be added code W11.
> A   initial encounter
> D   subsequent encounter
> S   sequela

✓x7th **W12 Fall on and from scaffolding**

> The appropriate 7th character is to be added code W12.
> A   initial encounter
> D   subsequent encounter
> S   sequela

✓4th **W13 Fall from, out of or through building or structure**

> The appropriate 7th character is to be added to each code from category W13.
> A   initial encounter
> D   subsequent encounter
> S   sequela

✓x7th **W13.0 Fall from, out of or through balcony**
> Fall from, out of or through railing

✓x7th **W13.1 Fall from, out of or through bridge**

✓x7th **W13.2 Fall from, out of or through roof**

✓x7th **W13.3 Fall through floor**

✓x7th **W13.4 Fall from, out of or through window**

> EXCLUDES 2   *fall with subsequent striking against sharp glass (W01.110)*

✓x7th **W13.8 Fall from, out of or through other building or structure**
> Fall from, out of or through viaduct
> Fall from, out of or through wall
> Fall from, out of or through flag-pole

✓x7th **W13.9 Fall from, out of or through building, not otherwise specified**

> EXCLUDES 1   *collapse of a building or structure (W20.-)*
> *fall or jump from burning building or structure (X00.-)*

✓x7th **W14 Fall from tree**

> The appropriate 7th character is to be added to code W14.
> A   initial encounter
> D   subsequent encounter
> S   sequela

✓x7th **W15 Fall from cliff**

> The appropriate 7th character is to be added to code W15.
> A   initial encounter
> D   subsequent encounter
> S   sequela

✓4th **W16 Fall, jump or diving into water**

> EXCLUDES 1   *accidental non-watercraft drowning and submersion not involving fall (W65-W74)*
> *effects of air pressure from diving (W94.-)*
> *fall into water from watercraft (V90-V94)*
> *hitting an object or against bottom when falling from watercraft (V94.0)*

> EXCLUDES 2   *striking or hitting diving board (W21.4)*

> The appropriate 7th character is to be added to each code from category W16.
> A   initial encounter
> D   subsequent encounter
> S   sequela

✓5th **W16.0 Fall into swimming pool**
> Fall into swimming pool NOS
> EXCLUDES 1   *fall into empty swimming pool (W17.3)*

✓6th **W16.01 Fall into swimming pool striking water surface**

✓7th **W16.011 Fall into swimming pool striking water surface causing drowning and submersion**
> EXCLUDES 1   *drowning and submersion while in swimming pool without fall (W67)*

✓7th **W16.012 Fall into swimming pool striking water surface causing other injury**

✓6th **W16.02 Fall into swimming pool striking bottom**

✓7th **W16.021 Fall into swimming pool striking bottom causing drowning and submersion**
> EXCLUDES 1   *drowning and submersion while in swimming pool without fall (W67)*

✓7th **W16.022 Fall into swimming pool striking bottom causing other injury**

✓6th **W16.03 Fall into swimming pool striking wall**

✓7th **W16.031 Fall into swimming pool striking wall causing drowning and submersion**
> EXCLUDES 1   *drowning and submersion while in swimming pool without fall (W67)*

✓7th **W16.032 Fall into swimming pool striking wall causing other injury**

EXCLUDES 1 Not coded here   EXCLUDES 2 Not included here   N Newborn Age: 0   P Pediatric Age: 0-17   M Maternity Age: 12-55   A Adult Age: 15-124

1070   ICD-10-CM 201

✓5ᵗʰ W16.1 Fall into natural body of water
    Fall into lake
    Fall into open sea
    Fall into river
    Fall into stream

    ✓6ᵗʰ W16.11 Fall into natural body of water striking water surface

        ✓7ᵗʰ W16.111 Fall into natural body of water striking water surface causing drowning and submersion
            EXCLUDES 1 drowning and submersion while in natural body of water without fall (W69)

        ✓7ᵗʰ W16.112 Fall into natural body of water striking water surface causing other injury

    ✓6ᵗʰ W16.12 Fall into natural body of water striking bottom

        ✓7ᵗʰ W16.121 Fall into natural body of water striking bottom causing drowning and submersion
            EXCLUDES 1 drowning and submersion while in natural body of water without fall (W69)

        ✓7ᵗʰ W16.122 Fall into natural body of water striking bottom causing other injury

    ✓6ᵗʰ W16.13 Fall into natural body of water striking side

        ✓7ᵗʰ W16.131 Fall into natural body of water striking side causing drowning and submersion
            EXCLUDES 1 drowning and submersion while in natural body of water without fall (W69)

        ✓7ᵗʰ W16.132 Fall into natural body of water striking side causing other injury

✓5ᵗʰ W16.2 Fall in (into) filled bathtub or bucket of water

    ✓6ᵗʰ W16.21 Fall in (into) filled bathtub
        EXCLUDES 1 fall into empty bathtub (W18.2)

        ✓7ᵗʰ W16.211 Fall in (into) filled bathtub causing drowning and submersion
            EXCLUDES 1 drowning and submersion while in filled bathtub without fall (W65)

        ✓7ᵗʰ W16.212 Fall in (into) filled bathtub causing other injury

    ✓6ᵗʰ W16.22 Fall in (into) bucket of water

        ✓7ᵗʰ W16.221 Fall in (into) bucket of water causing drowning and submersion

        ✓7ᵗʰ W16.222 Fall in (into) bucket of water causing other injury

✓5ᵗʰ W16.3 Fall into other water
    Fall into fountain
    Fall into reservoir

    ✓6ᵗʰ W16.31 Fall into other water striking water surface

        ✓7ᵗʰ W16.311 Fall into other water striking water surface causing drowning and submersion
            EXCLUDES 1 drowning and submersion while in other water without fall (W73)

        ✓7ᵗʰ W16.312 Fall into other water striking water surface causing other injury

    ✓6ᵗʰ W16.32 Fall into other water striking bottom

        ✓7ᵗʰ W16.321 Fall into other water striking bottom causing drowning and submersion
            EXCLUDES 1 drowning and submersion while in other water without fall (W73)

        ✓7ᵗʰ W16.322 Fall into other water striking bottom causing other injury

    ✓6ᵗʰ W16.33 Fall into other water striking wall

        ✓7ᵗʰ W16.331 Fall into other water striking wall causing drowning and submersion
            EXCLUDES 1 drowning and submersion while in other water without fall (W73)

        ✓7ᵗʰ W16.332 Fall into other water striking wall causing other injury

✓5ᵗʰ W16.4 Fall into unspecified water

    ✓×7ᵗʰ W16.41 Fall into unspecified water causing drowning and submersion

    ✓×7ᵗʰ W16.42 Fall into unspecified water causing other injury

✓5ᵗʰ W16.5 Jumping or diving into swimming pool

    ✓6ᵗʰ W16.51 Jumping or diving into swimming pool striking water surface

        ✓7ᵗʰ W16.511 Jumping or diving into swimming pool striking water surface causing drowning and submersion
            EXCLUDES 1 drowning and submersion while in swimming pool without jumping or diving (W67)

        ✓7ᵗʰ W16.512 Jumping or diving into swimming pool striking water surface causing other injury

    ✓6ᵗʰ W16.52 Jumping or diving into swimming pool striking bottom

        ✓7ᵗʰ W16.521 Jumping or diving into swimming pool striking bottom causing drowning and submersion
            EXCLUDES 1 drowning and submersion while in swimming pool without jumping or diving (W67)

        ✓7ᵗʰ W16.522 Jumping or diving into swimming pool striking bottom causing other injury

    ✓6ᵗʰ W16.53 Jumping or diving into swimming pool striking wall

        ✓7ᵗʰ W16.531 Jumping or diving into swimming pool striking wall causing drowning and submersion
            EXCLUDES 1 drowning and submersion while in swimming pool without jumping or diving (W67)

        ✓7ᵗʰ W16.532 Jumping or diving into swimming pool striking wall causing other injury

✓5ᵗʰ W16.6 Jumping or diving into natural body of water
    Jumping or diving into lake
    Jumping or diving into open sea
    Jumping or diving into river
    Jumping or diving into stream

    ✓6ᵗʰ W16.61 Jumping or diving into natural body of water striking water surface

        ✓7ᵗʰ W16.611 Jumping or diving into natural body of water striking water surface causing drowning and submersion
            EXCLUDES 1 drowning and submersion while in natural body of water without jumping or diving (W69)

        ✓7ᵗʰ W16.612 Jumping or diving into natural body of water striking water surface causing other injury

    ✓6ᵗʰ W16.62 Jumping or diving into natural body of water striking bottom

        ✓7ᵗʰ W16.621 Jumping or diving into natural body of water striking bottom causing drowning and submersion
            EXCLUDES 1 drowning and submersion while in natural body of water without jumping or diving (W69)

        ✓7ᵗʰ W16.622 Jumping or diving into natural body of water striking bottom causing other injury

✓5ᵗʰ W16.7 Jumping or diving from boat
    EXCLUDES 1 Fall from boat into water—see watercraft accident (V90-V94)

    ✓6ᵗʰ W16.71 Jumping or diving from boat striking water surface

        ✓7ᵗʰ W16.711 Jumping or diving from boat striking water surface causing drowning and submersion

        ✓7ᵗʰ W16.712 Jumping or diving from boat striking water surface causing other injury

    ✓6ᵗʰ W16.72 Jumping or diving from boat striking bottom

        ✓7ᵗʰ W16.721 Jumping or diving from boat striking bottom causing drowning and submersion

        ✓7ᵗʰ W16.722 Jumping or diving from boat striking bottom causing other injury

---

◼ Additional Character Required   ✓×7ᵗʰ Placeholder Alert   Unspecified Dx   Other Specified Dx   Manifestation   ▶◀ Revised Text   ● New Code   ▲ Revised Code Title

Chapter 20. External Causes of Morbidity *(side margin)*

✓5ᵗʰ **W16.8 Jumping or diving** into other water
    Jumping or diving into fountain
    Jumping or diving into reservoir

  ✓6ᵗʰ **W16.81 Jumping or diving into other water** striking water surface

    ✓7ᵗʰ **W16.811 Jumping or diving into other water striking water surface causing** drowning and submersion
        EXCLUDES 1 *drowning and submersion while in other water without jumping or diving (W73)*

    ✓7ᵗʰ **W16.812 Jumping or diving into other water striking water surface causing other injury**

  ✓6ᵗʰ **W16.82 Jumping or diving into other water** striking bottom

    ✓7ᵗʰ **W16.821 Jumping or diving into other water striking bottom causing** drowning **and** submersion
        EXCLUDES 1 *drowning and submersion while in other water without jumping or diving (W73)*

    ✓7ᵗʰ **W16.822 Jumping or diving into other water striking bottom causing other injury**

  ✓6ᵗʰ **W16.83 Jumping or diving into other water** striking wall

    ✓7ᵗʰ **W16.831 Jumping or diving into other water striking wall causing** drowning **and** submersion
        EXCLUDES 1 *drowning and submersion while in other water without jumping or diving (W73)*

    ✓7ᵗʰ **W16.832 Jumping or diving into other water striking wall causing other injury**

✓5ᵗʰ **W16.9 Jumping or diving into** unspecified **water**

  ✓x7ᵗʰ **W16.91 Jumping or diving into unspecified water causing** drowning **and submersion**

  ✓x7ᵗʰ **W16.92 Jumping or diving into unspecified water causing other injury**

✓4ᵗʰ **W17 Other fall from one level to another**

> The appropriate 7th character is to be added to each code from category W17.
> A   initial encounter
> D   subsequent encounter
> S   sequela

✓x7ᵗʰ **W17.0 Fall into well**

✓x7ᵗʰ **W17.1 Fall into storm drain or manhole**

✓x7ᵗʰ **W17.2 Fall into hole**
    Fall into pit

✓x7ᵗʰ **W17.3 Fall into empty swimming pool**
    EXCLUDES 1 *fall into filled swimming pool (W16.0-)*

✓x7ᵗʰ **W17.4 Fall from dock**

✓5ᵗʰ **W17.8 Other fall from one level to another**

  ✓x7ᵗʰ **W17.81 Fall down embankment (hill)**

  ✓x7ᵗʰ **W17.82 Fall from (out of) grocery cart**
    Fall due to grocery cart tipping over

  ✓x7ᵗʰ **W17.89 Other fall from one level to another**
    Fall from cherry picker
    Fall from lifting device
    Fall from mobile elevated work platform [MEWP]
    Fall from sky lift

✓4ᵗʰ **W18 Other slipping, tripping and stumbling and falls**

> The appropriate 7th character is to be added to each code from category W18.
> A   initial encounter
> D   subsequent encounter
> S   sequela

✓5ᵗʰ **W18.0 Fall due to bumping against object**
    Striking against object with subsequent fall
    EXCLUDES 1 *fall on same level due to slipping, tripping, or stumbling with subsequent striking against object (W01.1-)*

  ✓x7ᵗʰ **W18.00 Striking against unspecified object with subsequent fall**

  ✓x7ᵗʰ **W18.01 Striking against** sports equipment **with subsequent fall**

  ✓x7ᵗʰ **W18.02 Striking against** glass **with subsequent fall**

  ✓x7ᵗʰ **W18.09 Striking against other object with subsequent fall**

✓5ᵗʰ **W18.1 Fall from or off toilet**

  ✓x7ᵗʰ **W18.11 Fall from or off toilet** without subsequent striking against object
    Fall from (off) toilet NOS

  ✓x7ᵗʰ **W18.12 Fall from or off toilet** with subsequent striking against object

✓x7ᵗʰ **W18.2 Fall in (into) shower or empty bathtub**
    EXCLUDES 1 *fall in full bathtub causing drowning or submersion (W16.21-)*

✓5ᵗʰ **W18.3 Other and unspecified fall on same level**

  ✓x7ᵗʰ **W18.30 Fall on same level, unspecified**

  ✓x7ᵗʰ **W18.31 Fall on same level due to stepping on an object**
    Fall on same level due to stepping on an animal
    EXCLUDES 1 *slipping, tripping and stumbling without fa due to stepping on animal (W18.41)*

  ✓x7ᵗʰ **W18.39 Other fall on same level**

✓5ᵗʰ **W18.4 Slipping, tripping and stumbling without falling**
    EXCLUDES 1 *collision with another person without fall (W51)*

  ✓x7ᵗʰ **W18.40 Slipping, tripping and stumbling without falling, unspecified**

  ✓x7ᵗʰ **W18.41 Slipping, tripping and stumbling without falling d** to stepping on object
    Slipping, tripping and stumbling without falling due to stepping on animal
    EXCLUDES 1 *slipping, tripping and stumbling with fall d to stepping on animal (W18.31)*

  ✓x7ᵗʰ **W18.42 Slipping, tripping and stumbling without falling d** to stepping into hole or opening

  ✓x7ᵗʰ **W18.43 Slipping, tripping and stumbling without falling d** to stepping from one level to another

  ✓x7ᵗʰ **W18.49 Other slipping, tripping and stumbling without falling**

✓x7ᵗʰ **W19 Unspecified fall**
    Accidental fall NOS
    AHA: 2012, 4Q, 95

> The appropriate 7th character is to be added to code W19.
> A   initial encounter
> D   subsequent encounter
> S   sequela

Exposure to inanimate mechanical forces (W20-W49)

EXCLUDES 1 *assault (X92-Y08)*
    contact or collision with animals or persons (W50-W64)
    exposure to inanimate mechanical forces involving military or war operations (Y36-, Y37-)
    intentional self-harm (X71-X83)

✓4ᵗʰ **W20 Struck by thrown, projected or falling object**
    Code first any associated:
    cataclysm (X34-X39)
    lightning strike (T75.00)
    EXCLUDES 1 *falling object in machinery accident (W24, W28-W31)*
      falling object in transport accident (V01-V99)
      object set in motion by explosion (W35-W40)
      object set in motion by firearm (W32-W34)
      struck by thrown sports equipment (W21.-)

> The appropriate 7th character is to be added to each code from category W20.
> A   initial encounter
> D   subsequent encounter
> S   sequela

✓x7ᵗʰ **W20.0 Struck by falling object in cave-in**
    EXCLUDES 2 *asphyxiation due to cave-in (T71.21)*

✓x7ᵗʰ **W20.1 Struck by object due to collapse of building**
    EXCLUDES 1 *struck by object due to collapse of burning building (X00.2, X02.2)*

✓x7ᵗʰ **W20.8 Other cause of strike by thrown, projected or falling object**
    EXCLUDES 1 *struck by thrown sports equipment (W21.-)*

EXCLUDES 1 Not coded here   *EXCLUDES 2* Not included here   N Newborn Age: 0   P Pediatric Age: 0-17   M Maternity Age: 12-55   A Adult Age: 15-12

1072   ICD-10-CM 20

W21 Striking against or struck by sports equipment

> EXCLUDES 1   *assault with sports equipment (YØ8.Ø-)*
> *striking against or struck by sports equipment with subsequent fall (W18.Ø1)*

> The appropriate 7th character is to be added to each code from category W21.
> A   initial encounter
> D   subsequent encounter
> S   sequela

✓5th **W21.Ø Struck by hit or thrown ball**

   ✓x7th **W21.ØØ Struck by hit or thrown ball, unspecified type**

   ✓x7th **W21.Ø1 Struck by football**

   ✓x7th **W21.Ø2 Struck by soccer ball**

   ✓x7th **W21.Ø3 Struck by baseball**

   ✓x7th **W21.Ø4 Struck by golf ball**

   ✓x7th **W21.Ø5 Struck by basketball**

   ✓x7th **W21.Ø6 Struck by volleyball**

   ✓x7th **W21.Ø7 Struck by softball**

   ✓x7th **W21.Ø9 Struck by other hit or thrown ball**

✓5th **W21.1 Struck by bat, racquet or club**

   ✓x7th **W21.11 Struck by baseball bat**

   ✓x7th **W21.12 Struck by tennis racquet**

   ✓x7th **W21.13 Struck by golf club**

   ✓x7th **W21.19 Struck by other bat, racquet or club**

✓5th **W21.2 Struck by hockey stick or puck**

   ✓6th **W21.21 Struck by hockey stick**

      ✓7th **W21.21Ø Struck by ice hockey stick**

      ✓7th **W21.211 Struck by field hockey stick**

   ✓6th **W21.22 Struck by hockey puck**

      ✓7th **W21.22Ø Struck by ice hockey puck**

      ✓7th **W21.221 Struck by field hockey puck**

✓5th **W21.3 Struck by sports foot wear**

   ✓x7th **W21.31 Struck by shoe cleats**
      Stepped on by shoe cleats

   ✓x7th **W21.32 Struck by skate blades**
      Skated over by skate blades

   ✓x7th **W21.39 Struck by other sports foot wear**

✓x7th **W21.4 Striking against diving board**
   Use additional code for subsequent falling into water, if applicable (W16.-)

✓5th **W21.8 Striking against or struck by other sports equipment**

   ✓x7th **W21.81 Striking against or struck by football helmet**

   ✓x7th **W21.89 Striking against or struck by other sports equipment**

✓x7th **W21.9 Striking against or struck by unspecified sports equipment**

W22 Striking against or struck by other objects

> EXCLUDES 1   *striking against or struck by object with subsequent fall (W18.Ø9)*

> The appropriate 7th character is to be added to each code from category W22.
> A   initial encounter
> D   subsequent encounter
> S   sequela

✓5th **W22.Ø Striking against stationary object**

>   EXCLUDES 1   *striking against stationary sports equipment (W21.8)*

   ✓x7th **W22.Ø1 Walked into wall**

   ✓x7th **W22.Ø2 Walked into lamppost**

   ✓x7th **W22.Ø3 Walked into furniture**

   ✓6th **W22.Ø4 Striking against wall of swimming pool**

      ✓7th **W22.Ø41 Striking against wall of swimming pool causing drowning and submersion**
         EXCLUDES 1   *drowning and submersion while swimming without striking against wall (W67)*

      ✓7th **W22.Ø42 Striking against wall of swimming pool causing other injury**

   ✓x7th **W22.Ø9 Striking against other stationary object**

✓5th **W22.1 Striking against or struck by automobile airbag**

   ✓x7th **W22.1Ø Striking against or struck by unspecified automobile airbag**

   ✓x7th **W22.11 Striking against or struck by driver side automobile airbag**

   ✓x7th **W22.12 Striking against or struck by front passenger side automobile airbag**

   ✓x7th **W22.19 Striking against or struck by other automobile airbag**

✓x7th **W22.8 Striking against or struck by other objects**
   Striking against or struck by object NOS
>   EXCLUDES 1   *struck by thrown, projected or falling object (W2Ø.-)*

W23 Caught, crushed, jammed or pinched in or between objects

> EXCLUDES 1   *injury caused by cutting or piercing instruments (W25-W27)*
> *injury caused by firearms malfunction (W32.1, W33.1-, W34.1-)*
> *injury caused by lifting and transmission devices (W24.-)*
> *injury caused by machinery (W28-W31)*
> *injury caused by nonpowered hand tools (W27.-)*
> *injury caused by transport vehicle being used as a means of transportation (VØ1-V99)*
> *injury caused by struck by thrown, projected or falling object (W2Ø.-)*

> The appropriate 7th character is to be added to each code from category W23.
> A   initial encounter
> D   subsequent encounter
> S   sequela

✓x7th **W23.Ø Caught, crushed, jammed, or pinched between moving objects**

✓x7th **W23.1 Caught, crushed, jammed, or pinched between stationary objects**

W24 Contact with lifting and transmission devices, not elsewhere classified

> EXCLUDES 1   *transport accidents (VØ1-V99)*

> The appropriate 7th character is to be added to each code from category W24.
> A   initial encounter
> D   subsequent encounter
> S   sequela

✓x7th **W24.Ø Contact with lifting devices, not elsewhere classified**
   Contact with chain hoist
   Contact with drive belt
   Contact with pulley (block)

✓x7th **W24.1 Contact with transmission devices, not elsewhere classified**
   Contact with transmission belt or cable

W25 Contact with sharp glass

   Code first any associated:
      injury due to flying glass from explosion or firearm discharge (W32-W4Ø)
   transport accident (VØØ-V99)
> EXCLUDES 1   *fall on same level due to slipping, tripping and stumbling with subsequent striking against sharp glass (WØ1.1Ø)*
> *striking against sharp glass with subsequent fall (W18.Ø2)*

> The appropriate 7th character is to be added to code W25.
> A   initial encounter
> D   subsequent encounter
> S   sequela

W26 Contact with knife, sword or dagger

> The appropriate 7th character is to be added to each code from category W26.
> A   initial encounter
> D   subsequent encounter
> S   sequela

✓x7th **W26.Ø Contact with knife**
>   EXCLUDES 1   *contact with electric knife (W29.1)*

✓x7th **W26.1 Contact with sword or dagger**

W27 Contact with nonpowered hand tool

> The appropriate 7th character is to be added to each code from category W27.
> A   initial encounter
> D   subsequent encounter
> S   sequela

✓x7th **W27.Ø Contact with workbench tool**
   Contact with auger
   Contact with axe
   Contact with chisel
   Contact with handsaw
   Contact with screwdriver

✓ Additional Character Required   ✓x7th Placeholder Alert   Unspecified Dx   Other Specified Dx   Manifestation   ▶◀ Revised Text   ● New Code   ▲ Revised Code Title

√x 7ᵗʰ **W27.1 Contact with garden tool**
Contact with hoe
Contact with nonpowered lawn mower
Contact with pitchfork
Contact with rake

√x 7ᵗʰ **W27.2 Contact with scissors**

√x 7ᵗʰ **W27.3 Contact with needle (sewing)**
EXCLUDES 1   *contact with hypodermic needle (W46.-)*

√x 7ᵗʰ **W27.4 Contact with kitchen utensil**
Contact with fork
Contact with ice-pick
Contact with can-opener NOS

√x 7ᵗʰ **W27.5 Contact with paper-cutter**

√x 7ᵗʰ **W27.8 Contact with other nonpowered hand tool**
Contact with nonpowered sewing machine
Contact with shovel

√x 7ᵗʰ **W28 Contact with powered lawn mower**
Powered lawn mower (commercial) (residential)
EXCLUDES 1   *contact with nonpowered lawn mower (W27.1)*
EXCLUDES 2   *exposure to electric current (W86.-)*

> The appropriate 7th character is to be added to code W28.
> A   initial encounter
> D   subsequent encounter
> S   sequela

√ 4ᵗʰ **W29 Contact with other powered hand tools and household machinery**
EXCLUDES 1   *contact with commercial machinery (W31.82)*
contact with hot household appliance (X15)
contact with nonpowered hand tool (W27.-)
exposure to electric current (W86)

> The appropriate 7th character is to be added to each code from category W29.
> A   initial encounter
> D   subsequent encounter
> S   sequela

√x 7ᵗʰ **W29.0 Contact with powered kitchen appliance**
Contact with blender
Contact with can-opener
Contact with garbage disposal
Contact with mixer

√x 7ᵗʰ **W29.1 Contact with electric knife**

√x 7ᵗʰ **W29.2 Contact with other powered household machinery**
Contact with electric fan
Contact with powered dryer (clothes) (powered) (spin)
Contact with washing-machine
Contact with sewing machine

√x 7ᵗʰ **W29.3 Contact with powered garden and outdoor hand tools and machinery**
Contact with chainsaw
Contact with edger
Contact with garden cultivator (tiller)
Contact with hedge trimmer
Contact with other powered garden tool
EXCLUDES 1   *contact with powered lawn mower (W28)*

√x 7ᵗʰ **W29.4 Contact with nail gun**

√x 7ᵗʰ **W29.8 Contact with other powered hand tools and household machinery**
Contact with do-it-yourself tool NOS

√ 4ᵗʰ **W30 Contact with agricultural machinery**
INCLUDES   animal-powered farm machine
EXCLUDES 1   *agricultural transport vehicle accident (V01-V99)*
explosion of grain store (W40.8)
exposure to electric current (W86.-)

> The appropriate 7th character is to be added to each code from category W30.
> A   initial encounter
> D   subsequent encounter
> S   sequela

√x 7ᵗʰ **W30.0 Contact with combine harvester**
Contact with reaper
Contact with thresher

√x 7ᵗʰ **W30.1 Contact with power take-off devices (PTO)**

√x 7ᵗʰ **W30.2 Contact with hay derrick**

√x 7ᵗʰ **W30.3 Contact with grain storage elevator**
EXCLUDES 1   *explosion of grain store (W40.8)*

√ 5ᵗʰ **W30.8 Contact with other specified agricultural machinery**

√x 7ᵗʰ **W30.81 Contact with agricultural transport vehicle in stationary use**
Contact with agricultural transport vehicle under repair, not on public roadway
EXCLUDES 1   *agricultural transport vehicle accident (V01-V99)*

√x 7ᵗʰ **W30.89 Contact with other specified agricultural machinery**

√x 7ᵗʰ **W30.9 Contact with unspecified agricultural machinery**
Contact with farm machinery NOS

√ 4ᵗʰ **W31 Contact with other and unspecified machinery**
EXCLUDES 1   *contact with agricultural machinery (W30.-)*
contact with machinery in transport under own power or being towed by a vehicle (V01-V99)
exposure to electric current (W86)

> The appropriate 7th character is to be added to each code from category W31.
> A   initial encounter
> D   subsequent encounter
> S   sequela

√x 7ᵗʰ **W31.0 Contact with mining and earth-drilling machinery**
Contact with bore or drill (land) (seabed)
Contact with shaft hoist
Contact with shaft lift
Contact with undercutter

√x 7ᵗʰ **W31.1 Contact with metalworking machines**
Contact with abrasive wheel
Contact with forging machine
Contact with lathe
Contact with mechanical shears
Contact with metal drilling machine
Contact with milling machine
Contact with power press
Contact with rolling-mill
Contact with metal sawing machine

√x 7ᵗʰ **W31.2 Contact with powered woodworking and forming machines**
Contact with band saw
Contact with bench saw
Contact with circular saw
Contact with molding machine
Contact with overhead plane
Contact with powered saw
Contact with radial saw
Contact with sander
EXCLUDES 1   *nonpowered woodworking tools (W27.0)*

√x 7ᵗʰ **W31.3 Contact with prime movers**
Contact with gas turbine
Contact with internal combustion engine
Contact with steam engine
Contact with water driven turbine

√ 5ᵗʰ **W31.8 Contact with other specified machinery**

√x 7ᵗʰ **W31.81 Contact with recreational machinery**
Contact with roller coaster

√x 7ᵗʰ **W31.82 Contact with other commercial machinery**
Contact with commercial electric fan
Contact with commercial kitchen appliances
Contact with commercial powered dryer (clothes) (powered) (spin)
Contact with commercial washing-machine
Contact with commercial sewing machine
EXCLUDES 1   *contact with household machinery (W29.-)*
contact with powered lawn mower (W28)

√x 7ᵗʰ **W31.83 Contact with special construction vehicle in stationary use**
Contact with special construction vehicle under repair, not on public roadway
EXCLUDES 1   *special construction vehicle accident (V01-V99)*

√x 7ᵗʰ **W31.89 Contact with other specified machinery**

√x 7ᵗʰ **W31.9 Contact with unspecified machinery**
Contact with machinery NOS

EXCLUDES 1 Not coded here   EXCLUDES 2 Not included here   N Newborn Age: 0   P Pediatric Age: 0-17   M Maternity Age: 12-55   A Adult Age: 15-12

1074

ICD-10-CM 201

W32 Accidental handgun discharge and malfunction
> INCLUDES   accidental discharge and malfunction of gun for single hand use
> accidental discharge and malfunction of pistol
> accidental discharge and malfunction of revolver
> handgun discharge and malfunction NOS

> EXCLUDES 1   accidental airgun discharge and malfunction (W34.010, W34.110)
> accidental BB gun discharge and malfunction (W34.010, W34.110)
> accidental pellet gun discharge and malfunction (W34.010, W34.110)
> accidental shotgun discharge and malfunction (W33.01, W33.11)
> assault by handgun discharge (X93)
> handgun discharge involving legal intervention (Y35.0-)
> handgun discharge involving military or war operations (Y36.4-)
> intentional self-harm by handgun discharge (X72)
> Very pistol discharge and malfunction (W34.09, W34.19)

> The appropriate 7th character is to be added to each code from category W32.
> A   initial encounter
> D   subsequent encounter
> S   sequela

√x 7th   **W32.0 Accidental handgun discharge**

√x 7th   **W32.1 Accidental handgun malfunction**
> Injury due to explosion of handgun (parts)
> Injury due to malfunction of mechanism or component of handgun
> Injury due to recoil of handgun
> Powder burn from handgun

W33 Accidental rifle, shotgun and larger firearm discharge and malfunction
> INCLUDES   rifle, shotgun and larger firearm discharge and malfunction NOS
> EXCLUDES 1   accidental airgun discharge and malfunction (W34.010, W34.110)
> accidental BB gun discharge and malfunction (W34.010, W34.110)
> accidental handgun discharge and malfunction (W32.-)
> accidental pellet gun discharge and malfunction (W34.010, W34.110)
> assault by rifle, shotgun and larger firearm discharge (X94)
> firearm discharge involving legal intervention (Y35.0-)
> firearm discharge involving military or war operations (Y36.4-)
> intentional self-harm by rifle, shotgun and larger firearm discharge (X73)

> The appropriate 7th character is to be added to each code from category W33.
> A   initial encounter
> D   subsequent encounter
> S   sequela

√5th   **W33.0 Accidental rifle, shotgun and larger firearm discharge**

√x 7th   **W33.00 Accidental discharge of unspecified larger firearm**
> Discharge of unspecified larger firearm NOS

√x 7th   **W33.01 Accidental discharge of shotgun**
> Discharge of shotgun NOS

√x 7th   **W33.02 Accidental discharge of hunting rifle**
> Discharge of hunting rifle NOS

√x 7th   **W33.03 Accidental discharge of machine gun**
> Discharge of machine gun NOS

√x 7th   **W33.09 Accidental discharge of other larger firearm**
> Discharge of other larger firearm NOS

√5th   **W33.1 Accidental rifle, shotgun and larger firearm malfunction**
> Injury due to explosion of rifle, shotgun and larger firearm (parts)
> Injury due to malfunction of mechanism or component of rifle, shotgun and larger firearm
> Injury due to piercing, cutting, crushing or pinching due to (by) slide trigger mechanism, scope or other gun part
> Injury due to recoil of rifle, shotgun and larger firearm
> Powder burn from rifle, shotgun and larger firearm

√x 7th   **W33.10 Accidental malfunction of unspecified larger firearm**
> Malfunction of unspecified larger firearm NOS

√x 7th   **W33.11 Accidental malfunction of shotgun**
> Malfunction of shotgun NOS

√x 7th   **W33.12 Accidental malfunction of hunting rifle**
> Malfunction of hunting rifle NOS

√x 7th   **W33.13 Accidental malfunction of machine gun**
> Malfunction of machine gun NOS

√x 7th   **W33.19 Accidental malfunction of other larger firearm**
> Malfunction of other larger firearm NOS

√4th   **W34 Accidental discharge and malfunction from other and unspecified firearms and guns**

> The appropriate 7th character is to be added to each code from category W34.
> A   initial encounter
> D   subsequent encounter
> S   sequela

√5th   **W34.0 Accidental discharge from other and unspecified firearms and guns**

√x 7th   **W34.00 Accidental discharge from unspecified firearms or gun**
> Discharge from firearm NOS
> Gunshot wound NOS
> Shot NOS

√6th   **W34.01 Accidental discharge of gas, air or spring-operated guns**

√7th   **W34.010 Accidental discharge of airgun**
> Accidental discharge of BB gun
> Accidental discharge of pellet gun

√7th   **W34.011 Accidental discharge of paintball gun**
> Accidental injury due to paintball discharge

√7th   **W34.018 Accidental discharge of other gas, air or spring-operated gun**

√x 7th   **W34.09 Accidental discharge from other specified firearms**
> Accidental discharge from Very pistol [flare]

√5th   **W34.1 Accidental malfunction from other and unspecified firearms and guns**

√x 7th   **W34.10 Accidental malfunction from unspecified firearms or gun**
> Firearm malfunction NOS

√6th   **W34.11 Accidental malfunction of gas, air or spring-operated guns**

√7th   **W34.110 Accidental malfunction of airgun**
> Accidental malfunction of BB gun
> Accidental malfunction of pellet gun

√7th   **W34.111 Accidental malfunction of paintball gun**
> Accidental injury due to paintball gun malfunction

√7th   **W34.118 Accidental malfunction of other gas, air or spring-operated gun**

√x 7th   **W34.19 Accidental malfunction from other specified firearms**
> Accidental malfunction from Very pistol [flare]

√x 7th   **W35 Explosion and rupture of boiler**
> EXCLUDES 1   explosion and rupture of boiler on watercraft (V93.4)

> The appropriate 7th character is to be added to code W35.
> A   initial encounter
> D   subsequent encounter
> S   sequela

√4th   **W36 Explosion and rupture of gas cylinder**

> The appropriate 7th character is to be added to each code from category W36.
> A   initial encounter
> D   subsequent encounter
> S   sequela

√x 7th   **W36.1 Explosion and rupture of aerosol can**

√x 7th   **W36.2 Explosion and rupture of air tank**

√x 7th   **W36.3 Explosion and rupture of pressurized-gas tank**

√x 7th   **W36.8 Explosion and rupture of other gas cylinder**

√x 7th   **W36.9 Explosion and rupture of unspecified gas cylinder**

√4th   **W37 Explosion and rupture of pressurized tire, pipe or hose**

> The appropriate 7th character is to be added to each code from category W37.
> A   initial encounter
> D   subsequent encounter
> S   sequela

√x 7th   **W37.0 Explosion of bicycle tire**

√x 7th   **W37.8 Explosion and rupture of other pressurized tire, pipe or hose**

√ Additional Character Required   √x 7th Placeholder Alert   Unspecified Dx   Other Specified Dx   Manifestation   ▶◀ Revised Text   ● New Code   ▲ Revised Code Title

Chapter 20. External Causes of Morbidity

√x 7ᵗʰ **W38 Explosion and rupture of other specified pressurized devices**

> The appropriate 7th character is to be added to code W38.
> A   initial encounter
> D   subsequent encounter
> S   sequela

√x 7ᵗʰ **W39 Discharge of firework**

> The appropriate 7th character is to be added to code W39.
> A   initial encounter
> D   subsequent encounter
> S   sequela

√4ᵗʰ **W40 Explosion of other materials**

> EXCLUDES 1   assault by explosive material (X96)
> explosion involving legal intervention (Y35.1-)
> explosion involving military or war operations (Y36.0-, Y36.2-)
> intentional self-harm by explosive material (X75)

> The appropriate 7th character is to be added to each code from category W40.
> A   initial encounter
> D   subsequent encounter
> S   sequela

√x 7ᵗʰ **W40.0 Explosion of blasting material**
Explosion of blasting cap
Explosion of detonator
Explosion of dynamite
Explosion of explosive (any) used in blasting operations

√x 7ᵗʰ **W40.1 Explosion of explosive gases**
Explosion of acetylene
Explosion of butane
Explosion of coal gas
Explosion in mine NOS
Explosion of explosive gas
Explosion of fire damp
Explosion of gasoline fumes
Explosion of methane
Explosion of propane

√x 7ᵗʰ **W40.8 Explosion of other specified explosive materials**
Explosion in dump NOS
Explosion in factory NOS
Explosion in grain store
Explosion in munitions
> EXCLUDES 1   explosion involving legal intervention (Y35.1-)
> explosion involving military or war operations (Y36.0-, Y36.2-)

√x 7ᵗʰ **W40.9 Explosion of unspecified explosive materials**
Explosion NOS

√4ᵗʰ **W42 Exposure to noise**

> The appropriate 7th character is to be added to each code from category W42.
> A   initial encounter
> D   subsequent encounter
> S   sequela

√x 7ᵗʰ **W42.0 Exposure to supersonic waves**

√x 7ᵗʰ **W42.9 Exposure to other noise**
Exposure to sound waves NOS

√4ᵗʰ **W45 Foreign body or object entering through skin**

> EXCLUDES 2   contact with hand tools (nonpowered) (powered) (W27-W29)
> contact with knife, sword or dagger (W26.-)
> contact with sharp glass (W25.-)
> struck by objects (W20-W22)

> The appropriate 7th character is to be added to each code from category W45.
> A   initial encounter
> D   subsequent encounter
> S   sequela

√x 7ᵗʰ **W45.0 Nail entering through skin**

√x 7ᵗʰ **W45.1 Paper entering through skin**
Paper cut

√x 7ᵗʰ **W45.2 Lid of can entering through skin**

√x 7ᵗʰ **W45.8 Other foreign body or object entering through skin**
Splinter in skin NOS

√4ᵗʰ **W46 Contact with hypodermic needle**

> The appropriate 7th character is to be added to each code from category W46.
> A   initial encounter
> D   subsequent encounter
> S   sequela

√x 7ᵗʰ **W46.0 Contact with hypodermic needle**
Hypodermic needle stick NOS

√x 7ᵗʰ **W46.1 Contact with contaminated hypodermic needle**

√4ᵗʰ **W49 Exposure to other inanimate mechanical forces**
INCLUDES   exposure to abnormal gravitational [G] forces
exposure to inanimate mechanical forces NEC
> EXCLUDES 1   exposure to inanimate mechanical forces involving military or war operations (Y36.-, Y37.-)

> The appropriate 7th character is to be added to each code from category W49.
> A   initial encounter
> D   subsequent encounter
> S   sequela

√5ᵗʰ **W49.0 Item causing external constriction**

√x 7ᵗʰ **W49.01 Hair causing external constriction**

√x 7ᵗʰ **W49.02 String or thread causing external constriction**

√x 7ᵗʰ **W49.03 Rubber band causing external constriction**

√x 7ᵗʰ **W49.04 Ring or other jewelry causing external constriction**

√x 7ᵗʰ **W49.09 Other specified item causing external constriction**

√x 7ᵗʰ **W49.9 Exposure to other inanimate mechanical forces**

Exposure to animate mechanical forces (W50-W64)

> EXCLUDES 1   Toxic effect of contact with venomous animals and plants (T63.-)

√4ᵗʰ **W50 Accidental hit, strike, kick, twist, bite or scratch by another person**
Hit, strike, kick, twist, bite, or scratch by another person NOS
> EXCLUDES 1   assault by bodily force (Y04)
> struck by objects (W20-W22)

> The appropriate 7th character is to be added to each code from category W50.
> A   initial encounter
> D   subsequent encounter
> S   sequela

√x 7ᵗʰ **W50.0 Accidental hit or strike by another person**
Hit or strike by another person NOS

√x 7ᵗʰ **W50.1 Accidental kick by another person**
Kick by another person NOS

√x 7ᵗʰ **W50.2 Accidental twist by another person**
Twist by another person NOS

√x 7ᵗʰ **W50.3 Accidental bite by another person**
Human bite
Bite by another person NOS

√x 7ᵗʰ **W50.4 Accidental scratch by another person**
Scratch by another person NOS

√x 7ᵗʰ **W51 Accidental striking against or bumped into by another person**
> EXCLUDES 1   assault by striking against or bumping into by another person (Y04.2)
> fall due to collision with another person (W03)

> The appropriate 7th character is to be added to code W51.
> A   initial encounter
> D   subsequent encounter
> S   sequela

√x 7ᵗʰ **W52 Crushed, pushed or stepped on by crowd or human stampede**
Crushed, pushed or stepped on by crowd or human stampede with or without fall

> The appropriate 7th character is to be added to code W52.
> A   initial encounter
> D   subsequent encounter
> S   sequela

EXCLUDES 1 Not coded here   EXCLUDES 2 Not included here   N Newborn Age: 0   P Pediatric Age: 0-17   M Maternity Age: 12-55   A Adult Age: 15-12

W53 Contact with rodent

INCLUDES contact with saliva, feces or urine of rodent

The appropriate 7th character is to be added to each code from category W53.
A   initial encounter
D   subsequent encounter
S   sequela

✓5th **W53.0 Contact with mouse**
   ✓x7th **W53.01 Bitten by mouse**
   ✓x7th **W53.09 Other contact with mouse**

✓5th **W53.1 Contact with rat**
   ✓x7th **W53.11 Bitten by rat**
   ✓x7th **W53.19 Other contact with rat**

✓5th **W53.2 Contact with squirrel**
   ✓x7th **W53.21 Bitten by squirrel**
   ✓x7th **W53.29 Other contact with squirrel**

✓5th **W53.8 Contact with other rodent**
   ✓x7th **W53.81 Bitten by other rodent**
   ✓x7th **W53.89 Other contact with other rodent**

W54 Contact with dog

INCLUDES contact with saliva, feces or urine of dog

The appropriate 7th character is to be added to each code from category W54.
A   initial encounter
D   subsequent encounter
S   sequela

✓x7th **W54.0 Bitten by dog**

✓x7th **W54.1 Struck by dog**
   Knocked over by dog

✓x7th **W54.8 Other contact with dog**

W55 Contact with other mammals

INCLUDES contact with saliva, feces or urine of mammal
EXCLUDES1 animal being ridden—see transport accidents
     bitten or struck by dog (W54)
     bitten or struck by rodent (W53.-)
     contact with marine mammals (W56.-)

The appropriate 7th character is to be added to each code from category W55.
A   initial encounter
D   subsequent encounter
S   sequela

✓5th **W55.0 Contact with cat**
   ✓x7th **W55.01 Bitten by cat**
   ✓x7th **W55.03 Scratched by cat**
   ✓x7th **W55.09 Other contact with cat**

✓5th **W55.1 Contact with horse**
   ✓x7th **W55.11 Bitten by horse**
   ✓x7th **W55.12 Struck by horse**
   ✓x7th **W55.19 Other contact with horse**

✓5th **W55.2 Contact with cow**
   Contact with bull
   ✓x7th **W55.21 Bitten by cow**
   ✓x7th **W55.22 Struck by cow**
     Gored by bull
   ✓x7th **W55.29 Other contact with cow**

✓5th **W55.3 Contact with other hoof stock**
   Contact with goats
   Contact with sheep
   ✓x7th **W55.31 Bitten by other hoof stock**
   ✓x7th **W55.32 Struck by other hoof stock**
     Gored by goat
     Gored by ram
   ✓x7th **W55.39 Other contact with other hoof stock**

✓5th **W55.4 Contact with pig**
   ✓x7th **W55.41 Bitten by pig**
   ✓x7th **W55.42 Struck by pig**
   ✓x7th **W55.49 Other contact with pig**

✓5th **W55.5 Contact with raccoon**
   ✓x7th **W55.51 Bitten by raccoon**

   ✓x7th **W55.52 Struck by raccoon**
   ✓x7th **W55.59 Other contact with raccoon**

✓5th **W55.8 Contact with other mammals**
   ✓x7th **W55.81 Bitten by other mammals**
   ✓x7th **W55.82 Struck by other mammals**
   ✓x7th **W55.89 Other contact with other mammals**

W56 Contact with nonvenomous marine animal

EXCLUDES1 contact with venomous marine animal (T63.-)

The appropriate 7th character is to be added to each code from category W56.
A   initial encounter
D   subsequent encounter
S   sequela

✓5th **W56.0 Contact with dolphin**
   ✓x7th **W56.01 Bitten by dolphin**
   ✓x7th **W56.02 Struck by dolphin**
   ✓x7th **W56.09 Other contact with dolphin**

✓5th **W56.1 Contact with sea lion**
   ✓x7th **W56.11 Bitten by sea lion**
   ✓x7th **W56.12 Struck by sea lion**
   ✓x7th **W56.19 Other contact with sea lion**

✓5th **W56.2 Contact with orca**
   Contact with killer whale
   ✓x7th **W56.21 Bitten by orca**
   ✓x7th **W56.22 Struck by orca**
   ✓x7th **W56.29 Other contact with orca**

✓5th **W56.3 Contact with other marine mammals**
   ✓x7th **W56.31 Bitten by other marine mammals**
   ✓x7th **W56.32 Struck by other marine mammals**
   ✓x7th **W56.39 Other contact with other marine mammals**

✓5th **W56.4 Contact with shark**
   ✓x7th **W56.41 Bitten by shark**
   ✓x7th **W56.42 Struck by shark**
   ✓x7th **W56.49 Other contact with shark**

✓5th **W56.5 Contact with other fish**
   ✓x7th **W56.51 Bitten by other fish**
   ✓x7th **W56.52 Struck by other fish**
   ✓x7th **W56.59 Other contact with other fish**

✓5th **W56.8 Contact with other nonvenomous marine animals**
   ✓x7th **W56.81 Bitten by other nonvenomous marine animals**
   ✓x7th **W56.82 Struck by other nonvenomous marine animals**
   ✓x7th **W56.89 Other contact with other nonvenomous marine animals**

✓x7th W57 Bitten or stung by nonvenomous insect and other nonvenomous arthropods

EXCLUDES1 contact with venomous insects and arthropods (T63.2-, T63.3-, T63.4-)

The appropriate 7th character is to be added to code W57.
A   initial encounter
D   subsequent encounter
S   sequela

W58 Contact with crocodile or alligator

The appropriate 7th character is to be added to each code from category W58.
A   initial encounter
D   subsequent encounter
S   sequela

✓5th **W58.0 Contact with alligator**
   ✓x7th **W58.01 Bitten by alligator**
   ✓x7th **W58.02 Struck by alligator**
   ✓x7th **W58.03 Crushed by alligator**
   ✓x7th **W58.09 Other contact with alligator**

✓5th **W58.1 Contact with crocodile**
   ✓x7th **W58.11 Bitten by crocodile**
   ✓x7th **W58.12 Struck by crocodile**
   ✓x7th **W58.13 Crushed by crocodile**
   ✓x7th **W58.19 Other contact with crocodile**

◢ Additional Character Required   ✓x7th Placeholder Alert   Unspecified Dx   Other Specified Dx   Manifestation   ▶◀ Revised Text   ● New Code   ▲ Revised Code Title

Chapter 20. External Causes of Morbidity

W59–W73

✓4ᵗʰ **W59 Contact with other nonvenomous reptiles**
> EXCLUDES 1   contact with venomous reptile (T63.0-, T63.1-)

> The appropriate 7th character is to be added to each code from category W59.
> A   initial encounter
> D   subsequent encounter
> S   sequela

✓5ᵗʰ **W59.0 Contact with nonvenomous lizards**

✓x7ᵗʰ   **W59.01 Bitten by nonvenomous lizards**

✓x7ᵗʰ   **W59.02 Struck by nonvenomous lizards**

✓x7ᵗʰ   **W59.09 Other contact with nonvenomous lizards**
> Exposure to nonvenomous lizards

✓5ᵗʰ **W59.1 Contact with nonvenomous snakes**

✓x7ᵗʰ   **W59.11 Bitten by nonvenomous snake**

✓x7ᵗʰ   **W59.12 Struck by nonvenomous snake**

✓x7ᵗʰ   **W59.13 Crushed by nonvenomous snake**

✓x7ᵗʰ   **W59.19 Other contact with nonvenomous snake**

✓5ᵗʰ **W59.2 Contact with turtles**
> EXCLUDES 1   contact with tortoises (W59.8-)

✓x7ᵗʰ   **W59.21 Bitten by turtle**

✓x7ᵗʰ   **W59.22 Struck by turtle**

✓x7ᵗʰ   **W59.29 Other contact with turtle**
> Exposure to turtles

✓5ᵗʰ **W59.8 Contact with other nonvenomous reptiles**

✓x7ᵗʰ   **W59.81 Bitten by other nonvenomous reptiles**

✓x7ᵗʰ   **W59.82 Struck by other nonvenomous reptiles**

✓x7ᵗʰ   **W59.83 Crushed by other nonvenomous reptiles**

✓x7ᵗʰ   **W59.89 Other contact with other nonvenomous reptiles**

✓x7ᵗʰ **W60 Contact with nonvenomous plant thorns and spines and sharp leaves**
> EXCLUDES 1   contact with venomous plants (T63.7-)

> The appropriate 7th character is to be added to code W60.
> A   initial encounter
> D   subsequent encounter
> S   sequela

✓4ᵗʰ **W61 Contact with birds (domestic) (wild)**
> INCLUDES   contact with excreta of birds

> The appropriate 7th character is to be added to each code from category W61.
> A   initial encounter
> D   subsequent encounter
> S   sequela

✓5ᵗʰ **W61.0 Contact with parrot**

✓x7ᵗʰ   **W61.01 Bitten by parrot**

✓x7ᵗʰ   **W61.02 Struck by parrot**

✓x7ᵗʰ   **W61.09 Other contact with parrot**
> Exposure to parrots

✓5ᵗʰ **W61.1 Contact with macaw**

✓x7ᵗʰ   **W61.11 Bitten by macaw**

✓x7ᵗʰ   **W61.12 Struck by macaw**

✓x7ᵗʰ   **W61.19 Other contact with macaw**
> Exposure to macaws

✓5ᵗʰ **W61.2 Contact with other psittacines**

✓x7ᵗʰ   **W61.21 Bitten by other psittacines**

✓x7ᵗʰ   **W61.22 Struck by other psittacines**

✓x7ᵗʰ   **W61.29 Other contact with other psittacines**
> Exposure to other psittacines

✓5ᵗʰ **W61.3 Contact with chicken**

✓x7ᵗʰ   **W61.32 Struck by chicken**

✓x7ᵗʰ   **W61.33 Pecked by chicken**

✓x7ᵗʰ   **W61.39 Other contact with chicken**
> Exposure to chickens

✓5ᵗʰ **W61.4 Contact with turkey**

✓x7ᵗʰ   **W61.42 Struck by turkey**

✓x7ᵗʰ   **W61.43 Pecked by turkey**

✓x7ᵗʰ   **W61.49 Other contact with turkey**

✓5ᵗʰ **W61.5 Contact with goose**

✓x7ᵗʰ   **W61.51 Bitten by goose**

✓x7ᵗʰ   **W61.52 Struck by goose**

✓x7ᵗʰ   **W61.59 Other contact with goose**

✓5ᵗʰ **W61.6 Contact with duck**

✓x7ᵗʰ   **W61.61 Bitten by duck**

✓x7ᵗʰ   **W61.62 Struck by duck**

✓x7ᵗʰ   **W61.69 Other contact with duck**

✓5ᵗʰ **W61.9 Contact with other birds**

✓x7ᵗʰ   **W61.91 Bitten by other birds**

✓x7ᵗʰ   **W61.92 Struck by other birds**

✓x7ᵗʰ   **W61.99 Other contact with other birds**
> Contact with bird NOS

✓4ᵗʰ **W62 Contact with nonvenomous amphibians**
> EXCLUDES 1   contact with venomous amphibians (T63.81-R63.83)

> The appropriate 7th character is to be added to each code from category W62.
> A   initial encounter
> D   subsequent encounter
> S   sequela

✓x7ᵗʰ **W62.0 Contact with nonvenomous frogs**

✓x7ᵗʰ **W62.1 Contact with nonvenomous toads**

✓x7ᵗʰ **W62.9 Contact with other nonvenomous amphibians**

✓x7ᵗʰ **W64 Exposure to other animate mechanical forces**
> INCLUDES   exposure to nonvenomous animal NOS
> EXCLUDES 1   contact with venomous animal (T63.-)

> The appropriate 7th character is to be added to code W64.
> A   initial encounter
> D   subsequent encounter
> S   sequela

Accidental non-transport drowning and submersion (W65-W74)

> EXCLUDES 1   accidental drowning and submersion due to fall into water (W16.-)
> accidental drowning and submersion due to water transport acciden (V90.-, V92.-)
> EXCLUDES 2   accidental drowning and submersion due to cataclysm (X34-X39)

✓x7ᵗʰ **W65 Accidental drowning and submersion while in bath-tub**
> EXCLUDES 1   accidental drowning and submersion due to fall in (into) bathtub (W16.211)

> The appropriate 7th character is to be added to code W65.
> A   initial encounter
> D   subsequent encounter
> S   sequela

✓x7ᵗʰ **W67 Accidental drowning and submersion while in swimming-pool**
> EXCLUDES 1   accidental drowning and submersion due to fall into swimmir pool (W16.011, W16.021, W16.031)
> accidental drowning and submersion due to striking into wall swimming pool (W22.041)

> The appropriate 7th character is to be added to code W67.
> A   initial encounter
> D   subsequent encounter
> S   sequela

✓x7ᵗʰ **W69 Accidental drowning and submersion while in natural water**
> Accidental drowning and submersion while in lake
> Accidental drowning and submersion while in open sea
> Accidental drowning and submersion while in river
> Accidental drowning and submersion while in stream
> EXCLUDES 1   accidental drowning and submersion due to fall into natural body of water (W16.111, W16.121, W16.131)

> The appropriate 7th character is to be added to code W69.
> A   initial encounter
> D   subsequent encounter
> S   sequela

✓x7ᵗʰ **W73 Other specified cause of accidental non-transport drowning an submersion**
> Accidental drowning and submersion while in quenching tank
> Accidental drowning and submersion while in reservoir
> EXCLUDES 1   accidental drowning and submersion due to fall into other water (W16.311, W16.321, W16.331)

> The appropriate 7th character is to be added to code W73.
> A   initial encounter
> D   subsequent encounter
> S   sequela

EXCLUDES 1 Not coded here   EXCLUDES 2 Not included here   N Newborn Age: 0   P Pediatric Age: 0-17   M Maternity Age: 12-55   A Adult Age: 15-12

1078

ICD-10-CM 201

✗7ᵗʰ W74 Unspecified cause of accidental drowning and submersion
Drowning NOS

The appropriate 7th character is to be added to code W74.
A   initial encounter
D   subsequent encounter
S   sequela

Exposure to electric current, radiation and extreme ambient air temperature and pressure (W85-W99)

EXCLUDES 1   exposure to:
     failure in dosage of radiation or temperature during surgical and medical care (Y63.2-Y63.5)
     lightning (T75.0-)
     natural cold (X31)
     natural heat (X30)
     natural radiation NOS (X39)
     radiological procedure and radiotherapy (Y84.2)
     sunlight (X32)

✗7ᵗʰ W85 Exposure to electric transmission lines
Broken power line

The appropriate 7th character is to be added to code W85.
A   initial encounter
D   subsequent encounter
S   sequela

4ᵗʰ W86 Exposure to other specified electric current

The appropriate 7th character is to be added to each code from category W86.
A   initial encounter
D   subsequent encounter
S   sequela

✓✗7ᵗʰ **W86.0 Exposure to domestic wiring and appliances**

✓✗7ᵗʰ **W86.1 Exposure to industrial wiring, appliances and electrical machinery**
     Exposure to conductors
     Exposure to control apparatus
     Exposure to electrical equipment and machinery
     Exposure to transformers

✓✗7ᵗʰ **W86.8 Exposure to other electric current**
     Exposure to wiring and appliances in or on farm (not farmhouse)
     Exposure to wiring and appliances outdoors
     Exposure to wiring and appliances in or on public building
     Exposure to wiring and appliances in or on residential institutions
     Exposure to wiring and appliances in or on schools

4ᵗʰ W88 Exposure to ionizing radiation
EXCLUDES 1   *exposure to sunlight (X32)*

The appropriate 7th character is to be added to each code from category W88.
A   initial encounter
D   subsequent encounter
S   sequela

✓✗7ᵗʰ **W88.0 Exposure to X-rays**

✓✗7ᵗʰ **W88.1 Exposure to radioactive isotopes**

✓✗7ᵗʰ **W88.8 Exposure to other ionizing radiation**

4ᵗʰ W89 Exposure to man-made visible and ultraviolet light
INCLUDES   exposure to welding light (arc)
EXCLUDES 2   *exposure to sunlight (X32)*

The appropriate 7th character is to be added to each code from category W89.
A   initial encounter
D   subsequent encounter
S   sequela

✓✗7ᵗʰ **W89.0 Exposure to welding light (arc)**

✓✗7ᵗʰ **W89.1 Exposure to tanning bed**

✓✗7ᵗʰ **W89.8 Exposure to other man-made visible and ultraviolet light**

✓✗7ᵗʰ **W89.9 Exposure to unspecified man-made visible and ultraviolet light**

✓4ᵗʰ W90 Exposure to other nonionizing radiation
EXCLUDES 1   *exposure to sunlight (X32)*

The appropriate 7th character is to be added to each code from category W90.
A   initial encounter
D   subsequent encounter
S   sequela

✓✗7ᵗʰ **W90.0 Exposure to radiofrequency**

✓✗7ᵗʰ **W90.1 Exposure to infrared radiation**

✓✗7ᵗʰ **W90.2 Exposure to laser radiation**

✓✗7ᵗʰ **W90.8 Exposure to other nonionizing radiation**

✓✗7ᵗʰ W92 Exposure to excessive heat of man-made origin

The appropriate 7th character is to be added to code W92.
A   initial encounter
D   subsequent encounter
S   sequela

✓4ᵗʰ W93 Exposure to excessive cold of man-made origin

The appropriate 7th character is to be added to each code from category W93.
A   initial encounter
D   subsequent encounter
S   sequela

✓5ᵗʰ **W93.0 Contact with or inhalation of dry ice**

     ✓✗7ᵗʰ **W93.01 Contact with dry ice**

     ✓✗7ᵗʰ **W93.02 Inhalation of dry ice**

✓5ᵗʰ **W93.1 Contact with or inhalation of liquid air**

     ✓✗7ᵗʰ **W93.11 Contact with liquid air**
         Contact with liquid hydrogen
         Contact with liquid nitrogen

     ✓✗7ᵗʰ **W93.12 Inhalation of liquid air**
         Inhalation of liquid hydrogen
         Inhalation of liquid nitrogen

✓✗7ᵗʰ **W93.2 Prolonged exposure in deep freeze unit or refrigerator**

✓✗7ᵗʰ **W93.8 Exposure to other excessive cold of man-made origin**

✓4ᵗʰ W94 Exposure to high and low air pressure and changes in air pressure

The appropriate 7th character is to be added to each code from category W94.
A   initial encounter
D   subsequent encounter
S   sequela

✓✗7ᵗʰ **W94.0 Exposure to prolonged high air pressure**

✓5ᵗʰ **W94.1 Exposure to prolonged low air pressure**

     ✓✗7ᵗʰ **W94.11 Exposure to residence or prolonged visit at high altitude**

     ✓✗7ᵗʰ **W94.12 Exposure to other prolonged low air pressure**

✓5ᵗʰ **W94.2 Exposure to rapid changes in air pressure during ascent**

     ✓✗7ᵗʰ **W94.21 Exposure to reduction in atmospheric pressure while surfacing from deep-water diving**

     ✓✗7ᵗʰ **W94.22 Exposure to reduction in atmospheric pressure while surfacing from underground**

     ✓✗7ᵗʰ **W94.23 Exposure to sudden change in air pressure in aircraft during ascent**

     ✓✗7ᵗʰ **W94.29 Exposure to other rapid changes in air pressure during ascent**

✓5ᵗʰ **W94.3 Exposure to rapid changes in air pressure during descent**

     ✓✗7ᵗʰ **W94.31 Exposure to sudden change in air pressure in aircraft during descent**

     ✓✗7ᵗʰ **W94.32 Exposure to high air pressure from rapid descent in water**

     ✓✗7ᵗʰ **W94.39 Exposure to other rapid changes in air pressure during descent**

✓✗7ᵗʰ W99 Exposure to other man-made environmental factors

The appropriate 7th character is to be added to code W99.
A   initial encounter
D   subsequent encounter
S   sequela

✓ Additional Character Required   ✓✗7ᵗʰ Placeholder Alert   Unspecified Dx   Other Specified Dx   Manifestation   ▶◀ Revised Text   ● New Code   ▲ Revised Code Title

Exposure to smoke, fire and flames (X00–X08)

EXCLUDES 1   arson (X97)
EXCLUDES 2   explosions (W35–W40)
       lightning (T75.0-)
       transport accident (V01–V99)

✓4th X00   Exposure to uncontrolled fire in building or structure

INCLUDES   conflagration in building or structure
Code first any associated cataclysm
EXCLUDES 2   exposure to ignition or melting of nightwear (X05)
       exposure to ignition or melting of other clothing and apparel (X06.-)
       exposure to other specified smoke, fire and flames (X08.-)

The appropriate 7th character is to be added to each code from category X00.
A   initial encounter
D   subsequent encounter
S   sequela

✓x7th   **X00.0**   Exposure to flames in uncontrolled fire in building or structure
✓x7th   **X00.1**   Exposure to smoke in uncontrolled fire in building or structure
✓x7th   **X00.2**   Injury due to collapse of burning building or structure in uncontrolled fire
       EXCLUDES 1   injury due to collapse of building not on fire (W20.1)
✓x7th   **X00.3**   Fall from burning building or structure in uncontrolled fire
✓x7th   **X00.4**   Hit by object from burning building or structure in uncontrolled fire
✓x7th   **X00.5**   Jump from burning building or structure in uncontrolled fire
✓x7th   **X00.8**   Other exposure to uncontrolled fire in building or structure

✓4th X01   Exposure to uncontrolled fire, not in building or structure

INCLUDES   exposure to forest fire

The appropriate 7th character is to be added to each code from category X01.
A   initial encounter
D   subsequent encounter
S   sequela

✓x7th   **X01.0**   Exposure to flames in uncontrolled fire, not in building or structure
✓x7th   **X01.1**   Exposure to smoke in uncontrolled fire, not in building or structure
✓x7th   **X01.3**   Fall due to uncontrolled fire, not in building or structure
✓x7th   **X01.4**   Hit by object due to uncontrolled fire, not in building or structure
✓x7th   **X01.8**   Other exposure to uncontrolled fire, not in building or structure

✓4th X02   Exposure to controlled fire in building or structure

INCLUDES   exposure to fire in fireplace
       exposure to fire in stove

The appropriate 7th character is to be added to each code from category X02.
A   initial encounter
D   subsequent encounter
S   sequela

✓x7th   **X02.0**   Exposure to flames in controlled fire in building or structure
✓x7th   **X02.1**   Exposure to smoke in controlled fire in building or structure
✓x7th   **X02.2**   Injury due to collapse of burning building or structure in controlled fire
       EXCLUDES 1   injury due to collapse of building not on fire (W20.1)
✓x7th   **X02.3**   Fall from burning building or structure in controlled fire
✓x7th   **X02.4**   Hit by object from burning building or structure in controlled fire
✓x7th   **X02.5**   Jump from burning building or structure in controlled fire
✓x7th   **X02.8**   Other exposure to controlled fire in building or structure

✓4th X03   Exposure to controlled fire, not in building or structure

INCLUDES   exposure to bon fire
       exposure to camp-fire
       exposure to trash fire

The appropriate 7th character is to be added to each code from category X03.
A   initial encounter
D   subsequent encounter
S   sequela

✓x7th   **X03.0**   Exposure to flames in controlled fire, not in building or structure
✓x7th   **X03.1**   Exposure to smoke in controlled fire, not in building or structure
✓x7th   **X03.3**   Fall due to controlled fire, not in building or structure
✓x7th   **X03.4**   Hit by object due to controlled fire, not in building or structure
✓x7th   **X03.0**   Other exposure to controlled fire, not in building or structure

✓x7th X04   Exposure to ignition of highly flammable material

Exposure to ignition of gasoline
Exposure to ignition of kerosene
Exposure to ignition of petrol
EXCLUDES 2   exposure to ignition or melting of nightwear (X05)
       exposure to ignition or melting of other clothing and apparel (X06)

The appropriate 7th character is to be added to code X04.
A   initial encounter
D   subsequent encounter
S   sequela

✓x7th X05   Exposure to ignition or melting of nightwear

EXCLUDES 2   exposure to uncontrolled fire in building or structure (X00.-)
       exposure to uncontrolled fire, not in building or structure (X01.-)
       exposure to controlled fire in building or structure (X02.-)
       exposure to controlled fire, not in building or structure (X03.-)
       exposure to ignition of highly flammable materials (X04.-)

The appropriate 7th character is to be added to code X05.
A   initial encounter
D   subsequent encounter
S   sequela

✓4th X06   Exposure to ignition or melting of other clothing and apparel

EXCLUDES 2   exposure to uncontrolled fire in building or structure (X00.-)
       exposure to uncontrolled fire, not in building or structure (X01.-
       exposure to controlled fire in building or structure (X02.-)
       exposure to controlled fire, not in building or structure (X03.-)
       exposure to ignition of highly flammable materials (X04.-)

The appropriate 7th character is to be added to each code from category X06.
A   initial encounter
D   subsequent encounter
S   sequela

✓x7th   **X06.0**   Exposure to ignition of plastic jewelry
✓x7th   **X06.1**   Exposure to melting of plastic jewelry
✓x7th   **X06.2**   Exposure to ignition of other clothing and apparel
✓x7th   **X06.3**   Exposure to melting of other clothing and apparel

✓4th X08   Exposure to other specified smoke, fire and flames

The appropriate 7th character is to be added to each code from category X08.
A   initial encounter
D   subsequent encounter
S   sequela

✓5th   **X08.0**   Exposure to bed fire
       Exposure to mattress fire
    ✓x7th   **X08.00**   Exposure to bed fire due to unspecified burning material
    ✓x7th   **X08.01**   Exposure to bed fire due to burning cigarette
    ✓x7th   **X08.09**   Exposure to bed fire due to other burning material

✓5th   **X08.1**   Exposure to sofa fire
    ✓x7th   **X08.10**   Exposure to sofa fire due to unspecified burning material
    ✓x7th   **X08.11**   Exposure to sofa fire due to burning cigarette
    ✓x7th   **X08.19**   Exposure to sofa fire due to other burning material

✓5th   **X08.2**   Exposure to other furniture fire
    ✓x7th   **X08.20**   Exposure to other furniture fire due to unspecified burning material

---

EXCLUDES 1 Not coded here   EXCLUDES 2 Not included here   N Newborn Age: 0   P Pediatric Age: 0-17   M Maternity Age: 12-55   A Adult Age: 15-124

√x7ᵗʰ **X08.21**   **Exposure to other furniture fire due to** burning cigarette

√x7ᵗʰ **X08.29**   **Exposure to other furniture fire due to other burning material**

√x7ᵗʰ **X08.8**   **Exposure to other specified smoke, fire and flames**

Contact with heat and hot substances (X10-X19)

EXCLUDES 1   exposure to excessive natural heat (X30)
exposure to fire and flames (X00-X09)

4ᵗʰ **X10**   **Contact with hot drinks, food, fats and cooking oils**

The appropriate 7th character is to be added to each code from category X10.
A   initial encounter
D   subsequent encounter
S   sequela

√x7ᵗʰ **X10.0**   **Contact with hot** drinks

√x7ᵗʰ **X10.1**   **Contact with hot** food

√x7ᵗʰ **X10.2**   **Contact with** fats and cooking oils

4ᵗʰ **X11**   **Contact with hot tap-water**

INCLUDES   contact with boiling tap-water
contact with boiling water NOS

EXCLUDES 1   contact with water heated on stove (X12)

The appropriate 7th character is to be added to each code from category X11.
A   initial encounter
D   subsequent encounter
S   sequela

√x7ᵗʰ **X11.0**   **Contact with hot water** in bath or tub
    EXCLUDES 1   contact with running hot water in bath or tub (X11.1)

√x7ᵗʰ **X11.1**   **Contact with running hot water**
Contact with hot water running out of hose
Contact with hot water running out of tap

√x7ᵗʰ **X11.8**   **Contact with other hot tap-water**
Contact with hot water in bucket
Contact with hot tap-water NOS

7ᵗʰ **X12**   **Contact with other hot fluids**
Contact with water heated on stove
EXCLUDES 1   hot (liquid) metals (X18)

The appropriate 7th character is to be added to code X12.
A   initial encounter
D   subsequent encounter
S   sequela

4ᵗʰ **X13**   **Contact with steam and other hot vapors**

The appropriate 7th character is to be added to each code from category X13.
A   initial encounter
D   subsequent encounter
S   sequela

√x7ᵗʰ **X13.0**   **Inhalation of steam and other hot vapors**

√x7ᵗʰ **X13.1**   **Other contact with steam and other hot vapors**

4ᵗʰ **X14**   **Contact with hot air and other hot gases**

The appropriate 7th character is to be added to each code from category X14.
A   initial encounter
D   subsequent encounter
S   sequela

√x7ᵗʰ **X14.0**   **Inhalation of hot air and gases**

√x7ᵗʰ **X14.1**   **Other contact with hot air and other hot gases**

4ᵗʰ **X15**   **Contact with hot household appliances**

EXCLUDES 1   contact with heating appliances (X16)
contact with powered household appliances (W29.-)
exposure to controlled fire in building or structure due to household appliance (X02.8)
exposure to household appliances electrical current (W86.0)

The appropriate 7th character is to be added to each code from category X15.
A   initial encounter
D   subsequent encounter
S   sequela

√x7ᵗʰ **X15.0**   **Contact with hot** stove (kitchen)

√x7ᵗʰ **X15.1**   **Contact with hot** toaster

√x7ᵗʰ **X15.2**   **Contact with** hotplate

√x7ᵗʰ **X15.3**   **Contact with hot** saucepan or skillet

√x7ᵗʰ **X15.8**   **Contact with other hot household appliances**
Contact with cooker   Contact with light bulbs
Contact with kettle

√x7ᵗʰ **X16**   **Contact with hot heating appliances, radiators and pipes**

EXCLUDES 1   contact with powered appliances (W29.-)
exposure to controlled fire in building or structure due to appliance (X02.8)
exposure to industrial appliances electrical current (W86.1)

The appropriate 7th character is to be added to code X16.
A   initial encounter
D   subsequent encounter
S   sequela

√x7ᵗʰ **X17**   **Contact with hot engines, machinery and tools**

EXCLUDES 1   contact with hot heating appliances, radiators and pipes (X16)
contact with hot household appliances (X15)

The appropriate 7th character is to be added to code X17.
A   initial encounter
D   subsequent encounter
S   sequela

√x7ᵗʰ **X18**   **Contact with other hot metals**
Contact with liquid metal

The appropriate 7th character is to be added to code X18.
A   initial encounter
D   subsequent encounter
S   sequela

√x7ᵗʰ **X19**   **Contact with other heat and hot substances**

EXCLUDES 1   objects that are not normally hot, e.g., an object made hot by a house fire (X00-X09)

The appropriate 7th character is to be added to code X19.
A   initial encounter
D   subsequent encounter
S   sequela

Exposure to forces of nature (X30-X39)

√x7ᵗʰ **X30**   **Exposure to excessive** natural heat
Exposure to excessive heat as the cause of sunstroke
Exposure to heat NOS
EXCLUDES 1   excessive heat of man-made origin (W92)
exposure to man-made radiation (W89)
exposure to sunlight (X32)
exposure to tanning bed (W89)

The appropriate 7th character is to be added to code X30.
A   initial encounter
D   subsequent encounter
S   sequela

√x7ᵗʰ **X31**   **Exposure to excessive** natural cold
Excessive cold as the cause of chilblains NOS
Excessive cold as the cause of immersion foot or hand
Exposure to cold NOS
Exposure to weather conditions
EXCLUDES 1   cold of man-made origin (W93.-)
contact with or inhalation of dry ice (W93.-)
contact with or inhalation of liquefied gas (W93.-)

The appropriate 7th character is to be added to code X31.
A   initial encounter
D   subsequent encounter
S   sequela

√x7ᵗʰ **X32**   **Exposure to sunlight**

EXCLUDES 1   radiation-related disorders of the skin and subcutaneous tissue (L55-L59)
man-made radiation (tanning bed) (W89)

The appropriate 7th character is to be added to code X32.
A   initial encounter
D   subsequent encounter
S   sequela

√x7ᵗʰ **X34**   **Earthquake**

EXCLUDES 2   tidal wave (tsunami) due to earthquake (X37.41)

The appropriate 7th character is to be added to code X34.
A   initial encounter
D   subsequent encounter
S   sequela

☑ Additional Character Required   √x7ᵗʰ Placeholder Alert   Unspecified Dx   Other Specified Dx   Manifestation   ▶◀ Revised Text   ● New Code   ▲ Revised Code Title

√x7th **X35 Volcanic eruption**

     EXCLUDES 2   tidal wave (tsunami) due to volcanic eruption (X37.41)

     The appropriate 7th character is to be added to code X35.
     A   initial encounter
     D   subsequent encounter
     S   sequela

√4th **X36 Avalanche, landslide and other earth movements**

     INCLUDES   victim of mudslide of cataclysmic nature
     EXCLUDES 1   earthquake (X34)
     EXCLUDES 2   transport accident involving collision with avalanche or
                  landslide not in motion (V01-V99)

     The appropriate 7th character is to be added to each code from
     category X36.
     A   initial encounter
     D   subsequent encounter
     S   sequela

√x7th **X36.0 Collapse of dam or man-made structure causing earth movement**

√x7th **X36.1 Avalanche, landslide, or mudslide**

√4th **X37 Cataclysmic storm**

     The appropriate 7th character is to be added to each code from
     category X37.
     A   initial encounter
     D   subsequent encounter
     S   sequela

√x7th **X37.0 Hurricane**
     Storm surge
     Typhoon

√x7th **X37.1 Tornado**
     Cyclone
     Twister

√x7th **X37.2 Blizzard (snow)(ice)**

√x7th **X37.3 Dust storm**

√5th **X37.4 Tidalwave**

     √x7th **X37.41 Tidal wave due to earthquake or volcanic eruption**
            Tidal wave NOS
            Tsunami

     √x7th **X37.42 Tidal wave due to storm**

     √x7th **X37.43 Tidal wave due to landslide**

√x7th **X37.8 Other cataclysmic storms**
     Cloudburst
     Torrential rain
     EXCLUDES 2   flood (X38)

√x7th **X37.9 Unspecified cataclysmic storm**
     Storm NOS
     EXCLUDES 1   collapse of dam or man-made structure causing earth
                  movement (X39.0)

√x7th **X38 Flood**
     Flood arising from remote storm
     Flood of cataclysmic nature arising from melting snow
     Flood resulting directly from storm
     EXCLUDES 1   collapse of dam or man-made structure causing earth
                  movement (X39.0)
                  tidal wave NOS (X37.41)
                  tidal wave caused by storm (X37.2)

     The appropriate 7th character is to be added to code X38.
     A   initial encounter
     D   subsequent encounter
     S   sequela

√4th **X39 Exposure to other forces of nature**

     The appropriate 7th character is to be added to each code from
     category X39.
     A   initial encounter
     D   subsequent encounter
     S   sequela

√5th **X39.0 Exposure to natural radiation**
     EXCLUDES 1   contact with and (suspected) exposure to radon and
                  other naturally occuring radiation (Z77.122)
                  exposure to man-made radiation (W88-W90)
                  exposure to sunlight (X32)

     √x7th **X39.01 Exposure to radon**

     √x7th **X39.08 Exposure to other natural radiation**

√x7th **X39.8 Other exposure to forces of nature**

Accidental exposure to other specified factors (X52, X58)

√x7th **X52 Prolonged stay in weightless environment**
     Weightlessness in spacecraft (simulator)

     The appropriate 7th character is to be added to code X52.
     A   initial encounter
     D   subsequent encounter
     S   sequela

√x7th **X58 Exposure to other specified factors**
     Accident NOS
     Exposure NOS

     The appropriate 7th character is to be added to code X58.
     A   initial encounter
     D   subsequent encounter
     S   sequela

Intentional self-harm (X71-X83)

Purposely self-inflicted injury
Suicide (attempted)

√4th **X71 Intentional self-harm by drowning and submersion**

     The appropriate 7th character is to be added to each code from
     category X71.
     A   initial encounter
     D   subsequent encounter
     S   sequela

√x7th **X71.0 Intentional self-harm by drowning and submersion while in bathtub**

√x7th **X71.1 Intentional self-harm by drowning and submersion while in swimming pool**

√x7th **X71.2 Intentional self-harm by drowning and submersion after jump into swimming pool**

√x7th **X71.3 Intentional self-harm by drowning and submersion in natural water**

√x7th **X71.8 Other intentional self-harm by drowning and submersion**

√x7th **X71.9 Intentional self-harm by drowning and submersion, unspecified**

√x7th **X72 Intentional self-harm by handgun discharge**
     Intentional self-harm by gun for single hand use
     Intentional self-harm by pistol
     Intentional self-harm by revolver
     EXCLUDES 1   Very pistol (X74.8)

     The appropriate 7th character is to be added to code X72.
     A   initial encounter
     D   subsequent encounter
     S   sequela

√4th **X73 Intentional self-harm by rifle, shotgun and larger firearm discharge**
     EXCLUDES 1   airgun (X74.01)

     The appropriate 7th character is to be added to each code from
     category X73.
     A   initial encounter
     D   subsequent encounter
     S   sequela

√x7th **X73.0 Intentional self-harm by shotgun discharge**

√x7th **X73.1 Intentional self-harm by hunting rifle discharge**

√x7th **X73.2 Intentional self-harm by machine gun discharge**

√x7th **X73.8 Intentional self-harm by other larger firearm discharge**

√x7th **X73.9 Intentional self-harm by unspecified larger firearm discharge**

√4th **X74 Intentional self-harm by other and unspecified firearm and gun discharge**

     The appropriate 7th character is to be added to each code from
     category X74.
     A   initial encounter
     D   subsequent encounter
     S   sequela

√5th **X74.0 Intentional self-harm by gas, air or spring-operated guns**

     √x7th **X74.01 Intentional self-harm by airgun**
            Intentional self-harm by BB gun discharge
            Intentional self-harm by pellet gun discharge

     √x7th **X74.02 Intentional self-harm by paintball gun**

     √x7th **X74.09 Intentional self-harm by other gas, air or spring-operated gun**

EXCLUDES 1 Not coded here   *EXCLUDES 2* Not included here   N Newborn Age: 0   P Pediatric Age: 0-17   M Maternity Age: 12-55   A Adult Age: 15-124

1082   ICD-10-CM 201

☑7ᵗʰ **X74.8** **Intentional self-harm by other firearm discharge**
     Intentional self-harm by Very pistol [flare] discharge

☑7ᵗʰ **X74.9** **Intentional self-harm by unspecified firearm discharge**

7ᵗʰ **X75 Intentional self-harm by explosive material**

> The appropriate 7th character is to be added to code X75.
> A   initial encounter
> D   subsequent encounter
> S   sequela

7ᵗʰ **X76 Intentional self-harm by smoke, fire and flames**

> The appropriate 7th character is to be added to code X76.
> A   initial encounter
> D   subsequent encounter
> S   sequela

4ᵗʰ **X77 Intentional self-harm by steam, hot vapors and hot objects**

> The appropriate 7th character is to be added to each code from category X77.
> A   initial encounter
> D   subsequent encounter
> S   sequela

☑7ᵗʰ **X77.0** **Intentional self-harm by** steam **or hot** vapors

☑7ᵗʰ **X77.1** **Intentional self-harm by hot** tap water

☑7ᵗʰ **X77.2** **Intentional self-harm by other hot** fluids

☑7ᵗʰ **X77.3** **Intentional self-harm by hot** household appliances

☑7ᵗʰ **X77.8** **Intentional self-harm by other hot** objects

☑7ᵗʰ **X77.9** **Intentional self-harm by unspecified hot objects**

4ᵗʰ **X78 Intentional self-harm by sharp object**

> The appropriate 7th character is to be added to each code from category X78.
> A   initial encounter
> D   subsequent encounter
> S   sequela

☑7ᵗʰ **X78.0** **Intentional self-harm by sharp** glass

☑7ᵗʰ **X78.1** **Intentional self-harm by** knife

☑7ᵗʰ **X78.2** **Intentional self-harm by** sword or dagger

☑7ᵗʰ **X78.8** **Intentional self-harm by other sharp object**

☑7ᵗʰ **X78.9** **Intentional self-harm by unspecified sharp object**

7ᵗʰ **X79 Intentional self-harm by blunt object**

> The appropriate 7th character is to be added to code X79.
> A   initial encounter
> D   subsequent encounter
> S   sequela

7ᵗʰ **X80 Intentional self-harm by jumping from a high place**
     Intentional fall from one level to another

> The appropriate 7th character is to be added to code X80.
> A   initial encounter
> D   subsequent encounter
> S   sequela

4ᵗʰ **X81 Intentional self-harm by jumping or lying in front of moving object**

> The appropriate 7th character is to be added to each code from category X81.
> A   initial encounter
> D   subsequent encounter
> S   sequela

☑7ᵗʰ **X81.0** **Intentional self-harm by jumping or lying in front of** motor vehicle

☑7ᵗʰ **X81.1** **Intentional self-harm by jumping or lying in front of (subway)** train

☑7ᵗʰ **X81.8** **Intentional self-harm by jumping or lying in front of other moving object**

4ᵗʰ **X82 Intentional self-harm by crashing of motor vehicle**

> The appropriate 7th character is to be added to each code from category X82.
> A   initial encounter
> D   subsequent encounter
> S   sequela

☑7ᵗʰ **X82.0** **Intentional collision of motor vehicle with other motor vehicle**

☑7ᵗʰ **X82.1** **Intentional collision of motor vehicle with** train

☑7ᵗʰ **X82.2** **Intentional collision of motor vehicle with** tree

☑7ᵗʰ **X82.8** **Other intentional self-harm by crashing of motor vehicle**

4ᵗʰ **X83 Intentional self-harm by other specified means**
> **EXCLUDES 1**   *intentional self-harm by poisoning or contact with toxic substance—see Table of Drugs and Chemicals*

> The appropriate 7th character is to be added to each code from category X83.
> A   initial encounter
> D   subsequent encounter
> S   sequela

☑7ᵗʰ **X83.0** **Intentional self-harm by** crashing of aircraft

☑7ᵗʰ **X83.1** **Intentional self-harm by** electrocution

☑7ᵗʰ **X83.2** **Intentional self-harm by** exposure to extremes of cold

☑7ᵗʰ **X83.8** **Intentional self-harm by other specified means**

Assault (X92-Y08)

INCLUDES   homicide
     injuries inflicted by another person with intent to injure or kill, by any means
EXCLUDES 1   *injuries due to legal intervention (Y35.-)*
     injuries due to operations of war (Y36.-)
     injuries due to terrorism (Y38.-)

4ᵗʰ **X92 Assault by drowning and submersion**

> The appropriate 7th character is to be added to each code from category X92.
> A   initial encounter
> D   subsequent encounter
> S   sequela

☑7ᵗʰ **X92.0** **Assault by drowning and submersion while in** bathtub

☑7ᵗʰ **X92.1** **Assault by drowning and submersion while in** swimming pool

☑7ᵗʰ **X92.2** **Assault by drowning and submersion after push into** swimming pool

☑7ᵗʰ **X92.3** **Assault by drowning and submersion in** natural water

☑7ᵗʰ **X92.8** **Other assault by drowning and submersion**

☑7ᵗʰ **X92.9** **Assault by drowning and submersion, unspecified**

☑7ᵗʰ **X93 Assault by** handgun **discharge**
     Assault by discharge of gun for single hand use
     Assault by discharge of pistol
     Assault by discharge of revolver
> **EXCLUDES 1**   *Very pistol (X95.8)*

> The appropriate 7th character is to be added to code X93.
> A   initial encounter
> D   subsequent encounter
> S   sequela

4ᵗʰ **X94 Assault by** rifle, shotgun and larger firearm **discharge**
> **EXCLUDES 1**   *airgun (X95.01)*

> The appropriate 7th character is to be added to each code from category X94.
> A   initial encounter
> D   subsequent encounter
> S   sequela

☑7ᵗʰ **X94.0** **Assault by** shotgun

☑7ᵗʰ **X94.1** **Assault by** hunting rifle

☑7ᵗʰ **X94.2** **Assault by** machine gun

☑7ᵗʰ **X94.8** **Assault by other larger firearm discharge**

☑7ᵗʰ **X94.9** **Assault by unspecified larger firearm discharge**

4ᵗʰ **X95 Assault by other and unspecified firearm and gun discharge**

> The appropriate 7th character is to be added to each code from category X95.
> A   initial encounter
> D   subsequent encounter
> S   sequela

5ᵗʰ **X95.0** **Assault by** gas, air or spring-operated guns

     ☑7ᵗʰ **X95.01** **Assault by** airgun **discharge**
         Assault by BB gun discharge
         Assault by pellet gun discharge

     ☑7ᵗʰ **X95.02** **Assault by** paintball gun **discharge**

     ☑7ᵗʰ **X95.09** **Assault by other gas, air or spring-operated gun**

☑7ᵗʰ **X95.8** **Assault by other firearm discharge**
     Assault by Very pistol [flare] discharge

☑ Additional Character Required   ☑ₓ7ᵗʰ Placeholder Alert   Unspecified Dx   Other Specified Dx   Manifestation   ▶◀ Revised Text   ● New Code   ▲ Revised Code Title

CD-10-CM 2016   1083

√x7ᵗʰ **X95.9**   Assault by unspecified firearm discharge

√4ᵗʰ **X96**   **Assault by explosive material**
> **EXCLUDES 1**   incendiary device (X97)
> terrorism involving explosive material (Y38.2-)

> The appropriate 7th character is to be added to each code from category X96.
> A   initial encounter
> D   subsequent encounter
> S   sequela

√x7ᵗʰ **X96.0**   **Assault by antipersonnel bomb**
> **EXCLUDES 1**   antipersonnel bomb use in military or war (Y36.2-)

√x7ᵗʰ **X96.1**   **Assault by gasoline bomb**

√x7ᵗʰ **X96.2**   **Assault by letter bomb**

√x7ᵗʰ **X96.3**   **Assault by fertilizer bomb**

√x7ᵗʰ **X96.4**   **Assault by pipe bomb**

√x7ᵗʰ **X96.8**   **Assault by other specified explosive**

√x7ᵗʰ **X96.9**   **Assault by unspecified explosive**

√x7ᵗʰ **X97**   **Assault by smoke, fire and flames**
> Assault by arson
> Assault by cigarettes
> Assault by incendiary device

> The appropriate 7th character is to be added to code X97.
> A   initial encounter
> D   subsequent encounter
> S   sequela

√4ᵗʰ **X98**   **Assault by steam, hot vapors and hot objects**

> The appropriate 7th character is to be added to each code from category X98.
> A   initial encounter
> D   subsequent encounter
> S   sequela

√x7ᵗʰ **X98.0**   **Assault by steam or hot vapors**

√x7ᵗʰ **X98.1**   **Assault by hot tap water**

√x7ᵗʰ **X98.2**   **Assault by hot fluids**

√x7ᵗʰ **X98.3**   **Assault by hot household appliances**

√x7ᵗʰ **X98.8**   **Assault by other hot objects**

√x7ᵗʰ **X98.9**   **Assault by unspecified hot objects**

√4ᵗʰ **X99**   **Assault by sharp object**
> **EXCLUDES 1**   assault by strike by sports equipment (Y08.0-)

> The appropriate 7th character is to be added to each code from category X99.
> A   initial encounter
> D   subsequent encounter
> S   sequela

√x7ᵗʰ **X99.0**   **Assault by sharp glass**

√x7ᵗʰ **X99.1**   **Assault by knife**

√x7ᵗʰ **X99.2**   **Assault by sword or dagger**

√x7ᵗʰ **X99.8**   **Assault by other sharp object**

√x7ᵗʰ **X99.9**   **Assault by unspecified sharp object**
> Assault by stabbing NOS

√x7ᵗʰ **Y00**   **Assault by blunt object**
> **EXCLUDES 1**   assault by strike by sports equipment (Y08.0-)

> The appropriate 7th character is to be added to code Y00.
> A   initial encounter
> D   subsequent encounter
> S   sequela

√x7ᵗʰ **Y01**   **Assault by pushing from high place**

> The appropriate 7th character is to be added to code Y01.
> A   initial encounter
> D   subsequent encounter
> S   sequela

√4ᵗʰ **Y02**   **Assault by pushing or placing victim in front of moving object**

> The appropriate 7th character is to be added to each code from category Y02.
> A   initial encounter
> D   subsequent encounter
> S   sequela

√x7ᵗʰ **Y02.0**   **Assault by pushing or placing victim in front of motor vehicle**

√x7ᵗʰ **Y02.1**   **Assault by pushing or placing victim in front of (subway) train**

√x7ᵗʰ **Y02.8**   **Assault by pushing or placing victim in front of other movin object**

√4ᵗʰ **Y03**   **Assault by crashing of motor vehicle**

> The appropriate 7th character is to be added to each code from category Y03.
> A   initial encounter
> D   subsequent encounter
> S   sequela

√x7ᵗʰ **Y03.0**   **Assault by being hit or run over by motor vehicle**

√x7ᵗʰ **Y03.8**   **Other assault by crashing of motor vehicle**

√4ᵗʰ **Y04**   **Assault by bodily force**
> **EXCLUDES 1**   assault by:
> submersion (X92.-)
> use of weapon (X93-X95, X99, Y00)

> The appropriate 7th character is to be added to each code from category Y04.
> A   initial encounter
> D   subsequent encounter
> S   sequela

√x7ᵗʰ **Y04.0**   **Assault by unarmed brawl or fight**

√x7ᵗʰ **Y04.1**   **Assault by human bite**

√x7ᵗʰ **Y04.2**   **Assault by strike against or bumped into by another person**

√x7ᵗʰ **Y04.8**   **Assault by other bodily force**
> Assault by bodily force NOS

√4ᵗʰ **Y07**   **Perpetrator of assault, maltreatment and neglect**
> **NOTE**   Codes from this category are for use only in cases of confirmed abuse (T74.-)
> Selection of the correct perpetrator code is based on the relationship between the perpetrator and the victim
> **INCLUDES**   perpetrator of abandonment
> perpetrator of emotional neglect
> perpetrator of mental cruelty
> perpetrator of physical abuse
> perpetrator of physical neglect
> perpetrator of sexual abuse
> perpetrator of torture

√5ᵗʰ **Y07.0**   **Spouse or partner, perpetrator of maltreatment and neglect**
> **NOTE**   Spouse or partner, perpetrator of maltreatment and neglect against spouse or partner

   Y07.01   **Husband, perpetrator of maltreatment and neglect**

   Y07.02   **Wife, perpetrator of maltreatment and neglect**

   Y07.03   **Male partner, perpetrator of maltreatment and neglect**

   Y07.04   **Female partner, perpetrator of maltreatment and neglect**

√5ᵗʰ **Y07.1**   **Parent (adoptive) (biological), perpetrator of maltreatment and neglect**

   Y07.11   **Biological father, perpetrator of maltreatment and neglect**

   Y07.12   **Biological mother, perpetrator of maltreatment and neglect**

   Y07.13   **Adoptive father, perpetrator of maltreatment and neglect**

   Y07.14   **Adoptive mother, perpetrator of maltreatment and neglect**

√5ᵗʰ **Y07.4**   **Other family member, perpetrator of maltreatment and neglect**

√6ᵗʰ **Y07.41**   **Sibling, perpetrator of maltreatment and neglect**
> **EXCLUDES 1**   stepsibling, perpetrator of maltreatment an neglect (Y07.435, Y07.436)

   Y07.410   **Brother, perpetrator of maltreatment and neglect**

   Y07.411   **Sister, perpetrator of maltreatment and neglect**

√6ᵗʰ **Y07.42**   **Foster parent, perpetrator of maltreatment and neglect**

   Y07.420   **Foster father, perpetrator of maltreatment and neglect**

   Y07.421   **Foster mother, perpetrator of maltreatment and neglect**

√6ᵗʰ **Y07.43**   **Stepparent or stepsibling, perpetrator of maltreatment and neglect**

   Y07.430   **Stepfather, perpetrator of maltreatment and neglect**

EXCLUDES 1 Not coded here   **EXCLUDES 2** Not included here   **N** Newborn Age: 0   **P** Pediatric Age: 0-17   **M** Maternity Age: 12-55   **A** Adult Age: 15-124

1084   ICD-10-CM 201

Y07.432 Male friend of parent (co-residing in household), perpetrator of maltreatment and neglect

Y07.433 Stepmother, perpetrator of maltreatment and neglect

Y07.434 Female friend of parent (co-residing in household), perpetrator of maltreatment and neglect

Y07.435 Stepbrother, perpetrator or maltreatment and neglect

Y07.436 Stepsister, perpetrator of maltreatment and neglect

✓6th **Y07.49** Other family member, perpetrator of maltreatment and neglect

Y07.490 Male cousin, perpetrator of maltreatment and neglect

Y07.491 Female cousin, perpetrator of maltreatment and neglect

Y07.499 Other family member, perpetrator of maltreatment and neglect

✓5th **Y07.5** Non-family member, perpetrator of maltreatment and neglect

Y07.50 Unspecified non-family member, perpetrator of maltreatment and neglect

✓6th **Y07.51** Daycare provider, perpetrator of maltreatment and neglect

Y07.510 At-home childcare provider, perpetrator of maltreatment and neglect

Y07.511 Daycare center childcare provider, perpetrator of maltreatment and neglect

Y07.512 At-home adultcare provider, perpetrator of maltreatment and neglect

Y07.513 Adultcare center provider, perpetrator of maltreatment and neglect

Y07.519 Unspecified daycare provider, perpetrator of maltreatment and neglect

✓6th **Y07.52** Healthcare provider, perpetrator of maltreatment and neglect

Y07.521 Mental health provider, perpetrator of maltreatment and neglect

Y07.528 Other therapist or healthcare provider, perpetrator of maltreatment and neglect
Nurse, perpetrator of maltreatment and neglect
Occupational therapist, perpetrator of maltreatment and neglect
Physical therapist, perpetrator of maltreatment and neglect
Speech therapist, perpetrator of maltreatment and neglect

Y07.529 Unspecified healthcare provider, perpetrator of maltreatment and neglect

Y07.53 Teacher or instructor, perpetrator of maltreatment and neglect
Coach, perpetrator of maltreatment and neglect

Y07.59 Other non-family member, perpetrator of maltreatment and neglect

Y07.9 Unspecified perpetrator of maltreatment and neglect

✓4th **Y08** Assault by other specified means

The appropriate 7th character is to be added to each code from category Y08.
A   initial encounter
D   subsequent encounter
S   sequela

✓5th **Y08.0** Assault by strike by sport equipment

✓x7th **Y08.01** Assault by strike by hockey stick

✓x7th **Y08.02** Assault by strike by baseball bat

✓x7th **Y08.09** Assault by strike by other specified type of sport equipment

✓5th **Y08.8** Assault by other specified means

✓x7th **Y08.81** Assault by crashing of aircraft

✓x7th **Y08.89** Assault by other specified means

Y09 Assault by unspecified means
Assassination (attempted) NOS
Homicide (attempted) NOS
Manslaughter (attempted) NOS
Murder (attempted) NOS

Event of undetermined intent (Y21-Y33)

Undetermined intent is only for use when there is specific documentation in the record that the intent of the injury cannot be determined. If no such documentation is present, code to accidental (unintentional)

✓4th **Y21** Drowning and submersion, undetermined intent

The appropriate 7th character is to be added to each code from category Y21.
A   initial encounter
D   subsequent encounter
S   sequela

✓x7th **Y21.0** Drowning and submersion while in bathtub, undetermined intent

✓x7th **Y21.1** Drowning and submersion after fall into bathtub, undetermined intent

✓x7th **Y21.2** Drowning and submersion while in swimming pool, undetermined intent

✓x7th **Y21.3** Drowning and submersion after fall into swimming pool, undetermined intent

✓x7th **Y21.4** Drowning and submersion in natural water, undetermined intent

✓x7th **Y21.8** Other drowning and submersion, undetermined intent

✓x7th **Y21.9** Unspecified drowning and submersion, undetermined intent

✓x7th **Y22** Handgun discharge, undetermined intent
Discharge of gun for single hand use, undetermined intent
Discharge of pistol, undetermined intent
Discharge of revolver, undetermined intent
EXCLUDES 2 Very pistol (Y24.8)

The appropriate 7th character is to be added to code Y22.
A   initial encounter
D   subsequent encounter
S   sequela

✓4th **Y23** Rifle, shotgun and larger firearm discharge, undetermined intent
EXCLUDES 2 airgun (Y24.0)

The appropriate 7th character is to be added to each code from category Y23.
A   initial encounter
D   subsequent encounter
S   sequela

✓x7th **Y23.0** Shotgun discharge, undetermined intent

✓x7th **Y23.1** Hunting rifle discharge, undetermined intent

✓x7th **Y23.2** Military firearm discharge, undetermined intent

✓x7th **Y23.3** Machine gun discharge, undetermined intent

✓x7th **Y23.8** Other larger firearm discharge, undetermined intent

✓x7th **Y23.9** Unspecified larger firearm discharge, undetermined intent

✓4th **Y24** Other and unspecified firearm discharge, undetermined intent

The appropriate 7th character is to be added to each code from category Y24.
A   initial encounter
D   subsequent encounter
S   sequela

✓x7th **Y24.0** Airgun discharge, undetermined intent
BB gun discharge, undetermined intent
Pellet gun discharge, undetermined intent

✓x7th **Y24.8** Other firearm discharge, undetermined intent
Paintball gun discharge, undetermined intent
Very pistol [flare] discharge, undetermined intent

✓x7th **Y24.9** Unspecified firearm discharge, undetermined intent

✓x7th **Y25** Contact with explosive material, undetermined intent

The appropriate 7th character is to be added to code Y25.
A   initial encounter
D   subsequent encounter
S   sequela

✓ Additional Character Required   ✓x7th Placeholder Alert   Unspecified Dx   Other Specified Dx   Manifestation   ►◄ Revised Text   ● New Code   ▲ Revised Code Title

ICD-10-CM 2016   1085

Chapter 2Ø. External Causes of Morbidity

√x7ᵗʰ **Y26 Exposure to smoke, fire and flames, undetermined intent**

> The appropriate 7th character is to be added to code Y26.
> A   initial encounter
> D   subsequent encounter
> S   sequela

√4ᵗʰ **Y27 Contact with steam, hot vapors and hot objects, undetermined intent**

> The appropriate 7th character is to be added to each code from category Y27.
> A   initial encounter
> D   subsequent encounter
> S   sequela

√x7ᵗʰ **Y27.Ø Contact with steam and hot vapors, undetermined intent**
√x7ᵗʰ **Y27.1 Contact with hot tap water, undetermined intent**
√x7ᵗʰ **Y27.2 Contact with hot fluids, undetermined intent**
√x7ᵗʰ **Y27.3 Contact with hot household appliance, undetermined intent**
√x7ᵗʰ **Y27.8 Contact with other hot objects, undetermined intent**
√x7ᵗʰ **Y27.9 Contact with unspecified hot objects, undetermined intent**

√4ᵗʰ **Y28 Contact with sharp object, undetermined intent**

> The appropriate 7th character is to be added to each code from category Y28.
> A   initial encounter
> D   subsequent encounter
> S   sequela

√x7ᵗʰ **Y28.Ø Contact with sharp glass, undetermined intent**
√x7ᵗʰ **Y28.1 Contact with knife, undetermined intent**
√x7ᵗʰ **Y28.2 Contact with sword or dagger, undetermined intent**
√x7ᵗʰ **Y28.8 Contact with other sharp object, undetermined intent**
√x7ᵗʰ **Y28.9 Contact with unspecified hot objects, undetermined intent**

√x7ᵗʰ **Y29 Contact with blunt object, undetermined intent**

> The appropriate 7th character is to be added to code Y29.
> A   initial encounter
> D   subsequent encounter
> S   sequela

√x7ᵗʰ **Y3Ø Falling, jumping or pushed from a high place, undetermined intent**
> Victim falling from one level to another, undetermined intent

> The appropriate 7th character is to be added to code Y30.
> A   initial encounter
> D   subsequent encounter
> S   sequela

√x7ᵗʰ **Y31 Falling, lying or running before or into moving object, undetermined intent**

> The appropriate 7th character is to be added to code Y31.
> A   initial encounter
> D   subsequent encounter
> S   sequela

√x7ᵗʰ **Y32 Crashing of motor vehicle, undetermined intent**

> The appropriate 7th character is to be added to code Y32.
> A   initial encounter
> D   subsequent encounter
> S   sequela

√x7ᵗʰ **Y33 Other specified events, undetermined intent**

> The appropriate 7th character is to be added to code Y33.
> A   initial encounter
> D   subsequent encounter
> S   sequela

Legal intervention, operations of war, military operations, and terrorism (Y35-Y38)

√4ᵗʰ **Y35 Legal intervention**
> **INCLUDES**   any injury sustained as a result of an encounter with any law enforcement official, serving in any capacity at the time of the encounter, whether on-duty or off-duty. Includes injury to law enforcement official, suspect and bystander

√5ᵗʰ **Y35.Ø Legal intervention involving firearm discharge**

√6ᵗʰ **Y35.ØØ Legal intervention involving unspecified firearm discharge**
> Legal intervention involving gunshot wound
> Legal intervention involving shot NOS

√7ᵗʰ **Y35.ØØ1 Legal intervention involving unspecified firearm discharge, law enforcement official injured**
√7ᵗʰ **Y35.ØØ2 Legal intervention involving unspecified firearm discharge, bystander injured**
√7ᵗʰ **Y35.ØØ3 Legal intervention involving unspecified firearm discharge, suspect injured**

√6ᵗʰ **Y35.Ø1 Legal intervention involving injury by machine gun**
√7ᵗʰ **Y35.Ø11 Legal intervention involving injury by machine gun, law enforcement official injured**
√7ᵗʰ **Y35.Ø12 Legal intervention involving injury by machine gun, bystander injured**
√7ᵗʰ **Y35.Ø13 Legal intervention involving injury by machine gun, suspect injured**

√6ᵗʰ **Y35.Ø2 Legal intervention involving injury by handgun**
√7ᵗʰ **Y35.Ø21 Legal intervention involving injury by handgun, law enforcement official injured**
√7ᵗʰ **Y35.Ø22 Legal intervention involving injury by handgun, bystander injured**
√7ᵗʰ **Y35.Ø23 Legal intervention involving injury by handgun, suspect injured**

√6ᵗʰ **Y35.Ø3 Legal intervention involving injury by rifle pellet**
√7ᵗʰ **Y35.Ø31 Legal intervention involving injury by rifle pellet, law enforcement official injured**
√7ᵗʰ **Y35.Ø32 Legal intervention involving injury by rifle pellet, bystander injured**
√7ᵗʰ **Y35.Ø33 Legal intervention involving injury by rifle pellet, suspect injured**

√6ᵗʰ **Y35.Ø4 Legal intervention involving injury by rubber bullet**
√7ᵗʰ **Y35.Ø41 Legal intervention involving injury by rubber bullet, law enforcement official injured**
√7ᵗʰ **Y35.Ø42 Legal intervention involving injury by rubber bullet, bystander injured**
√7ᵗʰ **Y35.Ø43 Legal intervention involving injury by rubber bullet, suspect injured**

√6ᵗʰ **Y35.Ø9 Legal intervention involving other firearm discharge**
√7ᵗʰ **Y35.Ø91 Legal intervention involving other firearm discharge, law enforcement official injured**
√7ᵗʰ **Y35.Ø92 Legal intervention involving other firearm discharge, bystander injured**
√7ᵗʰ **Y35.Ø93 Legal intervention involving other firearm discharge, suspect injured**

√5ᵗʰ **Y35.1 Legal intervention involving explosives**

√6ᵗʰ **Y35.1Ø Legal intervention involving unspecified explosives**
√7ᵗʰ **Y35.1Ø1 Legal intervention involving unspecified explosives, law enforcement official injured**
√7ᵗʰ **Y35.1Ø2 Legal intervention involving unspecified explosives, bystander injured**
√7ᵗʰ **Y35.1Ø3 Legal intervention involving unspecified explosives, suspect injured**

EXCLUDES 1 Not coded here   **EXCLUDES 2** Not included here   N Newborn Age: 0   P Pediatric Age: 0-17   M Maternity Age: 12-55   A Adult Age: 15-124

1086   ICD-10-CM 2016

✓6th **Y35.11** **Legal intervention involving injury by dynamite**

   ✓7th **Y35.111** **Legal intervention involving injury by dynamite, law enforcement official injured**

   ✓7th **Y35.112** **Legal intervention involving injury by dynamite, bystander injured**

   ✓7th **Y35.113** **Legal intervention involving injury by dynamite, suspect injured**

✓6th **Y35.12** **Legal intervention involving injury by explosive shell**

   ✓7th **Y35.121** **Legal intervention involving injury by explosive shell, law enforcement official injured**

   ✓7th **Y35.122** **Legal intervention involving injury by explosive shell, bystander injured**

   ✓7th **Y35.123** **Legal intervention involving injury by explosive shell, suspect injured**

✓6th **Y35.19** **Legal intervention involving other explosives**
    Legal intervention involving injury by grenade
    Legal intervention involving injury by mortar bomb

   ✓7th **Y35.191** **Legal intervention involving other explosives, law enforcement official injured**

   ✓7th **Y35.192** **Legal intervention involving other explosives, bystander injured**

   ✓7th **Y35.193** **Legal intervention involving other explosives, suspect injured**

✓5th **Y35.2** **Legal intervention involving gas**
    Legal intervention involving asphyxiation by gas
    Legal intervention involving poisoning by gas

  ✓6th **Y35.20** **Legal intervention involving unspecified gas**

   ✓7th **Y35.201** **Legal intervention involving unspecified gas, law enforcement official injured**

   ✓7th **Y35.202** **Legal intervention involving unspecified gas, bystander injured**

   ✓7th **Y35.203** **Legal intervention involving unspecified gas, suspect injured**

  ✓6th **Y35.21** **Legal intervention involving injury by tear gas**

   ✓7th **Y35.211** **Legal intervention involving injury by tear gas, law enforcement official injured**

   ✓7th **Y35.212** **Legal intervention involving injury by tear gas, bystander injured**

   ✓7th **Y35.213** **Legal intervention involving injury by tear gas, suspect injured**

  ✓6th **Y35.29** **Legal intervention involving other gas**

   ✓7th **Y35.291** **Legal intervention involving other gas, law enforcement official injured**

   ✓7th **Y35.292** **Legal intervention involving other gas, bystander injured**

   ✓7th **Y35.293** **Legal intervention involving other gas, suspect injured**

✓5th **Y35.3** **Legal intervention involving blunt objects**
    Legal intervention involving being hit or struck by blunt object

  ✓6th **Y35.30** **Legal intervention involving unspecified blunt objects**

   ✓7th **Y35.301** **Legal intervention involving unspecified blunt objects, law enforcement official injured**

   ✓7th **Y35.302** **Legal intervention involving unspecified blunt objects, bystander injured**

   ✓7th **Y35.303** **Legal intervention involving unspecified blunt objects, suspect injured**

  ✓6th **Y35.31** **Legal intervention involving baton**

   ✓7th **Y35.311** **Legal intervention involving baton, law enforcement official injured**

   ✓7th **Y35.312** **Legal intervention involving baton, bystander injured**

   ✓7th **Y35.313** **Legal intervention involving baton, suspect injured**

  ✓6th **Y35.39** **Legal intervention involving other blunt objects**

   ✓7th **Y35.391** **Legal intervention involving other blunt objects, law enforcement official injured**

   ✓7th **Y35.392** **Legal intervention involving other blunt objects, bystander injured**

   ✓7th **Y35.393** **Legal intervention involving other blunt objects, suspect injured**

✓5th **Y35.4** **Legal intervention involving sharp objects**
    Legal intervention involving being cut by sharp objects
    Legal intervention involving being stabbed by sharp objects

  ✓6th **Y35.40** **Legal intervention involving unspecified sharp objects**

   ✓7th **Y35.401** **Legal intervention involving unspecified sharp objects, law enforcement official injured**

   ✓7th **Y35.402** **Legal intervention involving unspecified sharp objects, bystander injured**

   ✓7th **Y35.403** **Legal intervention involving unspecified sharp objects, suspect injured**

  ✓6th **Y35.41** **Legal intervention involving bayonet**

   ✓7th **Y35.411** **Legal intervention involving bayonet, law enforcement official injured**

   ✓7th **Y35.412** **Legal intervention involving bayonet, bystander injured**

   ✓7th **Y35.413** **Legal intervention involving bayonet, suspect injured**

  ✓6th **Y35.49** **Legal intervention involving other sharp objects**

   ✓7th **Y35.491** **Legal intervention involving other sharp objects, law enforcement official injured**

   ✓7th **Y35.492** **Legal intervention involving other sharp objects, bystander injured**

   ✓7th **Y35.493** **Legal intervention involving other sharp objects, suspect injured**

✓5th **Y35.8** **Legal intervention involving other specified means**

  ✓6th **Y35.81** **Legal intervention involving manhandling**

   ✓7th **Y35.811** **Legal intervention involving manhandling, law enforcement official injured**

   ✓7th **Y35.812** **Legal intervention involving manhandling, bystander injured**

   ✓7th **Y35.813** **Legal intervention involving manhandling, suspect injured**

  ✓6th **Y35.89** **Legal intervention involving other specified means**

   ✓7th **Y35.891** **Legal intervention involving other specified means, law enforcement official injured**

   ✓7th **Y35.892** **Legal intervention involving other specified means, bystander injured**

   ✓7th **Y35.893** **Legal intervention involving other specified means, suspect injured**

✓5th **Y35.9** **Legal intervention, means unspecified**

  ✓x 7th **Y35.91** **Legal intervention, means unspecified, law enforcement official injured**

  ✓x 7th **Y35.92** **Legal intervention, means unspecified, bystander injured**

  ✓x 7th **Y35.93** **Legal intervention, means unspecified, suspect injured**

✓4th **Y36** **Operations of war**
   INCLUDES   injuries to military personnel and civilians caused by war, civil insurrection, and peacekeeping missions
   EXCLUDES 1   *injury to military personnel occurring during peacetime military operations (Y37.-)*
    military vehicles involved in transport accidents with non-military vehicle during peacetime (V09.01, V09.21, V19.81, V29.81, V39.81, V49.81, V59.81, V69.81, V79.81)

   AHA: 2014, 3Q, 4

The appropriate 7th character is to be added to each code from category Y36.
A   initial encounter
D   subsequent encounter
S   sequela

✓5th **Y36.0** **War operations involving explosion of marine weapons**

  ✓6th **Y36.00** **War operations involving explosion of unspecified marine weapon**
    War operations involving underwater blast NOS

   ✓7th **Y36.000** **War operations involving explosion of unspecified marine weapon, military personnel**

   ✓7th **Y36.001** **War operations involving explosion of unspecified marine weapon, civilian**

☑ Additional Character Required   ✓x7th Placeholder Alert   Unspecified Dx   Other Specified Dx   Manifestation   ▶◀ Revised Text   ● New Code   ▲ Revised Code Title

ICD-10-CM 2016   1087

✓6th **Y36.01** War operations involving explosion of depth-charge

   ✓7th **Y36.010** **War operations involving explosion of depth-charge, military personnel**

   ✓7th **Y36.011** **War operations involving explosion of depth-charge, civilian**

✓6th **Y36.02** War operations involving explosion of marine mine

   War operations involving explosion of marine mine, at sea or in harbor

   ✓7th **Y36.020** **War operations involving explosion of marine mine, military personnel**

   ✓7th **Y36.021** **War operations involving explosion of marine mine, civilian**

✓6th **Y36.03** War operations involving explosion of sea-based artillery shell

   ✓7th **Y36.030** **War operations involving explosion of sea-based artillery shell, military personnel**

   ✓7th **Y36.031** **War operations involving explosion of sea-based artillery shell, civilian**

✓6th **Y36.04** War operations involving explosion of torpedo

   ✓7th **Y36.040** **War operations involving explosion of torpedo, military personnel**

   ✓7th **Y36.041** **War operations involving explosion of torpedo, civilian**

✓6th **Y36.05** War operations involving accidental detonation of onboard marine weapons

   ✓7th **Y36.050** **War operations involving accidental detonation of onboard marine weapons, military personnel**

   ✓7th **Y36.051** **War operations involving accidental detonation of onboard marine weapons, civilian**

✓6th **Y36.09** War operations involving explosion of other marine weapons

   ✓7th **Y36.090** **War operations involving explosion of other marine weapons, military personnel**

   ✓7th **Y36.091** **War operations involving explosion of other marine weapons, civilian**

✓5th **Y36.1** War operations involving destruction of aircraft

   ✓6th **Y36.10** War operations involving unspecified destruction of aircraft

     ✓7th **Y36.100** **War operations involving unspecified destruction of aircraft, military personnel**

     ✓7th **Y36.101** **War operations involving unspecified destruction of aircraft, civilian**

   ✓6th **Y36.11** War operations involving destruction of aircraft due to enemy fire or explosives

     War operations involving destruction of aircraft due to air to air missile

     War operations involving destruction of aircraft due to explosive placed on aircraft

     War operations involving destruction of aircraft due to rocket propelled grenade [RPG]

     War operations involving destruction of aircraft due to small arms fire

     War operations involving destruction of aircraft due to surface to air missile

     ✓7th **Y36.110** **War operations involving destruction of aircraft due to enemy fire or explosives, military personnel**

     ✓7th **Y36.111** **War operations involving destruction of aircraft due to enemy fire or explosives, civilian**

   ✓6th **Y36.12** War operations involving destruction of aircraft due to collision with other aircraft

     ✓7th **Y36.120** **War operations involving destruction of aircraft due to collision with other aircraft, military personnel**

     ✓7th **Y36.121** **War operations involving destruction of aircraft due to collision with other aircraft, civilian**

   ✓6th **Y36.13** War operations involving destruction of aircraft due to onboard fire

     ✓7th **Y36.130** **War operations involving destruction of aircraft due to onboard fire, military personnel**

     ✓7th **Y36.131** **War operations involving destruction of aircraft due to onboard fire, civilian**

   ✓6th **Y36.14** War operations involving destruction of aircraft due to accidental detonation of onboard munitions and explosives

     ✓7th **Y36.140** **War operations involving destruction of aircraft due to accidental detonation of onboard munitions and explosives, military personnel**

     ✓7th **Y36.141** **War operations involving destruction of aircraft due to accidental detonation of onboard munitions and explosives, civilian**

   ✓6th **Y36.19** War operations involving other destruction of aircraft

     ✓7th **Y36.190** **War operations involving other destruction of aircraft, military personnel**

     ✓7th **Y36.191** **War operations involving other destruction of aircraft, civilian**

✓5th **Y36.2** War operations involving other explosions and fragments

   EXCLUDES 1   war operations involving explosion of aircraft (Y36.1-)

     war operations involving explosion of marine weapons (Y36.0-)

     war operations involving explosion of nuclear weapons (Y36.5-)

     war operations involving explosion occurring after cessation of hostilities (Y36.8-)

   ✓6th **Y36.20** War operations involving unspecified explosion and fragments

     War operations involving air blast NOS

     War operations involving blast NOS

     War operations involving blast fragments NOS

     War operations involving blast wave NOS

     War operations involving blast wind NOS

     War operations involving explosion NOS

     War operations involving explosion of bomb NOS

     ✓7th **Y36.200** **War operations involving unspecified explosion and fragments, military personnel**

     ✓7th **Y36.201** **War operations involving unspecified explosion and fragments, civilian**

   ✓6th **Y36.21** War operations involving explosion of aerial bomb

     ✓7th **Y36.210** **War operations involving explosion of aerial bomb, military personnel**

     ✓7th **Y36.211** **War operations involving explosion of aerial bomb, civilian**

   ✓6th **Y36.22** War operations involving explosion of guided missile

     ✓7th **Y36.220** **War operations involving explosion of guided missile, military personnel**

     ✓7th **Y36.221** **War operations involving explosion of guided missile, civilian**

   ✓6th **Y36.23** War operations involving explosion of improvised explosive device [IED]

     War operations involving explosion of person-borne improvised explosive device [IED]

     War operations involving explosion of vehicle-borne improvised explosive device [IED]

     War operations involving explosion of roadside improvised explosive device [IED]

     ✓7th **Y36.230** **War operations involving explosion of improvised explosive device [IED], military personnel**

     ✓7th **Y36.231** **War operations involving explosion of improvised explosive device [IED], civilian**

   ✓6th **Y36.24** War operations involving explosion due to accidental detonation and discharge of own munitions or munitions launch device

     ✓7th **Y36.240** **War operations involving explosion due to accidental detonation and discharge of own munitions or munitions launch device, military personnel**

     ✓7th **Y36.241** **War operations involving explosion due to accidental detonation and discharge of own munitions or munitions launch device, civilian**

   ✓6th **Y36.25** War operations involving fragments from munitions

     ✓7th **Y36.250** **War operations involving fragments from munitions, military personnel**

EXCLUDES 1 Not coded here   EXCLUDES 2 Not included here   N Newborn Age: 0   P Pediatric Age: 0-17   M Maternity Age: 12-55   A Adult Age: 15-124

1088   ICD-10-CM 2016

✓7ᵗʰ **Y36.251** **War operations involving fragments from munitions,** civilian

✓6ᵗʰ **Y36.26** **War operations involving fragments of** improvised explosive device **[IED]**
War operations involving fragments of person-borne improvised explosive device [IED]
War operations involving fragments of vehicle-borne improvised explosive device [IED]
War operations involving fragments of roadside improvised explosive device [IED]

     ✓7ᵗʰ **Y36.260** **War operations involving fragments of improvised explosive device [IED],** military personnel

     ✓7ᵗʰ **Y36.261** **War operations involving fragments of improvised explosive device [IED],** civilian

✓6ᵗʰ **Y36.27** **War operations involving** fragments from weapons

     ✓7ᵗʰ **Y36.270** **War operations involving fragments from weapons,** military personnel

     ✓7ᵗʰ **Y36.271** **War operations involving fragments from weapons,** civilian

✓6ᵗʰ **Y36.29** **War operations involving** other explosions and fragments
War operations involving explosion of grenade
War operations involving explosions of land mine
War operations involving shrapnel NOS

     ✓7ᵗʰ **Y36.290** **War operations involving other explosions and fragments, military personnel**

     ✓7ᵗʰ **Y36.291** **War operations involving other explosions and fragments, civilian**

✓5ᵗʰ **Y36.3** **War operations involving** fires, conflagrations and hot substances
War operations involving smoke, fumes, and heat from fires, conflagrations and hot substances

     EXCLUDES 1   *war operations involving fires and conflagrations aboard military aircraft (Y36.1-)*
war operations involving fires and conflagrations aboard military watercraft (Y36.0-)
war operations involving fires and conflagrations caused indirectly by conventional weapons (Y36.2-)
war operations involving fires and thermal effects of nuclear weapons (Y36.53-)

✓6ᵗʰ **Y36.30** **War operations involving** unspecified **fire, conflagration and hot substance**

     ✓7ᵗʰ **Y36.300** **War operations involving unspecified fire, conflagration and hot substance, military personnel**

     ✓7ᵗʰ **Y36.301** **War operations involving unspecified fire, conflagration and hot substance, civilian**

✓6ᵗʰ **Y36.31** **War operations involving** gasoline bomb
War operations involving incendiary bomb
War operations involving petrol bomb

     ✓7ᵗʰ **Y36.310** **War operations involving gasoline bomb, military personnel**

     ✓7ᵗʰ **Y36.311** **War operations involving gasoline bomb, civilian**

✓6ᵗʰ **Y36.32** **War operations involving** incendiary bullet

     ✓7ᵗʰ **Y36.320** **War operations involving incendiary bullet, military personnel**

     ✓7ᵗʰ **Y36.321** **War operations involving incendiary bullet, civilian**

✓6ᵗʰ **Y36.33** **War operations involving** flamethrower

     ✓7ᵗʰ **Y36.330** **War operations involving flamethrower, military personnel**

     ✓7ᵗʰ **Y36.331** **War operations involving flamethrower, civilian**

✓6ᵗʰ **Y36.39** **War operations involving other fires,** conflagrations and hot substances

     ✓7ᵗʰ **Y36.390** **War operations involving other fires, conflagrations and hot substances, military personnel**

     ✓7ᵗʰ **Y36.391** **War operations involving other fires, conflagrations and hot substances, civilian**

✓5ᵗʰ **Y36.4** **War operations involving firearm discharge and other forms of conventional warfare**

✓6ᵗʰ **Y36.41** **War operations involving** rubber bullets

     ✓7ᵗʰ **Y36.410** **War operations involving rubber bullets, military personnel**

     ✓7ᵗʰ **Y36.411** **War operations involving rubber bullets, civilian**

✓6ᵗʰ **Y36.42** **War operations involving** firearms pellets

     ✓7ᵗʰ **Y36.420** **War operations involving firearms pellets, military personnel**

     ✓7ᵗʰ **Y36.421** **War operations involving firearms pellets, civilian**

✓6ᵗʰ **Y36.43** **War operations involving** other firearms discharge
War operations involving bullets NOS

     EXCLUDES 1   *war operations involving munitions fragments (Y36.25-)*
war operations involving incendiary bullets (Y36.32-)

     ✓7ᵗʰ **Y36.430** **War operations involving other firearms discharge, military personnel**

     ✓7ᵗʰ **Y36.431** **War operations involving other firearms discharge, civilian**

✓6ᵗʰ **Y36.44** **War operations involving** unarmed hand to hand combat

     EXCLUDES 1   *war operations involving combat using blunt or piercing object (Y36.45-)*
war operations involving intentional restriction of air and airway (Y36.46-)
war operations involving unintentional restriction of air and airway (Y36.47-)

     ✓7ᵗʰ **Y36.440** **War operations involving unarmed hand to hand combat, military personnel**

     ✓7ᵗʰ **Y36.441** **War operations involving unarmed hand to hand combat, civilian**

✓6ᵗʰ **Y36.45** **War operations involving combat using blunt or piercing object**

     ✓7ᵗʰ **Y36.450** **War operations involving combat using blunt or piercing object, military personnel**

     ✓7ᵗʰ **Y36.451** **War operations involving combat using blunt or piercing object, civilian**

✓6ᵗʰ **Y36.46** **War operations involving** intentional restriction of air and airway

     ✓7ᵗʰ **Y36.460** **War operations involving intentional restriction of air and airway, military personnel**

     ✓7ᵗʰ **Y36.461** **War operations involving intentional restriction of air and airway, civilian**

✓6ᵗʰ **Y36.47** **War operations involving** unintentional restriction of air and airway

     ✓7ᵗʰ **Y36.470** **War operations involving unintentional restriction of air and airway, military personnel**

     ✓7ᵗʰ **Y36.471** **War operations involving unintentional restriction of air and airway, civilian**

✓6ᵗʰ **Y36.49** **War operations involving** other forms of conventional warfare

     ✓7ᵗʰ **Y36.490** **War operations involving other forms of conventional warfare, military personnel**

     ✓7ᵗʰ **Y36.491** **War operations involving other forms of conventional warfare, civilian**

✓5ᵗʰ **Y36.5** **War operations involving** nuclear weapons
War operations involving dirty bomb NOS

✓6ᵗʰ **Y36.50** **War operations involving** unspecified **effect of nuclear weapon**

     ✓7ᵗʰ **Y36.500** **War operations involving unspecified effect of nuclear weapon, military personnel**

     ✓7ᵗʰ **Y36.501** **War operations involving unspecified effect of nuclear weapon, civilian**

✓6ᵗʰ **Y36.51** **War operations involving** direct blast **effect of nuclear weapon**
War operations involving blast pressure of nuclear weapon

     ✓7ᵗʰ **Y36.510** **War operations involving direct blast effect of nuclear weapon, military personnel**

✔ Additional Character Required   ✓x7ᵗʰ Placeholder Alert   Unspecified Dx   Other Specified Dx   Manifestation   ▶◀ Revised Text   ● New Code   ▲ Revised Code Title

Chapter 20. External Causes of Morbidity

Y36.511–Y37.040

✓7ᵗʰ **Y36.511** **War operations involving direct blast effect of nuclear weapon, civilian**

✓6ᵗʰ **Y36.52** **War operations involving indirect blast effect of nuclear weapon**
War operations involving being thrown by blast of nuclear weapon
War operations involving being struck or crushed by blast debris of nuclear weapon

    ✓7ᵗʰ **Y36.520** **War operations involving indirect blast effect of nuclear weapon, military personnel**

    ✓7ᵗʰ **Y36.521** **War operations involving indirect blast effect of nuclear weapon, civilian**

✓6ᵗʰ **Y36.53** **War operations involving thermal radiation effect of nuclear weapon**
War operations involving direct heat from nuclear weapon
War operation involving fireball effects from nuclear weapon

    ✓7ᵗʰ **Y36.530** **War operations involving thermal radiation effect of nuclear weapon, military personnel**

    ✓7ᵗʰ **Y36.531** **War operations involving thermal radiation effect of nuclear weapon, civilian**

✓6ᵗʰ **Y36.54** **War operation involving nuclear radiation effects of nuclear weapon**
War operation involving acute radiation exposure from nuclear weapon
War operation involving exposure to immediate ionizing radiation from nuclear weapon
War operation involving fallout exposure from nuclear weapon
War operation involving secondary effects of nuclear weapons

    ✓7ᵗʰ **Y36.540** **War operation involving nuclear radiation effects of nuclear weapon, military personnel**

    ✓7ᵗʰ **Y36.541** **War operation involving nuclear radiation effects of nuclear weapon, civilian**

✓6ᵗʰ **Y36.59** **War operation involving other effects of nuclear weapons**

    ✓7ᵗʰ **Y36.590** **War operation involving other effects of nuclear weapons, military personnel**

    ✓7ᵗʰ **Y36.591** **War operation involving other effects of nuclear weapons, civilian**

✓5ᵗʰ **Y36.6** **War operations involving biological weapons**

  ✓6ᵗʰ **Y36.6X** **War operations involving biological weapons**

    ✓7ᵗʰ **Y36.6X0** **War operations involving biological weapons, military personnel**

    ✓7ᵗʰ **Y36.6X1** **War operations involving biological weapons, civilian**

✓5ᵗʰ **Y36.7** **War operations involving chemical weapons and other forms of unconventional warfare**
  EXCLUDES 1   *war operations involving incendiary devices (Y36.3-, Y36.5-)*

  ✓6ᵗʰ **Y36.7X** **War operations involving chemical weapons and other forms of unconventional warfare**

    ✓7ᵗʰ **Y36.7X0** **War operations involving chemical weapons and other forms of unconventional warfare, military personnel**

    ✓7ᵗʰ **Y36.7X1** **War operations involving chemical weapons and other forms of unconventional warfare, civilian**

✓5ᵗʰ **Y36.8** **War operations occurring after cessation of hostilities**
War operations classifiable to categories Y36.0-Y36.8 but occurring after cessation of hostilities

  ✓6ᵗʰ **Y36.81** **Explosion of mine placed during war operations but exploding after cessation of hostilities**

    ✓7ᵗʰ **Y36.810** **Explosion of mine placed during war operations but exploding after cessation of hostilities, military personnel**

    ✓7ᵗʰ **Y36.811** **Explosion of mine placed during war operations but exploding after cessation of hostilities, civilian**

✓6ᵗʰ **Y36.82** **Explosion of bomb placed during war operations but exploding after cessation of hostilities**

    ✓7ᵗʰ **Y36.820** **Explosion of bomb placed during war operations but exploding after cessation of hostilities, military personnel**

    ✓7ᵗʰ **Y36.821** **Explosion of bomb placed during war operations but exploding after cessation of hostilities, civilian**

✓6ᵗʰ **Y36.88** **Other war operations occurring after cessation of hostilities**

    ✓7ᵗʰ **Y36.880** **Other war operations occurring after cessation of hostilities, military personnel**

    ✓7ᵗʰ **Y36.881** **Other war operations occurring after cessation of hostilities, civilian**

✓6ᵗʰ **Y36.89** **Unspecified war operations occurring after cessation of hostilities**

    ✓7ᵗʰ **Y36.890** **Unspecified war operations occurring after cessation of hostilities, military personnel**

    ✓7ᵗʰ **Y36.891** **Unspecified war operations occurring after cessation of hostilities, civilian**

✓5ᵗʰ **Y36.9** **Other and unspecified war operations**

  ✓x7ᵗʰ **Y36.90** **War operations, unspecified**

  ✓x7ᵗʰ **Y36.91** **War operations involving unspecified weapon of mass destruction [WMD]**

  ✓x7ᵗʰ **Y36.92** **War operations involving friendly fire**

✓4ᵗʰ **Y37** **Military operations**
  INCLUDES   injuries to military personnel and civilians occurring during peacetime on military property and during routine military exercises and operations
  EXCLUDES 1   *military aircraft involved in aircraft accident with civilian aircraft (V97.81-)*
military vehicles involved in transport accident with civilian vehicle (V09.01, V09.21, V19.81, V29.81, V39.81, V49.81, V59.81, V69.81, V79.81)
military watercraft involved in water transport accident with civilian watercraft (V94.81-)
war operations (Y36.-)

> The appropriate 7th character is to be added to each code from category Y37.
> A   initial encounter
> D   subsequent encounter
> S   sequela

✓5ᵗʰ **Y37.0** **Military operations involving explosion of marine weapons**

  ✓6ᵗʰ **Y37.00** **Military operations involving explosion of unspecified marine weapon**
Military operations involving underwater blast NOS

    ✓7ᵗʰ **Y37.000** **Military operations involving explosion of unspecified marine weapon, military personnel**

    ✓7ᵗʰ **Y37.001** **Military operations involving explosion of unspecified marine weapon, civilian**

  ✓6ᵗʰ **Y37.01** **Military operations involving explosion of depth-charge**

    ✓7ᵗʰ **Y37.010** **Military operations involving explosion of depth-charge, military personnel**

    ✓7ᵗʰ **Y37.011** **Military operations involving explosion of depth-charge, civilian**

  ✓6ᵗʰ **Y37.02** **Military operations involving explosion of marine mine**
Military operations involving explosion of marine mine, at sea or in harbor

    ✓7ᵗʰ **Y37.020** **Military operations involving explosion of marine mine, military personnel**

    ✓7ᵗʰ **Y37.021** **Military operations involving explosion of marine mine, civilian**

  ✓6ᵗʰ **Y37.03** **Military operations involving explosion of sea-based artillery shell**

    ✓7ᵗʰ **Y37.030** **Military operations involving explosion of sea-based artillery shell, military personnel**

    ✓7ᵗʰ **Y37.031** **Military operations involving explosion of sea-based artillery shell, civilian**

  ✓6ᵗʰ **Y37.04** **Military operations involving explosion of torpedo**

    ✓7ᵗʰ **Y37.040** **Military operations involving explosion of torpedo, military personnel**

EXCLUDES 1 Not coded here   EXCLUDES 2 Not included here   N Newborn Age: 0   P Pediatric Age: 0-17   M Maternity Age: 12-55   A Adult Age: 15-124

1090   ICD-10-CM 2016

✓7ᵗʰ **Y37.041** Military operations involving explosion of torpedo, civilian

✓6ᵗʰ **Y37.05** Military operations involving accidental detonation of onboard marine weapons

  ✓7ᵗʰ **Y37.050** Military operations involving accidental detonation of onboard marine weapons, military personnel

  ✓7ᵗʰ **Y37.051** Military operations involving accidental detonation of onboard marine weapons, civilian

✓6ᵗʰ **Y37.09** Military operations involving explosion of other marine weapons

  ✓7ᵗʰ **Y37.090** Military operations involving explosion of other marine weapons, military personnel

  ✓7ᵗʰ **Y37.091** Military operations involving explosion of other marine weapons, civilian

✓5ᵗʰ **Y37.1** Military operations involving destruction of aircraft

✓6ᵗʰ **Y37.10** Military operations involving unspecified destruction of aircraft

  ✓7ᵗʰ **Y37.100** Military operations involving unspecified destruction of aircraft, military personnel

  ✓7ᵗʰ **Y37.101** Military operations involving unspecified destruction of aircraft, civilian

✓6ᵗʰ **Y37.11** Military operations involving destruction of aircraft due to enemy fire or explosives

  Military operations involving destruction of aircraft due to air to air missile

  Military operations involving destruction of aircraft due to explosive placed on aircraft

  Military operations involving destruction of aircraft due to rocket propelled grenade [RPG]

  Military operations involving destruction of aircraft due to small arms fire

  Military operations involving destruction of aircraft due to surface to air missile

  ✓7ᵗʰ **Y37.110** Military operations involving destruction of aircraft due to enemy fire or explosives, military personnel

  ✓7ᵗʰ **Y37.111** Military operations involving destruction of aircraft due to enemy fire or explosives, civilian

✓6ᵗʰ **Y37.12** Military operations involving destruction of aircraft due to collision with other aircraft

  ✓7ᵗʰ **Y37.120** Military operations involving destruction of aircraft due to collision with other aircraft, military personnel

  ✓7ᵗʰ **Y37.121** Military operations involving destruction of aircraft due to collision with other aircraft, civilian

✓6ᵗʰ **Y37.13** Military operations involving destruction of aircraft due to onboard fire

  ✓7ᵗʰ **Y37.130** Military operations involving destruction of aircraft due to onboard fire, military personnel

  ✓7ᵗʰ **Y37.131** Military operations involving destruction of aircraft due to onboard fire, civilian

✓6ᵗʰ **Y37.14** Military operations involving destruction of aircraft due to accidental detonation of onboard munitions and explosives

  ✓7ᵗʰ **Y37.140** Military operations involving destruction of aircraft due to accidental detonation of onboard munitions and explosives, military personnel

  ✓7ᵗʰ **Y37.141** Military operations involving destruction of aircraft due to accidental detonation of onboard munitions and explosives, civilian

✓6ᵗʰ **Y37.19** Military operations involving other destruction of aircraft

  ✓7ᵗʰ **Y37.190** Military operations involving other destruction of aircraft, military personnel

  ✓7ᵗʰ **Y37.191** Military operations involving other destruction of aircraft, civilian

✓5ᵗʰ **Y37.2** Military operations involving other explosions and fragments

  EXCLUDES 1   military operations involving explosion of aircraft (Y37.1-)
       military operations involving explosion of marine weapons (Y37.0-)
       military operations involving explosion of nuclear weapons (Y37.5-)

✓6ᵗʰ **Y37.20** Military operations involving unspecified explosion and fragments

  Military operations involving air blast NOS
  Military operations involving blast NOS
  Military operations involving blast fragments NOS
  Military operations involving blast wave NOS
  Military operations involving blast wind NOS
  Military operations involving explosion NOS
  Military operations involving explosion of bomb NOS

  ✓7ᵗʰ **Y37.200** Military operations involving unspecified explosion and fragments, military personnel

  ✓7ᵗʰ **Y37.201** Military operations involving unspecified explosion and fragments, civilian

✓6ᵗʰ **Y37.21** Military operations involving explosion of aerial bomb

  ✓7ᵗʰ **Y37.210** Military operations involving explosion of aerial bomb, military personnel

  ✓7ᵗʰ **Y37.211** Military operations involving explosion of aerial bomb, civilian

✓6ᵗʰ **Y37.22** Military operations involving explosion of guided missile

  ✓7ᵗʰ **Y37.220** Military operations involving explosion of guided missile, military personnel

  ✓7ᵗʰ **Y37.221** Military operations involving explosion of guided missile, civilian

✓6ᵗʰ **Y37.23** Military operations involving explosion of improvised explosive device [IED]

  Military operations involving explosion of person-borne improvised explosive device [IED]
  Military operations involving explosion of vehicle-borne improvised explosive device [IED]
  Military operations involving explosion of roadside improvised explosive device [IED]

  ✓7ᵗʰ **Y37.230** Military operations involving explosion of improvised explosive device [IED], military personnel

  ✓7ᵗʰ **Y37.231** Military operations involving explosion of improvised explosive device [IED], civilian

✓6ᵗʰ **Y37.24** Military operations involving explosion due to accidental detonation and discharge of own munitions or munitions launch device

  ✓7ᵗʰ **Y37.240** Military operations involving explosion due to accidental detonation and discharge of own munitions or munitions launch device, military personnel

  ✓7ᵗʰ **Y37.241** Military operations involving explosion due to accidental detonation and discharge of own munitions or munitions launch device, civilian

✓6ᵗʰ **Y37.25** Military operations involving fragments from munitions

  ✓7ᵗʰ **Y37.250** Military operations involving fragments from munitions, military personnel

  ✓7ᵗʰ **Y37.251** Military operations involving fragments from munitions, civilian

✓6ᵗʰ **Y37.26** Military operations involving fragments of improvised explosive device [IED]

  Military operations involving fragments of person-borne improvised explosive device [IED]
  Military operations involving fragments of vehicle-borne improvised explosive device [IED]
  Military operations involving fragments of roadside improvised explosive device [IED]

  ✓7ᵗʰ **Y37.260** Military operations involving fragments of improvised explosive device [IED], military personnel

  ✓7ᵗʰ **Y37.261** Military operations involving fragments of improvised explosive device [IED], civilian

---

☑ Additional Character Required   ✓ˣ7ᵗʰ Placeholder Alert   Unspecified Dx   Other Specified Dx   Manifestation   ►◄ Revised Text   ● New Code   ▲ Revised Code Title

Chapter 20. External Causes of Morbidity

√6th **Y37.27** **Military operations involving fragments from weapons**

  √7th **Y37.270** **Military operations involving fragments from weapons, military personnel**

  √7th **Y37.271** **Military operations involving fragments from weapons, civilian**

√6th **Y37.29** **Military operations involving other explosions and fragments**

  Military operations involving explosion of grenade
  Military operations involving explosions of land mine
  Military operations involving shrapnel NOS

  √7th **Y37.290** **Military operations involving other explosions and fragments, military personnel**

  √7th **Y37.291** **Military operations involving other explosions and fragments, civilian**

√5th **Y37.3** **Military operations involving fires, conflagrations and hot substances**

  Military operations involving smoke, fumes, and heat from fires, conflagrations and hot substances

  EXCLUDES 1   *military operations involving fires and conflagrations aboard military aircraft (Y37.1-)*
    military operations involving fires and conflagrations aboard military watercraft (Y37.0-)
    military operations involving fires and conflagrations caused indirectly by conventional weapons (Y37.2-)
    military operations involving fires and thermal effects of nuclear weapons (Y36.53-)

√6th **Y37.30** **Military operations involving unspecified fire, conflagration and hot substance**

  √7th **Y37.300** **Military operations involving unspecified fire, conflagration and hot substance, military personnel**

  √7th **Y37.301** **Military operations involving unspecified fire, conflagration and hot substance, civilian**

√6th **Y37.31** **Military operations involving gasoline bomb**

  Military operations involving incendiary bomb
  Military operations involving petrol bomb

  √7th **Y37.310** **Military operations involving gasoline bomb, military personnel**

  √7th **Y37.311** **Military operations involving gasoline bomb, civilian**

√6th **Y37.32** **Military operations involving incendiary bullet**

  √7th **Y37.320** **Military operations involving incendiary bullet, military personnel**

  √7th **Y37.321** **Military operations involving incendiary bullet, civilian**

√6th **Y37.33** **Military operations involving flamethrower**

  √7th **Y37.330** **Military operations involving flamethrower, military personnel**

  √7th **Y37.331** **Military operations involving flamethrower, civilian**

√6th **Y37.39** **Military operations involving other fires, conflagrations and hot substances**

  √7th **Y37.390** **Military operations involving other fires, conflagrations and hot substances, military personnel**

  √7th **Y37.391** **Military operations involving other fires, conflagrations and hot substances, civilian**

√5th **Y37.4** **Military operations involving firearm discharge and other forms of conventional warfare**

√6th **Y37.41** **Military operations involving rubber bullets**

  √7th **Y37.410** **Military operations involving rubber bullets, military personnel**

  √7th **Y37.411** **Military operations involving rubber bullets, civilian**

√6th **Y37.42** **Military operations involving firearms pellets**

  √7th **Y37.420** **Military operations involving firearms pellets, military personnel**

  √7th **Y37.421** **Military operations involving firearms pellets, civilian**

√6th **Y37.43** **Military operations involving other firearms discharge**

  Military operations involving bullets NOS

  EXCLUDES 1   *military operations involving munitions fragments (Y37.25-)*
    military operations involving incendiary bullets (Y37.32-)

  √7th **Y37.430** **Military operations involving other firearms discharge, military personnel**

  √7th **Y37.431** **Military operations involving other firearms discharge, civilian**

√6th **Y37.44** **Military operations involving unarmed hand to hand combat**

  EXCLUDES 1   *military operations involving combat using blunt or piercing object (Y37.45-)*
    military operations involving intentional restriction of air and airway (Y37.46-)
    military operations involving unintentional restriction of air and airway (Y37.47-)

  √7th **Y37.440** **Military operations involving unarmed hand to hand combat, military personnel**

  √7th **Y37.441** **Military operations involving unarmed hand to hand combat, civilian**

√6th **Y37.45** **Military operations involving combat using blunt or piercing object**

  √7th **Y37.450** **Military operations involving combat using blunt or piercing object, military personnel**

  √7th **Y37.451** **Military operations involving combat using blunt or piercing object, civilian**

√6th **Y37.46** **Military operations involving intentional restriction of air and airway**

  √7th **Y37.460** **Military operations involving intentional restriction of air and airway, military personnel**

  √7th **Y37.461** **Military operations involving intentional restriction of air and airway, civilian**

√6th **Y37.47** **Military operations involving unintentional restriction of air and airway**

  √7th **Y37.470** **Military operations involving unintentional restriction of air and airway, military personnel**

  √7th **Y37.471** **Military operations involving unintentional restriction of air and airway, civilian**

√6th **Y37.49** **Military operations involving other forms of conventional warfare**

  √7th **Y37.490** **Military operations involving other forms of conventional warfare, military personnel**

  √7th **Y37.491** **Military operations involving other forms of conventional warfare, civilian**

√5th **Y37.5** **Military operations involving nuclear weapons**

  Military operation involving dirty bomb NOS

√6th **Y37.50** **Military operations involving unspecified effect of nuclear weapon**

  √7th **Y37.500** **Military operations involving unspecified effect of nuclear weapon, military personnel**

  √7th **Y37.501** **Military operations involving unspecified effect of nuclear weapon, civilian**

√6th **Y37.51** **Military operations involving direct blast effect of nuclear weapon**

  Military operations involving blast pressure of nuclear weapon

  √7th **Y37.510** **Military operations involving direct blast effect of nuclear weapon, military personnel**

  √7th **Y37.511** **Military operations involving direct blast effect of nuclear weapon, civilian**

EXCLUDES 1 Not coded here   EXCLUDES 2 Not included here   N Newborn Age: 0   P Pediatric Age: 0-17   M Maternity Age: 12-55   A Adult Age: 15-124

1092   ICD-10-CM 2016

✓6ᵗʰ **Y37.52 Military operations involving** indirect blast effect of **nuclear weapon**
Military operations involving being thrown by blast of nuclear weapon
Military operations involving being struck or crushed by blast debris of nuclear weapon

　　✓7ᵗʰ **Y37.52Ø Military operations involving indirect blast effect of nuclear weapon, military personnel**

　　✓7ᵗʰ **Y37.521 Military operations involving indirect blast effect of nuclear weapon, civilian**

✓6ᵗʰ **Y37.53 Military operations involving** thermal radiation effect of **nuclear weapon**
Military operations involving direct heat from nuclear weapon
Military operation involving fireball effects from nuclear weapon

　　✓7ᵗʰ **Y37.53Ø Military operations involving thermal radiation effect of nuclear weapon, military personnel**

　　✓7ᵗʰ **Y37.531 Military operations involving thermal radiation effect of nuclear weapon, civilian**

✓6ᵗʰ **Y37.54 Military operation involving** nuclear radiation effects **of nuclear weapon**
Military operation involving acute radiation exposure from nuclear weapon
Military operation involving exposure to immediate ionizing radiation from nuclear weapon
Military operation involving fallout exposure from nuclear weapon
Military operation involving secondary effects of nuclear weapons

　　✓7ᵗʰ **Y37.54Ø Military operation involving nuclear radiation effects of nuclear weapon, military personnel**

　　✓7ᵗʰ **Y37.541 Military operation involving nuclear radiation effects of nuclear weapon, civilian**

✓6ᵗʰ **Y37.59 Military operation involving** other effects of nuclear **weapons**

　　✓7ᵗʰ **Y37.59Ø Military operation involving other effects of nuclear weapons, military personnel**

　　✓7ᵗʰ **Y37.591 Military operation involving other effects of nuclear weapons, civilian**

✓5ᵗʰ **Y37.6 Military operations involving** biological weapons

　　✓6ᵗʰ **Y37.6X Military operations involving biological weapons**

　　　✓7ᵗʰ **Y37.6XØ Military operations involving biological weapons, military personnel**

　　　✓7ᵗʰ **Y37.6X1 Military operations involving biological weapons, civilian**

✓5ᵗʰ **Y37.7 Military operations involving** chemical weapons and other forms of unconventional warfare
　　EXCLUDES 1 military operations involving incendiary devices (Y36.3-, Y36.5-)

　　✓6ᵗʰ **Y37.7X Military operations involving** chemical weapons and other forms of unconventional warfare

　　　✓7ᵗʰ **Y37.7XØ Military operations involving chemical weapons and other forms of unconventional warfare, military personnel**

　　　✓7ᵗʰ **Y37.7X1 Military operations involving chemical weapons and other forms of unconventional warfare, civilian**

✓5ᵗʰ **Y37.9 Other and unspecified military operations**

　✓×7ᵗʰ **Y37.9Ø Military operations, unspecified**

　✓×7ᵗʰ **Y37.91 Military operations involving unspecified** weapon of mass destruction [WMD]

　✓×7ᵗʰ **Y37.92 Military operations involving** friendly fire

✓4ᵗʰ **Y38 Terrorism**
　　NOTE These codes are for use to identify injuries resulting from the unlawful use of force or violence against persons or property to intimidate or coerce a Government, the civilian population, or any segment thereof, in furtherance of political or social objective.
　Use additional code for place of occurrence (Y92.-)

　The appropriate 7th character is to be added to each code from category Y38.
　A　initial encounter
　D　subsequent encounter
　S　sequela

✓5ᵗʰ **Y38.Ø Terrorism involving explosion of marine weapons**
Terrorism involving depth-charge
Terrorism involving marine mine
Terrorism involving mine NOS, at sea or in harbor
Terrorism involving sea-based artillery shell
Terrorism involving torpedo
Terrorism involving underwater blast

　✓6ᵗʰ **Y38.ØX Terrorism involving explosion of** marine weapons

　　✓7ᵗʰ **Y38.ØX1 Terrorism involving explosion of marine weapons, public safety official injured**

　　✓7ᵗʰ **Y38.ØX2 Terrorism involving explosion of marine weapons, civilian injured**

　　✓7ᵗʰ **Y38.ØX3 Terrorism involving explosion of marine weapons, terrorist injured**

✓5ᵗʰ **Y38.1 Terrorism involving destruction of aircraft**
Terrorism involving aircraft burned
Terrorism involving aircraft exploded
Terrorism involving aircraft being shot down
Terrorism involving aircraft used as a weapon

　✓6ᵗʰ **Y38.1X Terrorism involving** destruction of aircraft

　　✓7ᵗʰ **Y38.1X1 Terrorism involving destruction of aircraft, public safety official injured**

　　✓7ᵗʰ **Y38.1X2 Terrorism involving destruction of aircraft, civilian injured**

　　✓7ᵗʰ **Y38.1X3 Terrorism involving destruction of aircraft, terrorist injured**

✓5ᵗʰ **Y38.2 Terrorism involving other explosions and fragments**
Terrorism involving antipersonnel (fragments) bomb
Terrorism involving blast NOS
Terrorism involving explosion NOS
Terrorism involving explosion of breech block
Terrorism involving explosion of cannon block
Terrorism involving explosion (fragments) of artillery shell
Terrorism involving explosion (fragments) of bomb
Terrorism involving explosion (fragments) of grenade
Terrorism involving explosion (fragments) of guided missile
Terrorism involving explosion (fragments) of land mine
Terrorism involving explosion of mortar bomb
Terrorism involving explosion of munitions
Terrorism involving explosion (fragments) of rocket
Terrorism involving explosion (fragments) of shell
Terrorism involving shrapnel
Terrorism involving mine NOS, on land
　　EXCLUDES 1 terrorism involving explosion of nuclear weapon (Y38.5)
　　　　terrorism involving suicide bomber (Y38.81)

　✓6ᵗʰ **Y38.2X Terrorism involving** other explosions and fragments

　　✓7ᵗʰ **Y38.2X1 Terrorism involving other explosions and fragments, public safety official injured**

　　✓7ᵗʰ **Y38.2X2 Terrorism involving other explosions and fragments, civilian injured**

　　✓7ᵗʰ **Y38.2X3 Terrorism involving other explosions and fragments, terrorist injured**

✓5ᵗʰ **Y38.3 Terrorism involving fires, conflagration and hot substances**
Terrorism involving conflagration NOS
Terrorism involving fire NOS
Terrorism involving petrol bomb
　　EXCLUDES 1 terrorism involving fire or heat of nuclear weapon (Y38.5)

　✓6ᵗʰ **Y38.3X Terrorism involving** fires, conflagration and hot substances

　　✓7ᵗʰ **Y38.3X1 Terrorism involving fires, conflagration and hot substances, public safety official injured**

　　✓7ᵗʰ **Y38.3X2 Terrorism involving fires, conflagration and hot substances, civilian injured**

✓7ᵗʰ **Y38.3X3** **Terrorism involving fires, conflagration and hot substances,** terrorist injured

✓5ᵗʰ **Y38.4** **Terrorism involving firearms**
Terrorism involving carbine bullet
Terrorism involving machine gun bullet
Terrorism involving pellets (shotgun)
Terrorism involving pistol bullet
Terrorism involving rifle bullet
Terrorism involving rubber (rifle) bullet

✓6ᵗʰ **Y38.4X** **Terrorism involving** firearms
✓7ᵗʰ **Y38.4X1** **Terrorism involving firearms,** public safety official injured
✓7ᵗʰ **Y38.4X2** **Terrorism involving firearms,** civilian injured
✓7ᵗʰ **Y38.4X3** **Terrorism involving firearms,** terrorist injured

✓5ᵗʰ **Y38.5** **Terrorism involving nuclear weapons**
Terrorism involving blast effects of nuclear weapon
Terrorism involving exposure to ionizing radiation from nuclear weapon
Terrorism involving fireball effect of nuclear weapon
Terrorism involving heat from nuclear weapon

✓6ᵗʰ **Y38.5X** **Terrorism involving** nuclear weapons
✓7ᵗʰ **Y38.5X1** **Terrorism involving nuclear weapons,** public safety official injured
✓7ᵗʰ **Y38.5X2** **Terrorism involving nuclear weapons,** civilian injured
✓7ᵗʰ **Y38.5X3** **Terrorism involving nuclear weapons,** terrorist injured

✓5ᵗʰ **Y38.6** **Terrorism involving biological weapons**
Terrorism involving anthrax
Terrorism involving cholera
Terrorism involving smallpox

✓6ᵗʰ **Y38.6X** **Terrorism involving** biological weapons
✓7ᵗʰ **Y38.6X1** **Terrorism involving biological weapons,** public safety official injured
✓7ᵗʰ **Y38.6X2** **Terrorism involving biological weapons,** civilian injured
✓7ᵗʰ **Y38.6X3** **Terrorism involving biological weapons,** terrorist injured

✓5ᵗʰ **Y38.7** **Terrorism involving chemical weapons**
Terrorism involving gases, fumes, chemicals
Terrorism involving hydrogen cyanide
Terrorism involving phosgene
Terrorism involving sarin

✓6ᵗʰ **Y38.7X** **Terrorism involving** chemical weapons
✓7ᵗʰ **Y38.7X1** **Terrorism involving chemical weapons,** public safety official injured
✓7ᵗʰ **Y38.7X2** **Terrorism involving chemical weapons,** civilian injured
✓7ᵗʰ **Y38.7X3** **Terrorism involving chemical weapons,** terrorist injured

✓5ᵗʰ **Y38.8** **Terrorism involving other and unspecified means**
Y38.8Ø **Terrorism involving unspecified means**
Terrorism NOS
✓6ᵗʰ **Y38.81** **Terrorism involving** suicide bomber
✓7ᵗʰ **Y38.811** **Terrorism involving suicide bomber,** public safety official injured
✓7ᵗʰ **Y38.812** **Terrorism involving suicide bomber,** civilian injured
✓6ᵗʰ **Y38.89** **Terrorism involving** other means
Terrorism involving drowning and submersion
Terrorism involving lasers
Terrorism involving piercing or stabbing instruments
✓7ᵗʰ **Y38.891** **Terrorism involving other means,** public safety official injured
✓7ᵗʰ **Y38.892** **Terrorism involving other means,** civilian injured
✓7ᵗʰ **Y38.893** **Terrorism involving other means,** terrorist injured

✓5ᵗʰ **Y38.9** **Terrorism, secondary effects**
NOTE This code is for use to identify injuries occurring subsequent to a terrorist attack, not those that are due to the initial terrorist attack.

✓6ᵗʰ **Y38.9X** **Terrorism,** secondary effects
✓7ᵗʰ **Y38.9X1** **Terrorism, secondary effects,** public safety official injured

✓7ᵗʰ **Y38.9X2** **Terrorism, secondary effects,** civilian injured

Complications of medical and surgical care (Y62-Y84)

INCLUDES complications of medical devices
surgical and medical procedures as the cause of abnormal reaction of the patient, or of later complication, without mention of misadventure at the time of the procedure

Misadventures to patients during surgical and medical care (Y62-Y69)

EXCLUDES 2 breakdown or malfunctioning of medical device (during procedure) (after implantation) (ongoing use) (Y7Ø-Y82)
surgical and medical procedures as the cause of abnormal reaction of the patient, without mention of misadventure at the time of the procedure (Y83-Y84)

✓4ᵗʰ **Y62** **Failure of** sterile precautions **during surgical and medical care**
Y62.Ø **Failure of sterile precautions during** surgical operation
Y62.1 **Failure of sterile precautions during** infusion or transfusion
Y62.2 **Failure of sterile precautions during** kidney dialysis and othe perfusion
Y62.3 **Failure of sterile precautions during** injection or immunization
Y62.4 **Failure of sterile precautions during** endoscopic examinatior
Y62.5 **Failure of sterile precautions during** heart catheterization
Y62.6 **Failure of sterile precautions during** aspiration, puncture and other catheterization
Y62.8 **Failure of sterile precautions during other surgical and medical care**
Y62.9 **Failure of sterile precautions during unspecified surgical and medical care**

✓4ᵗʰ **Y63** **Failure in** dosage **during surgical and medical care**
EXCLUDES 2 accidental overdose of drug or wrong drug given in error (T36-T5Ø)
Y63.Ø **Excessive amount of blood or other fluid given during transfusion or infusion**
Y63.1 **Incorrect dilution of fluid used during infusion**
Y63.2 **Overdose of radiation given during therapy**
Y63.3 **Inadvertent exposure of patient to radiation during medical care**
Y63.4 **Failure in dosage in electroshock or insulin-shock therapy**
Y63.5 **Inappropriate temperature in local application and packing**
Y63.6 **Underdosing and nonadministration of necessary drug, medicament or biological substance**
Y63.8 **Failure in dosage during other surgical and medical care**
Y63.9 **Failure in dosage during unspecified surgical and medical care**

✓4ᵗʰ **Y64** **Contaminated** medical or biological substances
Y64.Ø **Contaminated medical or biological substance,** transfused or infused
Y64.1 **Contaminated medical or biological substance,** injected or used for immunization
Y64.8 **Contaminated medical or biological substance administered by other means**
Y64.9 **Contaminated medical or biological substance administered by unspecified means**
Administered contaminated medical or biological substance NOS

✓4ᵗʰ **Y65** **Other misadventures during surgical and medical care**
Y65.Ø **Mismatched blood in transfusion**
Y65.1 **Wrong fluid used in infusion**
Y65.2 **Failure in suture or ligature during surgical operation**
Y65.3 **Endotracheal tube wrongly placed during anesthetic procedure**
Y65.4 **Failure to introduce or to remove other tube or instrument**
✓5ᵗʰ **Y65.5** **Performance of** wrong procedure (operation)
Y65.51 **Performance of wrong procedure (operation) on correct patient**
Wrong device implanted into correct surgical site
EXCLUDES 1 performance of correct procedure (operation) on wrong side or body part (Y65.53)

Y65.52 **Performance of procedure (operation) on** patient
not scheduled for surgery
Performance of procedure (operation) intended for
another patient
Performance of procedure (operation) on wrong
patient

Y65.53 **Performance of correct procedure (operation) on
wrong side or body part**
Performance of correct procedure (operation) on
wrong side
Performance of correct procedure (operation) on
wrong site

Y65.8 Other specified misadventures **during surgical and medical
care**

Y66 **Nonadministration of surgical and medical care**
Premature cessation of surgical and medical care
EXCLUDES 1   DNR status (Z66)
palliative care (Z51.5)

Y69 **Unspecified misadventure during surgical and medical care**

Medical devices associated with adverse incidents in diagnostic and therapeutic use (Y70-Y82)

INCLUDES   breakdown or malfunction of medical devices (during use) (after
implantation) (ongoing use)
EXCLUDES 1   misadventure to patients during surgical and medical care, classifiable
to (Y62-Y69)
later complications following use of medical devices without
breakdown or malfunctioning of device (Y83-Y84)

√4ᵗʰ **Y70 Anesthesiology devices associated with adverse incidents**
Y70.0 Diagnostic and monitoring **anesthesiology devices associated
with adverse incidents**
Y70.1 Therapeutic (nonsurgical) and rehabilitative **anesthesiology
devices associated with adverse incidents**
Y70.2 Prosthetic and other implants, **materials and accessory
anesthesiology devices associated with adverse incidents**
Y70.3 Surgical instruments, materials **and anesthesiology devices
(including sutures) associated with adverse incidents**
Y70.8 **Miscellaneous anesthesiology devices associated with
adverse incidents, not elsewhere classified**

√4ᵗʰ **Y71 Cardiovascular devices associated with adverse incidents**
Y71.0 Diagnostic and monitoring **cardiovascular devices associated
with adverse incidents**
Y71.1 Therapeutic (nonsurgical) and rehabilitative **cardiovascular
devices associated with adverse incidents**
Y71.2 Prosthetic and other implants, **materials and accessory
cardiovascular devices associated with adverse incidents**
Y71.3 Surgical instruments, materials **and cardiovascular devices
(including sutures) associated with adverse incidents**
Y71.8 **Miscellaneous cardiovascular devices associated with adverse
incidents, not elsewhere classified**

√4ᵗʰ **Y72 Otorhinolaryngological devices associated with adverse
incidents**
Y72.0 Diagnostic and monitoring **otorhinolaryngological devices
associated with adverse incidents**
Y72.1 Therapeutic (nonsurgical) and rehabilitative
**otorhinolaryngological devices associated with adverse
incidents**
Y72.2 Prosthetic and other implants, **materials and accessory
otorhinolaryngological devices associated with adverse
incidents**
Y72.3 Surgical instruments, materials **and otorhinolaryngological
devices (including sutures) associated with adverse incidents**
Y72.8 **Miscellaneous otorhinolaryngological devices associated
with adverse incidents, not elsewhere classified**

√4ᵗʰ **Y73 Gastroenterology and urology devices associated with adverse
incidents**
Y73.0 Diagnostic and monitoring **gastroenterology and urology
devices associated with adverse incidents**
Y73.1 Therapeutic (nonsurgical) and rehabilitative
**gastroenterology and urology devices associated with
adverse incidents**
Y73.2 Prosthetic and other implants, **materials and accessory
gastroenterology and urology devices associated with
adverse incidents**
Y73.3 Surgical instruments, materials **and gastroenterology and
urology devices (including sutures) associated with adverse
incidents**

Y73.8 **Miscellaneous gastroenterology and urology devices
associated with adverse incidents, not elsewhere classified**

√4ᵗʰ **Y74 General hospital and personal-use devices associated with
adverse incidents**
Y74.0 Diagnostic and monitoring **general hospital and personal-use
devices associated with adverse incidents**
Y74.1 Therapeutic (nonsurgical) and rehabilitative **general hospital
and personal-use devices associated with adverse incidents**
Y74.2 Prosthetic and other implants, **materials and accessory
general hospital and personal-use devices associated with
adverse incidents**
Y74.3 Surgical instruments, materials **and general hospital and
personal-use devices (including sutures) associated with
adverse incidents**
Y74.8 **Miscellaneous general hospital and personal-use devices
associated with adverse incidents, not elsewhere classified**

√4ᵗʰ **Y75 Neurological devices associated with adverse incidents**
Y75.0 Diagnostic and monitoring **neurological devices associated
with adverse incidents**
Y75.1 Therapeutic (nonsurgical) and rehabilitative **neurological
devices associated with adverse incidents**
Y75.2 Prosthetic and other implants, **materials and neurological
devices associated with adverse incidents**
Y75.3 Surgical instruments, materials **and neurological devices
(including sutures) associated with adverse incidents**
Y75.8 **Miscellaneous neurological devices associated with adverse
incidents, not elsewhere classified**

√4ᵗʰ **Y76 Obstetric and gynecological devices associated with adverse
incidents**
Y76.0 Diagnostic and monitoring **obstetric and gynecological
devices associated with adverse incidents** ♀
Y76.1 Therapeutic (nonsurgical) and rehabilitative **obstetric and
gynecological devices associated with adverse incidents** ♀
Y76.2 Prosthetic and other implants, **materials and accessory
obstetric and gynecological devices associated with adverse
incidents** ♀
Y76.3 Surgical instruments, materials **and obstetric and
gynecological devices (including sutures) associated with
adverse incidents** ♀
Y76.8 **Miscellaneous obstetric and gynecological devices
associated with adverse incidents, not elsewhere classified** ♀

√4ᵗʰ **Y77 Ophthalmic devices associated with adverse incidents**
Y77.0 Diagnostic and monitoring **ophthalmic devices associated
with adverse incidents**
Y77.1 Therapeutic (nonsurgical) and rehabilitative **ophthalmic
devices associated with adverse incidents**
Y77.2 Prosthetic and other implants, **materials and accessory
ophthalmic devices associated with adverse incidents**
Y77.3 Surgical instruments, materials **and ophthalmic devices
(including sutures) associated with adverse incidents**
Y77.8 **Miscellaneous ophthalmic devices associated with adverse
incidents, not elsewhere classified**

√4ᵗʰ **Y78 Radiological devices associated with adverse incidents**
Y78.0 Diagnostic and monitoring **radiological devices associated
with adverse incidents**
Y78.1 Therapeutic (nonsurgical) and rehabilitative **radiological
devices associated with adverse incidents**
Y78.2 Prosthetic and other implants, **materials and accessory
radiological devices associated with adverse incidents**
Y78.3 Surgical instruments, materials **and radiological devices
(including sutures) associated with adverse incidents**
Y78.8 **Miscellaneous radiological devices associated with adverse
incidents, not elsewhere classified**

√4ᵗʰ **Y79 Orthopedic devices associated with adverse incidents**
Y79.0 Diagnostic and monitoring **orthopedic devices associated
with adverse incidents**
Y79.1 Therapeutic (nonsurgical) and rehabilitative **orthopedic
devices associated with adverse incidents**
Y79.2 Prosthetic and other implants, **materials and accessory
orthopedic devices associated with adverse incidents**
Y79.3 Surgical instruments, materials **and orthopedic devices
(including sutures) associated with adverse incidents**
Y79.8 **Miscellaneous orthopedic devices associated with adverse
incidents, not elsewhere classified**

☑ Additional Character Required   ᵥₓ₇ᵗʰ Placeholder Alert   Unspecified Dx   Other Specified Dx   Manifestation   ►◄ Revised Text   ● New Code   ▲ Revised Code Title

Chapter 20. External Causes of Morbidity

✓4ᵗʰ Y80 Physical medicine devices associated with adverse incidents

Y80.0 Diagnostic and monitoring physical medicine devices associated with adverse incidents

Y80.1 Therapeutic (nonsurgical) and rehabilitative physical medicine devices associated with adverse incidents

Y80.2 Prosthetic and other implants, materials and accessory physical medicine devices associated with adverse incidents

Y80.3 Surgical instruments, materials and physical medicine devices (including sutures) associated with adverse incidents

Y80.8 Miscellaneous physical medicine devices associated with adverse incidents, not elsewhere classified

✓4ᵗʰ Y81 General- and plastic-surgery devices associated with adverse incidents

Y81.0 Diagnostic and monitoring general- and plastic-surgery devices associated with adverse incidents

Y81.1 Therapeutic (nonsurgical) and rehabilitative general- and plastic-surgery devices associated with adverse incidents

Y81.2 Prosthetic and other implants, materials and accessory general- and plastic-surgery devices associated with adverse incidents

Y81.3 Surgical instruments, materials and general- and plastic-surgery devices (including sutures) associated with adverse incidents

Y81.8 Miscellaneous general- and plastic-surgery devices associated with adverse incidents, not elsewhere classified

✓4ᵗʰ Y82 Other and unspecified medical devices associated with adverse incidents

Y82.8 Other medical devices associated with adverse incidents

Y82.9 Unspecified medical devices associated with adverse incidents

Surgical and other medical procedures as the cause of abnormal reaction of the patient, or of later complication, without mention of misadventure at the time of the procedure (Y83-Y84)

EXCLUDES 1   misadventures to patients during surgical and medical care, classifiable to (Y62-Y69)

✓4ᵗʰ Y83 Surgical operation and other surgical procedures as the cause of abnormal reaction of the patient, or of later complication, without mention of misadventure at the time of the procedure

Y83.0 Surgical operation with transplant of whole organ as the cause of abnormal reaction of the patient, or of later complication, without mention of misadventure at the time of the procedure

Y83.1 Surgical operation with implant of artificial internal device as the cause of abnormal reaction of the patient, or of later complication, without mention of misadventure at the time of the procedure

Y83.2 Surgical operation with anastomosis, bypass or graft as the cause of abnormal reaction of the patient, or of later complication, without mention of misadventure at the time of the procedure

Y83.3 Surgical operation with formation of external stoma as the cause of abnormal reaction of the patient, or of later complication, without mention of misadventure at the time of the procedure

Y83.4 Other reconstructive surgery as the cause of abnormal reaction of the patient, or of later complication, without mention of misadventure at the time of the procedure

Y83.5 Amputation of limb(s) as the cause of abnormal reaction of the patient, or of later complication, without mention of misadventure at the time of the procedure

Y83.6 Removal of other organ (partial) (total) as the cause of abnormal reaction of the patient, or of later complication, without mention of misadventure at the time of the procedure

Y83.8 Other surgical procedures as the cause of abnormal reaction of the patient, or of later complication, without mention of misadventure at the time of the procedure

Y83.9 Surgical procedure, unspecified as the cause of abnormal reaction of the patient, or of later complication, without mention of misadventure at the time of the procedure

✓4ᵗʰ Y84 Other medical procedures as the cause of abnormal reaction of the patient, or of later complication, without mention of misadventure at the time of the procedure

Y84.0 Cardiac catheterization as the cause of abnormal reaction of the patient, or of later complication, without mention of misadventure at the time of the procedure

Y84.1 Kidney dialysis as the cause of abnormal reaction of the patient, or of later complication, without mention of misadventure at the time of the procedure

Y84.2 Radiological procedure and radiotherapy as the cause of abnormal reaction of the patient, or of later complication, without mention of misadventure at the time of the procedure

Y84.3 Shock therapy as the cause of abnormal reaction of the patient, or of later complication, without mention of misadventure at the time of the procedure

Y84.4 Aspiration of fluid as the cause of abnormal reaction of the patient, or of later complication, without mention of misadventure at the time of the procedure

Y84.5 Insertion of gastric or duodenal sound as the cause of abnormal reaction of the patient, or of later complication, without mention of misadventure at the time of the procedure

Y84.6 Urinary catheterization as the cause of abnormal reaction of the patient, or of later complication, without mention of misadventure at the time of the procedure

Y84.7 Blood-sampling as the cause of abnormal reaction of the patient, or of later complication, without mention of misadventure at the time of the procedure

Y84.8 Other medical procedures as the cause of abnormal reaction of the patient, or of later complication, without mention of misadventure at the time of the procedure
AHA: 2014, 4Q, 24

Y84.9 Medical procedure, unspecified as the cause of abnormal reaction of the patient, or of later complication, without mention of misadventure at the time of the procedure

Supplementary factors related to causes of morbidity classified elsewhere (Y90-Y99)

NOTE   These categories may be used to provide supplementary information concerning causes of morbidity. They are not to be used for single-condition coding.

✓4ᵗʰ Y90 Evidence of alcohol involvement determined by blood alcohol level

Code first any associated alcohol related disorders (F10)

Y90.0 Blood alcohol level of less than 20 mg/100 ml

Y90.1 Blood alcohol level of 20-39 mg/100 ml

Y90.2 Blood alcohol level of 40-59 mg/100 ml

Y90.3 Blood alcohol level of 60-79 mg/100 ml

Y90.4 Blood alcohol level of 80-99 mg/100 ml

Y90.5 Blood alcohol level of 100-119 mg/100 ml

Y90.6 Blood alcohol level of 120-199 mg/100 ml

Y90.7 Blood alcohol level of 200-239 mg/100 ml

Y90.8 Blood alcohol level of 240 mg/100 ml or more

Y90.9 Presence of alcohol in blood, level not specified

✓4ᵗʰ Y92 Place of occurrence of the external cause

The following category is for use, when relevant, to identify the place of occurrence of the external cause. Use in conjunction with an activity code.

Place of occurrence should be recorded only at the initial encounter for treatment

✓5ᵗʰ Y92.0 Non-institutional (private) residence as the place of occurrence of the external cause

EXCLUDES 1   abandoned or derelict house (Y92.89)
home under construction but not yet occupied (Y92.6-)
institutional place of residence (Y92.1-)

✓6ᵗʰ Y92.00 Unspecified non-institutional (private) residence as the place of occurrence of the external cause

Y92.000 Kitchen of unspecified non-institutional (private) residence as the place of occurrence of the external cause

Y92.001 Dining room of unspecified non-institutional (private) residence as the place of occurrence of the external cause

Y92.002 Bathroom of unspecified non-institutional (private) residence single-family (private) house as the place of occurrence of the external cause

Y92.003 Bedroom of unspecified non-institutional (private) residence as the place of occurrence of the external cause

EXCLUDES 1 Not coded here   *EXCLUDES 2* Not included here   **N** Newborn Age: 0   **P** Pediatric Age: 0-17   **M** Maternity Age: 12-55   **A** Adult Age: 15-124

1096   ICD-10-CM 2016

Y92.007   Garden or yard of unspecified non-institutional (private) residence as the place of occurrence of the external cause

Y92.008   Other place in unspecified non-institutional (private) residence as the place of occurrence of the external cause

Y92.009   Unspecified place in unspecified non-institutional (private) residence as the place of occurrence of the external cause

Home (NOS) as the place of occurrence of the external cause

✓6ᵗʰ **Y92.01**   Single-family non-institutional (private) house as the place of occurrence of the external cause

Farmhouse as the place of occurrence of the external cause

EXCLUDES 1   *barn (Y92.71)*
chicken coop or hen house (Y92.72)
farm field (Y92.73)
orchard (Y92.74)
single family mobile home or trailer (Y92.02-)
slaughter house (Y92.86)

Y92.010   Kitchen of single-family (private) house as the place of occurrence of the external cause

Y92.011   Dining room of single-family (private) house as the place of occurrence of the external cause

Y92.012   Bathroom of single-family (private) house as the place of occurrence of the external cause

Y92.013   Bedroom of single-family (private) house as the place of occurrence of the external cause

Y92.014   Private driveway to single-family (private) house as the place of occurrence of the external cause

Y92.015   Private garage of single-family (private) house as the place of occurrence of the external cause

Y92.016   Swimming-pool in single-family (private) house or garden as the place of occurrence of the external cause

Y92.017   Garden or yard in single-family (private) house as the place of occurrence of the external cause

Y92.018   Other place in single-family (private) house as the place of occurrence of the external cause

Y92.019   Unspecified place in single-family (private) house as the place of occurrence of the external cause

✓6ᵗʰ **Y92.02**   Mobile home as the place of occurrence of the external cause

Y92.020   Kitchen in mobile home as the place of occurrence of the external cause

Y92.021   Dining room in mobile home as the place of occurrence of the external cause

Y92.022   Bathroom in mobile home as the place of occurrence of the external cause

Y92.023   Bedroom in mobile home as the place of occurrence of the external cause

Y92.024   Driveway of mobile home as the place of occurrence of the external cause

Y92.025   Garage of mobile home as the place of occurrence of the external cause

Y92.026   Swimming-pool of mobile home as the place of occurrence of the external cause

Y92.027   Garden or yard of mobile home as the place of occurrence of the external cause

Y92.028   Other place in mobile home as the place of occurrence of the external cause

Y92.029   Unspecified place in mobile home as the place of occurrence of the external cause

✓6ᵗʰ **Y92.03**   Apartment as the place of occurrence of the external cause

Condominium as the place of occurrence of the external cause

Co-op apartment as the place of occurrence of the external cause

Y92.030   Kitchen in apartment as the place of occurrence of the external cause

Y92.031   Bathroom in apartment as the place of occurrence of the external cause

Y92.032   Bedroom in apartment as the place of occurrence of the external cause

Y92.038   Other place in apartment as the place of occurrence of the external cause

Y92.039   Unspecified place in apartment as the place of occurrence of the external cause

✓6ᵗʰ **Y92.04**   Boarding-house as the place of occurrence of the external cause

Y92.040   Kitchen in boarding-house as the place of occurrence of the external cause

Y92.041   Bathroom in boarding-house as the place of occurrence of the external cause

Y92.042   Bedroom in boarding-house as the place of occurrence of the external cause

Y92.043   Driveway of boarding-house as the place of occurrence of the external cause

Y92.044   Garage of boarding-house as the place of occurrence of the external cause

Y92.045   Swimming-pool of boarding-house as the place of occurrence of the external cause

Y92.046   Garden or yard of boarding-house as the place of occurrence of the external cause

Y92.048   Other place in boarding-house as the place of occurrence of the external cause

Y92.049   Unspecified place in boarding-house as the place of occurrence of the external cause

✓6ᵗʰ **Y92.09**   Other non-institutional residence as the place of occurrence of the external cause

Y92.090   Kitchen in other non-institutional residence as the place of occurrence of the external cause

Y92.091   Bathroom in other non-institutional residence as the place of occurrence of the external cause

Y92.092   Bedroom in other non-institutional residence as the place of occurrence of the external cause

Y92.093   Driveway of other non-institutional residence as the place of occurrence of the external cause

Y92.094   Garage of other non-institutional residence as the place of occurrence of the external cause

Y92.095   Swimming-pool of other non-institutional residence as the place of occurrence of the external cause

Y92.096   Garden or yard of other non-institutional residence as the place of occurrence of the external cause

Y92.098   Other place in other non-institutional residence as the place of occurrence of the external cause

Y92.099   Unspecified place in other non-institutional residence as the place of occurrence of the external cause

✓5ᵗʰ **Y92.1**   Institutional (nonprivate) residence as the place of occurrence of the external cause

Y92.10   Unspecified residential institution as the place of occurrence of the external cause

✓6ᵗʰ **Y92.11**   Children's home and orphanage as the place of occurrence of the external cause

Y92.110   Kitchen in children's home and orphanage as the place of occurrence of the external cause

Y92.111   Bathroom in children's home and orphanage as the place of occurrence of the external cause

Y92.112   Bedroom in children's home and orphanage as the place of occurrence of the external cause

Y92.113   Driveway of children's home and orphanage as the place of occurrence of the external cause

Y92.114   Garage of children's home and orphanage as the place of occurrence of the external cause

✓ Additional Character Required   ✓x7ᵗʰ Placeholder Alert   Unspecified Dx   Other Specified Dx   Manifestation   ▶◀ Revised Text   ● New Code   ▲ Revised Code Title

ICD-10-CM 2016   1097

Y92.115 Swimming-pool of children's home and orphanage as the place of occurrence of the external cause

Y92.116 Garden or yard of children's home and orphanage as the place of occurrence of the external cause

Y92.118 Other place in children's home and orphanage as the place of occurrence of the external cause

Y92.119 Unspecified place in children's home and orphanage as the place of occurrence of the external cause

✓6ᵗʰ **Y92.12** Nursing home as the place of occurrence of the external cause

Home for the sick as the place of occurrence of the external cause

Hospice as the place of occurrence of the external cause

Y92.120 Kitchen in nursing home as the place of occurrence of the external cause

Y92.121 Bathroom in nursing home as the place of occurrence of the external cause

Y92.122 Bedroom in nursing home as the place of occurrence of the external cause

Y92.123 Driveway of nursing home as the place of occurrence of the external cause

Y92.124 Garage of nursing home as the place of occurrence of the external cause

Y92.125 Swimming-pool of nursing home as the place of occurrence of the external cause

Y92.126 Garden or yard of nursing home as the place of occurrence of the external cause

Y92.128 Other place in nursing home as the place of occurrence of the external cause

Y92.129 Unspecified place in nursing home as the place of occurrence of the external cause

✓6ᵗʰ **Y92.13** Military base as the place of occurrence of the external cause

EXCLUDES 1   military training grounds (Y92.83)

Y92.130 Kitchen on military base as the place of occurrence of the external cause

Y92.131 Mess hall on military base as the place of occurrence of the external cause

Y92.133 Barracks on military base as the place of occurrence of the external cause

Y92.135 Garage on military base as the place of occurrence of the external cause

Y92.136 Swimming-pool on military base as the place of occurrence of the external cause

Y92.137 Garden or yard on military base as the place of occurrence of the external cause

Y92.138 Other place on military base as the place of occurrence of the external cause

Y92.139 Unspecified place military base as the place of occurrence of the external cause

✓6ᵗʰ **Y92.14** Prison as the place of occurrence of the external cause

Y92.140 Kitchen in prison as the place of occurrence of the external cause

Y92.141 Dining room in prison as the place of occurrence of the external cause

Y92.142 Bathroom in prison as the place of occurrence of the external cause

Y92.143 Cell of prison as the place of occurrence of the external cause

Y92.146 Swimming-pool of prison as the place of occurrence of the external cause

Y92.147 Courtyard of prison as the place of occurrence of the external cause

Y92.148 Other place in prison as the place of occurrence of the external cause

Y92.149 Unspecified place in prison as the place of occurrence of the external cause

✓6ᵗʰ **Y92.15** Reform school as the place of occurrence of the external cause

Y92.150 Kitchen in reform school as the place of occurrence of the external cause

Y92.151 Dining room in reform school as the place of occurrence of the external cause

Y92.152 Bathroom in reform school as the place of occurrence of the external cause

Y92.153 Bedroom in reform school as the place of occurrence of the external cause

Y92.154 Driveway of reform school as the place of occurrence of the external cause

Y92.155 Garage of reform school as the place of occurrence of the external cause

Y92.156 Swimming-pool of reform school as the place of occurrence of the external cause

Y92.157 Garden or yard of reform school as the place of occurrence of the external cause

Y92.158 Other place in reform school as the place of occurrence of the external cause

Y92.159 Unspecified place in reform school as the place of occurrence of the external cause

✓6ᵗʰ **Y92.16** School dormitory as the place of occurrence of the external cause

EXCLUDES 1   reform school as the place of occurrence of the external cause (Y92.15-)

school buildings and grounds as the place of occurrence of the external cause (Y92.2-)

school sports and athletic areas as the place of occurrence of the external cause (Y92.3-)

Y92.160 Kitchen in school dormitory as the place of occurrence of the external cause

Y92.161 Dining room in school dormitory as the place of occurrence of the external cause

Y92.162 Bathroom in school dormitory as the place of occurrence of the external cause

Y92.163 Bedroom in school dormitory as the place of occurrence of the external cause

Y92.168 Other place in school dormitory as the place of occurrence of the external cause

Y92.169 Unspecified place in school dormitory as the place of occurrence of the external cause

✓6ᵗʰ **Y92.19** Other specified residential institution as the place of occurrence of the external cause

Y92.190 Kitchen in other specified residential institution as the place of occurrence of the external cause

Y92.191 Dining room in other specified residential institution as the place of occurrence of the external cause

Y92.192 Bathroom in other specified residential institution as the place of occurrence of the external cause

Y92.193 Bedroom in other specified residential institution as the place of occurrence of the external cause

Y92.194 Driveway of other specified residential institution as the place of occurrence of the external cause

Y92.195 Garage of other specified residential institution as the place of occurrence of the external cause

Y92.196 Pool of other specified residential institution as the place of occurrence of the external cause

Y92.197 Garden or yard of other specified residential institution as the place of occurrence of the external cause

Y92.198 Other place in other specified residential institution as the place of occurrence of the external cause

Y92.199 Unspecified place in other specified residential institution as the place of occurrence of the external cause

EXCLUDES 1 Not coded here   EXCLUDES 2 Not included here   N Newborn Age: 0   P Pediatric Age: 0-17   M Maternity Age: 12-55   A Adult Age: 15-124

✓5ᵗʰ Y92.2 School, other institution and public administrative area as the place of occurrence of the external cause
     Building and adjacent grounds used by the general public or by a particular group of the public

> EXCLUDES 1   building under construction as the place of occurrence of the external cause (Y92.6)
> residential institution as the place of occurrence of the external cause (Y92.1)
> school dormitory as the place of occurrence of the external cause (Y92.16-)
> sports and athletics area of schools as the place of occurrence of the external cause (Y92.3-)

✓6ᵗʰ Y92.21 School (private) (public) (state) as the place of occurrence of the external cause

Y92.210   **Daycare center as the place of occurrence of the external cause**

Y92.211   **Elementary school as the place of occurrence of the external cause**
     Kindergarten as the place of occurrence of the external cause

Y92.212   **Middle school as the place of occurrence of the external cause**

Y92.213   **High school as the place of occurrence of the external cause**
     AHA: 2012, 4Q, 108

Y92.214   **College as the place of occurrence of the external cause**
     University as the place of occurrence of the external cause

Y92.215   **Trade school as the place of occurrence of the external cause**

Y92.218   **Other school as the place of occurrence of the external cause**

Y92.219   **Unspecified school as the place of occurrence of the external cause**

Y92.22 Religious institution as the place of occurrence of the external cause
     Church as the place of occurrence of the external cause
     Mosque as the place of occurrence of the external cause
     Synagogue as the place of occurrence of the external cause

✓6ᵗʰ Y92.23 Hospital as the place of occurrence of the external cause

> EXCLUDES 1   ambulatory (outpatient) health services establishments (Y92.53-)
> home for the sick as the place of occurrence of the external cause (Y92.12-)
> hospice as the place of occurrence of the external cause (Y92.12-)
> nursing home as the place of occurrence of the external cause (Y92.12-)

Y92.230   **Patient room in hospital as the place of occurrence of the external cause**

Y92.231   **Patient bathroom in hospital as the place of occurrence of the external cause**

Y92.232   **Corridor of hospital as the place of occurrence of the external cause**

Y92.233   **Cafeteria of hospital as the place of occurrence of the external cause**

Y92.234   **Operating room of hospital as the place of occurrence of the external cause**

Y92.238   **Other place in hospital as the place of occurrence of the external cause**

Y92.239   **Unspecified place in hospital as the place of occurrence of the external cause**

✓6ᵗʰ Y92.24 Public administrative building as the place of occurrence of the external cause

Y92.240   **Courthouse as the place of occurrence of the external cause**

Y92.241   **Library as the place of occurrence of the external cause**

Y92.242   **Post office as the place of occurrence of the external cause**

Y92.243   **City hall as the place of occurrence of the external cause**

Y92.248   **Other public administrative building as the place of occurrence of the external cause**

✓6ᵗʰ Y92.25 Cultural building as the place of occurrence of the external cause

Y92.250   **Art Gallery as the place of occurrence of the external cause**

Y92.251   **Museum as the place of occurrence of the external cause**

Y92.252   **Music hall as the place of occurrence of the external cause**

Y92.253   **Opera house as the place of occurrence of the external cause**

Y92.254   **Theater (live) as the place of occurrence of the external cause**

Y92.258   **Other cultural public building as the place of occurrence of the external cause**

Y92.26 Movie house or cinema as the place of occurrence of the external cause

Y92.29 Other specified public building as the place of occurrence of the external cause
     Assembly hall as the place of occurrence of the external cause
     Clubhouse as the place of occurrence of the external cause

✓5ᵗʰ Y92.3 Sports and athletics area as the place of occurrence of the external cause

✓6ᵗʰ Y92.31 Athletic court as the place of occurrence of the external cause

> EXCLUDES 1   tennis court in private home or garden (Y92.09)

Y92.310   **Basketball court as the place of occurrence of the external cause**

Y92.311   **Squash court as the place of occurrence of the external cause**

Y92.312   **Tennis court as the place of occurrence of the external cause**

Y92.318   **Other athletic court as the place of occurrence of the external cause**

✓6ᵗʰ Y92.32 Athletic field as the place of occurrence of the external cause

Y92.320   **Baseball field as the place of occurrence of the external cause**

Y92.321   **Football field as the place of occurrence of the external cause**

Y92.322   **Soccer field as the place of occurrence of the external cause**

Y92.328   **Other athletic field as the place of occurrence of the external cause**
     Cricket field as the place of occurrence of the external cause
     Hockey field as the place of occurrence of the external cause

✓6ᵗʰ Y92.33 Skating rink as the place of occurrence of the external cause

Y92.330   **Ice skating rink (indoor) (outdoor) as the place of occurrence of the external cause**

Y92.331   **Roller skating rink as the place of occurrence of the external cause**

Y92.34 Swimming pool (public) as the place of occurrence of the external cause

> EXCLUDES 1   swimming pool in private home or garden (Y92.016)

Y92.39 Other specified sports and athletic area as the place of occurrence of the external cause
     Golf-course as the place of occurrence of the external cause
     Gymnasium as the place of occurrence of the external cause
     Riding-school as the place of occurrence of the external cause
     Stadium as the place of occurrence of the external cause

✓5ᵗʰ Y92.4 Street, highway and other paved roadways as the place of occurrence of the external cause

> EXCLUDES 1   private driveway of residence (Y92.014, Y92.024, Y92.043, Y92.093, Y92.113, Y92.123, Y92.154, Y92.194)

✓ Additional Character Required   ✕7ᵗʰ Placeholder Alert   Unspecified Dx   Other Specified Dx   Manifestation   ▶◀ Revised Text   ● New Code   ▲ Revised Code Title

✓6ᵗʰ **Y92.41** Street and highway as the place of occurrence of the external cause

    Y92.410 Unspecified street and highway as the place of occurrence of the external cause
         Road NOS as the place of occurrence of the external cause

    Y92.411 Interstate highway as the place of occurrence of the external cause
         Freeway as the place of occurrence of the external cause
         Motorway as the place of occurrence of the external cause

    Y92.412 Parkway as the place of occurrence of the external cause

    Y92.413 State road as the place of occurrence of the external cause

    Y92.414 Local residential or business street as the place of occurrence of the external cause

    Y92.415 Exit ramp or entrance ramp of street or highway as the place of occurrence of the external cause

✓6ᵗʰ **Y92.48** Other paved roadways as the place of occurrence of the external cause

    Y92.480 Sidewalk as the place of occurrence of the external cause

    Y92.481 Parking lot as the place of occurrence of the external cause

    Y92.482 Bike path as the place of occurrence of the external cause

    Y92.488 Other paved roadways as the place of occurrence of the external cause

✓5ᵗʰ **Y92.5** Trade and service area as the place of occurrence of the external cause
    EXCLUDES 1 *garage in private home (Y92.015)*
         schools and other public administration buildings (Y92.2-)

  ✓6ᵗʰ **Y92.51** Private commercial establishments as the place of occurrence of the external cause

    Y92.510 Bank as the place of occurrence of the external cause

    Y92.511 Restaurant or café as the place of occurrence of the external cause

    Y92.512 Supermarket, store or market as the place of occurrence of the external cause

    Y92.513 Shop (commercial) as the place of occurrence of the external cause

  ✓6ᵗʰ **Y92.52** Service areas as the place of occurrence of the external cause

    Y92.520 Airport as the place of occurrence of the external cause

    Y92.521 Bus station as the place of occurrence of the external cause

    Y92.522 Railway station as the place of occurrence of the external cause

    Y92.523 Highway rest stop as the place of occurrence of the external cause

    Y92.524 Gas station as the place of occurrence of the external cause
         Petroleum station as the place of occurrence of the external cause
         Service station as the place of occurrence of the external cause

  ✓6ᵗʰ **Y92.53** Ambulatory health services establishments as the place of occurrence of the external cause

    Y92.530 Ambulatory surgery center as the place of occurrence of the external cause
         Outpatient surgery center, including that connected with a hospital as the place of occurrence of the external cause
         Same day surgery center, including that connected with a hospital as the place of occurrence of the external cause

    Y92.531 Health care provider office as the place of occurrence of the external cause
         Physician office as the place of occurrence of the external cause

    Y92.532 Urgent care center as the place of occurrence of the external cause

    Y92.538 Other ambulatory health services establishments as the place of occurrence of the external cause

  Y92.59 Other trade areas as the place of occurrence of the external cause
     Office building as the place of occurrence of the external cause
     Casino as the place of occurrence of the external cause
     Garage (commercial) as the place of occurrence of the external cause
     Hotel as the place of occurrence of the external cause
     Radio or television station as the place of occurrence of the external cause
     Shopping mall as the place of occurrence of the external cause
     Warehouse as the place of occurrence of the external cause

✓5ᵗʰ **Y92.6** Industrial and construction area as the place of occurrence of the external cause

  Y92.61 Building [any] under construction as the place of occurrence of the external cause

  Y92.62 Dock or shipyard as the place of occurrence of the external cause
     Dockyard as the place of occurrence of the external cause
     Dry dock as the place of occurrence of the external cause
     Shipyard as the place of occurrence of the external cause

  Y92.63 Factory as the place of occurrence of the external cause
     Factory building as the place of occurrence of the external cause
     Factory premises as the place of occurrence of the external cause
     Industrial yard as the place of occurrence of the external cause

  Y92.64 Mine or pit as the place of occurrence of the external cause
     Mine as the place of occurrence of the external cause

  Y92.65 Oil rig as the place of occurrence of the external cause
     Pit (coal) (gravel) (sand) as the place of occurrence of the external cause

  Y92.69 Other specified industrial and construction area as the place of occurrence of the external cause
     Gasworks as the place of occurrence of the external cause
     Power-station (coal) (nuclear) (oil) as the place of occurrence of the external cause
     Tunnel under construction as the place of occurrence of the external cause
     Workshop as the place of occurrence of the external cause

✓5ᵗʰ **Y92.7** Farm as the place of occurrence of the external cause
   Ranch as the place of occurrence of the external cause
  EXCLUDES 1 *farmhouse and home premises of farm (Y92.01-)*

  Y92.71 Barn as the place of occurrence of the external cause

  Y92.72 Chicken coop as the place of occurrence of the external cause
     Hen house as the place of occurrence of the external cause

  Y92.73 Farm field as the place of occurrence of the external cause

  Y92.74 Orchard as the place of occurrence of the external cause

  Y92.79 Other farm location as the place of occurrence of the external cause

✓5ᵗʰ **Y92.8** Other places as the place of occurrence of the external cause

  ✓6ᵗʰ **Y92.81** Transport vehicle as the place of occurrence of the external cause
    EXCLUDES 1 *transport accidents (V00-V99)*

    Y92.810 Car as the place of occurrence of the external cause

    Y92.811 Bus as the place of occurrence of the external cause

    Y92.812 Truck as the place of occurrence of the external cause

    Y92.813 Airplane as the place of occurrence of the external cause

EXCLUDES 1 Not coded here   **EXCLUDES 2** Not included here   N Newborn Age: 0   P Pediatric Age: 0-17   M Maternity Age: 12-55   A Adult Age: 15-124

1100   ICD-10-CM 201

Y92.814   **Boat** as the place of occurrence of the external cause

Y92.815   **Train** as the place of occurrence of the external cause

Y92.816   **Subway car** as the place of occurrence of the external cause

Y92.818   **Other transport vehicle as the place of occurrence of the external cause**

✓6ᵗʰ **Y92.82**   **Wilderness area**

Y92.820   **Desert** as the place of occurrence of the external cause

Y92.821   **Forest** as the place of occurrence of the external cause

Y92.828   **Other wilderness area as the place of occurrence of the external cause**
     Swamp as the place of occurrence of the external cause
     Mountain as the place of occurrence of the external cause
     Marsh as the place of occurrence of the external cause
     Prairie as the place of occurrence of the external cause

✓6ᵗʰ **Y92.83**   **Recreation area** as the place of occurrence of the external cause

Y92.830   **Public park** as the place of occurrence of the external cause

Y92.831   **Amusement park** as the place of occurrence of the external cause

Y92.832   **Beach** as the place of occurrence of the external cause
     Seashore as the place of occurrence of the external cause

Y92.833   **Campsite** as the place of occurrence of the external cause

Y92.834   **Zoological garden (Zoo)** as the place of occurrence of the external cause

Y92.838   **Other recreation area as the place of occurrence of the external cause**

Y92.84   **Military training ground** as the place of occurrence of the external cause

Y92.85   **Railroad track** as the place of occurrence of the external cause

Y92.86   **Slaughter house** as the place of occurrence of the external cause

Y92.89   **Other specified places as the place of occurrence of the external cause**
     Derelict house as the place of occurrence of the external cause

Y92.9   **Unspecified place or not applicable**

✓4ᵗʰ **Y93**   **Activity codes**

NOTE   Category Y93 is provided for use to indicate the activity of the person seeking healthcare for an injury or health condition, such as a heart attack while shoveling snow, which resulted from, or was contributed to, by the activity. These codes are appropriate for use for both acute injuries, such as those from chapter 19, and conditions that are due to the long-term, cumulative effects of an activity, such as those from chapter 13. They are also appropriate for use with external cause codes for cause and intent if identifying the activity provides additional information on the event. These codes should be used in conjunction with codes for external cause status (Y99) and place of occurrence (Y92).

This section contains the following broad activity categories:

Y93.0   Activities involving walking and running
Y93.1   Activities involving water and water craft
Y93.2   Activities involving ice and snow
Y93.3   Activities involving climbing, rappelling, and jumping off
Y93.4   Activities involving dancing and other rhythmic movement
Y93.5   Activities involving other sports and athletics played individually
Y93.6   Activities involving other sports and athletics played as a team or group
Y93.7   Activities involving other specified sports and athletics
Y93.A   Activities involving other cardiorespiratory exercise
Y93.B   Activities involving other muscle strengthening exercises
Y93.C   Activities involving computer technology and electronic devices
Y93.D   Activities involving arts and handcrafts
Y93.E   Activities involving personal hygiene and interior property and clothing maintenance
Y93.F   Activities involving caregiving
Y93.G   Activities involving food preparation, cooking and grilling
Y93.H   Activities involving exterior property and land maintenance, building and construction
Y93.I   Activities involving roller coasters and other types of external motion
Y93.J   Activities involving playing musical instrument
Y93.K   Activities involving animal care
Y93.8   Activities, other specified
Y93.9   Activity, unspecified

✓5ᵗʰ **Y93.0**   **Activities involving walking and running**
   EXCLUDES 1   *activity, walking an animal (Y93.K1)*
               activity, walking or running on a treadmill (Y93.A1)

Y93.01   **Activity, walking, marching and hiking**
     Activity, walking, marching and hiking on level or elevated terrain
     EXCLUDES 1   *activity, mountain climbing (Y93.31)*

Y93.02   **Activity, running**

✓5ᵗʰ **Y93.1**   **Activities involving water and water craft**
   EXCLUDES 1   *activities involving ice (Y93.2-)*

Y93.11   **Activity, swimming**

Y93.12   **Activity, springboard and platform diving**

Y93.13   **Activity, water polo**

Y93.14   **Activity, water aerobics and water exercise**

Y93.15   **Activity, underwater diving and snorkeling**
     Activity, SCUBA diving

Y93.16   **Activity, rowing, canoeing, kayaking, rafting and tubing**
     Activity, canoeing, kayaking, rafting and tubing in calm and turbulent water

Y93.17   **Activity, water skiing and wake boarding**

Y93.18   **Activity, surfing, windsurfing and boogie boarding**
     Activity, water sliding

Y93.19   **Activity, other involving water and watercraft**
     Activity involving water NOS
     Activity, parasailing
     Activity, water survival training and testing

✓5ᵗʰ **Y93.2**   **Activities involving ice and snow**
   EXCLUDES 1   *activity, shoveling ice and snow (Y93.H1)*

Y93.21   **Activity, ice skating**
     Activity, figure skating (singles) (pairs)
     Activity, ice dancing
     EXCLUDES 1   *activity, ice hockey (Y93.22)*

Y93.22   **Activity, ice hockey**

Y93.23   **Activity, snow (alpine) (downhill) skiing, snow boarding, sledding, tobogganing and snow tubing**
     EXCLUDES 1   *activity, cross country skiing (Y93.24)*

Y93.24   **Activity, cross country skiing**
     Activity, nordic skiing

Y93.29 Activity, other involving ice and snow
    Activity involving ice and snow NOS

☑5ᵗʰ **Y93.3** Activities involving climbing, rappelling and jumping off
    EXCLUDES 1   activity, hiking on level or elevated terrain (Y93.01)
              activity, jumping rope (Y93.56)
              activity, trampoline jumping (Y93.44)

Y93.31 Activity, mountain climbing, rock climbing and wall climbing

Y93.32 Activity, rappelling

Y93.33 Activity, BASE jumping
    Activity, Building, Antenna, Span, Earth jumping

Y93.34 Activity, bungee jumping

Y93.35 Activity, hang gliding

Y93.39 Activity, other involving climbing, rappelling and jumping off

☑5ᵗʰ **Y93.4** Activities involving dancing and other rhythmic movement
    EXCLUDES 1   activity, martial arts (Y93.75)

Y93.41 Activity, dancing
    AHA: 2012, 4Q, 108

Y93.42 Activity, yoga

Y93.43 Activity, gymnastics
    Activity, rhythmic gymnastics
    EXCLUDES 1   activity, trampolining (Y93.44)

Y93.44 Activity, trampolining

Y93.45 Activity, cheerleading

Y93.49 Activity, other involving dancing and other rhythmic movements

☑5ᵗʰ **Y93.5** Activities involving other sports and athletics played individually
    EXCLUDES 1   activity, dancing (Y93.41)
              activity, gymnastic (Y93.43)
              activity, trampolining (Y93.44)
              activity, yoga (Y93.42)

Y93.51 Activity, roller skating (inline) and skateboarding

Y93.52 Activity, horseback riding

Y93.53 Activity, golf

Y93.54 Activity, bowling

Y93.55 Activity, bike riding

Y93.56 Activity, jumping rope

Y93.57 Activity, non-running track and field events
    EXCLUDES 1   activity, running (any form) (Y93.02)

Y93.59 Activity, other involving other sports and athletics played individually
    EXCLUDES 1   activities involving climbing, rappelling, and
                jumping (Y93.3-)
              activities involving ice and snow (Y93.2-)
              activities involving walking and running
                (Y93.0-)
              activities involving water and watercraft
                (Y93.1-)

☑5ᵗʰ **Y93.6** Activities involving other sports and athletics played as a team or group
    EXCLUDES 1   activity, ice hockey (Y93.22)
              activity, water polo (Y93.13)

Y93.61 Activity, American tackle football
    Activity, football NOS

Y93.62 Activity, American flag or touch football

Y93.63 Activity, rugby

Y93.64 Activity, baseball
    Activity, softball

Y93.65 Activity, lacrosse and field hockey

Y93.66 Activity, soccer

Y93.67 Activity, basketball

Y93.68 Activity, volleyball (beach) (court)

Y93.6A Activity, physical games generally associated   ℙ
    with school recess, summer camp and children
    Activity, capture the flag
    Activity, dodge ball
    Activity, four square
    Activity, kickball

Y93.69 Activity, other involving other sports and athletics played as a team or group
    Activity, cricket

☑5ᵗʰ **Y93.7** Activities involving other specified sports and athletics

Y93.71 Activity, boxing

Y93.72 Activity, wrestling

Y93.73 Activity, racquet and hand sports
    Activity, handball
    Activity, racquetball
    Activity, squash
    Activity, tennis

Y93.74 Activity, frisbee
    Activity, ultimate frisbee

Y93.75 Activity, martial arts
    Activity, combatives

Y93.79 Activity, other specified sports and athletics
    EXCLUDES 1   sports and athletics activities specified in
                categories Y93.0-Y93.6

☑5ᵗʰ **Y93.A** Activities involving other cardiorespiratory exercise
    Activities involving physical training

Y93.A1 Activity, exercise machines primarily for cardiorespiratory conditioning
    Activity, elliptical and stepper machines
    Activity, stationary bike
    Activity, treadmill

Y93.A2 Activity, calisthenics
    Activity, jumping jacks
    Activity, warm up and cool down

Y93.A3 Activity, aerobic and step exercise

Y93.A4 Activity, circuit training

Y93.A5 Activity, obstacle course
    Activity, challenge course
    Activity, confidence course

Y93.A6 Activity, grass drills
    Activity, guerilla drills

Y93.A9 Activity, other involving cardiorespiratory exercise
    EXCLUDES 1   activities involving cardiorespiratory exercise
                specified in categories Y93.0-Y93.7

☑5ᵗʰ **Y93.B** Activities involving other muscle strengthening exercises

Y93.B1 Activity, exercise machines primarily for muscle strengthening

Y93.B2 Activity, push-ups, pull-ups, sit-ups

Y93.B3 Activity, free weights
    Activity, barbells
    Activity, dumbbells

Y93.B4 Activity, pilates

Y93.B9 Activity, other involving muscle strengthening exercises
    EXCLUDES 1   activities involving muscle strengthening
                specified in categories Y93.0-Y93.A

☑5ᵗʰ **Y93.C** Activities involving computer technology and electronic devices
    EXCLUDES 1   activity, electronic musical keyboard or instruments
                (Y93.J-)

Y93.C1 Activity, computer keyboarding
    Activity, electronic game playing using keyboard or
        other stationary device

Y93.C2 Activity, hand held interactive electronic device
    Activity, cellular telephone and communication device
    Activity, electronic game playing using interactive
        device
    EXCLUDES 1   activity, electronic game playing using
                keyboard or other stationary device
                (Y93.C1)

Y93.C9 Activity, other involving computer technology and electronic devices

☑5ᵗʰ **Y93.D** Activities involving arts and handcrafts
    EXCLUDES 1   activities involving playing musical instrument (Y93.J-)

Y93.D1 Activity, knitting and crocheting

Y93.D2 Activity, sewing

Y93.D3 Activity, furniture building and finishing
    Activity, furniture repair

Y93.D9 Activity, other involving arts and handcrafts

☑5ᵗʰ **Y93.E** Activities involving personal hygiene and interior property and clothing maintenance
    EXCLUDES 1   activities involving cooking and grilling (Y93.G-)
              activities involving exterior property and land
                maintenance, building and construction (Y93.H-
              activities involving caregiving (Y93.F-)
              activity, dishwashing (Y93.G1)
              activity, food preparation (Y93.G1)
              activity, gardening (Y93.H2)

Y93.E1 Activity, personal bathing and showering

Y93.E2 Activity, laundry

EXCLUDES 1 Not coded here   *EXCLUDES 2* Not included here   ℕ Newborn Age: 0   ℙ Pediatric Age: 0-17   Ⓜ Maternity Age: 12-55   Ⓐ Adult Age: 15-124

Y93.E3   **Activity,** vacuuming

Y93.E4   **Activity,** ironing

Y93.E5   **Activity,** floor mopping and cleaning

Y93.E6   **Activity,** residential relocation
       Activity, packing up and unpacking involved in
           moving to a new residence

Y93.E8   **Activity, other** personal hygiene

Y93.E9   **Activity, other** interior property and clothing
       maintenance

✓5ᵗʰ   **Y93.F**   **Activities involving** caregiving
       Activity involving the provider of caregiving

Y93.F1   **Activity, caregiving,** bathing

Y93.F2   **Activity, caregiving,** lifting

Y93.F9   **Activity, other caregiving**

✓5ᵗʰ   **Y93.G**   **Activities involving food preparation, cooking and grilling**

Y93.G1   **Activity, food** preparation and clean up
       Activity, dishwashing

Y93.G2   **Activity,** grilling and smoking food

Y93.G3   **Activity,** cooking and baking
       Activity, use of stove, oven and microwave oven

Y93.G9   **Activity, other involving cooking and grilling**

✓5ᵗʰ   **Y93.H**   **Activities involving exterior property and land maintenance, building and construction**

Y93.H1   **Activity,** digging, shoveling and raking
       Activity, dirt digging
       Activity, raking leaves
       Activity, snow shoveling

Y93.H2   **Activity,** gardening and landscaping
       Activity, pruning, trimming shrubs, weeding

Y93.H3   **Activity,** building and construction

Y93.H9   **Activity, other involving exterior property and land maintenance, building and construction**

✓5ᵗʰ   **Y93.I**   **Activities involving roller coasters and other types of external motion**

Y93.I1   **Activity,** rollercoaster riding

Y93.I9   **Activity, other involving external motion**

✓5ᵗʰ   **Y93.J**   **Activities involving playing musical instrument**
       Activity involving playing electric musical instrument

Y93.J1   **Activity,** piano **playing**
       Activity, musical keyboard (electronic) playing

Y93.J2   **Activity,** drum and other percussion instrument **playing**

Y93.J3   **Activity,** string instrument **playing**

Y93.J4   **Activity,** winds and brass instrument **playing**

✓5ᵗʰ   **Y93.K**   **Activities involving** animal care
       EXCLUDES 1   activity, horseback riding (Y93.52)

Y93.K1   **Activity,** walking **an animal**

Y93.K2   **Activity,** milking **an animal**

Y93.K3   **Activity,** grooming and shearing **an animal**

Y93.K9   **Activity, other involving animal care**

✓5ᵗʰ   **Y93.8**   **Activities, other specified**

Y93.81   **Activity,** refereeing **a sports activity**

Y93.82   **Activity,** spectator **at an event**

Y93.83   **Activity,** rough housing and horseplay

Y93.84   **Activity,** sleeping

Y93.89   **Activity, other specified**

Y93.9   **Activity, unspecified**

   Y95   **Nosocomial condition**
       AHA: 2013, 4Q, 119

✓4ᵗʰ   **Y99**   **External cause status**
     NOTE   A single code from category Y99 should be used in conjunction with the external cause code(s) assigned to a record to indicate the status of the person at the time the event occurred.

Y99.0   Civilian **activity done for income or pay**
       Civilian activity done for financial or other compensation
       EXCLUDES 1   military activity (Y99.1)
             volunteer activity (Y99.2)

Y99.1   Military **activity**
       EXCLUDES 1   activity of off duty military personnel (Y99.8)

Y99.2   Volunteer **activity**
       EXCLUDES 1   activity of child or other family member assisting in compensated work of other family member (Y99.8)

Y99.8   **Other external cause status**
       Activity NEC
       Activity of child or other family member assisting in compensated work of other family member
       Hobby not done for income
       Leisure activity
       Off-duty activity of military personnel
       Recreation or sport not for income or while a student
       Student activity
       EXCLUDES 1   civilian activity done for income or compensation (Y99.0)
             military activity (Y99.1)
       AHA: 2012, 4Q, 108

Y99.9   **Unspecified external cause status**

Additional Character Required   ✓x7ᵗʰ Placeholder Alert   Unspecified Dx   Other Specified Dx   Manifestation   ▶◀ Revised Text   ● New Code   ▲ Revised Code Title

D-10-CM 2016   1103

Chapter 21. Factors Influencing Health Status and Contact with Health Services (Z00–Z99)

Chapter Specific Guidelines with Coding Examples

The chapter specific guidelines from the ICD-10-CM Official Guidelines for Coding and Reporting have been provided below. Along with these guidelines are coding examples, contained in the shaded boxes, that have been developed to help illustrate the coding and/or sequencing guidance found in these guidelines.

Note: The chapter specific guidelines provide additional information about the use of Z codes for specified encounters.

a. Use of Z codes in any healthcare setting

Z codes are for use in any healthcare setting. Z codes may be used as either a first-listed (principal diagnosis code in the inpatient setting) or secondary code, depending on the circumstances of the encounter. Certain Z codes may only be used as first-listed or principal diagnosis.

> Patient with middle lobe lung cancer admitted for initiation of chemotherapy
>
> **Z51.11**   **Encounter for antineoplastic chemotherapy**
>
> **C34.2**   **Malignant neoplasm of middle lobe, bronchus or lung**
>
> *Explanation:* A Z code can be used as first-listed in this situation based on guidelines in this chapter as well as chapter 2, "Neoplasms."

> Patient has chronic lymphocytic leukemia for which the patient had previous chemotherapy and is now in remission
>
> **C91.11**   **Chronic lymphocytic leukemia of B-cell type in remission**
>
> **Z92.21**   **Personal history of antineoplastic chemotherapy**
>
> *Explanation:* The personal history Z code is used to describe a secondary (supplementary) diagnosis to identify that this patient has had chemotherapy in the past.

b. Z Codes indicate a reason for an encounter

Z codes are not procedure codes. A corresponding procedure code must accompany a Z code to describe any procedure performed.

c. Categories of Z codes

1) Contact/exposure

Category Z20 indicates contact with, and suspected exposure to, communicable diseases. These codes are for patients who do not show any sign or symptom of a disease but are suspected to have been exposed to it by close personal contact with an infected individual or are in an area where a disease is epidemic.

Category Z77, Other contact with and (suspected) exposures hazardous to health, indicates contact with and suspected exposures hazardous to health.

Contact/exposure codes may be used as a first-listed code to explain an encounter for testing, or, more commonly, as a secondary code to identify a potential risk.

2) Inoculations and vaccinations

Code Z23 is for encounters for inoculations and vaccinations. It indicates that a patient is being seen to receive a prophylactic inoculation against a disease. Procedure codes are required to identify the actual administration of the injection and the type(s) of immunizations given. Code Z23 may be used as a secondary code if the inoculation is given as a routine part of preventive health care, such as a well-baby visit.

3) Status

Status codes indicate that a patient is either a carrier of a disease or has the sequelae or residual of a past disease or condition. This includes such things as the presence of prosthetic or mechanical devices resulting from past treatment. A status code is informative, because the status may affect the course of treatment and its outcome. A status code is distinct from a history code. The history code indicates that the patient no longer has the condition.

A status code should not be used with a diagnosis code from one of the body system chapters, if the diagnosis code includes the information provided by the status code. For example, code Z94.1, Heart transplant status, should not be used with a code from subcategory T86.2, Complications of heart transplant. The status code does not provide additional information. The complication code indicates that the patien is a heart transplant patient.

For encounters for weaning from a mechanical ventilator, assign a code from subcategory J96.1, Chronic respiratory failure, followed by code Z99.11, Dependence on respirator [ventilator] status.

The status Z codes/categories are:

Z14	Genetic carrier

    Genetic carrier status indicates that a person carries a gene, associated with a particular disease, which may be passed to offspring who may develop that disease. The person does not have the disease and is not at risk of developing the disease.

Z15	Genetic susceptibility to disease

    Genetic susceptibility indicates that a person has a gene that increases the risk of that person developing the disease.

    Codes from category Z15 should not be used as principal or first-listed codes. If the patient has the condition to which he/she is susceptible, and that condition is the reason for the encounter, the code for the current condition should be sequenced first. If the patient is being seen for follow-up after completed treatment for this condition, and the condition no longer exists, a follow-up code should be sequenced first, followed by the appropriate personal history and genetic susceptibility codes. If the purpose of the encounter is genetic counseling associated with procreative management, code Z31.5, Encounter for genetic counseling, should be assigned a the first-listed code, followed by a code from category Z15. Additional codes should be assigned for any applicable family or personal history.

Z16	Resistance to antimicrobial drugs

    This code indicates that a patient has a condition that is resistant to antimicrobial drug treatment. Sequence the infection code first.

Z17	Estrogen receptor status
Z18	Retained foreign body fragments
Z21	Asymptomatic HIV infection status

    This code indicates that a patient has tested positive for HIV bu has manifested no signs or symptoms of the disease.

Z22	Carrier of infectious disease

    Carrier status indicates that a person harbors the specific organisms of a disease without manifest symptoms and is capable of transmitting the infection.

Z28.3	Underimmunization status
Z33.1	Pregnant state, incidental

    This code is a secondary code only for use when the pregnanc is in no way complicating the reason for visit. Otherwise, a cod from the obstetric chapter is required.

Z66	Do not resuscitate

    This code may be used when it is documented by the provide that a patient is on do not resuscitate status at any time durin the stay.

Z67	Blood type
Z68	Body mass index (BMI)
Z74.01	Bed confinement status
Z76.82	Awaiting organ transplant status
Z78	Other specified health status

    Code Z78.1, Physical restraint status, may be used when it is documented by the provider that a patient has been put in restraints during the current encounter. Please note that this code should not be reported when it is documented by the provider that a patient is temporarily restrained during a procedure.

Z79	Long-term (current) drug therapy

    Codes from this category indicate a patient's continuous use o a prescribed drug (including such things as aspirin therapy) fo the long-term treatment of a condition or for prophylactic use It is not for use for patients who have addictions to drugs. Thi subcategory is not for use of medications for detoxification or maintenance programs to prevent withdrawal symptoms in patients with drug dependence (e.g., methadone maintenanc for opiate dependence). Assign the appropriate code for the drug dependence instead.

Assign a code from Z79 if the patient is receiving a medication for an extended period as a prophylactic measure (such as for the prevention of deep vein thrombosis) or as treatment of a chronic condition (such as arthritis) or a disease requiring a lengthy course of treatment (such as cancer). Do not assign a code from category Z79 for medication being administered for a brief period of time to treat an acute illness or injury (such as a course of antibiotics to treat acute bronchitis).

Z88	Allergy status to drugs, medicaments and biological substances

Except: Z88.9, Allergy status to unspecified drugs, medicaments and biological substances status

Z89	Acquired absence of limb
Z90	Acquired absence of organs, not elsewhere classified
Z91.0-	Allergy status, other than to drugs and biological substances
Z92.82	Status post administration of tPA (rtPA) in a different facility within the last 24 hours prior to admission to a current facility

Assign code Z92.82, Status post administration of tPA (rtPA) in a different facility within the last 24 hours prior to admission to current facility, as a secondary diagnosis when a patient is received into a facility and documentation indicates they were administered tissue plasminogen activator (tPA) within the last 24 hours prior to admission to the current facility.

This guideline applies even if the patient is still receiving the tPA at the time they are received into the current facility.

The appropriate code for the condition for which the tPA was administered (such as cerebrovascular disease or myocardial infarction) should be assigned first.

Code Z92.82 is only applicable to the receiving facility record and not to the transferring facility record.

Z93	Artificial opening status
Z94	Transplanted organ and tissue status
Z95	Presence of cardiac and vascular implants and grafts
Z96	Presence of other functional implants
Z97	Presence of other devices
Z98	Other postprocedural states

Assign code Z98.85, Transplanted organ removal status, to indicate that a transplanted organ has been previously removed. This code should not be assigned for the encounter in which the transplanted organ is removed. The complication necessitating removal of the transplant organ should be assigned for that encounter.

See section I.C19. for information on the coding of organ transplant complications.

Z99	Dependence on enabling machines and devices, not elsewhere classified

Note: Categories Z89-Z90 and Z93-Z99 are for use only if there are no complications or malfunctions of the organ or tissue replaced, the amputation site or the equipment on which the patient is dependent..

4) History (of)

There are two types of history Z codes, personal and family. Personal history codes explain a patient's past medical condition that no longer exists and is not receiving any treatment, but that has the potential for recurrence, and therefore may require continued monitoring.

Family history codes are for use when a patient has a family member(s) who has had a particular disease that causes the patient to be at higher risk of also contracting the disease.

Personal history codes may be used in conjunction with follow-up codes and family history codes may be used in conjunction with screening codes to explain the need for a test or procedure. History codes are also acceptable on any medical record regardless of the reason for visit. A history of an illness, even if no longer present, is important information that may alter the type of treatment ordered.

The history Z code categories are:

Z80	Family history of primary malignant neoplasm
Z81	Family history of mental and behavioral disorders
Z82	Family history of certain disabilities and chronic diseases (leading to disablement)
Z83	Family history of other specific disorders
Z84	Family history of other conditions
Z85	Personal history of malignant neoplasm

Z86	Personal history of certain other diseases
Z87	Personal history of other diseases and conditions
Z91.4-	Personal history of psychological trauma, not elsewhere classified
Z91.5	Personal history of self-harm
Z91.8-	Other specified personal risk factors, not elsewhere classified

Except: Z91.83, Wandering in diseases classified elsewhere

Z92	Personal history of medical treatment

Except: Z92.0, Personal history of contraception

Except: Z92.82, Status post administration of tPA (rtPA) in a different facility within the last 24 hours prior to admission to a current facility

5) Screening

Screening is the testing for disease or disease precursors in seemingly well individuals so that early detection and treatment can be provided for those who test positive for the disease (e.g., screening mammogram).

The testing of a person to rule out or confirm a suspected diagnosis because the patient has some sign or symptom is a diagnostic examination, not a screening. In these cases, the sign or symptom is used to explain the reason for the test.

A screening code may be a first-listed code if the reason for the visit is specifically the screening exam. It may also be used as an additional code if the screening is done during an office visit for other health problems. A screening code is not necessary if the screening is inherent to a routine examination, such as a pap smear done during a routine pelvic examination.

Should a condition be discovered during the screening then the code for the condition may be assigned as an additional diagnosis.

Prostate screening of healthy 50-year-old male patient; PSA noted to be elevated but normal digital rectal exam

Z12.5	**Encounter for screening for malignant neoplasm of prostate**
R97.2	**Elevated prostate specific antigen [PSA]**

Explanation: The patient had no signs or symptoms of any prostate-related illness prior to coming in for the screening. The screening code is appropriately used as the first-listed code to signify that this was for routine screening. The elevated PSA is reported as a secondary diagnosis to reflect that an abnormal lab value was found as a result of the screening procedure(s).

The Z code indicates that a screening exam is planned. A procedure code is required to confirm that the screening was performed.

The screening Z codes/categories:

Z11	Encounter for screening for infectious and parasitic diseases
Z12	Encounter for screening for malignant neoplasms
Z13	Encounter for screening for other diseases and disorders

Except: Z13.9, Encounter for screening, unspecified

Z36	Encounter for antenatal screening for mother

6) Observation

There are two observation Z code categories. They are for use in very limited circumstances when a person is being observed for a suspected condition that is ruled out. The observation codes are not for use if an injury or illness or any signs or symptoms related to the suspected condition are present. In such cases the diagnosis/symptom code is used with the corresponding external cause code.

The observation codes are to be used as principal diagnosis only. Additional codes may be used in addition to the observation code but only if they are unrelated to the suspected condition being observed.

Codes from subcategory Z03.7, Encounter for suspected maternal and fetal conditions ruled out, may either be used as a first-listed or as an additional code assignment depending on the case. They are for use in very limited circumstances on a maternal record when an encounter is for a suspected maternal or fetal condition that is ruled out during that encounter (for example, a maternal or fetal condition may be suspected due to an abnormal test result). These codes should not be used when the condition is confirmed. In those cases, the confirmed condition should be coded. In addition, these codes are not for use if an illness or any signs or symptoms related to the suspected condition or problem are present. In such cases the diagnosis/symptom code is used.

Additional codes may be used in addition to the code from subcategory Z03.7, but only if they are unrelated to the suspected condition being evaluated.

Codes from subcategory Z03.7 may not be used for encounters for antenatal screening of mother. *See Section I.C.21. Screening.*

For encounters for suspected fetal condition that are inconclusive following testing and evaluation, assign the appropriate code from category O35, O36, O40 or O41.

The observation Z code categories:

Z03   Encounter for medical observation for suspected diseases and conditions ruled out

Z04   Encounter for examination and observation for other reasons

       Except: Z04.9, Encounter for examination and observation for unspecified reason

7) Aftercare

Aftercare visit codes cover situations when the initial treatment of a disease has been performed and the patient requires continued care during the healing or recovery phase, or for the long-term consequences of the disease. The aftercare Z code should not be used if treatment is directed at a current, acute disease. The diagnosis code is to be used in these cases. Exceptions to this rule are codes Z51.0, Encounter for antineoplastic radiation therapy, and codes from subcategory Z51.1, Encounter for antineoplastic chemotherapy and immunotherapy. These codes are to be first-listed, followed by the diagnosis code when a patient's encounter is solely to receive radiation therapy, chemotherapy, or immunotherapy for the treatment of a neoplasm. If the reason for the encounter is more than one type of antineoplastic therapy, code Z51.0 and a code from subcategory Z51.1 may be assigned together, in which case one of these codes would be reported as a secondary diagnosis.

The aftercare Z codes should also not be used for aftercare for injuries. For aftercare of an injury, assign the acute injury code with the appropriate 7th character (for subsequent encounter).

The aftercare codes are generally first-listed to explain the specific reason for the encounter. An aftercare code may be used as an additional code when some type of aftercare is provided in addition to the reason for admission and no diagnosis code is applicable. An example of this would be the closure of a colostomy during an encounter for treatment of another condition.

Aftercare codes should be used in conjunction with other aftercare codes or diagnosis codes to provide better detail on the specifics of an aftercare encounter visit, unless otherwise directed by the classification. Should a patient receive multiple types of antineoplastic therapy during the same encounter, code Z51.0, Encounter for antineoplastic radiation therapy, and codes from subcategory Z51.1, Encounter for antineoplastic chemotherapy and immunotherapy, may be used together on a record. The sequencing of multiple aftercare codes depends on the circumstances of the encounter.

Certain aftercare Z code categories need a secondary diagnosis code to describe the resolving condition or sequelae. For others, the condition is included in the code title.

Additional Z code aftercare category terms include fitting and adjustment, and attention to artificial openings.

Status Z codes may be used with aftercare Z codes to indicate the nature of the aftercare. For example code Z95.1, Presence of aortocoronary bypass graft, may be used with code Z48.812, Encounter for surgical aftercare following surgery on the circulatory system, to indicate the surgery for which the aftercare is being performed. A status code should not be used when the aftercare code indicates the type of status, such as using Z43.0, Encounter for attention to tracheostomy, with Z93.0, Tracheostomy status.

The aftercare Z category/codes:

Z42   Encounter for plastic and reconstructive surgery following medical procedure or healed injury

Z43   Encounter for attention to artificial openings

Z44   Encounter for fitting and adjustment of external prosthetic device

Z45   Encounter for adjustment and management of implanted device

Z46   Encounter for fitting and adjustment of other devices

Z47   Orthopedic aftercare

Z48   Encounter for other postprocedural aftercare

Z49   Encounter for care involving renal dialysis

Z51   Encounter for other aftercare

8) Follow-up

The follow-up codes are used to explain continuing surveillance following completed treatment of a disease, condition, or injury. They imply that the condition has been fully treated and no longer exists. They should not be confused with aftercare codes, or injury codes with a 7th character for subsequent encounter, that explain ongoing care of a healing condition

or its sequelae. Follow-up codes may be used in conjunction with history codes to provide the full picture of the healed condition and its treatment. The follow-up code is sequenced first, followed by the history code.

A follow-up code may be used to explain multiple visits. Should a condition be found to have recurred on the follow-up visit, then the diagnosis code for the condition should be assigned in place of the follow-up code.

The follow-up Z code categories:

Z08   Encounter for follow-up examination after completed treatment for malignant neoplasm

Z09   Encounter for follow-up examination after completed treatment for conditions other than malignant neoplasm

Z39   Encounter for maternal postpartum care and examination

Follow-up for patient several months after completing a regime of IV antibiotics for recurrent pneumonia; lungs are clear and pneumonia is resolved

Z09   **Encounter for follow-up examination after completed treatment for conditions other than malignant neoplasm**

Z87.01   **Personal history of pneumonia (recurrent)**

Explanation: Code Z09 identifies the follow-up visit as being unrelated to a malignant neoplasm, and code Z87 describes the condition that has now resolved.

Follow-up for patient several months after completing a regime of IV antibiotics for recurrent pneumonia; pneumonia has recurred, and a new antibiotic regimen has been prescribed

J18.9   **Pneumonia, unspecified organism**

Explanation: Since the follow-up exam for pneumonia determined that the pneumonia was not resolved or recurred, code Z09 Encounter for follow-up examination after completed treatment for conditions other than malignant neoplasm, no longer applies. Instead the first-listed code describes the pneumonia.

---

9) Donor

Codes in category Z52, Donors of organs and tissues, are used for living individuals who are donating blood or other body tissue. These codes are only for individuals donating for others, not for self-donations. They are not used to identify cadaveric donations.

10) Counseling

Counseling Z codes are used when a patient or family member receives assistance in the aftermath of an illness or injury, or when support is required in coping with family or social problems. They are not used in conjunction with a diagnosis code when the counseling component of care is considered integral to standard treatment.

The counseling Z codes/categories:

Z30.0-   Encounter for general counseling and advice on contraception

Z31.5   Encounter for genetic counseling

Z31.6-   Encounter for general counseling and advice on procreation

Z32.2   Encounter for childbirth instruction

Z32.3   Encounter for childcare instruction

Z69   Encounter for mental health services for victim and perpetrator of abuse

Z70   Counseling related to sexual attitude, behavior and orientation

Z71   Persons encountering health services for other counseling and medical advice, not elsewhere classified

Z76.81   Expectant mother prebirth pediatrician visit

11) Encounters for obstetrical and reproductive services

See Section I.C.15. Pregnancy, Childbirth, and the Puerperium, for further instruction on the use of these codes.

Z codes for pregnancy are for use in those circumstances when none of the problems or complications included in the codes from the Obstetrics chapter exist (a routine prenatal visit or postpartum care). Codes in category Z34, Encounter for supervision of normal pregnancy, are always first-listed and are not to be used with any other code from the OB chapter.

Codes in category Z3A, Weeks of gestation, may be assigned to provide additional information about the pregnancy. The date of the admission should be used to determine weeks of gestation for inpatient admissions that encompass more than one gestational week.

The outcome of delivery, category Z37, should be included on all maternal delivery records. It is always a secondary code. Codes in category Z37 should not be used on the newborn record.

Z codes for family planning (contraceptive) or procreative management and counseling should be included on an obstetric record either during the pregnancy or the postpartum stage, if applicable.

Z codes/categories for obstetrical and reproductive services:

Z30	Encounter for contraceptive management
Z31	Encounter for procreative management
Z32.2	Encounter for childbirth instruction
Z32.3	Encounter for childcare instruction
Z33	Pregnant state
Z34	Encounter for supervision of normal pregnancy
Z36	Encounter for antenatal screening of mother
Z3A	Weeks of gestation
Z37	Outcome of delivery
Z39	Encounter for maternal postpartum care and examination
Z76.81	Expectant mother prebirth pediatrician visit

12) Newborns and infants

See Section I.C.16. Newborn (Perinatal) Guidelines, for further instruction on the use of these codes.

Newborn Z codes/categories:

Z76.1	Encounter for health supervision and care of foundling
Z00.1-	Encounter for routine child health examination
Z38	Liveborn infants according to place of birth and type of delivery

13) Routine and administrative examinations

The Z codes allow for the description of encounters for routine examinations, such as, a general check-up, or, examinations for administrative purposes, such as, a pre-employment physical. The codes are not to be used if the examination is for diagnosis of a suspected condition or for treatment purposes. In such cases the diagnosis code is used. During a routine exam, should a diagnosis or condition be discovered, it should be coded as an additional code. Pre-existing and chronic conditions and history codes may also be included as additional codes as long as the examination is for administrative purposes and not focused on any particular condition.

Some of the codes for routine health examinations distinguish between "with" and "without" abnormal findings. Code assignment depends on the information that is known at the time the encounter is being coded. For example, if no abnormal findings were found during the examination, but the encounter is being coded before test results are back, it is acceptable to assign the code for "without abnormal findings." When assigning a code for "with abnormal findings," additional code(s) should be assigned to identify the specific abnormal finding(s).

12-month-old boy admitted for well-child visit; pediatrician notices some eczema on the child's scalp and back of the knees

Z00.121   Encounter for routine child health examination with abnormal findings

L30.9   Dermatitis, unspecified

Explanation: The Z code identifying that this is a routine well-child visit is reported first. Because an abnormal finding (eczema) was documented, a code for this condition may also be appended.

Pre-operative examination and pre-procedural laboratory examination Z codes are for use only in those situations when a patient is being cleared for a procedure or surgery and no treatment is given.

The Z codes/categories for routine and administrative examinations:

Z00	Encounter for general examination without complaint, suspected or reported diagnosis
Z01	Encounter for other special examination without complaint, suspected or reported diagnosis
Z02	Encounter for administrative examination
	Except: Z02.9, Encounter for administrative examinations, unspecified
Z32.0-	Encounter for pregnancy test

14) Miscellaneous Z codes

The miscellaneous Z codes capture a number of other health care encounters that do not fall into one of the other categories. Certain of these codes identify the reason for the encounter; others are for use as additional codes that provide useful information on circumstances that may affect a patient's care and treatment.

Prophylactic Organ Removal

For encounters specifically for prophylactic removal of an organ (such as prophylactic removal of breasts due to a genetic susceptibility to cancer or a family history of cancer), the principal or first-listed code should be a code from category Z40, Encounter for prophylactic surgery, followed by the appropriate codes to identify the associated risk factor (such as genetic susceptibility or family history).

If the patient has a malignancy of one site and is having prophylactic removal at another site to prevent either a new primary malignancy or metastatic disease, a code for the malignancy should also be assigned in addition to a code from subcategory Z40.0, Encounter for prophylactic surgery for risk factors related to malignant neoplasms. A Z40.0 code should not be assigned if the patient is having organ removal for treatment of a malignancy, such as the removal of the testes for the treatment of prostate cancer.

Miscellaneous Z codes/categories:

Z28	Immunization not carried out
	Except: Z28.3, Underimmunization status
Z40	Encounter for prophylactic surgery
Z41	Encounter for procedures for purposes other than remedying health state
	Except: Z41.9, Encounter for procedure for purposes other than remedying health state, unspecified
Z53	Persons encountering health services for specific procedures and treatment, not carried out
Z55	Problems related to education and literacy
Z56	Problems related to employment and unemployment
Z57	Occupational exposure to risk factors
Z58	Problems related to physical environment
Z59	Problems related to housing and economic circumstances
Z60	Problems related to social environment
Z62	Problems related to upbringing
Z63	Other problems related to primary support group, including family circumstances
Z64	Problems related to certain psychosocial circumstances
Z65	Problems related to other psychosocial circumstances
Z72	Problems related to lifestyle
Z73	Problems related to life management difficulty
Z74	Problems related to care provider dependency
	Except: Z74.01, Bed confinement status
Z75	Problems related to medical facilities and other health care
Z76.0	Encounter for issue of repeat prescription
Z76.3	Healthy person accompanying sick person
Z76.4	Other boarder to healthcare facility
Z76.5	Malingerer [conscious simulation]
Z91.1-	Patient's noncompliance with medical treatment and regimen
Z91.83	Wandering in diseases classified elsewhere
Z91.89	Other specified personal risk factors, not elsewhere classified

15) Nonspecific Z codes

Certain Z codes are so non-specific, or potentially redundant with other codes in the classification, that there can be little justification for their use in the inpatient setting. Their use in the outpatient setting should be limited to those instances when there is no further documentation to permit more precise coding. Otherwise, any sign or symptom or any other reason for visit that is captured in another code should be used.

Nonspecific Z codes/categories:

Z02.9	Encounter for administrative examinations, unspecified
Z04.9	Encounter for examination and observation for unspecified reason
Z13.9	Encounter for screening, unspecified
Z41.9	Encounter for procedure for purposes other than remedying health state, unspecified
Z52.9	Donor of unspecified organ or tissue
Z86.59	Personal history of other mental and behavioral disorders
Z88.9	Allergy status to unspecified drugs, medicaments and biological substances status
Z92.0	Personal history of contraception

16) Z codes that may only be principal/first-listed diagnosis

The following Z codes/categories may only be reported as the principal/first-listed diagnosis, except when there are multiple encounters on the same day and the medical records for the encounters are combined:

Z00	Encounter for general examination without complaint, suspected or reported diagnosis
	Except: Z00.6
Z01	Encounter for other special examination without complaint, suspected or reported diagnosis
Z02	Encounter for administrative examination
Z03	Encounter for medical observation for suspected diseases and conditions ruled out
Z04	Encounter for examination and observation for other reasons
Z33.2	Encounter for elective termination of pregnancy
Z31.81	Encounter for male factor infertility in female patient
Z31.82	Encounter for Rh incompatibility status
Z31.83	Encounter for assisted reproductive fertility procedure cycle
Z31.84	Encounter for fertility preservation procedure
Z34	Encounter for supervision of normal pregnancy
Z39	Encounter for maternal postpartum care and examination
Z38	Liveborn infants according to place of birth and type of delivery
Z42	Encounter for plastic and reconstructive surgery following medical procedure or healed injury
Z51.0	Encounter for antineoplastic radiation therapy
Z51.1-	Encounter for antineoplastic chemotherapy and immunotherapy
Z52	Donors of organs and tissues
	Except: Z52.9, Donor of unspecified organ or tissue
Z76.1	Encounter for health supervision and care of foundling
Z76.2	Encounter for health supervision and care of other healthy infant and child
Z99.12	Encounter for respirator [ventilator] dependence during powe failure

Female patient seen at 32 weeks' gestation to check the progress of her first pregnancy

Z34.03   **Encounter for supervision of normal first pregnancy, third trimester**

Z3A.32   **32 weeks gestation of pregnancy**

Explanation: Category Z34 is appropriate as a first-listed diagnosis. Category Z3A helps to clarify at which point in the pregnancy the patient was provided supervision.

Chapter 21. Factors Influencing Health Status and Contact With Health Services (Z00-Z99)

NOTE Z codes represent reasons for encounters. A corresponding procedure code must accompany a Z code if a procedure is performed. Categories Z00-Z99 are provided for occasions when circumstances other than a disease, injury or external cause classifiable to categories A00-Y89 are recorded as "diagnoses" or "problems". This can arise in two main ways:

(a) When a person who may or may not be sick encounters the health services for some specific purpose, such as to receive limited care or service for a current condition, to donate an organ or tissue, to receive prophylactic vaccination (immunization), or to discuss a problem which is in itself not a disease or injury.

(b) When some circumstance or problem is present which influences the person's health status but is not in itself a current illness or injury.

This chapter contains the following blocks:

Z00-Z13	Persons encountering health services for examinations
Z14-Z15	Genetic carrier and genetic susceptibility to disease
Z16	Resistance to antimicrobial drugs
Z17	Estrogen receptor status
Z18	Retained foreign body fragments
Z20-Z28	Persons with potential health hazards related to communicable diseases
Z30-Z39	Persons encountering health services in circumstances related to reproduction
Z40-Z53	Encounters for other specific health care
Z55-Z65	Persons with potential health hazards related to socioeconomic and psychosocial circumstances
Z66	Do not resuscitate status
Z67	Blood type
Z68	Body mass index (BMI)
Z69-Z76	Persons encountering health services in other circumstances
Z77-Z99	Persons with potential health hazards related to family and personal history and certain conditions influencing health status

Persons encountering health services for examinations (Z00-Z13)

NOTE Nonspecific abnormal findings disclosed at the time of these examinations are classified to categories R70-R94.

EXCLUDES 1 examinations related to pregnancy and reproduction (Z30-Z36, Z39-)

Z00 Encounter for general examination without complaint, suspected or reported diagnosis

EXCLUDES 1 encounter for examination for administrative purposes (Z02.-)

EXCLUDES 2 encounter for pre-procedural examinations (Z01.81-)
special screening examinations (Z11-Z13)

✓5ᵗʰ **Z00.0 Encounter for general adult medical examination**
Encounter for adult periodic examination (annual) (physical) and any associated laboratory and radiologic examinations

EXCLUDES 1 encounter for examination of sign or symptom—code to sign or symptom
general health check-up of infant or child (Z00.12-)

Z00.00 Encounter for general adult medical examination without abnormal findings   PDx A
Encounter for adult health check-up NOS

Z00.01 Encounter for general adult medical examination with abnormal findings   PDx A
Use additional code to identify abnormal findings

✓5ᵗʰ **Z00.1 Encounter for newborn, infant and child health examinations**

✓6ᵗʰ **Z00.11 Newborn health examination**
Health check for child under 29 days old
Use additional code to identify any abnormal findings

EXCLUDES 1 health check for child over 28 days old (Z00.12-)

Z00.110 Health examination for newborn under 8 days old   PDx N
Health check for newborn under 8 days old

Z00.111 Health examination for newborn 8 to 28 days old   PDx N
Health check for newborn 8 to 28 days old
Newborn weight check

✓6ᵗʰ **Z00.12 Encounter for routine child health examination**
Encounter for development testing of infant or child
Health check (routine) for child over 28 days old

EXCLUDES 1 health check for child under 29 days old (Z00.11-)
health supervision of foundling or other healthy infant or child (Z76.1-Z76.2)
newborn health examination (Z00.11-)

Z00.121 Encounter for routine child health examination with abnormal findings   PDx P
Use additional code to identify abnormal findings

Z00.129 Encounter for routine child health examination without abnormal findings   PDx P
Encounter for routine child health examination NOS

Z00.2 Encounter for examination for period of rapid growth in childhood   PDx P

Z00.3 Encounter for examination for adolescent development state   PDx P
Encounter for puberty development state

Z00.5 Encounter for examination of potential donor of organ and tissue   PDx

Z00.6 Encounter for examination for normal comparison and control in clinical research program
Examination of participant or control in clinical research program

✓5ᵗʰ **Z00.7 Encounter for examination for period of delayed growth in childhood**

Z00.70 Encounter for examination for period of delayed growth in childhood without abnormal findings   PDx P

Z00.71 Encounter for examination for period of delayed growth in childhood with abnormal findings   PDx P
Use additional code to identify abnormal findings

Z00.8 Encounter for other general examination   PDx
Encounter for health examination in population surveys

✓4ᵗʰ **Z01 Encounter for other special examination without complaint, suspected or reported diagnosis**

INCLUDES routine examination of specific system

NOTE Codes from category Z01 represent the reason for the encounter. A separate procedure code is required to identify any examinations or procedures performed.

EXCLUDES 1 encounter for examination for administrative purposes (Z02.-)
encounter for examination for suspected conditions, proven not to exist (Z03.-)
encounter for laboratory and radiologic examinations as a component of general medical examinations (Z00.0-)
encounter for laboratory, radiologic and imaging examinations for sign(s) and symptom(s)—code to the sign(s) or symptom(s)

EXCLUDES 2 screening examinations (Z11-Z13)

✓5ᵗʰ **Z01.0 Encounter for examination of eyes and vision**

EXCLUDES 1 examination for driving license (Z02.4)

Z01.00 Encounter for examination of eyes and vision without abnormal findings   PDx
Encounter for examination of eyes and vision NOS

Z01.01 Encounter for examination of eyes and vision with abnormal findings   PDx
Use additional code to identify abnormal findings

✓5ᵗʰ **Z01.1 Encounter for examination of ears and hearing**

Z01.10 Encounter for examination of ears and hearing without abnormal findings   PDx
Encounter for examination of ears and hearing NOS

✓6ᵗʰ **Z01.11 Encounter for examination of ears and hearing** with abnormal findings

Z01.110 Encounter for hearing examination following failed hearing screening   PDx

Z01.118 Encounter for examination of ears and hearing with other abnormal findings   PDx
Use additional code to identify abnormal findings

Z01.12 Encounter for hearing conservation and treatment

✓5ᵗʰ **Z01.2 Encounter for dental examination and cleaning**

Z01.20 Encounter for dental examination and cleaning without abnormal findings   PDx
Encounter for dental examination and cleaning NOS

Z01.21 Encounter for dental examination and cleaning with abnormal findings   PDx
Use additional code to identify abnormal findings

Chapter 21. Factors Influencing Health Status and Contact with Health Services *(left margin)*

✓5ᵗʰ **Z01.3** **Encounter for examination of blood pressure**

    Z01.30 **Encounter for examination of blood pressure without abnormal findings** `PDx`
        Encounter for examination of blood pressure NOS

    Z01.31 **Encounter for examination of blood pressure with abnormal findings** `PDx`
        Use additional code to identify abnormal findings

✓5ᵗʰ **Z01.4** **Encounter for gynecological examination**
    EXCLUDES 2 *pregnancy examination or test (Z32.0-)*
        routine examination for contraceptive maintenance (Z30.4-)

    ✓6ᵗʰ **Z01.41** **Encounter for routine gynecological examination**
        Encounter for general gynecological examination with or without cervical smear
        Encounter for gynecological examination (general) (routine) NOS
        Encounter for pelvic examination (annual) (periodic)
        Use additional code:
          for screening for human papillomavirus, if applicable, (Z11.51)
          for screening vaginal pap smear, if applicable (Z12.72)
          to identify acquired absence of uterus, if applicable (Z90.71-)
        EXCLUDES 1 *gynecologic examination status-post hysterectomy for malignant condition (Z08)*
            screening cervical pap smear not a part of a routine gynecological examination (Z12.4)

        Z01.411 **Encounter for gynecological examination (general) (routine) with abnormal findings** `PDx` ♀

        Z01.419 **Encounter for gynecological examination (general) (routine) without abnormal findings** `PDx` ♀
          Use additional code to identify abnormal findings

    Z01.42 **Encounter for cervical smear to confirm findings of recent normal smear following initial abnormal smear** `PDx` ♀

✓5ᵗʰ **Z01.8** **Encounter for other specified special examinations**

    ✓6ᵗʰ **Z01.81** **Encounter for preprocedural examinations**
        Encounter for preoperative examinations
        Encounter for radiological and imaging examinations as part of preprocedural examination

        Z01.810 **Encounter for preprocedural cardiovascular examination** `PDx`

        Z01.811 **Encounter for preprocedural respiratory examination** `PDx`

        Z01.812 **Encounter for preprocedural laboratory examination** `PDx`
          Blood and urine tests prior to treatment or procedure

        Z01.818 **Encounter for other preprocedural examination** `PDx`
          Encounter for preprocedural examination NOS
          Encounter for examinations prior to antineoplastic chemotherapy

    Z01.82 **Encounter for allergy testing** `PDx`
        EXCLUDES 1 *encounter for antibody response examination (Z01.84)*

    Z01.83 **Encounter for blood typing** `PDx`
        Encounter for Rh typing

    Z01.84 **Encounter for antibody response examination** `PDx`
        Encounter for immunity status testing
        EXCLUDES 1 *encounter for allergy testing (Z01.82)*

    Z01.89 **Encounter for other specified special examinations** `PDx`

✓4ᵗʰ **Z02** **Encounter for administrative examination**

    Z02.0 **Encounter for examination for admission to educational institution** `PDx`
        Encounter for examination for admission to preschool (education)
        Encounter for examination for re-admission to school following illness or medical treatment

    Z02.1 **Encounter for pre-employment examination** `PDx`

    Z02.2 **Encounter for examination for admission to residential institution** `P`
        EXCLUDES 1 *examination for admission to prison (Z02.89)*

    Z02.3 **Encounter for examination for recruitment to armed forces** `P`

    Z02.4 **Encounter for examination for driving license** `P`

    Z02.5 **Encounter for examination for participation in sport** `P`
        EXCLUDES 1 *blood-alcohol and blood-drug test (Z02.83)*

    Z02.6 **Encounter for examination for insurance purposes** `P`

✓5ᵗʰ **Z02.7** **Encounter for issue of medical certificate**
    EXCLUDES 1 *encounter for general medical examination (Z00-Z01, Z02.0-Z02.6, Z02.8-Z02.9)*

    Z02.71 **Encounter for disability determination** `P`
        Encounter for issue of medical certificate of incapaci
        Encounter for issue of medical certificate of invalidit

    Z02.79 **Encounter for issue of other medical certificate** `P`

✓5ᵗʰ **Z02.8** **Encounter for other administrative examinations**

    Z02.81 **Encounter for paternity testing** `P`

    Z02.82 **Encounter for adoption services** `P`

    Z02.83 **Encounter for blood-alcohol and blood-drug test** `P`
        Use additional code for findings of alcohol or drugs blood (R78.-)

    Z02.89 **Encounter for other administrative examinations** `P`
        Encounter for examination for admission to prison
        Encounter for examination for admission to summe camp
        Encounter for immigration examination
        Encounter for naturalization examination
        Encounter for premarital examination
        EXCLUDES 1 *health supervision of foundling or other healthy infant or child (Z76.1-Z76.2)*

    Z02.9 **Encounter for administrative examinations, unspecified** `P`

✓4ᵗʰ **Z03** **Encounter for medical observation for suspected diseases and conditions ruled out**
    NOTE This category is to be used when a person without a diagnosis is suspected of having an abnormal condition, without signs or symptoms, which requires study, but after examination and observation, is ruled out. This category is also for use for administrative and legal observation status.
    EXCLUDES 1 *contact with and (suspected) exposures hazardous to health (Z77.-)*
        newborn observation for suspected condition, ruled out (P00-P04)
        person with feared complaint in whom no diagnosis is made (Z71.1)
        signs or symptoms under study—code to signs or symptoms

    Z03.6 **Encounter for observation for suspected toxic effect from ingested substance ruled out** `P`
        Encounter for observation for suspected adverse effect from drug
        Encounter for observation for suspected poisoning

    ✓5ᵗʰ **Z03.7** **Encounter for suspected maternal and fetal conditions rule out**
        Encounter for suspected maternal and fetal conditions not found
        EXCLUDES 1 *known or suspected fetal anomalies affecting management of mother, not ruled out (O26-, O35-, O36-, O40-, O41-)*

        Z03.71 **Encounter for suspected problem with amniotic cavity and membrane ruled out** `PDx` `M`
          Encounter for suspected oligohydramnios ruled out
          Encounter for suspected polyhydramnios ruled out

        Z03.72 **Encounter for suspected placental problem ruled out** `PDx` `M`

        Z03.73 **Encounter for suspected fetal anomaly ruled out** `PDx` `M`

        Z03.74 **Encounter for suspected problem with fetal growth ruled out** `PDx` `M`

        Z03.75 **Encounter for suspected cervical shortening ruled out** `PDx` `M`

        Z03.79 **Encounter for other suspected maternal and fetal conditions ruled out** `PDx` `M`

EXCLUDES 1 Not coded here   *EXCLUDES 2* Not included here   `N` Newborn Age: 0   `P` Pediatric Age: 0-17   `M` Maternity Age: 12-55   `A` Adult Age: 15-124   `PDx` Primary

1110   ICD-10-CM 20

✓5ᵗʰ Z03.8   Encounter for observation for other suspected diseases and conditions ruled out

✓6ᵗʰ Z03.81   Encounter for observation for suspected exposure to biological agents ruled out

Z03.810   Encounter for observation for suspected exposure to anthrax ruled out `PDx`

Z03.818   Encounter for observation for suspected exposure to other biological agents ruled out `PDx`

Z03.89   Encounter for observation for other suspected diseases and conditions ruled out `PDx`

Z04   Encounter for examination and observation for other reasons

`INCLUDES` encounter for examination for medicolegal reasons

`NOTE` This category is to be used when a person without a diagnosis is suspected of having an abnormal condition, without signs or symptoms, which requires study, but after examination and observation, is ruled-out. This category is also for use for administrative and legal observation status.

Z04.1   Encounter for examination and observation following transport accident `PDx`

`EXCLUDES 1` encounter for examination and observation following work accident (Z04.2)

Z04.2   Encounter for examination and observation following work accident `PDx`

Z04.3   Encounter for examination and observation following other accident `PDx`

✓5ᵗʰ Z04.4   Encounter for examination and observation following alleged rape

Encounter for examination and observation of victim following alleged rape

Encounter for examination and observation of victim following alleged sexual abuse

Z04.41   Encounter for examination and observation following alleged adult rape `PDx` `A`

Suspected adult rape, ruled out

Suspected adult sexual abuse, ruled out

Z04.42   Encounter for examination and observation following alleged child rape `PDx` `P`

Suspected child rape, ruled out

Suspected child sexual abuse, ruled out

Z04.6   Encounter for general psychiatric examination, requested by authority `PDx`

✓5ᵗʰ Z04.7   Encounter for examination and observation following alleged physical abuse

Z04.71   Encounter for examination and observation following alleged adult physical abuse `PDx` `A`

Suspected adult physical abuse, ruled out

`EXCLUDES 1` confirmed case of adult physical abuse (T74.-)

encounter for examination and observation following alleged adult sexual abuse (Z04.41)

suspected case of adult physical abuse, not ruled out (T76.-)

Z04.72   Encounter for examination and observation following alleged child physical abuse `PDx` `P`

Suspected child physical abuse, ruled out

`EXCLUDES 1` confirmed case of child physical abuse (T74.-)

encounter for examination and observation following alleged child sexual abuse (Z04.42)

suspected case of child physical abuse, not ruled out (T76.-)

Z04.8   Encounter for examination and observation for other specified reasons `PDx`

Encounter for examination and observation for request for expert evidence

Z04.9   Encounter for examination and observation for unspecified reason `PDx`

Encounter for observation NOS

Z08   Encounter for follow-up examination after completed treatment for malignant neoplasm

Medical surveillance following completed treatment

Use additional code to identify any acquired absence of organs (Z90.-)

Use additional code to identify the personal history of malignant neoplasm (Z85.-)

`EXCLUDES 1` aftercare following medical care (Z43-Z49, Z51)

Z09   Encounter for follow-up examination after completed treatment for conditions other than malignant neoplasm

Medical surveillance following completed treatment

Use additional code to identify any applicable history of disease code (Z86-. Z87-)

`EXCLUDES 1` aftercare following medical care (Z43-Z49, Z51)

surveillance of contraception (Z30.4-)

surveillance of prosthetic and other medical devices (Z44-Z46)

`AHA:` 2015, 1Q, 8

✓4ᵗʰ Z11   Encounter for screening for infectious and parasitic diseases

`NOTE` Screening is the testing for disease or disease precursors in asymptomatic individuals so that early detection and treatment can be provided for those who test positive for the disease.

`EXCLUDES 1` encounter for diagnostic examination—code to sign or symptom

Z11.0   Encounter for screening for intestinal infectious diseases

Z11.1   Encounter for screening for respiratory tuberculosis

Z11.2   Encounter for screening for other bacterial diseases

Z11.3   Encounter for screening for infections with a predominantly sexual mode of transmission

`EXCLUDES 2` encounter for screening for human immunodeficiency virus [HIV] (Z11.4)

encounter for screening for human papillomavirus (Z11.51)

Z11.4   Encounter for screening for human immunodeficiency virus [HIV]

✓5ᵗʰ Z11.5   Encounter for screening for other viral diseases

`EXCLUDES 2` encounter for screening for viral intestinal disease (Z11.0)

Z11.51   Encounter for screening for human papillomavirus (HPV)

Z11.59   Encounter for screening for other viral diseases

Z11.6   Encounter for screening for other protozoal diseases and helminthiases

`EXCLUDES 2` encounter for screening for protozoal intestinal disease (Z11.0)

Z11.8   Encounter for screening for other infectious and parasitic diseases

Encounter for screening for chlamydia

Encounter for screening for rickettsial

Encounter for screening for spirochetal

Encounter for screening for mycoses

Z11.9   Encounter for screening for infectious and parasitic diseases, unspecified

✓4ᵗʰ Z12   Encounter for screening for malignant neoplasms

`NOTE` Screening is the testing for disease or disease precursors in asymptomatic individuals so that early detection and treatment can be provided for those who test positive for the disease.

Use additional code to identify any family history of malignant neoplasm (Z80.-)

`EXCLUDES 1` encounter for diagnostic examination—code to sign or symptom

Z12.0   Encounter for screening for malignant neoplasm of stomach

✓5ᵗʰ Z12.1   Encounter for screening for malignant neoplasm of intestinal tract

Z12.10   Encounter for screening for malignant neoplasm of intestinal tract, unspecified

Z12.11   Encounter for screening for malignant neoplasm of colon

Encounter for screening colonoscopy NOS

Z12.12   Encounter for screening for malignant neoplasm of rectum

Z12.13   Encounter for screening for malignant neoplasm of small intestine

Z12.2   Encounter for screening for malignant neoplasm of respiratory organs

✓5ᵗʰ Z12.3   Encounter for screening for malignant neoplasm of breast

Z12.31   Encounter for screening mammogram for malignant neoplasm of breast

`EXCLUDES 1` inconclusive mammogram (R92.2)

`AHA:` 2015, 1Q, 24

Z12.39   Encounter for other screening for malignant neoplasm of breast

dditional Character Required   `✓x7ᵗʰ` Placeholder Alert   Unspecified Dx   Other Specified Dx   Manifestation   ►◄ Revised Text   ● New Code   ▲ Revised Code Title

-10-CM 2016   1111

Z12.4 **Encounter for screening for malignant neoplasm of** cervix ♀
Encounter for screening pap smear for malignant neoplasm of cervix
> **EXCLUDES 1** *encounter for screening for human papillomavirus (Z11.51)*
> *when screening is part of general gynecological examination (Z01.4-)*

Z12.5 **Encounter for screening for malignant neoplasm of** prostate ♂

Z12.6 **Encounter for screening for malignant neoplasm of** bladder

✓5ᵗʰ **Z12.7** **Encounter for screening for malignant neoplasm of** other genitourinary organs

    Z12.71 **Encounter for screening for malignant neoplasm of** testis ♂

    Z12.72 **Encounter for screening for malignant neoplasm of** vagina ♀
Vaginal pap smear status-post hysterectomy for non-malignant condition
Use additional code to identify acquired absence of uterus (Z90.71-)
> **EXCLUDES 1** *vaginal pap smear status-post hysterectomy for malignant conditions (Z08)*

    Z12.73 **Encounter for screening for malignant neoplasm of** ovary ♀

    Z12.79 **Encounter for screening for malignant neoplasm of other genitourinary organs**

✓5ᵗʰ **Z12.8** **Encounter for screening for malignant neoplasm of** other sites

    Z12.81 **Encounter for screening for malignant neoplasm of** oral cavity

    Z12.82 **Encounter for screening for malignant neoplasm of** nervous system

    Z12.83 **Encounter for screening for malignant neoplasm of** skin

    Z12.89 **Encounter for screening for malignant neoplasm of other sites**

Z12.9 **Encounter for screening for malignant neoplasm, site unspecified**

✓4ᵗʰ **Z13** **Encounter for screening for** other diseases and disorders
> **NOTE** Screening is the testing for disease or disease precursors in asymptomatic individuals so that early detection and treatment can be provided for those who test positive for the disease.
> **EXCLUDES 1** *encounter for diagnostic examination—code to sign or symptom*

Z13.0 **Encounter for screening for diseases of the** blood and blood-forming organs **and certain disorders involving the immune mechanism**

Z13.1 **Encounter for screening for** diabetes mellitus

✓5ᵗʰ **Z13.2** **Encounter for screening for nutritional, metabolic and other endocrine disorders**

    Z13.21 **Encounter for screening for** nutritional disorder

    ✓6ᵗʰ **Z13.22** **Encounter for screening for** metabolic disorder

      Z13.220 **Encounter for screening for** lipoid disorders
Encounter for screening for cholesterol level
Encounter for screening for hypercholesterolemia
Encounter for screening for hyperlipidemia

      Z13.228 **Encounter for screening for other metabolic disorders**

    Z13.29 **Encounter for screening for other suspected endocrine disorder**
> **EXCLUDES 1** *encounter for screening for diabetes mellitus (Z13.1)*

Z13.4 **Encounter for screening for certain** developmental **disorders in** childhood   Ⓟ
Encounter for screening for developmental handicaps in early childhood
> **EXCLUDES 1** *routine development testing of infant or child (Z00.1-)*

Z13.5 **Encounter for screening for** eye and ear **disorders**
> **EXCLUDES 2** *encounter for general hearing examination (Z01.1-)*
> *encounter for general vision examination (Z01.0-)*

Z13.6 **Encounter for screening for** cardiovascular **disorders**

✓5ᵗʰ **Z13.7** **Encounter for screening for** genetic and chromosomal anomalies
> **EXCLUDES 1** *genetic testing for procreative management (Z31.4-*

    Z13.71 **Encounter for nonprocreative screening for gene** disease carrier status

    Z13.79 **Encounter for other screening for genetic and chromosomal anomalies**

✓5ᵗʰ **Z13.8** **Encounter for screening for** other specified diseases and disorders
> **EXCLUDES 2** *screening for malignant neoplasms (Z12.-)*

    ✓6ᵗʰ **Z13.81** **Encounter for screening for** digestive system disorders

      Z13.810 **Encounter for screening for** upper gastrointestinal **disorder**

      Z13.811 **Encounter for screening for** lower gastrointestinal **disorder**
> **EXCLUDES 1** *encounter for screening for intestinal infectious dise (Z11.0)*

      Z13.818 **Encounter for screening for other digestive system disorders**

    ✓6ᵗʰ **Z13.82** **Encounter for screening for** musculoskeletal disorder

      Z13.820 **Encounter for screening for** osteoporo

      Z13.828 **Encounter for screening for other musculoskeletal disorder**

    Z13.83 **Encounter for screening for** respiratory disorder ▶
> **EXCLUDES 1** *encounter for screening for respiratory tuberculosis (Z11.1)*

    Z13.84 **Encounter for screening for** dental disorders

    ✓6ᵗʰ **Z13.85** **Encounter for screening for** nervous system disorders

      Z13.850 **Encounter for screening for** traumatic brain injury

      Z13.858 **Encounter for screening for other nerv system disorders**

    Z13.88 **Encounter for screening for disorder** due to exposure to contaminants
> **EXCLUDES 1** *those exposed to contaminants without suspected disorders (Z57-Z77-)*

    Z13.89 **Encounter for screening for other disorder**
Encounter for screening for genitourinary disorder

Z13.9 **Encounter for screening, unspecified**

Genetic carrier and genetic susceptibility to disease (Z14-Z15

✓4ᵗʰ **Z14** **Genetic carrier**

✓5ᵗʰ **Z14.0** Hemophilia A **carrier**

    Z14.01 Asymptomatic **hemophilia A carrier**

    Z14.02 Symptomatic **hemophilia A carrier**

Z14.1 Cystic fibrosis **carrier**

Z14.8 **Genetic carrier of other disease**

✓4ᵗʰ **Z15** Genetic susceptibility **to disease**
Confirmed abnormal gene
Use additional code, if applicable, for any associated family history of disease (Z80-Z84)
> **EXCLUDES 1** *chromosomal anomalies (Q90-Q99)*

✓5ᵗʰ **Z15.0** **Genetic susceptibility to** malignant neoplasm
Code first, if applicable, any current malignant neoplasm (C00-C75, C81-C96)
Use additional code, if applicable, for any personal history of malignant neoplasm (Z85.-)

    Z15.01 **Genetic susceptibility to malignant neoplasm of** breast

    Z15.02 **Genetic susceptibility to malignant neoplasm of** ovary

    Z15.03 **Genetic susceptibility to malignant neoplasm of** prostate

    Z15.04 **Genetic susceptibility to malignant neoplasm of** endometrium

    Z15.09 **Genetic susceptibility to other malignant neopla**

✓5ᵗʰ **Z15.8** **Genetic susceptibility to other disease**

    Z15.81 **Genetic susceptibility to** multiple endocrine neoplasia [MEN]
> **EXCLUDES 1** *multiple endocrine neoplasia [MEN] syndromes (E31.2-)*

    Z15.89 **Genetic susceptibility to other disease**

Resistance to antimicrobial drugs (Z16)

Z16 Resistance to antimicrobial drugs
> **NOTE** The codes in this category are provided for use as additional codes to identify the resistance and non-responsiveness of a condition to antimicrobial drugs.
>
> Code first the infection
> **EXCLUDES 1** *Methicillin resistant Staphylococcus aureus infection (A49.02)*
> *Methicillin resistant Staphylococcus aureus infection in diseases classified elsewhere (B95.62)*
> *Methicillin resistant Staphylococcus aureus pneumonia (J15.212)*
> *Sepsis due to Methicillin resistant Staphylococcus aureus (A41.02)*

√5ᵗʰ Z16.1 Resistance to beta lactam antibiotics
> **Z16.10 Resistance to unspecified beta lactam antibiotics**
> **Z16.11 Resistance to penicillins**
> > Resistance to amoxicillin
> > Resistance to ampicillin
> **Z16.12 Extended spectrum beta lactamase (ESBL) resistance**
> **Z16.19 Resistance to other specified beta lactam antibiotics**
> > Resistance to cephalosporins

√5ᵗʰ Z16.2 Resistance to other antibiotics
> **Z16.20 Resistance to unspecified antibiotic**
> > Resistance to antibiotics NOS
> **Z16.21 Resistance to vancomycin**
> **Z16.22 Resistance to vancomycin related antibiotics**
> **Z16.23 Resistance to quinolones and fluoroquinolones**
> **Z16.24 Resistance to multiple antibiotics**
> **Z16.29 Resistance to other single specified antibiotic**
> > Resistance to aminoglycosides
> > Resistance to macrolides
> > Resistance to sulfonamides
> > Resistance to tetracyclines

√5ᵗʰ Z16.3 Resistance to other antimicrobial drugs
> **EXCLUDES 1** *resistance to antibiotics (Z16.1-, Z16.2-)*
> **Z16.30 Resistance to unspecified antimicrobial drugs**
> > Drug resistance NOS
> **Z16.31 Resistance to antiparasitic drug(s)**
> > Resistance to quinine and related compounds
> **Z16.32 Resistance to antifungal drug(s)**
> **Z16.33 Resistance to antiviral drug(s)**
> **√6ᵗʰ Z16.34 Resistance to antimycobacterial drug(s)**
> > Resistance to tuberculostatics
> > **Z16.341 Resistance to single antimycobacterial drug**
> > > Resistance to antimycobacterial drug NOS
> > **Z16.342 Resistance to multiple antimycobacterial drugs**
> **Z16.35 Resistance to multiple antimicrobial drugs**
> > **EXCLUDES 1** *Resistance to multiple antibiotics only (Z16.24)*
> **Z16.39 Resistance to other specified antimicrobial drug**

Estrogen receptor status (Z17)

Z17 Estrogen receptor status
> Code first malignant neoplasm of breast (C50.-)
> **Z17.0 Estrogen receptor positive status [ER+]**
> **Z17.1 Estrogen receptor negative status [ER-]**

Retained foreign body fragment (Z18)

Z18 Retained foreign body fragments
> Embedded fragment (status)
> Embedded splinter (status)
> Retained foreign body status
> **EXCLUDES 1** *artificial joint prosthesis status (Z96.6-)*
> *foreign body accidentally left during a procedure (T81.5-)*
> *foreign body entering through orifice (T15-T19)*
> *in situ cardiac device (Z95.-)*
> *organ or tissue replaced by means other than transplant (Z96.-, Z97.-)*
> *organ or tissue replaced by transplant (Z94.-)*
> *personal history of retained foreign body fully removed (Z87.821)*
> *superficial foreign body (non-embedded splinter)—code to superficial foreign body, by site*

√5ᵗʰ Z18.0 Retained radioactive fragments
> **Z18.01 Retained depleted uranium fragments**
> **Z18.09 Other retained radioactive fragments**
> > Other retained depleted isotope fragments
> > Retained nontherapeutic radioactive fragments

√5ᵗʰ Z18.1 Retained metal fragments
> **EXCLUDES 1** *retained radioactive metal fragments (Z18.01-Z18.09)*
> **Z18.10 Retained metal fragments, unspecified**
> > Retained metal fragment NOS
> **Z18.11 Retained magnetic metal fragments**
> **Z18.12 Retained nonmagnetic metal fragments**

Z18.2 Retained plastic fragments
> Acrylics fragments
> Diethylhexylphthalates fragments
> Isocyanate fragments

√5ᵗʰ Z18.3 Retained organic fragments
> **Z18.31 Retained animal quills or spines**
> **Z18.32 Retained tooth**
> **Z18.33 Retained wood fragments**
> **Z18.39 Other retained organic fragments**

√5ᵗʰ Z18.8 Other specified retained foreign body
> **Z18.81 Retained glass fragments**
> **Z18.83 Retained stone or crystalline fragments**
> > Retained concrete or cement fragments
> **Z18.89 Other specified retained foreign body fragments**

Z18.9 Retained foreign body fragments, unspecified material

Persons with potential health hazards related to communicable diseases (Z20-Z28)

√4ᵗʰ Z20 Contact with and (suspected) exposure to communicable diseases
> **EXCLUDES 1** *carrier of infectious disease (Z22.-)*
> *diagnosed current infectious or parasitic disease—see Alphabetic Index*
> **EXCLUDES 2** *personal history of infectious and parasitic diseases (Z86.1-)*

√5ᵗʰ Z20.0 Contact with and (suspected) exposure to intestinal infectious diseases
> **Z20.01 Contact with and (suspected) exposure to intestinal infectious diseases due to Escherichia coli (E. coli)**
> **Z20.09 Contact with and (suspected) exposure to other intestinal infectious diseases**

Z20.1 Contact with and (suspected) exposure to tuberculosis

Z20.2 Contact with and (suspected) exposure to infections with a predominantly sexual mode of transmission

Z20.3 Contact with and (suspected) exposure to rabies

Z20.4 Contact with and (suspected) exposure to rubella

Z20.5 Contact with and (suspected) exposure to viral hepatitis

Z20.6 Contact with and (suspected) exposure to human immunodeficiency virus [HIV]
> **EXCLUDES 1** *asymptomatic human immunodeficiency virus [HIV] HIV infection status (Z21)*

Z20.7 Contact with and (suspected) exposure to pediculosis, acariasis and other infestations

√5ᵗʰ Z20.8 Contact with and (suspected) exposure to other communicable diseases
> **√6ᵗʰ Z20.81 Contact with and (suspected) exposure to other bacterial communicable diseases**
> > **Z20.810 Contact with and (suspected) exposure to anthrax**
> > **Z20.811 Contact with and (suspected) exposure to meningococcus**
> > **Z20.818 Contact with and (suspected) exposure to other bacterial communicable diseases**
> **√6ᵗʰ Z20.82 Contact with and (suspected) exposure to other viral communicable diseases**
> > **Z20.820 Contact with and (suspected) exposure to varicella**
> > **Z20.828 Contact with and (suspected) exposure to other viral communicable diseases**
> **Z20.89 Contact with and (suspected) exposure to other communicable diseases**

Z20.9 Contact with and (suspected) exposure to unspecified communicable disease

---

Additional Character Required   **√x7ᵗʰ Placeholder Alert**   Unspecified Dx   Other Specified Dx   Manifestation   ►◄ Revised Text   ● New Code   ▲ Revised Code Title

Z21 Asymptomatic human immunodeficiency virus [HIV] infection status
HIV positive NOS
Code first human immunodeficiency virus [HIV] disease complicating pregnancy, childbirth and the puerperium, if applicable (O98.7-)
EXCLUDES 1 *acquired immunodeficiency syndrome (B20)*
contact with human immunodeficiency virus [HIV] (Z20.6)
exposure to human immunodeficiency virus [HIV] (Z20.6)
human immunodeficiency virus [HIV] disease (B20)
inconclusive laboratory evidence of human immunodeficiency virus [HIV] (R75)

√4th **Z22 Carrier of infectious disease**
Colonization status
Suspected carrier

Z22.0 Carrier of typhoid

Z22.1 Carrier of other intestinal **infectious diseases**

Z22.2 Carrier of diphtheria

√5th **Z22.3 Carrier of** other **specified bacterial diseases**

     Z22.31 Carrier of bacterial disease due to meningococci

√6th   **Z22.32 Carrier of bacterial disease due to** staphylococci

         Z22.321 Carrier or suspected carrier of Methicillin susceptible **Staphylococcus aureus**
         MSSA colonization

         Z22.322 Carrier or suspected carrier of Methicillin resistant **Staphylococcus aureus**
         MRSA colonization

√6th   **Z22.33 Carrier of bacterial disease due to** streptococci

         Z22.330 Carrier of Group B **streptococcus**

         Z22.338 Carrier of other streptococcus

     Z22.39 Carrier of other specified bacterial diseases

Z22.4 Carrier of infections with a predominantly sexual mode of transmission

√5th **Z22.5 Carrier of** viral hepatitis

     Z22.50 Carrier of unspecified viral hepatitis

     Z22.51 Carrier of viral hepatitis B
     Hepatitis B surface antigen [HBsAg] carrier

     Z22.52 Carrier of viral hepatitis C

     Z22.59 Carrier of other viral hepatitis

Z22.6 Carrier of human T-lymphotropic virus type-1 [HTLV-1] **infection**

Z22.8 Carrier of other infectious diseases

Z22.9 Carrier of infectious disease, unspecified

Z23 Encounter for immunization
Code first any routine childhood examination
NOTE   Procedure codes are required to identify the types of immunizations given

√4th **Z28 Immunization not carried out and underimmunization status**
Vaccination not carried out

√5th **Z28.0 Immunization not carried out because of** contraindication

     Z28.01 Immunization not carried out because of acute illness **of patient**

     Z28.02 Immunization not carried out because of chronic illness **or condition of patient**

     Z28.03 Immunization not carried out because of immune compromised state **of patient**

     Z28.04 Immunization not carried out because of patient allergy to vaccine or component

     Z28.09 Immunization not carried out because of other contraindication

Z28.1 Immunization not carried out because of patient decision for reasons of belief or group pressure
     Immunization not carried out because of religious belief

√5th **Z28.2 Immunization not carried out because of patient decision for** other and unspecified **reason**

     Z28.20 Immunization not carried out because of patient decision for unspecified reason

     Z28.21 Immunization not carried out because of patient refusal

     Z28.29 Immunization not carried out because of patient decision for other reason

Z28.3 Underimmunization status
Delinquent immunization status
Lapsed immunization schedule status

√5th **Z28.8 Immunization not carried out for other reason**

     Z28.81 Immunization not carried out due to patient havir had the disease

     Z28.82 Immunization not carried out because of caregive refusal
     Immunization not carried out because of guardian refusal
     Immunization not carried out because of parent refusal
     EXCLUDES 1 *immunization not carried out because of caregiver refusal because of religious belief (Z28.1)*

     Z28.89 Immunization not carried out for other reason

Z28.9 Immunization not carried out for unspecified reason

Persons encountering health services in circumstances related t reproduction (Z30-Z39)

√4th **Z30 Encounter for contraceptive management**

√5th **Z30.0 Encounter for general counseling and advice on** contraception

√6th   **Z30.01 Encounter for** initial prescription **of contraceptive**
     EXCLUDES 1 *encounter for surveillance of contraceptive (Z30.4-)*

     Z30.011 Encounter for initial prescription **of contraceptive pills**

     Z30.012 Encounter for prescription of emergency **contraception**
     Encounter for postcoital contraception

     Z30.013 Encounter for initial prescription of injectable **contraceptive**

     Z30.014 Encounter for initial prescription of intrauterine **contraceptive device**
     EXCLUDES 1 *encounter for insertion of intrauterine contraceptive device (Z30.430, Z30.432)*

     Z30.018 Encounter for initial prescription of other contraceptives

     Z30.019 Encounter for initial prescription of contraceptives, unspecified

     Z30.02 Counseling and instruction in natural family planning **to avoid pregnancy**

     Z30.09 Encounter for other general counseling and advice on contraception
     Encounter for family planning advice NOS

Z30.2 Encounter for sterilization

√5th **Z30.4 Encounter for** surveillance **of contraceptives**

     Z30.40 Encounter for surveillance of contraceptives, unspecified

     Z30.41 Encounter for surveillance of contraceptive pills
     Encounter for repeat prescription for contraceptive

     Z30.42 Encounter for surveillance of injectable **contraceptive**

√6th   **Z30.43 Encounter for surveillance of** intrauterine **contraceptive device**

     Z30.430 Encounter for insertion **of intrauterine contraceptive device**

     Z30.431 Encounter for routine checking **of intrauterine contraceptive device**

     Z30.432 Encounter for removal **of intrauterine contraceptive device**

     Z30.433 Encounter for removal and reinsertion **of intrauterine contraceptive device**
     Encounter for replacement of intrauterine contraceptive device

     Z30.49 Encounter for surveillance of other contraceptives

Z30.8 Encounter for other contraceptive management
Encounter for postvasectomy sperm count
Encounter for routine examination for contraceptive maintenance
EXCLUDES 1 *sperm count following sterilization reversal (Z31.42)*
sperm count for fertility testing (Z31.41)

Z30.9 Encounter for contraceptive management, unspecified

√4th **Z31 Encounter for procreative management**
EXCLUDES 1 *complications associated with artificial fertilization (N98.-)*
female infertility (N97.-)
male infertility (N46.-)

Z31.0 Encounter for reversal of previous sterilization

EXCLUDES 1 Not coded here   EXCLUDES 2 Not included here   N Newborn Age: 0   P Pediatric Age: 0-17   M Maternity Age: 12-55   A Adult Age: 15-124   PDx Primary

✓5ᵗʰ Z31.4 Encounter for procreative investigation and testing
> EXCLUDES 1   postvasectomy sperm count (Z30.8)

Z31.41 Encounter for fertility testing
> Encounter for fallopian tube patency testing
> Encounter for sperm count for fertility testing

Z31.42 Aftercare following sterilization reversal
> Sperm count following sterilization reversal

✓6ᵗʰ Z31.43 Encounter for genetic testing of female for procreative management
> Use additional code for recurrent pregnancy loss, if applicable (N96, O26.2-)
> EXCLUDES 1   nonprocreative genetic testing (Z13.7-)

Z31.430 Encounter of female for testing for genetic disease carrier status for procreative management ♀

Z31.438 Encounter for other genetic testing of female for procreative management ♀

✓6ᵗʰ Z31.44 Encounter for genetic testing of male for procreative management
> EXCLUDES 1   nonprocreative genetic testing (Z13.7-)

Z31.440 Encounter of male for testing for genetic disease carrier status for procreative management ♂

Z31.441 Encounter for testing of male partner patient with recurrent pregnancy loss Ⓐ♂

Z31.448 Encounter for other genetic testing of male for procreative management Ⓐ♂

Z31.49 Encounter for other procreative investigation and testing

Z31.5 Encounter for genetic counseling

✓5ᵗʰ Z31.6 Encounter for general counseling and advice on procreation

Z31.61 Procreative counseling and advice using natural family planning

Z31.62 Encounter for fertility preservation counseling
> Encounter for fertility preservation counseling prior to cancer therapy
> Encounter for fertility preservation counseling prior to surgical removal of gonads

Z31.69 Encounter for other general counseling and advice on procreation

✓5ᵗʰ Z31.8 Encounter for other procreative management

Z31.81 Encounter for male factor infertility in female patient PDx ♀

Z31.82 Encounter for Rh incompatibility status PDx ♀
> AHA: 2014, 4Q, 17

Z31.83 Encounter for assisted reproductive fertility procedure cycle PDx ♀
> Patient undergoing in vitro fertilization cycle
> Use additional code to identify the type of infertility
> EXCLUDES 1   pre-cycle diagnosis and testing—code to reason for encounter

Z31.84 Encounter for fertility preservation procedure PDx
> Encounter for fertility preservation procedure prior to cancer therapy
> Encounter for fertility preservation procedure prior to surgical removal of gonads

Z31.89 Encounter for other procreative management Ⓜ

Z31.9 Encounter for procreative management, unspecified

◢ Z32 Encounter for pregnancy test and childbirth and childcare instruction

✓5ᵗʰ Z32.0 Encounter for pregnancy test

Z32.00 Encounter for pregnancy test, result unknown ♀
> Encounter for pregnancy test NOS

Z32.01 Encounter for pregnancy test, result positive Ⓜ♀

Z32.02 Encounter for pregnancy test, result negative ♀

Z32.2 Encounter for childbirth instruction

Z32.3 Encounter for childcare instruction
> Encounter for prenatal or postpartum childcare instruction

◢ Z33 Pregnant state

Z33.1 Pregnant state, incidental Ⓜ♀
> Pregnant state NOS
> EXCLUDES 1   complications of pregnancy (O00-O9A)

Z33.2 Encounter for elective termination of pregnancy PDx Ⓜ♀
> EXCLUDES 1   early fetal death with retention of dead fetus (O02.1)
> late fetal death (O36.4)
> spontaneous abortion (O03)

✓4ᵗʰ Z34 Encounter for supervision of normal pregnancy
> EXCLUDES 1   any complication of pregnancy (O00-O9A)
> encounter for pregnancy test (Z32.0-)
> encounter for supervision of high risk pregnancy (O09.-)
> AHA: 2014, 4Q, 17

✓5ᵗʰ Z34.0 Encounter for supervision of normal first pregnancy

Z34.00 Encounter for supervision of normal first pregnancy, unspecified trimester PDx Ⓜ

Z34.01 Encounter for supervision of normal first pregnancy, first trimester PDx Ⓜ

Z34.02 Encounter for supervision of normal first pregnancy, second trimester PDx Ⓜ

Z34.03 Encounter for supervision of normal first pregnancy, third trimester PDx Ⓜ

✓5ᵗʰ Z34.8 Encounter for supervision of other normal pregnancy

Z34.80 Encounter for supervision of other normal pregnancy, unspecified trimester PDx Ⓜ

Z34.81 Encounter for supervision of other normal pregnancy, first trimester PDx Ⓜ

Z34.82 Encounter for supervision of other normal pregnancy, second trimester PDx Ⓜ

Z34.83 Encounter for supervision of other normal pregnancy, third trimester PDx Ⓜ

✓5ᵗʰ Z34.9 Encounter for supervision of normal pregnancy, unspecified

Z34.90 Encounter for supervision of normal pregnancy, unspecified, unspecified trimester PDx Ⓜ♀

Z34.91 Encounter for supervision of normal pregnancy, unspecified, first trimester PDx Ⓜ

Z34.92 Encounter for supervision of normal pregnancy, unspecified, second trimester PDx Ⓜ

Z34.93 Encounter for supervision of normal pregnancy, unspecified, third trimester PDx Ⓜ

Z36 Encounter for antenatal screening of mother Ⓜ
> EXCLUDES 1   abnormal findings on antenatal screening of mother (O28.-)
> diagnostic examination—code to sign or symptom
> encounter for suspected maternal and fetal conditions ruled out (Z03.7-)
> suspected fetal condition affecting management of pregnancy—code to condition in Chapter 15
> EXCLUDES 2   genetic counseling and testing (Z31.43-, Z31.5)
> routine prenatal care (Z34)

✓4ᵗʰ Z3A Weeks of gestation
> NOTE   Codes from category Z3A are for use, only on the maternal record, to indicate the weeks of gestation of the pregnancy.
> Code first complications of pregnancy, childbirth and the puerperium (O00-O9A)
> AHA: 2014, 3Q, 17; 2014, 2Q, 9; 2013, 2Q, 33

✓5ᵗʰ Z3A.0 Weeks of gestation of pregnancy, unspecified or less than 10 weeks

Z3A.00 Weeks of gestation of pregnancy not specified Ⓜ♀

Z3A.01 Less than 8 weeks gestation of pregnancy Ⓜ♀

Z3A.08 8 weeks gestation of pregnancy Ⓜ♀

Z3A.09 9 weeks gestation of pregnancy Ⓜ♀

✓5ᵗʰ Z3A.1 Weeks of gestation of pregnancy, weeks 10-19

Z3A.10 10 weeks gestation of pregnancy Ⓜ♀

Z3A.11 11 weeks gestation of pregnancy Ⓜ♀

Z3A.12 12 weeks gestation of pregnancy Ⓜ♀

Z3A.13 13 weeks gestation of pregnancy Ⓜ♀

Z3A.14 14 weeks gestation of pregnancy Ⓜ♀

Z3A.15 15 weeks gestation of pregnancy Ⓜ♀

Z3A.16 16 weeks gestation of pregnancy Ⓜ♀

Z3A.17 17 weeks gestation of pregnancy Ⓜ♀

Z3A.18 18 weeks gestation of pregnancy Ⓜ♀

Z3A.19 19 weeks gestation of pregnancy Ⓜ♀

✓5ᵗʰ Z3A.2 Weeks of gestation of pregnancy, weeks 20-29

Z3A.20 20 weeks gestation of pregnancy Ⓜ♀

Z3A.21 21 weeks gestation of pregnancy Ⓜ♀

Z3A.22 22 weeks gestation of pregnancy Ⓜ♀

Z3A.23 23 weeks gestation of pregnancy Ⓜ♀

Z3A.24 24 weeks gestation of pregnancy Ⓜ♀

Z3A.25 25 weeks gestation of pregnancy Ⓜ♀

Z3A.26 26 weeks gestation of pregnancy Ⓜ♀

Z3A.27 27 weeks gestation of pregnancy Ⓜ♀

Z3A.28 28 weeks gestation of pregnancy Ⓜ♀

Additional Character Required   ✓x7ᵗʰ Placeholder Alert   Unspecified Dx   Other Specified Dx   Manifestation   ►◄ Revised Text   ● New Code   ▲ Revised Code Title

-10-CM 2016   1115

Z3A.29   **29 weeks gestation** of pregnancy   M♀

✓5ᵗʰ Z3A.3   **Weeks of gestation** of pregnancy, weeks 30-39

Z3A.30   **30 weeks gestation** of pregnancy   M♀
Z3A.31   **31 weeks gestation** of pregnancy   M♀
Z3A.32   **32 weeks gestation** of pregnancy   M♀
Z3A.33   **33 weeks gestation** of pregnancy   M♀
Z3A.34   **34 weeks gestation** of pregnancy   M♀
Z3A.35   **35 weeks gestation** of pregnancy   M♀
Z3A.36   **36 weeks gestation** of pregnancy   M♀
Z3A.37   **37 weeks gestation** of pregnancy   M♀
Z3A.38   **38 weeks gestation** of pregnancy   M♀
Z3A.39   **39 weeks gestation** of pregnancy   M♀

✓5ᵗʰ Z3A.4   **Weeks of gestation** of pregnancy, weeks 40 or greater
     AHA: 2014, 4Q, 23

Z3A.40   **40 weeks gestation** of pregnancy   M♀
Z3A.41   **41 weeks gestation** of pregnancy   M♀
Z3A.42   **42 weeks gestation** of pregnancy   M♀
Z3A.49   **Greater than 42 weeks gestation** of pregnancy   M♀

✓4ᵗʰ **Z37**   **Outcome of delivery**
     NOTE   This category is intended for use as an additional code to identify the outcome of delivery on the mother's record. It is not for use on the newborn record.
     EXCLUDES 1   *stillbirth (P95)*

Z37.0   **Single live birth**   M♀
     AHA: 2014, 2Q, 9
Z37.1   **Single stillbirth**   M♀
Z37.2   **Twins, both liveborn**   M♀
Z37.3   **Twins, one liveborn and one stillborn**   M♀
Z37.4   **Twins, both stillborn**   M♀

✓5ᵗʰ Z37.5   **Other multiple births, all liveborn**
Z37.50   **Multiple births, unspecified, all liveborn**   M♀
Z37.51   **Triplets, all liveborn**   M♀
Z37.52   **Quadruplets, all liveborn**   M♀
Z37.53   **Quintuplets, all liveborn**   M♀
Z37.54   **Sextuplets, all liveborn**   M♀
Z37.59   **Other multiple births, all liveborn**   M♀

✓5ᵗʰ Z37.6   **Other multiple births, some liveborn**
Z37.60   **Multiple births, unspecified, some liveborn**   M♀
Z37.61   **Triplets, some liveborn**   M♀
Z37.62   **Quadruplets, some liveborn**   M♀
Z37.63   **Quintuplets, some liveborn**   M♀
Z37.64   **Sextuplets, some liveborn**   M♀
Z37.69   **Other multiple births, some liveborn**   M♀

Z37.7   **Other multiple births, all stillborn**   M♀
Z37.9   **Outcome of delivery, unspecified**   M♀
     Multiple birth NOS
     Single birth NOS

✓4ᵗʰ **Z38**   **Liveborn infants according to place of birth and type of delivery**
     NOTE   This category is for use as the principal code on the initial record of a newborn baby. It is to be used for the initial birth record only. It is not to be used on the mother's record.

✓5ᵗʰ Z38.0   **Single liveborn infant, born in hospital**
     Single liveborn infant, born in birthing center or other health care facility
Z38.00   **Single liveborn infant, delivered vaginally**   PDx N
Z38.01   **Single liveborn infant, delivered by cesarean**   PDx N
Z38.1   **Single liveborn infant, born outside hospital**   PDx N
Z38.2   **Single liveborn infant, unspecified as to place of birth**   PDx N
     Single liveborn infant NOS

✓5ᵗʰ Z38.3   **Twin liveborn infant, born in hospital**
Z38.30   **Twin liveborn infant, delivered vaginally**   PDx N
Z38.31   **Twin liveborn infant, delivered by cesarean**   PDx N
Z38.4   **Twin liveborn infant, born outside hospital**   PDx N
Z38.5   **Twin liveborn infant, unspecified as to place of birth**   PDx N

✓5ᵗʰ Z38.6   **Other multiple liveborn infant, born in hospital**
Z38.61   **Triplet liveborn infant, delivered vaginally**   PDx N
Z38.62   **Triplet liveborn infant, delivered by cesarean**   PDx N
Z38.63   **Quadruplet liveborn infant, delivered vaginally**   PDx N
Z38.64   **Quadruplet liveborn infant, delivered by cesarean**   PDx N

Z38.65   **Quintuplet liveborn infant, delivered vaginally**   PDx
Z38.66   **Quintuplet liveborn infant, delivered by cesarean**   PDx
Z38.68   **Other multiple liveborn infant, delivered vaginally**   PDx
Z38.69   **Other multiple liveborn infant, delivered by cesarean**   PDx
Z38.7   **Other multiple liveborn infant, born outside hospital**   PDx
Z38.8   **Other multiple liveborn infant, unspecified as to place of birth**   PDx

✓4ᵗʰ **Z39**   **Encounter for maternal postpartum care and examination**
Z39.0   **Encounter for care and examination of mother immediately after delivery**   PDx
     Care and observation in uncomplicated cases when the deliv● occurs outside a healthcare facility
     EXCLUDES 1   *care for postpartum complication—see Alphabetic index*
Z39.1   **Encounter for care and examination of lactating mother**   PDx
     Encounter for supervision of lactation
     EXCLUDES 1   *disorders of lactation (O92.-)*
Z39.2   **Encounter for routine postpartum follow-up**   PDx

Encounters for other specific health care (Z40-Z53)

     NOTE   Categories Z40-Z53 are intended for use to indicate a reason for ca They may be used for patients who have already been treated for disease or injury, but who are receiving aftercare or prophylactic care, or care to consolidate the treatment, or to deal with a residu state.
     EXCLUDES 2   *follow-up examination for medical surveillance after treatment (Z08-Z09)*

✓4ᵗʰ **Z40**   **Encounter for prophylactic surgery**
     EXCLUDES 1   *organ donations (Z52.-)*
             therapeutic organ removal—code to condition

✓5ᵗʰ Z40.0   **Encounter for prophylactic surgery for risk factors related ● malignant neoplasms**
     Admission for prophylactic organ removal
     Use additional code to identify risk factor
Z40.00   **Encounter for prophylactic removal of unspecified organ**
Z40.01   **Encounter for prophylactic removal of breast**
Z40.02   **Encounter for prophylactic removal of ovary**
Z40.09   **Encounter for prophylactic removal of other organ**
Z40.8   **Encounter for other prophylactic surgery**
Z40.9   **Encounter for prophylactic surgery, unspecified**

✓4ᵗʰ **Z41**   **Encounter for procedures for purposes other than remedying health state**
Z41.1   **Encounter for cosmetic surgery**
     Encounter for cosmetic breast implant
     Encounter for cosmetic procedure
     EXCLUDES 1   *encounter for plastic and reconstructive surgery following medical procedure or healed injury (Z42.-)*
             encounter for post-mastectomy breast implantation (Z42.1)
Z41.2   **Encounter for routine and ritual male circumcision**
Z41.3   **Encounter for ear piercing**
Z41.8   **Encounter for other procedures for purposes other than remedying health state**
Z41.9   **Encounter for procedure for purposes other than remedying health state, unspecified**

✓4ᵗʰ **Z42**   **Encounter for plastic and reconstructive surgery following medical procedure or healed injury**
     EXCLUDES 1   *encounter for cosmetic plastic surgery (Z41.1)*
             encounter for plastic surgery for treatment of current injury—code to relevent injury
Z42.1   **Encounter for breast reconstruction following mastectomy**   PDx
     EXCLUDES 1   *deformity and disproportion of reconstructed breast (N65.1-)*
Z42.8   **Encounter for other plastic and reconstructive surgery following medical procedure or healed injury**

Z43 Encounter for attention to artificial openings

> **INCLUDES**   closure of artificial openings
> passage of sounds or bougies through artificial openings
> reforming artificial openings
> removal of catheter from artificial openings
> toilet or cleansing of artificial openings
>
> **EXCLUDES 1**   *artificial opening status only, without need for care (Z93.-)*
> *complications of external stoma (J95.0-, K94.-, N99.5-)*
>
> **EXCLUDES 2**   *fitting and adjustment of prosthetic and other devices (Z44-Z46)*

Z43.0   Encounter for attention to tracheostomy

Z43.1   Encounter for attention to gastrostomy

Z43.2   Encounter for attention to ileostomy

Z43.3   Encounter for attention to colostomy

Z43.4   Encounter for attention to other artificial openings of digestive tract

Z43.5   Encounter for attention to cystostomy

Z43.6   Encounter for attention to other artificial openings of urinary tract
> Encounter for attention to nephrostomy
> Encounter for attention to ureterostomy
> Encounter for attention to urethrostomy

Z43.7   Encounter for attention to artificial vagina

Z43.8   Encounter for attention to other artificial openings

Z43.9   Encounter for attention to unspecified artificial opening

Z44 Encounter for fitting and adjustment of external prosthetic device

> **INCLUDES**   removal or replacement of external prosthetic device
>
> **EXCLUDES 1**   *malfunction or other complications of device—see Alphabetical Index*
> *presence of prosthetic device (Z97.-)*

✓5ᵗʰ **Z44.0**   Encounter for fitting and adjustment of artificial arm

   ✓6ᵗʰ **Z44.00**   Encounter for fitting and adjustment of unspecified artificial arm

     Z44.001   Encounter for fitting and adjustment of unspecified right artificial arm

     Z44.002   Encounter for fitting and adjustment of unspecified left artificial arm

     Z44.009   Encounter for fitting and adjustment of unspecified artificial arm, unspecified arm

   ✓6ᵗʰ **Z44.01**   Encounter for fitting and adjustment of complete artificial arm

     Z44.011   Encounter for fitting and adjustment of complete right artificial arm

     Z44.012   Encounter for fitting and adjustment of complete left artificial arm

     Z44.019   Encounter for fitting and adjustment of complete artificial arm, unspecified arm

   ✓6ᵗʰ **Z44.02**   Encounter for fitting and adjustment of partial artificial arm

     Z44.021   Encounter for fitting and adjustment of partial artificial right arm

     Z44.022   Encounter for fitting and adjustment of partial artificial left arm

     Z44.029   Encounter for fitting and adjustment of partial artificial arm, unspecified arm

✓5ᵗʰ **Z44.1**   Encounter for fitting and adjustment of artificial leg

   ✓6ᵗʰ **Z44.10**   Encounter for fitting and adjustment of unspecified artificial leg

     Z44.101   Encounter for fitting and adjustment of unspecified right artificial leg

     Z44.102   Encounter for fitting and adjustment of unspecified left artificial leg

     Z44.109   Encounter for fitting and adjustment of unspecified artificial leg, unspecified leg

   ✓6ᵗʰ **Z44.11**   Encounter for fitting and adjustment of complete artificial leg

     Z44.111   Encounter for fitting and adjustment of complete right artificial leg

     Z44.112   Encounter for fitting and adjustment of complete left artificial leg

     Z44.119   Encounter for fitting and adjustment of complete artificial leg, unspecified leg

   ✓6ᵗʰ **Z44.12**   Encounter for fitting and adjustment of partial artificial leg

     Z44.121   Encounter for fitting and adjustment of partial artificial right leg

Z44.122   Encounter for fitting and adjustment of partial artificial left leg

Z44.129   Encounter for fitting and adjustment of partial artificial leg, unspecified leg

✓5ᵗʰ **Z44.2**   Encounter for fitting and adjustment of artificial eye

> **EXCLUDES 1**   *mechanical complication of ocular prosthesis (T85.3)*

Z44.20   Encounter for fitting and adjustment of artificial eye, unspecified

Z44.21   Encounter for fitting and adjustment of artificial right eye

Z44.22   Encounter for fitting and adjustment of artificial left eye

✓5ᵗʰ **Z44.3**   Encounter for fitting and adjustment of external breast prosthesis

> **EXCLUDES 1**   *complications of breast implant (T85.4-)*
> *encounter for adjustment or removal of breast implant (Z45.81-)*
> *encounter for initial breast implant insertion for cosmetic breast augmentation (Z41.1)*
> *encounter for breast reconstruction following mastectomy (Z42.1)*

Z44.30   Encounter for fitting and adjustment of external breast prosthesis, unspecified breast   ♀

Z44.31   Encounter for fitting and adjustment of external right breast prosthesis   ♀

Z44.32   Encounter for fitting and adjustment of external left breast prosthesis   ♀

Z44.8   Encounter for fitting and adjustment of other external prosthetic devices

Z44.9   Encounter for fitting and adjustment of unspecified external prosthetic device

✓4ᵗʰ **Z45 Encounter for adjustment and management of implanted device**

> **INCLUDES**   removal or replacement of implanted device
>
> **EXCLUDES 1**   *malfunction or other complications of device—see Alphabetical Index*
> *presence of prosthetic and other devices (Z95-Z97)*
>
> **EXCLUDES 2**   *encounter for fitting and adjustment of non-implanted device (Z46.-)*

✓5ᵗʰ **Z45.0**   Encounter for adjustment and management of cardiac device

   ✓6ᵗʰ **Z45.01**   Encounter for adjustment and management of cardiac pacemaker

> **EXCLUDES 1**   *encounter for adjustment and management of automatic implantable cardiac defibrillator with synchronous cardiac pacemaker (Z45.02)*

     Z45.010   Encounter for checking and testing of cardiac pacemaker pulse generator [battery]
> Encounter for replacing cardiac pacemaker pulse generator [battery]

     Z45.018   Encounter for adjustment and management of other part of cardiac pacemaker

   Z45.02   Encounter for adjustment and management of automatic implantable cardiac defibrillator
> Encounter for adjustment and management of automatic implantable cardiac defibrillator with synchronous cardiac pacemaker

   Z45.09   Encounter for adjustment and management of other cardiac device

Z45.1   Encounter for adjustment and management of infusion pump

Z45.2   Encounter for adjustment and management of vascular access device
> Encounter for adjustment and management of vascular catheters
>
> **EXCLUDES 1**   *encounter for adjustment and management of renal dialysis catheter (Z49.01)*

✓5ᵗʰ **Z45.3**   Encounter for adjustment and management of implanted devices of the special senses

Z45.31   Encounter for adjustment and management of implanted visual substitution device

   ✓6ᵗʰ **Z45.32**   Encounter for adjustment and management of implanted hearing device

> **EXCLUDES 1**   *Encounter for fitting and adjustment of hearing aide (Z46.1)*

     Z45.320   Encounter for adjustment and management of bone conduction device

     Z45.321   Encounter for adjustment and management of cochlear device

---

Additional Character Required   ✓x7ᵗʰ Placeholder Alert   Unspecified Dx   Other Specified Dx   Manifestation   ▶◀ Revised Text   ● New Code   ▲ Revised Code Title

Chapter 21. Factors Influencing Health Status and Contact with Health Services

Z45.328–Z48.Ø1

Z45.328 **Encounter for adjustment and management of other implanted hearing device**

✓5th **Z45.4** **Encounter for adjustment and management of implanted nervous system device**

Z45.41 **Encounter for adjustment and management of cerebrospinal fluid drainage device**
Encounter for adjustment and management of cerebral ventricular (communicating) shunt

Z45.42 **Encounter for adjustment and management of neuropacemaker (brain) (peripheral nerve) (spinal cord)**

Z45.49 **Encounter for adjustment and management of other implanted nervous system device**
AHA: 2014, 3Q, 19

✓5th **Z45.8** **Encounter for adjustment and management of other implanted devices**

✓6th **Z45.81** **Encounter for adjustment or removal of breast implant**
Encounter for elective implant exchange (different material) (different size)
Encounter removal of tissue expander without synchronous insertion of permanent implant
EXCLUDES 1 complications of breast implant (T85.4-)
encounter for initial breast implant insertion for cosmetic breast augmentation (Z41.1)
encounter for breast reconstruction following mastectomy (Z42.1)

Z45.811 **Encounter for adjustment or removal of ♀ right breast implant**

Z45.812 **Encounter for adjustment or removal of ♀ left breast implant**

Z45.819 **Encounter for adjustment or removal of ♀ unspecified breast implant**

Z45.82 **Encounter for adjustment or removal of myringotomy device (stent) (tube)**

Z45.89 **Encounter for adjustment and management of other implanted devices**
AHA: 2014, 4Q, 26-28

Z45.9 **Encounter for adjustment and management of unspecified implanted device**

✓4th **Z46** **Encounter for fitting and adjustment of other devices**
INCLUDES removal or replacement of other device
EXCLUDES 1 malfunction or other complications of device—see Alphabetical Index
EXCLUDES 2 encounter for fitting and management of implanted devices (Z45.-)
issue of repeat prescription only (Z76.Ø)
presence of prosthetic and other devices (Z95-Z97)

Z46.Ø **Encounter for fitting and adjustment of spectacles and contact lenses**

Z46.1 **Encounter for fitting and adjustment of hearing aid**
EXCLUDES 1 encounter for adjustment and management of implanted hearing device (Z45.32-)

Z46.2 **Encounter for fitting and adjustment of other devices related to nervous system and special senses**
EXCLUDES 2 encounter for adjustment and management of implanted nervous system device (Z45.4-)
encounter for adjustment and management of implanted visual substitution device (Z45.31)

Z46.3 **Encounter for fitting and adjustment of dental prosthetic device**
Encounter for fitting and adjustment of dentures

Z46.4 **Encounter for fitting and adjustment of orthodontic device**

✓5th **Z46.5** **Encounter for fitting and adjustment of other gastrointestinal appliance and device**
EXCLUDES 1 encounter for attention to artificial openings of digestive tract (Z43.1-Z43.4)

Z46.51 **Encounter for fitting and adjustment of gastric lap band**

Z46.59 **Encounter for fitting and adjustment of other gastrointestinal appliance and device**

Z46.6 **Encounter for fitting and adjustment of urinary device**
EXCLUDES 2 attention to artificial openings of urinary tract (Z43.5, Z43.6)

✓5th **Z46.8** **Encounter for fitting and adjustment of other specified devices**

Z46.81 **Encounter for fitting and adjustment of insulin pump**
Encounter for insulin pump instruction and training
Encounter for insulin pump titration

Z46.82 **Encounter for fitting and adjustment of non-vascular catheter**

Z46.89 **Encounter for fitting and adjustment of other specified devices**
Encounter for fitting and adjustment of wheelchair

Z46.9 **Encounter for fitting and adjustment of unspecified device**

✓4th **Z47** **Orthopedic aftercare**
EXCLUDES 1 aftercare for healing fracture—code to fracture with 7th character D

Z47.1 **Aftercare following joint replacement surgery**
Use additional code to identify the joint (Z96.6-)

Z47.2 **Encounter for removal of internal fixation device**
EXCLUDES 1 encounter for adjustment of internal fixation device fracture treatment—code to fracture with appropriate 7th character
encounter for removal of external fixation device—code to fracture with 7th character D
infection or inflammatory reaction to internal fixation device (T84.6-)
mechanical complication of internal fixation device (T84.1-)

✓5th **Z47.3** **Aftercare following explantation of joint prosthesis**
Aftercare following explantation of joint prosthesis, staged procedure
Encounter for joint prosthesis insertion following prior explantation of joint prosthesis
AHA: 2015, 1Q, 16

Z47.31 **Aftercare following explantation of shoulder joint prosthesis**
EXCLUDES 1 acquired absence of shoulder joint following prior explantation of shoulder joint prosthesis (Z89.23-)
shoulder joint prosthesis explantation status (Z89.23-)

Z47.32 **Aftercare following explantation of hip joint prosthesis**
EXCLUDES 1 acquired absence of hip joint following prior explantation of hip joint prosthesis (Z89.62-)
hip joint prosthesis explantation status (Z89.62-)

Z47.33 **Aftercare following explantation of knee joint prosthesis**
EXCLUDES 1 acquired absence of knee joint following prior explantation of knee prosthesis (Z89.52-)
knee joint prosthesis explantation status (Z89.52-)

✓5th **Z47.8** **Encounter for other orthopedic aftercare**

Z47.81 **Encounter for orthopedic aftercare following surgical amputation**
Use additional code to identify the limb amputated (Z89.-)

Z47.82 **Encounter for orthopedic aftercare following scoliosis surgery**

Z47.89 **Encounter for other orthopedic aftercare**
AHA: 2015, 1Q, 8

✓4th **Z48** **Encounter for other postprocedural aftercare**
EXCLUDES 1 encounter for follow-up examination after completed treatment (ZØ8-ZØ9)
EXCLUDES 2 encounter for attention to artificial openings (Z43.-)
encounter for fitting and adjustment of prosthetic and other devices (Z44-Z46)
AHA: 2015, 1Q, 6-7

✓5th **Z48.Ø** **Encounter for attention to dressings, sutures and drains**
EXCLUDES 1 encounter for planned postprocedural wound closure (Z48.1)

Z48.ØØ **Encounter for change or removal of nonsurgical wound dressing**
Encounter for change or removal of wound dressing NOS

Z48.Ø1 **Encounter for change or removal of surgical wound dressing**

EXCLUDES 1 Not coded here   EXCLUDES 2 Not included here   N Newborn Age: Ø   P Pediatric Age: Ø-17   M Maternity Age: 12-55   A Adult Age: 15-124   PDx Primary

1118   ICD-10-CM 2Ø

Z48.02   **Encounter for removal of** sutures
     Encounter for removal of staples

Z48.03   **Encounter for change or removal of** drains

Z48.1   **Encounter for planned** postprocedural **wound closure**
     EXCLUDES 1   *encounter for attention to dressings and sutures (Z48.0-)*

✓5th **Z48.2**   **Encounter for aftercare following** organ transplant

   Z48.21   **Encounter for aftercare following** heart **transplant**

   Z48.22   **Encounter for aftercare following** kidney **transplant**

   Z48.23   **Encounter for aftercare following** liver **transplant**

   Z48.24   **Encounter for aftercare following** lung **transplant**

   ✓6th **Z48.28**   **Encounter for aftercare following** multiple **organ transplant**

     Z48.280   **Encounter for aftercare following heart-lung transplant**

     Z48.288   **Encounter for aftercare following** multiple **organ transplant**

   ✓6th **Z48.29**   **Encounter for aftercare following** other **organ transplant**

     Z48.290   **Encounter for aftercare following** bone marrow **transplant**

     Z48.298   **Encounter for aftercare following other organ transplant**

Z48.3   **Aftercare following** surgery for neoplasm
     Use additional code to identify the neoplasm

✓5th **Z48.8**   **Encounter for other specified postprocedural aftercare**

   ✓6th **Z48.81**   **Encounter for surgical aftercare following** surgery on specified body systems

     NOTE   These codes identify the body system requiring aftercare. They are for use in conjunction with other aftercare codes to fully explain the aftercare encounter. The condition treated should also be coded if still present.

     EXCLUDES 1   *aftercare for injury—code the injury with 7th character D*
         aftercare following surgery for neoplasm (Z48.3)

     EXCLUDES 2   *aftercare following organ transplant (Z48.2-) orthopedic aftercare (Z47.-)*

     Z48.810   **Encounter for surgical aftercare following surgery on the** sense organs

     Z48.811   **Encounter for surgical aftercare following surgery on the** nervous system
         EXCLUDES 2   *encounter for surgical aftercare following surgery on the sense organs (Z48.810)*

     Z48.812   **Encounter for surgical aftercare following surgery on the** circulatory system
         AHA: 2012, 4Q, 96

     Z48.813   **Encounter for surgical aftercare following surgery on the** respiratory system

     Z48.814   **Encounter for surgical aftercare following surgery on the** teeth or oral cavity

     Z48.815   **Encounter for surgical aftercare following surgery on the** digestive system

     Z48.816   **Encounter for surgical aftercare following surgery on the** genitourinary system
         EXCLUDES 1   *encounter for aftercare following sterilization reversal (Z31.42)*

     Z48.817   **Encounter for surgical aftercare following surgery on the** skin and subcutaneous tissue

   Z48.89   **Encounter for other specified surgical aftercare**

■ **Z49**   **Encounter for care involving renal dialysis**
     Code also associated end stage renal disease (N18.6)

✓5th **Z49.0**   Preparatory care **for renal dialysis**
     Encounter for dialysis instruction and training

   Z49.01   **Encounter for fitting and adjustment of** extracorporeal dialysis catheter
     Removal or replacement of renal dialysis catheter
     Toilet or cleansing of renal dialysis catheter

   Z49.02   **Encounter for fitting and adjustment of** peritoneal dialysis catheter

✓5th **Z49.3**   **Encounter for** adequacy testing for dialysis

   Z49.31   **Encounter for adequacy testing for** hemodialysis

   Z49.32   **Encounter for adequacy testing for** peritoneal dialysis
     Encounter for peritoneal equilibration test

✓4th **Z51**   **Encounter for other aftercare**
     Code also condition requiring care
     EXCLUDES 1   *follow-up examination after treatment (Z08-Z09)*

   Z51.0   **Encounter for antineoplastic** radiation therapy   PDx

   ✓5th **Z51.1**   **Encounter for antineoplastic chemotherapy and immunotherapy**
     EXCLUDES 2   *encounter for chemotherapy and immunotherapy for nonneoplastic condition—code to condition*

     Z51.11   **Encounter for antineoplastic** chemotherapy   PDx

     Z51.12   **Encounter for antineoplastic** immunotherapy   PDx

   Z51.5   **Encounter for** palliative care

   ✓5th **Z51.8**   **Encounter for** other specified aftercare
     EXCLUDES 1   *holiday relief care (Z75.5)*

     Z51.81   **Encounter for** therapeutic drug level **monitoring**
     Code also any long-term (current) drug therapy (Z79.-)
         EXCLUDES 1   *encounter for blood-drug test for administrative or medicolegal reasons (Z02.83)*

     Z51.89   **Encounter for other specified aftercare**
     AHA: 2012, 4Q, 95-97

✓4th **Z52**   **Donors of organs and tissues**
     INCLUDES   autologous and other living donors
     EXCLUDES 1   *cadaveric donor—omit code examination of potential donor (Z00.5)*
     AHA: 2012, 4Q, 99

   ✓5th **Z52.0**   Blood donor

     ✓6th **Z52.00**   Unspecified **blood donor**

       Z52.000   **Unspecified donor,** whole **blood**   PDx

       Z52.001   **Unspecified donor,** stem cells   PDx

       Z52.008   **Unspecified donor, other blood**   PDx

     ✓6th **Z52.01**   Autologous **blood donor**

       Z52.010   **Autologous donor,** whole **blood**   PDx

       Z52.011   **Autologous donor,** stem **cells**   PDx

       Z52.018   **Autologous donor, other blood**   PDx

     ✓6th **Z52.09**   Other **blood donor**
       Volunteer donor

       Z52.090   **Other blood donor,** whole **blood**   PDx

       Z52.091   **Other blood donor,** stem **cells**   PDx

       Z52.098   **Other blood donor, other blood**   PDx

   ✓5th **Z52.1**   Skin **donor**

     Z52.10   **Skin donor, unspecified**   PDx

     Z52.11   **Skin donor,** autologous   PDx

     Z52.19   **Skin donor, other**   PDx

   ✓5th **Z52.2**   Bone **donor**

     Z52.20   **Bone donor, unspecified**   PDx

     Z52.21   **Bone donor,** autologous   PDx

     Z52.29   **Bone donor, other**   PDx

   Z52.3   Bone marrow **donor**   PDx

   Z52.4   Kidney **donor**   PDx

   Z52.5   Cornea **donor**   PDx

   Z52.6   Liver **donor**

   ✓5th **Z52.8**   **Donor of** other **specified organs or tissues**

     ✓6th **Z52.81**   Egg (Oocyte) **donor**

       Z52.810   **Egg (Oocyte) donor** under age 35, anonymous **recipient**   PDx M ♀
         Egg donor under age 35 NOS

       Z52.811   **Egg (Oocyte) donor** under age 35, designated **recipient**   PDx M ♀

       Z52.812   **Egg (Oocyte) donor** age 35 and over, anonymous **recipient**   PDx M ♀
         Egg donor age 35 and over NOS

       Z52.813   **Egg (Oocyte) donor** age 35 and over, designated **recipient**   PDx M ♀

       Z52.819   **Egg (Oocyte) donor, unspecified**   PDx M ♀

     Z52.89   **Donor of other specified organs or tissues**   PDx

   Z52.9   **Donor of unspecified organ or tissue**
     Donor NOS

■ Additional Character Required   ✓7th Placeholder Alert   Unspecified Dx   Other Specified Dx   Manifestation   ►◄ Revised Text   ● New Code   ▲ Revised Code Title

D-10-CM 2016   1119

✓4th **Z53 Persons encountering health services for specific procedures and treatment, not carried out**

  ✓5th **Z53.0 Procedure and treatment not carried out because of** contraindication

    Z53.01 Procedure and treatment not carried out due to patient smoking

    Z53.09 Procedure and treatment not carried out because of other contraindication

  Z53.1 Procedure and treatment not carried out because of patient's decision for reasons of belief and group pressure

  ✓5th **Z53.2 Procedure and treatment not carried out because of patient's decision for** other and unspecified reasons

    Z53.20 Procedure and treatment not carried out because of patient's decision for unspecified reasons

    Z53.21 Procedure and treatment not carried out due to patient leaving prior to being seen by health care provider

    Z53.29 Procedure and treatment not carried out because of patient's decision for other reasons

  Z53.8 Procedure and treatment not carried out for other reasons

  Z53.9 Procedure and treatment not carried out, unspecified reason

Persons with potential health hazards related to socioeconomic and psychosocial circumstances (Z55-Z65)

✓4th **Z55 Problems related to education and literacy**
  EXCLUDES 1 disorders of psychological development (F80-F89)

  Z55.0 Illiteracy and low-level literacy

  Z55.1 Schooling unavailable and unattainable

  Z55.2 Failed school examinations

  Z55.3 Underachievement in school

  Z55.4 Educational maladjustment and discord with teachers and classmates

  Z55.8 Other problems related to education and literacy
    Problems related to inadequate teaching

  Z55.9 Problems related to education and literacy, unspecified
    Academic problems NOS

✓4th **Z56 Problems related to employment and unemployment**
  EXCLUDES 2 occupational exposure to risk factors (Z57.-)
    problems related to housing and economic circumstances (Z59.-)

  Z56.0 Unemployment, unspecified

  Z56.1 Change of job   Ⓐ

  Z56.2 Threat of job loss

  Z56.3 Stressful work schedule

  Z56.4 Discord with boss and workmates

  Z56.5 Uncongenial work environment
    Difficult conditions at work

  Z56.6 Other physical and mental strain related to work

  ✓5th **Z56.8 Other problems related to employment**

    Z56.81 Sexual harassment on the job

    Z56.82 Military deployment status   Ⓐ
      Individual (civilian or military) currently deployed in theater or in support of military war, peacekeeping and humanitarian operations

    Z56.89 Other problems related to employment

  Z56.9 Unspecified problems related to employment
    Occupational problems NOS

✓4th **Z57 Occupational exposure to risk factors**

  Z57.0 Occupational exposure to noise

  Z57.1 Occupational exposure to radiation

  Z57.2 Occupational exposure to dust

  ✓5th **Z57.3 Occupational exposure to** other air contaminants

    Z57.31 Occupational exposure to environmental tobacco smoke
      EXCLUDES 2 exposure to environmental tobacco smoke (Z77.22)

    Z57.39 Occupational exposure to other air contaminants

  Z57.4 Occupational exposure to toxic agents in agriculture
    Occupational exposure to solids, liquids, gases or vapors in agriculture

  Z57.5 Occupational exposure to toxic agents in other industries
    Occupational exposure to solids, liquids, gases or vapors in other industries

  Z57.6 Occupational exposure to extreme temperature

  Z57.7 Occupational exposure to vibration

  Z57.8 Occupational exposure to other risk factors

  Z57.9 Occupational exposure to unspecified risk factor

✓4th **Z59 Problems related to housing and economic circumstances**
  EXCLUDES 2 problems related to upbringing (Z62.-)

  Z59.0 Homelessness

  Z59.1 Inadequate housing
    Lack of heating
    Restriction of space
    Technical defects in home preventing adequate care
    Unsatisfactory surroundings
    EXCLUDES 1 problems related to the natural and physical environment (Z77.1-)

  Z59.2 Discord with neighbors, lodgers and landlord

  Z59.3 Problems related to living in residential institution
    Boarding-school resident
    EXCLUDES 1 institutional upbringing (Z62.2)

  Z59.4 Lack of adequate food and safe drinking water
    Inadequate drinking water supply
    EXCLUDES 1 effects of hunger (T73.0)
      inappropriate diet or eating habits (Z72.4)
      malnutrition (E40-E46)

  Z59.5 Extreme poverty

  Z59.6 Low income

  Z59.7 Insufficient social insurance and welfare support

  Z59.8 Other problems related to housing and economic circumstances
    Foreclosure on loan
    Isolated dwelling
    Problems with creditors

  Z59.9 Problem related to housing and economic circumstances, unspecified

✓4th **Z60 Problems related to social environment**

  Z60.0 Problems of adjustment to life-cycle transitions
    Empty nest syndrome
    Phase of life problem
    Problem with adjustment to retirement [pension]

  Z60.2 Problems related to living alone

  Z60.3 Acculturation difficulty
    Problem with migration
    Problem with social transplantation

  Z60.4 Social exclusion and rejection
    Exclusion and rejection on the basis of personal characteristics such as unusual physical appearance, illness or behavior.
    EXCLUDES 1 target of adverse discrimination such as for racial or religious reasons (Z60.5)

  Z60.5 Target of (perceived) adverse discrimination and persecution
    EXCLUDES 1 social exclusion and rejection (Z60.4)

  Z60.8 Other problems related to social environment

  Z60.9 Problem related to social environment, unspecified

✓4th **Z62 Problems related to upbringing**
  Current and past negative life events in childhood
  Current and past problems of a child related to upbringing
  EXCLUDES 2 maltreatment syndrome (T74.-)
    problems related to housing and economic circumstances (Z59.-)

  Z62.0 Inadequate parental supervision and control

  Z62.1 Parental overprotection

  ✓5th **Z62.2 Upbringing away from parents**
    EXCLUDES 1 problems with boarding school (Z59.3)

    Z62.21 Child in welfare custody
      Child in care of non-parental family member
      Child in foster care
      EXCLUDES 2 problem for parent due to child in welfare custody (Z63.5)

    Z62.22 Institutional upbringing
      Child living in orphanage or group home

    Z62.29 Other upbringing away from parents

  Z62.3 Hostility towards and scapegoating of child

  Z62.6 Inappropriate (excessive) parental pressure

☑5ᵗʰ Z62.8   Other specified problems related to upbringing

   ☑6ᵗʰ Z62.81   Personal history of abuse in childhood

     Z62.810   Personal history of physical and sexual abuse in childhood
       EXCLUDES 1   current child physical abuse (T74.12, T76.12)
             current child sexual abuse (T74.22, T76.22)

     Z62.811   Personal history of psychological abuse in childhood
       EXCLUDES 1   current child psychological abuse (T74.32, T76.32)

     Z62.812   Personal history of neglect in childhood
       EXCLUDES 1   current child neglect (T74.02, T76.02)

     Z62.819   Personal history of unspecified abuse in childhood
       EXCLUDES 1   current child abuse NOS (T74.92, T76.92)

   ☑6ᵗʰ Z62.82   Parent-child conflict

     Z62.820   Parent-biological child conflict
       Parent-child problem NOS

     Z62.821   Parent-adopted child conflict

     Z62.822   Parent-foster child conflict

   ☑6ᵗʰ Z62.89   Other specified problems related to upbringing

     Z62.890   Parent-child estrangement NEC

     Z62.891   Sibling rivalry

     Z62.898   Other specified problems related to upbringing

   Z62.9   Problem related to upbringing, unspecified

Z63   Other problems related to primary support group, including family circumstances
   EXCLUDES 2   maltreatment syndrome (T74-, T76)
       parent-child problems (Z62.-)
       problems related to negative life events in childhood (Z62.-)
       problems related to upbringing (Z62.-)

   Z63.0   Problems in relationship with spouse or partner
     EXCLUDES 1   counseling for spousal or partner abuse problems (Z69.1)
         counseling related to sexual attitude, behavior, and orientation (Z70.-)

   Z63.1   Problems in relationship with in-laws

   ☑5ᵗʰ Z63.3   Absence of family member
     EXCLUDES 1   absence of family member due to disappearance and death (Z63.4)
         absence of family member due to separation and divorce (Z63.5)

     Z63.31   Absence of family member due to military deployment
       Individual or family affected by other family member being on military deployment
       EXCLUDES 1   family disruption due to return of family member from military deployment (Z63.71)

     Z63.32   Other absence of family member

   Z63.4   Disappearance and death of family member
     Assumed death of family member
     Bereavement
     AHA: 2014, 1Q, 25

   Z63.5   Disruption of family by separation and divorce
     Marital estrangement

   Z63.6   Dependent relative needing care at home

   ☑5ᵗʰ Z63.7   Other stressful life events affecting family and household

     Z63.71   Stress on family due to return of family member from military deployment
       Individual or family affected by family member having returned from military deployment (current or past conflict)

     Z63.72   Alcoholism and drug addiction in family

     Z63.79   Other stressful life events affecting family and household
       Anxiety (normal) about sick person in family
       Health problems within family
       Ill or disturbed family member
       Isolated family

   Z63.8   Other specified problems related to primary support group
     Family discord NOS
     Family estrangement NOS
     High expressed emotional level within family
     Inadequate family support NOS
     Inadequate or distorted communication within family

   Z63.9   Problem related to primary support group, unspecified
     Relationship disorder NOS

☑4ᵗʰ Z64   Problems related to certain psychosocial circumstances

   Z64.0   Problems related to unwanted pregnancy   M♀

   Z64.1   Problems related to multiparity   ♀

   Z64.4   Discord with counselors
     Discord with probation officer
     Discord with social worker

☑4ᵗʰ Z65   Problems related to other psychosocial circumstances

   Z65.0   Conviction in civil and criminal proceedings without imprisonment

   Z65.1   Imprisonment and other incarceration

   Z65.2   Problems related to release from prison

   Z65.3   Problems related to other legal circumstances
     Arrest
     Child custody or support proceedings
     Litigation
     Prosecution

   Z65.4   Victim of crime and terrorism
     Victim of torture

   Z65.5   Exposure to disaster, war and other hostilities   ▲
     EXCLUDES 1   target of perceived discrimination or persecution (Z60.5)

   Z65.8   Other specified problems related to psychosocial circumstances

   Z65.9   Problem related to unspecified psychosocial circumstances

Do not resuscitate status (Z66)

Z66   Do not resuscitate
   DNR status

Blood type (Z67)

☑4ᵗʰ Z67   Blood type

   ☑5ᵗʰ Z67.1   Type A blood
     Z67.10   Type A blood, Rh positive
     Z67.11   Type A blood, Rh negative

   ☑5ᵗʰ Z67.2   Type B blood
     Z67.20   Type B blood, Rh positive
     Z67.21   Type B blood, Rh negative

   ☑5ᵗʰ Z67.3   Type AB blood
     Z67.30   Type AB blood, Rh positive
     Z67.31   Type AB blood, Rh negative

   ☑5ᵗʰ Z67.4   Type O blood
     Z67.40   Type O blood, Rh positive
     Z67.41   Type O blood, Rh negative

   ☑5ᵗʰ Z67.9   Unspecified blood type
     Z67.90   Unspecified blood type, Rh positive
     Z67.91   Unspecified blood type, Rh negative

Body mass index [BMI] (Z68)

☑4ᵗʰ Z68   Body mass index [BMI]
   Kilograms per meters squared
   NOTE   BMI adult codes are for use for persons 21 years of age or older.
     BMI pediatric codes are for use for persons 2-20 years of age. These percentiles are based on the growth charts published by the Centers for Disease Control and Prevention (CDC).

   Z68.1   Body mass index [BMI] 19 or less, adult   ▲

   ☑5ᵗʰ Z68.2   Body mass index [BMI] 20-29, adult
     Z68.20   Body mass index [BMI] 20.0-20.9, adult   ▲
     Z68.21   Body mass index [BMI] 21.0-21.9, adult   ▲
     Z68.22   Body mass index [BMI] 22.0-22.9, adult   ▲
     Z68.23   Body mass index [BMI] 23.0-23.9, adult   ▲
     Z68.24   Body mass index [BMI] 24.0-24.9, adult   ▲
     Z68.25   Body mass index [BMI] 25.0-25.9, adult   ▲
     Z68.26   Body mass index [BMI] 26.0-26.9, adult   ▲
     Z68.27   Body mass index [BMI] 27.0-27.9, adult   ▲

Additional Character Required   **✓x7ᵗʰ** Placeholder Alert   Unspecified Dx   Other Specified Dx   Manifestation   ▶◀ Revised Text   ● New Code   ▲ Revised Code Title

Z68.28   Body mass index [BMI] 28.0-28.9, adult   Ⓐ
Z68.29   Body mass index [BMI] 29.0-29.9, adult   Ⓐ

√5ᵗʰ **Z68.3**   **Body mass index [BMI] 30-39, adult**

Z68.30   Body mass index [BMI] 30.0-30.9, adult   Ⓐ
Z68.31   Body mass index [BMI] 31.0-31.9, adult   Ⓐ
Z68.32   Body mass index [BMI] 32.0-32.9, adult   Ⓐ
Z68.33   Body mass index [BMI] 33.0-33.9, adult   Ⓐ
Z68.34   Body mass index [BMI] 34.0-34.9, adult   Ⓐ
Z68.35   Body mass index [BMI] 35.0-35.9, adult   Ⓐ
Z68.36   Body mass index [BMI] 36.0-36.9, adult   Ⓐ
Z68.37   Body mass index [BMI] 37.0-37.9, adult   Ⓐ
Z68.38   Body mass index [BMI] 38.0-38.9, adult   Ⓐ
Z68.39   Body mass index [BMI] 39.0-39.9, adult   Ⓐ

√5ᵗʰ **Z68.4**   **Body mass index [BMI] 40 or greater, adult**

Z68.41   Body mass index [BMI] 40.0-44.9, adult   Ⓐ
Z68.42   Body mass index [BMI] 45.0-49.9, adult   Ⓐ
Z68.43   Body mass index [BMI] 50-59.9, adult   Ⓐ
Z68.44   Body mass index [BMI] 60.0-69.9, adult   Ⓐ
Z68.45   Body mass index [BMI] 70 or greater, adult   Ⓐ

√5ᵗʰ **Z68.5**   **Body mass index [BMI] pediatric**

Z68.51   Body mass index [BMI] pediatric, less than 5th percentile for age   Ⓟ
Z68.52   Body mass index [BMI] pediatric, 5th percentile to less than 85th percentile for age   Ⓟ
Z68.53   Body mass index [BMI] pediatric, 85th percentile to less than 95th percentile for age   Ⓟ
Z68.54   Body mass index [BMI] pediatric, greater than or equal to 95th percentile for age   Ⓟ

Persons encountering health services in other circumstances (Z69-Z76)

√4ᵗʰ **Z69**   **Encounter for mental health services for victim and perpetrator of abuse**
Counseling for victims and perpetrators of abuse

√5ᵗʰ **Z69.0**   **Encounter for mental health services for child abuse problems**

√6ᵗʰ **Z69.01**   **Encounter for mental health services for parental child abuse**

Z69.010   Encounter for mental health services for victim of parental child abuse   Ⓟ
Z69.011   Encounter for mental health services for perpetrator of parental child abuse
> EXCLUDES 1   encounter for mental health services for non-parental child abuse (Z69.02-)

√6ᵗʰ **Z69.02**   **Encounter for mental health services for non-parental child abuse**

Z69.020   Encounter for mental health services for victim of non-parental child abuse   Ⓟ
Z69.021   Encounter for mental health services for perpetrator of non-parental child abuse

√5ᵗʰ **Z69.1**   **Encounter for mental health services for spousal or partner abuse problems**

Z69.11   Encounter for mental health services for victim of spousal or partner abuse
Z69.12   Encounter for mental health services for perpetrator of spousal or partner abuse

√5ᵗʰ **Z69.8**   **Encounter for mental health services for victim or perpetrator of other abuse**

Z69.81   Encounter for mental health services for victim of other abuse
Encounter for rape victim counseling
Z69.82   Encounter for mental health services for perpetrator of other abuse

√4ᵗʰ **Z70**   **Counseling related to sexual attitude, behavior and orientation**
Encounter for mental health services for sexual attitude, behavior and orientation
> EXCLUDES 2   contraceptive or procreative counseling (Z30-Z31)

Z70.0   **Counseling related to sexual attitude**

Z70.1   **Counseling related to patient's sexual behavior and orientation**
Patient concerned regarding impotence
Patient concerned regarding non-responsiveness
Patient concerned regarding promiscuity
Patient concerned regarding sexual orientation

Z70.2   **Counseling related to sexual behavior and orientation of third party**
Advice sought regarding sexual behavior and orientation of child
Advice sought regarding sexual behavior and orientation of partner
Advice sought regarding sexual behavior and orientation of spouse

Z70.3   **Counseling related to combined concerns regarding sexual attitude, behavior and orientation**

Z70.8   **Other sex counseling**
Encounter for sex education

Z70.9   **Sex counseling, unspecified**

√4ᵗʰ **Z71**   **Persons encountering health services for other counseling and medical advice, not elsewhere classified**
> EXCLUDES 2   contraceptive or procreation counseling (Z30-Z31)
>   sex counseling (Z70.-)

Z71.0   **Person encountering health services to consult on behalf of another person**
Person encountering health services to seek advice or treatment for non-attending third party
> EXCLUDES 2   anxiety (normal) about sick person in family (Z63.7)
>   expectant (adoptive) parent(s) pre-birth pediatrician visit (Z76.81)

Z71.1   **Person with feared health complaint in whom no diagnosis made**
Person encountering health services with feared condition which was not demonstrated
Person encountering health services in which problem was normal state
"Worried well"
> EXCLUDES 1   medical observation for suspected diseases and conditions proven not to exist (Z03.-)

Z71.2   **Person consulting for explanation of examination or test findings**

Z71.3   **Dietary counseling and surveillance**
Use additional code for any associated underlying medical condition
Use additional code to identify body mass index (BMI), if known (Z68.-)

√5ᵗʰ **Z71.4**   **Alcohol abuse counseling and surveillance**
Use additional code for alcohol abuse or dependence (F10.-)

Z71.41   Alcohol abuse counseling and surveillance of alcoholic
Z71.42   Counseling for family member of alcoholic
Counseling for significant other, partner, or friend of alcoholic

√5ᵗʰ **Z71.5**   **Drug abuse counseling and surveillance**
Use additional code for drug abuse or dependence (F11-F16, F18-F19)

Z71.51   Drug abuse counseling and surveillance of drug abuser
Z71.52   Counseling for family member of drug abuser
Counseling for significant other, partner, or friend of drug abuser

Z71.6   **Tobacco abuse counseling**
Use additional code for nicotine dependence (F17.-)

Z71.7   **Human immunodeficiency virus [HIV] counseling**

√5ᵗʰ **Z71.8**   **Other specified counseling**
> EXCLUDES 2   counseling for contraception (Z30.0-)
>   counseling for genetics (Z31.5)
>   counseling for procreative management (Z31.6-)

Z71.81   Spiritual or religious counseling
Z71.89   Other specified counseling

Z71.9   **Counseling, unspecified**
Encounter for medical advice NOS

Z72 Problems related to lifestyle
> EXCLUDES 2   problems related to life-management difficulty (Z73.-)
> problems related to socioeconomic and psychosocial circumstances (Z55-Z65)

Z72.0 Tobacco use
Tobacco use NOS
> EXCLUDES 1   history of tobacco dependence (Z87.891)
> nicotine dependence (F17.2-)
> tobacco dependence (F17.2-)
> tobacco use during pregnancy (O99.33-)

Z72.3 Lack of physical exercise

Z72.4 Inappropriate diet and eating habits
> EXCLUDES 1   behavioral eating disorders of infancy or childhood (F98.2- F98.3)
> eating disorders (F50.-)
> lack of adequate food (Z59.4)
> malnutrition and other nutritional deficiencies (E40-E64)

Z72.5 High risk sexual behavior
Promiscuity
> EXCLUDES 1   paraphilias (F65)

Z72.51 High risk heterosexual behavior

Z72.52 High risk homosexual behavior

Z72.53 High risk bisexual behavior

Z72.6 Gambling and betting
> EXCLUDES 1   compulsive or pathological gambling (F63.0)

Z72.8 Other problems related to lifestyle

Z72.81 Antisocial behavior
> EXCLUDES 1   conduct disorders (F91.-)

Z72.810 Child and adolescent antisocial behavior   P
Antisocial behavior (child) (adolescent) without manifest psychiatric disorder
Delinquency NOS
Group delinquency
Offenses in the context of gang membership
Stealing in company with others
Truancy from school

Z72.811 Adult antisocial behavior   A
Adult antisocial behavior without manifest psychiatric disorder

Z72.82 Problems related to sleep

Z72.820 Sleep deprivation
Lack of adequate sleep
> EXCLUDES 1   insomnia (G47.0-)

Z72.821 Inadequate sleep hygiene
Bad sleep habits
Irregular sleep habits
Unhealthy sleep wake schedule
> EXCLUDES 1   insomnia (F51.0-, G47.0-)

Z72.89 Other problems related to lifestyle
Self-damaging behavior

Z72.9 Problem related to lifestyle, unspecified

Z73 Problems related to life management difficulty
> EXCLUDES 2   problems related to socioeconomic and psychosocial circumstances (Z55-Z65)

Z73.0 Burn-out

Z73.1 Type A behavior pattern

Z73.2 Lack of relaxation and leisure

Z73.3 Stress, not elsewhere classified
Physical and mental strain NOS
> EXCLUDES 1   stress related to employment or unemployment (Z56.-)

Z73.4 Inadequate social skills, not elsewhere classified

Z73.5 Social role conflict, not elsewhere classified

Z73.6 Limitation of activities due to disability
> EXCLUDES 1   care-provider dependency (Z74.-)

Z73.8 Other problems related to life management difficulty

Z73.81 Behavioral insomnia of childhood

Z73.810 Behavioral insomnia of childhood, sleep-onset association type   P

Z73.811 Behavioral insomnia of childhood, limit setting type   P

Z73.812 Behavioral insomnia of childhood, combined type   P

Z73.819 Behavioral insomnia of childhood, unspecified type   P

Z73.82 Dual sensory impairment

Z73.89 Other problems related to life management difficulty

Z73.9 Problem related to life management difficulty, unspecified

Z74 Problems related to care provider dependency
> EXCLUDES 2   dependence on enabling machines or devices NEC (Z99.-)

Z74.0 Reduced mobility

Z74.01 Bed confinement status
Bedridden

Z74.09 Other reduced mobility
Chair ridden
Reduced mobility NOS
> EXCLUDES 2   wheelchair dependence (Z99.3)

Z74.1 Need for assistance with personal care

Z74.2 Need for assistance at home and no other household member able to render care

Z74.3 Need for continuous supervision

Z74.8 Other problems related to care provider dependency

Z74.9 Problem related to care provider dependency, unspecified

Z75 Problems related to medical facilities and other health care

Z75.0 Medical services not available in home
> EXCLUDES 1   no other household member able to render care (Z74.2)

Z75.1 Person awaiting admission to adequate facility elsewhere

Z75.2 Other waiting period for investigation and treatment

Z75.3 Unavailability and inaccessibility of health-care facilities
> EXCLUDES 1   bed unavailable (Z75.1)

Z75.4 Unavailability and inaccessibility of other helping agencies

Z75.5 Holiday relief care

Z75.8 Other problems related to medical facilities and other health care

Z75.9 Unspecified problem related to medical facilities and other health care

Z76 Persons encountering health services in other circumstances

Z76.0 Encounter for issue of repeat prescription
Encounter for issue of repeat prescription for appliance
Encounter for issue of repeat prescription for medicaments
Encounter for issue of repeat prescription for spectacles
> EXCLUDES 2   issue of medical certificate (Z02.7)
> repeat prescription for contraceptive (Z30.4-)

Z76.1 Encounter for health supervision and care of foundling   PDx

Z76.2 Encounter for health supervision and care of other healthy infant and child   PDx P
Encounter for medical or nursing care or supervision of healthy infant under circumstances such as adverse socioeconomic conditions at home
Encounter for medical or nursing care or supervision of healthy infant under circumstances such as awaiting foster or adoptive placement
Encounter for medical or nursing care or supervision of healthy infant under circumstances such as maternal illness
Encounter for medical or nursing care or supervision of healthy infant under circumstances such as number of children at home preventing or interfering with normal care

Z76.3 Healthy person accompanying sick person

Z76.4 Other boarder to healthcare facility
> EXCLUDES 1   homelessness (Z59.0)

Z76.5 Malingerer [conscious simulation]
Person feigning illness (with obvious motivation)
> EXCLUDES 1   factitious disorder (F68.1-)
> peregrinating patient (F68.1-)

Z76.8 Persons encountering health services in other specified circumstances

Z76.81 Expectant parent(s) prebirth pediatrician visit
Pre-adoption pediatrician visit for adoptive parent(s)

Z76.82 Awaiting organ transplant status
Patient waiting for organ availability

Z76.89 Persons encountering health services in other specified circumstances
Persons encountering health services NOS
AHA: 2014, 2Q, 10

☑ Additional Character Required   Placeholder Alert   Unspecified Dx   Other Specified Dx   Manifestation   ▶◀ Revised Text   ● New Code   ▲ Revised Code Title

Persons with potential health hazards related to family and personal history and certain conditions influencing health status (Z77-Z99)

Code also any follow-up examination (Z08-Z09)

☑4ᵗʰ Z77 Other contact with and (suspected) exposures hazardous to health

INCLUDES contact with and (suspected) exposures to potential hazards to health

EXCLUDES 2 contact with and (suspected) exposure to communicable diseases (Z20.-)
exposure to (parental) (environmental) tobacco smoke in the perinatal period (P96.81)
newborn (suspected to be) affected by noxious substances transmitted via placenta or breast milk (P04.-)
occupational exposure to risk factors (Z57.-)
retained foreign body (Z18.-)
retained foreign body fully removed (Z87.821)
toxic effects of substances chiefly nonmedicinal as to source (T51-T65)

☑5ᵗʰ Z77.0 Contact with and (suspected) exposure to hazardous, chiefly nonmedicinal, chemicals

☑6ᵗʰ Z77.01 Contact with and (suspected) exposure to hazardous metals

Z77.010 Contact with and (suspected) exposure to arsenic

Z77.011 Contact with and (suspected) exposure to lead

Z77.012 Contact with and (suspected) exposure to uranium

EXCLUDES 1 retained depleted uranium fragments (Z18.01)

Z77.018 Contact with and (suspected) exposure to other hazardous metals
Contact with and (suspected) exposure to chromium compounds
Contact with and (suspected) exposure to nickel dust

☑6ᵗʰ Z77.02 Contact with and (suspected) exposure to hazardous aromatic compounds

Z77.020 Contact with and (suspected) exposure to aromatic amines

Z77.021 Contact with and (suspected) exposure to benzene

Z77.028 Contact with and (suspected) exposure to other hazardous aromatic compounds
Aromatic dyes NOS
Polycyclic aromatic hydrocarbons

☑6ᵗʰ Z77.09 Contact with and (suspected) exposure to other hazardous, chiefly nonmedicinal, chemicals

Z77.090 Contact with and (suspected) exposure to asbestos

Z77.098 Contact with and (suspected) exposure to other hazardous, chiefly nonmedicinal, chemicals
Dyes NOS

☑5ᵗʰ Z77.1 Contact with and (suspected) exposure to environmental pollution and hazards in the physical environment

☑6ᵗʰ Z77.11 Contact with and (suspected) exposure to environmental pollution

Z77.110 Contact with and (suspected) exposure to air pollution

Z77.111 Contact with and (suspected) exposure to water pollution

Z77.112 Contact with and (suspected) exposure to soil pollution

Z77.118 Contact with and (suspected) exposure to other environmental pollution

☑6ᵗʰ Z77.12 Contact with and (suspected) exposure to hazards in the physical environment

Z77.120 Contact with and (suspected) exposure to mold (toxic)

Z77.121 Contact with and (suspected) exposure t harmful algae and algae toxins
Contact with and (suspected) exposure to (harmful) algae bloom NOS
Contact with and (suspected) exposure to blue-green algae bloom
Contact with and (suspected) exposure to brown tide
Contact with and (suspected) exposure to cyanobacteria bloom
Contact with and (suspected) exposure to Florida red tide
Contact with and (suspected) exposure to pfiesteria piscicida
Contact with and (suspected) exposure to red tide

Z77.122 Contact with and (suspected) exposure t noise

Z77.123 Contact with and (suspected) exposure t radon and other naturally occuring radiation

EXCLUDES 2 radiation exposure as the cause a confirmed condition (W88-W90, X39.0-)
radiation sickness NOS (T66)

Z77.128 Contact with and (suspected) exposure t other hazards in the physical environme

☑5ᵗʰ Z77.2 Contact with and (suspected) exposure to other hazardous substances

Z77.21 Contact with and (suspected) exposure to potentially hazardous body fluids

Z77.22 Contact with and (suspected) exposure to environmental tobacco smoke (acute) (chronic)
Exposure to second hand tobacco smoke (acute) (chronic)
Passive smoking (acute) (chronic)
EXCLUDES 1 nicotine dependence (F17.-)
tobacco use (Z72.0)
EXCLUDES 2 occupational exposure to environmental tobacco smoke (Z57.31)

Z77.29 Contact with and (suspected) exposure to other hazardous substances

Z77.9 Other contact with and (suspected) exposures hazardous to health

☑4ᵗʰ Z78 Other specified health status

EXCLUDES 2 asymptomatic human immunodeficiency virus [HIV] infection status (Z21)
postprocedural status (Z93- Z99)
sex reassignment status (Z87.890)

Z78.0 Asymptomatic menopausal state Ⓐ
Menopausal state NOS
Postmenopausal status NOS
EXCLUDES 2 symptomatic menopausal state (N95.1)

Z78.1 Physical restraint status
EXCLUDES 1 physical restraint due to a procedure - omit code

Z78.9 Other specified health status

☑4ᵗʰ Z79 Long term (current) drug therapy
INCLUDES long term (current) drug use for prophylactic purposes
Code also any therapeutic drug level monitoring (Z51.81)
EXCLUDES 2 drug abuse and dependence (F11-F19)
drug use complicating pregnancy, childbirth, and the puerperium (O99.32-)

☑5ᵗʰ Z79.0 Long term (current) use of anticoagulants and antithrombotics/antiplatelets
EXCLUDES 2 long term (current) use of aspirin (Z79.82)

Z79.01 Long term (current) use of anticoagulants

Z79.02 Long term (current) use of antithrombotics/antiplatelets

Z79.1 Long term (current) use of non-steroidal anti-inflammatories (NSAID)
EXCLUDES 2 long term (current) use of aspirin (Z79.82)

Z79.2 Long term (current) use of antibiotics

Z79.3 Long term (current) use of hormonal contraceptives
Long term (current) use of birth control pill or patch

Z79.4 Long term (current) use of insulin

☑5ᵗʰ Z79.5 Long term (current) use of steroids

Z79.51 Long term (current) use of inhaled steroids

Z79.52 Long term (current) use of systemic steroids

☑5ᵗʰ Z79.8 Other long term (current) drug therapy

☑6ᵗʰ Z79.81 Long term (current) use of agents affecting estrogen receptors and estrogen levels
Code first, if applicable:
    malignant neoplasm of breast (C50.-)
    malignant neoplasm of prostate (C61)
Use additional code, if applicable, to identify:
    estrogen receptor positive status (Z17.0)
    family history of breast cancer (Z80.3)
    genetic susceptibility to malignant neoplasm
      (cancer) (Z15.0-)
    personal history of breast cancer (Z85.3)
    personal history of prostate cancer (Z85.46)
    postmenopausal status (Z78.0)
    EXCLUDES 1   hormone replacement therapy
           (postmenopausal) (Z79.890)

Z79.810 Long term (current) use of selective estrogen receptor modulators (SERMs)
Long term (current) use of raloxifene
    (Evista)
Long term (current) use of tamoxifen
    (Nolvadex)
Long term (current) use of toremifene
    (Fareston)

Z79.811 Long term (current) use of aromatase inhibitors
Long term (current) use of anastrozole
    (Arimidex)
Long term (current) use of exemestane
    (Aromasin)
Long term (current) use of letrozole
    (Femara)

Z79.818 Long term (current) use of other agents affecting estrogen receptors and estrogen levels
Long term (current) use of estrogen
    receptor downregulators
Long term (current) use of fulvestrant
    (Faslodex)
Long term (current) use of
    gonadotropin-releasing hormone
    (GnRH) agonist
Long term (current) use of goserelin
    acetate (Zoladex)
Long term (current) use of leuprolide
    acetate (leuprorelin) (Lupron)
Long term (current) use of megestrol
    acetate (Megace)

Z79.82 Long term (current) use of aspirin

Z79.83 Long term (current) use of bisphosphonates

☑6ᵗʰ Z79.89 Other long term (current) drug therapy

Z79.890 Hormone replacement therapy (postmenopausal)   ♀

Z79.891 Long term (current) use of opiate analgesic
Long term (current) use of methadone for
    pain management
    EXCLUDES 1   methodone use NOS (F11.2-)
           use of methodone for treatment
           of heroin addiction (F11.2-)

Z79.899 Other long term (current) drug therapy

☑ Z80 Family history of primary malignant neoplasm

Z80.0 Family history of malignant neoplasm of digestive organs
Conditions classifiable to C15-C26

Z80.1 Family history of malignant neoplasm of trachea, bronchus and lung
Conditions classifiable to C33-C34

Z80.2 Family history of malignant neoplasm of other respiratory and intrathoracic organs
Conditions classifiable to C30-C32, C37-C39

Z80.3 Family history of malignant neoplasm of breast
Conditions classifiable to C50-

☑5ᵗʰ Z80.4 Family history of malignant neoplasm of genital organs
Conditions classifiable to C51-C63

Z80.41 Family history of malignant neoplasm of ovary

Z80.42 Family history of malignant neoplasm of prostate

Z80.43 Family history of malignant neoplasm of testis

Z80.49 Family history of malignant neoplasm of other genital organs

☑5ᵗʰ Z80.5 Family history of malignant neoplasm of urinary tract
Conditions classifiable to C64-C68

Z80.51 Family history of malignant neoplasm of kidney

Z80.52 Family history of malignant neoplasm of bladder

Z80.59 Family history of malignant neoplasm of other urinary tract organ

Z80.6 Family history of leukemia
Conditions classifiable to C91-C95

Z80.7 Family history of other malignant neoplasms of lymphoid, hematopoietic and related tissues
Conditions classifiable to C81-C90, C96-

Z80.8 Family history of malignant neoplasm of other organs or systems
Conditions classifiable to C00-C14, C40-C49, C69-C79

Z80.9 Family history of malignant neoplasm, unspecified
Conditions classifiable to C80.1

☑4ᵗʰ Z81 Family history of mental and behavioral disorders

Z81.0 Family history of intellectual disabilities
Conditions classifiable to F70-F79

Z81.1 Family history of alcohol abuse and dependence
Conditions classifiable to F10-

Z81.2 Family history of tobacco abuse and dependence
Conditions classifiable to F17-

Z81.3 Family history of other psychoactive substance abuse and dependence
Conditions classifiable to F11-F16, F18-F19

Z81.4 Family history of other substance abuse and dependence
Conditions classifiable to F55

Z81.8 Family history of other mental and behavioral disorders
Conditions classifiable elsewhere in F01-F99

☑4ᵗʰ Z82 Family history of certain disabilities and chronic diseases (leading to disablement)

Z82.0 Family history of epilepsy and other diseases of the nervous system
Conditions classifiable to G00-G99

Z82.1 Family history of blindness and visual loss
Conditions classifiable to H54-

Z82.2 Family history of deafness and hearing loss
Conditions classifiable to H90-H91

Z82.3 Family history of stroke
Conditions classifiable to I60-I64

☑5ᵗʰ Z82.4 Family history of ischemic heart disease and other diseases of the circulatory system
Conditions classifiable to I00-I52, I65-I99

Z82.41 Family history of sudden cardiac death

Z82.49 Family history of ischemic heart disease and other diseases of the circulatory system

Z82.5 Family history of asthma and other chronic lower respiratory diseases
Conditions classifiable to J40-J47
    EXCLUDES 2   family history of other diseases of the respiratory
           system (Z83.6)

☑5ᵗʰ Z82.6 Family history of arthritis and other diseases of the musculoskeletal system and connective tissue
Conditions classifiable to M00-M99

Z82.61 Family history of arthritis

Z82.62 Family history of osteoporosis

Z82.69 Family history of other diseases of the musculoskeletal system and connective tissue

☑5ᵗʰ Z82.7 Family history of congenital malformations, deformations and chromosomal abnormalities
Conditions classifiable to Q00-Q99

Z82.71 Family history of polycystic kidney

Z82.79 Family history of other congenital malformations, deformations and chromosomal abnormalities

Z82.8 Family history of other disabilities and chronic diseases leading to disablement, not elsewhere classified

☑4ᵗʰ Z83 Family history of other specific disorders
    EXCLUDES 2   contact with and (suspected) exposure to communicable
           disease in the family (Z20.-)

Z83.0 Family history of human immunodeficiency virus [HIV] disease
Conditions classifiable to B20

Z83.1 Family history of other infectious and parasitic diseases
Conditions classifiable to A00-B19, B25-B94, B99

Z83.2 Family history of diseases of the blood and blood-forming organs and certain disorders involving the immune mechanism
Conditions classifiable to D50-D89

Z83.3   **Family history of** diabetes mellitus
     Conditions classifiable to E08-E13

✓5ᵗʰ   Z83.4   **Family history of other endocrine, nutritional and metabolic diseases**
     Conditions classifiable to E00-E07, E15-E88

    Z83.41   **Family history of** multiple endocrine neoplasia [MEN] syndrome

    Z83.49   **Family history of other endocrine, nutritional and metabolic diseases**

✓5ᵗʰ   Z83.5   **Family history of eye and ear disorders**

    ✓6ᵗʰ   Z83.51   **Family history of** eye **disorders**
     Conditions classifiable to H00-H53, H55-H59
     EXCLUDES 2   *family history of blindness and visual loss (Z82.1)*

      Z83.511   **Family history of** glaucoma

      Z83.518   **Family history of other specified eye disorder**

    Z83.52   **Family history of** ear **disorders**
     Conditions classifiable to H60-H83, H92-H95
     EXCLUDES 2   *family history of deafness and hearing loss (Z82.2)*

Z83.6   **Family history of other diseases of the** respiratory system
     Conditions classifiable to J00-J39, J60-J99
     EXCLUDES 2   *family history of asthma and other chronic lower respiratory diseases (Z82.5)*

✓5ᵗʰ   Z83.7   **Family history of diseases of the digestive system**
     Conditions classifiable to K00-K93

    Z83.71   **Family history of** colonic polyps
     EXCLUDES 1   *family history of malignant neoplasm of digestive organs (Z80.0)*

    Z83.79   **Family history of other diseases of the digestive system**

✓4ᵗʰ   **Z84   Family history of other conditions**

    Z84.0   **Family history of diseases of the** skin and subcutaneous tissue
     Conditions classifiable to L00-L99

    Z84.1   **Family history of disorders of** kidney and ureter
     Conditions classifiable to N00-N29

    Z84.2   **Family history of other diseases of the** genitourinary system
     Conditions classifiable to N30-N99

    Z84.3   **Family history of** consanguinity

    ✓5ᵗʰ   Z84.8   **Family history of other specified conditions**

     Z84.81   **Family history of carrier of** genetic disease

     Z84.89   **Family history of other specified conditions**

✓4ᵗʰ   **Z85   Personal history of malignant neoplasm**
     Code first any follow-up examination after treatment of malignant neoplasm (Z08)
     Use additional code to identify:
      alcohol use and dependence (F10.-)
      exposure to environmental tobacco smoke (Z77.22)
      history of tobacco use (Z87.891)
      occupational exposure to environmental tobacco smoke (Z57.31)
      tobacco dependence (F17.-)
      tobacco use (Z72.0)
     EXCLUDES 2   *personal history of benign neoplasm (Z86.01-)*
              personal history of carcinoma-in-situ (Z86.00-)

    ✓5ᵗʰ   Z85.0   **Personal history of malignant neoplasm of** digestive organs

     Z85.00   **Personal history of malignant neoplasm of unspecified digestive organ**

     Z85.01   **Personal history of malignant neoplasm of esophagus**
      Conditions classifiable to C15

     ✓6ᵗʰ   Z85.02   **Personal history of malignant neoplasm of** stomach

      Z85.020   **Personal history of malignant** carcinoid **tumor of stomach**
       Conditions classifiable to C7A.092

      Z85.028   **Personal history of other malignant neoplasm of stomach**
       Conditions classifiable to C16

     ✓6ᵗʰ   Z85.03   **Personal history of malignant neoplasm of** large intestine

      Z85.030   **Personal history of** malignant carcinoid **tumor of large intestine**
       Conditions classifiable to C7A.022-C7A.025, C7A.029

      Z85.038   **Personal history of other malignant neoplasm of large intestine**
       Conditions classifiable to C18

     ✓6ᵗʰ   Z85.04   **Personal history of malignant neoplasm of** rectum, rectosigmoid junction, and anus

      Z85.040   **Personal history of malignant** carcinoid **tumor of rectum**
       Conditions classifiable to C7A.026

      Z85.048   **Personal history of other malignant neoplasm of rectum, rectosigmoid junction, and anus**
       Conditions classifiable to C19-C21

     Z85.05   **Personal history of malignant neoplasm of** liver
      Conditions classifiable to C22

     ✓6ᵗʰ   Z85.06   **Personal history of malignant neoplasm of** small intestine

      Z85.060   **Personal history of malignant** carcinoid **tumor of small intestine**
       Conditions classifiable to C7A.01-

      Z85.068   **Personal history of other malignant neoplasm of small intestine**
       Conditions classifiable to C17

     Z85.07   **Personal history of malignant neoplasm of** pancre
      Conditions classifiable to C25

     Z85.09   **Personal history of malignant neoplasm of other digestive organs**

    ✓5ᵗʰ   Z85.1   **Personal history of malignant neoplasm of** trachea, bronch and lung

     ✓6ᵗʰ   Z85.11   **Personal history of malignant neoplasm of** bronch and lung

      Z85.110   **Personal history of malignant** carcinoid **tumor of bronchus and lung**
       Conditions classifiable to C7A.090

      Z85.118   **Personal history of other malignant neoplasm of bronchus and lung**
       Conditions classifiable to C34

     Z85.12   **Personal history of malignant neoplasm of** trachea
      Conditions classifiable to C33

    ✓5ᵗʰ   Z85.2   **Personal history of malignant neoplasm of other** respirator and intrathoracic organs

     Z85.20   **Personal history of malignant neoplasm of unspecified respiratory organ**

     Z85.21   **Personal history of malignant neoplasm of** larynx
      Conditions classifiable to C32

     Z85.22   **Personal history of malignant neoplasm of** nasal cavities, middle ear, and accessory sinuses
      Conditions classifiable to C30-C31

     ✓6ᵗʰ   Z85.23   **Personal history of malignant neoplasm of** thymus

      Z85.230   **Personal history of malignant** carcinoid **tumor of thymus**
       Conditions classifiable to C7A.091

      Z85.238   **Personal history of other malignant neoplasm of thymus**
       Conditions classifiable to C37

     Z85.29   **Personal history of malignant neoplasm of other respiratory and intrathoracic organs**

    Z85.3   **Personal history of malignant neoplasm of** breast
     Conditions classifiable to C50.-

    ✓5ᵗʰ   Z85.4   **Personal history of malignant neoplasm of** genital organs
     Conditions classifiable to C51-C63

     Z85.40   **Personal history of malignant neoplasm of unspecified** female **genital organ**

     Z85.41   **Personal history of malignant neoplasm of** cervix uteri

     Z85.42   **Personal history of malignant neoplasm of other parts of uterus**

     Z85.43   **Personal history of malignant neoplasm of** ovary

     Z85.44   **Personal history of malignant neoplasm of other** female **genital organs**

     Z85.45   **Personal history of malignant neoplasm of unspecified** male **genital organ**

     Z85.46   **Personal history of malignant neoplasm of prostate**

     Z85.47   **Personal history of malignant neoplasm of** testis

     Z85.48   **Personal history of malignant neoplasm of epididymis**

     Z85.49   **Personal history of malignant neoplasm of other** male **genital organs**

    ✓5ᵗʰ   Z85.5   **Personal history of malignant neoplasm of** urinary tract
     Conditions classifiable to C64-C68

EXCLUDES 1 Not coded here   **EXCLUDES 2** Not included here   🅽 Newborn Age: 0   🅿 Pediatric Age: 0-17   🅼 Maternity Age: 12-55   🅰 Adult Age: 15-124   **PDx** Primary

1126   ICD-10-CM 20

Z85.50   **Personal history of malignant neoplasm of unspecified urinary tract organ**

Z85.51   **Personal history of malignant neoplasm of** bladder

☑6ᵗʰ **Z85.52**   **Personal history of malignant neoplasm of** kidney
> EXCLUDES 1   *personal history of malignant neoplasm of renal pelvis (Z85.53)*

     Z85.520   **Personal history of malignant carcinoid tumor of kidney**
         Conditions classifiable to C7A.093

     Z85.528   **Personal history of other malignant neoplasm of kidney**
         Conditions classifiable to C64

Z85.53   **Personal history of malignant neoplasm of** renal pelvis

Z85.54   **Personal history of malignant neoplasm of** ureter

Z85.59   **Personal history of malignant neoplasm of other urinary tract organ**

Z85.6   **Personal history of** leukemia
     Conditions classifiable to C91-C95
> EXCLUDES 1   *leukemia in remission C91.0-C95.9 with 5th character 1*

☑5ᵗʰ **Z85.7**   **Personal history of other malignant neoplasms of lymphoid, hematopoietic and related tissues**

Z85.71   **Personal history of** Hodgkin lymphoma
     Conditions classifiable to C81

Z85.72   **Personal history of** non-Hodgkin lymphomas
     Conditions classifiable to C82-C85

Z85.79   **Personal history of other malignant neoplasms of lymphoid, hematopoietic and related tissues**
     Conditions classifiable to C88-C90, C96
> EXCLUDES 1   *multiple myeloma in remission (C90.01)*
> *plasma cell leukemia in remission (C90.11)*
> *plasmacytoma in remission (C90.21)*

☑5ᵗʰ **Z85.8**   **Personal history of malignant neoplasms of other organs and systems**
     Conditions classifiable to C00-C14, C40-C49, C69-C79, C7A.098

☑6ᵗʰ **Z85.81**   **Personal history of malignant neoplasm of** lip, oral cavity, and pharynx

     Z85.810   **Personal history of malignant neoplasm of tongue**

     Z85.818   **Personal history of malignant neoplasm of other sites of lip, oral cavity, and pharynx**

     Z85.819   **Personal history of malignant neoplasm of unspecified site of lip, oral cavity, and pharynx**

☑6ᵗʰ **Z85.82**   **Personal history of malignant neoplasm of** skin

     Z85.820   **Personal history of malignant melanoma of skin**
         Conditions classifiable to C43

     Z85.821   **Personal history of** Merkel cell carcinoma
         Conditions classifiable to C4A

     Z85.828   **Personal history of other malignant neoplasm of skin**
         Conditions classifiable to C44

☑6ᵗʰ **Z85.83**   **Personal history of malignant neoplasm of** bone and soft tissue

     Z85.830   **Personal history of malignant neoplasm of bone**

     Z85.831   **Personal history of malignant neoplasm of soft tissue**
> EXCLUDES 2   *personal history of malignant neoplasm of skin (Z85.82-)*

☑6ᵗʰ **Z85.84**   **Personal history of malignant neoplasm of** eye and nervous tissue

     Z85.840   **Personal history of malignant neoplasm of eye**

     Z85.841   **Personal history of malignant neoplasm of brain**

     Z85.848   **Personal history of malignant neoplasm of other parts of nervous tissue**

☑6ᵗʰ **Z85.85**   **Personal history of malignant neoplasm of** endocrine glands

     Z85.850   **Personal history of malignant neoplasm of thyroid**

     Z85.858   **Personal history of malignant neoplasm of other endocrine glands**

Z85.89   **Personal history of malignant neoplasm of other organs and systems**

Z85.9   **Personal history of malignant neoplasm, unspecified**
     Conditions classifiable to C7A.00, C80.1

☑4ᵗʰ **Z86**   **Personal history of certain other diseases**
     Code first any follow-up examination after treatment (Z09)

☑5ᵗʰ **Z86.0**   **Personal history of in-situ and benign neoplasms and neoplasms of uncertain behavior**
> EXCLUDES 2   *personal history of malignant neoplasms (Z85.-)*

☑6ᵗʰ **Z86.00**   **Personal history of** in-situ neoplasm

     Z86.000   **Personal history of in-situ neoplasm of breast**

     Z86.001   **Personal history of in-situ neoplasm of** ♀ **cervix uteri**

     Z86.008   **Personal history of in-situ neoplasm of other site**

☑6ᵗʰ **Z86.01**   **Personal history of** benign neoplasm

     Z86.010   **Personal history of** colonic polyps

     Z86.011   **Personal history of benign neoplasm of the** brain

     Z86.012   **Personal history of benign** carcinoid tumor

     Z86.018   **Personal history of other benign neoplasm**

     Z86.03   **Personal history of** neoplasm of uncertain behavior

☑5ᵗʰ **Z86.1**   **Personal history of** infectious and parasitic diseases
     Conditions classifiable to A00-B89, B99
> EXCLUDES 1   *personal history of infectious diseases specific to a body system*
> *sequelae of infectious and parasitic diseases (B90-B94)*

     Z86.11   **Personal history of** tuberculosis

     Z86.12   **Personal history of** poliomyelitis

     Z86.13   **Personal history of** malaria

     Z86.14   **Personal history of** Methicillin resistant Staphylococcus aureus **infection**
         Personal history of MRSA infection

     Z86.19   **Personal history of other infectious and parasitic diseases**

Z86.2   **Personal history of diseases of the** blood and blood-forming organs **and certain disorders involving the** immune mechanism
     Conditions classifiable to D50-D89

☑5ᵗʰ **Z86.3**   **Personal history of** endocrine, nutritional and metabolic diseases
     Conditions classifiable to E00-E88

     Z86.31   **Personal history of** diabetic foot ulcer
> EXCLUDES 2   *current diabetic foot ulcer (E08.621, E09.621, E10.621, E11.621, E13.621)*

     Z86.32   **Personal history of** gestational diabetes   ♀
         Personal history of conditions classifiable to O24.4-
> EXCLUDES 1   *gestational diabetes mellitus in current pregnancy (O24.4-)*

     Z86.39   **Personal history of other endocrine, nutritional and metabolic disease**

☑5ᵗʰ **Z86.5**   **Personal history of** mental and behavioral disorders
     Conditions classifiable to F40-F59

     Z86.51   **Personal history of** combat and operational stress reaction   Ⓐ

     Z86.59   **Personal history of other mental and behavioral disorders**

☑5ᵗʰ **Z86.6**   **Personal history of diseases of the** nervous system and sense organs
     Conditions classifiable to G00-G99, H00-H95
> EXCLUDES 2   *personal history of anaphylactic shock (Z87.892)*

     Z86.61   **Personal history of** infections of the central nervous system
         Personal history of encephalitis
         Personal history of meningitis

     Z86.69   **Personal history of other diseases of the nervous system and sense organs**

☑5ᵗʰ **Z86.7**   **Personal history of diseases of the** circulatory system
     Conditions classifiable to I00-I99
> EXCLUDES 2   *old myocardial infarction (I25.2)*
> *personal history of anaphylactic shock (Z87.892)*
> *postmyocardial infarction syndrome (I24.1)*

☑6ᵗʰ **Z86.71**   **Personal history of** venous thrombosis and embolism

     Z86.711   **Personal history of** pulmonary **embolism**

◀ Additional Character Required   ⁰⁷ᵗʰ Placeholder Alert   Unspecified Dx   Other Specified Dx   Manifestation   ▶◀ Revised Text   ● New Code   ▲ Revised Code Title

Z86.718   **Personal history of other venous thrombosis and embolism**

Z86.72   **Personal history of thrombophlebitis**

Z86.73   **Personal history of transient ischemic attack (TIA), and cerebral infarction without residual deficits**
Personal history of prolonged reversible ischemic neurological deficit (PRIND)
Personal history of stroke NOS without residual deficits
> **EXCLUDES 1**   *personal history of traumatic brain injury (Z87.820)*
>   *sequelae of cerebrovascular disease (I69.-)*
> **AHA:** 2012, 4Q, 92

Z86.74   **Personal history of sudden cardiac arrest**
Personal history of sudden cardiac death successfully resuscitated

Z86.79   **Personal history of other diseases of the circulatory system**

✓4th Z87   **Personal history of other diseases and conditions**
Code first any follow-up examination after treatment (Z09)

✓5th Z87.0   **Personal history of diseases of the respiratory system**
Conditions classifiable to J00-J99

Z87.01   **Personal history of pneumonia (recurrent)**

Z87.09   **Personal history of other diseases of the respiratory system**

✓5th Z87.1   **Personal history of diseases of the digestive system**
Conditions classifiable to K00-K93

Z87.11   **Personal history of peptic ulcer disease**

Z87.19   **Personal history of other diseases of the digestive system**

Z87.2   **Personal history of diseases of the skin and subcutaneous tissue**
Conditions classifiable to L00-L99
> **EXCLUDES 2**   *personal history of diabetic foot ulcer (Z86.31)*

✓5th Z87.3   **Personal history of diseases of the musculoskeletal system and connective tissue**
Conditions classifiable to M00-M99
> **EXCLUDES 2**   *personal history of (healed) traumatic fracture (Z87.81)*

✓6th Z87.31   **Personal history of (healed) nontraumatic fracture**

Z87.310   **Personal history of (healed) osteoporosis fracture**
Personal history of (healed) fragility fracture
Personal history of (healed) collapsed vertebra due to osteoporosis

Z87.311   **Personal history of (healed) other pathological fracture**
Personal history of (healed) collapsed vertebra NOS
> **EXCLUDES 2**   *personal history of osteoporosis fracture (Z87.310)*

Z87.312   **Personal history of (healed) stress fracture**
Personal history of (healed) fatigue fracture

Z87.39   **Personal history of other diseases of the musculoskeletal system and connective tissue**

✓5th Z87.4   **Personal history of diseases of genitourinary system**
Conditions classifiable to N00-N99

✓6th Z87.41   **Personal history of dysplasia of the female genital tract**
> **EXCLUDES 1**   *personal history of malignant neoplasm of female genital tract (Z85.40-Z85.44)*

Z87.410   **Personal history of cervical dysplasia**   ♀

Z87.411   **Personal history of vaginal dysplasia**   ♀

Z87.412   **Personal history of vulvar dysplasia**   ♀

Z87.42   **Personal history of other diseases of the female genital tract**   ♀

✓6th Z87.43   **Personal history of diseases of the male genital organs**

Z87.430   **Personal history of prostatic dysplasia**   ♂
> **EXCLUDES 1**   *personal history of malignant neoplasm of prostate (Z85.46)*

Z87.438   **Personal history of other diseases of male genital organs**   ♂

✓6th Z87.44   **Personal history of diseases of the urinary system**
> **EXCLUDES 1**   *personal history of malignant neoplasm of cervix uteri (Z85.41)*

Z87.440   **Personal history of urinary (tract) infections**

Z87.441   **Personal history of nephrotic syndrome**

Z87.442   **Personal history of urinary calculi**
Personal history of kidney stones

Z87.448   **Personal history of other diseases of urinary system**

✓5th Z87.5   **Personal history of complications of pregnancy, childbirth and the puerperium**
Conditions classifiable to O00-O9A
> **EXCLUDES 2**   *recurrent pregnancy loss (N96)*

Z87.51   **Personal history of pre-term labor**
> **EXCLUDES 1**   *current pregnancy with history of pre-term labor (O09.21-)*

Z87.59   **Personal history of other complications of pregnancy, childbirth and the puerperium**
Personal history of trophoblastic disease

✓5th Z87.7   **Personal history of (corrected) congenital malformations**
Conditions classifiable to Q00-Q89 that have been repaired or corrected
> **EXCLUDES 1**   *congenital malformations that have been partially corrected or repaired but which still require medical treatment—code to condition*
> **EXCLUDES 2**   *other postprocedural states (Z98.-)*
>   *personal history of medical treatment (Z92.-)*
>   *presence of cardiac and vascular implants and grafts (Z95.-)*
>   *presence of other devices (Z97.-)*
>   *presence of other functional implants (Z96.-)*
>   *transplanted organ and tissue status (Z94.-)*

✓6th Z87.71   **Personal history of (corrected) congenital malformations of genitourinary system**

Z87.710   **Personal history of (corrected) hypospadias**

Z87.718   **Personal history of other specified (corrected) congenital malformations of genitourinary system**

✓6th Z87.72   **Personal history of (corrected) congenital malformations of nervous system and sense organs**

Z87.720   **Personal history of (corrected) congenital malformations of eye**

Z87.721   **Personal history of (corrected) congenital malformations of ear**

Z87.728   **Personal history of other specified (corrected) congenital malformations of nervous system and sense organs**

✓6th Z87.73   **Personal history of (corrected) congenital malformations of digestive system**

Z87.730   **Personal history of (corrected) cleft lip and palate**

Z87.738   **Personal history of other specified (corrected) congenital malformations of digestive system**

Z87.74   **Personal history of (corrected) congenital malformations of heart and circulatory system**

Z87.75   **Personal history of (corrected) congenital malformations of respiratory system**

Z87.76   **Personal history of (corrected) congenital malformations of integument, limbs and musculoskeletal system**

✓6th Z87.79   **Personal history of other (corrected) congenital malformations**

Z87.790   **Personal history of (corrected) congenital malformations of face and neck**

Z87.798   **Personal history of other (corrected) congenital malformations**

✓5th Z87.8   **Personal history of other specified conditions**
> **EXCLUDES 2**   *personal history of self harm (Z91.5)*

Z87.81   **Personal history of (healed) traumatic fracture**
> **EXCLUDES 2**   *personal history of (healed) nontraumatic fracture (Z87.31-)*

✓6th Z87.82   **Personal history of other (healed) physical injury and trauma**
Conditions classifiable to S00-T88, except traumatic fractures

Z87.820   **Personal history of traumatic brain injury**
> **EXCLUDES 1**   *personal history of transient ischemic attack (TIA), and cerebral infarction without residual deficits (Z86.73)*

EXCLUDES 1 Not coded here   **EXCLUDES 2** Not included here   N Newborn Age: 0   P Pediatric Age: 0-17   M Maternity Age: 12-55   A Adult Age: 15-124   PDx Primary D

1128   ICD-10-CM 20

Z87.821   **Personal history of** retained foreign body fully removed

Z87.828   **Personal history of** other (healed) physical injury and trauma

✓6th   **Z87.89**   **Personal history of** other specified conditions

Z87.890   **Personal history of** sex reassignment

Z87.891   **Personal history of** nicotine dependence
> EXCLUDES 1   *current nicotine dependence (F17.2-)*

Z87.892   **Personal history of** anaphylaxis
> Code also allergy status such as:
> allergy status to drugs, medicaments and biological substances (Z88.-)
> allergy status, other than to drugs and biological substances (Z91.0-)

Z87.898   **Personal history of other specified conditions**
> **AHA:** 2013, 1Q, 21

Z88   Allergy status to drugs, medicaments and biological substances
> EXCLUDES 2   *allergy status, other than to drugs and biological substances (Z91.0-)*

Z88.0   **Allergy status to** penicillin

Z88.1   **Allergy status to other** antibiotic **agents status**

Z88.2   **Allergy status to** sulfonamides **status**

Z88.3   **Allergy status to other** anti-infective **agents status**

Z88.4   **Allergy status to** anesthetic **agent status**

Z88.5   **Allergy status to** narcotic **agent status**

Z88.6   **Allergy status to** analgesic **agent status**

Z88.7   **Allergy status to** serum and vaccine **status**

Z88.8   **Allergy status to other drugs, medicaments and biological substances status**

Z88.9   **Allergy status to unspecified drugs, medicaments and biological substances status**

Z89   Acquired absence of limb
> INCLUDES   amputation status
> postprocedural loss of limb
> post-traumatic loss of limb
> EXCLUDES 1   *acquired deformities of limbs (M20-M21)*
> *congenital absence of limbs (Q71-Q73)*

✓5th   **Z89.0**   **Acquired absence of** thumb and other finger(s)

✓6th   **Z89.01**   **Acquired absence of** thumb

Z89.011   **Acquired absence of** right thumb

Z89.012   **Acquired absence of** left thumb

Z89.019   **Acquired absence of unspecified thumb**

✓6th   **Z89.02**   **Acquired absence of** other finger(s)
> EXCLUDES 2   *acquired absence of thumb (Z89.01-)*

Z89.021   **Acquired absence of** right finger(s)

Z89.022   **Acquired absence of** left finger(s)

Z89.029   **Acquired absence of unspecified finger(s)**

✓5th   **Z89.1**   **Acquired absence of** hand and wrist

✓6th   **Z89.11**   **Acquired absence of** hand

Z89.111   **Acquired absence of** right hand

Z89.112   **Acquired absence of** left hand

Z89.119   **Acquired absence of unspecified hand**

✓6th   **Z89.12**   **Acquired absence of** wrist
> Disarticulation at wrist

Z89.121   **Acquired absence of** right wrist

Z89.122   **Acquired absence of** left wrist

Z89.129   **Acquired absence of unspecified wrist**

✓5th   **Z89.2**   **Acquired absence of** upper limb above wrist

✓6th   **Z89.20**   **Acquired absence of** upper limb, unspecified level

Z89.201   **Acquired absence of** right upper limb, unspecified level

Z89.202   **Acquired absence of** left upper limb, unspecified level

Z89.209   **Acquired absence of unspecified upper limb, unspecified level**
> Acquired absence of arm NOS

✓6th   **Z89.21**   **Acquired absence of** upper limb below elbow

Z89.211   **Acquired absence of** right upper limb below elbow

Z89.212   **Acquired absence of** left upper limb below elbow

Z89.219   **Acquired absence of unspecified upper limb below elbow**

✓6th   **Z89.22**   **Acquired absence of** upper limb above elbow
> Disarticulation at elbow

Z89.221   **Acquired absence of** right upper limb above elbow

Z89.222   **Acquired absence of** left upper limb above elbow

Z89.229   **Acquired absence of unspecified upper limb above elbow**

✓6th   **Z89.23**   **Acquired absence of** shoulder
> Acquired absence of shoulder joint following explantation of shoulder joint prosthesis, with or without presence of antibiotic-impregnated cement spacer

Z89.231   **Acquired absence of** right shoulder

Z89.232   **Acquired absence of** left shoulder

Z89.239   **Acquired absence of unspecified shoulder**

✓5th   **Z89.4**   **Acquired absence of** toe(s), foot, and ankle

✓6th   **Z89.41**   **Acquired absence of** great toe

Z89.411   **Acquired absence of** right great toe

Z89.412   **Acquired absence of** left great toe

Z89.419   **Acquired absence of unspecified great toe**

✓6th   **Z89.42**   **Acquired absence of** other toe(s)
> EXCLUDES 2   *acquired absence of great toe (Z89.41-)*

Z89.421   **Acquired absence of other** right toe(s)

Z89.422   **Acquired absence of other** left toe(s)

Z89.429   **Acquired absence of other toe(s), unspecified side**

✓6th   **Z89.43**   **Acquired absence of** foot

Z89.431   **Acquired absence of** right foot

Z89.432   **Acquired absence of** left foot

Z89.439   **Acquired absence of unspecified foot**

✓6th   **Z89.44**   **Acquired absence of** ankle
> Disarticulation of ankle

Z89.441   **Acquired absence of** right ankle

Z89.442   **Acquired absence of** left ankle

Z89.449   **Acquired absence of unspecified ankle**

✓5th   **Z89.5**   **Acquired absence of leg below knee**

✓6th   **Z89.51**   **Acquired absence of** leg below knee

Z89.511   **Acquired absence of** right leg below knee

Z89.512   **Acquired absence of** left leg below knee

Z89.519   **Acquired absence of unspecified leg below knee**

✓6th   **Z89.52**   **Acquired absence of** knee
> Acquired absence of knee joint following explantation of knee joint prosthesis, with or without presence of antibiotic-impregnated cement spacer

Z89.521   **Acquired absence of** right knee

Z89.522   **Acquired absence of** left knee

Z89.529   **Acquired absence of unspecified knee**

✓5th   **Z89.6**   **Acquired absence of leg above knee**

✓6th   **Z89.61**   **Acquired absence of** leg above knee
> Acquired absence of leg NOS
> Disarticulation at knee

Z89.611   **Acquired absence of** right leg above knee

Z89.612   **Acquired absence of** left leg above knee

Z89.619   **Acquired absence of unspecified leg above knee**

✓6th   **Z89.62**   **Acquired absence of** hip
> Acquired absence of hip joint following explantation of hip joint prosthesis, with or without presence of antibiotic-impregnated cement spacer
> Disarticulation at hip

Z89.621   **Acquired absence of** right hip joint

Z89.622   **Acquired absence of** left hip joint

Z89.629   **Acquired absence of unspecified hip joint**

Z89.9   **Acquired absence of limb, unspecified**

✓4th   **Z90   Acquired absence of organs, not elsewhere classified**
> INCLUDES   postprocedural or post-traumatic loss of body part NEC
> EXCLUDES 1   *congenital absence—see Alphabetical Index*
> EXCLUDES 2   *postprocedural absence of endocrine glands (E89.-)*

✓5th   **Z90.0**   **Acquired absence of part of** head and neck

Z90.01   **Acquired absence of** eye

Z90.02   **Acquired absence of** larynx

Z90.09 **Acquired absence of other part of head and neck**
Acquired absence of nose
EXCLUDES 2 teeth (K08.1)

✓5ᵗʰ **Z90.1** **Acquired absence of** breast and nipple

Z90.10 **Acquired absence of unspecified breast and nipple**

Z90.11 **Acquired absence of** right breast and nipple

Z90.12 **Acquired absence of** left breast and nipple

Z90.13 **Acquired absence of** bilateral breasts and nipples

Z90.2 **Acquired absence of** lung [part of]

Z90.3 **Acquired absence of** stomach [part of]

✓5ᵗʰ **Z90.4** **Acquired absence of** other specified parts of digestive tract

  ✓6ᵗʰ **Z90.41** **Acquired absence of** pancreas
Use additional code to identify any associated:
insulin use (Z79.4)
diabetes mellitus, postpancreatectomy (E13.-)

    Z90.410 **Acquired** total absence **of pancreas**
Acquired absence of pancreas NOS

    Z90.411 **Acquired** partial absence **of pancreas**

  Z90.49 **Acquired absence of other specified parts of digestive tract**

Z90.5 **Acquired absence of** kidney

Z90.6 **Acquired absence of other** parts of urinary tract
Acquired absence of bladder

✓5ᵗʰ **Z90.7** **Acquired absence of** genital organ(s)
EXCLUDES 1 personal history of sex reassignment (Z87.890)
EXCLUDES 2 female genital mutilation status (N90.81-)

  ✓6ᵗʰ **Z90.71** **Acquired absence of** cervix and uterus

    Z90.710 **Acquired absence of** both cervix and uterus   ♀
Acquired absence of uterus NOS
Status post total hysterectomy

    Z90.711 **Acquired absence of uterus** with remaining cervical stump   ♀
Status post partial hysterectomy with remaining cervical stump

    Z90.712 **Acquired absence of cervix** with remaining uterus   ♀

  ✓6ᵗʰ **Z90.72** **Acquired absence of** ovaries

    Z90.721 **Acquired absence of ovaries,** unilateral   ♀

    Z90.722 **Acquired absence of ovaries,** bilateral   ♀

  Z90.79 **Acquired absence of other genital organ(s)**

✓5ᵗʰ **Z90.8** **Acquired absence of** other organs

  Z90.81 **Acquired absence of** spleen

  Z90.89 **Acquired absence of other organs**

✓4ᵗʰ **Z91** **Personal risk factors, not elsewhere classified**
EXCLUDES 2 contact with and (suspected) exposures hazardous to health (Z77.-)
exposure to pollution and other problems related to physical environment (Z77.1-)
personal history of physical injury and trauma (Z87.81, Z87.82-)
occupational exposure to risk factors (Z57.-)

✓5ᵗʰ **Z91.0** **Allergy status, other than to drugs and biological substances**
EXCLUDES 2 allergy status to drugs, medicaments, and biological substances (Z88.-)

  ✓6ᵗʰ **Z91.01** Food allergy status
EXCLUDES 2 food additives allergy status (Z91.02)

    Z91.010 **Allergy to** peanuts

    Z91.011 **Allergy to** milk products
EXCLUDES 1 lactose intolerance (E73.-)

    Z91.012 **Allergy to** eggs

    Z91.013 **Allergy to** seafood
Allergy to shellfish
Allergy to octopus or squid ink

    Z91.018 **Allergy to other foods**
Allergy to nuts other than peanuts

  Z91.02 **Food additives allergy status**

  ✓6ᵗʰ **Z91.03** Insect allergy status

    Z91.030 Bee allergy status

    Z91.038 **Other insect allergy status**

  ✓6ᵗʰ **Z91.04** **Nonmedicinal substance allergy status**

    Z91.040 Latex allergy status
Latex sensitivity status

    Z91.041 Radiographic dye allergy status
Allergy status to contrast media used for diagnostic X-ray procedure

Z91.048 **Other nonmedicinal substance allergy status**

Z91.09 **Other allergy status, other than to drugs and biological substances**

✓5ᵗʰ **Z91.1** **Patient's noncompliance with medical treatment and regimen**

Z91.11 **Patient's noncompliance with** dietary regimen

✓6ᵗʰ **Z91.12** **Patient's** intentional underdosing of medication regimen
Code first underdosing of medication (T36-T50) with fifth or sixth character 6
EXCLUDES 1 adverse effect of prescribed drug taken as directed—code to adverse effect poisoning (overdose)—code to poisoning

Z91.120 **Patient's intentional underdosing of medication regimen due to** financial hardship

Z91.128 **Patient's intentional underdosing of medication regimen for other** reason

✓6ᵗʰ **Z91.13** **Patient's** unintentional underdosing of medicatio regimen
Code first underdosing of medication (T36-T50) with fifth or sixth character 6
EXCLUDES 1 adverse effect of prescribed drug taken as directed—code to adverse effect poisoning (overdose)—code to poisoning

Z91.130 **Patient's unintentional underdosing of medication regimen due to** age-related debility

Z91.138 **Patient's unintentional underdosing of medication regimen for other** reason

Z91.14 **Patient's other noncompliance with medication regimen**
Patient's underdosing of medication NOS

Z91.15 **Patient's noncompliance with** renal dialysis

Z91.19 **Patient's noncompliance with other medical treatment and regimen**

✓5ᵗʰ **Z91.4** **Personal history of psychological trauma, not elsewhere classified**

  ✓6ᵗʰ **Z91.41** **Personal history of** adult abuse
EXCLUDES 2 personal history of abuse in childhood (Z62.81-)

    Z91.410 **Personal history of adult** physical and sexual abuse
EXCLUDES 1 current adult physical abuse (T74.11, T76.11)
current adult sexual abuse (T74.21, T76.11)

    Z91.411 **Personal history of adult** psychological abuse

    Z91.412 **Personal history of** adult neglect
EXCLUDES 1 current adult neglect (T74.01, T76.01)

    Z91.419 **Personal history of unspecified adult abuse**

  Z91.49 **Other personal history of psychological trauma, n◆ elsewhere classified**

Z91.5 **Personal history of self-harm**
Personal history of parasuicide
Personal history of self-poisoning
Personal history of suicide attempt

✓5ᵗʰ **Z91.8** **Other specified personal risk factors, not elsewhere classifi◆**

Z91.81 **History of falling**
At risk for falling

Z91.82 **Personal history of military deployment**
Individual (civilian or military) with past history of military war, peacekeeping and humanitarian deployment (current or past conflict)
Returned from military deployment

Z91.83 *Wandering in diseases classified elsewhere*
Code first underlying disorder such as:
Alzheimer's disease (G30.-)
autism or pervasive developmental disorder (F84.-)
intellectual disabilities (F70-F79)
unspecified dementia with behavioral disturbance (F03.9-)

Z91.89 **Other specified personal risk factors, not elsewher◆ classified**

EXCLUDES 1 Not coded here   *EXCLUDES 2* Not included here   N Newborn Age: 0   P Pediatric Age: 0-17   M Maternity Age: 12-55   A Adult Age: 15-124   PDx Primary

1130   ICD-10-CM 20

Z92 Personal history of medical treatment

EXCLUDES 2 postprocedural states (Z98.-)

Z92.0 **Personal history of contraception**

EXCLUDES 1 counseling or management of current contraceptive practices (Z30.-)
long term (current) use of contraception (Z79.3)
presence of (intrauterine) contraceptive device (Z97.5)

✓5th **Z92.2** **Personal history of drug therapy**

EXCLUDES 2 long term (current) drug therapy (Z79.-)

Z92.21 **Personal history of antineoplastic chemotherapy**

Z92.22 **Personal history of monoclonal drug therapy**

Z92.23 **Personal history of estrogen therapy**

✓6th **Z92.24** **Personal history of steroid therapy**

Z92.240 **Personal history of inhaled steroid therapy**

Z92.241 **Personal history of systemic steroid therapy**

Personal history of steroid therapy NOS

Z92.25 **Personal history of immunosupression therapy**

EXCLUDES 2 personal history of steroid therapy (Z92.24)

Z92.29 **Personal history of other drug therapy**

Z92.3 **Personal history of irradiation**

Personal history of exposure to therapeutic radiation

EXCLUDES 1 exposure to radiation in the physical environment (Z77.12)
occupational exposure to radiation (Z57.1)

✓5th **Z92.8** **Personal history of other medical treatment**

Z92.81 **Personal history of extracorporeal membrane oxygenation (ECMO)**

Z92.82 **Status post administration of tPA (rtPA) in a different facility within the last 24 hours prior to admission to current facility**

Code first condition requiring tPA administration, such as:
acute cerebral infarction (I63.-)
acute myocardial infarction (I21-, I22-)

AHA: 2013, 4Q, 124

Z92.83 **Personal history of failed moderate sedation**

Personal history of failed conscious sedation

EXCLUDES 2 failed moderate sedation during procedure (T88.52)

Z92.89 **Personal history of other medical treatment**

Z93 Artificial opening status

EXCLUDES 1 artificial openings requiring attention or management (Z43.-)
complications of external stoma (J95.0-, K94.-, N99.5-)

Z93.0 **Tracheostomy status**

AHA: 2013, 4Q, 129

Z93.1 **Gastrostomy status**

Z93.2 **Ileostomy status**

Z93.3 **Colostomy status**

Z93.4 **Other artificial openings of gastrointestinal tract status**

✓5th **Z93.5** **Cystostomy status**

Z93.50 **Unspecified cystostomy status**

Z93.51 **Cutaneous-vesicostomy status**

Z93.52 **Appendico-vesicostomy status**

Z93.59 **Other cystostomy status**

Z93.6 **Other artificial openings of urinary tract status**

Nephrostomy status
Ureterostomy status
Urethrostomy status

Z93.8 **Other artificial opening status**

Z93.9 **Artificial opening status, unspecified**

Z94 Transplanted organ and tissue status

INCLUDES organ or tissue replaced by heterogenous or homogenous transplant

EXCLUDES 1 complications of transplanted organ or tissue—see Alphabetical Index

EXCLUDES 2 presence of vascular grafts (Z95.-)

Z94.0 **Kidney transplant status**

Z94.1 **Heart transplant status**

EXCLUDES 1 artificial heart status (Z95.812)
heart-valve replacement status (Z95.2-Z95.4)

Z94.2 **Lung transplant status**

Z94.3 **Heart and lungs transplant status**

Z94.4 **Liver transplant status**

Z94.5 **Skin transplant status**

Autogenous skin transplant status

Z94.6 **Bone transplant status**

Z94.7 **Corneal transplant status**

✓5th **Z94.8** **Other transplanted organ and tissue status**

Z94.81 **Bone marrow transplant status**

Z94.82 **Intestine transplant status**

Z94.83 **Pancreas transplant status**

Z94.84 **Stem cells transplant status**

Z94.89 **Other transplanted organ and tissue status**

Z94.9 **Transplanted organ and tissue status, unspecified**

✓4th Z95 Presence of cardiac and vascular implants and grafts

EXCLUDES 1 complications of cardiac and vascular devices, implants and grafts (T82.-)

Z95.0 **Presence of cardiac pacemaker**

EXCLUDES 1 adjustment or management of cardiac pacemaker (Z45.0)
presence of automatic (implantable) cardiac defibrillator with synchronous cardiac pacemaker (Z95.810)

Z95.1 **Presence of aortocoronary bypass graft**

Z95.2 **Presence of prosthetic heart valve**

Presence of heart valve NOS

Z95.3 **Presence of xenogenic heart valve**

Z95.4 **Presence of other heart-valve replacement**

Z95.5 **Presence of coronary angioplasty implant and graft**

EXCLUDES 1 coronary angioplasty status without implant and graft (Z98.61)

✓5th **Z95.8** **Presence of other cardiac and vascular implants and grafts**

✓6th **Z95.81** **Presence of other cardiac implants and grafts**

Z95.810 **Presence of automatic (implantable) cardiac defibrillator**

Presence of automatic (implantable) cardiac defibrillator with synchronous cardiac pacemaker

Z95.811 **Presence of heart assist device**

Z95.812 **Presence of fully implantable artificial heart**

Z95.818 **Presence of other cardiac implants and grafts**

✓6th **Z95.82** **Presence of other vascular implants and grafts**

Z95.820 **Peripheral vascular angioplasty status with implants and grafts**

EXCLUDES 1 peripheral vascular angioplasty without implant and graft (Z98.62)

Z95.828 **Presence of other vascular implants and grafts**

Presence of intravascular prosthesis NEC

Z95.9 **Presence of cardiac and vascular implant and graft, unspecified**

✓4th Z96 Presence of other functional implants

EXCLUDES 2 complications of internal prosthetic devices, implants and grafts (T82-T85)
fitting and adjustment of prosthetic and other devices (Z44-Z46)

Z96.0 **Presence of urogenital implants**

Z96.1 **Presence of intraocular lens**

Presence of pseudophakia

✓5th **Z96.2** **Presence of otological and audiological implants**

Z96.20 **Presence of otological and audiological implant, unspecified**

Z96.21 **Cochlear implant status**

Z96.22 **Myringotomy tube(s) status**

Z96.29 **Presence of other otological and audiological implants**

Presence of bone-conduction hearing device
Presence of eustachian tube stent
Stapes replacement

Z96.3 **Presence of artificial larynx**

✓5th **Z96.4** **Presence of endocrine implants**

Z96.41 **Presence of insulin pump (external) (internal)**

Z96.49 **Presence of other endocrine implants**

Z96.5 **Presence of tooth-root and mandibular implants**

✓5th **Z96.6** **Presence of orthopedic joint implants**

Z96.60 **Presence of unspecified orthopedic joint implant**

Additional Character Required ✓x7th Placeholder Alert Unspecified Dx Other Specified Dx Manifestation ▶◀ Revised Text ● New Code ▲ Revised Code Title

-10-CM 2016 1131

✓6ᵗʰ **Z96.61 Presence of** artificial shoulder joint
    Z96.611 Presence of right **artificial shoulder joint**
    Z96.612 Presence of left **artificial shoulder joint**
    Z96.619 Presence of unspecified artificial shoulder joint

✓6ᵗʰ **Z96.62 Presence of** artificial elbow joint
    Z96.621 Presence of right **artificial elbow joint**
    Z96.622 Presence of left **artificial elbow joint**
    Z96.629 Presence of unspecified artificial elbow joint

✓6ᵗʰ **Z96.63 Presence of** artificial wrist joint
    Z96.631 Presence of right **artificial wrist joint**
    Z96.632 Presence of left **artificial wrist joint**
    Z96.639 Presence of unspecified artificial wrist joint

✓6ᵗʰ **Z96.64 Presence of** artificial hip joint
    Hip-joint replacement (partial) (total)
    Z96.641 Presence of right **artificial hip joint**
    Z96.642 Presence of left **artificial hip joint**
    Z96.643 Presence of artificial hip joint, bilateral
    Z96.649 Presence of unspecified artificial hip joint

✓6ᵗʰ **Z96.65 Presence of** artificial knee joint
    Z96.651 Presence of right **artificial knee joint**
    Z96.652 Presence of left **artificial knee joint**
    Z96.653 Presence of artificial knee joint, bilateral
    Z96.659 Presence of unspecified artificial knee joint

✓6ᵗʰ **Z96.66 Presence of** artificial ankle joint
    Z96.661 Presence of right **artificial ankle joint**
    Z96.662 Presence of left **artificial ankle joint**
    Z96.669 Presence of unspecified artificial ankle joint

✓6ᵗʰ **Z96.69 Presence of** other orthopedic joint **implants**
    Z96.691 Finger-joint replacement of right **hand**
    Z96.692 Finger-joint replacement of left **hand**
    Z96.693 Finger-joint replacement, bilateral
    Z96.698 Presence of other orthopedic joint implants

Z96.7 Presence of other bone and tendon implants
    Presence of skull plate

✓5ᵗʰ **Z96.8 Presence of other specified functional implants**
    Z96.81 Presence of artificial skin
    Z96.89 Presence of other specified functional implants

Z96.9 Presence of functional implant, unspecified

✓4ᵗʰ **Z97 Presence of other devices**
    EXCLUDES 1 complications of internal prosthetic devices, implants and grafts (T82-T85)
    fitting and adjustment of prosthetic and other devices (Z44-Z46)
    EXCLUDES 2 presence of cerebrospinal fluid drainage device (Z98.2)

Z97.0 Presence of artificial eye

✓5ᵗʰ **Z97.1 Presence of** artificial limb (complete) (partial)
    Z97.10 Presence of artificial limb (complete) (partial), unspecified
    Z97.11 Presence of artificial right **arm (complete) (partial)**
    Z97.12 Presence of artificial left **arm (complete) (partial)**
    Z97.13 Presence of artificial right **leg (complete) (partial)**
    Z97.14 Presence of artificial left **leg (complete) (partial)**
    Z97.15 Presence of artificial arms, bilateral **(complete) (partial)**
    Z97.16 Presence of artificial legs, bilateral **(complete) (partial)**

Z97.2 Presence of dental prosthetic device **(complete) (partial)**
    Presence of dentures (complete) (partial)

Z97.3 Presence of spectacles and contact lenses

Z97.4 Presence of external hearing-aid

Z97.5 Presence of (intrauterine) contraceptive device   Ⓜ♀
    EXCLUDES 1 checking, reinsertion or removal of contraceptive device (Z30.43)

Z97.8 Presence of other specified devices

✓4ᵗʰ **Z98 Other postprocedural states**
    EXCLUDES 2 aftercare (Z43-Z49, Z51)
    follow-up medical care (Z08- Z09)
    postprocedural complication—see Alphabetical Index

Z98.0 Intestinal bypass and anastomosis status
    EXCLUDES 2 bariatric surgery status (Z98.84)
    gastric bypass status (Z98.84)
    obesity surgery status (Z98.84)

Z98.1 Arthrodesis status

Z98.2 Presence of cerebrospinal fluid drainage device
    Presence of CSF shunt

Z98.3 Post therapeutic collapse of lung status
    Code first underlying disease

✓5ᵗʰ **Z98.4 Cataract extraction status**
    Use additional code to identify intraocular lens implant statu (Z96.1)
    EXCLUDES 1 aphakia (H27.0)
    Z98.41 Cataract extraction status, right **eye**
    Z98.42 Cataract extraction status, left **eye**
    Z98.49 Cataract extraction status, unspecified eye

✓5ᵗʰ **Z98.5 Sterilization status**
    EXCLUDES 1 female infertility (N97.-)
    male infertility (N46.-)
    Z98.51 Tubal ligation status
    Z98.52 Vasectomy status

✓5ᵗʰ **Z98.6 Angioplasty status**
    Z98.61 Coronary angioplasty status
      EXCLUDES 1 coronary angioplasty status with implant and graft (Z95.5)
    Z98.62 Peripheral vascular angioplasty status
      EXCLUDES 1 peripheral vascular angioplasty status wi implant and graft (Z95.820)

✓5ᵗʰ **Z98.8 Other specified postprocedural states**
    ✓6ᵗʰ **Z98.81 Dental procedure status**
      Z98.810 Dental sealant status
      Z98.811 Dental restoration status
       Dental crown status
       Dental fillings status
      Z98.818 Other dental procedure status
    Z98.82 Breast implant status
      EXCLUDES 1 breast implant removal status (Z98.86)
    Z98.83 Filtering (vitreous) bleb after glaucoma surgery status
      EXCLUDES 1 inflammation (infection) of postprocedur bleb (H59.4-)
    Z98.84 Bariatric surgery status
      Gastric banding status
      Gastric bypass status for obesity
      Obesity surgery status
      EXCLUDES 1 bariatric surgery status complicating pregnancy, childbirth, or the puerperium (O99.84)
      EXCLUDES 2 intestinal bypass and anastomosis status (Z98.0)
    Z98.85 Transplanted organ removal status
      Transplanted organ previously removed due to complication, failure, rejection or infection
      EXCLUDES 1 encounter for removal of transplanted organ—code to complication of transplanted organ (T86.-)
    Z98.86 Personal history of breast implant removal
    ✓6ᵗʰ **Z98.87 Personal history of in** utero procedure
      Z98.870 Personal history of in utero procedure during pregnancy
       EXCLUDES 2 complications from in utero procedure for current pregnancy (O35.7)
       supervision of current pregnan with history of in utero pr cedure during previous pr nancy (O09.82-)
      Z98.871 Personal history of in utero procedure while a fetus
    Z98.89 Other specified postprocedural states
      Personal history of surgery, not elsewhere classified

EXCLUDES 1 Not coded here   *EXCLUDES 2* Not included here   Ⓝ Newborn Age: 0   Ⓟ Pediatric Age: 0-17   Ⓜ Maternity Age: 12-55   Ⓐ Adult Age: 15-124   ᴾᴰˣ Primary

Z99   **Dependence on enabling machines and devices, not elsewhere classified**
     EXCLUDES 1   *cardiac pacemaker status (Z95.0)*

Z99.0   **Dependence on aspirator**

Z99.1   **Dependence on respirator**
     Dependence on ventilator

     Z99.11   **Dependence on respirator [ventilator] status**
         AHA: 2015, 1Q, 21

     Z99.12   **Encounter for respirator [ventilator]**   **PDx**
         dependence during power failure
         EXCLUDES 1   *mechanical complication of respirator [ventilator] (J95.850)*

Z99.2   **Dependence on renal dialysis**
     Hemodialysis status
     Peritoneal dialysis status
     Presence of arteriovenous shunt for dialysis
     Renal dialysis status NOS
     EXCLUDES 1   *encounter for fitting and adjustment of dialysis catheter (Z49.0-)*
              noncompliance with renal dialysis (Z91.15)
     AHA: 2013, 4Q, 125

Z99.3   **Dependence on wheelchair**
     Wheelchair confinement status
     Code first cause of dependence, such as:
         muscular dystrophy (G71.0)
         obesity (E66.-)

Z99.8   **Dependence on other enabling machines and devices**

     Z99.81   **Dependence on supplemental oxygen**
         Dependence on long-term oxygen
         AHA: 2013, 4Q, 129

     Z99.89   **Dependence on other enabling machines and devices**
         Dependence on machine or device NOS

Additional Character Required   **vx7th** Placeholder Alert   Unspecified Dx   Other Specified Dx   Manifestation   ▶◀ Revised Text   ● New Code   ▲ Revised Code Title

ppendix A: 10 Steps to Correct Coding

w the 10 steps below to correctly code encounters for health care services.

p 1: Identify the reason for the visit or encounter (i.e., a , symptom, diagnosis and/or condition).

medical record documentation should accurately reflect the patient's ition, using terminology that includes specific diagnoses and symptoms or ly states the reasons for the encounter.

sing the main term that best describes the reason chiefly responsible for ervice provided is the most important step in coding. If symptoms are nt and documented but a definitive diagnosis has not yet been rmined, code the symptoms. **For outpatient cases, do not code itions that are referred to as "rule out," "suspected," "probable," or stionable."** Diagnoses often are not established at the time of the initial unter/visit and may require two or more visits to be established. Code only is documented in the available records and only to the highest degree of inty known at the time of the patient's visit, unless it is an inpatient medical d, in which case uncertain diagnoses may be reported if documented at the of discharge.

p 2: After selecting the reason for the encounter, ays consult the alphabetic index before verifying code ction in the tabular section.

most critical rule is to begin code selection in the *alphabetic index*. Never first to the tabular list. The index provides cross-references, essential and ssential modifiers, and inclusion terms not found in the tabular list. To nt coding errors, always use both the alphabetic index (to identify a code) he tabular list (to verify a code), as the index does not include the important uctional notes found in the tabular list. An added benefit of using the lar list, which groups like things together, is that while looking at one code e list, a coder might see a more specific one that would have been missed he coder relied solely on the alphabetic index. Additionally, many of the s require a fourth, fifth, sixth, or seventh, character to be valid, and many of e characters can be found only in the tabular list.

p 3: Locate the main term entry.

alphabetic index is a listing of conditions, which may be expressed as nouns onyms, with critical use of adjectives. Some conditions known by several es have multiple main entries. Reasons for encounters may be located under ral terms such as admission, encounter, and examination. Other general s such as history of, status post, or presence (of) are used to locate factors encing health.

p 4: Read cross-references listed with the main term or subterm.

-references such as *"see"* and *"see also"* are identified by italicized type and ld always be checked to ensure that all alternative terms are researched.

p 5: Review entries for modifiers.

essential modifiers are the terms in parentheses following the main term . These parenthetical terms are supplementary words or explanatory mation that may or may not appear in the diagnostic statement and do not t code selection. The subterms listed under the main term are essential ifiers that do affect coding assignment. Each line of indent represents a specific code entry. The nonessential modifiers apply to the subterms wing a main term except when they are mutually exclusive, in which case ubterm takes precedence. For example, if "acute" is listed as a nonessential ifier but there is a subentry for "chronic," then the nonessential modifier of e" does not apply.

p 6: Interpret abbreviations, cross-references, default es, additional characters, and brackets.

bbreviation NEC (not elsewhere classified) that follows some main terms or erms indicates that there is no specific code for the condition even though nedical documentation may be very specific. The code next to the main is called the default code. It represents the condition most commonly ciated with the main term or the unspecified code for the main term. tional characters may be required to construct the code; the tabular list be referenced to determine what those specific characters should be. The abetic index uses brackets [] to enclose manifestation codes that can be

used only as secondary codes to the underlying condition code immediately preceding it. Both codes must be reported in this multiple-coding situation.

Step 7: Choose a potential code and locate it in the tabular list.

The coder must follow any Includes, Excludes 1 and Excludes 2 notes, and other instructional notes, such as "Code first" and "Use additional code," listed in the tabular list for the chapter, category, subcategory, and subclassification level of code selection that direct the coder to use a different or additional code. Any codes in the tabular range, A00.0- through T88.9-, may be used to identify the diagnostic reason for the encounter. The tabular list encompasses many codes describing disease and injury classifications (e.g., infectious and parasitic diseases, neoplasms, symptoms, nervous and circulatory system etc.).

Codes that describe symptoms and signs, as opposed to definitive diagnoses, should be used for reporting purposes when an established diagnosis has not been made (confirmed) by the physician. Chapter 18 of the ICD-10-CM code book, "Symptoms, Signs, and Abnormal Clinical and Laboratory Findings" (codes R00.--R99), contains many, but not all, codes for symptoms.

ICD-10-CM classifies encounters with health care providers for circumstances other than a disease or injury using codes in chapter 21, "Factors Influencing Health Status and Contact with Health Services" (codes Z00–Z99.8). Circumstances other than a disease or injury often are recorded as chiefly responsible for the encounter.

Step 8: Determine whether the code is at the highest level of specificity.

A code is invalid if it has not been coded to the full number of characters (greatest level of specificity) required. Codes in ICD-10-CM can contain from three up to seven alphanumeric characters. A three-character code is to be used only if the category is not further subdivided into four-, five-, or six-character codes. Placeholder character X is used both to allow for future expansion and as a placeholder for empty characters in a code that requires a seventh character but has no fourth, fifth, or sixth character. Certain categories require seventh characters that apply to all codes in that category. Always check the category level for applicable seventh characters for that category.

Step 9: Assign the code.

Having reviewed all relevant information concerning the possible code choices, assign the code that most completely describes the condition.

Repeat steps one through nine for all additional documented conditions that meet the following criteria:

- Conditions that currently exist at the time of the visit
- Conditions that require or affect patient care, treatment, or management

Step 10: Sequence codes correctly.

Sequencing is the order in which the codes are listed on the claim. List first the ICD-10-CM code for the diagnosis, condition, problem, or other reason for the encounter/visit, which is shown in the medical record to be chiefly responsible for the services provided. List additional codes that describe any coexisting conditions. Follow the official coding guidelines (see section II, "Selection of Principal Diagnosis"; section III, "Reporting Additional Diagnoses"; and section IV, "Diagnostic Coding and Reporting Guidelines for Outpatient Services") on proper sequencing of codes.

Coding Examples

Diagnosis: Anorexia

Step 1: The reason for the encounter was the condition, anorexia.

Step 2: Consult the alphabetic index.

Step 3: Locate the main term "Anorexia."

Step 4: There are no cross-references to check.

Step 5: Note that there are two possible subterms (essential modifiers), "hysterical" and "nervosa," neither of which is documented in this instance and therefore cannot be used in code selection. The code listed next to the main term is called the default code selection.

Step 6: There are no abbreviations, cross-references, additional character icons, or brackets.

Step 7: Turn to code R63.0 in the tabular list and read the instructional notes. In this case the Excludes 1 note indicates that anorexia nervosa and loss of appetite determined to be of nonorganic origin should be coded to a code from chapter 5. The diagnostic statement does not indicate nonorganic origin.

Step 8: There is no further division of the category past the fourth character subcategory. Therefore, the subcategory code level is the highest level of specificity.

Step 9: The default code, R63.0 Anorexia, is the correct code selection

Step 10: Since anorexia is listed as the chief reason for the health care encounter, the first-listed, or principal, diagnosis is R63.0. Note that this is a chapter 18 symptom code but can be assigned since the provider did not establish a more definitive diagnosis.

Diagnosis: Acute bronchitis

Step 1: The reason for the encounter was the condition, acute bronchitis.

Step 2: Consult the alphabetic index.

Step 3: Locate the main term "Bronchitis."

Step 4: There are cross-references to interpret.

Step 5: Review entries for modifiers. Since "acute" is not listed as a nonessential modifier, read past the "with" modifier until you find the subterm "acute or subacute" with a nonessential modifier of "with bronchospasm or obstruction," code J20.9.

Step 6: There are no abbreviations, cross-references, additional character icons, or brackets.

Step 7: Since there are no more appropriate subterms, turn to code J20.9 in the tabular list. The Includes note under category J20 does refer to other alternative terms for acute bronchitis. Note that the inclusion term list is not exhaustive but is only a representative selection of diagnoses that are included in the subcategory. The Excludes 1 note refers bronchitis and tracheobronchitis NOS to category J40. There are several Excludes 2 notes that, if applicable, can be coded in addition to this code.

Step 8: Note that the subcategories included in J20 represent acute bronchitis due to various infectious organisms that would be selected if identified in the documentation. In this case, the organism was not identified and there is no further division of the category past the fourth character subcategory. Therefore, the subcategory code level is the highest level of specificity.

Step 9: Assign code J20.9 Acute bronchitis, unspecified.

Step 10: Repeat steps 1-9 for any additional code assignments.

Diagnosis: Infectious diarrhea

Step 1: The reason for the encounter was the condition, infectious diarrhea.

Step 2: Consult the alphabetic index.

Step 3: Locate the main term "Diarrhea" in the alphabetic index.

Step 4: There are no cross-references to check.

Step 5: Review entries for modifiers. Note that the nonessential modifiers (in parentheses) after the main term do not include the term "infectious," which means that the coder should search the subterms for the term "infectious." The subterm "infectious" refers to code A09.

Step 6: There are no abbreviations, cross-references, additional character icons, or brackets.

Step 7: Locate code A09 in the tabular list, and read all instructional notes under the main category and subcategories. The Includes notes does not list the term "infectious diarrhea" under code A09; however, as instructed by the alphabetic index, you should code the condition to A09. The ICD-10-CM code book implies that infectious diarrhea is the same as infectious gastroenteritis, enteritis, and colitis.

Step 8: There is no further division of the category past the third-character category level. Therefore, the category code level is the highest level of specificity. The final code assignment would be A09.

Step 9: Assign code A09 Infectious gastroenteritis and colitis, unspecified.

Step 10: Since infectious diarrhea is listed as the chief reason for the health care encounter, the first-listed, or principal, diagnosis is A09.

Diagnosis: Decubitus ulcer of right elbow with skin loss and necrosis of subcutaneous tissue

Step 1: The reason for the encounter was the condition, decubitus ulcer.

Step 2: Consult the alphabetic index.

Step 3: Locate the main term "Ulcer" in the alphabetic index.

Step 4: There are no cross-references to check.

Step 5: This entry does not have any important nonessential modifier however, there are other terms such as ulcerated, ulcerating, etc., that included as main terms. Locate the subterm "decubitus" and note that there is an italicized cross-reference to "*see* Ulcer, pressure, by site." Go the subterm "pressure" and locate "elbow," which refers to code L89.0-

Step 6: Note that the code L89.0 is followed by a dash and an additio character icon, which indicate that more characters are required. From here, the tabular list can be consulted at code L89.0-.

Step 7: Locate code L89.0 in the tabular list, and check the category le L89 for any instructional, Includes, and Excludes 1 and 2 notes. Note th "decubitus" is an Includes note under L89 Pressure ulcer. Excludes 2 no indicate that if this were documented as a diabetic pressure ulcer, it w be necessary to use a code from chapter 4.

Step 8: Read through the subcategory codes under L89.0 and note th the fifth character describes laterality. Locate the right elbow at subcategory L89.01. See that an additional sixth character is now nee to complete the code. The sixth character specifies the stage of the ulc which can be determined either by the specific documentation of the stage (e.g., stage 1, stage 2) or in this case, a description that matches of the Includes notes that follow each stage code. For example, the description in this case of "skin loss and necrosis of the subcutaneous tissue" matches the Includes notes under L89.013 Pressure ulcer of rig elbow, stage 3.

Step 9: Assign code L89.013 Pressure ulcer of right elbow, stage 3

Step 10: Since the decubitus ulcer is listed as the chief reason for the health care encounter, the first-listed, or principal, diagnosis is L89.013 However, according to the Code first instructional note at the L89 cate level, gangrene would be sequenced before the pressure ulcer if it wer documented.

Diagnosis: First visit for bimalleolar fracture of the right ank due to trauma

Step 1: The reason for the encounter was the condition, bimalleolar fracture of the right ankle.

Step 2: Consult the alphabetic index.

Step 3: Locate the main term "Fracture" in the alphabetic index.

Step 4: Note that the first main term for Fracture is pathological with cross-reference to "*see also* Fracture, traumatic." Locate the main term "Fracture, traumatic."

Step 5: Review entries for nonessential modifiers. Locate the subterm "ankle," "bimalleolar." Note that "displaced" is a nonessential modifier following "bimalleolar," indicating that S82.84- is the default code unle the fracture is specified as nondisplaced.

Step 6: Note that code S82.84- is followed by a dash and an additiona character icon, both of which indicate that more characters are require From here, the tabular list can be consulted at code S82.84.

Step 7: Locate code S82.84 Bimalleolar fracture of lower leg, in the tab list and check the category level S82 for any instructional, Includes, an Excludes 1 and 2 notes. See the instructional notes indicating that fract not specified as displaced or nondisplaced default to displaced, and fractures not designated as open or closed default to closed. See also t list of appropriate seventh characters to be added to all codes from category S82.

Step 8: Read through the subcategory codes under S82.84, and note the sixth character specifies displaced or nondisplaced and laterality. Locate the displaced bimalleolar fracture of the right lower leg at code S82.841. See that an additional seventh character is still needed to complete the code. The seventh character specifies the type of encoun and whether the fracture is open or closed. Use character A listed in th box at the category level to describe initial encounter, closed fracture.

Step 9: Assign code S82.841A Displaced bimalleolar fracture of right lo leg, initial encounter for closed fracture.

Step 10: Since this is an injury code, code additionally any external ca place of occurrence, and activity codes, with the injury (fracture) sequenced first.

ppendix B: Valid 3-character ICD-10-CM Codes

9	Infectious gastroenteritis and colitis, unspecified
3	Tetanus neonatorum
4	Obstetrical tetanus
5	Other tetanus
6	Erysipelas
5	Chlamydial lymphogranuloma (venereum)
7	Chancroid
8	Granuloma inguinale
4	Unspecified sexually transmitted disease
5	Nonvenereal syphilis
Ø	Chlamydia psittaci infections
8	Q fever
6	Unspecified viral encephalitis
9	Unspecified viral infection of central nervous system
Ø	Dengue fever [classical dengue]
1	Dengue hemorrhagic fever
4	Unspecified arthropod-borne viral fever
9	Unspecified viral hemorrhagic fever
3	Smallpox
4	Monkeypox
9	Unspecified viral infection characterized by skin and mucous membrane lesions
Ø	Human immunodeficiency virus [HIV] disease
9	Unspecified mycosis
4	Unspecified malaria
9	Pneumocystosis
4	Unspecified protozoal disease
2	Dracunculiasis
5	Trichinellosis
9	Trichuriasis
Ø	Enterobiasis
6	Scabies
9	Unspecified parasitic disease
1	Sequelae of poliomyelitis
2	Sequelae of leprosy
1	Malignant neoplasm of base of tongue
7	Malignant neoplasm of parotid gland
2	Malignant neoplasm of pyriform sinus
9	Malignant neoplasm of rectosigmoid junction
Ø	Malignant neoplasm of rectum
3	Malignant neoplasm of gallbladder
3	Malignant neoplasm of trachea
7	Malignant neoplasm of thymus
2	Malignant neoplasm of vagina
5	Malignant neoplasm of uterus, part unspecified
8	Malignant neoplasm of placenta
1	Malignant neoplasm of prostate
3	Malignant neoplasm of thyroid gland
4	Benign neoplasm of thyroid gland
5	Polycythemia vera
2	Acute posthemorrhagic anemia
5	Disseminated intravascular coagulation [defibrination syndrome]
6	Hereditary factor VIII deficiency
7	Hereditary factor IX deficiency
1	Functional disorders of polymorphonuclear neutrophils
7	Other disorders of blood and blood-forming organs in diseases classified elsewhere
2	Subclinical iodine-deficiency hypothyroidism
5	Nondiabetic hypoglycemic coma
5	Disorders of endocrine glands in diseases classified elsewhere
Ø	Kwashiorkor
1	Nutritional marasmus
2	Marasmic kwashiorkor

E43	Unspecified severe protein-calorie malnutrition
E45	Retarded development following protein-calorie malnutrition
E46	Unspecified protein-calorie malnutrition
E52	Niacin deficiency [pellagra]
E54	Ascorbic acid deficiency
E58	Dietary calcium deficiency
E59	Dietary selenium deficiency
E6Ø	Dietary zinc deficiency
E65	Localized adiposity
E68	Sequelae of hyperalimentation
FØ4	Amnestic disorder due to known physiological condition
FØ5	Delirium due to known physiological condition
FØ9	Unspecified mental disorder due to known physiological condition
F21	Schizotypal disorder
F22	Delusional disorders
F23	Brief psychotic disorder
F24	Shared psychotic disorder
F28	Other psychotic disorder not due to a substance or known physiological condition
F29	Unspecified psychosis not due to a substance or known physiological condition
F39	Unspecified mood [affective] disorder
F42	Obsessive-compulsive disorder
F53	Puerperal psychosis
F54	Psychological and behavioral factors associated with disorders or diseases classified elsewhere
F59	Unspecified behavioral syndromes associated with physiological disturbances and physical factors
F66	Other sexual disorders
F69	Unspecified disorder of adult personality and behavior
F70	Mild intellectual disabilities
F71	Moderate intellectual disabilities
F72	Severe intellectual disabilities
F73	Profound intellectual disabilities
F78	Other intellectual disabilities
F79	Unspecified intellectual disabilities
F82	Specific developmental disorder of motor function
F88	Other disorders of psychological development
F89	Unspecified disorder of psychological development
F99	Mental disorder, not otherwise specified
GØ1	Meningitis in bacterial diseases classified elsewhere
GØ2	Meningitis in other infectious and parasitic diseases classified elsewhere
GØ7	Intracranial and intraspinal abscess and granuloma in diseases classified elsewhere
GØ8	Intracranial and intraspinal phlebitis and thrombophlebitis
GØ9	Sequelae of inflammatory diseases of central nervous system
G1Ø	Huntington's disease
G14	Postpolio syndrome
G2Ø	Parkinson's disease
G26	Extrapyramidal and movement disorders in diseases classified elsewhere
G35	Multiple sclerosis
G53	Cranial nerve disorders in diseases classified elsewhere
G55	Nerve root and plexus compressions in diseases classified elsewhere
G59	Mononeuropathy in diseases classified elsewhere
G63	Polyneuropathy in diseases classified elsewhere
G64	Other disorders of peripheral nervous system
G92	Toxic encephalopathy
G94	Other disorders of brain in diseases classified elsewhere
H22	Disorders of iris and ciliary body in diseases classified elsewhere
H28	Cataract in diseases classified elsewhere
H32	Chorioretinal disorders in diseases classified elsewhere
H36	Retinal disorders in diseases classified elsewhere

H42	Glaucoma in diseases classified elsewhere
I00	Rheumatic fever without heart involvement
I10	Essential (primary) hypertension
I32	Pericarditis in diseases classified elsewhere
I38	Endocarditis, valve unspecified
I39	Endocarditis and heart valve disorders in diseases classified elsewhere
I41	Myocarditis in diseases classified elsewhere
I43	Cardiomyopathy in diseases classified elsewhere
I52	Other heart disorders in diseases classified elsewhere
I76	Septic arterial embolism
I81	Portal vein thrombosis
I96	Gangrene, not elsewhere classified
J00	Acute nasopharyngitis (common cold)
J13	Pneumonia due to Streptococcus pneumoniae
J14	Pneumonia due to Hemophilus influenzae
J17	Pneumonia in diseases classified elsewhere
J22	Unspecified acute lower respiratory infection
J36	Peritonsillar abscess
J40	Bronchitis, not specified as acute or chronic
J42	Unspecified chronic bronchitis
J60	Coalworker's pneumoconiosis
J61	Pneumoconiosis due to asbestos and other mineral fibers
J64	Unspecified pneumoconiosis
J65	Pneumoconiosis associated with tuberculosis
J80	Acute respiratory distress syndrome
J82	Pulmonary eosinophilia, not elsewhere classified
J90	Pleural effusion, not elsewhere classified
J99	Respiratory disorders in diseases classified elsewhere
K23	Disorders of esophagus in diseases classified elsewhere
K30	Functional dyspepsia
K36	Other appendicitis
K37	Unspecified appendicitis
K67	Disorders of peritoneum in infectious diseases classified elsewhere
K77	Liver disorders in diseases classified elsewhere
K87	Disorders of gallbladder, biliary tract and pancreas in diseases classified elsewhere
L00	Staphylococcal scalded skin syndrome
L14	Bullous disorders in diseases classified elsewhere
L22	Diaper dermatitis
L26	Exfoliative dermatitis
L42	Pityriasis rosea
L45	Papulosquamous disorders in diseases classified elsewhere
L52	Erythema nodosum
L54	Erythema in diseases classified elsewhere
L62	Nail disorders in diseases classified elsewhere
L80	Vitiligo
L83	Acanthosis nigricans
L84	Corns and callosities
L86	Keratoderma in diseases classified elsewhere
L88	Pyoderma gangrenosum
L99	Other disorders of skin and subcutaneous tissue in diseases classified elsewhere
N08	Glomerular disorders in diseases classified elsewhere
N10	Acute tubulo-interstitial nephritis
N12	Tubulo-interstitial nephritis, not specified as acute or chronic
N16	Renal tubulo-interstitial disorders in diseases classified elsewhere
N19	Unspecified kidney failure
N22	Calculus of urinary tract in diseases classified elsewhere
N23	Unspecified renal colic
N29	Other disorders of kidney and ureter in diseases classified elsewhere
N33	Bladder disorders in diseases classified elsewhere
N37	Urethral disorders in diseases classified elsewhere
N51	Disorders of male genital organs in diseases classified elsewhere
N61	Inflammatory disorders of breast
N62	Hypertrophy of breast
N63	Unspecified lump in breast
N72	Inflammatory disease of cervix uteri
N74	Female pelvic inflammatory disorders in diseases classified elsewhere
N86	Erosion and ectropion of cervix uteri
N96	Recurrent pregnancy loss
O68	Labor and delivery complicated by abnormality of fetal acid-base balance
O76	Abnormality in fetal heart rate and rhythm complicating labor and delivery
O80	Encounter for full-term uncomplicated delivery
O82	Encounter for cesarean delivery without indication
O85	Puerperal sepsis
O94	Sequelae of complication of pregnancy, childbirth, and the puerperium
P09	Abnormal findings on neonatal screening
P53	Hemorrhagic disease of newborn
P60	Disseminated intravascular coagulation of newborn
P84	Other problems with newborn
P90	Convulsions of newborn
P95	Stillbirth
Q02	Microcephaly
R05	Cough
R12	Heartburn
R17	Unspecified jaundice
R21	Rash and other nonspecific skin eruption
R32	Unspecified urinary incontinence
R34	Anuria and oliguria
R37	Sexual dysfunction, unspecified
R42	Dizziness and giddiness
R51	Headache
R52	Pain, unspecified
R54	Age-related physical debility
R55	Syncope and collapse
R58	Hemorrhage, not elsewhere classified
R61	Generalized hyperhidrosis
R64	Cachexia
R69	Illness, unspecified
R75	Inconclusive laboratory evidence of human immunodeficiency virus [HIV]
R81	Glycosuria
R99	Ill-defined and unknown cause of mortality
T07	Unspecified multiple injuries
Y09	Assault by unspecified means
Y66	Nonadministration of surgical and medical care
Y69	Unspecified misadventure during surgical and medical care
Y95	Nosocomial condition
Z08	Encounter for follow-up examination after completed treatment for malignant neoplasm
Z09	Encounter for follow-up examination after completed treatment for conditions other than malignant neoplasm
Z21	Asymptomatic human immunodeficiency virus [HIV] infection state
Z23	Encounter for immunization
Z36	Encounter for antenatal screening of mother
Z66	Do not resuscitate

ppendix C: Pharmacology List 2016

s section enables the coder to quickly review drugs, drug actions, and indications that are often associated with overlooked or undocumented diagnoses.
e coder should review the patient's medication record and know what condition the physician is treating with the prescribed medication based on
cumentation in the medical record. When documentation is lacking, the coder can reference this section to locate the drug, determine the drug action,
nfirm drug indications, and when necessary query the physician.

rug	Drug Action	Indications
:cupril [quinapril]	ACE inhibitor; antihypertensive	Congestive heart failure; essential hypertension
:etaminophen and codeine :cetominophen/codeine phosphate]	Analgesic	Pain, moderate to severe
:temra [tocilizumab]	Antirheumatic	Rheumatoid arthritis
:tonel [risedronate]	Electrolytic and renal agent; bone resorption inhibitor	Decrease bone loss in multiple myeloma patients; Paget's disease; hyperparathyroidism; osteoporosis
dalat CC [nifedipine]	Calcium channel blocker	Vasospastic angina; chronic stable angina; essential hypertension
dactone [spironolactone]	Cardiovascular agent; antihypertensive agent; diuretic; electrolytic and renal agent	Treatment of severe heart failure; ascites associated with cirrhosis; hypokalemia
legra [fexofenadine/ hydrochloride seudoephedrine]	Antihistamine	Seasonal allergic rhinitis
lopurinol [allopurinol]	Antigout	Gouty arthritis, renal calculus, hyperuricemia, hyperuricemia secondary to leukemia, hyperuricemia secondary to lymphoma
phagan P [brimonidine]	Antiglaucoma agent (ophthalmic) antihypertensive, ocular	Open angle glaucoma or another condition in which pressure in the eye is too high (ocular hypertension)
prazolam [alprazolam]	Antianxiety; sedative/hypnotic	
tace [ramipril]	ACE inhibitor; antihypertensive	Congestive heart failure, essential hypertension
maryl [glimepiride]	Blood glucose regulator	Diabetes mellitus
mbien [zolpidem]	Sedative/hypnotic	Insomnia
oilify [aripiprazole]	Antipsychotic	Depression, bipolar disorder, schizophrenia, autism symptoms
mikacin [amikacin sulfate]	Aminoglycoside antibiotic	Active in treatment of gram-negative bacterial infections such as *Pseudomonas, Escherichia coli (E. coli), Proteus, Klebsiella-Enterobacter-Serratia*
minophylline [aminophylline]	Bronchodilator, pulmonary vasodilator, smooth muscle relaxant	Relief and/or prevention of symptoms from asthma and reversible bronchospasms in bronchitis and emphysema
mitriptyline hydrochloride mitriptyline hydrochloride]	Anorexiant/CNS stimulant; antidepressant	Depression
moxicillin, Amoxil [amoxicillin]	Penicillin	Effective for infections with a broad spectrum of bactericidal activity against many gram-positive and gram-negative micro-organisms; otitis media, gonorrhea, skin, respiratory, gastrointestinal, and genitourinary infections
mrix [cyclobenzaprine hydrochloride]	Muscle relaxant	Adjunct to rest and physical therapy for muscle spasms
ncef [cefazoline sodium]	Semisynthetic cephalosporin antibiotic	Respiratory tract infections due to *Streptococcus pneumoniae, Klebsiella species, Haemophilus influenzae (H. influenzae), Staphylococcus aureus*, and group A betahemolytic streptococci; urinary tract infections due to *E. coli*, Proteus mirabilis, Klebsiella species and some strains of Enterobacter and enterococci; skin and skin structure infections, biliary tract infections, bone and joint infections, genital infections, septicemia, and endocarditis
ntabuse [disulfiram]	Alcohol treatment	Alcoholism
nzemet [dolasetron mesylate]	Antiemetic/ antinauseant	Management of nausea/vomiting following surgery or from effects of chemotherapy or cancer
ranesp [darbepoetin alfa]	Erythropoiesis-stimulating agent (ESA)	Treat lower than normal blood cells (anemia) from disorders such as CKD and neoplasms
ricept [donepezil hydrochloride]	Acetylcholine sterase inhibitor	Symptoms of mild to moderate Alzheimer's disease; can improve thinking ability in some patients
rthrotec [diclofenac/misoprostol]	Analgesic	Treatment of patients with arthritis who may develop stomach ulcers from taking nonsteroidal anti-inflammatory drugs (NSAIDs) alone; used to help relieve some symptoms of arthritis, such as inflammation, swelling, stiffness, and joint pain

Drug	Drug Action	Indications
Atenolol [atenolol]	Antianginal; antihypertensive; beta blocker	Chronic stable angina pectoris; essential hypertension; reduces cardiovascular mortality in those with definite or suspected acute myocardial infarction
Ativan [lorazepam]	Antianxiety; sedative/hypnotic	Anxiety disorder associated with depressive symptoms; controls tension, agitation, irritability, and insomnia
Atrovent [ipratropium bromide]	Antiasthmatic/bronchodilator	Chronic bronchitis, emphysema; bronchial asthma
Augmentin [amoxicillin/clavulanate]	Antibacterial	Middle ear, lower respiratory, sinus, skin and skin structures, and urinary tract infections
Avapro [irbesartan]	Antihypertensive	Hypertension
Axid [nizatidine]	Histamine H2-receptor antagonist	Acid/peptic disorder; gastroesophageal reflux; duodenal, gastric, and peptic ulcers
Bactrim [sulfamethoxazole trimethoprim]	Antibacterial	Treatment of urinary tract infections, acute otitis media, acute exacerbation of chronic bronchitis, shigellosis, and pneumocystis carinii
Bactroban [mupirocin]	Dermatologic; topical anti-infective	Topical treatment of impetigo
Beconase AQ [beclomethasone dipropionate monohydrate]	Corticosteroids; antiasthmatic	Bronchial asthma, prevention of nasal polyps, perennial allergies, seasonal allergies and vasomotor rhinitis
Betoptic [betaxolol hydrochloride]	Cardioselective beta-adrenergic receptor blocking agent	Lowers intraocular pressure; also used for treatment of ocular hypertension and chronic open-angle glaucoma
Biaxin [clarithromycin]	Macrolide	Acid/peptic disorder or ulcer, acute exacerbation chronic bronchitis, human immunodeficiency virus, lower and upper respiratory tract infection, sinus infection, prophylaxis mycobacterium avium complex, pharyngitis, pneumonia, tonsillitis
Buspirone [buspirone hydrochloride]	Antianxiety	Generalized anxiety disorder
Butorphanol Tartrate [butorphanol tartrate]	Narcotic analgesic	Moderate to severe postsurgical pain
Calan [verapamil hydrochloride]	Antianginal; antiarrhythmic, antiarthritic, antihypertensive, calcium channel blocker	Angina pectoris at rest and chronic stable, arrhythmia, atrial fibrillation, atrial flutter, paroxysmal supraventricular tachycardia, ventricular arrhythmia, essential hypertension
Cardizem CD, Tiazac [diltiazem hydrochloride]	Antianginal, antiarrhythmic, antihypertensive, channel blocker, coronary vasodilator	Chronic stable angina, atrial fibrillation, atrial flutter, essential hypertension, paroxysmal supraventricular tachycardia
Cardura [doxazosin mesylate]	Antihypertensive	Benign prostatic hyperplasia, essential hypertension
Catapres, Clonidine [clonidine]	Antihypertensive	Hypertension
Ceftin [cefuroxime axetil]	Antibiotic: second generation cephalosporins	Acute exacerbation and chronic bronchitis, middle ear infection, sexually transmitted gonorrhea infection, upper respiratory tract infection, urinary tract infection, pharyngitis, tonsillitis
Cefprozil [cefprozil]	Antibiotic: second generation cephalosporins	Acute exacerbation and chronic bronchitis, lower respiratory tract infection, upper respiratory tract infection, pharyngitis, tonsillitis
Celebrex [celecoxib]	Antirheumatic, nonsteroidal anti-inflammatory	Relief of some symptoms caused by arthritis, such as inflammation, swelling, stiffness, and joint pain
Celexa [citalopram hydrobromide]	Antidepressant	Depression
Chantix [varenicline]	Smoking cessation aid	Nicotine addiction, smoking
Cipro [ciprofloxacin]	Anti-infective; quinolone	Cystitis, infectious diarrhea, gonorrhea, bone and joint infection, gastrointestinal tract infection, lower and upper respiratory tract infection, sinus infection, urinary tract infection, nosocomial pneumonia, chronic prostatitis
Claritin [loratadine/ pseudoephedrine sulfate]	Antihistamine	Seasonal allergic rhinitis, chronic idiopathic urticaria
Clonazepam, Klonopin [clonazepam]	Anticonvulsant	Absence, akinetic and myoclonic epilepsy, Lennox-Gastaut syndrome
Cogentin [benztropine mesylate]	Antiparkinsonism	Parkinson's disease
Colace [docusate sodium]	Gastrointestinal agent; laxative, stool softener	Constipation
Combivent [ipratropium bromide/albuterol sulfate]	Antiasthmatic/bronchodilator	Chronic bronchitis, emphysema; bronchial asthma
Compro [prochlorperazine] suppository form only	Antiemetic, antipsychotic	Nausea, vomiting, and manic phase of bipolar syndrome or schizophrenia

g	Drug Action	Indications
tisporin [hydrocortisone tate/neomycin sulfate]	Topical anti-infective, topical steroid	Dermatosis
madin [warfarin sodium]	Thrombolytic agent/anticoagulant	Prophylaxis and treatment of venous thrombosis, treatment of atrial fibrillation with embolization (pulmonary embolism), arrhythmias, myocardial infarction, and stroke prevention
aar [losartan]	Antihypertensive	Essential hypertension
stor [rosuvastatin calcium]	HMG-CoA reductase inhibitor (statin)	Hypercholesterolemia, hyperlipidemia, hyperproteinemia
xivan [indinavir sulfate]	HIV inhibitor	HIV, asymptomatic HIV
omel [liothyronine sodium]	Thyroid hormone	Treatment of hypothyroidism or prevention of euthyroid goiters
pro [oxaprozin]	Nonsteroidal anti-inflammatory drug (NSAID)	Osteoarthritis and rheumatoid arthritis
akote [divalproex]	Anticonvulsant	Bipolar affective disorder; complex absence, complex partial and mixed pattern epilepsy; migraine headache
ogen [desogestrel/ethinyl estradiol]	Contraceptive; estrogen/progestin	Contraception
rol [tolterodine tartrate]	Muscarinic receptor antagonist	Overactive bladders in patients with urinary frequency, urgency, or urge incontinence
ucan [fluconazole]	Antifungal agent	Oropharyngeal and esophageal candidiasis and cryptococcal meningitis in AIDS patients
oxin [digoxin]	Cardiotonic glycoside	Heart failure, atrial flutter, atrial fibrillation, and supraventricular tachycardia
antin [phenytoin sodium]	Anticonvulsant	Control of grand mal and psychomotor seizures
van [valsartan]	Ace inhibitor	Essential hypertension
xor XR [venlafaxine]	Antidepressant	Depression
nephrine [epinephrine]	Bronchodilator, cardiotonic	Most commonly used to relieve respiratory distress due to bronchospasm and to restore cardiac rhythm in cardiac arrest
vir, Epivir-HBV [lamivudine]	HIV and HBV inhibitor	HIV, hepatitis B (HBV), asymptomatic HIV
-TAB [erythromycin]	Acne product; macrolide; ocular anti-infective; topical anti-infective	Acne vulgaris, intestinal amebiasis, infectious conjunctivitis, diphtheria, endocarditis, prevention, erythrasma treatment of infections: endocervical, gynecologic, lower and upper respiratory tract; ophthalmic, rectal; skin and skin structures, and urethral; Legionnaires' disease, pelvic inflammatory disease, pertussis, pneumonia, rheumatic fever, prophylaxis, syphilis
race [estradiol]	Estrogen therapy	Vaginal cream used to treat vaginal and vulvar atrophy
raderm, Climara [estradiol]	Estrogen therapy	Osteoporosis prevention and to treat menopausal symptoms, vaginal and vulvar atrophy, hypoestrogenism, ovarian failure
sta [raloxifene hydrochloride]	Estrogen receptor modulator, selective osteoporosis prophylactic	Prevention of thinning of the bones (osteoporosis) only in postmenopausal women
voxate hydrochloride [flavoxate rochloride]	Urinary tract spasmolytic	Relief of dysuria, urgency, nocturia, suprapubic pain, frequency, and incontinence associated with cystitis, prostatitis, urethritis, and urethrocystitis/urethrotrigonitis
max [tamsulosin hydrochloride]	Benign prostatic hypertrophy therapy agent	Signs and symptoms of benign enlargement of the prostate (benign prostatic hyperplasia or BPH)
nase [fluticasone propionate]	Corticosteroid-inhalation/nasal; topical steroid	Corticosteroid-responsive dermatosis; perennial allergic and seasonal allergic rhinitis
vent HFA [fluticasone propionate]	Corticosteroid-inhalation/nasal; topical steroid	Corticosteroid-responsive dermatosis, perennial allergic and seasonal allergic rhinitis
amax [alendronate sodium]	Calcium metabolism	Osteoporosis; Paget's disease
sinopril sodium [fosinopril sodium]	ACE inhibitor; antihypertensive	Essential hypertension
cophage [metformin hydrochloride]	Blood glucose regulator	Diabetes mellitus antihyperglycemic drug used in the management of non-insulin-dependent diabetes mellitus (NIDDM)
cotrol [glipizide]	Oral blood-glucose-lowering agent	Adjunct to diet for the control of hyperglycemia in patients with noninsulin dependent diabetes mellitus (NIDDM, type II)
buride (micronized) [glyburide]	Blood glucose regulator	Diabetes mellitus
parin sodium [heparin sodium]	Anticoagulant	Prophylaxis and treatment of venous thrombosis, pulmonary embolism; prevention of cerebral thrombosis, and treatment of consumptive coagulopathies

Drug	Drug Action	Indications
Hydrochlorothiazide [hydrochlorothiazide]	Diuretic, antihypertensive	Management of hypertension and in adjunctive therapy for ede associated with congestive heart failure, hepatic cirrhosis, corticosteroid, and estrogen therapy
Hydrocodone bitartrate and acetaminophen [acetaminophen/ hydrocodone bitartrate]	Analgesic, general; analgesic-narcotic; antitussive/expectorant	Pain, moderate to severe
Hyzaar [hydrochlorothiazide/ losartan/potassium]	Antihypertensive	Hypertension
Imitrex [sumatriptan succinate]	Antimigraine	Migraine headache
Inderal [propranolol hydrochloride]	Beta-adrenergic blocking agent	Management of hypertension, long-term management of angi pectoris due to coronary atherosclerosis, cardiac arrhythmias
Isordil [Isosorbide dinitrate]	Smooth muscle relaxant	Acute anginal attacks
Isuprel [isoproterenol hydrochloride]	Adrenergic agent	Bronchodilator for asthma, chronic pulmonary emphysema, bronchitis, and other conditions accompanied by bronchospasr can be used in cardiogenic shock cases
K-Tab, Klor-Con [potassium chloride]	Replaces potassium and maintains potassium level	Hypokalemia
Keflex [cephalexin]	Antibacterial	Bone, middle ear, skin and skin structures, upper respiratory tra and urinary tract infections; acute prostatitis
Klonopin [clonazepam]	Anticonvulsant, anxiolytic - benzodiazepine	Epilepsy, seizures, panic disorder
Lamisil [terbinafine hydrochloride]	Antifungal	*Tinea cruris* (jock itch), *T. pedis* (athlete's foot), *T. corporis* (ringworm)
Lanoxin [digoxin]	Cardiotonic glycoside	Congestive heart failure
Lasix [furosemide]	Antihypertensive; diuretic	Management of edema associated with congestive heart failure renal disease, including nephrotic syndrome and hypertension
Lescol [fluvastatin]	HMG-CoA reductase inhibitor (statin)	Hypercholesterolemia; hyperlipidemia; hyperlipoproteinemia
Levaquin [levofloxacin]	Fluoroquinolone antibacterial	Acute exacerbation chronic bronchitis; cellulitis; furuncle; impeti infections of the lower and upper respiratory tract, sinus, skin ar skin structures, and urinary tract; pneumonia, community-acquired; pyoderma
Levoxyl [levothyroxine sodium]	Synthetic thyroid hormone	Euthyroid goiter; hypothyroidism
Lexapro [escitalopram oxalate]	Antidepressant—selective serotonin reuptake inhibitor (SSRI)	Depression, anxiety
Librium [chlordiazepoxide hydrochloride]	Antianxiety agent	Acute withdrawal symptoms, especially from alcohol, or for othe anxiety-producing conditions
Lidocaine [lidocaine hydrochloride]	Antiarrhythmic	Management of ventricular arrhythmias or during cardiac manipulation, such as cardiac surgery
Lipitor [atorvastatin calcium]	HMG-CoA reductase inhibitor (statin)	Hypercholesterolemia, hyperlipidemia, hyperproteinemia
Lithium [lithium carbonate]	Antimanic	Control of manic episodes in bipolar disorders
Lomotil [diphenoxylate hydrochloride with atropine]	Antidiarrheal	Treatment of symptoms of chronic and functional diarrhea
Lopid [gemfibrozil]	Lipid regulating agent	Hypercholesterolemia, hyperlipidemia, hyperlipoproteinemia, hypertriglyceridemia
Lopressor [metoprolol tartrate]	Antihypertensive, betablocker antianginal; antihypertensive; betablocker	Essential hypertension therapy, angina pectoris, and myocardial infarction
Lorazepam [lorazepam]	Antianxiety; sedative/hypnotic	Anxiety disorder associated with depressive symptoms; controls tension, agitation, irritability, and insomnia
Lotensin [benazepril]	ACE inhibitor; antihypertensive	Essential hypertension
Lotrel [amlodipine/benazepril]	Antihypertensive	Hypertension
Lotrisone [clotrimazole/ betamethasone]	Antifungal-corticosteroid	Relief of redness, swelling, itching, and other discomfort of fung infections
Lovastatin [lovastatin]	HMG-CoA reductase inhibitor (statin)	Hypercholesterolemia; hyperlipidemia, hyperlipoproteinemia
Macrodantin [nitrofurantoin]	Antibacterial	Urinary tract infection; prophylaxis
Meclinzine hydrochloride [meclizine hydrochloride]	Antihistamine	Management of nausea and vomiting, and dizziness associated with motion sickness

rug	Drug Action	Indications
edrol [methylprednisolone]	Glucocorticoid; anti-inflammatory	Acute/chronic adrenal insufficiency, congenital adrenal hyperplasia, adrenal insufficiency secondary to pituitary insufficiency; nonendocrine disorders include arthritis, rheumatic carditis, bronchial asthma, cerebral edema, and allergic, collagen, intestinal tract, liver, ocular, renal, and skin diseases
ethergine [methylergonovine maleate]	Oxytocic agent	Routine management of postpartum hemorrhage after delivery of placenta
iacalcin [calcitonin salmon]	Calcitonin; a peptide hormone	Hypercalcemia, osteoporosis, postmenopausal symptoms, Paget's disease
onoket [isosorbide mononitrate]	Antianginal; coronary vasodilator, nitrate	Angina pectoris
otrin [ibuprofen]	Analgesic, general; analgesic, non-narcotic; antiarthritic; antigout; antipyretic; NSAID	Osteoarthritis and rheumatoid arthritis, dysmenorrhea, fever; pain, mild to moderate
ultaq [dronedarone]	Cardiac rhythm regulator	Treatment of patients with recent episodes of atrial fibrillation or atrial flutter
abumetone [nabumetone]	Non-steroidal anti-inflammatory drug (NSAID)	Osteoarthritis and rheumatoid arthritis
aprosyn [naproxen]	Anti-inflammatory analgesic, general; analgesic, non-narcotic; antiarthritic; antigout; NSAID	Rheumatoid, gouty arthritis and osteoarthritis; ankylosing spondylitis; bursitis; dysmenorrhea; pain, mild to moderate; tendonitis
efazodone hydrochloride [nefazodone ydrochloride]	Antidepressant	Depression
embutal sodium [pentobarbital odium]	Sedative; hypnotic	Adjunct medication in diagnostic procedures or for emergency use with convulsive disorders
eurontin [gabapentin]	Anticonvulsant	Epilepsy, partial
exium [esomeprazole magnesium]	Proton pump inhibitor	Gastroesophageal reflux disease (GERD), erosive esophagitis
itropress [sodium nitroprusside]	Vasodilator	Potent, rapid action in reducing blood pressure in hypertensive crisis or for controlling bleeding during anesthesia by producing controlled hypotension
itrostat [nitroglycerin]	Muscle relaxant antianginal; antihypertensive; coronary vasodilator	Prophylaxis and treatment of angina pectoris; heart failure associated with myocardial infarction; hypertension, perioperative; surgery, adjunct
orpace [disopyramide]	Antiarrhythmic	Coronary artery disease, for prevention, recurrence and control of unifocal, multifocal, and paired PVCs
orvasc [amlodipine besylate]	Calcium channel blocker	Hypertension, chronic stable angina, and vasospastic angina
nglyza [saxagliptin]	Blood glucose regulator	Adjunct to diet and exercise for the control of hyperglycemia in patients with noninsulin-dependent diabetes mellitus (NIDDM, type II)
rphenadrine citrate [orphenadrine itrate]	Muscle relaxant	Acute spasms, tension, and post-trauma cases
rtho-Novum [norethindrone/ethinyl stradiol]	Contraceptive; estrogen/progestin	Contraception
xazepam [oxazepam]	Antianxiety	Anxiety, tension, and alcohol withdrawal
avabid [papaverine hydrochloride]	Vasodilator	Relief of cerebral and peripheral ischemia
axil [paroxetine]	Antidepressant	Anxiety with panic disorder and depression; obsessive-compulsive disorder
enicillin-VK [penicillin V potassium]	Natural penicillin	Chorea, prevention; endocarditis, prevention, secondary to tooth extraction; erysipelas; infections of the skin and skin structures, upper respiratory tract; rheumatic fever, prophylaxis; scarlet fever; Vincent's gingivitis; Vincent's pharyngitis
epcid [famotidine]	Histamine H2-receptor inhibitor	Acid/peptic disorder; adenoma, secretory; gastroesophageal reflux; duodenal and gastric ulcer; Zollinger-Ellison syndrome
ercocet, Roxicet [oxycodone and cetaminophen]	Analgesic, general; analgesic-narcotic	Pain, moderate to severe
ersantine [dipyridamole]	Platelet inhibitor	Therapy for chronic angina pectoris, preventing clots post heart valve surgery
henobarbital [phenobarbital sodium]	Barbiturate	Grand mal epilepsy
itocin [oxytocin]	Synthetic oxytocin	Induction or stimulation of labor at term

Drug	Drug Action	Indications
Plasmanate [plasma, plasma protein fraction]	Blood volume expander	Hypovolemic shock, burn patients, and hemorrhages when whole blood is unavailable
Plavix [clopidogrel bisulfate]	Antithrombotic platelet aggregation inhibitor	Lessening of the chance of heart attack or stroke
Plendil [felodipine]	Antihypertensive; calcium channel blocker	Essential hypertension
Pravachol [pravastatin]	HMG-CoA reductase inhibitor (statin)	Hypercholesterolemia, hyperlipidemia, hyperlipoproteinemia
Prednisone [prednisone]	Adrenocorticoid, corticosteroid	Used for its immunosuppressant effects and for relief of inflammations; used in arthritis, polymyositis and other systemic diseases
Pregnyl [chorionic gonadotropin]	Gonadotropic hormone	Prepubertal cryptorchidism, hypogonadism, corpus luteum insufficiency and infertility
Premarin [conjugated estrogens]	Antineoplastic; estrogen	Vasomotor symptoms associated with menopause; atrophic vaginitis; kraurosis vulvae, female hypogonadism; primary ovarian failure
Prempro [conjugated estrogens/medroxyproges- terone]	Estrogen/progestin	Menopause, osteoporosis, atrophic vaginitis
Prevacid [lansoprazole]	Proton pump inhibitor (PPI)	Acid/peptic disorder, erosive esophagitis, duodenal ulcer, Zollinger-Ellison syndrome
Prinivil [lisinopril]	Synthetic peptide derivative, long-acting angiotensin converting enzyme inhibitor	Congestive heart failure, essential hypertension
Prilosec [omeprazole]	Proton pump inhibitor	Acid/peptic disorder; endocrine adenoma; erosive esophagitis; systemic mastocytosis; gastroesophageal reflux; duodenal, peptic and gastric ulcer; Zollinger-Ellison syndrome
Procardia [nifedipine]	Antianginal agent; calcium channel blocker	Management of vasospastic angina and chronic stable angina, essential hypertension
Promethazine hydrochloride [promethazine hydrochloride]	Anesthesia, adjunct to; antiemetic; antihistamine; antitussive/expectorant; sedative/hypnotic; vertigo/motion sickness/vomiting	Anesthesia; adjunct; angioedema; conjunctivitis; dermographism; hypersensitivity, motion sickness; pain; perennial, seasonal, and allergic rhinitis; sedation, obstetrical; urticaria
Protonix [pantoprazole]	Proton pump inhibitor (PPI)	Short-term treatment and maintenance therapy of erosive esophagitis associated with gastroesophageal reflux disease (GERD)
Proventil-HFA [albuterol sulfate]	Antiasthmatic/bronchodilator	Asthma
Provera/Depo-Provera [medroxyprogesterone acetate]	Antineoplastic; contraceptive; progestin	Amenorrhea; carcinoma, endometrium, adjunct; carcinoma, renal, contraception; hemorrhage
Prozac [fluoxetine hydrochloride]	Serotonin reuptake inhibitor	Bulimia nervosa; depression; obsessive-compulsive disorder
Qnasl [beclomethasone dipropionate]	Corticosteroid	Perennial allergies, seasonal allergies, and vasomotor rhinitis
Quinidine gluconate [quinidine gluconate]	Antiarrhythmic	Management of cardiac arrhythmias
Qvar [beclomethasone dipropionate]	Corticosteroids; antiasthmatic	Prevention and control of symptoms related to asthma
Restoril [temazepam]	Sedative/hypnotic	Insomnia
Retrovir [zidovudine]	Antiretroviral agent	Indicated in symptomatic HIV infection
Risperdal [risperidone]	Antipsychotic/antimanic	Schizophrenia; bipolar I disorder
Ritalin [methylphenidate hydrochloride]	Central nervous system (CNS) stimulant	Treatment of depression and hyperkinetic activity in children
Sabril [vigabatrin]	Anticonvulsant	Refractory complex partial seizures
Septra [sulfamethoxazole trimethoprim]	Antibacterial	Treatment of urinary tract infections, acute otitis media, acute exacerbations of chronic bronchitis, and shigellosis
Serevent [salmeterol xinafoate]	Bronchodilator	Asthma
Sinemet [carbidopa, levodopa]	Antiparkinsonian	Parkinson's disease
Singulair [montelukast]	Antiasthmatic, leukotriene receptor antagonist	Treatment of mild to moderate asthma to decrease the symptoms of asthma and the number of acute asthma attacks
Soltamox [tamoxifen citrate]	Antineoplastic; hormonal/biological response modifier	Breast cancer
Solu-Medrol [methylprednisolone sodium succinate]	Adrenocorticosteroid	Anti-inflammatory and antiallergenic for shock and ulcerative colitis
Synthroid, Levothroid [levothyroxine sodium]	Thyroid hormone	Treatment of hypothyroidism

g	Drug Action	Indications
amet [cimetidine]	Acid reducer	Treatment of active duodenal ulcer, short-term treatment of active, benign gastric ulcer, and treatment of pathological hypersecretory conditions
retol [carbamazepine]	Anticonvulsant; analgesic	Epilepsy, especially with complex symptomatology; specific analgesic for trigeminal neuralgia
ormin [atenolol]	Antianginal; antihypertensive; beta blocker	Treatment of hypertension; lowering blood pressure lowers the risk of fatal and nonfatal cardiovascular events, primarily strokes and myocardial infarctions
azosin hydrochloride [terazosin rochloride]	Alphablocker; antihypertensive; diuretic	Benign prostatic hypertrophy; essential hypertension
radex [tobramycin and amethasone]	Aminoglycoside ocular anti-infective; anti-inflammatory	Infectious conjunctivitis; dermatosis, corticosteroid-responsive with secondary infection; foreign body in eye; corneal inflammation; uveitis
rol-XL [metoprolol succinate]	Antianginal antihypertensive beta blocker	Angina pectoris, essential hypertension
zodone hydrochloride [trazodone rochloride]	Antidepressant	Depression
amterene and hydrochlorothiazide amterene/ hydrochlorothiazide]	Antihypertensive, diuretic	Edema; essential hypertension
methoprim [trimethoprim]	Antibacterial	Acute exacerbation chronic bronchitis; travelers' diarrhea; infections of the middle, lower respiratory tract, and urinary tract; pneumonia, pneumocystis; shigellosis
ora-28 [ethinyl estradiol/ onorgestrel]	Contraceptive, estrogen/progestin	Contraception
ram [tramadol]	Analgesic, non-narcotic	Pain, moderate to moderately severe
phyl [theophylline]	Bronchodilator, pulmonary vasodilator, smooth muscle relaxant	Treatment of bronchial obstruction in asthma and chronic obstructive pulmonary disease
ium [diazepam]	Antianxiety, muscle relaxant, anticonvulsant	Anxiety, tension, withdrawal from alcohol, muscle spasms and anticonvulsant therapy; epilepsy, generalized tonic-clonic; status epilepticus; stiff-man syndrome; tetanus
otec [enalaprilat]	ACE inhibitor, antihypertensive	Congestive heart failure; essential hypertension
tolin HFA [albuterol, albuterol fate]	Antiasthmatic/bronchodilator	Asthma
apamil HCL, Calan [verapamil rochloride]	Antianginal, antiarrhythmic, antiarthritic, antihypertensive, calcium channel blocker	Angina pectoris, chronic stable angina, atrial fibrillation, atrial flutter, paroxysmal supraventricular tachycardia, ventricular arrhythmia, essential hypertension
gra [sildenafil citrate]	Phosphodiesterase-5 (PDE5) inhibitor	Erectile dysfunction
toza [liraglutide recombinant]	Glucagon-like peptide-1 (GLP-1) receptor agonist	Adjunct to diet and exercise for the control of hyperglycemia in patients with noninsulin-dependent diabetes mellitus (NIDDM, type II)
taril [hydroxyzine pamoate]	Antianxiety agent, antiemetic	Treatment of nausea and vomiting, for reducing narcotic requirement in surgery and as tranquilizer for tension, anxiety, or agitation states
llbutrin SR, Welbutrin XL [bupropion drochloride]	Antidepressant; CNS	Depression; smoking cessation
latan [latanoprost]	Prostaglandin F2α analogue	Glaucoma, open-angle; ocular hypertension
nax, Xanax XR [alprazolam]	Antianxiety; sedative/hypnotic	Anxiety disorders with panic disorder and depression
ris [drotrecogin alfa]	Biologic response modifier	Severe sepsis
ntac [ranitidine hydrochloride]	Histamine H2-receptors inhibitor	Acid/peptic disorder, erosive esophagitis, gastrointestinal hypersecretion, mastocytosis, gastroesophageal reflux, peptic ulcer, Zollinger-Ellison syndrome
storetic [lisinopril and drochlorothiazide]	ACE inhibitor; antihypertensive	Congestive heart failure; essential hypertension
stril [lisinopril]	ACE inhibitor; antihypertensive	Congestive heart failure; essential hypertension
c [bisoprolol fumarate/ drochlorothiazide]	Antihypertensive	Essential hypertension
hromax [azithromycin]	Macrolide	Infections of the cervix, lower respiratory tract, skin and skin structures, urethra, nongonococcal; mycobacterium avium complex; pharyngitis, streptococcal pneumonia; tonsillitis

Drug	Drug Action	Indications
Zocor [simvastatin]	HMG-CoA reductase inhibitor (statin)	Hypercholesterolemia, hyperlipidemia, hyperlipoproteinemia, hypertriglyceridemia
Zoloft [sertraline hydrochloride]	Antidepressant	Anxiety with panic disorder and depression; obsessive-compuls disorder
Zovirax [acyclovir]	Antiviral	Genital herpes and herpes zoster infections
Zyloprim [allopurinol]	Antigout	Gouty arthritis, renal calculus, hyperuricemia, hyperuricemia secondary to leukemia, hyperuricemia secondary to lymphoma
Zyprexa [olanzapine]	Antipsychotic/antimanic	Psychotic disorders; schizophrenia
Zyrtec [cetirizine hydrochloride]	Antihistamine	Perennial allergic and seasonal allergic rhinitis; chronic urticaria

ppendix D: Z Codes for Long-Term Drug Use with Associated Drugs

.Ø1 Long term (current) use of anticoagulants
Arixtra
Coumadin
Eliquis
Heparin
Jantoven
Lovenox
Pradaxa
Warfarin
Xarelto

.Ø2 Long term (current) use of antithrombotics/antiplatelets
Aggrenox
Aggrastat
Clopidogrel
Clopidogrel bisulfate
Effient
Persantine
Plavix
Pletal
Pradaxa
Ticlid

.1 Long term (current) use of non-steroidal anti-inflammatories (NSAID)
Advil
Aleve
Anaprox
Celebrex
Clinoril
Daypro
Feldene
Ibuprofen
Indocin
Lodine
Motrin
Nalfon
Naprosyn
Orudis
Ponstel
Relafen
Tolectin
Toradol
Voltaren

.2 Long term (current) use of antibiotics
Amikin
Amoxicillin
Amoxil
Ampicillin
Ancef

Augmentin
Azactam
Azithromycin
Bactrim
Cefaclor
Ceftriaxone
Cephalexin
Cephalosporin
Cipro
Ciprofloxacin
Clarithromycin
Cleocin
Clindamycin
Co-trimoxazole
Daptomycin
Dificid
Doxycycline
Ertapenem
ERYC
Erythromycin
Factive
Flagyl
Flucloxacillin
Gentamicin
Isoniazid
Invanz
Keflex
Levaquin
Macrobid
Merrem
Metronidazole
Minocin
Nitrofurantoin
Omnipen
Ornidazole
Penicillin G
Penicillin V
Polycillin
Primaxin
Rifampicin
Rocephin
Septra
Streptomycin
Tazicef
Tazocin
Tetracycline HCl
Timentin
Trimethoprim
Tobramycin
Unipen
Vancocin
Vancomycin
Vibramycin

Zinacef
Zithromax
Zosyn
Zyvox

Z79.3 Long term (current) use of hormonal contraceptives
Oral
   Combined oral contraceptive
   Progestin-only pills
Patch
   Ortho Evra
Injectable
   DMPA—depo medroxyprogesterone acetate
Vaginal Ring
   NuvaRing
Implantable rods
   Implanon

Z79.4 Long term (current) use of insulin
Apidra
Humalog
Humulin
Lantus
Levemir
Novolin
NovoLog
Velosulin

Z79.51 Long term (current) use of inhaled steroids
Advair
Aerospan
Alvesco
Asmanex Twisthaler
Dulera
Flovent
Pulmicort
Qvar
Symbicort

Z79.52 Long term (current) use of systemic steroids
Cortef
Cortisone acetate
Depo-Medrol
Dexamethasone
Hydrocortisone
Kenalog
Medrol
Methylprednisolone
Prednisolone
Prednisone
Solu-Medrol

Z79.810 Long term (current) use of selective estrogen receptor modulators (SERMs)
Evista
Fareston
Nolvadex
Osphena
Raloxifene
Soltamox
Tamoxifen
Toremifene

Z79.811 Long term (current) use of aromatase inhibitors
Anastrozole
Arimidex
Aromasin
Exemestane
Femara
Letrozole

Z79.818 Long term (current) use of other agents affecting estrogen receptors and estrogen levels
Eligard
Faslodex
Fulvestrant
Lupron
Megace
Supprelin La
Synarel
Trelstar
Vantas
Viadur
Zoladex

Z79.82 Long term (current) use of aspirin
Bayer
Ecotrin
Bufferin

Z79.83 Long term (current) use of bisphosphonates
Actonel
Aredia
Atelvia
Binosto
Boniva

Didronel
Fosamax
Reclast
Zometa

Z79.890 Hormone replacement therapy (postmenopausal)
Activella
Alora
Angeliq
Climara
Enjuvia
Estrace
Estratest
EstroGel
Femring
Femtrace
Menostar
Premarin
Provera
Vivelle

Z79.891 Long term (current) use of opiate analgesic
Astramorph
Avinza
Buprenex
Buprenorphine
Codeine
Demerol
Dilaudid
Duragesic
Duramorph
Fentanyl
Fentora
Fioricet with codeine
Hydrocodone
Hydromorphone
Kadian
Lorcet
Lortab
Methadone HCL
Methadose
Morphine
MS Contin
Norco
Oxycodone

OxyContin
Percocet
Roxicodone
Sublimaze
Tylenol with codeine
Ultram

Z79.899 Other long term (current) drug therapy]
Actimmune
Antineoplastic/chemotherapy
Astagraf XL
Avonex
Cellcept
Cyclosporin
Envarsus XR
Gengraf
Imuran
Interferon
Monoclonal antibodies
Neoral
Orthoclone OKT3
Peginterferon
Prograf
Protopic
Rapamune
Rebif
Sandimmune
Simulect
Sirolimus
Sylatron
Tacrolimus
Torisel
Zenapax

ppendix E: Z Code Only as Principal Diagnosis List

0.00	Z01.20	Z02.3	Z03.810	Z34.00	Z38.4	Z51.11	Z52.4
0.01	Z01.21	Z02.4	Z03.818	Z34.01	Z38.5	Z51.12	Z52.5
0.110	Z01.30	Z02.5	Z03.89	Z34.02	Z38.61	Z52.000	Z52.6
0.111	Z01.31	Z02.6	Z04.1	Z34.03	Z38.62	Z52.001	Z52.810
0.121	Z01.411	Z02.71	Z04.2	Z34.80	Z38.63	Z52.008	Z52.811
0.129	Z01.419	Z02.79	Z04.3	Z34.81	Z38.64	Z52.010	Z52.812
0.2	Z01.42	Z02.81	Z04.41	Z34.82	Z38.65	Z52.011	Z52.813
0.3	Z01.810	Z02.82	Z04.42	Z34.83	Z38.66	Z52.018	Z52.819
0.5	Z01.811	Z02.83	Z04.6	Z34.90	Z38.68	Z52.090	Z52.89
0.70	Z01.812	Z02.89	Z04.71	Z34.91	Z38.69	Z52.091	Z76.1
0.71	Z01.818	Z02.9	Z04.72	Z34.92	Z38.7	Z52.098	Z76.2
0.8	Z01.82	Z03.6	Z04.8	Z34.93	Z38.8	Z52.10	Z99.12
1.00	Z01.83	Z03.71	Z04.9	Z38.00	Z39.0	Z52.11	
1.01	Z01.84	Z03.72	Z31.81	Z38.01	Z39.1	Z52.19	
1.10	Z01.89	Z03.73	Z31.82	Z38.1	Z39.2	Z52.20	
1.110	Z02.0	Z03.74	Z31.83	Z38.2	Z42.1	Z52.21	
1.118	Z02.1	Z03.75	Z31.84	Z38.30	Z42.8	Z52.29	
1.12	Z02.2	Z03.79	Z33.2	Z38.31	Z51.0	Z52.3	

Peripheral Nervous System

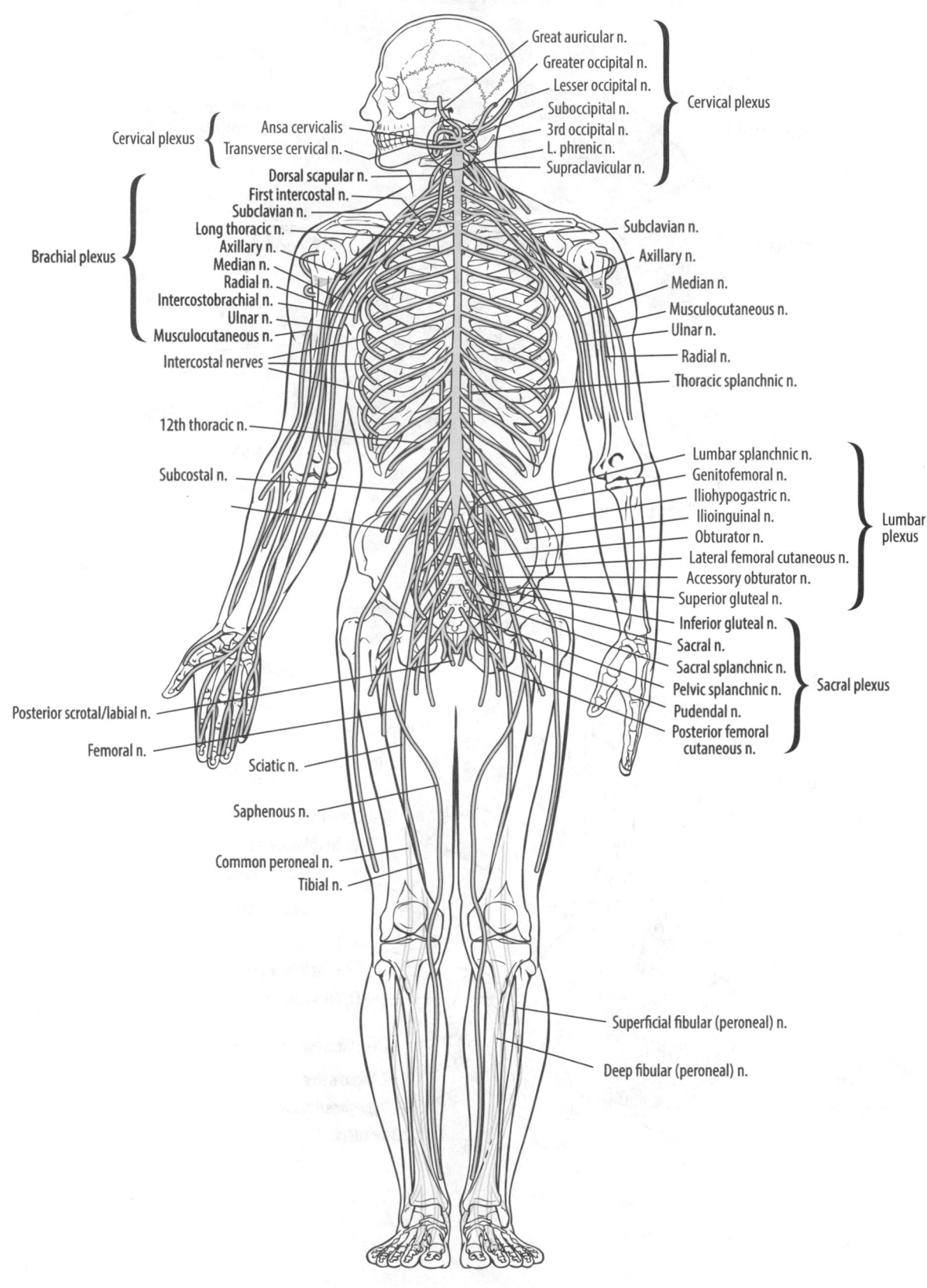

Great auricular n.
Greater occipital n.
Lesser occipital n.
Suboccipital n.
3rd occipital n.
L. phrenic n.
Supraclavicular n.

Cervical plexus

Cervical plexus
Ansa cervicalis
Transverse cervical n.

Dorsal scapular n.
First intercostal n.
Subclavian n.
Long thoracic n.
Axillary n.
Median n.
Radial n.
Intercostobrachial n.
Ulnar n.
Musculocutaneous n.

Brachial plexus

Intercostal nerves

12th thoracic n.

Subcostal n.

Subclavian n.
Axillary n.
Median n.
Musculocutaneous n.
Ulnar n.
Radial n.
Thoracic splanchnic n.

Lumbar splanchnic n.
Genitofemoral n.
Iliohypogastric n.
Ilioinguinal n.
Obturator n.
Lateral femoral cutaneous n.
Accessory obturator n.
Superior gluteal n.

Lumbar plexus

Inferior gluteal n.
Sacral n.
Sacral splanchnic n.
Pelvic splanchnic n.
Pudendal n.
Posterior femoral cutaneous n.

Sacral plexus

Posterior scrotal/labial n.

Femoral n.

Sciatic n.

Saphenous n.

Common peroneal n.
Tibial n.

Superficial fibular (peroneal) n.

Deep fibular (peroneal) n.

Brain

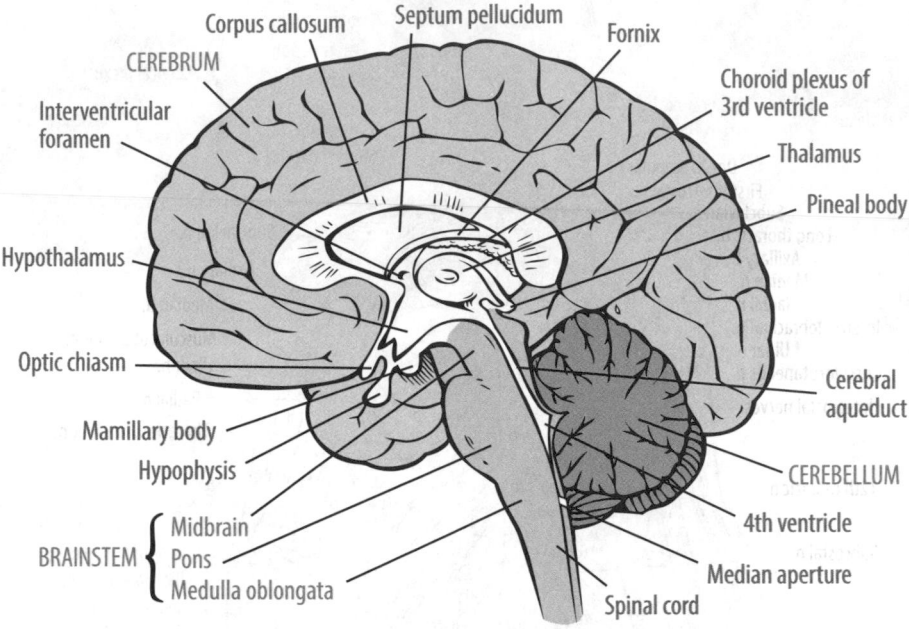

Corpus callosum · Septum pellucidum · Fornix

CEREBRUM

Interventricular foramen

Hypothalamus

Optic chiasm

Mamillary body

Hypophysis

BRAINSTEM { Midbrain
Pons
Medulla oblongata

Choroid plexus of 3rd ventricle

Thalamus

Pineal body

Cerebral aqueduct

CEREBELLUM

4th ventricle

Median aperture

Spinal cord

Cranial Nerves

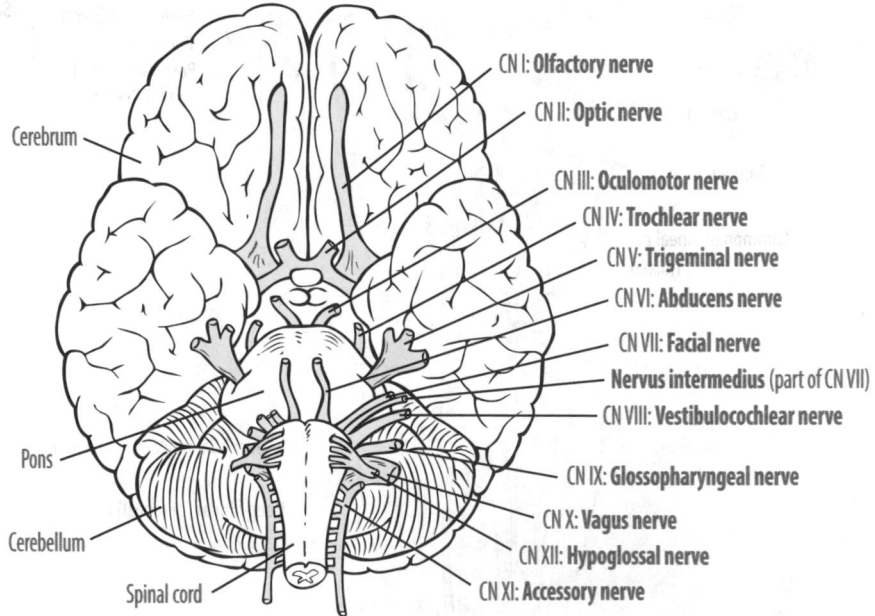

Cerebrum

Pons

Cerebellum

Spinal cord

CN I: **Olfactory nerve**

CN II: **Optic nerve**

CN III: **Oculomotor nerve**

CN IV: **Trochlear nerve**

CN V: **Trigeminal nerve**

CN VI: **Abducens nerve**

CN VII: **Facial nerve**

Nervus intermedius (part of CN VII)

CN VIII: **Vestibulocochlear nerve**

CN IX: **Glossopharyngeal nerve**

CN X: **Vagus nerve**

CN XII: **Hypoglossal nerve**

CN XI: **Accessory nerve**

Eye

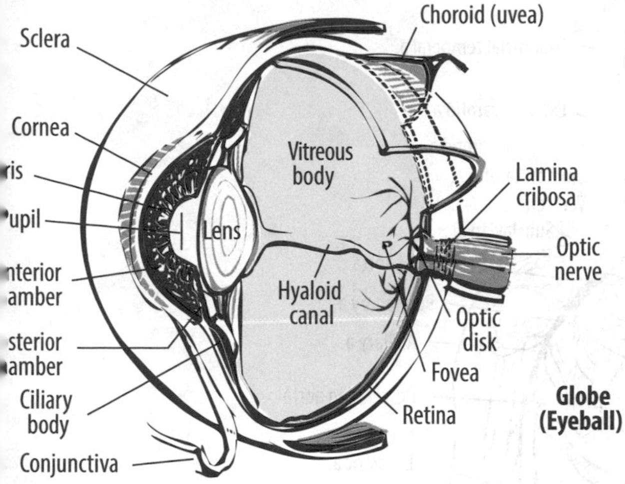

Sclera
Cornea
Iris
Pupil
Anterior chamber
Posterior chamber
Ciliary body
Conjunctiva

Choroid (uvea)
Vitreous body
Lamina cribosa
Lens
Optic nerve
Hyaloid canal
Optic disk
Fovea
Retina

Globe (Eyeball)

Lacrimal System

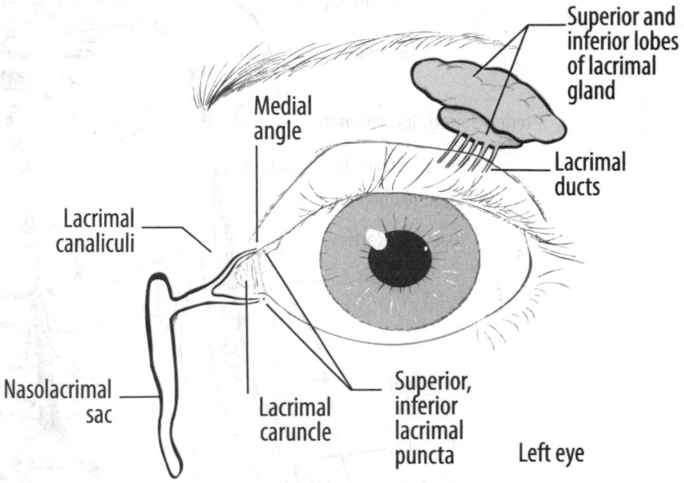

Superior and inferior lobes of lacrimal gland
Medial angle
Lacrimal ducts
Lacrimal canaliculi
Nasolacrimal sac
Lacrimal caruncle
Superior, inferior lacrimal puncta

Left eye

Posterior Pole of Globe

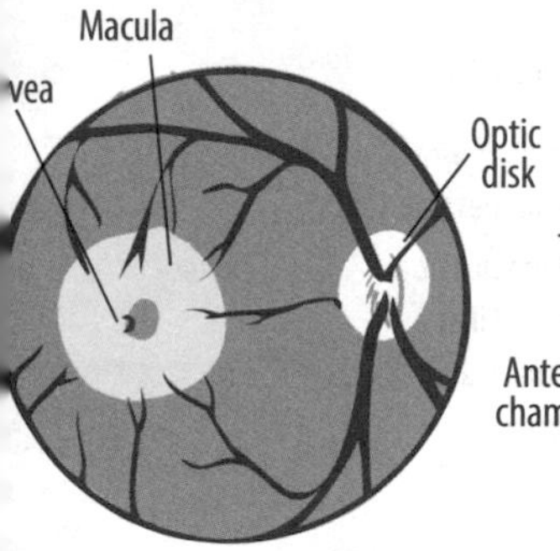

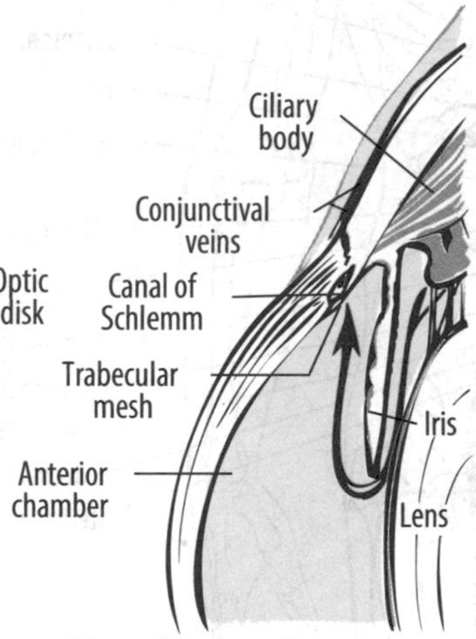

Macula
Fovea
Optic disk

Ciliary body
Conjunctival veins
Canal of Schlemm
Trabecular mesh
Anterior chamber
Iris
Lens

Flow of Aqueous Humor

Ear and Mastoid

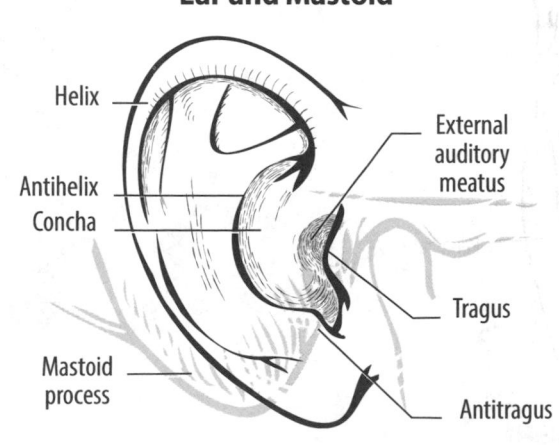

Helix
Antihelix
Concha
Mastoid process
External auditory meatus
Tragus
Antitragus

Middle Ear

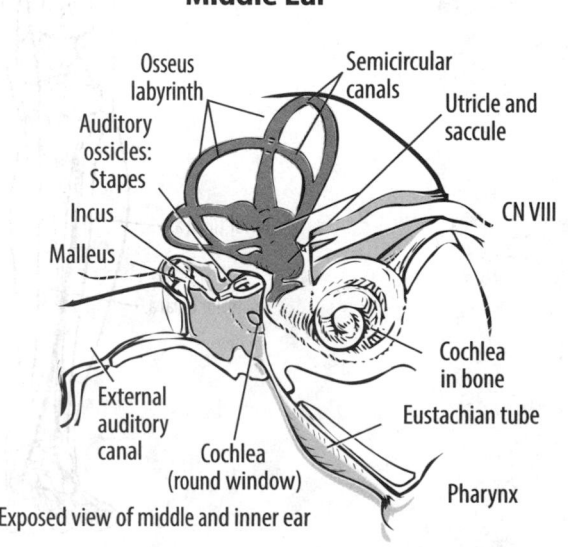

Osseus labyrinth
Auditory ossicles: Stapes
Incus
Malleus
Semicircular canals
Utricle and saccule
CN VIII
Cochlea in bone
Eustachian tube
External auditory canal
Cochlea (round window)
Pharynx

Exposed view of middle and inner ear

Arteries

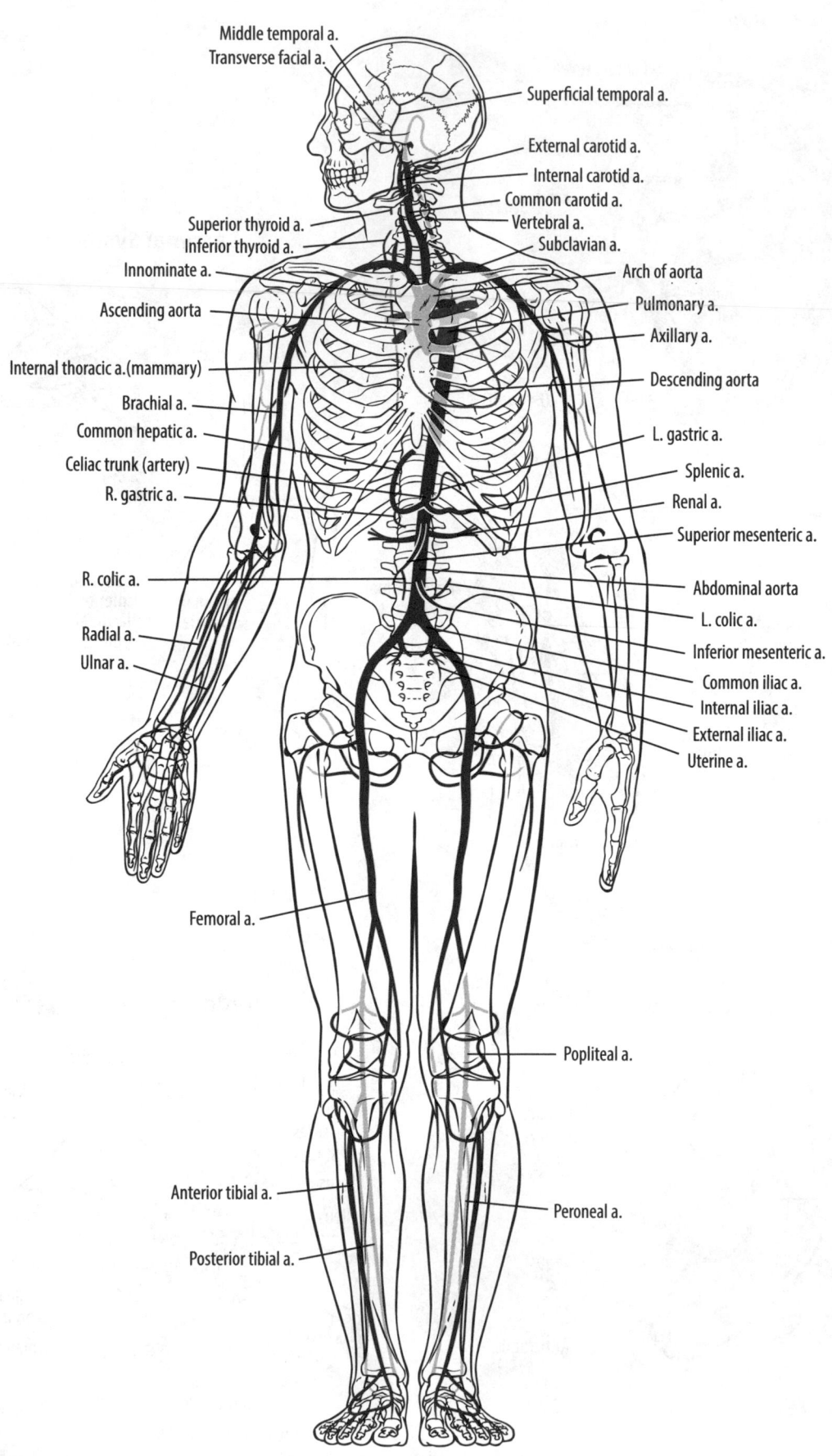

Middle temporal a.
Transverse facial a.
Superficial temporal a.
External carotid a.
Internal carotid a.
Common carotid a.
Superior thyroid a.
Vertebral a.
Inferior thyroid a.
Subclavian a.
Innominate a.
Arch of aorta
Ascending aorta
Pulmonary a.
Axillary a.
Internal thoracic a.(mammary)
Descending aorta
Brachial a.
Common hepatic a.
L. gastric a.
Celiac trunk (artery)
Splenic a.
R. gastric a.
Renal a.
Superior mesenteric a.
R. colic a.
Abdominal aorta
L. colic a.
Radial a.
Inferior mesenteric a.
Ulnar a.
Common iliac a.
Internal iliac a.
External iliac a.
Uterine a.
Femoral a.
Popliteal a.
Anterior tibial a.
Peroneal a.
Posterior tibial a.

Veins

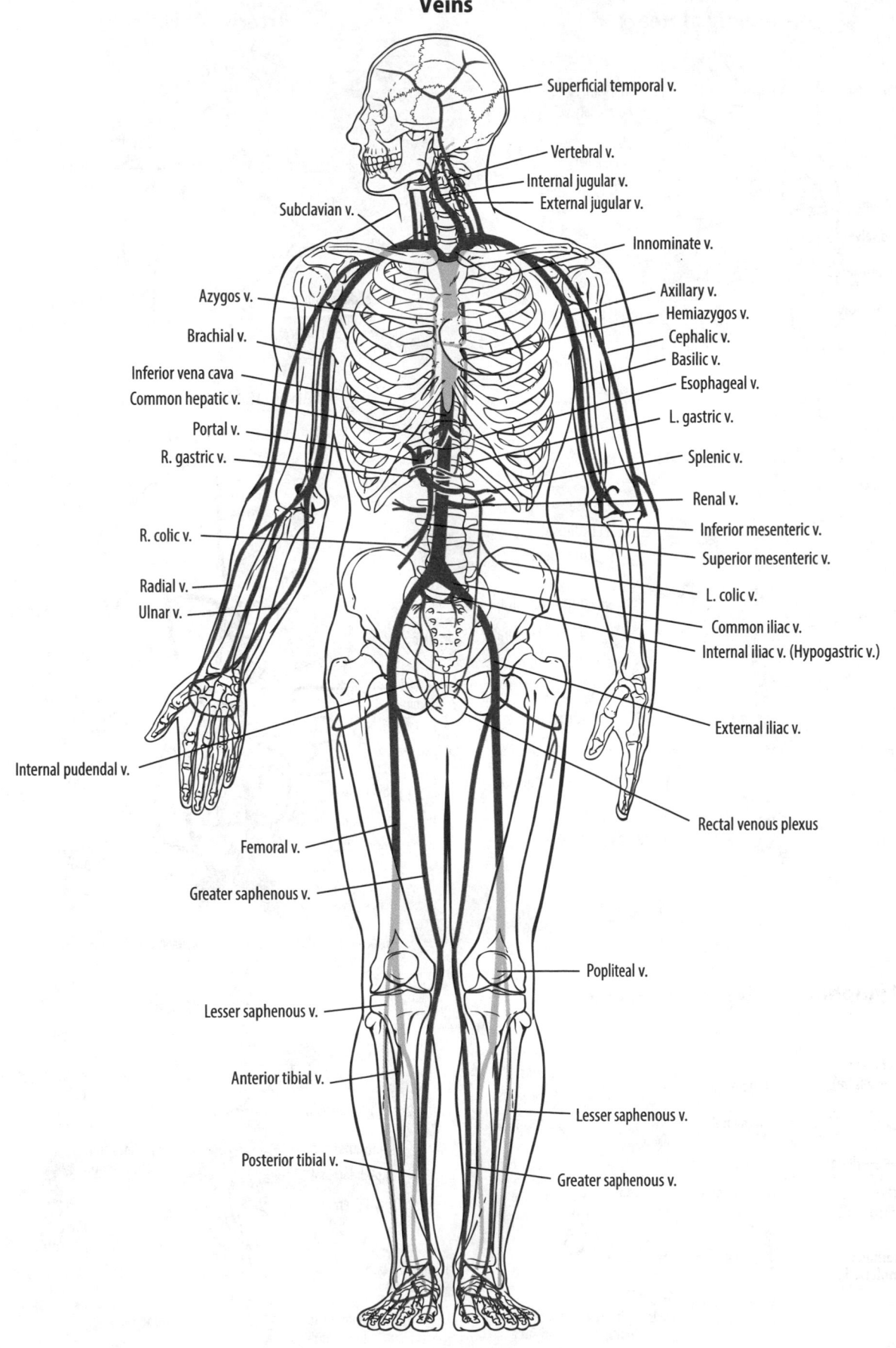

Superficial temporal v.

Vertebral v.

Internal jugular v.

External jugular v.

Subclavian v.

Innominate v.

Axillary v.

Azygos v.

Hemiazygos v.

Brachial v.

Cephalic v.

Basilic v.

Inferior vena cava

Esophageal v.

Common hepatic v.

L. gastric v.

Portal v.

R. gastric v.

Splenic v.

Renal v.

R. colic v.

Inferior mesenteric v.

Superior mesenteric v.

Radial v.

L. colic v.

Ulnar v.

Common iliac v.

Internal iliac v. (Hypogastric v.)

External iliac v.

Internal pudendal v.

Rectal venous plexus

Femoral v.

Greater saphenous v.

Popliteal v.

Lesser saphenous v.

Anterior tibial v.

Lesser saphenous v.

Posterior tibial v.

Greater saphenous v.

Anatomy of Heart

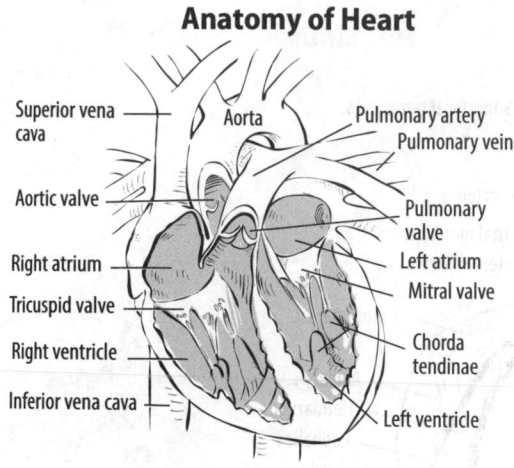

Arteries of Heart

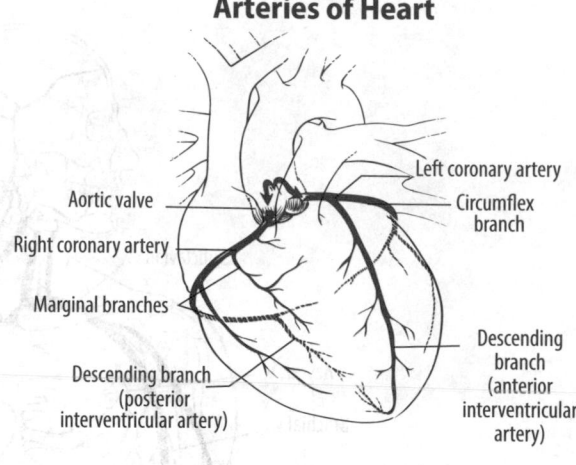

Cerebrovascular Arteries

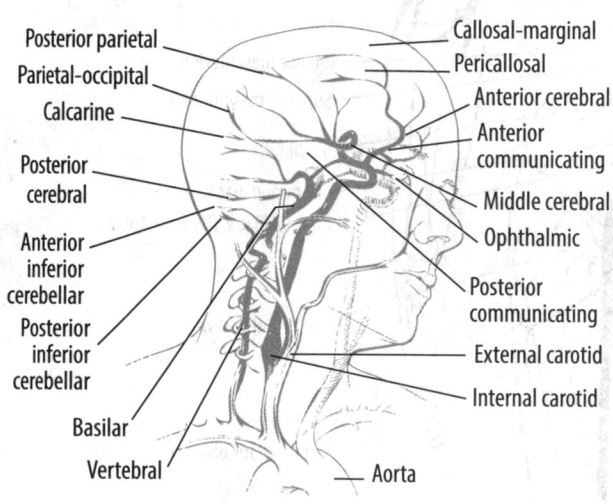

Veins of Head and Neck

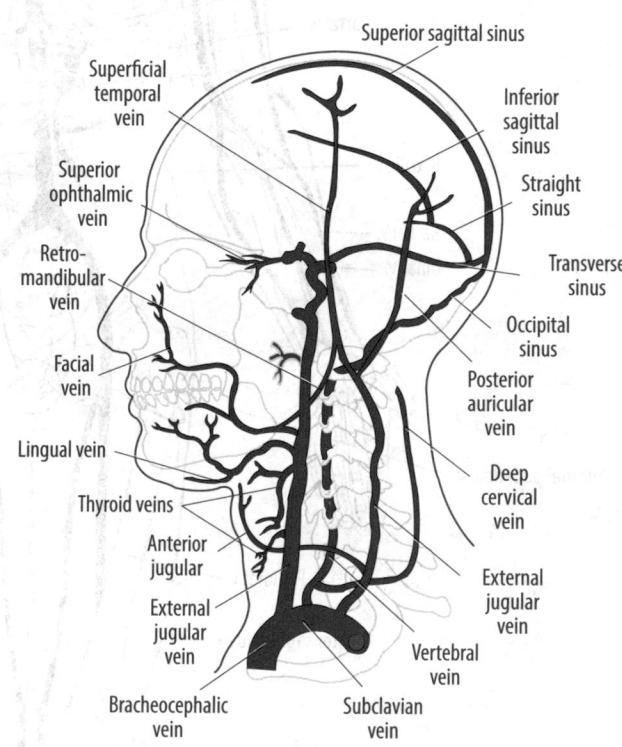

Lymphatic System of Head and Neck

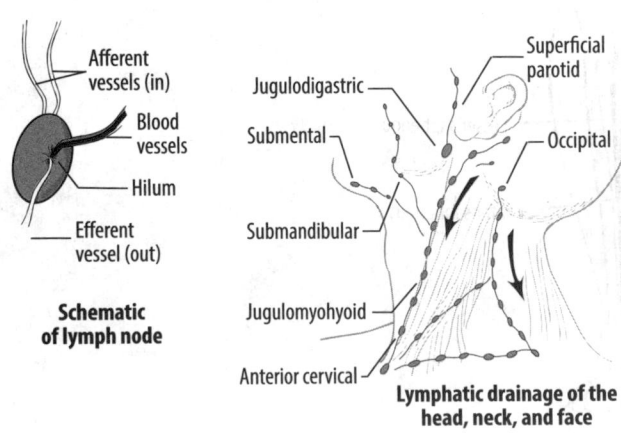

Schematic of lymph node

Lymphatic drainage of the head, neck, and face

Lymph Nodes

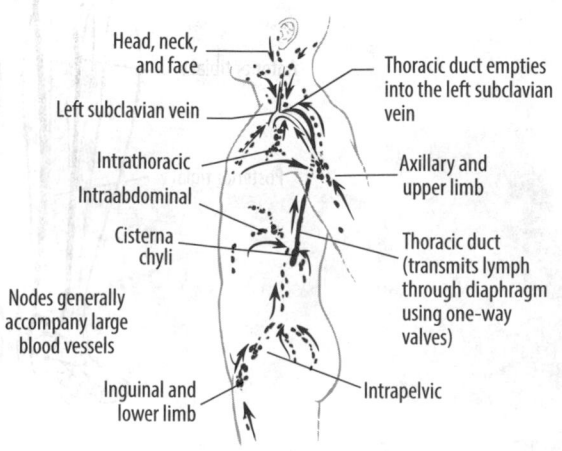

Respiratory System

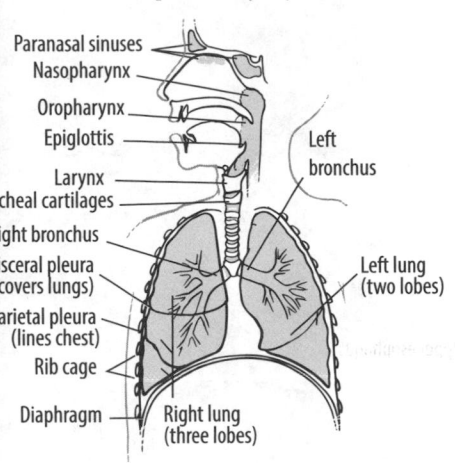

Paranasal sinuses
Nasopharynx
Oropharynx
Epiglottis
Larynx
Tracheal cartilages
Right bronchus
Visceral pleura (covers lungs)
Parietal pleura (lines chest)
Rib cage
Diaphragm
Left bronchus
Left lung (two lobes)
Right lung (three lobes)

Paranasal Sinuses

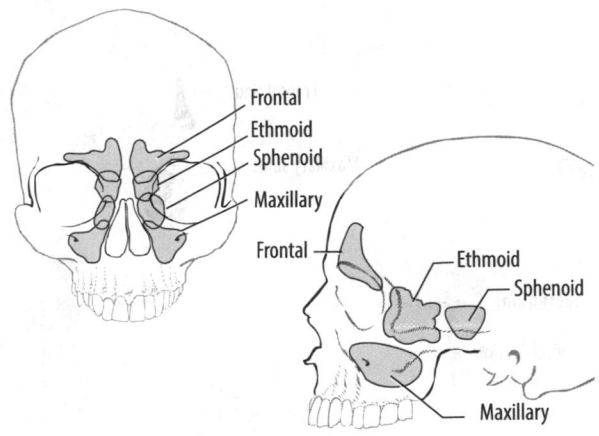

Frontal
Ethmoid
Sphenoid
Maxillary
Frontal
Ethmoid
Sphenoid
Maxillary

Oral Cavity

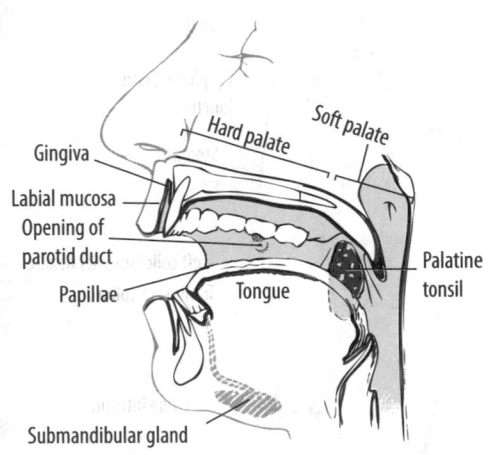

Gingiva
Labial mucosa
Opening of parotid duct
Papillae
Submandibular gland
Hard palate
Soft palate
Tongue
Palatine tonsil

Pancreas

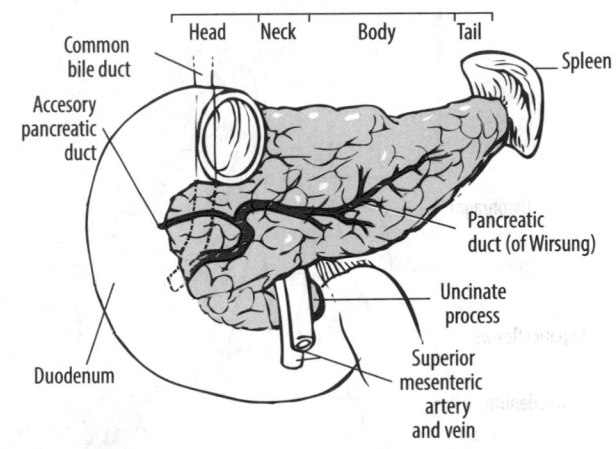

Head   Neck   Body   Tail
Common bile duct
Accesory pancreatic duct
Duodenum
Spleen
Pancreatic duct (of Wirsung)
Uncinate process
Superior mesenteric artery and vein

Gallbladder and Bile Ducts

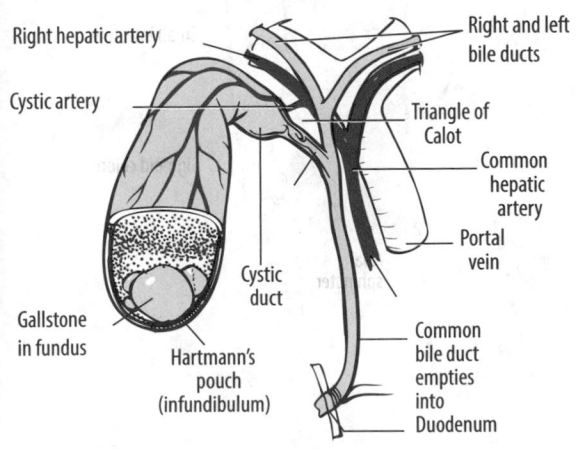

Right hepatic artery
Cystic artery
Gallstone in fundus
Hartmann's pouch (infundibulum)
Cystic duct
Right and left bile ducts
Triangle of Calot
Common hepatic artery
Portal vein
Common bile duct empties into Duodenum

Liver

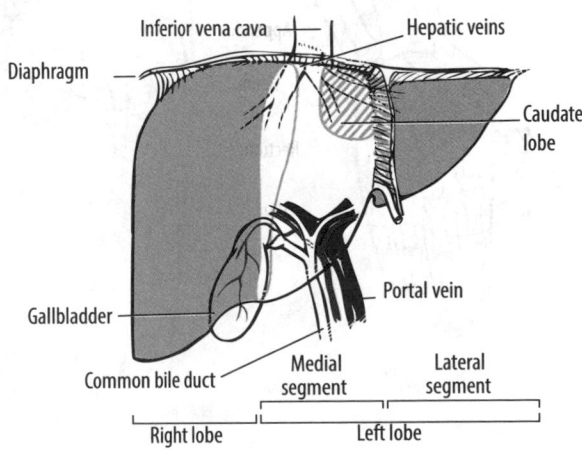

Inferior vena cava
Diaphragm
Gallbladder
Common bile duct
Hepatic veins
Caudate lobe
Portal vein
Medial segment
Lateral segment
Right lobe
Left lobe

Gastrointestinal System

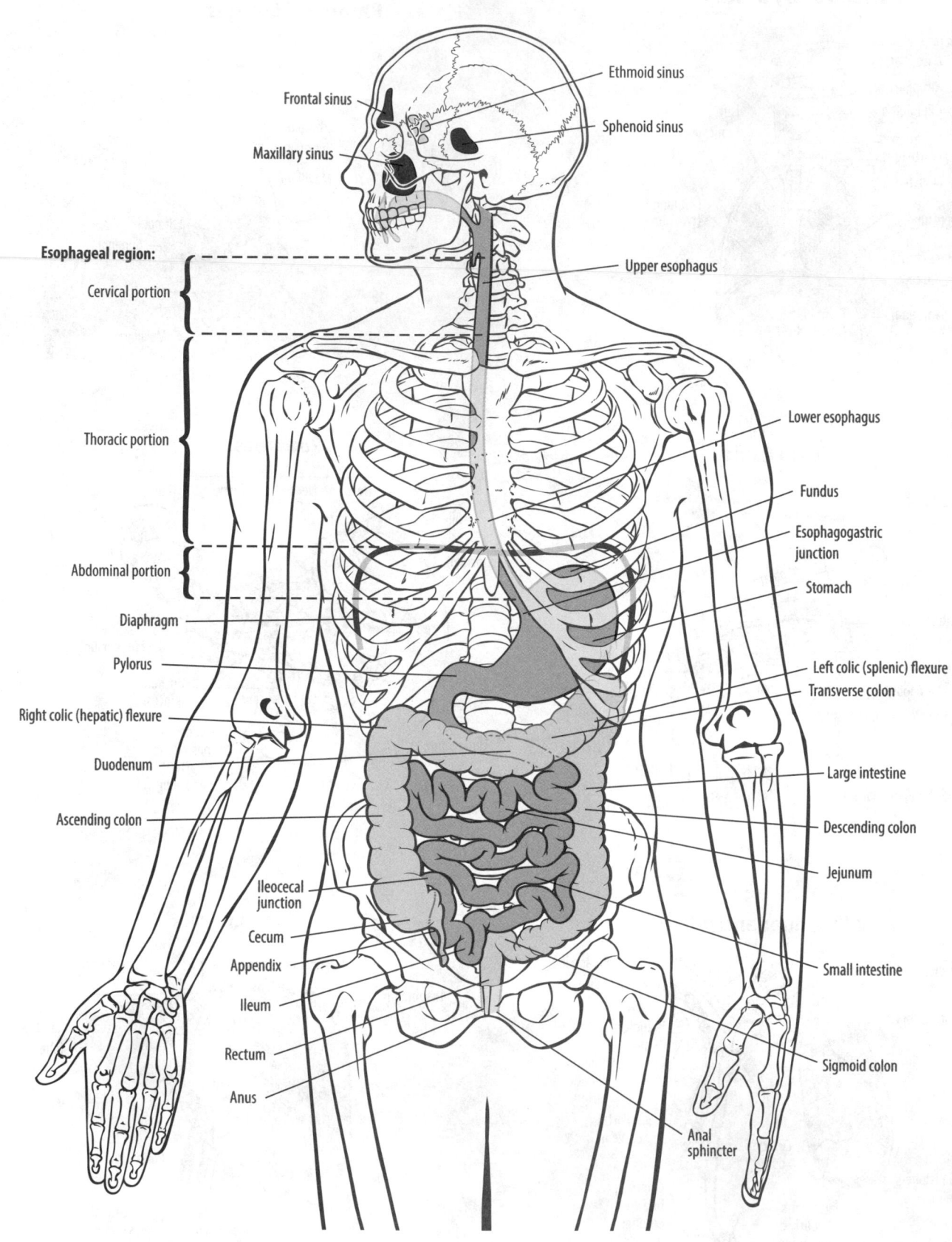

Frontal sinus

Maxillary sinus

Ethmoid sinus

Sphenoid sinus

Esophageal region:

Cervical portion

Thoracic portion

Abdominal portion

Diaphragm

Pylorus

Right colic (hepatic) flexure

Duodenum

Ascending colon

Ileocecal junction

Cecum

Appendix

Ileum

Rectum

Anus

Upper esophagus

Lower esophagus

Fundus

Esophagogastric junction

Stomach

Left colic (splenic) flexure

Transverse colon

Large intestine

Descending colon

Jejunum

Small intestine

Sigmoid colon

Anal sphincter

Endocrine System

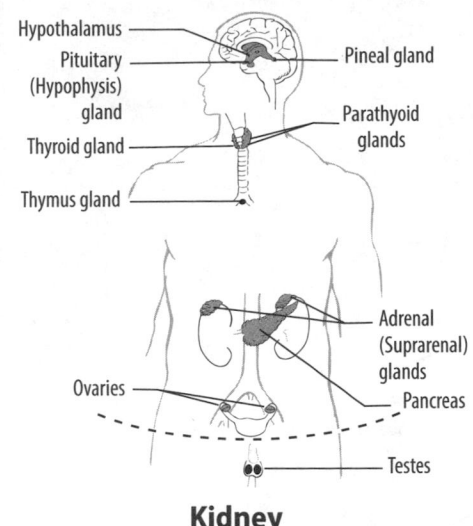

Hypothalamus
Pituitary (Hypophysis) gland
Pineal gland
Parathyroid glands
Thyroid gland
Thymus gland
Adrenal (Suprarenal) glands
Ovaries
Pancreas
Testes

Dorsal View of Parathyroid Gland

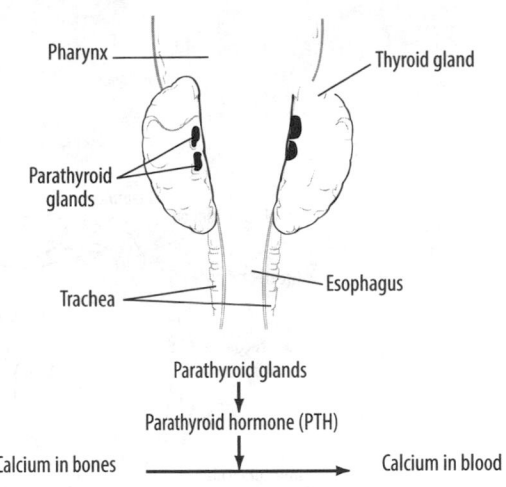

Pharynx
Thyroid gland
Parathyroid glands
Trachea
Esophagus

Parathyroid glands
↓
Parathyroid hormone (PTH)
↓
Calcium in bones → Calcium in blood

Kidney

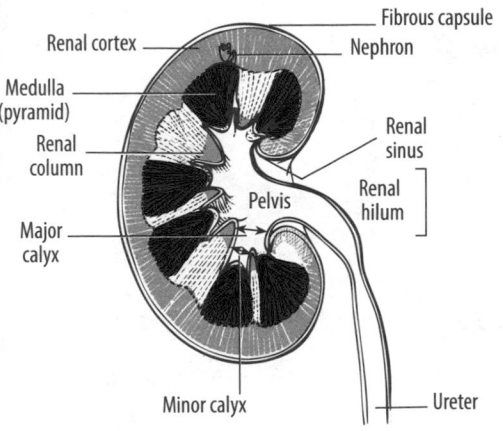

Renal cortex
Fibrous capsule
Nephron
Medulla (pyramid)
Renal column
Renal sinus
Major calyx
Pelvis
Renal hilum
Minor calyx
Ureter

Urinary System

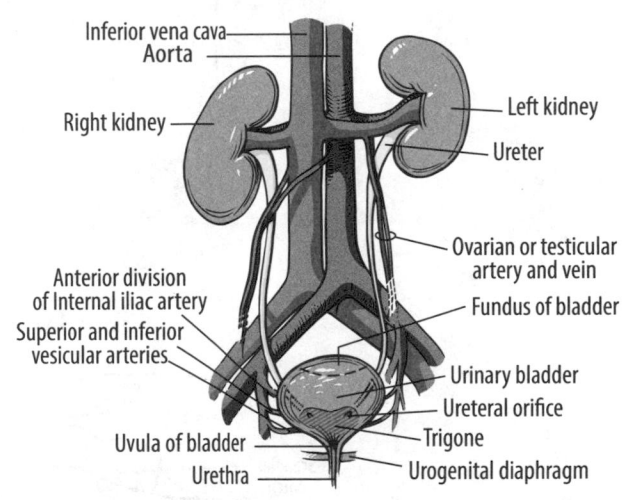

Inferior vena cava
Aorta
Right kidney
Left kidney
Ureter
Anterior division of Internal iliac artery
Superior and inferior vesicular arteries
Ovarian or testicular artery and vein
Fundus of bladder
Urinary bladder
Ureteral orifice
Trigone
Uvula of bladder
Urethra
Urogenital diaphragm

Male Pelvic Organs

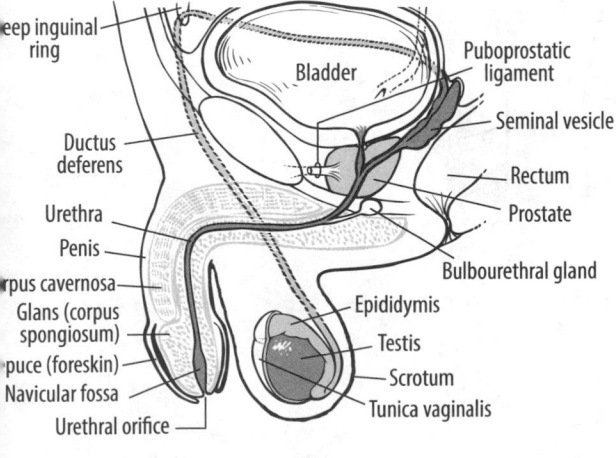

Deep inguinal ring
Bladder
Puboprostatic ligament
Seminal vesicle
Ductus deferens
Rectum
Prostate
Urethra
Penis
Bulbourethral gland
Corpus cavernosa
Epididymis
Glans (corpus spongiosum)
Testis
Prepuce (foreskin)
Scrotum
Navicular fossa
Tunica vaginalis
Urethral orifice

Female Genitourinary System

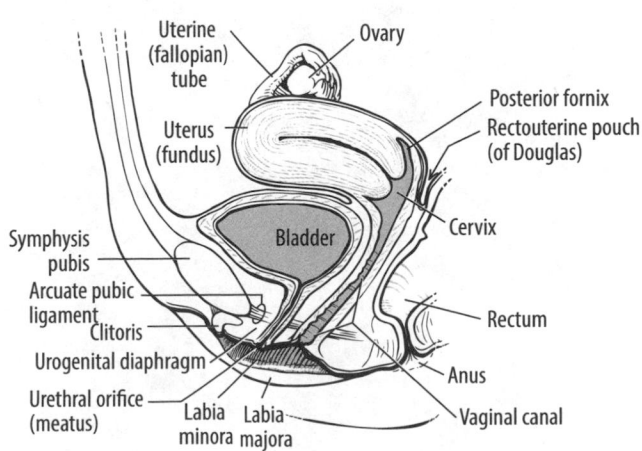

Uterine (fallopian) tube
Ovary
Uterus (fundus)
Posterior fornix
Rectouterine pouch (of Douglas)
Symphysis pubis
Bladder
Cervix
Arcuate pubic ligament
Clitoris
Rectum
Urogenital diaphragm
Urethral orifice (meatus)
Labia minora
Labia majora
Anus
Vaginal canal

Joints

Shoulder (Anterior View)

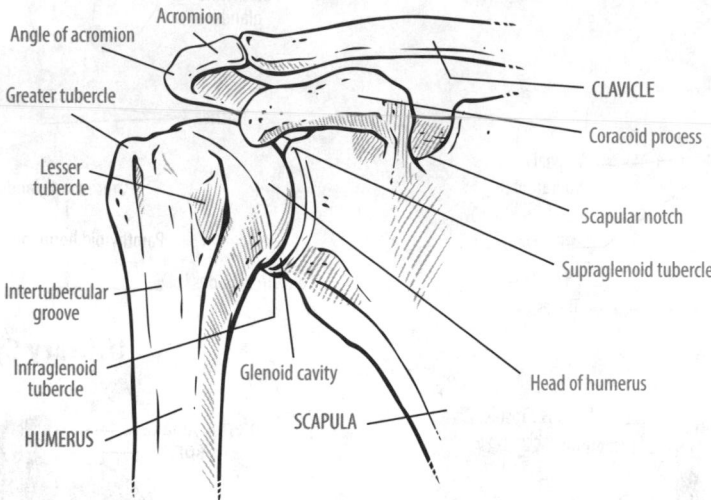

Angle of acromion
Acromion
Greater tubercle
Lesser tubercle
CLAVICLE
Coracoid process
Scapular notch
Supraglenoid tubercle
Intertubercular groove
Infraglenoid tubercle
Glenoid cavity
Head of humerus
HUMERUS
SCAPULA

Shoulder (Posterior View)

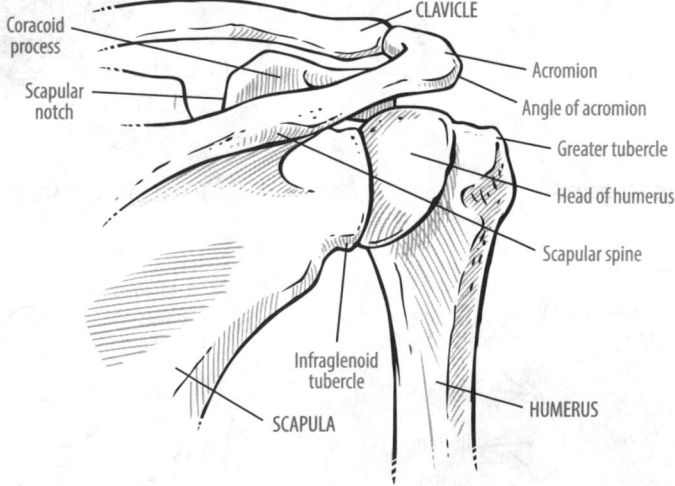

Coracoid process
Scapular notch
CLAVICLE
Acromion
Angle of acromion
Greater tubercle
Head of humerus
Scapular spine
Infraglenoid tubercle
SCAPULA
HUMERUS

Joints
Elbow (Anterior View)

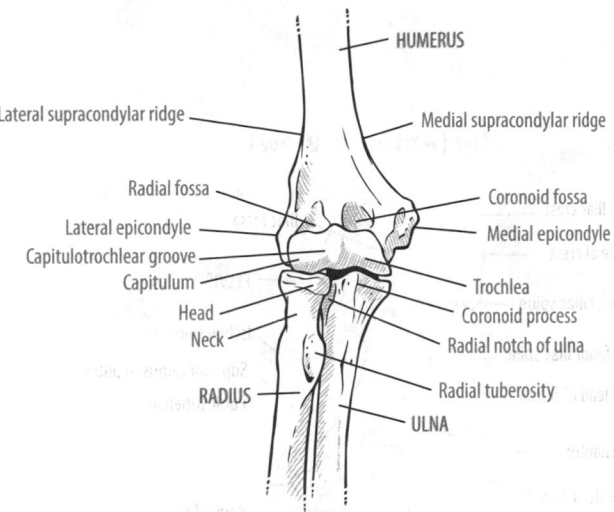

HUMERUS

Lateral supracondylar ridge

Medial supracondylar ridge

Radial fossa

Coronoid fossa

Lateral epicondyle

Medial epicondyle

Capitulotrochlear groove

Capitulum

Trochlea

Head

Coronoid process

Neck

Radial notch of ulna

RADIUS

Radial tuberosity

ULNA

Elbow (Posterior View)

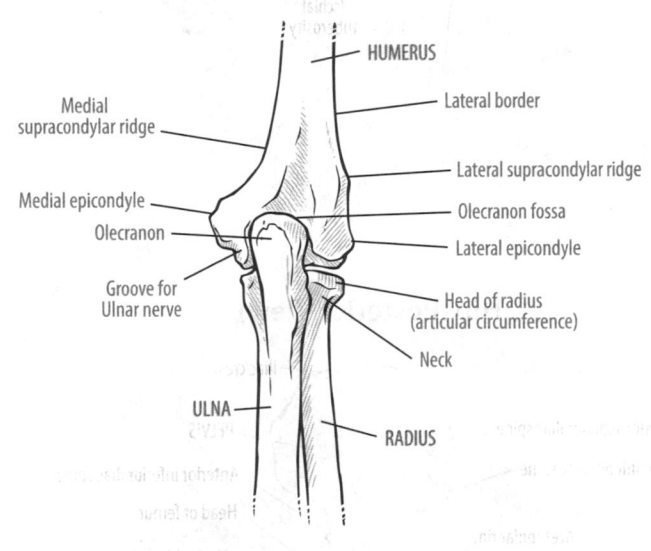

HUMERUS

Medial supracondylar ridge

Lateral border

Lateral supracondylar ridge

Medial epicondyle

Olecranon fossa

Olecranon

Lateral epicondyle

Groove for Ulnar nerve

Head of radius (articular circumference)

Neck

ULNA

RADIUS

Hand

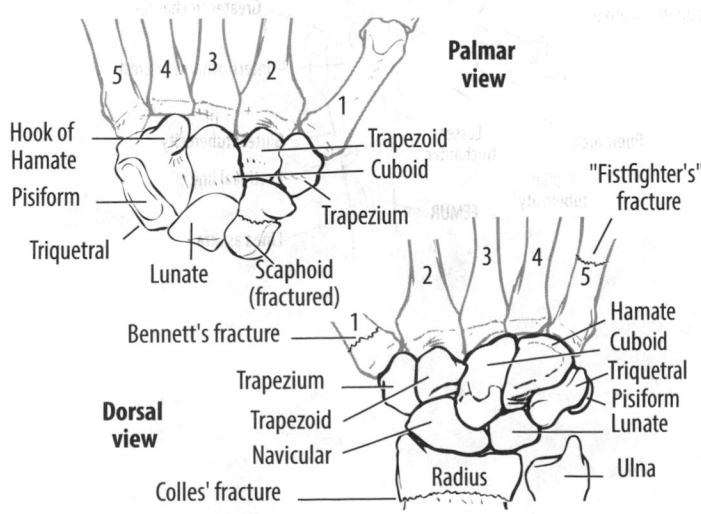

Palmar view

5   4   3   2

1

Hook of Hamate

Trapezoid

Pisiform

Cuboid

Triquetral

Trapezium

Lunate

Scaphoid (fractured)

"Fistfighter's" fracture

3   4   5

Bennett's fracture

2

1

Hamate

Cuboid

Trapezium

Triquetral

Trapezoid

Pisiform

Navicular

Lunate

Dorsal view

Radius

Ulna

Colles' fracture

Joints

Hip (Anterior View)

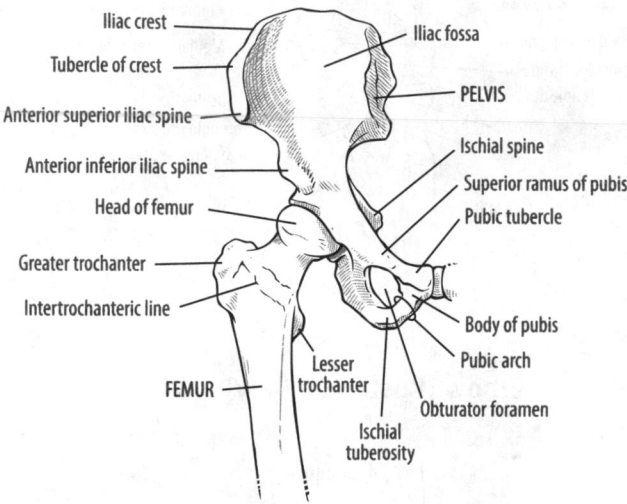

Iliac crest

Tubercle of crest

Anterior superior iliac spine

Anterior inferior iliac spine

Head of femur

Greater trochanter

Intertrochanteric line

FEMUR

Lesser trochanter

Ischial tuberosity

Iliac fossa

PELVIS

Ischial spine

Superior ramus of pubis

Pubic tubercle

Body of pubis

Pubic arch

Obturator foramen

Hip (Posterior View)

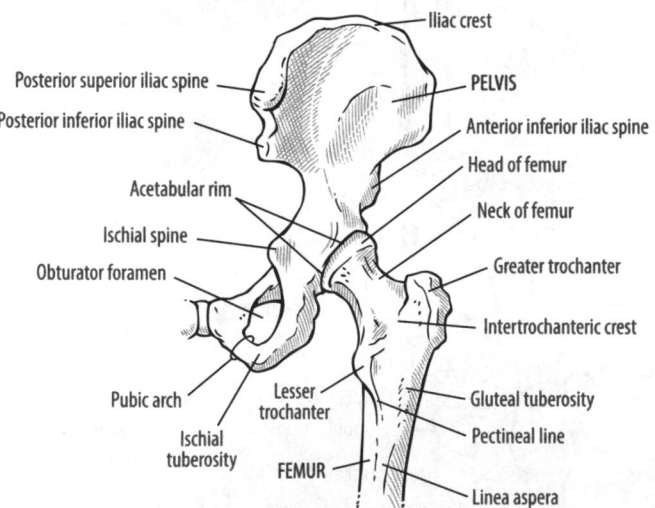

Iliac crest

Posterior superior iliac spine

Posterior inferior iliac spine

Acetabular rim

Ischial spine

Obturator foramen

Pubic arch

Ischial tuberosity

Lesser trochanter

FEMUR

PELVIS

Anterior inferior iliac spine

Head of femur

Neck of femur

Greater trochanter

Intertrochanteric crest

Gluteal tuberosity

Pectineal line

Linea aspera

Joints

Knee (Anterior View)

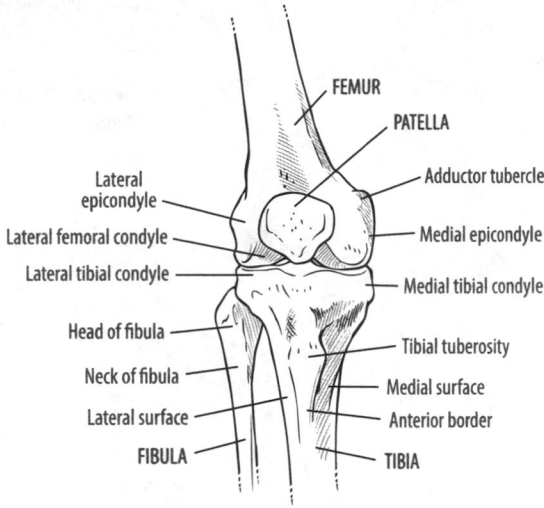

FEMUR

PATELLA

Lateral epicondyle

Adductor tubercle

Lateral femoral condyle

Medial epicondyle

Lateral tibial condyle

Medial tibial condyle

Head of fibula

Tibial tuberosity

Neck of fibula

Medial surface

Lateral surface

Anterior border

FIBULA

TIBIA

Knee (Posterior View)

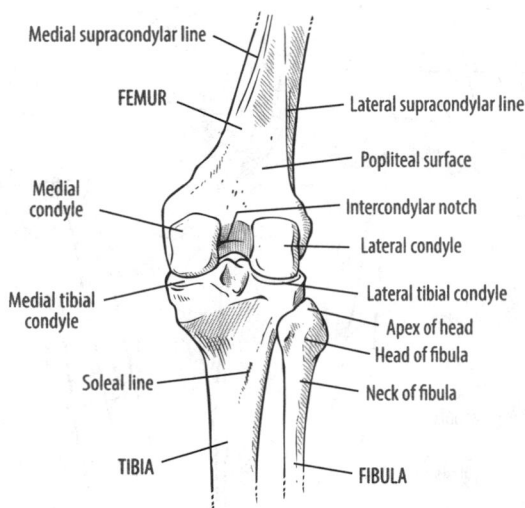

Medial supracondylar line

FEMUR

Lateral supracondylar line

Popliteal surface

Medial condyle

Intercondylar notch

Lateral condyle

Medial tibial condyle

Lateral tibial condyle

Apex of head

Head of fibula

Soleal line

Neck of fibula

TIBIA

FIBULA

Right Foot

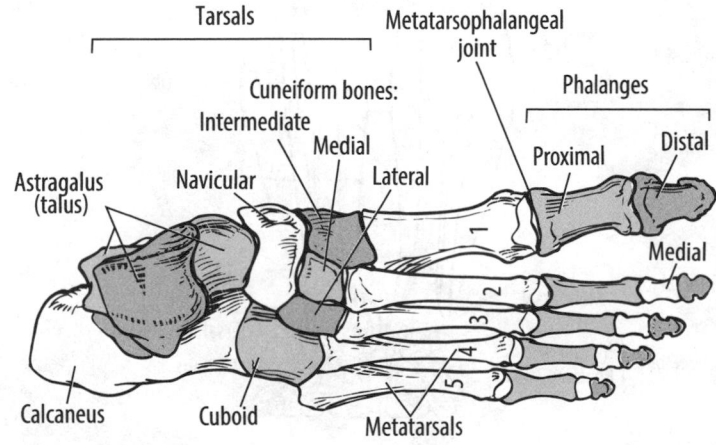

Tarsals

Metatarsophalangeal joint

Cuneiform bones:

Phalanges

Intermediate

Medial

Proximal

Distal

Astragalus (talus)

Navicular

Lateral

Medial

Calcaneus

Cuboid

Metatarsals

Bones/Joints

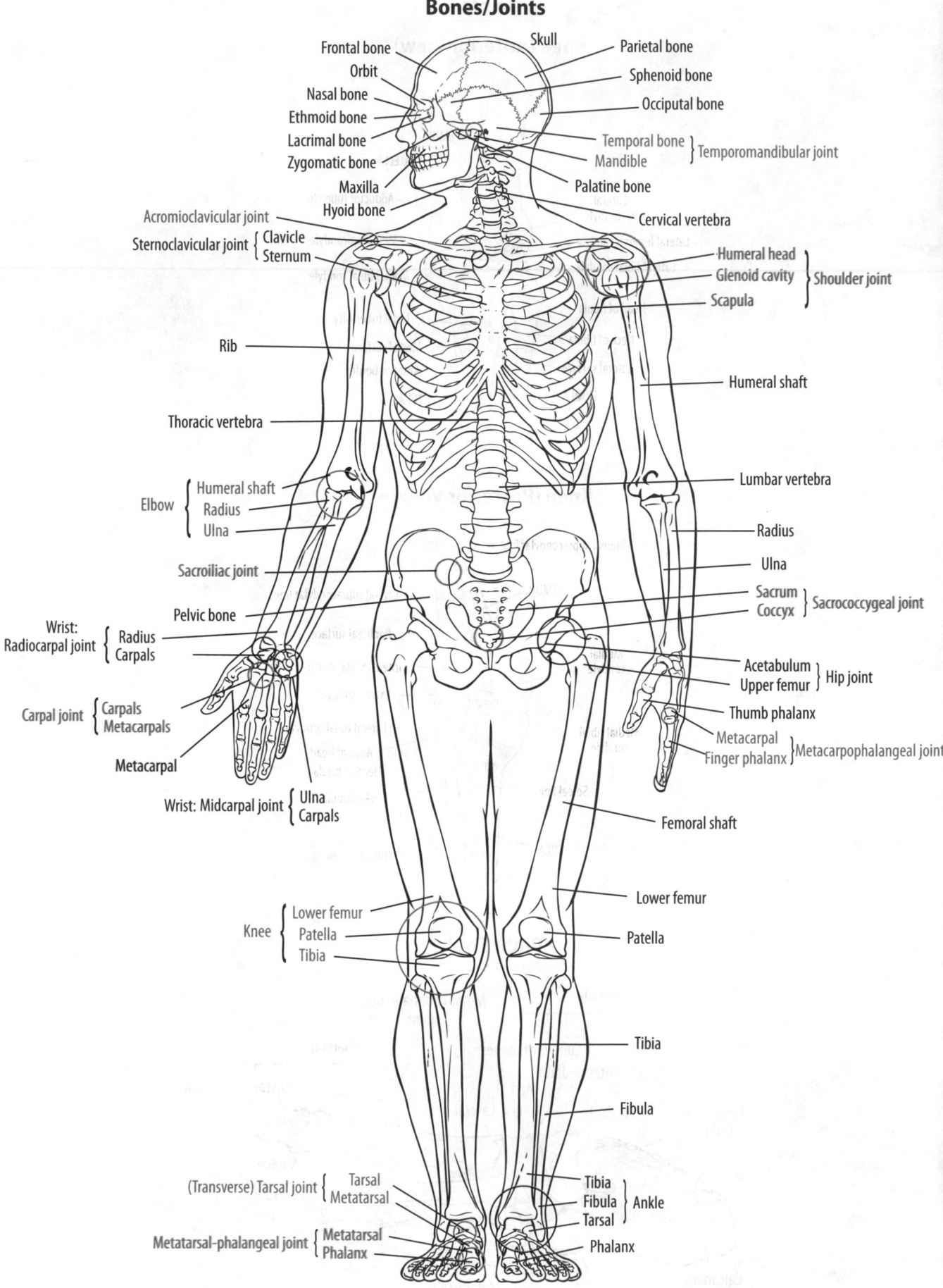

Muscles

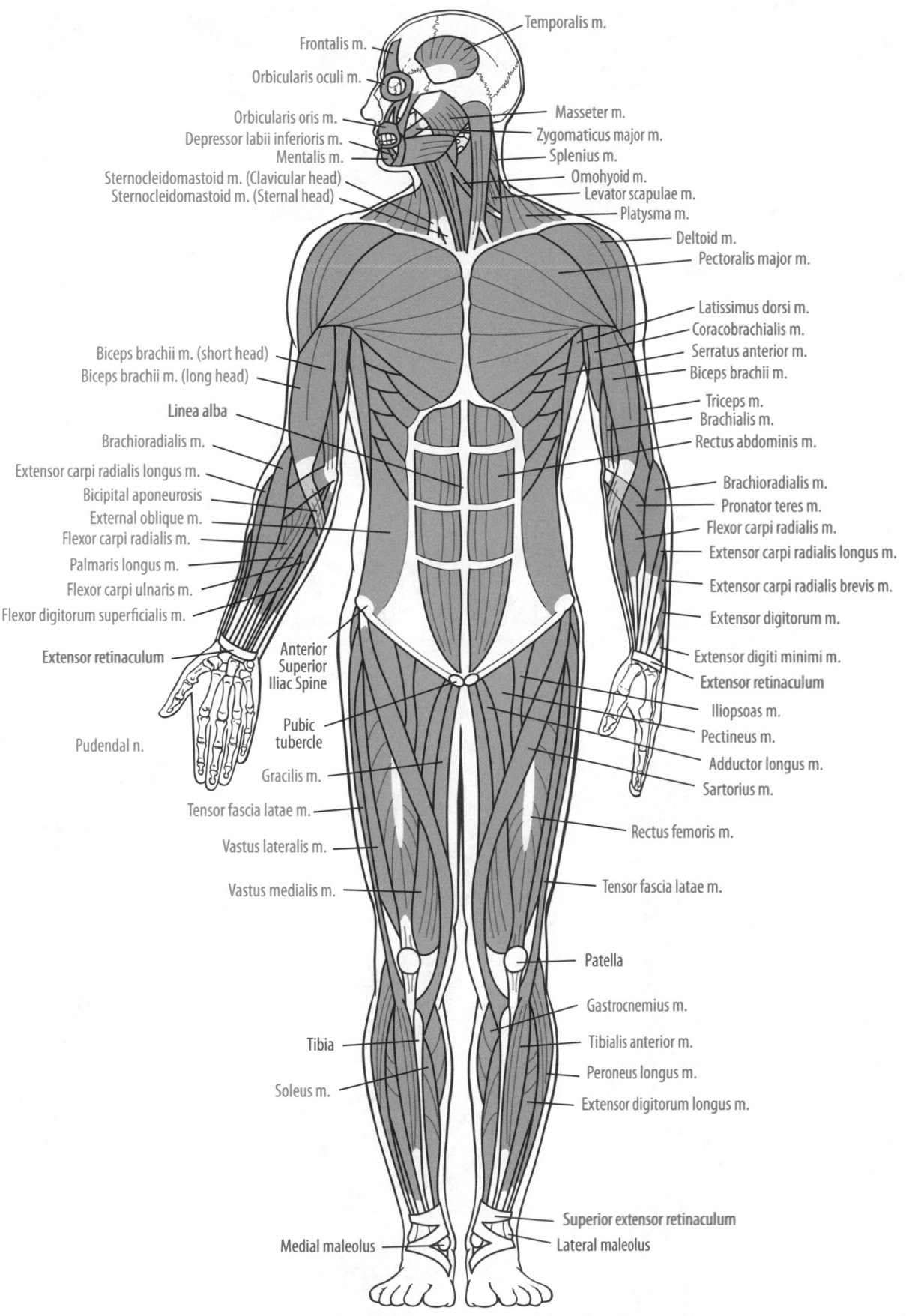

Frontalis m.

Temporalis m.

Orbicularis oculi m.

Orbicularis oris m.

Masseter m.

Depressor labii inferioris m.

Zygomaticus major m.

Mentalis m.

Splenius m.

Sternocleidomastoid m. (Clavicular head)

Omohyoid m.

Sternocleidomastoid m. (Sternal head)

Levator scapulae m.

Platysma m.

Deltoid m.

Pectoralis major m.

Biceps brachii m. (short head)

Latissimus dorsi m.

Biceps brachii m. (long head)

Coracobrachialis m.

Serratus anterior m.

Biceps brachii m.

Linea alba

Triceps m.

Brachialis m.

Brachioradialis m.

Rectus abdominis m.

Extensor carpi radialis longus m.

Brachioradialis m.

Bicipital aponeurosis

Pronator teres m.

External oblique m.

Flexor carpi radialis m.

Flexor carpi radialis m.

Extensor carpi radialis longus m.

Palmaris longus m.

Extensor carpi radialis brevis m.

Flexor carpi ulnaris m.

Flexor digitorum superficialis m.

Extensor digitorum m.

Extensor retinaculum

Extensor digiti minimi m.

Anterior
Superior
Iliac Spine

Extensor retinaculum

Iliopsoas m.

Pubic
tubercle

Pectineus m.

Pudendal n.

Adductor longus m.

Gracilis m.

Sartorius m.

Tensor fascia latae m.

Rectus femoris m.

Vastus lateralis m.

Tensor fascia latae m.

Vastus medialis m.

Patella

Gastrocnemius m.

Tibia

Tibialis anterior m.

Peroneus longus m.

Soleus m.

Extensor digitorum longus m.

Superior extensor retinaculum

Medial maleolus

Lateral maleolus